Principles and Practice of Nursing

Principles and Practice of Nursing

SIXTH EDITION

Virginia Henderson, R.N., A.M.

Research Associate Emeritus, Yale University School of Nursing, New Haven, Connecticut. Formerly Associate Professor of Nursing Education, Teachers College, Columbia University, New York City; Instructor in the School of Nursing, Norfolk Protestant Hospital, Norfolk, Virginia, and the School of Nursing, University of Rochester, and Strong Memorial Hospital, Rochester, New York

Gladys Nite, R.N., A.M.

Coordinator of Nursing Studies, Veterans Administration Hospital, Houston, Texas. Formerly Professor of Medical-Surgical Nursing, Texas Woman's University College of Nursing, Houston, Texas; Associate Professor of Nursing, University of Washington School of Nursing, Seattle, Washington; Director of Nursing Research, Community Studies, Kansas City, Missouri; and Professor and Director, Graduate Programs in Nursing, University of Texas School of Nursing, Galveston, Texas

MACMILLAN PUBLISHING CO., INC.
New York

COLLIER MACMILLAN PUBLISHERS
London

Copyright © 1978, Macmillan Publishing Co., Inc.

Printed in the United States of America

Earlier editions entitled *Text-book of the Principles and Practice of Nursing,*
by Bertha Harmer, copyright 1922, 1928, and 1934 by Macmillan Publishing Co., Inc.
Earlier editions entitled *Textbook of the Principles and Practice of Nursing,*
by Bertha Harmer and Virginia Henderson, copyright 1939 and © 1955 by Macmillan Publishing Co., Inc.
Copyright renewed 1950, 1956, 1962, 1967.

Macmillan Publishing Co., Inc.
866 Third Avenue, New York, New York 10022

Collier Macmillan Canada, Ltd.

Library of Congress Cataloging in Publication Data

Henderson, Virginia.
    Principles and practice of nursing

    Editions for 1922–1955 by B. Harmer published
under title: Textbook of the principles and practice of nursing; 4th ed. (1939) by B. Harmer and
V. Henderson and 5th ed. (1955) rev. by V. Henderson.
    Includes bibliographies and index.
    1. Nursing.   I. Nite, Gladys, joint author.
II. Harmer, Bertha. Textbook of the principles and
practice of nursing.   III. Title. [DNLM:
1. Nursing care. WY100 H497p]
RT41.H24   1978   610.73   76–17020

ISBN 0-02-353580-6

Printing: 1 2 3 4 5 6 7 8   Year: 8 9 0 1 2 3 4

Preface to the Sixth Edition

Like the fifth edition, this book is intended as a guide for instructors and students of nursing and as a reference for practicing nurses. It is a reference also for those who want to guard their own or their family's health or take care of a sick relative or friend. We hope it will be useful to those who teach health in schools other than nursing. The language is deliberately free from medical jargon and most technical terms are defined parenthetically. The responsibility every person has for his or her health—the importance of being informed and self-reliant—is stressed. A list of national self-help organizations is given as an appendix. Our position is that a great deal is known about how to prevent disease, and that the spiraling cost of health care will be reversed only when people value health sufficiently to acquire and apply this knowledge in healthful living.

As in earlier editions, health and therapeutic practices are suggested following a review of research and expert opinion on which the recommended practice is based. However, conflicting data are often cited and the difficulty of selecting a method is acknowledged. Attention is called to the rapidity with which the body of scientific knowledge is expanding. Continuing study throughout the working life of health personnel is recognized as essential.

The entire book has been rewritten by the two authors and seventeen clinical nurse contributors. Although the overall plan is like that of the fifth edition, it has been revised in certain respects to conform to the curriculum design suggested in the first author's booklet, *The Nature of Nursing.*

Part I, "The Place of Nursing in Health Service," defines nursing and discusses the process of nursing and the theory underlying it; it also discusses the education of nurses—initial, graduate, in-service, and continuing programs. Preparation of the nurse for increasingly independent practice is discussed, stressing the importance of interdisciplinary education of health workers. Health service in the United States is, to some extent, compared with that in other countries, as are the independent and collaborative roles of nurses,

physicians, and other health workers. A chapter is devoted to the major settings in which nurses work. There are new materials, particularly in occupational, school, and prison nursing in this chapter. Part II, "The Role of the Nurse in Health Evaluation and Planning Patient Care or Meeting Patients' Health Needs," describes the nurse's expanded function in observing, reporting, and recording, in conducting physical examinations, and in helping physicians with health assessment—physical, mental, and emotional. Two chapters cover the nurse's role in making certain diagnostic tests and measurements, or helping others to make them. The admission of well clients and sick patients to health services is discussed, also planning care and rehabilitation and terminating care. Part III, "Fundamentals of Nursing Care—Helping Others Provide for Their Basic Needs," stresses underlying principles and describes in detail how nurses help clients with the activities of daily living—breathing, eating, eliminating, moving, resting and sleeping, keeping well groomed, dressing and undressing, controlling the environment, communicating with others, learning, working, playing, and worshiping. The discussion of communicating, or relating to others, is greatly expanded as is the discussion of worship. The chapter on worship includes a brief description of the major living religions, since an understanding of a person's religion seems essential to understanding the person. Part IV, "Therapeutic Measures," is really a reference section for the entire book. It describes procedures used in the fundamentals of care and in symptomatic nursing. The chapter on selection of method includes new material on research in nursing —its development, the uses of research, current emphases, and the protection of human rights in clinical research. Part V, "Common Problems—Symptomatic Nursing," deals with the modifications of fundamental nursing care when there are abnormalities in breathing, eating, eliminating, moving, resting, sleeping, communicating, or any other aspects of daily living. Part V includes the care of people with such problems as acute oxygen want, nutritional disorders, hyperactivity and hypoactivity, unconsciousness, depression, infection (local and generalized), blindness, deafness, and intractable pain. It also describes the general nursing of patients before and after surgery, nursing of those in shock or during a hemorrhage, and, finally, the care of those who are dying.

Although most common nursing problems (those encountered in all clinical services and in many settings) were discussed in the fifth edition, there is more complete coverage in this edition. There is new material throughout the book, but in Part V a number of chapters are new or expanded. In the fifth edition there were a chapter on shock and one on accidents and emergencies. The materials in those chapters have been distributed among chapters within Part V. The treatment of topics such as burns and asphyxia is so much enlarged that the chapters in which they appear seem new. The chapters on hypoactivity and hyperactivity contain almost entirely new content, as do the chapters on disturbance of consciousness and orientation, anxiety and depression, disorders of communication, and the management of pain. The chapter on death and dying is greatly enlarged to stress the consideration of the entire family, the management of pain and other symptoms in terminal illness, also the kind of care that emphasizes living until the end—the support offered the terminally ill in hospices and specialized services, not only support for the patient but support for the family that extends into the period of bereavement.

Throughout the book we have assumed that nursing is a service to the well and the sick and that prevention and therapy can rarely be separated. As in the fifth edition, we have stressed the interdependence of physical, emotional, mental, and spiritual aspects of living and the inescapable conclusion that the medical and surgical nurse must know how to care for the psyche and that the psychiatric nurse must know how to care for the soma. There is no attempt to deal separately with any clinical specialty in nursing either according to the age or the clinical diagnosis of the client or patient. An effort has been made to identify some of the particular needs according to sex and age. Rehabilitation is treated as an aspect of the care of all sick and disabled persons from the time they are admitted to a health service until their care is terminated. Although the necessity for the patient's depending on health workers, families, and friends is recognized, the emphasis is on helping people to acquire optimum independence as soon as possible.

References, such as tables of abbreviations, measurements, diets, and lists of addresses, are in the Appendix. Metric and apothecary equivalents are given throughout the book.

References cited and additional suggested readings are given for each chapter. We intended to include for each chapter suggested audiovisual, or nonprint, learning materials in addition to books and journal articles. Instead these materials will be described in a separate publication.

We wish we could mention all those who have helped revise materials in the fifth edition or helped prepare new materials. The contributors have greatly enriched the content of this book. We are grateful to them and to those who have read and criticized certain parts of it. All of these are acknowledged at the ends of the chapters on which they worked.

We are grateful to those associated with the Macmillan Publishing Co., Inc., particularly Thomas Patrick McConahay, for their help and their patient support and encouragement during the prolonged preparation of this book.

Special thanks are due Elsie S. Mowe, who has not only typed nearly all of the manuscript but has helped with editing it and coordinating the efforts of the many persons involved in its preparation. Laura C. McCarthy has also helped with the typing, with library searches, and with preparing a file of nonprint materials.

Many illustrations are new and we thank all individuals, institutions, and firms that have supplied charts, diagrams, tables, drawings, or photographs. We also thank authors and publishers who have allowed us to quote from their works.

An effort has been made to see health care, and particularly nursing, worldwide. Descriptions of health services on every continent have been read; some have been cited and some quoted. It would be presumptuous to suggest that this work will be equally useful to nurses and others within and without the United States, but we hope that everybody concerned with health care, particularly nursing, will find something of interest within the covers of this book.

V. H.
G. N.

Preface to the Fifth Edition

This text is intended as a guide to instructors and students of nursing, and as a general reference for nurses practicing in hospital or clinic, office or home. I am persuaded that the best way to meet the needs of student and graduate alike is first to present the scientific principles that underlie practice and then to suggest the methods that embody these principles, rather than merely to recommend any one method of a particular institution or agency. Where I have found conflicts in experimental evidence and expert opinion, they are reported; in such cases the recommended method may represent, in certain respects, my own weighing of evidence or opinion. Actually no claim is made for any procedure that it is the best possible practice. I have emphasized the tentative nature of the scientists' conclusions, hoping that the nurse reader will be stimulated to continue to think of herself as a student and of her practice as subject to modification with every major advance in the biological and social sciences.

While virtually the entire text has been rewritten, the organization remains essentially unchanged. Part I, "The Place of Nursing in Health Service," is a definition of nursing as I interpret it, and a discussion of the preparation of the nurse and of her place in current health programs. Part II, "Fundamentals of Nursing Care," while stressing underlying principles, shows in detail how to help a person meet his fundamental health needs. Part III, "The Role of Nursing in Health Evaluation and Diagnostic Techniques," describes the nurse's role in assessing the patient's nursing needs and his physical and emotional status, and in assisting him with the diagnostic measures prescribed by the physician. Part IV, "The Role of Nursing in Therapeutic Measures," deals with the nurse's role in giving, or assisting patients with, prescribed therapy. Finally, in Part V, "Common Problems in Nursing Practice," are discussed selected problems that the nurse commonly encounters, such as the following: How to care for a person with a local or systemic infection; how to nurse the patient who is about to undergo surgery or who is recovering from it; and how to nurse

the unconscious or the dying. Those chapters in Part V of the fourth edition that described nursing care in specific diseases have been omitted. Although in some cases they were used to illustrate a disease category or a larger problem, their inclusion may have suggested to the reader a broader scope for the book than in fact it had. Students and practitioners in each clinical service will prefer, I believe, to consult specialized texts for help in meeting the particular needs of the person with diabetes, for instance, or heart disease, or scarlet fever, or the one undergoing a brain operation or a thyroidectomy.

An early chapter is devoted to planning nursing care around the requirements of the individual. The importance of understanding what the patient's illness means to him and his family is stressed. This clearly demands of the nurse, as well as of other medical workers, considerable knowledge of the cultural and social settings in which their patients live.

Throughout the text I have proceeded on the premise that nursing is a service to both well and sick; and that all branches of medicine have their preventive and therapeutic aspects. I have tried also to indicate the concepts that mind and body are inseparable, that structure and function affect each other, and that physical and emotional health are interdependent. For this reason I abandoned an earlier intention to include a section on the "psychiatric aspects of general nursing." Instead, I have tried to point out that every aspect of nursing has an emotional, or psychological, component. This is an inescapable conclusion if one believes that every thought or emotion has its physical expression even though the manifestation is often too minute or fleeting for measurement. I believe that, if this concept were applied, it would convert all general nursing into a preventive psychiatric service which might materially reduce the incidence of fully developed mental disorder.

Rehabilitation as an aspect of nursing is another pervasive idea that refused to be confined to any part of the text, although one chapter is devoted to a summarization of the subject. If the aim of *all* medical care is to help *every* patient to increase his emotional and physical independence, rehabilitation is a psychosocial and physical process which should begin as soon as anyone comes under treatment for disease or disability. Unless medical workers look upon rehabilitation as applicable to every person in all stages of illness (except the final one), the patient may develop in an early stage unnecessary helplessness that must be painfully relinquished when later the medical staff and his family and friends expect him to be self-reliant. This does not mean that the value of sympathy with the unavoidable, and sometimes healing, dependence of the sick and injured should be ignored.

All material of a strictly referable nature, such as lists of abbreviations and tables of measurement, have been placed in the Appendix. For the convenience of the reader who may be familiar with the metric but not the apothecaries' system, or vice versa, equivalents have been given throughout the text.

Since women predominate in the occupation of nursing and men in that of medicine, the nurse is referred to as "she" and the doctor as "he." I hope this will offend neither the man nurse nor the woman physician.

I wish I could mention each person who has helped me revise this text. It is impossible, however, to gauge all I have learned from the graduate nurses with whom I, as a teacher, have been associated, nor has it been practicable to list under "References" all the written works of others that I have consulted in preparing the manuscript.

To those who have revised certain chapters, or parts of them, I am deeply grateful: to Dr. John Hampden Hobart for preparing Chapter 19; to Miss Margaret Gibson for her work on Chapter 24; to Miss Virginia Dericks for revising Chapter 39; and, particularly, to Miss Barbara Russell, not only for revising Chapters 27, 42, and parts of others, but for her competence and understanding as the publisher's editor. To Mr. W. Holt Seale and Macmillan Publishing Co., Inc., who have been embarrassed by the delays in publication, I wish to express my appreciation of their continued support and patience.

The major burden of typing and initial editing of the manuscript was borne by my sister, Miss Lucy R. Henderson, and Mrs. Joseph E. Johnson contributed, with the same generosity, these invaluable services; to both of them I am particularly indebted. Mrs. Richard Landon, Miss Bessie Carroll, and Mr. Wilbur Baily also assisted in typing; Mrs. Jan van Tijn aided with the typing and some of the library research; Miss Marion D. Cleveland, Miss Cecile Covell, and Dr. David V. Habif read and criticized various chapters.

The total number of illustrations has been increased, and the majority are new. The Clay-Adams Company of New York City has made for this text, or supplied from their stock of purchasable medical Kodachromes (Medichromes), illustrations, many of them photographs. I thank Mr. Edgar Nebel, of this firm, for his expert photography and also the administration of the Columbia-Presbyterian Medical Center, who put their facilities at my disposal when the photographs were taken. I acknowledge the kindness of the American Hospital Supply Corporation and Becton, Dickinson and Company in lending many of the items of improved equipment shown in some of these photographs.

For the original figure drawings in this volume, I am indebted to Miss Lalah Durham and Mr. Scaisbrooke L. Abbot; for some of the diagrams to Mr. Harry Guillaume; and for the architectural scheme in Chapter 7 to Mr. Jesse L. Orrick.

To the authors and publishers who have allowed me to quote or to use illustrations from their works, I extend my thanks, as well as to the manufacturers who have provided illustrations of their equipment.

The economics of textbook publishing imposes limits to size and scope. Regretting that this is so, I nevertheless take full responsibility for the text. Likewise, I am responsible for any errors it may contain.

May, 1955   V. H.

Contributors

Faye G. Abdellah, R.N., Ed.D., F.A.A.N., Assistant Surgeon General, Chief Nurse Officer, Public Health Service; and Director, Office of Long Term Care, Department of Health, Education, and Welfare, Washington, D.C.

Carol Dawn Davis, R.N., M.S.N., M.P.H., Assistant Professor of Community Nursing, Yale University School of Nursing, New Haven, Conn.

Rhetaugh Graves Dumas, R.N., Ph.D., Acting Deputy Director, Division of Manpower and Training Programs, National Institute of Mental Health, Alcohol, Drug Abuse, and Mental Health Administration, Department of Health, Education, and Welfare, Rockville, Md.

Mimi Dye, R.N., M.S.N., Associate Professor and Chairman, Psychiatric-Mental Health Nursing Program, Yale University School of Nursing; and Clinical Specialist in Psychiatric Nursing, Connecticut Mental Health Center, New Haven, Conn.

Catherine K. Forrest, R.N., M.S.N., Assistant Professor of Psychiatric Nursing, Yale University School of Nursing, New Haven, Conn.

LaNelle E. Geddes, R.N., Ph.D., Associate Professor, Assistant Department Head, Purdue University Department of Nursing, West Lafayette, Ind.

Dorothy D. Harrison, R.N., Ph.D., Assistant Dean and Director of Undergraduate Programs, School of Nursing, State University of New York at Stony Brook, Stony Brook, N.Y.

Angela Barron McBride, R.N., M.S.N., Formerly Assistant Professor of Psychiatric Nursing, Yale University School of Nursing, New Haven, Conn.

Shirley M. Morrison, R.N., M.S., Clinical Coordinator, Veterans Administration Hospital, Houston, Tex.

Katherine R. Nelson, R.N., Ed.D., Formerly Associate Professor of Nursing Education, Teachers College, Columbia University, New York, N.Y.

Roberta S. O'Grady, R.N., M.A., Assistant Professor of Pediatric Nursing, Yale University School of Nursing; and Nurse Clinician, Yale–New Haven Hospital, New Haven, Conn.

Julina P. Rhymes, R.N., M.S.N., Assistant Professor of Nursing, Yale University School of Nursing, New Haven, Conn.

Roberta K. Spurgeon, R.N., M.S.N., J.D., Formerly Chairman, Psychiatric Nursing Program, Yale University School of Nursing; and Director of Nursing, Connecticut Mental Health Center, New Haven, Conn.

Eleanor Taggart, R.N., M.S.N., Assistant Professor of Medical-Surgical Nursing, Yale University School of Nursing, New Haven, Conn.

Catherine Temple, R.N., M.A., Rehabilitation Specialist, Regional Office, International Rehabilitation Associates, Inc., Dallas, Tex.

Florence S. Wald, R.N., M.N., M.S., Associate Clinical Professor of Nursing, Yale University School of Nursing, New Haven, Conn.

Patience Wilson, R.N., M.S., Assistant Professor of Community Health Nursing, Yale University School of Nursing, New Haven, Conn.; and Clinical Nurse Practitioner, Veterans Administration Hospital, West Haven, Conn.

Contents

PART IV. THERAPEUTIC MEASURES, PROCEDURES, OR TECHNIQUES THAT NURSES PERFORM OR HELP PATIENTS, THEIR FAMILIES, AND MEDICAL WORKERS (OTHER THAN NURSES) PERFORM

PART V. COMMON PROBLEMS—SYMPTOMATIC NURSING

Principles and Practice of Nursing

PART I

The Place of Nursing in Health Service

CHAPTER 1

The Practice of Nursing and Preparation of the Nurse

1. NURSING AS AN ASPECT OF HEALTH CARE

The Goal of All Health Care. What is nursing and what is the function of the nurse? These are questions with which society should be concerned; but those who practice, administer, teach, study, conduct research on, or legislate for nursing *must* answer these questions since consciously or unconsciously they operate under some concept of nursing and the function of the nurse. If the concept is clear and valid, it can guide them to consistent and constructive action; if it is confused and uninformed, it can lead to inconsistent, ineffective, or even harmful action. These questions could be asked and statements made about any health occupation and its members. In the last analysis, all health workers are trying to promote the health and happiness of the individual and the preservation of the species. Each category of health worker must try to define its role in this joint effort.

All organisms behave instinctively to preserve their lives. For some, this instinctive, protective behavior is sufficient, and such organisms (the simpler forms of life) are independent of their parents throughout their separate existence; complex organisms (the higher forms of life) require parental protection and teaching. Generally speaking, the more complex the organism, the longer the period of dependency on adults.[1]

As a species develops communal life, or a society, all members, not only parents, may protect, teach, and nurture the young and protect the sick and helpless; or special members of the community may be assigned these functions. Studies of insect and animal life, as well as studies of human life, show such divisions of labor, or specialized helping functions. Communities of ants, for example, are said to have "nurses" and "sanitarians," the latter disposing of dead bodies. Bees have comparable specialists within the hive.[2,3]

Human societies allow the young shorter or longer periods of dependence on parents, nurses, and teachers according to the particular culture. Even today, in different parts of the world, the dependence of the young man lasts only through puberty or well into adulthood. The dependency of children, the very old, and the sick has been such a threat to the survival of some peoples, particularly nomads, that infanticide and euthanasia were practiced.*

In some cultures, the *care* of the young, the sick, and the infirm has been the responsibility of all women rather than designated members; the treatment of disease, or *cure,* has usually been assigned to designated men, sometimes priests, sometimes "medicine men." The "cures" of the latter supplemented the "care" given the sick by women.

As societies increase in size and organiza-

* Eike-Henner Kluge's *The Practice of Death* is a treatise on the extent to which past and present-day cultures practice abortion, infanticide, suicide, and genocide. (Yale University Press, New Haven, Conn., 1975.)

tion, these basic functions of caring for (nurturing or nursing), teaching about, and curing disease (doctoring) are again subdivided. The assignment of their component functions to groups of men or women depends to a large extent on the status of males and females in the society, and on differences in their education and roles. If there is no agreement among the major categories of workers and their subdivisions as to who does what, there is chaos. If nurses, teachers, or doctors (or any of their subdivisions) get too numerous or too powerful in a society, or develop practices inimical to the welfare of the population, they may make the society as a whole unduly dependent on them or they may pervert the instinctive behavior that preserves the individual and protects the species. If the different categories or subdivisions of workers have ill-defined functions and are competitive, they may develop along the lines of self-interest rather than in ways that will further the common good. It is for these reasons, among others, that the functions of nurses, teachers, and doctors, and the subdivisions of these essential health workers, must be considered *interdependently* and their roles in society continually studied in relationship to each other rather than as separate entities. Common goals for health workers, a certain amount of common knowledge, and cooperative relationships are essential to effective health care. This is particularly true for nurses and doctors, who are the oldest and largest groups of specialized health workers in most societies.

There are many indications today that health workers, especially nurses and doctors, are realizing the necessity of cooperation and that they are trying to identify the commonalities in their practice and the particular roles of each in health care. In order to understand the difficulties they face in changing their roles and relationships, it is necessary to know something about the history of medicine and the history of nursing. A thorough study of each is rewarding, and full-length works are included among the suggested readings at the end of this chapter. The following historical sketch does nothing more than give some of the significant differences in the origins and concepts of nurses and doctors.

Medicine and Nursing. Their Origins, the Public's Image of Doctors and Nurses, Their Preparation and Cultural Influences. Any study of medicine and nursing involves a study of cultural settings. Henry E. Sigerist makes the following statement:

Medical theories always represent one aspect of the general civilization of a period. . . .

If we attempt to see the theories of medicine as products of their time . . . then we understand the religious character of Babylonian medicine. We understand why the Greek physicians interpreted the phenomena of health and disease in philosophic terms.*

Fielding Garrison explains the omniscience of the "medicine man":

Primitive medicine is inseparable from primitive modes of religious belief. . . . the diagnosis and treatment of disease, . . . was only one phase of a set of mystic processes designed to promote human well-being, such as averting the wrath of angered gods or evil spirits, fire-making, making rain, purifying streams or habitations, fertilizing soil, improving sexual potency or fecundity, preventing or removing blight of crops and epidemic diseases. These powers, originally united in one person, were he god, hero, king, sorcerer, priest, prophet, or physician, formed the savage's generic concept of "making medicine". . . .†

Primitive healers still function among North and South American Indians and have their equivalents in other tribal societies on every continent today. Physicians practicing modern Western medicine in such cultures may collaborate with the indigenous "healers." ‡ Prevention of disease in primitive systems is thought to depend on placating the omnipresent spirits. If this belief is disregarded, the "scientific" treatment may be ineffective. Anthropologists note that individuals in primitive societies who believe they are doomed to die may respond negatively to a scientific regimen that would under other circumstances be life-saving.

Egyptians are said to have refined primitive medicine and, in observing the dead body, which they prepared elaborately for entry into the next world, derived explanations for many illnesses. Babylonian medicine, as has been noted, was essentially religious, with metaphysical "cures." Ancient Chinese medicine was influenced by Confucian philosophy which taught that Yang—the masculine element— and Yin—the feminine—are balanced in health. This principle still influences Chinese

---

* Sigerist, Henry E.: *A History of Medicine.* Volume 1. *Primitive and Archaic Medicine.* Oxford University Press, New York, 1951, p. 11.

† Garrison, Fielding H.: *An Introduction to the History of Medicine,* 4th ed. W. B. Saunders Co., Philadelphia, 1960, p. 20.

‡ Mike Samuels, a physician, calls the body "a three million year old healer." In his book, *The Well Body Book,* written with Hal Bennett for the public and designed to help people stay healthy, Samuels gives credit to Rolling Thunder (an American Indian) "who taught me healing." (Random House/Bookworks, New York, 1973, p. vi.) A nurse, R. S. Bryan, writes about "My Friends the Witchdoctors," *Nurs. Times,* **68:**1220, (Sept. 28) 1972.

health care and may be the Eastern counterpart of the Western concept of balance in the negatively and positively charged elements of the fluid-electrolyte system of the body, accepted as essential to health. Traditional Eastern and modern Western medicine are practiced side by side in China today. Research in both ancient and modern practice is encouraged in the People's Republic of China.[4]

V. Djukanovic and E. P. Mach, reporting a joint UNICEF-WHO study under the title *Alternative Approaches to Meeting Basic Health Needs in Developing Countries* (WHO, Geneva, 1975), suggest the extent to which primitive concepts persist and are combined in currently effective health programs on various continents.

Sigerist dates "the new epoch" of medicine from the Indo-European peoples. He says, "the parallelism in the development of Greek and Indian medicine is striking, both in chronology and in content." He believes that "we glorify the Greeks" and disregard other ancient medical systems except as precursors of Greek medicine and this approach to history is "utterly naive and viciously wrong." A thorough study, he thinks, shows that "Western and Indian medicine were closely related and equally effective not only in antiquity but also in the Middle Ages." * It is interesting that one of the effective UNICEF-WHO health programs is based on the 3000-year-old Ayurvedic medicine of India, which, according to those reporting the study, is used by most peoples living in India and neighboring countries. They say that "as an integral part of Indian culture it cannot be ignored." † Indian physicians (400,000 of them) are trained to use this ancient system which includes a psychosomatic approach to health in preventive and curative aspects. Medical research in India, as in China, is focused on indigenous as well as Western medicine.

As Sigerist notes, most historians say that "Western medicine" is derived from Greek medicine, because both are based on critical analysis of observation. Hippocrates is called "the father of medicine," and most medical students of today take the Hippocratic Oath at graduation. The Greeks saw humans as differentiated from the rest of nature by their capacity for thought or reason; they recognized that emotions affected the body and believed that man had a "soul." Being healthy was a Greek virtue. Vern and Bonnie Bullough[5] say that the rudiments of health were common

knowledge, and self-care rather than constant recourse to health workers characterized the Greek citizen.* Relatively little is known about nursing in Greece, as distinct from medicine. Physicians had trained helpers and some say they were nurses. Edwin B. and Myra E. Levine[6] suggest that Hippocrates is "father" to both medicine and nursing.

The Greeks emphasized exercise, rest, and diet rather than medication. Their health spas were also temples where there were statues of the gods of medicine and health—Asclepius (or Aesculapius, Roman spelling) † and his daughters Hygeia, the goddess of health, and Panakeia, the goddess of healing.

Edgar Jackson[7] says that Aesculapius was thought to restore disordered function, while Hygeia symbolized the quality of wholeness, or health. Some see this distinction as typified today by the work of doctors on one hand and nurses on the other. Mack Lipkin says:

Hygeia, the guardian of health, symbolized that blessed state achieved by living a sane life in a good environment. Her sister was reputed to heal by her great knowledge of drugs and manipulations. As [R. J.] Dubos [*Mirage of Health*, Harper & Row, New York, 1959, p. 182] points out, ever since there has been an oscillation between the two points of view of medicine. . . . Since the teachings of Hygeia require self-discipline, they are commonly ignored. The help of the healer, Panakeia, is sought more often.‡

Fielding H. Garrison credits the Romans with advancing surgery "including obstetrics and ophthalmology." He says it "reached a stage of perfection which it was not to reach again before the time of Ambroise Paré (sixteenth century)." §

According to Edmund D. Pellegrino, "Many of the Roman ideas of disease were corruptions of the Greek." || One of their methods of treatment depended on "keeping the pores of the skin open." The Roman baths were a com-

---

* Self-help is thought by many to be our best hope today. Keith E. Sehnert titles an article "Miracle Drugs and Lifesaving Machines May Make Headlines But It's the Individual Who Is the Cornerstone of a Sound Medical System," (*Fam. Health*, **7**:41, [Nov.] 1975).

† Beatrice J. Kalisch, in an article titled "Of Half Gods and Mortals: Aesculapian Authority," suggests that this influence persists, leading some wag to say that "M.D. stands for Minor Diety." (*Nurs. Outlook*, **23**:22, [Jan.] 1975).

‡ Lipkin, Mack: *The Care of Patients: Concepts and Tactics*. Oxford University Press, New York, 1974, p. 55.

§ Garrison, Fielding H.: *op. cit.*, p. 108. (The erroneous concept that obstetrics is a branch of surgery is deeply rooted in the literature.)

|| Pellegrino, Edmund D.: "Medicine, History, and the Idea of Man," *Ann. Am. Acad. Pol. Sci.*, **346**:9, (Mar.) 1953.

---

* Sigerist, Henry E.: *op. cit.*, p. 3.

† Djukanovic, V., and Mach, E. P. (eds.): *op. cit.*, p. 3.

bination of clubhouse and spa. The "baths" or "watering places," so numerous in many countries throughout the nineteenth and early part of the twentieth centuries, had these characteristics also. The people of Japan today put great emphasis on communal bathing, and the Scandinavian sauna is popular around the world. But hydrotherapy as such is not typical of the present age.

Judaeo-Christian thought dominated the Western world following the decline of the Roman Empire and throughout the Middle Ages, the latter sometimes called "The Age of Faith." * Its monotheistic philosophy emphasized the worth and uniqueness of the individual, the unity of body and soul, or the total personality. Christians were, to some extent, resigned to suffering in this world but stressed heaven as the reward of a well-spent life. One road to heaven was succoring the sick and helpless. Nursing became a Christian virtue and hospitals and hospices flourished in the Middle Ages. Some of the best-known men and women of the early Christian centuries were made famous, or even raised to sainthood, by a selfless devotion to the sick, the poor, and the unfortunate. Highborn persons often joined religious orders that owned and operated hospitals or hospices, or they cared for the sick and helpless at home. Groups whose chief work was nursing were formed all over the known Western world. While some were secular, many were religious. During the Crusades, military chivalric nursing orders were founded, and it was not unmanly to belong to them, although the members of these orders treated as well as nursed the sick, or combined medicine and nursing.[8] Some hospitals and hospices established in the Middle Ages and a number of nursing orders founded then are still functioning today. Lucie Young Kelly identified the latter in a 1975 publication.[9]

Arabian medicine, practiced during the Middle Ages within the Moslem Empire, was based on translations of the Greeks and was enhanced by rigorous study of chemistry, physiology, and pharmacy. Arabian physicians developed a rational system of medical care and were respected members of society. The Mohammedan religion embraced the teachings of some of the major contemporary religions, so Moslem learning was broad rather than narrow. A strict hygienic regimen was part of religious practice. Arabic-Hebraic medicine was the most enlightened of any during the Middle Ages, and it kept alive some of the advances made by the Greeks. However, because dissection of the human body was prohibited by the Mohammedan religion, misconceptions of anatomy and physiology persisted.

During the Renaissance, there was an intense interest in learning, rediscovery of the classics, and the study of man. This period was marked by geographic exploration and by the development of libraries and universities. Schools of medicine, theology, philosophy, and law were included in the Renaissance universities, although there were medical schools in the universities at Boulogne, Montpellier, and Paris during the Middle Ages.[10]

While Renaissance medicine was based largely on translations of Greek texts, dissection of the human body and experimentation were introduced, and this led to important changes in thought and practice. Pellegrino makes the following observation:

Modern man was born sometime in the Renaissance at that indefinite but crucial point when his thought turned from a primary interest in philosophy and theology to the investigation of himself and his world with the tools of experimentation and mathematics.*

While medicine from the Middle Ages onward has had a place in the university, the preparation of physicians and surgeons and their social status have varied. As late as the nineteenth century, many of them learned the medical arts through an apprenticeship. Hospitals controlled some medical schools and others might be operated for profit. Vernon W. Lippard [11] says that the British system was dominated by the hospital schools of London. He maintains that the medical school in the United States had its roots not only in the British system but also in the German system centered in universities. As a whole, medical education in the United States rated below that in Europe at the time of the Flexner Report (1910).[12] Not until after this report on American medicine were proprietary medical schools and correspondence courses eliminated in the United States. Today, American medical schools are within universities and doctors have a uniform, rigorous, and costly preparation. At present, medicine is more scientific and technical than humanistic.

This trend toward the development of a medical technology from a science is not new. Hans Peter Dreitzel says:

This conception of medicine as a science developed during the Enlightenment. It was Paracelsus who, still in the Middle Ages, first effectively re-

---

* Dates given by authorities for the Middle Ages and the European Renaissance vary. They range roughly from 400 to 1500 for the former and 1300 to 1700 for the latter.

[d] Pellegrino, Edmund D.: *op. cit.*

jected theological and magical conceptions of illness and opened the way to the modern development of medicine.*

Medical historians attribute to René Descartes, French philosopher of the seventeenth century (sometimes called "the Age of Reason"), a trend toward a mechanistic view of man and life, for, instead of seeing the human body and soul as one, Descartes thought the soul pure spirit and the body pure matter. Cartesian thought was widely discussed and had a profound effect on many aspects of life in France and elsewhere.† Pellegrino says that, while Descartes finally admitted his defeat, he tried to develop a theory of medicine "based on infallible demonstrations." Pellegrino attributes reintroduction of the notion of disease as a total disturbance to Immanuel Kant, German philosopher of the eighteenth century and his followers, who emphasized "transcendental, subjective, imaginative systems." This encouraged study of psychology and psychiatry.

In an article titled "Educating the Humanist Physician," Pellegrino calls this "an ancient ideal reconsidered." He makes the following observation:

In the growing litany of criticism to which our profession is increasingly exposed, there is one that in many ways is more painful than all the rest. It is the assertion that physicians are no longer humanists and that medicine is no longer a learned profession. Our technical proficiency is extolled, but in its application we are said to be insensitive to human values. We are, in short, presumed to be wanting as educated men and as responsive human beings.‡

Actually, medicine based on the scientific method of investigation, or "modern medicine," is historically still young. Except for psychiatry, it is largely an application of the physical and biologic sciences.

The microscope, developed by Anton van Leeuwenhoek (1632–1723), made it possible to study the structure and function of the cell. Claude Bernard's [13] nineteenth-century concept of keeping the lymph around the cell (relatively) constant, or in physiologic balance, revolutionized the practice of medicine. Now the scanning electron microscope has ushered in a new era in the study of microbiology, histology, and cell physiology. Lennart Nilsson and Jan Lindberg make the following comparison between the capabilities of the ordinary microscope and the scanning electron microscope:

The common laboratory microscope uses light rays to illuminate an object. Anything smaller than the wavelength of visible light, i.e., smaller than half a thousandth of a millimeter, is beyond the capacity of the light microscope and cannot be reproduced. This limitation does not apply to the scanning electron microscope, which uses a beam of electrons instead of visible light. Magnetic fields are used to direct and focus the beam so that it behaves like a ray of light. The "camera" of the electron microscope picks up the activity of the electron beam as it scans the preparation to be studied and produces a picture on a screen in somewhat the manner of a television camera.

The definition in depth of the scanning electron microscope is up to five hundred times greater than that of the light microscope. For this reason, this type of microscope is used to study and photograph surface structures. Its magnifying power varies between 20,000 and 60,000.*

It is hard to imagine the full effect that use of electronic photography will have on study of cell structure and function and ultimately on public understanding of health and disease; and there are other recent technologic developments that may greatly alter health care. Bioelectric medicine, the collaboration of engineers and physicians, is radically changing diagnostic procedures; the laser beam may drastically alter surgery; and modern methods of communicating make health discoveries common knowledge. Nilsson's and Lindberg's book, *Behold Man,* [14] Lewis Thomas's *The Lives of a Cell,* [15] and the film "The Incredible Machine" (the last shown first on public television in 1975) can give even a child a clearer picture of the microscopic structure of tissues and of some body functions than great scientists had in earlier decades.

While contemporary medicine is largely a technical application of physiology, this cannot be said of modern psychiatry, which is based largely on psychology, anthropology, and sociology. With the exception of psychiatry, modern medicine is criticized for being too dependent on technology. The *art of medicine,* as opposed to the *science of medicine,* has its roots in human values. Modern medicine is believed by some critics to overempha-

* Dreitzel, Hans Peter (ed.): *The Social Organization of Health*. Recent Sociology No. 3. Macmillan Publishing Co., Inc., New York, 1971, p. vii.

† Descartes' writings were the subject of conversation in the fashionable as well as the intellectual world. There are many references to such conversations in Madame de Sévigné's letters to her daughter from the court of France in Paris. (de Sévigné, Marie de Rabutin-Chantal: *The Letters of Madame de Sévigné*. Carnavelet Ed. W. T. Morrell and Co., London, 1928.)

‡ Pellegrino, Edmund D.: "Educating the Humanist Physician," *J.A.M.A.*, **227:**1288, (Mar. 18) 1974.

* Nilsson, Lennart: *Behold Man—A Photographic Journey Inside the Body*. In collaboration with Jan Lindberg. Little, Brown & Co., Boston, 1974, p. 248.

size its science and underrate its art.* Contemporary medicine is even thought by some critics to do more harm than good. Ivan Illich develops this theory under the title *Medical Nemesis. The Expropriation of Health* (Pantheon Books, New York, 1976) and Rick J. Carlson under the title *The End of Medicine* (John Wiley & Sons, New York, 1975). They consider the people of many countries exploited by industrialized health care which, unevenly distributed but universally sought, is making people unrealistic in their expectation of escaping pain and incapable of self-care. Its spiraling cost is believed by many to put a disproportionate burden on society. While a full explanation of the aggrandizement of medical science as opposed to its art would be presumptuous at this point, some reasons are clear to the most superficial student. Through technical research, the causes of many diseases have been identified and the development of cures and preventive methods established; anesthesia has been developed; and, through animal experimentation, surgery has progressed to the point where surgeons daily perform life-saving operations that would, until this century, have been thought impossible. Surgery was, until this age, quite rightly feared and distrusted, as was the surgeon. Only in this century has the surgeon in Europe enjoyed the same social acceptance as the physician. The technical accomplishments of this era have fostered pride in medical "progress" rather than self-criticism.†

Organized medicine in many countries, most particularly the United States, has opposed rather than supported attempts to distribute health care equally—attempts to make it as universally available as education. Tax-supported education has been rooted in value systems and dominated by social science; tax-supported health care is often referred to as the largest, or next to the largest, "industry";

it is technologic and dominated by the physical and biologic sciences.

While nursing has been greatly influenced by and in some instances is inseparable from medicine, its history—its development in most cultures—is different. The fact that physicians were usually men and nurses were usually women may partially explain the difference. Vern and Bonnie Bullough's study, *The Subordinate Sex—A History of Attitudes Towards Women* [16] and Jo Ann Ashley's work, *Hospitals, Paternalism, and the Role of the Nurse* [16a] show some of the ways in which attitudes toward women have affected nursing and medicine. Margaret Mead,[17] an anthropologist, frequently observes that most cultures tend to assume that the woman's share of the work is easier and less intellectually demanding than the man's. It is only in this century that nursing has been accepted in any country as a university discipline, whereas medicine has had a place in universities since the latter began.* Nursing as an art is as old as the art of medicine; nursing as a science is much younger than medicine as a science. The humanistic element in nursing still dominates the scientific.

It is hard to identify the beginning of the science of nursing. If enough was known about the early training programs, it might be seen that some nurses were introduced to the science of the time and place, but Anne L. Austin,[18] whose *History of Nursing Source Book* is a compilation of excerpts from writings on nurses and nursing from ancient to modern times, dates the "profession of nursing" from the Nightingale era. The existence of nursing science may even now be questioned by some, but there are courses of study in nursing science here and in Europe.[19-21]

Like medicine, nursing can be traced to primitive cultures, and in some form has existed in all cultures. The art of nursing has flowered in religious communities throughout the centuries and in some secular and military orders. Like medicine, it has been influenced by dominant philosophies. Since nursing has usually been seen as woman's work, woman's status has affected nursing's status, just as man's status has affected medicine's status.

---

* See, for example, Jan Howard and Anselm Strauss, *Humanizing Health Care* (John Wiley & Sons, New York, 1975) and articles such as that of John P. Geyman, "On Depersonalization in Medicine," (*J. Fam. Practice,* 3:239, [June] 1976).

† Many critics of health care point out that even though technically excellent care is available in a country, it will not affect the health indices materially until a political system is developed that makes necessary care available to all citizens and that provides them with adequate food and a healthful environment. Health is said to be a social problem and the organization of health care a political task. Roger Hurley maintains that a failure to provide a satisfactory organization should be attributed to a society (in this case American) rather than to its medical profession. (Hurley, Roger: "Health Crisis of the Poor," in Dreitzel, Hans Peter [ed.]: *The Social Organization of Health.* Macmillan Publishing Co., Inc., New York, 1971, p. 113 [Recent Sociology No. 3].)

---

* Even in Sweden where nursing is generally thought to have flourished, its schools are under the National Board of Education, while medical schools are under the office of the chancellor of the Swedish universities. Responsibility for training physical therapists, in contrast, comes under both. (Tengstam, Anders: *Patterns of Health Care and Education in Sweden.* Centre for Educational Research and Innovation [CERI], Organisation for Economic Co-operation and Development, Paris, France, 1975, p. 27.)

Even today, a doctor is usually referred to as "he," a nurse as "she."

In some societies, however, there is no sharp distinction between medicine and nursing, between doctors and nurses. Margaret Read, discussing traditional systems of care in sickness and the role of the traditional practitioners, says:

Health personnel and anthropologists have distinguished several kinds of healer. First, there are the women, whose skills in the use of home remedies, widespread across the world, are shared by countless others. Women's techniques include such practices as the use of purgatives and emetics, poulticing, inducing sweating by various processes, and all the traditional birth practices.*

In a 1957 study of Navaho Indians cited by Read, among 73 diagnosticians, 43 were men and 30 were women. In countries such as India, where women led sheltered lives, men performed the functions of nurses outside the home, most particularly the functions that necessitated touching the bodies of adult males.

Differentiation of function between doctors and nurses, between the practice of medicine and nursing, is especially difficult in military services. The barber surgeons of the Middle Ages, attached to European armies, both treated and cared for the sick and injured.[22] Schools for Russian feldshers, military and civil, that have existed since the eighteenth century, today offer 3- to 4-year programs that combine medicine and nursing, as the latter are conceived in the United States. Today's feldshers are taught by doctors and nurses. The recently established schools for physician's assistants in the United States are following the feldsher pattern to some extent.[23,24]

To understand "modern nursing," the nurse's function and status, it should be stressed that nursing schools did not (like medical schools) originate in the universities. While there were apprenticeship training programs for nurses in a variety of settings in many countries, the independent Nightingale School of Nursing (with St. Thomas's Hospital in London used as its practice field) is generally considered the first true school of nursing. Established under the influence of Florence Nightingale, it reflected her philosophy. She was deeply religious and committed to the service of her fellow man. She thought the life of a nurse "the happiest of any." Like the Greeks, she trusted in cleanliness, fresh air, good food, rest, sleep, and (with less emphasis) exercise as support

for nature's curative forces. She seems to have feared the physician's interference with nature and to have believed both physicians and nurses ignorant about the fundamentals of health. She decried their overriding interest in disease and their relative indifference to helping people achieve good health.[25] Mrs. Cecil Woodham-Smith,[26] whose biography of Florence Nightingale is one of the more definitive, concluded that her work in nursing was the greatest of all her contributions to society. She said Miss Nightingale saw nursing as helping people to live; she saw the body and soul as inseparable; she looked upon the patient as a member of a family and a community and upon nursing as an expression of the nurse's citizenship and religion. Florence Nightingale was a competent mathematician and statistician. She was one of the first to use health statistics as leverage in effecting health legislation for England and other parts of the British Empire. In this age, Miss Nightingale might have been called a sociologist and economist as well as a statistician.

Women who have shaped nursing since the Nightingale era have, like her, tended to emphasize the psychosocial aspects of nursing—to see nursing as significant in changing the social order. Ethel Bedford Fenwick in England and Lillian Wald, Lavinia Dock, and Annie W. Goodrich in the United States are examples of those who believed nursing to be a complex and creative social service growing out of the needs of contemporary society. Miss Goodrich entitled her collective works *The Social and Ethical Significance of Nursing.*[27] These women worked in the Women's Suffrage movement. Lillian Wald persuaded President Theodore Roosevelt to create the US Children's Bureau, which, among other functions, controlled child labor.[28] Public health nurses (community nurses) have always considered the family rather than the individual as the patient, or client, and have responded to a wide range of social needs.* In recent years, psychiatric nurses have developed the psychosocial aspects of care to a high degree. Most nurses in many countries give at least lip service to the concept of family-centered health care.

While institutional nursing is often impersonal and may seem to be dominated by technological medicine, nursing as a whole has

---

* Read, Margaret: *Culture, Health and Disease. Social and Cultural Influences on Health Programs in Developing Countries.* J. B. Lippincott Co., Philadelphia, 1966, p. 16.

* Some of the developing countries are giving health care high priority and nurses are playing a significant role in planning and giving health care. F. O. Okedigi discusses the "Economics of Health Care Delivery" in "Nigeria's Second National Plan 1970–1974" in its "Sociological Perspective" (*Niger Nurse,* **5:**31, [Apr.–June] 1973).

remained a service derived from the universal human needs of the very young, the helpless, and the sick. Certain branches of nursing have concentrated on health teaching, on promotion of health, and on prevention of disease. Later in this chapter, the roles of doctors, nurses, and teachers and their overlapping functions are discussed.* Chapter 3 is a description of nursing in the various settings in which it is practiced.

The points made in the preceding historical review are the following: Health care is an integral part of every culture or is affected by the philosophy and the social values of the culture. Looking at health care worldwide, all stages of its development can be found today, from the primitive to so-called "modern medicine." Both Occidental, or "Western medicine," and Oriental, or Eastern medicine, are derived from many cultures. Primitive and ancient practices may survive intact, they may be blended with newer methods, or they may subtly influence practice and the public image of the health worker. "Modern" Western medicine, while not even today free from the occult or from mysticism, derives from classic (Greek) medicine (according to Sigerist, from the Indo-Grecian culture), and has been, in certain countries, a university discipline since the Middle Ages. Western medicine in this age is based largely on the application of the physical sciences and is influenced to a high degree by institutional technology. Eastern medicine puts more emphasis on the totality of man and on the metaphysical aspects of treatment.

Nursing as a profession dates from the latter half of the nineteenth century, but generic nursing has existed in every culture. The founder of modern nursing and subsequent leaders have conceived of "professional" nursing as a social service with revolutionary capabilities. While influenced by its association with domestic service, with religious and military groups, and more recently with institutional technology, nursing remains essentially a nurturing, family-centered service. Nursing has based much of its practice on the applica-

tion of the biologic sciences of physiology and bacteriology but, to a greater extent than medicine, on the social sciences—on psychology, human development, sociology, and economics. Nursing research (discussed in Chapter 19) is most often derived from the social sciences. While the following may be an oversimplification, it would seem that Western medicine has been focused on disease control and research in the physical and biologic sciences; nursing on meeting the human needs of the very young, the old, the sick, and the helpless, drawing on the psychosocial sciences in an effort to improve the lot of mankind. Nursing has been, more than has medicine, a substitute for self-care.

All health care in every culture is affected by the dominant religions or ethics, especially as they relate to the protection of the very young, the old, the sick, and the helpless. The World Health Organization has taken the position that health care is a universal right. Most nations are trying to achieve this goal. New categories of health workers have been created, and functions and responsibilities among established categories of health workers have been redistributed. The current emphasis in medicine on primary care and family practice and in nursing on physical assessment and clinical research suggests a trend toward overlapping functions, common goals and shared responsibility.

As both medicine and nursing emphasize prevention, and as doctors and nurses recognize the importance of self-help by the client or patient, the interdependence of physicians and nurses with health educators will be as apparent as the interdependence of physicians and nurses. Each society must answer the following questions: What should all citizens know about health? When should they learn it? Who should teach it? Where should it be taught?

Medicine, Nursing, Health Education, and Social Service. Assuming that promotion of health and prevention of disease are more important to human welfare and less costly to society than the cure of disease (both are generally conceded), it would seem that there is no limit to what the average citizen might profitably know about health promotion and disease prevention. However, people should not only learn how to be healthy and avoid disease, but they must *want to be healthy*. Health must be valued—a sought after ideal or goal. Healthy habits must be acquired, and the earlier in life the better, for unhealthy habits are hard to break. The single most important condition in promoting health is that the individual *wants to be healthy*.

---

* The differentiation of the doctor's and nurse's roles is difficult in every age and every country. Dr. Charles Harris, an eminent American surgeon of this century who gave a million-dollar endowment to the Harris College of Nursing at the Texas Christian University, Fort Worth, made this observation to the writer in 1959. He said that doctors of the Eastern United States did not know how hard nursing was because they had never had to do it. He, on the other hand, if he wanted a man to survive an amputation performed on the kitchen table at a Western ranch, had been obliged to stay and nurse the patient for two or three days. Dr. Harris remarked that he did not know which was more difficult—the surgery or the nursing.

Knowledge of health is constantly unfolding, so, if the general public is to profit by the growing body of knowledge, people must continue to learn throughout the life span, and acquire the ability to change habitual behavior in applying new knowledge. The preceding statements suggest that there should be no fence around knowledge on which to base health practice, that acquiring this knowledge is a lifetime quest.

It is not easy to outline how to inculcate health values, goals, and ideals. Current theories of learning are discussed in Chapter 16 and have direct bearing on this question. Few persons of any schools of thought doubt that family, clan, tribal, or societal influences contribute toward the development of values, goals, and ideals. In childhood, individuals are most likely to adopt the values of parents; in adolescence, they accept the values of their age group or of adult role models; and later, they are more susceptible to the values of the social class to which they belong. Only in maturity are people relatively free to create a highly individualized pattern of behavior. These statements suggest that health motivation is a widely shared responsibility and that actions contributing to it pervade all aspects of life.

Promotion of health and prevention of disease are indeed everybody's business, as many have said. Mark Van Doren,[29] studying liberal education in 1943, concluded that health was one of its goals, that good health is characteristic of the "liberally" educated. Those who agree with him must see doctors and nurses and all other health workers as sharing with educators of all age groups the responsibility for teaching health promotion and disease prevention. Carlson [29a] and others suggest that a health dollar spent on education is more effective than one spent on medical care.

The word doctor comes from *docere,* meaning to teach, and some persons see teaching as the principal service the physician performs. John B. Dillon,[30] a physician, decries the overemphasis on research and technologic medicine and on specialization. Speaking of the reform in medical education stemming from Abraham Flexner's study, he says that Flexner considered prevention of disease through education of the public the physician's most important function and that he deeply regretted what happened to medical education in this century.

With the tendency toward specialization in American medicine and with the increasing importance attached to medical research, physicians have had less and less time to know their patients and to teach them, even in the unstudied manner of the family practitioner.[31,*] The inadequacy of the health care system, especially as it relates to disease prevention, is widely discussed. Most developed countries have organized or reorganized health care in recent decades, stressing its preventive aspects and giving the recipients of care more influence. James O. and Donna M. Hepner,[32] calling for reorganization of health care in the United States, refer to "the new consumerism."

Chapter 2 is devoted to the subject of health programs in the United States and elsewhere. Some of the ways in which different countries are providing health services for all citizens are discussed; for example, the system in the People's Republic of China, where military, industrial, and rural workers are trained to teach health, give preventive and remedial care, and to collaborate with more thoroughly trained professional nurses, doctors, and others, distributing the task of health education among a wide variety of workers; also the Russian network of health services, designed to bring preventive and remedial services to all citizens; and the nationalized health service of Great Britain. In Britain, one or more general medical practitioners, working with one or more district nurses, a health visitor, and a health officer, constitutes one of the building units for the national health service. These workers are available to every citizen of the area they serve, and they offer health education and preventive and remedial services (see Figures 1-1 and 1-2).

In all these and other countries that have nearly eliminated a private fee-for-service system of medical care and established a tax-supported health service, preventive and curative services are available to all, and health teaching is an integral part of the service. In such national plans, the physician shares the responsibility for health teaching with other workers.

In the United States, some segments of the population have tax-supported health care that is preventive as well as remedial. There is a general trend toward universal health insurance, or prepaid preventive and remedial care. While the United States is almost, if not the only, developed country that does not have a national health program comparable to that of

---

* The reader should not assume that there is any intention to belittle the importance of research in the field of health. It is only when the cause of disease is established that the best preventive program can be designed; it is only possible to teach the optimum diet when controlled experiments demonstrate its essentials. Chapter 19 is devoted to a discussion of research as a basis for designing and evaluating health practices with special reference to nursing.

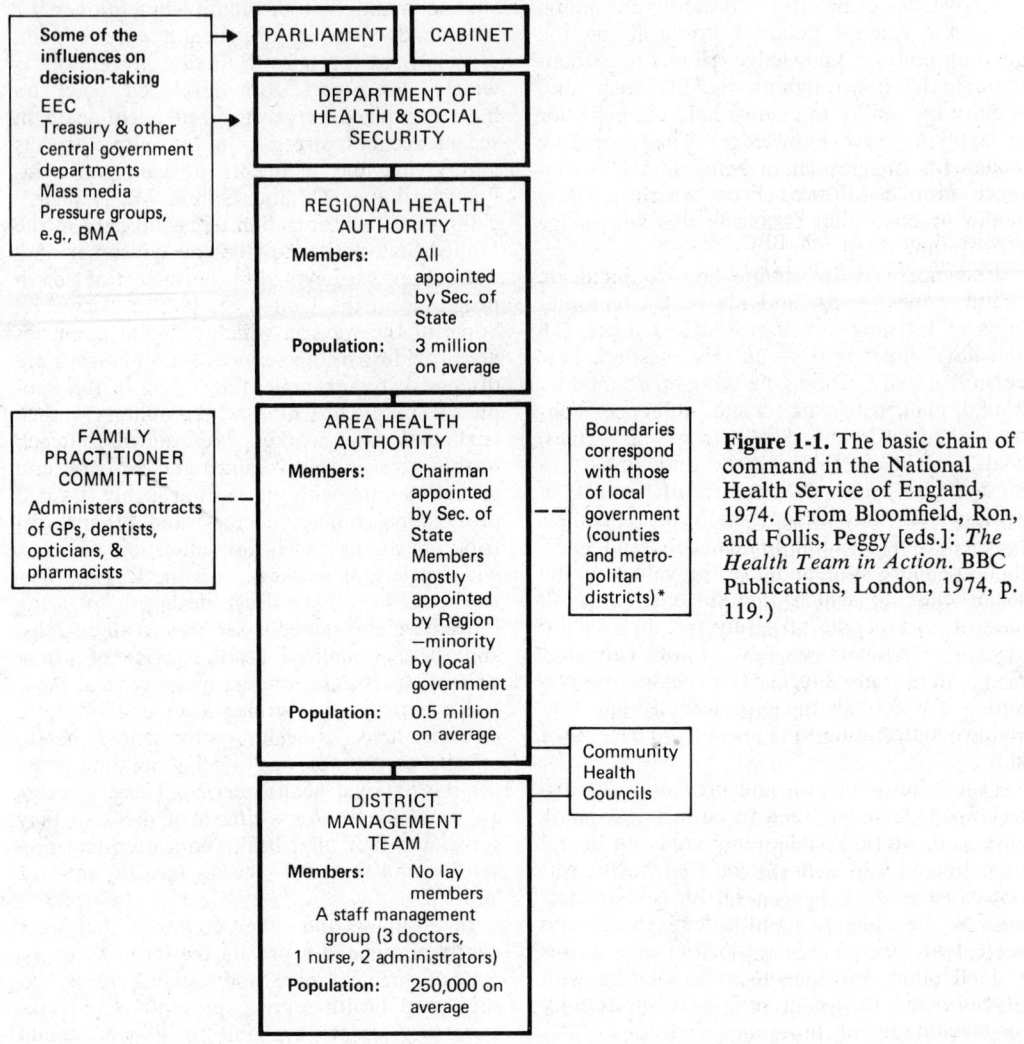

Figure 1-1. The basic chain of command in the National Health Service of England, 1974. (From Bloomfield, Ron, and Follis, Peggy [eds.]: *The Health Team in Action*. BBC Publications, London, 1974, p. 119.)

*Arrangements in Scotland, Wales, and Northern Ireland are somewhat different.

the British Isles or the (provincial) programs in Canada, in the USSR, mainland China, or the Scandinavian countries, it is generally believed that some plan of national health insurance will be adopted in the near future. When this happens, teaching people to be healthy and to avoid disease will be essential on economic as well as humane grounds.

The extent to which health workers have collaborated and should collaborate with teachers interested in health education in primary and secondary education is hard to assess. Many eminent health educators in the schools have been physicians; joint commissions, composed of members of national health organizations and national educational organizations, have provided guidelines for practice; physicians, nurses, and other health workers

employed in school health and college health systems have tried, and are trying, to answer the questions, Who teaches what about health? To whom, and where? *

There has been a tendency in the past for physicians to think "a little knowledge [of medicine] is a dangerous thing"; a tendency to guard medical secrets, to expect patients to trust physicians to prescribe the right drug, the proper treatment. Nurses have been taught to refer to physicians any questions from patients

* In 1973, the first international conference on "education in the health sciences" was held. Such meetings should encourage the development of common objectives and help to remove interdisciplinary barriers. ("A 'First'—An International Conference on Education in the Health Sciences" [News], *Int. Nurs. Rev.*, **20:**71, [May–June] 1973.)

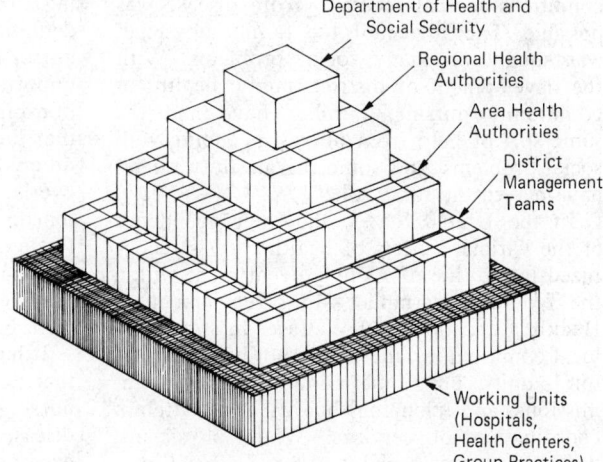

Department of Health and
Social Security

Regional Health
Authorities

Area Health
Authorities

District
Management
Teams

Working Units
(Hospitals,
Health Centers,
Group Practices)

Figure 1-2. Organization of health services in Great Britain. (From Bloomfield, Ron, and Follis, Peggy [eds.]: *The Health Team in Action.* BBC Publications, London, 1974, p. 121.)

on diagnosis, prognosis, or therapy. These beliefs and practices, limiting what was taught patients and who taught it, are now challenged. Books and journals about all major diseases written for the general public are available, as are films, television programs, and multisensory media of all sorts. Widely distributed "bills" listing the "rights of patients" include their right to be informed. Patients can and do bring suit against practitioners who treat them without explaining the purpose and the risks of treatment. It is no longer feasible for physicians, or any other therapists, to avoid educating patients, and with the kind of information now available to the general public, teaching must be increasingly sophisticated. Knowledge needed by a newspaper science editor to write a good article on open heart surgery, nuclear medicine, or treatment of leprosy may equal or exceed that of the average physician; the same statement might be made about producers of films and other multisensory teaching aids in the field of health. While the practice of medicine increases in complexity, the mysterious elements are disappearing, and the public is almost demanding that the sources of information be available to everybody.

Medical libraries have been traditionally open to physicians only. Gradually, they were opened to nurses and other health workers. Now, in the United States, medical libraries that accept funds from public sources must be open to the public.* Libraries in universities,

once called "medical," are now called "health science libraries or information centers," and they serve the entire university community. Many persons believe all "medical" libraries (national, provincial, state, or local community) should be renamed to more accurately describe the scope of the contents and to invite the broadest possible usage.

There is an implication in what has been said so far that health may be promoted, disease prevented, cured, or controlled, if there are health workers and others to teach patients and their families and to give supportive care and remedial treatment. While these are the services stressed in this book, none is effective if patients or clients lack an adequate diet, shelter, and the other necessities of healthful living.* Many religious orders giving health care have provided a variety of social services; hospitals and other institutions employ social workers to help patients and their families with socioeconomic problems and in some countries, in certain eras, nurses, particularly those in community nursing, were prepared for both nursing and social work. Family physicians were once, in a more personal culture, also friends and often helped a family alter living

to patients or potential patients. The health occupations should have no "trade secrets," no "private" source of information. It is the mark of professionals to share their knowledge and to make those they serve independent of them. Lucie Young Kelly, writing about "the patient's right to know" and the laws enforcing this right, expresses the opinion that "this movement may have a much more dramatic impact on health care than any series of exotic scientific discoveries." (*Nurs. Outlook,* **24**:26, [Jan.] 1976.)

* It must be recognized that the provision of health care is an economic, a political, issue. Victor R. Fuchs, an economist, expresses this in the title of a 1974 publication, *Who Shall Live? Health, Economics, and Social Choice,* Basic Books, Inc., New York, 1974.

* Some medical centers and hospitals set up patients' libraries as separate from the library that serves the health workers. (See Collen, F. Bobbie, and Soghikian, Krikor: "A Health Library for Patients," Health Services Reports, **29**:236, [May–June] 1974.) While librarians especially prepared to help the general public seem to me to promise better service, the writer believes that the entire range of the literature should be available

conditions so that recovery from disease was possible. The advice of the family physician was sought on many social problems. With the development of district, public health, or community nursing, families have had the same sort of help from nurses in coping with social problems, and some private duty nurses have played the same role.

In the United States, the interdependence of the various aspects of health care is recognized in the title of a single department within the federal government—the Department of Health, Education, and Welfare. In states and local communities, there may not be this structural unity but joint committees or commissions and planning boards may attempt coordination of services. While physicians, dentists, nurses, social workers, clinical psychologists, health educators, and other health workers must concentrate their energies on performance of their respective functions, their efforts may be relatively ineffective if they work in isolation and are unconcerned with other aspects of health care. Critics of health care available in the United States see a lack of planning, inadequate coordination, overlapping functions among workers, and unfulfilled needs of the people. Critics also say that health care imposes an unsupportable burden on most families. Contemporary articles on health care suggest a rapidly changing scene with terms such as ferment, crisis, chaos, transition, conflicting roles, emerging concepts, issues, new directions, and a new era appearing in titles of books and articles.[33-41]

Chapter 2 is devoted to health programs and the nurses' part in promoting optimum health service. There, and in this chapter, the importance of flexibility is stressed so that in each age, in each place, health needs of people may be served most effectively with resources available. No plan that sacrifices the welfare of the receivers of care to those who give it or the other way around will be tolerated by a society indefinitely.*

It may seem that, for a book about nursing, undue attention has been paid so far to the practice of medicine and the practice of teach-

ing. The next topic to be discussed is the definition of nursing and the function of the nurse. Before discussing this subject, it seems important to emphasize nursing's close relationship to medicine particularly; to point out that the functions of doctors and nurses have differed from one era to another, have often overlapped, and in some cases have been combined; and to stress that nursing, as a profession, is much younger and less established than medicine. The public image of the nurse has been less prestigious than that of the physician, but not in all eras less sympathetic.

It has been suggested in the preceding pages that teaching is inherent in both medicine and nursing, that promoting health and preventing disease is largely a matter of teaching, and that even remedial medicine depends for its efficacy upon the informed self-help of patients and their families. The functions, roles, and responsibilities of health workers and health educators are described as interdependent; coordinated planning is essential if the goal of an effective health service for all citizens is to be reached. Every community, state, and nation is trying to establish its health goals, assess its resources, and develop the services essential to the realization of its health objectives. This process of cooperative planning is much more established and more effective in some countries than in others. It can drastically change the functions and relationships of health workers with patients, and with each other.[42-46]

Regardless of the rapidly changing scene, it is helpful to review efforts in the past to define nursing and to also give the *working definition of nursing* on which the content of this book is based. The following definition, as expressed in a booklet, *ICN Basic Principles of Nursing,** has been accepted by the International Council of Nurses as its working definition of nursing. The heart of this definition, which will be discussed in more detail later, is as follows:

Nursing is primarily assisting individuals (sick or well) with those activities contributing to health, or its recovery (or to a peaceful death) that they perform unaided when they have the necessary strength, will, or knowledge; nursing also helps individuals carry out prescribed therapy and to be independent of assistance as soon as possible.

Health care should be considered as a whole, even though working definitions of the roles of each class of practitioners are useful, in fact,

---

* Everett Hughes, a sociologist, compared health care to the task a group of workers faces who must get a load of faggots up a mountain—every one of them. To accomplish this, he said that if any worker dropped a faggot another worker must pick it up. In like manner, if physicians or nurses or dietitians drop any of the tasks they have traditionally performed, some other worker must pick them up. His point was that no one health group should feel free to define its function or change its established role until it is assured that related groups are willing to change their roles so that the health care goals can still be reached. (Hughes, Everett, *et al.: Twenty Thousand Nurses Tell Their Story,* J. B. Lippincott Co., Philadelphia, 1958.)

* This booklet, written in 1960 and revised in 1969, which is now distributed by national nursing organizations and by the ICN, has been translated into 22 languages.

necessary. Health workers must be generalists as well as specialists. Nursing can never be defined for all time and for all ages and without reference to the roles and numbers of physicians and medical technicians, dentists and dental hygienists, social workers, pharmacists, physical therapists, health educators, sanitarians, clinical psychologists, and others. In every age, every community, and every health agency, an attempt should be made to understand and cope with the over-all problem of providing health care. The services needed and the numbers and competences of available workers should determine what each does. The resulting plan may demand a willingness on the part of all those concerned to forget traditional roles to some extent, to abrogate privileges, and to share functions and responsibilities.*

2. DEFINING NURSING AND THE FUNCTION OF THE NURSE

Some Definitions of Nursing and Nurses by Individuals from the Nightingale Era to the Present. Nurses, physicians, and others have been defining nursing for many years. Florence Nightingale seems to have looked upon both physicians and nurses (if they functioned effectively) as nature's colleagues. In the conclusion of her small volume, *Notes on Nursing, What It Is and What It Is Not,* she makes the following statement:

It is often thought that medicine is the curative process. It is no such thing; medicine is the surgery of functions, as surgery proper is that of limbs and organs. Neither can do anything but remove obstructions; neither can cure; nature alone cures. Surgery removes the bullet out of the limb, which is an obstruction to cure, but nature heals the wound. So it is with medicine; the function of an organ becomes obstructed; medicine, so far as we know, assists nature to remove the obstruction, but does nothing more. *And what nursing has to do in either case, is to put the patient in the best condition for nature to act upon him.*† [italics ours]

Nightingale thought all disease "at some period or other of its course, . . . a reparative process, not necessarily accompanied with suffering. . . ." * The writer has heard nurses of this era say that they thought the Nightingale definition of 1860 the most helpful. In any event, the Nightingale philosophy dominated nursing well into the twentieth century. She is regarded as a genius by nurses and nonnurses alike, and her concept of the body as self-healing is generally accepted today.

With the evolution of medical science, development and proliferation of medical and nursing schools, and enactment of medical and nursing legislation, definitions of medicine and nursing that would clearly differentiate the practice of doctors and nurses were needed, although each was referred to as an art rather than a science until recently. W. S. Thayer, an eminent physician, referred in 1919 to medicine as an art, and said, "it is difficult to overstate the contribution of the trained nurse." He spoke of the nurse's function as "wholly complementary" [to medicine] and said that without the nurse "the proper practice of the art of therapy is inconceivable." †

Sir William Osler, speaking to nurses, commented on the "art of nursing" and its roots in prehistoric practices. He said:

Nursing as an art to be cultivated, as a profession to be followed, is modern: nursing as a practice originated in the dim past, when some mother among the cave-dwellers cooled the forehead of her sick child with water from the brook, or first yielded to the prompting to leave a well-covered bone and a handful of meal by the side of a wounded man left in the hurried flight before an enemy.‡

In 1934, writing about the nature of nursing, Effie J. Taylor accepted the idea that it was "adapting prescribed therapy and preventive treatment to the specific physical and psychic needs of the individual." However, she said "The real depths of nursing can only be made known through ideals, love, sympathy, knowledge, and culture, expressed through the practice of artistic procedures and relationships." §

In 1946, Annie W. Goodrich published the following statement that stressed the nurse as an activator of medical and social sciences. She suggested the range of service but seemed to accept the idea that the nurse was "di-

* Discussing the proposed 1970 revision of the British National Health Service, the Ministry of Health spokesman said, "The establishment of an integrated Health Service will make it necessary to consider how far particular specialised training programmes are still appropriate, whether existing personnel can with further training undertake wider functions, and *whether new forms of generic training need to be developed.*" (Ministry of Health: *The National Health Service—the Administrative Structure of the Medical and Related Services in England and Wales,* H. M. Stationery Office, London, 1968, Section 106.)
† Nightingale, Florence: *Notes on Nursing, What It Is and What It Is Not.* (Republication of first American edition published by D. Appleton & Co., 1860.) Dover Publications, Inc., New York, 1969, p. 133.

* Nightingale, Florence: *op. cit.,* p. 7.
† Thayer, W. S.: "Nursing and the Art of Medicine," *Am. J. Nurs.,* **20:**187, (Dec.) 1919.
‡ Osler, Sir William: *Aequanimitas and Other Addresses.* Blakiston Co., Philadelphia, 1925, p. 163.
§ Taylor, Effie J.: "Of What Is the Nature of Nursing?" *Am. J. Nurs.,* **34:**476, (May) 1934.

rected" by a "qualified" instructor. In the following paragraph, the reader is left wondering who gave this direction:

Nursing is that expression of social activities that seeks under qualified instruction and direction to interpret through action the findings of the medical and social sciences in relation to bodily ills, their care, cure and prevention, including all factors, personal and environmental, that bear upon the achievement of the desired objective, a healthy citizenry.*

Following World War II, there was a demand for a reevaluation of the nurse's function. J. C. Meakins, a Canadian physician, joined the chorus with an article entitled "Nursing Must Be Defined." [47]

In 1947, Esther Lucile Brown, who was conducting a nationwide investigation of nursing in the United States, asked a nationally selected committee of nurses to produce a statement on the "probable nature of nursing in the latter half of this century." She cited it as follows in her report, Nursing for the Future:

. . . the professional nurse will be one who recognizes and understands the fundamental [health] needs of a person, sick or well, and who knows how these needs can best be met. She will possess a body of scientific nursing knowledge which is based upon and keeps pace with general scientific advancement, and she will be able to apply this knowledge in meeting the nursing needs of a person and a community. She must possess that kind of discriminative judgment which will enable her to recognize those activities which fall within the area of professional nursing and those activities which have been identified with the fields of other professional or nonprofessional groups.†

While this statement suggests a vital role for nursing, it fails to specify the difference between nursing and other health services. The phrases "health needs," "nursing needs," and "how these needs can best be met" must be explained if the statement is to help readers who are trying to differentiate between the practice of nursing and other medical arts and sciences.

During the late 1940s, an advanced course in medical-surgical nursing at Teachers College, Columbia University, in New York City, was organized around common nursing problems (for example, adapting care to age needs and to preoperative and postoperative states or the communicability of the patient's disease) rather than around diseases of body systems, which was at that time the common pattern. In

the fifth edition of The Principles and Practice of Nursing, Part V was entitled "Common Problems in Nursing Practice," and an explanation was given of this problem-solving approach.* In 1951, R. Louise McManus, in a study emanating from Teachers College, Columbia University, offered the following definition of nursing function:

. . . the unique function of the professional nurse may be . . . : (1) the identification or diagnosis of the nursing problem and the recognition of its interrelated aspects; (2) deciding upon a course of nursing actions to be followed for the solution of the problem, in light of immediate and long-term objectives of nursing, with regard to prevention of illness, direct care, rehabilitation, and promotion of highest standards of health possible for the individual.†

In 1960, Faye G. Abdellah and her associates published Patient-Centered Approaches to Nursing [48] which presented 21 problems as a foundation on which to build a nursing program; in 1970, Mae M. Johnson and Mary Lou C. Davis presented a text on method entitled Problem Solving in Nursing Practice.[48a] Parenthetically, since 1970, Lawrence L. Weed has promoted the "problem-oriented" approach to medical practice, including medical records. Many nurses have participated in this movement and adapted their records accordingly. (See Chapter 4.) While the problem approach has been gaining acceptance by teachers of nursing and the importance of nursing research has been recognized, the hunt for a satisfying definition of nursing goes on.

Between 1953 and 1955, the writer visited 27 states interviewing nurses, student nurses, physicians, social scientists, and others to find out what studies of nursing and nurses had been made in these states and what studies were thought needed. In answer to the second question, the usual response was "Investigations to more clearly establish the function of the nurse." [49]

In 1961, Ida Jean Orlando, in connection with a USPHS-funded "project" on integrating mental health with other aspects of the basic curriculum, published The Dynamic Nurse-Patient Relationship. In discussing the "task of the professional nurse," she differentiated

---

* Goodrich, Annie W.: A Definition of Nursing (privately printed, 1946); also in the "Report of the Biennial," Am. J. Nurs., 46:741, (Nov.) 1946.
† Brown, Esther Lucile: Nursing for the Future. Russell Sage Foundation, New York, 1948, p. 73.

* Attention was called in this discussion to the work of William R. Houston, who, in The Art of Treatment (Macmillan, 1936), advocated the organization of medical courses around the principal method of therapy (the medical problem) rather than around diseases of body systems.
† McManus, R. Louise: "Assumptions of Functions of Nursing," in Regional Planning for Nursing and Nursing Education. Teachers College, Columbia University, New York, 1951, p. 54.

between *nursing* [a cold] and *doctoring* [a cold]. The latter, she thought, implied using "the products of medical science—pills, inhalers and the like." She made the following statement:

The *purpose of nursing is to supply the help a patient requires in order for his needs to be met.* The nurse achieves her purpose by initiating a *process* [italics ours] which ascertains the patient's immediate need and helps to meet the need directly or indirectly. She meets it directly when the patient is unable to meet his own need; indirectly when she helps him obtain the services of a person, agency, or resource by which his need can be met.

. . .

The nurse, in achieving her purpose contributes simultaneously to the mental and physical health of her patient. This is so because in helping him she affects for the better his sense of adequacy or well-being. These may be small changes but they are helpful at the moment and may have cumulative value. Nursing in its professional character does not add to the distress of the patient. Instead the nurse assumes the professional responsibility of seeking out and obviating impediments to the patient's mental and physical comfort. In order for the nurse to develop and maintain the professional character of her work she must know and be able to validate how her actions and reactions help or do not help the patient or know and be able to validate that the patient does not require her help at a given time.*

Orlando's description of nursing as a *process* has had wide acceptance. Her insistence that nurses ask patients to confirm or correct their (the nurses') perceptions of patients' needs has also had wide acceptance as part of the "nursing process." Validating the effect of nursing is also accepted as part of the process.†

Margaret M. Lamb, who was at the time chairman of the General Nursing Council for Scotland, asked in 1970 "Nursing Is What?" and answered the question in part by saying that:

The nurse exists . . . to nourish or cherish the patient. . . . The bulk of nursing *is* physical care. . . . I submit that nursing yesterday, today and tomorrow is caring for people and that unless it is built on an ideal of service to others it is built on shifting sand. . . .‡

M. L. Badouaille,[50] a New Zealand nurse, explained in 1973 why she thought nursing was "different" from other health services. If time and space allowed citations of books and articles from around the world, it would be apparent that there is a universal and continuing effort to define nursing.

Most recently, definitions of nursing have tended to stress the nurse's interest in health promotion, in contrast with the cure of disease. Rozella M. Schlotfeldt in 1972 wrote as follows:

My purpose here is to set forth a straightforward and unambiguous conceptualization of nursing in terms of the profession's goal and the phenomena with which nurses must be concerned if they are to fulfill their social responsibilities. Simply stated, *the goal of nursing as a field of professional endeavor is to help people attain, retain, and regain health.* The phenomena with which nurses are concerned are man's health-seeking and coping behaviors as he strives to attain health. Nurses are independent, professional practitioners whose field of work is health care.*

Marjorie Ramphal, as president, addressing the ANA's Congress on Nursing Practice, made this statement in her summary:

The goal of nursing is to help the patient, as needed, in pursuit of his goal of behavioral integrity. Behavioral integrity means that the patient's interrelated behavioral patterns directed toward fulfilling major needs result and are likely to continue to result in biological, psychological and social health.†

In a pamphlet published in 1976 by the National League for Nursing, Shirley Chater, a nurse educator, gave the following definition of nursing as compared with medical practice:

Nursing is a process through which *care* is provided to individuals, families, or community groups *primarily* around circumstances and situations that arise from health-related problems. Medical practice, on the other hand, is primarily cause- and cure-oriented. It is important in the above definition to stress the word *primarily,* for settings, numbers, and other circumstances can change the degree of overlapping functions between the nursing and medical professions. For instance, in remote areas nurses often come closer to practicing medicine than nursing. Similarly, a physician may sit beside his patient in the recovery room caring for the subtle circumstances that arise during the postoperative course, prac-

---

* Orlando, Ida Jean: *The Dynamic Nurse-Patient Relationship.* G. P. Putnam's Sons, New York, 1961, pp. 8, 9.

† In 1972, Orlando elaborated on her concept of the nursing process and reported an evaluative study entitled *The Discipline and Teaching of Nursing Process* (G. P. Putnam's Sons, New York).

‡ Lamb, Margaret M.: "Nursing Is What?" *Int. Nurs. Rev.,* **17**:373 (No. 4) 1970.

* Schlotfeldt, Rozella M.: "This I Believe . . . Nursing Is Health Care," *Nurs. Outlook,* **30**:245, (Apr.) 1972.

† Ramphal, Marjorie: "Further Thoughts re Scope [of Nursing]." Paper addressed to Congress on Nursing Practice, Pleasantville, N.Y., Jan. 21, 1972, p. 16 (mimeographed).

ticing something more akin to nursing than to medicine.*

There is a consensus that nursing function, like all other aspects of health service, should derive from the needs of the patients, or clients. Janet M. Kraegel and her associates,[51] studying the appropriate use of nurses at St. Mary's Hospital, Milwaukee, Wisconsin (under a USPHS grant), identified 22 "patient needs" and classified them as physical, socio-psychological, and environmental. They showed how the structure and organization of a patient care unit could be organized around these needs.

While the call for a definition of nursing has been loud and clear, some persons think too much time and energy have been devoted to a question that answers itself. For example, Frances Storlie, an American nurse, writing in 1970, expressed the following opinion: "Nursing need never be defined. . . . The danger of definition is loss of mystery, loss of aura, and diminishing beauty. The substance of nursing will resist being reduced to so-called facts no matter how precise the research." †

The foregoing definitions of nursing by individuals that have been cited are just a few of those that might be included. Definitions used in official and legal documents, discussed in the following pages, may have, in the last analysis, more effect on nursing practice than the opinions of individuals, although they too must be arrived at by a consensus of individuals.

Some Definitions of Nursing and Nurses by Organizations. Organizations have found it necessary to define nursing for many reasons. Internationally, nationally, and by state and province, nurses have sought cooperation based on a definition of the nature of nursing, on an ethical code, on legislation, and on the scope of practice, or on nursing curricula.

The International Council of Nurses has based its membership on the assumption that in each country represented in the Council there was an association of "trained nurses" whose constitution and by-laws were "in harmony with those of the Council." ‡ The Council stands for self-government by nurses in their associations. At first it was assumed that

"a trained nurse" meant the same thing world-wide, but it was soon apparent that this was not so. With the development of *nurse registration* in the United States, the international effort to define nursing can be traced in Daisy Caroline Bridges' *A History of the International Council of Nurses, 1899–1964*,[52] in its official journal, the *International Nursing Review*, and in reports of ICN Congresses.

The following definition of "a nurse" was adopted by the ICN's Council of Nurse Representatives in 1975.

A nurse is a person who has completed a programme of basic nursing education and is qualified and authorised in her/his country to practice nursing. Basic nursing education is a formally recognised programme of study which provides a broad and sound foundation for the practice of nursing and for post-basic education which develops specific competency. At the first level, the educational programme prepares the nurse, through study of behavioural, life and nursing sciences and clinical experience, for effective practice and direction of nursing care, and for the leadership role. The first-level nurse [professional nurse] is responsible for planning, providing and evaluating nursing care in all settings for the promotion of health, prevention of illness, care of the sick and rehabilitation; and functions as a member of the health team. In countries with more than one level of nursing personnel, the second-level programme prepares the nurse, through study of nursing theory and clinical practice, to give nursing care in co-operation with and under the supervision of a first-level nurse.*

Efforts within the ICN to keep the definition of a nurse sufficiently explicit to have meaning and sufficiently general to make it possible for countries with different patterns of nurse education to be members of the Council have persisted.

In 1973, the Council of National Representatives (CNR) of the ICN approved the following statements on the "professional nurse" and the "auxiliary nurse" to be forwarded to the International Labour Organization in hopes that it would use them in its next edition of the *International Standard Classification of Occupations:*

Workers in this unit group [professional nurses] assist individuals, families, groups and communities in the promotion and preservation of health as

* Chater, Shirley: *Operation Update: The Search for Rhyme and Reason.* National League for Nursing, New York, 1976, pp. 5, 6.

† Storlie, Frances: "Nursing Need Never Be Defined," *Int. Nurs. Rev.,* **17**:255, (No. 3) 1970.

‡ Bridges, Daisy Caroline: *A History of the International Council of Nurses, 1899–1964. The First Sixty-Five Years.* Pitman Medical Publishing Co., Ltd., London, 1967, p. 234.

* International Labour Office: *Employment and Conditions of Work and Life of Nursing Personnel.* Report VII (2), International Labour Conference, 61st Session, 1976. The Office, Geneva, 1976, p. 84. (Response of the ICN to questionnaire from the ILO.) See also "ICN Adopts Definition of 'a Nurse,'" *Int. Nurs. Rev.,* **22**:163, (Nov.–Dec.) 1975.

well as contributing to recovery and rehabilitation in illness.

They participate in the development and implementation of the therapeutic and educational plans of the health team.

Their functions include: (1) carrying out the therapeutic programme, including personal services concerned with hygiene and comfort as they cover the range of basic human needs; (2) creating and maintaining a physical and psychological environment, conducive to health improvement, convalescence, recovery, or the achievement of a dignified death; (3) enlisting the interest of the patient and his family in seeking the conditions necessary to attain recovery, rehabilitation and optimal self-maintenance; (4) counselling people, sick and well, in measures promoting physical, mental and social well-being; (5) instituting measures of, and encouraging the pursuit of, disease prevention; (6) developing goals for nursing activities and coordinating them with those of all other members of the health team in order to achieve the broadest health care benefits for those involved; (7) participating in the teaching of nursing and other health personnel; (8) assisting in the administration of the delivery of health care in institutional or community settings.

[Professional nurses] have successfully completed a recognized nursing education programme qualifying them to be registered or licensed as a nurse by the appropriate authority.

. . . the professional nurse, specialized [is] one who provides specialized nursing in a particular branch of nursing practice: consultation, administration, teaching or research, applied to nursing; has recognized preparation in the field of specialization.

Auxiliary nurses . . . provide care which does not require the training and theoretical knowledge of a professional nurse. They work in an organized health service which provides guidance and supervision.*

The passage of a Nurse Practice Act in each state began when laws were enacted by New Jersey, New York, North Carolina, and Virginia. Such acts incorporate statements on the function of the nurse, or the nature and scope of nursing practice. The ANA, through its Council of State Boards, has defined nursing and constructed model Nurse Practice Acts. In 1937, the following definition of nursing, published by the ANA, is reflected even today in Nurse Practice Acts:

A blend of intellectual attainment, attitudes and mental skills based upon the principles of scientific medicine acquired by means of a prescribed course in a school of nursing affiliated with a hospital, recognized by the state and practiced in conjunction with curative and preventive medicine by an individual licensed to do so by the state.*

Other definitions, such as that in the 1937 *A Curriculum Guide for Schools of Nursing*,[53] said that nursing was, in effect, helping people to keep well, or regain their health when ill. Although these definitions were, in a sense, official definitions, there is considerable evidence that they were neither specific nor broad enough to satisfy everyone.

During the 1950s, the American Nurses' Association spent $400,000 studying the functions of the nurse. Twenty-one separate studies in 17 states were reported by Everett C. Hughes and his associates in *Twenty Thousand Nurses Tell Their Story*.[54] While this exhaustive nationwide study threw light on what nurses were doing (one study identified more than 400 activities) and what nurses themselves and the public then thought of the nurse, it failed to define nursing to everybody's satisfaction. People have continued to ask what is unique about nursing and what is the function of the nurse.

In 1967, the National Commission for the study of Nursing and Nursing Education, organized by the American Nurses' Association and the National League for Nursing, began its work under grants from the Mellon (then Avalon) and Kellogg Foundations and an anonymous donor. It continued its work under continued support from these and additional sources. In its first major publication, *An Abstract for Action,* Jerome P. Lysaught reviewed the development of nursing in America and noted the relationship of nursing and medical care. He seemed to think that the development of "nursing science" is "retarded," that "nursing has many miles to go before it can reach full professional status." † While recognizing that nursing had a unique role, no one definition seems to be favored in the Commission's report. Recommendations in this report and the subsequent papers published as a volume under the title *Action in Nursing: Progress in Professional Purpose*[55] (1974) are mentioned later, but the emphasis throughout is on the importance of the nurse's role, on unity of purpose among nurses, on essential steps in becoming a full-blown profession, on the necessity of assuming the responsibilities of a profession but, at the same time, cooperating with other categories of health workers.

---

* "CNR Approves Definition for International Standard Classification of Occupations" (news), *Int. Nurs. Rev.,* **20**:153, (No. 5) 1973. (The proposed definition was prepared by the ICN Professional Services Committee.)

* "Professional Nursing Defined" (editorial), *Am. J. Nurs.,* **37**:518, (May) 1937.

† National Commission for the Study of Nursing and Nursing Education: *An Abstract for Action.* (Jerome P. Lysaught, Director.) McGraw-Hill Book Co., New York, 1970, p. 44.

Not only in the Commission's report but in many critiques of health care, there is increasing recognition of overlapping roles of nurses, physicians, and others (discussed later in more detail) and of the importance of legislation that permits overlapping roles. In 1972, a Joint Commission on Practice with representatives of the ANA and the AMA was appointed. It is funded by the two associations and the W. K. Kellogg Foundation. A study of Nurse Practice Acts and Medical Practice Acts was initiated by the Joint Commission. In the report *Statutory Regulation of the Scope of Nursing Practice—A Critical Survey*,[56] Virginia Hall, an attorney, seemed to conclude that nurses were then practicing medicine, as so defined, as well as nursing, as so defined, and that they must continue to do so if the needs of the public are to be met. In any event, Hall instanced and commented on the varying definitions in Nurse Practice Acts and suggested that instead of modifying existing Nurse Practice Acts, an over-all solution might be to exempt professional nurses from the prohibition against the practice of medicine in Medical Practice Acts. (See also page 65 for discussion of Nurse Practice Acts.)

It is safe to say that in no other era has there been such wide disagreement on the definition of nursing and the function of the nurse.*

The effort to differentiate between the practice of nursing and other health practices and to differentiate between nursing research and other health-related research has led to a study of nursing "theory" and nursing "concepts." The following is a brief review of some efforts along these lines. Nursing conferences in past decades tended to focus on function, and later on research. In recent years they were more apt to deal with theory and concepts. Curricula are planned to reflect a particular philosophy on, or concept of, nursing.

Philosophies, Concepts, Theories, and Systems Underlying Definitions of Nursing and the Function of the Nurse. All health services are influenced by prevailing philosophies or cultural values, by political environments in which they exist. Nursing, like all other health services, is affected by attitudes toward sex, age, color, race, religious beliefs, physical fitness, intellectual ability, creative ability, educational achievement, self-expression, self-discipline, equality of opportunity, respect for authority, and respect for life—human and nonhuman. To be specific, a culture that values the young more than the old is likely to provide better health care for infants and children than for the aged and dying; a society committed to equal opportunity is more likely to make health service universally available than one that is not; a people who look for reward in an afterlife may put less emphasis on health care than one that looks for its reward on this earth; and a culture committed to protecting animal and insect life has a different system of health care (including diet) from one that makes the welfare of other forms of life dependent on what that particular culture believes best for humans.

Some nurse educators, nurse researchers, and others have emphasized the importance of identifying goals or stating the philosophy underlying nursing. Mildred A. E. Newton's study, *Florence Nightingale's Philosophy of Life and Education* (Ed.D. dissertation, Stanford University, Palo Alto, Calif., 1949), showed the extent to which her values affected nursing for many years; the *Curriculum Guide*,[57] prepared under the sponsorship of the National League of Nursing Education in 1937, stressed educational philosophy; its proposed curriculum was dominated by the concept of adaptation as an educational goal. In 1962, Sister Madeleine Clémence Vaillot[58] discussed existentialism as a philosophy of commitment and its meaning for her in nursing.* Other examples might be given to show that throughout its history nursing has identified its philosophic base. There is, however, considerable evidence that the *insistence* on identifying philosophy, concepts, theories, or systems in which nursing operates is new. Of 1464 master's theses and papers written between 1930 and 1955, there were only a few that dealt with philosophic, political, cultural, or ethnic questions.[59] Martha M. Brown,[60] a nurse reporting a study in 1969 on "nurses, patients, and social systems," makes the categorical statement that, conceptually, nursing is a "primitive discipline." The profession is, perhaps, overly sensitive to such criticism. In any event, faculties of schools of nursing seeking accreditation know they had better state the philosophy or the concept of nursing on

---

* Although the discussion here focuses on the United States, uncertainty about the scope of nursing practice, or the function of the nurse, is worldwide. A Finnish publication puts the problem in the same terms that might be used here: "The objectives of social policy and health policy determine the needs which nurses have to meet. At the present time nurses are uncertain what needs are their particular responsibility, due to poor definition of the field of responsibility, quality of education, etc." (Vainio, Aune: "A Review of the Activities of the Development Seminar on Nursing Care/Health Science," *Sairaanhoidon Vuosikirja* [*Helsinki*], 11:53, 1974.)

---

* Sister Madeleine quotes Rollo May as saying all science needs a philosophical base—and she agrees.

which they base their curricula, and research proposals must often embody a philosophic statement, a concept or theory of nursing. National regional conferences focus on such topics, as do journal articles and full-length books.[61-76]

Theory comes from the Greek *theōria*, a beholding, spectacle, contemplation, speculation. Webster's gives six meanings other than these, but the following is the sense in which it is used here:

The general or abstract principles of any body of facts real or assumed; pure, as distinguished from applied, science or art; as, the *theory* of music or of medicine.

Ernest Nagle[77] calls a theory "an intellectual tool." Using it in this sense, the following questions must be asked: Has nursing, as distinct from other branches of health practice, "a body of facts real or assumed?" Is research in nursing (from which such a body of facts would be derived) different in content and method from research in health education, in psychology, chemistry, physics, physiology, pathology, microbiology? Medicine, interpreted as diagnosis and therapy—whose research might be assumed to most closely resemble nursing research—not only borrows from all these sciences but collaborates in its research with scientists in these fields. This idea of borrowing from other fields seems to be rejected by some nurses. Gean Mathwig says:

. . . I endorse the philosophy that by definition of a profession, the theoretical knowledge of a profession evolves from that profession. . . .
. . . the theoretical core of nursing knowledge evolves not from administration, anthropology, biology, psychology, sociology, nor any other discipline, but rather from the field of nursing per se.*

Florence Wald, a nurse, and Robert Leonard, a sociologist,[78] described the development of "nursing practice theory" as distinct from the theory of practice in any other health field.

M. Isabel Harris accepted the definition of theory as a "more or less plausible or scientific acceptable principle to explain phenomena." She saw it as "a conceptual structure built for a purpose" † which, in nursing, was practice. She traced the development of nursing theory from Florence Nightingale in whose writings she thought theory *implicit;* she thought *explicit* theory recent.

Rosemary Ellis discussed the characteristics of a significant theory and said it was "one that enlightens us about the patient and what happens to him." * She said *studies of nurses* might or might not contribute to the development of significant theories for nursing, and she proposed that practitioners were the theorists in nursing.

Imogene M. King reviewed the literature, "synthesized ideas," and concluded that "the essential characteristics of nursing were those properties that had persisted in spite of environmental changes." She said, "If nursing is a science, then the body of knowledge taught, learned, and used by professional nurses is characterized by certainty, structure and generalizations." † (She thought these the characteristics of science.)

King presented a series of diagrams to clarify her concepts of how nurses work with individuals, groups, and social systems to help individuals and groups "attain, maintain, and restore health." In the following definition of nursing, King seems to synthesize the positions of Virginia Henderson, Ida Orlando, Hildegard Peplau, and Martha E. Rogers:

Nursing is a process of action, reaction, interaction and transaction whereby nurses assist individuals of any age and socioeconomic group to meet their basic needs in performing activities of daily living and to cope with health and illness at some particular point in the life cycle.‡

Margaret A. Newman made the following statement about nursing theory, implying that the borrowing phase is over:

Nursing theory has evolved through several phases: borrowing theory from other disciplines; analyzing nursing practice situations to seek conceptual relationships; and developing a conceptual framework.§

Dorothy E. Johnson took another position in a paper entitled "Theory in Nursing: Borrowed and Unique." She said:

It is extremely hazardous to attempt to differentiate between borrowed and unique theory in nursing. It is hazardous first of all because the man-made, more or less arbitrary division between the sciences are neither firm nor constant. It appears there is an essential unity in knowledge, corresponding to a unity in nature, which defies established boundaries, and continuously presses

* Mathwig, Gean: "Nursing Science—The Theoretical Core of Nursing Knowledge," *Image,* **4:**20, (No. 1) 1971.
† Harris, M. Isabel: "Theory Building in Nursing. A Review of the Literature," *Image,* **4:**6, (No. 1) 1972.

* Ellis, Rosemary: "The Practitioner as Theorist," *Am. J. Nurs.,* **69:**1434, (July) 1969.
† King, Imogene M.: *Toward a Theory for Nursing: General Concepts of Human Behavior.* John Wiley & Sons, New York, 1971, pp. IX, 15.
‡ King, Imogene M.: *op. cit.,* p. 25.
§ Newman, Margaret A.: "Nursing's Theoretical Evolution," *Nurs. Outlook,* **20:**449, (July) 1972.

for the larger, more cohesive view. Moreover, knowledge does not innately "belong" to any field of science. It is not exactly happenstance that a given bit of knowledge is discovered by one discipline rather than another, but the fact of discovery does not confer the right of ownership. Viewed in this light borrowed and unique have no real permanence, nor any real meaning.*

(Johnson's position on theory in nursing seems eminently reasonable to the writer and it is one with which she concurs.)

It seems to be useful to many persons to express concepts of nursing schematically—as systems. For instance, Martha Rogers [78a] used the coiled spring to express the concept of continuing change, continuing interaction between the nurse and the client. College courses are built around the idea of systems analysis, and almost any activity can be diagrammed as either a closed or open system.[79,80] Ludwig Von Bertalanffy made the following distinction between open and closed systems:

From the physical point of view, the characteristic state of the living organism is that of an open system. A system is closed if no material enters or leaves it; it is open if there is import and export and, therefore, change of the components. Living systems are open systems, maintaining themselves in exchange of materials with environment, and in continuous building up and breaking down of their components.†

Reference has been made to King's diagrammatic exposition of nursing theory as a system. Kraegel and her associates reported a study at St. Mary's Hospital, Milwaukee, Wisconsin, in which the management of patient care was revised to meet basic human needs. The plan was described and diagrammed as a system.[81,82] Figure 1-3 shows the definition of nursing used in this book by Virginia Henderson and Gladys Nite and a similar definition used by Dorothea Orem and her associates, diagrammed by them as "systems."

The following are some of the *concepts* of the registered nurse that have been discussed during this century:

The professional registered nurse is (1) nature's helper in restoring the body to health; (2) a mother substitute—the professional mother; (3) the physician's assistant in caring for the ill and preventing disease; (4) the physician's complement—the physician concentrating on *cure*, the nurse on *care;* (5) a substitute for the physician; (6) a coordinator

of the services of all health workers; (7) a manipulator of the environment and a trainer and director of personnel with less preparation than that of the professional nurse; (8) a health educator; (9) someone who, through the nursing process, enables the client or patient to make the best use of health resources; (10) someone who applies "nursing science" for the betterment of mankind; (11) someone who "intervenes" in the client's or patient's behalf in a crisis or time of need; (12) the patient's and family's helper in meeting their health needs.[83-97]

These concepts are not mutually exclusive. Many persons would combine two or more in giving their idea of a nurse. In the United States, Canada, and some other countries, all nurses are, at least theoretically, health educators as well as caregivers. In England, a health visitor is a community nurse who is primarily a health educator, while a district nurse is primarily a caregiver. Many persons recognize the overlapping functions of professional nurses and physicians and admit that nurses, especially public health nurses, have always been substitutes for the physician in situations where the latter's services were unavailable.

Throughout this chapter, the concept of a physician as a healer or a worker interested in cure of disease has been stressed, as has been the concept of the nurse as a caretaker or as a worker more interested than the physician in promoting health. However, if health workers listen to current criticism of medical care or health care, or if they note the growth of the self-help movement, the concept of what constitutes "good" health care might change radically, and with it, the concept of the way nurses and physicians function.[98-104] At present, their respective functions are overlapping, confused, and sometimes in conflict with those of other health workers.

The Overlapping and Collaborative Roles of Nurses, Physicians, and Other Health Workers. Some people see nurses and physicians as having separate and distinct functions; others see both as responding to the health needs of individuals in every situation according to the worker's particular competence and according to competences of the health manpower available. While the latter view has always influenced health care, there seems to be more discussion of the relationship of nursing and medicine now than in the past, and since the demand for health service is mounting, the question is increasingly critical.

The prevailing point of view is that health care should be universally available. In most people's minds, this entails periodic visits to (or from) health workers from conception to the grave. Illich [105] thinks that this concept

---

* Johnson, Dorothy E.: "Theory in Nursing: Borrowed and Unique," *Nurs. Res.,* 17:206, (May–June) 1968.

† Von Bertalanffy, Ludwig: "The Theory of Open Systems in Physics and Biology," in Emery, F. E. (ed.): *Systems Thinking.* Penguin Books, Ltd., Harmondsworth, Eng., 1969, p. 70.

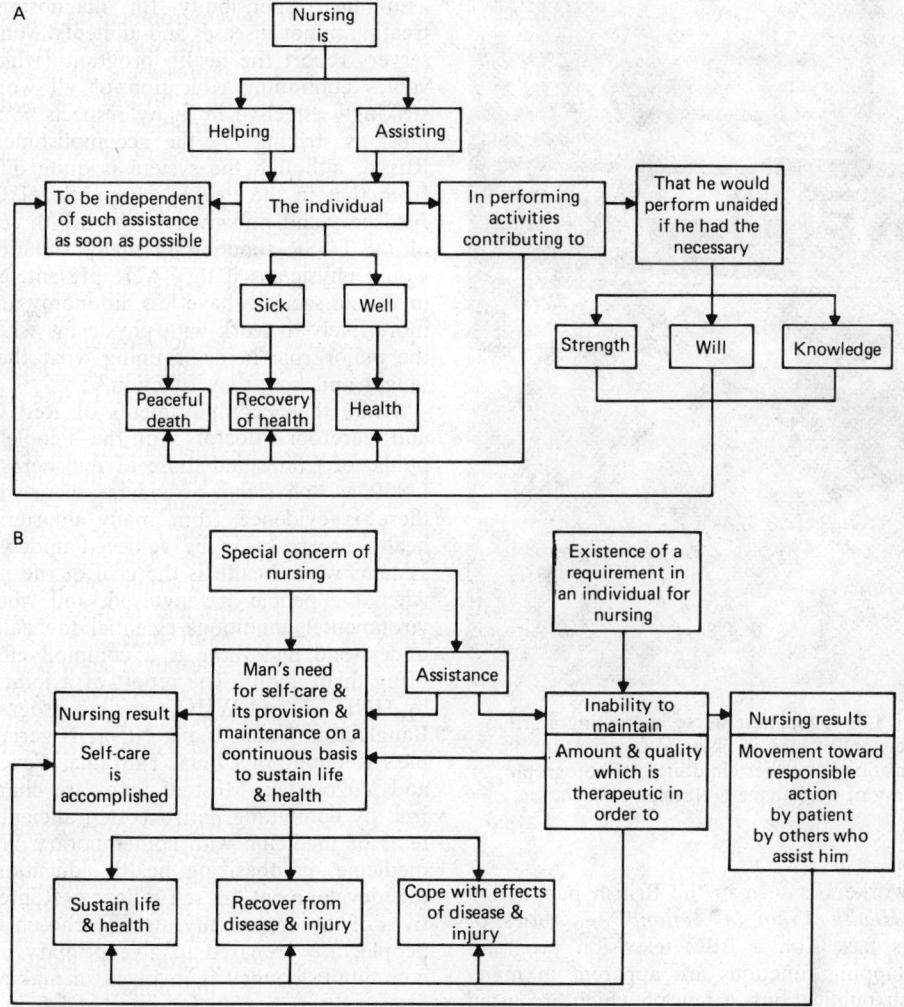

Figure 1-3. Diagrams showing (*A*) Virginia Henderson's concept of nursing; (*B*) Dorothea Orem's concept of nursing. (From Nursing Development Conference Group: *Concept Formalization in Nursing: Process and Product.* Little, Brown and Co., Boston, 1973, pp. 56, 57.)

makes "patients" of well people throughout life and prevents development of "normal" or desirable self-reliance. Others might concur in this opinion, but the trend toward spending more and more of the gross national product (GNP) on health has not been reversed nor has the trend toward developing more and more categories of workers. Physicians seem to be increasingly willing for nurses and others to assume a greater share of responsibility for health assessment, for supervision of "well" children and the chronically ill, and for almost total care of the aged. While some physicians seem to want to claim that they "supervise" nurses in all these roles, others believe this is neither practical nor desirable and are willing

for nurses to be legally, and in every other way, accountable for their practice even though it encompasses functions that are generally considered the domain of medicine.

The question of the overlapping roles of doctors, physician's assistants, feldshers, nurses, and other health workers is apparent in the discussions at two recent conferences with an international focus. One was in England, the report of which is entitled *The Greater Medical Profession*,[106] and the other was in the United States, the report of which is *Intermediate-Level Health Practitioners*.[107] The overlapping functions of private medical practitioners, health officers, nurses (district nurses, health visitors, and nurse-midwives), and so-

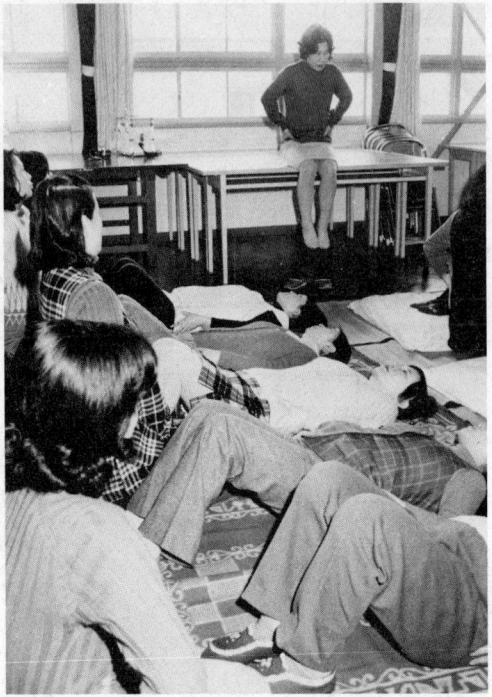

Figure 1-4. A Japanese nurse instructing a group of pregnant women in physical exercises in preparation for easier childbirth. (Photograph courtesy of the Japanese Nursing Association.)

cial workers is seen in the British publication *The Health Team in Action* [108]—a series of essays based on a BBC television program. Overlapping functions are apparent in many British publications, a few of which are listed among the references for this chapter. [109-113]

In Canada, nurses, physicians, and others are studying the function of the nurse. Under the sponsorship of the Department of National Health and Welfare, a study has been in progress on the function of the nurse since 1971. Doctors, nurses, and others are making task analyses in six universities of nursing practice, particularly that in Northern outposts. The resulting documents clearly show the extent to which nurses carry out diagnostic and therapeutic procedures that traditionally lie within the province of medicine. [114-120] (The Canadian study is discussed in more detail under the next subhead—"The Nurse as Therapist (The Extended Role).")

In the People's Republic of China, health care has undergone radical revision. There, "barefoot" and "Red Guard doctors" (workers with far less preparation than registered nurses in the United States or feldshers in Russia) are in factories, rural communes, and elsewhere assuming responsibility for diagnosing and treating minor diseases and ailments. Many observers report the health program (which involves continuing education of all workers) strikingly effective in many respects. [121-123] Almost as striking are the accomplishments in Russia, although the system is quite different from that in the People's Republic of China. Feldshers and midwives in the health services of the USSR function in many situations as would physicians if they were present. Nurses in Russia seem to have less autonomy and are more likely to work with physicians who play the major role in determining what they are taught and how they function. [124-126]

While the accomplishments of Red Guard and barefoot "doctors" in the People's Republic of China and those of feldshers in the USSR as "physician extenders" seem striking, there is evidence from many quarters that health progress can be achieved under many systems when health is the goal of the people, when the people are involved, and when environmental conditions essential to health are understood and there is a common effort to bring them about. The report of a joint study by UNICEF and WHO describes programs in Bangladesh, Cuba, India, Niger, Nigeria, People's Republic of China, Tanzania, Venezuela, and Yugoslavia. Most of them are characterized by combining native (often ancient) systems of medicine with contemporary Western medicine, emphasizing health education and the development of self-reliance. Representatives of the community, usually chosen by the people, are prepared to give primary care; a community council is involved in making and implementing a plan for improved living conditions and developing self-reliance in health and other aspects of social welfare. The point is made in the report that "Organizing the delivery of health care so that part of it 'belongs' to those it is designed to serve has enormous advantages." * The primary caregivers are known to and trusted by the people they serve. They share the lot of the people and often toil with them in farming or other manual labor.

In summary, if health care is studied internationally, it is clear that not only do doctors' and nurses' roles overlap but that the roles of both are filled by a wide variety of workers. Nevertheless, the extended (or expanded) role of the nurse is the most widely discussed topic in nursing meetings and in nursing journals. The following is an attempt to suggest the na-

---

* Djukanovic, V., and Mach, E. P. (eds.): *Alternative Approaches to Meeting Basic Health Needs in Developing Countries. A Joint UNICEF-WHO Study.* World Health Organization, Geneva, 1975, p. 16.

ture and range of the discussion, especially in the United States and Canada.

The Nurse as Therapist (The Extended Role). While the term "extended" or "expanded" role is new, some people maintain that the "trained" nurse of the Nightingale era often functioned in this capacity as it is now described and that some doctors then treated nurses as collaborators rather than as "hand-maidens" as is so often implied by critics of the doctor-nurse relationship. Private duty nurses, caring for patients in their homes, undoubtedly worked in partnership with physicians. It is interesting to find in a 1902 directory of trained nurses in four major cities of the Eastern seaboard an article by a doctor on the ideal nurse and another on what doctors "owe trained nurses." [127] A 1923 directory lists, in one small pamphlet, the nurses and physicians of New Haven County, Connecticut.[128]

The extended role involves assessing clients' health status, diagnosing, and prescribing treatment or giving primary care, which means admitting clients or patients to the health care system. Barbara G. Schutt,[129] in 1972, reviewed the history of "primary care nursing" and concluded that nurses have always been "in the primary care business but haven't cared to talk about it." She noted the following terms used for nurses giving primary care in 1972: pediatric nurse practitioner *; pediatric nurse associate *; family nurse practitioner (PRIMEX); clinical associate (of the family physician); adult health practitioner; medical nurse practitioner; nurse midwife; nurse practitioner. To these might now be added psychiatric nurse practitioner, geriatric nurse practitioner, school nurse practitioner, and industrial nurse practitioner. "Clinical specialist" and "nurse clinician" are other terms used to denote postbasic preparation that prepares the worker for the extended role.†

Schutt studied the Frontier Nursing Service

in Kentucky, noting that its staff had been giving primary health care for 40 years.[130] As evidence of this, the nurse-midwifery service there delivered its first 1000 babies with only one death,[131] which is a demonstration of excellent primary maternal and newborn care. Although the Frontier Nursing Service operates under *Medical Directives* (7th ed., the Service, Wendover, Ky., 1975), which can be interpreted as delegation of authority from medical advisers or consultants, it is clear that its staff nurses have, since the inception of the Service, been functioning independently in giving primary care.*

It bears repeating that the functions of all health workers vary from place to place and from one decade to another. Their functions depend on the public's concept of health, what it expects from trained workers, the numbers and varieties of workers available, and the services they are prepared to give. No category of workers can be considered in isolation. The report of a 1976 international conference on nursing contains the following statements:

. . . the legal and professional problems inherent in the changing role of nursing have recently been . . . the subject of close study in collaboration with other health disciplines at the policy level.

The part played by nurses has expanded . . . professional nurses have been taking over some of the duties traditionally reserved for the doctor.

. . . summary definitions [of nursing] seem inadequate since nurses are increasingly called upon to do work which puts them in danger of being accused of practising medicine.†

Laws regulating practice affect function, but when they are in conflict with human needs, people tend to disregard them. The fact that almost everybody accepts the United Nations dictum that health care is a universal human right is forcing people to accept professional nurses as givers of primary care.‡ As noted, national prepaid health insurance is the rule rather than the exception in developed countries, and some developing countries have adopted it. Even in most countries that have no national health insurance, all citizens assume that health care is a right.

---

* Some patients call them "the lady pediatrician."

† In the opinion of the writer, such titles should not suggest that it is the exception for nurses to be in practice, to be involved in clinical nursing, or to be concerned with the family, or even functioning as a physician's associate, since all of these conditions should be the rule rather than the exception. Titles should rather indicate the clinical field (as maternal and child health, psychiatry, surgery, or medicine) and the length and depth of the nurse's preparation. For example, a "surgical nurse specialist" should mean that the nurse has studied surgical nursing in a postbasic program. Eventually, as nursing education is upgraded, this should imply the completion of a graduate program in a university. In some institutions, nurses are numbered or lettered as Nurse 1, Nurse 2, or Nurse 3, or Nurse A, Nurse B, or Nurse C to designate different levels of competence or different functions. This has the disadvantage of requiring interpretation.

---

* For the first time in 1975, the Frontier Nursing Service had a physician as a director.

† International Labour Office: *Employment and Conditions of Work and Life of Nursing Personnel.* International Labour Conference, 61st Session, 1976, Report VII (1). The Office, Geneva, 1976, pp. 12, 16, 24.

‡ United Nations: *Universal Declaration of Human Rights.* "It is a fundamental human right for every person to have a standard of living adequate for the health and well-being of himself and his family including food, clothing, housing and medical care and necessary social services."

If the peoples of this earth are to receive health care as a basic human right, a wide variety of systems is necessary, since the kinds and numbers of health workers vary from country to country. Physicians and "trained" nurses are almost nonexistent in some parts of the world. It is reported, for instance, that in Tanzania there was in 1972 one physician for every 28,000 of the population "with a correspondingly low ratio of other health professionals and auxiliaries." In rural India, the ratio of physicians may fall lower than one to 11,000, while it may be as high as 1:1200 in cities.[132] In the United States, Canada, Great Britain, Scandinavia, and other economically favored parts of the world, the ratio of physicians to the population in cities may be as high as one physician to every 500 of the population and one to 1000 in some rural areas, and in the USSR, the ratio is reported to be about one physician to every 370 inhabitants.[133] In economically favored countries, the supply of nurses has increased rapidly; the ratio of registered nurses may range from 1:250 to 1:400. At the turn of the century, it is variously reported that the ratio of physicians to the population equalled or exceeded the ratio of "trained

nurses" in the United States; in 1976, the ratio of registered nurses *far exceeded* that of physicians and the ratio of auxiliary nursing personnel to the population exceeded that of registered nurses. While the worldwide goal of one professional nurse to 5000 inhabitants and one health auxiliary for every 1000 inhabitants has not been reached, the ratio of professional nurses exceeds the ratio of physicians on every continent except Asia.[134,135] It seems obvious that the system of meeting the health needs must vary from country to country and even from decade to decade and that in this era nurses are almost forced to give primary care.

Nursing journals from all over the world carry articles on the extended role of the nurse. In June, 1972, the International Council of Nurses released the following statement on the "developing role of the nurse":

In the light of scientific and social change and the goals of social and health policy to extend health services to the total population, nursing and other health professions are faced with the need to adapt and expand their roles. In planning to meet health needs it is imperative that nurses and physicians collaborate to promote the development and optimum utilization of both professions. A

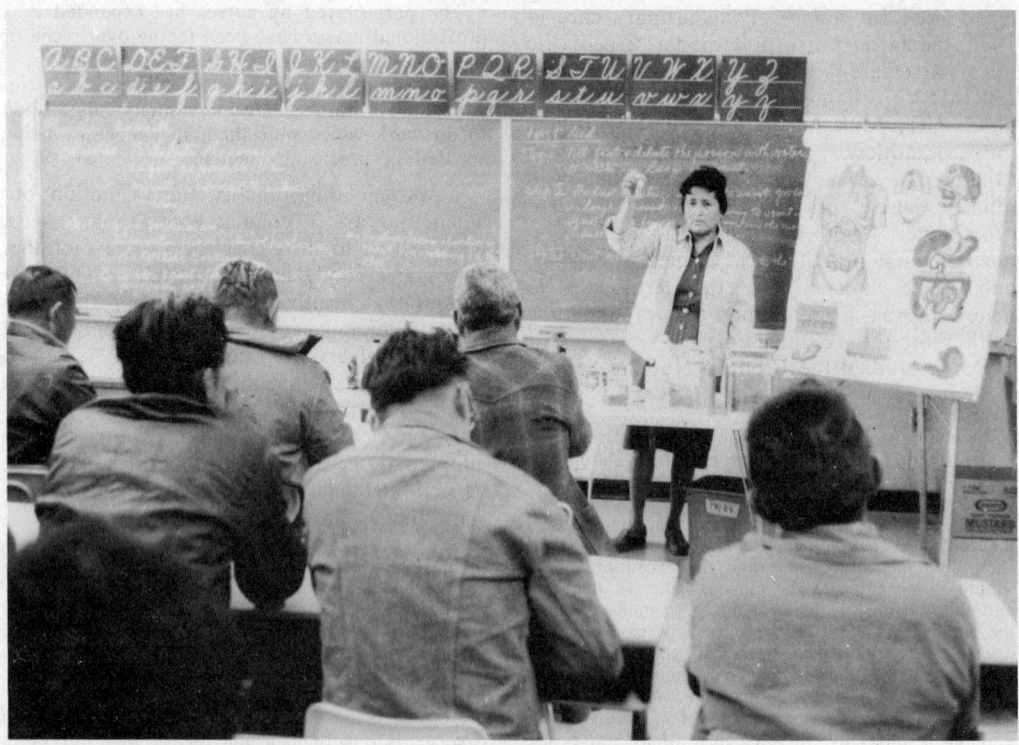

Figure 1-5. An American Indian nurse teaching a class in household poisons to a group of adults on the Navajo reservation in Arizona. (Photo courtesy of the PHS Indian Hospital, Winslow, Arizona, and the Indian Health Service.)

variety of practices may evolve in different settings including the creation of new categories of health workers. Although this may require nurses to delegate some of their traditional activities and undertake new responsibilities, the core of their practice and their title should remain distinctly nursing and education programmes should be geared to prepare them for their duly recognized role.*

In 1970, the American Medical Association's Committee on Nursing published a position statement supporting increased numbers of nurses, expansion of role, preparation of nursing at "all levels," increased involvement of nurses in direct medical care of patients, and collaboration of medicine and nursing.[136] The Canadian Nurses' Association and the Canadian Medical Association issued a joint statement on the interdependent role of nursing and medicine and agreed upon an experimental approach in developing an extended role for the nurse.[137,138] While physicians in the United States have also developed physician's assistants as "extenders" of medical care, physicians in Canada have not done so.

Since the Canadian experience is more contained and easier to follow, it might be described before that in the United States. Canadians seem to have realized for years that many nurses, but particularly those in the medical services of the North, were practicing a combination of nursing and medicine. Articles in nursing journals for decades reported the broad scope of the community nurse's practice in northern outposts. Nurses serving Indians and Eskimos may be the only professionals in health stations for months, and while they may be able to consult physicians by telephone, it has been impracticable for nurses to consult them every time they had to decide whether and how to treat a sick patient or whether to have the patient flown to an appropriate hospital. (See Figures 1-5 and 1-6.)

Ruth E. May, describing the Canadian experience of a university nursing school and medical school collaborating in preparation of graduate students for outpost nursing, said it had its roots in a 1964 investigation of the Royal Commission on Health Services. This involved visits by a medical educator to the Canadian Arctic and other remote areas.[139] A resulting program at Dalhousie University Medical School, Halifax, Nova Scotia, is the prototype of those established later in other universities.

A study made by a Committee on Clinical Training of Nurses for Medical Services in the

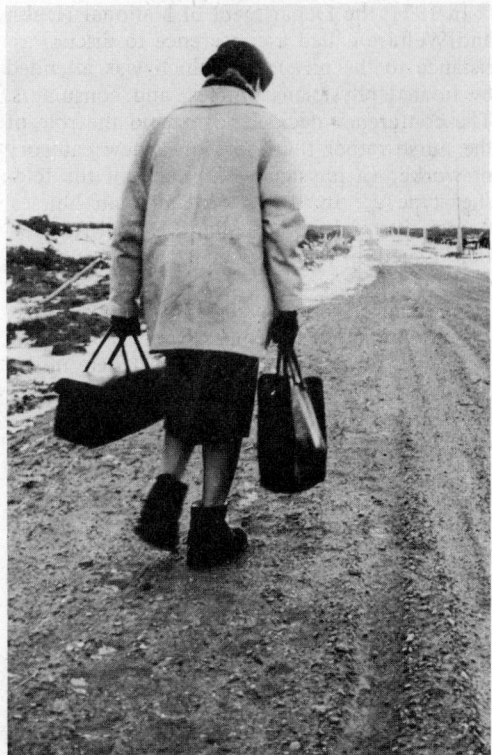

Figure 1-6. Registered nurse, working at a Canadian Red Cross Society outpost hospital in the province of New Brunswick, sets out to visit a patient at home. (Photograph by Dugal Bichan in Handbury, Eric: *Nurse.* McClelland & Stewart, Ltd., Toronto, Ont., 1975. Sponsored by the Registered Nurses Association of Ontario for the celebration of its 50th Anniversary. Courtesy of Canadian Red Cross Society.)

North, appointed by the Department of National Health and Welfare, was reported by its chairman, Dorothy J. Kergin, in 1970.[140] As a result of the findings of this committee, clinical courses of study for graduate nurses were begun in the Universities of Alberta, McGill, Manitoba, Ontario, Toronto, Sherbrooke, and Western Ontario to improve the competence of nurses in isolated nursing stations in the North.[141] With the exception of the course at Ontario University, they were funded by the Medical Services Branch of the Department of National Health and Welfare and it was stipulated that the universities were obligated to evaluate the effectiveness of the courses. This led to a "task analysis" of nursing in these stations, or the skills the Kergin report indicated were needed. A list of these skills clearly showed that nurses were functioning within the traditional scope of medicine as well as in the traditional scope of nursing.[142]

---

* International Council of Nurses: News Release. Statement on the Developing Role of the Nurse. No. 9–73, June 1972.

In 1971, the Department of National Health and Welfare called a conference to discuss assistance to the physician, which was attended by invited physicians, nurses, and consumers. The conference decided to expand the role of the nurse rather than develop a new category of worker (a physician's assistant of the feldsher type).[143] In 1973, the Canadian Nurses' Association and the Canadian Medical Association issued a joint statement endorsing this decision.[144]

At each of the universities mentioned above, a "validating panel" consisting of a nurse, a physician, and a content specialist determined whether a course objective (a skill) was necessary for a "clinically trained nurse." The hundreds of "objectives" (procedures) identified are reported in a 600-page document with the following 30 chapter headings: History and Physical Examination; Laboratory Procedures; X-ray Procedures; Pharmacology; Fluids and Electrolytes; Nutrition; Growth and Development; Obstetrics and the Newborn; Gynaecology; Ophthalmology; Otorhinolaryngology; Dentistry; Respiratory System; Cardiovascular System; Gastro-intestinal System; Genitourinary System; Central Nervous System; Musculoskeletal System; Dermatology; Haematology; Deficiency and Metabolic Disorders; Endocrine System; Psychiatry; Communicable Diseases and Immunization; Immunology and Allergies; Burns; Accidents; Surgical Procedures; Adult Flowsheets; Pediatric Flowsheets.*

From the evidence just cited, it is clear that a broad scope of nursing practice is recognized in Canada and it would seem that doctors and nurses accept an overlapping function. Because the health programs of each province are different, generalizations may be challenged. It is not possible to review the recent legislation affecting the legal scope of nursing practice throughout Canada. It is interesting, however, that the unified health legislation of Quebec, which in 1973 promulgated the Professional Code (S.Q. 1973, ch. 43), brought 38 "professional corporations" under an umbrella act. Nicole Du Mouchel and Odile LaRose reported that 21 professions had exclusive right to practice "as well as reserved title" and 17 had reserved title only. Nursing is one of the 21 exclusive professions, each of which is governed by a special act. The Nurses Act (S.Q. 1973, ch. 48) defines the practice of the profession as follows:

Every act the object of which is to identify the health needs of persons, contribute to methods of diagnosis, provide and control the nursing care required for the promotion of health, prevention of illness, treatment and rehabilitation, and to provide care according to a medical prescription constitutes the profession of nursing.

A nurse may in practising the profession inform the population on health problems.*

From this definition, the Order of Nurses of Quebec has developed the philosophy, objectives, and functions of nurses in maternal, infant, preschool, school, adult, and aged health services which were published in 1974 under the title *Community Health Nursing*. It is perhaps significant that the Centre within the [International] Organization for Economic Cooperation and Development (OECD), Paris, got a "Group of Experts" to study the "Ontario Experience" in educating health professions "in the context of the health care system." The 1975 report of this study (financed by the Josiah Macy, Jr. Foundation) suggests complete acceptance of an extended role for the nurse.[145]

While the preceding discussion of primary care by nurses in Canada is obviously simplistic and incomplete, it does suggest that physicians and nurses are collaborating effectively in planning and implementing plans.

In the United States, recognition of the ability of nurses to give primary care seems to have come from a number of centers during the 1960s. In 1964, Pellegrino, in "Nursing and Medicine; Ethical Implications in Changing Practice," urged "joint discussion" in the readjustment of functions.[146] Since this time, in his work at several medical centers, he has promoted reexamination of the functions of health personnel. During a 1972 conference on interdisciplinary education in the health professions, Pellegrino made the following observation:

A major deterrent to our efforts to fashion health care that is efficient, effective, comprehensive, and personalized is our lack of a design for the synergistic interrelationship of all who can contribute to the patient's well-being. We face, in the next decade, a national challenge to redeploy the functions of health professions in new ways, extending the roles of some, perhaps eliminating others, but more closely meshing the functions of each than ever before.†

Barbara Bates, another physician, who was associated with Pellegrino in the Department

---

* Hazlett, C. B.: "Task Analysis of the Clinically Trained Nurse (C.T.N.)," *Nurs. Clin. North Am.*, **10**:699, (Dec.) 1975.

* Du Mouchel, Nicole, and LaRose, Odile: "Community Health Nursing in Quebec," **10**:721, (Dec.) 1975.

† Pellegrino, Edmund D.: "Interdisciplinary Education in the Health Professions: Assumptions, Definitions, and Some Notes on Teams." Reprinted from *Report of a Conference: Educating for the Health Team*. National Academy of Sciences, Institute of Medicine, Washington, D.C., October 1972.

of Medicine at the University of Kentucky Medical Center, began her study there of the working relationships of physicians and nurses which she has, with nursing participation, continued at the University of Rochester. In 1970, Bates wrote:

Medicine and nursing have common goals: the preservation and restoration of health. Yet their roles in achieving these objectives are not identical and may be visualized as two overlapping circles, each with its own content but sharing a common ground. The primary [chief] role of medicine comprises diagnosis and treatment—the "cure" process described by Schulman, Mauksch and others. In contrast, the primary [chief] role of nursing lies in the "care" process, expressive in nature, and consisting of caring, helping, comforting and guiding. Neither role is an exclusive domain. Both professions feel responsible for trying to meet patients' psychologic needs. Furthermore, as technology advances, a steadily enlarging area of overlapping roles is made up of tasks instrumental to diagnosis and treatment, delegated by doctor to nurse.*

Few would question the statement by Bates that neither role is an exclusive domain; however, some would question the premise that nurses can only perform a diagnostic or treatment "task" if it is delegated by a doctor. Can the doctors, then, only perform "caring, helping, comforting and guiding" tasks if delegated by a nurse? † Bates and others have shown the overlapping functions of health workers with overlapping circles (see Fig. 1-7). It may be useful to stress here that, according to the kind of help people need and according to the persons available to give this help, the physician, the nurse, the social worker, the physical therapist, the prosthesis maker, the vocational counselor, or others may be the most valuable or major helper. In 1966, the writer tried to show with a series of "pie graphs" (see Fig. 1-8) the fallacy of assuming that any one health worker was always the dominant member, or the appropriate "captain," of the team.

Sir George Godber, discussing "The Greater Medical Profession," in 1975 commented on "the undoubted decline in understanding between the medical and nursing professions, as the right of the latter to share in decision making is too little realised. . . . I am a doctor and I believe that the medical role in health

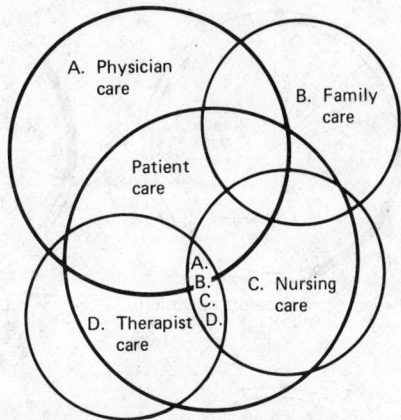

Figure 1-7. Diagram showing overlapping of (*A*) physician care, (*B*) family care, (*C*) nursing care, and (*D*) therapist care. (Adapted from National Commission for the Study of Nursing and Nursing Education: *An Abstract for Action.* Jerome P. Lysaught, director. McGraw-Hill Book Co., New York, 1970, p. 39.)

care is central, but coordinating rather than dominant. Some of the other professional contributions can be, at times, more important and they are quite distinct from that which the physician can make." *

While the health care available in medical centers within the United States tends to establish a standard of care (possibly because most health workers are trained in these centers), many nurses in recent decades have reminded their colleagues and the public that in remote and sparsely populated areas they, like the Canadian nurses, are forced to substitute for all other health workers, including physicians.

Any study of the extended role of the nurse takes into account nurse-midwifery (already mentioned in connection with the Frontier Nursing Service) and the care of infants and children by pediatric nurses.

Henry Silver, a physician, in association with Loretta Ford, a nurse, is credited with having inaugurated at the University of Colorado in 1965 the first Pediatric Nurse Practitioner Program.[147] Nurses with baccalaureate degrees who were given special preparation saw well infants and children and treated minor illnesses and conditions in consultation with physicians. This program received so much attention that *Time Magazine* ran a feature article in 1966 entitled "Where Doctors Don't Reach" (**88:**71, July 22).

In 1969, Silver, collaborating with the

* Bates, Barbara: "Doctor and Nurse: Changing Roles and Relations," *N. Engl. J. Med.,* **283:**129, (July 16) 1970.
† It can hardly be denied that every adult and many children "diagnose" and treat aches and pains, injuries, and dysfunction of all sorts daily. More nonprescription than prescription drugs are sold in most countries. Why should not nurses advise people on self-help when they are the only, or the most informed, persons available?

* Godber, Sir George: "Ira V. Hiscock Lecture, 1975. The Greater Medical Profession," *Yale J. Biol. Med.,* **49:**137, 1976.

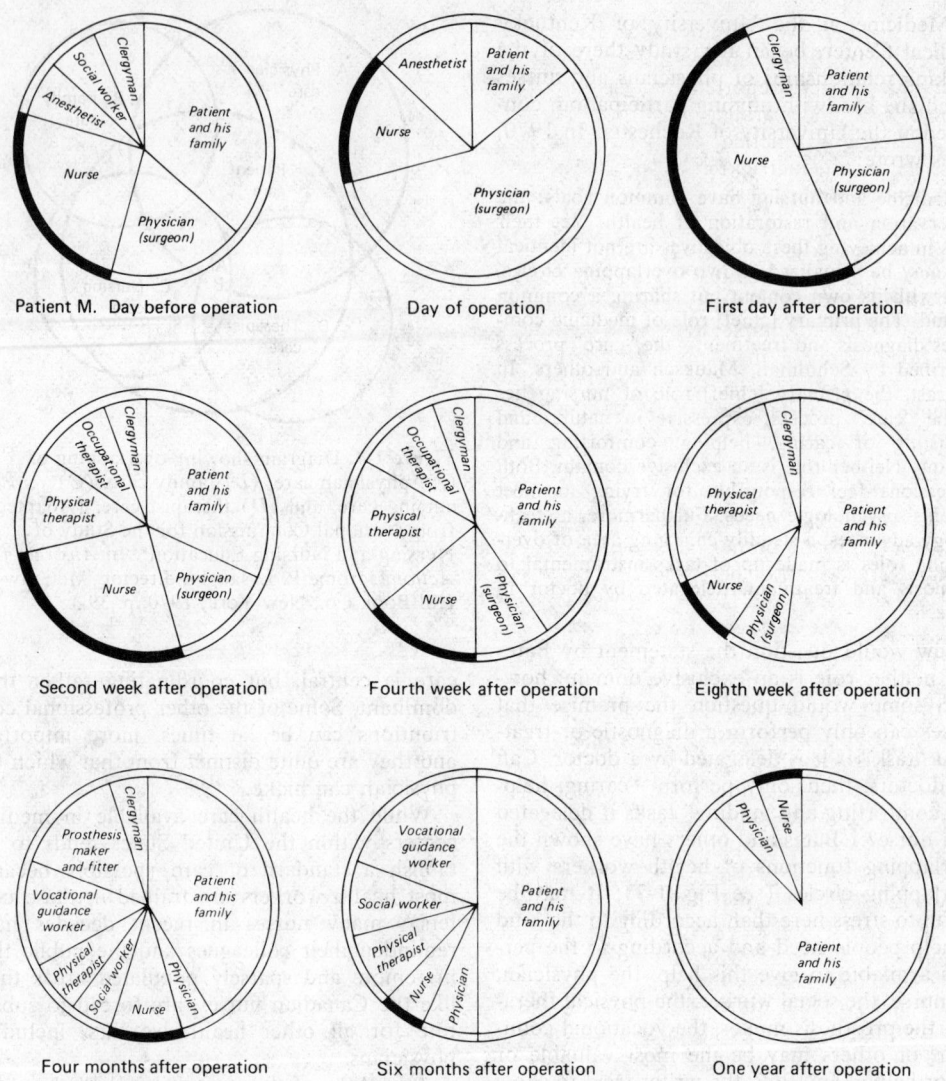

Figure 1-8. Diagrams that show the changing dominance in the roles of patients and their families, physicians, nurses, and other health workers during the various phases of illness and rehabilitation. (Adapted from Henderson, Virginia: *The Nature of Nursing.* Macmillan Publishing Co., Inc., New York, 1966.)

School of Nursing, University of Colorado, established the Child Health Associate Program which enabled graduates to "practice pediatrics under close physician supervision" as defined under a new Colorado law. These child health associates came into the program with 2 years of college and had 3 years of professional studies that included a 1-year internship.[148,149]

Many programs similar to those in Colorado have been instituted and assessments made of graduates. A few reports of each are listed at the end of this chapter.[150-163]

The Maternal and Child Health Service,

Health Services Administration, US Department of Health, Education, and Welfare, has funded a 3-year study by the American Nurses' Association to develop research methods for evaluating the impact of pediatric nurse practitioner (PNP) programs and their graduates on the health care of children.[164]

The nurse-midwife was probably the first nurse accepted as giving primary care in the United States; the pediatric nurse practitioner and the child health associate were perhaps the next to be accepted. However, some psychiatric nurses have functioned as therapists for decades. In the review of nursing research reported by Leo W. Simmons and Virginia Henderson in 1964,[165] more studies of nursing in psychiatry were reported than in any other clinical field and parallel upgrading of their preparation and practice was noted. For decades, some psychiatric nurse specialists have been giving primary care in private practice, in clinics, and in hospitals.[166-169]

While the extended role of the pediatric nurse was being developed at the University of Colorado, C. E. Lewis, a physician, and Barbara Resnick, a nurse, developed a primary role for the nurse in a medical ambulatory service at the University of Kansas. This experience was reported in journals and as a final report in 1968 to the US Public Health Service, the funding agency.[170-173] Barbara R. Noonan [174] has reported on 8 years in a medical nurse clinic at the Massachusetts General Hospital in Boston and on her changing role as she assumed a caseload of her own.

In the decade of the 1970s, the primary care role of the nurse has been developed in almost every clinical setting—maternal and child care, medical nursing, and psychiatry and in most of the occupational settings discussed in Chapter 3—hospitals, clinics, nursing homes, offices, industries, schools, private homes. In 1973, Mary H. Browning and Edith P. Lewis compiled articles on the expanded role of the nurse in a volume which was published by the American Journal of Nursing Company.[175] While most articles indicate that patients, nurses, and physicians respond positively to an extended role for the nurse, change in human relationships is not easy, and nurses in this role describe many of the difficulties they encounter. Robert Galton, a physician, and his associates make the following comment:

The movement toward a physician-nurse team care of patients with complementary roles has not developed as quickly as was originally projected. Both patients and physicians are loathe to have anything interfere with the traditional relationship. Physicians have expressed anxiety about losing their patients to nurses.*

Throughout the 1960s and 1970s, the US Department of Health, Education, and Welfare has sponsored studies of the extended role. The Secretary's Committee to Study Extended Roles for Nurses published a report in 1971. The Committee was composed of 11 physicians and 10 nurses, and the staff director was Faye G. Abdellah. The report stated that "health care should reflect patient needs rather than professional prerogatives, and those who provide

health care should work as a team whenever the needs of the patient and his family warrant. . . . Nursing practice . . . may be compartmentalized under . . . primary care, acute care, and long-term care." Primary care, as used in the report, was defined as "(a) a person's first contact in any given episode of illness with the health care system that leads to a decision of what must be done to help resolve his problem; and (b) the responsibility for the continuum of care, i.e., maintenance of health, evaluation and management of symptoms, and appropriate referrals." * This report carried weight and, perhaps more than any other publication in the United States, established the extended role as an accomplished fact. By 1975, there were 74 "nurse practitioner" programs in 34 states that awarded a B.S. degree and/or certificate and 53 programs in 34 states that awarded a master's degree.[176]

The conclusions and recommendations of the Secretary's Committee are very much in line with those in the report of the National Commission for the Study of Nursing and Nursing Education.[177] The American Nurses' Association took a similar stand on the extended role and collaborated with the National Commission in activating its recommendations. The ANA's ongoing Joint Practice Commission with the American Medical Association to study the functions of nurses and physicians and their overlapping functions is a model for state and local commissions of this sort.[178]

The development of the *physician's assistant* by the medical profession in the United States and their role as primary care providers must be considered in even a brief discussion of the nurse's extended role. Just as feldshers were developed in Russia during the seventeenth century to nurse (and treat) sick and wounded soldiers and sailors, medical technicians were developed in most countries to nurse (and treat) military personnel or to "extend" the services of physicians and professional nurses. Patrick B. Storey prepared a report on USSR feldshers for the National Institutes of Health in 1972.[178a] The contribution of Russian feldshers to health care is described in greater detail in a pamphlet prepared by the Ministry of Health of the USSR for, and distributed by, the World Health Organization in 1974. By 1956, there were almost 300,000 employed feldshers. In the 1970s, they belong to categories such as feldsher-generalist, midwife, sanitarian, laboratory technician, and dental

---

* Galton, Robert, et al.: "Observations on the Participation of Nurses and Physicians in Chronic Care," *Bull. N.Y. Acad. Med.*, 49:112, (Feb.) 1973.

* US Department of Health, Education, and Welfare: *A Report of the Secretary's Committee to Study Extended Roles for Nurses.* US Government Printing Office, Washington, D.C., 1971, pp. 2, 4, 8.

assistant or dental mechanic. The formal feld-sher training programs began in the seventeenth century, some for physician's assistants in civil life and some for military feldshers, the latter being longer and more rigorous programs. They now have 8 years of primary education and the feldsher curriculum is about 4 years in length. Students are taught by physical, bio-logic, and social scientists, physicians, nurses, and others.[179] Generally speaking, feldshers function more independently in the USSR than registered nurses do in the United States.[180] Feldsher programs are said to prepare gradu-ates to give medical care in the absence of the physician. In the USSR, both feldshers and nurses are classified as "middle-level medical personnel"; both are taught by physicians (who administer the schools), and both, if they show special ability, may later study medicine with-out having to pass an entrance examination to medical school.[181]

In World War I, but more particularly in World War II, a wide variety of medical aides were developed in the United States military forces, with preparation that ranged from weeks to months or even years. Some medical technicians remained in military service to function in this capacity; others went into schools of nursing in civil life; others were in-terested in becoming assistants to physicians rather than becoming nurses. Physicians in the United States who had found them helpful in military service and other physicians who were impressed with the work of feldshers in Russia promoted the creation of physician's assistants. Eugene A. Stead, a physician of Duke Univer-sity, Durham, North Carolina is credited with leadership in initiating such programs. With K. G. Andreoli, he reported the progress of the Duke program in 1967.[182] In 1968, Thelma Ingles, a nurse who had worked with Stead, also described the program which welcomed nurses as applicants.[183]

In 1970, Ernest B. Howard, vice-president of the American Medical Association, speculated that 100,000 nurses who could be "quickly trained" to expand physicians' abilities to serve patients could relieve the physician shortage, including the resumption of house calls.[184] This unilateral action excited a negative response from organized nursing and tended to discour-age recruitment of nurses into the physician's assistant programs that had by 1974, 48 AMA-accredited programs.[185] The programs may be called physician's assistant, physician's asso-ciate, or MEDIC or MEDEX programs—the latter being programs for military personnel with medical experience. They are under the direction of medical schools, community col-leges, public or private universities, or hos-

pitals. About 1000 graduates are now produced annually, the total by September, 1975, was estimated as 3000—the ratio of male to fe-males being 7:3. Thirty-six states had, by the end of 1975, legislation sanctioning physician's assistants or MEDEX.* [186]

There is considerable disagreement on the extent to which the functions of nurses and physician's assistants overlap and on the pro-fessional relationship of nurses and physician's assistants. A great variety of opinion ex-ists.[187-190] While their numbers are few, physi-cian's assistants are organized and have an of-ficial publication (*The P.A. Journal—A Journal for New Health Practitioners*). At present, their numbers, the length of training, their role in health care, and their relationship to nursing are quite different from those of feldshers in Russia. Alfred M. Sadler and his associates, discussing the independence and de-pendence of health workers and the expanding roles of physician's assistants, speak of the "legally dependent and flexible status" of physi-cians' assistants in contrast to the status of nurses who are "striving for an independent function." [191] Whatever the difference, it is as necessary for nurses in the United States to have effective working relationships with physi-cian's assistants as it is for nurses in the USSR to have effective working relationships with feldshers.

Whether or not there is one body of knowl-edge on health and disease or whether it can be parceled out as psychology, physiology, health education, medicine, dentistry, phar-macy, nursing, nutrition, and so on, is de-batable. The fragmentation of health care and the elaboration of health workers goes on and on. And within each category of health worker, as, for instance, medicine and nursing, special-ization results in further fragmentation of health care.

Some physicians still seem to think that everyone entering the health care system should see an internist, a diagnostician, a family health physician, or a primary care physician. Texts such as Mack Lipkin's *The Care of Patients, Concepts and Tactics,*[192] addressed to medical students, barely mentions nurses (or physi-cian's assistants), and Robert E. Rakel, a phy-sician writing on "Primary Care—Whose Re-sponsibility?",[193] seems to say that the answer lies in training a sufficient number of primary care physicians. Admitting the value of thor-ough training and seasoned clinical judgment, this goal is unattainable in even the most eco-nomically favored countries even if their com-

---

* Programs that prepare nurses to give primary care are called PRIMEX programs.

plements of doctors were equally distributed.

In 1972, the National Joint Practice Commission of the American Nurses' Association and the American Medical Association was initiated with equal numbers of physician and nurse practitioners. Shirley A. Smoyak has described its origin and purpose.[194] At its 1974 conference, *Building for the Future*, such subjects were discussed as the roles of physician's assistants and expanded roles of nurses, interdisciplinary education, and legal aspects of joint practice.[195] The Commission is studying medical and nursing practice acts [196] and has published a bibliography with abstracts on joint practice.[197]

Private foundations are sponsoring studies of primary care and roles of physicians, nurses, physician's assistants, and others. Two conferences funded by the Josiah Macy, Jr. Foundation were reported under the titles *The Greater Medical Profession,* 1973 (held in England) and *The Intermediate-Level Health Practitioners,* 1974 (held in the United States). The Josiah Macy, Jr. Foundation funded a study by the Secretary-General of the [International] Organization for Economic Cooperation and Development, reported in 1975 under the title *New Directions in Education for Changing Health Care Systems.* The Foundation also financed for the Center for Educational Research and Innovation (CERI) the study *The Ontario Experience,* referred to on page 28.* Support for the development of physician's assistants has come from a number of foundations—the Carnegie Corporation, the Commonwealth Fund, the Rockefeller Foundation, and the Robert Wood Johnson Foundation, as well as from the US Department of Health, Education, and Welfare.

In all these conferences and publications, the unequal distribution of health manpower is stressed, as are the wasteful use of expensively prepared workers in some places, the insupportable cost of health care, the overuse of resources in some countries, with consequent fostering of dependence, and the effectiveness of community involvement and indigenous health workers who understand the people's problems and who have their trust.

There can be little doubt that the role of the physician is changing, as is that of the nurse.

In a WHO conference on health economics, it is noted that one way of "containing costs" is to "ensure that the degree of technical complexity involved [in the workers' preparation] is appropriate for the task to be performed." * Because their education is the most lengthy and costly, doctors are advised to turn over to other health workers any tasks the latter can safely perform. This principle, and the fact that there are not enough physicians to give the care the peoples of the world believe to be their right, is forcing physicians in every country to relinquish many of their traditional functions. A collaborative role for physicians and nurses is essential if the goal of providing a universal health service is to be reached.†

In the writer's opinion, every health institution would profit by the creation of *an interdisciplinary committee on practice to assess the needs of the clientele to be served and the available health manpower, and the allocation of functions and responsibilities among the available workers.* All categories of clinical health professionals should retain some direct service to the client or patient, for without this human interaction, the service loses its chief reward and the opportunity for the worker to sense the patient's problem, the kinds of research needed, and possible changes that might be made to improve the service.

Albert Schweitzer, who left successful musical and theological careers to be a medical missionary, said he wanted to be able:

. . . to work without having to talk. For years I have been giving myself out in words and it was with joy that I had followed the calling of theological teacher and preacher. But this new form of activity [the practice of medicine] I couldn't represent to myself as being talking about the religion of love but only as an actual putting it into practice.‡

He quotes Goethe's *Faust,* "In the beginning was the Deed." Nursing is a service primarily of deeds. Annie W. Goodrich used to say there was no such thing as a "menial act," but that a person could have a menial attitude toward

---

* The World Health Organization has designated the Center for Educational Development, University of Illinois College of Medicine, as a "WHO Collaborating Institute in Medical Education." In 1973, it published a collection of papers under the title *Development of Educational Programmes for the Health Professions* [198] which suggests an international trend toward interdisciplinary education and collaborative practice.

* World Health Organization: *Health Economics.* Report on a WHO Interregional Seminar. The Organization, Geneva, 1975, p. 16 (Public Health Papers No. 64).

† Many studies of nurses in extended roles and of physician's assistants have been reported. E. D. Cohen et al. prepared a bibliography of such reports in 1974. (*An Evaluation of Policy Related Research on New and Expanded Roles of Health Workers: Annotated Bibliography.* Yale University School of Medicine, Office of Regional Activities and Continuing Education, New Haven, Conn.)

‡ Schweitzer, Albert: *Out of My Life and Thought.* (Translated by C. T. Campion.) Henry Holt & Co., New York, 1933, p. 114.

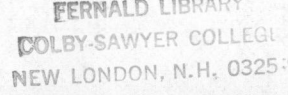

any kind of work. Esther A. Werminghaus in her biographical sketch of Annie W. Goodrich says:

Gradually a new symbol is emerging. . . . Miss Goodrich has referred to her as "the complete nurse." A few schools can produce a good many complete nurses, but it is Miss Goodrich's unfaltering contention that all nurses must be complete nurses before we can expect to realize the great social potentialities of professional nursing.*

An Operational Definition of Nursing Used in This Book.† Admitting the importance of theory, of identifying values and goals, and of unifying these into a system which might also be called a philosophy, the writer believes it still necessary to have a specific operational definition of nursing. And because so many health workers would claim the over-all goals for nursing that have been cited, it is helpful to define nursing so that it is differentiated from health education, the practice of medicine, clinical psychology, or social service. In fact, it is necessary, even in an age of rapid change, as long as students in these fields are educated in different programs and their respective practice is regulated by separate laws and regulations.

Under any health care system, each category of worker should be recognized as having a peculiar or *unique* function, no matter how many functions they have in common with others. Certainly the members of each vocational group should be more competent in performing some activities than are the workers in any other vocation. So the questions must be asked: What *is nursing* that is not also medicine, physical therapy, social work, etc.?; and What is *the unique function of the nurse?* The writer assumes responsibility for the following analysis but cannot take full credit for it since association with hundreds of nurses and others interested in nursing has contributed to clarification of these concepts—right or wrong. They are presented in the hope that they may help others, whether they agree or disagree, to develop a working concept of the place of nursing in society.

Nursing is primarily helping people (sick or well) in the performance of those activities contributing to health, or its recovery (or to a peaceful death) that they would perform un-

aided if they had the necessary strength, will, or knowledge. It is likewise the unique contribution of nursing to help people to be independent of such assistance as soon as possible. Nursing has a part in other activities that contribute to the accomplishment of what Goodrich refers to as "a healthy citizenry," just as medicine, whose unique function is diagnosing disease and prescribing therapy, may be engaged cooperatively in all activities concerned with health in its fullest meaning. From the preceding definition of nursing, the definition of the *unique* function of nurses follows: *To help people, sick or well, in the performance of those activities contributing to health or its recovery (or to a peaceful death) that they would perform unaided if they had the necessary strength, will, or knowledge. It is likewise the function of nurses to help people gain independence as rapidly as possible.* This part of their work nurses initiate and control; of this they are masters. In addition (or as part of this defined function if it is broadly interpreted), nurses help patients carry out therapeutic plans as initiated by physicians. Nurses also, as members of a cooperative health team, help its other members, as they in turn may help nurses, to plan and carry out with patients and their families the total program of care. No member of the team should make such heavy demands on other members that they are unable to perform their special or unique function. Nor should any member of the team be diverted by nonmedical activities such as cleaning, clerking, and filing, as long as their unique task must be neglected. All members of the team should consider the person (patient) served as the central figure, and should realize that primarily they are all *assisting him or her.* If patients do not understand, accept, and participate in planning the program of care, the effort of the health team is largely wasted. The sooner people recognize the nature of their health problems, the reasons they are ill, the rationale of treatment, the sooner they can care for themselves—even carry out their own treatments—the better off they are.

This concept of the nurse as a substitute for what patients lack to make them "complete," "whole," or "independent," be it the lack of physical strength, will, or knowledge, may seem limited to some who read this.* The more one thinks about it, however, the more complex is the nurse's function, as so defined. Think how

---

*Werminghaus, Esther A.: *Annie W. Goodrich; Her Journey to Yale.* Macmillan Publishing Co., Inc., New York, 1950, p. 7.
†Eileen Pearlman Becknell and Dorothy M. Smith in *System of Nursing Practice, A Clinical Nursing Assessment Tool* (F. A. Davis Co., Philadelphia, 1975) use this definition and show how it can be implemented in a problem-oriented system of care and problem-oriented record (see Chapter 4).

*Dorothea Orem and her associates subscribe to this concept of nursing but they call this lack of knowledge, will, or strength the client's "health deficit." They think it is the nurse's function to make up this deficit.

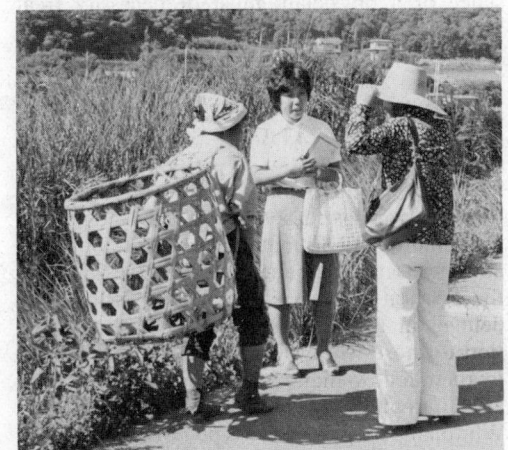

A

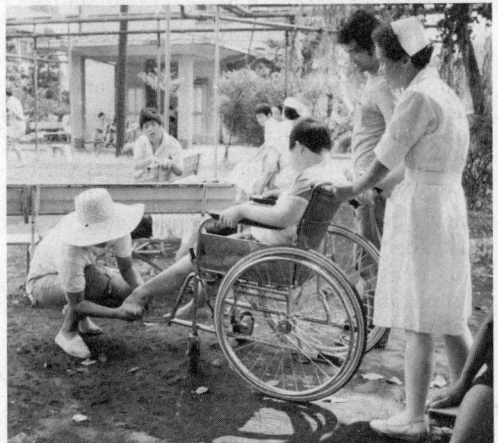

B

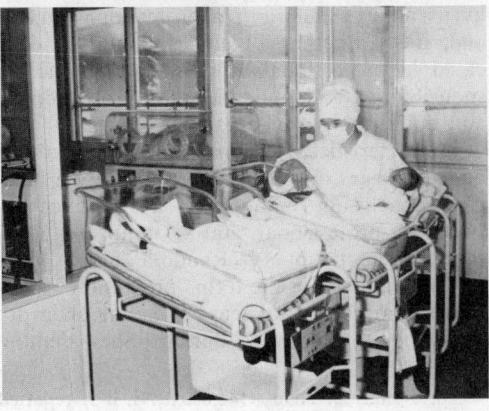

C

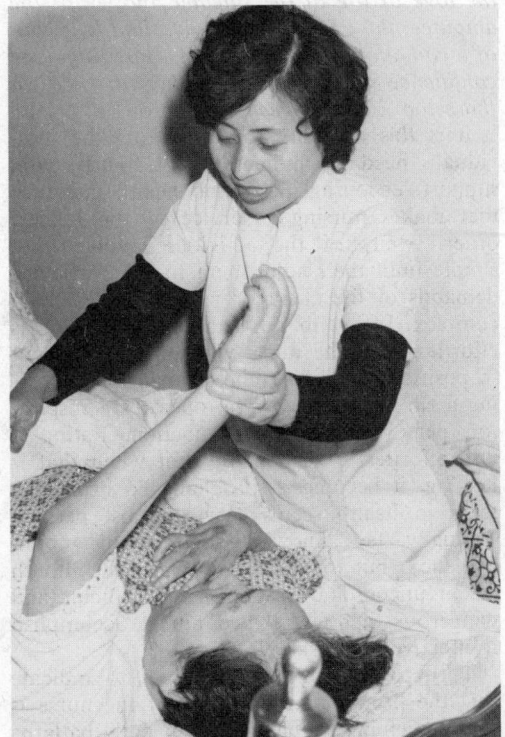

D

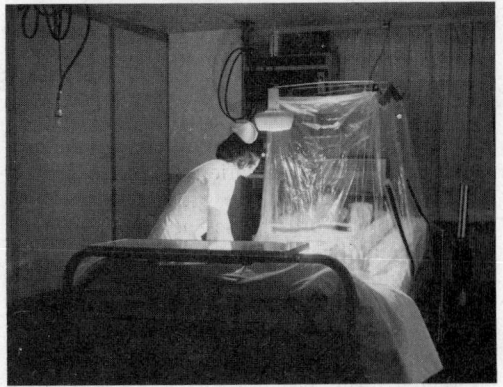

E

Figure 1-9. Nursing in a variety of settings.
A. A community health nurse. *B.* At a hospital
for mentally and physically handicapped children.
C. In the newborn nursery. *D.* Visiting nurse
helping a bedfast man at home. *E.* Night duty in
an intensive care unit. (All photos courtesy of
the Japanese Nursing Association.)

rarely one sees independence, completeness, or
wholeness of mind and body! To what extent
good health is a matter of heredity, to what
extent it is acquired, is controversial, but it is
generally admitted that intelligence and education, by and large, tend to parallel health status.

If, then, most people find "good health" a difficult goal to reach, how much more difficult
it is for health workers to help others reach it.
Nurses must, in a sense, get "inside the skin"
of each patient in order to know what help he
or she needs from them. *The nurse is tempo-*

rarily the consciousness of the unconscious, the love of life of the suicidal, the leg of the amputee, the eyes of the newly blind, a means of locomotion for the newborn, knowledge and confidence for the young mother, a voice for those too weak to speak, and so on.

It is this necessity for estimating the individual's need for momentary or hourly care, support, encouragement, and health guidance that makes nursing a service of the highest order. Many of the activities involved are simple until their adjustment to the particular demands of the client or patient makes them complex. In health, for example, breathing is effortless; but the nurse who places a patient in position for proper chest expansion following a rib resection, or who operates a respirator, performs a complex function. Eating is also effortless with appetite; but when that is lacking, it becomes a problem. To brush the teeth in health seems easy to most persons (actually few know enough about mouth hygiene); but to thoroughly clean the mouth of an unconscious patient is so difficult and dangerous that few skilled nurses accomplish it effectively and safely.

Perhaps enough has been said to indicate that the primary responsibility of the nurse is that of helping people with their daily patterns of living, or with the following activities that they ordinarily perform without assistance: breathing, eating, eliminating, resting, sleeping and moving, cleaning the body and keeping it warm and properly clothed. Nurses also help provide for those activities that make life more than a vegetative process, namely, social intercourse, learning, occupations that are recreational and those that are productive in some way. In other words nurses help people maintain or create health regimens that, were they strong, knowing, and filled with the love of life, they would carry out unaided. It is this intimate, demanding, and yet inexpressibly rewarding service that nurses are best prepared to render. And because nurses are the most numerous of all health workers in most countries, and nursing service in most institutions is the only 24-hour service, nursing is the only service organized to give this most essential help.

In addition to this unique function of nurses, they help patients identify and express their health needs; they help them find and use the health resources of the community and carry out such treatments prescribed by therapists, or physicians, as they cannot perform unaided. And in the absence of physicians and other licensed therapists, nurses may function in these capacities. While nurses are not primarily therapists, as defined in this book, nursing may

include therapy, since everybody, in the absence of a physician, must of necessity treat himself or herself.

3. NURSING AND WHAT IT OFFERS AS AN OCCUPATION

Vocational Motivation. People choose vocations for various reasons; they may seek spiritual, emotional, or material rewards, but usually they are compelled by ideals as well as the necessity of earning a living. Nursing as defined in this text offers immediate satisfaction to those who want to give a direct service to their fellow man. It is interesting that men as different as Mahatma Gandhi and Walt Whitman sought this type of satisfaction through nursing, as have thousands in almost all periods of recorded history. Undoubtedly, many persons have adopted this vocation with idealistic as well as materialistic motives.*

The leaders of modern nursing, by and large, believe that if nursing is to attract able men and women in sufficient numbers, it must offer not only the satisfaction of a vital service, but also the belief that the service is valued by society, and that society is willing to pay as much for it as for comparable services in rival fields. Most students of human behavior think it is possible for people to serve others most sympathetically and effectively when they are themselves happy and secure in public esteem.

The extent to which nursing offers personal satisfaction and security depends to some extent on whether it is accepted as a profession. There is a difference of opinion as to whether, by its nature, nursing is a professional service and, if so, whether all nurses should be educated in professional schools, assume the responsibilities and obligations of professionals, and enjoy their privileges.

Characteristics, Responsibilities, Obligations, and Privileges of a Profession. It is *not* a foregone conclusion that there is a difference between a professional and a nonprofessional service. One dictionary (Random House) gives seven meanings for the term "profession" stemming from its general sense of laying claim to, declaring, or affirming.† Bernard Shaw demon-

---

* In a study of almost 141,000 RNs, it is reported "Almost all participants had chosen nursing as a career because they wanted to help others . . ." (Knopf, Lucille: *RN's One and Five Years After Graduation. A Report of the Nurse Career-Pattern Study.* National League for Nursing, New York, 1975, p. 4 (Pub. No. 19–1535).

† 1. A vocation requiring knowledge of some department of learning or science: *the profession of teaching.* . . . 2. Any vocation or business. 3. The body of persons engaged in an occupation or calling: *to be re-*

strated his contempt for the term with the title of his play, *Mrs. Warren's Profession.* Mrs. Warren was a "madam," or ran a house of prostitution. Reference is often made to prostitution as "the oldest profession."

Many students of occupations have attempted to list the criteria of a profession. The following, laid down by Abraham Flexner in his 1915 study of social work, are often cited:

1. They [professions] involve essentially intellectual operations accompanied by large undivided responsibility.
2. They are learned in nature and their members are constantly resorting to the laboratory and seminar for a fresh supply of facts.
3. They are not merely academic and theoretical, however, but are definitely practical in their aims.
4. They possess a technique capable of communication through a highly specialized educational discipline.
5. They are self-organized, with activities, duties and responsibilities which completely engage their participants and develop group consciousness.

6. They are likely to be more responsible to public interest than are unorganized and isolated individuals, and they tend to become increasingly concerned with the achievements of social ends.*

William J. McGlothlin in 1964 presented criteria which overlap with but differ from Flexner's. He said a profession:

1. Deals with matters of great urgency and significance.
2. Is directed to human benefit and is guided by ethical standards.
3. Is learned.
4. Undertakes tasks which require the exercise of judgment in applying knowledge to the solution of problems and accepts responsibility for results.†

McGlothlin showed graphically the comparative length of preparation for 16 "professions" in 1964 (see Fig. 1-10).

Alfred North Whitehead differentiated crafts and professions. He said a craft is "an avocation based upon customary activities and modified by the trial and error of individual practice"; a profession is "an avocation whose activities are subject to theoretical analysis and

spected by the medical profession. 4. Act of professing; avowal; a declaration, whether true or false: *professions of dedication.* 5. The declaration of belief in or acceptance of religion or a faith: *the profession of Christianity.* 6. A religion or faith professed. 7. The declaration made on entering into membership of a church or religious order. (*The Random House Dictionary of the English Language.* Random House, New York, 1966, p. 1148.)

* Flexner, Abraham: "Is Social Work a Profession?" *Proceedings of the National Conference of Charities and Corrections,* Chicago, Ill., 1915, p. 578.
† McGlothlin, William J.: *The Professional Schools.* Center for Applied Research in Education, New York, 1964, p. 3.

Figure 1-10. Length of preparation for 16 professional fields in 1964, showing medicine with the longest preparation time and 7 professions (including nursing) with the shortest. (From McGlothlin, William J.: *The Professional Schools.* Center for Applied Research in Education, Inc., New York, 1964, p. 46.)

Field	1	2	3	4	5	6	7	8	9	10	11	12
Agriculture												
Architecture												
Business administration												
Dentistry												
Engineering												
Forestry												
Home economics												
Law												
Medicine												
Nursing												
Optometry												
Pharmacy												
Psychology												
Social work												
Teaching												
Veterinary medicine												

KEY: College of arts and sciences
Professional school
Internship
Residency

are modified by theoretical conclusions derived from that analysis." *

Collectively, these criteria include measurable attributes and hard-to-measure attitudes. Applying them, it is clear that some highly educated workers are "unprofessional" in practice and those who may be largely self-taught practice professionally. While few would question the desirability of health workers having Flexner's and McGlothlin's attitudes and attributes, many deplore the intellectual snobbery underlying the rigid hierarchy in hospitals and other health agencies that has interfered with the interchange of information and opinion essential to effective patient care.†

The International Council of Nurses defines the term *nurse* in such a way as to imply that nursing *is* a profession (see page 18). The Council states that entry requirements for admission to schools of nursing should be in line with those for entry into "other comparable professions in each country," and it holds that "nurse educators should be prepared in post-basic and postgraduate programs [university based] which provide advanced study in nursing practice." ‡

Because the ICN is a body representing nursing organizations of 84 countries (in 1975) whose educational systems vary, its statements are less specific than those of component organizations. However, since one or more basic collegiate programs have been instituted in most of the ICN member countries, it is clear that there is an international trend toward collegiate education for nursing. In most cultures, the *upgrading of education goes hand in hand with professionalization of any occupation.*

In the United States, there is growing recognition of nursing as a profession. McGlothlin, measuring it against his criteria, said in 1961: "At long last, then, I reach the conclusion that nursing has established its own place among the professions." § He also said, with respect

to "learning," nursing is "in the process of becoming." Since then he notes that nursing has recognized its obligation to advance knowledge by assessing its members in support of research. The pyramidal Figure 1-11 shows the very small percentage of nursing personnel with a college degree of any sort. McGlothlin's reference to nurses who qualify as professionals (who meet his criteria) is obviously related to a few at the top of the pyramid. Jerome P. Lysaught, director of the National Commission for the Study of Nursing and Nursing Education, on the other hand, is less inclined to accord nursing professional status than was McGlothlin. In the conclusion of the Commission's 1970 report, he says:

During the months of this study, the commission and staff have lived with the problems, the frustrations, and the triumphs of our American health system. In particular, we have become intimately acquainted with the history and the disappointments, as well as the great joys, of nursing. Out of this has come the recognition that nursing is not only important, but crucial to the future of health care in America.

Yet nursing has been and is a troubled occupation. It is an occupation that fails in every characteristic to achieve the status of a full profession, despite the fact that its best practitioners are professional in every sense of that word. It is an occupation that has never controlled its own destiny, but has suffered severe consequences when it has failed to meet the demands imposed by our society. It is an occupation fraught with paradox and promise—and it holds within itself the key to whether or not the vast majority of our people will receive quality health care.

Nursing cannot continue to be the stepchild of the health professions.*

The American Nurses' Association is more specific than the ICN about the professional status of nursing. The Association, believing that nurses need the kind of preparation for their work that in this country is available only within colleges and universities, adopted the position that higher education is where basic programs in professional nursing belong.[199] The New York State Nurses Association is proposing legislation that will provide two kinds of nursing education programs leading to licensure after 1984: the baccalaureate degree for nursing and the associate degree for practical nursing.[200] However, in spite of the official position of nursing on the essentially professional nature of its service, the question is still debated.

Using the criteria cited, some nurses and

* Whitehead, Alfred North: *Adventures of Ideas.* Pelican Books, London, 1948, p. 73.

† To show the difficulty of defining a profession we might note that Henry E. Sigerist said: "the history of medicine is first of all the history of a γέχνη, of a craft." (*A History of Medicine.* Volume 1. *Primitive and Archaic Medicine.* Oxford University Press, New York, 1951, p. 28)

‡ International Council of Nurses: *Statement on Nursing Education. Nursing Practice and Service and the Social and Economic Welfare of Nurses.* The Council, Geneva, 1969, p. 3; and World Health Organization: *World Directory of Post-Basic and Post-Graduate Schools of Nursing.* The Organization, Geneva, 1965.

§ McGlothlin, William J.: "The Place of Nursing Among the Professions," *Nurs. Outlook,* 9:214, (Apr.) 1961.

* National Commission for the Study of Nursing and Nursing Education: *An Abstract for Action.* (Jerome P. Lysaught, Director.) McGraw-Hill Book Co., New York, 1970, p. 163.

some critics of nursing say that only the administration and teaching of nursing represent a professional service; others say that to this should be added nursing service to the individual patient where there is a high component of teaching, such as is found in so-called public health or community nursing, and also the nursing care in a clinical specialty for which the nurse has had special preparation. Another point of view is that all nursing, as defined in this chapter, is essentially complex, depending for its full expression on a profound knowledge of the nature of man and familiarity with a large body of health science. The latter view is comparable to the position educators take that all teaching, even the teaching of children in nursery school, is a service of a professional nature that demands professional preparation. Educators say that all teachers should have an understanding of children and should be able to apply this in trying to meet the varying needs of children. Such an hypothesis leads us to assume that the preparation for nursing will eventually, like the preparation for all the vocations that demand an understanding of the total personality, move into the colleges and universities. While there is unquestionably a worldwide movement in this direction, it is most apparent in the United States and Canada.

The term *professional nurse* is generally applied to the graduates of recognized basic or initial nursing programs of from 2 to 4 years who have met the requirements for registered nurses in a state, province, or country in which they are licensed to practice (see page 18 for the ICN's statement). All such schools in the United States now require the candidate to be at least a high school graduate or the equivalent. It has often been proposed (and New York State wants a law to enforce it) that the term "professional nurse" be reserved for graduates of nursing schools affiliated with colleges and universities that can claim to meet standards of other professional schools. It is most likely that with upgrading of nursing schools, as with upgrading of medical schools, no attempt will be made in any country to take away from graduates of schools known in their day as "professional," a title in common usage.

Different types of educational programs will be described in this chapter. The difference between professional and technical nursing has been so widely debated that Shirley Chater and associates [201] prepared in 1972 an annotated bibliography on the subject. Sister Dorothy Sheahan,[202] in an article on "professional" and "technical" nursing, says that there are several levels of nursing education but only *one level of nursing practice* (italics ours). She believes that decision-making power is inherent in

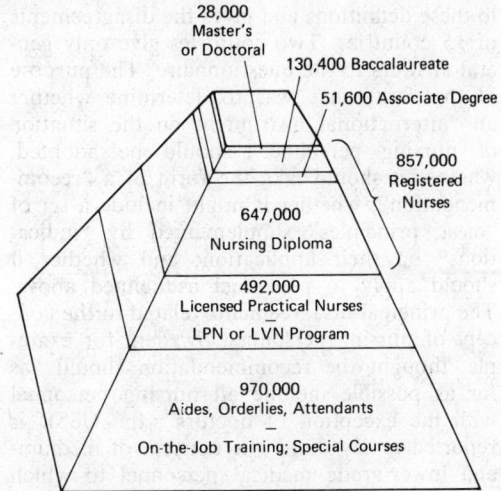

Figure 1-11. Active nursing personnel in the United States by educational preparation, January 1974. (From Hudson, Helen H., and McCarthy, Margaret D.: *Source Book—Nursing Personnel*. US Government Printing Office, Washington, D.C., 1974, p. 4.)

nursing and that professional nursing practice demands a certain type of nurse-patient relationship and nursing authority.

As nursing takes its place beside the more established professions, and as the colleges assume responsibility for the education of nurses, it is possible that the titles associate, bachelor, master, and doctor of nursing will be used to designate, as in other professions, the thoroughness of nurses' preparation for their work. This will be far less confusing than current terms, such as *registered nurse, technical nurse, nurse practitioner,* and *clinical specialist,* that fail to tell the public what it has a right to know about the length and depth of the worker's preparation.

The assumption that nursing education will eventually take its place in colleges and universities is justified for the United States and Canada where this trend is so obvious. The report of a 1976 study by the International Labour Office, *Employment and Conditions of Work and Life of Nursing Personnel,*[203] in which 53 countries replied to a questionnaire, suggests that the concept of nursing varies greatly from one continent to another and even between adjacent countries. While there is a noticeable international trend toward upgrading nursing education, it is quite clear that conditions in the United States and Canada are more atypical than otherwise.

The ILO report defines (1) *the professional nurse,* (2) *the auxiliary nurse,* and (3) *the aide;* the report lists the 36 countries that agree to these definitions and gives the disagreements of 15 countries. Two countries give only general answers to the questionnaire. The purpose of the conference was to determine whether an "international instrument on the situation of nursing personnel" should be adopted; whether it should take the form of a "recommendation"; whether it might include a set of "basic principles" supplemented by "indications" on their application; and whether it should apply to personnel as defined above. The principal disagreements related to the concept of nursing personnel. Sweden, for example, thought the recommendation should "as far as possible include all nursing personnel with the exception of doctors"; the USSR is reported to say that "The concept of medium- and lower-grade medical personnel to which the instrument should apply could be broader than that reflected in the definitions formulated by the ILO-WHO Joint Meeting. In the USSR, this concept covers not only nurses and aides but also the *feldsher* (doctors' assistants), midwives, laboratory technicians and other personnel." Japan thought it difficult to formulate a "precise definition of the aide" and this

should be left to the "discretion of the member states." While 44 of the responding 53 countries approved the adoption of an international instrument, Japan thought it would be "premature." Yugoslavia thought "the instrument should apply to all nursing personnel." These responses suggest the complexity of discussing nursing as an occupation from an international standpoint.[204]

Types of Nursing Personnel Other Than Professional Nurses. In many countries, nursing personnel with less than "professional" education equal or exceed in number the professional nurses. Such nursing personnel in the United States include practical nurses, nurse's aides, attendants, and orderlies. There were in 1972 1,127,547 registered nurses, of which 780,000 were reported by the ANA to be employed. There were also 427,000 employed licensed practical nurses and 900,000 nurses' aides, orderlies, and attendants.[205] The preparation of allied personnel or auxiliaries varied from a 2-year planned program to none at all. (See Fig. 1-12 for graph showing rapid increase in allied personnel or auxiliaries in the United States from 1950–1974, and Figure

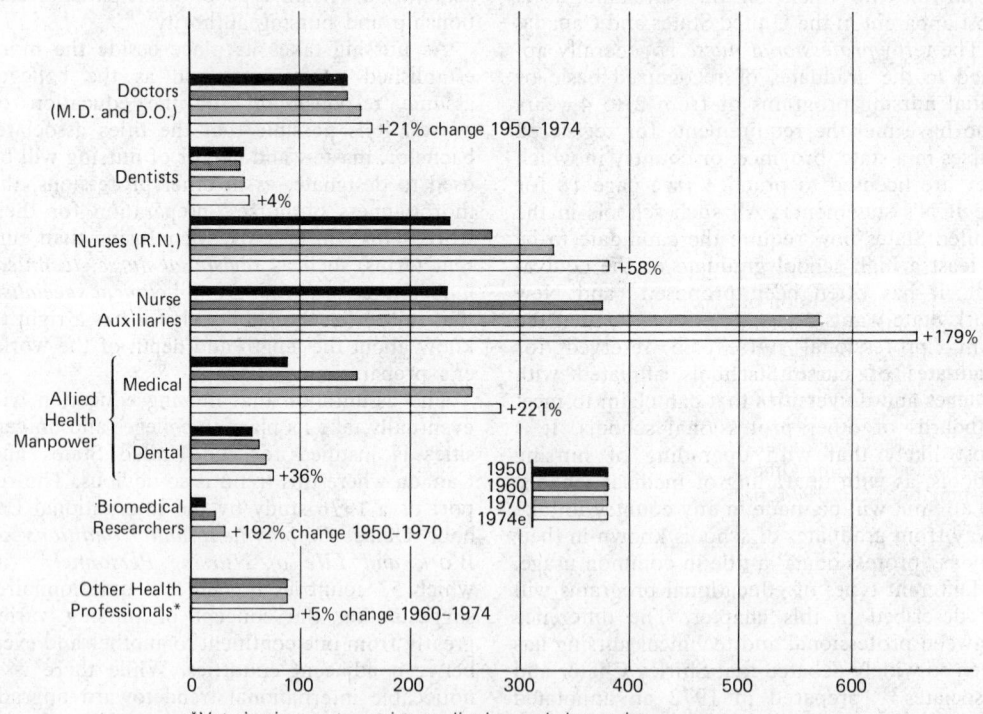

*Veterinarians, optometrists, podiatrists, and pharmacists.

Figure 1-12. Number of active health professionals per 100,000 population in United States 1950, 1960, 1974, showing marked increase in fields of medicine and nursing. (From Center for Health Policy Studies, National Planning Association: *Chartbook of Federal Health Spending 1949–74.* The Association, Washington, D.C., 1974, p. 22.)

1-13 for distribution of registered nurses and licensed practical nurses in the United States.) Few people other than nurses can accurately differentiate between categories of nursing personnel; few know how they are prepared or the nature of their intended function.

Later in this chapter preparation for nursing is discussed and attention is called to the growing acceptance of the "ladder principle"—the idea that educational programs should be designed so that a person can progress from the most elementary to the most advanced program.

In addition to the "professional" and "auxiliary" nursing personnel whose numbers *can* be counted, there are women and men all over the country whose numbers *cannot* be estimated who are giving nursing care in private homes where no trained workers of any sort are available.

How the Public Sees Nursing and How Nurses See Themselves. The literature abounds in statements that the public does not see nurses as nurses see themselves.* The public is obviously confused by the variety of workers in the occupation. This is sometimes said to be a major source of dissatisfaction among nurses. Nursing organizations have in various ways tried to tap public opinion and also give the public what they believe to be "facts" about nursing. There is a biennial statistical publication with this title, and pamphlets such as *Your Career in Nursing* and *Husband-Father-Humanitarian-Specialist—NURSE* (the latter describes opportunities for men in nursing), which are made available to the public by the American Nurses' Association. The National

---

* The "literature" here refers to books and articles on nursing. There have been numerous studies, however, on the public image of nursing as shown in novels, poetry, and drama. A recent annotated bibliography by Joanne Trautman and Carol Pollard, *Literature and Medicine* (Society for Health and Human Values, Philadelphia, 1975) includes publications that reflect writers' concepts of nurses from classical to modern times.

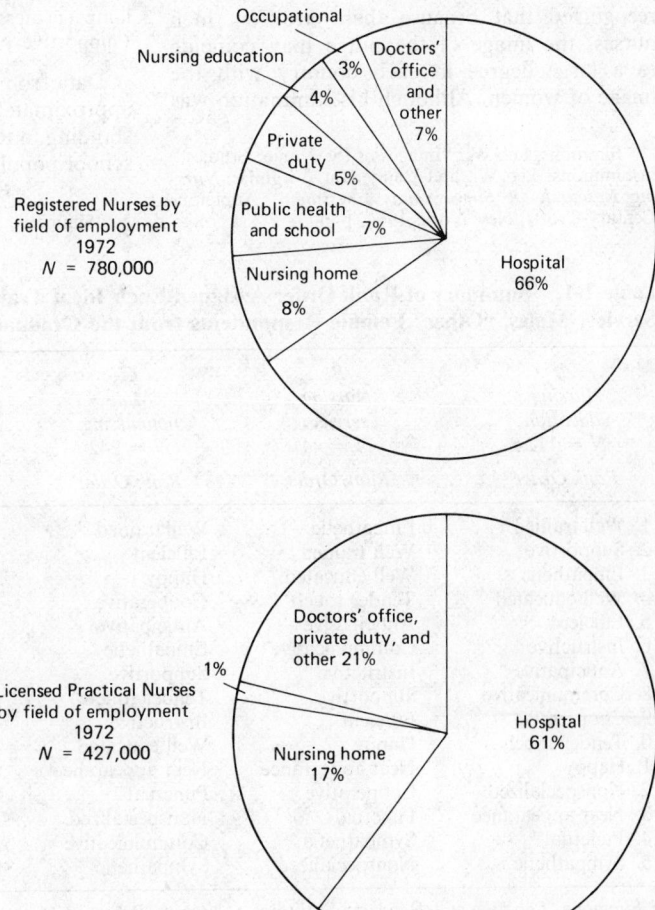

Figure 1-13. Distribution of registered nurses and licensed practical nurses by field of employment in the United States. (From Hudson, Helen H., and McCarthy, Margaret D.: *Source Book—Nursing Personnel.* US Government Printing Office, Washington, D.C., 1974, p. 61.)

League for Nursing has publications describing the various educational programs in nursing.

There is, of course, not one homogeneous public, but many, and studies of "the image of the nurse" have assessed the opinions of nurses themselves, of physicians and other health workers, and of different socioeconomic classes.

Leo W. Simmons, reviewing the image and profile studies, makes the following observation:

While extremes of idealized and derogatory opinions of the nurse are replete in the literature, balanced and representative views of her are notably lacking until near the middle of the twentieth century. The chief exceptions to this general statement is the halo-like image of the nurse inspired by biographical sketches of a few famous women and the training school dicta on what a nurse *should* be and do. Neither of these image constructs could be said to reflect the realistic views of any differentiated publics.*

Simmons tabulates in rank order the ideal traits as given by nurses and by nonnursing males and females (see Table 1-1). Simmons recognized that because there are few men nurses, the image of the nurse may coincide to a large degree in each country with the image of women. Although his summation was

* Simmons, Leo W.: "Images of the Nurse: Studies," in Simmons, Leo W., and Henderson, Virginia: *Nursing Research. A Survey and Assessment.* Appleton-Century-Crofts, New York, 1964, p. 173.

published in 1964, it is doubtful whether the gains made under the women's liberation movement of this decade would materially alter the following statement:

Granting a high level of technical competence as essential in the ideal nurse, the findings suggest considerable respondent agreement that she should also be personally alert, concerned, and responsive. The inference could be drawn from this that potential patients, including nurses, have been and will be more ready to share with nurses than with most other professionals an intimate personal relationship. . . . that people cherish this closeness to the nurse; and herein may lie for her a golden opportunity, for it casts her in a significant supportive and therapeutic role—within easy access to the patient. . . .

. . .

The way forward for nursing tends, also, toward the "human side" of patient care. Thus, the ideal image of the nurse for the future would appear to call for a special blending of the old and warm Nightingale spirit with the new and cool professional skills. Perhaps the lamp as a symbol of nursing can still serve its purpose—providing nurses can come to combine with the light of the lamp (professional skills) the warmth of the light (supportive personal response).*

Data from a recent "career-pattern" study of approximately 13,852 nurses show 10,493 with standing in top or next-to-top fourth of the high school population. This suggests an intellectual

* Simmons, Leo W.: *op. cit.,* p. 223.

Table 1-1. Summary of Rank Order Assigned Each Ideal Trait by Nursing Education, Nursing Service, Males, "Other" Female Respondents from the Graduate Student Study—As Adapted *

A Nursing education N = 112 Rank Order	B Nursing service N = 44 Rank Order	C Male nonnursing N = 242 Rank Order	D Female nonnursing N = 280 Rank Order	E All groups combined N = 678 Rank Order
1. Well trained	Empathetic	Well trained	Well trained	Well trained
2. Supportive	Well trained	Efficient	Efficient	Empathetic
3. Empathetic	Well educated	Happy	Tender touch	Efficient
4. Well educated	Tender touch	Cooperative	Anticipative	Anticipative
5. Efficient	Anticipative	Anticipative	Empathetic	Supportive
6. Instructive	Communicative	Empathetic	Happy	Tender touch
7. Anticipative	Instructive	Supportive	Supportive	Well educated
8. Communicative	Supportive	Tender touch	Cooperative	Happy
9. Cooperative	Efficient	Instructive	Well educated	Cooperative
10. Tender touch	Happy	Well educated	Neat appearance	Instructive
11. Happy	Neat appearance	Neat appearance	Communicative	Communicative
12. Nonspecialized	Cooperative	Punctual	Instructive	Neat appearance
13. Neat appearance	Punctual	Nonspecialized	Punctual	Punctual
14. Punctual	Sympathetic	Communicative	Nonspecialized	Nonspecialized
15. Sympathetic	Nonspecialized	Sympathetic	Sympathetic	Sympathetic

* Simmons, Leo W., and Henderson, Virginia: *Nursing Research. A Survey and Assessment.* Appleton-Century-Crofts, New York, 1964, p. 221.

Table 1-2. High School Academic Standing of Nurse Career-Pattern Study Participants, by Type of Program: All Years Combined *

High School Standing	Associate Degree		Diploma		Baccalaureate	
	No.	%	No.	%	No.	%
Top fourth	4,901	35.4	7,467	48.3	8,367	62.4
Second fourth	5,592	40.4	5,922	38.3	3,672	27.4
Third fourth	2,032	14.7	1,422	9.2	836	6.2
Bottom fourth	237	1.7	106	0.7	118	0.9
No response	1,090	7.9	551	3.6	417	3.1
Total	13,852	100.0	15,468	100.0	13,410	100.0

* Knopf, Lucille: *Graduation and Withdrawal from RN Programs.* (A Report of the Nurse Career-Pattern Study.) US Government Printing Office, Washington, D.C., 1975, p. 110 (DHEW Pub. No. [HRA] 76–17).

capacity above the average for the majority (see Table 1-2). The father's social index indicates that the percentage of nurses from class one ranges from 3.4 to 10.1 per cent according to the type of program from which they graduated (diploma, associate degree, or baccalaureate). The percentage from class five ranges from 11.1 to 6.0 according to type of program, with the highest percentages coming from classes three and four (see Table 1-3). See also Tables 1-4 and 1-5 on occupations of fathers and family income showing clustering of nurse sampling around so-called middle-class categories. These data indicate that the majority of nurses come from those with average or below average social and economic advantages. Graduates of baccalaureate programs come from more favored homes. With an increase in collegiate programs, the socioeconomic profile of the nurse will change.

While nurses are predominantly women and the image of nursing is confused with the concept of what a woman should be, recent and current legislation freeing nurses to function as independent health-care givers must sooner or later affect the self- and public image of the nurse. As more women study medicine and more men study nursing, the influence of sex on the status of both will be affected. As the length of preparation for medicine and for nursing more nearly approximate each other, the image of the nurse will change, and finally, if, as in the USSR, all health workers form a single occupational group characterized by lateral and vertical mobility of the various categories, the current image of nurses may change materially.* In fact, titles and functions may change to such an extent that the findings of studies cited here are no longer relevant. In any age, what nurses do affects their self-image and the public's opinion of them. Activity, or functional, analyses of nursing are among the earliest occupational studies.

* See Bonnie and Vern L. Bullough "Sex Discrimination in Health Care," as presently affecting both those who give and those who receive care. (*Nurs. Outlook,* **23**:40, [Jan.] 1975.)

Table 1-3. Social Index Classification of Fathers of Nurse Career-Pattern Study Participants by Type of Program: All Years Combined. *

Father's Social Index	Associate Degree		Diploma		Baccalaureate	
	No.	%	No.	%	No.	%
One	612	4.4	529	3.4	1,357	10.1
Two	1,471	10.6	1,472	9.5	2,635	19.6
Three	2,169	15.7	3,220	20.8	2,846	21.2
Four	4,908	35.4	6,498	42.0	3,981	29.7
Five	1,307	9.4	1,713	11.1	808	6.0
Undetermined and no response	3,385	24.4	2,036	13.2	1,783	13.3
Total	13,852	100.0	15,468	100.0	13,410	100.0

* Knopf, Lucille: *Graduation and Withdrawal from RN Programs.* (A Report of the Nurse Career-Pattern Study.) US Government Printing Office, Washington, D.C., 1975, p. 110 (DHEW Pub. No. [HRA] 76–17).

Table 1-4.   Occupations of Fathers of Nurse Career-Pattern Study Participants by Type of Program: All Years Combined. *

Father's Occupation	Associate Degree		Diploma		Baccalaureate	
	No.	%	No.	%	No.	%
Physician	165	1.2	149	1.2	461	3.4
Medically oriented professional and nonprofessional	309	2.2	293	1.9	413	3.1
Service including clergy	786	5.7	777	5.0	1,068	8.0
Professional or semiprofessional†	1,557	11.2	1,580	10.2	2,536	18.9
Sales or clerical	2,837	20.5	3,597	23.2	3,074	22.9
Farmer or outdoor	1,125	8.1	1,340	8.6	991	7.4
Military officer or enlisted	237	1.7	255	1.6	433	3.2
Skilled worker	3,108	22.4	3,987	25.8	2,326	17.3
Semiskilled and unskilled	1,454	10.5	2,027	13.1	930	6.9
Not working or not identified	800	5.8	548	3.5	376	2.8
No response	1,474	10.6	915	5.9	802	6.0
Total	13,852	100.0	15,468	100.0	13,410	100.0

* Knopf, Lucille: *Graduation and Withdrawal from RN Programs.* (A Report of the Nurse Career-Pattern Study.) US Government Printing Office, Washington, D.C., 1975, p. 109 (DHEW Pub. No. [HRA] 76–17).

† Includes owner of large business and executive.

Activity Analyses of Nursing. One of the earliest studies was made at Bellevue Hospital in New York City by Ethel Johns and Blanche Pfefferkorn for the Committee on the Grading of Nursing Schools of the National League of Nursing Education in 1934.[206] It was part of a nationwide educational study. While this activity analysis was a notable achievement, it was a study of how student nurses, rather than graduates, were functioning and it was limited to one setting.* As part of the ANA's study of the function of the nurse, this type of

analysis was made by Louis J. Kroeger Associates in 40 California hospitals during 1952. This study identified 434 hospital staff nursing activities.[207]

Studies of clinical services like orthopedics and tuberculosis care gave a more complete list within a specialty. Nell Beeby,[208] almost 40 years ago, showed some of the more intangible aspects of the nurse's work by listing the problems or "situations" the nurse finds in obstetrics. Her analysis indicated the variety and complexity of the nurse's work. Other analyses have differentiated between activities that required more and those that required less knowledge, judgment, or skill. Such lists are a basis for differentiating between the functions of the better and less prepared nurse or for assigning

* In that era, student nurses were giving nearly all the care offered hospital patients unless the patients were very ill or wealthy, in which case they were nursed by "private duty" registered nurses.

Table 1-5.   Family Income of Nurse Career-Pattern Study Participants at Time of Entrance to Nursing School, by Type of Program: All Years Combined *·†

Reported Income	Associate Degree		Diploma		Baccalaureate	
	No.	%	No.	%	No.	%
Below $5,000	2,804	20.2	3,415	22.1	1,947	14.5
$5,000–$9,999	5,920	42.7	7,022	45.4	4,844	36.1
$10,000–$14,999	2,878	20.8	2,764	17.9	3,390	25.3
$15,000 and over	1,083	7.8	842	5.4	1,819	13.6
Ambiguous or no response	1,167	8.4	1,425	9.2	1,410	10.5
Total	13,852	100.0	15,468	100.0	13,410	100.0

* Knopf, Lucille: *Graduation and Withdrawal from RN Programs.* (A Report of the Nurse Career-Pattern Study.) US Government Printing Office, Washington, D.C., 1975, p. 109 (DHEW Pub. No. [HRA] 76–17).

† Data gathered 1962, 1965, 1967.

nursing personnel to patients demanding more or less complex care. The weakness in this practice lies in the questionable assumption that the patient's needs are static. If they are assumed to be changing and unpredictable, we see that each time nurses help patients with any aspect of health or their therapeutic programs, they may have an opportunity to teach or encourage them to acquire increasing independence—in other words, to rehabilitate them. This teaching requires clinical judgment, and the personality of the nurse is in itself a therapeutic factor. What nurses say, the interest they show in people, the understanding of their problems, or the hopefulness of their attitude, may have as great an influence on patients' recoveries as what they actually do for them.

If the practice of medicine and the practice of nursing are fine arts, as this writer believes, the kind of persons doctors or nurses are is of great importance. Lin Yutang expressed this idea, with reference to the fine arts, in the following statement:

Here we are faced with the central problem of art, the problem of personality in art. The achievement of a special atmosphere is like achieving a special outlook in philosophy or a special style in writing. The atmosphere, the outlook, the style must come from the personality and must be a natural outgrowth from it. It is not something that can be imposed from the outside by any trickery in technique. Hence, in training an artist, the Chinese always insist on the cultivation of a high moral personality. The final test of a great art is, according to the Chinese, does it show a high personality? The technique may be flawless and yet the personality may be lacking.*

In like manner, the technique of nurses may be flawless, while their performances are lacking in character. Practiced sympathetically, nursing, like all the medical arts, makes heavy demands, if sympathy is correctly interpreted as "the willingness to suffer with another." Florence R. Weiner,[209] who wrote about empathy, thought the interest (or love) shown patients by nurses the most essential element of their service.

In an effort to arrive at a sound basis on which to build a curriculum, the National League of Nursing Education [210] in 1937 listed qualities or traits nurses should have, as well as what they should do. It is generally agreed that personality cannot be reduced to a formula, and that it is a mistake to ask all nurses to behave in the same way; nevertheless, there seems to be some reason to believe that successful nurses have certain characteristics in common, and that these characteristics can be cultivated. Table 1-1 lists in rank order the ideal traits identified by nurses and nonnurses. Attempts to identify the qualities associated with success in nursing persist even today.

In 1964, Simmons reviewed major *functional studies* in the following categories: general studies, staff nurse, private duty and industrial nursing; also descriptive and experimental ward studies and studies of the function of ancillary nursing personnel. He concluded that:

. . . the patient-centered, goal-determined, variable-controlled, and experimental studies in nursing functions hold much more promise for the future of nursing than do the staff-centered, time-activity, survey-type studies of which there have been so many.*

This summarization by Simmons of functional studies is useful to the reader who wants to know more about this subject. Hughes and his associates summarized the functional studies sponsored by the ANA between 1950 and 1955 under the title *Twenty Thousand Nurses Tell Their Story*.†[211] Readers interested in studies of the activities of public health nurses will find abstracts of them in *Nursing Research* (**8**:42, Spring 1959). Since 1960, *Nursing Research* has included abstracts of all types of nursing studies, including those of nursing functions. Chapter 19 is devoted to a discussion of nursing research, its history, types of studies, and its importance in all aspects of professional progress.

Presently, the role of the nurse is changing so rapidly that activity analyses and studies of ideal traits made in the 1950s and 1960s are poor guides for the profession and those entering nursing schools who want to picture their future. The Canadian study of functions, discussed on page 24 in connection with the extended role of the nurse, might give an up-to-date picture, as does the ANA's "sample survey of pediatric nurse practitioners" in 1974.[212] In this chapter, the writer has tried to stress the essential nature of nursing as an occupation. More and more often in the Western world nursing is referred to as "the cornerstone of health care delivery." In the field of maternal and child health, nurse-midwives and

---

* Yutang, Lin: "East to West in Art," *Magazine of Art,* **31**:70, (Feb.) 1938.

* Simmons, Leo W.: "Studies in Nursing Functions," in Simmons, Leo W., and Henderson, Virginia: *Nursing Research. A Survey and Assessment.* Appleton-Century-Crofts, New York, 1964, p. 277.

† Between 1950 and 1955, about $400,000 was invested in this research. Most of the money was contributed by nurses themselves as Clara A. Hardin says in the report of the studies in 17 states that she edited under the title *Nurses Invest in Patient Care* (American Nurses' Association, Kansas City, Mo., 1956).

pediatric nurse specialists are assuming wider responsibilities. In psychiatry, nurses may be assigned to patients as principal therapists; in medicine and surgery, nurses in intensive care units play the life-saving role because it is they who watch the monitoring devices and, when no physician is present, institute immediate resuscitation if this is indicated. The family health nurse practitioner meets many of the needs the family doctor used to meet.

In most countries, wherever health services exist, the nurse is found—in homes, hospitals, clinics, and nursing homes; in schools and colleges; in industry and services for transient labor; on ships, planes, and trains; in penal institutions; in camps; in research institutes; and in experimental health services for travel in space or life under the oceans. In all clinical settings, nurses may be giving primary care. Nurses are employed in their own organizations, in hundreds of health organizations such as the American Lung Association and the American Cancer Society, and in agencies and institutions with worldwide influence such as the United Nations, the World Health Organization, the International Red Cross, or the Peace Corps.* Nursing organizations in most countries publish pamphlets on nursing careers and occupational opportunities and some state or provincial nursing organizations provide regional data. Mary W. Searight's *Your Career in Nursing* [213] discusses the work of the nurse —the varied opportunities and rich rewards in nursing; Eugenia Spalding and Lucille E. Notter, writing for the initiated in *Professional Nursing. Foundations, Perspectives and Relationships,* [214] go more deeply into career choices. Lucie Young Kelly's *Dimensions of Professional Nursing* [215] provides a wealth of occupational information, as does Edith P. Lewis's compilation of journal articles entitled *Changing Patterns of Nursing Practice.* [216]

Nurses as "Change Agents." Annie Warburton Goodrich was ahead of her time in seeing the impact that the socially experienced and well-prepared nurse might have. In 1932, she published her collected papers under the title *The Social and Ethical Significance of Nursing.* [217] While she didn't call the nurse a "change agent," she saw the nurse as one who could effect change. Storlie, in her book *Nursing and the Social Conscience,* makes it clear that she thinks nurses have not lived up to the opportunities Goodrich believed they had. Storlie asks nurses to question their

role in society; to see whether they are as concerned with promoting health as with curing disease. She asks whether they can

. . . enlarge their concern for the hospital sick to the social sick, strive less to treat anemia and more to put meat on our children's plates; whether they can stretch their arms to the helpless, the feeble, the aged and infirm, the troubled and torn, the protester, the prostitute and the very poor? *

Activity, or functional, studies are efforts to find out what nurses are doing. Evaluative studies have about the same history. They are particularly important today when all health care is under scrutiny, as is the division of responsibility for its quality between the givers and recipients of care.

Evaluation of Nursing—Qualitative and Quantitative Standards. In January, 1974, the Institute of Medicine in the National Academy of Sciences held a Conference on Regulation in the Health Industry. In the report, *Controls on Health Care,* [218] legislation on certification of need, regulation of fees to providers, and other regulatory legislation were discussed. The point was made in the report that the cost of health care was exceeding reasonable limits and that, if public funds were to be used in paying providers, the agencies, institutions, and individuals that gave care must produce evidence that the receivers needed the care and that it met qualitative standards.

There is general recognition, at least in the United States, that health care is unequally distributed, that it is uneven in quality, that services are over-utilized in some respects and under-utilized in others, and that costs are uncontrolled. Nevertheless, Roger G. Noll, an economist, said at this conference, "The health care delivery system is among the most extensively regulated sectors of the American economy." † Robert M. Ball, former Commissioner of Social Security in the US Department of Health, Education, and Welfare, noted that regulations covered "a great range of activities"; they involved more than 7000 hospitals, more than 20,000 nursing homes and other institutions and agencies, 325,000 active physicians, 100,000 active dentists, more than 750,000 professionally active nurses, (an unspecified number of) allied health personnel with more

---

* In 1973, there were 130 Peace Corps volunteer nurses in 37 countries. (American Nurses' Association: *Facts About Nursing 74–75.* The Association, Kansas City, Mo., 1976, p. 36.)

* Storlie, Frances: *Nursing and the Social Conscience.* Appleton-Century-Crofts, New York, 1970, p. ix.

† National Academy of Sciences, Institute of Medicine: *Controls on Health Care.* Papers of the Conference on Regulation in the Health Industry, Jan. 7–9, 1974. The Academy, Washington, D.C., 1975, pp. 25, 5, 6.

than 400 titles, and about 40,000 drugstores.*

In Chapter 3, there is some discussion of regulating hospitals, nursing homes, and home health agencies; in the following discussion, an effort is made to suggest some of the more significant ways in which nursing is evaluated quantitatively and qualitatively, particularly in the United States.

Countries with universal health insurance and national or provincial health programs have established quantitative and qualitative standards, and some have gone through the planning on which the United States is embarking under the recent Health Planning Act (see Chapter 2, page 157). Committees established in each state under this Act are assessing health needs and resources. Nurses as members of these committees must know what data is available, what standards have been established, and what studies are in progress.

During the twentieth century, federal governments have assumed increasing responsibility for establishing quantitative and qualitative standards of health care since they increasingly finance it (see Fig. 1-14). No attempt can be made here to compare methods or standards worldwide. Obviously, the totalitarian states such as the USSR and the People's Republic of China are examples of countries in which there is thoroughgoing standard-setting for health service and the preparation of health workers. Great Britain and the Commonwealth countries have established national health services since World War II with resulting standards and systems of evaluation. Canada has a national health service that is administered province by province, and the provincial plans differ.

The [US] National Health Planning and Resource Development Act of 1974 (Public Law 93–641, enacted January 4, 1975) which has created planning state by state may result in state programs in the United States that will, in many respects, resemble the Canadian provincial plans. In any event, study of the British and Canadian health services should be especially useful to nurses in this country. The ANA in a 1974 resolution supported the concept of a health program that guarantees coverage of all people for the full range of comprehensive health service.† This more or less commits the profession to a continuous assessment of needs and resources within the United

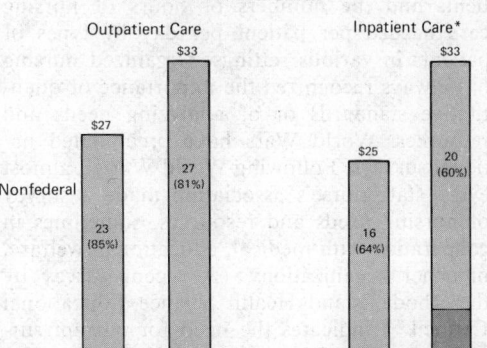

*Includes long-term care outlays.

Figure 1-14. Federal government share of national health care costs for outpatient and inpatient care, 1969 and 1974, in billions of 1969 dollars. (From Center for Health Policy Studies, National Planning Association: *Chartbook of Federal Spending 1969–74.* The Association, Washington, D.C.,1974, p. 33.)

States. Under the next topic in this chapter, "Utilization of Nurses," certain aspects of nursing evaluation are discussed that are not included here under qualitative and quantitative standards.

If, in the United States, federal funds for health care are allocated state by state, the amount will depend in part on data accumulated by surveys and other research techniques. The allocation of public funds for education of health workers also depends upon data from studies of needs and resources. For these and other reasons, organized nursing is presently concentrating on establishing quantitative and qualitative standards.

Evaluation of nursing goes back to Florence Nightingale when she showed statistically the effect of nursing care on the recovery rate of soldiers in the military hospitals of the Crimea. Carlson, discussing the "impact of medicine," says: "the determinations of the quality of care are made [by researchers] without reference to the actual outcomes of care to the patient"; but he gives Florence Nightingale as one of two exceptions to this generalization.*

Simmons [219] noted the early and persistent attempts in this century to develop quantitative

---

* *Ibid.*

† At the Annual Meeting of the ANA's American Academy of Nursing, Jan. 20–21, 1975, papers were presented which were published under the title *Models for Health Care Delivery; Now and For the Future,* representing concepts of three members of the Academy. (The Association, Kansas City, Mo., 1975.)

* Carlson, Rick J.: *The End of Medicine.* John Wiley & Sons, New York, 1975, p. 6.

standards—the proper ratio of nurses to pa-tients and the numbers of hours of nursing care needed per patient per day by types of patients in various settings. Organized nursing has always recognized the importance of quan-titative standards or of analyzing needs and resources. World Wars have precipitated na-tional surveys. Following World War II, almost every state nurse's association made a survey of nursing needs and resources, sometimes in cooperation with medical, educational, welfare, or other organizations. (A recent survey by the Rhode Island Health Science Educational Council [220] indicates the need for current sur-veys.) Personnel from the National League for Nursing or the Division of Nursing Resources, USPHS,* might be lent to conduct or par-ticipate in these state surveys. Since 1949, the ANA has conducted periodic surveys of reg-istered nurses and reported its findings in *Facts About Nursing*. The numbers of nurses by county and urban area have been reported since 1972.† Inventories of registered nurses were conducted in 1949, 1951, 1956–58, 1966, and 1972, the Division of Nursing, USPHS, partially funding the inventories.[221,222] Repre-

* Division of Nursing Resources, USPHS, was or-ganized in 1949 and renamed the Division of Nursing in 1960.
† The National Health Council's 1973 annotated bibliography, *Distribution of Health Manpower* (The Council, New York) lists the survey reports available, state by state, up until April 1973.

sentatives of this federal agency, with ANA and NLN representatives, formed in 1953 the Interagency Conference on Nursing Statistics (ICONS). Since 1954, it has prepared biennial estimates of registered nurses. (Earlier esti-mates were available from other sources on nurses in hospitals and in public health.) The US Health Resources Administration publishes a *Decennial Census Data for Selected Health Occupations* and in 1976 published *Health Manpower Issues*.[223,224]

Beginning with the first World War, the fed-eral government has increased the number of nurses by helping to finance nursing education. The Army School of Nursing [225,226] recruited hundreds of students and by its high standards affected nursing education wherever it set up civil affiliations. However, the effect of this school was minimal compared to that of the Cadet Nurse Corps established in World War II. Under the Bolton Act of 1943, $184 million was spent by the USPHS within 6 years on nursing education, with 85 per cent of the nursing schools in the country participating.[227] Since then, the government has been ever more deeply involved in financing the preparation of health workers—physicians, nurses, physician's assistants, medical technicians, and others. (Note Figure 1-15 showing that 0.7 billion dol-lars was spent by the federal government for health manpower "training" in 1969, 1.1 bil-lion in 1974.)

In 1976, under a contract from the Division

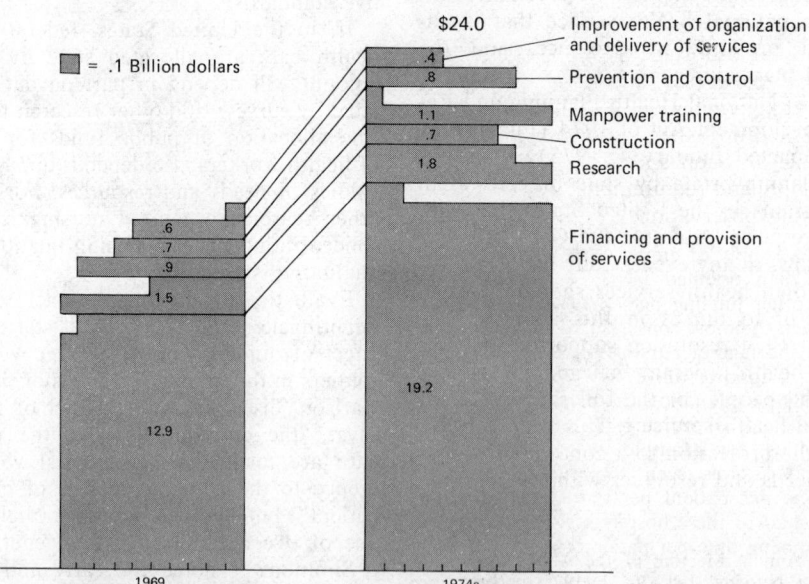

Figure 1-15. Total federal health outlays by activity, 1969 and 1974, showing increase in every category except construction. (From Center for Health Policy Studies, National Planning Association: *Chartbook of Federal Spending 1969–74.* The Association, Washington, D.C., 1974, p. 4.)

of Nursing, Health Resources Administration, Department of Health, Education, and Welfare, the Western Interstate Commission for Higher Education (WICHE) is conducting a national study, Analysis and Planning for Improved Distribution of Nursing Personnel and Services.[228] Its purpose is to develop analytical models that can be used in planning for numbers and distribution of nursing personnel and services and to prepare nurses to do such planning. WICHE published a newsletter in August, 1976, on "Analysis and Planning for Improved Distribution of Nursing Personnel and Services," or "Project Update," which describes the nature of the study. Emphasis on minority issues in nursing education is included in the project. The Southern Regional Education Board has studied the development of potential manpower in nursing which is reported as follows: Vol. 1, *Selected Workshop Presentations;* Vol. 2, *An Annotated Bibliography for Special Programs in Nursing;* Vol. 3, *Final Report.* (*Developing Potential Manpower in Nursing,* the Board, Atlanta, 1975.)

Quantitative standards, such as numbers of nurses and numbers of hours of nursing care needed, are not absolutes that can be set once and for all, so the obejctive today is to develop a method to be used by planning boards. Standards depend upon the other workers available, the population served, the health facilities, the economic status of the country (the money available to pay health workers), and other conditions.

The National League for Nursing in 1957 published *Nurses for a Growing Nation,*[228a] which reported a shortage of nurses and recommended the goal for 1970 as a ratio of 1 nurse for every 286 population. This was based on the highest ratios then existing in favored states. Jessie M. Scott and Eugene Levine, discussing supply and requirements in 1976, made the following observation:

While the supply of employed registered nurses has more than doubled in the past twenty-five years and other nursing personnel have increased fivefold, even the most conservative estimates indicate that a shortage of nurses still exists. Demands for nursing manpower have paralleled the growth in supply. One explanation for this is the intensification in the use of nursing personnel. In short-term hospitals, for example, where the optimal staffing pattern was seen to be 3.5 hours of nursing time per patient per day in 1950, today more than half of these hospitals average nearly 6 hours of nursing time per patient.*

Lippard makes the following distinction between "demand" and need for physicians in the 1950s:

It was realized that estimates of physician requirements based on demand alone, without consideration of need, were not reliable. Demand was interpreted as the amount of medical service people ask for spontaneously and can afford to pay for; need was defined as the amount of medical service, preventive and curative, necessary to provide optimal care for all the people. While few reliable studies of need had been made, isolated experiences indicated that when service was made available demand increased and more nearly approached need.*

Lippard's statement holds true for any health worker. Ultimately, society must decide how much it wants to pay for health care, how much help it can afford from professionals, how much help is useful, and the point at which help discourages self-reliance. Society must decide whether health care shall be available to all citizens. Parenthetically, in the nineteenth century when the state governments decided to make education universally available —compulsory for children and youth—they assumed responsibility for the preparation of teachers, mainly through tax-supported normal schools and state teachers colleges. By 1944, Karl Bigelow [229] reported that, of 1,093,000 teachers in the United States, 85 per cent were college graduates. Obviously the United States has not made the same commitment to health care. Of the 778,470 registered nurses in the United States in 1972, 80.5 per cent were *not* college graduates.[230] (See Fig. 1-11.)

Stuart H. Altman, in his 1971 report to the US Department of Health, Education, and Welfare, *Present and Future Supply of Registered Nurses,* the result of a 4-year study, said that the professional nurse has "been the backbone of the health industry" particularly in hospitals, and that "The number of practicing registered nurses will grow from the 1970 level of 700,000 to . . . between 864,-000 and 924,000 by 1980." He thought then that the supply would continue to grow faster than the population in the United States so that there would be "between 379 and 406 RNs available for every 100,000 residents in 1980 . . . as compared with 341 in 1970." † D. C. Jones and associates, summarized a later study and gave the following figures: "The 1980 projected supply of registered nurses under four different sets of assumptions ranged from

---

* Scott, Jessie M., and Levine, Eugene: "Nursing Manpower Analysis: Its Past, Present and Future," in Hiestand, Dale L., and Ostow, M. (eds.): *Health Manpower Information for Policy Guidance.* Ballinger Publishing Co., Cambridge, Mass., 1976, p. 35.

* Lippard, Vernon W.: *A Half-Century of American Medical Education, 1920–1970.* Josiah Macy, Jr. Foundation, New York, 1974, p. 17.
† Altman, Stuart H.: *Present and Future Supply of Registered Nurses.* US Government Printing Office, Washington, D.C., 1971, p. 5.

941,000 to 1,034,000. The 1985 projections ranged from 964,000 to 1,168,000 for the same four sets of assumptions." * The Interagency Conference on Nursing Statistics (ICONS) reported in April 1975 that there was in 1974 an increase in practicing nurses. When corrected for the number of part-time workers in the total 857,000 active nurses, it gave a ratio of 347 full-time nurses per 100,000 population in 1974 as compared with 333 per 100,000 in 1973 (or one nurse for every 287 population in 1974 as opposed to one nurse to

300 population in 1973).[231] Just what the ratio should be no one really knows. Presently, nurses are poorly distributed. For example, in 1972, there was one public health nurse to 1476 residents of the District of Columbia and one public health nurse to 2383 residents in Alaska.*[232] See Figures 1-16, and 1-17 for graphic presentations of nursing and related health manpower from 1900 to 1967 and distribution of registered nurses in 1972.

The National Commission for the Study of

---

* Jones, D. C., et al.: *Trends in Registered Nurse Supply. Health Manpower References.* US Government Printing Office, Washington, D.C., 1976, p. 3 (DHEW Pub. No. [HRA] 76–15).

* The 1970 Emergency Health Personnel Act (PL 91–623) was designed to relieve the maldistribution of health service by sending doctors, dentists, nurses, and supporting personnel to critical areas. Such personnel are designated the National Health Service Corps.

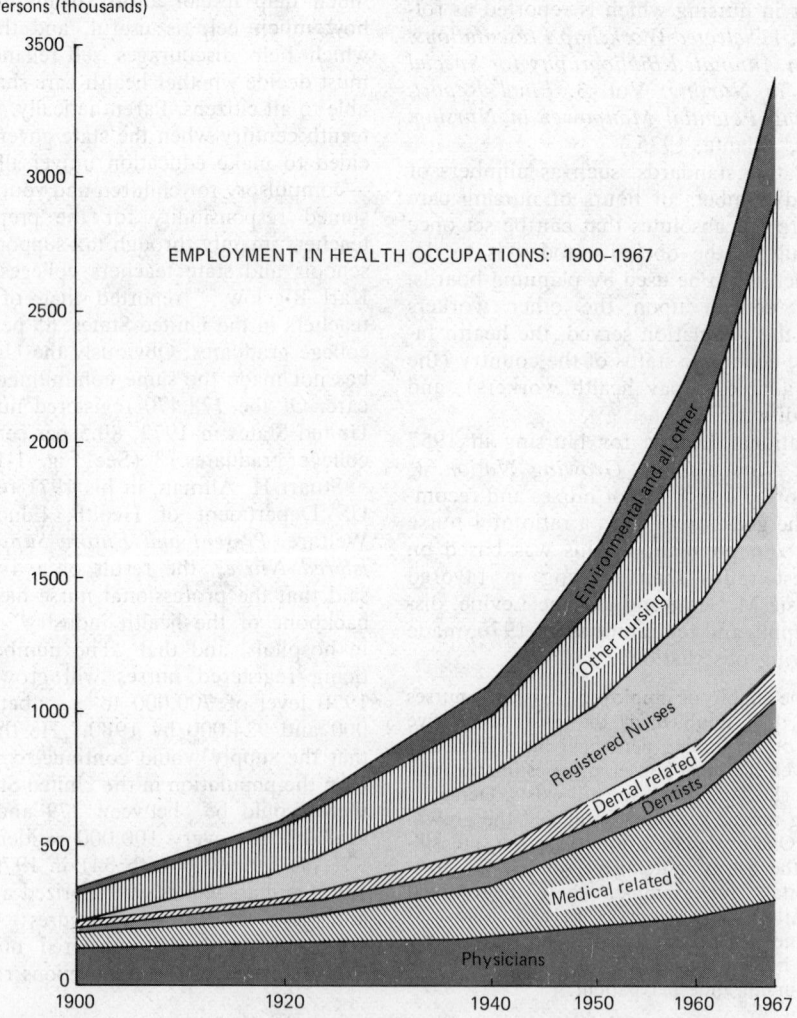

Figure 1-16. Graph showing rapid increase in number of registered nurses and other nursing personnel as compared with physicians and dentists, 1900–1967. (From US Public Health Service: *Health Manpower Source Book, Sec. 21. Allied Health Manpower, 1950–80,* p. 21.)

Nursing and Nursing Education questions the "shortage of nurses"; it does *not* question the misuse of nurses, the need for more qualified nurses, and the need for conditions that discourage dropouts from the profession and the turnover in employment.[233]

In Chapter 3, where nursing in various settings is discussed, data is given to show that there is crying need for more nurses in nursing homes, in correctional institutions, in homes for the mentally retarded and for the mentally ill, and in certain underserved geographical areas.

As countries accept the rights of human beings to health care as well as to education, more public funds are made available for the preparation of health workers, and to hold workers in health occupations, their economic security is increased, as are the intangible occupational rewards. Altman noted that state and local governments are assuming more and more responsibility for "training professional nurses" and he noted "rapidly rising salaries." However, he thought that it was "the nonpecuniary attributes, such as prestige and service to humanity, that appear to be greater for nursing than for other occupations frequently selected by high school graduates." He said "Thus nursing has retained its popularity . . . [with girls]." *

It is obvious from the preceding discussion that quantitative standards cannot be "scientific" absolutes. Even those most poorly served areas of the United States have more nurses, and more thoroughly prepared nurses, than most nations of the world. In the International Labour Office's report (see page 19), the statement is made that in "almost all countries . . .

* Altman, Stuart H.: *op. cit.*, pp. 5, 3.

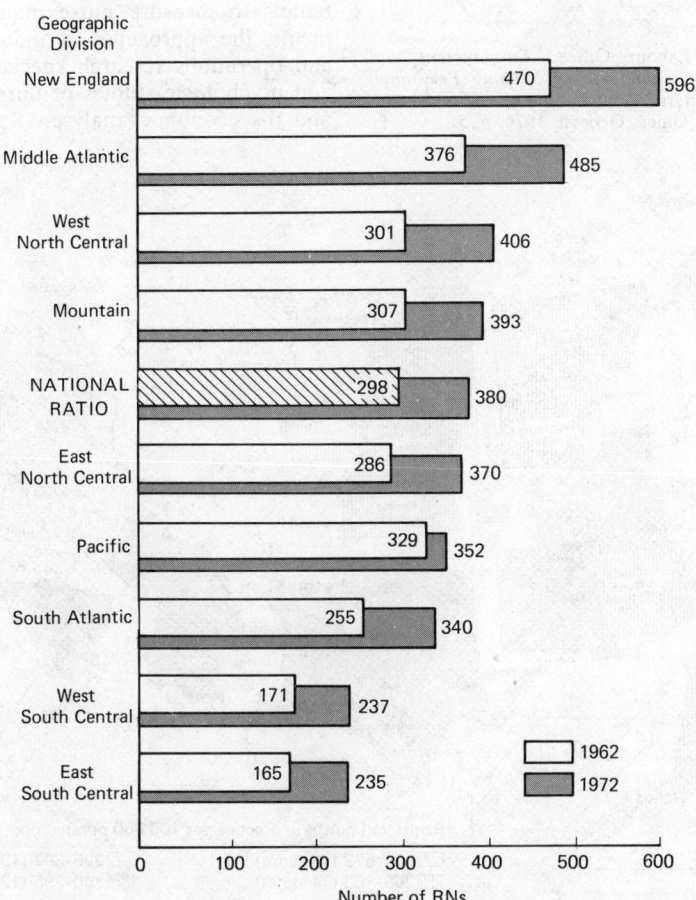

Figure 1-17. Distribution of registered nurses per 100,000 population in geographic regions of United States, 1962 and 1972. (From Hudson, Helen H., and McCarthy, Margaret D.: *Source Book—Nursing Personnel*. US Government Printing Office, Washington, D.C., 1974, p. 8.)

nursing personnel have been inadequate . . . to satisfy even the modest aims set for the First and Second Development Decades of one nurse for every 5,000 inhabitants and one health auxiliary for every 1,000." * Obviously, the emphasis in the United States should be on qualitative standards and on the best use of available nursing personnel. Those who take an international view may say that the United States should encourage health personnel to work in underserviced areas of the world.

Special efforts are made in some countries to hold needed health workers; to prevent migration to areas where conditions of work are better or more inviting. Those parts of the world that offer the most desirable conditions for practice tend to have the best opportunities for study, but programs in developed countries may not prepare students for work in undeveloped countries. Foreign students may therefore tend to stay in the country where they have studied. Some graduates of the better

* International Labour Office: *Employment and Conditions of Work and Life of Nursing Personnel.* Report VII (1), International Labour Conference, 61st Session, 1976. The Office, Geneva, 1976, p. 5.

schools abroad may be attracted to countries where they think they can practice as they are taught. For instance, Hossain A. Ronaghy and associates [234] report that 32.1 per cent of the graduates of the Nemazee School of Nursing in Iran have emigrated to the United States. Iran has one physician for every 3652 inhabitants, and health care under these circumstances cannot compare with that in the United States. The US Department of Health, Education, and Welfare has published an annotated bibliography, *International Migration of Physicians and Nurses* (US Government Printing Office, Washington, D.C., 1975 [DHEW Pub. No. (HRA) 75–281]).

In the volume *Health Manpower Information for Policy Guidance,* edited by Dale L. Hiestand and M. Ostow, Jessie M. Scott and Eugene Levine have a chapter "Nursing Manpower Analysis: Its Past, Present, and Future." They review the early studies, the state surveys, the national data collection systems, the attempts to measure nurse manpower requirements, the approaches of industrial engineers and operations research specialists, the social and psychologic studies of nursing manpower, and the economic analyses. Scott and Levine

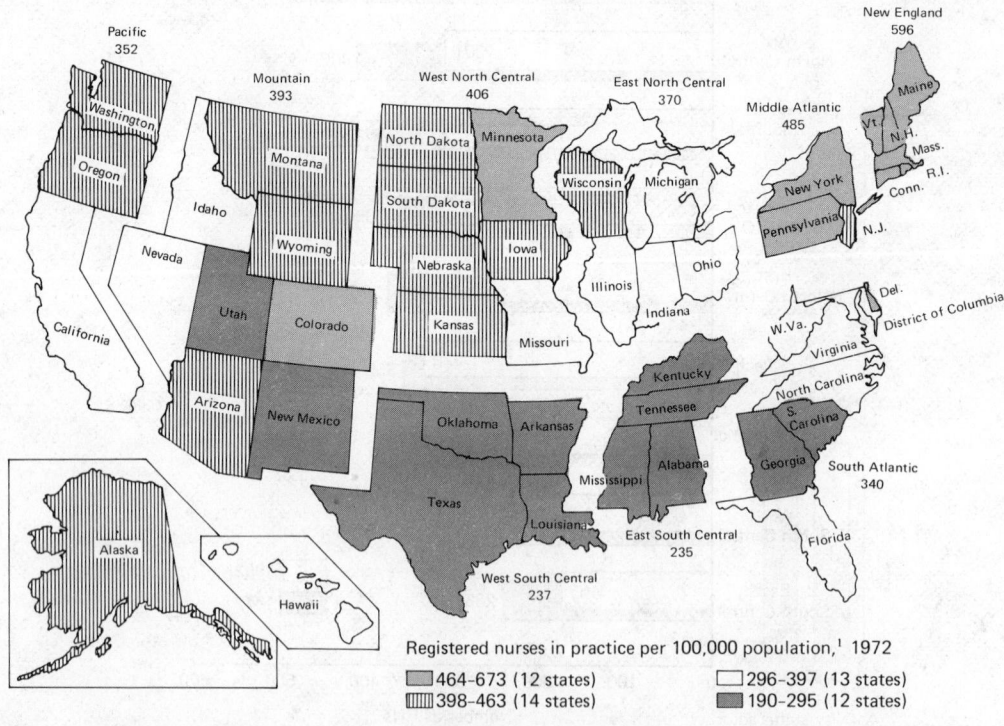

Registered nurses in practice per 100,000 population,[1] 1972

☐ 464–673 (12 states)   ☐ 296–397 (13 states)
▨ 398–463 (14 states)   ■ 190–295 (12 states)

[1] Excludes armed forces overseas.

Figure 1-18. Ratio of employed nurses to population, 1972. (From American Nurses' Association: *Facts About Nursing 72–73.* The Association, Kansas City, Mo., 1974, p. 11.)

also summarize "What we know about nursing manpower"—about supply, requirements, education, and utilization of nursing personnel. They also summarize the fallacies in the use of manpower information—the failure to distinguish nursing roles, the tendency to see nursing as only a series of tasks, the failure to account for the organized nature of nursing (to account for the time spent in administrative tasks), and the tendency to base estimates on the status quo. The conclusion is reached that inadequate terminology and concepts have been used and that even a "cursory review of the many studies . . . will frequently reveal a negative bias, conscious or unconscious, toward nursing." The authors express the opinion that "Determination of the total health care needs of the population, those receiving care and those not, would indeed result in a reexamination of the relationship between nurse supply and demand." *

Those who want to pursue the subject of quantitative and to some extent qualitative measurements will find the review of Scott and Levine invaluable, as is the Division of Nursing's *Source Book—Nursing Personnel* (US

* Scott, Jessie M., and Levine, Eugene: *op. cit.,* pp. 34, 42.

Government Printing Office, Washington, D.C., 1974 [DHEW Pub. No. (HRA) 75–43]).

Qualitative assessment of nursing is, if anything, more subtle and difficult than quantitative assessment. An account of an ANA-sponsored conference in December, 1975, is reported under the heading "Measures of Quality Nursing Care? Experts Agree Valid Approach Not Yet Found." [234a] Another report of the conference in ANA's newspaper is headed "Assessment Difficult. Individual Concepts Affect Quality Measures." [235] Avedis Donabedian (whose nationally recognized work on appraisal techniques in the structure, process, and outcome in health work is discussed in Chapter 19) makes the point that all three of the above—structure, process, and outcome—must be studied (see Fig. 1-20). He thinks a knowledge of their relationships the only basis for corrective or preventive action to safeguard quality. At the above conference, Kathleen Sward reviewed an 80-year record of ANA's "involvement in quality assurance." The Technical Advisory Group to ANA's Professional Services Review Organization are considering, among others, the following questions: What level of health care is society willing to accept and pay for? What role will society legitimatize for the nurse? How can nursing gain some con-

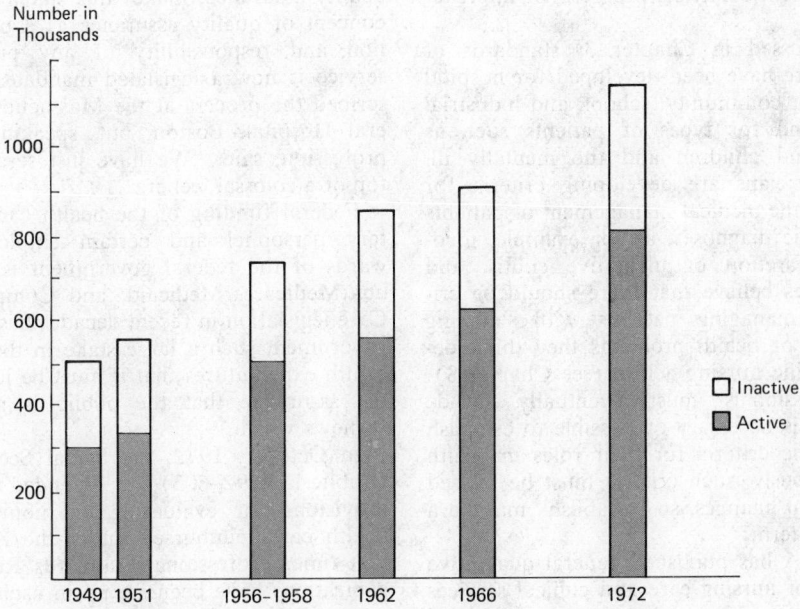

Activity status adjusted for nonresponse.

Figure 1-19. Active and inactive registered nurses, 1949–1972, showing trend toward higher proportion of active nurses. (From American Nurses' Association: *The Nation's Nurses: 1972 Inventory of Registered Nurses.* Prepared by Aleda V. Roth and Alice R. Walden. The Association, Kansas City, Mo., 1974, p. 125.)

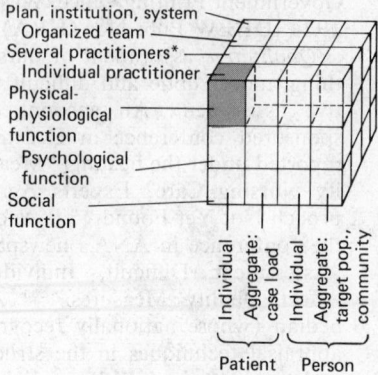

Plan, institution, system
Organized team
Several practitioners*
Individual practitioner
Physical-physiological function
Psychological function
Social function

Individual
Aggregate: case load
Individual
Aggregate: target pop., community

Patient   Person

Cubical figure *used by Avedis Donabedian as framework for discussing assessment of quality. On one side of the cube are three aspects in concept of health: physical-physiological function, psychological, and social. Another side shows aggregates of subjects of care, ranging from individual to community. Distinction is made between patient, who has access to some care, and person, who does not. The third side shows providers, from individual practitioner to plan or system. Simplest to consider is shaded area of one patient, one practitioner, and physiological function.*

*Of the same profession or different professions.

Figure 1-20. Level and scope of concern as factors in the definition of quality. (From "Measures of Quality of Nursing Care? Experts Agree Valid Approach Not Yet Found," *Am. J. Nurs.,* **76:**186, [Feb.] 1976.)

trol over patients' entry and exit points into nursing services, which few nurses now have? Which criteria really measure nursing impact?

In reviewing qualitative studies, Henderson [236] noted in 1964 that quality has been measured by assessing opinions of clients, or patients and those of nurses and other medical personnel; by analyzing patient-nurse interaction, its nature and extent; and by analyzing patient behavior, progress, or improvement.

As discussed in Chapter 3, standards of nursing care have been developed for hospital nursing, for community, school, and industrial nursing, and for types of patients such as mothers and children and the mentally ill. Some physicians are developing criteria for evaluating the medical management of patients with specific diagnoses, as for example, myocardial infarction or ulcerative colitis, and some nurses believe that there should be criteria for managing patients with "nursing diagnoses" or health problems they think demand specific nursing action (see Chapter 8). All professionals must eventually decide whether it is necessary or possible to establish such specific criteria for their roles in health care. Obviously, such criteria must be revised as treatment changes, so "establish" may be a misleading term.

The ANA has published general qualitative standards of nursing care and clinical services (as, for example, nursing in maternal and child care or nursing in psychiatric or orthopedic services), some of which are discussed in Chapter 3.[237-239] The Association has also published its plan for implementing its standards of nursing practice.[240] It is not within the scope of this chapter to discuss all these plans, but interested readers can study the publications listed among the references for this chapter.

The National League for Nursing has been equally concerned with quality assessment and quality assurance, and its publications are also listed among the references for this chapter.[241,242] Mary E. MacDonald, in one of the papers presented at a 1975 NLN forum on quality assurance, makes this statement: "The concept of quality assurance as a basic function and responsibility of any professional service is now a legislated mandate." She described the process at the Massachusetts General Hospital, Boston, but, speaking for the profession, said, "We have just scratched the top of a colossal iceberg. . . ." *

Federal funding of the health care of military personnel and certain employees and wards of the federal government is not new, but Medicare, Medicaid, and Comprehensive Care legislation in recent decades has given the government such a large stake in the national health expenditures that it must be justified by the assurance that the public is getting its money's worth.

In October, 1972, the Social Security Act (Public Law 92–603) was amended to include provisions for evaluating or monitoring all health care reimbursed under the Act. Since that time, Professional Standards Review Organizations have been set up in each state for

* National League for Nursing, Department of Baccalaureate and Higher Degree Programs: *Quality Assurance—A Joint Venture.* Papers presented at an Open Forum, NLN Convention, New Orleans, 1975. The League, New York, 1975, pp. 2, 6 (Pub. No. 15–1595).

this purpose. Each official professional organization of health workers establishes standards for the care given by representatives of that profession and for supplying PSROs with standards by which the services of doctors, dentists, osteopaths, nurses, social workers, speech therapists, and others can be measured. While PSROs have been composed of physicians in most states who base their evaluation chiefly on study of medical records, some of them include other health professionals, and ultimately they will be true interdisciplinary bodies. (See also Chapters 3 and 19 for discussions of PSROs.)

Richard C. Jelinek and associates of the US Department of Health, Education, and Welfare, have published *A Methodology for Monitoring Quality of Nursing Care,*[243] and the Department sponsored a recent conference on Assessment of Nursing Services.[244] There are numerous full-length publications on this much discussed subject.[245-247] The creation of a unified national health service in the United States might eliminate much of the present duplication of effort and piecemeal evaluation that goes on in the United States.

While nurses in organizations and in administrative positions help make decisions that affect qualitative and quantitative standards, nurses everywhere should have the habit of evaluating their work. There are few nurses working in hospitals who have not heard of or participated in "nursing audits." [248] Karolyn Klammer Hanna, discussing a process used at the Mercy San Juan Hospital, Carmichael, California (see Fig. 1–21), said: "Any method which systematically examines the quality of nursing care could be termed a nursing audit." * The method Hanna described is based on a model developed by the California Medical Association and the California Hospital Association and endorsed by the California Nurses Association. This method is designed to assess the total care of the patient rather than the nursing or the medical care separately. The evaluation is based on review of a sample of discharged patients' charts. Criteria are developed for patients with a specific condition by the institutional staff. See Figures 1-21*A* and *B* showing a sample audit for a patient with angina pectoris and an analysis of the audit.

While this type of "audit" is the most common evaluative procedure currently used by nurses in institutions, it is only one type of evaluation. If it is true, as many believe, that

less and less care will be given in institutions, audits must be devised that are suited to all settings in which nurses function.[249,250] Above all, methods of evaluation must be developed that are practical or productive. Methods that are so time-consuming that they appreciably reduce the hours of nursing care available to clients or patients are self-defeating.

Assessing the effectiveness of nursing is part of the process of nursing, and the search for better measurements will continue indefinitely, if for no other reason than that new knowledge changes health care and the functions of workers. It is hard to conceive of static criteria or static functions for caregivers.

Utilization of Nurses—Staffing Patterns. The unequal distribution of health workers throughout the world has been stressed repeatedly in this chapter. Even within an economically favored country, such as the United States, it has been shown that the ratio of nurses to the population differs from state to state. For instance, in the District of Columbia it is more than three times that in the State of Alaska, and the ratio of nurses to patients in hospitals is equally uneven.

Generally speaking, nurses, like doctors, tend to prefer urban to rural practice and to go where there are other health workers and the facilities they grew accustomed to as students. For these reasons, to control the cost of health care and to promote the satisfaction of all concerned, it is important to make the best possible use of the nursing personnel available.

In discussing the "extended role of the nurse," the point was made that the nurse's function changes in accordance with the ratio of physicians and other health personnel available to the population served. Tabulated data from the World Health Organization in 1975 gave figures on numbers of physicians, dentists, and pharmacists in most countries. Data on other categories of health personnel—midwives, medical assistants, nurses, and nursing auxiliaries is less complete. Comparisons are difficult, but the uneven distribution of doctors as well as nurses is obvious. Canada is reported to have had, in 1972, a total of 34,509 physicians and 114,349 nurses, while India with 121,990 physicians in 1972 had (in 1973) only 82,300 nurses; Egypt in 1973 had 23,501 physicians and only 7528 nurses; Kenya in 1973 had 766 physicians and 1578 nurses; the Congo had 154 physicians and 246 nurses.[251] These figures have more meaning if they are accompanied by data on medical and nursing assistants and other health workers, but they illustrate the question under discussion—poor distribution of nurses, and an unequal ratio of

---

* Hanna, Karolyn Klammer: "Nursing Audit at a Community Hospital," *Nurs. Outlook,* **24**:33, (Jan.) 1976.

SAMPLE NURSING AUDIT

Patient # _____ Age _____ Sex _____ Admitted _____ Discharged _____ L.O.S. _____

ON PATIENT'S CHART, THERE SHALL BE EVIDENCE OF:

Criteria	Yes	No	Expected Compliance Level	Actual Compliance Level
1. Admission note which includes patient's history of chest pain.	23	___	85%	92%
2. Physical assessment of the patient at least *q4h during the first 24 h* including *3 of the following:* a. Quality of vital signs _____ b. Apical *and* radial pulse _____ c. Temperature of skin _____ d. Color of skin _____	0	___	90%	0%
3. At least *once per shift* there shall be a statement regarding presence *or* absence of pain. (If pain is present, the statement shall include a description of the pain, its onset and duration, location, and effect of medications and/or O_2.)	1	___	95%	4%
4. At least *once per shift* there shall be a statement giving the nurse's assessment of the patient's emotional state (such as reaction to pain and/or illness, reaction to visits of family members, reaction to hospital routine, etc.)	1	___	80%	4%
5. Prior to discharge, the patient and family or significant others shall verbalize an understanding of: a. Factors that prevent anginal attacks (such as regulation of activities; cessation of smoking; loss of weight, if applicable; avoidance of stressful situations)	0	___	90%	0%
b. What to do to curb an anginal attack once it has begun (includes how and when to take nitroglycerin, resting, etc.)	0	___	90%	0%

Based on 25 cases
Discharges July 1973 through June 1974

A

nurses to physicians. Uneven distribution is intensified by the fact that countries such as the United States that have relatively high ratios of both physicians and nurses to the population attract health workers from less well supplied countries who come to study but often remain to practice. Lippard, discussing what was thought to be underproduction of doctors in American schools between 1920 and 1970, said this was "balanced to some extent by the emigration to European universities of American students . . . and by the immigration of foreign physicians." * The United States, with a relatively high ratio of nurses to the population, issued 6824 licenses to registered nurses from 81 foreign countries in 1971

* Lippard, Vernon W.: *op. cit.*, p. 116.

and 1972 (3116 of these to nurses of the Philippines, 1020 to those of Canada, and 798 to those of England).[252] It seems obvious that countries with high nurse-population ratios will use "nursepower" differently from those with low ratios and that their use will be affected by high and low ratios of other categories of health personnel. A survey of nursing in India was made in 1974 in an effort partly to explain unemployment of nurses in India and their migration to other countries. James S. Tong, Director of the Study and Executive Secretary for the Coordinating Agency for Health Planning, reporting the unemployment, made the following observation: "Simultaneously voluntary hospital societies in India, realizing the great shortage of nurses, were appealing to funding agencies for grants to build new nurs-

ANALYSIS OF SAMPLE NURSING AUDIT

Problem: Poor performance on all criteria except #1.

Solutions

Analysis

1. Even though criterion #1 had a high level of compliance, it was not a good measure because it is broad and vague.

2. a. Criterion #2 is too confining by specifying q4h.
   b. Often two of the items were mentioned but not all three. Color and temperature of skin not charted unless they were unusual.
   c. Some staff may not know how to take an apical pulse and/or may not realize the importance of doing so.

3. a. Staff may not realize importance of documenting descriptions of pain 1 q shift.
   b. Format of criteria on #3 may be difficult to follow.

4. Once per shift may be an unrealistic expectation especially if the patient sleeps most of the shift.

5. a. Some nurses may not be doing adequate patient and/or family teaching re angina pectoris.
   b. Nurses may be hesitant to initiate patient teaching without a specific physician order, and forget or are reluctant to ask the doctor to write an order.
   c. Nurses may be doing patient teaching but are not documenting the patient's response.

1. Change criterion #1 to read "Admission note with history of symptoms including all of these:
   a. Onset of pain
   b. How long pain lasts
   c. Effect of medication
   d. How patient relieves symptoms."

2. a&b. Change criterion #2 to read, "Physical assessment of patient *twice each shift during the first* 24 h, including *two of these:*
   a. Quality of vital signs
   b. Apical *and* radial pulse
   c. Temperature *and* color of skin."
   c. Conduct team conferences on all units on angina pectoris and review the procedure and rationale for taking an apical pulse.

3. a. Review all aspects of care of patients with angina pectoris in team conferences.
   b. Revise criterion #3 to read, "At least *once per shift* there shall be a statement of presence or absence of pain. If pain present, include:
   (1) Description of pain
   (2) Onset & duration
   (3) Location of pain
   (4) Effects of medication and/or O_2."

4. Change item #4 to read, "*once every 24 hours.*"

5. a. Organize a teaching program for angina patients at the hospital. Use pamphlets available from American Heart Association.
   b. Encourage nurses to develop better dialogue with physicians regarding early initiation of teaching for patients with angina.
   c. Encourage nursing staff to observe and document the patient's response to teaching.

B

Figure 1-21. *A*. Sample nursing audit for patient with angina pectoris. *B*. Analysis of sample audit. (From Hanna, Karolyn Klammer: "Nursing Audit at a Community Hospital," *Nurs. Outlook,* **24**:33, [Jan.] 1976.)

ing schools. The unemployment was rather obviously due to lack of budget to pay them [rather] than to any surplus of nurses." *

The proliferation of nursing personnel within the United States, creating a bewildering hierarchy, has made utilization studies especially pertinent but also difficult. Repeated attempts have been made to classify nursing activities or functions into "professional" and "technical" categories. It is hard to discuss the studies of utilization or staffing, because nursing personnel is so heterogeneous.

Eugene Levine and Henry D. Kahn, in a chapter of the volume, *Operations Research in*

Health Care by Larry J. Shuman and R. D. Speas, Jr. (Johns Hopkins University Press, Baltimore, 1975), review related nursing studies. They give the history of such research, reaching back to the time and motion studies of Frank Gilbraith in the early 1900s. They review many efforts to establish staffing standards and they categorize the operations research applications to health manpower. The categories include studies that (1) redistribute tasks among nursing personnel according to perceived levels of skill; (2) simplify work; (3) substitute capital for labor (using computers and other forms of automation); (4) improve work schedules; (5) reduce time spent in movement by improving architectural designs; (6) improve organization of patient care services; (7) improve knowledge and skills of

* Coordinating Agency for Health Planning with the Trained Nurses Association of India: *Nursing Survey in India.* The Agency, New Delhi, 1974 (I).

health manpower; (8) improve supervision; and (9) improve the administrative climate. Much of the research was conducted by industrial or management engineers, systems analysts, psychologists, economists, and other social scientists, at the Universities of Pittsburgh, Iowa, Michigan, Ohio State, and Johns Hopkins. Levine and Kahn make the following summary statement:

If we date the origins of modern applications of operations research to health manpower problems to the latter part of the 1950s, it is fair to say that the amount of progress that has been achieved is not commensurate with the amount of time that has been available for the application of operations research techniques. Health care costs continue to rise, gaps in services are widespread, and deficiencies in quality are reported.

In defense of operations research, however, it must be said that the operations research effort in the health manpower field has been rather small in comparison to the magnitude of the problems needing solutions. Moreover, there have been a number of constraints on the fruitful application of operations research techniques to health manpower problems.*

Levine and Kahn list and comment on the "constraints": their fragmentation (no over-all design into which the studies fit); their limited scope in some cases; inadequate attention to psychosocial aspects of management; the complexity of the health care institution; communication barriers between researchers and health personnel; studies confined to hospitals with few in other care settings and to one aspect of the operation rather than the whole setting; emphases on the existing system rather than anticipating change; lack of controls; and, perhaps of most importance, lack of sensitive measuring devices, especially the measurement of quality of performance.

While the recent and extensive studies of utilization of health manpower have, generally speaking, been directed by social scientists, some nurses have been deeply involved in research of this nature, beginning with Blanche Pfefferkorn's activity and cost analyses in the 1930s and 1940s.[253,254] After the establishment of the Division of Nursing Resources in 1949 in the USPHS, its staff encouraged and often participated in research of this sort. It published a manual How to Study Nursing Activities in a Patient Unit [255] which was revised in 1964. Viola Bredenberg's and Marion Wright's studies of team nursing were reported

in the 1950s.[256,257] Virginia Walker's work, begun in the 1950s, culminating in a volume Nursing and Ritualistic Practice,[258] questioned the value of certain aspects of nursing practice; and Marguerite E. Kakosh's method of studying utilization of nursing personnel was reported in 1959.[259] In 1964, Faye G. Abdellah and Eugene Levine reported an extensive study under the title Patients and Personnel Speak,[260] dealing with patient and personnel satisfaction according to staffing. It and the investigation by Myrtle K. Aydelotte and M. E. Tener,[261] reported in 1960, have been widely cited. In 1973, Aydelotte provided researchers with a review of the literature on nurse staffing methodology.[262] In this list of utilization studies with major nurse direction or participation should be mentioned the reorganization of a nursing unit around patient needs, reported by Janet M. Kraegel and associates in 1972 (see Fig. 1-22).[263] Marie Manthey's study of assigning nurses to patients in hospitals (called by her and her associates "primary nurses") should also be mentioned in this connection.[264] All have influenced hospital staffing.

As practical nurses and home health aides in the United States play an increasingly important role in home care agencies, there will be more studies such as that of D. D. Doster, "Utilization of Available 'Nurse Power' in Public Health." [265] It might be expected that studies will be made to measure the effect on client welfare of various categories of nursing personnel in every setting. No attempt can be made in this chapter to mention more than examples of staffing studies, but the reviews cited should enable interested readers to make fairly complete reviews of work in the United States to 1976.

In an effort to use available nurse power, there have been many attempts to differentiate between nursing services that require a greater or lesser degree of nursing judgment and skill, assigning different grades of services to better and less well prepared persons. One method of doing this is assigning the "professional nurse" to the patients whose care is thought to present the more difficult problems, while assigning the "practical nurse," the "attendant," the "nurse's aide," or some other member of the auxiliary nursing group to those whose care is believed to be less complex.

A second plan for spreading the "professional nurse" power is to have the "professional nurse" supervise the care of all patients, and/or carry out the more complex activities involved. Other categories of nursing personnel work with the "professional nurse" to give each patient total nursing care, each nurse performing her or his relatively more complex or

* Levine, Eugene, and Kahn, Henry D.: "Health Manpower Models," in Shuman, Larry J., and Speas, R. D., Jr.: Operations Research in Health Care. Johns Hopkins University Press, Baltimore, 1975, p. 347.

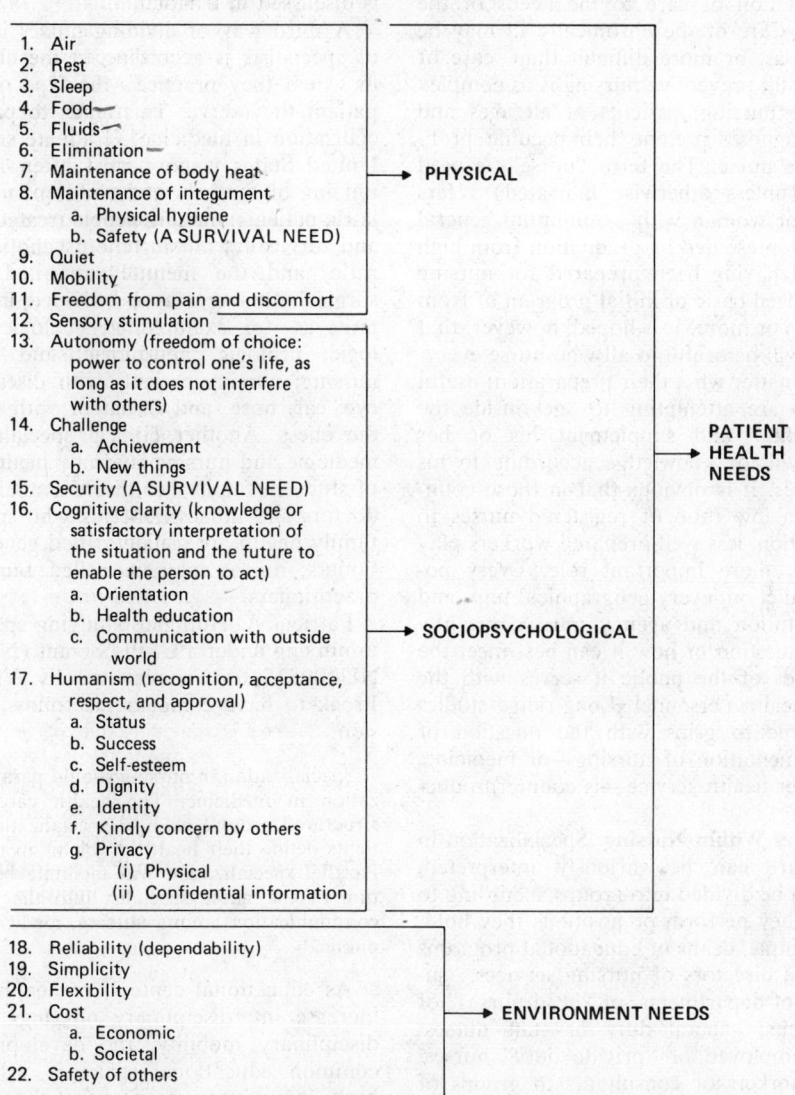

PATIENT NEEDS

1. Air
2. Rest
3. Sleep
4. Food
5. Fluids
6. Elimination
7. Maintenance of body heat
8. Maintenance of integument
   a. Physical hygiene
   b. Safety (A SURVIVAL NEED)

→ PHYSICAL

9. Quiet
10. Mobility
11. Freedom from pain and discomfort
12. Sensory stimulation
13. Autonomy (freedom of choice:
    power to control one's life, as
    long as it does not interfere
    with others)
14. Challenge
    a. Achievement
    b. New things
15. Security (A SURVIVAL NEED)
16. Cognitive clarity (knowledge or
    satisfactory interpretation of
    the situation and the future to
    enable the person to act)
    a. Orientation
    b. Health education
    c. Communication with outside
       world

→ SOCIOPSYCHOLOGICAL

→ PATIENT HEALTH NEEDS

17. Humanism (recognition, acceptance,
    respect, and approval)
    a. Status
    b. Success
    c. Self-esteem
    d. Dignity
    e. Identity
    f. Kindly concern by others
    g. Privacy
       (i) Physical
       (ii) Confidential information

18. Reliability (dependability)
19. Simplicity
20. Flexibility
21. Cost
    a. Economic
    b. Societal
22. Safety of others

→ ENVIRONMENT NEEDS

Figure 1-22. Patient needs as seen by Janet M. Kraegel and her associates in a study of a system of patient care based on their needs. (From Kraegel, Janet M., et al.: *Patient Care Systems.* J. B. Lippincott Co., Philadelphia, 1974.)

less complex role. In other words, each patient has an assigned "team" of nursing personnel and all members contribute to the planning and execution of care. Some persons insist that under any plan the nursing care of *all* patients should be "supervised" by the "professional nurse" when it is given by the nonprofessional worker. A third, and widely accepted, method of conserving nurse power is to assign all nonnursing functions once performed by nursing personnel to ward clerks and other nonnurse workers, as, for example, housekeepers, maids, porters, clerks, and unit managers. Nursing personnel now rarely order, clean and sterilize supplies, or serve diets as they did in the past. Many agencies are trying to eliminate from the functions of graduate nurses everything that is not a service to the person (mind and body) of the patient or client. Administering, teaching, and keeping the records of this service (nursing care) are, however, considered integral parts of the nursing function.

The position is taken in this book that *all* "nursing care" as defined in this chapter is essentially complex because it involves constant adaptation of care to the needs of the individual. Care of the chronically ill may be as difficult as, or more difficult than, care of the acutely ill; preventive nursing is as complex as curative nursing; patients of all ages and with all diagnoses present their peculiar problems to the nurse. The term "nurse" as used hereafter (unless otherwise indicated) refers to a man or woman with a minimum general education represented by graduation from high school and having been prepared for nursing in a recognized basic or initial program of from 2 to 4 years or more. It is hoped, however, that this book will be useful to all who nurse everywhere, no matter what their preparation; useful to all who are attempting to "get inside the patient's skin" and supplement his or her strength, will, or knowledge according to his or her needs. It is obvious that in those countries with a low ratio of registered nurses to the population, less well-prepared workers play a relatively more important role. Every political jurisdiction, every geographical unit, and every institution and agency must constantly study the question of how it can best meet the health needs of the public it serves with the available health personnel. Long-range studies should come to grips with the question of when fragmentation of nursing—or medicine, or any other health service—is counterproductive.

Specialties Within Nursing. Specialization in nursing care can be variously interpreted. Nurses can be divided into groups according to functions they perform or positions they hold, as, for example, deans of educational programs or teachers; directors of nursing services, "supervisors" of departments, or "head nurses" of smaller units; general duty or staff nurses; privately employed or "private duty" nurses; research workers or consultants to groups of institutions or agencies.

In certain eras and in some countries, postbasic courses were, and still are, built around the functions of administering, supervising, teaching, consulting, and researching.*

A second way of interpreting specialization is according to the setting in which nurses function, as, for example, hospital nurses, community nurses, school nurses, industrial nurses,

and prison nurses. This type of specialization is discussed in Chapter 3.

A third way of dividing nurses into groups of specialists is according to the clinical area in which they practice—the type of client or patient they serve. This tends to parallel specialization in medicine. Graduate study in the United States is now most often focused on nursing of mothers and children; nursing geriatric patients; nursing people treated medically and surgically; nursing the psychotic, the neurotic, and the mentally retarded. Medical-surgical nursing may be divided into smaller units as, for example, gynecologic, dermatologic, urologic, neurologic, and orthopedic nursing; nursing patients with diseases of the eye, ear, nose, and throat or with diseases of the chest. Another clinical specialty in both medicine and nursing is family health. Courses of study in family health are available to both doctors and nurses. Doctors who specialize in family health are usually called general practitioners; nurses may be called family health practitioners.

Patricia A. Hummel, studying specialization in nursing under a USPHS grant (No. 1–D10–NU–09535–01) is reported by Valencia N. Prock to have come to the following conclusion:

Specialization in nursing should parallel specialization in medicine. The health care system is structured around medical specialization, and patients define their health problems in those terms. Parallel specialization will facilitate both integration of the nurse specialist into the system and communication among nursing, medicine, and the public.*

As educational centers for health personnel increase interdisciplinary offerings and interdisciplinary mobility, the development of a common educational structure will facilitate both. It is easy to see now that the preparation of obstetricians and nurse-midwives has much in common. It is very likely that the education of pediatricians and pediatric nurse specialists should have a common core and that the same is true for psychiatrists and psychiatric nurses, for internists and medical nurses, for orthopedists and orthopedic nurses, and so on.

Lippard, in a history of medical education from 1920 to 1970, makes the following observation in his Epilogue:

---

* The following statement from the *Nurse Training Act of 1975. Fact Sheets* (Division of Nursing, Bureau of Health Manpower, Health Resources Administration, Bethesda, Md., Sept. 1975) shows the difficulty in defining specialties in nursing: "Traineeship support for the advanced training of registered nurses is extended and is now authorized for the preparation of nurse practitioners, as well as nurse teachers, administrators, supervisors, and nurse specialists."

* Prock, Valencia N.: "Implications of Change for Nursing Practice and Education," in Roberts, Doris E., and Freeman, Ruth B. (scientific eds.): *Redesigning Nursing Education for Public Health. Report of The Conference, May 23–25, 1973.* US Government Printing Office, Washington, D.C., 1973, p. 93 (DHEW Pub. No. [HRA] 75–75).

The roles of various health professionals and the interrelationship of these roles are also changing. One result of this trend may be that the discrete organization of the medical faculty will cease to exist and be absorbed into a much broader faculty concerned with the education of health workers with a spectrum of backgrounds and interests. The traditional departmental organization is threatened as the boundaries between the disciplines become less distinct and interdisciplinary instruction more common.*

Fifty years ago, most people all over the world entered the health care system through the doctor's office or a division of a hospital or clinic where they were examined by a physician. Today, more and more people in the United States are seen first, or given primary care, by nurses or physician's assistants. Health workers giving primary care must be able to conduct a physical examination, to identify the person's needs or health problems, and to make appropriate referrals to other health workers. Nurses in all clinical specialties are now being prepared in the United States and Canada for the expanded role or to give primary care.

Clinical specialization in nursing all over the world now implies assuming what is called an expanded role. As noted earlier, international, national, state, provincial, and local organizations are stating their positions on this subject. Since the expanded role involves assumption by nurses of functions once thought to be medical, the position papers may be statements made jointly by nursing and medical organizations.

The expanded role of nurses whose educational preparation has extended beyond the initial program into some specialty has necessitated changes in Nurse Practice Acts. This in turn has necessitated changes in Medical Practice Acts. In some states, doctors and nurses work together so that a nursing act won't allow a practice prohibited by a medical act, or vice versa. In the United States, where the physician's assistant, numerous medical technicians, and types of nursing personnel complicate the nurse-physician relationship, the definition of roles and the enactment of enabling legislation is difficult. In the following pages an effort is made to describe the various ways in which society provides nursing personnel (especially registered nurses) with credentials that assure the public of their competence and that protect the public and the competent nurse from those who are unprepared to give nursing care.

Licensure and Other Credentials for Nursing Personnel. In a program to ensure the quality of health care, nothing exceeds in importance the steps taken to ensure the competence of health workers. Before discussing these steps, the terms used to describe them should be defined. The following definitions are taken from *A Proposal for Credentialing Health Manpower* (US Department of Health, Education, and Welfare, Public Health Service, Health Resources Administration, Washington, D.C., June 1976, p. 1).*

Credentialing: The formal recognition of professional or technical competence. As used in this report, "credentialing" is a generic term referring to the processes of accreditation, certification, and licensure.
Accreditation: The process by which an agency or organization evaluates and recognizes an institution or program of study as meeting certain predetermined criteria or standards.
Certification: The process by which a nongovernmental agency or association grants recognition to an individual who has met certain predetermined qualifications specified by that agency or association.
Licensure: The process by which an agency of government grants permission to an individual to engage in a given occupation upon finding that the applicant has attained the minimal degree of competency necessary to ensure that the public health, safety, and welfare will be reasonably well protected.

Those who have effected changes in nursing education, practice, and research have recognized the importance of understanding the political process, knowing the laws controlling or affecting nurses and nursing, and knowing how to promote new legislation or modify existing laws. Florence Nightingale, Ethel Bedford Fenwick, Lillian Wald, Lavinia Dock, M. Adelaide Nutting, Annie W. Goodrich, and Shirley Titus were all politically effective. A few nurses have earned law degrees so that they could play more active roles in nursing jurisprudence or the larger field of health legislation. State boards of nurse examiners have met regularly throughout this century to discuss legal problems; texts and articles by nurses on nursing jurisprudence go back many decades and are proliferating rapidly.[266-276] The literature on medical jurisprudence contains discussions of nursing-related questions. In 1970, the International Council of Nurses sponsored a 6-day International Seminar on Nursing Legislation in Warsaw, Poland.[277] With the Florence Nightingale International Foundation, the ICN in 1974 sponsored a second seminar in Bogota, Colombia.[277a] National or-

---

* Lippard, Vernon W.: *op. cit.*

* In this publication, the terms "health occupations," "health professions," and "health disciplines" are used interchangeably and are said to extend to the "entire range of health manpower."

ganizations have legislative committees, councils, or departments, as do state and provincial organizations. Some have offices in national, state, or provincial capitals, with a program for informing members and working with legislators.

In 1969, the ICN published thirteen "principles" to guide nursing organizations in promoting new nursing legislation or revising existing laws on nursing education and practice.[278] As Betty D. Pearson [279] pointed out, nations may choose to accept or reject international rules, but these rules have a potent influence. The ICN's code of ethics, while not legally binding, affects laws, since nurses try to design legislation that is consistent with their ethical codes. National nursing codes of ethics are, by and large, patterned after the international code.[280-282]

In 1974, the Nurses Coalition for Action in Politics (N-Cap) was established in the United States.[283] In the same year, Louisiana formed a federation of eight nursing organizations, largely for political purposes, to "unify the voice of nursing." [284] While individuals have been effective politically, nurses have not spoken with one voice nor, considering their numbers and the critical nature of their service, have they had nearly as much influence on health legislation as they might. Some persons attribute this not only to nursing's having been a women's occupation, but also to a hierarchical health care system that has discouraged the nurse's initiative.

Preparation of nurses has not been comparable in length or depth to that of physicians, and this may also have made them less assertive. The official nursing organization in many a country has represented too few of those who might belong to it.* In many cases leadership has been divided between several or many organizations rather than concentrated in the official body.

Katherine B. Nuckolls in an article titled "Who Decides What the Nurse Can Do?" says:

At present, most nurses who are practicing in "expanded roles" function, in part, under standing orders, with authority delegated by physicians. Although state laws, with their associated rules and regulations, are the ultimate determinants of the legal scope of practice, other factors have a more immediate effect. To a large extent, what the nurse can do is determined by the employing agency, her co-workers in that agency, the consumer of health care and, most of all, by the nurse herself.

. . .

In our highly complex society, the provision of health care is necessarily a shared responsibility rather than the prerogative of a single group. Medicine and nursing are interdependent professions, with overlapping areas of competence. In such relationships, decisions as to who does what must be mutually agreed upon. Both professions must accept the challenge of role change.*

In discussing the legal status of nurses, it should be noted that the first consideration is their legal *status as a citizen*. Laws that discriminate on the basis of sex, color, race, religion, education, or economic class affect nursing.† Nurses who are citizens of a country have a different legal status from those who are aliens. It is not within the scope of this book to discuss the legal status of women versus men, of whites versus blacks, or any other contrasting groups, but it is obvious that these questions are involved in the legal status of the nurse.‡ Throughout its history, the nursing literature includes publications on sex, ethnic, racial, and religious discrimination.[285-290]

Nurses are affected by labor laws—*their status as workers*. The International Labour Office (ILO) is one of the organizations with which the ICN and the WHO have worked most closely. At the request of the WHO, the ILO is considering the preparation of an "international instrument on the employment and conditions of work of nursing personnel." The "proposed conclusions" in 1976 are that the instrument will take the form of a "Recommendation" to include policy statements on nursing services and nursing personnel; education, or training; laws affecting practice; participation in decision making; reasonable career prospects; remuneration commensurate with needs, qualifications, experience, and responsibilities; working time and rest periods; occupational health protection; social security; special employment arrangements; protection of student rights; and provision for international cooperation.[290a]

Protective labor legislation in a country can apply to any health worker. The fact that all categories of health personnel, including doc-

---

* Nuckolls, Katherine B.: "Who Decides What the Nurse Can Do?" *Nurs. Outlook*, **22**:626, (Oct.) 1974.

† The ANA has had committees for many years to promote fair treatment for minorities. The creation in 1976 of a Commission on Human Rights within the organization is the latest and most sweeping act. This step may be attributed to the work of the Association's Affirmative Action Task Force.

‡ Virginia S. Cleland has called "Sex Discrimination: Nursing's Most Pervasive Problem" (*Am. J. Nurs.*, **71**:1542, [Aug.] 1971), but nurses in earlier decades were even more harassed by sex discrimination. Annie W. Goodrich said "Eighteen years of this struggle has made a woman suffragist out of me." (*Am. J. Nurs.*, **9**:962, [Sept.] 1909.)

---

* Of more than 1 million registered nurses in the United States in 1974, only 196,000 belonged to the ANA. (*Facts about Nursing, op. cit.*, p. 221).

tors, belong to one union in the USSR is the extreme example of this principle. National, provincial, and state nursing organizations have social security programs designed largely to protect the rights of nurses as workers—rights to sick leaves, vacations, retirement pay or pensions, fair remuneration and hours of work, and bargaining rights, for example. In the United States, social security programs of the ANA and state nurse associations have been increasingly effective in protecting rights of nurses as workers.

As mentioned earlier, "professional" workers in most societies are accorded certain rights or a special legal status. Physicians cannot, for instance, be required to divulge the confidence of patients, nor clergymen the confidence of their parishioners. This right to privacy affects the nurse-patient relationship and nurses have sought in this, and other respects, to be accorded the legal status of professionals. Eric Springer, a participant in a 1973 symposium on the accountability of the nurse, answered affirmatively the question as to whether nurses are professionals. He includes the following observations:

I suggest that you will have to ask these questions continually: what are we, who are we, what do we do, how do we do it? As science grows so does your profession grow.

. . .

The courts have uniformly said that the nurse has a duty to call important problems to a doctor's attention. If the physician subsequently fails to act, the nurse must call it to someone else's attention: the director of nursing, the chief of staff, the administrator of the hospital, someone who can intervene. Why? To take the necessary steps to provide quality care of the patient. The nurse has a professional duty, if you will, "to blow the whistle" on a malpracticing physician, because the law considers the nurse a professional. This is one of the elements involved in any discussion of accountability and responsibility.*

The educational rights of all citizens obviously affect nursing. Countries vary greatly in the amount of "free" or tax-supported education available to residents and even more in laws that make it compulsory for parents to send their children to school. Where education through college, and even continuing education, is tax supported, education for nursing is obviously affected positively just as it is affected negatively by a private and discrimina-

tory system. Legislation designed to ensure the quality of educational institutions and programs affects nursing just as do laws requiring graduates to pass licensure examinations if they wish to practice and laws that require continued study if they wish to maintain this licensure. Legislation to protect the status of students in colleges and universities affects students in nursing programs within the system.

Licensing laws stipulate who shall design and administer licensing examinations. The extent to which the occupation controls these processes and the extent to which institutions and the individuals who use their services control them is under debate.

In 1971, the US Department of Health, Education, and Welfare asked for a moratorium on licensure of additional categories of health manpower and established a subcommittee on health manpower "credentialing" under the aegis of the USPHS Health Manpower Coordinating Committee. Harris S. Cohen, chairman, with Lawrence H. Miike, brought out reports in 1971 and 1973.[291,292] These reports were followed by DHEW-sponsored studies and conferences. The subcommittee's third report in the form of a proposal in June 1976 [293] includes recommendations * that: (1) a (nonfederal) national council on certification be formed to develop and evaluate criteria and policies, help develop national standards, and apprise the federal government of the certification organizations approved; (2) national standards for selected occupations be continually evaluated by interested parties, including representatives of the federal government, the proposed national council (above), professional organizations, appropriate educational institutions, accrediting agencies, employers and employees, and state governments; such standards to be adopted by the proposed national council and state licensing occupations; (3) *federal reimbursement financing programs* be limited to services rendered by health professionals who are licensed by state boards adopting national standards or certified by organizations adopting national standards and approved by the national certification council; (4) criteria be established by states designed to make licensure of additional health personnel deliberate and cautious; (5) accountability and effectiveness of licensing boards be strengthened by states; (6) effective competency measures as a requirement for credentialing be recognized and promoted by certification, licensure and accrediting bodies; (7) requirements and procedures to assure

* Springer, Eric: "Who Said Nurses Are Professionals?" in *Accountability of the Nurse. Are There Legal Barriers to Assuming Full Professional Responsibility?* (Speeches presented during the 48th Convention, American Nurses' Association.) The Association, Kansas City, Mo., 1973, p. 7.

* These recommendations apply to the entire range of health manpower categories.

continued competence of health personnel be adopted by certification organizations, licensure boards, and professional organizations.

These recommendations were, in 1976, under consideration. They were designed to promote geographic and career mobility and to provide government funding agencies and others with national standards for public protection. Whether or not these recommendations are accepted and activated, they will certainly influence future quality controls.

The foregoing discussion is an attempt to show that nurses are controlled by the laws affecting all members of the society in which they live and the laws affecting all workers, all health workers, and all "professionals." As citizens, they are responsible for the passage and periodic revision of such laws.

At present, the *legal status of the nurse* is differentiated from that of other health workers in the United States by *state nurse practice acts*. Since nurse practice acts should differentiate nursing from the practice of medicine, dentistry, or social work, they should be consistent with practice acts in related fields. As mentioned earlier nurses and physicians of the United States established a National Joint Practice Commission in 1972 to make recommendations on the "congruent" roles of physicians and nurses; most states have a comparable body.* Under the sponsorship of the NJPC and grants from the AMA, ANA, and the W. K. Kellogg Foundation, Virginia C. Hall, an attorney, assembled and analyzed for their "efficacy" and "probable effects" the medical and nursing acts of the states and the District of Columbia. She noted that so many acts are in the process of revision that almost any opinion on them found in print is out of date. The Introduction to Hall's report includes the following statements:

It has become apparent that nurses functioning in what has become known as an "expanded role" can significantly decrease the cost of health maintenance and health care without sacrificing quality, and that this is a result which is socially beneficial and should be encouraged. At the same time, there has been an equal recognition that the assumption by some nurses of new medical responsibilities must be responsibly monitored, in order to protect the public from practitioners who purport to act in a sphere outside their competence.

In response to these sentiments, an increasing

number of States have amended their nurse practice acts in attempts to free the nursing profession from unwarranted restrictions and at the same time subject it to responsible control.

. . .

It should be noted that new methods of health care delivery have not raised any comparable questions for physicians of the legality of their practice under the various medical practice acts, all of which have remained substantially unchanged since their passage with respect to the nature of medical practice. Medicine has traditionally been and still is thought of as consisting essentially of providing health care through the three functions of diagnosis, treatment and prescription; almost all medical practice acts have either a definition of the practice of medicine or a prohibition against the unlicensed practitioner which incorporates these concepts. Although the accepted methods of performing these functions have changed drastically since the medical practice acts were first passed, the concept of medical practice as comprising them has not; therefore no change in the medical practice acts has been necessary, even though new discoveries and technology have revolutionized the practice. By contrast, new concepts of health care have called for educating certain nurses to assume responsibility for acts which may arguably be called diagnosis, treatment or prescription, all of which are outside the traditional ambit of nursing, and have traditionally required a license to practice medicine.*

In concluding, Hall recommended that those contemplating a statutory amendment consider the following questions:

. . . does the proposed amendment restrict nursing to something other than medicine? Does it assume or explicitly provide for a dependent role in the performance of medical acts? Does it speak in particularized terms which themselves create ambiguities and which, if not already outdated, may well be so in a few years? Does it rely on implementation by rules and regulations or on a meaningful, self-executing criterion? And is it consistent with the other practice acts? †

She thought that whatever the statutory change, the law should be "flexible in permitting new professional developments, and at the same time responsible to the public. Only then . . . can nursing feel free to devote its full attention to what should and must be its primary concern: determining what role it can best fill in the delivery of health care now and in the future." ‡

In the body of her report, Hall dealt with acts based on the "traditional" definition of the practice of professional nursing (see page 19) by the ANA. She noted that 13 states had acts incorporating this definition "unaltered"; 11

---

* The Joint Practice Commission adopted the following statement June 6, 1975: "Joint practice is nurses and physicians collaborating as colleagues to provide patient care." (Hall, Virginia C.: *Statutory Regulation of the Scope of Nursing Practice—A Critical Survey*, National Joint Practice Commission, Chicago, 1975, frontispiece.)

* Hall, Virginia C.: *op. cit.*, pp. 3, 5.
† *Ibid.*, p. 43.
‡ *Ibid.*

states had slightly modified it; four states used a similar definition; and two had abbreviated it. Additional "acts" (activities of nurses) were authorized by 13 states; five states stipulated that the medical and nursing professions must recognize the "additional acts" as "proper"; ten states provided that nurses be trained to perform the additional acts and two states stipulated that "diagnosis of illness or prescription of therapeutic or corrective measures" must be "delegated" by a physician. The New York State definition and variants of it in seven states were discussed separately, as was the California law. Those of Maryland and Minnesota were considered together. Provisions in six states dealing with nurse anesthetists were discussed, as was the provision in New Hampshire directed toward the "advanced registered nurse practitioner." In an ANA-sponsored conference, reported in 1975, Hall suggested that the simplest approach is to exempt nursing from prohibition of medical practice. She said:

In the final analysis, given the best of all possible worlds, the simplest and I feel best approach statutorily to the changing role of nursing vis-a-vis medicine would probably be to repeal the definition of nursing entirely and to exempt nursing from the prohibitions of the medical practice act. The law would then of necessity be forced to rely on professional opinion, which is the best standard anyway for determining what a nurse should and should not do, and both professions would be free to devote their complete attention to ways in which they can best serve the public without being worried about the content and effect of abstract concepts like "treatment," "diagnosis," and "prescription." *

* Hall, Virginia C.: "Legal Problems Stemming from the Nurse and Medical Practice Acts," in American

The above data indicate a shifting scene and are a source of confusion for nurses who tend to move frequently. Even the terminology is confusing. Licensure is required for health workers who practice legally. (See Table 1-6 for per cent passing licensure examinations 1963–1972.)

In the United States (except in California and Texas where they are called vocational nurses), practical nurses who have passed the mandatory state practical nurse examination and are licensed use the title Licensed Practical Nurse or L.P.N. after their names; in California and Texas, L.V.N.

Certification or registration is defined by DHEW as

. . . the process by which a nongovernmental agency or association grants recognition to an individual who has met certain predetermined qualifications specified by that agency or association. Such qualifications may include (a) graduation from an accredited or approved program; (b) acceptable performance on a qualifying examination or series of examinations; and/or (c) completion of a given amount of work experience.*

Between 1903 and 1923, all of the 48 existing United States passed nurse practice acts and established state boards of examiners that inspected schools and administered mandatory state board (licensing) examinations for grad-

Nurses' Association: *Building for the Future.* (Papers presented at a Conference, Kansas City, Mo., Sept. 20–22, 1974.) The Association, Kansas City, Mo., 1975, p. 42.

* US Department of Health, Education, and Welfare: *op. cit.,* p. 7.

Table 1-6. Licensing Data on United States Registered Nurses, 1963–1972 *

Year	Licenses Issued to US† Registered Nurses for the First Time by Examination	Per Cent Passing Examination		New US Graduates	Licensure Ratio‡
		First Time	Subsequently		
1963–64	32,916	85.7	62.8	35,259	93.4
1964–65	33,417	85.8	63.3	34,686	96.3
1965–66	33,968	85.6	58.5	35,125	96.7
1966–67	37,884	85.3	58.2	38,234	99.1
1967–68	41,155	84.6	58.3	41,555	99.0
1968–69	41,665	84.3	57.7	42,196	98.7
1969–70	42,866	83.2	53.8	43,639	98.2
1970–71	45,419	—	—	47,001	96.6
1971–72	48,070	81.8	52.5	51,784	92.8

* Jones, D.C., et al.: *Trends in Registered Nurse Supply.* US Government Printing Office, Washington, D.C., 1976, p. 83 (DHEW Pub. No. [HRA] 75–15).

† Excludes RNs from foreign countries.

‡ Licensure ratio-licenses issued in year *T*/new US graduates in year *T*.

uates of approved schools of nursing.* Those who pass are entered in a state register of nurses and may use the title "Registered Nurse" or R.N. after their names. In the United States, the terms "registered" and "licensed" are used to designate those nurses who have passed licensing examinations administered by a governmental agency. "Registered" is arbitrarily used for the "professional" nurse, "licensed" for the "practical" or "vocational" nurse.

Licensing laws may be mandatory or permissive. A mandatory or compulsory law requires all who nurse for monetary compensation to be licensed. A permissive or voluntary law allows nurses to practice for compensation but not to use the title "registered nurse" or "licensed practical nurse." The ANA is promoting mandatory licensure in all states.

In the United States, nurse-midwives are certified by the American College of Nurse Midwifery. While such certification is voluntary, the requirement may be part of a state law on the practice of nurse-midwifery.

In 1973, the ANA established a program of voluntary certification. The Executive Committees of the five Divisions of Practice and the Certification Boards appointed by them are responsible for designing and implementing the program; the ANA's Congress for Nursing Practice is responsible for the uniformity of criteria and it has developed guidelines to be used by the certifying bodies.†[294] Certification of specialists is voluntary but it may come to have as much weight in nursing as certification by specialty boards has in medicine. In 1975, the ANA published a *Directory of Certified Nurses*.[295] The numbers of certified nurses will be increased by the decision in 1976 to certify nurses in each clinical division of practice on specialist and generalist levels. (See American Nurses' Association: *House of Delegates Reports 1974–1976, 50th Convention, ANA, June 1976.* The Association, Kansas City, Mo., 1976.)

There is a wealth of publications on the subject of licensure, registration, certification, and "credentialing," or providing a worker with credentials. The summary treatment of "Licensure—the Legal Basis of Nursing Practice," in Kelly's *Dimensions of Professional Nursing,* gives a brief history of licensure in the United States and a description of current practices.[296]

Nurses were the first of the health professions in the United States to have an examination that is used nationwide to judge a candidate's competence and right to be licensed. Since 1976, the examination is given twice a year on the same day in every state.[297] It is administered statewide as part of the state's right to assure its citizens of qualified practitioners and to protect workers. Great strides have been made in establishing national standards through the State Board Test Pool Examination used in all United States jurisdictions, although each state retains the right to set the passing grade or score. This has facilitated interstate licensing, or reciprocity. Many persons would like to see the acceptance of national standards to further facilitate reciprocity, or even an international licensure that would reduce the difficulties for nurses who want to practice in foreign countries. The latter question is under discussion by the International Council of Nurses.

In discussing the legal status of the nurse as a health practitioner, mention should be made of their legal accountability. *Malpractice suits* against nurses are relatively few in number but Helen Creighton made the following observations in 1974:

Earlier in this century a malpractice suit was uncommon, and very seldom did a nurse or other health care provider find herself the defendant in a lawsuit by a dissatisfied patient. Many factors have contributed to the increase that began in California and spread rapidly to other jurisdictions such as New York, Texas, Ohio, and the District of Columbia and has left no state untouched. Today more people than ever receive medical and nursing care, and this increases the exposure to incidents that can lead to suits. Concurrently innovations in medical and nursing care—new procedures, new drugs, and new treatments—while representing advances still bring with them new risks of injury. Many clients or patients do not appreciate either the hazard or complexity of modern nursing and medical practice. They assume negligent conduct when the outcome fails to meet expectations, and this increases the number of malpractice claims.*

Creighton goes on to trace the changes in nursing practice, in medical care, in social conditions, and public attitudes that have increased lawsuits against health practitioners. She gives definitions of malpractice and negligence but concludes that "professional negligence is synonymous with malpractice." Creighton says that "the consistent practice of her profession is her strongest safeguard

---

* The first nurse practice law was passed by North Carolina in 1903 and the last state or territory to enact this legislation was Guam in 1952. (American Nurses' Association: *Facts About Nursing 72–73.* The Association, Kansas City, Mo., 1974, p. 59.)

† ANA Divisions are Community Health Nursing, Geriatric Nursing, Maternal and Child Health Nursing, Medical-Surgical Nursing, Psychiatric and Mental Health Nursing.

* Creighton, Helen: "The Malpractice Problem," *Nurs. Clin. North Am.,* 9:425, (Sept.) 1974.

against suits for damages" but she quotes others as saying that all nurses should carry malpractice insurance. Nurses proved guilty by court proceedings or those whose behavior conflicts with the nursing profession's code of ethics may be reprimanded or have their license to practice revoked.

Texts on nursing and the law and symposia such as that reported in the September, 1974, issues of *Nursing Clinics of North America* discuss the particular problems of independent nurse practitioners in community nursing, in schools, in industry, in prisons, in maternal and child health nursing, and in emergency and critical care nursing.

Inez G. Hinsvark, discussing "the implications for action" in the expanded practice of nursing, comments on the need for a legislative base—the necessity, for example, of changing nurse practice acts, as the State of Washington has done, to make nurses responsible for their decisions and actions. She makes the following observation:

All of the existing nursing and medical practice acts ought to be reviewed and changed to give the nurse the right to practice as an independent practitioner. Almost all laws permit this by default but only a few laws give nurses the right to such practice. Washington has a new law that does just that.*

Hinsvark, commenting on the relatively passive role of nurses, thinks that they must change their self-image and public image, they must modify their education to foster independent and creative thought, and they must take a more effective part in their organizations.

Luther Christman, a nurse educator and sociologist, is among those who stress the interdependence of health workers. He thinks new organizational models are needed that will foster interdisciplinary study, interdisciplinary committees, shared power, and the freedom of each health worker to intervene in the patient's or client's behalf according to his or her competence to act. Christman believes that if workers are accountable for their acts, they will not be tempted to intervene unless they are prepared.[297a] He thinks "Interdependence between professional persons likely will emerge as a state of balance of power based on individual competence." †

The Economic Status of the Nurse. The material reward for nursing differs substantially

from country to country, but it is safe to say that it rates low on the scale of nursing's occupational advantages. Reference was made on page 18 to the 1976 International Labour Conference on Employment and Conditions of Work and Life of Nursing Personnel. The report of this conference called attention to the expansion of health services, the fact that nurses are the largest group that deal with health, the "enormous demand" for nurses, and the inadequacy of the supply (in quantity and quality). The report suggested a critical situation in the following terms:

Studies of what can only be called a crisis have shown that it is due both to the economic and social situation of nurses and to their morale and the general conditions of the profession. The chief causes of concern are the following: pay; working hours, rest periods and holidays; health protection; social security; initial and further training facilities; staffing practices; the organisation of work; rights of defence in disciplinary matters; career possibilities; the participation of nurses in the fixing of their conditions in general; and, more broadly, everything contributing to job satisfaction. Despite progress in these fields, it is widely recognised that nurses are often in a situation that accords ill with the importance of their role and of their responsibilities in the raising of the general level of health and well-being throughout the world.*

The report noted a "prevailing discontent," referring to strikes of nurses in recent years to defend "their occupational, moral or economic interests" in Canada, Denmark, France, Israel, Japan, Switzerland, the United Kingdom, and the United States. Discussing careers and opportunity for "advancement," the report concluded that "broadly speaking" the "best paid jobs—the most highly considered"—are those in which there is least direct contact with patients or the community, although they noted a recent trend toward increasing salaries for clinical work. Reviewing varying "career systems," the report noted that in the USSR nurses and feldshers are "middle-level" medical personnel. Nurses there have less opportunity for independent practice (or "advancement" within the system) than feldshers but both, after several years' experience, may, if qualified, study medicine and thereby improve their economic status. Canada, the United States, and the United Kingdom were mentioned as countries that offer greater opportunities for advancement; France as a country where opportunities for advancement are "limited." In developing countries, opportunities

---

* Hinsvark, Inez G.: "Implications for Action in the Expanded Role of the Nurse," *Nurs. Clin. North Am.,* **9:**411, (Sept.) 1974.

† Christman, Luther: "Where Are We Going?" (Paper presented at the Annual Meeting of the Delaware Nurses Association, Wilmington, Del., Nov. 3, 1973.)

* International Labour Office: *op. cit.*

for nursing personnel improve as health services expand. In countries that are not economically developed, nurses are in the employ of the government. The report gives comparative figures on salaries showing the wide range from country to country and even within a country. ILO recommendations apply to nurses as well as to all workers. Attention is called, however, to an ILO recommendation on Hours of Work in Hospitals that dates from 1930 and the recommendations from an Ad Hoc Meeting on Conditions of Work and Employment of Nurses in Geneva in 1958.[298]

As previously noted the ILO is working jointly with the WHO on the current study of employment and conditions of work and life of nursing personnel. The ICN is promoting optimum nurse participation in the drafting of the final "instrument" which the Council believes should be "unique" to nursing and should deal with the fundamental concerns of nursing and not with the "narrow issues of employment which are common to all working people." *

A Permanent Committee of Nurses in Liaison with European Economic Community, composed of representatives of national nursing organizations, was organized in 1974 to discuss and evolve recommendations and lobby for legislation affecting the economics of nursing.[299]

It is not within the scope of this book to review economic nursing research—even that within the United States. National investigations, most often focused on nursing education, have included something on nurses' earnings. A report of the Committee on the Grading of Nursing Schools, *Nurses, Patients and Pocketbooks,* gave considerable data on this subject. Since this report reflects what 67,938 nurses, physicians, hospital administrators, and patients said, as well as data from other sources, the findings were of great interest, but because the study was made during a serious depression (1928) they have been used guardedly.[300,301] Harold F. Clark's 1937 report, *Life Earnings,*[302] was especially useful since it compared selected professional occupations. It showed nurses, for example, earning less than teachers or social workers but it also showed that nurses earned more or less in relation to the time and money invested in their preparation. D. C. Jones and associates, in a recent study, reported the ratio of earnings of registered nurses to public school teachers 1960

to 1972 showing a rise of 15 per cent in this period. (See Fig. 1-23).

The report of the National Commission for the Study of Nursing and Nursing Education in 1970 noted the paradox of a shortage of nurses, a high percentage of inactive nurses, and relatively low salaries.

In *Facts About Nursing,* now published biennially by the American Nurses' Association, data on salaries of nurses are available to the public. It is obvious that there is a steady advance in the earnings of nurses in the United States, but unless this advance is studied in relation to the advance in the cost of living and in comparison with comparable occupations, it means very little. Knopf's study, *RN's One and Five Years After Graduation,*[303] shows that economic reasons for moving from one position to another were not dominant in the group studied and that 78 to 87 per cent of the respondents said their salary expectations had been met. Frank A. Sloan's[304] study involving 5000 nurses (see Table 1-7) shows baccalaureate and graduate study reflected in higher salaries but "the increase is small"; the length of employment in one hospital has a greater impact on earnings than the measure of general experience. The fact that from 65 to 85 per cent of nurses, according to the country, are employed by hospitals has a standardizing effect on earnings, geographically. Hospitals tend to cooperate * in regulating salaries, which has, from the standpoint of economics, a monopolistic effect and may account for the unusual occurrence of an oc-

* This cooperation may take the form of a collective "memorandum of agreement."

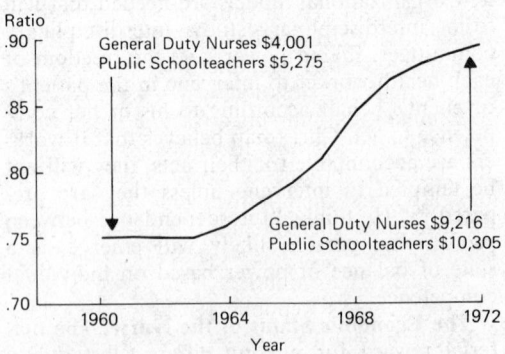

Figure 1-23. Ratio of earnings of registered nurses to public schoolteachers, 1960 to 1972, showing rise of almost 15 per cent in 12 years. (Adapted from Jones, D. C., *et al.: Trends in Registered Nurse Supply.* [DHEW Pub. No. HRA 75–15.] US Government Printing Office, Washington, D.C., 1976.)

* Communication from Adele Herwitz, Executive Director, International Council of Nurses, to Presidents of ICN member associations, Mar. 1976, on Second ILO Report on Employment and Conditions of Work and Life of Nursing Personnel (Report VII [2]).

Table 1-7. Reasons for Refusing Employment in Rural and Poor Sections of Central Cities: Marital Status, Training, and Ethnicity *

Reasons	Marital Status			Type of Education			Ethnicity	
	Single	Married	Other	A.A.	B.A.	Diploma	White	Black
Small community								
Inadequate transportation	7.7	3.5	4.6	3.1	5.0	4.7	3.9	7.8
Transportation time	11.9	8.2	7.3	9.3	8.1	9.1	8.3	13.2
Personal danger	4.8	2.1	2.4	2.6	2.2	2.8	2.3	3.9
Types of patients	7.8	2.6	2.8	3.9	6.4	3.2	3.6	6.2
Spouse would oppose it	—	17.2	—	8.9	9.6	13.2	11.9	11.6
Poor schools	2.6	4.1	3.6	3.8	3.5	3.7	3.5	4.7
Poor sections								
Inadequate transportation	9.3	6.9	6.9	6.9	7.9	7.5	7.5	4.7
Transportation time	15.4	13.6	12.5	14.8	12.4	14.1	14.2	9.3
Personal danger	28.8	18.2	16.1	18.9	21.2	20.4	20.8	15.5
Types of patients	12.3	6.7	6.7	8.9	9.2	7.4	18.0	6.2
Spouse would oppose it	—	30.3	—	18.7	20.0	22.8	22.4	12.4
Poor schools	9.0	14.7	13.3	13.7	12.3	13.6	13.6	13.2

* Sloan, Frank A.: *The Geographic Distribution of Nurses and Public Policy. Health Manpower References.* US Government Printing Office, Washington, D.C., 1975, p. 152 (DHEW Pub. No. [HRA] 75–53).

cupation with a shortage of workers and a relatively low economic status.

The fact that nursing has attracted few men helps explain its low economic status (see Fig. 1-24). Organized nursing is now trying to bring more men into the profession but, of the 1,127,657 registered nurses in 1972, only 14,625 were men. Of the 85,077 admissions to 1377 initial programs, 5170 (6.1 per cent) were men and only 1693 (3.8 per cent) graduated.[305] Still, this represents an upward trend from 1.7 per cent graduations in 1965–66. Another significant trend is the increasing number of men appointed to prestigious positions in nursing, as, for example, deanships of collegiate programs, directors of nursing services, and officers in nursing organizations. While women seem to have preempted the field of nursing in this age, there is no reason to believe that this situation will persist. Making the occupation of nursing attractive to educated men and women and to all national, ethnic, and religious groups is essential if desirable qualitative and quantitative standards of nursing are to be met, including adequate remuneration.

In totalitarian countries such as the USSR and the People's Republic of China, the remuneration of health workers is strictly regulated; in countries such as Great Britain that have a national health service or Canada that has a national scheme with modifying provincial programs, salary scales for health workers are prepared and published by national commissions, councils, or committees. Remuneration of health workers in the United States is not regulated to the same extent, although the federal and state programs of Medicare and Medicaid provide a measure of control. The Blue Cross Association, with the American Hospital Association, must be mentioned as a controlling force in the private sector.

The failure of public and private agencies to satisfactorily control the costs of health care is widely discussed. A report of Isidore S. Falk in 1973, one from the National Academy of Sciences in 1975, and Sylvia A. Law's report of 1976 might be cited in this connection.[306-308] Study of these sources will show that "third-party" payment (the third party being the insuring agency) has not affected the earnings of nurses as it has the earnings of physicians. Cathryne A. Welch's [309] review of health care financing in the United States and the limited recognition of the nature and value of nursing services as distinct from those of medicine explains why health insurance in the United States has so little affected the earnings of nurses. She says that nursing is seeking entry into the "reimbursement system" at a time when the public is "sensitive to the need for reorganization of the health care delivery system and its enabling financial mechanisms" and that nursing "faces severe challenges." Payment of health workers on a fee-for-service basis is under question even for physicians, so legislation to enable nurses to charge on this basis will meet with opposition in many quarters.

The American Nurses' Association has a Commission on Economic and General Welfare, with counterparts in state nurses' associa-

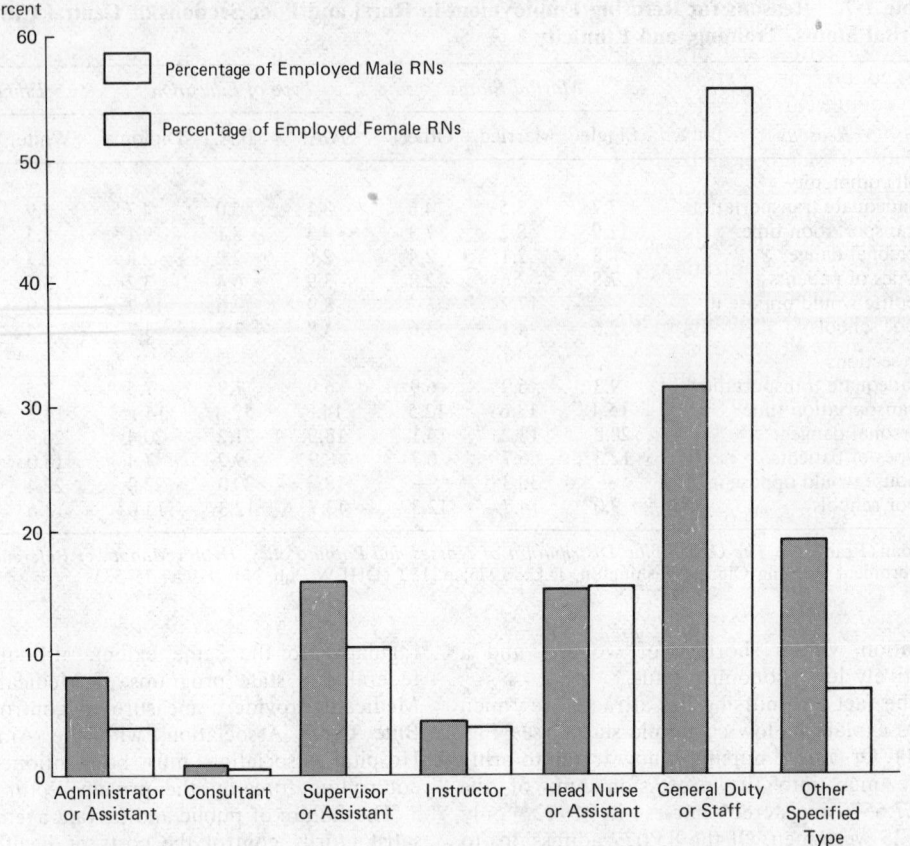

Figure 1-24. Percentage distribution of employed men registered nurses and women registered nurses by type of position, 1972. (From American Nurses' Association: *The Nation's Nurses: 1972 Inventory of Registered Nurses.* The Association, Kansas City, Mo. 1974, p. 125.)

tions. Under the National Labor Relations Act, the collective bargaining rights of nurses have been recognized. The ANA's national commission "has established and maintains representation on the board of directors of the Coalition of American Public Employees, Federal Mediation and Conciliation Service's Task Force on the Health Care Industry, and ANA's Task Force on Manpower." *

It is the goal of the Commission to represent the economic and professional interests of nurses, and to help any state nurses' association develop and maintain effective programs that will attract and retain members and will give nurses a "strong voice in determining the scope and quality of health care in this country." The Commission has issued statements on na-

tional health insurance and on third-party payments for registered nurses.

While nurses deserve and should have a material reward that is commensurate with the value of their services and in line with the expenditure of time and money in preparation for their work, the extent to which those in an occupation are not *primarily* motivated by material gain is a measure of its professionalism.

Nursing Organizations. Like all major occupations, nursing has official organizations that represent it internationally, regionally, nationally, by states or provinces, or locally. Most official organizations publish journals, newspapers, or both. In addition to official nursing organizations designed to represent all nurses of a geographical or political unit, there are hundreds of organizations representing groups of nurses with common interests. There are a few "nursing organizations" that have non-nurse members and there are thousands of health organizations that have nurse members

* American Nurses' Association: *House of Delegates Reports 1974–1976. 50th Convention American Nurses' Association, June 1976.* The Association, Kansas City, Mo., 1976, p. 44.

who may or may not form nursing committees, councils, or divisions.

Major international organizations have national counterparts; national organizations have state counterparts (some have regional subdivisions), and they may have district components. Nursing organizations on all levels collaborate with health organizations on corresponding levels.

It is obviously impossible to list here, much less discuss, all organizations that might be of interest to nurses.*

Health workers, moving to new communities in the United States, can usually get a list of health agencies and organizations from local health departments or chambers of commerce. Readers will find international, national, and local directories of health organizations and agencies published yearly in official journals. The *American Journal of Nursing* (see April 1976) includes a yearly Directory of International, National, Federal Government and State Nursing and Related Organizations. The *Nursing Outlook* also has an official directory (see March 1976). The following pages mention only a few of those listed in these directories.

While the public's image of the worker, and the accomplishments of an occupation, depend ultimately on the performance of individual members, the effectiveness of its organizations determine how much collective progress it can make. Education of the workers, their services and conditions of work, would be chaotic without its organizations. Members of an occupation who do not belong to its official organizations are, in a sense, given a "free ride" by those who do, and lose their best chance to effect change and to learn from their peers.

The oldest *international* nursing organization is the International Council of Nurses (with which is associated the Florence Nightingale International Foundation) representing 74 official nursing organizations in 1975. It had then a total membership of 601,754.[310] Nurses who belong to their official national nursing organization automatically belong to the ICN. A national nursing organization must meet certain ICN requirements to be eligible for membership in the ICN. Revision of these requirements, written into the constitution and by-laws of the ICN, that have the effect of excluding some current national nursing organizations, are periodically considered by the Council. Organized regional groups such as the Asian Nurses Federation, the Northern Nurses Federation, the Pan-American Nurses Federa-

tion, and the West European Nursing Group, now have a formal relationship with the ICN.

The Council dates from 1899. Its headquarters was in London until 1966, when it moved to Geneva, Switzerland. At its Congress every 4 years, held in various large cities around the world, and at interim Council and committee meetings, international standards of ethics, education, service, and research have been developed that have had a universal effect on nursing.

Officers and staff members have given consultation service, have organized and sponsored international seminars or conferences, and have published guides on the structure of nursing organizations and on getting experience in foreign countries. With the FNIF, the ICN has published international lists of educational programs in nursing, Congress proceedings and papers, and its official journal, whose present title is *The International Nursing Review*. The ICN works with international health and welfare organizations including the International Labour Office (ILO), International Committee of the Red Cross, International Confederation of Midwives, International Hospital Federation, League of Red Cross Societies, Union of International Associations, United Nations, United Nations Educational, Scientific and Cultural Organization (UNESCO) and International Children's Emergency Fund (UNICEF), World Health Organization, and World Medical Association.[311]

Katherine Densford Dreves called the ICN a "fact-finding, standard-making coordinating body . . ."; Marie Madeleine Bihet said the ICN "has been an incentive for all countries in the world to create, improve, and promote professional nursing." *

Margrethe Kruse was involved for many years in economic and welfare programs for nurses before assuming the ICN presidency. Attending the 5th Congress of the Trade Unions International of Public and Allied Employees in 1973 while president of the ICN, she reported that 60 countries were represented, with the ILO the only international organization represented. She explored the possibility of contacts between Russian and other nurses of the world (Russian nurses were not represented in the ICN). Kruse noted that, of the 8,000,000 members of the Health Service Workers Union in Russia, 2,500,000 were nurses.[312] As noted earlier, the ILO, in 1974,

---

* See Appendix for list of selected organizations and agencies.

* Bridges, Daisy Caroline: *A History of the International Council of Nurses, 1899–1964.* [Introductory Statements.] Pitman Medical Publishing Co., Ltd., London, 1967.

urged by the ICN, agreed to consider in a 1976 conference an international "instrument" for nurses that "if implemented" would upgrade the status and working conditions for nurses around the world." [313]

In an article entitled "ICN at the Crossroads," Kruse urged a more influential role for students and for the Council by allowing more national nursing organizations to be members and by allowing responsible involvement for six regional groups—Northern [European] Nurses Federation (1920), Western European Nursing Group (1946), Caribbean Nurses Organization (1957), Pan-American Nurses Federation (1966), East African Federation (1970), and Asian Federation of Nurses Associations (1972). [314] Kruse [315] also urged that nurses substitute internationalism for nationalism. Recent decisions of the Council of National Representatives suggest that the ICN is moving in these directions advocated by its former president.

The Council has encouraged international study and exchange of experience for nurses. In 1974, 5358 professional nurses and medical trainees were admitted as immigrants to the United States. [316] Emory University School of Nursing, Atlanta, Georgia, has an International Nursing Center that offers a 10-week course for international nurses. [317] Many countries work closely with the ICN and make special provisions for foreign students.

Roman Catholic nurses have had an International Catholic Federation of Nurses and an International Catholic Nurses Guild. The current and most representative organization is the International Committee of Catholic Nurses, with headquarters (1975) in Brussels, Belgium.

A very recent organization is the World Federation of Neurosurgical Nurses, with headquarters in Manchester, England. If all clinical nursing specialists decide that they should have international organizations, the WFNN will have many counterparts. Most international bodies organized around clinical specialties have nurse members who may form committees, councils, or divisions. An example of such a body is the International Federation of Midwives or International Confederation of Midwives which holds the International Congress of Midwives at 2-year intervals.

The World Health Organization is an example of an international health agency of which nursing is an integral part. Until recently, it has had a division of nursing with a nurse as chief officer; nursing is now distributed among the various divisions of the organization headquarters and its regional offices. Standards set by WHO have influenced health care around the world, as have regional nursing seminars on education, service, and research sponsored by WHO.

All developed countries have *national* nursing organizations, one of which officially represents the nurses of that country. Most adhere to a constitution and by-laws that qualifies them for membership in the ICN; most are counterparts of the official organizations of other health workers such as doctors, dentists, and social workers whose memberships are composed of persons qualified to practice in the respective professions. In the case of the ANA, members must be "nurses" as defined by the Association. (See page 18 for the current ICN definition which covers first- and second-level nurses as recommended to the ICN's Council of National Representatives by the Professional Services Committee in 1975.) [318]

The official national nursing organization in the United States is the American Nurses' Association whose structure continues to change. Founded in 1897 as the Nurses Associated Alumnae of the United States and Canada, it was renamed the American Nurses' Association in 1911. It had no paid staff nor headquarters office until 1920 when the ANA and the National League of Nursing Education took over the offices of the American Red Cross Bureau of Information, set up to help nurses returning from military assignments to readjust to civil life.* In 1921, the ANA, the NLNE, and the National Organization for Public Health Nursing established a joint headquarters in New York City under the same roof as the National Health Council. [319-322]

The ANA had its various headquarters in New York until 1972 when it moved to Kansas City, Missouri. In 1976, the Association had 26 administrative units staffed by 176 persons. [322a] This staff worked with members of the ANA in the Congress for Nursing Practice, the four Commissions (Economic and General Welfare Human Rights, Nursing Education, Nursing Research, and Nursing Services), the five divisions (Community Health Nursing, Geriatric Nursing, Maternal and Child Health Nursing, Medical-Surgical Nursing, and Psychiatric and Mental Health Nursing), and the Academy of Nursing.† The staff also worked in the Association's Membership Activities Division (Membership, Affirmative

* The ANA raised its dues from 15 to 50 cents to finance a headquarters office!

† The Academy, initiated in 1973 with 36 Charter Fellows designated by the ANA Board of Directors, admits 26 newly elected members at the annual meeting. (American Nurses' Association: *Facts About Nursing 74–75.* The Association, Kansas City, Mo., 1976, p. 223; "Academy of Nursing Admits New Fellows," *Nurs. Outlook,* **23:**138, [Mar.] 1975.)

Action, Statistics, and Economic and General Welfare), in the Business and Personnel Administration, with the Board of Directors, in the Government Relations Division, and on special projects. The titles just given suggest the Association's range of activities and its major concerns. The ANA has an office in Washington, D.C., which furnishes the membership with news about health legislation. From this office, members of the ANA promote legislation and lobby for or against legislative proposals. The Association owns the American Journal of Nursing Company which publishes *The American Nurse,* the *American Journal of Nursing,* and other publications.

Along with five other national nursing organizations, the ANA was reorganized in 1953, and its structure and function continues to change. In the 1950s, there was a movement to amalgamate national nursing organizations —to strengthen and unify the voice of nursing; today, proliferation of organizations is so marked that only through some federation of organizations could unity be achieved.

At one time, the NLNE was considered the educational arm of the ANA. However, when the NLNE and the NOPHN were disbanded, the NLN formed, and the program of the ANA revised, the latter was restructured in 1953 to assume more responsibility for educational standards. Its concern for education has steadily increased. The Association has now assumed major responsibility for continuing education. It is currently investigating credentialing and the whole process of quality assurance, with special reference to education. During the 1974–76 biennium, the ANA's Commission on Education held three conferences on accreditation of basic and graduate education and is conducting a study of the subject. The NLN was invited to co-sponsor the study but it declined.[323-325]

Student nurses play an increasingly active role in the affairs of the occupation. The National Student Nurses' Association, founded in 1953 as an autonomous organization, has its headquarters in New York City. Those in prenursing programs in colleges and universities, those in state-approved programs preparing for registered nurse licensure, and registered nurses in programs leading to baccalaureate degrees in nursing are eligible for membership. Its conventions are often held at the same time and at the same place where registered nurses are convening, and joint sessions provide opportunities for students and graduates to discuss common concerns. The Association has an official journal, *Imprint.* In 1975, the NSNA published *The Bill of Rights for Students of Nursing.* Its activities

have also included the promotion of minority recruitment, federal funding of nursing education, and study of self-assessment and career choices.

There are numerous national nursing organizations based on special clinical interests or specialized preparation. Some examples are the American Association of Critical Care Nurses, American Association of Neurosurgical Nurses, American Association of Nurse Anesthetists, American College of Nurse Midwives, and the Orthopedic Nurses Association.

Other national nursing organizations are based on the place where the nurse practices. Two examples are the American Association of Industrial Nurses and the Association of Operating Room Nurses. National organizations are also based on a function of the nurse, for example, the Association of Rehabilitation Nurses; others are based on the common ethnic background of members, for example, the American Indian Nurses Organization or the National Black Nurses Association; and there are honor societies, for instance, Alpha Tau Delta and Sigma Theta Tau. There are a few national nursing organizations devoted to special aspects of nursing education. One is the American Association of Colleges of Nursing; another is Nurses Educational Funds.

A national nursing organization may be devoted to another function, for example, research. While promoting or conducting research is a function of many nursing organizations, the American Nurses' Foundation was established by the ANA in 1950 as an independent body to receive grants for and promote or conduct research. Its headquarters was moved from New York City to Kansas City in 1974. Between 1950 and 1955, the Foundation funded 27 studies of nursing function; between 1955 and 1973, it funded 69 projects, many of them doctoral studies.[326] The Foundation published a *Directory of Nurses with Earned Doctoral Degrees* in 1969, with later supplements and a new directory in 1973; it publishes a quarterly newsletter, *Nursing Research Report.*

Since 1962, the Foundation has conducted an abstracting service with its abstracts published in *Nursing Research.* (See also Chapter 19 for a discussion of ANF.)

Almost all of the foregoing organizations have memberships confined to registered nurses. There are, however, national nursing organizations that admit both registered nurses and licensed practical nurses or that confine their membership to the licensed practical nurse. The National Federation of Licensed Practical Nurses, founded in 1949, with its headquarters in New York City, serves licensed practical nurses in the same way that the ANA serves registered nurses. Its membership is composed entirely of licensed practical nurses. Its official journal is *Nursing Care.*

Besides the organizations whose memberships are confined to one or two categories of nurses, there are national nursing organizations that admit nonnurses as well as nurses. The largest of these organizations is the National League for Nursing whose membership is so open and whose concerns are so broad that it might be called a "national league for health," although its stated purpose is to see that the "nursing needs" of the people are met.* In 1953, when the National League of Nursing Education and the National Organization for Public Health Nursing † were disbanded, many aspects of their programs were taken over by the newly formed NLN. The League has its headquarters in New York City; it has regional

---

* Its "primary function is to work with health care agencies of which nursing services are a basic component, with nursing educational institutions and with communities to improve health care services and nursing education programs needed by society through services in accreditation, consultation, testing, continuing education, research and publications." (National League for Nursing: *Statement of Purpose.* The League, New York, May 1975.) The NLN had more than 15,000 individual members in 1975 and over 1800 agency members. Anna Fillmore *et al.* said "The NLN is Everybody's Business" (*Nurs. Outlook,* **1:**22, [Jan.] 1953).

† The NLNE was founded in 1893 as the American Society of Superintendents of Training Schools for Nurses of the United States and Canada. The National Organization for Public Health Nursing was founded in 1912.

offices and constituent state leagues. The League has individual and agency members and a division of each with an Interdivisional Coordinating Committee. Within the Division of Agency Members there are six councils (see Fig. 1-25).[327,328]

The NLN's Division of Measurement has developed tests used by the State Board Test Pool that have gone a long way toward establishing national standards for nursing. The NLN took over the NLNE's responsibility for accrediting nursing education programs that the NLNE assumed in 1938. The NLN has been recognized by the US Commissioner of Education as the accrediting agency for educational programs in nursing. It periodically publishes complete lists of accredited programs, state by state, in the August issue of its official magazine, *Nursing Outlook,* with a supplementary list in March. Partial lists may appear in other issues. Since 1973, the League has also, with the American Public Health Association, accredited community nursing services.[329,330]

While the NLN is concerned with the education of licensed practical nurses as well as the education of registered nurses, the National Association for Practical Nurse Education and Service, organized in 1941 under the title Association of Practical Nurse Schools, was the first agency to accredit practical nursing programs. NAPNES is recognized by the US Commissioner of Education as one of the accrediting bodies for practical nurse education. The membership of this organization includes both registered nurses and licensed practical nurses.

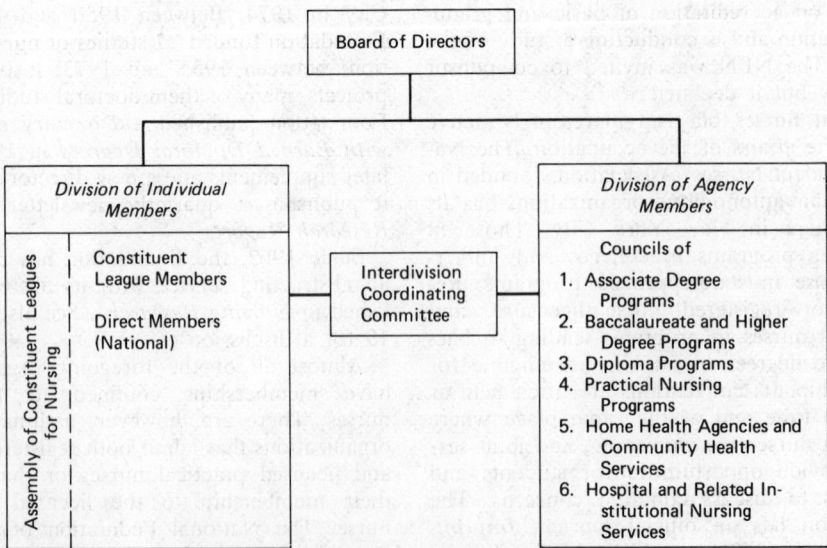

Figure 1-25. Organizational chart of National League for Nursing.

Many national health organizations have nursing components. Examples are the National Nurses Society of Alcoholism which is a [provisional] member of the National Council on Alcoholism; the Council on Cardiovascular Nursing that is a component of the American Heart Association; or the Nurses Association of the American College of Obstetricians and Gynecologists. Other organizations have a nursing division, for example, the American Hospital Association, or a committee on nursing, for instance, the American Medical Association. Some national health organizations have nursing consultants, national and regional. The American Cancer Society is an example.

Regional nursing organizations are component parts of some national nursing organizations. The NLN, for example, has regional offices. The Southern Regional Education Board, the Western Interstate Commission for Higher Education, and the New England Board of Higher Education, with their nursing components, have all influenced the development of nursing education in the geographic areas they serve—particularly graduate and continuing education. The Midwest Continuing Professional Education for Nurses was organized recently for the latter purpose.

State nursing organizations in the United States and provincial nursing organizations in Canada have structures that tend to follow those of the parent national bodies—the American Nurses' Association and the Canadian Nurses' Association. The directory for the United States, published in the April 1976 issue of the *American Journal of Nursing,* gives the officers of the state organizations and the addresses of state headquarters. State nursing organizations (like state medical associations) have *district nursing organization* components. Representatives of district nursing organizations, particularly official organizations participating in local health councils, can help coordinate and promote the quality of health care in the area served. District nursing organizations that include large cities like New York, Chicago, and San Francisco may have more members than state organizations in sparsely populated states. Whether or not the district nursing organization is large or small, it has great potential usefulness. All of the organizations mentioned can furnish readers with lists of their publications which include statements on function or purpose, and that often list histories of the organizations. Readers who would like detailed information on nursing organizations should consult such sources.

An effort has been made in this section to discuss some of the characteristics of nursing as an occupation; its claim to being a profession; the public and self-image of a nurse; nurses as accountable practitioners; the guarantees they offer society for the reliability of their practice; the extent to which they control their practice; the effectiveness with which nurse manpower is utilized; and the rewards for practice—material and spiritual or emotional. The National Commission on Nursing and Nursing Education has been quoted as saying that nursing has been and is "a troubled occupation" (see page 38). It is certainly a rapidly growing and changing one. This is reflected in its proliferating organizations on whose programs nurses must depend for the resolution of many of their occupational problems. The remainder of this chapter is devoted to nursing education, which also reflects the ferment in nursing. Nurse leaders, with reference to nursing education, refer to this ferment as "chaos" (see page 90).

4. PREPARATION FOR GENERAL NURSING—SOME INITIAL, OR BASIC, PROFESSIONAL PROGRAMS

Preparation of Nursing Personnel. It is not within the scope of this book to discuss in any detail the preparation of the various workers giving nursing care throughout the world, or even all those in the United States. The following pages are devoted mainly to the preparation in North America of the registered "professional" nurse as defined by the International Council of Nurses (see page 18). The registered "professional" nurse is the worker referred to as "the nurse" throughout this book. There is no intention of disregarding or underestimating the contribution to health care of licensed practical nurses, nurse's assistants, nurse's aides, orderlies, and nursing personnel with other titles. The current trend toward identifying information and skills all health workers should acquire is, we believe, constructive. Making it possible for students to move from one educational program to another is also thought desirable by the writer. Nursing, as discussed here, will, we hope, interest all those who practice it regardless of their titles.

In 1975, Dorothy Ozimek[331] of the National League for Nursing, reviewing current studies, summarized recent changes and predicted the future of nursing education, noting major social trends that affect its future. Nothing characterizes nursing in this era more than experimentation in nursing education and rapid changes in curricula. Many institutions and agencies in the United States and elsewhere are trying to individualize student programs and to encourage independent study that allows a student to progress at his or her own pace.[332] Admission requirements have been liberalized so that young men and women with dissimilar social and ethnic backgrounds have equal opportunity to enter the nursing occupations, though minorities do not presently have proportional representation.* The "open curriculum" and the "ladder concept" in nursing education are widely discussed and encouraged by grants that make demonstration projects possible. Even a doctoral degree may be acquired from "the University without walls." [333,334] See Tables 1-8 and 1-9 for data on students enrolled in open curricula in 1974.

The idea that continuing education will be available to all health workers makes the concept of watertight, dead-end programs obsolete. In the USSR and the People's Republic of China, radically new and productive systems of health care have been developed in surprisingly short time periods. These countries use health workers with relatively brief training programs. Since, however, these workers come from, live beside, and understand the needs of the people, and since in both countries continuing education and the ladder concept are

* The US Department of Health, Education, and Welfare reports that of 700,000 employed nurses in 1970 3.6 per cent (25,000) were black and 0.06 per cent (450) were American Indians. (Bureau of Health Resources Development, Health Resources Administration, US Department of Health, Education, and Welfare: *Nursing Student Loan Programs.* The Bureau, Bethesda, Md., p. 1.)

Table 1-8. Educational Background of Students in Open Curricula by Type of Program in Which They Were Enrolled Oct. 15, 1974. *

Educational Background	Diploma	Associate Degree	Bacca- laureate
Registered nurses	—	—	7,511
Previously enrolled in RN school	636	1,020	1,311
LPN/LVNs	680	2,659	355
Medical corpsmen	28	150	123
Aides, orderlies	71	255	139
Other health	52	71	146
Some college, not health	2,988	3,093	6,122
College completed, not health	339	448	874

* National League for Nursing, Division of Research: "Educational Preparation for Nursing—1974," (Report prepared by Walter L. Johnson.) *Nurs. Outlook,* **23:**578, (Sept.) 1975.

Table 1-9. Students Enrolled in Open Curricula of Basic RN Programs, Oct. 15, 1974 *

	Diploma	Associate Degree	Bacca- laureate
Total enrollments	64,083	85,452	104,532
Number of open curriculum students	4,707	7,785	16,581
Percent of open curriculum students	7	9	16

* National League for Nursing, Division of Research: "Educational Preparation for Nursing—1974," (Report prepared by Walter L. Johnson.) *Nurs. Outlook,* **23:**578, (Sept.) 1975.

part of the system, health workers with a limited initial training can make good use of what they know and can go as far as their innate ability allows them since they return again and again for additional study and experience in health centers. Health education programs for the public encourage self-help and effective use of all types of health workers and facilities.

Certain countries, for example, Canada, have discouraged the proliferation of health workers, even rejecting the idea of "intermediate" health workers as exemplified by the feldshers of the USSR or the physician's assistants of the United States. Claude Castonguay expressed the prevalent view when he said, with reference to proposed legislation, "Nurses . . . will as a group remain what is justly called the 'backbone' of the health establishment." He rejected the physician's assistant (feldsher type) because he thought no category of health worker should be an assistant "forever." *

Some students of health care systems in the United States and elsewhere believe that proliferation of health workers makes for fragmentation of care and they would like to see fewer varieties, each prepared to give a wider range of services or more effective service. To modify the present hierarchical system of health care in the United States, it has been suggested that new terms or titles be used that would do away with the present public and self-image of doctors, nurses, and others, for current images may be barriers to good working relationships and hence barriers to effective health care.

Suggestions for a single health profession, or for fewer or new kinds of health workers in

* "ANPQ [Association of Nurses of the Province of Quebec] Hears Claude Castonguay on Proposed Legislation," *Can. Nurse,* **68:**13, (Dec.) 1972.

Province	Type of Institution	Control
British Columbia	Community Colleges	Boards of School Trustees Department of Education
	Technical Institute (BCIT)	Department of Education but under the Director of Technical and Vocational Training
Alberta	Junior Colleges	Department of Advanced Education
Saskatchewan	Institutes of Applied Arts and Sciences	Department of Continuing Education
Manitoba	Community College	Department of Colleges and University Affairs
Ontario	Colleges of Applied Arts and Technology (CAAT)	Council of Regents, Ministry of Colleges and Universities
Quebec	General and Vocational Colleges (CEGEP)	Direction Generale de l'Enseignement Collegial, Ministry of Education

Figure 1-26. Type of control of educational institutions within which diploma programs (formerly under hospital control) are now established in Canadian Provinces. (From Alberta Task Force on Nursing Education: *Report of The Alberta Task Force on Nursing Education, September 1975.* The Task Force, Alberta, Canada, Sept. 1975, p. 189.)

the United States imply such radical changes in educational programs that no attempt can be made to identify them here. However, the practice in some North American universities of offering interdisciplinary courses for medical and nursing students and students in other health fields is a step in this direction, as is the requirement of continuing education for all health workers. Many students in one health occupation now take, as electives, courses designed primarily for those in a different occupation; nursing faculties include nonnurses such as physicians, social workers, and clinical psychologists, while medical faculties include many nonphysicians—sometimes nurses. The overlapping functions and responsibilities of physicians, nurses, social workers, health educators, and others is increasingly recognized and is modifying their preparation for practice. Much of this argument has been presented in the discussion of the extended role of the nurse.

Because rapid change characterizes this era, defining types of nursing personnel and their preparation must be tentative. Statements from the World Health Organization and the ICN on page 18 may soon be of historical interest only. Both indicate, however, that registered

nurses should be so prepared that they can offer a professional service.

In most countries, nursing personnel whose preparation is most like that of the registered nurse are prepared in a 1-year to 2-year planned program under educational or hospital auspices. In the United States, this category of worker is called a "licensed practical nurse" and in Canada a "qualified nursing assistant," although a 1976 Canadian publication refers to practical nursing schools.

The second category of nursing personnel with less preparation than that of the registered nurse was described as follows by the WHO:

Nursing personnel able to perform specified tasks related to patient care that require considerably less use of judgment. They should be able to relate well to patients and to carry out dependably, under supervision, the tasks for which they have been trained.*

While in many countries, such workers are given in-service training which ranges considerably in length and thoroughness, the

* World Health Organization: *Fifth Report of the Expert Committee on Nursing.* The Organization, Geneva, Switzerland, 1966 (Tech. Report Series No. 347).

American Nurses' Association recommends short, intensive courses in vocational service institutions rather than on-the-job training.

In the United States, the ANA calls both categories just discussed "allied nursing personnel," saying that the licensed practical nurse is a distinct occupational group and that nurse's aides, orderlies, and home health aides constitute another group. In Canada, nursing personnel with less preparation than the registered nurse are called "auxiliary nursing personnel."

In the United States, the estimated numbers of employed allied nursing personnel (including practical nurses) in 1972 totalled 1,327,-000, a considerably larger number than the 780,000 employed registered nurses and even more than the 1,127,657 registered nurses. In Canada, the licensed auxiliary nursing personnel totalled 45,945 in 1972, considerably less than the total 114,349 employed registered nurses in that country. However, since some auxiliary nursing personnel are not licensed, this comparison may be misleading.[335,336]

Allied or auxiliary nursing personnel are obviously giving a great deal of the nursing care in these (and other) countries, so it is of the utmost importance that their preparation be upgraded. While this question is not discussed here, it is recognized as part of the over-all aspect of nursing education.

Historical Background. Nursing education today is, like practice, changing rapidly, and these changes can be understood best by those who know its history. It has been the subject of more published volumes, more doctoral dissertations, and more journal articles than has any other nursing topic. National surveys of nursing schools and critical analyses of the system of nursing education in the United States date from Adelaide M. Nutting's study in 1912 to that of the current National Commission for the Study of Nursing and Nursing Education. At least five other major studies were reported in the intervening years. All of these reports have recommended that nursing schools be put under educational auspices rather than under hospitals, which are primarily service institutions, and that the preparation of nurses be comparable to that of other professionals, for example, teachers, doctors, and lawyers. In the United States, this means putting nursing schools in colleges and universities. Some individuals saw the desirability of this even in the nineteenth century. For example, Abby H. Woolsey,[337] the Civil War, self-taught nurse, in 1876 recommended the equivalent of a normal school education for nurses. (Normal schools of that day were in some respects like community colleges of today. They prepared most

teachers in the United States at that time.) Isabel A. Hampton made ardent appeals for a liberalized education for nurses, but she did not, according to Mary Roberts,[338] see the necessity of getting them out from under hospital control. In 1901, Mrs. Bedford Fenwick[339] of England gave four reasons behind her "plea for the higher education of trained nurses." Some physicians supported these nursing leaders. Among them was Richard C. Cabot,[340] who, in 1906, reported a local study showing the exploitation of nursing students by hospitals. One hospital earned $12,845.36 from payment to the hospital for services of student nurses to patients in their homes.* In 1910, Richard Olding Beard,[341] a physician, described the creation of a nursing school under university auspices at the University of Minnesota.

In 1912, Annie W. Goodrich,[342] in an article, "The Complete Nurse," discussed the complexity of nursing and the importance of social experience and a thorough education for the nurse. Hers was a life-long struggle to get schools of nursing into the universities. In 1921, Ethel Johns,[343] a Canadian nurse, presented the logic of placing nursing schools in universities and she described one degree program offered nurses in four of the Canadian universities.

In 1931, Dean E. P. Lyon[344] of the University of Minnesota Medical School read a paper at several state nurses' association meetings entitled "Taking the Profit Out of Nursing Education." He reported that at the University Hospital connected with the Schools of Medicine and Nursing, pupil nurses saved the hospital "around $20,000" a year. He called on nursing to follow the example of the medical profession, which, after the Flexner Report and through the AMA Council on Medical Education, no longer countenanced a medical school "connected with a profit-making college." Lyon's article was duplicated in nonmedical journals which showed some public interest in the question. Martha Dreiblatt,[345] for example, asked "Shall We Have Cheap Labor or Good Nurses?"

In 1937, a British physician, Harold Balme,[346] recommended the closing of non-approved schools and the inauguration of a "model college of nursing." In effect, he approved the position of nursing leaders in England and in North America, but college education for nurses in Great Britain has made

---

* In most educational systems, students can decide whether they will work to pay for their tuition; student nurses in the early schools had no choice; they all paid for their "training" by giving nursing service, or they worked their way through training.

comparatively little progress. In 1976 Roslyn Emblin and Michael J. Hill compiled descriptions of 14 degree courses in England, Scotland, and Wales. They made the following introductory statement: "Degree Courses in Nursing have evolved over a period of 15 years in this country and are therefore comparative newcomers to the scene of British Nurse Education." *

Isabel M. Stewart traced the evolution of collegiate nursing education in her monograph, *The Education of Nurses.*[347] Charles L. Russell, in 1958, reported a careful study of "Liberal Education and Nursing,"[348] showing the overwhelming support the ideas of such persons as have been mentioned received throughout their lives; he also showed the forces that held back the movement.

In 1965, the American Nurses' Association published its first "Position on Education for Nursing." It included the following statements:

The education for all those who are licensed to practice nursing should take place in institutions of higher education; minimum preparation for beginning professional nursing practice at the

present time should be baccalaureate degree education in nursing; minimum preparation for beginning technical nursing practice at the present time should be associate degree education in nursing; education for assistants in the health service occupations should be short, intensive preservice programs in vocational education institutions rather than on-the-job training programs.*

While the US President's Commission on Higher Education had made similar recommendations in 1947 and national studies of nursing education had repeatedly made some of these recommendations, the fact that the ANA's House of Delegates supported this position paper carried great weight.† In 1975, the ANA's Commission on Nursing Education issued *Standards for Nursing Education* covering graduate, basic (programs leading to baccalaureate and to associate degrees and to diplomas), and continuing education. The Commission claims "the responsibility for developing standards and devising methods for

---

* Emblin, Roslyn, and Hill, Michael J. (comps.): *Degree Courses in Nursing.* Nursing and Hospital Course Information Centre, London, and Association of Integrated and Degree Courses in Nursing, Guildford (Surrey), England, 1976, p. 1.

* American Nurses' Association, Committee on Education: "American Nurses' Association First Position on Education for Nursing," *Am. J. Nurs.,* **65:**106, (Dec.) 1965.

† The US President's Commission on Higher Education's *Higher Education for American Democracy* (US Government Printing Office, Washington, D.C., 1948, 6 pam.) included the discussion of educating practical nurses in junior colleges and of educating professional nurses in universities.

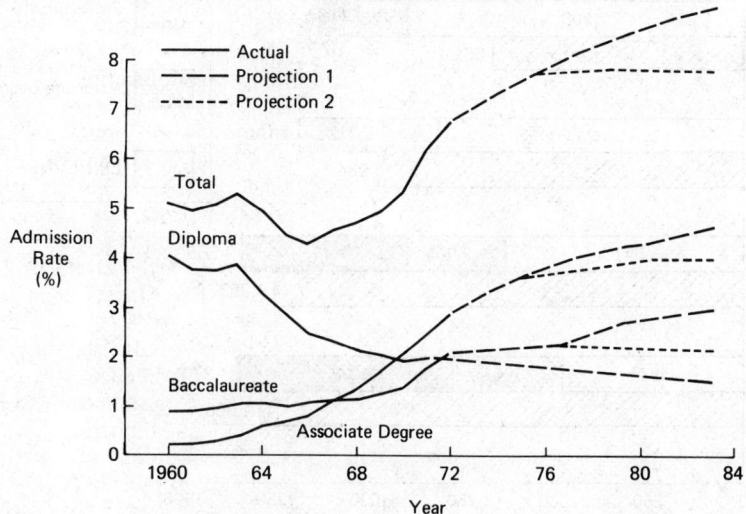

Note: Projection 1 assumes *W* increases to 1.00 in 1980–81. Projection 2 assumes *W* constant at 0.9 from 1973–74 to 1980–81.

Figure 1-27. Admissions to professional nursing schools as a per cent of female high school graduates by type of program. (From Jones, D. C., *et al.: Trends in Registered Nurse Supply.* US Government Printing Office, Washington, D.C., 1976, p. 75.)

gaining acceptance and implementation through appropriate channels." * The ANA's increasing concern for the education of nurses and for quality assurance is indirectly affecting all programs.

Regional and state commissions on higher education have had a marked effect on nursing education. They have promoted interdisciplinary understanding, joint planning, joint study, and sharing of facilities. They have promoted all collegiate education, baccalaureate and graduate, and have stimulated research.

Most states have now formed *statewide planning bodies* that are committed to "phasing out" diploma programs under hospital control. In fact, this has been accomplished in many states. In the Canadian provinces, diploma programs are no longer under hospital control (see

* American Nurses' Association, Commission on Nursing Education: *Standards for Nursing Education.* The Association, Kansas City, Mo., 1975, p. 33.

Fig. 1-26 showing the Canadian system of control). The National Commission for the Study of Nursing and Nursing Education [349] noted that, in the United States between 1958 and 1968, nearly 200 diploma programs closed and 350 associate and baccalaureate degree programs were established. The changing patterns of nursing education in the United States are shown in Figures 1-27 and 1-28 and Table 1-10.

Nursing education programs are undeniably moving out from under hospital control in the United States and other countries. There seems to be a parallel worldwide move to experiment in curriculum content, methods of teaching, length of programs, and a flexibility that enables students and practitioners to move from one program to another and from one type of health service to another. Health careers and *career ladders,* or career mobility, are the subjects of many articles here and abroad.[350-354] The Russian and Chinese patterns that facili-

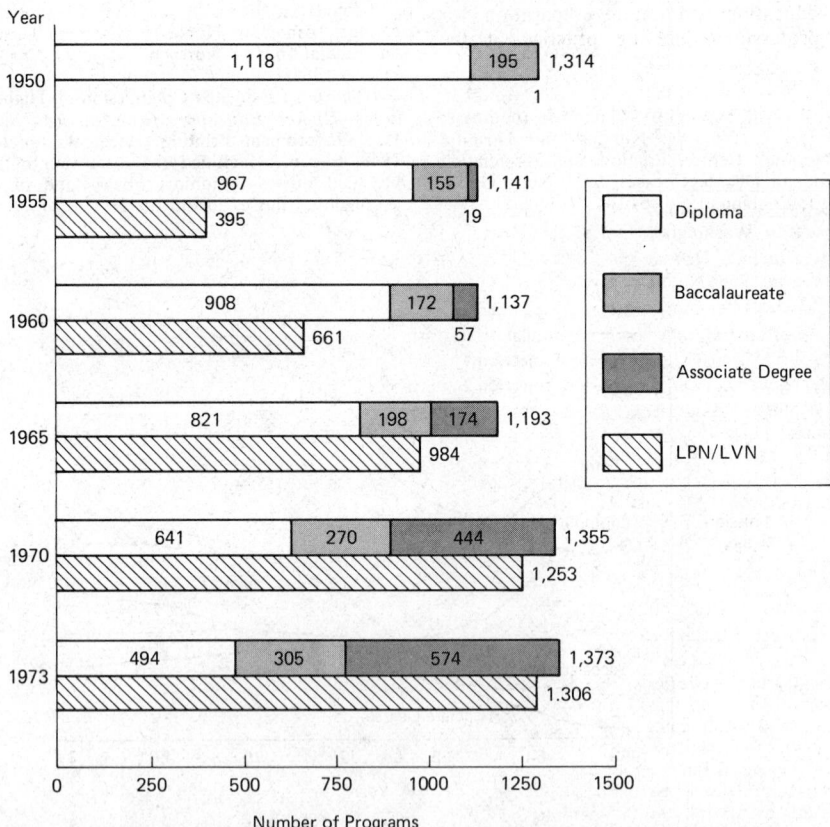

Figure 1-28. The changing patterns of nursing education from 1950 to 1973, showing rapid rise in number of LPN/LVN programs from 1955 on, increasing number of associate degree programs from 1950 on, a steady increase in baccalaureate degree programs, and rapid decline in diploma programs. (From Hudson, Helen H., and McCarthy, Margaret D.: *Source Book—Nursing Personnel.* US Government Printing Office, Washington, D.C., 1974, p. 75.)

Table 1-10.   State-Approved Schools of Nursing (RN) by Type of Program: 1950–73 *

Year †	Number of Schools	Number of Programs ‡			
		Total	Baccalaureate §	Diploma	Associate Degree
January:					
1950	1190	1314	195	1118	1
1952	1155	1263	198	1065	4
1953	1125	1236	198	1017	21
1954	1124	1237	215	992	30
1955	1129	1161	146	981	34
October:					
1955	1125	1141	155	967	19
1956	1115	1137	161	956	20
1957	1118	1138	166	944	28
1958	1125	1145	172	935	38
1959	1119	1137	171	918	48
1960	1123	1137	172	908	57
1961	1118	1126	174	883	69
1962	1128	1136	178	874	84
1963	1142	1148	183	860	105
1964	1153	1158	188	840	130
1965	1191	1193	198	821	174
1966	1219	1225	210	797	218
1967	1262	1269	221	767	281
1968	1287	1293	235	728	330
1969	1328	1339	254	695	390
1970	1343	1355	270	641	444
1971	1350	1363	285	587	491
1972	1363	1377	293	543	541
1973	1359	1373	305	494	574

* Hudson, Helen H., and McCarthy, Margaret D.: *Source Book—Nursing Personnel.* US Government Printing Office, Washington, D.C., 1974, p. 95.

† All years include Hawaii and Puerto Rico, Virgin Islands beginning 1965, Guam beginning 1966, and Alaska in 1968. Numbers include only schools with students enrolled on reporting date.

‡ Some schools offer more than one program.

§ Includes initial program leading to a master's degree.

SOURCES: National League for Nursing Education. *State-Approved Schools of Nursing.* New York, The League, 1950, 77 pp.

American Nurses' Association. *Facts About Nursing: A Statistical Summary.* New York, The Association, Annual eds.: 1952, p. 62; 1953, p. 64; 1954, p. 68; 1955–56, p. 89; 1957, p. 83; 1958, p. 86; 1959, p. 87; and 1965, p. 102.

National League for Nursing. *State-Approved Schools of Nursing—R.N.* New York, The League, Annual eds.: 1965–1974.

tate movement from one health specialty to another are under study in many countries.*

In the United States, the creation of the

* In Russia, *all* health workers belong to the same trade union, from the Minister of Health to the ward maids. There are 3 main categories of medical personnel: (1) higher—physicians and dentists; (2) middle—feldshers or physician's assistants, nurses (the most numerous), midwives, assistant sanitarians; (3) orderlies, porters, domestics, and "outside workers." In Russia, the most able student nurses and feldshers are encouraged to study medicine. The functions of both are limited and prescribed and they are taught by physicians. Nursing is not in every sense a separate profession in the USSR, and it is noted by nurse observers that physicians (who are proponderantly women in Russia) perform many functions that nurses in the United States perform.[355-357]

Federation of Associations of the Schools of the Health Professions should promote mobility, coordination of health careers, and emphasis on common knowledge and goals for health workers.[358] The National Commission for the Study of Nursing and Nursing Education urged the nursing profession to *experiment* in nursing education and to base change on such research. In 1973, the Commission identified as "emergent forces" *individualization, articulation,* and *concentration.*[359] The Division of Nursing in the US Public Health Service has funded a number of such experiments and the development of theoretical models.

While recognizing the need for experimentation, there are international, national, state, and provincial organizations and agencies that establish *standards* and some that *certify, qualify,* or *license* graduates of programs of specified length and content. In the United States, the National League for Nursing is now recognized as the agency that *accredits* programs nationally and the state boards approve schools within a state and also license graduates. This, however, is an oversimplification, for nursing programs in colleges and universities are also affected by regional accrediting bodies for all higher education. In 1974, the ANA House of Delegates passed a resolution to examine the feasibility of accrediting basic and graduate education programs. Later, the proposal was expanded to the study of all credentialing mechanisms in nursing (accreditation, certification, and licensure) and providing "quality assurance" to the public served and to recommend future directions for credentialing. The ANA contracted with the Center for Health Research, College of Nursing, Wayne State University, Detroit, Michigan, for a study proposal. (As stated earlier, the NLN considered joining the ANA in this study but finally decided not to do so.) [360]

Financing Nursing Education. Some of the most extensive research in nursing has focused on the philosophical question of who shall pay for nursing education, and on surveys showing who is paying for it. It is not practicable to attempt a systematic review of such studies in this chapter, but a number have been cited. If the question is discussed from an international standpoint it is soon obvious that some governments with national health insurance for all citizens have assumed the financial responsibility for preparing health personnel, including nurses, to provide care. Governments with national health insurance for only segments of the population are likely to assume less than total financial responsibility for preparing health workers.

In the United States, funds for the education of health personnel come from both public and private sectors. Parents, for example, may pay the full cost of medical or nursing education for their sons and daughters; scholarships and fellowships are available from a wide variety of private foundations, professional organizations, commissions, agencies, and institutions, and from commercial sources. However, funds from the federal government have been available for nursing education since World War I and World War II, as is pointed out on page 42. State funds are also used for the educa-

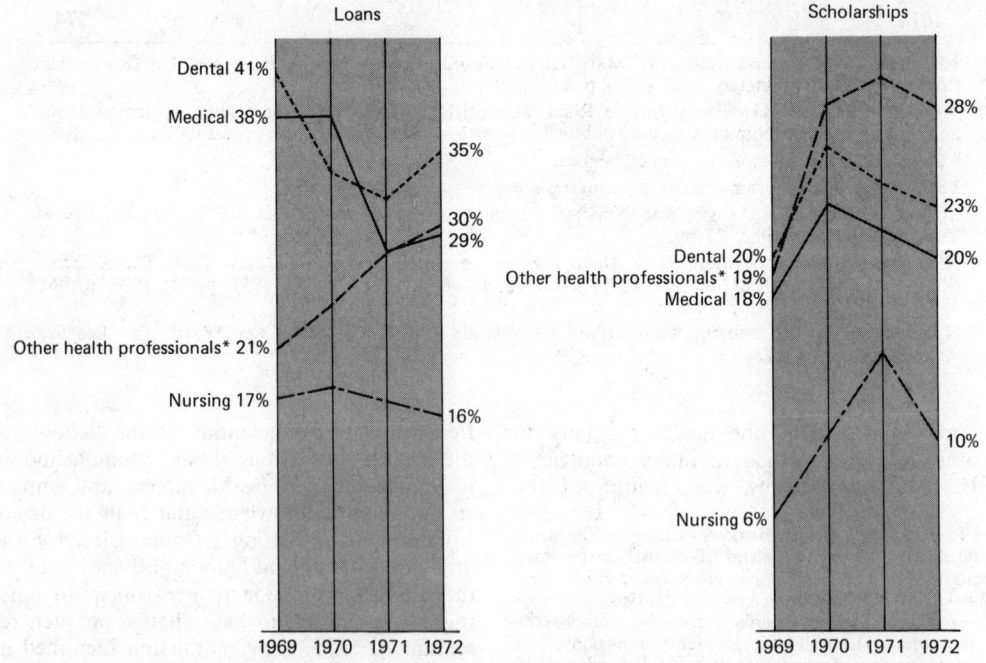

*Includes students of optometry, pharmacy, podiatry, and veterinary medicine only.

Figure 1-29. Percentage of health professions students receiving federal funds for loans and scholarships, 1969–72. (From Center for Health Policy Studies, National Planning Association: *Chartbook of Federal Health Spending 1969–74.* The Association, Washington, D.C., 1974, p. 27.)

tion of health personnel since they support state colleges, universities, and vocational institutes that assume a large proportion of the cost of educating their students. States may have scholarships and loan funds for students.

Table 1-11 shows the federal funds spent on nursing education by agency from 1968 to 1974. The total spent increased from $60,539,-000 in 1969 to $127,243,000 in 1974. Figure 1-30 shows comparative data on federal funds for education of selected health professions, 1969 and 1974. More funds were available for research personnel than for physicians, more for physicians than for nurses, and less for dentists than for either of the latter. The remainder for "other health professionals and nondegree noncertificate training" constituted 44 per cent of the whole in 1974. The total manpower training budget increased 54 per cent from 1969 to 1974 and rose to $1,385,-000,000 "current dollars." Figure 1-31 shows percentage of students of health professions receiving federal funds for loans and scholarships 1969–1972 (from the Bureau of Health Manpower Education).

Since federal funding is dependent in all countries on politics, such figures as shown here represent past but not necessarily future policy. It is obvious that the trend is in the direction of greater public support of nursing education in the United States, but this trend could be reversed at any time.

There is in both private and public sectors an effort to draw more students from minorities into programs for health workers. Data on minority students is given in a 1974 publication of the US Department of Health, Education, and Welfare, *How to Pay for Your Health Career Education. A Guide for Minority Students* (Pub. No. [HRA] 74–8). Based on a 1969 survey, the total average expenditures for nursing school students were given as follows: $4128 for a 3-year diploma program; $4142 for a 2-year associate degree program; and $9744 for a 4-year baccalaureate program. The cost for 1973 was estimated as 3 per cent higher (see Table 1-12).

For readers who want detailed information on financing nursing education, the following publications of the NLN might be consulted: *Financial Management for Schools of Nursing; The Cost of Nursing Education* (1974); *A Preliminary Report on Methodological Problems* (1975); *Scholarships, Fellowships, Educational Grants and Loans for Registered Nurses* (1975). Such publications are available from comparable nursing organizations in other countries.

Length and General Nature of the Curricula in Basic, or Initial, Programs. All registered nurses in the United States must currently complete a basic course of study that measures up to standards set by a state board of nurse examiners. Comparable boards or bodies have this regulating function in the provinces of Canada, in Great Britain, and in other countries.

In Chapter 3, there is further discussion of the development of nursing education. It is pointed out there that chaotic conditions in the

Table 1-11. Federal Funds for Nursing Education by Agency, Fiscal Years 1968–74 in Thousands of Dollars *

Agency	1968	1969	1970	1971	1972	1973	1974
Total	—	$60,539	$71,884	$80,496	$95,482	$128,819	$127,243
Department of Health, Education and Welfare	$43,772	46,644	59,851	66,778	76,557	112,063	109,503
HSA: Health Services	393	408	485	468	1,034	847	1,227
HSA: Indian Health Service	70	74	128	134	97	101	105
HRA: Bureau of Health Manpower Education	31,891	35,690	47,143	54,516	58,255	99,198	99,569
Alcohol, Drug Abuse, and Mental Health Administration	10,399	9,394	10,980	10,624	13,292	7,726	4,380
Social and Rehabilitation Service	508	486	500	420	160	181	145
Office of Education	—	—	—	—	3,090	3,090	3,105
Other HEW †	511	592	615	616	629	920	972
Appalachian Regional Commission	NA	105	398	327	398	478	279
Department of Defense	NA	11,892	9,307	10,775	15,487	12,710	13,351
Veterans Administration	NA	1,898	2,328	2,616	3,040	3,568	4,110

* Russell, Louise B., et al.: *Federal Health Spending 1969–74.* Center for Health Policy Studies, National Planning Association, Washington, D.C., 1974, p. 35.

† Howard University, Freedman's Hospital and/or St. Elizabeth's Hospital.

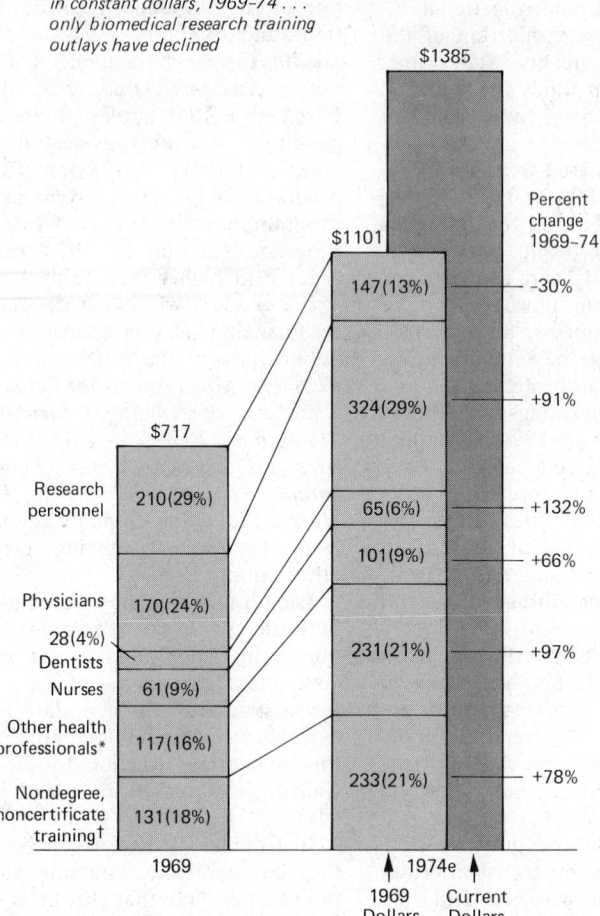

Health manpower training budget increased 54% in constant dollars, 1969–74 . . . only biomedical research training outlays have declined

*Students of optometry, podiatry, veterinary medicine, pharmacy, public health, and allied health professions.
†Short-term and refresher courses for health professionals, public education programs, and training of federal agency staff.

Figure 1-30. Comparative data on federal funds for education of selected health professionals, 1969 and 1974. (From Center for Health Policy Studies, National Planning Association: *Chartbook of Federal Health Spending 1969–74. The Association*, Washington, D.C., 1974, p. 20.)

rapidly increasing number of schools under hospital ownership in the United States led to publication by the National League of Nursing Education in 1917 of *The Standard Curriculum*. It gave the length of the program, the total numbers of hours of organized or classroom instruction, the clinical hospital services (medicine and surgery and their specialties, obstetrics and pediatrics) on which students should have experience, and even the disease conditions they should have seen and the nursing skills, arts, techniques, or procedures they should be able to perform.

The concept of rigid standards was gradually modified and it is now replaced by the en-

couragement of flexibility and experimentation.*

The following description of initial nursing programs or curricula is based on a study of selected current bulletins or catalogues from 17 schools offering initial (Registered Nurse) baccalaureate programs in the north, south, east, and west of the United States. Bulletins of diploma and associate degree programs were

---

* The present dissimilarity in initial programs and the varied and often ambiguous titles of courses (especially nursing courses) may lead to another effort on the part of national nursing organizations and concerned citizens to clearly define the purpose and nature of the preparation for general nursing.

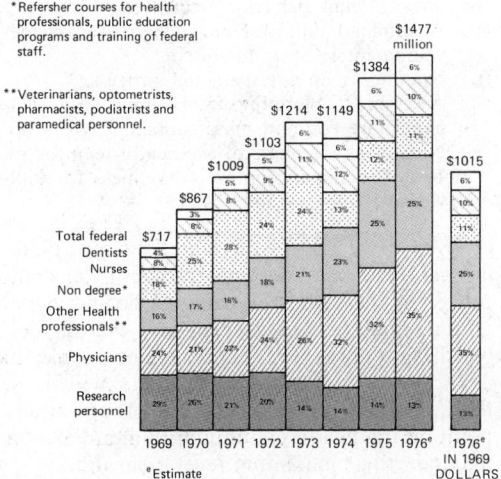

* Refersher courses for health professionals, public education programs and training of federal staff.

** Veterinarians, optometrists, pharmacists, podiatrists and paramedical personnel.

Total federal
Dentists
Nurses
Non degree*
Other Health professionals**
Physicians
Research personnel

1969 1970 1971 1972 1973 1974 1975 1976° 1976°
°Estimate IN 1969 DOLLARS

Figure 1-31. Federal outlays (in millions of dollars) for training of health professionals (physicians, dentists, nurses, and others). (From Koleda, Michael S., et al.: *The Federal Health Dollar: 1969–1976; A Chartbook of Analysis of Activities Supported and Strategies Pursued in Federal Expenditures for Health.* Center for Health Policy Studies, National Planning Association, Washington, D.C., 1977, p. 47.)

also studied, but less data on them is given here.

Diploma programs under hospital auspices are usually 3 years in length, associate degree programs in junior colleges 2 years in length, and baccalaureate programs 4 years in length, although nursing content may be concentrated in the last 2 years. Some initial nursing programs in universities may require a bachelor's degree from an academic program as an admission requirement. In such cases the program is usually 2 years in length and in several schools the student is awarded a master's degree in nursing.

Of 1372 initial (R.N.) programs in the

Table 1-12. Average Expenses for Nursing School Students in Initial Programs According to a 1969 Survey (in 1973 the estimated increase was 5 per cent and by 1978 might be 10 per cent) *

Program	*Average Expenses for Nursing School Students*	
	One Year Expenses All Classes All Schools	Total Expenses During Program
Diploma	$1376	$4128 (3 years)
Associate Degree	2071	4142 (2 years)
Baccalaureate	2436	9744 (4 years)

Costs in 1973 are estimated to be about 5 per cent higher for the nursing education programs than when the survey was made.

* US Department of Health, Education, and Welfare: *How to Pay for Your Health Career Education. A Guide for Minority Students.* US Government Printing Office, Washington, D.C., 1974, p. 5 (DHEW Pub. No. [HRA] 74–8).

United States in 1974, 461 were diploma, 598 were associate degree, and 313 were baccalaureate (see Tables 1-13). However, of the total students admitted to these programs in the fall of 1974, 26,943 were admitted to diploma programs, 48,596 to associate degree programs, and 32,672 to baccalaureate programs.[361] Study of available data shows the number of graduations from diploma programs decreasing and the numbers of associate degree and baccalaureate programs increasing and graduations from them increasing. The highest growth rate in graduations is from the baccalaureate programs.

Purpose of Initial Programs. Most nursing school bulletins of this decade that were consulted gave the school's philosophy, and the goals or purposes growing out of the philosophy, which usually contains a definition of

Table 1-13. Number of Programs That Prepare Registered Nurse and Practical Nurse Graduates for Beginning Practice for the Years 1970–74 *

Academic Year	Associate Degree	Diploma	Bacca-laureate	Total Basic R.N. Programs	Practical or Vocational	Grand Total
1970	444	641	270	1355	1253	2608
1971	491	587	285	1363	1291	2654
1972	541	543	293	1377	1310	2687
1973	574	494	305	1373	1306	2679
1974	598	461	313	1372	1315	2687

* National League for Nursing, Division of Research: "Educational Preparation for Nursing—1974." (Report prepared by Walter L. Johnson.) *Nurs. Outlook,* **23:**578, (Sept.) 1975.

nursing. The following statement is from the Faculty of Nursing of Syracuse University:

Professional nursing is a deliberative process of human interaction designed to promote, maintain, and restore the health of individuals, families, and communities. This is achieved through the provision of care and comfort while assisting in the channeling of energies for maximum use of extrinsic and intrinsic resources to cope with stress in order to move toward a state of effective adaptation, including a peaceful and dignified death.*

The University of Texas System School of Nursing (with branches in six cities) defined nursing in the following terms:

Professional nursing practice involves assessing health needs, and planning, providing, directing, and evaluating nursing care for individuals and groups in a variety of settings. It is a scientifically-based process devoted to helping individuals, families, and groups make maximum use of their resources in meeting their respective health needs. It further incorporates the individualities of nurse and patient/client and is most effective when the thoughts, feelings, and values of both are recognized; therefore, a high degree of communication skill and sensitivity in interpersonal situations is required. The obligation to improve nursing practice encompasses the use of knowledge and skills as well as the systematic study of the effects of this practice on human health.†

This university system listed seven "beliefs and knowledge" which the graduate of the baccalaureate program would have, sixteen "skills" they would have in assessment, planning, implementation, and practice, and four characteristics of their practice. The purpose of the programs was to help students acquire these skills and characteristics.

The Faculty of the School of Nursing at the University of Rochester, in describing its basic program, said:

The faculty believe that nursing is a useful occupation, a service rendered by one human being for another, or for a group, in which knowledge is drawn from the health sciences and applied to the maintenance and restoration of physical and mental well-being of persons and in that the nurse acts in the interests of the person or persons being served.‡

The University of Oregon School of Nursing defined nursing as "a process of interaction with the following characteristics":

(a) Nursing contributes to and makes use of the physical and behavioral sciences.
(b) An understanding of normal growth and development is basic to nursing.
(c) Nursing is an interpersonal process.
(d) Assessment, planning, intervention, and evaluation are components of nursing.
(e) Nurses, as members of the health team, work toward achieving optimum wellness for individuals, families and society.*

The University of Maryland School of Nursing said the baccalaureate program "is committed to the total well-being of an individual and demonstrates a respect for the dignity, worth, autonomy and uniqueness of people. In a variety of settings, the graduate will assist the individual and selected small groups at any point on the health continuum to attain and/or maintain their maximum level of health." †

The Faculty of the Frances Payne Bolton School of Nursing of Case Western Reserve University stated its "concept of professional nursing practice" as a collaborative process:

Professional nursing shares with other health professionals responsibility for meeting the health needs of society. Nursing, as an integral part of the health care delivery system, shares responsibility for working collaboratively toward attaining optimal health for all members of society.‡

In a lengthy statement the following paragraphs showed the emphasis placed on health as opposed to disease:

Professional nursing is responsible for the promotion, restoration and maintenance of an optimal state of health for individuals, families, groups and the community. Professional nursing practice includes nursing actions which assist persons to cope with physiological, psychological, and socio-cultural threats to health.

Professional nursing is responsible for formulating a nursing diagnosis based upon systematic collection of data about the health status of the individual. The plan of care and subsequent nursing actions are goal directed, derived from the nursing diagnosis and based upon knowledge of social, behavioral, biological, physical, medical and nursing sciences. Nursing actions which are performed humanely and competently, are also based upon the creation of interpersonal relationships and an environment conducive to optimal functioning. These actions and plan of care are eval-

* Syracuse University: Bulletin, School of Nursing. The University, Syracuse, N.Y., Dec. 1971, p. 6.
† University of Texas System School of Nursing: 1975–1976 Catalogue. The University, Austin, El Paso, Fort Worth, etc., p. 52.
‡ University of Rochester: Official Bulletin, University of Rochester, 1974–1975, Undergraduate Studies. The University, Rochester, N.Y., p. 217.

* University of Oregon: Bulletin. University of Oregon School of Nursing, Portland, 1974–1975. The University, Portland, p. 12.
† University of Maryland: School of Nursing, University of Maryland at Baltimore, 1974–1975. The University, Baltimore, p. 27.
‡ Case Western Reserve University: Frances Payne Bolton School of Nursing Bulletin: 1974–1975. The University, Cleveland, p. 8.

uated continually and systematically in terms of the stated goals and the person's responses.*

Later in the bulletin, under "Philosophy of Undergraduate Education," the purpose of the basic nursing education was briefly and clearly expressed:

Baccalaureate education in nursing at Case Western Reserve University constitutes the essential minimal preparation for the beginning professional nurse practitioner, who is a generalist. The educational program prepares nurse practitioners to engage in primary, acute and long-term care of people of all ages and in a variety of settings.†

The preceding statements taken from six recent university nursing school bulletins from the north, south, west, east, and middle of the United States suggest diversity rather than unanimity of thinking about basic programs, although the diversity may be more a matter of style than substance. At least the statements show that these initial baccalaureate nursing programs were designed to prepare graduates to give nursing care to people of all ages and in all settings.

"Nursing" was obviously believed to include promotion of health and prevention of disease as well as care of the sick. Some faculties saw the basic program as preparing "nurse generalists" and "nurse practitioners" to give "primary, acute, and long-term care."

Statements on philosophy and purpose in the bulletins of hospital diploma programs tended to be less elaborate than those of baccalaureate programs, and those consulted did not claim to prepare "nurse practitioners" for giving primary, acute, and long-term care.‡ All types of initial programs were said to prepare graduates for further study, either continuing education, admission to baccalaureate programs for diploma graduates, or admission to graduate (master's) programs.

Main Divisions of the Initial (Basic) Nursing Programs. According to their current bulletins the curricula of 17 initial baccalaureate nursing programs listed courses that might be classified into (1) *the humanities,* (2) *biological and physical sciences,* (3) *social sciences, and* (4) *medical and nursing arts and sciences.*

Programs leading to a baccalaureate degree in nursing were usually 4 years in length. Nursing courses might be concentrated in the last 2 years or might be distributed. Nursing courses were based on the assumption that the student

had some knowledge of the humanities and sciences.

Of the 17 schools whose bulletins were analyzed, about half used the blanket term *humanities,* but all specified courses in English literature and composition (or "speech communication" or "nature of language"); a few specified ethics, philosophy, logic, religion, history, and music appreciation.

Physical and biologic sciences were universally required, either as an element in the nursing curriculum or as prerequisites. These courses were listed under 20 different titles. All programs included human anatomy and physiology, either as separate or combined courses. Pathology might be combined with physiology and called pathophysiology. All programs examined included chemistry; two, biochemistry; one, nutritional biochemistry; one, biophysics and biochemistry; one, chemistry and physics of life; one program recommended but did not require physics; several listed zoology and biology; one offered a course entitled "Science, Elegance, and Discovery." All programs included microbiology, or bacteriology (the more common term); one listed advanced microbiology and immunology. Only ten programs listed nutrition—normal and therapeutic; one, food and nutrition; one, nutrition and dietetics. Physical education was listed as a requirement in five programs. While the above titles vary, there seems to be far more uniformity in thinking about the biologic and physical sciences than any other aspects of initial nursing curricula.

Required or recommended *social sciences* were listed under 43 different titles, some so vague or ambiguous, even in the course description, as to defy classification under any traditional terms. All programs included straight sociology, although the following titles might belong under this heading: Social Change, American Society, Social Systems Analysis, and Marriage and Family. Psychology was included in all 17 programs, and the following courses, either required or recommended, might fall under psychology: Human Life Cycle, Growth Development, Human Development, Deviations in Growth and Development, Abnormal Psychology, Group Dynamics, Psychological Adaptation in Health and Illness, Behavioral Science, Human Behavior, Behavioral Social Science, Child Psychology, and Adolescent and Adult Psychology.

Anthropology was required in eight programs, and some courses mentioned above, for instance, American Society, might fall under this heading rather than sociology.

There was little indication that schools of nursing were trying to help their graduates

---

* *Ibid.*
† *Ibid.,* p. 13.
‡ For definitions of these terms, see pages 31 and 32. Bulletins using these terms would do well to define them since they presently have different meanings.

understand political forces underlying health care systems, or how to effect changes in them. However, one program included Principles of Management, one included Health and Illness in American Society, another Social Systems Analysis, and another Health Care Systems. Statistics, required in four programs, and Man and the Computer required in one, might be mentioned in this connection, although these courses are probably more related to the conduct of research in health and disease, health sciences, or medical and nursing arts and sciences than to the politics of health care.

Courses here classified as *nursing or medical arts and sciences* were listed under 140 titles in 17 bulletins analyzed and it is hard to group them under such traditional terms as hygiene, epidemiology, public health, pathology, therapeutics, maternal and child care (obstetrical and pediatric nursing), geriatric nursing, mental health, or neurologic and psychiatric nursing. Nor can they be classified under nursing in various settings such as hospitals, clinics, schools, homes, or industries. Some designers of nursing programs were obviously trying to get away from emphasis on the hospital setting and were stressing health promotion rather than care of the ill. Medical terminology seems to be rejected in part but not totally.

Studying current bulletins, it is hard to find how much experience students have in any setting, although most state board requirements are still relatively specific about the clinical experience students must have, so this information may be available in the school's records.

The following is an attempt to show the main subdivisions of the category which we, in this analysis, arbitrarily call *Medical and Nursing Arts and Sciences*, since, as courses are now titled, it is impossible to separate them. Nursing students were once introduced to health promotion and the prevention of disease in courses with titles such as hygiene, sanitation, epidemiology, and public health. Such terms seem to be in disuse, but the following titles may be related to them. Introduction to Public Health Science, Principles of Epidemiology and Research, Health and Society, Health Care Delivery, Health Promotion, Human Awareness in the Health Professions, Comprehensive Health Planning, and Public Health Fundamentals. Such courses are sometimes tied to the students' experience in so-called community (extra-hospital) nursing, which, in some form, is probably common to all baccalaureate programs.

Nursing students were formerly or traditionally introduced to pathology and therapeutics under courses so titled or, perhaps, called Introduction to Medical Sciences. Two schools listed a course entitled Pathology, but some other courses listed in the 17 bulletins analyzed that might relate to pathology and therapeutics included the following: Medical Science, Biomedical Science, Pathophysiology, Pathophysiological Basis of Nursing Practice (two programs), Basic Nursing Science, Clinical Nursing Science, Systemic Investigation, Introduction to Basic Concepts of Illness, and possibly an interdisciplinary course entitled Patient, Professional, and Society.

Nursing students were traditionally introduced to nursing practice or the science and art of nursing by giving aspects of care to selected patients on medical, surgical, and maternal and child care services of the hospital, with an accompanying course that emphasized the acquisition of basic nursing skills. An obvious effort is now made to offer students early experiences that are not hospital- or sickness-dominated and that may be creative rather than technical. The words "procedures," "skills," and "techniques" are used infrequently. Some schools build the nursing curriculum around such concepts as Man and Health, Man and Stress, Man and Adaptation, Health Issues Affecting Family and Community Life, Dynamics of Nursing, the Nursing Process, Nursing in Health Crises, Nursing Intervention in Health Crises, Crisis Theory. One school listed seven courses under the over-all title of Nursing Science; another listed four courses under Foundations of Nursing. One school offered a course that reviewed or studied current concepts or theories of nursing, and many listed courses in Nursing Process, although course descriptions suggested that this term meant different things to different faculties.

Some schools had titles for beginning nursing courses that were quite specific. For example, five schools listed Introduction to Nursing, four listed Nursing Fundamentals, one listed Health Skills, another Principles of Nursing Care, another Basic Nursing Sciences and Clinical Nursing Science. It is not easy to find out where students participate in the care of either well clients or sick patients.

Obviously, all schools offered study of and experience in care of mothers and children, but even here terminology was far from uniform. The following are titles that specifically related to maternal and child care: Maternal Child Nursing (six programs offered this course), Maternal and Newborn Nursing, Nursing of Children, Nursing in the Beginning of Life Cycle, Nursing in the Evolving Life Cycle, Nursing with Individual Families and Groups in Health and Illness. Other related titles included Family and Community Patterns in

Health and Illness, Growth and Development, Obstetrical Nursing and Clinical Experience in Obstetrical Nursing (two programs), Maternity Nursing, Pediatric Nursing (two programs), and Clinical Experience in Pediatric Nursing, Nursing Care of Adults and Children, Family Centered Adult-Child Nursing, Health Issues Affecting Family and Community Life. Only one bulletin listed the course Human Sexuality.

Geriatric nursing was not listed as such and mentioned only once under Care of Adult Patients (Medical-Surgical Geriatrics), but might be included in many of the courses that were organized around the development of man from birth to death. Specific preparation in the care of the dying did not seem to have been considered by faculties of the baccalaureate programs sampled except to be mentioned as a topic in several course descriptions.

There is little doubt that all nursing students in these schools have experience in the units of a hospital where patients are treated medically and surgically. In graduate programs medical-surgical nursing courses were commonly listed but in the 17 bulletins that described baccalaureate programs, only four listed Medical and Surgical Nursing, or Medical-Surgical Nursing. However, six schools listed Pharmacology, one listed Introduction to the Administration of Medications, one listed Operating Room-Continuous Care Experience, and one listed Care of the Chronically Ill.

Psychiatric Nursing was listed in five bulletins, Psychiatric and Mental Health Nursing in two programs. Courses under the following titles are probably substitutes for or related to psychiatric nursing: Modern Concepts in Psychiatric Nursing, Reading in Psychiatric Nursing, Communication and Interviewing, Crises Theory, Dynamics of Interpersonal Relationships, Behavioral Concepts in Nursing, Dynamics of Nursing, Human Behavior, Human Relations, Psychopathology, Man and Stress, Man and Adaptation, Intervention in Crises Throughout Life, Therapeutic Strategies of Mental Health, Therapeutic Communication and Psychopathology, Psychosocial Dynamics in Nursing, Nursing Communications (two programs), and Dynamics of Human Relations.

In only three bulletins was Public Health Nursing listed; two bulletins listed Community Health Nursing. It is quite clear, however, that most schools offered nursing experience in and related study of health care outside the hospital. Some courses that suggested this include the following: Family and Community Patterns in Health and Illness, Nursing in the Social Order, Ecology of Nursing, Nursing with Individual Families, Group Concepts in

Health and Illness, Comprehensive Health Planning, Public Health Fundamentals, Nursing in Society, Introduction to Public Health Science, Family and Community Nursing, Family Counselling, Rural County Nursing, and Nursing in Health Care Systems. The nature and scope of extra-hospital nursing experience offered students is hard to assess, but programs seem quite dissimilar in this respect.

Seven bulletins listed Independent Study and a number said that students might elect to concentrate on an "area"; one listed Senior Clinical Nursing, others Advanced Nursing, Individual Study in Nursing, Advanced Clinical Experience in Nursing, Advanced Nursing Process in Major Health Areas, and Senior Seminar (supporting independent study, specialized topics in nursing). Courses entitled Nursing Research were offered in four programs, but Explorations in Nursing, Directed Reading or Research, and Senior Honors Thesis were other titles suggesting that students were introduced to research. It is obvious that many baccalaureate programs were trying to prepare graduates for the (admittedly ill-defined but much-discussed) "expanded role." Two schools listed Nursing Assessment, one school listed Health Assessment, another Process of Clinical Judgment, another Concepts of Illness, another Clinical Health Skills, one Physical Examination, and another Systemic Investigation. Descriptions of clinical courses and independent study stress the intent of helping the student acquire independence in making clinical judgment. One bulletin listed courses, Introduction to Primary Health Care and Introduction to Secondary Health Care.

Initial or basic nursing programs traditionally included courses in nursing history, current trends, and problems and opportunities within the profession. Only one bulletin listed History of Nursing, but three listed Issues and Trends in Nursing and Health Care; two listed Legal Aspects of Health Care, one Nursing in the Social Order, three Nursing Leadership and Management in Nursing, one Principles of Administration and Leadership, one Nursing in the Changing Order, one Study of the Nursing Profession, one Nursing in Society, one Background for Nursing, one Patterns of Organization for Nursing Leadership, one Perspectives in Nursing, one Leadership Responsibilities in Nursing, and one Principles of Management and Leadership.

Differences in Baccalaureate Programs. For those unfamiliar with nursing in the United States, the preceding pages must present a confused picture. It is an indication that the selected schools represented here are experimenting and trying to develop a new pattern of nursing education. Nursing *is* a new profession and nursing education in the United States *is* obviously floundering. Nurse educators Claire M. Fagin, Margaret McClure, and Rozella Schlotfeldt, in the January, 1976, issue of the *American Journal of Nursing,* try to answer the question "Can We Bring Order Out of the Chaos of Nursing Education?" They noted that three programs ranging from 2 to 4 years in length prepared graduates to write state board examinations enabling them to be registered nurses. Functions or competences of associate degree (2-year), diploma (3-year), and baccalaureate (4-year) graduates have never been satisfactorily differentiated, and Fagin thinks the public is unaware of the differences. (Actually, in the writer's opinion, the public finds difficulty in differentiating between the registered nurse and the practical nurse in the United States.)

Fagin and McClure concluded that registered "professional" nurses should be at least graduates of baccalaureate programs in universities and that practical nurse programs should be merged with associate degree programs in junior colleges to prepare a second category of nursing personnel. They pointed out that this conclusion was reached repeatedly in national studies of nursing education from 1948 on. They would retain the two nursing licenses since new ones would only add to public confusion. The baccalaureate program would prepare persons licensed as the professional nurse (RN) who is capable of "self-directed" work and the associate degree program would prepare the "technical" or practical nurse. Both writers admitted the drawbacks in these terms and they failed, in our opinion, to clearly state the difference between the role of the technical or practical nurse and that of the professional nurse.

Schlotfeldt took a different position. She said professional nurses should be as thoroughly prepared for their special function as are physicians for theirs, and she recommended a doctor of nursing (D.N.) as the initial degree. She thinks the promotion of health and the prevention of disease—the nurses' special contribution—as important and as difficult as treatment, which is the physician's special province, and she aligned her position on the nurse's role with that of Florence Nightingale's, the founder of "modern" nursing. She put her position in the following terms:

Nursing's right to create a future in which nurses can provide people with the kind of care that promotes healthy, productive, rewarding, and happy lives inheres in its magnificent heritage.

It was Florence Nightingale, the brilliant and visionary founder of modern nursing, who, over a century ago, explicated the nature of nursing in terms of its goals and outcomes. She clearly established nursing's practice focus to be that of assessing and promoting the health status, health assets, and health potential of human beings of all ages, all nationalities, all races, and all varieties of human circumstances.*

The New York State Nurses' Association has proposed legislation to make a baccalaureate base mandatory for professional nurse licensure. The American Association of Colleges of Nursing has developed a model licensure law that makes a B.S. a base for "nurse" licensure and the junior college degree a base for the "nursing associate." Even these proposals are meeting with opposition, so it would be difficult to implement the Schlotfeldt recommendations in the near future, even if nurses, physicians, and the public could accept the assumption that health promotion and prevention of disease is a function separate from the cure of disease. While it may be generally accepted that the nurse is more expert in care than is the physician and the physician more expert in cure than is the nurse, these two workers presently perform both functions. As long as there are situations in which nurses are the best prepared health workers available to the public, they are forced into the curing role, and, in rare cases, when there is no nurse available, physicians must assume the caring role or their patients will die.

Nursing education has for many years accepted medical education as its model. The care of patients has usually been organized, patients actually housed, around the physician's diagnosis and treatment plan. Patients of all ages with tuberculosis or with cancer were once segregated, for example, or patients to undergo surgery were often segregated according to the region of the body or the surgical specialist performing the operation, for example, the orthopedic surgeon or the neurosurgeon. Diseases have been classified under the *systems* affected and formal instruction organized this way. Nursing State Boards have required a certain number of weeks' experience in hospital divisions established to a large extent for the convenience of physicians and surgeons under the systems classification.

It has been, and still is, most convenient for urologists to have all their patients in one place, although they are of both sexes and all ages; some bedfast, others ambulatory. The same thing holds for the cardiologist, the ophthalmologist, or the dermatologist. In recent

* Schlotfeldt, Rozella: "Can We Bring Order Out of the Chaos of Nursing Education? Rozella Schlotfeldt says . . . ," *Am. J. Nurs.,* **76:**105, (Jan.) 1976.

years, this system of segregating patients has been questioned and other schemes substituted. Some medical centers have, for example, segregated patients according to the amount of help they need from the institution's staff. People who come to the center for diagnosis and can take care of themselvs may stay in a unit that is run very much like an inn or hotel; those who are ambulatory but need some help are housed in another unit and so on until those who need most help are in intensive care units. Some large state neuropsychiatric hospitals have been broken down into small autonomous units that house patients according to the county, city, or town of which they are residents. Infants and children may or may not be segregated.

This reassembling of patients is one reason why some faculties believe that medical-surgical nursing and pediatric nursing are no longer valid courses in the curriculum. Another reason that these courses are questioned is that they have been hospital-oriented and disease-oriented. Nurse educators are trying to give students experience as observers or participants in extra-hospital health services, for example, private homes, schools, industries, neighborhood health maintenance units, and even penal institutions, and are searching for terminology in describing courses that will convey the prevalent philosophy that health care is an inherent right of all people everywhere.

The multiplicity of nursing courses, or titles used to describe them, suggests that, while faculties are striving to break the hospital- and disease-oriented mold that has dominated both nursing and medical education, it is not easy to identify a new pattern for the current initial or basic program.

While the traditional pattern of nursing education seems to be under fire, all the 17 baccalaureate programs examined have not relinquished it. The Frances Payne Bolton School of Nursing at Case Western Reserve University gives the following courses in "a typical program plan": General Chemistry, Organic Chemistry, General Biology, Anatomy, Human Physiology, Microbiology, Sociology or Anthropology, Growth and Development, Introduction to Basic Concepts of Illness, Pharmacology, Nutrition, Statistics, Fundamentals of Nursing, Medical and Surgical Nursing, Maternal and Newborn Nursing, Nursing of Children, Nursing in the Social Order, Public Health Nursing, Psychiatric Nursing, and Senior Clinical Nursing.*

Because this section has presented such a confusing picture of current basic or initial

curricula, the writer offers in the next sections some curricula suggestions. It is hoped that among other concepts they may encourage interdisciplinary study, emphasize helping people everywhere with health problems (rather than nursing the acutely ill in hospitals), and encourage the self-reliance of patients or clients (rather than fostering dependence).

5. SUGGESTIONS FOR INITIAL, OR BASIC, NURSING CURRICULA

An Interdisciplinary Approach. The Division of Health Manpower Development in the World Health Organization seems to recognize the interrelation of education for health workers. Two of its publications are entitled *Development of Educational Programmes for the Health Professions* (1973) [362] and *Educational Strategies for the Health Professions* (1974). [363] Various contributors to these publications discuss program planning, educational objectives, curricula design, preparation of faculty, and methods of teaching. Most of the studies reported were conducted at the Center for Educational Development, University of Illinois College of Medicine, which has been made a WHO Collaborating Institute; most focus on the education of medical students, but Tamaś Fülöp, director of the Division of Health Manpower Development in WHO, stresses the organization's "comprehensive, co-ordinated long-term programs for teachers of medical and allied health sciences." * Lippard was quoted on page 61 as saying that the medical school faculty as an entity might cease to exist. Pellegrino, [364] in 1972, discussed the Carnegie Commission's recommendation that 126 area health education centers be established to "improve education in the health professions." As its Dean, Pellegrino described the health "consortium" at the New York State University Center at Stony Brook—the "Health Science Center-Medical School" which is an implementation of this concept. There students of "medicine, dentistry, nursing, allied health, basic health sciences and social work" can study together in many courses and use the same facilities. Since we believe this to be the prototype of future schools for health workers, a nursing curriculum is suggested in the following pages that seems to the writer to fit into a health-science center. The prerequisite

---

* Case Western Reserve University: *op. cit.*

* Miller, George E., and Fülöp, Tamaś (eds.): *Educational Strategies for the Health Professions.* World Health Organization, Geneva, 1974, p. 89 (Public Health Paper No. 61).

courses could be taken with students in any other discipline, and the third phase of nursing, which is focused on adapting care to the needs of patients with particular disease or conditions, could be studied in part with medical students in "clinical clerkships." In studying certain aspects of care, students of social work, physical therapy, clinical psychology, and even dentistry might participate. Since graduates of all these schools must collaborate as practitioners if patients are to be well served, it seems highly desirable that they study together.

Courses Prerequisite to or Supporting the Nursing Courses. Either as prerequisite to the study of nursing or included in the initial program there should be courses in the *humanities* that ensure students' ability to use language effectively, to consider the present in the light of history, and to have some understanding of logic and the dominant philosophies and religions of the world.* It is certainly desirable that nursing students have some art appreciation, including music appreciation, and have an opportunity to continue to cultivate any special artistic talents they may have. Among the *social sciences,* psychology is of outstanding importance—developmental psychology (human development from birth to death) especially. The study of sociology and anthropology provides a background that is almost essential to the understanding of society. It is desirable that students in the health professions know about governmental processes, not only the governmental systems within their own country but those in other parts of the world, including international law. It is especially important that they understand the ways in which governments promote the welfare of citizens—their education and health care. This may involve an introduction to economics and political theory.

There is little question that nursing students profit by a strong background in the *biologic and physical sciences.* In the opinion of the writer, this cannot be too strong. Whether these courses are taught separately or combined, they should include chemistry, physics, anatomy, and physiology. Physiology is particularly important. Knowledge of cell structure and function has been so enhanced by use of the electron microscope and special photographic techniques that students now entering nursing schools may bring with them more advanced concepts of anatomy and physiology than were held by experts before recent techniques were developed. Certainly the physiology made

available to nursing students should include cell physiology and some of the theories of electronic balance within the cell.

The physiology of nutrition is usually singled out for emphasis in a special course because good nutrition is so essential to health but it is possible that the same emphasis should be put on neuromotor physiology and other essential functions modifiable by daily living habits and by medical treatment. It is desirable that students in the health field understand man's relationship to other living organisms, and for this reason general courses in biology and zoology are recommended. The study of microorganisms should include the essential nature of microscopic life as well as its role in causing disease—epidemic and sporadic.

In the 1955 revision of this book, an effort was made to suggest an *ordering of nursing education* around the needs of clients or patients. The ideas expressed there were elaborated on in *The Nature of Nursing* (Macmillan Publishing Co., Inc., New York, 1966). The following is, to some extent, a synthesis of the discussion in these two sources. It constitutes an effort to show the implications for initial or basic nursing education in the definition of nursing underlying nursing practice given in this chapter (see page 34).

Adaptation of Treatment and Nursing Care to the Needs of the Patient as an Over-all Goal. Those who see the skill and confidence of successful physicians and nurses often marvel at their ability to adapt treatment and nursing care to the particular needs of their patients, no matter how ill they are, what disease they have, or what age they may be. Obviously, even those medical workers with the widest experience have not always seen similar conditions, and since each personality is unique, each client or patient, presents a unique problem. The success of health workers must therefore lie in a knowledge of guiding principles and in their ability to study patients and provide the care and treatment that each demands.* The development of this ability should be the major aim of all nursing curricula. Nursing faculties are constantly trying to find satisfactory answers to the following question: How much and what kind of experience is necessary to enable the graduate to adapt nursing care to particular patients and situations?

* Nursing students will find it useful to know languages other than their own but this should probably not be a prerequisite or a requirement.

* Vernon W. Lippard, discussing medical education, said that "all thought of total coverage" has been abandoned. Basic concepts are stressed, "the mechanisms of disease; continuing self-education; the development of a scientific critique; the cultivation of skills; and the inculcation of ideals." (*A Half Century of American Medical Education: 1920–1970.* Josiah Macy, Jr. Foundation, New York, 1974, p. 17.)

Classification and Organization of Subject Matter and Its Influence on Medical and Nursing Thought. Courses in nursing and medicine in the past were most often based on anatomic classifications of disease. For example, units of clinical study might be entitled "Treatment and Nursing Care of Diseases of the Respiratory System," or of the genitourinary system or the nervous system. A great effort was formerly made to enable medical and nursing students to see as many operations, conditions, or diseases as they could and to take part in the care of these patients. It is no wonder that students of both professions, brought up under such an educational plan, tended to refer to "the cardiac in Bed 2," or "the hysterectomy in Room 15." With emphasis on the disease or the operation rather on the individual with certain symptoms and difficulties, it is not surprising that students of both medicine and nursing were likely to assume that all persons with the same disease should be treated in the same way.

There are today marked changes in medical as well as nursing education. There is, for example, the effort to stress health promotion and disease prevention, to develop awareness in the medical student of people's needs as they see them, and to individualize care. Developing the public's self-reliance is stressed. This is often expressed as "the self-help movement." The fact that physicians are required to get "informed consent" for treatment implies knowledge of disease and the rationale of treatment on the part of the public. Television programs are making everyone aware of the signs of cancer, drug addiction, venereal disease, depressive psychoses, and many other forms of pathology and means of preventing them.

In spite of this emphasis on health education and the prevention of disease, the medical curricula in most American universities are still focused on the physician's functions of diagnosis, prognosis, and therapy. Diagnosis is based on a physical examination of the anatomic systems of the body. It is often called a "systems' review." Diseases are classified under systems, and texts and courses are organized under systems. William R. Houston,[365] a physician of long experience writing in 1936, expressed the opinion that this was *not* the most effective way to teach therapy. In his *Art of Treatment,* he pointed out, for example, that grouping a deviated nasal septum or pharyngitis with lung cancer did not facilitate learning, even though all these conditions might be diseases or defects of the respiratory system. He suggested grouping diseases around the main lines of therapy, which he identified as

administration of specifics, psychotherapy, limiting or modifying the living pattern, altering the physiology, supplying nursing, or giving supportive care (where there was no other effective therapy), and using an experimental or tentative approach.

Recently, some medical schools, trying to develop a health-centered, individualized approach to medicine, have assigned beginning medical students to families in their homes when a baby is to be born to the parents.* Students study psychologic and physiologic problems associated with pregnancy and seek help from appropriate resources within the medical school as they work with the families and the nurses and social workers who are also interested in the families. But whether or not the medical curriculum is didactic and planned or grows out of assigned experience, it is usually focused on the physician's principal functions. The nursing curriculum, whether planned or growing out of assigned experience, should, it seems to the writer, focus on the nurse's principal functions. Where the functions of doctors and nurses overlap, joint study seems appropriate. For example, medical and nursing students need the same knowledge of the health care system, the health resources of the country and the smaller community where they work; both medical and nursing students must be able to assess health or conduct health examinations effectively. While medical students need a broader knowledge of diagnostic procedures, nurses are now using or requesting the more common ones. Medical students study pathologic changes ("pathophysiology") in greater depth, but nursing students must have considerable knowledge of them and may elect to study them intensively. It is not possible for either medical or nursing students to study the hundreds of diseases affecting humans; it is possible to study disease processes, for example, the body's response to a bacterial invasion, prolonged emotional stress, vitamin or protein deficiency, blood loss, or oxygen want.

While therapy is the main focus of the medical curriculum, nursing curricula that prepare graduates to give primary care must also offer students an opportunity to study therapeutics. In order to help patients carry out therapy

* Vernon W. Lippard described the curriculum of the medical school of Case Western Reserve University as follows: "The four-year curriculum was divided into three phases: the first, lasting one year, was concerned with normal structure, function, growth and development; the second, lasting one-and-a-half years, was concerned with alterations of normal structure, function, and development and the study of disease; the third, also lasting one-and-a-half years, was devoted to clinical application of the knowledge previously acquired." (*Ibid.,* p. 18.)

prescribed by physicians, nurses have always needed an understanding of therapeutics, but their present need is even greater. The extent to which the study of therapeutics should be interdisciplinary is debatable. Obstetricians and nurse-midwives need common knowledge and skills, as do pediatricians and pediatric nurses, psychiatrists and psychiatric nurses. Physicians and nurses in medical services, especially those serving the elderly and the chronically ill, also have common needs. Only on surgical services is the preparation of a surgeon quite different from the preparation of a surgical nurse.

If and when medical and nursing students study diagnosis and therapy on an interdisciplinary basis, faculties should make an effort to classify or organize the content of such courses into units that have meaning for both, that emphasize causes and prevention as well as cure, that give guiding principles rather than rules, and that stress the treatment of the person rather than the condition or the disease.

It is suggested that the nursing courses in the initial curriculum be organized into the three following blocks representing three stages of learning: *Basic Nursing Care* (see Fig. 1-32); *Symptomatic Nursing, or Common Problems in Nursing* (see Fig. 1-33); *and Disease-Oriented Nursing* and *Mother, Infant, and Child Care* (see Fig. 1-34). All focus on the nurse's principal function of supplementing the patient's strength, will, or knowledge in performing his or her daily activities or carrying out prescribed therapy, with the ultimate goal of independence or rehabilitation for the client or patient when this is possible and an ability to cope with incurable chronic disease or achieve a "good death" (see Chapter 50) when neither a cure nor "coping" is possible.

The first block of experience (Nursing I. Basic Nursing Care) and related instruction is organized around helping people with their daily activities or providing conditions that enable them to perform them without help. This

1. Breathe normally.
2. Eat and drink adequately.
3. Eliminate by all avenues of elimination.
4. Move and maintain desirable posture (walking, sitting, lying, and changing from one to the other).
5. Sleep and rest.
6. Select suitable clothing, dress and undress.
7. Maintain body temperature within normal range by adjusting clothing and modifying the environment.
8. Keep the body clean and well groomed and protect the integument.
9. Avoid dangers in the environment and avoid injuring others.
10. Communicate with others in expressing emotions, needs, fears, questions, and ideas.
11. Worship according to his faith.
12. Work at something that provides a sense of accomplishment.
13. Play, or participate in various forms of recreation.
14. Learn, discover, or satisfy the curiosity that leads to "normal" development and health.

This includes making a plan for such assistance, taking into consideration the following factors always present that affect the person's needs.

1. Age: newborn, child, youth, adult, middle-aged, aged, and dying.
2. Temperament, emotional state, or passing mood:
   a. "Normal" or
   b. Euphoric and hyperactive
   c. Anxious, fearful, agitated, or hysterical or
   d. Depressed and hypoactive

3. Social or cultural status:
   A member of a family unit with friends and status or a person relatively alone and/or maladjusted, destitute.

4. Physical and intellectual capacity:
   a. Normal weight
   b. Underweight
   c. Overweight
   d. Normal mentality
   e. Subnormal mentality
   f. Gifted mentality
   g. Normal sense of hearing, sight, equilibrium, and touch
   h. Loss of special sense
   i. Normal motor power
   j. Loss of motor power

Figure 1-32. Nursing I. Basic Nursing Care. Content of course organized around the fundamental needs of man, around planning care, and the nurse's unique function of helping patients with their daily activities. (From Henderson, Virginia: *The Nature of Nursing.* Macmillan Publishing Co., Inc., New York, 1966, p. 49.)

1. Marked disturbance of intake and output of gases demanding medical intervention such as administration of oxygen.

2. Marked disturbance of nutrition, fluid and electrolyte balance, starvation, obesity, pernicious vomiting, diarrhea.

3. Marked disturbance of elimination with constipation, suppression or retention of urine, incontinence of urine or feces.

4. Motor disturbance limiting motion; also prescribed immobilization.

5. Hyperactivity, with or without convulsions or hysteria.

6. Fainting, dizziness (loss of equilibrium), transitory and prolonged coma, or unconsciousness, disorientation, delirium.

7. Insomnia, anxiety, depression.

8. Hyperthermia or hypothermia as a result of exposure to environmental temperatures or as prescribed treatment.

9. Local injury, or wound, with infection.

10. A systemic infection, a communicable condition transmitted by various channels, with or without febrile states.

11. Shock, or collapse, with or without hemorrhage.

12. Disorders of communication attributable to congenital defects of sight, hearing, or speech (including deafness and mutism), and such handicaps when imposed by illness or treatment.

13. Preoperative state.

14. Postoperative state.

15. Persistent, or intractable pain.

16. Dying state.

Figure 1-33. Nursing II. Symptomatic Nursing, or Common Problems in Nursing. Content organized around symptoms, syndromes, or states (common to many diagnoses) encountered by nurses in many settings. (From Henderson, Virginia: *The Nature of Nursing*. Macmillan Publishing Co., Inc., New York, 1966, p. 52.)

experience is available in almost any health service or clinical unit of the hospital, in nursing homes, or in private homes. The needs of clients or patients are analyzed according to age, temperament, social or cultural status, and physical and intellectual capacity (see Fig. 1-32). In this first phase of the curriculum, there is no emphasis on the patient's diagnosis or the therapeutic plan, although students with inquiring minds will learn a good deal about both. During this stage of learning, students are participant observers or assistants to more experienced students or to graduates who are helping patients with daily activities and prescribed treatment. At the end of Nursing I. Basic Nursing Care, the student should have acquired many skills, as well as the ability to plan with patients for the 14 daily functions listed in Figure 1-32 to help them with their activities as they need help, and to become independent of help as soon as possible.

The second phase of the suggested clinical, or nursing, curriculum is Nursing II. Symp-

tomatic Nursing. Student experience is focused on helping patients meet their momentary, hourly, daily, or future needs when there are marked disturbances of one or more of the 14 functions listed in Figure 1-32. These disturbances, regardless of the disease diagnosis, constitute problems for patients and those who nurse them, and they demand modifications in daily living that must be made by the patient or the nurse, or both, if the symptom is to be relieved or made tolerable. Figure 1-33 lists 16 symptoms or disturbances of function that create problems for patients and nurses. They may occur in both sexes, in all ages, and in almost any setting, although in order to have experience with these common nursing problems, students may have to be assigned to a number of services, including the emergency, medical, surgical, psychiatric, and pediatric services. Patients are chosen for the specific symptoms or states they present; the student studies the pathologic changes in patient physiology and the rationale of therapy prescribed

ON MEDICAL SERVICES	
Therapy related to general conditions such as:	Therapy related to special diseases such as:
Long-term illness Metabolic disorders Endocrine disorders Functional disorders Neoplasms Infections Degenerative processes	Arthritis Osteomalacia Addison's disease Anemia Leukemia Tuberculosis Cardiovascular diseases
ON SURGICAL SERVICES	
Therapy related to general conditions such as:	Therapy related to specific diseases such as:

Preoperative state, operative, and postoperative state in
        Head and neck
        Chest
Areal surgery Abdomen
        Pelvis
        Extremities
	Brain tumor removal
	Thyroidectomy
	Lobectomy (lung)
	Colostomy
	Nephrectomy
	Reduction and fixation of fracture of an extremity

ON MATERNAL AND CHILD CARE SERVICES	
Therapy related to general states such as:	Therapy related to specific diseases such as:
Prenatal Natal Postnatal Newborn Infancy Preschool children Middle childhood Adolescence	Eclampsia Cesarean birth Mastitis Erythroblastosis fetalis Eczema Cerebral palsy Poliomyelitis Rheumatic fever
ON NEUROPSYCHIATRIC SERVICES	
Therapy related to general conditions such as:	Therapy related to specific diseases such as:
Mental deficiency Pathological personality development Anxiety states—psychoneuroses Acute depression with suicidal tendencies Maniacal states Paranoid states	Hydrocephalus Alcoholism and drug addiction Manic-depressive psychoses Schizophrenia

Figure 1-34. Nursing III. Disease-Oriented Nursing and Mother, Infant, and Child Care. Content organized around prescribed therapy and the modification of daily activities indicated by disease or physiologic developmental states. (From Henderson, Virginia: *The Nature of Nursing.* Macmillan Publishing Co., Inc., New York, 1966, p. 54.)

to relieve symptoms or make them tolerable. Some of the common nursing problems, for instance, the care of those who have intractable pain or those who are dying, are extremely complex. Volumes are written on these subjects, and health workers are devoting their lives to the study of these states. Students in the initial or basic program cannot be expected to learn all there is to know about them, but society expects every registered nurse to be able to help people cope with them and so every basic program should offer an opportunity to do just this. Faculties may very well identify other or different aberrations of body functions, human states, or common nursing problems with which students should have experience. Faye G. Abdellah and her associates in *Patient-Centered Approaches to Nursing* [366] in 1961 listed 21 problems with which they thought students should have experience.*

It is obviously desirable for students to help people with these commonly encountered problems in settings outside as well as inside hospi-

* Olga Andruskiw and Betsy L. B. Battick in 1964 studied two of these problems (oxygen want and electrolyte imbalance) and identified diseases and conditions in which they occur. ("Identification of Nursing Problems," *Nurs. Res.,* **13:**75, [Winter] 1964.)

tals and clinics where all kinds of experts, equipment, and supplies are available. It is desirable that the skills patients and nurses (one or both) must learn in order to cope with these problems be identified and efforts made to help nursing students acquire these skills. It is a common criticism of present-day registered nurses that they lack certain skills that employers expect them to have.* It is even more disturbing that graduates of some basic programs lose their self-confidence, finding themselves lacking in the ability to give patients the kind of help they would like to be able to give them, including the ability to perform, or teach patients to perform, necessary procedures. For example, while it is essential that nurses understand the physiology of respiration and the common pathology involved in oxygen want, it is also essential that they be able to use the mechanical devices and teach patients or their families to use mechanical devices that increase the oxygen supply to the patient; knowledge of the causes of coma, the pathology involved, are certainly necessary for those who nurse the unconscious patient, but skill in cleaning their mouths, in moving and lifting them, and in preventing pressure sores is also essential. While this second phase of the nursing curriculum focuses on symptomatic treatment, it includes helping the patient with the 14 daily activities stressed in the first phase of the curriculum and all the skills, abilities or competences essential to both the first and second phase. In this phase, nursing students might study with medical students but, most particularly, with students of physical, occupational, and speech therapy who also help patients with activities of daily living.

The third phase of the suggested clinical, or nursing, curriculum is Nursing III. Disease-Oriented Nursing and the Care of Mothers, Infants, and Children (see Fig. 1-34). Here, the focus is on the modification of care demanded, or on the particular problem patients face because of a specific disease or an operation that requires special preparation or postoperative care or because they are in a phase of reproduction or a growth cycle that makes them dependent.

There have been many attempts to identify the diseases, the conditions, and the operations with which nursing (and medical) students should have some experience. As noted earlier, it is obviously impossible for either to study the care of patients with all the diseases, conditions, and operations they may encounter as physicians or nurses. It is therefore suggested that educators stress the care and therapy associated with *types* of conditions, as shown in Figure 1-33. On medical services, some types are long-term illness, metabolic, endocrine, and functional disorders, neoplasms, infections, and degenerative processes. Experience can be provided students in the care of some patients with conditions of each type. Patients should be selected so that students have experience in the care of males and females of all ages. Experience in maternal and child care should include the normal and abnormal. While previous phases of the clinical curriculum should have stressed developmental needs, special emphasis should be put on them in this phase of the curriculum. Some faculties may offer a special course in geriatrics, as they do in pediatrics. It seems even more important to take a developmental approach in all clinical courses, helping students to see that every patient has to make adjustments in care and treatment imposed by his or her age.

In this third phase of the clinical curriculum, "classes" (discussions, seminars, conferences) are around particular patients. Lippard,[367] with reference to medical teaching, says patient-centered clinical teaching is never "behind the times" since the student is learning about the diseases and treatments of the day. Christman,[368] describing the new nursing program at Rush University, Chicago, emphasizes the importance of the practitioner-teacher who teaches students around "his or her own set of patients."

On surgical services, experience can be provided in the care of patients with each category of regional surgery since there are, for example, commonalities in the care of all patients having abdominal surgery or operations on the extremities. In maternal, infant, and child nursing, experience can be offered in the care of patients with representative pathologic conditions in the prenatal, natal, and postnatal states, in infancy and childhood, and through adolescence. In neuropsychiatric services, students might have experience in the care of patients in all age groups, in mental deficiency, in abnormal personality development, in anxiety states or psychoneuroses, in depression or suicidal states, in maniacal and paranoid states. In the second column (Fig. 1-34), *examples* of diagnosis falling within these general categories are given, but they are examples only. It is not our intention to suggest either the most common or the most important examples. The experience available and the judgment of faculty and interests of students

* Eleanor Gill, dean of the School of Nursing at the University of Connecticut, told the writer in 1975 that the faculty of this school has "gone back" to the practice of having a checklist of skills, procedures, or techniques with which students must have experience.

will determine in every school the assignment to patients in hospitals, clinics, nursing homes, home care programs, and other settings.

In this third phase of the student nurse's clinical program, he or she should have the opportunity to help patients with all aspects of care, including planning: in other words, an opportunity to practice nursing as students as they will be expected to practice as graduates. Presently, this includes conducting physical examinations, assessing health, determining the diagnostic procedures and referrals to other health workers that are indicated, and in some cases suggesting a plan of therapy.

Students should have an opportunity to give the best care of which they are capable, and to study thoroughly the prescribed therapy and the patient's responses to it. Experience should be planned so that students can follow at least some patients through all stages of treatment, for example, preoperative, operative, and postoperative care or prenatal, natal, and postnatal care. If students are to graduate with a concept of family-centered nursing, it is important that they visit patients before hospitalization, that they care for hospital patients when they go home, and that they make home visits with community, school, industrial, or prison nurses and hospital nurses assigned to home care programs.

In this third phase of the clinical nursing program, students should have an opportunity to give as nearly "ideal" nursing care as possible to both sexes and all ages; at the same time, they should learn the realities of health service as it exists today and should see some effective efforts made to maintain the better services or improve the inadequate ones. If students see only ideal conditions, they may be unfitted for work in existing agencies and institutions. Obviously, as long as students are students, the faculty is responsible for the judgments they make and the care they give. At any point where either is contrary to the patient's welfare, the faculty must so advise students and help them make appropriate changes, or themselves make the decision or give the care for which the student is unprepared.

Clinical nursing curricula—however they are organized, however they are taught—should foster an inquiring attitude toward practice. While students need the assurance that the care they learn to give is safe and effective in the light of present knowledge, they should accept the fact that the boundaries of knowledge are constantly expanding, that health workers, in fact, everyone, should be open to new ideas —ready to modify practice as new findings in the physical, biologic, and social sciences invalidate current practice.

Nursing students must be able to find pertinent research, read it, evaluate it, and apply it as they seek answers to clinical problems. Therefore, they need a course that introduces them to the scientific method of investigation if their prenursing education has not included research experience. It is desirable that the initial nursing program include some experience in conducting a clinical study, and possibly a course in statistics and the use of computers. However, students are not likely to think of nursing research as the basis on which changes are made in nursing practice unless they see this happening in the centers where they study nursing.

Finally, the initial nursing curriculum should prepare graduates to play a constructive role as members of a major health profession. They can understand the current opportunities, obligations, and problems of nursing only if they have some knowledge of the history of health care in general and of nursing in particular. Nursing students should have firsthand experience as active members, associate members, or observers in nursing and other health organizations, as well as the opportunity to see and discuss the work of those who are maintaining effective services or helping to bring about change in the health structure. Knowledge of medical and nursing ethics and jurisprudence is increasingly important. If students have an opportunity to see health legislation in the making or participate in efforts to enact legislation, they are more likely as graduates to help effect change in a variety of ways.* Health care is presently accepted all over the world as a human right. The United States occupies a unique position among the developed nations in its fee-for-service system. Nurses who believe that health opportunities should be equalized and wish to work toward that end must be knowledgeable in the governmental and legal processes inherent in a national health insurance system that covers all citizens. For nurses who believe the United States should remain unique in retaining its fee-for-service system, knowledge of governmental and legal processes will also serve their needs.

A basic curriculum, however designed, is only the beginning of a lifetime of study for the practicing nurse; the succeeding sections describe postbasic study, graduate programs, and continuing and staff education.

---

* There is considerable evidence that nurses are helping to effect change. A survey conducted by the ANA in 1975 through the state nurses' associations showed 15 RNs in 13 state legislatures, nine of whom were serving on health or social service committees. ("15 Nurse Legislators Reported in 13 States," *Am. Nurse,* 7:5, (May) 1975.

6. BACCALAUREATE PROGRAMS FOR REGISTERED NURSES WITH DIPLOMAS OR ASSOCIATE DEGREES IN NURSING

Need for Baccalaureate Programs for Registered Nurses with Diplomas or Associate Degrees. In discussing initial nursing programs, it was noted that there is a movement, which is gaining momentum in the United States and other countries, to make a baccalaureate degree essential to the licensure of the professional registered nurse. If this becomes fact, and if the requirement should be made retroactive (which is most unlikely), registered nurses who graduated from initial diploma and associate degree programs must go to institutions offering baccalaureate degrees to registered nurses. (See Figure 1-35 for proportion of nurses with baccalaureate and higher degrees in the United States.)

Perhaps more important is the growing demand by employers for degree-holding nurses,

or nurses prepared to work independently and creatively. An over-all shortage of nurses may be debatable, but few question the undersupply of well-prepared nurses. Some hospitals are closing in the United States and Canada because hospital occupancy is falling and there is a realization that there may be too many hospitals. This may result in unemployed nurses and create an impression of a surplus. In any economically depressed country, nurses, like all other workers, fear unemployment. A thorough preparation for work (if it is not accompanied by a demand for a disproportionate rise in salary) is the best guarantee against unemployment. It is economically desirable in North America for graduate nurses to hold a baccalaureate degree which makes them more effective in generalized nursing, makes possible subsequent preparation for specialized nursing in graduate programs, and promotes economic security.

Of the 778,470 registered employed nurses in the United States in 1972, 626,857 (or 80.5

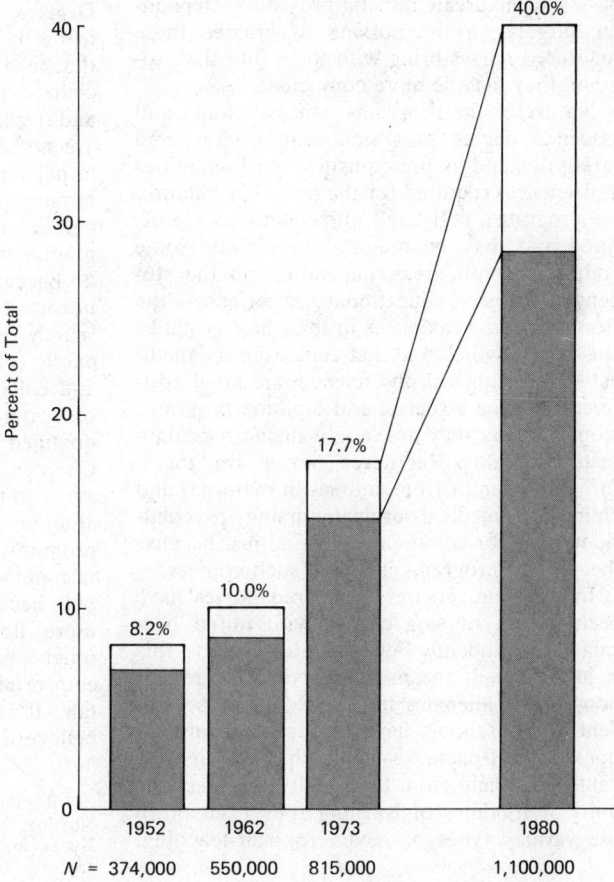

Figure 1-35. Proportion of registered nurses with baccalaureate and higher degrees, 1952, 1962, and 1973, with estimate for 1980. (From Hudson, Helen H., and McCarthy, Margaret D.: *Source Book—Nursing Personnel.* US Government Printing Office, Washington, D.C., 1974.)

per cent) had less than a baccalaureate degree. In the fall of 1972, there were 15,967 graduate nurses enrolled in colleges and universities for full-time and part-time study. In 1970–1972, 2337 graduate nurse students were granted baccalaureate degrees from 258 colleges and universities.* [369] By 1974, the NLN reported 3003 registered nurses receiving baccalaureate degrees from 226 programs. Almost certainly, these numbers will continue to increase until most of the younger nurse graduates with diplomas or associate degrees have a bachelor's degree.[370]

The Purpose of Baccalaureate Programs for Registered Nurses. The goal of all baccalaureate programs for registered nurses is to give them the learning opportunities offered by initial baccalaureate programs that they have missed as students in diploma or associate degree programs. It is not easy to identify these opportunities, so baccalaureate programs for registered nurses in the United States vary considerably. Colleges and universities offering such programs expect their graduates to be at least as competent as graduates of initial or basic baccalaureate nursing programs. Depending largely on the nursing experience these registered nurses bring with them into the program, they may be more competent.

Nature of the Programs. Since diploma and associate degree programs cannot offer, and rarely demand as prerequisites, the humanities and sciences required for the initial baccalaureate programs, registered nurse students are offered and may be required to include some courses in both areas, depending on the student's former educational experience—the strengths and weaknesses in their backgrounds. It is generally believed that courses in the medical and nursing arts and sciences are taught differently in the associate and diploma programs from the way they are taught in the baccalaureate programs. Registered nurses are, therefore, not exempt from courses in maternal and child care, medical-surgical nursing, psychiatric nursing, or community nursing just because their initial programs included such courses.

In some universities, registered nurses have been put in nursing classes with initial baccalaureate students. Few educators believe this is justifiable. It means a great deal of repetition, which alienates the registered nurse student. Most schools have exemption examinations or self-pacing systems that enable students, with help from the faculty, to select the units or modules of learning they need or to use various types of media for self-teaching.

Many schools offer special clinical courses designed especially for the registered nurse student. Because they are at home in the clinical setting and have usually learned the basic nursing skills, the clinical experience (sometimes called "the practicum") can be of a different nature from that of the student in the initial baccalaureate program. Experienced and able registered nurse students may be allowed more electives, may have more independent study assignments, or may be able to follow their special clinical interests to a greater extent than students in the initial or basic baccalaureate program. Courses of study should be individually planned so that students see them as opportunities for useful and interesting learning rather than the fulfillment of a stereotyped requirement.

7. PREPARATION FOR SPECIALIZED NURSING—GRADUATE PROGRAMS

Need for Nurse Specialists with Graduate Degrees. The major national nursing surveys in the United States have for decades stressed the need for nurses with preparation in specialized practice, for teaching, administration, and research. Initial baccalaureate programs are not designed to prepare specialists in maternal and child health, medical and surgical nursing or any of its subspecialties, or in psychiatric nursing, although many are preparing graduates for generalized primary nursing. Nor do baccalaureate programs offer more than an introduction to teaching, administration, or research, or to the special problems of nursing in public (or community) health agencies, schools and colleges, industries, penal institutions, and other settings.* There is a demand for well-qualified nurses in all the settings discussed in Chapter 3 and for nurses who have advanced study in the care of patients in every age group and clinical category. Most graduates of initial programs take staff nursing positions in hospitals not only because they are needed there but because most initial programs provide more hospital nursing experience than any other kind, and graduates from them feel more comfortable nursing inside than outside hospitals. It is also true that many new graduates believe they profit by additional experience in

---

* There were 63 institutions that had no graduates in 1972, and three institutions offering programs that had no enrollment.

* Beginning in 1974, the Yale University School of Nursing, New Haven, Connecticut offered an initial 3-year master's program for college graduates that prepares these men and women to give generalized primary care, to function as specialists in a field of their choice, and "to gain basic skills in research in nursing practice." This was said, in 1974, to be the only such program in existence.

giving nursing care in hospitals, even the fundamentals of care, and by more practice in the basic skills.

The rising rate at which nurses with baccalaureate degrees are entering and graduating from master's programs and later doctoral programs indicates an established demand in the United States for nurses with more thorough preparation for their work (see Table 1-14). In 1952, there were only 1449 graduations from programs of advanced study of practice, teaching, or administration in nursing. In 1969–70, there were 1988 graduations from nursing programs leading to a master's degree; in 1973–74, there were 2643 graduations from such programs. Simmons and Henderson [372] reported a total of 80 dissertations earned by nurses in the 25 years between 1928 and 1955.* In the 2-year period of 1973–74, the NLN reported 46 graduations from doctoral programs (see Table 1-16). The American Nurses' Foundation has continued the search for nurse holders of earned doctoral degrees. It reported the first doctoral degree earned by a nurse in 1927; in 1973, 964 nurses of the United States held doctoral degrees, and 1019 held doctoral degrees worldwide.[373]

Nursing, like all new professions, has found it difficult to provide its schools with faculties whose educational preparation was comparable to that of faculties in the established professional schools and, therefore, to establish graduate programs. Of the 28,820 nurses employed in schools of nursing in 1972, 7128 (24.7 per cent) had less than a baccalaureate education; 8953 (31.1 per cent) had a baccalaureate degree; 9810 (35 per cent) had a master's degree in nursing or another field; and 601 (2.1 per cent) had a doctoral degree.[374] In 1974 there were 7924 students enrolled in master's programs and 312 in doctoral programs.[375]

Until nurses on the faculties of college and university schools of nursing have master's or doctoral degrees, there will be a crying need for nurses with graduate degrees, and until nurses in administrative positions, in research, and in specialized clinical practice have master's or doctoral degrees, opportunities for graduate study should be increased; Rozella Schlotfeldt [376] would say until all "professional" nurses can study in a graduate program leading to a doctoral degree, they should be increased (see page 90). Margaret A. Newman [377] takes the same position.

* The doctoral dissertation of Edith S. Bryan is cited by Simmons and Henderson as the first written by a nurse. The date is 1928; the American Nurses' Foundation also cites this as the first, but gives the date as 1927.

Table 1-14. Graduations from Nursing Programs Leading to Master's and Doctoral Degrees, 1969–70 Through 1973–74 *

Academic Year	Master's Programs	Doctoral Programs
1969–70	1988	27
1970–71	2083	41
1971–72	2135	27
1972–73	2446	49
1973–74	2643	46

* National League for Nursing, Division of Research: "Educational Preparation for Nursing—1974," (Report prepared by Walter L. Johnson.) *Nurs. Outlook*, **23**:578, (Sept.) 1975.

The Purpose and Nature of Master's Programs. In 1972, there were 86 colleges and universities in the United States offering master's programs for graduate nurse students.[377a] The evolution of master's programs for graduate nurses is discussed in Chapter 3, where it is observed that before the late 1940s they did not differ very much from the baccalaureate programs for graduate nurses. Both offered preparation for teaching or administration or for public health nursing, and in some cases school or industrial nursing. There were a few postbasic programs offering courses on nurse midwifery, and later still, nursing of children, medical and surgical nursing, tuberculosis and cancer nursing. If the graduate nurse student had earned a baccalaureate nursing degree, the clinical courses might be built into a master's program, but they might also be part of a baccalaureate program. Until midcentury, advanced preparation in clinical nursing was far less common than advanced preparation for the functions of teaching and administration.

In the late 1940s, the NLN issued a series of publications on advanced clinical courses, stressing the need for them and suggesting the form they might take. By 1969, the ANA gave as the "major purpose of graduate . . . study in nursing":

. . . the preparation of nurse clinicians capable of improving nursing care through the advancement of nursing theory and science. . . . Traditionally, graduate education in nursing has been considered as preparation for particular functions and positions—primarily teaching and administration. This emphasis, unfortunately has tended to devalue nursing care and practice by suggesting that there is no more nursing knowledge than can be encompassed in the initial, undergraduate preparation.*

* American Nurses' Association: *Statement on Graduate Education in Nursing.* The Association, Kansas City, Mo., 1969, p. 2.

The following statement by the NLN in 1974 emphasizes advanced clinical courses and preparation for research in both master's and doctoral programs:

Graduate study is education pursued beyond the baccalaureate degree in an institution of higher learning. The characteristics of graduate education in nursing include specialization in a clinical area of interest, mastery of knowledge in that area, freedom of inquiry in the pursuit of knowledge and the acquisition of skills, and competence in research. The programs are organized according to a conceptual scheme and culminate in the awarding of a master's or a doctoral degree in a chosen area of study. . . .*

While the current need is for nurses who are able and accountable in specialized clinical nursing, master's programs for graduate nurses in the United States offer a wide variety of courses. The University of Maryland in 1974–75, for example, offered more than 50 courses; the University of Texas in 1975–76 offered more than 40 courses.[378,379] Some programs offer courses in nursing history, nursing concepts, and nursing process on a graduate level. Not every master's program has developed all the clinical specialties—maternal and infant health, child health, medical-surgical nursing, and psychiatric nursing, but the current bulletins examined indicated that the trend was in this direction. Some programs offered developmental nursing, or study of the nursing care of infants, children, young adults, the middle-aged, and the aged. "Intradisciplinary nursing" and "liaison nursing" are courses providing opportunity to study the mental health aspects of nursing in any clinical department or health service.

Courses in nursing according to the setting in which the nurse functions were uncommon except for community health nursing, which may still be called public health nursing and which is sometimes called family health nursing.† In describing the "practicum" or the experience offered in connection with the various clinical specialties, there was the implication in some bulletins that students might elect to have it in a wide variety of health institutions and agencies.

Community health nursing included nursing in industry and schools and might include nursing in penal institutions. Study of nursing in these settings, however, tends to be neglected, although the ANA reports that of the 308 master's programs in public health nursing, nine "focused" on school nursing.[380] Community health programs emphasized the function of the nurse in state, county, and city health departments and in visiting nurse agencies. If there was a school of public health in the university, its courses were available to students in master's programs in nursing, or the nursing school might itself offer such courses as epidemiology and public health administration.

While few master's programs were focused on the functions of teaching, administration, or research, many offered courses in educational and managerial theory and systems analysis and some offered experience in teaching or administration, or both. As indicated earlier, employers expect nurses holding master's degrees to be familiar with the scientific method of investigation, to be able to read research reports, and to apply the findings of research. Most master's programs include experience in conducting a study of some sort, usually leading to a master's thesis. Courses in statistics and the use of computers are common.

Master's programs studied included a wide variety of electives. Graduate nurse students were urged to take courses in other schools or departments in the university—the schools of public health, education, medicine, law, or management, and the departments of biologic and physical sciences and social sciences. If and when the United States develops out of the present chaos a well-defined and effective pattern of health service, all universities may develop interdisciplinary courses in those aspects of the service that can be studied profitably by all health professionals.

The Purpose and Nature of Doctoral Programs. The purpose and nature of doctoral programs in nursing have been and remain controversial. As noted, the first nurse from the United States to earn a doctoral degree is believed to be Edith S. Bryan, who earned a Ph.D. in psychology. Her dissertation, submitted to Johns Hopkins University in 1928, is titled "A Psychological Study of the Reactions of the Newborn." [381] It was not until 1946 that nurses were offered an opportunity in two universities to get doctoral degrees in nursing; before 1946, they were obliged to get a doctorate in education, philosophy, law, a biologic or physical science, public health, or some other area of study. Simmons and Henderson found that of the 80 doctoral degrees earned by nurses (other than M.D.'s earned by nurses) between 1928 and 1955, there were four types distributed as follows: Ed.D. 46;

---

* National League for Nursing: *Characteristics of Graduate Education in Nursing.* The League, New York, 1974.

† The terminology is questionable when it only applies to extra-hospital nursing, since, ideally, nurses in all health services, including those in hospitals, clinics, and nursing homes, work with patients as members of a family.

Ph.D. 32; Jur.D. 1; and Sci.D. 1.* [382] When the US Department of Health, Education, and Welfare reported the *Conference on Future Directions of Doctoral Education for Nurses,* it showed that in 1969, 25 kinds of doctoral degrees were being awarded nurses, which included Doctor of Nursing (D.N.), Doctor of Nursing Science (D.N.Sc. or D.N.S.), Doctor of Public Health Nursing (D.P.H.N.), and Doctor of Nursing Education (D.N.Ed.).[383]

Publications of the NLN and ANA, cited earlier, encourage graduate nurse students to take programs leading to doctoral degrees in nursing, although few question the value of advanced study in related fields. Susan Taylor and her associates, reporting on nurses with earned doctoral degrees by 1971, gave the following figures: 47 per cent held degrees in the behavioral sciences, 33.8 per cent in education, 8.3 per cent in the biological sciences, 6.4 per cent in nursing, 1.9 per cent in epidemiology and public health, and 2.6 per cent in other fields.†

For both master's and doctoral students, the NLN in 1974 gave the following characteristics as cited by Kelly:

The nurse in the advanced professional program (1) pursues an area of clinical specialization; (2) elects an area of role development; (3) develops and tests nursing theories; (4) advances knowledge in the field through systematic observation and experimentation; (5) relates basic science theories to the development of knowledge in the clinical and functional areas; (6) identifies and implements nursing's leadership role within the health care delivery system; and (7) engages in a collaborative role with others interested in health care.‡

Rozella Schlotfeldt [384] and Margaret A. Newman [385] maintain that the nurse is the worker most available to the public and most interested in and able to give primary health care, particularly the service directed toward health promotion and disease prevention. They believe preparation on a doctoral level is needed to qualify nurses for this function and to give them the public recognition and authority of other major health professionals.

The assumption that professional nurses are particularly interested in "care," in the psychosocial problem of patients, as opposed to "cure" and the technical aspects of treatment said by some to be typical of the associate degree graduate and/or the practical nurse, seems to be borne out by a number of recent studies. However, Bonnie Bullough and Colleen Sparks [386] questioned the "care-cure dichotomy." They think this distinction, expressed in the ANA's position paper of 1965, may be creating a difference in initial nursing programs "contrived" by nurse educators or theorists. They suggested that by creating two types of graduates who function differently, upward mobility for the "cure" nurse may be blocked and the nurse who is primarily concerned with "care" may be frustrated in real life situations where the nurse is expected to function in both capacities. Marlene Kramer [387] questioned whether professional nurses are being prepared in present-day schools to meet the public's expectations and to satisfy their own desire to practice effectively. Dorothy A. Mereness [388] suggested that "evidence of ability to practice professionally" be a prerequisite to acceptance of nurses as candidates for master's degrees.

The effort in Canada to identify specific functions that nurses in each clinical area should learn to perform, the competences they should demonstrate in an educational program (see page 27), is one practical approach to the question of whether care and cure can or should be separated, and whether the preparation of professional nurses should be comparable in length, depth, and breadth to that of physicians and dentists.

William K. Selden, who has directed educational research in various fields, says that problems in graduate nursing education are not unique. He made the following observation:

As nursing fosters and supports more educational offerings in academic institutions in contrast to education in service agencies, it should be more discriminating than it appears to have been in adopting the pedagogical mores of higher education. It should select only those educational practices that will assist its practitioners to improve their competencies in the delivery of health care.*

Selden applauded one institution's "lucid and direct . . . statement of philosophy" from which the following was excerpted: "The primary purpose of the doctoral program is the enhancement of clinical competence through the development of a body of nursing knowledge upon which a sound practice of nursing is based." †

* The holders of these doctoral degrees were at the time, or afterwards became, citizens of the United States.

† Taylor, Susan, et al.: "Doctoral Degrees," *Nurs. Res.,* **20:**415, (Sept.–Oct.) 1971.

‡ Kelly, Lucie Young: *Dimensions of Professional Nursing,* 3rd ed. Macmillan Publishing Co., Inc., New York, 1975, p. 179.

* Selden, William K.: "Are Problems in Graduate Nursing Education Unique?" *Nurs. Outlook,* **23:**622, (Oct.) 1975.

† *Ibid.*

Regional commissions on higher education have for decades promoted graduate programs for nursing. Interstate planning has resulted in less duplication of programs and the development of better programs. Funds from private foundations and the USPHS have supported a variety of projects. Cooperative graduate education in nursing, in which twelve universities in California and Nevada are participating, was in progress under a 5-year USPHS grant (1971–1976). This has demonstrated the feasibility of a master's student taking courses in several universities simultaneously.[389]

Patricia A. Moxley and Dorothy T. White [390] discussed "Fitting the Graduate Program to the Student" at the School of Nursing, Medical College of Georgia, and "removing barriers to admission." A volume, Open Learning and Career Mobility in Nursing, edited by Carrie B. Lenburg, asks for "diversity for a learning society." She reviewed the current efforts to fit initial and graduate programs to the needs of the people. She noted that "Open learning is not a phenomenon unique to the United States; it is an international movement, with institutions around the globe. . . ." She noted that "The University of London developed an external degree program in 1836 and has been meeting the education needs of working students for more than 138 years." *

A doctoral degree is now awarded in the United States by the Union Graduate School —a union for experimenting colleges and universities, which had 31 member institutions in October, 1975. The Ph.D. program (a non-campus graduate program initiated in 1969) "now enrolls over 300 students and has more than 200 graduates." †

While graduate programs of study in nursing in the United States do not seem to the writer to present as confused a picture as do initial programs, they are far from stable, and the developments just mentioned suggest some of the differing directions they are taking. Depending on what happens in the development of health service and the role nurse practitioners play in it, graduate education may continue to change drastically, as it has throughout this century.

Postbasic education at the beginning of the century consisted at first of blocks of experience in hospitals and health agencies that differed little from the experiences of nurses employed in them except that the "postgraduate student" was paid little or nothing. The program for hospital nurse administrators established at Teachers College, Columbia University, New York City, was at the time a great innovation. This program for administrators was duplicated for teachers. Soon, programs were developed to prepare graduate nurses to function in special settings. Finally, programs were designed to prepare clinical specialists and researchers. In one setting, the latter includes research historians.[391,392] Today, the major emphasis in graduate education is on the preparation of clinical specialists.

While the preceding pages have stressed the development of opportunities for graduate study in nursing in the United States, opportunities in Canada are also increasing. There were, in 1969, eight institutions offering master's degrees, with 18 graduations [394]; in 1972, there were eleven institutions offering master's degrees, with 45 graduations and 159 students enrolled; [395] in 1974 the number of master's programs increased to sixteen.[395a] In 1954, the Florence Nightingale International Foundation published an international list of advanced programs in nursing education and has since brought out supplements.[393]

Study beyond the initial nursing program may take many forms. All major nursing investigations have stressed the need for nurses with broad social experience and higher degrees. The report of a 1973 conference is entitled Redesigning Nursing Education for Public Health (Division of Nursing, Public Health Service, Health Resources Administration, US Department of Health, Education, and Welfare, Bethesda, Md., [1975] (DHEW Pub. No. [HRA] 75–75). Conferences on education in other fields might properly suggest comparable changes.

8. IN-SERVICE EDUCATION

Definition. The American Nurses' Association defines in-service education as follows: "An instructional or training program provided by an employing agency in the work setting and designed to increase competence in a specific area of practice. In-service education is one aspect of staff development, but the terms are not interchangable." * The inclusive term "staff development" is defined by the

---

* Lenburg, Carrie B. (ed.): Open Learning and Career Mobility in Nursing. C. V. Mosby Co., St. Louis, 1975.

† The Union Graduate School consists of The Union Graduate School—I, The Center for Minority Studies, The Union Graduate School—Elementary and Secondary Education, The Union Research Institute, and The Union Graduate School—West. [Prospectus 1975.]

* American Nurses' Association: Continuing Education in Nursing. Guidelines for Staff Development. The Association, Kansas City, Mo., 1976, p. 11.

ANA as: "A term describing the total process which includes both formal and informal learning opportunities. The focus of the process is on assisting individuals to perform competently in fulfillment of role expectations within a specific agency. Resources both within and outside the agency are utilized to facilitate the process." *

The Need for In-Service Education. Health service, if ineptly given, is potentially dangerous. Agencies offering it are liable, to a greater or lesser extent, for the mistakes of their employees, although workers may also suffer the consequences of their acts. However, the welfare of those served, those operating the agency, and the workers themselves is dependent upon the competence of the workers. In-service education is a necessity regardless of the quality of the worker's preparation since the purpose and programs of agencies, conditions of work, personnel, facilities, and equipment differ. New employees need orientation, and all workers need ongoing programs to keep them abreast of developments within the institution or agency. Without some planned program, the service lacks unity, and its quality may suffer to a dangerous degree.

Myrtle Aydelotte [396] reported in 1968 that of 1172 hospitals surveyed, 84 per cent had planned in-service programs. The director of such programs is often an assistant administrator of the nursing service, whether this is in a hospital or a community nursing agency. In 1975, Stephen A. Treffman, associate director of the Hospitalwide Education and Training Project, Hospital Research and Educational Trust, Chicago, estimated that "7,000 nurses are working full-time on in-service [education]" (an increase of 115 per cent over a decade) in 50 per cent of the nation's hospitals.† Treffman called attention to the practice in some hospitals of establishing a centralized education department which provides in-service education for all hospital employees, including nurses. He said that in any centralized program, "Nurses, without any doubt, will play a very large role in this next period and . . . hospitalwide programming may yet prove to be a significant opportunity for nurses to exert a broad positive effect on the health care delivery system." ‡

In-service education will depend upon the opportunities for continuing education which is the next topic discussed in this chapter.

Nature of In-Service Programs. The great variety of in-service programs makes describing a typical program difficult. Most, if not all, include an orientation of new employees to the physical setting, the goals of the institution or agency, its organizational structure, its resources. Skills may be demonstrated, and observational and practice periods provided. Films and other audiovisual media are often used. Industry has highly efficient on-the-job training methods which have been successfully adapted to the needs of health agencies, but any method of teaching (or learning) may be used in the program. The staff may play an active role in determining content and conduct, or a staff committee may be given the responsibility for planning, on the assumption that such persons are more likely to know the needs and interests of the staff than are administrators. As continuing education offerings increase, they may affect the character of in-service programs; this is especially true if they are well organized units around clinical functions and if continuing education is mandatory.

Nurse administrators in two hospitals and a community health agency, discussing "quality assurance," emphasize the importance of continuing study. Delanne A. Simmons says a vital component is ". . . a stimulating, dynamic staff development program designed to meet the needs of staff and provide skills which will meet the agency's program objectives." *

9. CONTINUING EDUCATION

Definitions. Continuing education can be described as any education following the basic preparation for a person's chosen occupation. H. J. Alford,[397] in a text devoted to the subject, says it can include all knowledge and apply to all mankind. Some persons use the term interchangeably with "adult education."

The International Council of Nurses, urging all member associations to initiate and promote a national system of continuing education, says it includes "a wide spectrum of educational activities such as self-directed individual study, in-service programmes, formal postbasic courses, and post-graduate academic studies." †
The American Nurses' Association defines continuing education as:

* Ibid.
† Treffman, Stephen A.: "The Role of the Hospital in Continuing Education," in *Outdate, Update, Continuing Education: Who, What, Where, When, How?* National League for Nursing, New York, 1975, p. 27.
‡ Ibid., p. 33.

* Simmons, Delanne A.: "Quality Assurance in a Home Health Agency," in National League for Nursing: *Quality Assurance. A Joint Venture.* The League, New York, 1975, p. 9 (Pub. No. 15–1595).
† "Continuing Education for Nurses Vital for Effective Nursing Care" (news), *Int. Nurs. Rev.,* **22:**163, (Nov.–Dec.) 1975.

. . . planned learning experiences beyond a basic nursing education program. These experiences are designed to promote the development of knowledge, skills, and attitudes for the enhancement of nursing practice, thus improving health care to the public.*

The National Commission for the Study of Nursing and Nursing Education defined continuing education in the following terms:

Formalized learning experiences or sequences designed to enlarge the knowledge or skills of practitioners. As distinct from *advanced education,* continuing education courses tend to be more specific, of generally shorter duration and may result in certificates of completion or specialization, but not in formal academic degrees.†

Enid Goldberg uses this last, more specific, definition in an NLN-sponsored conference in 1974, reported under the title *Outdate Update, Continuing Education: Who, What, Where, When, How.* (The League, New York, 1975, p. 2.)

The Need for Continuing Education. Although many people have not recognized it, there has always been a need for continuing education in any occupation. This is particularly true for the health occupations based on a developing body of scientific knowledge and a rapidly expanding technology. Pellegrino made the following observations:

Next to integrity, competence is the first and most fundamental moral responsibility of all the health professions.

. . .

The uniqueness of a "profession" is its declaration that it possesses special knowledge of use to individuals and society. When we truly embrace that knowledge and can use it for optimal solution of a health problem, we are competent practitioners. When we do not, we are guilty of pretense and hypocrisy.

. . .

Continuing education is the only guarantee of continuing competence and the ultimate protection for the patient of the quality of care he receives. It is too important to be left as an individual responsibility. We must make it a corporate responsibility by imposing it as a requirement for all members of the health professions through their professional organizations.

Only in this way can we forestall restrictive legislation and only in this way can we really meet our own responsibility for maintenance of competence—which I wish to iterate, as I did at the outset, is now a moral responsibility.*

As a "corporate responsibility," continuing education has been more or less accepted by a number of professions; nursing is in the process of accepting it.

Goldberg [398] maintains that (voluntary) continuing education is not "new" in nursing. She cites Florence Nightingale's statement, "Let us never consider ourselves as finished nurses. . . . We must be learning all our lives." Mentioning some early programs, Goldberg dates the current emphasis from the first National Conference on Continuing Education for Nurses in Williamsburg, Va., in 1969, which was instituted by "concerned nurses" from the School of Nursing at the Medical College of Virginia in Richmond and attended by representatives of 46 colleges and universities and 19 regional medical programs representing 37 states. However, in 1967 and 1968, the ANA had issued two pamphlets—*Avenues for Continued Learning* and *Continued Education in Nursing: Tools and Techniques,* indicating concern within the Association.

The National Conference Group on Continuing Education in Nursing had initiated *The Journal of Continuing Education in Nursing* in 1970, and in 1971 asked the ANA to develop an "appropriate mechanism to incorporate one group." [399] The ANA announced in November, 1971 (*Am. J. Nurs.,* **71:**2071), that it would have a Council on Continuing Education which is now under the Commission on Education. The first Council meeting was held in 1973, and from then on, according to Alice Price,[400] the "voluntary [conference] groups became a part of the professional nursing organization."

At first, the question of whether continuing education should be voluntary or compulsory was hotly debated. Gertrude Gibbs,[401] nurse educator, discussing this question in 1971, compared policies and practices in medicine, dentistry, dietetics, and nurse anesthesiology. In 1973, Cohen and Miike [402] noted continuing education was a requirement for relicensure in some states for chiropractors, dentists, nursing home administrators, osteopaths, pharmacists, physicians, physician's assistants and dental assistants, podiatrists, and veterinarians.

The Division of Nursing in the USPHS funded a study of continuing education in five states under the direction of Signe S. Cooper and Helen Hestad Byrns, the report of which was published in 1973.[403] This study has re-

* American Nurses' Association: *Continuing Education in Nursing. An Overview.* The Association, Kansas City, Mo., 1976, p. 1.
† National Commission for the Study of Nursing and Nursing Education: *Continuing Education in Nursing: Necessity and Opportunity.* The Commission, Rochester, N.Y., [1971], p. 4.

* Pellegrino, Edmund D.: "Continuing Education in the Health Professions," *Am. J. Pharm. Educ.,* **33:**712, (Dec.) 1969.

sulted in a wide range of offerings at the universities of these states.

While the ANA's House of Delegates rejected mandatory continuing education in 1972, it passed a resolution in 1974 that supported "establishing participation in continuing education approved by state nurses' associations as one prerequisite for continuing registration of the license to practice the profession of nursing." *

At its 1975 convention, the NLN appointed a task force to review the League's role in continuing education. In 1974 the League stated its belief that "a continuing education requirement as a requisite for renewal of licensure of nurses will promote the delivery of optimum care" † and, in 1975, supported "gradual and carefully planned implementation of such a requirement." ‡

Mandatory continuing education for relicensure in nursing requires legislative changes, state by state. California was the first state to enact such legislation. In 1971, it adopted a compulsory system, with initial "certification and recertification" for nurses and practical nurses every five years beginning in 1973.[404] Utah in 1971 made continuing education a requisite of membership in the state nurses' association.[405]

Any listing of legislation on continuing education is out of date by the time it is printed. One recent newsletter of a state nurses' association made the following observation:

Non-credit continuing education has been the fastest growing segment of education since the close of World War II. The upsurge in non-credit educational offerings can be traced directly to: (1) the rapid expansion of knowledge, and (2) the obsolescence of its long term utility. These two factors have contributed substantially to the demand for non-credit continuing education directed toward the rehabilitation and retraining of the existing worker force.§

In 1974, the ANA's Council on Continuing Education published *Standards for Continuing Education in Nursing;* in 1975, an Ad Hoc Committee of the Council prepared *Accreditation of Continuing Education in Nursing— State Nurses Associations, National Specialty Nursing Organizations, Federal Nursing Serv-* *ices, State Boards of Nursing.* The latter publication, approved by the Council, is a guide for all those involved in such programs. Appendices include forms used in applying for "accreditation," for "approval of continuing education activity." Another publication of the Ad Hoc Committee in 1976 is *Continuing Education in Nursing, An Overview.* See Figure 1-36 for a diagram showing the structure under which continuing education programs are accredited.

Laws and professional regulations on continuing education stipulate a unit of measurement. In the United States, the nationally accepted Continuing Education Unit (CEU), which requires six CEUs for every 2-year relicensing period, is used in the California law. A CEU represents 10 "contact-hours" of participation in an organized continuing education experience under responsible sponsorship, capable direction, and qualified instruction.[406] It was developed by a National Task Force on the CEU initiated in 1968.[407] Many students of the subject doubt whether an unfocused program of study—simply a collection of Continuing Education Units—will materially improve the effectiveness of the health worker. Nursing organizations agree that the quality of continuing education should be guaranteed. The NLN takes the position that continuing education courses offered by accredited nursing programs in colleges and universities are automatically accredited. The League's official magazine, *Nursing Outlook,* in the November 1975 issue, listed continuing education courses in nine · universities, the American Academy of Medical Administrators, and the American Academy of Orthopedic Surgeons. The ANA's official organ, *American Journal of Nursing,* in the January 1976 issue, listed continuing education programs under eight universities alone or in conjunction with related hospitals, one international health organization, six national health organizations, one polytechnic institute and hospital, and one hospital. Many state nursing organizations have devised or are developing systems for assignment of credit toward a continuing education requirement using guidelines issued by the NLN and ANA.* Special guidelines on short-term continuing education programs for nursing specialties will evolve, for example, the program for Pediatric Nurse Associates issued by the Division of Maternal and Child Health Nursing Practice of the ANA and the American Academy of Pedi-

---

* American Nurses' Association: *Statement on Continuing Education.* The Association, Kansas City, Mo., 1974.

† National League for Nursing: *NLN's Role in Continuing Education in Nursing.* The League, New York, 1974.

‡ "NLN's Board Reviews Statement on Continuing Education Issues," *NLN News,* **23:**3, (June–July) 1975.

§ Connecticut Nurses' Association: "Continuing Education," *Nurs. News,* **48:**3, (May) 1975.

* No national or state organization is proposing credit toward a degree, or the earning of a degree as mandatory for relicensure.

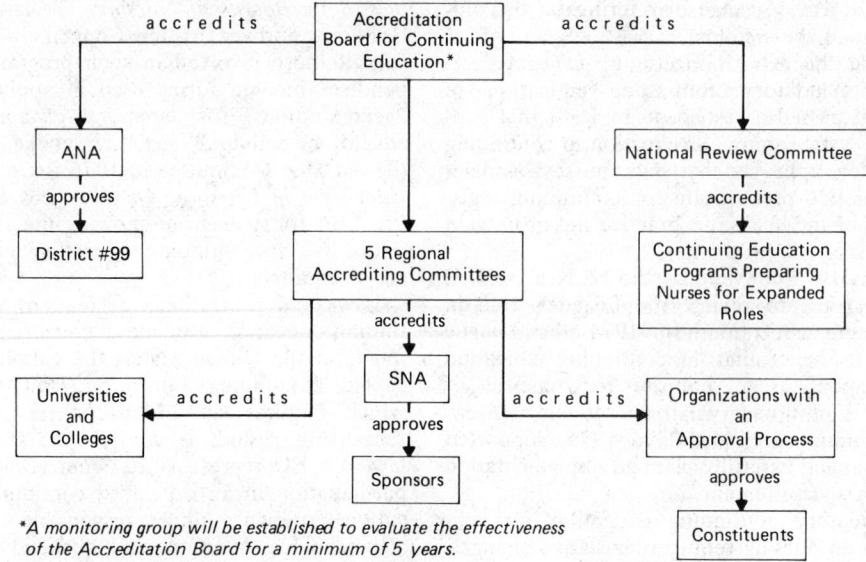

Figure 1-36. ANA accreditation mechanism for continuing education in nursing. (From "ANA Setting Up National Accreditation of Continuing Education Programs," *Am. J. Nurs.*, **75:**1249, [Aug.] 1975.)

atrics in 1971.[408] In 1975, a "Blue Ribbon Commission" composed of representatives from ANA Division on Maternal-Child Health Nursing Practice, National Foundation-March of Dimes, American Board of Pediatrics, American Academy of Pediatrics, Health Services Administration, American Association of Colleges of Nursing, American College of Obstetricians and Gynecologists, American Board of Obstetrics and Gynecology, and clinical specialists in each area produced the following: *Guidelines for Short-Term Continuing Education Programs for the Nurse Clinician in Intensive Neonatal Care and the Nurse Clinician in Intensive Maternal-Fetal Care.* The Commission was sponsored by the National Foundation.[409]

All nursing organizations will eventually be concerned with legislation on and professional awards or recognition for continued study; they will also be involved in planning and devising more effective programs and methods. The subject is so much discussed that statements made today are out of date tomorrow. Students of nursing cannot afford to neglect this question, and will find ample information on it in current nursing journals.

SUMMARY

Nursing is shown in this chapter to be an essential health service that attracts increasing numbers of men and women, although women still dominate the profession and, in the United States, minorities do not have proportionate representation in nursing. Types of nursing personnel continue to increase, with numbers of "allied" or "auxiliary" workers exceeding registered nurses in number in this and some other countries. One authority on international standards for health workers is quoted as saying that 400 categories are involved. Coordination of health care is increasingly difficult, with fragmentation and impersonalization of care common complaints of the public.

Because the roles of health workers overlap and vary from place to place and from one era to another, an understanding of the development of nursing depends upon some knowledge of the development of medicine. And since health workers share with other general educators the responsibility for health education of the public, this relationship must be recognized. Health education is especially pertinent today when the loudest critics of health care stress putting more emphasis than there is at present on prevention and the development of self-help, or self-reliance, in matters of health.

The role of the registered nurse has unquestionably "expanded," but there is currently more recognition than in the past of the extent to which registered nurses have always been "extenders of medical care"—a role now shared with feldshers in Russia and physician's assistants in this and some other countries.

While nurses, physicians, special therapists,

medical social workers, and all health personnel have the same goal in raising health standards and reducing unnecessary suffering, each category has a function or role in which it is most proficient. Various definitions of the nurse's function are recognized and have been noted, but the concept dominating this book is stressed—namely, that nurses are uniquely qualified to help people perform those functions (related to health) that they would perform unaided if they had the strength, the will, or the knowledge, and to give people this help in such a way that they gain their independence as soon as possible, learn to cope with a health handicap that cannot be eliminated, or die in dignity when death is inevitable.* When physicians are unavailable, and just as in emergencies when any citizen may treat the victim, nurses may prescribe therapy; they regularly help patients with the therapeutic regimen prescribed by physicians. The extent to which nursing is a profession is examined in this chapter, the independent nurse practitioner is recognized, and the conclusion is reached that all registered nurses are legally accountable for their acts.

If nursing is studied as an occupation, it is seen in most countries to be the largest in the health field. Certain social scientists have noted that the public image and self-image of nurses are different and that there is a lag in the public's understanding of the role nurses are playing in health care. Whether or not there is a national (tax-supported) health service available to all citizens or a mixture of private and public services, there is a pervasive feeling in many countries that the cost of health care is too high. In the United States, current studies are in progress to establish quantitative and qualitative standards to facilitate planning and act as controls on health care, although some critics say the present system in the United States is beyond salvage with any contemplated controls. While the cost of health care in the United States, Canada, Great Britain, Sweden, and other countries is burdensome for the taxpayer or the individual (according to the system), international and national studies show that there is less economic reward for nursing than for other occupations, such as teaching, with which it might be compared.

Registered nurses who graduate from initial or basic programs may hold diplomas in nursing, or associate, baccalaureate, or master's degrees in nursing. In a postbasic program, registered nurses earn baccalaureate degrees, and in graduate programs, they earn master's

and doctoral degrees. Allied or auxiliary nursing personnel are prepared in a variety of programs and function under a variety of titles. Some reasons why nursing education is said to be "chaotic" are shown in this chapter. In-service programs are discussed briefly and continuing education is discussed in more detail.

While the emphasis is on the role of the registered nurse in the United States and Canada, there are many references to related health personnel and to health care in other parts of the world.

The work of nurses is vital and varied in its character; because of its variety and impelling interest, it appeals to many different natures. A study of successful nurses seems to show they have a number of common characteristics, but this does not mean that the successful nurse is "a type." There is the science of nursing, but equally important, there is the art of nursing. In its highest form, nursing calls for the same qualities that are found in most persons who work successfully in other professional fields—sensitiveness to people and their moods, insight into human nature, an ability to distinguish what is true from what is false, the capacity for sustained effort, and the mastery of the techniques involved.

REFERENCES

1. Frazer, James George: *The Golden Bough.* Macmillan Publishing Co., Inc. New York, 1926.
2. Topoff, Howard F.: "The Social Behavior of Army Ants," *Sci. Am.,* **227:**71, (Nov.) 1972.
3. Wilson, Edward O.: "Animal Communication," *Sci. Am.,* **227:**53, (Sept.) 1972.
4. Sidel, Victor W., and Sidel, Ruth: *Serve the People. Observations on Medicine in the People's Republic of China.* Beacon Press, Boston, 1973.
5. Bullough, Vern, and Bullough, Bonnie: *Emergence of Modern Nursing.* Macmillan Publishing Co., Inc., New York, 1969.
6. Levine, Edwin B., and Levine, Myra E.: "Hippocrates, Father of Nursing, Too?" *Am. J. Nurs.,* **65:**86, (Dec.) 1965.
7. Jackson, Edgar: *The Pastor and His People.* Channel Press, Manhasset, N.Y., 1963.
8. Hume, Edgar Erskine: *Medical Work of the Knights Hospitalers of Saint John of Jerusalem.* Johns Hopkins Press, Baltimore, 1940.
9. Kelly, Lucie Young: *Dimensions of Professional Nursing,* 3rd ed. Macmillan Publishing Co., Inc., New York, 1975, p. 21.
10. Hastings, Randall: *The Universities of*

* The fact that the ICN uses this definition makes it of special interest.

Europe in the Middle Ages. Clarendon Press, Oxford, 1895.

11. Lippard, Vernon W.: *A Half-Century of American Medical Education 1920–1970.* Josiah Macy, Jr. Foundation, New York, 1974, p. 3.

12. Flexner, Abraham: *Medical Education in the United States and Canada. A Report to the Carnegie Foundation for the Advancement of Teaching.* The Foundation, New York, 1910.

13. Bernard, Claude: *Introduction to the Study of Experimental Medicine.* (Translated by Henry C. Greene.) Macmillan Publishing Co., New York, 1927.

14. Nilsson, Lennart: *Behold Man—A Photographic Journey Inside the Body.* In collaboration with Jan Lindberg. Little, Brown & Co., Boston, 1974.

15. Thomas, Lewis: *The Lives of a Cell. Notes of a Biology Watcher.* Viking Press, New York, 1974.

16. Bullough, Vern, and Bullough, Bonnie: *The Subordinate Sex—A History of Attitudes Towards Women.* University of Illinois Press, Urbana, 1973.

16a. Ashley, Jo Ann: *Hospitals, Paternalism, and the Role of the Nurse.* Teachers College Press, New York, 1976.

17. Mead, Margaret: *Male and Female.* William Morrow & Co., New York, 1949.

18. Austin, Anne L.: *History of Nursing Source Book.* G. P. Putnam's Sons, New York, 1957, p. 257.

19. National League for Nursing: *Extending the Boundaries of Nursing Education—The Preparation and Role of the Nurse Scientist.* Papers and summary from second conference of Council of Baccalaureate and Higher Degree Programs, Cleveland, Mar., 1968. The League, New York, 1968 (Pub. No. 15–342).

20. National League for Nursing: *Doctoral Programs in Nursing/Nurse Scientist Graduate Training Grants Program—1973.* The League, New York, 1973 (Pub. No. 15–1558).

21. Eriksson, Katie: "Sairannhoidon Kehittäminen Oppiaineena," (An Approach—How to Develop Nursing Science.) *Sairaanhoidon Vuosikirja* **XI**:9 (Helsinki) 1974.

22. Henderson, Virginia: "Barber Surgeons of France in the Sixteenth Century." Teachers College, Columbia University, New York, 1931 (unpublished study).

23. World Health Organization: *The Training and Utilization of Feldshers in the USSR.* A Review Prepared by the Ministry of Health of the USSR for the World Health Organization. The Organization, Geneva, 1974, pp. 9, 18.

24. Sadler, Alfred M., et al.: *The Physician's Assistant Today and Tomorrow. Issues Confronting New Health Practitioners,* 2nd ed. Ballinger Publishing Co., Cambridge, Mass., 1975.

25. Nightingale, Florence: *Notes on Nursing.* Dover Publications, New York, 1969. (Republication of first American edition, 1860.)

26. Woodham-Smith, Mrs. Cecil: *Florence Nightingale, 1820–1910.* Constable & Co., Ltd., London, 1950.

27. Goodrich, Annie W.: *The Social and Ethical Significance of Nursing.* Macmillan Publishing Co., Inc., New York, 1932.

28. "The National Children's Bureau" (editorial), *Am. J. Nurs.,* **9:**389, (Mar.) 1909.

29. Van Doren, Mark: *Liberal Education.* Henry Holt, New York, 1943.

29a. Carlson, Rick J.: *The End of Medicine.* John Wiley & Sons, New York, 1975.

30. Dillon, John B.: "How Did it Happen?" *Calif. Med.,* **113:**86, (Aug.) 1970.

31. Carnegie Commission on Higher Education: *Higher Education and the Nation's Health—Policies for Medical and Dental Education.* McGraw-Hill Book Co., New York, 1970.

32. Hepner, James O., and Hepner, Donna M.: *The Health Strategy Game. A Challenge for Reorganization and Management.* C. V. Mosby Co., St. Louis, 1973.

33. "Nursing in the Decade Ahead," *Am. J. Nurs.,* **70:**2115, (Oct.) 1970.

34. Brodt, Dagmar E.: "Excellence or Obsolescence: The Choice for Nursing," *Nurs. Forum,* **9:**19 (No. 1) 1970.

35. Christman, Luther: "What the Future Holds for Nursing," *Nurs. Forum,* **9:**12, (No. 1) 1970.

36. Somers, Anne R.: *Health Care in Transition: Directions for the Future.* Hospital Research and Educational Trust, Chicago, 1971.

37. National League for Nursing: *Crisis in Nursing—Changing Roles.* Papers presented at 1973 NLN Biennial Convention. The League, New York, 1973 (Pub. No. 20–1503).

38. Roe, Anne, and Sherwood, Mary: *Nursing in the Seventies.* John Wiley & Sons, New York, 1973.

39. Taffe, P.: "Nursing Today—A Profession —A Vocation—A Job?" *Aust. Nurses J.,* **2:**31, (Oct.) 1973.

40. Dyson, R.: "Changes in Professional Roles —Implications for the Future," *Can. J. Psychiatr. Nursing,* (Jan.–Feb.) 1973.

41. National League for Nursing: *Current Issues in Nursing Education.* Papers presented at 11th Conference of Council of Baccalaureate and Higher Degree Programs, Kansas City, Mo., Nov. 1973. The League, New York, 1974.

42. Bowman, Rosemary Amason, and Culpepper, Rebecca Clark: "National Health Insurance: Some of the Issues," *Am. J. Nurs.,* **75:**2017, (Nov.) 1975.

43. Gartner, A.: "Health Systems and New

Careers," *Health Serv. Res.,* **88:**124, (Feb.) 1973.

44. National League for Nursing: *Goals for a National Health Insurance Program.* The League, New York, 1974.

45. Broussean, B. L.: "The Transfer of Functions Between Health Professions," *Can. Hosp.,* **49:**44, (Sept.) 1972.

46. Wagner, D. L.: "Issues in the Provision of Health Care for All," *Am. J. Public Health,* **63:**481, (June) 1973.

47. Meakins, J. C.: "Nursing Must Be Defined," *Am. J. Nurs.,* **48:**622, (Oct.) 1948.

48. Abdellah, Faye G., et al.: *Patient-Centered Approaches to Nursing.* Macmillan Publishing Co., Inc., New York, 1960.

48a. Johnson, Mae M., and Davis, Mary Lou C.: *Problem Solving in Nursing Practice,* 2nd ed. William C. Brown, Dubuque, Iowa, 1975.

49. Simmons, Leo W., and Henderson, Virginia: *Nursing Research. A Survey and Assessment.* Appleton-Century-Crofts, New York, 1964, p. 33.

50. Badouaille, M. L.: "Why Nursing Is Different," *N.Z. Nurs. J.,* **66:**29, (July) 1973.

51. Kraegel, Janet M., et al.: *Patient Care Systems.* J. B. Lippincott Co., Philadelphia, 1974.

52. Bridges, Daisy Caroline: *A History of the International Council of Nurses, 1899–1964. The First Sixty-Five Years.* Pitman Medical Publishing Co., Ltd., London, 1967.

53. National League of Nursing Education, Committee on Curriculum: *A Curriculum Guide for Schools of Nursing.* The League, New York, 1937, p. 20.

54. Hughes, Everett C., et al.: *Twenty Thousand Nurses Tell Their Story.* J. B. Lippincott Co., Philadelphia, 1958.

55. Lysaught, Jerome P. (ed.): *Action in Nursing; Progress in Professional Purpose.* (A collection of 33 articles and pamphlets related to work of National Commission for the Study of Nursing and Nursing Education.) McGraw-Hill Book Co., New York, 1974.

56. Hall, Virginia: *Statutory Regulation of the Scope of Nursing Practice—A Critical Survey.* National Joint Practice Commission, Chicago, 1975.

57. National League of Nursing Education, Committee on Curriculum: *op. cit.*

58. Vaillot, Sister Madeleine Clémence: *Commitment to Nursing. A Philosophical Investigation.* J. B. Lippincott Co., Philadelphia, 1962, p. 27.

59. Simmons, Leo W., and Henderson, Virginia: *op. cit.,* p. 119.

60. Brown, Martha M.: *Nurses, Patients and Social Systems. The Effect of Skilled Nursing Intervention upon Institutionalized Older Patients.* University of Missouri Press, Columbia, 1969, p. 96 (University of Missouri Studies Vol. XLVI).

61. Fielo, Sandra B.: *A Summary of Integrated Nursing Theory,* 2nd ed. McGraw-Hill Book Co., New York, 1975.

62. Harris, M. Isabel: "Theory Building in Nursing. A Review of the Literature," *Image,* **4:**6, (No. 1.) 1972.

63. Jacox, Ada: "Theory Construction in Nursing: An Overview," *Nurs. Res.,* **23:**4, (Jan.–Feb.) 1974.

64. Johnson, Dorothy E.: "Theory in Nursing: Borrowed and Unique?" *Nurs. Res.,* **17:**206, (May–June) 1968.

65. King, Imogene M.: *Toward a Theory for Nursing.* John Wiley & Sons, New York, 1971.

66. Ketefian, Shake (ed.): *Translation of Theory into Nursing Practice and Education with a Bibliography on Change.* Proceedings of 7th Annual Clinical Sessions, New York, Apr. 27, 1974. New York University, Division of Nurse Education, New York, 1974.

67. Kintzel, Kay Corman (ed.): *Advanced Concepts in Clinical Nursing.* J. B. Lippincott Co., Philadelphia, 1971.

68. Mathwig, Gean: "Nursing Science—The Theoretical Core of Nursing Knowledge," *Image,* **4:**20, (No. 1) 1971.

69. Mitchell, Pamelia (ed.): *Concepts Basic to Nursing.* McGraw-Hill Book Co., New York, 1973.

70. Murphy, Juanita F.: *Theoretical Issues in Professional Nursing.* Appleton-Century-Crofts, New York, 1971.

71. Murray, Ruth, and Zeniner, Judith: *Nursing Concepts for Health Promotion.* Prentice-Hall, Inc., Englewood Cliffs, N.J., 1975.

72. Newman, Margaret A.: "Nursing's Theoretical Evolution," *Nurs. Outlook,* **20:**449, (July) 1972.

73. Nursing Development Conference Group: *Concept Formalization in Nursing Process and Product.* Little, Brown & Co., Boston, 1973.

74. Riehl, J. P., and Roy, Sister Callista: *Conceptual Models for Nursing Practice.* Appleton-Century-Crofts, New York, 1974.

75. Rogers, Martha E.: *An Introduction to the Theoretical Basis of Nursing.* F. A. Davis Co., Philadelphia, 1970.

76. Strauss, Anselm: "The Structure and Ideology of American Nursing: An Interpretation," in David, Fred (ed.): *The Nursing Profession: Five Sociological Essays.* John Wiley & Sons, New York, 1966.

77. Nagle, Ernest: *The Structure of Science.* Harcourt, Brace & World, New York, 1961, p. 106.

78. Wald, Florence, and Leonard, Robert: "Toward Development of Nursing Practice Theory," *Nurs. Res.,* **13:**309, (Fall) 1964.

78a. Rogers, Martha E.: *op. cit.*

79. Santayana, George: "The Process of Nursing as an Open System," in Kintzel, Kay Corman (ed.): *Advanced Concepts in Clin-*

ical Nursing. J. B. Lippincott Co., Philadelphia, 1971.

80. Von Bertalanffy, Ludwig: *General Systems Theory.* George Brazillier, New York, 1968.

81. Kraegel, Janet M.: "A System of Patient Care Based on Patient Needs," *Am. J. Nurs.,* **72:**257, (Apr.) 1972.

82. Kraegel, Janet M., et al.: *Patient Care Systems.* J. B. Lippincott Co., Philadelphia, 1974.

83. Bowar-Ferres, Susan: "Loeb Center and Its Philosophy of Nursing," *Am. J. Nurs.,* **75:**810, (May) 1975.

84. University of Kansas Medical Center, Department of Nursing Education: *Case Studies of Nursing Intervention.* McGraw-Hill Book Co., New York, 1974.

85. Giblin, Elizabeth S.: "Symposium on Assessment as Part of the Nursing Process," *Nurs. Clin. North Am.,* **6:**113, (Mar.) 1971.

86. Henderson, Virginia: "Is the Role of the Nurse Changing?" *Weathervane,* **27:**12, (Oct.) 1968.

87. Jamann, JoAnn Shafer: "Providing for the Maintenance of Health," in Kintzel, Kay Corman (ed.): *Advanced Concepts in Clinical Nursing.* J. B. Lippincott Co., Philadelphia, 1971, p. 14.

88. Marriner Ann: *The Nursing Process: A Scientific Approach to Nursing Care.* C. V. Mosby Co., St. Louis, 1975.

89. Mauksch, Hans O.: "The Nurse: Coordinator of Patient Care," in Skipper, James K., Jr., and Leonard, Robert C.: *Social Interaction and Patient Care.* J. B. Lippincott Co., Philadelphia, 1965.

90. Nightingale, Florence: *op. cit.*

91. Orlando, Ida Jean: *The Dynamic Nurse-Patient Relationship.* G. P. Putnam's Sons, New York, 1961.

92. Rogers, Martha E.: *op. cit.*

93. Sand, René: "The Nurse—Sentinel of Health," *Aust. Nurses J.,* **52:**80, (Apr.) 1954.

94. Schulman, S.: "Basic Functional Roles in Nursing: Mother Surrogate and Healer," in Jaco, E. G. (ed.): *Patients, Physicians and Illness: Sourcebook on Behavioral Science and Medicine.* Free Press, Glencoe, Ill., 1958.

95. Sobol, Evelyn G., and Robischon, Paulette: *Family Nursing; A Study Guide.* C. V. Mosby Co., St. Louis, 1975.

96. Sutterley, Doris Cook, and Donnelly, Gloria Ferraro: *Perspectives in Human Development—Nursing Throughout the Life Cycle.* J. B. Lippincott Co., Philadelphia, 1973.

97. Woolley, F. Ross, et al.: *Problem-Oriented Nursing.* Springer Publishing Co., New York, 1974.

98. Dubos, René: *Mirage of Health.* Doubleday & Co., Garden City, N.Y., 1959.

99. Cochrane, A. L.: *Effectiveness and Efficiency: Random Reflections on Health Services.* Nuffield Provincial Hospitals Trust, London, 1972.

100. Illich, Ivan: *Medical Nemesis; The Expropriation of Health.* McGlelland & Stewart, London, 1975.

101. Malleson, Andrew: *Need Your Doctor Be So Useless?* George Allen & Unwin, London, 1973.

102. Meador, Clifton: "The Art and Science of Non-Disease," *N. Engl. J. Med.,* **272:**92, (Jan. 14) 1965.

103. Shey, Herbert H.: "Iatrogenic Anxiety," *Psychiatr. Q.,* **45:**343, (No. 1) 1971.

104. Vayda, Eugene: "A Comparison of Surgical Rates in Canada and in England and Wales," *N. Engl. J. Med.,* **289:**1224, (Dec. 6) 1973.

105. Illich, Ivan: *op. cit.*

106. Royal Society of Medicine, and Josiah Macy, Jr. Foundation: *The Greater Medical Profession.* The Foundation, New York, 1973.

107. Josiah Macy, Jr. Foundation: *Macy Conference on Intermediate-Level Health Personnel in the Delivery of Direct Health Services. Intermediate-Level Health Practitioners.* The Foundation, New York, 1973.

108. Bloomfield, Ron, and Follis, Peggy (eds.): *The Health Team in Action.* BBC Publications, London, 1974.

109. Anderson, J. A. D., et al.: "Attachment of Community Nurses to General Practices: A Follow-up Study," *Br. Med. J.,* **4:**103, (Oct. 10) 1970.

110. Anderson, Evelyn R.: *The Role of the Nurse.* Royal College of Nursing, London, 1973.

111. "Reorganization—1974 or 1984? Where the Nurses Will Stand," *Br. Med. J.,* **2:**603, (June 9) 1973.

112. Moore, M. F., et al.: "First Contact Decisions in General Practice. A Comparison Between a Nurse and Three General Practitioners," *Lancet,* **1:**817, (Apr. 14) 1973.

113. Wilson, Barnett J.: "A Description of the Working Environment and Work of the Unit Nursing Officer," *Int. J. Nurs. Studies,* **10:**185, (Aug.) 1973.

114. Apitzer, W. O., et al.: "Nurse Practitioners in Primary Care. 3. Southern Ontario Randomized Trial," *Can. Med. Assoc. J.,* **108:**1005, (Apr. 21) 1973.

115. Canada. Department of National Health and Welfare, Committee on Clinical Training of Nurses for Medical Services in the North: *Report.* (Chairman, D. Kergin.) The Department, Ottawa, 1970.

116. Canadian Nurses' Association: *Joint CMA/CNA/CHA Conference, Health Action, Sept. 23–24, 1972.* Canadian Nurses' Association, Ottawa, 1972.

117. Carpenter, Helen: "The Canadian Scene," *Int. Nurs. Rev.,* **21:**43, (Mar–Apr.) 1974.

118. DeMarsh, Kathleen G.: "Red Cross Out-

post Nursing in New Brunswick," *Can. Nurse,* **69:**24, (June) 1973.

119. Hazlett, C. B.: "Task Analysis of the Clinically Trained Nurse," *Nurs. Clin. North Am.,* **10:**699, (Dec.) 1975.

120. Jones, Phyllis E.: "A Program in Continuing Education for Primary Care," *Nurs. Clin. North Am.,* **10:**691, (Dec.) 1975.

121. Bowers, John A., and Purcell, E. F. (eds.): *Medicine and Society in China.* Report of a Conference sponsored jointly by National Library of Medicine and Josiah Macy, Jr. Foundation. The Foundation, New York, 1974.

122. Kessen, William (ed.): *Childhood in China.* Yale University Press, New Haven, Conn., 1975.

123. Sidel, Victor W., and Sidel, Ruth: *op. cit.*

124. Maxwell, R.: *Health Care: The Proving Dilemma; Needs Versus Resources in Western Europe, the U.S. and U.S.S.R.* McKinsey & Co., New York, 1974.

125. Quinn, Sheila M.: "Nursing in the Soviet Union," *Int. Nurs. Rev.,* **15:**75, (Jan.) 1968.

126. Seldon, Mark: *China: Revolution and Health.* Health Policy Advisory Center, New York, 1972.

127. Simon, Carlton (ed.): *Shobers Directory of Trained Nurses. Being a Selected List of Names and Addresses of Competent Graduated Trained Nurses Practicing in the Cities of Greater New York, Boston, Philadelphia, Baltimore and Washington.* Chober-Cornell Publishing Co., New York, 1902.

128. *Nurses' and Physicians' Directory and Health Book of New Haven County.* City Printing Co., New Haven, Conn., 1923.

129. Schutt, Barbara G.: "Spot Check on Primary Care Nursing," *Am. J. Nurs.,* **72:**1996, (Nov.) 1972.

130. ————: "Frontier's Family Nurses," *Am. J. Nurs.,* **72:**903, (May) 1972.

131. "Frontier Nurses of Kentucky Set an Enviable Record," *Mod. Hosp.,* **39:**60, (Sept.) 1932.

132. Djukanovic, V., and Mach, E. P. (eds.): *Alternative Approaches to Meeting Basic Health Needs in Developing Countries. A Joint UNICEF/WHO Study.* World Health Organization, Geneva, 1975.

133. World Health Organization: *The Training and Utilization of Feldshers in the U.S.S.R.* The Organization, Geneva, 1974, p. 7.

134. American Nurses' Association: *Facts About Nursing 74–75.* The Association, Kansas City, Mo., 1976, p. 165.

135. International Labour Office: *Employment and Conditions of Work and Life of Nursing Personnel.* International Labour Conference, 61st Session, 1976, Report VII (1). The Office, Geneva, 1976, pp. 5, 17.

136. American Medical Association, Committee on Nursing: "Medicine and Nursing in the 1970s: A Position Statement," *J.A.M.A.,* **213:**1881, (Sept. 14) 1970.

137. "The Expanded Role of the Nurse. A Joint Statement of CNA/CMA," *Can. Nurse,* **69:**23, (May) 1973.

138. "Canadian Nurses, Doctors Develop Statement of Policy on Expanded Role," *Int. Nurs. Rev.,* **21:**28, (Jan.–Feb.)1974.

139. May, Ruth E.: "Programme in Outpost Nursing," in International Council of Nurses: *Focus on the Future.* Proceedings of 14th Quadrennial Congress, Montreal, 1969. The Council, Geneva, 1970, p. 326.

140. Canada. Department of National Health and Welfare: [*Report of*] *Committee on Clinical Training of Nurses for Medical Services in the North.* (Chairman, Dorothy J. Kergin.) The Department, Ottawa, 1970.

141. Jones, Phyllis E.: "A Program in Continuing Education for Primary Health Care," *Nurs. Clin. North Am.,* **10:**691, (Dec.) 1975.

142. Hazlett, C. B.: "Task Analysis of the Clinically Trained Nurse (C.T.N.)," *Nurs. Clin. North Am.,* **10:**699, (Dec.) 1975.

143. Splane, Verna Huffman: "Foreword. Symposium on Community Nursing in Canada," *Nurs. Clin. North Am.,* **10:**687, (Dec.) 1975.

144. "The Expanded Role of the Nurse. A Joint Statement of CNA/CMA," *Can. Nurse,* **69:**23, (May) 1973.

145. Charron, K. C.: *Education of the Health Professions in the Context of the Health Care System: The Ontario Experience.* Organization for Economic Cooperation and Development, Paris, 1975.

146. Pellegrino, Edmund D.: "Nursing and Medicine; Ethical Implications in Changing Practice," *Am. J. Nurs.,* **64:**110, (Sept.) 1964.

147. Silver, Henry: "The Pediatric Nurse Practitioner Program," *J.A.M.A.,* **204:**298, (Apr. 22) 1968.

148. ————: "New Allied Health Professionals: Implications of the Colorado Child Health Associate Law," *N. Engl. J. Med.,* **284:**304, (Feb. 11) 1971.

149. Sadler, Alfred M., Jr., et al.: *The Physician's Assistant Today and Tomorrow; Issues Confronting New Health Practitioners,* 2nd ed. Ballinger Publishing Co., Cambridge, Mass., 1975, p. 8.

150. American Nurses' Association, and American Academy of Pediatrics: *Guidelines on Short-Term Continuing Education Programs for Pediatric Nurse Associates (A Joint Statement).* The Association, Kansas City, Mo., 1971.

151. American Nurses' Association: *Pediatric Nurse Practitioners—Their Practice Today.* The Association, Kansas City, Mo., 1975.

152. Brown, Marie S., et al.: "The Maternal-Child Nurse Practitioner," *Am. J. Nurs.,* **75:**1298, (Aug.) 1975.

153. Charney, Evan, and Kitzman, Harriet: "The Child-Health Nurse (Pediatric Nurse Practitioner) in Private Practice: A Con-

trolled Trial," *N. Engl. J. Med.,* **285:**1353, (Dec. 9) 1971.

154. Chappell, James A., and Drogos, Patricia A.: "Evaluation of Infant Health Care by a Nurse Practitioner," *Pediatrics,* **49:**871, (June) 1972.

155. Day, L. R., et al.: "Acceptance of Pediatric Nurse Practitioners," *Am. J. Dis. Child.,* **119:**204, (Mar.) 1970.

156. Freeman, B. L., et al.: "How Do Nurses Expand Their Roles in Well Child Care?" *Am. J. Nurs.,* **72:**1866, (Oct.) 1972.

157. Metzler, J., et al.: *A Pediatric Nurse Practitioner and Three Pediatricians Collaborate in Private Practice.* National League for Nursing, New York, 1973.

158. Hilmer, N. A., et al.: "The School Nurse Practitioner and Her Practice: A Study of Traditional and Expanded Health Care Responsibilities for Nurses in Elementary Schools," *J. Sch. Health,* **43:**431, (Sept.) 1973.

159. Lees, R. E.: "Physician Time-Saving by Employment of Expanded-Role Nurses in Family Practice," *Can. Med. Assoc. J.,* **108:**871, (Apr. 7) 1973.

160. Macah, R. C., et al.: "Patients' Attitudes Towards the Nurse as Physician Associate in Pediatric Practice," *Can. J. Public Health,* **64:**121, (Mar.) 1973.

161. Nuckolls, Katherine B., et al.: *Pediatric Nurse Practitioner Preparation in a Graduate Program.* National League for Nursing, New York, 1975 (Pub. No. 15–1563).

162. Stein, R., et al.; "A New Primary Care Medical Practitioner," *Am. J. Dis. Child.,* **126:**298, (Sept.) 1973.

163. Stone, F. M.: "Child Health Associates and Pediatric Nurses: Their Competence," *Pediatrics,* **52:**307, (Aug.) 1973.

164. Poirer, Brooke: "Impact of PNP Programs to be Studied by ANA," *Am. Nurse,* **7:**1, (May) 1975.

165. Simmons, Leo W., and Henderson, Virginia: *op. cit.*

166. Colbert, L.: "The Psychiatric Nurse Clinical Specialist Works with Nursing Service," *J. Psychiatr. Nurs.,* **9:**21, (July–Aug.) 1971.

167. Peplau, Hildegard E.: "Educating the Nurse to Function in Psychiatric Services," in *Nursing Personnel for Mental Health Programs.* Report of a Conference sponsored by the Southern Regional Program on Mental Health Training and Research, Wagoner, Okla., Mar. 27–29, 1957. Southern Regional Education Board, Atlanta, Ga., 1958.

168. Tudor, Gwen E.: "A Sociopsychiatric Nursing Approach to Intervention in a Problem of Mutual Withdrawal on a Mental Ward," *Psychiatry,* **15:**193, (May) 1952.

169. Ruell, Virginia M.: "Nurse-Managed Care for Psychiatric Patients," *Am. J. Nurs.,* **75:**1156, (July) 1975.

170. Lewis, C. E., and Resnik, Barbara: "Nurse Clinics and Progressive Ambulatory Care,"

N. Engl. J. Med., **277:** 1236, (Dec. 7) 1967.

171. ———: "The Nurse Clinic: Dynamics of Ambulatory Care—New Roles for Old Disciplines," *J. Kans. Med. Soc.,* **68:**123, 1967.

172. Lewis, C. E., et al.: "Activities, Events and Outcomes in Ambulatory Patient Care," *N. Engl. J. Med.,* **280:**645, (Mar. 20) 1969.

173. Lewis, C. E.: *Dynamics of Nursing in Ambulatory Care.* (Final Report of Study under USPHS Grant NU-00145). US Government Printing Office, Washington, D.C., 1968.

174. Noonan, Barbara R.: "Eight Years in a Medical Nurse Clinic," *Am. J. Nurs.,* **72:**1128, (June) 1972.

175. Browning, Mary H., and Lewis, Edith P. (comps.): *The Expanded Role of the Nurse.* American Journal of Nursing Co., New York, 1973 (Contemporary Nursing Series).

176. Sadler, Alfred M., Jr., et al.: *The Physician's Assistant Today and Tomorrow; Issues Confronting New Health Practitioners,* 2nd ed. Ballinger Publishing Co., Cambridge, Mass., 1975.

177. National Commission for the Study of Nursing and Nursing Education: *Abstract for Action.* (Report prepared by Jerome P. Lysaught.) McGraw-Hill Book Co., New York, 1970.

178. "AMA Endorses Expanded Role for Nurses. Seeks Study of R.N. and P.A. Functions" (news), *Am. J. Nurs.,* **72:**1365, (Aug.) 1972.

178a. Storey, Patrick B.: *The Soviet Feldsher as a Physician's Assistant.* National Institutes of Health, Bethesda, Md., 1972 (DHEW Pub. No. [NIH] 72–58).

179. World Health Organization: *The Training and Utilization of Feldshers in the U.S.S.R.* The Organization, Geneva, 1974.

180. Quinn, Sheila M.: *op. cit.*

181. International Labour Office: *Employment and Conditions of Work and Life of Nursing Personnel.* International Labour Conference, 1976, 61st Session, Report VII (1). The Office, Geneva, 1976, p. 72.

182. Andreoli, K. G., and Stead, Eugene A.: "Training Physician's Assistants at Duke," *Am. J. Nurs.,* **67:**1442, (July) 1967.

183. Ingles, Thelma: "A New Health Worker," *Am. J. Nurs.,* **68:**1059, (May) 1968.

184. "AMA Unveils Surprise Plan to Convert R.N. into Medic" (news), *Am. J. Nurs.,* **70:**691, (Apr.) 1970.

185. Sadler, Alfred M., Jr., et al.: *The Physician's Assistant Today and Tomorrow; Issues Confronting New Health Practitioners,* 2nd ed. Ballinger Publishing Co., Cambridge, Mass., 1975, p. 153.

186. Sadler, Alfred M., Jr., et al.: *op. cit.,* p. 106.

187. Lambertsen, Eleanor C.: "Perspective on the Physician's Assistant," *Nurs. Outlook,* **20:**32, (Jan.) 1972.

188. Bergman, A.: "Physician's Assistants Be-

long in the Nursing Profession," *Am. J. Nurs.,* **71:**975 (May) 1971.

189. deTornyay, R.: "Expanding the Nurse's Role Does Not Make Her a Physician's Assistant," *Am. J. Nurs.,* **71:**974, (Sept.) 1971.

190. "Nurse Groups Ask R.N.–M.D. Dialogue, Some Get It," *Am. J. Nurs.,* **70:**953, (May) 1970.

191. Sadler, Alfred M., Jr., et al.: *op. cit.,* p. 106.

192. Lipkin, Mack: *The Care of Patients, Concepts and Tactics.* Oxford University Press, New York, 1974.

193. Rakel, Robert E.: "Primary Care—Whose Responsibility?" *J. Fam. Pract.,* **2:**429, (Dec.) 1975.

194. Smoyak, Shirley A.: "Origin, Purpose and Thrust of the National Joint Practice Commission," in *Building for the Future.* Papers presented at ANA Conference, Sept., 1974. The Association, Kansas City, Mo., 1975.

195. Ford, Loretta: "Interdisciplinary Education for Nurses in the Expanded Role: The Way of the Future," in *Building for the Future.* Papers presented at ANA Conference, Sept., 1974. The Association, Kansas City, Mo., 1975.

196. Hall, Virginia: *Statutory Regulation of the Scope of Nursing Practice—A Critical Survey.* National Joint Practice Commission, Chicago, 1975.

197. Devlin, M. M.: *Selected Bibliography with Abstracts on Joint Practice.* National Joint Practice Commission, Chicago, 1975.

198. World Health Organization: *Development of Educational Programmes for the Health Professions.* (Prepared by Center for Educational Development, University of Illinois College of Medicine.) The Organization, Geneva, 1973 (Public Health Papers No. 52).

199. American Nurses' Association, Committee on Education: "ANA's First Position Paper on Education for Nursing," *Am. J. Nurs.,* **65:**106, (Dec.) 1965.

200. Schorr, Thelma M.: "The New York Plan." (editorial), *N.Y. State Nurses Assoc. J.,* **6:**4, (Dec.) 1975.

201. Chater, Shirley, et al.: *Differentiation Between Technical and Professional Nursing—An Annotated Bibliography.* National League for Nursing, New York, 1972 (League Exchange No. 97).

202. Sheahan, Sister Dorothy: "The Game of the Name," *Nurs. Outlook,* **20:**440, (July) 1972.

203. International Labour Office: *Employment and Conditions of Work and Life of Nursing Personnel.* International Labour Conference, 1976, 61st Session, Report VII (2). The Office, Geneva, 1976, p. 10.

204. Schafer, Morris: *Joint Meeting on Conditions of Work and Life of Nursing Personnel.* World Health Organization, Geneva, 1974 (Public Health Papers No. 59).

205. American Nurses' Association: *Facts About Nursing 74–75.* The Association, Kansas City, Mo., 1976, pp. 3, 157, 165.

206. Johns, Ethel, and Pfefferkorn, Blanche: *An Activity Analysis of Nursing.* National League of Nursing Education, New York, 1934.

207. California State Nurses' Association: *Nursing Practice in California Hospitals; A Report Based on a Study of Actual Practice in Forty California Hospitals.* (Conducted by Louis J. Kroeger Associates.) The Association, San Francisco, 1953, processed.

208. Beeby, Nell: "Where and What Shall We Teach," *Am. J. Nurs.,* **37:**64, (Jan.) 1937.

209. Weiner, Florence R.: "Professional Consequences of the Nurse's Occupational Status," *Am. J. Nurs.,* **51:**614, (Oct.) 1951.

210. National League of Nursing Education, Committee on Curriculum: *A Curriculum Guide for Schools of Nursing.* The Association, New York, 1937.

211. Hughes, Everett C., et al.: *op. cit.*

212. American Nurses' Association, Department of Nursing Practice and Department of Statistics: *Pediatric Nurse Practitioners. Their Practice Today.* (Report prepared under direction of Barbara E. Bishop and Aleda V. Roth.) The Association, Kansas City, Mo., 1975 (Pub. No. MCH-5 IM 9/75).

213. Searight, Mary W.: *Your Career in Nursing.* Julian Messner, New York, 1970.

214. Spalding, Eugenia, and Notter, Lucille E.: *Professional Nursing. Foundations, Perspectives, and Relationships,* 8th ed. J. B. Lippincott Co., Philadelphia, 1970.

215. Kelly, Lucie Young: *Dimensions of Professional Nursing,* 3rd ed. Macmillan Publishing Co., Inc., New York, 1975.

216. Lewis, Edith P. (comp.): *Changing Patterns of Nursing Practice.* American Journal of Nursing Co., New York, 1971 (Contemporary Nursing Series).

217. Goodrich, Annie Warburton: *The Social and Ethical Significance of Nursing.* Macmillan Publishing Co., Inc., New York, 1932.

218. National Academy of Sciences, Institute of Medicine: *Controls on Health Care.* Papers of the Conference on Regulation in the Health Industry, Jan. 7–9, 1974. The Academy, Washington, D.C., 1975.

219. Simmons, Leo W., and Henderson, Virginia: *op. cit.,* p. 143.

220. Rhode Island Health Science Education Council: *Nursing Needs and Resources in Rhode Island.* The Council, Cranston, R.I., 1975.

221. American Nurses' Association: *The Nation's Nurses: 1972 Inventory of Registered Nurses.* (Prepared by Aleda V. Roth and Alice R. Walden.) The Association, Kansas City, Mo., 1974.

222. Scott, Jessie M., and Levine, Eugene: "Nursing Manpower Analysis: Its Past,

Present and Future," in Hiestand, Dale L., and Ostow, M. (eds.): *Health Manpower Information for Policy Guidance*. Ballinger Publishing Co., Cambridge, Mass., 1976.

223. US Health Resources Administration: *Decennial Census Data for Selected Health Occupations; United States, 1970*. The Administration, Rockville, Md., 1975 (DHEW Pub. No. [HRA] 76–1231).

224. US Health Resources Administration: *Health Manpower Issues. A Presentation at the White House, Nov. 13, 1975*. The Administration, Rockville, Md., 1976 (DHEW Pub. No. [HRA] 76–40).

225. Roberts, Mary: *American Nursing; History and Interpretation*. Macmillan Publishing Co., Inc., New York, 1954, p. 141.

226. Condé, Marlette: *The Lamp and the Caduceus. The Story of the Army School of Nursing*. Army School of Nursing Alumni Association, [Washington, D.C.], 1975.

227. Kalisch, Beatrice, and Kalisch, Philip A.: "Nurses in American History. The Cadet Nurse Corps in World War II," *Am. J. Nurs.*, **76**:240, (Feb.) 1976.

228. Western Interstate Commission for Higher Education: "Analysis and Planning for Improved Distribution of Nursing Personnel and Services" (memorandum). The Commission, Boulder, Colo., Dec. 19, 1975.

228a. National League for Nursing: *Nurses for a Growing Nation*. The League, New York, 1957.

229. Bigelow, Karl: *Teachers for Our Time*. American Council on Education, Washington, D.C., 1944, p. 12.

230. American Nurses' Association: *Facts About Nursing 72–73*. The Association, Kansas City, Mo., 1974, p. 10.

231. "1974 Shows Increase in Practicing Nurses" (news), *Nurs. Outlook*, **23**:200, (Apr.) 1975.

232. American Nurses' Association: *Facts About Nursing 74–75*. The Association, Kansas City, Mo., 1976, p. 22.

233. Lysaught, Jerome P.: *Action in Nursing, Progress in Professional Purpose*. McGraw-Hill Book Co., New York, 1974, p. 29.

234. Ronaghy, Hossain A., et al.: "Migration of Iranian Nurses to the U.S.: A Study of One School of Nursing in Iran," *Int. Nurs. Rev.*, **22**:87, (May–June) 1975.

234a. "Measures of Quality Nursing Care? Experts Agree Valid Approach Not Yet Found" (news), *Am. J. Nurs.*, **76**:186, (Feb.) 1976.

235. "Assessment Difficult. Individual Concepts Affect Quality Measures," *Am. Nurse*, **8**:1, (Jan. 16) 1976.

236. Henderson, Virginia: "Studies of Nursing Care," in Simmons, Leo W., and Henderson, Virginia: *Nursing Research. A Survey and Assessment*. Appleton-Century-Crofts, New York, 1964, p. 282.

237. American Nurses' Association: *Standards*

for Nursing Services in Hospitals, Community Health Agencies, Nursing Homes, Industry, Schools, Ambulatory Services, and Related Health Care Organizations*. The Association, Kansas City, Mo., 1973.

238. American Nurses' Association, Division of Medical-Surgical Nursing Practice, and Orthopedic Nurses' Association: *Standards of Orthopedic Nursing Practice*. ANA, Kansas City, Mo., 1975.

239. Association of Operating Room Nurses, and American Nurses' Association, Division of Medical-Surgical Nursing Practice: *Standards of Nursing Practice—Operating Room*. ANA, Kansas City, Mo., 1975.

240. American Nurses' Association: *A Plan for the Implementation of the Standards of Nursing Practice. A Report of the Congress for Nursing Practice of the American Nurses' Association*. The Association, Kansas City, Mo., 1975.

241. National League for Nursing: *Quality Assessment and Patient Care*. Presentations at Fall 1974 Forum for Nursing Service Administrators in the West. The League, New York, 1975.

242. ————: *Quality Assessment; Programs and Process*. Sponsored by Western Regional Assembly of Constituent Leagues. The League, New York, 1975.

243. Jelinek, Richard C., et al.: *A Methodology for Monitoring Quality of Nursing Care*. US Government Printing Office, Washington, D.C., 1974.

244. US Department of Health, Education, and Welfare: *Assessment of Nursing Services. Report of the Conference*. US Government Printing Office, Washington, D.C., 1975.

245. Horswill, Kay: *A Study of Nursing Quality Assurance Programs in Wisconsin*. University of Wisconsin Extension, Madison, 1975.

246. Mayers, Marlene, et al.: *Quality Assurance for Patient Care: Nursing Perspectives*. Appleton-Century-Crofts, New York, 1976.

247. Ertel, Paul Y., and Medical Advances Institute: *Quality Criteria for Automated Peer Review: Theory and Practice*. C. V. Mosby Co., St. Louis, 1976.

248. Benedikter, Helen: *The Nursing Audit— A Necessity. How Shall It Be Done?* National League for Nursing, New York, 1973 (Pub. No. 20–1501).

249. Rubin, C. W., et al.: "Nursing Audit— Nurses Evaluating Nurses," *Am. J. Nurs.*, **72**:916, (May) 1972.

250. Benedikter, Helen: *op. cit.*

251. World Health Organization: *World Health Statistics Report*, Vol. 28, No. 3, 1975.

252. American Nurses' Association: *Facts About Nursing 72–73*. The Association, Kansas City, Mo., 1974, p. 53.

253. Pfefferkorn, Blanche, and Rovetta, C. A.: *Administrative Cost Analysis for Nursing Service and Nursing Education*. American

Hospital Association and Illinois League of Nursing Education, Chicago, 1940.

254. Pfefferkorn, Blanche: "Measuring Nursing, Quantitatively and Qualitatively," *Am. J. Nurs.*, **32:**80, (Jan.) 1932.

255. US Public Health Service, Division of Nursing: *How to Study Nursing Activities in a Patient Unit,* rev. ed. US Government Printing Office, Washington, D.C., 1964 (PHS Pub. No. 570).

256. Bredenberg, Viola: *Nursing Service Research: Experimental Studies with the Nursing Team.* J. B. Lippincott Co., Philadelphia, 1951.

257. Wright, Marion: *Improvement of Patient Care.* G. P. Putnam's Sons, New York, 1954.

258. Walker, Virginia: *Nursing and Ritualistic Practice.* Macmillan Publishing Co., Inc., New York, 1967.

259. Kakosh, Marguerite E.: "A Method of Studying the Utilization of Nursing Personnel in Veterans Administration Hospitals," *Nurs. Res.,* **6:**79, (Oct.) 1959.

260. Abdellah, Faye G., and Levine, Eugene: *Patients and Personnel Speak,* rev. ed. US Government Printing Office, Washington, D.C., 1964 (PHS Pub. No. 527).

261. Aydelotte, Myrtle K., and Tener, M. E.: *An Investigation of the Relation Between Nursing Activity and Patient Welfare.* State University of Iowa, Iowa City, 1960.

262. Aydelotte, Myrtle K.: *Nurse Staffing Methodology: A Review and Critique of Selected Literature.* US Government Printing Office, Washington, D.C., 1973 (DHEW Pub. No. [NIH] 73–433).

263. Kraegel, Janet M., et al.: *Patient Care Systems.* J. B. Lippincott Co., Philadelphia, 1974.

264. Manthey, Marie: "Primary Nursing Is Alive and Well in the Hospital," *Am. J. Nurs.,* **73:**83, (Jan.) 1973.

265. Doster, D. D.: "Utilization of Available 'Nurse Power' in Public Health," *Am. J. Public Health,* **60:**25, (Jan.) 1970.

266. Bernzweig, Eli P.: *The Nurse's Liability for Malpractice. A Programmed Course,* 2nd ed. McGraw-Hill Book Co., New York, 1975.

267. Bullough, Bonnie: *The Law and the Expanding Nursing Role.* Appleton-Century-Crofts, New York, 1975.

268. Creighton, Helen: *Law Every Nurse Should Know,* 3rd ed. W. B. Saunders Co., Philadelphia, 1975.

269. ———, et al.: "Symposium on Current Legal and Professional Problems," *Nurs. Clin. North Am.,* **9:**391, (Sept.) 1974.

270. Deloughery, Grace L., and Gebbie, Kristine M.: *Political Dynamics: Impact on Nurses and Nursing.* C. V. Mosby Co., St. Louis, 1975.

271. Health Law Center, and Streiff, Charles J. (eds.): *Nursing and the Law,* 2nd ed. Aspen System Corp., Rockville, Md., 1975.

272. Walsh, Margaret E.: *The Health Professional Education Organization and the Governmental Process.* National League for Nursing, New York, 1974 (Pub. No. 14–1541).

273. Roemer, R.: *Legal Regulations of Modern Nursing Practice.* National League for Nursing, New York, 1973 (Pub. No. 15–22).

274. Schaefer, M. J.: "The Political and Economic Scene in the Future of Nursing," *Am. J. Public Health,* **63:**887, (Oct.) 1973.

275. Speller, S. R.: *Law Notes for Nurses,* 7th ed. Royal College of Nursing and National Council of Nurses of the United Kingdom, London, 1972.

276. Van Rokeghem, S.: "The Nurses Are Fed Up with Living Outside the Law," *Nurs. Mirror,* **136:**30, (Apr. 20) 1973.

277. International Council of Nurses: *Report of International Seminar on Nursing Legislation, Warsaw, Poland, July 6–16, 1970.* The Council, Geneva, 1972.

277a. Pearson, Betty D.: "Nursing Legislation: The International Dimension," *Nurs. Clin. North Am.,* **9:**535, (Sept.) 1974.

278. International Council of Nurses: *Principles of Legislation for Nursing Education and Practice. A Guide to Assist National Nurses Associations.* The Council, Geneva, 1969.

279. Pearson, Betty D.: *op. cit.*

280. International Council of Nurses: "Professional Services Committee Prepares Proposals on Current Nursing Issues," *Int. Nurs. Rev.,* **22:**819, (Jan.–Feb.) 1975.

281. International Council of Nurses: *Code for Nurses.* The Council, Geneva, 1973. (Adopted 1953; revised 1965 and 1973.)

282. Bergman, Rebecca: "Ethics—Concepts and Practice," *Int. Nurs. Rev.,* **20:**140, (Sept.–Oct.) 1973.

283. "N-Cap Offers Nurses New Opportunities to Work Toward Legislative Goals" (news), *Am. J. Nurs.,* **74:**1213, (July) 1974.

284. "New Federation Formed to Unify Nursing Voice" (news), *Am. J. Nurs.,* **74:**1229, (July) 1974.

285. Bullough, Bonnie, and Bullough, Vern L.: "Sex Discrimination in Health Care," *Nurs. Outlook,* **23:**40, (Jan.) 1975.

285a. American Nurses' Association: *Affirmative Action Programming for the Nursing Profession Through the American Nurses' Association.* The Association, Kansas City, Mo., 1975.

286. Cleland, Virginia S.: "To End Sex Discrimination," *Nurs. Clin. North Am.,* **9:**563, (Sept.) 1974.

287. Johnson, Walter L.: "Admission of Men and Ethnic Minorities to Schools of Nursing," *Nurs. Outlook,* **22:**45, (Jan.) 1974.

288. "Sex Barrier Falls," *Nurs. Times,* **69:**224, (Feb. 26) 1971.

289. Vaz, D.: "High School Senior Boys' At-

titudes Toward Nursing as a Career," *Nurs. Res.*, **17**:533, (Nov.–Dec.) 1968.

290. Williams, R. A.: "Characteristics of Male Baccalaureate Students Who Selected Nursing as a Career," *Nurs. Res.*, **22**:520, (Nov.–Dec.) 1973.

290a. International Labour Office: *Employment and Conditions of Work and Life of Nursing Personnel.* International Labour Conference, 1976, 61st Session, Report VII (2). The Office, Geneva, 1976, p. 69.

291. US Public Health Service, Health Manpower Coordinating Committee, Subcommittee on Health Manpower Credentialing: *Report on Licensure and Related Health Personnel Credentialing.* (Prepared by Harris S. Cohen and Lawrence H. Miike.) US Government Printing Office, Washington, D.C., 1971 (DHEW Pub. No. [HSM] 72–11).

292. US Bureau of Health Services Research and Evaluation: *Developments in Health Manpower Licensure.* (Prepared by Harris S. Cohen and Lawrence H. Miike.) US Government Printing Office, Washington, D.C., 1973 (DHEW Pub. No. [HRA] 73–3101).

293. US Public Health Service, Health Manpower Coordinating Committee, Subcommittee on Health Manpower Credentialing: *A Proposal for Credentialing Health Manpower.* US Government Printing Office, Washington, D.C., 1976.

294. Dunkley, Pearl H.: "The ANA Certification Program," *Nurs. Clin. North Am.* **9**:485, (Sept.) 1974.

295. American Nurses' Association: *Directory of Certified Nurses.* The Association, Kansas City, Mo., 1975.

296. Kelly, Lucie Young: *op. cit.*

297. Schorr, Thelma M.: "Securing Licensure" (editorial), *Am. J. Nurs.*, **75**:1131, (July) 1975.

297a. Christman, Luther: "Problems of Role Definition in the Health Care Team." (Paper presented at 102nd Annual Forum of National Conference on Social Welfare, San Francisco, Calif., May 11, 1975.)

298. International Labour Office: *Employment and Conditions of Work and Life of Nursing Personnel.* International Labour Conference, 1976, 61st Session, Report VII (1). The Office, Geneva, 1976, pp. 6, 72, 73, 1.

299. Florin, Marie-Paule: "The Nursing Profession and the European Economic Community," *Int. Nurs. Rev.*, **21**:184, (Nov.–Dec.) 1974.

300. Burgess, May Ayres: *Nurses, Patients and Pocketbooks.* Committee on the Grading of Nursing Schools, New York, 1928.

301. Committee on the Grading of Nursing Schools: *Nurses, Production, Education, Distribution, and Pay.* The Committee, New York, 1930.

302. Clark, Harold F.: *Life Earnings.* Harper and Row, New York, 1937.

303. Knopf, Lucille: *RN's One and Five Years After Graduation.* National League for Nursing, New York, 1975, p. 26.

304. Sloan, Frank A.: *The Geographic Distribution of Nurses and Public Policy.* US Government Printing Office, Washington, D.C., 1975, p. 211 (DHEW Pub. No. [HRA] 75–53).

305. American Nurses' Association: *Facts About Nursing 72–73.* The Association, Kansas City, Mo., 1974, pp. 16, 17.

306. Falk, Isadore S.: "Medical Care in the U.S.A.—1932–1972," *Milbank Mem. Fund Q.*, **51**:1, (Winter) 1973.

307. National Academy of Sciences, Institute of Medicine: *Controls on Health Care.* Papers of the Conference on Regulation in the Health Industry, Jan. 7–9, 1974. The Academy, Washington, D.C., 1975.

308. Law, Sylvia A.: *Blue Cross. What Went Wrong?* 2nd ed. (Prepared by the Health Law Project, University of Pennsylvania.) Yale University Press, New Haven, Conn., 1976.

309. Welch, Cathryne A.: "Health Care Distribution and Third-Party Payment for Nurses' Services," *Am. J. Nurs.*, **75**:1844, (Oct.) 1975.

310. Cornelius, Dorothy: "Report of the ICN President, 1973–1975," *Int. Nurs. Rev.*, **22**:168, (Nov.–Dec.) 1975.

311. American Nurses' Association: *Facts About Nursing 74–75.* The Association, Kansas City, Mo., 1976, p. 231.

312. "ICN President Attends Congress [5th Congress of the Trade Unions International of Public and Allied Employees]; Meets Nurses in Moscow" (news), *Int. Nurs. Rev.*, **20**:5, (Jan.–Feb.) 1973.

313. "ICN Successful in Urging ILO to Take Action on International Instrument for Nurses" (news), *Int. Nurs. Rev.*, **21**:135, (Sept.–Oct.) 1974.

314. Kruse, Margrethe: "ICN at the Crossroads," *Int. Nurs. Rev.*, **20**:42, (Mar.–Apr.) 1973.

315. Kruse, Margrethe: "A World of Unity. From Nationalism to Internationalism," *Imprint*, **20**:14, (Apr.) 1973.

316. American Nurses' Association: *Facts About Nursing 74–75.* The Association, Kansas City, Mo., 1976, p. 77.

317. "U.S. University Offers Courses for International Nurses," *Int. Nurs. Rev.*, **21**:188, (Nov.–Dec.) 1974.

318. "Professional Services Committee Prepares Proposal on Current Nursing Issues" (news), *Int. Nurs. Rev.*, **22**:4, (No. 1) 1975.

319. Fitzpatrick, M. Louise: *The National Organization for Public Health Nursing 1912–1952: Development of a Practice Field.* National League for Nursing, New York, 1975 (Pub. No. 11–1510).

320. Pfefferkorn, Blanche: "Nursing Organizations in the United States, Their Origin,

Purpose and Some of Their Results," *Mod. Hosp.,* **8:**131, (Feb.) 1917.

321. "National Headquarters Established" (editorial), *Am. J. Nurs.,* **20:**869, (Aug.) 1920.

322. "An Announcement [from ANA]," *Am. J. Nurs.,* **11:**771, (July) 1911.

322a. Jacobi, Eileen M.: "Executive Director's Report," in *ANA Convention. House of Delegates Reports, 1974–1976.* The Association, Kansas City, Mo., 1976.

323. American Nurses' Association, Commission on Nursing Education: "Report," in *ANA Convention, House of Delegates Reports, 1974–1976.* The Association, Kansas City, Mo., 1976, p. 45.

324. American Nurses' Association: *Licensure and Credentialing. Proceedings of the ANA Conference for Members and Professional Employees of State Boards of Nursing and ANA Advisory Council, Apr. 27–28, 1972.* The Association, Kansas City, Mo., 1974.

325. "Credentialing Trends Cited," *NLN News,* **23:**2, (June–July) 1975.

326. Kelly, Lucie Young: *op. cit.,* p. 376.

327. Freeman, Ruth B.: "NLN at Twenty: Challenge and Change," *Nurs. Outlook,* **20:**376, (June) 1972.

328. National League for Nursing: *This Is the National League for Nursing.* The League, New York, 1975 (Pub. No. 41–1532).

329. National League for Nursing, Department of Baccalaureate and Higher Degree Programs: "Baccalaureate and Master's Degree Programs in Nursing Accredited to NLN, 1975–76," *Nurs. Outlook,* **23:**391, (June) 1975.

330. National League for Nursing, Department of Home Health Agencies and Community Health Agencies: "Community Nursing Services Accredited by NLN-APHA April 1974," *Nurs. Outlook,* **22:**270, (Apr.) 1974.

331. Ozimek, Dorothy: *The Future of Nursing Education.* National League for Nursing, New York, 1975 (Pub. No. 15–1581).

332. Ruffin, Janice: "Issues for the Black Nurse Today. Competence and Commitment," in National League for Nursing, Council of Baccalaureate and Higher Degree Programs: *Current Issues in Nursing Education.* The League, New York, 1974.

333. Lenburg, Carrie, and Johnson, Walter: "Career Mobility Through Nursing Education," *Nurs. Outlook,* **22:**266, (Apr.) 1974.

334. American Nurses' Association, Council of State Boards of Nursing: *Boards of Nursing—Open Curriculum. Proceedings of the ANA Conference for Members and Professional Employees of State Boards of Nursing, June 7, 1974.* The Association, Kansas City, Mo., 1975.

335. American Nurses' Association: *Facts About Nursing 72–73.* The Association, Kansas City, Mo., 1974, pp. 6, 167, 181.

336. Canadian Nurses' Association: *Countdown 1973.* The Association, Ottawa, 1974, p. 114.

337. Woolsey, Abby H.: "Hospitals and Training Schools," in *A Century of Nursing.* G. P. Putnam's Sons, New York, 1950, p. 133.

338. Roberts, Mary: *American Nursing; History and Interpretation.* Macmillan Publishing Co., Inc., New York, 1954, p. 22.

339. Fenwick, Ethel Gordon: "A Plea for the Higher Education of Trained Nurses," *Am. J. Nurs.,* **2:**4, (Oct.) 1901.

340. Cabot, Richard C.: "A Statistical Study of the Educational Opportunities Offered in the Massachusetts Training School for Nurses," *Am. J. Nurs.,* **6:**438, (Apr.) 1906.

341. Beard, Richard Olding: "The University Education of the Nurse," *Teach. Coll. Rec.,* **11:**28, (May) 1910.

342. Goodrich, Annie Warburton: "The Complete Nurse," *Am. J. Nurs.,* **12:**799, (July) 1912.

343. Johns, Ethel: "The University in Relation to Nursing," *Public Health J. Can.,* **12:**6, (Jan.) 1921.

344. Lyon, E. P.: "Taking the Profit Out of Nursing Education," *Mod. Hosp.* **37:**122, (Nov.) 1931.

345. Dreiblatt, Martha: "Shall We Have Cheap Labor or Good Nurses?" *Am. Mercury,* Apr. 1931.

346. Balme, Harold: *A Criticism of Nursing Education with Suggestions for Constructive Reform.* Oxford University Press, London, 1937.

347. Stewart, Isabel M.: *The Education of Nurses. Historical Foundations and Modern Trends.* Macmillan Publishing Co., Inc., New York, 1943.

348. Russell, Charles H.: "Liberal Education and Nursing," *Nurs. Res.,* **7:**116, (Oct.) 1958.

349. National Commission for the Study of Nursing and Nursing Education: *Individualization, Articulation, Concentration: Emergent Forces in Nursing Education.* The Commission, Rochester, N.Y., [1973].

350. "Ladder System Outlined, Aide to R.N.," *Am. J. Nurs.,* **68:**1743, (Aug.) 1968.

351. Bullough, Bonnie, and Bullough, Vern R.: "A Career Ladder in Nursing. Problems and Prospects," *Am. J. Nurs.,* **71:**1938, (Oct.) 1971.

352. Drage, Martha O.: "Core Courses and a Career Ladder," *Am. J. Nurs.,* **71:**1356, (July) 1971.

353. Ramphal, Marjorie: "Needed: A Career Ladder in Nursing," *Am. J. Nurs.,* **68:**1234, (June) 1968.

354. Wilbur, Dwight L.: "Total Manpower Needs and Resources—Medicine and Nursing," *Nurs. Outlook,* **17:**32, (Dec.) 1969.

355. Quinn, Sheila M.: *op. cit.*

356. Ingles, Thelma: "An American Nurse Visits the Soviet Union," *Am. J. Nurs.,* **70:**754, (Apr.) 1970.

357. World Health Organization: *The Training and Utilization of Feldshers in the U.S.S.R.*

A Review Prepared by the Ministry of Health of the U.S.S.R. for the World Health Organization. The Organization, Geneva, 1974.

358. "Health Professions Schools Form Federation," *Am. J. Nurs.,* **68:**1196, (June) 1968.

359. National Commission for the Study of Nursing and Nursing Education: *Individualization, Articulation, Concentration: Emergent Forces in Nursing Education.* The Commission, Rochester, N.Y., [1973].

360. "NLN to Reconsider Joining ANA Credentialing Study" (news), *Am. J. Nurs.,* **76:**137, (Jan.) 1976.

361. National League for Nursing, Division of Research: "Educational Preparation for Nursing—1974," *Nurs. Outlook,* **23:**578 (Sept.) 1975.

362. World Health Organization: *Development of Educational Programmes for the Health Professions.* The Organization, Geneva, 1973 (Public Health Paper No. 52).

363. Miller, George E., and Fülöp, Tamás (eds.): *Educational Strategies for the Health Professions.* World Health Organization, Geneva, 1974 (Public Health Paper No. 61).

364. Pellegrino, Edmund D.: "The Regionalization of Academic Medicine: The Metamorphosis of a Concept," *J. Med. Educ.,* **48:**119, (Feb.) 1973.

365. Houston, William R.: *Art of Treatment.* Macmillan Publishing Co., Inc., New York, 1936.

366. Abdellah, Faye G., et al.: *Patient-Centered Approaches to Nursing.* Macmillan Publishing Co., Inc., New York, 1960.

367. Lippard, Vernon W.: *A Half-Century of American Medical Education 1920–1970.* Josiah Macy, Jr. Foundation, New York, 1974, p. 11.

368. Christman, Luther: "The Practitioner-Teacher: A Working Paper," unpublished, 1973. (Rush University, Chicago.)

369. National League for Nursing, Division of Research: "Educational Preparation for Nursing—1974," *Nurs. Outlook,* **23:**578, (Sept.) 1975. (Report prepared by Walter L. Johnson.)

370. *Ibid.*

371. *Ibid.*

372. Simmons, Leo W., and Henderson, Virginia: *op. cit.,* p. 122.

373. American Nurses' Foundation: *International Directory of Nurses with Doctoral Degrees.* The Foundation, New York, 1973.

374. American Nurses' Association: *Facts About Nursing 72–73.* The Association, Kansas City, Mo., 1974, p. 10.

375. National League for Nursing, Division of Research: *op. cit.*

376. Schlotfeldt, Rozella: "Can We Bring Order Out of the Chaos of Nursing Education?" *Am. J. Nurs.,* **76:**105, (Jan.) 1976.

377. Newman, Margaret A.: "The Professional Doctorate in Nursing: A Position Paper," *Nurs. Outlook,* **23:**704, (Nov.) 1975.

377a. American Nurses' Association: *Facts About Nursing 72–73.* The Association, Kansas City, Mo., 1974, p. 116.

378. University of Maryland: *School of Nursing, University of Maryland at Baltimore, 1974–1975.* The University, Baltimore, p. 27.

379. *University of Texas System School of Nursing: 1975–1976 Catalogue.* The University, Austin, El Paso, Forth Worth, etc., p. 52.

380. American Nurses' Association: *Facts About Nursing 72–73.* The Association, Kansas City, Mo., 1974, p. 119.

381. *Ibid.*

382. Simmons, Leo W., and Henderson, Virginia: *op. cit.,* p. 124.

383. US Department of Health, Education, and Welfare: *Future Directions of Doctoral Education for Nurses. Report of a Conference.* US Government Printing Office, Washington, D.C., 1971, p. 6.

384. Schlotfeldt, Rozella: *op. cit.*

385. Newman, Margaret A.: *op. cit.*

386. Bullough, Bonnie, and Sparks, Colleen: "Baccalaureate vs. Associate Degree Nurses. The Care-Cure Dichotomy," *Nurs. Outlook,* **23:**688, (Nov.) 1975.

387. Kramer, Marlene: *Reality Shock Why Nurses Leave Nursing.* C. V. Mosby Co., St. Louis, 1974.

388. Mereness, Dorothy A.: "Graduate Education, As One Dean Sees It," *Nurs. Outlook,* **23:**638, (Oct.) 1975.

389. Chater, Shirley S.: "COGEN: Cooperative Graduate Education in Nursing," *Nurs. Outlook,* **23:**630, (Oct.) 1975.

390. Moxley, Patricia A., and White, Dorothy T.: "Fitting the Graduate Program to the Student," *Nurs. Outlook,* **23:**625, (Oct.) 1975.

391. Roberts, Mary M.: "The Story of the Department of Nursing and Health, Teachers College, New York," *Am. J. Nurs.,* **21:**518, (May) 1921.

392. "The Contribution of Teachers College to Nursing Education," *Teach. Coll. Rec.,* **16:**71, (May) 1915.

393. Florence Nightingale International Foundation: *An International List of Advanced Programmes in Nursing Education, 1951–1952.* International Council of Nurses, Geneva, 1958.

394. Canadian Nurses' Association: *Countdown 1970.* The Association, Ottawa, 1970, p. 79.

395. Canadian Nurses' Association: *Countdown 1972.* The Association, Ottawa, 1972, pp. 84, 89.

395a. Personal communication, Aug. 25, 1976, Canadian Nurses' Association.

396. Aydelotte, Myrtle: *Survey of Hospital Nursing Services.* National League for Nursing, New York, 1968, p. 4.

397. Alford, H. J.: *Continuing Education in Action.* John Wiley and Sons, New York, 1967, p. 1.

398. Goldberg, Enid: "The Implications of Continuing Education in Nursing," in National League for Nursing: *Outdate Update, Continuing Education: Who, What, Where, When, How.* The League, New York, 1975, p. 1.

399. *Ibid.,* p. 2.

400. Price, Alice: "Professional Control of Continuing Education," in National League for Nursing: *Outdate Update, Continuing Education: Who, What, Where, When, How.* The League, New York, 1975, p. 23.

401. Gibbs, Gertrude E.: "Will Continuing Education Be Required for License Renewal?" *Am. J. Nurs.,* **71**:2175, (Nov.) 1971.

402. US Bureau of Health Services Research and Evaluation: *op. cit.,* p. 42.

403. Cooper, Signe S., and Byrns, Helen Hestad: *A Plan for Continuing Education in Five North Central States: Michigan, Minnesota, Montana, North Dakota and Wisconsin.* Department of Nursing, University of Wisconsin Extension, Madison, 1973.

404. "California Assembly Passes Continuing Education Bill" (news), *Am. J. Nurs.,* **71**:1498, (Aug.) 1971.

405. "Utah Nurses See Their New Certification Plan as Purely Professional Responsibility" (news), *Am. J. Nurs.,* **71**:1298, (July) 1971.

406. Phillips, Louis E.: "The Origin and Evolution of the Continuing Education Unit," in National League for Nursing: *Outdate Update, Continuing Education: Who, What, Where, When, How.* The League, New York, 1975.

407. National Task Force on the CEU: *The Continuing Education Unit. Criteria and Guidelines.* National University Extension Association, Washington, D.C., 1974.

408. American Nurses' Association, Division of Maternal and Child Health Nursing Practice, and American Academy of Pediatrics: "Guidelines on Short-Term Continuing Education Programs for Pediatric Nurse Associates," *Am. J. Nurs.,* **71**:509, (Mar.) 1971.

409. "Guidelines for Short-Term Continuing Education Programs for the Nurse Clinician in Intensive Neonatal Care and the Nurse Clinician in Intensive Maternal-Fetal Care," *Am. Nurse,* **7**:13, (May) 1975.

Virginia Henderson

CHAPTER 2

Health Programs and Nursing Relationships; The Nurse's Part in Promoting Optimum Health Services

1. VALUE OF HEALTH AND HUMAN LIFE
2. CONDITIONS AFFECTING COMMUNITY HEALTH
3. OUTSTANDING ACCOMPLISHMENTS IN DISEASE CONTROL AND HEALTH PROMOTION
4. ORGANIZATION OF HEALTH CARE
5. INTERNATIONAL AGENCIES; NATIONAL, STATE, AND LOCAL HEALTH AGENCIES IN THE UNITED STATES
6. PLACE OF HOSPITALS, NURSING HOMES, AND HOSPICES IN HEALTH PROGRAMS
7. NURSE'S ROLE IN PROMOTING HEALTH PROGRAMS

1. VALUE OF HEALTH AND HUMAN LIFE

Human life, or capital, exceeds in economic value all other material resources of a nation. A healthy population, in its broadest sense, is the best measure of a people's prosperity. Its value in terms of human happiness is immeasurable. In the preamble of the charter of the World Health Organization, health is defined as "a state of complete physical, mental and social well-being and not merely the absence of disease or infirmity." *

René Dubos, in defining health, emphasizes man's continual adaptation to the stresses of life. Dubos says, "the states of health or disease are the expressions of the success or failure experienced by the organism in its efforts to respond adaptively to environmental challenges." † Still another way of defining health is expressed by Halbert L. Dunn as "an integrated method of functioning which is oriented toward maximizing the potential of which the individual is capable. It requires that the individual maintain a continuum of balance and purposeful direction within the environment where he is functioning." ‡

There is a growing realization that this "nat-

ural wealth" is the *quality of health* rather than life itself, that margin of mental and physical vigor that allows a person to work most effectively and to reach his highest potential level of satisfaction in life. Abraham Maslow [1] and others call this self-realization. Arriving at this state, they think, is the ultimate expression of maturity.

In a publication called *Improvements in the Quality of Life; Estimates of Possibilities in the U.S., 1974–1983,* Nestor R. Terleckyi [2] indicates that the average life expectancy at birth in 1973 (71.3 years) would increase by 1.4 years in a decade, and that the disabled population would decrease from 17.5 per cent to 16.8 per cent in 1983, if we made fundamental changes in health-related habits and living patterns. He cites as important factors the following: reduction in smoking, improvement in nutrition and general fitness, prevention of accidents, reduction of the abuse of alcohol and other drugs, improved cancer diagnosis and treatment, mental health care, treatment of arthritis, expanded services for the poor, expanded care for mothers and children, and establishment of additional neighborhood recreational facilities. Table 2-1 points out the effects of certain activities on cost, life expectancy, and disability.

People of different cultures attach importance to health in varying degrees. In spite of our growing knowledge of and interest in health, we in the United States apparently do not yet consider it of primary importance. A

---

* Parran, Thomas: "Charter for World Health," *J.A.M.A.*, **131**:1207, (Aug. 10) 1946.

† Dubos, René: *Man Adapting.* Yale University Press, New Haven, Conn., 1965, p. xvii.

‡ Dunn, Halbert L.: *High-Level Wellness.* R. W. Beatty, Ltd., Arlington, Va., 1961, p. 4.

Table 2-1.   Effects of Activities on Average Life Expectancy and the Number of Persons Disabled *

Activity and Percent of Relevant Population Affected	Total Cost 1974–83 (billions of 1973 dollars)	Average Life Expectancy (years)	Percent of Population Disabled
Base 1973	—	71.3	17.5%
Base 1983	—	72.7	16.8%
Changes in health-related habits & patterns	$ 64	+5.3	−3.3%
(a) Elimination of smoking (90%)	5	+1.8	−0.4
(b) Improvement of nutrition & fitness (70%)	35	+3.8	−1.6
(c) Prevention of accidents (50%)	1	+0.6	−0.2
(d) Reduction of alcoholism and alcohol abuse (33%)	17	+0.3	−1.3
(e) Reduction of drug abuse (90%)	6	+0.1	−0.5
Health services related to specific conditions	66	+1.7	−3.1
(a) Cancer: R&D, diagnostic and treatment expansion (50%)	6	+1.0	−0.1
(b) Mental health treatment (30%)	54	+0.7	−1.9
(c) Arthritis prevention & treatment (70%)	6	+0.0	−1.1
Special health services for vulnerable population groups	91	+2.5	−1.0
(a) The poor (100%)	73	+2.2	−1.0
(b) Maternal and child services (100%)	18	+0.6	—
Recreation facilities in neighborhoods	127	+1.1	−0.4
Combined Effects			
Health-related habits; recreational facilities	191	+5.5	−3.4
Health-related habits; health services	130	+6.8	−5.9
Health-related habits; special health services	155	+7.3	−4.1
Health services; special health services	157	+4.1	−3.9
Special health services; recreational facilities	218	+3.5	−1.3
Health-related habits; health services; special health services	221	+8.7	−6.7
Total, All Activities	$348	+8.9	−6.8%

* Terleckyi, Nestor R.: *Improvements in the Quality of Life; Estimates of Possibilities in the U.S., 1974–1983*, National Planning Association, Washington, D.C., 1975, p. 88.

series of national conferences in this country, beginning with the National Conservation Commission in 1909, have made "Reports to the President," calling attention to the tangible and intangible waste that results from our failure to apply what is known about health conservation. These reports are concerned with such topics as nutrition, children and youth, environmental control, and heart disease, cancer, and stroke, to mention just a few. One of the late conferences was on aging.[3] It is generally recognized that many cultures not only provide inadequately for the physical and emotional needs of the elderly but also waste the unique service this segment of the population is prepared to give. Reading such reports, we cannot escape the conclusion that the health of the population and the social conditions of the nation are interdependent. Throughout the world, health resources are part of social security programs; this is true in developing countries as well as in those with the most advanced technology. For example, the US Department of Health, Education, and Welfare,

in a publication called *Social Security Programs Throughout the World, 1971*,[4] has compiled information on the principal features of the social security systems of 125 nations. These data are useful for comparison of one country's system with another and for persons interested in determining exactly what their rights or obligations are under the existing legislation of a country.

As United States citizens the writers tend to stress North American conditions, organizations, agencies, and institutions. It should be recognized, however, that even among the "Western" nations the United States is atypical. For example, its population, which is 6 per cent of the world's population of 3500 million, is reported by Ansley J. Coale[5] to use 30 per cent of the world's resources. Although it has the highest ratio of doctors to the population, compared with Sweden, another example of an economically favored Western nation (see Table 2-2), its life expectancy in 1973, its provision of hospital beds, its stay in hospitals, its health expenditures, and its total tax burden

Table 2-2. A Profile of Two Health Systems*

	Sweden	United States
	Population 8,000,000	208,000,000
Life expectancy Men	75.44	67.4
(in years) Women	79.42	74.9
Infant mortality (per 1000 population)	13	18.5
Doctors (per 100,000 population)	135	172
Hospital beds (per 1000 population)	18	7.4
Average length hospital stay (in days)	11.9	7.9
Health expenditures (as % of G.N.P.)	8	7.6
Total tax burden (as % of G.N.P.)	41.4	30.2

* The *New York Times*, Dec. 23, 1973.

are all lower. On the other hand, its infant mortality (often cited as an indicator of the excellence of health care) is higher, or 18.5 per 1000 population as compared to Sweden's 13 per 1000 population.

As will be pointed out later, the United States' lack of a unified health care system is unusual in this age among the developed nations and partially explains why, although the country is economically favored, its system of health care and its health status are not what might be expected.

J. Fry, comparing medical care in the United States with that in the Union of Soviet Socialist Republics and the United Kingdom in 1970, says: "Modern medical care is expensive and beyond the means of the ordinary family. . . . All systems . . . must be planned to make the best use of resources, and government subsidization and involvement are inevitable. The form and nature of the three systems mirror national philosophies and attitudes." * His diagrams showing the flow of medical care in the three societies (see Fig. 2-1) are instructive, although recent changes in these systems would modify his statements were they made today.

Ruth Lubic,[6] a nurse who visited the U.S.S.R. with a medical delegation, in discussing what she saw and heard in 1974 commented on what seemed to be a universal interest in and knowledge of health, even among children: the control of insects, the eradication

* Fry, J.: "Medical Care in Three Societies," *Int. J. Health Services,* 1:121, (Nov. 2) 1971.

of many communicable diseases, the universal availability of health care, and the effective working relationship of health personnel.

Faye G. Abdellah,[7] following an observation visit to the U.S.S.R., listed the basic principles of the Soviet Health Services as follows: (1) health care is a responsibility of the government; (2) no direct charges should be made to the patient for health care; (3) health services should be unified, centrally directed, and accessible to all; (4) science should be the foundation for health care; (5) prevention of disease should receive major emphasis; and (6) efforts should be made to improve the health knowledge of the population. Abdellah notes the high degree of centralized planning in that country and stresses the availability of care there. For example, in an emergency, any citizen can dial a number and a skilled operator, with a physician consultant if indicated, sends the necessary personnel and equipment to the needy citizen. The coordinated hospital system and the preparation of health workers that gives them a common core of knowledge and an opportunity to move out of one health category into another are described. Both Abdellah and J. E. Muller et al.[8] discuss features of the Soviet system that might be tried in other countries—particularly in the United States.

G. E. W. Wolstenholme,[9] a British physician keenly aware of universal human needs, advocates a World Health Service as a step toward man's well-being and toward a world society. He calls attention to the world of the "have-nots," where a single capsule of gentamicin costs what two people might have to spend on their health care in a year. He notes that the "haves" tend to double their population in 70 years, the "have-nots" in 30 years, which, of course, compounds all social problems, including health.

Readers interested in a global view of health should bear in mind that the data in this chapter, so often based on the North American experience, are not highly representative.

Andrew Malleson,[10] a Canadian physician, discussing "our right to survive," systems for "delivering health," and the difference between what he considers constructive and destructive health care, doubts whether the quality of care and the money spent on it have risen proportionately in the Western world. He notes that in 1950 the United States spent 4.6 per cent of its Gross National Product (G.N.P.) on health; in 1971 it spent 7.4 per cent; in England and Wales the National Health Service spent in 1970 over 6 times as much as it did in 1950; and yet he thinks that the outlook for our future health is "gloomy." On the other hand, all

FLOW OF MEDICAL CARE IN THE U.S.S.R.

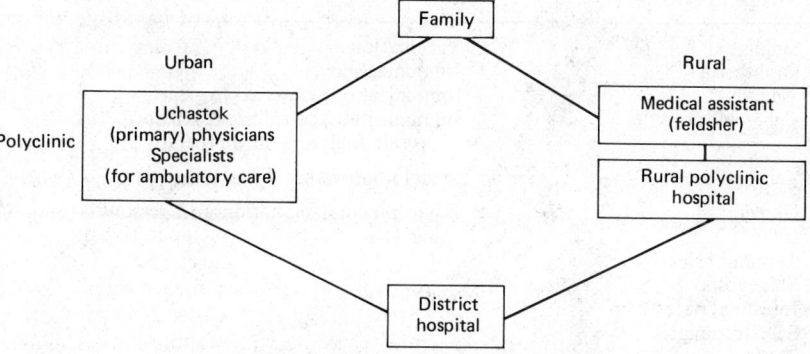

FLOW OF MEDICAL CARE IN THE UNITED KINGDOM

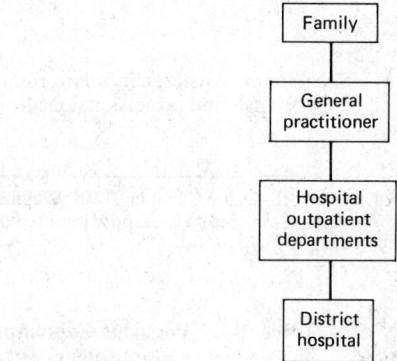

FLOW OF MEDICAL CARE IN THE UNITED STATES

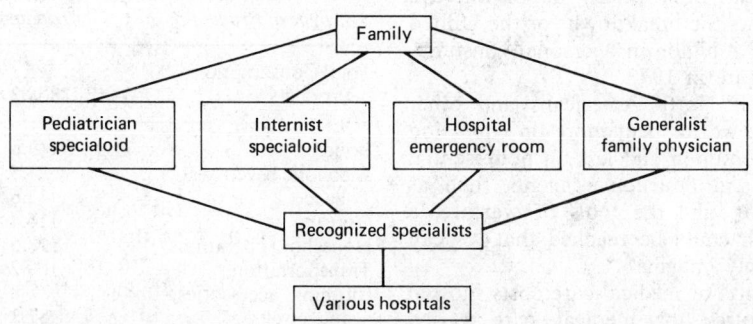

Figure 2-1. Flow of medical care in three societies in 1970. (Adapted from Fry, J.: "Medical Care in Three Societies," *Int. J. Health Services,* **1:**121, [No. 2] 1971.)

reports on countries, as, for example, China, that have effected population control, eradication of communicable disease, and widespread health education do seem to show tangible results for health expenditures and a promising future. Frederick F. Kao,[11] an American physician who visited China in 1972, enumerating some of its outstanding accomplishments, refers to diseases that have been stamped out, eradicated, or brought under control. He refers to the marked "zeal" of medical personnel to serve the people, to the disappearance of "elitism" in medical professionals, and to the controlled birth rate. The chief means of attack on selected major diseases by the Chinese are listed in Table 2-3.

Health economics is a specialized field and it cannot be treated in scope or depth in this

Table 2-3.   Selected Major Diseases in China in 1949, and Chief Means of Attack *

Smallpox	Vaccination
Diphtheria	Immunization
Tetanus	Immunization; maternal hygiene
Tuberculosis	Immunization; social improvement; case finding; and chemotherapy
Venereal disease	Social improvement; chemotherapy
Cholera	Environmental sanitation and personal hygiene
Typhoid fever	"
Shigellosis	"
Intestinal parasitism	"
Schistosomiasis	"
Typhus	"
Malaria	Eliminate breeding; kill infected mosquitoes; chemoprophylaxis and therapy

Some Other Problems
Malnutrition
Maternal and infant mortality
Heart diseases   } Social improvement; education; trained personnel; and professional facilities
Cancer
Mental diseases

* Heller, Peter S.: "The Strategy of Health-Sector Planning," in Wegman, Myron E., et al. (eds.): *Public Health in the People's Republic of China.* Josiah Macy, Jr. Foundation, New York, 1973, p. 76.

chapter but it merits study by all providers of health care. For those working in the United States the comparison of what is spent on medical (or health) care with what is spent on other needs and desires may be of interest. Table 2-4 shows the breakdown for the United States of $615.8 billion in "personal consumption" expenditure in 1973.

Obviously, if North Americans and other peoples of the world spent more on education and health promotion and less on nonessential commodities and destructive agents such as tobacco, liquor, and the tools of warfare, a level of health could be reached that we can now only barely imagine.

Earlier reports of medical care costs showed that expenditures for medical care varied greatly, depending on family income; today there is no clear relationship between the cost of care and income, except that families reporting incomes of $15,000 or more per year report the greatest expenses.[12] Yet, it is known that families with low incomes have a greater need for care. The cost of illness for the poor is magnified by increased disability, lost wages (as a result of holding jobs that have no sick leave), lack of access to health services, discrimination, and such a fragmented and faulty system of health care that it is often called a "no-system." Some persons believe that ad-

Table 2-4.   Personal Consumption Expenditures, by Product, United States, 1973 *

Type of Product	Expenditures (in billions of dollars)	Per Cent of Total
Total Consumption—All Products	805.2	100.0
Food	143.6	18.0
Alcoholic beverages	21.5	3.0
Tobacco	13.6	2.0
Housing	116.4	14.5
Household operations	117.5	14.6
Transportation	109.2	13.6
Clothing, accessories, and jewelry	81.3	10.1
Medical Care Expenses	62.7	7.8
Recreation	52.3	6.5
Personal business	45.2	5.6
Private education and research	13.2	}
Religious and welfare activities	10.8	} 3.7
Foreign travel and other	5.6	}
Personal care	12.3	1.5

* Table adapted from US Department of Commerce, Bureau of the Census: *The 1976 U.S. Fact Book, The American Almanac, Statistical Abstract of the U.S.* Grosset & Dunlap, Inc., New York, 1976, p. 383.

equate funds are spent on health and welfare but that the *way* they are spent accounts for the unsatisfactory results.

When United States President Lyndon B. Johnson convened the National Conference on Medical Costs in 1967, he did so because the price of medical services was rising so rapidly. In a report of this conference, the following statement was made:

This Nation possesses both the medical know-how and the wealth that makes possible provision of quality medical care for all.

Yet the blunt truth is that all Americans do not yet enjoy the benefits of this progress. The increases in medical prices that have taken place have denied many Americans access to vitally needed medical care.

Private consumer expenditures for medical care have risen from $8½ billion in 1950 to $28.1 billion in 1965; about $6 billion of this increase in consumer expenditures has been consumed by the rise in medical prices during these same years.

Between 1956 and 1966 the prices of all items included in the consumer price index rose 19 per cent while the index of medical care prices rose 42 percent.*

The distribution of the federal budget for the years 1969–1972 by income function is shown in Figure 2-2. As can be seen, health

* US Department of Health, Education, and Welfare: *Report of the National Conference on Medical Costs.* US Government Printing Office, Washington, D.C., 1967, p. xiii.

and income security expenditures comprise 31 per cent of the budget, second only to national defense.

The growth in medical care spending has greatly surpassed that of the economy in general. Much of the increased share of the Gross National Product (G.N.P.) is due to higher *costs* of medical care (see Figs. 2-3 and 2-4). Just where medical care prices have risen most is in the areas of hospital daily service charge and physicians' fees (see Fig. 2-4).

Rapidly increasing costs affect most drastically those segments of the population who can least afford it—the poor, aged, and chronically ill; but they affect also *all* Americans who pay for medical care through insurance plans or directly through out-of-pocket payments. Medicare and Medicaid payments alone account for 71 per cent of health services spending.

In 1949, it was estimated that the average private expenditure for medical care in the United States was $54.00 per capita. In 1970, personal out-of-pocket medical expenses averaged $183.00 per person.[13] Additional sums were spent by the military services, the Veterans Administration, and other federal agencies on medical care and research. Even these figures give no correct impression of the total cost of illness. Federal funding for health services in 1974 and 1975 is shown in Table 2-5.

It has often been said that the people of the United States have the best medical care in the world, but it is now generally accepted that the

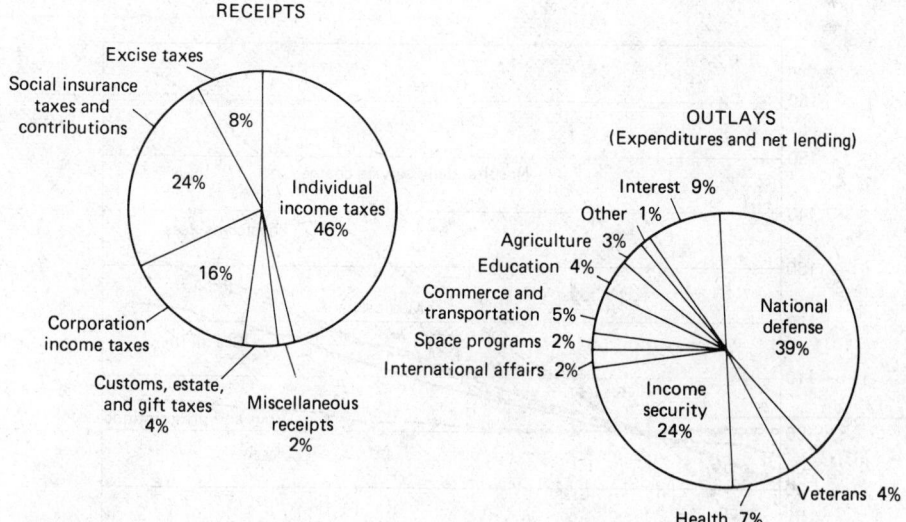

Figure 2-2. Annual federal budget, 1969 to 1972, showing average annual per cent distribution, by function, for fiscal years ending June 30. (Source: U.S. Department of Commerce, Bureau of the Census: *The 1973 American Almanac. The U.S. Book of Facts, Statistics, and Information.* Grosset & Dunlap, Inc., New York, 1973, p. 384.)

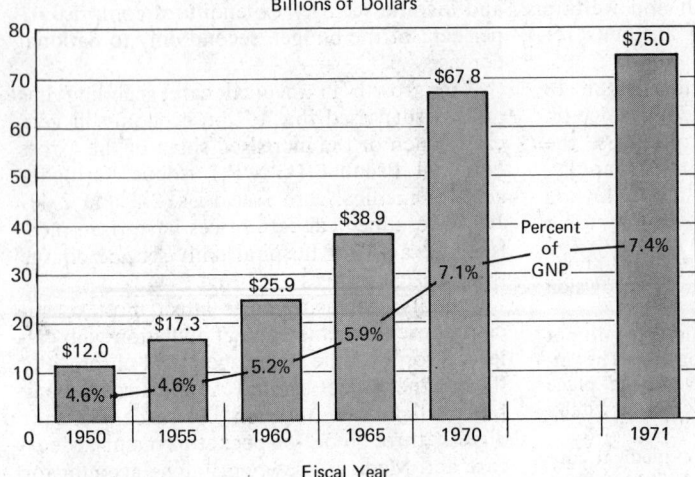

Figure 2-3. National health expenditures as a per cent of gross national product, selected fiscal years, 1950–71. (Source: US Department of Health, Education, and Welfare: *Cost of National Medical Care, 1973.* US Government Printing Office, Washington, D.C.)

quantity and quality of care are uneven and even the wealthy in some areas are unable to get the care they think they need.

Nancy Milio [14] makes the point very clear in her book, *Care of Health in Communities,* that physicians, dentists, and specialists are more plentiful in the more affluent states, as are nurses and other health personnel.

It is clear that larger and larger sums are being spent on health in the United States. With the rapidly rising cost of medical care it is hard to use money as an index of improvement in the national health program (if the United States can be said to have one), and sometimes the gains in the program seem to be offset by unfavorable environmental conditions or other destructive forces. There is considerable evidence that the level of health is not what it should, or might, be. For example, 22.1 per cent of the draftees examined for military service in 1960 were medically disqualified (not including those who failed mental tests), and by 1973 this percentage had jumped to 43.0.[15] In 1967 infant mortality in the United States was high compared with that in 13 other nations (see Fig. 2-5), and venereal disease was on the increase, as was drug addiction. Infant mortality rates by age and color in the United States are shown in Table 2-6. But by comparing the present with the past, most au-

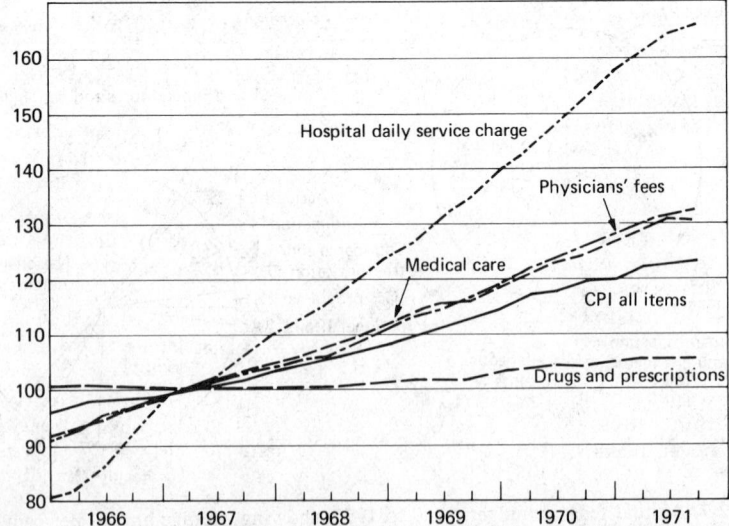

Figure 2-4. Quarterly index of consumer and medical care prices, 1966–1971. (Source: US Department of Health, Education, and Welfare: *Cost of National Medical Care, 1973.* US Government Printing Office, Washington, D.C.)

Table 2-5.   Federal Funding for Health Services *

	($ in thousands)			
	1974 Appropriation	1975 Appropriation	1976 Budget Request	1976 CHF Minimum
Health Services Administration				
Community Health Services	343,233	314,150	174,390	410,000
Maternal and Child Health	270,208	294,868	211,422	339,750
Family Planning	103,225	100,615	79,435	135,000
Health Maintenance Organizations	60,000	79,200	18,612	25,000
National Health Service Corps	13,000	13,000	12,529	20,000
Quality Assurance (PSROs)		37,000	54,682	54,682
Patient Care and Special Health Services	116,961	112,684	115,468	115,468
Indian Health Service	234,210	293,153	310,999	350,000
Buildings and Facilities	21,000	1,300	13,229	13,229
Regional Office Central Staff	5,602			
Program Direction	5,470	31,825	29,569	30,000
Emergency Medical Services	27,000	37,000	25,100	37,000
Totals for HSA	1,199,909	1,314,795	1,045,435	1,530,129
Alcohol, Drug Abuse, and Mental Health Administration				
Mental Health (NIMH)	427,022	420,239	306,063	491,400
Drug Abuse (NIDA)	243,276	219,899	221,858	235,200
Alcoholism (NIAAA)	144,921	145,915	114,199	184,500
Office of the Administrator	8,443	9,555	11,564	10,511
Totals for ADAMHA	819,764	795,608	653,684	915,611

* "Health Coalition Offers Alternate Proposal to Administration Budget for Health Programs" (news), *Am. J. Nurs.*, **75:**1041, (June) 1975.

thorities would probably agree that the average man of this generation has become increasingly aware of the importance of health. He knows more about the way he functions and about the prevention and cure of disease. He is willing to spend each year larger and larger sums to "buy" health. Man's life span is increasing steadily,* and the key has been found to control of disease caused by many microorganisms, even though chronic diseases are on the increase and admissions to general hospitals and psychiatric outpatient clinics mount rapidly. Although man may be more aware of the importance of health, there are other dangers confronting the average citizen of which he may be entirely unaware.

General texts on health, as, for example, *Health and Modern Man* by Donald A. Read and Walter H. Greene,[16] and *Health; Man in a Changing Environment* by Benjamin A. Kogan,[17] emphasize the stress of rapid change. While life has never been static, few would

* Life expectancy at birth in 1920 was 54.1 years; in 1940, 62.9 years; in 1960, 69.7 years; and in 1973, 71.3 years. (US Department of Commerce, Bureau of the Census: *The 1976 U.S. Fact Book, The American Almanac, Statistical Abstract of the U.S.* Grosset & Dunlap, New York, 1976, p. 59.)

question the statement that there has never been such a rapid rate of change.

Stanley J. Matek [18] points to the space program as an example of "synergism," a process in which the results of the combination of technologies (developed in that undertaking) achieved a greater magnitude than the sum of its component technologies. The space program also produced dramatic changes in food products, electronics, communications, education, and medicine. Communications, for example, have increased in volume and intensity recently because the message sender has to compete for more attention via commercials, headlines, and advertising. This increases individual stress, of course.

Most persons are vaguely or specifically aware of the constant demand on their powers of adaptation, the threat to mental health or peace of mind, the extent of the "generation gap." All of this accounts for the popularity of books such as Alvin Toffler's *Future Shock* [19] and *Things to Come* by Herman Kahn and B. Bruce-Briggs.[20] The latter is said to be "an organizational product" of the Hudson Institute, which in recent years has been engaged in the study of the future ("futurology"). *Mankind 2000* [21] is another such book dealing

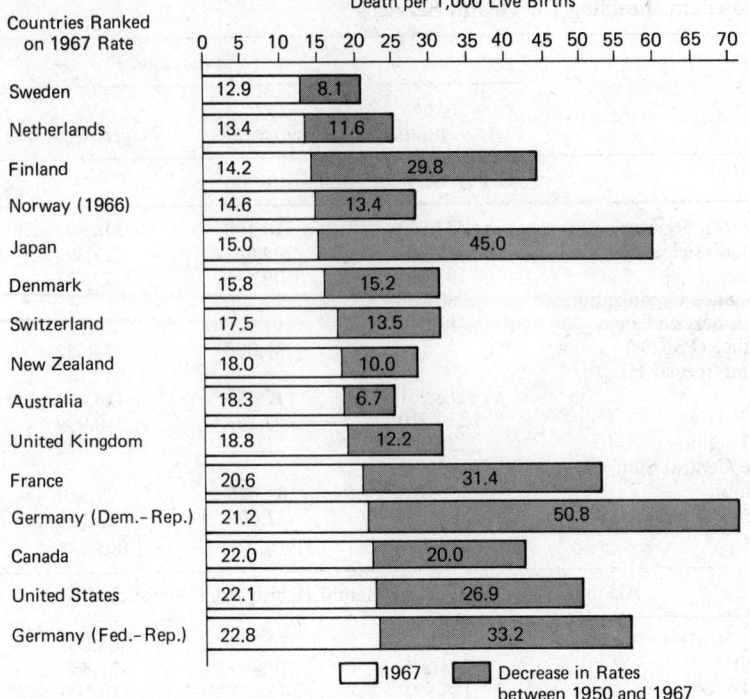

Figure 2-5. Infant mortality rate for selected countries, 1950 and 1967. (Source for 1950: United Nations, *Demographic Yearbook,* Ninth Issue, Special Topic: Mortality Statistics. New York, 1957, pp. 200–209. Source for 1967: United Nations, *Demographic Yearbook, 1969,* 21st Issue, Special Topic: Mortality Statistics, Table 42. New York, 1970, pp. 575–81.)

Table 2-6.   Infant Mortality Rates by Age and Color: United States *

(For 1974, based on a 10 per cent sample of deaths; for all other years, based on final data. Rates per 1,000 live births)

Year	Total			White			All Other		
	Under 1 Year	Under 28 Days	28 Days to 11 Months	Under 1 Year	Under 28 Days	28 Days to 11 Months	Under 1 Year	Under 28 Days	28 Days to 11 Months
1974 (est.)	16.5	12.1	4.4	14.7	11.1	3.6	24.6	16.6	8.0
1973	17.7	13.0	4.8	15.8	11.8	3.9	26.2	17.9	8.3
1972	18.5	13.6	4.8	16.4	12.4	4.0	27.7	19.2	8.5
1971	19.1	14.2	4.9	17.1	13.0	4.0	28.5	19.6	8.9
1970	20.0	15.1	4.9	17.8	13.8	4.0	30.9	21.4	9.5
1969	20.9	15.6	5.3	18.4	14.2	4.2	32.9	22.5	10.4
1968	21.8	16.1	5.7	19.2	14.7	4.5	34.5	23.0	11.6
1967	22.4	16.5	5.9	19.7	15.0	4.7	35.9	23.8	12.1
1966	23.7	17.2	6.5	20.6	15.6	5.0	38.8	24.8	13.9
1965	24.7	17.7	7.0	21.5	16.1	5.4	40.3	25.4	14.9
1964	24.8	17.9	6.9	21.6	16.2	5.4	41.1	26.5	14.6
1963	25.2	18.2	7.0	22.2	16.7	5.5	41.5	26.1	15.4
1962	25.3	18.3	7.0	22.3	16.9	5.5	41.4	26.1	15.3
1961	25.3	18.4	6.9	22.4	16.9	5.5	40.7	26.2	14.5
1960	26.0	18.7	7.3	22.9	17.2	5.7	43.2	26.9	16.4
1950	29.2	20.5	8.7	26.8	19.4	7.4	44.5	27.5	16.9

* Cranley, Mecca S.: "When a High-Risk Infant Is Born," *Am. J. Nurs.,* **75:**1696, (Oct.) 1975.

with long-range prospects of mankind. These three books attempt to identify trends and countertrends, the prevailing culture and the counterculture, or counterreformation—the influence of "the Establishment" and that of the dissidents. *Mankind 2000* is a collection of papers by scientists ("futurologists") presented at a conference in Oslo, Norway, in 1967. It examines technology, so often equated with "progress," analyzes its positive and negative values, and questions whether man can control or reverse current trends. Herman Kahn and B. Bruce-Briggs [22] in *Things to Come* discuss man's disillusionment with progress, some of its "mixed blessings," and some aspects of privacy threatened by technology. They list areas that by 1985 are likely to give rise to "special dangers":

1. Intrinsically dangerous technology
   Modern means of mass destruction
   Nuclear reactors—fission or fusion
   Nuclear explosives, high-speed gas centrifuges, etc.
   Research missiles, satellite launchers, commercial aircraft, etc.
   Biologic and chemical "progress"
   Molecular biology and genetics
   "Mind control"
   New techniques for insurgency, criminality, or ordinary violence
   New techniques for counterinsurgency or imposition of order
   New "serendipities" and synergisms
2. Gradual and/or national contamination or degradation of the environment
3. Spectacular and/or multinational contamination or degradation of the environment
4. Dangerous internal political issues
5. Upsetting international consequences
6. Dangerous personal choices
7. Bizarre issues

Although some of the technologic dangers may not seem to bear directly on health, they constitute a shapeless, nameless aura of anxiety surrounding the life of all those who read, or even those who see filmed programs dealing with such dangers. Fear and anxiety are as threatening to health as the more tangible dangers of chemical poisons or pathogenic microorganisms.

In summary, it seems that modern man recognizes the value of human life (economists give a specific figure for the value of an infant, an adult, and a middle-aged man), but he has not learned to control those forces that are inimical to health, particularly mental health; and even in the United States the people have not yet spent enough money and effort—but

particularly effort—or distributed them well enough, to take full advantage of the enormous store of knowledge that biologic, social, and medical scientists have accumulated. Further discussion of the subject is beyond the scope of this book. This chapter describes conditions affecting health and indicates some outstanding health achievements and problems, and some plans for improving health; it outlines the organization, or the machinery, for health promotion, and the place of hospitals and other institutions in health care; and it points out the particular place of the nurse in this program.

2. CONDITIONS AFFECTING COMMUNITY HEALTH

Many factors contribute toward establishing a high standard of health within a community. In the United States there are areas where the death and sickness rates are extremely low, and others where the rates are appallingly high, as compared with the rates for the country as a whole or the rates in other countries. It is possible here to suggest only some of the outstanding causes.

An economic status that provides an adequate diet, shelter, medical service, and other minimal health essentials is almost certainly the most important contributing factor in producing a high standard of health in any geographical area. Recent data from the National Health Survey * show that those with low incomes are at most disadvantage when it comes to health. Families with an annual income of less than $5000 in 1971 had more limitation of activity, more disability, and more hospitalization than the total population. Within this group, recipients of public aid had higher illness rates than nonrecipients—often twice as high.[23] Bonnie Bullough and Vern L. Bullough,[24] in reporting on the health problems of the poor, stated that a California survey in 1970 showed that 44 per cent of the children in families receiving Aid to Families with Dependent Children had gone without food one or more days during the year because of insufficient funds.

Education is another important factor, the effect of which is difficult to isolate and mea-

---

* The National Health Survey is a continuous, nationwide survey conducted by the National Center for Health Statistics, US Department of Health, Education, and Welfare. Each week a representative sample of households around the country is visited to obtain information about the health of each family member. During the year approximately 42,000 interviews are conducted concerning the health of 134,000 persons.

sure, since the economic status tends to rise with the educational level and more intelligent persons tend to get the best education. There can be little doubt that a knowledge of the essentials of health and familiarity with community resources are a protection for the individual.

Rodger Hurley,[25] in "Health Crisis of the Poor," notes that reports on school health examinations and screening tests show that the lower the educational level of the family the less likely it is to seek corrective measures for the child's defects. This in turn increases the child's absence from school and lowers his or her achievement. So, there is a vicious circle that is hard to break. Few would challenge the statement, however, that as the level of general education rises in a community the morbidity and mortality rates fall. However, education will be effective only if it stimulates *interest* in health. As long as people value wealth, power, or pleasure more than mental and physical health, knowledge alone will not protect them. Motivation is essential and it does not necessarily accompany knowledge.

The provision of *health services and facilities* is a third factor on which the health status depends. The World Health Organization at its founding in 1948 stated that "enjoyment of the highest attainable standard of health is one of the fundamental rights of every human being without distinction of race, religion, political belief, economic or social condition." While some countries even before this had highly developed social security systems that included health care, the WHO pronouncement has undoubtedly hastened the establishment of national health schemes on every continent that are designed to provide for all human beings their "fundamental right" to health care.

The disparity in the distribution of health resources has been hinted at already. It is impossible to do much more than this. According to Nancy Milio,[26] the United States shares with other wealthy countries (and with poor countries, too) the maldistribution of health services.

The publication, *Social Security Programs Throughout the World, 1971,*[27] gives the salient features of existing national health schemes. Many peoples live in countries where no such scheme can be said to exist. Most, but not all, health schemes are centralized. The organization of health programs by province in Canada is an example of a national scheme that is administered through smaller units. In Quebec, a reorganization of health care programs under a 1972 bill grouped all health and social service systems into four large categories: social service centers, local community service centers,

hospital centers, and reception centers, in an effort to improve the quality and distribution of health care.[28,29]

The distribution of health programs throughout various departments in the federal government in the United States is shown in Figure 2-6 and discussed later in this chapter. This country has not fully embraced the WHO pronouncement but the 1966 Public Law 89–749 was a step in this direction for its aim was "promoting and assuring the highest level of health attainable for every person. . . ." *

In recent years there has been a proliferation of federal programs in the United States for the establishment of a variety of health facilities. Figure 2-6 illustrates this trend.

It has been pointed out that persons with higher incomes by and large need less medical care and receive more, while the underprivileged families have greater need for medical service and receive less. In any fee-for-service system, this will be true and is, of course, an argument for the extension of tax-supported medical service, not only for the sake of the so-called underprivileged but also for the sake of the population as a whole, since any society benefits from an improved health status of its members.

Anne R. Somers in *Health Care in Transition; Directions for the Future* [30] writes about the new hazards of affluence. While she concedes that the incidence of serious illness is two or three times higher for the poor as for the total population, she calls attention to some of the effects of plenty—overeating and drinking, underexercising, and misuse of drugs. She believes that higher income and educational levels lead to more demand (if not need) for health services.

The passage of legislation in the 1960s—particularly programs benefiting the medically indigent under 65 years, those over 65 years, and the poor—is evidence that the United States government recognized the need for a more equitable distribution of health services.†

The ratio of physicians to the population has been and still is considered a vital factor in providing health services. The World Health Organization proposed a target ratio of doctors to the population of 1:10,000. Wolsten-

---

* *United States Statutes at Large, 1966,* Vol. 80. Part 1, *Public Laws and Reorganization Plans.* US Government Printing Office, Washington, D.C., 1967, p. 1180.

† The Social Security Amendments of 1965 (Public Law 89–97) provided medical insurance for the needy under age 65 in a section of the law called Title 19 (Medicaid) and for those over 65 years in Title 18 (Medicare). Other parts of the amendments provided money for the construction of neighborhood health centers to benefit the poor.

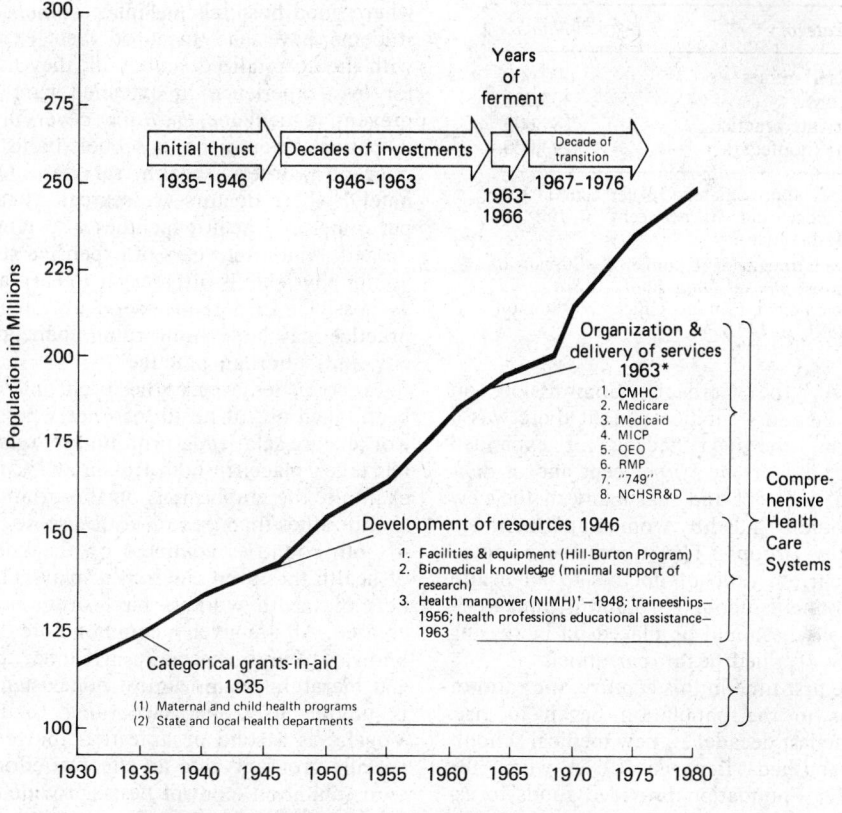

*(1) Community Mental Health Centers (CMHC); (2) Title
XVIII, Social Security Act of 1965 (Medicare); (3) Title
XIX, Social Security Act of 1965 (Medicaid); (4) Maternal
and Infant Care Projects (MICP); (5) Neighborhood Health
Centers (OEO); (6) Regional Medical Programs, (RMP); (7)
Comprensive Health Planning — "The Partnership for Health"
(749); and (8) National Center for Health Services Research
and Development (NCHSR and D).

†National Institute of Mental Health

Figure 2-6. Major health programs of the federal government—transition to
comprehensive health-care systems. (From Kissick, William L.: "Health-Policy
Directions for the 1970's," *N. Engl. J. Med.*, **282:**1345, [June 11] 1970. Based on
National Advisory Commission on Health Facilities: *A Report to the President,
December 1968.* US Government Printing Office, Washington, D.C., 1968.)

holme,[31] noting the unequal distribution worldwide, says this would mean that Africa would
immediately need 24,000 doctors and could absorb a 10-year output of doctors in Great
Britain, but by this time Great Britain would
have employed 10,000 and the United States
36,000 doctors from Asia and Africa (because
of doctor migration).

The United States has throughout this century had a comparatively low ratio of physicians to the population. In 1900 there was one
physician to every 578 persons. Bernard H.
Stern[32] says the proportion increased until
1949, when there was one physician to every

741 persons, but if only those in active practice
were considered there was one physician to
every 982 persons in the population of the
United States. According to Louis I. Dublin,[33]
in 1963 there was a further decline of physicians in active practice to one per 1082 persons. The ratio was higher in large cities having
better medical facilities and higher economic
levels than it was in rural areas not possessing
these incentives.

In 1969 the following health workers—
nurses, physicians, and dentists—were actively
practicing their professions in the United
States:

Category	Number
Registered nurses	680,000
Physicians	303,000
In private practice	184,000*
Dentists (nonfederal)	93,000

* Includes approximately 30 per cent in general practice and 70 per cent in full-time specialty practice.
(US Department of Commerce, Bureau of the Census: *Pocket Data Book, U.S.A. 1971.* US Government Printing Office, Washington, D.C., 1971, p. 147.)

In 1970, the Carnegie Commission on Higher Education [34] indicated that there was a need during the next decade for expanded training of doctors by 50 per cent and of dentists by 20 per cent and that many of the new places should be filled by women and members of minority groups. The Commission noted that the current ratio of doctors to all health care personnel is about 1:10 and it thinks primary emphasis should be placed on increasing the supply of allied health personnel.

For the first time in this century, the ratio of physicians to the population began to rise. During the last decade, 20 new medical schools were established. Between 1922, when the Rockefeller Foundation provided funds to establish the School of Hygiene and Public Health at Johns Hopkins University in Baltimore, and the 1950s, 21 schools of public health in the United States and abroad were opened to help improve the health of the public.[35]

Somers [36] in *Health Care in Transition; Directions for the Future* devotes a chapter to the physician. In it she stresses the over-all shortage, the uneven distribution, the high earnings, but also the price they and the public pay for their rising productivity. While doctors saw about 50 patients a week in 1940, they averaged 132 per week in 1970. One survey reported that the average length of time spent with the patient was 6.1 minutes. The establishment in the United States in 1969 of the medical specialty called Family Practice is one effort to combat the high rate of specialization among physicians (70–75 per cent) and the common criticism that medical care is too impersonal and technical.

In spite of such data as have been presented, some physicians in the United States still maintain there is no shortage of doctors and, judging by world averages, the ratio is very high; everybody, however, admits that there is poor distribution. Students learn to practice medicine in a center where the facilities and equipment are excellent. They become dependent on these conditions and are unwilling to practice

where good hospitals are inaccessible. Medical students have had most of their experience with the hospitalized acutely ill; they have had far less experience in extended care and in preventive medicine; they may never have been in patients' homes or in school, industrial, or migrant workers' health services. Unfortunately, where doctors are scarce, other health personnel and health facilities also tend to be limited. And after years of expensive study the young physician is often eager to earn as much as possible. In a fee-for-service system, rural practice may be less rewarding financially than city and suburban practice.

In countries where the profit motive has been taken out of health care, or where health workers are salaried, a profound reorganization has taken place. In both Russia and China, for example, the emphasis is on the promotion of health rather than treatment of disease. Visitors to both countries comment on the knowledge of health that even children display. The numbers of health workers have dramatically increased. All are given a common core of health knowledge and, especially in China, the medical hierarchy seems almost nonexistent. What is unique to China, according to Ezra F. Vogel,[37] is a solid organization that combines specific programs into an effective effort to extend sanitation, control pests, provide immunizations, and perform other practices that extend public health and medical care in a country that is not even industrialized.

Higher-, intermediate-, and lower-level health workers are reported to work as a team. (See China's demand and supply for these health workers in Table 2-7.) Vertical communication among hospital personnel, medical brigades, clinics, peasant doctors, and other health workers is enhanced by the movement of individuals up and down and by rotation of assignments. There is shared responsibility among Chinese health workers for providing preventive measures, direct services, training, and health committee work.[38]

Kao in his review "China, Chinese Medicine and the Chinese Medical System," says, "The laboratory is now located where the patients are. Teachers in mobile units travel to teach medical workers in the field. Confusing and pedantic educational methods have been abolished or transformed." He says they avoid "ivory towerism." Kao reports that China has 200,000 "professional" doctors, 200,000 nurses, 100,000 pharmacists, and 1,000,000 "barefoot doctors" (and Red Guard doctors) who are close to the people, know them, and act as "a filter system in the over-all health care delivery system." *

* Kao, Frederick F.: *op. cit.*

Table 2-7. A Trial Balance Sheet of Demand and Supply for Higher and Intermediate Medical Manpower in 1957, 1966, and 1971 *

Category	Demand	Supply	Deficiency
1957 [1]			
Higher-level medical personnel	254,000	74,000	180,000
Intermediate medical personnel	597,000	261,000	336,000
1966 [2]			
Higher-level medical personnel			
1.5% growth in population	290,000	210,000	80,000
2% growth in population	303,000	210,000	93,000
Intermediate medical personnel			
1.5% growth in population	680,000	520,000	160,000
2% growth in population	712,000	520,000	192,000
1971 [3]			
Higher-level medical personnel			
1.5% growth in population	314,000	267,000	47,000
2% growth in population	335,000	267,000	68,000
Intermediate medical personnel			
1.5% growth in population	738,000	620,000	118,000
2% growth in population	787,000	620,000	167,000

* Cheng, Chu-Yuan: "Health Manpower: Growth and Distribution," in Wegman, Myron E., et al. (eds.): *Public Health in the People's Republic of China.* Josiah Macy, Jr. Foundation, New York, 1973, p. 151.

Sources: (1) Population in 1957, *T'ung-chi Kung-tso* (*Statistical Work*) no. 11 (June 1957): 25; (2) Population for 1966 is calculated on the basis of 1957 official data. At 1.5 per cent growth rate the population was 728 million; at 2 per cent growth rate, 758.8 million; (3) population for 1971, calculated at 1.5 per cent growth rate, was 783 million; at 2 per cent growth rate, 837 million.

The intermediate-level health practitioner was the focus of attention in a conference sponsored by the Josiah Macy, Jr. Foundation in 1973. In this conference and another on the greater medical profession sponsored jointly by the Foundation and the Royal College of Medicine in London, many entrenched ideas were challenged. The ratio of doctors to the population as an indicator of effective health service was, for example, under question. Victor W. Sidel [39] pointed to the fact that German field barbers, the forerunners of feldshers in Russia, have been for centuries the main dependence of the rural population. There were schools for feldshers as early as 1864, and in 1967 more feldshers were graduated than physicians. He says they outnumbered physicians in 1914 before the current upsurge in the production of physicians began. He reports that the Soviets wish to phase out the feldsher and hope to have 800,000 physicians by 1980, which will give them a ratio of 1:300 in their 250 million population. Sidel also cites the effectiveness of the intermediate health workers in China (barefoot, Red Guard, and "worker" doctors).

E. D. Acheson,[40] a British physician, discussing the educational consequences of accepting the concept of the greater medical profession, feels that doctors constitute only a small minority of skilled personnel who work together in the health service. (See Figure 3-1 in Chapter 3, showing that, in Great Britain today, doctors and dentists represent only 15 per cent of "the greater medical profession," nurses and midwives 75 per cent, and other professional and technical workers 12 per cent.)

Vernon W. Lippard,[41] a physician, in an introduction to the conference report on the greater medical profession, says that physicians outnumbered other health professionals in the United States at the beginning of the twentieth century by a ratio of 2:1, whereas 70 years later "auxiliaries" outnumbered physicians by a ratio of 13:1.

Sir George Godber, Chief Medical Officer of Health and Social Security of England, says, "I believe the greater medical profession consists not of doctors, not even predominantly of doctors, but of a group of people who between them can deploy all medical and related skills that any patient at some time may need. There are scores of kinds of doctors in this, plus lots of different kinds of nurses, technicians and scientists. . . . I do not think his [the physician's] position is dominant although sometimes he may lead." Godber notes that while the numbers of doctors and nurses working in hospitals have doubled in the last 25 years, "other professional and technical staffs have increased by over 150 per cent." *

Robert S. Morison, a biologist, says, "First, I would like to think about paramedical personnel from the standpoint of *improving* on what the doctor is already doing. Most discussions of the subject seem to assume . . . that the ideal way to deliver medical care is through the services of excellently trained physicians. . . . at most we [in the United States] are asking ourselves what parts of the doctors' job can be done *just as well* by other people. I believe it is time we took a more positive approach, and ask what might be done better." †

Malleson [42] in *Need Your Doctor Be So Useless?* has written chapters on "The Uses of Sickness and the Sick-Making Society," "Help Can Be Lethal," and "Healthy Doctoring." He makes a strong plea for health education, for encouragement of the self-help movement as exemplified by Alcoholics Anonymous, Synanon, and Weight Watchers, and for the development of self-reliance as opposed to dependency.

Many students of sociology have called attention to the close relationship among poverty, sickness, vice, and crime. Some doubt may exist as to what is cause and what is effect, but whether sickness results from poverty or poverty from sickness it is plain to see that the total social picture has to be taken into consideration if health conditions of the community are to be materially improved.

John Knowles,[43] Medical Director of the Rockefeller Foundation, has listed the major deterrents to effective health care as follows: (1) unemployment, (2) poverty, (3) inadequate housing, (4) civil injustice and prejudice, (5) maldistribution of wealth, (6) dissipation of energy resources, (7) environmental pollution, (8) urban density, and (9) overpopulation. Knowles thinks a strong stand against these barriers must be taken if we are to make changes in our health care system.

In summary, the conditions that have a direct effect on a community's health are its economic status, the educational level of its members, the provision of adequate health services and facilities, and the ratio of health care workers to the population, particularly

physicians. The experience of China and Russia and their organizations for health care have been discussed.

3. OUTSTANDING ACCOMPLISHMENTS IN DISEASE CONTROL AND HEALTH PROMOTION

While few countries are satisfied with their health services or the health status of their peoples, there is no doubt that the means of controlling disease and improving health are immeasurably greater in this age than at any other period of history. Except in the remaining "primitive" societies, *medical practice has emerged from an art that was based on a meager body of knowledge and vague theories of "fluxes" and "humors" into a science growing out of present knowledge of cell physiology* especially, although atomic medicine and the electric field theory promise further enlightenment. The microscope, microphotography, x-rays, and modern laboratory methods in chemistry and physics have revolutionized the study of anatomy and physiology and, consequently, the practice of medicine. Claude Bernard's [44] pronouncement that, in effect, health consists of keeping the lymph constant around the cell is so simple that many persons hear it and assume that they have always known it. He pointed out that all vital mechanisms of the body, varied as they are, have but one object: to preserve the constant conditions of life in the internal environment. Actually it is a most profound observation, and in it medicine and nursing have one sure guide. Disease is a state in which components or conditions of the cell and its fluids are out of equilibrium; temperature, water, chemicals, nutrients, gases, hormones, enzymes, and other components may change. The constancy of the fluid around the cell may be disturbed, for example, by the presence of bacteria, viruses, or abnormal cells, and the effects of their activity. The cell fluids may be invaded or changed by substances, or there may be a disequilibrium of fluids on either side of the cell membrane that prevents the free flow of fluids, which helps maintain the "constancy." The electron microscope that makes it possible to televise microscopic activity in tissues and individual cells will still further revolutionize the knowledge of anatomy and physiology. Television programs for the general public will develop levels of understanding that were impossible before the development of the electron microscope and television.

Some persons believe that so-called mental disease is as much a disturbance of this in-

* Godber, George: "Manpower Problems on Either Side of the Atlantic," in The Royal Society of Medicine and the Josiah Macy, Jr. Foundation: *The Greater Medical Profession*. The Foundation, New York, 1973, pp. 133, 22.

† Morison, Robert S.: "Manpower Problems on Either Side of the Atlantic. In the United States," in The Royal Society of Medicine and the Josiah Macy, Jr. Foundation: *The Greater Medical Profession*. The Foundation, New York, 1973, p. 29.

ternal environment as is so-called physical disease. Emotions can produce a disequilibrium in components or conditions of the cell and cell fluids just as completely as can toxic substances that are swallowed, or growths that interfere with normal physiology, and emotions can demonstrably change the body's electric fields. The work of Harold Saxton Burr has not been applied as has that of Bernard but the studies that have been made show great promise (see Chapters 5 and 31).

The realization that health consists of this equilibrium of the fluid surrounding body cells does not endow us, however, with the ability to maintain it. Disease will not be conquered until the answers are found to the problems involved and until man is able and willing to control emotions, to eat a balanced diet, to avoid living and nonliving toxic agents and mechanically injurious agents, and to adapt to the constantly changing environment. Science has provided the best tools yet devised, but man has not learned to use them except in specific and limited areas. The greatest failure is in the realm of the spirit, the mind, or the emotions. Increased mental illness suggests that with all the new methods available for the maintenance of nutritional equilibrium, for the removal of disequilibrium of body fluids, for the destruction of invading organisms, little has been learned about the control of injurious psychic forces. Hope lies in the fact that so many people recognize this great need. Most doctors, nurses, and others who work in education, the ministry, and medicine are now provided with some psychological and psychiatric training; and the medical and theological schools in the United States cannot accommodate all the well-prepared applicants who intend to work for spiritual, mental, or emotional harmony through medicine and the ministry.

Dubos, a biologist, is deeply concerned about the human being's *response to stress and to environmental and social change.* In his book, *Man Adapting,* he says, "Living organisms never submit passively to the impact of environmental forces; however primitive they may be, all of them attempt to respond adaptively to these forces, each in its own manner," and, he goes on to say, at a "cruel price in terms of human values." * Dubos' concern is mirrored again in his book *So Human an Animal.* He says, "Each human being is unique, unprecedented, unrepeatable." † Yet, he warns, we face the danger of losing this humanness

to our mechanized surroundings. He further states:

If it is true, as it appears to be, that our environment and way of life profoundly affect our attitudes and those of following generations, nothing could be more distressing for our immediate and distant future than the decadence and ugliness of our great urban areas, the breakdown in public means of transportation, the overwhelming accent on materialistic and selfish comfort, the absence of personal and social discipline, the sacrifice of quality to quantity in production as well as in education. The lack of creative response to these threats is particularly discouraging because all thinking persons are aware of the situation and are anxious to do something to correct it. But common action cannot be mustered because it demands a common faith that does not exist. It is because we need a common faith that the search for significance is the most important task of our times.*

In spite of the concern about the present and the future as expressed by Dubos and others, health scientists are proud of a lengthened *life expectancy.* The average life span in 1973 was 71.3 years in the United States, in contrast to 49.2 years in 1900. It is true that the gain is largely due to saving the lives of infants and small children through better environmental conditions (clean food and water especially), improved maternal and child health services, and the control of infectious diseases. Advances in scientific medicine are currently most dramatic in saving the acutely ill and injured, but there has been little progress in the arrest of chronic diseases.† It is clear, too, that the gains in the United States are much greater among white people than nonwhites. In 1973, the life expectancy of nonwhite males was 61.9 years as compared with 68.4 for white males, and 70.1 for nonwhite females as compared with 76.1 for white females.[45] These racial differences in longevity are, however, lessening as the earnings and education of nonwhites more nearly approach those of whites. The average length of life is influenced by the daily per capita consumption of food. Countries that have a consistent food shortage have the lowest life expectancy, and countries with a high life expectancy have a more nearly adequate national diet. Current world population estimates and estimated

---

* Dubos, René: *op. cit.,* pp. 256, 275.
† Dubos, René: *So Human an Animal.* Charles Scribner's Sons, New York, 1968, p. viii.

* *Ibid.,* p. 180.
† The picture of chronic disease has changed, not so much because it is on the increase, but because more persons live to be middle-aged or elderly to contract disease. In its Statistical Bulletin for May 1969 (p. 4), the Metropolitan Life Insurance Company says that the chances of a male eventually dying from chronic disease are 83 in 100 for the United States compared with 52 in 100 at the beginning of this century.

Table 2-8. World Population Estimates in Millions *†

Africa	391
Northern Africa	96
Western Africa	113
Eastern Africa	111
Middle Africa	44
Southern Africa	27
Asia	2,208
Southwest Asia	86
Middle South Asia	818
Southeast Asia	315
East Asia	989
North America	235
Canada	22.5
United States	211.9
Latin America	316
Middle America	76
Caribbean	27
Tropical South America	175
Temperate South America	38
Europe	469
Northern Europe	81
Western Europe	152
Eastern Europe	106
Southern Europe	131
USSR	253
Oceania	21
World	3,893

Source: Information Service, Population Reference Bureau, Inc., Washington, D.C.

* Manisoff, Miriam: "Family Planning Democratized," *Am. J. Nurs.,* **75:**1665, (Oct.) 1975.

† As of mid-1974; based on interpolation of the mid-1970 population estimate and the mid-1975 "medium variant" projection by the United Nations using the projected rate of growths for the 1970–1975 period.

world populations by continent to the year 2000 are shown in Tables 2-8 and 2-9.

Quoting figures for 1960, Dublin [46] said that only in Australia, New Zealand, Norway, Sweden, Denmark, and The Netherlands does the average length of life exceed that in the United States. Somers, however, concludes that there is a reversal in the long-range improvement in life expectancy in the United States. She says:

Although the change is small, it appears to be significant, especially for men—both white and black—in their most productive middle years and especially when compared to the experience of other nations. According to a study by the National Advisory Commission on Health Manpower, based on data mostly from the late 1950s and early 1960s, 17 nations are reported to have longer life expectancy, at birth, for males, than the United States. Our comparative position appears to have worsened rather than improved during the last two decades.*

Most authorities attribute the saving of maternal and child life to the *control of infections* —the most conspicuously successful accomplishment of health science. Actually, bacteriologists and sanitarians, lawmakers and law enforcement workers, may have played as important roles as doctors and nurses. If the findings of geneticists are ever common knowledge and applied by the people, improvement in the quality of life and extension of the life span might assume undreamed-of proportions.

Diseases caused by microorganisms usually produce *acute* illness. In 1900, such diseases were responsible for more than two-fifths of the deaths in the United States. Today nearly three-quarters of the deaths that occur yearly are caused by diseases ordinarily classed as *chronic* (see Table 2-10). Students of public health believe that chronic disease is not necessarily increasing, however. They call attention to the fact that more persons are now living past middle age, when tumorous growths and degenerative processes are most likely to manifest themselves. Although the birth rate in the United States has markedly diminished since 1945, the death rate shows little change.

It has been demonstrated that when the cause and mode of transmission are known and a protective serum, or specific drug, is available, a communicable disease can be practically wiped out. Smallpox, malaria, typhoid fever, poliomyelitis, and diphtheria are examples of such diseases. Their occurrence in any numbers is considered something of a disgrace in a developed country with a well-organized health service. Almost any communicable condition, regardless of what is known about the causative organism, can be controlled by isolation of the infected persons so that epidemics of all sorts are less and less common. If properly treated, persons with some infectious diseases need not be isolated. But in spite of all these methods of control the goal of preventing communicable disease has not been reached in any country, even in China, where remarkable progress has been made.

* Somers, Anne R.: *Health Care in Transition; Directions for the Future.* Hospital Research and Educational Trust, Chicago, 1971, p. 18. (Data are based on National Advisory Commission on Health Manpower: *Report,* Vol. 1, pp. 91–92; Rutstein, D.: *The Coming Revolution in Medicine.* Massachusetts Institute of Technology Press, Cambridge, Mass., 1967, pp. 15–28.)

Table 2-9.   Estimated World Population: A.D. 1000–A.D. 2000 *

Continent	Population at given times (in millions)						
	1000	1600	1800	1900	1960	1975 (est.)	2000 (est.)
Asia and Oceania	165	279	599	921	1,700	2,231	3,900
Europe, including Russia	47	102	192	423	641	751	947
Africa	50	90	90	120	244	303	517
Americas	13	15	25	144	407	543	904
Total	275	486	906	1,608	2,992	3,828 †	6,268

Source: Annabelle Desmond, "How Many People Have Ever Lived on Earth?" from *The Population Crisis and the Use of World Resources* (The Hague, 1964), p. 39, abstracted from *The Future Growth of World Populations; Population Studies, No. 28* (New York, 1958), p. 23.

* Kogan, Benjamin A.: *Health: Man in a Changing Environment.* Harcourt, Brace & World, New York, 1970, p. 440.

† More recent projections indicate that world population will pass the 4 billion mark by 1975 (Population Reference Bureau press release, April 1969).

Although deaths from pneumonia and influenza have been falling since 1900 when these diseases were the leading causes of death in the United States, they still rank sixth on the 1960 list (see Table 2-10). Whereas we tend to think that modern health care controls communicable disease, there has been a marked increase in viral and nosocomial (hospital-acquired) infections in recent years because new organisms have emerged and older organisms have developed virulent strains. (This is discussed in Chapter 15.) Tuberculosis and nephritis are no longer among the ten leading causes of death but have been replaced by congenital malformations and cirrhosis of the liver. Alcoholism, because it is the underlying cause of accidents, cardiovascular disease, and cirrhosis of the liver, and also because it often goes unrecognized and unreported, is considered by many authorities in the field to rank as one of the three leading causes of death today. There has always been a fluctuation in the incidence of venereal disease, worldwide. Wars, for example, tend to increase the number of cases. In the United States a higher rate is found, generally speaking, among military men, in nonwhites, and in families with low incomes. The means of arresting and preventing the spread of venereal disease are so well established that many countries had practically eliminated these infections before World War II, and it is reported that China has virtually no venereal disease. In the United States, there was a drop in the incidence of primary and secondary syphilis until the early 1960s, when it rose again. By 1970, reported cases increased beyond the 20,000 mark, and even with exist-

ing programs it is estimated that there are still over 500,000 latent or late-stage syphilitics who have not received any treatment or whose treatment has been inadequate.[47] This poses a serious threat to the people of the United States.

Currently there is an epidemic of gonorrhea in the United States, in England and Wales, and in the Scandinavian countries. Some of the explanations for the rapid rise in the incidence of this disease are the increased and rapid means of travel, the existence of a permissive society, relaxation of the restraining influences of religion and family standards of behavior, and changed public opinion. The improvement of contraceptives[48] has removed much of the fear from sexual activity and thus has tended to increase the disease.

Rapid and effective methods for treating syphilis and gonorrhea with antimicrobial agents have been developed, just as they have for almost every other infectious disease. A deterrent to effective treatment, however, is the increasing resistance of the gonococcus organism to antibiotics, particularly penicillin. Current studies indicate the possibility of scientists' developing prophylactic measures by means of (1) a blood test to detect gonorrhea (there has long been a blood test to detect syphilis), and (2) a vaccine to prevent syphilis. There is presently no vaccine to prevent any venereal disease.[49]

In this brief review of progress in combating communicable disease there is great risk of being misleadingly simplistic. The conquest of communicable disease in North America and Europe and recently in China is not a

Table 2-10.   The Ten Leading Causes of Death in the United States, 1900 and 1960 *

Rank	Cause of Death	Death Rate per 100,000 Population	Per Cent of Deaths from All Causes
	1960		
	All causes	955	100.0
1	Diseases of heart	369	38.7
2	Cancer	149	15.6
3	Cerebral hemorrhage	108	11.3
4	Accidents	52	5.5
5	Premature birth	37	3.9
6	Pneumonia and influenza	37	3.9
7	Arteriosclerosis	20	2.1
8	Diabetes	17	1.8
9	Congenital malformations	12	1.3
10	Cirrhosis of the liver	11	1.2
	First ten causes	812	85.3
	1900		
	All causes	1719	100.0
1	Pneumonia and influenza	202	11.8
2	Tuberculosis	194	11.3
3	Diarrhea and enteritis	143	8.3
4	Diseases of heart	137	8.0
5	Cerebral hemorrhage	107	6.2
6	Nephritis	89	5.2
7	Accidents	72	4.2
8	Cancer	64	3.7
9	Diphtheria	40	2.3
10	Meningitis	34	2.0
	First ten causes	1082	63.0

* Dublin, Louis I.: *The Facts of Life from Birth to Death,* 2nd ed. Macmillan Publishing Co., Inc., New York, 1965, p. 103.

global phenomenon. For example, in a series of articles published under the title *The Social Organization of Health,* Charles C. Hughes and John M. Hunter [50] discuss "the mantle of disease" in Africa. They speak of the "incessant morbidity and premature mortality" with, they say, sickness as the norm, and they cite a study showing that there are, on the average, two infections per man. Bilharziasis, filariasis, yaws, leprosy, malaria, and hookworm are all common. As these African countries are "developed," newcomers with no immunity will be particularly susceptible to these diseases and the natives will, in turn, be equally susceptible to infections brought in by inhabitants of other continents. In every country, the effort to control communicable disease should be continuous and unending.

Modern obstetrics has *reduced maternal and infant mortality.* Childbirth is far less hazardous for both mother and infant than it was years ago. Birth control pills and other agents to prevent unwanted pregnancies, diagnosis of intrauterine conditions by amniocentesis (withdrawal of amniotic fluid for analysis), electronic fetal monitoring, treatment with intrauterine transfusions, rubella antibody testing, immunization of the mother to prevent Rh disease in the infant, and radical surgery in the treatment of cancer all have effected changes in the practice of obstetrics and gynecology. The maternal death rate (number of maternal deaths per 100,000 live births) in the United States in 1973 was 15.2, a decline from the 1940 rate of 376.0.[51] This fact alone indicates that safe and skillful medical and nursing care is available to those members of the population. To illustrate what good medical supervision and nursing care can accomplish in reducing the infant death rates, the work of the nurse-midwives at the University of Mississippi, as reported by Marie C. Meglen,[52] reduced the rate of one rural Mississippi county from a 1969 high of 39.1 deaths per 1000 live births to 21.3 in

1971.* The infant death rate over-all in the United States in 1973 was 17.7 deaths per 1000 live births.[53] Great strides have been made in reducing this rate both here and abroad, and yet the United States still ranks fourteenth among the countries of the world in infant mortality. A recent survey found a strong correlation between infant death and low socioeconomic status of the parents. Those reporting the study state that nearly 50 per cent of these deaths might have been prevented because they were due to such things as ignorance about child care and failure to seek professional care.[54]

Developments in the field of nutrition should certainly receive honorable mention in even the briefest review of medical progress. Not only have dietary measures been discovered for nutritional disorders such as celiac disease, nontropical sprue, and lactose intolerance, but also in almost every branch of medicine and surgery, therapy has been improved by more scientific methods of feeding. Improved feeding patterns and widespread recognition of the significance of vitamins in the diet have saved infants, children, and adults from true nutritional diseases such as scurvy, rickets, beriberi, and pellagra. Yet iron-deficiency anemia remains a major nutritional problem in the United States in infants and young children.[55] In developing countries, protein-calorie malnutrition and vitamin deficiency diseases continue to be major sources of early deaths. Food shortages are acute in many parts of the world and famine is a specter that haunts thoughtful people in this decade.

Experiments with animals and studies of regional and national diets have helped establish nutritional requirements for various ages, for women during pregnancy, and for conditions such as obesity or hyperlipidemia (excess of fats in the bloodstream). (See Chapters 10 and 36.) Some evidence is accumulating that learning skills of children may be grossly impaired by faulty diets.[56]

The diet in the United States as a whole is often said to be more adequate and varied than that of any other nation. Students from other countries come here to study feeding methods in hospitals and schools. In spite of this fact, there are large areas of the country in which the diet of the average family is deficient in certain essentials. Of recent interest is the preference of many people for a diet composed exclusively of "natural" foods. The danger with this diet is that necessary vitamins and minerals may be eliminated inadvertently. Experimentation with diets is widespread, especially among young people. Many are vegetarians as well as devotees of natural foods.

When economic conditions limit food selection, few families know enough about nutrition to provide the essential food elements. There is a great deal to be done through health education and further discoveries through research. The chemistry of nutrition is relatively new; its students consider they have barely scratched the surface of this science and some nutritionists accuse health workers themselves of knowing little about it. Much is being done to correct this situation through extensive education of professionals and the public.

The development of *asepsis* and modern *anesthesia* and *surgical technique* has entirely altered the outlook for those who must undergo operations. A hundred years ago, surgeons expected wounds to become infected, whereas today an infected wound in considered preventable. The use of chemotherapeutic agents and antibiotics has still further reduced the incidence and duration of surgical infections. Prior to the middle of the last century, operations were performed without an anesthetic as the term is now understood. In some cases the patient would be made drunk with alcohol or drugged with opium or mandrake. Surgery performed under these conditions could not fail to produce the shock of any painful and fearful experience. Anesthesia has been made progressively more effective, less dangerous, and less unpleasant from the patient's point of view. Surgical treatment has been improved in so many ways that the hazards are enormously reduced and the person is returned to normal living much sooner. Extended knowledge of acupuncture as a substitute for chemical anesthesia is adding a new dimension to surgery both in the East and West. It is discussed in Chapters 47 and 49.

Organ transplants, developments in the field of immunology, open-heart surgery, burn therapy, angiography, and hemodialysis, and the use of special equipment to monitor cardiac, brain wave, and other vital signs have all revolutionized modern *medical and surgical care.* The control of endocrine disorders, such as diabetes with oral hypoglycemic agents, and the effective treatment of other metabolic diseases with glandular secretions in a purified or a synthetic form are among the great blessings modern medicine has brought to mankind. The idea of treating disease with secretions of the body and organs of animals is not new, however. Medical historians call attention to the

---

* An even more striking example of skilled nurse-midwifery is the loss of only one mother in the first 1000 deliveries of the Frontier Nursing Service in Kentucky as reported by Louis I. Dublin in *Public Health Nurs.*, **24**:582, (Oct.) 1932.

ancient practice of compounding remedies from the spinal cords or brains of animals and from the urine and blood of human beings.

Improved diagnostic methods make it possible to treat many patients more accurately than has ever before been possible. The use of radioactive isotopes to diagnose diseases of the thyroid, lung, bones, or brain through scanning procedures and the discovery of the effect of steroids on inflammatory diseases have been of great significance in the control of many chronic illnesses. As effective agents are discovered for treating and arresting previously debilitating and fatal diseases, the lives of more and more ill persons are saved.

In no area of health have conditions changed more radically than in the *management of mental disorders* or antisocial behavior, although it is a question whether what is generally believed to be improved managment has reduced the incidence, length, or severity of mental illness. Given a boost by legislation passed in 1963 and 1965 to establish community mental health centers, the field of psychiatry has greatly changed in the past 20 years. The use of chemicals, but particularly tranquilizing drugs, and early discharges to community after-care facilities have changed the care formerly received by institutionalized patients. John J. Hanlon says:

Each year in the United States over 1 million persons, including 4,000 children and youths, are treated in mental hospitals. While only about 2 per cent of all hospital admissions are for psychiatric disorders, about one half of the hospital beds in the nation are occupied by mentally ill patients. In addition, 1.5 million adults and children visit outpatient clinics and private physicians for psychiatric diagnosis and treatment each year. It has been estimated that about one half of all children and adults who consult private physicians for any reason have some kind of emotional disorder. Similarly it is estimated that of the 20 million patients who go to general hospitals for physical ailments each year about 6 million have illnesses caused by emotional disturbances.*

The very definition of mental disease is in question, while alcoholics and other drug addicts who were punished for their addictions are now treated for their "illnesses." Many persons writing about the United States and other countries refer to their "drugged societies"; others say society is schizophrenic—that it teaches a set of values it disregards in practice. R. D. Laing[57] (a controversial figure among psychiatrists) says, "There is little conjunction of truth and social reality." This

Scottish psychiatrist questions the idea that successful treatment of the mentally ill should always be directed toward helping them adapt to the world as it is. He questions who is "normal," remarking that "Normal men have killed perhaps 100,000,000 of their fellow normal men in the last fifty years."

The writings of Erik Erikson, Sigmund Freud, Kazimierz Dabrowski, James Hillman, Sidney J. Jourard, R. D. Laing, Abraham Maslow, Rollo May, and many other physicians and social scientists have introduced generations of college students to the psychiatric vocabulary and what is known or conjectured about mental health and psychiatric treatment. Since Clifford Beers' epoch-making book *The Mind That Found Itself* (1908), descriptions of psychiatric treatment are increasingly popular in the United States. Psychiatric hospitals are the setting for plays, films, and television programs. *The Snake Pit* (1946) and *I Never Promised You a Rose Garden* (1964) were best sellers, and *One Flew Over the Cuckoo's Nest* was a popular book and film (1976). Newspapers and weekly and monthly journals in many countries have carried so many articles about therapy and conditions in psychiatric institutions that both are well known.

Addiction to mind-altering drugs, including alcohol, has increased so alarmingly that it has led to the study of drug addiction by millions of professionals and laymen all over the world. Helping groups for addicts, such as Alcoholics Anonymous and Synanon, are increasingly active in the United States and elsewhere. Although nonprofessional, they have their roots in psychology, human development, psychiatric theory, ethics, and mysticism.

Narcotics, mainly heroin, have been reported to be the leading cause of death in New York City among those 15 to 35 years old.[58] It is estimated that there are between 9 and 10 million alcoholics in the United States, and that alcoholism is related to over half the accidental deaths and to many suicides.[59,60] The homicide rate has risen 60 per cent in the United States since 1950. According to Somers,[61] in 1969 the rate was over 7 per 100,000. Prisons are overcrowded, and the treatment in most of them is brutalizing rather than rehabilitative. Health professionals such as Karl Menninger are questioning the social value of prisons.[62] In 1972, the Department of the Solicitor General in Canada and the American Medical Association in the United States reported surveys of the health services in each country's respective penal institutions.[63,64] While surveys focus on the availability to prisoners of health care comparable to that available to the unincarcerated elements of society,

* Hanlon, John J.: *Principles of Public Health Administration.* C. V. Mosby Co., St. Louis, 1969, p. 425.

such services might include research on the cause of crime and the question of whether antisocial behavior is a form of mental illness or mental retardation. Jessica Mitford's [65] study of prisoners and the parole system in the United States, *Kind and Usual Punishment,* presents data supporting the conclusions that the "corrective system" is not corrective. Kogan, in *Health; Man in a Changing Environment,* takes the position that antisocial behavior is a symptom of the imbalance of man and the environment. He says, "Man is in trouble. He is trapped in the web of his own technological triumphs. Never before has he known so much of both his inner mechanisms and his outer world. Yet never before has he been so oppressed by the imbalances between them" * Rollo May,[66] in *Power and Innocence. A Search for the Sources of Violence,* makes the point that violence is the way in which persons deprived of power seek to assert themselves. He speaks of violence as a kind of communication or self-assertion by those who feel alienated from their environments. Withdrawal (perhaps through drugs) he thinks is another form of communication.

Taking the broadest view of mental illness and mental retardation, it is very difficult to define either state. The point made here is that not only health professionals but also large segments of society have ceased to believe that every person is either "sane" or "insane," "normal" or "retarded," "innocent" or "criminal," even though for legal purposes individuals must be declared so by the courts.

More and more persons accept the premise that physical disease has an emotional, or mental, component and vice versa; most persons have heard the term "psychosomatic" and recognize the interrelationship of mind and body. This has led to the establishment of services for patients with psychosomatic disorders in psychiatric units in general hospitals.[67] More and more often there are special units for the treatment of alcoholism and other forms of drug addiction in general hospitals. Such units treat patients admitted to them but they also supply the consultation services of doctors, nurses, and other health professionals on their staffs from other divisions of the hospital or medical center. While mental hospitals housing thousands of patients still exist in many countries, there is a movement to eliminate them and include psychiatric services in general hospitals or medical centers, and to provide patients in them with the same comprehensive inpatient and outpatient services provided throughout the center, and to provide home care on the same equal basis.

Attempts to combat some of the disadvantages of very large psychiatric hospitals include dividing them into small autonomous units where patients and staff from the same geographic area are segregated so that each unit may resemble a small local institution. Psychiatric hospitals may offer care during the day only, or care at night only, or continuing support for patients who are gainfully employed outside the hospital. Psychiatric patients now go into the community not only to work but also for recreation and study. Placement of psychiatric patients in foster homes has taught the public a great deal about psychiatric care. This practice is centuries old in some countries, new in others.

For several years attention has been directed toward developing a "bill of rights" for mentally ill patients. Some ideas for the institutionalized patient that have been suggested are the right to receive treatment, refuse treatment, be protected from harm, be paid for institution-maintaining labor, be placed in the least restrictive form of treatment, receive legal counsel, have limitations on the length of involuntary hospitalization, have privacy, free communication, and the opportunity to vote, have access to citizen advocates and ombudsmen, and to be provided decent living conditions, regular outdoor exercise, and adequate medical care.[68] One state in the United States, New Jersey, enacted such a law in 1975 to guarantee the rights of the mentally ill.[69]

During the 1950s, many American states established commissions on mental health and most have been made aware of their strengths and weaknesses. While the creation of mental hospitals has historically been hailed as a major health achievement because they proclaimed the status of inmates as sick persons rather than persons who menaced society and had to be incarcerated, the spirit of "bedlam" has not been entirely exorcised. Erving Goffman [70] published a study of mental hospitals in 1961 under the title *Asylums.* He concluded that most psychotics still live under the power structure and "norms" of a community of prisoners. While the atmosphere is decried and many persons are trying to eradicate it, few would deny the validity of Goffman's statement, even today. Bruno Bettelheim, whose book *Love Is Not Enough* (1950) introduced many readers to effective treatment of emotionally disturbed children, says in a 1974 publication:

There was never any proper reason or excuse for the dreadful places where mental patients are kept; nor for the neglect and outright mistreatment that camouflages itself as their therapy. Our

---

* Kogan, Benjamin A.: *Health; Man in a Changing Environment.* Harcourt, Brace & World, New York, 1970, p. ix.

mental institutions are shameful, festering sores of society which break shockingly into public awareness, only to be quickly forgotten before they seriously disturb our consciences. Not so long ago [1946] the image of the snake pit shook many into realizing how inhumanly we treat the mentally ill. Yet the treatment of these wretched people is no better today, even though every year or two there is this great public outcry when the utter degradation of mental patients is discovered in some institution, as if such conditions were not typical of mental hospitals all over the world.*

Malleson [71] is skeptical about a great deal of current psychiatric treatment, observing that the passivity induced by drugs in contemporary hospitals is more destructive than the efforts in "asylums" of yesterday to channel patients' energies into the work of maintaining the institution or operating its surrounding farm. Douglas H. Bennett,[72] discussing the treatment of mental disorders in Great Britain and the United States, notes a certain disillusionment of young psychiatrists with treatment. He cites as the main development in Britain the "social psychiatry" in treatment of the hospitalized psychotic and the "dynamic psychiatry" in treating ambulatory neurotics in the United States.

Bennett notes the benefit to the British patient of the 1974 reorganization of the National Health Service "in which all the inpatient, day patient, general practitioner or local authority services jointly form a comprehensive service to patients . . . in which the emphasis is on rehabilitation, in the preservation of the patients' personal relationships and contacts with the local community." He says, "The aim is to transfer the care of the psychiatric patient from the old mental hospital to his local community where it will be undertaken with the support of the psychiatric unit and the social service department." Bennett notes that between 1949 and 1967 psychiatric hospital admissions more than trebled and outpatient department referrals more than doubled. He makes a plea for effective partnerships, decrying descriptions of teams composed of a psychiatrist and *"his* medical staff," *"his* nurses" etc., saying that the expression is destructive to partnerships and noting that the World Health Organization has "recently barred all references to the 'paraprofessional worker.' " † He says that successful care of the psychotic depends upon successful inter-

vention by the person who is present, not on the work of any one profession. In the British system the plan is to provide 120 "day places" for every 100 beds.

Although many believe there has been an over-all improvement in the delivery of mental health services, again Malleson [73] questions this. He notes the rising admissions to psychiatric hospitals in Canada as well as England and the United States. He thinks treatment in psychiatry and some other areas tends to foster dependency rather than self-reliance. The effort to integrate mental health care into all health services, however, seems to be generally accepted as a constructive move.

Psychiatry and psychiatric nursing make excessive demands on the imagination of the health worker. They require to a greater extent than any other branch of medicine a thorough understanding of human nature. Although treatment is often long and drawn out and recovery is slow, the field has attracted many dedicated health workers. There is a need, however, for more general knowledge of the early symptoms of mental disease, for a recognition of the value of early treatment and preventive care, and for a more hopeful outlook and open manner in dealing with psychiatric conditions.

This summary of the progress that has been made in raising health standards touches upon only a few of the outstanding achievements. The suggested health problems facing medical workers and the public at large are only a sampling of the total list, but in all these, as in nearly every aspect of therapy and health education, *nurses* have taken an active part. In the control of communicable disease, it is the nurse who most constantly applies the principles of microbiology in preventing the transfer of disease-producing organisms from one individual to another. In hospitals, homes, schools, industry, prisons, and in private practice, and as the representatives of official and voluntary health agencies, nurses teach those with communicable conditions to care for themselves in such a way that they will not be a menace to others. Nurses administer protective and curative therapies prescribed by themselves or the physician, and make and record observations, which are an essential part of the study of all disease.

In the maternity program nurses have been especially conspicuous. In clinics and in homes they work with physicians and other members of the health care team in teaching and supervising antepartal, intrapartal, postpartal, and interconceptional (between pregnancies) care. Insofar as possible, nurses attempt to provide patients and families with near optimum con-

---

* Bettelheim, Bruno: *A Home for the Heart.* Alfred A. Knopf, New York, 1974, p. 3.
    † Bennett, Douglas H.: "Mental Disorders. In Great Britain," in The Royal Society of Medicine and the Josiah Macy, Jr. Foundation: *The Greater Medical Profession.* The Foundation, New York, 1973, p. 83.

ditions in which to give birth to their infants. More than anybody else, nurses protect the newborn from harmful elements in their environments. They protect the mother after delivery from microorganisms that many years ago attacked and killed one out of every two women. The fall in the infant and maternal death rates is probably due as much to the nurse's contributions as to the increased skill of the obstetrician.

The nurse-midwife has played an important role in the British Commonwealth and other countries during a large part of this century. Many nurses certified in other areas of practice elect to be certified in midwifery also. In recent years in the United States, certified nurse-midwives have grown in popularity and respect with both professionals and lay persons alike. Their services include care of families throughout normal pregnancy, delivery, and in-hospital care, and the provision of postpartal and family planning services. They teach mothers about their own and their infant's care during the childbearing cycle. With available physician consultation and functioning under approved standing orders, nurse-midwives prescribe appropriate treatments and medications, and attend and assist the mother throughout the delivery when no complications occur. Nurse-midwives also examine and manage the care of the newborn infant. In clinics they take histories, carry out breast, abdominal, and pelvic examinations (sometimes complete physical examinations), perform tests, prescribe medications, and provide complete family planning services. In all of the nurse-midwives' activities they are responsible for providing expert nursing care and extending the nursing role into the area of management of care whenever the circumstances meet the criteria for "normal."

Pediatric nurse practitioners, or specialists, continue the care initiated by nurse-midwives. Their services include the complete management of the well child and management of many common pediatric illnesses and maturational problems and the supervision of childhood growth and development. They also conduct physical examinations, prescribe medications and treatments, teach and counsel children and their parents, and provide expert nursing care. Both the certified nurse-midwife and the pediatric nurse practitioner may, in many instances, engage in research as an ongoing part of their work.

Psychiatric nursing specialists who are prepared to give psychotherapy share with the psychiatrist the responsibility for providing therapy in one-to-one relationships or in group interaction. By initiating and monitoring drug therapy, brief treatment in emergencies, preventive programs, and day hospital care, the psychiatric nursing specialist has an independence in practice once undreamed of. It is only in places where excellent nursing is available that such harmful practices as physical restraint, confinement, and widespread use of drugs to quiet violent persons (chemical restraint) are reduced or eliminated entirely. The improvement in care of the mentally ill lies partly in the work of psychiatric liaison nurses who work in hospitals or in visiting nurse associations and health departments to coordinate care of patients before and after they are discharged to their homes in the community.

Family nurse practitioners combine the skills of pediatric and medical nurse practitioners with the generalized approach of the community health nurse. They are primary care providers who often work with family physicians in ambulatory or community health settings to assist families to achieve the highest level of health possible. By adding medical diagnostic and management skills to community nursing skills, these nurses are able to include all levels of preventive care. They work in collaboration with health and social agencies to meet the needs of the individual, the family, and the community.[74]

Medical-surgical nurse practitioners provide specialized care to clients throughout both the acute and chronic phases of their illnesses. Adult and medical nurse practitioners, nurse clinicians, clinical nurse specialists, and public health nurse coordinators all make invaluable contributions to the care of clients. As with other specialists, nursing research is frequently an important aspect of their work.

Progress in nutrition has resulted from the combined efforts of nutritionists, chemists, physiologists, laboratory technicians, physicians, nurses, and social workers. A nurse does not ordinarily supervise the preparation of food in institutions. Everyone, but particularly nurses, should have some knowledge of this art, however. Nurses are often responsible for food selection within the range allowed by the prescribed diet; they help in and teach the patient or the family about food selection and budgeting and about funds or stamps available for food purchasing. Nurses help plan a nutritional diet and help patients eat when they need such assistance. In this, as in all fields of medical research, they participate by their constant observation of the patient and by recording and reporting these observations, and, in some instances, nurses may even initiate and conduct nutritional research.

The authors' emphasis here is on *nursing* because this text is for nurses, and the purpose of this discussion is to impress students and members of this profession with the relationship of nurses to the total health program. It is essential, however, that each group appreciate the need for understanding and cooperating with other groups, and so the total program is discussed in some detail.

In summary, the outstanding accomplishments in disease control and health promotion include a lengthened life expectancy, the control of communicable diseases, modern obstetric and midwifery care, developments in nutrition, improved medical and surgical care, and improved diagnostic methods. Attention has been drawn to changes in the care of the mentally ill and the development of new nursing roles.

4. ORGANIZATION OF HEALTH CARE

Responsibility for Health Care Worldwide. The World Health Organization's twentieth-century pronouncement that health care is a universal human right seems to go undisputed. The American Nurses' Association 1971 *Statement on the Essential Elements of a Health Care System* strongly supports this view.[75] The nineteenth-century concept that education is a universal human right also goes undisputed. Some governments take the responsibility for providing, through taxation, for making health care and education available to all residents. Mentioned earlier in this chapter is the US Department of Health, Education, and Welfare's analysis of the social security programs throughout the world.[76] Published in 1971, it lists laws (with dates) and types of programs under the following headings and subheadings that suggest the interrelation of health with other aspects of social welfare: (1) *Old Age, Invalidity and Death*—Social Insurance System; (2) *Sickness and Maternity*—Social Insurance System; (3) *Work Injury*—Social Insurance System; (4) *Unemployment;* (5) *Family Allowances*—Unemployment Related Systems. This analysis shows that laws under "Sickness and Maternity" date from 1883 (in Germany) and that tax-supported health care, in most countries that have it, dates as recently as the 1940s onward. Some "undeveloped" countries still have none. Many undeveloped countries of Africa do not have legal programs under "Sickness and Maternity." Large countries, such as the United States and Canada, may have state or provincial health programs that vary in nature and may antedate national programs. Only 12 countries of the world were said in 1971 to have medical benefits that

cover "all residents," * but if the People's Republic of China were included (extent of coverage said to be "unknown"), there would be 13 countries. One country (Canada) has hospitalization programs that cover "all residents" and provincial medical-care programs cover 95 per cent of all residents according to this publication.

Women and industrial workers have had more protection than other categories of society, by and large, and employed women more protection than unemployed. Programs may be administered by departments of labor, but when a country has a ministry of health, medical benefits are under its jurisdiction. Some countries also have social security departments or institutes that administer sickness insurance funds.

According to the US Department of Health, Education, and Welfare's analysis of sickness and maternity "laws and types of programs," the "first and current laws" for the United States were P.L. 89–97, the medical benefits of the Social Security Amendments of 1965 (Medicare and Medicaid), and cash benefits in six states for certain workers dating from 1942 to 1969. In the United States in 1971 medical benefits were under the "general supervision" of the Department of Health, Education, and Welfare, and the cash benefits were variously administered in the states.

The United Kingdom of Great Britain and Northern Ireland is a good example of a country that has not only universal health insurance (under the National Health Service Act of 1946 and the National Insurance Act of 1965) but also, under its reorganization plan of 1974, a highly unified and comprehensive health program. The previously tripartite service (public health, hospital, and private practitioner) has been coordinated and services administered locally by area health authorities. In a 1973 publication, J. J. A. Reid's[77] prediction was that these health areas will range in population from 200,000 to about 1.5 million. The chief medical officer will be a specialist in community medicine. There will be primary care teams, groups of GPs (general practitioners), and attached to them a number of local health authority nurses, usually comprising a range of

---

* These countries are Denmark (all residents must become "active" or passive members of a local sickness fund), Finland, Iceland, Japan, New Zealand, Norway, Sweden, United Kingdom, Union of Soviet Socialist Republics. The countries of Ceylon, Malaysia, and Singapore indicate coverage of "all residents within limit of facilities available." For the People's Republic of China, extent of coverage was reported as "unknown," but recent information makes the authors believe it is universal.

qualifications and skills from the health visitor, through the state-registered and state-enrolled levels of nursing, to the nursing auxiliary. "Health centres" under the reorganization plan in Great Britain are multiplying rapidly, and, although they vary in size and quality, the aim of each is to provide a coordinated service to all residents of a given area. According to Vernon W. Lippard,[78] if the United States had followed the lead of Great Britain in the 1940s and established a national health scheme, the decline of the general practitioner might have been forestalled.

Most of those consulted seem to think the British reorganization is promising. Sir George Godber,[79] Chief Medical Officer of Health and Social Security, claimed in 1973 that the British system had not realized its potential mainly because organization had not kept up with scientific advance; the 1974 reorganization was an attempt to correct this imbalance. Colin T. Dollery,[80] a pharmacist and educator, referring to the reorganization to effect "an integrated area service," was skeptical, however, and claimed that the drift in the National Health Service was undoubtedly "toward a more centralized and authoritarian system." Others question the separation of health and social services. A. L. Cochrane, Director of the Epidemiological Unit of the Medical Research Council, commenting on changes in acute hospitals that, he thinks, will have "reduced intake, reduced length of stay" and "pruning of . . . auxiliary services," says, "There will be two other centres of power in the integrated service, growing partly at the expense of the acute hospital—the general practitioner and his team, and the director of social services and his team." * Muriel Skeet,[81] a British nurse, thinks that the 1970 Local Authority Social Service Act of Great Britain which provided a single door through which the patient might reach any social agency his situation demanded, was praiseworthy, but, she says, "most problems in the field have both health and social elements." However, there seems to be a consensus in Great Britain that the access of every resident to a health center where he or she will be seen by general practitioners and "attached" nurses, and from which he or she will be referred to a hospital or any other health agency as indicated by need, has created a unity of care since all these services are actually one organization or administratively related. Each local health authority is, in effect,

responsible for delivering health services to the residents of the area.

Many of those who write and speak on health care in the United States refer to its "no-system." Eugene Stead, an American physician, says, "In the United States no one is responsible for rendering personal health service to all the people. A doctor is licensed by the state and this gives him the legal right. . . . Insurance programs . . . encourage the use of hospitals and . . . discourage the development of systems for giving ambulatory care. . . . The doctors have little incentive to make changes in the present system. They are busy, well paid, and enjoy high social prestige. . . ." He thinks they are "unmoved" when people can't get medical care and when "the cost is prohibitive." *

Efforts have been made in the United States to establish unified health services for a community. Edmund D. Pellegrino, 20 years later, describes the program of the Hunterdon Medical Center in New Jersey, where the community hospital was established in 1953 "that really belonged to the community." It had a preventive and curative program and most of the health services of the community centered in the hospital. "All Hunterdon patients, regardless of ability to pay, had an attending physician responsible for their care as individuals." [82]

But Pellegrino takes a pessimistic view of the organization of health care in the United States as a whole. He says, "American medicine today has the capability, and American society the resources, to make a full measure of health available to all our citizens. The expenditure of $75 billion annually and the employment of 4 million health workers attest to our interest in achieving this end. What is lacking, however, is a clear matching of this massive endeavor with the common and universal needs of the population." Pellegrino says the health care system "resembles a huge renegade planet" launched on a course that seems "bent to the autonomous needs of the system" rather than on satisfying the health needs of the people. He thinks the solution lies in primary care centers with primary, secondary, and tertiary care articulated.†

Malleson, a Canadian physician, also calls

* Cochrane, A. L.: "Acute and Chronic Illness. In Great Britain," in The Royal Society of Medicine and the Josiah Macy, Jr. Foundation: *The Greater Medical Profession.* The Foundation, New York, 1973, p. 57.

* Stead, Eugene: "Roles, Accountability and Leadership. In the United States," in The Royal Society of Medicine and the Josiah Macy, Jr. Foundation: *The Greater Medical Profession.* The Foundation, New York, 1973, p. 151.

† Pellegrino, Edmund D.: "Delivery of Medical Care—By Whom? In the United States," in The Royal Society of Medicine and the Josiah Macy, Jr. Foundation: *The Greater Medical Profession.* The Foundation, New York, 1973, pp. 58, 63.

for unification of health services and believes the present "chaotic" health care can be "tidied up" by the creation of "community health centres" that provide all the medical and social care services for the community. He refers to the Peckham Experiment [83] in England as a model *de luxe*. There, families, not individuals, were enrolled and the center offered a wide range of health and social services.

Malleson stresses the importance of health education, the development of self-reliance, and the involvement of the average citizen. He thinks everybody has the "right to survive," but he thinks in its present form professional health service in Great Britain, Canada, and the United States offers "baby help" that degrades. As mentioned earlier, he calls attention to the effectiveness of the self-help movements exemplified by Alcoholics Anonymous, Al-Anon, Synanon, Weight Watchers, and Ostomy Clubs, and thinks the principle might be more generally applied, that the capacity for growth or healing resides in every human being and that groups with the same health or social problem can help each other. Malleson decries the spiraling cost of health care and suggests that funding as it now exists is demoralizing to physicians and patients alike since it fosters the perpetuation of dependency and a "health industry" that tends to expand and protect its interests rather than those of the people it serves.

Anne R. Somers,[84] in the study earlier described, *Health Care in Transition; Directions for the Future,* made for the Hospital Research and Educational Trust, Chicago, discusses the proposed health programs for the United States. While she points to effectiveness of the Kaiser-Permanente model described by Sidney R. Garfield (see pages 149 and 150), she seems to think it most likely that the hospital will be the hub, or the unifying force, or the agency in the United States around which all health care will be organized.

Regardless of the administrative structure, or in what offices or agencies most power is invested, there is a trend toward unifying all health services within a geographic area, a trend toward stressing a comprehensive, continuous health and sickness service, and a trend toward giving the patient—or the public—a more important role in policy-making and actual operation of health services.

Responsibility for Health Care in the United States. Health promotion and medical care of the sick have always been decentralized and divided in the United States. Bureaus concerned with health have been and still are scattered through many departments of the United States government in contrast to the centralized ministry of health found in many national governments. State health departments have set up regulations and established standards but have left the county or city health department free to provide service to the individual without much interference as to kind, quantity, and quality. In general, the services of the public health (tax-supported) agencies have been educational or of a nature designed to protect the citizenry from dangers in the environment. This has been interpreted to include hospitalization of persons with communicable and chronic diseases and mental illness. Tax-supported care has grown to include (in principle) all kinds of medical care for American Indians, Alaska natives, migrant workers, military and government personnel, and war veterans. Although in the past the government has been slow to develop ways to deliver health services, it has begun now to include such activities as health planning, health maintenance organization services, preparation of health manpower, and health research. In addition, the government has studied or fostered certain developments such as neighborhood health centers, prepaid group medical practices, participation of the consumer in health care, and licensing of health personnel. Gradually the general medical care of the indigent has come to be included in the list of tax-supported services. In some states, facilities formerly used for tuberculosis patients have been converted to provide care for indigents with other diseases.

In contrast to these tax-supported "public health services," there are medical care and health promotion services for the major part of the population that have been, and still are, private, or voluntary. Private, or voluntary, health services are furnished by individual practitioners and by private or voluntary health agencies on a fee-for-service basis.

To sum up, the task of maintaining a healthy people is accepted by some countries as the responsibility of the central government, although the authority to deliver health service may be delegated to local units. The governments of other countries have not accepted this responsibility or may divide it among so many poorly coordinated departments that the effect is chaotic. In the United States the first big division of the task is between public (tax-supported) and private (voluntary) agencies. The functions of the two groups are not always clear-cut, but even when they are there is so much overlapping and so inadequate a system of getting the individual to the proper agency, or practitioner, that his or her need often goes unanswered.

The responsibility of the state for providing

an education for everyone has been accepted by the people of the United States, and every state has the machinery for providing it. Federal aid for education is advocated by some as a nationwide means of improving the quality of education; it is feared by others who believe that federal aid will mean interference with the right of the state to control its educational system. There is considerable evidence that the United States is moving toward the same concept of public responsibility for the health of the individual that has been assumed for education. Many persons believe that federal aid is necessary in order to provide adequate health services in certain areas. Whether or not it is universally acceptable, the federal government has played an increasingly important role in health promotion. The major proposals for a national health program are discussed in the following section.

Health Legislation. A vivid account of public health legislation in the 1960s is told by Richard Harris in *A Sacred Trust*.[85] In the early 1970s, the federal government had before its legislative committees a wide variety of *health insurance plans* that would substantially reorganize health care in the United States. There may have been as many as 30 plans written during this time. Many people believe that none of these plans offers the people full health protection. Unless the country adopts *a national health services system* that guarantees health care to every United States citizen regardless of age, geographic location, and economic or social status, there will be continuing citizen dissatisfaction.

The Health Policy Advisory Center (HEALTH PAC) in San Francisco, California, said in 1973, after analyzing the major health insurance proposals, "National health insurance, then, is not a massive popular movement for better health care. Nineteen seventy's-style national insurance is mainly the creation of large health businesses to insure their economic well-being. So profits can be expected to have a clear edge over service in deciding health care priorities," * George A. Silver is quoted by HEALTH PAC as saying, "those insured under a national health insurance act will be physicians and hospitals, not patients; that the guarantee will be of payment to the provider, not of service to the patient. . . ." †
HEALTH PAC adds that "As long as a small, underfinanced public system coexists with a large, wealthy private one, the private system will successfully compete for paying patients, doctors, money and power." *

Sidney R. Garfield,[86] one of the most active proponents of a reorganized health care delivery system, thinks the separation of sick people and well people is an essential aspect of reorganization. Because health insurance eliminates the fee barrier, Garfield says, such health systems get overloaded. He believes it is important, however, that well people seek health services so that they may be guided away from sick care to a meaningful preventive health care program. An innovative diagram of a new system was constructed by Garfield and is shown in Figure 2-7. It shows a *health-testing and referral center* separating the well and worried well from the sick and early sick and directing these four groups to the *health-care center* or the *sick-care center*, with both having access to a *preventive-maintenance service*. Both services and centers use a central computer service and people can be referred from one to the other. It may serve as a model for planners of health care in the future.

Madeleine Leininger, a nurse, has proposed a client-centered model of health care delivery that also recognizes the need to integrate a wellness-oriented system with an illness-oriented system (see Fig. 2-8). This model may also be useful for future health care planners.

Health Insurance Proposals. Almost everyone now believes that health insurance with universal coverage in the United States is a foregone conclusion. The main question is how it will be administered, what agency or agencies will control it, and whether it will meet the people's needs. Eveline M. Burns,[87] in a thoughtfully written article, questioned not the existence of health insurance but the *kind* of protection to be offered to citizens.

Table 2-11 summarizes selected health legislation affecting home/community health as of September 1975.

Although no one of these bills has been passed as of June 1, 1976, or these plans acted upon, most persons believe that the United States will adopt some form of universal health insurance in the near future comparable to the health insurance systems of the "developed" and some of the "undeveloped" countries. While each of these plans has its advocates, the Medical Committee for Human Rights questions the adequacy of each. While it has no counterproposal, some of its members have offered the following principles as those that should underlie any health care system in America:

---

* Health Policy Advisory Center: *Who Will Pay Your Bills? A HEALTH PAC Special Report on National Health Insurance.* The Center, San Francisco, 1973, p. 22.

† *Ibid.,* p. 23. [From Silver, George A.: "Insurance Is Not Enough," *Nation,* (June 8) 1970, p. 680.]

* *Ibid.,* p. 24.

1. All Americans are equally entitled to complete and preventive health care, with no charge at the time of service. Health services should be easily accessible in every community.
2. Health care should be paid for by a progressive national tax on total wealth—a tax without loopholes that makes the very rich pay their share.
3. No one should gain profit from the sickness, misery, and death of others. There should be an end to profit-making in health care.
4. Health care institutions should be locally con-

trolled by representatives of patients and health workers.
5. Race and sex discrimination should be ended for health workers. Minorities, women, and the poor should be justly represented in all health jobs.*

* Medical Committee for Human Rights, San Francisco Bay Area Chapter: *Billions for Band-Aids. An Analysis of the U.S. Health Care System and of Proposals For its Reform.* The Chapter, San Francisco, 1972, p. 118.

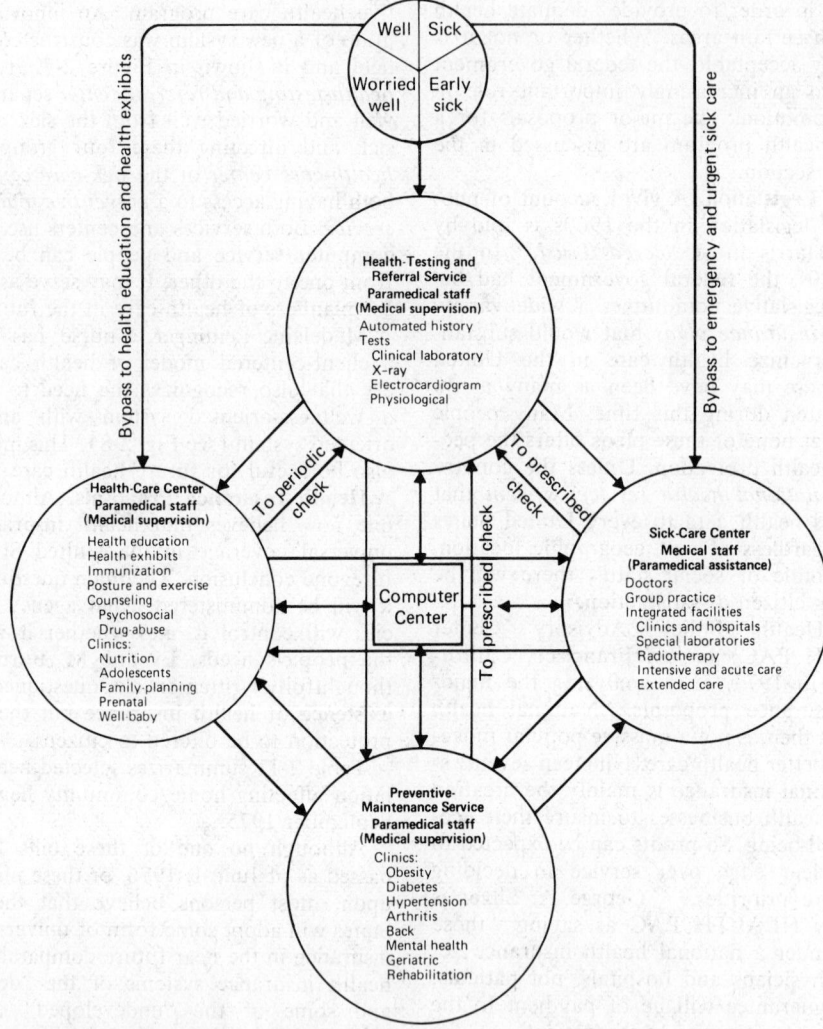

Figure 2-7. New delivery system proposed by Sidney R. Garfield would separate the sick from the well by establishing a new method of entry, the health-testing service, to perform the regulating function that has been performed, more crudely, by the fee for service. After testing the patient would be referred for sick care, health care, or preventive maintenance as required and would be transferred among the services as his condition changed. The computer center would regulate the flow of patients and information among the units, coordinating the entire system, which would depend heavily on paramedical personnel to save doctors' time. (From Garfield, Sidney R.: "The Delivery of Medical Care," *Sci. Am.,* **222:**22, [Apr.] 1970.)

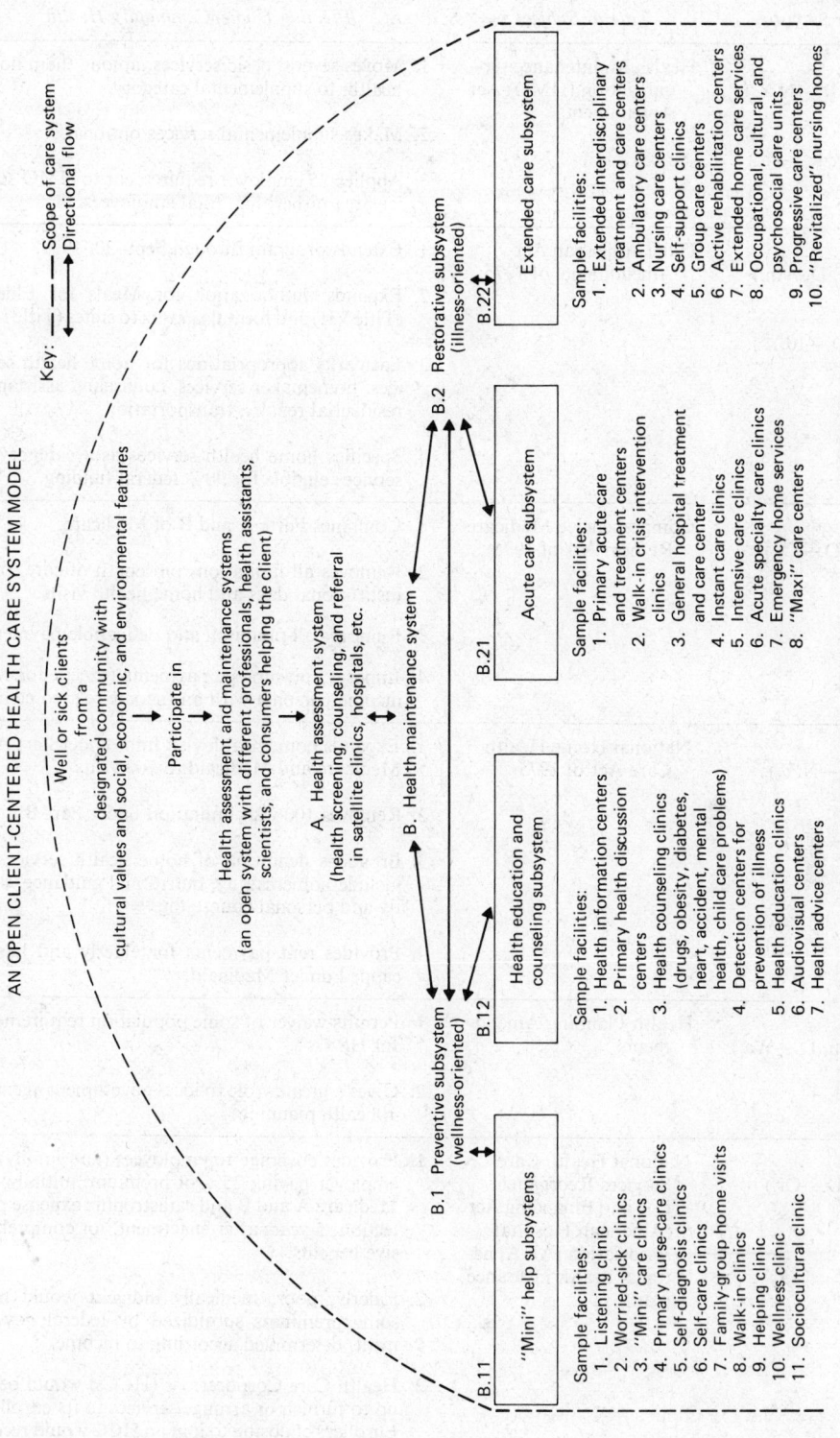

Figure 2-8. A proposed model to allow clients various entry and exit routes to and from the health care system. (From Leininger, Madeleine: "An Open Health Care System Model," *Nurs. Outlook,* **21**:171, [Mar.] 1973.)

The figure contains the following text:

AN OPEN CLIENT-CENTERED HEALTH CARE SYSTEM MODEL

Key:
———— Scope of care system
- - - - Directional flow

Well or sick clients
from a
designated community with
cultural values and social, economic, and environmental features

Participate in

Health assessment and maintenance systems
(an open system with different professionals, health assistants,
scientists, and consumers helping the client)

A. Health assessment system
(health screening, counseling, and referral
in satellite clinics, hospitals, etc.)

B. Health maintenance system

Preventive subsystem
(wellness-oriented)

Restorative subsystem
(illness-oriented)

B.1

B.2

B.11

B.12

B.21

B.22

"Mini" help subsystems

Sample facilities:
1. Listening clinic
2. Worried-sick clinics
3. "Mini" care clinics
4. Primary nurse-care clinics
5. Self-diagnosis clinics
6. Self-care clinics
7. Family-group home visits
8. Walk-in clinics
9. Helping clinic
10. Wellness clinic
11. Sociocultural clinic

Health education and
counseling subsystem

Sample facilities:
1. Health information centers
2. Primary health discussion centers
3. Health counseling clinics (drugs, obesity, diabetes, heart, accident, mental health, child care problems)
4. Detection centers for prevention of illness
5. Health education clinics
6. Audiovisual centers
7. Health advice centers

Acute care subsystem

Sample facilities:
1. Primary acute care and treatment centers
2. Walk-in crisis intervention clinics
3. General hospital treatment and care center
4. Instant care clinics
5. Intensive care clinics
6. Acute specialty care clinics
7. Emergency home services
8. "Maxi" care centers

Extended care subsystem

Sample facilities:
1. Extended interdisciplinary treatment and care centers
2. Ambulatory care centers
3. Nursing care centers
4. Self-support clinics
5. Group care centers
6. Active rehabilitation centers
7. Extended home care services
8. Occupational, cultural, and psychosocial care units
9. Progressive care centers
10. "Revitalized" nursing homes

Table 2-11. Overview of Selected Legislation as of September 26, 1975 *

Bill Number and Major Sponsor	Title or Subject	Major Provisions Affecting Home/Community Health
H.R. 9019 (Hastings, R.—N.Y.) S. 1926 (Schweiker, R.—Pa.)	Health Maintenance Organization (HMO) Act Amendments	1. Moves several basic services, among them home health, to supplemental category. 2. Makes supplemental services optional. 3. Applies 25 employee requirement to HMO service area rather than total employees.
H.R. 3922 (Brademas, D.—In.) S. 1426 (Church, D.—Id.)	Older American Act Amendments of 1975	1. Extends program through Sept. 30, 1979. 2. Expands authorization for Meals for Elderly (Title VII) and formula grants to states (Title III). 3. Earmarks appropriations for home health services, homemaker services, counseling assistance, residential repairs, transportation. 4. Specifies home health services as a category of services eligible for 90% federal funding.
S. 1456 (Ribicoff, D.—Ct.)	Comprehensive Medicare Reform Act of 1975	1. Combines Parts A and B of Medicare. 2. Removes all limitations on length of care, both institutional days and home health visits. 3. Removes all premium and deductible payments. 4. Imposes coinsurance payments (except for low-income persons) with an income-related ceiling.
H.R. 4772 (Koch, D.—N.Y.) S. 1163 (Moss, D.—Ut.)	National Home Health Care Act of 1975	1. Expands home health visit limit under Part A of Medicare and Medicaid to 200 visits. 2. Removes 100 visit limitation under Part B. 3. Broadens definition of home health services to include homemaking, nutritional guidance, family and personal counseling. 4. Provides rent payments for elderly and handicapped under Medicaid.
S. 1905 (Magnuson, D.—Wa.)	Health Planning Amendments	1. Permits waiver of some population requirements for HSAs. 2. Gives a greater role to local government agencies in health planning.
H.R. 1 (Ullman, D.—Or.)	National Health Care Services Reorganization and Financing Act (American Hospital Association [AHA] national health insurance plan)	1. Provides coverage to employees (and family) by employer paying 75% of premium: initially, for Medicare A and B and catastrophic expense protection; 5 years after enactment, for comprehensive benefits. 2. Elderly, poor, medically indigent would have some premiums subsidized by federal government, determined according to income. 3. Health Care Corporations (HCCs) would be set up to furnish or arrange services to its enrollees. Enrollees choosing to join an HCC would receive a 10% federal subsidy of premium but would pay a capitation rate.

Table 2-11   (Continued)

Bill Number and Major Sponsor	Title or Subject	Major Provisions Affecting Home/Community Health
		4. Home health care services limited to 200 days in any benefit period and defined to include three levels of care: intensive, intermediate and basic. Each visit would have a $2.00 copayment.
		5. Health Cards would be issued to each covered person; any copayment, deductible, or cost sharing would be settled between patient and carrier, rather than provider.
		6. Home health care programs eligible for grants, loans, and loan guarantees during implementation phase of the program.
H.R. 21 (Corman, D.—Ca.) S. 3 (Kennedy, D.—Ma.)	Health Security Act (Committee on National Health Insurance plan)	1. Financed by employer payroll taxes (3.5%), 1% tax on employee wages, self-employed income taxes (2.5%), and contributions from federal general revenues equal to total amount collected through above listed taxes.
		2. Entire population would be covered; Medicare would be terminated and all other federal programs, such as Medicaid, vocational rehabilitation, maternal and child health would cease except if benefits of such programs are broader than Health Security.
		3. All providers would be compensated directly by the program; no private health insurance organizations would be used.
		4. Unlimited home health visits.
		5. Requires that after 2 years of enactment, a home health agency will be a qualified provider only if it has an affiliation agreement with a participating hospital or group practice organization under which the medical staff of the hospital or organization will assume responsibility for the professional services furnished by the home health agency.
		6. Provides grants to home health agencies to test feasibility of home maintenance care for chronically ill or disabled.
H.R. 5990 (Burleson, D.—Tx.) S. 1438 (McIntyre, D.—N.H.)	National Health Care Act (Health Insurance Association of America [HIAA] national health insurance plan)	1. Voluntary health insurance under three programs all with same benefits: employer-employee plans (sharing cost of premiums); individual plans (full cost of premium tax deductible); poor and uninsurable (state would pay premium).
		2. 270 home health agency services per year.
		3. 20% copayment rate: some deductible. Total of copayment and deductible would have a maximum per year.
		4. Financed entirely by premiums except for poor and uninsurable which would be shared by state and federal government (federal share to be between 70 and 90%).

Table 2-11   (Continued)

Bill Number and Major Sponsor	Title or Subject	Major Provisions Affecting Home/Community Health
H.R. 6222 (Fulton, D.—Tn.)	Comprehensive Health Care Insurance Act of 1975 (American Medical Association [AMA] national health insurance plan)	1. Coverage provided through private insurance under programs for the employed, nonemployed, and others: Employers required to furnish coverage to employees and families; employee participation elective (employer pays 65% of premium); nonemployed and self-employed eligible for federal contribution to cost of protection depending on income (100% for poor and between 10 and 99% for others). 2. Elderly continue with Medicare plus can purchase supplemental coverage to bring protection up to benefit level of under 65 population. 3. Unlimited home health services subject to 20% coinsurance. The coinsurance is applicable only up to $500 worth of such services.

* Courtesy of Council of Home Health Agencies and Community Health Services, National League for Nursing, New York City.

These principles have the endorsement of the Health Policy Advisory Center in Washington, an agency that also questions the value to the public of any proposed legislation to date (see page 152).

Historical Events in the Growth of Health Services in the United States. A brief listing of events since the turn of the century shows that the United States has moved toward (1) concentration of health functions in one federal department; (2) extension of the functions of federal, state, and local tax-supported health agencies; (3) interpretation of the function of the tax-supported agency as that of promoting the health of the individual by all types of service; (4) districting of the nation into regional health units; (5) coordination of the work of all health agencies, public and private, by national, state, district, and local health councils; and (6) distribution of the cost of medical care by a system of insurance.

It is not practicable to do more than list some of the following historical events in this book.* Nurses will find it profitable to study

* It might be noted, however, that it is difficult for texts to reflect the most recent change in thought and practice. William H. Stewart says, "While public health textbooks abound on the subject of public health administration their content is built around the older classical model of public health. The conventional wisdom of the management of a structure of health services in an efficient and economical manner has not been developed. It is still emerging. . . . It hasn't arrived at that stage of consensus . . . to allow it to be captured in textbooks." (Stewart, William H.: "Preventive Medicine in the United States," in The Royal Society of Medicine and the Josiah Macy, Jr. Foundation: *The Greater Medical Profession*. The Foundation, New York, 1973, p. 128.)

them through the writings of such authorities as George Rosen,[88] John J. Hanlon,[89] Edwin D. Kilbourne, and Wilson G. Smillie,[90] and I. S. Falk.[91]

1909   Report to President Theodore Roosevelt by the National Conservation Commission on National Vitality: Its Waste and Conservation.
First White House Conference on Children and Youth held.

1912   Public Health and Marine Hospital Service became United States Public Health Service.
Children's Bureau signed into law by President William H. Taft.

1921   Formation of the National Health Council with the objective of coordinating the activities of the member agencies, official (public) and voluntary (private).
First continuing program of federal grants-in-aid to state health agencies for direct services to individuals established by the Maternity and Infancy (Sheppard-Towner) Act of 1921.

1930   White House Conference on Child Health and Protection called by President Herbert Hoover.

1933   Publication of *Costs of Medical Care*—a study made by I. S. Falk under the auspices of the American Medical Association and other national health agencies that showed adequate medical care was not universally available, nor was it economically possible for a large proportion of the population. This gave impetus to the development of sickness insurance.

1935   Report to President Franklin D. Roosevelt by the Committee on Economic Security, including recommendations on health and welfare, that served as a basis for the *Social Security Act* adopted by Congress in this same year. The bill provided for assistance to the aged, the unemployed, the blind, and the crippled, and for grants-in-aid to improve maternal and child care. It also extended public health services and provided for increase in trained health personnel.

1935–1936   "The Health Survey"—the first of several periodic studies made by the US Public Health Service incorporating a house-to-house canvass of 3 million people in 19 states. On the basis of the data collected, the conclusion was reached that the incidence of illness was higher in low-income groups and that where the need was greatest the care was least adequate.

1938   The National Health Conference, held as an Interdepartmental Committee to coordinate health and welfare activities.

1939   Federal Security Agency established by President Franklin D. Roosevelt to bring together a large part of the health, welfare, and educational services of the federal government.

1940–1950   Expansion of voluntary health insurance plans purchased by the population.

1943   First proposal for compulsory national health insurance introduced by Senator Robert Wagner *et al.* Reintroduction of proposals throughout President Harry S. Truman's administration, all defeated by Congress.

1944   Public Health Service Act reorganized the US Public Health Service and expanded biomedical research through several Institutes.

1946   Hospital Survey and Construction Act (Hill-Burton) program helped develop patterns for national health activities utilizing local initiative, state review, and federal sharing in support.

1946–1948   Creation of a World Health Organization by the United Nations of which the United States became a member in 1948.

1949   First Hoover Commission recognized a need for coordination of various federal programs. The Housing Act, passed by Congress, established a long-range federal program for slum clearance, urban development, and low-rent housing.

1950   Mid-Century White House Conference on Children and Youth widened support for child health and welfare programs. National Conference on Aging highlighted needs of the elderly.

1953   Establishment of the Department of Health, Education, and Welfare (DHEW) coordinated the activities of many federal health agencies in one department.

1945–1960   Rapid growth in federal support for biomedical research and establishment of many Institutes of the National Institutes of Health (NIH) in Washington.

1960   Kerr-Mills Act passed to provide medical assistance to the needy. (Later to be incorporated into the Medicare-Medicaid legislation of 1965.) A series of Public Laws on health were passed in the 1960s, a decade of unprecedented health legislation.

1961–1962   Legislation passed to promote accident prevention, vaccination assistance, aid to migrant workers, and community health services.

1962   Department of Labor health-manpower expansion program for training semiskilled and paraprofessionals.

1963   Mental Retardation Facilities and Community Mental Health Construction Act of 1963 (Public Law 88–164).* Health Professions Educational Assistance Act of 1963 (88–129). Clean Air Act (88–206).

1964   Graduate Public Health Training Amendments of 1964 (88–497). Nurse Training Act of 1964 (88–581). Child Abuse Prevention and Treatment Act of 1964. Hospital and Medical Facilities Amendment of 1964 (88–443). Civil Rights Act of 1964. Office of Economic Opportunity (OEO) established.

1965   Social Security Amendments of 1965 (89–97). Title 18 (Medicare) provided medical insurance for persons over 65 years. Title 19 (Medicaid) provided medical insurance to the needy under 65 years. Child Health and Welfare Amendments provided programs for

* Legislation passed by the US Congress is identified by a Public Law number, the first number indicating the session of Congress in which the bill became law and the second being an identifying number assigned to it.

maternal and child health, crippled children, child welfare, and the mentally retarded, and special project grants for preschool and school child health services, and for neighborhood health centers.

Drug Abuse Control Amendments of 1965 (89–74).

Heart Disease, Cancer, and Stroke Amendments of 1965 (89–239) provided an opportunity for regionalization of medical programs and research.

Vocational Rehabilitation Act Amendments of 1965 (89–333).

Community Health Services Extension Amendments of 1965 (89–109).

Mental Retardation Facilities and Community Mental Health Centers Construction Act Amendments of 1965 (89–105).

Appalachian Regional Development Act of 1965 (89–4).

Federal Cigarette Labelling and Advertising Act (89–92).

Air Pollution and Solid Waste Disposal Act (89–272).

Medical Library Assistance Act (89–291).

Older Americans Act of 1965.

Water Quality Act (89–234).

1966   Allied Health Professional Personnel Training Act of 1966 (89–751).

Comprehensive Health Planning and Public Health Services Amendments of 1966 (89–749). This law expanded the capabilities of local areas to plan, develop, and provide public health services.

National School Lunch and Child Nutrition Act of 1966.

Narcotic Rehabilitation Act of 1966 (89–793).

Demonstration Cities and Metropolitan Development Act of 1966 (89–754).

1967   Partnership for Health Amendments of 1967 (90–174).

Child Health Act increased the availability of family planning services.

Air Quality Act (90–148).

1968   Health Manpower Act of 1968 (90–490).

1969   White House Conference on Food, Nutrition, and Health.

1970   Amendment to the Public Health Service Act (91–519) required a report identifying the problems and making recommendations for licensure and certification of health personnel.

Seventh White House Conference on Children.

Comprehensive Alcohol Abuse and Alcoholism Prevention, Treatment, and Rehabilitation Act of 1970.

Comprehensive Drug Abuse Prevention and Control Act (91–513).

Health Training Improvement Act (91–519).

Heart Disease, Cancer, Stroke, and Kidney Disease Amendments (91–515).

Emergency Health Personnel Act of 1970.

Occupational Safety and Health Act of 1970.

Mental Retardation Facilities (91–517) and Mental Health Centers (91–211).

1971–1976   National Health Insurance proposals debated in Congress.

1971   Nurse Training Act of 1971.

Comprehensive Health Manpower Training Act of 1971 (92–157).

White House Conference on Aging.

National Cancer Act of 1971 (92–218).

National Health Service Corps established.

Drug Listing Act of 1971 (92–387).

1972   Social Security Amendments of 1972 ordered the creation of Professional Standards Review Organizations (PSRO) for the review of medical care provided to Medicare and Medicaid recipients (92–603).

Commission on Marijuana and Drug Abuse Act (92–13).

Nutrition Program for Aged (92–258).

Action Office for Drug Abuse and Prevention Act (92–255).

Communicable Diseases Control Act (92–449).

National Sickle-Cell Anemia Prevention Act (92–294).

Cooley's Anemia Control Act (92–414).

A National Institute of Arthritis, Metabolism, and Digestive Disease established within the National Institutes of Health.

Maternal and Child Health Projects extended.

1973   Reorganization of the Department of Health, Education, and Welfare concentrated public health services in six agencies: Alcohol, Drug Abuse, and Mental Health Administration, Center for Disease Control, Food and Drug Administration, Health Resources Administration, Health Services Administration, and the National Institutes of Health.

Health Maintenance Organization Act of 1973 (93–222).

Emergency Medical Services Systems Act of 1973.

Veterans Health Care Expansion Act of 1973.

1974 National Health Planning and Resources Development Act of 1974 (93–641). This law provided for the development of a network of Health Systems Agencies responsible for health planning and development in designated health service areas (HSA).

Nurse Training Act of 1974.

National Center on Child Abuse and Neglect established within DHEW.

Narcotic Addict Treatment Act of 1974.

Comprehensive Alcohol Abuse and Alcoholism Prevention, Treatment, and Rehabilitation Amendments of 1974.

National Institute on Aging established within the National Institutes of Health. Research on Aging (93–296).

1975 Special Health Revenue Sharing Act of 1975. Extended family planning, community mental health centers, migrant health, community health centers, National Health Service Corps, nurse training, and other health services.

Education for All Handicapped Children Act (94–142).

1976 Swine Flu Immunization (94–266).

Medical Device Safety Act (94–295).

National Health Promotion and Disease Prevention Act (94–317).

Health Professions Educational Assistance Act (94–484) amended the Nurse Training Act to provide funds for nurse practitioners who return to their home areas of shortage to practice.

Indian Health Care (94–437) improved and expanded federal health programs for Indians.

HEW Inspector General (94–505) to coordinate investigations of fraud and abuse in Medicare and Medicaid programs.

Veterans Omnibus Health Care Act (94–581).

Obviously, what has been accomplished so far would not have been possible without the *organized* efforts of medical and nonmedical workers. The fall in the nation's death rate is an example, it is to be emphasized, of the co-operation of doctors, nurses, allied health workers, sanitarians, laboratory technicians, legislators, public health officials, and citizens. The control of disease, too, is a result of the cooperative efforts of many individuals, especially those farsighted legislators who have provided the means to combat these conditions that plague mankind. Much depends on, or will depend on, the extent to which the resources for combatting disease are organized and the degree to which cooperation exists among the various groups of health workers.

In 1965 the National Commission on Community Health Services,[92] in its report *Health is a Community Affair,* outlined a number of recommendations for communities to follow to achieve a better balance between what is known scientifically about health care and what is done to prevent the hazards that threaten man. The positions taken by the Commission relate to such areas as (1) the delivery of health services across political jurisdictions, (2) comprehensive personal health services, (3) the changing role of the personal physician, (4) comprehensive environmental health services, (5) control of man's environment, (6) accident prevention, (7) family planning, (8) urban design and health, (9) education, (10) health manpower, (11) hospital care, (12) organization and administration of official agencies, (13) voluntary citizen participation, and (14) action-planning for community health services.

In spite of the opposition that persists in some quarters to so-called socialized medicine, the functions of official health organizations—that is, tax-supported agencies—are constantly enlarging and the volume of work is increasing. A system of disease control that leaves everything to private enterprise has never adequately protected the health of either the privileged or underprivileged. Private or voluntary institutions and individual workers are learning to value cooperation with public agencies more highly.

Communities have organized health councils whose functions are to collect and apportion funds for the support of the voluntary agencies represented, and to study the needs of the community, the facilities, and the activities of the various public and voluntary agencies and how they might be coordinated. Such a study serves as a basis for planning more adequate and less wasteful health service. In many places there is unnecessary duplication of effort in some directions and uncared-for needs in others. The most satisfactory type of community health organization is one in which there is some central control and direction, so that all agencies, public and private, are working together. Even in countries where government-funded health services are available to all residents and the coordination of the work of public and private agencies is a minor problem, local health councils are still useful. It will always be ultimately the public's responsibility to see that its health needs are met.

The Nurse's Role. Jessie M. Scott,[93] in a 1973 report of a conference, said that nursing must confront the issue of what kind of nursing system should be developed to fit into the health care delivery system of the future. She said that the federal government has maintained a special role in helping nursing find its new place by supporting research in expansion of nursing practice and education.

Nurses as citizens and nursing organizations have tended to play a passive role in the development of health programs, national, state, or local. They have been followers rather than leaders with some notable exceptions, as, for example, Florence Nightingale, Annie W. Goodrich, and Lillian Wald. Most persons attribute this passive role to the fact that nursing has been a woman's occupation or that nurses have not been prepared on a professional level or that nursing is an emerging rather than an established profession.

Frances Storlie,[94] in *Nursing and the Social Conscience,* asks nurses to examine their purpose and their profession. She thinks they can play an effective role in determining the direction for health programs and makes the following statement:

Nursing moves slowly. Nursing is a mature profession. Maturity is to be valued so long as it is not used as a shield to keep from making crucial decisions. It is possible for one to weigh the issues so long, that he forgets what the issues are. Now is the time for the nursing profession to proclaim a stand on issues, on legislation, on inequality of economics and health care.*

On the occasion of the seventy-fifth anniversary of the *American Journal of Nursing,* a roundtable discussion [95] by notable nursing leaders was held and reported on in a special anniversary issue. The discussants confronted a wide range of important issues in nursing and faced many controversial questions of concern to nurses. They seemed, however, not to emphasize enough the need for a unified health system in this country. It is the opinion of the authors that more discussion should focus on the experience of other countries of the world, on the limitations or disadvantages of the fee-for-service system, on the importance of reducing the different types of health workers and of personalizing care, on the fostering of the self-help movement that puts more respon-

sibility on individuals, on the universal provision of essential health services, and on the reversal of the spiraling cost of care.

Nurses who hope to take an intelligent part in the community health program should know and be able to use the existing machinery for health promotion. They should be able to promote the establishment of, and work in, community health agencies. It is part of their professional obligation to be informed about the health needs of the community and to further legislation which they believe will help supply these needs.

Further discussion of the nurse's role in health programs is presented in Chapter 3.

In summary, this section has presented data on the organization of health care and health programs worldwide and has contrasted the British and other health systems with the fragmented or "no-system" in the United States. Our responsibilities in this country for health care through health legislation and health insurance programs were pointed out, and a chronological listing of historical events in the growth of health services in this country was presented. The importance of nurses' participation in all facets of health care was emphasized. The next section includes information on the organization of international health agencies and of those in the United States on national, state, and local levels.

5. INTERNATIONAL AGENCIES; NATIONAL, STATE, AND LOCAL HEALTH AGENCIES IN THE UNITED STATES

There are many books on public health or community health that give a full account of the origin, control, aims, and functions of the more important health agencies. Such detailed information goes beyond the scope of this book. The following is nothing more than a bird's-eye view of the subject, and may be supplemented by some of the texts listed at the end of the chapter. No attempt is made to discuss health agencies outside the United States.

John J. Hanlon [96] estimated that by 1974 there were approximately 100,000 separate categorical voluntary health or disease-related agencies in the United States, and in 1966 there were 1712 full-time official local health agencies of one type or another. On the state level, in addition to the state department of health, and also on a national level, there are many different kinds of health agencies.

Classifications of health agencies are based on (1) control, (2) scope or area served by the agency, (3) function or type of service ren-

---

* Storlie, Frances: *Nursing and the Social Conscience.* Appleton-Century-Crofts, New York, 1970, p. x.

dered, and (4) the class of persons served. Control depends upon the source from which the organization receives its support, and, since this is such an important factor in determining both scope and function, agencies are usually classified according to whether they are (1) public or official, that is, supported by tax funds, or (2) voluntary or private, meaning that they are supported by private funds.

It would not be practical here to give a long list of categories of agencies according to their function or class of persons served as used in directories of social agencies. A classification of this kind includes headings such as family counseling, adoption and foster home care, rehabilitation, legal aid services, and housing authorities. The system of classification that places agencies under the group of persons served includes such headings as senior citizens' programs, veterans' medical services, and juvenile detention homes.

The following classification gives types of agencies according to the scope or area they serve, and their control:

Classification of Health and Welfare Agencies According to Scope and Control

A. International

1. PUBLIC OR OFFICIAL. Those supported by public funds from the national governments represented. *Example*—World Health Organization.
2. PRIVATE OR VOLUNTARY. Those supported by private funds * from sources such as membership fees and endowments, and engaged in activities that are international in their scope. *Examples*—International Council of Nurses, Rockefeller Foundation.

B. National

1. PUBLIC OR OFFICIAL. Those administered by appointees of the federal government and supported by funds from federal taxes, and engaged in activities that are national in their scope. Example—US Department of Health, Education, and Welfare (includes the US Public Health Service, the Social Security Administration, and others).
2. PRIVATE OR VOLUNTARY. Those supported by private funds from sources

such as membership fees and endowments, and engaged in activities that are national in their scope. *Examples*— American Nurses' Association, American Cancer Society.

C. State

1. PUBLIC OR OFFICIAL. Those administered by appointees of the state government represented, supported by funds from the state treasury, and engaged in activities that are statewide in their scope. *Examples*—North Carolina State Board of Health.
2. PRIVATE OR VOLUNTARY. Those supported by private funds from sources such as membership fees and endowments, and engaged in activities that are statewide in their scope. *Example*— Massachusetts Heart Association.

D. Local (County, Township, Municipal)

1. PUBLIC OR OFFICIAL. Those administered by appointees of county, township, or municipal governments, and engaged in activities affecting one of these local areas. *Example*—Allegheny County Health Department, Pennsylvania.
2. PRIVATE OR VOLUNTARY. Those supported by private funds from sources such as gifts, endowments, and membership or patients' fees, and engaged in activities affecting a county, town or city, or a section of one of these. *Example*—Visiting Nurse Service of New York.

Ernest L. Stebbins [97] dates the beginning of *international health organizations* from the efforts of the Egyptian Quarantine Board in 1831 to control the spread of plague in Europe. In 1851 the first formal International Health Council was held in Paris; this Health Council finally succeeded in establishing an International Office of Public Health in Paris in 1909. It continued to function until 1947, when it was absorbed by the World Health Organization.

In 1902, the International Sanitary Conference of American Republics met in Washington, D.C., to establish the International Sanitary Bureau, which became the Pan-American Sanitary Bureau in 1924 and later was to become a regional office of the Health Section of the League of Nations. Still later, this office was to become known as the Pan American Health Organization and now is a regional

---

* Public funds are in some cases allocated to private organizations when they perform some service that is recognized as a public responsibility. A good example of this is the payment of public funds to a private hospital that undertakes the care of public charges (welfare clients) in the community.

office of the World Health Organization, with headquarters in Washington, D.C.*

The work of the Health Section of the League of Nations and the health work of the United Nations Relief and Rehabilitation Administration (1943) were taken over by the World Health Organization, established in 1948 as a specialized agency of the United Nations.

The purposes of the World Health Organization are

1. To assist governments upon request in strengthening health services.
2. To promote improved standards of teaching and training in health, medical, and related professions.
3. To provide information, counsel, and assistance in the field of health.
4. To promote, in cooperation with other specialized agencies where necessary, the improvement of nutrition, housing, sanitation, recreation, economic or working conditions, and other aspects of environmental hygiene.
5. To promote cooperation among scientific and professional groups which contribute to the advancement of health.
6. To promote maternal and child health and welfare; to foster the ability to live harmoniously in a changing total environment.
7. To foster activities in the field of mental health, especially those affecting the harmony of human relations.
8. To promote and conduct research in the field of health.
9. To study and report, in cooperation with other specialized agencies where necessary, administrative and social techniques affecting public and medical care from preventive and curative points of view, including hospital services and social security.†

By 1972, there were 135 member states, making the World Health Organization the largest of the United Nations' specialized agencies.[98] The official budget was $132,665,000 in

* Headquarters of the parent World Health Organization is in Geneva, Switzerland. Its regional offices are in Washington, D.C., for the Americas, in Copenhagen for European countries, in Brazzaville for Africa, in Alexandria for the Eastern Mediterranean countries, in New Delhi for Southeast Asia, and in Manila for the Western Pacific member countries.

† Stebbins, Ernest L.: "International Health Organization," in Sartwell, Philip E. (ed.): *Maxcy-Rosenau Preventive Medicine and Public Health*, 9th ed. Appleton-Century-Crofts, New York, 1965, p. 1040.

1975,[99] financed largely by contributions from members; over half its resources were devoted to communicable disease control, environmental health, public health services, health protection and promotion, and education and training.[100] Willard L. Thorp[101] commented on the inadequacy of the funding for the many tasks of the agency. Because the organization is still developing and is very limited by its budget, it has concentrated its efforts on a few health problems in what might be called "trouble spots." Priority is given to malaria, tuberculosis, venereal disease, and yaws, and, recently, to smallpox eradication, to child and maternal health and nutritional programs, and to the improvement of environmental conditions in places where they are thought to be responsible for a "significant proportion of deaths." It is generally agreed that such programs can succeed only where there are funds and technical assistance provided.

National or federal health work in the United States has been carried on in a number of federal agencies under cabinet secretaries, administrators, or commissioners (see Fig. 2-9). In most countries there is a Ministry of Health just as there is a Ministry of the Treasury, of Agriculture, and of Commerce, from which all health work emanates. In the United States the National Health Board, established in the latter part of the last century as part of the plan to control a yellow fever epidemic, was an abortive attempt to centralize federal health work. It was not possible to accomplish much in the way of reorganization of health since the Board was discontinued in 1882. Transference of important health bureaus from other departments to the Federal Security Agency in 1939 and to the Department of Health, Education, and Welfare in 1953 was a successful effort to centralize federal health work, although it is still distributed among a dozen departments or divisions of the United States government, as can be seen in Figure 2-9. In Canada and Great Britain and many other countries, health care is organized around a central health ministry and board and every citizen is entitled to care provided by the government of that country.

The work of the Public Health Service is the most extensive and varied of any health agency in the United States government. Since World War II, the Veterans Administration's health

Figure 2-9. [OPPOSITE] Administrative plan of the chief federal agencies concerned with health and related programs, 1972–73. (Based on data from United States Government *Organization Manual, 1972–73*. Federal Register Office, National Archives and Records Service, General Services Administration, Washington, D.C., revised as of July 1972; and on reorganization plans released in July 1973 by US Department of Health, Education, and Welfare.)

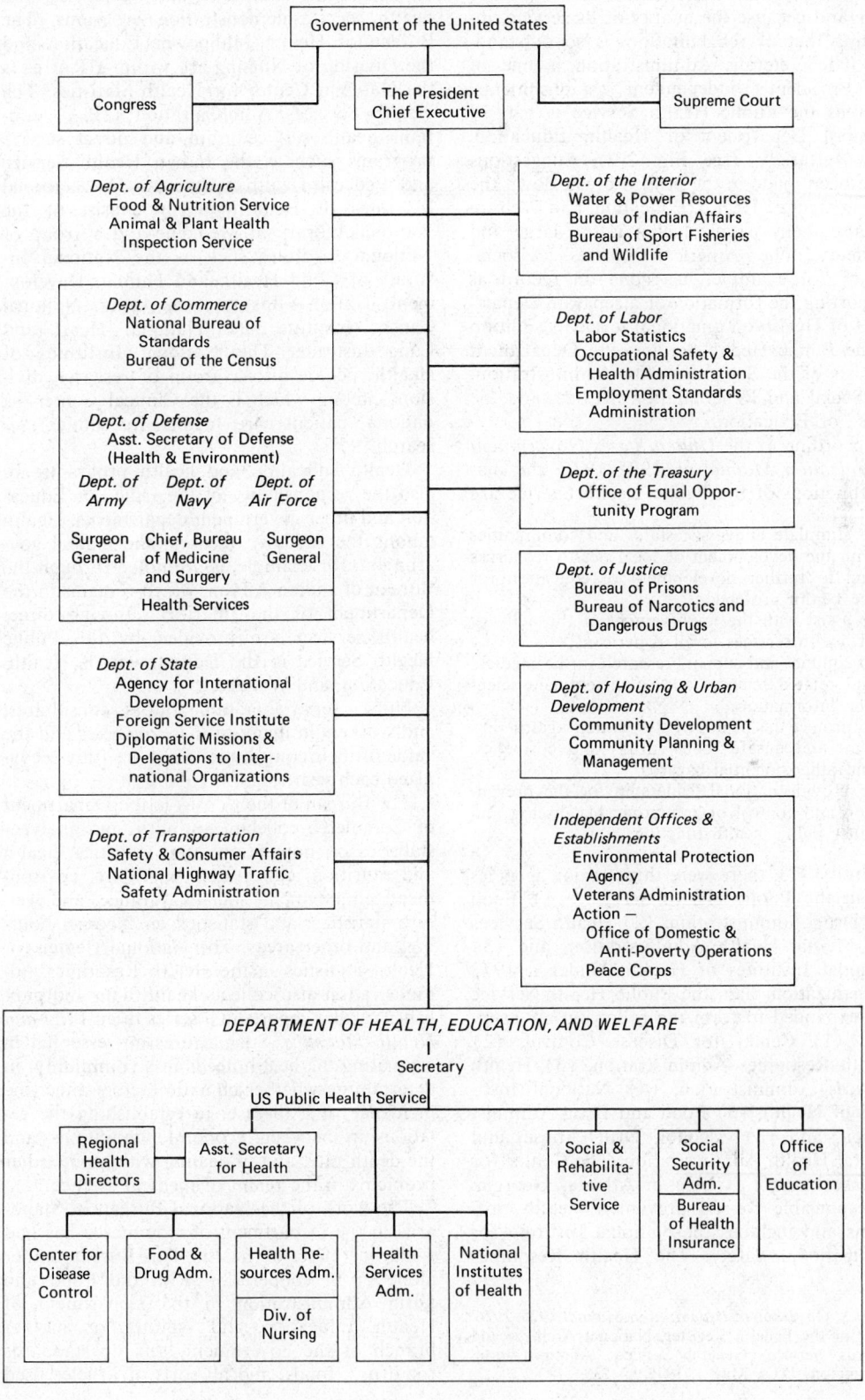

service has also assumed great importance because the number of veterans served is so large and because the quality of its service, including that of rehabilitation, is so outstanding. The Veterans Administration is one of the President's independent establishments, whereas the Public Health Service is part of the vast Department of Health, Education, and Welfare [102] (see Fig. 2-9). Suggestions have been made in the past to break down the Department of Health, Education, and Welfare because many people feel it is too large and unwieldy. The American Nurses' Association,[103] for example, has gone on record as supporting the formation of a separate Department of Health on a national level. In addition to the Public Health Service, the Department consists of the Social Security Administration, the Social and Rehabilitation Service, and the Office of Education.

According to the *United States Government Organization Manual* of 1975/1976, the major functions of the Public Health Service are

1. to stimulate and assist states and communities with the development of local health resources and to further development of education for the health professions;
2. to assist with the improvement of the delivery of health services to all Americans;
3. to conduct and support research in the medical and related sciences and to disseminate scientific information;
4. to protect the health of the Nation against impure and unsafe foods, drugs and cosmetics, and other potential hazards;
5. to provide national leadership for the prevention and control of communicable disease and other public health functions.*

Until 1973, there were three major agencies within the Public Health Service: (1) Food and Drug Administration, (2) Health Services and Mental Health Administration, and (3) National Institutes of Health. Under a 1973 reorganization plan, the Public Health Service was expanded to form the following six agencies: (1) Center for Disease Control, (2) Health Resources Administration, (3) Health Services Administration, (4) National Institutes of Health, (5) Food and Drug Administration, and (6) Alcohol, Drug Abuse, and Mental Health Administration. The Center for Disease Control (CDC) in Atlanta, Georgia, is responsible for all preventive health programs and includes the National Institute for Occupational Safety. The Health Resources

Administration (HRA) contains programs of data gathering and surveillance activities, and health service demonstration programs. The Bureau of Health Manpower Education and the Division of Nursing are within HRA, as is the National Center for Health Statistics. The Health Services Administration (HSA) contains health service grant and direct service programs such as the Indian Health Service and Federal Health Programs. The National Institutes of Health (NIH) consist of the National Library of Medicine and a group of National Institutes such as the National Institute of Child Health and Human Development, National Institute on Aging, National Cancer Institute, and National Heart and Lung Institute. The National Institutes of Health include also a group of research divisions among which is the Clinical Center—a national patient care facility for clinical research.[104,105]

Health education and health programs are also the responsibility of the Office of Education and other government departments. Health among the Indians, wards of the federal government, for example, is promoted through the Bureau of Indian Affairs, which remains in the Department of the Interior, although direct health services are provided by the Public Health Service in the Department of Health, Education, and Welfare.

Nurses serve as administrators, consultants, and workers in many of these agencies and the value of their contributions is more fully recognized each year.

The Bureau of the Census in the Department of Commerce collects, compiles, and analyzes statistics on population; vital statistics; health and nutrition, education, geography, environment, employment, social insurance, and welfare statistics; and statistics on income, housing, and other areas. The National Center for Health Statistics in the Health Resources Administration also collects health data and publishes regular reports in a series titled *Vital and Health Statistics*. Such figures are essential in estimating the health needs in a community, in determining whether climatic factors affect the incidence of a disease, in establishing the relationship between economic conditions and the death rate, and in dealing with many other problems in the realm of medical science.

The work of the National Bureau of Standards in the Department of Commerce has had a marked effect on health. This Bureau, either alone or in cooperation with the Food and Drug Administration in the Department of Health, Education, and Welfare, or another branch of the government, sets up standards for drugs, foods, and all sorts of articles used

---

* *U.S. Government Organization Manual 1975/1976.* Office of the Federal Register, National Archives and Records Service, General Services Administration, Washington, D.C., May 1, 1975, p. 235.

in hospitals, clinics, and the home care of the sick. "U.S.P." on a drug container means that the preparation is made according to the formula in the *United States Pharmacopoeia*.* When a manufacturer advertises a product as "made according to US government specifications," it is a recommendation of quality. The establishment of universally recognized standards is designed to protect the public from injurious or ineffective products and harmful pharmaceuticals.

Through the Departments of Agriculture and Interior, plant and animal diseases that affect man's health are studied and controlled so that the public may be protected, for example, from contaminated fish and dairy products. The Food and Nutrition Service of the Department of Agriculture carries on a program of instruction that helps raise health standards in the home and community.

A study of the functions of the federal health services shows that they are so organized as to allow the states freedom in planning and conducting their programs. The federal government provides medical care to certain of its personnel including those in the armed services, veterans, Indians, and other groups; it operates to prevent the spread of communicable disease from abroad and between states; it tests, publishes reports of, and controls the manufacture of biological products; and it also gathers statistics. Other portions of its program consist of allocating funds for research and demonstration projects, education of personnel and the public, environmental protection and safety programs, and social and health insurance programs, and furnishing technical assistance and consultation service to state health officials.

As has been noted, the federal government, working through state governments and agencies, is taking a more and more active part in the nation's health program, and most commentators believe the tempo of this trend will increase rapidly.

A *state health department* serves the people in that state largely by assisting the local health organizations. When a local organization (for example, a city or county health department) is not prepared to deal with the health problems in the community, the state department may send workers to help the local health officers or it may even take charge of the program. In certain instances, the Center for Disease Control may send specially qualified epidemiologists to an area where an outbreak of in-

fectious disease is a serious threat to the health of the community.

H. Denny Donnell, Jr.,[106] Director of the Bureau of Communicable Diseases in the Division of Health of Missouri, thinks that nurses, especially those in public health work, should think and act as independent professionals rather than waiting for orders in the case of an epidemic. He thinks that nurses should understand how to conduct investigations and know what kinds of procedures are involved in examining and tracking down a disease of public health concern, without specific guidance from a state or municipal epidemiologist.

The authority of the state usually is supreme, although the state may delegate considerable authority to a large local health department or it may bow to the authority of the national government. Lenor S. Goerke and Ernest L. Stebbins call attention to the relationship of a state government to the federal government with respect to control over health matters in the following statement:

The states have broad powers to organize their own government, to generate programs to meet social needs, and to raise revenues to support these programs. They also have the power to organize *local* governments and to authorize the levy of local taxes. The federal government intervenes in state activities when foods, drugs, and biologic products are sold in interstate commerce or when certain problems arise that are beyond the control of an individual state. A good example is the interstate pollution of common waterways by cities and industries. When cities and states pollute water or use an inequitable amount of any natural resources to the detriment or disadvantage of surrounding states, the federal government has the power to intervene for mutual protection of all population groups.*

A comparison of a state and a local health organization shows that they have approximately the same divisions or sections; for example, there is a division of public health nursing in the state and there is likewise a division, bureau, or department of public health nursing in the local health organization. The same is true of departments of maternal and child health, preventive medicine, environmental health, vital statistics, laboratory, and other aspects of health work. The administrative plans of all the 50 state health departments are not identical; however, many of them are similar to the Department of Health of the State of California, shown diagramatically in Figure 2-10, and some are very different.

---

* The *U.S. Pharmacopoeia* is published by the U.S.P. Convention, Inc., a private corporation that stands under the force of Congressional law.

* Goerke, Lenor S., and Stebbins, Ernest L.: *Mustard's Introduction to Public Health*, 5th ed. Macmillan Publishing Co., Inc., New York, 1968, p. 49.

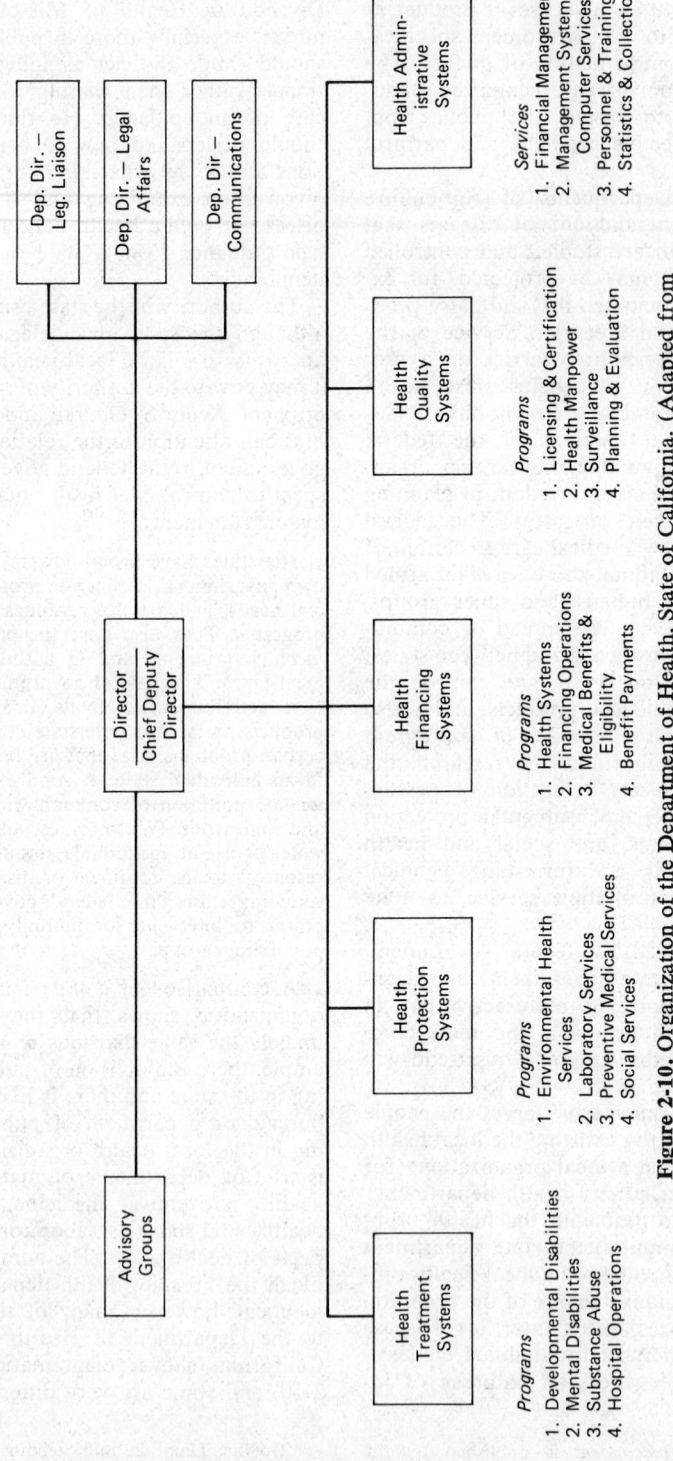

CALIFORNIA STATE DEPARTMENT OF HEALTH

Figure 2-10. Organization of the Department of Health, State of California. (Adapted from *Summary Organization Chart*, Department of Health, State of California, Sacramento, July 2, 1973.)

Dep. Dir. — Leg. Liaison

Dep. Dir. — Legal Affairs

Dep. Dir. — Communications

Director
Chief Deputy Director

Advisory Groups

Health Treatment Systems

Programs
1. Developmental Disabilities
2. Mental Disabilities
3. Substance Abuse
4. Hospital Operations

Health Protection Systems

Programs
1. Environmental Health Services
2. Laboratory Services
3. Preventive Medical Services
4. Social Services

Health Financing Systems

Programs
1. Health Systems
2. Financing Operations
3. Medical Benefits & Eligibility
4. Benefit Payments

Health Quality Systems

Programs
1. Licensing & Certification
2. Health Manpower
3. Surveillance
4. Planning & Evaluation

Health Administrative Systems

Services
1. Financial Management
2. Management Systems & Computer Services
3. Personnel & Training
4. Statistics & Collection

The official *local health organization* may be a county, a town, or a city health department. Its functions vary with the community and the funds available for health work. The efficiency of the organization and type of men and women appointed as officers and staff also affect the quantity and quality of health service given by this agency. Hanlon lists the following as fundamental *responsibilities* of a local health organization as recommended by the American Public Health Association: (1) to determine the health status and health needs of the people within its jurisdiction; (2) to determine the extent to which these needs are being met by effective measures currently available; and (3) to take steps to see that the unmet needs are satisfied." * A summary of Hanlon's necessary *functions* of a local health department follows:

1. Recording and analyzing health data— births, deaths, marriages, divorces, and notifiable diseases; maintaining registers of persons with long-term diseases and impairments; conducting surveys; collecting morbidity data from clinics, hospitals, industrial and other facilities; maintaining records on health personnel and health services; and evaluating community health needs and services.
2. Educating and informing—or stimulating the public to recognize health problems; cooperating with community organizations and groups in developing health programs; providing individual instruction in the care of well children, those with communicable disease, and those with chronic disease; organizing materials and resources for special classes and courses; using mass media for health education; and developing professional education programs.
3. Supervising and regulating—or protecting food, water, and milk supplies; controlling nuisances, disposing of waste in a sanitary way, controlling air and water pollution; preventing occupational diseases and accidents; controlling sources of infection; enforcing housing regulations; and inspecting and licensing health facilities.
4. Providing environmental health services (as necessary)—or constructing pit privies; treating mosquito-breeding areas; controlling rodents and insects.
5. Administering personal health services—or instituting immunization measures, advisory health maintenance service as in child health conferences, prenatal clinics, parents' classes, and public health nursing visits;

conducting case-finding surveys of the population; and providing diagnostic services to physicians and diagnostic and treatment services for specific diseases.
6. Operating health facilities—or engaging in those activities necessary for operating health centers, clinics, and hospitals.
7. Coordinating activities and resources—or providing effective leadership in recognizing and meeting health needs; encouraging agencies to avoid overlapping of activities, and participating on boards dealing with all phases of health care.

As mentioned several times in this chapter, the federal government has played an increasingly important role in health affairs. The major proposals for national health insurance for this country (described on page 152) suggest some of the future trends in public health. Many of the concepts in these proposals are designed to improve the administration of community health services. It will be necessary for knowledgeable health workers to shape the future of health care through careful planning for, and better distribution of, health services. The creation of effective programs, according to William L. McKissick,[108] requires an assessment of health problems, judgment on the effectiveness of the program in improving the population's health, and the realization of maximal health services from available resources so as to influence the consumer's health behavior and utilization of services.

Health Maintenance Organizations (HMOs) are considered by many persons to be the chief or primary mechanism for the delivery of health care and as such they merit particular attention. The Health Maintenance Organization Act of 1973 (93–222) provided monies for the establishment of such centers. Beverlee A. Myers describes the four elements of an HMO in the following terms:

1. An organized health delivery system, which includes health manpower and facilities capable of providing or at least arranging for all the health services a population might require.
2. An enrolled population, consisting of individual persons and groups who contract with the delivery system for provision of a range of health services which the system assumes responsibility to make available.
3. A financial plan which incorporates underwriting the costs of the agreed upon set of services on a prenegotiated and prepaid per person or per family basis.
4. A managing organization which assures legal, fiscal, public, and professional accountability.*

* Myers, Beverlee A.: "Health Maintenance Organizations: Objectives and Issues," *HSMHA Health Rep.*, **86**:585, (July) 1971.

* Hanlon, John J.: *op. cit.*, p. 295.

Community mental health programs, neighborhood health centers, and prepaid group practice plans all embrace some of these elements. The Kaiser-Permanente program in California and the Health Insurance Plan of Greater New York are two of the earliest programs to incorporate all of these elements. They are in effect Health Maintenance Organizations but not financed by public funds.

Community and regional health care delivery systems were given a boost through legislation passed in the 1960s for Heart Disease, Cancer, and Stroke (P.L. 89–239), Comprehensive Health Planning (P.L. 89–749) and the Partnership for Health Amendments (P.L. 90–174). Public Law 89–239 established 55 Regional Medical Programs (RMPs) that were directed first toward the control of cardiovascular disease and cancer but soon acquired a more general focus toward a variety of medical illnesses; their scope also varied from one geographical area to another. A "region" as described in the legislation creating Regional Medical Programs might be a state or several states or parts of several states and a regional program might be comprised of a few or many projects. They might concentrate on the improvement of inpatient or ambulatory services or the coordination of services; they might include educational projects, or the improvement of library services. These heavily funded programs produced a greater awareness of the need to merge the ideas of service and educational institutions in the planning process and to involve lay and professional persons in the "grass-roots" delivery of health care.[109-114] From the concept of RMPs came the National Health Planning and Resources Development Act of 1974 (P.L. 93–641). This law provided for the development of a network of Health Systems Agencies responsible for health planning and development in designated Health Service Areas (HSAs).

Another area of importance in the development of health projects is the emergence of *consumer participation*. The average consumer, according to Margaret C. Olendzki,[115] is a reasonable individual, slow to criticize his own health care but able to denounce physicians and hospitals in general, ready to accept more of a partnership role, not opposed to innovation, hopeful for some long-term solution to the complexities of health care, and possessing commonsense notions about health and medical care. Certainly consumers can be allies for nurses and nursing in the struggle for a better health care system. Nurses must learn from their patients and from citizens what they as recipients of care need to know in order to preserve their own and their families' health.[116]

Consumer participation became a viable issue in the creation of new health programs. G. M. Hochbaum says the growth of consumer participation in health planning and decision-making is not based so much on demonstrable and objective evidence as on its results. He also says the trend toward more lay involvement in health matters "could irrevocably change our health care and even our entire social system." * Reference has been made elsewhere to the importance Malleson [117] attaches to the self-help movement and to the development of self-reliance.

Programs of local health units are unequal in their extent and in the quality of service given. In many areas, especially in rural and sparsely settled areas, health organization is extremely poor. The American Public Health Association backs the recommendation of Hanlon [118] that a local health unit serve an area with a population of not less than 50,000 persons. The staff should include at least one full-time medical officer for 50,000 population, one sanitarian for 15,000 population, one staff nurse for 5000 population (2500 if bedside nursing is included), one administrative and teaching nurse for six to eight staff nurses, one office worker for 15,000 population, and other specialized personnel as problems demand and funds are available.

As improved health units are organized, health councils are formed to study and provide for the health needs of the district. All health agencies, including hospitals, are considered in the planning. There is a trend in the United States toward coordinating under one administration all public agencies, hospitals, clinics, and bureaus giving educational, preventive, and curative services.

As has been mentioned, recent federal and state appropriations have considerably extended most health services. Tax-supported health agencies have gradually taken over a great deal of what was formerly done by voluntary agencies. Nursing care of the sick in their homes is one of the few functions that is still almost entirely in the hands of private visiting nurse associations. With increasing change in public opinion on the government's responsibility for the protection of people's health, there is every reason to suppose that there will continue to be an increase in "socialized medicine" or the health service given by official agencies, which already has been extended to include home nursing by both official

---

* Hochbaum, G. M.: "Consumer Participation in Health Planning: Toward a Conceptual Clarification," *Am. J. Public Health,* **59:**1698, (Sept.) 1969.

and voluntary organizations, certified as "home health agencies."

Private, or Voluntary, Health Agencies. Because of the growing confusion and complexity of services provided by voluntary agencies, the National Health Council * in 1962 issued a statement called *Voluntaryism and Health*.[119] In it the Board of Directors defined national voluntary health agencies as (1) composed of both lay and professional persons; (2) organized voluntarily and democratically on a national basis with the primary purpose of combatting a particular disease, disability, or group of these; (3) supported by the public's voluntary contributions; and (4) engaged in research, education, and service to individuals and communities in their particular area of interest.

Voluntary health agencies are more properly designed to perform the services not supplied by official agencies. Until recently they have offered the major share of the person-to-person health service in this country. It is not so easy to say this now, however, with the extension of service in recent years by official agencies. While the services of public agencies have expanded, voluntary agencies have proliferated phenomenally. As noted earlier in this section, Hanlon [120] estimates that there are now about 100,000 voluntary health agencies in the United States and that they draw their support from and serve literally millions of persons. The difficulties growing out of such rapid expansion were recognized early. In 1913 a committee was formed to study functions and relationships of agencies. This led to the development in 1921 of a permanent coordinating organization, the National Health Council.

In a comprehensive study in 1945 of voluntary health agencies in the United States by Selskar M. Gunn and Philip S. Platt,[121] the authors recommended that each community establish *one* unified central voluntary health agency with a board and an executive director to supervise the work of special divisions such as tuberculosis, mental health, and others. The tendency of interested persons to form a health agency for the control of one disease, or *cause*, resulted in a duplication of effort in fund raising, administration, and actual service to the public. The Gunn and Platt recommendation was in line with the emphasis on the treatment of a person, and complete health service to a family, in contrast to the treatment of a disease. Some health and welfare agencies are very successful in providing a total centralized health, recreational, and welfare service to families, but others lag behind.

Gunn and Platt in 1945 listed eight basic functions of voluntary health agencies:

1. Exploring or surveying, in search of needs not being served and new methods of meeting recognized needs.
2. Demonstrating practical methods for improving the public health, and for their wider application by official or other agencies.
3. Educating in a broad sense, in which all agencies engage more or less energetically and effectively.
4. Supplementing health departments with personnel or facilities not yet available through public funds.
5. Serving as guardians of citizen interest in maintaining the effectiveness of health departments.
6. Guarding and advancing legislation bearing on health.
7. Coordinating efforts with those of other agencies and groups having related purposes.
8. Developing well-rounded community health programs.*

An Ad Hoc Committee on voluntary health and welfare agencies in the United States, directed by Robert H. Hamlin, studied these agencies in 1961. The Committee thought that resolution of the problems of voluntary agencies would come about through the following changes:

1. Stronger voluntary agency leadership.
2. Higher standards for local affiliates.
3. Increased participation in organized planning.
4. Better reporting of programs and accomplishments.
5. Greater emphasis on research and the application of new knowledge.†

Two major recommendations of this Committee were (1) to appoint a National Commission on Voluntary Health and Welfare Agencies and (2) to develop uniform accounting and financial reporting for voluntary agencies.[122] Some progress has been made in achieving the latter recommendation.

It is clear that public and private health agencies often give the same kind of service. The scope of each is a controversial question which cannot be discussed here in any detail, but today the services provided by voluntary agencies in the United States are indispensable.

Like official agencies, voluntary agencies are classified according to the area served, as inter-

---

* The National Health Council is a national coordinating body for voluntary health agencies; official agencies may work in the Council in an advisory capacity.

* Gunn, Selskar M., and Platt, Philip S.: *Voluntary Health Agencies*. Ronald Press, New York, 1945, p. 55.
† Hamlin, Robert H.: *Voluntary Health and Welfare Agencies in the United States*. Schoolmasters' Press, New York, 1961, p. 50.

national, national, state, and local, and may be grouped in various ways according to their degree of specialization, scope of services, or persons served. Some agencies are concerned with specific diseases, as, for example, the American Diabetes Association; some with a specific organ or structure of the body, as, for instance, the American Lung Association; some with a special group of persons, as the Easter Seal Society for Crippled Children and Adults; and others with a particular phase of health care, as the Planned Parenthood—World Population.

Large foundations represent another type of voluntary agency that may be partially or exclusively concerned with health programs. They are financed by private philanthropy. Examples are the W. K. Kellogg Foundation, the Milbank Memorial Fund, and the Robert Wood Johnson Foundation. Other voluntary agencies concerned with health care are associations of health workers such as the American Medical Association and the American Nurses' Association.* Other groups engaged in health work are integrating agencies such as United Funds, Community Chests and Councils, and Health Councils. Increasingly, commercial firms—drug companies, life insurance companies, manufacturers of baby products—engage in health activities, but since their primary goal is monetary profit the products and services they offer must be carefully evaluated for scientific merit and benefit to the human being before they are used.

National voluntary agencies may join forces to form an *international organization*. The International Council of Nurses and the World Federation of Neurological Nurses are two examples in nursing. All established health workers have national organizations. Some examples are the American Dietetic Association, the American Academy of Pediatrics, the American Public Health Association, and the National Association of Social Workers.

* The following are some of the national nursing associations listed in the *American Journal of Nursing* Directory: American Association of Colleges of Nursing, American Association of Critical-Care Nurses, American Association of Industrial Nurses, American Association of Nephrology Nurses and Technicians, American Association of Neurosurgical Nurses, American Association of Nurse Anesthetists, American College of Nurse-Midwives, American Nurses' Association, Association of Operating Room Nurses, Emergency Department Nurses' Association, National Association for Practical Nurse Education and Service, National Black Nurses' Association, National Federation of Licensed Practical Nurses, National League for Nursing, National Student Nurses' Association, Nurses' Association of the American College of Obstetricians and Gynecologists. (*Am. J. Nurs.,* **74:**151, [Jan.] 1974.)

The agencies that have been mentioned differ greatly in their functions. Some are service organizations; others raise funds with which they help either official or nonofficial agencies administer a health service; many of them put all their efforts into health education and research. Altogether they play an important part in the total health program.

Since it is difficult to administer any sort of service on a national scale, it will be seen that most of the private national health organizations operate through *state organizations*. In some cases the work started within the state and spread throughout the country, and in other instances the original organization was a national one and from its membership the state chapters, committees, or associations were formed. All established health workers have state organizations. Membership dues for state organizations ordinarily include the fee for membership in the national organization. National organizations tend to form state units, and state units are again broken up into *local units*. In nursing, for example, the American Nurses' Association has state branches, and state associations have district branches; these district organizations may cover an area of from one to ten or more counties. The American Medical Association has the same type of organization, and the National Association for Mental Health, for example, has state and local chapters as well as a national organization.

Besides the local health agencies that are a part of a parent organization, there are many independent local agencies, some of which are hospitals, clinics, visiting nurse associations, extended care and nursing care facilities,* and diagnostic laboratories.

All communities need a coordinating council of social agencies. Many people feel that a systematic exchange of data on families served by health and welfare agencies is an important help in the referral process. Some local areas are finding an information and referral service of great benefit to patients and their families in helping them locate the appropriate agency to meet their needs. Effective methods of referring families to agencies are also essential. As alluded to earlier, health associations, community chests, and community health councils are increasing not only in number and usefulness but, it is to be hoped, in this aspect of coordinating services, also.

It is difficult to distinguish between the organizations that are designed primarily to promote health and those that indirectly affect the health of the people in a community. Hanlon

* For definitions of these terms, see page 170.

puts the multifaceted relationships of health and *public health* in the following statement:

Health is a state of total effective physiologic and psychologic functioning; it has both a relative and an absolute meaning, varying through time and space, in both the individual and in the group; it is the result of the combination of many forces, intrinsic and extrinsic, inherited and contrived, individual and collective, private and public, medical, environmental, and social; and it is conditioned by culture and economy, and by law and government.*

Accepting such a statement and the implication that health means more than the absence of disease, it is easy to see that almost all social institutions have some effect on health. For instance, a vocational placement service may help the handicapped to establish maximum potential mental health just as truly as a physical therapy service helps the client regain the use of his muscles. Schools for the deaf and the blind are of more use to such persons than hospitals; juvenile and family relation courts often supply help to the mentally ill; and nursery and prekindergarten programs provide expert guidance for young children and help prevent some physical and emotional abnormalities. All of these agencies and many others play such an important part in the total health program of the community that nurses cannot afford to be ignorant of them or to ignore their own responsibility for cooperation with such agencies.

The American Medical Association [123] publishes a *Directory of National Voluntary Health Organizations* which lists and gives the functions of the most important national agencies. This national directory is a useful tool, and is available without charge from the Association. Every health worker should have for reference also a directory of the social agencies in his or her state and local community. Agencies are usually grouped according to function and the functions are listed alphabetically, so that if a physician or a nurse wants to refer a patient to a social agency it is a simple matter to find a suitable one. All those concerned with nursing should learn to help others make the most effective use of the facilities at their disposal.

In summary, the classification of health and social agencies by scope and control and their functions have been described for international, national, state, and local agencies, both official and voluntary. The role of the World Health Organization and other agencies, consumer participation, and the emergence of Health Maintenance Organizations have been

* Hanlon, John J.: *op. cit.,* p. 4.

mentioned in this section on health agencies. The place of hospitals, nursing homes, and hospices in the health care system will be described next.

6. PLACE OF HOSPITALS, NURSING HOMES, AND HOSPICES IN HEALTH PROGRAMS

Hospital and Nursing Homes. In developed countries, *hospitals* play a major role in health care. Earlier in this chapter, in discussing the delivery of health care, it was pointed out that some authorities believe the hospital is and should be the critical agency or the principal provider of health care; others believe that, as in Great Britain, the hospital, the local health unit, and private practitioners, the latter operating from local offices or community health centers, should form a coordinated unit under one area health authority.

In the U.S.S.R., there is a highly structured health service of which the hospital is an integral part. The 15 Republics (each with its own Ministry of Health) are divided into provinces or *oblasts* and each *oblast* has a health department. The largest hospitals are *oblast* hospitals with about 600 to 1200 beds. *Oblasts* are subdivided into *rayons* with populations of around 40,000. *Rayon* hospitals have 100 to 300 beds and provide acute general and specialized care. *Rayons* are divided into *uchastoks,* or local districts with populations of about 4000. *Uchastok* hospitals have from 35 to 100 beds. Staffs of the larger *uchastok* hospitals may have six physicians and one or more surgeons. Such hospitals may give some specialized care. There are other hospitals attached to research institutes that treat patients with conditions under study by the institutes. Throughout Russia there are health stations, the smallest administrative health unit. This unit is called a *punkt* and is manned by the feldsher-midwife who treats patients or sends them to an appropriate *uchastok, rayon,* or *oblast* hospital.[124]

Faye G. Abdellah, who, after visiting Russia, gave the preceding description of the hospital network, says about nursing homes, "Many times our delegation asked to see health facilities for the aged, expecting to find numerous institutions like our nursing homes. Eventually we saw a home for invalids and the aged but found that only 1 per cent of those over 65 reside in such homes, compared with 4 per cent in the United States. A law that assigns responsibility to the children for care of their aged parents may account for part of this difference, but other factors are also important."

She goes on to say that "certain classes of pensioners . . . receive full retirement income in addition to full pay for work" and that "Others help their working children by caring for those children's children." *

Hospitals in the United States, with their related ambulatory and extended care facilities, are the principal providers of health care, but they function much more independently of other agencies than those in countries with government-controlled health services such as Great Britain and the U.S.S.R. The American Hospital Association publishes annually a volume of information on hospitals and nursing homes with the inclusive title *Guide to the Health Care Field*.[125] The 1973 publication lists 7061 AHA-registered hospitals in the United States in 1972 in the following classifications: (1) federal; (2) nonfederal psychiatric; (3) nonfederal tuberculosis; (4) nonfederal long-term general and other special; (5) nonfederal short-term general and other special; (6) nongovernmental not-for-profit short-term general and other special; (7) for-profit short-term general and other special; and (8) state and local governmental short-term general and other special. In this Guide are reported, per category, the number of beds, the admissions, the daily census, per cent occupancy, average length of stay, the expense per patient day, and other data. The average daily census in these 7061 hospitals is 1,209,000. This Guide also lists the 59 US government hospitals in 22 countries outside the United States and the long-term care facilities accredited by the Joint Commission on Accreditation of Hospitals (January 1973). These long-term care facilities include (1) *extended care facilities,* defined as establishments with organized medical staffs and with continuous professional nursing service that are established to provide comprehensive inpatient care (which is usually postacute hospital care), for the most part of relatively short duration, and to serve convalescent patients who are not in an acute episode of illness or who are in a stable stage of illness and who have a variety of medical conditions; (2) *nursing care facilities,* defined as establishments with medical staffs or a medical staff equivalent and with continuous nursing service under professional nurse direction. They provide, usually, long-term inpatient care (not necessarily posthospital) to patients who have a variety of medical conditions requiring service; and (3) *resident care facilities,* defined as establishments providing safe, hygienic, sheltered living

for residents not capable of or desiring fully independent living. They furnish regular and frequent but not continuous medical and nursing services and they furnish continuous supportive, restorative, and preventive health services. Most health professionals and the public call these three categories of long-term care facilities *nursing homes.*

Mary Adelaide Mendelson [126] gives the estimated number of nursing homes (using this inclusive definition) as 23,000, more than three times the number of hospitals in the United States.* Estimates on the number of inmates in nursing homes vary greatly, but since nursing homes are generally small as compared with hospitals the total numbers of beds in nursing homes and hospitals may not be too far apart. However, it is generally believed that there are more people in the nursing homes of the United States than in its hospitals.

While the following statement might be challenged, most patients in hospitals are, generally speaking, acutely ill and receive treatment, while patients in nursing homes are chronically ill, old, and dependent on help, or merely homeless, and receive custodial care. Some types of hospitals, such as large mental hospitals and hospitals for veterans, have populations that include the chronically ill and helpless—comparable to nursing home populations. Hospitals may have nursing home units within their walls or in separate plants but administratively related. Comparatively few hospitals (a small proportion of hospital beds) are proprietary or profit-making; nursing homes are, by and large, operated for profit, although county and municipal homes for the indigent might be said to represent tax-supported and nonprofit nursing home beds, and homes owned by religious bodies and fraternal organizations are also nonprofit institutions.

The availability of government funds under the Hill-Burton Act has led to increased hospital construction. Since hospital occupancy is reported by the AHA [127] as 78 per cent, some authorities say beds are available in excess of the country's needs. This, in turn, has unnecessarily increased the cost of hospital care, since patients who occupy beds are, in effect, paying for the maintenance of empty beds. Of the 7061 hospitals listed by the American Hos-

---

* Abdellah, Faye G.: "Nursing and Health Care in the U.S.S.R.," *Am. J. Nurs.,* **73:**2096, (Dec.) 1973.

* This figure for nursing homes includes 4057 extended care facilities licensed to receive Medicare payments, 6500 skilled nursing homes, and 12,000 intermediate care facilities. The latter are licensed to receive Medicaid payments. The AHA's *Guide to the Health Care Field* (1973) lists 1485 extended care facilities as institutions accredited by the Joint Commission on Accreditation of Hospitals.

pital Association in 1972, only 738 (10.4 per cent) are classified as "for-profit." Of the 1,550,000 hospital beds in the United States, 57,000 (3.7 per cent) are in the "for-profit" (proprietary) hospitals. In contrast, most nursing homes are proprietary, or commercial, the chief exceptions being those as mentioned owned by and operated under the auspices of religious or fraternal organizations. The profit in owning and operating nursing homes and the relatively less stringent regulations governing their operation than for operating hospitals have led to a rapidly expanding "industry." *

The concept of the hospital's function has changed so rapidly and hospitals differ so much in character from one country to another and within each country that it is hard to describe the position of the average present-day hospital in the community and harder still to say what it will be in years to come. Most people in the United States think of a hospital as concerned primarily with the care of the sick; others are also accustomed to think of it as a practice field in which to learn the medical arts.† The functions of research, preventive medicine, health education, and total rehabilitation of the chronically ill and handicapped are not so generally expected by the public and assumed by the hospital, but they will be in the future if more hospitals expand their functions to include these aspects of health care. The typical nonprofit voluntary hospital of the past in the United States, and even of the present, is more or less autonomous, pays no taxes, and receives its support from health insurance reimbursements, patient fees, some state and federal funds, and voluntary community and individual contributions.

In those countries with national health insurance that provide benefits for all residents, hospitals and nursing homes are usually government owned and operated. Even such countries, however, may allow private organizations and individuals to operate private or voluntary institutions. But where an effective national health plan exists, comparatively few people want to go to private institutions since their taxes are helping to support the public in-

stitutions, and the services they offer are the right of every taxpayer.

In countries that have no comprehensive health service or health insurance with benefits for all residents, as, for example, the United States, many hospitals may also be owned and operated by the national, state, county, or municipal governments. Since they tend to be large hospitals, it is not surprising to find that of the 1,550,000 hospital beds in the United States 349,000 (22.5 per cent) are in tax-supported federal hospitals or state and local short-term hospitals. There are 457,000 beds (29.5 per cent) in nonfederal psychiatric hospitals, many of which are also tax supported.[128] The United States government provides hospitals for the armed forces in this country and overseas, for veterans, for US Public Health Service employees, and for Indians, who are wards of the government. States have provided hospitals for the mentally ill, and counties and municipalities have owned and operated hospitals for the indigent and those with certain communicable diseases that might menace society.

Although "expense" per hospital bed, or care for the acutely ill, has risen steeply since World War II,* short-term hospitals operating for profit have increased from 39 in 1946 to 57 in 1972. However, nursing homes offering a custodial or less costly type of care have increased with inordinate rapidity in this period.[130] In fact, little was heard about nursing homes before this period.

Since federal health insurance in the form of Medicare and federal and state aid in the form of Medicaid can be applied to the cost of hospital or nursing home care in the United States, governmental agencies are requiring health institutions and agencies to meet minimum standards if they want patients to be eligible for Medicare and Medicaid payments. *Accreditation* of hospitals was started by the American College of Surgeons 30 years ago. There is now a Joint Commission on Accreditation of Hospitals (JCAH) (sponsored by the American Medical Association, the American Hospital Association, the American College of Physicians, and the American College of Surgeons), which not only accredits hospitals but also has begun to accredit nursing homes. By the end of 1973, it had accredited 2300 nursing homes.[131,132] Interdisciplinary teams visit and evaluate hospitals and nursing homes. Quality assurance programs have recently been established to evaluate patient care, largely

---

* Any fee-for-service system of health care is in danger of being dominated by the profit motive. It is unfortunate that in the United States all health care is commonly referred to as "the health industry" rather than "the health service."

† A common criticism of health workers—doctors, nurses, and others—is that they learn to practice in the hospitals where the population consists of sick people, most of them very sick. Students in the health field are theoretically taught preventive medicine, or health care, but have little or no opportunity to practice it.

---

* The American Hospital Association reports that the total expense of hospitals per patient day was $7.98 in 1950, $16.46 in 1960, and $73.89 in 1972.[129]

through the study of records.[133-135] The Social
Security Amendment of 1972 was of great interest to the health professions because of its
mandate to establish Professional Standards
Review Organizations (PSROs). Bonnie Bullough[136] is one of those who thinks this program will initiate the eventual establishment
of adequate health care for all. Yet Paul J.
Sanozaro and his associates[137] in an article on
"research and development in quality assurance" call the Professional Standards Review
Organization program "experimental." *

The accreditation of hospitals has a long
and relatively successful history, partly because medical educators, who have found it
necessary to know whether they are suitable as
practice fields for medical students, interns,
and residents, have stood behind the program.
The accreditation of nursing homes in the
United States has, by comparison, limited influence on the quality of patient care, partly
because they have, by and large, no connection
with educational programs. H. M. Parrish[138]
writes about the need for an academic health
center affiliation for the nursing home. Those
of the American Nursing Home Association
are discussing peer review and, as stated earlier, the Joint Commission on Accreditation of
Hospitals has made a start on accrediting nursing homes.[139]

Much has been written about the problems
of nursing homes. The most significant influences on nursing homes of the United States
are the state programs of licensure, certification, and surveillance, usually by the state
health department, but the department of welfare or a special unit may be made responsible.[140] A British nurse describes the registration and inspection of nursing homes in 1973
by the deputy medical officer of health and the
director of nursing services as a satisfying
function.[141] This may be because nursing
homes in Great Britain seem to provide a more
satisfying service to patients than those in the
United States.

In 1963, Rita P. Kelliher and Mary E.

Shaughnessy[142] reported a survey of nursing
homes in Massachusetts that showed the institutions' limitations; a 1970 quantitative
measure of nursing service in homes in Colorado also revealed some deficiencies.[143] By
this time people were sporadically aroused, and
some young women who called themselves
Ralph Nader's Study Group, directed by Claire
Townsend, published a report of a nationwide
survey under the title *Old Age: The Last
Segregation,* known also as *The Nader Report.*[144] *Time Magazine* termed it "a passionate
indictment" and during the mid-1970s many
investigations of nursing home practices appeared with titles such as "The Nursing Home
Scandal." The Nader group set up specific
criteria by which they evaluated nursing
homes. Referring to the lack of opportunity
for social activity, they reported that only one
out of 20 homes visited appeared to offer an
environment where elderly people lived meaningful, full, and productive lives.[145] A 1970
study by Dorothea Jaeger and Leo W. Simmons of *The Aged Ill,*[146] while not a study of
nursing homes primarily, showed their baleful
effects on inmates.

A nationwide survey of nursing homes conducted by Faye G. Abdellah, Director of the
Office of Nursing Home Affairs, US Public
Health Service, showed in 1975 that there was
a significant degree of noncompliance with the
rules and regulations of Medicare and Medicaid programs in visits to nearly 300 skilled
nursing facilities.[147]

The conclusions reached in all these studies
are reinforced by a 1974 publication, *Tender
Loving Greed,*[148] which describes "how the in-
credibly lucrative nursing home industry is
exploiting America's old people and defraud-
ing us all." Mary Adelaide Mendelson, who
spent almost 10 years on a nationwide investigation during which she visited 200 homes in
different areas, describes the proliferation of
nursing homes since 1940 and the entrance of
the federal government into the nursing home
business with the Amendments to the Social
Security Act (P.L. 89–97) that provide direct
payments to nursing homes for the care of the
elderly. When Title 18 (Medicare) and Title
19 (Medicaid) of the Act were passed in 1965,
very large amounts of public money flowed
into the nursing home industry—a system that
in 1972 had an estimated income of $3.5
billion.[149] With 20 million Americans over 65
and the number rising by 300,000 to 400,000
per year, "the nursing home industry" if not
regulated, according to Mendelson, promises
ever greater profit.[150] She places the blame
squarely on the government for pumping so
much money into a system incapable of po-

---

* Some critics of the Professional Standards Review
Organization legislation question having health workers
alone evaluate care, believing that the receivers of
care should be on national or state review organizations. In most states the PSROs are composed of
physicians; in a few states nurses are also members.
Review presently emphasizes treatment by the physician. Marjorie Ramphal reports that "the American
Nurses' Association is developing guidelines for use
in the initiation of peer review within agencies." She
adds, "Peer review is seen as one means of implementing the Standards for Nursing Practice which
were developed under the aegis of the ANA Congress
for Nursing Practice and the five ANA Divisions on
Practice." (Ramphal, Marjorie: "Peer Review," *Am.
J. Nurs.,* **74**:63, [Jan.] 1974.)

licing itself. Much of the new money, she claims, went into higher costs instead of more service to those in need of it.

With the availability of so much public money, most of which came from Medicaid,* Mendelson says greed was inevitable. She thinks it was this greed that caused owners, operators, and businessmen already in the industry to see an opportunity for a quick way to make huge profits at the expense of the sick by buying cheap food, hiring low-quality help, accepting healthy clients, and buying off inspectors and caseworkers. Because operators were suspected of making a great deal of money, one financial study was done in Cleveland by GEOMET, Inc., of Rockville, Maryland. It showed that a large nursing home operator could make an annual pretax return of 76 per cent on an initial investment if all the patients were on Medicaid's maximum rate. The Connecticut Hospital Commission estimated that it was possible for the owners of an average 40-bed home to earn an annual return of 39 per cent on their investment.[151]

The crisis in "the nursing home industry" exists partly, according to Mendelson, because new legislation has not corrected abuses. New laws have been passed and new legislation written, but fundamentally nothing has changed in the industry. The government, she says, has failed to take any meaningful action and "so long as enforcement continues to lag far behind legislation, the new laws, like the old, will merely create the illusion of progress without its substance." † Mendelson thinks the solution involves forcing the government to answer some basic questions about the industry, publicizing the results of independent studies of profiteering and of the quality of life in nursing homes, and finally the acceptance by all United States citizens of some responsibility for the human beings in these institutions.[152]

Marie Callender, a nurse who is Special Assistant for Nursing Home Affairs in the US Department of Health, Education, and Welfare, would probably challenge some of Mendelson's conclusions. In 1972, she wrote an article titled "Washington Creates a Climate for Responsible Change in the Nation's Nursing Homes," [153] and another titled "National Approach to Long-Term Care." [154] In both she points out that fragmented policy and programs have been brought together under

HEW's Office of Nursing Home Affairs, whose director is Faye Abdellah, the highest ranking nurse in the US Public Heath Service; that states have moved to upgrade survey and certification programs; that 500 nursing homes not meeting standards have been "decertified" or have voluntarily withdrawn requests for Medicaid payments; that more than half of the state Medicaid inspectors have received federally sponsored training; that nursing home ombudsman units have been established under HEW contracts with the National Council of Senior Citizens in four states; that more than 40,000 nurses, physicians, activity directors, and administrators "will be reached" during 1973 through training courses funded by HEW and "fashioned by" the ANA, the AMA, the American Nursing Home Association, and the Association of University Programs in Hospital Administration. She says, "Finally, HEW, in close cooperation with other federal agencies, the states, the professions, and the health care industry, has embarked on an historic study of the uses, standards, abuses, practices, and potential of long-term care." * In the years since Callender's statement, the Senate Subcommittee on Long-Term Care in 1975 issued a five-year report condemning nursing home care and the Office of Nursing Home Affairs also in 1975 issued its report on conditions in nursing homes.[154a,154b]

In 1975, after over a year's work by the American Nurses' Association's Committee on Skilled Nursing Care, a major paper called *Nursing in Long-Term Care: Toward Quality Care for the Aging* made recommendations to Senator Frank E. Moss, Chairman of the US Senate Subcommittee on Long-Term Care. These recommendations concerned (1) the right of the elderly to receive high-quality care; (2) the need for a national policy on care of the aging, and for national health insurance for all citizens; (3) the need for availability of supportive services such as home care, out-of-home day care, and nursing home care for the elderly; (4) the deletion of the term "skilled nursing" in federal standards as it is unmeasurable; and (5) the strengthening of nursing education programs by including more gerontological and geriatric nursing.[155] This paper and other studies of care to the elderly in institutions should lead to eventual improvement in the treatment of our aged citizens. (For further discussion of nursing homes, see Chapter 3.)

As was touched on earlier, what is called the "consumer revolution" is significantly changing

---

* Medicaid allows unlimited nursing home stays for the poor of any age, whereas Medicare permits only up to 100 days in a nursing home for those over 65 provided that this stay follows a hospitalization. (Mendelson, Mary Adelaide: *Tender Loving Greed.* Alfred A. Knopf, New York, 1974, p. 36.)

† Mendelson, Mary Adelaide: *op. cit.,* p. XII.

* Callender, Marie: "National Approach to Long-Term Care," *Nurs. Outlook,* 21:22, (Jan.) 1973.

health care everywhere, but particularly institutional care. Nancy Quinn and Anne R. Somers,[156] writing on "The Patient's Bill of Rights" as a significant aspect of the consumer revolution, think that the first of such documents was the National League for Nursing's [157] 1959 publication *What People Can Expect of Modern Nursing Service*. In 1973, the American Hospital Association [158] issued a *Patient's Bill of Rights* prepared in 1972. State legislatures are considering effective uses of this document. Minnesota, for example, has required a similar statement to be given every patient on admission to the hospital, and the Insurance Commission of Pennsylvania has drawn up a bill going further than that of the AHA, and, as mentioned earlier, New Jersey has already passed a law for mental patients' rights. The International Council of Nurses reports that the Council of Europe has been asked to adopt a European Declaration of the Rights of the Sick.[158a] The last point of the AHA document contains the following statement: "12. *Consumer Advocacy*. The public has a right to expect a hospital to behave as a consumer advocate rather than as a business headquarters for doctors and hospital officials." * Such publications and the effect of the work of the US Department of Health, Education, and Welfare Secretary's Commission on Medical Malpractice [159] should materially affect the role of hospitals, regardless of the form national health insurance takes in the next few years. Whether or not hospitals, community health workers, or Health Maintenance Organizations are the primary unit or "hub" of the system, the public seems determined that they shall offer services that meet human needs at a price it can afford. The Commission on Medical Malpractice concludes that effective consumer participation improves health care and increases patient satisfaction.

Perhaps the greatest injustice to the patient is, however, the fact that hospital and nursing home care, conceived as a humane service, has been converted into an "industry," some think, dominated by the profit motive. The Health Policy Advisory Center said in 1973:

Of the $83 billion that Americans spent for health in 1972, at least 10% went directly for profits. Drug companies earn over $600 million in profits each year and spend 1.5 billion more in advertising. The health insurance industry collected $20 billion in premiums in 1970 and paid out only $17 billion in health care benefits. . . . Nursing homes, proprietary hospitals, and medical supply companies together earn $600 million in profits . . . each year $8 billion . . . leaves the health care system as profits and profit-creating advertising and administration. . . . Approximately 20% of the total national expenditures for health, personal health services, is wasted, down the drain of unnecessary hospitalization, needless surgery, duplication of facilities, fragmentation and duplication of administrative cost. (This 20% amounted to $16.6 billion in 1972.) *

Basil S. Georgopoulos,[160] discussing the hospital at a meeting devoted to research on the organization of health institutions, calls the hospital a specialized and internally differentiated system for the purpose of solving human problems; he also calls it a "work-performing sociotechnical system," an "adaptive system," a "complex social system," and a "living system." The modern hospital is a highly organized institution that exists for human beings to help other human beings. It is to be hoped that those who operate hospitals will find ways to make them more humane, more responsible to the psychosocial needs of those they serve.

Hospitals have in the past played an important role in the education of health personnel. Except for orientation and on-the-job training, educational programs are moving out of hospitals into schools, colleges, and universities. Recently some persons in the management of United States hospitals and specialists in licensure have advocated that hospitals license and establish credentials, or qualifications, for all health practitioners in the hospital.[161] The American Nurses' Association has publicly opposed *institutional licensure* with respect to nursing personnel. Those who write on the nature and purpose of professions usually include licensure as one of their rights or obligations. William J. McGlothlin, for example, makes the following statement:

Once a profession is awarded legal status. . . . It licenses or certifies appropriately trained members of the profession and excludes the rest. It has an obligation to police its own ranks, to make certain that those who wear the name and display the license are in fact ethical and competent practitioners.†

It is not likely that any of the health professions will readily give up this widely recognized prerogative, but public participation in the licensing of health workers is widely discussed by nurses and others and is demanded in some quarters.[162-169]

The spiraling cost of hospital care in the

---

* Denenberg, H. S.: *Citizen's Bill of Hospital Rights: What the Patient and Public Can and Should Expect from Our Hospitals*. Pennsylvania Insurance Department, Harrisburg, 1973.

* Health Policy Advisory Center: *op. cit.,* p. 20.
† McGlothlin, William J.: *The Professional Schools*. Center for Applied Research in Education, Inc., New York, 1964, p. 10.

United States and in other countries alluded to earlier is well known, although the United States leads all others in this respect. According to *The 1976 U.S. Fact Book,*[170] in 1970 the average hospital expense per patient day in the United States was $83.67 and each person spent an average of $178.88 yearly for hospital care. In a report of a study over 15 months by Cancer Care, Inc.[171] (New York City), it is stated that a catastrophic illness can reduce a family of medium means to poverty in less than 2 years, the average cost being $21,718. In one case in 1973, hospital costs were $45,000, and 73 per cent of United States families had hospital bills exceeding $5000.

Both proprietary hospitals (those owned and operated for profit) and governmental hospitals and other nonprofit hospitals have faced extraordinary increases in operating expenses, as noted earlier. Many persons believe ways must be found to lower the cost of hospital operations and also to reduce the use of hospitals to the minimum that is consistent with actual health needs. The views of Garfield, Malleson, and others were cited earlier in this chapter, that the public should have access to local health centers or Health Maintenance Organizations where families are registered and known to the staff of the center. This staff would determine the patient's need for hospitalization and often provide treatment that would make it unnecessary. Effective home care programs and extended care facilities coordinated with health centers and hospitals can also shorten the time spent in high-cost acute care general hospitals.

In any health program, and regardless of which organization or institutional unit is the primary one (or the hub of the wheel), everyone agrees that hospitals should be interlocking parts of a regional plan for providing a total or comprehensive health service. They should not function in isolation but in a carefully worked out relationship with smaller or larger hospitals, specialized hospitals, and other health institutions and agencies. Such regional planning often crosses state boundaries. Ultimately, such regional or area planning should include nursing homes or long-term facilities.

An example of regional planning in this country is embodied in the 911 system for handling emergency telephone calls. This system, in use in England for 30 years, gives the population of a town or a group of towns or an entire city quick access to a communications center in an emergency. Calling a central telephone office operator results in the dispatch of appropriate emergency equipment and personnel to the scene of an emergency. Figure 2-11 shows the concept of the 911 system. Co-operation of public health officials, public safety organizations, and the public itself is essential for success of the system.[172]

Another regional plan involving health institutions is depicted in Figure 2-12 showing a school of health sciences, three types of hospitals, and their relationships. Surrounding this hospital network are other health institutions and agencies from which people may be referred to the hospitals or to which hospitals may refer people. The medical center (often connected with university-based schools of health sciences) offers all kinds of medical care with its various special therapies, sophisticated equipment, health education of the public, medical education for personnel, services of the public health department, and rehabilitation including vocational placement. Patients receive care in the hospital and clinic, but from this center many kinds of workers may be sent to the home to provide the care the person needs. Smaller secondary hospitals may surround this medical center, giving such care as they are prepared to give with the help that can be gotten from the larger institution. Likewise, these smaller secondary or "district hospitals" are surrounded by emergency, often rural units that can give a very limited service but that, nevertheless, are valuable. Since they are articulated with community hospitals and the medical center, they can transfer and refer patients promptly to those institutions prepared to give them the help they need.

Forty years ago John Ellis, writing on the place of the hospital in the community said:

Few will disagree with the thesis that the hospital will increasingly be the central and strategic factor in medical care and medical education. Not many will deny that the hospital of the future is bound to be an important center of consultation service. . . .

In their external affairs, the hospitals must lose their intense individualism and become part of a broad social welfare program. They must realize that they are only one element in the community resources for the care of the sick. They must be integrated with other similar health services.*

One effect of this unification of medical service, of particular interest to nurses, is the wiping out of the line between what are now called public health nursing and institutional nursing. Many visiting nurse organizations, both public and private, have offices in hospitals, most often in the outpatient department. As medical centers develop home care pro-

---

* Ellis, W. John: "How Shall the Hospital Develop to Meet the Demand of the Future?" *Hospitals,* **11:**49, (Oct.) 1937.

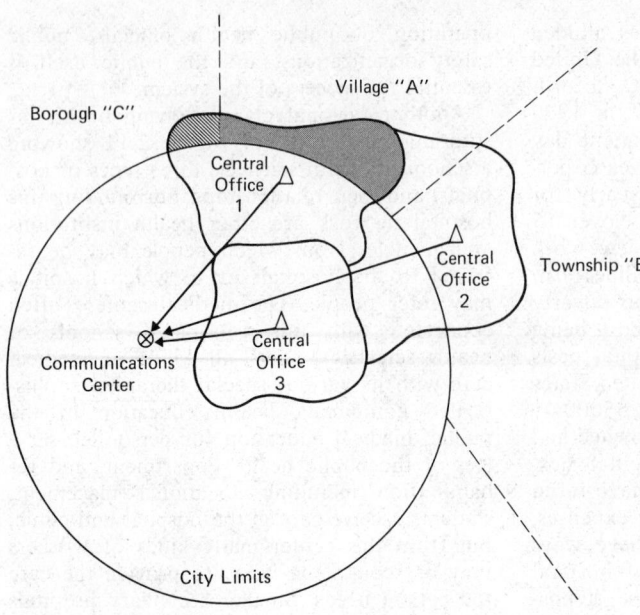

Figure 2-11. 911 regional concept. (US Department of Health, Education, and Welfare: *Emergency Medical Services Communications Systems.* US Government Printing Office, Washington, D.C., 1972, p. 22. DHEW Pub. No. [HSM] 73–2003.)

grams, physicians, nurses, and other workers will visit patients in their homes. It will also be necessary to prepare institutional nurses for home nursing or to bring about a more thorough amalgamation of the various nursing groups in the community. This seems altogether desirable, since institutional workers will in this way become more conscious of the public's need for health teaching and the adjustment of social problems; the public health worker will, through contact with a hospital, tend to keep in closer touch with the field of medical science. Home care programs such as that of Montefiore Hospital in New York City have pioneered in these efforts.[173,174]

In discussing hospitals, nursing homes, and hospices, mention should be made of the Loeb Nursing Center connected with Montefiore Hospital in New York City. Conceived and directed by the late Lydia Hall, a nurse, and now under the direction of Genrose Alfano, it offers a unique service. Patients are admitted to this institution, usually from the hospital, who have not achieved the independence that would enable them to live at home but for whom nursing has much and medicine little to offer. Graduate nurses plan programs of care with patients and their families and call in physicians as consultants when needed.[175-180]

Visitors to the Center are impressed with the helpful atmosphere; with the rapid progress patients make in developing independence or coping with handicaps. They are also impressed with the satisfaction staff nurses find in working at the Center, where they can give high quality nursing care and are held accountable for the welfare of their assigned patients.

The success of the Loeb Nursing Center's program has been widely recognized, and it must have occurred to many observers that certain aspects of the program, if adopted by nursing homes, might materially improve the services they offer.

During the Middle Ages, *hospices* were established along the route to the Holy Land to serve those making pilgrimages. Travelers stayed at these hospices until they were able to continue their journey, or they might die in a hospice. In the 1971–1972 Annual Report of St. Christopher's Hospice in London, Cicely Saunders, medical director, discussing the medieval use of the word hospice, says:

The word [hospice] continued to be used in France and was extended to hospices for the elderly, the incurable and for foundlings. . . . Mother Mary Aidenhead then took up the title when she founded the Irish Sisters of Charity in the middle of the last century, although the Hospice at Harold's Cross, Dublin, was only dedicated especially to the care of dying patients 67 years ago. Her foundation has long extended to several Hospices, mainly concerned with the care of the dying and the long term sick. St. Joseph's Hospice, Hackney, was founded in 1905 but before it opened its doors the Sisters were visiting the sick in their homes, thus foreshadowing the domiciliary work we have now started at St. Christopher's over the past three years.*

St. Christopher's Hospice was opened in 1967. It serves people of all ages who need more extended nursing or more personal care than is available in hospitals and those who

* St. Christopher's Hospice Annual Report, 1971–1972.

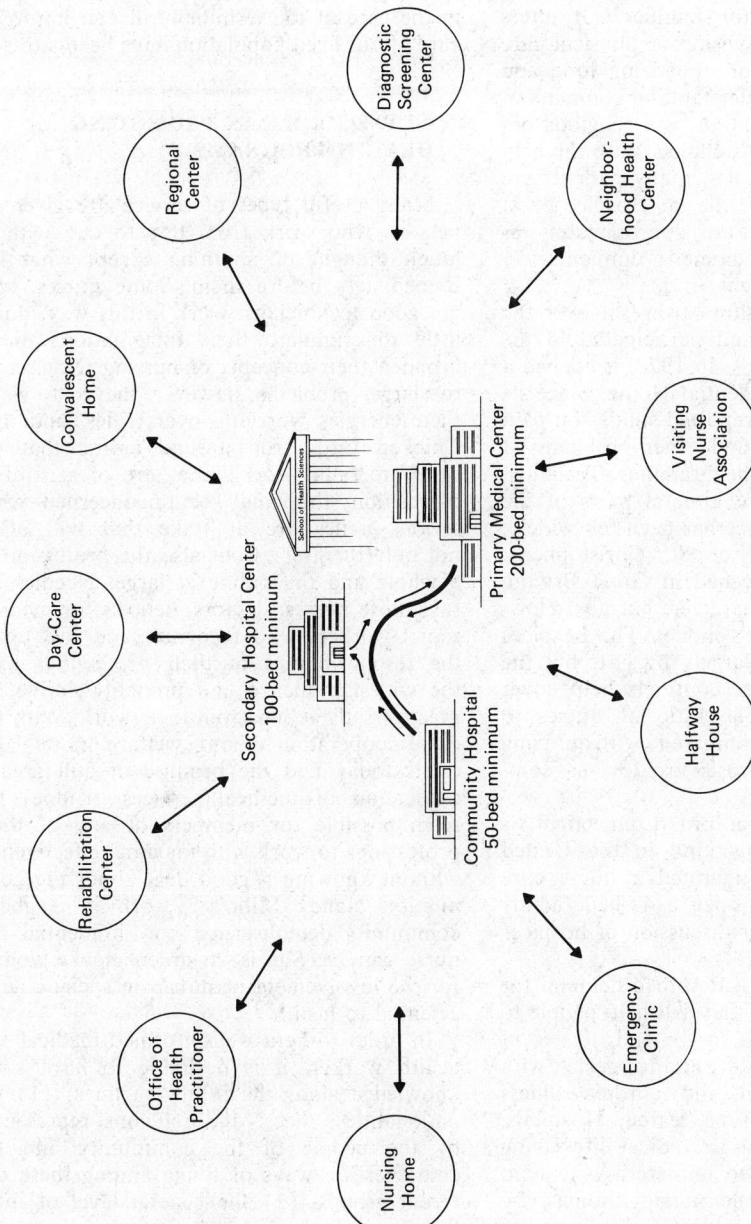

Figure 2-12. Relationships of health care facilities in a regionalized medical system. Primary Medical Center contains a full range of specialty services and technical facilities backed up by the research and educational system of a School of Health Sciences. The Secondary Hospital Center contains basic specialty services and some educational programs and facilities. The Community Hospital is equipped to provide general services on a limited basis. All hospitals refer to and receive services from a wide variety of community supportive agencies.

need specialized treatment for chronic pain or other forms of distress. It offers "a community" made up of patients, relatives and friends, paid staff, volunteers, and relatively well elderly who occupy a special "residents' wing" and, during the day, children of workers in the "Play Group" or nursery school. It is described as "a family, caring for families." It offers control of pain, the provision of physical care with special emphasis on appetizing food and continued mobility, understanding companionship, occupation, recreation, and religious observances of the patient's choice. With the help given patients and families, many patients are able to live, and finally die, at Hospice or at home. Presently there are approximately as many patients on the home ("domiciliary") service as on the inpatient service.

Several thousand visitors from all over the world have observed and participated in the work at St. Christopher's. In 1973, it opened a Study Centre and Residential Home. Since its founding, the staff has reported studies on pain control, bereavement, and other problems of the terminally ill and their families. Teaching, study, and research are integral parts of the program and its influence has been felt widely.

Since the founding of St. Christopher's, other hospices have opened in Great Britain, each having its own character, but all following the St. Christopher's model. The hospices in Britain are funded largely by gifts but the National Health Service contracts help cover the "running cost." The ratio of nurses to patients is high as compared with nursing homes but treatment costs are low as compared with hospitals.

Hospice, Inc., in Branford, Connecticut, is the first agency of this kind in the United States. In 1974 it inaugurated a home care service and expects to open a 44-bed facility in 1978.[181] (For further discussion of hospices see Chapters 3 and 50.)

There is presently a widespread demand for a facility and a service that will help people to live as fully as possible to the end, to accept death when it is inevitable, and to meet it with dignity—making death and chronic illness something that needn't be feared. Hospitals, with their commitment to radical life-saving treatment, often seem to unmercifully extend the dying process, while nursing homes, by and large, offer little incentive to live whether the inmates are sick or well.

To sum up, the use of hospitals in the United States as contrasted with that in the Union of Soviet Socialist Republics points out the importance of regional health planning and organization of units in an interlocking network. The high cost of health care in this country versus its low yield of improved health of the population demands changes. The deplorable conditions in nursing homes, the recognition of patients' rights, the accreditation of hospitals and nursing homes, and the licensing of health personnel have all been discussed in this section. The place of hospices in the care of the terminally ill and improved care of our aged population have been stressed.

7. NURSE'S ROLE IN PROMOTING HEALTH PROGRAMS

Many useful types of service are given by persons who work from day to day without much thought of anything except what lies immediately before them. Some nurses, who are good technicians, work in this way, doing little to stimulate their imaginations or to broaden their concepts of nursing. Not seeing the larger problems, however, they may waste their energies worrying over trifles, and, like Chicken Little, run around crying that the skies are falling; or, if they are of a carefree disposition, they may be unconcerned when serious issues are at stake that will affect not only themselves but also the profession as a whole and the public at large. Needless to say, those nurses, doctors, dentists, or medical social workers who recognize and live up to the responsibilities of their professions have the widest influence and probably derive the greatest satisfaction from their work. With the close cooperation among welfare groups that exists today and the promise of still greater unification of medical services, it does not seem possible for members of any of these professions to work with maximal effectiveness without knowing a good deal about the community. Nancy Milio's[182] work in a ghetto community demonstrated how influential one nurse can be. She is an ardent spokeswoman for the involvement of nurses in social change essential to health.

In order to be a well-informed medical and health worker, it is desirable to have some knowledge along the following lines: (1) the nationalities, races, and religions represented by the people of the community and the characteristic ways of living among these different groups; (2) the general level of intelligence and the interest of people in, and their knowledge of, laws governing healthful living; (3) the economic status of persons living in different districts of the community; (4) the social agencies and the health facilities available to the people; (5) the local health government and its relationship to the state and national government; and (6) the machinery for the passage of health legislation and the ways in which the individuals in the community may make their influence felt when questions affecting the health and welfare of the community are up for discussion before bodies of lawmakers. Nurses should welcome opportunities to keep up, through the daily newspapers and through regular reference to nursing journals and other professional journals, with what is going on locally and nationally; to observe the work of other health workers and agencies; to take part in discussions of current health problems; to work on coordinating committees and in agencies; to participate in professional and other health-related meetings; to initiate or participate in research on health care; and to write about their activities in professional and other publications. The patterns of nursing practice are constantly changing. The well-informed nurse who is professionally active or inactive is always in a position to promote the health of the population wherever he or she lives and works. Chapter 3 describes more fully the nurse's role in various health settings.

SUMMARY

In estimating the resources of a nation, human life and the health of the people are said to exceed all other economic resources. While a growing health consciousness is apparent in the United States and in many other countries, our knowledge of how to prevent and control disease far exceeds its application. The average life span has been increased by more than 20 years since 1900, and the incidence of many diseases has been materially reduced, but conditions for which the means of early detection and treatment are well known still rank high among the common causes of death. Health care costs have markedly increased in the 1960s and 1970s, and our expenditures for better health care have proportionately increased. In order to raise health standards, however, the main problems seem to be the establishment of an economic status that provides people with the necessities of life, a general education that will stimulate a desire for and knowledge of health, and the provision of adequate medical service and other health facilities. Some countries have national health schemes that make health care universally available, just as is education. In the United States, universal coverage has not been effected, but new programs have provided many groups of people with health care or with the opportunity to have it.

An important aspect of health programs has been the improvement and extension of all kinds of nursing service. The part that nursing care plays in raising health standards is recognized and has added not only to the dignity but to the interest of the nurse's work. Some of the changes in nursing that have enhanced the profession are the growth of nurse-midwifery and the enlarged role of nurse practitioners and clinical nurse specialists. Nurses in all specialties today are credited in many circles with being sensitive to the social causes of disease and to the possibilities of prevention and treatment with a comprehensive approach to health. This may be the single most significant development in nursing.

Some outstanding accomplishments in disease control and the promotion of health through scientific and technical advances in medicine that have brought progress in raising health standards are the control of infectious diseases, modern obstetrical and surgical care, an increase in nutritional knowledge, and the changes brought about in psychiatric care. Social scientists working with health professionals have helped improve the psychological and sociological components of health care.

The importance of organization in health care is reflected in the numbers of official and voluntary health agencies. International, national, state, and local health agencies are organized to carry on a variety of programs that are interrelated in their work. The differing functions of tax-supported and voluntary agencies provide services to expand the availability of health care to large numbers of people.

The government's responsibilities in health work have grown since the early 1900s. Some countries have developed a national health service that provides universal coverage. The service, though nationalized, may be administered through smaller geographic units, as in Canada through provincial governments. The United States has *not* developed a national health service but has created services that provide health care to certain groups, as, for example, the aged, indigent children, Indians, the military, veterans, and certain government employees. The United States government's interest in health care has greatly increased. Proposals for national health insurance have made the public aware that "socialized medicine" or tax-funded medical care is believed by most of the world to be a human right. Current plans embody such concepts as Health Maintenance Organizations, comprehensive health planning, consumer participation in health affairs, and the regionalization of medical care.

The hospital's role in the community health program is an important and crucial one, and most persons see hospitals as part of a regional plan for health care rather than as autonomous, isolated institutions. Systems for preventing hospitalization, such as prepaid group practice plans, screening and diagnostic centers, and health education centers, are taking on added importance as the care provided in most hospitals is economically unsupportable. Extended care and nursing care facilities must be considered part of the health care system also. It is hoped that their services will be more effectively integrated and the quality more adequately ensured than they are presently. As they are developed, hospices will also be a part of the system.

All types of agencies are recognizing their interdependence and the importance of a more unified family health service. Health workers are urged to study the people, the conditions, and the health facilities within their communities in order that they may give the best possible service to persons in their care. In almost every community, better planning, closer coordination, and simplification of health services are needed.

There are few, if any, public or private agencies that do not consider nurses essential members of their staffs. They have taken an active part in all health programs and in all aspects of research. It is significant that the period of time in which professional nursing has existed is also the period in which greatest advances have been made in medical science.

Nurses are credited by many observers as being especially sensitive to human needs. Wolstenholme suggests that "at this moment of human tumult, lost faith, and economic bewilderment, the greater medical profession, the doctors and nurses and all who share their care, concern, and curiosity in the relief of unnecessary suffering could inspire a critical mass of mankind with the determination to give every one in the world an opportunity to enjoy a life worth living." *

REFERENCES

1. Maslow, Abraham H.: *Motivation and Personality.* Harper & Row, New York, 1970.
2. Terleckyi, Nestor R.: *Improvements in the Quality of Life; Estimates of Possibilities in the U.S., 1974–1983.* National Planning Association, Washington, D.C., 1975, pp. 73–89.
3. *White House Conference on Aging, 1971.* (Various Reports.) US Government Printing Office, Washington, D.C., 1971–.

* Wolstenholme, G. E. W.: *op. cit.,* p. 261.

4. US Department of Health, Education, and Welfare, Social Security Administration: *Social Security Programs Throughout the World, 1971.* US Government Printing Office, Washington, D.C., 1972 (DHEW Pub. No. [SSA] 72–11802).
5. Coale, Ansley J.: "Man and His Environment," *Science,* **170:**132, (Oct.) 1970.
6. Lubic, Ruth: Personal communication, 1974.
7. Abdellah, Faye G.: "Nursing and Health Care in the U.S.S.R.," *Am. J. Nurs.,* **73:** 2096, (Dec.) 1973.
8. Muller, J. E., et al.: "The Soviet Health System—Aspects of Relevance for Medicine in the United States," *N. Engl. J. Med.,* **286:**693, (Mar. 30) 1972.
9. Wolstenholme, G. E. W.: "Outline of a World Health Service as a Step Towards Men's Well-Being and Towards a World Society," in Ciba Foundation Symposium: *Health of Mankind.* J. & A. Churchill, London, 1969, p. 227.
10. Malleson, Andrew: *Need Your Doctor Be So Useless?* George Allen & Unwin, Ltd., London, 1973, p. 192.
11. Kao, Frederick F.: "China, Chinese Medicine, and the Chinese Medical System," *Am. J. Chinese Med.,* **1:**1, (Jan.) 1973.
12. US Department of Health, Education, and Welfare, National Center for Health Statistics: *Health Interview Survey—Provisional Data.* Monthly Vital Statistics Report, Vol. 22, No. 1 (Supplement), Apr. 2, 1973, p. 2.
13. *Ibid.,* p. 3.
14. Milio, Nancy: *Care of Health in Communities.* Macmillan Publishing Co., Inc., New York, 1975.
15. US Department of Commerce, Bureau of the Census: *The 1976 U.S. Fact Book, The American Almanac, Statistical Abstract of the U.S.* Grosset & Dunlap, New York, 1976, p. 330.
16. Read, Donald A., and Greene, Walter H.: *Health and Modern Man.* Macmillan Publishing Co., Inc., New York, 1973.
17. Kogan, Benjamin A.: *Health; Man in a Changing Environment.* Harcourt, Brace & World, New York, 1970.
18. Matek, Stanley J.: "Some Key Features in the Emerging Context for Future Health Policy Decision in America," in US Department of Health, Education, and Welfare, Division of Nursing: *Redesigning Nursing Education for Public Health.* Report of the Conference, May 23–25, 1973. The Department, Bethesda, Md., 1973, p. 28 (DHEW Pub. No. [HRA] 75–75).
19. Toffler, Alvin: *Future Shock.* Bantam Books, New York, 1970.
20. Kahn, Herman, and Bruce-Briggs, B.: *Things To Come. Thinking About the Seventies and Eighties.* Macmillan Publishing Co., Inc., New York, 1972.
21. Jungk, Robert, and Galtung, Johan (eds.):

Mankind 2000. George Allen & Unwin, Ltd., London, 1969.

22. Kahn, Herman, and Bruce-Briggs, B.: *op. cit.,* p. 211.

23. US Department of Health, Education, and Welfare, National Center for Health Statistics: *Health Characteristics of Low-Income Persons.* Series 10, No. 74. US Government Printing Office, Washington, D.C., 1972, p. 2.

24. Bullough, Bonnie, and Bullough, Vern L.: *Poverty, Ethnic Identity, and Health Care.* Appleton-Century-Crofts, New York, 1972, p. 117.

25. Hurley, Rodger: "Health Crisis of the Poor," in Drietzel, Hans Peter (ed.): *The Social Organization of Health.* Macmillan Publishing Co., Inc., New York, 1971, p. 92.

26. Milio, Nancy: *op. cit.,* p. 81.

27. US Department of Health, Education, and Welfare, Social Security Administration: *op. cit.*

28. Enterline, P. E., et al.: "The Distribution of Medical Services Before and After Free Medical Care; The Quebec Experience," *N. Engl. J. Med.,* **289:**1174, (Nov. 29) 1973.

29. Arcand, Lisette: "New Health Programs in Quebec—A Trend for the Future," *Can. Nurse,* **68:**27, (Dec.) 1972.

30. Somers, Anne R.: *Health Care in Transition; Directions for the Future.* Hospital Research and Educational Trust, Chicago, 1971, p. 21.

31. Wolstenholme, G. E. W.: *op. cit.,* p. 227.

32. Stern, Bernard H.: *American Medical Practice in the Perspectives of a Century.* Commonwealth Fund, New York, 1945, p. 108.

33. Dublin, Louis I.: *Factbook of Man from Birth to Death.* Macmillan Publishing Co., Inc., New York, 1965, p. 88.

34. Carnegie Commission on Higher Education: *Higher Education and the Nation's Health. Policies for Medical and Dental Education.* McGraw-Hill Book Co., New York, 1970, p. 5.

35. Lippard, Vernon W.: *A Half-Century of American Medical Education 1920–1970.* Josiah Macy, Jr. Foundation, New York, 1974, p. 108.

36. Somers, Anne R.: *op. cit.,* p. 5.

37. Vogel, Ezra F.: "Organization of Health Services," in Wegman, Myron E., et al. (eds.): *Public Health in the People's Republic of China.* Josiah Macy, Jr. Foundation, New York, 1973, p. 51.

38. Chin, Robert: "The Changing Health Conduct of the 'New Man,'" in Wegman, Myron E., et al. (eds.): *Public Health in the People's Republic of China.* Josiah Macy, Jr. Foundation, New York, 1973, p. 121.

39. Sidel, Victor W.: "Feldshers and Feldsherism," *N. Engl. J. Med.,* **278:**934 (Apr. 25) 1968.

40. Acheson, E. D.: "Educational Consequences. In Great Britain," in The Royal Society of Medicine and the Josiah Macy, Jr. Foundation: *The Greater Medical Profession.* The Foundation, New York, 1973, p. 192.

41. Lippard, Vernon W.: "Introduction," in The Royal Society of Medicine and the Josiah Macy, Jr. Foundation: *The Greater Medical Profession.* The Foundation, New York, 1973, p. ix.

42. Malleson, Andrew: *op. cit.*

43. Knowles, John: Public address, 1971.

44. Bernard, Claude: *Introduction to the Study of Experimental Medicine* (trans. by Henry C. Greene). Macmillan Publishing Co., Inc., New York, 1927.

45. US Department of Commerce, Bureau of the Census: *op. cit.,* p. 59.

46. Dublin, Louis I.: *op. cit.,* p. 392.

47. *The VD Crisis. Proceedings of the International Venereal Disease Symposium, St. Louis, Mo., 1971.* Pfizer Laboratories Division, Pfizer, Inc., New York, 1971, p. 8.

48. *Ibid.,* p. 13.

49. *Ibid.,* pp. 15, 75.

50. Hughes, Charles C., and Hunter, John M.: "Disease and 'Development' in Africa," in Drietzel, Hans Peter (ed.): *The Social Organization of Health.* Macmillan Publishing Co., Inc., New York, 1971, p. 151.

51. US Department of Commerce, Bureau of the Census: *op. cit.,* p. 63.

52. Meglen, Marie C.: "A Prototype of Health Services for Quality of Life in a Rural County," *Bull. Am. Coll. Nurse-Midwives,* **17:**103, (No. 4) 1972.

53. US Department of Commerce, Bureau of the Census: *op. cit.,* p. 63.

54. "Underdevelopment in the U.S.," *Sci. Am.,* **227:**45, (Aug.) 1972.

55. Wilson, Patience: "Iron-deficiency Anemia," *Am. J. Nurs.,* **72:**502, (Mar.) 1972.

56. Cravioto, Joaquin: "Nutritional Deficiencies and Mental Performance in Childhood," in Glass, David C. (ed.): *Environmental Influences.* Rockefeller University Press and Russell Sage Foundation, New York, 1968, p. 23.

57. Laing, R. D.: *The Politics of Experience.* Ballantine Books, New York, 1967, p. I (Introduction), p. 28.

58. National Commission on Marihuana and Drug Abuse: *Drug Use in America: Problem in Perspective. Second Report.* US Government Printing Office, Washington, D.C., 1973, p. 194.

59. Kessel, N., and Grossman, G.: "Suicide in Alcoholics," *Br. Med. J.,* **2:**1671, 1971.

60. Campbell, E. O'F.: "Alcohol Involvement in Fatal Motor Vehicle Accidents," *Mod. Med. Can.,* **26:**7, (Nov. 7) 1971.

61. Somers, Anne R.: *op. cit.,* p. 19.

62. Menninger, Karl: *The Crime of Punishment.* Viking Press, New York, 1960.

63. Canada, Department of the Solicitor General: *Health Care Services in the Canadian Penitentiary Service.* The Department, Ottawa, May 1972 (Report No. 35).

64. American Medical Association: *Medical Care in U.S. Jails—A 1972 AMA Survey.* The Association, Chicago, 1973.
65. Mitford, Jessica: *Kind and Usual Punishment.* Alfred A. Knopf, New York, 1973.
66. May, Rollo: *Power and Innocence. A Search for the Sources of Violence.* W. W. Norton & Co., New York, 1972.
67. Gentry, J. T., et al.: "Provision of Mental Health Services by Community Hospitals and Health Departments, A Comparative Analysis," *Am. J. Public Health,* **63:**863, (Oct.) 1973.
68. Carini, Esta, et al.: *The Mentally Ill in Connecticut: Changing Patterns of Care and the Evolution of Psychiatric Nursing, 1636–1972.* Connecticut Department of Mental Health, Hartford, 1974, p. 518.
69. "Mental Patients' Rights Guaranteed in Jersey Under Law," *Am. J. Nurs.,* **75:**1210, (July) 1975.
70. Goffman, Erving: *Asylums. Essays on the Social Situation of Mental Patients and Other Inmates.* Doubleday Anchor Books, New York, 1961.
71. Malleson, Andrew: *op. cit.*
72. Bennett, Douglas H.: "Mental Disorders. In Great Britain," in The Royal Society of Medicine and the Josiah Macy, Jr. Foundation: *The Greater Medical Profession.* The Foundation, New York, 1973.
73. Malleson, Andrew: *op. cit.*
74. Januska, Charlotte, et al.: "Development of a Family Nurse Practitioner Curriculum," *Nurs. Outlook,* **22:**103, (Feb.) 1974.
75. American Nurses' Association: *Statement on the Essential Elements of a Health Care System.* The Association, Kansas City, Mo., 1971.
76. US Department of Health, Education, and Welfare, Social Security Administration: *op. cit.*
77. Reid, J. J. A.: "Preventive Medicine. In Great Britain," in The Royal Society of Medicine and the Josiah Macy, Jr. Foundation: *The Greater Medical Profession.* The Foundation, New York, 1973, p. 119.
78. Lippard, Vernon W.: *op. cit.,* p. 92.
79. Godber, George: "Manpower Problems on Either Side of the Atlantic," in The Royal Society of Medicine and the Josiah Macy, Jr. Foundation: *The Greater Medical Profession.* The Foundation, New York, 1973, p. 29.
80. Dollery, Colin T.: "Prologue," in The Royal Society of Medicine and the Josiah Macy, Jr. Foundation: *The Greater Medical Profession.* The Foundation, New York, 1973, p. 10.
81. Skeet, Muriel: "Roles, Accountability, and Leadership," in The Royal Society of Medicine and the Josiah Macy, Jr. Foundation: *The Greater Medical Profession.* The Foundation, New York, 1973, p. 141.
82. Pellegrino, Edmund D.: "Hunterdon—Ideas Before Their Time," in a Symposium *Twenty Years After,* sponsored by Hunterdon Medical Center and Princeton University at Woodrow Wilson High School, Princeton, N.J., 1973.
83. Malleson, Andrew: *op. cit.,* p. 207.
84. Somers, Anne R.: *op. cit.*
85. Harris, Richard: *A Sacred Trust.* The New American Library, New York, 1966; Pelican Books, Inc., New York, 1969.
86. Garfield, Sidney R.: "The Delivery of Medical Care," *Sci. Am.,* **225:**15, (Apr.) 1970.
87. Burns, Eveline M.: "Health Insurance: Not if, or When, but What Kind," *Am. J. Public Health,* **61:**2164, (Nov.) 1971.
88. Rosen, George: *A History of Public Health,* MD Publications, New York, 1958.
89. Hanlon, John J.: *Public Health Administration and Practice,* 6th ed. C. V. Mosby Co., St. Louis, 1974, p. 8.
90. Kilbourne, Edwin D., and Smillie, Wilson G. (eds.): *Human Ecology and Public Health,* 4th ed. Macmillan Publishing Co., Inc., New York, 1969, p. 109.
91. Falk, I. S.: "Medical Care: Its Social and Organizational Aspects," *N. Engl J. Med.,* **270:**22, (Jan. 2) 1964.
92. *Health Is a Community Affair. Report of the National Commission on Community Health Services.* Harvard University Press, Cambridge, Mass., 1967, p. 196.
93. Scott, Jessie M.: "Opening Remarks," in US Department of Health, Education, and Welfare, Division of Nursing: *Redesigning Nursing Education for Public Health.* Report of the Conference, May 23–25, 1973. The Department, Bethesda, Md., 1973, p. 28 (DHEW Pub. No. [HRA] 75–75).
94. Storlie, Frances: *Nursing and the Social Conscience.* Appleton-Century-Crofts, New York, 1970.
95. "Nurses and Nursing's Issues—A Round-Table Discussion," *Am. J. Nurs.,* **75:**1848, (Oct.) 1975.
96. Hanlon, John J.: *op. cit.,* pp. 293, 310.
97. Stebbins, Ernest L.: "International Health Organization," in Sartwell, Philip E. (ed.): *Maxcy-Rosenau Preventive Medicine and Public Health,* 9th ed. Appleton-Century-Crofts, New York, 1965, p. 1036.
98. World Health Organization: *Basic Documents,* 23rd ed. The Organization, Geneva, 1973, p. 143.
99. US Department of Commerce, Bureau of the Census: *op. cit.,* p. 865.
100. World Health Organization: *Album.* The Organization, Geneva, 1966, p. 32.
101. Thorp, Willard L.: "New International Programs in Public Health," *Am. J. Public Health,* **40:**1479, (Dec.) 1950.
102. *US Government Organization Manual, 1975/1976.* Office of the Federal Register, National Archives and Records Service, General Services Administration, Washington, D.C., May 1, 1975.
103. *The American Nurse,* **4:**1, (May–June)

1972. (Newspaper published by the American Nurses' Association.)

104. *US Government Organization Manual, 1975/1976, op. cit.,* p. 234.

105. "HEW Changes Causing Some Anxiety Among Agencies," *Am. J. Nurs.,* **73:**1139, (July) 1973.

106. Donnell, H. Denny, Jr.: Personal communication, Sept. 15, 1972.

107. Hanlon, John J.: *op. cit.,* p. 295.

108. McKissick, William L.: "Health-Policy Directions for the 1970's," *N. Engl. J. Med.,* **282:**1343, (June 11) 1970.

109. US Department of Health, Education, and Welfare: *Fact Book on Regional Medical Programs.* US Government Printing Office, Washington, D.C., Aug. 1971.

110. Castle, C. Hilmon: "The Regional Medical Program: The Unicentral (Rural) Region," *Med. Clin. North Am.,* **54:**19, (Jan.) 1970.

111. Paul, Oglesby: "The Regional Medical Program: The Multicentral (Urban) Area," *Med. Clin. North Am.,* **54:**29, (Jan.) 1970.

112. Komaroff, Anthony L.: "Regional Medical Programs in Search of a Mission," *N. Engl. J. Med.,* **284:**758, (Apr. 8) 1971.

113. Conley, Veronica L., and Olson, Stanley W.: "Regional Medical Programs," *Am. J. Nurs.,* **68:**1916, (Sept.) 1968.

114. Craytor, Josephine K.: "The Nurse in the Regional Medical Program," in *ANA Regional Clinical Conferences, 1967.* Appleton-Century-Crofts, New York, 1968, p. 12.

115. Olendzki, Margaret C.: "Concerns of the Consumer," in US Department of Health, Education, and Welfare, Division of Nursing: *Redesigning Nursing Education for Public Health.* Report of the Conference, May 23–25, 1973. The Department, Bethesda, Md., 1973, p. 77 (DHEW Pub. No. [HRA] 75–75).

116. Prock, Valencia N.: "Implications of Change for Nursing Practice and Education," in US Department of Health, Education, and Welfare, Division of Nursing: *Redesigning Nursing Education for Public Health.* Report of the Conference, May 23–25, 1973. The Department, Bethesda, Md., 1973, p. 84 (DHEW Pub. No. [HRA] 75–75).

117. Malleson, Andrew: *op. cit.*

118. Hanlon, John J.: *op. cit.,* p. 297.

119. National Health Council: *Voluntaryism and Health. The Role of the National Voluntary Health Agency.* The Council, New York, 1962, p. i.

120. Hanlon, John J.: *op. cit.,* p. 310.

121. Gunn, Selskar M., and Platt, Philip S.: *Voluntary Health Agencies.* Ronald Press, New York, 1945, p. 302.

122. Hamlin, Robert H.: *Voluntary Health and Welfare Agencies in the United States.* Schoolmasters' Press, New York, 1961, p. 34.

123. American Medical Association: *American Medical Association Directory of National Voluntary Health Organizations,* 1971 ed. The Association, Chicago, 1971.

124. Abdellah, Faye G.: "Nursing and Health Care in the U.S.S.R.," *Am. J. Nurs.,* **73:**2096, (Dec.) 1973.

125. American Hospital Association: *Guide to the Health Care Field.* The Association, Chicago, 1973 (published annually).

126. Mendelson, Mary Adelaide: *Tender Loving Greed.* Alfred A. Knopf, New York, 1974, p. 88.

127. American Hospital Association: *op. cit.,* p. 7.

128. *Ibid.*

129. *Ibid.*

130. *Ibid.*

131. Porterfield, John D.: "Nursing Home Accreditation," *Nurs. Homes,* **22:**27, (June) 1973.

132. Holle, Henry A.: "The Meaning of Accreditation," in Jacobs, H. L., and Morris, Woodrow W. (eds.): *Nursing and Retirement Home Administration.* Iowa State University, Ames, 1966, p. 267.

133. Donabedian, Avedis: "Promoting Quality Through Evaluating the Process of Patient Care," *Med. Care,* **6:**181, 1968.

134. Payne, Beverly C.: *Quality Assurance of Medical Care.* Regional Medical Programs Service, US Department of Health, Education, and Welfare, Washington, D.C., Feb. 1973.

135. Williamson, John W.: "Evaluating Quality of Patient Care—A Strategy Relating to Outcome and Process Assessment," *J.A.M.A.,* **218:**565, (Oct.) 1971.

136. Bullough, Bonnie: "The Medicare-Medicaid Amendments," *Am. J. Nurs.,* **73:**1926, (Nov.) 1973.

137. Sanozaro, Paul J., et al.: "Research and Development in Quality Assurance; The Experimental Medical Care Review Organization Program," *N. Engl. J. Med.,* **287:**1125, (Nov. 30) 1972.

138. Parrish, H. M.: "Nursing Home—Academic Health Center Affiliation Is Needed," *Mod. Nurs. Home,* **30:**10, (June) 1973.

139. Erickson, J.: "Does ANHA's Peer Review Concept Work? Yes," *J. Mod. Nurs. Home,* **30:**28, (Apr.) 1973.

140. Freeman, Ruth B.: *Community Health Nursing Practice.* W. B. Saunders Co., Philadelphia, 1970, pp. 343, 355, 360.

141. Keywood, O.: "The Registration and Inspection of Nursing Homes," *Nurs. Times,* **69:**544, (Apr.) 1973.

142. Kelliher, Rita P., and Shaughnessy, Mary E.: *Fact-Finding Survey of Massachusetts Nursing Homes.* Boston College School of Nursing, Boston, 1963.

143. McKnight, Eleanor M.: *Nursing Home Research Study. Quantitative Measurement of Nursing Services.* US Department of Health, Education, and Welfare, Public Health Service, National Institutes of Health, Washington, D.C., 1970.

144. Townsend, Claire: *Old Age: The Last Segregation.* Grossman Publishers, New York, 1971.
145. *Ibid.,* p. 130.
146. Jaeger, Dorothea, and Simmons, Leo W.: *The Aged Ill: Coping with Problems in Geriatric Care.* Appleton-Century-Crofts, New York, 1970.
147. *Long-Term Care Facility Improvement Study; Interim Report.* US Public Health Service, Office of Nursing Home Affairs, Rockville, Md., 1975.
148. Mendelson, Mary Adelaide: *op. cit.*
149. *Ibid.,* p. 36.
150. *Ibid.,* p. 34.
151. *Ibid.,* p. 30.
152. *Ibid.*
153. Callender, Marie: "Washington Creates a Climate for Responsible Change in the Nation's Nursing Homes," *Nurs. Homes,* 21:7, (Nov.) 1972.
154. ———: "National Approach to Long-Term Care," *Nurs. Outlook,* 21:22, (Jan.) 1973.
154a. US House of Representatives, Select Committee on Aging, Subcommittee on Health and Long-term Care: *New Perspectives in Health Care for Older Americans. (Recommendations and Policy Directions of the Subcommittee on Health and Long-Term Care.)* US Government Printing Office, Washington, D.C., Jan. 1976 (Pub. No. 66–559).
154b. US House of Representatives, Select Committee on Aging, Subcommittee on Health and Long-Term Care: *Long-Term Care, Facility Improvement Study; Interim Report.* US Government Printing Office, Washington, D.C., Jan. 1976.
155. "ANA and Senate Subcommittee Air Long-Term Care Recommendations," *Am. J. Nurs.,* 75:921, (June) 1975.
156. Quinn, Nancy, and Somers, Anne R.: "The Patient's Bill of Rights. A Significant Aspect of the Consumer Revolution," *Nurs. Outlook,* 22:240, (Apr.) 1974.
157. National League for Nursing, Committee to Draft a Patient's Bill of Rights: *What People Can Expect of Modern Nursing Service.* The League, New York, 1959.
158. American Hospital Association: *Implementation and Information Program for a Patient's Bill of Rights.* The Association, Chicago, 1973.
158a. "Council of Europe Asked to Adopt a European Declaration of the Rights of the Sick," *Int. Nurs. Rev.,* 22:16, (Nov. 1) 1975.
159. US Department of Health, Education, and Welfare, Secretary's Commission on Medical Malpractice: *Medical Malpractice.* US Government Printing Office, Washington, D.C., 1973 (DHEW Pub. No. [OS] 73–88).
160. Georgopoulos, Basil S.: "The Hospital as an Organization and Problem-Solving System," in Georgopoulos, Basil S.: (ed.): *Organization Research on Health Institutions.* Institute for Social Research, University of Michigan, Ann Arbor, 1972, p. 9.
161. US Department of Health, Education and Welfare: *Report on Licensure and Related Health Personnel Credentialing.* US Government Printing Office, Washington, D.C., June 1971, pp. 65, 77.
162. Agree, B. C.: "The Threat of Institutional Licensure," *Am. J. Nurs.,* 73:1758, (Oct.) 1973.
163. Forni, P. R.: "Trends in Licensure and Certification," *J. Nurs. Admin.,.* 3:17, (Sept.–Oct.) 1973.
164. Kelly, Lucie Young: "Institutional Licensure," *Nurs. Outlook,* 21:566, (Sept.) 1973.
165. Miike, L. H.: "What Is Institutional Licensure?" *Superv. Nurse,* 4:39, (Aug.) 1973.
166. Pennell, Maryland Y., et al.: *Accreditation and Certification in Relation to Allied Health Manpower.* US Department of Health, Education, and Welfare, Bureau of Health Manpower, Bethesda, Md., 1971.
167. Hagen, C.: "HEW Requests 2 Year Moratorium on Licensing of Health Professionals," *ASHA,* 13:731, (Dec.) 1971.
168. Roemer, R.: *Legal Regulations of Modern Nursing Practice.* National League for Nursing, New York, 1973.
169. Schrader, E. S.: "Nurses Battle Institutional Licensure" (editorial), *AORN J.,* 18:1089, (Dec.) 1973.
170. US Department of Commerce, Bureau of the Census: *op. cit.,* pp. 71, 81.
171. Cancer Care, Inc.: *The Impact, Costs, and Consequences of Catastrophic Illness on Patients and Families.* National Cancer Foundation, New York, 1973.
172. US Department of Health, Education, and Welfare: *Emergency Medical Services Communications Systems.* US Government Printing Office, Washington, D.C., 1972, pp. 32–36.
173. Henderson, Cynthia, et al.: "Can Nursing Care Hasten Recovery?" *Am. J. Nurs.,* 64:80, (June) 1964.
174. "More Care, Fewer Patients," *Med. World News,* Nov. 20, 1964.
175. Hall, Lydia E.: "A Center for Nursing," *Nurs. Outlook,* 11:806, (Nov.) 1963.
176. ———: "Nursing—What Is It?" *Can. Nurse,* 60:150, (Feb.) 1964.
177. ———, and Alfano, Genrose: "Incapacitation or Rehabilitation?" *Am. J. Nurs.,* 64:C20, (Nov.) 1964 (Special Supplement).
178. ———: "Another View of Nursing Care and Quality," in Straub, Kathleen M., and Parker, Kitty S. (eds.): *Continuity of Patient Care: The Role of Nursing.* Catholic University of America Press, Washington, D.C., 1966, p. 47.
179. Alfano, Genrose: "Whom Do You Care For?" in *ANA Clinical Conferences, 1969.* Appleton-Century-Crofts, New York, 1970.
180. ———: *Long-Term Effects of an Experimental Nursing Process.* (Research in progress at Montefiore Hospital and Medical Center, New York City, 1972.)
181. Hospice, Inc.: (Notices and Reports.) New Haven, Conn., 1974.

182. Milio, Nancy: *9226 Kercheval. The Store-front That Did Not Burn.* University of Michigan Press, Ann Arbor, 1971.

Additional Suggested Reading

Aime, D. J.: "Philosophy and Structure of a Day Treatment Center," *J. Psychiatr. Nurs.,* **11:**27, (July–Aug.) 1973.

American Public Health Association: "The State Public Health Agency. Policy Statement," *Am. J. Public Health,* **55:**2011, (Dec.) 1965.

――――: "The Local Health Department—Services and Responsibilities. Policy Statement," *Am. J. Public Health,* **54:**131, (Jan.) 1964.

Arnstein, Sherry: "A Ladder of Citizen Participation," *J. Am. Inst. Planners,* **35:**7, (July) 1969.

Bean, Margaret A.: "The Nurse-Midwife at Work," *Am. J. Nurs.,* **71:**949, (May) 1971.

Begg, N. C.: *The Plunket Society of New Zealand.* The Society, Dunedin, 1968.

Bonn, Ethel M.: "Day Care: A Vital Link in Services," *Hosp. Community Psychiatry,* **23:**41, (May) 1972.

Brown, Esther Lucile: *Nursing Reconsidered: A Study of Change,* Parts 1 and 2. J. B. Lippincott Co., Philadelphia, 1971.

Changing Patterns of Nursing Practice. Contemporary Nursing Series. American Journal of Nursing Co., New York, 1971.

Coleman, Jules V.: "Research in Walk-in Psychiatric Services in General Hospitals," *Am. J. Psychiatry,* **124:**1668, (June) 1968.

Community Health Centre in Canada. Report of the Community Health Center Project to the Health Ministers. Information Canada, Ottawa, 1972.

Dickey, Frank G.: "Accreditation—What About the Public?" *Nurs. Outlook,* **19:**668, (Oct.) 1971.

Duhl, Leonard J.: "Health—2000 A.D.," *Am. J. Public Health,* **59:**1809, (Oct.) 1969.

Evans, Frances M. C.: *The Role of the Nurse in Community Health.* Macmillan Publishing Co., Inc., New York, 1968.

Freidson, Eliot: *Profession of Medicine—A Study of the Sociology of Applied Knowledge.* Dodd, Mead & Co., New York, 1973.

Graber, J. B.: "Preventing Dependency: Protective Health Services," *Am. J. Public Health,* **59:**1413, (Aug.) 1969.

Hargreaves, Anna, et al.: "A Day Hospital for Psychiatric Patients," *Am. J. Nurs.,* **62:**80, (Sept.) 1962.

Harris, David, et al.: "Nurse Midwifery in New York City," *Am. J. Public Health,* **61:**64, (Jan.) 1971.

Hauser, Philip M.: "The Census of 1970," *Sci. Am.,* **225:**17, (July) 1971.

Herman, Harold, and McKay, Mary Elizabeth: *Community Health Services.* Municipal Management Series. International City Managers' Association, Washington, D.C., 1968.

Hinkle, L. E., Jr., and Wolf, H. G.: "Health and the Social Environment: Experimental Investigations," in Leighton, A. H., et al. (eds.): *Ex-plorations in Social Psychiatry.* Basic Books, Inc., New York, 1957.

Kaufman, Edward, and Klagsbrun, Samuel: "An Emergency Room Changes (Impact of Psychiatric Walk-in Clinic on Emergency Room of General Hospital)," *Dis. Nerv. Syst.,* **33:**231, (Apr.) 1972.

Kidd, C. B., and Zorbas, Anthony: "From Out-Group to In-Group. The Introduction of a Psychiatric Unit to a General Hospital," *Int. J. Soc. Psychiatry,* **17:**101, (Spring) 1971.

Kirkpatric, W. J.: "The In and Out Nurse: Thoughts on the Role of the Psychiatric Nurse in the Community and the Preparation Required," *J. Nurs. Studies,* **4:**225, (Aug.) 1967.

Knollmueller, Ruth N.: "A Column of Health," *Nurs. Outlook,* **21:**457, (July) 1973.

Krieger, George: "Issues Facing Federal Mental Hospitals in the Seventies," *Hosp. Community Psychiatry,* **23:**43, (Aug.) 1972.

Kudo, Yoshio: "Psychiatric Service in the General Hospital in Japan," *Int. J. Soc. Psychiatry,* **16:**216, (Summer) 1970.

Lee, Philip R.: "Role of the Federal Government in Health and Medical Affairs," *N. Engl. J. Med.,* **279:**1139, (Nov. 21) 1968.

Porterfield, J. D.: "Accreditation Problems. Medical Care Evaluation: The JCAH System," *Hospitals,* **47:**26, (Oct. 16) 1973.

Read, Margaret: *Culture, Health, and Disease.* Tavistock Publications, London; J. B. Lippincott Co., Philadelphia, 1966.

Rice, Dorothy P., and Cooper, Barbara S.: "The Economic Value of Human Life," *Am. J. Public Health,* **57:**1954, (Nov.) 1967.

Rosen, George: "Historical Trends and Future Prospects in Public Health," in McLachlan, G., and McKeown, T. (eds.): *Medical History and Medical Care.* Oxford University Press, London, 1971.

Sidel, R.: "The Role of Revolutionary Optimism in the Treatment of Mental Illness in the People's Republic of China," *Am. J. Orthopsychiatry,* **43:**732, (Oct.) 1973.

Szasz, T.: *The Myth of Mental Illness.* Harper & Row, New York, 1961.

Tinkham, C. W., and Voorhies, E. F.: *Community Health Nursing, Evolution and Process.* Appleton-Century-Crofts, New York, 1972.

US Congress, Committee on Ways and Means: *Basic Facts on the Health Industry.* US Government Printing Office, Washington, D.C., 1972.

Volker, J. F.: "New Commission for Study of Accreditation of Selected Health Education Programs," *J.A.M.A.,* **218:**238, (Oct. 11) 1971.

Weiss, James M. A. (ed.): *Nurses, Patients, and Social Systems.* University of Missouri Press, Columbia, 1969.

World Health Organization: *Planning of Public Health Services.* The Organization, Geneva, 1961 (Tech. Report Series No. 215).

――――: *Vector Control in International Health.* The Organization, Geneva, 1972.

Patience Wilson
Virginia Henderson

CHAPTER 3

Settings in Which the Nurse Functions

1. INTRODUCTION

Nursing as a Constant Factor in Health Services. In most countries it is rare to find a health service that doesn't involve the *nurse*. Care of the sick, the injured, and the helpless has always involved *nursing,* although families, friends, religious or military personnel, and physicians may have given this care. In 1900 physicians outnumbered "trained" nurses and were the most constant factor in health service; now nurses and midwives outnumber them in most countries. E. D. Acheson, speaking for Great Britain, said:

It is a fact . . . that doctors now constitute only a small minority of the skilled personnel who work together in the health service. Medical and dental staff are small fry, numerically, compared with nurses, midwives, and the professional and technical health service staff; they account for approximately 15 per cent of the total. . . . If such an analysis had been carried out in 1858, the year of the first medical act that delineated the roles, responsibilities, and education of the "smaller medical profession," doctors and dentists, with the help of a few apothecaries, would have been shown to be virtually alone in the field.*

Figures for other European countries, especially Scandinavia, the United States and Canada, Australia, and New Zealand now show a

* Acheson, E. D.: "Educational Consequences. In Great Britain," in the Royal Society of Medicine, and the Josiah Macy, Jr. Foundation: *The Greater Medical Profession.* The Foundation, New York, 1973, p. 192.

comparable preponderance of nurses among health workers. Feldshers in the USSR are also very numerous, as are barefoot and Red Guard doctors in China. They are to be found in these countries in some positions that would be filled by nurses elsewhere. In this chapter, no attempt is made to discuss the settings in which nurses function country by country. Throughout this book, the emphasis is on nursing practice in the United States, with occasional comparisons with Canada, the British Commonwealth, and other parts of the world. Figure 3-1 shows for the 1970s the predominance of nurses (and nurse-midwives) in "The Greater Medical Profession" in Great Britain.*

* From such accounts as the writer has found, nurses in the Union of Soviet Socialist Republics and the People's Republic of China have a role that is different from their roles in the United States, Canada, and the British Commonwealth. Feldshers in Russia, and "assistant doctors" ("Red Guard," "barefoot," and other) who are graduates of "secondary medical schools," outnumber "nurses" and "first-level" doctors so they are possibly the most constant factor in health services. It is believed, however, that in both countries where open curricula, continuing education, and upgrading of all health workers is part of the system the proportion of assistant doctors to first-level doctors and nurses may be reduced. Victor and Ruth Sidel reported in 1973 that in Shunyi County, with 450,000 members of 19 communes, there were 676 "medical workers (excluding barefoot doctors and health workers) . . . 312 doctors, sixty-five nurses and 299 pharmacists and technicians." In the Shanghai countryside there were 4500 barefoot doctors and 29,000 peasant health workers. (Sidel, Victor W., and Sidel, Ruth: *Serve the People. Observations on Medicine in the People's Republic of China.* Beacon Press, Boston, 1973, pp. 79, 95.)

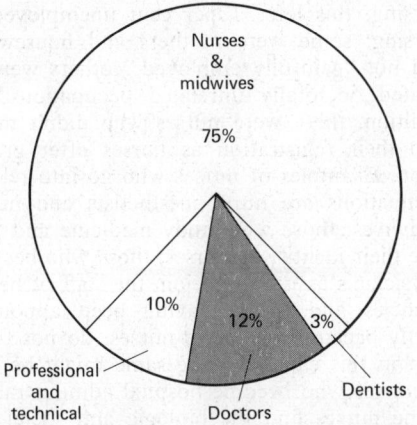

Figure 3-1. "The Greater Medical Profession" of Great Britain. (Acheson, E. D.: "Educational Consequences. In Great Britain," in the Royal Society of Medicine and the Josiah Macy, Jr. Foundation: *The Greater Medical Profession*. The Foundation, New York, 1973, p. 192.)

Settings in Which Nurses Are Employed.
Nurses are employed almost anywhere that a health service exists, and it is difficult to make an exhaustive list of settings. Full statistical data in the American Nurses' Association's *Facts About Nursing*[1] are available for eight "fields"; other data come under "other specified field" or "field not stated." The specified fields or settings for the United States are hospital, nursing home, school of nursing, private duty, public health, school nurse, industrial nurse, and office nurse. For Canada the fields are hospital/other institutions (which includes nursing homes), public health agency, occupational health, home care/visiting care agency, community health centre, physicians'/dentists' offices, educational institution, and private practice.[2] While complete data are available only in these fields, nursing in the following additional fields will be discussed: hospices; community health centers and health maintenance type organizations; offices of the private practitioner of nursing; college health services; and jails, prisons, and other correctional institutions. Nursing in ships, planes, and space transport operations and in health agencies and organizations have brief mention. Another way to classify nursing is according to functions nurses perform, or positions they hold.*

* It will be noted that much information on nurses and nursing has been attributed to either the ANA publication *Facts About Nursing 72–73* or *Facts About Nursing 74–75*. The reason for this is that the 74–75 publication does not in every case give or update the information in the 72–73 edition. *Countdown*

Specialization of Nursing According to Function or Position. After graduation from a school of nursing and taking a licensing examination, nurses may elect to (1) practice nursing; (2) administer a nursing service, agency, or organization; (3) teach nursing; (4) act as a consultant, which is perhaps a form of teaching; (5) conduct research; or (6) write about nursing. Many nurses go beyond the basic program in preparation for any of these functions and, as discussed in Chapter 1, continuing education may become a requirement for annual nurse registration, in which case nurses functioning in any capacity will continue to study. It is not feasible in this book to give data on the numbers of nurses according to function or position. As might be expected, registered nurses in practice far exceed those performing any other function.

Specialization According to Clinical Entity. Either by study, years of experience, or both, nurses specialize in the care of age groups, as, for example, child care (pediatrics) or care of the aged (geriatrics). Even with such specialties, there may be subspecialties such as the care of infants or adolescents. Nurses specialize in maternal care, becoming obstetrical nursing specialists or assuming more responsibility and becoming nurse-midwives; others elect to specialize in the care of patients treated medically or surgically or combine these to become medical-surgical nursing specialists. Within surgery and medicine there are many subspecialties. Nurses, for example, become neurosurgical, orthopedic, urologic or gynecologic, ocular, otologic, or dermatologic nurses; they may specialize in the care of patients with one type of surgery and be, for example, an "ostomy nurse"; they may elect to care for patients with a disease, as, for example, cancer (oncologic nursing), heart disease (cardiac nursing), arthritis, tuberculosis, or a group of related diseases such as infections (communicable disease) or metabolic disorders. Surgical nursing can be divided into subspecialties according to the stage of surgery—some nurses electing to care for patients before and during recovery from surgery, others to work with surgeons during the operation, and still others to care for patients in the immediate postanesthesia period in the "recovery room." Surgical nurses may study anesthesia and become nurse-anesthetists. Medical nursing could be divided into almost the same subspecialties. Many nurses elect to work in intensive care units, others in short-term acute care hospital units,

1974 was the last compendium on Canadian nursing available to the writer in 1976. However, the Canadian Nurses' Association staff has given us late data in some cases.

and others in ambulatory and long-term care institutions and health agencies.

Nursing care of those with behavior disorders comprises one of the major clinical specialties—psychiatric nursing. Nursing the mentally defective is a related (and neglected) specialty. Psychiatric nurse specialists may be divided into those who care for children and those who care for adults and, as in obstetric nursing, some psychiatric nurses elect to assume more responsibility and after certain programs of graduate study call themselves "nurse therapists." Psychiatric nurses in some institutions and agencies spend their time working with other nurses on behavioral problems of patients in nonpsychiatric settings. They are often called "liaison nurses." Lisa Robinson entitles a 1974 text *Liaison Nursing: Psychological Approach to Patient Care.* (F. A. Davis Company, Philadelphia, 1974).

Organizations for Specialists. As pointed out in Chapter 1, every country belonging to the International Council of Nurses must have an official national nursing organization composed of registered nurses whose preparation conforms to a standard articulated by the ICN.[3] In the United States, the official nursing organization is the American Nurses' Association. To provide for the needs of nurses with special interests, national nursing organizations provide departments, divisions, councils, or commissions. Their character and titles vary from one era to another as specialties in nursing evolve and disappear or change in character. University-sponsored postbasic programs in the first decade of this century prepared graduate nurses to administer or to teach; they might have emphasized working in a setting such as the community ("public health") or in schools or industry. In some countries, the emphasis may still be on role and function, or the setting in which service is given; in the United States, the current emphasis is on preparation for nursing in a clinical field. Because divisions within the American Nurses' Association and the National League for Nursing (and their state and local counterparts) have not, perhaps, adequately supplied the needs of specialists, many groups have formed national, state, and even local nursing organizations around special interests. (See the Appendix for a list of such organizations.) Any published list of nursing organizations in the United States is incomplete because they are proliferating so rapidly. Readers who are interested in any nursing specialty should consult indexes to current periodical literature.

Nursing in Related Fields. In the United States, the 1972 inventory of registered nurses shows that 69 per cent were employed in nursing; this left 31 per cent unemployed in nursing; some were mothers and housewives and not "gainfully employed," others were in related or totally unrelated occupations.[4] In addition, there were nurses who didn't maintain their registration as nurses after graduation. Examples of nurses who go into related occupations are nurse-anesthetists and nurse-midwives; those who study medicine and thus lose their identity as nurses; those who become physician's assistants or join the staff of health agencies and, while having been appointed partly because they were nurses, do not function in this capacity. The same might be said of nurses who become hospital administrators. Some nurses find the biologic and social sciences interesting, get higher degrees in them, and teach or conduct research in the science of their choice. A few nurses have studied law, believing that only through legislation can health conditions be materially improved; others go into local, state, or federal government for the same reason. The multiform careers in nursing cannot be fully discussed in a book of this general nature. Histories of nursing, such as Vern and Bonnie Bullough's text *The Emergence of Modern Nursing,*[5] full-length descriptions of the field of nursing, such as Lucie Young Kelly's *Dimensions of Professional Nursing,*[6] and current articles in nursing journals help inform the public and help students and recent graduates make wise occupational choices. A report on a nurse career study conducted by the National League for Nursing and reported by Lucille Knopf in 1975 might be consulted. Data were collected by a questionnaire answered by almost 6000 respondents.[7] Recent publications of the ANA and the NLN provide accurate data for those making career decisions.

One of the attractions in nursing is the wide range of opportunities it offers. Never have they been more numerous. Rola Pratt, chief nursing officer in the Federal Ministry of Health, Nigeria, writes about "new horizons for nursing" in an article, "The Challenge of Nursing in Developing Countries." She urges creativeness and quotes the well-known poem "New occasions teach new duties/Time makes ancient good uncouth/She must still be up and onward/Who would keep abreast of truth." *

While it is impractical in this chapter to attempt a discussion of the established and emerging specialties in nursing, the major settings in which nurses are employed are described briefly in the following pages. It should

---

* Pratt, Rola: "The Challenge of Nursing in Developing Countries," *Int. Nurs. Rev.,* **17:**158, (No. 2) 1970.

be borne in mind that nurses may practice, administer, teach, or conduct research in most of these settings, and that in many of them clinical specialists may be employed.

An attempt will be made in this chapter to answer the following questions: (1) Do nurses work in this setting all over the world, and what proportion of American and Canadian nurses are found in it? (2) What is the setting like—what are the facilities and resources? (3) What functions do nurses perform in the setting? (4) Have standards of nursing service been established for it? (5) What are the difficulties and the special satisfactions and rewards of working in the setting?

2. HOSPITALS

Employment of Nurses in Hospitals. In Great Britain, Canada, Australia, New Zealand, Scandinavia, the United States, and other countries, there are more nurses employed in hospitals than in any other setting. There are few hospitals in *any* country that do not employ nurses. Some exceptions will be mentioned later, as, for example, hospitals in United States federal prisons that, by and large, employ only physician's assistants, and some military hospitals that may be staffed by nonnurse medical personnel.

Of the 857,000 employed professional registered nurses in the United States in 1974, 529,677 (62 per cent) were employed in hospitals.[1] (In 1972, 8646 of these were men nurses.[1a]) Of the 128,675 professional nurses registered in Canada and employed in nursing in 1974, 107,769 (84 per cent) were employed in hospitals.[2] Data on employment of nonprofessional nursing personnel show the same concentration in hospitals and other institutions. Of the 427,000 licensed practical nurses in the United States in 1972, 260,000 were employed in hospitals; of the estimated 900,000 nurses' aides, orderlies, and attendants, 565,000 were employed in hospitals.[3] This means there were, in 1972, about one-third more nonprofessional than professional nursing personnel in hospitals.

Nature of the Hospital. The words *hospice, hotel,* and *hospital* are derived from the same root—*hospes*—which means host. Hospitals have in different countries and different eras had different functions. They have sheltered the indigent and homeless as well as the sick. In this age, hospitals chiefly provide care and treatment for the sick. In addition, they provide society with a practice field where a variety of workers learn the medical arts and sciences; a place where students, patients, and workers can learn to prevent disease and promote health; and a setting for research.

In Chapter 2, it was pointed out that hospitals may be an integral part of a total health or medical service for the residents of a given geographic area, as is the case, for example, in Great Britain, the USSR, and mainland China. In some countries, hospitals may be autonomous units, as is ordinarily the case in the United States.* However, even here, according to its ownership or control, a hospital's services may be coordinated with those in other types of health and welfare agencies in a given area or with the services of other hospitals having the same ownership and control. To illustrate the first case, a municipal hospital may be required to admit its sick indigent and to conduct certain laboratory tests for and report births, deaths, and morbidity data to the county or city health department, or it may purchase certain supplies from factories operated under the municipal prison system; in the second case, United States Veterans, Army, Navy, or Air Force hospitals coordinate their programs to facilitate transfer of patients, personnel, records, equipment, and supplies from one institution to another throughout the country.

Most hospitals in the United States have outpatient departments, clinics, and emergency rooms offering a variety of services to both well and sick. The obstetric clinic, for example, serves well parents who want to be prepared for the prenatal, natal, and postnatal periods, including the care of their newborn. Many hospitals have well-child clinics. The sick and "worried well," as Sidney Garfield calls them, flock to medical clinics as the cost of a physician's house call rises and as fewer doctors make them.

In Great Britain, private practitioners and the "team" of health workers associated with them, the public health service, and the hospital coordinate their services for a geographical area, as was pointed out in Chapter 2. Discussing the delivery of health care with special

---

* In its pamphlet, *History of the American Hospital Association's Position on Planning,* the Association claims that, in 1912, it recognized the need to avoid duplication of hospitals; during World War II, it appointed a Post War Planning Committee; in 1960, the Board voted to establish a joint committee with the US Public Health Service to "develop principles for areawide health facility planning," and in 1969, it published its *Statement on the Financial Requirements of Health Care Institutions and Services,* which called upon all health care institutions to participate in planning. "Up until this time, [1960] hospitals did their own planning within their own four walls. . . ." Statewide commissions that by 1972 evolved from these efforts to avoid duplication and other abuses are discussed on p. 195.

reference to preventive medicine, J. J. A. Reid makes the following concluding statement which shows the integrated role played by hospitals in Great Britain:

The practice of preventive medicine in Great Britain has undergone substantial change in recent years and is no longer an isolated activity of the public health service. It is increasingly becoming the concern of general practitioners and their primary care teams; *hospital* [italics ours] staffs are likewise involved, particularly in its secondary and tertiary phases. Public health doctors now commonly look upon themselves as being primarily concerned with the provision of help and support for their colleagues in the other two branches of the NHS and thus have been able to make the work of the latter both more efficient and more effective. In less than two years the present public health services, which have evolved over a period of more than a century, will cease to exist; their staffs will join with their general practitioner and hospital colleagues in the administratively unified NHS.

The principle of administrative unification is entirely logical, although the detailed structures of the new service will be the subject of continuing debate. Only through unification will it be possible at all levels, and especially locally, to look synoptically at overall needs and at total resources, and arrive at a sensible order of priorities. Members of the former public health services will have even broader scope to develop their skills within this wider framework than they have had in the past, and although 1974 will bring greater changes to them than to their *hospital* [italics ours] and general practitioner colleagues, they are ready to face the challenge and to make their contribution within the developing discipline of community medicine.*

Recognizing the fragmentation of care in the United States and the desirability of reducing hospitalization to a minimum, numerous hospitals have home care programs, as was noted in Chapter 2. Dating from the 1940s when Martin Cherkasky[5-7] started a program at the Montefiore Hospital in New York City, these programs allow sick patients who wish to go home, either intermittently or permanently, to remain on the hospital's rolls, to rent or borrow hospital equipment, and to be visited by physicians and other categories of hospital personnel who attended them as inpatients. Hospital-based nurses may give care in the home, or patients may be referred to the visiting nurse agency.[8,9] In 1972, the American Hospital Association surveyed 243 nonfederal hospital-administered home care

programs.[10] It found that the services of 12 of the 16 categories of hospital health personnel examined were available to patients, the exceptions being those of occupational therapists, social work assistants, volunteers, and psychiatrists. Hospital-employed and private physicians were most often available: 98 per cent of the programs provided services of registered nurses, 90 per cent provided services of physical therapists, and about this percentage of the programs provided medical supplies to patients. By and large, the programs (82 per cent) were certified by the US Social Security Administration for Medicare payments.

Doctors, nurses, and others in special services within hospitals recognize the economic waste of keeping patients in the hospital until they have no further need for help. Giving the necessary help at home not only reduces the cost of care to the patient but releases hospital beds in specialized units that may be in great demand. Patricia Calleia and John A. Boswick[11] describe a home care nursing program for burn patients in which hospital-based nurses spend half of their time helping patients with home care. Celia Moss Hailperin[12] reports a 5-year demonstration to determine the need for hospital services to the chronically ill child at home; T. T. Friedman and associates[13] in 1964 reported a 5-year experience with a psychiatric home treatment service, and in 1970, C. R. Blagg and associates[14] wrote that training for helping patients with home dialysis was generally recognized.

The dangers and disadvantages of fragmented care and the value of continued care have long been recognized and today go undisputed. In an effort to promote continuity, some visiting nurse services have for decades maintained an office or center in one or more hospitals. During the 1940s in Barry County, Michigan, one physical plant housed all major health agencies for that county, including a hospital and a visiting nurse service.[15] Sharon Taylor[16] described in 1970 an "initiation and development of a hospital-based home health agency" in South Dakota. Claire F. Ryder and associates,[17] reporting a study in 1969 of home health services "past, present, and future," showed that of the 1543 certified * participating agencies in 1966, 79 agencies (5.1 per cent) reported hospital-based home care programs, while in 1969, 173 of the 1543 agencies (7.9 per cent) reported hospital-based home health services.

As health workers from the hospital find themselves serving patients in their homes, it

---

* Reid, J. J. A.: "Delivery of Health Care: Preventive Medicine. In Great Britain," in the Royal Society of Medicine, and the Josiah Macy, Jr. Foundation: *The Greater Medical Profession.* The Foundation, New York, 1973, p. 123.

* Certified by the US Social Security Administration for Medicaid and Medicare payments.

is inevitable that they will see the patient's problems as related to the total family welfare and that their service will grow more and more into a family health service, combining preventive and morbidity aspects. In his 1945 monograph, *Patients Have Families,* Henry B. Richardson,[18] analyzing the effectiveness of the medical service given a family in a big metropolitan hospital, traced a large part of the illness in the mother and daughters to an uncorrected physical condition of the father. His conclusion that patients must be treated as members of the family, or a social unit, now goes unchallenged, although this goal has by no means been reached. Recent works, such as Jan de Hartog's *The Hospital,*[19] Michael Crichton's *Five Patients,*[20] or the study by Raymond S. Duff and August B. Hollingshead, *Sickness and Society,*[21] show how far representative hospitals in the United States come from giving humane family-centered care. Elizabeth Barnes' 1961 report[22] of a study of hospital care in nine countries gave some worldwide data. Actually, there are so many books and articles critical of hospital care that it seems fruitless to mention these few examples. However, in spite of this widespread criticism, the life-saving value of hospitals and society's dependence upon them is generally accepted. As more hospitals in the United States assume responsibility for home care programs and as hospital-employed nurses divide their time between care of inpatients, clinic patients, and home patients, the differences between hospital nursing and public health nursing (community or visiting nursing in the United States and district nursing and health visiting in Great Britain) may disappear. Under such circumstances, all nurses will tend to be versed in the highly developed technical aspects of hospital care and at the same time be able to help people cope with the problems of daily living at home that are imposed by illness.

While hospitals exist primarily as settings in which treatment may be given the sick and wounded, where infants may be born and they and their mothers cared for, hospitals also provide a setting in which physicians, nurses, dietitians, social workers, physical therapists, hospital administrators, and others learn much of what they must know in order to practice their professions. Without hospitals or their equivalents, it would be impossible to give an adequate preparation for almost any type of modern health service.*

As pointed out in Chapter 1, hospitals at one time in some countries owned and operated medical schools. Medical schools are now university based and hospitals offer a practice field for medical students. The majority of professional nursing schools in most countries are still owned and operated by hospitals but gradually they also, like medical schools, are moving into the mainstream of education. For degree-granting nursing programs, hospitals, under contractual arrangements with universities or colleges, offer a practice field for nursing students just as they do for medical students. Regardless of whether hospitals own and operate educational programs, *education of health workers and of patients* is one of the services they offer society. With their laboratory facilities, trained personnel, numbers of patients, accumulation of records, and libraries, hospitals offer health workers opportunities for investigation that are unavailable elsewhere. This *research* is thought to be such an important factor in the successful practice of medicine and in the advancement of medical science that all physicians seek, and are urged to make, some connection with a hospital.

It has been pointed out that there is a trend toward the establishment of close association between the small rural hospitals and research centers and between all hospitals and other community health organizations in order that their personnel may have access to adequate research, and to diagnostic, therapeutic, and library facilities. The free flow of patients and workers to and from these research centers and district hospitals should foster all kinds of medical research.

Types and Numbers of Hospitals. Hospitals in the United States are grouped or classified in a variety of ways as, for example, the following: (1) according to type of service offered; (2) according to ownership and control; and (3) as accredited and nonaccredited hospitals.

Hospitals classified according to service offered fall into two main groups—general hospitals that admit patients with many types of disease or conditions to be treated in a variety of ways, and special hospitals. The latter include the following: maternity; children's; convalescent; chronic; eye, ear, nose, and throat; tuberculosis; orthopedic; skin and cancer; neurologic; and psychiatric hospitals.

Hospitals classified according to control or ownership fall into two main classes—govern-

---

* Since most patients in hospitals are sick, and students in the hospital have little association with well clients, the preventive aspects of health care are relatively neglected. It is likely that in the future students in the health field will spend less time than they now spend in hospitals and more time where preventive medicine is practiced.

mental and nongovernmental. Governmental hospitals are those owned by the federal government, that is, the hospitals of the Army, Navy, or Air Force, the US Public Health Service, the Bureau of Indian Affairs, and the Veterans Administration, and those owned by the state, city, or county governments. Governmental hospitals are sometimes called *public hospitals*. They may offer one or many types of clinical service.

Nongovernmental hospitals are owned by churches, fraternal orders, individuals, or groups of individuals in partnership, corporations, or industries such as mines and railroads. If hospitals depend upon their earnings for support and are organized to make a profit on their services, they are designated as for-profit, or *proprietary,* hospitals. Of the 1,550,-000 hospital beds in the United States in 1972, 57,000 (3.7 per cent) were in proprietary hospitals.[23] These hospitals are usually small as compared with nonprofit hospitals. Public hospitals tend to be large as compared with private hospitals in the United States. However, with the advent of Medicare and Medicaid in 1965 and the payment (or partial payment) of the cost of care in any accredited hospital with forms of federal health insurance, the distinction between public and private hospitals blurs to some extent.

As mentioned in Chapter 2, the American Hospital Association's *Guide to the Health Care Field* (published annually) classifies the AHA-registered hospitals in the following groups: (1) federal; (2) nonfederal psychiatric; (3) nonfederal tuberculosis; (4) nonfederal long-term general and other special; (5) nonfederal short-term general and other special which include (6) nongovernmental not-for-profit short-term general and other special; (7) for-profit short-term general and other special; and (8) state and local governmental short-term general and other special.[24] Table 3-1 is based on some of the data in this publication. Study of the table shows striking differences in size from one classification to another.

Standardization, Certification, and Regulation of Hospitals. The Joint Commission on Accreditation of Hospitals * representing the American Hospital Association, the American Medical Association, the American College of Physicians, and the American College of Surgeons publishes lists of accredited hospitals. The medical profession has for decades recognized the necessity of evaluating hospitals to determine whether they were suitable practice fields for residents, interns, and medical students. Standards were established for the plant and for the organization, administration, personnel and services (including nursing service), records, and other criteria. The program was first called the Standardization Program and it was under the American College of Surgeons which, in 1946, published its *Manual of Hospital Standardization.*[25] In 1950, the American Hospital Association and the National League of Nursing Education, both cooperating with the American College of Surgeons, published the *Hospital Nursing Service Manual.*[26] Evaluation of nursing service was then a part of the "standardization" procedure and it continues as part of the certification process. A nurse is a member of the evaluating team. During the 1950s and 1960s, there were numerous studies of nurse staffing in hospitals. A classic study by Faye G. Abdellah and Eugene Levine (*Effect of Nurse Staffing on Satisfactions with Nursing Care,* Hospital Monograph Series No. 4, American Hospital Association, Chicago, 1958) is an example. Another classic study is that by Myrtle [Kitchell] Aydelotte and Marie Tener (*An Investigation of the Relation Between Nursing Activity and Patient Welfare,* Final Research Report, GN 4786 and GN 8570, University of Iowa, Iowa City, 1960). Levine has continued to study nursing needs and resources, and Aydelotte made a survey, *Hospital Nursing Services,* (National League for Nursing, New York, 1948). Her "Review and Critique of Selected Literature" on *Nurse Staffing Methodology* (US Government Printing Office, Washington, D.C., 1973 [DHEW Pub. No. (NIH) 73–433]) is a guide to the work in this field.

With the advent of Medicare and Medicaid in 1965, federal and state funds were available for third-party payment of hospital care. It followed that the government must assume responsibility for the way the funds were spent —that is, for measuring the quality of care given by hospitals. Instead of using existing machinery for evaluation, a professional review organization was set up in each state according to a regulation of the Social Security Administration (see Chapter 19). Termed peer "review," the emphasis was on review of medical, rather than total, care, and on review by physicians of their "peers" (other physicians). In 1972, the ANA House of Delegates resolved "That in every health care facility there be provision for nurses to participate in utilization review and other arrangements for monitoring health care practice." * The role of nurses in

---

* The American Nurses' Association is currently (1976) asking for representation on this Commission.

* Orme, June Y., and Lindbeck, Rosemary S.: "Nurse Participation in Medical Peer Review," *Nurs. Outlook,* **22:**27, (Jan.) 1974.

Table 3-1. Trends in Hospital Utilization, Personnel, and Finances for Selected Years 1950–1974 * (Data do not include figures for 59 US Government hospitals in 22 countries outside the United States)

Classification	Year	Hospitals	Beds in Thousands	Admissions in Thousands	Average Daily Census in Thousands	Per cent Capacity	Personnel Numbers in Thousands	Personnel per 100 Census	Payroll in Millions	Expenses per Patient Day
United States totals	1950	6,788	1,456	18,483	1,253	86.0	1,058	84	2,191	7.98
	1960	6,876	1,658	25,027	1,402	84.6	1,598	114	5,588	16.46
	1974	7,174	1,513	35,506	1,167	77.2	2,919	250	23,821	97.23
1. Federal	1950	414	189	1,284	152	80.4	169	111	520	12.77
	1960	435	177	1,476	154	87.2	186	120	921	20.11
	1974	387	136	1,841	109	80.7	244	223	2,651	99.44
2. Nonfederal psychiatric	1950	533	620	293	607	97.9	147	24	305	2.43
	1960	488	722	362	672	93.1	238	35	848	4.91
	1974	543	383	585	307	80.0	308	100	2,669	33.12
3. Nonfederal tuberculosis	1950	398	72	79	62	86.1	45	74	91	7.22
	1960	238	52	68	39	75.4	39	99	128	13.37
	1974	46	8	21	5	63.2	9	184	69	54.39
4. Nonfederal long-term general and other special	1950	412	70	164	60	85.7	34	57	72	5.39
	1960	308	67	151	58	86.9	55	95	192	12.82
	1974	221	54	106	45	82.5	69	154	571	53.44
5. Nonfederal short-term general and other special†	1950	5,031	505	16,663	372	73.7	662	178	1,203	15.62
	1960	5,407	639	22,970	477	74.7	1,080	226	3,499	32.23
	1974	5,977	931	32,943	701	75.3	2,289	326	17,861	128.05
6. Nongovernmental not-for-profit short-term general and other special	1950	2,871	332	11,629	247	74.4	473	191	848	16.89
	1960	3,291	446	16,788	341	76.6	792	232	2,561	33.23
	1974	3,381	650	23,374	506	77.8	1,634	323	12,858	127.33
7. For-profit short-term general and other special	1950	1,218	42	1,661	26	61.9	41	161	72	15.32
	1960	856	37	1,550	24	65.4	48	196	143	31.07
	1974	775	70	2,553	47	67.5	133	283	952	119.81
8. State and local governmental short-term general and other special	1950	942	131	3,374	99	75.6	148	149	282	12.56
	1960	1,260	156	4,632	112	71.6	241	215	796	29.43
	1974	1,821	211	7,016	148	70.2	522	351	4,025	133.13

* Based on data in American Hospital Association: *Guide to the Health Care Field*. The Association, Chicago, 1975, p. 17.

† The data in this box are totals for the data in the last three classifications.

Medical Peer Review varies from state to state, but they are increasingly active, and even when nurses are not members of state PROs, they may be employed by physicians of the organization to make the assessment or conduct the reviews.

Roger G. Noll, economist, discussing the consequences of public utility regulation of hospitals at the Institute of Medicine, National Academy of Sciences, January, 1974, made the following statement:

The health care delivery system is among the most extensively regulated sectors of the American economy. Professional licensure, hospital accreditation and certification, qualification requirements for federal subsidies, and governmental oversight of the third-party payer system constitute a complex set of institutional constraints on the structure and performance of the hospital industry. Beginning about a decade ago, serious demands have been made—notably by some of the trade associations and professional societies in the industry—to complete the circle of regulation by establishing administrative agencies, at either the state or federal level, to subject the industry to "public utility" regulation. These pressures have yielded results: Most states have either established hospital regulation, or are considering legislation that would accomplish that end.*

Noting the failure of the regulatory mechanisms to stem inflation in hospital costs, Noll goes on to question the current model, as do many critics of the hospital "industry." Many recommend a larger role for users ("consumers") in the evaluative and regulatory process. Clark C. Havighurst, lawyer, says:

For example, PSROs, the so-called foundations for medical care, and other self-regulatory programs may also be analyzed as cartels which, though undeniably dedicated to improving existing conditions somewhat, ultimately will stop well short of delivering to the public all the benefits that a well-organized competitive market (or an appropriately regulated system) would yield. Indeed, it is not inaccurate to view the fundamental health policy choice as being between, on the one hand, a system controlled directly or indirectly by organized providers who accommodate their public responsibilities with their own self-interest and, on the other hand, a system of social control by impersonal market forces, allowing cost-conscious consumers a larger impact and assigning government a less intrusive role.†

Standards that actually measure the value of care to patients, their families, and society are still evolving. Nurses, like all professional workers, assume responsibility for the quality of their service. For nursing, the hours per day of care by nursing personnel according to type ("professional" or "registered," licensed practical or assistant nurses, and nurse's aides) has been used because it was an available measure; it is now, however, recognized as a crude and largely quantitative measure rather than a qualitative one.‡ The ANA's *Standards for*

Nursing Services (*In Hospitals, Community Health Agencies, Nursing Homes, Industry, Schools, Ambulatory Services, and Related Health Care Organizations*) have replaced this measure. Prepared by the Commission on Nursing Services, the pamphlet gives the following twelve "standards" with "guidelines" to show how these standards are implemented:

Standard I. Nursing administration has a philosophy and objectives which reflect the purposes of the health care organization and give direction to the nursing care program.

Standard II. Nursing administration has the responsibility and authority for the quality of nursing practice within the health care organization.

Standard III. A nursing service has a designated leader who is a qualified Registered Nurse and a member of the operational policy-making bodies of the health care organization.

Standard IV. The nursing care program is integrated into the total program of the health care organization.

Standard V. Nursing administration determines the budget necessary to carry out the nursing care program and administers the approved budget.

Standard VI. A nursing service organization plan delineates the functional structure of the department and shows established relationships among nursing personnel and with other services.

Standard VII. The nursing administration has written personnel policies which assist in recruiting and maintaining a qualified staff.

Standard VIII. Nursing administration shall detail guidelines for utilization of nursing personnel.

Standard IX. The nursing administration provides programs for orientation and continued learning of nursing personnel.

Standard X. A nursing service has the responsibility to participate in the education of students in the health care field.

Edward J. Halloran made the point that the most cited studies of staffing and the most used standards of nursing hours needed per patient per day are based on measurements of care that are task centered and assumed to result in adequate, even good or excellent, nursing care but that haven't been measured by any stated qualitative criteria. He believed that if the findings of qualitative studies of nursing care or any of the leading concepts or theories of nursing purpose were used as a basis for quantitative measurements they might alter some commonly accepted quantitative standards as, for example, those arrived at by the CASH (Commission for Administrative Services in Hospitals) program in Southern California or the Hospital Systems Improvement Program at the University of Michigan. Halloran concluded that a "restructuring of nursing care on inpatient units which is patient centered is called for"; he doubts whether this will provide a "formula" for staffing but he thinks the accumulation of this sort of data will enable nurses to deal more effectively with the problem of staffing. (Halloran, Edward J.: *Nurse Staffing Issues and An Analysis of A Task Oriented Staffing Methodology.* Unpublished master's thesis, Yale University School of Medicine, Department of Epidemiology and Public Health, New Haven, Conn., 1975.)

---

* Noll, Roger G.: "The Consequences of Public Utility Regulation of Hospitals," in *Controls on Health Care.* Papers of the Conference on Regulation in the Health Industry, Jan. 7–9, 1974. National Academy of Sciences, Institute of Medicine, Washington, D.C., 1975, p. 25.

† Havighurst, Clark C.: "Regulation of Health Institutions," in *Controls on Health Care.* Papers of the Conference on Regulation in the Health Industry, Jan. 7–9, 1974. National Academy of Sciences, Institute of Medicine, Washington, D.C., 1975, p. 81.

‡ In a study entitled *Nurse Staffing Issues and an Analysis of a Task Oriented Staffing Methodology,*

Standard XI. A nursing service supports research in the health care field.

Standard XII. A nursing service evaluates its clinical and administrative practices.*

In Chapter 1, attention was called to the International Council of Nurses' effort, through the Nursing Service Committee, to establish *standards of nursing practice*. This resulted in a series of publications during the 1950s and 1960s. In the first report of the World Health Organization's Expert Committee on Nursing, the following statement was made in 1950: "In many countries where medicine is highly developed and nursing is not, the health status of the people does not reflect the advanced stage of medicine." Citing this, Daisy Bridges, in an introduction to an ICN publication, said: "This . . . stresses how essential it is to evaluate our own standards, and to do so in line with modern trends and changes in medical practice." †

National, state, and local nursing organizations have taken steps in this direction, and the published standards of the American Nurses' Association Congress for Nursing Practice influence over-all evaluation of nursing care in any setting. General standards relate to (1) collecting, communicating, and recording client/patient data and making it accessible; (2) making a nursing "diagnosis" or assessment; (3) planning nursing care derived from this assessment and from desired goals; (4) establishing priorities and measures to achieve goals; (5) providing for client/patient participation in promoting, maintaining, and restoring health; (6) helping client/patient maximize his or her health capabilities; (7) determining the client's/patient's progress (or lack of it) toward goals set by him or her with the nurse; and (8) reassessing, reordering priorities and goals and revising plans of nursing care.[27]

The foregoing standards apply to all patients and are variously paraphrased for different settings and clinical services. A special standard for maternal-child health nursing practice is that it provide for using and coordinating all services that help individuals "prepare for responsible sexual roles"; a specific standard for geriatric nursing is that it promote communication and social interaction of "aged persons with individuals, family, and other groups"; and a specific standard for psychiatric-mental health nursing practice is that it provide psychotherapeutic intervention to help clients "achieve their maximum development." [28-30]

As nurses evaluate, or help certify, hospitals (and other health agencies) these standards, published by official nursing organizations, directly or indirectly affect their evaluations.*

Commissions have been appointed in some states to exercise certain controls over hospitals and other health agencies. Such commissions are designed to assess the supply of, and demand for, services—statewide and local. Any individual or group wishing to build or expand a facility or materially change a service must have a commission's approval.† The commission may set up conditions under which approval is given.‡ While the average daily occupancy of 78 per cent for hospital beds in the United States as a whole suggests an oversupply, hospital facilities are unevenly distributed and certain elements of society are more adequately served than others. Standards such as 12 beds per 1000 population set by the US Public Health Service in 1949,[32] used as one basis of determining the use of funds under the 1946 Hospital Survey and Construction Act, must be continually examined in the light of current needs and demands.

Because the percentage of beds occupied has dropped from 86 in 1950 to 78 in 1972, there is reason to believe that hospital facilities exceed the need. The numbers of hospitals and hospital beds have not increased so greatly, but the decrease in the average length of stay accounts for the increase in admissions from 18,483,000 in 1950 to 33,265,000 in 1972. The numbers of personnel employed in hos-

---

* Standards of nursing care have tended to stress hours of care per patient; more recently, for patients classified as requiring maximum care, partial care, or able to be independent, or care for themselves. Marie J. Zimmer reports that the American Academy of Nursing in 1973 stated that nurses should be included in "quality assurance review organizations," and she presents a series of articles illustrating the point that unless the desired outcomes of health care are defined it is not possible to establish satisfactory standards. (Zimmer, Marie J.: "Quality Assurance for Outcomes of Patient Care," *Nurs. Clin. North Am.,* **9:**305, [June] 1974.)

† The American Hospital Association gives the following definition of certification of need: ". . . the process whereby the state grants permission to health care providers to change the scope of their services, or, in the case of prospective providers, permission to introduce new services." (American Hospital Association: *Guidelines for Implementation of Certification of Need for Health Care Facilities and Services.* The Association, Chicago, 1972, p. 2.)

‡ In 1975, Clark C. Havighurst said that 23 states have certification-of-need laws.[31]

---

* American Nurses' Association, Commission on Nursing Services: *Standards for Nursing Services (In Hospitals, Community Health Agencies, Nursing Homes, Industry, Schools, Ambulatory Services, and Related Health Care Organizations).* The Association, Kansas City, Mo., 1973.

† Henderson, Virginia: *ICN Basic Principles of Nursing Care.* International Council of Nurses, Geneva, 1963, p. iii.

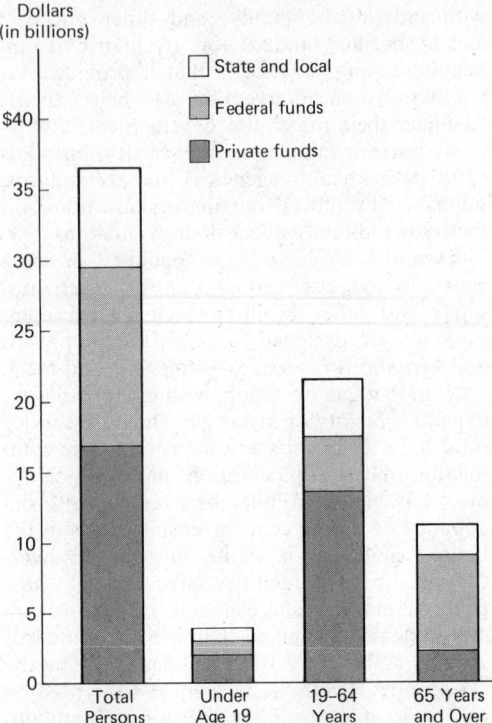

Figure 3-2. Estimated personal expenditures for hospital care, by source of funds and age, fiscal year 1973. (Source: US Department of Health, Education, and Welfare, Social Security Administration, Office of Research and Statistics, *Social Security Bull.*, May 1974; and American Nurses' Association: *Facts About Nursing 74–75*. The Association, Kansas City, Mo., 1976, p. 212.)

pitals more than doubled from 1950 to 1972, the numbers of personnel per 100 patients rising from 84 to 221. The expense per patient per day is reported to be $7.98 in 1950 and $73.89 in 1972.[33]

While the current "expense" to the hospital of patient care and the cost to the public has, certainly in the United States, risen out of proportion to that of general living costs, no end seems to be in sight. Andrew Malleson[34] and others suggest that under a fee-for-service system and as long as it is easier to collect third-party payment of fees for health services given in hospital and other institutions than in homes, it is difficult or impossible to reverse the trend. (See Fig. 3-2.)

The visionary Florence Nightingale is often quoted as saying that hospitals may some day be unnecessary. As preventive and home health services improve, and as community health centers develop and people learn to use them, it seems inevitable that the need for hospitalization will eventually be reduced, even if elimination now seems "the impossible dream." *

Undoubtedly the technical aspects of hospital construction, equipment, supplies, organization, administration, and service have been improved. The establishment of standards, certification, and peer review procedures have all promoted this improvement, but skepticism about the regulatory processes so far devised remains. The amount of public dissatisfaction with hospitals indicates that the problems of protecting people from unwanted, unnecessarily expensive, inadequate, and even dangerous treatment have not been solved. Community participation and clarification of the patient's role and rights are receiving more and more attention as the public expresses its dissatisfaction more vehemently.

The Rights of Patients—Their Position in the Hospital. Responsible adults go to and leave the hospital of their own free will. Exceptions to this are the psychiatric patient who is committed to an institution and the person who is under legal custody. Children and temporarily irrational patients are brought to hospitals by parents or guardians. If such patients leave the institution when the results of this step are injurious or disastrous, the institution may be sued for negligence. In case a patient demands a discharge from the hospital against the advice of the physician and refuses to sign a statement to this effect, the physician should tell the patient in the presence of several persons what the results may be. For the protection of the medical staff and the hospital, the patient's record should contain the physician's witnessed statement of the circumstances and what was said. Patients with certain communicable diseases are subject to public health regulations, and may not be free to leave the hospital except under conditions that give full protection to others (see Chapter 44).

Treatment cannot be legally forced on a rational adult patient nor can parents be made to agree, in most instances, to have their child treated in any manner of which they disapprove. When patients or guardians show lack of confidence in the prescribed treatment, however, physicians usually prefer to give up the case. For the protection of the surgeon and the

---

* S. S. Goldwater, a physician, in an article written in 1930, "Seeing Hospitals with Florence Nightingale," (*Mod. Hosp.*, **35:**57, [Sept.] 1930) said: "Florence Nightingale's 'Notes on Hospitals' is a document that every student of hospitals should be required to read at least once a year, not because all of its doctrines are either perfectly sound in the light of modern knowledge or quite applicable to present conditions, but because for boldness of aim, warmth of expression and breadth of view it has no equal in hospital literature."

hospital, the patient or guardian always signs a statement of informed consent to any operation. It is only in a life-threatening emergency that a surgeon assumes responsibility for operating without this written permission.

The position of patients in the hospital is that of paying guests. Even if they are indigent, tax funds finance their hospitalization; the hospital staff itself is not, therefore, "giving" its services.

Hospitals are organized to serve the public —they depend upon patients for their existence, and their personnel should try to make these institutions what the thoughtful members of the community want them to be. The average person going to a hospital expects, primarily, adequate attention from the various professional groups concerned; in addition, he or she expects the same provision for physical comfort and protection afforded by a good hotel. In some cases this may be as much as the individual wants or needs, but in many instances, it is not. Sick persons are often thrown off their balance—they are dependent, sensitive, frightened, and emotional, so that they want and need the kindness, consideration, and support they would get from their family and friends if they were at home. This element in hospital care, which is neither technical competence nor efficient institutional management, is what makes the patient's position in the institution a difficult one to define. The recognition of this element by the hospital staff, or their failure to recognize it, accounts in a large measure for the popularity of some hospitals and the unpopularity of others. Many persons have noted that each institution has a distinct "feeling" or personality. It is almost as if the attitudes of the administrative officers toward the staff and patients, or clients, were contagious and affected everyone within the institution.

Hospitals have solicited patient opinion in a variety of ways, with varying success. During hospitalization, many patients fear retaliation if they are critical; after discharge, they may want to forget any unhappy experiences they had, and so neglect answering a questionnaire. Most health workers realize that patients or clients want to be thought reasonable and cooperative but do not know what is expected of them or what their rights are. Most hospitals have a leaflet that answers patients' potential questions. The University [of Western Ontario] Hospital, London, Canada, has an eye-catching 23-page, indexed graphic pamphlet, *Patient Information Handbook*, covering 68 topics. On leaving, patients are given a questionnaire.

In some of the United States, all hospitals are required to give every patient a copy of *A*

Patient's Bill of Rights, published by the American Hospital Association in 1972. Its implementation is widely discussed by hospital administrators, doctors, nurses, and others (see Fig. 3-3).[35-38] In some states, there is a special document on the rights of mental patients.* [39,40]

Organized nursing, from the International Council of Nurses to local groups, is backing not only the public's right to health care but also the right to have a voice in the kind of care it receives.[41-43] In a recent interdisciplinary study of a patient unit of St. Mary's Hospital, Milwaukee, Wisconsin,[44] the traditional administrative pattern was replaced by one designed to meet basic human needs as enunciated by Abraham H. Maslow. Popular literature abounds in titles such as "The Plight of the U.S. Patient," [45] "Experiencing Dehumanization in the Role of a Patient" [46] (description by a physician of his own experience), and "Sociological Sheep Shearing," [47] which describes the patient's loss of rights when he or she enters a hospital.

As these protests get more numerous, so do articles with titles such as "Consumer Choice, Consumer Control in Service Delivery" [48] and "Health Is Everybody's Business." [49] Hospitals for the chronically ill (particularly psychiatric hospitals) establish some form of patient government that gives them an active voice in decisions affecting such questions as hours for meals, quiet hours, home leaves, and regulations for visitors. One British hospital reported that each hospital unit, staff, and patients "formulates its own policy for administration, for the selection, admission, and treatment of patients, and for the meetings and discussions it will hold. There is an overall expectation that patients will take part in the daily work of the unit. . . . Eventually the patients of one unit were given complete responsibility for providing servery service for all patients. . . ." †

Optimum patient participation is important primarily because it discourages inactivity and dependence. Practiced widely and judiciously, it could be a form of health education and at the same time reduce the cost of hospital care. Bruno Bettelheim,[50] describing the program of

---

* A psychiatric nurse consultant, in a 1974 letter to the writer, speaks of how interesting but how frustrating the work is—"I am free to do what I like in getting about and talking to nurses. But the system and the way it maintains the psychiatric patient as a second class citizen becomes harder and harder to justify. I feel much of what *I* do has only a superficial impact on what *really* happens to an individual patient. . . ."

† Gazdar, E. Jeanette: "Patient-Staff Activities in Medical Units," in Barnes, Elizabeth (ed.): *Psychosocial Nursing.* Tavistock Publications, London, 1968, p. 88.

BILL OF RIGHTS FOR PATIENTS

In the interest of "more effective patient care and greater satisfaction for the patient, his physician, and the hospital organization," the American Hospital Association has adopted a "Patient's Bill of Rights" as a national policy statement and distributed it to its member hospitals throughout the country. Intended to "give the consumer something to go by," the 12 rights, in summary, are:

1. The patient has the right to considerate and respectful care.

2. The patient has the right to obtain from his physician complete current information concerning his diagnosis, treatment, and prognosis in terms the patient can be reasonably expected to understand.

3. The patient has the right to receive from his physician information necessary to give informed consent prior to the start of any procedure and/or treatment.

4. The patient has the right to refuse treatment to the extent permitted by law, and to be informed of the medical consequences of his action.

5. The patient has the right to every consideration of his privacy concerning his own medical care program.

6. The patient has the right to expect that all communications and records pertaining to his care should be treated as confidential.

7. The patient has the right to expect that within its capacity a hospital must make reasonable response to the request of a patient for services.

8. The patient has the right to obtain information as to any relationship of his hospital to other health care and educational institutions insofar as his care is concerned.

9. The patient has the right to be advised if the hospital proposes to engage in or perform human experimentation affecting his care or treatment.

10. The patient has the right to expect reasonable continuity of care.

11. The patient has the right to examine and receive an explanation of his bill regardless of source of payment.

12. The patient has the right to know what hospital rules and regulations apply to his conduct as a patient.

Figure 3-3. The American Hospital Association's Bill of Rights for Patients (summary form). (From *Nurs. Outlook,* 21:82, [Feb.] 1973.)

---

a psychiatric hospital for children and young adults in Chicago in a volume entitled *A Home for the Heart,* shows, perhaps, the ultimate limit to which the principle of patient choice may be carried. Nurses in any sort of hospital would profit from a study of the methods used in these two psychiatric hospitals. They might also find it instructive to learn how peoples in certain cultures protect patients from loneliness by sending a member of the family to stay with them throughout the period of hospitalization. The family member participates in the care of the patient and provides companionship, even at night. Hospitals worldwide often' admit parents with infants and small children, but the constant attendance of relatives or friends is discouraged in most hospitals for adults.

Location, Physical Plans, and Furnishings of Hospitals. Because they should be accessible to the people they serve, hospitals are usually found in cities and towns. Psychiatric and convalescent hospitals are sometimes built in the suburbs or country to make it economically possible to provide ample grounds for outdoor life and the therapeutic effect of a beautiful setting. If the hospital is inaccessible, the hospital may operate a bus for patients, staff, and visitors, to and from a nearby center.

The location, design, and structure of hospitals depends on their function. General and special hospitals for the treatment of short-term acute illness, where the patient's average stay is about 7 days and where the average daily cost to the patient is around $100, are designed for functional efficiency. They tend to be vertical structures which, even in congested cities, give all rooms access to light and a view from the windows. They are compactly built, with elevator and service areas centrally located, while patients' rooms or units, each provided with its own bathroom, are on the periphery. (See Chapter 15 for discussion of space for equipment or "nurservers" and other details of the hospital environment.) With the current emphasis on rehabilitation and the fear of even short periods of inactivity, all hospitals are more and more likely to provide for some communal living.

Hospitals for long-term care may be of vertical design, but often comprise a series of low buildings or pavilions connected by corridors, all having easy access to the outdoors or an inner court. In some instances, each pavilion may be autonomous and offer the attractions of a small hospital, but usually patients are admitted and discharged through one department, operations are performed in one suite of operating rooms, physical therapy is concentrated as much as possible in a centrally located department, diets are prepared in one main kitchen, equipment is sterilized in one place, and supplies are issued from one storeroom. The rambling pavilion type of hospital obviously presents a more difficult problem in the transportation of patients and supplies to and from these central departments than does the vertical plan in which elevator service provides a rapid means of transportation. (See Figs. 3-4 and 3-5.)

The general scheme, decoration, and furnishing of the building are affected by the funds available. In highly endowed institutions, handsome accommodations may be found for patients and staff. Where hospital grounds are limited, as in metropolitan areas, roof gardens are seen as substitutes. Buildings are sometimes constructed so that practically every patient has access to a porch or balcony. Sitting rooms furnished with recreational facilities are provided on each corridor for patients and their visitors. Suites may be available for persons who wish to have a member of their family stay with them, and dining rooms for convalescent patients and their visitors are provided. Many types of recreation rooms are found in hospitals for convalescents and those not acutely ill. Diagnostic units where patients are

ambulatory and require little if any nursing care may seem like small hotels. It is not unusual in children's hospitals to see nursery schools and classrooms for older children. Psychiatric hospitals are essentially schools where people learn to change their behavior. One for children and young adults is called the Orthogenic School of the University of Chicago and it has little resemblance to the average psychiatric hospital.

General hospitals now usually provide for the care and treatment of medical, surgical, maternal and child, and neuropsychiatric patients. Some hospitals have units for the care and treatment of communicable diseases. Each of these categories of patients may occupy a separate floor or building; each group may be divided into units for subspecialties.

Another way of grouping patients is according to the amount of attention they require. Patients progress from intensive to intermediate to self-help units that are more like hotels.

As patients are encouraged to move about the hospital and to acquire or maintain their independence, the following conditions and facilities should be provided: (1) sufficient space between beds or other furnishings to make it possible for patients in wheelchairs or on crutches to move about freely; (2) doorways, even those to bathroom cubicles and telephone

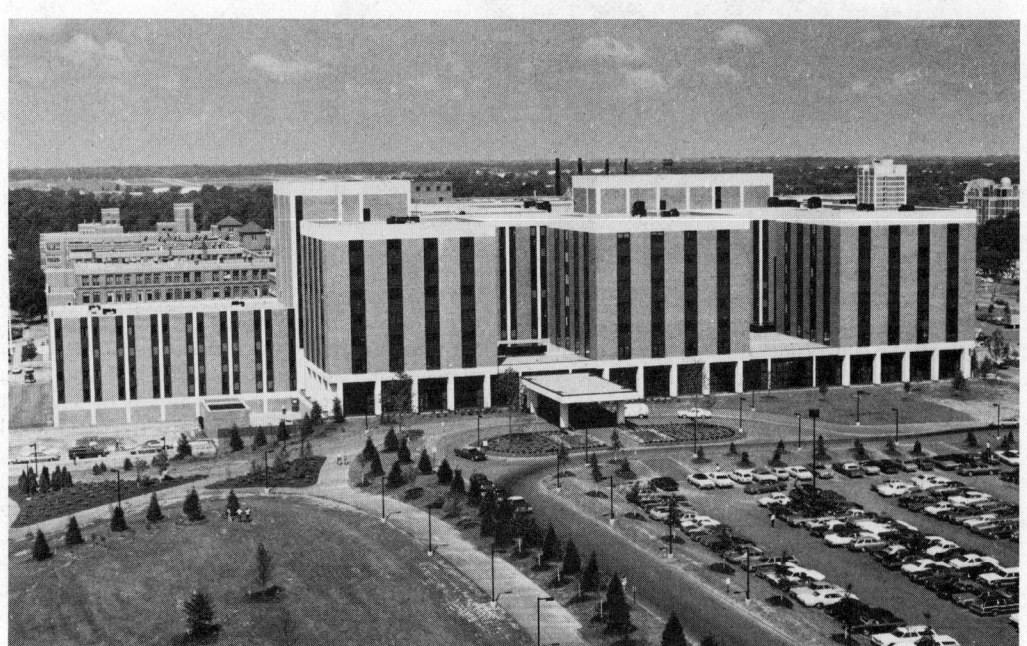

Figure 3-4. Example of a vertical structure for the care of the acutely ill, having two floors below ground and eight above with 698 beds. Patient units have a radial arrangement with patient-care station in the center. (Courtesy of Strong Memorial Hospital of the University of Rochester, Rochester, N.Y.)

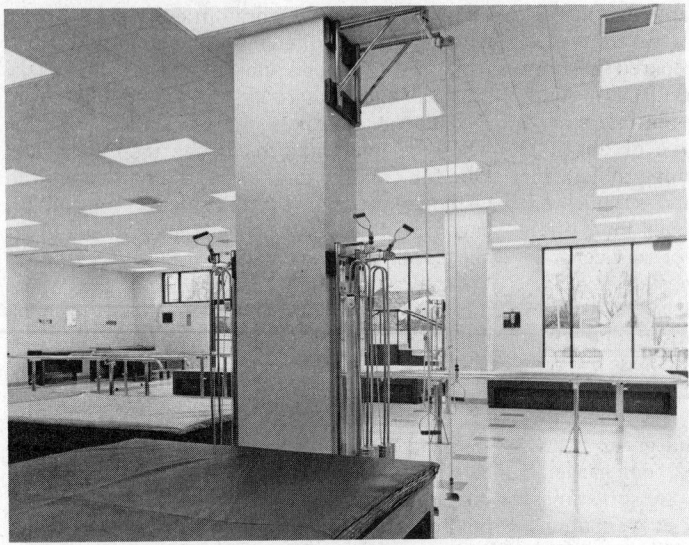

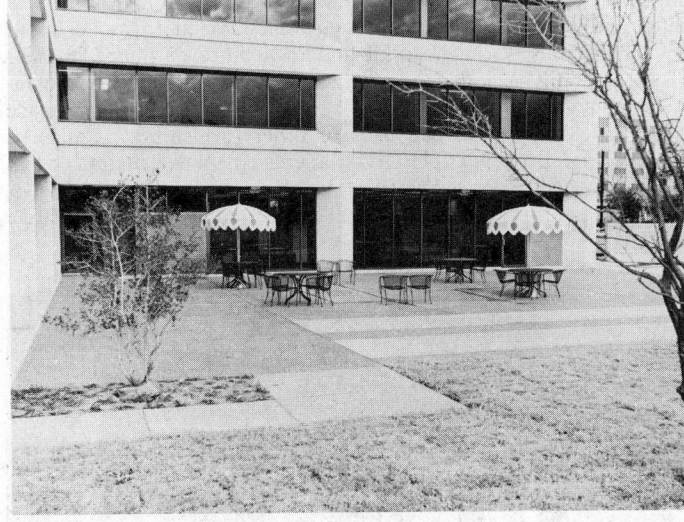

Figure 3-5. Indoor and outdoor views of the Carr P. Collins Rehabilitation Hospital, Baylor University Medical Center, Dallas, Texas, showing easy access to the outdoors from an exercise room. (Courtesy of Baylor University Medical Center, Dallas, Tex.)

booths, large enough to admit a wheelchair *; (3) ramps as substitutes for steps; (4) railings along corridors, as well as beside toilets and bathtubs; (5) greatly increased bathroom facilities with tubs so arranged that those helping a patient with a bath can stand on either side of the tub; (6) tubs provided with seats so that weak and elderly patients can sit during a bath and a surgical patient with an abdominal dressing can take a tub bath and keep the dressing dry; (7) improved facilities for washing the hair and cleaning the mouth and for all aspects of the toilet; (8) conference rooms where groups of patients may assemble for the discussion of common health problems; (9) one

or more rooms equipped so that patients can learn to launder clothing, use a stove and a refrigerator, get across a street, or mount a bus with whatever handicap illness or accident may have brought them; and (10) recreational facilities such as game rooms, libraries, radios, television, movies, pianos, and studios and shops for arts and crafts and even for learning certain trades. Pedestal tables in libraries, shops, recreational, dining, and other communal rooms make it possible for patients in wheelchairs to work, eat, and enjoy association with others.

Most large hospitals have a system providing a two-way voice communication between the patient and the nurse or another worker at the nurse's station; at the same time, the customary signal light over the door of the pa-

---

* Wall telephones can be placed so that persons in wheelchairs can reach them.

tient's room and a corresponding light in the nurse's floor station flashes on. Such an intercommunication system is reassuring to patients because they know that their call will receive immediate attention. The system saves time, since a clerk or unit manager may be able to answer the patient's question. If a nurse is needed, he or she may often be able to collect necessary equipment before going to the patient's room. Intercommunication systems are made so that patients can turn off the mechanism to ensure privacy when they have visitors.

With the necessity for conserving the time of highly prepared workers, centralized workrooms are provided, as in hotels, where equipment may be cared for and dispensed by personnel employed for this purpose. Utility rooms are constructed to make the best known use of labor-saving machinery and to encourage the employment of nonnursing personnel for cleaning, sorting, and dispensing linen, clothing, toilet articles, and medical supplies.

The most carefully planned institutions provide ample and convenient working space for personnel and at the same time arrange workrooms so that they cannot be seen by patients and visitors; likewise, business offices are detached from the main lobby of the hospital. Space is allocated for hostesses, information clerks, and messengers at entrances to the hospital and to the clinical divisions, not only to provide attention and direction for patients and visitors but also to prevent the interruption of work by medical and nursing personnel. In the clinical divisions, offices are provided for the medical and nursing staffs; in some cases there is a separate room for reporting and recording. Stairways and elevator shafts are often enclosed for the control of noise and fire. Sitting rooms and dressing rooms for the nursing staff on the clinical division are not unusual. Clinical classrooms and conference rooms on each service facilitate the instruction of patients and any students there may be in the hospital.

The *protection of patients and personnel* is safeguarded in modern hospitals as it never has been in the past. Buildings are constructed almost entirely of fireproof materials and incorporate the various means of preventing and controlling fire discussed in Chapter 15 which deals with the environment. Hospital windows are designed so that they will not open far enough to allow anyone to fall through them, elevators will not move while the doors are open, and in many other ways hospital buildings have been improved to protect occupants. (See also Chapter 15 for prevention of mechanical injury, and a discussion of lighting and air conditioning.)

Interior decoration of hospitals has undergone a marked change during this century. In the first decades, sanitation was the keynote. William Ernest Henley, in a poem called *In Hospital,* refers to it as "cold, naked, clean—half work-house and half jail." * Typical hospitals were bare and usually white; tiles and painted iron furniture were everywhere. Carbolic acid and formaldehyde odors were so pervasive that everything and everyone in the hospital smelled of them. Henley said, "The atmosphere suggests the trail of a ghostly druggist." Outside the institution, staff members were often told, to their surprise, on introduction: "You must be a doctor," or "You must be a nurse." In an effort to make the hospital "sanitary," curtains, rugs, pictures, and unnecessary objects were removed from the patients' rooms and even from the entrance halls, dining rooms, and corridors.† The average hospital was a very austere place. Lately there has been a reaction against the forbidding appearance of such institutions. *Color* is used freely in walls, floor coverings, and draperies; windows are treated more or less as they are in homes. Many hospitals have so far departed from the "sanitary tradition" as to have pictures on the walls of patients' rooms. (It is interesting to note in this connection that Florence Nightingale suggested changing the pictures in rooms for the sick as a diversion for the patients.) Hospitals for the well-to-do and a few private psychiatric hospitals look like fine inns or hotels.

But the costliest hospitals are not necessarily the most pleasing to look at or the most convenient. Efficiency is achieved through wise planning and organization; beauty, by good proportions, harmonious color combinations, and suitable furnishings. All that is essential to the recovery of the patient, as a matter of fact, may be provided in very simple surroundings. There is a good deal of danger that health workers who learn to take care of patients, and some patients who recover, in luxurious hospitals, may be poorly prepared to deal with the problem of sickness in the average home. In hospital planning, as in all phases of health work, essentials should be stressed and provided before attention is given or money spent on nonessentials. Nurses and all other major groups of the hospital staff should be represented on planning committees.

---

* Henley, William Ernest: *In Hospital.* Thomas B. Mosher, Portland, Maine, 1908, pp. 3, 5.

† While infection remains a hazard for patients and staff, odorless disinfectants and improved methods of cleaning and air-conditioning make odors unnecessary. However, habits persist. The author visited a hospital in 1974 that reeked of carbolic, a condition that cannot be justified today.

Organization and Administration of the Hospital. In countries where hospitals are an integral part of a regional health service, organizational plans differ from plans in autonomous hospitals, as is typical in the United States. Here the organization varies according to the ownership and to control by governments, churches, universities, industries, and individuals. There are, however, the following common features.

A governing board, which theoretically represents the interests of the patients or clients, or the citizens who own the facility, determines policy with relation to needs; sees that certain standards of care are maintained; coordinates the professional, administrative, and financial interests of the hospital with the consumers' or community's needs; directs administrative personnel to carry out policies; and sees that there is an adequate income to make these activities possible.

Much of this work may be accomplished through committees. This central or governing board may delegate authority to its committees, to the medical staff, and to the chief executive officer. This officer or director administers the policies of the board of directors and is responsible to them for the successful management of the institution. Since it is impossible for one person to be an authority in all departments of the hospital, each aspect of the work is under a director of that division, and the hospital administrator delegates to division directors the authority that enables them to operate their departments effectively. There are two main divisions of hospital work: the first is concerned with "business management," and the second with the "professional care of patients." Auditing, purchasing, issuance of supplies, engineering, housekeeping, laundry, supervision of buildings and grounds, and other aspects that have to do with providing a setting for health care come under business administration. Each department is under the management of a supervisor who may be responsible to the business director or, in smaller institutions, to the director of the hospital. The medical, nursing, dietary, and social service departments are jointly concerned with the professional care of patients. Each of these departments has a director, and under each departmental director are varying numbers of assistants who administer smaller divisions of work within the department.*

Students of medicine, nursing, physical ther-

---

* It is fashionable to call administrators "facilitators" to stress the point that it is their function to create a setting in which a group of persons can work effectively.

apy, occupational therapy, social service, or hospital administration, and students of other health occupations, may all be found in hospitals. There are many hospitals, however, in which there are no students of any kind. If there are students, the organization of the hospital and the organization of the schools it controls, or with which it is affiliated, should be separate and distinct, and the relationship of the two organizations clearly defined.

The director of any one of the professional schools may be a person who holds no hospital appointment. In many cases, however, the director is at the head of one of the departments of the hospital. For example, the director of the nursing school may also be the director of the nursing service. In this case he or she has two distinct functions. As director or dean of the school, he or she is responsible to the governing board of the school; as the director of the nursing service, he or she is responsible to the director of the hospital. The director of the school has various administrative and teaching assistants or instructors. Some of these instructors also may be members of the hospital staff. When such persons hold joint appointments, they are responsible to the director of the nursing service for the performance of their hospital duties and to the director of the school for the performance of their educational function.

Students may pay a fee to the hospital for its use as a practice field, the benefits to the institution may be thought to cancel the benefits to the students, or the hospital may pay students for their services during the learning period. If students are paid members of the hospital staff, the institution must assume responsibility for their work and may demand a reasonably high standard of performance and conformity to hospital regulations. Because hospital work is of a serious nature, there is in all cases a distinct understanding between the hospital and school authorities that students' activities are to be confined to those that they can perform without danger to others, that students use methods acceptable to the institution, and that they work under the supervision of the hospital staff when adequate direction is not provided by the school.

Functions, Satisfactions, Rewards, and Difficulties in Hospital Nursing. The fact that, in 1974, 62 per cent of the employed registered nurses in the United States and 84 per cent of those in Canada were in hospitals, nursing homes, and related institutions suggests that nurses fill an important role in such institutions and that the satisfactions and rewards of institutional nursing far outweigh its dissatisfactions.[51,52]

Nurses administer nursing services, teach, conduct research, and practice nursing in hospitals, or they may combine any two or more of these functions. Until recent decades, nurses in the British Commonwealth, the United States, and other countries often filled the post of hospital director or "superintendent." * In this era, hospital administration is considered a specialty in itself; persons appointed to these posts who may have had no previous health training are prepared in university-based programs. Nurses and doctors who graduate from such programs and become hospital directors lose their identity as nurses and doctors to a large extent.

The director of the nursing service holds a key position. He or she has often had advanced programs in nursing, as well as in the art and science of management. Assistant administrators in charge of the nursing service in various hospital divisions are usually nurse specialists who have managerial skills.

The director of the nursing service may also be the director of the hospital-owned school or dean of a university-based school of nursing that uses the hospital as a practice field for its students. Assistant nursing service directors may also hold joint appointments for teaching or research, or both. Some people think this dual commitment to service and education (or triple commitment if research is included) is insupportable. The writer agrees with those who think this is desirable practice and that there is a trend in this direction. A recent demonstration at Case-Western Reserve University illustrates this point (see Fig. 3-6).[53] Practice changes so rapidly in the health field that unless nurse educators remain active in the clinical field it is difficult for them to teach current theory and practice. Pertinent clinical research, the findings of which can lead to improvement in practice, most often derives from the practitioner's experience; hence the logic of the dual or triple commitment.

Many of the satisfactions and rewards of hospital nursing are obvious. Patients in hospitals are there because they need help; if the help they think they need is supplied, their appreciation is rewarding. If patients recover from an illness, learn to cope with a handicap, or die peacefully, the nurse has a deep professional satisfaction. Hospitals, particularly large medical centers, provide almost unlimited resources for care and treatment. Nurses enjoy the opportunity of working in a community of expert health workers of all types, particularly working with medical specialists, few of whom practice outside hospitals. There is a wide salary range, but highly qualified nursing service administrators command top salaries, and the average beginning staff nurse's salary is not far below that of the average staff nurse salary in public health agencies, even though the latter is educationally better qualified.[54,55]

Hospital nursing care is under considerable criticism for a variety of reasons. It is often seen to be impersonal, fragmented, and inadequate in kind and amount. In the first decades of this century, for the sake of efficiency, hospital nursing was divided into tasks or functions. Later, case (patient) assignment was advocated, with the consistent use of a written plan of care for each patient. With the elaboration of nursing personnel, the assignment of a nursing team to a patient was promoted. In this decade, "primary nursing" is the term used in hospitals for the assignment of *a* nurse to each patient as a means of personalizing care and increasing the satisfaction of the patient and the nurse. Authority for decisions about nursing care is decentralized. Decisions are made by this "primary" nurse who knows the patient best. Daren Ciske calls "primary nursing" "An Organization that Promotes Professional Practice," (*J. Nurs. Admin.,* **4**:28, [Jan.–Feb.] 1974). After 3 years' experience with primary nursing at the University of Minnesota Hospital, Marie Manthey writes about it under the title "Primary Care Is Alive and Well in the Hospital," (*Am. J. Nurs.,* **73**: 83, [Jan.] 1973). She is credited with having developed this type of patient assignment into a currently workable system.

There is a realization by spokesmen for nursing that funding of nursing service by government is dependent on quality assurance and measurement of nursing needs and resources. An example of a study of monitoring quality of nursing care, under a grant from the US Department of Health, Education, and Welfare (Public Health Service, Health Resources Administration, Bureau of Health Manpower, Division of Nursing) is in progress in nineteen hospitals in various parts of the United States. The criteria master list used in monitoring quality includes the following:

1. The plan of nursing care is formulated
2. The physical needs of the patient are attended
3. The nonphysical needs (psychological, emotional, mental, social, spiritual) of the patient are attended
4. Achievement of nursing care objectives is evaluated
5. Unit procedures are followed for the protection of all patients

* During the 1920s, the writer worked with one such nurse who not only administered a 250-bed hospital, its nursing service, and nursing school, but relieved the dietitian when she was on vacation and often gave anesthetics in emergencies.

6. The delivery of nursing care is facilitated by administrative and managerial services.*

These are only a few examples of recent studies of hospital nursing. In the last three decades, hospital nursing in the United States has been studied extensively and, in some cases, exhaustively.[56-61] It is impossible to summarize in a few paragraphs what was

* Haussmann, R. K. Dieter, et al.: *Monitoring Quality of Nursing Care. Part II. Assessment and Study of Correlates*. US Department of Health, Education, and Welfare, Public Health Service, Health Resources Administration, Bureau of Health Manpower, Division of Nursing, Bethesda, Md., July, 1976 (DHEW Pub. No. [HRA] 76-7).

learned about the satisfactions, advantages, dissatisfactions, and disadvantages of hospital nursing. The satisfactions just enumerated are derived from this research; the disadvantages are diffuse and hard to define. The outstanding objection to hospital nursing expressed by nurses is that "the system" does not enable them to fully exercise nursing judgment, to nurse creatively, or, in many cases, to give effective or even safe care, and that "the system" forces them to waste their time on nonnursing functions. In hospitals with interns and residents, medical "orders" are often written for what nurses believe to be nursing care rather than medical treatment. Many hospital

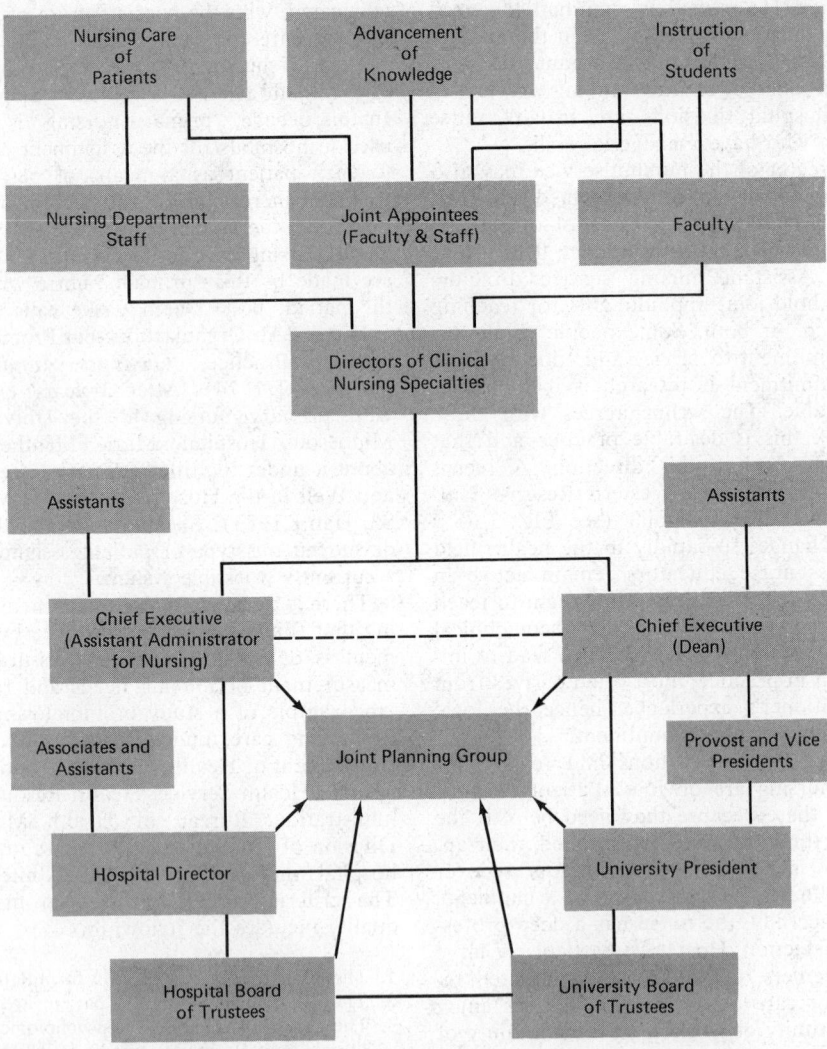

Figure 3-6. Organizational scheme for nursing at the University Medical Center, Cleveland, Ohio. (From Schlotfeldt, Rozella M., and MacPhail, Jannetta: "An Experiment in Nursing. Part I: Rationale and Characteristics," in Lewis, Edith P. [comp.]: *Changing Patterns of Nursing Practice*. American Journal of Nursing Co., New York, 1971, p. 280.)

nurses believe there is insufficient collaboration between doctors, nurses, and social workers, and most particularly, insufficient patient and family participation in decision making. While there have been, and still are, many experiments designed to humanize patient care, the functional assignment system (as opposed to the patient assignment system) that exists in many hospitals makes it impossible for staff nurses to fully identify with any patients, to see enough of them and to do enough for them to know the patients' needs, or to estimate their own effectiveness as nurses. Hospitals using a patient assignment system in small, relatively autonomous nursing units, that recognize the overlapping functions of professional health workers, and that have an appropriate machinery to help them function as colleagues overcome the principal disadvantages of hospital nursing.[62-67]

3. NURSING HOMES—"EXTENDED CARE FACILITIES"

Employment of Nurses in Nursing Homes. It was reported by the American Nurses' Association in 1975 that there were 65,235 registered nurses employed in nursing and personal care homes in the United States, and 280,000 aides and orderlies who "give 80 to 90 per cent of the care."[1] In 1972, there were 73,000 licensed practical nurses employed in nursing homes and 280,000 aides, orderlies, and attendants. These figures indicate that there were then about 7 to 8 times as many nonprofessional as professional nursing personnel in nursing homes.[1a] (See Fig. 3-7.)

Nature, Types, and Numbers of Nursing Homes. The term "nursing home" is used collectively for a variety of institutions. In Chapter 2, the American Hospital Association's

breakdown into (1) Extended Care Facilities, (2) Nursing Care Facilities, and (3) Resident Care Facilities was noted. The first two categories have medical staffs or equivalents, and nursing staffs under the direction of professional nurses. The American Nurses' Association divides nursing homes into (1) Nursing Care [homes], (2) Personal Care [homes] with nursing, (3) Personal Care [homes] without nursing, and (4) Domiciliary Care [homes]. The first two categories offer nursing care, the third offers personal care but no nursing, and the fourth offers domiciliary care only.[2]

These categories suggest a wide range of institutions, but even the term "nursing home" has a different (and happier) connotation in Great Britain where they, by and large, offer far more safety and comfort than they do in the United States.

In 1974, Mary Adelaide Mendelson,[3] who made a 10-year study of nursing homes in the United States, reported that there were 24,000 nursing homes in "the industry." The ANA[4] reported 22,004 for 1971, which indicates how rapidly these institutions multiplied in this period. Most nursing homes are small. In 1971, 8266 had less than 25 beds and 16,145 had less than 100 beds; 16,439 provided nursing care, 5369 personal care without nursing, and 196 domiciliary care only.[5]

Since "nursing homes" offer such a wide range of facilities and services, it is almost impossible to describe one that might be called typical. The Joint Commission on Accreditation of Hospitals in its *Lists of Health Care Institutions* reported 1485 accredited Extended Care Facilities (in the 50 states) for January 1973.[6] Mendelson reported the following data:

. . . [the nation's nearly 23,000 nursing homes are] divided into three categories, according to the amount of medical care they are supposed to provide. In descending order of amount of care, there

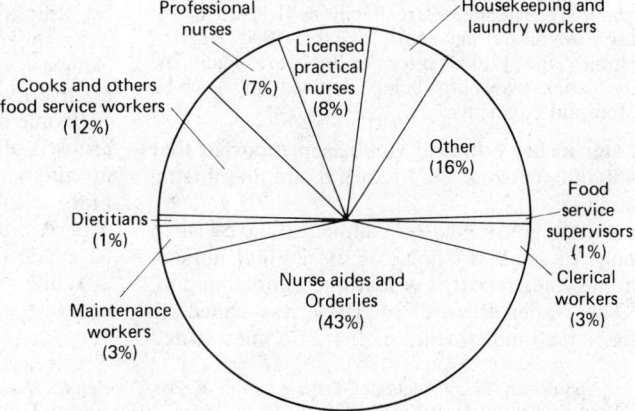

Figure 3-7. Occupational composition of employment in surveyed nursing homes and related health facilities. (From US Senate, Special Committee on Aging, Subcommittee on Long-Term Care: *Nursing Home Care in the United States: Failure in Public Policy.* US Government Printing Office, Washington, D.C., 1974, p. 23.)

Professional nurses

Housekeeping and laundry workers

Licensed practical nurses (8%)

Cooks and others food service workers (12%)

(7%)

Other (16%)

Dietitians (1%)

Food service supervisors (1%)

Clerical workers (3%)

Nurse aides and Orderlies (43%)

Maintenance workers (3%)

Table 3-2.   Registered Nurses Employed in Nursing and Personal Care Homes, 1971 *

State	Number of Registered Nurses		State	Number of Registered Nurses	
	Full-Time	Part-Time		Full-Time	Part-Time
Total	40,160	26,274			
Alabama	340	110	Missouri	693	382
Alaska	54	17	Montana	270	128
Arizona	284	148	Nebraska	302	212
Arkansas	254	140	Nevada	87	12
California	4,580	2,390	New Hampshire	329	241
Colorado	754	406	New Jersey	1,695	1,163
Connecticut	1,521	1,351	New Mexico	94	28
Delaware	91	78	New York	4,004	2,899
District of			North Carolina	536	239
Columbia	113	41	North Dakota	164	141
Florida	1,337	615			
Georgia	564	208	Ohio	1,872	1,295
Hawaii	138	49	Oklahoma	470	205
Idaho	146	79	Oregon	517	265
Illinois	2,044	1,218	Pennsylvania	2,687	1,885
Indiana	1,019	565	Rhode Island	261	154
Iowa	864	586	South Carolina	295	144
Kansas	438	251	South Dakota	233	212
Kentucky	356	165	Tennessee	248	109
Louisiana	401	137	Texas	931	365
Maine	310	185	Utah	128	60
Maryland	541	391	Vermont	194	157
Massachusetts	2,235	2,172	Virginia	478	309
Michigan	1,365	894	Washington	1,160	656
Minnesota	1,340	1,358	West Virginia	104	80
Mississippi	170	69	Wisconsin	1,087	1,271
			Wyoming	62	39

Source: U.S. Department of Health, Education and Welfare, Public Health Service, Health Resources Administration, National Center for Health Statistics, Division of Health Resources Statistics; 1971 Master Facility Inventory. Unpublished data.

* American Nurses' Association: *Facts About Nursing 72–73*. The Association, Kansas City, Mo., 1974, p. 30.

are 4,057 Extended Care Facilities licensed to receive Medicare payments, 6,500 Skilled Nursing Homes and 12,000 Intermediate Care Facilities, the latter two both being licensed to received Medicaid payments.*

Later in her critique, Mendelson reported that 450,000 persons on Medicaid are in nursing homes.[7]

Although Mendelson claimed to have visited only "a small fraction" of the 24,000 nursing homes, her report is a scathing condemnation. "The Nader Report" of 1970 was called "a passionate indictment" of the 20 homes visited

by Ralph Nader's Study Group: "only one . . . appeared to offer an environment where elderly people lived meaningful, full, and productive lives." *

People of the United States seem thoroughly aroused about and ashamed of the care given in nursing homes. It is not possible to cite more than a few of the investigations now in progress, but that of the Gray Panthers might be added to those already mentioned.

While some may claim that most reports exaggerate the defects of nursing homes, the

* Mendelson, Mary Adelaide: *Tender Loving Greed*. Alfred A. Knopf, New York, 1974, p. 23.

* Townsend, Claire: *Old Age. The Last Segregation. Ralph Nader's Study Group Report on Nursing Homes*. Grossman Publishers, New York, 1971, p. 130.

Introductory Report. Nursing Home Care in the United States. Failure in Public Policy[8] prepared by the US Senate Special Committee on Aging is, if anything, more damaging than those of private individuals and groups. It is based on a study begun in 1959, which will result in a 12-volume series on nursing home problems.[8a] The care received by millions of Americans is said to have been not only unsafe but in some cases inhuman; nursing home inmates are said to have been exposed to fire hazards, unsanitary conditions, poor food, overtranquilization, and medication errors. Some were injured, even fatally. Homes that provide good care do exist, but these are in the minority. Medicaid is said to be paying 60 per cent and Medicare 7 per cent of the nation's $3.7 billion nursing home bill in 1974. (Federal support was $500 million in 1960.) For the first time in 1972, Medicaid expenditures for nursing home care exceeded those for surgical and general hospital care. The average monthly cost for nursing home care is reported as $600. Altogether, the report painted a sad picture.

At the request of the Senate's Subcommittee on Long-Term Care of the Special Committee on Aging, the ANA's Committee on Skilled Nursing Care made a study of the report which was published in 1975 under the title *Nursing and Long-Term Care. Toward Quality Care for the Aging.* (It is included as Supporting Paper No. 4 in the Subcommittee Report.) * The ANA involved 22 national organizations concerned with long-term care in its task forces. Testimony cited in the ANA report confirms the conclusions reached in the other investigations that have been mentioned. Noting that Americans spend more on health care than any other nation, and that the average American works approximately one month of the year to support the health industry, the Committee notes neglect of health needs in various quarters. It specifically notes 5 per cent of the population over 65 are in long-term care facilities in the United States as compared with 1 per cent in the United Kingdom. The Committee notes the dearth of day care centers, of provision for home care (home care should be "fashionable"), and of adequately prepared personnel. The ANA made the following recommendations, given here in the briefest form: (1) That a national policy on care of the aging be developed; (2) That a plan for national health insurance be developed

that ensures health care for all citizens; (3) That a wide range of services be made available so that elderly citizens can live in their own homes as well as institutions; (4) That "skilled" be deleted from skilled nursing care in federal standards; (5) That all "professional persons" and "workers" in long-term care in any setting have a background in basic care of the aging.[8b]

While these multifarious institutions are, in common parlance, lumped under one term, "nursing homes," they range all the way from the equivalent of an accredited hospital for the chronically ill to "convalescent homes" and old-fashioned boarding houses. They are inextricably tied in the public's mind to the care of the aged, and most persons in the United States fear them as a point of no return. They feel "committed" when they go to them, as they might to life incarceration in a prison.

The Subcommittee on Health and Long-Term Care of the Select Committee on Aging, US House of Representatives, shows the breakdown of $118.5 billion spent in fiscal year 1975 for medical costs (private, $68,552 billion; public, $49,948 billion) (see Table 3-3). The Subcommittee notes that despite the fact that expenditures for Medicare almost doubled between 1972 and 1974, home health care received a "miniscule" portion of national health expenditures. The expenditure on nursing home care was less than that spent on drugs and drug sundries.*

In a brief discussion of nursing homes, it is hard to avoid oversimplification. Because the evidence that has been found is so damaging, it is impossible to present this setting for health care as anything but a problem for, and a challenge to, society and more particularly to lawmakers and those in the health occupations.

Certification-Regulation of Nursing Homes. Unlike the program of standardization and certification of hospitals that has been in existence for decades, the regulation of nursing homes is relatively new. There was almost no curb on the opening of nursing homes or regulations that ensure quality until 1967 when Medicare and Medicaid payments became effective for nursing home residents.[9] The federal government must now assume responsibility for determining whether the care given by health agencies justifies the use of federal funds. Mendelson's report, just cited, that a total of

---

*US Senate. Special Committee on Aging, Subcommittee on Long-Term Care: *Nursing Home Care in the United States: Failure in Public Policy.* US Government Printing Office, Washington, D.C., April, 1975.

* US House of Representatives. Select Committee on Aging, Subcommittee on Health and Long-Term Care: *New Perspectives in Health Care for Older Americans. (Recommendations and Policy Directions of the Subcommittee on Health and Long-Term Care.)* US Government Printing Office, Washington, D.C., Jan., 1976, p. 14 (Pub. No. 66–559).

Table 3-3.   Medical Expenses in the United States 1975 in Billions *

	Billions
Health services and supplies	$111.250
Physician services	22.100
Dentist	7.500
Other professional services	2.180
Drugs and drug sundries	10.600
Eyeglasses and appliances	2.300
Nursing home care	9.000
Expenses for prepayment and administration	4.593
Government public health activities	3.457
Other health services	3.000
Research and medical facilities construction	7.250

* US House of Representatives. Select Committee on Aging, Subcommittee on Health and Long-Term Care: *New Perspectives in Health Care for Older Americans.* (*Recommendations and Policy Directions of the Subcommittee on Health and Long-Term Care.*) US Government Printing Office, Washington, D.C., Jan. 1976, p. 14 (Pub. No. 66–559).

22,557 institutions were licensed in 1973 to receive Medicare and Medicaid payments, suggested that either the federal standards were inadequate or were unenforced. Regulatory programs under state health departments in the United States have existed for many years but they have varied in their effectiveness. The US Senate's Subcommittee on Long-Term Care of the Senate Special Committee on Aging criticizes the Department of Health, Education, and Welfare and the majority of state governments for lax and unenforced standards. HEW's "new standards" were said to be so vague as to defy enforcement.[10] Federal and state standards or requirements are available and should be studied by nurses.[11-17] In 1971, President Nixon announced an eight-point program in response to the problems of substandard nursing homes, and the Office of Nursing Home Affairs was established. In 1972 and 1973, Marie Callender, a nurse who was special assistant for nursing home affairs, US Department of Health, Education, and Welfare, and others associated with nursing homes held out promise of an effective national program.[18]

In 1973, Faye G. Abdellah was appointed director of the ONHA, and in 1974, was made the Public Health Service coordinator for aging. Abdellah, in a statement on the historical development of the ONHA, USPHS, and DHEW, includes the following statement:

In April 1974, the Secretary, DHEW, rearranged responsibilities both centrally and regionally to facilitate the enforcement of health and safety standards for long-term care facilities participating in the Medicare and Medicaid programs. Regional Directors were delegated responsibility for survey and certification. . . . New Offices of Long-Term Care Standards Enforcement were established in each region. . . .*

The ONHA works with these regional offices in matters of legislative authorities and federal standards, their guidelines, application, and enforcement. An Advisory Committee on Home Health Services under the chairmanship of ONHA, established in 1974, has the responsibility for coordinating and monitoring home health service activities and for program development for DHEW. Currently involved in aspects of long-term care and aging are ten agencies within the Department and five in other federal departments.

In 1974, the Research on Aging Act was signed into Public Law 93–296 which authorized the establishment of a National Institute on Aging as a component of the National Institutes of Health. The NIA is now (in 1976) under the direction of Robert Butler, a physician.

Effects of this concentrated effort within the federal government to upgrade nursing homes and all services to the aging should soon be measurable. As all who watch television and read news media know, parallel upgrading programs are going forward in the private sector.

The Rights of Nursing Home Inmates. Inmates of nursing homes should have the same rights as hospital patients, but in the United States, as noted earlier, they have not been nearly as well protected. The rights of patients in Skilled Nursing Facilities as established by the Social Security Administration, October, 1974, are described below.

For patients receiving Medicare benefits, the Social Security Administration requires that the facility establish written policies that are made available to residents and guardians or next of kin. The policies ensure the following conditions for each inmate:

1. Is fully informed, as evidenced by the patient's written acknowledgement . . . of these rights and all rules and regulations . . . ;
2. Is fully informed . . . of services available . . . and of related charges . . . ;
3. Is fully informed, by a physician, of his medical condition . . . and afforded opportunity to participate in planning . . . treatment and

* Abdellah, Faye G.: *Accomplishments (Fiscal 1974) and Objectives of the Office of Nursing Home Affairs (Fiscal 1975 and 1976).* Department of Health, Education, and Welfare, Public Health Service, Office of Nursing Home Affairs, Rockville, Md., Oct. 9, 1974, p. 2, processed.

to refuse to participate in experimental research;

4. Is transferred or discharged only for medical reasons, or for his welfare or that of other patients, or for nonpayment for his stay (except as prohibited by titles XVIII or XIX of the Social Security Act and is given reasonable . . . notice . . . and such actions are documented in his medical record;

5. Is encouraged and assisted . . . to exercise his rights as a patient and as a citizen and . . . may voice grievances and recommend changes in policies and services to facility staff . . . ;

6. May manage his personal financial affairs, or is given at least a quarterly accounting of financial transactions . . . ;

7. Is free from mental and physical abuse, and free from chemical and (except in emergencies) physical restraints except as authorized in writing by a physician . . . ;

8. Is assured confidential treatment of his personal and medical records . . . ;

9. Is treated with consideration, respect, and full recognition of his dignity and individuality, including privacy in treatment and in care for his personal needs;

10. Is not required to perform services for the facility that are not included for therapeutic purposes in his plan of care;

11. May associate and communicate privately with persons of his choice and send and receive his personal mail unopened, unless medically contraindicated . . . ;

12. May meet with, and participate in activities of, social, religious, and community groups at his discretion, unless medically contraindicated . . . ;

13. May retain and use his personal clothing and possessions as space permits . . . ;

14. If married, is assured privacy for visits by his/her spouse; if both are inpatients in the facility, they are permitted to share a room, unless medically contraindicated (as documented by the attending physician in the medical record).*

Some of the more common and shocking reports are that inmates are held in institutions against their will; sick inmates are not seen by doctors or other professional health workers; incoming and outgoing mail is opened and sometimes intercepted; starvation diets and inedible foods are served; bathing and toilet facilities are inadequate; and physical restraints and the use of tranquilizers are grossly abused.[19-27]

The US Department of Health, Education, and Welfare has had Nursing Home Ombudsman [patient advocate] Demonstration projects since 1972 that by 1974 had received "1,196 individual complaints," most of which were investigated.* Giving nursing home residents a feeling that someone will listen to reports of unmet needs or actual abuse and will try to see that their needs are met, or rights accorded them, cannot fail to help, whether patients' advocates are from the public or private sector. Pennsylvania's Nursing Home Ombudsman Demonstration Project has published a *Consumer's Handbook on Nursing Homes,* and the Gray Panthers, with headquarters in Philadelphia, include an ombudsman program in their Nursing Home Project.†

Responsibility for the mistreatment of nursing home inmates must be shared by families and friends who fail to visit inmates or to get involved in what is happening to them. The care of the chronically ill and aged will be humane when the average citizen believes it is his or her right and when society provides the conditions that make this not only possible but mandatory.

Location, Physical Plans, and Furnishings of Nursing Homes. Nursing homes are found in large cities, towns, suburbs, and in the country. A few are well designed, well furnished, and equipped to provide care and rehabilitation; most are converted private dwellings or structures built for other purposes. Old mansions with handsome exteriors offer deceptive luxury, for the interior is usually unsuitable for communal living. New structures are often cheaply built and furnished with little to offer from the standpoint of health or esthetics. In Great Britain, some nursing homes offer the ultimate in comfort, but this is rare in the United States. Here, large nursing homes are more likely to be found in cities, small ones in the country. Small homes are more likely to be operated for profit than large ones.

In an issue of *The Nursing Clinics of North America,* half of which was devoted to geriatric nursing standards, Gertrude B. Ujhely had this to say about nursing homes in 1972:

Nursing homes, especially if they are public institutions, are frequently erected on available government property, which is often too far removed for any type of meaningful integration of the older person with the surrounding community. Patients, or residents, . . . are taken on oc-

---

* US Department of Health, Education, and Welfare, Social Security Administration: *Skilled Nursing Facilities. Federal Register,* Vol. 39, No. 193, Oct. 3, 1974, pp. 35775.

* Forman, Allan: "The Nursing Home Ombudsman Demonstration Program," *Health Serv. Rep.,* **89:**128, (Mar.–Apr.) 1974.

† Commonwealth of Pennsylvania: *Consumer's Handbook on Nursing Homes.* Pennsylvania Nursing Home Ombudsman Demonstration Project, Governor's Office for Human Resources, [Harrisburg], Dec. 1973; Gray Panthers: *Nursing Home Project.* Gray Panthers, Philadelphia, Oct., 1974, processed.

casional bus trips to department stores or special community festivities which literally swamp the older person's receptor system with overwhelming numbers of stimuli. Within the nursing home the older person frequently finds himself to be an isolated dot in a sea of vast corridors and identical rooms, all painted in uniform white, so that it takes more skill than he could possibly have at his disposal to orient himself.

Given these circumstances, it is no wonder that older people often withdraw into the security of their own being and that they decline and regress much faster than their physiologic condition would lead one to expect.

Add to this picture other factors that are familiar to most nurses who have had any professional contact with the aged. There is, for instance, the mixture of well oriented and utterly deteriorated patients on one and the same ward. There is the constantly blaring television set that is out of focus. There are the belittling attitudes on the part of the staff and last, but not least, the well balanced but usually unchewable meals which land in the wastebasket more often than in the patient's stomach.*

Organization and Administration of Nursing Homes. Some accredited extended care facilities are organized under a board of directors and administered by a qualified hospital administrator, as might be expected of a hospital for the chronically ill; many small nursing homes are owned and administered by the same individuals, who may in some cases be doctors or nurses. They may also be lawyers, or industrialists, or others whose training and experience in no way fits them for operating a health agency. The lack of consumer participation and control is conspicuous.[28,29] Specialized texts on the organization and operation of nursing homes describe currently accepted practices, but there are many deviations from them. While society seems to be aroused by the publicity given neglect of the aged and the scandalous conditions in nursing homes in the United States, Mendelson charges the public with slipping back into apathy after each exposé. F. N. Elliott,[30] in an article "Goals for Quality Must be Based on Values Derived from Changing Society," made the point that health care personnel cannot effect changes until they have the backing of consumers and until the system of health care makes reform possible.

Functions, Satisfactions, Rewards, and Difficulties for Nurses in Nursing Homes. The potential functions of nurses in nursing homes are those of nurses in hospitals, although Sheldon Ornstein writes "a nursing home is not a hospital."[31] In accredited extended care facilities with adequate and organized medical and nursing staffs, the functions of nurses and physicians are quite like those in hospitals. In nursing homes where physicians make only brief weekly or monthly visits, the nursing staff may assume much more decision-making responsibility than it would in most hospitals. Nurses may operate under "standing orders" from physicians that enable them to use their judgment in giving a wide range of drugs and other treatments. In many homes, decisions are forced on nursing personnel that they are inadequately prepared but often too willing to make.

Nathan Hershey[32] discussed some of the legal issues in the care of nursing home patients, as these institutions were operated in 1973, partly with reference to the dearth of professional personnel. The US Senate's Special Committee on Aging has been concerned with legal problems in nursing home care.[33]

The American Nurses' Association has studied nursing care of the aged in this and other settings and one of its annual awards in 1974 went to Virginia Stone for her leadership in geriatric nursing. Lois N. Knowles has led conferences on geriatric nursing and was chairman of the ANA committee that published *Standards for Geriatric Nursing Practice.*[34,35] National nursing organizations in the United States are cooperating with federal and state agencies to bring about needed changes. Publications from Canada and Europe suggest that many countries are baffled by the problems imposed by the extended life span and the breakdown in family life.[36-39] Nursing and nursing home journals show an awareness of the need for improving the facilities and services. Bibliographies on geriatric nursing are lengthy.[40] A selection of 36 articles from the *American Journal of Nursing,* entitled *Nursing and the Aging Patient,* is one of the *Contemporary Nursing Series.*[41] Texts and studies of geriatric nursing and care of nursing home patients reflect a hopeful concern for the elderly but, in the writer's opinion, a depressing picture of current institutions and agencies.[42-54]

Well-prepared nurses who have participated in high-quality health care find employment in the average nursing home in the United States unsatisfying because, under the present conditions in such an institution, they find it impossible to meet basic human needs and they are also forced to see sick patients inadequately treated from the medical standpoint.

Because the medical profession has devoted so little time, comparatively, to the nursing home population, some nurses see the care of these patients as a particular challenge to nurs-

---

* Ujhely, Gertrude B.: "The Environment of the Elderly," *Nurs. Clin. North Am.,* 7:281, (June) 1972.

ing and as an opportunity to prove the value of nursing to society. Well nursed, or nursed with the intent to rehabilitate, many inmates of nursing homes could be returned to independent living and life with their families. The disorientation of many nursing home residents is completely unnecessary. Carolyn Chambers,[55] analyzing the behavior of an elderly patient, asked whether he is suffering from "senility or deprivation." A. O. Rossi and associates,[56] discussing the care of nursing home inmates, concluded that "treating old people like children can bring on mental breakdown." In any event, the segregation of the aged in nursing homes is questionable. R. L. Wolk and R. B. Seiden [57] call old age "a contagious disease," and V. Sulds [58] notes that "when the children come so does laughter."

General neglect, inadequate diet, inactivity with a lack of sensory stimulation, displacement from familiar surroundings and companions lead to disorientation, introversion, and behavior that may brand the elderly as psychotic. Returned to familiar surroundings, to the stimulation of family life with relatives and friends, the supposedly psychotic behavior disappears.[59] J. A. Whitehead [60] called attention to "myths of mental illness in the elderly"; D. S. Wilkiemeyer [61] wrote about affection as "the key to care for the elderly." It is doubtful whether this can be supplied in satisfying amounts by the employees of even the best institutions.

In Great Britain, where better provision has been made for helping the aged to be independent than in most countries, the return of patients to their own homes, or to the homes of family members, seems to be the aim of institutional care.[62-64] There is, however, a good deal in the literature to suggest that nurses everywhere reject the uncritical acceptance of custodial care as the lot of the elderly.[65-69] E. L. Farnsworth [70] reports a survey made in nursing homes purporting to show that "rehabilitation is becoming routine." The "homemaker services" and "meals-on-wheels" are current efforts to give the sick and elderly the help they need if they are to live at home. Margaret Wilson [71] described a guide to public health nurses in helping the elderly achieve functional tasks at home. The well-known work of Doris Schwartz, in association with other nurses, physicians, and social workers, in ambulatory services at the New York Hospital, New York City, has focused on the maintenance of independence for the chronically ill and elderly, or the ability to "cope." [72,73]

In a society that makes full use of the potential value of the older population, the care of the aged could offer high rewards and great satisfaction. At present, nurses in settings where geriatric nursing is practiced are not highly rewarded materially or professionally.

S. H. May [74] has written about old age as "the crowning years" but most references to the end of life, if so designated, are derisive. Patricia Kinsella's [75] article "Geriatric Nursing: It Can Be Rewarding, Fulfilling, Exciting" is a sincere statement of one nurse's viewpoint. More often there is the feeling that nurses who work in institutions and agencies for the elderly are "second-class nurses," [76,77] B. R. Tuck [78] in 1972 called the geriatric nurse "a pioneer in a new specialty." Hopefully, these "pioneers" can reverse the trend toward neglect of the elderly and find in doing so as great a satisfaction as can be found in any other setting for nursing practice.

4. HOSPICES

"Hospice" is a new term to many. In Chapter 2, it was pointed out that hospices date from the Middle Ages and that currently the term has been adopted for institutions designed to meet special needs of the terminally ill. Reference was made to the development of Hospice, Inc., in Branford, Connecticut, as the first American hospice. It started an outpatient service in 1974 and hopes to open an inpatient service in 1979.

The commitment of physicians to prolonging life at any cost to patients and their families, and the development of technology that makes it possible to keep people alive long after the capacity for enjoying life has ceased, leads many to dread death in the hospital. The title of an article in *Medical World News* in 1972 made the following statement and asked the following question: "The Problems Created by Medical Progress. What Do You Do for the Aged—and When Do You Stop Doing It?" [1] Jeanne C. Quint, who reported in 1967 a full-length study, *The Nurse and the Dying Patient*,[2] made this statement in an article discussing obstacles to helping the dying:

Perhaps we need to remind ourselves from time to time that patients who are dying are not just dying. They are also living. Whether or not they have the opportunity to live this final human experience to the fullest—each in his own way—is influenced in great measure by us who take care of them.*

Hospices are designed to eliminate the obstacles of physical and psychologic suffering, to provide a setting that gives the dying an

---

* Quint, Jeanne C.: "Obstacles to Helping the Dying," *Am. J. Nurs.*, **69**:1568, (July) 1969.

opportunity to live as fully as possible, and to provide health personnel with the facilities and resources that enable them to give patients and their families optimum help. Hospice services are particularly effective with patients who are in advanced stages of cancer. Much of the literature focuses on care of patients terminally ill with cancer but all dying persons deserve special consideration.

Religious orders throughout the centuries have offered the dying a refuge; present-day hospices, notably those in Great Britain in secular institutions, offer spiritual and physical comfort, with care based on current knowledge of social, physical, and biologic sciences.*

Because there are so few hospices, no figures are available on the numbers of nurses working in them.† Hospice, Inc., in Branford, Connecticut, that is modeled largely on hospices in England, will be classified as a chronic disease hospital, and the staffing will be comparable with respect to professional nurses, licensed practical nurses, and nurse's aides, except that since all patients need critical care, the professional nurse ratio will be high. The salary range is also comparable. The plan is for nurses to rotate through home care and inpatient care services. Volunteers will play a more important role than in most hospitals. Nursing personnel, physicians, social workers, pharmacists, the clergy, special therapists, maintenance personnel, volunteers, patients, and their families will form "a community" that is supportive to all its members. As in England, a nursery school for caregivers' children will be a part of the facility. This means that all ages will be represented under Hospice's roof.

Figure 3-8 shows some of the features of the first hospice built in the United States—the accessibility of the outdoors to all patients, the provision of communal recreational and dining areas, the central location of a non-denominational place of worship and spiritual replenishment, areas for study and research by the staff, and overnight accommodations for a family member of a patient who is very near death or who for other reasons needs special support.

Hospices everywhere are subject to the same regulatory processes as other health care institutions, and while most are autonomous agencies with support from private funds, they also have contractural arrangements with private and public sources of third-party reimbursement. The rights of patients are the same as those in other hospitals.

Most hospices and nursing homes for the terminally ill in England are located in cities and towns so that they are accessible by public transportation to families and friends who are encouraged to spend as much time with patients as is mutually desirable.

The organization and administration of hospices are less formal than in most hospitals. In annual reports of St. Christopher's Hospice in London, modeled to some extent on St. Joseph's Hospice, a wing of St. Joseph's 150-bed hospital in London, the staff is said to be "a family caring for families."

The writings of Cicely Saunders, a social worker-nurse-physician who founded St. Christopher's, give some idea of the functions, rewards, and difficulties of nursing in a hospice.[3-5] Pictures taken and films made at St. Christopher's show the satisfactions so vividly that nurses from many countries have been attracted and gone there in recent years for experience.[6] Florence Wald (coauthor of Chapter 50 on death and dying in this book), one of the founders of Hospice, Inc., in Branford, Connecticut, has, with Joan Craven, described some of the satisfactions in hospice nursing, with special reference to the Connecticut program which Edward F. Dobihal has also described.[7,8]

The body of literature on thanatology (the study of the phenomena of somatic death) is growing so rapidly that nurses and other health workers specializing in the care of the dying patient cannot keep up with it. Conferences on the care of the dying atract those in the health occupations and the ministry. As facilities develop that make a peaceful, dignified death possible, nurses will find employment in them especially rewarding. For further discussion of hospices, see Chapter 50.

5. PUBLIC HEALTH AGENCIES

Employment of Nurses in Public Health Agencies. The American Nurses' Association in *Facts About Nursing 74–75* reported that in

---

* Secular leaders in the current hospice movement rarely fail to mention the influence of the Irish Sisters of Charity, a Roman Catholic order, in St. Joseph's Hospice in London, England, but students of history will recall many instances of royal deaths in convents and monasteries.

† In the American Nurses' Association report *Nursing and Long-Term Care,* the following statement indicates the need for institutions that provide terminal care: "A setting that is virtually nonexistent is one that provides for the care of an individual who is in a terminal phase of illness, who is severely disabled, or who is in a transitional phase of illness." (American Nurses' Association, Committee on Skilled Nursing Care: *Nursing and Long-Term Care. Toward Quality Care for the Aging.* The Association, Kansas City, Mo., 1975, p. 34.) These observations suggest that not only hospices but institutions providing *any* kind of terminal care are rare.

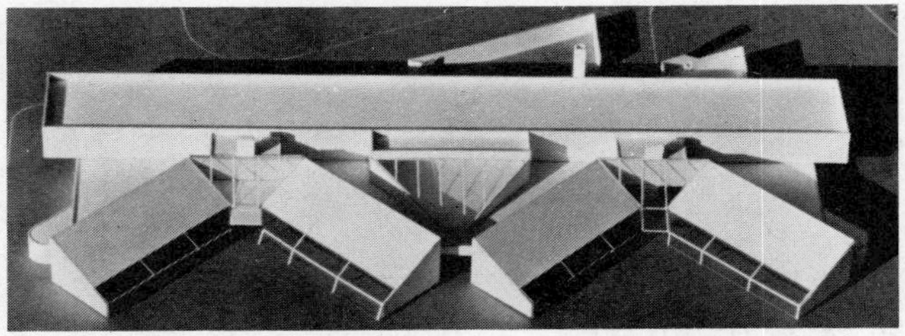

Figure 3-8. *A.* Photograph of architect's model of Hospice, Branford, Conn. Four 10-bed patient units open on to triangular terraces in front and corridors behind leading to work-rooms, bathrooms, conference and reading rooms. In the center of the building is a chapel that opens on a central corridor through which can be reached, at the back of the building, the admissions office, home care office, pharmacy, kitchen, staff dining room, crafts room, and room for day care of children of staff members. *B.* A floor plan of the main floor. The upper floor (not shown) contains offices, storage space, room where families can be with the body after death, staff lounge, and staff lockers. (Courtesy of Lo-Yi Chan of Prentice and Chan, Ohlhausen, architects, New York.)

Staff dining

Crafts

Day care

Kitchen

Staff

Nook

Hair-dressing

Trash, etc.

Main corridor

Commons

Living room

Chapel

Pharmacy

Home care staff

X-ray

Exam

Admissions

Entry

Home care conference

N

Toilets, bath linens, utility, etc.

Conf. room

W. C. and lav

Reading room

Single rooms

Green house corridor

Terrace

Three 4-bedded wards

A

B

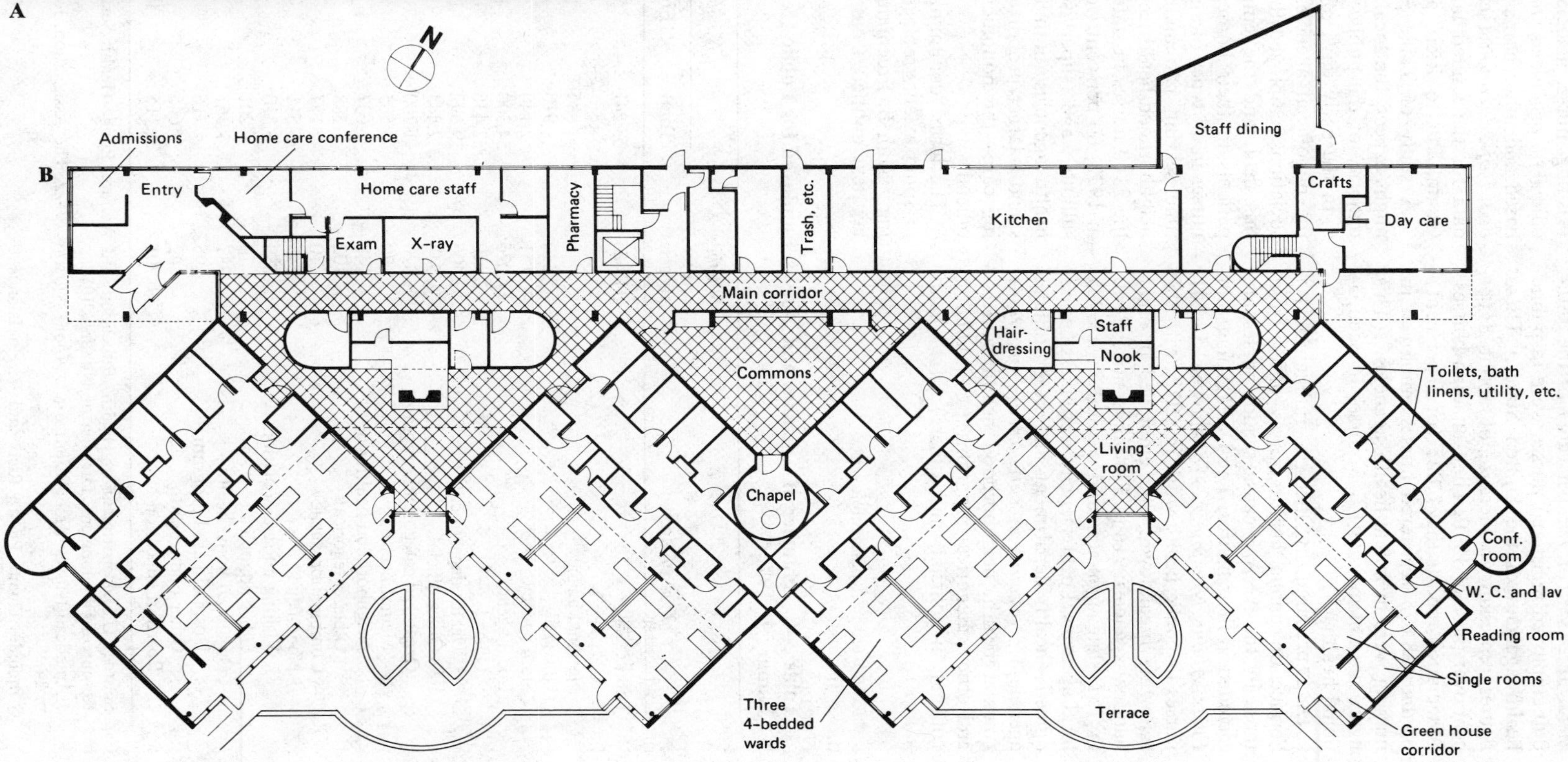

1972, 58,241 * (or 7½ per cent) of the 780,-000 employed registered nurses were in public health agencies of the United States.[1] These figures represent an increase of about 8 per cent over those of 1970. The Canadian Nurses' Association reports that 6,025 (or 5 per cent) of the 128,675 registered nurses employed in nursing were in public health agencies.[2] (This figure did not include 1,603 nurses in occupational health.)

Data prepared by the US Public Health Service on public health nurses differ from those by the ANA because school nurses are included in their figures. The USPHS figure in *Facts About Nursing 72–73* showed 58,241 nurses in public health work in 1972, with the following breakdown: 885 employed in eight national agencies; 916 in 270 universities; 2140 in 151 state agencies; and 54,300 in 11,025 local agencies. Local agencies were classified as *official* (health department and other official agencies); *organized categorical programs* (mental health, neighborhood health centers, and other categorical programs); *combination* (official, nonofficial, and others); *nonofficial*

(visiting nurse associations and other nonofficial); *organized home health* (hospital-based and other home health programs); and *board of education* (school programs).[3] Cited data for the United States included nurses in Guam, Puerto Rico, and the Virgin Islands.

A study of Table 3-4 shows that, as one might expect, the local agencies employed the majority of the public health nurses.

In the early days of public health nursing, the nonofficial agencies, or visiting nurse associations, employed the bulk of the nurses in this field, and the emphasis was on care of patients in their homes; today, public health nurses in all types of agencies may spend more time serving patients in offices, clinics, and neighborhood health centers than in homes. Of the 2140 nurses in state public health agencies in 1972, 60 per cent were administrators, consultants, and supervisors.[4] Nurses in local health agencies, both official and nonofficial, spend a larger proportion of their time in giving care—the nonofficial more time than the official.

The term "community health nursing" has, to some extent, replaced "public health nursing." Ruth B. Freeman, in the 1970 edition of her text entitled *Community Health Nursing*

* 7255 were part-time employees.

Table 3-4.   Number of Agencies and Nurses Employed for Public Health Work, as of January 1, 1972 *

Type of Agency	Number of Agencies	Number of Nurses		
		Total	Full-Time	Part-Time
Total †	11,455	58,241	50,986	7,255
National agency	8	885	835	50
University	270	916	789	127
State agency	151	2,140	2,060	80
Local agency	11,026	54,300	47,302	6,998
Official	2,950	22,436	19,277	3,159
Health department	2,406	19,592	17,006	2,586
Other official	544	2,844	2,271	573
Organized categorical program	320	1,700	1,476	224
Mental health	70	505	459	46
Neighborhood health center	148	607	509	98
Other categorical	102	588	508	80
Combination agency	70	2,177	1,997	180
Nonofficial	648	5,511	4,247	1,264
Visiting nurse association	578	5,310	4,113	1,197
Other nonofficial	70	201	134	67
Organized home health	337	1,361	950	411
Hospital based program	195	716	530	186
Other home health	142	645	420	225
Board of education	6,701	21,115	19,355	1,760

Source: U.S. Department of Health, Education and Welfare, Public Health Service, Bureau of Health Resources Development, Division of Nursing, 1972.

* American Nurses' Association: *Facts About Nursing 72–73*. The Association, Kansas City, Mo., 1974, p. 34.

† Includes Guam, Puerto Rico, and Virgin Islands.

Practice, had the following to say about this branch of nursing:

Dramatic changes in the technical and social nature of health services are demanding equally dramatic changes in professional practice in all of the health disciplines.

. . .

Community health nursing is seen as a population-based obligation, realized through a multidisciplinary, ecologically oriented effort and utilizing concepts and skills that derive both from generic nursing and from public health practice. It focuses on nursing the community, in contradistinction to nursing *in* the community. Family nursing care is seen as an essential aspect of health care of the population, and the community health nurse's responsibility is seen as encompassing but not being limited to this aspect of the program.*

The American Nurses' Association, in *Standards. Community Health Nursing Practice,* gave the following definition:

Community Health Nursing is a synthesis of nursing practice and public health practice applied to promoting and preserving the health of populations. The nature of this practice is general and comprehensive. It is not limited to a particular age or diagnostic group. It is continuing, not episodic. The dominant responsibility is to the population

as a whole. Therefore, nursing directed to individuals, families or groups contributes to the health of the total population. Health promotion, health maintenance, health education, coordination and continuity of care are utilized in a holistic approach to the family, group, and community. The nurse's actions acknowledge the need for comprehensive health planning, recognize the influences of social and ecological issues, give attention to populations at risk and utilize the dynamic forces which influence change.*

The ANA listed and elaborated on the following standards by which community health nursing practices were evaluated:

(1) The collection of data about the health status of the consumer is systematic and continuous. The data are accessible, communicated and recorded; (2) Nursing diagnoses are derived from health status data; (3) Plans for nursing service include goals derived from nursing diagnoses; (4) Plans for nursing service include priorities and nursing approaches or measures to achieve the goals derived from diagnoses; (5) Nursing actions provide for consumer participation in health promotion, maintenance and restoration; (6) Nursing actions assist consumers to maximize health potential; (7) The consumer's progress toward goal achievement is determined by the consumer and the nurse; (8) Nursing

---

* Freeman, Ruth B.: *Community Health Nursing Practice.* W. B. Saunders Co., Philadelphia, 1970, p. iii.

* American Nurses' Association: *Standards. Community Health Nursing Practice.* The Association, Kansas City, Mo., 1973, p. 2.

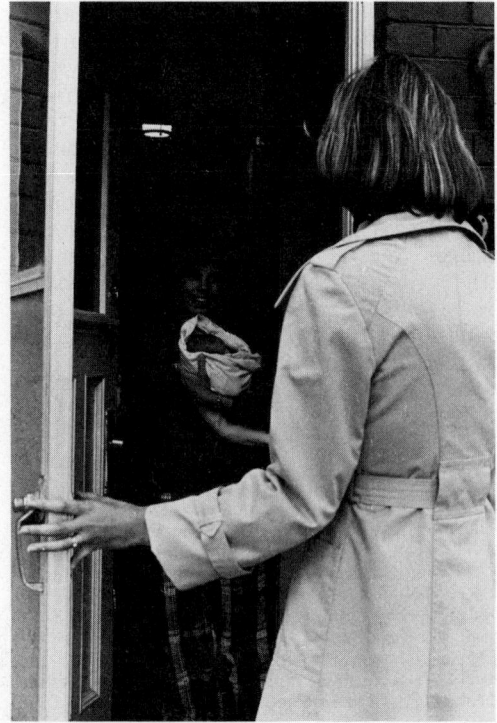

Figure 3-9. Public health nurse (Toronto District) carries out home visiting program for mother with newborn. (Photograph by Dougal Bichan in Handbury, Eric: *Nurse.* McClelland & Stewart, Ltd., Toronto, Ont., 1975. Sponsored by the Registered Nurses Association of Ontario for the celebration of its 50th Anniversary.)

actions involve ongoing reassessment, reordering of priorities, new goal setting and revision of the nursing plan.*

In Great Britain, public health nurses are divided into health visitors and district nurses. The former teach health and concentrate on prevention, while the district nurses devote more time to nursing the sick in their homes. In 1971, the Royal College of Nursing and the National Council of Nurses of the United Kingdom published a pamphlet on *The Role of the Health Visitor.* The following is the last of 44 conclusions: "The health visitor, uncertain of her role in the past, should now meet the challenge of the present and look forward to a different but richly satisfying future as a unique and important full member of the community health team." † In 1973, the College and the Council, in the *RCN Comment on the Report of the Committee on Nursing,* made the following recommendation: "There should be a continuing distinction of functions and qualifications between nurses engaged in family clinical (home nursing) and family health (visiting) services." ‡ They go on to say that retaining the present title of "district nurse" [under the reorganization of the health service] would "cause confusion." There is said to be "considerable feeling" among the membership that the titles should not be changed.

There is a difference of opinion on the division of responsibility "in public health nursing," but Helen McCarrick [5] thinks the health visitor in Great Britain is "the key figure of the future." Hers is but one of many articles indicating that this is a period of analysis of and marked change in community health services, including the nursing component.[6-16]

In Great Britain, community nurses (district nurses and health visitors) and physicians form teams to serve a geographical area or population. They may operate from a physician's office or from a neighborhood health center.§ The work in such offices or centers is coordinated with the programs of hospitals and other health agencies in the area under one central medical authority. In Canada and the United States, various experiments along these lines have been reported.[17-26]

* American Nurses' Association: *ibid.,* p. 3.
† Royal College of Nursing and National Council of Nurses of the United Kingdom: *The Role of the Health Visitor.* The College and the Council, London, 1971, p. 17.
‡ Royal College of Nursing and National Council of Nurses of the United Kingdom: *RCN Comment on the Report of the Committee on Nursing.* The College and the Council, London, 1973, p. 36.
§ See Chapter 2, page 148, for reference to The Peckham Experiment as the *de luxe* model for such health centers in England and Canada.

Barbara Schutt,[26a] evaluating the program of the Frontier Nurses of Kentucky, calls it 40 years' experience in giving primary health care in the mountains of this state.

As neighborhood health centers or health maintenance type organizations develop, more effective coordinating systems than now exist undoubtedly will be sought in all countries. The Kaiser-Permanente pattern is often mentioned as the most effective one at present in the United States.[27,28]

Standardization and Certification of Public Health Nursing Services. Public health nursing in the United States has a long history of attempts to standardize practice and ensure its quality. In 1909, Yssabella Waters,[29] a statistician, reported data from, and a directory of, state and city visiting nurse services sponsored by "businesses," churches, hospitals, and voluntary and official agencies and associations. This was the first major national nursing survey in America. The wide variation in practice shown by the Waters' report hastened the development of a national organization that could, among other things, set standards for practice. The National Organization for Public Health Nursing, organized in 1912, was the first national nursing organization to have a headquarters office with a paid staff.[30,31] From its founding, the organization upgraded and standardized practice and published annual data based on a questionnaire sent to agencies. The data was published in the Association's journal in a Yearly Review. Dorothy E. Wiesner and Margaret M. Murphy[32] of the NOPHN reported a summary of similarities and variations in programs in 1942 that is of historical interest. Later, the US Public Health Service collaborated with the NOPHN in the collection and publication of data on public health nursing. Since the disbanding of the NOPHN, the USPHS and other federal agencies have collaborated with the ANA's Statistics Department in collecting information on nursing, but they prepare the most complete data on public health nursing.

The ANA's Congress for Nursing Practice, through the Association's divisions of nursing practice, has prepared a series of pamphlets, one of which is *Standards* [for] *Community Health Nursing Practice,*[33] designed to establish, maintain, and improve standards, to educate the public, and to protect members of the profession.

The American Public Health Association in the United States and its equivalent in other countries have directly and indirectly influenced public health nursing worldwide. Since 1966, in the United States, the National League for Nursing and the American Public Health

Association have sponsored a voluntary program of Accreditation of Community Nursing Services. This involves a periodic review at 5-year intervals. By April 1974, 200 agencies had applied for accreditation and 72 community nursing services had been accredited. The program is being broadened to include other disciplines. Representatives from the American Dietetic Association, American Occupational Therapy Association, American Physical Therapy Association, American Speech and Hearing Association, National Association of Social Workers, National Council of Homemakers, Home Health Aide Services, Inc., and medical representation from the APHA's Medical Care Section are collaborating with nurse members of the Association's Accreditation Standards and Review Committee to develop criteria to use in the broadened program.[34]

Since public health nursing agencies are now receiving third-party payment for their services, they, like hospitals, nursing homes, and other health agencies, must meet standards set by the US Social Security Administration for the disbursement of Medicare and Medicaid funds. What has been said under Hospitals and Nursing Homes about the federal government's role in certification of agencies need not be repeated here. There is a *Directory of Home Health Agencies Certified as Medicare Providers* published by the National League for Nursing.[34a]

The Rights of Patients in Public Health Agencies. It has been more difficult in the past for institutionalized patients to protect themselves from unwanted, or what they believed to be inappropriate or harmful, services than it has for those in outpatient clinics or home care programs. Institutional care is provided under policies set by the boards or trustees that govern the institution, and, while boards and trustees also establish policies for ambulatory services, the workers seem to have more influence in them than in institutions. As hospitals offer more ambulatory services and as community nurses and other public health personnel operate more often from doctors' offices, community health centers, and hospital-based home care programs, the differences diminish. Only in their homes can patients or clients fully protect themselves by simply refusing to admit the health worker to the home. Actually, this has never been entirely possible, since certain patients, such as those with some communicable diseases and those declared legally insane, have had their liberties curtailed even when they are in their homes.

Most of what was said about patients' rights on page 197 applies here. There must be "in-formed consent" to treatment, patients' right to refuse treatment must be recognized, and the privacy of records must be safeguarded. Problem-oriented records may be used in a home health agency. A Family Data and Problem Index put out by the National League for Nursing in 1973 is shown in Figure 3-10.

Organization and Administration of Public Health Nursing Services. Public health nurses may be employed in international agencies such as the World Health Organization; in national agencies such as (in the United States) the US Public Health Service, the Veterans Administration, or the Indian Health Service; in state agencies such as a state health department; or in local agencies such as a city health department or a visiting nurse agency, or a combination agency formed by a public and private agency. Public health nurses may also be college health or school nurses employed by educational institutions; they may be psychiatric nurses in mental health centers; they may be specialists in occupational health and be employed by industries; or they may be in the field of prison health and employed by federal, state, county, or city correctional institutions. In this brief treatment of the topic, it is not possible to show the wide range of organizations, agencies, and institutions employing public health nurses. Recent texts, symposia, and journal articles may be consulted by the interested reader.[35-46]

As noted earlier, public health nurses from local health authorities in Great Britain are regularly assigned to work with private practitioners serving a geographical area, and there are experimental programs along these lines elsewhere. In many countries, public health nurses work in mobile units supplying health care—especially health education and preventive services—to people where they live or work. Visitors to the USSR and the People's Republic of China are impressed with this aspect of their health programs. In an article entitled "We Care Enough To Come To You," Lilja A. Snyder[47] describes a mobile unit (one of the sporadic attempts in the United States to employ this principle) that serves Polk County, Minnesota. This unit was initiated by the Polk County Nursing Service and financed by the Northlands Regional Medical Program.

Public health nurses may even be employed by hospitals to facilitate their work with other health agencies, or they may be employed by schools of nursing and medicine to help students practice a family-centered service. Public health nurses are employed in health programs for Indians and Eskimos (native Americans and Canadians) and in programs for migratory laborers. Clinical specialists in public health

FAMILY NAME _____

FAMILY I.D. No. _____

**FAMILY DATA
AND PROBLEM INDEX**

DATE	ADDRESS	DIRECTIONS–C/O–NEAR	APT/FLOOR	TELEPHONE	HEALTH AREA

FAMILY ROSTER

NAME	BIRTH DATE	MARITAL STATUS
Man:		☐S ☐M ☐W ☐D ☐SEP.
Woman:	Maiden Name:	☐S ☐M ☐W ☐D ☐SEP.

Comments:

CHILDREN	BIRTH DATE	SEX	COMMENTS
1			
2			
3			
4			
5			
6			
7			
8			

OTHERS IN HOUSEHOLD	BIRTH DATE	SEX	RELATIONSHIP	COMMENTS

RECORD OF SERVICE

NAME	DATE Adm.	DATE Disch.	PRIMARY DIAGNOSIS	NAME	DATE Adm.	DATE Disch.	PRIMARY DIAGNOSIS

FORM 21-FDPI   DHHA/CHS   ©1973 National League for Nursing

Figure 3-10. Problem-oriented record advocated by the National League for Nursing to be used in community nursing. (Courtesy of National League for Nursing, New York, N.Y.)

FAMILY HISTORY
physical, functional, nutritional, etc.

ENVIRONMENTAL FACTORS
housing, sanitation, transportation, safety, etc.

FAMILY ADJUSTMENTS
social, emotional, cultural, vocational, religious, etc.

Date   Signature and title

Figure 3-10. (Continued)

	OTHER AGENCIES ACTIVE				
DATE	FAMILY MEMBER	AGENCY	NAME OF WORKER	TELEPHONE NUMBER	DATE INACTIVE

FAMILY PROBLEM INDEX

List all potential, current, or significant past problems which affect the family as a group. Include the date of onset or identification and the date of resolution for each problem.

PROBLEM NO.	FAMILY PROBLEMS POTENTIAL/CURRENT-ACTIVE	DATE OF ONSET	DATE RESOLVED	FAMILY PROBLEMS SIGNIFICANT PAST-INACTIVE

CONTINUE ON REVERSE SIDE

Figure 3-10. (Continued)

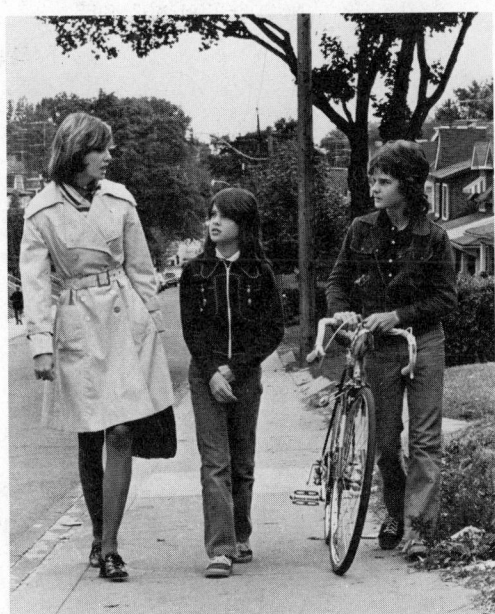

Figure 3-11. Public health nurse (Toronto District) chats with neighborhood children who attend one of the schools in her area where she is the "school nurse." (Photograph by Dougal Bichan in Handbury, Eric: *Nurse.* McClelland & Stewart, Ltd., Toronto, Ont., 1975. Sponsored by the Registered Nurses Association of Ontario for the celebration of its 50th Anniversary.)

agencies may function as consultants within the agency, to other agencies, to nursing homes, to hospitals, or to other institutions.[48-58]

Because the settings in which public health nurses function are so varied, it is not possible to discuss here the organizational structures and administrative patterns under which they operate. Most who consider themselves public health, or community, nurses would probably claim that they function more independently than nurses in hospital practice. However, it is the writer's opinion that differences have greatly diminished in recent years and that organizational structures and administrative patterns under which nurses function everywhere are beginning to offer well-prepared nurses the opportunity to practice professionally, or to use professional judgment. In 1975, Sarah E. Archer and Ruth P. Fleshman, reporting a study of the "typology" of practice in community health nursing, try to identify distinguishing characteristics of public health nurses (in this case, 81 "community nurse practitioners"). They note that nurses in other areas of practice have been moving into the community and that nurse educators are integrating community concepts throughout nursing curricula. Admitting that the adage "whatever every one knows and does is no longer a specialty" is particularly applicable to community nursing, they still consider it a special field of practice.[58a] (Archer and Fleshman are editors of *Community Health Nursing. Patterns and Practice,* Duxbury Press, North Scituate, Massachusetts, 1975.)

The June, 1975, issue of *Nursing Outlook* is devoted to community nursing. Its editor, Edith P. Lewis, suggests that as "manners make the man," the setting may make the nurse. She thinks there remains "something special" about community nurses. She thinks they are "people oriented," "health oriented," and that they provide "the bulk of the primary, preventive, individualized care that the public is so desperately seeking." *

Functions, Satisfactions, Rewards, and Difficulties in Public Health Nursing. The functions of public health or community health nursing have been defined by the American Public Health Association,[59] the Canadian Public Health Association,[60] and the American Nurses' Association.[61] These statements are in line with the World Health Organization's[62] statement of functions as given in its "technical report" on public health nursing in 1959. This report lists (and elaborates on) the following seven functions: (1) to provide and promote comprehensive nursing service to families; (2) to use nursing as a channel for strengthening family life and for promoting personal or family development and self-realization; (3) to participate in disease control by preventing and identifying disease early, providing and supervising care to reduce effects of disease; (4) to work with appropriate personnel in special settings in planning and implementing nursing phases of health programs; (5) to plan and evaluate nursing service for population groups to maximize nursing care benefits and relate it to the services of other health workers; (6) to contribute toward agency and community decisions; and (7) to contribute to the extension of knowledge in nursing and health care by surveys, studies, and research.

In the writer's opinion, public health nurses take more satisfaction in their work than do most nurses. This may be because their preparation is above average. While only 12.1 per cent of the total number of nurses in the United States held bachelor's degrees in 1972, 27.4 per cent of the public health nurses held bachelor's degrees; while only 2.2 per cent in the total nursing population held master's degrees, 4.9 per cent of the public health nurses

* Lewis, Edith P.: "They Still Make House Calls" (editorial), *Nurs. Outlook,* **23:**257, (June) 1975.

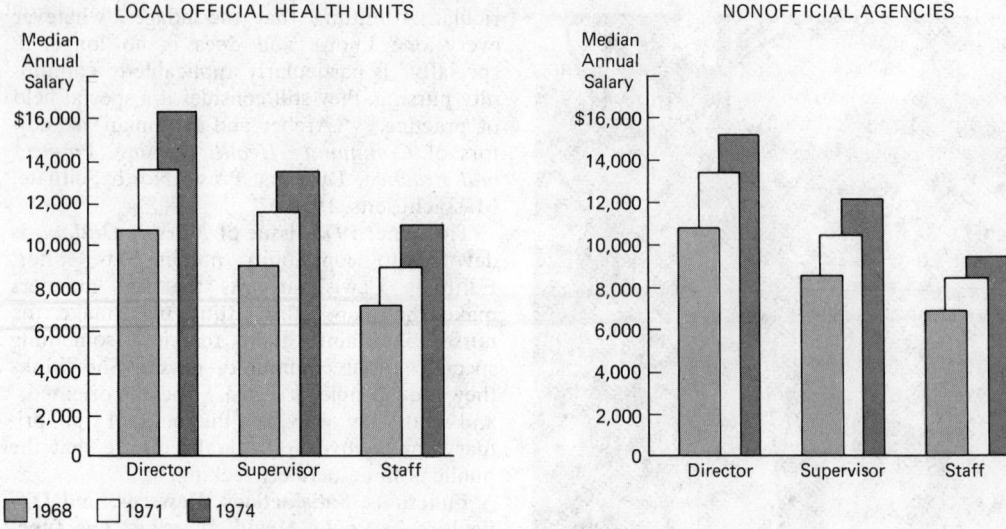

Figure 3-12. Median annual salaries of nurses in selected community health agencies, 1968, 1971, and 1974. (Source: National League for Nursing. From: American Nurses' Association: *Facts About Nursing 74–75*. The Association, Kansas City, Mo., 1976, p. 119.)

held master's degrees.[63] (The only category of American nurses with better academic preparation were those who administered and taught in schools of nursing.) Another source of satisfaction is the extent to which public health nurses are self-directed.* The extrainstitutional setting forces them to rely on their own judgment rather than to defer to others; they are also able to evaluate their service since they serve patients, clients, or families over long periods. Community nurses work under a patient-assignment rather than a functional-assignment system, and they consistently serve families rather than individuals.†

Because public health nurses are asked to assume considerable responsibility and their preparation is better than average, the salaries of public health staff nursing personnel in 1972 were proportionately higher than those of hospital staff nurses, for example.[64,65] However, as the preparation of all professional nurses moves into colleges and universities, as their functions expand in all settings, as public

* Nurse-midwives are, as a class, highly qualified and, in the writer's opinion, they also take more than average satisfaction in their work. They may function in offices, hospitals, clinics, public health agencies, and other agencies and institutions.

† As the costs of home visits by community nurses escalate in the United States, much of the actual nursing care in homes is given by home health aides. The registered nurse may do little more than "supervise" the care given by the aide. Under these circumstances, the satisfaction to nurse and family of a close helping relationship may be greatly diluted.

health nurses are employed in a greater variety of settings, the differences between public health and other types of nursing will be less noticeable. The writer believes that the unification of health services in manageable geographical units, as has been effected in some countries and proposed in others, will, in a sense, convert all nursing into "community nursing." In the United States, free neighborhood clinics, neighborhood health centers, and health maintenance type organizations are all steps in the direction of providing a unified, family-centered comprehensive service.[66-75]

6. OFFICES OF PRIVATE PRACTITIONERS

Employment of Nurses in Offices of Private Practitioners. The "office" setting differs according to the health care system. For example, general medical practitioners in Great Britain are salaried under the National Health Service; public health nurses and nurse-midwives are also salaried under this service and some are assigned to work with general practitioners in serving a geographical area. Nurses and nurse-midwives may function in a traditional office setting or in community health centers staffed with medical specialists as well as generalists, and with other health personnel such as social workers, physical therapists, and nutritionists.[1-13] Office nursing in any country with a national health service designed to serve all citizens has some of these characteristics. In the United States and in other countries where physicians operate under a fee-for-service system, the physician is the employer of most nurses who work in offices, and the physician's concept of the "office nurse's" role and function affects what they are asked to do. In 1970, E. V. Kuenssberg,[14] writing in England on "The Management of Staff in General Practice," asks "The Nurse—A Luxury or a Necessity in General Practice?" However, speaking of the British system in 1972, J. J. A. Reid, County Medical Officer of Health and Principal School Medical Officer, Buckinghamshire County Council, Aylesbury, at a Conference on the Greater Medical Profession, made the following comments that include a comparison of the British and United States systems:

As far as general practice is concerned, the attachment of public health staff, including health visitors, district nurses, and midwives, is leading to the development of a team approach to patient care, and the GP [general practitioner] is increasingly assuming the role of leader of the team rather than remaining an isolated entrepreneur with little effective support. Such teamwork is being enhanced by the provision by local health authorities of health centres, thus bringing GPs and public health staff together to provide preventive care and cure; in the case of the larger ones, hospital staff may also be involved.

. . .

In Britain public health is no longer in competition with the general practitioner and hospital services. . . .

Later, discussing the over-all problem of health manpower, he says:

So far as the United States is concerned, the physician's assistant does one thing that is potentially dangerous: He is the creature of the physician and it is his job to perpetuate what the physician has always done. Miss Skeet [a British nurse participant at the Conference] and I agree that we do not require that kind of person in this country. I think one of the great roles of the nurse in attachment schemes is first, to complement the doctor's work, and, second to challenge it. . . . They have infiltrated general practice and they are challenging existing methods.*

Reid's comparison suggests that office nursing is one type of service when physicians, nurses, and other health workers have a common employer; it is a different type of service when the physician employs the nurse or other health worker. However, as physicians in the United States employ pediatric nurse specialists (called here pediatric nurse practitioners or pediatric associates) and as obstetricians employ, or take into partnership, nurse-midwives, such nurses work in the peer relationship im-

plied in Reid's comments. Some are offered proportionate earnings of the group practice rather than a salary.* When there is a peer relationship, the distinction between "office nursing" in Great Britain and the United States no longer holds. Medical and nursing students, physicians, and nurses working in free clinics, neighborhood health centers, and some health maintenance type organizations are trying to establish conditions that make it possible for all workers to realize their full potential for service.[15-21]

Numbers and Types of Offices and Number of Nurses Employed in Office Nursing. In 1972, there were said to be 333,259 active physicians in the United States; of these, 22 per cent were in general practice, while 78 per cent had "primary specialization other than general practice." Of the active physicians, 199,000 (60 per cent) were nonfederal physicians in office-based practice.[22] Since there were only 52,390 registered nurses employed in office nursing (6.7 per cent of the 778,470 employed registered nurses), it is obvious that some physicians then had no registered nurses associated with their office practice,[23] although some physicians shared the services of a registered nurse.† The Canadian Nurses' Association reports that 2,958 (2.3 per cent) of the 128,675 registered nurses employed in nursing were in physicians' or dentists' offices.[24] No figures were found on other types of nursing personnel in this setting, but the numbers would undoubtedly exceed those for professional nurses.

It is hard to describe a typical or average physician's office; there may be one or many rooms; the physician may practice alone or in association with other physicians. Groups of physicians may have large suites or a building, meager furnishings and equipment or elaborate furnishings and technologically advanced equipment. A physician or group of physicians may have a single employee or a large staff of professional and clerical workers.

A recent and arresting development is the increasing number of registered nurses who are setting up an office practice of their own and functioning as independent practitioners. However, while they operate in offices, this type of independent practitioner, discussed on pages 25 to 39, is not what is usually meant by an "office nurse."

The practice by physicians in the United

---

* Reid, J. J. A.: *op. cit.,* pp. 114, 154.

* Physicians in the United States are employing physician's assistants as well as nurses to assume some of their responsibilities in office practice, but no attempt is made here to discuss this topic.

† ANA *Facts About Nursing 74–75* (p. 33) gives an estimated 55,617 offices nurses in 1973.

States of employing nursing personnel with less preparation than the registered nurse, or assistants with no nursing preparation, is common. *In the Doctor's Office. The Art of the Medical Assistant* [25] was written in the early 1950s by Esther Jane Parsons, a nonnurse who taught in the Paine Hall School of Medical Assistants in New York City. In 1958, the Dean of Women in the Eastern School for Physician's Aides, in New York City, wrote a comparable book, but its title, *The Medical Assistant; A Guide for the Nurse, Secretary, and Technician,* [26] makes it plain that she is writing for all groups. More recently, two physician's assistants have published *A Textbook for Medical Assistants* [27] that stresses work in the office setting for this type of health worker.

Standardization, Certification, and Regulation of Office Nursing. In Britain, where district nurses, health visitors, and nurse-midwives are attached to general practitioners, and in all countries where health workers are salaried under a national health service, the regulations designed to protect the public and the worker apply to office nursing just as they do to nursing in any setting. In the United States, office nursing is one of the least regulated types of nursing. In 1954, committees of the reorganized American Nurses' Association developed statements of functions, standards, and qualifications of practice which were based on data and opinions collected from thousands of nurses and others, and these statements included one on office nursing.[28] About this time, Johnnye G. Schick,[29] chairman of the ANA's Office Nurses' Conference Group, wrote "Office Nurses Are On Their Way," citing as evidence their activity in ANA's Special Group Section, the Association's preparation of a "Model Form for Minimum Employment Standards for Office Nurses," and the fact that state nursing associations' economic security programs had adopted minimum employment standards for office nurses on a state level.

In 1951, office nurses in Washington State reported "the first" study of this type of nursing—a survey of salaries and employment conditions.[30] In 1958, the Research and Statistics Unit of the ANA published a *Survey of Employment Conditions of Professional Registered Office Nurses.*[31] Currently, some of this data is reported biennially in *Facts About Nursing,* but it is less detailed than information on hospital staff nurses or public health nurses. For example, salaries for office nurses are not given.

As a summary statement, it seems fair to say that nursing in the American office setting is not standardized or regulated, that the personnel in physicians' offices perform a very wide range of functions in the name of nursing, and that those the public looks upon as "nurses" in physicians' offices may have no preparation in nursing or may, in rare instances, hold a graduate degree in nursing.

The Rights of Patients and Their Position in the Offices of Private Practitioners. While the writer has found no such statement, she believes that the rights of patients under treatment by general practitioners and medical specialists in offices parallel those stated for hospital patients (see page 197). Office nurses might be guided by the rights of patients to nursing care as stated there. Since health practitioners in offices are not, in the United States, so subject to review of their work by their peers, patients do not have the same protection they have in hospitals or community agencies where there is systematic assessment; on the other hand, people who do not get the help they seek in physicians' offices are free to go elsewhere for treatment. Nurses employed by physicians who often question the physician's prescribed treatment and patient management are likely to terminate their association with the physician, just as physicians who question the effectiveness of the relationship between a nurse and patients are likely to terminate that nurse's employment.

Organization and Administration of the Offices of Private Practitioners. In countries where physicians and nurses in office settings are salaried under a national health scheme, the organizational and administrative plan can be shown and the authority, function, and responsibility of nurses can be clearly stated. This is true even for physicians and nurses in offices and health centers operating in the United States under such health insurance plans as the Health Insurance Plan of Greater New York or the Kaiser-Permanente Medical Care Program on the West Coast. Most nurses in office practice in the United States are, however, employed by physicians (a few by dentists) who depend almost entirely on oral contracts and on the development of a personally effective working relationship. Some office nurses may prefer this unstructured setting; those who do not may ask their employer for a contract that specifies the conditions of employment.

Functions, Satisfactions, Rewards and Difficulties in Office Nursing. The ANA's 1954 statement on the functions of office nurses includes three types of functions: (1) direct nursing service, (2) indirect nursing service, and (3) administration of the office. As defined in 1954, the direct service involves giving drugs prescribed by the physician or treatment "under the direction of the physician"; indirect nursing service includes such things as maintaining supplies and equipment, teaching nonprofessional employees, and arranging patient transfers and referrals; office administration involves being responsible for maintaining patient records, handling correspondence, bookkeeping, banking, and making appointment schedules.[32]

According to the philosophy and wishes of the employers of office nurses, the direct nursing service given by office nurses today might include more independent functions than is suggested by the 1954 statement. Physicians may elect to work with office nurses as associates or as assistants for whose acts they assume responsibility. Registered nurses in offices may give almost no direct service but work through others in teaching and "supervising" the nursing care given by personnel with less preparation than their own; they may also function almost solely as office managers.

One satisfaction in office nursing may be its diversity; another may be the freedom of the nurse and her employer, usually a physician, to develop a mutually helpful relationship. Close association with patients and the opportunity to follow and influence their treatment and recovery is almost certainly, for some nurses, the greatest satisfaction in office nursing. Since nursing in the office setting rarely involves night or weekend service, the nurse with family responsibilities finds adapting to the work schedule easier than adapting to a hospital schedule.

Employers of office nurses may not want or demand academically well-prepared nurses. Of the 52,390 office nurses in 1972, only 11.3 per cent had a baccalaureate or higher degree. Industry is the only other major setting in the United States in which registered nurses are less prepared academically.[33] In Canada, of the 2958 professional registered nurses in offices, only 2.3 per cent held baccalaureate degrees.[34]

Annual salaries for 75 per cent of office nurses in 1973 ranged from under $5000 to $10,000; the remaining 25 per cent ranged from $10,000 to an undetermined figure.[35] Salaries tend to parallel preparation for nursing. It might be assumed that the economic return for office nursing is not one of its major attractions. Nurse specialists who are prepared to work with physicians as colleagues and who share the income from the office practice on a proportional basis may have a relatively high income. This is one setting in which physicians and nurses of the United States and Canada are most free to develop programs in line with their personal viewpoints on health care; in countries with tax-supported health care, or under certain health insurance plans in any country, office practice may come under central control.

7. HOMES AND HOSPITALS (AS "PRIVATE DUTY" NURSES)

Employment of "Private Duty" or "Private Practice" Nurses in Homes and Hospitals. "Private duty" or "private practice" is the oldest occupational specialty for registered nurses. Private duty nurses, as the term is used in ANA's *Facts About Nursing 74–75,* or private practice nurses as they are called in Canada, are those who are employed by a patient to care for him or her exclusively or by two or three patients who share the "special nurse's" time.

The Royal College of Nursing and the National Council of Nurses of the United Kingdom apply the title "the privately employed nurse" to private nurses, practising midwives, private visiting nurses, nurses specially engaged for "last offices," "staffs in private homes, convalescent homes, rest homes, nurses in independent schools" and in "agencies for the supply of nurses" [registries].* In other words, the "privately employed" are all those who are not employed in the National Health Service but are in "the private sector."

As nurses of this era adopt the role of "independent nurse practitioners" (an "expanded role") and set up an office practice, alone or with other nurses, there is some question as to whether they are also "private duty" or "private practice'" nurses. The *International Nursing Index* for 1971 has three entries under *Nursing, Private Duty,* all dealing with private duty in the traditional sense; in 1972 and 1973, the few articles under this heading include several on the independent nurse practitioner and an article on private duty nursing entitled "Update or Outdate." In 1974, under *Nursing, Private Duty,* there were two entries, and under *Private Practice,* eight articles. In 1975, under *Nursing, Private Duty,* there were twelve entries (one "In Defense of the Private Duty Nurse"), and under *Private Practice,* 14 entries.

In 1934, Maurice Dubin[1] asked "Special Nursing—Is It a Necessity or a Luxury?" In 1946, Kenneth A. Brent[2] reported a questionnaire study asking whether private duty nurses should be "barred," which helps explain an article in 1944 by Elsa Gidlow,[3] "Private Duty

---

* Royal College of Nursing and National Council of Nurses of the United Kingdom: *The Privately Employed Nurse: Recommended Fees and Condition of Service.* The College and the Council, London, 1973.

Fights for Its Life." Martha Dudley,[4] in 1959, asked "Is Private Duty Nursing on the Way Out?"

It is evident that some persons look upon private duty nursing in the traditional American sense as outmoded. However, contrary to the idea that they are a "vanishing species," the American Nurses' Association in *Facts About Nursing 72–73* reports private duty nurses as the fifth largest group. Of the 778,470 employed registered nurses in the United States reported for 1972, 38,923 (5 per cent) were classified by the ANA as private duty nurses including 365 men nurses so classified. Of 128,675 employed professional registered nurses 614 (0.5 per cent—"the smallest group") are reported by the Canadian Nurses' Association as being in "private practice."[5,6] Obviously, the nursing profession must clarify the meanings of these terms and finally resolve the ambiguity in practice.

At the turn of the century, more private duty nurses were found in homes than in hospitals; today they are seldom found in homes. Mary M. Roberts[7] said that there was serious unemployment among private duty nurses from 1915 until after World War I. Since this time, national nursing surveys have attempted to identify the supply of and demand for private duty nurses. In spite of periods of unemployment during economic recessions, the figures just cited for the United States and Canada seem to show that many patients and related medical personnel see the private duty nurse as a valued, or in some cases, an essential, member of the health team. At the same time, some hospital administrators have thought that the hospital nursing staff should furnish the care all patients need. The character of private duty nursing may change so that the functions of private duty nurses and private practitioners in the "expanded role" will merge.

When health insurance is available to all citizens under a national health plan, it affects all health workers. Bergilot Larsson,[8] then President of the Norwegian Nurses' Association, disagreeing with the American viewpoint on "Private Nursing" in 1925, commented on its future if and when it is a service provided by public taxation.

Standardization, Certification, and Regulation of Private Duty Nursing. Since patients rather than institutions and agencies have been, for the most part, employers of private duty nurses in America, they have been subjected to few standardizing or regulating influences. Hospitals in which the nurse practices have set up regulations to which private practitioners must conform. Registries have regulations that must be observed by those who seek employ-

ment through them. Residences and clubs for private duty nurses had very stringent regulations in the early decades. Early journal articles dwelt on the need for standards (as in the Sara Elizabeth Parsons[9] article "Why Private Nurses Should Organize") and on the stultifying effects of regulations that left nurses with little freedom. The development of private practice in the United States in the first decade of this century can be traced in Isabel McIsaac's department in the *American Journal of Nursing,* "Practical Points on Private Nursing," later "Problems in Private Nursing," and in Katharine DeWitt's[10] text *Private Duty Nursing.*

After the Private Duty Section of the American Nurses' Association was formed in 1916, it was the spokesman for this group. The development of standards for private duty nurses of the United States can be traced in the reports of this section at ANA Conventions from 1916 on.[11] With the reorganization of the ANA in 1952, a Committee on Functions, Standards, and Qualifications for Practice was established within each section. The Committee's report appeared in the Proceedings and in the *American Journal of Nursing.*[12] This statement has influenced regulations set up by state and district organizations.

Standards affect preparation for practice, licensure, hours of employment, fees, and other conditions. States set up regulations on licensure and reciprocity and on employment conditions and ethical conduct of all nurses. Increasingly, states are setting up requirements for continuing education which means that, for the first time, private duty nurses must add something beyond the basic nursing course to their preparation for practice. The American Nurses' Association in 1974 approved the resolution that it establish a system of accreditation of continuing education programs and consider the "feasibility" of accrediting basic and graduate education. The Association, in its official newspaper, reported in January, 1975, as follows:

The Commission on Nursing Education has now completed final details of a mechanism to approve nurse practitioner programs which are non-degree granting.

. . . .

Clinical content . . . for expanded role programs has been developed by respective Divisions on Practice [in specified areas] . . . and are now being developed in other areas . . ." *

Accreditation of nondegree programs in continuing education and definition of the clinical

* "Non-Degree Approval Ready to Go," *Am. Nurse,* 7:1, (Jan.) 1975. See also "ANA Holds 1st Accreditation Conference," same issue.

content of programs to prepare nurses for expanded roles provide a mechanism for upgrading, standard-setting, and certification in private practice that has not been available to United States nurses before. (See Chapter 1 for discussion of continuing education.)

In the United Kingdom, the Nurses and Midwives Whitley Council negotiates agreements with the National Health Service on salaries and conditions of service for all those employed by the Service; it publishes "recommended fees and conditions of service" for the privately employed nurse. Nurses are encouraged to demand contracts with private employers that provide salaries and conditions of service comparable to those under which nurses work who are employed in the public sector.[13]

The Rights of Patients in Private Duty Nursing. Since patients are usually the private duty nurses' employers, they are in a position to discontinue the services whenever they, the patients, believe them to be useless or harmful. However, there is a long history of efforts to establish public understanding of what it should and should not expect from the private duty nurse. Private duty nurses themselves, hospitals, registries, and nursing organizations have developed statements for the mutual protection of the patient and the nurse which the nurse can give the patient on accepting "the case."

Since, historically, professional private duty nurses supplanted relatives, friends, neighborly nurses, and domestic servants in taking care of the sick at home, their position in the home has been especially anomalous. Some patients expected nurses to do exactly what they asked; others expected nurses to do what the physician "ordered"; and some patients thought private duty nurses would do what they, as professional medical workers, believed was in the best interests of the patient.*

If, in the future, private duty nursing or "specialing" is part of a prepaid national health service, the rights of patients in hospitals, that guide hospital staff nurses, and the rights of patients in their homes, that guide public health or community nurses, will also guide private duty nurses. To some extent, this is true today. Nurses in all settings are guided by the profession's ethical code.

Organization and Administration of Private Duty Nursing. Nurses who elect private practice are perhaps by nature persons who like to work as individuals rather than as a member of a group. They may prefer an unstructured working environment and prefer employment by an individual or a family to employment by an institution, organization, or community. In any event, although they have been and still are a large element of the nursing population, they have tended to be the least organized and the most opposed to change.

The Private Duty Nursing Section of the ANA was created in 1916 and was retained in subsequent reorganizations of the Association. The Private Duty Nursing Forum is in 1976 one of the ten occupational forums of the Association.[14] However, in studying the history of nursing, the writer gets the impression that nurse administrators and educators, as for example Ethel Bedford Fenwick in Great Britain and Annie W. Goodrich, Sara Elisabeth Parsons, Lavinia Dock, and Louise Darche in the United States, saw, even more clearly than did private duty nurses themselves, the need to organize. They promoted residence clubs with answering services and other types of registries and they promoted sections or departments within official nursing organizations that would provide protection for the public and the private duty nurse in this branch of practice.[15-23]

In Europe, graduates who wished to go into private practice often lived in residences operated and controlled by their hospital schools of nursing, by their alumnae associations, or by nursing organizations. In the United States and Canada, nurses in private practice were more likely to live alone or in small groups, but they did develop clubhouses.[24-26] Their employment was dependent on their accessibility to the public, and they had to be listed in directories or registries so that hospitals, doctors, and patients could reach them. Occasionally, private duty nurses were kept busy by one or more doctors and never used a registry, but they were the exceptions.[27-30] Such nurses might have the complete confidence of the physician and might function in what would be considered now an "expanded role."

In the nineteenth century, there were few nurses available for private duty, but by the first decade of the twentieth century, the supply exceeded the demand. There was keen competition for patients. The leisure that private duty nurses had was hard to enjoy fully, since they were tied to a telephone that might call them to their next "case."

The current emphasis on the nurse's expanded role and the nurse as an independent health practitioner or a private practitioner makes the study of "private duty" especially timely. (The independent nurse practitioner is discussed in Chapters 1 and 5.) As stated

---

* The writer, on the third day after the operation, paid a man recovering from a herniotomy a friendly visit. A special nurse was feeding him his dinner, forkful by forkful. When, later, I asked him whether the doctor had told him not to feed himself, he said "Oh no, but considering what I'm paying a special nurse I figure she can feed me."

earlier, private duty was the first, and for a while, almost the only setting in which graduate nurses actually practiced nursing. Those employed in hospitals were administrators and teachers. It is not possible here to do more than mention some of the main events influencing the organization and administration of private duty nursing in the United States and to suggest their relationship with current events.

As the early schools of nursing produced "graduate" or professional nurses, the hospitals administering the schools tended to operate registries that would ensure the employment of their graduates. However, in 1879 the New York Agency for Trained Nurses was organized. It was a central headquarters sponsored by the Philomena Society. Roberts said this society was the first organization of graduate nurses in the United States, but it was short-lived. According to Roberts, Adelaide Mabie organized this registry at the urging of the mayor of New York who told her the people of that city should have a central place where they could find nurses. After the Philomena Society "died of inanition in 1887," the registry "was continued as a commercial venture by one of the nurse members of Philomena." *

From this time on, nursing leadership urged the development of central registries operated for the benefit of nurses and the public under the control of the profession. This principle is generally accepted today, although some hospitals still operate nurse registries. The May 1974 issue of the *American Journal of Nursing* (p. 968) carried a list of registries in 29 states which, with a few exceptions, were owned and operated by state and district nurses' associations.

There have been sporadic, but mostly unsuccessful, attempts in the United States to develop national, state, and local nurse *directories* comparable to those for physicians. Historically, it is interesting to find in the US Library of Congress a combined directory of physicians and nurses in New Haven County (Conn.) printed in 1923 by the New Haven City Printing Company.[31] It was evidently developed for the mutual benefit of the public and medical and nursing practitioners, and was probably financed commercially by the firms and agencies that advertised in it. In 1902, the Shober-Cornell Publishing Company put out the *Directory of Trained Nurses,* which was a "Selected List of Names and Addresses of Competent Graduated Trained Nurses Practicing in the Cities of Greater New York, Boston, Philadelphia, Baltimore, and Washington." [32]

In Great Britain in 1892, the Matron's' Council of Great Britain and Ireland began to sponsor a *Nursing Directory* for all nurses in England, Scotland, Wales, and Ireland, and for residents abroad. It was published annually by the *Nursing Record* of London.[33] *Burdett's Official Nursing Directory* was said in 1900 to be something of a Nurse's *Who's Who.*[34] In 1908, there was a report on the background of, and opposition to, an Official Directory Bill which was to be sponsored by the Hospital Council for London.[35]

The nurse registration movement and the publication of lists of registered nurses (licensed to practice) should not be confused with the development of registries for private duty nurses. The fact that British nurses had for decades a published registry (or directory) of all registered nurses licensed to practice simplified the making of directories of nurses in any clinical or occupational specialty. In fact, the British nurses' registry was a series of volumes, one for each occupational specialty. Ethel Bedford Fenwick, the leader of the movement for nurse registration in England, was presented a copy of "the first Statutory Register" by the National Council of Nurses of Great Britain and Ireland in 1923.[36] In America, in headquarters offices of state nurses' associations, there are lists of nurses registered in that state, but these lists are not readily available to the profession or the public at large and are not collated into a national directory.

Private duty, or "specialing," was not confined to graduate nurses. With the expansion of hospital schools of nursing from 1900 to 1930, students assumed the major role in hospital nursing and even functioned as head nurses. In some hospitals, they were assigned to "special" patients and even to "special" patients in their homes. In 1906, Richard C. Cabot, a physician, reported data from 48 Massachusetts hospitals showing that 18 of them collected substantial funds for student nursing in homes.* [37]

Because many persons who need constant nursing care cannot afford the fees of private duty nursing, there have been many efforts to make the necessary care available to all. Dur-

---

* Roberts, Mary M.: *American Nursing; History and Interpretation.* Macmillan Publishing Co., Inc., New York, 1954, pp. 120, 121.

* Since the majority of nurses went into private-duty nursing, some hospital administrators and even some nurse educators justified this practice, although it was believed by others to exploit students. Alfred Worcester, a physician of the Waltham (Mass.) Hospital, was the main proponent of having students learn to nurse in homes. While most educators thought there was merit in guided experience for students in home nursing, Cabot denounced their employment for hospital gain, and Lavinia Dock was so opposed to it that she wrote scathing editorials criticizing the system and those who promoted it.

ing World War II, some hospitals began to employ private duty nurses on a monthly basis, assigning them to patients who needed more attention than could be given by staff nurses and students. This salaried private duty nurse might care for two or three patients, according to the patients' conditions. This was called "group nursing," for patients shared the cost and the nurse's attention.[38-40] Some private duty nurses did group nursing on their own, charging patients accordingly. "Team nursing" was developed in the 1940s with the hope that various categories of nursing personnel working as a team could more nearly meet patients' needs.[41-43] Now, the nursing staffs of intensive care units in hospitals provide the constant observation formerly provided by private duty nurses, and this system of "progressive patient care" has reduced the demand for private nursing. "Primary [hospital] nursing" of today, which involves patient assignment so that every patient has "his (or her) nurse," was discussed on page 203.

In summary, private nursing as interpreted in America is probably less organized than any other occupational specialty. This is particularly true when the nurse is employed by patients to care for them at home. When patients employ the private duty nurse in the hospital, they must conform to regulations established by the hospital. Private duty nurses employed by the hospital and assigned to patients by its administration operate as staff nurses with special assignments.

Functions, Satisfactions, Rewards, and Difficulties in Private Duty or Private Practice. Nurses in private practice are more able than those in any other setting to function as the patient's alter ego: to help these patients with those activities contributing to health or its recovery (or to a peaceful death) that they would perform unaided if they had the strength, will, or knowledge, and to attain independence as rapidly as possible. The fact that the private duty nurse has all the time there is to devote to a patient and can nurse as well as she knows how to nurse is the chief reason that this occupational specialty still attracts thousands of nurses.

When patients (the employers) and physicians (the co-workers) have had confidence in private nurses, they have functioned in an expanded role. In 1917, Carolyn E. Gray and Marie T. Lockwood,[44] writing on the relationship of private duty nurses to the public, noted that they were teachers and social workers as well as nurses. S. Lillian Clayton[45] wrote on their "social training," since it was important that they be able to form an effective helping relationship with all classes and fit into any home setting. In 1936, Nell V. Beeby[46] reviewed the literature on health teaching and reported on "the private duty nurse as a teacher."

In the 1930s, partly to relieve the unemployment of nurses in private practice, hospitals employed them as staff nurses. For the first time, the care of ward patients by student nurses was shared by graduates. With the employment of graduate nurses as staff nurses, private nurses felt less necessary and, as has been shown, they felt threatened. One volume of the Grading Committee's Report in 1932, *Nurses, Patients and Pocketbooks,*[47] concentrated on the self-image and the public image of nurses. More than 38,000 nurses answered the questionnaires sent out in this investigation. The report on private practice reinforced the opinion commonly held that the nurses' rewards came from their independence and their relationships with patients rather than from their professional associates, although some nurses did report satisfaction in working with physicians whose therapeutic skill they admired.

The earnings of nurses in private practice have always been low as compared with the earnings of nurses in teaching and administration.[48-54] Even today, the private duty nurses who graduated last month get the same fees as those with 20 years' experience. There is no system of financial advancement. In discussing private duty, Roberts made the following observation in 1954:

The ANA has worked continuously to secure improvement in the conditions under which nurses practice their profession, but no method has been devised for rewarding, financially or socially, the nurse who becomes an expert practitioner. Those who take academic or other postgraduate courses therefore do not commonly remain in the field of nursing practice.

The question of a sliding scale of fees for private duty nurses had been considered and rejected early in the century in connection with the problem of providing care for patients of moderate means. Would a sliding scale of fees for private duty nurses provide an answer to two needs; that of patients for care and that of private duty nurses for a tangible incentive to develop expertness in their chosen field? Why, said the exponents of a sliding scale, shouldn't Mrs. Millions pay a nurse more than Mrs. Modest Purse? The system worked well for doctors, why not for nurses, they argued. Why should recently graduated nurses receive the same compensation for a day or a week or a month on duty as would the nurses who had already demonstrated their professional competence and personal adaptability? A professional person, it was argued, continues to add to her knowledge and skills and should, therefore, be able to command a higher fee. The basic problems in the administration of such a scheme, it was pointed out, would inevitably be: How shall a

Table 3-5. Standard Fees Recommended by State Nurses' Associations for Private Duty Nurses, January 1974 *

State or Territory	Date of Standards	Basic 8-Hour Fee	Hourly Rate for Overtime After 8 Hours	Hourly Nursing Rate		Two Patient 8-Hour Fee
				First Hour	Thereafter	
Alabama	1974	$32.50	(†)	$10.45	$5.20	$55.70
Alaska ‡	—	—	—	—	—	—
Arizona	1974	39.67	5.64	10.18	10.18	56.71
Arkansas	1973	34.95	—	8.75	4.37§	52.45
California ‖	—	—	—	—	—	—
Colorado	1973	36.75	6.85	10.00	5.00	52.50
Connecticut ‡	—	—	—	—	—	—
Delaware	1974	42.00	(†)	7.50	7.50	63.00
District of Columbia	1974	44.00	6.60	—	—	66.00
Florida	1969	36.00	6.75	9.00	6.50	54.00
Guam	1973	40.00	—	—	—	—
Georgia	1973	40.90	(†)	—	—	62.00
Hawaii ‡	—	—	—	—	—	—
Idaho	1970	35.00	7.50	7.50	5.00	50.00
Illinois	1974	40.25	(†)	14.80	7.40	70.44
Indiana	1972	32.00	5.00	10.00	5.00	48.00
Iowa	1970	35.00	5.00	7.00	5.00	50.00
Kansas	1973	40.00	7.50	10.00	5.00	60.00
Kentucky	1974	40.00	—	17.50	4.35	52.50
Louisiana	1974	35.06	7.00	8.00	4.00	40.00
Maine	1974	34.75	(†)	8.70	8.70	52.20
Maryland ‡	—	—	—	—	—	—
Massachusetts	1974	39.70	(†)	9.64	4.94	59.54
Michigan	1972	32.00–40.00	(†)	—	—	—
Minnesota	1974	40.00	(†)	6.00	5.00	53.00
Mississippi	1971	33.00–35.00	(#)	4.25	—	45.00
Missouri ‖	—	—	—	—	—	—
Montana	1974	31.75	(†)	7.00	7.00	—
Nebraska	1968	35.00	—	8.75	4.40	52.50
Nevada **	—	—	—	—	—	—
New Hampshire	1974	36.29 ††	—	8.68 ††	8.68 ††	52.00
New Jersey	—	—	—	—	—	—
New Mexico	1974	34.70	—	—	—	—
New York	1973	38.00–45.50	(‖)	(‖)	(‖)	(‖)
North Carolina	—	—	—	—	—	—
North Dakota	1974	32.00	4.00	5.00	4.00	48.00
Ohio ‖	—	—	—	—	—	—
Oklahoma	1974	35.00	—	—	—	—
Oregon	1974	45.00	8.85	8.40	6.30	—
Pennsylvania ‡	—	—	—	—	—	—
Rhode Island	1973	36.93	—	—	—	—
South Carolina	1970	30.00	3.75	—	—	38.00
South Dakota	1971	30.00	5.63	7.50	4.50	—
Tennessee ‡	—	—	—	—	—	—
Texas ‡	—	—	—	—	—	—
Utah ‡	—	—	—	—	—	—
Vermont	1970	35.00	(†)	8.50	4.35	52.50
Virgin Islands ‡	—	—	—	—	—	—
Virginia ‡	—	—	—	—	—	—
Washington ‡	—	—	—	—	—	—

230

Table 3-5   (Continued)

State or Territory	Date of Standards	Basic 8 Hour Fee	Hourly Rate for Overtime After 8 Hours	Hourly Nursing Rate		Two Patents 8-Hour Fee
				First Hour	Thereafter	
West Virginia	1974	33.00	—	10.50	5.20	59.50
Wisconsin	1972	33.50	(†)	7.80	4.20	44.67
Wyoming ‡	—	—	—	—	—	—

* American Nurses' Association: *Facts About Nursing 74–75*. The Association, Kansas City, Mo., 1976, p. 103.
† Overtime is paid at the rate of time and one-half.
‡ No standard fees recommended.
§ Fee applies to first 4 hours.
‖ Fee varies by district.
One-half-day fee under 4 hours.
** No report.
†† Fee applies to state nurses' association members only.
Source: American Nurses' Association, Statistics Department, "State Nurses' Associations' Report to American Nurses' Association as of March, 1974."

nurse's competence be evaluated? How shall the patient's ability to pay be determined? Most nurses believe a sliding scale undesirable. Their decision might have been stated in Gertrude Stein fashion—a nurse is a nurse is a nurse.*

Since private practitioners were for many years the largest group in ANA's membership, they strived, if with little success, to improve their lot. Janet Geister's studies between 1926 and 1948 gave eloquent testimony to their accomplishments and difficulties.[55-57] Her *Hearsay and Facts in Private Duty Nursing* was catalytic, leading to other studies. She showed that nurses returning from military service after World War I seldom wanted to go back into private practice. Susan C. Francis,[58] commenting on the accomplishments of the Private Duty Section of the ANA in 1936, wrote hopefully on "The Private Duty Nurse in a New Era." In 1939, Margaret C. Klem [59] studied, for the ANA, the employment of private duty nurses. This is only one of the many studies dealing with the economics of private nursing. In the 1950s, when the ANA sponsored a nationwide series of studies on the function of nursing, several of these concentrated on the nurse in private practice. One study, *Human Relations in Private Duty Nursing*,[60] reported in 1957, showed that seeing the patient get better was still the private practitioner's chief reward. Other studies in this series reinforce this conclusion.[61,62]

While a modest and uncertain income has been and remains one of the chief deterrents to private practice, long hours of employment have been another source of dissatisfaction. In

the nineteenth century, private practitioners might be "on duty" for 24 hours, with a few hours off in the afternoon if there was someone to relieve them. Well into the twentieth century, these nurses could be found sleeping on a cot or a chair beside the patient. Early texts on this specialty had suggestions for dealing with this problem which had, of course, its health hazards. For example, the fresh air cure for pneumonia, thought at the time to be a boon to patients, was always a problem for nurses who had to remain in the room but couldn't surround themselves with the blankets and hot-water bottles that kept the patient warm.

Gradually, nurses and the public came to realize that they should adopt reasonable working hours. The literature of the 1930s includes many studies of the 8-hour day for private practitioners.[63-67] By 1940, the 8-hour day was widespread in the United States.[68]

The development of private practice spans the same time period in which professional nursing has existed, and to summarize what has been said about it is difficult. Private practice represents nursing at its best because the conditions under which nurses in it practice do not limit what nurses can do for patients. When, on the other hand, private practitioners cease to study, when they are unfamiliar with current therapy, and, most particularly, when they foster dependence in patients rather than independence, their service can actually do harm.* The continuing education movement, the em-

* The concept of starting the patient's rehabilitation from the onset of illness or the time of injury has not even now pervaded medical and nursing care, but private duty nurses in particular have been criticized for fostering dependency.

* Roberts, Mary M.: *op. cit.*, p. 118.

phasis in the ANA on recognizing clinical competence, the development of the independent nurse-practitioner in the expanded role, and the prospect of universal health insurance with a national health plan through which it will be administered promises to change the nature of private practice materially.

8. SCHOOL AND COLLEGE HEALTH SERVICES

Employment of Nurses in School and College Health Services. Because children (chiefly) are involved in one service and adolescents in another, school and college health services are considered quite different by some persons—especially those who work in these settings. Both groups belong to the ANA, but school nurses may also belong to the National Council for School Nurses, the School Health Section of the American Public Health Association, the Department of School Nurses under the National Education Association, the American School Health Association, or, if they are residents of the state, the California School Nurse Association or the New York State School Nurse-Teachers Association. Nurses in health services of colleges and universities in the United States belong to the American College Health Association, which has a nursing section.

The American Nurses' Association in its *Facts About Nursing 72–73* has no title such as College Health Nurses or Nursing, nor does it include data on school and college health, but lists only "School Nurses." (*Facts About Nursing 74–75* does not include school nurses in the index or in any tabulated data found.)

The ANA reported that of 778,470 employed registered nurses in the United States in 1972, 29,849 (3.8 per cent) were "school nurses." [1] The Canadian Nurses' Association has no "school nurse" category and includes these nurses under "public health." [2]

This age takes for granted the presence of registered (trained or professional) nurses in public schools—actually, in all schools of any size. School nursing is a development of the twentieth century in the United States. Teresa E. Christy [3] said that Lillian D. Wald and Lina Rogers established the first system for public school nursing in the United States. Roberts said that Miss Wald was "familiar with school nursing as it had developed in London before 1900," * which suggests that her 1-month "experiment" in 1902 in the New York schools which resulted in the employ-

ment of school nurses citywide was based on the British experience. This is substantiated by Honnor Morton's report in 1901 on "Progressive Movements. The London [Eng.] Public School Nurse." [4] The nursing journals of the Western world during the two decades of the twentieth century carried many articles on school nursing. It was, and still is, considered one of the most important health services. Health practices developed in childhood and youth affect a person throughout life, making health education and health care in schools a critical service. There are annual state and local conferences in most countries devoted to school and college health that attract participants from a wide variety of professions and agencies. In 1954, the World Health Organization sponsored a European school health conference with 20 countries participating. [5]

Nature of School and College Health Services. The nature of school and college health services varies greatly and depends on the size of the institution, the economic resources, and whether students are day students or boarders. It may depend even more on the concepts of what the service should be as held by governing boards, administrators, and staffs of the health services.

The history of physicians' services in schools antedates the provision of nurses' services. Presently, schools and colleges provide a wide variety of health services. On a full-time or part-time basis, they may employ—besides doctors and nurses—dentists, clinical psychologists, nutritionists, social workers, specialists in guidance or counseling, physical therapists, speech therapists, and other health experts.

In boarding schools, colleges, and universities, there are infirmaries or small hospitals. Doctors and nurses may also serve sick or injured students who remain in their own rooms. Most schools and colleges transfer acutely ill students or those who need surgery to nearby hospitals. While some school health services are like office practice for pediatricians and pediatric nurses, and health services in school infirmaries are like a hospital service, school nurses are often classified as public health or community nurses because they work with students and families in their homes and make referrals to community agencies.

In day schools, the emphasis is on health teaching, prevention, and the care of the pupil or student as a member of a family. With pupils living nearby, school nurses make home visits and utilize community health resources. Doris S. Bryan said: "The school nurse works with parents and other community workers as necessary and often bridges the gap between the school and the home and between the

* Roberts, Mary M.: *op. cit.,* p. 85.

school and various community organizations and health resources." *

In boarding schools, the health service is a combination of that in offices and hospitals, since the infirmary is like a small hospital. The same comparison might be made for health services in some colleges; however, certain universities in the United States are providing a comprehensive health service for students, faculty, and staff and their families which might be compared with the Kaiser-Permanente or the Health Insurance Plan of Greater New York health maintenance services. In such cases, the service may employ health workers in the different clinical specialties, and nurses who can function in the so-called expanded role. Facilities for such comprehensive services may include offices, clinics (with emergency and first aid services), and nonacute inpatient (infirmary or hospital) services. (See Fig. 3-13.) If a comprehensive university health plan is to meet the requirements of a health maintenance type organization under the recently enacted

legislation, it must offer a wide range of services, including home care. For boarding students, this may mean seeing them in their dormitory rooms; for day students, faculty, and staff, it may mean visits to homes. As university health plans in the United States begin to qualify as health maintenance type organizations, they must meet federal requirements for such organizations as stated in Public Law 93–222 and its evolving regulations.*

In the British Commonwealth, the evolution of the University Health Service into a comprehensive service seems established. The Royal College of Nursing, London, says that university health services have changed "radically" in the last two decades. Larger institutions are moving toward a "comprehensive

---

* Bryan, Doris S.: *School Nursing in Transition.* C. V. Mosby Co., St. Louis, 1973, p. 185.

* Title XIII Health Maintenance Organizations reads: "Sec. 1301. (a) For purposes of this title, the term 'health maintenance organization' means a legal entity which (1) provides basic and supplemental health services to its members in the manner prescribed by subsection (b), and (2) is organized and operated in the manner prescribed by subsection (c)." (US Congress: *Public Law 93–222, 93rd Congress, S.14, December 29, 1973.*)

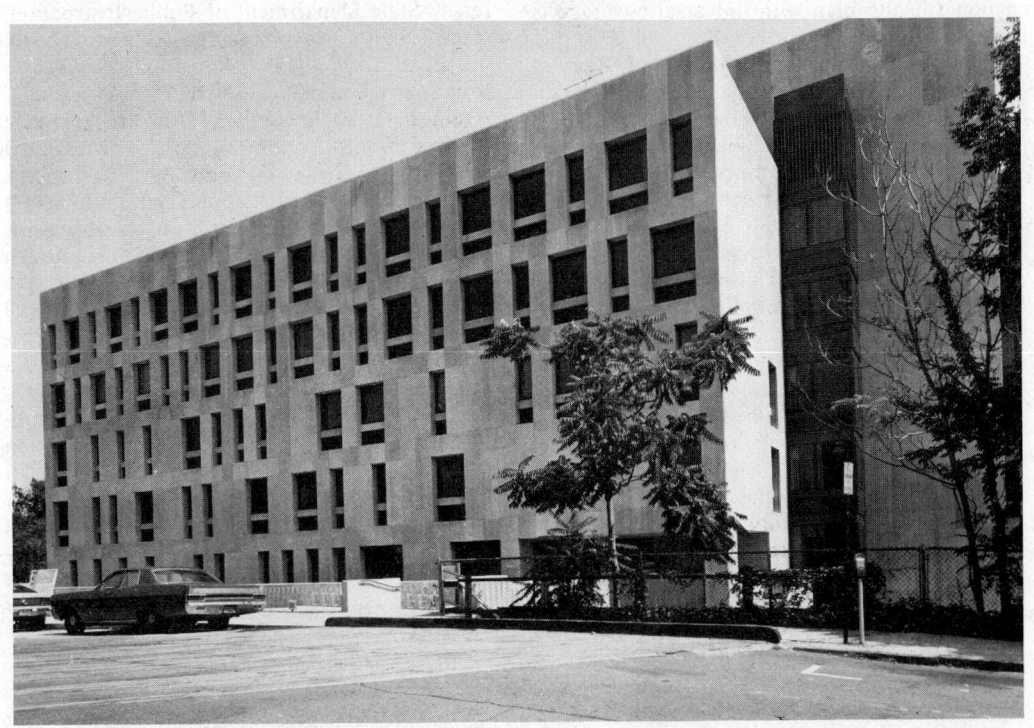

Figure 3-13. Building housing student and employee health service and prepaid voluntary comprehensive health service for the (nonstudent) Yale University community, New Haven, Conn. Facility includes laboratory, physical therapy unit, pharmacy, and 36-bed in-patient unit for hospitalization of Yale community members with illness requiring intermediate level of care. (Courtesy of Yale University Health Services, New Haven, Conn.)

service . . . providing treatment facilities for students and staff eligible for registration within the National Health Service combined with an occupational health function available for the whole community. Smaller units may provide a general practitioner service for students only and others an occupational health service similar to that in industry." The Royal College of Nursing, in defining a university health service, however, gives it the broadest meaning —"A service to promote and protect the health of the university community." *

In recent years, British journals have carried many articles describing the change in school and college health services. Articles in nursing journals emphasize the change in what the nurse does and how the school and college health services fit into the reorganized National Health Service.[6-9] Recent American journals have also published a great deal on change in school and college health services. One writer asks as the title of her article, "College Health Services—Demise or Rebirth?"[10] Articles in nursing journals emphasize the expanded role of the nurse.[11-21] In any country where nurses assume more responsibility in school and college health services, the implementation of a national health plan with universal coverage is facilitated.

Standardization, Certification, and Regulation of School and College Health Services. Since school nurses may be employees of state, county, or municipal school systems or state, county, or municipal health departments which, under contract with the school system, work within the schools giving care to school-age children as part of a generalized nursing service, and since they may also be employees of private institutions, the organizations and agencies that set standards, that certify and regulate them, are varied (see Fig. 3-14). College health nurses are also subject to a number of regulating agencies since some are employed by public institutions, others by private colleges and universities.

If school nurses in the United States are employees of city, county, or state health departments or if they are employees of visiting nurse agencies and working in schools under contract, what was said on page 216 about standardizing, certifying, and regulating community nursing services applies here. If school nurses are employed by boards of education or boards of supervisors, such boards can set up their own regulations. These vary from state to state.

Bryan made the following observation in 1973:

School nurses have the most varied education and the most varied requirements and titles of any group within the nursing profession. Some states have no certification requirements for school nurses; others require a year of study beyond the baccalaureate degree. . . . The Division of Health Services of the Denver Public Schools in the 1970 to 1971 report discusses . . . a . . . training project for school nurses to become school nurse practitioners.*

Bryan suggested a classification for "levels" of school nursing personnel eligible for certification or "credentialing" † that included consultants in school nursing, directors of school nursing, school nursing educators, supervisors, coordinators and practitioners, and school-community nursing. She listed five other categories of nursing personnel, including volunteers working under nursing supervision, who are not eligible for certification or "credentialing."

Certification of school nurses and standards for their performance have a long history and only a few of the studies can be mentioned here. In 1930, Lula P. Dilworth, of the New Jersey State Department of Public Instruction, made a nationwide survey of certification and published data in the *Public Health Nurse* from questionnaires answered by 44 states.[22] Again in 1950 and 1958, Dilworth reported surveys of certification practices in the United States.[23-25] In 1938, the Education Committee of the National Organization for Public Health Nursing published minimum qualifications for nurses appointed to school nursing positions. In 1947, a Committee on Qualifications of the Nurse in the School was set up in the School Nursing Section of the NOPHN that, at the request of the Education Committee, presented a statement on functions and related abilities.[26,27] In 1959, the School Nurses Branch of the Public Health Nurses Section of the American Nurses' Association prepared a leaflet, *Essential Considerations for Certification of School Nurses Employed by Boards of Education,* which included a statement on purpose, suggested procedure, and types of certification.[28] In the early 1950s when the ANA set up a commit-

---

* Bryan, Doris S.: *op. cit.,* p. 5.

† *Certification,* according to Bryan, is giving evidence of completion of professional preparation for satisfactory performance in a specialized field. She says "The school nurse who obtains the basic education in professional nursing by completing a baccalaureate degree in nursing may be eligible for a credential in school nursing. In several states nurses now take up to an additional year of graduate study before being eligible for a school nurse credential." (Bryan, Doris S.: *op. cit.,* p. 20.)

---

* Royal College of Nursing, and National Council of Nurses of the United Kingdom: *University Health Nursing Structure.* The College and the Council, London, 1972, pp. 4, 5.

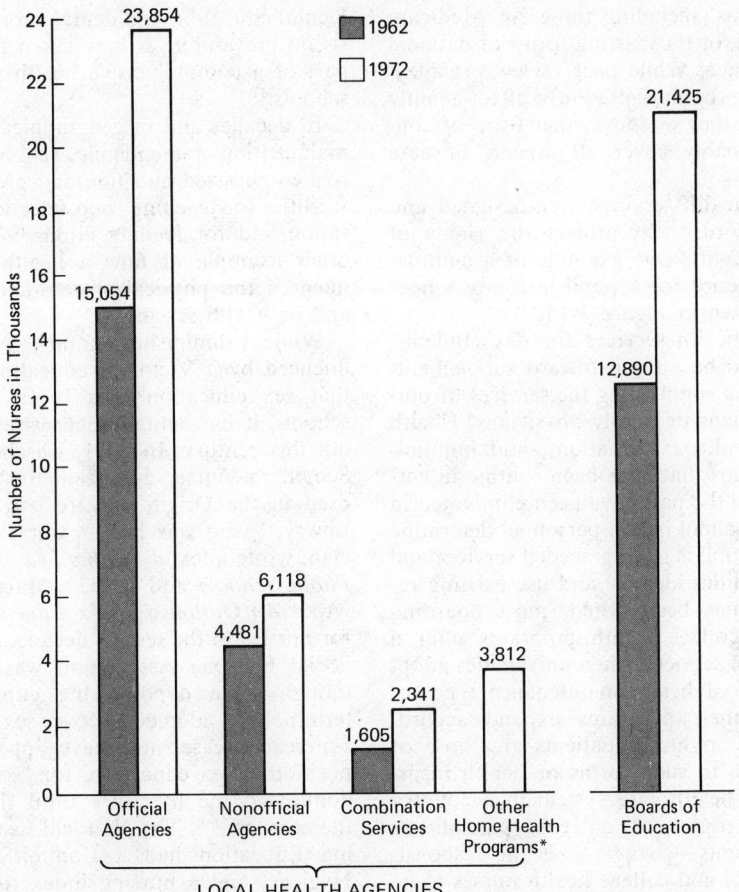

Figure 3-14. Registered nurses employed for public health work in local health agencies and boards of education in 1962 and 1972. (Hudson, Helen M., and Mc-Carthy, Margaret D.: *Source Book—Nursing Personnel*. US Department of Health, Education, and Welfare, Division of Nursing, Bethesda, Md., 1974.)

tee to study functions, standards, and qualifications for practice in various settings, school nurses were included in the statement on public health nursing. While employment standards are established by state agencies, the ANA in 1954 issued a "Model Form for SNA Schedules of Minimum Employment Standards for Public Health Nurses." [29]

Programs for School Nurse Practitioners, such as that at the University of Colorado Medical Center, are fitting nurses for the "expanded role" in this setting and will almost certainly help raise standards. The American Nurses' Association and the American School Health Association have issued a joint statement recommending the educational preparation and a definition of the expanded role and functions of the School Nurse Practitioner. [30]

The Rights of Patients in School and College Health Services. While most of what has been said under this heading for other settings also applies to students, faculty, and staffs of schools, colleges, and universities, there are specific legal aspects of nursing in schools and colleges. There is, for example, the right of students to appropriate health instruction, treatment, and care, but there is also the right of well students to be protected from sick students with threatening conditions or communicable disease. School and college health nurses should study educational, health, and safety codes of the states in which they are employed. If a university health service wishes to qualify as a health maintenance type organization, nurses associated with it should be familiar with federal and state standards affecting patients, including those for Medicare and Medicaid, or the existing forms of national health insurance. While peer review organization (PRO) programs presently affect mainly medical care, they or some other form of control will probably cover all aspects of care eventually.

As in all health services, well-designed and well-kept records help protect the rights of clients or patients. One example of a cumulative health record for a pupil in a city school system is shown in Figure 3-15.

In school health services for day students, there seems to be a trend toward supplementing rather than supplanting the services of outside pediatricians or family physicians. Health inspection, health examinations, and immunization programs that have been routine in certain schools in the past have been eliminated in many cases. School health personnel determine whether the pupil is getting needed services and they help families identify and use existing resources. As has been noted, most boarding schools and college health programs offer a wider range of service. When universities adopt the programs of health maintenance type organizations, their programs expand accordingly, and the rights of patients are those of all subscribers to such forms of health insurance. As the health care system in a country changes, the rights of citizens—patients or potential patients—change. It is the responsibility of school and college health nurses to be informed about, and in fact promote, health legislation affecting the rights of givers and recipients (providers and providees) of care. Helen Creighton and G. Marjorie Squires have reviewed the legal aspects of the school nurse's work in a recent issue of *Nursing Clinics of North America.*[31]

Location and Physical Plans of School and College Health Services. Since the health service for a school may operate from one or two small rooms or from a large building (see Fig. 3-13), it is hard to describe a typical setting in which school and college health nurses function. Facilities vary with the times, the place, and the health problems of the era. For example, when school health personnel in the early decades of this century were combating infectious disease, sanitation was stressed, and schools might have open-air schoolrooms for tuberculous children.[32-34] During the first three decades, dental facilities were developed in schools. The work of dental hygienists (called school dental nurses) in New Zealand was used as a model around the world.[35-42] (This emphasis was reflected in 1929 in a "suggested outline of lectures on dentistry to nurses in training" by Isabel M. Stewart.)[43]

Dental education and dental care, with emphasis on prevention, is now taken for granted as part of a comprehensive health service in the schools.[44,45]

In decades and in geographical areas where malnutrition was endemic, school health services emphasized nutrition and provided special facilities for teaching food selection and preparation and for feeding pupils.[46-53] This is another example of how a health problem influences the physical structure of the school and its health service.

While a diminishing number of persons, influenced by a Victorian education, may think that sex education is a recent emphasis in schools, it has actually been stressed throughout this century. In 1911, Elisabeth Robinson Scovil,[54] a nurse, discussed "Instructing Children in the Origin of Life," in 1914, E. B. Lowry,[55] who was both a nurse and a physician, wrote a text *Teaching Sex Hygiene in the Public Schools,* and in 1921, Mary Lee Barry[56] wrote *An Outline for Sex Education* designed for nurses. In the second decade, the American Social Hygiene Association was formed. Although some opposed the euphemism, this terminology, adopted to cover sex behavior and venereal disease, may have appeased the opposition to sex education, for "social hygiene" dominated the literature until the middle of the century.[57-63] The National League of Nursing Education had a Committee on Social Hygiene, and a nursing index for this period gives *Sex—See Social Hygiene.*[64,65] Today, sex behavior and sexually transmitted diseases are discussed frankly, although one writer in 1974 asked "What Place Does Sex Education Have in the Schools?"[66] A nurse in 1972 expressed "concern" over the high school student's lack of factual knowledge of venereal disease, and others emphasized the inadequacy of current sex education.[67-70]

Few question the statement that with more general knowledge of birth control, with increased use of drugs that weaken inhibitions, and with less public censure of extramarital sex, the incidence of venereal disease and extramarital pregnancy has increased.

The interrelationship of drug abuse (including alcoholism), venereal disease, and pregnancy in schools is often noted.[71,72] School health programs may include facilities for counseling, testing, and treating students faced with any one or a combination of these problems. Schools may even provide separate classrooms for pregnant girls.[73-83]

Cultural or ethnic groups vary in their attitudes toward extramarital pregnancy and to children born out of wedlock. Current programs designed to enable young people to

CUMULATIVE HEALTH RECORD CARD

Birthdate _____

	Last Name		First Name		Mid. Initial		Mo.	Day	Yr.
SCHOOL									
ROOM									
GRADE									
DATE									

Father's Name & Address at Work   Mother's Name & If Working, Where

Tel. No:

No.	ADDRESS	CITY OR TOWN	SCHOOL	HOME TELEPHONE	PHYSICIAN	DENTIST

PLEASE: Check (X) all available answers and date of occurrence. Explain items and complications under "NOTES"

Family Health History

Disease	Yes	No	Observations
1. Allergies			
2. Blood Diseases			
3. Congenital Defects			
4. Diabetes			
5. Epilepsy			
6. Mental and Nervous			
7. Rheumatic Fever			
8. Syphilis			
9. Tuberculosis			
10. Other familial diseases			

Prenatal Birth - Infancy History

	Normal	Complication
Pregnancy		
Delivery		
Condition at Birth		
Newborn		
Infancy		
Nutrition		
Development		
Growth		
Other		
Birth Weight	lb	oz

ADDITIONAL INFORMATION OBTAINED   YES   NO
(V.N.A. File or other)

Please check Yes or No if the child has or has had the following conditions:

PUPIL'S PAST AND PRESENT DISEASES OR CONDITIONS

	Yes	No	Date		Yes	No	Date
1 - Allergies				10 - Kidney Disease			
2 - Anemia				11 - Meningitis			
3 - Convulsions				12 - Obesity			
4 - Diabetes				13 - Pneumonia			
5 - Ear Infections				14 - Rheumatic Fever			
6 - Hearing defects				15 - Skin conditions			
7 - Heart disease				16 - Speech defects			
8 - Intestinal Parasites				17 - Tonsilitis			
9 - Hernia				18 - Other			

COMMUNICABLE DISEASES

1 - Chicken pox				6 - Roseola			
2 - German measles				7 - Scarlet fever			
3 - Measles				8 - Whooping Cough			
4 - Mumps				9 - Other			
5 - Poliomyelitis				10 - Complications			

	KIND	OBSERVATIONS	DATE
OPERATIONS			
ACCIDENTS			

Please check the following:

Finger Sucking	Yes	No		Normal Appetite	Yes	No	Other
Nail Biting	Yes	No		Normal Sleep	Yes	No	
Bedwetting	Yes	No		Behavior Problems	Yes	No	

IMMUNIZATIONS

Type	1st	2nd	3rd	Booster	Booster	Booster
DPT Triple						
DT (or TD)						
Influenza						
Salk Poliovaccine						
Sabin Poliovaccine Trivalent		1st	2nd	3rd	Booster	
Sabin Poliovaccine Monovalent	Type I	Type II	Type III			
Measles Vaccine	K'lled ▢	Live ▢	Date			
Gamma Globulin	Yes ▢	No ▢	Date			

TESTS

Type	Date	Result
Schick		
Tuberculin (Kind of Test)		
Other		

SMALLPOX VACCINATION

Date	Result	Date	Result

OTHER SCREENING   DATES

Hemoglobin	Gms.	
Urinanalysis	S A Alb.	
Other		

Figure 3-15. Record form used in New Haven (Conn.) School Health Program. (Courtesy of Department of Health, New Haven, Conn.)

Name _____ Address _____ Tel. Number _____

I authorize the school physician to give needed immunization and perform the following tests: hemoglobin, Tine test and urinalysis.

Information obtained by _____ Date _____ Signature of Parent _____

EVALUATION AND SCREENING RECORD

School															
Grade	Pre-Kg.	Kg	1	2	3	4	5	6	7	8	9	10	11	12	
Mo. Yr.															
Age															
WEIGHT (lb.)															
Month															
HEIGHT (inches)															
Month															
VISION With Glass R/L															
Without Glass R/L															
Both Eyes															
Date															
HEARING NORMAL R/L															
ABNORMAL R/L															
Report included															
Date															
TEETH (use code)															
Date															
SPEECH (use code)															
Date															

Last Name _____ First Name _____ Mid. Initial _____ Birthdate _____ Mo _____ Day _____ Yr. _____

	Pre-Kg Kg Gr I	Code	Gr IV	Code	Gr VII	Code	Gr X	Code
Indicate place where P.E. was done								
GRADE								
CURRENT HISTORY OR REASONS FOR PHYSICAL EXAM.								
General Physical appearance								
Eyes - Strabismus								
Ears								
Nose - Sinus								
Mouth - Pharynx								
Teeth - Gums								
Skin - Scalp								
Lymph Nodes								
Neck - Thyroid								
Chest - Breast								
Cardio-Vascular								
Lungs and Resp. System								
Back & Spine								

Figure 3-15. (Continued)

Genitals										
Extremities Posture										
Nervous System Habits Behavior										
OTHER FINDINGS										
Development Nutrition										
Comment on Abnormal Findings										
Referrals: 1-										
2-										
3-										
Physician										
Nurse										
Date										
Relative Present										
Follow-up 1-										
2-										
3-										

(see also Health Counseling Memoranda)

CODE:
- 0 - NO defect
- 1 - Slight deviation NOT requiring correction
- 2 - Defect REQUIRING attention
- 3 - Irremediable defect

In addition to above, please indicate if:
- N - New defect
- K - Known defect
- UC - Under care
- C - Corrected

SCHOOL NURSE NOTES: ILLNESS-ACCIDENT

Date	Absence	Cause	Duration

HEALTH COUNSELING MEMORANDA

Date		Date	

Figure 3-15. (Continued)

make an informed choice about sex behavior and the use of drugs should promote healthy sex and reduce unwanted pregnancy, drug abuse, and venereal disease.

While those unfamiliar with comprehensive school health programs may still think of school health services as housed in one or two rooms presided over by *a* nurse, most school health personnel reject this stereotype. They point out that a modern school health service requires a suite of rooms or a building designed and equipped so that the staff can participate in the health education program, offer health counseling, practice disease prevention, and give a range of services to the sick and injured depending on their needs and the resources available in the community. According to the size and location of the school, college, or university, and its related resources, the health program may require a few rooms in a building, an entire building or buildings, or in some cases, substations scattered over a large campus.

Organization and Administration of School and College Health Services. It seems necessary and yet repetitious to say that the organization and administration of school and college health services depend upon the ownership and control of the institution. Schools and colleges may be controlled by national, state, provincial, county, or municipal governments; by religious and other organizations; by corporations or individuals.

Health services in public schools may be the responsibility of boards of health or boards of education, or these boards may be jointly responsible. During the first decade of this century, "medical inspection" was used almost interchangeably with school health service.[83] The *American Journal of Nursing,* in a 1906 editorial on Lina Rogers' report of school nursing in New York City, refers to nurses as "inspectors."[84] S. Weir Newmayer, a physician, entitled his text on school health, first published in 1913, *Medical and Sanitary Inspection of Schools for the Health Officer, the Physician, the Nurse and the Teacher.*[85]

Control of communicable disease being the overriding problem of that era, it is no wonder that the sanitarian and the board of health had such important roles to play. However, throughout its history the organization and administration of health services in public schools has been a joint responsibility and presents a confusing picture. In 1913, Louis W. Papeer[86] described the reorganization of health provisions in school systems. In some states, provinces, counties, or municipalities, educational boards might be totally responsible for health service; in others, the boards of health might

make the policies and supply the personnel; and in still others, there was joint control.

In the United States, national policy guidelines were published by joint committees of the National Education Association and the American Medical Association.[87,88] At a world conference on education in 1924, the Federation of Education Associations was formed, with a Health Section sponsored by the American Child Health Association.[89] The ACHA became very influential in school health.

With the development in the United States of official, private, and later combined public health nursing agencies in most communities, it was possible for schools to contract with these agencies for nursing service. In 1933 and 1949, *Public Health Nursing* carried articles on administering school nursing on a generalized basis.[90,91] Later, the administration of school nursing was included as a topic in the National Organization for Public Health Nursing's Annual Review.[92,93] It is not surprising to find articles with titles such as "School Health —Whose Job Is It?"[94] or "A School Health Program is a Community Enterprise."[95] Actually, the latter is true, since students and parents, educators and health workers all have a role to play and a heavy stake in the product. Parent-teacher associations have influenced decisions about school health questions, as, for example, how sex education is taught. As teachers, school nurses have worked within the educational structure; as nurses, they have worked within the organizational structure of a health service.

N. G. Hawkins,[96] a sociologist, who in 1971 reviewed portions of the literature and conducted a limited investigation with 20 nurses in Pennsylvania, asked "Is There a School Nurse Role?" He urged leaders of the nursing profession to study the role confusion. He said that school nurses "cannot assume independent direction of any segment of their activity," being "in conflict with" or "subordinate to" health instructors, psychologists, and others who may have a formally qualified claim on various areas of responsibility in which nurses also function. While many school nurses would probably say that Hawkins exaggerates the anomaly of their role, as early as 1909 articles by school nurses were published on "the obstacles" in their paths,[97] and Bryan's[98] recent text entitled *School Nursing in Transition* suggests a recognition of the need for change.

The organization and administration of health services in private schools have been less confusing than in public schools. However, since each school can set up its own service with few controls, these services are highly individual. Nurses in private schools have more opportunity to influence the nature of their service than those in public schools.

In countries such as Great Britain, where school health services may qualify as one aspect of a National Health Service, its structure and standards or requirements influence the nature of the school health services, and they may come under regional or area boards.

The organization and administration of college and university health services are less confusing than those of school health services but, like the latter, are different in public and private institutions. All of them are subject to policies established by governing boards of the particular college or university, but public institutions are more subject to pressures from elected state, provincial, or municipal bodies that set standards and appropriate funds. As indicated earlier, college and university health services, whether in public or private institutions, seeking third-party payments from health insurance systems, are vitally affected by their organizational and administrative requirements. That these services are changing few would question. Already cited is R. H. Woody's article, "College Health Services—Demise or Rebirth?" [99]

The role of the nurse in the administrative and organizational structure of college and university health services of the United States can be traced in books and articles dating from 1914.[100-109] In 1962, John S. Hathaway, James S. Davie, and Helene Fitzgerald, in separate articles, gave a progress report on a study of "The Role of the Nurse in a University Health Service." [110-112] While the effect of the nurse's expanded role on the organization and administration of the service was not spelled out (the study was designed to measure its effectiveness by student usage of the service and the numbers of health problems identified by nurses), it obviously necessitated changes. Nurses in the new role were obliged to make decisions they had not previously made.

Governing boards of large universities may appoint a director of health affairs who is sometimes a vice president, and the university health service in such cases comes within his or her purview. Under any system, there is a medical director of the school, college, or university health service. The director's concept of administration and health service determines, to a large extent, the roles of the various health professionals functioning in the service, including nurses. The program may be based on arbitrary administrative decisions or on group decisions. Directors of nursing in school and college health services may initiate and administer these services under liberal and flexible policies and legislation that enables nurses to function interdependently with other health professionals, or they may be cast in unprofessional and dependent roles. Traditionally, school and college health nurses have been forced to exercise more clinical judgment and make more decisions than hospital nurses because so few school and college health services have employed physicians full time. In any event, delegated authority and "standing orders" from physicians have enabled nurses to function more independently than an organizational chart would suggest. There is every reason to believe that nurses in schools and colleges function most effectively and derive most satisfaction from their work when a role commensurate with their ability is clearly defined and when the school or university health service is organized so that they can fulfill this role.

Functions, Satisfactions, Rewards, and Difficulties in School and College Health Services. From what has been said under other headings, most readers will have formed some opinions on the functions of nurses in school and college health services, their rewards and difficulties.

At the turn of the century, nurses went into the schools in a crusading spirit. While they were sometimes called "nurse inspectors" and the emphasis was on controlling and eradicating communicable disease, including parasitic infestations, early studies showed that school nurses taught health (often called "hygiene") to teachers as well as pupils and were greatly concerned with correcting or helping pupils to cope with defects of hearing, vision, speech, posture, mobility, and other handicaps. In 1908, Thomas F. Harrington,[113] reviewing the history of health services ["medical inspection"] in Boston, Massachusetts, schools, from its inception in 1894, reported that since 1906 [when nurses were appointed to the service], they (nurses) had made 22,292 home visits.

It was the hope of many school nurses that the service to children and the health practices taught them would improve the health status of the whole family. This idea was expressed by many persons, as, for example, Jane Addams, a social worker, and Thomas D. Wood, M. Adelaide Nutting, and Isabel M. Stewart, medical and nursing educators.[114,115] School attendance and dealing with truancy have always been problems, and it was soon recognized that the presence of nurses in the school improved attendance. It was one of the functions of nurses to determine the cause of the pupil's absence and, if possible, remove it.

A review of articles on what school nurses did and texts by experts showing what was expected of them gives a reasonably accurate picture of both during the first half of this century.[116-130] Following World War II, the function of the nurse in every setting was questioned and studied. In studying the nursing needs and resources of a state, school nursing was analyzed to see, for example, whether the preparation of nurses was wasted on nonnursing tasks.[131] School nursing was the subject of at least two doctoral dissertations by nurses during the 1950s, and in 1963, by a nonnurse.[132-134] A doctoral study of guidelines on their preparation was made in 1961.[135]

The psychosocial aspect of every branch of nursing has been stressed in recent decades. The mental health component of school and college nursing has been discussed in publications since 1950, and is reflected in guidelines, statements on functions, standards, and qualifications, and in texts on school health.[136-148] Hawkins[149] said health counseling was, in 1971, the school nurse's most useful function. The nurse must now be prepared to work with "the exceptional child," the "hyperactive child," and it is even suggested by one writer that, along with physicians and "health educators," school nurses must know something about transcendental meditation.[150,151] In other words, they must be able to work with currently recognized interests and problems of students.

Bryan, in her 1973 description *School Nursing in Transition,* divided school nurse practice into direct child care and health education. She also saw the school nurse as a liaison agent between the school and the community and as a participant in planning and evaluating the health program.

The chief reward of school and college health nursing is, rather obviously, direct service to those in need. However, for nurses who enjoy teaching, this setting offers a signal opportunity to teach students and their families, faculty, and staff. For nurses who are asked or want to teach but who are unprepared for this function, their work can be anything but satisfying.

It was stated at the beginning of this section that nurses of the United States and Canada who work in the school setting have the highest academic standing except for those who are employed in schools of nursing and in public health agencies.

While there are reports of lectures given for school nurses in earlier decades, the first postbasic programs probably date from the early 1930s. Thomas D. Wood, a physician, worked with M. Adelaide Nutting and Isabel M. Stewart in developing a postbasic program at Teachers College, Columbia University, to pre-

pare school nurses for the dual function of health care and health education. Mary Ella Chayer, whose 1931 text *School Nursing—A Contribution to Health Education*[152] established her leadership in this branch of nursing, directed the program. Her analysis and later studies represent efforts to find out how to prepare school nurses. Most, until recently, have been prepared as public health nurses, but there is a conviction held by many that certification of school nurses means that they are qualified health educators. Courses in hygiene have given way to courses in the life sciences, with a concerted effort to build them around the students' needs. This concept may have been carried to its ultimate conclusion in a current service program described in 1974 by Mary Anne Lewis,[153] a school nurse. She is experimenting with "child-initiated care," where children are encouraged to decide when they need care and to help decide how to handle their health problems. This program is worth emphasizing, for many thoughtful writers such as Ivan Illich and Andrew Malleson suggest that self-reliance and self-help must be encouraged to combat the excessive dependence on health service and the spiraling cost of health care.

School nursing has changed, just as public health nursing has changed. It must be adjusted to those it serves. Through exposure to mass media and more sophisticated library resources and learning tools, the school population is more knowledgeable about health.

There seems to be a consensus that school nurses must be prepared for "an expanded role." The American Nurses' Association and the American School Health Association have issued a joint statement approving the expansion of their role so that they function as "school nurse practitioners" who "work collaboratively with physicians and other health professionals, educators and parents to provide comprehensive assessment and remedial action. . . ." *

Bryan,[154] in *School Nursing in Transition,* says that, while school nurses are among the best-prepared nurses and have more satisfaction in their work than most nurses, a barrier for them is the misunderstanding of their function by school administrators and even other nurses. Bryan's statement on preparation is substantiated by figures in ANA's *Facts About Nursing 72–73.* Their educational status is reflected in salaries that are comparable to those for public health nurses.[155]

---

* Connecticut Nurses' Association: "Expanded Role for School Nurses Spelled Out by Major Health Organizations," *Nurs. News,* **45:**4, (Oct.) 1973.

As college health services come to offer comprehensive care, college nursing offers a wide variety of satisfactions or rewards. Jane Foster [156] reported on "the first meeting of nurses in college health" in 1940, at which a Subcommittee on College Health Nursing of the School Nursing Section of the NOPHN was formed; in this same year, Fern A. Goulding,[157] the chairman of the School Nursing Section, reported a survey of college nursing services in 6, north central colleges. While college health nurses have worked through nursing organizations, they have also been a part of variously titled organizations on health in colleges. There is a nursing section of the American College Health Association. At the Annual National Conference on Health in Colleges, dating from 1950 (first called Conference on College Hygiene), nurses have had an opportunity to discuss college health services with students, physicians, and other health workers. Some contemporary college health services employ a variety of clinical nurse specialists and offer them the opportunity to practice with other health specialists a high quality of preventive and curative service. College health nursing, in addition, offers qualified nurses the satisfaction of membership in a college or university community.

9. OCCUPATIONAL HEALTH SERVICES— INCLUDING THOSE IN INDUSTRY

Definitions. The all-inclusive term *occupational health* has to some extent, since 1950, replaced the restricted terms *industrial health* and *industrial hygiene*. In a 1964 symposium on occupational health in industry, David H. Goldstein and Leo Orris, discussing diseases of white collar workers, make the following statement:

> The legal definition of an occupational disease varies in each State, depending on the scope of its workmen's compensation law. For the purposes of this study, an occupational disease is defined as a compensable disease that arises out of and in the course of employment.*

They distinguish between occupational diseases, which represent 3 per cent of all occupationally caused disabilities, and accidental injuries, which are responsible for 97 per cent of the occupationally caused disabilities.† The

---

* Goldstein, David H., and Orris, Leo: "Diseases of White Collar Workers," *Public Health Rep.*, **79:**958, (Nov.) 1964.

† In 1968, the US Public Health Service published a leaflet, *Occupational Disease—The Silent Enemy*.[1] It pointed out that in California, where the law makes occupational disease as well as injury reportable, there were 27,000 cases reported in 1965. Projected na-

point in citing their definition is the fact that it hinges on the condition entitling the person to compensation from the employer. Such an interpretation explains why physicians employed by hospitals to work in radiology departments who acquire skin cancer that "arises out of and in the course of their employment" are just as eligible for compensation from the hospital as are workers in a watch factory who acquire skin cancer "that arises out of and in the course of their employment." Nurses who acquire tuberculosis in the course of their employment in a hospital and soldiers who acquire the disease in military service are as eligible for compensation as are the miners who acquire lung disease in mining.

Occupational health services, therefore, include not only industrial health services, but other health services as well, and the term takes on new meaning. A 1970 publication of the USPHS is entitled *Community Health Nursing for Working People*.[2] This expresses the current concepts that occupational health nursing is a community service and that it is for all who work rather than just for those who work in industry. Nevertheless, the older concept persists, and it is hard to avoid misleading statements in writing about this "setting" because two terms with different meanings are so often used interchangeably. The 1966 *International Nursing Index*, following, as far as possible, the terminology of the National Library of Medicine, carried the following headings: *Industrial Medicine, Industrial Nursing, Occupational Diseases;* the 1974 INI added *Occupational Health Services.* A list of selected references prepared in 1973 by the Canadian Nurses' Association is titled *Occupational Health Nursing.*

Employment of Nurses in Occupational Health Services. It is hard to give accurate figures under this heading. The American Nurses' Association *Facts About Nursing 72–73* listed the number of employed registered "industrial nurses" as 19,403 in 1972.[3] This is 2½ per cent of the total of 778,470 employed registered nurses.* However, the index of this publication under the heading *Industrial Nursing* says See *Occupational Health Nursing.* The reader wonders whether the numbers of industrial nurses include those who, for example, work in the occupational health services of hospitals. The Canadian Nurses' Association uses "occupational health" only and gives the total number of employed registered

---

tionally for 75,000,000 employed, this would make an estimated 336,000 cases of reportable disease or injury.

* If the working population is estimated at 82,000,000 in 1972, this makes a ratio of about one nurse to 4200 workers.

nurses as 1,603, or 1.2 per cent of the total of 128,675 registered nurses employed in nursing.[4] Again, whether these figures represent nurses employed in industry only or include those employed in services for hospital workers or for workers in organizations such as the United Nations is hard to determine. In 1972, there were 264 men nurses in industry in the United States, about half of these in administrative positions. Here and in other countries, the dangerous trades such as mining attract men nurses.[5,6] Feldshers in Russia play a major role in the health centers of mines.[7]

Origins of Occupational Health Nursing. Books and articles on the history of occupational health medicine and occupational health nursing suggest that they have been neglected and, perhaps more than most health services, are dependent on political, social, cultural, and economic conditions. Jean Spencer Felton and his associates, tracing the "historic events in occupational medicine," noted that manual labor was performed by slaves in ancient Egypt, Greece, and Rome. Free men, or citizens, were forbidden to "ply a trade." They made the following observations:

Unable to control the hazards of work, the ruling classes of Egypt, Rome and Greece chose to banish them [activities which maimed and destroyed] from civilized society.

. . .

It proved a costly method of adjustment . . . as the number of slaves and free workers [artisans of great talent] alike grew larger, they sank deeper into poverty and disease, and . . . flourishing cities were overwhelmed by their own impoverished populations.*

Civilizations that have their roots in Egyptian, Greek, and Roman culture may still be influenced by their ancient attitudes toward labor. In any event, occupational disease was seldom mentioned in medical literature until recently. Felton and his associates noted occasional references to the diseases of miners and other workers in the Middle Ages and earlier. They identified physicians of the sixteenth, seventeenth, and eighteenth centuries who interested themselves in the welfare of workers. They attributed to Bernardino Ramazzini, an Italian physician who "examined the conditions of work and the diseases of most of the occupations of his time," the practice of including in every diagnostic case history an answer to the question "Of what trade are you?" †

The technology of the eighteenth century

and the formation of guilds that protected and regulated the lives of their members changed the public's attitude toward manual labor. Felton and his associates said that Denis Diderot, in his *Encyclopédie* (1751–65), "systemized and lifted the artisans from the prejudice they had suffered for centuries." * Percivall Pott wrote on occupational cancer. His publications on the scrotal cancer of chimney sweeps led to the Chimney-Sweepers Act of 1788, which is often cited as the first law to protect laborers.[8]

The Industrial Revolution replaced cottage industries with factories and the development of machines. Skilled craftsmen were replaced by women and children who could be hired at the lowest wages. Factories were soon surrounded by slums which persisted until automobiles and higher wages made it unnecessary for workers to walk to work.

The social abuses in England described by Charles Dickens were soon duplicated in the United States and other industrialized countries. They led to the creation of trade unions to protect workers and to reforms initiated by humanitarians. Robert Owen in 1799 stopped the employment of children in a factory he bought in Manchester, England, and established sickness and old age insurance. He helped draft the Factory Act of 1819, which was one of a series of acts during this century. The 1878 Act that established a "centralized system of factory inspection with a chief investigator" was perhaps the most important.†

Irene H. Charley,[9] in *The Birth of Industrial Nursing*, says that Philippa Flowerday, a district nurse who was employed in 1878 by the Carrow Works of the J. and J. Coleman Company in England to work in the factory and tend the sick in their homes, was the first industrial nurse. According to Mary Louise Brown,[10] the first industrial nurse in the United States was Ada Mayo Stewart [Markolf] who was employed by the Vermont Marble Company in 1895 to visit sick workers in their homes and to teach health to children in the schools. Stewart, much later, described her work in a nursing journal.[11] In 1897, the John Wanamaker Company of New York City was the first store in the United States to employ a nurse,[12] and the *Trained Nurse* carried an article in 1912 about "The Department-Store Nurse." [13] According to Brown, by 1900, 21 companies were known to have employed nurses.[14]

It is often said that the Industrial Revolution of the eighteenth and nineteenth centuries initiated protective legislation for workers and

---

* Felton, Jean Spencer, et al.: *Man, Medicine and Work. Historic Events in Occupational Medicine.* US Government Printing Office, Washington, D.C., 1964, p. 7.

† Felton, Jean Spencer, et al.: *op. cit.,* p. 20.

* Felton, Jean Spencer, et al.: *op. cit.,* p. 23.

† Felton, Jean Spencer, et al.: *op. cit.,* p. 39.

their families. T. Owen Edwards [15] thinks this is too narrow a view of industry, for he identifies "industrial legislation" in the medieval period.

Most occupations can be viewed as potentially hazardous. Even the seemingly safe work of a tailor imposes the dangers of a sedentary life; the building trades, on the other hand, and others that involve the use of heavy machinery, are obviously more risky. Firemen and many policemen live very dangerously.* By 1800, Robert Owen had seen the need for protective legislation for factory workers, but society at large came to believe that those who reap the profits and enjoy the products of industry should pay for injuries arising out of and in the course of employment. Later, society accepted the responsibility for family allowances, for sustaining workers through periods of unemployment, and for women during maternity leaves.† National, state, and provincial social security programs were first designed for the working population and only gradually have been extended in some countries to include all citizens (see Chapter 2). The US Department of Health, Education, and Welfare [17] reviewed social security programs in 1971 and among other data gave the year of the first work injury law in each country. The study shows that Germany's and Poland's were the first laws (1884). By 1900, 12 countries had passed work injury laws. Of the 126 countries included in the report, Ethiopia was the last to pass such a law (1960) except for the emerging states that tend to enact a variety of social security measures at once—work injury, work benefits, maternity legislation, sickness, unemployment, and old age insurance.

Since the employer has been forced to assume a large share of the cost of work injuries, and, later, disease arising out of and in the course of employment, it was soon obvious that it was in the employer's interest to prevent occupational injury and disease and to provide effective first aid and even home care for the injured and sick. The employment of "industrial hygienists," sanitary engineers, physicians, industrial psychologists, and nurses satisfied

* Some philosophers see industrialization as the chief threat to human happiness.
† While in most countries, work injury legislation preceded other forms of social security, there are exceptions. For example: Hungary had legislation to protect mothers (1891) before it passed work injury legislation (1907); New Zealand passed old age assistance legislation (1898) before its work injury benefits law (1908); Sweden had sickness and maternal legislation (1891) before its work injury law (1901); Denmark had sickness and maternity legislation (1892) and old age benefit legislation (1891) before its work injury law (1898); and Spain had sickness and maternity legislation (1929) and old age benefits (1919) before its work injury laws (1932). [16]

the social conscience, but it also proved to be "good business." Studies of industrial nursing have shown, for example, that, after the employment of nurses, work injuries and absenteeism decrease. Lillian D. Wald persuaded the Metropolitan Life Insurance Company to provide its policyholders with a visiting nurse service because it was in their interest to do so. [18] She is also credited with initiating the Children's Bureau that was largely responsible for curtailing child labor in the United States where its effects were deplorable.

World Wars I and II with their dependence on industry stimulated the employment of industrial nurses in all warring countries. The number of industrial nurses in the United States increased from 5512 in 1941 to 11,200 in 1943. This number, almost doubled by 1972, still failed to provide nursing service to all workers of this country. [19,20]

The Nature of Occupational Health Services. Like school health services, occupational health services range from a part-time service given by a doctor and a nurse in one or several rooms to a comprehensive program with health stations, clinics, home care, and hospital services such as those offered by the Kaiser-Permanente System.

The most constant element of an occupational health service may be a first-aid service. Workers are taught to give first aid because health service personnel may not be available when needed and because so many accident victims require immediate treatment if their life is to be saved or permanent disability avoided. Another fairly constant element is the preemployment examination. Health workers collaborate with management, sanitarians, and engineers in identifying and minimizing hazards in the work environment, including communicable disease. Most occupational health services offer an educational program of some sort. A few occupational health services provide a full range of diagnostic, preventive, and therapeutic services, including ambulatory, hospital, and home care programs, and fewer still provide evaluative or research services. The development of American industrial nursing is well documented in the literature. [21-36] Nursing journals in North America and the British Commonwealth carry an occasional article on occupational health nursing in foreign countries but persons especially interested in a country should review its publications. [37-46] R. V. Bolyard points to some of the "lessons from the past" in occupational health. [47] Nurses in this as in all settings profit from a knowledge of how the service developed.

Standardization, Certification, and Regulation of Occupational Health Nursing. Generally speaking, occupational health nurses have not been under pressure from specialized regulatory bodies in most countries. This is reflected in the fact that in the United States, in 1972, they had the least educational preparation among nurses in identified fields of employment except that of private duty. While 12.1 per cent of the total 778,470 employed registered nurses had a baccalaureate degree, only 7.2 per cent of the 19,403 industrial nurses had a baccalaureate degree.[48] In Canada, only 4.7 per cent of the 1603 occupational health nurses have baccalaureate degrees, with only private duty and office nurses having less preparation.[49]

It seems to have been assumed by many that occupational health nursing is not so much a specialty as one form of public health nursing. Jean Gray in 1967, discussing the desirability of defining occupational health nursing, said:

Efforts in the past to prepare nurses for work in occupational health have become lost or so diffused they are out of focus. . . . Whereas graduate programs for specialized preparation in most nursing fields are increasing in numbers and quality, there are none in occupational health nursing.*

Mildred Walker,[50] a Canadian nurse, in 1965 said: "Occupational health nursing is not unique." She said it was only the setting in which it is practiced that made it different. However, she did not imply that it was less demanding. She said the principal functions of the occupational health nurse are making health estimates, giving emergency care, supervising the environment, teaching, and counseling. All of these are complex services.

In 1972, Mary E. Scanlon, writing on the work of an industrial visiting nurse outside the plant, said: "The popular concept of an industrial visiting nurse as a police officer is obsolete. She can and should function as a member of the occupational health staff and act as a liaison between the sick or injured employee and the company." †

The first occupational nurse in England was a district nurse. There, in Canada, and in the United States, occupational health nurses were from the first associated with public health nursing as contrasted with institutional nursing. Some early articles referred to the occupational nurse as "the welfare nurse," which suggested a high component of social work in his or her function. The chief personnel officer

in a British industry wrote in 1957 about "the industrial nurse's relationship with other social workers." [51-57] So the concept persists.

International agencies have, in the last three decades, influenced occupational health standards. There is a nursing session at International Congresses of Industrial Medicine; the work of the Joint ILO/WHO Committee on Occupational Health includes consideration of the nurse's role; both the International Labour Office and the World Health Organization have sponsored seminars on the nurses' preparation for or role in industry, and the Permanent Commission and International Association on Occupational Health is concerned with the nurse's contribution.[58-66] Since 1958, when the ILO worked with the ICN at the Council's request in studying the conditions of work and employment of nurses around the world, these two agencies have had a cooperative relationship which has indirectly influenced all branches of nursing.[67,68] Margrethe Kruse was the chief investigator for the ILO study, and later was president of the ICN.

British nurses seem to have been aware in the early decades of the importance of special preparation for occupational health nursing. Irene H. Charley, who wrote a history of this field, directed the Industrial Nurses' Bureau of Great Britain. In 1932, she addressed a conference on "postgraduate" nursing education.[69] The Occupational Health Section of the Royal College of Nursing, organized in 1952, has not only made surveys, set standards, and backed certification of occupational health nurses, but has taken the initiative in promoting a uniform national health service for workers.[70-73] In 1968, an Occupational Health Committee of the Royal College of Nursing published *Occupational Health Nursing* and *Occupational Health Nursing Structure*,[74,75] and in 1969, they published *A National Occupational Health Service*.[76] The first two spell out the preparation, functions, and role of nurses; the third presents the objectives, functions, responsibility, structure, and method of financing a national occupational health service. The Committee reached the following conclusion:

The RCN considers that in the interest of the health of employees and subsequently the efficiency of industry and commerce and the economy of the country, steps should be taken to protect all employees from health risks arising from their work and environment and to promote a high degree of well-being of all employed persons.

To achieve such aims, the national health service should be extended to provide a total health service by the inclusion of a national occupational health service.

It is recommended that the organisation, ad-

---

* Gray, Jean: "Why Define Occupational Health Nursing?" *Nurs. Outlook*, 15:52, (Oct.) 1967.

† Scanlon, Mary E.: "An Industrial Visiting Nurse. Occupational Health Outside the Plant," *Nurs. Clin. North Am.*, 7:143, (Mar.) 1972.

ministration, and coordination of all health services, including occupational health should be undertaken by Area Health Boards as recommended by the Review of Medical Services Committee, or by the Area Boards as proposed in the Green Paper.*

With the reorganization of the British National Health Service, occupational health became an integral part of the health programs administered under area health boards. A central regulatory mechanism exists for all areas. This is only practicable when there is a national health service with universal coverage.

It is not possible to comment even briefly on the regulations of occupational health services in other countries, but Finland might be cited with Great Britain as having regulated occupational health nursing. Ruth Säynäjärvi,[77] consultant to the Institute of Occupational Health, Helsinki, as early as 1957, described the occupational health content that all public health nurses must study.

In the United States, standards for occupational health nursing have been influenced by the committees, subcommittees, bureaus, or divisions for occupational health in the following national organizations and agencies: National Organization for Public Health Nursing, National League of Nursing Education and National League for Nursing, American Nurses' Association, American Association of Industrial Nurses, American Public Health Association, American Medical Association, US Public Health Service, and, tangentially, the US Department of Labor, the US Department of the Interior (Bureau of Mines), the American Foundation of Occupational Health, and the American Conference of Governmental Industrial Hygienists (Subcommittee on Plant Records). Occupational health nursing, like all health care, is affected by federal legislation. The fact that so many agencies and organizations have been concerned with occupational health nursing in the United States may account for its difficulty in establishing and enforcing high standards of preparation and practice.

Formation of the Industrial Nursing Section in the NOPHN in 1930 gave the profession what might have been a standard-setting agency. It and the Industrial Nurses Section of the ANA, established in 1942,[78,79] undoubtedly improved the quality of occupational health nursing. The Committee on Professional Education of the APHA made a stab in this direc-

tion in 1939 when it published "Desirable Qualifications of Nurses Appointed to Public Health Nursing Positions in Industry." [80] Existing organizations must have failed to meet the needs of occupational health nurses of this era, for the American Association of Industrial Nurses was formed in 1942, and it was hailed as a great event in the journal *Industrial Medicine*.[81,82] In 1945, the AAIN published *Qualifications, Duties, Personnel Policies, and Educational Programs for Industrial Nurses* (revised in 1949).[83] This publication and the Association's *Guide for the Preparation of an Industrial Nursing Manual* [84] offered models that had a standardizing influence. In 1951, the Association offered *Recommended Qualifications for Industrial Nurses Working with Nursing Supervision*.[85]

When, during the Structure Study (1949–1953), the existing national nursing organizations combined to form six organizations, the AAIN decided to maintain its identity.[86,87] However, the ANA retained its Industrial Nurses Section. These events necessarily divided the leadership in this branch of nursing.

In the early 1950s, the ANA conducted a far-flung research project on the function of nursing which included the function of industrial nurses.[88] These investigations were paralleled by the creation in the ANA of a Committee on Functions, Standards, and Qualifications for Practice.[89] Each section of the ANA prepared a statement which was widely distributed.[90] The ANA statement first published in 1956 was revised in 1958, 1960, and 1968. In 1955, the AAIN published its statement on the "duties and responsibilities of the professional nurse in an industrial medical service,"[91] and the NLN Exchange published *Educational Responsibilities of Occupational Health Nurses* in 1956.[92]

In 1943, the American Medical Association's Council on Occupational Health published standing orders for industrial nurses, a statement revised in 1962 under the title "Medical Directives for Occupational Health Nurses."[93] In 1955, this association's Council on Industrial Health published *Guiding Principles and Procedures for Industrial Nurses*.[94] Since few industries have ever had full-time physicians, they have, through standing orders, delegated considerable responsibility for diagnosis and treatment to nurses. In 1959, the Committee on Industrial Nursing of the Council on Industrial Health made a statement on the legal scope of industrial nursing practice.[95]

In 1960, the USPHS published a statement on an occupational health program for hospital employees.[96] In 1962 and 1963, the ANA published "guides" on developing an employee

* Royal College of Nursing and National Council of Nurses of the United Kingdom: *A National Occupational Health Service*. The College and the Council, London, 1969, p. 14.

health program,[97,98] and in 1968, the ANA's Division of Community Health Practice published *Functions and Qualifications for an Occupational Health Nurse in a One-Nurse Service*.[99] In 1965, the AAIN issued a statement, *Standards and Criteria for Evaluating an Occupational Nursing Service*.[100]

The Department of Public Health Nursing of the NLN collaborated with the USPHS in preparing the pamphlet *Community Health Nursing for Working People. A Guide for Voluntary and Official Health Agencies To Provide Part-Time Occupational Health Nursing Services* (1970) [101] which replaced *Nursing Part-Time in Industry* (1965).

The Social Security Act of 1935 stimulated the program of the Division of Industrial Hygiene (later the Division of Occupational Health) in the USPHS and made grants-in-aid available to states to promote industrial health. The Occupational Safety and Health Act of 1970 [102] is a fresh stimulus to promoting higher standards of occupational health. A flyer giving the highlights of this legislation includes the following statement:

The Occupational Safety and Health Act of 1970 seeks to provide American workers with protection against personal injury and illness resulting from hazardous working conditions. Under its terms, the Federal Government is authorized to develop and set mandatory occupational safety and health standards applicable to any business affecting interstate commerce. The responsibility for promulgating and enforcing occupational safety and health standards rests with the Department of Labor.

The Department of Health, Education, and Welfare is responsible for conducting research on which new standards can be based, and for implementing education and training programs for producing an adequate supply of manpower to carry out the purposes of the Act. HEW's responsibilities are carried out by the National Institute for Occupational Safety and Health.

Mary Louise Brown, formerly Chief, Occupational Health Nurses Training, Occupational Safety and Health Branch, Environmental Control Administration, US Department of Health, Education, and Welfare, was in 1975 Chief, Nurses Training, Division of Occupational Safety and Health Training, National Institute for Occupational Safety and Health. In these and former positions, she has studied the preparation of the occupational health nurse. In 1964, the Nursing Section of the Bureau of Occupational Safety and Health (later the National Institute for Occupational Safety and Health) made a survey involving 10,000 occupational health nurses.[103,104] This study was followed by an experimental course

in Employee Mental Health and Industrial Nursing Practice.[105] It was conducted by Jean Gray and cosponsored by the USPHS and the Industrial Hygiene Foundation of America (now the Industrial Health Foundation of America).

In 1971, Marjorie Keller and W. Theodore May [106] published a report of a study of the occupational health content (based on meeting human needs) in baccalaureate nursing education conducted at the University of Tennessee under a grant from the USPHS. Brown, in 1971, discussing the extended role of the nurse in occupational health nursing, reviewed these and other current programs developed under USPHS sponsorship, including that of the American Institute for Research for the Industrial Health Foundation. She concluded that "Training opportunities to increase the nurse's knowledge and to develop her skills in occupational mental health are available." * While no one would challenge this general statement, it does not alter the conclusion that, on the whole, educational programs for occupational health nurses have been inadequate in numbers and quality. Brief series of lectures, educational institutes, symposia, conferences, workshops, and projects have been sponsored by organizations, agencies, universities, and individuals, but these have not established a pattern of basic or postbasic preparation for occupational nursing in the United States. There is a growing consensus that undergraduate and graduate programs should include participation or experience in occupational health services rather than observation.[107-119]

The preceding discussion of standardization, certification, and regulation of industrial nursing practice and preparation for practice in the occupational health setting must present a confused picture to the reader. There is no escaping the conclusion that nurses in this setting in the United States have looked for guidance and direction from many sources but that, perhaps for this very reason, they have failed to establish clear-cut standards of practice which might lead to a sufficient number of effective educational programs. However, as organized nursing in the United States and other countries develops continuing education requirements for the certification of all nurses, this requirement will lead to the establishment of short-term programs described by Brown and graduate programs such as those at the University of North Carolina. While few nurses favor retroactive regulations, many oc-

---

* Brown, Mary Louise: "The Extended Role of the Nurse in Occupational Mental Health Programs," *Ind. Med.,* **40:**17, (Dec.) 1971.

cupational health nurses commend certification as a means of upgrading the quality of nursing practice.[120-122] This should lead to higher standards of practice and preparation and eventually to a sufficient number of educational programs to meet the needs of nurses in occupational health. Mandatory continuing education will, of course, affect nurses in the occupational setting as well as other specialties (see page 106).

The Rights of Patients (Workers). As pointed out on page 198, compensation legislation for workers is of long standing and is now almost universal. While in some countries compensation laws vary with the state or province, they are relatively specific if the worker has a compensable injury or disease. Laws regulating the environment to prevent injury or disease are less specific, and laws specifying the number and types of health personnel, the hours of service, and the types of facilities are even less so. In 1966, Margaret F. McKiever[123] wrote that of an estimated 80,000,-000 workers in the United States plants only 15,000,000 had some sort of health service available. The remainder had only minimal protection from injury and disease. It seems to be generally conceded that the smaller the industry, the less protection for the worker.

Occupational health nurses should, of course, be familiar with publications cited in the preceding section describing their role in the occupational health program; they should also study official descriptions of the total program and be familiar with federal, state (or provincial), and local laws that affect the health care of workers. For example, the National Institute for Occupational Safety and Health in the USPHS publishes *Safety Standards*[124]; the US Department of Labor (Wage and Labor Standards Administration) published *State Workmen's Compensation Laws*[125] and their Women's Bureau published *1969 Handbook on Women Workers*[126]; and the US Department of the Interior (Bureau of Mines) published *State Compensatory Provisions for Occupational Diseases.*[127] The American Public Health Association's pamphlet, *Local Health Officials' Guide to Occupational Health,*[128] and *Basic Facts on the Health Industry,*[129] prepared by the Committee on Ways and Means of the US Congress, are instructive, as is the American National Standards Institute's *Methods of Recording and Measuring Work Injury Experience*[130] and the AMA's statement *Scope, Objectives, and Functions of Occupational Health Programs.*[131]

Helen Creighton, a nurse and lawyer, Lorice Ede, a lawyer, and David H. Goldstein, a lawyer, have written useful articles for occu-pational health nursing on laws affecting practice.[132-134] Theoretically, workers have a right to optimum protection from hazards in the working environment, to health education and other preventive services, to first aid, acute long-term care, and rehabilitation. Workers also have a right to monetary compensation for injury or disease arising out of and in the course of employment and, in some cases, family support. McKiever[135] describes the special rights of women who work.

As industrial health programs become integral parts of a national health service, centrally administered for a geographic area, the rights of patients may be more nearly the same in all settings. For nurses in the United States, the *President's Report on Occupational Safety and Health* (1972)[136] offers a summary of present strengths and weaknesses in the program and future directions. Health care is often referred to as one of the "largest industries" in developed countries. If health care is "industrial," the protection of its workers should come under the same kind of laws and regulations protecting miners and factory workers; if it is an essential public service, they should have the same protection as firemen and policemen. As more and more people come to believe that all workers have the same right to health care, the distinction between the services available to "industries" and "professions" will diminish and vanish. The literature suggests that there is a marked trend in this direction.[137-157] Health services for employees in factories, in hospitals, and at the UN headquarters all come under the blanket title of occupational health. When nurses who serve the space program, who are members of a ship's crew, or who minister to all those in need at race tracks or airports are classified as occupational health workers, the term "environmental health" seems an appropriate substitute for "occupational health." If everyone has a right to protection from hazards of the environment, a definition under this heading is extremely difficult.

Location and Physical Plans of Occupational Health Services. Like school health services, occupational health services may be quartered in one or two rooms or may be housed in a large suite, a building, a series of buildings, or in a network of buildings if a comprehensive health service is provided for the employees of a far-flung industry or for members of a union.

Most industries are small, employing less than 50 workers. Most, therefore, have one or two rooms in which part-time doctors and nurses function. The idea of buildings or hospitals to serve industrial workers is not new, however. In 1904, W. B. Lowman,[158] a physician, discussed the "importance and necessity of industrial hospitals" as a humanitarian step and a good business investment. He described a hospital attached to the Cambria Iron Company in Pennsylvania.

A system of hospitals operated by railroads dates from the first decades of this century, and the Miners' Hospitals of this era are outstanding.[159-161] The hospitals, clinics, and health maintenance units of the Kaiser-Permanente health care system are famous.* The Slough Industrial Health Service established in England in 1947 under the sponsorship of the Nuffield Foundation, Nuffield Provincial Hospitals Trust, and Slough Estates, Ltd., to serve 178 firms and 17,324 persons, has had comparable resources.[163]

In *Community Health Nursing for Working People*, Jane A. Lee, Occupational Health Nurse Consultant in the USPHS, refers to "the health unit" and states that the space allotted it is determined by the number of employees on the largest shift.[164] The significance of a name for this space is discussed in an article contrasting "Employee Health Service" with "First Aid Room."[165] Some small industries have so little health service that the first aid given the injured by other workers is about all that is regularly available.[166] In such cases "First Aid Room" is an accurate title.

Mary E. Scanlon gives the following description of the medical department of the Gillette Safety Razor Company, South Boston, Massachusetts, which she says is a highly automated light industry employing about 3000 workers in a three-shift operation:

The . . . facility . . . opened in July, 1963 . . . is . . . in the center of the plant. It includes an x-ray department with a full-time x-ray technician, a laboratory with a full-time registered laboratory technician, a physiotherapy room, a small operating room . . . , a[n] . . . eye department, a sound-proof audio-test unit, a cardiac room with electrocardiograph machine, oxygen, monitor, and defibrillator, eight examining rooms, and a large general treatment room.†

Some industries that contract for service to workers with health departments, visiting nurse agencies, clinics, and hospitals use the agencies' facilities for preemployment examinations and ambulatory and inpatient treatment and care.

Mobile health units are used extensively for occupational health services in the Union of Soviet Socialist Republics and the People's Republic of China, the principle in both these countries being to take health care to people where they live and work. In Great Britain and the United States, mobile health units have been and are currently used to bring health services to agricultural districts, especially to migrant laborers.

Migrant health is a subject that deserves special attention because, generally speaking, services and facilities for migrant labor have been totally lacking or inadequate. But the service, such as it is, is not new. As early as 1907, the *British Journal of Nursing* described the work of nurses for hop-pickers [167]; in 1925, a public health nurse in the United States described public health nursing in "hop yards." [168] In 1932 and 1939, there were descriptions of "health problems among California migrants" and "nursing among the migrants." [169,170] These are isolated examples of earlier concern for this type of worker.

The "dust bowl" disaster in the 1930s focused public attention on the plight of migrant workers in the United States. John Steinbeck's *Grapes of Wrath* had a wide audience and ever since its publication more people in the United States have been aware of the hardship of migrant labor.

During the 1960s and early 1970s, there was a concentrated effort to relieve rural poverty and to provide certain areas with the needed health facilities and services. The Economic Research Service of the US Department of Agriculture made a survey reported under the title *Domestic Migratory Farm Workers, Personal and Economic Characteristics* [171]; and for a US Senate committee it prepared a report on *Economic and Social Conditions of Rural America in the 1970's*.[172] The US President's National Advisory Commission on Rural Poverty in the United States was established in 1968.[173] The American Friends Service Committee made a special report in 1971 on child labor in agriculture.[174] A number of states developed programs and conducted studies. The Occupational Health and Environmental Epidemiology Bureau of the California Public Health Department, for example, investigated the relationship of occupational disease related to the use of pesticides and other agricultural chemicals.[175]

Oklahoma and West Virginia ("Appalachia") have had, perhaps, most public attention as a result of rural poverty and the sorry plight of migrant workers, but states using migrant labor extensively have had programs funded under the Federal Migrant

---

* Anne R. Somers, describing the Kaiser-Permanente Medical Care Program, reported that, in 1970, it had about 2,000,000 members and that it operated a network of hospitals, clinics, and medical groups in the West Coast states, in Colorado, and Hawaii.[162]

† Scanlon, Mary E.: "An Industrial Visiting Nurse," *Nurs. Clin. North Am.,* 7:143, (Mar.) 1972.

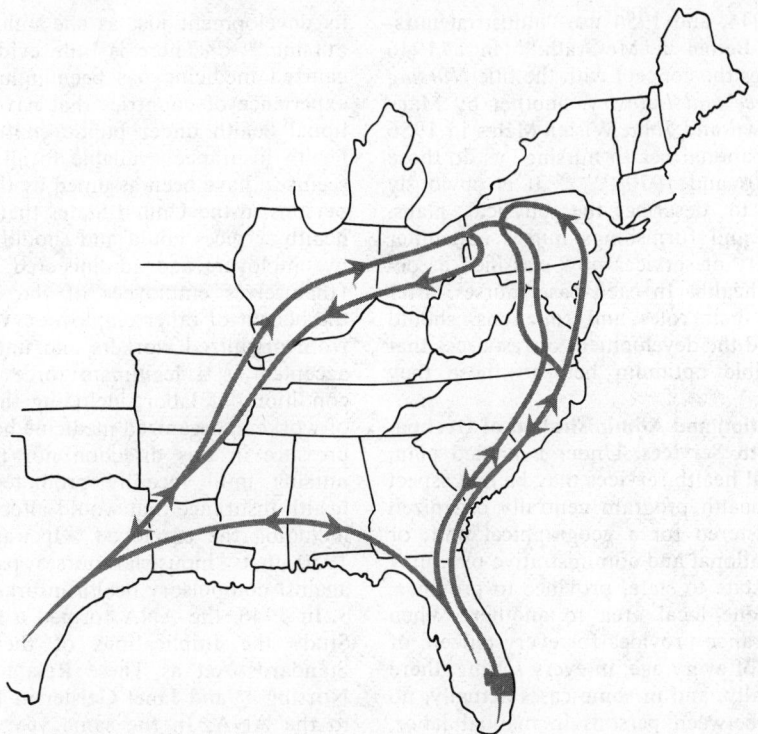

Figure 3-16. The migrant stream in the eastern United States. (Johansson, Mabel S.: "A Migrant Referral System for Continuity of Health Care," *Nurs. Clin. North Am.,* 8:133, [Mar] 1972, p. 135.)

Health Grant of 1963, and under grants from other agencies. Mabel S. Johansson, a public health nurse, in 1972 described a migrant health service referral system cooperatively developed by the Florida State Board of Health and the Planned Parenthood Federation of America to ensure continuity of service. She reported that between 1964 and 1968 "85 per cent of all contact referrals resulted in the provision of health service." She stated that "Public health nurses working in official and voluntary health agencies have been the determining factor in the initiation and completion of these referrals." * California with its Medi-Cal program has tried to provide full coverage for migrant workers.[176] Cesar Chavez of the AFL-CIO United Farm Workers of America has been active in this state and has influenced the health program. Marion Moses,[177] a nurse, described a 5-year experience as a volunteer in a mobile clinic in the San Joaquin Valley.† Frances Storlie, in *Nursing*

and the Social Conscience, has a chapter on health care for migrants. She includes a description of a visit to Marion Moses in her "trailer clinic" that served 250 farm workers and their families. She spoke of how troubled Marion Moses was: "She would almost demand of me 'Where are the nurses? Where are the doctors? The need is here but where are they?' " *

Those who think "industrial nursing" see the nurse functioning as a physician's assistant or surrogate in the health unit of a typical industry or factory equipped primarily for first aid, physical examinations, and treatment of minor ailments; those who think "occupational health nursing" and "environmental health nursing" are more likely to see the nurse in a wide variety of settings—mines, oil fields, farms, hotels, stores, theaters, space operation headquarters, transportation terminals, organization headquarters, and even racetracks.

Articles written in 1913 and 1936 on "factory nursing" suggest that the authors equated this term with industrial nursing.[178,179] Texts

* Johansson, Mabel S.: "A Migrant Referral System for Continuity of Health Care," *Nurs. Clin. North Am.,* 8:133, (Mar.) 1972.

† In 1973, Marion Moses was studying medicine with the hope of serving migrant workers more effectively.

* Storlie, Frances: *Nursing and the Social Conscience.* Appleton-Century-Crofts, New York, 1970, p. 79.

in 1920, 1944, and 1954 use "industrial nursing."[180-182] Bethel J. McGrath,[183] in a 1946 text, enlarges the concept with the title *Nursing in Commerce and Industry;* another by Mary Louise Brown and John Wister Meigs in 1956 uses "occupational health nursing" as do those in the 1960s and 1970s.[184-186] It is obviously impossible to describe the physical plans, equipment, and furnishings nurses encounter in the variety of services now classified as occupational health. In each case, nurses, after identifying their roles and functions, should work toward the development of resources that make possible optimum help to those they serve.

Organization and Administration of Occupational Health Services. Under a unified plan, occupational health services may be one aspect of a total health program centrally organized and administered for a geographical unit; or the organizational and administrative plan may vary from state to state, province to province, and from one local area to another. When health insurance provides for every citizen, of both sexes, of every age, in every setting, there is theoretically, and in some cases actually, no distinction between persons in manual labor, in management, in domestic employment, in the arts, in professional services, and in all other kinds of employment. The USSR and mainland China are representative of such countries. Great Britain has a National Health Service that provides health insurance for all, including the employed. The Occupational Health Section of the Royal College of Nursing (with its official journal) and the National Council of Nurses of the United Kingdom seem throughout their existence to have supported, and even taken the initiative in proposing, legislation to provide a unified and adequate occupational health program. In this decade they recommend, among other conditions, that all who practice occupational health nursing have a special course of training in occupational health nursing and that nurses with administrative responsibilties study management.[187,188]

In countries where health insurance and health services are fragmented, as in the United States, occupational health services have been neglected.[189-190] This is especially serious in the United States where such health insurance as exists under Social Security (Medicaid and Medicare) is not designed primarily to protect those who are of an age to be gainfully employed. Occupational health nurses in the United States and those who consider employment in this setting might find it profitable to study the record for this country beginning with articles by Lillian D. Wald, who influenced

its development just as she influenced school nursing.[191-202] There is little evidence that organized medicine has been influenced by the experience of countries that have put occupational health under public control and made health insurance available to all citizens.[203] It seems to have been assumed by the majority of persons in the United States that occupational health services could and should be organized by employers and administered by physicians (themselves employees of the industry) for the benefit of other employees. While pressure from organized workers and unions has been accepted as a legitimate force in improving conditions of labor, including the health care of workers, organized medicine has not exerted pressure in this direction nor has organized nursing until recently promoted a national health insurance that would affect all residents including the employed.* It was reported in 1950 that "industrial nurses pass resolution against compulsory health insurance." †

In 1946, the ANA formed a Committee to Study the Implications of the Fair Labor Standards Act as These Relate to Industrial Nursing[204] and Janet Geister in 1950 reported to the ANA. In the same year Margaret C. Klem[205] reported on nursing opportunities in medical care insurance. The ANA was then concerned that such insurance cover nursing but it did not oppose the AMA's negative position on national health insurance.[206] While it is certain that all countries, including the United States, will ultimately implement WHO's position that health care is a "human right," some studies show that a small per cent of the industrial working force in the United States has adequate protection.

In a survey of 1293 plants in the late 1950s, a first-aid service was available in only 24 plants.[207] Most small industries contracted with individual physicians, a health department, a visiting nurse service, a health maintenance type organization, a clinic, or a hospital for service. Most occupational health services have been provided through some form of insurance with "management" and "labor" sharing the cost. Unions, or other workers' organizations, may, however, take over the responsibility of providing health care for their members. As some of the trades that in 1971 had well-developed health insurance plans through their unions, Anne R. Somers[207a] (in *Health Care in Transition; Directions for the Future*) men-

---

* Individuals and minority groups within medical and nursing organizations have supported comprehensive national health insurance.
† "Industrial Nurses Pass Resolution Against Compulsory Health Insurance" (news), *Arch. Ind. Med. Occup. Med.,* **2:**101, (July) 1950.

tions miners, longshoremen, steel, automobile, building, and clothing workers. Somers comments that since almost all developed countries have comprehensive national health programs the United States is unique in having its "model" health insurance program [the Kaiser-Permanente program] under industrial management. Bea W. Graves,[208] in 1917, described her "first aid work in the Seattle Construction and Dry Dock Company" where the service was managed and paid for by the employees.

Nurses in the occupational health setting in any country, but particularly in a country that has no central control, should study the organizational and administrative structure within which they must function since their usefulness and the satisfaction they take in their work is directly affected by the structure.

In the United States, the AAIN has worked closely with the AMA's Council on Industrial Health. Since there are few industries with full-time physicians, nurses must teach and give first aid, meet emergencies and treat minor ailments, and teach workers to do this when they are not present. Industrial nurses, like school nurses, operate under standing medical directives. World War II, with its health manpower shortages, stimulated the transfer of medical responsibilities to nurses.[209,210] Suggested sets of standing orders are revised periodically, but the "legal scope" of occupational nursing, its organization and administration, must, of necessity, change with time and place or the needs of the recipients and providers of care.[211,212]

While the health care system in the United States is often referred to as "a no-system," or as "laissez faire," federal, state, and municipal health departments have occupational health bureaus. One was organized in Cleveland, Ohio, as early as 1916.[213] In 1934, a physician reported a 7-year health demonstration when four small industries in Philadelphia employed nurses of the city's visiting nurse association.[214] Increasingly, public health nursing agencies, voluntary and official, provide part-time occupational health nursing services.[215-218] The organizational and administrative plans under which nurses function are shown within the contract. The USPHS published a guide in 1965 (revised in 1970) entitled *Community Health Nursing for Working People. A Guide for Voluntary and Official Health Agencies to Provide Part-Time Occupational Health Services.*[219]

Functions, Satisfactions, Rewards, and Difficulties in Occupational Health Nursing. In 1959, in International Labour Organization's Recommendation 112 defined occupational health as follows:

(a) protecting the workers against any health hazard which may arise out of their work or the conditions in which it is carried on;

(b) contributing towards the physical and mental adjustment, in particular by the adaptation of the work to the workers and the assignment to jobs for which they are suited;

(c) contributing to the establishment and maintenance of the highest degree of physical and mental well-being of the workers.*

The responsibility of nurses for planning, carrying out, and evaluating any program to promote occupational health depends on the wishes of those who employ them or those who administer the service; on the resources in the setting; on the nurses' concepts of their functions; and on the willingness of clients or workers to accept the nurses' help. As in all health services, what nurses do depends to a large extent on whether they are the only health workers in the setting or whether they are members of a team of health workers. In small industries, as in small schools, there may be only one nurse, and he or she may give only part-time service.

The Royal College of Nursing and the National Council of Nurses of the United Kingdom recommend the following seven grades of occupational health nurses within "the new health structure" for occupational health: Chief Nursing Officer, Principal Nursing Officer, Senior Nursing Officer, Nursing Officer, Assistant Nursing Officer (all State Registered Nurses), Senior Nurse, and Nurse (State Enrolled Nurses). They specify the responsibilities of each grade.[220]

In the United States, the ANA's Industrial Nurses Section in 1956 made very specific statements on *functions* and *standards* under the following five headings: Administration and Operation of the Health Service Department; Nursing Care—Health Maintenance; Safety Education; Health and Welfare Benefits; and Community Health and Welfare. *Qualifications* were listed under Professional, Personal Competence, Essential Knowledge and Skills.[221] The ANA's 1968 publication, *Functions and Qualifications for an Occupational Health Nurse in a One-Nurse Service,*[222] divided functions into Collaborative Functions and Nursing Care Functions. In the first section, there are 21 functions distributed under six subheadings on collaboration with management and one on collaboration with management and the physician. In the second section, under Nursing Care, there are 39

---

* Royal College of Nursing, and National Council of Nurses of the United Kingdom: *Occupational Health Nursing Structure*. The College and the Council, London, 1971, p. 7.

functions distributed under ten subheadings as follows: defining nursing responsibilities; administering nursing care; coordinating medical and nursing responsibilities in the health evaluation (examination) program; developing a framework for health education and counseling; helping employees "cope" with problems; developing and maintaining a manual; developing and maintaining a system of records and reports consistent with existing systems in the plan; establishing relationships with community agencies; cooperating with education institutions in providing experience for students and faculty; and evaluating the administrative and nursing practices.

Twelve qualifications of an occupational health nurse in a one-nurse service are listed under the following headings: Legal, Education, and Qualities and Proficiencies. It is specified that the nurse have a baccalaureate degree in nursing with "additional study" in business administration, industrial relations, and principles of insurance.

The following statement by Mary Louise Brown in 1969 helps explain why the educational qualification is not more specific for nursing in this setting: "Since there is no formal, prescribed occupational health nursing curriculum, their [occupational health nurses] training and education must be discussed in the context of nursing education in general." * She said that while baccalaureate education was "considered . . . the preparation of choice . . . less than one occupational nurse in a hundred" had a college degree. She described four "job-oriented" training courses then offered by the Bureau of Occupational Safety and Health in the Environmental Control Administration of the US Department of Health, Education, and Welfare. The development of these courses, the occupational health content of the baccalaureate nursing program at the University of Tennessee,[223] and the graduate programs at the University of North Carolina[224] show a greater differentiation between the functions of occupational health nurses and nurses in other settings.

Whether or not the functions of occupational health nurses as described in such publications as those cited are unique may be debatable. It is, however, unique that occupational health nurses serve primarily employed, well adults.

The services of occupational health nurses to victims of trauma is very much like that of nurses in other emergency services except that the compensation laws involved are more specific. Their work with families of the employed is like that of most community health nurses. The nurse's function in preventing accidents, in teaching and giving first aid and emergency treatment, has been and is still stressed, and some of the best texts on these subjects have been developed for industry. The occupational nurse's role in accident prevention is unique in its scope and emphasis. (See also Chapter 43.)

It is not possible to mention all the emphases in the occupational health nurse's function, but some are outstanding. Preemployment health examinations and periodic assessments are a major element in occupational health services since so much depends on whether the worker has what the job or position demands. Nurses have always worked with physicians in conducting examinations, but more and more often, nurses perform the examinations.[225-231] In 1971, Josephine Cippola and Gilbearth Collings,[232] a nurse and physician with the New York City Telephone Company, described a 24-session course in the physical examination presented to nurses there. Nurses so prepared function in this capacity.

Preemployment and periodic examinations identify all sorts of strengths and weaknesses, or handicaps, but those of sight and hearing have been considered especially important. Regulations to protect eyes have been stressed in safety programs.[233-236] Regulations to protect hearing have also been stressed, for it is generally recognized that the noise of certain industries is their chief danger. Industrialization is thought to account largely for the increasing incidence of deafness in developed countries.[237-240] Programs to identify and help drug abusers are not new, but there is a recent emphasis on them.[241-245] The industries that have made continued employment for addicts contingent on attendance at meetings of self-help organizations have enviable records for rehabilitation of alcoholics. Some industries finance for certain employees a stay of several weeks or months in centers operated by recovered addicts.

Rehabilitation is, of course, the objective in all health services, but it seems particularly important in industrial nursing where the welfare of a family may depend on the rehabilitation of its employed adult members. Industry is encouraged to employ the handicapped and many take pride in their reputation for this.[246-248]

Record keeping by occupational health nurses has always been one of their most essential functions. Accurate and complete records protect the employer, the employee, and the health worker. Compensation hinges on them and this makes knowledge by the nurse

* Brown, Mary Louise: "Occupational Health Nursing in the United States; Training and Education," *Occup. Health Nurs.* (*N.Y.*) **17**:11, (Nov.) 1969.

of protective legislation necessary. All texts on occupational health nursing stress the function of record keeping from the legal angle and as a basis for occupational health research. As preparation of nurses in this specialty improves, they will play a more active role in research.

Whole libraries could be filled with books and articles on industrialization and its effect on man—the machine doing the physical work for man but depriving him of the full use of his body and all the faculties that go into creation of a hand-made product. Most recent publications stress the effect of automation. While the effect of piece work deprived workers of the satisfaction in creating and putting their imprints on finished products, and the operation of machines was often boring and potentially hazardous, the effects of automation are almost more striking. "Before and after" photographs show a plant full of heavy machinery studded with workers operating it, and the same plant, with even heavier machinery, empty of workers except for one person at a control booth operating the machinery. Some of the meanings for health workers are obvious. Since workers aren't near the machinery, they are protected from potential boredom and accidents, but they may lose their employment or fear losing it. Operation of a control board substitutes mental for physical effort and still further removes the workers from the satisfaction of seeing the products they are making. Whatever the reason, the mental health of the worker is receiving more and more attention. Health counseling, but especially mental health counseling, is stressed as a major function of occupational health workers.[249-257]

The satisfactions in occupational health nursing are obvious when nurses have an opportunity to help make decisions about plant design, furnishings, and equipment, about food service, work programs, and personnel policies; when they participate in preemployment and periodic health examinations, health education and counseling, first aid, and treatment programs for workers and their families. The extent to which management or employers and medical directors of occupational health services see nurses as collaborators and the extent to which they are prepared to function as colleagues affects the nature of their work and the satisfaction they take in it. Most studies found on occupational health nursing indicate that while management recognized the value of nurses and often expressed the opinion that they should have a voice in policy-making and other high-level activities, they did not provide them with the outward "status" symbols, as,

for example, membership on key committees and salaries commensurate with decision-making responsibility. The annual average salary of nurses employed in industry in the United States in 1973 was $9308. This was lower than the average earnings of staff nurses in hospitals ($10,512) as reported by the ANA in *Facts About Nursing 74–75.*[*][258] (Comparable figures for Canada were not found.) It should be recognized, however, that occupational health nurses are not as well prepared as public health nurses. And it is also suggested in some studies that industrial nurses with no postbasic preparation, often carrying major responsibility for the care of their families, do not expect or want a decision-making role. However, as more and more industries contract with public health nursing agencies for nursing service on a part-time basis, the difference between industrial nursing and public health nursing will diminish.

Reports of studies should be consulted by those interested in detailed analyses of functions, roles, responsibilities, working conditions, satisfactions, and difficulties in occupational health nursing throughout this century.[259-268] One nurse, writing in 1970, calls it "a varied, interesting nursing career."[269] It is certainly a critical one in the total health program of any developed country since occupational health nurses serve the most productive element of society.

10. SCHOOLS OF NURSING AND OTHER EDUCATIONAL INSTITUTIONS (AS TEACHERS AND ADMINISTRATORS)

Employment of Nurses as Teachers and Administrators in Schools of Nursing and Other Educational Institutions. Of the total 778,470 employed registered nurses in the United States in 1972, the American Nurses' Association reported that 28,820 (including 361 men nurses) were in schools of nursing as administrators or assistants (2800), consultants (243), supervisors (640), instructors (22,859), head nurses (350), general duty or staff (1019), other specified types (214), and not reported (695).[1] Of the total 128,675 nurses registered in Canada and employed in nursing in 1974, the Canadian Nurses' Association reported that 3,678 were employed in educational institutions as "directors or assistants" (211) and instructors (3,467).[2]

---

* Some United States industries have plants in foreign countries and may employ United States personnel. In such cases they may offer comparatively higher salaries as an inducement to doctors, nurses, and others.

To anyone familiar with the history of nursing education, these are impressive figures. However, almost 4 per cent of the budgeted positions in professional schools of nursing of the United States were unfilled in 1974, so contemporary nurse educators here see these figures as inadequate.[3]

While teaching is inherent in all nursing practice and nurses may be employed for the sole purpose of teaching patients, such teaching is not the focus of this section, but rather the teaching of nursing by nurses.

Nursing education was discussed in Chapter 1 and the observation made that more has been written about, and more studies made on, nursing education than on any other subject related to the occupation. In Chapter 1, the focus is on the nature of nursing education; here it is on the nature of employment in educational programs, but it seems impossible to avoid repetition. Here, as in Chapter 1, readers are referred to the many surveys, reports, and, for those interested in the development of nursing education in the United States, to Mary M. Roberts' *American Nursing, History and Interpretation* (Macmillan, 1954), to M. Adelaide Nutting's *A Sound Economic Basis for Schools of Nursing* (Putnam, 1926), Annie W. Goodrich's *The Social and Ethical Significance of Nursing* (Macmillan, 1932), and Isabel M. Stewart's *The Education of Nurses* (Macmillan, 1922). The more that present-day nurse educators know about the history of nursing schools, the more understandable the contemporary scene.

Writing in 1943, Stewart divided the history of professional nursing education into its development (1870–1900), its expansion (1900–1930), and its analysis or study—a period beginning in 1930 and continuing beyond the publication of her record.

As pointed out in Chapter 1, during the period of development a few schools followed the Nightingale pattern, which was an independent school using St. Thomas' Hospital in London as a practice field. However, hospital administrators and boards soon saw the advantage of having students to nurse their patients, and even before the period of expansion many "schools" were established under hospital ownership and control. These hospital-controlled "schools" (which in the United States increased in number from 432 in 1900 to 1843 in 1930) rarely justified the name.[4] They were apprenticeship training programs dominated by service needs. Nurses who administered the programs and taught students were primarily responsible for patient care; doctors who taught student nurses were rarely paid to do so. Few schools operated under a budget separate from that of the hospital. The fact that teachers were heavily committed to service meant that they were often late for classes or cancelled them without prior notice. Charlotte A. Aiken's text *Hospital Training School Methods and the Head Nurse*[5] published in 1907 emphasized the close relationship of teaching and service.

Nutting entitled her collected papers *A Sound Economic Basis for Schools of Nursing* because she thought the lack of a sound basis was the chief deterrent to effective nursing education. But even in the early days a few schools employed nurses for the sole purpose of teaching. In 1905, Goodrich[6] reported on "the introduction of salaried instruction in the training schools" over a 20-year period. At one time, nursing leadership thought the employment of full-time faculty the most important step in improving nursing education. The separation of teaching and service was sufficiently established in 1919 to make members of state boards of nurse examiners realize, however, that it had its disadvantages as well as its advantages. Parmelia Murman Doty,[7] of the New York board, discussed "the need for cooperation between the head nurse and the instructor." As long as they were one and the same person, this was not a problem.

The extent to which, and the conditions under which, teachers and students should practice has been a question for all schools that prepare health and welfare workers; it has been a problem throughout the history of nursing education. Asking an overburdened nursing service staff to teach and expecting nursing students doing the work of staff nurses to learn the science underlying practice was recognized as unreasonable and was questioned by nurse leaders, doctors, educators, and others, and expecting patients to be willing subjects for students in the health field will always be debatable. As early as 1904, Anne Steward Russell,[8] a British nurse who wrote on "the shortcomings of the teaching and methods of present training schools from the standpoint of the graduate nurse in institutional work," suggested that the solution might lie in a 3-year nursing program *preceded* by college.* In most countries, the solution was sought in the employment of full-time teachers, in having students learn basic skills in a laboratory, and in freeing students from service demands.

Recently, there is a trend toward joint ap-

---

* In 1975, schools of nursing at the Universities of Tennessee (Nashville), St. Louis (Mo.), and Creighton (Omaha, Nebr.), are experimenting with a 1-year initial nursing program for college graduates, and there are several longer initial programs for college graduates.

pointments, with the faculty committed to service as well as teaching and, in some cases, to research. The joint appointment is reflected in the figures cited at the beginning of this section. Nurses employed in schools of nursing are also supervisors, head nurses, and staff nurses.

Having nursing service in the related hospital directed by the faculty is the pattern under which the Schools of Nursing at Yale University (New Haven, Conn.) and the University of Florida (at Gainesville), for example, were established and is now consistently exemplified by the School of Nursing at Case-Western Reserve University (Cleveland, Ohio). However, there is no denying the gulf that still lies between practitioners and educators in nursing, although, in the writer's opinion, it is slowly closing. Regional conferences cosponsored by all six councils of the National League for Nursing in 1975 were designed "to encourage a more effective dialogue between nurse service and nursing education." * M. M. Pierik's [9] article, "Joint Appointment: Collaboration for Better Patient Care" and Myrtle K. Aydelotte's [10] "Nursing Education and Practice: Putting It All Together" speak for what we presume to designate the *avant-garde* of this decade. As nursing education emphasizes prevention, faculty holding joint appointments will be found in home health, school, industrial, prison, and other community health services as well as in hospital services that are geared to critical remedial care.

The Nature and Location of Nursing Schools and Other Educational Programs. There are few occupations whose schools and educational programs offer such a wide range of programs. They differ from one nation to another and within each country. As noted in Chapter 1, the International Council of Nurses defines two grades of nurses based on the nature of their preparation—registered professional nurses and assistant nurses—called variously, according to the country, enrolled nurses, assistants, and practical nurses.

Mary Beard, Mary M. Roberts, and Isabel M. Stewart in 1932 compared systems of nursing education in many countries during a symposium on international aspects of nursing education.[11] Since that time, differences from one country to another have, we think, diminished, due largely to increased mobility of populations as well as the unifying influence of the International Council of Nurses, Florence Nightingale International Foundation, World Health Organization, and other international bodies that have regional counterparts and that have held meetings all other the world. However, a French educator, C. Mordacq, at a 1972 Symposium on Higher Education in Nursing convened by the Regional Office for Europe of the WHO, made the following observation on differences in nursing careers:

Anyone who has visited several European countries, met African nurses and been to the United States and Canada cannot fail to be astonished at the differences between nursing careers in the respective countries. For example, in one country, nurses perform subordinate tasks with only one or two levels of responsibility, whereas in a neighbouring country, they have ten different types of responsibility, at all the levels of the country's health services.*

Mordacq suggested three "measures" to combat the "problem" of "function." With relation to "training," she suggested that it should prepare nurses to make decisions:

This assumes that the organization of the professional training is open and based on the analysis of situations, communication, written or oral, through dialogue and group discussions, and on a methodology which makes it possible to acquire knowledge and solve problems.†

In welcoming the conference, W. B. Gerritsen, Director-General of Public Health of the Dutch Government, reminded participants of the "historical accident which in many countries of Europe had established nursing as a service to medicine rather than to patients." The conclusions reached by the conference included the following:

The education of nursing personnel should be provided for in the general education system of a country. Students of nursing should have the same rights and responsibilities as all other students.

In transferring from a traditional pattern of nursing education to one within the general system of education, care should be taken to ensure that the teaching of nursing and the direct administration of the educational programme are the responsibility of nurses.

University education for nurses should have the same financial support as other educational programmes within the system of general education.‡

In Great Britain and, to some extent in other countries, registered professional nurses were at one time prepared in basic or initial pro-

---

* National League for Nursing, Council of Baccalaureate and Higher Degree Programs: *Memo to Members*. The League, New York, January 1975, p. 5.

* Mordacq, C.: "Constraints and Opportunities in a Nursing Career," in *Higher Education in Nursing. Report on a Symposium.* Regional Office for Europe, World Health Organization, Copenhagen, 1973, p. 20.
† Mordacq, C.: *op. cit.,* p. 24.
‡ *Higher Education in Nursing. Report on a Symposium.* Regional Office for Europe, World Health Organization, Copenhagen, 1973, p. 14.

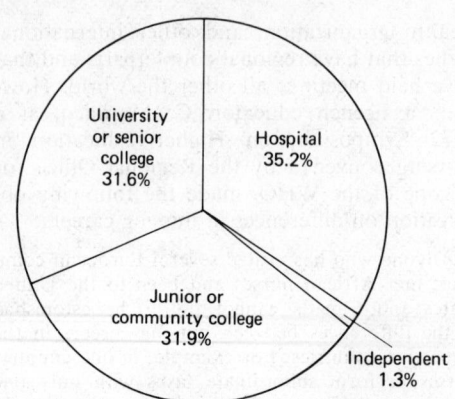

Figure 3-17. Schools of nursing offering initial professional programs, by type of control, Oct. 15, 1973. (Source: National League for Nursing. From: American Nurses' Association: *Facts About Nursing 74–75.* The Association, Kansas City, Mo., 1976, p. 82.)

grams to practice in specialized fields such as psychiatric nursing, child nursing, or even nursing patients with communicable disease. But even in England where separate registries were once maintained, all nurses now have a basic, generalized program that includes experience in medical, surgical, obstetric, child, and psychiatric services. Training programs for nurses who work with the mentally subnormal are the only exception. Recommendations of the Royal College of Nursing and the National Council of Nurses of the United Kingdom in 1967 imply current recognition of this difference, but advocate changes in the program, and imply that there may soon be a sweeping "reform" in all nurse preparation.[12,13]

Programs in the United States in which nurses may teach nursing include basic (initial) diploma and practical nurse programs offered by hospitals; basic associate degree programs offered by junior colleges; basic and postbasic baccalaureate, basic and postbasic master's, doctoral, and continuing education programs offered by colleges and universities; and in-service programs in hospitals and other health institutions and agencies.

The American Nurses' Association reported that of 1359 initial nursing programs in 1973 in the United States, 479 were controlled by hospitals, 429 by universities or senior colleges, 43ɔ by junior or community colleges, and 17 were independently owned and controlled.[13a] (See Figures 3-17 and 3-18.)

Degree-granting programs for graduate nurses in 1971 and 1972 included baccalaureate programs in 233 colleges and universities, master's programs in 86 colleges and universi-

ties, and doctoral programs in eight universities.[14] The establishment of continuing education programs in colleges and universities is a relatively recent development. They are increasing so rapidly that available figures are almost meaningless.

The Canadian Nurses' Association reported that in 1974 there were 130 initial programs— 108 diploma, 22 baccalaureate. Of the 108 diploma programs, 70 were within the general education system at the postsecondary level and 38 were under hospital control. For graduate nurses, there were 45 postbasic programs in 19 universities. Of these, eight were "diploma-certificate," 21 were baccalaureate, and 16 were master's degree programs.[15] Collegiate nursing education in Canada is also increasing rapidly. In fact, in 1975, nursing education was virtually under the control of senior and community colleges throughout Canada. In 1974, McGill University opened a 3-year basic (initial) program for college graduates.* Col-

---

* Schools of nursing reported for Canada in 1972 do not include junior college programs as such. The Ministry of Colleges and Universities in Ontario published in 1973 *Questions and Answers Relating to the Transfer of Nursing Education from Hospitals to Community Colleges* (The Ministry, [Toronto], 1973).

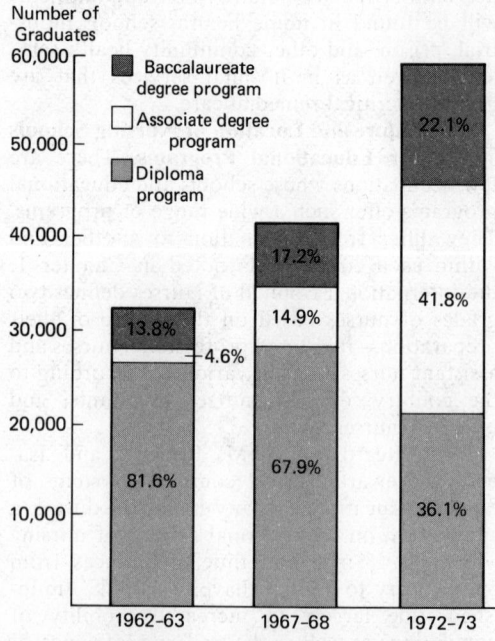

Figure 3-18. Students graduated from initial programs of nursing education—R.N. Academic years 1962–63, 1967–68, 1972–73. (Source: National League for Nursing; and American Nurses' Association: *Facts About Nursing 74–75.* The Association, Kansas City, Mo., 1976, p. 67.)

legiate nursing schools are more common in the United States and Canada than elsewhere but most countries, even the developing countries, have some collegiate programs.[16,17] In fact, it may be easier to establish collegiate nursing schools in countries where hospital nursing schools aren't entrenched institutions. The Royal College of Nursing and the National Council of Nurses of the United Kingdom, in a 1964 report titled *A Reform of Nursing Education,* said:

There is a widely held opinion that . . . nursing, . . . is a suitable subject for study at university level. The close collaboration reflected in courses already associated with universities is encouraging; it is hoped that the establishment of a degree course in nursing will not be long deferred.*

Under "The means of reform," they say "University degrees in nursing should be established." Appendices of this publication describe programs at the University of Manchester and the University of Edinburgh. The report on the *Function, Scope and Training of Nurses in England and Wales for the Mentally Subnormal* [18] mentions "a proposed experimental course" between Greaves Hall Hospital, Southport, and Harris College, Preston, to train teacher-nurses for the mentally subnormal. Reference was made in Chapter 1 (p. 79) to a 1976 report on 14 degree courses in England, Scotland, and Wales. The following observation is taken from a report of a 1972 World Health Organization conference:

The participants were in full agreement that the nurse, as already defined, should be educated in universities or in equivalent institutions of higher education. The rich resources of the university are of unique value in preparing the student nurse for the level and scope of nursing demanded in modern health care and for a future career that requires flexibility and the capacity to adapt to change and to the unknown. It is within the university/higher education environment that the habit of independent life-long learning, analytical thinking and systematic investigation basic to the nursing process can be fostered. Human relations and communication skills, often acquired with considerable difficulty in the hospital-based education model, are more easily developed in the university where all disciplines meet and think together. In addition, the universities provide a wealth of reference, research and other materials so often lacking in the hospital based school.†

* Royal College of Nursing, and National Council of Nurses of the United Kingdom: *A Reform of Nursing Education.* The College and the Council, London, 1964, p. 26.

† *Higher Education in Nursing. Report on a Symposium: op. cit.,* p. 8.

History of collegiate nursing education often begins with the address of Richard Olding Beard in 1909 to the American Society of Superintendents of Training Schools for Nurses.[19] As pointed out in Chapter 1, the basic program established in this year at the University of Minnesota is, in this connection, cited as the first collegiate program even though it did not grant a degree until 1919. Roberts [20] says that the John Sealy Hospital School of Nursing, but under the auspices of the Medical Department of the University of Texas in 1896, may well be the first university-affiliated school of nursing. The 1-year course in hospital economics offered at Teachers College, Columbia University, New York City, initiated in 1899, is almost certainly the first postbasic university program for nurses.

Those with a special interest in the development of collegiate schools will find Charles H. Russell's study a guide to what was written up until 1957.[21] He showed the early dreams; the interruption of progress by World War I; the influence of the 1923 *Report of the Committee for the Study of Nursing Education in the United States,* which resulted in the establishment of basic collegiate programs at Yale University, Western Reserve University, and Vanderbilt University; the influence of the National League of Nursing Education founded in 1893, and the Association of College Schools of Nursing founded in 1932; the effect of the Grading Committee's reports and those of the National Commission for the Improvement of Nursing Services and the National Nursing Council following World War II.[22-25] The current National Commission for the Study of Nursing and Nursing Education, in *An Abstract for Action* [26] and related reports, has reinforced the findings of all previous studies that advocated the placement of professional nursing education within colleges and universities.

As basic (initial) nursing programs moved into 4-year colleges and universities, the difficulty for hospitals of meeting a higher standard of nursing education was apparent. Harriet M. Gillett,[27] for example, in 1922 asked what the future was for schools of nursing without university affiliation. Central schools and hourly instructors that could supply a group of schools with needed courses were thought to be one answer.[28] Community or junior colleges were a resource for prenursing programs and centralized teaching. In 1932, Robert L. Harris [29] reported on "three years of new type college training" in a California junior college with nursing as one of the "semiprofessional" curricula. Other reports during the 1930s and 1940s showed some use by nursing of junior colleges.[30-34] Mildred L. Montag's [35] *The Education of Nursing Technicians* in 1951 advocated the full utilization of junior colleges to prepare graduates who would qualify as registered nurses. It was assumed that these graduates would not be interested in positions demanding more than an associate degree. Experimental junior college programs followed rapidly. A study by Montag and Lassar G. Gotkin [36] of the 2-year associate degree graduates comparing them with 3-year diploma graduates lent support to substituting junior college programs for hospital diploma programs. By 1974, they exceeded in numbers the hospital diploma programs. The title of "nurse technician" has not, however, had wide acceptance, and the prevailing "ladder concept" means that junior college programs must be coordinated with senior college programs. The NLN's Department of Diploma and Associate Degree Programs, constituted in 1955, attested to the wide and early acceptance of these schools in the United States. With the reorganization of the League into the Division of Individual Members and the Division of Agency Members, six separate councils were formed within the second division; one of these is the Council on Associate Degree Programs, with a separate Council for Diploma Programs.

Open curricula and career mobility are, however, recognized by the League as desirable. Publications on these subjects are numerous and some are distributed by the League.[36a-38] D. K. Story's monograph *Career Mobility; Implementing the Ladder Concept in Associate Degree and Practical Nurse Curricula* [39] shows how completely rejected in some quarters is the idea of terminal curricula. The continuing education movement is further evidence of the rejection of terminal curricula. While mandatory continuing education for relicensure for certification and for membership in professional organizations is variously regarded in the United States, nurses around the world are recognizing its importance [40-47] or the necessity of study as long as they practice nursing.

As junior college programs and initial baccalaureate nursing programs increased in the United States, hospital diploma programs had, by 1973, been "phased out" in 12 states or areas (Alaska, Arizona, Arkansas, Hawaii, Idaho, Nevada, New Mexico, Utah, Vermont, Wyoming, Guam, and the Virgin Islands). There were then 14 states with one to three schools that will soon have only initial associate, baccalaureate, or master's programs. However, the total diploma programs in 1973 exceed the junior college programs and the degree programs.[48] (See Fig. 3-18.) The influence of the hospital diploma programs on collegiate programs may last many years in all the countries they have dominated. As has been noted elsewhere, the hospital-based practical nurse program embodies many of the features of the hospital diploma program. Nursing schools, by and large, prepare their graduates to nurse inside rather than outside hospitals. While many health professionals claim to be equally concerned with preventive and remedial care, the fact that students have most of their experience in hospitals means that teachers are chosen for their remedial nursing competence, and the curricula they set up reflect this.

Facilities of nursing schools, by and large, leave much to be desired. In the early days of professional nursing education, it was sometimes hard to differentiate the "school's" facilities. Although there was usually a nurses' residence, students and faculty might be housed in a part of the hospital. There might have been classrooms in the residence or hospital but students might also have met for instruction in dining rooms, treatment rooms, or patients' sitting rooms. Classrooms on clinical services were rare and are still inadequate; libraries were often nonexistent and are even now below the standard for most professional schools.* Science laboratories were found in only the best nursing schools in the early decades. Unless the nursing school uses the facilities of an associated medical school, science laboratories and libraries are usually inadequate.[49]

With the introduction of preliminary periods of instruction, most nursing schools developed adequate, often excellent, "nursing arts" laboratories in which students could learn a wide range of nursing skills using dolls or each other as subjects. The injustice to patients and students of allowing the latter to have their initial practice in the clinical situation was recognized. As schools enlarged and full-time faculty found themselves more at home with students in classrooms than with patients, elaborate educational units were built, most of the instruction was moved out of the hospital, and students were forced to adapt methods learned in classrooms to the clinical situation.

Currently, the facilities of the nursing schools more nearly parallel those of other health professions, and, as noted in Chapter 1, with the movement toward joint curricula, students in the health sciences share all resources. Students in collegiate nursing schools

---

* The library of the Boston College School of Nursing is, as far as the writer knows, as good as if not better than any other nursing library. It contains approximately 30,000 volumes. The better medical school libraries may contain more than 300,000 volumes.

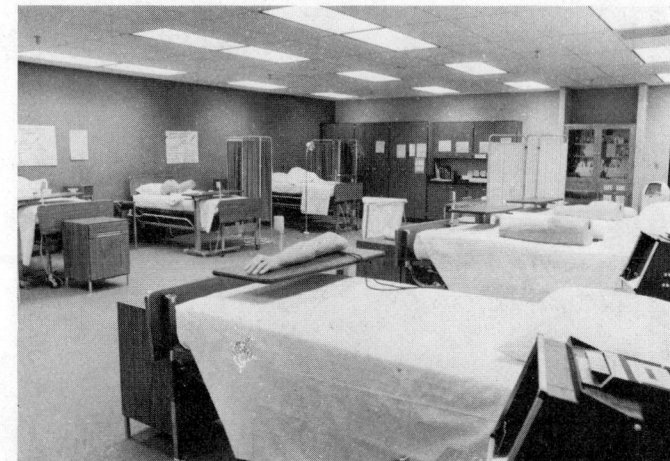

Figure 3-19. *A*. Self-instruction laboratory for practice of special procedures with anatomical models and video instruction facilities available. *B*. Main self-instruction laboratory with anatomical models and video instruction facilities available. (Hoose, David C.: "A Model for a Nursing Media Center," *Nurs. Outlook,* **24:**104, [Feb.] 1976.)

A

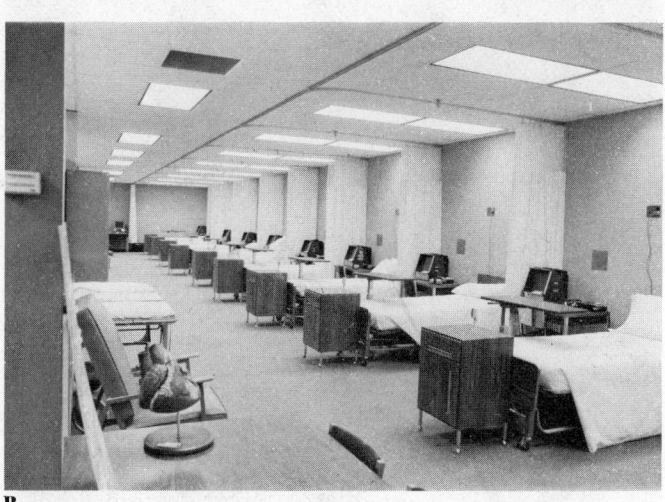

B

live in dormitories with students of other disciplines. They use the health science library with other students in the field of health and very often use the same science laboratories and classrooms on clinical services. Nursing schools in the United States that require or favor joint faculty and service appointments are most apt to have teaching space within clinical services.* In such schools, students see their teachers practice, and get direct help

* Study of Susan Crawford's report "Health Science Libraries in the United States: A Five-Year Perspective" (*Bull. Med. Lib. Assoc.,* **63:**7, [Jan.] 1975) shows the trend toward interdisciplinary use of library facilities. A nurse and physician of the Kaiser-Permanente Medical Care Program describe "A health education library for patients initiated in 1969 in Oakland, California, that has steadily grown in contents, service, and usage and that holds promise for the future (Collen, F. Bobbie, and Krikor, Soghkian: "A Health Library for Patients," *Health Services Reports,* **89:**236, [May–June] 1974).

from them on patient units which function as learning laboratories where patients are protected by the presence of expert practitioners. The so-called nursing arts laboratory is used less in teaching by instructors and more by students who want a place where they can practice at their own pace (see Fig. 3-19*A, B*).

Many nursing schools have exceptionally good audiovisual facilities, equipment, and supplies. Professional nurses, pressured by society throughout most of their existence to increase their numbers, have recognized the economy of teaching large groups with audiovisual aids. Some nursing schools have audiovisual departments that house, repair, distribute, and make films. Such departments house and operate the machinery or "hardware" and provide cubicles and rooms where faculty and students can use such learning materials.[50] (See Fig. 3-20 *A, B*.)

With the current emphasis on preventive and comprehensive health care, many educa-

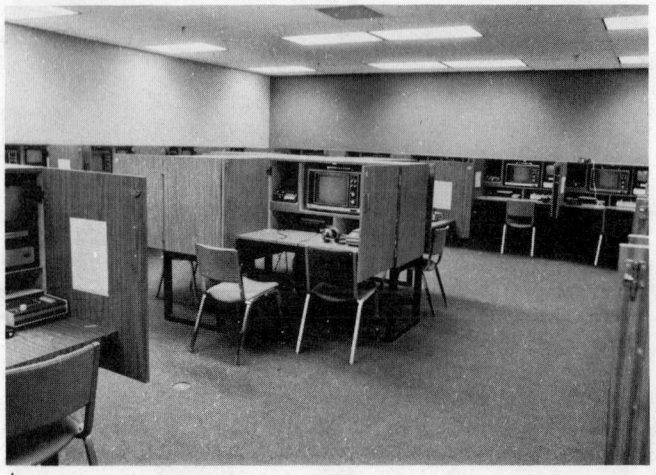

A

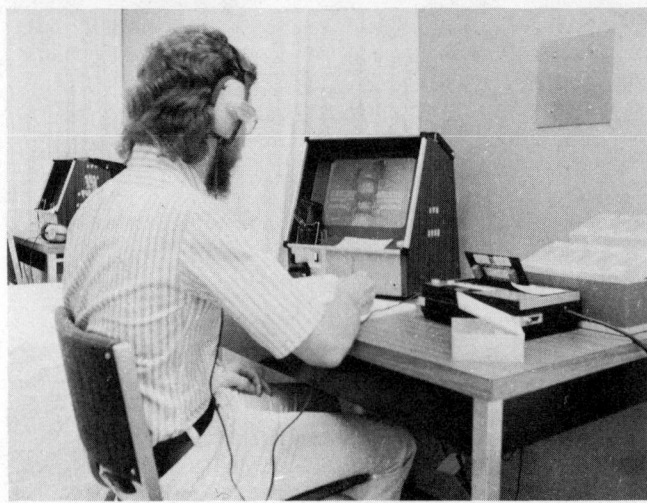

B

Figure 3-20. *A*. Carrels in self-instruction laboratory where students can use "responsive TV," or get answers to questions from programmed units, at School of Nursing, University of Wisconsin. *B*. Student using filmstrip and cassette player in self-study unit of learning media center's library at School of Nursing, University of Wisconsin. (Hoose, David C.: "A Model for a Nursing Media Center," *Nurs. Outlook,* **24**:104, [Feb.] 1976.)

tors doubt whether nurses, doctors, and other health workers can be adequately prepared to practice as long as their learning experience is almost entirely within hospitals. Nursing schools have for decades offered students experience in visiting nurse agencies, which has afforded them the opportunity to care for people in their homes. A few medical schools are offering some home care experience. As indicated in other parts of this chapter and in Chapter 1, nursing students may also have experience in nursing homes, in schools, in industry, in health maintenance organizations, and in other settings. Health services for the mentally retarded and for those in jails and other correctional institutions might improve more rapidly if students in the health professions had some experience in them. This recommendation recurs again and again in the studies of prison health services.[51]

Standardization and Certification of Nursing Schools. During the developing stage of nursing education, "training" schools answered every description. There was no uniformity. Before World War I, more than one third of the schools were in hospitals of less than 50 beds.[52] Students were accepted almost any time they applied. There might be one student known as the senior student in a school. Each hospital might establish its own prerequisites —race, sex, age, health, educational, and marital status. Few schools accepted men, minority races, married women, or those with physical handicaps. While a high moral character and a "good education" were generally thought desirable, several letters of recommendation might suffice in the first case and one or two years of high school or its equivalent might be adequate in the second.

On admission, students were often assigned

immediately to a clinical service where the head nurse was either interested in teaching or believed to be "a good influence." Often students had to be assigned to a clinical unit where it was known that they got little help. While the better programs had a sequence of experiences for students, their rotations through the various services were often haphazard. If a "curriculum" existed, it might take the form of a list of lectures or demonstrations or both. Until the passage of state nurse practice acts giving the basis for licensure and school accreditation (between 1903 and 1919 in the United States), there was no way of enforcing standards advocated by nurse leaders who, from the earliest days of professional nursing, saw the importance of establishing standards.

Before 1900, nurses in Great Britain, the United States, and other developed countries saw the necessity of regulating organizations and agencies. Elizabeth C. Burgess, in giving the history of registration, noted the resolution relating to it in the ICN Congress of 1901.[53] In 1907, a collecton of Isabel Hampton Robb's addresses was published under the title *Educational Standards for Nurses with Addresses on Nursing Subjects,*[54] and in 1909, she addressed the ICN Congress on this topic.[55] An educational committee of the Council was established in 1912 which, in 1934, under the direction of Isabel M. Stewart, produced an international guide, *The Educational Programme of the School of Nursing.*[56,57]

Publications of the Council such as *The Basic Education of the Professional Nurse,*[58] *Principles of Legislation for Nursing Education and Practice,*[59] and *Statement on Nursing Education, Nursing Practice and Service and the Social and Economic Welfare of Nurses.*[60] have helped establish international standards. The courses conducted under the sponsorship of the Florence Nightingale International Foundation, affiliated with the ICN, should be mentioned in this connection.[61] Meetings and publications of the World Health Organization since 1950 have also promoted international standards of nursing education, only a few of which can be cited.[62-70]

In the United States and for Canada in the early years, the creation of the American Society of Superintendents of Training Schools for Nurses (1893) provided a standard-setting agency. When it became the National League of Nursing Education in 1912, Canadian membership ceased.

M. Adelaide Nutting, and later Isabel M. Stewart, as chairmen of the League's Education Committee, were in the forefront of the standard-setting movement. The League's headquarters was at Teachers College, Columbia University, New York City, until 1920 when a National Headquarters was established for it, the ANA (before 1911 the Nurses' Associated Alumnae of the United States), and the NOPHN. Even before this move, the NLNE was considered the educational arm of the ANA. Its Education Committee published the *Standard Curriculum for Schools of Nursing* in 1917. A revision was published in 1929 under the title *A Curriculum for Schools of Nursing* and the last revision in 1937 was *A Curriculum Guide for Schools of Nursing.*[71]

Parenthetically, the first World War interrupted the progress of nursing education under the leadership of the League, but it provided an opportunity to raise standards. The Army School of Nursing, conceived by Annie W. Goodrich, was established with the blessing of a nursing committee that was the precursor of the National Nursing Council for War Service. It had branches at military centers throughout the United States and had 10,000 applicants; it graduated, in 1921, 512 students from two units who, within an initial nursing program, had had not only medical and surgical, pediatric and maternal nursing experience, but also psychiatric and public health experience.[72-75] Many graduates had one or more years of college before entering the school and some had a prenursing course at the Vassar Training Camp. Since students of this school had affiliations in civil hospitals throughout the country, their curriculum affected many programs.

The NLNE was involved in the nationwide survey of education in 1923 and 1929–32, previously mentioned, that so greatly affected standards of education and service. In 1933, the League published *The Nursing School Faculty—Duties, Qualifications and Preparation,* revised in 1946[77]; in 1936, it published *Essentials of a Good School of Nursing,*[78] revised in 1942. Both set national standards. The last curriculum revision, published in 1937, represented the work of nurse specialists in every geographical area. For the first time, experience in psychiatric nursing was recommended nationally as an aspect of all basic preparation.

The extent to which an initial program could prepare graduates for first-level staff nursing in public health agencies has been debated throughout the life of this branch of nursing. The Yale University School of Nursing curriculum was designed to test the hypothesis that a university school of nursing could do this. Dean Goodrich's description of the program emphasizes this feature.[79,80] While the League was the dominant factor in setting national standards for nursing education, the NOPHN was equally if not more concerned about the preparation of public health nurses. In conjunction with the USPHS, it studied the content of basic, postbasic, and graduate programs in public health nursing. Their joint committee reports and related studies established national standards for the preparation of public health nurses.[81-83] Public health nurses were added to basic nursing faculties and there were conferences and reports on integration of preventive health concepts and practices throughout the curriculum.[84]

A Department of Studies was established in the League in 1932, with Blanche Pfefferkorn as director. It collected annual data on schools that provided a factual basis for standard setting. The Curriculum Committee of the NLNE also continued its data-gathering and standard-setting function even after the second World War, but there was no longer any thought of having a single curriculum guide.[85,86]

During World War II, there was again the pressing need for increased health manpower. Instead of an Army School of Nursing, the US Cadet Nurse Corps program, approved by the National Nursing Council for War Service (on which were represented all major national nursing organizations), provided federal funds to students and approved schools of nursing. Lucile Petry, Director, Division of Nurse Education, USPHS, reported periodically on the accelerated program designed to produce 65,000 new students in about 2 years.[87] It affected basic collegiate and hospital schools but, since Cadet funds were available only to schools meeting certain minimum standards, all schools tried to qualify and were affected.

The National League of Nursing Education established a special committee on educational problems in wartime. The League published a series of bulletins on accelerating but safeguarding the preparation of nurses. Some were addressed to collegiate, others to hospital, schools.[88,89]

Throughout the life of professional nursing, a lack of prepared faculties has been a major problem. Commenting on the "fervent" search for professional status since the late 1800s, the Nursing Curriculum Project staff of the Southern Regional Education Board made the following observation: "The most serious gap in matching expectation to reality is a vast shortage of nursing expertise. The lack of nurses educationally prepared for college teaching, clinical specialization, administration, and research is appalling." *

* Southern Regional Education Board, Nursing Curriculum Project: *Nursing Education in the South 1973—Pathways to Practice, Vol. 1.* The Board, Atlanta, Ga., 1973, p. 4.

The first courses for graduate nurses in hospitals offered those who took them little more than staff nursing in their chosen fields. However, the program started at Teachers College, Columbia University, for administrators was soon followed by programs for teachers and supervisors in other universities in the United States and abroad,[90-96] and finally by programs to prepare clinical specialists.

The ICN, the League of Red Cross Societies, and, after its founding in 1934, the Florence Nightingale International Foundation (which took over the educational program of the LORCS) promoted postbasic education. The Foundation maintains an international directory of such programs which are now taking their place as established courses of study in colleges and universities.[97-101] During the 1940s, the NLNE had a committee to study and promote advanced clinical programs in universities. Increasingly, since that time, graduate programs focus on a clinical field rather than on a function such as administration, supervision, or teaching.[102-105] In the United States, since 1950, three regional boards of higher education have supported the development of graduate nursing programs, especially advanced clinical programs, and those programs preparing nurses for research.[106-111]

Of the 4324 nurses enrolled in graduate programs in the United States in 1972, 1439 were preparing to teach. Of the 2340 focusing on advanced clinical practice, many will undoubtedly teach full-time or part-time.[111a]

While the NLNE, the NOPHN, and to some extent the USPHS established national standards of nursing education during the first half of this century, the standards set up by state boards of nurse examiners were even more important since they had the force of law. Only graduates from schools approved by state boards could take state licensing examinations. During the first half of this century, as states passed nurse registration acts and established state licensing boards, the latter set up minimum standards and licensing examinations. Four states enacted laws in 1903, the majority within the first decade, but Alaska's first Nursing Practice Act was in 1941 and the Virgin Islands' in 1945.[112] Requirements in some states were higher than in others, those in New York State, for example, being especially high. Reports from its board during the incumbency of Annie W. Goodrich were especially analytic, detailed, and explicit in showing the board's efforts to promote higher standards.[113,114]

In 1914, the ANA set up a National Bureau of Legislation and Information which emphasized licensing laws; in 1934, it established a Bureau of State Boards of Nurse Examiners, later a Committee of State Boards of Nursing which is, currently in 1976, a Council of State Boards of Nursing. These bodies have had a unifying and standardizing effect, although Bernice E. Anderson's studies of interstate movement of registered nurses in 1950 showed how much divergence remained then.[115]

In the early days, many state boards were dominated by physician members; they have tended to be conservative bodies that have discouraged rather than encouraged experimental programs. More recently, these boards have had all nurse members and in many states they have encouraged experimentation. In Chapter 1, the subject of licensure was discussed and the threat to organized nursing (as seen by it) of proposed institutional licensure and proposed boards to license a variety of health workers, including nurses.[116-125]

While two world wars undoubtedly interrupted the development of nursing education, they have encouraged cooperative efforts to mobilize the health resources of the affected countries. National Nursing Councils for War Service in the United States certainly had this effect. The Council of World War II was the parent of several bodies sponsoring national studies of nursing organizations, nursing service, and nursing education.[126-130]

The so-called Structure Study resulted in the elimination of certain national nursing organizations and the realignment of functions in the remaining six. The National League of Nursing Education, the Association of Collegiate Schools of Nursing, and the National Organization for Public Health Nursing were among the organizations that disbanded. The National League for Nursing, formed in 1952, absorbed the resources and programs of the following organizations and committees: National League of Nursing Education, National Organization for Public Health Nursing, Association of Collegiate Schools of Nursing, Joint Committee on Practical Nurses and Auxiliary Workers in Nursing Services, Joint Committee on Careers in Nursing, National Committee for the Improvement of Nursing Services, and National Nursing Accrediting Service.[131] Realignment of functions within and between the ANA and the League has continued and both, in 1975, functioned as standard-setting agencies.

The NLN was established in 1952 with a Division of Nursing Service and a Division of Nursing Education. Within the latter were Departments of Diploma and Associate Degree Programs and Baccalaureate and Higher Degree Programs. The Division of Nursing Education of the NLN sponsored activities related to all nursing education as, for example, the

study of objectives of educational programs or how to improve the long-term illness content of the nursing curricula and the study of nurse faculty members in basic schools. It sponsored a series of regional conferences on curricula. The departments in the Division of Nursing Education took over activities related to the types of schools each represented. These activities and the Division's publications have been a unifying and standardizing force.[132-140]

In 1967, the NLN was reorganized. In 1975, there was a Division of Individual Members (who join through constituent state leagues) and a Division of Agency Members with an Interdivisional Coordinating Committee. The Division of Agency Members has six councils as follows: Home Health Agencies and Community Health Services; Hospital and Related Institutional Nursing Services; Baccalaureate and Higher Degree Programs; Diploma Programs; Associate Degree Programs; and Practical Nursing Programs.*

As nursing programs moved into colleges and universities, standards and evaluative processes of higher education have been adopted by nursing in the United States. Six national nursing organizations that were conducting accrediting activities formed a joint committee on accreditation. In 1949, the Committee published a *Manual of Accrediting Educational Programs in Nursing,*[141] and released a list of approved programs by states. The National Nursing Accrediting Service supplanted other accrediting programs which, in the case of the NLNE, preceded it by more than a decade.[142-150] The NLN, formed in 1952, took over the accrediting function of the NNAS. The following statement showed the League's importance as a national standard-setting agency:

Through its Division of Measurement, NLN offers achievement tests to schools of nursing, and examinations for use in the admission, guidance, and placement of students in registered nurse and practical nurse programs. In cooperation with the ANA Council of State Boards of Nursing and its Committees, it also prepares licensing examinations for use by state boards of nursing. The National League for Nursing is recognized as the accrediting agency for masters, baccalaureate and associate degree nursing programs by the National Commission on Accrediting and is approved for accreditation of masters, baccalaureate, associate degree, diploma and practical nursing programs by the U.S. Office of Education. Accreditation of community nursing services is a jointly spon-

---

* American Nurses' Association: *Facts About Nursing 74–75.* The Association, Kansas City, Mo., 1976, p. 225.

sored program of the American Public Health Association and the National League for Nursing.*

While accreditation by the League is not compulsory, certain funds and other benefits accrue only to accredited programs, and few faculties are indifferent to the advantages of national accreditation.†

"Standard" curricula are no longer stressed. There are, however, guides for faculties in every type of nursing program. Experimentation rather than standardization is characteristic of this era. Open curricula, joint curricula, and the ladder concept in the preparation of health workers with continuing education lead to diverse programs.[151-158]

The American Nurses' Association, reorganized following the Structure Study of 1952, had an Educational Administrators, Consultants, and Teachers Section. Its 1956 statement on functions, standards, and qualifications for practice was an official call for degree-holding faculties, and in 1959 it published a *Guide for the Development of Standards of Employment for Teachers in Nursing*.[159,160] The ANA also worked through special committees and councils to set up guidelines for state examining boards.[161]

Like the League, the ANA has again been reorganized. Four commissions now develop and implement the policies established by the board of directors. One of the stated purposes of the ANA is to promote the professional and educational advancement of nurses. The Commission on Nursing Education has the following program:

. . . develops standards for nursing education. The Commission evaluates scientific and educational developments as well as changes in health needs and practices to determine implications for nursing education. The encouragement and stimulation of research in all areas of nursing education and the formulation of policy recommendations concerning federal and state legislation in the field of education are also responsibilities of the Commission. The Council on Continuing Education, under the aegis of the Commission, develops standards of continuing education and works toward their implementation; formulates and recommends policies and programs to fulfill the Association's responsibility in relation to continuing education; and provides a means of communication among nurses with primary interest and responsibility in continuing education in nursing.‡

* American Nurses' Association: *ibid.*, p. 259.

† Of 1377 initial programs in 1972, 855 were reported by the National League for Nursing as accredited. Nursing schools in colleges and universities must also meet standards established for such institutions of higher education.

‡ American Nurses' Association: *ibid.*, p. 252.

The Commission's (then a Committee) "position paper" on nursing education put the official nursing organizations behind a collegiate preparation for all professional nurses, and state associations were quick to adopt comparable positions.[161a]

In spite of a consensus on standards, this category of nurses (nurses employed in schools of nursing), conceded to be the best academically prepared of any, have not reached the goal stated in the ANA position paper. Of the total 16,794 nurse faculty members reported for 1972, almost half, 7672, held diplomas only. Of the 1260 nurse administrators in diploma programs, 545 held diplomas only.[162] The lack of faculties that could meet the standards of higher education has been the most serious deterrent in developing and expanding collegiate programs and in the general improvement of nursing education.

Organization and Administration of Schools of Nursing. Since there is such a diversity of educational programs in nursing in the United States and other countries, it is hard to discuss their organization and administration briefly. Volumes have been written on the subject. They include analyses of then existing programs and the application to nursing of principles of educational administration; many books and articles focus on cost and who should own and operate the school—who should pay for nursing education.[163-178] In this chapter and in Chapter 1, data was presented to support the conclusion reached by international and national bodies that nursing education should be within the educational framework of the country; in the United States, "professional nursing" should be within the system of higher education. In 1972, hospitals were still very much in the business of educating health workers. They owned and controlled 524 of the 1363 programs to prepare registered "professional" nurses and almost half of the 1310 programs to prepare licensed practical or "vocational" nurses.[179] In schools of nursing owned and operated by hospitals, the policies are made by the hospital's governing board and carried out by the school's director who is, almost without exception, a nurse, but the non-nurse hospital administrator may exercise certain control over the school. The hospital board often establishes a subcommittee on the school of nursing or an accessory advisory committee. Some hospital schools, and in fact some university schools, have been under, or a department of, a medical board. University schools of nursing usually have their own deans and are as independent units within the university, as are the other professional schools such as those for law, education, or medicine.

Nurses considering appointments in nursing schools will find it helpful to know the history of the school; how it is organized and administered; its purpose; its role in the community; its relationships with other institutions and agencies; the composition of the policy-making body; the decision-making role of the faculty; the source of funds and the size of the budget. Organization charts clarify some of these points. Many institutions avoid making them, some claiming that they tend to ossify relationships that should be dynamic.

In countries with a national health service, personnel to staff it may be prepared with public funds. This is true in the Union of Soviet Socialist Republics and the People's Republic of China and has been true for physicians in some parts of the British Commonwealth.* In the report of a special committee of the Royal College of Nursing and the National Council of Nurses of the United Kingdom on the reform of nursing education, it is recommended that a school of nursing should be governed by a School Council (of not more than 15 members) appointed by the Regional Council after consultation with appropriate bodies. The School Council should submit a budget and receive money from the Regional Council to cover running costs. The report recommends relieving students of service demands and providing educational grants for the first and second years from public funds.[180]

While the education of health workers in the United States is not generally thought to be the public's responsibility, the federal and state governments are assuming an ever larger share. Jerome P. Lysaught[181] noted that about $250,000 in federal funds for nursing education was appropriated in 1950, while $80,000,000 in federal funds was spent on basic professional ("R.N.") programs in 1970. He thought this amount should be increased to from $110,000,000 to $125,000,000. Noting that states contributed $140,000,000 directly or indirectly to medical education in 1967, Lysaught thought it reasonable to conclude that they should contribute at least half of this amount to nursing education.†

In earlier decades, student nurses generally paid for their training by service to the hospital. As hospital schools improved, student fees and federal or state stipends have helped reduce the cost of operating hospital programs. It is generally accepted that the use of patient fees for the operation of educational programs in hospitals is unsound since it taxes the sick, rather than the total population. Each generation must strive to establish what Nutting called a "sound economic basis for nursing education." But the economic aspect is only one part of nursing administration. Most authorities believe there is a science and art of administration. It is highly desirable that directors of nursing programs be qualified administrators.

Functions, Satisfactions, Rewards, and Difficulties in Administering and Teaching in Schools of Nursing and Other Educational Institutions. Administration of nursing schools and educational programs was, in the early decades, highly authoritative; today, administrators are called "facilitators," to suggest a democratic approach. They are, in effect, chair-

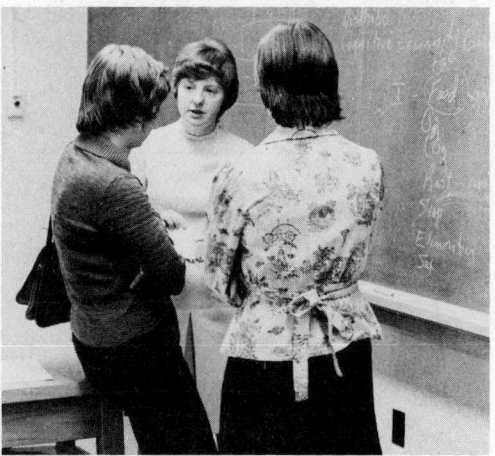

Figure 3-21. Assistant professor, Faculty of Nursing, University of Western Ontario, discusses course assignment with two students in the B.Sc.N. program. (Photograph by Dougal Bichan in Handbury, Eric: *Nurse.* McClelland & Stewart, Ltd., Toronto, Ont., 1975. Sponsored by the Registered Nurses Association of Ontario for the celebration of its 50th Anniversary.)

---

* A prominent medical dean in the United States made the following statement in 1974: "The country may eventually realize that the education of health personnel, like the provision of medical care for all segments of the population, is a national responsibility." (Lippard, Vernon: *A Half-Century of American Medical Education 1920–1970.* Josiah Macy, Jr. Foundation, New York, 1974, p. 130.) This suggests that health personnel are in a class by themselves. Some would argue that a good society is dependent on an adequate preparation of all essential workers.

† The US Public Health Service has provided stipends for students in basic (or initial), postbasic, and

graduate programs. It has made grants to supply or improve facilities and to finance educational research. Many nursing leaders of this era have been and are associated with the Service. Faye Abdellah, Margaret Arnstein, Ava Dilworth, Pearl McIver, Lucile Petry, Jessie Scott, Ellwynne Vreeland, and many others have directly and indirectly affected the structure, the conduct, and the resources of educational programs.

men of faculties, the other members of which share with the administrator the responsibility for decisions reached. However, it remains questionable whether administrators without vision—those who act merely as spokesmen for their faculties—perform their function adequately.

The dean or director of a nursing school or educational program should be competent as a nurse and as an administrator. Few professional health schools, including nursing schools, are directed by persons from other disciplines, and it is generally conceded that nurses should administer nursing schools. Administrators and teachers in university programs of the United States are the best academically prepared nurses in the country. Over half the nurses with earned doctoral degrees in 1972 (601 of the 1106) were in schools of nursing and 9810 of the 24,885 nurses holding earned master's degrees were in schools of nursing.[182] Their salaries were proportionately high, we believe, although specific figures have not been found for the United States. In Canada, full-time nurse faculty members in 1974 totalled 2395. Of these, 476 had no degrees, 1533 had baccalaureate, 350 master's, and 36 doctoral degrees. Of the 36 holding doctoral degrees, 33

were in university programs, and 247 of the 350 holding master's degrees were in university programs. Salaries for full-time faculty in university programs were higher than salaries of faculty in diploma programs.[183] Employment in universities and colleges in any country offers the many advantages, tangible and intangible, of work in an academic setting.

Full-time teaching that has given nurses no time for practice has been unsatisfying to those who find association with patients their chief reward. Joint appointments with schools and service agencies provide the satisfaction of helping students learn to nurse and patients learn to keep well, recover from or cope with disease, or accept death when this is inevitable. Some teaching positions offer joint faculty appointments in teaching and service, teaching and research, or in some cases all three.

Generally speaking, the nursing school setting has offered professional status and economic security. When administrators and teachers are inadequately prepared or assume positions without knowing the organizational and administrative limitations within which they must function, the disadvantages may outweigh the advantages of their work. Since faculties greatly influence the attitudes and

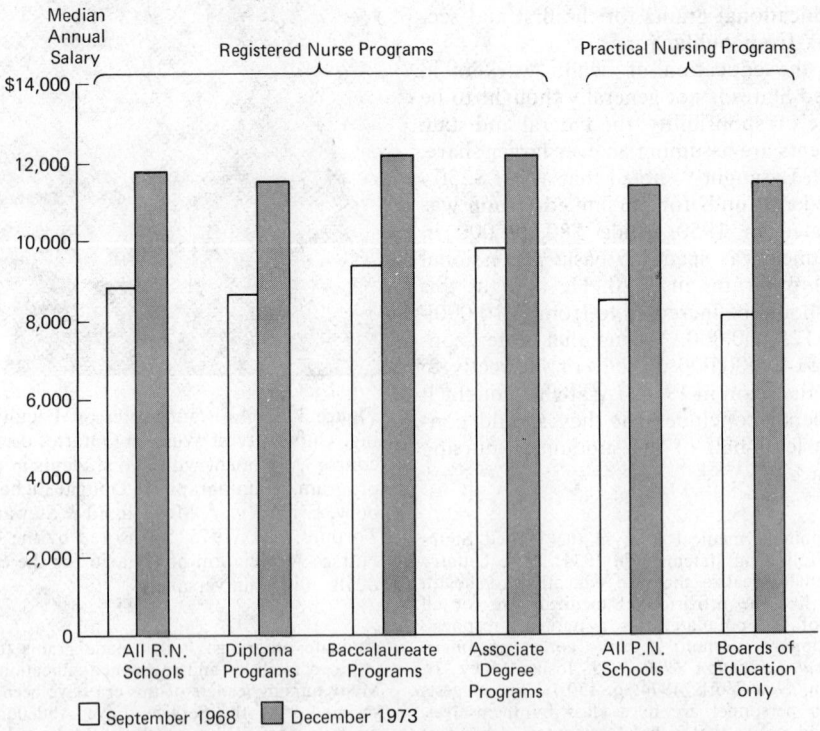

Figure 3-22. Median annual salaries of full-time R.N. faculty members in nursing educational programs in the United States, Sept. 1968 and Dec. 1973. (From American Nurses' Association: *Facts About Nursing 74–75*. The Association, Kansas City, Mo., 1976, p. 129.)

competence of future generations of nurses, it is important that they continue to attract the best prepared nurses. It is also important that students see their teachers as role models for practice rather than as classroom instructors with theoretical concepts of health service, which, with protracted separation from service, get more and more unrealistic. At the same time, it is crucial that nursing faculties be able to see what is ineffective and inequable in existing health services and be able to promote changes that will make services more nearly meet the needs of the citizenry.

11. JAILS, PRISONS, AND OTHER CORRECTIONAL INSTITUTIONS

Definitions. In spite of the rising "crime" rate, most people live within the law of the land, are never incarcerated, and give little thought to *penology*—the study of punishment for wrongdoing. They may never have wondered to what extent humans are born with criminal tendencies or commit crimes because their environments are inducive to antisocial (illegal) behavior; they may never have wondered whether punishment is a deterrent and whether the "criminal" can be "reformed." Some persons may never have studied the various ways in which different cultures treat those whose behavior is sufficiently deviant to make them "deserve punishment" or merit "reforming."

Philosophers, anthropologists, sociologists, psychologists, and those whose novels and essays constitute social comment clearly show that acts praised by one culture are condemned by others. Montaigne's essay on cultures is a miniature treatise on this subject.[1] For those who expect to work in health services connected with penal institutions, some basic questions for which they must find satisfying answers are: What constitutes antisocial behavior? Who shall mete out punishment? and How can the punishment be made to fit the antisocial behavior? Should the punishment deter crime, prevent crime, or should it "reform" or rehabilitate? Should society seek to change itself so that people do not want to act antisocially or should it seek to change those who do? Not only health workers but responsible citizens need guiding principles if they are to play a role in reducing crime, and both should study some representative views on penology.[2-7]

In most societies, offenses for which people are deprived of their property or liberty, or both, range in seriousness from *misdemeanors* to *felonies* to *crimes*. All are subject to court action. When apprehended, suspected felons or criminals are jailed until tried in the courts unless they can post bail. *Bail* is property (usually in the form of money) given as surety that a person released from custody will return at an appointed time. In affluent societies, most suspected felons and criminals post bail and are free until they are tried and convicted or found innocent. For this reason, the majority of jail inmates in the United States are reported to be unemployed, poor, young, from minority groups in cities, and relatively powerless.[8-10]

Jail is the term used for buildings where persons convicted of minor offenses are held for very short periods or where suspected (indicted) persons are detained or deprived of their liberty until they are tried. During "crime waves" when court calendars are overcrowded, suspects may await trial for months or years, which means that jail populations include many innocent persons. *Prisons* are buildings housing a few persons awaiting trial but most inmates of prisons are those serving a sentence following a conviction.

"Prison" is the more inclusive term. One encyclopedia did not even list the term "jail." However, in studying the history of detention for offenses against society, the statement is often made that "prison" is the newer term, as is the concept of prolonged incarceration with an attempt to reform or make the offender "penitent" * or a constructive member of society. These are the ostensible aims of most prisons, although this could hardly be claimed in the case of military and political prisons.

Lewis E. Lawes,[11] a former warden of Sing Sing Prison, writing an historical sketch of prisons in 1958, said that they developed from *work houses* that incarcerated paupers, vagrants, and debtors, but not felons or criminals. According to Lawes, the death penalty was used indiscriminately for almost every offense until the middle of the eighteenth century when corporal punishment, the galleys, and banishment began to supplant it. The papal prison of Clement XI around 1700 is said to be the first prison, and there were none in the United States until 1773. Until the nineteenth century, according to Lawes, prisoners existed in "disease breeding" wards or cells, the silent system prevailed, food was "hardly fit for swine," recreation was unheard of, prisoners were literally worked to death, and hospital and medical facilities were, of course, inadequate or nonexistent.†

John Howard, a Bedfordshire sheriff, was

---

* Hence the term *penitentiary* for prisons.

†A state or county that did not want to spend the money to maintain the prison might lease it to outsiders who operated the prison as a labor camp.

so appalled by the condition of prisons in nineteenth-century England that he devoted his life to prison reform.* Following Howard"s exposé of prison conditions, Parliament asked him to suggest reform measures. These were afterward written into law. The Quakers in England and the United States took an active role in prison reform. Elizabeth Fry of England was particularly effective in working with women prisoners. Philadelphia Quakers formed the Society for Alleviating the Miseries of Public Prisons.

In the hope of making prisoners penitent and giving them a chance to reform, Philadelphia prisons introduced cells that inmates rarely left and where they had nothing to read but the Bible and no visitors but a chaplain. A system known as the *Pennsylvania System* was developed and some of its elements persist. In New York State, the *Auburn System* introduced dividing prisoners into three groups, keeping the most serious "criminals" in solitary confinement, but allowing the other two groups to live and work together during the day, although locked in cells at night.

Lawes [12] observed that "methods utilized to reclaim offenders were indeed illogical." † He maintained that if antisocial conduct were largely a consequence of objectionable habits acquired because of an unfavorable environment and improper association, the following conditions in prison prevented the formation of desirable habits: all types of offenders housed together; men separated from women for months or years and deprived of normal sex relations; visits from relatives and friends restricted and mail censored; prisoners idle much of the time so they could not develop good work habits and deprived of initiative and stimulating experience.‡ He listed the following as "recent" reforms: civil service examinations that guards must pass; abolishment of silence; destruction or renovation of unsanitary buildings; work, recreational, and educational programs introduced, with radio announcements and news broadcasts to keep

inmates informed; psychiatrists assigned to prisons; and hospital facilities provided.

With the hope of changing antisocial to acceptable behavior came a new terminology and new types of management of houses of detention. *Reformatories* for minors were introduced in 1825 and called in New York City and Boston "houses of refuge." In 1840, a reformatory for men was established in New York State. This Brockway Reformatory had much in common with a military school, and the *indeterminate sentence* was introduced. The latter meant that the inmate was released at the discretion of the reformatory authorities. Brockway operated under the following assumptions: treatment should be individual; reform through education is possible; there should be cooperation between inmates and officials; and the length of the sentence should be determined by the inmate's behavior, as judged by the correctional staff.

Concepts of penology vary greatly from nation to nation, within nations from one state or province to another, and from age to age. In 1970, the Fourth United Nations Congress on Prevention of Crime and Treatment of Offenders reaffirmed The Standard Minimum Rules, drawn up in 95 statements, on all aspects of care and treatment. Statements 22 through 25 on medical services recommend that the medical services be organized in close relationship to the general health administration of the community or nation and that prisoners who require special treatment should be sent to hospitals outside prisons. The rules mention "medical officer" and "medical services," including psychiatric service, and "dental officer," but no mention is made of nursing.[13] However, the ICN has published the following statement on the "Role of the Nurse in the Care of Detainees and Prisoners," with emphasis on political prisoners and the UN 1971 Declaration of Human Rights: *

Whereas, the ICN *Code for Nurses* specifically states that
1. "The fundamental responsibility of the nurse is fourfold: to promote health, to prevent illness, to restore health and to alleviate suffering.
2. "The nurse's primary responsibility is to those people who require nursing care.
3. "The nurse when acting in a professional capacity should at all times maintain standards of personal conduct which reflect credit upon the profession.
4. "The nurse takes appropriate action to safeguard the individual when his care is en-

* The I.C.N., in 1929, gave the "minimum standards" for prisons submitted by the Howard League for Penal Reform to the League of Nations, calling it an International Charter for Prisoners. ("Current Events of International Interest. International Charter for Prisoners," *I.C.N.*, 4:75, [Jan.] 1929.)
† The amount of *recidivism* is often cited as proof of the failure of the prison system. This is the chronic tendency toward repetition of criminal or antisocial behavior. To what extent this is inborn or acquired remains a question, but many penologists think prison life *unfits* the inmate for a self-directed life and that the freed inmate in some cases invites arrest so that he or she can return to the security of prison life.
‡ Lawes noted that in Russia wives were allowed to live with their husbands in prison camps.

* "ICN Statement on the Role of the Nurse in the Care of Detainees and Prisoners," in *ICN Policy Statements.* International Council of Nurses, Geneva, 1976; *Int. Nurs. Rev.*, 22:182, (Nov.–Dec.) 1975.

dangered by a co-worker or any other person," and

Whereas, in 1973 ICN reaffirmed support for the Red Cross Rights and Duties of Nurses under the Geneva Conventions of 1949, which specifically state that, in case of armed conflict of international as well as national character (i.e., internal disorders, civil wars, armed rebellions):

1. Members of the armed forces, prisoners and persons taking no active part in the hostilities
   (*a*) shall be entitled to protection and care if wounded or sick,
   (*b*) shall be treated humanely, that is:
   —they may not be subjected to physical mutilation or to medical or scientific experiments of any kind which are not justified by the medical, dental or hospital treatment of the prisoner concerned and carried out in his interest,
   —they shall not be wilfully left without medical assistance and care, nor shall conditions exposing them to contagion or infection be created,
   —they shall be treated humanely and cared for by the Party in conflict in whose power they may be, without any adverse distinction founded on sex, race, nationality, religion, political opinion, or any other similar criteria.
2. The following acts are and shall remain prohibited at any time and in any place whatsoever with respect to the above-mentioned persons:
   (*a*) violence to life and person, in particular murder of all kinds, mutilation, cruel treatment and torture,
   (*b*) outrages upon personal dignity, in particular humiliating and degrading treatment.

Whereas, in 1971 ICN endorsed the United Nations Universal Declaration of Human Rights and, hence, accepted that

1. "Everyone is entitled to all the rights and freedoms, set forth in this Declaration, without distinction of any kind, such as race, colour, sex, language, religion, political or other opinion, national or social origin, property, birth or other status (Art. 2),
2. "No one shall be subjected to torture or to cruel, inhuman or degrading treatment or punishment (Art. 5)"; and

Whereas, in relation to detainees and prisoners of conscience, interrogation procedures are increasingly being employed which result in ill effects, often permanent, on the person's mental and physical health;

Therefore be it resolved, that ICN condemns the use of all such procedures harmful to the mental and physical health of prisoners and detainees; and

Further be it resolved, that nurses having knowledge of physical or mental ill-treatment of detainees and prisoners take proper action, including reporting such information to appropriate national and/or international bodies; and

Further be it resolved, that nurses participate in clinical research carried out on prisoners, only if the freely given consent of the patient has been secured after a complete explanation and under-

standing by the patient of the nature and risk of the research; and

Finally be it resolved, that the nurse's first responsibility is towards her patients, notwithstanding considerations of national security and interest.

While this international code and those relating specifically to military and political prisoners are widely used in cases dealing with abuse or neglect of prisoners, the philosophy of national, state, and local authorities who control the penal institutions largely determines their character. Commissioners and wardens, or directors, may believe in an authoritarian system, a benevolent despotism, a republic or a democracy, or any combination of these. Modern institutions that curtail the inmates' liberties may be called *road camps, schools, boys' republics, boys' towns,* or *work farms. Guards* are often called *custodial* or *correctional officers. Concentration camps* are guarded compounds for the detention or imprisonment of aliens or political opponents rather than felons or criminals.

While many believe that the changing penal terminology reflects efforts to improve the system, Jessica Mitford doubts this and makes the following observation:

To find one's way around the modern prison system one must first master the new terminology. Notable advances have recently been made in this area. The authors of the Attica Commission Report, evaluating the work of a special committee appointed by the governor in 1965 to study the treatment of prisoners, concluded that the committee's major accomplishment after five years of labor was to change the names of all the state's maximum security prisons: "Effective July 8, 1970 . . . there were no more prisons; in their places, instead, stood six maximum security 'correctional facilities.' The prison wardens became 'institutional superintendents' . . . and the old-line prison guards awakened that morning to find themselves suddenly 'correctional officers.' No one's job or essential duties changed, only his title. Certainly the institutions themselves did not change. . . . To a man spending 14 to 16 hours a day in a cell being 'rehabilitated,' it was scarcely any comfort and no reassurance to learn that he was suddenly 'an inmate in a correctional facility' instead of a convict in a prison." In the same spirit some prisons are now called "therapeutic correctional communities," convicts are "clients of the correctional system," solitary confinement and punishment cells have become "adjustment centers," "seclusion," or, in Virginia, "meditation." *

In describing her study of "the prison business" Mitford explained why she omitted "jails" in her investigation, saying:

---

* Mitford, Jessica: *Kind and Usual Punishment. The Prison Business.* Alfred A. Knopf, New York, 1973, p. 6.

The jails have no apologists, they are universally recognized to be hellish places.

I decided to forego these pockets of iniquity [she excepted a woman's jail in the District of Columbia] and instead to travel the broad highway of prison reform, to look mainly at those large, well-ordered, highly financed prison systems that have incorporated as their stated policy reforms fought for over the decades: rehabilitation as opposed to punishment, utilization of the latest scientific therapy techniques, classification of prisoners based on their performance in prison, a chance for every offender to return to the community as soon as he is ready.*

Mitford interviewed many prisoners and concluded, as did Eugene Victor Debs [14] and Bertrand Russell [15] (both of whom served prison terms), that they (prisoners) were on the average like the rest of us. In discussing whether to reform or abolish prisons, she said she shared the conviction of Federal District Judge James Doyle of Wisconsin, whom she quoted as saying:

I am persuaded that the institution of prison probably must end. In many respects it is as intolerable within the United States as was the institution of slavery, equally brutalizing to all involved, equally toxic to the social system, equally subversive of the brotherhood of man, even more costly by some standards, and probably less rational.†

For the benefit of those who might like to join the "fight for prisoners' rights," Mitford, in an appendix, gave the names and addresses of 212 organizations in 49 states "engaged in various aspects of this fight." She also listed nine periodicals devoted to this cause.

Volumes have been written on crime, punishment, and correction. In recent years national committees and commissions have studied civil disorders, crime, and correction in many countries. In 1967, the (US) President's Crime Commission made its report, *The Challenge of Crime in a Free Society*.[15a] Leo Tolstoy, George Bernard Shaw, Karl Menninger, and many others have questioned the right of one person to punish another, using "the crime of imprisonment" and "the crime of punishment" as catch phrases.[16,17] No attempt can be made in this chapter to even mention the salient points for and against a prison system. Mitford reviews the conclusions of national commissions, beginning with one appointed by President Hoover in 1929 calling for drastic reforms or abolishment of prisons, and conclusions of individuals such as Eugene Debs, Frank Tannenbaum, Ramsey Clark, and many others who would abolish them.[18-20] She

* *Ibid.,* p. 5.
† *Ibid.,* p. 273.

quotes Carl Rauh, advisor to the deputy attorney general of Washington, D.C., who showed the futility of prisons with the following figures:

Of the 100 major crimes, 50 are reported to the police. For 50 incidents reported, 12 people are arrested. Of the 12 arrested, 6 are convicted of anything—not necessarily of the offense reported. Of the 6 who are convicted, 1.5 go to prison or jail.*

In the same context, Mitford said that the President's Commission on Causes and Prevention of Violence reported that, of an estimated 9,000,000 crimes committed in the United States in a recent year, only 1½ per cent of the perpetrators were imprisoned.

In the last analysis, the citizens of every governmental unit are responsible for its judicial system, its penal code, and the treatment of those who commit misdemeanors, felonies, or crimes. But as long as prisons, by any name, exist, the health of the inmates is the responsibility of the health care system.†

Employment of Nurses in Jails, Prisons, and Other Correctional Institutions. The numbers of nurses employed in jails, prisons, and related institutions are not reported by the American Nurses' Association in *Facts About Nursing* nor by the Canadian Nurses' Association in *Countdown*.[21,22] Some data is available that leads this writer to believe that in the United States in 1976 professional nurses employed in prisons may number less than 2000. The Federal Prison System with 43 institutions and approximately 23,000 inmates (convicted federal offenders) reported only 35 "nurses" employed November 30, 1972.‡ Most of these

* *Ibid.,* p. 276.
† The Law Enforcement Assistance Administration reported a 1970 National Jail Census showing 153,063 adults and 7800 juveniles in 4037 locally administered jails (not including federal and state prisons or correctional institutions, those used exclusively for juveniles, state-operated jails of Connecticut, Delaware, and Rhode Island, "drunk tanks," "lock-ups," and other facilities holding people for less than 2 days). Of the 160,863 persons in the 4037 jails, 5 per cent were females, 52 per cent were pretrial detainees or "otherwise not convicted," two-thirds of the juveniles falling in this category. Medical facilities exist in slightly more than half of the nation's jails. (Law Enforcement Assistance Administration: "National Jail Census 1970. National Criminal Justice Information Statistics Service, Series SC No. 1," in American Bar Association, and American Medical Association: *Medical and Health Care in Jails, Prisons, and Other Correctional Facilities. A Compilation of Standards and Materials,* 3rd ed. American Bar Association, Washington, D.C., 1974, p. 141.)
‡ The Federal Prison System includes (1973) six long-term adult institutions; six intermediate-term adult institutions with women's facilities in 2 of them; six short-term adult institutions; six young adult insti-

were in the prison for women only or in the women's division of other prisons.* [23,24] No such total count has been found for all state and local prisons.

In 1972, the American Medical Association, in cooperation with the American Bar Association, made a questionnaire survey of 2930 United States jails, the reported findings representing 1159 usable responses.[25] While professional medical service on some basis was available in 69.9 per cent of the jails and dental service in about 37.8 per cent, "nurses" were reported as available in only 18.6 per cent and social service in 15.2 per cent. The usable responses showed 326 physicians regularly scheduled, 132 on call, 158 dentists, 174 social workers, 192 psychologists, 135 "unspecified" health workers, and 189 "nurses." A survey of prisons rather than jails might have shown a higher ratio of nurses to other types of health workers. A 1976 survey of jails and prisons would undoubtedly show a higher count for nurses than the 1972 surveys.

Since 1965, a number of studies of medical services in state, county, and municipal penal systems and in specific jails and prisons have been reported. They show a mounting interest in prison health. In the 1971 Massachusetts report, nurses were on the survey team, and the findings and recommendations include nursing. The number of nurses in the system was, however, not specified.[26] The 1959 Illinois report had little information on nursing, but since Cook County Jail was reported as having five full-time nurses and the Chicago House of Correction eight full-time and five on-call nurses, the reader might assume that nurses did not, in 1969, play a very important role in the health service of Illinois jails.[27]

A 1973 Survey of Penal Institutions by the Medical and Chirurgical Faculty of the State of Maryland gives no data on numbers of nurses but the following statements indicate more than average nurse involvement: "All physicians interviewed were pleased with the quality of nursing care . . . all . . . declared . . . more nurses needed." "Nurses interviewed seemed generally satisfied with their working conditions . . . but all felt they could do a better job if they had more help." Inmates in some cases "felt that nurses were overworked. . . . sick call is conducted very rapidly by a nurse who screens each patient. . . . Approximately 10–20% of all patients on sick call see the physician." * In Maryland, funds for more nurses were requested in 1972, 1973, and 1974 budgets by the Medical Director of the Department of Correction, which suggests that the need for nursing care was at least recognized. Some survey reports suggested that nurses, or at least women nurses, were not thought suitable health personnel for prisons.

In 1974, a Task Force of the Kentucky Public Health Association, in cooperation with the American Public Health Association, reported a survey of "penitentiaries, reformatories, farms, juvenile detention centers, and city and county jails," all referred to by the generic term "prison." The number of nurses employed in prisons was not given in the report available to the writer but the recommendations indicated that nurses in the health service were seen as essential. The use of inmate nurses was not approved. It was suggested that nurses "or medics" perform screening tests and "triage" procedures. The comment was made that, while nurses were already functioning in these capacities in some juvenile centers, such roles "could be greatly expanded." The following is one of the concluding recommendations:

Medical students, interns, and nurses from the University of Louisville and University of Kentucky should rotate through the penal health care system. They could appropriately provide services at Type I, II, III and VI institutions. Closer cooperation is needed with the medical centers at Louisville on referrals and follow-up.†

(Parenthetically, it was reported in 1972 that 54 of the 103 medical schools in the United States were providing health care services to a state prison or local detention center.[28] No comparable data has been found on nursing schools.)

The California Department of Corrections

---

tutions; three youth and juvenile institutions, one having a woman's facility; one woman's institution; one medical center; and 14 Community Treatment Centers.

* The Division of Health Service of the US Bureau of Prisons employed 185 medical technical assistants as of November, 1972. Even in some hospitals connected with federal prisons that were accredited by the Joint Commission on Accreditation of Hospitals, there were no registered nurses employed.

* Medical and Chirurgical Faculty of the State of Maryland: "Report of the Ad Hoc Committee on Medical Care in State Penal Institutions," in American Bar Association, and American Medical Association: *Medical and Health Care in Jails, Prisons, and Other Correctional Facilities. A Compilation of Standards and Materials*, 3rd ed. American Bar Association, Washington, D.C., 1974, pp. 142aa, 142ee.

† Task Force on Prison and Jail Health, Kentucky Public Health Association and American Public Health Association: "The Captive Patient: Prison Health Care. A Report of Task Force. . . ," in American Bar Association, and American Medical Association: *Medical and Health Care in Jails, Prisons, and Other Correctional Facilities. A Compilation of Standards and Materials*, 3rd ed. American Bar Association, Washington, D.C., 1974, pp. 142z.

in 1973 spent almost $5000 per inmate annually.[29] This should provide better-than-average conditions in prisons. The findings of a 1973 study of health care services in the San Diego County Jail by Rita Judd Stokes,[30] a social worker, suggests, however, "grave deficiencies in health care service." For example, prisoners were not adequately screened for communicable disease, and evaluation at sick call averaged one minute. Stokes reported that there were two "experienced RN's on duty around the clock" but she concluded that they were poorly utilized and bogged down with paper work.

A report in 1973 from the Commissioner of Correction in New York City described a contract with the Montefiore Hospital which, when fully operative, he thought would provide ". . . the finest medical services for inmates [of Riker's Island Prisons] in the country." * In 1975, Rena Murtha,[31] then Director of Nursing Service since July 1973 in the Prison Health Service of New York City, described the service for nine institutions in the boroughs

* Malcolm, Benjamin J.: "New York City Inmate Medical Services Contract with Montefiore Hospital," in American Bar Association, and American Medical Association: *Medical and Health Care in Jails, Prisons, and Other Correctional Facilities. A Compilation of Standards and Materials,* 3rd ed. American Bar Association, Washington, D.C., 1974, p. 302.

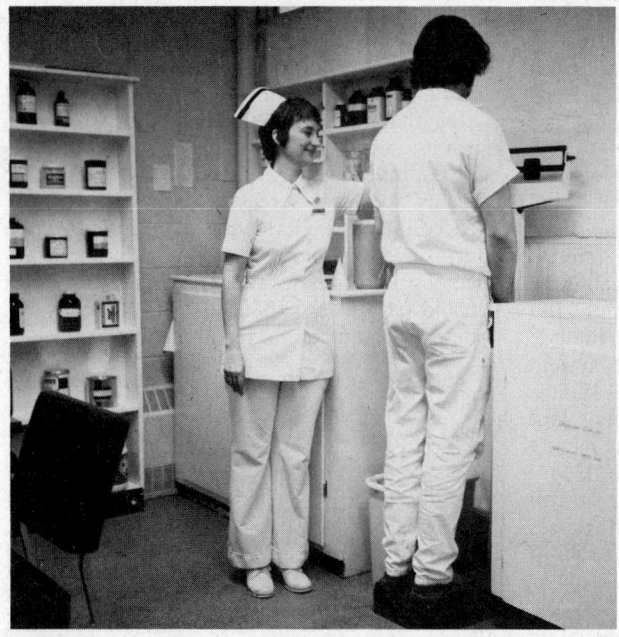

A

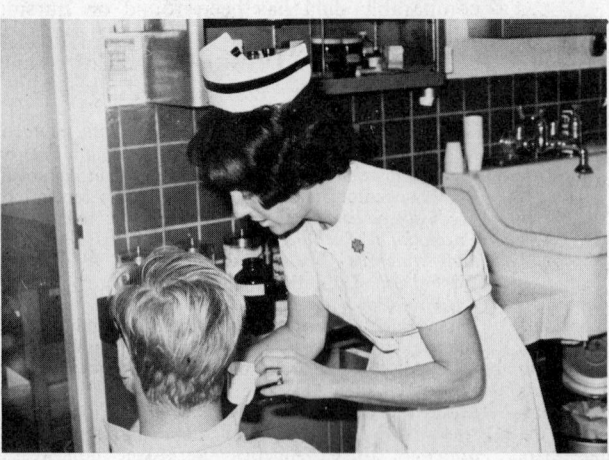

B

Figure 3-23. Nurses and patients in treatment unit of (*A*) Adult Centre; (*B*) Juvenile Training Centre. (Courtesy of Ministry of Correctional Services, Toronto, Ontario.)

of Bronx, Brooklyn, and Queens. For about 10,000 inmates * (not quite half the total inmate population of Federal prisons), there were 104 registered nurses, 118 practical nurses, and 12 nurse's aides. If this approximate ratio of one professional nurse to 100 inmates was maintained for the total prison population of the United States, there would be far more than 2000 registered nurses in the country's prison health system.

Satisfactory data on nurses in the Canadian Penitentiary Service have not been available to the writer. In 1972, the Management Consulting Service, at the request of the Director of Medical Services, Department of the Solicitor General, prepared a report on *Health Care Services in the Canadian Penitentiary Service.* A "nursing advisor" was mentioned several times; otherwise, nurses at that time seemed to have no part in the Service. The following substantiates that observation:

These services are brought to the 7,600 inmates in 39 different locations across Canada by a staff of 60 professionals and 170 hospital officers at a cost of $4,000,000 per year ($550 per inmate). The 60 professionals are psychiatrists, physicians, dentists and surgeons employed full-time, part-time, on contract or on a fee basis. To this list must be added medical specialists (e.g. ophthalmologist, E.N.T.) who visit the institution when required usually on a fee basis.†

As in the United States and other developed countries, Canada has had many surveys of prison health services by boards of inspectors or commissions. A Correctional Planning Committee proposed "The Ten Year Plan" of constructing new penitentiaries, which was begun in 1963. The Committee recommended construction of regional medical centers, each with a psychiatric facility.

While nursing has apparently played a negligible role in the Canadian prison health service until very recently, the preceding report suggests that in Canada there has been since World War II an effort to segregate psychiatric inmates and give them appropriate care. In 1971, the Solicitor General of Canada appointed an Advisory Board of Psychiatric Con-

sultants to study psychiatric services in "Federal correctional services in Canada." The Board's report was published in 1972.[32] Among other conditions, the report showed that, in 1971, 10.2 per cent of the penitentiary population required psychiatric care and treatment. Federal prisons were said to have progressively deteriorating facilities for the care of psychiatric patients and were finding it "unacceptable" in nearly every province to transfer psychiatric prisoners to outside provincial health services. After reviewing the systems in some other countries, the Board recommended the creation of five Regional Psychiatric Centers under the Canadian Penitentiary Service. Psychiatrists making this recommendation showed the nurse in a major role. They recommended a ratio of one psychiatrist to 20 patients, one psychologist to 30, one social worker to 30, and 80 nursing personnel to 100 patients.[33]

Writing in *Discussion,* the staff magazine of the Canadian Penitentiary Service in Ottawa, A. R. Arrowsmith, the nurse advisor to the Service at that time, in an article titled "Nurses Answer Another Challenge," made the following observations:

In 1972 the Commissioner of penitentiaries appointed a Nursing Advisory Committee* . . . empowered to study all aspects of nursing in federal penitentiaries, and to recommend training and improvement of service. . . .

. . .

This year [1973] the advisory committee visited most penitentiaries in Ontario.

. . .

Most of the recommendations affecting nursing made in the report of the Solicitor General's management consulting service have been acted on.

. . .

The penitentiary hospital has become a health care center and hospital officers are now health care officers. . . .

. . .

Nursing in C.P.S. has long been unrecognized in penal and outside nursing circles.

. . .

A large percentage of decisions by health care officers are made in the absence of a physician. Therefore, nursing knowledge and skills must be at a high level.†

Carl I. Archer, a nurse of the Regional Medical Center, Abbotsford, British Columbia, described its program where registered psychi-

---

* Murtha reports that "About 85 per cent are detainees, or persons who have been charged but cannot post bail and are therefore 'detained' until their trials; 15 per cent have been convicted and are serving sentences of one year or less." (Murtha, Rena: "Health Care in Prison: Change in One City's System. It Started with a Director of Nursing," *Am. J. Nurs.,* **75:**421, [Mar.] 1975.)

† [Canadian] Department of the Solicitor General: *Health Care Services in the Canadian Penitentiary Service.* Report to the Department by Management Consulting Service. The Department, [Ottawa], May 1972 (Report No. 35).

* The Committee includes a representative from the Canadian Nurses' Association, Health and Welfare Canada, and the Canadian Forces Medical Services, plus the director of medical services and nursing advisor of medical services, Canadian Penitentiary Service.

† Arrowsmith, A. R.: "Nurses Answer Another Challenge," *Discussion,* **1:**12, (Dec.) 1973.

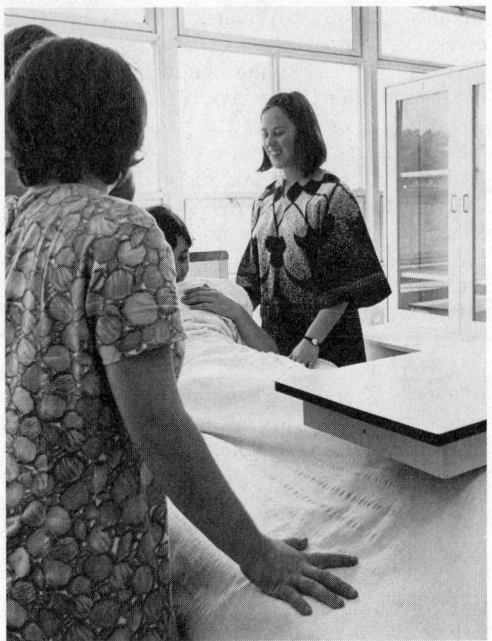

Figure 3-24. Home nursing course in progress at Girls' Training School. (Courtesy of Ministry of Correctional Services, Toronto, Ontario.)

atric nurses functioned as therapists. About this service a physician said:

> The goal . . . is not just to treat the number of patients who will be admitted, but to influence the entire penitentiary service to bring the concept of healing arts into the care of the mentally ill offender. . . . Instead of developing a vertical hierarchy we are developing horizontally so that nurses are the centre of our activities.*

Nora J. Earle, a nurse of the Ministry of Correctional Services of Ontario, gives the following information for this province: 131 nurses employed in "the various institutions"; five are men nurses, one of these a "nurse practitioner'"; 75 are full-time, the others "casuals"; our "largest jail of 800 inmates requires 24 hours service with a roster of 21 nurses (which we have yet to achieve)." † If these figures are representative, the ratio of nurses to prisoners in the provinces of Canada may be higher than in the United States. As the philosophy of nursing in the Regional Psychiatric Centres dominates nursing in all aspects of the prison service, undoubtedly a higher ratio of nurses to inmates will eventually be found throughout the program.

* Archer, Carl I.: "Nurses with a Unique Role in Treatment," *Discussion,* **1:**14, (Dec.) 1973.
　† Letter from Nora J. Earle to Virginia Henderson, May 1975.

Although the preceding data on nursing in prisons of the United States and Canada suggest that progress is of recent origin, nursing in this setting has a longer history than most persons may be aware of.

Janet Whitney [34] wrote a biography entitled *Elizabeth Fry, Quaker Heroine.* Elizabeth Fry devoted her mature years to prison reform, teaching inmates to care for the sick and, before the Nightingale period, organized the Protestant Sisters of Charity who were often called "Fry Nurses." In 1909, Ethel Gordon Fenwick,[35] in England, proposed an Elizabeth Fry League to train men and women for prison nursing. Elizabeth S. Haldane,[36] in 1908, gave working conditions, civil service requirements, and salaries of nurses as prison matrons and "warders." An anonymous author,[37] in 1902, discussed the need for nurses in a home for 250 "truant boys" of 7 to 14 years. Mrs. Maxwell St. John,[38] member of the Howard Penal Reform League, in 1914 described prison nursing at two large prisons. In 1919, the League sent a deputation to the Home Secretary stressing conditions of juvenile offenders and recommending the employment of qualified nurses in jails. Under Beatrice Kent's leadership, five nurses were assigned to Holloway Prison that year.[39-41]

In England, many women, a number of them socially prominent, were sent to prison during the suffrage movement.* Some nurses were active suffragists and a few wrote exposés of prison conditions.[42,43] This may account to some extent for the fact that the writer has found more in nursing journals on prison nursing in England than any other country. Influential conscientious objectors and men and women war protesters throughout most of this century in many countries have questioned the penal system in the United States and abroad.[44-51] Jane A. Kennedy, a nurse war protester, in 1975 described 14 months in "one of the best women's prisons in the country." She said:

> I conclude that prison corrects nothing. It rehabilitates no one, nor does it restore the individual's ability to work. . . . The ultimate irony is that of all those who commit crimes only 1.5% are imprisoned and they are the poor and members of the minority groups . . . it does one thing well. Prison punishes.†

* Lady Constance Lytton, an ardent suffragist, was imprisoned but treated with special consideration as a person of rank. She took the name Jane Warton and dressed as a working girl to see how unknowns would be treated. She described this in *Prisons and Prisoners; Some Personal Experiences.* (Heinemann, London, 1914.)
　† Kennedy, Jane A.: "Health Care in Prison. A View from Inside," *Am. J. Nurs.,* **75:**417, (Mar.) 1975.

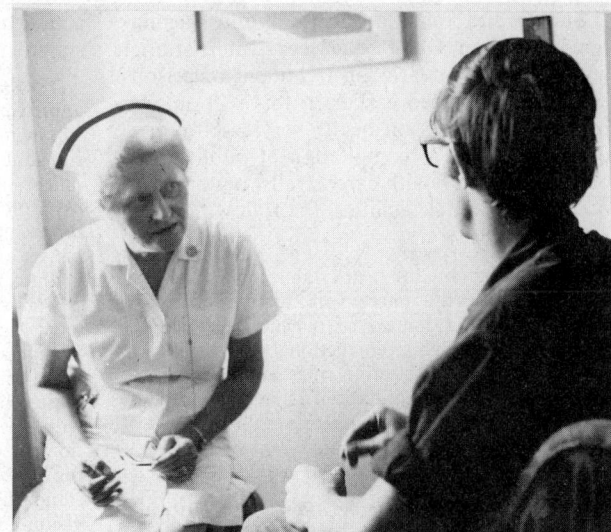

Figure 3-25. Nurse talking with inmate of Neuro-Psychiatric Unit, Guelph Correction Centre. (Courtesy of Ministry of Correctional Services, Toronto. Ontario.)

While Kennedy questioned the social worth of imprisonment, she thought "prisons would feel immediate, significant relief if professionals in health, education, and religion insisted that prisoners should leave prisons and come to them for care, for knowledge, for worship." * As described by Kennedy, prison nurses gave no "relief."

Neither "nurses" nor "nursing" is indexed in Jessica Mitford's *Kind and Usual Punishment*. The only mention found in this volume of either is in the chapter on research, titled "Cheaper Than Chimpanzees." Here, she said that inmate technicians and nurses who staff laboratories were reported to be getting a feeling of self-respect from participating in the research. In one experiment, their "wages" ranged "from 30¢ a day for a nurse to $1.25 a day for chief technicians." † There are numerous reports of inmate training programs for subprofessional nursing but many persons writing on prison health condemn health care by any inmate personnel.

Nature of a Prison Health Service. As stated earlier, some jails have no health services; some may boast little more than a first-aid kit in the sheriff's office. Medical personnel who are on call may bring with them a bag of instruments and supplies. Jails claiming a health service with full- or part-time health personnel may have several rooms or a floor within the jail; others may have a hospital (called a "health care centre" in Canadian penitentiaries) that is a part of the jail or prison. Hospitals for the criminally insane may constitute one of the prisons in a national, state, or municipal penal system. In both the United States and Canada, psychiatric hospitals outside prisons may establish units for the criminally insane and contract with prisons for treatment of inmates. Prison inmates are nearly always sent to hospitals outside prisons for major surgery or for diagnosis and treatment of obscure and serious medical conditions. Pregnant women are sent to outside hospitals for delivery of their babies. (If a baby is born in a prison, the fact is not entered on the birth certificate.)

Since most prisoners cannot move freely about the penal institution but must be escorted by custodial staff (a "corrections officer"), there may be a health station on every tier of cells to reduce time spent in escort duty. Because health workers can be subpoenaed to give testimony in court, their relationship with prisoner-patients is not the same as it is with patients outside prisons when there is privileged communication between physician and patient or nurse and patient. And, because the corrections officer is either present or within earshot, the prisoner is not tempted to have a confidential relationship with the health worker. Even when prison inmates are sent to civil hospitals for treatment, a prison guard may be assigned whose presence or proximity changes the nature of the health service. "Prison health centers" such as those described in the Canadian Penitentiary Service, and health services in "junior republics" more nearly approximate health services in industry or schools as described elsewhere in this chapter. Figures 3-23, 3-24, and 3-25 show some representative prison health facilities.

* *Ibid.*
† Mitford, Jessica: *op. cit.*, p. 156.

Standardization, Certification, and Regulation of Prison Health Services. International and national standards on treatment of prisoners have been cited earlier in this section. All include statements on health services for prisoners. In the 1974 compilation of publications on medical and health care in jails, prisons, and other correctional facilities, the following comment is made:

It should be noted that the standards and recommendations presented here were, for the most part, developed in the context of a general consideration of inmate rights, correctional programs and organization, administrative rules and procedures, and the goals of rehabilitation. In many instances, successful and workable controls on the delivery of medical services will be contingent on how well these broader issues have been addressed.*

The American Correctional Association's 1966 *Manual of Correctional Standards* has a chapter on "Health and Medical Services"; the National Advisory Commission on Criminal Justice in its 1973 report includes among its *Standards* one on medical care; the National Sheriff Association's 1970 *Manual on Jail Administration* has a chapter on health services; the US Bureau of Prisons in its 1971 *The Jail—Its Operation and Management* includes material on health in the chapter on "Special Prisoners"; and the American Academy of Pediatrics issued in 1973 *Health Standards for Juvenile Court Residential Facilities.*

It is noteworthy that, with the exception of the Academy's statement,

. . . none of the standards and recommendations presented have been the work product of medical or health groups and organizations, (although consultation and contributions by medical authorities and practitioners has been relied on in most of these issuances). This suggests a potential public service contribution for refinement, elaboration and improvement of the concepts articulated which might be undertaken within the medical and public health professions.†

The fact that some federal prison hospitals with no registered nurses on their staffs are accredited by the Joint Commission on Accreditation of Hospitals of the American Hospital Association and the American Medical Association suggests that prison health services are not measured by the same standards as those outside prisons. The American Correctional Association in its chapter on "Health and Medical Services" makes the following statements under staff allocation:

The basic medical staff for a penal institution of approximately 500 inmates should include the following: one full-time chief medical officer, one full-time psychiatrist, serving as assistant medical officer, one full-time dental officer, one full-time psychologist, five full-time medical technicians representative of the technical specialties described above and a suitable complement of consultants in the various medical and surgical specialties.

For every additional 500 to 1,000 inmates at least one additional medical officer and medical technician should be added. An additional dental officer is required for each 1,000 additional inmates. In large institutions of over 1,500 inmates, with hospitals having 40 or more beds, consideration should be given to the inclusion of trained registered nurses to insure that the highest nursing standards are maintained with adequate supervision of the operating room as well as the intensive treatment areas. Experience has shown that female nurses can function effectively in the performance of these duties. In smaller institutions, adequate nursing services can be provided by suitably trained medical technicians. However, hospitals depending upon this type of nursing service should have continuous training programs including suitable refresher courses to insure that the nursing skills of the technicians are maintained at an acceptable level.*

While the ACA goes on to approve the supplementation of "regular full-time hospital employees" with "suitably trained inmates" for "paramedical services," other groups condemn this practice.

Organized nursing in the United States has not, to the writer's knowledge, developed standards for nursing in correctional institutions. There are no divisions, sections, departments, or commissions in national nursing organizations for nurses employed in the penal system that might assume this responsibility. However, Murtha is encouraged by recent interest in prison nursing expressed by official nursing in the United States. She made the following observation: "The ANA's 1974 Resolution on Health Care in Correctional Institutions confirms that what we and other prison nurses are doing is not in vain." †

Every one interested in prison health in the United States must be heartened by any recognition of its importance by organized nursing,

* American Bar Association, and American Medical Association: *Medical and Health Care in Jails, Prisons, and Other Correctional Facilities. A Compilation of Standards and Materials,* 3rd ed. American Bar Association, Washington, D.C., 1974, p. 2.
† American Bar Association, and American Medical Association: *op. cit.,* p. 6.

* American Correctional Association: "Manual of Correctional Standards," in American Bar Association, and American Medical Association: *Medical and Health Care in Jails, Prisons, and Other Correctional Facilities. A Compilation of Standards and Materials,* 3rd ed. American Bar Association, Washington, D.C., 1974, p. 11.
† Murtha, Rena: "Health Care in Prison: Change in One City's System. It Started with a Director of Nursing," *Am. J. Nurs.,* **75:**421, (Mar.) 1975.

but more is needed than an expression of concern. Nursing in a penal system requires specialized knowledge and competence. Murtha, speaking of the need for specialized preparation, says that the continuing education program for nurses in the New York City Prison Health Service

. . . deals with suicide prevention, group dynamics, interview techniques, history and physical assessment, mental health nursing, cardiopulmonary resuscitation, pharmacology, alcoholism and drug abuse, leadership/management, and, through assistance from the NYC Corrections Academy, with correctional orientation, the use and abuse of tear gas, and what to do in case of riot.*

Patricia Winstead-Fry, psychiatric nurse-consultant to the New York City Prison Health Service, discussing the role development of nurses with special reference to suicide prevention, contrasts the tendency of nurses in the past to say that they could take care of inmates if correction officers would leave them alone with the current recognition that "many of the needed changes in correction and inmate subsystems must come from court and prison reform, a profound change that nurses as citizens can influence." † Nurses who know little or nothing about the prison system are, obviously, in no position to influence its "reform."

Statements by organized nursing on the functions, standards, and qualifications for practice in prison health services might not only improve nursing in this setting but encourage all nurses to use their influence as citizens to promote prison reform.

The Rights of Prisoners. Statements listed under the previous discussion of standards bear on the rights of prisoners. However, there is almost no topic in the literature on penal reform that does not directly or indirectly relate to prisoners' rights. Civil Liberties Unions, Friends Service Committees, lawyers, guilds, and law student organizations, Medical Committees on Human Rights, and many other agencies are studying the question. Chapter 1 of Mitford's *Kind and Usual Punishment* begins with the following statement:

My involvement with prisons came about almost by accident. Early in 1970 I was asked by the American Civil Liberties Union if I would prepare an article on prisoners' rights to be published in a national magazine as part of the ACLU's fiftieth anniversary program. ("That's an easy assignment," observed a criminologist with whom

I discussed the project. "Just turn in a sheaf of blank papers—they *haven't* any rights.") *

Mitford cited case after case in which the courts ruled that prisoners' rights were disregarded. She noted riots based on the infringement of rights and quoted an associate warden of San Quentin Prison as saying that riots by prisoners rose in that prison from about 50 in 1960 to 5000 in 1970.[52] More and more law students and established lawyers are supporting prisoners' rebellions at "the unfettered discretion'" of corrections officers. A bill of rights evolved from the Attica riots.[53]

Some of the rights listed in prisoners' demands and those argued in court cases include the following: the right to survive; to the necessities of life—adequate food, shelter, clothing, cleanliness, exercise, rest and sleep; to companionship; to medical or health care, to protection from communicable disease; to education and vocational training; to worthwhile jobs at prevailing union wages; to be treated with human dignity; freedom to exercise self-determination; the right to counsel and to due process if there is infringement of a substantial right. Protection of prisoners from exploitation in medical research (discussed later) has been extensively studied by law students and others.

While health personnel are most concerned with prisoners' rights to health care during incarceration, in halfway houses, and in ambulatory services during parole, other rights are so essential to health that they cannot be considered separately. If and when prison health is brought into the mainstream of the health service system, physicians, nurses, social workers, clinical psychologists, and other health workers may be in the forefront of the struggle for prisoners' rights. This struggle may materially alter or destroy the present penal system of prisons and parole—a system based on the theory of constructive custody.

Location and Physical Plans and Furnishings of Prison Health Services. Prisons range in size from one-room lockups to institutions housing thousands. Courthouses have locked facilities that are part of the prison system. Prisons are found in crowded cities, in towns, and in remote rural areas. For greater "security," they may be concentrated on islands as, for instance, the prisons of New York City are concentrated on Riker's Island.† While

---

* Murtha, Rena: *op. cit.*
† Winstead-Fry, Patricia: "Health Care in Prison: Change in One City's System. Mental Health Nursing of Inmates," *Am. J. Nurs.,* **75**:425, (Mar.) 1975.

* Mitford, Jessica: *op. cit.,* p. 3.
† Since a person on foot might be mistaken for an escaping prisoner, workers and visitors on Riker's Island are forbidden to go from one institution to another except by car. This gives the whole island a strange forsaken appearance. There are roads but no sidewalks or footpaths.

"correction" or "rehabilitation" is said to be the dominant purpose of the penal system, most critics of it think that punishment is the dominant if unconscious motive of society and of those who operate the system. Possibly for this reason, prisons are usually grim and forbidding. Prisoners and their visitors in some prisons have nothing to sit on as they look at each other through a murky glass window and talk to each other over a telephone. Furnishings of health services look as if they might be objects discarded when certain hospitals were renovated decades earlier. While the maintenance of some prisons is excellent, in others, it is intolerable. Buildings are dark inside because windows are coated with grime and the human odor of crowded quarters is masked in some cases by the reek of carbolic disinfectants, an aspect of hospital life that has long since been corrected in most countries. It would almost seem as if society were trying to punish visitors and those who staff prisons as well as the prisoners themselves.

If, as Jane A. Kennedy and others recommend, prisoners go outside prisons for health service, the physical plan and furnishings of the health facility may not differ from those for free citizens. Units for the criminally insane in psychiatric hospitals look like any other unit offering "maximum security"; the presence of correction officers may be conspicuous or they may be almost unnoticeable. Health personnel, if employed in sufficient numbers and if given a voice in policy-making on the administration of prisons, could materially affect not only the design and furnishing of the health service units but that of the entire prison or correctional institution.

Organization and Administration of Prison Health Services. Since imprisonment is the result of court action, prisons have been organized and administered by national, state, county, and municipal justice departments. In the United States, there is a Bureau of Prisons within the Department of Justice. Under a 1930 Act (4.6 Stat 273; 18 USC 4005), the US Public Health Service provides health services to federal prisoners.* Within the Bureau of Prisons, there is a medical director who is a Public Health Service officer. Until 1972, all Federal Prison Medical Service personnel were members of the Public Health Service Commissioned Corps or Civil Service. Since June 1972, all Civil Service employees have been under the Bureau of Prisons in the Department of Justice.[54]

The 1972 study, *Health Care Services in the Canadian Penitentiary Service,* a study made within the Department of the Solicitior General, contains the following statement:

The health care services provided to inmates are similar to those provided to the general public, the difference lies in the method of delivery of these services.

The health care services required by an inmate are obtained through different types of health care centres either in the institution where he resides or in another institution, D.N.D. facilities, D.V.A. hospitals, or public institutions, depending on the nature of the services.

Usually the health care centre in an institution is under the direction of a Senior Hospital Officer who reports to an Assistant Deputy Warden for administrative purposes but who receives his medical direction from the institution medical officer and various other medical professionals dispensing medical care within the institution. The institution Medical Officer theoretically reports to the same person and supervises the Senior Hospital Officer, but in fact most of them enjoy a great deal of autonomy and do very little supervision. This is in part due to the fact that many of these professionals are at the institutions only a few half days a week while some part-time and contract professionals often attend only one half day per week.*

In 1973, the Solicitor General of Canada appointed an Advisory Board of Psychiatrist Consultants to advise him on the treatment of mentally ill inmates.† This followed a 1960–1970 study by the Canadian Committee on Corrections that emphasized the need for greatly improved psychiatric facilities under the concept of a "just society."[55]

The Advisory Board recommended five Regional Psychiatric Centres in the CPS and a "unified psychiatric service . . . under the professional direction of a regional psychiatrist who would assign the professional staff to provide the range of services required on a priority basis." ‡

While the (Canadian) Management Consulting Service appears to accept in the federal prison system the division of responsibility for health service between the warden (or

* In 1931, Lucy Minnigerode, Superintendent of Nursing in the USPHS, described nursing in Federal prisons. (*Am. J. Nurs.,* **31**:1056, [Sept.] 1931.)

* [Canadian] Department of the Solicitor General: *op. cit.,* p. 2.

† This Advisory Board noted that Canada appears to be unique in having a correctional system split into federal and provincial jurisdictions based on *severity of sentence.* They compared this with the United States federal and state correctional systems based on the *nature of the crime.*

‡ Advisory Board of Psychiatric Consultants: *The General Program for the Development of Psychiatric Services in Federal Correctional Services in Canada.* Report of Advisory Board to Solicitor General of Canada. Department of Solicitor General, Ottawa, 1973, p. 24.

the correctional officer) and the medical director as well as the care of inmates by "paramedical" hospital officers,* the Advisory Board of Psychiatric Consultants recommends that responsibility for the kind and quality of care be in the hands of the medical (psychiatric) director and that, out of a total of 119 professionals, 92 be "nurses." [56]

The difficulty of generalizing on the organizational and administrative patterns of prison health services seems obvious, since even within these two federal systems, recent changes have occurred and radical changes have been recommended. State systems vary within the United States and provincial systems within Canada. For example, in Connecticut, Rhode Island, and Delaware, all adult correctional facilities including county jails are under the jurisdiction of the State Department of Correction. In New York State, the New York City prisons contract with the City Health Department for prison health services. Rena Murtha's position as Director of Prison Nursing Services is sufficiently unusual to merit emphasis. However, the Massachusetts Medical Advisory Committee on State Prisons recommends that all prison health services be under the control of an agency separate from the Department of Correction and that a position be created for a director of the dental program and a central nursing administrative section be set up.[57]

Nurses and all health workers who accept positions in prison health services should know to what extent they can control the amount and quality of care, for what they are responsible, and to whom they are accountable. Wardens motivated by the idea of rehabilitation and democratic concepts of administration may provide a setting in which health service personnel can develop highly effective health services; wardens motivated by the idea of punishment and authoritarian concepts of administration may provide a setting in which effective health service is impossible. This is the danger of having health service personnel accountable to the correctional staff. If, on the other hand, health services and correctional or custodial services are completely separate, a lack of communication and understanding between them may be mutually destructive. An ideal organizational and administrative plan is one that makes it possible for all within the penal system and its institutions to establish

and try to reach a common goal.* It might be noted that nurses in Great Britain and the United States have functioned as "matrons." While their work seems to be largely that of nurses, as matrons they are part of the custodial staff.[58,59]

The cost of operating a penal system was reported to be about $5000 per inmate per year in 1972 in the federal system of the United States and in California—a state believed to have one of the best systems.[60,61] From $500 to $550 is spent on health care per inmate per year in the federal and California systems. No satisfactory explanation has been given of how little of the millions spent on the prison program goes toward humane care and rehabilitation of inmates. However, Mitford, among others, suggests that the cost of "security," the salaries of correctional personnel, is proportionately high. She concludes that products of prison labor represent a lucrative business. Prisoners may produce uniforms and a wide variety of supplies for the military; they may staff laundries and bakeries that supply state or municipal institutions. Health personnel should be informed about the economics of the penal system if they are to play an effective role in improving it.

Functions, Satisfactions, Rewards, and Difficulties in Prison Nursing. Although no official figures were found on the total numbers of nurses in prison health in any country, enough was available for the United States and Canada to justify the statement that registered nurses in prison health are few in number. Adult male prisoners in the federal prisons of the United States are cared for by medical technicians and male inmates with nursing preparation or experience; women prisoners in federal prisons are cared for by a few registered nurses, by licensed practical nurses, attendants, and female inmates with some nursing preparation or experience. Adult prisoners in the federal penitentiaries of Canada appear to be cared for by paramedical personnel (variously called "hospital officers," "health care officers," "health service officers"), with varied preparation and experience. Registered nurses are employed in psychiatric units in prison health centers and in psychiatric hospitals for the criminally insane. Psychiatrists advising the Canadian Solicitor General recommend a

---

* "Hospital officers" in Canada, just as medical technicians in the United States, appear to play the major role in the federal prison health services. The school of experience is largely responsible for their preparation in both cases.

* J. D. Sullivan, in an article entitled "Without Authority," described her experience in a hospital for "mentally ill male offenders" where she thought she effected "more positive and lasting change in viewpoints" through guidance than could have been effected through "transcendent authoritative directive." (*Am. J. Nurs.*, **69**:2654, [Dec.] 1969.)

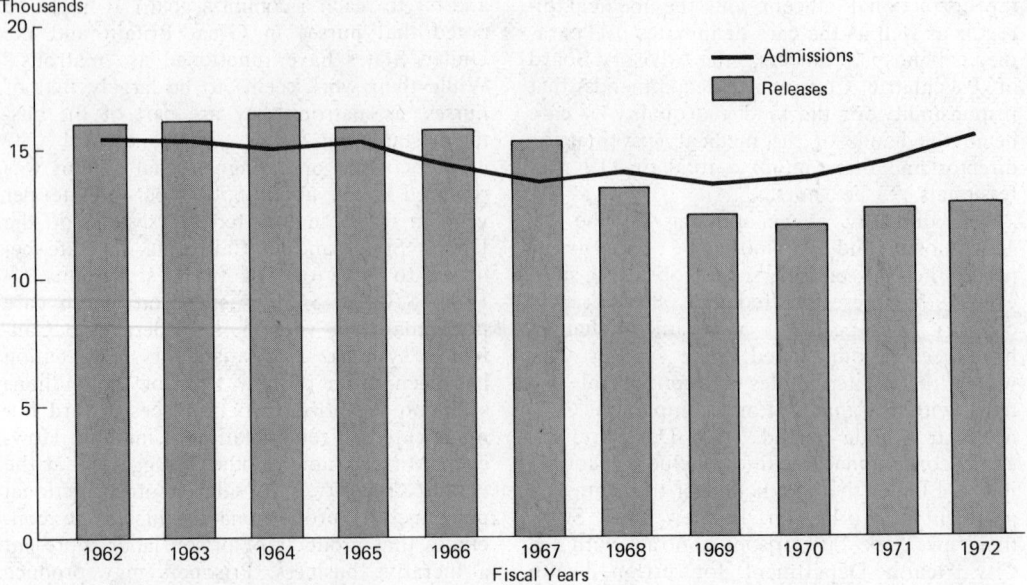

Figure 3-26. Admissions and releases, federal institutions, 1962–1972. (From US Department of Justice, Bureau of Prisons: *A Look at the Federal Prison System*. The Bureau, Washington, D.C., 1973, p. 3.)

high ratio of "professional" psychiatric nurses. The writer gets the impression from the literature that more interest is currently shown in prison health by psychiatric nurses than by nurses in any other clinical specialty. In recent years, prisons have been more likely to have full-time resident psychiatrists and clinical psychologists than any other professional medical workers, which may help to explain the interest of psychiatric nurses in prison health. Psychiatrists, of course, support professional psychiatric nurses who wish to work with inmates on the psychosocial aspects of health.

The close relationship between crime and mental illness is obvious; in fact, many persons believe both are forms of antisocial behavior. Prisons are an obvious setting for research on the causes of crime, on the so-called "psychopathic personality," on drug abuse, on traits such as aggression, on homosexuality, and on all types of behavior for which people are imprisoned. Many believe that prison populations have been exploited in this kind of research, but there has been even more exploitation in pharmacologic research. Prisoners "volunteer" as subjects for research on drugs for a variety of reasons. They may think it will help shorten their sentences, they may think that for a while they may get better food or live more comfortably, or they may want the small sums paid them in certain cases.

While professional nurses might very well be interested in the preceding types of re-

search, the writer has found no evidence of it. Some psychiatric nurses have, however, studied the effect of group therapy in prisons and have found the work rewarding.[62-66]

The principal satisfaction in prison nursing must lie in the hope of helping those who are guilty of or charged with antisocial behavior and are undergoing the punishment society metes out to those who cannot pay fines and stand bail. Psychiatric nurses, like psychiatrists, are students of behavior, and antisocial behavior may be of special interest. Pediatric nurses may elect employment in reformatories, state farms for juveniles, and junior republics because they find the emotionally disturbed and antisocial youth especially interesting or in greater need of help than those who have no such problems.

Nurses in prison health have not enjoyed an enviable status either within or without the profession, although people who have seen or read records of dedicated prison nurses serving inmates cannot fail to be impressed.[67-76] Data on salaries for prison nursing are meager and the figures found may not be representative. However, the fact that so many studies of prison health call for higher salaries for all health personnel, and in some cases for nurses specifically, suggests that nurses who have dependents may be deterred from employment in prisons by the low salaries. The experience of Jane A. Kennedy,[77] a nurse inmate, suggests that even though the salaries are low some nurses work in this setting for no other reason than that they are motivated by the desire to serve a powerless population.

The more obvious difficulties and dissatisfactions in prison nursing have been implied. Some prison health services are so organized that the custodial staff or correction officers make policies and control health workers. What the nurse can do, therefore, depends more on the philosophy of the wardens than that of medical directors. The latter may be part-time employees, and nurses may act as their deputies under standing orders that give them neither the opportunity to exercise the professional competence that the needs of inmates demand nor the legal protection nurses need if they do exercise professional judgment. When prison health services are controlled by city, county, state, or federal bodies that are centrally located and far removed from prison operation, they may not be able to give prison nurses the understanding, advice, and support they need.

When prison nurses play a negligible role in policy-making, they are frustrated in their attempts to achieve prison reform as they see it. Only when prison nurses or their nurse representatives are members of top administrative committees, boards, or councils is it possible for them to materially affect the kind and quality of the prison health service. While this condition has been mentioned several times, it is worth repeated emphasis that, since a correction officer is, in most prison settings, present or within earshot, nurses cannot have the normal, confidential, helping nurse-patient relationship to which they are accustomed. This condition must be changed and legal sanction given for holding in confidence what the inmate tells them if prison nurses are ever to practice as effectively as they might.

Prison nurses usually function in gloomy, sometimes grimy, and foul-smelling environments. To the extent that they identify with inmates they suffer for them as well as for themselves. Personnel and prisoners live during working hours in a locked and sometimes isolated institution lacking many of life's usual amenities.

Actually, the attitude of society toward prison inmates inevitably colors the attitude of health personnel. Various cultures have imprisoned, among others, political opponents of current governments (including women or ethnic groups demanding suffrage or other equal rights); persons who couldn't pay their debts (including men divorced from wives demanding alimony); "vagrants" who are jobless and without a residence; those possessing personality-altering drugs (excluding alcohol);

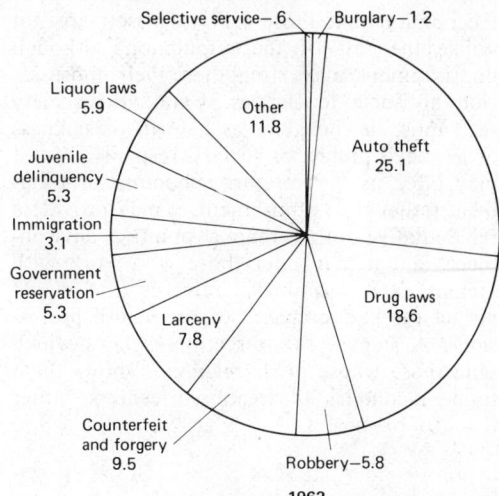

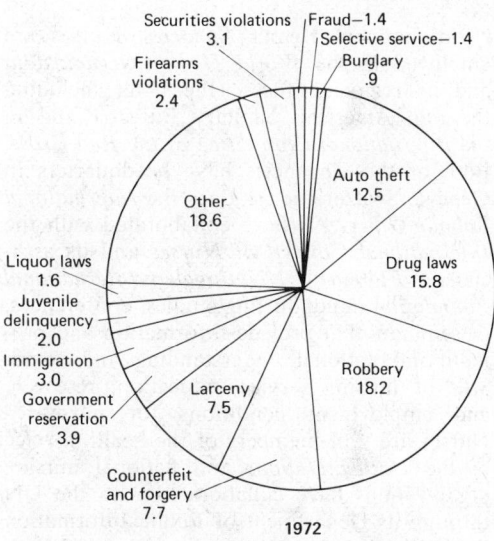

Figure 3-27. Percent of inmates confined in Bureau of Prisons' institutions, by offense, 1962 and 1972. (From US Department of Justice, Bureau of Prisons: *A Look at the Federal Prison System.* The Bureau, Washington, D.C., 1973, p. 3.)

those intoxicated by or unconscious from the use of drugs (including alcohol); those "indecently exposed"; those using obscene language; homosexuals molesting minors; perjurers; rapists; extortionists; thieves; and murderers (excepting those who kill in self-defense or those in the government services who kill political enemies of the state). Prisons (using the term in its broadest sense) in the United States are at least half full of persons suspected but not yet convicted of these "felonies" or "crimes."

Eugene Debs and other social critics who have spent months or years in prison express the opinion that those sent to prison are not unlike the rest of the population, although imprisonment may strengthen their most serious antisocial tendencies. If and when society sees antisocial behavior as a form of sickness or as social protest or social irresponsibility, it may offer its perpetrators schooling or treatment rather than punishment; it may provide a rehabilitative rather than a punitive environment; and it may offer those who work with "felons" and "criminals" rewards that would attract the best prepared of the health professions. A step in this direction is laws which send those whose public behavior shows them to be alcoholics to treatment centers rather than to prisons.

12. OTHER SETTINGS

International Health Agencies. Nurses are employed in the *World Health Organization* and its regional offices (the latter including the Pan American Sanitary Bureau) and in the *International Committee of the Red Cross.* Both of these agencies have headquarters in Geneva, Switzerland, as does the *International Labour Office.* All have collaborated with the *International Council of Nurses* and its associated *Florence Nightingale International Foundation* in conducting studies, conferences, or seminars that provide information and promote international understanding and standards of nursing service, education, research, and employment conditions for nurses.[1-10] Nurses are staff members of the health service of the *United Nations* and national nursing organizations have collaborated with the UN through its Department of Public Information in the Section for Non-Governmental Organizations.[11] Nurses played a very important role in the United Nations Relief and Rehabilitation Administration (UNRRA) following World War II.[12]

Because nursing is an essential element of most health services, nurses may be employed as staff members of or consultants to all international health agencies. No attempt is made here to find the number of nurses on the staffs of international health agencies or to assess their roles, satisfactions, and difficulties, but there is every indication that highly qualified members of the nursing profession are sought for work with international agencies and that positions in them are peculiarly satisfying to nurses with broad interests in health or human welfare.[13-17]

Missions. During the last quarter of the nineteenth century and the first quarter of the twentieth century, the Western pattern of nursing was carried to all continents and many nations by missionary nurses, but the number of journal articles on missionary nursing has steadily declined since then. Some representative articles are given at the end of this chapter.[18-26] The conditions under which missionary nurses worked have been so diverse that it is hard to give typical roles and functions. Today, health personnel, including nurses, from developed countries are more likely to be employed as consultants to governments of developing countries than to serve as missionaries. Such consultants try to help each nation develop a program suited to its peculiar culture rather than to promote the adoption of a program with which the consulting health worker is most familiar but which might be entirely unsuited to the needs of the developing country. Such work demands unusual professional competence, an understanding of the essential elements of health service, education, and research, a knowledge of the "politics of health," and an ability to work with people of different cultures. Norman Bethune, a Canadian physician, is a hero in the People's Republic of China because he helped develop a mobile system of health care suited to the needs of that country. In the 1930s, Mao Tsetung wrote an essay "In Memory of Norman Bethune" which is said to be read by most Chinese people.* [27]

Foundations. In 1967, the Russell Sage Foundation published a directory of more than 7000 agencies.[28] In a 1955 directory of 4289 foundations, from the American Foundations Information Service, 771 were listed as social welfare agencies.[29] As members of foundation staffs or as consultants to foundations concerned with health, nurses have greatly influenced nursing service, education, and research in the United States and abroad. The Commonwealth Fund, Robert Wood Johnson Foundation, W. K. Kellogg Foundation, Josiah Macy, Jr. Foundation, Milbank Memorial Fund, and Rockefeller Foundation are outstanding examples. The evolution of western medicine, including nursing, in many undeveloped or war-torn countries, owes a great debt to foundations with international programs. Foundation support is often sought within each country for new or experimental programs. Nurses on foundation staffs have a peculiar opportunity to initiate change and to

---

* Norman Bethune established a school of nursing at Chang Yu and organized a "practical work week" when doctors and nurses together bathed patients and cleaned the wards to help break down the hierarchical system and to dignify work with the hands as opposed to intellectual work.

interpret nursing to other health professionals and to the public.

Federal Government Agencies. Nurses are employed in the following federal agencies of the United States: Air Force; Army; Navy; Action/Peace Corps; Civil Service Commission; Public Health Service (within the Department of Health, Education, and Welfare) which has within it an Office of International Health, Regional Offices, the Indian Health Service, the National Institutes of Health, the Bureau of Health Resources Development, the Center for Disease Control, the Alcohol, Drug Abuse and Mental Health Administration, the Bureau of County Health Services, and other important branches; Office of Education (in the Department of Health, Education, and Welfare); Social and Rehabilitation Service (in the Department of Health, Education, and Welfare); Department of State; and Veterans Administration.* The American Nurses' Association in *Facts About Nursing 74–75* reported a total of 26,938 registered nurses employed by "selected Federal Government Agencies" in October, 1973.[29a] (In Chapter 2, page 161, Figure 2-9 shows the chief United States federal agencies concerned with health and related programs.)

The ANA divides these federal agencies into the following *executive departments:* Department of Agriculture; Department of Commerce; Department of Defense—Air Force, Army, Navy, other; Department of Health, Education, and Welfare—Health Services, Mental Health Administration, National Institutes of Health, other; Department of the Interior; Department of Justice; Department of Labor; Department of State—Agency for International Development, other; Department of Transportation; and Department of the Treasury. Nurses are also employed in the following *independent* federal agencies: Atomic Energy Commission; Canal Zone Government; Environmental Protection Agency; General Services Administration; National Aeronautics and Space Administration; Panama Canal Company; United States Postal Service; Veterans Administration; "all other agencies." † Comparable lists of federal agencies employing nurses might be given for other countries and attempts made to characterize roles of nurses in federal agencies, but both go beyond the scope of this book. However, it would be

graceless to leave the topic of nursing in federal agencies in the United States without acknowledging the influential roles they have played, and are playing. Nurses in the US Public Health Service have had far-reaching influence on nursing service, nursing education, and research. Chosen from among the best-prepared members of the profession, Public Health Service nurses have interpreted the needs of nursing, made or helped with surveys of nursing needs and resources, conducted research of various types, and influenced the allocation of federal funds for health work. Nurses within the National Institutes of Health and the Clinical Center in Bethesda have been and are participants in many health demonstrations. Nurses are increasingly found in administrative roles in federal agencies whose programs involve a total health service rather than nursing service alone.

Nurses of the Air Force, Army, Navy, and Veterans Administration care for a large segment of the population in outpatient and inpatient services and have played a significant role in promoting and conducting research.* In peacetime, their clinics, hospitals, and home care services are not very different from nonfederal institutions and agencies; during wars, nurses who serve with combatant units in field installations work under most unusual and threatening circumstances. The work of nurses in military and veterans' services has been described in books and articles, only a few of which can be listed at the end of this chapter. Standard texts on nursing history have chapters on military and war-time nursing. Descriptions of the diversified roles of nurses in the Peace Corps are also available to those who may be considering employment in its ranks.[29b-42]

Commercial Transportation. Commercial transport companies have health services for their employees. Nurses who work in such services might be said to be in occupational health nursing, which has been described. Many transport companies, in the past or currently, also employ nurses to serve their passengers as well as their crews. Nurses have served passengers in ships, trains, planes, and buses.

Ocean liners may employ a physician as well as one or more registered nurses and other health personnel. While commercial planes of this era rarely employ nurses, the first stewardesses were registered nurses, and nurses are

---

* A detailed directory of these agencies with the names of nurse administrators or consultants is published annually in the August issue of the *American Journal of Nursing.*

† American Nurses' Association: *Facts About Nursing 74–75.* The Association, Kansas City, Mo., 1976, p. 35.

* Nurses in the Space Program take part in a particularly interesting program of research on the effect of space on body function and the maintenance of life under laboratory conditions simulating those in outer space.

still found on hospital planes or airlifts for the sick and injured and on buses used to transport such passengers. Nurses are employed in many mobile medical units; they are rarely employed in ambulances these days, although they often had "ambulance duty" in the past. Nurses employed to serve passengers should be especially competent in managing emergencies and, when physicians are unavailable, they must be able to make diagnostic and therapeutic decisions. Because physician's assistants seem more willing to function in these capacities, they may be preferred by the commercial transport companies to registered nurses with a longer and, in some respects, more thorough preparation.

Nursing Organizations. The role of nursing organizations in developing and promoting standards of service, education, research, and employment conditions has been stressed throughout this chapter. Nursing organizations are *international, national, state* (or *provincial*), and *local*. They are initiated or founded by nurses. When the organization is small and new, the founders may volunteer their services, the budget may be negligible, and members may meet in their homes. As the membership, the budget, and the programs grow, headquarters offices are rented or bought and a paid staff is employed. Staffs of nursing organizations include nurses as well as non-nurses, although nurse boards, officers, and committees volunteering their services usually establish policies and plan programs to be activated by the staff. Nursing organizations that have extensive programs may provide any combination of the following services: publications, a library service, an occupational placement service, a collective bargaining service, a testing bureau; they may conduct research and a variety of educational or promotional meetings; they may conduct an information bureau; participate in joint or liaison committees; provide consultant or advisory services; and certify their members. Professional health organizations in some countries maintain offices in national or state capitals to study health legislation, to inform their memberships, and to see that their representatives are heard when bills are discussed that affect their services, preparation, employment conditions, or research.

Nurses employed on the staffs of nursing organizations occupy singularly responsible positions. They are (or should be) chosen for a broad knowledge of the health needs of the area (international, national, state or provincial, or local); the role of nursing in its relation to other health services; the characteristics of effective health services; a knowledge of health politics; an ability to collaborate with other health workers and the public and to interpret nursing in speaking and writing. According to the position a nurse occupies in the organization, other highly specialized abilities may be demanded. Officers and executive directors of official nursing organizations affect the public image of the nurse and should, if for no other reason, be appointed and elected with care; they carry a heavy burden of work, responsibility, and accountability; they deserve the gratitude of the membership as expressed in the intangibles of status. Employed staff merit but do not necessarily receive relatively high salaries; all have the satisfaction of knowing that they are in a position to influence the kind of health service available to the population they represent.

SUMMARY

Nursing is seen as the most constant factor in the health services of most countries and its function as having depended largely in every era on the presenting needs of patients. The overlapping roles of nurses, physicians, social workers, health educators, and others is believed to have existed throughout the life of professional nursing, but attention is called to the current emphasis on the nurse's "expanded role" and efforts to legalize it. The following ten settings in which nurses are employed are discussed in some detail: hospitals; nursing homes—"extended care facilities"; hospices; public health agencies; offices of private practitioners; private homes and hospitals where private duty nurses are employed; school and college health services; occupational health services; schools of nursing; and jails, prisons, and other correctional institutions. The settings are described, the numbers of nurses in the United States and Canada employed in the setting given when the figures were available, standards of nursing care noted, the rights of patients discussed, the organization and administration of nursing services in the setting described, and some attempt made to assess the functions, satisfactions, rewards, and difficulties in each setting. Nursing in international health agencies, missions, foundations, federal government agencies, commercial transportation, and nursing organizations is discussed briefly. The emphasis throughout this chapter is on nursing in the United States, but an effort has been made to compare practices in this country with those in Canada and other parts of the world and to suggest sources that might enable interested readers to go beyond the scope of this work.

REFERENCES *

It will be noted that much information on nurses and nursing has been attributed to either the ANA publication *Facts About Nursing 72–73* or *Facts About Nursing 74–75.* The reason for this is that the 74–75 publication does not in every case give or update the information in the 72–73 edition. *Countdown 1974* was the latest compendium of data on Canadian nursing available to the writer in 1976.

Introduction

1. American Nurses' Association: *Facts About Nursing 72–73.* The Association, Kansas City, Mo., 1974.
1a. American Nurses' Association: *Facts About Nursing 74–75.* The Association, Kansas City, Mo., 1976.
2. Canadian Nurses' Association: personal communication, Aug. 25, 1976.
3. Bridges, Daisy C.: *A History of the ICN 1899–1964.* Pitman Medical Publishing Co., London, 1967, p. 312.
4. American Nurses' Association: *The Nation's Nurses. 1972 Inventory of Registered Nurses.* The Association, Kansas City, Mo., 1974, p. 125.
5. Bullough, Vern, and Bullough, Bonnie: *The Emergence of Modern Nursing,* 2nd ed. Macmillan Publishing Co., Inc., New York, 1969.
6. Kelly, Lucie Young: *Dimensions of Professional Nursing,* 3rd ed. Macmillan Publishing Co., Inc., New York, 1975.
7. Knopf, Lucille: *RN's One and Five Years After Graduation.* National League for Nursing, Division of Research, New York, 1975 (Pub. No. 19–1535).

Hospitals

1. American Nurses' Association: *Facts About Nursing 74–75.* The Association, Kansas City, Mo., 1976, pp. 1, 12.
1a. ———: *Facts About Nursing 72–73.* The Association, Kansas City, Mo., 1974, p. 17.
2. Canadian Nurses' Association: Personal communication, Aug. 25, 1976.
3. American Nurses' Association: *Facts About Nursing 74–75.* The Association, Kansas City, Mo., 1976, pp. 158, 159, 164, 165.
4. Garfield, Sidney R.: "The Delivery of Medical Care," *Sci. Am.,* 222:15, (Apr.) 1970.
5. Cherkasky, Martin, and Randall, Marian G.: "A Community Home Care Program," *Am. J. Nurs.,* 49:650, (Oct.) 1949.
6. Cherkasky, Martin: "The Montefiore Hos-

pital Home Care Program," *Am. J. Public Health,* 39:163, (Feb.) 1949.
7. ———: "A Community Home Care Program," *Can. Hosp.,* 25:48, (Sept.) 1948.
8. Hilbert, Hortense: "Extending Hospital Care to the Home," *Public Health Nurs.,* 41:378, (July) 1949.
9. Richter, Lorraine, and Gonnerman, Alice: "Hospital-Administered Home Care Programs," *Hospitals,* 46:40, (May 1) 1972.
10. American Hospital Association: *The Hospital and the Home Care Program.* The Association, Chicago, 1972.
11. Calleia, Patricia, and Boswick, John A., Jr.: "A Home Care Nursing Program for Patients with Burns," *Am. J. Nurs.,* 72:1442, (Aug.) 1972.
12. Hailperin, Celia Moss: *Hospital Services for the Child at Home.* Montefiore Hospital Association of Western Pennsylvania, Pittsburgh, 1969.
13. Friedman, T. T., et al.: "The Psychiatric Home Treatment Service: A Preliminary Report of Five Years of Clinical Experience," *Am. J. Psychiatry,* 120:782 (Feb.) 1964.
14. Blagg, C. R., et al.: "The Importance of Patient Training in Home Hemodialysis," *Ann. Intern. Med.,* 73:841, (Nov.) 1970.
15. Slee, Vergil N., Director, Barry County Health Center, Hastings, Mich. Personal correspondence with the author, 1953.
16. Taylor, Sharon: "The Initiation and Development of a Hospital-Based Home Health Agency," in *ANA Clinical Conferences, 1969.* Appleton-Century-Crofts, New York, 1970.
17. Ryder, Claire F., et al.: "Home Health Services—Past, Present, Future," *Am. J. Public Health,* 59:1720, (Sept.) 1969.
18. Richardson, Henry B.: *Patients Have Families.* Commonwealth Fund, New York, 1945.
19. de Hartog, Jan: *The Hospital.* Atheneum Publishers, New York, 1964.
20. Crichton, Michael: *Five Patients. The Hospital Explained.* Alfred A. Knopf, New York, 1970.
21. Duff, Raymond S., and Hollingshead, August B.: *Sickness and Society.* Harper and Row, New York, 1968.
22. Barnes, Elizabeth (ed.): *People in Hospital.* Macmillan and Co., Ltd., London, 1961.
23. American Hospital Association: *Guide to the Health Care Field.* The Association, Chicago, 1973, p. 7. (Published annually.)
24. *Ibid.,* p. 7.
25. American College of Surgeons: *Manual of Hospital Standardization.* The College, Chicago, 1946.
26. American Hospital Association, and National League of Nursing Education: *Hospital Nursing Service Manual.* The League, New York, 1950.
27. American Nurses' Association, Congress for Nursing Practice: *Standards; Nursing Prac-*

---

* References for this chapter are organized under the chapter subheadings.

tice. The Association, Kansas City, Mo., 1973.

28. ———: *Standards of Maternal-Child Health Nursing Practice.* The Association, Kansas City, Mo., 1973.

29. ———: *Standards of Geriatric Nursing Practice.* The Association, Kansas City, Mo., 1973.

30. ———: *Standards of Psychiatric-Mental Health Nursing Practice.* The Association, Kansas City, Mo., 1973.

31. Havighurst, Clark C.: "Regulation of Health Institutions," in *Controls on Health Care.* Papers of the Conference on Regulation in the Health Industry, Jan. 7–9, 1974. National Academy of Sciences, Institute of Medicine, Washington, D.C., 1975, p. 78.

32. US Public Health Service: *The Nation's Needs for Hospitals and Health Centers.* US Government Printing Office, Washington, D.C., 1949.

33. American Hospital Association: *op. cit.,* p. 7.

34. Malleson, Andrew: *Need Your Doctor Be So Useless?* George Allen and Unwin, Ltd., London, 1973, p. 144.

35. American Hospital Association: *A Patient's Bill of Rights.* The Association, Chicago, 1972.

36. American Hospital Association: *Implementation and Information Program for a Patient's Bill of Rights.* The Association, Chicago, 1973.

37. "Bill of Rights for Patients," *Nurs. Outlook,* **21**:82, (Feb.) 1973. (See also editorial comment, p. 21, same issue.)

38. Carnegie, M. Elizabeth: "The Patient's Bill of Rights," *Nurs. Clin. North Am.,* **9**:557, (Sept.) 1974.

39. Rosner, S. S.: "The Rights of Mental Patients. The New Massachusetts Law," *Ment. Hyg.,* **56**:117, (Winter) 1972.

40. Roith, A. I.: "Rights of Mental Patients," *Lancet,* **1**:1389, (June 24) 1972.

41. International Council of Nurses, Council of National Representatives: "The CNR Resolution on Human Rights," *Int. Nurs. Rev.,* **19**:51, (No. 1) 1972.

42. "Health Care Coalition Proposed by ANA as Consumer Voice," *Am. J. Nurs.,* **71**:1500, (Aug.) 1971.

43. Kramer, Marlene: "The Consumer's Influence on Health Care," *Nurs. Outlook,* **20**:574, (Sept.) 1972.

44. Kraegel, Janet M., et al.: "A System of Patient Care Based on Patient Needs," *Nurs. Outlook,* **20**:247, (Apr.) 1972.

45. "The Plight of the U.S. Patient," *Time Magazine,* Feb. 21, 1969, p. 53.

46. Smith, Gary M.: "Experiencing Dehumanization in the Role of a Patient," *Ment. Hyg.,* **56**:75, (Winter) 1972.

47. Taylor, Carol Dickinson: "Sociological Sheep Shearing," *Nurs. Forum,* **1**:80, (Feb.) 1962.

48. Meenaghan, T. M., and Mascari, M.:

"Consumer Choice, Consumer Control in Service Delivery," *Social Work,* **16**:50, (Oct.) 1971.

49. Henderson, Virginia: "Health Is Everybody's Business," *Can. Nurse,* **67**:31, (Mar.) 1971.

50. Bettelheim, Bruno: *A Home for the Heart.* Alfred A. Knopf, New York, 1974.

51. American Nurses' Association: *Facts About Nursing 74–75.* The Association, Kansas City, Mo., 1976, p. 12.

52. Canadian Nurses Association: personal communication, Aug. 25, 1976.

53. Schlotfeldt, Rozella M., and MacPhail, Jannetta: "An Experiment in Nursing. Part 1: Rationale and Characteristics," *Am. J. Nurs.,* **69**:1018, (May) 1969; Part 2: "Introducing Planned Change," **69**:1247, (June) 1969; Part 3: "Implementing Planned Change," **69**:1475, (July) 1969.

54. American Nurses' Association, *Facts About Nursing 72–73.* The Association, Kansas City, Mo., 1974, p. 10.

55. Canadian Nurses Association: *Countdown 1974.* The Association, Ottawa, 1974. p. 12.

56. Abdellah, Faye G., and Levine, Eugene: *Patients and Personnel Speak. A Method of Studying Patient Care in Hospitals.* US Government Printing Office, Washington, D.C., 1957.

56a. Corwin, Ronald: "The Professional Employee. A Study of Conflict in Nursing Roles," *Am. J. Sociology,* **66**:604 (May) 1961.

57. Dodge, Joan S.: "Nurses' Sense of Adequacy and Attitudes Toward Keeping Patients Informed," *J. Health Human Behavior,* **2**:213, (Fall) 1961.

58. Johnson, Miriam M., and Martin, Harry W.: "A Sociological Analysis of the Nurse Role," *Am. J. Nurs.,* **58**:373, (Mar.) 1958.

59. Reissman, Leonard, and Rohrer, John H.: *Change and Dilemma in the Nursing Profession. Studies of Nursing Services in a Large General Hospital.* G. P. Putnam's Sons, New York, 1957.

60. Skipper, James K.: "The Role of the Hospital Nurse: Is It Instrumental or Expressive?" in Skipper, James K., and Leonard, Robert C.: *Social Interaction and Patient Care.* J. B. Lippincott Co., Philadelphia, 1965.

61. Nuffield Provincial Hospitals Trust: *The Work of Nurses in Hospital Wards.* The Trust, London, 1953.

62. Bates, Barbara: "Comprehensive Medicine; A Conference Approach with Inpatient Emphasis," *J. Med. Educ.,* **40**:778, (Apr.) 1965.

63. ———: "Doctor and Nurse: Changing Roles and Relations," *N. Engl. J. Med.,* **283**:129, (July 16) 1970.

64. ———, and Kern, M. Sue: "Doctor-Nurse Teamwork: What Helps? What Hinders?" *Am. J. Nurs.,* **67**:2066, (Oct.) 1967.

65. ———: "Nurse-Physician Teamwork," *Med. Care,* **4**:69, (Apr.–June) 1966.
66. Christman, Luther: "Nurse-Physician Communication in the Hospital," *J.A.M.A.,* **194**:539, (Nov. 1) 1965.
67. Dilworth, Ava S.: "Joint Preparation for Clinical Nurse Specialists," *Nurs. Outlook,* **18**:22, (Sept.) 1970.

Nursing Homes—"Extended Care Facilities"

1. American Nurses' Association, Committee on Skilled Nursing Care: *Nursing and Long-Term Care. Toward Quality Care for the Aging.* (Sister Marilyn R. Schwab, Chairman.) The Association, Kansas City, Mo., 1975, p. xvii.
1a. American Nurses' Association: *Facts About Nursing 74–75.* The Association, Kansas City, Mo., 1976, p. 158.
2. ———: *Facts About Nursing 72–73.* The Association, Kansas City, Mo., 1974, p. 224.
3. Mendelson, Mary Adelaide: *Tender Loving Greed.* Alfred A. Knopf, New York, 1974, p. XI.
4. American Nurses' Association, *op. cit.,* p. 226.
5. *Ibid.*
6. American Hospital Association: *Guide to the Health Care Field.* The Association, Chicago, 1973, p. 239.
7. Mendelson, Mary Adelaide: *op. cit.,* p. 237.
8. US Senate, Special Committee on Aging: *Introductory Report. Nursing Home Care in the United States. Failure in Public Policy.* US Government Printing Office, Washington, D.C., 1974.
8a. *US Congressional Record. Proceedings and Debates of the 93rd Congress, Second Session. Senate.* Vol. 120, No. 163, Nov. 22, 1974.
8b. American Nurses' Association, Committee on Skilled Nursing Care: *Nursing and Long-Term Care. Toward Quality Care for the Aging.* (Sister Marilyn R. Schwab, Chairman.) The Association, Kansas City, Mo., 1975, pp. 45, 26, 19, xix.
9. US Department of Health, Education, and Welfare: *Conditions of Participation; Extended Care Facilities.* The Department, Washington, D.C. (Code of Federal Regulations, HIR-11 Feb. 1968.)
10. US Senate, Special Committee on Aging: *op. cit.*
11. Aspen Systems Corporation: *Nursing Home Law Manual: The Legal Guide for Long-Term Care Institutions.* The Corporation, Pittsburgh, 1971.
12. Coggeshall, John H.: *Management of Retirement Homes and Long-Term Care Facilities.* C. V. Mosby Co., St. Louis, 1973.
13. US National Center for Health Statistics: *Nursing Homes, a County and Metropolitan Area Data Book Reported by National Center for Health Statistics.* US Government Printing Office, Washington, D.C., 1970.
14. US Community Services Administration: *Compilation of Federal Requirements for Skilled Nursing Homes.* US Government Printing Office, Washington, D.C., 1972.
15. US Public Health Service: *Hospitals and Nursing Home Equipment Planning Guide.* The Service, Washington, D.C., 1967 (PHS Pub. No. 930-D-4).
16. Braverman, Jordan: *Nursing Home Standards. A Tragic Dilemma in American Health; An Analysis by State of Nursing Home Standards Under Federal Medicine and State Licensure Programs.* American Pharmaceutical Association, Washington, D.C., 1970.
17. US Senate, Special Committee on Aging: *Alternatives to Nursing Home Care: A Proposal with Discussion of Deficiencies in Federally-Assisted Programs for Treatment of Long-Term Disability.* US Government Printing Office, Washington, D.C., 1971.
18. Callender, Marie: "Improved Nursing Home Care: National Approach to Long-Term Care," *Nurs. Outlook,* **21**:22, (Jan.) 1973.
19. Lieberman, M. A.: "Relationship of Mortality Rates to Entrance to a Home for the Aged," *Geriatrics,* **16**:515, (Oct.) 1961.
20. Marshall, D.: "A Geriatric Nursing Program for the Community," *Nurs. Clin. North Am.,* **6**:549, (Sept.) 1971.
21. Mendelson, Mary Adelaide: *op. cit.*
22. Moss, F. D.: "Is the Quality of Care Adequate in Nursing Homes? Has the Tranquilizer Replaced TLC?" *Bedside Nurse,* **5**:11, (Sept.) 1972.
23. Nichols, Lynn Wernett: "A Study of Sociopsychologic Needs of Institutionalized Chronically Ill and Aging Patients," in *ANA Clinical Conferences, 1970.* Appleton-Century-Crofts, New York, 1970.
24. Routh, Thomas A.: *Nursing Homes: A Blessing or a Curse.* Charles C Thomas, Publisher, Springfield, Ill., 1968.
25. Stotsky, B. A., and Dominick, J. R.: "Mental Patients in Nursing Homes. I. Social Deprivation and Regression," *J. Am. Geriatr. Soc.,* **17**:1, (Jan.) 1969.
26. ———: "Mental Patients in Nursing Homes. IV. Ethnic Influences," *J. Am. Geriatr. Soc.,* **17**:1, (Jan.) 1969.
27. Townsend, Claire: *Old Age. The Last Segregation. Ralph Nader's Study Group Report on Nursing Homes.* Grossman Publishers, New York, 1971.
28. Mendelson, Mary Adelaide: *op. cit.*
29. Townsend, Claire: *op. cit.*
30. Elliott, F. N.: "Goals for Quality Must Be Based on Values Derived from Changing Society," *Mod. Nurs. Home,* **27**:33, (July) 1971.
31. Ornstein, Sheldon: "Improving Nursing Home Care. Pt. 3. A Nursing Home Is Not

a Hospital," *Nurs. Outlook,* **21**:28, (Jan.) 1973.

32. Hershey, Nathan: "Issues in the Care of Nursing Home Patients," *J. Nurs. Adm.,* **3**:30, (Jan.–Feb.) 1973.

33. US Senate, Special Committee on Aging: *Legal Problems Affecting Older Americans.* US Government Printing Office, Washington, D.C., 1971.

34. Knowles, Lois N.: *Maintaining High Level Wellness in Older Years.* University of Florida Press, Gainesville, 1965.

35. American Nurses' Association: *Standards for Geriatric Nursing Practice.* The Association, Kansas City, Mo., 1973.

36. Egeday, H.: ["We Should Not Run Away from Our Responsibility,"] *Sygeplejersken,* **72**:15, (June 8) 1972.

37. "VON [Victorian Order of Nurses] Coordinates Health Care for Seniors," *Can. Nurse,* **69**:44, (Feb.) 1973.

38. Riley, Matilda White, et al.: *Aging and Society,* Vols. I, II, III. Russell Sage Foundation, New York, 1968–1972.

39. "New Hope for the Aged," *World Health,* (Apr.) 1972 (Special Issue).

40. Brantl, Virginia M., and Brown, Sister Marie Raymond; *Readings in Gerontology.* C. V. Mosby Co., St. Louis, 1973.

41. Browning, Mary H. (comp.): *Nursing and the Aging Patient.* American Journal of Nursing Co., New York, 1974 (Contemporary Nursing Series).

42. Anderson, Helen C.: *Newton's Geriatric Nursing,* 5th ed. C. V. Mosby Co., St. Louis, 1971.

43. Birchenall, Joan, and Streight, Mary E.: *Care of the Older Adult.* J. B. Lippincott Co., Philadelphia, 1973.

44. Blumberg, Jeanne E., and Drummond, Eleanor E.: *Nursing Care of the Long-Term Patient.* Springer Publishing Co., New York, 1971.

45. Brickner, Philip W. (ed.): *Care of the Nursing Home Patient.* Macmillan Publishing Co., Inc., New York, 1971.

46. Brown, Martha M.: "Personalization of the Institutionalized Older Patient," in *ANA Clinical Conferences, 1969.* Appleton-Century-Crofts, New York, 1970.

47. Burnside, Irene Mortenson: *Psychosocial Nursing; Care of the Aged.* McGraw-Hill Book Co., New York, 1973.

48. Caldwell, Esther, and Hegner, Barbara R.: *Geriatric Nursing; A Study of Maturity and Instructor's Guide.* Delmar Publishers, Albany, N.Y., 1972.

49. Callahan, Catherine L.: "The 1971 White House Conference on Aging," *Nurs. Outlook,* **20**:96, (Feb.) 1972.

50. Jaeger, Dorothea, and Simmons, Leo W.: *The Aged Ill. Coping with Problems in Geriatric Care.* Appleton-Century-Crofts, New York, 1970.

51. Moe, Mildred I.: *For Patient's Sake; A Book for All Personnel Who Care for the Aged.* Geriatric Care, Minneapolis, 1972.

52. Rudd, T. N.: *The Nursing of the Elderly Sick,* 5th ed. Faber & Faber, Ltd., London, 1966.

53. Schwenger, C. W., and Sayers, L. A.: "A Canadian Survey by Public Health Nurses of the Health and Living Conditions of the Aged," *Am. J. Public Health,* **61**:1189, (June) 1971.

54. *White House Conference on Aging. Background and Issues.* (Various reports). US Government Printing Office, Washington, D.C., 1971–.

55. Chambers, Carolyn: "Senility of Deprivation," in *ANA Clinical Sessions, 1966.* Appleton-Century-Crofts, New York, 1966.

56. Rossi, A. O., et al.: "Treating Old People Like Children Can Bring on Mental Breakdown," *Mod. Nurs. Home,* **29**:62, (Sept.) 1972.

57. Wolk, R. L., and Seiden, R. B.: "A Contagious Disease: Old Age," *J. Am. Geriatr. Soc.,* **13**:343, (Apr.) 1965.

58. Sulds, V.: "When the Children Come So Does Laughter," *Mod. Nurs. Home,* **30**:45, (Apr.) 1973.

59. Loud, M. S., et al.: "From Apathy to Involvement," *Nurs. Homes,* **20**:19, (Jan.) 1971.

60. Whitehead, J. A.: "Myths of Mental Illness in the Elderly," *Nurs. Mirror,* **133**:18, (Aug. 28) 1971.

61. Wilkiemeyer, D. S.: "Affection: Key to Care for the Elderly," *Am. J. Nurs.,* **72**:2166, (Dec.) 1972.

62. Wilson, E. H., et al.: "From Hospital to Community," *Nurs. Mirror,* **135**:17, (Aug. 18) 1972.

63. ———: "Integration of Hospital and Local-Authority Services in the Discharge of Patients from a Geriatric Unit," *Lancet,* **2**:864, (Oct. 16) 1971.

64. US Senate, Special Committee on Aging: *Making Services for the Elderly Work: Some Lessons from the British Experience.* US Government Printing Office, Washington, D.C., 1971.

65. Jacobs, S. E.: "Older Patients Get More Care: AHA Nursing Activity Study Questions Equity of Medicare Reimbursement Formula," *Hospitals,* **43**:68, (Dec.) 1969.

66. Kramer, C. H.: "The Next Step—Total Therapeutic Care," *Geriatric Institutions,* **6**:12, (Fall) 1964.

67. Ornstein, Sheldon: "A Program of Staff-Resident Interaction to Diminish the Negative Effects of Institutionalization of the Aged Person," in *ANA Clinical Sessions, 1970.* Appleton-Century-Crofts, New York, 1971.

68. Rapelje, Douglas H.: "A Home for the Aged Where People Live," *Can. Nurse,* **64**:45, (Nov.) 1968.

69. Tuck, B. R.: "Telling It Like It Was . . .

and Like It Is Now," *Nurs. Homes,* **10**:20, (Oct.) 1970.

70. Farnsworth, E. L.: "Rehabilitation Is Becoming Routine, Survey Shows," *Mod. Nurs. Home,* **50**:4, (Jan.) 1973.

71. Wilson, Margaret: "A Guide for the Public Health Nurse to Assist Elderly Patients in the Achievement of Selected Functional Tasks at Home," *Int. J. Nurs. Studies,* **7**:243, (Nov.) 1970.

72. Schwartz, Doris: "Nursing Care of the Aged," in Rossman, Isadore (ed.): *Clinical Geriatrics.* J. B. Lippincott Co., Philadelphia, 1971.

73. ———, et al.: *The Elderly Ambulatory Patient. Nursing and Psychosocial Needs.* Macmillan Publishing Co., New York, 1964.

74. May, S. H.: *The Crowning Years.* J. B. Lippincott Co., Philadelphia, 1969.

75. Kinsella, Patricia: "Geriatric Nursing: It Can Be Rewarding, Fulfilling, Exciting," *Hosp. Adm. Can.,* **14**:52, (Dec.) 1972.

76. Nelson, J.: "Second-Class Nurses," *Nurs. Mirror,* **134**:20, (May 12) 1972.

77. Winston, W. A.: "What Do the Professionals Think and Say About Geriatric Nurses?" *AAMA Executive,* **11**:5, (Jan.) 1972.

78. Tuck, B. R.: "The Geriatric Nurse, A Pioneer in a New Specialty," *RN,* **35**:35, (Aug.) 1972.

Hospices

1. "The Problems Created by Medical Progress. What Do You Do for the Aged—and When Do You Stop Doing It?" *Med. World News,* **13**:42, (Apr. 7) 1972

2. Quint, Jeanne C.: *The Nurse and the Dying Patient.* Macmillan Publishing Co., Inc., New York, 1967.

3. Saunders, Cicely: "The Last Stages of Life," *Am. J. Nurs.,* **65**:70, (Mar.) 1965.

4. ———: *Care of the Dying.* Macmillan Co., Ltd., London, 1966.

5. ———: "A Therapeutic Community: St. Christopher's Hospice," in Schoenberg, Bernard, et al. (eds.): *Psychosocial Aspects of Terminal Care.* Columbia University Press, New York, 1972.

6. St. Christopher's Hospice: *Annual Reports.* The Hospice, London.

7. Craven, Joan, and Wald, Florence: "Hospice Care for Dying Patients," *Am. J. Nurs.,* **75**:181, (Oct.) 1975.

8. Dobihal, Edward F., Jr.: "Talk or Terminal Care?" *Conn. Med.,* **38**:364, (July) 1975.

Public Health Agencies

1. American Nurses' Association: *Facts About Nursing 74–75.* The Association, Kansas City, Mo., 1976, pp. 3, 19, 20.

2. Canadian Nurses' Association: personal communication, Aug. 25, 1976.

3. American Nurses' Association: *Facts About Nursing 72–73.* The Association, Kansas City, Mo., 1974, pp. 34, 36.

4. *Ibid.,* p. 33.

5. McCarrick, Helen: "Careers in Nursing: Key Figure of the Future—the Health Visitor," *Nurs. Times,* **67**:1243, (Oct. 7) 1971.

6. Butterworth, J.: "The Community Nursing Services; The Need for Change," *J. Health Visit.,* **45**:353, (Nov.) 1972.

7. Clark, June: "The 'New Breed' Health Visitor," *Nurs. Times,* **68**:121, (Aug. 3) 1972.

8. Collière, M. F.: "The Functions of the Public Health Nurse," *Int. Nurs. Rev.,* **18**:6, (Jan.) 1971.

9. "The Start of a New Era for the National Health Service," *Dist. Nurs.,* **15**:261, (Mar.) 1974.

10. Driscoll, B.: "The Changing Face of Public Health Nursing in Great Britain Today and the SSAFA Nursing Service," *Health Visit.,* **43**:277, (Aug.) 1970.

11. Royal College of Nursing, and National Council of Nurses of the United Kingdom: *District Nursing—Functions, Training and Opportunities.* The College and Council, London, 1975.

12. Hagger, H.: "A Day in the Life of an English Health Visitor," *Aust. Nurses J.,* **2**:8, (June) 1973.

13. Hunt, Maura: "The Dilemma of Identity in Health Visiting," *Nurs. Times,* **68**:17, (Feb. 3) 1972.

14. Kergin, Dorothy J.: "Symposium on Community Nursing in Canada," *Nurs. Clin. North Am.,* **6**:463, (Sept.) 1971.

15. Subhadra, V., et al.: "An Evaluation of Public Health Nursing Services at an Urban Health Centre," *Int. J. Nurs. Studies,* **7**:257, (Nov.) 1970.

16. Thorpe, E.: "Health Visiting Objectives and the Role of the Health Visitor. A Need for Organizational Research," *Health Visit.,* **46**:156, (May) 1973.

17. Anderson, J. A. D., et al.: "Attachment of Community Nurses to General Practices: A Follow-up Study," *Br. Med. J.,* **4**:103, (Oct. 10) 1970.

18. Day, J. J., et al.: "A Study of the Effect of Collaboration Between Family Physician and Public Health Nurse," *Can. Fam. Physician,* **15**:65, (Aug.) 1969.

19. Davis, E. J.: *Public Health Nurse with Group Practice.* National League for Nursing, New York, 1972.

20. Heaton, Peter, and Fleet, Darlene: "The Doctor and the Community Health Nurse," *Can. Fam. Physician,* **17**:71, (Aug.) 1971.

21. Rosser, W. W., and Barrie, Brenda: "The Role of the Municipally Employed Public Health Nurse in a Family Practice Unit," *Can. J. Public Health,* **63**:165, (Mar.—Apr.) 1972.

21a. Milne, Barbara: "A Public Health Nurse in a Family Medical Center," *Can. Fam. Physician,* **19:**99, (Jan.) 1973.

22. Helmer, L. S.: "A Public Health Nurse's Activities in a Private Physician's Practice. A Report of a Pilot Project," *Nurs. Clin. North Am.,* **5:**233, (June) 1970.

23. Hutchison, D. A., and Mumby, Dorothy M.: "Public Health Nurses Work with Family Physicians," *Can. Nurse.,* **66:**28, (Jan.) 1970.

24. Shannon, Iris R.: "More Nursing per Square Mile; A Neighborhood Center Provides a Pivotal Point for Extending Health Care to Indigent Residents of an Inner City," *Nurs. Outlook,* **18:**42, (Apr.) 1970.

25. Smiley, Olga Roman: "The Family-Centered Approach—A Challenge to Public Health Nurses," *Can. J. Public Health,* **63:**424, (Sept.–Oct.) 1972.

26. Victorian Order of Nurses, Richmond-Vancouver Branch: *The Victorian Order Nurse Associate. A Descriptive Study of the Attachment of a Victorian Order Nurse to a Selected Group of Family Physicians.* The Order, Vancouver, 1971.

26a. Schutt, Barbara: "Frontier's Family Nurses," *Am. J. Nurs.,* **72:**903, (May) 1972.

26b. Bernal, Henrietta: "Power and Interorganizational Health Care Projects," *Nurs. Outlook,* **24:**418, (July) 1976.

27. Garfield, Sidney R.: "The Delivery of Medical Care," *Sci. Am.,* **222:**15, (Apr.) 1970.

28. Somers, Anne R.: *Health Care in Transition: Directions for the Future.* Hospital Research and Educational Trust, Chicago, 1971.

29. Waters, Yssabella: *Visiting Nursing in the United States.* Charities Publication Committee, New York, 1909.

30. Gardner, Mary Sewall: "The National Organization for Public Health Nursing," *Visiting Nurse Q.,* **4:**13, (July) 1912.

31. Roberts, Mary M.: *American Nursing—History and Interpretation.* Macmillan Publishing Co., Inc., New York, 1954, p. 83.

32. Wiesner, Dorothy E., and Murphy, Margaret M.: "Similarities and Variations in Programs." *Public Health Nurs.,* **34:**100, (Feb.) 1942.

33. American Nurses' Association: *Standards. Community Health Nursing Practice.* The Association, Kansas City, Mo., 1973.

34. "Community Nursing Services Accredited by NLN-APHA, April 1974," *Nurs. Outlook,* **22:**270, (Apr.) 1974.

34a. National League for Nursing: *Directory of Home Health Agencies Certified as Medicare Providers.* The League, New York, 1975.

35. Arcand, Lisette: "New Health Programs in Quebec—A Trend for the Future," *Can. Nurse,* **68:**27, (Dec.) 1972.

36. Ebert, B., et al.: "A Study of the Ac-

tivities of Nursing Personnel in Ten Health Units and One City Health Department in the Province of Alberta, 1968," *Can. J. Public Health,* **61:**126, (Mar.–Apr.) 1970.

37. Davies, Brian Meredith: *Community Health and Social Services.* English Universities Press, London, 1972.

38. Gareau, Olivette: "Public Health Nurses in Quebec and the Castenguay-Nepveu Report," *Can. J. Public Health,* **62:**339, (July–Aug.) 1971.

39. Kergin, Dorothy J.: "Symposium on Community Nursing in Canada," *Nurs. Clin. North Am.,* **6:**463, (Sept.) 1971.

40. Leahy, Kathleen M., et al.: *Community Health Nursing.* McGraw-Hill Book Co., New York, [1972].

41. National League for Nursing, Department of Home Health Agencies and Community Health Services: *Community Health—Strategies for Change.* (Papers presented at 1972 Regional Meeting of Council of Home Health Agencies and Community Health Services.) The League, New York, 1973.

42. ———: *The Community Health Nurse Is Where You Need Her.* (Council of Home Health Agencies and Community Health Services.) The League, New York, 1975 (Pub. No. 21–1601).

43. McLachlan, Dorothy: "A New Look in Public Health Nursing," *Can. J. Public Health,* **63:**527, (Nov.–Dec.) 1972.

44. Smiley, O. R.: "The Core Committee—A New Model for Decision Making Within Public Health Units," *Can. J. Public Health,* **64:**290, (May–June) 1973.

45. Stinson, Shirley M.: "New and Changing Roles in Public Health Nursing," *Can. J. Public Health,* **61:**317, (July–Aug.) 1970.

46. Tinkham, Catherine W., and Voorhies, Eleanor F.: *Community Health Nursing; Evolution and Process.* Appleton-Century-Crofts, New York, [1972].

47. Snyder, Lilja A.: "We Care Enough to Come to You," *Nurs. Outlook,* **22:**168, (Mar.) 1974.

48. Afek, Luella Barron, and Hickey, Jane: "Health Classes for Migrant Workers' Families," *Am. J. Nurs.,* **72:**1296, (July) 1972.

49. Barckley, V.: "Cancer Consultant to Nursing Homes," *Am. J. Nurs.,* **70:**804, (Apr.) 1970.

50. Archer, Sarah E., and Fleshman, Ruth P. (eds.): *Community Health Nursing: Patterns and Practice.* Duxbury Press, North Scituate, Mass., 1975.

51. Chladek, Marian: "Nursing Service for Agricultural Migrants," *Am. J. Nurs.,* **65:**62, (June) 1965.

52. Downey, Dorothy: "Public Health Nurses' Attitudes Toward Patients with a Psychiatric Diagnosis," *Nurs. Res.,* **18:**244, (May–June) 1969.

53. Keywood, O.: "Night Nursing on the Dis-

trict," *Nurs. Times,* **69:**974, (July 26) 1973.

54. Mitch, A. D., and Kaczala, S.: "Public Health Nurse Coordinator in a General Hospital," *Nurs. Outlook,* **16:**34, (Feb.) 1968.

55. MacArthur, M. Christine: "Visiting Nursing North of the Border," *Nurs. Clin. North Am.,* **4:**333, (June) 1969.

56. Turner, Lettie: "The Nurse Specialist or Clinician in Public Health Nursing," *Can. J. Public Health,* **64:**196, (Mar.) 1973.

57. Wright, Ora: "The Mental Health Component in a Public Health Nursing Caseload," *Can. J. Public Health,* **63:**427, (Sept.–Oct.) 1972.

58. "In Indian Health Services Nurses Play Key Role," *Your Health,* **55:**7, (July–Aug.) 1969.

58a. Archer, Sarah E., and Fleshman, Ruth P.: "Community Health Nursing: A Typology of Practice," *Nurs. Outlook,* **23:**358, (June) 1975.

59. American Public Health Association, Committee on Professional Education: "Educational Qualifications of Public Health Nurses," *Am. J. Public Health,* **52:**501, (Mar.), 1962.

60. Canadian Public Health Association: *A Statement of Functions and Qualifications for the Practice of Public Health Nursing in Canada.* The Association, Toronto, 1967.

61. American Nurses' Association: *Functions and Qualifications in the Practice of Public Health Nursing.* The Association, Kansas City, Mo., 1964.

62. World Health Organization: *Public Health Nursing. Fourth Report of the Expert Committee on Nursing.* The Committee, Geneva, 1959 (Tech. Series No. 167).

63. American Nurses' Association: *Facts About Nursing 72–73.* The Association, Kansas City, Mo., 1974, p. 10.

64. *Ibid.,* pp. 132, 147.

65. Brock, L.: "Salaries in Community Health Services, 1973," *Nurs. Outlook,* **21:**785, (Dec.) 1973.

66. Arcand, Lisette: "New Health Programs in Quebec—A Trend for the Future," *Can. Nurse,* **68:**12, (Dec.) 1972.

67. Bates, Barbara: "Nursing in a Health Maintenance Organization," *Am. J. Public Health,* **62:**991, (July) 1972.

68. Berger, Michael, et al.: "A Case Study in Professional Collaboration," *Nurs. Outlook,* **20:**714, (Nov.) 1972.

69. Brown, Douglas R.: "Community Health Planning or Who Will Control the Health Care System?" *Am. J. Public Health,* **62:**1336, (Oct.) 1972.

70. Canadian Public Health Association: "Council Policy on Regionalization of Health Services," *Can. J. Public Health,* **63:**368, (July–Aug.) 1972.

71. Hastings, John E. F.: "For the Well-Being of Canadians—Community Health Centers?" *Can. Welfare,* **48:**4, (Mar./Apr.) 1972.

72. Jones, Phyllis E., and Bondy, Doreen M.: "Family Health Service: The P.H.N. and the G.P.," *Can. Nurse,* **65:**38, (Sept.) 1969.

73. Stinson, Shirley M.: "New and Changing Roles in Public Health Nursing," *Can. J. Public Health,* **61:**317, (July–Aug.) 1970.

74. Truscott, Lionel B.: "Health Care Delivery in the Community," *J.A.M.A.,* **221:**289, (July 17) 1972.

75. Wallace, J. D.: "The Community Health Center Project Report," *Can. J. Public Health,* **63:**381, (Sept.–Oct.) 1972.

Offices of Private Practitioners

1. Dugale, N.: "Midwifery and the Integration of Health Services," *Midwives Chron.,* **83:**400, (Dec.) 1970.

2. Gold, E. M.: "Public Health Aspects of Future Ob-Gyn Services," *Obstet. Gynecol.,* **41:**461, (Mar.) 1973.

3. Grimm, L. M.: "Changed Patterns of Obstetric Care: Maternity Continuity Clinic," *Am. J. Nurs.,* **73:**1723, (Oct.) 1973.

4. Harris, M.: "The Work of a 'Nurse Practitioner.' Experience of Two Years in a West Midlands Group Practice," *Nurs. Times,* **66:**1402, (Oct. 29) 1970.

5. Lees, R. E.: "Physician Time-Saving by Employment of Expanded-Role Nurse in Family Practice," *Can. Med. Assoc. J.,* **108:**871, (Apr. 7) 1974.

6. Murata, J. E.: "The Nurse as a Family Practitioner," *Am. J. Nurs.,* **74:**254, (Feb.) 1974.

7. "Nurses in General Practice," *Lancet,* **2:**1350, (Dec. 26) 1970.

8. Milio, Nancy: "Getting Resources for Innovation in Health Care," *J. Nurs. Adm.,* **1:**40, (May–June) 1971.

9. "Nurses and the New Health Service. Details and Aims of the Reorganization," *Nurs. Times,* **68:**1166, (Sept 14) 1972.

10. Pang, H.: "An Approach to Primary Care. The Role of the General Practitioner and the General Practice Nurse," *Aust. Nurs. J.,* **2:**18, (Feb.) 1973.

11. Smith, R. A.: "MEDEX—An Operational and Replicated Manpower Program: Increasing the Delivery of Health Services," *Am. J. Public Health,* **62:**1563, (Dec.) 1972.

12. *Working Together. A Study of Coordination and Cooperation Between General Practice, Public Health and Hospital Services.* King Edward's Hospital Fund, London, 1968.

13. Wieler, A.: "Physician's Substitute—the Role of the Nurse in the North," *Can. J. Public Health,* **62:**333, (July–Aug.) 1971.

14. Kuenssberg, E. V.: "The Management of Staff in General Practice. The Nurse—A Luxury or a Necessity in General Prac-

tice?" *J. R. Coll. Gen. Pract.,* **19:**(Suppl) 34, (June) 1970.

15. Abrams, Herbert K.: "Neighborhood Health Centers," *Am. J. Public Health,* **61:**2236, (Nov.) 1971.

16. Bates, Barbara: "Nursing in a Health Maintenance Organization," *Am. J. Public Health,* **62:**991, (July) 1972.

17. Levy, B. S., et al.: "Reducing Neonatal Mortality Rate with Nurse-Midwives," *Am. J. Obstet. Gynecol.,* **109:**50, (Jan. 1) 1971.

18. McCormack, R. C., et al.: "Family Doctors' Use of Office Assistants and Opinions Regarding Nurses in Primary Care," *South. Med. J.,* **64:**415, (Apr.) 1971.

19. Mauksch, Ingeborg G., and Young, Paul D.: "Nurse-Physician Interaction in a Family Medical Care Center," *Nurs. Outlook,* **22:**108, (Feb.) 1974.

20. Record, Jane Cassels, and Cohen, H. R.: "The Introduction of Midwifery in a Prepaid Group Practice," *Am. J. Public Health,* **62:**354, (Mar.) 1972.

21. Silver, H. K., et al.: "Time-Motion Study of Pediatric Nurse Practitioners: Comparison with 'Regular' Office Nurses and Pediatricians," *J. Pediatr.,* **79:**331, (Aug.) 1971.

22. American Nurses' Association: *Facts About Nursing 72–73.* The Association, Kansas City, Mo., 1974, p. 227.

23. *Ibid.,* p. 10.

24. Canadian Nurses' Association: personal communication, Aug. 25, 1976.

25. Parsons, Esther Jane: *In the Doctor's Office. The Art of the Medical Assistant,* 2nd ed. J. B. Lippincott Co., Philadelphia, 1956.

26. Bredow, Miriam: *The Medical Assistant; A Guide for the Nurse, Secretary, and Technician for the Doctor's Office.* McGraw-Hill Book Co., New York, 1958.

27. Lawton, M. Murray, and Foy, Donald F.: *A Textbook for Medical Assistants,* 2nd ed. C. V. Mosby Co., St. Louis, 1971.

28. American Nurses' Association: "Statement of Functions," [Functions of Office Nurses prepared by Office Nurses Conference Group.] *Am. J. Nurs.,* **54:**994, (Aug.) 1954.

29. Schick, Johnnye C.: "Office Nurses Are on Their Way," *Am. J. Nurs.,* **54:**429, (Apr.) 1954.

30. Long, Elizabeth, and Young, Matilda L.: "Office Nurses Make History—'the First' in the United States," *Nurs. World,* **125:**334, (Aug.) 1951.

31. American Nurses' Association, Research and Statistics Unit: *Survey of Employment Conditions of Professional Registered Office Nurses.* The Association, Kansas City, Mo., 1958.

32. American Nurses' Association: "Statement of Functions," op. cit.

33. American Nurses' Association: *Facts About Nursing 72–73.* The Association, Kansas City, Mo., 1974, p. 10.

34. Canadian Nurses' Association: personal communication, Aug. 25, 1976.

35. American Nurses' Association: *Facts About Nursing 74–75.* The Association, Kansas City, Mo., 1976, p. 131.

Homes and Hospitals (as "Private Duty" Nurses)

1. Dubin, Maurice: "Special Nursing—Is It a Necessity or a Luxury?" *Mod. Hosp.,* **42:**89, (Mar.) 1934.

2. Brent, Kenneth A.: "Should Private Duty Nurses Be Barred? Majority in Hospital Poll Says 'No'," *Hosp. Manage.,* **61:**70, (Mar.) 1946.

3. Gidlow, Elsa: "Private Duty Fights for Its Life," *R.N.,* **7:**34, (Jan.) 1944.

4. Dudley, Martha: "Is Private Duty Nursing on the Way Out?" *R.N.,* **22:**46, (June) 1959.

5. American Nurses' Association: *Facts About Nursing 72–73.* The Association, Kansas City, Mo., 1974, pp. 10, 17.

6. Canadian Nurses' Association: personal communication, Aug. 25, 1976.

7. Roberts, Mary M.: *American Nursing—History and Interpretation.* Macmillan Publishing Co., New York, 1954, p. 120.

8. Larsson, Bergilot: "Private Nursing," *Am. J. Nurs.,* **25:**895, (Nov.) 1925.

9. Parsons, Sara Elizabeth: "Why Private Nurses Should Organize," *Am. J. Nurs.,* **16:**299, (Jan.) 1916.

10. DeWitt, Katharine: *Private Duty Nursing.* J. B. Lippincott Co., Philadelphia, 1913.

11. American Nurses' Association, Private Duty Section: Annual and Biennial Reports, 1916–28, in *Proceedings, 19th–26th Conventions.* The Association, New York, 1916–28.

12. American Nurses' Association: "Functions, Standards, and Qualifications for Practice of Private Duty Nursing," *Am. J. Nurs.,* **56:**1030, (Aug.) 1956.

13. Royal College of Nursing, and National Council of Nurses of the United Kingdom: *The Privately Employed Nurse. Recommended Fees and Conditions of Service.* The College and the Council, London, 1973.

14. Roberts, Mary M.: *op. cit.,* p. 117.

15. Thornton, Mary E.: "The Organization and Management of Clubs and Homes for Graduate Nurses," *Am. J. Nurs.,* **1:**378, (Feb.) 1901.

16. Fenwick, Ethel Gordon: "Private Nursing," *Nurs. Record,* **28:**349, (May 3) 1902.

17. "New York Hospital [School of Nursing] Graduated Nurses' Clubs," *Am. J. Nurs.,* **5:**169, (Dec.) 1905.

18. Russell, Martha A.: "Club-houses," *Am. J. Nurs.,* **5:**802, (Aug.) 1905.

19. Foster, Reba Thelin: "The Organization of Nurses' Clubs and Directories Under State Associations," *Am. J. Nurs.,* **9:**247, (Jan.) 1909.

20. "Central Club [New York, N.Y.] for Nurses," *Mod. Hosp.,* **14:**36, (Jan.) 1920.

21. Beatle, Alice C.: "The Isabel Hampton

Robb Memorial Club, Cleveland, Ohio," *Am. J. Nurs.,* **13:**436, (Mar.) 1913.

22. "Pittsburgh [Pa.] Opens its Nurses' Club," *Am. J. Nurs.,* **27:**11, (Jan.) 1927.

23. "General Nursing Council of Scotland—The Register of Nurses," *Br. J. Nurs.,* **71:**280, (Nov. 3) 1923.

24. Correl, Carrie B.: "The Industrial Nurses' Club of Cleveland, Ohio," *Public Health Nurse,* **12:**116, (Feb.) 1920.

25. "The College of Nursing Club in Birmingham [Eng.]," *Nurs. Mirror,* **38:**9, (Oct. 6) 1923.

26. Richardson, Linna G.: "Reasons for Central Registries and Club Houses," *Am. J. Nurs.,* **9:**983, (Sept.) 1909.

27. Burgess, Elizabeth C.: "The Future of the Central Registry," *Am. J. Nurs.,* **15:**1033, (Aug.) 1915.

28. Rein, Anna: "The Relation of the Private Nurse to the Registry," *Am. J. Nurs.,* **14:**831, (July) 1914.

29. Rutley, Sophia L.: "Private Duty Nurses and Their Relationship to the Directory," *Am. J. Nurs.,* **15:**939, (Aug.) 1915.

30. "Official Registries and Professional Progress," *Am. J. Nurs.,* **26:**91, (Feb.) 1926.

31. *Nurses' and Physicians' Directory and Health Book of New Haven County [Conn.].* New Haven City Printing Co., New Haven, 1923.

32. Simon, Carlton (ed.): *Shobers Directory of Trained Nurses. Being a Selected List of Names and Addresses of Competent Graduated Trained Nurses Practicing in the Cities of Greater New York, Boston, Philadelphia, Baltimore and Washington.* Shober-Cornell Publishing Co., New York, 1902.

33. Matron's Council of Great Britain and Ireland: *Nursing Directory for 1901. 10th Annual Issue.* Nursing Record, London, 1901.

34. "Burdett's Official Nursing Directory," *Hosp. (Lond) Nurs. Mirror,* **27:**195, (Jan. 13) 1900.

35. "Official Directory Bill," *Br. J. Nurs.,* **40:**245, (Mar. 28); 330, (Apr. 25); 352, (May 2); 371, (May 9); 389, (May 16) 1908.

36. "Presentation of the First Statutory Register to Mrs. Bedford Fenwick," *Br. J. Nurs.,* **70:**390, (June) 1923.

37. Cabot, Richard C.: "A Statistical Study of the Educational Opportunities Offered in the Massachusetts Training Schools for Nurses," *Am. J. Nurs.,* **6:**438, (Apr.) 1906.

38. Littauer, David, and Swenson, Vada C.: "Everybody Benefits by Menorah Hospital's Plan of Group Nursing Service," *Mod. Hosp.,* **76:**69, (May) 1951.

39. Pastore, Evelyn: "Share the Nurse Plan," *Nurs. World,* **126:**17, (July) 1952.

40. Wellenkamp, Jeanne: "All Groups Benefit by Group Nursing Plan," *Mod. Hosp.,* **92:**67, (Apr.) 1959.

41. Bredenberg, Viola Constance: *A Functional Analysis of the Nursing Service Team.* Catholic University of America Press, Washington, D.C., 1949.

42. Berger, Harriett, and Johnson, Marjorie: "Developing the Nursing Team at St. Luke's Hospital, Chicago, Ill.," *Am. J. Nurs.,* **49:**442, (July) 1949.

43. Jones, Elizabeth, and Ellsworth, Joan Grube: "An Experiment in Team Assignment," *Am. J. Nurs.,* **49:**146, (Mar.) 1949.

44. Gray, Carolyn E., and Lockwood, Marie T.: "The Relation of the Private Duty Nurse to the Public, as an Educator, as a Social Worker," *Am. J. Nurs.,* **17:**1193, (Sept.) 1917.

45. Clayton, S. Lillian: "The Social Training of the Private Duty Nurse," *Am. J. Nurs.,* **17:**506, (Mar.) 1917.

46. Beeby, Nell V.: "The Private Nurse as a Teacher," *Am J. Nurs.,* **36:**778, (Aug.) 1936.

47. Burgess, May Ayres: *Nurses, Patients, and Pocketbooks.* Committee on the Grading of Nursing Schools, New York, 1928.

48. Bickel, Elsie: "Remuneration of Private Duty Nursing," *Am. J. Nurs.,* **13:**278, (Jan.) 1913.

49. McMillan, Clara Barton: "Private Duty Nursing," *Am. J. Nurs.,* **19:**7, (Oct.) 1919.

50. Ott, Frances M.: "Private Duty, Past and Present," *Trained Nurse,* **80:**696, (June) 1928.

51. "Results of Study of Private Duty Nursing in New York Shows Nurses in State Earned Only 49 Cents Per Hour During Week of February 21 to 28, About Even with Charwomen, Servants and Unskilled Workers," *Public Health J. (Can.),* **17:**413, (Aug.) 1926.

52. Burgess, Mary Ayres: "The Generosity of Nurses," *Am. J. Nurs.,* **27:**931, (Nov.) 1927.

53. Luck, Mary Gorringe: "The Cost of Living of the Private Duty Nurse," *Pac. Coast J. Nurs.,* **26:**573, (Sept.) 1930.

54. Scott, Alma Ham, and Best, Ella: "Schemes for Supervision and Regular Allowances for Private Duty Nurses," *Int. Nurs. Rev.,* **9:**110, (Jan.) 1934.

55. Geister, Janet M.: "Hearsay and Facts in Private Duty," in American Nurses' Association: *Proceedings, Twenty-Fifth Convention. 1926.* The Association, Kansas City, Mo., 1926.

56. ———: "Private Duty Nursing Then—and Now," *Trained Nurse,* **100:**383, (Apr.) 1938.

57. ———: "—And What of Private Duty," *R.N.,* **11:**34, (Jan.) 1948.

58. Francis, Susan C.: "The Private Duty Nurse in a New Era," *Am J. Nurs.,* **36:**773, (Aug.) 1936.

59. Klem, Margaret C.: "Who Purchase Private Duty Nursing Services?" *Am. J. Nurs.,* **39:**1069, (Oct.) 1939.

60. Couey, Fred, and Couey, Elizabeth D.

Human Relations in Private Duty Nursing. Atlanta Mail Advertising, Atlanta, Ga., 1957.

61. American Nurses' Association: *Nurses Invest in Patient Care.* The Association, Kansas City, Mo., 1956.
62. Hardin, Clara A.: "Twenty Studies of Nursing Functions," *Am. J. Nurs.,* **54:**1378, (Nov.) 1954.
63. "The Eight-Hour Day," *Am. J. Nurs.,* **34:**162, (Feb.) 1934.
64. Baker, Madalene: "The Eight-Hour Day in Ontario, Can.," *Can. Nurse,* **33:**329, (July) 1937.
65. Johnson, Sally: "A Trial of the Eight-Hour Day for Hospital Special Nurses," *Bull. Am. Hosp. Assoc.,* **9:**123, (Jan.) 1935.
66. Parsons, Anne F.: "Eight-Hour Duty for Private Duty Nurses," *Am. J. Nurs.,* **36:**915, (Sept.) 1936.
67. Tracy, Margaret Anthony: "The Eight-Hour Day for Special Nurses at the University of California Hospital," *Am. J. Nurs.,* **35:**29, (Jan.) 1935.
68. American Nurses' Association: *Hospitals in the United States Having an Eight-Hour (or Less) Day Schedule for Private Duty Nurses, as Reported to the ANA Headquarters, June 1940.* New York, the Association, 1940.

School and College Health Services

1. American Nurses' Association: *Facts About Nursing 72–73.* The Association, Kansas City, Mo., 1974, p. 10.
2. Canadian Nurses' Association: personal communication, Aug. 25, 1976.
3. Christy, Teresa E.: "Portrait of a Leader. Lillian D. Wald," *Am. J. Nurs.,* **70:**50, (Mar.) 1970.
4. Morton, Honnor: "Progressive Movements. The London Public School Nurse," *Am. J. Nurs.,* **1:**274, (Jan.) 1901.
5. "School Health Services in Europe; WHO Conference," *Chron. WHO,* **9:**269, (Aug.) 1955.
6. Chanlry-Price, A.: "An Insight into University Health Nursing," *Nurs. Times,* **68:**1609, (Dec. 21) 1972.
7. "The Future of the School Health Service," *Health Visitor,* **45:**273, (Sept.) 1972.
8. Murrell, J.: "Health Visitors and Teaching in Schools," *Health Visitor,* **46:**41, (Feb.) 1973.
9. Smith, M. C., et al.: "School Health in the Reorganized British National Health Service," *J. Sch. Health,* **43:**629, (Dec.) 1973.
10. Woody, R. H.: "College Health Services— Demise or Rebirth?" *J. Sch. Health,* **43:**442, (Sept.) 1973.
11. Abdellah, Faye G.: "School Nurse Practitioner—An Expanded Role for Nurses," *J. Am. Coll. Health Assoc.,* **21:**423, (June) 1973.

12. Anspach, Ellen, et al.: "Johnny and the School Nurse Practitioner," *Am. J. Nurs.,* **74:**1099, (June) 1974.
13. Chinn, P. A.: "Relationship Between Health and School Problems: A Nursing Assessment," *J. Sch. Health,* **43:**85, (Feb.) 1973.
14. Drake, Richard E.: "The School as a Locus of Community Health Services," *Nurs. Clin. North Am.,* **5:**657, (Dec.) 1970.
15. Ford, Loretta C.: "The School Nurse Role —A Changing Concept in Preparation and Practice," *J. Sch. Health,* **40:**1, (Jan.) 1970.
16. Fulford, Dorothy: "Needed: A School-Based Health Center for Children," *Can. Nurse,* **68:**25, (June) 1972.
17. Hilmar, M. A., et al.: "The School Nurse Practitioner and Her Practice; A Study of Traditional and Expanded Health Care Responsibilities for Nurses in Elementary Schools," *J. Sch. Health,* **43:**431, (Sept.) 1973.
18. Lampe, J. M.: "New Approaches to Delivery of Health Care to School Children as Instituted by Denver, Colorado, Public Schools," *J. Sch. Health,* **42:**272, (May) 1972.
19. McAtee, P. A.: "Nurse Practitioners in our Public Schools? An Assessment of Their Expanded Role as Compared with School Nurses," *Clin. Pediatr.,* **13:**360, (Apr.) 1974.
20. Saltarelli, J., et al.: "A Look at the Status of School Health Nursing—Past-Present-Future," *J. N.Y. State Sch. Nurs. Health Assoc.,* **5:**17, (Fall) 1973.
21. Silver, Henry K.: "The School Nurse Practitioner Program," *J.A.M.A.,* **216:**1332, (May 24) 1971.
22. "Certification of School Nurses," *Public Health Nurse,* **23:**185, (Apr.) 1931.
23. "Study of Certification of School Nurses in U.S.," *J. Sch. Health,* **20:**55, (Jan.) 1950.
24. Dilworth, Lula P.: "Study of Certification of School Nurses by State Departments of Education," *J. Sch. Health,* **28:**63, (Mar.) 1958.
25. "Certification of School Nurses," *Public Health Nurs.,* **43:**32, (Jan.) 1951.
26. National Organization for Public Health Nursing, Education Committee: "Minimum Qualifications for Nurses Appointed to School Nursing Positions," *Public Health Nurs.,* **30:**108, (Feb.) 1938.
27. National Organization for Public Health Nursing, School Nursing Section, Committee on Qualifications of the Nurse in the School: "The Nurse in the School Health Program," *Public Health Nurs.,* **39:**185, (Apr.) 1947.
28. American Nurses' Association, Public Health Nurses Section, School Nurses Branch: *Essential Considerations for Certification of School Nurses Employed by Boards of Education.* The Association, New York, 1959.

29. "Model Form Issued by ANA for Employment Standards for Public Health Nurses" (News About Nursing), *Am. J. Nurs.,* **54:**344, (Mar.) 1954.

30. American Nurses' Association, and American School Health Association: "Joint Statement Recommendations on Educational Preparation and Definition of the Expanded Role and Functions of the School Nurse Practitioner," *J. Sch. Health,* **43:** 594, (Nov.) 1973.

31. Creighton, Helen, and Squires, G. Marjorie: "School Nurses: Legal Aspects of Their Work," *Nurs. Clin. North Am.,* **9:**467, (Sept.) 1974.

32. Rose, Frederick: "Nurse in the Open-Air School," *Br. J. Nurs.,* **43:**415, (Nov. 20) 1909.

33. Badger, S. C., and Hawes, John B.: "Open-Air Rooms and Hospital Schools," *Boston Med. Surg. J.,* **165:**791, (Nov. 23) 1911.

34. Baker, S. Josephine: "The Control of Communicable Diseases in Schools," *Am. J. Public Health,* **6:**1078, (Oct.) 1916.

35. Davis, William R.: "The Nurse and Teacher in a Public Health Dental Program," *J. Am. Dent. Assoc.,* **15:**1156, (June) 1928.

36. Doherty, W. H.: "A Brief History of Dental Inspection and School Dental Clinics in Toronto," *Public Health J. (Can.)* **5:**139, (Mar.) 1914.

37. Durban, Emma: "Oral Hygiene in Los Angeles County (Calif.) Health Department," *Pacif. Coast J. Nurs.,* **21:**140, (Mar.) 1925.

38. Fones, Alfred C.: "The Public School Hygienist," *J. Am. Dent Assoc.,* **11:**229, (Mar.) 1924.

39. Great Britain Ministry of Health, United Kingdom Dental Mission: *New Zealand School Dental Nurses.* His Majesty's Stationery Office, London, 1950.

40. Henshaw, Charles H.: "Dental Hygiene in the Health Program of the Public Schools," *J. Am. Dent. Assoc.,* **14:**359, (Feb.) 1927.

41. New York Association for Improving the Condition of the Poor: *Community Oral Hygiene. A Four Year Report of the Mulberry Health Center, (New York City).* The Association, New York, 1924.

42. Saunders, J. Llewellyn: "The New Zealand School Dental Nurse—Comments on Recent Reports," *J. Am. Dent. Assoc.,* **43:**472, (Oct.) 1951.

43. Stewart, Isabel Maitland: "Suggested Outline of Lectures on Dentistry to Nurses in Training," *Am. J. Nurs.,* **29:**862, (July) 1929.

44. Boffa, J., et al.: "Development and Testing of a Junior High School Oral Hygiene Education Program," *J. Sch. Health,* **40:**567, (Dec.) 1970.

45. Cocker, Charles F.: "Current Trends in Dental Care Delivery Systems: Comprehensive Health Service for Children and Youth," *Am. J. Public Health,* **59:**909, (June) 1969.

46. Eichelberger, Marietta: "The Hot School Lunch," *J. Am. Diet. Assoc.,* **8:**339, (Nov.) 1932.

47. Kiess, Susan E.: "Thank You Mr. Rat," *Public Health Nurs.,* **41:**549, (Oct.) 1949.

48. Hart, Winifred A.: "Teaching Diet to School Children," *J. Am. Dent. Assoc.,* **10:**1029, (Nov.) 1923; **11:**634, (July) 1924.

49. Hubbell, H. L.: "Nutritional Experiment in Mt. Kisco (N.Y.) High School," *Public Health Nurse,* **11:**732, (Sept.) 1919.

50. Kearns, Mildred H., and Allen, Sarah Grant: "Breakfast in the Classroom—An Experiment in Nutrition Education at the Elementary Level," *J. Sch. Health,* **13:**187, (Oct.) 1943.

51. McLaughlin, Margaret: "A Nutritional Appraisal Program," *Public Health Nurs.,* **40:**15, (Jan.) 1948.

52. Pugh, Jeanette E.: "Warm Lunches for Rural Schools," *Public Health Nurse,* **18:**4, (Jan.) 1926.

53. Warnes, Mary B.: ["Problem of Hot School Lunches,"] *Trained Nurse,* **94:**446, (May) 1935.

54. Scovil, Elisabeth Robinson: "Instructing Children in the Origin of Life," *Am. J. Nurs.,* **12:**11, (Oct.) 1911.

55. Lowry, E. B.: *Teaching Sex Hygiene in the Public Schools.* Forbes & Co., Chicago, 1914.

56. Barry, Mary Lee: "An Outline for Sex Education," *Public Health Nurse,* **13:**247, (May) 1921.

57. Brown, Adelaide: "An Outline for Instruction of Pupil Nurses on Social Hygiene," *Am. J. Nurs.,* **16:**215, (Dec.) 1915.

58. Wheeler, Claribel A.: "The Role of the Nurse in the Social Hygiene Movement," *J. Soc. Hyg.,* **11:**402, (Oct.) 1925.

59. Yarros, Rachelle S.: "Moscow Revisited; Social Hygiene 1930–1936," *J. Soc. Hyg.,* **23:**200, (Apr.) 1937.

60. Goldberg, Jacob A.: "How Can the Social Hygiene Society Cooperate with Medical, Nursing and Social Work Groups?" *J. Soc. Hyg.,* **25:**437, (Dec.) 1939.

61. Gruenberg, Benjamin C.: *High Schools and Sex Education.* US Public Health Service, Washington, D.C., 1940 (Education Pub. No. 7).

62. Taylor, Jane Barbara, and Wills, Mildred F.: "The Contribution of the Nurse in the Schools to Venereal Disease Control," *J. Ven. Dis. Infect.* **28:**271, (Dec.) 1947.

63. Goldberg, Jacob A., and Tauber, Miriam E.: "Social Hygiene in the Nursing School Curriculum," *Am. J. Nurs.,* **49:**296, (May) 1949.

64. National League of Nursing Education, Committee on Social Hygiene: "Annual Report, 1931," in National League of Nursing Education: *Annual Report, 1931, and Record of Proceedings of 35th Con-*

vention. The League, New York, 1931.

65. *Nursing Studies Index,* Vol. I. J. B. Lippincott Co., Philadelphia, 1972.

66. Gordon, S. J.: "What Place Does Sex Education Have in the Schools?" *J. Sch. Health,* **44:**186, (Apr.) 1974.

67. Hammond, E.: "A Nurse's Concern Regarding Factual Knowledge of V.D. in a Regional High School," *J. Sch. Health,* **42:**599, (Dec.) 1972.

68. Brown, M. A.: "Adolescents and VD," *Nurs. Outlook,* **21:**99, (Feb.) 1973.

69. Bernfield, W. K.: "Sexually Transmitted Diseases," *Nurs. Mirror,* **135:**18, (Dec. 24) 1972.

70. McGrath, P., et al.: "Level of Basic Venereal Disease Knowledge Among Junior and Senior High School Nurses in Massachusetts: A Survey," *Nurs. Res.,* **23:**31, (Jan.–Feb.) 1974.

71. Benell, F. B.: "Drug Abuse and Venereal Disease Misconceptions of a Selected Group of College Students," *J. Sch. Health,* **43:**584, (Nov.) 1973.

72. Connaught, J. F.: "Health Care for Pregnant Heroin Addicts," *Aust. Nurses J.,* **1:**18, (July) 1972.

73. Davis, L., et al.: "Anticipatory Counseling of Unwed Pregnant Adolescents," *Nurs. Clin. North Am.,* **6:**581, (Dec.) 1971.

74. Mary Caroline, Sister: "Why Students Take Drugs," *Nurs. J. India,* **63:**387, (Nov.) 1972.

75. Klaus, H.: "Experience with Teenage Pregnancy," *Bull. Am. Coll. Nurse Midwives,* **17:**114, (Nov.) 1972.

76. Fulton, G. B.: "Current Assessment of Marihuana: A Rebuttal," *J. Sch. Health,* **43:**60, (Jan.) 1973.

77. Fox, V.: "Alcoholism in Adolescence," *J. Sch. Health,* **43:**32, (Jan.) 1973.

78. Chafetz, M. E.: "Problems of Reaching Youth," *J. Sch. Health,* **43:**40, (Jan.) 1973.

79. Bender, S. J.: "Sex and the College Student," *J. Sch. Health,* **43:**278, (May) 1973.

80. Wake, F. R., et al.: "Nurses, Smoking and School Children," *Can. Nurse,* **69:**19, (July) 1973.

81. Shimek, M. L.: "Pregnancy Testing in a High School," *J. Sch. Health,* **43:**622, (Dec.) 1973.

82. Kappelman, M., et al.: "A Unique School Health Program in a School for Pregnant Teenagers," *J. Sch. Health,* **44:**303, (June) 1974.

83. Harrington, Thomas F.: "Medical Inspection," *J. Educ.,* **67:**289, (Mar. 12) 1908.

84. "Nurse Inspector of New York City Schools" (editorial), *Am. J. Nurs.,* **6:**360, (Mar.) 1906.

85. Newmayer, S. Weir: *Medical and Sanitary Inspection of Schools for the Health Officer, the Physician, the Nurse and the Teacher.* Lea and Febiger, Philadelphia, 1913.

86. Papeer, Louis W.: "The Reorganization of Health Provisions in School Systems," *J. Educ.,* **77:**228, (Feb. 27) 1913.

87. Joint Committee on Health Problems in Education of the National Education Association and the American Medical Association: *Minimum Health Requirements for Rural Schools.* AMA, Chicago, 1922.

88. ———: *The Nurse in the School—An Interpretation.* NEA, Washington, D.C., 1940.

89. Jammé, Anna C.: "Report of the World's Conference on Education," in American Nurses' Association: *Proceedings, Thirty-Fourth Convention,* 1924. The Association, New York, 1924.

90. "Administering School Nursing on a Generalized Basis," *Public Health Nurs.,* **25:**507, (Sept.) 1933.

91. Irish, Eleanor M.: "The School Health Program in a Generalized Service," *Public Health Nurs.,* **41:**236, (Apr.) 1949.

92. Weisner, Dorothy E., and Swanson, Marie: "Some Administrative Procedures in School Nursing," *Public Health Nurs.,* **41:**668, (Dec.) 1949.

93. National Organization for Public Health Nursing, School Nursing Section: "School Nursing in the United States in 1952," *Public Health Nurs.,* **44:**563, (Oct.) 1952.

94. Brake, Charles E.: "School Health—Whose Job Is It?" *Public Health Nurs.,* **38:**66, (Feb.) 1946.

95. Moir, Berta H.: "A School Health Program Is a Community Enterprise," *Nurs. Outlook,* **3:**342, (June) 1955.

96. Hawkins, N. G.: "Is There a School Nurse Role?" *Am. J. Nurs.,* **71:**744, (Apr.) 1971.

97. Kefauver, Christine R.: "Obstacles in the Path of the School Nurse," *Am. J. Nurs.,* **9:**815, (Aug.) 1909.

98. Bryan, Doris S.: *School Nursing in Transition.* C. V. Mosby Co., St. Louis, 1973.

99. Woody, R. H.: *op. cit.*

100. Mills, D. Elva: "Work of a Resident Nurse in a College," *Am. J. Nurs.,* **14:**721, (June) 1914.

101. "Organization and Activities of a University Health Service," *School Soc.,* **4:**343, (Sept. 2) 1916.

102. Krusey, Effie M.: "College Nursing," *Am. J. Nurs.,* **23:**554, (Apr.) 1923.

103. Michigan, University. Division of Hygiene and Public Health: *Health Service in American Colleges and Universities.* The University, Ann Arbor, 1926.

104. Eby, Florence O.: "Dormitory Nursing at the University of Michigan," *Am. J. Nurs.,* **32:**393, (Apr.) 1932.

105. Griswold, Don M., and Spicer, Hazel I.: *University Student Health Services.* University of Chicago Press, Chicago, 1932.

106. Goulding, Fern A.: "A Modern College Health Program," *Public Health Nurs.,* **31:**264, (May) 1939.

107. Diehl, Harold S., and Shepard, Charles E.: *The Health of College Students.* American

Council on Education, Washington, D.C., 1939.

108. Goulding, Fern A.: "A Study of College Nursing Services," *Public Health Nurs.,* **32:**319, (Mar.) 1940.

109. Moore, Norman S., and Summerskill, John: *Health Services in American Colleges and Universities.* Cornell University, Ithaca, N.Y., [1954.]

110. Hathaway, John S.: "The Role of the Nurse in a University Health Service. The Research Plan," *Nurs. Outlook,* **10:**533, (Aug.) 1962.

111. Davie, James S.: "The Role of the Nurse in a University Health Service. How Students Viewed Their Health Service," *Nurs. Outlook,* **10:**534, (Aug.) 1962.

112. Fitzgerald, Helene: "The Role of the Nurse in a University Health Service. A New Dimension to the Nurse's Role," *Nurs. Outlook,* **10:**535, (Aug.) 1962. (See also editorial, same issue.)

113. Harrington, Thomas F.: *op. cit.*

114. Addams, Jane: "The Visiting Nurse and the Public School," *Am. J. Nurs.,* **8:**918, (Aug.) 1908.

115. Wood, Thomas D., et al.: *The Ninth Yearbook of the National Society for the Study of Education. Part II. The Nurse in Education.* University of Chicago Press, Chicago, 1911.

116. Pearse, Helen L.: "School Nursing," *Br. J. Nurs.,* **51:**210, (Sept. 13) 1913.

117. MacDonald, Isabel: *School Children; Their Care and Nursing.* Scientific Press, London, 1916.

118. Struthers, Lina Rogers: *The School Nurse: A Survey of the Duties and Responsibilities of the Nurse in the Maintenance of Health.* G. P. Putnam's Sons, New York, 1917.

119. Kelly, Helen W., and Bradshaw, Mabel C.: *A Handbook for School Nurses.* Macmillan Publishing Co., Inc., New York, 1918.

120. Ging, Zia: "School Nursing," *Q. J. Chinese Nurses,* **7:**10, (July) 1926.

121. Long, Harvey L.: "What Do School Nurses Do?" *Public Health Nurs.,* **21:**13, (Jan.) 1929.

122. Chayer, Mary Ella: "Nursing in the High Schools—A Study," *Public Health Nurs.,* **26:**245, (May) 1934.

123. Cromwell, Gertrude: "Preliminary Report on What Does a School Superintendent Expect of a School Nurse?" *J. Sch. Health,* **14:**224, (Nov.) 1944.

124. Brown, Jean E.: "Nursing and Health Education in Rural Communities. II. Health Teaching in the Rural Schools of Canada," *ICN,* **1:**172, (July) 1926.

125. Chayer, Mary Ella: "Changing Conceptions of School Nursing," *Public Health Nurs.,* **28:**385, (June) 1936.

126. *School Nursing—A Contribution to Health Education.* G. P. Putnam's Sons, New York, 1931.

127. Rogers, James Frederick: "Health Educa-

tion and Health Service in Schools," *J.A.M.A.,* **109:**842, (Sept.) 1937.

128. Walker, W. Frank, and Randolph, Carolina R.: *School Health Services.* Commonwealth Fund, New York, 1941.

129. Cromwell, Gertrude E.: *The Health of the School Child.* W. B. Saunders Co., Philadelphia, 1946.

130. Swanson, Marie: "Reasons for Lack of Treatment of Physical Defects of High School Pupils," *J. Sch. Health,* **19:**174, (Sept.) 1949.

131. Illinois Department of Public Instruction: *Functions of the Nurse in the School Health Program.* (Edited by Helen Lyon and Hazel O'Neal.) The Department, Springfield, 1953.

132. Poe, Nancy Margaret: *Functions of a School Nurse.* Ed.D. Dissertation, Boston University, Boston, 1957 (typed).

133. Stobo, Elizabeth C.: *Relating Theory and Nursing Practice in the School Health Program.* Ed.D. Dissertation, Teachers College, Columbia University, New York, 1957 (typed).

134. Eidens, C. O.: *The Work of the School Nurse-Teachers as Perceived by Selected Public School Staff Personnel.* Ed.D. Dissertation, Teachers College, Columbia University, New York, 1963 (typed).

135. Stobo, Elizabeth C.: *Findings of a Study Designed to Assist in the Development of Guidelines for the Preparation of Nurses for School Health Work.* National League for Nursing, New York, 1961.

136. Cree, Margaret A.: "Present-Day Views on School Nursing," *Am. J. Public Health,* **42:**818, (July) 1952.

137. Oberteuffer, Delbert: *School Health Education; A Textbook for Teachers, Nurses and Other Health Personnel,* 2nd ed. Harper and Row, New York, 1954.

138. Wilson, Dorothy (ed.): "School Health Records in Health Counseling of Children and Parents," *Nurs. Res.,* **4:**90, (Oct.) 1955.

139. Smiley, Lyda: "Report of Questionnaire Sent to Members of the Committee on School Nursing Policies and Practices, American School Health Association, August 1955," *J. Sch. Health,* **26:**174, (June) 1956.

140. Tipple, Dorothy C.: "The Future of School Nursing," *J.A.M.A.,* **171:**59, (Sept. 5) 1959.

141. Cromwell, Gertrude E.: *Nurse in the School Health Program.* W. B. Saunders Co., Philadelphia, 1963.

142. American Nurses' Association: *Functions and Qualifications for School Nurses.* The Association, New York, 1966.

143. "Symposium on the Nurse in the School Health Program; Guidelines for School Nursing," *J. Sch. Health,* **37**(Suppl):19, (Feb.) 1967.

144. American School Health Association, School Nursing Committee: "The Nurse

in the School Health Program; Guidelines for School Nursing," *J. Sch. Health,* **37:**1, (Feb.) 1967 (Special Issue).

145. National Education Association: *Standards for School Nurse Services.* The Association, Washington, D.C., 1970.
146. Crosby, Marian H.: "The Study of Mental Health and the School Nurse," *J. Sch. Health,* **40:**7, (Sept.) 1970.
147. Murphy, M. L.: "Values and Health Problems," *J. Sch. Health,* **43:**23, (Jan) 1973.
148. Newman, I. M., et al.: "Community Health Problems and the School's Unrecognized Mandate," *J. Sch. Health,* **43:**562, (Nov.) 1973.
149. Hawkins, N. G.: *op. cit.*
150. Tipple, D.: "The School Nurse Works with the Exceptional Child," in *ANA Regional Clinical Conferences, 1965.* Appleton-Century-Crofts, New York, 1966.
151. Bright, D., et al.: "What School Physicians, Nurses and Health Educators Should Know About Transcendental Meditation," *J. Sch. Health,* **43:**192, (Mar) 1973.
152. Chayer, Mary Ella: *School Nursing—A Contribution to Health Education.* G. P. Putnam's Sons, New York, 1931.
153. Lewis, Mary Ann: "Child-Initiated Care," *Am. J. Nurs.,* **74:**652, (Apr.) 1974.
154. Bryan, Doris S.: *op. cit.,* p. 7.
155. American Nurses' Association: *Facts About Nursing 72–73.* The Association, Kansas City, Mo., 1974, pp. 10, 153.
156. Foster, Jane: "College Nursing Round Table," *Public Health Nurs.,* **32:**692, (Nov.) 1940.
157. Goulding, Fern A.: "A Study of College Nursing Services," *Public Health Nurs.,* **32:**319, (May) 1940.

Occupational Health Services—Including Those in Industry

1. US Public Health Service: *Occupational Disease—The Silent Enemy.* The Service, Washington, D.C., 1968 (PHS Pub. No. 68–10258).
2. ———: *Community Health Nursing for Working People.* (Prepared by Jane A. Lee.) US Government Printing Office, Washington, D.C., 1970 (PHS Pub. No. 1295).
3. American Nurses' Association: *Facts About Nursing 72–73.* The Association, Kansas City, Mo., 1974, p. 10.
4. Canadian Nurses' Association: personal communication, Aug. 25, 1976.
5. American Nurses' Association: *op. cit.,* p. 17.
6. Felton, Jean Spencer, and Pleasants, Iva: "Men in Occupational Health Nursing," *Occup. Health Nurs. (NY),* **18:**9, (Jan.) 1970.
7. Kolesnikov, B. D.: "Organizational Format and Work Methods Used at the Mine

Health Centers," *Feldsher Akush.,* **38:**7, (Aug.) 1973.
8. Felton, Jean Spencer, et al.: *Man, Medicine and Work. Historic Events in Occupational Medicine.* US Government Printing Office, Washington, D.C., 1964, p. 27.
9. Charley, Irene H.: *The Birth of Industrial Nursing: Its History and Development in Great Britain.* Bailliere, Tindall and Cox, London, 1954, p. 49.
10. Brown, Mary Louise: "Nursing in Occupational Health," *Public Health Rep.,* **79:**967, (Nov.) 1964.
11. Markolf, Ada Mayo Stewart: "Industrial Nursing Begins in Vermont," *Public Health Nurs.,* **37:**125, (Mar.) 1945.
12. Brown, Mary Louise: *op. cit.*
13. Donnell, Jennie T.: "The Department-Store Nurse," *Trained Nurse,* **49:**75, (Aug.) 1912.
14. Brown, Mary Louise: *op. cit.*
15. Edwards, T. Owen: "Summary of Industrial Legislation from the Mediaeval Period," *J. Roy. San. Inst.,* **29:**553, (Nov.) 1908.
16. US Department of Health, Education, and Welfare, Social Security Administration: *Social Security Programs Throughout the World, 1971.* US Government Printing Office, Washington, D.C., 1971.
17. *Ibid.*
18. Charley, Irene H.: "Industrial Nursing," *Irish Nurs. World,* **2:**10, (Nov.) 1932.
19. Dingman, R.: "The Catherine R. Dempsey Lecture—Occupational Health Nursing: Tomorrow? Or Tomorrow," *Occup. Health Nurs. (NY),* **21:**9, (June) 1973.
20. Henriksen, Heide L.: "Health Care of Workers in the United States," *Nurs. Outlook,* **16:**32, (May) 1968.
21. Anderson, Eva S.: "The Work of an Industrial Visiting Nurse," *Public Health Nurse Q.,* **5:**38, (Apr.) 1913.
22. Kesner, Fannie: "The Public Health Nurse in Industry," *Am. J. Nurs.,* **15:**379, (Feb.) 1915.
23. King, Jeanette D.: "The Industrial Nurse in Relation to Public Health," *Public Health Nurse,* **11:**100, (Feb.) 1919.
24. Bailey, Harriet: "Nurse in Industry," *Int. J. Public Health,* **2:**212, (Mar.–Apr.) 1921.
25. MacKay, Muriel: "The Trained Nurse in Industry," *Can. Nurse,* **19:**466, (Aug.) 1923.
26. Butzerin, Eula B.: "Is Industrial Nursing Keeping Pace?" *Public Health Nurse,* **21:**81, (Feb.) 1929.
27. Hodgson, Violet H.: "The Nurse in Industry," *Public Health Nurse,* **21:**597, (Nov.) 1929.
28. Devlin, Winifred: "Industrial Nursing Consultant—Where Is She Going?" *Ind. Med.,* **18:**301, (Oct.) 1949.
29. Brown, Mary Louise: *op. cit.*
30. Kingston, Irene: "Occupational Health Services in Canada," *Occup. Health Rev.,* **19:**17, (Mar.–Apr.) 1967.
31. Hunter, W., et al.: "Modern Role of the

Occupational Health Nurse," *Nurs. Mirror,* **129:**39, (July 25) 1969.

32. Brown, Mary Louise: "A Profile of Occupational Health Nursing," *Am. Assoc. Ind. Nurses J.,* **18:**16, (Feb.) 1970.

33. Slaney, B.: "Broad Aspects of Occupational Health Nursing," *Occup. Health (London),* **21:**256, (Sept.–Oct.) 1969.

34. Block, D. L.: "Current Trends in Occupational Health Nursing," *Occup. Health Nurs. (NY),* **19:**7, (June) 1971.

35. MacArthur, M. C.: "New Challenges for Visiting Nurses," *Nurs. Clin. North Am.,* **6:**467, (Sept.) 1971.

36. Brown, Mary Louise: "Trends for the Future of Occupational Health Nursing," *Occup. Health Nurs. (NY),* **21:**7, (Aug.) 1973.

37. Donovan, J.: "Occupational Health Nursing in Great Britain," *Occup. Health (London),* **18:**223, (Sept.–Oct.) 1966.

38. Knabe, H.: "The Occupational Health Nurse in the German Democratic Republic," *Occup. Health (London),* **20:**252, (Sept.–Oct.) 1968.

39. Courtenay, Irene: "Occupational Health Nursing," *Can. Nurse,* **64:**36, (Apr.) 1968.

40. Junel, I.: "Education of the Occupational Health Nurse in Sweden," *Occup. Health (London),* **21:**81, (Mar.–Apr.) 1969.

41. Blakeley, Mary: "The Specialty of Occupational Health and the Nurse's Role Within It," *Aust. Nurses J.,* **67:**241, (Nov.) 1969.

42. Säyänjärvi, R.: "Education of the Occupational Health Nurse in Finland," *Occup. Health (London),* **21:**87, (Mar.–Apr.) 1969.

43. Samra, G. H.: "Remarks on State of Occupational Health Services in the Philippines," *Phil. J. Nurs.,* **39:**23, (July–Sept.) 1970.

44. Allan, M. C.: "The Work of the OH Nurse in Holland," *Occup. Health (London),* **23:**197, (June) 1971.

45. Radwanski, Dorothy: "Occupational Health Services in Nigeria," *Int. Nurs. Rev.,* **19:**283, (No. 3) 1972.

46. Brigstoke, H.: "Nurses Break the Ice," *Can. Nurse,* **70:**38, (Apr.) 1974.

47. Bolyard, R. V.: "Lessons from the Past," *Occup. Health (London),* **26:**3, (Jan.) 1974.

48. American Nurses' Association: *Facts About Nursing 72–73.* The Association, Kansas City, Mo., 1974, p. 10.

49. Canadian Nurses' Association: personal communication, Aug. 25, 1976.

50. Walker, Mildred: "Today's Occupational Health Nurse," *Nurs. Outlook,* **13:**62, (Nov.) 1965.

51. Dickinson, May Bliss: "Factory Welfare Work," *Am. J. Nurs.,* **11:**941, (Aug.) 1911.

52. Koch, Felix J.: "Nurses of Mercy to the Lone Fur-Trappers," *Br. J. Nurs.,* **47:**322, (Oct. 21) 1911.

53. Friedlander, Miss: "The Welfare Nurse," *Pac. Coast J. Nurs.,* **9:**448, (Oct.) 1913.

54. "Industrial Welfare Nursing," *Nurse,* **1:**348, (Nov.) 1914.

55. Crandall, Ella Phillips: "Industrial Welfare Nursing," *Public Health Nurse Q.,* **8:**32, (Apr.) 1916.

56. McCormac, Alice H.: "Industrial Nursing. Welfare Work and Nursing Service of the Metropolitan Life Insurance Company," *Am. J. Nurs.,* **17:**234, (Dec.) 1917.

57. Wilmore, M.: "The Industrial Nurse's Relationship with Other Social Workers," *J. Ind. Nurses,* **9:**24, (Spring) 1957.

58. Simpson, H. M.: "Naples Congress. The Nursing Session at the XI International Congress on Industrial Medicine," *Nurs. Times,* **50:**1130, (Oct. 15), 1954.

59. "International Review in Industrial Nursing," *Nurs. Times,* **54:**160, (Feb. 7) 1958.

60. World Health Organization: *Joint ILO/WHO Committee on Occupational Health. Third Report.* The Organization, Geneva, 1955.

61. "The Nurse in Industry," *J. Ind. Nurses,* **9:**187, (Winter) 1957.

62. Gillion, J. J.: *Occupational Health Services in Small Factories in France.* Joint WHO/ILO Seminar on Health Service in Small Factories, 1963. The Organization, Geneva, 1963.

63. Symposium on the Training of Occupational Health Nurses, Geneva, 1969: *The Occupational Health Nurse.* International Labour Office, Geneva, 1970.

64. World Health Organization: *The Nurse in Industry. Report of a Seminar.* The Organization, Copenhagen, 1957.

65. Stoves, V.: "The I.L.O. Symposium on the Training of Occupational Health Nurses," *Occup. Health (London),* **21:**89, (Nov.–Dec.) 1969.

66. Permanent Commission and International Association on Occupational Health: *The Nurse's Contribution to the Health of the Worker.* 1969

67. International Labour Organization: *Conditions of Work and Employment of Nurses.* The Organization, Geneva, 1958.

68. International Council of Nurses: "News from ICN House; ILO Study on Working Conditions of Nurses," *Int. Nurs. Rev.,* **5:**41, (Apr.) 1958.

69. Charley, Irene H.: "Industrial Nursing," *Nurs. Mirror,* **56:**152, (Nov. 19) 1932.

70. Doherty, I. Gwendoline: "The Occupational Health Section of the Royal College of Nursing," *J. Ind. Nurses,* **4:**185, (Winter) 1952.

71. "Conditions of Service. Comments on the Results of a Survey," *J. Ind. Nurses,* **8:**185, (Winter) 1956.

72. "The Factory Bill, 1958, Royal College of Nursing Memorandum," *J. Ind. Nurses,* **11:**106, (Summer) 1959.

73. Royal College of Nursing, Occupational

Health Section: "Salary Scales for State-Registered Nurses in Industry," *J. Ind. Nurses*, **11**:101, (Summer) 1959.

74. Royal College of Nursing, and National Council of Nurses of the United Kingdom: *Occupational Health Nursing, 1968*. The College and the Council, London, 1968.

75. ———: *Occupational Health Nursing Structure*. The College and the Council, London, 1968 (revised 1971).

76. ———: *A National Occupational Health Service*. The College and the Council, London, 1969.

77. Säyänjärvi, Ruth: "The Professional Education of the Occupational Health Nurse in Finland," *J. Ind. Nurses*, **9**:133, (Summer) 1957.

78. American Nurses' Association, Industrial Nurses Section: "Biennial Reports, 1946–48," in *Proceedings, 33rd–36th Conventions, 1946–48*. The Association, New York, 1946–48.

79. National Organization for Public Health Nursing, Industrial Nursing Section: "Biennial Reports," *Public Health Nurse*, 22, 1930–.

80. American Public Health Association, Committee on Professional Education: "Desirable Qualifications of Nurses Appointed to Public Health Nursing Positions in Industry," *Am. J. Public Health*, **29**:789, (July) 1939.

81. Stralko, Victoria C.: "National Organization for Industrial Nurses," *Ind. Med.*, **11**:243, (May) 1942.

82. Dempsey, Catherine R.: "Introducing . . . the A.A.I.N.," *Trained Nurse*, **108**:440, (June) 1942.

83. American Association of Industrial Nurses: *Qualifications, Duties, Personnel Policies, and Educational Programs for Industrial Nurses*. The Association, New York, 1945–49.

84. ———: *Guide for the Preparation of an Industrial Nursing Manual*. The Association, New York, 1950.

85. ———: *Recommended Qualifications for Industrial Nurses Working with Nursing Supervision*. The Association, New York, 1951.

86. Brown, Mary Louise: "Industrial Nursing's Place in the New Structure," *Nurs. World*, **126**:176, (Apr.) 1952.

87. "AAIN's Decision of 1952" (editorial), *Am. Assoc. Ind. Nurses J.*, **7**:9, (Mar.) 1959.

88. Hughes, Everett, et al.: *Twenty Thousand Nurses Tell Their Story*. J. B. Lippincott Co., Philadelphia, 1958.

89. American Nurses' Association, Industrial Nurses Section, Committee on Functions, Standards, and Qualifications for Practice: "Biennial Report to Section, 1952–54," in *Proceedings, 39th Convention, 1954*. The Association, New York, 1954.

90. ———: "ANA Statements of Functions, Standards, and Qualifications," *Am. J. Nurs.*, **56**:899, (July) 1956.

91. "Duties and Responsibilities of the Professional Nurse in an Industrial Medical Service," *Am. Assoc. Ind. Nurses J.*, **2**:13, (June) 1955.

92. National League for Nursing: *Educational Responsibilities of Occupational Health Nurses*. The League, New York, 1956 (League Exchange No. 19).

93. American Medical Association, Council on Occupational Health: "Medical Directives for Occupational Health Nurses," *Arch. Environ. Health*, **5**:631, (Dec.) 1962.

94. American Medical Association, Council on Industrial Health: *Guiding Principles and Procedures for Industrial Nurses*. The Association, Chicago, 1955.

95. American Medical Association, Council on Industrial Health, Committee on Industrial Nursing: "The Legal Scope of Industrial Nursing Practice," *J.A.M.A.*, **169**:1072, (Mar. 7) 1959; *Am. J. Nurs.*, **59**:996, (July) 1959.

96. US Public Health Service: *An Occupational Health Program for Hospital Employees*. US Government Printing Office, Washington, D.C., 1960 (PHS Pub. No. 725).

97. American Nurses' Association: *Guide for the Development of an Employee Health Program for Nurses*. The Association, New York, 1962.

98. ———: *Guide for the Development of a Manual for an Employee Health Program*. The Association, New York, 1963.

99. American Nurses' Association, Division of Community Health Practice: *Functions and Qualifications for an Occupational Health Nurse in a One-Nurse Service*. The Association, New York, 1968.

100. American Association of Industrial Nurses: *Standards and Criteria for Evaluating an Occupational Nursing Service*. The Association, New York, 1965.

101. US Public Health Service: *Community Health Nursing for Working People*. (Prepared by Jane A. Lee.) US Government Printing Office, Washington, D.C., 1970 (PHS Pub. No. 1295).

102. US Congress: *Occupational Safety and Health Act of 1970*. Public Law 91–596, 91st Congress, S2193, Dec. 29, 1970. US Government Printing Office, Washington, D.C., 1972 (759–453/302).

103. Brown, Mary Louise: "Highlights of the Occupational Health Nursing Study," *Am. Assoc. Ind. Nurses J.*, **13**:50, (May) 1965.

104. US Public Health Service, Division of Occupational Health: *Occupational Health Nurses: An Initial Survey*. (Prepared by Mary Louse Brown and Mary L. Bauer.) US Government Printing Office, Washington, D.C., 1966 (PHS Pub. No. 1470).

105. Industrial Hygiene Foundation of America: *Employee Mental Health and Industrial Nursing Practices, An Experimental Course*.

The Foundation, Pittsburgh, 1965 (Nursing Series Bull. No. 1).

106. Keller, Marjorie, and May, W. Theodore: *Occupational Health Content in Baccalaureate Nursing Education*. US Department of Health, Education, and Welfare, Public Health Service, National Institute for Occupational Safety and Health, Cincinnati, 1971.

107. Hills, Mary Grace: "An Institute for Industrial Nurses," *Public Health Nurse*, **13:** 33, (Jan.) 1921.

108. American Foundation of Occupational Health: *Medical Services in Industry*. The Foundation, Chicago, 1952.

109. Symposium on Industrial Nursing, Boston College, Chestnut Hill, Mass., Oct.–Nov. 1953: *Proceedings*. Liberty Mutual Insurance Co., Boston, 1953, Processed.

110. National League for Nursing: *Guide for the Orientation of Newly Employed Occupational Health Nurses*. The League, New York, 1956 (League Exchange No. 16).

111. Workshop in Industrial Nursing, Oklahoma City, Mar. 29–30, 1957: *Contemporary Developments in Occupational Health Nursing*. University of Oklahoma, Oklahoma City, 1957.

112. Workshop on Occupational Health Nursing, Yale University, New Haven, Sept. 12–14, 1956: *Report*. National League for Nursing, New York, 1957 (League Exchange No. 19).

113. Henriksen, Heide L.: *Curriculum Study of the Occupational Health Aspects of Nursing. An Adventure in Cooperation*. Minnesota League for Nursing, Minneapolis, 1959.

114. "Industrial Nurses Endorse Two Certifications" (News and Reports), *Nurs. Outlook*, **23:**611, (Oct.) 1975.

115. Roberts, L.: "Educational Opportunities for Industrial Nurses," *Am. Assoc. Ind. Nurses J.*, **14:**17, (Oct.) 1966.

116. Klutas, E. M.: *Occupational Health Nursing for the Basic Nursing Student*. National League for Nursing, New York, 1966.

117. Summers, Virginia M.: "An Occupational Health Nursing Study," *Nurs. Outlook*, **15:** 64, (July) 1967.

118. Hausman, D. M.: "Community Health Nursing Includes Occupational Health Nursing Experience," *Occup. Health Nurs. (NY)*, **21:**11, (Nov.) 1973.

119. Keller, M. J.: "Nursing Education and the Occupational Health Setting," *Occup. Health Nurs. (NY)*, **22:**14, (Jan.) 1974.

120. Benoit, J. N.: "Occupational Health Nurse Certification," *Occup. Health Nurs. (NY)*, **19:**22, (Apr.) 1971.

121. Harris, A. M.: "Certification of Occupational Health Nurses," *Occup. Health Nurs. (NY)*, **21:**21, (Nov.) 1973.

122. Slaney, B. M.: "Why Take the Occupational Health Nursing Certificate?" *Nurs. Mirror*, **123:**221, (Dec. 9) 1966.

123. McKiever, Margaret F.: *National Health Survey Findings of Occupational Health Interest*. US Government Printing Office, Washington, D.C., 1966 (PHS Pub. No. 1418).

124. US Public Health Service, National Institute for Occupational Safety and Health: *Safety Standards, Vol. 20, May–June 1971*. US Government Printing Office, Washington, D.C., 1971.

125. US Department of Labor, Wage and Labor Standards Administration: *State Workmen's Compensation Laws*. US Government Printing Office, Washington, D.C., 1969 (Revision of 1964 Bull. No. 161).

126. US Department of Labor, Women's Bureau: *1969 Handbook on Women Workers*. US Government Printing Office, Washington, D.C., 1969 (Women's Bur. Bull. No. 294).

127. US Department of the Interior, Bureau of Mines: *State Compensatory Provisions for Occupational Diseases*. US Government Printing Office, Washington, D.C., 1967 (Bull. No. 623).

128. American Public Health Association: *Local Health Officers' Guide to Occupational Health*. The Association, Washington, D.C., 1970.

129. US Congress, Committee on Ways and Means: *Basic Facts on the Health Industry*. US Government Printing Office, Washington, D.C., 1971.

130. American National Standards Institute: *Method of Recording and Measuring Work Injury Experience*. The Institute, New York, 1967.

131. American Medical Association: *Scope, Objectives and Functions of Occupational Health Programs*. The Association, Chicago, 1971.

132. Creighton, Helen: "The Nurse and the Law in Occupational and Public Health," *Okla. Nurse*, **44:**7, (Nov.) 1969.

133. Ede, Lorice: "Legal Relations in Nursing," *Am. Assoc. Ind. Nurses J.*, **17:**9, (Dec.) 1969.

134. Goldstein, David H.: "The Occupational Safety and Health Act of 1970," *Am. J. Nurs.*, **71:**1535, (Aug.) 1971.

135. McKiever, Margaret F.: *The Health of Women Who Work*. US Government Printing Office, Washington, D.C., 1965 (PHS Pub. No. 1314).

136. *President's Report on Occupational Safety and Health*. US Government Printing Office, Washington, D.C., 1972.

137. "Does the Fair Labor Standards Act Apply to Nurses?" *Am. J. Nurs.*, **41:**185, (Feb.) 1941.

138. American Nurses' Association: "Industrial Nurses and the Wage and Hour Law," *Am. J. Nurs.*, **44:**467, (May) 1944.

139. US Public Health Service: *An Occupational Health Program for Hospital Employees*. US Government Printing Office, Washington, D.C., 1960 (PHS Pub. No. 725).

140. Scheffler, Gustave: "The Nurse's Role in Hospital Safety," *Nurs. Outlook,* **10:**680, (Oct.) 1962.

141. Gafafer, W. M. (ed.): *Occupational Diseases, A Guide to Their Recognition.* US Government Printing Office, Washington, D.C., 1964.

142. Fleming, A. J.: "The Many Faces of Occupational Health," *J. Occup. Med.,* **8:**201, (Apr.) 1966.

143. Sturgis, K. R.: "Implications of Current Social Changes for the Nurse in Occupational Health," *Am. Assoc. Ind. Nurses J.,* **15:**12, (Oct.) 1967.

144. Saller, D. M.: "The Varied Role of the Industrial Nurse," *Am. Assoc. Ind. Nurses J.,* **16:**13, (Dec.) 1967.

145. Johnson, D. R.: "Today and Tomorrow. The Occupational Health Nurses' Broadening Responsibility," *Am. Assoc. Ind. Nurses J.,* **16:**17, (June) 1968.

146. Hutchins, J.: "Orientation of the Aerospace Nurse to Occupational Health," *Am. Assoc. Ind. Nurses J.,* **16:**7, (July) 1968.

147. O'Brien, Mary E.: "Widening Horizons in Occupational Health Nursing," *Int. Nurs. Rev.,* **15:**280, (July) 1968.

148. Levinson, Harry: "Emotional Toxicity of the Work Environment," *Arch. Environ. Health,* **19:**239, (Aug.) 1969.

149. Skrimshire, M.: "The New Occupational Health Nursing Structure," *Occup. Health (London),* **21:**4, (Jan.–Feb.) 1969.

150. Schilling, R. S. F.: "Changing Concepts in Occupational Health," *Am. J. Public Health,* **59:**1366, (Aug.) 1969.

151. Mayers, Mary R.: *Occupational Health Hazards of a Work Environment.* Williams and Wilkins Co., Baltimore, 1969.

152. Keller, M. J.: "An Overview of Occupational Health Nursing in an Era of Change," *Occup. Health Nurs. (NY),* **18:**19, (Apr.) 1970.

153. Russo, Angela M.: "The Focus of the Occupational Health Nurse in a Changing Environment," *Am. Assoc. Ind. Nurses J.,* **17:**18, (July) 1970.

154. Fisher, E. D.: "The Health Care of Personnel in the New York Hospital–Cornell Medical Center," *Int. Nurs. Rev.,* **18:**113, (No. 2) 1971.

155. Holcomb, F. W., Jr.: "IBM's Health Screening Program and Medical Data System," *J. Occup. Med.,* **15:**863, (Nov.) 1973.

156. Bridgman, R. F., and Roemer, M. I. (eds.): *Interrelationships Between Health Programmes and Socio-Economic Development.* American Public Health Association, Washington, D.C., 1973.

157. Berry, C. M.: "Occupational Health and the Health Maintenance Organization," *Occup. Health Nurs. (NY),* **22:**7, (Jan.) 1974.

158. Lowman, W. B.: "The Importance and Necessity of 'Industrial Hospitals'," *Trained Nurse,* **32:**107, (Feb.) 1904.

159. Ainsworth, F. K.: "The Southern Pacific Company's Railroad Hospital," *Mod. Hosp.,* **4:**295, (May) 1915.

160. McNeil, A. W.: "What a Hospital Does for 22,000 Men and Women in a Great Manufacturing Plant," *Pac. Coast J. Nurs.,* **26:** 501, (Aug.) 1920.

161. Drach, Gustave: "The Hospital of the Tennessee Coal, Iron and Railroad Company," *Mod. Hosp.,* **17:**95, (Aug.) 1921.

162. Somers, Anne R. (ed.): *The Kaiser-Permanente Medical Care Program: Proceedings of a Symposium.* Commonwealth Fund, New York, 1971.

163. Challen, P. J. R., and Hickish, D. W.: "Occupational Hygiene and Its Development at Slough," *J. Ind. Nurses,* **10:**86, (Summer) 1958.

164. US Public Health Service: *Community Health Nursing for Working People.* (Prepared by Jane A. Lee.) US Government Printing Office, Washington, D.C., 1970 (PHS Pub. No. 1295).

165. Travers, D.: "The Significance of a Name. Employee Health Service *vs.* First Aid Room," *Am. Assoc. Ind. Nurses J.,* **14:**20, (Feb.) 1966.

166. Dingman, R.: "Occupational Health Nursing Participation in the Development of Part-Time Nursing Services to Small Industries," *Occup. Health Nurs. (NY),* **22:**10, (Jan.) 1974.

167. "Work of Nurses for Hop-Pickers," *Br. J. Nurs.,* **39:**126, (Aug. 17) 1907.

168. Douglas, Ruth Huff: "Public Health Nursing in Hop Yards," *Public Health Nurse,* **17:**20, (Jan.) 1925.

169. Barnes, H. Eva: "Health Problems Among California Migrants," *Public Health Nurs.,* **24:**616, (Nov.) 1932.

170. Engelin, Margaret, and Volin, Jeanne: "Nursing Among the Migrants," *Pac. Coast J. Nurs.,* **35:**597, (Oct.) 1939.

171. US Department of Agriculture, Economic Research Service: *Domestic Migratory Farm Workers, Personal and Economic Characteristics.* US Government Printing Office, Washington, D.C., 1967.

172. US Senate, Government Operations Committee: *Economic and Social Conditions of Rural America in the 1970's.* (Prepared by Economic Research Service, Department of Agriculture, 92nd Congress, 1st Session, Part 1, May 1971.) US Government Printing Office, Washington, D.C., 1971.

173. President's National Advisory Commission on Rural Poverty: *Rural Poverty in the United States.* US Government Printing Office, Washington, D.C., 1968.

174. American Friends Service Committee: *Child Labor in Agriculture, Summer 1970; A Special Report.* The Committee, Philadelphia, 1971.

175. California Public Health Department, Occupational Health and Environmental Epidemiology Bureau: *Occupational Disease in*

California Related to Pesticides and Other Agricultural Chemicals, 1967. The Department, Sacramento, 1968.

176. Storlie, Frances: *Nursing and the Social Conscience.* Appleton-Century-Crofts, New York, 1970.

177. Moses, Marion: "Viva La Causa," *Am. J. Nurs.,* **73:**842, (May) 1973.

178. Thwing, Mary Dunning: "Factory Nursing," *Public Health Nurse Q.,* **5:**28, (Apr.) 1913.

179. "The First Factory Nurse," *Nurs. Mirror,* **63:**31, (Apr. 11) 1936.

180. Wright, Florence Swift: *Industrial Nursing for Industrial, Public Health, and Pupil Nurses and for Employers of Labor.* Macmillan Publishing Co., New York, 1920.

181. MacDonald, M. Gray: *Handbook of Nursing in Industry.* W. B. Saunders Co., Philadelphia, 1944.

182. Charley, Irene H.: *The Birth of Industrial Nursing: Its History and Development in Great Britain.* Bailliere, Tindall and Cox, London, 1954.

183. McGrath, Bethel J.: *Nursing in Commerce and Industry.* Commonwealth Fund, New York, 1946.

184. Brown, Mary Louise, and Meigs, John Wister: *Occupational Health Nursing.* Springer Publishing Co., New York, 1956.

185. Tyer, F. H.: *Occupational Health Nursing.* Bailliere, Tindall and Cox, London, 1961.

186. Copplestone, John F., et al.: *Preventive Aspects of Occupational Health Nursing.* Williams and Wilkins Co., Baltimore, 1968.

187. Royal College of Nursing, and National Council of Nurses of the United Kingdom: *Occupational Health Nursing Structure.* The College and the Council, London, 1968 (revised 1971).

188. ————: *A National Occupational Health Service.* The College and the Council, London, 1969.

189. Kerr, L. E.: "The Neglect of Occupational Health," *Natl. Tuberc. Resp. Dis. Assoc. Bull.,* **58:**11, (Oct.) 1972.

190. Felton, Jean Spencer, et al.: *Man, Medicine and Work. Historic Events in Occupational Medicine.* US Government Printing Office, Washington, D.C., 1964.

191. Wald, Lillian D.: "The Doctor and the Nurse in Industrial Establishments," *Am. J. Nurs.,* **12:**403, (Feb.) 1912.

192. ————: "The Sanitary Control of an Industry by the Industry Itself," *Public Health Nurse,* **5:**13, (Apr.) 1913.

193. Wright, Florence Swift: "The Responsibilities and Opportunities of the Industrial Nurse," *Public Health Nurse,* **11:**854, (Nov.) 1919.

194. ————: "Development and Present Scope of Industrial Nursing in the United States," *Int. J. Public Health,* **2:**43, (Jan.–Feb.) 1921.

195. Whitlock, Olive M., et al.: *Nursing Practices in Industry.* US Government Printing Office, Washington, D.C., 1944 (PHS Bull. No. 283).

196. McGrath, Bethel J.: "Fifty Years of Industrial Nursing in the United States," *Public Health Nurs.,* **37:**119, (Mar.) 1945.

197. ————: *Nursing in Commerce and Industry.* Commonwealth Fund, New York, 1946.

198. Brown, Mary Louise, and Meigs, John Wister: *Occupational Health Nursing.* Springer Publishing Co., New York, 1956.

199. Lucal, Margaret W.: "Industrial Nursing—A History," *Am. Assoc. Ind. Nurses J.,* **6:**14, (Feb.) 1958.

200. Brown, Mary Louise, and Goldstein, David: *Nursing Education and Occupational Health Nursing. Report to Committee on Industrial Nursing, Council on Industrial Health, American Medical Association, March 15, 1959* (Processed).

201. Felton, Jean Spencer: "Medical Direction in Occupational Health Nursing," *Am. J. Nurs.,* **66:**2019, (Sept.) 1966.

202. Keller, Marjorie J.: "An Overview of Occupational Health Nursing in an Era of Change," *Occup. Health Nurs. (NY),* **18:**19, (Apr.) 1970.

203. Burgeson, E. C.: "Sixty-two Years Later the Philosophy and Principles Are the Same—Only the People Have Changed," *Occup. Health Nurs. (NY),* **18:**18, (Aug.) 1970.

204. American Nurses' Association, Committee to Study the Implications of the Fair Labor Standards Act as These Relate to Industrial Nursing: "Biennial Report, 1946," in *Proceedings, 35th Convention, 1946.* The Association, New York, 1946.

205. Klem, Margaret C.: "Nursing Opportunities in Medical Care Insurance," *Public Health Nurs.,* **43:**8, (Jan.) 1951.

206. "Health Plans By-Pass Nursing," *R.N.,* **14:**41, (Sept.) 1951.

207. Guida, Miriam: "Occupational Health Nursing for Small Industry," in *ANA Regional Clinical Conferences, 1967.* Appleton-Century-Crofts, New York, 1968.

207a. Somers, Anne R.: *Health Care in Transition. Directions for the Future.* Hospital Research and Educational Trust, Chicago, 1971.

208. Graves, Bea W.: "First Aid Work in the Seattle Construction and Dry Dock Company," *Pac. Coast J. Nurs.,* **13:**293, (May) 1917.

209. "Standing Orders for Nurses in Industry," *J.A.M.A.,* **122:**1247, (Aug. 28) 1943.

210. Tabershaw, I. R., and Hargreaves, Margaret S.: "Function of Standing Orders for the Nurses in Industry," *Am. J. Public Health,* **37:**1430, (Nov.) 1947.

211. American Medical Association, Council on Industrial Health, Committee on Industrial Nursing: "The Legal Scope of Industrial Nursing Practice," *J.A.M.A.,* **169:**1072, (Mar. 7) 1959.

212. Rosati, J.: "The Case of the Industrial Nurse," *Can. Occup. Safety Mag.*, **7**:16, (Sept.) 1969.

213. Perry, Florence: "A Municipal Occupational Disease Bureau," *Public Health Nurse Q.*, **8**:73, (Oct.) 1916.

214. Everts, Glenn S.: "Public Health Nursing Service in Small Industries," *Public Health Nurs.*, **26**:590, (Nov.) 1934.

215. Blaisdell, Leah M.: "We Offer Nursing Service to Industry," *Public Health Nurs.*, **34**:550, (Oct.) 1942.

216. Fillmore, Anna M.: "Part-Time Nursing Service to the Small Plant," *Public Health Nurs.*, **37**:130, (Mar.) 1945.

217. Dingman, R.: "Occupational Health Nursing Participation in the Development of Part-Time Nursing Services to Small Industries," *Occup. Health Nurs. (NY)*, **22**:10, (Jan.) 1974.

218. Metcalf, Wendell O.: *Health Maintenance Programs for Small Business Management.* US Government Printing Office, Washington, D.C., 1964.

219. US Public Health Service: *Community Health Nursing for Working People.* (Prepared by Jane A. Lee.) US Government Printing Office, Washington, D.C., 1970 (PHS Pub. No. 1295).

220. Royal College of Nursing, and National Council of Nurses of the United Kingdom: *Occupational Health Nursing Structure.* The College and the Council, London, 1968 (revised 1971).

221. American Nurses' Association, Industrial Nurses Section: "ANA Statement of Functions, Standards, and Qualifications," *Am. J. Nurs.*, **56**:899 (July) 1956.

222. American Nurses' Association: *Functions and Qualifications for an Occupational Health Nurse in a One-Nurse Service.* The Association, Kansas City, Mo., 1968.

223. Keller, Marjorie J., and May, W. Theodore: *Occupational Health Content in Baccalaureate Nursing Education.* US Public Health Service, Cincinnati, 1970.

224. University of North Carolina: *Graduate Preparation in Occupational Health Nursing.* The University, Chapel Hill, [197–].

225. Mathew, G. G.: "The Nurse's Role in Initial Health Examinations," *Occup. Health (London)*, **18**:275, (Nov.–Dec.) 1966.

226. Flynn, Eileen D.: "Barriers to Utilization of Multiphasic Screening—The Nurse's Role," *Am. Assoc. Ind. Nurses J.*, **17**:19, (July) 1967.

227. Brogan, M. M.: "Training and Retraining of Nurses in Routine Physical Examinations," *Bull. N.Y. Acad. Med.*, **45**:1353, (Dec.) 1969.

228. Bews, D. C., et al.: "Preplacement Health Screening by Nurses," *Am. J. Public Health*, **59**:2178, (Dec.) 1969.

229. Munro, L. B.: "Preplacement Health Screening by Nurses in Industry," *Can. Nurse*, **66**:29, (Nov.) 1970.

230. Burkeen, O. E.: "The Role of the Occupational Nurse in Performing Health Examinations," *Occup. Health Nurs. (NY)*, **21**:22, (May) 1973.

231. Byrd, C. A.: "The Nurse and Employee Health—Efficiency and Stability: Job Placement," *Occup. Health Nurs. (NY)*, **22**:9, (Mar.) 1974.

232. Cippola, Josephine, and Collings, Gilbearth, Jr.: "Nurse Clinicians in Industry," *Am. J. Nurs.*, **71**:1530, (Aug.) 1971.

233. Drysdale, R. S.: "Safety-Care of the Eyes," *Occup. Health (London)*, **23**:23, (Jan.) 1971.

234. Lee, J. A.: "Eye Health and Safety Programs," *Occup. Health Nurs. (NY)*, **18**:7, (Oct.) 1970.

235. Tyler, I. C.: "A Glaucoma Screening and Study by Nurses," *Occup. Health Nurs. (NY)*, **19**:11, (Sept.) 1971.

236. Ure, A. W.: "Vested Interest in Visual Welfare," *Occup. Health (London)*, **23**:85, (Mar.) 1971.

237. Rintelmann, W. F., et al.: "A Survey of Hearing Conservation Programs in Representative Aerospace Industries, I. Prevalence of Programs and Monitoring Audiometry," *Am. Ind. Hyg. Assoc. J.*, **28**:372, (July–Aug.) 1967.

238. Murphy, A. J.: "Hearing Conservation in Industry; An Overview," *Am. Assoc. Ind. Nurses J.*, **16**:15, (May) 1968.

239. ———: "The Identity of the Nurse in an Industrial Hearing Conservation Program," *Occup. Health Nurs. (NY)*, **17**:32, (May) 1969.

240. Burns, W.: *Hearing and Noise in Industry.* H. M. Stationery Office, London, 1970.

241. Trice, H. M., et al.: "Identifying and Confronting the Alcoholic Employee: Role of the Industrial Nurse," *Am. Assoc. Ind. Nurses J.*, **13**:7, (Oct.) 1965.

242. Hine, C. H.: "The Role of the Industrial Nurse in the Detection and Prevention of Drug Abuse," *Occup. Health Nurs. (NY)*, **17**:15, (Apr.) 1969.

243. Sohn, D., et al.: "Drug Screening in Industrial Nursing," *Occup. Health Nurs. (NY)*, **18**:7, (Aug.) 1970.

244. Millsap, Mary: "Occupational Health Nursing in an Alcohol Addiction Program," *Nurs. Clin. North Am.*, **7**:121, (Mar.) 1972.

245. Sandin, Don: "Al-Anon: A Resource for Labor and Management Alcoholism. A Family Disease," *National Council on Alcoholism, Labor-Management Alcoholism Newsletter,* Vol. 2, No. 5, (Mar.–Apr.) 1973.

246. Tibbs, T.: "Rehabilitating Laryngectomies," *Am. Assoc. Ind. Nurses J.*, **16**:23, (Feb.) 1968.

247. Martin, N.: "The Rehabilitation Process. A Challenge to Nursing," *Occup. Health Nurs. (NY)*, **18**:13, (Nov.) 1970.

248. Watrous, W. B.: "Rehabilitation Nurse: Counselor and Coordinator," *Occup. Health Nurs. (NY)*, **21**:16, (Dec.) 1973.

249. Burgeson, Ethel C.: "The Industrial Nurse as a Health Counselor in Industry," *Am. J. Public Health*, **39**:777, (June) 1949.

250. Peplau, H. E.: "Interpersonal Relations and the Work of the Industrial Nurse," *Am. Assoc. Ind. Nurses J.*, **15**:7, (Nov.) 1967.

251. Illich, Ivan: *Medical Nemesis. The Expropriation of Health*. McClelland and Stewart, London, 1975.

252. Felton, Jean Spencer: "Care, Compassion and Confrontation—The Correctives in the Occupational Mental Health of the Future," *J. Occup. Med.*, **10**:331, (July) 1968.

253. Levenson, Harry: "Various Approaches to Understanding Man at Work," *Arch. Environ. Health*, **22**:612, (May) 1971.

254. Galli, E. A.: "The Occupational Health Nurse and Mental Health," *S.A. Nurs. J.*, **38**:35, (Apr.) 1971.

255. Brown, Mary Louise: "The Extended Role of the Nurse in an Occupational Mental Health Program," *Occup. Health Nurse (Auckland)*, **19**:13, (May) 1971.

256. Keenan, E. W.: "Industrial Health Counseling Service. A Pilot Project of the National Institute of Industrial Gerontology," *Occup. Health Nurs. (NY)*, **19**:7, (July) 1971.

257. Noland, R. L. (ed.): *Industrial Mental Health and Employee Counseling*. (Management Training Series.) Behavioral Publications, New York, 1973.

258. American Nurses' Association: *Facts About Nursing 74–75*. The Association, Kansas City, Mo., 1976, pp. 137, 105.

259. US Public Health Service: *Studies of the Medical and Surgical Care of Industrial Workers*. (Prepared by Clarence D. Selby.) US Government Printing Office, Washington, D.C., 1919.

260. Frankel, Lee K.: "Industrial Nursing as a Means of Fighting Tuberculosis," *Public Health Nurse*, **14**:3, (Jan.) 1922.

261. American Public Health Association, Public Health Nursing Section: "A Study of Industrial Nursing Services," *Public Health Nurs.*, **32**:631, (Oct.) 1940.

262. Whitlock, Olive M., et al.: *Nursing Practices in Industry*. US Government Printing Office, Washington, D.C., 1944.

263. Barschak, Erna: *Today's Industrial Nurse and Her Job*. G. P. Putnam's Sons, New York, 1956.

264. Smith, Wendell I.: *The Industrial Nurse: An Analysis of Her Functions*, Bucknell University, Lewisburg, Pa., 1957.

265. Brown, Mary Louise: "Data on Occupational Health Nurses," *Am. J. Nurs.*, **65**:120, (May) 1965.

266. ——: "Factors Related to Job Satisfactions of Nurses Working in Occupational Health," *Occup. Health (London)*, **19**:85, (Mar.–Apr.) 1967.

267. Hendricksen, Heide L.: "Health Care of Workers in the United States," *Nurs. Outlook*, **16**:32, (May) 1968.

268. Wetzel, Fonda C.: "Management's Appraisal of the Nurse in Industry," *Nurs. Outlook*, **13**:65, (Nov.) 1965.

269. Smith, V. L.: "Industrial Nursing. A Varied, Interesting Nursing Career," *Bedside Nurse*, **3**:20, (Dec.) 1970.

Schools of Nursing and Other Educational Institutions (as Teachers and Administrators)

1. American Nurses' Association: *Facts About Nursing 72–73*. The Association, Kansas City, Mo., 1974, pp. 10, 14, 17.

2. Canadian Nurses' Association: personal communication, Aug. 25, 1976.

3. American Nurses' Association: *Facts About Nursing 74–75*. The Association, Kansas City, Mo., 1976, p. 25.

4. Roberts, Mary M.: *American Nursing; History and Interpretation*. Macmillan Publishing Co., Inc., New York, 1954, p. 110.

5. Aikens, Charlotte A.: *Hospital Training School Methods and the Head Nurse*. W. B. Saunders Co., Philadelphia, 1907.

6. Goodrich, Annie Warburton: "The Introduction of Salaried Instruction in the Training Schools," in American Society of Superintendents of Training Schools for Nurses: *Annual Report, 1905, and Proceedings of 11th Convention Including Report of First Meeting of American Federation of Nurses*. J. M. Furst, Baltimore, 1905.

7. Doty, Parmelia Murnan: "The Need of Cooperation Between the Head Nurse and the Instructor," in National League of Nursing Education: *Annual Report 1919 and Proceedings of 25th Convention*. Williams and Wilkins Co., Baltimore, 1919.

8. Russell, Anne Steward: "The Shortcomings of the Teaching and Methods of Present Training Schools from the Standpoint of the Graduate Nurse in Institutional Work," *Am. J. Nurs.*, **4**:267, (Jan.) 1904.

9. Pierik, M. M.: "Joint Appointment: Collaboration for Better Patient Care," *Nurs. Outlook*, **21**:576, (Sept.) 1973.

10. Aydelotte, Myrtle K.: "Nursing Education and Practice: Putting It All Together," *J. Nurs. Educ.*, **11**:21, (Nov.) 1972.

11. Columbia University, Teachers College, Department of Nursing Education: *International Aspects of Nursing Education*. Bureau of Publications, Teachers College, New York, [1932].

12. Royal College of Nursing, and National Council of Nurses of the United Kingdom: *The Function, Scope and Training of Nurses in England and Wales for the Mentally Subnormal*. The College and the Council, London, 1967.

13. ——: *A Reform of Nursing Education*.

The College and the Council, London, 1964, p. 38 (reprinted 1969, 1970).

13a. American Nurses' Association: *Facts About Nursing 74–75.* The Association, Kansas City, Mo., 1976, p. 89.

14. American Nurses' Association: *Facts About Nursing 72–73.* The Association, Kansas City, Mo., 1974, pp. 98, 113, 116.

15. Canadian Nurses' Association: personal communication, Aug. 25, 1976.

16. Vaughan-Richards, A.: "Education and Preparation of the Nurse to Meet the Health Needs of the Nation [Nigeria]," *Niger. Nurse,* **4:**21, (Jan.–Mar.) 1972.

17. Jibneze, M. W.: "Continuing Education for Nurses in Nigeria," *Niger. Nurse,* **5:**39, (Apr.–June) 1973.

18. Royal College of Nursing, and National Council of Nurses of the United Kingdom: *op. cit.*

19. Beard, Richard Olding: "The University Education of the Nurse," in American Society of Superintendents of Training Schools for Nurses: *Annual Report, 1909, and Proceedings of 15th Convention Including Report of Second Meeting of American Federation of Nurses.* J. H. Furst, Baltimore, 1910.

20. Roberts, Mary M.: *op. cit.,* p. 66.

21. Russell, Charles H.: *Liberal Education and Nursing.* Bureau of Publications, Teachers College, Columbia University, New York, 1959; *Liberal Education and Nursing, A Bibliography.* Institute of Higher Education, Teachers College, Columbia University, New York, [1957], processed.

22. Committee for the Study of Nursing Education in the United States: *Report of the Committee . . . and Report of a Survey by Josephine Goldmark, Secretary.* Macmillan Publishing Co., New York, 1923.

23. Committee on the Grading of Nursing Schools: *Nursing Schools—Today and Tomorrow.* The Committee, New York, 1934.

24. West, Margaret, and Hawkins, Christy: *Nursing Schools at the Mid-Century.* National Commission for the Improvement of Nursing Services, New York, 1950.

25. Brown, Esther Lucile: *Nursing for the Future.* Russell Sage Foundation, New York, 1948.

26. National Commission for the Study of Nursing and Nursing Education: *An Abstract for Action.* (Prepared by Jerome P. Lysaught.) McGraw-Hill Book Co., New York, 1970.

27. Gillett, Harriet M.: "The Future of Teaching in Schools of Nursing Without University Affiliation," in National League of Nursing Education: *Annual Report, 1921, and Proceedings of 27th Convention.* Williams and Wilkins Co., Baltimore, 1922.

28. Robinson, Grace C.: "The Hourly Instructor," *Pac. Coast J. Nurs.,* **17:**165, (Mar.) 1921.

29. Harris, Robert L.: "Three Years of New Type College Training," *Junior Coll. J.,* **3:**19, (Oct.) 1932.

30. Bradley, H. Lenore: "Central Schools for Rural Areas," *Am. J. Nurs.,* **43:**447, (May) 1943.

31. Ringheim, Alice: "A Study of Nursing Education in Twenty-five Junior Colleges," *Am. J. Nurs.,* **32:**971, (Sept.) 1932.

32. Newton, Mildred E.: "Nursing Courses in Junior Colleges," *Junior Coll. J.,* **4:**82, (Oct.) 1933.

33. Faville, Katharine: "Nursing Needs Challenge Junior College," *Junior Coll. J.,* **13:**76, (Oct.) 1942.

34. Seyffer, Charlotte: "Pre-nursing Curriculums in 116 Junior Colleges in the United States," *Junior Coll. J.,* **20:**23, (Sept.) 1949.

35. Montag, Mildred L.: *The Education of Nursing Technicians,* Ed.D. dissertation, Columbia University, Teachers College, New York, 1951.

36. ———, and Gotkin, Lassar G.: *Community College Education for Nursing; An Experiment in Technical Education for Nursing.* McGraw-Hill Book Co., New York, 1959.

36a. Lenburg, Carrie B.: *Open Learning and Career Mobility in Nursing.* C. V. Mosby Co., St. Louis, 1975.

37. Lenburg, Carrie B., et al.: *Directory of Career Mobility Opportunities in Nursing.* National League for Nursing, New York, 1973.

38. Collins, B.: *An Experiment in Open Curriculum.* National League for Nursing, New York, 1972.

39. Story, D. K.: *Career Mobility; Implementing the Ladder Concept in Associate Degree and Practical Nursing Curricula.* C. V. Mosby Co., St. Louis, 1974.

40. Kroman, L. M.: "Continuing Education in the Non-University Setting," *Can. Hosp.,* **49:**42, (Jan.) 1972.

41. "California's Continuing Education Law," *Calif. Nurse,* **69:**3, (May) 1973.

42. Cooper, Signe S.: "A Brief History of Continuing Education in Nursing in the United States," *J. Continuing Educ. Nurs.,* **4:**5, (May–June) 1973.

43. ———: "Should Continuing Education Be Required for Licensure's Renewal," *Occup. Health Nurs. (N.Y.),* **27:**7, (June) 1974.

44. McGraff, E. P.: "Continuing Education in Nursing," *Nurs. Clin. North Am.,* **8:**325, (June) 1973.

45. Egelston, E. M.: "Continuing Education: A Requirement for Professional Membership or a Necessity for Relicensure," *J. Continuing Educ. Nurs.,* **5:**12, (May–June) 1974.

46. Rhee, J. C.: *Accreditation—Certification . . . Continuing Education.* National League for Nursing, New York, 1974.

47. Whitaker, Judith G.: "The Issue of Mandatory Continuing Education," *Nurs. Clin. North Am.,* **9:**475, (Sept.) 1974.

48. American Nurses' Association: *Facts About Nursing 74–75.* The Association, Kansas City, Mo., 1976, p. 84.
49. Henderson, Virginia: "Library Resources in Nursing—Their Development and Use," *Int. Nurs. Rev.,* Vol. 15, Nos. 2, 3, 4, 1968.
50. Hoose, David C.: "A Model for a Nursing Media Center," *Nurs. Outlook,* **24:**104, (Feb.) 1976.
51. American Bar Association, and American Medical Association: *Medical and Health Care in Jails, Prisons and Other Correctional Facilities. A Compilation of Standards and Materials,* 3rd ed. American Bar Association, Washington, D.C., 1974.
52. Roberts, Mary M.: *op. cit.,* p. 106.
53. Burgess, Elizabeth C.: "Recent Progress in Nursing Legislation," *Can. Nurse,* **22:**409, (Aug.) 1926.
54. Robb, Isabel Hampton: *Educational Standards for Nurses with Addresses on Nursing Subjects.* Koeckert, Cleveland, 1907.
55. ———: "An International Education Standard for Nurses," *Br. J. Nurs.,* **43:**231, (Sept. 18) 1909.
56. Nutting, M. Adelaide, and Stewart, Isabel M.: "Report of the Committee on Education, ICN," in International Council of Nurses: *Fifth Regular Meeting, Helsingfors, Finland, July 20–25, 1925.* The Council, Geneva, [1926].
57. International Council of Nurses, Education Committee: *The Educational Programme of the School of Nursing.* (Prepared by Isabel Maitland Stewart.) The Council, Geneva, 1934.
58. International Council of Nurses, Committee on Education: *The Basic Education of the Professional Nurse,* 3rd ed. The Council, Geneva, 1952 (revised 1958 by Frances S. Beck as *Basic Nursing Education; Principles and Practices of Nursing Education*).
59. International Council of Nurses: *Principles of Legislation for Nursing Education and Practice; A Guide to Assist National Nurses' Associations.* The Council, Geneva, 1969.
60. ———: *Statement on Nursing Education, Nursing Practice and Service and the Social and Economic Welfare of Nurses.* The Council, Geneva, 1970.
61. Florence Nightingale International Foundation: *International Courses; Prospectus.* The Foundation, Geneva, 1936; 1937; 1938; 1939; [1947].
62. World Health Organization, Expert Committee on Nursing: *First Report,* 1950 (Tech. Report Series No. 22): *Fifth Report,* 1966 (Tech. Report Series No. 347). The Organization, Geneva.
63. WHO Seminar on Nursing Education, Taipei, Taiwan, Nov. 1952: *Report of the . . . .* World Health Organization, Geneva, 1953.
64. World Health Organization: "Conference in Kampala [Uganda, Autumn 1953]; Nursing Education in Africa," *Chron. WHO,* **8:** 276, (Sept.) 1954.
65. World Health Organization, Regional Office in Europe: *Basic Nursing Curriculum in Europe.* The Organization, Geneva, 1956.
66. World Health Organization, Expert Committee on Professional and Technical Education of Medical and Auxiliary Personnel: *Third Report.* The Organization, Geneva, 1956.
67. World Health Organization: *Nursing in Intensive Care.* Report of Seminar Convened by Regional Office for Europe of WHO, Copenhagen, Nov. 10–14, 1969. The Organization, Geneva, 1971.
68. *Higher Education in Nursing. Report on a Symposium.* Regional Office for Europe, World Health Organization, Copenhagen, 1973.
69. World Health Organization: *Development of Educational Programmes for the Health Professions.* The Organization, Geneva, 1973 (Public Health Papers No. 52).
70. World Health Organization: *Directory of Schools of Nursing in the European Region.* The Organization, Geneva, 1971.
71. National League of Nursing Education, Education Committee: *Standard Curriculum for Schools of Nursing.* The League, New York, 1917 (revised 1929 as *A Curriculum for Schools of Nursing;* 1937, *A Curriculum Guide for Schools of Nursing*).
72. Goodrich, Annie Warburton: "The Contribution of the Army School of Nursing," in National League of Nursing Education: *Annual Report, 1919, and Proceedings of 25th Convention.* Williams and Wilkins Co., Baltimore, 1919.
73. Stewart, Isabel Maitland: "The Army School of Nursing Established on a Permanent Basis," *Am. J. Nurs.* **20:**555, (Apr.) 1920.
74. "The Proposed Army School of Nursing," *School Soc.,* **7:**732, (June 22) 1918.
75. Roberts, Mary M.: *op. cit.,* p. 140.
76. Condé, Marlette: *The Lamp and the Caduceus.* Army School of Nursing Alumni Association [Washington, D.C.], 1975.
77. National League of Nursing Education, Committee on Revision of the Faculty Pamphlet: *Faculty Positions in Schools of Nursing and How to Prepare for Them.* The League, New York, 1946 (revision of *The Nursing School Faculty—Duties, Qualifications and Preparation,* 1933).
78. National League of Nursing Education, Committee on Standards: *Essentials of a Good School of Nursing.* The League, New York, 1936 (revised 1942).
79. Goodrich, Annie Warburton: "Yale University School of Nursing," *Am. J. Nurs.,* **25:**360, (May) 1925.
80. ———: "The School of Nursing and the Future," *Am. J. Nurs.,* **32:**675, (Jan.) 1932.
81. McIver, Pearl: *An Analysis of First Level Public Health Nursing in Ten Selected*

Organizations. National Organization for Public Health Nursing, New York, 1935.

82. Joint Committee of the National Organization for Public Health Nursing and the U.S. Public Health Service [on Curriculum]: *The Public Health Nursing Curriculum Guide.* The Organization, New York, 1942.

83. Wilson, Dorothy: *Summary Report of the Initial Yearly Reviews for the Academic Year 1941–1942 of 29 of the 31 Programs of Study in Public Health Nursing Accredited by NOPHN as of June 1942.* National Organization for Public Health Nursing, New York, 1943.

84. Joint Committee on Integration of the Social and Health Aspects of Nursing in Basic Curriculum: "Faculty Preparation in the Health and Social Components of Nursing," *Am. J. Nurs.,* 45:564, (July) 1945.

85. National League of Nursing Education, Committee on Nursing Curricula: *A Check List on Abilities Needed by Nurses with Suggestions for Continued Curriculum Study.* The League, New York, 1951.

86. Shields, Mary: "An Opinion Study on Purposes of Schools of Nursing," *Nurs. Outlook,* 2:30, (Jan.) 1954.

87. Petry, Lucile: "The U.S. Cadet Nurse Corps—A Summing Up," *Am. J. Nurs.,* 45:1027, (Dec.) 1945.

88. National League of Nursing Education: *Nursing Education in War-Time. Complete Series of Fourteen Bulletins, 1942–1945.* The League, New York, 1945.

89. National League of Nursing Education, Committee on Educational Problems in Wartime: *Problems of Collegiate Schools of Nursing Offering Basic Professional Programs.* The League, New York, 1945.

90. Nutting, M. Adelaide: "The Nurse as an Educator," *Am. J. Nurs.,* 13:927, (Sept.) 1913.

91. "Current Events of International Interest. Finland. Post-Graduate Course for Supervisory and Teaching Nurses in Schools of Nursing," *ICN,* 1:219, (July) 1926.

92. Hillyers, G. V.: "Nursing Education and the Universities in Great Britain. 1. The Sister Tutor's Course, King's College, University of London," *ICN,* 3:12, (Jan.) 1928.

93. Florence Nightingale International Foundation, Committee of Management: [*Facilities for Advanced Nursing Education in London and Future Educational Policy of FNIF.*] The Foundation, Geneva, 1936.

94. Stewart, Isabel Maitland: "[Postgraduate Education]," *Am. J. Nurs.,* 33:361, (Apr.); 583, (June) 1933.

95. Ashline, Sister Rosaline: *An Investigation of the Curricula in Nursing Education as Constructed in 130 Institutions of Higher Learning.* Catholic University of America, Washington, D.C., 1935.

96. Oates, Louise: "Advanced Professional Curricula," *Am. J. Nurs.,* 38:909, (Aug.) 1938.

97. Florence Nightingale International Foundation: *International Courses; Prospectus.* The Foundation, Geneva, 1936; 1937; 1938; 1939; [1947].

98. International Council of Nurses, Committee on Education: *Developing Graduate Nurse Education.* The Council, Geneva, 1951.

99. Florence Nightingale International Foundation: *An International List of Advanced Programmes in Nursing Education, 1951–1952.* International Council of Nurses, Geneva, 1954 (Supplement, 1958).

100. ———: *Directory of Graduate Nurse Programs in United States and Canada, 1954–1956.* International Council of Nurses, Geneva, 1956.

101. Schroeder, Yvonne: *Post-Basic Nursing Education; Principles of Administration as Applied to Advanced Programmes in Nursing Education.* International Council of Nurses, Geneva, 1957, 2 vol.

102. National League of Nursing Education, Committee to Study Post Graduate Clinical Nursing Courses: "[Advanced Courses in Clinical Nursing]," *Am. J. Nurs.,* 41:945, (Aug.) 1941; 43:1120, (Dec.) 1943; 44:579, (June); 683, (July); 1162, (Dec.) 1944; 45:645, (Aug.) 1945; 46:332, (May); 859, (Dec.) 1946; 47:177, (Mar.) 1947.

103. National League of Nursing Education: *Clinical Nursing Courses Offered to Graduate Professional Nurses.* The League, New York, 1951.

104. National League for Nursing, Division of Nursing Education: "Educational Resources for the Preparation of Nurses. 2. Preparation for Advanced Positions in Professional Nursing," *Nurs. Outlook,* 6:86, (Feb.) 1958.

105. ———: "A Report on Progress in Nursing Education. 2. Graduate Education," *Nurs. Outlook,* 6:397, (July) 1958.

106. Work Conference on Regional Planning for Nursing and Nursing Education, Plymouth, N.H., June 12–13, 1950: *Report on the . . .* Bureau of Publications, Teachers College, Columbia University, New York, 1950.

107. Coulter, Pearl Parvin: *The Winds of Change. A Progress Report of Regional Cooperation in Collegiate Nursing Education in the West, 1956–1961.* Western Interstate Commission for Higher Education, Boulder, Colo., 1963.

108. Bixler, Genevieve K., and Simmons, Leo W.: *The Regional Project in Graduate Education and Research in Nursing.* Southern Regional Education Board, Atlanta, 1960.

109. Belcher, Helen C.: *The SREB Project in Nursing Education.* Southern Regional Education Board, Atlanta, 1972.

110. Henderson, Virginia: *Report on NECHEN Past and Present and Some Suggestions for the Future.* For New England Council on Higher Education for Nursing, New Eng-

land Board of Higher Education, 1969, processed.

111. Task Force, New England Council on Higher Education for Nursing, New England Board of Higher Education: *Report of the Task Force on Purpose, Structure, and Functions of the New England Council on Higher Education for Nursing.* The Board, Wellesley, Mass., 1969, processed.

111a. American Nurses' Association: *Facts About Nursing 72–73.* The Association, Kansas City, Mo., 1974, p. 114.

112. American Nurses' Association: *Facts About Nursing 72–73.* The Association, Kansas City, Mo., 1974, pp. 58–61.

113. Goodrich, Annie Warburton: "A General Presentation of the Statutory Requirements of the Different States," *Am. J. Nurs.,* **12:** 1001, (Sept.) 1912.

114. ———: "Some State Regulations upon the Appointment of Faculties of Nursing Schools, Their Number, Preparation and Status," *Am. J. Nurs.,* **13:**950, (Sept.) 1913.

115. Anderson, Bernice E.: *The Facilitation of Interstate Movement of Registered Nurses.* J. B. Lippincott Co., Philadelphia, 1950.

116. New York (State) University: [Course of Study and Syllabus for the Guidance of Nurse Training Schools in the Preparation of Students for the Examinations of the Board.] University Bull. No. 498, July 1, 1911 (revised periodically after this date).

117. Pennsylvania State Board of Examiners for Registration of Nurses: *Curricula of the Pennsylvania State Board . . . for the Training Schools of the State of Pennsylvania.* State Printer, Harrisburg, 1916.

118. West, Roberta M.: "Uniform Statutory Requirements for Schools of Nursing and Licensure to Practice Nursing," *Am. J. Nurs.,* **20:**846, (July) 1920.

119. Kandel, Phoebe Miller: "Standardizing Agencies and State Boards of Nurse Examiners," in National League of Nursing Education: *Annual Report, 1932, and Record of Proceedings of 36th Convention.* The League, New York, 1932.

120. American Nurses' Association: *Nurse Practice Acts and Board Rules: A Digest.* The Association, New York, 1940, 1948 (supplement 1949).

121. New York (State) University, and State Education Department, Division of Professional Education: *Experimental Programs in Nursing Curriculums; New York State.* The Department, Albany, 1957.

122. Agree, B. C.: "The Threat of Institutional Licensure," *Am. J. Nurs.,* **73:**1758, (Oct.) 1973.

123. Hall, C. M.: "Who Controls the Nursing Profession? Role of the Professional Association," *Niger. Nurse,* **5:**30, (July–Sept.) 1973.

124. American Nurses' Association, Council of State Boards of Nursing: *Licensure and Credentialing.* Proceedings of ANA Con-

ference for Members and Professional Employees of State Boards of Nursing and ANA Advisory Council, Detroit, Mich., Apr. 27–28, 1972. The Council, New York, 1974.

125. ———: *Licensure to Practice Nursing.* The Council, New York, 1974.

126. National Nursing Council for War Service, and Association of Collegiate Schools of Nursing: *A Guide for Organization of Collegiate Schools of Nursing.* The Council, New York, 1942.

127. Brown, Esther Lucile: *op. cit.*

128. West, Margaret, and Hawkins, Christy: *op. cit.*

129. National Nursing Council: *A Thousand Think Together; A Report of Three Regional Conferences Held in Connection with the Study of Schools of Nursing.* The Council, New York, 1948.

130. National Committee for the Improvement of Nursing Services, Subcommittee on School Data Analysis: "The School Data Survey," *Am. J. Nurs.,* **49:**636, (Oct.) 1949.

131. American Nurses' Association: *Facts About Nursing 72–73.* The Association, Kansas City, Mo., 1974, p. 258.

132. National League for Nursing, Division of Nursing Education: *Objectives of Educational Programs in Nursing.* The League, New York, 1955.

133. Fritz, Edna L.: *Toward Better Nursing Care of Patients with Long-Term Illness.* National League for Nursing, New York, 1956.

134. National League for Nursing, Division of Nursing Education: *Ten Thousand Nurse Faculty Members in Basic Professional Schools of Nursing.* The League, New York, 1953.

135. National League for Nursing, Department of Diploma and Associate Degree Programs: *Criteria for the Evaluation of Educational Programs in Nursing Leading to a Diploma.* The League, New York, 1958.

136. ———: *Self-Evaluation Guide for Schools of Nursing Offering Programs Leading to a Diploma.* The League, New York, 1957 (supplement, 1958).

137. National League for Nursing, Division of Nursing Education, Department of Baccalaureate and Higher Degree Programs: *Self-Evaluation Guide for Collegiate Schools of Nursing.* The League, New York, 1954.

138. ———: *Some Statistics on Nursing Education, 1958* The League, New York, 1959.

139. National League for Nursing, Department of Diploma and Associate Degree Programs: *Report on Hospital Schools of Nursing, 1957.* The League, New York, 1959.

140. Elliott, Florence E.: "Regional Conferences on Curriculum in 1957," *Nurs. Outlook,* **6:**173, (Mar.) 1958.

141. [Joint] Committee of the Six National Nursing Organizations on Unification of Accrediting Activities: *Manual of Accrediting Educational Programs in Nursing.* National Nursing Accrediting Service, New York, 1949.

142. Hawkinson, Nellie X.: "The National League of Nursing Education's Plan for the Accrediting of Schools of Nursing," *Hospitals,* **10:**22, (Sept.) 1936.

143. Burgess, Elizabeth C.: "General Plan for Accrediting Schools of Nursing," *Hosp. Manage.,* **51:**41, (Jan.) 1941.

144. "Catholic Schools of Nursing Approved by the Council of Nursing Education and Accredited by the Catholic Hospital Association," *Hosp. Prog.,* **23:**1, (Jan.) 1942.

145. National League of Nursing Education, Committee on the Administration of the Accrediting Program: *Statement of Policy for the Accreditation of Schools of Nursing.* The League, New York, 1939 ed.; 1944 ed.

146. Schwitalla, Alphonse M.: "A Single Accrediting Body in Nursing in Relation to the Catholic Schools of Nursing," *Hosp. Prog.,* **27:**315, (Oct.) 1946.

147. Petry, Lucile: "We Hail an Important 'First'," *Am. J. Nurs.,* **49:**630, (Oct.) 1949.

148. Nahm, Helen: "Accreditation of Programs in Public Health Nursing," *Public Health Nurs.,* **43:**692, (Dec.) 1951.

149. National League for Nursing, Division of Nursing Education: *Report on the Program of Temporary Accreditation of National Nursing Accrediting Service.* The League, New York, 1952, 2 vol., processed.

150. "Educational Programs in Nursing Approved by National Nursing Accrediting Service—1952," *Am. J. Nurs.,* **52:**216, (Feb.) 1952.

151. National League for Nursing: *Proceedings —Open Curriculum Conference I: A Project of the NLN Study of the Open Curriculum in Nursing Education.* The League, New York, 1974.

152. Walsh, Margaret E.: *The Health Profession Education Organization and the Governmental Process.* National League for Nursing, New York, 1974.

153. National League for Nursing: *The Problem-Oriented System—A Multidisciplinary Approach,"* The League, New York, 1974.

154. ———: *Developing Nursing Programs in Institutions of Higher Education—1974.* The League, New York, 1974.

155. ———: *Masters Education in Nursing; Route to Opportunity in Contemporary Nursing—1974–75.* The League, New York, 1974.

156. National League for Nursing, Department of Baccalaureate and Higher Degree Programs: *Current Issues in Nursing Education.* Papers presented at Tenth Conference of Council of Baccalaureate and Higher Degree Programs, St. Louis, Mo., Nov. 15–17, 1972. The League, New York, 1973.

157. National League for Nursing: *Baccalaureate Education in Nursing: Key To a Professional Career in Nursing—1974–75.* The League, New York, 1974.

158. ———: *Associate Degree Education for Nursing; Current Issues 1974.* Papers presented at Seventh Conference of Council of Associate Degree Programs. The League, New York, 1974.

159. American Nurses' Association, Educational Administrators, Consultants and Teachers Section: "ANA Statements of Functions, Standards, and Qualifications," *Am. J. Nurs.,* **56:**1586, (Dec.) 1956.

160. ———: *Guide for the Development of Standards of Employment for Teachers in Nursing.* The Association, New York, 1959.

161. American Nurses' Association, Special Committee of State Boards of Nursing: *Progress Report of the Subcommittee on the Preparation of Education Standards to Be Used as a Guide by State Boards.* The Association, New York, 1956.

161a. American Nurses' Association, Committee on Education: "American Nurses' Association First Position on Education for Nursing," *Am. J. Nurs.,* **65:**106, (Dec.) 1965.

162. American Nurses' Association: *Facts About Nursing 72–73.* The Association, Kansas City, Mo., 1974, p. 42.

163. Nutting, M. Adelaide: *A Sound Economic Basis for Schools of Nursing.* G. P. Putnam's Sons, New York, 1926.

164. Goodrich, Annie Warburton: *The Social and Ethical Significance of Nursing.* Macmillan Publishing Co., New York, 1932.

165. Rockefeller Foundation: *Methods and Problems of Medical Education. Nursing Education and Schools of Nursing.* The Foundation, New York, 1932.

166. Davis, Michael M.: "Public Responsibility for the Education of Nurses," *Am. J. Nurs.,* **33:**694 (July) 1933.

167. Petry, Lucile: "Basic Professional Curricula in Nursing Leading to Degrees; a Study," *Am. J. Nurs.,* **37:**287, (Mar.) 1937.

168. Davis, Helen E.: *Fifty Schools of Nursing Education; A Study of Administrative Practices.* National League of Nursing Education, New York, 1939.

169. Pfefferkorn, Blanche, and Rovetta, Charles A.: *Administrative Cost Analysis for Nursing Service and Nursing Education.* American Hospital Association, Chicago, and National League of Nursing Education, New York, 1940.

170. National League of Nursing Education: *Fundamentals of Administration for Schools of Nursing.* The League, New York, 1940.

171. Petry, Lucile: "Nursing Education in Higher Institutions of the North Central Association," *North Central Assoc. Q.,* **15:**400, (Apr.) 1941.

172. Williams, Dorothy Rogers: *Administration of Schools of Nursing.* Macmillan Publishing Co., New York, 1950.

173. Thielbar, Frances C.: *Administrative Organization of Collegiate Schools of Nursing.* Ph.D. dissertation, University of Chicago, Chicago, 1951.

174. Bridgman, Margaret: *Collegiate Education for Nursing.* Russell Sage Foundation, New York, 1952.

175. Bixler, Roy W., and Bixler, Genevieve K.: *Administration of Nursing Education.* G. P. Putnam's Sons, New York, 1954.

176. Buechel, J. F. Marvin: *Principles of Administration in Junior and Community College Education for Nursing.* G. P. Putnam's Sons, New York, 1956.

177. Rowe, H. R., and Flitter, Hessel H.: *Study of Cost of Nursing Education.* National League for Nursing, New York, 1965.

178. National Commission for the Study of Nursing and Nursing Education: *op. cit.*

179. American Nurses' Association: *Facts About Nursing 72–73.* The Association, Kansas City, Mo., 1974, pp. 98, 186.

180. Royal College of Nursing, and National Council of Nurses of the United Kingdom: *A Reform of Nursing Education.* The College and the Council, London, 1964, pp. 17, 33 (reprinted 1969, 1970).

181. Lysaught, Jerome P.: "Costs of Nursing Education and a Case for Its Great Support," in Lysaught, Jerome P. (ed.): *Action in Nursing.* McGraw-Hill Book Co., New York, 1974, pp. 304, 306.

182. American Nurses' Association: *Facts About Nursing 72–73.* The Association, Kansas City, Mo., 1974, p. 10.

183. Canadian Nurses' Association: personal communication, Aug. 25, 1976.

Jails, Prisons, and Other Correctional Institutions

1. Montaigne, Michel E. de: *Essayes.* Modern Library, Random House, New York, 1928.

2. Black, Hugo: Quoted in Minton, Jr., Robert J. (ed.): *Inside Prison American Style.* Random House, New York, 1971.

3. Brown, J. W.: "The Increase of Crime in the United States," *The Independent,* 1907; quoted in Sarbin, Theodore R.: *The Myth of the Criminal Type.* Wesleyan University Press, Middletown, Conn., 1969.

4. Ohlin, L. E. (ed.): *Prisoners in America.* Prentice Hall, Englewood Cliffs, N.J., 1973.

5. Schwitzgebel, Ralph K.: *Crime and Delinquency Issues: A Monograph Series.* US Government Printing Office, Washington, D.C., 1971 (PHS Pub. No. 2056).

6. Johnston, Norman, et al. (eds.): *The Sociology of Punishment and Correction,* 2nd ed. John Wiley and Sons, New York, 1970.

7. Hawkins, Gordon: *The Prison—Policy and Practice.* University of Chicago Press, Chicago, 1976.

8. Mitford, Jessica: *Kind and Usual Punishment. The Prison Business.* Alfred A. Knopf, New York, 1973, p. 9.

9. Murtha, Rena: "Health Care in Prison: Change in One City's System. It Started with a Director of Nursing," *Am. J. Nurs.,* **75:**421, (Mar.) 1973.

10. American Medical Association, Center for Health Services: *Medical Care in U.S. Jails. A 1972 AMA Survey.* The Association, Chicago, 1973.

11. Lawes, Lewis E.: "Prisons," in *The Encyclopedia Americana.* Americana Corp., New York, 1958, p. 605.

12. Ibid., p. 607.

13. "Fourth United National Congress on Prevention of Crime and Treatment of Offenders," in American Bar Association, and American Medical Association: *Medical and Health Care in Jails, Prisons, and Other Correctional Facilities. A Compilation of Standards and Materials,* 3rd ed. American Bar Association, Washington, D.C., 1974.

14. Debs, Eugene Victor: *Walls and Bars.* Socialist Party, Chicago, 1927, pp. 19, 25.

15. Russell, Bertrand: *The Autobiography of Bertrand Russell, 1914–1944.* Little, Brown and Co., Boston, 1968, p. 30.

15a. President's Crime Commission: *The Challenge of Crime in a Free Society. A Report by the President's Commission on Law Enforcement and Administration of Justice.* U.S. Government Printing Office, Washington, D.C., 1967.

16. Shaw, George Bernard: *The Crime of Imprisonment.* The Philosophical Library, New York, 1946.

17. Menninger, Karl: *The Crime of Punishment.* Viking Press, New York, 1969.

18. Debs, Eugene Victor: *op. cit.*

19. Tannenbaum, Frank: *Wall Shadows.* Oxford University Press, New York, 1948.

20. Clark, Ramsey: *Crime in America.* Simon and Schuster, New York, 1970.

21. American Nurses' Association: *Facts About Nursing 72–73.* The Association, Kansas City, Mo., 1974.

22. Canadian Nurses' Association: *Countdown 1974.* The Association, Ottawa, 1975.

23. US Department of Justice, Bureau of Prisons: "Federal Prison Medical Program," in American Bar Association, and American Medical Association: *Medical and Health Care in Jails, Prisons, and Other Correctional Facilities. A Compilation of Standards and Materials,* 3rd ed. American Bar Association, Washington, D.C., 1974.

24. US Department of Justice: *A Look at the Federal Prison System.* The Department, Washington, [1973], p. 2.

25. American Medical Association, Center for Health Services: *op. cit.,* pp. 11, 20.

26. [Massachusetts] Medical Advisory Committee on State Prisons: "Report of the Committee," in American Bar Association, and American Medical Association: *Medical and Health Care in Jails, Prisons, and Other Correctional Facilities, A Compilation of Standards and Materials,* 3rd ed.

American Bar Association, Washington, D.C., 1974.

27. Mattick, Hans W., and Sweet, Ronald P.: "Illinois Jails. Challenge and Opportunity for the 1970's," in American Bar Association, and American Medical Association: *Medical and Health Care in Jails, Prisons, and Other Correctional Facilities. A Compilation of Standards and Materials,* 3rd ed. American Bar Association, Washington, D.C., 1974.

28. "Datagram," J. Med. Educ., **47**:831, (Oct.) 1972.

29. Mitford, Jessica: *op. cit.,* p. 181.

30. Stokes, Rita Judd: "Health Care Services in the San Diego Jail," in American Bar Association, and American Medical Association: *Medical and Health Care in Jails, Prisons, and Other Correctional Facilities. A Compilation of Standards and Materials,* 3rd ed. American Bar Association, Washington, D.C., 1974.

31. Murtha, Rena: *op. cit.*

32. [Canadian] Advisory Board of Psychiatric Consultants: *The General Program for the Development of Psychiatric Services in Federal Correctional Services in Canada.* Report of Advisory Board to Solicitor General of Canada. Department of Solicitor General, Ottawa, 1973, p. 11.

33. *Ibid.,* pp. 21, 36, 59.

34. Whitney, Janet: *Elizabeth Fry, Quaker Heroine.* Little, Brown and Co., Boston, 1937.

35. Fenwick, Ethel Gordon: "Elizabeth Fry League." *Br. J. Nurs.,* **43**:495, (Dec. 18) 1909.

36. Haldane, Elizabeth S.: "Nurses as Prison Matrons and Warders," *Br. J. Nurs.,* **40**:128, (Feb. 15) 1908.

37. Anonymous: "Nursing in Penal Institutions," *Trained Nurse,* **28**:17, (Jan.) 1902.

38. St. John, Mrs. Maxwell: "Nursing in Prisons," *Br. J. Nurs.,* **53**:95, (Aug. 1) 1914.

39. "Royal British Nurses Supplement. Penal Reform League," *Br. J. Nurs.,* **63**:231, (Apr. 5) 1919.

40. Dock, Lavinia L.: "Foreign Department. Nursing in Prisons," *Am. J. Nurs.,* **20**:318, (Jan.) 1920.

41. Kent, Beatrice: "Trained Nursing in Prisons," *I.C.N.,* **1**:194, (July) 1926.

42. "Release of Nurse [Ellen] Pitfield," *Br. J. Nurs.,* **48**:310, (Apr. 20) 1912.

43. "The Nursing Outlook. Nurses for Women Prisoners," *Nurs. Mirror,* **8**:183, (Dec. 19) 1908.

44. Bennett, James V.: *I Chose Prison.* Alfred A. Knopf, New York, 1970.

45. Clark, Ramsey: *op. cit.*

46. Debs, Eugene Victor: *op. cit.*

47. Ellis, Desmond: *Violence in Prisons.* Lexington Books, D. C. Heath Co., Boston, 1973.

48. Fox, Vernon: *Violence Behind Bars.* Vantage Press, New York, 1956.

48a. Greenberg, David F., and Stender, Fay: "The Prison as a Lawless Agency," *Buffalo Law Rev.,* **21**:799, 1972.

49. Hirschkop, Philip J., and Milleman, Michael A.: "The Unconstitutionality of Prison Life," *Virginia Law Rev.,* **55**:795, 1969.

50. Shaw, George Bernard: *op. cit.*

51. Wallerstein, James, and Wylie, C. J.: "Our Law-abiding Law-breakers," *Probation,* 1947; quoted in American Friends Service Committee: *Struggle for Justice. A Report on Crime and Punishment in America.* Hill and Wang, New York, 1971.

52. Mitford, Jessica: *op. cit.,* p. 255.

53. Badillo, Herman, and Haynes, Milton: *A Bill of Rights: Attica and the American Prison System.* Outerbridge and Lazard, New York, 1972.

54. US Department of Justice, Bureau of Prisons: *op. cit.*

55. [Canadian] Advisory Board of Psychiatric Consultants: *op. cit.,* p. 12.

56. *Ibid.,* pp. 24, 60.

57. [Massachusetts] Medical Advisory Committee on State Prisons: *op. cit.*

58. Haldane, Elizabeth S.: *op. cit.*

59. Holly, Helen: "Jail Matron, R.N.," *Am. J. Nurs.,* **72**:1621, (Sept.) 1972.

60. US Department of Justice, Bureau of Prisons: *op. cit.*

61. Mitford, Jessica: *op. cit.,* p. 173.

62. Gunn, A. D.: "Vulnerable Groups. 4. A Life with Bars. The Medico-Social Problems of Imprisonment," *Nurs. Times,* **64**:499, (Apr. 12) 1968.

63. Hargreaves, Anne G.: "The Nurse Group Therapist in a Variety of Settings: Community, Hospital, School and Prison," in *ANA Regional Clinical Conferences, 1967.* Appleton-Century-Crofts, New York, 1968.

64. Protzel, Mary Sue: "Nursing Behind Bars," *Am. J. Nurs.,* **72**:505, (Mar.) 1972.

65. Smyth, A. A., et al.: "Relationship Between Type of Offender and Reasons for Seeking Medical Care in a Correctional Setting," *Nurs. Res.,* **19**:456, (Sept.–Oct.) 1970.

66. Schrag, C.: "Conference on the Nature and Science of Nursing. Science and the Helping Professions," *Nurs. Res.,* **17**:486, (Nov.–Dec.) 1968.

67. Archer, C. I.: "Psychiatric Nursing Behind an Iron Fence," *Can. J. Psychiatr. Nurs.,* **14**:6, (Sept.–Oct.) 1973.

68. Arrowsmith, A. R.: "Psychiatric Nursing in the Canadian Penitentiary Service. A New Philosophy," *Can. J. Psychiatr. Nurs.,* **14**:1, (Sept.–Oct.) 1973.

69. Alperin, Shirley Hope: "Nursing at Sing Sing," *Nurs. World,* **14**: (July) 1959.

70. McNiff, M. A.: "Nursing in a Psychiatric Prison Service," *Am. J. Nurs.,* **73**:1586, (Sept.) 1973.

71. "[We Should Not Forget the Prison

Nurses]," *Sairaanh. Vuosik.,* **48:**198, (Mar. 10) 1972.

72. McCarrick, H.: "Nursing Behind Bars. 2. The Surgical Unit at Wormwood Scrubs," *Nurs. Times,* **65:**158, (Dec. 11) 1969; "3. Pucklechurch Remand Centre," **65:**162, (Dec. 18) 1969.

73. McCarrick, H.: "M. M. Prison, Holloway," *Nurs. Times,* **65:**15, (Dec. 4) 1969.

74. Norens, G.: "Nurses in Prison," *Can. Nurse,* **67:**37, (May) 1971.

75. Ryan, J. W.: "The Wynne Treatment Center," *Can. J. Psychiatr. Nurs.,* **8:**11, (Apr.) 1967.

76. Walton, A.: "Working 'Inside' Prison," *Occup. Health Nurse,* **1:**1, (Oct.) 1967.

77. Kennedy, Jane A.: "Health Care in Prisons: A View from Inside," *Am. J. Nurs.,* **75:**417, (Mar.) 1975.

Other Settings

1. International Council of Nurses: *Basic Documents.* The Council, Geneva, revised 1970.

2. ———: *Statement on Nursing Education, Nursing Practice and Service and the Social and Economic Welfare of Nurses.* The Council, Geneva, 1970.

3. ———: *Guidelines for Drafting a Constitution and Regulations of a National Nurses Organization.* The Council, Geneva, 1971.

4. International Council of Nurses, Florence Nightingale International Foundation: *Report of an International Seminar on Nursing Legislation, Warsaw, Poland.* The Council, Geneva, 1971.

5. World Health Organization: *Directory of Schools of Nursing in the European Region.* WHO, Regional Office for Europe, Copenhagen, 1971.

6. ———: *Planning and Programming for Nursing Services.* The Organization, Geneva, 1971 (WHO Public Health Papers No. 44).

7. ———: *Family Planning in the Education of Nurses and Midwives.* (Edited by L. M. Turnbull and Helena Pizurki.) The Organization, Geneva, 1973 (WHO Public Health Papers No. 53).

8. ———: *Nursing Manpower Development— a Review of Methods.* (Prepared by Nursing Unit, WHO Headquarters for Scientific Group on Development of Studies in Health Manpower Conference held in Geneva, 1970.) The Organization, Geneva, 1970.

9. Brown, B. S., and Torrey, E. F. (eds.): *International Collaboration in Mental Health.* US Department of Health, Education, and Welfare, Washington, D.C., 1973 (DHEW Pub. No. [HSM] 73–9120).

10. Bridgman, R. F., and Roemer, M. I.: *Hospital Legislation and Hospital Systems.*
World Health Organization, Geneva, 1973 (WHO Public Health Papers No. 50).

11. Orrick, James B.: *Participation of Non-Governmental Organizations in United Nations Activities.* American Nurses' Association, New York, 1949.

12. United Nations Relief and Rehabilitation Administration: *The Story of U.N.R.R.A.* The Administration, Washington, D.C., 1948.

13. Columbia University, Teachers College: *International Aspects of Nursing.* Bureau of Publications, Teachers College, New York [1932], processed.

14. Gochanour, Eleanor: "Nursing: An International Experience," *Public Health Nurs.,* **39:**132, (Mar.) 1947.

15. Bridges, Daisy Caroline: *A History of the International Council of Nurses.* Pitman Medical Publishers, London, 1967.

16. Hämelin, Ingrid: "The Operations and Importance of the ICN," *Sairaanhoidon Vuosikirja,* **8:**192, 1971.

17. Kruse, Margrethe: "The International Council of Nurses in Close-Up," *Sairaanhoidon Vuosikirja,* **8:**192, 1971.

18. Bewer, Alice C.: "The Medical Missionary Association of Turkey," *Am. J. Nurs.,* **9:**118, (Nov.) 1908.

19. "Nursing in Mission Stations. Moravian Missions for Lepers," *Am. J. Nurs.,* **9:**667, (June) 1909.

20. DeWitt, Katharine: "Letters from Missionary Nurses," *Am. J. Nurs.,* **14:**867, (July) 1914.

21. Gage, Nina D.: "Nursing in Mission Stations. Nursing in China," *Am. J. Nurs.,* **18:**797, (June) 1918.

21a. Neuschwanger, Thomas: "The Medical Mission Field in Africa," *Hosp. Prog.,* **5:**38, (Jan.) 1924.

22. Hyde, K. J.: "Missionary Nurses in Ovamboland," *Nurs. Mirror,* **135:**30, (Dec. 8) 1972.

23. Noyes, Clara D.: "Red Cross Nurses in India," *Am. J. Nurs.,* **24:**1055, (Oct.) 1924.

24. Withrington, Kathleen: "Health Among All Nations," *Nurs. Times,* **47:**1179, (Nov. 24); 1203, (Dec. 1) 1951.

25. Hewitt, S.: "Nursing with the Church in Malawi," *Nurs. Mirror,* **132:**24, (Jan. 29) 1971.

26. Helgestad, H.: "[Nurse's Work in the Mission Field]," *Tidsskr. Sygepl.,* **71:**82, (Feb.) 1971.

27. Sidel, Victor W., and Sidel, Ruth: *Serve the People. Observations on Medicine in the People's Republic of China.* Beacon Press, Boston, 1973.

28. Lewis, Marianna O. (ed.): *The Foundation Directory,* 3rd ed. Russell Sage Foundation, New York, 1967.

29. Rich, Wilmer Shields: *American Foundations and Their Fields,* 7th ed. American Foundations Information Service, New York, 1955.

29a. American Nurses' Association: *Facts About Nursing 74–75.* The Association, Kansas City, Mo., 1976, pp. 34, 36.

29b. Hay, Ian: *One Hundred Years of Army Nursing. The Story of the British Army Nursing Services From the Time of Florence Nightingale to the Present Day.* Cassell and Co., Ltd., London, 1953.

30. Zeller, Dorothy N.: "Recent Advances in Military Nursing," *Milit. Surg.,* **114:**126, (Feb.) 1954.

31. McLeod, Agnes: "Military and Veteran Care Nursing," *Can. Nurse,* 51:213, (Mar.) 1955.

32. Haynes, Inez: "Broader Opportunities for Military Nurses," *Nurs. World,* **132:**21, (Feb.) 1958.

33. Martin, Anita M.: "We Earn Our Wings," *Am. J. Nurs.,* 57:894, (July) 1957.

34. Jackson, Wilma Leona: "We've Reached the Golden Years [in the U.S. Navy Nurse Corps]," *Am. J. Nurs.,* 58:671, (May) 1958.

35. Bowe, Ethel J., and McRae, Charlotte: "Nursing in the Australian Military Service," *Am. J. Nurs.,* 58:378, (Mar.) 1958.

36. "Army Nursing History," *Nurs. Times,* **55:**623, (May 29) 1959.

37. Lay, Frances I.: "Next Stop—Outer Space," *Am. J. Nurs.,* **59:**971, (July) 1959.

38. Dovotny, Dorothy R.: "Aerospace Nursing," in *ANA Regional Clinical Conferences, 1969.* Appleton-Century-Crofts, New York, 1970; and International Council of Nurses: *Focus on the Future. Proceedings of 14th Quadrennial Congress, Montreal, June 1969.* ICN, Geneva, 1970.

39. Piper, Doris Ann, and Corrado, Vivien P.: "Space Age Nursing," *Int. Nurs. Rev.,* **15:**368, (Oct.) 1968.

40. Ricks, M. C.: "Continuing to Care—Even in the Air," *Can. Nurse,* 66:11, (Nov.) 1970.

41. O'Connor, Valeria: "Nursing Link with Those Men in Their Flying Machines," *Nurs. Times,* 67:45, (Nov. 11) 1971.

42. Culcissure, D. F.: "Medical Benefits from Space Research," *Am. J. Nurs.,* **74:**275, (Feb.) 1974.

Virginia Henderson

The Role of the Nurse in Health Evaluation and Planning Patient Care or Meeting Patients' Health Needs

CHAPTER 4

Observing, Reporting, and Recording

1. IMPORTANCE OF OBSERVATION IN ALL MEDICAL SCIENCES
2. RESPONSIBILITY OF THE NURSE
3. HOW AND WHAT THE NURSE OBSERVES
4. METHODS OF REPORTING AND RECORDING
5. THE PATIENT'S RECORD

1. IMPORTANCE OF OBSERVATION IN ALL MEDICAL SCIENCES

Observation is described by Abraham Kaplan[1] as a deliberate search, carried out with care and forethought. People observe their surroundings constantly, but these acts are largely passive, rather than deliberate or planned. Often they cannot be recalled or communicated to others. It is the deliberation and control of the process of observation that is distinctive of science in general and health sciences in particular. The aim of observation is to get information that will play a part in subsequent phases of inquiry or diagnosis, to order the observations, to formulate a problem, to intervene or institute therapy, and to evaluate the intervention.

R. D. Judge and G. D. Zuidema list three major sources of inaccurate observation and ways to overcome them:

. . . the three major sources of inaccurate observation are (1) oversight, (2) forgetting, (3) bias. Oversights are minimized by habituation to method and by fractionating observations into logical, sequential small units. Forgetting is minimized by jotting down immediate notes . . . and by transferring the information to the permanent record as promptly as possible. Bias is a life long challenge. It may be lessened by understanding how it distorts. By repeated self analysis . . . you may minimize the tendency, but . . . you will fall prey to your prejudices. We all do, unfortunately.*

Many of the problems inherent in the observation of people, which is a major activity of nurses, stem from what Kaplan calls the "shared humanity of the scientist and his sub-

ject matter." * In other words, the act of observation affects both the observer and the person observed. Behavior has meaning to the person engaging in it as well as to the observer, and the two meanings may not necessarily coincide. Ida Jean Orlando describes this duality as it affects the process of patient care:

It is . . . exceedingly important for the nurse to distinguish between her understanding of general principles and the meanings which she must discover in the immediate nursing situation in order to help the patient. In making the distinction, the nurse first attempts to understand the meaning to the patient in a time and place context of what she observes and how she can exercise her professional function in relation to it. She also becomes aware of how the patient is affected by what she says or does.†

2. RESPONSIBILITY OF THE NURSE

All those who contribute to the care of patients develop the ability to learn about them by listening to them and studying their appearance and actions. The sum total of their findings and the continuous analysis of their observations are the basis for the initial and evolving plan of care. Diagnosis, prognosis, and therapy are steps in the process of giving care which the physician, nurse, psychologist, social worker, and special therapist all employ. Definitions of these acts in relation to specific professionals are found in every American jurisdiction in the practice acts for a specific professional group. The *International Digest of Health Legislation* is published quarterly by the World Health Organization in two editions

* Judge, R. D., and Zuidema, G. D. (eds.): *Physical Diagnosis: A Physiological Approach to the Clinical Examination,* 2nd ed. Little, Brown & Co., Boston, 1968, p. 38.

* Kaplan, Abraham: *The Conduct of Inquiry.* Chandler Publishing Co., San Francisco, 1964, p. 126.
† Orlando, Ida Jean: *The Dynamic Nurse Patient Relationship: Functions, Process, and Principles.* G. P. Putnam's Sons, New York, 1961, p. 1.

English and French, and contains a selection of health laws and regulations and studies in comparative health legislation. This journal is a valuable resource for the study of practice acts and educational programs for specific health workers.*

The beginning practitioner will note that there is a continual realignment of professional functions of physician, nurse, and others. The statutes governing the practice of nursing define professional nursing in general terms that permit practice to advance into areas of increasing complexity. It need only be shown that the newly assumed nursing function is predicated on the practitioner's ability to draw on knowledge of physical, biologic, and social sciences.[2] (See also Chapters 1 and 5 for further discussion of the legal status of nursing practice.)

There can be no question that nurses observe symptoms and reactions and interpret these observations. Only then are they able to take intelligent and humane action with or on behalf of their patients.

Florence Nightingale, who probably saw the nurse's function more clearly than had any one before her, said that without the habit of ready and correct observation nurses are useless, no matter how devoted. She also pointed out that otherwise nursing becomes a mechanical routine often inimical to the patient's interests.[3] It is of interest to note in the *Nursing Studies Index, Vol. I (1900-1929)*,[4] that there are nine titles listed referring to articles on the responsibility of the nurse to observe, interpret, and record signs and symptoms of illness. More recently, Katherine Kelly states:

The observational function is now conceived to be a process that includes three specific operations: . . .
1. Observation—the recognition of signs and symptoms presented by the patient.
2. Inference—making a judgment about the state of the patient and/or the nursing needs of the patient.
3. Decision-making—determining the action which should be taken that will be of optimal benefit to the patient.†

Throughout the discussion in this chapter of observation, reporting, and recording, one must keep in mind the ways in which the nurse's

observational function varies according to the education and experience of the nurse, the needs of patients, and the settings in which care is provided in health and illness. Institutional nurses may corroborate or correct their judgment with other members of the medical team continuously, because of the proximity of various professionals in the institutional setting. Nurses working in homes have to depend more completely on their own observations. A great deal of the success of a community health program is the result of the nurse's ability to detect early signs of disease. Community nurses need specific knowledge of "norms" in all ages so that they can recognize deviations. They should also be able to observe environmental conditions adversely affecting health, since correction by a health agency is often in response to a request from the nurse.*

Medical and nursing research is dependent on observations accurately made and recorded. Such sciences as physiology, medicine, and nursing are built on observations. Observing, recording, analyzing, and making deductions are the essential steps in scientific inquiry.

Of all the patients' medical attendants, nurses are with them most constantly. For this reason the quality of their observations and reports, written and oral, are of utmost importance. Their observations guide them primarily in assessing the patients' temporary and permanent limitations so that they may give adequate nursing care, but because nurses are in touch with the institutionalized patients around the clock, all other medical attendants have come to depend upon their observations. It is they who watch patients in danger of hemorrhage, checking the pulse and blood pressure at brief intervals; they note the signs and symptoms during labor, and it is they who get the obstetrician when needed; it is their vigilance and judgment that prevent self-destruction in the suicidal; it is they who watch the heavily anesthetized postoperative patient. These examples suggest crises of a more or less exceptional nature; it is, on the other hand, impossible to enumerate the kinds of observations nurses must make, nor can any limit be set to their value in the role of observer. Two nurses may be equally skillful with their hands; yet the first is outstanding in clinical judgment and the other is a technician who, when she or he looks at the patient, notices only a small frac-

* For example, see the following issues of the *International Digest of Health Legislation,* published by the World Health Organization, Geneva: "Nursing: A Survey of Recent Legislation," 4:463–497, 1952–1953; "Midwives: A Survey of Recent Legislation," 5:433–480, 1954; "Auxiliary Personnel in Nursing," 17:198–229, 1966; "Medical, Dental and Pharmaceutical Auxiliaries," 19:4–129, 1968.

† Kelly, Katherine: "Clinical Inference in Nursing. I. A Nurse's Viewpoint," *Nurs. Res.,* 15:23, (Winter) 1966.

* Nervi Ahla, studying the cooperation between the visiting nurse and the social caseworker, calls attention to the strategic position of the nurse in observing and reporting "family social disintegrations." She concludes that when many different nurses are assigned to one family, the referral of the family to social case workers is likely to be delayed. ("Briefs," *Nurs. Res.,* 1:37, [June] 1952.)

tion of what the first nurse sees. The beginning practitioner must realize that *there is no substitute for continuing education and experience in actual nursing.* The capacity for detecting disabilities and perceiving slight changes in the patient's physical or emotional state, the ability to discriminate between the significant and inconsequential remark, and the art of reporting accurately and succinctly are built up gradually and increase with every year of nursing experience. Nurses can add to the value of experience by listening to what their patients tell them about the impact of illness, by going to medical and nursing clinics, when they can see highly trained and experienced observers at work, and by comparing their observations with those of veteran nurses and doctors. Signe S. Cooper [5] describes the need for continuing education in nursing and the variety of educational opportunities available to practicing nurses. She says, however, that "self directed learning is the most significant aspect of continuing education." *

Nurses must be guided in everything they do for patients by what they believe to be their needs; the estimate of patients' needs is, of course, based on observation. Nurses cannot carry out prescribed treatments effectively unless they observe intelligently. They do not, for example, continue ruthlessly to apply cold applications when they see signs of a circulatory stasis in the area, nor do they continue to give a prescribed drug when toxic symptoms appear. Nurses who can most nearly distinguish between normal and abnormal behavior—physical, emotional, and mental—and can describe such behavior contribute in largest measure to determining patients' diagnoses. Obviously, this capacity knows no bounds. The physician is particularly dependent upon the nurse in treating infants and children, the irrational and unconscious, but the observations of an able nurse contribute toward effective medical care in any case.

Nurses learn to observe gradually and unconsciously. The technique of observation, like others used in nursing, is based on knowledge, interest, attention, and the empathy that enables nurses to put themselves in the position of the patient. The trained mind is essential. Louis Pasteur said: "In the field of observation, chance favors only the mind that is prepared." A patient often will tell the nurse important facts which he or she "did not like to tell the doctor," "did not want to bother the doctor with," or "did not think it important enough" to tell the doctor. Such symptoms should always be listened to attentively, and, if impor-

tant, reported in the words of the patient as far as possible.

Symptoms may be misleading in various ways. They may be exaggerated by the patient's imagination, or minimized by shyness and dislike of giving trouble. Often patients are unable to describe symptoms, or they may report those having little bearing on their condition and neglect to mention those most important. Patients may be too ill to concentrate on what the doctors or nurses are saying, or they may be confused by the questions asked and give answers that they know to be misleading. Skillful questioning on the part of the professional is always necessary to draw from patients the subjective symptoms bearing on the case, and the answers must be supplemented by their observations.

Moreover, symptoms may be misleading because they frequently manifest themselves in some part of the body remote, or seemingly not connected, with the seat of the disease; for instance, such symptoms as difficult breathing or coughing and spitting may be caused not by disease of the lungs but of the heart; a cough may be the result of an abscess in the ear that is pressing on a nerve connected with that supplying the lungs, and so giving rise to a "reflex cough." Pain is often a misleading symptom, because it may be "referred" or felt in a spot far from the seat of trouble. Physical signs must frequently be relied on in making a correct diagnosis. The fact that certain symptoms may be misleading is all the more reason that they should be reported fully, accurately, and at the time of their occurrence; a symptom by itself may seem to be of no importance, but when associated with others, a group of symptoms may be very significant indeed.

Directed observations made by the patients or their families, as well as those by nurses, contribute to making the diagnosis. For example, nurses may ask patients in their homes to take their temperature once or twice a day and keep a record of it for a period of a week or more. Patients are sometimes taught to make estimates and records of their blood pressure. The American Cancer Society recommends that women make a monthly self-examination of the breasts. The Society says: "The nurse should encourage women to examine their breasts once a month just after the menstrual period and, equally important, at regular monthly intervals after the cessation of menses." * This society is teaching every one the "seven danger signals of cancer": (1) Any sore that does not heal; (2)

* Cooper, Signe S.: "Why Continuing Education in Nursing," *Cardiovasc. Nurs.*, **9**:13, (May–June) 1973.

* American Cancer Society: *A Breast Check—So Simple . . . So Important.* The Society, New York, 1973.

a lump or thickening in the breasts or elsewhere; (3) unusual bleeding or discharge; (4) any change in a wart or mole; (5) persistent indigestion or difficulty in swallowing; (6) persistent hoarseness or cough; and (7) any change in normal bowel habits. Likewise the National Tuberculosis and Respiratory Disease Association, the American Heart Association, and other health agencies are educating the public to recognize signs of disease and to seek immediate medical advice. Nurses must be alert to the patient's particular need for guidance in making effective observations. Busy physicians rarely give full explanations or complete demonstrations of the procedures involved. In both hospitals and homes, nurses must assume the responsibility for teaching patients and their families to make certain health estimates.

To summarize: nurses are responsible for observations that (1) guide them in constant adaptation of nursing care to meet the patient's changing needs; (2) serve as a basis for diagnosis, prognosis, and treatment; (3) guide others, such as social workers or rehabilitation officers, in their services to the patient; (4) contribute toward their own knowledge and the accumulation of data on which the development of medical science depends; and (5) assist patients or their families to make effective observations.

3. HOW AND WHAT THE NURSE OBSERVES

While observation usually means what one sees, the term as used in medicine includes the discoveries made with all the senses. Certainly the nurse, like the physician, looks, listens, feels, and smells in making a continuous estimate of the patient's condition. Any impairment in the sense of sight, sound, touch, or smell would seriously handicap either a physician or a nurse.

Symptoms are usually divided into the subjective—those felt or experienced by patients, of which they may or may not complain, such as pain or itching; and the objective—those that may be seen, felt, heard, or smelled by others, as, for example, pallor, swelling, coughing, or fetid breath. Although the terms "physical sign" and "symptom" are often used interchangeably, the former is more properly used for objective symptoms detected by such special methods of examination as listening with a stethoscope, manipulating a part, or measuring body temperature with a thermometer.

The most effective nurses observe the patient in every aspect of his or her being. They realize that "mind," "spirit," "intellect," and body

of the person are interdependent and inseparable, even if disease is put by some persons into categories of mental, functional, and organic, as if "mind" might be separated from the body and an organ from its function. The experienced observer tries first to estimate the temperament, or the habitual pattern of moods, and the general appearance; in other words to get an over-all picture. No accurate idea of the patient's condition can be formed, however, without a long period of observation and study; even then our knowledge of others is always relatively incomplete. The necessity for continued observation cannot be overstressed.

Observation in nursing is inseparable from the development and application of questions or hypotheses about events. All observations are made within a set of basic assumptions that delimit and determine that which is to be observed. This set of assumptions is modified as the constant interplay of observing, asking, and resolving questions in nursing care proceeds. Basic assumptions in nursing practice come from many sources and are often a synthesis from related social and physical sciences. With the continued reporting of case studies in nursing and research in clinical practice, one can expect a synthesis of old concepts and a discovery of new relationships for understanding and explaining what takes place in patient care.

The following is intended to suggest the scope of the nurse's observations and to serve as a limited guide in the terminology of reporting. This chapter should be read in conjunction with Chapter 5 on the health examination, and texts on psychiatric and physical diagnosis should be consulted for more detailed help. It is intentional that no separation is made here between psychic and physical behavior. By observation, nurses attempt to assess the general physical and emotional make-up. They try to determine how normally people function in expressing their interests, needs, desires, and affection; how normally they function in working, playing, learning, breathing, eating, excreting, regulating body temperature, moving, maintaining muscle tone and normal posture, resting and sleeping. Nurses also try to recognize indications that are, but may not seem, part of the abnormality of the functions just listed. Examples of such symptoms are pain, tenderness, itching, burning, tingling, swelling, hypertrophy, atrophy, discoloration of any visible tissues, the presence of a discharge from a normally moist or dry area, the presence of a growth, a lesion, and a rash.

1. General Appearance. It is natural to make an over-all estimate of a person by noting his or her physical make-up. Common terms used in describing a physique are tall, medium height, short, emaciated, thin, well nourished, fat, and obese. The description may indicate whether the person is symmetrically and normally developed for his or her age or the opposite. (A discussion of predominantly feminine or "gynic" and predominantly male or "andric" shapes is found in Chapter 5, on page 389.) The observer notes any missing members, prostheses (artificial parts), or obvious blemishes. The muscle tone, posture, and gait contribute to the general impression of personality and state of health. They may express excitement, vigor, interest, lassitude, acute fatigue, dejection, depression, anxiety, and other emotions.

Levels of consciousness are also indicated by posture and muscle tone. Facial expression is no less a part of the general appearance. One may note signs of cheerfulness, anxiety, exhaustion, or anger. The symmetry of the face is important. Long-standing effects of happiness or unhappiness, productivity or frustration may be reflected in the facial lines, as well as chronologic age and apparent age.[6] Throughout their association with patients nurses should be acutely aware of their general appearance.

2. Temperament, Mental or Emotional Life, Feeling, "Affect," or Psychic Condition. Temperament is the characteristic phenomenon of a person's emotional nature, including susceptibility to emotional stimulation, customary strength and speed of response, the quality of his or her prevailing mood, and fluctuations and intensity of mood. A person may be described as habitually interested in others and expressing interest and affection, or as withdrawn, or self-centered. When a person's moods are of normal intensity but usually under control and when his or her behavior is consistent, he or she is said to be "well-balanced" or "well-adjusted." To form any reasonably accurate estimate of temperament, it is necessary to study a person's relationship to family, friends, acquaintances, and strangers; to note behavior in work and play; and to take account of participation in the activities of their immediate environment, and those of the larger community. Nurses can learn a great deal about peoples' interests, occupation and education, family and social life from the medical history, but everything they do for, or with, patients gives them additional opportunity to study the personality. Nursing care and treatment are affected by the nurse's ability to recognize varying states of alertness, interest, enthusiasm, excitement, apathy, aggressiveness, passivity, irritability, anxiety, fear, resignation, and acceptance.

3. Gender Identity and Sexuality. The health status cannot be fully understood without knowledge of the individual's gender, his or her sexual identity, and its pattern of expression. Observations can be made to determine the relative degree to which an individual's sexual impulses are integrated with the realities of the environment and the relative degree of acceptance of responsibility for their own sexuality.

There are many illnesses that result in changes of physical capacity for sexual expression or in which the individual perceives that his or her sexual identity and behavior will be changed. Cynthia Scalzi[7] describes aggressive sexual behavior in the cardiac patient and the meaning it may have in the total situation. Milton J. Senn and Albert J. Solnit[8] describe the young child's awareness of sexuality and sex differences. The anxious feelings that children have when undergoing intrusive and operative procedures in the hospital can often be attributed to their concern about their bodies and fear of genital injury.

Sexuality is expressed not only through heterosexual and homosexual intercourse but also through friendship, ideals, parent-child affection, love of abstractions, and self-love. A lack of knowledge about the patient's view of his or her sexuality makes it impossible to meet the total needs for care. George Griffith[9] makes an urgent appeal that health care practitioners know more about the meaning of sexual behavior in the lives of patients who must change their sexual behavior to achieve a healthy state or learn about their sexual capacities following severe illness. As in all caregiving activities, understanding of one's own sexuality is essential to helping another individual whose sexuality and sexual function are a source of stress.

4. Relationships to Other Persons, Places, and Things. To find meaning and significance as a person is to mean something to someone else, to be acknowledged by someone, to have life in the thoughts and feelings of another, and to be reflected in another's existence in an understanding and affectionate way. There is a human need to belong and to participate in a unit thought greater than the self.

Nurses will learn from individuals in their care what other persons and activities are important to them—in what situations they enjoy a sense of well-being and in what situations they lose the feeling of self-worth. Most persons wish to be of service to another, a group, or a cause. They seek an experience of mutuality in interaction with persons or things. They are accustomed to a certain role or reciprocal modes of behavior between themselves and others. The experience of illness can temporarily or permanently change a person's role within the family or community. Symptoms of disrupted relationships may be persistent feelings of separateness and isolation, inability to trust a professional person, inability to communicate needs, and failure to respond appropriately, both physically and psychologically, to treatment.

Seeing that persons who seek care have the companionship of those people who are most important to them and those objects they treasure will promote their sense of identity and self-worth.

5. Consciousness, Awareness of Surroundings, Sleep. Since the help patients must have from nurses is so dependent on their state of consciousness and their interpretation of time, place, and people, it is especially important that the nurse be able to make an accurate estimate of the patient's orientation.

The condition of normal persons when fully awake is such that they are responsive to psychologic stimuli and indicate by their behavior and speech that they are aware of themselves and their environment. Sleep is a state of physical and mental inactivity from which the person may be aroused to normal consciousness. Sleeping persons give little evidence of being aware of themselves or their environment, yet they differ from comatose patients in that they may still respond to unaccustomed stimuli and be capable of mental activity in the form of dreams. Observation of sleep should indicate the time of day or night and the duration. This is so important in some cases that a graphic sleep chart is kept in order that the physician can see the sleep pattern at a glance. The depth or soundness of the sleep should be noted.

Inattentiveness or confusion implies that the individual does not take into account all the elements of the immediate environment. He or she is usually unable to do more than carry out a few simple instructions; capacity for speech may be limited to a few words or phrases; and there is little awareness of the surrounding activity.

Reduced states of consciousness are described as stupor—a state in which the person can still be aroused—and coma—a state in which he or she cannot be aroused. Reporting certain signs and their change gives a more exact description of the level of consciousness. The signs that are reported are the predominant posture of the body, the position of the head and eyes, the rate, depth, and rhythm of respiration, the pulse, and the temperature. The state of responsiveness is the reaction when the name is called and the ability to execute simple directions or to respond to painful stimuli. By grading these responses, both the degree of coma and the changes from hour to hour can be evaluated. Chapter 40 deals in more detail with states of consciousness.

6. Loss or Impairment of Special Senses. The patient who is handicapped in speaking or hearing, seeing, maintaining equilibrium, or interpreting tactile sensations requires special help from the nurse; the loss of the sense of smell, or ability to differentiate common odors, is less serious but should be noted.

The condition of the eyes is particularly significant. Signs of disease may be evident in the face and eyelids, the prominence of the eyes, and their expression.[10] The pupils may fail to respond to light or distance; there may be *photophobia* (sensitiveness to moderate light) and abnormal eye movements. *Nystagmus* is an example of the latter. Failure to interpret objects correctly should be reported. This may be a defect of vision or a misinterpretation.

Speech is affected by normal moods and almost always reflects the mental, if not the physical, condition. What the person says and how he or she says it should be noted. Some disease conditions produce aphasia (inability to arrange words into a meaningful sentence); others produce mutism, tremulous speech, subspeech (grunts), blocking (pausing), irrelevancy, echolalia (repetition of what others say), incoherency, and speech that is explosive, slurring, whispering, or hoarse. The mentally ill may go from one subject to another so rapidly and disconnectedly that they are said to have a "flight of ideas." In reporting the content of a patient's speech, samples of exact words should be given.

Indications of deafness should be reported as they occur. Inattention to what is said may or may not be the result of deafness. Ringing in the ears or any tenderness in or around the ears should be noted. Impairment of equilibrium is often not apparent when the person can compensate by sight. Dizziness, swaying, and falling when the eyes are closed are serious symptoms.

Disease may affect the nerve endings in the skin or the centers in the brain that interpret sensation of touch or heat and cold. Complete failure to respond or failure to respond normally to such stimuli should be reported. Sensory impairments are discussed in Chapters 40 and 46.

7. Abnormalities in Sensation or Interpretation of Stimuli; Abnormality in the Realm of Thought. The systematic examination of intelligence, mood, memory, and judgment, which are affective and cognitive functions, permits the observer to reach certain conclusions about the mental status of the patient.[11] Without these data, errors will be made in evaluating the reliability of the patient's history or in diagnosing neurologic or psychiatric disease.

People are said to be confused when there is a general reduction in alertness, attentiveness, and perception of environmental stimuli. They may also be slow and inefficient in thinking and fail to remember.

Loss of memory should always be noted, and a differentiation made between loss of memory for the immediate and distant past.

Fabrication is a term used to describe the practice of making statements contrary to fact if there is reason to believe that the memory is intact.

Delirium describes a disorder of consciousness characterized by excessive alertness, sleeplessness, and frenzied excitement. (This condition is discussed in Chapters 39 and 40.)

A person is said to have an illusion when an object in his or her environment is incorrectly interpreted—a sick man may think his wife is sitting in a chair when it is only a coat thrown over the chair. When a woman with a high fever hears nonexistent voices or feels rats running over her while nothing is touching her but her own bedding or clothing, she is said to have hallucinations—sensations without external stimuli. Delusions are common symptoms of psychoses. Deluded persons hold a belief that has no basis in fact. They have what might be called pathological experiences in thought. They often think they are someone they are not, rich when they are poor, a holder of high office when they hold none; or they may believe they are being persecuted and that their friends, family, or the medical personnel are menacing them. Often these ideas are systematically worked out, and in describing the grandiose position or persecution, they will be very convincing. It is important for the nurse to report *exactly what they say.*

Phobias—unreasonable fears and compulsions resulting in acts the person feels compelled to perform—are not uncommon, nor are obsessions—thoughts from which the person cannot rid himself or herself. Sometimes the mentally ill will say they feel unreal or that an outside force controls their actions.

Thinking may be defined as selective ordering of symbols for problem-solving and the capacity to reason and form sound judgments. In a general way, the thinking processes may be examined for speed and efficiency, conceptual content, coherence and logical relationship of ideas, quantity and quality of association to a given idea, and appropriateness of feeling and behavior in relation to the idea.[12]

These features of the thought process may be examined by analyzing the person's spontaneous speech and by engaging him or her in conversation. Disorders of thought are frequent in delirium and in degenerative and other types of cerebral disease. Fragmentation, repetition, and perseverance may characterize the organization of thoughts. Criticizing and rationalizing is a type of thinking seen in depressive psychoses. The flight of ideas, in which a person moves from one idea to another, with numerous and loosely linked associations, is a common feature of hypomanic and manic states. A poverty of ideas combined with gloomy thoughts is found in depression.[13]

8. Motor Activity—Posture and Symptoms of Impaired Motor Function. The activity of the neuromuscular system may be studied by inspection, by touch, and by moving parts of the body to determine range-of-motion. The physician and nurse are particularly interested in muscle tone as a health index.

Posture is studied for signs of weakness, such as continuously slipping down from an erect sitting posture. Posture may indicate pain, as when the legs are flexed to relax muscles over a distended abdomen, or when a side-lying position is assumed to limit the expansion of the chest, as in pleurisy. When any position is assumed habitually it should be noted as should any unusual position.

The condition of the muscles of the eyes, of swallowing, and of respiration and that of the urethral and rectal sphincters are studied in order to determine the normality of specific body areas. Disease, including highly emotional states, may produce hyperactivity or hypoactivity. The normal amount of activity differs with the personality so that the nurse should describe the behavior rather than designate it as hyper- or hypoactive. The gait should be noted in terms such as rapid, slow, hesitant, dragging, rolling, rocking, running, tottering, or staggering. Any rigidity, or tension of the whole body or part thereof, is significant, as are paralysis and difficulty or discomfort in moving an extremity, eyes, or eyelids, in speaking, swallowing, breathing, defecating, or voiding. Rhythmic, stereotyped, or automatic motions, tremors, convulsions, and unnatural flexibility are motor symptoms that should be reported.

9. Breathing. Respiration is an automatic function, but its rate and depth are nevertheless affected by emotional states, exercise, drugs, and anything that alters the body's need of oxygen. Mechanical interference with respiration also affects the rate and depth. The nurse should note the character of the respiration; the symmetry of structure and movements of the chest, abdomen, and nose; the sounds accompanying respiration; the patient's position, expression, and change in color; and actual complaints indicating difficult breathing.

Through auscultation the nurse learns the normal sounds of air moving through the nose, throat, and lungs, as well as abnormal respiratory murmurs arising from disease. Considerable experience in listening to the wide range of normal breath sounds is necessary before abnormal sounds can be distinguished. Some characteristics of abnormal breathing are noisy or musical sounds (rhonchi). These are caused by movement of exudate in the bronchial tubes or inflammation or narrowing of the bronchial tubes. There may be a grating sound from the rub of an inflamed serous surface or a crackling sound (rale) which indicates the presence of fluid or inflammation within the respiratory tract. Judge and Zuidema [14] present a useful classification of breath sounds and methods of listening to the chest. Variations in respiration are characterized by the following descriptions and may indicate physical disease or emotional stress: sensation of difficult breathing or shortness of breath is called *dyspnea,* and increased depth of respiration is called *hyperpnea.* A more common term to describe increased depth of respiration is *hyperventilation.* Inability to breathe comfortably while lying down is *orthopnea,* and an increased rate of respiration is *tachypnea. Stridor* is difficult respiration characterized by high-pitched crowing sounds in inspiration. *Apnea* is a temporary suspension of breathing. *Cyanosis* is the term used to describe the bluish tint of the lips, nail beds, or skin resulting from inadequate oxygenation of the blood. Breathing with the mouth open habitually is abnormal and should be reported.

10. Eating and Drinking. Reva Rubin [15] describes food not only as a source of nutrition and physical sustenance but also as the source of nurturance, the interactive and interpersonal matrix in which we learn about ourselves and others. M. F. K. Fisher takes the same position in a book titled *The Gastronomical Me:*

It seems to me that our three basic needs, for food and security and love, are so mixed and mingled and entwined that we cannot straightly think of one without the others.*

Food has many symbolic meanings and one's response to offered food is influenced by how one feels about oneself in the situation or relationship. [16] In helping the person who is seeking health care or being treated for illness, the social and cultural significance of food and ways of eating must be considered before at-

tempts at feeding or teaching nutritional needs can succeed. Food intake is usually balanced with the caloric demands of the body. As a rule, people eat what they need and no more. Nevertheless, habits of eating continue beyond the necessity for them and appetite becomes related to desire more than need. [17] Overeating may be a response to a nonspecific emotional tension, a substitute gratification, or a symptom of emotional illness. Undernutrition, or a progressive weight loss without obvious explanation, should be treated as a symptom of illness and receive serious consideration in the over-all assessment of the person. [18]

It is obvious that health and recovery from disease are dependent on food intake. Unless patients are aware of their nutritional needs and are able and willing to meet them, the burden of seeing that they get adequate nourishment rests largely upon nurses. They should observe signs of appetite or its lack, food likes, cravings, dislikes, idiosyncrasies, and phobias. If patients do not enjoy their meals, nurses should try to discover the cause. Actually they may be hungry, but eating may be for some reason painful or uncomfortable. Sore mouth, ill-fitting dentures, difficulty in swallowing, or weakness may interfere with the satisfaction of eating. The mentally ill may think themselves unworthy of food, they may believe the food is poisoned, or it may represent an object that is unfit for consumption. Food habits are discussed further in Chapter 10 on nutrition, and disorders of nutrition are discussed in Chapter 36.

11. Elimination. Individuals defecate, urinate, and dispose of excreta in ways that meet physiologic demands of their bodies, are satisfying to them, and are compatible with cultural expectations. Acts of elimination are invested with feelings about control of self and environment. In Western cultures the prevalent attitudes toward excreta are ones of distaste, if not revulsion. The odors are considered unpleasant, and it is expected that body parts associated with elimination be covered. Self-care during elimination is highly valued and is taught to the child in Western cultures at an early age, often with little regard for the physiologic readiness to urinate and defecate voluntarily.

Cultural values vested in elimination are those of regularity, cleanliness, conformity, obedience, privacy, and modesty. An individual is interested in elimination as a subjective index of the integrity of the body. For the adult and child, the acts of elimination can be a vehicle for the expression of emotions. For example, a child may develop constipation as a way of expressing his or her feelings about

---

* Fisher, M. F. K.: *The Gastronomical Me.* Duell, Sloan & Pearce, New York, 1943, p. vii.

events that he or she cannot understand, such as a new place in the family when a brother or sister is born.

Reports on the amount, frequency, and nature of elimination are included in all patient observations. If people are rational and ambulatory, they may assume the responsibility for reporting to the nurse or doctor any irregularity in defecation, urination, and sweating; if they are not able to assume this responsibility, nurses note the character of the excretions and the frequency of defecation and urination. If pain or discomfort accompanies these acts, this should be noted. Attention should be called at once to cessation of these functions. Sweating or abnormal dryness of the skin and the body areas affected should be reported. If the sweat has an unusual odor, as of urine, it should be noted. The balance between fluid taken in and eliminated cannot be too greatly upset without serious consequence. A record is therefore kept as a basis for estimating how nearly intake and output tally. Sunken eyes, dry mouth, loose skin, and concentrated urine are characteristic of dehydration and are danger signs. Any indication that fluid is held in the tissues is also significant. Puffy eyes, clubbed fingers, swollen hands and feet (edema), or accumulation of fluid in the tissues of the back when the patient is sitting should be noted. *Ascites* is the term used when free fluid distends the abdominal cavity. Occasionally, with the use of certain drugs, or in the case of poisoning, excretions are discolored or have an unusual odor. Drugs may be deposited in the tissues and give the mucous membranes, skin, or the sclera of the eye an unnatural appearance that should be noted and described. In Chapter 11 there is a discussion of elimination and in Chapter 37 a discussion of its disorders.

12. Regulation of Body Temperature. Maintenance of body temperature within the normal range is accomplished by a number of physiologic processes involving both chemical and physical transfer of heat. The operation of these mechanisms is mediated by the central nervous system.

The principal source of body heat is combustion of food in the body. Heat produced by muscular activity maintains a uniform body temperature, the activity readily increasing or decreasing according to need. Heat is eliminated by the processes of radiation, vaporization, and convection. Fever is an elevation of temperature due to disease or exposure to high environmental temperatures. Evaluation of the significance of fever requires knowledge of temperature control and the various ways in which the control can be disturbed.[19]

The oral or rectal glass and mercury thermometer is available to anybody who wants to measure his or her body temperature. This is the most common instrument for measuring body temperature in homes and in ambulatory and inpatient services. A portable electronic thermometer will measure oral or rectal temperature within seconds, as against minutes with the traditional instrument, and displays the temperature reading simultaneously on a screen on the instrument. The electronic thermometer has disposable covers for the temperature probe. This instrument is the most practical to use where there are large groups of individuals who need periodic measurement of their temperature.

The measurement of body temperature differs depending on the area of the body where the measurement is taken.[20] For example, oral temperature is not considered to be the best reflection of deep body temperature. Knowing the deep body temperature is important in critical illness and certain surgical procedures. Therefore, in critical care hospital units various devices for the continuous measurement of body temperature are available which are introduced into the rectum or esophagus to measure deep body temperature.

Abdominal skin temperature is monitored in the premature or sick infant, as the temperature at this site most closely approximates the deep body temperature.[21] Failure to provide an optimal environment (thermoneutral) for newborn infants will subject them to such metabolic difficulties as oxygen deprivation and metabolic acidosis.[22] The thermoneutral environment for newborns is that environment in which they can maintain abdominal skin temperature or axillary temperature between 36.6° and 37.5°C (97° and 99°F).

The measurement and control of body temperature will undoubtedly become more convenient and comfortable for the individual and more precise for the collection of data on health and disease processes than they are today. Nevertheless, close observation of other signs of disturbance in body temperature will never be negated by technologic developments in equipment. The condition of the skin may be described as hot, flushed, cold, or clammy. There may be an obvious chill or a sensation of which the person complains. If the patient has a dry nose and mouth, which makes swallowing difficult, the lips get cracked and parched and the tongue appears coated and discolored. All of these are signs of dehydration accompanying fever that the nurse can see and should record. For further discussion of body temperature and thermometry, see Chapters 6 and 42.

13. Noting Gross Disease Processes. Abnormal functioning of the body constitutes disease, but there are pathologic processes the nurse should note that have not been emphasized under the functional headings just used. For example, any signs of inflammation—redness, heat, swelling, discomfort, or pain—should be reported. Note and report any discoloration of the skin or mucous membranes, swelling, hypertrophy, any sign of a growth, break in the tissues, discharges from body orifices or lesions, abnormal odors, tenderness as the body is manipulated, and all subjective symptoms of which the patient complains. Examples are pain, tenderness, itching, burning, tingling, prickling, numbness, throbbing, chilliness or a sensation of being overheated, headache, nausea, dizziness, spots before the eyes, ringing in the ears (tinnitus), deafness, a sense of fullness, pressure, or a "gone" or weak feeling. All of these should be reported in the patient's own words with the sensation localized when it is local and characterized as the patient describes it. Patients may say that they have a "gnawing pain that comes and goes" in the stomach and that "it is relieved by food," or they "feel as if there is a heavy weight" on the chest, or they "can't get their breath." Since such comments may have a different significance for any two medical attendants, a verbatim report is desirable.

Feelings or emotions are expressed in such questions or statements as "Isn't the doctor coming soon?" "Does the doctor think my condition is serious?" "I know it isn't cancer." "There's no danger in a blood pressure of 180, is there?" or "Do you think I'll get well?" When the nurse thinks that a question indicates any emotional state that markedly affects the patient's diagnosis, prognosis, or treatment, it is wise to record it in the patient's words. All symptoms are important, though not equally so; therefore, a selection must be made from the patient's acts, including speech, that seem significant. Anything a patient does is an indication of what concerns him or her, of the effectiveness or ineffectiveness of the care given, and of the nature of the illness.

4. METHODS OF REPORTING AND RECORDING

Observation of the patient is continuous, as has been said repeatedly, and serves as a basis for the hourly and daily modification of nursing care. Since it is obviously impossible for nurses to record all their observations, some guide is necessary in making a selection of items that may be helpful to patients, nurses, physicians, social workers, and special therapists.

Nurses should report any signs of disorientation, unconsciousness, anxiety, fear, or any strong emotion and particularly instability of mood, deterioration of the patient's relationship with others, or any marked change in the personality. They should report any handicap or limitation of function as soon as it is noted. In general, symptoms should be reported that have any of the following characteristics: (1) are intense or severe in character, as severe pain; (2) are prolonged, even though not severe; (3) are a departure from normal, as an increase or decrease in pulse rate; (4) tend to recur, as pain between meals; (5) show progressive development, as loss of weight; (6) are known danger signals, as a sharp abdominal pain in perforated peptic ulcer; (7) indicate a complication, as coughing following an operation; (8) point to the onset of a disease, as a rash; (9) cannot be relieved by nursing measures, as failure to eat or sleep, void, or defecate; (10) show faulty hygiene or health habits that cannot be corrected by nursing care, as neglected teeth, the need of eyeglasses, or a more balanced diet; (11) indicate a disturbance in function of any organ or part of the body; and (12) show a change for the better or for the worse.

Reports are made orally, by notation on the patient's chart, or both ways. Anything that is serious or that requires immediate attention should be reported promptly, both orally and on the medical record—the patient's chart. The written report must never be omitted, for this helps to ensure notice of the condition and to protect medical personnel from accusations of negligence. Patient-centered conferences among nurses, doctors, nutritionists, social workers, rehabilitation officers, and special therapists offer an invaluable opportunity to exchange such observations and opinions as are difficult to report fully in writing. The beginning practitioner of nursing should err on the side of being overzealous in reporting to the nurse in charge of the service or to the physician responsible for the patient's medical program any observation that he or she thinks may even possibly have serious consequences. Ninety-nine times the caution may be unnecessary, the nurse's judgment questioned, but the hundredth time he or she may save a life.

The patient's record, or chart, is still the most commonly used medium for reporting observations (signs and symptoms of patient behavior). The value of nurses' notations is a fairly good index of their nursing ability. Gradually nurses build up a technique of observing and recording. Before going to the patient, they regularly review what others have written on the record and the treatment prescribed by the physician. Nurses get whatever oral reports they can from others, they welcome the opinions of the patient's family and friends; then, after observation made while they care for the patient, they report and record whatever they think is significant. Such records are made daily, hourly, or at less frequent intervals, according to the patient's needs and the time available for nursing care.

5. THE PATIENT'S RECORD

Observing, reporting, and recording are almost inseparable processes in the medical world.

The medical record is a concise account of the health history of the patient and his or her family, a report of the findings on examination, the signs and symptoms occurring while the patient is under medical observation, the treatment and progress of the disease, if one is involved. (A medical record is made for every patient who has a health examination.) Besides the data that bear directly on the medical problem, there is sociologic information that may indirectly affect diagnosis and treatment and that is necessary for identification of the patient and the administration of the hospital or health service.

A record for each patient is kept by physicians in private practice and by all groups of medical workers associated with health agencies. The hospital record is the one emphasized here, but it has many features in common with that used by private physicians, visiting nurse organizations, and other community health and medical services as indicated by Figures 4-1*A-C* and 4-2.

The *Accreditation Manual for Hospitals* [23] states that while form and detail of the medical record vary, all medical records must contain (1) identification data and consent forms, except when unobtainable; (2) history of the patient; (3) report of the physical examination; (4) diagnostic and therapeutic orders; (5) observations; (6) reports of actions and findings; and (7) conclusions. The reader is referred to the Manual for a full explanation of each of these categories. The Manual also provides for the confidentiality, currency, and accuracy of records, the qualifications of the registered record administrator, and the management of the medical record department. The Manual requests that hospital records be sufficiently detailed to provide for effective, continuing care, and for consultant opinion. The data contained in the record should be such that another practitioner could give care at any time. In summary, the record must identify the patient clearly, justify the diagnosis and treatment, and document the results. Innovations for improvement both in content and organization of the record by a standing committee (see page 358) are encouraged.

The order of the parts of the hospital record varies according to whether the record is structured by source or by the patient's problems. The record that is structured by source ("source oriented" or traditional medical record) contains the information about the patient's plans for treatment and evaluation of care according to the personnel (sources) who supply the information. Each section of the record is labeled according to these personnel. For example, the notations made by the physician on the patient's history, physical examination, and progress in the medical plan of care are found in one section of the record. The notations of nursing personnel, the laboratory, social service, and any other types of workers who provided care to the patient are found in subsequent sections. Within each section the data are arranged in chronologic sequence. Each professional worker who uses the record is obligated to study the plans and findings of other contributors in order to coordinate the treatment for the patient and maintain a unified appraisal of existing needs and difficulties of the patient. The diverse problems and data recorded by the many "source" personnel must be integrated by a single person.[24] In the hospital, this integrator is usually the responsible physician. In clinic, office, and home settings, this integrative function is performed by the person who gives primary care. This may be the nurse as often as it is the physician. Nurses who are independent practitioners keep records, as do nurses in visiting nurse agencies, that have no other "sources."

Parts of the source-structured hospital record are usually arranged in the chart cover in the following way: (1) graphic chart of temperature, pulse, and respiration; other items of information may also be shown on this sheet such as blood pressure, the number of evacuations, and volume of fluid intake and output; (2) orders for treatment written by the physician; (3) nurse's plan of care, record of care, and report of observations; (4) reports of laboratory findings and special examinations; (5) reports of anesthesia, operation, physical therapy, occupational therapy, social service, and any special treatment; (6) family history, record of present illness, and health habits, findings of the physical examination, medical progress notes, a summary made at the time of

[*Text continued on page 334.*]

FAMILY IDENTIFICATION RECORD				Family Folder No. _____			
				District _____ Interpreter _____			
Family Name				Referred by _____			

Date	Address	Floor & Apt.	Date	Address		Floor & Apt.

Telephone   Religion:

Race / Members in Household	Sex	Date of Birth	Place of Birth	Marital Status	Socio-Economic Factors		Service & Classification	Date Adm.	Date Disc.
					Education	Occupation			
Man									
Woman									
Children									
Others in Family & Relationship									

Name, Address, Telephone of Relative or Friend (State relationship)

Date	Agency To Which Known	Telephone	Name of Agency Worker	Problem and/or Identification Number

Form 1N-3-74-10M LP   VNA OF HARTFORD, INC.

Figure 4-1. Forms used by a visiting nurse organization. (Courtesy of Visiting Nurse Association of Hartford, Hartford, Conn.) *A*. Family identification record.

NAME .... F.F. # ....

FAMILY HEALTH HISTORY

Place an X under appropriate heading or headings where there is positive history.	Adult Male	Adult Female	Adult Male's Relatives	Adult Female's Relatives	Children	COMMENTS
Allergies (medicines, food, pollen)						
Birth defects						
Blood disease (hemophilia, sickle cell anemia, leukemia, etc.)						
Bone or joint disorders						
Breathing problems (chronic bronchitis, asthma, emphysema, etc.)						
Cancer or tumors						
Diabetes						
Drugs – Alcohol abuse						
Ear and hearing disorders						
Eye & vision disorders (glaucoma, cataracts, etc.)						
Heart trouble (rheumatic fever, angina, etc.)						
High Blood Pressure						
Kidney or urinary disease						
Mental retardation						
Muscle disease (weakness, poor control, etc.)						
Nerve disease (cerebral palsy, epilepsy, etc.)						
Obesity						
Parasites						
Pica						
Psychiatric condition						
Stomach trouble - ulcers						
Stroke						
Tuberculosis						
Venereal disease						
Other						
No Significant Health Problems						

Form 1FH-5M-3-74 LP

VNA OF HARTFORD, INC.

Figure 4-1. *B*. Health history.

REHABILITATION NURSING ASSESSMENT: BASELINE DATA

Name _____ Birth Date _____ Date _____ F.F. # _____

Diagnoses _____

Adaptive Equipment _____

Orthetic/Prosthetic Appliances _____

Patient Assessment

Activities: bed	
chair	
standing/walking	
sleep	
Posture/positioning	
Deformities	
ROM: upper extremities	
lower extremities	
Personal hygiene: bathing	
hair	
mouth care	
foot care	
Dressing	
Transfer: bed	
furniture	
toilet	
Ambulation: indoors	
stairs	
outdoors	
Elimination: bladder	
bowels	
routines	
special devices	
ostomy	
Respiration:	
special devices	

Form 1RNA-5M-3-74-LP   VNA OF HARTFORD, INC.

Figure 4-1. *C*. Assessment for patient care.

Yale University
Health Services Visit Record

Date

Social Security #

Name

Sex — Male ☐ Female ☐

Birthdate — Mo ☐☐ Da ☐☐ Yr ☐☐

Membership

	Head	Dep		Head	Dep
Undergraduate	☐	☐	Employee	☐	☐
Graduate	☐	☐	Associate	☐	☐
Faculty	☐	☐	Non-member	☐	

Staff Code ☐☐☐ **Staff Code 2** ☐☐☐ **Department Code** ☐☐

Visit — Walk-in ☐ Appointment ☐ Referral ☐ Home Visit ☐

In Time ☐☐ : ☐☐ AM/PM

Out Time ☐☐ : ☐☐ AM/PM

Non-member Payment — Address ______ Telephone ______ Medicare ☐ Subrogation ☐ Fee for Service ☐

Employee Health — Job Related-Yale ☐ Job Related-Other ☐

Organized Sports — Freshman ☐ Junior Varsity ☐ Varsity ☐ Intercollege ☐ Other ☐

Presenting Problem

Tentative Dx this visit

Primary Dx if any

Gp ICDA

Reason for Visit (one only)

- Illness: initial visit ☐ return visit ☐
- Injury: initial visit ☐ return visit ☐
- Physical Exam: initial visit ☐ return visit ☐ Eye ☐ Gyn ☐
- Pre/Post Natal: ☐
- Well Baby/Child: ☐
- Immunization: ☐

Disposition

- Consultation/Referral ☐
- No Follow up Necessary ☐
- Telephone Follow up ☐
- Return Appointment ☐
- Return Prn ☐
- ICF ☐
- Hospital ☐
- Other: ______

Consultation/Referral

Department	In YHS	Outside
Athletic Medicine	☐	☐
Dentistry	☐	☐
Dermatology	☐	☐
Dietitian	☐	☐
Fam. Plan./Sex Couns.	☐	☐
Genetics	☐	☐
Immunology	☐	☐
Internal Medicine	☐	☐
Mental Hygiene/Psych.	☐	☐
Neurology	☐	☐
Ob/Gyn	☐	☐
Ophthamology	☐	☐
Orthopedics	☐	☐
Otolaryngology	☐	☐
Pediatrics	☐	☐
Physiotherapy	☐	☐
Radiotherapy	☐	☐
Student Medicine	☐	☐
Surgery	☐	☐
Urology	☐	☐
Other: ______	☐	☐

Laboratory

- Hematology ☐
- Urinalysis ☐
- Chemistry ☐
- Microbiology ☐
- Blood Typing ☐
- Serology ☐
- Papanicolaou ☐
- Pulmonary Function ☐
- EKG ☐
- Special Procedures ☐

Radiology

- Plain Films ☐
- Contrast Studies ☐
- Special Procedures ☐

Provider Signature

Figure 4-2. A record of a visit to a community health service. A health history and a record of a physical examination would also be part of a patient's record in a community health service or private physician's office. (Courtesy of Yale University Health Services, New Haven, Conn.)

discharge, operative permit, autopsy permit, and a report of the autopsy (obviously, all these records vary according to the treatment and the outcome of a disease); and (7) statistical and social data. In many institutions this last sheet contains the medical summary. (Figures 4-3A–D are examples of record forms used in source-structured records.)

There are many variations of this basic arrangement of the source-structured record. When the patient is discharged from a health care agency, the record is filed and the order of its parts may be changed so that the record can be used more easily as a research tool. Edna K. Huffman [25] describes the methods of storage and retrieval of records and what the health professional can expect in the future practice of maintaining a complete health record. The development of microfilm has made it possible to store information in a very small space so a person can have a lifelong health record on microfilm.[26] As people move from one community—even one country—to another, more and more often this provision assumes considerable importance. The public may be expected some day to demand that they own a copy of medical records, including x-ray films and photographs, for which they have often paid dearly.

The order of arrangement of the parts of the medical record is different when the "problem-oriented record system" is used. Instead of being arranged according to the sources of information, the data are recorded according to the series of problems identified by physicians, nurses, and others.[27] The first part of the record is the initial data base, that is, all the information necessary to determine the patient's problems. In general, for the hospitalized patient the elements include (1) the chief complaint; (2) a patient profile (a description of how he or she spends his or her average day) and related social data; (3) present illness or illnesses; (4) past history and review of body systems based on a series of explicit and related questions, logically arranged in a branching pattern; (5) physical examination; and (6) baseline laboratory examination. The information defined as adequate for a data base varies markedly within departments of a hospital and among health care agencies.[28]

The criteria for the selection of information to be included in the data base is determined by the problems for which a population is "at risk" (health problems common in a given sex, age, race, or occupational group). For example, women 18 to 60 years of age are "at risk" for cervical cancer. The laboratory test that must be included in the data base for this group of persons is the examination of ex-foliated cells of the cervix which are stained in a special manner to detect the presence of a malignant process (Papanicolaou's smear or "pap" smear).

Following the data base is the numbered problem list. It is a table of contents and index combined, and the care with which it is constructed determines the quality of the whole record.[29] The problems are identified through the collection of the defined data base. They are numbered and titled as they are discovered, and include socioeconomic, demographic, psychologic, and physical problems. Problems are further labeled as active or inactive. There may be no further notation made on an inactive problem other than to list it in the table of contents. Problems are defined at the level they are understood. For example, a woman may have the following problems: vaginal itching (pruritus), insatiable thirst (polydipsia), and sugar present in the urine (glycosuria). After further study, diabetes may be defined as the active problem.

The plans for each active problem consist of three aspects—a statement of further information needed to delineate the problem, appropriate therapeutic measures, and patient instruction or guidance.[30]

Progress notes are found under appropriate problems to which they refer. Each professional worker who cares for the patient submits narrative notes, lists of parameters that are being followed simultaneously (flow sheets), and teaching or discharge plans under the appropriate problem. The parts of the record for physician's, nurse's, or other professional's notations are therefore not separate as in the "source-oriented" or traditional record.

Figures 4-4A–F illustrate a patient's record in which the data, assessment, and treatment are organized according to the problem-oriented system.*

Those who use the problem-oriented record system see the system not only as an improved way to organize the data in the patient's record but also as a system that has implications for the delivery of health care to patients and the education of those giving care. For example,

* Figures 4-4A–F illustrate the problem-oriented record as it would be written by the professional workers caring for the patient. Figures 4-5A–F illustrate the problem-oriented record which has been "printed out" by a computer. This is an actual patient record which has been stored in a computer system and can be retrieved instantly by the user of the record, displayed either on a screen or in printed form. The authors wish to thank the University of Vermont, College of Medicine, for the records printed by computer. These records are the first efforts of a continually developing system.

[*Text continued on page 351.*]

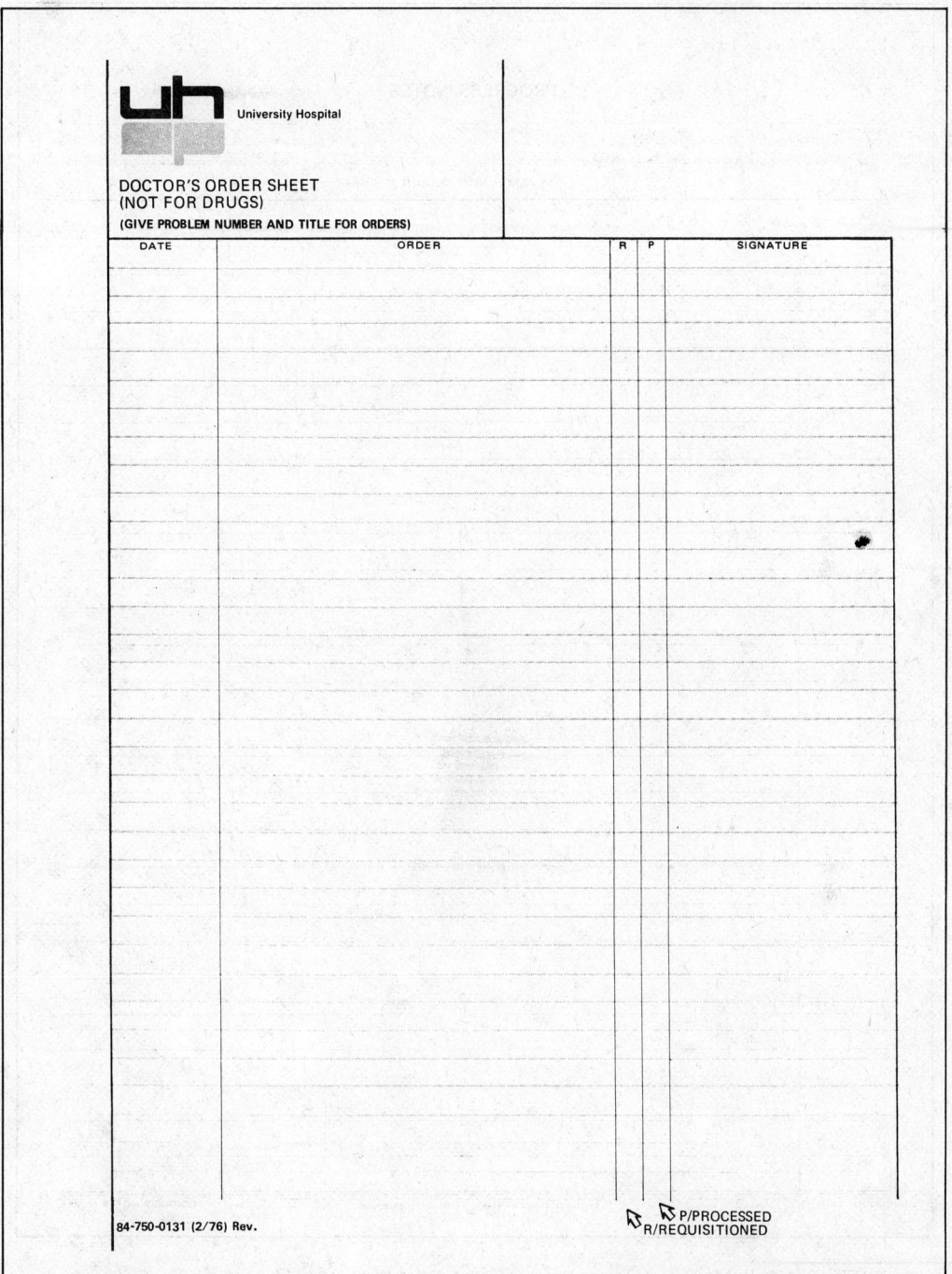

Figure 4-3. Forms for a source-structured record. *A*. Orders for treatment written by the physician. (Courtesy of University Hospital, University of Western Ontario, London, Ont.)

PROGRESS NOTES

Family Name	First Name	File No.
DATE	EACH NOTE SHOULD BE SIGNED	

FORM NH-241   PHYSICIANS' RECORD CO., BERWYN, ILLINOIS - PRINTED IN U.S.A.   PROGRESS NOTES (OVER)

Figure 4-3. *B*. Medical progress notes. (Courtesy of Physicians' Record Co., Berwyn, Ill.)

NURSES' PROGRESS NOTES

Family Name	First Name	File No.

DATE	NURSING CARE NOTES	SIGNATURE

FORM NH-242   PHYSICIANS' RECORD CO., BERWYN, ILLINOIS · PRINTED IN U.S.A.   NURSES' PROGRESS NOTES (OVER)

Figure 4-3. *C.* Nurse's record of care and report of observations. (Courtesy of Physicians' Record Co., Berwyn, Ill.)

SUMMARY SHEET

Family Name	First Name	Middle Name	Home- Phone	Room No.	Hosp. No.

Address	City	Zone	State	Sex M F	Civil Status M S W D Sep.	Religion

Age—Yrs.	Birth Date Mo. Day Year	Birthplace	Nationality	How Many Years in City County State U.S.	Ever in Military Service	Soc. Sec. No.

Occupation	Employer or Employer of Spouse	Address of Employer—Phone

Name of Husband or Maiden Name of Wife	Address if Other Than Above	Birthplace

Notify in Case of Emergency	Relationship	Address	Phone

Name of Father	Birthplace	Maiden Name of Mother	Birthplace

Name of Blue Cross and/or Blue Shield Plan	Group No.	Contract No.	Effective Date	Subscriber ☐ Dependent ☐	Family Member ☐ Comprehensive Coverage ☐

Other hospitalization insurance	Name	Address	Cert. or Policy No.	Group No.	Effective Date

Attending Physician	Date of Last Admission	Admission Date A.M. P.M.	Discharge Date A.M. P.M.

Provisional Diagnosis (to be completed within 24 hours after admission):

On admission, patient or qualified person must sign authorization for Medical and/or Surgical Treatment on reverse side

Final Diagnosis: Code No.

Secondary Diagnosis or Complications:

Operation:

Discharged Alive: ☐   Died: ☐ Under 48 hours   ☐ Over 48 hours   Autopsy: ☐ Yes   ☐ No

_____ M.D., Attending Physician

FORM A-145   PHYSICIANS' RECORD CO., BERWYN, ILLINOIS - PRINTED IN U.S.A.   SUMMARY SHEET (OVER)

Figure 4-3. *D*. Statistical and social data and medical summary. (Courtesy of Physicians' Record Co., Berwyn, Ill.)

MEDICAL CENTER HOSPITAL OF VERMONT

CLINICAL RECORD

(Date)   Data Base

Admission Vital Signs - General Appearance

White female, appears chronically ill, very obese,

alert, talkative, appears anxious.

Temperature - 37.3 C orally.

Pulse - 96/min., strong and regular

Respirations - 16/min. - no distress

Blood pressure - 160/90 rt arm, sitting

Weight - 260 lbs.

Height - 5 feet

Patient Profile

Allergies - none known

Present Medications - none

Family - single, childless, lives with elderly parents

and brother on farm.

Occupation - school teacher

Personal Habits - can care for self.

Diet - Diabetic - no allergies to food.

Elimination - no problems

Attitude/concerns - casual, offhand manner when discussing

health problems. Concerned about care of aged parents

and farm responsibilities. Accepts surgery as necessary.

Typical Day - very active, many responsibilities, teaches,

cares for elderly parents and also a brother who has

been ill. Cares for sheep and cattle - does farm chores,

rises at 4 a.m. - retires at 9 p.m.

(Signed) R.N.

FORM #768-008 (12-71)

Figure 4-4. The problem-oriented record as it would be written by the professional workers caring for the patient. All information becomes part of the data base from which the patient's problems are discerned. (All illustrations of problem-oriented records shown are courtesy of Medical Center Hospital of Vermont, Burlington, Vt.)

A. The patient interview.

MEDICAL CENTER HOSPITAL OF VERMONT
BASELINE PHYSICAL EXAMINATION

PATIENT:
DATE:
PHYSICIAN:
GENERAL APPEARANCE: (Describe)

		NOR.	ABN.	NOT EXAM.	DESCRIBE OR MEASURE
SKIN:	Rash:	X			
	Texture:	X			
	Hair:	X			
	Local Lesion:	X			
	Pigmentation:	X			
	Scars:	X			
HEAD:		X			
EYES:	Lids:	X			
	Conjunctiva:	X			
	Cornea:	X			
	Sclera:	X			
	Pupils:	X			Round, equal, react to light.
	EOM:				
	Fundi:				
	Arter.		X		Nicking
	Veins	X			
	Retina	X			
	Discs	X			
	Media/Lens	X			
	Gross Visual Fields	X			
EARS:	Hearing:	X			
	Canals:		X		cerumen present
	MT's:	X			
NOSE:	Septum:	X			
	Turbinates:	X			
	Sinuses:	X			
MOUTH:	Lips:	X			
	Teeth:		X		edentulous
	Gums:	X			
	Tongue:	X			
	Buccal mucosa:	X			
	Pharynx:	X			
	Tonsils/Pillars:	X			
NECK:	Trachea:	X			midline
	Thyroid:	X			
	Mobility:	X			
NODES:	Cervical:	X			
	Supraclavicular:	X			
	Axillary:	X			
	Epitrochlear:	X			
	Inguinal:	X			
CHEST:	Configuration:	X			
	Excursions:	X			
BREASTS:	RIGHT LEFT	X			
	Nipples:	X			
	Masses:	X			
	Symmetry:	X			
	Discharge:	X			none

Form # 768-012 (5/72)   1 of 4

Figure 4-4. *B*. The physical examination.

BASELINE PHYSICAL EXAMINATION

		NOR.	ABN.	NOT EXAM.	DESCRIBE OR MEASURE
LUNGS:	Percussion:	X			resonant throughout
	Auscultation:		X		wheezing - course rhonchi both bases
HEART:	Precordium:	X			
	PMI:	X			
	Percussion:	X			
	Auscultation:	X			
	Jugular pulses:	X			
	Venous pressure:			X	
B.P.:	Arm:	160/100			supine
	Leg:			X	
PERIPHERAL VESSELS:					
	Carotids: R L	X			
	Femorals: R L	X			
	Popliteals: R L	X			
	DP's: R L	X			
	PT's: R L	X			
ABDOMEN: Shape:			X		obese, markedly
	Venous pattern:	X			
	Percussion:	X			
	Tenderness:	X			
	Organ Enlrg.	X			
	Masses:	X			
	Bruits:	X			
	Hernias:	X			
	Scars:		X		rt upper quadrant, well healed
	Bowel sounds:	X			
MALE GENITALIA:					
	Penis:				
	Testes:				
	Discharge:				
RECTAL:	Anus:		X		external hemorrhoid, small
	Sphincter:	X			
	Prostate:				
	Masses, etc.:	X			
	Bimanual:	X			
	Sigmoidoscopy:			X	
PELVIC:	Vulva:	X			
	Urethra:	X			
	Vagina/Disch:	X			
	Cervix:	X			nulliparous, mucosa pink
	Fundus:		X		midline, large
	Adnexa:			X	nonpalpable bilaterally
	Rectovaginal:	X			
	Pap done:	X			
	Culture/Trich:			X	
MUSCULOSKELETAL:		X			
	Spine:				
	Pelvis:	X			
	Extremities:	X			
	Joints:	X			
	Subc. nodules:	X			

Form #768-012 (5/72) 2 of 4

Figure 4-4. *B.* (continued).

MEDICAL CENTER HOSPITAL OF VERMONT
BASELINE PHYSICAL EXAMINATION

Patient:

	NOR.	ABN.	NOT EXAM.	DESCRIBE OR MEASURE
NEUROMUSCULAR:	X			
General cerebral				
function:				
Cranial nerves:				
I:			X	
II:	X			visual fields norm to confrontation
III, IV, VI:	X			
V:	X			
VII:	X			
VIII:			X	
IX, X:	X			
XI:	X			
XII:	X			
Motor Function:				
Gait:	X			
Muscle Strength:	X			
Atrophy:				
Tremor:				
Cerebellar:				
Sensory:				
Position:	X			
Vibratory:	X			
Handedness:	rt			
Reflexes:				
KJ's:	X			
AJ's:	X			
Babinski:	X			
Biceps:	X			
Triceps:	X			
OTHER: Leg veins:	X			
Edema:		X		slight, non pitting, ankle, bilaterally
Support devices:				

(Use space below and reverse side for additional observations)

....
Signature M.D.

Form #768-012 (5/72)   3 of 4

Figure 4-4. *B*. (continued).

BASELINE PHYSICAL EXAMINATION

Form #768-012 (5/72)   4 of 4

Figure 4-4. *B*. (continued).

MEDICAL CENTER HOSPITAL OF VERMONT

Please Check: MFU ☐   DU ☐

PROBLEM LIST

(Attending and House Staff Physicians should
Formulate Single Problem List within 24 Hours
of Admission)

DATE ONSET	ACTIVE PROBLEMS	DATE RESOLVED	INACTIVE OR RESOLVED PROBLEMS
1970	CHIEF COMPLAINT: #1 Perimenopausal menometrorrhagia --> uterine leiomyoma --> total abdominal hysterectomy - BSO		
8-13-73			
noted 1963	#2 Diabetes Mellitus		
child-hood	#3 Obesity		
1958	#4 Smoker - 2 1/2 pack/15 yrs.		
1973	#5 Household management problems		
	#6 -------------------------------------->	1972	Cholecystectomy
? (noted 1972)	#7 Hypertension		

STRUCTURED BY A:

1. Medical Problem:
   a. A "Diagnosis"
   b. Physiological Abnormality
   c. Symptom or Physical Finding
   d. Laboratory Abnormality
2. Psychiatric Problem
3. Socioeconomic Problem
4. Demographic Problem

FORM #768-007 (12/71)

Figure 4-4. *C.* The problem list derived from the data base.

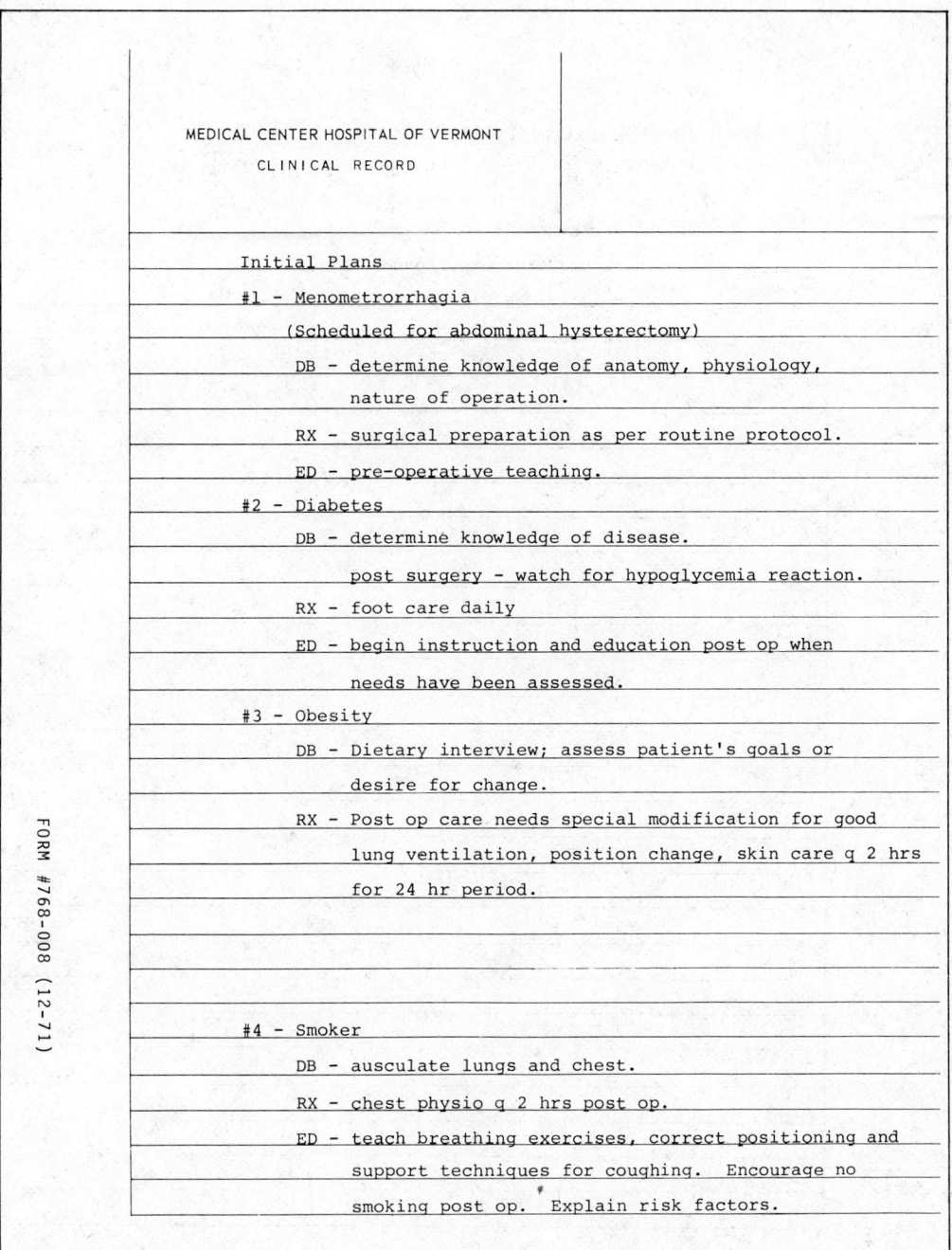

MEDICAL CENTER HOSPITAL OF VERMONT

CLINICAL RECORD

Initial Plans

#1 - Menometrorrhagia

  (Scheduled for abdominal hysterectomy)

  DB - determine knowledge of anatomy, physiology,
      nature of operation.

  RX - surgical preparation as per routine protocol.

  ED - pre-operative teaching.

#2 - Diabetes

  DB - determine knowledge of disease.
      post surgery - watch for hypoglycemia reaction.

  RX - foot care daily

  ED - begin instruction and education post op when
      needs have been assessed.

#3 - Obesity

  DB - Dietary interview; assess patient's goals or
      desire for change.

  RX - Post op care needs special modification for good
      lung ventilation, position change, skin care q 2 hrs
      for 24 hr period.

#4 - Smoker

  DB - ausculate lungs and chest.

  RX - chest physio q 2 hrs post op.

  ED - teach breathing exercises, correct positioning and
      support techniques for coughing. Encourage no
      smoking post op. Explain risk factors.

FORM #768-008 (12-71)

Figure 4-4. *D*. Initial plans formulated by the nurse and based on the identified problems of the patient.

MEDICAL CENTER HOSPITAL OF VERMONT

CLINICAL RECORD

Initial Plans, con't

#5 - Household management problem

    DB - Social service consultation.

#7 - Hypertension

    DB - BP QID post op period.

                     (Signed) R.N.

FORM #768-008 (12-71)

Figure 4-4. *D.* (continued).

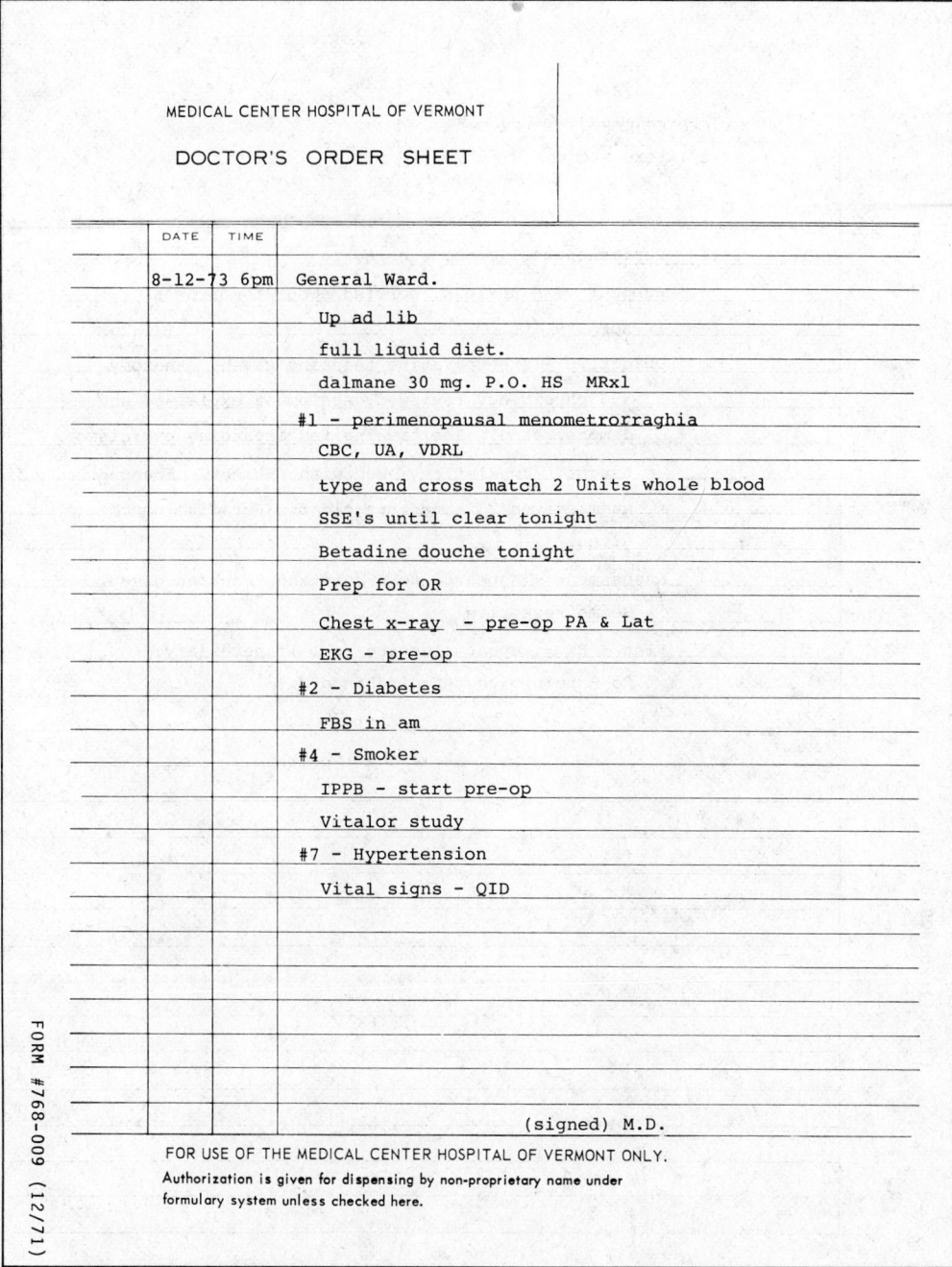

Figure 4-4. *E.* The relationship between the patient's problems and the physician's plans for care are clearly evident when the orders are written according to each of the patient's problems.

MEDICAL CENTER HOSPITAL OF VERMONT

CLINICAL RECORD

(date)   #1 - Perimenopausal menometrorrraghia

      Subjective - anxious, worried about tomorrow's surgery.

      Objective - pre-operative teaching given. Anatomy and physiology reviewed, equipment explained and demonstrated. Positioning and breathing exercises taught. Booklet reviewed with patient. Soapsuds enema given X2 - returns clear. Betadine douche given.

      Assessment - Appeared to understand teaching given. Seems receptive.

      Plan - Rx - repeat sleeping med. if necessary. Ed - reinforce teaching in a.m.

                   (Signed) R.N.

FORM #768-008 (12-71)

Figure 4-4. *F*. Narrative notes written for a problem-oriented record.

MEDICAL CENTER HOSPITAL OF VERMONT

CLINICAL RECORD

(date)   #1 - Total Hysterectomy

Post-op Day 5

Subjective - nothing

Objective - Surgical wound dressing removed. Retention

suture sites cleansed with H_2O_2. Bottom two retention

sutures are deeply imbedded in roll of adipose

tissue. These areas are quite moist with some loss

of good skin color (area being more grey than

anything else). Small areas of skin breakdown noted

along creases. Telfa strip inserted.

Output - one moderate brown formed stool/shift.

Voiding without difficulty in moderate amounts.

Assessment - Improving overall. Feel that the biggest

problem now is wound care and unless vigorous

treatment is initiated, wound breakdown could be

the result.

Plan Rx - (1) Cleanse retention suture sites with

H_2O_2 BID, once on days and once on evenings.

(2) Use heat lamp on bottom two retention suture

sites BID and more frequently if possible. (3) Insert

telfa strip in fat folds.

(Signed) R.N.

FORM #768-008 (12-71)

Figure 4-4. *F.* (continued).

MEDICAL CENTER HOSPITAL OF VERMONT

CLINICAL RECORD

(Date)   10 a.m. #2 - Diabetes

Symptomatic - weakness, dizziness, sweating, "heart
pounding." Describes feelings as resembling
hypoglycemic reaction which she has had frequently
in past. Is accustomed to carrying chocolate bars.
Objective - vs P120 R24. Skin pale, moist. Given
orange juice with sugar added.
Assessment - hypoglycemic reaction; patient in need
of diabetic data base to ascertain teaching needs.
Plan - M.D. notified. Remain with patient for 15 min.
continue ingestion of high calorie drink.

(Signed) R.N.

FORM #768-008 (12-71)

Figure 4-4. *F.* (continued).

Figure 4-5*A* shows a history that was completed by a patient and Figure 4-5*F* shows a teaching program organized according to the problems jointly identified by the patient and professional staff. The plan prepared by the nurse and "printed out" by the computer is given directly to the patient. Figure 4-5*D* shows the thinking behind a plan of care, which makes it possible to evaluate the nurse's practice, not only on what was accomplished but also on the knowledge that went into making the plan.

The merit of the medical record is not dependent on the method by which patient data are arranged. Regardless of the method, a good record reflects the value that health practitioners attach to the patient's ability to report his needs and problems, the way that professional workers communicate with each other and the patient for the patient's benefit, and the way that each worker defines and follows clinical problems and systematically records and solves them.

It is likely that medical records will undergo a marked change in the near future. Those in current use do not make it clear to medical workers that they should (1) provide the psychologic or social aspects of care during illness; (2) treat the patient so that the best interests of his or her family or household are served; and (3) rehabilitate him or her through the combined resources of the community.

If the present trend in emphasizing social aspects of medical care continues, all health agencies will develop records that, for the average patients, give a more complete picture of their living and working situations, their insight or understanding of their health problems, and their independence or dependence in carrying out the essential activities of daily living. Forms will also be developed that will still further facilitate exchange of information between health agencies and pooling services in the interests of a family. Jesse B. Aronson[31] points out that improvement in preventive medicine and "case finding" in syphilis, tuberculosis, and other diseases is dependent on better family health records and exchange of data.

A. R. Feinstein[32] discusses some current problems in medical records and traces their sources. He gives instances where medical problems are dealt with out of context, progress notes are sparse, isolated, and uninformative. He cites the absence of a meaningful "audit" (see page 55 for further discussion of the audit) in the practice of medicine, due in part, he thinks, to withdrawal or apathy of the more experienced physicians who are now more often engrossed in laboratory research. Lawrence L. Weed,[33] on the other hand, thinks that the absence of a meaningful "audit" in the practice of medicine is not due to withdrawal or apathy of the more experienced physicians, but to the haphazard way in which data are recorded in the "source-oriented" record. He believes that the problem-oriented medical record documents the thinking, planning, and observations of the person making the record which can then be examined or "audited" for completeness and content, thoroughness, reliability, analytic sense, and efficiency.

A development that seems inevitable is the automation of medical records. This will require that medical, nursing, and all other health professions establish uniform terminology and standards of measurement. Weed[34] states that every phase of medical action will benefit from computerization and that the "data base phase" can profit immediately. The patient may interact directly with a television terminal that is the point of computer input. For example, he or she gives a health history by answering questions presented on a touch-sensitive cathode ray tube terminal (see Fig. 4-6). That data, structured by the computer, can be printed out in ordinary language and in narrative form for the health professional's use (see Figs. 4-5*A–F*).

Making the Record. In private practice, the record may be made by the physician, the independent nurse practitioner, a nurse who assists a physician, or a clerical worker. Patients contribute to their health record by completing their health history. The Cornell Medical Index Health Questionnaire (see Fig. 4-7) is an example of a record that is completed by the patient.

In hospitals, many persons contribute toward making the record. On admission of the patient to the institution, an *admitting officer* records certain statistical, administrative, and social data, such as name, address, age, nationality, religion, and occupation. The physician or the nurse prepares a history of the health of the patient and his or her family, and also the history of the present illness. The professional worker who examines the patient will record the physical findings. This may be the nurse who has been prepared to make a physical examination. The nurse in collaboration with the patient will develop a plan of care and will write the appropriate directives for nursing measures. The physician will write directives for the plan of medical management. Nurses in private practice and in some clinics take complete responsibility for the plan of care. The physician may be called in as a consultant, or, if the nurse believes it is necessary,

[*Text continued on page 354.*]

<HISTORY & LAB DATA BASE>

/UN026/ 12:09 11/02/73

NAME: @PATIENT'S NAME@

SOCIAL PROFILE:
   LIVES WITH PARENTS.
   4 IN HOUSEHOLD.
   SINGLE.
   PROBS W/RELATIVES.   [P/A]
   ILLNESS IN FAMILY PAST YR.[NOTE REL. TO PT.]
   PROBS W/WORK CONDITIONS.   [P/A]
   CURRENTLY SUPPORTED BY SELF.
   RESPONSIBLE FOR SUPPORT OF 3 OTHER PEOPLE.
   WORKING/EMPLOYED.
   WORKS 34-40 HRS./WEEK.
   WORKING HOURS/SCHEDULE UNSATISFACTORY.
   HIGHEST GRADE IN SCHOOL: GRADUATE WORK OR DEGREE.
   SATISFIED W/ CURRENT MEDICAL CARE.
   FOLLOWS SPECIAL DIET.
   USUAL YEARLY VACATION >2 WEEKS.
   DOESN'T HAVE ENOUGH LEISURE TIME.
   HEALTH INTERFERES WITH NORMAL LIFE PATTERN.
   HAS NOT MADE OUT WILL.   [P.ED]
   DOES NOT WEAR SEAT BELTS IN THE CAR.   [P.ED]
   MOUTH-TO-MOUTH RESUSCITATION TECHNIQUE NOT KNOWN.   [P.ED]
   IN CASE OF MEDICAL EMERGENCY DOESN'T KNOW WHAT TO DO.   [P.ED]
   FOR ACCIDENTAL POISONING DOESN'T KNOW WHAT TO DO.   [P.ED]

IMMUNIZATIONS:
   ORAL POLIO VACCINE: NOT IMMUNIZED.   [P.ED]
   POLIO SHOTS: NOT IMMUNIZED.
   RUBELLA: NOT IMMUNIZED.   [P.ED]
   FLU VACCINE NOT OBTAINED PAST 2 YRS.
   DPT: IMMUNIZED
   LAST TETANUS BOOSTER - W/IN 2 YRS.

FAMILY HISTORY/GENETIC:
   LIVING BROTHERS/SISTERS: 1.   [I]

ALLERGY:
   TO PENICILLIN- RASH/HIVES.   [PL]
   DOESN'T WEAR ID TAG STATING ALLERGIES.   [P.ED]
   TO FOOD, POLLEN, FUR OR ANIMALS.   [PL]
   TO DETERGENTS, SOAPS OR SHAMPOOS.   [PL]
   TO COSMETICS, HAIR DYES OR PERMANENT WAVES.   [PL]

DERMATOLOGY:
   POTENTIAL:
   SELF-EXAM OF BREAST NOT PERFORMED REGULARLY.   [P.ED]

EYES:
   NEGATIVE.

EARS:
   NEGATIVE.

NOSE:
   NEGATIVE.

DENTAL:
   POTENTIAL:
   DENTAL FLOSS NOT USED.   [P.ED]

MOUTH/THROAT/LARYNX:
   NEGATIVE.

HEMATOPOIETIC:
   NEGATIVE.

Figure 4-5. Problem-oriented record printed out by a computer. (All illustrations courtesy of Medical Center Hospital of Vermont, Burlington, Vt.)

A. A history completed by a patient according to a predefined set of questions formulated by health workers, stored in the computer, and answered by the patient at a computer terminal.

```
RESPIRATORY:
  POTENTIAL:
    SMOKES CIGARETTES 1-2 PACKS DAILY.                          [P.ED]
    SMOKED 10-15 YEARS.                                            [I]

CARDIOVASCULAR:
  CURRENT - IN PAST YR:
    RESTRICTED SALT INTAKE ON ADVICE.                           [P/A]
    ANTI-HYPERTENSIVES TAKEN.                                     [M]
  POTENTIAL:
    SMOKES CIGARETTES.                                          [P.ED]
    DRINKS 5 OR MORE CUPS OF COFFEE DAILY.                      [P.ED]
    HAS BEEN TOLD BLOOD PRESSURE IS HIGH.           [P. ED/CHECK BP]
    FEELS PRESSURED MOST OF THE TIME.                          [P.ED]
    THOUGHT TO BE OVERCRITICAL BY OTHERS.                         [I]

GASTROINTESTINAL:
  CURRENT - IN PAST YR:
    RECURRENT RECTAL ITCH, BURNING OR PAIN.                     [P/A]
  PAST - HX OF:
    GALL BLADDER SURG.                                           [PL]

MUSCULO-SKELETAL:
  NEGATIVE.

ENDOCRINE:
  CURRENT - IN PAST YR:
    WEIGHT PROBLEM.                                             [P/A]
    DIABETES MEDS TAKEN.                                          [M]
  PAST - HX OF:
    DIABETES MELLITUS.                                          [PL]
    BLOOD SUGAR ABNORMAL.                                       [PL]

OBSTETRICS:
  NEGATIVE.

GYNECOLOGY:
  CURRENT - IN PAST YR:
    LMP APPROXIMATELY 0-1 MONTH AGO.                             [I]
    IRREGULAR PERIODS.                                            [I]
    EXCESSIVE FLOW WITH PERIODS.                              [I;P/A]
    HEADACHES, DEPRESSION W/PERIODS.                          [I;P/A]
    BIRTH CONTROL BY NO METHOD.                             [I/P.ED]
  PAST - HX OF:
  NO PAP IN PAST YEAR.                                  [PAP SMEAR]

GENITO-URINARY/RENAL:
  NEGATIVE.

NEUROLOGY:
  NEGATIVE.

PSYCHIATRY:
  CURRENT:
    LESS ABLE TO CONCENTRATE ON OWN ACTIVITY.
    FEELS CONSTANTLY UNDER STRAIN MORE THAN USUAL.
    FEELS DIFFICULTIES CAN'T BE OVERCOME.
    ENJOYING NORMAL DAY TO DAY ACTIVITIES LESS THAN USUAL.
    LESS ABLE TO FACE UP TO PROBLEMS.
    UNHAPPY AND DEPRESSED MORE THAN USUAL.
    ALL THINGS CONSIDERED, FEELING LESS HAPPY THAN USUAL.
  * GHQ SCORE >1.  ATTENTION WARRANTED. .  [P/A]
    FEELS DEPRESSED OR LONELY OFTEN.                            [P/A]
  POTENTIAL:
    TOO MANY RESPONSIBILITIES.                                 [P.ED]

SUMMARY STATISTICS:
  INTERVIEW COMPLETED.
   67 PRINTING RESP.
   232 TOTAL RESP.
```

Figure 4-5. *A.* (continued).

```
-- COMPUTERIZED POMR --   SN 9 /UN026/  8/30/73  10:56   PAGE   2

PATIENTS NAME PRO-UVM 000-000-0 F 42 SERVICE


                    <PATIENT PROFILE>
          --------------------------------
                                      /UN026/  9:21  8/28/73
ADMITTED: AMBULATORY.
CONDITION OF PATIENT: CHRONICALLY ILL
DURATION THIS ILLNESS: 20 YEARS.
PAST ILLNESSES:
    HOSPITALIZATIONS: @CHOLECYSTECTOMY 1972, T&A AS CHILD,
        DIABETES 1966@
    @OBESITY, ELEVATED BLOOD PRESSURE, @
    EXPERIENCE WITH HOSPITALIZATIONS FAVORABLE.
EFFECT OF HOSPITALIZATION
    CREATES PROBLEMS:
        FAMILY: DEPENDENT RELATION AT HOME,
GENERAL ATTITUDE: @CASUAL AND OFF HAND MANNER WHEN DISCUSSING
        HEALTH PROBLEMS. CONCERNED ABOUT CARE OF AGED PARENTS
        AND FARM RESPONSIBILITIES, REALIZES SURGERY IS GREAT
        UNDERTAKING FOR HER. HAS GOOD ATTITUDE TOWARD MEDICAL
        SUPERVISION.@
PLACE IN FAMILY:
    THE PATIENT IS CHILDLESS, IS SINGLE THE PATIENT LIVES:
        W/FAMILY. OCCUPATION:  @SCHOOL TEACHER, @
PERSONAL HABITS:
    MOUTH CARE: BRUSHES TEETH.
    BATHING: BY SELF, LIKES SHOWERS, FACILITIES FOR BATH,
        SHOWER,
    SLEEP/NAPS:
        USUALLY ARISES AT 4 A.M.
        USUALLY RETIRES AT 9 P.M.
    EATING HABITS/PATTERN:
        EATS 3 REGULAR MEALS/DAY. SNACKS IRREGULARLY,
        FOOD 'ALLERGIES': @NONE@
        DISLIKES:
        SPECIAL DIET: DIABETIC,
    SMOKES: CIGARETTES, 30/DAY :
    EXERCISE: @FARM WORK@ DAILY.
    URINARY: NO PROBLEMS.
    BOWELS: REGULAR MOVEMENTS
TYPICAL DAY: @VERY ACTIVE WOMAN WITH MANY RESPONSIBILITIES,
        TEACHES, CARES FOR ELDERLY PARENTS AND ALSO A BROTHER
        WHO HAS BEEN ILL, CARES FOR SHEEP AND CATTLE, DOES
        FARM CHORES. @
ALLERGIES: NONE KNOWN.
PRESENT MEDICATIONS: NONE.
MEDICAL CARE:
    DOCTOR: MOST RECENT: @BLANK@
```

Figure 4-5. *B.* Patient profile or nursing history. The nurse interviews a patient and stores this information in the computer.

the patient is referred to a physician or other health professional. (See also Chapters 1 and 5 for discussion of this subject.)

On the patient's discharge, a summary report is written by the physician, the nurse who is in independent practice, or the physician and nurse together, explaining the patient's condition, progress of the disease, success or failure of the treatment, further care required, and plans for teaching or rehabilitation. In hospitals, medical aspects of the record are written by medical students, or medical clerks,

```
\3513->22\
  -- COMPUTERIZED POMR --    SN 9 /UN026/  8/30/73  10:56    PAGE   1

   PATIENTS NAME PRO-UVM 000-000-0 F 42 SERVICE


               <ACTIVE PROBLEM LIST>

1.->TOTAL HYSTERECTOMY: W/BILATERAL           /UN026/ 13:27  8/01/73
             SALPINGOOOPHORECTOMY FOR UTERINE LEIOMYOMA.

2.DIABETES MELLITUS MATURITY ONSET, W/O COMPLICATIONS. 13:11

3.OBESITY OF CHILDHOOD ONSET: SEVERE ASSOC.W/ ENVIRONMENTAL FACTORS.

4.SMOKING: 2.5 PACKS/DAY FOR 15 YEARS.

5.HOUSEHOLD MANAGE.PROBS,

7.HYPERTENSION: COMBINED: MILD,                      9:58  8/28/73

    (TEMPORARY PROBLEMS)

A.HEADACHE, OCCIPITAL, CONTINUOUS,                   9:19
               <TOTAL PROBLEM LIST>

1.PERIMENOPAUSAL MENOMETRORRHAGIA              13:11  8/01/73
   ->UTERINE LEIOMYOMA:                        13:26
   ->TOTAL HYSTERECTOMY: W/BILATERAL           13:27
             SALPINGOOOPHORECTOMY FOR UTERINE LEIOMYOMA.

2.DIABETES MELLITUS MATURITY ONSET, W/O COMPLICATIONS. 13:11

3.OBESITY OF CHILDHOOD ONSET: SEVERE ASSOC.W/ ENVIRONMENTAL FACTORS.

4.SMOKING: 2.5 PACKS/DAY FOR 15 YEARS.

5.HOUSEHOLD MANAGE.PROBS,

6.H/O BILIARY SURGERY: CHOLECYSTECTOMY. BY HISTORY    9:16  8/28/73
             (1972)
   H/O BILIARY SURGERY: CH* ->RES/INACT              9:18

7.HYPERTENSION: COMBINED: MILD,                      9:58

    (TEMPORARY PROBLEMS)

A.HEADACHE, OCCIPITAL, CONTINUOUS,                   9:19
```

Figure 4-5. *C*. List of patient problems derived from the data and printed out by the computer.

interns, medical residents, and attending and consulting physicians. Reports of special examinations, including autopsy reports, are made by physicians in charge of diagnostic laboratories and by *technicians* who act as their assistants.

Records of special treatments may be written by *dietitians, physical therapists, occupational therapists,* and *medical social workers,* as well as physicians and nurses. A relatively large part of the average patient's record is made by *nurses*. Although *clerks* may be employed to help them in some mechanical details, they are responsible for the graphic rec-

```
        POST-OP DAY 5:                              /UN051/ 15:04
           SURGICAL WOUND:
              DRESSING: REMOVED.
              SUTURES: RETENTION SITE CLEANSED WITH: HYDROGEN PEROXIDE.
                 @BOTTOM TWO RETENTION SUTURES ARE DEEPLY IMBEDDED IN
                 ROLL OF ADIPOSE TISSUE. THESE TWO AREA WERE QUITE
                 MOIST WITH SOME LOSS OF GOOD SKIN COLOR (AREA BEING
                 MORE GREY THAN ANYTHING ELSE). SMALL AREAS OF SKIN
                 BREAKDOWN ALONG CREASES NOTED. TELFA STRIP INSERTED.@
           OUTPUT:
              STOOL: CONSISTENCY: FORMED. COLOR: BROWN. AMOUNT:
                 MODERATE. 1 PER SHIFT.
              VOIDING: WITHOUT DIFFICULTY. IN MODERATE AMOUNTS.
ASMT:
   IMPROVING OVERALL.
           @FEEL THAT BIGGEST PROBLEM NOW IS WOUND CARE AND UNLESS
                 VIGOROUS TREATMENT IS INITIATED, WOUND BREAKDOWN COULD
                 BE THE RESULT.@
PLN-PRO:
   @CLEANSE RETENTION SUTURE SITES WITH H2O2 BID. ONCE ON DAYS. ONCE
                 ON EVENINGS.@
   @USE HEAT LAMP TO BOTTOM TWO RETENTION SUTURE SITES BID AND MORE
                 FREQUENTLY IF POSS.@
   @INSERT TELFA STRIP IN FAT FOLD@
```

Figure 4-5. *D*. A narrative note written by a nurse at a computer terminal and printed by the computer.

```
                              <PROG NOTES>
                     ----------------------------

           (TEMPORARY PROBLEMS)

   A.HEADACHE, OCCIPITAL, CONTINUOUS.
     SX:
           HEADACHE                           /UN026/ 10:04  8/28/73
              ONSET: SUDDEN (ABRUPT).
              COMMENCED: 2 HOURS AGO.
              SEVERITY AT WORST: SEVERE REQUIRING RX, CANNOT CONTINUE
                    USUAL ACTIVITY.
              AMOUNT EACH TIME: OF VARIABLE INTENSITY.
              PRECIPITATED BY: @SURGERY@
              PRECEDED BY: NOTHING.
              QUALITY: ACHING.
              LOCATION: OCCIPITAL, NECK/SHOULDER, BILATERAL.
              RELIEVED BY: POSITION: LYING DOWN, COLD.
              NOT RELIEVED BY: SPECIFIC MEDIC., ANALGESICS.
              MADE WORSE BY: POSITION: STANDING UP.
              ASSOCIATED WITH: ASS W/KNOWN DX OR H.O.: DIABETES MELLITUS.
              ASSOCIATED WITH: @SPINAL ANESTHESIA@
              OVERALL COURSE: UNCHANGED.
              PATIENT'S ATTITUDE: IS DEPRESSED. ACCEPTS STATEMENT OF
                    PROBLEM.
     ASMT:
        STAYING SAME OVERALL.
           @HEADACHE PROBABLY DUE TO SPINAL ANESTHESIA@
     PLN-DDA:
        @OFFER SALTY BROTH. EXTRA SALT WITH MEALS. ENCOURAGE FLUIDS. @
                    FLUIDS AD LIB.
        PT.ACT: PT.ACT: @FLAT AS MUCH AS POSSIBLE@

                        -- RETRIEVAL REQUEST --

           ENTIRE RECORD

- - - - - - - - - - - - - - - - - - - - - - - - - - - - - - - - - -
```

Figure 4-5. *E*. The computer prints the symptoms, assessment, and plan which have been written by nurse or physician.

```
   2.DIABETES MELLITUS MATURITY ONSET, W/O COMPLICATIONS.
   ASMT:
              @CONTROLED BY DIET AND MADE WORSE BY   /MD164/  17:30   7/15/73
                   OBESITY.@
   PLN-DR:
      FBS  X1
      @COMPLETE DIABETIC DATA BASE WHEN POST OP    /UN050/   8:14   7/16/73
                   CODITION PERMITS: DURING POST OP PERIOD-CAREFUL
                   SURVEILLANCE FOR HYPER OR HYPOGLYCEMIC REACTIONS@
   SX:
         NAUSEA                                    /UN221/  16:00   7/23/73
         WEAKNESS
              ONSET: GRADUAL (INSIDIOUS). 1
              COMMENCED: 6 HOURS AGO.
              SEVERITY AT WORST: @SYMPTOMS BECAME MORE PROMINENT AROUND
                   12NOON.@
              RELIEVED BY: REST.
              ASSOCIATED WITH: DIDN'T DETERMINE.
              OVERALL COURSE: NOW COMPLETELY SUBSIDED.
              PATIENT'S ATTITUDE: TO PAST SIMILAR ILLNESS/SX: UNDERSTANDS
                   SIGNIFICANCE. ACCEPTS STATEMENT OF PROBLEM.
   OBJ:
      @PT. APPEARED DIAPHORETIC AND RESTLESS.@  @URINE TESTED N/N.@
   ASMT:
              @HYPOGLYCEMIC REACTION.@
   PLN-MGT:
      @TEST FRAC. URINE A.C. AND H.S. CALL M.D. IF PT. EXPERIENCES ANY
                   FURTHER REACTIONS. ATTEMPT TO OBTAIN DATA-BASE ON
                   DIABETES FROM PT.@
   SX:
         DIABETES MELLITUS                         /UN050/  10:45   7/24/73
              ONSET: SUDDEN (ABRUPT).
              COMMENCED: 10 YEARS AGO. AT AGE 32
              TYPE OF ONSET:
                   SYMPTOMATIC ONSET: LASSITUDE/FATIGUE,
              SEVERITY AT WORST: COULDN'T DETERMINE.
              QUALITY: STABLE.
              MADE WORSE BY: EMOTIONAL STRESS,
              ASS.W/
                   SX/SIGNS/FINDINGS: OBESITY, SINCE CHILDHOOD
                   CARDIOVASC.SX/SIGN: HYPERTENSION,
              ASS.W/ GENETIC FACTORS: F/H DIABETES MELLITUS: MOTHER F/H
                   OBESITY: MOTHER FATHER SIBLINGS 1
              OVERALL COURSE: FLUCTUATING.
              PATIENT'S ATTITUDE: UNDERSTANDS SIGNIFICANCE. @DOES NOT
                   FOLLOW DIET@ CDN'T DETERMINE DEGREE OF ACCEPTANCE OF
                   PROBLEM.
      @EXPERIENCES FREQUENT EPISODES OF HYPOGLYCEMIA MANIFESTED BY
                   WEAKNESS. DIZZINESS, SWEATING, PALPITATIONS: CARRIES
                   CHOCALATE BARS: DOES NOT CARRY IDENTIFICATION: IS A
                   COMPULSIVE EATER. AND IS EXTREMELY ACTIVE AT HARD
                   PHYSICAL LABOR: TESTS URINE FOR GLUCOSE ONLY
                   SPORADICALLY (MAYBE 2X/WEEK): GOES BAREFOOT: KNOWS
                   FOOD EXCHANGES BUT DOESN'T ABIDE BY THEM@
   ASMT:
              @IS UNABLE TO REALLY COMMIT HERSELF TO DIETARY
                   CONSIDERATIONS OF DISEASE@
```

Figure 4-5. *E.* (continued).

ord of the temperature, pulse, and respiration, the report of other physical functions such as the amount of food and fluids taken, the elimination of feces and urine, or abnormal elimination by profuse sweating or vomiting. Nurses are responsible for recording treatments and nursing care given by them and often by others and for making written reports of the patient's behavior that they think might affect diagnosis, medical treatment, nursing care, or rehabilitation.

In many cases the *patients* may contribute something or even a great deal toward the medical record. They may write portions of

```
DISCHARGE TEACHING: HYSTERECTOMY:        /UN050/ 10:37
      ACTIVITY: DRIVING--ONLY IF ABSOLUTELY NECESSARY. MAY GO
         OUTSIDE WITHIN 1 WEEK. MINIMAL ACTIVITY FOR 1-2 WEEKS.
         STAIRS--AVOID. MAY CLIMB 2-3 TIMES A DAY. NO
         PUSHING-PULLING, STANDING LONG PERIODS. GRADUAL RETURN
         TO NORMAL ACTIVITY. ELEVATE LEGS WHEN SITTING AVOID
         CROSSING LEGS.
      DIET/FLUIDS: HI PROTEIN, IRON RICH, FLUIDS--2 QUARTS A
         DAY. SPECIAL DIET DISCUSSED: @IS ON DIABETIC DIET@
      HYGIENE: SHOWER OR TUB BATH PERMITTED. NO DOUCHING,
         TAMPON, INTERCOURSE UNTIL SEEN BY MD. EXERCISE
         ACCORDING TO DOCTOR'S ORDERS.
      BOWELS: MAY TAKE MILK OF MAGNESIA OR MINERAL OIL.
         ROUGHAGE IN DIET AND FLUID INTAKE IMPORTANT.
      SIGNS/SX TO REPORT: FEVER, EXCESSIVE,BRIGHT RED FLOW,

      ABDOMINAL PAIN, BURNING ON URINATION, FLANK/LEG/CHEST
         PAIN.
      MEDICATIONS: HORMONES: HOW TO TAKE: @PREMARIN 1.25 MG
         ONCE DAILY FOR 25 CONSECUTIVE DAYS OF EACH MONTH:
         ADVISED TO TAKE AT NIGHT TO AVOID STOMACH UPSET@ IRON:
         HOW TO TAKE: @3 TIMES DAILY BETWEEN MEALS@ SIDE
         EFFECTS: @CONSTIPATION@ @DARVON COMPOUND AS NEEDED FOR
         PAIN@
      FOLLOW-UP: @TO RETURN TO DR SIMS OFFICE NEXT WEEK FOR
         STAY SUTURE REMOVAL@
      PATIENT CONCERNS: @WOUND CARE-DIFFICULT FOR HER TO
         VISUALIZE OR CARE FOR AREA: WILL GET ASSIST FOR TWICE
         A DAY CLEANSING WITH SOAP AND WATER: TO PLACE DRY
         GAUZE IN LOWER  ABDOMINAL CREASE TO KEEP DRY@
      PATIENT UNDERSTANDING: RECEPTIVE, UNDERSTANDS,
```

Figure 4-5. *F.* The guide for patient instruction at the time of discharge has been stored in the computer. The nurse selects the proper information and the computer prints it onto a form which is given to the patient to take home.

the social data, take psychometric tests, keep a diary, write a personal history, answer a questionnaire, and sign statements signifying permission for operation or treatments involving risks, and in certain conditions their writings or drawings may be included in the record as evidence of symptoms or attitudes.

A standing committee on records composed of representatives of all departments concerned should exist in every health agency. The most useful medical record can be developed only through joint endeavor. Each professional group may have its own committee, but none of these can function satisfactorily without representation on the central committee. In many cases, representatives of cooperating agencies should be consultants on the committee. The possibility of consumer participation in the development of medical records should be explored. Certainly a record should be available to which patients contribute and that can remain in their possession.

Weed states:

There are those who fear the patient will panic if he owns and understands his own health record. But what of the confusion, bad medicine and suffering that result directly from the present practice of keeping source oriented records unavailable to patients and families just when they need them most. . . . It may be the most effective weapon we have against over-utilization of medical care. . . . If you want to protect yourself against bad health practices and develop a mature and helpful philosophy about maintaining your health, you need to understand the means by which physicians' clinical judgments are made and tested.*

Progress Notes. Notes on the progress of the patient written by nurses vary with the responsibility that the nurse has for the patient and the type of record he or she is using. For example, nurses who give primary care in an office or clinic may be responsible for recording the patient's history, the physical examination, the conclusions, evaluation, and plan of care. Nurses caring for patients whose needs require the services of several medical specialists may be responsible for recording more specific data related to their progress.

Progress notes are written by each person who cares for the patient and are relevant to their particular area of patient responsibility

---

* Weed, Lawrence L.: *Your Health Care and How to Manage It.* PROMIS Laboratory, University of Vermont, Burlington, 1975, p. 51.

[*Text continued on page 369.*]

Table 4-1.   The Computerized Problem-Oriented Medical Record * : Key to Symbols for Figure 4-5A–F

POMR	Problem-oriented medical record	*	Asterisks appear when something
SN 9	Station number from which the retrieval of this record was requested		has been truncated in the record
		T & A	Tonsillectomy and adenoidectomy
		Post-Op	Postoperatively
Patient's name		ASMT	Assessment
PRO-UVM		PLN—PRO	Plan for procedure
000–000–0 F 42		H_2O_2	Hydrogen peroxide
Service	Identification data	BID	Twice a day
/UN026	Unit nurse with identifying number	Poss	Possible
		PROG	Progress
MD 164	Physician with identifying number	S_x	Symptoms
12:09 11/02/73	Date and time of retrieval	R_x	Treatment
@	Appears before and after information that was entered from the keyboard, rather than from the structured information on the displays	Medic	Medication
		Ass W/	Associated with
		Dx	Diagnosis
		H.O.	History of
		PLN—DDA	Plan for treatment (drug, diet, or activity)
PROBS	Problems		
w/	With	Pt. Act.	Patient activity
[P/a]	Use as an attribute of present illness—an action to be taken from the responses in the history	W/O	Without
		PLN—DB	Plan for data base
		F B S	Fasting blood sugar
[P. ED]	Educate the patient—an action to be taken from the response in the history	X1	Once or one time
		Obj	Objective information (see definition in text)
[I]	Information	N/N	Urine negative for sugar and acetone
[PL]	Put on problem list		
Hx	History	PLN—MGT	Plan for management
[M]	Medication	Frac. urine A.C. and H.S.	Test samples of urine for sugar and acetone before meals and at bedtime
LMP	Last menstrual period		
Pap	Papanicolaou smear—a test for cervical cancer		
		F/H	Family history
GHQ	General health questionnaire, a psychiatric screening questionnaire	2x	Twice or two times
		Q	Every

* Courtesy of Medical Center Hospital of Vermont, Burlington, Vt.

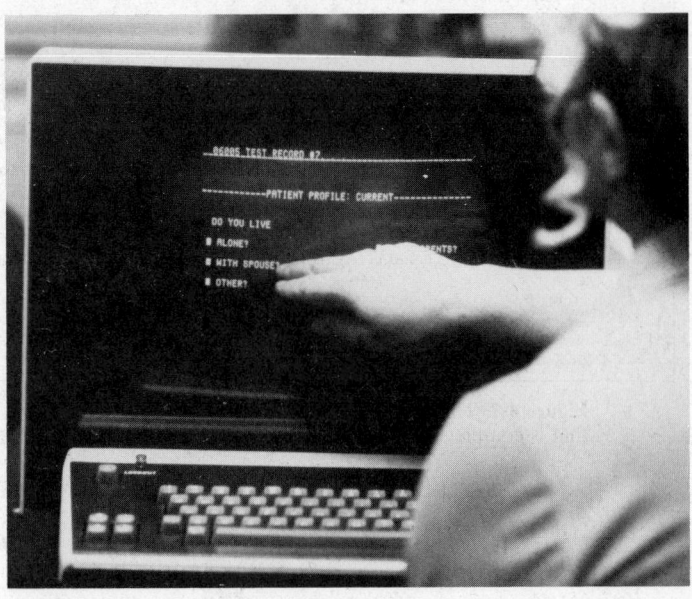

Figure 4-6. The patient gives a health history by answering questions presented on a touch-sensitive cathode ray tube terminal. (Courtesy of Medical Center Hospital of Vermont, Burlington, Vt.)

(WOMEN)

History Number

100 DISEASES EDITION

CORNELL MEDICAL INDEX

Date_____

HEALTH QUESTIONNAIRE

Print
Your
Name_____

Your
Home
Address_____

How Old Are You?_____ Circle If You Are . . Single, Married, Widowed, Separated, Divorced.

Circle the Highest
Year You Reached
In School | 1 2 3 4 5 6 7 8 | | 1 2 3 4 | | 1 2 3 4 |
Elementary School   High   College

What Is Your
Occupation?_____

Directions: This questionnaire is for **WOMEN ONLY.**

If you can answer **YES** to the question asked, put a circle around the (Yes)

If you have to answer **NO** to the question asked, put a circle around the (No)

Answer all questions. If you are not sure, guess.

A. HEAD

1. Do you suffer from frequent severe headaches? Yes No
2. Does constant pressure in your head and neck make life miserable? .... Yes No
3. Do you often feel dizzy and faint? .... Yes No

B. NECK

4. Do you usually have pain or stiffness in your neck? .... Yes No
5. Do you get sharp pains when you suddenly turn or bend your neck? .... Yes No
6. Has your neck become enlarged or swollen? Yes No

C. EYES

7. Do you wear glasses? .... Yes No
8. Is your eyesight blurred even when you wear glasses? .... Yes No
9. Do you suffer from constant eyestrain? .... Yes No
10. Is your eyesight rapidly getting worse? .... Yes No
11. Has your eyesight often blacked out completely? .... Yes No
12. Do you often have severe pains in your eyes? Yes No
13. Do your eyes continually blink or water? Yes No
14. Are you troubled with burning or itching of your eyes? .... Yes No
15. Do you sometimes see colored rings around lights? .... Yes No
16. Do you often see double? .... Yes No
17. Is one of your eyes turned in or turned out? Yes No

D. EARS

18. Are you hard of hearing? .... Yes No
19. Do you hear constant noises in your ears? . Yes No
20. Do you often have severe pains in your ears? Yes No
21. Have you ever had a running ear? .... Yes No

E. MOUTH

22. Do you have cavities or decay in any of your teeth? .... Yes No
23. Are any of your teeth loose or broken? .... Yes No
24. Do you often have severe toothaches? .... Yes No
25. Do you have a painful swelling in your gums or jaw? .... Yes No

F. NOSE

26. Do you usually find it hard to breathe through your nose? .... Yes No
27. Is one side of your nose always stuffed up? Yes No
28. Do you suffer from a constantly running nose? .... Yes No

G. THROAT

29. Do you have to clear your throat frequently? Yes No
30. Do you get many attacks of severe sore throat? .... Yes No
31. Did a doctor say that your tonsils are enlarged? .... Yes No
32. Is swallowing difficult or painful? .... Yes No

759
Copyright 1949
Printed in U. S. A.

Cornell University Medical College
1300 York Avenue, New York 21, N. Y.

OPEN TO NEXT PAGE

Figure 4-7. The Cornell Medical Index, Health Questionnaire, an example of a record that is completed by a patient. (Courtesy of the New York Hospital, New York)

H. RESPIRATORY SYSTEM

33. Do you often catch severe head colds?   Yes   No

34. Do you suffer from heavy chest colds?   Yes   No

35. When you catch a cold, do you always have to go to bed?   Yes   No

36. Are you troubled by constant coughing?   Yes   No

37. Do you cough up large amounts of sputum (phlegm)?   Yes   No

38. Have you often coughed up blood?   Yes   No

I. CARDIAC SYSTEM

39. Does every little effort leave you short of breath?   Yes   No

40. Do you sometimes get out of breath just sitting still?   Yes   No

41. Do you sleep propped up in bed?   Yes   No

42. Are you often bothered by thumping of the heart?   Yes   No

43. Does your heart often race like mad?   Yes   No

44. Do you have pains in the heart or chest?   Yes   No

45. Are your ankles often greatly swollen?   Yes   No

J. VASCULAR SYSTEM

46. When you walk, do you get pains in the calves of your legs?   Yes   No

47. Does your face often become red and flushed?   Yes   No

48. Do you sweat a great deal even in *cool* weather?   Yes   No

49. Do you generally feel chilly even in *warm* weather?   Yes   No

K. DIGESTIVE SYSTEM

50. After eating, do you always belch a lot?   Yes   No

51. Do you suffer from indigestion (upset stomach)?   Yes   No

52. Are you often nauseated (sick to your stomach)?   Yes   No

53. Do you often vomit (throw up)?   Yes   No

54. Did you ever vomit blood?   Yes   No

55. Do severe pains in the abdomen (belly) often double you up?   Yes   No

56. Do you suffer from constant intestinal trouble?   Yes   No

57. Are you always constipated?   Yes   No

58. Do you often get diarrhea (frequent loose bowel movements)?   Yes   No

59. Are your bowel movements ever pitch black in color?   Yes   No

60. Are your bowel movements often whitish gray in color?   Yes   No

61. Are your bowel movements usually full of mucus (slime)?   Yes   No

62. Are your bowel movements sometimes bloody?   Yes   No

63. Do you often have severe pain when you move your bowels?   Yes   No

64. Have you ever had jaundice (yellow eyes and skin)?   Yes   No

L. URINARY SYSTEM

65. Do you have to get up every night and urinate (pass water)?   Yes   No

66. During the day, do you urinate frequently?   Yes   No

67. Do you sometimes lose control of your water?   Yes   No

68. Do you often have severe burning pain when you urinate?   Yes   No

69. Is your urine always cloudy?   Yes   No

70. Have you ever passed blood when urinating?   Yes   No

M. GENITAL SYSTEM

71. Have your menstrual periods been extremely painful?   Yes   No

72. Have you always felt weak or sick with your periods?   Yes   No

73. Do you sometimes have bleeding when it is not your period?   Yes   No

74. Has a doctor ever said that you have tumors in your womb?   Yes   No

75. Has a doctor ever said that your womb is fallen or twisted?   Yes   No

76. Do you usually have a dragging down feeling in your abdomen?   Yes   No

77. Are you troubled by a constant vaginal discharge or itching?   Yes   No

78. Did you have the change of life?   Yes   No

79. Have you noticed a lump in your breasts?   Yes   No

80. Do your breasts frequently become painful?   Yes   No

GO TO NEXT PAGE

Figure 4-7. (continued).

N. MUSCULOSKELETAL SYSTEM

81. Do your muscles and joints constantly feel stiff? .... Yes   No
82. Do you usually have severe pains in your joints? .... Yes   No
83. Are your joints often painfully swollen? ...... Yes   No
84. Does moving your shoulder cause severe pain? .... Yes   No
85. Do weak or painful feet make life miserable? Yes   No
86. Do pains in the back constantly trouble you? Yes   No
87. Does coughing or sneezing cause sharp pains in your back? .... Yes   No
88. Is your back bent or twisted? .... Yes   No

O. SKIN

89. Do you have an eruption or rash on your skin? .... Yes   No
90. Has any part of your skin become red or inflamed? .... Yes   No
91. Do you often get hives (raised red spots)? Yes   No
92. Are you bothered by severe itching? .... Yes   No
93. Do you have acne (pimples on your face)? .. Yes   No
94. Do you break out in boils? .... Yes   No
95. Is any skin on your fingers red and sore? .... Yes   No
96. Do you have an itching rash between your toes (athlete's foot)? .... Yes   No
97. Has your skin become dry and rough? ...... Yes   No
98. Does the skin on your scalp constantly flake off (dandruff)? .... Yes   No
99. Do you have a scaly rash on your elbows or knees? .... Yes   No
100. Have you developed a mole or a wart on your skin? .... Yes   No
101. Do you have growths or lumps on your body? .... Yes   No
102. Do you have a cyst (swelling) at the bottom of your backbone? .... Yes   No

P. NERVOUS SYSTEM

103. Is your walking unsteady? .... Yes   No
104. Was any part of your body ever paralyzed (without power)? .... Yes   No
105. Do you have numbness or tingling in any part of your body? .... Yes   No
106. Do your hands shake constantly? .... Yes   No
107. Did you ever have spells of unconsciousness (complete blackout)? .... Yes   No

Q. PAST HISTORY

Did you ever have

108. Migraine headaches? .... Yes   No
109. Chronic sinusitis (in your head)? .... Yes   No
110. Hay fever? .... Yes   No
111. Asthma? .... Yes   No
112. A goiter (in your neck)? .... Yes   No
113. Heart trouble? .... Yes   No
114. High blood pressure? .... Yes   No
115. Peptic ulcers (stomach ulcers)? .... Yes   No
116. Liver or gallbladder disease? .... Yes   No
117. Gallstones? .... Yes   No
118. Kidney or bladder disease? .... Yes   No
119. Kidney stones? .... Yes   No
120. A hernia (rupture)? .... Yes   No
121. Hemorrhoids (piles)? .... Yes   No
122. Varicose veins (swollen veins)? .... Yes   No
123. Arthritis (rheumatism)? .... Yes   No
124. Severe anemia (thin blood)? .... Yes   No
125. Epilepsy (fits or convulsions)? .... Yes   No
126. Rheumatic fever or growing pains? .... Yes   No
127. Diabetes (sugar disease)? .... Yes   No
128. Syphilis (bad blood)? .... Yes   No
129. A tumor or cancer? .... Yes   No
130. A nervous breakdown? .... Yes   No

R. FAMILY HISTORY

Did any of your blood relatives ever have

131. Hay fever or asthma? .... Yes   No
132. Heart trouble? .... Yes   No
133. High blood pressure? .... Yes   No
134. Diabetes (sugar disease)? .... Yes   No
135. Cancer? .... Yes   No
136. Obesity (very much overweight)? .... Yes   No
137. A nervous breakdown? .... Yes   No

TURN TO NEXT PAGE

Figure 4-7. (continued).

S. HABITS

138. Are you always thirsty for water? .... Yes No

139. Do you take two or more alcoholic drinks a day? .... Yes No

140. Do you smoke more than 20 cigarettes a day? .... Yes No

141. Are you troubled with insomnia (difficulty in sleeping)? .... Yes No

142. Do you often take medicines? .... Yes No

143. Do you always feel hungry? .... Yes No

144. Are you very much *overweight*? .... Yes No

145. Have you recently *lost* much weight? .... Yes No

T. GENERAL HEALTH

146. Do you always feel weak and without energy? .... Yes No

147. Do you suffer from constant exhaustion and fatigue? .... Yes No

148. Does every little effort entirely wear you out? .... Yes No

149. Do you get up tired and worn out in the morning? .... Yes No

150. Do you have severe nervous exhaustion? .... Yes No

151. Are you continually troubled with aches and pains? .... Yes No

152. Are you frequently ill in bed? .... Yes No

153. Does illness make you constantly miserable? Yes No

154. Do you wear yourself out worrying about your health? .... Yes No

FEELING REACTIONS

U.

155. Do you always find it hard to make up your mind? .... Yes No

156. Would you like to have someone always at your side to advise you? .... Yes No

157. Do you sweat and tremble during examinations or questioning? .... Yes No

158. Do you get all nervous and shaky when approached by a superior? .... Yes No

159. Does your work fall to pieces when a superior watches you? .... Yes No

V.

160. Do you often get directions and orders wrong? .... Yes No

161. Do you constantly make mistakes? .... Yes No

162. Do you have many small accidents or injuries? .... Yes No

163. Must you do things slowly in order to do them correctly? .... Yes No

164. Has your thinking become slow? .... Yes No

165. Do you get mixed up when you have to do things quickly? .... Yes No

W.

166. Do you constantly worry? .... Yes No

167. Are you often scared? .... Yes No

168. Do frightening thoughts keep troubling you? Yes No

169. Do you often have nightmares? .... Yes No

170. Are you considered a nervous person? .... Yes No

X.

171. Do you usually feel discouraged or depressed? .... Yes No

172. Are you always unhappy and blue? .... Yes No

173. Do you constantly feel all alone and sad? .... Yes No

174. Do you often cry? .... Yes No

175. Does life look entirely hopeless? .... Yes No

176. Do you wish you were dead and away from it all? .... Yes No

Y.

177. Do people constantly criticize you without reason? .... Yes No

178. Do people often try to harm you? .... Yes No

179. Are messages being sent through the air to fool or trap you? .... Yes No

180. Do you sometimes suddenly hear voices talking to you? .... Yes No

181. Do you often feel violent fights going on inside you? .... Yes No

Z.

182. Do people often annoy or irritate you? ...... Yes No

183. Are you a touchy person? .... Yes No

184. Are you always keyed up and jittery? .... Yes No

185. Do you go to pieces if you don't constantly control yourself? .... Yes No

Figure 4-7. (continued).

(MEN)

History Number

100 DISEASES EDITION

CORNELL MEDICAL INDEX

Date

HEALTH QUESTIONNAIRE

Print
Your
Name_____

Your
Home
Address_____

How Old Are You?_____   Circle If You Are . . Single, Married, Widowed, Separated, Divorced.

Circle the Highest
Year You Reached
In School | 1 2 3 4 5 6 7 8 | | 1 2 3 4 | | 1 2 3 4 |
              Elementary School   High   College

What Is Your
Occupation?_____

Directions: This questionnaire is for **MEN ONLY.**

If you can answer **YES** to the question asked, put a circle around the (Yes)

If you have to answer **NO** to the question asked, put a circle around the (No)

Answer all questions. If you are not sure, guess.

A. HEAD

1. Do you suffer from frequent severe headaches?   Yes   No
2. Does constant pressure in your head and neck make life miserable? ....   Yes   No
3. Do you often feel dizzy and faint? ....   Yes   No

B. NECK

4. Do you usually have pain or stiffness in your neck? ....   Yes   No
5. Do you get sharp pains when you suddenly turn or bend your neck? ....   Yes   No
6. Has your neck become enlarged or swollen?   Yes   No

C. EYES

7. Do you wear glasses? ....   Yes   No
8. Is your eyesight blurred even when you wear glasses? ....   Yes   No
9. Do you suffer from constant eyestrain? ....   Yes   No
10. Is your eyesight rapidly getting worse? ....   Yes   No
11. Has your eyesight often blacked out completely? ....   Yes   No
12. Do you often have severe pains in your eyes?   Yes   No
13. Do your eyes continually blink or water? ....   Yes   No
14. Are you troubled with burning or itching of your eyes? ....   Yes   No
15. Do you sometimes see colored rings around lights? ....   Yes   No
16. Do you often see double? ....   Yes   No
17. Is one of your eyes turned in or turned out?   Yes   No

D. EARS

18. Are you hard of hearing? ....   Yes   No
19. Do you hear constant noises in your ears? ..   Yes   No
20. Do you often have severe pains in your ears?   Yes   No
21. Have you ever had a running ear? ....   Yes   No

E. MOUTH

22. Do you have cavities or decay in any of your teeth? ....   Yes   No
23. Are any of your teeth loose or broken? ....   Yes   No
24. Do you often have severe toothaches? ....   Yes   No
25. Do you have a painful swelling in your gums or jaw? ....   Yes   No

F. NOSE

26. Do you usually find it hard to breathe through your nose? ....   Yes   No
27. Is one side of your nose always stuffed up?   Yes   No
28. Do you suffer from a constantly running nose? ....   Yes   No

G. THROAT

29. Do you have to clear your throat frequently?   Yes   No
30. Do you get many attacks of severe sore throat? ....   Yes   No
31. Did a doctor say that your tonsils are enlarged? ....   Yes   No
32. Is swallowing difficult or painful? ....   Yes   No

Cornell University Medical College
1300 York Avenue, New York 21, N. Y.

OPEN TO NEXT PAGE

Figure 4-7. (continued).

H. RESPIRATORY SYSTEM

33. Do you often catch severe head colds? .... Yes No

34. Do you suffer from heavy chest colds? .... Yes No

35. When you catch a cold, do you always have to go to bed? .... Yes No

36. Are you troubled by constant coughing? ...... Yes No

37. Do you cough up large amounts of sputum (phlegm)? .... Yes No

38. Have you often coughed up blood? .... Yes No

I. CARDIAC SYSTEM

39. Does every little effort leave you short of breath? .... Yes No

40. Do you sometimes get out of breath just sitting still? .... Yes No

41. Do you sleep propped up in bed? .... Yes No

42. Are you often bothered by thumping of the heart? .... Yes No

43. Does your heart often race like mad? .... Yes No

44. Do you have pains in the heart or chest? ...... Yes No

45. Are your ankles often greatly swollen? .... Yes No

J. VASCULAR SYSTEM

46. When you walk, do you get pains in the calves of your legs? .... Yes No

47. Does your face often become red and flushed? Yes No

48. Do you sweat a great deal even in *cool* weather? .... Yes No

49. Do you generally feel chilly even in *warm* weather? .... Yes No

K. DIGESTIVE SYSTEM

50. After eating, do you always belch a lot? ...... Yes No

51. Do you suffer from indigestion (upset stomach)? .... Yes No

52. Are you often nauseated (sick to your stomach)? .... Yes No

53. Do you often vomit (throw up)? .... Yes No

54. Did you ever vomit blood? .... Yes No

55. Do severe pains in the abdomen (belly) often double you up? .... Yes No

56. Do you suffer from constant intestinal trouble? .... Yes No

57. Are you always constipated? Yes No

58. Do you often get diarrhea (frequent loose bowel movements)? Yes No

59. Are your bowel movements ever pitch black in color? Yes No

60. Are your bowel movements often whitish gray in color? Yes No

61. Are your bowel movements usually full of mucus (slime)? Yes No

62. Are your bowel movements sometimes bloody? Yes No

63. Do you often have severe pain when you move your bowels? Yes No

64. Have you ever had jaundice (yellow eyes and skin)? Yes No

L. URINARY SYSTEM

65. Do you have to get up every night and urinate (pass water)? Yes No

66. During the day, do you urinate frequently? Yes No

67. Do you sometimes lose control of your water? Yes No

68. Do you often have severe burning pain when you urinate? Yes No

69. Is your urine always cloudy? Yes No

70. Have you ever passed blood when urinating? Yes No

M. GENITAL SYSTEM

71. Do you have trouble starting your stream when urinating? Yes No

72. Is your stream very weak? Yes No

73. Do you have trouble emptying your bladder? Yes No

74. Did a doctor say that you have prostate trouble? Yes No

75. Has your prostate been removed? Yes No

76. Did you ever have anything seriously wrong with your genitals (privates)? Yes No

77. Did you ever have treatment for your genitals? Yes No

78. Do you have a swelling in or near your genitals? Yes No

79. Is there a lump on your testicles (balls)? Yes No

80. Are your testicles often painful or sore? Yes No

GO TO NEXT PAGE

Figure 4-7. (continued).

N. MUSCULOSKELETAL SYSTEM

81. Do your muscles and joints constantly feel stiff? .... Yes   No

82. Do you usually have severe pains in your joints? .... Yes   No

83. Are your joints often painfully swollen? ...... Yes   No

84. Does moving your shoulder cause severe pain? .... Yes   No

85. Do weak or painful feet make life miserable? Yes   No

86. Do pains in the back constantly trouble you? Yes   No

87. Does coughing or sneezing cause sharp pains in your back? .... Yes   No

88. Is your back bent or twisted? .... Yes   No

O. SKIN

89. Do you have an eruption or rash on your skin? .... Yes   No

90. Has any part of your skin become red or inflamed? .... Yes   No

91. Do you often get hives (raised red spots)? Yes   No

92. Are you bothered by severe itching? .... Yes   No

93. Do you have acne (pimples on your face)? .. Yes   No

94. Do you break out in boils? .... Yes   No

95. Is any skin on your fingers red and sore? .... Yes   No

96. Do you have an itching rash between your toes (athlete's foot)? .... Yes   No

97. Has your skin become dry and rough? .... Yes   No

98. Does the skin on your scalp constantly flake off (dandruff)? .... Yes   No

99. Do you have a scaly rash on your elbows or knees? .... Yes   No

100. Have you developed a mole or a wart on your skin? .... Yes   No

101. Do you have growths or lumps on your body? .... Yes   No

102. Do you have a cyst (swelling) at the bottom of your backbone? .... Yes   No

P. NERVOUS SYSTEM

103. Is your walking unsteady? .... Yes   No

104. Was any part of your body ever paralyzed (without power)? .... Yes   No

105. Do you have numbness or tingling in any part of your body? .... Yes   No

106. Do your hands shake constantly? .... Yes   No

107. Did you ever have spells of unconsciousness (complete blackout)? .... Yes   No

Q. PAST HISTORY

Did you ever have

108. Migraine headaches? .... Yes   No

109. Chronic sinusitis (in your head)? .... Yes   No

110. Hay fever? .... Yes   No

111. Asthma? .... Yes   No

112. A goiter (in your neck)? .... Yes   No

113. Heart trouble? .... Yes   No

114. High blood pressure? .... Yes   No

115. Peptic ulcers (stomach ulcers)? .... Yes   No

116. Liver or gallbladder disease? .... Yes   No

117. Gallstones? .... Yes   No

118. Kidney or bladder disease? .... Yes   No

119. Kidney stones? .... Yes   No

120. A hernia (rupture)? .... Yes   No

121. Hemorrhoids (piles)? .... Yes   No

122. Varicose veins (swollen veins)? .... Yes   No

123. Arthritis (rheumatism)? .... Yes   No

124. Severe anemia (thin blood)? .... Yes   No

125. Epilepsy (fits or convulsions)? .... Yes   No

126. Rheumatic fever or growing pains? .... Yes   No

127. Diabetes (sugar disease)? .... Yes   No

128. Syphilis (bad blood)? .... Yes   No

129. A tumor or cancer? .... Yes   No

130. A nervous breakdown? .... Yes   No

R. FAMILY HISTORY

Did any of your blood relatives ever have

131. Hay fever or asthma? .... Yes   No

132. Heart trouble? .... Yes   No

133. High blood pressure? .... Yes   No

134. Diabetes (sugar disease)? .... Yes   No

135. Cancer? .... Yes   No

136. Obesity (very much overweight)? .... Yes   No

137. A nervous breakdown? .... Yes   No

TURN TO NEXT PAGE

Figure 4-7. (continued).

S. HABITS

138. Are you always thirsty for water? .... Yes   No

139. Do you take two or more alcoholic drinks a day? .... Yes   No

140. Do you smoke more than 20 cigarettes a day? .... Yes   No

141. Are you troubled with insomnia (difficulty in sleeping)? .... Yes   No

142. Do you often take medicines? .... Yes   No

143. Do you always feel hungry? .... Yes   No

144. Are you very much *overweight*? .... Yes   No

145. Have you recently *lost* much weight? ...... Yes   No

T. GENERAL HEALTH

146. Do you always feel weak and without energy? .... Yes   No

147. Do you suffer from constant exhaustion and fatigue? .... Yes   No

148. Does every little effort entirely wear you out? .... Yes   No

149. Do you get up tired and worn out in the morning? .... Yes   No

150. Do you have severe nervous exhaustion?   Yes   No

151. Are you continually troubled with aches and pains? .... Yes   No

152. Are you frequently ill in bed?   Yes   No

153. Does illness make you constantly miserable?   Yes   No

154. Do you wear yourself out worrying about your health? .... Yes   No

FEELING REACTIONS
U.

155. Do you always find it hard to make up your mind? .... Yes   No

156. Would you like to have someone always at your side to advise you? .... Yes   No

157. Do you sweat and tremble during examinations or questioning? .... Yes   No

158. Do you get all nervous and shaky when approached by a superior? .... Yes   No

159. Does your work fall to pieces when a superior watches you? .... Yes   No

V.

160. Do you often get directions and orders wrong? .... Yes   No

161. Do you constantly make mistakes? .... Yes   No

162. Do you have many small accidents or injuries? .... Yes   No

163. Must you do things slowly in order to do them correctly? .... Yes   No

164. Has your thinking become slow? .... Yes   No

165. Do you get mixed up when you have to do things quickly? .... Yes   No

W.

166. Do you constantly worry? .... Yes   No

167. Are you often scared? .... Yes   No

168. Do frightening thoughts keep troubling you?   Yes   No

169. Do you often have nightmares? .... Yes   No

170. Are you considered a nervous person?   Yes   No

X.

171. Do you usually feel discouraged or depressed? .... Yes   No

172. Are you always unhappy and blue? ...... Yes   No

173. Do you constantly feel all alone and sad?   Yes   No

174. Do you often cry? .... Yes   No

175. Does life look entirely hopeless? .... Yes   No

176. Do you wish you were dead and away from it all? .... Yes   No

Y.

177. Do people constantly criticize you without reason? .... Yes   No

178. Do people often try to harm you? ...... Yes   No

179. Are messages being sent through the air to fool or trap you? .... Yes   No

180. Do you sometimes suddenly hear voices talking to you? .... Yes   No

181. Do you often feel violent fights going on inside you? .... Yes   No

Z.

182. Do people often annoy or irritate you? ...... Yes   No

183. Are you a touchy person? .... Yes   No

184. Are you always keyed up and jittery? ...... Yes   No

185. Do you go to pieces if you don't constantly control yourself? .... Yes   No

Figure 4-7. (continued).

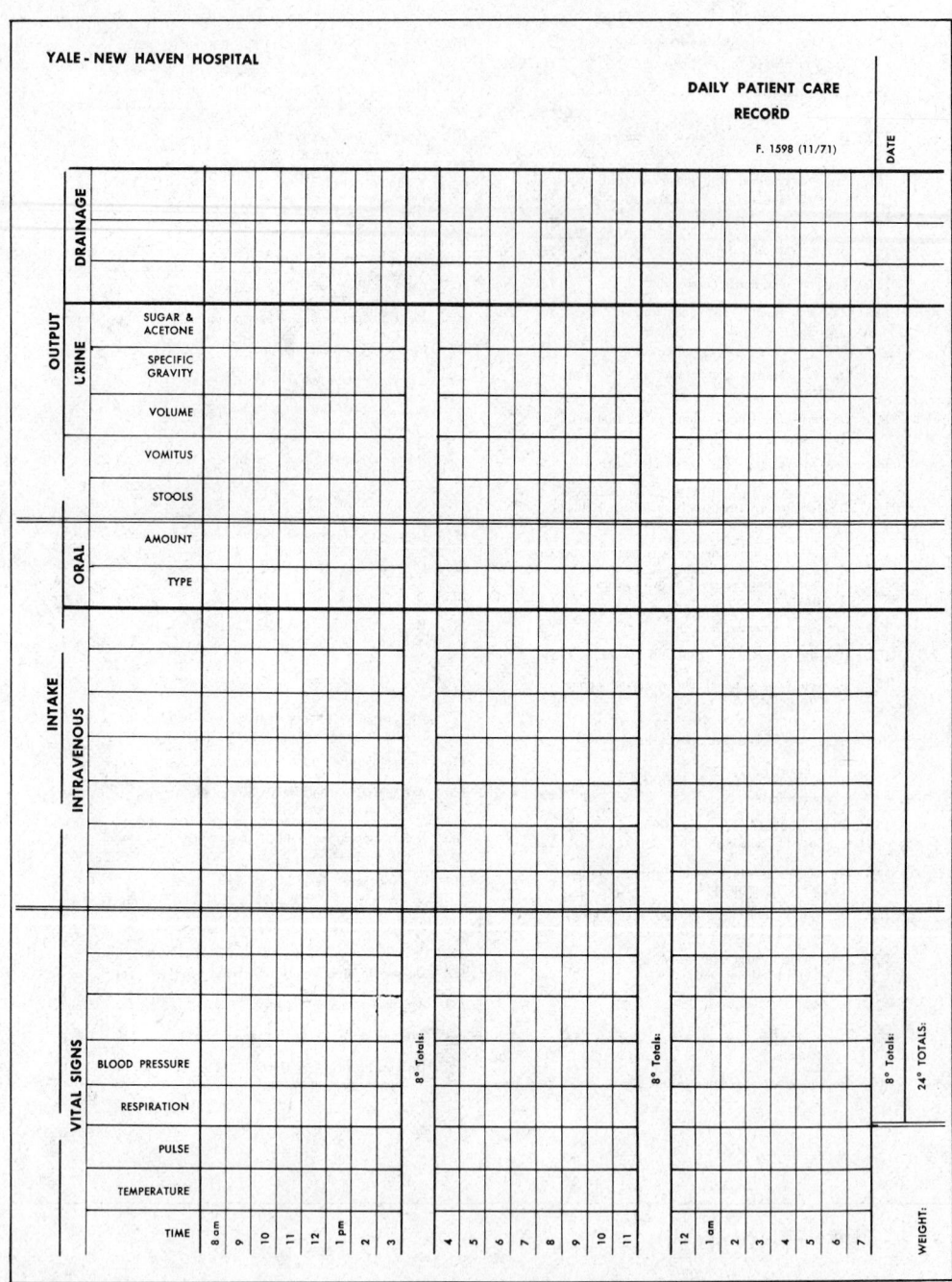

Figure 4-8. An example of a flow sheet used for recording vital signs and intake and output. (Courtesy of Yale–New Haven Hospital, New Haven, Conn.)

and therapy.[35] Weed believes that, in the future, physicians and other health professionals will assume an integrated and easily audited role in solving the patient's problems, and each will avoid the possibility of dealing with one problem isolated from the other problems.[36] Figure 4-4F is an example of a patient's progress note written by a nurse. Progress note forms may be used by both physician and nurse; actually, by all professional caretakers. The preoperative teaching program is carefully integrated with the plans for physical preparation.

In both the "source-oriented" and "problem-oriented" patient records, two types of progress notes are used. One shows several variables occurring at a given time. These are called flow sheets. The most common examples are the records of vital signs or medications (see Fig. 4-8). Two different flow sheets are described by Mary Woody and Mary Mallison [37] that show the value of constructing a flow sheet appropriate for the unit in which it is to be used. The time intervals on flow sheets may be minutes or months and may show changes in physiologic, behavioral, or social phenomenon. Flow sheets are used in place of narrative notes when it is essential to follow several variables at once in order to understand and predict a patient's progress.[38]

The other type of progress note is called a narrative note. This is a factual account of an incident or series of happenings characterized by a tracing of causes and effects and by an attempt to estimate, evaluate, and interpret the patient's signs, symptoms, diagnosis, and response to treatment. Figure 4-9 shows a narrative note written for a source-oriented record. The narrative note in the problem-oriented record is written somewhat differently. The number and the title of the problem are written first, and the note is divided into four parts. The first part is titled "subjective information" or, more commonly, "subjective." The subjective information includes how the patient describes his or her symptoms, feelings, and concerns about the problem. When the patient is an infant or child or for any reason cannot give an account of his or her problem, recollections of a parent or other responsible person make up the subjective information. The subjective information also includes questions asked by the professional worker that help him or her understand the nature of the problem. Depending on the problem, questions may be asked about the functions of digestion, elimination, vision and hearing, mental status, and sexual activity. In the case of infants and children, questions are asked about growth and development.

The second section of the narrative note in the problem-oriented medical record is called "objective information" and consists of measurements related to the problem. Examples of objective information are the findings from the physical examination, developmental examination (for infant or child), and the mental status examination. Results of laboratory tests and radiographic examinations, description of living conditions as observed by the professional worker (such as the public health nurse in the home), or financial statements gotten during an interview are also objective information, depending on the nature of the problem identified.

The third section of the narrative note is the assessment or what the professional worker thinks about the problem. This is usually a short statement that is clearly based on or is logically derived from the subjective or objective data. The assessment or "impression" may be the diagnosis, a statement that the patient is or is not improving, the medication is having an appropriate or inappropriate effect, or the pathophysiology or psychodynamics of the problem is more clearly understood or remains obscure. Woody and Mallison [39] think the interpretation of the observations or assessment portion of the narrative note is the most difficult aspect of recording for nurses. Actually, assessment is the intellectual processing of an event and is a difficult task for everyone. In some cases, the assessment is that the patient data are insufficient to permit a conclusion or interpretation or that the recorder does not know the conclusion to be drawn from the data. To write "do not know" is acceptable if true.

The final section of the narrative note for the problem-oriented record is the plans. These are directives for the patient, a parent, another relative or friend, or another professional worker to carry out. They may be descriptions of how more information about the patient's problem will be gotten or descriptions of teaching programs for the patient and family. The plans state as exactly as possible the future self or parental care, medical or surgical therapy, nursing care, and social or psychologic intervention required to solve the problem.

The narrative note in the problem-oriented medical record is written only when progress, or lack of progress, has occurred and not at times set by an arbitrary time schedule, such as once in 8 hours, or once a day. Figure 4-4F shows a narrative note written for a problem-oriented record.

When writing a narrative note for either the source- or problem-oriented patient record,

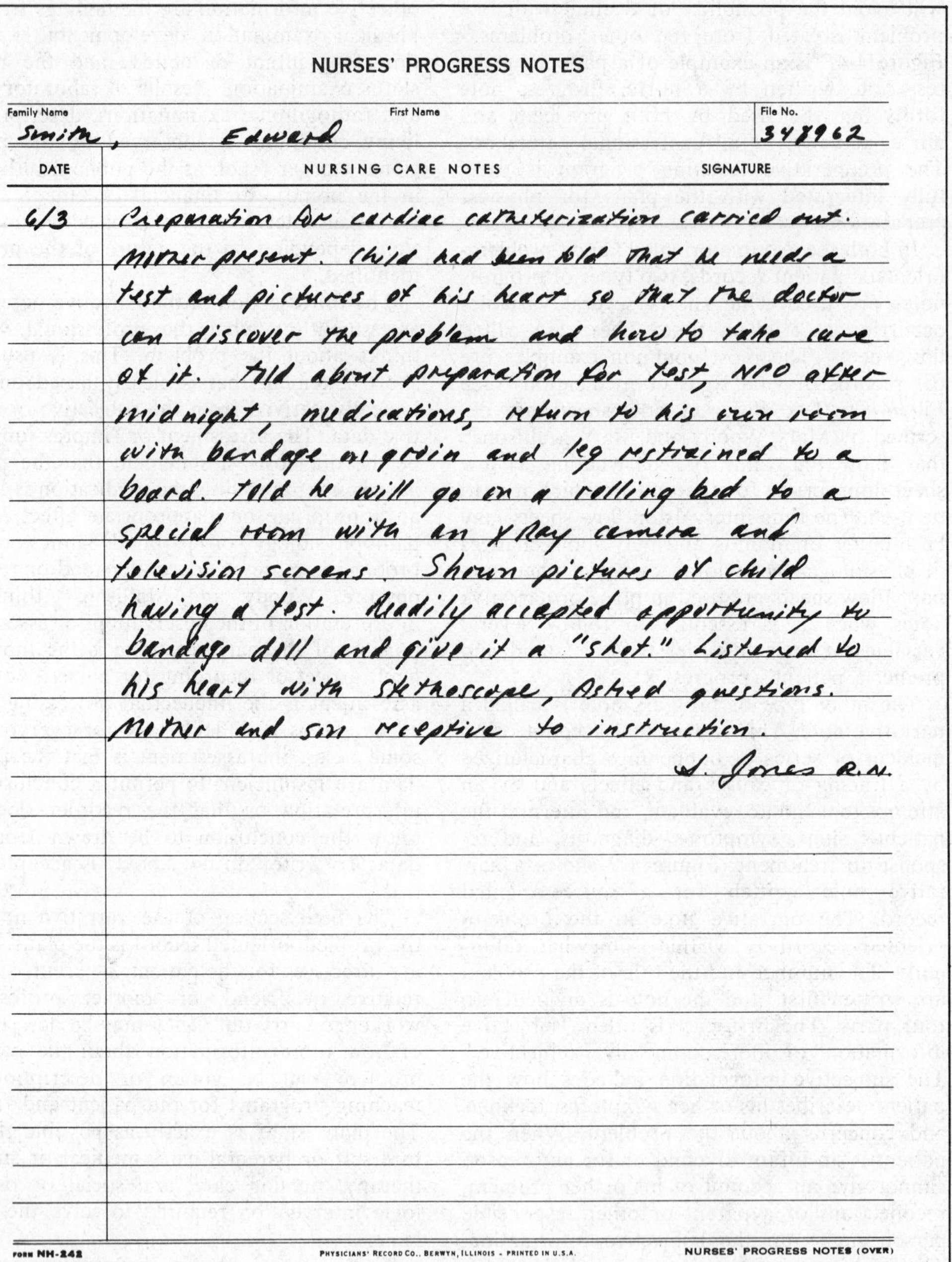

NURSES' PROGRESS NOTES

Family Name	First Name	File No.
Smith,	Edward	348962

DATE	NURSING CARE NOTES	SIGNATURE

6/3 Preparation for cardiac catheterization carried out. Mother present. Child had been told that he needs a test and pictures of his heart so that the doctor can discover the problem and how to take care of it. Told about preparation for test, NPO after midnight, medications, return to his own room with bandage on groin and leg restrained to a board. Told he will go on a rolling bed to a special room with an xray camera and television screens. Shown pictures of child having a test. Readily accepted opportunity to bandage doll and give it a "shot." Listened to his heart with stethoscope. Asked questions. Mother and son receptive to instruction.

S. Jones R.N.

FORM NH-242   PHYSICIANS' RECORD CO., BERWYN, ILLINOIS · PRINTED IN U.S.A.   NURSES' PROGRESS NOTES (OVER)

Figure 4-9. A narrative note written for a source-oriented record. (Courtesy of Physician's Record Co., Berwyn, Ill.)

effort must be made by the nurse and other professional workers to record significant information and to avoid producing a bulky report containing irrelevant material. For example, a recording may be that the patient, a man, is talking incoherently and does not answer questions. This statement describes the behavior precisely, whereas the statement "patient is irrational" does not describe his behavior so that it is understood by everyone. A note stating that the patient, a woman, slept from 11:00 to 1:00 and from 3:30 to 5:30 describes actual events. "The patient slept badly" is a value judgment by the recorder and not an event experienced by her. An infant boy may be described as lying on his right ear, groaning from time to time and putting his hand to his ear. The interpretation that the infant may be suffering from pain in the ear is then a logical conclusion, and any other professional reading this record will understand how the conclusion was reached.

Common flaws in narrative notes are that comments tend to be confined to physical manifestations and that abnormalities and pathologic signs are recorded, whereas moods, attitudes, favorable signs, and normal behavior are neglected.

A discharge summary is also part of the patient's record, whether it is "source" or "problem" oriented. All professional workers who cared for the patient contribute to it. The historical, physical, behavioral, social, and laboratory information necessary to the future analysis and management of a problem is included. Goals of the patient's care are developed with the patient and his or her family. A teaching program may be outlined or the amount and type of information given the patient and the family recorded. The discharge summary can be an excellent way to demonstrate how well the patient, family, and health workers have worked together and which areas of care each will be responsible for in the future.

The first part of this chapter is a discussion of what and how to observe. The patient's progress notes constitute a written report of the most significant of these observations.

The nurse, like the physician, should develop a simple, direct, and lucid style. A technical vocabulary is necessary, but the use of medical terms can be greatly overdone. Abbreviations and hospital slang are to be avoided. Symbols are convenient and proper in certain cases but are likely to be used indiscriminately. Only standard abbreviations and symbols, such as those given by Morris Fishbein,[40] should be used. In computerized records, abbreviations are freely employed but it is to be hoped that these will be nationally,

or internationally, standardized to facilitate universal interpretation of records and collection and publication of health statistics.

No mechanical aspects of record keeping, such as constructing forms, should be assigned to highly trained health personnel that are in short supply. A constant effort should be made to eliminate wasted time. The use of machine-made rather than handmade forms, rubber stamps for uniform entries, color coding to make it easy to find parts of a record, and a good system of filing are helpful.

Adequate space in a quiet place for recording should be provided. Effective recording requires concentration as well as other mental qualities. Above all else the record should be accurate; therefore, keen powers of observation and complete honesty are prime requisites in all those who contribute to this document.

Accuracy in Medical Records. It is so essential that medical records be exact and correct that each person who has a part in making them signs any notations he or she makes, using the full name rather than initials only. Insofar as possible, the record should consist of facts rather than opinions. The physician, the nurse, and others should report what they see, hear, smell, or feel, rather than what they deduce, although opinions cannot be avoided in some cases. The contributor to a patient's record accepts legal responsibility for what he or she has written and for the reports of persons whom he or she has delegated to complete certain parts of the record.

Data from the records of patients are compared with standards of care expected of the professional staff. This process is called the "audit" and is carried out with the assistance of the director of medical records.[41] The quality of care received by the patient is reflected in the medical record. As the notations are evaluated, techniques of care that were used and whether or not they were helpful are discussed. The audit protects the patient, it protects the institution from liability or legal action, and it educates those who make the audit. All levels of nursing personnel benefit from studying written records by nurses of positive approaches to patient care, and such study helps them learn to record observations more meaningfully.[42] The evaluation of health care by "peer review" is discussed in Chapters 1 and 19.

Uses of the Record. It has been pointed out that a number of professional workers are usually coordinating their various services. It is essential that each one of them knows what the others plan to do, are doing, and have done for the patient. The medical record is one means of making such information available to all concerned. *In any health organization all pro-*

fessional workers should have access to the record. The record is filed so that during any subsequent illness members of the same institution, other institutions, or private physicians may refer to the record or get a copy of the significant parts. Without the record, effective treatment and nursing care are nearly impossible, for few have memories sufficiently accurate for matters of this kind; nor would it be practicable to try to get verbal information about patients from many persons concerned with their care. Mention has been made of the desirability of giving patients copies of their records.

Items of information about the patient's age and occupation, the date of his or her admission and discharge or death, the nature of the medical treatment, and the space he or she occupied are the bases for computing charges for medical care and preparing annual reports for the work of the institution. While some of these data are reported elsewhere than in the medical record, the patient's chart is an indispensable item in the administration of a health service. Data taken from patients' records provide a base on which local, state, national, and international health services are planned.

A large part of the education of physicians and other medical personnel is based on a study of patients' records. They are used in all case conferences and clinics. Students of medicine, nursing, dietetics, social work, and other health specialties would be immeasurably less well prepared if during their period of study they were denied the use of medical records. They study not only the history of the patients under their observation but also the records of those who have been discharged or those who have died. All *medical research* would be sadly hampered, and many kinds of research would be impossible without such sources of data.

The Record as an Aid in Legal Justice. Cases occur in which the patient, his or her family, the medical worker, or the administrative staff of the institution believe that they have received unfair treatment. A complaint may be brought against the hospital administration, or the physician or nurse may be charged with malpractice. Such cases are often settled out of court, but many of them are brought to trial. In either case, the medical record is usually referred to, and if made by competent and conscientious workers, it can be a means of arriving at a fair judgment. Emanuel and Jonathan Hayt describe in detail the admissibility of hospital records as evidence in court:

The legislatures of many states have met the problem of using hospital records as evidence by enacting statutes which enable business entries and records of all kinds, made in the regular course of business, to be used in evidence. Hospital records which relate to diagnosis, prognosis or treatment or which are otherwise helpful in understanding of the medical aspects of the hospitalization are admissible in evidence.*

The doctrine of "privileged communication" is a rule that may prevent the use of the patient's record or bar the testimony of the physician or nurse.[43] In states that have a confidential communication statute the physician, and in some states the nurse, is not required by law to divulge the personal details of the patient's life which he or she shared with in confidence, just as a wife is freed from obligation to testify against her husband, or a man against himself. In such states the patient's record cannot be subpoenaed into court; but if the subpoena is accepted by the authorities of the institution, they are then obliged to send a representative of the staff to court with the record. The person selected to do this should be someone who can interpret the record effectively. Some state laws require public institutions to submit patients' records, or certified copies, for legal purposes, but exempt private institutions from this regulation.

In certain cases, such as claims for compensation, patients may ask to have their medical history used as evidence. (See Fig. 4-10*A-B* for forms permitting review of medical records and release of medical information.) Leo P. Dolan[44] makes the point that the patient should read his or her record before he or she makes this request, because there may be facts in the history, of which the patient is unaware, that are detrimental to the patient's interests.

Generally speaking, medical records are used legally to refresh the memory of the physician or nurse in testifying, but the data contained therein are not considered conclusive proof. It seems to be a common practice to call on living witnesses to give verbal testimony rather than to use written statements they have made as evidence. In case the observations of dead nurses or physicians are needed, the medical record is more likely to be used. A qualified person must identify the signatures of the deceased.

It is repeatedly stated that insurance companies have no legal right to demand access to medical records. On a written request from the patient, the hospital may give the company certain information from the record. If the case is taken to court, the laws of the par-

* Hayt, Emanuel, and Hayt, Jonathan: *Legal Aspects of Medical Records.* Physicians' Record Co., Berwyn, Ill., 1964, p. 165.

AUTHORIZATION FOR REVIEW OF MEDICAL RECORDS

Hospital No._____

To_____Hospital   _____19_____

_____

You are hereby authorized to allow_____

to review and make a copy of the   ☐ complete record of my hospitalization

☐ record of my hospitalization from_____19_____ to_____19_____

Signed_____
(PATIENT)

Signed_____
(NEAREST OF KIN)

Signed_____
(ATTENDING PHYSICIAN)   _____
(RELATIONSHIP)

*Authorization must be signed by the patient, or by the nearest relative in the case of a minor;
or when patient is physically or mentally incompetent, and also by the attending physician.*

FORM C-404   PHYSICIANS' RECORD CO., BERWYN, ILLINOIS   PRINTED IN U.S.A.

AUTHORIZATION FOR RELEASE OF INFORMATION

To_____ Hospital Number_____
(NAME OF HOSPITAL)

You are hereby authorized to furnish such professional information, in accordance with the policy of your hospital, as may be

necessary for the completion of my hospitalization claims by_____
(NAME OF THIRD PARTY)

_____ from the medical records compiled during my hospitalization
(NAME OF THIRD PARTY)

from_____19_____to_____19_____ and are

hereby released from all legal liability that may arise from the release of the information requested.

Date _____   Signed_____
(PATIENT OR NEAREST OF KIN)

Signed_____   _____
(PARTY INSPECTING RECORD)   (RELATIONSHIP IF SIGNED BY OTHER THAN PATIENT)

Date of inspection of record_____19_____   Signed_____
(ATTENDING PHYSICIAN)

*Authorization must be signed by the patient, or by the nearest relative in
the case of a minor or when patient is physically or mentally incompetent.*

FORM C-409   PHYSICIANS' RECORD CO., BERWYN, ILLINOIS   PRINTED IN U.S.A.

Figure 4-10. Patients give permission to another professional person or health care
agency to review, copy, or release information from their medical records.
(Courtesy of Physician's Record Co., Berwyn, Ill.)

ticular state involved regulate the decision as to the use made of the record. The executors of an estate may be allowed to use the medical record to the extent that is necessary in their service to the patient and his or her legatees.

Hospital officers and medical workers should get legal advice before allowing anyone, other than a professional person in attendance upon the patient, to have access to the chart. While students and research workers in the medical field are allowed to use such records, they are bound by a strict ethical code to hold all such information in confidence. Some institutions codify medical records for filing purposes, removing the names entirely so that they may be used in research without identification of individuals.

Use Influences Nature of Record. The use to which the medical record is put should influence the way data are collected and recorded. For example, in states that make medical histories "admissible evidence in legal cases," physicians may withhold certain confidences of the patient that they would not hesitate to make a part of the record in a state where such data are inviolate. As shown by Huffman,[45] the use to which the medical record is put is determined by custom, statute, and the particular situation.

Care of Medical Records. Since the patient's chart is unquestionably a valuable document, it should be made on paper of good quality and protected from soiling, tearing, and blurring. Hinged aluminum covers are commonly used in hospitals. Chart backs that leave the front page exposed also are used. They may be kept in a special rack on wheels or hung in a chart room near the nurse's station and transferred to a conveyor for clinics and "rounds." Parts of the patient's record may be kept with him or her in a hospital or may be left permanently in the patient's possession. An example of the latter is the record of immunizations that a mother keeps for her child. Some hospitals give to the mother at the birth of an infant a health record in book form that she makes for the child until he or she is old enough to keep a life health record.

In the hospital, selected record forms may be kept at the bedside, dependent on several factors, such as convenience for the person who is recording and the involvement of the patient in his or her care. An example of the former is the flow sheet of physiologic data for a patient in a critical care unit. This is kept near the patient so that the person who measures and records these data does not have to leave the bedside in the course of caring for someone so seriously ill. An example of the latter is the parent who is staying with her child in the hospital (rooming-in) and who keeps the record of food and fluid consumed and amount and type of elimination. While the patient may ultimately be told everything that the record contains, for his or her own sake the time for telling certain things should be wisely chosen. In the case of responsible adults, they are free to withhold any information about their illness from their family or friends, and the institution has no right to make their charts accessible without the patient's permission.

Lucie Young Kelly, writing about changes in common and statutory law that give patients their legal right to know (that has always been their moral right), discusses differing positions in health agencies on the use of the medical record. The Given Health Care Center in Burlington, Vt., makes patients part of the team, their records are available to them, and they "share" the record with health providers. Kelly says: "Most physicians and health administrators . . . greet this record-sharing with open hostility," but she thinks

The time in which there is a choice in the matter of sharing the record may be ending. While it is legally recognized that the patient's record is the property of the hospital or physician (in his office), the information that the record contains is not similarly protected. Currently, only nine states allow patients access to their records, either through the patient's attorney (California, Illinois, and Utah) or directly (Massachusetts, Wisconsin, New Jersey, Louisiana, Mississippi and Connecticut).

. . .

A sign of the future may be seen in federal legislation passed at the end of 1974: new amendments strengthening the 1967 Freedom of Information (FIA) Act and the Privacy Act of 1974 (PL 93-579). The FIA was passed as a result of pressure for more openness in government, and the general purpose was to give the public access to files maintained by the executive branch of the government.*

It is possible that in the future records may be designed and kept with a view to patient understanding (or to health education) and that a copy will be given the person. In this age of mobility, of frequent change of employment, it is highly desirable that a health record go with the patient from one locality to another.

Each hospital is responsible for developing patient record forms to fit its needs. Neither the American Hospital Association nor the Joint Commission on Accreditation of Hospi-

---

* Kelly, Lucie Young: "The Patient's Right to Know," *Nurs. Outlook,* **24**:26, (Jan.) 1976.

tals recommends specific forms.[46] As has been noted, health care agencies and hospitals usually have a committee responsible for designing patient record forms, reviewing proposed forms, and revising or discontinuing forms no longer needed.

It is usual to find a registered record administrator in charge of a department devoted to the care of medical records. Records are sometimes microfilmed after 10 years or more to reduce storage space.[47] Briefs or abstracts also may be substituted for very old medical histories.[48] Records are usually filed by the number given the patient on admission to the hospital or clinic. An index system should enable the record administrator to find the corresponding name and the diagnosis of the patient.

In some record departments there are desks for those who want to use the record. In some cases it is permissible to sign for the record and use it in other parts of the institution, but individuals are not allowed to take the record away from the hospital or clinic except under very unusual circumstances, as, for example, on an order from a court of law.

Since the welfare of a patient, even life itself, may depend on the accessibility of a medical record, it is easy to see why such stringent regulations are made to protect it from destruction, loss, and injudicious handling.

Automated data-processing techniques, employing complex computer programs and expensive equipment, are being developed for the storage and retrieval of patients' records.[49] This raises certain legal questions about security and reliability of the medical record.[50] Some states require a written record and authentication by signature of the responsible professional persons who wrote the record. Questions on the requirements that records must be written and signed will probably be resolved soon on a state-by-state basis.[51,52]

In the view of many, the most significant problem related to the development of automated patient record systems is that of privacy.[53] The installation of an automated system has the potential of making confidential records more readily available to a greater number of persons. Eric W. Springer[54] reviews ways in which the invasion of privacy can occur when automated patient records are used. At this time it is crucial for all health professionals to increase their understanding of the way in which health records of the future will be compiled and maintained. Only in this way will these methods achieve their highest potential for the improvement of health care, and, at the same time, assure the authenticity of the record and the privacy of the individual.

REFERENCES

1. Kaplan, Abraham: *The Conduct of Inquiry.* Chandler Publishing Co., San Francisco, 1964, p. 126.
2. Murchison, Irene A., and Nichols, Thomas S.: *Legal Foundations of Nursing Practice.* Macmillan Publishing Co., New York, 1970, p. 82.
3. Nightingale, Florence: *Notes on Nursing: What It Is, and What It Is Not* (facsimile of 1859 ed.). J. B. Lippincott Co., Philadelphia, 1946.
4. *Nursing Studies Index, Vol. I (1900–1929).* Prepared by Yale University School of Nursing Index Staff under the direction of Virginia Henderson. J. B. Lippincott Co., Philadelphia, 1972.
5. Cooper, Signe S.: "Why Continuing Education in Nursing," *Cardiovasc. Nurs.,* **9:**13, (May–June) 1973.
6. Judge, R. D., and Zuidema, G. D. (eds.): *Physical Diagnosis: A Physiologic Approach to the Clinical Examination,* 2nd ed. Little, Brown & Co., Boston, 1968.
7. Scalzi, Cynthia: "Nursing Management of Behavioral Responses Following an Acute Myocardial Infarction," *Heart Lung,* **2:**62, (Jan.–Feb.) 1973.
8. Senn, Milton J., and Solnit, Albert J.: *Problems in Child Behavior and Development.* Lea & Febiger, Philadelphia, 1968, p. 65.
9. Griffith, George: "Sexuality and the Cardiac Patient," *Heart Lung,* **2:**70, (Jan.–Feb.) 1973.
10. Judge, R. D., and Zuidema, G. D. (eds.): *op. cit.,* p. 81.
11. Wintrobe, Maxwell M., et al. (eds.): *Harrison's Principles of Internal Medicine,* 6th ed. McGraw-Hill Book Co., New York, 1970, p. 185.
12. *Ibid.,* p. 187.
13. *Ibid.,* p. 187.
14. Judge, R. D., and Zuidema, G. D. (eds.): *op. cit.,* p. 131.
15. Rubin, Reva: "Food and Feeding, A Matrix of Relationships," *Nurs. Forum,* **6:**195, (No. 2) 1967.
16. *Ibid.*
17. MacBryde, Cyril M., and Blacklow, Robert S. (eds.): *Signs and Symptoms: Applied Pathologic Physiology and Clinical Interpretation,* 5th ed. J. B. Lippincott Co., Philadelphia, 1970, p. 864.
18. *Ibid.,* p. 874.
19. *Ibid.,* p. 451.
20. *Ibid.,* p. 454.
21. Korones, Sheldon B., et al.: *High Risk Newborn Infants: The Basis for Intensive Nursing Care.* C. V. Mosby Co., St. Louis, 1972, p. 61.
22. *Ibid.,* p. 61.
23. *Accreditation Manual for Hospitals, 1970.* Hospital Accreditation Program, Joint Commission on the Accreditation of Hospitals, Chicago, p. 93.
24. Feinstein, A. R.: "The Problems of the 'Prob-

lem Oriented Medical Record,' " *Ann. Intern. Med.,* **78**:751, 1973.

25. Huffman, Edna K.: *Medical Record Management,* 6th ed. Physicians' Record Co., Berwyn, Ill., 1972, p. 175.

26. *Ibid.,* p. 126.

27. Weed, Lawrence L.: *Medical Records, Medical Education, and Patient Care.* Press of Case-Western Reserve University, Cleveland (distributed by Year Book Medical Publishers, Chicago), 1971, p. 54.

28. *Ibid.,* p. 16.

29. *Ibid.,* p. 25.

30. *Ibid.,* p. 25.

31. Aronson, Jesse B.: "The Family Record in the Red Hook-Gowanus Health Center District," *Am. J. Public Health,* **40**:1230, (Oct.) 1950.

32. Feinstein, A. R.: *op. cit.*

33. Weed, Lawrence L.: *op. cit.,* p. 109.

34. *Ibid.,* p. 109.

35. *Ibid.,* p. 54.

36. *Ibid.,* p. 54.

37. Woody, Mary, and Mallison, Mary: "The Problem Oriented System for Patient Centered Care," *Am. J. Nurs.,* **73**:1168, (July) 1973.

38. *Ibid.*

39. *Ibid.*

40. Fishbein, Morris: *Medical Writing: The Technique and the Art,* 4th ed. Charles C Thomas, Publisher, Springfield, Ill., 1972, p. 46.

41. Huffman, Edna K.: *op. cit.,* p. 504.

42. Dunn, Helen W., and Morgan, Elizabeth M.: *The Nursing Audit.* (League Exchange No. 84.) National League for Nursing, Department of Hospital Nursing, New York, 1968.

43. Hayt, Emanuel, and Hayt, Jonathan: *Legal Aspects of Medical Records.* Physicians' Record Co., Berwyn, Ill., 1964, p. 173.

44. Dolan, Leo P.: "The Patient's Record—A Sacred Document," *Hospitals,* **11**:68, (June) 1937.

45. Huffman, Edna K.: *op. cit.,* p. 121.

46. *Ibid.,* p. 51.

47. *Ibid.,* p. 201.

48. Hayt, Emanuel, and Hayt, Jonathan: *op. cit.,* p. 50.

49. Huffman, Edna K.: *op. cit.,* pp. 126, 414.

50. *Ibid.,* pp. 414, 418.

51. *Ibid.*

52. Springer, Eric W.: *Automated Medical Records and the Law.* The Health Center, Aspen Systems Corporation, Pittsburgh, 1971, p. 119.

53. *Ibid.,* p. 55.

54. *Ibid.,* p. 69.

Additional Suggested Reading

Anderson, John, and Forsythe, John M. (eds.): *Information Processing of Medical Records.* Proceedings of the International Federation for Information Processing TC4 Working Conference on Information Processing of Medical Records, Lyons, France, April 1970. North Holland Publishing Co., London and Amsterdam, 1970.

Carlson, Carolyn (ed.): *Behavioral Concepts and Nursing Intervention.* J. B. Lippincott Co., Philadelphia, 1970.

Chinn, Peggy L.: *Child Health Maintenance: Concepts in Family Centered Care.* C. V. Mosby Co., St. Louis, 1974.

———, and Leitch, Cynthia J.: *Child Health Maintenance: A Guide to Clinical Assessment.* C. V. Mosby Co., St. Louis, 1974.

Hurst, J. Willis, and Walker, H. Kenneth (eds.): *The Problem-Oriented System.* Medcom Press, New York, 1972.

Illingworth, R. S.: *Common Symptoms of Disease in Children,* 5th ed. Blackwell Scientific Publications, Oxford, 1975.

Little, Dolores, and Carnevali, Doris: *Nursing Care Planning.* J. B. Lippincott Co., Philadelphia, 1969.

Masters, William H., and Johnson, Virginia E.: *Human Sexual Response.* Little, Brown & Co., Boston, 1966.

Morgan, William L., Jr., and Engel, George L.: *The Clinical Approach to the Patient.* W. B. Saunders Co., Philadelphia, 1969.

Sadler, Alfred, et al.: *The Physician's Assistant —Today and Tomorrow.* Yale University Press, New Haven, Conn., 1972.

Schultz, Jan, et al.: "An Initial Operational Problem-Oriented Medical Record System—For Storage, Manipulation and Retrieval of Medical Data," in American Federation of Information Processing Societies Conference Proceedings, Vol. 38. AFIPS Press, Montvale, N.J., 1971.

Wu, Ruth: *Behavior and Illness.* Prentice-Hall, Englewood Cliffs, N.J., 1973.

Roberta O'Grady
Virginia Henderson

CHAPTER 5

The Health Examination

1. THE ART AND SCIENCE OF HEALTH ASSESSMENT

Health Assessment Is Everybody's Business. Universal greetings such as "How are you?" and "How do you do?" and farewells such as "Keep well" suggest a universal concern for the health of others which is expressed daily, even hourly. Those unduly preoccupied with their own health are called hypochondriacs, but knowledge of what constitutes health and the ability to use it characterize superior individuals and cultures. Certainly the "high-level wellness" described by Halbert R. Dunn[1] in his radio talks of 1961 (later published as a book) is a measure of superiority and can only be achieved by the knowledgeable and disciplined—those who develop the habit of consciously or unconsciously measuring their health behavior against demanding standards. They and persons whom Abraham H. Maslow[2] describes as "self-realized" would be prepared to know when such behavior (mental, emotional, and physical) is substandard, when they can modify it unaided, or when they need help from others. They would also know the kind of health worker to seek out.

But the concept "health" is also elusive. René Dubos[3] speaks of the "mirage of health." He thinks it is an ideal state we seek but never reach. Others say health is not freedom from disease but the ability to cope with life. Just as it is virtually impossible to find a "perfect" flower, a "perfect" leaf, or a flawless biologic specimen, just so is it impossible to find an anatomically and physiologically "perfect" human being, assuming that perfection can be defined.

If the above generalizations are true, health assessments can never be standardized, mechanized procedures, the sole responsibility of any one element of society, nor can they be divorced from the individual's concept of health, his attitudes toward life, his total being.

The Nature of Health Assessment as Discussed Here. While it is suggested that health assessment is a conscious or unconscious function of living for everybody, and an on-going process in all health care, this chapter describes only what is variously called "the health examination," "the health assessment," "the medical examination," "the physical examination," and "the diagnostic process." Chapter 4 discusses on-going observing, reporting, and recording; Chapters 6 and 7 deal with health indicators, or diagnostic measurements and tests; and many other chapters refer to "normal" and "abnormal" values. This chapter, however, focuses on the sessions and procedures devoted especially to mass screening programs, to initial and periodic health appraisals, and to diagnostic examinations. The difference in emphasis and in the methods used in assessing health, identifying hidden disease, and diagnosing, or discovering, the cause of symptoms from which a patient is suffering are discussed.

An Historical Note on Health Assessment. The Development of Current Practices. The art of health assessment is ancient and has existed in some form in all cultures; the science is newer and has been so highly developed in this age in Western countries that it has tended to diminish or obscure the art.

Since time immemorial, assessors, appraisers, or examiners have used their senses of sight, hearing, smell, and touch to measure the health status of clients. Today these senses have been extended and objective measurements substituted for subjective assessments by a wide variety of instruments or machines. The unaided senses are to some extent distrusted in this age.

In other ages health assessments tended to be estimates of the general state of the body or mind and this tendency persists in some cultures today. In primitive societies the "sick" person is usually thought to be made sick by forces outside the body. A man is ill because the gods are angry with him; a woman may be under a spell or curse; sickness might be attributed to "the dark of the moon" or to the change of seasons. The baleful force, whatever it is, must be bought off, or appeased. Medicine men, priests, and other assessors and healers are in some cultures appeasers or go-betweens; mystic powers are attributed to them. These concepts exist full-blown in certain primitive cultures today and some medical historians say that vestiges of them persist in all cultures.[4-6] For example, it is not unusual to find people in any country looking upon illness as punishment. They cry "O God, what did I do to deserve this?" And the practicing physician is thought to have almost magic powers. An obviously dying child is brought to a doctor and the parents say, "Doctor, *do* something!"

Another ancient, but more rational, approach to health assessment was taken by the Chinese at least 5000 years ago when they attributed sickness to an imbalance between the Yin-Yang * principle *within* the body rather than a force from without acting on it. This approach, although modified, is still used in China today. The editors of the *American Journal of Chinese Medicine* say, "Chinese medicine can . . . be seen as a nexus of ideas; the philosophical is inseparable from the physiological, myth from fact, theory from practice." †

Edith Hamilton [6a] and other classics scholars writing about Greece say that the Greeks made our (Western) world and so it is not surprising that Hippocrates is often called the father of Western medicine. Like the Chinese, he attributed health to an internal balance rather than to outside forces, but instead of Yin-Yang principles he sought a balance in the "humors" within the body.

Modern Western medicine has been, in this century, based largely on Claude Bernard's [7] dictum that health depends on the constancy

of the intercellular fluid, or the cell's environment. Walter B. Cannon [8] in his much-quoted *Wisdom of the Body* elaborates on this concept and stresses homeostasis * as the physiologic goal.

Psychiatrists and clinical psychologists tend to take the over-all view of health and disease. While most acknowledge the influence of the genetic endowment and recognize the physiologic basis of mental health, they also stress forces from without acting on the personality to change its structure. Sidney M. Jourard, for example, says he sees sickness "whether physical or mental" as "a form of protest against a way of life society seems to have demanded." He looks upon illness as "the last and loudest protest of a violated organism against the destructive way of life that he has lived." †

Also in this age are certain religious groups that look upon illness as a failure to think right. The Christian Science healer's assessment, for example, is general rather than specific and the "cure" is a metaphysical process.

Another approach to assessing health on an over-all basis, which is of this age, is the measurement of the electromagnetic field of the body. In Chapter 19, page 1072, there is a brief description of a proposed interdisciplinary study along these lines to be directed by Dorothy Harrison, a nurse and anthropologist. It is based on the work of Harold Saxton Burr, his contemporary associates, and subsequent workers who have used his thesis. Electrometric study of the healing of wounds and of ovulation has demonstrated the clinical practicability of Burr's original investigations.[9-14] The philosophic implications of Burr's theory are discussed by Edward W. Russell, a journalist, in a popular work, *Design for Destiny: Science Reveals the Soul.* He calls it a "Layman's Guide to Harold S. Burr's Remarkable Discoveries and to Their Revolutionary Implications for Medicine and Psychiatry." ‡ Burr himself relates his scientific work to philosophy and religion in his book *The Nature of Man and the Meaning of Existence,*[15] and earlier in an article with F. S. C. Northrop, a philosopher, "The Electro-Dynamic Theory of Life." [16] Leonard J. Ravitz [17] used Burr's theory and method in testing mood swings in psychiatric patients and he thought it an ob-

---

* Yin = shady side, earth, moon, night, female, negative, death, destroying, etc. Yang = sunny side, heaven, sun, day, male, life-creating, hot, etc.

† (Editorial), *Am. J. Chinese Med.,* 1:viii, (Jan.) 1973.

* Homeostasis is the condition in which the circulatory system is supplying the cells with necessary nutrients and is removing cell secretions and excretions, all of which maintain the constancy of inter- and intracellular fluids.

† Jourard, Sidney M.: *Disclosing Man to Himself.* Van Nostrand & Reinhold Co., New York, 1968, p. 38.

‡ Russell, Edward W.: *Design for Destiny: Science Reveals the Soul.* Ballantine Books, New York, 1971.

jective and reliable method as opposed to depending on what clients or patients say, since the latter are influenced by what they want the examiner to know.

It is interesting to speculate on the possibility that Burr's "scientific" approach to assessing the disease process by measuring the balance between positively charged and negatively charged particles (anodes and cathodes) with a voltmeter is close kin to the ancient Chinese medical concept of Yin-Yang balances. Burr presents a chart plotting the electromagnetic fields within the body; Chinese medicine that embodies the Yin-Yang concept and uses acupuncture as one of its principal diagnostic and therapeutic modes has traced "the loci and meridians of the body along which Ch'i or vital energy travels." * For example, Frederick F. Kao, discussing "the new Chinese medicine"—a marriage of ancient Eastern philosophy and Western science—says "Disease occurs when Ch'i is locally excessive or deficient. Acupuncture therapy is thought to correct energetic imbalance by removing obstructions or sedating excess and thereby restoring bodily function to its normal state." † (See Chapter 31 for further discussion of this bioelectric phenomenon.)

In contrast to these over-all concepts of health and the cause of "dis-ease," there is the idea of specificity. The discovery in the nineteenth century that microorganisms caused many diseases, each with its characteristic group of symptoms, introduced a new medical era. The writings of Louis Pasteur, Robert Koch, Ignaz Semmelweis, and others were revolutionary. Since it was found that infectious disease could be prevented, controlled, or cured when the causative organism was isolated, and when a specific vaccine, toxin, antitoxin, or drug was developed that acted on the organism, specificity in diagnosis, prevention, and treatment came to be the goal. (Some chemicals effective in the treatment of diseases caused by microorganisms had, of course, been used pragmatically for centuries before microscopic life was demonstrated. Cinchona bark and its derivative quinine were, for example, used to treat malaria before the discovery of the plasmodium and its mode of transmission. No one, however, knew exactly how the drug acted.)

The importance attached to identifying the specific disease of microbial origin seems to have carried over into general medical practice. Medical education is still focused largely on

the process of making *the* diagnosis, or treating "the chief complaint." Making *the* diagnosis is the major aim in taking the "medical history" and doing a physical examination.[18-20] Some believe that this is at least partially responsible for impersonalized health care and for categorizing, even segregating, patients according to diagnosis, or the body area or the body system receiving major attention. Treatment units still admit exclusively patients with tuberculosis, heart disease, or hemiplegia; or "chest cases," "head injuries," or "abdominal surgery"; or conditions of the skin, the urologic system, or the nervous system. In spite of the criticism of this practice, patients are still referred to as "the craniotomy in Ward B," "the pemphigus case in Room 221," or "the muscular dystrophy in Cubicle 3." Even people who are mentally ill are diagnosed as schizophrenics, manic-depressives, or involutional melancholics. In all but psychiatric practice, the laboratory tests or technologic aspects of health assessment are relied on heavily. In some mass screening programs, physicians, or principal examiners, don't see patients until health measurements have been made by others and the laboratory findings are available. Then they discuss principally with the patient the meaning of test results. Some persons attach so much importance to computerized analysis of test data that they prophesy increasingly accurate diagnoses arrived at by computers in technologically developed countries.

But even in the most highly scientific circles there is a reaction to purely technologic and disease-centered medical care. There is currently an emphasis on the problem-oriented system of health care (discussed in Chapter 4) where an attempt is made to identify all the health problems of the patient, not just the "chief complaint"; there is emphasis on preventive care, or health maintenance, on health education, on public involvement in health care, and on comprehensive care. Patients in treatment units are now more likely to be segregated according to age, their need for care (self-help deficit), than on the basis of diagnosis. For example, people are assigned to intensive care units, intermediate ambulatory services, or half-way houses. In large psychiatric hospitals, patients may be assigned to cottages or wards, not according to diagnosis, but according to the city, town, or county in which they live. In such large state hospitals, health personnel are assigned on the same basis, the assumption being that a sense of community is therapeutic and that treatment is more likely under such circumstances to be comprehensive and family-centered than fragmented and technical.

* Kao, Frederick F.: "Part III—The New Chinese Medicine 'Chung Kuo I Hsueh' (1949 to Present)." *Am. J. Chinese Med.*, 1:26, (Jan.) 1973.
    † *Ibid.*

The philosophy of care in the health agency or health practitioner's office influences the nature of the health examination and the roles played by patients, parents, physicians, and others. The numbers and availability of health workers in the area also determine the roles played by the various workers. If it were possible to review practices on an international basis it would be obvious that the dominant political philosophy influences the availability and nature of the process by which people enter the health care system; it also influences the numbers, distribution, or availability of health workers. These questions are discussed to some extent in this chapter but the particular practices described reflect chiefly those within the United States.

2. ROLES OF PATIENTS, PARENTS, PHYSICIANS, NURSES, AND OTHERS IN ASSESSING HEALTH

The Health Examination as an Introduction to the Health Care System. Since the health examination in some form is part of the introduction to the health care system, it is essential that a way of conducting such examinations evolves that doesn't block admission to the system. Entry into the system is sometimes called *primary care,** although other meanings are also assigned the term.

In Chapters 1 and 2 there is some discussion of "primary care," of national, state, and local

* The report of the US Department of Health, Education, and Welfare Secretary's Committee to Study Extended Roles for Nurses gives the following definition of primary care:
　　(a) a person's first contact in any given episode of illness with the health care system that leads to a decision of [on] what must be done to help resolve his problem; and
　　(b) the responsibility for the continuum of care— that is, maintenance of health, evaluation and management of symptoms, and appropriate referrals. (US Department of Health, Education, and Welfare: *Extending the Scope of Nursing Practice. A Report of the Secretary's Committee to Study Extended Roles for Nurses.* US Government Printing Office, Washington, D.C., 1972; "Extending the Scope of Nursing Practice," *Nurs. Outlook,* **20:**46, [Jan.] 1972.)
The Canadian Nurses' Association and the Canadian Medical Association have agreed jointly on the following description of primary care:
　　. . . all of those health services which are provided for individuals mainly on an ambulatory basis in the community or in their homes . . . preventive and health maintenance services in the community; diagnostic and therapeutic services offered in physicians' offices, in clinics, or in health centers; home care services for those who are ill; and rehabilitative services. ("Extended Role of Nurse and Preparation for it as Defined in Canadian R.N. and M.D. Statement," *Am. J. Nurs.,* **73:**964, [June] 1973.)

programs—the health services available to the people—and the nurse's part in promoting such programs, especially in North America. Attention is called to the worldwide acceptance of the principle that health care is a basic human right. In Chapters 1 and 2 the point is made that available health personnel must be used as effectively as possible if this goal is to be reached and that the public must be more knowledgeable, more able to prevent disease, more able to treat minor ailments, and more able to use health personnel effectively.

Supply of Health Manpower as It Affects the Conduct of Health Examinations. In the United States and many other countries, there aren't enough doctors to examine all those who want a health assessment, either as a basis for preventive care or for diagnosis and treatment of disease. Some persons suggest that the shortage of physicians can be overcome through their redistribution and reorganization; others think that many of the physician's current functions must be turned over to "intermediate-level" health practitioners; some writers suggest that machines, and the technicians who operate them, can provide computerized data that will sufficiently facilitate the physician's work to make it possible to keep health assessment and diagnosis in their hands; and others believe that the cost of medical care can only be brought within bounds by teaching the public to be more self-reliant in assessing and treating itself.[21-28] In the United States the incidence of disease goes down as the family income goes up.[29] Frances Storlie [30] and Nancy Milio [31] are nurses who have urged social action to prevent poverty as the most effective means of upgrading health.

Sidney R. Garfield, writing in 1970 on admission of people to the health care system and on delivery of health care, says: "Any realistic solution to the medical-care problem must . . . begin by facing up to the facts about the [inadequate] supply of physicians." * Garfield thinks the self-sustaining prepaid group practice, patterned after the Kaiser-Permanente program (which he started) is a step in the right direction but far from the entire answer. He believes that at the point of entry into the health care system clients must be divided into "(1) the well; (2) the worried well; (3) the early sick; and (4) the sick." He believes the fee for service keeps all but the sick away from the doctor since, as he puts it, nobody wants to pay for unneeded medical care. Garfield thinks health insurance, paid in a lump sum, induces "the well," "the worried well,"

* Garfield, Sidney R.: "Delivery of Medical Care," *Sci. Am.,* **225:**15, (Apr.) 1970.

and "the early sick" to seek treatment but it also overtaxes our present system. Garfield describes and illustrates a system of health testing (see page 149) designed to identify the categories of clients just itemized, to fully utilize technology and technicians, and to demand the minimum time of physicians.*

While Garfield's suggestions have been widely acclaimed, many persons believe that admission to the health care system should not depend solely on the availability of the physician for either maximum or minimum participation. They point out reasons why the physician has "guarded the entrance to the health care system" and why this concept is outmoded.

At the beginning of this century most persons with a physical or mental health problem, if they sought help, consulted a family doctor. Some might instead or in addition consult the clergy, a public health nurse, the corner druggist, or a neighbor. But traditionally and officially, the physician guarded the entrance to

---

* Ivan Illich (a nonmedical critic of health care systems) thinks the routine health assessment harmful. He maintains that periodic health examinations make every person a patient and turn the well into the worried well. He says: "Effective health care depends on self-care: this fact is currently heralded as if it were a discovery. . . . The medicalization of early diagnosis not only hampers and discourages preventative health care but it also trains the patient-to-be to function in the meantime as an acolyte to his doctor. He learns to depend on the physician in sickness and in health. He turns into a life-long patient." (Illich, Ivan: *Medical Nemesis. The Expropriation of Health.* McClelland & Stewart, Ltd., Toronto, 1975, p. 50.)

Lewis Thomas, a physician, agrees with Illich on some but not all points. Discussing "your very good health," he decries the terms "health industry" and "health maintenance organizations," and the implication that if adequately "maintained" enough is known to prevent all disease. On the other hand, he thinks too little emphasis is put on the capacity of the body to resist disease. He says, "Meanwhile, we are paying too little attention, and respect, to the built-in durability and sheer power of the human organism. Its surest tendency is toward stability and balance. It is a distortion, with something profoundly disloyal about it, to picture the human being as a teetering, fallible contraption, always needing watching and patching, always on the verge of flapping to pieces; this is the doctrine that people hear most often, and most eloquently, on all our information media. We ought to be developing a much better system for general education about human health, with more curricular time for acknowledgment, and even some celebration, of the absolute marvel of good health that is the real lot of most of us, most of the time."

Thomas says that none of his internist friends have routine physical examinations, that "almost all have resisted surgery," and that "laboratory tests for anyone in the family are extremely rare." He thinks doctors' families "seem a normal, generally healthy lot, with a remarkably low incidence of iatrogenic illness." (Thomas, Lewis: *The Lives of a Cell. Notes of a Biology Watcher.* Viking Press, New York, 1974, pp. 83, 84, 85.)

---

health care services. Public health nurses, for instance, had the policy of paying only two or three visits to a family if there was no physician in attendance. Until recently only the dentist accepted patients for treatment without referral from the physician. The corner druggist, the bonesetter, the chiropractor, the faith healer, and others stepped into the breach left by an inadequate supply of physicians, but their advice and treatment was given outside the pale of *the* medical care system. To this day medical practice acts make diagnosis and treatment by persons other than physicians (and dentists) illegal. Many persons recognize the necessity of modifying these acts, for the picture is changing and many physicians realize that they cannot supply all the primary care needed, or all "first contacts with the health care system."

The categories and numbers of health workers prepared under the auspices of higher education and qualifying as "professionals" have multiplied. Clinical psychologists, psychotherapists, social workers, nutritionists, physical, occupational and speech therapists, health educators, nurse-midwives and other nurse practitioners qualify as professionals under most accepted criteria. And while the public still recognizes the physician's preeminence in the diagnosis and treatment of disease, it is relying more and more on its own knowledge and it recognizes the special competence of other health workers. For example, the public often turns to nutritionists for advice on the selection and preparation of food; to marriage counsellors for advice on sex; to the physical culturist for help in muscular development; to the speech therapist for advice on language development; and to the nurse for help with a wide range of health problems including, for example, infant and child feeding, obesity, skin care, postural defects, fatigue, insomnia, constipation, depression, contraception, and family planning.* Health workers with preparations that qualify them as "professionals" are effectively promoting legislation that enables them to serve the public without referral from physicians.

Actually health workers with less than professional preparation and people not classified as health workers but with special life experiences may be able to give certain kinds of help that most physicians and nurses either cannot give or are not interested in giving. Recovered alcoholics and other rehabilitated drug abusers staff and operate highly effective treatment centers. Alcoholics Anonymous, Synanon,

---

* In Chapters 1 and 3 there is a discussion of nurses who have private offices and practice independently.

Reach for Recovery, and Weight Watchers are examples of nonmedical agencies that have been uniquely successful in helping individuals and groups of "patients," or clients, with stubborn health problems.*

Physicians themselves are questioning their traditional roles, alerting the public to iatrogenic disease (disease resulting from treatment), and urging everyone to accept more responsibility for their own health. Works in this category are Halbert R. Dunn's *High-Level Wellness,*[32] Michael Crichton's *Five Patients. The Hospital Explained,*[33] Mike Samuels' and Hal Bennett's *The Well Body Book,*[34] and Andrew Malleson's *Need Your Doctor Be So Useless?*[35]

Outside the United States, Canada, and the other countries where typically "Western medicine" is practiced, there are different kinds of health care "systems," and ways of entering them. In Chapters 1 and 2 the preparation and function of feldshers in Russia were discussed as were the roles of "barefoot" and "Red Guard" doctors in China. The latter outnumber physicians (whose preparation is comparable to medical education in the United States) and they examine and treat certain categories of patients in certain situations. Kao says:

> Common recurrent diseases, e.g., common cold, respiratory infections, skin diseases and gastrointestinal disorders are . . . treated by barefoot doctors in the commune, red guard doctors in the factories and health officers in the PLA and the hospitals. Propaganda teams are efficient in educating the public. . . . As a matter of fact, the emphasis in the treatment of disease is on prevention. . . .†

In any successful national, state, provincial, or local health planning, who does what in assessing health and treating disease must depend on the numbers and types of workers available, the effective use made of them, the way society sees their functions, the customary and legal scope of their practice, and how much money the people of the area elect to spend on health care.

The Client's or Patient's Role in Health Examinations. In health examinations, as in most aspects of health care, the client's or patient's role is the most important; or in the case of infants and small children the parent's role. They decide when to seek help; whether to use primary preventive measures such as immunization, or whether to wait for alarming symptoms before consulting a health worker. Samuels and Bennett wrote *The Well Body Book* as a "tool" to help youths and adults examine their own bodies and develop their own "practical system of healing and preventive medicine using the physician as a consultant." They say "Your body is a three million year healer." * They think most people know far too little about the structure and function of the body but could learn enough about anatomy and physiology, about normal health values, to examine their own body or that of a friend. Malleson, author of *Need Your Doctor Be So Useless?*[36] thinks that people are increasingly knowledgeable and that only when they do assume optimum responsibility for preventing illness and treating minor ailments can the "cancer" of spiraling health care costs be controlled. He notes legislation in the United States that requires physicians to have "informed consent" from the patient for treatment. This means that the physician must explain the prescribed treatment, the benefits, risks, and alternatives. We believe, however, that there are even now people like the Victorian lady who said to her doctor as he tried to explain the nature of constipation "Oh, don't tell me, doctor, I like to think of myself as lined with pink crepe de chine!"

Arlene and Howard Eisenberg,[37] two journalists, describe a course in "self-help preventive medicine" in Reston, Va., said to be the first of its kind in the United States. It is sponsored by Georgetown University Community Health Plan's Department of Community Medicine and is taught by nine physicians who are said to encourage people to save money by attending to minor problems or by becoming "activated" patients. Those taking the course are referred by one doctor to a 1734 text by Dr. John Tennent, *Everyman His Own Doctor or The Poor Planter's Physician.*[38] Students are taught to use the sphygmomanometer, to take temperature, pulse, and respiration, to look at eardrums with otoscopes, what to do in emergencies, and how to treat some less serious ailments. While this course has much in common with those taught for many years under Red Cross auspices, the significant feature of it, as related to this chapter, is that doctors are now teaching the public certain skills of health evaluation, diagnosis, and treatment that have until recently been reserved for the physician's use.

Beside the importance of the subject's role in knowing how his or her body should function, how to deal with minor ailments, and when to seek help, a great deal depends upon

---

* Many groups of former hospital patients are organizing themselves to help each other, as, for example, psychiatric and neurotic patients, and people who have had colostomies or laryngectomies.

† Kao, Frederick F.: "China, Chinese Medicine and the Chinese Medical System," *Am. J. Chinese Med.,* **1:**1, (Jan.) 1973.

* Samuels, Mike, and Bennett, Hal: *The Well Body Book.* Random House, New York, 1973, pp. x, 1.

the ability of patients to give a clear and accurate account of their health practices and the signs and symptoms of disease. With babies and young children, the health worker, of course, depends on the ability of parents or guardians to do this. Types of records to be kept—forms to be filled in, questionnaires to be answered by patients or parents are shown and discussed later in the chapter. Some autobiographies describe the subject's feelings and behavior so accurately that physicians reading the descriptions centuries later can say with assurance that they suffered from such and such a disease. Health examiners depend heavily on what patients tell them, how honestly they answer the questions put to them, and on how highly motivated they are to be healthy, to correct defects, and to eliminate disease.

Roles of Physicians, Nurses, and Other Health Workers in Conducting Health Examinations. The roles of various types of health examiners depend on the setting, the type of examination, and the personnel available. *Physicians* in their private offices may conduct the entire examination with minimum help from nurses or other attendants although they seldom take simple measurements such as the temperature, pulse, and respiration or make the laboratory tests or take x-rays that are a part of the health examination. Some physicians have professional nurses associated with them in their private practice who may conduct most health examinations or most aspects of the examination. Pediatricians especially are turning over the health assessments of well infants and children to professional nurses, and obstetricians who have professional nurses and nurse-midwives working with them may ask these nurses and nurse-midwives to carry out the initial health examination.

In health screening units and agencies with optimum technologic facilities and processes, physicians may not see patients until a series of health measurements and tests have been made and until patients themselves have answered an extensive questionnaire. If physicians practice as a group or offer a comprehensive health service, several may meet with the patient, or patients and their families, after the initial screening process to discuss the health problems identified during the examination and to suggest a corrective program, or a treatment regimen.

In large hospitals—especially those with medical schools—residents, interns, and medical students usually examine the patient and discuss their findings with the attending physician. The latter may then repeat certain aspects of or the whole examination. When patients are very ill or when the cause of the illness is obscure, not only one but several physicians may examine them.

Professional nurses in independent practice examine their patients, or clients, in the nurse's office with or without assistance from other workers. Nurse-midwives and public health nurses in clinics conduct health examinations on certain categories of patients and health examinations are made by community nurses in patients' homes. Professional nurses in ambulatory services of hospitals are more and more frequently conducting health examinations. This is particularly true in services for children, the chronically ill, and the elderly. Most nurses conducting health examinations have had post-basic preparation and acquire differentiating titles.* It is, however, increasingly common in the United States to include training for and experience in physical diagnosis in basic collegiate nursing programs.

It is recognized that nurses have, actually, for many years in certain geographical areas and in certain agencies made health assessments.[39-44] Community nurses ("public health nurses") have throughout this century assumed considerable responsibility for health assessment. Figure 5-1 shows nurses, as judged by the clothing, examining immigrants to the United States as they go through the Health Service on Ellis Island (New York City) in the first decade of this century. Canadian nurses in the Indian Health Service, nurses on certain islands where there are no physicians, and nurses of the Frontier Nursing Service in Kentucky are other examples. The relative unavailability of medical care in the latter areas has obliged them to make assessments and institute treatment, using physicians as consultants when necessary, and arranging for transportation to large treatment centers for the most seriously ill and injured.

In all settings where there are physicians and nurses, both may be cast in their "traditional" roles—physicians carrying out most steps in the physical examination and discussing their findings with the patient; nurses helping patients get ready for the examination, explaining the procedure to those who are unfamiliar with it, adjusting positions, clothing, and covering, and giving such reassurance as seems needed. In most settings, nursing personnel make certain measurements such as body temperature, pulse and respiratory rates, weight and height, and see that a specimen of urine is available for analysis. These are the

---

* In the United States the terminology is confusing, as noted in Chapter 1. Nurses prepared to assume an "expanded role" may be called variously "family nurse practitioners," "primary care nurses," "pediatric nurse practitioners," "pediatric associates," "clinical specialists," or by other titles.

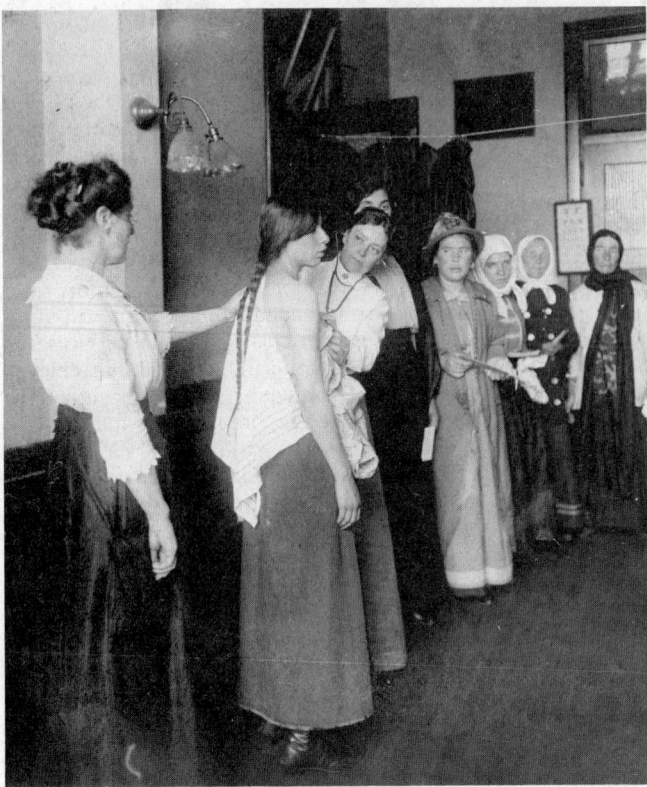

Figure 5-1. Public health nurses examining immigrants on arrival at Ellis Island (New York City) about 1912. (Photograph from Brown Brothers, Sterling, Pa.)

usual procedures, but they may make other measurements and get other specimens. Nurses may stay with the patient and physician throughout the examination, providing as much comfort for the patient as is possible, often holding an infant if the mother is not present. If the patient and doctor are of the same sex, the nurse may not be present during the entire examination, but in the case of a female patient and male physician, the presence of a woman nurse during the pelvic examination is a protection for both the patient and the physician. After the examination, nurses answer patients' questions, reinforce the physician's directions for follow-up, and carry out any other forms of health teaching that are indicated.

Physician's assistants may conduct health examinations under (almost) the same circumstances as do professional nurses. *Feldshers* in Russia are surrogates for the physician and examine patients just as physicians do. They are more likely to be found in satellite hospitals, ambulatory services, and mobile units than in the large teaching hospitals.[45,46] Barefoot and Red Guard doctors in the People's Republic of China have comparable responsibilities.[47]

In the United States *clinical psychologists* and other specialists, as, for instance, the *phys-*

ical therapist, may conduct special aspects of the health examination. The psychologist may administer psychometric tests and the physical therapist tests for motor power and motor skills. The *vocational guidance expert* in a rehabilitation center may administer a battery of tests to measure potentialities for employment; the *speech therapist* in such a center or in the stroke program of a hospital may give a series of tests to determine the nature of the speech impairment and the possibility of improving or restoring normal speech.

With the improvement of health services, which must come if the needs of the people are to be met, the health examination will vary according to the problems presented by the patient and the examination will be made by a team of workers, the composition of which is determined by the patient's needs, the purpose of the examination, and the available health manpower.

3. PURPOSES AND TYPES OF HEALTH EXAMINATIONS

Assessments, or examinations, are made because parents or guardians want the health of infants or children evaluated periodically or disease diagnosed when they note signs and symptoms of it; well adults want accurate knowledge of their health status; adults who are well, but, as Garfield puts it, "worried well," want reassurance; and adults who have signs and symptoms of illness want to be diagnosed and treated. Some persons may live and die without having had a health examination but this happens less and less often since most schools require examination of students before or immediately after admission and, in many cases, at periodic intervals thereafter. Employers, commercial insurance companies, and all prepaid health care providers may have similar requirements. Research on certain diseases and studies on the health problems within a nation, state, province, community, institution, or social group often demand complete or partial health examinations as a means of collecting data. In some cases, as in studies of incipient and early cancer, the examination is far more thorough than the average mass screening procedure, while examinations to detect tuberculosis may include only a single procedure. The Framingham (Mass.) investigation [48] of cardiovascular disease with a 16-year follow-up is an excellent example of research whose validity and reliability depend on the effectiveness of the health assessment procedure.

It is impossible in a general work to describe all types of health examinations; the following is only a brief description of the major types according to purpose. It is assumed here that any one of a number of types of workers may conduct the examination, that it may be in a home, a doctor's or nurse's office, a health maintenance organization, the health service of a school, an industry or correctional institution, a clinic, a nursing home, or a hospital. It is also assumed in this chapter that everyone is responsible for assessing their own health status and repeated reference will be made to this. In describing health assessment it is taken for granted that essential laboratory and x-ray services are available and some uses made of computers. Ideally, all health services will eventually offer facilities, including computers, that will make available to the public health assessment processes comparable to those available to the 2 million subscribers of the Kaiser-Permanente Plan. [49] According to Victor W. Sidel and Ruth Sidel, [49a] the national health service of mainland China has provided an assessment service for its population which, although not as highly developed technologically in all its aspects as the above, is, at least, universally available.

Health Examinations in Qualifying for Admission to a School, an Employing Agency, or an Agency Providing Health Care. Health being one of a person's chief assets, an estimate of it is, naturally, of interest to those who administer schools and admit students; and to other types of institutions, agencies, and industries when they employ workers. The standard of health required by institutions, agencies, organizations, and industries varies greatly. For example, some private schools rule out applicants with physical or mental defects. While public school systems in most countries cannot do this, they try to identify pupils' health deficits and provide special programs for handicapped pupils. Some schools, as, for example, schools for the blind or deaf, are designed for only those so handicapped and their admission examinations rule out all who can see or hear well enough to get along in other systems. Agencies and organizations, in establishing health standards, consider their special needs. Physical strength and stamina may be very important if the worker must endure long hours of work or travel great distances, as do, for example, the nurse-midwives of the Frontier Nursing Service in Kentucky, nurses who care for Indians and Eskimos in the north of Canada, or nurses who serve sparsely settled regions of Australia's "bush" country or "outback." Mental and emotional health may be the prime requirement in workers who apply for administrative positions in many agencies and organizations. In such cases personality and psychometric tests or measurements are stressed in the health examinations for applicants.

Industries vary greatly in the health measurements of prospective employees that concern them especially—which seems quite obvious. The results of psychometric measurements might be of major interest if the prospective employee is to work with the design or repair of computers; while personality tests, physical measurements, and other attributes that please or displease the eye are important if the prospective employee is to work as a steward, a stewardess, or a model.

Institutions, agencies, organizations, and industries usually have a form or forms to guide the examiner. They may have one form which the applicant's physician fills in; most have forms used by their own health services in conducting health examinations, initially and periodically. Nurses on the staffs of such services may help design these forms and conduct, or take part in conducting, the examinations. Eileen D. Flynn, [50] in a symposium on multiphasic screening, discusses one industrial nurse's role. In general, such examinations are more like health screening procedures and periodic health examinations than the examination to diagnose the cause of signs and symptoms troubling the patient. No attempt can be made here to differentiate between health examinations in schools, other institutions, agencies, organizations, and industries, or to point out differences within these categories.

Multiphasic Health Screening. Periodic Health Examinations. The Health Examination as a Tool in Research on Health. Health screening and the periodic health examination differ from examinations made to determine the cause of pathologic symptoms chiefly in purpose, which is to detect disease in its embryonic stage as a basis for early, and consequently more successful, treatment. It is the foundation stone of preventive medicine when the examination is made by competent health workers who combine it with health guidance. If disease is detected, the savings in human life and happiness are obvious; if the findings are negative, the person usually profits by an increased sense of well-being. Nurses are in a position to promote (or discourage) periodic health examinations by their own example and by discussing their possible value (or, according to Illich, possible harm) with others.

The more complete the examination, the greater its value as a preventive measure but, as in all aspects of health care, its quality is affected by the availability of personnel and facilities. Most texts describing health (medical) histories and physical examinations outline a traditional procedure which, if followed in annual "check-ups" for the total population, would, we believe, consume more highly trained health manpower time than is available in any country for this aspect of health care. Multiphasic health screening processes have therefore been devised that make optimum use of questionnaires answered by patients and technologic tests and measurements made by technicians. Some of these are described later in this chapter. While a history-taking interview and the traditional steps as described for the diagnostic examination (see pages 391 and 401) might ideally be used in all periodic health examinations, the latter should include at least the following: health (medical) history; health and social family history; personal and social history; physical examination; mental health status or psychiatric assessment; and laboratory tests.

Histories taken by interview in periodic health assessments, preemployment health assessments, and for admissions to schools follow the procedure described in detail in later sections of this chapter. Histories taken by questionnaires can be quite thorough although an interview by the person making the physical examination has obvious advantages. The physical examination should include inspection of the entire body; examination of organs of the head, chest, abdomen, and pelvis; examina-

tion of the genitalia and the extremities; measurements of pulse rate, blood pressure, respiration, height and weight, and vision and hearing. Chest x-ray films should be made. Laboratory tests on blood and urine are essential. Blood tests for hemoglobin, cell count, and syphilis are routine, and some authorities believe that laboratory tests should include tests for sugar and cholesterol.[51] Urine is always tested for the presence of sugar and albumin. Tests for certain microorganisms in the body are indicated for persons in occupations where there is special danger of disease transmission. For example, a stool culture may be required in examinations of food handlers, or throat cultures for health workers assigned to nurseries.

In periodic health assessments of infants and children, special attention is paid to measurement of growth and development. Actually, assessment at any age might include this measurement. Doris Cook Sutterley and Gloria Ferraro Donnelly have written a thought-provoking system-oriented nursing text entitled *Perspectives in Human Development; Nursing Throughout the Life Cycle.** Esther Lucile Brown in a foreword says "The authors have attempted nothing less than to look at human beings in their totality." This should certainly be the aim in health assessment, or in health or diagnostic examinations. They should include measurements of physical growth or maturation and estimates of mental and emotional growth and stability. Psychiatric, psychometric, or mental status measurements are included in all complete health examinations just as are orthopedic, neurologic, and other "specialty measurements."

Keeve Brodman and his associates[52] described the Cornell Medical Index-Health Questionnaire as a diagnostic instrument in 1951. This 4-page leaflet containing 195 questions, stated in simple language, has been a model for other such questionnaires. In its present form, as used at the New York Hospital, it is called "The Patient's Medical History." Admitted patients are asked to fill in the form as part of their initial examination, allowing the physician to concentrate on the "more significant points in the history" (see Fig. 4-7). The questions are designed to uncover emotional as well as physical disorders of all sorts. Those who constructed and have used this questionnaire believe that it is an extremely helpful instrument bringing to light many con-

* Sutterley, Doris Cook, and Donnelly, Gloria Ferraro: *Perspectives in Human Development; Nursing Throughout the Life Cycle.* J. B. Lippincott Co., Philadelphia, 1973, p. vii.

ditions that may be overlooked in the ordinary medical examination. Patients seem to take satisfaction in filling in the form, and this has the added advantage of saving the examiner's time. A brief study of the patients' answers to such questions as "Are you depressed and blue much of the time?" "Are you . . . keyed up and jittery?" "Are your feelings easily hurt?" "Do you bite your fingernails?" "Do you cry easily?" and "Do you have frightening thoughts?" shows emotional disturbances that otherwise might only be discovered after a long period of observation. In 1950, A. L. Chapman[53] advocated multiple screening as a means of combatting chronic diseases and he expressed the opinion that the Cornell Index would go a long way toward uncovering their signs and symptoms.

Figure 4-6 in Chapter 4 shows a patient at a computer terminal at the University of Vermont Medical Center answering questions like those in the Cornell Index that will go into the computerized data base. This is also comparable to the data collected in the Kaiser-Permanente system with punch cards.

Health examinations may vary according to the prevalence of disease in the region or in age or ethnic groups represented by clients, or patients. A good example is tuberculosis which is not feared in the United States as it once was because the rate has dropped (from 53.0 per 100,000 in 1953 to 24.4 per 100,000 in 1966.) The peak prevalence has shifted, however, from the young adult to the aged in the last 30 years. In 1953, 37.4 per cent occurred in age range of 25 to 44, in 1966 the percentage dropped to 28, while the percentage for age 65 or more was 50.4 per cent. Tuberculosis in nonwhites comprised 35 per cent of all new cases in 1968.[54] In health examinations greater stress might be put on detection of tuberculosis in the susceptible groups than in those that are comparatively immune.

With the increase in venereal disease, the prevalence of drug addiction, including alcoholism, in the United States and many other countries, health examinations should be designed to detect them. Demography (the science of people collectively considered) influences the nature and frequency of health appraisals. Reliable demographic health data are dependent on effective health examinations and accurate reporting. It also dictates any number of variations in the health examination. Obviously those conducting or participating in health examinations should know the purposes for which they are made.

For instance, Garfield[55] gives the following steps in health testing in the Kaiser-Permanente Multitest Laboratory, Oakland, Calif.:

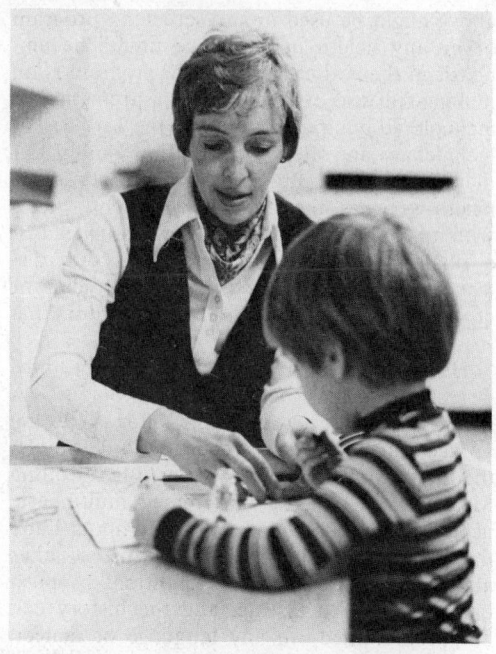

Figure 5-2. Assistant Nursing Director of the Borough of East York Health Unit (Toronto area) conducts testing to determine child's motor development. (Photograph by Dougal Bichan in Handbury, Eric: *Nurse.* McClelland & Stewart, Ltd., Toronto, Ont., 1975. Sponsored by the Registered Nurses Association of Ontario for the celebration of its 50th Anniversary.)

(1) the patient registers; (2) the patient is assigned a dressing room where he or she partially undresses and dons a paper gown; (3) an electrocardiogram is made and the pulse and blood pressure are measured; (4) height and weight are recorded; (5) fat is measured with a skinfold test on the back over the scapula; (6) a tendon reflex on the ankle is checked; (7) the chest is x-rayed, and the breasts, if the patient is a woman (mammography); (8) the patient dresses and drinks a glucose solution in preparation for a blood test an hour later; (9) visual acuity is measured; (10) eyes are checked for glaucoma with a tonometer; (11) lung capacity is measured; (12) hearing is tested electronically; (13) the patient is given punch cards for a self-administered medical questionnaire; (14) a blood sample is taken for analysis; (15) a urine sample is collected for study; (16) the patient is given another set of cards for a psychologic test; (17) the patient talks with a doctor [in a later session] after the doctor has seen and studied the data collected by others and processed in the computer center.

The procedure as described in the steps listed

above might be used in any screening program or by any health maintenance unit. The emphasis in the Kaiser-Permanente program is on making full use of tests and measurements, of technologic equipment, and of the services of technicians and clerks, so that minimum demands are made on the physician. In some health services the client, or patient, meets with a group of health professionals instead of a single physician or nurse. The group discusses the findings and any treatment or changes in the person's living pattern that seem indicated.

Health care is often referred to as the third largest "industry" in the United States.* A number of commercial firms offer a testing service and a system of records. For example, the International Health Systems, Inc. (Rolling Meadows, Ill.) has an automated multiphasic health testing system (called Computa-Lab) that includes an automated health-history-taker allowing patients to answer questions by push button at their own rate, and the history can be "programmed" in any language or dialect. Tests include 12-lead ECG, pulmonary function, blood pressure, tonometry, audiometry, vision, heart rate, anthropometry, and temperature. Computer printouts eliminate paper work; testing requires less than 1 hour and two people can be tested simultaneously with the system.[56]

While it can be expected that these time-saving automated processes will increase they are presently an exception in most health examinations. And no matter how data is collected, by machines or by people, health workers must interpret the findings or data to patients and their families, so the process of health testing can never be totally automated.

If nurses in their offices as private practitioners, in a school, in industry, or any other setting make the health assessment without participation by the physician, nurses discuss the findings with clients, or patients, and any changes in health management they suggest. If treatment by a physician, a dentist, or any other health specialist is indicated, nurses make the referral at this time.

In mainland China, where universal medical care is a comparatively recent achievement, Kao[57] says that it has been accomplished because about 45,000 "mobile medical workers" have cooperated with peasants, workers, and

soldiers in bringing services and health teaching to rural and other "needy areas." Medical workers went to the people with "mobile units" instead of expecting the people to come to health centers.* It is reported that the birth rate is under control; that smallpox, cholera, kala-azar, and schistosomiasis japonica were stamped out by 1958; and that plague and venereal disease were brought under control by 1959. Ruth Watson Lubic,[58] a nurse who went on a health survey visit to China in 1973, remarked on its freedom from insect disease carriers and on the healthy appearance and vigor of children and adults. Universally available health assessment with health teaching is an essential component of public health programs that achieve such results.

An Examination to Find the Explanation for Signs and Symptoms of Disease as a Basis for Treatment. In illness, the health, or medical, examination is modified according to the patient's symptoms. Diagnostic examinations, therefore, vary considerably even though all of them include the elements of the periodic health examination just described, unless some such appraisal has just been made and the record is available. Diseases are not always limited to the area in which the pain or discomfort appears. In an extensive text edited by Cyril M. MacBryde and Robert Stanley Blacklow,[59] titled *Signs and Symptoms,* a chapter is devoted to "Back Pain." It is noted that this symptom may indicate disease in the chest, abdomen, or pelvis; or in the legs or feet; or it may be caused by fatigue resulting from any number of systemic diseases, as well as from diseases of the spinal column itself.

A thorough diagnostic examination is a long procedure, often requiring the services of many professional health workers and technicians and many tests. Chapter 7 is devoted to the more common ones. In some instances patients go to a community health center or a clinic where physicians, nurses, and others practice in a group, giving the patient the advantage of their varied preparations and combined judgments. In other instances the entire examination is made by one physician in an office, a home, or a hospital. Physicians of the present day, practicing in and outside institutions, depend heavily on help from laboratory technicians and pathologists in making diagnoses.

Medical practitioners who are convinced that mind and body cannot be thought of sep-

---

* As pointed out in Chapter 2, health care institutions and agencies are appropriately called "industries" if they are privately owned and if the owners, or the health care providers, make a profit. Almost all nursing homes and some hospitals are privately owned; they and nearly all practitioners who charge a fee-for-service are profit-making.

* Health services are available, however, in schools, industries, in rural communes, and in the headquarters of military brigades. "Barefoot" and Red Guard doctors, who have minimal preparation originally, are increasingly competent because continuing education for all health workers is the rule.

arately, and certainly not studied independently, make an analysis of the personality development of the patient. They record data on his relationships with family, friends, and associates, and the way he lives and works; they note his behavior and his general appearance. George Draper and associates,[60] Ernst Kretschmer,[61] William H. Sheldon and S. S. Stevens,[62] S. Gluek and E. Glueck,[63] and others who wrote extensively on genetics and medicine, believe that the person's appearance, shape, and size are, in themselves, a clue to his ailment. W. J. Gradpaille [64] reports in 1972 a review of research into the physiology of maleness and femaleness. Findings from studies of nonhumans show the same range of dominant male, dominant female, and mixed types. R. Goldschmidt [65] reports on intersexuality in gypsy moths which is demonstrated by different shades of gray, white, and black moths in the same species. A chapter is devoted to the "Mosaic of Androgyny" in the book by Draper and associates, *Human Constitution in Clinical Medicine.* They say:

So far as one knows, the actual phenomenon of reproduction is achieved through the genital organs alone. A person's other task of survival depends upon adequate adjustment to a complex environment, which includes human relations. The impulse to survive is expressed extragenitally by the man in manly fashion, and by the woman in womanly ways. The opposite and special endowments for these purposes are in general well known, and are displayed by differences between man and woman in morphology, physiology, immunity, and psychology—or as cellular sex in the total organism. This composite structure of masculine and feminine characters has been called "the mosaic of androgyny" ($\alpha\nu\delta\rho os$ = male; $\gamma\upsilon\nu\dot{\eta}$ = female).

The term is used because the nongenital qualities appropriate to each sex are never complete in a given woman to the exclusion of some evidence of the counterpart.* Thus, traits that are ordinarily judged to be the man's may appear in the woman to form kaleidoscopic patterns with her own; the reverse is likewise true. The contrasting qualities have to do not only with outward design, structure, and function, but even more significantly with the extragenital dynamics of the whole person. *So far as the relation of human constitution to disease is concerned, the androgynous phase of sex seems to be of greater significance than the genital.** And it is for this reason that the terms "andric" and "gynic" (adjectives formed from the joint word's component parts) have been chosen to designate the divergent organismal aspects of man and woman.†

Sheldon and Kretschmer use different terminology to designate structural types, but both believe that there is a characteristic emotional make-up associated with each of the following: the stocky figure with a large visceral cavity and a tendency to fat; the contrasting type, the asthenic, whose trunk is slender; and the athletic type, whose skeletal and muscular systems are well developed. These constitutional patterns are predisposed to different kinds of emotional disorders or so-called mental disease. According to some psychiatrists they have different interests, capacities, and need for affection, approval, and so on (see Fig. 5-3).

Gordon W. Allport, in *Pattern and Growth in Personality,* examines the work of Kretschmer, Sheldon, Glueck, and others. He concludes that there is something in their formulations, but he says "To preserve the doctrine of empirical types at all it is necessary to say that most people are mixed types." * While physicians are not in agreement on the relationship that has just been suggested between constitution and disease, the "gallbladder type," with feminine or "gynic" characteristics predominating, and the "ulcer type," with the pronounced "andric" characteristics, are a part of medical language.

Draper's point of view is in harmony with the concepts of psychosomatics, which is another way of saying that organic, or somatic, disease has psychic or emotional origin. The physiologic explanation is that strong emotion and anxiety states either affect the endocrine system or in fact are actually our interpretation of their activity. It is easy to see that organic disease can result from a lack of balance in glandular physiology with its all-powerful and pervasive influence over the rest of the body.

Mimi Dye and Richard Charlat [66] say that it is important to understand that everyone has ways of dealing with life's usual problems or stress—for maintaining or reestablishing equilibrium with the internal and external environment. Roy Shafer,[67] writing about internalization, says there are the following *personality types* (along a continuum): the rigid (rigidly integrated and highly self-conscious); the flexible (appropriately flexible); and the fluid (too readily seek satisfaction and reassurance in fantasy or through inappropriate impulsive behavior).

Dye and Charlat maintain that illnesses, whether mainly psychic or mainly somatic, are essentially disturbances in the adaptive func-

---

* The italics are the writer's.
† Draper, George, et al.: *Human Constitution in Clinical Medicine.* Paul B. Hoeber, New York, 1944, p. 75.

* Allport, Gordon W.: *Pattern and Growth in Personality.* Holt Rinehart & Winston, New York, 1965, p. 350.

A

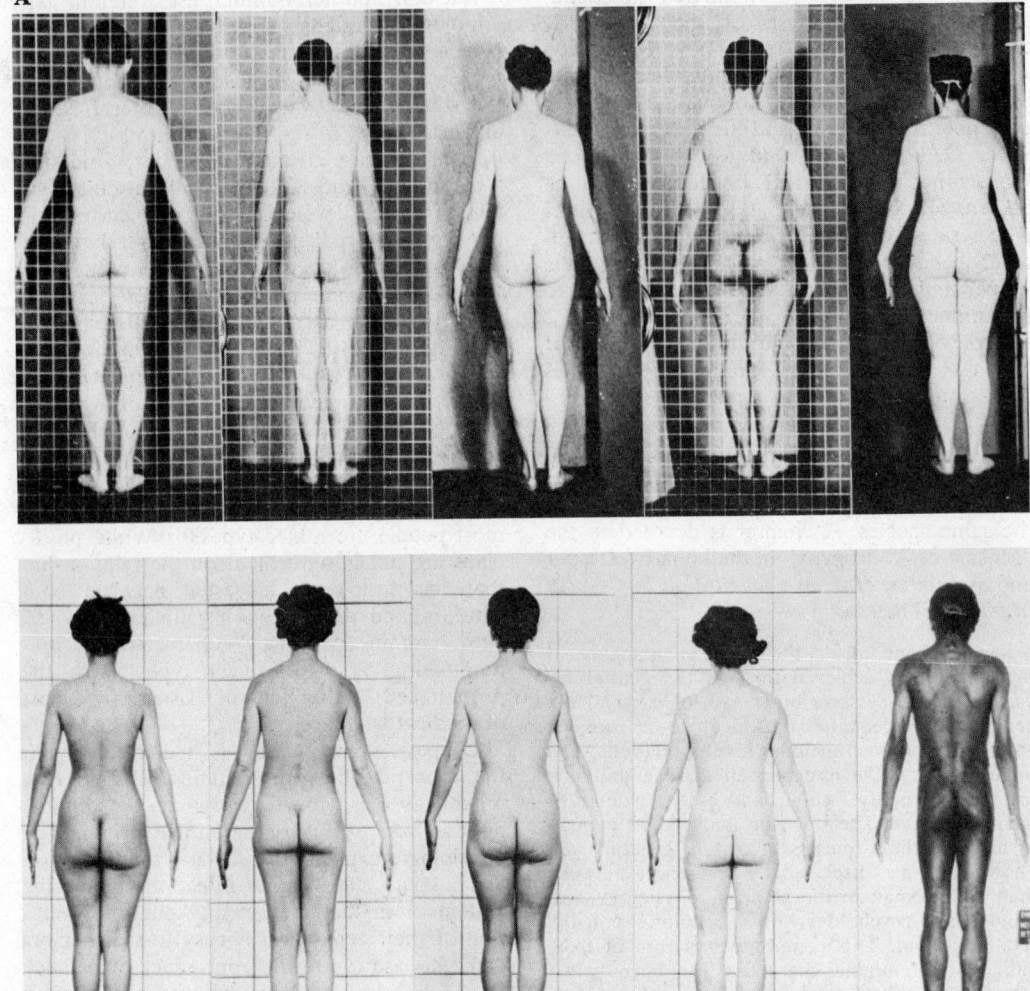

B

Figure. 5-3. *A*. Comparison of the male morphology when male, or andric, factors predominate (left) and when female, or gynic, factors predominate (right). (From Sheldon, William H., and Stevens, S. S.: *The Varieties of Temperament: A Psychology of Constitutional Differences.* Harper & Brothers, New York, 1942.) *B*. Comparison of the female morphology when female, or gynic, factors predominate (left) and when male, or andric, factors predominate (right). (Courtesy of Dr. William H. Sheldon and associates.)

tions of the organism. Heinz Hartmann [68] says that healthy adaptation involves a reciprocal relationship between the person and the environment. Numerous studies have shown the relationship between life events and symptoms of stress, or physical and mental illness.[69-72] The wise family doctor has in all ages recognized a relationship between temperament, environment, and illness. Our present concepts

are more scientific, and their application more necessary, as the patients often find themselves treated by a group of specialists, none of whom know them or their family. Draper and his associates [73] said that the medical history holds the key to diagnosis. Any thorough diagnostic examination takes into account the psychologic or emotional aspects of disease. If the symptoms suggest a marked emotional disturbance, the examination may include an extensive psychiatric investigation.

John A. Prior and Jack S. Silberstein, in their text *Physical Diagnosis. The History and Examination of the Patient,* stress the importance of the mental examination as part of every health assessment. They say:

Traditionally, the mental examination has been considered a procedure only for psychiatrists, to be used in determining whether or not a patient might be mentally ill—that is, sane or insane, responsible or irresponsible, neurotic or "normal." Today we know that such a limited concept of the use of the mental examination is no longer valid. In reality the mental examination is one part of the total examination of the patient, just as is the neurologic, cardiac, or pelvic examination. No patient can be considered as having been completely studied if the mental examination has been omitted. The mental examination can make many valuable contributions to the understanding of all patients and their illnesses.

To be sure, the mental examination is concerned with the patient's mind and its function. Also, it is concerned with the patient's attitudes, thoughts, and feelings. It is concerned with whether or not the patient is mentally ill in the strictest sense of the word. However, the mental examination also has other concerns that have deep significance for the physician other than the psychiatrist. A person's attitudes, thoughts, and feelings are not isolated phenomena. They have an influence on physiologic processes throughout the body. Consequently, it is important that they are taken into consideration whenever one is evaluating symptoms and disorders in various parts of the body.*

Moreover, Dye and Charlat[74] believe that every health examination should include a psychiatric assessment. They believe the examiner should find out about the person's current environment and how he or she looks upon the interview with the examiner in order to understand his or her behavior and the symptoms presented. They stress the importance of describing symptoms or problems in the patient's language because this says how he or she perceives them. They think to ignore the patient's perceptions jeopardizes a constructive relationship between examiners and patients, which is essential to continuing assessment. To facilitate a thorough and accurate assessment, patients should feel comfortable. What patients tell the examiner, or how the two relate, is itself symptomatic.

There seems to be some confusion in the terminology used to describe the psychic, mental and/or emotional aspects of the health examination. Ian Stevenson and William M. Sheppe, Jr.,[75] writing in 1959 on the psychiatric examination in the *American Handbook of Psychiatry,* list the following aspects of the "mental status examination": (1) appearance, attitude, and activity; (2) thought processes; (3) thought content; (4) emotional state; and (5) sensorium. Edward A. Strecker,[76] writing in 1947, includes all of these and adds *insight.* Oscar Diethelm,[77] writing in 1949 on the evaluation of a psychiatric examination, warns against thinking of it in the "narrow terms" of mental status. He described an examination that is a study of a patient over a period of days which he called a group of experiments. He attached little importance to the findings from psychologic tests made when the person is in a state of anxiety.

Bruno Bettelheim,[78] describing first meetings of patients in the Orthogenic School (a psychiatric hospital for autistic, schizophrenic, and suicidal children and adults up to 25 years of age), stresses their reception in a "living room," as a guest would be received; he describes the repeated visits that give the staff an opportunity to make an adequate assessment and the patient a chance to decide whether he or she wishes to come to live in the school, for he says what the patient thinks of the therapist is more important than the reverse. He might agree with Howard F. Hunt,[79] who said in 1950, discussing "psychodiagnostics," that the emphasis is shifting from more objective to more subjective methods.

Extensive examinations made by specialists —urologists, obstetricians, neurologists and psychiatrists, for example—are not described in this text. Interested readers will find descriptions of them in cited references and suggested readings at the end of this chapter. A fairly specific suggested procedure for the mental status examination, or the general psychiatric assessment, to be included in all health examinations, is described on pages 423 and 424.

4. THE HEALTH HISTORY—ITS NATURE AND PURPOSE

Nature of the Health History. Its Purpose and Importance. Elmer L. DeGowin and Richard L. DeGowin *define* the health history as "an account of the events in the patient's life that have relevance to his mental and physical health. Much more than the patient's unprompted narrative, it is a specialized literary form in which the physician [or other] composes and writes an account based upon facts supplied by the patient or other informants offered spontaneously or secured by skillful

---

* Prior, John A., and Silberstein, Jack S.: *Physical Diagnosis. The History and Examination of the Patient.* C. V. Mosby Co., St. Louis, 1973, p. 27.

probing. Items are accepted for the record only after rigorous evaluation by the physician, who employs his knowledge of the natural history of diseases to secure pertinent details and establish the sequence of events." *

Richard D. Judge and George D. Zuidema [80] say in effect that the *objectives* (or purposes) in history-taking are the following: (1) getting to know and understand the patient and his or her environment; (2) eliciting diagnostic information; (3) helping the physician to know what to focus on in the physical examination; (4) learning the patient's functional disabilities; (5) suggesting appropriate laboratory studies; (6) sowing "the seeds of future therapy." History-taking also gives the patient a chance to "size up" the physician.

In any type of health examination the subject's health history is of the *greatest importance*. MacBryde and Blacklow quote a "master diagnostician" as saying "Let me take the history and I will accept any good intern's word on the physical findings." †

Prior and Silberstein [81] say that while it is both "possible" and "probable" that computerized health histories will "become routine," the personal interview method of history-taking must be learned and used for the present. This involves listening, observing, synthesizing, and integrating the information the patient provides. All information recorded in the past about the patient, whether it is physical or laboratory findings, is part of the patient's history and is important information to incorporate in his or her record.

Nurses, social workers, medical students when present, and nonmedical personnel, as well as physicians, elicit and record the client's, or patient's, health history. Patients themselves and relatives and parents or guardians of infants and children give the information, and, as noted earlier, use is often made of automated systems of data collection.

George L. Engel and William L. Morgan, Jr. [82] say that questions about symptoms (current symptoms especially) should be asked so that the respondent will give the following information: (1) where the symptom is *located* in the body; (2) its *quality*—what it is like; (3) its *quantity*, or how intense it is; (4) its *chronology*—when it began and the course it has followed; (5) *the setting*—under what circumstances it occurs; (6) what *aggravates* or *relieves* it; and (7) what other symptoms or *phenomena* are *associated with it*.

While many physicians, discussing the health history, say that the process of "taking" it establishes rapport with the patient which is hard to establish in any other way, they recognize that writing a health history is time-consuming and admit that few busy doctors can write extensive histories for all their patients. Some ways of conserving the physician's time are (1) to use preprinted health history forms to reduce the amount of writing necessary; (2) to dictate histories into recorders and have them typed by nonmedical personnel; (3) to have nonphysician health personnel interview patients and write the histories; (4) to use automated devices for data gathering; and (5) to have patients themselves answer questionnaires.

Records Made by Patients, or Clients, and by Parents or Guardians. Booklets are sometimes presented to mothers of newborn infants in which it is suggested that they keep a health record until the boy or girl is able to keep the record. Such books provide a health history that can be used throughout the individual's lifetime. It has also been suggested that health agencies give people Xeroxed or microfilmed copies of their medical records so that this mobile generation can always carry the record with them as they move from place to place. Such records can be wallet size.[83] Some communities are establishing communication systems with computerized data banks that make information available by teletype on request from professional health workers in certain types of health institutions and agencies. There is some inherent danger in this practice, however, because confidential information is no longer confidential and the patient loses control over the information disseminated.

The Patient's Medical History based on a questionnaire has been discussed and is shown on page 360. These questions, answered by the patient, constitute a health history of a sort. They are designed to help the health examiners concentrate on the more significant points, or on the patient's problems. The questionnaire answered by the patient on a conventional punch card in the Kaiser-Permanente System and that answered by the patient sitting at a computer terminal used in the Weed System (see page 359) are all parts of, or forms of, health histories. In the Weed System, described in Chapter 4, the history is part of what is called the "data base" on which all aspects of care and treatment are planned and given. The use of data supplied by the patient in response to written questions seems to be gaining ground. D. P. Goldberg's [84] monograph, *The*

* DeGowin, Elmer L., and DeGowin, Richard L.: *Bedside Diagnostic Examination*, 3rd ed. Macmillan Publishing Co., Inc., New York, 1976, p. 12.

† MacBryde, Cyril M., and Blacklow, Robert Stanley (eds.): *Signs and Symptoms: Applied Pathologic Physiology and Clinical Interpretation*, 5th ed. J. B. Lippincott Co., Philadelphia, 1970, p. xi.

Detection of Psychiatric Illness by Question-naire (1972), is an example of the acceptance of this practice.

Health Histories for the Use of All or Different Types of Health Workers. Health histories (and data bases) vary greatly in value. Written questionnaires and forms filled in by patients may or may not elicit the kind and amount of information the physician, the nurse, the clinical psychologist, or the social worker think they need in order to give the particular help each of these workers believes they are uniquely prepared to give. When this is the case, each class of worker may collect supplementary information, or data.

Some nurses, who find histories taken by physicians an inadequate base for planning nursing care, advocate a separate "nursing history" for each patient [85]; Dorothy M. Smith [86] calls a nursing history guide a "clinical nursing tool." An outline for a nursing history is shown in Chapter 8, page 582. The writer of this chapter believes that the best interests of both patients and workers are served by having a common data base that all health workers contribute to and use. The writer also thinks, however, that full patient participation is desirable and that nurses, as well as doctors, can be prepared to interview effectively and write health histories when questionnaires answered by patients are unavailable or do not supply the needed information.*

Any discussion of the health history and who should elicit the information must take into account the patient's attitude toward and ability to reveal himself or herself in an interview. A health history necessitates for the client, or patient, answering very personal questions. Health histories should give those who

refer to them mental pictures of the subjects —their appearance and attitude, their mental status, their positions in the family or the social groups to which they belong, their places in the community, their occupations and major interests, their economic and educational status, their past and present health status and particularly their reasons for seeking help. In asking and recording questions that elicit such information, interviewers establish a relationship with respondents that can be an asset or a deterrent in subsequent decision making on treatment. The person who expects to play the leading role in diagnosis and therapy may well demand the privilege of "taking" the health history.

Maria C. Phaneuf [87] has summarized years of experience and research in evaluating nursing on the basis of records in a volume entitled *The Nursing Audit: Profile for Excellence.* With Mabel A. Wandelt, Phaneuf [88] describes three instruments for measuring the quality of nursing care that have items ranging from 50 to 85 in number. Evaluating care, as described by records in community health nursing agencies and hospitals, has impressed Phaneuf and Wandelt with the inadequacy of the data bases nurses themselves develop in public health nursing services and with the failure to make appropriate use (or any use) of the health (or medical) histories in hospitalized patients' records. Phaneuf asks "What is most conducive to the health and well-being of patients?" and gives the following answer:

For nurses, the answer to that question must rest on a demonstrated clinical base which is associated with explicit nursing judgments recorded on patients' charts. Experience with auditing suggests that more nursing emphasis on data and on explicit judgments, combined with a more disciplined intellectual nursing approach to care and to physicians—who also have their problems of quality appraisal—will facilitate the urgently needed changes in health care and health services delivery systems.*

Information Collected by Interviewing. It is so generally thought that health and welfare workers invade the privacy of those they try to help that books, plays, and cartoons parody the subject. Interviewing is an art that all health workers must cultivate. While some personalities intuitively invite trust or confidence, and avoid offending, the science of interviewing is based on a knowledge of personality development and psychotherapy. The writings of Gordon W. Allport, [88a] Erik H. Erikson, [89] Sid-

---

* The value of a health history taken during an interview with a nurse was demonstrated in the University Health Service at Yale University, New Haven, Conn. A physician (John S. Hathaway), a social scientist (James S. Davie), and a nurse (Helene Fitzgerald) report a 4-year study in which three ways of assessing the health status of new students were evaluated as well as the students' subsequent use of the University Health Service. One group of first-year students had a "screening-health interview" with a nurse, the second had a physical examination by a physician, and the third had both. The interview by the nurse was more effective than the physical examination alone and about as effective as the examination with the interview as judged by the number of health problems identified (referrals made), the students' satisfaction with the Health Service, and the subsequent use made of it. (Hathaway, John S.: "A Report of the Four-Year Study Conducted at Yale's Department of University Health on the Role of the Nurse in a University Health Service," *Nurs. Outlook,* **10:**533, [Aug.] 1962; Davie, James S.: "How Students Viewed Their Health Service," *Nurs. Outlook,* **10:**534, [Aug.] 1962; Fitzgerald, Helene, et al.: "A New Dimension to the Nurse's Role," *Nurs. Outlook,* **10:**535, [Aug.] 1962.)

* Phaneuf, Maria C.: *The Nursing Audit: Profile for Excellence.* Appleton-Century-Crofts, New York, 1972, p. 109.

ney M. Jourard,[90,91] Carl Jung,[92] R. D. Laing,[93] Abraham H. Maslow,[94,95] Rollo May,[96] Carl R. Rogers,[97-99] and Harry Stack Sullivan [100] are cited often throughout this text; study of such works will help develop interviewing competence. Psychiatric nurses, as for instance Florence G. Blake,[101] Florence Erickson,[102] Joan King,[103] Hildegard E. Peplau,[104-106] and Gwen E. Tudor [107] have applied theories of human development and therapeutic counseling to nursing. Nursing journals abound in articles on *interviewing* and Loretta Sue Bermosk and Mary Jane Mordan [108] have a monograph on the subject. Jon C. Marshall (an educator) and Sally Feeney [109] (a nurse) report a comparative study of structured versus intuitive interviews. Ethel K. Gozzi and Marie J. Morris (nurses) and Barbara M. Korsch [110] (a physician) identified gaps and blocks in doctor-patient communication and what made for noncompliance with advice. Some of the blocks were interrupting; making vague or argumentative comments; ignoring or switching the subject of the person's remarks; continuing to talk after asking a question; failing to respond to a question; deprecating or challenging the subject's comment; using jargon; and failing to definitely open an interview, state its purpose, and close it. All health personnel tend to block communication in these ways and must make a conscious effort to avoid them. William C. Fowkes, Jr., and Virginia K. Hunn,[111] among many others, say that there is a tendency on the part of medical care providers to approach patients in an authoritarian way, which is inappropriate and tends to stimulate a childish response from the patient. Malleson [112] says "help can be lethal" and says "the baby help" we give fosters dependency.

Jourard, in his volume *Disclosing Man to Himself* (which is addressed to experimental psychologists and psychotherapists) and in his article "The Bedside Manner" (addressed to nurses), makes a plea for naturalness and spontaneity in the interviewer. He believes a person will disclose himself to another if he is convinced that it will help him or her and that the information is to be used for his or her benefit and not for the benefit of an institution the interviewer is serving. A nonjudgmental attitude on the part of the interviewer is essential. Jourard believes that people are more likely to reveal themselves to those who are themselves open. Discussing "the dyadic effect" he says:

Research in self-disclosure has shown that what a person will disclose to another is a function of many variables, including the subject matter to be disclosed, characteristics of the person, the setting in which disclosure is to take place, and—more important—characteristics of the audience-person. The most powerful determiner of self-disclosure appears to be the willingness of the audience [listener] to disclose *himself* to the subject to the same extent that he expects the subject to confide his experience . . . "disclosure begets disclosure." *

A physician or nurse getting a health history from a person whom they can see eats too much or one whom they suspect drinks too much often get denials, whereas the obese patient will be honest at a Weight Watchers meeting and the alcoholic will talk freely about how much and why he or she drinks when talking with members of Alcoholics Anonymous.

People are said to give "a good history" if they answer questions honestly, but the interviewer must realize that fear of disapproval makes this honesty difficult for the patient. People are, generally speaking, ashamed of or guilty about illness and disability. Face to face with the health expert—physician, clinical psychologist, nurse, or other type of worker— they are more likely to belittle than exaggerate signs and symptoms of disease. Jourard says:

Healthy personality is manifested by a mode of being that we can call authenticity, or more simply honesty. Less healthy personalities, people who function less than fully, who suffer recurrent breakdowns or chronic impasses, may usually be found to be *liars*. They say things they do not mean. Their disclosures have been chosen more for cosmetic value than for truth. . . .

One of the reasons less healthy personalities are so selfconscious, so deliberate in their choice of word and action before others, is that they dread letting something slip out that truly expresses their being, something which will get them into trouble. They are, as it were, idolators of the state of artificial grace known as "staying out of trouble." †

Jourard believes that if people are sufficiently "sensitive," "imaginative," and "courageous," they recognize signals, such as pain, fatigue, boredom, anxiety, depression, or feeling of futility that suggest a change of life that might prevent a breakdown. But, Jourard says, change takes courage, and he thinks the capacity for self-awareness and other life-saving qualities are "usually trained out of people" while growing up. After the person has broken down, the medical profession "springs to action to repair the damage so the person again can take his place in a system that is crushing him" but he will sicken again.

Jourard also believes that physicians "persist

* Jourard, Sidney M.: *op. cit.,* p. 24.
† *Ibid.,* p. 41.

in treating symptoms of illness with a drug or knife" rather than "inquiry into the patient's way of life." He thinks psychiatrists have followed the examples of their medical colleagues and that most health workers and ministers fall in with the medical view. He says "I think that the healing professions have not addressed themselves wholeheartedly to the task of healing, but rather to the task of repairing people for more bad use of themselves." * Malleson,[113] a physician, in the monograph *Need Your Doctor Be So Useless?* presents a similar argument and is especially persuasive in making the point that drugs are prescribed injudiciously and as a result of superficial histories or study of the patient's problems.

Effective history-taking begins with simple courtesy. The examiner's manner is of great importance. A too hearty or too cheerful welcome suggests that he or she is unaware that the patient is anxious, frightened, or in pain. Bettelheim [113a] makes the point that with the emotionally disturbed patient, especially, he or she should be allowed to stay at a "social distance" from the interviewer. Examiners should introduce themselves and should greet patients by name. According to the culture from which patients come they should use the appropriate form of address, as, for example, "Mr.," "Miss," "Doctor," or "Father"; they should *not* ordinarily call youths and adults by their first names. Examiners should ask family members or friends of adolescents, youths, and adults to participate in the interview only after discussing this with the subject. The person or persons to be interviewed should be made comfortable in a sitting or recumbent position (according to their condition) and as much privacy assured as is possible in the available setting. When the examiner does not speak the client's language an interpreter of the same sex and comparatively the same age as an adult client should be used if available.

A *few rules for interviewing* might include the following: Greet the client, or patient (and companions if possible) by name, using the appropriate forms of address for youths and adults as "Mr.," "Miss," and "Mrs." or other, as above; introduce yourself and give your function (a nurse † for example); seat patients comfortably facing the interviewer or have

them lie down if their condition indicates it; watch clients and try to adjust the wording of questions to their level of comprehension and, to some extent, to their cultural bias. Use a written guide in interviewing, and take notes or record responses unless this seems to inhibit the respondent. Clients may be struggling against fear, embarrassment, anger, reserve, skepticism, or surprise about the health worker's need for knowing so much about them. In contrast, some people are delighted to have the opportunity to tell someone about their medical problems. Try to understand patients' difficulties and conduct the interview in such a way as to overcome them if possible. If using a tape recorder, be sure that the patient understands and accepts its purpose and the way the tape is to be used. The patient's permission to record the interview on tape must be recorded on the tape.

The Family as the Client or Patient. It is generally accepted that effective health care depends upon seeing and treating individuals as members of a family or a social unit of some sort. To make the point, public health nurses say "the family is the patient." Catherine W. Tinkham and Eleanor F. Voorhies,[114] in their text *Community Health Nursing: Evolution and Process,* show a 7-page questionnaire to be used as a guide to "Family Data Collection" by the nurse. Some questions could be answered in writing by the head of a household but they are constructed principally as a guide to the nurse. Questions are grouped under the following headings: I. Family Characteristics; II. Socioeconomic and Cultural Factors; III. Environmental Factors; IV. Health and Medical History; and V. Summary. The questions under Summary are: "What are the family health problems?" "To which of the family health problems *can* nursing make a contribution?" "To which of the family health problems *should* nursing make a contribution? Why?" "Which of the family health problems should nursing *leave alone?* Why?" and "What are the family nursing needs that you will give first priority? Second priority? Third priority? and so forth."

The Peckham Experiment: A Study of the Living Structure of Society is the title under which a family health experiment in England was reported. Innes Pearse and Lucy H. Crocker [115] described the work in a health center where the family (never the individual) registered and where the family was interviewed as a group by the health workers on admission to the program. The report of the experiment had great influence, as did Henry B. Richardson's [116] family health study in Baltimore, Md., reported by him under the title

---

* *Ibid.,* pp. 39, 40.

† When nurses in physicians' offices, hospitals schools, industries, or other places take over health assessment procedures with patients who are accustomed to having doctors perform this function, the change should be explained to them—possibly by the doctors of that staff or health service. It is especially important for the nurse to clarify his or her role to avoid having the client assume he or she is a physician.

Patients Have Families. Both studies showed the effect on health of human relationships and the waste of effort in treating symptoms without identifying and, if possible, eliminating their causes. Malleson [117] uses the Peckham experiment as the prototype of the community health centers that he thinks are the essential building block of a health care delivery system.

According to the purpose of the health examination and whether the client or patient is an individual or a family, the forms selected for health histories vary. Some types are shown in the following pages.

5. STEPS IN HISTORY-TAKING AND SOME HEALTH HISTORY FORMS

The traditional steps in collecting information or writing a health (or medical) history seem to have influenced the forms used, or the sequence of topics. Identifying data comes first on all forms. The "chief complaint" and "present illness" are likely to follow, and to precede the past health history, the personal and "social history," and the "family history"; also, "the review of systems," or the review of functions.

Medical care in the United States and many "Western" countries has focused on curative rather than preventive medicine and it may be that the forms used for health (or medical) histories are designed primarily to meet the needs of the most critically ill. The doctor or other medical worker questioning the patient, the child's parent or guardian, the adolescent youth, or the adult wants to know the "chief complaint" and "present illness" because emergency measures may be demanded. If patients are hemorrhaging, for example, or if they have an extremely high fever, or if they are delirious or comatose, it may be desirable to institute therapy before getting the necessary social and family history for a complete therapeutic regimen. In practicing preventive medicine it might, on the other hand, be desirable to get the social and family history before going into the history of past illnesses and such current health problems as the patients or parents are able to identify.

The Cornell Medical Index-Health Questionnaire, now called simply The Medical History (see page 360), emphasizes a nontraditional or preventive approach, as does the multiphasic screening process at the Kaiser-Permanente program discussed in this chapter (see page 380). In both cases the physician, or health consultant, is given a wealth of data supplied by the patient. This data is studied before the

health consultant or giver of "primary care" questions the client or patient.

In Lawrence L. Weed's system of medical management, discussed in Chapter 4, and illustrated with a patient study and the forms used in the Medical Center of the University of Vermont at Burlington, a computerized problem-oriented type of data base is shown. It should be reviewed under this topic. In this chapter several of the problem-oriented types of records recommended by the National League for Nursing for community health nursing are shown (see Chap. 3, Fig. 3-10). Forms used for health histories in schools and industrial health services vary greatly in design and scope. The ones shown on pages 219 and 237 are not necessarily typical.

Health (or medical) histories used in most hospitals still follow the traditional pattern. The outlines given by DeGowin and DeGowin and by Morgan and Engel and others are very similar. The following is a composite of the categories under which data is traditionally organized in the medical interview:

1. *Present illness*—refers to those recent changes in health that led the patient to seek health care and should describe the patient's symptoms in succinct, chronologic terms.
2. *Past health*—refers to an over-all appraisal of the patient's general health and includes an orderly review of all previous illnesses (both childhood and adult), hospitalizations, operations, accidents, injuries, obstetric history, psychiatric illnesses, allergies, immunizations, and bleeding tendency.
3. *Family health*—covers the health of the immediate family (parents and siblings) of the patient with age and health or age at death and causes. Particular attention is paid to diseases of recognized familial importance.
4. *Personal and social history*—includes birthplace and residence of the patient, marital status and children, education, military service, occupational history, economic status, leisure activities, and habits with regard to use of drugs, coffee, alcohol, and tobacco.
5. *Review of systems*—outlines the salient features and positive findings under each "system."

The "systems review," a term commonly used, really includes questions designed to identify pathology or abnormal functions in organs and areas of the body as well as in whole systems or even a combination of systems (see Fig. 5-4). The following symptoms are usually considered under each "system," according to

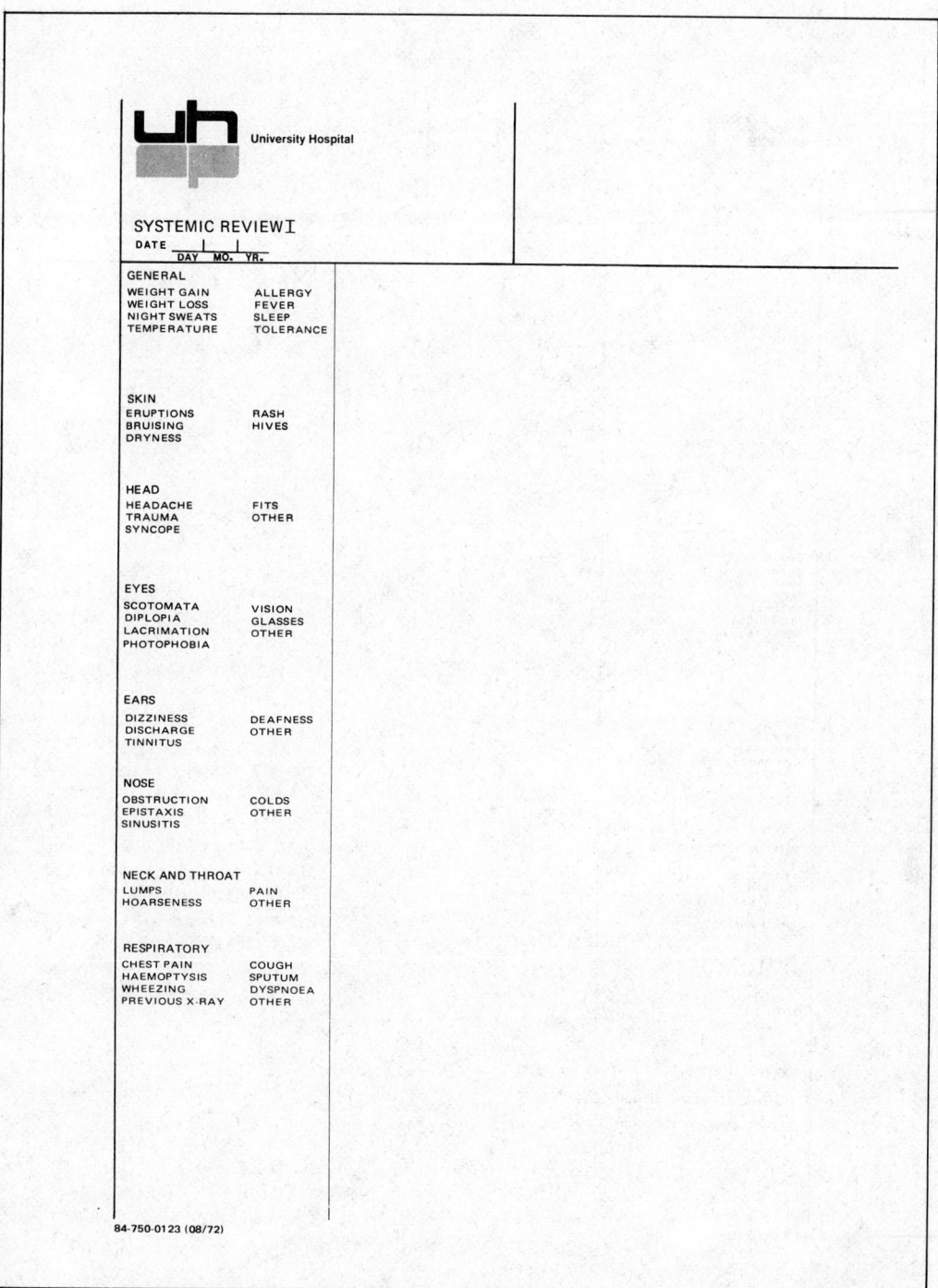

Figure 5-4. Examples of "systems review" recording form. (Courtesy of University Hospital, University of Western Ontario, London, Ont.)

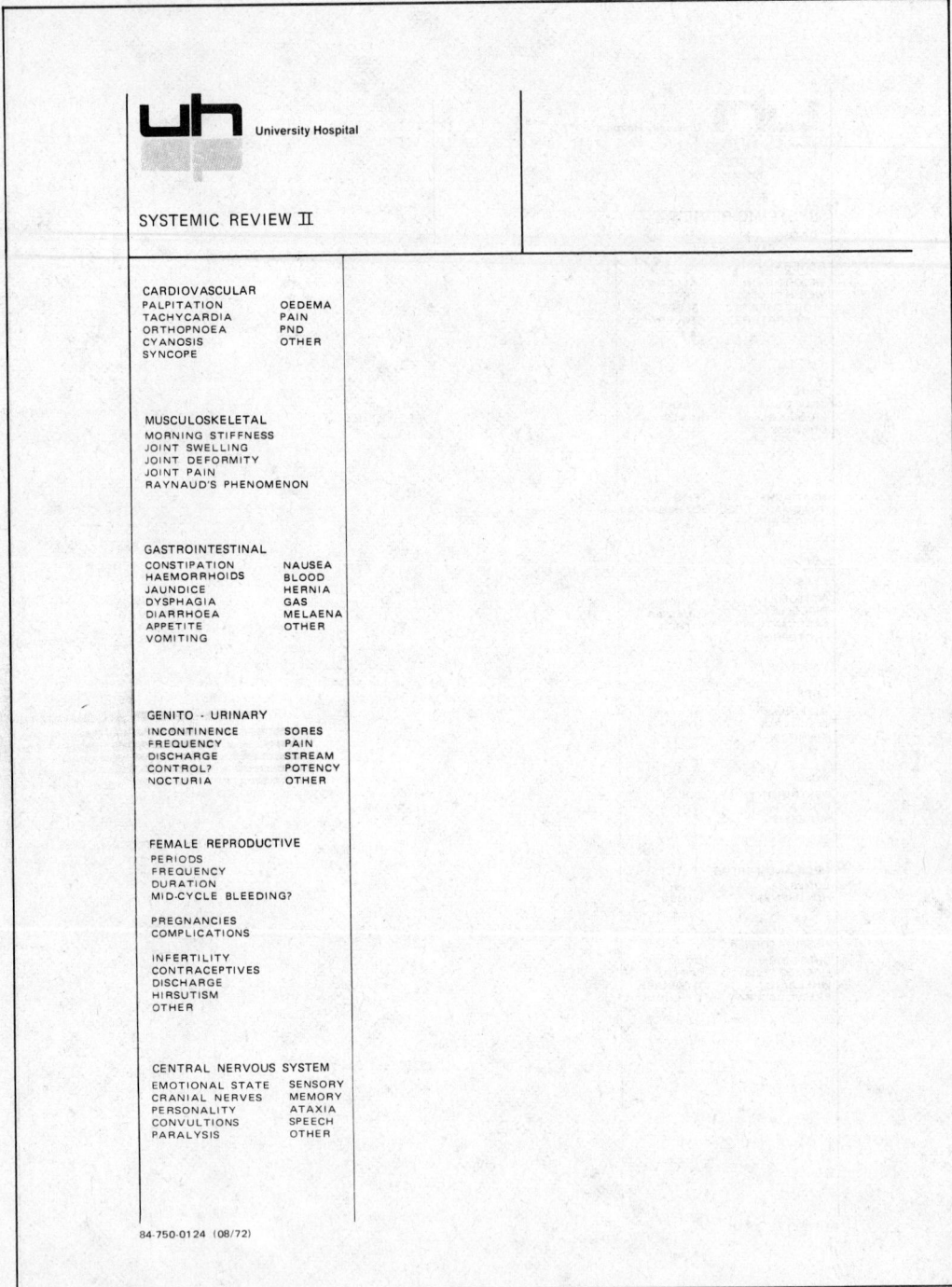

University Hospital

SYSTEMIC REVIEW II

CARDIOVASCULAR
PALPITATION   OEDEMA
TACHYCARDIA   PAIN
ORTHOPNOEA   PND
CYANOSIS   OTHER
SYNCOPE

MUSCULOSKELETAL
MORNING STIFFNESS
JOINT SWELLING
JOINT DEFORMITY
JOINT PAIN
RAYNAUD'S PHENOMENON

GASTROINTESTINAL
CONSTIPATION   NAUSEA
HAEMORRHOIDS   BLOOD
JAUNDICE   HERNIA
DYSPHAGIA   GAS
DIARRHOEA   MELAENA
APPETITE   OTHER
VOMITING

GENITO - URINARY
INCONTINENCE   SORES
FREQUENCY   PAIN
DISCHARGE   STREAM
CONTROL?   POTENCY
NOCTURIA   OTHER

FEMALE REPRODUCTIVE
PERIODS
FREQUENCY
DURATION
MID-CYCLE BLEEDING?

PREGNANCIES
COMPLICATIONS

INFERTILITY
CONTRACEPTIVES
DISCHARGE
HIRSUTISM
OTHER

CENTRAL NERVOUS SYSTEM
EMOTIONAL STATE   SENSORY
CRANIAL NERVES   MEMORY
PERSONALITY   ATAXIA
CONVULTIONS   SPEECH
PARALYSIS   OTHER

84-750-0124 (08/72)

Figure 5-4 (*continued*).

Morgan and Engel, Sherman and Fields, and others:

Skin—color changes, itching (pruritus), bruising, petechiae, birthmarks, moles, infections, rashes; hair loss or changes; and changes in nails.

Hematopoietic—anemia; transfusions, and reactions, with dates; spontaneous or excessive bleeding after tooth extraction, tonsillectomy, minor injury, or excessive bruising; enlarged, tender, or suppurative nodes.

Head and face—headache, facial pain, trauma.

Ears—pain; discharge; ringing, roaring, hissing (tinnitus); deafness; dizziness (vertigo).

Eyes—vision; glasses (date last checked); pain, inflammation, infections; double vision (diplopia); blurring, spots before the eyes (scotomata).

Nose and sinuses—bleeding (epistaxis), obstruction, discharge, postnasal drip, sinus pain.

Mouth, pharynx, and larynx—sores, bleeding gums, teeth (abscesses, extractions, dentures, date last checked); sore tongue; sore throat; hoarseness; difficulty in swallowing.

Breasts—discharge from nipples; lumps; pain.

Respiratory tract—cough, change in chronic cough; sputum—nature, amount, presence of blood (hemoptysis); wheeze; pleuritis pain; night sweat; date of last chest film.

Cardiovascular system—chest pain on exertion; difficult breathing (dyspnea) on exertion; nocturnal dyspnea; position for sleep; dependent edema; palpitation; high blood pressure; known murmur; pain on exertion (especially calf); varicosities.

Gastrointestinal system—appetite, thirst; nausea, vomiting; bleeding (hematemesis); food idiosyncrasies; gas, belching, sour eructations; trouble swallowing food; heartburn; abdominal pain; jaundice; bowel movements (frequency, diarrhea, constipation, presence of blood, dark [tarry] stools, change in bowel habits, use of laxatives); hemorrhoids; presence of hernia.

Urinary tract—difficult or painful urination (dysuria); unusual color; excessive amount (polyuria); frequency, urgency, nocturia; burning; blood in urine (hematuria); stones; trouble with stream; incontinence, bed-wetting (enuresis); retention; generalized edema.

Genital tract (male)—blood in urine; penile discharge or lesion; history of syphilis (positive serology); testicular pain or swelling.

Genital tract (female)—menstrual history (age of onset, characteristics of first periods, frequency, regularity, duration of flow, pads or tampons per day, date of last period, associated symptoms); intermenstrual or postmenopausal bleeding, discharge; itching (pruritus); contraceptive pills or devices; menopause (age and symptoms); evidence of venereal disease (abscess, genital lesion, positive serology).

Skeletal system—pain in extremities, back, or neck; stiffness; limitation of motion; joint swelling, heat, redness; grating sound on movement (crepitation); sprains; deformity.

Nervous system—convulsions, fainting (syncope), dizziness, vertigo; tremor, ataxia, speech difficulty; muscle atrophy or tenderness, limp, weakness or paralysis; perversions of feeling—crawling, tingling, burning (paresthesia); loss of feeling (anesthesia).

Endocrine system—goiter; tremor; intolerance of heat or cold, sweating; protruding eyes (exophthalmos); voice change; excessive eating (polyphagia); excessive voiding (polyuria); excessive thirst or drinking (polydysia); change in body contour; change in glove or shoe size or hair distribution; infertility.

Psychologic status—nervousness, irritability; memory loss; depression; phobias; insomnia, nightmares; impotence, frigidity; sexual disturbances; criminal or other sociopathic behavior.

The questions designed to assess the psychologic or mental status, the intelligence, and emotional stability of the individual might be considered a part of the history, but in this chapter they are discussed more specifically as part of the examination.

Henry K. Silver and his associates,[118] outlining the health or medical history for the pediatrician, include the headings "Development," "Nutrition," "Personality History," and "Habits." It is possible that these topics also have bearing on the health of adults. In getting a child's, adolescent's, or youth's history it is important to let the subject speak for himself or herself as much as possible. As stated earlier in the chapter, adolescents and youths should be asked whether they want parents, guardians, or friends with them during any part of health examinations.

While the "systems review" headings may remain in their traditional form for many years, they may some day be replaced with a list of functions, such as those given in Chapter 8.

William Houston [119] questioned the systems approach in his *Art of Treatment* (1933) and made a good case for organizing therapeutics around the main line of treatment, as, for example, specific drugs, psychotherapy, limitation of living, and nursing care. (The last category included treatment of patients with diseases of unknown origin for which supportive nursing care is the only recognized means of helping patients recover.) The "system," as used here, is an anatomic and static concept as compared with function, which is physiologic—psychologic and dynamic. Functions involve more than one system and hence relationships. The function, for instance, of communicating, or relating to others, involves speech and hearing, thought, touch, and other processes. This function, so essential to health, is hard to translate into the list of systems involved. Then, questions about a function have the merit of being immediately understood by patients and give them an opportunity to identify the health problem associated with it. The question "Have you trouble breathing?" for example may be answered with information about frequent colds, blocked air passages, shortness of breath, or chest pains. The question "Have you any problems in personal relationships, in communicating with, or relating to others?" may be answered with information about hearing or speech, about shyness, hostility, irritability, or withdrawal.

Since many nurses think of their role as that of helping patients with functions or activities of daily living, they may, when they take health histories, naturally ask such questions and identify self-help deficits under functional headings, either in addition to or as a substitute for the traditional "systems review." Whatever approach is used to history-taking the person collecting the data should, throughout the process, be making *estimates of the client's* insight and his or her capacity for self-care and need for help from health workers.

Joan E. Lynaugh, a nurse, and Barbara Bates, a physician, write about the two languages of nursing and medicine.* They say the "Central questions of the profession" are, for nursing, "What are the patient's problems, how is he coping with them and what help does he need?"; for medicine, "What is the patient's diagnosis and what treatment does he need?" "Phenomena" that nurses deal with are "discomfort, patient concern, vision, hearing, mobility, elimination, the patient with tuberculosis, the patient with disease of bones and joints"; phenomena that the physician deals with are "symptom, disease, eyes, ears, musculoskeletal and neurological systems, disease of the colon and rectum, diseases due to mycobacteria, diseases of joints." The "process of improving the patient's future health," as

nurses see it, is "promotion of health care and well-being, health care supervision"; this "process as the physician sees it is preventive medicine."

Lynaugh and Bates speak of the "person orientation" of nursing and the "disease orientation" of the physician. They say the doctor may be reluctant to dilute his hard-won scientific professional self-image with the "softer" orientation of the nurse. They say, however, that mutual understanding is "essential" and they reaffirm the folk-saying of their common purpose "To care sometimes, to relieve often, to comfort always." *

As nurses assume more and more responsibility for health assessment they may adopt the medical pattern uncritically and follow it slavishly. It is this writer's opinion that they should capitalize on their more "personal" and "softer" (psychosocial?) approach to facilitate the individualized, patient-problem-oriented type of health care advocated by so many critics of the present health care system.

Nurses have much to learn from physicians about health assessment but they might in turn help develop a procedure that is less anxiety-producing, more comfortable physically, more revealing of patient problems, and a learning experience for patients and families.

Engel and Morgan suggest the use of a family tree diagram (see Fig. 5-5) when considering familial transmission of disease. The family tree indicates the health history of each member of the family, whether living or dead, the age and any known illnesses, and the date and cause of death. It is important to include those illnesses not responsible for the deaths when there is a question of contagion, congenital influence, a genetic factor, or the psychologic impact of a parent's or sibling's illness. If sufficiently detailed or expanded, this family tree might be used later as an adjunct in *genetic counseling* of clients or patients on prospective or potential parenthood (see page 401).

Health histories may be taken in demographic † studies and the particular purpose of the study may determine the information sought. For example, a study of alcoholism may be designed to measure the relationship between the character of the alcoholism, the alcoholic's cultural background, economic

---

* Even this saying, attributed variously to Hippocrates and Maimonides, is questioned by certain therapists who make the point that, for some persons, profoundly disturbing them is the only way to help them give up a destructive way of living.

† Demography is the statistical study of human life and is concerned with data that describes the population's level, its housing, income, education, race, family size, vital statistics, and morbidity data.

---

* Lynaugh, Joan E., and Bates, Barbara: "The Two Languages of Nursing and Medicine," *Am. J. Nurs.,* **73:**66, (Jan.) 1973.

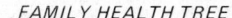

FAMILY HEALTH TREE

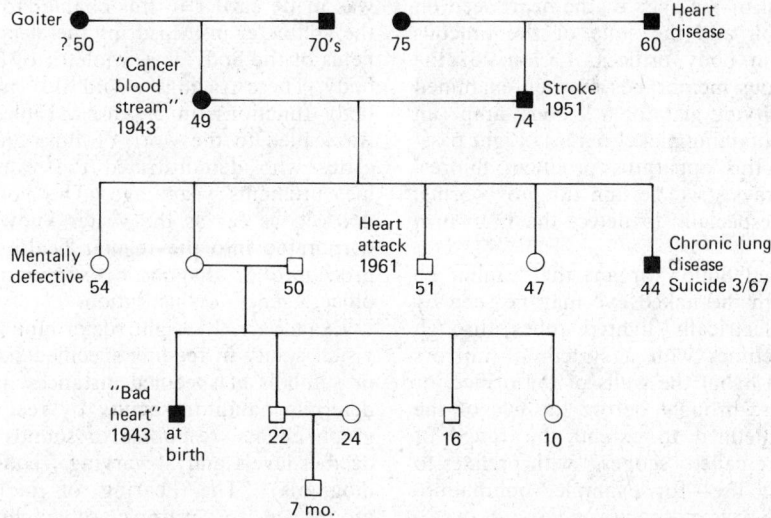

Figure 5-5. A family health tree. (From Morgan, William L., and Engel, George L.: *Interviewing the Patient*. W. B. Saunders Co., Philadelphia, 1973, p. 118.)

status, religious affiliation, position with relation to siblings, or his or her diet. Studies of alcoholism may also focus on liver damage and cardiovascular changes; studies of smoking on cardiovascular and respiratory signs and symptoms; while studies of schizophrenia would emphasize psychosocial aspects of the health history.

One of the commonest criticisms of current health services is their emphasis on episodic illness, on care and cure of the ill, as opposed to health guidance for the well—or preventive medicine. If the latter is ever given the attention it deserves, the health histories and the whole assessment process and the forms used may be materially altered to make them instructive for patients and families.

6. THE PHYSICAL EXAMINATION —ITS NATURE AND PURPOSE

Methods. Examiners, as one might expect, use their senses of sight, feeling, hearing, and even smell * in making judgments during health examinations, although natural powers of sight and hearing have been extended by instruments and laboratory analyses for judgments that might have been based at one time on odors from the body or its excretions.

* While current texts have very little to say about the use of smell in health examination, a recent article in a nursing journal raises and answers the question "What's the Meaning of That Patient's Odor?" (*Nurs. Update,* 2:12, [Apr.] 1971.)

Terms used in medical parlance for these universal functions of seeing, feeling, and hearing are inspection, palpation, percussion, and auscultation. In Chapter 4 the importance of observation was stressed, and Florence Nightingale was cited as saying that without the habit of "ready and correct observation" nurses would be "useless" with all their "devotion." In this chapter, the methods are defined and described and the observations made by anyone conducting a health examination, including a nurse, are discussed in the order in which they are traditionally made and recorded.

The term *Inspection* is used by Prior and Silberstein and by others to designate "a series of accurate and meaningful observations" which they say "involves the use of at least four of one's special senses—sight, hearing, touch, and to a lesser degree, smell." * In this chapter, inspection is used to mean observing with the naked eye or with lenses that magnify the object or area of inspection. The examiner notes by inspection the general behavior, the size of the body and its contour, posture, body movements, gait, state of nutrition, skin color,† presence of rashes, swelling, scars, and other visible signs of health and

* Prior, John A., and Silberstein, Jack S.: *op. cit.,* p. 47.

† Lora B. Roach, in an article "Assessment—Color Changes in Dark Skin," (*Nursing '72,* 2:19, [Nov.] 1972) says that judgments are not reliable unless the observer knew the "normal" appearance of the skin. She thinks that changes in the color of nailbeds and the sclera of the eyes may be of especial significance in the dark-skinned patient.

pathology. By inspection, the examiner also notes a thrust of the apex of the heart seen on the chest wall and the state of the mucous membranes in body orifices. Lesions of the skin or mucous membranes may be examined with a magnifying glass or a Woods lamp (an apparatus containing nickel oxide). Light passing through this apparatus produces fluorescence when rays strike certain fungi or worms; this is used especially to detect the ringworm (tinea).

Cavities and hollow organs that cannot be inspected with the naked eye may be seen by means of electrically lighted tubes through which (sometimes with a system of mirrors reflecting the light) the walls of the orifice, or the organ, are brought before the eye of the examiner. Intended to extend the range of sight, they are called "scopes," with prefixes to indicate their use—for example, ophthalmoscope for the eye, otoscope for the ear, cystoscope for the bladder, bronchoscope for the bronchi, and proctoscope for the rectum. Irmgard Belinsky and associates [119a] describe a flexible "fiberoptic colonoscope" that enables the examiner to see the colon as far as the ileocecal junction.

Tissues in any part of the body are made visible, in a sense, *by x-rays.* The outlines of dense tissues, for example, bones, are most easily seen in roentgenograms, and hollow organs can be filled with opaque substances and made more visible. Certain deductions can be made about soft tissues by their radio image on x-ray. *Microscopic photographs* extend the powers of sight to include objects invisible to the naked eye. When polarized light (light made to vibrate in a single plane) is thrown on an object under the microscope, internal structures within living and dead tissues are seen in a wide range of colors. This development in the microscopic examination of tissue makes it possible to learn far more than was learned from staining techniques used in the past for identification of cell and tissue structure. Thomas E. Everhart and Thomas L. Hayes [120] describe and illustrate in *Scientific American* the dramatic and varied uses of the *scanning electron microscope* (see also Chapter 6).

The value of *ultrasound* in producing pictures is said in some instances to provide better information than x-rays. It has been demonstrated in the laboratory and has been put to clinical use in obstetrics, for example, at Yale-New Haven Hospital, to identify the location of the placenta, to diagnose multiple pregnancy, a hydatidiform mole, or tumors, or to locate remnants after an abortion.

Machines are available that trace electric charges within the heart and brain, making their function to some extent visible. Reference was made earlier in this chapter to the use of the voltmeter in measuring the electromagnetic fields of the body as a whole or of parts of the body. These tracings would also make certain body functions, in a sense, visible. Attention was called to the work of Burr and his associates who demonstrated the value of such measurements years ago. The voltmeter has not yet, as far as the writer knows, been incorporated into the regular health assessment procedure or diagnostic examination of any office, agency, or institution.

Examiners, by sight, determine the client's visual acuity in reading specified sizes of types or symbols at specified distances; just as they determine auditory acuity by recording on a graph clients' responses to sounds at various decibel levels and at varying frequencies (audiograms). The hearing of individuals in groups, as, for example, schoolchildren, may be tested by having them put into writing what they hear of recorded language. This is believed to be a crude measurement as compared to others described here and for this reason is seldom if ever used. Chapter 7, dealing with diagnostic tests, describes many of the procedures mentioned here in more detail, as do some references listed at the end of this chapter.

Palpation is the medical term for feeling with the hands. Examiners by palpation determine the rate and character of the pulse, the vibrations transmitted through the chest wall, the size and position of lymph nodes in the neck and of organs of the abdomen and pelvis that can be felt through the abdominal wall or through the rectum or vagina. Some of the organs are always palpable and any changes in size, shape, and location can usually be felt; others are palpable only when enlarged or displaced, or when diseased.

By palpation the examiner can get a fairly accurate idea of the body's muscular tone. The tension on walls of blood vessels and hollow organs exerted by their contents can be roughly estimated by palpation. The tonometer is an instrument used to measure the intraocular pressure more accurately than it can be measured by feeling the eyeball through the closed lid.

Before *thermometers* were invented the body's temperature was estimated by how warm it felt. While experienced clinicians might make fairly accurate estimates of fever, thermometry has almost universally replaced assessment by feeling. The rise and fall of the chest can be both seen and felt in determining respiratory rate and the latter method is commonly used. During periods of critical illness, the temperature, heart and respiratory rates, blood pressure, and even the electric activity of the brain and heart may be monitored constantly so that changes can be seen immediately by tracings on the monitor. (For further discussion of this, see Chapter 6.)

Percussion is the tapping of a body area to determine the character of the internal part by the sounds produced (see Fig. 5-17). It is therefore dependent on the examiner's hearing and especially the technique used. The middle finger of one hand is held flat on the area to be examined with the other fingers held *off* the skin. Prior and Silberstein [121] say the examiner should strike the base of the distal phalanx of the middle finger with a short quick blow from the tip of the middle finger of the other hand. The entire action should come from the wrist, the forearm uninvolved. Jacques L. Sherman and Sylvia Kleiman Fields [122] show "blunt percussion" used to detect tenderness of the liver and kidney. One hand is laid flat on the skin over the area and the back of the hand struck with the fist of the other hand.

Percussion is particularly useful in examining the thorax or chest. It is by no means a new method, for it was discovered in 1761 by a physician named Auenbrugger. He, however, was the only one to use it. And so it had almost disappeared when, according to Howard W. Haggard [123] in *The Doctor in History*, a French physician, Corvisart, revived its use and wrote a book on the subject many years later. Since then, it has been an indispensable part of every examination. Percussion is based on the fact that a hollow organ such as the lung, if filled with air, gives a characteristic sound when tapped, but if consolidated or if there are areas of imperfect expansion (atelectasis), it gives a duller sound. Therefore, it is possible to find out whether the lungs are well aerated, imperfectly expanded, or congested.

Auscultation is the medical term for listening to sounds in the body. The ear may be held against the body, but it is more common to use a stethoscope (*stethos*—breast or chest, and *skopein*—see, look). According to Haggard, Rene Laennec invented this instrument quite by accident. He had been unable to hear sounds through the chest wall of an obese patient. One day he saw some children tapping on a wooden beam and listening to the sounds produced at the other end. Seeing that the same principle could be used to solve his difficulty, he rolled a paper, put one end on a patient's chest and his ear to the other. He could hear the sounds very well. The modern stethoscope consists of two rubber tubes, one end of each being connected to a small earpiece, the other end to a disk or cone- or bell-shaped device through which the sounds are transmitted. Auscultation is used in examination of the heart, lungs, arteries, and abdomen where variations in sounds are important. The stethoscope is simply a device to facilitate hearing. Because the sounds are often faint and the difference between them slight, the room should be very quiet during auscultation and both bell- or cone-shaped ends for the stethoscope available.

Sister Janet Lehman, a cardiovascular nursing specialist, makes the following comment about the use of the disc and cone or bell stethoscope in an article on auscultation of heart sounds:

The ability to hear these sounds on the chest wall depends both on the intensity and frequency of the vibrations and on the use of the stethoscope. The diaphragm of the stethoscope is used to hear high-pitched sounds, which include both components of the first heart sound, both components of the second heart sound, and the ejection clicks [extra heart sounds early in systole] and opening snaps of the heart valves. The bell of the stethoscope is used to hear low-pitched sounds, which include third and fourth heart sounds and most murmurs.*

Machines used for health assessment, designed to extend or make more accurate the examiner's measurements by their unaided senses, are being developed daily. It is almost impossible to keep up with them. Other machines are discussed in Chapter 7.

The role of *laboratory tests* in making health estimates and diagnosing disease is increasingly prominent. On page 386 the tests commonly advocated for periodic health examinations were listed. Those used in diagnostic examination would include all these and additional tests according to the suspected pathology. It should be noted, however, in this connection that a common criticism of current-day Western medicine is the indiscriminate and costly use of laboratory tests and x-rays, the latter and some of the former involving risks to the patient.† Certain tests on urine and blood are routine; tests on feces of food handlers are obligatory in some areas. The contents of body cavities, discharges from wounds, and pieces of living tissue are examined by a variety of methods, the more frequently used of which are described in Chapter 7. Actually it is impossible in anything but a specialized text to give a true picture of the range of diagnostic methods now available.

---

* Lehman, Sister Janet: "Auscultation of Heart Sounds," *Am. J. Nurs.*, **72:**1242 (July) 1972.
† Particulary "scans."

Providing for the Client's or Patient's Comfort and That of Family Members or Friends. It is customary for the same person who takes the health history to do the physical examination. In such cases, *introductions,* and possibly *explanations,* have already been made. However, as pointed out earlier, there are various ways of collecting the data base and many persons and machines may be involved. If the person who conducts the physical examination is not the person who "took" the history, introductions and explanations must be made afresh and, even though he or she has studied the history (the data base), the examiner may find it necessary to repeat, for clarification, some of the questions previously asked the patient as the examination progresses. It should be stated emphatically that it is desirable for the same health worker to take the history and conduct the physical examination both from the patient's and examiner's viewpoints.

Parents or guardians usually stay with infants and small children during the physical examination to answer questions and reduce the psychologic trauma of the experience; adolescents, youths, and adults ordinarily prefer to exclude relatives and friends. The comfort of the patient must always be considered when deciding who does which part of the examination. When the examiner does not speak the client's language, an interpreter is, of course, necessary.

Physicians conducting physical examinations may want nursing personnel present throughout. If the physician is a man and the patient a woman, a nurse (or woman health worker of some sort) should be present during the pelvic examination for the patient's comfort and for the legal protection of both patient and physician, as has been noted.

Generalizations are always subject to question, but few would dispute the statement that a physical examination makes the subject apprehensive, and it is embarrassing to those unaccustomed to exposure of the entire body.[124] The promptness with which the client or patient is seen and the care with which the examination is carried out reduces the patient's anxiety, but the examiner's manner, and his or her sensitivity, is even more important. *Minimal* body exposure consistent with an effective examination is desirable. Only the area under examination should be exposed. Assuring patients of as much *privacy* as possible and making them physically as *comfortable* as possible are ways of expressing consideration for them, but both actually reduce tension, which is one source of their discomfort. *Warmth* also reduces tension, as does freedom from alarming or repellent sights, sounds, and odors. Warming the blankets covering the patient and the examiner's hands and warming instruments used, especially instruments inserted into body cavities, decreases discomfort. Psychologically, warmth can be provided with color in the furnishings of the room. Music may divert infants and children during parts of the physical examination.* Many informed and fastidious patients are reassured if they see examiners wash their hands before beginning examinations and at their termination. *Cleanliness* is not only important in preventing infection but in giving the patient a sense of security.

Facilities and Equipment. A *room* that will insure privacy is highly desirable; when this is not possible the space used for the examination can be made private to some extent with movable screens, sliding walls, or curtains. A dressing room or cubicle should adjoin the examining space with access for workers to handwashing facilities and for the patient to a toilet as well as a hand basin. A free-standing examining table or bed should enable the examiner (who may be either right- or left-handed) to work on either side in a comfortable position. Since most persons are right-handed, the examiner usually works from the right side. It is very desirable that the table be adjustable in height or, if not, a footstool attached, so that the patient can get on it easily. The examiner may sit for a part of the examination, as, for example, the pelvic examination. If the patient is examined in bed, a stool that will not tip must be available to enable short patients to get on and off the bed comfortably. Whether a table or bed, it should be so constructed that the patient can be supported in any position that may be essential to a satisfactory examination.

A cabinet for storing instruments is necessary and a movable table, or stand, on which are placed the articles used in the examination. A heating unit in the table or stand top to keep instruments warm is a comfort measure. A warming cabinet to store cotton blankets used to cover the patient should also be provided.

There should be space in the examining room or area for the patient to walk around so that the examiner can see whether the gaits, movements, or posture are normal. Eye examinations may require space but they are often conducted in a special area. An abbreviated eye examination may be done with the patient less than 20 ft away from the visual acuity chart, if a special chart designed

---

* I was impressed with the great beauty of a doctor's visiting and examining rooms in Florence, Italy. The walls were hung with paintings, the rooms spacious and elegantly furnished, the "clinical" objects reduced to a minimum. I couldn't but think that a physical examination in such surroundings might be quite different from one in the typical cold and sparse setting. [V. H.]

for this purpose is used. Chairs or stools should be available for the examiner and a parent of infants or children who may want, or be asked, to sit down during some parts of the examination.

Positions of Patients During Examinations. The initial position of the patient for examination is upright on the side of the examining table or bed with the examiner facing the patient for a general inspection, vital signs, and examination of the head and neck, thorax and lungs, breasts, axillary regions, and heart. Very ill persons may need support in a sitting position and in some cases the examiner may allow them to stay recumbent. Patients may lie on the back with legs extended or slightly flexed for comfort and to relax abdominal muscles for the next part of the examination. Flexion of the legs is especially important during the abdominal examination. A small pillow under the head is preferred by most persons. This is called the *horizontal recumbent* (supine) position.

The *dorsal recumbent* position is like the horizontal recumbent except that the legs are separated and flexed with the soles of the feet resting on the table or bed. If the female patient is on a table with no stirrups available, a pelvic examination may be performed in this position. The buttocks are brought to the very edge of the table while the feet rest on it. The vagina, internal organs, and rectum can be examined with the patient in this position.

Patients should be covered with a lightweight washable blanket except in hot weather when a sheet may be preferred. For a pelvic examination two blankets, sheets, or disposable paper sheets should be placed over the patient then separated so that both cover the trunk and each covers a leg, leaving the genitalia exposed.* Another method is to use one blanket or sheet over the lower part of the body with the middle part of the sheet raised and pushed back to expose the genitalia, while leaving the legs covered. For some patients, it is important to reduce exposure to a minimum because it decreases their embarrassment, but for everyone warmth is important since it relaxes muscles and facilitates the work of the examiner.

The following positions as described here and illustrated in Figure 5-6 may be occasionally or rarely used in examinations. For convenient reference the complete list is given:

The *dorsal lithotomy* position is the same as the dorsal recumbent except that the legs are

well separated and the thighs are acutely flexed on the abdomen and the legs on the thighs. The buttocks are brought to the extreme edge of the table or a little beyond. To maintain this position and further separate the legs, upright rods with stirrups attached are fastened to the sides of the table and the legs supported in the stirrups. The word lithotomy comes from two Greek words (*litho*—stone, and *tome*—incision). The position was so called because it was used in the operation for removing stones from the bladder. It is now used for cystoscopic examinations, examinations and operations on the perineum, vagina, cervix, bladder, and rectum. The draping is essentially the same as for the dorsal recumbent position.

In the *Sims*, or *left lateral-prone*, position the patient lies on the left side obliquely across the bed or table with one small pillow under the head, the left cheek resting on it. The left arm is drawn behind the body and the body inclined forward so that some of its weight is on the chest. The right arm may be in any position comfortable for the patient. The thighs are flexed, the right sharply against the abdomen and the left less sharply. This position is frequently used for the rectal examination of the male patient and might possibly be used for certain vaginal and rectal examinations and treatments. The anus or vaginal orifice may be exposed by folding back a small portion of the blanket or sheet covering the patient.

The *knee-chest*, or *genupectoral*, position as the term implies means that the patient rests on the knees and chest. The head is turned to one side with the cheek on a pillow. The arms should be extended on the bed or table, flexed at the elbows and resting to partially support the patient; they should not be under the patient. The weight of the body should rest mainly on the chest and knees, which are flexed so that the thighs are at right angles to the legs as they rest on the bed or table. A small pillow may be placed under the chest, but the abdomen is unsupported. The position is often used for examinations of the rectum with the anoscope and sigmoidoscope and less often for examination of the vagina. (It is also used as an exercise for postpartum patients.) During examinations two sheets are put over the patient, one for the upper and one for the lower part of the body, leaving an opening over the anus. One large sheet with a hole (a "fenestra") in the center is more satisfactory than two sheets.

The *Trendelenburg* position is not used for examinations but is sometimes used in the operating room during pelvic surgery in order to displace the intestines from the pelvis into the upper abdomen. A special table is required,

---

* The use of paper on examining tables and as drapery for patients provides less comfort for patients than cotton fabrics and adds to the problem of waste disposal. It is therefore recommended only in those situations where adequate laundry service is unavailable.

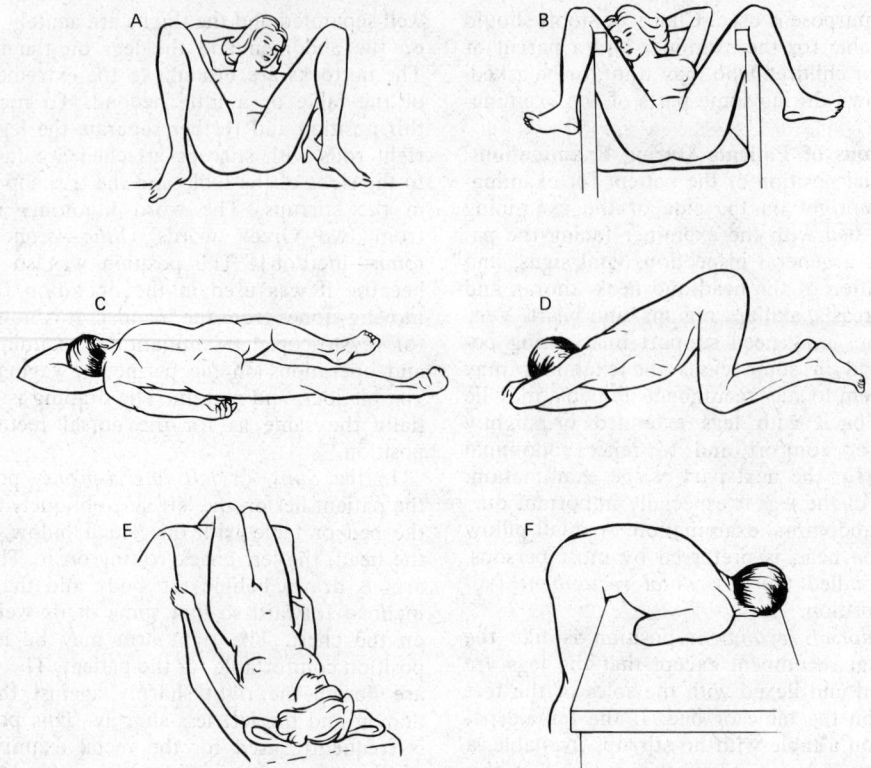

Figure 5-6. Positions used in examinations and treatments: *A.* Dorsal-recumbent position with knees flexed. *B.* Lithotomy, or dorsal-recumbent, position with knees supported, or heels in stirrups. *C.* Lateral or Sims' position (position may be right or left lateral). *D.* Knee-chest or genupectoral position. *E.* Trendelenburg position. *F.* Jackknife position. For illustrative purposes the positions are shown without drapes. However, it is important to remember that drapes should always be used. See text for explanation.

one that can be adjusted so that the patient's head is low, the body on an inclined plane, and the knees flexed over the adjustable lower section of the table, which is lowered. The patient is carefully supported to prevent slipping. Draping depends on the kind of operation to be performed.

The *standing,* or *erect,* position, which describes itself, is used in judging posture, equilibrium, and when testing gait. It is also used in examination of the male genitalia and for detecting inguinal herniae.

The *jackknife* position is used for rectal examination in the male. The patient stands on the floor, bending at the hips over a table or bed. Few men would want or expect covering over the legs during this examination but with old and debilitated patients it may be desirable. If used for rectal surgery the angle is reduced, the patient lies on the stomach, well supported by a gatched table, with a footrest. Covering should be provided above and below the anus

to keep the body warm and, as in all surgery, to provide a sterile field.

Instruments and Supplies. The following items should be available to the examiner: blood pressure apparatus, stethoscope, thermometer, scales, watch, tuning fork, bell or rattle for a child, small hammer with rubber tip, sterile needle, cotton pledgets, oto-ophthalmoscope, tape measure, pen-shaped flashlight, tongue blades (spatulas), gloves, lubricant, vaginal specula of various sizes, applicators and glass slides for making vaginal smears (Papanicolaou tests) and smears of discharges from the penis, and paper and pencil to note abnormal findings. (If a microscopic examination is made for syphilis, the material from the genital or mouth lesion [chancre] must be fresh so that the spirochetes are seen in motion under the microscope. For this reason the test is usually made in a laboratory). Snellen charts and Rosenbaum pocket charts are used for testing visual acuity and the tuning fork to test hearing; these may be in the examining room or in another area. In hospitals, urine and stool specimens are sent to the laboratory but the urine may be "screened" with a multitest dip-stick and the stool tested for the presence of blood with a reagent (benzidine or hemoccult test).

The Denver Developmental Screening Kit and Manual * or some comparable developmental testing equipment should be available for children. Forms for psychometric and psychiatric tests should also be available (see also p. 423).

7. STEPS IN THE PHYSICAL EXAMINATION AND SOME PHYSICAL EXAMINATION FORMS

This section gives the "steps" in making a physical examination. The sequence depends to some extent on the age and sex of the client or patient, whether they are in-patients or ambulatory, whether they are well, slightly, moderately, or very ill. An attempt is made here to give the steps in the most usual sequence. The description of the steps is necessarily brief. The text *A Guide to Physical Examination* by Barbara Bates (1974),[124a] a physician who has worked closely with nurses for decades, is especially helpful. A wealth of photographs clearly show the steps involved. Nurses will find the text *Clinical Assessment for the Nurse Practitioner* (1973) by William C. Fowkes, Jr., and Virginia K. Hunn [125] (a nurse) geared to their particular interests, as is *Guide to Patient Evaluation* (1974) by Jacques L. Sherman and Sylvia Kleiman Fields [126] (a nurse). The latter "guide" includes history-taking, physical examination, and the problem-oriented method. It and *The Physical Assessment, A Programmed Unit of Study for Nurses* (1974) by Marie M. Seedor [127] show how to drape the patient for minimal exposure during the examination. *The Clinical Approach to the Patient* (1969) by William L. Morgan, Jr., and George L. Engel,[128] and *Interviewing the Patient* (1973) by Engel and Morgan [128a] while addressed to the medical student, are equally useful to nurses who are making health assessments, especially for the technique of taking a history. Elmer L. DeGowin's and Richard L. DeGowin's [129] *Bedside Diagnostic Examination* (1976) and Richard D. Judge's and George D. Zuidema's [130] *Methods of Clinical Examination; A Physiological Approach* (1974) are written for medical students but useful to any examiner. However, the numbers and ex-

cellence of the photographs in John A. Prior's and Jack S. Silberstein's [131] *Physical Diagnosis. The History and Examination of the Patient* (1973) make it especially valuable to learners, as does the Bates text cited earlier. Pediatric, obstetric, orthopedic, neurologic and psychiatric texts should be consulted for modifications of the general method given here. In this book it is not possible to give the details to be found in the texts listed above.

"Steps" in the physical examination are based on the position assumed by the patient and the examiner and the area exposed for examination. The sequence has been worked out to avoid unnecessary change of position for the patient—to expedite the examination. However, the sequence is not always the same. In examining infants, for example, the painful aspects of the examination are done last so that crying will interfere as little as possible with auscultation.

The steps in the physical examination, as shown in Figure 5-7, represent a suggested procedure to be modified according to the age and condition of the patient, the facilities, and the health personnel available. It presupposes that a health history has been taken by questionnaire or interview or a combination of the two. The physical examination and history should complement rather than duplicate each other. The history is extremely important and should help the examiner know what to look for in the examination.

The health worker taking the history or the person conducting the physical examination (one person customarily does both) makes an *over-all assessment* or sizes up the person and decides whether he or she is well developed physically, mentally, and emotionally, able to tolerate the usual procedure for the physical examination, able to sit up and walk around for parts of it or whether the examination should be carried out in bed with as much dispatch as possible with perhaps certain aspects omitted. The steps listed in Figure 5-7 are those that would be used for a person who is able to tolerate the complete procedure and who wishes or is willing to have one.

Parenthetically, when admitting patients, health personnel should note a chain around the arm or neck with a plaque that says *Medic Alert* (see Fig. 5-8). This means that the patient belongs to the Medic Alert Foundation International, a charitable, nonprofit organization that encourages people to inform the public, or their caretakers, about their medical problems or physiologic characteristics, as, for example, diabetes, epilepsy, a heart condition, an implanted pacemaker, asthma, allergies, drugs being taken (such as anticoagulants),

* Available from LaDoca Co., Denver, Colo.

Step	Positions of Patient and Examiner				Areas, Organs, "Systems" Examined and Special Measurements	Methods of Examination
	Ambulatory Patient		Bedfast (Prostrated) Patient			
	Male	Female	Male	Female		
1	Sitting, lying, standing	Sitting, lying, standing	Lying	Lying	Overall assessment—weight, height, temperature	Inspection Weighing and measuring Thermometry
2	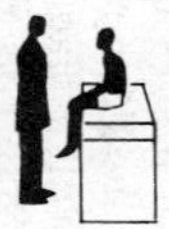	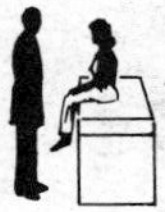	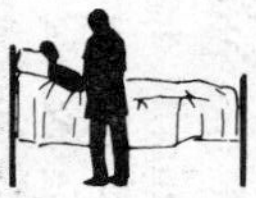	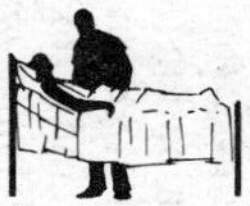	Head (eyes, ears, nose, mouth, cranial nerves) Arms, axillae, hands Blood pressure in arm Radial pulse Anterior Chest or in Breasts Step 4 Heart	Inspection, gross, and with help of ophthalmoscope, otoscope Palpation Percussion Auscultation with help of stethoscope and sphygmomanometer
3	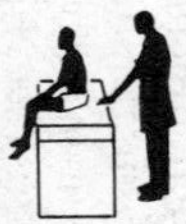	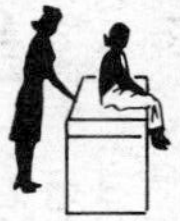	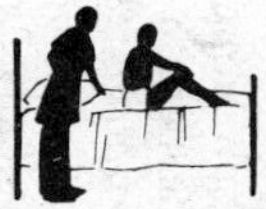	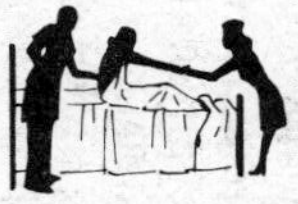	Neck (posterior) Chest (posterior) Back–spine	Inspection Palpation Percussion Auscultation with help of stethoscope
4	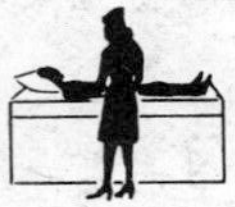	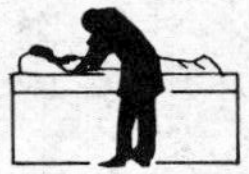	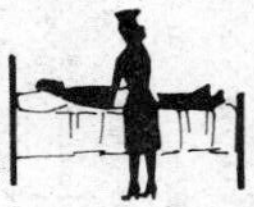	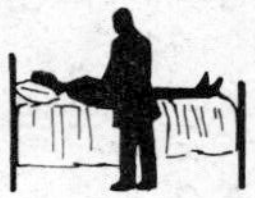	Breasts Anterior chest or in with heart Step 2 and lungs Abdomen Lower extremities	Inspection Palpation Percussion Auscultation with help of stethoscope
5	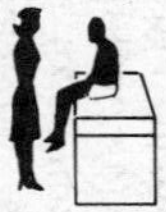		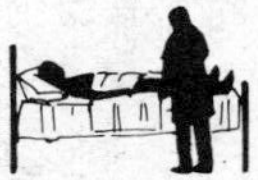		Lower extremities (knee and ankle) reflexes	Inspection Percussion with help of hammer
6	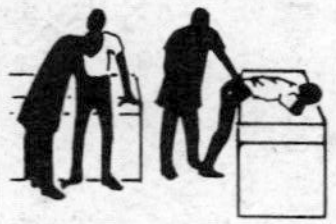	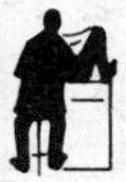	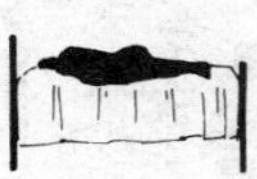	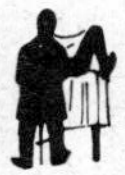	Genitalia (for males includes examination of groin for inguinal hernia) Rectum	Inspection (with help of proctoscope in some cases) Palpation
7	Standing	Standing	–	–	Overall assessment of gait and equilibrium	Inspection
8	Sitting	Sitting	Lying	Lying	Overall assessment of personality	Psychometric and psychiatric written tests and interviews

Figure 5-7. Steps in general physical examination. (Adapted from Morgan, William L, and Engel, George L.: *The Clinical Approach to the Patient.* W. B. Saunders Co., Philadelphia, 1969.)

glaucoma, and the use of contact lenses. Persons wearing a Medic Alert bracelet or necklace have reported such data to the Foundation whose headquarters is in Turlock, Calif. Collect calls to the central file (209–634–4917) make such information available. The Foundation is endorsed by one hundred organizations including the American Nurses' Association.[131a]

Ambulatory patients are asked to undress and put on a special garment that enables the examiner to expose different areas of the body in turn. They may be provided with disposable slippers or asked to wear their shoes into the examining area. For the neurologic and orthopedic aspects of the examination, the gown may be dispensed with and a covering for only the genitalia provided, and sometimes a bib or brassiere to cover the breasts. Bedfast, prostrated patients wear the usual hospital gown.

Before beginning the inspection the patient is weighed,* infants entirely without clothing. Infants and children are always measured; for some adults it may be important. The body temperature is taken and the patient asked to void in an appropriate receptacle so that a specimen of urine may be sent to the laboratory for analysis and so that the bladder is empty during the examination of the abdomen and pelvis. The rectum should also be empty. If a specimen of feces is required the patient is asked to bring one. (See Chapter 7 for appropriate containers and for special cleaning of the rectum when the physical examination is to include a proctoscopy.)

If the physician is conducting the physical examination the preparation and Step 1 (as outlined in Fig. 5-7) are usually carried out by nursing personnel. When the professional nurse is conducting the physical examination he or she may or may not have assistance from other categories of nursing personnel. Regardless of the sequence of steps, examiners look at the eyes, listen to chest sounds, and feel the abdomen with certain criteria of health, or normal values, in mind. The following is a suggested procedure for examining each area, organ, or system, giving briefly what the examiner is trying to discover. Examiners can make the procedure a learning experience for patients if they explain the purpose of each step before or as they take it.† The person's

* Virginia Bennett Moore in "In-Bed Weighing" (*Nursing '72,* **2:**13, [July] 1972) describes three devices for weighing bed patients who cannot stand on a scale. Most institutions have a specified technique suited to their equipment and furnishings.

† Attention has been called to *The Well Body Book* by Samuels and Bennett in which the authors describe and illustrate the steps in the physical examination as performed by nonmedical persons.

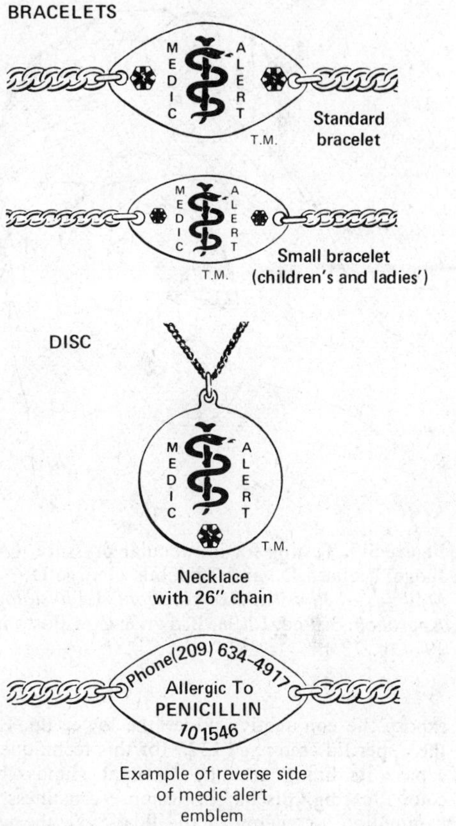

Figure 5-8. Bracelets and necklace with Medic Alert emblem. (Courtesy of Medic Alert Foundation International, Turlock, Calif.)

strengths as well as his or her weaknesses should be identified just as they should be noted in taking a history. Health programs should capitalize on clients' strengths and, if possible, eliminate or minimize their weaknesses.

Suggested Procedure (Steps in the Physical Examination)

Head and Face as a Whole. Inspect the shape and size in relation to the body, the expression—whether symmetrical, mobile, or masklike; note the temperature and color of the *skin,* texture, pigmentation, moisture, rashes, lesions, or scars. Feel lesions to determine size, tenderness, consistency, and whether superficial or attached to deeper tissues. Palpate the skull for any bony abnormalities.

Hair. Notice its texture and distribution, color, loss of hair (alopecia) or oily and scaly scalp (seborrhea), scalp lesions, and signs that the patient scratches the scalp, pulls out, or neglects the hair.

Eyes. Inspect the *conjunctiva, sclera, cornea,* and *iris* of each eye. Using a flashlight, pull downward on the lower lid just below the eyelashes to

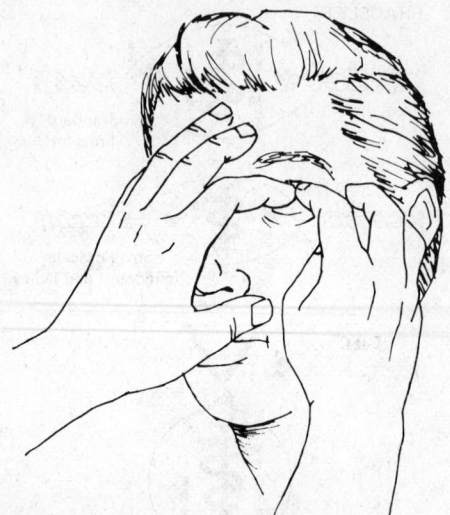

Figure 5-9. Testing for intraocular pressure. (After Judge, Richard D., and Zuidema, George D.: *Methods of Physical Examination: A Physiologic Approach,* 3rd ed. Little, Brown & Co., Boston, 1974, p. 72.)

expose the conjunctiva under the lower lid. Evert the upper lid (see page 1325 for this technique) to expose its lining and the lacrimal glands. Note color, tearing, discharge, lesions, crustiness, inflammation, or edema of the lids. Note the width of the openings between the lids when patient is looking upward and straight ahead. (Inequality in the palpebral fissures indicates a ptosis of the lid.) Test intraocular pressure by gently indenting the upper eye with the fingers or use the tonometer (see Fig. 5-9).*

After asking the patient to stare at a dark wall, note the size and shape of the *pupils,* then the reaction to the flashlight as it is moved laterally toward each eye. Note also whether the pupils respond the same way when the patient looks at a distant and then a near object (accommodation). *Accommodation* may also be tested by asking the patient to watch the tip of the examiner's finger as it is moved from a distance to a point near the eyes. Note changes in the size of the pupils in each case. Test the *extraocular muscles*

* David N. Cohen, physician, of the Spokane (Wash.) Eye Clinic, has been using the Carotid Compression Tonography Test (CCT) to detect carotid occlusion which carries with it the threat of stroke. He uses an electric tonometer connected with a graphic recorder to show changes in intraocular pressure induced by pressure on the carotid artery. Robert Northrop, engineer, of the University of Connecticut, Storrs, is developing a system to detect carotid occlusions through no-touch ocular pulse measurements. The instrument will use "continuous-wave *ultrasound* reflected from the cornea . . ." (Correspondence with Dr. Cohen and Mr. Northrop, Jan. 1976. See also Cohen, D. N., et al.: "Correlation with Bilateral Carotid Arteriography in the Diagnosis of Extracranial Carotid Occlusion Disease," *Stroke,* **6**:257, 1975.)

(EOMs) by asking the patient to hold the head still and follow the examiner's moving finger through the "six cardinal directions" as described by Prior and Silberstein [132] (points on an imaginary circle around the patient's head). Note jerky movement, crossed eye movement (nystagmus), or inability to follow examiner's directions (see Fig. 5-10). Test the *visual fields* by covering the eye not being tested and then have the patient look at the examiner's nose. In this position have the patient indicate when he sees the examiner's moving finger come into his field of vision. This test is also conducted in each of the six cardinal positions.

Visual acuity is tested most accurately with a Snellen chart with standard size letters at a distance of 20 ft, or it may be tested with a Rosenbaum pocket vision screener * held at a distance of 14 inches. A rough estimate of the vision in each eye can also be made by asking the patient, with the other eye closed, to read newspaper print at about 2 ft.†

Next darken the room and carefully inspect each eye with the ophthalmoscope. Because successful ophthalmoscopic examination requires a great deal of patience and practice on the part of the examiner, the reader is referred to any one of the standard texts on physical examination listed at the end of this chapter. DeGowin and DeGowin [133] describe the process more or less as follows: In general, the examiner's right eye examines the patient's right, and his left examines the patient's left, so that the examiner's nose

* Available from Smith, Miller, and Patch, Inc., New Brunswick, N.J.

† If patients wear glasses, visual acuity tests should be made with the glasses in place.

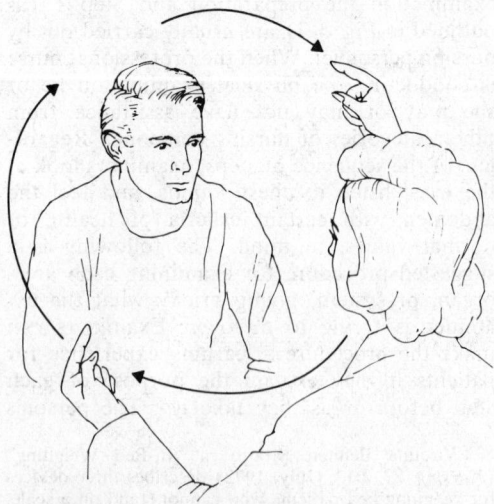

Figure 5-10. Testing the extraocular muscles and visual field. (After Judge, Richard D., and Zuidema, George D.: *Methods of Physical Examination: A Physiologic Approach,* 3rd ed. Little, Brown & Co., Boston, 1974, p. 344.)

parallels the patient's cheek. The media is inspected with a +8 lens held about 12 in. from the patient's eye. The examiner's forefinger changes the lenses of the ophthalmoscope and the opposite hand rests on the patient's head with the thumb gently retracting and holding the upper lid to prevent excessive blinking. As the examiner moves toward the patient, reducing the lens gradually to zero, the cornea, lens, vitreous, and retina may be seen successively. The optimal direction of gaze for the patient is temporally and about 20 degrees upward to enable the examiner to visualize the optic disc (nerve). Note the size, shape, color, and margins of the disc. Examination of the retina includes an evaluation of the arteries and veins radiating outward from the disc. Note their color, size—in relationship to each other—pulsations, appearance of the arteriolar-venous crossings, and the presence of hemorrhages, exudates, or pigmentation.

Ears. Examine the external ear for growths, lesions, or cartilaginous changes. Inspect the canal after straightening it by pulling the ear lobe up and back (with infants and small children pull down). The largest speculum that fits the canal is selected to expose the canal and eardrum, and the otoscope is used to throw an intense light on the eardrum. The eardrum is inspected for color, bulging, inflammation, retractions, scars, perforations, anatomic landmarks, and light reflex. Note wax that blocks the canal (some wax is normal), any lesion or growth, and any sign of irritation or discharge from the canal and ear lobe. Hold one ear closed while testing hearing in the other. Whisper a phrase or sentence and ask the patient to repeat it, speaking louder each time until it is correctly repeated, or move a watch toward the ear on a line with the examiner's so that the latter can judge the patient's hearing by his or her own. The Weber test is made with a tuning fork struck and placed on the middle of the patient's forehead. Normally the sound is perceived as originating in the middle of the forehead. The Rinne test is also done with a tuning fork. This test com-

pares bone conduction with air conduction. The fork is struck and placed on the mastoid process until the patient no longer detects conduction of sound by the bone. Then it is placed next to the patient's ear to allow further detection of the sound by air conduction. Normally air conduction exceeds bone conduction by a ratio of 2:1.

Nose. Inspect the nose for deformities and scars. Ask the patient to tilt the head backward, push up the tip of the nose and, using a flashlight and nasal speculum, look up and back into the nasal cavity. The nasal mucosa should be pink and moist. Note swollen, bluish, or red mucosa, deviated septum, or any discharge or growths. (Nasal polyps are likely to be high up in the nasal cavity.) Ask the patient to close one nostril and breathe through the other to test the *patency of the airway.* Palpate face over frontal and maxillary sinuses for tenderness.

Mouth and Pharynx. Inspect the lips for color, moisture, and the presence of ulcers, fissures, growths, crusts, or pigmentation. Ask the patient to open the mouth wide and by palpation note any abnormal action of the temporomandibular joint. When dentures are worn ask the patient to put them in a denture cup or paper towel. Study the oral cavity, using a flashlight and a wooden tongue blade to retract the cheek and make it possible to see the *tongue, teeth, gums, mucous membranes, palate,* and *salivary gland ducts* (see Fig. 5-13). Note any lesions, pigmentation, scars, or white patches in the mouth or on the tongue; note swollen, glistening, discolored, or retracted gums, missing and carious teeth; note odor of the breath. If a growth or lesion is seen, palpate it with a gloved hand. Ask the patient to stick the tongue out and note any tremor, abnormal movements, or lateral deviation; ask the patient to move the tongue up and down and to each side and note any difficulty with these movements. After the tongue is withdrawn ask the patient to open the mouth wide and say "Aaah" while a tongue blade is pressed firmly on the lateral posterior surface of the tongue. Note the rise of the *uvula* in the mid-

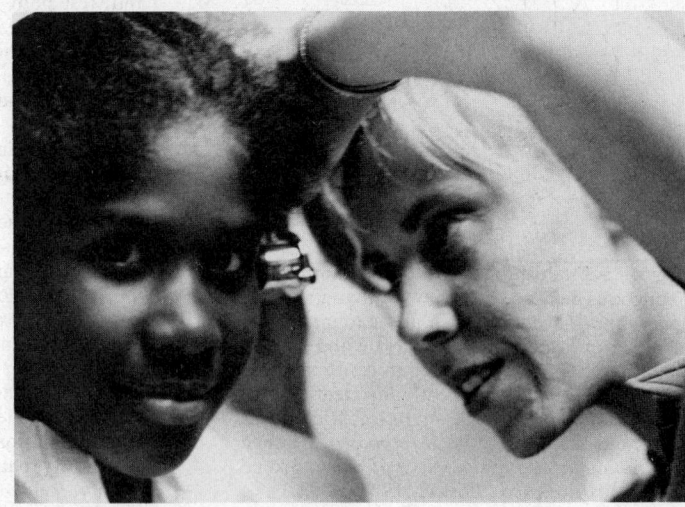

Figure 5-11. Nurse examining the ear using otoscope. (Courtesy of Yale University School of Nursing, New Haven, Conn.)

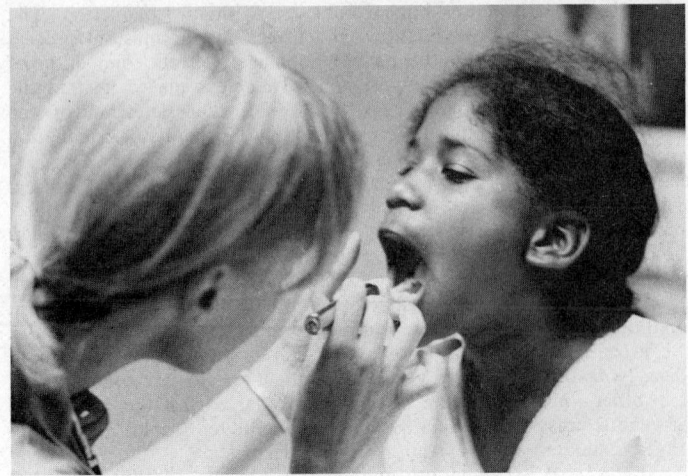

Figure 5-12. Nurse examining mouth of child using longer blade and flashlight. (Courtesy of Yale University School of Nursing, New Haven, Conn.)

line or any deviation. Inspect the *posterior pharynx* and *tonsil area.* Tonsils are proportionately larger in childhood. This is not a sign of pathology. In adults they may be too shrunken to see. Test the gag reflex by touching each side of the pharynx gently, warning the patient first.

In the procedures described so far, some of the twelve cranial nerves have been tested; those that have not are I (olfactory), V (trigeminal), VII (facial), and XI (accessory). The following procedures complete this aspect of the neurologic phase of the general examination. (See Fig. 5-14).

Completing Cranial Nerve Tests. The *olfactory nerve* (I) is rarely tested but if a neurologic

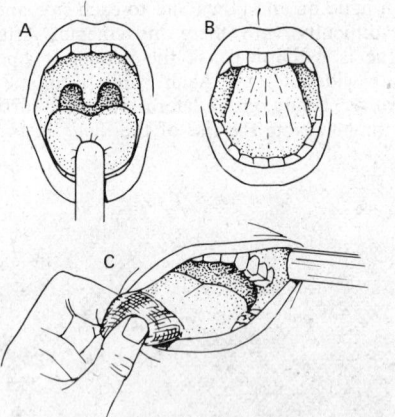

Figure 5-13. Positions for mouth examination. *A.* Tongue is depressed for view of uvula, palate, and pharynx. *B.* Mouth is open and patient raises tongue for inspection of underside and floor of the mouth. *C.* Tongue is grasped in gauze sponge and cheek is retracted to inspect gums, teeth, and mucous membranes. (After Judge, Richard D., and Zuidema, George D.: *Methods of Physical Examination: A Physiologic Approach,* 3rd ed. Little, Brown & Co., Boston, 1974, p. 82.)

condition is suspected patients may be asked to discriminate between fragrant, fetid, and acrid odors by use of such materials as coffee, vanilla, menthol, and tobacco. The ophthalmic branch of the *trigeminal nerve* (V) is tested by touching the central edge of the cornea with a wisp of cotton as the lower lid is pulled down and as the patient gazes laterally. Normally the patient blinks; note absence of this reflex. Test the three sensory divisions of V on the face on both sides by touching it at different points with warm and cold objects, or with sharp and dull objects, or with a wisp of cotton. Patients are asked to close their eyes and say what they feel. Test the motor division of V by asking patients to open and close the mouth and clench the teeth. Palpate the masseter muscles and note any pulling to one side. Test the *facial nerve* (VII) by noting asymmetry when asked to smile, grimace, frown, squeeze the eyes closed, and wrinkle the brow. Test the *spinal accessory nerve* (XI) by asking the patient to turn the head to the side and hold it in that position against the resistance offered by the examiner's hand; test both right and left sternocleidomastoid muscles. To test the trapezius muscle put both hands on the shoulders of the patient, ask him or her to rise against this resistance and note strength or weakness and any inequality between the strength of the two sides.

Some examiners complete the sensory and motor aspects of the neurologic examination over the entire body at this point or they may include such tests in the remaining "steps" of the examination.

Neck. Standing before the patient, inspect the *skin* and underlying *muscular-bony structure.* Note color, texture, scars, pulsations of *blood vessels,* size and visibility of *glands.* Test the range-of-motion in the neck by asking the patient to move the head backward and forward and from side to side both with and without resistance, noting limitations of motion, stiffness, weakness, or pain. By palpation note the distribution, size, mobility, and tenderness of *lymph nodes* and

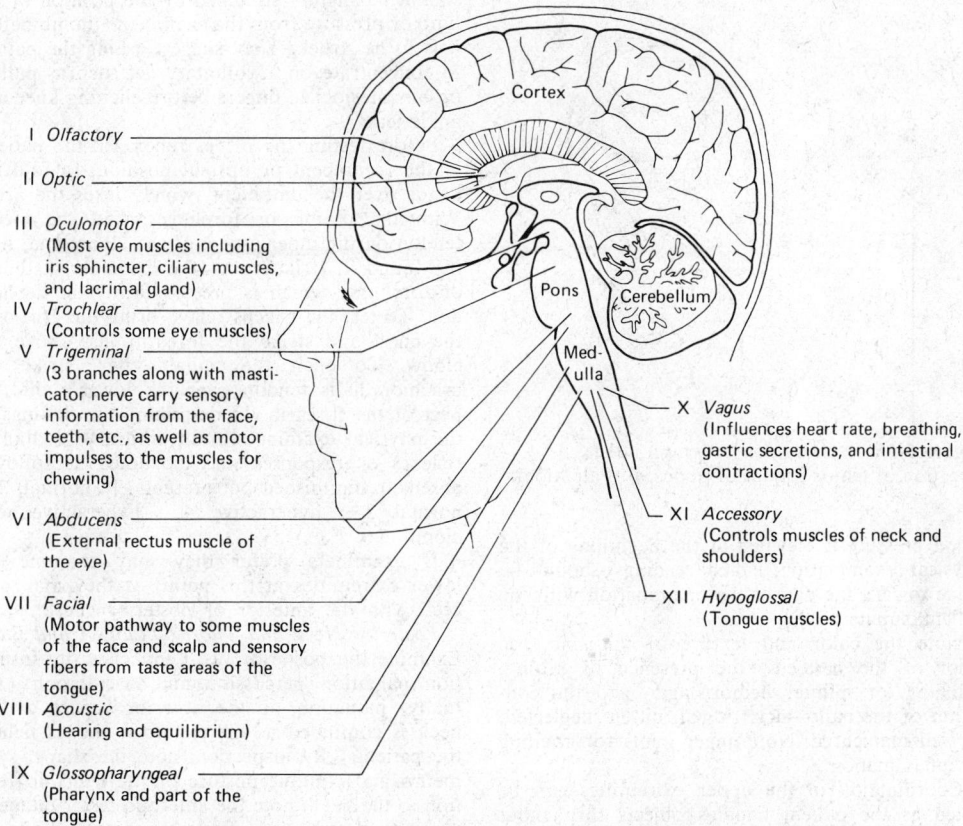

I *Olfactory*

II *Optic*

III *Oculomotor*
(Most eye muscles including
iris sphincter, ciliary muscles,
and lacrimal gland)

IV *Trochlear*
(Controls some eye muscles)

V *Trigeminal*
(3 branches along with masti-
cator nerve carry sensory
information from the face,
teeth, etc., as well as motor
impulses to the muscles for
chewing)

VI *Abducens*
(External rectus muscle of
the eye)

VII *Facial*
(Motor pathway to some muscles
of the face and scalp and sensory
fibers from taste areas of the
tongue)

VIII *Acoustic*
(Hearing and equilibrium)

IX *Glossopharyngeal*
(Pharynx and part of the
tongue)

Cortex

Pons   Cerebellum

Med-
ulla

X *Vagus*
(Influences heart rate, breathing,
gastric secretions, and intestinal
contractions)

XI *Accessory*
(Controls muscles of neck and
shoulders)

XII *Hypoglossal*
(Tongue muscles)

Figure 5-14. Diagram showing the approximate areas of origination for the cranial
nerves, their distribution, and functions they affect. The neurologic examination includes tests for these functions.

salivary glands. Actually, normal lymph nodes are hard to feel, and especially so unless the patient is relaxed (see Fig. 5-15). Note the position of the *trachea.* Inspect the *thyroid gland* with the examiner standing behind and the patient sitting, or, if supine, with the head of the bed raised. Ask the patient to swallow a small amount of water so that the gland, lying low in the neck below the cricoid, can be palpated gently as it rises and falls under the examiner's fingers. Note contour, symmetry, mobility, tenderness, and nodules. If the gland is greatly enlarged listen for the "bruit" (noise or roar) of increased vascularity. Examination by palpation of the thyroid gland with both hands is completed when the examiner stands behind the patient to examine the posterior thorax. Note enlargement, masses, tenderness, nodules, and immobility of the gland on swallowing with the neck slightly extended.

Inspect and palpate the *jugular veins* and *carotid arteries* and listen for bruits over the carotids (bruits are extracardiac blowing sounds resulting from turbulence in stenosed vessels, usually arterial). Examine the neck for a distended jugular vein when the patient is semirecumbent and with head elevated. Distention when the

patient is sitting or has the head elevated 45 degrees indicates elevated venous pressure.

Hands and Arms. Examine the upper extremities by inspection and palpation. The *skin, lymph nodes, muscles, bones and their joints, blood vessels,* and *nerves* are examined. Ask the patient to extend both arms, to hold them steady with outstretched fingers and with palms up and palms down. Note asymmetric and weak movements, drifting, gross, or fine tremors. Ask the patient to grasp examiner's crossed hands and compare the strength of the grip of each hand. Ask the patient to hold the arms flexed while the examiner tries to straighten the arm. This tests the *motor strength* of the extremity. It is desirable to put each extremity through its full range-of-motion. Test coordination by asking the patient to extend his or her arm and touch the nose with the finger, both with eyes open and closed. Palpate arm, noting swelling, tenderness, lesions or enlarged axillary nodes, and pulsating arteries. Count pulsations in the radial artery, noting rate, rhythm, and character of the pulsations. Measure the blood pressure (usually in the left arm) with the sphygmomanometer. (See Chapter 6 for detailed discussion of pulse and blood pressure.) If the

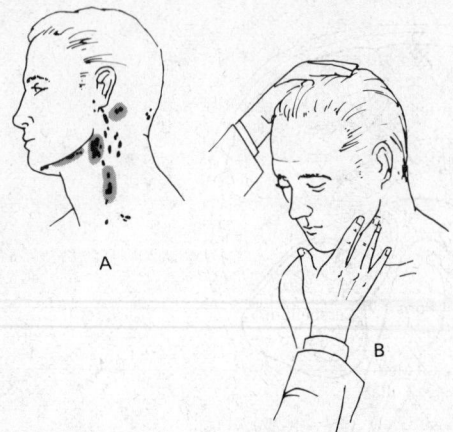

Figure 5-15. Examination of lymph nodes. *A*. Location of major groups of nodes. *B*. Palpation.

blood pressure is elevated at the beginning of the physical examination, other readings should be made toward the end of the examination with the patient supine.

Note the color and texture of the skin, the color of the nailbeds, the presence of pitting, clubbing, or splinter hemorrhages, and the condition of the nails—dry, ridged, bitten, neglected, or well manicured. Note finger joints for swelling or inflammation.

Coordination in the upper extremities can be noted as the patient handles objects throughout the physical examination and in the finger-to-nose test. *Sensory responses* can be elicited on the arms (or any part of the body) as on the face with a sterile needle for sharp and dull pain discrimination, a wisp of cotton for light touch. Fowkes and Hunn [134] say that since pain and temperature are mediated through the same pathways, it is unnecessary to test both. However, some examiners may want patients to show that they can discriminate between hot and cold objects as well as between the dull and sharp. Unless neurologic pathology is suspected, however, these tests may not be made over the entire body. *Vibratory sensation* is usually tested by holding the end of a vibrating tuning fork against distal bones of the hands and feet, asking patients first to close their eyes and describe their sensations as the vibrating fork is held on distal and proximal bony prominences. (For a description of a thorough neurologic examination that includes other discriminatory tests, the reader should consult special texts listed at the end of this chapter.)

The deep tender reflexes (DTRs) are tested by using the rubber hammer and holding it loosely so that it falls heavily against the tendon and elicits a characteristic reflex response. Test the biceps, triceps, and radial (brachioradialis) reflexes. Since comparison of the response right and left is important, test the biceps reflex on both sides before testing the triceps and so on. The patient should be relaxed when the reflex is tested but DeGowin and DeGowin [135] say the muscle should be slightly stretched by the position of the limb or pressure from the examiner's thumb before it is to be struck. They suggest asking the patient to concentrate on a voluntary act such as pulling on his interlocked fingers before eliciting knee and ankle jerks.

Before testing the biceps reflex ask the patient, in the recumbent or upright position, to fold the hands over the umbilicus, which flexes the arms. With the thumb or forefinger, find the biceps tendon on the inner aspect of the elbow and, having found it, strike your (the examiner's) thumb or forefinger which is pressed firmly on the tendon. To test the triceps reflex, bring the arm over the chest and strike the forearm just above the elbow. To elicit the radial reflex, strike the brachioradialis tendon over the lower radial aspect of the forearm. In describing the findings of the physical examination, an arbitrary grading of reflexes or responses may be noted as follows: absent 0; diminished but present 1+; normal, 2+; normal 3+; hyperactive 4+; hyperactive with clonus 5+.[136]

If examiners prefer they may examine the lower extremities at this point, or they may proceed with the anterior or posterior chest.

Posterior Neck and Thorax (Lungs) and Back. Examine the posterior neck and chest by inspection, palpation, percussion, and auscultation. (Actually, palpation of the anterior aspect of the neck is continued as the examiner moves behind the patient.) By inspection, note the shape, symmetry, and contour posture of the trunk in relation to the head; note the anteroposterior diameter and any deformities; note asymmetric chest elevation, expansion, or bulging and retraction during respiration. A common way to estimate symmetry and degree of expansion is to grasp the lower rib cage with both hands, pointing the thumbs toward the spine with their tips equidistant from the spinal column. As the patient inspires and the examiner's thumbs move laterally see whether the distance between them and the spinal column is the same on both sides of the body. Note spinal curvatures and palpate bony prominences, although spinal abnormalities and posture can be judged more effectively if the patient can stand and move.

Feel, or palpate, the neck and posterior thorax for tenderness and swelling. Ask the patient to say, with resonance, "ninety-nine" or "one, two" and feel the vibrations with the palmar aspect of the fingers or ulnar surface of the hand, comparing the "tactile fremitus" in the same areas on either side of the thorax from the apex of the lungs to the diaphragm. Note intensity or absence of vibration.

Before percussing * the posterior chest, ask the patient to bend forward with (in the sitting position) the elbows and forearms on the thighs (see Fig. 5-17). This spreads the scapulae and gives maximum exposure of lung fields. To determine the level of the diaphragm ask the patient to take a

---

* The vibration felt during percussion by an experienced examiner is as informative as the sounds heard.

deep breath and hold it; then percuss downward in a vertical line below the tip of the scapula until a dull sound is elicited. Ask the patient to exhale, or release the breath, then continue percussing upward 3 to 5 cm (1 to 1½ inches) until a new level of dullness is heard as the lungs deflate. The distance between the two levels of dullness measures the descent of the diaphragm. This process is repeated on the opposite side and findings compared. Listen to breath sounds * in the lungs using a stethoscope (auscultation) and note the loudness and pitch of the sounds heard on inspiration or expiration. The patient is again asked to say "ninety-nine" and "one, two" and the same sounds are whispered. According to DeGowin and DeGowin,[137] a modification in the voice sounds, or bleating (egophony) is useful in detecting plural effusion and occasionally consolidation. Ask the patient to say "E" repeatedly and if there is effusion the sound will be heard as "A" when the stethoscope crosses the upper level of effusion.

Anterior Chest (Breasts, Lungs, and Heart). Expose the entire chest (male and female) leaving the upper abdomen covered. Inspect the skin again for color, pigmentation, varicosities, pulsations, circumscribed areas of pigmentation or vascularization (nevi), hair distribution, scars, lesions, and masses. Note the contour and symmetry of the chest and record the rate and depth

* It takes considerable experience to differentiate between "vesicular" sounds (over the lower lungs), "bronchovesicular" (over the thoracic portion of the trachea) and bronchial sounds (over the bronchi), and tracheal or harsh sounds (over the trachea). Accidental, acquired, foreign (adventitious) sounds include wheezes, rales (abnormal sounds that may be described as moist or dry, fine or coarse), and rhonchi (described as coarse, sibilant, sonorous, or by other adjectives). Classification of these sounds may be found in any of the texts on physical examination listed at the end of this chapter.

of respirations at rest. As in examination of the posterior chest, palpation, percussion, and auscultation are used to examine the *lung fields,* remembering that the heart obscures more of the left than the right lung sounds and that the right bronchus is directed more anteriorly than the left. Palpate, percuss, and auscultate from above downward in midclavicular, anterior axillary, and midaxillary lines. Percuss and auscultate the apices of the lungs carefully, including the area above the clavicle, since these can't be reached posteriorly. Any suspicious area found in the lungs is, of course, examined with special care.

Examine the *breasts* and *axillary region* by inspection and palpation. The size,* contour, and symmetry of the breasts are seen best with patients, particularly women, in the sitting position. Inspect nipples for bleeding or other discharge, ulceration, inversion, or tumor. Ask the patient to raise the arms above the head and also to contract the pectoral muscles by pressing the hands on the hips or pressing the palms of both hands together. In these positions note any skin retraction or dimpling that may indicate an underlying growth. Palpate the breasts with the patient in the upright and in the supine position, feeling each quadrant systematically with the palmar aspect of the fingertips using a rotary motion and pressing down gently against the chest wall. Mammary glands feel lumpy, or lobular; tumors and cysts in the glands are harder and may feel fixed, but their differentiation is no simple matter. While women are more likely than men to have growths in the breasts, both should be examined for them.

Ask the patient to raise the arms above the head and inspect the axillae for rashes, pigmentation, and furuncles. Palpate the axillae deeply for enlarged lymph nodes with the arms lowered

* Inequality in the size of the breasts is common and by itself does not indicate pathology, but irregularity of contour suggests the possibility of an underlying mass.

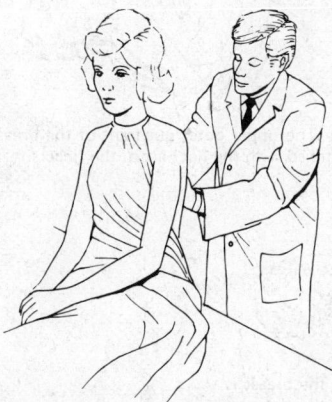

Figure 5-16. Proper positioning of the patient for examination of the lungs. (After Judge, Richard D., and Zuidema, George D.: *Physical Diagnosis: A Physiologic Approach to the Clinical Examination,* 2nd ed. Little, Brown & Co., Boston, 1963.)

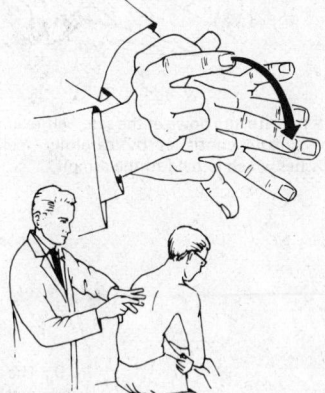

Figure 5-17. Method for percussion of the chest. (After Judge, Richard D., and Zuidema, George D.: *Physical Diagnosis: A Physiologic Approach to the Clinical Examination,* 2nd ed. Little, Brown & Co., Boston, 1963.)

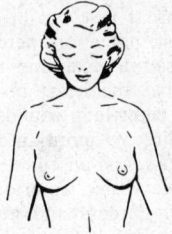

1. Careful examination of the breasts before a mirror for symmetry in size and shape, noting any puckering or dimpling of the skin or retraction of the nipple.

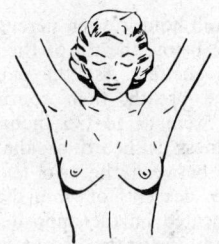

2. Arms raised over head, again studying the breasts in the mirror for the same signs.

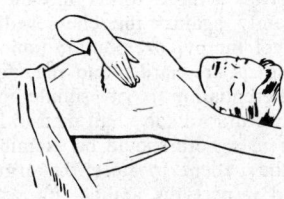

3. Reclining on bed with flat pillow or folded bath towel under the shoulder on the same side as breast to be examined.

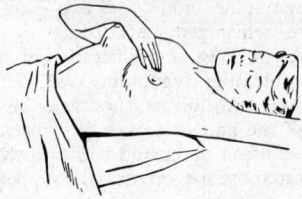

4. To examine the inner half of the breast, the arm is raised over the head. Beginning at the breastbone and, in a series of steps, the inner half of the breast is palpated.

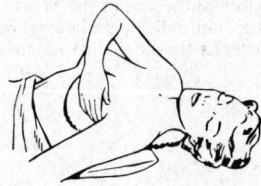

5. The area over the nipple is carefully palpated with the flat part of the fingers.

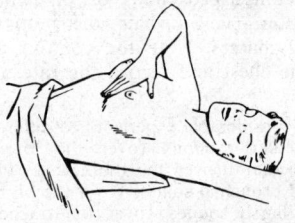

6. Examination of the lower inner half of the breast is completed.

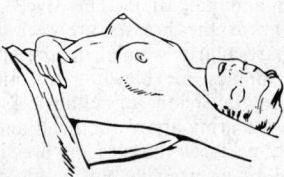

7. With arm down at the side, self-examination of breasts continues by carefully feeling the tissues which extend to the armpit.

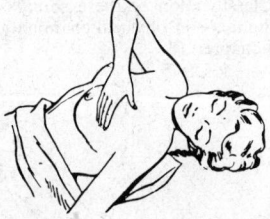

8. The upper outer quadrant of the breast is examined with the flat part of the fingers.

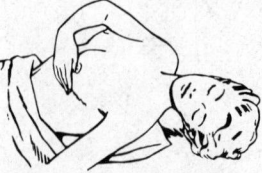

9. The lower outer quadrant of the breast is examined in successive stages with the flat part of the fingers.

Figure 5-18. Breast self-examination. (*The Nurse and Breast Self-Examination.* American Cancer Society, Inc., New York, N.Y., 1952.)

and slightly withdrawn from the body and also palpate the supraclavicular area for nodes.

Inspect the *cardiac region;* palpate, percuss, and auscultate it. Make this examination with the patient sitting upright part of the time and for its completion have the patient supine and turned on the left side. This brings the heart as close as possible against the thoracic wall and enables the examiner to hear heart murmurs most clearly. The cardiac examination is designed less to show the size and position of the heart than it is to learn as much as can be determined about its function.

Inspecting *the chest,* note bulging on either side of the thorax that may be caused by distended veins; note pulsations, and with the examining fingers identify the point of maximum impulse (PMI) or apical pulse, which, if the heart is not enlarged or displaced, lies near the left mid-clavicular line in the fifth intercostal space. Ask the patient to hold the breath in expiration to bring the heart and blood vessels close to the thoracic wall (after asking a woman with a large breast to lift it) and palpate the apical pulse which may or may not be visible, and note a thrill (palpable vibration) if present. In any event, the PMI should be verified later by auscultation. With the patient in the upright position palpate the cardiac region to determine if there is a heave under the hand or a thrill. Prior and Silberstein [138] say that the skills of a cardiac examination must be practiced repeatedly and that we "must educate our eyes to observe, our ears to listen, our hands to feel, and our minds to concentrate." Nothing is more true than this of the cardiac examination because, next to the ophthalmic examination of the eye, the heart is the most complicated organ to examine.

Percussion has very limited use in estimating the heart's size, since the sternum obscures some portions of the heart. Cardiac fluoroscopy or chest x-ray is generally far more precise in delineating the size and contour of the heart.

Auscultation or listening to the heart is difficult under ideal circumstances and requires a quiet room and intense concentration on the part of the examiner. The heart's cycle, or sequential contractions, can be heard and the closure of the mitral and tricuspid valves produces the first heart sound (S_1) and the closure of the aortic and pulmonic valves produces the second heart sound (S_2). See Figure 5-19 for the following auscultation areas: aortic area (2nd intercostal space just to the right of the sternum); pulmonic area (2nd intercostal space to the left of the sternum); mitral area (at the cardiac apex or PMI); and tricuspid area (to the left of the low sternum). Some authorities suggest listening to these areas in the order listed or in reverse order including auscultation along the left sternal border. Both examiner and patient should be comfortable and the room quiet. Use the diaphragm of the stethoscope for most of the examination but low-pitched sounds (apical diastolic murmurs, for example) are heard best with the bell stethoscope.

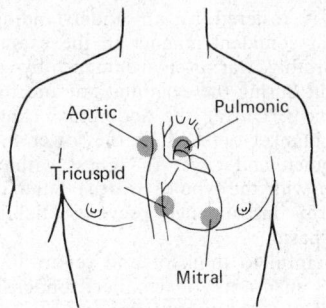

Figure 5-19. Auscultation points for heart sounds. (After Judge, Richard D., and Zuidema, George D.: *Methods of Physical Examination: A Physical Approach,* 3rd ed. Little, Brown & Co., Boston, 1974, p. 151.)

The sound of a heart beat at the apex or in the mitral area can be described as *"lubb,* dup; *lubb,* dup; *lubb,* dup . . . "—the second sound higher in pitch and sharper or more emphatic. The reverse is true in the aortic and pulmonic areas where the second sound is more emphatic. Identify these two sounds, note their rate, rhythm (whether irregularity is related to respiration), the equality of the sounds from one cycle to the next, their intensity, any splitting of the sounds, and sounds heard between "lubb, *dup"* (S_1 and S_2). Focus on systole and then on diastole and listen for and describe any extra sounds heard between these two and any hissing or rumbling sounds (murmurs). Certain murmurs, whether functional or pathologic, are heard best in different positions that the patient may assume. If murmurs are heard, listen for the shape, length, and quality of the murmur and whether it radiates to another part of the precordium or axilla. Examiners should learn to draw graphically in the patient's record the heart sounds and any murmurs they have heard. While the whole physical examination demands knowledge and skill, the examination of the heart is, perhaps, the most demanding. Specialized texts should be used in developing competence in this area of health assessment and disease diagnosis.*

Abdomen. With the patient supine and relaxed (if possible) inspect, auscultate, percuss, and palpate the abdomen, superficially and deeply. Re-

---

* Just as diagnosis by sight is extended with a variety of instruments that include macro- and microphotography, the ultrasound machine is used to extend normal hearing. See Chapter 7 for discussion of the uses of macro- and microphotography and diagnostic ultrasound.

In a symposium on approaches to the study of nursing questions and development of nursing science (*Nurs. Res.,* **21:**482, (Nov.–Dec.) 1972) Elizabeth L. McKinnon-Mullett discussed clinical capillary microscopy as a tool in evaluating the effect of nursing. She noted that the Microcirculatory Society, Inc., was organized in 1942, and in 1972 boasted international membership with three nurse scientist members.

laxation is fostered by an understanding, courteous, and confident manner in the examiner; by a comfortably warm environment; by diverting the patient during the examination; and by flexion of the knees. During the abdominal examination fold the blanket or sheet to the lower margin of the abdomen and cover the chest with a towel. Palpation with the whole (warm) hand or hands and warm instruments prevents tickling and muscle spasm.

It is helpful to think of and report findings in the four quadrants or smaller topographic divisions of the abdomen. It is essential that examiners visualize the position of the abdominal and pelvic organs in each area and learn how to feel the abdomen so that they can identify their margins or contours through the abdominal wall (see Fig. 5-20). Competent examiners can feel the

sigmoid colon, the liver, possibly the right kidney, and the abdominal aorta. The normal spleen, left kidney, empty bladder, and uterus cannot be felt on abdominal examination but if enlarged they can. Masses or growths in the abdomen can be felt. This is one of the main objects in examining the abdomen, although areas of tenderness can also suggest pathology. Decide upon a series of steps in palpation and follow them methodically. Texts on the physical examination differ slightly in the suggested sequence but deep palpation, which can cause discomfort or pain, is always left until the last.

Inspect the symmetry and shape of the abdomen, any distention or bulging. Note the muscle tone and subcutaneous fat. Note scars, abrasions, eruptions, any skin lesions, pigmentation, striae, capillary hemorrhages, and distended veins. Ask

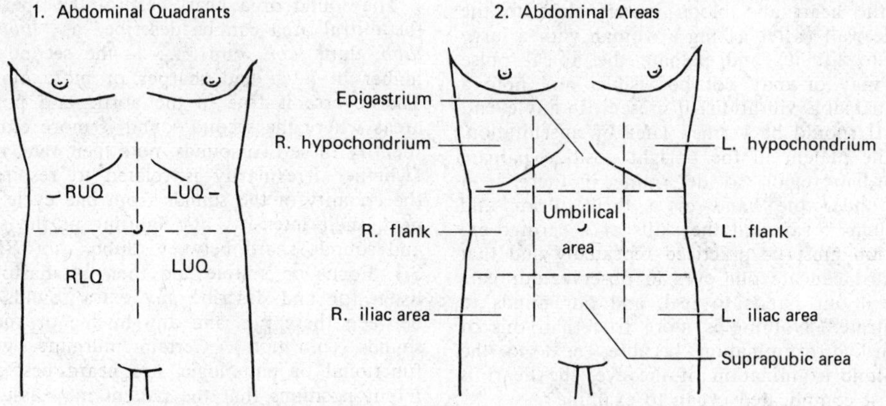

1. Abdominal Quadrants

RUQ | LUQ
RLQ | LUQ

2. Abdominal Areas

Epigastrium
R. hypochondrium — L. hypochondrium
R. flank — Umbilical area — L. flank
R. iliac area — L. iliac area
Suprapubic area

Utilizing the quadrant map, the examiner can visualize the following organs in each quadrant:

Right Upper Quadrant (RUQ)
  Liver and gallbladder
  Pylorus
  Duodenum
  Head of pancreas
  Right adrenal gland
  Portion of right kidney
  Hepatic flexure of colon
  Portions of ascending and
    transverse colon

Left Upper Quadrant (LUQ)
  Left lobe of liver
  Spleen
  Stomach
  Body of pancreas
  Left adrenal gland
  Portion of left kidney
  Splenic flexure of colon
  Portions of transverse and
    descending colon

Right Lower Quadrant (RLQ)
  Lower pole of right kidney
  Cecum and appendix
  Portion of ascending colon
  Bladder (if distended)
  Ovary and salpinx
  Uterus (if enlarged)
  Right spermatic cord
  Right ureter

Left Lower Quadrant (LLQ)
  Lower pole of left kidney
  Sigmoid colon
  Portion of descending colon
  Bladder (if distended)
  Ovary and salpinx
  Uterus (if enlarged)
  Left spermatic cord
  Left ureter

Loops of small bowel are found in all quadrants.

Figure 5-20. *1.* Abdomen divided into quadrants, with a list below of organs in each quadrant. *2.* Abdomen divided into smaller topographic units with terms used in describing location of signs and symptoms. (Adapted from DeGowin, Elmer L., and DeGowin, Richard L.: *Bedside Diagnostic Examination,* 2nd ed. Macmillan Publishing Co., Inc., New York, 1969, p. 452.)

the patient to raise the head and look for herniation around scars at the umbilicus or between the rectus muscles. It is customary to *auscultate* the abdomen next for bruits and bowel sounds.

If bowel obstruction is suspected, Morgan and Engel [139] suggest that examiners should auscultate the abdomen before palpating it since the latter can decrease or increase peristalsis and interfere with the diagnosis. They caution against confusing bowel sounds with those from the heart, transmitted from the chest, or from abdominal blood vessels. They suggest holding the diaphragm of the stethoscope on the abdomen for several minutes in two or three places to identify the sounds of peristalsis. Auscultation of the abdomen can identify one important physical finding, an abdominal bruit, indicating vascular pathology.

Palpate the abdomen lightly, watching the patient's face. Look for tenderness, muscle spasm, or resistance from an underlying mass. If there is tenderness, estimate the degree and localize the area of irritation; if within the wall, grasping a fold of subcutaneous tissue is painful; if in the peritoneum, pain follows the quick release of pressure exerted by the examiner's two fingers on the tender spot. If the irritation is in an underlying organ or mass (tumor), compressing the area between both hands is painful.

Repeat the light palpation with gentle but deeper palpation using a rotary motion. Hard feces in the sigmoid colon in the lower left quadrant may be mistaken for a mass. Masses may represent enlarged organs or lymph nodes, growths or lesions on or in organs. Masses should be studied for their location, size, shape, consistency, tenderness, mobility, and whether they pulsate. There are specific skills in palpating the liver, spleen, kidney, colon, aorta, enlarged bladder, and uterus which should be studied in texts that describe the physical examination in more detail. Percussion as well as auscultation and palpation is used to determine the location and character of abdominal organs, particularly the liver and spleen, lesions, and masses. Generally speaking, a healthy abdomen is soft and no masses are felt. Percussing the normal abdomen produces a hollow sound; a dull sound suggests an enlarged organ, fluid, or a solid mass of some sort. Areas of tenderness also suggest pathology and indicate the need for special diagnostic tests. Before leaving the abdomen, lightly stroke the four quadrants in turn to elicit abdominal reflexes to complete the routine neurologic examination. Also, palpate the femoral arteries in both inguinal regions.

Lower Extremities. After examining the abdomen, the genitalia and rectum may be examined or the legs. Some operators prefer to examine the legs after examining the arms. Whatever the sequence, the procedure is the same for the extremities, comparing muscle strength and status right and left and the reflexes in arms, hands, legs, and feet. When examining the legs, rearrange the blanket or sheet covering the patient to expose the legs, but cover the pubic area. *Inspect* the color and condition of the skin and *feel* its temperature. Inspect the nails, blood vessels, muscles, joints, and lymph nodes. Note any lesions, edema, muscle atrophy, or tremors. Note enlarged or deformed joints (bunions) on the feet; also corns (clavus) and calluses. Test for edema by pressing over the anterior tibial area of the ankle for about 5 seconds to see whether tissues pit or return promptly to normal appearance. If one leg seems larger than the other, it may be desirable to measure the circumference of the calves.

Note any areas of inflammation or tenderness on the lower extremities, and palpate the dorsalis pedis, the posterior tibial and popliteal pulses, comparing them in the two extremities. Palpate the soles of the feet for plantar warts or for calluses, the latter suggesting fallen transverse arches. Test the joints of hip, knee, ankle, and those of the toes for range-of-motion. Test for muscle strength by asking the patient to raise each leg, hold position for about 20 seconds, and lower slowly. Inability to hold the leg up and move smoothly indicates weakness, as does an effort to move one leg with leverage exerted by the other leg. Patients may also demonstrate strength by pushing as hard as they can against the examiner's hand. Muscle strength may be graded as follows: 0 means no visible muscle contraction; 1 means contraction but no movement of joint; 2, complete motion with no help from gravity; 3, barely complete motion against gravity; 4, complete motion against gravity and some resistance; 5, "normal" movement against gravity and full resistance.[140]

The neurologic tests for the lower extremities parallel those for the hands and arms. In fact, a reason for examining the lower extremities immediately after examining the upper extremities is to compare their reflexes. When the extremities are examined in the same "step" it is advisable to begin the examination of the lower extremities with testing the knee and ankle jerks and the plantar reflex.

Ask the supine subject to relax; support the lower thighs by passing one hand under both legs, which flexes the knees slightly. Strike the tendon immediately below the patella with the percussion hammer. It is much easier, however, to test the patellar reflex with the patient sitting upright with legs dangling. To test the ankle reflexes, place each foot in turn on the opposite shin and, with the examiner holding the patient's foot, strike the Achilles tendon with the flat part of the percussion hammer above the heel. Absence of a "jerk" is in both cases abnormal. Before testing the plantar reflex, tell the patient that a rough object, such as a key or a broken tongue blade, will be drawn across the lateral plantar surface of each foot from the heel to the ball of the big toe, which will feel slightly painful like a scratch. The motion must be firm enough not to tickle. Note the initial response of the big toe to this stroke. Dorsiflexion of the big toe and fanning of the other toes are abnormal responses. Reflexes of the legs as well as the arms are graded from 0 to 4+.

To evaluate coordination, ask the supine patient to put a heel on the knee of the other leg and run it down the shin to the ankle; ask the

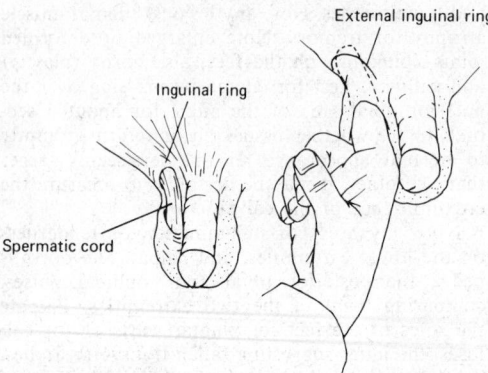

Figure 5-21. Technique of examining inguinal canal. (After Judge, Richard D., and Zuidema, George D.: *Methods of Physical Examination; A Physiologic Approach,* 3rd ed. Little, Brown & Co., Boston, 1974, p. 256.)

person to sit up motionless without support and notice wavering. Ask the patient to tap the thighs rapidly with both hands, palmar surfaces down, then up (rapid alternating movement); if the patient can sit up, ask him to tap the ground rapidly with first one foot and then the other; ask the patient to stand, feet together and eyes closed, with arms extended (Romberg test). The examiner must stand in front of and close to the patient when conducting this test in order to catch the patient should he waver. Notice the patient's gait and ability to walk in tandem steps forward and backward or to balance on one foot. Toe-walking and heel-walking may also be used to test gait.

Sensory tests for touch, pain, and temperature are made as described for the arms, as is the test for *vibratory sensation. Position sense* can be tested by flexing and extending both big toes and asking patients, who have been told to shut their eyes, the direction in which their toes are moved.

Genitalia and Pelvic Organs. This examination can follow the abdominal examination or examination of the lower extremities. Examine the *male genitalia* and *pelvic organs* by inspection and palpation. If the patient is ambulatory, he may stand in slippers or on a paper square, with the gown turned up at the waist or he may be supine. If he is bedfast, he is in the supine position with the blanket or sheet turned down to expose the genitalia. It is desirable to wear gloves while examining the genitalia to protect the examiner from possible infection and as a deterrent to erotic stimulation. Inspect the genitalia and surrounding area for swelling, inflammation, lesions, or asymmetry. Palpate the scrotum, comparing the two sides. Identify the testis, epididymis, and spermatic cord in each hemisphere. Note the size, contour, and sensitivity. The testes are sensitive and even mild pressure produces discomfort. Note the smoothness of the testis and the postlateral attached epididymis. If fluid is felt around the testis, it can be confirmed by darkening the room,

pressing a flashlight against the scrotum, and noting by transillumination a less dense area. Feel the spermatic cord, which contains the vas deferens, with thumb and forefinger. Note character of the vas, which should be smooth. Note any beading, varicosities, cysts, or other masses. Palpate the penis gently and firmly. Retract, or ask the patient to retract, the foreskin if present and inspect the glans, noting the position and size of the urethral meatus. Note presence and character of urethral discharge and any scarring of the glans or coronal sulcus. (A slide for microscopic examination or a culture may be made at this time or the material for study collected later by a laboratory worker.) After replacing the foreskin (if retracted), palpate penile shaft, noting its smoothness and that of contained urethra which can be felt as it leaves the upper part of the scrotum and passes through the perineum and prostate gland to the bladder. (The prostate is palpated through the rectal wall.)

While examining the genitalia, look for inguinal hernias. With the male in a standing or supine position, ask him to "bear down" and note any bulging in the groin. If there is a bulge, palpate the inguinal canal, explaining the uncomfortable, or slightly painful, procedure before doing it.* Ask the patient to evert the leg on the side to be examined. Find the external inguinal ring on the side of the scrotum (see Fig. 5-21). Then, carrying the loose skin of the scrotum and groin up into the canal with the forefinger (use the little finger for a small boy), follow the spermatic cord to the internal ring. Holding the pad of the finger against the ring, ask the patient to bear down, or cough. A bulge is felt against the finger and a hernia as a soft mass entering the canal. A hernia is less easily felt with the patient in the supine position but the procedure is the same.

It is best to prepare the patient carefully for the rectal examination by inquiring whether or not this is a new procedure for him. Suggest that he breathe through the mouth and explain that a lubricant (K-Y jelly) will be applied around the anus to decrease the discomfort when the finger is inserted in the anus.

After putting on a glove, examine the rectum by inspection and palpation. Examine the *rectum of the male,* if he is ambulatory, as he leans at a right angle over the examining table; or, if he is bedfast or if the examination is done following the abdominal examination, ask him to turn on his side (away from the examiner) in the Sims, or left lateral position (see Fig. 5-22). Spread the buttocks to expose the anus, the perineal area, and the sacrococcygeal or pilonidal sinus region where the opening of a pilonidal cyst, if present, will be seen. Note the skin color, pigmentation, inflammation, anal fissures, and any other lesions or growth. Varicosities of the lower rectum and anus (hemorrhoids) can be seen and felt. Note and record the position as if the anus was a clock with 12 pointing to the symphysis pubis. Be sure

---

* Most authorities think all physical examinations should include this procedure.

there is ample lubrication before introducing the forefinger into the rectum. Put the finger beside the anus for a few seconds before entering the rectum, giving the patient time to relax from the instantaneous reaction of contracting the anal sphincter. Also ask the patient to bear down to relax the rectal sphincter; introduce the finger slowly and gently, pointing toward the umbilicus. Note the tone of the sphincter, the crypts of the lower rectum, any tenderness, masses, or thrombosed internal hemorrhoids that feel like cords. Note the presence of blood or pus.

Palpate the male rectum for both lobes of the prostate and the medial sulcus which can be felt under the anterior wall, noting size, contour, smoothness of the borders, presence of nodules, and tenderness. Since the rectal examination is very uncomfortable, even painful, it is hard to be sure that the hurt expressed by the patient as the prostate is palpated is due to its tenderness.

Morgan and Engel [141] say that masses can be felt in the upper rectum if the examiner introduces the finger as far as possible, rotating the forearm so that the forefinger "sweeps" the rectal circumference. This procedure is most effective if the patient can bear down and can squat during it whether the patient is male or female; both bring the lower part of the rectal sigmoid within reach of the finger. (Some examiners depend regularly on anoscopic and proctoscopic explorations for identifying rectal masses or lesions.) In palpating, a fecal mass can be identified by its free movement as contrasted with a polyp or tumor which is attached to the rectum. Withdraw the examining finger slowly. If there is feces on the glove it may be spread on filter paper and tested for the presence of blood. Anoscopic and proctoscopic examinations are described in Chapter 7. They are performed with patients (male or female) in the knee-chest position and usually after special preparation that clears the rectum of feces. After any rectal examination, wipe the anus with a tissue or provide patients with one so that they may do so.

Examination of the female genitalia and pelvic organs follows either the examination of the abdomen or the lower extremities. Being sure that the patient's bladder and rectum have been emptied, put the patient on an examining table in the dorsal recumbent position with the knees flexed, the feet in stirrups or braced against extensions of the table, and the edge of the buttocks at the edge of the table. Bedfast patients can lie across the bed so that the buttocks are near the edge and the knees flexed. If the patient is very weak or ill, the flexed legs should be supported by pillows, and some examiners want the buttocks elevated with pillows. Obviously this examination is more easily made with the patient on a table than in a bed. Drape the patient with a blanket so that only the genitalia and perineum are exposed and cover this area with a towel. If the examiner is male, female nursing personnel prepare the patient and stay with her during the examination. (For discussion of this, see page 384 and see page 422 for a discussion of the circumstances under which pelvic examinations are omitted in

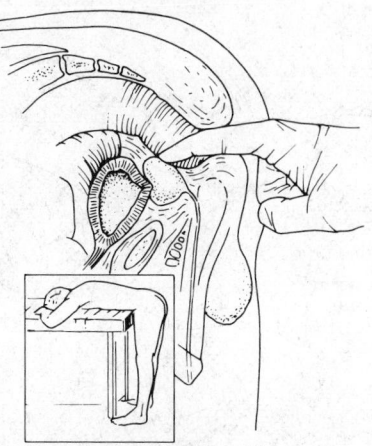

Figure 5-22. Examination of the prostate gland. Inset shows best position, with patient bending over examining table. (After Judge, Richard D., and Zuidema, George D.: *Methods of Physical Examination: A Physiologic Approach,* 3rd ed. Little, Brown & Co., Boston, 1974, p. 245.)

health assessment and diagnosis of disease.) Have a good light directed on the genitalia and sit on a stool in front of or slightly to the side of the area to be examined.

Put on gloves, and before removing the towel and inspecting the external genitalia, ask the patient to draw the knees apart. With the gloved thumb and fingers spread the labia to expose the clitoris and urethral and vaginal openings. Note the character of the pubic hair, the structures just mentioned, the perineum, muscular support, and anus. Look for inflammation, pigmentation or discoloration, lesions, scars, cysts, and discharges. To test the strength of the supporting tissues ask the patient to bear down. Bulging of the anterior vaginal wall indicates a cystocele and urethrocele and bulging of the posterior wall a rectocele. If the uterus is prolapsed the cervix may be seen at or near the vaginal orifice (introitus). Gently palpate the lesser vestibular or Skene's glands and the greater vestibular or Bartholin's glands.

To examine the vagina and cervix, gently introduce sideways a warm closed speculum of the proper size (lubricated with water only) exerting pressure toward the rectum (see Fig. 5-23). When in place, open and lock the blades and inspect the vagina, cervix, and cervical opening (os) for color, swelling, erosions or lesions, masses, and bleeding or other discharge, noting, of course, whether blood is bright red or darker menstrual blood. At this point most pelvic examinations of the female include the collection of specimens from the cervix or vagina for culture, microscopic study, or cytology. After inspecting the area and collecting the specimen or specimens (see Chapter 7), close and remove the speculum, being careful not to pinch the vaginal wall.

To estimate the size, consistency, position,

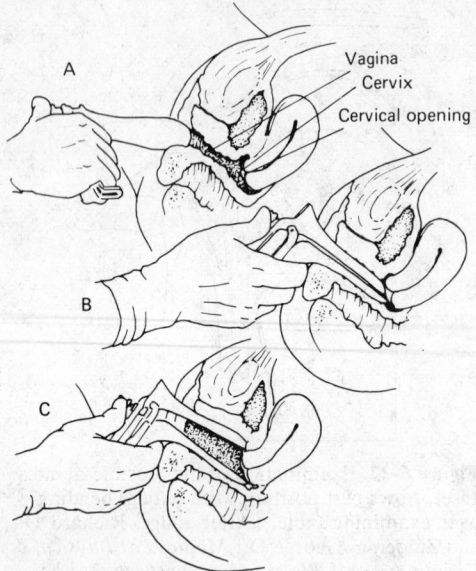

Figure 5-23. Insertion of vaginal speculum. *A*. Blades held obliquely on entering vagina. *B*. Blades rotated to the horizontal position as they pass introitus. *C*. Blades separated by depressing thumbpiece and elevating handle. (After Judge, Richard D., and Zuidema, George D.: *Methods of Physical Examination: A Physiologic Approach*, 3rd ed. Little, Brown & Co., Boston, 1974, p. 277.)

shape, mobility, and tenderness of the cervix, uterus, ovaries, cul-de-sac, and surrounding areas, palpate them with one hand (the right if right-handed), pressing down on the lower abdomen, with the first and second fingers of the other gloved hand well-lubricated and gently inserted into the vagina. This brings the organs and areas under examination between the two hands (see Fig. 5-24). This part of the physical examination is

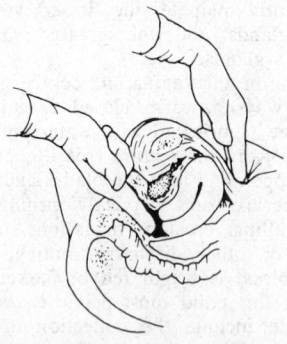

Figure 5-24. Two-handed pelvic examination. The abdominal hand brings the pelvic contents to the intravaginal fingers. (After Judge, Richard D., and Zuidema, George D.: *Methods of Physical Examination: A Physiologic Approach*, 3rd ed. Little, Brown & Co., Boston, 1974, p. 279.)

uncomfortable and even painful. A virginal vagina may not admit more than one finger and even this may stretch the hymen. If pathology is suspected in the cul-de-sac or the tissues between the vagina and rectum, tenderness in the area or the structures may be felt by introducing the forefinger in the vagina and the middle finger (of the same hand) in the rectum. This procedure is used to determine the various positions of the uterus. Opinions differ on the importance of including a vaginal examination of virgins unless pathology is suspected, but it is essential for all women to have a yearly Papanicolaou test. Some women would prefer not to have a pelvic examination during menstruation, but it is not contraindicated medically, and this is the usual time for an intrauterine contraceptive device to be inserted. For detailed description of the technique of the pelvic examination the reader is again referred to any of the standardized texts on physical examination or obstetrics.

Variations in the Foregoing Procedure and Specialized Examinations. An examination such as the one just described may not be possible or advisable when emergency treatment, such as surgery, is indicated. It is not possible when patients are comatose, too weak to move, disoriented, or unwilling to cooperate. The examiner may need one or more assistants. The necessity of an interpreter for those who do not speak the examiner's language has been mentioned, as has the value of support from family members and friends.

When the general physical examination identifies serious pathology or when the examiner wants another opinion, an appropriate specialist may be asked to act as a consultant; he or she may then conduct a more thorough examination of the body "systems," or body areas, involved. There are texts in every medical field with descriptions of these specialized examinations that cannot be included in a general work such as this. Each medical publisher is apt to have a systemic monograph, as, for instance, one on examination of the neurologic system,[142-144] or of an organ or organs such as the heart [145] or the colon, rectum, and anus,[146] or a function such as motor strength and coordination.[147] All examiners should make full use of detailed sources as needs arise.

Modifications of the steps in the physical examination for infants, children, and adolescents is essential. All newborn infants should have an assessment, and Virginia Apgar has suggested a mnemonic device (see Fig. 5-25), with special reference to potential asphyxiation, that may be scored. The Apgar Score for the newborn is very commonly used.[148,149] The use of this checking device immediately after birth is helpful but does not determine the need for certain procedures such as suctioning nose and mouth, suctioning with administration of oxy-

Sign	Score		
	0	1	2
A Appearance (color)	Blue; pale	Body pink, extremities blue	Completely pink
P Pulse	Absent	Below 100	Over 100
G Grimace (reflex irritability in response to stimulation of the sole of the foot)	No response	Grimace	Cry
A Activity (muscle tone)	Limp	Some flexion of extremities	Active motion
R Respiration (respiratory effort)	Absent	Slow, irregular	Good strong cry

Figure 5-25. Apgar score used to determine need for resuscitation of newborn infant. (From Silver, Henry K., et al.: *Handbook of Pediatrics,* 10th ed. Lange Medical Publications, Los Altos, Calif., 1973, p. 119.)

gen by face mask, or, in the severely depressed newborn with scores of 0 to 3, intubating and administering positive pressure with a self-inflating breathing bag (see Chapter 20).

Silver and his associates [150] say that if the newborn is vigorous at birth, a complete physical examination can be delayed for 6 to 12 hours; it may be necessary to examine prematurely born infants in stages to avoid tiring them. A pediatric text should be consulted for details of the examination of the newborn, but this examination should disclose, among other things, skeletal and neuromotor defects (cleft palate and spina bifida, for example) and imperforate openings to the body cavities such as the bladder or rectum.

Most authorities think that every child should have a complete physical examination at regular intervals. The order of steps is different for children and adults. It is desirable, for example, to start with examination of the heart and chest before the child starts crying, which makes auscultation impossible. It is suggested that steps that hurt, as, for example, palpating the abdomen and examining the ears, be postponed to the end of the examination. The examiner should make an effort to interest and entertain the children but never patronize them or seem hesitant and ill-at-ease, or rush at them. George H. Lowry, writing in Judge and Zuidema,[151] says "proceed nonchalantly" and with "confidence."

Children up to 4 years of age may be held in the mother's lap during most of the examination; the mother should be allowed to undress the child and take the temperature of the small child. The child is undressed in stages as necessary. Toys, music, and conversation may be used to divert small children and the understanding of older children should be elicited since the examination can be interesting and instructive to them. The examiner sits during most of the examination and, in general, tries to work at eye level with the child.

Many children are shy and embarrassed if required to undress in the presence of others, especially strangers. A sheet or a special garment should be provided that spares them experiences that may make them dread physical assessments all their lives. Adolescents are especially sensitive but physicians should not omit examination of the genitalia unless there is some indication for this. Specialized publications listed at the end of this chapter should be used by those who are studying the physical examination of infants, children, and adolescents.[152-155]

Laboratory Tests. There are routine tests, such as those listed for periodic health examinations (see page 386), that are also regularly included in diagnostic examinations. Additional tests that might be included are too numerous to even mention here. Chapter 7 is devoted to a description of types of tests and a description of individual tests thought most commonly used.

Mental Status, or Psychiatric Examination. Earlier in this chapter (see page 389) the point was made that every health examination include some assessment of mental and emotional health—the person's psychic, as well as his or her physical, development. It was pointed out that the data or information may be elicited by questionnaires (written or by touch terminals) or by interviews, or by combining these methods. The mental, or emotional, data may be integrated with the physical data sought or it may be separated. Complete separation is actually impossible because people's postures, movements, expressions, the way they dress, and what they say tell something about their mental state. The health history and the physical examination, as described in the preceding pages, may give the examiner sufficient data to make portions of the following test unnecessary. But whether the content of the test is integrated or covered separately either before or after the physical examination, it should include certain evaluations. The following description is based largely on the work of Dye and Charlat [156] and Edward S. Tucker.[157]

Dye and Charlat say there are three main types of observations to be made: the *immediate data*—major complaints or problems; their symptoms and what precipitated them; the mental state, use of drugs and general physical condition; *external data* or psychosocial environment and any history of past illnesses or use of drugs; and *characteristic way of behaving,* or interacting, with others.

Ideally, mental status or psychiatric examinations should not be threatening or anxiety-provoking. The examiner, who is interviewing or administering a questionnaire, should try to put the subject at ease, assuring him or her that the questions are a part of every health examination—a means of organizing and recording observations. Patients should be interviewed in privacy, and if ambulatory, either before they have undressed for the physical examination or after it is over and they are again dressed. Data may be recorded under the following headings (Tucker suggests having all parts of a mental status test written and all answers recorded as given):

1. *Appearance, manner* in responding to the examiner or the nonverbal behavior.
2. *Speech,* noting its quality (tone, inflection, pronunciation, continuity); quantity (free, monosyllabic, or other); and organization (coherent, logical, relevant, disorganized, or other).
3. *Orientation,* as judged by answers to questions on time, place, and person. (Such questions are inappropriate if the person's orientation is obviously normal.)
4. *Thought processes,* noting spontaneity, coherence, continuity; the ease or difficulty with which questions are answered, any "flight of ideas," or unwanted recurring thoughts (obsessions), any strange experiences or thoughts (delusions or hallucinations), and any feeling of being the subject of talk by others.
5. *Short-term memory* is tested by asking the person to immediately repeat a sentence with a theme and numbers and then repeat it in about 10 minutes. This is auditory recall. Visual recall may be tested by asking the subjects after 10 minutes to name objects shown them.
6. *Registration, immediate recall, and ability to organize* can be tested by asking subjects to repeat a simple series of numbers forward and backward, being sure first that the patients understand what they are to do. Tucker says that most persons can repeat 7 numbers forward and 5 backward.
7. *Attention and concentration* can be tested by asking subjects to subtract a series of 7s from 100 (as 93, 86, 79, etc.) until 8 to 10 calculations have been made.
8. *General information* (or general intelligence) * can be assessed by asking questions increasingly difficult to answer, as, How many days in a week? How many things in a dozen? Who invented the airplane? What's the capital of Ohio? Why does oil float? What is a hieroglyph? Who wrote Paradise Lost? What is a prime number?
9. *Abstraction* or ability to conceptualize can be tested by asking subjects to interpret a well-known proverb, making sure that there are no language or cultural barriers. Another exercise is to ask people to say in what way two things are alike, as, for example, a dog and a cat, an apple and a plum, a flute and a piano, a verb and a noun, and a train and an airplane.
10. *Judgment* may be tested by asking questions about the social order, laws, customs, or personal relations, as, for example, Why must an automobile be licensed? What would you do if you discovered a fire in a public building? Why should promises be kept? What do you do if you find you have offended a person unintentionally?
11. *Emotional state* is judged by the appropriateness of the ideas expressed, the range of emotions, mood swings (emotional lability), pervasive elation, undue optimism (euphoria), pessimism, and depression.

Robert A. McKinnon and Robert Michels [158] say that suicidal intentions should be investigated in all depressed persons. They recommend asking people whether they want to live. If they say "No," ask them whether they have suicidal thoughts or plans and if so what they are. McKinnon and Michels think that talking

* When subjects' responses to these and other questions suggest a discrepancy between their educational levels and intelligence, a detailed psychologic test such as the Wechsler Adult Intelligence Scale (WAIS) may be administered by specialists.

about them is more likely to prevent than to precipitate suicide, as is commonly believed. Planning is a serious symptom, especially if the means are at hand. Dye and Charlat think the existence of a plan for suicide is the single most significant symptom.

There is a higher incidence of suicide in males than females and in older than younger persons. Other related conditions are recent stress or loss of a beloved relative or friend, psychosis—especially severe depression, schizophrenia, agitation, a serious physical illness, hopelessness, alcoholism or other drug addiction, homosexuality—and extreme poverty or destitution. For more information on suicide and sources of help, see Chapter 41.

Health workers in emergency units or ambulatory services may often be confronted with the necessity of intervening in a crisis. The general examination just described may be inappropriate for acutely ill psychotic persons. For further study of this subject, consult specialized works.[159-164]

8. DIAGNOSIS AND DECISION-MAKING; HEALTH COUNSELING

Definition, Various Meanings of "Diagnosis." Diagnosis is a word that can be used specifically or generally. It is a Greek word derived from verbs meaning to distinguish and to know. Webster gives the first meaning of diagnosis as "the art or act" of recognizing disease from its symptoms and also "the decision reached"; its second meaning as "scientific determination, critical scrutiny or its resulting judgment." If "scientific determination" and "critical scrutiny" are accepted as legitimate meanings, clearly the term can be used not only in the specific sense of recognizing disease from its symptoms but in the very general sense of critical scrutiny and scientific determination in solving any problem, whether or not it is in the field of health.

Role of Patient, Family, and Friends in Diagnosis and Decision-Making in Matters of Health. Usually when people think that they are functioning abnormally, or, most particularly, if they have pain or discomfort, they want to know why, or "what's wrong." Sometimes, as in the case of infants or small children, it is the parent or guardian who notices malfunction or signs of pain and wants to know "what's wrong." Occasionally a change in function may be so gradual that it is unrecognized by the subject; he or she is shocked to have a relative or friend say "Why are you so short of breath?" or "When did you get so deaf?" But usually those affected realize they

are sick or disabled and by the time they take the problem to someone who they believe more knowledgeable than themselves—be it the corner druggist, the tribal medicine man, the physician, the nurse, or some other health worker—they have one or more "diagnoses" in mind. They may, in fact, have been quietly treating themselves on the assumption that they did know what was wrong. Many a person, for example, has attributed pain in the area of the stomach to "too much acid" and has used bicarbonate of soda to cure their "dyspepsia," or "acid-indigestion," only to find, after being correctly diagnosed as having pernicious anemia, that their indigestion could be relieved by taking an acid (hydrochloric) after each meal instead of the alkaline salt they thought they needed. On the other hand, a man with an alcoholic wife may know subconsciously that his indigestion has an emotional origin but, not wanting to admit his problem to himself or to a doctor, may never be correctly diagnosed or treated.

Effective treatment depends, therefore, on many things, including an accurate health history, a thorough examination (physical and mental or psychologic), a correct diagnosis, and upon the acceptance of the diagnosis and treatment by patients and families. So it is important for health workers to begin the diagnostic process by identifying what patients and families believe to be the health problem or problems and what steps they have taken to solve it or them. With the "neurotic" and "hypochondriac," self-knowledge is essential to improvement; for everyone, understanding of the problem, participation in solving it, or decision-making, is most important.

Reference was made earlier in this chapter to the present-day legal stress on "informed consent" from the patient before instituting treatment. But this is only the beginning. The patient's participation in decision-making is almost necessary if he or she is to be fully rehabilitated or regain independence.

Some physicians clearly recognize the necessity of self-diagnosis and self-treatment and have written many home remedy texts designed to help the layman recognize and treat common diseases. A 1973 publication, *The Well Body Book*,[165] by Mike Samuels (a physician) and Hal Bennett (an educator), has been mentioned several times in this chapter. It tells laymen how to examine their own or a friend's body and how to recognize and treat conditions such as acne, scabies, impacted ear wax, influenza, hay fever, hemorrhoids, lower back pain, varicose veins, and infectious mononucleosis. The authors tell the layman how to use the doctor as a "consultant" and in some cases

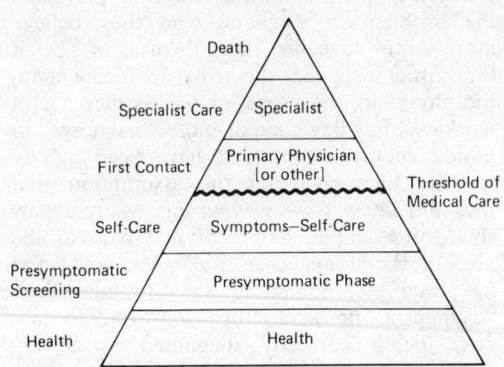

Figure 5-26. The iceberg of health and disease. (From Fry, J.: "Medical Care in Three Societies. Common Problems and Dilemmas in the U.S.S.R., U.S.A., and U.K.," *Int. J. Health Services,* **1:**121, [No. 2] 1971.)

what tests the patient might ask the doctor to make, or what drugs or type of drug the doctor might be asked to prescribe. Obviously, the authors expect the patient to play a leading role in preventing, diagnosing, and treating disease. See also Figure 5-26 for a graphic illustration of treatment that goes on below the threshold of medical care.

References in this and other chapters have been made to the role of nurses and other health workers in diagnostic and decision-making processes. Practice varies greatly from country to country, from state to state (or province), and from one institution to another. The following discussion is an attempt to identify trends in varied and rapidly changing roles.

Role of the Physician. Of all health workers, physicians are best prepared to diagnose disease. Diagnosis and treatment of disease are the functions that organized medicine values most, although some physicians spend their professional lives in preventing disease while others specialize in research. The wording of medical practice acts limits the right to diagnose and treat disease to physicians (and dentists).* This has been and still is a roadblock in the delivery of health care in those countries with so few, such poorly distributed, or such specialized physicians that they cannot provide primary medical care for the entire population. Organized medicine in many countries is moving toward compromise, toward changes in medical practice acts that enable physicians to share with other health workers the responsibility for diagnosis and treatment.

* See Chapter 1 for further discussion of this question and the suggestion that professional nurses be exempted from this prohibition.

State medical associations have endorsed nurse practice acts that include "diagnosis" and "decision-making" as nursing functions. Eliot Freidson,[166] in his monograph *Professional Dominance*, expresses the opinion that the competition doctors are now experiencing is "healthy"; Barbara Bates,[167-172] a physician, who has worked for years with nurses as colleagues, expresses the opinion that doctors must accept the fact that as other health professionals assume some of their traditional functions, they must necessarily compete for "the health dollar," for working space, and for institutional privileges. She and her colleagues make a strong plea for colleague relationships and shared responsibility, presenting diagrams that show the overlapping functions of doctors and nurses. Lynaugh and Bates[173] point out differences in medical and nursing emphases and terminology, suggesting that a doctor and a nurse looking at the same problem can suggest a better solution than either might suggest working alone.

Western medicine has, until very recently, concentrated on diagnosis of disease rather than assessment of health and disease prevention. DeGowin and Degowin give the following meanings of diagnosis:

The name of the patient's disease or state of altered function is termed *the diagnosis* or *a diagnosis.* . . . But the act of searching for or determining the patient's disease is commonly referred to as *diagnosis* (without the article), . . . *

Judge and Zuidema say the elements of diagnostic logic may be identified as observation, description, interpretation, verification, diagnosis, and action. They say, "diagnosis . . . involves applying the final label. *The decision:* which disease or diseases account for the illness." Under action, they say that "This involves determining a course based on the diagnosis. *The decision:* selecting the proper treatment, whether it be surgical or nonsurgical." † Engel and Morgan say "The diagnostic process is the mental operation through which *the disease* [italics ours] is identified and the illness evaluated." ‡ Engel[174] in 1960 had called for a unified concept of health and disease.

Alvin R. Feinstein,[175] in *Clinical Judgment,* urges doctors to make diagnoses more "patient centered," saying that the care of the patient

* DeGowin, Elmer L., and DeGowin, Richard L.: *op. cit.,* p. 1.
† Judge, Richard D., and Zuidema, George D.: *Physical Diagnosis, A Physiologic Approach to the Clinical Examination,* 2nd ed. Little, Brown & Co., Boston, 1968, p. 9.
‡ Engel, George L., and Morgan, William L.: *Interviewing the Patient.* W. B. Saunders Co., Philadelphia, 1973, p. 16.

is the ultimate specific act that characterizes a clinician, but he says diagnosis is that "which gives the disease a name and tells what is wrong."

Recently Weed [176] has led a movement away from the kind of diagnostic process that focuses on *the* diagnosis; that is, naming *the* disease or condition from which the patient suffers and is to be treated. The problem-oriented medical care management he advocates is discussed and illustrated in Chapter 4. Under this plan of medical management many problems may be identified by physicians and others. The patient may get help with some or all of them but all problems are recorded and progress in solving them assessed.

The problem-oriented system of medical management is receiving wide attention and support from many quarters, as noted in Chapter 4. It is in line with the observation of the Carnegie Commission on Higher Education [177] that emphasis in medical education is changing from naming the disease to helping families with health problems and recognizing that assessing behavior is as important as assessing physical symptoms. It was noted in Chapter 1 that John B. Dillon,[178] a physician, in an article decrying the overemphasis on technologic research in medical education, entitled "How Did It Happen?", pointed out that Abraham Flexner, whose report of 1910 "reformed" medical education, actually considered preventive medicine and teaching the patient essential aspects of medical practice.

Medicine has invested an inordinate amount of time in identifying and categorizing diseases, as evidenced by many publications.[179,180] Several hundred years of effort have culminated in an *International Classification of Diseases* [181] prepared under the auspices of, and published by, the World Health Organization. The tabulation of diseases and surgical operations in the following categories fills a volume of 671 pages in its 8th edition (1963).

Tabular List of Inclusions and Fourth-Digit Subcategories

Infective and Parasitic Diseases; Neoplasms; Endocrine, Nutritional, and Metabolic Diseases; Diseases of the Blood and Blood-Forming Organs; Mental Disorders; Diseases of the Nervous System and Sense Organs; Diseases of the Circulation System; Diseases of the Respiratory System; Diseases of the Digestive System; Diseases of the Genitourinary System; Complications of Pregnancy, Childbirth, and the Puerperium; Diseases of the Skin and Subcutaneous Tissue; Diseases of the Musculoskeletal System and Connective Tissue; Congenital Anomalies; Certain Causes of Perinatal Morbidity and Mortality; Symptoms and Ill-Defined Conditions; Accidents, Poisonings, and Violence (External Cause).

Surgical Operations, Diagnostic and Other Therapeutic Procedures

Neurosurgery; Ophthalmology; Otorhinolaryngology; Operations on Thyroid, Parathyroid, Thymus, and Adrenals; Vascular and Cardiac Surgery; Thoracic Surgery; Abdominal Surgery; Proctologic Surgery; Urologic Surgery; Breast Surgery; Gynecologic Surgery; Obstetric Procedures; Orthopedic Surgery; Plastic Surgery; Oral and Maxillofacial Surgery; Dental Surgery; Biopsy; Diagnostic Endoscopy; Diagnostic Radiography; Radiotherapy and Related Therapies; Physical Medicine and Rehabilitation; Other Nonsurgical Procedures.

Uniform nomenclature is essential for morbidity and mortality statistics—international, national, state or province, county, city, and institutional.

Physicians who see the diagnostic and decision-making process as a matter of deciding on *the* disease or condition from which the patient is suffering and *the* treatment for it are more likely to think of the doctor's role as *the* diagnostician; physicians who see diagnosis and decision-making as a matter of identifying the health problems of individuals and families and helping them cope with them are more likely to see diagnosis and decision-making as a collaborative procedure. Bates [182,183] and Karen F. Pridham [184] are among the physicians who have tried to show, in some cases writing with nurses, just how collaboration with nurses works.

In hospitals and clinics with medical students, interns, and residents and highly qualified nurses, the physical examination is very often made by one of them with attending physicians repeating the whole, parts of, or no part of the procedure but discussing the findings with the examiner; in hospitals and nursing homes where there is no resident medical personnel, the patient's physician has usually made some sort of examination before asking that the patient be admitted. In schools and industries, practices vary greatly in the quality of the health services they provide, but in most, if not all of them, nurses and other health workers conserve the physicians' time by carrying out such aspects of the physical examination as the physicians do not elect to carry out themselves.[185-189] This is also true in the health screening processes in military recruitment centers, health maintenance units, and comparable services. As has been described by Garfield,[190] health screening services depend heavily on technology, with the physician's role being that of an analyzer of data collected by technicians and machines, an interpreter of the findings to the client, and a consultant to him or her on following up or correcting defects identified during the health assessment.

Role of the Nurse. The circumstances under which nurses practice have always affected their roles in diagnosis and decision-making. Nurses working on islands and in remote rural areas where there are no doctors have been forced by the urgent needs of those they served to take histories, do physical examinations, analyze their findings, "diagnose" or label the "presenting problem" or problems, and institute action or "treatment," and they have often been very effective. For example, the success of nurse-midwives working independently of physicians most of the time in the Kentucky mountains is relatively well documented.[191-193] The effectiveness of nurses working with minimal recourse to medical collaboration in the health services for Eskimos and Indians in Canada and the United States has been recognized.[194-198] Nurses in schools, in industry, in corrective institutions (and in many hospitals where doctors are not readily available at night) must of necessity make "diagnoses" and decide on courses of action. J. J. A. Reid, a British medical officer of health, says there is still an argument as to whether the nurse should have a role in diagnosis, but he thinks much depends on what is meant by the term. He says:

District nurses have for many years been accustomed to . . . the public consulting them about minor ailments and . . . being asked for advice on whether the condition is serious enough to warrant consulting a doctor. In the hospital . . . the ward sister or night superintendent has always had to decide on whether a doctor should be called because of some change in a patient's condition. Similarly the . . . occupational health nurse has long been used to assessing whether a patient . . . with a minor ailment or injury should be treated on the spot or whether he should be referred to his general practitioner or to the hospital . . . emergency department. There is ample precedent for involvement of nurses in the diagnostic process.*

Jane Henderson, a Canadian nurse, is quoted as follows in a news item: " . . . as we broaden the definition of care from one centered on pathology to one concerned with life style and environment we simultaneously broaden the definition of diagnosis." † A diagram of "the iceberg of health and disease" by J. Fry (see Fig. 5-26) makes a similar point

that most health problems are not brought to the physician or a surrogate for solution but are actually "diagnosed" by the person who has the symptoms, or by the family.

While people intimately associated with health services know that nurses everywhere have been forced by circumstances to fill the role of diagnostician and decision-maker the function has never been written into nurse practice acts until this decade, nor have history-taking and methods of physical (or clinical) assessment been taught in basic nursing curricula. They have been taught, however, in some form in graduate programs.

Since 1972, when the New York State Nurse Practice Act was amended to include the following description of nursing practice, other states have followed suit or have committees working on amendments to their practice acts:

The practice of the profession of nursing as a registered professional nurse is defined as diagnosing and treating human responses to actual or potential health problems through such services as casefinding, health teaching, health counseling, and provision of care supportive to or restorative of life and well-being, and executing medical regimens prescribed by a licensed or otherwise legally authorized physician or dentist. A nursing regimen shall be consistent with and not vary any existing medical regimen.*

A Bill to amend Sections 2725 and 2726 of the Business and Professions Code relating to nurses was referred to the Committee on Health of the California legislature in February 1974. It reads, in part, as follows:

The practice of nursing within the meaning of this chapter means those functions helping people cope with difficulties in daily living which are associated with their actual or potential health or illness problems or the treatment thereof which require a substantial amount of scientific knowledge or technical skill, and includes all of the following:

(a) Direct and indirect patient care services that insure the safety, comfort, personal hygiene, and protection of patients; and the performance of disease prevention and restorative measures.

(b) Direct and indirect patient care services, including, but not limited to, the administration of medications and therapeutic agents, necessary to implement a treatment, disease prevention, or rehabilitative regimen prescribed by a physician, dentist, or podiatrist.

(c) The performance of basic health care, testing, and prevention procedures, including, but not limited to, skin tests, immunization

---

* Reid, J. J. A.: "Preventive Medicine. In Great Britain," in the Royal Society of Medicine and the Josiah Macy, Jr. Foundation: *The Greater Medical Profession.* The Foundation, New York, 1973, p. 111.

† "Basic Health Care Changes Needed, Nurse Tells Physicians' Meeting," *Can. Nurse,* **69:**7, (Nov.) 1973.

* New York State, Senate-Assembly: *An Act to Amend the Law in Relation to the Practice of Nursing, 1972.* N.Y. Ed. Law Section 6902.

techniques, and the withdrawal of human blood from veins and arteries.

(d) Observation of signs and symptoms of illness, reactions to treatment, general behavior, or general physical condition, and (1) determination of whether such signs, symptoms, reactions, behavior, or general appearance exhibit abnormal characteristics; and (2) implementation, based on observed abnormalities, of appropriate reporting, or referral, or standardized procedures, or changes, in treatment regimen in accordance with standardized procedures, or the initiation of emergency procedures.

Using the words "diagnosis" or "diagnose" and "treatment" in proposed nurse practice acts seems to delay enactment and to elicit opposition from organized medicine. However, if modifying terms that limit the nurse's role in diagnosis and treatment are used, the opposition is overcome. Eileen M. Jacobi, analyzing nurse practice acts in 1973 and responses to a questionnaire on the expanded role of the nurse, noted that "In two states, the definition of nursing practice has been modified (1) to permit diagnosis and treatment under emergency or special conditions, including special training, and (2) by rules and regulations promulgated jointly by the board of nursing and the board of medicine." * Jacobi questioned whether definitions of nursing practice in the laws of the United States were flexible enough to allow nurses to expand their role. She noted that definitions in 18 states restricted the right of nurses to diagnose and prescribe treatment. In Chapter 1, the study for the National Joint Practice Commission by Virginia C. Hall, *Statutory Regulation of the Scope of Nursing Practice—A Critical Survey,* was cited. She made the following observation:

The only way to permit expansion of the independent practice of nursing into medicine, and at the same time retain in the law the traditional notion of the distinct nature of the independent practice of the two, is to adopt a theory that whatever is nursing cannot, by definition, *because* it is nursing, fall within the scope of what is medical, even if it includes acts which if performed by a physician would concededly be medical—in other words, that the nature of the practitioner determines the nature of the act. This theory seems much too metaphysical to be credible. In addition, it proves too much, because in effect it obliterates any exclusive province of medicine and by its terms would permit the expansion of nursing into all of medicine. Any express or implicit statutory prohibition against acts of medical diagnosis or other medical acts would simply be irrelevant as applied to nursing.

Even in the unlikely event that some such theory of interpretation is judicially accepted in some States, it would still amount to a highly circuitous and unnecessarily complex way to achieve the desired result. There is no reason why the traditional medicine/nursing dichotomy should be retained where it is no longer realistic. Therefore, except where political realities dictate otherwise, it should be discarded entirely and, optimally, be replaced by an explicit recognition of the overlap of the independent practice of the professions of nursing and medicine.*

Hall thinks that exempting nurses from the prohibition against the practice of medicine in medical practice acts the simplest way to solve the legal problems involved in the expanded role of the nurse, as mentioned in Chapter 1.

Lucie Young Kelly, also studying nurse practice acts, said in 1974:

The silent conspiracy among hospital administrators, nurses, and physicians to allow nurses to perform services that were desired by and convenient to all concerned, under the guise of overall physician supervision and medical protocol, continued as it had for a hundred years, although in a more sophisticated manner. It was obvious that nurses practiced effectively in ICU's and saved countless lives. What else could anyone ask? †

Fowkes, and Hunn,[199] discussing "legal considerations" in clinical assessment for the nurse practitioner in 1973, express the opinion that proposed revision in state nurse practice acts will define "areas of responsibility" and "provide legal coverage."

In Canada, a joint statement of the Canadian Nurses' Association and the Canadian Medical Association on the expanded role of the nurse included the following:

. . . priority should be given to expanding the role of nurses who work in direct and close association with physicians in the field of primary health care. . . .
. . . primary health care . . . refers to . . . services . . . provided for individuals mainly on an ambulatory basis in the community or in their homes and includes . . . diagnostic and therapeutic services offered in physicians' offices, in clinics or in health centres. . . .

The Joint Committee concluded that the roles of nurses and physicians are "interdependent," that the associative role is an "evolving one,"

---

* Jacobi, Eileen M.: "Accountability of the Nurse." "Are There Legal Barriers to Assuming Full Professional Responsibility?" (Speeches presented during the 48th Convention of the American Nurses' Association.) The Association, Kansas City, Mo., 1973, p. 1.

* Hall, Virginia C.: *Statutory Regulation of the Scope of Nursing Practice—A Critical Survey.* National Joint Practice Commission, Chicago, 1975, pp. 21–22.
† Kelly, Lucie Young: "Nursing Practice Acts," *Am. J. Nurs.,* **74:**1310, (July) 1974,

and that the "mix of professionals working in a setting will influence what a nurse would regularly do." The Joint Committee said that the "ultimate responsibility for diagnosis and establishment of a medical therapeutic plan will remain with the physician." The Canadian report seemed to suggest that with special preparation, graduates of 2-year or 3-year basic nursing programs might take over "selected responsibilities now tending to be handled by physicians" if the nurse is working "in association with the physician." *

In a period of rapid social change—and no one questions that this is one of them—it is understandable that roles of the doctors and nurses change and that change alters their relationship. As nurses take over in certain institutions and agencies the function of health assessment for all or groups of patients, it may be expected that they will bring to it the emphasis of nursing, which has been on how people cope with life, or the daily activities of living, rather than on the existence within them of a particular disease.† For this reason, nursing has welcomed Weed's approach to medical management, since it emphasizes identification of patients' problems rather than the identification of a particular disease or *the* diagnosis.[200,201,201a] Mack Lipkin, whose text *The Care of Patients, Concepts and Tactics* (Oxford University Press, New York, 1974) is as helpful to nurses as to physicians, makes the following comment on the Weed system:

Its advantages are numerous and important. Properly used, it produces better data, better organized. It encourages a clearer appreciation of the patient's problems and their logical evaluation. It has been a powerful stimulus to changing the existing pattern of devoting more teaching time to pathophysiology than to the needs of the patient (p. 108).

Because certain nurses have thought that they needed something more than the medical diagnosis to guide them in giving nursing care, they propose that nurses make a "nursing diagnosis" for each patient. They see the nurse's diagnosis as something apart from the physician's diagnosis.

Kristine Gebbie and Mary Ann Lavin, in a report of the First National Conference on the Classification of Nursing Diagnoses held at St.

Louis University, October, 1973, gave the following "Tentative List of [34] Nursing Diagnoses," * which are listed alphabetically because the conference participants couldn't agree on a classification system:

Alterations in faith
Altered relationships with self and others
Altered self-concept
Anxiety
Body fluids, depletion of
Bowel function, irregular
Cognitive functioning, alteration in the level of
Comfort level, alterations in
Confusion (disorientation)
Deprivation
Digestion, impairment of
Family's adjustment to illness, impairment of
Family process, inadequate
Fear
Grieving
Lack of understanding
Level of consciousness, alterations in
Malnutrition
Manipulation
Mobility, impaired
Motor incoordination
Noncompliance
Pain
Regulatory function of the skin, impairment of
Respiration, impairment of
Respiratory distress
Self-care activities, altered ability to perform
Sensory disturbances
Skin integrity, impairment of
Sleep-rest pattern, ineffective
Susceptibility to hazards
Thought process, impaired
Urinary elimination, impairment of
Verbal communication, impairment of

Most of these diagnoses are psychosocial problems in coping with which the patient presumably needs help from nurses. Gebbie and Lavin note that it has taken the medical profession 300 years to develop the "sophisticated" *International Classification of Diseases and Systematized Nomenclature of Pathology;* they suggest that nursing should "learn from other disciplines" but they imply that it should develop a parallel list of nursing diagnoses. It may be that nursing will take this direction or it may be that nursing and medicine will develop a thoroughly collaborative role in which the patient will benefit from the medical emphasis on specific pathology and the nurse's sensitivity to the psychosocial needs of the patient. The latter approach has been taken in

---

* "The Expanded Role of the Nurse: A Joint Statement of CNA/CMA," *Can. Nurse,* **69:**23, (May) 1973; "Extended Role of the Nurse and Preparation for It as Defined in Canadian RN–MD Statement," *Am. J. Nurs.,* **73:**964, (June) 1973.

† Joan E. Lynaugh and Barbara Bates, a nurse and physician, discussing "The Two Languages of Nursing and Medicine," (*Am. J. Nurs.,* **73:**66, [Jan.] 1973) note that, among the contrasting emphases, nurses talk about patients' problems and how nurses can help them deal with them; physicians talk about the diagnosis and treatment.

* Gebbie, Kristine, and Lavin, Mary Ann: "Classifying Nursing Diagnoses," *Am. J. Nurs.,* **74:**250 (Feb.) 1974.

this text and seems to be suggested by the writings of Weed and other physicians, who say that all professional health workers may identify patient problems, and by Bates and her associates, who call attention to the improvement of patient care through "nurse-physician teamwork." [202-204]

Just as diagnosis or patient problems may be identified collaboratively by the patient, the physician, the nurse (and other health professionals), the decision-making, treatment, or course of action is most likely to be effective if it is arrived at jointly.

In the report of a study of the nurse's role made by Evelyn R. Anderson for the Royal College of Nursing and the National Council of Nurses of the United Kingdom, it is noted that "the doctor is most concerned with the technical aspects of the nurse's work," but later Anderson says "Nurses must not stress technical competence at the expense of continuing to give emotional support that is so strongly needed, as *evidenced by patient comments* [italics ours]. Therefore the training of doctors and nurses should include methods of dealing with the emotional problems of hospitalized patients." In another context Anderson says "Doctor/nurse partnerships in the form of health teams in the community are being advanced. The nurse in 1980 may be moving freely between home and hospital, being responsible for family groups in a role similar to that of the family [medical] practitioner. This changing role will require much adaptation from the nursing profession." *

The role of the nurse in health assessment, diagnosis, and decision-making is under discussion around the world, as evidenced by programs at the 1973 International Council of Nurses' Quadrennial Meeting in Mexico. The Josiah Macy, Jr. Foundation sponsored two conferences on the roles of various health workers in delivering health care in various countries.[205-206] The National Science Foundation in the United States sponsored the preparation of a critical annotated bibliography of research on new health practitioners [nurse practitioners, physician's assistants, and others]. By 1974, about 200 studies had been identified.[207]

There is general agreement that the nurse's actual role has, throughout this century, often been a more independent one than is reflected in nurse practice acts; that nurse practice acts should be amended to enable nurses to legally practice more independently and to be ac-

countable for their acts. It is also believed by many that nursing education must regularly prepare professional nurses for independent practice—most especially for clinical assessment, diagnosis, and decision-making.

As indicated throughout this chapter, the decision, or plan of care, is always, in the final analysis, the right of the adult, or, for the infant or child, the right of the parents or guardian. The "decision" of the health worker can take the form of health counseling or prescribing treatment but either can be accepted or rejected by the patient or the parents or guardian.

If prevention of disease is really more important than its cure, and many writers say that more "health dollars" should be spent on prevention than on cure, it follows that health counseling is more important than treatment. Malleson,[208] in his critique of medical care titled *Need Your Doctor Be So Useless?* seems to come to this conclusion. He believes no system yet devised is really effective; he thinks "treatment can be lethal," and he believes drugs are overused by doctors. He cited studies indicating that doctors spend so little time with patients that they can't possibly know enough about patients' conditions to prescribe drugs, particularly dangerous drugs and ones that demand close medical supervision. Malleson attributes much of the abuse of drugs to the fact that the public expects, even demands, drug prescriptions from the doctor. Whatever treatment medical workers give, Malleson makes the over-all judgment that it tends to produce dependency rather than self-reliance, which should be the goal of therapy. Like Samuels and Bennett,[209] Ivan Illich,[209a] and Rick J. Carlson [209b] Malleson sees the concerned, educated, independent patient as the only hope for reversing the unfortunate consequences of much of the present-day spiraling medical care and its spiraling cost.

Health counseling begins with population control—preventing the birth of unwanted children and diseased or defective children. The increasing incidence of "the battered child syndrome" is, according to some writers, a symptom of overpopulation. Preventing the birth of unwanted children is certainly one effective approach to abolishing child abuse. Another way of attacking the problem is to prevent the birth of defective infants by genetic counseling,* for defective children are most likely to be abused.

---

* Anderson, Evelyn R.: *The Role of the Nurse. Views of the Patient, Nurse and Doctor in Some General Hospitals in England.* The Study of Nursing Care Project Reports, Series 2, Number 1. Royal College of Nursing, London, 1973.

* In genetic counseling, someone with special knowledge of genetics (physician, nurse, physiologist, or other) discusses the inheritance of defects and diseases with parents, or potential parents, and its implications for birth control, abortion, treatment during pregnancy, and family planning.

Genetics is a rapidly developing science and the significance of DNA (deoxyribonucleic acid) has received wide attention in professional and popular journals. As everyone knows, this global subject involves controversy. The very titles of recent works on the subject suggest it: *Brave New Baby; Promise and Peril of the Biological Revolution* (David M. Rorwik, 1971) [210]; *Fabricated Man. The Ethics of Genetic Control* (Paul Ramsey, 1970) [211]; *Early Diagnosis of Human Genetic Defects; Scientific and Ethical Considerations* (M. Harris, ed., 1971) [212]; and *Moral Dilemmas in Contraceptive Developments* (R. F. R. Gardner, 1973).[213] There are general texts on genetics such as *The Genetics of Human Populations* (L. L. Cavalli-Sforza and L. L. Bodmer, 1971) [214]; *Principles of Genetics* (E. J. Gardner, 1971) [215]; and general works on genetic counseling such as that by Alan C. Stevenson and his associates [216] and James R. Sorenson [217]; and genetics in medical practice by M. Bartolos.[218] In some general works on nursing, as for example *Advanced Concepts in Clinical Nursing* by Kay Corman Kintzel, there is a chapter on genetics and the nurse.[219] Since 1966 articles have been appearing in nursing journals that point out opportunities nurses have for genetic counseling.[220-223]

In 1971, Theodore Friedmann [224] published, in *Scientific American,* an article, "Prenatal Diagnosis of Genetic Disease," in which he said that over 1600 diseases are known to be genetically determined. Examples are cystic fibrosis, sickle cell anemia, and phenylketonuria. (The last condition has had, perhaps, most attention.) [225-227] Forty diseases, according to Friedmann, can be diagnosed prenatally from samples of amniotic fluid. Pregnant women over 35, many persons believe, should have genetic evaluations and be counseled according to the findings. Figure 5-27 shows the report of a chromosome study given a patient by the staff of the Department of Human Genetics at Yale University, New Haven, Conn.

Claire O. Leonard and associates [228] evaluated the effectiveness of genetic counseling by physicians, giving "the consumer's view." Their findings reinforce the conclusion that this is a complex problem with which few health professionals are prepared to help people effectively and it is a problem few parents will face. Nursing education programs should provide opportunities for nurses who assume the role of genetic counselors to make a special study of the subject. Nurses may be employed in genetic clinics and specialize in this field. Considering the improvement in plants and animals that has resulted from the application of genetic principles, it seems as if humans might learn how to apply genetic principles to the improvement of the human race. Under health histories, the desirability of making a family tree as a basis for counseling was discussed on page 401 (see Fig. 5-5).

Actually, all health counseling is as specialized as clinical practice, and while all nurses

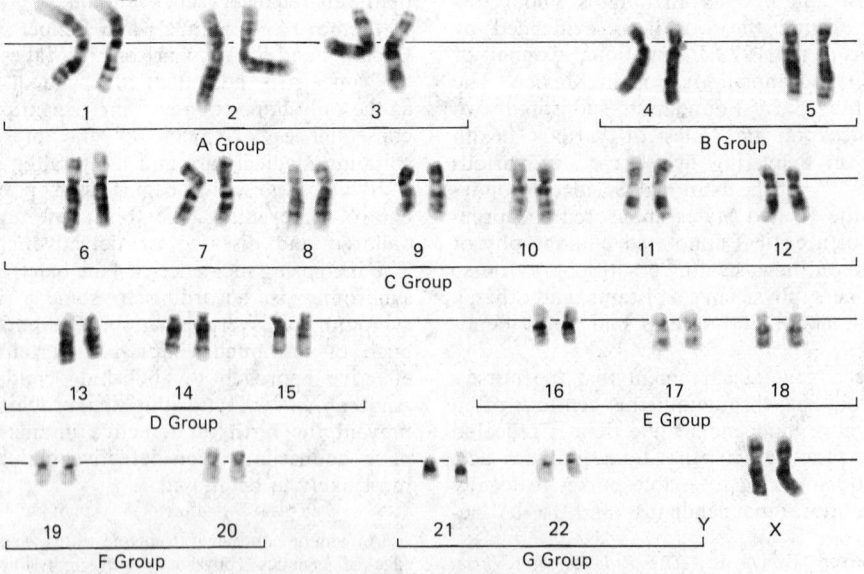

Figure 5-27. A normal female karyotype. (Courtesy of Department of Human Genetics, Yale University School of Medicine, New Haven, Conn.)

might be expected to give generalized help, the most effective counseling on child care comes from pediatric nurses and counseling on problems of the aged from geriatric nurses. Following examinations in which disease is diagnosed, the patient with cancer, for example, should get the best help from the oncologic nurse; the patient with heart disease from the cardiac nurse; and the patient with tuberculosis from the nurse who has specialized in chest disease.

The nurse's role in diagnosis and decision-making always involves patients and families; most often nurses are members of a team of health workers. They participate in these processes with other professionals in helping the client or patient. In some cases, when other health workers are unavailable or when nurses assume responsibility for giving primary care, act as principal therapists or as private practitioners, they may play as independent a role as the physician, the dentist, the clinical psychologist, or the marriage counselor. There are hundreds of articles that might be cited dealing with this old but newly-articulated function of the nurse. Reference has been made to published bibliographies and to those in preparation and to specific reports.[229-237] Chapter 8 is devoted to planning patient care. The discussion of the nurse's function in it and how he or she collaborates with patients, their families, and other health workers is discussed in some detail in that chapter.

REFERENCES

1. Dunn, Halbert R.: *High-Level Wellness.* Mt. Vernon Publishing Co., Washington, D.C., 1961.
2. Maslow, Abraham H.: *Religions, Values, and Peak Experiences.* Ohio State University Press, Columbus, 1964.
3. Dubos, René: *Mirage of Health.* Doubleday Anchor Books, Garden City, N.Y., 1961.
4. Haggard, Howard W.: *The Doctor in History.* Yale University Press, New Haven, Conn., 1934.
5. ———: *Devils, Drugs and Doctors.* Harper & Row, New York, 1929.
6. Sigerist, Henry E.: *A History of Medicine.* Oxford University Press, New York, 1951.
6a. Hamilton, Edith: *The Echo of Greece.* W. W. Norton & Co., New York, 1957.
7. Bernard, Claude: *Introduction to the Study of Experimental Medicine.* Macmillan Publishing Co., Inc., New York, 1927.
8. Cannon, Walter B.: *The Wisdom of the Body.* W. W. Norton & Co., New York, 1939.
9. Burr, Harold Saxton: *The Electric Fields of Life.* Ballantine Books, New York, 1972.

(Originally published by Neville Spearman, London, 1935.)
10. ———, and Northrop, F. S. C.: "The Electro-Dynamic Theory of Life," *Q. Rev. Biol.,* **10:**322, (Sept.) 1935.
11. ———, et al.: "An Electrometric Study of the Healing of Wounds in Man," *Yale J. Biol. Med.,* **12:**483, (May) 1939.
12. ———, et al.: "A Bioelectric Record of Human Ovulation," *Science,* **86:**312, (Oct.) 1937.
13. Geddes, L. A., et al.: "Continuous Measurement of Ventricular Stroke Volume by Electrical Impedence," *Cardiovasc. Res. Cent. Bull.,* **4:**118, (Apr.–June) 1966.
14. Pressman, A.: *The Electromagnetic Fields of Life.* Plenum Press, New York, 1970.
15. Burr, H. S.: *The Nature of Man and the Meaning of Existence.* Charles C Thomas, Publisher, Springfield, Ill., 1962.
16. ———, and Northrop, F. S. C.: *op. cit.*
17. Ravitz, Leonard J.: "Electrodynamic Field Theory in Psychiatry," *South. Med. J.,* **46:**650, (July) 1953.
18. Carnegie Commission on Higher Education: *Higher Education and the Nation's Health —Policies for Medical and Dental Education.* McGraw-Hill Book Co., New York, 1970.
19. Lynaugh, Joan E., and Bates, Barbara: "The Two Languages of Nursing and Medicine," *Am. J. Nurs.,* **73:**66, (Jan.) 1973.
20. Weed, Lawrence L.: *Medical Records; Medical Education and Patient Care.* Press of Case-Western Reserve University, Cleveland, 1970.
21. Carnegie Commission on Higher Education: *op. cit.*
22. Dillon, John B.: "How Did It Happen?" *Calif. Med.,* **113:**86, (Aug.) 1970.
23. Dunn, Halbert R.: *op. cit.*
24. Engel, George L.: "A Unified Concept of Health and Disease," *Perspect. Biol. Med.,* **3:**459, (Summer) 1960.
25. The Royal Society of Medicine and the Josiah Macy, Jr. Foundation: *The Greater Medical Profession.* The Foundation, New York, 1973.
26. Samuels, Mike, and Bennett, Hal: *The Well Body Book.* Random House, New York, 1973.
27. Kao, Frederick F.: "China, Chinese Medicine and the Chinese Medical System" *Am. J. Chinese Med.,* **1:**1, (Jan.) 1973.
28. Malleson, Andrew: *Need Your Doctor Be So Useless?* George Allen & Unwin, Ltd., London, 1973.
29. US Department of Health, Education, and Welfare: *Human Investment Program. Delivery of Health Services for the Poor.* US Government Printing Office, Washington, D.C., 1968.
30. Storlie, Frances: *Nursing and the Social Conscience.* Appleton-Century-Crofts, New York, 1970.
31. Milio, Nancy: *9226 Kercheval. The Store-*

front That Did Not Burn. University of Michigan Press, Ann Arbor, 1970.

32. Dunn, Halbert R.: *op. cit.*

33. Crichton, Michael: *Five Patients. The Hospital Explained.* Alfred A. Knopf, New York, 1970.

34. Samuels, Mike, and Bennett, Hal: *op. cit.*

35. Malleson, Andrew: *op. cit.*

36. *Ibid.*

37. Eisenberg, Arlene, and Eisenberg, Howard: "A New Teaching Program. How to Be Your Own Doctor—Sometimes," *New Haven Register,* (Feb. 24) 1974, p. 11.

38. Tennent, John: *Everyman His Own Doctor or The Poor Planter's Physician* [1734].

39. Gregg, Elinor D.: *The Indians and the Nurse.* University of Oklahoma Press, Norman, 1965.

40. McNicholas, Ellen L.: "International Nurse-Practitioner Committees," *Int. Nurse Rev.,* **16**:279, (No. 3) 1969.

41. Quinn, S.: "The Immediate Past, the Urgent Present, and Focus on the Future," *Niger Nurse,* **2**:6, (July) 1970.

42. Thomas, B.: "Mountaineering with Nursing," *AORN J.,* **12**:11, (Oct.) 1970.

43. US Public Health Service, Health Services and Mental Health Administration: *Nursing Careers in the Indian Health Service.* US Government Printing Office, Washington, D.C., 1971.

44. Weber, C. V.: "The Value of the Nurse's Role in Innovation of Care," in *Continuity of Care—Can or Should the Nurse Innovate Change.* Papers presented at the Nursing Sessions of the National Tuberculosis and Respiratory Disease Association 1970 Annual Meeting. National League for Nursing, New York, 1970.

45. Andreoli, Kathleen G.: "A Look at the Physician's Assistant," *Am. J. Nurs.,* **72**:710, (Apr.) 1972.

46. World Health Organization: *Report of the Travelling Seminar on Nursing in the U.S.S.R.* The Organization, Geneva, 1967.

47. Kao, Frederick F.: *op. cit.*

48. *The Framingham Study. An Epidemiological Investigation of Cardiovascular Diseases. Section 26, Some Characteristics Related to the Incidence of Cardiovascular Disease and Death; Framingham Study, 16-year Follow-up.* US Government Printing Office, Washington, D.C., 1971.

49. Garfield, Sidney R.: "Delivery of Medical Care," *Sci. Am.,* **222**:15, (Apr.) 1970.

49a. Sidel, Victor W., and Sidel, Ruth: *Serve the People. Observations on Medicine in the People's Republic of China.* Beacon Press, Boston, 1973.

50. Flynn, Eileen D.: "Barriers to Utilization of Multiphasic Screening. The Nurse's Role," (Symposium on Multiphasic Screening), *J. Occup. Med.,* **11**:361, (July) 1969.

51. "Experts Ask Routine Blood Lipid Testing," *Am. J. Nurs.,* **73**:34, (Jan.) 1973.

52. Brodman, Keeve, et al.: "The Cornell Medical Index-Health Questionnaire. II. As a Diagnostic Instrument," *J.A.M.A.,* **145**:152, (Jan. 20) 1951.

53. Chapman, A. L.: "Multiple Screening for a Variety of Diseases," *Hospitals,* **24**:37, (May) 1950.

54. US Public Health Service: *Reported Tuberculosis Rates 1966.* US Government Printing Office, Washington, D.C., 1968 (USPHS Pub. no. 638).

55. Garfield, Sidney R.: *op. cit.*

56. "Automated Multiphasic Health Testing," *Am. J. Nurs.,* **73**:880, (May) 1973.

57. Kao, Frederick F.: *op. cit.*

58. Lubic, Ruth Watson: Personal Communication.

59. MacBryde, Cyril M., and Blacklow, Robert Stanley (eds.): *Signs and Symptoms; Applied Pathologic Physiology and Clinical Interpretation,* 5th ed. J. B. Lippincott Co., Philadelphia, 1970, p. 203.

60. Draper, George, et al.: *Human Constitution in Clinical Medicine.* Paul B. Hoeber, New York, 1944.

61. Kretschmer, Ernst: *Physique and Character: An Investigation of the Nature of Constitution and the Theory of Temperament,* 2nd ed. rev. Humanities Press, New York, 1951.

62. Sheldon, William H., and Stevens, S. S.: *The Varieties of Temperament: A Psychology of Constitutional Differences.* Harper & Row, New York, 1942.

63. Glueck, S., and Glueck, E.: *Physique and Delinquency.* Harper & Row, New York, 1956.

64. Gradpaille, W. J.: "Research into the Physiology of Maleness and Femaleness," *Arch. Gen. Psychiatry,* **26**:193, (Mar.) 1972.

65. Goldschmidt, R.: "Analysis of Intersexuality in the Gypsy Moth," *Q. Rev. Biol.,* **6**:125, (Mar.) 1931.

66. Dye, Mimi, and Charlat, Richard: *Initial Assessment of Psychiatric Patients: A Clinical Model.* In preparation.

67. Shafer, Roy: *Aspects of Internalization.* International Universities Press, New York, 1968, p. 108.

68. Hartmann, Heinz: *Ego Psychology and the Problem of Adaptation.* International Universities Press, New York, 1958.

69. Myers, Jerome K., et al.: "Life Events and Psychiatric Impairment," *J. Nerv. Ment. Dis.,* **152**:149, (Mar.) 1971.

70. Paykel, Eugene S., et al.: "Life Events and Depression," *Arch. Gen. Psychiatry,* **21**:753, (Dec.) 1969.

71. Schmale, A. H., Jr.: "Relationship of Separation and Depression to Disease," *Psychosom. Med.,* **20**:259, (July–Aug.) 1958.

72. Wyler, A. R., et al.: "Magnitude of Life Events and Seriousness of Illness," *Psychosom. Med.,* **33**:115, (Mar.–Apr.) 1971.

73. Draper, George, et al.: *op. cit.*

74. Dye, Mimi, and Charlat, Richard: *op. cit.*

75. Stevenson, Ian, and Sheppe, William M.,
Jr.: "The Psychiatric Examination," in
Arieti, Silvano (ed.): *American Handbook
of Psychiatry I*. Basic Books, Inc., New
York, 1959, p. 215.

76. Strecker, Edward A.: *Fundamentals of Psychiatry*, 4th ed. J. B. Lippincott Co., Philadelphia, 1947.

77. Diethelm, Oscar: "The Evaluation of a
Psychiatric Examination," *Am. J. Psychiatry*, **105**:606, (Feb.) 1949.

78. Bettelheim, Bruno: *A Home for the Heart*.
Alfred A. Knopf, New York, 1974, pp.
131, 174.

79. Hunt, Howard F.: "Clinical Methods: Psychodiagnostics," *Annu. Rev. Psychol.*, **1**:
207, 1950.

80. Judge, Richard D., and Zuidema, George
D. (eds.): *Methods of Clinical Examination; A Physiologic Approach*, 3rd ed. Little,
Brown & Co., Boston, 1974, p. 7.

81. Prior, John A., and Silberstein, Jack S.:
Physical Diagnosis. The History and Examination of the Patient. C. V. Mosby Co., St.
Louis, 1973, p. 3.

82. Engel, George L., and Morgan, William L.,
Jr.: *Interviewing the Patient*. W. B. Saunders, Philadelphia, 1973, p. 35.

83. "Wallet Size Medical Record Now Available," *Am. J. Nurs.*, **71**:2000, (Oct.) 1971.

84. Goldberg, D. P.: *The Detection of Psychiatric Illness by Questionnaire*. Oxford
University Press, New York, 1972.

85. McPhetridge, L. Mae: "Nursing History;
One Means to Personalize Care," *Am. J.
Nurs.*, **68**:68, (Jan.) 1968.

86. Smith, Dorothy M.: "Clinical Nursing
Tool; Nursing History Guide," *Am. J.
Nurs.*, **68**:2384, (Nov.) 1968.

87. Phaneuf, Maria C.: *The Nursing Audit:
Profile for Excellence*. Appleton-Century-
Crofts, New York, 1972, p. 89.

88. Wandelt, Mabel A., and Phaneuf, Maria
C.: "Three Instruments for Measuring the
Quality of Nursing Care," *Hosp. Top.*,
150:20, (Aug.) 1972.

88a. Allport, Gordon W.: *Pattern and Growth
in Personality*. Holt, Rinehart & Winston,
New York, 1965.

89. Erikson, Erik H.: *Childhood and Society*,
2nd ed. W. W. Norton & Co., New York,
1963.

90. Jourard, Sidney M.: "The Bedside Manner," *Am. J. Nurs.*, **60**:63, (Jan.) 1960.

91. ———: *Disclosing Man to Himself*. Van
Nostrand-Reinhold Co., New York, 1968.

92. Jung, Carl: *The Undiscovered Self*. Kegan
Paul, London, 1958.

93. Laing, R. D.: *The Politics of Experience*.
Ballantine Books, New York, 1967.

94. Maslow, Abraham H.: *The Farther Reaches
of Human Nature*. Viking Press, New
York, 1972.

95. ———: *Motivation and Personality*. Harper
& Row, New York, 1954.

96. May, Rollo: *Psychology and the Human
Dilemma*. Van Nostrand-Reinhold Co., New
York, 1967.

97. Rogers, Carl R.: "The Characteristics of
a Helping Relationship," *Personnel Guidance J.*, **37**:6, (Sept.) 1958.

98. ———: *Counseling and Psychotherapy*.
Houghton Mifflin Co., New York, 1942.

99. ———, and Rothelsberger, F. J.: "Barriers
and Gateways to Communication," *Harvard
Business Rev.*, 1952.

100. Sullivan, Harry Stack: *The Interpersonal
Theory of Psychiatry*. W. W. Norton &
Co., New York, 1953.

101. Blake, Florence G., et al.: *Nursing Care
of Children*, 8th ed. J. B. Lippincott Co.,
Philadelphia, 1970.

102. Erickson, Florence: "The Nurse in Modern
Pediatrics," *Int. J. Nurs. Studies*, **2**:139,
(No. 2) 1965.

103. King, Joan: "The Initial Interview: Basis
for Assessment in Crisis Intervention,"
Perspect. Psychiatr. Care, **9**:247, (Nov.–
Dec.) 1971.

104. Peplau, Hildegard E.: *Basic Principles of
Patient Counseling*, 2nd ed. Smith, Kline &
French Laboratories, Philadelphia, 1964.

105. ———: *Interpersonal Relations in Nursing*.
G. P. Putnam's Sons, New York, 1952.

106. ———: "Talking With Patients," *Am. J.
Nurs.*, **60**:964, (July) 1960.

107. Tudor, Gwen E.: "A Sociopsychiatric Nursing Approach to Intervention in a Problem
of Mutual Withdrawal on a Mental Hospital
Ward," *Psychiatry*, **15**:193, (May) 1952.

108. Bermosk, Loretta Sue, and Mordan, Mary
Jane: *Interviewing in Nursing*. Macmillan
Publishing Co., Inc., New York, 1973.

109. Marshall, Jon C., and Feeney, Sally: "Structured Versus Intuitive Intake Interview,"
Nurs. Res., **21**:269, (May–June) 1972.

110. Gozzi, Ethel K., et al.: "Gaps in Doctor-
Patient Communication; Implications for
Nursing Practice," *Am. J. Nurs.*, **69**:529,
(Mar.) 1969.

111. Fowkes, William C., Jr., and Hunn, Virginia K.: *Clinical Assessment for the Nurse
Practitioner*. C. V. Mosby Co., St. Louis,
1973, p. 9.

112. Malleson, Andrew: *op. cit.*, p. 113.

113. *Ibid.*

113a. Bettelheim, Bruno: *op. cit.*, p. 174.

114. Tinkham, Catherine W., and Voorhies,
Eleanor F.: *Community Health Nursing:
Evolution and Process*. Appleton-Century-
Crofts, New York, 1972.

115. Pearse, Innes, and Crocker, Lucy H.: *The
Peckham Experiment: A Study of the
Living Structure of Society*. Yale University
Press, New Haven, Conn., 1944.

116. Richardson, Henry B.: *Patients Have Families*. Commonwealth Fund, New York,
1945.

117. Malleson, Andrew: *op. cit.*, p. 200.

118. Silver, Henry K., et al.: *Handbook of Pediatrics*. Lange Medical Publications, Los
Altos, Calif., 1973, p. 2.

119. Houston, William: *Art of Treatment.* Macmillan Publishing Co., Inc., New York, 1933.

119a. Belinsky, Irmgard, et al.: "Colonofiberoscopy: Technique in Colon Examination," *Am. J. Nurse.,* **73:**306, (Feb.) 1973.

120. Everhart, Thomas E., and Hayes, Thomas L.: "The Scanning Electron Microscope," *Sci. Am.,* **226:**55, (Jan.) 1972.

121. Prior, John A., and Silberstein, Jack S.: *op. cit.,* p. 184.

122. Sherman, Jacques L., and Fields, Sylvia Kleiman: *Guide to Patient Evaluation.* Medical Examination Publishing Co., Flushing, N.Y., 1974, pp. 163, 174.

123. Haggard, Howard W.: *The Doctor in History.* Yale University Press, New Haven, Conn., 1934, p. 331.

124. Johnson, J. E.: "Cognitive Processes Underlying Emotional and Instrumental Behavior During a Medical Examination," in *Science and Direct Patient Care.* Fourth Annual Nurse Scientist Conference, University of Colorado Medical Center, Denver, Colo., 1971.

124a. Bates, Barbara: *A Guide to Physical Examination.* J. B. Lippincott Co., Philadelphia, 1974.

125. Fowkes, William C., Jr., and Hunn, Virginia K.: *op. cit.*

126. Sherman, Jacques L., and Fields, Sylvia Kleiman: *op. cit.*

127. Seedor, Marie M.: *The Physical Assessment. A Programmed Unit of Study for Nurses.* Teachers College Press, New York, 1974.

128. Morgan, William L., Jr., and Engel, George L.: *op. cit.*

128a. Engel, George L., and Morgan, William L., Jr.: *op. cit.*

129. DeGowin, Elmer L., and DeGowin, Richard L.: *Bedside Diagnostic Examination,* 3rd ed. Macmillan Publishing Co., Inc., New York, 1976.

130. Judge, Richard D., and Zuidema, George D. (eds.): *op. cit.*

131. Prior, John A., and Silberstein, Jack S.: *op. cit.*

131a. Medic Alert Foundation: *Why? Medic Alert.* The Foundation, Turlock, Calif.

132. Prior, John A., and Silberstein, Jack S.: *op. cit.,* p. 90.

133. DeGowin, Elmer L., and DeGowin, Richard L.: *op. cit.,* pp. 81–126.

134. Fowkes, William C., Jr., and Hunn, Virginia K.: *op. cit.*

135. DeGowin, Elmer L., and DeGowin, Richard L.: *op. cit.,* p. 790.

136. *Ibid.,* p. 771.

137. *Ibid.,* p. 300.

138. Prior, John A., and Silberstein, Jack S.: *op. cit.,* p. 245.

139. Morgan, William L., Jr., and Engel, George L.: *op. cit.,* p. 132.

140. DeGowin, Elmer L., and DeGowin, Richard L.: *op. cit.,* p. 305.

141. Morgan, William L., Jr., and Engel, George L.: *op. cit.,* p. 161.

142. Mayo Clinic, Department of Neurology: *Clinical Examinations in Neurology,* 4th ed. W. B. Saunders Co., Philadelphia, 1971.

143. Alpers, B. J.: *Essentials of the Neurological Examination.* F. A. Davis Co., Philadelphia, 1971.

144. Delong, R.: *The Neurologic Examination.* Harper & Row, New York, 1967.

145. Liusada, A. A., and Sainani, G.: *Primer of Cardiac Diagnosis.* Warner & Green, Inc., St. Louis, 1968.

146. Kellogg, Cal S.: *Diseases of the Anus, Rectum, and Colon. Family Practice.* W. B. Saunders Co., Philadelphia, 1973.

147. Kendall, H. O.: *Muscles, Testing and Function.* Williams & Wilkins Co., Baltimore, 1971.

148. Apgar, Virginia: "Evaluation of the Newborn Infant—Second Report," *J.A.M.A.,* **168:**1985, (Dec. 13) 1958.

149. Apgar, Virginia, and Bergsma, Daniel: *Birth Defects.* National Foundation—March of Dimes, New York, 1964.

150. Silver, Henry K., et al.: *op. cit.*

151. Judge, Richard D., and Zuidema, George D. (eds.): *op. cit.,* p. 369.

152. Barness, Lewis A.: *Manual of Pediatric Physical Diagnosis,* 4th ed. Yearbook Medical Publishers, Chicago, 1972.

153. Frankenburg, William K., et al.: *Denver Developmental Screening Test.* University of Colorado Medical Center, Denver, 1970.

154. Gentry, Elizabeth, and Paris, Lulu Mae: "Tools to Evaluate Child Development," *Am. J. Nurs.,* **69:**2544, (Dec.) 1969.

155. Illingworth, R. S.: *Common Symptoms of Diseases in Children,* 4th ed. Blackwell Scientific Publications, Oxford, 1973.

156. Dye, Mimi, and Charlat, Richard: *op. cit.*

157. Tucker, Edward S.: Formal Mental Status Testing. Yale University School of Medicine, New Haven, Conn., 1974, 2 lv, processed.

158. McKinnon, Roger A., and Michels, Robert: *The Psychiatric Interview in Clinical Practice.* W. B. Saunders Co., Philadelphia, 1971, p. 205.

159. Anderson, E. W., and Trethowan, W. H.: *Psychiatry,* 3rd ed. Bailliere, Tindall & Cox, London, 1973.

160. Cadoret, Remi J., and King, Lucy J.: *Psychiatry in Primary Care.* C. V. Mosby Co., St. Louis, 1974.

161. Cooper, J. E.: *Psychiatric Diagnosis in New York and London.* Oxford University Press, New York, 1972.

162. Gill, Merton, et al.: *The Initial Interview in Psychiatric Practice.* International Universities Press, New York, 1954.

163. Travelbee, Joyce: *Intervention in Psychiatric Nursing,* 2nd ed. F. A. Davis Co., Philadelphia, 1971.

164. Russell, G. F. M., and Walton, H. J.: *The Training of Psychiatrists. Proceedings of*

Conference on Post Graduate Psychiatric Education, Mar. 1969, Royal Medico-Psychological Association. Headley Bros., Ltd., Ashford, Kent, Eng., 1970.

165. Samuels, Mike, and Bennett, Hal: *op. cit.*

166. Freidson, Eliot: *Professional Dominance: The Social Structure of Medical Care.* Aldine-Atherton, Inc., Chicago, 1970.

167. Bates, Barbara: "Comprehensive Medicine; a Conference Approach With Inpatient Emphasis," *J. Med. Educ.,* **40:**778, (Apr.) 1965.

168. ———: "Nurse-Physician Teamwork," *Med. Care,* **4:**69, (Apr.–June) 1966.

169. ———, and Kern, M. Sue: "Doctor-Nurse Teamwork: What Helps? What Hinders?" *Am. J. Nurs.,* **67:**2066, (Oct.) 1967.

170. ———: "Doctor and Nurse: Changing Roles and Relations," *N. Engl. J. Med.,* **283:**129, (July 16) 1970.

171. ———, and Chamberlin, Robert W.: "Physician Leadership as Perceived by Nurses," *Nurs. Res.,* **19:**534, (Dec.) 1970.

172. "Nursing in a Health Maintenance Organization. Report on the Harvard Community Health Plan," *Am. J. Public Health,* **62:**991, (July) 1972.

173. Lynaugh, Joan E., and Bates, Barbara: *op. cit.*

174. Engel, George L.: *op. cit.*

175. Feinstein, Alvin R.: *Clinical Judgment.* Williams & Wilkins Co., Baltimore, 1967, p. 25.

176. Weed, Lawrence L.: *op. cit.*

177. Carnegie Commission on Higher Education: *op. cit.*

178. Dillon, John B.: *op. cit.*

179. US Department of Health, Education, and Welfare; Regional Council for International Education: *The Dynamics of Interinstitutional Cooperation in International Education.* US Government Printing Office, Washington, D.C., 1971.

180. Surawicz, Frida, and Sandifer, M. G.: "Cross Cultural Diagnosis: A Study of Psychiatric Diagnosis Comparing Switzerland, the United States and the United Kingdom," *Int. J. Soc. Psychiatry,* **16:**232, (Summer) 1970.

181. World Health Organization: *International Classification of Diseases,* 8th ed. The Organization, Geneva, 1963, Vol. 1.

182. Bates, Barbara, and Kern, M. Sue: *op. cit.*

183. Bates, Barbara: "Doctor and Nurse: Changing Roles and Relations," *N. Engl J. Med.,* **283:**129, (July 16) 1970.

184. Aradine, Carolyn R., and Pridham, Karen F.: "Model for Collaboration," *Nurs. Outlook,* **21:**655, (Oct.) 1973.

185. Silver, Henry K., et al.: "Pediatric Nurse-Practitioner Program; Expanding the Role of the Nurse to Provide Increased Health Care for Children," *J.A.M.A.,* **204:**298, (Apr. 22) 1968.

186. deCastro, Fernando J., and Rolfe, Ursula T.: *The Pediatric Nurse Practitioner,* 2nd ed. C. V. Mosby Co., St. Louis, 1976.

187. Pinder, J. E.: "A Reply to the Role Conflicts of the New Breed Health Visitor," *Health Visitor,* **44:**188, (June) 1971.

188. O'Boyle, Catherine: "A New Era in Emergency Service," *Am. J. Nurs.,* **72:**1392, (Aug.) 1972.

189. Sheedy, Susan Gerberding: "Medical Nurse Practitioner in a Neighborhood Clinic," *Am. J. Nurs.,* **72:**1416, (Aug.) 1972.

190. Garfield, Sidney R.: *op. cit.*

191. Poole, Ernest: *Nurses on Horseback.* Macmillan Publishing Co., Inc., New York, 1932.

192. "Family Nurse Practitioner Program," *Frontier Nurs. Serv. Q. Bull.,* **47:**31, (Summer) 1971.

193. Schutt, Barbara G.: "Frontier's Family Nurses," *Am. J. Nurs.,* **72:**903, (May) 1972.

194. Bain, H. W., and Goldthorpe, Garey: "The University of Toronto Sioux Lookout Project: A Model of Health Care Delivery," *Can. Med. Assoc. J.,* **107:**523, (Sept. 23) 1972.

195. DeMarsh, Kathleen G.: "Red Cross Outpost Nursing in New Brunswick," *Can. Nurse,* **69:**24, (June) 1973.

196. Hazlett, C. B.: "Task Analysis of the Clinically Trained Nurse (C.T.N.)," *Nurs. Clin. North Am.,* **10:**699, (Dec.) 1975.

197. Keith, Catharine W.: *Role and Preparation of the Outpost Nurse (Canada).* (Paper prepared for Pan American Conference on Health Manpower Planning, Ottawa, Sept. 1973). Processed.

198. Sutherland, Ruth, and Besner, Jeanne: "Community Nursing in a Northern Setting," *Nurs. Clin. North Am.,* **10:**731, (Dec.) 1975.

199. Fowkes, William C., Jr., and Hunn, Virginia K., *op. cit.,* p. 5.

200. Weed, Lawrence L.: "Medical Records That Guide and Teach, Parts 1 and 2," *N. Engl. J. Med.,* **278:**593, (Mar. 14); **278:**652, (Mar. 21) 1968.

201. ———: *Medical Records; Medical Education and Patient Care.* Press of Case-Western Reserve University, Cleveland, 1970.

201a. ———: *Your Health Care and How to Manage It.* Promis Laboratory, University of Vermont, Burlington, 1975.

202. Bjorn, J. C., and Cross, H. D.: *Problem-Oriented Private Practice of Medicine; System for Comprehensive Health Care.* Modern Hospital Press, McGraw-Hill Publications Co., New York, 1970.

203. Bates, Barbara: "Nurse-Physician Teamwork," *Med. Care,* **4:**69, (Apr.–June) 1966.

204. ———, and Kern, M. Sue: *op. cit.*

205. The Royal Society of Medicine and the Josiah Macy, Jr. Foundation: *The Greater Medical Profession.* The Foundation, New York, 1973.

206. Lippard, Vernon W., and Purcell, Elizabeth R. (eds.): *Intermediate-Level Health*

Practitioners. Josiah Macy, Jr. Foundation, New York, 1973.

207. Cohen, Eva D. (ed.): *Evaluation of Research on New Health Practitioners.* (Under a grant from the National Science Foundation, Office of Regional Activities and Continuing Education.) Yale University School of Medicine, New Haven, Conn., 1974.

208. Malleson, Andrew: *op. cit.*

209. Samuels, Mike, and Bennett, Hal: *op. cit.*

209a. Illich, Ivan: *Medical Nemesis. The Expropriation of Health.* McClelland & Stewart, Ltd., Toronto, 1975.

209b. Carlson, Rick J.: *The End of Medicine.* John Wiley & Sons, New York, 1975.

210. Rorwik, David M.: *Brave New Baby; Promise and Peril of the Biological Revolution.* Doubleday & Co., Garden City, N.Y., 1971.

211. Ramsey, Paul: *Fabricated Man. The Ethics of Genetic Control.* Yale University Press, New Haven, Conn., 1970.

212. Harris, M. (ed.): *Early Diagnosis of Human Genetic Defects; Scientific and Ethical Considerations.* US Government Printing Office, Washington, D.C., 1971.

213. Gardner, R. F. R.: *Moral Dilemmas in Contraceptive Developments.* CMF Publications, London, [1973].

214. Cavalli-Sforza, L. L., and Bodmer, L. L.: *The Genetics of Human Populations.* W. H. Freeman, San Francisco, 1971.

215. Gardner, E. J.: *Principles of Genetics,* 4th ed. John Wiley & Sons, New York, [1971].

216. Stevenson, Alan C., et al.: *Genetic Counseling.* J. B. Lippincott Co., Philadelphia, 1970.

217. Sorensen, James R.: *Genetic Counseling.* Princeton University, Princeton, N.J., 1971.

218. Bartolos, M. (ed.): *Genetics in Medical Practice.* J. B. Lippincott Co., Philadelphia, 1968.

219. Kintzel, Kay Corman, and Lake, Dolores: "Medical Genetics and the Nurse," in Kintzel, Kay Corman (ed.): *Advanced Concepts in Clinical Nursing.* J. B. Lippincott Co., Philadelphia, 1971.

220. Forbes, N.: "The Nurse and Genetic Counseling," *Nurs. Clin. North Am.,* **1**:679, (Dec.) 1966.

221. Hillman, G. M.: "Genetics and the Nurse," *Nurs. Outlook,* **14**:34, (Jan.) 1966.

222. Nitowsky, Harold M.: "Prenatal Diagnosis of Genetic Abnormality," *Am. J. Nurs.,* **71**:1551, (Oct.) 1971.

223. Ragsdale, N., and Koch, R.: "Phenylketonuria: Detection and Therapy," *Am. J. Nurs.,* **64**:90, (Jan.) 1964.

224. Friedmann, Theodore: "Prenatal Diagnosis of Genetic Disease," *Sci. Am.,* **225**:34, (Nov.) 1971.

225. Lake, D.: "Nursing Implications from an Investigation of Mothering, Diet and Development in Two Groups of Children with Phenylketonuria," in *ANA Clinical*

Sessions, 1968. Appleton-Century-Crofts, New York, 1968.

226. US Health Services and Mental Health Administration, Maternal and Child Health Service: *State Laws Pertaining to Phenylketonuria as of November 1970.* US Government Printing Office, Washington, D.C., 1971.

227. ——: *What Do You Know About PKU?* US Government Printing Office, Washington, D.C., 1972.

228. Leonard, Claire O., et al.: "Genetic Counseling: A Consumer's View," *N. Engl. J. Med.,* **287**:443, (Aug. 31) 1972.

229. Mundinger, Mary O'Neill: "Primary Nurse —Role Evaluation," *Nurs. Outlook,* **21**:642, (Oct.) 1973.

230. Mussallem, Helen K.: "The Changing Role of the Nurse," *Am. J. Nurs.,* **69**:514, (Mar.) 1969.

231. National Commission for the Study of Nursing and Nursing Education: *Nurse Clinician and Physician's Assistant: The Relationship Between Two Emerging Practitioner Concepts.* The Commission, Rochester, [1971].

232. Perry, Lesley: *The Nurse as a Primary Health Provider and the Nurse Practitioner; An Annotated Bibliography.* Genesee Valley Nurses' Association, Rochester, N.Y., 1971.

233. Pranulis, Maryann F., and Roth, Oscar: "Medical and Legal Aspects of the Role of the Nurse in Coronary Care," in *Yearbook of Legal Medicine.* Appleton-Century-Crofts, New York, 1972.

234. Reed, D. E., et al.: "Acceptability of an Expanded Nurse Role to Nurses and Physicians," *Med. Care,* **9**:372, (July–Aug.) 1971.

235. Sheedy, Susan Gerberding: *op. cit.*

236. Sheldon, Alan, and Hope, Penelope K.: "Developing Role of the Nurse in a Community Mental Health Program," *Perspect. Psychiatr. Care,* **5**:272, (Nov.–Dec.) 1967.

237. Stolar, Vera, and Rubenstain, Reva: "Developing the Science Component in a PRIMEX Program," *Nurs. Outlook,* **21**:325, (May) 1973.

Additional Suggested Reading

Abramson, J. H.: "The Cornell Medical Index as an Epidemiological Tool," *Am. J. Public Health,* **56**:287, (Feb.) 1966.

Aguilera, Donna C., et al.: *Crisis Intervention: Theory and Methodology.* C. V. Mosby Co., St. Louis, 1970.

Apple, L. E.: *Distance Vision and Perceptual Training.* American Foundation for the Blind, New York, [1971].

Barnard, Kathryn, and Douglas, H.: *Child Health Care Assessment, Part 1: A Literature Review.* US Government Printing Office, Washington, D.C., 1974 (DHEW Pub. No. [HRA] 75–30).

Beck, Aaron T.: *The Diagnosis and Management*

of Depression. University of Pennsylvania Press, Philadelphia, 1967.

Bell, R. W., et al.: "A Rating System for the Assessment of Hyperactive and Withdrawn Children in Preschool Samples," *Am. J. Orthopsychiatry*, (Jan.) 1972.

Berg, Robert L. (ed.): *Health Status Indexes. Proceedings of a Conference Conducted by Health Services Research, Tucson, Ariz., Oct. 1972.* Health Services Research, Tucson, Ariz., 1973.

Bonkowsky, Marilyn L.: "Adapting the POMR to Community Child Health Care," *Nurs. Outlook,* **20**:515, (Aug.) 1972.

Braverman, Irwin M.: *Skin Signs of Systemic Disease.* W. B. Saunders Co., Philadelphia, 1970.

Brown, William J.: "Acquired Syphilis: Drugs and Blood Tests," in *Human Sexuality: Nursing Implications.* American Journal of Nursing Co., New York, 1973 (Contemporary Nursing Series).

Caird, F. I., and Judge, T. G.: *Assessment of the Elderly Patient.* Sir Isaac Pitman & Sons, Ltd.; available from J. B. Lippincott Co., Philadelphia, 1974.

Canadian Nurses Association: *An Investigation of the Approach to Early Detection of Breast Cancer.* (Prepared by the Registered Nurses Association of British Columbia.) CNA, Ottawa, 1975.

Chinn, P. L., and Leitch, C. J.: *Child Health Maintenance; A Guide to Clinical Assessment.* C. V. Mosby Co., St. Louis, 1974.

Cippola, Josephine, and Collings, Gilbearth, Jr.: "Nurse Clinicians in Industry," *Am. J. Nurs.,* **71**:1530, (Aug.) 1971.

Collen, Frances Bobbie, et al.: "Kaiser-Permanente Experiment in Ambulatory Care," *Am. J. Nurs.,* **71**:1371, (July) 1971.

Conference on a Critical Analysis of the Cost-Effectiveness of Multiphasic Screening, Seattle, Wash., 1971: *Proceedings . . . .* Medical Computer Services Association, Seattle, 1972.

Copp, Laurel Archer: "Professional Change: Which Trends Do Nurses Endorse?" *Int. J. Nurs. Studies,* **10**:55, 1973.

——: "The Spectrum of Suffering," *Am. J. Nurs.,* **74**:491, (Mar.) 1974.

Duncan, Burris, et al.: "Comparison of the Physical Assessment of Children by Pediatric Nurse Practitioners and Pediatricians," *Am. J. Public Health,* **61**:1170, (June) 1971.

Ehrenreich, Barbara, and English, Deirdre: *Witches, Midwives, and Nurses—A History of Women Healers.* The Feminist Press, Old Westbury, N.Y., 1973 (Glass Mountain Pamphlet No. 1).

Farberow, Norman L., and Shneidman, Edwin S. (eds.): *The Cry for Help.* McGraw-Hill Book Co., New York, 1965.

Farberow, Norman L., et al.: "Evaluation and Management of Suicidal Persons," in Shneidman, Edwin S., et al. (eds.): *The Psychology of Suicide.* Science House, New York, 1970.

Ford, E. H. R.: *Human Chromosomes.* Academic Press, New York, 1973.

Frankenburg, W. M., and Dodds, J. B.: "The Denver Developmental Screening Test," *J. Pediatr.,* **71**:181, 1967.

Freeman, Barbara L., et al.: "How Do Nurses Expand Their Roles in Well Child Care?" *Am. J. Nurs.,* **72**:1866 (Oct.) 1972.

Hobson, L. B.: *Examination of the Patient; A Text for Nursing and Allied Health Personnel.* McGraw-Hill Book Co., New York, 1975.

Holmstrom, Lynda L., and Burgess, Ann W.: "Assessing Trauma in the Rape Victim," *Am. J. Nurs.,* **75**:1288, (Aug.) 1975.

Hurst, J. Willis, and Schlant, R. C.: "Auscultation of the Heart," in Hurst, J. Willis, and Logue, R. Brace (eds.): *The Heart.* McGraw-Hill Book Co., New York, 1970.

Jackson, Edgar B., Jr.: "In the Screening Clinic. Guidelines to the Appraisal of Some Common Problems," *Am. J. Nurs.,* **72**:1398, (Aug.) 1972.

Kadushin, Charles: *Why People Go to Psychiatrists.* Atherton Press, New York, 1969.

Keough, Gertrude, and Niebel, Harold N.: "Oral Cancer Detection—A Nursing Responsibility," *Am. J. Nurs.,* **73**:684, (Apr.) 1973.

Knobloch, Hilda, and Pasamanich, Benjamin (eds.): *Gessell and Amatruda's Development Diagnosis,* 3rd ed. Harper & Row, New York, 1974.

Larson, L. A. (ed.): *Fitness, Health and Work Capacity; International Standards for Assessment.* Macmillan Publishing Co., Inc., New York, 1974.

Lieb, Julian, et al.: *The Crisis Team.* Harper & Row, New York, 1973.

Litman, Robert E.: "Suicide as Acting Out," in Shneidman, Edwin S., et al. (eds.): *The Psychology of Suicide.* Science House, New York, 1970.

——, and Farberow, Norman L.: "Emergency Evaluation of Suicidal Potential," in Shneidman, Edwin S., et al. (eds.): *The Psychology of Suicide.* Science House, New York, 1970.

Littman, David: "Stethoscopes and Auscultation of Heart Sounds," *Am. J. Nurs.,* **72**:1239, (July) 1972.

McGurn, Wealtha Collins: "The Heart: Principles of Function, Pathophysiology and Nursing Goals," in Kintzel, Kay Corman (ed.): *Advanced Concepts in Clinical Nursing.* J. B. Lippincott Co., Philadelphia, 1971.

Murray, Ruth, and Zentner, Judith: *Nursing Assessment and Health Promotion Through the Life Span.* Prentice-Hall, Englewood Cliffs, N.J., 1975.

Myers, Jerome K., et al.: "Life Events and Psychiatric Impairment," *J. Nerv. Ment. Dis.,* **152**:149, 1971.

National Academy of Sciences: *Genetic Screening. Procedural Guide and Recommendations.* The Academy, Washington, D.C., 1975.

Offer, Daniel, and Sabshin, Melvin: *Normality: Theoretical and Clinical Concepts of Mental Health.* Basic Books, New York, 1966.

Rosen, Emmanuel S., and Savir, Hannah: *Basic Ophthalmoscopy. Ophthalmoscope Diagnosis in*

Systemic Disorders. Appleton-Century-Crofts, New York, 1972.

Rothberg, June S.: "Nurse and Physician's Assistant: Issues and Relationships," *Nurs. Outlook,* **21:**154, (Mar.) 1973.

Sadler, Alfred M., et al.: *The Physician's Assistant Today and Tomorrow. Issues Confronting New Health Practitioners,* 2nd ed. Ballinger Publishing Co., Cambridge, Mass., 1975.

Sana, J. M., and Judge, R. D. (eds.): *Physical Appraisal Methods in Nursing Practice.* Little, Brown & Co., Boston, 1975.

Sedlock, Stephanie Ann: "Detection of Chronic Pulmonary Disease," *Am. J. Nurs.,* **72:**1407, (Aug.) 1972.

Seward, C. M.: *Bedside Diagnosis.* Williams & Wilkins Co., Baltimore, 1971.

Sherman, Jacques L., Jr., and Fields, Sylvia Kleiman: *Guide to Patient Evaluation: History Taking, Physical Examination and the Problem-Oriented Method.* Medical Examination Publishing Co., New York, 1974.

Snyder, Mariah, and Baum, Rebecca: "Assessing Station and Gait," *Am. J. Nurs.,* **74:**1256, (July) 1974.

Society for Advanced Medical Systems: *Automated Multiphasic Health Testing.* US Federal Health Programs Service, Washington, D.C., 1971.

Stevenson, Ian: *The Psychiatric Examination.* Little, Brown & Co., Boston, 1969.

Taylor, R. B.: *A Primer of Clinical Symptoms.* Harper & Row, New York, 1973.

US Department of Health, Education, and Welfare: *Current Estimates from the Health Interview Survey, United States—1970.* US Government Printing Office, Washington, D.C., 1972.

————: *Interviewing Methods in the Health Interview Survey.* US Government Printing Office, Washington, D.C., 1972.

US Health Services and Mental Health Administration, Division of Health Care Services: *A Conceptual Model of Organized Primary Care and Comprehensive Community Health Services.* US Government Printing Office, Washington, D.C., 1970.

US Health Services and Mental Health Administration, Division of Emergency Health Services: *Emergency Health Services: Selected References.* US Government Printing Office, Washington, D.C., 1972.

US Health Services and Mental Health Administration, Federal Health Programs Service: *Vision Screening on Your Health Unit.* US Government Printing Office, Washington, D.C., 1972.

US National Center for Health Services Research and Development: *Provisional Guidelines for Automated Multiphasic Health Testing and Services,* Vol. 3. US Government Printing Office, Washington, D.C., 1970.

US Public Health Service: *Reported Tuberculosis Data 1969.* US Government Printing Office, Washington, D.C., 1971 (PHS Pub. No. 2180).

————: *Screening Children for Nutritional Status; Suggestions for Child Health Programs.* US Government Printing Office, Washington, D.C., 1971 (PHS Pub. No. 2158).

Weiss, Jay M.: "Psychological Factors in Stress and Disease," *Sci. Am.,* **226:**104, (June) 1972.

Wilson, Patience: "Evaluating Chest Films," *Nurse Pract.* **2:**6, (Jan.–Feb.) 1977.

Wong, Donna M.: "Providing Experience in Physical Assessment for Students in Basic Programs," *Am. J. Nurs.,* **75:**974, (June) 1975.

World Health Organization: *Principles and Practice of Screening for Disease.* (By J. M. G. Wilson and G. Jung.) The Organization, Geneva, 1968.

Virginia Henderson

The author gratefully acknowledges the critical reading of this chapter by Mimi Dye and Patience Wilson (both contributors of other chapters) and their help in the preparation of certain sections.

CHAPTER 6

Temperature, Respiration, Pulse, Blood Pressure, and Electrocardiography as Health Indicators

1. THE CARDINAL SYMPTOMS
2. BODY TEMPERATURE
3. RESPIRATION
4. THE PULSE
5. BLOOD PRESSURE
6. ELECTROCARDIOGRAPHY
7. IMPLANTED PACEMAKERS

1. THE CARDINAL SYMPTOMS

Temperature, pulse rate, and respiration rates are so constant and in health conform with such regularity to a standard that we speak of the "normal" temperature, pulse, and respiration. Mechanisms that govern them are so finely adjusted that a marked change or departure from normal rates is looked upon as a symptom of disease; consequently, "taking" the temperature, pulse, and respiration is one of the first means of assessing a person's condition. As long as the patient is in the hospital or under nursing care in a home they are usually taken at least twice during each 24 hours, although in some cases this may amount to a meaningless and unjustifiable routine. If there is marked departure from normal, measurements are made and recorded every 4 hours, or more frequently. The pulse, respiration, and blood pressure, are watched constantly in critical conditions by electric monitors in intensive care units and in some instances in the general clinical areas of the hospital. Although the temperature may not be taken when it might disturb the patient, a nurse is on the alert to note signs of temperature elevation, such as flushing of the face; hot, dry skin; hot and tremulous hands; dry, parched, and tremulous lips; rapid breathing; and mental confusion.

Again, so important are changes in temperature, pulse, and respiration, so typical of certain diseases, and of certain stages in the disease, that a special "temperature sheet" is kept, indicating numerically and graphically by means of dots and lines the temperature and pulse curves and the relation of one to the other (see Fig. 6-1).

This temperature sheet is usually the first on the patient record so that the doctor sees it at a glance. From this alone in some diseases he or she is able to judge the patient's condition. The temperature is a symptom that may be accurately determined by even an inexperienced person. Since it is accompanied by and runs parallel with the other symptoms of injury to the nervous system not so easily recognized by the inexperienced, a record of the temperature over a 24-hour period may give the nurse and physician a valuable clue to the patient's condition during that time.

These signals of distress held out by nature must be closely and accurately observed; nurses must never record a temperature, pulse, or respiration carelessly taken or one of which they are in doubt.

A full understanding of the temperature, pulse, and respiration as discussed in the following pages comes only with a thorough knowledge of anatomy and physiology and with wide experience. For a more complete treatment of these subjects the reader is referred to the texts listed at the end of this chapter.

2. BODY TEMPERATURE

Normal Body Temperature. Body temperature is usually measured by placing a thermometer in one of the body orifices. This is usually a glass instrument containing a column of mercury that expands, or rises, as it is

441

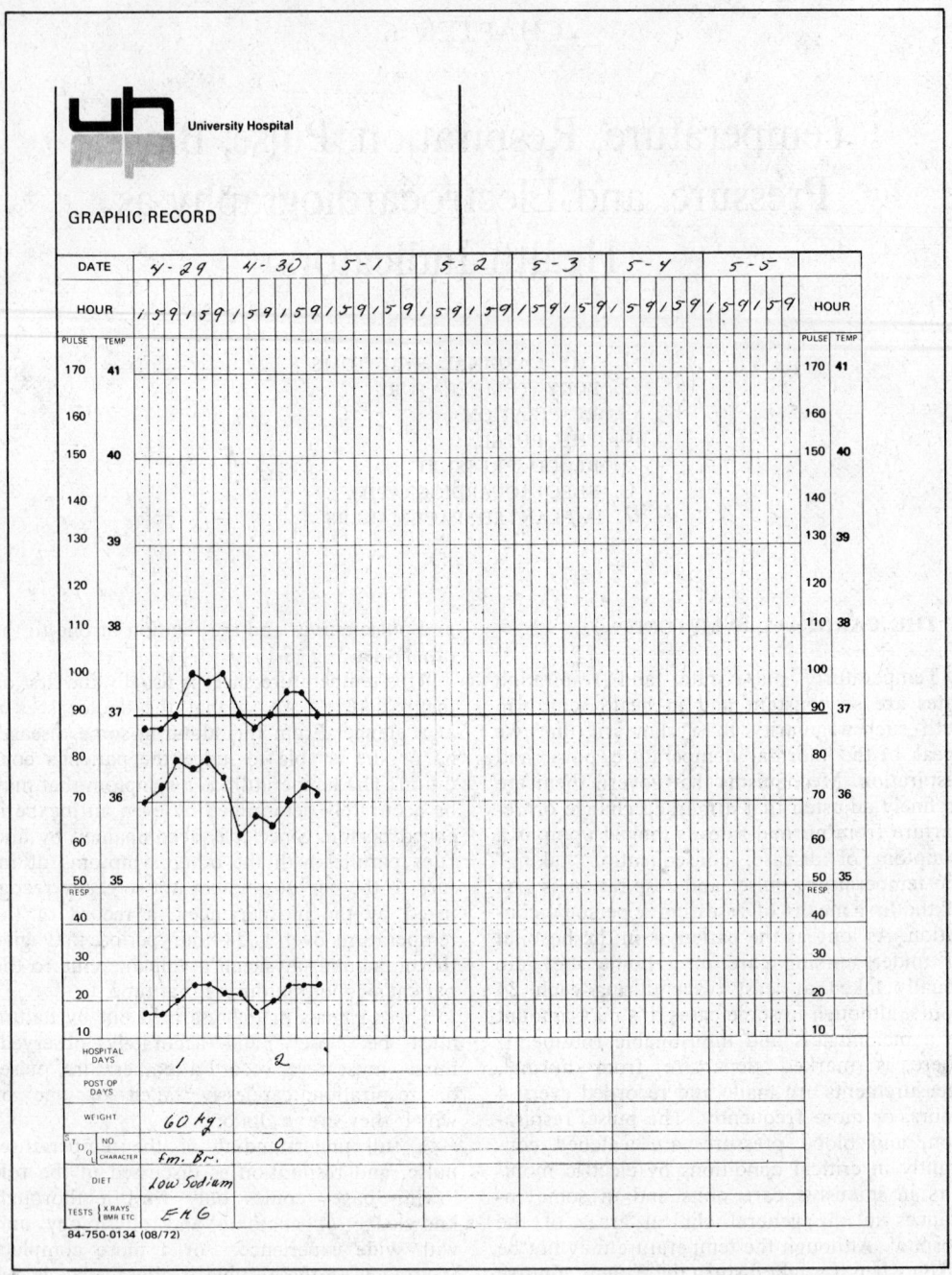

Figure 6-1. One example of a graphic record, showing temperature, pulse, respiration, and other important information. (Courtesy of University Hospital, University of Western Ontario, London, Ont.)

heated. Electronic thermometers, however, are used in most intensive care units and throughout some hospitals in the United States and elsewhere. For each cavity there is a range of measurements that may be termed normal. Eugene F. DuBois suggests that thermometers should be made to show these ranges (see Fig. 6-2). At present they have arrows at 37°C or 98.6°F, and deviations from these points are unfortunately believed by the average person to indicate disease. DuBois emphasizes the range of temperatures in different areas of the body. In extreme conditions, he says, it may range from 38°C (100.4°F) (in the interior or

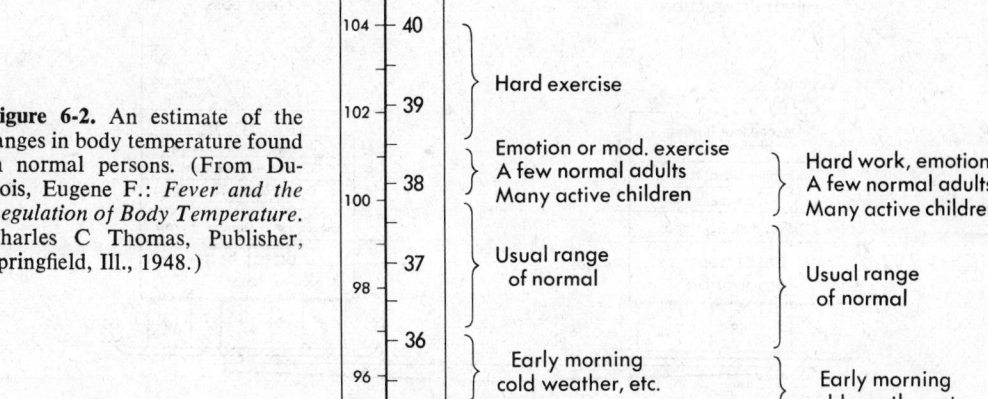

Figure 6-2. An estimate of the ranges in body temperature found in normal persons. (From DuBois, Eugene F.: *Fever and the Regulation of Body Temperature.* Charles C Thomas, Publisher, Springfield, Ill., 1948.)

core) to 0°C (32°F) (in the skin). "There is no one body temperature, but a series of gradients." * The liver, according to him, is the warmest part of the body. John R. Brobeck[1] places the temperature of the liver at about 37.8°C (100°F); the normal average mouth temperature at 37°C (98.6°F); the rectal temperature at 37.3°C (99.2°F); and the axillary skin temperature at 36.4°C (97.6°F).

George Brengelmann and Arthur C. Brown[2] say that for the heat produced in the deep organs (such as the liver, heart, viscera, and brain) to be lost these organs "must be warmer than the perfusing blood or the surrounding tissue." According to W. I. Cranston and associates,[3] the temperature of a tissue depends on several variables—the temperature and rate of blood flow through it, local heat production, and the exchange of heat with its surroundings. Skin temperatures vary widely with climatic conditions, with the clothing covering the area, and with the structure of the underlying tissues. DuBois says under ordinary conditions they range from 34°C (93.2°F) to 37°C (98.6°F). Temperature varies during the day, and there are also individual differences according to the way of life. A sedentary person is likely to have a lower temperature than the one living an active outdoor life. Temperature is lowest between 2 and 6 A.M., rising gradually during the day and reaching the maximum between 5 and 7 P.M., and again falling during the night.[4] This change in normal body temperature during the 24-hour period is called the *circadian thermal rhythm.* Currently it is thought that a "circadian clock" located in the region of the hypothalamus is responsible for the rhythmic variation in the body.[5] Although work and social habits as well as other external rhythmic factors play an important part in maintaining the 24-hour rhythm, this body temperature rhythm is reversed (after a 1- to 3-week period) in persons who sleep during the day and work at night.[6,7] The difference between the early morning and evening temperatures may be 1.11°C (2.0°F) or even 1.67°C (3.0°F).[8] For accurate comparison, it should be measured for each patient at the same hours each day, and one of these measurements should be made at 6 P.M., the peak of the circadian thermal rhythm.[9]

The average temperature also varies slightly with age, that of an infant or child being less stable and usually 0.56°C (1°F) higher than that of an adult. After age 30 the temperature is said to fall about 1°F, while in very advanced age it rises 1°F. The temperature is also affected by temperament. Emotion may produce a fever. As the relationship between the endocrines and metabolism is more clearly demonstrated, the statement that fever can have an emotional origin is more generally accepted.

Production of Heat. Body heat is produced continuously as a by-product of metabolism and is lost continuously to the environment. A person is said to be in heat balance when the rate of heat production is equal to that of heat loss (see Fig. 6-3). W. W. Tuttle and Byron A. Schottelius say:

Increasing or decreasing of the body temperature is brought about in two ways:
1. Regulating the loss of heat (thermolysis), that is, physical heat regulation.
2. Regulating the production of heat (thermogenesis), that is, chemical heat regulation.*

* DuBois, Eugene F.: *Fever and the Regulation of Body Temperature.* Charles C Thomas, Publisher, Springfield, Ill., 1948, p. 33.

* Tuttle, W. W., and Schottelius, Byron A.: *Textbook of Physiology,* 17th ed. C. V. Mosby Co., St. Louis, 1973, p. 468.

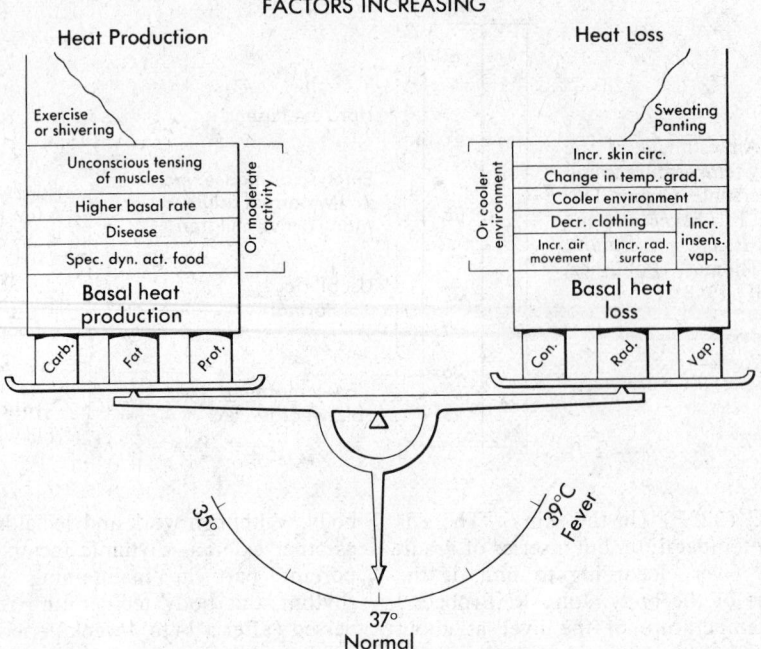

FACTORS INCREASING

Heat Production   Heat Loss

Figure 6-3. Balance between factors increasing heat production and heat loss. (From DuBois, Eugene F.: *Fever and the Regulation of Body Temperature.* Charles C Thomas, Publisher, Springfield, Ill., 1948.)

Body heat is the result of cell activity, particularly contraction of muscle cells, and for this and all other metabolic processes food is essential. For this reason the body has been compared, perhaps erroneously, to a furnace where the foods we eat, if burned, produce heat. Because the heat that food will produce is more easily measured than other forms of energy transformation, such as muscle activity or cell division, the value of food is reckoned in terms of the heat unit.

The calorie is the heat unit and is the amount of heat necessary to raise 1 gm of water 1°C. One large calorie (C) is the quantity of heat necessary to raise the temperature of 1000 gm of water 1°C. Each food has its specific caloric yield. The following are averages commonly given:

1 gm protein (heat value)
    = 4100 calories (4.1 C)
1 gm carbohydrate (starch)
    = 4100 calories (4.1 C)
1 gm fat   = 9305 calories (9.3 C)

These figures therefore represent the amount of energy, in the form of either heat or mechanical work, these foods are capable of supplying to the body. In this way the quantitative value of any diet may be estimated.

Food in the body, however, will not pro-duce heat without oxygen. Just as there are drafts in a furnace to regulate the oxygen entering according to the heat desired, so in the body in order to burn food and produce heat, there must be oxygen and a means of supplying it as needed. This is provided by the respiratory apparatus—air rich in oxygen is inhaled, and carbon dioxide, excess heat, and other waste products are exhaled in air now poor in oxygen. Thus there is a definite relation between body temperature and respiration, and they should be considered together.

Production of heat in the body is the result of activity in all its cells, but most of the heat is produced in certain organs. The more active the organ, the more food it burns and the more heat it produces. This heat is distributed by blood in its vessels to cooler parts of the body so that while the temperature of both external and internal parts may vary, their temperature is nearly uniform. A cold environment, however, may bring the skin temperature which usually ranges from 37° to 34°C (98.6° to 93.2°F) as low as 0°C (32°F).[10]

The muscles and secreting glands are the furnaces where most heat is generated. All know that when they are cold, *exercise* warms them. Strenuous exercise is said by some authorities to raise the body temperature from

0.56° to 2.24°C (1° to 4°F) or more.[11] *Shivering* is one of nature's means of producing heat when the body is chilled. Infections are characterized by chills with subsequent fever. This production of heat by muscular activity is a matter of common experience, and in warm climates people avoid exercise and diets rich in energy-producing foods—fats and carbohydrates. In cold climates the opposite conditions prevail.

It is generally known that eating increases body temperature. The maximal increase occurs about 1½ hours after meals. *Strong emotions,* which are the psychic response to glandular activity, also increase body temperature, and therefore the familiar expression "keep cool," when what is really meant is "don't get excited or angry."

A definite relation between body temperature and endocrine activity in health is demonstrated in women during the childbearing period. If a rectal temperature is taken daily in the morning before arising, most women show a characteristic variation during the menstrual cycle. Just before menstruation the temperature falls 0.40°C (0.8°F) below its previous level and remains low until ovulation, which is about the thirteenth or fourteenth day of the cycle. After the rupture of the graafian follicle and the escape of the ovum, the temperature rises 0.28°C (0.5°F) to 0.40°C (0.8°F) and remains at the higher level until the next menstruation.[12] Parenthetically, this knowledge of temperature fluctuation is used as a means of controlling conception, since it indicates the time at which the ovum may be penetrated by a spermatozoon. Thyroxin, norepinephrine, and epinephrine increase the metabolic rate of all tissues of the body and hence the production of body heat.[13]

Exposure to extremes of temperature in the surroundings—air or water—may also increase body temperature by radiation, convection, and conduction. *Brief exposure to cold* stimulates the body to produce more heat to protect itself. *A very high external temperature* upsets the balance of heat regulation by direct action on the heat-regulating center in the brain, it is thought, and may therefore produce a high temperature; for instance, a sunstroke may increase the body temperature to 41.7° or 43.3°C (107° or 110°F).

It is important for nurses to have some knowledge of the physiology of heat regulation. It is not enough to take the temperature; they must know when the temperature is above normal, what measures will prevent a further elevation, when it is subnormal, and what measures will increase the temperature. For instance, when the temperature is above normal, nurses should regulate the temperature of the surrounding air and the amount and kind of bedclothes; they should prevent all possible excitement or exertion on the part of patients and encourage them to rest as much as possible. In addition, patients should be given a diet low in protein and fat as well as an increased amount of water to drink. Sponge baths may also be given if drug therapy prescribed by the physician does not remove the cause and control the fever.

When the temperature is markedly subnormal, it may indicate that the patient is in a state of collapse, and nursing measures must be instituted to increase heat production. Unless the decrease in the blood supply to the skin is a protective mechanism, as in shock, the nurse should try to warm the body by applying heated blankets, rubbing, and giving warm drinks. (Care of the patient in shock is discussed in Chapter 45.)

Loss of Heat. If all the heat produced by cell activity were stored up in the tissues, such an accumulation would destroy the body. According to Brobeck:

The total quantity of heat lost in twenty-four hours must, of course, just equal the amount produced; otherwise, the body temperature would rise or fall. The heat production of an average man doing light work is about 3000 calories. The proportions of this which are dissipated through the various channels at ordinary room temperature are given in the following table, in approximate figures.

	Calories	Per Cent
(a) Radiation, convection and conduction	1950	65
(b) Evaporated from skin and lungs, and liberation of CO_2	900	30
(c) Warming inspired air	90	3
(d) Urine and feces (i.e., heat of these excreta over that of the food and water)	60	2
Total daily heat loss	3000	100*

* Brobeck, John R.: "Control Systems That Establish Regulations," in Brobeck, John R., et al. (eds.): *Best and Taylor's Physiological Basis of Medical Practice,* 9th ed. Williams & Wilkins Co., Baltimore, 1973, pp. 9–130.

As this tabulation shows, 65 per cent of heat is lost from the skin by radiation, convection, and conduction; however, the amount lost depends on external and internal conditions. The external conditions are the temperature and humidity of the air, velocity of air currents, and temperature of surrounding objects. Consequently, a person may regulate the loss of body heat voluntarily to a certain extent by protecting the body by clothing and shelter, by eating warm food and liquids, and by warming the air. The reader should consult Chapter 42 for a detailed discussion of this subject. Regulation of body heat by involuntary means is brought about by the vasomotor mechanism and by perspiration. For example, when a thinly clothed person is resting in an environmental temperature of 25° to 29.4°C (77° to 85°F), the vasomotor mechanism is operating, solely; below 25°C the body temperature drops; sweating begins at 29.4°C; and when the temperature rises above 29.4°C, the sweating mechanism is more important while the vasomotor mechanism is progressively less important. The *physiologically economic range of temperature of man* is from 25° to 35°C (77° to 95°F) where the loss of heat is the least and metabolism is at a minimum.[14]

Anything that reduces activity *decreases* heat production. The temperature falls during sleep, shock, and unconscious states. Sedatives lower body temperature; and vasodilators, such as alcohol, lower the temperature of the blood by bringing a greater blood volume to the skin, where it is cooled.

Heat Regulation. Normal body temperature is the balance maintained between heat produced and heat loss. In warm-blooded animals this balance is set at a standard normal for that particular species. The so-called cold-blooded animals, such as the frog or fish, are those whose temperature varies with that of the surrounding air or water. The warm-blooded animals are those that maintain a relatively constant temperature summer and winter, practically independent of the temperature of their surroundings. This is accomplished by a heat-regulating mechanism, and in man partly by clothing—an artificial means of preventing excess loss of heat through the skin by radiation and conduction.

The most important means of controlling loss of heat from the body is, therefore, by controlling that lost through the skin. This is accomplished by sympathetic centers of the posterior hypothalamus that control the circulation of blood and the secretion of sweat. The arteries in the skin subdivide into an enormous number of minute capillaries and thus increase the amount of blood exposed to the influence of the surrounding cooler air. Through these vessels flows a very large volume of warm blood from the muscles and glands, giving off some of its heat to the cooler atmosphere before returning to the interior of the body.

When the surrounding temperature is very cold, the *heat-sensitive neurons* located in the preoptic area of the anterior hypothalamus cause the blood vessels in the skin to contract so that less blood flows through the skin and less heat is lost. The production of sweat also is checked so that less heat is lost. The *temperature receptors in the skin* transmit impulses to the hypothalamus and the process of producing heat is begun; shivering may result, and the appetite is stimulated so that more food is eaten. Heat production is increased by increased output of thyroxin, epinephrine, and norepinephrine (called *chemical thermogenesis*). When the surrounding air is warmer, the opposite effect occurs—the blood vessels in the skin dilate, more blood flows through them, more heat is lost, sweating increases, and activity and appetite are diminished. Skin temperature receptors (both for heat and cold) transmit impulses into the spinal cord and then to the hypothalamus region of the brain to help control the temperature of the body.

It is thought that the regulating centers (preoptic area and adjacent regions of the anterior hypothalamus) act like the regulator or thermostat connected with a furnace or oven. In health the thermostat is set for a temperature around 37°C (98.6°F). The temperature control mechanisms struggle against any marked change from the normal temperature until they themselves are exhausted. If there is an infection, the thermostat seems to be set at a higher figure. Fever and related nursing care are discussed in Chapters 28 and 44.

Variations within the limits shown in Figure 6-2 are ordinarily not significant. Mouth temperatures above 38°C (100.4°F) or below 36°C (96.8°F) usually indicate pathology. Temperatures above normal are called febrile; those below, subnormal. The elevation of temperature is not always an index of the seriousness of the disease, for it may be higher in the shorter, less serious infections than in the most fatal. For instance, the temperature in tonsillitis is frequently higher than in diphtheria, and in some fatal infections there may be no elevation at all. A prolonged high temperature is always serious because it can destroy brain cells.

Temperatures above Normal—Fever. Elisha Atkins defines "fever" as "an elevation of the body temperature due to disease." * He makes it clear, however, that a person in health may have a rectal temperature of 40°C (104°F) as

---

* Atkins, Elisha: "Fever," in MacBryde, Cyril Mitchell, and Blacklow, Robert Stanley (eds): *Signs and Symptoms: Applied Pathologic Physiology and Clinical Interpretation,* 5th ed. J. B. Lippincott Co., Philadelphia, 1970, p. 451.

a result of exercise or an elevated mouth temperature from chewing gum. *Pyrexia* is another term for fever, and *hyperpyrexia* and *hyperthemia* for temperatures of 40.6°C (105°F) or above.

Fever is an imbalance between heat production and elimination. The origin of the imbalance is explained by several theories, but none has been established. William Boyd [15] says laboratory studies have shown that polymorphonuclear leukocytes contain a *pyrogen*. He thinks that when cells are injured they give off their own pyrogen which excites the production of fever. It is believed that substances causing fever act on the thermoregulatory centers of the brain. Some students of fever have attributed it to adrenal activity. Atkins says that this theory is disproven by the fact that animals without adrenals can be made febrile, while those without a hypothalamus cannot. There is good evidence that the activity of the thermoregulatory centers is "modified by some product or products of tissue injury." * He lists as causes of fever: infections; diseases of the nervous system; certain malignant neoplasms; blood diseases, such as leukemia and severe pernicious anemia; embolism and thrombosis; heat stroke from exposure to hot environments; dehydration; paroxysmal tachycardia and congestive heart failure, with and without known accompanying infections; surgical trauma and crushing injuries; possibly the gum injury in teething babies; peptic ulcer; skin abnormalities that interfere with normal heat loss; serums containing an irritating foreign protein and intravenous solutions containing pyrogens; and he lists some drugs that may cause fever. Atkins discusses "habitual hyperthermia" and cites Hobart A. Reimann's [16] study of rare persons whose temperature seems to be set slightly above the average level. He thinks "most physicians are convinced that under certain conditions an emotional stimulus may induce an elevation of temperature." † He cites the slight rise of temperature so commonly seen in hospital admissions and army draftees, and Frank B. Wynn's [17] observation of 0.33°C (0.6°F) average rise in body temperature among nurses about to write state-board examinations. Prolonged pain is believed to cause a temperature rise, which might be the result of tissue injury or of the fear that accompanies pain.

Treatment of fever (discussed in Chapter 44) depends upon the cause, its severity, and duration. It is a symptom, not a disease. DuBois asks, "Fever—friend or foe?" and is

inclined to say in most cases "friend." Its value has been established in neurosyphilis and in certain types of infections, and there is clinical evidence that if persons with a severe infection do not develop fever the prognosis may be grave. Fever does not seem to serve any useful purpose in noninfectious conditions and may even be harmful, as for example in malignant diseases and following myocardial infarction.[18] Extreme fever is always dangerous and should be reduced if possible. Fever of 41.1°C (106°F) or higher in adults is believed to be spurious.[19]

Ward J. MacNeil [20] gives 46°C (114.8°F) as the upper limit beyond which irreversible changes in tissues take place. Very high temperatures cause delirium and convulsions, showing injury of the central nervous system. While moderate temperatures are not combatted as they once were, the hyperpyrexia of heatstroke, which may well be fatal, is reduced by every available means. Convulsions often accompany a sudden onset of fever in children, whose heat-regulating mechanism is unsteady until puberty or thereabouts.

With every degree of body temperature there is believed to be a 7 per cent increase in the metabolic rate, just as all chemical reactions are speeded by heat. At a temperature of 40.6°C (105°F) metabolism is about 50 per cent above normal.[21] This suggests the danger of protracted temperatures where the food intake, for one reason or another, cannot be raised in proportion to the metabolic rate.

Course of the Fever, or Temperature Curve. Fever usually runs a typical course, characteristic of a particular disease; so it is commonly said, "The fever must run its course." In some diseases the temperature curve, or the diagrammatic representation on the chart of the course of the fever, is so typical that the diagnosis is suggested at a glance. When the course of the disease is arrested by a drug, as it often is now, the fever curve will of course not be so characteristic.

The *onset* or *invasion* may be sudden, as in pneumonia and scarlet fever, or it may be gradual, as in typhoid. After the temperature has reached its maximum, it usually remains elevated for a few days to 2 or 3 weeks or longer unless the course of the disease is arrested by treatment. This period of high fever is called the *fastigium* or *stadium*. (*Stadium*, from the Greek, a measure of distance in races, and *fastigium* from the Latin, the ridge of a roof.)

Fever may subside suddenly, the temperature falling 2.24° or 2.8°C (4° or 5°F) within a few hours and reaching normal or below in from 12 to 24 hours, accompanied by a

---

* Atkins, Elisha: *op. cit.*, p. 458.
† *Ibid.*, p. 458.

marked improvement in the patient's condition; or it may subside gradually. When the temperature subsides suddenly, as in unarrested lobar pneumonia, the drop is called the *crisis.* It is not so much the drop in temperature, but the lessened severity of symptoms that marks the true crisis. A sudden fall in the temperature not accompanied by an improvement in the general condition is not a true crisis. It may indicate the body's inability to combat the infection, or approaching death. In such cases the drop in temperature is a danger signal and not a sign of improvement.

Fever is said to subside by *lysis* when, as in typhoid, the temperature falls step by step in a zigzag manner for two or three days or a week before reaching normal. During this time the other symptoms also gradually disappear.

Types of Fever. (1) *Habitual hyperthermia* is a term used for the consistent elevation of temperature slightly above normal levels found in occasional individuals. (2) *Constant fever* describes one that remains near the same elevation throughout a period of days or weeks. (3) *Remittent fever* has wide variations in the temperature level morning and evening, but never falls to normal. (4) *Intermittent* or *quotidian fever* is one in which the body temperature rises and returns to normal daily. When the difference between the high and low points is very great, the fever is called *hectic* or *septic.* (5) *Relapsing fever* is one in which there are brief febrile periods followed by one or more days of normal temperature.

During convalescence from fever there may be a recrudescence. The temperature elevation may be merely temporary, due to excitement, as from the visits of friends or to some unusual exertion. Such a recurrence, however, should receive careful attention, as it may mean a return of the infection that must again run its course, or it may indicate complications.

Subnormal Temperatures. The body must maintain a certain degree of heat in order to carry on vital processes. Subnormal temperatures may be caused by (1) excessive heat elimination, as from profuse sweating, severe hemorrhage, or loss of other body fluids; (2) lessened heat production, as in starvation and lowered vitality; (3) extreme depression of the nervous system, as in shock or collapse; and (4) long exposure to cold environments. Studies in the past have shown that man can survive subnormal temperatures for a surprising length of time. The purpose and effects of induced hypothermia are discussed in Chapter 42.

Clinical Thermometer. The Fahrenheit self-registering clinical thermometer was the instrument commonly used in the United States, Canada, and Great Britain for measuring body temperature, but the continental centigrade scale or the metric system is coming into general use in all the countries. The clinical thermometer is a glass bulb containing mercury and a stem in which the mercury can rise. On the stem is a graduated scale representing degrees of temperature. The lowest temperature registered is 35°C or 95°F; the highest 43.3°C or 110°F, because body temperatures below or above these points are exceedingly rare. The stem usually has a curved surface that magnifies the lines and figures on the scale and a flattened back with a sharp ridge that makes it easier to read the scale, prevents rolling, and lessens the danger of breakage.

Thermometers are made with bulbs of different sizes and shapes. The greater the surface of glass surrounding the mercury, the more rapidly the mercury heats and therefore the more rapidly the thermometer registers. Mouth thermometers with long, slender bulbs may register more rapidly than rectal thermometers with short bulbs. A slender bulb must not be used in the rectum as it is likely to injure the mucosa. Both mouth and rectal thermometers are made with short, fat bulbs and are probably less easily broken than the slender type, but it is esthetically important to have different instruments for these two methods of taking the temperature. Rectal thermometers often have colored bulbs. Pigment used in making the temperature scale is gradually removed with use, but manufacturers of high-grade thermometers will furnish pigment with which to replace the scale. Different shapes and methods of marking thermometers are shown in Figure 6-4 and various types with cases are shown in Figure 6-5. One type of electronic thermometer is shown in Figure 6-6.

The principle upon which the use of the thermometer is based is that mercury expands with heat, the height to which the column rises depending upon the intensity, which it therefore accurately registers, because in the self-registering thermometer the mercury stays at this height until shaken down. Needless to say, the thermometer must not be used for anything hotter than 43.3°C (110°F), for the mercury would continue to expand and break the stem. Before using the thermometer, see that the mercury registers about 35°C (95°F). To shake the mercury down, grasp the thermometer securely by the upper end (never hold it by the bulb), flex the hand, and give a quick movement of the wrist as when snapping the fingers or cracking a whip. Do not shake the mercury below 35°C (95°F), as it may be difficult to get it up again. Be careful not to let the thermometer fall or strike against anything.

The reliability of oral and rectal glass clini-

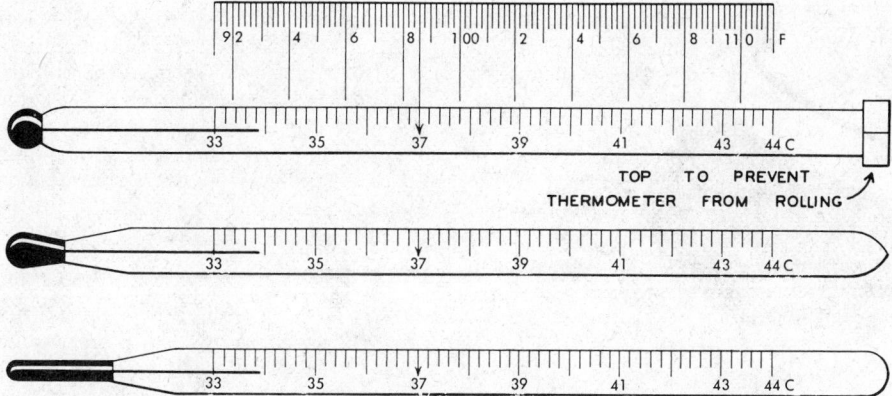

Figure 6-4. Three shapes of thermometers and corresponding Fahrenheit-centigrade conversion scale.

cal thermometers is largely dependent on their accuracy. E. G. Diamond and M. H. Andrews [22] (1954) report that when 465 glass clinical thermometers were tested, 78 per cent had variations of less than 0.28°C (0.5°F), 22 per cent had errors greater than 0.28°C (0.5°F), and 7 per cent had errors of 0.56°C (1°F). Herbert A. Knapp [23] (1966) compared the inaccuracies of 12 standard glass oral thermometers (randomly selected from a hospital) and the probes of two electronic thermometers. The findings showed that glass thermometers had an average error of 0.14°C (0.25°F) and with maximum errors approaching 0.22°C (0.4°F); whereas in a bath temperature of 40.6°C (105°F) the errors in glass thermometers were larger, with the maximum approaching 0.39°C (0.7°F). When two electronic thermometers were similarly tested, the maximum error was only 0.08°C (0.15°F). Gayle Tate Ferguson and associates [24] report a 0.11°C (0.2°F) error in the electronic thermometer over the 35° to 40.6°C (95° to 105°F) range tested. When the accuracies of the two types of thermometers are compared, the electronic thermometer obviously is more accurate than the glass clinical thermometer. Its accuracy is attributed to the fact that it can be *calibrated* while the glass thermometer can-

not. Electronic thermometers are being used for patients in whom accurate temperature measurement is crucial.

Instruments of special design are available for determining skin temperatures, a thermocouple giving the most accurate measurement. In a skin thermometer the same principles of construction are observed as those for the mouth and rectal thermometers except that the bulb is flattened to facilitate skin contact. Special infant temperature monitor tapes applied directly to the abdomen are available and are said to accurately monitor rectal temperatures of newborn infants. They are in common use in some parts of the United States. The degree of temperature is reflected in varying colors of the tape.

Suggested Method of "Taking Temperature." Body temperature may be determined by putting the thermometer in the mouth or rectum. Sometimes the axilla or groin is used and occasionally the vagina, but the last site is particularly undesirable.[25] The temperature sought is that of the interior of the body uninfluenced by contact with clothing, air, or moisture. Therefore, the thermometer must be placed where it can be completely surrounded by body tissues and where there are large blood vessels near the surface. The nearer these conditions

Figure 6-5. Various types of clinical thermometers and cases. (Courtesy of Becton, Dickinson & Co., Rutherford, N.J., and Clay-Adams Co., New York, N.Y).

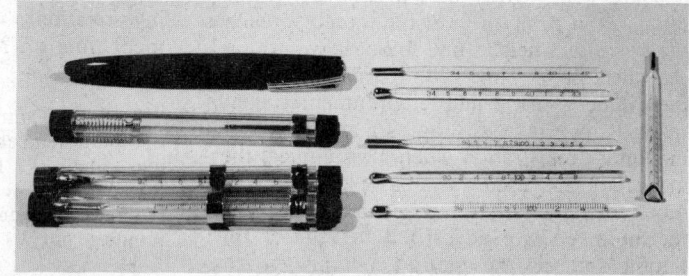

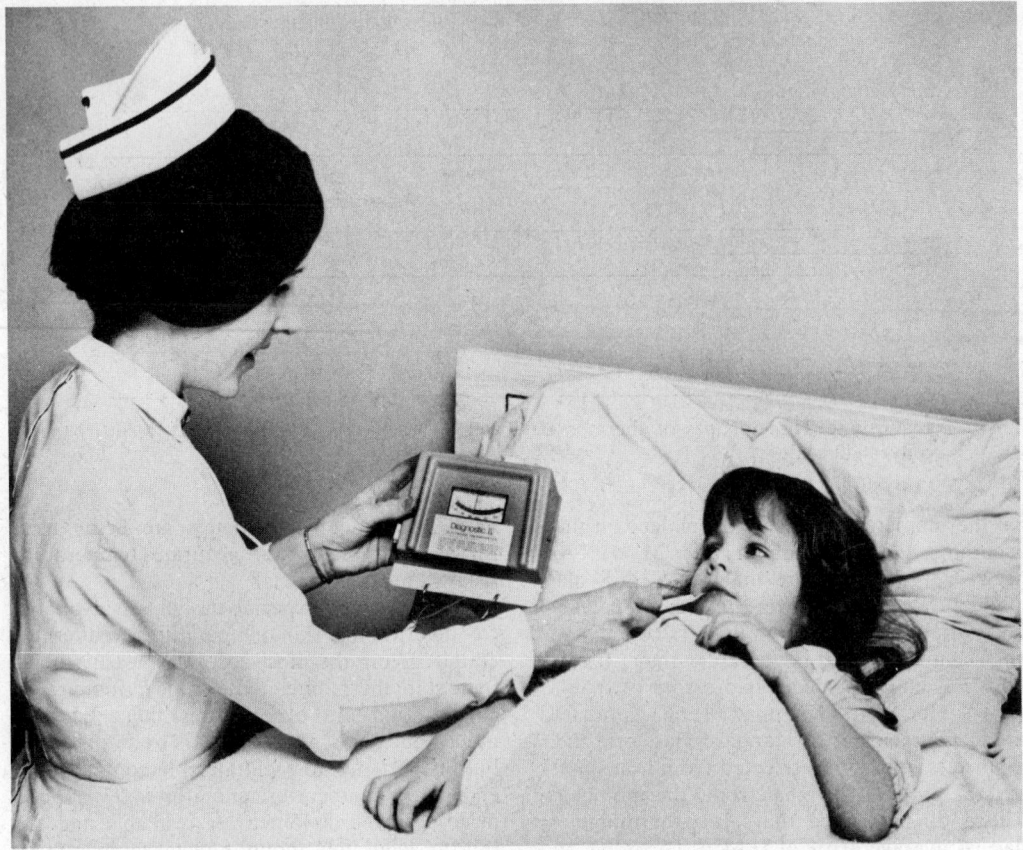

Figure 6-6. One type of electronic thermometer. This instrument measures body temperature in 15 seconds by means of a temperature-sensitive resistor called a thermistor. Most electronic thermometers require calibration at specific intervals and require a prewarming period for accurate measurement. The risk of cross contamination is virtually eliminated by use of disposable patient probes. (Courtesy of Diagnostic, Inc., Indianapolis, Ind.)

are approached, the more accurate the measurement.

In taking the *temperature by mouth,* place the end of the thermometer containing the mercury under the tongue, because here it will be close to large blood vessels. (When using an electronic thermometer, place the disposable sheath over the probe and then place the end of the probe under the tongue.) See that the lips are kept tightly closed. Leave the thermometer in position until the mercury reaches the maximum height, but do not leave it longer than necessary. Time required depends on the thermometer used and environmental conditions; it may take as long as 8 minutes to get maximum registration when glass clinical thermometers are used, whereas electronic thermometers take only a few seconds. High-grade thermometers are advertised to register in 1 minute, but as the mouth contains environmental air the lips must remain tightly closed for 8 minutes to warm the air to body temperature. When taking temperatures of patients on cold porches, allow 10 minutes for registration of the thermometer. During the past decade a large number of studies have been conducted by nurses for the purpose of determining accurate measurement of body temperature. Glennadee A. Nichols and Deloros H. Kucha, following an analysis of data from six investigations [26-31] of oral thermometer placement time on 390 subjects, report the following:

Subjects required 1 to 11 minutes to reach their optimum temperature readings—maximum readings minus 0.2°F. It required 8 minutes for at least 90 per cent of the subjects to attain optimum readings, making the optimum placement time 8 minutes, not 3 or 5.

. . .

The 8-minute readings ranged from 0.2° to 1.6°F higher than the 3-minute readings with the average difference being 0.57°F.*

Subjects 18 to 39 years required 8 minutes for optimum readings but those over 40 years required 7 minutes; men required 7 minutes, women 8 minutes. Environmental temperature also affects oral temperature recordings in men and women—men 8 minutes, and women 9 minutes in rooms of temperature 18.3° to 23.9°C (65° to 75°F), but in rooms 24.4° to 30°C (76° to 86°F) "optimum placement time is 7 minutes for all adults."

Febrile children (boys and girls age 7 to 13) are reported to require an optimum placement time of 7 minutes [32] (see Table 6-1).

Katharine Brim and Betty A. Chandler (1948) conducted one of the first studies of the effects on oral temperature recordings of drinking hot and cold liquids, smoking cigarettes, and chewing gum. According to them:

Hot liquids caused a deviation from the control temperature for from twenty to eighty minutes, whereas following the drinking of cold liquids, the temperatures of the majority of test subjects returned to the original level in from five to ten minutes. However, in some cases, the temperature taken ten to twenty minutes after the drinking of cold liquids had not only reached the control temperature but had surpassed it by as much as 1.4°F. Ten minutes after drinking hot liquids, twenty-four individuals' temperatures were still one degree Fahrenheit above their control temperatures.

Both the chewing of gum and smoking may raise or lower the oral temperature, but the chewing of gum seems to have a more prolonged effect than does smoking.†

In a study of 50 afebrile men who drank 150 ml of hot tea 48.9°–51.7°C (120°–125°F), Cynthia A. Logan [33] reports 10 to 15

---

* Nichols, Glennadee A., and Kucha, Deloros H.: "Taking Adult Temperatures; Oral Measurements," *Am. J. Nurs.*, **72**:1091, (June) 1972.

† Brim, Katharine, and Chandler, Betty A.: "Changes in Oral Temperature," *Am. J. Nurs.*, **48**:772, (Dec.) 1948.

---

minutes was required for the subjects' temperatures to return to levels near their baseline, but the temperatures of 11 of the 50 subjects (22 per cent) had not returned to within 0.11°C (0.2°F) of their baseline levels at the end of 30 minutes. According to studies of Ellen A. Woodman and associates,[34] drinking cold liquids can affect the accuracy of the oral temperature as much as 0.89°C (1.6°F), and Brenda Forster and associates [35] report its duration as 15 minutes. Some studies report that smoking and chewing gum did not affect oral temperature recordings.[36,37]

While C. Rosendorff and W. I. Cranston [37a] (1968) report that salicylates given orally or intravenously to 12 afebrile adults had no effect on body temperature, Evelyn Satinoff [37b] (1972) found that 64 afebrile rats given intraperitoneal injections of salicylates showed a decline in rectal temperature as much as 5.5°C (41.9°F) when placed in a 5°C (41°F) environment. She says evidence from these experiments suggests that antipyretic agents do affect normal temperature regulation.

It is far from simple to get an accurate estimate of the temperature of any body area. The nurse should be aware of and take into account the difficulties involved.

Contraindications for Mouth Temperatures. The mouth is the most convenient place for taking the temperature, but should not be used immediately after the patient has smoked, chewed gum, or had hot or cold drinks or food, when he or she is breathing through the mouth or when having cold or hot applications to the face or throat. Mouth thermometers should not be used when the patient has difficulty in breathing from any cause or when the mouth cannot be closed for the required time: for instance, when the patient has an acute head cold or an inflamed obstructed respiratory tract; when sneezing or coughing; or when the mouth falls open from extreme weakness. They must not be used when the mouth is dry, parched, or inflamed; never used for very young children or for restless, delirious, unconscious, or irrational patients because of the

---

Table 6-1. Time and Optimum Oral Temperatures *

Minutes	1	2	3	4	5	6	7	8	9	10	11	12
Number of subjects	41	53	53	55	60	39	44	24	11	7	3	0
Percentage	10.5	13.6	13.6	14.1	15.4	10.0	11.2	6.2	2.8	1.8	0.8	
Cumulative percentage	10.5	24.1	37.7	51.8	67.2	77.2	88.4	94.6	97.4	99.2	100	

* How thermometers registered minute by minute for 390 study subjects. (Nichols, Glennadee A., and Kucha, Deloros H.: "Taking Adult Temperatures; Oral Measurements," *Am. J. Nurs.*, **72**:1091, [June] 1972.)

danger of biting and breaking the thermometer and swallowing the glass and mercury. Mouth thermometers are rarely used on psychiatric services. The mercury, if swallowed, would probably do no harm because in its metallic form it is almost inert.* If such an accident occurs, however, it should be reported at once. The doctor may prescribe white of egg, milk, or another antidote for mercury. The broken particles of glass, if swallowed, might perforate the mucosa. If a thermometer should accidentally be broken, all particles of glass should be removed from the mouth. If any glass has been swallowed, eating bread or some other soft food may help to prevent injury to the lining of the esophagus.

Should the temperature taken by mouth seem unusually low, or should there be any doubt of its accuracy, take it over again, take it with another thermometer, or take it by rectum. While most studies of body temperature have been made with self-registering rectal thermometers and many clinicians favor this route, taking the temperature by mouth has many advantages. The chief argument for oral temperatures is that they are physically and psychologically so much more acceptable to the patient. They should be used unless the measurement is critical or conditions prohibit it.

The temperature is sometimes taken by axilla when it cannot be taken by mouth, because it is convenient and hygienic and occasions little exertion for the patient, although many persons find it difficult to hold one posture for as long as is required. Before putting the thermometer in the axilla, see that it is free from perspiration, but do not rub the part because friction may increase the skin temperature and make the reading misleading. Place the bulb securely in the axilla, surround it with body tissues by placing the arm over the chest with the fingers on the opposite shoulder, and leave it 10 minutes. Do not allow the clothing to come in contact with the thermometer.

For infants the groin temperature is sometimes taken and the temperature of the skin of the abdomen. The thigh must be well flexed over the abdomen. Ten minutes is required for registration. Jane T. Torrance,[37e] following a study of 120 premature infants, says 4 minutes was required for stabilized temperature readings in 95 per cent of the babies.

Axillary and groin temperatures are usually 0.56°C (1°F) lower than that of the mouth.

Contraindications for Rectal Temperatures. The *rectal temperature* is generally used for the very ill and for infants, children, and irrational patients. Since exposure of the pubic and anal regions is generally distasteful, rectal temperatures should be taken only when necessary. These areas are contaminated after rectal operations or when the rectum is diseased, inflamed, or impacted with feces. Bacteria are always present in fecal matter, causing decomposition and consequent heat production. The presence of fecal matter therefore probably increases the rectal temperature and interferes with accurate measurement. DuBois says: "Although the rectal temperature usually changes in the same direction as the average body temperature, it may change in the opposite direction. . . . It is well to remember that in a man who exercises the rectal temperature rises while the oral temperature remains constant or falls." *

In taking a rectal temperature it is important to have the thermometer well lubricated not only because it is more comfortable but also because irritation stimulates the muscles of the rectum to expel the instrument. Insert the bulb about 1½ inches and leave it in position for at least 2 minutes (see Table 6-2). Some studies show that as much as 4 minutes is required.[37d-37f] Because the rectum is a closed cavity, less affected by external conditions than the mouth, its temperature is from 0.28° to 0.56°C (½ to 1°F) higher.

Never leave children or irrational adults alone with a thermometer, no matter what method is used, for their restless movements are likely to displace or break it. Patients occasionally try to mislead the nurse into thinking that their temperature is elevated when it is not. They may have a second thermometer

* DuBois, Eugene F.: *op. cit.*, p. 47.

Table 6-2. Time and Optimum Rectal Temperatures *

Minutes	1	2	3	4	5	6
Number of subjects	315	58	21	8	1	0
Percentage	78.2	14.4	5.2	2.0	0.2	
Cumulative percentage	78.2	92.6	97.8	99.8	100	

* Several physicians report cases of broken thermometers with no ill effects from the swallowed mercury. Harry Gold says, "the mercury released from the broken bulb of the thermometer may be ignored with impunity." (Gold, Harry [ed.]: *Cornell Conferences on Therapy*, Vol. 4. Macmillan Publishing Co., Inc., New York, 1952, p. 5.)

* Time and optimum rectal temperature studies using 403 subjects showed that rectal thermometers don't need a full 5 minutes to register, and the author concluded 3 minutes is enough. (Nichols, Glennadee A.: "Taking Adult Temperatures; Rectal Measurements," *Am. J. Nurs.*, **72:**1092, [June] 1972.)

which they substitute for the one given them, or they may heat the mercury by friction in the hand, the mouth, or the rectum. Virginia Hale and Olga Evseichick report a case of "fraudulent fever," in which the patient made the thermometer register several degrees above the body temperature by "repeated contraction of the anal sphincter muscles." * MacNeil suggests the following procedure when it is suspected that the patient is using tricks to elevate the registration. Make "simultaneous observations of the temperature . . . by one or more thermometers in each axilla, another beneath the tongue, and another in the rectum, the stem of each instrument being held steadily by the hand of the observer and never entrusted to the patient." † He believes that "reasonable agreement" of these readings indicates reliability. He suggests as a check testing the temperature of freshly voided feces and urine. Malingerers hope by running a fever to get more attention or to prolong hospitalization. They should always be considered and treated as psychiatric problems.

Care of Thermometers. Thermometers should be clean and free from infectious material when used or stored. They should be tested and compared at regular intervals with a standard thermometer, because, unless seasoned, the glass gradually contracts, and after a time the readings are inaccurate, being slightly high. Manufacturers of good-grade thermometers claim, however, that their instruments remain accurate until broken.

Most hospitals in the United States provide individual thermometers which are kept in the patient's unit. They should be washed with soap and water and dried after use. To prevent breakage, they should be kept in a covered box, cylinder, or other suitable container. There is no more reason for keeping the patient's individual thermometer in a disinfectant solution than there is his toothbrush. Before the instrument is used for another person, it must be disinfected chemically. When the same thermometer is used from day to day by two or more patients, it is disinfected each time it is used.

Margaret Welsh and Martha E. Erdman [37g] and Elisabeth Ryan and Virginia B. Miller [37h] in two similar series of tests on disinfectants commonly used for thermometers found bichloride of mercury in a solution of 1:1000 the most efficient of the solutions tested. In both sets of tests, destruction of microorganisms was more nearly complete and rapid when organic material from the mouth or rectum

was removed from the instrument by wiping and washing in soap and water before disinfection. A later study showed excellent results when, after a thorough cleaning with a mixture of equal parts of tincture of green soap and 95 per cent ethyl alcohol, thermometers were immersed for 10 minutes in 1.0 per cent solutions of iodine in 70 per cent isopropyl alcohol ("rubbing alcohol") or 70 per cent ethyl alcohol. When 70 per cent ethyl or isopropyl alcohol without iodine was used, the results were almost equally satisfactory. Soap is available in homes and usually some sort of alcohol. Mercury compounds were not included in the study because, according to the authors of the report, "Previous work has demonstrated that its action is inhibited by organic material and it is a bacteriostatic rather than a bacteriocidal substance." *

3. RESPIRATION

The underlying physiology of respiration and some of the factors affecting it in "healthy" persons are discussed in Chapter 9. Emphasis is put on personal and community responsibility for maintaining respiratory health in all persons. Because normal respiratory function is complex and difficult to understand, some of the major concepts discussed in Chapter 9 are summarized in this section. We believe that when *complex* concepts are discussed in different (but not conflicting) ways, the learner is helped to understand the subject. Chapter 35 deals with marked disturbances of respiration.

Vital Importance of Respiration. As noted in Chapter 9, respiration is the exchange of gases between an organism and its environment and is one of the characteristics common to all living entities. It is essential for the chemical changes of metabolism on which life depends. The human body can survive for only a matter of minutes without oxygen.

Oxygen and food are required by each body cell in order to maintain life and function. They must be carried to the cells, where they can be utilized in cell metabolism. Carbon dioxide is one of the resulting waste products, so it is important that the body be provided with a system that will not only supply the tissues with oxygen but also rid them of carbon dioxide; otherwise, each cell would, in a sense, suffocate. When we speak of a person's strangling or smothering to death, we really mean

* Hale, Virginia, and Evseichick, Olga: "Fraudulent Fever," *Am. J. Nurs.,* **43:**992, (Nov.) 1943.

† MacNeil, Ward J.: "Hyperthermia, Genuine and Spurious," *Arch. Intern. Med.,* **64:**800, (Oct.) 1939.

* Sommermeyer, Lucille, and Frobisher, Martin, Jr.: "Laboratory Studies on Disinfection of Oral Thermometers," *Nurs. Res.,* **1:**32, (Oct.) 1952.

that his cells are smothering. The greater the activity of the cell, the more oxygen required and the greater the amount of carbon dioxide eliminated.

Provision for this exchange of gases is made in man by the respiratory and circulatory systems. Air containing roughly 20 per cent oxygen and 0.4 per cent carbon dioxide is drawn into the lungs. Here oxygen is absorbed by and carbon dioxide given off from the capillaries. The expired air contains 16.3 per cent oxygen and 4 per cent carbon dioxide. By means of the circulatory system, the oxygen absorbed in the lungs is conveyed to the tissues, and carbon dioxide is conveyed from the tissues to the lungs to be exhaled. Both the respiratory and circulatory systems are a means to an end, the end being the absorption of oxygen by the cells, and elimination by the cells of carbon dioxide and other waste products of metabolism. Because the cells are so remote from the oxygen supply, the exchange of gases must take place both between the blood and the air in the lungs and between the blood and the tissue cells. The former is called *external or pulmonary respiration* and the latter, *internal or tissue respiration*. However, *diffusion and transport of gases* is the term commonly used to describe tissue respiration because of its accuracy.

Regulation of Respiration. Rhythmic movements of respiration are regulated by the respiratory center, nerve fibers of the autonomic nervous system, and the chemical composition of the blood.

The respiratory center is in the medulla and coincides in position with the sensory center of the vagus. It was called the "vital knot" by its discoverer, Flourens, because he found that when it is destroyed, respiration ceases and death follows. This center sends out motor nerves that supply the muscles of respiration. It is essentially automatic—that is, it sends out impulses to the muscles independently of any impulses sent to it; however, it is also affected by sensory stimuli from all parts of the body. Sensory fibers travel to it through the vagus from the lungs and larynx. Sensory fibers also travel to it from the cerebrum so that stimulation of any sensory nerves in the body, through the cerebrum, may stimulate the respiratory center reflexively and thus affect the rate and character of breathing. Because there is this connection between the cerebrum and the respiratory center and because the muscles of respiration are voluntary, a person can, to a limited degree, control respiration. When singing or speaking a person regulates the depth and rate of respiration; most of the time, however, respiration is rhythmic and involuntary. The effort to "hold the breath" is soon over-

come by exhaustion, accumulation of carbon dioxide, and lack of oxygen.

Stimulation of the sensory fibers of the vagus from the lungs and larynx is thought to regulate the respiratory rhythm; the center starts respirations, but *messages from the lungs regulate* them. This explains why a patient (when the respiratory center is not paralyzed) may often be revived by artificial respiration (see pages 1492–93). Stimulation of sensory nerves in the nose, pharynx, larynx, or bronchial tubes by foreign bodies will check respiration, and the glottis will close to protect the lungs.

The temperature and chemical composition of the blood regulate the rate and depth of the respirations by stimulation of the respiratory center. The rate and depth of respiration increase or decrease in relation to the increase and decrease in temperature and three chemicals—carbon dioxide, hydrogen ion, and oxygen. Increases in carbon dioxide and the hydrogen ion act on the respiratory center to stimulate the rate and depth of respiration, whereas decreases in oxygen act in a similar manner.

Normal respiration consists in a rhythmic rising and falling of the chest wall and of the walls of the abdomen, which occurs in a resting adult about 18 times per minute. It is quiet and effortless, or automatic.

Suggested Method of "Taking" the Respiration. As in taking the pulse, the patient should be at rest. Allow any effect of exertion or excitement to subside, for these will increase the rate and alter the character of breathing. Even the consciousness of being watched will change the rate and rhythm; therefore, respirations should be counted without the patient's knowledge. After counting the pulse, with the fingers on the wrist as though still engaged in counting the pulse, watch the rise and fall of the chest or upper abdomen; or, better still, if it causes no discomfort to the patient, when counting the pulse, allow the patient's arm to rest lightly on the lower thorax and without watching him feel the chest and abdomen rising and falling. In this way the respirations can be counted without a person's knowledge. In noisy breathing the count may be made by listening. There are certain characteristics, however, that can be noted only by watching the movements of the chest and abdomen. Counting for 1 minute is desirable, although the ½-minute count may be made and doubled.

What to Observe When Assessing the Respiration. A nurse must observe the *rate* and *character* of the respirations, *the movements and expansion of the chest and abdomen, the color of the patient,* and *the position* he may instinctively assume.

Rate and Depth of Respiration. The average rate for a healthy adult is from 14 to 18 respirations per minute; it is more rapid in childhood (20 to 25) and in infancy (30 to 40). In health there is a fairly uniform relation of one respiration to four or five pulse beats. In disease the respirations and pulse are usually increased, but not always in the one to four or five relationship. In disorders of the lungs and air passages the respirations may increase out of proportion to the increase in the pulse, while in other diseases (and this is more common) the pulse increases out of proportion to the respiratory rate.

Conditions Affecting the Rate and Depth of Respiration. Some of the conditions affecting man's respiratory health are discussed in Chapter 9; these conditions (or factors) include smoking, obesity, emotion, environmental pollution, and age. The reader should refer to this material when studying the following. *Certain changes in the atmospheric pressure increase the respiratory rate.* In high altitudes, such as are encountered in flying or in mountain climbing, the pressure of oxygen in the atmosphere is very low so that not enough oxygen is absorbed by the blood. The result is "mountain sickness," characterized by great weakness, and "air hunger" because the tissue cells have insufficient oxygen. At sea level, air is 20 per cent oxygen, and this is ample to meet the body needs and provide a sufficient margin of safety. When the proportion is reduced to 10 per cent, this margin of safety is removed. In high altitudes there is only a slight margin. It has been demonstrated that if the climb is sufficiently gradual, the normal respiratory and circulatory mechanisms can make the necessary adjustments. The altitude at which oxygen must be added to the atmosphere to make it safely habitable for man is discussed in Chapter 15.

Anything that increases the metabolic rate, or the oxygen used, and anything that interferes with an adequate supply *increase the rate and/or the depth of respiration.* As many authorities say in discussing dyspnea, increased demand for oxygen by the tissues must be met by an increased supply. *Exertion of any sort* increases the metabolic rate and stimulates respiration. Dressing may increase metabolism as much as 60 per cent; swimming or housework, as much as 200 per cent above the basal level. There must be a proportionate increase in the oxygen supply. *Exposure to cold* increases the oxygen need as the body moves to keep warm, shivers, or goes into a chill; cold applied to the body may stimulate reflex centers affecting respiration. Fever increases metabolism and hence the respiratory rate. It is possible that the same chemicals in the blood, thought to set the temperature center at a higher level, may act in a similar fashion on

the respiratory center. *Drugs* increase the rate and depth of respiration in various ways. They may increase the metabolic rate, they may stimulate reflex centers, or they may be absorbed by the bloodstream and act directly on the respiratory center. The exertion of eating and *ingested food* increase metabolism, the need for oxygen, and hence the respiratory rate. Almost all emotion increases oxygen need. Everyone can recognize the smothering sensation that accompanies fright. Anxiety is really a low-grade and protracted fear that, like intense fear, stimulates adrenal activity, and increases metabolism and oxygen need. Air hunger of the neurotic state is one of its greatest afflictions. The long sigh of the anxious, depressed, fearful person is an effort to supply the needed oxygen. Elation, however, as well as fear, increases metabolism and oxygen needs.[38-40]

Most diseases increase the respiratory rate. Endocrine disorders, particularly thyroid disease, raise the metabolic, pulse, and respiratory rates. *Anything that reduces blood volume or the oxygen-carrying elements of the blood* increases the respiratory rate. An example of the first is hemorrhage, and of the second, anemia, or carbon monoxide poisoning when the hemoglobin that ordinarily carries oxygen combines with the carbon monoxide. *Any condition that obstructs the air passages* mechanically increases the respiratory rate because less air is inhaled with each inspiration.[40a] Because dehydration (water deprivation) has been shown to increase airway obstruction in normal subjects, it is thought that dehydration in acute asthma is likely to contribute to difficult and increased respiration.[41] A common cold, pneumonia, lung abscess, tuberculosis, bronchitis, fluid in the lungs, asthma, adenoids, or enlarged tonsils all increase the respiratory rate. *Anything that cuts down the functioning lung area* increases the respiratory rate. A collapse of a lung or a part of it, inflammation of the pleura or covering of the lung, and fluid in the abdominal cavity that makes pressure on the diaphragm reduce lung expansion and force the person to breathe more rapidly in order to get an adequate oxygen supply.

Conditions that increase the carbon dioxide content of the blood increase the depth or rate of respiration, although the excessive stimulation of the respiratory center may finally exhaust and paralyze it. *Brain pathology* affects the respiratory rate and is most likely to slow it.

From the discussion of what increases the rate and depth of respiration it is comparatively easy to see what will *decrease* it. *Atmospheres rich in oxygen, lowering the metabolic rate, rest and sleep, warm (not overheated) environments, normal body temperatures, respiratory depressant drugs, a calm state of mind, adequate intake of fluids, normal blood, and normal conditions of the respiratory tract* all reduce the rate and depth of respiration or keep it within the normal range for the individual. As has been noted, pathology usually results in an increased rate. The exception to this is brain pathology. When there is intercranial pressure from tumors, infections, or fractures sufficient to affect the respiratory center, the result is usually a slow rate of respiration. Narcotics and sedatives, especially opium and its derivatives, are respiratory depressants, and morphine, for example, is sometimes fatal as a result of this action. It might be safe to say that most respiratory stimulants, such as carbon dioxide, can in too large doses overstimulate and so exhaust the muscles of respiration. When the respiratory rate falls below 8 or rises above 40 per minute, the outlook is grave.

Character of Respiration. A normal average man at rest inspires and exhales about 500 cc of air with each respiration. If considerably more than this quantity of air passes in and out of the lungs, the respiration is said to be deep; if considerably less, it is called shallow. A normal sedentary man of average size has an estimated "vital capacity" of 4500 cc of air. (It must be estimated because he cannot force out all the air. If he did, his lungs would collapse.) An athletic person has a greater vital capacity than a sedentary one, and men's vital capacity is naturally greater than women's.[42,43]

Any disease that reduces the vital capacity, that interferes with the exchange of gases by the blood, or that increases the need for oxygen beyond the body's capacity to supply it causes *hyperpnea* (Greek, *hyper* = beyond, above, over; *pnoia* = breath), hard or deep breathing; *polypnea* (Greek, *polys* = many), very rapid breathing; or *dyspnea* (Greek, *dys* = bad or difficult) labored or difficult breathing. Vigorous exercise necessitates an increase in the depth and rate of respiration. The level of activity provoking dyspnea varies from person to person according to age, sex, body size, and physical training. Daniel S. Lukas says, "Dyspnea indicates disease only when it occurs at levels of activity below those expected to be normally tolerated." * It is usually defined as a consciousness of the necessity for increased respiratory effort. Whereas the need for more rapid or deeper respiration is felt briefly during health and easily met by

compensatory mechanisms, oxygen need in sickness is likely to be protracted and fearsome to patients because they sense that their compensatory mechanisms cannot cope with it.

Nurses should observe carefully for signs of *dyspnea*. The patient's position is telling. If the expansion of a lung is painful, the patient will lie on the affected side to splint it and to allow the unaffected side free movement. During abdominal pain the abdomen is held rigid, and the patient takes rapid, shallow breaths to prevent deep excursions of the diaphragm that make pressure on the abdomen. Shallow respirations must of necessity be rapid in order to pass sufficient air through the lungs. This type of respiration often results in extreme muscular fatigue. Patients in any clinical setting (in or outside the hospital) should be questioned about their present tolerance of their usual activities. For example, patients previously may have been able to walk a considerable distance without discomfort but they now are unable to walk more than one or two city blocks without shortness of breath.

Usually a dyspneic person has a rapid, labored respiration that makes a distinct sound; the lips are blue or dusky (cyanotic); the expression is anxious, and the eyes seem prominent. If the dyspnea is severe, muscles not ordinarily used are forced into action; the nostrils dilate, the upper chest is greatly expanded by the action of the neck muscles that stand out on either side of the throat, and as the diaphragm contracts forcibly the abdominal walls protrude. Each breath is drawn with heavings of the chest and abdomen. Dyspnea is discussed in great detail in Chapter 35.

When respiration is very difficult, a person may instinctively sit up to relieve the pressure the abdominal content makes on the diaphragm and the organs of the chest. This condition, called *orthopnea* (Greek, *orthos* = straight), is typical of the dyspnea of heart disease.

When dyspnea is prolonged and severe and the patient weak and exhausted, the breathing is frequently irregular and gasping. Dyspnea may affect inspiration or expiration, or the whole act of breathing may be a struggle.

Dyspnea is often accompanied by generalized cyanosis. The bluish cast of cyanosis noticed first about the lips and in severe cases in the extremities, under the nails, and finally over the whole body.

Apnea (*a* = not) means absence or complete cessation of breathing. It occurs when there is an increase of oxygen in the blood and a decrease of carbon dioxide which is the normal stimulus to the respiratory center. *Cheyne-Stokes respirations* (named after the two men who first described them) consist of periods of dyspnea preceded and followed by

---

* Lukas, Daniel S.: "Dyspnea," in MacBryde, Cyril Mitchell, and Blacklow, Robert Stanley (eds.): *Signs and Symptoms; Applied Pathologic Physiology and Clinical Interpretation,* 5th ed. J. B. Lippincott Co., Philadelphia, 1970, p. 341.

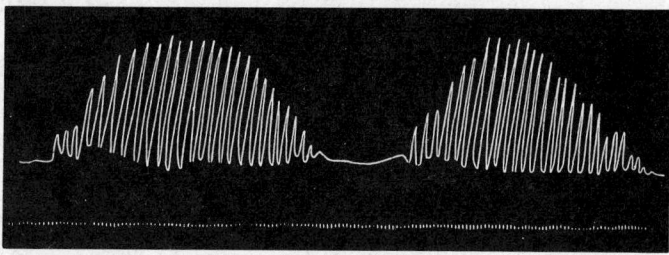

Figure 6-7. Stethograph tracing of a Cheyne-Stokes respiration in a man; the time is marked in seconds in the lower white line. (From Kimber, D. C., Gray, C. E., Stackpole, C. E. and Leavell, L. C.: *Textbook of Anatomy and Physiology,* 13th ed. Macmillan Publishing Co., Inc., New York, 1955.)

periods of apnea and occurring in a rhythmic cycle, each paroxysm lasting from 30 to 60 seconds (see Fig. 6-7). The period of dyspnea begins with short, shallow, almost imperceptible respirations; but each respiration increases in rate, depth, and sound until a maximum of dyspnea is reached, when they gradually decrease in rate, depth, and sound until they finally cease altogether and the apneic period begins. The latter may last from 1 to 10 seconds, when the whole cycle begins again. During the period of apnea, patients may drop off to sleep for a few seconds, but during the period of dyspnea they are likely to be restless, even when they appear to sleep.

Although Cheyne-Stokes respirations may sometimes occur in healthy children and adults, when asleep, particularly when lying flat on the back, in disease it is usually a grave symptom. Patients in whom this symptom has been marked have recovered, but in acute illness it is usually a sign of approaching death. This form of breathing is most common in severe heart diseases, in uremia, and in cerebral diseases with increased intracranial pressure.

Auscultation of the chest for breath sounds has been an important part of medical practice for more than a century, but only in the past decade have nurses begun to use it in health examinations and in the care of the acutely ill. Authorities consulted say that it takes consistent practice over a period of time to become skilled in this technique or to identify the many abnormalities of respiration. Earle B. Weiss and C. Jeffrey Carlson [44] describe a system for recording breath sounds on an instrument that can be used in learning to assess them. The reader should consult references listed at the end of this chapter, as well as appropriate medical texts, for a detailed description of auscultation of the chest and methods used.

4. THE PULSE

Definition. The distention or pulsation of the blood vessels produced by the wave of blood forced into them as the heart's left ventricle contracts is called "the pulse." Ordinarily, the term refers to the pulsation of the arteries. Each time the heart beats, it forces approximately 70 ml of blood at a pressure of about 120 mm Hg into the aorta and from there into the systemic arteries. The increased pressure within the arteries forces the column of blood onward, distending the vessels in a wave that diminishes as it extends into the capillaries. With proper instruments, the pulse wave can be detected in these microscopic tubes. The wave of dilation and the recoil are felt in the elastic arteries at whatever point they can be compressed against a bone. An upward curve of the pulse wave is felt that corresponds to the contraction, or *systole* of the heart, and a recoil or downward curve that corresponds to the relaxation, or the *diastole,* of the heart. These two periods constitute "the pulse" and represent one heartbeat. In the average adult about 5 liters of blood is ejected from the left ventricle every minute, which is called cardiac output (the output is the product of stroke volume times heart rate). For example, in a healthy adult (at rest) the stroke volume is about 70 ml and normal heart rate is about 70 per minute; consequently, 4900 ml of blood is ejected every minute, a little less than the volume of blood (6 liters) in the circulatory system.

Nurses are rarely asked to note it, but the venous pulse is visible in the large veins of the neck and is the pulsation caused by the rhythmic partial emptying of these veins with each cardiac cycle. However, since these veins respond to the alternating pressure in the chest during respiration, it is difficult to get an accurate count of the venous pulse.

Dependence of the Pulse on Heart Action, Blood Pressure, Volume, and Viscosity. No part of the circulatory system functions independently. Heart action, the tone of the blood vessels, and the nature and quantity of the circulatory fluids are in every case dependent on all the others. The circulatory system is in turn affected by all the other systems of the body so that any discussion of its function is complicated. Although the knowledge of physiology in this area is complex and incomplete, nurses, as well as other health workers, should recognize that the more understanding they have of the subject, the more effectively they can care for themselves and others.

Heart action and blood pressure are not under man's control.* His behavior, however, is

* Instances of individuals having the power to increase the heart rate and the ability of certain practitioners of yoga in India to stop the heart voluntarily have been reported. Gerald Jonas, in his book *Visceral Learning* (Viking Press, New York, 1972), describes some of the early works of Dr. Neal Miller, an experimental psychologist, and others who contributed so much to the development of psychophysiology, a young discipline concerned with the complex and interfused relationships between mind and body. Through the use of biofeedback, attempts are being made to teach humans to control body functions—heart rate, blood pressure, salivation, respiration, and others. For a recent summary of research in this area see Brown, Barbara B. (ed.): *The Biofeedback Syllabus; A Handbook for the Psychophysiologic Study of Biofeedback* (Charles C Thomas, Publisher, Springfield, Ill., 1975).

reflected in them just as it is in respiration and, to a less extent, in the temperature of the body. This is partially understood even by those who have no knowledge of physiology as shown in the expressions: "My heart stood still," "My heart sank," "My heart leapt with joy," and "That made my blood pressure rise." The cardiac and vasomotor centers are in the medulla oblongata, and intercranial pressure affects the heart rate as it does the respiratory rate. There are nerve cells or ganglia outside the medulla that also influence the heart rate and the size of the blood vessels.

Figure 6-8 shows the nerve supply to the heart. It diagrams two sets of motor nerves: the inhibitory fibers of the vagus that act as a check rein (the parasympathetic division of the autonomic system) and the accelerator nerve fibers that pass to the heart by way of the spinal cord through the cardiac nerves and

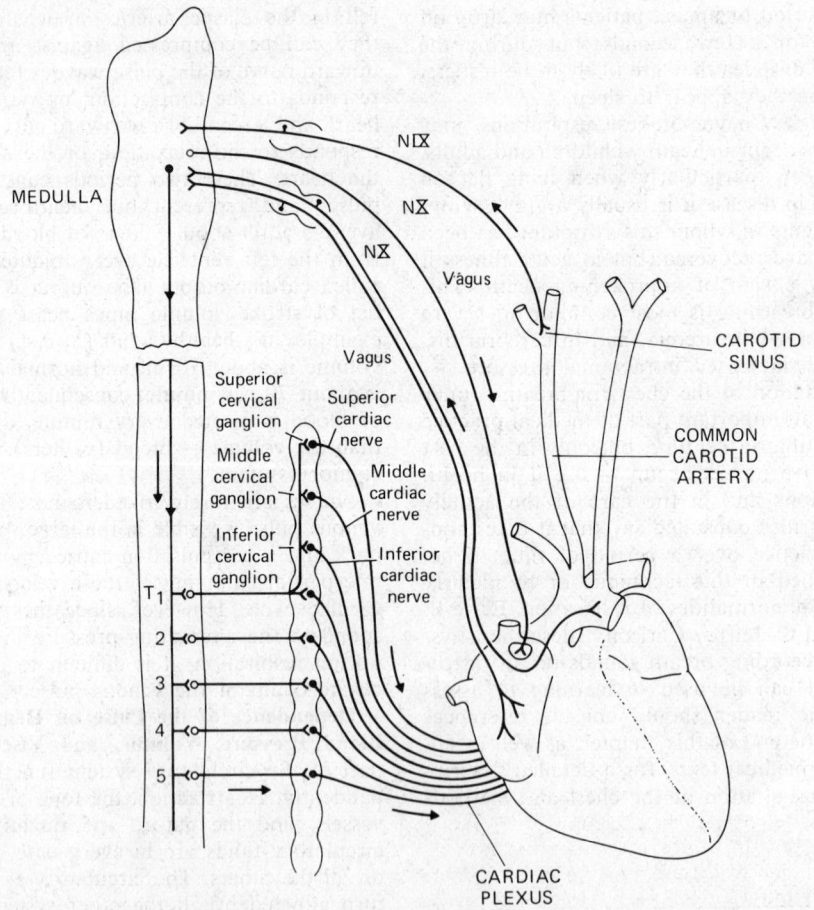

Figure 6-8. Nerve supply of the heart. *NIX,* fiber of the glossopharyngeal nerve; *NX,* vagus nerve; *T,* thoracic nerves. (From Miller, M. A.; Drakontides, A. B.; and Leavell, L. C.: *Kimber-Gray-Stackpole's Anatomy and Physiology,* 17th ed. Macmillan Publishing Co., Inc., New York, 1977.)

through visceral branches of the five thoracic spinal nerves (the sympathetic division of the autonomic system).

These two antagonistic sets of motor, or efferent, fibers have their counterpart in two antagonistic sets of sensory, or afferent, fibers arising in the heart and blood vessels called *depressor* (inhibiting) and *pressor* (accelerator) fibers. With this complex nerve supply—that is, nevertheless, a simple system of checks and balances—the rate of the heartbeat and the blood pressure stay within a normal range unless the body taxes itself unduly or it is attacked by disease.

Everyone knows that heart action, and therefore the pulse, is affected by emotion. Whereas the statement that every thought or emotion is reflected in the activity of the circulatory system is hard for many persons to grasp, exaggerated examples of the interaction of the psyche and the soma are recognized. Almost all persons, if awakened from a sound sleep by frightening noises, instantly feel their heart pound and their respirations increase in depth and frequency, and they have a sense of weight on the chest. With the contraction of the smooth muscles in the skin, goose flesh appears, and the skin will blanch. These effects are brought about through increased cardiac action and changes in the vessels through impulses acting on the cardiac and vasomotor centers in the medulla and liberation of epinephrine from the medulla of the adrenal glands into the circulation to reinforce the action of the sympathetic system and to prepare affected persons for defensive action. The heart rate has increased greatly, and the contractions are forceful; blood pressure has risen to 200 mm systolic and 105 mm diastolic (in some instances) with the vascular changes associated with crisis—dilation of vessels in the heart and voluntary muscles and vasoconstriction elsewhere; the blood sugar level has risen to supply fuel for muscular activity; respirations have increased in rate and depth, and the spleen has discharged more red blood cells to accommodate the increased oxygen needed; the pupils have dilated for far vision; and coagulation time of the blood has shortened for protection in case of injury.[45]

The reaction just described is an exaggerated one, characteristic of fear, but these changes in a less marked degree accompany other emotions. No health worker can assess the vital signs intelligently or understand the psychic origin of pathology in the circulatory mechanism unless he or she has some understanding of its relationship to the interdependent endocrine and autonomic nervous systems. The rate and force of the heart, the caliber of the blood vessels, the character and quantity of the circulatory fluids, all vary with emotional, or glandular, behavior.

Muscles of the heart and blood vessels respond to chemicals other than endocrine hormones (epinephrine, norepinephrine, aldosterone, and thyroxin). The "chemoreceptors" (carotid and aortic bodies) are responsive to changes in oxygen, carbon dioxide, and hydrogen ion concentration in the blood. Other "thermoreceptors" are sensitive to temperature changes.

This sensitiveness of the heart makes the pulse a valuable index of the condition of the body. The sphygmomanometer, the electrocardiograph, and x-ray, all developed in the past century, enable the present-day physician to assess the condition of the heart and blood vessels far more accurately than could doctors in the past, who had little more than the pulse and heart sounds to go by. In the last two decades cardiac monitors have been developed and currently are used by nurses and physicians, especially in cardiovascular and in intensive care units, to continuously assess cardiac function, for example, cardiac rhythm (electrocardiograph) and pulse rate. The importance of this equipment in determining various arrhythmias cannot be overemphasized. However, since most nurses in general units of the hospitals as well as in other health settings do not have the equipment or training for using it, it is still important for them as well as for physicians to be able to form judgments on feeling the pulse.

Frequency with Which the Pulse Is Noted. The pulse of a sick patient is usually assessed with the temperature and respiration twice during the 24 hours or every 4 hours in some cases; when the patient's condition is critical the pulse rate and quality should be noted almost constantly. With monitors, constant surveillance is possible. The pulse may be taken before, during, and after many activities requiring mental or physical strain that are likely to overtax the heart.

Where the Pulse Can Be Taken. The character of the arterial pulse tracings taken from the aorta to the peripheral arteries varies considerably, but for practical purposes any large superficial artery that lies directly over a bone against which it can be compressed is used for taking the pulse (see Fig. 6-9). The radial artery is most commonly palpated. It is convenient and compressible since it lies just underneath the skin of the inner surface of the wrist and directly over the radius. The temporal, facial, carotid, femoral, or dorsalis pedis arteries can be used when the wrist is covered by dressings, a plaster cast, or splint.

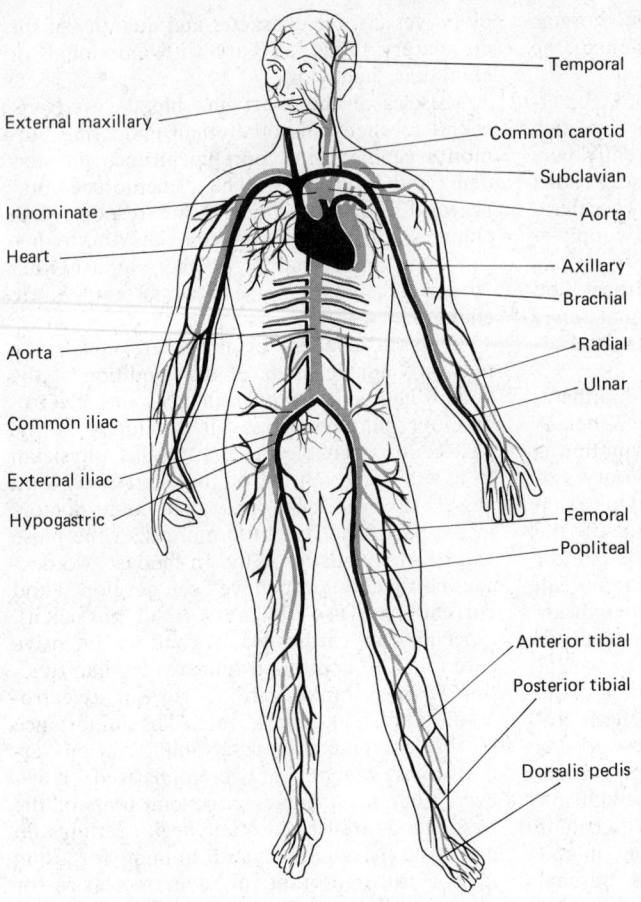

External maxillary

Innominate

Heart

Aorta

Common iliac

External iliac

Hypogastric

Temporal

Common carotid

Subclavian

Aorta

Axillary

Brachial

Radial

Ulnar

Femoral

Popliteal

Anterior tibial

Posterior tibial

Dorsalis pedis

Figure 6-9. A general diagram of the circulation, showing the course of the major arteries and suggesting pressure points at which the pulse may be felt. (From Kimber, D. C., Gray, C. E., Stackpole, C. E., and Leavell, L. C.: *Textbook of Anatomy and Physiology*, 13th ed. Macmillan Publishing Company, Inc., New York, 1955.)

Sometimes the temporal artery may be used with least disturbance to the patient, and it must be used during packs, when the body is wrapped in blankets or sheets and when the patient is in a respirator. The carotid arteries, although not lying over bones, are large, near the surface, and quite close to the heart so that pulsations may be felt here when imperceptible at the wrist. In some diseases, pulsations may be seen and counted in the temporal and carotid arteries without touching the patient. There may be a palpable pulse in the femoral artery when none can be felt in the radial. In shock or collapse and in approaching death, it may be possible to count the weakened cardiac contractions only by listening to the heart through a stethoscope. When the radial pulse is irregular, the physician may want the pulse taken by two persons simultaneously, one counting the pulsations at the wrist and the other listening to the heart sounds at its apex. The difference between the apical and radial counts, which must be made simultaneously, is called the *pulse deficit*. It is the result of two beats of the heart that come so close together

that the second beat pumps little blood, if any, because the left ventricle does not have enough time to fill between the two beats. Ordinarily, the greater the rate of pulse deficit the more serious the arrhythmia.[46]

Slight differences in the pulse can always be detected most easily if the pulse is counted at the same place each time.

Suggested Procedure in Counting the Arterial Pulse. See that the person is at rest and, usually, recumbent. If the pulse is assessed following exertion or excitement, the fact should be noted. In fearful persons the heart rate may be increased just because the pulse is being counted. Nurses should try to put patients at ease and divert their attention if possible. Place the tips of the first, second, and third fingers on the artery, exerting such pressure as does not obliterate but makes the pulsation most distinct. With three fingers rather than one, the character of the artery and the shape of the pulse wave are more easily felt. The thumb should never be used because the pulsation of its artery may be mistaken for the patient's pulse. A full-minute count should be made, and longer periods may be necessary to judge regularity in some cases.

When taking the radial pulse, support the forearm in a semipronated position. With a new patient, check the pulsations in both wrists or verify the count at two pressure points. If there is any doubt about the count, get a more experienced person to repeat the procedure before recording the pulse.

The pulse count is graphed on the same sheet with the temperature and respiration. In hospitals this mechanical recording should be done by a clerk from figures given by the nurse, who in turn should write any necessary comments on the quality of the pulse under "Nurse's Notes" or other record forms that may be used.

What to Note in Taking the Arterial Pulse. The most important measurement is the *rate* of the pulse, and the next, its *rhythm*, or regularity. In addition, and according to her ability, the nurse notes the *tension*, or compressibility, *of the artery* and the *volume of the pulse,* or the shape of the pulse wave. All of these qualities can be seen in the sphygmographic tracing of a pulse or by the trained eye in the electrocardiograph. Nurses will better understand what they feel in the arterial pulse and what they hear in listening to the heartbeat if they study tracings similar to the one illustrated in Figure 6-10.

An electrocardiogram, called an ECG (EKG), is a graphic record, taken from the body surfaces, of the electric potential differences due to cardiac action. Record of a normal pulse shows 6 waves. The first, called the P wave, is due to excitation of the atria (auricles); Q, R, and S to excitation of the ventricles; T to repolarization of the ventricles; and U is a diastolic wave of unknown origin (see Fig. 6-22).

A sphygmographic tracing of a pulsation is made on a revolving drum by a stylus attached by a delicate spring to a mechanism that, when fixed over a pressure point, responds to the pulsation of the artery. The upward curve represents the expansion of the artery caused by the sudden inflow of blood during the contraction of the left ventricle. This measures the force of the heartbeat. A forceful heartbeat and a soft arterial wall give the upward curve height. An inelastic or sclerosed, artery cannot be distended by a strong contraction of the ventricle. In hemorrhage there is less blood forced into the arteries with each heartbeat, and this lowers the height of the upward curve. While the upward curve is smooth, the broken line in the downward curve represents several pulsations of the artery. Normally these pulsations or waves on the downward curve are all imperceptible to the examining finger. In some diseases the middle, or dicrotic, wave is so pronounced, however, that the pulse is spoken of as the "dicrotic pulse," and it is necessary that nurses recognize and understand it.

It will be noticed that in the normal pulse the downward curve is much more gradual than the upward. This is because the upward

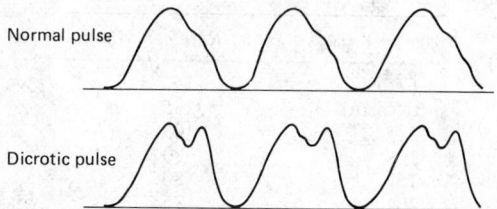

Figure 6-10. A sphygmographic recording of the pulse. (After DeGowin, Elmer L., and DeGowin, Richard L.: *Bedside Diagnostic Examination*, 3rd ed., Macmillan Publishing Co., Inc., New York, 1976, p. 394.)

curve is due to the forceful heartbeat, whereas the downward is brought about by the elastic recoil of the walls of the artery. The upward curve represents the systole of the heart when blood is streaming into the arteries and the artery rises against the finger; it is then the pulse is counted. The downward curve represents the diastole of the heart in which the semilunar valves are closed; blood has ceased to flow into the aorta; the elastic walls are returning to their original size, pressing constantly and steadily on the blood and sending it onward; and the artery seems to fall away gradually from the fingers. The dicrotic wave is caused by the closure of the semilunar valves. The elastic wall of the aorta as it recoils drives the blood in two directions—onward and back against the closed semilunar valves, which it strikes with considerable force, depending upon the original force of the heartbeat. From this wall of resistance and sudden check to its flow, it rebounds, and this rebound causes the expansion of the artery called the dicrotic wave. When the tone of the blood vessel is very low, it dilates abnormally at this point, and the dicrotic wave is felt almost as distinctly as the primary curve. This condition should be reported, but the dicrotic wave must not be counted as a heartbeat.

The "Normal" Pulse. Since the heart rate and blood pressure vary in health with age, size, sex, and emotional and physical activity, there can be no one heart rate or blood pressure that is normal. On the other hand, measurements made of healthy persons of both sexes and all ages give averages that are considered normal. It would be more nearly correct, however, to think of a range in heart rate and blood pressure that seems characteristic of the healthy state.

The following are average resting *heart rates* for man at different ages.*

* Heymans, Corneille: *Introduction to the Regulation of Blood Pressure and Heart Rate.* Charles C Thomas, Publisher, Springfield, Ill., 1950, p. 8.

Age in Years	Heart Rate per Minute
Fetus	150
0 (birth)	135
5	105
10	90
15	80
20	75
25–40	70
80	75

It is apparent that the heart rate, like the respiratory rate, decreases with size. The heart rate of a canary is about 1000 per minute; that of a mouse, 700; that of the elephant, around 25. Size partly accounts for the fact that a man's average heart rate is several counts lower than a woman's. Muscular exercise temporarily increases the pulse rate, but muscular development ultimately decreases the resting rate. Best and Taylor say that a healthy athlete may have a resting pulse as low as 50 or 60. A pulse rate of 55 to 60 is found during sleep in some healthy adults.[47] The pulse rate increases during health, however, from 20 to 60 counts or more to meet the needs of the body during physical and emotional activity. The heart is stimulated chemically by the endocrine secretions, hormones, and by their effect on the blood vessels. It is now known that a normal heart rate is dependent upon the proportion of sodium, potassium, and calcium ions in the extracellular and intracellular fluids.

A normal pulse has a regular *rhythm*. The beats are felt by the fingers at regular intervals, in a one-two-three-four fashion, and seem to be of equal force. The artery feels elastic, neither hard nor soft, under the fingers. Because even in health arteries tend to lose their elasticity, the judgment of normal tension, or *compressibility*, must take the person's age into consideration. The *volume* of the pulse is thought normal if the artery feels full to the touch and the pulsations strong with a normal interval between them.

Abnormal Conditions of the Pulse. Mental and physical disease, drugs, and exposure to harmful environments may result in abnormalities of rate, rhythm, tension, and volume of the pulse, as has been indicated in this chapter.

To judge whether a person's resting heart rate is rapid or slow, one must know the normal range for sex and age. The habitual pulse rate of the individual in health should also be considered. A resting pulse over 100 in an adult in comfortable environments, under no apparent emotional strain, is usually, but not always, an indication of disease; a very rapid pulse (*tachycardia; tachys* = swift) is the term used for a heart rate over 150. The rate may

rise to 250. When the rate is so fast that it cannot be counted it is described as "running." In organic and functional heart diseases the contractions of the heart may be so rapid and weak that the heart is said to "fibrillate," which means to quiver. Under such circumstances the pulse cannot be counted; a very low blood volume as in hemorrhage, and many other conditions, can result in such a weak and rapid pulse that it is even impalpable.

A pulse rate of less than 60 is usually, but not always, considered a sign of disease. *In certain conditions a pulse below 60 is a danger sign.*

Following brain injury or whenever there is a possibility of an increase in intercranial pressure, the pulse should be counted frequently, and *any slowing of the rate reported at once.* Under such circumstances a fall below 60 is a grave symptom that may indicate pressure on the nerve center in the medulla supplying the inhibitory fibers of the vagus nerve. Drugs given to slow the heart, such as digitalis, are discontinued when the pulse falls to 60. Occasionally, a very slow pulse (*bradycardia; bradys* = slow) indicates organic heart disease of a serious nature. Nurses who would report a rapid pulse at once often fail to understand that a decrease in the heart rate may be equally serious.

Irregularities of rhythm are called *arrhythmias*. The intervals between beats may be of different lengths, or the beats may be of unequal force. Common irregularities in rate and rhythm include premature beats, pauses, tachycardia, bradycardia, and chaotic pulse (see Fig. 6-11). These conditions are seen in many apparently healthy persons, and in some cases the heart action is normal but in others this evidence indicates a serious arrhythmia. The nurse must report such changes in the rate and rhythm to the physician and at the same time include additional information (gathered after noting changes in rate and rhythm) such as blood pressure reading, chest pain, dyspnea, apprehension (and other changes in the patient's mental state), change in skin color, and headache.[48] An electrocardiogram should be made to determine the origin of the irregularity.

Tension, or compressibility, of the artery is measured with the sphygmomanometer, and determination of blood pressure is a part of every medical examination. Softness and rigidity of the artery can be felt, however, and the nurse should note both conditions. A degree of softness is typical of the pulse in youth, but when that factor is taken into account, arterial pulsation that can be obliterated means very low blood pressure. This may occur when any-

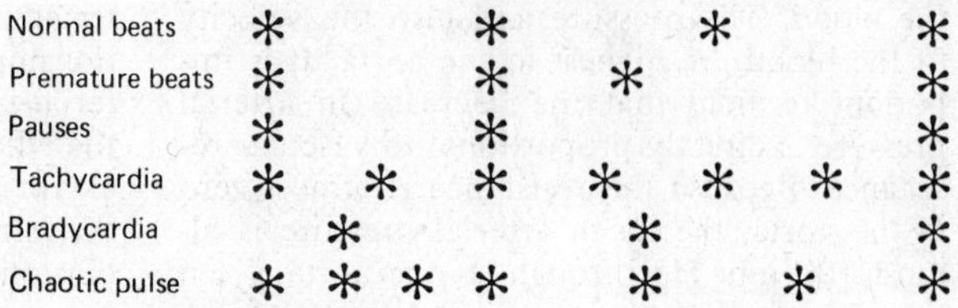

Figure 6-11. Schematic representation of normal and arrhythmic pulse beats.

Normal beats	✳		✳		✳	✳
Premature beats	✳		✳	✳		✳
Pauses	✳		✳			✳
Tachycardia	✳	✳	✳	✳	✳ ✳	✳
Bradycardia		✳			✳	✳
Chaotic pulse	✳ ✳ ✳			✳	✳	✳

thing interferes with vasoconstriction, as in a sympathectomy, or when the blood volume is low, as in hemorrhage. A hard artery that can be rolled under the fingers like a cord, sometimes called a pipestem, or one that feels tortuous or knotted indicates disease of the vessels —arteriosclerosis. A tracing of such a pulse shows a shortening or straightening of all the curves seen in the normal pulse.

If the *volume* of blood is normal and the heartbeat strong, a very soft artery will give its pulsation a bounding quality. The tracing of such a pulse shows a high primary wave. Such a pulse is described as bounding, large, or full. If, on the other hand, there has been loss of blood as in hemorrhage, or redistribution of body fluids, as in shock, the decrease in volume is felt in the small, weak, or even flickering pulse, a tracing of which would show a lower primary curve.

Nurses who hope to give maximum help to their patients will study the pulse and by specialized reading add to the limited information supplied in a general discussion of this sort.

5. BLOOD PRESSURE

Definition. Blood pressure is the lateral pressure exerted by the blood on the walls of the vessels. The term "blood pressure" usually refers to the pressure of blood on the wall of the artery, so "arterial blood pressure" is the more accurate term. Again, this is so general as to be misleading because the blood pressure within the artery varies during the cardiac cycle. So we should say the "systolic," the "diastolic," or the "mean" arterial blood pressure. Corneille Heymans describes these as follows:

The arterial pressure in the large arteries is characterized by a *systolic pressure,* an increase of pressure induced by the systolic contraction of the left heart ventricle, and by a *diastolic pressure,* a drop of arterial pressure occurring during the diastolic arrest of the heart between two contractions. The *mean arterial pressure* represents the average between the systolic rise and the diastolic fall of pressure.*

* Heymans, Corneille: *Introduction to the Regulation of Blood Pressure and Heart Rate.* Charles C Thomas, Publisher, Springfield, Ill., 1950, p. 8.

While in clinical practice blood pressure is usually measured in the arteries, it can be measured anywhere in the vascular system, and within recent years clinicians have used measurement of the venous pressure as a diagnostic aid.

Historical Note. Arthur Ruskin [49] and Arthur M. Master et al. [49a] credit Stephen Hales with the first actual measurement of blood pressure in 1733. The measurement was made on a horse. Hales, a minister with scientific leanings, found that the blood rose 8 ft in a tube inserted into the femoral artery. Since then, there have been many experiments and studies with animals and human beings leading to the development of more accurate instruments. The mercury sphygmomanometer (*sphygmos* = pulse), developed by Riva-Rocci in 1896, was based on the same principles as the instrument now in common use. Recent investigations have shown that when the width of the cuff of this instrument is not modified according to the diameter of the extremity to which it is applied, its measurements are inaccurate. It is likely that other refinements of sphygmomanometry will follow.

The same principles for measuring arterial pressure apply to venous pressure, but a more sensitive device than the air cuff must be placed over the vein and a water manometer substituted for a mercury scale. Mercury, being 13.5 times heavier than water, will not be lifted high enough in the manometer by venous pressure to be easily read. Clinical measurements of venous pressure have been used only within the past 25 years; present procedures require the introduction of a needle into a vein and considerable judgment in the use of such instruments as are available. Venous pressure measurements are therefore seldom made, and when they are, the physician makes them.

Physiology of Blood Pressure. Blood is confined under pressure in the blood vessels. *Pressure varies from a positive pressure in the arteries to a gradually diminishing and finally a negative pressure just as the blood is returned to the heart by the large veins.* Blood pressure depends on the cardiac output (quantity of blood pumped into the aorta each minute), the peripheral resistance, the elasticity (or tone) of the vessels, and the volume and viscosity of the blood. The pressure and also the velocity of the blood are highest in the aorta. It is important to note that the decrease in arterial pressure is directly proportional to vascular resistance. Because the resistance is almost zero in the aorta, the mean arterial pressure is almost 100 mm Hg throughout the aorta; from the end of the aorta to the beginning of the arterioles the pressure drops to 85 mm Hg. On the other hand, as the blood passes from the arterial to the capillary end of the arterioles the pressure falls to 30 mm Hg because the resistance of the arterioles to the blood is the greatest encountered in any part of the systemic circulation, according to Guyton.[50] As the blood passes through the capillaries into the venules the pressure is about 10 mm Hg, a drop of 20 mm Hg which shows that the capillary resistance is about two fifths that of the arterioles.

As the arterioles divide into myriads of microscopic capillaries, their walls offer a resistance that slows the stream. Again the velocity increases as capillaries combine to form venules, and as venules are joined to form veins. With each beat of the heart the force of negative pressure is exerted on the veins emptying into it. Positive venous pressure is highest in the peripheral veins and lowest in those near the heart. Zero pressure is believed to be reached by the time the blood reaches the atrium.

If readers study the figures just given, they can understand that the tone of the arterioles is very important since they act as a check, or regulating force, between the high-pressure system of the arteries and the low-pressure system of the veins. The heartbeat sends the blood into the arteries in great waves; the arterioles slow and steady the stream so that it flows into the vast network of capillaries as water flows from a river into a lake. While blood is in the capillaries, some of which are just large enough in diameter to accommodate a single blood cell, the exchange of nutrients, regulators, and wastes between the blood and the other body elements occurs. If the blood were said to run through the arteries, it would amble through the capillaries. It was formerly thought that normally pulsation was lost in the capillaries, but according to Best and Taylor it is found in healthy young persons although it cannot be induced in the aged. Health depends on keeping pressures in all parts of the vascular system within normal ranges.

Blood pressure may be measured in any accessible part of the circulatory mechanism at any moment in the cardiac cycle. To the physiologist "blood pressure" usually suggests the mean pressure; to the layman, the systolic arterial pressure; and to the clinician, the relationship between the systolic and diastolic arterial pressures. Most authorities consulted say the efficiency of the circulation is shown by the extent to which the heart raises the pressure of the stream of blood in systolic above the diastolic, or back pressure. This difference is known as the *pulse pressure* and represents the volume output of the left ventricle. The importance of pulse pressure is emphasized by George E. Burch and Nicholas P. DePasquale:

In patients with diseases of the myocardium that impair the ability of the heart to act as a pump, the systolic pressure decreases in association with a decrease in cardiac output. The fall in cardiac output is associated with a compensatory increase in peripheral resistance and a rise in diastolic pressure with a resultant decrease in pulse pressure.*

Nothing could be more vital than normal capillary conditions, but estimates of their status are difficult to make and interpret. In discussing heart action (see page 457) it was necessary to include *regulation of blood pressure* since the heart is only a specialized section of what might be diagramed as a continuous vascular tube. Anything that affects the heart also affects the blood vessels. Both are under the control of the autonomic system, and both respond to thermal and chemical stimuli. Both are safeguarded by a multiple nerve supply so that if one set of fibers or one group of cells is destroyed, other fibers and other cells eventually take on their function.

Burch and DePasquale, in speaking of the regulation of arterial blood pressure by the neurohumoral phenomena, say:

The vasomotor center located within the midbrain is constantly receiving impulses from pressoreceptors (baroreceptors) and chemoreceptors located in the heart, lungs and aortic arch, at the bifurcation of the carotid arteries and many other vessels, and from higher centers located in the hypothalamus and cerebral cortex. These impulses reach the vasomotor center through the vagus and glossopharyngeal nerves and through intracentral nerve pathways. The impulses are integrated in the vasomotor center and are translated into "correcting" impulses that reach the heart and blood vessels through autonomic nerve pathways to adjust the heart rate, cardiac output, tone of the vessels, and peripheral resistance. The purpose of such a system of reflexes is to maintain the arterial blood pressure at a relatively constant level to meet the needs of the circulation. For example, if the peripheral resistance suddenly increases due to emotional stimulation, the blood

---

* Burch, George E., and DePasquale, Nicholas P.: *Primer of Clinical Measurement of Blood Pressure.* C. V. Mosby Co., St. Louis, 1962, p. 116.

pressure will suddenly rise and the rate of impulse formation in the pressoreceptors of the aortic arch will increase. The vasomotor receives these afferent impulses and translates them into inhibitory efferent impulses that buffer the increase in cardiac rate, cardiac output, and peripheral arteriolar constriction.*

Since the caliber of blood vessels changes in response to the percentage of oxygen, carbon dioxide, electrolytes, hormones (epinephrine, norepinephrine, aldosterone), and enzymes (produced by the kidneys) in the blood, it is easy to see why blood pressure varies with emotional and physical activity. Some scientists believe the action of the enzymes is limited to conditions where blood supply is limited to the kidneys. Master and associates,[51] in the report of an extensive study, say blood pressure tends to increase with weight. Homer Wheelon illustrates the effect of exercise on blood pressure with the following measurements made on a young person †:

	Blood Pressure	Pulse Pressure
Lying down	116/75	41
Sitting	120/76	44
Standing	122/82	40
After 5-minute exercise	139/86	53

Since the diastolic pressure does not rise in proportion to the systolic, the pulse pressure, or the volume output of the ventricles, varies sufficiently to provide the adaptation of the blood supply necessary for the varying demands of the body. Blood pressure is lowered in health during periods of sleep, physical rest, and freedom from emotional excitement. The systolic blood pressure drops as much as 20 mm mercury during sleep. The diastolic drop is not so great. However, the blood pressure does not decrease if sleep is disturbed by restlessness including dreams. Geraldene Felton, in a study of 32 healthy subjects, reports that "systolic blood pressure was lowest in the early morning, rose to a high in the late morning, and then began to decline. The systolic blood pressure appeared to reflect the social-cultural pattern of activity." ‡

Blood pressure, like heart rate, varies with sex but much more markedly with age. Henry I. Russek et al., studying about 5000 men, concluded that the old but then discredited dictum that the systolic pressure should be 100 plus the age of the individual is fairly reliable. They said, however: "Essential hypertension cannot be defined solely in terms of the systolic pressure. It is the diastolic level alone that determines the existence of disease." *

Heymans in 1950 gave the following averages for normal persons at five periods, or ages.†

Age	Systolic Pressure	Diastolic Pressure
Infancy	75 to 90 mm	Around 50 mm first
Childhood	90 to 110 mm	5 years of life
About puberty	100 to 120 mm	After that remains
Adults	125 to 130 mm	fairly constant at
Old people	140 to 150 mm	60 to 80 mm

Master and his associates, studying the records of 15,706 men and women between the ages of 16 and 65, taken by random sampling from 74,000 records, concluded in 1952 that normal ranges for the middle-aged and elderly should be raised from the commonly accepted standards to those shown in Table 6-3.

From this study the conclusion was reached that women tend to have a slightly lower blood pressure before the age of 40, but after 50 it is slightly higher than men's. Master and his associates thought that the limit of 150 mm of mercury that has been erroneously set on "normal" systolic blood pressure has aroused needless fear among healthy patients. They said: "There exists a high incidence of so-called hypertension in the normal population. . . . The need for upward revision of the commonly accepted limits of blood pressure . . . for each age group and for both sexes is, therefore, clear." ‡ Blais Moia [52] in 1959 said a blood pressure of 150 mm Hg systolic and 90 mm Hg diastolic is widely accepted as "normal" for persons at age 40. It should be noted that individuals differ greatly in the capacity of their blood vessels to tolerate pressure.

Pathologic Changes Affecting Blood Pressure. Disease in any part of the circulatory system may cause abnormal blood pressure. Pathology of the endocrine glands, particularly

* Ibid., p. 46.

† Wheelon, Homer: "The Interpretation of Blood Pressure Variations; with Observations on Normal Pressure Variations and Relation of the Adrenals and the Autonomic Nervous System to the Production of Blood Pressure," NY State J. Med., 113:505, (Apr.) 1921.

‡ Felton, Geraldene: "Effect of Time Cycle Change on Blood Pressure and Temperature in Young Women," Nurs. Res., 19:48, (Jan.–Feb.) 1970.

* Russek, Henry I., et al.: "The Influence of Age on Blood Pressure," Am. Heart J., 32:468, (Oct.) 1946.

† Heymans, Corneille: op. cit., p. 1.

‡ Master, Arthur M., et al.: Normal Blood Pressure and Hypertension; New Definitions. Lea & Febiger, Philadelphia, 1952, p. 83.

Table 6-3. Average or Normal Blood Pressure in Middle and Old Age *

Age and Sex	Normal Range		Borderline Hypertension	
	Systolic	Diastolic	Systolic	Diastolic
Males 55 years	115–165	70–98	165–180	98–108
Males 65 years	115–170	70–100	170–190	100–110
Females 55 years	110–170	70–100	170–185	100–108
Females 65 years	115–175	70–100	175–190	100–110

* Adapted from Master, Arthur M., et al.: *Normal Blood Pressure and Hypertension; New Definitions.* Lea & Febiger, Philadelphia, 1952, p. 83.

the adrenals, whose hormones so greatly affect the cardiovascular mechanism, alters blood pressure. The kidneys secrete a pressor substance (renin-angiotensin system), it is believed, which is largely responsible for the cardiovascular involvement found in nephritis. This group of symptoms is akin to the uremia of abnormal pregnancy, characterized by blood pressure elevation. Drugs and bacterial poisons can constrict the arterioles just as these endotoxins do.

Most students of *hypertension* support the view that temperament can predispose to high blood pressure. The ambitious person who has drives, perhaps beyond his capacity, for achievement and who represses resentment against those who, in his opinion, thwart him is an oversimplified characterization of the type. Hypertension in such persons can often be relieved by severing the sympathetic (vasoconstrictor) fibers largely responsible for elevation of blood pressure seen in emotional states. Such a condition is called neurogenic hypertension and is a functional rather than an organic disease. W. S. Peart says there is no recognizable cause for about two thirds of all the cases seen; the condition is called essential or idiopathic. There are many classifications of hypertension and various terms are used to differentiate the outlook for persons with this condition. Peart believes "The term 'benign' should be abandoned because it is a poor description for a condition that leads to death by stroke, myocardial infarct, and renal failure." *

Hypertension is a serious problem in the United States, affecting people in all socio-economic groups.[52a,b]

The fact that certain peoples, such as the Chinese, who eat high-carbohydrate diets are generally free from hypertension has led to the theory that the American and European diet may be a predisposing factor in high blood pressure. Animal experimentation and clinical experience have, in some cases, substantiated this theory. Cholesterol found in fats has been identified in deposits of the coronary vessels; consequently many patients with hypertension are now treated with low-fat, high-carbohydrate diets. Studies conducted throughout the world show a direct relationship between high blood pressure and obesity. It is thought that hypertension is the cause of the increased death rate of obese persons.[53] Figure 6-12 shows the difference between a normal artery and one with atherosclerotic deposits.

Joseph A. Wilber and J. Gordon Barrow [54] in a community survey of two counties in Georgia report that 1050 persons with hypertension were found; some were under the care of a physician while others were not. They suggest that the physician should tell each patient that hypertension is the "major cause of stroke, heart failure and kidney failure"; that a person cannot determine the need for medication by the way he or she feels; that blood pressure must be checked the rest of a person's life once it is found to be high; and that antihypertensive drugs must be taken daily. Emphasis is put on giving the person a booklet on high blood pressure as is done with the diabetic. Attempts should be made to teach those with severe or moderate hypertension to take their own blood pressure. Some physicians believe that no home should be without devices for measuring blood pressure and heartbeat and they ask their patients with hypertension to keep regular records, making notes of any unusual happening that precedes a high reading; other physicians disagree. Neighborhood hypertensive clinics are opening in various parts of the country, staffed by doctors and nurses, who find, treat, and educate people with high blood pressure.

In a study of 89 male subjects (31 normals and 58 with chronic obstructive pulmonary

* Peart, W. S.: "Arterial Hypertension," in Beeson, Paul B., and McDermott, Walsh (eds.): *Cecil-Loeb Textbook of Medicine,* 13th ed. W. B. Saunders Co., Philadelphia, 1971, p. 1058.

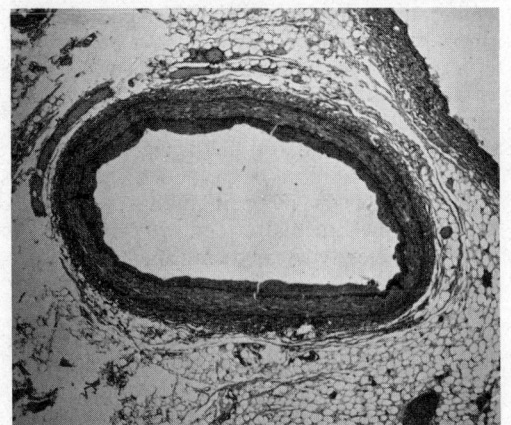

A

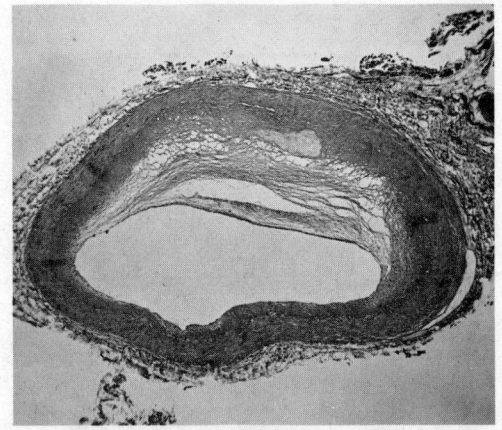

B

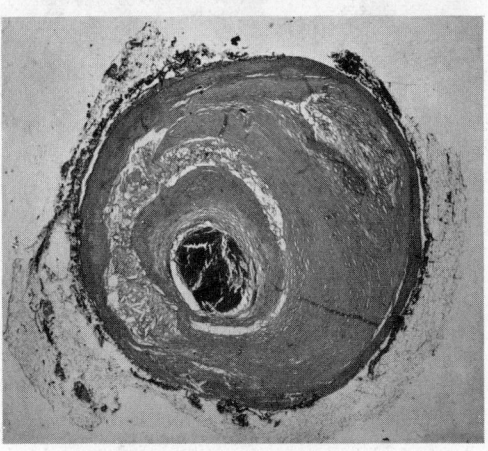

C

Figure 6-12. A normal artery (*A*), an artery with atherosclerotic deposits in the inner lining (*B*), and an artery narrowed by atherosclerotic deposits and now blocked by a blood clot, the dark inner circle (*C*). (From Robinson, C., and Lawler, M.: *Normal and Therapeutic Nutrition*, 15th ed., Macmillan Publishing Co., Inc., New York, 1977. Photos courtesy, American Heart Association.)

disease between the ages of 30 and 70 years), Mary Ann K. Surprenant reports that the results demonstrated the following:

(1) chronic obstructive pulmonary diseases are associated with a significant respiratory blood pressure, fluctuation of the systemic blood pressure; (2) the magnitude of the respiratory blood pressure fluctuation reflects the severity of ventilatory obstruction; and (3) inaccurate blood pressure levels may be recorded in patients who exhibit a marked respiratory fluctuation.*

The danger of hemorrhage from a ruptured blood vessel is always present with an excessive blood pressure. Since there is less room for expansion of vessels in the cranial cavity than in any other part of the body, a hemorrhage is most likely to occur there. Intercranial pressure from any cause affects the vasomotor center in the medulla. A most important function of the

* Surprenant, Mary Ann K.: "Respiratory Blood Pressure Fluctuation: An Unrecognized Index of Pulmonary Diseases," in *ANA Clinical Sessions, 1968.* Appleton-Century-Crofts, New York, 1969, p. 243.

nurse in the care of a patient with a cranial injury or operation is to check blood pressure at intervals of 10 to 30 minutes. Marked deviations of any sort should be reported at once to the physician. Early recognition of blood pressure changes may save a life.

Hypotension, or low blood pressure, may be habitual, temporary, or primary. Most authorities say a consistent systolic pressure below 100 mm Hg is no cause for concern and that low blood pressure often is associated with old age free of illness. Secondary hypotension following disease is a symptom that disappears with the condition if it is successfully treated. Hypotension is seen in Addison's disease (chronic adrenal cortical insufficiency), in extreme malnutrition, and following acute and chronic infection. The marked drop in blood pressure accompanying anesthesia, traumatic shock, hemorrhage, heart disease, as for example myocardial infarction, insulin shock, and other crises is dangerous and should be corrected as quickly as possible. In some cases it is necessary to give blood or its substitutes continuously for several days. Saline and glucose are

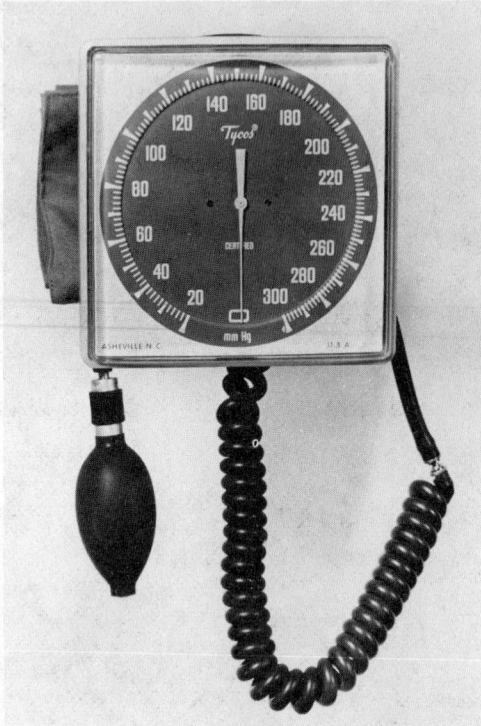

Figure 6-13. An aneroid manometer. (Courtesy of Taylor Instrument, Consumer Products Division, Arden, N.C.)

not effective because they rapidly filter into the tissues.

The importance of making accurate estimates of blood pressure cannot be overestimated. Both systolic and diastolic readings must be taken and recorded. When nurses are not sure of their findings, they should have them checked by a more experienced worker.

Types of Apparatus Used in Measuring Blood Pressure. For measuring *arterial blood pressure* the mercury manometer is usually employed because it is considered reasonably accurate and more easily kept in good condition than certain other devices. Some physiologists think the mercury manometer less sensitive than the aneroid type, which is an instrument with a dial on which pressure is shown by an indicator, or pointer, attached to a spring mechanism (see Fig. 6-13). Obviously, both these instruments must be connected by rubber tubing to a rubber cuff that is placed over an artery of the arm or leg. Reading the oscillation of the mercury column and the spring indicator is no longer thought to be a reliable means of estimating blood pressure. Listening to the sounds over the artery at the

obliteration of pulsation and after pulsation returns is now thought essential, so a stethoscope is a necessary part of the equipment. A variety of cuffs should be available so that one may be chosen that is 20 per cent wider than the diameter of the arm or leg (see Fig. 6-14).

Blood pressure also can be measured by palpation, that is, by maintaining tactile contact with the brachial artery while the sphygmomanometer cuff is being deflated.[55] Arlene M. Putt [56] suggests the use of palpatory determinations in place of auscultatory (use of stethoscope) ones when the nurse has hearing problems or when there are excessive noises in the environment.

For measuring central venous pressure, a water manometer is used. Because mercury is a heavy liquid, the venous pressure may not be sufficient to make visible changes in the level of a column of mercury in a manometer. The manometer is attached by a three-way stopcock to a venous catheter and to sterile tubing attached to intravenous fluid (see Fig. 6-15). The apparatus, because it comes in contact with fluid that enters the bloodstream, should be sterile. Central venous pressure (CVP) monitoring is used to measure the venous pressure in the vena cava or the right atrium (usually in conjunction with arterial blood pressure and hourly urine output), as a guide for determining the amount and rate of intravenous fluid being given. It should be monitored in all patients with circulatory failure if there is difficulty stabilizing circulatory dynamics or if there is doubt about the cause, according to Charles E. Eastridge and associates. They write:

Situations in which C.V.P. monitoring have been helpful are: (1) shock in which the usual measures have failed to improve circulation; (2) conditions in which rapid or large quantities of replacement fluids are required, especially for elderly patients having known or unsuspected heart disease; (3) shock in which multiple factors contribute to an unknown extent to the circulatory disturbance; and (4) septic shock.*

Special methods have been developed to measure peripheral local blood pressure, especially in the fingers and toes, for the purpose of evaluating arterial insufficiency. Jorgen Gundersen [57] says minicuffs made for fingers and toes and mercury-in-rubber strain gauges are used to detect the pulse. The gauges are connected to an electrocardiograph machine which records the pressure of the cuff. A

* Eastridge, Charles E., et al.: "Central Venous Pressure Monitoring, a Useful Aid in the Management of Shock," *Am. J. Surg.,* **114:**648, (Nov.) 1967.

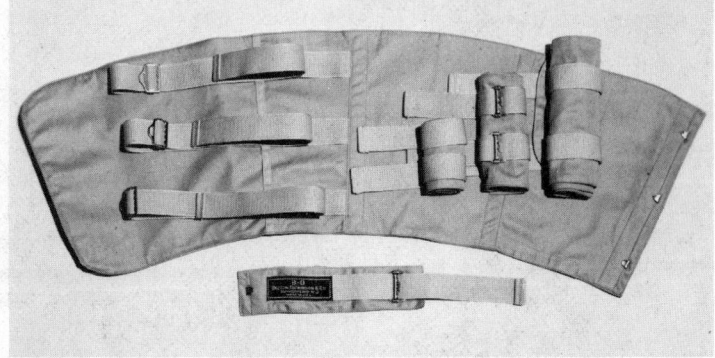

Figure 6-14. Various sizes and types of blood pressure cuffs. The largest are used over the adult thigh; the smallest is designed for an infant's arm. (Courtesy of Becton, Dickinson, & Co., Rutherford, N.J., and Clay-Adams Co., New York, N.Y.)

new automated "do-it-yourself" machine has been developed for use in public buildings, schools, hospitals and other agencies (see Fig. 6-16A). People can also be taught to use the regular spring type sphygmomanometer themselves (see Fig. 6-16B).

Capillary tension is judged by the changes in skin color following immersion of hands or feet in hot and cold water; or it may be assessed by the appearance of the skin during and after manual pressure with a glass slide.

When to Measure Blood Pressure. Master contrasts the "basal blood pressure"—measurements following a 10- to 12-hour fast and rest—and the "casual blood pressure"—measurements made during an office visit or without special preparation. If the former measurement is used in order to rule out the effects of exertion and food, the operator may try also to eliminate the effect of fear by repeating the

readings at 10-minute intervals for four or five times in order to accustom the patient to the test and to his presence. When "casual" measurements are made, they should also be repeated to minimize the effect of anxiety. If the tests are made in rapid succession, the reading is less likely to be distorted by a spasm of the artery, sometimes induced by the pressure of the cuff.

Suggested Procedure in Taking Measurements of Arterial Blood Pressure. Have the patient in a comfortable horizontal or sitting position, preferably the former, with the arm or leg to be used supported. If the patient must lie in the lateral position for some reason, it should be remembered that the readings may be incorrect.[58] Measurements may be made in either arm or leg, but repeated readings should be taken in the same extremity, since structural differences may affect the findings. Blood pressure is most often meas-

Figure 6-15. Positioning of patient and manometer is crucial for accurate central venous pressure measurement. The patient lies supine and quiet, with the head of the bed flat. The manometer is set so that the zero mark lies at the level of the midaxillary line (level of the right atrium), as shown. The physician positions the patient initially. The patient may be turned or positioned in some other fashion between measurements, but the nurse returns him to the supine position and aligns the manometer again before each subsequent measurement is taken. (From Russell, Margaret W., and Maier, Willis P.: "The ABC's of C.V.P. Measurement," *RN*, 32:35, [Mar.] 1969.)

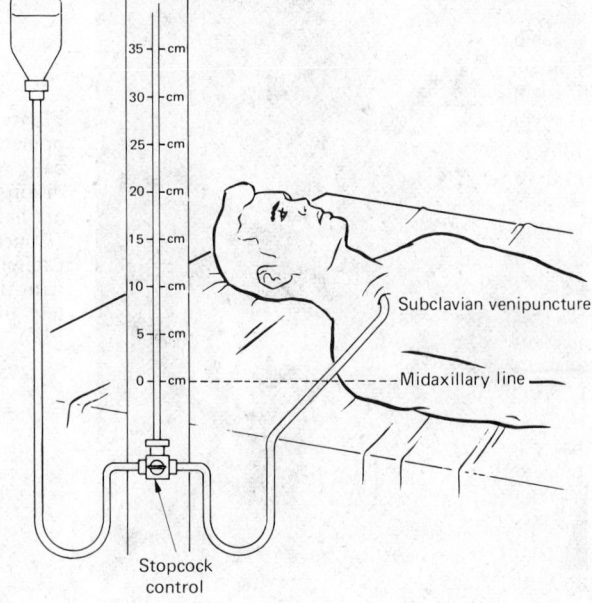

A

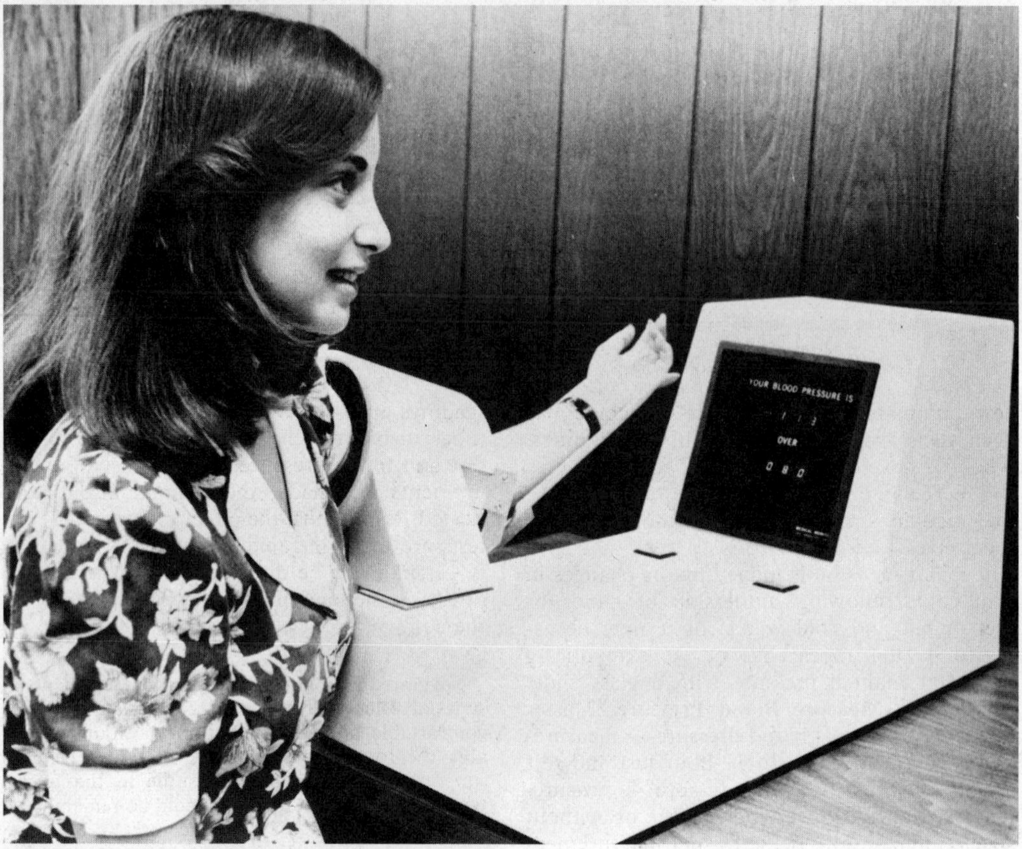

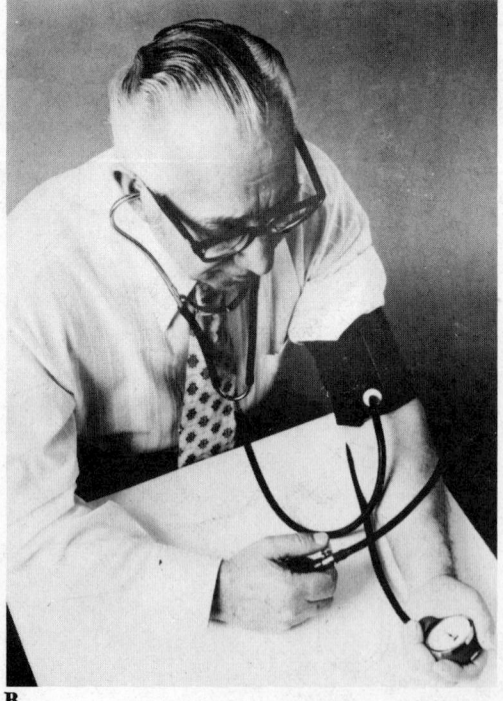

B

Figure 6-16. *A.* Automatic electronic sphygmomanometer (a microcomputer unit) which automatically records blood pressure without human supervision. Within 60 seconds, blood pressure figures are flashed accurately on the machine's digital dial. (Courtesy of Medical Monitors, Inc., Los Angeles, Calif.) *B.* A man taking his own blood pressure with the Manoscope Blood Pressure Unit. (Courtesy of Micro Mechanisms, Inc., Tarpon Springs, Fla.)

ured in the left arm. Paul L. Mitchell and associates advocate the "forearm at the horizontal level of the fourth intercostal space at the sternum." *

Explain the procedure, and in every way try to prevent excitement and anxiety or see that the patient is physically and mentally quiet. Expel any air in the cuff and adjust it comfortably around the arm above the elbow so that the tubes from it will not be over the point of the brachial artery where the stethoscope is placed. When measurements are made on the leg, place the cuff above the knee and the stethoscope over the popliteal artery in the popliteal space. Before inflating the cuff, find the pulsation of the brachial artery (the inner aspect of the bend of the arm), and place the stethoscope exactly over this point. Inflate the cuff with the rubber bulb until the pulsation of the artery that has become audible during the inflation of the cuff is no longer heard. Then allow the air to escape very slowly until the first sounds appear (the beginning of the first phase) and record as the *systolic blood pressure*. This first reappearance of sound is the blood being forced through the partially compressed vessel during systole. The pressure in the cuff at this point (the reading of the manometer) is almost equal to the systolic pressure within the blood vessel.

Having taken the systolic reading, gradually de-

flate the cuff and the sounds will change from a sharp thud (phase one) to a swishing or blowing sound (the second phase); then to a softer thud than phase one (third phase); then to a blowing sound of relatively low intensity (fourth phase); and gradually to a fainter sound which disappears altogether (the fifth phase).* Record the *diastolic arterial pressure* at the fifth phase, as recommended by the American Heart Association. However, some physicians prefer to use the readings at the fourth phase while others ask that both (diastolic) pressures be recorded (see Fig. 6-17).

Taking blood pressure readings accurately and expeditiously requires understanding and skill acquired through experience. Health workers should practice this procedure with individuals who provide normal or typical sounds as well as those with unusual or atypical sounds. In learning the skill emphasis should be placed on listening to the character of the sounds rather than noting the pressure. Films are helpful to the learner as are programmed instructions.[59,59a] Standardization of the procedure has been shown to contribute to accuracy of nurses, students, and nursing assistants in measuring blood pressure recordings.[60]

Suggested Procedure in Taking Central Venous Pressure Measurements. Whether central venous pressure measurements are made continuously or on one occasion as a supplement to other diagnostic techniques, the physician inserts the central

---

* Mitchell, Paul L., et al.: "Effect of Vertical Displacement of the Arm on Indirect Blood-Pressure Measurement," *N. Engl. J. Med.*, **271:**72, (July 9) 1964.

* The sounds as described in this paragraph are called the "Korotkoff sounds" because a doctor by this name first described them (in 1905).

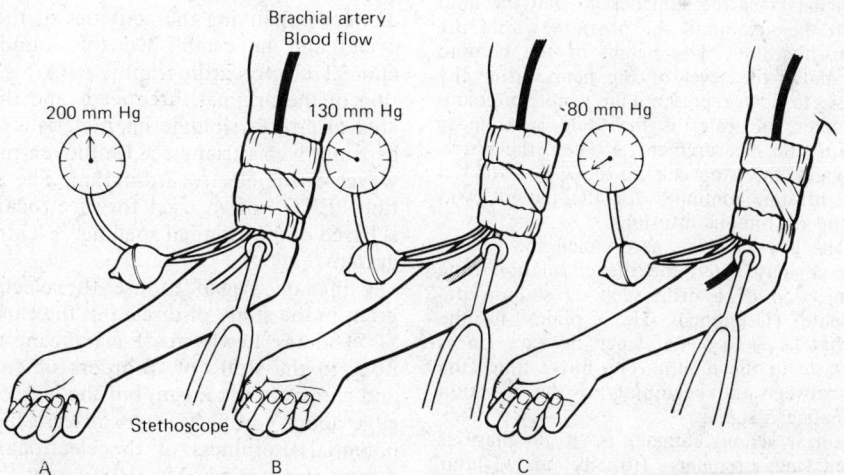

Figure 6-17. Steps in taking arterial blood pressure. *A.* Inflate the cuff to approximately 200 millimeters of mercury (200 mm Hg), thereby fully occluding the brachial artery. At this point, no sound is heard through the stethoscope. *B.* Slowly deflate the cuff until the first sounds are heard. The pressure reading at this point represents the systolic blood pressure. *C.* Continue slowly deflating the cuff, noting the changes in sound intensity. The point at which the sound once again disappears is recorded as the diastolic blood pressure. In this illustration, the blood pressure is recorded as 130/80, and the pulse pressure is 130 − 80 or 50 mm Hg. (See text for explanation of physiologic factors in blood pressure measurement.)

venous catheter (intracath).* In most hospitals the equipment is prepared and supplied by the central supply department if commercially pre-packaged sterile sets are not used; in some places the nurse may be responsible for sterilizing the equipment, for preparing the patient psychologi-cally and physically, and for working with the physician as he or she makes the test. The manom-eter, three-way stopcock, syringes, and a large-bore needle should be sterilized by steam under pressure. The venous catheter (intracath) is steri-lized commercially. The manometer, a calibrated cylinder, is supported by a suitable stand. Sterile physiological saline must be provided for the manometer.

Because the position of the patient and manom-eter are crucial for accurate venous pressure measurement, have the patient lie supine with the head of the bed flat. Tell the patient to lie quiet. Before the catheter is placed in the selected vein (external jugular, subclavian, cephalic, or basilic vein), prepare the skin as for any needle puncture. The physician inserts the needle, re-moves the cannula, and advances the catheter through the needle into the superior vena cava or the right atrium, then removes the needle and secures the catheter to the patient and at-taches it to the manometer. The sterile tubing from the saline (or other appropriate intravenous fluid) is attached to the manometer by the three-way stopcock, also. After setting the manom-eter so the zero mark lies at the level of the midaxillary line (which is the level of the right atrium) and starting the intravenous flow, the physician adjusts the stopcock so that the solution flows into the manometer rather than the pa-tient. When the manometer level reaches 30 cm, the physician turns the stopcock so that the fluid flows into the vein until the pressure within the vein stops the flow. The height of the column of fluid above the level of the heart, after the fluid ceases to flow, represents the venous pressure in millimeters of water if the scale is a linear scale. After the measurement is taken, the physi-cian changes the stopcock to flow position so that the infusion continues for the patient who is receiving continuous infusions.

After the physician has ascertained the venous pressure, he may determine the circulation time by an injection of a drug such as sodium de-hydrocholate (Decholin). He explains to the patient that he is to signal when he experiences a bitter taste in the mouth. The nurse times the interval between the beginning of the injection and the patient's signal.

The central venous catheter is left in place if subsequent measurements (usually at ½-hour or 1-hour intervals) are prescribed; the nurse takes these measurements following the steps as described above for the physician.

---

* In some intensive and coronary care units, nurses are permitted to place central venous catheters for monitoring of central venous pressure. (Whipple, Gerald H., et al.: *Acute Coronary Care*, Little, Brown & Co., Boston, 1972, p. 137.)

Record the measurement each time it is taken. Report to the physician significant changes in the level of venous pressure; he or she usually indicates the level at which venous pressure is to be maintained. The normal range is 5 to 12 cm of water pressure.

6. ELECTROCARDIOGRAPHY

Definition. The electrocardiogram is a graphic representation of the electric events occurring in the cardiac cycle reflected by a series of waves or deflections that correspond to a particular aspect of cardiac activity.[61] The conductive system of the heart generates elec-tric impulses producing a weak electric current that spreads throughout the body. This current may be recorded by placing electrodes on the skin surface and connecting these to an elec-trocardiograph machine. The graphic recording indicates the strength and direction of the cur-rent and is an important diagnostic tool.

Historical Development. The first human electrocardiogram was reported in a publica-tion in 1887 by Augustus D. Waller. He de-veloped a capillary electrometer that showed a dampened but clearly recognizable P-QRS-T. Dissatisfied with the lack of sensitivity of Wal-ler's capillary electrometer, William Einthoven developed a technique that has hardly been improved upon throughout the years. He de-vised a sensitive and responsive instrument that could record the minute changes in volt-age accompanying the activities of the cardiac cycle, and he established the foundation of clinical electrocardiography with his descrip-tion of the original three leads and the associ-ated electrophysiologic characteristics (known as Einthoven's triangle). Einthoven named the waves of the electrocardiogram. The abbrevia-tion "EKG" often used for electrocardiogram is based on his original spelling, "elektrokardio-gramm."

Clinicians began to use the electrocardio-gram in the study of disease in the early 1900s. Sir Thomas Lewis made significant contribu-tions to the study of disorders of conduction and cardiac mechanism, but the lack of knowl-edge about coronary artery disease limited the potential usefulness of the electrocardiogram during this period. The 1930s saw the devel-opment of better and more reliable instruments and advancements in the theory of cardiac electrophysiology. Contributions by Frank N. Wilson and his associates improved the role of the electrocardiogram in the study of disease. As the knowledge of coronary artery disease increased, differences among theory, tech-nique, instrumentation, and practice were defined. Since World War II the electrocardiogram has been a useful diagnostic tool for all physicians and medical students. Each day new insights are gained on cardiovascular disease and there is increasing usefulness of the electrocardiogram, but the basic principles of electrophysiology of the heart have changed little over the past 60 years.[62]

Conduction System of the Heart. To interpret the graphic recording of the electrocardiogram, it is necessary to understand the mechanical and electrochemical events that produce each heartbeat.

Electric impulses generated in special tissues of the heart cause the heart to automatically and rhythmically contract, producing a normal heartbeat. These impulses normally originate in an area of specialized tissue in the right atrium, the sinoatrial node (SA node). Many areas of the heart muscle, however, have the potential ability to spontaneously discharge electric impulses, but the sinus node usually discharges more rapidly than other areas and is the pacemaker. An electric impulse occurs rhythmically at 60 to 100 times per minute under normal conditions. If the pacemaker fails or if impulses are discharged too slowly, other areas in the heart will assume the function of pacing the heart, but usually at a rate slower than the SA node. The route of the impulse is illustrated in Figure 6-18. The impulse is transmitted from the SA node through the atria (making the atria contract) to the atrioventricular (AV) node and passes down the bundle of His into the left and right bundle branches, terminating in the Purkinje fibers of

the ventricle and stimulating ventricular contraction. Following contraction, the heart muscles rest while the ventricles fill with blood. The next impulse normally arrives when filling is complete and contraction of the ventricles occurs again.[63,64]

The actual contraction and relaxation of the heart muscle are preceded by certain electrochemical events. In the fluid, both inside and outside the cell membranes, there are electrolyte solutions containing positive and negative ions. When the heart is active, the current will flow from the negative ions in the intracellular fluid to the positive ions in the extracellular fluid. As seen in Figure 6-19, when the muscles of the heart are at rest, the extracellular fluid is positively charged and the intracellular fluid is negatively charged. There is no flow of current. When the muscle is stimulated, as in Figure 6-19, the normal negative potential inside the cell is changed. There is a flow of current until all the cells in the muscle fiber have been stimulated to change from negative to positive. This is the process of *depolarization*. A fraction of a second after depolarization, there is another reversal of potential and the positive ions again go to the outside of the cell, as seen in Figure 6-19. This return of the cells of the muscle fiber to the resting state is the process of *repolarization. This movement of the charged particles across the membranes of the myocardial cells produces the deflections on the electrocardiogram.*[65,66]

Because the electric current moves in several directions simultaneously, it is necessary to record the flow of current in different planes.

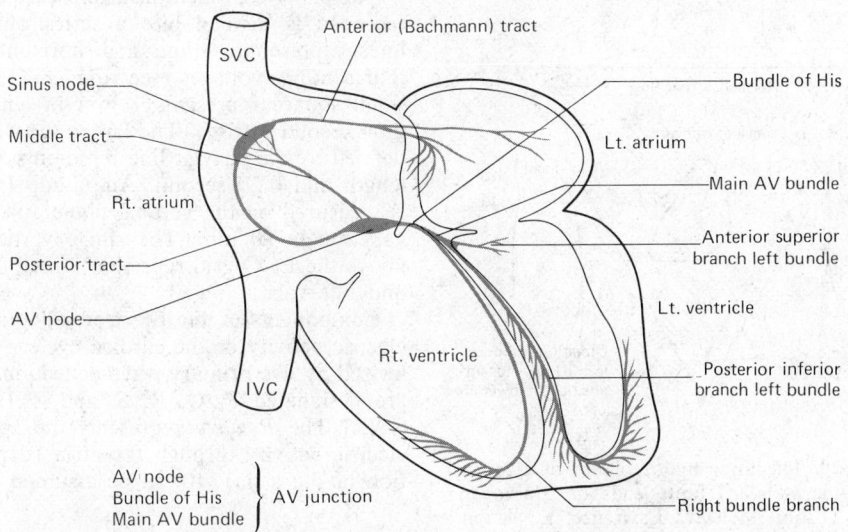

Figure 6-18. The conduction system of the heart. (From Bilitch, Michael: *A Manual of Cardiac Arrhythmias.* Little, Brown & Co., Boston, 1971, p. 4.)

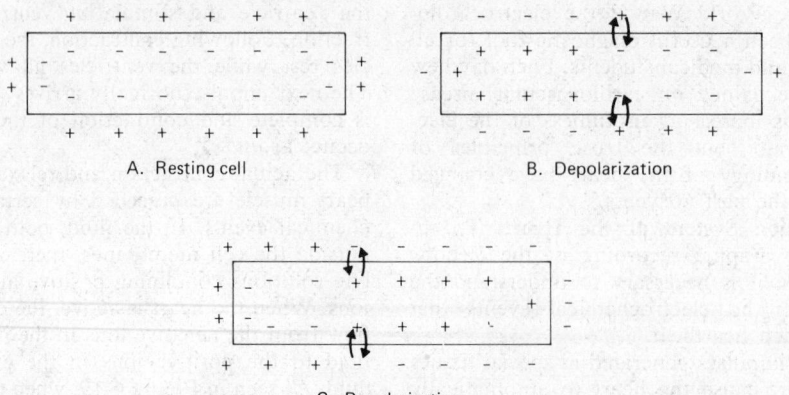

A. Resting cell

B. Depolarization

C. Repolarization

Figure 6-19. The heart muscle at rest, during depolarization, and repolarization. (From Zalis, Edwin G., and Conover, Mary H.: *Understanding Electrocardiography.* C. V. Mosby Co., St. Louis, 1972, p. 11.)

This is essentially what the 12-lead electrocardiogram does.

There are three major planes of electric activity detected with electrodes placed on the right arm, the left arm, and the left leg (as seen in Fig. 6-20). These three points form Einthoven's original triangle with the heart the center point. These are the standard limb leads (leads I, II, III) that measure the difference between two points (bipolar). Henry J. L. Marriott says "about 80 to 90 per cent accuracy in diagnosis can be achieved by inspecting these leads alone. Most arrhythmias and most types of heart block are easily diagnosed from these leads alone." * Lead I connects the two arms at the wrist; lead III connects the left arm at the wrist with the left leg at the ankle; and lead II connects the right arm at the wrist with the left leg at the ankle (the hypotenuse of the triangle). As a matter of convenience, the electrodes are connected at the wrist and ankle. In addition to the three standard leads, there are three augmented unipolar leads (aVR, aVL, aVF) that record the difference in potential between the limb and the center of the heart and six pericardial, or chest, leads (V1–V6) that provide views of the heart from different angles and are used to determine how far anteriorly or posteriorly the electrical forces are directed.[67,68]

The paper on which the electrocardiogram is recorded is divided into a series of vertical lines representing time and horizontal lines representing voltage (see Fig. 6-21). Each small square represents 1 mm in length and 0.04 second in time. The larger square that is defined by the heavier line represents 5 mm in length and 0.20 second. Amplitude (voltage) is measured on the vertical plane and 1 millivolt equals 10 mm. The single vertical lines above the ECG grid represent 3-inch or 3-second intervals.

Components of the Electrocardiogram. The electric activity of the cardiac cycle is characterized by five primary wave deflections. These are designated P, Q, R, S, and T (see Fig. 6-22). The *P wave* represents the spread of electric activity through the atria (depolarization of the atria). It can be assumed that the

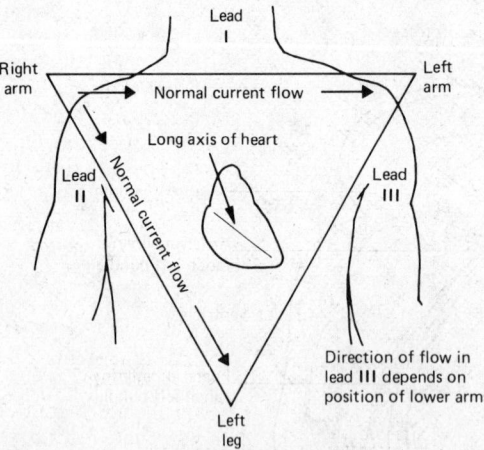

Figure 6-20. The three major planes of electrical activity—the standard limb leads or Einthoven's triangle. (From Meltzer, Lawrence E., et al.: *Intensive Coronary Care: A Manual for Nurses.* Coronary Care Unit Fund of Presbyterian Hospital, Philadelphia, 1965, p. 128.)

* Marriott, Henry J. L.: *Practical Electrocardiography,* 3rd ed. Williams & Wilkins Co., Baltimore, 1962, p. 1.

impulse began in the SA node if P waves are present and are of normal size and shape. If these waves are absent or not normal, it implies that the impulse began outside the SA node. The *P-R interval* is the period from the beginning of the P wave to the beginning of the QRS complex. This interval represents the time taken for the original impulse to spread through the atria and cross the AV node, and usually does not exceed 0.20 second. If the P-R interval is prolonged, there is a delay in the conduction through the AV node. In certain instances the P-R interval may be shorter than normal (less than 0.10 second) due to the impulse reaching the ventricle outside the normal conductive tissues. The *QRS complex* represents the activation of the ventricles as the impulse passes through the bundle of His, the bundle branches, and the Purkinje fibers. There is an initial downward deflection (Q wave), followed by an upright deflection (R wave), and another downward deflection (S wave). Normally the duration of this complex is less than 0.12 second and prolongation of these waves indicates that the ventricles have been stimulated in a delayed or abnormal manner. The *S-T segment* follows the QRS complex and indicates the period between completion of depolarization of the ventricles and recovery of the ventricular muscles. This segment is normally on the baseline and either an elevation or depression may be indicative of muscle injury or diminished blood supply (ischemia). The *T wave* represents the return of the ventricles to a resting state following contraction (repolarization of the ventricles). Alterations in the direction, height, or shape of the T wave may be indicative of muscle injury or electrolyte imbalances.[69]

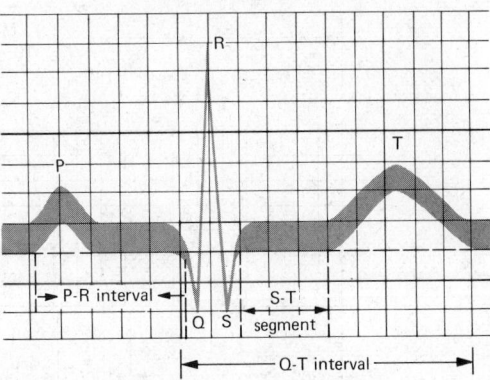

Figure 6-22. Graphic representation of the electrical activity of the cardiac cycle.

There are several methods of measuring or approximating heart rate by using the readings of the electrocardiogram. One of the most common is to count the number of cycles in 5, 6, or 10 seconds and then multiply this by 12, 10, or 6. This is quite accurate if the rate is irregular. Another common method is to count the number of large squares between R waves and to divide this into 300, based on the assumption that 300 large squares equal 1 minute. This method is accurate enough for all practical purposes, and the slower the rate, the more accurate the approximation. It is the method probably used most often by nurses and physicians. A third, and very accurate method, is to count the number of small squares between R waves and divide this into 1500 (1500 small squares in 1 minute) [70] (see Fig. 6-23).

The electrocardiogram is a useful diagnostic tool but must be viewed in conjunction with other clinical findings as the ECG "does not depict the actual physical state of the heart nor its functions, only disturbances in the electrical forces." * A patient with organic heart disease may have an electrocardiogram that appears normal unless the disease process has disturbed the electrical forces and a normal individual may show nonspecific abnormalities on an electrocardiograph tracing. The most important use of the electrocardiogram has been in the diagnosis of coronary heart disease and disturbances in heart rhythm. Analysis of the electrocardiogram can provide a great deal of indirect information about the heart and has proved valuable in metabolic and electrolyte disturbances, the study of effects of certain drugs (such as digitalis and quinidine), inflam-

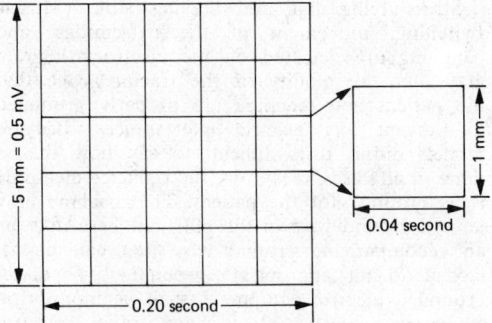

Figure 6-21. Graphic grid of the electrocardiogram with vertical lines representing voltage and horizontal lines representing time. The interval between two heavy lines is .20 second. (From Andreoli, Kathleen G., et al.: *Comprehensive Cardiac Care,* C. V. Mosby Co., St. Louis, 1971, p. 71.)

---

* Meltzer, Lawrence E., et al.: *Intensive Coronary Care: A Manual for Nurses.* Coronary Care Unit Fund of the Presbyterian Hospital, Philadelphia, 1965, p. 132.

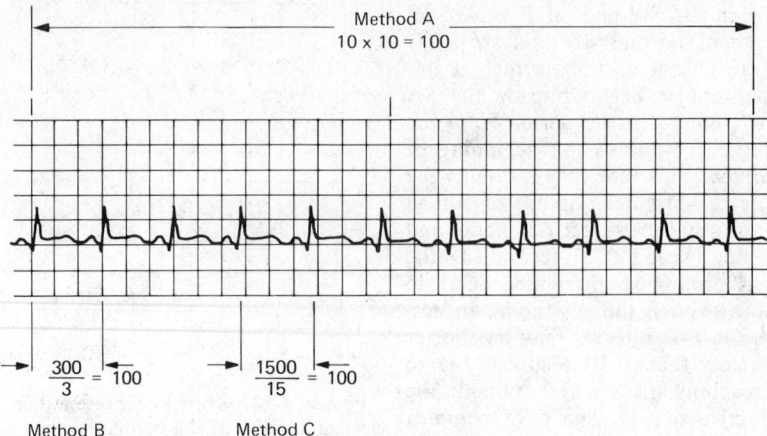

Figure 6-23. Calculation of heart rate. Method A—Count the number of cardiac cycles (P, Q, R, S, T configurations) in a six-second cycle, then multiply that by the number of six-second intervals in a minute (10 cycles × 10 six-second intervals = 100 beats per minute). Method B—Count the number of large squares between two R waves and divide that into 300. Method C—Count the number of small squares and divide this into 1500. (From Bilitch, Michael: *A Manual of Cardiac Arrhythmias.* Little, Brown & Co., Boston, 1971, p. 16.)

mation of the pericardial sac, hypertrophy of the chambers of the heart, and systemic diseases that affect cardiac function.[71] Interpretation of the electrocardiogram must be made in conjunction with other clinical findings.

Authorities agree that the electrocardiogram tracings may be affected by a variety of factors; and consequently it is important that nurses be aware of these whether or not they are taking the electrocardiogram themselves. There must be good contact between the patient's skin and the electrodes. This can be assured by applying electrode jelly to the skin where the electrode is attached. The patient's position is also important and can affect the tracing. He or she should be lying flat and as relaxed as possible because any movements or muscular twitching is recorded by the machine and alters the tracing. It is important that the patient and the machine be properly grounded to prevent interference in the recording (see Suggested Procedure). There are specific positions for the placement of the chest leads and the nurse should know what they are. Improper placement of the chest leads can greatly distort the tracing and alter the diagnostic conclusions. (For this proper placement, see Suggested Procedure.) Finally, it is important that the machine instructions, included in a manual furnished by the manufacturer, be properly standardized.

In many clinical settings (such as intensive and coronary care units) it is the responsibility of the nurse to make the electrocardiogram, interpret the findings, and institute treatment

accordingly. In community clinics, physicians' offices, general units of the hospital, and other health settings a technician may perform this function, but in some instances the nurse does. However, it is important that the nurse know how to make an electrocardiogram because in emergency situations, when an immediate electrocardiogram is required for diagnosis and treatment, the technician may be unavailable.

Suggested Procedure in Taking Electrocardiogram Tracings.[72,73] Ask patients whether they have had the test; if not, explain what an electrocardiogram is, why it is being made, and how they can cooperate. Assess each patient and provide the information appropriate to that individual.

Stress lying flat and staying still. (Muscle twitching, movement of the extremities, and coughing are detected on the electrocardiogram and alter the quality of the tracing.) See that the patient and machine are properly grounded to prevent any electric interferences. Because models differ, it is difficult to say how this is done in all cases. Generally the right leg electrode is a "ground" for the patient. The machine may have a ground wire in the plug, or there may be an accompanying ground wire that can be attached to an appropriate grounding. No nongrounded electric equipment such as monitoring equipment, electric beds, and other electric apparatus should be used in the monitoring area.

Apply electrode jelly to the skin before attaching an electrode. Place the electrodes on the right arm, left arm, right leg, and left leg as shown in Figure 6-24. If the patient is especially thin, move the electrodes up the extremity to an area that is least bony.

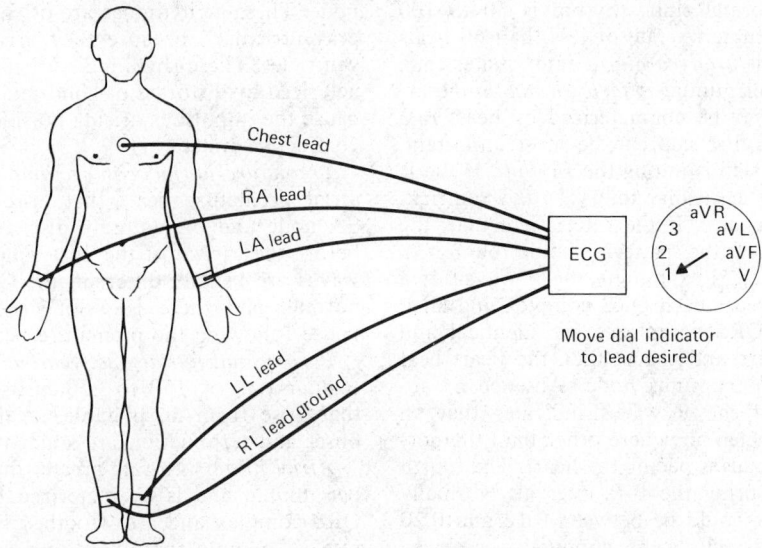

Figure 6-24. Electrocardiogram machine with leads attached. (Goldman, Mervin J.: *Principles of Clinical Electrocardiography,* 9th ed. Lange Medical Publications, Los Altos, Calif., 1976, p. 4.)

Before making an electrocardiogram, check the machine for proper standardization. When the standardization button is pressed there should be a deflection of 10 mm on the graph paper. This means that the spike made will be two large squares in height. Interpretation of the electrocardiogram is based on this standardization, so it is important that this be checked and properly adjusted.

Label the tracing with the patient's name, the date, and usually the beginning time. There is an indicator dial that has a position for the various leads (leads I, II, III, aVR, aVL, aVF); adjust the dial for the appropriate lead. This technique, as well as the labeling of each lead, varies with the equipment. Some of the more

modern machines make simultaneous recordings of more than one lead at a time.

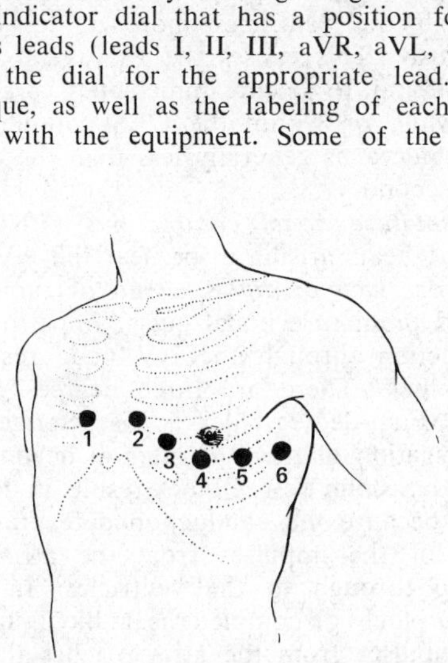

There is a marking on the indicator dial for the chest (V) leads and the placement of these leads is illustrated in Figure 6-25. The location of V_1 is the fourth intercostal space to the left of the sternum, V_2 in the fourth intercostal space to the right of the sternum, V_3 midway between V_2 and V_4, V_4 in the fifth intercostal space below the nipple, and V_5 and V_6 in the same horizontal positions on the lateral aspect of the chest.

The Electrocardiogram and Disturbances of Rate and Rhythm. Normal sinus rhythm is characterized by the following:

1. P wave preceding each QRS complex.
2. P-R interval not more than 0.20 second.
3. P waves all alike in size and shape.
4. Heart rate 60 to 100 beats per minute.
5. QRS complex not greater than 0.12 second.

If these conditions do not prevail, then there is a disturbance in the normal heart rhythm, or an *arrhythmia.** As previously mentioned, one of the most important uses of the electrocardiogram has been the identification of rhythm disturbances.

For a meaningful interpretation, the electrocardiographic tracing must be approached in an orderly manner. The first step is looking at

Figure 6-25. Placement of precordial (chest) leads. (Goldman, Mervin J.: *Principles of Clinical Electrocardiography,* 9th ed. Lange Medical Publications, Los Altos, Calif., 1976, p. 9.)

* *Dysrhythmia* is used by some medical workers instead of *arrhythmia.* Both mean essentially "without rhythm," or "disturbance of rhythm."

the rate. Normal sinus rhythm is 60 to 100 beats per minute. A rate of less than 60 beats per minute is *bradycardia;* a rate greater than 100 beats per minute is *tachycardia.* Some arrhythmias may be characterized by heart *rate* only, so this first step can be most important. The second step is noting the *rhythm.* If the R waves occur at regular intervals, the ventricular rate is regular. If the rate is irregular, the consistency of the pattern should be noted. The third step is examining the P waves. If a P wave precedes each QRS complex and all P waves and QRS complexes are identical and normal in size and shape, then the heart beat originates in the sinus node. Absence or abnormality of the P waves indicates that an ectopic (situated anywhere other than the normal pace) focus is pacing the heart. The fourth step is measuring the P-R interval. Normally this interval should be between 0.12 and 0.20 second. A defect in the conductive pathway will prolong or reduce the interval.

The fifth and last step is measuring the QRS complex. Normally this value is less than 0.12 second, usually 0.04 to 0.11 second. If the width of the QRS complex is greater than 0.12 second, this indicates a defect in the intraventricular conduction system. After these observations are made, it is necessary to classify the arrhythmia and institute the appropriate treatment. The reader should consult specialized texts for a more detailed discussion of reading electrocardiograms and instituting treatment.

Disorders of Cardiac Function Showing in the Electrocardiogram. *Cardiac arrhythmias,* or disorders of the rate and rhythm, may be classified in a variety of ways, but one of the commonest and most easily understood is according to anatomic site, or origin. First, there are the disturbances originating in the sinus node. They are characterized by the P wave and the QRS complex occurring in a 1:1 relationship.

Sinus tachycardia is a rapid rate over 100 beats per minute and may be associated with exercise, eating, pain, fever, thyrotoxicosis, and infection. It is also a common reaction to heart disease, heart failure, and drugs.

Sinus bradycardia is a slow rate less than 60 beats per minute and is a physiologic reaction to vagal stimulation, sleep, and certain cardiotonic drugs. This may be a common finding in the well-trained athlete.

Sinus arrhythmia is a variation in rhythm that corresponds to the respiratory cycle. It is a normal finding, especially in children.

Sinus arrest occurs when the sinus node fails to emit one or more impulses.

Atrial arrhythmias arise from an irritable focus within the atria other than the sinus node. These arrhythmias are often termed "supraventricular" because they arise above the ventricles. These rhythm disturbances are characterized by distorted or abnormal P waves because the impulse is arising outside the normal conductive system.

Premature atrial contractions (PAC) are atrial premature beats that arise outside the SA node and prematurely discharge the atria before the arrival of the next sinus impulse. P waves are usually different, the QRS complex normal, and there is a longer than normal pause following the premature beat.

Paroxysmal atrial tachycardia is a rapid, regular rate of 150 to 250 beats per minute that arise from an irritable atrial focus. The onset and termination are sudden and abrupt.

Atrial flutter is a rate greater than 250 beats per minute and is characterized by a normal QRS complex and a sawtoothed baseline. The rate is so rapid that every impulse cannot be transmitted to the ventricles, so the ventricles will respond to every second, third, or fourth (and so on) impulse.

Atrial fibrillation is an irregular and ineffective rhythm at an excessively rapid rate (more than 350 beats per minute). There is the absence of P waves and instead only coarse fibrillating waves.

In certain instances and under various conditions, the atrioventricular (AV) node may act as the pacemaker for the heart with its own intrinsic rate of 35 to 60 beats per minute. When the impulse arises in the AV node, the pathway it travels is altered and the impulse will travel up through the atria and down through the ventricles more or less simultaneously. This causes the P wave to be inverted and to occur immediately preceding, following, or within the QRS complex. The P-R interval is generally less than the normal 0.12 second.

Premature nodal contractions (PNC) are ectopic beats arising in or near the AV node.

Nodal tachycardia is a run of rapidly repeated premature nodal beats. Impairment of conduction through the AV node results in AV block. There are three degrees of AV block. First-degree block is characterized by a prolongation of the P-R interval beyond 0.20 second. Second-degree block results in dropped beats because the conduction defect prevents some of the impulses from the atria from getting through to the ventricles. In third-degree block, or complete heart block, none of the impulses from the atria reaches the ventricles. A ventricular pacemaker stimulates the ventricles at a slow rate, usually 20 to 45 beats per minute.

Ventricular arrhythmias arise from an ectopic focus in the wall of the ventricle and produce a distorted and prolonged QRS complex because of the altered conduction pathway.

The *premature ventricular contraction* is probably the most easily recognized arrhythmia due to its bizarre QRS. It is further characterized by a long pause (compensatory pause) before the next normal beat. Premature ventricular contractions are dangerous if frequent (more than 5 to 6 per minute), occur in groups, appear to come from more than one ectopic foci, or fall on the T wave.

Ventricular tachycardia is a run of rapidly repeated premature ventricular beats. This is a serious arrhythmia that requires prompt treatment.

Ventricular fibrillation is a terminal arrhythmia predisposing death. It is easily recognized by the absence of formed ventricular responses and requires immediate defibrillation or emergency measures to prevent death.[74-77]

The observations of nurses caring for cardiac patients are extremely important, for often it is the nurse at the bedside who first detects a change in rate or rhythm. They should document the abnormal rate or arrhythmia with a full electrocardiographic tracing and note the frequency of any ectopic beats. Although nurses who are not trained to detect and diagnose arrhythmias may not know the significance of a rhythm disturbance, they can assess the patient's condition and vital signs to determine if the arrhythmia has compromised cardiac output or cardiopulmonary status. But invaluable to them and the physician is the electrocardiogram in the treatment of a malfunctioning heart.

Well-prepared nurses in mobile units, in intensive care divisions of the hospital, and everywhere that critically ill persons are treated are reducing the death rate markedly by the initiation and maintenance of cardiac monitors and appropriate therapy. Cardiac surgery is almost commonplace. More and more surgical nurses must be prepared to give preoperative, operative, and postoperative care. Implants and temporary and permanent pacemakers are no longer rarities; all nurses should know something about them and should appreciate the importance of special study when they are responsible for giving care or guidance to persons who have special cardiac surgery, implants, and pacemakers.

7. IMPLANTED PACEMAKERS

Artificial Pacing.[78,79,79a] Normally, the sinus node paces the heart with regular, rhythmic impulses. Certain physiologic changes and defects in the conductive system may disturb the normal heart rate, rhythm, or conduction. Many of these disturbances may be corrected with an electronic pacemaker, which delivers an electric current to the heart through electrodes that are in contact with the heart muscle (see Fig. 6-26). Artificial pacing may be instituted on a permanent or temporary basis. Indications for electronic pacing include:

1. Heart block, whether a chronic condition of low cardiac output or acute ischemia.
2. Supraventricular and ventricular arrhythmias.
3. Myocardial infarction when there is transient block, sinus slowing, or complications of failure, shock, or arrhythmias.
4. Prophylactically during or following surgery.
5. For slow ventricular rates that produce serious problems.

Types of Pacemakers. The *continuous asynchronous* (fixed rate) pacemaker fires at a set rate regardless of the patient's own intrinsic rhythm.

The *demand pacemaker* fires only if the patient's own rate falls below a preset level. It functions by determining the P-R interval and evaluating this electronically. There are several types of demand units and catheters may be placed in either atrium or ventricle.

The *synchronized pacemaker* is synchronized with the patient's P wave, or, if there is no P wave, the pacer will fire automatically. There may be electrodes in both the atrium and the ventricle or just in the ventricle. This mode of pacing creates an approximation of normal synchronous cardiac function and the atrioventricular contraction is preserved.

Methods of Insertion.[80] In *transvenous* insertion, the electrode catheter is placed into either the right atrium or ventricle via a cutdown of a peripheral vein. The catheter is advanced under fluoroscopy until the catheter tip is in contact with the wall of the heart (endocardium). For a permanent unit, the battery is surgically inserted into a pocket of subcutaneous tissue. With the temporary units, the electrodes are attached to the external battery and firmly anchored to the patient's arm.

Transthoracic insertion is an emergency procedure in which the electrodes are inserted directly into the ventricle through the chest wall. External pacing may also be accomplished by delivering a shock across the chest wall.

For *epicardial* insertion, the chest is opened and the electrodes are sutured directly on the outer wall of the atrium or ventricle (epicardium). The pulse generator is inserted into the subcutaneous tissue and the electrodes connected.

If the pacemaker electrode is to function

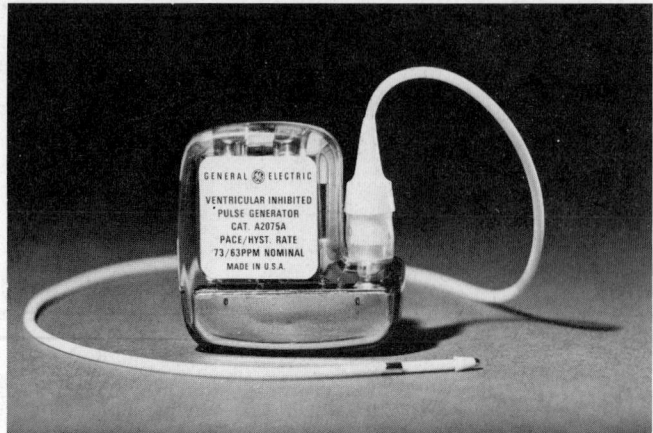

Figure 6-26. Implantable standby pacemaker with intracardiac catheter electrode. (Courtesy of Medical Systems Department of General Electric Co., Milwaukee, Wis.)

properly in delivering the stimulus to the heart muscle, the electrode must be in contact with the myocardium, the battery functioning properly, the electrode wire intact, and the threshold potential of the myocardial cells not greater than that delivered by the pacemaker. These conditions must be met if proper pacing is to be achieved.

Complications of Artificial Pacing.[81-83a] There are several complications with electronic pacing. It is important that the nurse be alert to signs of malfunction.

There may be premature failure of the pacemaker battery. Failure is indicated by either an increase or a decrease in pulse rate, a decrease in the amplitude on the ECG, absence of a pacemaker stimulus when a discharge is expected, convulsions or fainting, and failure of a stimulus to depolarize the heart. Battery replacements are advised every 18 to 24 months.

Fracture of the electrode wire is another complication of artificial pacing. This problem is less frequent with alloys and coiled wire but is likely to occur if the wire is too angulated.

In some instances, there may be malplacement or displacement of the transvenous electrode. This is an early complication following the insertion of the pacemaker and is not common after a few days. Perforation of the ventricle may occur with artificial pacing but is rare.

Following the insertion of a pacemaker, there is fibrosis around the tip of the catheter. This may insulate the heart and prevent the stimulus from pacing. With an external pacemaker, it is usually the nurse's responsibility to increase the milliamperage sufficiently for the pacemaker to "capture." Infection may be a problem following the insertion of a pacemaker. There may be cellulitis, phlebitis, pericardial inflammation, or pressure necrosis.

Competition between the patient's normal spontaneous rhythm and the paced rhythm may occur. There is less competition with the synchronous type of pacemaker.

In caring for patients with a pacemaker, nurses should have certain information. Immediately following the insertion, they should get some baseline values of pacemaker function such as escape interval, refractory period, current or voltage delivered by pacemaker, mode of pacing, reason for insertion, set rate, and pulse amplitude. They should know what a paced beat looks like and should determine if the pacemaker stimulation results in a ventricular response each time. On the electrocardiogram, the pacer spike from a unipolar electrode is large, and one from a bipolar electrode is small. Pulse rate and quality should be checked for a full minute. The patient's position is important with an external (temporary) pacemaker, and it should be determined whether pacemaker function is altered by changes in position. Measures should be instituted to prevent infection and if possible to monitor rhythm so that any dysfunction or ectopic beats can be recognized immediately.

Patient Teaching. Patient teaching is an important step in rehabilitation of the patient with a pacemaker, especially in dealing with his or her feelings and fears. A teaching program should be designed to meet each patient's specific needs, but generally should include information about the physiology and function of the heart, the function of the pacemaker and methods of checking it. It is advised that the patient at home check the pulse twice daily. Checking involves testing the pacemaker battery with a transistor radio. The signal the pacemaker sends out can be heard on a transistor radio when the dial is placed at 550 kilocycles and the radio placed over the battery. The patient can then feel the pulse at the wrist and note if there is a clicking from the radio with each beat. Demand pacemakers can be checked with a magnet that is placed over the battery that makes the pacemaker function at a fixed rate.

It is important to remember that a pacemaker only corrects a symptom; it does not change the pathologic condition. Patients therefore need guidance on diet, medications, and activity. They should be taught about electric equipment also. Patients may use most household appliances but large power tools must be properly grounded. Working directly over a running engine should be avoided as well as high-frequency sources such as electrocautery, diathermy, and microwave ovens.

REFERENCES

1. Brobeck, John R.: "Control Systems That Establish Regulations," in Brobeck, John R., et al. (eds.): *Best and Taylor's Physiological Basis of Medical Practice,* 9th ed. Williams & Wilkins Co., Baltimore, 1973, p. 9–128.

2. Brengelmann, George, and Brown, Arthur C.: "Temperature Regulation," in Ruch, Theodore C., and Patton, Harry D.: *Physiology and Biophysics,* 19th ed. W. B. Saunders Co., Philadelphia, 1965, p. 1057.

3. Cranston, W. I., et al.: "Oral, Rectal and Oesophageal Temperatures and Some Factors Affecting Them in Man," *J. Physiol.,* **126**:355, (Nov.) 1954.

4. Selle, W. A.: *Body Temperature: Its Changes with Environment, Disease and Therapy.* Charles C Thomas, Publisher, Springfield, Ill., 1952, p. 9.

5. Mills, J. N.: "Human Circadian Rhythms," *Physiol. Rev.,* **46**:128, (Jan.) 1966.

6. Sharp, G. W.: "Reversal of Diurnal Temperature Rhythms in Man," *Nature,* **190**:146, (Apr.) 1961.

7. Mills, J. N.: "Circadian Rhythms During and After Three Months in Solitude Underground," *J. Physiol.,* **174**:217, (Nov.) 1964.

8. Brobeck, John R.: *op. cit.,* pp. 9–128.

9. DeRisi, Lucy: "Body Temperature Measurements in Relation to Circadian Rhythmicity in Hospitalized Male Patients," in *ANA Clinical Sessions, 1968.* Appleton-Century-Crofts, New York, 1969, p. 251.

10. DuBois, Eugene F.: *Fever and the Regulation of Body Temperature.* Charles C Thomas, Publisher, Springfield, Ill., 1948, p. 31.

11. Tuttle, W. W., and Schottelius, Byron A.: *Textbook of Physiology,* 17th ed. C. V. Mosby Co., St. Louis, 1973, p. 467.

12. Best, Charles H., and Taylor, Norman B.: *The Physiological Basis of Medical Practice,* 8th ed. Williams & Wilkins Co., Baltimore, 1966, p. 1626.

13. Guyton, Arthur C.: *Textbook of Medical Physiology,* 5th ed. W. B. Saunders Co., Philadelphia, 1976, p. 963.

14. Tuttle, W. W., and Schottelius, Byron A.: *op. cit.,* p. 470.

15. Boyd, William: *A Textbook of Pathology: Structure and Function in Disease,* 8th ed. Lea & Febiger, Philadelphia, 1970, p. 59.

16. Reimann, Hobart A.: "The Problem of Long Continued, Low Grade Fever," *J.A.M.A.,* **107**:1089, (Oct. 3) 1936.

17. Wynn, Frank B.: "The Psychic Factor as an Element in Temperature Disturbance," *J.A.M.A.,* **73**:31, (Oct. 5) 1919.

18. Atkins, Elisha: "Fever," in MacBryde, Cyril Mitchell, and Blacklow, Robert Stanley (eds.): *Signs and Symptoms; Applied Pathologic Physiology and Clinical Interpretation,* 5th ed. J. B. Lippincott Co., Philadelphia, 1970, p. 461.

19. Lee, Richard V., and Atkins, Elisha: "Spurious Fever," *Am. J. Nurs.,* **72**:1094, (June) 1972.

20. MacNeil, Ward J.: "Hyperthermia, Genuine and Spurious," *Arch. Intern. Med.,* **64**:800, (Oct.) 1939.

21. Atkins, Elisha: *op. cit.,* p. 459.

22. Diamond, E. G., and Andrews, M. H.: "Clinical Thermometers and Urinometers: Determination of Their Accuracy," *J.A.M.A.,* **156**:125, (Sept. 11) 1954.

23. Knapp, Herbert A.: "Accuracy of Glass Clinical Thermometers Compared to Electronic Thermometers," *Am. J. Surg.,* **112**:130, (July) 1966.

24. Ferguson, Gayle Tate, et al.: "The Advantages of the Electronic Thermometer," *Hospitals,* **45**:62, (Aug. 1) 1971.

25. Tompkins, Pendelton S.: "Danger in Securing Vaginal Temperatures," *Fertil. Steril.,* **1**:543, (Nov.) 1950.

26. Nichols, Glennadee A., et al.: "Oral, Axillary, and Rectal Temperature Determinations and Relationships," *Nurs. Res.,* **15**:307, (Fall) 1966.

27. ———, and Verhonick, Phyllis J.: "Placement Time for Oral Thermometers; a Nursing Study Replication," *Nurs. Res.,* **17**:159, (Mar.–Apr.) 1968.

28. ———: "Time and Temperature," *Am. J. Nurs.,* **67**:2304, (Nov.) 1967.

29. Verhonick, Phyllis J., and Nichols, Glennadee A.: "Temperature Measurement in Nursing Practice and Research," *Can. Nurse,* **64**:41, (June) 1968.

30. Nichols, Glennadee A., et al.: "Taking Oral Temperatures of Febrile Patients," *Nurs. Res.,* **19**:448, (Sept.–Oct.) 1967.

31. ———, and Kunst, Mildred E.: "Geriatric Patients Temperatures," 1967. (Unpublished manuscript.)

32. ———, et al.: "Measuring Oral and Rectal Temperatures of Febrile Children," *Nurs. Res.,* **21**:261, (May–June) 1972.

33. Logan, Cynthia A.: Duration of Effect of a Hot Liquid on the Oral Temperature," August, 1972. (Unpublished Master's thesis,

Texas Woman's University, Houston, Tex.)

34. Woodman, Ellen A., et al.: "Sources of Unreliability in Oral Temperatures," *Nurs. Res.,* **16:**276, (Summer) 1967.

35. Forster, Brenda, et al.: "Duration of Effects of Drinking Iced Water on Oral Temperatures," *Nurs. Res.,* **19:**169, (Mar.–Apr.) 1970.

36. Woodman, Ellen A., et al.: *op. cit.*

37. Verhonick, Phyllis J., and Werley, Harriet H.: "Experimentation in Nursing Practice in the Army," *Nurs. Outlook,* **11:**305, (Mar.) 1963.

37a. Rosendorff, C., and Cranston, W. I.: "Effects of Salicylate on Human Temperature Regulation," *Clin. Sci.,* **35:**81, 1968.

37b. Satinoff, Evelyn: "Salicylate: Action on Normal Body Temperature in Rats," *Science,* **176:**532, (May) 1972.

37c. Torrance, Jane T.: "Temperature Readings of Premature Infants," *Nurs. Res.,* **17:**312, (July–Aug.) 1968.

37d. Nichols, Glennadee A.: "Time Analyses of Afebrile and Febrile Temperature Readings," *Nurs. Res.,* **21:**463, (Sept.–Oct.) 1972.

37e. ———, and Glor, Beverly A. K.: "A Replication of Rectal Thermometer Placement Studies," *Nurs. Res.,* **17:**360, (July–Aug.) 1968.

37f. ———, et al.: "Rectal Thermometer Placement Times for Febrile Adults," *Nurs. Res.,* **21:**76, (Jan.–Feb.) 1972.

37g. Welsh, Margaret, and Erdman, Martha E.: "Studies in Thermometer Techniques," *Nurs. Ed. Bull.,* No. 11, Bureau of Publication, Teachers College, Columbia University, New York, 1929.

37h. Ryan, Elisabeth, and Miller, Virginia B.: "Disinfection of Clinical Thermometers," *Am. J. Nurs.,* **32:**197, (Feb.) 1932.

38. Dunbar, Helen F.: *Emotions and Bodily Change,* 3rd ed. Columbia University Press, New York, 1946, pp. 170, 239.

39. Stevenson, Ian: "Physical Symptoms During Pleasurable Emotional States," *Psychosom. Med.,* **12:**98, (Mar.–Apr.) 1950.

40. Jacobs, Martin A., et al.: "Life Stress and Respiratory Illness," *Psychosom. Med.,* **32:**233, (May–June) 1970.

40a. Traver, Gayle A.: "Living with Chronic Respiratory Disease," *Am. J. Nurs.,* **75:**1777, (Oct.) 1975.

41. Govindaraj, M.: "The Effect of Dehydration on the Ventilatory Capacity in Normal Subjects," *Am. Rev. Resp. Dis.,* **105:**842, 1972.

42. West, Howard F.: "Clinical Studies on the Respiration; A Comparison of Various Standards for the Normal Vital Capacity of the Lungs," *Arch. Intern. Med.,* **25:**306, (Mar.) 1920.

43. Foley, Mary F.: "Pulmonary Function Testing," *Am. J. Nurs.,* **71:**1136, (June) 1971.

44. Weiss, Earle B., and Carlson, C. Jeffrey: "Recording of Breath Sounds," *Am. Rev. Resp. Dis.,* **105:**835, 1972.

45. Detweiler, David K.: "Regulation of Systemic and Pulmonary Circulation," in Brobeck, John R., et al. (eds.): *Best and Taylor's Physiological Basis of Medical Practice,* 9th ed. Williams & Wilkins Co., Baltimore, 1973, p. 3–189.

46. Guyton, Arthur C.: *op. cit.,* p. 242.

47. Best, Charles H., and Taylor, Norman B.: *op. cit.,* p. 795.

48. Storlie, Frances: "Pulse," *Nursing '71,* **1:**34, (Nov.) 1971.

49. Ruskin, Arthur: *Classics in Arterial Hypertension.* Charles C Thomas, Publisher, Springfield, Ill., 1956, p. 1.

49a. Master, Arthur M., et al.: *Normal Blood Pressure and Hypertension; New Definitions.* Lea & Febiger, Philadelphia, 1952, pp. 11, 28.

50. Guyton, Arthur C.: *op. cit.,* p. 238.

51. Master, Arthur M., et al.: *op. cit.*

52. Moia, Blais: "The Range of Normal Blood Pressure," in Luisado, Aldo A. (ed.): *Cardiology.* McGraw-Hill Book Co., New York, 1959, p. 15.

52a. US Department of Health, Education, and Welfare: *Hypertension; The Silent Killer.* Nursing Clinical Conference presented by the Nursing Department of the Clinical Center, National Institutes of Health. US Government Printing Office, Washington, D.C., 1975 (DHEW Pub. No. [NIH] 76–708).

52b. Stamler, Jeremiah: *High Blood Pressure in the United States.* US Government Printing Office, Washington, D.C., 1974 (DHEW Pub. No. [NIH] 75–755).

53. Albrink, Margaret J.: "Obesity," in Beeson, Paul B., and McDermott, Walsh (eds.): *Cecil-Loeb Textbook of Medicine,* 13th ed. W. B. Saunders Co., Philadelphia, 1971, p. 1451.

54. Wilber, Joseph A., and Barrow, J. Gordon: "Hypertension—A Community Problem," *Am. J. Med.,* **52:**653, (May) 1972.

55. Enselberg, Charles D.: "Measurement of Diastolic Blood Pressure by Palpation," *N. Engl. J. Med.,* **265:**272, (Aug. 10) 1961.

56. Putt, Arlene M.: "A Comparison of Blood Pressure Readings by Auscultation and Palpation," *Nurs. Res.,* **15:**311, (Fall) 1966.

57. Gundersen, Jorgen: "Diagnosis of Arterial Insufficiency with Measurement of Blood Pressure in Fingers and Toes," *Angiology,* **22:**101, 1971.

58. Foley, Mary F.: "Variations in Blood Pressure in the Lateral Recumbent Position," *Nurs. Res.,* **20:**64, (Jan.–Feb.) 1971.

59. Wilcox, Jane: "Observer Factors in Measurement of Blood Pressure," *Nurs. Res.,* **10:**4, (Winter) 1961.

59a. "Correcting Common Errors in Blood Pressure Measurement; Programmed Instruction," *Am. J. Nurs.,* **65:**133, (Oct.) 1965.

60. Glor, Beverly A. K., et al.: "Reproducibility of Blood Pressure Measurements; A Replication," *Nurs. Res.,* **19:**170, (Mar.–Apr.) 1970.

61. Goldman, Mervin J.: *Principles of Clinical*

Electrocardiography, 7th ed. Lange Medical Publications, Los Altos, Calif., 1970, p. 1.

62. Blake, Thomas M.: *Introduction to Electrocardiography*, 2nd ed. Appleton-Century-Crofts, New York, 1972, p. 7.

63. Meltzer, Lawrence E., et al.: *Intensive Coronary Care: A Manual for Nurses.* Coronary Care Unit Fund of the Presbyterian Hospital, Philadelphia, 1965, p. 126.

64. Zalis, Edwin G., and Conover, Mary H.: *Understanding Electrocardiography.* C. V. Mosby Co., St. Louis, 1972, p. 3.

65. Andreoli, Kathleen G.: *Comprehensive Cardiac Care.* C. V. Mosby Co., St. Louis, 1971, p. 52.

66. Zalis, Edwin G., and Conover, Mary H.: *op. cit.,* p. 10.

67. Marriott, Henry J. L.: *Practical Electrocardiography*, 3rd ed. Williams & Wilkins Co., Baltimore, 1962, p. 2.

68. Andreoli, Kathleen G., et al.: *op. cit.,* p. 61.

69. Marriott, Henry J. L.: *op. cit.,* p. 16.

70. Kernicki, Jeanette, et al.: *Cardiovascular Nursing.* G. P. Putnam's Sons, New York, 1970, p. 339.

71. Goldman, Mervin J.: *op. cit.,* p. 1.

72. Marriott, Henry J. L.: *op. cit.,* p. 31.

73. Goldman, Mervin J.: *op. cit.,* pp. 5, 10, 16.

74. Committee on Coronary Care Units and Cardiopulmonary Resuscitation: *Introduction to Arrhythmia Recognition.* California Heart Association, San Francisco, 1968.

75. Meltzer, Lawrence E., et al.: *op. cit.,* p. 126.

76. Bilitch, Michael: *A Manual of Cardiac Arrhythmias.* Little, Brown & Co., Boston, 1971.

77. Andreoli, Kathleen G., et al.: *op. cit.,* p. 70.

78. Sowton, Edgar: "Cardiac Pacemaker and Pacing," *Mod. Concepts Cardiovasc. Dis.,* **36:**31, (June) 1967.

79. Andreoli, Kathleen G., et al.: *op. cit.,* p. 112.

79a. Winslow, Elizabeth Hahn, and Marino, Lynne Brooks: "Temporary Cardiac Pacemakers," *Am. J. Nurs.,* **75:**586, (Apr.) 1975.

80. Zalis, Edwin G., and Conover, Mary H.: *op. cit.,* p. 144.

81. Andreoli, Kathleen G., et al.: *op. cit.,* p. 102.

82. Kernicki, Jeanette, et al.: *op. cit.,* p. 360.

83. Bain, Barbara: "Pacemakers and the People Who Need Them," *Am. J. Nurs.,* **71:**1582, (Aug.) 1971.

83a. Klingemaier, C. H., et al.: "A Method of Computer-Assisted Pacemaker Surveillance from a Patient's Home Via Telephone," *Comput. Biomed. Res.,* **6:**327, (Aug.) 1973.

Additional Suggested Reading

Anderson, Bernice: "Legal Aspects of Nursing Care for Cardiac Patients," *Cardiovasc. Nurs.,* **5:**5, (Mar.–Apr.) 1969.

Aslam, P. A.: "A Simple Method of Flushing Arterial Catheters," *Ann. Thorac. Surg.,* **11:**61, (Jan.) 1971.

Ayres, Stephen M., and Lagerson, Joanne: "Pulmonary Physiology at the Bedside: Oxygen and Carbon Dioxide Abnormalities," *Cardiovasc. Nurs.,* **9:**1, (Jan.–Feb.) 1973.

Barstow, Ruth E.: "Nursing Care of Patients with Pacemakers," *Cardiovasc. Nurs.,* **8:**7, (Mar.–Apr.) 1972.

Bell, Shirley: "Early Morning Temperatures?" *Am. J. Nurs.,* **69:**764, (Apr.) 1969.

Blainey, Carol Gohrke: "Site Selection in Taking Body Temperature," *Am. J. Nurs.,* **74:**1859, (Oct.) 1974.

Broch, Ole J.: "Calibrated Hypoxemia Test in Normal Subjects and Coronary Patients," *Acta Med. Scand.,* **191:**185, (Mar.) 1972.

Callard, George M., and Jude, James R.: "Cardiopulmonary Resuscitation in the Cardiac Care Unit," *Nurs. Clin. North Am.,* **7:**573, (Sept.) 1972.

Chung, Donald K., and Chung, Edward K.: "A Pulse Deficit—Important Findings in Patients with Artificial Pacemakers," *J.A.M.A.,* **219:**1468, (Mar. 13) 1972.

Clark, F. J., and von Euler, C.: "On the Regulation of Depth and Rate of Breathing," *J. Physiol. (Lond.),* **222:**267, (Apr.) 1972.

Cohn, Jay N.: "Central Venous Pressure as a Guide to Volume Expansion," *Ann. Intern. Med.,* **66:**1283, (June) 1967.

Conover, Mary H.: *Cardiac Arrhythmias; Exercises in Pattern Interpretation.* C. V. Mosby Co., St. Louis, 1974.

Conte, Andrea, et al.: "Group Work with Hypertensive Patients," *Am. J. Nurs.,* **74:**910, (May) 1974.

Cross, K. W., et al.: "Lack of Temperature Control in Infants with Abnormalities of Central Nervous System," *Arch. Dis. Child.,* **46:**437, (Aug.) 1972.

Culclasure, David F.: "Medical Benefits from Space Research," *Am. J. Nurs.,* **74:**275, (Feb.) 1974.

Curtin, B. Colleen, and Reick, Kay L.: "Effects of Bodily Position on the Systolic Blood Pressure Response to Valsalva's Maneuver," *Nurs. Res.,* **18:**119, (Mar.–Apr.) 1969.

Dahm, Lida S., and James, L. Stanley: "Newborn Temperature and Calculated Heat Loss in the Delivery Room," *Pediatrics,* **49:**504, (Apr.) 1972.

Delano, Alice, et al.: "Monitoring the Acutely Ill Cardiac Patient," *Cardiovasc. Nurs.,* **7:**61, (Jan.–Feb.) 1971.

Dowd, Judith, and Jenkins, Leonard C.: "The Lung in Shock: A Review," *Can. Anaesth. Soc. J.,* **19:**309, (May) 1972.

Downes, John J., et al.: "Acute Respiratory Failure in Infants and Children," *Pediatr. Clin. North Am.,* **19:**423, (May) 1972.

Doyle, Margaret, and Jordon, Lila E.: "A Comparison of Pulse Deficit Readings by Serial and Simultaneous Measurement," *Nurs. Res.,* **17:**460, (Sept.–Oct.) 1968.

Dyer, Elaine, and Bagnell, Howard K.: "Local Tissue and General Temperature Changes in

Dogs Produced by Temperature Applications," *Nurs. Res.,* **19**:37, (Jan.–Feb.) 1970.

Federspill, Billie: "Renin and Blood Pressure," *Am. J. Nurs.,* **75**:1462, (Sept.) 1975.

Felton, Geraldine: "Effect of Time Cycle Change on Blood Pressure and Temperature in Young Woman," in Downs, Florence S., and Newman, Margaret A. (eds.): *A Source Book of Nursing Research.* F. A. Davis Co., Philadelphia, 1973.

Forsberg, S. A., et al.: "Validity of Blood Pressure Measurement with Cuff in the Arm and Forearm," *Acta Med. Scand.,* **188**:389, 1970.

Geselowitz, D. B.: "Electric and Magnetic Fields of the Heart," *Annu. Rev. Biophysics,* 1973.

Gilbo, Dona: "Nursing Assessment of Circulatory Function," *Nurs. Clin. North Am.,* **3**:53, (Mar.) 1968.

Goldreyer, Bruce N.: "Intracardiac Electrocardiography in the Analysis and Understanding of Cardiac Arrhythmias," *Ann. Intern. Med.,* **77**:117, (July) 1972.

Gorman, M. Leah: "Conscious Repatterning of Human Behavior," *Am. J. Nurs.,* **75**:1752, (Oct.) 1975.

Graas, Suzanne: "Thermometer Sites and Oxygen," *Am. J. Nurs.,* **74**:1862, (Oct.) 1974.

Groom, Dale: "Comparative Efficiency of Stethoscopes," *Am. Heart J.,* **68**:220, (Aug.) 1964.

Hagerman, Charles W.: "Electronic Thermometers," *Nursing '71,* **1**:21, (Nov.) 1971.

Hargest, Thomas S.: "Start Your Count with Zero," *Am. J. Nurs.,* **74**:887, (May) 1974.

Hochberg, Howard M., and Salomon, Harvey: "Accuracy of an Automated Ultrasound Blood Pressure Monitor," *Curr. Ther. Res.,* **13**:129, (Feb.) 1971.

Hurst, J. Willis, and Myerburg, Robert J.: *Introduction to Electrocardiography,* 2nd ed. McGraw-Hill Book Co., New York, 1973.

Indyk, Leonard: "Monitoring in Children—II. Temperature and Blood Pressure," *Clin. Pediatr.,* **11**:157, (Mar.) 1972.

James, Paul M., and Myers, Richard T.: "Central Venous Pressure Monitoring: Misinterpretation, Abuses, Indications and a New Technique," *Ann. Surg.,* **175**:693, (May) 1972.

Johns, Lois A.: "An Experimental Approach to Vigilance in Nursing-Patient Monitoring," in Downs, Florence S., and Newman, Margaret A. (eds.): *A Source Book of Nursing Research.* F. A. Davis Co., Philadelphia, 1973.

Kafka, Heinz L., and Oh, William: "Direct and Indirect Blood Pressure Measurements in Newborn Infants," *Am. J. Dis. Child.,* **122**:426, (Nov.) 1971.

Kannel, William B., and Dawber, Thomas R.: "Atherosclerosis as a Pediatric Problem," *J. Pediatr.,* **80**:544, (Apr.) 1972.

Keller, Margaret R., and Truscott, B. Lionel: "Transient Ischemic Attacks," *Am. J. Nurs.,* **73**:1330, (Aug.) 1973.

Krueger, Jean M.: *Monitoring Central Venous Pressure.* Springer Publishing Co., New York, 1972.

Lahira, Sukhamay, et al.: "Ventilation in Man During Exercise at High Altitude," *J. Appl. Physiol.,* **32**:766, (June) 1972.

Lee, Gertrude M.: "A Rural Hypertension-Control Program," *Am. J. Nurs.,* **74**:1450, (Aug.) 1974.

Lehmann, Sister Janet: "Auscultation of Heart Sounds," *Am. J. Nurs.,* **72**:1242, (July) 1972.

Leonard, James J., and Kroestz, Frank W.: "Lessons Learned Through Intracardiac Phonocardiography," *Mod. Concepts Cardiovasc. Dis.,* **35**:69, (Feb.) 1966.

Lewis, F. John, et al.: "Continuous Patient Monitoring with a Small Digital Computer," *Comput. Biomed. Res.,* **5**:411, (Aug.) 1972.

Liebert, Peter S.: "Central Venous Catheters in Children—Their Placement and Care," *Clin. Pediatr.,* **10**:218, (Apr.) 1971.

Littman, David: "Stethoscopes and Auscultation," *Am. J. Nurs.,* **72**:1238, (July) 1972.

McInnes, Betty: *The Vital Signs, with Related Clinical Measurements: A Programmed Presentation.* C. V. Mosby Co., St. Louis, 1975.

Modell, Jerome H., and Moya, Frank: "Postoperative Pulmonary Complications—Incidence and Management," *Anesth. Analg.,* **45**:432, (July–Aug.) 1966.

Neal, Mary, and Nauen, Claire: "Ability of Premature Infant to Maintain His Own Body Temperature," *Nurs. Res.,* **17**:396, (Sept.–Oct.) 1968.

Neely, William A., et al.: "Postoperative Respiratory Insufficiency: Physiological Studies with Therapeutic Implications," *Ann. Surg.,* **171**:679, (May) 1970.

Nielson, M. A.: "Intra-arterial Monitoring of Blood Pressure," *Am. J. Nurs.,* **74**:48, (Jan.) 1974.

Parsons, Edward F., et al.: "Effect of Positive Pressure Breathing on Distribution of Pulmonary Blood Flow and Ventilation," *Am. Rev. Resp. Dis.,* **103**:356, (Mar.) 1971.

Phibbs, B., et al.: "Transient Myocardial Ischemia: The Significance of Dyspnea," *Am. J. Med. Sci.,* **256**:210, (Oct.) 1968.

Phillips, Raymond E., and Feeney, Mary Kay: *The Cardiac Rhythms. A Systematic Approach to Interpretation.* W. B. Saunders Co., Philadelphia, 1973.

Russin, Ann Woolbert: "Electronic Monitoring of the Fetus," *Am. J. Nurs.,* **74**:1294, (July) 1974.

Schmitt, Yvonne, et al.: "Armchair Treatment in the Coronary Care Unit: Effect on Blood Pressure and Pulse," *Nurs. Res.,* **18**:114, (Mar.–Apr.) 1969.

Singer, B., et al.: "Monitoring of Core Temperature Through the Skin: A Comparison with Esophageal and Tympanic Temperatures," *Bull. N.Y. Acad. Med.,* **51**:947, (Sept.) 1975.

Sitzman, Judith: "Respiratory Problems and the Nurse's Changing Responsibilities," *Cardiovasc. Nurs.,* **6**:41, (May–June) 1970.

Sparrks, Coleen: "Peripheral Pulses," *Am. J. Nurs.,* **75**:1132, (July) 1975.

Strong, William B., et al.: "The Normal Adolescent Electrocardiogram," *Am. Heart J.,* **83:** 115, (Jan.) 1972.

Tate, Gayle, et al.: "Correct Use of Electric Thermometers," *Am. J. Nurs.,* **70:**1898, (Sept.) 1970.

Varady, Paul D., and Maxwell, Morton H.: "Assessment of Statistically Significant Changes in Diastolic Blood Pressures," *J.A.M.A.,* **221:** 365, (July 24) 1972.

Westfall, Una Elizabeth: "Electrical and Mechanical Events in the Cardiac Cycle," *Am. J. Nurs.,* **76:**231, (Feb.) 1976.

Wilber, Joseph A., and Barrow, J. Gordon: "Reducing Elevated Blood Pressure," *Minn. Med.,* **52:**1303, (Aug.) 1969.

Williams, M. Henry, and Shim, Chang S.: "Ventilatory Failure," *Am. J. Med.,* **48:**477, (Apr.) 1970.

Wilson, John N., and Owens, J. Cuthbert: "Continuous Monitoring of Venous Pressure in Optimal Blood Volume Maintenance," *Surg. Forum,* **40:**94, 1965.

Winslow, Elizabeth Hahn: "Digitalis," *Am. J. Nurs.,* **74:**1062, (June) 1974.

Winter, Peter M., and Lowenstein, Edward: "Acute Respiratory Failure," *Sci. Am.,* **221:**23, (Nov.) 1969.

Wood, David W., et al.: "A Clinical Scoring System for the Diagnosis of Respiratory Failure," *Am. J. Dis. Child.,* **123:**227, (Mar.) 1972.

Zipes, Douglas P.: "Interpretation and Significance of Supraventricular Arrhythmia with Abnormal QRS Complex," *Nurs. Clin. North Am.,* **7:**491, (Sept.) 1972.

Gladys Nite
Virginia Henderson

The authors acknowledge the assistance of Dorothy Cumby, R.N., M.S., Instructor of Medical-Surgical Nursing, College of Nursing, Medical University of South Carolina, Charleston, in the preparation of two sections: Electrocardiography and Implanted Pacemakers.

CHAPTER 7

Other Diagnostic Tests and Measurements

1. GENERAL USES

Diagnostic tests and measurements may be used to identify suspected disease or to assess the health status of an individual, a family, a group within a community, or the residents of any geographic unit. The process of health assessment when no disease is suspected is termed "screening." The difference between examinations for health assessment and disease diagnosis is discussed in Chapter 5. Chapter 6 describes the most common health measurements—body temperature, respiration, pulse, blood pressure, and electrocardiography—and they will not be discussed in this chapter even though they are of primary importance in assessing health and diagnosing disease.

Almost any test or measurement discussed in this or other chapters can be used to screen (separate those with specified pathology from those without it) and some may be used to diagnose a disease in a person with signs and symptoms.

Regardless of its purpose, a test will be of most value to the subject, or patient, if the following steps are taken: establishing the need for the test by collecting the necessary data; explaining the need to the patient, parent, or guardian and getting an informed consent (giving such information as may be needed for a wise decision); after selecting the appropriate procedure, explaining it to the subject and preparing him or her for it; providing for infants and children, and others in need of it, a supporting presence when tests are painful or frightening; performing the tests skillfully and expeditiously; analyzing and reporting the test results to the subject and to the health workers involved in the care of the patient; arriving at conclusions and planning further tests if indicated; and, finally, initiating appropriate treatment.

Patients who are frightened or sick and particularly those who are in pain are often relieved to be having diagnostic tests; those who feel well may resist them. Before instituting multiphasic screening it may be necessary to have an educational program to get public acceptance of it.

Screening Tests. Robert M. Thorner defines screening as "the presumptive identification of *unrecognized disease or defect* by the application of tests, examinations or other procedures that can be applied rapidly to sort out apparently well persons who probably have a disease from those who probably do not." * Screening was originally developed to protect the public from the spread of communicable disease and to protect the whole population rather than the individual. Whenever communicable disease control is a problem, mass screening may still be used for this purpose and mass screening techniques are being applied regularly for the

---

* Thorner, Robert M.: "Whither Multiphasic Screening?" *N. Engl. J. Med.,* **280:**1038, (May 8) 1969.

early detection of certain chronic noncommunicable diseases. Health officials all over the world use screening tests along with other investigative methods. Health surveys provide information needed for planning, developing, and implementing health programs that monitor disease trends and patterns in the community. In mass screening programs, those with previously undetected or unreported health problems are identified (as, for example, those with venereal disease by blood tests and those with diabetes by urine tests) and can then be treated. In some instances a screening program is instituted for the protection of a community of people. For example, throat cultures are made on a population exposed to streptococcal disease. Those who have positive cultures are then asked to undergo a medical evaluation and any necessary treatment for protection of the population.

In mass screening programs tests are made once or repeated at specified time periods. An example of a single mass screening program might be that of giving a tuberculin test to a school population exposed to tuberculosis. An example of repeated screening is that of the yearly Papanicolaou test for cervical cancer. One of the objectives of mass screening is to prevent disease, as, for example, when a tuberculin-positive person is discovered, the drug isoniazid is often given for 1 year; another is to alter the outcome of predisposing disease in a community, a group, a family, or an individual, as, for example, when treatment is instituted for an abnormally high reading on glaucoma screening examination. Thus, screening tests are used to make possible early treatment and preventive programs. Another example is blood pressure screening to identify hypertensive individuals and initiate treatment early in the disease to prevent the development of cardiac, renal, and central nervous system complications.

Thus, mass screening tests are made for the purpose of early detection of chronic noncommunicable diseases with a view to their prevention, reversal, or arrest by treatment as well as for the control of communicable disease. How mass screening examinations will be used in the future will depend on scientific and technical development in the world and the evolution of disease patterns. At the present time, the use of mass screening techniques is dependent on safe, simple procedures, the availability of health personnel, the ability to get the test to the desired population, and costs within the reach of the population. Indiscriminate use of screening or diagnostic tests cannot be justified. The present cost of medical care is attributable in part to the number of tests prescribed for an annual health examination.*

Automated procedures promise to revolutionize many kinds of mass screening. Grace A. Cononi and Mildred Siler [1] have described the application of medical electronics to patient care in the hospital. A patient is admitted to the Multitest Center in Waltham, Mass., and receives a broad spectrum of tests beginning with a self-administered medical history. Figure 4-6 in Chapter 4 shows a patient responding to a comparable Medical Questionnaire Console. In Chapter 5 health assessments are discussed that include a comparable battery of tests.

The cost of such a multiphasic screening in 1968 was analyzed at two centers in California by Morris F. Collen and his associates.[2] Examining 500 patients per week in each center was found to cost only $21.32, but this figure may bear little relation to current costs. Personnel staffing for one multiphasic laboratory is shown in Table 7-1.

Another Multiphasic Screening Center sponsored by the Rhode Island Department of Health and located adjacent to Rhode Island Hospital in Providence was described by Herbert R. Constantine [3] in 1968. Its purpose, as a public health facility, is to demonstrate how such a program could be integrated into the existing community health service structure. The floor plan of this unit is shown in Figure 7-1.

Diagnostic Tests. The purpose of diagnostic testing is to get information that will contribute to the determination of the health status of an individual and to diagnose health as well as disease. Jacques Wallach [4] says that laboratory testing may play an important role in the following: discovery of occult disease; prevention of irreparable damage; early diagnosis after onset of signs or symptoms; differential diagnosis of various possible diseases; determining the stage of the disease; estimating the activity of the disease; detecting the recurrence of disease; measuring the effect of therapy; genetic counseling in familial conditions; and solving medicolegal problems such as paternity suits. Although diagnostic testing may either precede or follow the clinical evaluation, it supplements—but does not replace—a carefully taken history, a thorough physical examination, and continuing clinical observation of the individual.

To identify an abnormal finding from a diag-

---

* It is the opinion of the third author that in countries where the fee-for-service system of medical care prevails the expense of diagnostic procedures incident to almost any visit to a doctor often deters many persons from seeking medical advice.

Table 7-1. Personnel Staffing for One Multiphasic Laboratory *

Phase	No.	Type
Registration	2	Receptionists
Electrocardiography	2	Aides
Electrocardiography (file & process)	1	Clerk
Chest x-ray examination	1	Aide
Mammography	2	Aides
(X-ray develop & file)	1	Clerk
Glucose administration	1	Aide
Anthropometry	1	Aide
Blood pressure	1	Nurse aide
Visual acuity	1	Nurse aide
Tonometry	1	Nurse
Respirometry	1	Nurse aide
Ankle test	1	Nurse aide
Hearing	1	Nurse aide
Medical	1	Nurse
questionnaire	1	Nurse aide
Immunization	1	Nurse
Clinical laboratory	5	Technologists
Retinal photography	1	Aide
Retinal photography (file)	½	Clerk
Return appointments	1	Receptionist
Data-input operator	1	Clerk
Supervisor	1	Nurse
Relief	1	Nurse
Appointments	1	Clerk
M.D. supervisor	(25%)	M.D.
Electrocardiographic M.D. reader	(20%)	M.D.
X-ray M.D. reader	(20%)	M.D.
Eye M.D. reader	(20%)	M.D.

* Collen, Morris F., et al.: "Cost Analysis of a Multiphasic Screening Program," *N. Engl. J. Med.*, **280:**1043, (May 8) 1969, p. 1044.

nostic test, it is necessary to define what is normal. In diagnostic testing this is done by making a series of measurements on healthy individuals. For tests in which the results are expressed numerically, these measurements must be made for every single test in order to set up a range of normal values to guide the clinician in his or her interpretation. There may be a wide variation in the normal values due to age, sex, geographic location of the population, the method used to establish values, the equipment used, the expertise of the individuals performing the test, and a number of other unknown variables.

Each laboratory establishes its own set of normal values for every test it performs and for every method used in performing it. This is done by making repeated tests on a number of healthy individuals within a given population. The average spread of scores for 95 per cent of that population is then calculated. These scores are considered to be within the normal range for that laboratory making

that test by its specific method. A value within the normal range can, however, be abnormal for the individual tested, and, conversely, an abnormal value can be normal for the individual tested. Those are judgments made by the clinician responsible for the patient, taking all factors into consideration.[5] (Tables of normal values are given in the Appendix.)

Elihu M. Schimmel [6] conducted a 1964 study among 29 patients in a large teaching hospital and identified 10 minor, 6 moderate, and 13 major reactions to diagnostic tests that resulted in 4 deaths. (See Tables 7-2 and 7-3.) He noted in the following statement that modern medicine had introduced methods that were very effective but also potentially harmful:

To seek absolute safety is to advocate diagnostic and therapeutic nihilism at a time when the scope of medical care has grown beyond previous imagination and power. The dangers of new measures must be accepted and are generally warranted by their benefits, and should not preclude their useful employment. Until safer procedures evolve, however, physicians will best serve their patients by weighing each measure according to its goals and risks, by choosing only those that have been justified, and by remaining prepared to alter the procedures when imminent or actual harm threatens to obliterate their good. *

Paul F. Griner and Benjamin Liptzin,[7] reporting on the overuse of the laboratory in a 1971 study, also in a teaching hospital, indicated that the cost of diagnostic testing amounted to approximately 25 per cent of the average hospital bill. This study also showed that some of the testing led to unnecessary duplication of information. Factors contributing to overuse included concern over missing a diagnosis or changes in the patient's condition, medicolegal considerations, curiosity, the need to do a complete "workup" to satisfy other physicians, and adherence to already established routines that did not relate to the needs of the patient.

Role of Nursing in Screening and Diagnostic Tests. Because everybody knows something about health and is capable of making observations on his or her state of health and the health of others, all persons at one time or another are active participants in health assessment. Individuals and families as guardians of their own health, and all citizens as guardians of the health of their communities share in the responsibility for health assessment with the providers of direct health care and those community health officials who serve the providers. To whatever extent they may be knowledgeable about health, the members of a community are the front-line observers and

* Schimmel, Elihu M.: "The Hazards of Hospitalization," *Ann. Intern. Med.*, **60:**109, (Jan.) 1964.

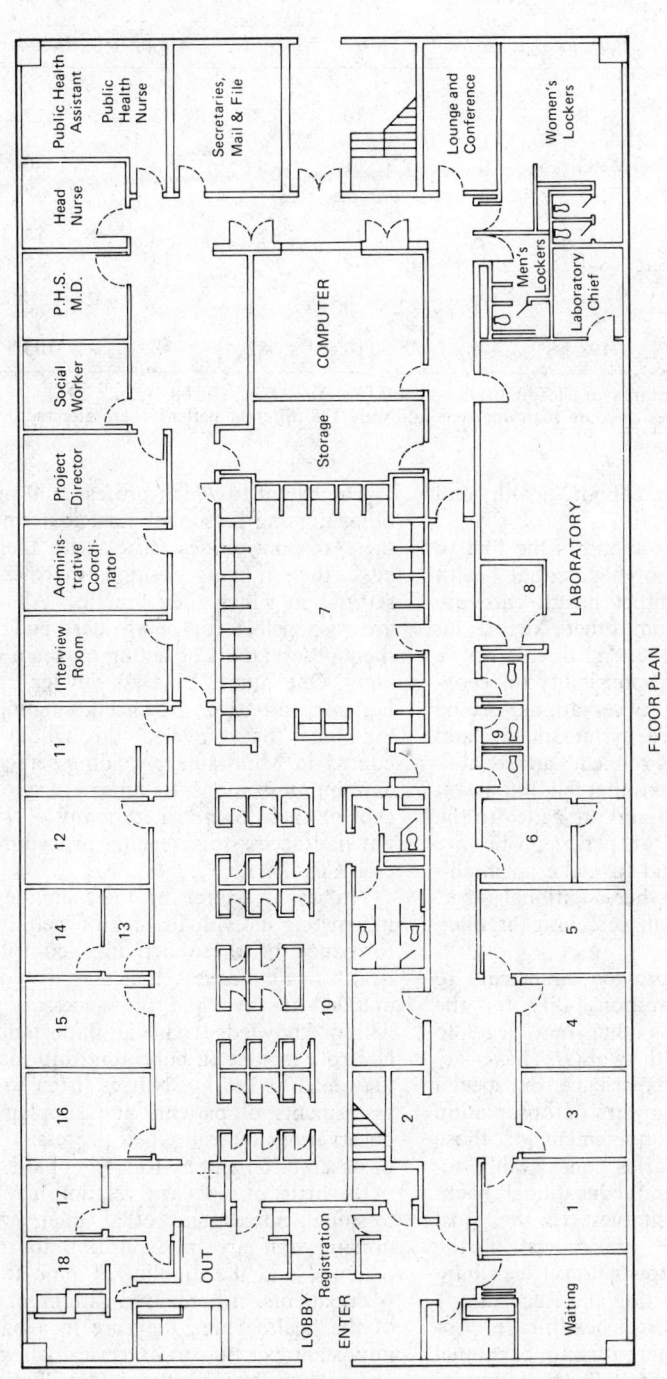

Figure 7-1. Floor plan of Rhode Island Hospital Multiphasic Screening Unit, Providence, R.I.

FLOOR PLAN

Rhode Island Hospital Multiphasic
Screening Unit
Providence, Rhode Island

1. Visual Acuity
2. Glucose Tolerance
3. Achilles Tendon
4. Spirometry
5. Tonometry
6. Audiometry
7. Medical History
8. Blood Drawing
9. Urine Collection
10. Dressing Room
11. Chest X-ray
12. Blood Pressure
13. Height & Weight
14. Retinal Photography
15. Peripheral Vascular
16. Electrocardiogram
17. Mammography
18. Pap Test

489

Table 7-2. Type and Severity of Episodes *

Type of Episode	Number of Patients	Number of Episodes	Number of Episodes of Each Grade			Number of Persistent Episodes	Number of Deaths
			Minor	Moderate	Major		
Reactions to diagnostic procedures	29	29	10	6	13	17	4
Reactions to therapeutic drugs	103	119	61	44	14	46	4
Reactions to transfusions	24	31	17	11	3	9	0
Reactions to other therapeutic procedures	24	24	11	11	2	14	2
Acquired infections	21	23	2	7	14	15	6
Miscellaneous hospital hazards	13	14	9	3	2	4	0
Totals	198 †	240	110	82	48	105	16

* Schimmel, Elihu: "The Hazards of Hospitalization," *Ann. Intern. Med.*, **60**:100, (Jan.) 1964.
† Several patients had episodes of more than one type and only 198 *different* patients were affected.

reporters of information about health and illness.

Although citizens are sometimes the first to detect a health problem or a potential health problem, providers of direct health care are usually the ones to whom others report information. Whoever discovers disease or a health problem has the responsibility to recognize the significance of observations; seeing that the observations are systematically and scientifically confirmed, refined, and elaborated; and making certain that all important observations are recorded and are called to the attention of the person or persons who are able to interpret them and to make an intelligent judgment about whether additional information obtainable through screening or diagnostic testing is needed.

Health workers who provide direct care to people have a special responsibility for the collection of information that may lead to testing because all health workers have acquired through either experience or special preparation heightened powers of observation in health matters. The refinement of those powers of observation varies considerably according to experience and educational background, but from the simplest to the most complex observation, all are crucial in the gathering of necessary information. (See Chapter 4 on Observing, Reporting and Recording.)

Among providers of direct health care, professional nurses and other nursing personnel are particularly important. Because nurses are the largest group of health workers and have many contacts with individuals and families, they are in a unique position to recognize the need for screening and diagnostic tests.

The extent to which professional nurses and other nursing personnel participate in fulfilling these responsibilities varies with their knowledge, their nursing positions or roles, and the settings in which they practice. All, however, are responsible for being alert and reporting their observations or acting on them appropriately. One nurse, Lilja A. Snyder,[8] acting on her own initiative, organized a mobile screening unit that traveled throughout a rural county in Minnesota providing screening tests and immunizations to an average of 39 per cent of each town visited, many of whom had not had access to screening procedures before (see Fig. 7-2).

Nurses, in exercising their unique function in assisting individuals, sick or well, in the performance of those activities contributing to health or its recovery that they would perform unaided if they had the necessary strength, will, or knowledge, have an important and special role to play in collecting information that may lead to testing. Nurses listen to the self-assessments of patients and supplement their observations by using their professional powers of observation and by following patients' leads.

By virtue of the warm relationships that professional nurses and other members of the nursing staff are in a position to form with patients, and the amount of time they spend with patients, as compared with other members of the health team, they are in a particularly important position to exercise their powers of observation in collecting data. Patients may feel more comfortable relating some kinds of self-observations to them. Nurses with their special skills and knowledge may enlarge that observation and rephrase it so that even if the

Table 7-3. Reactions to Diagnostic Procedures *

Agent or Procedure	Manifestation
Test Drugs	
Sulfobromophthalein (BSP)	Shock
Sulfobromophthalein (BSP)	Shock
Sulfobromophthalein (BSP)	Infiltration
Dehydrocholic acid (Decholin)	Infiltration
Histamine	Shock
Endotoxin	Fever and herpes
Premedications	
For bronchoscopy	Shock
For liver biopsy	Shock
Endoscopy	
Esophagoscopy	Perforation
Esophagoscopy	Perforation
Esophagoscopy	Shock
Cystoscopy	Cardiac arrest
Cystoscopy	Pyelonephritis
Bronchoscopy	Dysphagia
Biopsy	
Liver	Hemorrhage
Liver	Peritonitis
Stomach	Perforation
Lymph node	Fistula
Muscle	Paresthesia
Radiography	
Barium enema	Cardiac arrest
Barium enema	Shock
Carotid arteriogram	Hematoma
Carotid arteriogram	Hematoma
Pneumoencephalogram	Fever
Miscellaneous Procedures	
Venous catheterization	Phlebitis
Venous catheterization	Cellulitis
Lumbar puncture	Headache
Reflex percussion	Hemarthrosis
Rebuck test	Dermatitis

* Schimmel, Elihu M.: "The Hazards of Hospitalization," *Ann. Intern. Med.,* **60:**100, (Jan.) 1964.

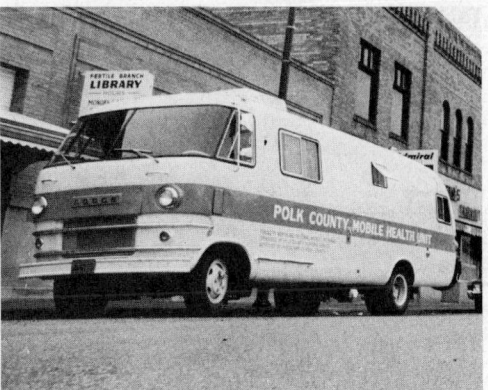

Figure 7-2. A mobile health unit. (From Snyder, Lilja A.: "We Care Enough to Come to You," *Nurs. Outlook,* **22:**168, [Mar.] 1974.)

nurse does not make the interpretation herself, the information can be meaningfully relayed to someone else.

Many diagnostic tests are made entirely by nurses. Their responsibility varies greatly according to the nature of the test and the particular situation. In many cases they are responsible for the preparation of the patient, preparation of the equipment to be used, and frequently collection of specimens. In addition, it may be the nurse's function to see that specimens are properly labeled and transported to the laboratories where they are analyzed. The findings are recorded by those who make the analysis, but nurses usually note on the pa-

tient's record the fact that the test was made.

Labels for specimens should contain the following items of information: the patient's name, his or her address, identifying number, nursing unit, the date and sometimes the hour of collection, the nature of the specimen and type of analysis, and the name (and sometimes the address) of the physician.

Not only are patients interested in the results of the diagnostic tests, but also, according to a small study reported by Alice Dlouhy,[9] 50 per cent or more wanted to know why and how the test would be made, on what part of the body the test was to be made, what they could do to help with the test, what the results of the test would indicate, when and who would tell them the results of the test, if the person performing the test was competent, and if more tests were necessary. (See Table 7-4.)

Jean E. Johnson [10] reports in a study of patients who were to have an endoscopy that stress was significantly reduced if they were given accurate descriptions of the sensations they might expect during the test. Giving preparatory information describing these sensations was more effective than the usual nursing practice of simply describing the procedure.

To reduce some of the stress associated with diagnostic tests, Marjorie H. Bartlett and her associates [11] describe a Dial Access Library–Patient Information Service initiated at four hospitals in Madison, Wisconsin. By dialing, the patient could listen to an authoritative 5-minute message on hospital personnel, diagnostic procedures, general medical subjects, x-ray studies, financial matters, and other subjects. This service enabled the patient to listen repeatedly, if necessary, to information he or she was not able to get from busy hospital staff members. Among the highly selective re-

Table 7-4. Total Response of 96 Patients to Statements on "What Patients Want to Know about Their Medical-Surgical Diagnostic Procedures" *

	Number of Patients Wanting Information				
Statements	All of the Time	Most of the Time	Some of the Time	Never	*No Answer*
I wanted to know					
1. Why the test was being done	72	10	7	6	1
2. Where in the hospital the test would be done	38	13	15	29	1
3. How the test would be done	50	11	17	16	2
4. Who would do the test	41	13	16	26	—
5. How long the test would take	39	12	22	22	1
6. What I could do to help with the test	61	5	13	16	1
7. If I would be uncomfortable	37	14	21	24	—
8. If the test would hurt	44	12	20	20	—
9. If I would be asleep during the test	39	7	21	29	—
10. The results of the test	83	6	5	2	—
11. What the results of the test would mean	84	5	6	1	—
12. When I would be told the results of the test	66	8	12	10	—
13. If this test is done on all hospital patients	11	6	14	62	3
14. What equipment would be used for the test	25	10	20	40	1
15. If the person who would do the test was competent	53	3	4	33	3
16. If the person who would do the test was nice	26	6	8	54	2
17. If the test would interrupt my daily hospital schedule	20	7	15	52	2
18. If I would have to be in a special position	23	9	14	47	3
19. On what part of the body the test was to be done	55	10	12	18	1
20. If I would be able to eat before the test	42	5	21	27	1
21. Who would tell me the results of the test	56	5	12	22	1
22. If more tests would be necessary	61	6	15	14	—
23. How much the test would cost	29	11	15	40	1
24. If the test would lengthen my hospital stay	38	9	15	33	1

* Dlouhy, Alice, et al.: What Patients Want to Know About Their Diagnostic Tests," *Nurs. Outlook,* **11**:266, (Apr.) 1963.

quests from patients were tapes on bladder and kidney x-rays, liver scan, and the myelogram.

Ruth B. Freeman [12] has identified the responsibilities of the community health nurses in motivating people to participate in health screening programs as using all available communication methods to inform people; trying to reach the neediest population through group discussions and home visiting; uncovering people's fears about health screening; facilitating participation by assisting with arrangements and helping to provide follow-up care; and learning more about nonparticipation in health screening. A public health nurse may, for example, note that a number of buildings in a neighborhood have lead-based paint. This may be the initial observation leading to a screening program for lead poisoning. Or a nurse may find an unusual number of infants with diarrhea in a particular geographic area. That observation might be responsible for screening a selected population to identify persons infected with or carriers of shigella. An occupational nurse through contacts with an employee may be responsible for the early detection of an occupationally related illness or a contagious condition defined or confirmed by special testing.

In providing follow-up care after a testing program, Freeman [13] suggests that the nurse's activities include: the provision of health counseling; referral to sources for further study or care; the interpretation to the public of the meaning of the screening examination; and reporting on follow-up outcomes and other data useful in evaluation of the screening activity. She believes that nurses should be so familiar with the screening procedure that they can determine: how *sensitive* and how *specific* were the tests used; what were the criteria for the referral of care; and what can be done to deal with the disease or the subclinical condition discovered.

2. EXAMINATION OF URINE

General Considerations. G. Mary Bradley and Ellis S. Benson state that "Inspection of the urine for diagnostic purposes has been practiced for centuries and probably represents the oldest of laboratory procedures used in medicine today." *

The composition of urine is influenced by the nutritional and metabolic state of the body and by the ability of the kidneys to filter blood, at the same time keeping substances needed for normal functioning and excreting those that are not. Because so many processes are reflected in the composition of urine, urine tests are usually included in every routine health assessment and often are among the first tests to be ordered when disease is present or suspected.

Nursing personnel are often responsible for collecting and temporarily storing urine specimens; for performing certain laboratory tests on them and interpreting the results; and, whenever feasible, for teaching patients how to do these things themselves. Knowledge of the proper techniques and skill in carrying them out are crucial in getting reliable results. A routine urinalysis form is shown in Figure 7-3.

Collection of the Single Urine Specimen. A single urine specimen is the amount passed in one voiding, all of which may or may not be sent to the laboratory for examination. From 100 to 120 ml of urine is sufficient for the usual tests, although much less is needed for most and only a few drops for some. All receptacles used in the collection and transfer of

* Bradley, G. Mary, and Benson, Ellis S.: "Examination of the Urine," in Davidsohn, Israel, and Henry, John H. (eds.): *Todd-Sanford Clinical Diagnosis by Laboratory Methods,* 15th ed. W. B. Saunders Co., Philadelphia, 1974, p. 15.

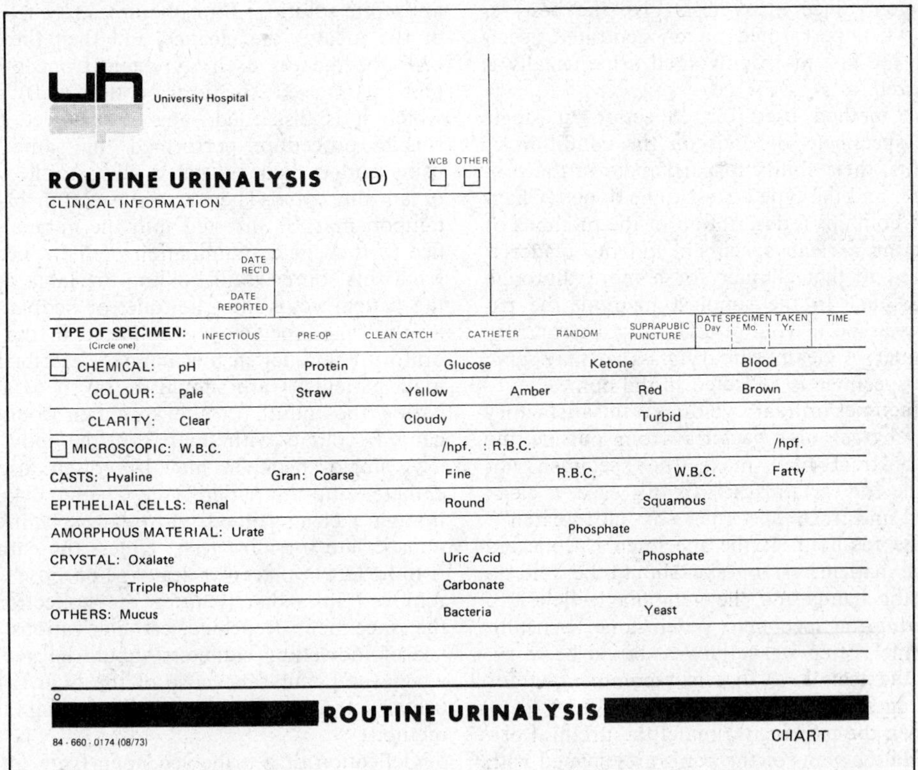
University Hospital

ROUTINE URINALYSIS (D) WCB ☐ OTHER ☐

CLINICAL INFORMATION

DATE REC'D

DATE REPORTED

TYPE OF SPECIMEN: (Circle one) INFECTIOUS PRE-OP CLEAN CATCH CATHETER RANDOM SUPRAPUBIC PUNCTURE | DATE SPECIMEN TAKEN Day Mo. Yr. | TIME

☐ CHEMICAL: pH Protein Glucose Ketone Blood

COLOUR: Pale Straw Yellow Amber Red Brown

CLARITY: Clear Cloudy Turbid

☐ MICROSCOPIC: W.B.C. /hpf. : R.B.C. /hpf.

CASTS: Hyaline Gran: Coarse Fine R.B.C. W.B.C. Fatty

EPITHELIAL CELLS: Renal Round Squamous

AMORPHOUS MATERIAL: Urate Phosphate

CRYSTAL: Oxalate Uric Acid Phosphate

Triple Phosphate Carbonate

OTHERS: Mucus Bacteria Yeast

ROUTINE URINALYSIS

84-660-0174 (08/73) CHART

Figure 7-3. A routine urinalysis form. (Courtesy of University Hospital, University of Western Ontario, London, Ont.)

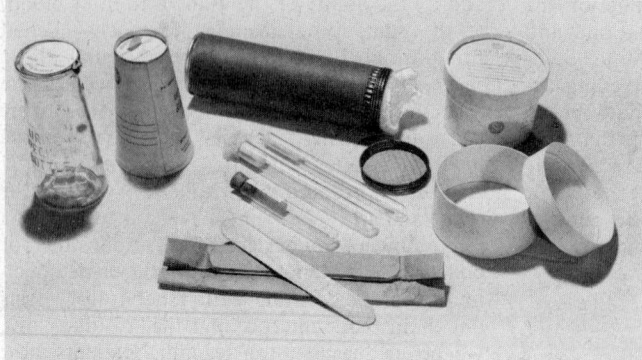

Figure 7-4. Specimen containers. (*Left to right*) A glass and a paper bottle for urine with space on the cap for writing patient's name, etc.; a carton in which a specimen can be mailed; two paper feces containers. Sterile spatulas are used to transfer feces from the bedpan to the paper cup for bacteriologic tests. In the center are sterile test tubes for smears and blood samples. (Courtesy of Clay-Adams Co., New York, N.Y.)

the specimen should be scrupulously clean and dry. A covered transfer container of glass or of disposable plastic should be labeled clearly with the patient's name and identification number, the date, and the tests desired. (For illustrations of specimen containers, see Fig. 7-4). Since urine should be examined while fresh, it should be taken to the laboratory immediately after collection. When delay is unavoidable, the specimen should be refrigerated, or a preservative, such as toluol or thymol, should be added to prevent deterioration of the specimen. Since many tests give the best results when performed on concentrated specimens, the first morning voided urine usually is preferred.

The method used for collection of single urine specimens depends on the condition of patients, their ability to participate in the procedure, and the type of test to be done. (Chapter 24 contains a description of the methods of collecting a clean specimen and the reader is referred to that chapter for a more thorough discussion.) In the simplest method, the patient is asked to void directly into a clean, dry container. A clean ordinary glass jar may serve if the specimen is collected in the home.

Sometimes ordinary voiding is unsatisfactory as discharges and bacteria from outside the urinary tract may make the specimen unsuitable for certain tests. In this case, a clean voided midstream specimen (or "clean catch") may be required. If the specimen is collected by the patient, he or she should be told to wash the hands and the genitalia well before collecting the specimen. When done by health personnel, often sterile gloves should be worn. (For the technique that is recommended for applying sterile gloves, see Chapter 15.)

When the patient is a male, the urethral orifice and the glans of the penis are cleaned with pads containing a mild antiseptic solution and then dried with sterile pads. Next the patient empties the bladder without interrupting the urinary stream. The first and last parts of the stream are allowed to escape into a toilet or urinal, and a small amount of the middle part is collected for analysis in a sterile laboratory container.

When the patient is a female, the cleaning procedure is done while standing over a toilet bowl or kneeling or squatting over a bedpan. The labia minora are separated widely with one hand, and, with the opposite hand, the urethral meatus and the area around it are cleaned with sterile cotton balls saturated with soap or an antiseptic solution. First the areas to each side of the meatus are cleaned and then the area over the meatus itself. A single front-to-back motion is used for each cotton ball, after which it is discarded. This is followed by a rinsing procedure performed the same way using cotton balls saturated with sterile water or an antiseptic. Then a sterile cotton ball or tampon may be inserted into the vaginal orifice to prevent contamination of the specimen from this source. Still holding the labia apart, the patient voids into the toilet or bedpan and a midstream specimen is collected in the laboratory container in the manner described for male patients. Care should be taken to avoid letting the mouth of the specimen container come in contact with any part of the body.

A single specimen may be gotten also by catheterizing the patient (see Chapter 24), although a clean voided midstream specimen is appropriate for most tests. Unless the catheter is to be left in place for drainage purposes, it is removed immediately after the collection of the specimen. Repeated catheterizations and use of indwelling catheters should be avoided whenever possible because of the high risk of urinary tract infection accompanying these methods.

Collection of a urine specimen from infants may be a difficult problem, especially with infant girls. In recent years, the use of pediatric collection bags made of disposable sterile plastic has simplified this procedure. John G. Keuhnelian and Virginia E. Sanders [11] describe this as follows: Single urine specimen bags are open at one end and closed at the other. An adhesive substance surrounds the opening. Bags for collection of multiple voidings are open at both ends, the second opening being attached to tubing that leads to a collection container. Before putting the collecting bags in place, the external genitalia and perineum are washed and dried, and compound tincture of benzoin is spread over the skin where the adhesive surface will be applied. These measures reduce the chances of contaminating the specimen and help protect the skin as well as keep the bag in place. With infant girls, the adhesive surface is put on the outside of the labia majora over the clitoris, urethral meatus, and vaginal orifice. For infant boys, the penis is drawn through the bag opening, and the adhesive surface is secured to the skin around the penis. The scrotum may be drawn through the opening as well as the penis if this can be done easily and without causing constriction. After the bag is in place, a loose fitting diaper is put on the child to help keep the bag in place.

When disposable collecting devices, such as those just described, are not available, a specimen may be collected from a male infant in a test tube held in place with a T-binder having an opening through which the tube is passed. For infant girls, glass vessels that fit over the vulva can be held in place with a T-binder. A simple way of collecting a specimen from a female infant is to place a small tray or shallow pan under the buttocks. The buttocks only rest on the tray. The gown may be turned back or otherwise arranged so that it will not rest on the tray. The edge of the tray, or pan, is padded, and the infant supported and placed in a comfortable position over the pan with pillows and soft restraining cloths until a sufficient amount of urine is collected.

Since collection of urine specimens from babies is difficult, many methods have been tried. At the time the rectal temperature is to be taken, nurses may get an appropriate glass container and, holding a thermometer in the rectum, place the test tube or glass vessel over the penis or vulva. Frequently, the baby voids while the thermometer is in the rectum. In this case the nurse is able to collect the urine specimen *without* the restraining binder. Another method is to apply a cellophane diaper so that there is a collecting portion between the legs. After the baby has voided, the diaper is removed carefully; the nurse then cuts the end of the cellophane diaper so that the urine runs into an appropriate container. Keuhnelian

and Sanders [15] say that, when available, a special mattress with a hole in its center and a collecting container under it may be used instead of the cellophane diaper.

When patients are to collect a specimen and bring it to the laboratory for examination, instructions should state the method of collection, the hour of collection, the amount necessary, and the kind of container to use. Generally speaking, a container with a screw top is preferable to one with a cork. State and city departments of health often provide containers and cartons for mailing, if the specimen is to be examined in their laboratories. This equipment may include a receptacle for collecting the specimen as well. In this instance the urine specimen cannot be examined while fresh, so a preservative is provided in the container.

Collection of a Timed Urine Specimen. A timed urine specimen is collected when it is desirable to make a quantitative rather than a qualitative analysis. While the qualitative urine specimen shows the constituents of the urine, only the timed specimen—the total amount secreted by the kidneys over a timed interval, usually 24 hours—will show what substances the kidneys are eliminating and the quantity of each. The diagnosis, diet, and general treatment of the patient may to a large extent be based on the findings of this examination; therefore, extreme care should be exercised in the collection of the specimen to ensure that it represents all urine voided during the specified period. The collection of the specimen is frequently started before breakfast at 8:00 A.M., as this seems to be a convenient hour to begin and end collection. If this time period is adopted, the patient should void at 8 o'clock the first morning and discard the urine. (This urine may have been excreted and then stored in the bladder for a considerable length of time before the 24-hour collection period.) After this, all urine voided up to and including 8:00 A.M. of the following morning must be collected in the specimen container and sent to the laboratory. It is important that the patient void at exactly 8:00 A.M. on the second morning to complete the collection of all the urine excreted by the kidneys in the 24-hour period and to make possible an accurate estimate of their function.

A 24-hour urine specimen is collected in a large container (usually a glass bottle) properly labeled and stoppered as suggested for the single specimen. To prevent deterioration of the specimen, a preservative, usually toluol, is added to the container at the beginning of the collection period or the container is refrigerated until sent to the laboratory. The equipment used to collect each voiding should be dry and clean to avoid diluting the specimen, adding to its volume, or introducing contaminants.

If possible, patients should not void at the same time as they defecate. Collecting the urine first in a separate container will make sure the specimen is not contaminated. If by accident urine should be lost or mixed with fecal matter, a note should be made of this on the specimen container and on the patient's chart.

Reagent Tablets, Papers, and Dip Sticks. In recent years, many tablets, papers, and dip sticks containing test reagents have been developed. This has made it possible for nonlaboratory health personnel, and in some cases patients and their families, to perform a variety of urine and other tests easily, quickly, and economically. Regardless of who uses these testing materials, it is essential that the manufacturer's directions be followed carefully to get accurate results. Since the principles for using the reagent strips are the same for many tests, a basic procedure for their use is described in the following and is taken from material in *Todd-Sanford Clinical Diagnosis by Laboratory Methods* edited by Israel Davidsohn and John H. Henry.[16]

Dip sticks are strips of nonreactive material that contain reactive chemicals or reagents impregnated on paper at one end. When this part is moistened with urine or other body fluids, the chemicals change color or remain the same depending on the composition of the fluid. Some dip sticks contain only one reagent strip and are used to test the presence of only one substance, while others contain several reagent strips and may be used to test for several substances at the same time. Only the number of dip sticks needed are removed from the container at the time of testing and the container cover is replaced immediately. Care is taken not to touch the reagent end and to avoid contaminating it with solid, liquid, or volatile substances in the testing area. A clean sheet of paper on a clean, dry surface may be used should it be necessary to put the dip stick down before using it. The entire reagent end is dipped in the specimen and is removed immediately. Excess fluid is removed by gently touching the stick against the mouth of the specimen container. After the length of time designated by the manufacturer has passed, the reagent end is held close to the manufacturer's color chart to read the results. Readings should be made only under good lighting conditions. To prevent loss of sensitivity, dip sticks should be kept in tightly capped containers in a cool —but not cold—dry place. If the reagent end of the dip stick is discolored, it should not be used.

Tests Made on Single Specimens. A *routine urinalysis* consists of many tests that are routinely made on a single urine specimen. Because a large amount of valuable information about the over-all functioning of the body can be gotten easily and inexpensively from a routine urinalysis, it usually is included as a screening measure in the health examination, upon admission to a hospital, before an operation, and in many other instances. Although there is variation from one laboratory to another, a routine urinalysis usually includes inspection of its appearance; determination of pH and specific gravity; test for the presence, or absence, of glucose, ketones, and protein; and microscopic examination of the sediment. These and the other commonly performed urine tests as described below are based on Davidsohn and Henry [17] unless another source is cited.

The appearance of normal urine is clear amber, although it may be pale yellow when fluid intake is high or dark yellow when it is low. Certain diseases, foods, and drugs also may influence the color of urine. For example, cloudy urine may be caused by the presence of white blood cells and bacteria, which usually indicates infection. Bleeding from the urinary tract, eating beets or rhubarb, or taking cascara may be the cause of red urine; or this may be the result of bleeding from the female genital tract, as in menstruation. Abnormal excretion of bilirubin, such as occurs in hepatitis and other biliary tract diseases, may turn urine various shades of yellow, orange, or brown.

The *odor* of freshly voided urine in health is usually faintly sweet. Unpleasant or strange-smelling urine may be one of the first indications of disease. An early sign of urinary tract infection, for example, may be voided urine with a strong, unpleasant odor. Certain foods may also affect the smell of urine. Asparagus, for example, produces a characteristically strong, unpleasant-smelling urine. Because nursing personnel often help patients with elimination, careful observation of the appearance and odor of urine is an important screening function which they may exercise whether specimens are collected or not.

The *pH* of urine refers to whether it is acid or alkaline and is a rough measure of the ability of the kidneys to regulate the acid-base balance of the body. Although in healthy individuals the pH may vary between 4.6 and 8, urine is usually acid. The average pH is 6.3, because on a mixed, or average, diet more foods are eaten that on metabolism yield acid waste products than yield alkaline products. The reaction, however, may vary somewhat with diet.

The urinary pH may affect the natural course of some conditions and their treatment. Some kinds of kidney stones, for example, form more easily in acid than alkaline urine, while the reverse is true for others; the sulfonamides and certain antibiotics used to treat urinary tract infections are found to be more effective when the urine is acid. A diet high in meat or in certain fruits, such as cranberries, produces acid urine, while a predominantly vegetable diet or one high in citrus fruits produces an alkaline urine. Certain drugs also affect the urinary pH. Ammonium chloride, for example, produces an acid urine and acetazolamide (Diamox) produces an alkaline urine. Most often, indicator paper is used to estimate pH, but more precise measurement may be made by other means.

The *specific gravity* of urine depends on the amount of solids in it in proportion to the amount of water. It is based on water as a standard—1 liter of water at a certain temperature weighs 1000 gm and has a specific gravity of 1.000. Urine is heavier than water because of the solids contained in it. The specific gravity of randomly obtained, normal urine varies from 1.016 to 1.022 when fluid intake is normal.

A urinometer or hydrometer is commonly used to measure specific gravity. The large end of the urinometer is inserted with a spinning motion into a test-tube-like container three quarters full of urine. The instrument should not touch the sides or bottom of the container. The reading is taken from the calibrated end of the urinometer at the bottom of the meniscus formed by the urine at its surface. The more concentrated the urine, the more the urinometer is buoyed up above the urine, giving a higher specific gravity reading, and the reverse is true for dilute urine.

Specific gravity may also be estimated by using a refractometer, an instrument that measures how much light rays are bent when they are shown through a special glass container holding a few drops of urine. The principle of the test is that the solids in urine bend light more than the water in it. The more concentrated the urine, therefore, the more it will bend the light rays, indicating a higher reading.

When a more precise measure of urine concentration is desired, *urine osmolality* is calculated. As the number of molecules and ions in a solution influence its properties, the same properties of different solutions may be compared using water as a base. Tests for urine osmolality make use of this principle. For example, in one commonly used method, the osmolality of a urine specimen is determined by measuring its freezing point. As it is known

that 1 milliosmole * (mosmol) of solute per kilogram (kg) of water will lower the freezing point of a solution 1.67°C (35°F) below that of water 0°C (32°F), measuring the freezing point of urine makes it possible to calculate its osmolality. For a normally hydrated, healthy adult on a normal diet, urine osmalality varies between 500 and 850 mosmol per kg of water.

Protein circulates in the blood to supply the cells and forms a necessary constituent of all body cells. Normally in the urine there is a small amount of protein but not enough to be detected by the ordinary tests used. In inflammation of any part of the urinary tract—kidneys, ureters, or bladder—an abnormal amount of protein, usually albumin, may be present in the urine. Inflammation may occur as a result of bacterial invasion, poisoning, or circulatory disturbances. Some people are said to have a functional disturbance of the kidneys; that is, the urine contains protein without having inflammation of the kidneys whenever fever is present, when there is emotional stress, after a cold bath or excessive exercise, or when eating a high-protein diet. The presence of protein in the urine, however, often is an indication of serious kidney disease which is important to recognize in its early stages. This fact is so generally accepted that no life insurance policy is granted without testing the urine for protein.

Tests for protein may be made with reagent strips containing bromphenol. Color changes occur in the presence of clinically significant amounts of urinary protein at a pH of 3 or more. Results are reported as "trace," or 1+ to 4+, depending on the amount of protein present. Positive tests should be confirmed in the laboratory by the heat and acetic acid test which is more sensitive than reagent strips. Calculation of the total protein excreted in 24 hours may be made from 24-hour urine specimens when even more accurate estimates are desired. If abnormal amounts of protein are detected in urine, an additional test is needed to find out if Bence Jones protein † is present. This type of protein is excreted in urine of half the patients with the disease multiple myeloma, a type of bone cancer; in only a few other disease states is it found.

Glucose is present in small amounts in normal urine and is not detectable by standard screening tests. Eating a large amount of carbohydrates or being excited or in pain may

* A milliosmole (mosmol) is defined as one thousandth of an osmole, the standard unit used in measuring osmotic pressure.
† So named for the English physician Henry Bence Jones (1813–1873).

temporarily cause a marked increase of sugar in the urine in a perfectly healthy person. Some healthy people have a particularly low renal threshold for glucose. The presence of detectable amounts, however, usually indicates that the patient is suffering from a very serious disease—diabetes mellitus. In this disease body cells are unable to burn the normal amount of sugar supplied them as fuel, and so they have difficulty producing the necessary heat and energy for normal body processes. If sugar taken in as food cannot be used fully by the diabetic, the level of glucose in the blood becomes abnormally high and exceeds the renal threshold so glucose is eliminated through the urine. Urinary tract infections are a frequent complication of diabetes, although it is believed that factors other than glycosuria provide a favorable growth media for bacteria which may account for the high incidence of infections in patients with diabetes mellitus. Chronic kidney disease often also occurs as a complication of diabetes mellitus, but high amounts of glucose in the urine do not necessarily indicate that this complication is present. Indeed, chronic kidney disease may cause an elevation of the renal threshold for glucose and thus lower or eliminate detectable glucose in the urine.

There are several commonly used screening tests for urinary glucose based on color changes of the reagent or tape or in solution. The glucose oxidase paper strip method, Testape,* is the easiest and most specific method available. Two other tests used are Benedict's and the Clinitest † tablet methods. Both are based on the fact that glucose is a reducing agent; that is, it will precipitate or separate copper from its compounds. These tests are less specific than the glucose oxidase paper strip method because the reagents are reduced by nonglucose sugars, uric acid, creatinine, and other substances in the urine. Ascorbic acid, a drug frequently given therapeutically or as a stabilizer in some antibiotics, will delay color changes in glucose-positive urines, and acetylsalicylic acid given in high doses may also give falsely low results.

To perform *Benedict's test,* put 5 ml of the reagent and 8 drops of urine in a test tube. Put the tube in a rack in a water bath of boiling water and keep the water boiling. At the end of exactly 5 minutes, remove the tube. Care must be taken to point the tube away from the face as rapid boiling often shoots the fluid out. If the fluid is opaque, it indicates the presence of sugar. If no sugar is present, the fluid re-

* Eli Lilly and Company, Indianapolis, Ind.
† Ames Company, Elkhart, Ind. (Clinitest)

mains clear or only a faint turbidity due to urates results. The color reactions are shown in the package insert.

For the *Clinitest* method, put 5 drops of urine and 10 drops of water in a test tube; add one reagent tablet. Do not shake the test tube during the reaction or for 15 seconds after boiling inside the test tube has stopped. Then shake the test tube gently and compare the color of the solution with the color scale to determine the presence and amount of sugar in the urine. In this test external heat has been eliminated, since the reagent tablet generates heat. The color scale of the Clinitest reaction is shown as an insert in the package.

Ketones are formed when fat metabolism is incomplete. When fat replaces carbohydrate as the main source of energy for the body, as, for example, in diabetes mellitus or starvation, ketones are detectable in the urine. Because excessive amounts of sodium and potassium are excreted with ketones, the buffering system of the body is altered. Ketoacidosis, which may be fatal if severe and untreated, can result. Other conditions in which ketones may be detectable in urine include those in which the patient has a fever, vomiting, or diarrhea, or after excessive exercise or exposure to cold. Reagent tablet and dip stick tests are based on the principle that sodium nitroprusside reacts with one type of ketones in the presence of a base.

The urine of diabetics often is tested four times a day for glucose and ketones. Specimens are collected before breakfast and 2 to 3 hours after each meal. To be certain that the specimens contain only urine excreted near the time of collection, a "double-voided" technique is usually adopted. With this technique, the patient is instructed to void half an hour before the time specified for collection and to discard the urine; to void again in 30 minutes and have this specimen tested. However, Jerome M. Feldman and Francine L. Lebovitz [18] have reported evidence that this method of urine collection may give misleading results if two or more glasses of water are drunk during the half hour before the test specimen is collected as significant overreading may occur with dilute urine.

Susan M. Williams,[19] in a study of glucose and ketone tests made by nursing personnel, found that 36 per cent of the tests were interpreted incorrectly. She found that there were a significant number of errors when the people making the tests performed them more than three times a week and when they knew the results of the patients' previous tests. Because the primary reason for testing the urine of a diabetic is to find out if adjustment of medication is needed, such a high frequency of errors in interpretation is very serious. Too much or too little medication may be prescribed on the basis of inaccurate test information and may result in life-threatening complications. The need for strict discipline in carrying out testing procedures correctly and interpreting the results with strict objectivity is obvious.

The *urinary sediment* is examined microscopically after centrifuging a specimen and pouring off the supernatant fluid. This examination should be made only on very fresh, concentrated urine. If the specimen cannot be analyzed immediately it should be refrigerated; but even this procedure may not prevent the loss of valuable information if there is a delay of 1 hour or more. Normally urinary sediment includes epithelial cells, inorganic crystals, and a *very* small number of blood cells and protein casts of the renal tubules. In the presence of disease, however, these constituents may increase. The entire urinary tract is lined with epithelium, some cells of which are constantly being worn out and shed into the urine (just as cells of the outer skin are shed), so that epithelial cells will normally be found in urine. Epithelial cells shed from the genital tract also appear as contaminants in urine, especially urine from women. The number of epithelial cells found in urine increases in various kinds of diseases of the kidney and urinary tract; therefore, it is especially important for women to use the vaginal tampon technique to increase the reliability of the urinalysis.

Many types of crystals are found in normal urine but are not usually noted in the urinalysis report unless there is a predominance of one kind, an abnormal type is seen, or the specimen comes from a patient prone to kidney stone formation and the laboratory has a special request. Little is known about the mechanism by which red and white blood cells enter the urine. Both types of cells may be increased in number in either renal or lower urinary tract disease. An increased number of renal casts is usually indicative of kidney disease be they red blood cell or white blood cell casts; hyaline and epithelial casts may not indicate disease.

Microorganisms are not found in normal urine unless they are contaminants from feces, the genital tract, or other sources. In a specimen collected by clean catch, catheterization, or direct bladder puncture their presence usually indicates urinary tract infection.

When red blood cells cannot be seen by microscopic methods, *occult blood and hemoglobin* can be detected in urine by reagent tablets and strips containing orthotolidine. False positive results occur when specimens contain potassium iodide, large numbers of bacteria, or myoglobin—a protein excreted in urine when skeletal muscle is damaged. False negative results occur when large amounts of ascorbic acid are present.

Bilirubin, present in normal urine at about 0.02 mg in 100 ml of urine, is increased in certain liver and biliary tract diseases. Specimens containing large amounts of bilirubin may be various shades of dark yellow, orange, or brown; and when shaken, they will produce yellow foam. The diazo method * is convenient for screening. Using this method, put 5 drops of urine on an asbestos-cellulose mat and place a reagent tablet on the moistened area. Put 2 drops of water on the tablet and observe the color in 30 seconds. A blue or purple ring on the mat around the tablet indicates a positive result, a pink or red color a negative result. The reagent tablets should be protected from moisture, prolonged exposure to light, and temperatures of 37.8°C (100°F) or more.

Phenylpyruvic acid, an intermediate product of metabolism of the essential amino acid, phenylalanine, is not found in normal urine; but it can be detected in the urine of people with phenylketonuria (PKU), an inborn error of phenylalanine metabolism. As this disease usually results in mental retardation when not detected and treated early, Richard Ravel [20] says that some states require screening tests to be made on all newborns.

A convenient screening test is available in which a reagent strip is dipped in urine or pressed against a wet diaper and then compared with a color chart. Because the test may be negative until 3 to 6 weeks after the birth of a phenylketonuric infant, when some brain damage may already have occurred, a blood screening test (the Guthrie test), which becomes positive earlier, is preferred, according to Ravel.[21]

Tests for pregnancy are based on the fact that chorionic gonadotropin, a hormone that is produced by living placental tissue shortly after the implantation of the fertilized ovum, is excreted in the urine. It may be detected readily in the urine by a number of biologic and immunologic tests. Though not infallible, the tests are highly accurate and are of value when it is desirable to make an early diagnosis of pregnancy. The principle on which the biologic tests are based is that when urine containing chorionic gonadotropin is injected into female mice, rabbits, or rats, characteristic anatomic changes occur in their ovaries. Davidsohn and Henry [22] describe the test de-

---

* Icotest made by Ames Co., Elkhart, Ind.

veloped by Selmar Aschheim and Bernhard Zondek (*A-Z test*) whose original method has been modified by others to decrease the time required, and to increase the convenience and simplicity. A more commonly used test is the *Friedman test.* A morning urine specimen is collected after restriction of fluids from 8:00 P.M. the evening before, and of salicylates and sedatives for at least 48 hours. Ten milliliters of the specimen is injected into the ear vein of a nongravid mature female rabbit. Forty-eight hours after injection the rabbit is killed and the ovaries explored for the presence of hemorrhagic ruptured follicles, which is a positive reaction, or indicates that the injected urine was from a pregnant woman.

Some immunologic tests for pregnancy are cheaper and faster than biologic tests and are based on the principle that human urine containing chorionic gonadotropin will react with specific antibodies. Thus some even newer urine tests for the early diagnosis of pregnancy can give the answer after only a short wait in the physician's office or clinic.

Both biologic and immunologic tests may detect chorionic gonadotropin in urine in very early pregnancy, but false negatives are common until 20 days after the last normal menstrual period and during the second and third trimesters of pregnancy. Both kinds of tests are positive in the presence of ectopic pregnancy, hydatidiform mole, and some types of ovarian and testicular tumors. They are used as diagnostic aids when these conditions are suspected.

Cytologic studies of cells sloughed from the lining of the urinary tract are of value in detecting carcinoma of the bladder. To make this test, part of a single urine specimen is combined with an equal amount of 70 per cent alcohol. A slide of the centrifuged sediment is prepared with Papanicolaou stain and the cells are examined for malignant characteristics.

Tests Made on Timed Urine Specimens. The following descriptions of tests are also based on Davidsohn and Henry.[23]

The *volume* of urine excreted over a 24-hour period is a simple and often used test of kidney function. The test is made by collecting in a large container all urine eliminated during a timed interval and then measuring the total. Normal adult 24-hour values range between 600 and 2000 ml, with an average of 1200 to 1500 ml. When urine excretion exceeds 2000 ml a day, the condition is called "polyuria." This may occur when fluid intake is excessive; when diuretic substances such as coffee, alcohol, or chlorothiazide are taken; and when certain diseases are present. In diabetes mellitus, for example, the kidney excretes large amounts of water to reduce the concentration of glucose present in the urine. In diabetes insipidus, a disease in which the secretion of an antidiuretic hormone by the posterior pituitary is disturbed, the ability of the kidneys to reabsorb water is decreased, with resulting polyuria. In some chronic kidney diseases, the kidneys lose their ability to concentrate urine. When less than 50 ml of urine is excreted in 24 hours, the condition is called "oliguria." This occurs in severe dehydration, shock, transfusion reactions, and some kidney diseases such as acute glomerulonephritis and severe chronic nephritis.

Creatinine, an end-product of muscle metabolism, is excreted in the urine by normal kidneys at a fairly constant rate regardless of the metabolic status of the body, urine volume, and diet. With kidney damage, the ability of the kidneys to clear the blood of creatinine is decreased. Thus, measurement of *creatinine clearance* is a useful test of kidney function, specifically of the glomerular filtration rate (GFR). Careful collection of all urine excreted over 24 hours is crucial in obtaining accurate results. Normal 24-hour values for men are 1000 to 1900 mg and for women are 800 to 1700 mg, assuming average weight.

Kidney function can also be measured by the *urea clearance test* in which the total urea excreted over a certain period, usually 2 hours, is measured. This test, however, is considered unreliable and is almost never done.

When the concentration, i.e., the specific gravity (as determined by hydrometer or refractive index) or osmolality (as determined by freezing point depression) of a specimen is abnormal, a *dilution* or *concentration test* may be made. These tests are based on the principle that the normal kidney adjusts the specific gravity according to the state of hydration of the patient. For example, with an increased fluid intake, more water will be excreted, and the urine will be dilute, and will have a low specific gravity; if water is withheld, the urine will become concentrated. Dilution and concentration tests measure the functional capacity of the kidneys, submitting them to extreme conditions. The second category of tests gives more information about kidney function than the first. In a convenient concentration test used today, the patient is allowed to eat supper, after which he or she is permitted nothing by mouth. Urine specimens passed during the evening and the first specimen of urine voided the next morning are discarded. The second voided morning specimen is tested for specific gravity or osmolality. If that specimen is normal, fluids are restricted for another 6 hours and a second specimen is collected and tested. Specific gravity values below 1.026 or osmolality values below 850 mosmol per kilogram indicate impaired concentrating ability of the kidneys. This test is dangerous when done in the presence of the disease diabetes insipidus.

A useful test for determining renal blood flow is the *phenolsulfonphthalein excretion test* (PSP). To administer this test to adults, 6 mg of phenolsulfonphthalein, which is a dye excreted only by the kidneys, is given intravenously and the exact time is noted. Urine is collected at 15, 30, 60, and 120 minutes. An instrument known as a colorimeter is used to determine the amount of dye excreted in the urine. Thirty minutes before the dye is given, patients drink 600 ml (three glasses) of water to make sure they can void at the specified times. For reliable results, at least 40 ml of urine must be voided each time it is collected, and additional hydration during the test may be necessary to get this volume. All the urine collected at each voiding is saved in separate containers and sent to the laboratory for examination. Normally, 20 to 50 per cent of the dye is eliminated in the 15-minute voiding, 16 to 24 per cent in the 30-minute voiding, 9 to 17 per cent in the 60-minute voiding, and 3 to 10 per cent in the 120-minute voiding. The amount of dye excreted in the first specimen is the most sensitive indicator of renal blood flow. Although the rapid hydration required for the test is usually tolerated well, it may dangerously overload the circulatory system of patients with conditions where there is severely limited renal blood flow, as in advanced vascular and kidney diseases.

The *Addis count* is a useful test for following the course of certain kidney diseases, such as acute glomerulonephritis. Urine is collected overnight for 6, 9, or 12 hours during a period of food and fluid restriction. During the collection period, all voidings are stored, unrefrigerated, in a container that has been rinsed with 10 per cent formaldehyde. The number of red and white blood cells and casts are estimated by microscopic examination of a centrifuged sample of the total. Normal 12-hour values for adults are 0 to 1,800,000 white cells, 0 to 500,000 red blood cells, and 0 to 5,000 casts.

Urobilinogen, a reduced product of bile, is found in normal urine in the amount of 0.5 to 2.5 mg in 24 hours. The amount is increased in the hemolytic anemias (those in which red blood cell destruction occurs) and in liver diseases. With complete bile duct obstruction, it may be absent. Although single and 24-hour specimens may be tested for urobilinogen, a 2-hour test is more often used. As urinary urobilinogen excretion is thought to be highest in the afternoon, specimens are collected exactly at the beginning and the end of a 2-hour afternoon interval, commonly 1:00 and 3:00 P.M. The first specimen is discarded and the second is sent to the laboratory for the test. Should

the patient have to void during the interval, this urine is collected and tested, also. To get accurate results, the specimens should be analyzed within 30 minutes after the collection period. Twenty-four-hour specimens require refrigeration as well as the addition of a preservative during the collection period.

Inorganic salts are most often measured in plasma, but sometimes it is important to know the quantities being excreted in urine. *Sodium* and *potassium* urine levels vary with diet, but when dietary intake is normal, 24-hour values are 80 to 180 mEq for sodium and 80 to 180 mEq for potassium. In adrenal cortex dysfunction, the ratio between sodium and potassium excretion may be altered drastically. *Chloride* excretion varies with sodium and potassium excretion as well as with other urine constituents. When the amount of *calcium* in the diet is normal, 50 to 300 mg of calcium is excreted in the urine. This amount is increased in some endocrine diseases, for example, hyperthyroidism and hyperparathyroidism, and in osteoporosis. Low urine calcium is seen in hypoparathyroidism and vitamin D deficiency.

17-Ketosteroids and *17-hydroxycorticoids* are hormones excreted by the adrenal cortex and eliminated in the urine. Twenty-four-hour urine measurements of these hormones may be made when primary or secondary diseases of the adrenal cortex are suspected. Specimens are stored in the refrigerator with a preservative during the collection period. Normal 24-hour 17-ketosteroid values for men are 8 to 15 mg and for women 6 to 11.5 mg. The normal values of 17-hydroxycorticoids range from 5.5 to 14.5 mg for men and 4.9 to 12.9 mg for women although these values may be various among different laboratories. Drugs, particularly tranquilizers, interfere with these tests and should be stopped 48 hours before specimen collection begins.

Several methods for evaluating the function of the adrenal medulla are available. *Catecholamines*—epinephrine and norepinephrine—are hormones secreted by the adrenal medulla and eliminated in the urine. Measurements of these substances in the urine along with their metabolites, such as *vanillymandelic acid* (VMA) may be made when catecholamine-producing tumors, such as pheochromocytomas, are suspected. As these tumors may cause hypertension, one or more of these tests may be included in the laboratory work-up of hypertensive patients. Twenty-four-hour specimens are collected in a brown bottle * containing 1 ml of concentrated hydrochloric acid. Values for catecholamines above 100 mcg and

---

* A brown bottle is used to avoid exposure of the specimen to light rays that may alter the test result.

for VMA above 7 mg are abnormal for adults. Coffee, chocolate, vanilla, fruits, and drugs should be eliminated from the diet 48 hours before VMA specimen collection begins, as these substances will distort the results.

3. EXAMINATION OF BLOOD

Methods of Getting Specimens. The method of getting blood for examination depends on the type of test to be made. Venous, capillary, or arterial blood may be used. For most tests the required amount of blood is aspirated from a vein by venipuncture. Except for a few tests that require a fasting sample, blood usually is collected following breakfast. Unless otherwise indicated, the following methods of getting blood specimens are based on Davidsohn and Henry.[21]

A commercially prepared unit of needle holder, sterile disposable double-ended needle, and vacuumized test tube (see Fig. 7-5) is commonly used in the United States. When such a unit is unavailable, a sterilized needle and syringe may be used instead. In this case if the equipment is to be reused, it should be sterilized as described in Chapter 32. Commercially prepared media and containers into which blood is injected for blood culture are also available.

When using the sterile disposable unit shown in Figure 7-5, a venipuncture is made while loosely holding the vacuumized test tube in the tube holder. (For the suggested technique for venipuncture, see Chapter 22.) After entering the vein with the long end of the double needle, the needle is held securely and the test tube is pushed firmly toward the head of the tube holder so that the short end of the double needle below its hub punctures the rubber top of the test tube. This breaks the vacuum inside the test tube and blood is drawn into it. When the filling stops, the test tube is removed; if more specimens are needed, additional test tubes are inserted into the holder in the same way and removed; the needle and holder may then be removed from the vein.

When an ordinary needle and syringe are used, the total amount of blood needed is collected in the syringe before removing the needle from the vein. The appropriate amount of blood is then injected slowly into sealed test tubes, avoiding air contact in the case of blood cultures and hemolysis in other cases by first removing the needle from the syringe and slowly injecting the blood into the tube.

If whole blood or blood plasma is required for a test, an anticoagulant such as potassium and ammonium oxalate, trisodium citrate, ethylene diamine tetraacetic acid (EDTA), or heparin is placed in the test tube to keep the blood from clotting; if serum is desired, the blood is placed in an empty test tube and allowed to clot. Immediately after the blood has been collected in a container with anticoagulant, it should be mixed thoroughly by *gently* rotating the container in order to prevent clotting. If no anticoagulant is present in the container, it should be allowed to remain undisturbed at room temperature for 15 to 20 minutes so that it clots properly. Shaking whole blood promotes hemolysis which makes most specimens useless for many tests.

Veins in the inner aspect of the elbow (antecubital fossa) and on the back of the hand are commonly used for venipuncture; but veins in other places, such as the feet, or, in infants, the scalp, may be used when blood cannot be gotten from the arm or hand. When it is thought that the patient may need multiple blood transfusions, the larger veins in the antecubital fossa should be saved for that purpose and if at all possible should not be used for the collection of blood specimens.

Immediate complications of venipuncture include bleeding into the tissues with hematoma formation and fainting. The former often can

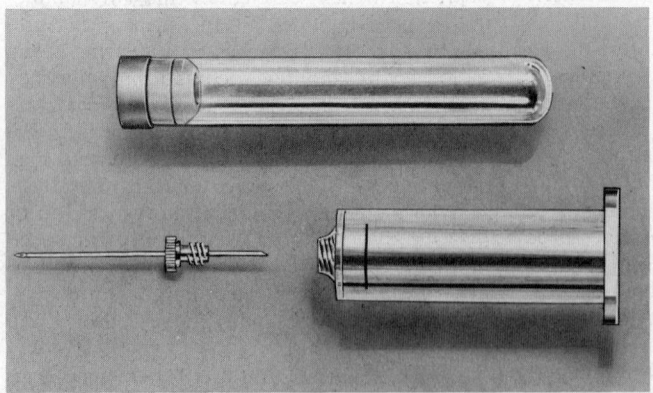

Figure 7-5. Commercially available unit consisting of vacuumized test tube (*top*), sterile double ended needle, and needle holder (*bottom*). (Courtesy of Becton, Dickinson and Co., Rutherford, N.J.)

be avoided by using the venipuncture technique described in Chapter 22 during the collection of the specimen, and by the immediate application of gentle pressure to the puncture site and elevation of the part immediately after the needle has been withdrawn. Although rare, fainting may occur during or shortly after venipuncture. For this reason the procedure should never be done with the patient standing or even sitting on a high stool. If the patient faints, he or she should be put in a recumbent position and a physician notified. Delayed complications include infection, phlebitis, and thrombosis. A systemic infection or even one in a distant organ may result from poor aseptic technique or unsterile equipment. Drug addicts commonly get hepatitis from sharing needles, but improperly sterilized equipment used in health services may be responsible for transmitting this disease also.

For tests that require a very small amount of blood, such as leukocyte, erythrocyte, and differential counts, a sufficient amount may be obtained by puncturing the lobe of the ear or the tip of the finger (see Fig. 7-6 for instrument used). In infants, the bottom of the heel or great toe frequently is used. In such cases the skin is cleaned, and a quick stab is made with a sterile sharp needle, lancet, or scalpel. After wiping away the first drop of blood, the blood is collected in a pipette as it oozes from this puncture. If the blood is to be examined microscopically, a smear slide is prepared immediately by collecting a small drop of blood directly from the puncture site onto a clean glass slide, not letting the slide touch the skin. If the instrument used for the puncture is not disposable and is to be reused, it should be sterilized as described in Chapter 32.

Blood collected from puncture wounds gives false laboratory values if taken from a site that is congested, edematous, cold, or cyanotic. False values also occur if the blood is forcefully squeezed from the puncture site, if the first drop of blood that oozes from the puncture is used, or if the skin around the puncture site is not dry.

Arterial punctures are usually made to get specimens for arterial blood-gas studies. A 20-gauge needle, attached to an air-free sterile syringe, the inside of which has been rinsed with a small amount of heparin, is used to take blood preferably from the brachial or radial artery and from the femoral only in emergencies. The appropriate artery is located by feeling for its pulse. Once the pulse is felt, the skin over it is cleaned with an antiseptic solution and the needle is inserted into the artery. The position of the patient during the procedure and the angle at which the needle is inserted varies with the puncture site. After at least 5 ml of blood enters the syringe, the needle is withdrawn, the tip of it is inserted rapidly into an air-tight cork or stopper, and the specimen is mixed by rolling. Then the syringe is immersed in a container of ice to preserve the specimen. Analysis should take place immediately. As soon as the needle has been withdrawn, a sterile bandage is put over the puncture site and held there with firm pressure for a minimum of 5 minutes. More time may be needed if oozing persists. After the oozing has stopped, a firm pressure bandage is applied to the puncture site. The bandage should be checked within 30 minutes and periodically thereafter for hemorrhage. At the same time, the pulse, temperature, and color below the puncture site of the extremity should be checked and compared with the same observations on the opposite extremity. Compli-

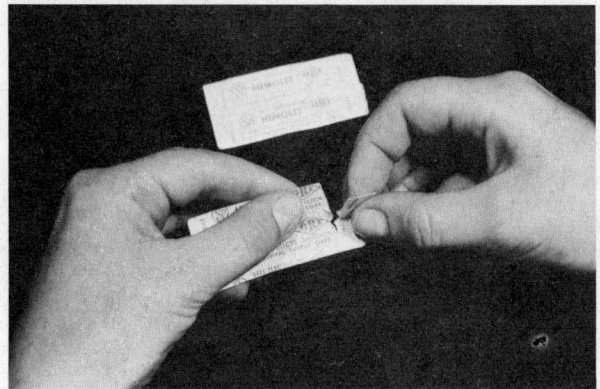
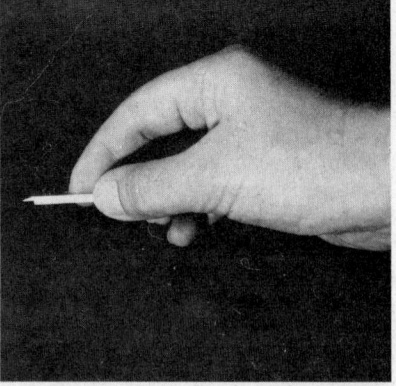

Figure 7-6. Sterile disposable instrument used to pierce the finger or ear lobe when collecting a small blood specimen. (Courtesy of Becton, Dickinson and Co., Rutherford, N.J.)

cations of arterial puncture include hemorrhage, hematoma formation, arterial spasm, arterial thrombosis, and injury to the nerves or other structures near the puncture site.

Hematologic Tests. Davidsohn and Henry emphasize that

The results of hematologic examinations forming what we call the "blood picture," are an essential part of the clinical description of practically every disease. A normal number and distribution of cells and a normal hemoglobin concentration in the blood are so important as physiologic constants that the absence of disease can scarcely be asserted until these observations have been made. That certain diseases do not produce significant changes in the blood is often a valuable point in differential diagnosis. Most hematologic changes are the result of pathologic processes not primarily affecting the blood or blood-forming tissues. . . .*

For these reasons, a leukocyte and differential count and a hemoglobin estimate or hematocrit determination often are included routinely in health examinations. If abnormal values are found, additional hematological tests are made. A hematology report form is shown in Figure 7-7.

The *leukocyte* or *white blood cell count* (WBC) is of considerable importance clinically, because there is a change in the number of leukocytes in response to many disease processes. The normal leukocyte count varies from about 5000 to 10,000 per cubic millimeter of blood. An increase in the white cell count, called "leukocytosis," may occur when the blood-forming organs produce an unusually large number of cells, according to the disease process and the body's ability to fight it. In leukemia, a disease often marked by an increase in white cells and a decrease in red cells, the number of white cells may increase tremendously, sometimes to 1,000,000 per cubic millimeter of blood. When infection is present, it is generally believed that a high leukocyte count indicates that the individual is reacting to the infection. The leukocyte count may not be increased if the individual is offering little or no resistance to the disease or if the infection is unthreatening. Leukopenia, or a marked decrease in white cells, may be a sign of overwhelming infection or may be due to agranulocytosis, a condition in which the bone marrow fails to make granulocytes.

Leukocyte (WBC) counts may be made by an electronic counter or by microscopic examination of an unstained smear. The electronic method requires anticoagulated venous blood, and the microscopic method requires fresh, unclotted capillary blood or anticoagulated venous blood.

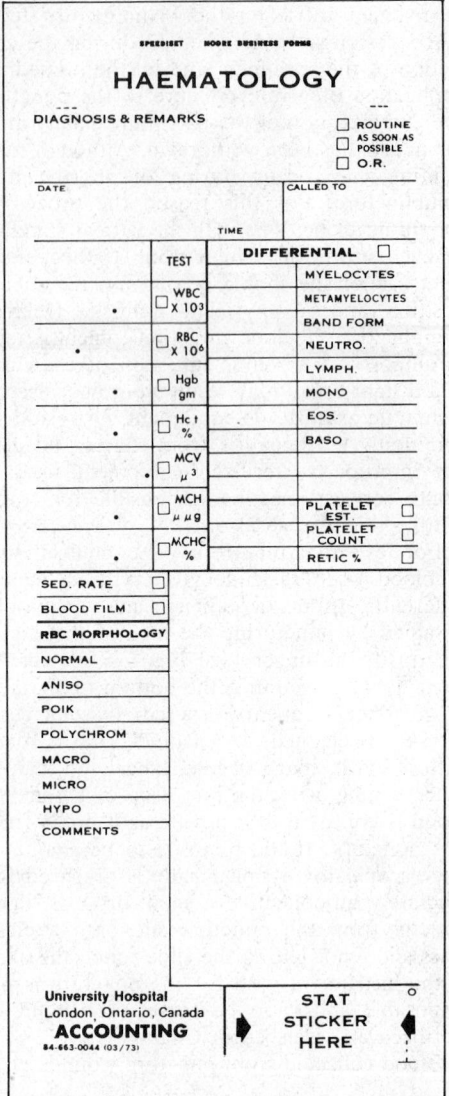

Figure 7-7. A hematology report form. (Courtesy of University Hospital, University of Western Ontario, London, Ont.)

The *differential count,* or the differentiation of the kinds of leukocytes, is as important as the total leukocyte count, if not more so. It is made by preparing a stained blood smear by one of several means. According to Davidsohn and Henry, of the total number of leukocytes, 20 to 40 per cent normally are lymphocytes; 2 to 6 per cent monocytes; 50 to 70 per cent polymorphonuclears; 1 to 4 per cent eosino-

* Davidsohn, Israel, and Henry, John H. (eds.): *Todd-Sanford Clinical Diagnosis by Laboratory Methods,* 15th ed. W. B. Saunders Co., Philadelphia, 1974, p. 180.

uh University Hospital

HAEMATOLOGY REPORTS

NOTE: (1) USE THIS FORM ONLY FOR <u>ROUTINE</u>
              <u>HAEMATOLOGY</u> (Long Form) REPORTS
       (2) FOR OTHER HAEMATOLOGY REPORTS, PLEASE
              USE LABORATORY REPORT SHEET.

1	2	3	4	5

84-750-0181 (09/72)

Figure 7-7 (*continued*)

phils; and 0.25 to 0.50 per cent basophils. In certain diseases, such as pernicious anemia, lymphocytic leukemia, pertussis, and exophthalmic goiter, the lymphocyte count is increased. In other diseases there is a change in the number of other kinds of leukocytes, as, for example, the monocyte count is high in malaria and typhoid fevers, and the polymorphonuclear cells are increased in many serious bacterial infections. Infection and inflammation will increase the total count of neutrophils and show production of some immature forms of cells. A so-called "shift to the left" has been named after the maturation sequence of Schilling whose diagram indicated the more mature forms going toward the right and the immature forms progressing toward the left. Eosinophilia, an increase in eosinophils, is characteristic of parasitic and allergic diseases. Myelogenous leukemia may produce a 500 per cent or more increase in polymorphonuclear leukocytes with many immature forms, constituting a definite diagnostic aid. Because the different kinds of leukocytes vary in number in certain diseases as already shown, a differential count is often exceedingly valuable.

Hemoglobin is a protein compound having a great affinity for oxygen. It is found in red blood cells, and its amount is usually proportional to the number of red cells. Normally hemoglobin is present in the blood as 16 gm plus or minus 2 gm per 100 ml of blood in the adult male, and 14 gm plus or minus 2 gm per 100 ml in the adult female. The use of the absolute value of hemoglobin, rather than a percentage, is the preferred way of expressing the hemoglobin level. An increase—that is, a hemoglobin above normal limits—is uncommon and may not be important except in polycythemia. On the other hand, a decrease is both common and significant.

Davidsohn and Henry state that, for practical purposes, anemia is present when there is fewer than 12 gm of hemoglobin in 100 ml of blood. Anemia may be a sign or a complication of a wide variety of diseases. Pernicious anemia and sickle cell anemia are forms of anemia in which less than 12 gm of hemoglobin occurs, but each is a distinct disease with a different cause, treatment, and prognosis.

Hemoglobin level is estimated in various ways using either micro- or macromethods. The specimen submitted for analysis may be either venous or capillary blood mixed with an appropriate anticoagulant.

Hematocrit, or packed cell volume, is the volume of red blood cells in a given quantity of whole blood expressed as a per cent, making this estimate the easiest, fastest, and most accurate method for detecting anemia. Normal values are 47 plus or minus 7 per cent for males and 42 plus or minus 5 per cent for females. Hematocrit may be substituted for hemoglobin determinations when accurate methods for estimating the latter are not available, or it may be used in conjunction with the red blood cell count and hemoglobin level, and certain blood indices for differentiating between types of anemia. As in hemoglobin determination, the hematocrit may be estimated by micro- or macromethods using venous or capillary blood samples mixed with an appropriate anticoagulant.

The *erythrocyte or red cell count* is one of the tests most commonly made in conjunction with the health examination. It is made by essentially the same methods as the leukocyte count. The average healthy man has about 5,000,000 red cells per cubic millimeter of blood. The number for women is about 4,500,000. There may at times be an increase in the number of red cells, such as in the disease polycythemia vera or in renal tumors. Individuals who live in the higher altitudes habitually have higher red cell counts. A decrease in the red cell count is commoner and more significant than an increase. The change in the red cell count is usually accompanied by a change in hemoglobin, but they need not necessarily correspond. A low red cell count is present in almost all the anemias. Leukemia often is characterized by a marked decrease in the red cell count.

When the presence of anemia has been determined by abnormal hemoglobin or hematocrit values, determination of the *red blood cell indices* may help identify the disease causing the anemia. These include the mean corpuscular volume (MCV), or average size of red blood cells; the mean corpuscular hemoglobin (MCH), or average weight of hemoglobin in the cells; and the mean corpuscular hemoglobin concentration (MCHC), or average hemoglobin concentration per red cell. Red cell indices are mathematically calculated from various combinations of values of erythrocyte count, hemoglobin measurement, and hematocrit determination. The normal value for the MCV is 87 plus or minus 5 cubic microns per cell; for the MCH, 29 plus or minus 2 micromicrograms per cell; and for the MCHC, 34 plus or minus 2 per cent.

The direct microscopic *examination of the bone marrow* is a valuable method of diagnosing many diseases of the blood and blood-forming organs since blood cells form in the bone marrow. Bone marrow specimens are usually taken from the iliac crest, the posterior superior iliac spine, or the sternum. Under local anesthesia, a needle is introduced into the marrow cavity of the bone and a small amount of marrow is aspirated. Some of the aspirate is smeared on glass slides which are stained and studied histologically. The remainder is fixed and sectioned for further histological study. After the needle has been withdrawn, a dry sterile dressing is applied to the puncture site and is firmly attached to the skin by adhesive tape. This technique is called *bone marrow aspiration*. It may be performed in an outpatient service; or if performed on an inpatient service, the person is not required to stay overnight. When done properly, it carries about the same degree of risk as venipuncture. As only the aspiration phase is painful, patients should be forewarned that it might hurt briefly. The technique for performing this aspiration biopsy is discussed in more detail in Chapter 22. A bone marrow report form is shown in Figure 7-8.

Another bone marrow study is *trephine biopsy*. A segment of marrow is taken just as in aspiration, except that a special, large-bore needle is used that removes a small cylinder of tissue. As with bone marrow aspirates, stained smears and histologic sections are prepared. This method is generally used when repeated aspirations have proved unsatisfactory or when the type of tissue wanted for examination cannot be withdrawn by aspiration. Trephine biopsy is more difficult than needle aspiration and the procedure is more painful for the patient. Both tests are used to diagnose blood diseases such as leukemia, pernicious anemia, and aplastic anemia. They may also help in the diagnosis of metastatic neoplasms; since the specimen is small, however, such lesions may not appear in it, so a negative biopsy may not rule out the condition. A complication of convulsions may occur during aspiration or biopsy if the patient has a seizure disorder or hyperventilates during the procedure. When the sternal puncture is performed improperly, the heart can be punctured and death may result from the collection of blood in the pericardial sac (tamponade).

The *platelets,* or *thrombocytes,* are the smallest formed element in the blood, with a diameter of less than one-half a red blood cell.* Their chief function is related to blood clotting, the agglutination of platelets being essential to it. Because of their small size and tendency to agglutinate, direct counting is difficult, and there is considerable variation in

* The average diameter of a red blood cell is 7.2 microns or 7.2 one-thousandth of a millimeter. (Ham, Thomas H.: *A Syllabus of Laboratory Examinations in Clinical Diagnosis.* Harvard University Press, Cambridge, Mass., 1950, p. 109.)

what are considered normal values. Levels between 50,000 and 100,000 are, however, generally considered critically low. The number of platelets may be estimated from the blood smear used for the differential count. Decreased numbers of platelets result in a tendency to bleed easily, particularly under the skin, producing a hemorrhagic rash, or purpura. The platelets may be decreased in diseases of the bone marrow, such as leukemia, or extensive metastatic carcinoma. Platelets may be decreased without obvious reason, as in idiopathic thrombocytopenic purpura.

The time required for a puncture wound to stop bleeding is called the *bleeding time*. Normal values vary with the method used. In the Duke method, an ear lobe puncture is made with a sterile lancet and blood is permitted to flow freely onto a filter paper. As the bleeding flows, the puncture site is blotted gently with a clean piece of filter paper every 30 seconds until blood stops staining it. Bleeding lasting less than 6 minutes is considered normal. In the Ivy method, an area of the forearm where there there are no obvious veins is used. A puncture wound is made after having applied a blood pressure cuff to the upper arm and inflating it to 40 mm of mercury. The wound is blotted with clean filter paper every 30 seconds from the time the puncture wound is made until blood stops staining the paper. A normal value by this method is 2 to 3 minutes. *Coagulation*, or *clotting time,* is the time necessary for the blood to clot after it has been removed from the vein and put in a glass container. Normal values for the clotting time are between 5 and 8 minutes.

The bleeding or clotting time, or both, may be abnormally elevated in diseases of the blood-clotting mechanism, such as hemophilia. The danger of trauma or surgery without proper preparation of such patients is self-evident.

Another useful test of the clotting mechanism is measurement of the *prothrombin time* (PT). This is a measure of the level of prothrombin and other factors in the body expressed in seconds. Prothrombin and other coagulation factors are circulating enzymes that take part in the process of clotting. Both the coagulation time and prothrombin time are valuable tests for following patients undergoing oral anticoagulation therapy, so that desirable levels may be maintained without decreasing the blood coagulability to dangerous levels. The prothrombin time should be about 11 to 13 seconds normally and 20 to 25 seconds therapeutically when bishydroxycoumarin (Dicumarol), crystalline sodium wafarin (Coumadin), or other vitamin K antagonist

uh University Hospital

BONE MARROW REPORT

CLINICAL HISTORY AND DIAGNOSIS   LAB. NO. _____

_____

_____

_____

_____

PERIPHERAL BLOOD

Hb_____ gm% HCT_____% RBC_____x10^6 MCV_____u^3 MCH_____uug MCHC_____%

WBC _____x 10^3 DIFFERENTIAL _____

PLATELETS _____RETICS _____% BLOOD FILM_____
_____

BONE MARROW

SITE _____ QUALITY _____ CELLULARITY _____

M/E RATIO _____

ERYTHROPOIESIS _____
_____

GRANULOPOIESIS _____
_____

MEGAKARYOCYTES _____

OTHER CELLS _____
_____

IRON STAIN _____
_____

OPINION _____
_____
_____
_____

84-663-0041

Figure 7-8. A bone marrow report form. (Courtesy of University Hospital, University of Western Ontario, London, Ont.)

anticoagulants are given. Because heparin affects coagulation in a different way, different tests are needed to determine its effects. Usually whole blood coagulation times or activated partial thromboplastin times (PTT) are used. In both tests, a patient's blood sample is compared with a control sample known to be normal and the values are expressed in seconds.

Most authorities recommend that for maximum therapeutic effect the coagulation time of patients on heparin should be two to three times as long as the control.[25] They say the prothrombin time of patients on bishydroxycoumarin should be two to two and one-half times as long as the control. Immediately after starting these drugs, tests are usually done once a day but may be performed more frequently if needed, or less frequently when the appropriate dosage has been determined. A special form used to report coagulation, screening and special tests is shown in Figure 7-9.

The *erythrocyte sedimentation rate* (ESR) employs the principle that red blood cells will settle to the bottom of the container in which blood is allowed to stand. Blood, collected by venipuncture, is mixed with an appropriate anticoagulant and is allowed to stand. The speed with which the cells settle is then measured. Various factors, such as the number and size of red blood cells, the protein content of the blood, and the viscosity of the blood, influence the rate of sedimentation. Westergren's method is simple and accurate but time consuming and so is rarely used to measure the sedimentation rate. In this test, diluted blood is put in long glass tubes calibrated in millimeters. The rate at which sedimentation normally occurs with the Westergren method is usually stated as less than 15 mm in 1 hour for men and 20 mm for women. The normal values for both sexes increase with age. The Wintrobe method uses short tubes and is somewhat faster but may produce a falsely elevated ESR in the presence of anemia. The sedimentation rate is a nonspecific test which may be altered by many disease processes, much like the body temperature. A high sedimentation rate usually reflects the presence of an inflammatory process, although it does not necessarily indicate its severity. A sedimentation test is of special value in following the activity of certain diseases such as rheumatic fever and rheumatoid arthritis and to detect occult organic disease.

Serologic Tests. Tests for syphilis are made on the blood serum to detect the presence of an antibody complex which is present in patients who have the disease. The first test of this nature was described by Wassermann, and since then many variations in the test have been developed. Besides the *Wassermann test,* there are the *Kolmer test,* the *Kahn test,* the *Mazzini test,* and the *VDRL* (*Venereal Disease Research Laboratory*) *test,* and many others. While these are good screening tests for syphilis, they are not entirely specific. Certain other diseases may produce false positive reactions. One or another form of serologic test is usually done as part of every routine examination, requiring about 5 ml of clotted blood taken by venipuncture.

Since 1949, a number of highly specific tests have been developed that detect a specific antibody in a patient's blood, which is capable of reacting with the spirochete *Treponema pallidum,* the etiologic agent of syphilis. Examples of these include the *fluorescent treponemal antibody absorption test* (FTA-ABS), the *Reiter protein complement fixation test* (RPCF), and the *Treponema pallidum immobilization test* (TPI). One of the first two mentioned above should be used to confirm the results of any of the standard screening tests, whether they are reactive or nonreactive, if clinical evidence suggests present or past syphilitic infection. If these tests are nonreactive but past or present infection is still suspected, a *Treponema pallidum* immobilization test is recommended.[26] These specific examinations are elaborate and expensive and so are not practical for large numbers of screening examinations.

Blood Cultures. Blood cultures are made to determine the presence or absence of bacteremia or to diagnose the cause of sepsis, and therefore should be taken by venipuncture under careful aseptic conditions. A recommended modified venipuncture technique is

1. Prepare the skin at proposed puncture site: Cleanse a wide area with iodine. Cleanse again with 70 per cent isopropanol.
2. Perform venipuncture using sterile syringe and needle.
3. Withdraw approximately 8 ml of blood.
4. Remove needle and transfer blood to culture bottle, using care not to touch neck of bottle.
5. Do not shake bottle or disturb interface on the broth of cultures drawn for anaerobic bacteria.
6. Label specimens with name, date, time, and number of culture.*

Blood cultures may also be made using a vacutainer tube containing sterile media. The procedure is like that described earlier in this chapter for venipuncture. Careful preparation of the skin is essential for both methods. After the blood is added to culture media and incu-

---

* Plumer, Ada Lawrence: *Principles and Practice of Intravenous Therapy.* Little, Brown & Co., Boston, 1970, p. 204.

uh University Hospital

COAGULATION
SCREENING AND SPECIAL TESTS

CLINICAL INFORMATION

DATE _____

TIME _____

1 SCREENING TESTS OF ABNORMAL HEMOSTATIC FUNCTION	PATIENT	CONTROL	NORMAL RANGE
PROTHROMBIN TIME (PRO TIME)	SEC.	SEC.	SEC.
ACTIVATED PARTIAL THROMBOPLASTIN TIME (APTT)	SEC.		SEC.
THROMBIN CLOTTING TIME (TCT)	SEC.	SEC.	
	SEC.	SEC.	
PLATELET COUNT	/mm³		/mm³
BLEEDING TIME (IVY-TEMPLATE)	MIN.		MIN.
PROTHROMBIN CONSUMPTION TEST	SEC.	SEC.	SEC.
EUGLOBULIN LYSIS TIME	MIN.	MIN.	MIN.
FIBRIN-FIBRINOGEN DEGRADATION PRODUCTS F D P	μ g/ml	μ g/ml	μ g/ml
FIBRINOGEN	mg%		mg%

2. COAGULATION FACTOR ASSAYS

3. SPECIAL TESTS OF PLATELET FUNCTION	PATIENT (%)	NORMAL RANGE(%)
PLATELET ADHESIVENESS TO GLASS		
PLATELET AGGREGATION ON EXPOSURE TO:	NORMAL	ABNORMAL
COLLAGEN		
ADRENALINE		
ADP		

4. OTHER STUDIES

5. COMMENTS

84-663-0039 (08/72)

CHART

Figure 7-9. A coagulation, screening, and special tests report form. (Courtesy of University Hospital, University of Western Ontario, London, Ont.)

bated, the culture is examined daily, frequently for as long as 2 weeks. Some of the organisms that can be demonstrated by blood culture are the *typhoid bacilli, pneumococci, staphylococci,* and *streptococci.*

Blood Typing and Crossmatching. Because certain types of blood are incompatible, it is necessary to type and crossmatch the blood used in transfusion with the blood of the recipient so that the bloods of both are compatible. Untoward reactions and sometimes death of the patient will result if incompatible bloods are combined. A blood transfusion report form is shown in Figure 7-10. A single specimen of venous blood, or capillary blood if micromethods are to be used, is taken from the recipient for crossmatching tests with many units of blood. When more than 24 hours passes between blood transfusions, a new crossmatching test must be performed. This is necessary because each blood transfusion could stimulate the formation of large amounts of incompatible substances within the blood of the recipient that were not there before in detectable or clinically significant amounts when the original crossmatch was made. These substances could cause a serious reaction to blood from the same donor 24 hours later. This problem is discussed more completely in Chapter 22.

Other uses of blood typing include exclusion of parentage in paternity suits, anthropologic classification, and identification of women with potential for delivering babies with erythroblastosis fetalis. Studies of blood groups and their genetic mechanisms yield increasingly important information about inheritance in man.

Blood Chemistry. Many chemical determinations are made on the blood when indicated. Chemical tests usually require 5 to 10 ml of blood collected by venipuncture. Capillary blood may often be used for tests if analyses are made by micromethods; and some tests, such as blood-gas studies, may require arterial blood. In most instances, patients need not fast before blood samples are drawn. Mentioned below are a few of the more frequently performed tests for blood chemistries along with a few examples of each of the common conditions and diseases in which deviations from the normal range occur. Normal ranges are found in the Appendix. Unless other citations have been made, Davidsohn and Henry have been consulted for the descriptions that follow.[27]

Measurements of serum or plasma *electrolytes,* including *sodium, potassium, chloride,* and *carbon dioxide,* are among the most frequently performed blood chemistry tests. The amount of sodium ion in the blood plays a crucial part in the maintenance of water balance in the body, and careful monitoring of this ion is particularly important in caring for patients who require fluid replacement. Normal potassium, chloride, and carbon dioxide blood concentrations are critical in maintaining acid-base balance, which may be assessed directly by measurement of the arterial or venous blood *pH.*

Arterial *blood-gas studies,* including the partial pressures of *carbon dioxide* (pCO_2) and *oxygen* (pO_2) and *oxygen saturation,* may be done along with arterial blood pH determinations when varying degrees of respiratory failure—which can drastically alter acid-base relationships—are known or suspected.

Blood urea nitrogen (BUN) and *creatinine tests* measure kidney function; these values are elevated as kidney function deteriorates in conditions such as shock, congestive heart failure, and various kidney diseases. A 50 per cent decrease in renal function usually occurs, however, before the BUN is elevated above the normal range. The creatinine level rises even more slowly as the kidneys decompensate.

Total protein and *protein electrophoresis* studies are made frequently to detect and monitor certain kidney and liver diseases. In such diseases, decreased albumin concentrations and alterations in the ratios between the various serum proteins frequently are found.

Values for *fasting blood glucose, 2-hour postprandial blood glucose,* and *oral and intravenous glucose tolerance tests* are elevated in diabetes mellitus. Each of the first two tests requires a single blood sample. A fasting specimen is needed for the former and a specimen taken 2 hours after eating for the latter. Oral and intravenous glucose tolerance tests require collections of both blood and urine while in the fasting state. As soon as these are collected, the patient drinks a solution containing 500 gm of glucose within a period of 5 minutes or eats a high-carbohydrate meal. Blood and urine are collected at 30 minutes and at 1-, 2-, 3-, and 4-hour intervals.

Protein-bound iodine (PBI), *triiodothyronine* (T_3), and *thyroxin* (T_4) tests are used commonly to measure thyroid function. These tests usually show abnormally high values in hyperthyroidism and abnormally low values in hypothyroidism. The PBI reflects the amount of thyroid hormone bound to protein in the peripheral blood. About 90 per cent of the PBI represents T_4 and 5 per cent T_3. Of the latter two, T_4 is often considered the test of choice because it is a direct measure of the major circulating thyroid hormone.[28]

Cholesterol and *triglyceride* measurements are used to detect disorders of lipid metabolism. Abnormally high cholesterol levels have been implicated as a causative factor in atherosclerosis and a contributor to coronary artery and cerebrovascular disease.

Normal *uric acid* blood levels vary with age and sex. They are increased in starvation, high fat diets, and gout. Alterations in the concentrations of *calcium* and *phosphorous* in the blood occur in bone, parathyroid, nutritional, and malabsorption diseases.

A variety of blood chemistry tests are used for evaluating liver function and for detecting extrahepatic biliary disease. *Total serum bili-*

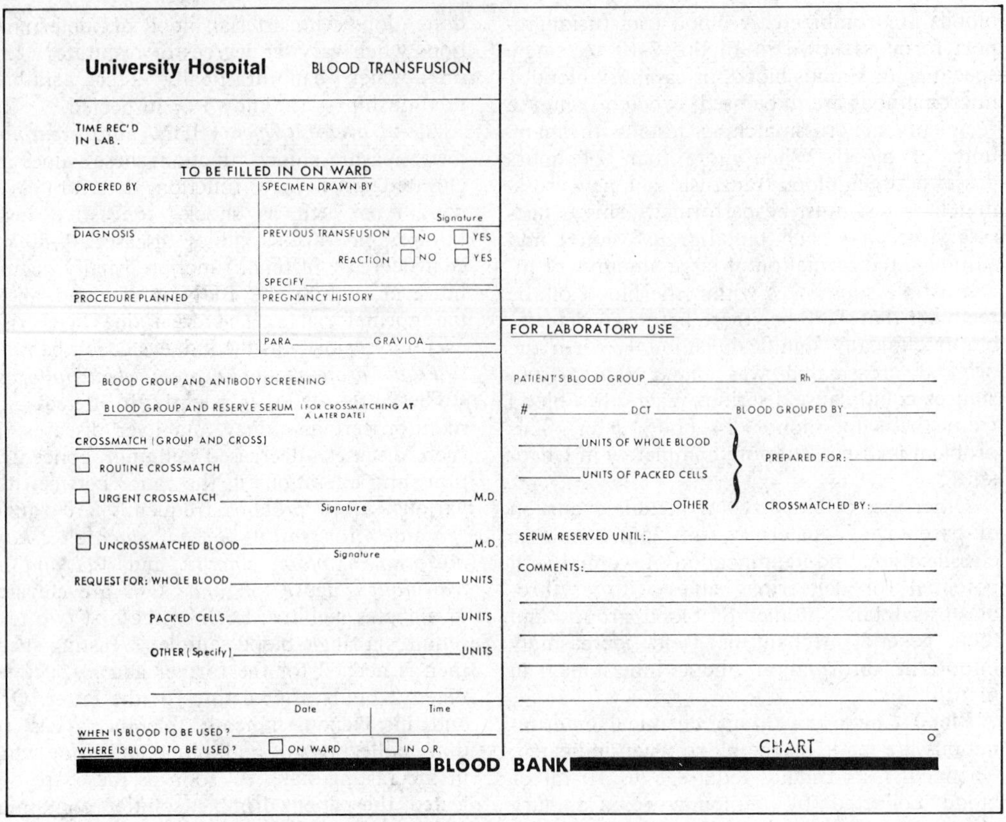
University Hospital BLOOD TRANSFUSION

TIME REC'D IN LAB.

TO BE FILLED IN ON WARD

ORDERED BY

SPECIMEN DRAWN BY

Signature

DIAGNOSIS

PREVIOUS TRANSFUSION ☐ NO ☐ YES

REACTION ☐ NO ☐ YES

SPECIFY

PROCEDURE PLANNED

PREGNANCY HISTORY

PARA GRAVIDA

☐ BLOOD GROUP AND ANTIBODY SCREENING

☐ BLOOD GROUP AND RESERVE SERUM (FOR CROSSMATCHING AT A LATER DATE)

CROSSMATCH (GROUP AND CROSS)

☐ ROUTINE CROSSMATCH

☐ URGENT CROSSMATCH M.D.

Signature

☐ UNCROSSMATCHED BLOOD M.D.

Signature

REQUEST FOR: WHOLE BLOOD UNITS

PACKED CELLS UNITS

OTHER (Specify) UNITS

Date Time

WHEN IS BLOOD TO BE USED?

WHERE IS BLOOD TO BE USED? ☐ ON WARD ☐ IN O.R.

FOR LABORATORY USE

PATIENT'S BLOOD GROUP Rh

DCT BLOOD GROUPED BY

UNITS OF WHOLE BLOOD

UNITS OF PACKED CELLS

OTHER

PREPARED FOR:

CROSSMATCHED BY:

SERUM RESERVED UNTIL:

COMMENTS:

CHART

BLOOD BANK

Figure 7-10. Blood transfusion report form. (Courtesy of University Hospital, University of Western Ontario, London, Ont.)

rubin is increased in conditions manifested by jaundice and it is measured to assess the severity of jaundice. *Direct* and *indirect bilirubin* determinations are helpful in the differential diagnosis of jaundice. Direct bilirubin will be high in instances of obstructive jaundice caused by a stone or carcinoma, whereas indirect bilirubin will be high when there is hemolysis or increased breakdown of red blood cells. The *icteric index,* also an indication of the presence or absence of liver impairment, may be measured in place of total serum bilirubin when the latter test is unavailable. *Cephalin flocculation* and *thymol turbidity* tests help to differentiate between liver disease, in which they are both abnormally high, and obstructive jaundice, in which values are within normal limits. The *sulfobromphthalein* (*BSP*) *excretion* test is the most sensitive indicator of liver function available. When BSP dye is administered intravenously, the liver removes the dye and excretes it. The rate of excretion is measured by drawing a blood sample 45 minutes after the injection of the dye to measure its concentration and then drawing repeated samples to measure the residual dye. With normal functioning of the liver, less than 5 per cent of the dye is retained after about 45 minutes. Correspondingly, if there is any abnormality present in the liver, the excretion of the dye is delayed in proportion to the degree of abnormality. The BSP test is a particularly useful test for patients who are not jaundiced and who are being evaluated for liver disease. Other tests that assess liver function are mentioned later in the subsection on serum enzymes and in the sections on urine and feces.

As mentioned earlier, the *Guthrie test* is a popular method for detecting phenylketonuria (PKU) in newborns. According to Ravel,[29] blood obtained by heel puncture is put on a filter paper and allowed to dry. This in turn is put on a culture medium containing *Bacillus subtilis* and a substance which, in the absence of phenylalanine, normally will inhibit the growth of this bacillus. If the Guthrie test is positive, that is, if there is bacterial growth, the serum phenylalanine level is measured. Normal serum values are less than 2 mg per cent. If blood for the Guthrie test is obtained before a newborn with phenylketonuria has been on a protein diet (milk) for at least 4 days, the test may be falsely negative. If the newborn is discharged from the hospital 3 or 4 days after birth, this blood test must be made soon after discharge.

Serum Enzyme Tests. Serum enzymes are altered in a wide variety of illnesses. When tested serially and in various combinations, serum enzyme studies provide important information that may be used in making a diagnosis or in monitoring a disease process. Increased levels of *serum glutamic oxaloacetic transaminase* (SGOT), *serum glutamic pyruvic transaminase* (SGPT), and *alkaline phosphatase* occur regularly in conditions of the hepatobiliary tract. Abnormally high levels of alkaline phosphatase are also found in bone diseases and in certain other disorders. Assays for 5'-nucleotidase are high in situations of high alkaline phosphatase caused by liver disease but normal when alkaline phosphatase is elevated because of bone disease. Myocardial infarction is characterized initially by elevated *creatinine phosphokinase* (CPK), and later by elevated SGOT and *lactic dehydrogenase* (LDH) values. Abnormally high enzyme values can also occur in diseases of skeletal muscle, such as dermatomyositis, in pulmonary infarction, in malignancy, and in anemias. An elevated *acid phosphatase* level is a prominent finding in cancer of the prostate that has metastasized. High levels of serum *lipase* and *amylase* are usual findings in pancreatitis.

4. EXAMINATION OF OTHER BODY FLUIDS AND DISCHARGES

General Principles. Body fluids are examined grossly and microscopically. They are examined for blood, bile, certain chemicals, and other substances; and for number and kinds of cells present in the fluid. The presence of certain bacterial and viral organisms is detected by taking a smear and by culturing the fluid.

Certain procedures are carried out almost universally in the examination of body fluids and discharges. A small quantity of the secretions of any body cavity open to the body's exterior may be taken by means of cotton applicators and transferred to a sterile glass tube. After the applicators are saturated with the material to be examined, they are carefully inserted into the tube without touching its sides. Speed is of utmost importance in transferring the specimens to the laboratory for a bacteriologic or viral smear and culture, although in many settings transport media are used, in which case more time may be taken in transporting the specimens. If the material is allowed to dry before examination, the organisms cannot be transferred to the slide and to the culture media adequately. Extreme care should be taken to prevent contamination of specimen handlers and the environment because very often body secretions are laden with virulent bacteria.

Smears and cultures are taken from many different parts of the body, including eyes, ears, nose, throat, urethra, vagina, and rectum. Urethral smears are particularly valuable in the presumptive diagnosis of gonorrhea in the male, while endocervical and rectal cultures for gonorrhea are required for diagnosis in the female. When wounds and abscesses are present, smears made from them may also be studied bacteriologically. Slide smears are generally made in conjunction with cultures; they are stained by appropriate methods, then examined microscopically for bacteria, in an effort to make a specific diagnosis. A wet-mounted smear may be made to view organisms in the living state, such as trichomonas, a vaginal inhabitant.

In order to determine the nature of a bacterial infection in any person, a sample of body secretions or material from a wound is transferred to a culture medium that encourages the growth of microorganisms. That growth, after a suitable period of time in an incubator with an appropriate oxygen–carbon dioxide environment, is studied under the microscope. In the laboratory the secretions may be applied to a blood agar plate or, when gonorrhea is suspected, directly to a chocolate agar plate, or Thayer-Martin medium, immediately after examining the patient. The culture may also be grown in a liquid medium. When this is done, it is essential that the applicator and tube of broth be protected from all contamination. Antimicrobial sensitivity tests are usually carried out on bacteriological specimens by using discs on the culture plate impregnated with various drugs, and evaluating which of the drugs has inhibited growth of the organisms.

Cultures of blood, urine, sputum, and spinal and other body fluids are made by subjecting them to certain media. Specimens must be collected under strict aseptic conditions for bacteriologic examination. Cultures of wounds and of infected throats, eyes and ears, and other body orifices are commonly made for diagnostic purposes. The specimen may be collected by the physician, the nurse, the epidemiologist, or others, all of whom must be thoroughly familiar with the principles and procedures. In the collecting of body fluids for microscopic examination, the laboratory slip should always indicate the *source* of the secretions to be studied and any pertinent clinical information, such as the antimicrobial agents the patient is receiving. If a particular organism is suspected, indicating this fact is an important guide to laboratory personnel in selecting appropriate media.

It should be pointed out that test results of many clinical laboratory examinations may be affected by a variety of factors including the time in the disease process the specimen is collected, the laboratory method, the age, sex, nutritional state, and diet of the patient, emotional factors, exercise factors, and, very commonly, drugs. A booklet called *Drug Induced Modifications of Laboratory Test Values —Revised 1973* and published by Norman V. Constantino and Hugh F. Kabat includes a tabulation of known interferences to diagnostic tests. They have compiled an exhaustive listing of reports of alterations in laboratory tests as a result of biologic, physical, or chemical mechanisms.*

The following discussion of the examination of other body fluids and discharges is based on Chapters 16, 17, 24, 25, 27, and 28 in Davidsohn and Henry.[30]

Sputum. Specimens of sputum for examination are collected by having the patient cough up material from the bronchi or lungs and expectorate into a special container. Sputum may also be obtained by having the patient use an aerosol sputum-inducing machine, or by placing the patient in one of several positions for postural drainage. The container most commonly used for sputum collection is a sterile, waterproof, disposable container of glass † or plastic that is wide-mouthed and contains a firm cork stopper or a cardboard cap. Care should be taken to prevent the contamination of the inside of the container. Specimens are usually collected first thing in the morning before breakfast. The mouth should be free of saliva and food particles before the sputum is collected because food particles in the material can confuse the laboratory examination. The patient must be instructed to raise material from the lungs by coughing and not simply expectorating saliva or the discharges of the nose and throat.

The most commonly collected specimen is the single morning one that is examined for

* Available from American Society of Hospital Pharmacists, 4630 Montgomery Avenue, Washington, D.C. 20014.

† When this type of container is used, the nurse covers the outside of the container with a paper towel, fastened in place with tape, so that the contents are not visible to patients and their visitors.

organisms by direct smear and culture. According to Davidsohn and Henry,[31] studies indicate that a single morning specimen is superior to the pooled 24-hour or 72-hour specimen because of the lower contamination rate. Occasionally, however, the physician may wish to examine the total sputum expectorated in a 24-hour or 72-hour period and so a complete collection is made. State and city health departments have containers available for patients who require periodic sputum tests. These containers are suitable for mailing specimens when there are no convenient laboratory facilities at hand.

The healthy person does not expectorate sputum; and, in a disease in which there is sputum produced, the amount may vary from a small quantity to several hundred milliliters. The measurement of this amount should be approximated. A simple way to estimate the quantity of sputum is to fill a similar container with water to approximately the same level as the sputum, and then measure the water. If sputum is not saved for laboratory examination, great care should be taken to dispose of it safely.

The sputum color is observed, and this, as well as the amount, varies considerably. Blood may be detected in sputum by its bright red color if it is of recent origin; if it is dark, this is an indication that it has been present in the lungs for some time. In pneumonia the sputum has a rusty color, whereas in lung abscesses, bronchiectasis, and carcinoma, the sputum may be greenish. In gangrenous conditions of the lung, the color is usually brown. Sputum may also be colorless or it may be gray or yellow in some lung infections. The consistency of sputum varies from a thin watery liquid to a thick purulent material. It may have no odor at all or may have a fetid odor, as, for example, in lung abscesses.

Sputum is examined by microscope and by culture to determine the presence of specific bacteria, fungi, viruses, and cells. If acid-fast bacilli (AFB) are found on the direct smear and if on culture these organisms have the morphologic characteristics of tubercle bacilli, the diagnosis of active tuberculosis is generally made. In pneumonia the organism causing the disease may be seen, and the type of pneumonia determined; many fungi cause lung diseases and their identity is also revealed through sputum smears and cultures.

Feces. Stool specimens are collected for laboratory examination for parasites, and occult blood, and for chemical analyses and culture. In the hospital, the stool is collected in a clean bedpan and transferred with wooden spatulas into a waterproof container in which it is sent to the laboratory. The container is usually made of heavily waxed paper. A sterile 2-ounce jar with screw top may be used for ambulatory patients. Care must be taken in transferring the specimen to avoid contaminating the outside of the container. The specimen should not be mixed with urine; it is wise to have the bed patient void first into one bedpan, replacing that with a clean one before defecating. Stools should be sent to the laboratory when fresh. When an examination for parasites (except ova and the cystic forms of parasites) is to be made, the stool should be sent to the laboratory while warm and kept warm during the examination, so that the movements of the organisms may be seen. Sometimes it is necessary to give a cleansing enema to collect the specimen. If this is done the solution to be used is preferably saline or tap water, because other solutions may affect the stool.

Stool specimens may also be sent to the laboratory by mail in specially prepared containers for examination by state health department technicians. A preservative of some kind is usually added to these containers, but when the patient is hospitalized and the specimen is examined in the hospital laboratory, a preservative may not be needed.

The amount of specimen usually required is small, but occasionally the whole stool is saved for observation. Such an examination is ordinarily a gross one, observing that which can be seen with the naked eye, as, for example, worms, blood, changes in stool color, and appearance or consistency. A 72-hour stool specimen may be necessary, and it is often collected by using inert, nonabsorbable stool markers taken by mouth to indicate the beginning and the end of the collection period. All stools are saved from the time the dye first appears in the stool until the time the second dose marker appears.

Examinations of stool specimens are made to identify viruses, bacteria, and fungi and to test for the presence of various substances in the intestinal tract. Leukocytes may be evident by microscopic examination if there are infections or ulcers of the lower intestinal tract. Cysts and eggs of the various intestinal parasites may also be seen this way. Many small worms cannot be seen except through the microscope. The stool may also be examined for fat and enzyme activity by chemical means. Fat may be present in abnormal amounts in certain diseases of the gastrointestinal tract, for example, celiac disease and sprue. A deficiency of pancreatic digestive enzymes may be seen in carcinoma of the pancreas.

Microbiologic examination of feces is made to identify certain pathogenic organisms that are present and that grow on special culture media. Acording to Davidsohn and Henry, the most common bacterial organisms that cause disease are *Salmonella,* including the typhoid bacillus, *Shigella,* enteropathogenic *Escherichia coli, Vibrio cholerae,* and *Staphylococcus aureus,* all of which can be identified by stool culture.[32]

One of the most important tests of the feces is for *blood.* Blood in large quantities can usually be noted, but traces of blood are harder to detect and often are much more important. The diagnoses of carcinoma of the esophagus, stomach, colon, and rectum and of gastric ulcers are often made as a result of finding traces of blood in the stool. The guaiac, benzidine, or orthotolidine tests are commonly used for this purpose. Tests for the presence of urobilinogen in the stool are rarely made because when bile flow obstruction is suspected a test of the urine for urobilinogen is preferred.

Gastric and Duodenal Contents. The examination of the contents of the stomach was one of the most widely used means of determining pathology of the stomach before other techniques such as gastroscopy, x-rays, and gastric cytology came into common use. Gastric analysis is still used, however, to determine if the patient can secrete gastric (hydrochloric) acid, as, for example, in pernicious anemia; to measure the amount of acid produced in a patient with peptic ulcer; to reveal a hypersecretory state characteristic of the Zollinger-Ellison syndrome; and to determine the effectiveness of a vagotomy.

Gastric fluid is obtained for examination by introducing a tube into the stomach and aspirating the contents. All procedures should be carefully explained to patients, but in this case it is essential to have their full cooperation and to minimize apprehension. A Levin tube, usually chilled with ice to reduce nausea, is passed through the nose to the stomach, or a Rehfuss tube may be passed through the mouth. Sometimes it is necessary to adjust the tip of the tube with fluoroscopic visualization. The tube remains in place taped to the patient's face for as long as needed to complete the aspiration of gastric fluid. The gastric contents are observed for bile, mucus, and "coffee-ground" appearance, the last being a condition resulting from blood of significant amount remaining in the acid-secreting stomach. The gastric contents are examined microscopically for various kinds of cells, yeasts, and bacteria, and chemically for hydrochloric acid, occult blood, and bile.

The *1-hour basal gastric secretion test* is the standard method of measuring gastric function. Following an overnight fast, four 15-minute samples are aspirated through the tube and analyzed. Other tests may be made such as the *augmented histamine test,* the *infusion histamine test,* the *Histalog test,* the *insulin hypoglycemia test,* or a *gastrin secretory test.* All of these tests stimulate gastric secretion and require special techniques. The *Diagnex Blue Test* is a tubeless gastric analysis test requiring the patient to take a gastric stimulant and then to ingest a dye which is secreted in the urine. This is an indirect test to indicate the stomach's ability to secrete hydrochloric acid.

Gastric contents may be aspirated for culture of acid-fast bacilli (AFB) in patients who are suspected of having pulmonary tuberculosis but who are unable to produce sputum. This test is often used with young children but must be made in a fasting state immediately upon awakening. Many investigators do not consider this to be a reliable test for tuberculosis.

The contents of the duodenum may be examined in a similar manner to that of the stomach. A double-lumened Diamond, Lagerlöf, or Dreiling tube is introduced and the patient is placed in different positions as the tube is maneuvered into the duodenum, again, possibly checking its position with a fluoroscope. Secretions are collected with a continuous vacuum-pump suction and are analyzed microscopically and chemically. Bile production may be stimulated by the introduction of magnesium sulfate to promote relaxation of the duodenum and drainage of the biliary tree. The usefulness of this test lies in the fact that three different kinds of bile come from three different parts of the biliary tract (common duct, gall bladder, and hepatic ducts) and various tests of the bile secreted can help in the diagnosis of disorders of the hepatobiliary system.

Spinal Fluid. Cerebrospinal fluid (CSF) for examination is usually obtained by inserting a lumbar puncture needle into the space between the third and fourth lumbar vertebrae, or lower, to avoid damage to the spinal cord. This sterile procedure, a lumbar puncture or spinal tap, is described in Chapter 26 and is carried out chiefly for the detection of organic central nervous system disease or to introduce radiographic contrast media or drugs. It is not without its dangers, and a lumbar puncture should not be done if increased intracranial pressure is suspected unless meningitis risks are of overriding concern. A detailed description of the procedure may be found in neurology textbooks, but the following are the essential steps: a two-way stopcock is attached to the spinal needle and the pressure is measured in a manometer before a small amount of fluid, usually 2 ml, is collected in each of three test tubes. The first fluid may contain red blood cells as a result of slight injury to the tissues from the needle, so it is important to carefully label the tubes sequentially. Pressure variations occur with respiration, jugular venous pressure, and straining or breath-holding (due to fear).

Normally cerebrospinal fluid is crystal clear and has a volume of 90 to 150 ml and a pressure of 70 to 150 mm of CSF, with the patient lying on his or her side. It has an alkaline reaction and a specific gravity of 1.006 to 1.008. CSF contains a few leukocytes, protein, glucose, and electrolytes as well as minute amounts of other constituents. A cell count of 0 to 8 is often normal, and it is important that this examination and that for bacteria be made as soon as possible after collecting the specimens because cells disintegrate (lyse) on prolonged standing.

When there is inflammation of the meninges (meningitis), the CSF may show turbidity and an increase in pressure with more protein and leukocytes and a decreased amount of glucose. In early pneumococcal meningitis, the CSF may have bacteria without cell increase. In an acute infection, the specific organism causing the infection may be identified in the CSF and may cause the cell count to markedly increase. Pure pus may be present in the fluid, especially in acute bacterial meningitis, causing it to be very turbid. In tumors of the brain, hemorrhage, and encephalopathy due to lead poisoning, the fluid may be under great pressure. Blood, usually dark in color, or an orange to yellowish color in the supernatant of centrifuged CSF suggests subarachnoid or intracerebral hemorrhage. Protein is usually increased in late neurosyphilis and in any lesion causing injury to the cerebral tissue.

In addition to gross examination of the CSF, pressure measurement, cell count, and protein and glucose determinations, microscopic examination for the presence of organisms such as meningococci, *Hemophilus influenzae,* tubercle bacilli, pneumococci, and others is made. A presumptive diagnosis is possible if any of these organisms is found; further substantiation of the diagnosis of syphilis of the central nervous system is possible when the CSF has a positive VDRL. A fungal infection, often by the cryptococcus organism, may yield yeast cells when special staining techniques are employed.

The importance of the blood-CSF barrier lies in the fact that different solutes diffuse between blood and CSF at different rates, some moving across more rapidly than others. Because large proteins do not diffuse readily unless there is injury to the barrier, the CSF protein electrophoresis pattern may change according to certain central nervous system abnormalities and is a reliable indicator of disease. Lange's colloidal gold test is not a routine test but may be made to evaluate CSF protein abnormalities, chiefly in multiple sclerosis, when electrophoresis is not feasible.

The cell count usually includes a differential as well as a white cell count. The few leukocytes that may normally be seen in the fluid are lymphocytes. An increase in leukocytes, chiefly neutrophils, is usually seen with meningitis. Acute purulent meningitis may have a cell count of from several hundred up to 20,000, almost all of which are neutrophils. The spinal fluid sugar is markedly decreased in both tuberculosis and bacterial meningitis, a finding that serves as another valuable diagnostic aid in the differential diagnosis of such conditions.

Synovial, Pleural, Pericardial, and Peritoneal Fluids. Synovial, pleural, pericardial, and peritoneal fluids are all examined in much the same way as discussed in the preceding section. *Synovial* or joint fluid may be aspirated from the large joints of the shoulder, elbow, wrist, hip, knee, or ankle. Normally only 1 to 4 ml of fluid is present but may be increased or altered in various forms of arthritis. Joint aspiration may be carried out to relieve pain, to get material for culture and analysis, and to instill drugs. Synovial fluid is examined for its appearance, viscosity, mucin clot, cell count, sugar, and protein.

Pleural fluid accumulates as a pleural effusion and is seen in bacterial, fungal, or viral infections, aseptic inflammation, and malignant tumors. A thoracentesis may be performed to obtain the fluid by which to determine the etiologic agents through microscopic examination and culture; to relieve dyspnea; to instill drugs; and to remove blood and pus when hemothorax or empyema is present.

Normally the *pericardial* sac contains 20 to 50 ml of fluid, but it may increase suddenly up to 200 ml to produce cardiac tamponade, an emergency condition when immediate aspiration is indicated. In the nonemergency situation, excess pericardial fluid can be removed to determine the etiology of and treat such a condition, to examine purulent fluid, and to instill drugs into the pericardium.

Peritoneal fluid may be examined after removing it by means of a paracentesis for treatment of ascites, possible abdominal trauma, or pain of unknown cause, and also to instill drugs.

Exfoliative Cytology. George Papanicolaou developed the technique for exfoliative cytology for the study of malignant disease. Body fluid and tissue cells are examined microscopically for the presence of tumor cells in various stages of growth. The term *exfoliative cytology* indicates that cells have sloughed off tissue, a constant and naturally occurring event. The following staging, originally reported by Papanicolaou, with some refinements, is in general use today: class I—normal cells; class II—atypical, but nonneoplastic cells; class III—cells suggestive of malignant tumor; class IV—cells strongly suggestive of malignant tumor; class V—conclusive evidence of malignant tumor cells.

The most valuable and extensively used test is the *Papanicolaou cervical and vaginal smear* for the detection of carcinoma of the cervix. The smear is taken during a periodic routine vaginal examination. The external os of the cervix and the posterior vagina are scraped with a wooden spatula and the material is placed on glass slides which are then sprayed with a fixative solution or placed in a bottle with fixative. Properly identified specimens are sent to the laboratory where the cytology examination is performed. Bronchial secretions and washings, gastric washings, urine sediment, pleural and peritoneal fluid sediment, and mammary gland discharge may all have the Papanicolaou test performed for the diagnosis of malignancy.

Seminal Fluid. A seminal fluid examination is most often made to help resolve infertility problems. This analysis may also be done to examine vaginal secretions or clothing stains for the presence of semen in cases of suspected rape. Seminal fluid normally consists of 3.5 ml of fluid per ejaculation and is a highly viscid, opaque, whitish liquid that may have a musky or acrid odor. It is usually collected following a 3-day period of continence, and is best collected in the physician's office or laboratory. If collected in the home, the fluid is ejaculated into a condom through normal intercourse and placed in a clean wide-mouthed jar. It is then transported to the laboratory for examination within 2 to 3 hours, avoiding any chilling that would damage the sperm. A sperm count is made with a hemocytometer and a motility study is completed before Papanicolaou staining, to determine abnormalities of the spermatozoa. Special tests are necessary for the examination of semen in vaginal secretions, on hair, and on clothing.

Amniotic Fluid. The removal of amniotic fluid from the uterus (amniocentesis) is done under strict aseptic conditions at 14 to 16 weeks' gestation by puncturing the uterus transabdominally with a special needle and withdrawing 10 to 20 ml of fluid.

Amniocentesis is not without its risks to both the fetus and the mother. Major maternal risks include bleeding and infection, and fetal risks include abortion, puncture, and induced malformation. Much of the danger has been reduced by use of ultrasonic scanning to locate accurately the position of the fetus in utero before amniocentesis is performed.

Amniotic fluid is usually clear or light yellow and consists of 98 per cent water and 1 to 2 per cent solids. About half the solids are organic, and half of these are protein. There is evidence that the constituents of amniotic fluid maintain a dynamic equilibrium with the maternal extracellular fluid, and vary in number, characteristic, and morphology during the course of pregnancy. Examination of amniotic fluid is made separately on the supernatant fluid and on the cellular portion. The cells, which are fetal in origin, are grown in special tissue culture media for a period of 10 to 14 days or longer for chromosomal analysis (karyotyping).*

Most commonly the leukocyte cells in the amniotic fluid are studied when they reach the metaphase stage of mitosis. At this stage of cell replication, the chromosomes are lined up singly. After chemical treatment and staining, they are microphotographed. The prints are enlarged and the chromosomes are matched according to size and morphology. The resulting pattern is a karyotype, and from special analysis the genetic sex pattern and certain genetic defects can be ascertained. (See Fig. 5-27.) Interpreters should remember that genetic sex may not match the patient's social, physical, or psychologic sex, and the last three are more important.

5. DIAGNOSTIC X-RAY

X-ray examinations are rarely painful, although the introduction of contrast media involves discomfort and sometimes pain. The responsibility for the explanation of these procedures to the patient, as well as the reason for the x-ray examination, lies not only with the physician but also with nurses and x-ray technicians who usually amplify the explanations and directions to the patient by conference and written instructions. If medical workers put themselves in the place of the patient, they will realize that these tests are often frightening. The patient may fear the discovery of a dread disease, and the machinery in the x-ray department can look very intimidating. Patients are asked to undress and

to put on a thin gown. Then they are asked to assume positions that may be very uncomfortable or, when some conditions are present, extremely painful. The hard, cold x-ray tables may add to their discomfort considerably. Nurses and x-ray technicians who are sensitive to the fears and distress associated with these x-ray procedures are often in a position to minimize them.

Since the discovery of x-ray in 1895 by Wilhelm Roentgen of Wurtzburg, Germany, its use in diagnosis has come to be widespread.* According to Lester W. Paul and John H. Juhl, x-rays "are a form of electromagnetic energy of very short wave length . . . . Because of their short wave lengths they have the ability to penetrate matter and it is this characteristic that makes them of use in the study of tissues." †

X-ray dosages are usually measured in units called "rads." Other terms sometimes used to measure the amount of x-rays absorbed are roentgens (R) and "rems." E. James Potchen and associates [33] say that for practical purposes each is equivalent to the rad. When x-rays are used for diagnostic purposes rather than for treatment, the doses are very low and range from a few millirads (1 millirad = 0.001 rad) to 10 rads delivered to a limited area of the body. Lethal doses occur when 300 or more rads are delivered to the entire body in a single x-ray.‡

Principles. The applicability of x-ray lies in the fact that various tissues and substances differ in their resistance to the passage of x-rays or roentgen rays. Radiologists recognize x-ray densities or increasing resistance to x-ray penetration in the following order: by air, fat, blood, muscle, and bone. In much the same way that camera film turns dark when exposed to light, x-ray film darkens when exposed to x-rays and to x-ray-induced light from fluorescent material on both sides of the film. When penetration is high, or resistance to x-rays is low, the x-ray film is dark, as in an x-ray of air in the lungs. Since the film registers the amount of x-rays that penetrate the tissues, the greater the penetration, the darker the film. Conversely, the lesser the penetration (the higher the resistance), the lighter the film, as in an x-ray of the bone.

It should be remembered that an x-ray film

---

* Chromosomal analysis and sex chromatin testing are part of the rapidly growing field of cytogenetics. Specialists in this field study human chromosomes and their abnormalities.

* For a discussion of x-ray as therapy, see Chapter 31.

† Paul, Lester W., and Juhl, John H.: *The Essentials of Roentgen Interpretation*, 3rd ed. Harper & Row, New York, 1972, p. 1.

‡ There is, however, considerable discussion of the possible danger of even diagnostic x-ray if used too often.

is viewed as a three-dimensional projection of the varying densities of the tissues, rather than an actual "picture" of the various organs, tissues, and bones. Correct interpretation of the shadows requires knowledge, skill, and experience. The technique of "plain" x-ray is used for the study of bones, their diseases, fractures, maturity, and size; for the study of the chest; and, to a certain extent, for the abdomen. Plain films are also taken of the skull, its sinuses, and the larynx and pharynx. A form used to report x-ray findings is shown in Figure 7-11.

The following discussion is based on the text *The Essentials of Roentgen Interpretation* by Lester W. Paul and John H. Juhl [34] unless other citations are indicated.

Usually two x-ray views are taken at right angles to each other. If only one view is taken, tissue of low density underlying a structure of high density may not show up on the film; while a second view will often show it. The anteroposterior (AP or frontal view) and right angle or lateral views are often taken. An anteroposterior view of the skull, for example, is taken with the patient facing the direction from which the x-rays are traveling and the back of the head against the film holder (cassette). In this position, the x-rays pass through the front of the skull (anterior) to the back of the skull (posterior). X-rays that are not absorbed by the body penetrate the film holder.

A posteroanterior (PA) view of the chest is just the opposite because the patient faces away from the x-ray beam and the chest is against the film holder. The x-rays pass through the back of the chest (posterior) to the front of the chest (anterior). For a left lateral view of the chest, the patient's left side is placed against the film holder and his or her right side faces the x-ray machine. For a right anterior oblique film, the front of the patient's right chest is placed against the film holder and the x-rays penetrate the right side of the back at a 45-degree angle. All x-rays are doubly reversed negatives so what is seen on the film is what would be seen if one were to imagine the examiner facing the patient directly.

Stereoradiography, a special technique used only occasionally, is one in which two slightly different views of the same part of the body are taken simultaneously. The two views are examined at the same time using special viewing equipment. A three-dimensional image is seen by the examiner. This technique is used for studying particularly complicated structures such as the base of the skull. The technique is also used when it is difficult or impossible to get views from more than one position.

Tomography (also called laminography, planigraphy, stratigraphy, and body section radiography) is a special technique that permits examination of a single layer of tissue. This is accomplished by blurring the image of the tissues above and below the layer to be examined at the time the x-ray is taken. Tomograms may be taken when an abnormality is seen on plain films or when a suspected abnormality cannot be seen on plain films. Tomograms of the chest, for example, are particularly helpful in examining patients with pulmonary tuberculosis, emphysema, and carcinoma of the lung.

Standard *fluoroscopy* is a method of x-ray in which the image, instead of being recorded on a film, is focused on a radiosensitive screen, and the shadows are studied directly by the radiologist who is in a room with the patient. Because a continuous stream of x-rays may be used with this technique, the dynamics of the body may be studied; for example, the action of the heart, the motion of the diaphragm, and the motility of the gastrointestinal tract.

Because the intensity of the light on the screen is poor, the procedure must take place in a dark room; there is usually also a waiting period of 20 minutes to allow the eyes of the radiologist to adapt to the darkness. However, if an image intensifier * is used, both the darkened room and the waiting period are unnecessary and the image can be studied in much greater detail. The radiation dose to the patient and the radiologist is high during fluoroscopy, particularly if an intensifier is not used. For this reason, it should be performed as rapidly as possible. The radiologist and other viewers if present should wear lead gloves and aprons for protection. E. M. McIlrath [35] says that when equipment is available, fluoroscopic procedures may be televised, making it possible for many people outside the x-ray room to view it by closed-circuit television. Videotapes may also be made for later and repeated viewings.

Unless other citations are made, the following discussion is based on the text. *Principles of Diagnostic Radiology* by E. James Potchen et al.[36]

In *photofluorography,* the image projected on the screen during fluoroscopy is photographed—producing a miniature film for study. If abnormalities are seen, full-sized x-ray films

---

* A special device which in some cases can increase the intensity of the light on the screen by more than 1000 times.

X-RAY REPORT

Family Name	First Name	Middle Name	Room No.	Hosp. No.

☐ Treatment of ☐ Examination	Name—Part		Sex M F	Age—Years	X-Ray No.
Attending Physician			Date		O.P.D. No.

Specify date, site, roentgens per minute, exposure time and operator when reporting fluoroscopic examinations

Report:

_____
SIGNATURE OF ROENTGENOLOGIST

FORM D-1912   PHYSICIANS RECORD CO., BERWYN, ILLINOIS - PRINTED IN U.S.A.   X-RAY REPORT

Figure 7-11. An x-ray report form. (Courtesy of Physicians' Record Co., Berwyn, Ill.)

are indicated. The procedure was developed and used extensively in mass screening programs for tuberculosis case-finding during World War II. It is a rapid and cheap method for screening many people, but total x-ray exposure is higher than with plain x-rays.

Mammography is a radiographic technique for examining the breast for either benign or malignant tumors. There is some controversy over when to use mammography, but it is thought that detecting deep lesions and evaluating multiple breast nodules are among its most important uses. Each breast is x-rayed in a cranial-caudal view with the nipple in profile and in a lateral view taken with the film placed well under the breast. *Thermography* is another diagnostic technique used to detect breast tumors. It is based on the fact that heat is generated at the site of any inflammatory lesion, dysplasia, or neoplasm. S. Cochrane Shanks and Peter Kerley,[37] in their text, describe a thermographic camera employing infrared radiation. A thermogram should be made of both breasts, producing a permanent image of areas of normal and increased heat emission.

Contrast Studies. The introduction of either air or opaque chemicals into the body to provide contrast has greatly increased the value of x-rays in the study of specific organs or organ systems. Contrast agents—compounds of iodine or barium—absorb more roentgen rays than soft tissues and are commonly used in contrast studies. Other contrast agents, such as carbon dioxide and air, are less dense and absorb fewer x-rays; they are not used as often as the opaque chemicals.

The many ways of diagnosing disease by use of x-ray contrast media are time consuming and complex. Lucy F. Squire,[38] who describes these procedures, cautions that while some contrast studies are nearly harmless, others may be dangerous and are contraindicated under some circumstances. Any patient who is suspected of having a large bowel obstruction, for example, should not take barium sulfate by mouth. Often the x-ray procedure itself is extremely tiring. It can be dangerous when the patient is acutely ill. The risk, however, must be taken if treatment depends on diagnostic x-rays. Proper preparation and thorough explanation to patients are essential to assure their cooperation. Without it, adequate x-ray films are not possible. (See Table 7-3 for radiographic reactions.)

Air Contrast Studies. Air can be introduced into the subarachnoid space of the brain through a spinal tap between the third and fourth lumbar vertebrae to provide contrast media for study of the skull. The air rises in the spinal canal and, if not obstructed, will fill the ventricles of the brain. X-rays may then be taken to visualize certain lesions because growths in adjacent areas will distort the symmetry of the ventricles. This procedure, a *pneumoencephalogram,* is particularly useful in diagnosing tumors impinging on the ventricles and those in the brain stem. A *ventriculogram* is in principle like a pneumoencephalogram, and is made when a pneumoencephalogram either is thought to be unsafe or cannot be done satisfactorily. Ventriculography is the direct introduction of air into the ventricles, and—except in infants, when the needle can be inserted through a fontanel—it requires making two small holes in the cranium through which the needles may be inserted. Air is then injected directly into the ventricles, and x-ray films are taken and interpreted as with the pneumoencephalogram. The air casts darker shadows on the x-ray film because it is less dense than the fluid normally filling the ventricles and less dense than the surrounding brain tissue. In the presence of "space-taking masses," part of the air-filled ventricular system will appear to be displaced. The ventricle is also distorted if a lesion destroys brain tissue and leaves a cavity near the ventricle.[39]

In *pelvic pneumography,* the pelvic structures of the female are outlined by a contrast gas, usually 100 per cent carbon dioxide or USP nitrous oxide. The gas is introduced into the uterus through the vagina or transabdominally and, because it is highly soluble, is rapidly absorbed. The resulting x-rays permit study of the uterus, ovaries, tubes, and ligaments for any defects, masses, or postinflammatory pathology.

Excretory and Secretory Contrast Studies. Chemical contrast agents can be introduced into a hollow organ or viscus such as those of the gastrointestinal tract, the biliary tract, the cardiovascular system, the bronchial tree, the spinal canal, the lymphatic system, and the genitourinary system. Many, but not all, of these procedures are described below. In general, they may be classified as either excretory or secretory contrast studies.

Excretory Studies. Excretory studies utilize the ability of certain organs, as, for example, the gallbladder and kidneys, to excrete radiopaque iodine-containing dyes. To see the gallbladder by x-ray, a dye may be given by mouth or intravenously (*oral cholecystogram* or *intravenous cholecystogram*).[40] The dye is excreted selectively by the liver with the bile, and is then concentrated by the gallbladder. When filled with the radiopaque dye, the shape and size of the gallbladder can be seen. The dye is usually given orally in tablet form after a light supper. After the patient fasts all night and the next morning, the colon is emptied using plain water enemas to clean it and to prevent shadows on the film from feces in the colon in the right upper quadrant. If the gallbladder is not well seen, the test may be repeated the next day or after a high-fat diet which removes old bile in the organ. When the common duct is injected with dye at surgery or postoperatively through a drainage tube, the procedure is called a *cholangiogram*. The common duct can be seen fluoroscopically and on x-ray immediately. Sometimes the dye is given intravenously and the common duct and gallbladder may be seen in 1 to 4 hours, unless there are abnormalities prohibiting visualization.

Intravenous urography (also called intravenous pyelography or IVP) is probably the most important x-ray examination of the urinary tract. A plain film of the kidneys, ureters, and bladder (KUB film) is taken prior to the intravenous injection of a radiopaque dye. Then the dye, or contrast material, is injected and is rapidly excreted by the kidneys. X-rays are taken at 4, 8, 12, and 15 minutes after injection of the dye. If the patient has hypertension, they are taken at 1, 2, 3, and 4 minutes to show differences between the kidneys in their ability to excrete urine. Intravenous urography carries few hazards, and the use of high-dose contrast media makes it more practical than *retrograde urography,* a procedure consisting of direct introduction of dye into the renal pelvis by catheter and cystoscopy. There is risk with this procedure of introducing or spreading infection and puncturing the ureter, so it is reserved usually for cases in which there is inadequate visualization of the renal collecting system by other means and especially where there is unexplained acute anuria. *Cystourethrography* carries little risk, however, and is often used for children with repeated urinary tract infections. The urethra and bladder are visualized after instillation of a dye directly into the bladder by catheter, and the x-rays are taken during voiding. It is obvious that for any of these excretory tests to be most successful and acceptable to the patient, as stated earlier, careful preparation and explanation are important.

Secretory Studies. The latter two studies described above may be considered secretory. The direct introduction of a contrast medium into various body cavities allows visualization of their hollow structures and interpretation of shadows cast by mucosal irregularities before the medium is secreted. Minimal amounts of opaque material are introduced and extend out over the surface of the mucosa of the cavity for study during fluoroscopy; spot x-ray films also demonstrate the material before it is secreted. For example, the upper gastrointestinal tract may be studied after proper fasting by having the patient swallow barium sulfate, an inert, nonabsorbable, tasteless contrast material. The esophagus alone may be studied (*esophagram*) or the stomach and duodenum (*upper GI series*). Fluoroscopy allows the physician or radiologist to observe the process of swallowing, diaphragmatic movements, peristaltic activity, and gastroesophageal spasm. A series of spot x-ray films during each of these activities is made in different positions for later study (see Fig. 7-12).

A *small bowel series* of films may be made in combination with an upper gastrointestinal examination, although this area is hard to examine radiographically because of the constant motion of bowel loops. X-ray films are taken serially to record progress of the barium through the bowel for later evaluation. The large intestine may be outlined by filling it with barium sulfate given by enema (*barium enema*). After proper emptying and cleaning of the bowel,* the contrast material is introduced by rectal catheter and the entire colon is outlined. A double-contrast study entails the injection of air to distend the colon further if necessary to confirm earlier findings. Abnormalities of the entire gastrointestinal tract may be visualized radiographically—tumors, ulcerations, lesions, filling defects, and areas of constriction or distention.

Other organs may likewise be visualized through the introduction of radiopaque dye with special catheters or instruments. *Myelography* is an x-ray examination of the spinal cord and its canal after injection of a radiopaque substance into the spinal canal through a lumbar puncture needle. The spinal canal may then be visualized by fluoroscopy and x-ray films, localizing tumors and certain other disorders of the spinal cord; external pressure on the cord from tumors, herniated disks, or bone fractures may also be demonstrated.

The cervical canal, uterine cavity, and fallopian tubes may be outlined by injecting the contrast agent through the cervix into the uterus. The resulting film, called a *hysterosalpingogram,* is sometimes used in determining uterine abnormalities and evaluating tubal patency in sterility problems. A *bronchogram* permits visualization of the tracheobronchial tree and is particularly helpful in the diagnosis

---

* Methods of emptying and cleaning the bowel differ with the radiologist and the institution. Printed instructions are usually given ambulatory patients. For inpatients the staff follows a prescribed routine in preparing the patient.

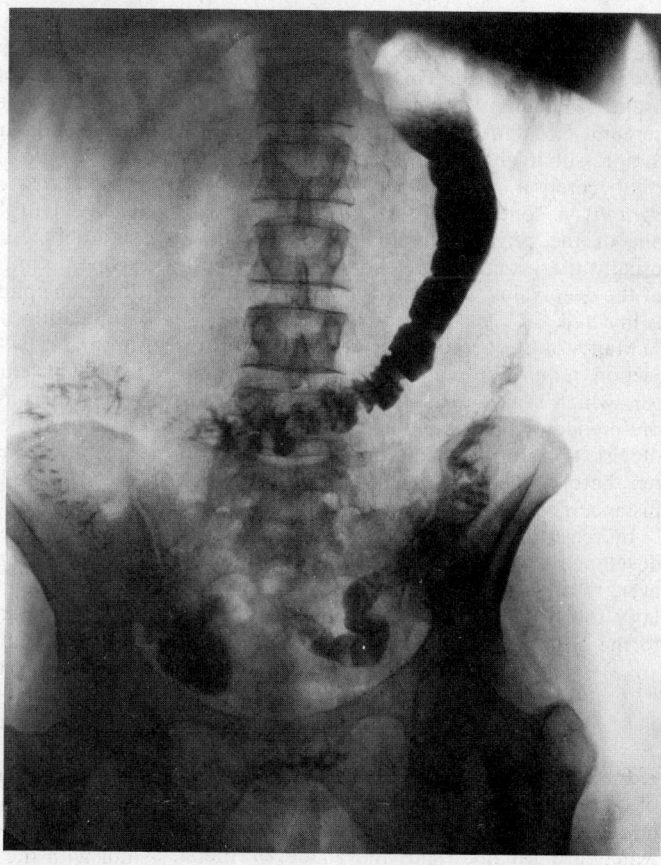

Figure 7-12. X-ray of intestines after the administration of barium sulfate. This is one of a series in the x-ray examination. (Courtesy of Columbia-Presbyterian Medical Center, New York, N.Y.)

of bronchiectasis and obstructive lesions. A *laryngogram* provides a means of studying the nature and extent of known or suspected lesions in the larynx and pharynx. Groups of lymph nodes may be visualized through *lymphoangiography* by injecting dye into lymph channels and filming portions of the entire nodal system. This technique is useful in diagnosis and therapeutic management of patients with lymphomas. Occasionally the extent of sinus tracts and cutaneous fistulas is studied by injecting dye directly into the opening and then making x-ray films to determine the need for surgery. In all of these studies, the contrast material is subsequently removed by the body.

Cardiovascular X-ray Studies. Radiographic visualization of the cardiovascular system is one of the most important advances in the use of contrast agents for the study of blood vessels, the heart, the brain, and other organs. *Angiocardiography* is usually done in conjunction with cardiac catheterization. In angiocardiography a dye is injected into the cardiac catheter so that the chambers of the heart and large vessels can be studied. To get a satisfactory angiocardiogram, several methods are used. A motion picture film (*cineangiography*)

is made to study the motions of the chambers and valves of the heart after injection of the dye. *Serial film angiocardiography* is also used to get a number of films in rapid sequence for later detailed study of the complex heart function. In *coronary angiography* a radiocontrast material is injected into the coronary vessels after the cardiac catheter has been inserted into an axillary or femoral vein. Cineangiography is also used with this procedure to study the coronary arteries.

In *pulmonary angiography* the vessels in the pulmonary vascular bed are demonstrated. Angiograms of the liver, spleen, and kidney can also be made for diagnostic purposes. When the arteries of the kidney are made visible as in *renal angiography*, the dye is injected by direct needle puncture of the abdominal aorta (*aortography*) or by introduction of a catheter through the femoral artery into the aorta. In selective renal arteriography, to diagnose various kinds of kidney disease, the catheter tip is placed in the renal artery.

Cerebral angiography is a method of injecting a water-soluble dye into the carotid (*carotid arteriogram*) or, less often, into the brachial or vertebral arteries. By taking a series of x-ray films at short intervals after the injection, the arterial, capillary, and venous systems are outlined. This examination is very useful in demonstrating abnormalities of the cerebral circulation and also the presence of a tumor, subarachnoid hermorrhage, or insufficient cerebral vascular circulation. In *venography* a contrast substance is injected into one of the peripheral veins of an extremity, usually the lower, for detection of thrombosis of the deep veins; with *arteriography* the artery is injected.

Many of the procedures described in this section require special preparation, directions for which vary with the examination and preference of the individual physician or radiologist; therefore, specific orders may be written before the examination, or, in certain instances, standing orders may be followed.

In recent years, contrast agents have been developed with a wide margin of safety; however, there is still great risk involved, particularly that of idiosyncratic or allergic reaction to the contrast agent.

6. ENDOSCOPY

Endoscopy is the direct visual examination of certain natural body openings or cavities by means of hollow lighted instruments or tubes which are usually rigid and made of metal. Recently developed flexible fiberoptic instruments * have considerably extended the practice of endoscopy, for they make it possible to see more of body cavities with less discomfort to the patient. They have, in some instances, made it possible to see and remove foreign bodies that formerly might have required surgery for their removal.

Not many years ago, the only internal openings available for routine inspection by the clinician were the mouth, throat, and rectum. Later, the development of the speculum made it possible to examine the vagina. The development of lighted instruments with mirrors and magnifying devices made possible an examination of the interior of the eyes, ear canal, nose, and larynx.

Cystoscopy and *urethroscopy* are procedures for viewing the inside of the bladder, the ure-

teral orifices, and the lining of the urethra by means of lighted instruments. Stones, growths, trauma, or other abnormalities can be seen in this way. Biopsies can be made and electrodesiccation of tissue through these scopes or tubes is possible.

The use of fiberoptic instruments has changed urology (and other specialties) considerably. According to S. Vincent,[41] the fiberscope permits better lighting of the bladder so that cinephotographs can be made during stimulation of the bladder. Where there is abnormal function of the bladder, these photographs produce a picture of the abnormality to guide the physician's or radiologist's diagnosis. A fiberoptic pyeloureteroscope provides a means of directly examining the calyceal surfaces of the kidney. This is another advance in the diagnostic evaluation of patients with urological problems.

Often *esophagoscopy* alone is performed to detect esophageal pathology, or it may be done in combination with *gastroscopy*. Bleeding sites, inflammations, tumors, ulcers, or erosions can often be detected much more easily by direct visual examination of the esophagus and stomach than with other diagnostic procedures. In the past, the patient may have been given a general anesthetic when a rigid gastroscope was passed down the esophagus to inspect the mucosa and to get tissue for a biopsy, but with the new fiberoptic gastroscope, which is so much more comfortable to the patient, only local anesthesia is used. The flexibility of the tube also permits visualization of the duodenum and of many formerly blind areas of the stomach.

Examination of the lower alimentary tract is variously called by the region into which the viewing instrument passes: *anoscopy* (anus), *proctoscopy* (rectum), *sigmoidoscopy* (sigmoid colon), and *colonoscopy* (upper colon). *Colonofiberoscopy* is a technique of colon examination using the fiberoptic colonoscope to view portions of the colon beyond that visible with the short, rigid sigmoidoscope. William I. Wolff and Hiromi Shinya [42] have developed a method of removing polyps of the colon with this instrument, a procedure that formerly required major abdominal surgery. Tissue can be taken for diagnostic biopsies through the fiberscope from the rectum to the cecum. The lowered cost to the patient and the savings in time for both patient and medical workers are great advantages of the fiberoptic colonoscope. There is also less risk of complications incident to all major surgery. All told, there is far less discomfort for the patient. The biopsy and even the removal of polyps can be done on an ambulatory basis in 10 to 30 minutes, and, ac-

---

* Not only is the fiberoptic instrument for endoscopic examinations extremely flexible, but it also permits biopsies and aspirations to be done. With a camera attachment it provides excellent color photographs of the internal parts of the body. The basic principle of the instrument is to transmit the image along very thin glass fibers in the form of minute spots of light that bounce off the sides of the tube no matter how flexed the tube becomes.

cording to Irmgard Belinsky and associates,[43] no medication of the patient may be necessary. Other workers, however, may use diazepam or meperidine hydrochloride as needed for amnesia and pain control, respectively.

The fiberoptic technique is also used in other ways to reduce costs and save time. A *laporoscopy* for achieving a tubal ligation enables a woman to resume normal activity twice as fast as after abdominal surgery for the same procedure.[44] Alastair M. Connell, writing in Alex T. Elder and Desmond W. Neill's text,[45] says that fiberoptic endoscopes have also been developed to inspect the peritoneal cavity and liver for diagnostic purposes—*peritoneoscopy*.

Bronchoscopy is the direct examination of the bronchial tree by inspection of the main bronchi and their branches. Using the older rigid bronchoscope presented many difficulties; its passage through the larynx and the trachea was painful and required anesthesia. The more flexible bronchoscopes that have been developed recently permit direct visualization of even the smallest bronchi. Specimens of fluid and cells taken by bronchial brushings provide information often unattainable in any other way for diagnosing lung disease and making the most effective treatment possible.

Mediastinoscopy is done by incising the supraclavicular region or the suprasternal fossa to permit passage of a lighted tube so as to examine the organs of the mediastinum. This procedure is particularly valuable for the observation and biopsy of mediastinal lymph nodes in diagnosing tumors of the lung.[46]

7. TESTS INVOLVING RADIOACTIVE ISOTOPES

Techniques involving radioactive substances are now widely used in modern hospital practice for clinical diagnosis, investigation, and treatment.* E. H. Belcher, writing in Elder and Neill's text,[47] describes their use in measuring aspects of body composition and function, in scanning organs and tissues of the body for disease, and in making assays in the laboratory on blood and other specimens.

Radioisotopes. The field of nuclear medicine has recently grown enormously and rapidly. This specialty uses radioisotopes (radionuclides) whose nuclei give off radiation energy. A radioisotope or radionuclide is considered an unstable form of an element. According to Ruth M. French,[48] it is a form of a given

---

* For another discussion of radioactive isotopes, especially as used in therapy, see Chapter 31.

element that is like it in its chemical reactions but differs from it in its mass number or atomic weight. In an effort to achieve stability, the radioisotope emits small particles of radiation over varying periods of time ranging from a few minutes to many years. It is this characteristic that determines its usefulness in clinical practice. As a tracer, a minute quantity is given by mouth or injected. The amount of radioactivity present in organs, tissues, or body fluids can then be measured. Various counters or scintiscanners have been designed to pick up the radiation in different ways. The exact concentration in each area of the body or the amount in a specimen can then be determined. Often the radiation counter is passed in close parallel paths across an organ or gland to pick up the radioactivity.

Modern scintillation counters and other nuclear radiation detection devices are used to scan small radiation particles, and, unlike a scintiscanner, they do not move across the organ but record the whole field from one position. The machine directs the computer to print a picture on paper, film, or magnetic tape.[49] The picture consists of a series of dots or x's in shades of white, gray, or black, depending on how much radiation is present. The picture produced on a cathode-ray oscilloscope is photographed with a Polaroid camera to preserve the image as a permanent record.

Thyroid Function. One of the most important radioisotopes or radionuclides in use today, both for diagnosis and treatment, is radioiodine (^{131}I). A good example of its use is in the study of the thyroid gland. When the ^{131}I *thyroid uptake test* is administered, a measured dose of ^{131}I is given to the patient by mouth. The activity of the gland is then measured by the amount of iodine taken up by the thyroid. High uptake is associated with hyperthyroidism and low uptake with hypothyroidism. If the gland is capable of handling iodine normally, the picture produced by the counter, scintiscanner, or gamma camera will be a homogeneously dark cluster of dots or x's in the shape of a thyroid gland. When there is a nonfunctioning adenoma present, the area, by contrast, will show up as a clear or "cold" spot. An overactive gland or a thyroid tumor will produce a local dark or "hot" spot. The chief advantage of the ^{131}I thyroid uptake test and other radioisotopic studies is that organ structure and function are simultaneously checked. Often this test is accompanied by measurement of a 24-hour urine for the amount of ^{131}I excreted. In hypothyroidism more than 24 hours is needed to clear the body of radioiodine, and in hyperthyroidism the reverse is true. Quantitative counts of thyroid uptake at periodic intervals up to 24 hours can also indicate hyper- or hypoactivity of the gland. The thyroid uptake test can be invalidated if the patient is being treated with Lugol's solution or thyroid medication, or is receiving thyroid radiation treatments.[50]

A common screening test to measure thyroid function employs radioactive material in the laboratory. The T_3 (*triiodothyronine*) *red blood cell uptake test* is made in vitro * and measures the amount of hormone taken up by the cell after the patient's blood is incubated with radioactive thyroid hormone (^{131}I [radioiodine] labeled T_3). As in the ^{131}I thyroid uptake test, the higher values are found in hyperthyroid patients and lower values in those with hypothyroidism.[51]

Radioisotopes in Diagnosis. In the investigation of body composition and organ function there are many applications of radioactive tracer techniques available. The kind of radioactive agent used varies with the particular organ under study. Table 7-5 lists some important diagnostic applications in the field of nuclear medicine and the radioisotopes frequently used as described by Belcher.

Radiochromium (^{51}Cr) is commonly used in measuring red blood cell survival to detect certain kinds of anemias, and in determining blood volume for assessing transfusion requirements. Radioiron (^{59}Fe) is also used to diagnose anemias by measuring the turnover of iron and the body's utilization of it. The inert gas xenon (^{133}Xe) is widely used in blood circulation studies, especially for the measurement of cerebral blood flow to detect brain tumors or subdural hematomas. It is also used for the study of pulmonary function in certain lung diseases when there is decreased ventilation or perfusion from such causes as pulmonary emboli or tumors. Radiocobalt (^{57}Co, ^{58}Co) is commonly used to differentiate pernicious anemia from other causes of faulty vitamin B_{12} absorption. The Schilling test is used to measure urinary excretion of radiocobalt after the patient is given a minute quantity of the radiopharmaceutical by mouth followed by a vitamin B_{12} injection. Liver function studies with radioactive agents can detect primary tumors or metastases. Kidney function studies using radioactive tracer techniques can determine altered renal blood flow due to vascular disease or transplant rejection.[52]

Treatment. Valuable as are radioisotopes in diagnosis, their use in treatment has some significance also. This is discussed more fully in Chapter 31.

Scanning. Scanning of organs is perhaps one

of the most widely practiced of all the radioactive diagnostic and treatment procedures. Many clinically useful applications of scanning techniques are available to permit both an outline of the organ or tissue under study and to detect space-occupying lesions within them.[53]

Because radioactive measurements are made so frequently within the hospital, medical personnel may forget that most patients are unfamiliar with these tests. Since people tend to associate radioactivity only with cancer, nurses should try to get them to express their fears. It may be possible to reduce or dispel the anxiety. In some cases the fear is justified but in all cases the nurse's understanding can minimize it.

In addition to thyroid scanning, discussed previously, there are many other areas of the body that can be scanned: the bones, bone marrow, brain, heart, kidney, liver, lungs, pancreas, parathyroids, placenta, and spleen. Special radiopharmaceuticals labeled with generator-produced radioisotopes that are especially suitable for scanning techniques are listed in Table 7-6.

Bone scans with radiostrontium (^{85}Sr) are used to detect bone metastases and tumors earlier than with any other procedures. Space-occupying lesions can be found with brain scans. A cardiac blood pool scan matched to a standard chest x-ray pericardial silhouette can help identify pericardial effusion. A kidney scan indicates a lesion of that organ when there is a "cold" or clear spot on the computer picture. This is true, of course, of liver and other organ scans. A liver scan is useful to help identify the site for getting biopsy specimens.[54]

Many other studies are possible, but often interpretation is so difficult as to render them almost useless. A new brain lesion detection device, the EMI scanner, was recently developed by Godfrey Hounsfield,[55] a British computer engineer. This sophisticated machine permits visualization of the brain in cross section. The picture produced by the scanner provides much greater detail than in conventional x-rays and scans. The hope has been expressed that machines of this sort can be developed in the future to study all organs, enhancing diagnosis and reducing the discomfort and costs of many hospital procedures.

8. DIAGNOSTIC ULTRASOUND

The application of the principle of reflected sound is the basis of ultrasonic diagnosis. As Donald A. Forbes explains it, "Just as the ship on the surface of the ocean can detect a

---

* Within an artificial environment, as in a test tube.

Table 7-5.   Applications of Radioactive Tracer Techniques in the Investigation of Body Composition and Organ Function*

Field	Application	Radiopharmaceuticals Used
Body composition studies	Measurement of total body water	^{3}H-water ^{125}I-, ^{131}I-iodoantipyrine
	Measurement of extracellular fluid volume	^{35}S-sulfate ^{77}Br-, ^{82}Br-bromide
	Measurement of total exchangeable sodium	^{22}Na, ^{24}Na
	Measurement of total exchangeable potassium	^{42}K, ^{43}K
Blood volume and red cell survival studies	Measurement of plasma volume	^{125}I-, ^{131}I-, ^{132}I-albumin
	Measurement of red cell volume	^{32}P-phosphate ^{51}Cr-chromate
	Study of red cell survival	^{32}P-diisopropyl phosphorofluoridate ^{51}Cr-chromate
	Measurement of gastrointestinal blood loss	^{51}Cr-chromate
Blood circulation studies	Radiocardiography	^{131}I-albumin
	Measurement of coronary blood flow	^{42}K ^{84}Rb, ^{86}Rb
	Measurement of peripheral blood flow	^{22}Na, ^{24}Na ^{51}Cr-chromate ^{85}Kr ^{125}I-, ^{131}I-albumin ^{133}Xe
	Measurement of cerebral blood flow	^{85}Kr ^{133}Xe
Kidney function studies	Renography	^{125}I-, ^{131}I-o-iodohippurate
	Measurement of glomerular filtration rate	^{51}Cr-ethylenediamine tetraacetate ^{57}Co-, ^{58}Co-vitamin B_{12} ^{125}I-, ^{131}I-allylinulin
	Measurement of renal plasma flow	^{125}I-, ^{131}I-o-iodohippurate
Liver function studies	Measurement of polygonal cell function	^{125}I-, ^{131}I-rose bengal
	Measurement of hepatic blood flow	^{125}I-, ^{131}I-albumin micro-aggregates ^{198}Au-colloid
Lung function studies	Study of distribution of ventilation and perfusion	^{85}Kr ^{133}Xe
Thyroid function studies	Study of thyroid hormone secretion	^{123}I-, ^{125}I-, ^{131}I-, ^{132}I-iodide
	Study of thyroid hormone utilization	^{125}I-, ^{131}I-thyroxine
Gastrointestinal absorption studies	Measurement of vitamin B_{12} absorption	^{57}Co-, ^{58}Co-vitamin B_{12}
	Measurement of iron absorption	^{55}Fe, ^{59}Fe
	Measurement of calcium absorption	^{45}Ca, ^{47}Ca
	Measurement of fat absorption	^{14}C-labeled fats ^{125}I-, ^{131}I-triolein ^{125}I-, ^{131}I-oleic acid
Turnover studies	Study of iron turnover	^{59}Fe
	Study of calcium turnover	^{47}Ca
	Study of plasma protein turnover	^{125}I-, ^{131}I-labeled proteins ^{51}Cr-chromate ^{51}Cr-albumin
	Measurement of gastrointestinal protein loss	^{125}I-, ^{131}I-albumin ^{125}I-, ^{131}I-polyvinyl pyrolidone

* A wide range of applications of radioactive tracer techniques relate to the investigation of various aspects of body composition and organ functions. Some important applications in this category are listed above. (Belcher, E. H.: "Diagnostic Applications of Radioisotopes," in Elder, Alex. T., and Neill, Desmond W. [eds.]: *Biomedical Technology in Hospital Diagnosis.* Pergamon Press, New York, 1972, p. 307.)

Table 7-6.   Applications of Scintigraphic Techniques *

Organ or Tissue	Radiopharmaceuticals Used
Bone	^{18}F ^{47}Ca ^{68}Ga ^{85}Sr ^{87m}Sr
Bone marrow	^{52}Fe ^{99m}Tc-sulphur colloid ^{198}Au-colloid
Brain	^{74}As-arsenate ^{99m}Tc-pertechnetate ^{131}I-albumin ^{197}Hg-, ^{203}Hg-chlormerodrin
Heart	^{99m}Tc-albumin ^{113m}In-transferrin ^{131}I-albumin ^{137m}Ba
Kidney	^{99m}Tc-iron complex ^{131}I-o-iodohippurate ^{197}Hg-, ^{203}Hg-chlormerodrin
Liver	^{99m}Tc-albumin microaggregates ^{99m}Tc-sulphur colloid ^{113m}In-colloids ^{131}I-Rose Bengal ^{198}Au-colloid
Lung	^{99m}Tc-albumin macroaggregates ^{113m}In-iron hydroxide particles ^{131}I-albumin macroaggregates
Pancreas	^{75}Se-selenomethionine
Parathyroid	^{75}Se-selenomethionine
Placenta	^{51}Cr-labelled red cells ^{11m}Tc-albumin ^{113m}In-transferrin ^{131}I-albumin ^{132}I-albumin
Spleen	Heat-treated ^{51}Cr-labelled red cells ^{197}Hg-, ^{203}Hg-bromomercurihydroxy-propane-treated red cells
Thyroid	^{99m}Tc-pertechnetate ^{125}I-iodide ^{131}I-iodide

* Belcher, E. H.: "Diagnostic Applications of Radioisotopes," in Elder, Alex. T. and Neill, Desmond W. (eds.): *Biomedical Technology in Hospital Diagnosis.* Pergamon Press, New York, 1972, p. 312.

submarine many fathoms below by listening to echos, so can the clinician receive information about many deep-lying body structures."*

When ultrasound, or sound that travels at frequencies greater than 20,000 cycles per second, strikes an object, part of it passes through, part of it is absorbed, and part of it is reflected. The extent to which each of these events takes place depends on the frequency of the ultrasonic sound waves and the ability of the different layers of the object to impede them. All the tissues of the body interact with ultrasound in the same way according to Forbes.[56] This makes it possible to observe certain structures which cannot be seen by x-ray; and since ultrasound, as employed diagnostically, is believed to be harmless, it can be used in some situations (pregnancy for example) in which x-ray carries a high risk.[57]

High levels of ultrasound are destructive to tissues. This characteristic has been used surgically, for example, in destroying the labyrinth of the ear in Meniere's disease. Although there is no direct evidence suggesting that ultrasound, as used in obstetric practice, is harmful to the fetus, there have been a few reports of studies where tissue cultures subjected to ultrasound showed more chromosomal abnormalities than tissue cultures that were not. C. J. Dewhurst [58] recommends that the safety of ultrasonic diagnostic techniques used in obstetrics and elsewhere be firmly established before their adoption.

A diagnostic ultrasonic machine consists of a transducer and an oscilloscope screen. The transducer, an object about 1 inch in diameter which generates ultrasound, is applied to the lubricated skin of the patient and is moved about over the area to be examined. Most of the ultrasound waves are reflected from the surface of the body. The remainder penetrate the skin and continue on until they reach a layer of tissue that will not allow the waves to penetrate it. Sound waves, when impeded by the skin and other tissues, echo along their original paths and are recaptured by the transducer. The transducer converts the sound energy into electric energy, amplifies it, and transmits it to an oscilloscope where a tracing of the structures scanned is displayed. The procedure is not painful, and generally causes no discomfort to the patient.[59]

Lele [60] says that diagnostic ultrasound was first used about 20 years ago to detect changes in the position of the midline of the brain

* Forbes, Donald A.: "The Use of Ultrasonics in Diagnosis," in Elder, Alex. T. and Neill, Desmond W.: (eds.): *Biomedical Technology in Hospital Diagnosis.* Pergamon Press, New York, 1972, p. 121.

which occur in some diseases. Since then, its use as a diagnostic aid has spread to many specialties. It has been used extensively in obstetrics to measure the fetal head, to locate the placenta, to detect twins, and to diagnose many obstetric and gynecologic problems. Cardiologists use ultrasound to study the structure and function of heart valves and to detect pericardial effusions. Ophthalmologists using ultrasound are able to examine parts of the eye hidden by cataracts, hemorrhage, and the retina. It is even being used to check blood pressure through the use of a new machine called an Arteriosonde; this bounces ultrasonic frequencies off the walls of a patient's artery, is extremely accurate, and can be used on patients in severe shock.[61]

Included in the preceding are only a few of the ways that diagnostic ultrasound has been used; improvement of present techniques and new ones is constantly being sought. That diagnostic ultrasound shows promise for replacing some kinds of invasive x-ray procedures is encouraging.

The use of ultrasound in therapy (sonar therapy) is discussed in Chapter 31.

9. GRAPHIC STUDIES

Cardiologists and neurologists use a number of special diagnostic tests, many of which have been discussed in previous sections. In addition, there are highly important graphic studies of heart function and of the nervous system that are invaluable to the clinician. Graphic studies are based on the fact that small electric impulses, given off by the active heart, brain, and muscles can be recorded on special paper and interpreted in such a way as to aid in the diagnosis of many diseases. The chief graphic studies are the electrocardiogram (ECG), the phonocardiogram (PCG), the omnicardiogram (OCG), the His bundle electrogram (HBE), the photoanalysis of the implanted cardiac pacemaker, the electroencephalogram (EEG), and the electromyelogram (EMG). The responsibility for explaining these procedures to the patient lies largely with nurses, who, in special instances, may carry out some of these tests themselves.

Electrocardiogram. The electrocardiogram is discussed in detail in Chapter 6 so that only a brief mention of it is made here. A sample reporting form is shown in Figure 7-13. Electrocardiographic tracings are made permanently on a long moving strip of paper by sending magnified electric impulses into a voltmeter whose indicator arm, an electrically heated stylus, is deflected upward or downward according to the direction of the charge. The heated stylus burns through a white gelatin coating on an otherwise black paper strip, producing a permanent record of the electric activity of the heart for interpretation by the clinician.

In intensive care and coronary care units, tracings are made semipermanently for direct visual monitoring on the fluorescent screens of cathode-ray oscilloscope heart monitors, but the convenience of monitors is somewhat balanced by a very high sensitivity to extraneous electric interference. Suspicions of arrhythmias and myocardial disease noted on monitors should be checked quickly by standard tracings. It should be remembered that electrocardiographic interpretation requires considerable skill and experience on the part of the clinician. It is an immeasurably valuable adjunct in the diagnosis of cardiac disorders when interpretations are made by the expert.

David Littmann summarizes the value of the ECG:

Of all laboratory cardiac procedures the electrocardiogram provides the most information for the effort involved. It is completely noninvasive, without risk, modest in expense, and can be performed by the physician, nurse, technician, or student. In fact, it can often be interpreted by any of them. The electrocardiogram provides information about heart rate, rhythm, state of the myocardium, the presence or absence of hypertrophy, ischemia or necrosis, abnormalities of conduction, and distribution. The electrocardiogram also reflects the presence of various drugs and the effects of disturbed electrolytes. Relatively specific abnormalities accompany pericarditis, and even malignant disease of the heart is sometimes detected. Perhaps most importantly, although a normal electrocardiogram may be found in the presence of a variety of chronic disorders of the heart, it is rarely seen with acute, serious disease.*

Omnicardiogram. R. W. Brancato and J. R. Levitt [62] have described a new method of cardiac recording called the omnicardiograph (OCG). This technique changes the conventional ECG pattern from a linear to a two-circle format, and provides a more complete recording of the electric activity of the heart. The OCG machine enables the clinician to see more easily all of the abnormalities of the heart on a single circular graph. According to the authors, physicians may be able to identify those persons who have incipient coronary artery disease long before myocardial infarction occurs. Figure 7-14 depicts normal and abnormal OCG patterns.

* Littmann, David: *Examination of the Heart. Part 5. The Electrocardiogram.* American Heart Association, New York, 1973, p. 1.

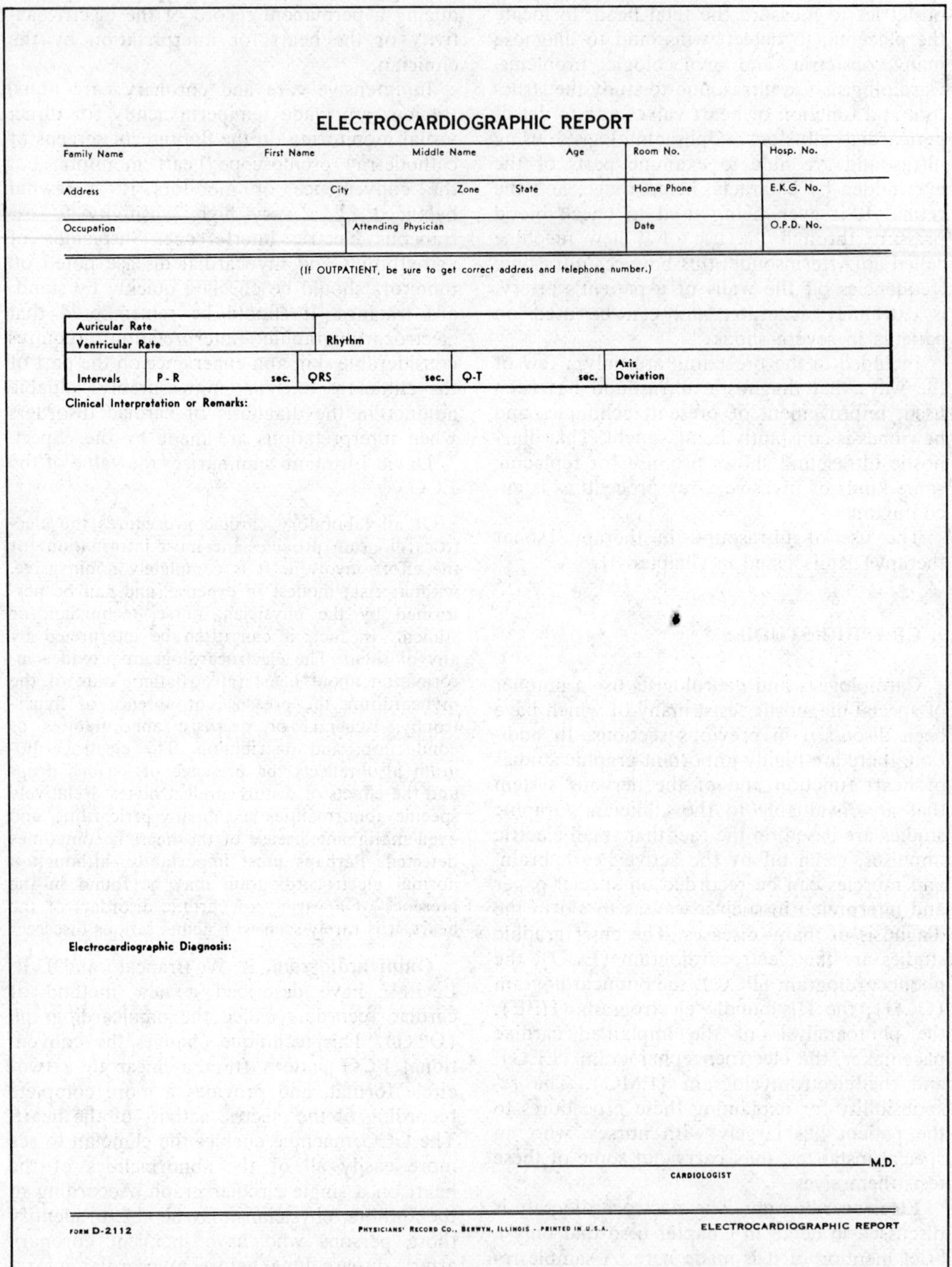

ELECTROCARDIOGRAPHIC REPORT

Family Name	First Name	Middle Name		Age	Room No.	Hosp. No.
Address		City	Zone	State	Home Phone	E.K.G. No.
Occupation		Attending Physician			Date	O.P.D. No.

(If OUTPATIENT, be sure to get correct address and telephone number.)

Auricular Rate						
Ventricular Rate		Rhythm				
Intervals	P - R sec.	QRS sec.	Q-T sec.	Axis Deviation		

Clinical Interpretation or Remarks:

Electrocardiographic Diagnosis:

_____ M.D.
CARDIOLOGIST

FORM D-2112   PHYSICIANS' RECORD CO., BERWYN, ILLINOIS · PRINTED IN U.S.A.   **ELECTROCARDIOGRAPHIC REPORT**

Figure 7-13. An electrocardiographic report form. (Courtesy of Physicians' Record Co., Berwyn, Ill.)

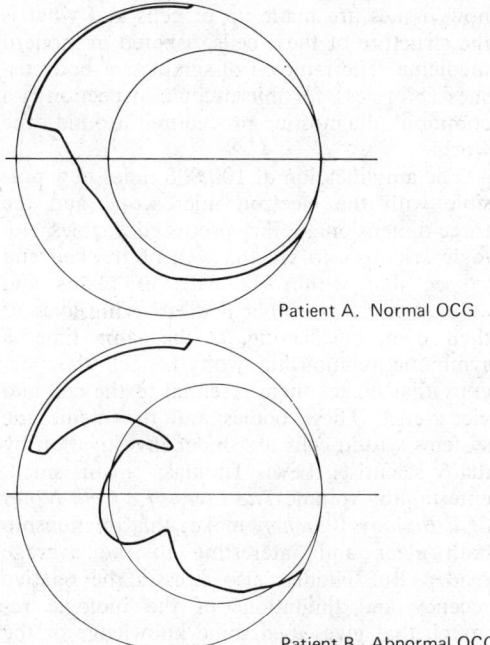

Patient A. Normal OCG

Patient B. Abnormal OCG

Figure 7-14. Normal and abnormal omnicardiographic recordings. (From Brancato, R. W., and Levitt, J. R.: The Omnicardiogram," *Med. Electronics & Data,* **5:**52, [July–Aug.] 1974.)

Phonocardiogram. Another cardiac graphic study that may be ordered is the phonocardiogram (PCG). This is a graphic representation of the sounds and murmurs that originate in the heart and great vessels. The sounds are picked up from the surface of the body and correspond with what the clinician hears through the stethoscope. They are amplified and traced on a graph to provide a permanent record of the events occurring in the cardiac cycle. The greatest value of the PCG is in its depiction of the precise timing and sequence of the heart sounds and murmurs.[63]

The sounds produced by the carotid artery can also be displayed graphically by means of a *carotid phonoangiogram* to detect carotid occlusive disease as a precursor of stroke. Another noninvasive technique is *oculoplethysmography,* which employs sensors on the corneas to record ocular pulses. A delay indicates significant reduction in carotid artery blood flow.[64]

His Bundle Electrogram. A His bundle electrogram (HBE) is another graphic record which can be made only during cardiac catheterization. After insertion through the brachial artery, the cardiac catheter lies next to the atrioventricular node and the bundle of His inside the heart and records electric activity at that junction. Edwin G. Zalis and Mary H. Conover [65] in describing this test say that it

is a significant one for determining the exact times of the progress of the current through the heart.

Photoanalysis of the Implanted Cardiac Pacemaker. Photoanalysis of the impulse from a cardiac pacemaker has been possible since 1965. G. J. Schmutzer [66] describes this method in discussing implanted pacemakers. The patient with an implanted cardiac pacemaker must return for frequent examinations in special clinics to detect early failure of this device. At this visit the nurse or technician uses a cathode-ray oscilloscope machine to record the pacemaker impulse pattern. This pattern is displayed graphically on the oscilloscope machine and is photographed with a Polaroid camera to obtain a permanent record of the impulse pattern. The clinician may make an immediate interpretation of the status of the pacemaker by comparing it with the patient's previous pacemaker impulse patterns. This examination enables the clinician to evaluate immediately the need for replacement of pacemaker batteries.

Electroencephalogram. The electroencephalogram (EEG) may be compared with the electrocardiogram in that electrodes are placed over the skull in many areas, and then the electric activity of the various segments of the brain is recorded. Like the electrocardiogram, the test is made by a trained technician and then read by a specialist. Quiet patients as subjects in well-insulated laboratories are necessary for good results. Like the electrocardiogram, the procedure is entirely painless.

The scalp electrodes, held in place by means of adhesive material, are good conductors of electric impulses from the brain. The EEG machine is a sophisticated electronic amplifier that changes the small scalp voltages into voltages capable of activating multichannel recording pens, which write in ink on paper moving at a speed of 2.5 cm per second. The origin of the recorded patterns is often unclear but, if correlated with the clinical picture, is reliable enough to make the EEG a standard, noninvasive, and safe technique for evaluating brain pathology, as, for example, tumors, abscesses, or epilepsy.

EEGs serve best to identify seizure disorders by type and area of origin within the brain. Often a patient will have no seizure activity during a single study, so repeat studies are ordered. Sometimes the patient is asked to breathe deeply for several minutes to produce alkalosis, a seizure-activating measure. Occasionally sleep deprivation is used as a seizure-inviting stress, or sleep may be induced by drugs or naturally to record activity during that state. Photostimulation such as flashing lights may also be a useful additional stress that can evoke a seizure. The purpose of these procedures is not to produce a convulsion but to induce diagnostically important abnormalities.

Brain tumors, abscesses, infarcts, and subdural hematomas may also cause abnormalities on EEG tracings. Unfortunately, the precise location achieved for such anatomic problems by EEG is usually not quite as good as that suggested by neurologic examination and brain scanning techniques, and never so good as the location achieved by cerebral arteriography or pneumoencephalography. The EEG is almost always abnormal in conditions where there is some impairment of consciousness: the more profound the loss, the greater the abnormality. According to Raymond D. Adams and Robert R. Young,[67] the EEG is used in the neurosurgical operating room to record activity of the exposed brain (*electrocorticogram*) and more recently to signify clinical death of a patient before the excision of an organ for transplant.

Electromyelogram. The electromyelogram (EMG) is a systematic recording of the electric currents given off by nerves and muscles. An EMG is done by inserting needle electrodes directly into the bodies of different muscles in turn and then observing their electric activity, both at rest and when active, by means of an electronic recording apparatus. The cathode-ray oscilloscope is the recording instrument of the EMG. After insertion of the needles, the examiner waits for all muscular activity to become electrically silent. When the muscle is voluntarily contracted by the patient, action potentials appear on the screen of the instrument. With a weak muscle having few contracting fibers, there will be a smaller total potential produced. The EMG is a useful aid in the diagnosis of peripheral nerve disorders such as amyotrophic lateral sclerosis, muscular dystrophy, myasthenia gravis, and myotonia; it also will diagnose fibrillation and fasiculations, which are spontaneous muscular activities during relaxation, and are an indication of diseased muscles.[68]

All of the graphic studies just described must be evaluated carefully by the clinician since each procedure is subject to technical error and misinterpretation. As has been mentioned before, all diagnostic laboratory tests to be of optimum value must be viewed against the background of clinical findings.

10. MICROPHOTOGRAPHY AND MACROPHOTOGRAPHY

The development of the microscope, enabling physiologists and pathologists to see how tissues are made up of cells and what is the structure of these cells, ushered in modern medicine. The removal of samples of body tissues (biopsies) for microscopic inspection is a common diagnostic procedure around the world.

The amplification of 100,000 times now possible with the electron microscope and the three-dimensional effect produced enables biologic scientists to see the wall of the cell and to see that within the cells of plants and animals there are other bodies having lives of their own, but having, at the same time, a symbiotic relationship with the cell they occupy that makes them essential to the cell and vice versa. These bodies and the membrane systems within cells are under investigation by many scientists. Lewis Thomas,[69] in his small, entertaining volume *The Lives of a Cell; Notes of a Biology Watcher,* makes this relationship both clear and interesting to the average reader. But Thomas also stresses the relative recency and limitations of the biologic research that gives men some knowledge of the microscopic system of the cell. He sees the study of biologic interdependence as supremely important.

Television programs and articles in popular journals have made the structure of nerve, muscle, and cancer cells familiar to even nonmedical people in technologic societies. Televised surgeons can be seen spending as much as 10 hours operating on a square inch of tissue as they refer to the microscopic structures of the operative site shown on a monitor. The effectiveness of treatment of lupus affecting the kidney can be determined by electron microscopic studies of the glomeruli, the material for study removed by needle biopsies.[70]

Genetics has entered a new era now that the electron microscope has taken much of the guesswork out of the study of chromosomes.[71]

It is not within the scope of this book to review or even mention the possible diagnostic uses of *microphotography,* particularly the newer form of electron microphotography, but a text such as that of Mariano F. LaVia and Rolla B. Hill, Jr.[72] suggests its importance in the study and treatment of inflammatory disease, neoplasia, and hereditary conditions. What may soon be learned about microscopic anatomy could upset many established concepts of etiology and therapy.

Macrophotography of the body, its parts, or areas has been widely used to show lesions, growths, or postural defects and their progression. It may also be employed to show stages in repair, correction, or cure.[72a] A photographic silhouette showing abnormal posture may do more than words to persuade a person to seek treatment, just as a photograph that shows progress from corrective exercises will encourage their continued use.

Plastic and dental surgeons use photography in diagnosis and as a record of therapeutic progress. "Before and after" photographs persuade many persons to have cosmetic surgery. Photographs can also be used in seeking consultation on treatment. They are an important element in some patients' permanent records.

11. PULMONARY FUNCTION TESTS

Many tests are available to measure disturbances of respiratory function. There are simple tests to measure vital capacity as well as complicated tests requiring special equip-

ment and intricate computation. The terms used in pulmonary function testing may appear confusing, but each has special meaning in the diagnosis and treatment of various forms of chronic obstructive and restrictive lung disease. Table 7-7 lists the common tests used to measure respiratory function.

The effect of any restriction of air flow to the lungs is best evaluated by means of a time-volume relationship. Vital capacity (VC)* and forced vital capacity (FVC) are not measured according to time, for example, but forced expiratory volume (FEV) and maximal voluntary ventilation (MVV) are calculated against a given time interval. Figure 7-15 is a graphic

* Abbreviations are often used in expressing measurements of pulmonary function.

Table 7-7.   Ventilatory Function Tests *

Description	Term Used	Symbol	Remarks
The largest volume measured on complete expiration after the deepest inspiration without forced or rapid effort.	Vital capacity.	VC	This may be normal or even high in COPD patients and is *of little value by itself.*
The vital capacity performed with expiration as forceful and rapid as possible.	Forced vital capacity.	FVC	This volume is often significantly reduced in COPD due to air trapping, and is an important standard measurement.
Volume of gas exhaled over a given time interval during the performance of forced vital capacity.	Forced expiratory volume (qualified by subscript indicating the time interval in seconds).	FEV_T ($FEV_{1.0}$)	If below predicted normal values, this is a valuable clue to the severity of the expiratory airway obstruction.
FEV_T expressed as a percentage of the forced vital capacity: $FEV_{T \times 100}$ FVC	Percentage expired (in T seconds).	$FEV_{T\%}$	This time-volume relationship is another way of expressing the presence or absence of airway obstruction.
The average rate of flow for a specified portion of the forced expiratory volume, usually between 200 and 1200 ml.	Forced expiratory flow.	$FEF_{200-1200}$	Formerly called maximum expiratory flow rate (MEFR). A slowed rate is an early manifestation of COPD.
Average rate of flow during the middle half of the forced expiratory volume.	Forced mid-expiratory flow.	$FEF_{25-75\%}$	Formerly called maximum mid-expiratory flow rate. This is slowed early in the course of ventilatory impairment.
Volume of air which a subject can breathe with voluntary maximal effort for a given time.	Maximal voluntary ventilation.	MVV	Formerly called maximum breathing capacity. Another valuable test, usually correlating well with the patient's complaint of dyspnea.

* National Tuberculosis and Respiratory Disease Association: *Chronic Obstructive Pulmonary Disease, A Manual for Physicians,* 3rd ed. The Association, New York, 1972, p. 42.

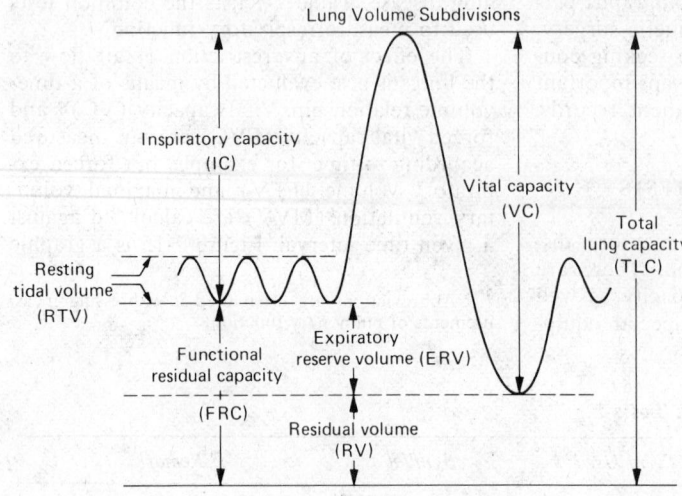

Figure 7-15. Diagram of lung volume subdivisions. Inspiratory capacity (IC) is the maximal volume inspired from a resting expiratory level; expiratory reserve volume (ERV) is the maximal volume expired from a resting expiratory level; vital capacity (VC) is the maximal volume expelled by complete expiration after a maximal inspiration; functional residual capacity (FRC) is the volume of gas in the lungs at the resting expiratory level; residual volume (RV) is the volume of gas in the lungs after a maximal expiration; total lung capacity (TLC) is the volume of gas in the lungs after a maximal inspiration, i.e., the VC plus the RV; resting tidal volume (RTV) is the volume of gas inspired or expired during each breathing cycle. (From National Tuberculosis and Respiratory Disease Association: *Chronic Obstructive Pulmonary Disease, A Manual for Physicians*, 3rd ed. The Association, New York, 1972, p. 44.)

representation of the lung volume subdivisions.

The technicians who carry out these tests may use many types of spirometers to measure respiratory volume and time-volume relationships. The usual laboratory instrument is a recording, belltype machine with a soft-tipped pen to produce the spirometric tracing or spirogram. After computations are made, the results are compared with predicted values found in standard spirometric tables for persons of the same sex, age, and height as the patient. The results are also expressed as a percentage of normal values.[73]

Differentiation of obstructive airway disease from restrictive airway disease is often possible with these tests. Restrictive impairment, or interference with the bellows action of the lungs, includes such conditions as congestive failure, pulmonary fibrosis, lung resection, and compression of the lung by air or fluid. There is obstructive impairment in bronchitis, bronchiolitis, and emphysema. Because there are wide normal variations in pulmonary function tests, especially for FEV rates, repeated tests on the same patient are of value and increase the reliability of the spirometry. Therapy may often be based almost exclusively on changes seen in pulmonary function tests. Often when the FEV is repeated after isoproterenol

(Isuprel) has been inhaled, there is an increase in the rate, indicating a positive effect of the bronchodilator and an element of reversibility in the disease. According to the authors of a Manual[74] published by the National Tuberculosis and Respiratory Disease Association (now called the American Lung Association), there can be reversibility in asthma and sometimes bronchitis but not usually in emphysema.

Patients who are asked to perform pulmonary function tests must understand the importance of making a maximal effort in order to get the best results. Even the most cooperative patient requires some coaching to enable him or her to have clinically valuable spirograms.

12. SKIN TESTS

The usefulness of skin testing in the diagnosis of certain illnesses depends on the purpose for which each is intended. Skin tests can be divided into at least three types according to their purposes: (1) those tests that indicate susceptibility or resistance to an infection; (2) those that produce a delayed skin reaction and indicate either a past or present experience with an infectious agent; and (3) those that indicate a hypersensitivity reaction to environmental allergens.

In the first category are the *Schick test* to identify individuals who may be susceptible to diphtheria and the *Dick test* to determine susceptibility to scarlet fever. Although not used extensively now because of the decreased incidence of these diseases, a positive reaction to a dilute toxin administered intradermally indicates a need for prophylactic measures against either diphtheria or scarlet fever. A *mumps antigen* has been developed to determine whether or not a person is resistant to the mumps virus. If the skin test is positive, there are antibodies present and the individual most likely will not get the disease; if it is negative, there are no antibodies present and he or she will be susceptible to the mumps virus. The test is also used to check for generalized anergy.

In the second group, by far the most common skin test to produce a delayed skin reaction is the *tuberculin test*. It is a widely used diagnostic and screening test. Useful in epidemiologic surveys to indicate the incidence of infection in a population and to detect new cases of the disease, the tuberculin test may be given intradermally (Mantoux test), or with a four-pronged tuberculin-impregnated disc (tine test), or by means of a jet-injection gun. Skin reaction to a very small amount of purified protein derivative (PPD) means that the individual has at some time become infected with the tubercle bacilli. A positive reaction in an individual known to have been nonreactive previously is a good indication of the presence of the disease. The positive tuberculin skin test will persist for life usually, although after the tuberculous lesion becomes inactive the test occasionally may revert to negative. Persons with a negative tuberculin reaction are commonly found to be in the advanced stages of tuberculosis, to have acute miliary tuberculosis, or to be on steroid therapy.

Whereas the tine test is frequently used as a screening test, the *Mantoux* or *intradermal skin test* is always given following a positive tine test. The usual method of performing the Mantoux is to inject 0.1 ml intradermally of a specially prepared dilute tuberculin on the inner (volar) aspect of the forearm. After 48 to 72 hours, an area of induration (not erythema) of 8 mm or more indicates a positive reaction. The usual initial intradermal tuberculin test is made with intermediate-strength PPD; however, there are a weaker first-strength PPD and a stronger second-strength PPD that are sometimes used.[75]

The *tine test* is administered by pressing four small tuberculin-impregnated tines on a plastic disc into the forearm skin for 1 second and evaluating the induration around each of the four puncture sites 2 to 3 days later by consulting a tine test reaction chart.

A positive tuberculin test may not necessarily indicate an infection with *Mycobacterium tuberculosis* but the reaction may be caused by one of the atypical mycobacteria. The classification by Ernest H. Runyon[76] subdivides the atypicals into four groups depending on their growth and colony characteristics (see Table 7-8). In general, the atypical mycobacteria produce a milder skin test reaction than does the *M. tuberculosis*. There are available specific skin tests for each of these groups to help in the clinical diagnosis; the tests are made in situations where the organism is resistant to the usual antituberculous drugs.[77]

Persons with calcified lesions in their lungs resembling those resulting from tuberculosis, but with negative tuberculin tests, may be found to have been infected with the fungus *Histoplasma capsulatum*. Mass testing programs indicate that many persons in certain geographic areas react positively to the histoplasmosis skin test. Other skin tests to identify mycotic or fungal infections have been developed for blastomycosis, coccidioidomycosis, and other diseases caused by fungi. The tests are often deceptive and usually interfere with more accurate serum antibody tests.

Bacterial infections can often also be identified through skin testing as an adjunct to other clinical investigations. Antigens are available to test for brucellosis, a disease frequently infecting meat packers and veterinarians; for tularemia, a disease of hunters and fur handlers; and for chancroid, leprosy, and glanders.

Table 7-8. Classification of the Atypical Mycobacteria *

Group I	Photochromogens (*M. kansasii* and others)
Group II	Scotochromogens (*M. scrofulaceum* and others)
Group III	Nonphotochromogens (*M. xenopii* and others)
Group IV	Rapid growers (*M. fortuitum* and others)

* Adapted from Ravel, Richard: *Clinical Laboratory Medicine,* 2nd ed. Year Book Medical Publishers, Chicago, 1973, p. 170. The original classification of the atypical mycobacteria was suggested by Ernest H. Runyon in *Am. Rev. Tuberc. Pulm. Dis.* (Correspondence), **72**:866, (June) 1955. Group I mycobacteria, the photochromogens, turn bright yellow when exposed to light; group III, the nonphotochromogens, do not; group II, the scotochromogens, are identified by their yellowish-orange pigmentation; group IV mycobacteria are identified by their characteristically rapid growth after incubation.

The *Frei test* is a widely used test to diagnose a viral disease called lymphogranuloma venereum. Skin tests for certain parasitic diseases such as echinococcosis, trichinosis, schistosomiasis, filariasis, and others have been developed but are not considered sufficiently specific to assure a diagnosis.

The *Kveim test* may be used to diagnose sarcoidosis. Ground-up human sarcoid tissue is diluted and prepared as an antigen, then injected intradermally. After 4 to 6 weeks, if positive, a papule at the injection site is biopsied and then examined histologically for the typical granulomas of sarcoidosis. The Kveim test is considered a highly specific test for this disease.

The third type of skin testing is that done for hypersensitivity reactions to environmental allergens such as pollen, spores, dander, food, drugs, and other substances. Known as atopic reactions, they are usually manifested as hay fever, asthma, coryza, urticaria, and gastrointestinal upsets. The most useful way to detect allergy to certain substances is through patch testing with dilute extracts of a wide variety of substances under suspicion. Intradermal injections of extracts of materials can be used as well as sun sensitivity patch tests to determine the offensive environmental agent. Because *allergy skin testing* is so complicated and potentially unsafe, it is best handled by specialists in allergic diseases.[80]

13. VISION, HEARING, AND SPEECH TESTS

There are many diagnostic and screening tests for children and adults with visual, hearing, and speech problems. Only a few are discussed in this section. Information on signs, symptoms, and ways to help patients with these defects is discussed in Chapter 46.

Vision Screening. Authorities seem to agree that careful measurement of central distance visual acuity is the single most important vision test. Reduced acuity determines the presence of many diseases as well as a need for refractive correction with glasses or contact lenses.

The standard Snellen chart and the Snellen E chart are commonly used to screen both adults and children. This chart consists of lines of letters or E symbols of varying sizes; well lighted, it is placed 20 ft from the patient. Acuity is recorded as a fraction with the numerator representing the distance to the chart and the denominator the distance at which a normal eye can read the line. A reading of 20/50 in one eye indicates that at 20 ft the patient can see the letters that a normal eye sees at 50 ft. Each eye is tested separately, while the opposite eye is covered with a card.[78] A new method of vision screening was recently reported by Aran Safir and his associates [78a] in which an instrument (Ophthalmetron) is used by technicians to automatically measure refraction characteristics of the eye.

For a more comprehensive visual examination, school-aged children may be given the *Massachusetts Vision Test* in three parts—a Snellen E chart test, a plus-lens test for hyperopia, and a muscle imbalance test. The Massachusetts Vision Test and the Snellen test have been reported to correlate best with findings on ophthalmoscopic examination.[79]

Color vision may be evaluated by using books with special designs in various colors. These color plates are available from optical companies and are called *Hardy-Rand-Rittler Pseudoisochromatic Plates* (H.R.R.) and the *Ishihara Test*.[80]

Preschool children can be screened with the Snellen E chart if they are able to comprehend directions. The following tests also have been reported to be useful in evaluating central distance vision of preschool children: the *Sjogren Hand Test,* the *Landolt Broken Ring Test,* the *California Clown Test* (Do-As-I-Do Vision Test), and the *Michigan Junior Vision Screening Test.* Some screening tests for very young children are based only on the child's ability to recognize forms and shapes and consist of matching letter tests, picture tests, a *Symbol Test,* and a *Miniature Toy Test.*[81]

For adults over 35 years of age with or without eye complaints, most ophthalmologists recommend tonometry screening. Early detection of glaucoma makes it possible to treat this condition and prevent blindness. There are many tonometers available and in use today, but the one most frequently used in screening programs is the Schiotz. It records anterior ocular pressure by measuring the resistance of the conjunctiva and sclera to indentation by the instrument's weighted plunger. After instillation of a topical anesthetic into each eye, the examiner holds the instrument vertically so the plunger is freely movable. While the patient's eye is held open, the plunger's lower tip touches and rests on the eye for a second or two. A reading is taken from the scale and later converted to millimeters of mercury (mm Hg). Applanation tonometers are newer and are most often used in diagnostic ophthalmoscopy. They are more accurate and cause less scleral indentation than does the Schiotz but are more expensive.[82] A still newer and more expensive machine measures eye pressures and then graphically records the readings on a moving strip of paper, much like an ECG recording. With any of these methods, however, intraocular pressure readings should not exceed 20 mm Hg. Beyond this level, a diagnosis of glaucoma may be suspected but not confirmed until a complete ophthalmologic examination is made.

Tests for Hearing. When hearing loss is suspected, there are a number of ways to evaluate the loss and determine the type of impairment. Chief among these methods is the careful assessment of the person's response to sound stimuli with a pure tone audiometer. In general, the quieter the environment, the more valid the test. Before donning earphones patients are asked to point to the ear in which the high- or low-frequency sounds are first perceptible. An alternative method is for patients to activate a light switch as soon as the sound is heard.

An audiometer is a pure frequency oscillator capable of delivering stimuli by air conduction (earphones) or bone conduction (bone oscillator) from 250 Hz* through 8000 Hz and at intensity levels from −10 dB † through +110 dB. Most screening audiometers have only air conduction capabilities and so offer a reduced frequency range. Sounds at various intensity levels and at various frequencies are presented to each ear. The examiner either determines the patient's threshold or conducts a screening test at an acceptable intensity level for the particular noise level of the room in which the test is performed. Most school screening tests are given at about 20 to 30 decibels.

The individual's response to the test when the signal is presented by air conduction indicates the integrity of the entire auditory system (outer ear, middle ear, and inner ear). Response to the test when the signal is presented by a bone oscillator is an indication of the integrity of the inner ear (cochlea) only. Comparison of the responses when the signal is presented by these two methods can help determine the type of hearing impairment. If there is no hearing loss when the signal is presented by air conduction, testing with the bone oscillator is unnecessary. An audiogram, a graph of the test results, is made for the patient's permanent record and interpreted by the audiologist or otologist.[83] An audiogram form is shown in Figure 7-16.

The earlier hearing impairment in a child is found, the greater are his or her chances

for rehabilitation, or the more possible is a normal life (see Fig. 7-17). Screening programs have been developed to identify the infant with a hearing problem. In a study by Marion P. Downs and Graham M. Sterritt [84] it was estimated that one newborn in 2000 to 3000 (if tested) would be found to have a hearing loss. Testing high-risk infants is desirable, but the high false positive rate makes mass screening of all newborns an unacceptable procedure.

In Chapter 46 the ways in which the nurse can recognize behavioral changes at different stages of growth, indicating defective hearing, are discussed. When hearing loss in an infant is suspected, cortical audiometry can be used. A computerized form of brain wave analysis, it is similar to the electroencephalogram. It involves sedating the child and then sending sounds through earphones to each ear and recording the response through EEG tracings.[85] The efficacy of the EEG hearing test has not been established, and its clinical use is debated by many health workers.

Older preschool children can be screened by presenting familiar sounds at certain designated frequencies. Children are asked to point to a picture representing the sound they hear and, if they "fail" are given a threshold audiogram with the pure tone audiometer.[86]

Group audiometry, requiring paper and pencil responses to sound stimuli, is rarely used to identify those who need attention. The Committee on Identification Audiometry of the American Speech and Hearing Association [87] says that periodic individual tests are preferable to group tests.

An acoustic impedance meter is a new device for indirectly determining the integrity of the auditory system. It requires no voluntary response on the part of the patient, but provides information on the condition of the middle ear and the performance of the various middle ear components. An ear probe unit is inserted into the ear to create an airtight system. Flexible rubber tubing is attached to the impedance meter to record various middle ear pressure changes. Interpretation of the impedance and compliance measurements and the condition of the ear structures is made when the readings are plotted on a graph.[88] Examples of various types of impedance curves are shown in Figure 7-18.

Because many hearing problems can be job-associated, industrial medical departments often require regular evaluations of each employee's hearing. Sample forms to record the worker's hearing history and audiometric data are shown in Figures 7-16 and 7-19. Many large industries have adopted the use of the von

---

* Hz stands for *Hertz* and is a symbol used to indicate the number of cycles per second (cps) of the sound.

† dB stands for *decibel* and indicates the intensity of the sound relative to zero, the normal hearing threshold.

MOBIL OIL CORPORATION
MEDICAL DEPARTMENT
AUDIOMETRIC DATA SHEET

SOCIAL SECURITY NO. _____

JOB TITLE _____

EMPLOYMENT DATE _____

NAME _____

BIRTH DATE _____

LOCATION _____

DATE	DAY OF WEEK		TIME
AUDIOMETER CALIBRATION:	☐ ANSI	☐ ISO	CALIBRATION DATE

TECHNICIAN'S NAME _____

PHYSICAL EXAMINATION OF EARS

ITEM		RIGHT	LEFT
EXTERNAL EAR	CERUMEN		
EXTERNAL CANAL	INFECTION		
DRUM	PERFORATION		
	REDNESS		
NASAL BLOCKAGE			

HEARING MEASUREMENTS

RECORD db	500	1000	2000	3000	4000	6000	
							RIGHT
							LEFT

HEARING READINGS   X = LEFT EAR

(0 = RIGHT EAR)

	500	1000	2000	3000	4000	6000
-10						
0						
10						
20						
26						NORMAL LEVEL (ANSI)
30						
40						
50						
60						
70						
80						
90						
100						

PHYSICAL HISTORY

1. Employee's evaluation of own hearing: ☐ GOOD ☐ FAIR ☐ POOR

2. Has employee noticed any change in hearing since last exam?
☐ NO ☐ YES   EXPLAIN _____

3. Since the last exam has employee had any of the following?

CONDITION					
EARACHE	☐ NO	☐ YES	FREQUENT COLDS	☐ NO	☐ YES
EAR INFECTION	☐ NO	☐ YES	HEAD INJURY	☐ NO	☐ YES
DIZZINESS	☐ NO	☐ YES	NASAL ALLERGIES (HAY FEVER)	☐ NO	☐ YES
			RINGING IN EAR	☐ NO	☐ YES
EXCESSIVE FATIGUE	☐ NO	☐ YES	SINUS INFECTION	☐ NO	☐ YES

4. Is the employee presently being treated for any medical condition?
☐ NO ☐ YES   WHAT? _____

5. Is the employee presently taking any medication?
☐ NO ☐ YES   WHAT? _____

6. Does the employee now have hobbies which expose him to excessive noise?
(loud music, firearms, hunting, motorcycles, planes, etc.)
EXPLAIN (HOW OFTEN ETC.) _____

COMMENTS _____

JOB HISTORY

If applicable answer questions 7 – 12   ☐ NOT APPLICABLE

7. How long has employee been in present job? _____

8. Estimate of hours spent per day working in noisy area? _____

9. Describe type of noise: (machinery, turbines, steam, etc.) _____

10. Does employee wear hearing protection while in noisy area? ☐ NO ☐ YES

11. How long since most recent exposure to excessive noise? _____

12. Duration of exposure to that excessive noise? _____

Figure 7-16. Form showing worker's audiometric data. (Courtesy of Mobil Oil Corp., Medical Department, New York, N.Y.)

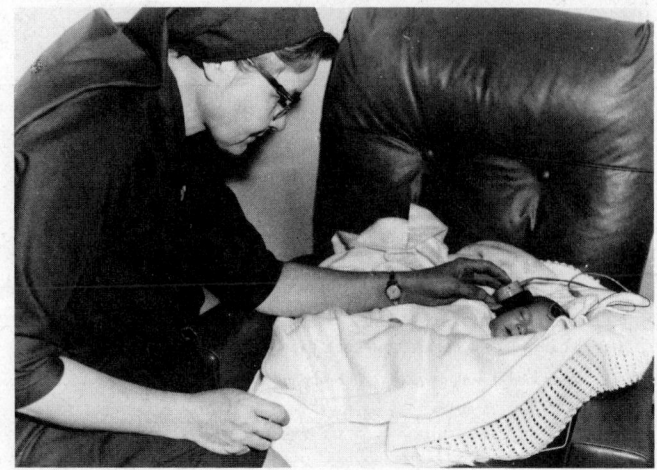

Figure 7-17. Infant asleep in an acoustically and electrically shielded room. Sound is delivered through earphones. The brain wave response is picked up by three skin electrodes attached to the scalp. (From Linnell, Craig, et al.: "The Hearing-Impaired Infant, Diagnosis and Rehabilitation," *Nurs. Clin. North Am.,* **5:** 511, [Sept.] 1970.)

Békésy self-administered audiogram, which involves listening to a machine and pressing and releasing a button to increase or decrease the intensity of certain tones to make them audible. A graph is produced by the machine, but interpretation by a specialist is required.[89]

Speech audiometry testing differs from pure tone audiometry in that words rather than sounds are used. It was developed during World War II to compare the efficiency of different communication systems. It is used in the United States to test the individual's ability to hear a series of standardized two-syllable words and to hear running speech delivered by a live voice or recording. The procedure is like that of pure tone audiometry except that the examiner sits in one room and the patient in a separate soundproof room. The test results are recorded on a speech audiogram for each ear. Such items as speech reception threshold, most comfortable loudness, tolerance level, dynamic range, and discrimination are recorded.[90]

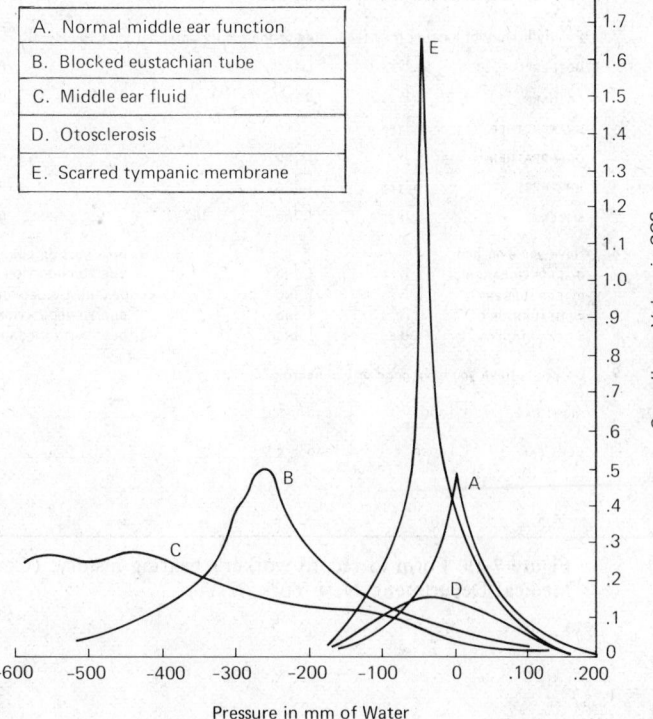

Figure 7-18. Pressure compliance curves relating to middle ear function. (From Taylor, Ian G.: "Audiometry," in Elder, Alex. T., and Neill, Desmond W. (eds.): *Biomedical Technology in Hospital Diagnosis.* Pergamon Press, New York, 1972, p. 139.)

A. Normal middle ear function
B. Blocked eustachian tube
C. Middle ear fluid
D. Otosclerosis
E. Scarred tympanic membrane

CO-4113 (2-73)

MOBIL OIL CORPORATION
MEDICAL DEPARTMENT
HEARING INFORMATION HISTORY

NAME _____   SOCIAL SECURITY NO. _____

BIRTH DATE _____   JOB TITLE _____

LOCATION _____   EMPLOYMENT DATE _____

READ CAREFULLY – PLEASE COMPLETE EACH ITEM

1. What kind of work do you do? Describe in your own words: _____
_____
_____

2. Are you ever in a noisy area?   ☐ Yes   ☐ No

   How long are you in a noisy area at one time? _____

3. How long during a 24-hour period are you in a noisy area? _____

4. Is ear protection equipment such as earmuffs, ear plugs, etc., provided for you?   ☐ Yes   ☐ No

5. Do you regularly wear the protection equipment provided?   ☐ Yes   ☐ No

6. Have you had previous hearing tests?   ☐ Yes   ☐ No

   WHEN _____   WHERE _____

   WHY _____

   ANY PROBLEMS _____
   _____

   Have you ever been advised to wear a hearing aid?   ☐ Yes   ☐ No

7. Family history of hearing loss (your side of the family only, not your spouse's).

   MOTHER   ☐ YES   ☐ NO   IF YES, WHAT AGE _____
   FATHER   ☐ YES   ☐ NO   IF YES, WHAT AGE _____
   GRANDMOTHER   ☐ YES   ☐ NO   IF YES, WHAT AGE _____
   GRANDFATHER   ☐ YES   ☐ NO   IF YES, WHAT AGE _____
   BROTHERS   ☐ YES   ☐ NO   IF YES, WHAT AGE _____
   SISTERS   ☐ YES   ☐ NO   IF YES, WHAT AGE _____

8. Have you ever had:
   a. BROKEN EARDRUM   ☐ YES   ☐ NO
   b. EAR SURGERY   ☐ YES   ☐ NO
   c. HEAD INJURY   ☐ YES   ☐ NO
   d. EAR INJURY   ☐ YES   ☐ NO

   e. DEAFNESS OR RINGING IN EARS
      DUE TO INFECTION OR INJURY   ☐ YES   ☐ NO
   f. DEAFNESS OR RINGING IN EARS
      DUE TO MEDICATION   ☐ YES   ☐ NO
   g. DEFORMITY OF EAR   ☐ YES   ☐ NO

9. Do you believe you have good or bad hearing?

   RIGHT EAR: ☐ GOOD   ☐ BAD   WHY _____

   LEFT EAR: ☐ GOOD   ☐ BAD   WHY _____

Figure 7-19. Form to record worker's hearing history. (Courtesy of Mobil Oil Corp., Medical Department, New York, N.Y.)

10. Do you have difficulty hearing on the telephone? ☐ Yes ☐ No

11. Do you have to turn up the T.V. or radio? ☐ Yes ☐ No

12. Can others hear sounds that you cannot ☐ Yes ☐ No

13. Have you ever worked in a noisy environment? ☐ Yes ☐ No

WHERE _____

14. Have you ever flown airplanes or worked around them, e.g., military or maintenance?

☐ Yes ☐ No WHERE AND HOW LONG _____

_____

15. How often do you use firearms? HOBBY _____

HUNTING _____ SKEET _____

TRAP _____ TARGET PRACTICE _____

16. If you were in the service, what were your duties?

_____

_____

_____

17. How frequently are you exposed to the following noise?

	NEVER	OCCASIONALLY	FREQUENTLY		NEVER	OCCASIONALLY	FREQUENTLY
AIR HAMMERS	☐	☐	☐	MOTORCYCLES	☐	☐	☐
AIRPLANES	☐	☐	☐	NOISY MACHINERY	☐	☐	☐
COMPRESSORS	☐	☐	☐	RIFLE RANGE	☐	☐	☐
EXPLOSIVES	☐	☐	☐	RIVETING	☐	☐	☐
HOBBY	☐	☐	☐	TRUCKS	☐	☐	☐
LOUD MUSIC	☐	☐	☐	OTHER	☐	☐	☐

18. Have you ever received treatment for tuberculosis? ☐ Yes ☐ No ☐ ☐ ☐

WHEN _____

WHERE _____

DATE _____ EMPLOYEE'S SIGNATURE _____

INTERVIEWER'S SIGNATURE _____

Figure 7-19 (*continued*)

Speech (and Language) Tests. Testing children for speech disorders is common in most large school systems and in speech and hearing departments of most major hospitals. The child with dysarthria or articulation disability may be tested with the *Denver Articulation Screening Examination*. This test, developed in Denver, Colorado, in 1973 for economically disadvantaged children to screen them for articulation problems, employs 30 sound elements in certain test words such as *t*able, *shirt, door,* and mo*t*her. Nurses and other health workers, and teachers, can administer this test and refer to a speech pathologist those children who score below an established cutoff point.[91]

The *Peabody Picture Vocabulary Test* (PPVT) measures vocabulary comprehension of children from 2½ to 18 years by measuring the child's hearing vocabulary. Because the individual tested is not required to read and need only point to one of four pictures in response to a verbal stimulus, this test is appropriate for both verbal and nonverbal children. The PPVT contains illustrations with clean, bold lines. It may be given in 10 to 15 minutes by someone with minimal preparation.[92]

To examine children with language problems the *Illinois Test of Psycholinguistic Abilities* (ITPA) or the *Utah Test of Language Development* may be used. Developed originally to help evaluate the mentally retarded, the ITPA deals with communication abilities of children from 2 to 10 years, with the psychologic processes involved, and with their levels of organization.[93] The Utah test is a measure of both expressive and receptive verbal language skills in the normal or handicapped child. It gives the examiner an idea about the growth and change of the child below 14½ years, about individual differences, and about exaggerated deviations that might be found in the child who is either communicatively gifted or handicapped.[94]

Aphasic and dysphasic patients are usually tested with the *Minnesota Test for Differential Diagnosis of Aphasia* developed by Hildred Schuell in 1955. Designed to identify the level at which language performance breaks down, this test attempts to show how language disruptions occur.[95] A newer, popular test for aphasics, developed by Bruce E. Porch in 1967, is called the *Porch Index of Communicative Ability* (PICA). It consists of a multidimensional scale to score responses to the naming of objects, colors, numbers, and other items.[96]

All of these speech and language tests are most often administered by speech clinicians who are familiar with the design, reliability, and procedure for each test. These specialists also interpret the results and institute remedial instruction or teach others how to help the child or adult with speech or language problems.

14. PSYCHOLOGIC TESTS

Psychologic testing is a useful adjunct in diagnosing and planning therapy for psychiatric patients but may be used for many persons not suspected of having a psychosis. Psychologic tests are, for example, used regularly in assessing applicants to schools or candidates for jobs or appointments. Many tests evaluate intellectual ability and personality; some can be used to identify psychogenic or organic brain dysfunction. The most important of these tests are described in the following paragraphs.

Since many of these examinations are often administered individually by clinical psychologists, nurses may not be involved; however, nurses should know their nature and purpose and the significance of the findings. Many persons react adversely when asked to take a test, thinking that they may not be able to "pass" the test or that they will be judged "insane" or neurotic. Nurses can help explain the value of these tests and can supplement what the psychologist may have told the patient and the family.

Most tests require verbal or written responses, but manual dexterity may also be evaluated in a performance (manipulative) test. Because it is important to watch the subject's behavior during some of the tests, the examination is carried out in privacy and in a quiet room, free from interruptions. Results are valid only under such conditions.

The interpretation of some tests is based on the results of testing a large series of individuals, both normal and abnormal. Such results have been compiled, and tables defining the range of normal and abnormal responses have been prepared from these data. The evaluation of the individual examination is made by the examining psychologist both on the basis of the responses of the patient, as compared with the normal scale, and also on the patient's reactions during the examination.

History. According to Lee J. Cronbach,[97] individual differences were first evaluated systematically in 1796 in the Greenwich (England) Observatory. This evaluation was made because an astronomer, who had been employed to record the precise instant that certain stars crossed the telescopic field, was found consistently to record his observations eight tenths of a second later than his superior who recorded his observations of the same phenomena. More careful study of reaction times some years later showed that differences in the records made by astronomers were the result of different speeds with which these scientists were capable of responding to stimuli. Gradually it was recognized that such differences were not only a source of confusing scientific data but also evidence of a significant fact about human nature.

During the nineteenth century a strong interest developed in differentiating between the insane and mentally retarded, in order to provide appropriate care for each. Two French physicians, Jean E. D. Esquirol (1838) and Edouard Séguin (1866) studied verbal ability and motor control of these two groups. Their work was the basis for that of early experimental psychologists who became interested in describing and measuring behavior. Using rigorous laboratory methods, they tested human reactions to visual, auditory, and other stimuli. Some pioneers in the psychologic testing movement were Sir Francis Galton in England, whose belief was that tests of sensory discrimination were a means of judging an individual's intellectual capacity, and James Cattell in America, who developed a series of tests given to college students to determine their intellectual level.[98]

Intelligence Tests. Toward the end of the nineteenth century a French psychologist, Alfred Binet, who was not happy with what were then called "mental tests," proposed new ones from which evolved the well-known *Binet intelligence scales.* Having gone through many revisions since Binet's original test in 1916, the 1960 Stanford-Binet is widely used in the United States to measure childhood intellectual ability and, particularly, to predict a child's school performance. Strongly weighted verbally, this test measures mental abilities at different ages, and, as with other tests, the score can be influenced by personality, emotions, or even environmental conditions.[99]

Other important tests that measure intellectual ability are those developed by David Wechsler in 1939. Highly reliable, these tests consist of both verbal and performance scales. They include the *Wechsler Adult Intelligence Scale* (WAIS), published in 1955 for ages 16 and up, the *Wechsler Intelligence Scale for Children* (WISC), developed in 1950 for ages 5 to 15, and the *Wechsler Preschool and Primary Scale of Intelligence* (WPPSI), published in 1967. The WAIS includes six subtests of verbal ability (information, comprehension, arithmetic, similarities, digit span, and vocabulary), and five subtests of performance (digit symbol, picture completion, block design, picture arrangement, and object assembly). The WAIS is primarily a measure of how well the adult has acquired intellectual skills taught in schools; it draws largely upon a fund of experience common to most adults.[100]

While it is obvious that native intelligence cannot be measured completely free of the influence of education, some tests have reduced to a minimum the effect of education on test results.

Personality Tests. Certain tests designed to study nonintellectual aspects of behavior include the measurement of such characteristics as emotional adjustment, interpersonal relations, motivation, interests, and attitudes. One of the most frequently used self-report personality tests is the *Minnesota Multiphasic Personality Inventory* (MMPI). It was developed originally to get at commonly disabling personality traits. The MMPI covers such areas as health, psychosomatic symptoms, neurologic and motor disturbances; sexual, religious, political, and social attitudes; educational, occupational, family and marital items; and common manifestations of neurotic and psychotic behavior. Self-administered questionnaires used in health assessments where there is no suspected psychosis or emotional disorder elicit information, however, that may fall under any of these headings (see Chapter 5).

The MMPI consists of 550 statements to which the individual responds with "true," "false," or "cannot say." Scores are then computed for various categories or scales: hypochondriasis, depression, hysteria, psychopathic deviate, masculinity-femininity, paranoia, psychasthenia, schizophrenia, hypomania, and social introversion. The MMPI is a complex test but is an important tool for the clinician in identifying seriously disturbed individuals.[101] Over the past few years psychologists have developed computer programs for this test that print out written descriptors of the patient's personality to simulate the clinical interpretation of the MMPI. These fully automated computerized profiles save time in the diagnostic workup.[102]

Other personality tests measure interests and attitudes and help an individual select an occupation; they represent an important dimension of psychologic testing. Special aptitude and occupational tests may help a person choose a career, and interest tests may help him or her plan a specific educational or recreational program. The most important of these tests are the *Strong Vocational Interest Blank* (SVIB) and the *Kuder Preference Record-Vocational.*

First developed in 1920 by E. K. Strong, Jr., the SVIB in its 1966 version consists of 399 items to which an individual responds with "like," "indifferent," or "dislike." The statements pertain to occupations, school subjects, amusements, and activities, associated with different sexes and types of people.* The subject's scores are compared with those of persons successfully engaged in approximately 86 occupations. Research on the SVIB has shown that it has high reliability and validity.

The *Kuder test*, often used by educational and vocational counselors, shows the subject's interest in a number of broad areas rather than specific occupations. The items are arranged so that the person must choose which activity he or she likes most and least. Scores in ten areas are then computed on outdoor, mechanical, computational, scientific, persuasive, artistic, literary, musical, social service, and clerical scales.[103]

Tests of Intellectual Impairment. According to Anne Anastasi,[104] psychologists often test patients to differentiate the retarded from persons with progressive deterioration in intellectual functioning as a result of brain damage, psychotic disorders, or other pathologic conditions. Brain dysfunction can have an organic cause or can be the result of cultural-familial deprivation, while psychotic disorders represent a decline from a higher level of functioning. Psychologists may analyze the patterns of subtest scores in the Wechsler series to study these patients and may also use other tests to measure intellectual impairment.

The *Benton Visual Retention Test* consists of ten cards with geometric designs, each of which is shown to the patient for a specified number of seconds. The patient must then draw the design on a sheet of paper. This test is useful in detecting brain-injured children and is also used to study emotionally disturbed children and mentally retarded, schizophrenic, or elderly patients.

The *Bender-Gestalt* is a psychological test of visual-motor behavior, which is used to study personality and measure intelligence, and to diagnose brain damage. Nine designs are presented to the patients one by one and they are asked to copy the design with the sample in front of them. Various scoring systems have been designed to differentiate "normal" from "abnormal" drawings, but some psychologists prefer to interpret the results by using the original descriptive analyses by Lauretta Bender (1938). According to Eugene

Byrd[105] and Elizabeth M. Koppitz,[106] this test has also been used to study children in need of psychotherapy and those with learning disturbances.

According to Joseph D. Matarazzo,[107] the *Memory-for-Designs Test* (*Graham-Kendall Test*) is also used when brain damage is suspected. This test requires patients to reproduce 15 designs on paper after viewing each for 5 seconds. All of these visual-motor tests are helpful to the psychiatrist in evaluating patients with impaired intellectual functioning.

Projective Techniques. There are many tests to study the responses of patients to a particular stimulus such as an ink blot, a picture, or a drawing. This unstructured method of testing, called projective testing, requires patients to "project" their thought processes onto a stimulus. By giving their imagination free play, the individuals allow fundamental aspects of their psychologic functioning to be revealed in their responses. Projective methods are used primarily by the clinician to uncover not only emotional, motivational, and interpersonal characteristics but also general intellectual level, originality, and problem-solving. The best known of these tests are the Rorschach Test, the Thematic Apperception Test (TAT), and the Machover Draw-a-Person Test (DAP).

The *Rorschach Test* consists of a series of ten standard ink blot patterns, each of which is presented to patients who are asked to describe what they see in the pattern. This test varies with individuals depending on their mental and emotional processes and intelligence. The more intelligent person may see things represented that would not occur to the mind of the less imaginative; a person with disturbed thoughts or emotions may, on the other hand, describe the images in terms of his or her subconscious fears or phobias. Herman Rorschach, a Swiss psychiatrist, developed this testing method in 1942 and was the first to apply such a technique to the study of the patient's total personality. The Rorschach Test has an elaborate scoring system that includes the following major categories into which responses may fall: the *location* (the part of the ink blot the patient describes); the *determinants* (form, color, shading, and "motion"); and the *content* (animals, human figures, various objects, or symbols). Despite problems in scoring, the Rorschach remains one of the most popular techniques in psychological testing.[108]

The *Thematic Apperception Test* consists of a series of 19 pictures which are shown to patients who are then asked to describe each picture, and then to write on a blank form a brief story of the action suggested by the pic-

---

* A new form of the SVIB has been published as the *Strong-Campbell Interest Inventory* and uses the same form for men and women.

ture. Persons with markedly disturbed function may not describe the picture accurately, while those with less severe abnormalities may indicate the nature of an abnormal attitude by the story the picture suggests to them.

Developed at Harvard University in 1938, the TAT also has been widely used in clinical practice and is usually administered in two 1-hour sessions. The interpretation of the themes is also complex and requires analysis according to a list of "needs" such as achievement, affiliation, and aggression and a list of "press" items, referring to environmental forces that interfere with the satisfaction of needs. According to Bernard I. Murstein,[109] the TAT indicates material that a person cannot or will not reveal about himself or herself and is a strong predictor of neurotic behavior.

According to Anastasi,[110] the *Draw-a-Person Test* is one of a group of expressive tests that is therapeutic as well as diagnostic because it allows the patient free expression through drawing. Not only may it reveal the patient's emotional problems, but it may also relieve them somewhat. In this examination, the patient is asked to "draw a person," then is asked to draw one of the opposite sex, and to make up a story about each. The examiner asks a list of specific questions about the characters in the story. Scoring is based on these responses as well as on many items such as size of the figures and their parts, and the style, quality, and characteristics of the drawing.

All of the tests described in these pages illustrate only some of the many forms of psychologic tests available, most of which are designed to test the patient's reactions to stimuli, to study his or her personality, and to evaluate his or her intelligence.

Robert R. Holt[111] says there seems to be a decline in psychologic testing now as a result of the assumption of many more functions by psychologists and a loss of confidence in the definitive diagnostic value of these tests. He thinks, however, that they have a brighter future because the newer tests are better and because new data and new methods of working with old tests as well as new ways of making inferences from data are available. He also predicts the development of a separate professional discipline—psychometrists—who will free psychodiagnosticians from testing and will allow them to concentrate on the more subtle aspects of their work. While it might be hard to get agreement in medical and educational circles on the value of psychologic testing, and the merit of specific tests, the process has an established place in diagnosis of disease, in health assessment, and in educational and vocational counseling.

REFERENCES

1. Cononi, Grace A., and Siler, Mildred: "Automated Multiphasic Health Testing in the Hospital Setting," *J. Nurs. Adm.*, **2**:70, (Nov.–Dec.) 1972.
2. Collen, Morris F., et al.: "Cost Analysis of a Multiphasic Screening Program," *N. Engl. J. Med.*, **280**:1043, (May 8) 1969.
3. Constantine, Herbert R.: "Adult Health Protection Through an Automated Multiphasic Screening Center," *RI Med J.*, **51**:258, (Apr.) 1968.
4. Wallach, Jacques: *Interpretation of Diagnostic Tests.* Little, Brown & Co., Boston, 1970, p. vii.
5. Davidsohn, Israel, and Henry, John H. (eds.): *Todd-Sanford Clinical Diagnosis by Laboratory Methods,* 15th ed. W. B. Saunders Co., Philadelphia, 1974, p. 2.
6. Schimmel, Elihu M.: "The Hazards of Hospitalization," *Ann. Intern. Med.*, **60**:100, (Jan.) 1964.
7. Griner, Paul F., and Liptzin, Benjamin: "Use of the Laboratory in a Teaching Hospital," *Ann. Intern. Med.*, **75**:157, (Aug.) 1971.
8. Snyder, Lilja A.: "We Care Enough to Come to You," *Nurs. Outlook*, **22**:168, (Mar.) 1974.
9. Dlouhy, Alice, et al.: "What Patients Want to Know about Their Diagnostic Tests," *Nurs. Outlook*, **11**:265, (Apr.) 1963.
10. Johnson, Jean E.: "Effects of Structuring Patients' Expectations on Their Reactions to Threatening Events," *Nurs. Res.*, **21**:499, (Nov.–Dec.) 1972.
11. Bartlett, Marjorie H., et al.: "Dial Access Library–Patient Information Service," *N. Engl. J. Med.*, **288**:994, (May 10) 1973.
12. Freeman, Ruth B.: *Community Health Nursing Practice.* W. B. Saunders Co., Philadelphia, 1970, p. 368.
13. *Ibid.*, p. 374.
14. Keuhnelian, John G., and Sanders, Virginia E.: *Urologic Nursing.* Macmillan Company, London, 1970, p. 78.
15. *Ibid.*, p. 78.
16. Davidsohn, Israel, and Henry, John H. (eds.): *op. cit.*, pp. 18–21.
17. *Ibid.*, pp. 15–80.
18. Feldman, Jerome M., and Lebovitz, Francine L.: "Tests for Glucosuria; An Analysis of Factors That Cause Misleading Results," *Diabetes*, **22**:115, (Feb.) 1973.
19. Williams, Susan M.: "Diabetic Urine Testing by Hospital Nursing Personnel," *Nurs. Res.*, **20**:444, (Sept.–Oct.) 1971.
20. Ravel, Richard: *Clinical Laboratory Medicine,* 2nd ed. Year Book Medical Publishers, Chicago, 1973, p. 397.
21. *Ibid.*, p. 397.
22. Davidsohn, Israel, and Henry, John H. (eds.): *op. cit.*, pp. 1280–1281.
23. *Ibid.*, pp. 39, 46, 62, 88, 718, 740, 773.
24. *Ibid.*, pp. 100, 437, 522.

25. Goodman, Louis S., and Gilman, Alfred (eds.): *The Pharmacological Basis of Therapeutics,* 5th ed. Macmillan Company, London, 1975, p. 1458.
26. Davidsohn, Israel, and Henry, John H. (eds.): *op. cit.,* p. 1220.
27. *Ibid.,* pp. 516, 577, 772, 811, 837.
28. Ravel, Richard: *op. cit.,* p. 334.
29. *Ibid.,* p. 397.
30. Davidsohn, Israel, and Henry, John H. (eds.): *op. cit.*
31. *Ibid.,* p. 1240.
32. *Ibid.,* p. 955.
33. Potchen, E. James, et al.: *Principles of Diagnostic Radiology.* McGraw-Hill Book Co., New York, 1971, p. 1.
34. Paul, Lester W., and Juhl, John H.: *The Essentials of Roentgen Interpretation,* 3rd ed. Harper & Row, New York, 1972, pp. 7, 9, 10, 747.
35. McIlrath, E. M.: "Radiological Diagnosis Techniques and Image Intensifiers," in Elder, Alex. T., and Neill, Desmond W. (eds.): *Biomedical Technology in Hospital Diagnosis.* Pergamon Press, New York, 1972, p. 271.
36. Potchen, E. James, et al.: *op. cit.,* pp. 24, 32, 49, 59, 65, 90, 140.
37. Shanks, S. Cochrane, and Kerley, Peter (eds.): *A Textbook of X-Ray Diagnosis,* Vol. VI, 4th ed. W. B. Saunders Co., Philadelphia, 1971, p. 817.
38. Squire, Lucy Frank: *Fundamentals of Roentgenology,* rev. ed. Harvard University Press, Cambridge, Mass., 1975, p. 244.
39. *Ibid.,* p. 332.
40. *Ibid.,* p. 277.
41. Vincent, S.: "The Engineering Approach to the Study of Bladder Control," in Elder, Alex. T., and Neill, Desmond W. (eds.): *Biomedical Technology in Hospital Diagnosis.* Pergamon Press, New York, 1972, p. 457.
42. Wolff, William I., and Shinya, Hiromi: "Polypectomy via the Fiberoptic Colonoscope," *N. Engl. J. Med.,* **288:**329, (Feb. 15) 1973.
43. Belinsky, Irmgard, et al.: "Colonofiberoscopy: Technique in Colon Examination," *Am. J. Nurs.,* **73:**306, (Feb.) 1973.
44. "Fiberoptics: Morbidity and Cost" (editorial), *N. Engl. J. Med.,* **288:**368, (Feb. 15) 1973.
45. Connell, Alastair M.: "Exploring Inside the Body," in Elder, Alex. T., and Neill, Desmond W. (eds.): *Biomedical Technology in Hospital Diagnosis.* Pergamon Press, New York, 1972, p. 444.
46. Jepsen, Otto: *Mediastinoscopy.* Munksgaard, Copenhagen, 1969, p. 12.
47. Belcher, E. H.: "Diagnostic Applications of Radioisotopes," in Elder, Alex. T., and Neill Desmond W. (eds.): *Biomedical Technology in Hospital Diagnosis.* Pergamon Press, New York, 1972, p. 277.
48. French, Ruth M.: *The Nurse's Guide to Diagnostic Procedures,* 4th ed. McGraw-Hill Book Co., New York, 1975, p. 313.
49. *Ibid.,* p. 319.
50. *Ibid.,* p. 321–23.
51. *Ibid.,* p. 159.
52. Belcher, E. H.: *op. cit.,* p. 306.
53. *Ibid.,* p. 311.
54. French, Ruth M.: *op. cit.,* p. 330.
55. Altman, Lawrence K.: "New Brain X-Ray Device May Transform Therapy," *New York Times,* Aug. 26, 1973, p. 1.
56. Forbes, Donald A.: "The Use of Ultrasonics in Diagnosis," in Elder, Alex. T., and Neill, Desmond W. (eds.): *Biomedical Technology in Hospital Diagnosis.* Pergamon Press, New York, 1972, p. 121.
57. Lele, Padmakar P.: "Application of Ultrasound in Medicine" (editorial), *N. Engl. J. Med.,* **286:**1317 (June 15) 1972.
58. Dewhurst, C. J.: "The Safety of Ultrasound," *Proc. R. Soc. Med.,* **64:**996 (Sept.) 1971.
59. Forbes, Donald A.: *op. cit.,* pp. 121, 124.
60. Lele, Padmakar P.: *op. cit.*
61. Robinson, Donald: "The Newest Advances in Hospital Care. 6. Ultrasound," *Parade, New Haven Register,* Oct. 27, 1974.
62. Brancato, R. W., and Levitt, J. A.: "The Omnicardiograph," *Med. Electronics & Data* **5:**52 (July–Aug.) 1974.
63. Ross, John, Jr., and O'Rourke, Robert: "Indirect Methods of Examination of the Heart," in Wintrobe, Maxwell M., et al. (eds.): *Harrison's Principles of Internal Medicine,* 7th ed. McGraw-Hill Book Co., New York, 1974, p. 1094.
64. Kartchner, Mark M., et al.: "Noninvasive Detection and Evaluation of Carotid Occlusive Disease," *Arch. Surg.,* **106:**528, (Apr.) 1973.
65. Zalis, Edwin G., and Conover, Mary H.: *Understanding Electrocardiography,* 2nd ed. C. V. Mosby Co., St. Louis, 1976, p. 7.
66. Schmutzer, G. J.: "The Analysis of Implanted Cardiac Pacemakers," *Biomed. Eng.,* **4:**58, (Feb.) 1969.
67. Adams, Raymond D., and Young, Robert R.: "Diagnostic Methods in Neurology," in Wintrobe, Maxwell M., et al. (eds.): *Harrison's Principles of Internal Medicine,* 7th ed. McGraw-Hill Book Co., New York, 1974, p. 1716.
68. Young, Robert R., et al.: "Laboratory Aids in the Diagnosis of Neuromuscular Diseases," in Wintrobe, Maxwell M., et al. (eds.): *Harrison's Principles of Internal Medicine,* 7th ed. McGraw-Hill Book Co., New York, 1974, p. 1914.
69. Thomas, Lewis: *The Lives of a Cell; Notes of a Biology Watcher.* Viking Press, New York, 1974.
70. Kashgarian, Michael, et al.: *Renal Disease.* Upjohn Co., Kalamazoo, Mich., 1974.
71. McGehee, Harvey A., et al. (eds.): *The Principles and Practice of Medicine,* 18th ed. Appleton-Century-Crofts, New York, 1972, pp. 470–71.

72. LaVia, Mariano F., and Hill, Rolla B., Jr. (eds.): *Principles of Pathobiology*, 2nd ed. Oxford University Press, New York, 1975.

72a. Longacre, J. J. (ed.): *Craniofacial Anomalies: Pathogenesis and Repair*. J. B. Lippincott Co., Philadelphia, 1968.

73. *Chronic Obstructive Pulmonary Disease. A Manual for Physicians*, 3rd ed. National Tuberculosis and Respiratory Disease Association, New York, 1972, p. 41.

74. *Ibid.*, pp. 46, 52.

75. Stead, William W.: "Tuberculosis," in Wintrobe, Maxwell M., et al. (eds.): *Harrison's Principles of Internal Medicine*, 7th ed. McGraw-Hill Book Co., New York, 1974, p. 865.

76. Runyon, Ernest H.: "Veterans Administration–National Tuberculosis Association Cooperative Study of Mycobacteria" (correspondence), *Am. Rev. Tuberc. Pulm. Dis.*, **72:**866, (June) 1955.

77. Ravel, Richard: *op. cit.*, p. 169.

78. Prior, John A., and Silberstein, Jack S.: *Physical Diagnosis; The History and Examination of the Patient*, 4th ed. C. V. Mosby Co., St. Louis, 1973, p. 78.

78a. Safir, Aran, et al.: "A New Method of Vision Care Delivery," *Health Serv. Rep.*, **88:**405, (May) 1973.

79. Lin-Fu, Jane S.: *Vision Screening of Children*. US Department of Health, Education, and Welfare, Public Health Service, Health Services and Mental Health Administration, Maternal and Child Health Service, Washington, D.C., 1971, p. 8.

80. *Ibid.*, p. 8.

81. *Ibid.*, p. 12.

82. Weinstock, Frank J.: "Tonometry Screening," *Am. J. Nurs.*, **73:**656, (Apr.) 1973.

83. Newby, Hayes A.: *Audiology*, 3rd ed. Appleton-Century-Crofts, New York, 1972, pp. 71, 100.

84. Downs, Marion P., and Sterritt, Graham M.: "A Guide to Newborn and Infant Hearing Screening Programs," in Ventry, Ira M., et al. (eds.): *Hearing Measurement; A Book of Readings*. Appleton-Century-Crofts, New York, 1971, p. 372.

85. Linnell, Craig, et al.: "The Hearing-Impaired Infant, Diagnosis and Rehabilitation," *Nurs. Clin. North Am.*, **5:**507, (Sept.) 1970.

86. Downs, Marion P., and Doster, Mildred E.: "A Hearing Testing Program for Pre-School Children," in Ventry, Ira M., et al. (eds.): *Hearing Measurement, a Book of Readings*. Appleton-Century-Crofts, New York, 1971, p. 381.

87. American Speech and Hearing Association, Committee on Identification Audiometry: "Identification Audiometry for School-Age Children: Basic Procedures," in Ventry, Ira M., et al. (eds.): *Hearing Measurement, a Book of Readings*. Appleton-Century-Crofts, New York, 1971, p. 388.

88. Taylor, Ian G.: "Audiometry," in Elder, Alex. T., and Neill, Desmond W. (eds.): *Biomedical Technology in Hospital Diagnosis*. Pergamon Press, New York, 1972, p. 135.

89. *Ibid.*, p. 146.

90. Newby, Hayes A.: *op. cit.*, pp. 69, 116.

91. Drumwright, Amelia, et al.: "The Denver Articulation Screening Exam," *J. Speech Hear. Disord.*, **38:**3 (Feb.) 1973.

92. Dunn, Lloyd M.: *Expanded Manual for the Peabody Picture Vocabulary Test*. American Guidance Service, Inc., Minneapolis, 1965.

93. Kirk, Samuel A., et al.: *Examiner's Manual, Illinois Test of Psycholinguistic Abilities*, rev. ed. University of Chicago Press, Chicago, 1968.

94. Mecham, Merlin J., et al.: *Utah Test of Language Development*, rev. ed. Communication Research Associates, Inc., Salt Lake City, 1967.

95. Schuell, Hildred: *Differential Diagnosis of Aphasia with the Minnesota Test*. University of Minnesota Press, Minneapolis, 1965.

96. Porch, Bruce E.: *Porch Index of Communicative Ability*. Consulting Psychologists Press, Inc., Palo Alto, Calif., 1967.

97. Cronbach, Lee J.: *Essentials of Psychological Testing*, 2nd ed. Harper & Row, New York, 1949, p. 157.

98. Anastasi, Anne: *Psychological Testing*, 3rd ed. Macmillan Company, London, 1968, p. 5.

99. *Ibid.*, pp. 9, 189, 210.

100. *Ibid.*, p. 271.

101. *Ibid.*, pp. 16, 441.

102. Gravitz, Melvin A.: "A New Computerized Method for the Fully Automated Printout of MMPI Graphic Profiles," *J. Clin. Psychol.*, **23:**101, (Jan.) 1967.

103. Anastasi, Anne: *op. cit.*, p. 466.

104. *Ibid.*, pp. 295, 302, 303.

105. Byrd, Eugene: "The Clinical Validity of the Bender-Gestalt Test with Children: A Developmental Comparison of Children in Need of Psychotherapy and Children Judged Well Adjusted," in Murstein, Bernard I. (ed.): *Handbook of Projective Techniques*. Basic Books, Inc., New York, 1965, p. 751.

106. Koppitz, Elizabeth M.: "The Bender-Gestalt Test and Learning Disturbances in Young Children," in Murstein, Bernard I. (ed.): *Handbook of Projective Techniques*. Basic Books, Inc., New York, 1965, p. 767.

107. Matarazzo, Joseph D.: *Wechsler's Measurement and Appraisal of Adult Intelligence*, 5th ed. Williams & Wilkins Co., Baltimore, 1972, p. 421.

108. Anastasi, Anne: *op. cit.*, p. 493.

109. Murstein, Bernard I. (ed.): *Handbook of Projective Techniques*, preface to Murray, Henry A.: "Uses of the Thematic Apperception Test." Basic Books, Inc., New York, 1965, p. 425.

110. Anastasi, Anne: *op. cit.*, p. 507.

111. Holt, Robert R.: "Editor's Foreword," in Rapaport, David, et al.: *Diagnostic Psychological Testing*, rev. ed. International Uni-

versities Press, New York, 1968, pp. 24, 38, 42.

Additional Suggested Reading

Adler, Francis H.: *Textbook of Ophthalmology,* 8th ed. W. B. Saunders Co., London, 1969 (revised by Harold G. Scheie and Daniel M. Albert).

Allison, Joel, et al.: *The Interpretation of Psychological Tests.* Harper & Row, New York, 1968.

Andreoli, Kathleen G., et al.: *Comprehensive Cardiac Care,* 3rd ed. C. V. Mosby Co., St. Louis, 1975.

Beeson, Paul B., and McDermott, Walsh (eds.): *Textbook of Medicine,* 14th ed. W. B. Saunders Co., Philadelphia, 1975.

Keys, John W., et al.: *CRC Manual of Nuclear Medicine Procedures,* 2nd ed. CRC Press, Cleveland, 1973.

Belcher, E. H., and Vetter, R. (eds.): *Radioisotopes in Medical Diagnosis.* Thornton Butterworth, Ltd., London, 1971.

Bogoch, Abraham (ed.): *Gastroenterology.* McGraw-Hill Book Co., New York, 1973.

DeJong, Russell N.: *The Neurologic Examination; Incorporating the Fundamentals of Neuroanatomy and Neurophysiology,* 3rd ed. Harper & Row, New York, 1967.

Felson, Benjamin: *Chest Roentgenology.* W. B. Saunders Co., Philadelphia, 1973.

Frankel, Sam, et al. (eds.): *Gradwohl's Clinical Laboratory Methods and Diagnosis,* 7th ed. C. V. Mosby Co., St. Louis, 1970.

Frankenburg, W. K., et al.: "The Revised Denver Developmental Screening Test: Its Accuracy as a Screening Instrument," *Pediatrics,* **79:**988, (Dec.) 1971.

Fraser, Robert G., and Paré, J. A. Peter: *Diagnosis of Diseases of the Chest; An Integrated Study Based on the Abnormal Roentgenogram.* W. B. Saunders Co., Philadelphia, 1970.

Friedman, T.: "Prenatal Diagnosis of Genetic Disease," *Sci. Am.,* **225:**34, (Nov.) 1971.

Gershon-Cohen, Jacob: "Thermography," *Sci. Am.,* **216:**94, (Feb.) 1967.

Grinker, Roy R., and Sahs, Adolph L.: *Neurology,* 7th ed. Charles C Thomas, Publisher, Springfield, Ill., 1976.

Hurst, J. Willis (ed.): *The Heart: Arteries and Veins,* 3rd ed. McGraw-Hill Book Co., New York, 1974.

Jenkins, James J., et al.: *Schuell's Aphasia in Adults; Diagnosis, Prognosis, and Treatment,* 2nd ed. Harper & Row, New York, 1975.

MacLean,, M. A.: "Cytology Screening—A Program That Works," *Can. Nurse,* **65:**40, (May) 1969.

Miller, J., et al.: "Endoscopy Review," *AORN J.,* **16:**146, (Nov.) 1972.

Provisional Guidelines for Automated Multiphasic Health Testing and Services. Report of the AMHTS Advisory Committee to the National Center for Health Services Research and Development. US Department of Health, Education, and Welfare, Public Health Service, Health Services and Mental Health Administration, Washington, D.C., 1971.

Sataloff, Joseph: *Hearing Loss.* J. B. Lippincott Co., Philadelphia, 1966.

Skydell, B., and Crowder, A. S.: *Diagnostic Procedures.* Little, Brown & Co., Boston, 1975.

Smith, A. M., et al.: "Serum Enzymes in Myocardial Infarction," *Am. J. Nurs.,* **73:**277, (Feb.) 1973.

Stradling, Peter: *Diagnostic Bronchoscopy, An Introduction.* E. & S. Livingstone, Ltd., Edinburgh and London, 1968.

Sutton, Audry L.: *Bedside Nursing Techniques,* 2nd ed. W. B. Saunders Co., Philadelphia, 1969.

Tavel, Morton E.: *Clinical Phonocardiography and External Pulse Recording,* 2nd ed. Year Book Medical Publishers, Chicago, 1972.

Travis, Lee Edward: *Handbook of Speech Pathology and Audiology.* Appleton-Century-Crofts, New York, 1971.

Van Riper, Charles, and Irwin, John V.: *Voice and Articulation.* Prentice-Hall, Englewood Cliffs, N.J., 1958.

Wagner, H. N., Jr. (ed.): *Principles of Nuclear Medicine.* W. B. Saunders Co., Philadelphia, 1968.

Watson, E. M.: "Clinical Laboratory Procedures," *Can. Nurse,* **70:**25, (Feb.) 1974.

White, Wilma L., et al.: *Practical Automation for the Clinical Laboratory,* 2nd ed. C. V. Mosby Co., St. Louis, 1972.

Williams, William J., et al.: *Hematology.* McGraw-Hill Book Co., New York, 1972.

Wilson, Patience: "Evaluating Chest Films," *Nurse Pract.,* **2:**6, (Jan.–Feb.) 1977.

Patience Wilson
Carol Dawn Davis
Virginia Henderson

Sections on Hearing and Speech and Language Testing were prepared in consultation with Robert Nagel, Ph.D., Assistant Clinical Professor of Otolaryngology, Yale–New Haven Hospital, New Haven, Conn.

The section on Psychological Testing was prepared in consultation with Donald Quinlan, Ph.D., Associate Professor of Psychology, Yale University School of Medicine, New Haven, Conn.

The entire chapter was critically reviewed by David B. Melchinger, M.D., Assistant Clinical Professor of Medicine, Yale University School of Medicine; Lecturer, Yale University School of Nursing; and Physician, University Health Services, New Haven, Conn. The authors gratefully acknowledge his contributions.

CHAPTER 8

Receiving the Patient; Planning Care and Rehabilitation; Terminating Care

1. RECEIVING ("ADMITTING") PATIENTS TO HEALTH SERVICES

Types of Health Services. Clients, or patients, are "admitted" to the services of a variety of health agencies and organizations. Some of these organizations provide service to prevent illness or to maintain health, while others provide service to relieve or cure disease. For example, admission officers, who are often nurses, "admit" clients to school health services, physicians' offices, health department clinics, and industry's health services to help prevent illness or maintain health. They "admit" clients to satellite clinics, hospital outpatient clinics, emergency rooms, general or special hospitals, and nursing homes generally for the purpose of relief or cure. Nurses may "admit" persons to health stations directed and operated by nurses and to the nurse's private practice. (The extent to which nurses are assuming responsibility for primary care is discussed in Chapters 1, 3, and 5.)

In all types of health service it is usually the nurse who initially gets information from patients about their health needs, who gives information about the health setting and the services it provides. Nurses may institute preliminary diagnostic procedures. While admitting personnel differ in training and background, nurses are often the ones who make sure that patients can be identified whether conscious or unconscious and who see that their personal belongings are protected. Nurses often transport or guide patients to the clinical division and see that they have the necessary clothing if they aren't prepared to stay in a hospital, nursing home, or other institution.

Routes by Which People Enter the Health Care System and Varieties of Admission Procedures. While the question of route of entry has been included in Chapters 1, 2, and 5, it is inherent in any discussion of admission procedures. Traditionally in the United States, and in fact in most countries, physicians guard the entry to the health care system. Diagnosing and prescribing treatment have been their sole prerogatives.* The number of physicians has therefore determined the number of persons who gain entrance to the health care system, get diagnosed, and are treated. In the United States—and many other countries—there is a growing tendency to prepare other types of health workers for health evaluation, diagnosis of health problems, treatment of some, and referral of patients to physicians. (See Chapters 1, 2, and 5 for more details.)

Nurses are opening offices for private practice and manning health stations to which people may apply for help on problems with which nurses are prepared to cope, or for referral to other health services—including those given by physicians. Dentists, family health counselors, clinical psychologists, and others have established their independence in offering their special services, and it is likely that other categories of workers such as physical therapists will do likewise.

Sidney R. Garfield,[1] a physician of the Kaiser Foundation Medical Care Program, believes that the benefits of the physician-patient relationship should be preserved but medical care extended by more effective use of other health workers and by the use of technology. He describes the Kaiser health maintenance program and the computerized multiphasic

---

* Attention has been called elsewhere to the help given unofficially by the corner druggist, by bone-setters, podiatrists, opticians, chiropractors, and many others who practice on the fringe of medicine; also to the help given in medical emergencies by any informed citizen and the role played by nurses whenever they find themselves the most prepared health worker available to the patient.

screening, diagnostic, and treatment processes. He says that the process may involve 60 interdependent health workers in the case of a person who is having an organ transplant with parallel elaboration of laboratory tests and computerization of findings.

Procedures for admitting an individual to a health care system differ greatly. They depend on the health workers, the facilities, and the technology available and, of course, on the consumer's knowledge of how to use the system.

In some hospitals all patients enter through the clinics of the outpatient department or an admitting office stationed within this department. Here it is determined where the patient should be treated and the admission procedure begins.

Because the emergency rooms in many hospitals provide services on a 24-hour basis and have excellent diagnostic and treatment facilities, more and more persons are using the hospital emergency room. They not only seek help for emergency and "crisis" health problems from these services but also come with health problems that are not emergencies in the usual sense.* In order to provide appropriate help for any person coming to the emergency department, some hospitals have a "triage" system for an initial appraisal of patients.[2,3] The triage system has been widely used in disasters and war zones. It also is used in home care for the elderly.[3a] It means the sorting and classifying of casualties to determine priority of need for care and assignment of appropriate place or person for treatment. (*Triage*, a culling, selecting, sifting, comes from *trier*, "to pick out," and has been used in France for the process of grading fruits and vegetables.) Figure 8-1 is an example of a form that is used in the emergency room.

The "triage nurse" receives the patient, gets a brief history, evaluates the patient's condition, and determines the priority, the place he or she should be sent, and the person who will give care. For example, the nurse may refer the patient to a private physician or an outpatient clinic; the nurse may send the patient to a "walk-in" clinic (so named because an appointment is not necessary); or the nurse may see that the patient has immediate medical treatment in the emergency room. In some

cases, the patient is later admitted to a clinical division for continuing treatment, while in others the patient is released with appointments to the outpatient department or ambulatory services. Figure 8-2 shows a form used to ensure continuity of patient care.

Frequently *maternity* patients are admitted directly to the clinical division and the necessary social, medical, and financial information is gotten later from the husband, other relative, or friend. When a patient in labor is admitted, the nurse focuses on the progress of labor and preparation for delivery. However, unless delivery is imminent it is usually possible to get other information from the patient that is essential for planning nursing care during the labor and delivery process, as well as planning for the postpartal period.

Identification of the *newborn* is an important aspect of the infant's admission to the hospital nursery. Both the American Hospital Association and the American Academy of Pediatrics recommend that immediately after delivery two * identification wristlets or anklets be put on the baby having the mother's name and hospital record number, the infant's sex ("boy" or "girl" rather than "male" or "female"), and date and time of birth. Later the mother's and infant's name bands are checked each time the baby is brought to the mother.[4,5]

In addition to name bands, a fingerprint of the mother and a footprint of the baby may be made while they are in the delivery room. Although the footprints or fingerprints cannot be used in daily identification of infant and mother, when properly made they are valuable when there is a legal question of identity. According to J. Edgar Hoover,[6] properly made footprints, as well as fingerprints, identify individuals throughout their lives. To be usable, a footprint or fingerprint must be clear enough so that the skin ridge characteristics can be easily seen with a magnifying glass.

To make the infant's footprint, the foot must be clean, dry, and *warm*. The foot is touched to the ink pad until a thin film of color is transferred to the sole of the foot. The specially prepared paper is placed on a smooth, firm surface and touched gently to the baby's foot. Care should be taken to keep the foot and paper steady to prevent smudging the print.

Another routine admission procedure for newborn infants is prophylactic treatment of

---

* Some commentators say that the 24-hour service of the hospital emergency department has assumed the load carried in the past by general practitioners, who not only had very long office hours but paid house calls during the day and night; others report that patients use the emergency departments as they might a club where they get comfort from companionship of other patients as well as help from health professionals.

* At the time of discharge of mother and baby, the identification bands are checked by the mother and nurse. One is removed and attached to the infant's hospital record while the other stays with the baby.

the eyes to reduce the possibility of infection by the gonococcus. One drop of a 1 per cent solution of silver nitrate is placed in each eye and washed out with normal saline solution; or a small amount of penicillin ointment (100,000 units per gram) is put in each eye.[7] The following statement is made in Waldo E. Nelson's *Textbook of Pediatrics:* "Although numerous methods of ophthalmic prophylaxis with sulfonamide or antibiotic preparations have been advocated, the instillation of 1% silver nitrate drops remains the best proved and only universally lawful method." *

Receiving the Patient. First impressions are likely to be vivid and not easily erased. Therefore, it is especially important at the time of admission to an agency, clinic, or institution that patients and those with them receive the most courteous attention, and patients the most effective initial health service. Many pediatric hospitals or departments are arranging "orientation" parties for children who are to be hospitalized. Before their admission, the children and their parents are given a tour of the hospital and meet nurses and other health workers. The children are given an opportunity to handle some of the equipment, such as a tongue blade, thermometer, stethoscope, syringe, and blood pressure cuff that will be used during their hospitalization.[8-9a] Nurses tend to forget that in every health service setting there are potentially distressing elements for clients. Each person brings unique experiences and problems that affect his or her reaction to the situation. A hypercritical attitude toward health workers, misconceptions about treatment, fear of hospitals, or morbid sensitiveness that often accompanies illness may turn a short delay, a moment of inattention, or a careless remark by health personnel into a real grievance.

If visiting nurses or health clinic nurses fail to make favorable impressions during their first meeting with clients, they may find it difficult to gain access to the home the next time they call, or patients may fail to keep clinic appointments; institutional nurses and the hospital admitting staff, however, are less likely to discover their failures. Patients usually wait until they leave the hospital to criticize it. They are, after all, at the mercy of hospital personnel and fear that criticism may invite disfavor. Unexpressed resentment, however, often makes patients uncooperative, taciturn, or irritable. Since patients base their estimates of an agency or institution on the sum total of their impressions, every contact they have with members of the staff may indirectly affect their reaction to the program of care.

Reception of the patients in a hospital is recognized to be of so much importance that many institutions employ hostesses and clerks who are especially qualified by virtue of their general poise and courteous manner to meet strangers and make them feel at ease. Such hostesses or clerks may ask patients or their families for certain social data and escort or direct them to the proper department. If there is a physician in charge of the patient's care, he or she is immediately notified of the patient's arrival.

Individualized Admissions. An unfortunate term used in hospitals is *the admission routine,* which has an equally unfortunate counterpart in practice; that is, it happens too often that there is a stereotyped way of greeting people followed by a series of procedures to which everyone is required to submit, regardless of temperament and physical needs. Sociologists, social anthropologists, and psychiatrists have commented on "dehumanizing" aspects of admission routines and hospital procedures.[10-12] Carol D. Taylor, for example, calls them "sociological sheep shearing" * and explains how "people are 'stripped' to patients."

The American Hospital Association has recognized this difficulty and has written *A Patient's Bill of Rights,*[12a] now used by many hospitals and given to patients when they are admitted, that stresses individualized care. The "Bill" describes the patient's right to complete and understandable information about his health problem; to informed consent for all treatment (including the use of experimental procedures); to privacy and confidentiality; to a full explanation of costs; and to refuse treatment. In addition, hospitals are adding to their staffs "patient representatives" whose goals are to see that the patient's rights are fulfilled. (In certain agencies such persons are called "ombudsmen.")

In 1951–1952, Leo W. Simmons, an anthropologist, directed a series of studies on the interpersonal relationships of patients, their relatives and friends, doctors, nurses, and auxiliary personnel. Although his report was made two decades ago, it is still pertinent and should help the nurse understand the reaction of the average person to a hospital admission. Simmons emphasizes the healing power of good relationships. He writes:

In our American traditions, a man's home is still his fortress, if not his castle, and even though

---

* Nelson, Waldo E. (ed.): *Textbook of Pediatrics,* 9th ed. W. B. Saunders Co., Philadelphia, 1969, p. 357.

* Taylor, Carol D.: "Sociological Sheep Shearing," *Nurs. Forum,* **1:**79, (Spring) 1962.

EMERGENCY ROOM RECORD

Family Name / First Name / Middle Name	Home Phone	Admission Date A.M. P.M.	Hosp. No.
Address / City / State / Zip	Age	Date of Birth / / · Sex M F · Civil Status M S W D Sep.	Religion
Employer	Address		Compensation Yes ☐ No ☐
Relative or Friend; Parent or Guardian if a Minor	Address		Phone
Name of Blue Cross and/or Blue Shield Plan · Group No.	Contract No.	Effective Date	Subscriber ☐ Dependent ☐ · Family Member ☐ Comprehensive ☐
Other Hospitalization Insurance · Name · Address	Cert. or Policy No.	Group No.	Effective Date
Family Doctor · Notified Yes ☐ No ☐ · Brought By Relative ☐ Self ☐ Police ☐ Fire ☐ Other ☐	Type of Service: Lab. ☐ XR ☐ PH ☐ PT ☐ Other ☐		S.S. No.
☐ Medicare Patient · Medicare No. and Other Information			

BRIEF HISTORY

If accident state where, when and how injured; if illness describe:________

NOTIFIED: Relative ☐ Police ☐ Coroner ☐ By Whom:

Nurse's Signature ____ R.N. · Officer's Signature · Star · District · Time A.M. P.M.

PHYSICIAN'S REPORT

CONDITION ON ADMISSION

Good ☐ Fair ☐ Poor ☐ Shock ☐ Hemorrhage ☐ Coma ☐ Temp.____ Oral Rectal P.____ R.____ B. P.____/____

Treatment: Tetanus Toxoid____cc. Tetanus Antitoxin Test____ Tetanus Antitoxin____units

Diagnosis:____

Disposition of Case:____

Referred to Dr.____ Date____

INSTRUCTIONS TO PATIENT____

____ PATIENT'S SIGNATURE · ____ DATE · ____ TIME .M. · ____ ATTENDING PHYSICIAN M.D.

EMERGENCY ROOM CHARGES (Does Not Include Fee of Attending Physician)

ITEM	CHARGE	ITEM	CHARGE	ITEM	CHARGE
Emergency Room		Drugs		Cast Room	
Anesthetic		Oxygen		Examining Room	
Antiseptics		Sutures			
Dressings		Tetanus Antitoxin			

OTHER SERVICES RENDERED: X-ray ☐ Laboratory ☐ Physical Therapy ☐ ☐ ☐ ☐

FORM D-2311 PHYSICIANS' RECORD CO., BERWYN, ILLINOIS - PRINTED IN U.S.A. AUTHORIZATIONS ON REVERSE SIDE

MEDICAL RECORD

Figure 8-1. Emergency room record. (Courtesy of Physicians' Record Co., Berwyn, Ill.)

he becomes a "patient" there, he still retains a proprietary sense of his rights and privileges, and he can insist on being treated on his own terms. . . .

In contrast the sick man's personal prerogatives undergo very important changes when he is moved out of *his* home and *his* bed and into *our* hospital and into *one of our* beds. Whereas at home he retained his work-a-day apparel and accoutrements which provided a sense of competence and self-sufficiency, in the hospital all this equipage and the associated symbols of power are stripped

AUTHORIZATION FOR EMERGENCY TREATMENT

The undersigned has been informed of the emergency treatment considered necessary for the patient whose name appears on the reverse hereof and that the treatment and procedures will be performed by physicians, members of the house staff and employees of the hospital. Authorization is hereby granted for such treatment and procedures.

The undersigned understands that a personal physician is to be selected by or on behalf of the patient within 24 hours if hospitalization or further treatment is required, or immediately if complications arise.

The undersigned has read the above authorization and understands the same and certifies that no guarantee or assurance has been made as to the results that may be obtained.

Date_____ Time_____ A.M. P.M.   Signed_____
                                                                PATIENT

Witness_____   Or_____
                                                                AUTHORIZED PERSON

                                              Relationship to Patient_____

> Both authorizations must be signed by the patient, or by an authorized person in the case of a minor or when patient is physically or mentally incompetent.

AUTHORIZATION FOR RELEASE OF INFORMATION

Authorization is hereby granted to release to the_____
                                                    NAME OF INSURANCE COMPANY OR COMPANIES
such information as may be necessary for the completion of my hospitalization claims.

Date_____   Signed_____
                                                                PATIENT

                                              Or_____
                                                                AUTHORIZED PERSON

                                              Relationship to Patient_____

Figure 8-1. (continued)

from him and locked away out of his sight and reach—or even sent back home.

Moreover, at home physical surroundings were familiar and afforded a sense of security, while hospital surroundings are very different, strange and disquieting to say the least. The contrast between the physical environment of the home and of the hospital may be regarded even by the physician as sufficiently upsetting to justify some prescribed sedation, just to numb the patient's sensitivity to the disturbing ward activity, especially at night. Added to this is the general impression which a patient can easily acquire that something very serious is about to take place to call for such an important move.

The social environment changes even more radically. Members of the hospital staff begin to rule this man's life, and, not infrequently, they

PATIENT INFORMATION AND TRANSFER FORM

Name_____
        (LAST)   (FIRST)

Age_____Sex_____Religion_____ Social Security No._____
                           (PREFIX)   (NUMBER)

Public Aid Number_____ Medicare Number_____

Relative or Guardian_____
                       (RELATION)

Relative or Guardian's Address_____ Tel._____

From_____ Admission_____

Address_____

Marital Status M☐ S☐ W☐ D☐ Sep. ☐

Address of Patient Prior to Hospitalization_____

Physician in Charge at Time of Transfer_____ M.D.

Date of Transfer_____

Transferred to_____
               (HOSP., NURSING HOME, AGENCY)

Address_____

Clinic Appt._____

Date and Time_____

(ATTACH CLINIC OR MEDICAL APPOINTMENT CARD)

Will this Physician care for Patient after Admission to Nursing Home?_____

II. MAJOR DIAGNOSES

DIET, DRUGS, AND OTHER THERAPY
at Time of Discharge

(Check if present)

Disabilities	Incontinence
Amputation	Bladder
Paralysis	Bowel
Contracture	Saliva
Decub. Ulcer	Activity Tolerance Limitations
Impairments	None Moderate Severe
Mentality	Patient knows diagnosis?
Speech	
Hearing	
Vision	
Sensation	

IMPORTANT MEDICAL INFORMATION
(State allergies if any)

Chest X-ray date_____ result_____
C. B. C. date_____ result_____
Serology date_____ result_____
Urinalysis date_____ result_____

SUGGESTIONS FOR COMPLETING FORM

1. The purpose of this form is to insure continuity of care in transfer from hospital to home or home to hospital.
2. The form is not intended to supply information of long-term nature.
3. Original should accompany patient with transfer. Carbon retained in patient's record.

Signature of Physician or Nurse_____ Date_____

FORM A-450 (REVISED JAN. 1970)   PHYSICIANS' RECORD CO., BERWYN, ILLINOIS   PRINTED IN U.S.A.

Figure 8-2. Patient information and transfer form. (Courtesy of Physicians' Record Co., Berwyn, Ill.)

appear to hold his life, if not his death, in their hands. The resident physician can become nearly all powerful, and a little head nurse is the boss of the place in all but major matters. . . .
. . . The social characteristics of the hospital (or its culture) tend to stimulate a considerable amount of dread and apprehension in the patient.

To an ill-prepared and apprehensive person, some of the needed treatments can seem to be not far short of unfriendly intent and sometimes even torture. However well-meaning the staff, and however justifiable the treatment, if a patient worries about explanations which are never given or fails to understand them if they are, if he is full of

III. PATIENT INFORMATION

SELF-CARE STATUS
(Check level of ability. Write S in space if needs supervision only. Draw line across if inapplicable.)

	Independent	Needs Assistance	Unable to do	
Bed Activity				Turns
				Sits
Personal Hygiene				Face, Hair, Arms
				Trunk & Perineum
				Lower Extremities
				Bladder Program
				Bowel Program
Dressing				Upper Extremities
				Trunk
				Lower Extremities
				Appliance, Splint
Feeding				
Transfer				Sitting
				Standing
				Tub
				Toilet
Loco-motion				Wheelchair
				Walking
				Stairs

BED Low_____Mattress: Firm_____Reg._____

Other _____

Side Rails: Yes_____No_____

BEHAVIOR

Alcoholic_____Belligerent_____Noisy_____

Senile_____Suspicious_____Withdrawn_____

May Wander_____

MENTAL STATUS

Alert_____Forgetful_____Confused_____

COMMUNICATION ABILITY   Yes   No

Can speak   ___ ___

Can write   ___ ___

Understands speaking   ___ ___

Understands writing   ___ ___

Understands gestures   ___ ___

Understands English   ___ ___

If no, state language spoken:_____

DIET

Regular_____Low Salt_____Diabetic_____

Bland_____Low Residue_____

PATIENT USES

Appliance_____Catheter_____Colostomy_____

Cane_____Crutches_____Prosthesis_____

Walker_____Chair_____

OTHER EQUIPMENT _____

ADDITIONAL PERTINENT INFORMATION
(Explain necessary details of care, diagnosis, medications, treatments, prognosis, teaching, habits, preferences, etc. Therapists and social workers add signature and title to notes.)

It is expected that the recipient's condition within the next 6 months will improve_____
remain static_____deteriorate_____

Rehabilitation potential: Is the recipient at his maximum level of functioning?   Yes_____No_____

If not, what improvements are expected in his functional capacity and self-care ability?

(a) Level of function to be attained_____

(b) Length of time it is expected to take to arrive at this_____

IV. SOCIAL INFORMATION (Adjustment to disability, emotional support from family, motivation for self-care, socializing ability, financial plan, family health problem, etc.)

SOCIAL ACTIVITIES

Encourage group_____individual_____

within_____outside_____home.

Transport: Ambulance_____Car_____

Car for handicapped_____Bus_____

Social Welfare Agencies Active_____   Signature_____   Title:_____Date:_____

Figure 8-2. (continued)

misgivings and emotional sets against the procedure, and if he feels that he has been tricked or coerced into something more severe than was necessary, then stressful interpersonal relationships have already complicated the situation, and they may affect the course of treatment.

... Sometimes it is easy to conclude that "headaches" and "heartaches" in our modern hospitals now surpass the physical pains, thanks perhaps to the almost miraculous "pain-killers." This accounts substantially, in my mind, for the increasing importance of the cultivation of improved interpersonal relationships in the very highly controlled hospital environment. . . .

There is in the sick man a *person* as well as a body. There are powers of personality within him for healing and for health, and also for sickness and death. Associated with him are other persons equally endowed with such powers. We know that the relationship of these persons to one another and to the patient are laden with both constructive and destructive possibilities. Every physician and nurse knows the difference it can make in a sick person to feel rejected and without interest in the fight for life on the one hand, or warmly wanted and stimulated to live on the other. . . .

In our attempts to explore the therapeutic possibilities of the interpersonal relationships in the treatment of disease, we have deliberately chosen to concentrate on certain of the key characters: the patient, his fellow patients, the physician, the staff nurse, the auxiliary help, the relatives and friends. . . .

. . . Traditionally the nurse has been a servant at the bedside, not really a co-worker in the patient's care and therapy.* But when the patient is treated seriously as a person instead of as a case, and therapy is boldly extended to utilize the resources of the personality, then the modern nurse is, both by training in our better schools of nursing and by the fact that she can spend so much more time with the patient, at some real advantage over the hurried and harried intern in her understanding of the patient as a person. . . .

Perhaps the most important [element] of all [in the hospital system] is the human resources latent in the nurse. . . .†

Simmons has been quoted at length in order to emphasize the therapeutic value he places on a sympathetic relationship between patients and nurses. There is no time at which this is more easily established, or more needed, than during admission procedures. The interest in the patient must be genuine if it is to be effective. It should be immediately apparent to patients that their care is to be individualized.

To individualize care, including the admission process, health workers should know how age, social, cultural, racial, and economic backgrounds of clients, or patients, affect their understanding of their situation and their reactions to it.[13-17a] For instance, studies have shown that when nurses in a mental hospital, emergency room, and surgical unit explored the patients' "perceptions" of hospitalization, determined whether they were in distress and what they saw as the cause of distress, and acted to relieve distress, the patients' blood pressure readings and pulse and respiration rates (all indicators of stress) decreased. In addition, patients in the experimental samples thought more often than did those in the control group that nursing care at the time of admission surpassed their expectations.[18,19] When a group of school-age children and their parents were admitted to the hospital using an admission method designed to take into account the children's developmental level of self-mastery, their eagerness to learn and participate, their self-esteem, safety, and "belonging" needs (as well as their parents' feelings), the anxiety of the children, as measured by the Palmar Sweat Test, decreased dramatically.[20]

Those who admit patients should make a consistent effort to put themselves in the patient's position. With experience and genuine interest comes an ability to recognize signs of fear, excitement, embarrassment, pain, depression, and loneliness. These emotions are often cloaked by an air of indifference or even false cheerfulness. Throughout this book the interrelationship of mind and body has been stressed; also the impossibility of saying that a person has a total physical or a total mental illness. G. Canby Robinson,[20a] in his study reported in 1939 as The Patient as a Person, concluded that more than half the persons treated in the medical service of a famous hospital were suffering from conditions with emotional origins. R. S. Duff and A. B. Hollingshead,[20b] in Sickness and Society, a report of a 1968 study, suggest that too often the patient's major health problem, as he or she sees it, remains untreated while the "chief complaint" or physician's diagnosis is the focus of attention. In Chapters 4 and 5, problem-centered patient management (often referred to as the "Weed System") is described. It is an attempt to take into consideration the total health problems presented by the client, or patient. The listening, interpreting, evaluating, and reporting abilities of admitting personnel can help identify problems and direct patients to the attention of those best qualified to care for them in the given situation.

There are certain administrative and diagnostic procedures that should be carried out for all patients, but there are many ways in which the reception and initial treatment should differ. The day laborer who is losing his or her job or means of livelihood because of facing an indefinite period of hospitalization may have a sense of impending doom, and therefore should receive a different type of psychologic treatment than the wealthy person with a similar disease condition whose economic status is not threatened. From the standpoint of the physical care of the patient, it is likewise obvious that fastidious persons who have prepared themselves with a careful toilet for admission should not be subjected to the same procedures for cleaning the skin, hair, mouth, and nails that are necessary when

* The author wrote this in 1951. Few would deny now that nurses are rapidly acquiring a collaborative relationship with physicians and also practicing as independent health workers. (See Chapter 1.)

† Simmons, Leo W.: "The Manipulation of Human Resources in Nursing Care," Am. J. Nurs., 51:452, (July) 1951.

dirty, untidy persons are admitted. Institutional regulations that deprive any patient, even temporarily, of his personal possessions, regardless of the patient's desire to have them or of his ability to take care of them, are open to criticism. Storage space to which the patient has free access should be provided on every clinical service. In fact, no one should be reduced to the status of a bed patient if it is good for him or her to remain ambulatory.

Courteous attention should always be given to the family or friends of the sick person. Introductions should be made as in a home, and waiting children given toys, or adults something to read. Relatives or friends who bring the patient to the hospital usually like to go with him or her to the clinical service. They often want to meet and talk to the physician and nurse who will be in charge of the patient's program of care. If they wait in order to learn what is discovered in the initial examination of the patient, they should be made as comfortable as the facilities allow. Their cooperation in the care of the patient should be enlisted, and institutional regulations, such as visiting hours, should be explained to them, as well as to the patient. Leaflets should be available to give them. This early meeting of the medical staff and the family or friends may establish a relationship that is badly needed if the care planned for the patient throughout his illness is to take the family situation into account. Early planning for joint conferences is desirable.

Standardization of equipment and method results, as a rule, in a saving of time and money, and for this reason poorly financed and inadequately staffed institutions and agencies are likely to give least consideration to the individual. When standardization is forced on an institution by economic necessity, an attempt should be made to explain to patients that regulations objectionable to them have been set up for the good of the majority.

In the plan for admission of the patient to an institution or agency, provision must be made for (1) getting preliminary medical and social data (sometimes called demographic * data); (2) guiding and transporting the patient to the proper clinical division if in a hospital; (3) safeguarding the patient's, or client's, possessions and providing suitable clothing if necessary; (4) orienting the patient to the physical environment of the clinical division of a hospital, nursing home, or other institution; (5) taking the vital signs and making pertinent observations; (6) getting an admission interview or history; and (7) preparing the patient for the examination which in some cases is made by the physician or nurse or through their collaboration. Figure 8-3 shows a record that may be used after all information, including the physician's prescriptions, has been written. Medical and nursing students may participate and special tests made by a variety of health personnel.

Bruno Bettelheim,[20c] in *A Home for the Heart,* describes in detail the highly individualized reception of patients to the Orthogenic School (a psychiatric hospital for children and young adults) associated with the University of Chicago. They are received in a living room, as one would receive a guest in a home. As one example of individualized treatment, the patient finds a gift, selected by the staff, on the bed to which he or she is assigned.

Getting Preliminary Social and Medical Data. The administrative department of an institution is responsible for recording certain data essential for identification and payment of fees. An admission officer from this department gets from the patient or his family the patient's name and address, telephone number, and the name and address of the nearest relative, friend, or guardian. If employed, the patient's employment is noted, his or her business address, and in certain cases the name of the employer. In some institutions, prepayment of fees is required; in others, a statement as to how the patient plans to meet the cost, including the use of health insurance. Patients too ill to answer questions should be admitted immediately and the necessary data supplied by family or friends at the first opportunity. These preliminary data may be recorded in the admission department of a hospital, or in the clinical service where the admission procedure is completed. A member of the business administration staff may come to the clinical division to get the information from the patient, but other kinds of personnel, including nurses, may be asked to act for him or her. Medical social workers frequently take part in the patient's admission in order that problems requiring their help may have immediate attention. Types of health histories are discussed later in this chapter, and Chapters 4 and 5 can be consulted for further details. Some are long questionnaires answered by the patient or a parent. They may or may not be automated. Many institutions and agencies are automating the process of getting, storing, and retrieving all types of information about patients.*

---

* Demography is the science of vital and social statistics, as of the births, deaths, diseases, marriages, etc., of populations.

* See Chapter 5 for a description of a bracelet or necklace ("Medic Alert") that provides vital information about wearers of the device in case they are unconscious, confused, or too weak to talk.

NURSING DEPENDENCY FORM

Name_____   Hosp._____
No._____ Day_____   Ward_____
Age_____   Date_____

Section A			X	Office use only	
				O	X
Mobility	Walk without assistance	1			
	Walk with assistance	2			
	Up in chair — Does not walk	3			
	Completely bedfast				
Toilet	Self — any time	1			
	When out of bed, self	2			
	When out of bed, assistance	3			
	Once daily, self	4			
	Once daily, assistance	5			
	Bedpan/commode	6			
Period up	All day, as desired	1			
	6 hours or more	2			
	3 hours but less than 6 hours	3			
	1 hour but less than 3 hours	4			
	Less than 1 hour	5			
	Does not get out of bed	6			
Bathing	Bathroom — self	1			
	Bathroom — assistance	2			
	Bedside — self	3			
	Bedside — assistance	4			
Feeding	Self	1			
	Assistance when necessary	2			

Section B					
Turning (Bedfast patients only)	Not needed	1			
	Turn 4 hourly	2			
	Turn 2 hourly	3			
Observations	T.R.P. — 4 hourly	1			
	Pulse — 4 hourly	2			
	Pulse — 2 hourly	3			
	Blood pressure — daily	4			
	Blood pressure — 4 hourly	5			
	Blood pressure — 2 hourly	6			
		7			
Treatment	Oxygen	1			
	IV therapy	2			
	Blood transfusion	3			
	Suction	4			
	Drainage	5			
Mental state	Unconscious	1			
	Confused, emotionally disturbed	2			
	Reassurance more than normal	3			

Dependency group

1
2
3
4
5

Figure 8-3. Form used to show patient's need for help from nurse (or others). (Courtesy of Royal College of Nursing, London.)

Getting the Patient to the Appropriate Therapist or Department. Patients in health, and those who are not very ill, walk into the hospital and are escorted to the admitting department, if there is one, or directly to the clinical division by a hostess, a porter, or a nurse from the clinical service. Wheelchairs should be available for those who are too sick, weak, or lame to walk. Patients brought to the hospital in ambulances usually enter by a special door and are taken to the admitting department or clinical service on a stretcher and put to bed immediately. Stretchers also should be ready for very ill patients who are brought to the hospital in private conveyances. As noted elsewhere, many patients are admitted to hospitals from the emergency service.

Safeguarding the Institutionalized Patient's Possessions and Providing Suitable Clothing. In giving patients any help they may need in undressing, nothing should be done to indicate that the nurse is aware of shabby or soiled clothing. The worse its condition the less likely it is that the patient can afford to have it carelessly handled. Lost articles must be replaced by the institution or agency. Negligence in handling patients' belongings brings criticism upon the institution and makes the personnel and other patients liable to suspicion. Hospitals and nursing homes are sometimes sued for loss of dentures, jewelry, and other possessions of value to the owner.

In private and semiprivate rooms, closets and chests of drawers are provided for clothing and other belongings, and their care presents comparatively little difficulty. If the patient is assigned to a service where inadequate provision is made for care of clothing, it is advisable to have relatives or friends return to the patient's home immediately any clothes not to be used in the hospital, and especially any valuables, such as papers, jewelry, or money. If this is done, the person assuming the responsibility should sign a list of the articles received. A complete itemized list of everything belonging to the patient to be retained in the hospital must be made in duplicate. This list should be checked with the patient, if not too sick, and the patient should verify and sign it. The valuable articles should be tied up in a separate package with one copy of the list and the patient's name, the unit number, the date, and the nurse's signature on it; then the package should be given to the head nurse or unit manager, who will transfer it to the safe that is kept for that purpose. The duplicate list is given to the patient or kept by the head nurse or unit manager.

Whether patients are in wards or in private rooms, they should be discouraged from keeping money, jewelry, or valuable papers with them. When they are not very ill and wish to keep a watch, fountain pen, some money, rings, or other effects, they do so at their own risk. If, later on, the patient's condition changes and he or she cannot be held responsible, a list of the articles must be made and it, with the articles, sent to the office for safekeeping. The person in charge of valuables is usually bonded to protect the institution. In ward services, where everything belonging to the patient is stored in a bedside cabinet, it is not practical for a patient to keep many personal belongings. Those that he or she will usually want or need are a dressing gown, bedroom slippers, night clothes, toilet articles, writing materials, a few books, a watch, and in some cases a photograph, a piece of jewelry, or an object that is cherished for sentimental reasons. If the patient is unprepared for admission to the hospital,

suitable clothing should be provided. Chapter 14 discusses kinds of clothing.

Increasingly, institutions are providing lockers for each patient in multibed units or providing a room for each person. It is unfortunate that so many hospitals have, in the past, made such inadequate provision for patients' belongings.

Before the clothing is put away, it should be examined for lice or other vermin if there is any reason to expect their presence. Pubic lice (crab lice) may spread to other hairy areas, or there may be body lice, both evidenced by scratches or scars on the skin from scratching. While pediculosis is rare in the United States, a school nurse's inspection of all children in a primary school in Armaugh, Ireland, in 1972 showed that about 3 per cent of the boys and about 8 per cent of the girls had lice or nits on their hair.[20d]

If lice are found on clothing, the condition is reported to the doctor, who prescribes a delousing procedure. "Standing orders" for this exist in some health agencies. (Delousing methods are discussed in Chapter 15.) In some cases when clothing is infested, or *very* dirty, it is advisable to burn it. This must first be explained to the patient or, if he or she is very sick, to relatives. The social service will, if necessary, supply substitute garments.

Care of clothing varies in different health institutions. In some a special room is provided for the storage and protection of clothing. If necessary, the clothing is cleaned. All outer garments such as coats and dresses are covered and hung. Scrupulous care of the clothing while in a health institution plays an important part in the program of health education and rehabilitation of the individual. It is said that "the way to keep a man out of the mud is to blacken his shoes." (Part of the rehabilitation of people in corrective agencies and institutions is to provide them with decent clothing and help them to look well-groomed.) The clothing of a patient with an infectious disease is put in special bags and containers, plainly marked, listed, and decontaminated, before it is stored (see Chapter 15).

Restrictive regulations for care of personal belongings must be carefully explained because patients often resent the fact that so many of their possessions are taken from them. It is understandable that deprived of his or her outer clothing a person feels a prisoner, or like a small child who is sent to bed for punishment. Depressed persons may have all sharp instruments (scissors, razors, even nail files) taken from them and this may be very disturbing. If patients understand that they can have their clothes or other possessions any time they need them and that the storage of their belongings is made necessary by a lack of storage space or other condition, they are not so likely to be resentful.

While the nurse or nursing assistant is helping the patient undress and arrange his or her possessions, he or she should be able to get some idea as to whether the person has good habits of cleanliness. As mentioned above, the presence of body lice can usually be detected. *Admission baths and shampoos* are not given unless there is some reason to believe that they are indicated, either as preparation for the physical examination or for the patient's comfort. If the patient is to have a bath on admission and his or her condition permits it, a tub bath or shower is given. This is particularly desirable if parts of the body are noticeably dirty or if the treatment the patient is to receive will make it impossible for him or her to get into a tub for some time. Bed baths should be given to any patients who are very weak or ill.

Among patients admitted to the hospital or nursing home, many will have established desirable habits of cleanliness and will be uncomfortable if these habits are disrupted. A few will object to the bath and particularly to the admission bath. Some object because they think it unnecessary and are rather insulted at the suggestion; others think too many baths bad for them, or fear they will catch cold. Some patients do not object to the bath, but from modesty or reserve dislike being bathed if they need this help. A nurse should be tactful in overcoming objections, and must be tolerant of prejudices. The person will soon learn to appreciate the comfort of the bath. The admission toilet does not differ in any respect from the daily attention to personal cleanliness (discussed in Chapter 14), except that in cases of neglect the cleansing process must be more thorough.

Brushing and combing the hair offer the nurse an opportunity to examine the scalp and the hair itself for pediculi and nits (eggs). If pediculi are present, which is rare in most communities, treatment is prescribed by the physician and instituted immediately. (For a discussion of this topic and illustration of lice, see Chapter 15.)

Orienting the Institutionalized Patient to the Environment. Patients who have not been hospitalized or those entering any institution for the first time should have an explanation of its layout, furnishings, equipment, and regulations. Specifically, in a hospital the call light and intercommunication system should be explained; patients should be told how to get a telephone, television set, or radio. Arrangements for meals and visiting hours should be explained; also the locations of day rooms, solariums, or bathrooms; and provisions for getting newspapers and other reading materials. Many hospitals provide patients with booklets that give this and other information, but even with this help most patients benefit from an explanation by the admitting person, especially if he or she encourages the patient to ask questions.

When people are admitted to extended care institutions that will be "home" to them for weeks, months, or years, it is important that they see the entire institution, meet the staff, and understand its organizational plan. Blodwen Wigley [20e] describes the patient community organization at the Cassel Hospital in London that is frequently found in psychiatric hospitals and occasionally in hospitals for the chronically ill and in nursing homes. It is obvious that independence is fostered by patient participation in the policy-making and operation of the institution.

Because institutional personnel usually wear name tags, they frequently assume that patients know who they are and therefore neglect to introduce themselves or to tell patients the name of key personnel (such as head nurse, team leader, and other nurses who will contribute to their care, and doctors who will attend them) on the division. Nurses often fail to introduce patients who are roommates, which to many persons seems a breach of common courtesy. Many patients comment on the lack of courtesy and individualization of the admission process.[21]

While some believe that ideally the professional nurse should admit patients to a clinical division, this is often impossible. If nursing assistants admit patients, the nurse should still feel responsible for seeing that the patient's needs are met.

Clients who are admitted to ambulatory health services should be introduced to the physical environment and agency personnel just as those admitted to inpatient services. Room arrangement, the location of various departments, and the functions of all staff should be explained. Color-coded wall signs or colored markings on the floor are used in some clinics to help people find their way in a large and busy place.

Taking Vital Signs and Observing the Patient. Because the temperature, pulse, respiration rate, and blood pressure readings give important information about a patient's condition, these are usually made at the time of admission. This information provides a baseline for subsequent measurements. (Chapters 6, 9, and 35 discuss vital signs in healthy and sick persons in detail.) A nursing assistant may in some cases measure and record the "vital signs" so that the readings are available to the physician or the nurse examining the patient.

In Chapter 4 observing, reporting, and recording are discussed in detail; here we note some specific observations that should be made on admission. Without making it obvious that they are doing so, nurses should note the general appearance of vigor, lassitude, or prostration in the patient and should also note color and expression—all of which indicate whether a person is in comparative health, mildly or acutely ill, and should limit exerting the patient accordingly.

All health workers who admit patients, but particularly nurses who are with them most, should be alert to handicaps or limitations. A sensitive person notices signs of deafness, blindness, or muteness, and tries to protect the patient from psychic and physical trauma; the same is true in motor disabilities or in disturbances of equilibrium. Nurses should be familiar with the literature on the handicapped. In every case they should try to supply the person's particular needs. For example, the deaf appreciate distinct rather than overloud speech and care on the part of others to announce their presence; or a written list of the members of the staff. The blind need a thorough introduction to the environment with attention to the regular placement of everything they use; they also need complete verbal explanations and descriptions and the opportunity to feel as many objects as possible. The blind are peculiarly responsive to sounds and will judge their attendant's liking or sympathy by the tone of voice; they will likewise suffer from noise or meaningless sounds. Persons with serious speech difficulties should be provided with paper and pencil or a "magic" slate so that they can write their wants and with cards on which are printed routine needs such as "drinking water" or "more covering." Those with motor disabilities may need canes, wheelchairs, crutches, handles suspended over the bed, guide ropes, special utensils for eating or writing, and other aids. (See Chapter 46 for further discussion of the needs of those with sensory handicaps and Chapter 38 for discussion of the needs of those with neuromotor disability or prescribed hypomobility.)

Above all their physical needs, the handicapped want the understanding treatment that minimizes their disabilities. A blind practicing physician, writing in 1952 under a pseudonym in *When Doctors Are Patients,* spoke for all those who have handicaps when he said:

Despite my best efforts to attain a serenity of spirit, I am still given to outbursts of irritability and to moods of depression, during which those I love are most likely to suffer. I own too that I have not been able entirely to overcome my aversion to those people whose efforts at patronizing kindness conceal but poorly the blend of smug pity and repugnance which lies beneath. Greatly to be cherished is the friend who keeps his pity buried deep and whose kindness does not cloy, but is kept faintly acid with the tang of humor and wit. The indulgence of a sense of humor is of great therapeutic value to those among the sightless so fortunately endowed; Thurber and *The New Yorker* are excellent substitutes for an appointment with the psychiatrist.*

It is obvious that when health personnel cannot speak the patient's language an interpreter is needed. In Chapter 4 the advantages of a self-administered health history are discussed, one of them being that it can be translated into many languages. Figure 4-6 shows an automated process in which the patient answers the question by touching the screen.

Interviewing and Getting the Health History. Lawrence L. Weed,[22] who has developed the Problem-Oriented System of Medical Care (for the benefit of the patient but also to improve medical education), calls the initial collection of information "the data base." He says the questions or topics under which data are collected are designed to gather whatever *specific* information is necessary to provide effective health care for a *particular* population of patients. He says, in addition, that those offering care should decide what the content of the questions or topics should be. This approach is demonstrated by a patient's record in Chapter 4 presented by Donna Gane, who is closely associated with Dr. Weed in the use and development of automation for this system at the Medical Center of the University of Vermont. There, both nurses and physicians identify patients' problems, they collaborate in working out with patients ways of coping with, or solving, their problems, and both nurses and physicians write progress notes related to the identified problems. This system promotes a partnership among patients, physicians, and nurses, and a unified medical record (which may or may not be automated). This unity and partnership among health workers we believe highly desirable. The "Weed System" may also, if automated, build up a bank of information on management of specific problems that, since the information can be retrieved, is immediately available in helping other patients with the same problems as, for example, inconti-

* Pinner, Max, and Miller, Benjamin F. (eds.): *When Doctors Are Patients.* W. W. Norton & Co., New York, 1952, p. 55.

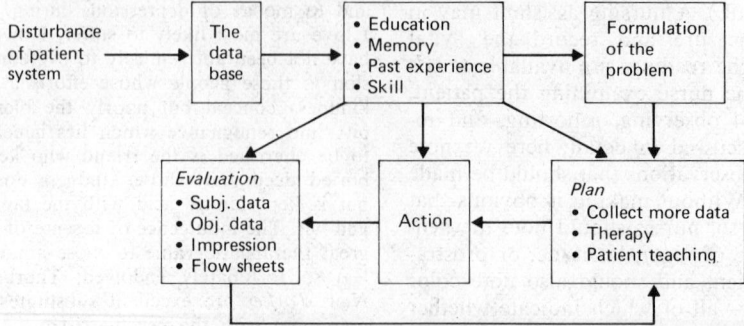

Figure 8-4. A model depicting feedback mechanisms inherent in Weed's approach to utilization of a problem-oriented patient record for education and patient care. The proper use of this method for analyzing and recording data creates a limited cybernetic model for each problem listed. Coding the data for use in writing computer programs would follow. (From Kinney, Anna Belle, and Blount, Mary: "Systems Approach to Myasthenia Gravis," *Nurs. Clin. North Am.*, **6:**435, [Sept.] 1971.)

nence, contractures, hiccups, salivation, dizziness, depression, or aphasia (see Fig. 8-4).

The "Weed System" has had such wide acclaim that commercial firms have found it profitable to produce all the necessary forms to activate the problem-centered approach.* As automated record systems spread, standardized records will facilitate the transfer of information from one agency or institution to another. A characteristic of this age is the mobility of the population, frequent moves of families, and change of position for the wage earners. In Chapter 4 the possibility of providing each person with a copy of his or her health history and medical record, which he or she carries through life, is mentioned. In this chapter the traditional and the problem-oriented types of histories are both discussed.

The problem approach to patient care is not new to nursing. "Problems" or "situations" with which the nurse might help the patient were discussed by Nell Beeby [22a] as early as 1937; Virginia Henderson, in the 1955 edition of this text (see Chapter 34), called attention to the possibility of teaching and practicing nursing with the problem approach; in 1960 Faye G. Abdellah and her associates [22b] published *Patient-Centered Approaches to Nursing;* and in 1964 Gladys Nite with Frank N. Willis, Jr.[22c] described the care of cardiac patients organized around their problems.

Because, in many health services, medical care is still organized around a diagnosis or a "chief complaint," nurses have found it necessary to collect data themselves on which to base a plan of nursing care. Nurses recognize that they can no longer leave to chance the collection of pertinent information for planning nursing care and have developed a variety of forms for collecting the information, each of which is useful in a particular institution or for a particular group of patients. Most of these admission interview forms or guides, however, contain questions about patients' socioeconomic and cultural background; patients' perceptions of their health problems; and patients' preferences and requirements for daily activities such as diet, rest and sleep, elimination, bathing, work, and recreation. In addition, many forms include questions about physical and psychologic aspects of patients' environment that are comforting or necessary.[23-25a] June S. Rothberg [26] believes that the information gathered through "the nursing history" and other sources of information about the patient leads to the identification of the patient's resources and "self-help deficits" whether they are intrinsic (within the patient) or extrinsic (outside the patient). The Nursing Development Conference Group [26a] coined the phrase "self-help deficits" and they plan nursing care around them. These identified resources and "deficits" of the patient indicate his or her specific needs for nursing, which in turn become the basis for planning nursing care. In Chapter 1 we use the homely phrase of trying to "get inside the patient's skin" to see what help he or she needs.

Since it is rarely possible at the time of admission to get all the information that would be required to develop a complete and final plan of care, some questions or topics may be left for a later session. For instance, questions

* Rocom, Darien, Conn., is an example of one such firm.

about individual or family health practices, the health status of family members, and their experiences and feelings about health care may be explored after admission and used to modify the initial plan.*

The health setting and its purpose of care will govern the focus of the questions and the emphasis given to certain topics in the history. For example, in the home, a nurse may ask questions to elicit information about family health goals and problems; in a nursing home, questions about the sensory perceptions and social relationships of the elderly; in a well-child clinic, questions about a child's developmental level and play activities.[26b, c] However, any form used by nurses should ask only for information that is not being collected by other health personnel and that is critically needed by nurses to plan and give effective care.

In some situations, such as well-child services in hospitals and community centers, health services, industrial health departments, and screening clinics, nurses are responsible for completing the client's, or patient's, physical examination at the time of admission to the service, and for making necessary referrals to physicians.[27-32] When a patient is admitted to a hospital clinical division, the physician usually examines the patient. Chapter 5 describes physical examinations as carried out by physicians and others in a variety of settings.

A word should be said here about the privacy of the patient and the confidentiality of information he or she may voluntarily give or be asked to give during the interview, and the requirement of sharing necessary information with members of the nursing or health team.[33] If a patient understands the purpose and ways that information is shared, he or she has the opportunity of deciding what to divulge. Throughout their association with patients, nurses should try to avoid giving the impression that they are idly curious. What should and should not be said to patients is a subject about which it is impossible to make hard and fast rules. In the last analysis, the judgment of the nurse will have to guide him or her. In this case, nurses will do well to remember that most individuals respond to a genuine professional interest in their condition by volunteering information that they think will be helpful; they

are not likely to resent questions if they are told why the questions are asked, and if the reasons seem to them to be good ones.

It is a tradition of the health professions that workers hold in confidence information volunteered by the patients as well as what they may have discovered while attending them. In most states the courts cannot force the doctor, the priest, or the nurse to divulge this information. Anything they learn about the patient is to be used solely as a means of giving better service. Health workers who consistently observe this principle are the ones in whom the patients are most likely to confide. A nurse who criticizes, ridicules, or betrays the confidence of one patient to another will thereby make her listener fear that he will be the subject of her conversation with someone else.

If the nursing and medical histories are separate, of course, the record made by the physician is, of course, a source of information for nurses as are written reports of other professional workers and the results of laboratory tests. All of this information and the "nursing history" (if it is separate) are kept together and called the patient's chart. However, as data-processing equipment is used by more and more hospitals to store information about patients, nurses will become more and more skillful in retrieving information about the patient at a computer terminal rather than from a chart.

A third source of information the nurse may use is the indirect help he or she gets from studying records of patients who have had similar conditions, or by studying appropriate literature, including textbook descriptions. In this way the nurse may learn symptoms the patient is likely to have, their significance, the cause of the condition, if known, and the usual treatment. Nurses caring for well persons should know the physiologic range in development or function and how normal development or function is maintained. The bank of information on how to deal with patient problems that is being developed by the computerized "Weed System" has been mentioned.

There is, of course, danger in trying to fit the care of the patient into the textbook picture or in assuming that treatment for one patient's problems will work for another, even though as fed into a data bank they seem to be of the same nature. Patients differ in their reaction to disease; the determination of patients to get well may hasten their recovery or a loss of interest in life retard it. A Spartan spirit or an inability to express themselves may mask symptoms of disease and make diagnosis difficult. In many cases, patients' conditions are incorrectly diagnosed. For these and other reasons, nurses must constantly remember that

---

* Self-administered health histories (such as that developed at Cornell Medical Center, New York City) or that developed in the "Weed System" include a wide range of information. They are discussed in Chapter 4. Again, we would stress that the best possible data base should be available to *all health workers* and that the unified approach to care is what we should strive for.

they are caring for individuals and not a symptom or disease, and must adjust the care to patients' changing condition and needs.

Observation of the patients is, of course, one of the prime sources of information about them. The nurse should observe for general appearance, body language, motor activity, and interpersonal interactions to name some of the more important foci (see Chapter 4).

Preparing the Patient for the Physical Examination. Nurses' observations should enable them to determine whether a person needs immediate medical attention and what preparation should be made for the physical examination. The rational patient should have a suitable explanation of the procedure unless he or she is familiar with it. An effort should be made to relieve, insofar as it is possible, the fear that so often accompanies the examination.

2. PLANNING CARE AND REHABILITATION

Meaning and Purpose. Everybody has some sort of design for living, and the concept of a health plan as part of this design is not confined to the medical world. All persons as they grow up deliberately or unconsciously develop a life pattern that is an adaptation of their native culture to their particular needs and desires. Different as these individual patterns often seem, the underlying needs, or urges, are similar. All human beings want security (food, clothing, and shelter) and desire love and approval; they also crave variety, adventure, and achievement, including learning, and, in varying degree, they search for the ultimate good, the ethical force that man sees in his God, or his religion.

Various types of health workers in every age have seen the difficulty, or even impossibility, of separating from the total life pattern those activities affecting health. It is generally believed now that the extent to which, and the way in which, man satisfies basic cravings is a measure of health. Health care that ignores any of man's fundamental needs is unconsciously fighting nature, an unconquerable force, an incomparable ally. The plan of patient care should therefore be made with the recognition that the person under treatment is constantly longing for security, approval, love, adventure, accomplishment, learning or diversion, and a renewal of his faith in God or a universal ethical principle. Health workers cannot provide patients with all this, but they can help them create an environment and set up a plan that makes possible the satisfaction of these cravings. The sick are suffering not so

much from a disease as from its threat to their economic security, to their relationships with others, and to those activities that bring variety, entertainment, or pleasure into their lives. Sickness may also threaten the patient's faith in the ultimate "goodness" of life; he or she cannot believe in a God that lets such terrible things happen. The sick may fear that they have lost favor in the sight of God, considering illness a punishment for real or imagined sins. (For more on this subject see Chapter 18.)

The pattern of living each person develops depends on intelligence, knowledge, economic resources, and the value he or she puts on health. Ideally, each person would develop a pattern that enables him or her to realize optimum usefulness and happiness; actually, this rarely happens. Because habitual ways of dressing, bathing, eating, eliminating, exercising, resting, and sleeping, as well as working and playing, tend to get so fixed and so essential to physical comfort and peace of mind that interruptions of the day's routine cause vague, or even acute, discomfort, a patient is often unable or unwilling to scrap his or her established pattern of living for a totally new one. Wise doctors and nurses will, therefore, learn as much as they can about the individual's habits so that, in helping him or her to make a new plan, they can build on the foundation of that person's established pattern.

Henrik L. Blum and associates suggest that health is more frequently sought as the basis for, or means of, "pursuing the critical needs of sustenance and of satisfaction" * than as an end in itself. This would seem to be true for many persons who ask for help with their health care only when disability, pain, or discomfort interferes with their capacity to fulfill their basic needs. On the other hand, increasing numbers of persons look for health guidance in order to maintain a state of independence. In either case, individuals or families expect help with modifying, to a varying degree, their way of living so that illness will be prevented, health maintained or restored, or, if a cure is impossible, suffering relieved. They finally seek help in postponing death or, when this is impossible, making death easy.

The purpose of health care and a health care plan is the modification of the individual's pattern of living, and the provision of any help necessary in carrying out a mutually agreed upon modification. The development of such

---

* Blum, Henrik L., et al.: *Health Planning 1969.* Western Regional Office, American Public Health Association, San Francisco, 1969, p. 304.

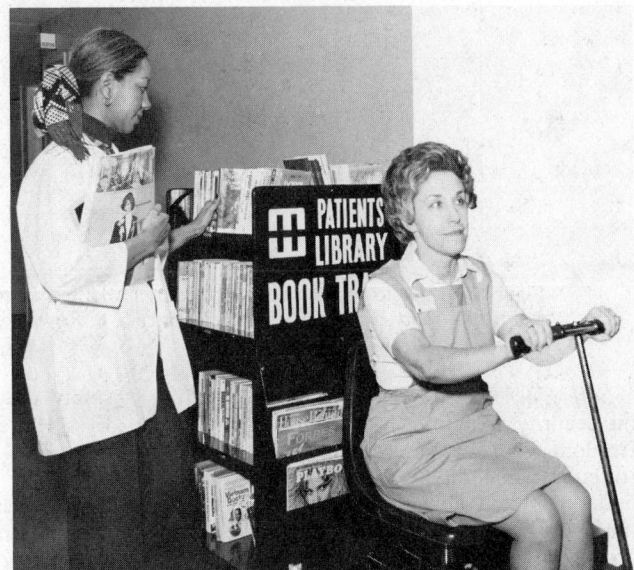

Figure 8-5. Motorized cart used to transport books and periodicals to clinical units. (Courtesy of Harper Hospital, Detroit, Mich.)

a plan requires that the health worker be constantly aware of the basic human needs (physiologic, psychologic, social, and spiritual). It requires knowledge and understanding of a number of factors that influence the person's established regimen as well as the modification that is possible. It requires knowledge and understanding of the ways that patterns of daily living reinforce an unhealthy condition or disrupt a healthy one and appreciation of internal and external conditions that cause illness, disease, or disability. It also requires knowledge and understanding of the purpose and probable effects of drugs, treatments, or health practices, and, finally, it requires knowledge and understanding of the functions and responsibilities of other professional persons and the community resources that can help the individual reach the agreed-upon health goals.

Some plans of care may be carried out by the patients themselves under direction of the physician or a nurse. More often they require the cooperation of others, as, for example, the family, the nutritionist, the physical therapist, the occupational therapist, the social worker, the minister, the vocational adviser, the psychologist, or others. Obviously, it is important that all those who help carry out the plan have a common understanding of the goals of therapy.

Basic Human Needs. The subject of basic human needs has been studied and organized in various ways by numerous social scientists since the middle of the last century.[33a] Describing a concept of a hierarchy of human needs in his theory of human motivation, Abraham H. Maslow says:

> This theory is, I think, in the functionalist tradition of James and Dewey, and is fused with the holism of Westheimer, Goldstein, and Gestalt psychology, and with the dynamism of Freud, Fromm, Horney, Reich, Jung, and Adler. This integration or synthesis may be called a holistic-dynamic theory.*

Basic human needs may be organized into a hierarchy of relative prepotency; that is, when lower needs, such as physiologic hungers, are satisfied, new (and higher) needs emerge, as, for example, the need for belonging and for love. Maslow categorizes basic needs in order of priority as shown in Figure 8-6.

To make a list of fundamental *physiologic needs* (the lowest needs) is impossible as well as useless because, as Maslow says, they can come to almost any number, depending on the degree of specificity of description. Some of the more basic are the need for air, food, water, oxygen, sleep, and sexual expression (not to be confused with the need to love and be loved). Physiologic or biologic needs are experienced by all human beings at all age levels and according to Maslow are the most prepotent of all. If a person is dominated by hunger, he has no other interest but food, and, in fact, his whole philosophy of the future tends to change. Ghandi, the mystic, said, in effect, that religion meant nothing to a starving man.

* Maslow, Abraham H.: *Motivation and Personality,* 2nd ed. Harper & Row, New York, 1970, p. 35.

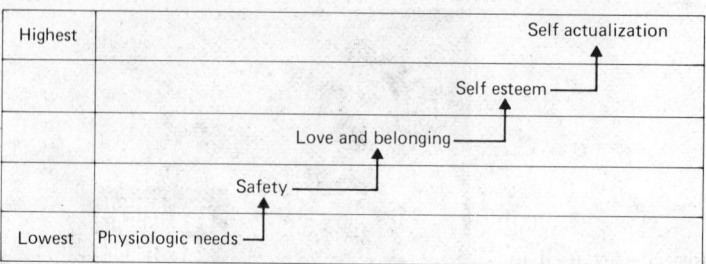

Figure 8-6. Maslow's hierarchy of needs. (Adapted from Maslow, Abraham H.: *Motivation and Personality,* 2nd ed. Harper & Row, New York, 1970.)

Safety needs (the second category), including security, stability, protection, dependency, freedom from fear and anxiety, and need for structure and limits, emerge when physiologic needs are relatively gratified. These needs are more easily seen in infants and children, who do not inhibit their reactions, than in adults who have learned to mask their reactions. All types of illness, and in fact anything that disrupts the child's routine or rhythm, make him or her feel unsafe. Parents and other family members have the central role in meeting a child's safety needs. Parental outbursts or threats of punishment, harsh words, or physical punishment may induce panic and terror. A child's fear of losing parental love is believed a part of this terror because the completely rejected child may be seen "clinging" to the "hating parents" apparently for sheer protection rather than as an expression of love or as a plea for love. The average child who is confronted with new, unfamiliar, and strange situations will frequently react in terror. It is well documented by the works of psychologists, psychotherapists, and teachers that permissiveness within limits, rather than unrestricted permissiveness, is preferred as well as *needed* by children. And most adults as well as children in our society prefer a safe, orderly, and predictable world and people who shield them from harm in situations over which they have little control. All too frequently in hospitals, adults already under stress are expected to learn new methods for solving problems and expected to adapt themselves to radical changes in life without showing their fears. A good example is the person who must accept the mutilation of a colostomy and learn to regulate bowel movements through an abdominal opening. Evidence of safety needs are not as obvious in the adult as in the child; however, most adults obviously prefer familiar rather than unfamiliar things and often show fear of the unknown.[33b]

While some may think that the average person in contemporary society feels safe (has his safety needs met), others think the opposite. Eric Hoffer,[33e] for instance, in his book *The Ordeal of Change,* discusses the profoundly disturbing effect of the rapid change in man's environment characteristic of this age. Benjamin A. Kogan,[33d] in *Health: Man in a Changing Environment,* expresses the opinion that the rise in the crime rate and in the use of drugs and the breakdown in family life and other signs of a sick society are the result of man's inability to keep pace internally with external change. René Dubos,[33e] in *So Human an Animal,* is expressing this same idea. Not only is rapid change threatening but so is the fear of cataclysmic warfare. While every era has its dangers, historians agree that some are more fearsome than others.

The extent to which fear is producing illness in this age and the degree to which illness not caused by fear is complicated by a fear-engendering society cannot be explored here. But health workers must realize that because this is not a peaceful era they can expect to see many adults behave like frightened children. Many so-called healthy adults in hospitals cannot get well because nurses and physicians fail to provide an emotionally safe environment for them and their families. They not only fail to understand these generalized fears but also fail to help them deal with the specified fears of illness. For example, they do not discuss the diagnosis, treatment plan, and prognosis with the patient or encourage patient and family participation in planning care.

Although research on the need to *belong* and the need to give and receive expressions of *love* is comparatively recent, love has been the central theme in poems, autobiographies, novels, and plays for many years. Sociologic and psychologic literature now abounds in reports of such studies.[34-37] When the lower needs (discussed above) are fairly well satisfied, the need for love, affection, and belongingness emerges.

Children who are forced to move from one city to another, from one neighborhood to another, or to leave their friends or family members (for any reason) suffer psychologically. Human beings and animals have a tendency "to herd, to flock, to join, to belong." Because it is not possible to discuss these concepts in detail, readers should consult special references at the end of this chapter.[38,39] (Chapter 16, dealing with communication, discusses the subject of emotional needs.) Thwarting the need to belong, to love and be loved, results in an unsatisfied hunger for human contact and intimacy, causing feelings of alienation, aloneness, strangeness, and loneliness so prevalent in all groups, especially youths. Maslow believes that today's mobility, scattering of family members, urbanization, and breakdown of traditional groupings, has resulted in a shallowness of American friendships and other relationships. This is seen in all types of health services where patients, families, and personnel remain relative strangers. Patients often are angry because health personnel do not relate to them as *real* people, or as personalities.

Volumes have been written on the many kinds of love, Eric Fromm's writings being among those most often cited. The word has different meanings for different people; to some it is synonymous with sex. Since a person cannot be dissociated from his or her sexuality, there will always be an argument as to whether a loving response to others is entirely unconditioned by sex, but the position is taken in this chapter that there can be sex expression with or without love and that love is not necessarily an expression of sex. Perhaps because nursing, as we know it, was developed in the Victorian period with its sex taboos, great stress was put on the objective, nonemotional, "professional" manner, or attitude, of the nurse. Also, the difficulty of behaving rationally under the influence of a strong emotion has been an argument for the health worker's avoiding "involvement" with the patient. And the drain on health workers if they live day in and day out watching people they "love" suffer is another argument for noninvolvement.

It is the opinion of the authors that in spite of the arguments for objectivity, or noninvolvement, health workers *should* love their patients and can express it in ways that do not suggest a sexual attachment or an untherapeutic interdependence. Real love means *not* using the patient to make the health worker feel better or important. Finally, it should be emphasized that love involves both giving and receiving love.

The need for *esteem* is felt by everyone in our society. This includes self-respect and esteem from others. These needs include the following: (1) desire for strength, adequacy, achievement, mastery, competence, independence and freedom, and confidence, and (2) desire for reputation or prestige (defined by other people), status, fame, and glory, recognition, attention, importance, and dignity. When the need for self-esteem is met, a person feels self-confident, worthy, capable, strong, and useful; whereas when these needs are thwarted a person feels helpless, inferior, and weak. Carried far enough, this can result in a neurosis.[40] Healthy self-esteem is based on *deserved* respect from others rather than unwarranted celebrity or external fame, according to Maslow. Self-esteem is a desirable goal. People who depend on others' approval will always feel incompetent. Nurses and physicians who allow patients to be "in charge" of their own health and treatment are doing a great deal to help them develop competency and self-esteem.

The highest need as listed by Maslow is for *self-actualization,* or self-fulfillment. If all the "lower" needs are fairly well met, man has a desire to do what he is best fitted for. A person may aspire to being an ideal parent, an artist, a physician, a nurse, a writer, a poet. Maslow thinks self-actualization is a product of maturity. While great accomplishments of young persons, as, for example, Joan of Arc, John Keats, and Alexander the Great, come to mind, Maslow's comments on contemporary society are worth noting:

In our culture at least, youngsters have not yet achieved identity, or autonomy, nor have they had time enough to experience an enduring loyal, post-romantic love relationship, nor have they generally found their calling, the altar upon which to offer themselves. Nor have they worked out their *own* system of values; nor have they had experience enough (responsibility for others, tragedy, failure, achievement, success) to shed perfectionistic illusions and become realistic; nor have they generally made their peace with death; nor have they learned how to be patient; nor have they learned enough about evil in themselves and others to be compassionate; nor have they had time to become post-ambivalent about parents and elders, power and authority; nor have they generally become knowledgeable and educated enough to open the possibility of becoming wise. . . .*

Although man's potential may have been realized only by the "mature, fully human, self-actualizing" person, this does not mean that human beings at any age are unhealthy; but it does mean that they are in a state of "growth-toward-self-actualization" which can

* Maslow, Abraham H.: *op. cit.,* p. XX.

be either "good" (promising) or "poor" (unpromising).

Socioeconomic Influences. Nurses should have such knowledge as shows them what kind of nursing care patients need. They must know the *sex* and *age* of patients; they should know their *race, nationality,* and *religion* in order to understand their language difficulties and the way they think and feel about many things. Orthodox Jews, for instance, will not want to eat meat unless the animal was killed under conditions prescribed by their faith. Many aspects of treatment, such as circumcision, have a religious significance for certain peoples. Nurses must understand and show respect for religious and racial customs if they hope to give the highest type of service. It is also useful for health workers to know the susceptibility of races to certain diseases or what to expect when a person comes from the "culture of poverty" or from the affluent culture. Health workers will find it is useful to compare local and national morbidity figures.

Physiologic differences between men and women, children and adults, racial groups, and people from very different geographic areas are known, and some of these differences affect the kind of nursing care planned. For instance, except during pregnancy, women have a lower metabolic rate than men, and, from 10 years of age onward during the childbearing period, a greater need for iron than do men.[41] This suggests the need for special dietary planning for women. Young children with their immature kidneys have a smaller margin of safety with fluid loss than do adults and they lose a greater proportion of body weight than adults.[42] The nurse should therefore plan careful weighing, recording, and comparing of an ill infant's daily weight. Some racial and geographic groups have a greater tendency toward certain blood disorders than do others.[43] Nurses should plan with persons from these groups to have any necessary blood tests and possibly genetic counseling.

Few studies have been made of the sex difference in response to stress, illness, or changing life patterns; however, the woman who has had a stroke or heart attack usually needs a different plan for rehabilitation than that for a man. Both men and women need the kind of planning, beginning early in their care, that helps them, on leaving the hospital, return to their desired and appropriate roles, as far as is possible.

The *age* of the person obviously influences the plan of care. There are innumerable studies on the reactions of children, both physiologic and psychologic, to illness and hospitalization, and on their health needs at various ages.[44-50] Our knowledge about needs of, and reactions to, health care in the elderly person has greatly increased; fewer systematic studies have been found on the needs of young and middle-aged adults.[51-54] Table 8-1 lists changes in physiologic processes common to aging.

Physiologic and psychologic differences between children and adults account for the fact that certain diseases are more serious or more prevalent at different ages. Pneumonia, for instance, in a child under 2 or an elderly person is much more serious and requires more nursing and surveillance than it does for the older child or a younger adult with pneumonia. Some communicable diseases for which no immunizing sera have been developed (scarlet fever, for example) occur more frequently in the school-age child than in other age groups.

Different periods of life also have, according to Erik Erikson, a central "crisis" of personality development. Erikson defines "crisis" as a "turning point, a crucial period of increased vulnerability and heightened potential," * rather than a catastrophic event. He theorizes that from birth to death personality development can be viewed as having eight stages, each of which can be roughly correlated with a chronologic age, and each stage has a central "crisis" that when resolved becomes a basis for the next stage (see Fig. 8-7). Erikson also says that while each central issue has a "best" time for its resolution that issue is not to be considered "secured once and for all at a given state." † He suggests, for example, that the sense of *basic trust* in infancy may or may not evolve into what is called *faith* in the aging.

The first four stages follow rapidly after one another and are most crucial in the first 10 to 12 years of life. Nurses caring for children and their mothers should plan nursing care for infants that increases development of basic trust; care for toddlers and 2-year-olds that promotes autonomy within healthy limitations; care for preschoolers that allows children the opportunity to use imagination (but with constant reminders of what is imaginative and what is real); and care for school children that allows them to "make things" for which they receive recognition and approval. At the same time the nurse is planning for the infant or child she should be planning for the parents who may be in any one of the next three

---

* Erikson, Erik: *Identity: Youth and Crisis.* W. W. Norton & Co., New York, 1968, p. 96.

† Erikson, Erik: *Childhood and Society,* 2nd ed. W. W. Norton & Co., New York, 1963, p. 273.

Table 8-1. Summary of Changes in Physiological Processes Common to Aging [*,†]

Nervous System	*Metabolic or Digestive Processes*	*Lungs*
Structural changes in CNS	Metabolism decreases	Constancy of body fluid in relation to oxygen and CO_2 and in buffer system
Impaired perception, loss of sensitivity → cutaneous and protopathic (sense of pain affected less)	Nutritional needs according to individual variations	Temperature regulation more difficult to adjust
Decrease in size and number of cells	Decrease in secretion of salivary glands → and % of enzymes	Loss in subcutaneous tissue → less efficient insulation of skin
Impulses decrease → slow down speed of action and reaction	Diminished taste	
Decrease in myelin sheath	Stomach may decrease in volume, enzyme action, and HCl	*Skin*
Possibly fewer brain cells in frontal lobe	Tone of large intestine may be impaired	Decrease in regenerative and growth power
		Sebaceous, sweat glands decrease → loss of elasticity
Mental Processes	*Heart and Blood Vessels*	
Impaired circulation, anoxia, hypoxia, nutritional impairment, fluid and electrolyte disturbance may all cause change in mental process	Capacity of heart to increase in rate and strength of beat during physical work is diminished	*Special Senses*
	Blood pressure increase (now believed to be due to disease process)	Decrease in visual perception, visual acuity (narrowing visual field)
Cognition or intelligence not necessarily affected by age—more likely due to disease process or deficiency as noted above	Change in blood flow, if any, would affect rhythm and rate	Hearing loss gradual (high notes first—low notes later)
	Decline in glucose tolerance (now believed due to age per se, not disease)	Taste less acute, less discriminating
Hormones	*Renal Function*	*Bone and Joint and Muscle Unit*
Decline in hormone production in all endocrine glands →	Reduction in renal blood flow to compensate for declining cardiac output (adaptive change)	Osteoporosis → atrophy or degenerative changes in joint structure (secretions?) loss of muscle tone—slowing of neuromuscular excitability increase in connective tissue → atrophy of muscle cells
Reduced rate of thyroxine utilization reflecting a loss of mainly muscle tissue		

[*] Sutterley, Doris Cook, and Donnelly, Gloria A.: "Meeting Nursing Needs Throughout the Life Cycle," in Kintzel, Kay Corman (ed.): *Advanced Concepts in Clinical Nursing.* J. B. Lippincott Co., Philadelphia, 1971, p. 62.

[†] Not necessarily age specific or the result of the aging process without disease (subject of current research).

stages, that is, identity vs. role confusion (adolescence); or intimacy vs. isolation (young adulthood); or generativity vs. stagnation (adulthood). In each of these three stages the first characteristic named is the goal of "well-being" for that stage. The last of the eight stages, ego integrity vs. despair, suggests that the nurse should plan both directly and indirectly to help the elderly find ego integrity in the present and satisfaction in recalling the past.

The *nationality* of patients and their *cultural* background influence their thinking, feeling, and behavior, and are therefore important factors in developing nursing plans.[55,56] Madeleine M. Leininger[57] suggests that nurses can develop "cultural awareness" by watching and listening to a person of another culture; by considering how the behavior of a "difficult" patient may reflect a cultural response to illness. Nurses can, of course, increase their knowledge of cultures by studying anthropology.

Much information has been accumulated on socioeconomic subcultures in the United States through recent studies. While it is impossible to report or apply the findings of these studies, some general characteristics of the groups surveyed can be described.

The term "culture of poverty" [*] was introduced by Oscar Lewis in the early 1960s and has since been used by anthropologists, sociologists, psychologists, educators, and others in describing patterns of living among the very poor that are passed down from generation to generation. Certain aspects of these patterns directly or indirectly affect the health care and health care planning for members of these groups. For instance, persons from a low-income group often have had less education than those more economically advantaged and therefore have less knowledge and understanding of the terminology, practices, or availability of health care. Many have grown up in environments where communication has

[*] Lewis, Oscar: *Anthropological Essays.* Random House, New York, 1970, p. 67.

POSITIVE VERSUS NEGATIVE DEVELOPMENT

	1	2	3	4	5	6	7	8
8 Maturity								Ego integrity vs. Despair
7 Adulthood							Generativity vs. Stagnation	
6 Young adulthood						Intimacy vs. Isolation		
5 Puberty and adolescence					Identity vs. Role confusion			
4 Latency				Industry vs. Inferiority				
3 Locomotor-genital			Initiative vs. Guilt					
2 Muscular-anal		Autonomy vs. Shame, doubt						
1 Oral sensory	Basic trust vs. Mistrust							

Stages

Figure 8-7. Eight stages of personality development correlated with chronological age. (Erik H. Erikson: *Childhood and Society,* 2nd ed. W. W. Norton Co., New York, 1963, p. 273.)

been limited to body language, facial expressions, and shouting or monosyllabic responses, and where childhood urges to explore and satisfy curiosity have been disciplined harshly. Individuals from low-income groups may therefore fail to understand questions or directions from health personnel, and hesitate to ask questions or ask for understandable explanations. Their feeling about persons in authority frequently interferes with their ability or willingness to carry out health regimens. In addition, their economic situation may prevent planning for the future; a long-range health plan has little meaning for the very poor and uneducated and reaching even short-term health goals is difficult unless these are somehow made pleasurable and nonfrustrating.[58-60]

According to Bonnie and Vern Bullough, "folk medicine" is still an important force among newly arrived Spanish-speaking immigrants to the United States and the poor of the "barrios." In their opinion, health workers should know folk medicine in order to understand its meaning to client, or patient. They also say that "Since available information suggests that the folk methods are often effective, it might well be that a creative cooperation between the two groups [American health practitioners and Spanish folk healers] would

improve the delivery of health services." * In Chapter 1 studies made under the auspices of WHO are cited that show the effectiveness of health services that are quite different from "Western medical care."

Regardless of whether the health worker is deeply religious, agnostic, or atheistic, he or she can accept the position taken by the social scientist that patients' religion is part of their culture and the source of many, sometimes most, of their ideas and attitudes. These may come through the religion of their forebears and associates, and patients may be relatively unconscious of their source and influence.

A number of religious and ethical questions are currently asked about some of the "traditional" ways of solving health problems. The legal availability of abortion is one example; the right of the dying patient to refuse additional treatment, the effects of birth control methods, artificial insemination, and organ transplants are other problematic topics. To understand patients and their responses to these and other health problems, some knowledge of their ethical values is essential to the nurse and, in fact, to all health workers. Religious advisers—ministers, rabbis, and priests

* Bullough, Bonnie, and Bullough, Vern L.: *Poverty, Ethnic Identity, and Health Care.* Appleton-Century-Crofts, New York, 1972, p. 85.

—on the therapeutic team can make an important contribution to the planning and implementation of the patient's care.*

If we accept the thesis that each man has a faith he lives by, it follows that he finds comfort in the presence and counsel of a representative of this faith, especially in the stress of birth, illness, and death. A man's faith or "religion" may be so unorthodox, so individual, that it is difficult to find "a representative" of his school of thought, but even such a person often recognizes that he is strengthened or calmed by the spirituality of another, although their faiths are dissimilar. The Joint Commission on Mental Illness and Health in *Americans View Their Mental Health* [61] reports that more people go to clergymen for counseling than to all the mental health professions combined. While Chapter 18 is devoted to worship and religious questions, it is hoped that what is said here emphasizes the importance of the clergy as a member of the therapeutic team and the obligation of health personnel to make possible the observation of those religious practices that are significant to each patient.

Daily Living Activities and Health Practices.
It is usually the nurse who helps the clients, or patients, temporarily or permanently modify their daily activities of living when, as carried out, they interfere with maintaining or acquiring a state of well-being. Such activities include eating, eliminating, resting and sleeping, working and playing, exercising, dressing and keeping clean, learning, communicating with others, and forms of worship if the person is religious. When patients are hospitalized, these habits are almost always modified. Ideally, they would be modified according to patients' physical and emotional needs; actually, patients are more likely to have their habits adjusted to institutional routines or the lives of those upon whom they become dependent. To the extent that it is within their power, health workers, including nurses, should try to help patients and their families work out plans that are best for *them* and that take into consideration previous patterns of living. Baths can be given in the evening as well as the morning, breakfast can often be delayed for the habitual late sleeper, or a snack can be served to the early riser who is on a nonrestricted diet. Habitual naptime and bedtime rituals, at least in part, can be observed when a child is the patient.

While the plan of care should be developed with patients who usually resist drastic changes in their daily regimens, the plan should also reflect the efforts health "experts" make in teaching health. It may be through changes in a daily regimen only that a person recovers from the condition that made him or her seek treatment. Poor eating habits, lack of exercise, and misuse of drugs are, for example, common causes of ill health. Old habits should be broken and new ones acquired, although this may necessitate changes in the family's economic status. This seems self-evident and is amply documented in the literature.

In a study of 401 women from all income levels, Lois Pratt [62] reports that there was a significant relationship between lack of exercise, poor nutrition, and inadequate dental care and a low level of health and low income. While a high per cent of the women in the low-income group failed to eat breakfast or to get sufficient exercise, a considerable number of women in the higher-income groups also neglected these areas of health practice. Pratt concludes, in part, that health programs should focus on teaching specific health practices since the study also showed that good health practices can be carried out without much knowledge of complex or abstract principles of health. When nurses know the patient's current health habits and background, they should plan with him or her how to change the undesirable or inadequate practices. An example of step-by-step planning is given in the pamphlet *How to Stop Smoking!* written by Donald T. Fredrickson [63] and distributed by the American Heart Association.

Diagnosis and Plan of Therapy. The nurse in private practice, the nurse in centers where there are no doctors, and nurses in some clinics and hospital services may be helping clients cope with certain health problems that do not demand the attention of the physician and in such cases base the plan of care on their assessment. Usually the plan of care is designed around the diagnosis, or identification, of patient problems by the physician and his or her prescribed treatment. Whether the plan of care is directed toward prevention of future illness, promotion of better health and development of independence, coping with a handicapping condition, or provisions for a peaceful death, the nurse should know the *direct* and *indirect* causes of the condition for which the patient is treated. It is important to know not only the *diagnosis* but also the *severity of the condition*. Persons with mild heart conditions may be able to take their own baths, assume almost any position in bed with comfort, exercise moderately, and talk to friends for several hours without being tired by the exertion. Those with acute or severe cardiac disease, however, should often be

* The forms of spoken address for the clergy are given in Chapter 18.

spared the slightest effort; they may be comfortable only when supported in a sitting posture, and absolute quiet may be essential to recovery.

The Patient and His Family, or Life Setting. All of us grow up in a family or a reasonable substitute for one, and often are unaware of the ways in which current experiences and reactions are influenced by early learning. As most literate persons know, family values and ways are so much a part of a child that it is difficult to determine whether the kind of person he or she is can be traced to genetic influences or the social influences of the family. Studies of identical twins, separated at birth, have attempted to answer this question. Theodore Lidz says, "Subsequent influences will modify those of the family, but they can never undo or fully reshape these early core experiences." * Nurses frequently make assumptions about the families of patients or about patients themselves that are negative and overly moralistic because of the kind of family values and perceptions they (nurses) hold. Some psychiatric nurses, for instance, are unable to work with and help alcoholic patients because of their own experiences with a parent or close relative who was alcoholic; some maternity nurses cannot understand or be helpful to the unwed mother who elects to raise her infant and some pediatric nurses condemn mothers who are unable to be with their young children during hospitalization.

The concepts of "family developmental tasks" and "family homeostasis" are suggested for nurses trying to help families. "Family developmental tasks"—the first concept—are "those that must be accomplished by a family in a way that will satisfy (1) biologic requirements, (2) cultural imperatives, and (3) personal values, if the family is to continue and grow as a unit." †

A generally used scheme is Evelyn W. Duval's [64] eight stages in the family life cycle, with developmental tasks shown for each family member during each stage. These stages are as follows: stage 1—married couples (without children); stage 2—childbearing families (oldest child birth to 30 months); stage 3—families with preschool children (oldest child 2½ to 6 years); stage 4—families with school children (oldest child 6 to 13 years); stage 5—families with teenagers (oldest child 13 to 20 years); stage 6—families as launching centers (first child gone to last child's leaving home); stage 7—middle-aged parents (empty nest to retirement); stage 8—aging family members (retirement to death of both spouses) (see Table 8-2).

According to the second concept of "family homeostasis," family members act so that a balance of relations is achieved among them, and if this balance is disrupted through "trouble," such as illness, the family as a unit may disintegrate, temporarily break down, and then recover, or may grow and become a better-integrated unit.[65,65a] E. James Anthony and Cyrille Koupernik [66] suggest that helpful, protective, and "saving" agents foster growth and recovery of the family.

It is impossible here to discuss in detail family developmental stages, their related developmental tasks, or the many ways a family regains equilibrium after a crisis. Readers are therefore urged to increase their knowledge about families through use of the references listed at the end of this chapter.

Institutional Policies As They Affect Care. The kind of nursing care planned for a patient is also influenced by variations in institutional policies. For example, in many pediatric units or hospitals mothers room with their children during illness and nursing care plans reflect this. Studies show that all mothers want information about what is happening and about the purposes of diagnostic tests; and they want to know what they can do for their children. If children are admitted to a day hospital for surgery, the nursing plan should include an orientation for them and their families as well as instruction for presurgical preparation and postsurgical care at home. Day care units and night care units for psychiatric patients, progressive care units, and extended care units are other policy variations that influence the kind of nursing care planned. In psychiatric day care hospitals, activities are relatively informal and the nurse has a large responsibility for planning ways by which a psychotherapeutic atmosphere and relationships can be maintained. In progressive care units and extended care units, ways to enhance the patient's independence should be carefully planned.[67-73]

In critical care units, such as coronary care and surgical intensive care, emphasis is placed on life-saving efforts by many experts and intervention in acute states of panic, depression, and grief. Visits to patients are planned according to their needs to see or experience the presence (that is, through touch or voice) of a member of their family or persons close to them. Visits are also planned according to the needs of the family—such as the need to

---

* Lidz, Theodore: *The Person.* Basic Books, Inc., New York, 1968, p. 47.

† Hill, Reuben: "Interdisciplinary Workshop on Marriage and Family Research," *Marriage and Family Living,* **13**:2, (Feb.) 1951. Quoted in Duval, Evelyn Willis: *Family Development,* 4th ed. J. B. Lippincott Co., Philadelphia, 1971, p. viii.

Table 8-2. Stage-Critical Family Developmental Tasks Through the Family Life Cycle *

Stage of the Family Life Cycle	Positions in the Family	Stage-Critical Family Developmental Tasks
1. Married couple	Wife Husband	Establishing a mutually satisfying marriage Adjusting to pregnancy and the promise of parenthood Fitting into the kin network
2. Childbearing	Wife-mother Husband-father Infant daughter or son or both	Having, adjusting to, and encouraging the development of infants Establishing a satisfying home for both parents and infant(s)
3. Preschool-age	Wife-mother Husband-father Daughter-sister Son-brother	Adapting to the critical needs and interests of preschool children in stimulating, growth-promoting ways Coping with energy depletion and lack of privacy as parents
4. School-age	Wife-mother Husband-father Daughter-sister Son-brother	Fitting into the community of school-age families in constructive ways Encouraging children's educational achievement
5. Teenage	Wife-mother Husband-father Daughter-sister Son-brother	Balancing freedom with responsibility as teenagers mature and emancipate themselves Establishing postparental interests and careers as growing parents
6. Launching center	Wife-mother-grandmother Husband-father-grandfather Daughter-sister-aunt Son-brother-uncle	Releasing young adults into work, military service, college, marriage, etc., with appropriate rituals and assistance Maintaining a supportive home base
7. Middle-aged parents	Wife-mother-grandmother Husband-father-grandfather	Rebuilding the marriage relationship Maintaining kin ties with older and younger generations
8. Aging family members	Widow/widower Wife-mother-grandmother Husband-father-grandfather	Coping with bereavement and living alone Closing the family home or adapting it to aging Adjusting to retirement

* Duval, Evelyn Willis: *Family Development*, 4th ed. J. B. Lippincott Co., Philadelphia, 1971, p. 151.

be reassured that the patient is alive.* The length of time and frequency of family visits are determined by mutual discussion and planning between staff and family.

Roles of Major Health Workers. If patients are rational, their understanding, interest, and cooperation are of the greatest importance in both planning and carrying out the program of care. While they are in an institution, it may be possible to force a regimen upon them, but even in the hospital cooperation is essential to successful therapy; ultimately, the health of individuals will depend on their ability to care for themselves. Plans, therefore, should be made with the assistance, the suggestion, and certainly the approval, or acceptance, of patients. They, after all, are more concerned than others with their condition and welfare.

* Visits are often of crucial importance immediately after the death to help the family recognize the reality of what has happened.

In order to help patients realize the importance of a suggested regimen, it may be necessary to give them considerable guidance. Blind faith in the wisdom of their health advisers may be sufficiently powerful to induce patients to follow plans made for them; but most individuals prefer to say what they will do or have done for them, when it shall be done, and who shall do it. If patients do not agree to the conditions that health advisers believe to be *essential* to effective therapy, the advisers may refuse to treat them. This they seldom do and then not until every effort has been made to help the patients understand the reasons for the proposed treatment. More and more it is believed that plans for health care should be made also in consultation with the *relatives* (or friends) involved. Ultimately the patient or the family must take the initiative in planning and the final stage of recovery depends on independence in planning.

In the British Peckham Experiment, re-

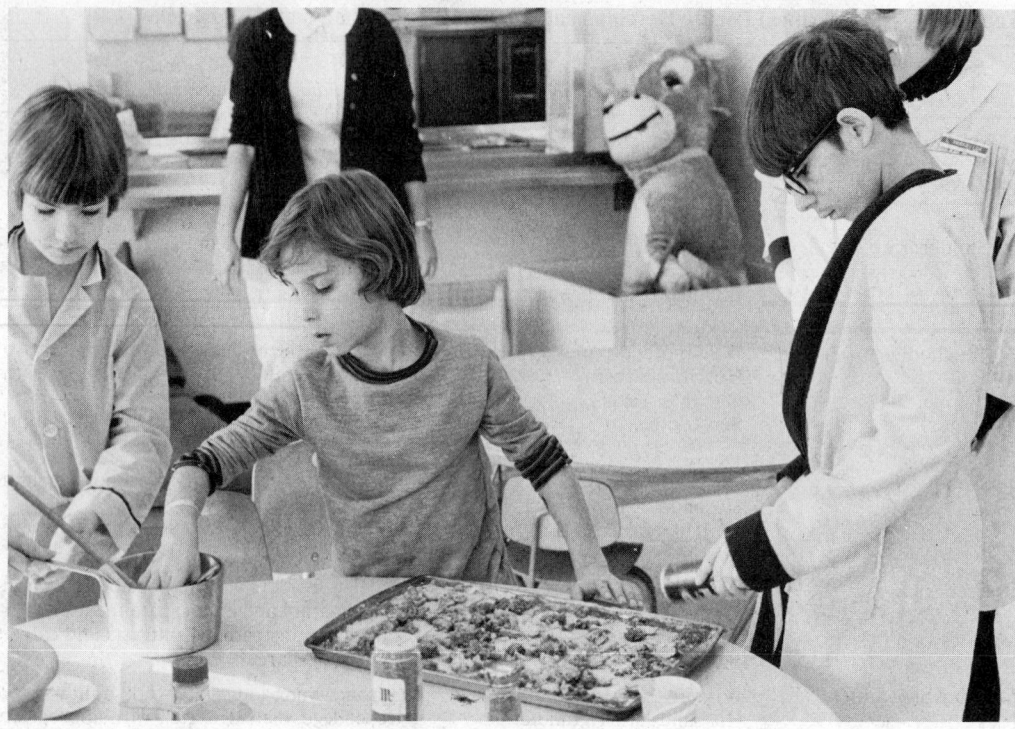

Figure 8-8. Young patients making pizza in the hospital playroom. (Courtesy of Children's Memorial Hospital, Chicago, Ill.)

ported in 1944, the relationship of illness to family structure was thoroughly investigated. Families, not individuals, were registered and were given a comprehensive health service.[74] Margaret L. Shetland,[75] in 1943, reported a study of family health service given by the Community Service Society of New York City,

and, in 1945, Henry B. Richardson,[76] in his text *Patients Have Families,* showed the wasted effort in treating a patient without consideration of the family situation. The importance of the *family's participation in planning care* for an individual and the importance of considering the family as the unit to be served are com-

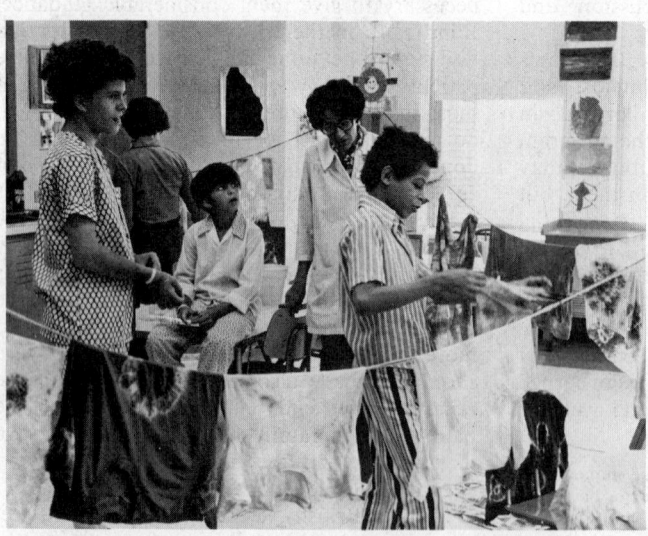

Figure 8-9. Children learning in the hospital playroom to get effects with tie-dyeing clothing. (Courtesy of Children's Memorial Hospital, Chicago, Ill.)

monplace statements in the health literature of today—especially in the writing of community ("public health," "district," or "visiting") nurses and "health visitors." Chapter 5 includes a guide for collecting "family data" designed to help nurses work more effectively with families.

George G. Reader, a physician, and Doris R. Schwartz, a nurse, associated for years in the study of care for the chronically ill and elderly in ambulatory services say:

Joint planning is here to stay as part of the present scene of patient care. Starting with the patient's nurse and physician it may be expected to extend to include many other health workers: the patient's family, social workers, physical and occupational therapists, dietitians, administrators and community planners, as well as a host of others who will be identified in the future. . . . Working together and planning together helps to define roles, diminish conflicts, and enhance the support the physician and nurse provide the patient and each other.*

Actually it is impossible to make rules about who should plan a person's care since it depends on his or her condition (whether the patient is an infant or a rational adult, whether he or she is conscious or unconscious, for example); the situation (whether the patient is at home or in a tent hospital, for instance); and those available to care for him or her. The person may be without family or friends, there may be no physician available, or the patient may be asking advice on a health problem from a physician or nurse in private practice. The following are generalizations that represent, perhaps, the most common practice.

Diagnostic and therapeutic procedures are usually prescribed by physicians. Certain of these they carry out themselves with patients, their families, nurses, or special therapists, but many are left entirely to others. Those who perform therapeutic procedures prescribed by the physician might be called in legal terms, the doctor's agents. This, however, is an oversimplification of a rather complex problem which is discussed also in Chapter 1. If other workers act as agents, physicians might be responsible for supervising and training them, but actually this is not the case. In practice, physicians prescribe physical and occupational therapy carried out by independent professional workers, and many of the therapeutic procedures physicians prescribe are so consistently performed by nurses that doctors consider them nursing procedures. The over-

lapping of medicine and nursing is obvious, with, at present, a marked trend toward increasing the scope of nursing responsibility.

Ordinarily doctors leave only the most general prescription for "bed rest" or "general diet" and expect nurses to arrange feedings, periods of sleep, rest, and diversion around their plans for therapy. Doctors may indicate the time at which treatments are to be given and diagnostic tests made; they always indicate their frequency; often they leave the timing to others. When physicians have no other professional workers associated with them in the care of the patient, they will necessarily have many more problems and carry greater responsibility in making and executing the total plan of care than when they are working in a modern hospital situation.

Medicine is so highly specialized that most medical programs are the result of collaboration among a number of doctors. One physician or one surgeon is usually in charge, and others act as consultants, unless doctors practice as a group and arrange to share the responsibility for all patients. With the growing belief that mind and body are inseparable and that disease affects both aspects—the psyche and the soma—the *psychiatrist's* help is more often sought. It is increasingly difficult to say one person is physically and another mentally ill. In some cases, physical symptoms may be more noticeable and more measurable, and in others the personality changes may stand out, but both are present in some degree. The plan of therapy is and should often be the product of the pooled judgment of physicians, nurses, and others. Patients and the guardians of minors can, of course, reject the plan of therapy if they believe it inappropriate or too risky.

In assessing the psychic component of illness and the potential abilities of patients, *psychologists* and *sociologists* are valuable members of the therapeutic team. As residents or consultants, clinical psychologists are employed in most psychiatric services and in rehabilitation centers. Their help is sought increasingly where psychometric tests are indicated, and where interviewing and counseling are needed. Many long-term plans of care include provision for the psychologist's participation through one or more of these channels.

E. Gartley Jaco [77] says that social epidemiology, the study of disease and its possible social causes, is a significant specialty in community health practice. He believes that *social and behavioral scientists* with their knowledge of life styles, value systems, and social processes will increasingly add to the understanding of disease.

* Reader, George G., and Schwartz, Doris R.: "Joint Planning for Patient Care," *J.A.M.A.,* **201**:364, (Aug. 7) 1967.

Physicians prescribe patients' diets, but if an expert in this field is available they rely on him or her to estimate quantities, to plan appetizing combinations of food, to get variety and balance in the diet, and to supervise its preparation. *Nutritionists* are often expected to guide patients in purchasing, planning, and preparing foods; they cooperate with physicians, nurses, and patients and their families in arranging suitable hours for feedings and in selecting foods. They may play an important role in the rehabilitation of some patients.

It was remarked earlier that the threat to economic security made by illness may involve far more suffering than the pain connected with the disease. Worry over finances, disrupted family relationships, or unemployment not only delays recovery but also may be the underlying cause of organic pathology. While physicians and nurses should have a sufficient knowledge of the community resources to enable them to advise the patient and his family, their burden will be lightened if *specialists in social work and vocational guidance* are participating in the patient's care. They give patients expert assistance in financial problems, in job placement, in finding and being admitted to health and welfare agencies, in securing housekeeping and other services demanded by sickness, and in other health problems too numerous to list.

Health care encompasses such a wide range of skills that experts have been developed to take over certain elements from the doctor and nurse. So, in a fully staffed medical center, there are *physical, occupational, recreational,* and *special therapists* as well as numerous *technicians*. The special therapists mentioned have professional standards of selection and preparation. Without their participation, the plan and execution of patient care are often incomplete, for no other workers are so highly trained in their specialties. The technician is a key worker in many situations. The man who makes a wearable leg for an amputee or an artificial eye for a patient who has just lost a natural one holds an important place on the rehabilitation team. As specialties multiply, however, the task of coordination and cooperation enlarges, and the service to the patient grows less personal. Morton A. Seidenfeld,[78] in 1949, discussing the psychologic aspects of medical care, made a plea for helping the patient to understand his illness and for orienting health personnel to a patient-centered program where his psychologic needs are recognized and met as carefully as his physical; but he doubted that a "platoon" of workers could be oriented to a patient's emotional problems. When the disadvantages of segmented care are recognized as outweighing its advantages, we will begin to prepare fewer types of workers more thoroughly, each of whom will give a wider variety of services. Some medical schools are offering students a variety of "tracks," one of which is general practice. This is in recognition of the need for generalists in medicine.

The clergy and the roles they play as health workers in planning for and assisting the patient are stressed in Chapters 18 and 50.

3. CURRENT EMPHASES AND FORMS FOR PLANS OF CARE

Importance of a Unified Plan. The importance of having a plan of care (including nursing care) for the patient in a hospital or nursing home is now recognized by the Joint Commission on Accreditation of Hospitals and the Social Security Administration of the United States government.[79,80] Both of these organizations require that institutions include a written care plan as part of the complete patient record for purposes of accreditation and certification for public funding. However, it would be misleading to imply that written plans of patient care, as interpreted by the authors, with stated goals for therapy and rehabilitation can be found in all or even the majority of health agencies. Rudy L. Ciuca,[81] in 1972, reported that a survey of 235 randomly chosen nursing care plans from six hospitals on the West Coast showed that almost 75 per cent of the notations were concerned with functional duties such as medications given, treatments completed, the monitoring of vital signs, intake and output (how much fluid the patient takes in and eliminates), and diagnostic studies. Only 1.7 per cent of the notations on the nursing care plans related to rehabilitation or planning for discharge.

One of the many reasons why nursing care plans have been inadequately used is that they are of necessity complex, and a single, universally acceptable form has not yet been developed. *It is hard to imagine anything requiring more insight, knowledge, skill, and cooperative effort on the part of the sick person, the family, and health workers than making a plan of care as interpreted here.*

When several workers are responsible for planning and giving care to a patient, it goes without saying that some means must be devised to coordinate their efforts and direct them toward a common goal. In some institutions and health agencies, regular time is set aside for discussing the care and progress of patients. These meetings, called *"case,"* or *patient conferences,* may be attended by doctors, nurses, dietitians, social workers, and others. In some of them, patients and their families are invited into the conference so that they can contribute to it and learn from the discussion how to take care of themselves when they go home. If patients and families participate, health workers can learn far more about how they can help patients change their patterns of living to meet their health needs than they can otherwise. Mental health agencies are perhaps most likely to ask patients and families to participate in conferences and encourage patients to set their own goals so the most constructive use may be made of the agency and its personnel. *Nursing rounds* that include all nursing personnel with perhaps a nurse specialist, a head nurse, or a team leader are used in some hospitals as a way of identifying patients' problems, discussing nursing plans, and coordinating nursing care of patients. The "rounds" are conducted at the bedside.[82,83] For people who have roommates it is desirable to take them to a conference room since patients rarely like to discuss their problems within the hearing of other patients. Some method for exchange of information and planning of care should be used; otherwise, many of the patient's needs may not be considered and therapy for these may go unplanned.

Although many nurses believe that gathering necessary information about a patient and writing a plan for comprehensive care require too much time from a schedule that is already full, others, who have used various tools for these purposes, have found that time is simply put to a better use when they make a plan. L. Mae McPhetridge[84] found that most "nursing history" interviews required about 30 minutes to complete, and while the information gathered might also have been acquired over a period of several days, having it early in the patient's hospital stay was considered a great advantage. Philothea R. Sweet and Irmagene Stark[85] say that when a Nursing Information Record was developed for obstetric patients and used on initial contact and accompanied them throughout their prenatal parturient, and postnatal periods (with all nurses using the information and adding to it) there was less duplication of information and therefore less duplication of effort by various health workers in planning for and caring for these women. Also, patients were better informed, seemed less apprehensive about their pregnancies, and were better prepared for motherhood. Continuity of care was assured.

Effective nursing has always involved problem-solving, planning, and evaluation. As pointed out in Chapter 1, there has been a concerted effort in recent decades to establish a definition of nursing, a theory (or theories) of nursing, and a science of nursing. Some persons find it helpful to use the term "the nursing process." In 1961, Ida Jean Orlando presented *The Dynamic Nurse-Patient Relationship; Function, Process and Principles.* She says, "A nursing situation is comprised of three basic elements: (1) the behavior of the patient, (2) the reaction of the nurse, and (3) the nursing actions which are designed for the patient's benefit. *The interaction of these elements with each other is nursing process."* * Obviously she looks upon the term as explaining the essential momentary, hourly, and daily activity of anyone who nurses analytically. Her most helpful contribution to the development of nursing is, in our opinion, the insistence that nurses tell the patient what their reactions are and how they interpret the patient's behavior. This gives the patient a chance to correct the nurses' interpretation before it is acted upon.

In 1973 the Nursing Development Conference Group presented *Concept Formalization in Nursing; Process and Product,*[85a] in which are discussed and diagrammed "dominant themes" in concepts of nursing from Florence Nightingale to contemporary concepts. Looking at the index of this book under "Nursing Process" one finds *"See* Practice of Nursing." So, "nursing" is an adequate term for some, "nursing process" more helpful for others, and "nursing practice" may be synonymous with both.

Other nurses [86,87] have described steps or phases within the process of planning patient care: (1) taking a history; (2) identifying health problems; (3) setting goals with and for the client, or patient; (4) describing nursing action (or intervention); and (5) evaluating the client's, or patient's, progress (by use of selected criteria) both concurrently and when care is terminated.

One way to see how these steps in the process of planning patient care are employed jointly by all members of a health care team is to study the patient care plans reported in Chapter 4. This plan was devised using Weed's Problem-Oriented System which is described in Chapter 4. In some institutions where the problem-oriented medical record (POMR) is used, nurses help to build the data base. The nursing history may be separate from or com-

---

* Orlando, Ida Jean: *The Dynamic Nurse-Patient Relationship; Function, Process, and Principles.* G. P. Putnam's Sons, New York, 1961, p. 36.

bined with the medical and psychosocial history. In the POMR system, progress notes for the client, or patient, include, in chronologic order, the reports and observations of all professional personnel involved in caring for the patient.[88-92] Whether this particular method helps the nurse evaluate or audit nursing care as separate from medical care has not been determined.

Health Problems and Determining the Patient's Need for Nursing. A *health problem* has been defined as an interruption in the individual's ability to meet a need, and a *nursing need* has been defined as whatever the person requires in knowledge, will, or strength to perform his or her daily activities and to carry out treatments prescribed for him or her, or as a "requirement of the patient which, if supplied, relieves or diminishes his [or her] . . . distress or improves his [or her] . . . sense of adequacy or well-being." *

When identifying an individual's health problems and needs, nurses must analyze the information they got through observations and interviewing, and call upon all their knowledge about people's behavior that can inhibit or improve their functioning. A number of models for the organization of problems and needs have been proposed and may be helpful. The sources for discussions of these models are listed at the end of this chapter.[93-98d]

Setting Goals. The establishment of goals or objectives as part of the patient's plan of care not only gives the nurse and patient a specific point to be reached but also provides a basis for evaluating the patient's progress and the care given by nurses, physicians, and other health workers. Some goals for patient care are formulated by nurses based on their areas of expertise and interest and some are complex goals requiring that a team of health workers confer on the appropriate statement of the goal and the means to reach it. Berniece M. Wagner[99] urges that goals be stated as patient behavior (not as nursing action); they are to be stated in specific terms and should deal with the patient's future as well as the present. She thinks nurses should not hesitate to state them in physiologic or pathologic terms. Marlene G. Mayers[100] makes the point that too often the established goals, particularly those that are short-term, are not assigned a time deadline. She believes that saying when the goal should be reached is one way of determining the patient's progress. If the goal is not being reached, a revision of nursing action may be necessary.

Dolores E. Little and Doris L. Carnevali[101]

caution that in some cases a too specific or narrow goal focuses attention on only a small part of the problem when a somewhat more general goal might help the patient more and permit a greater diversity of nursing action. For instance, the nursing objective for a 4-year-old boy hospitalized with pneumonia and there without his mother was "To decrease crying by using operant conditioning." * A more general objective, but one that focused on the basic problem, might have been "To relieve fears of abandonment and punishment."

Whatever objectives or goals (with their related problems) are established, the order in which they will be met should also be considered by the patient, family, and nurse. Fay L. Bower[103] says that problems that threaten the life and integrity of an individual, family, or community should have the highest priority; problems that threaten a destructive change in the individual, family, or community the next priority; and problems that affect normal growth of the individual, family, or community the next priority.

As goals or objectives are met in a priority order, short-term and long-term goals become apparent. New goals may develop as more is learned about the person, or, as immediate goals are reached, those with a lower priority in the initial plan may advance to a higher priority. Nurses also should consider that more than one goal can be reached in a single situation. For instance, when giving a preschool child an oral medication the goal of helping the child grow in self-mastery and carry out distasteful tasks can be met at the same time.

Long-term illness, or one that is chronic, threatening to life, or threatening to the body image, often increases *dependency*. The nurse should therefore help the person develop specific objectives early in the nursing care plan that will foster independence.

Types of Plans and Forms Used. The plan of care for patients includes an immediate and a long-term program designed with reference to each patient's problems and needs and the conditions under which he or she lives. In some cases, the latter type is all that is needed. The program or plan is made by the physician in collaboration with the patient and his or her family or possibly a friend, the nurse, the dietitian, the social worker, special therapists, and

---

* Orlando, Ida Jean: *op. cit.,* p. 5.

* Operant conditioning also called reinforcement therapy, and sometimes behavior modification, is based on B. F. Skinner's work in the psychology of learning. Briefly, the basic tenets are that behavior is learned; learning is the result of reinforcement; behavior that is rewarded becomes pleasurable and is repeated; and behavior that is ignored or not rewarded gradually fades and finally stops.[102]

other health workers associated in care of the patient; in some cases, the clergyman may play a significant role. The person for whom the plan is made, if he or she is not too sick and has reached the age of reason, participates in making and executing the plan, since the patient's acceptance of the plan is essential to its success. It is important that all concerned with the program of care should know the central therapeutic aim and related goals. It is equally important that there should be a schedule of care for the patient, known to all those who are responsible for its execution, in order to prevent omissions and overlapping.

There are differing opinions about the amount of detail that should be in a written plan.[104-106] Some experienced nurses believe that with a patient objective such as "Increase oral fluid intake to 1500 ml daily," details about the kinds of drinks enjoyed by the patient, whether he needs or wants help with drinking, whether he abhors paper cups or cannot use a cup of any kind, or whether he needs constant, consistent reminding about taking fluids should be in the written plan. Others believe this kind of information should be found in the health history or obtained in nursing conferences and believe writing this information consumes unnecessary time and creates an inflexible plan. But the inclusion of details increases the continuity of care and gives patients assurance that the nursing staff considers them as individuals since they are not repeatedly questioned about likes and dislikes, or abilities and disabilities.

Usually the nurse, or other health worker, has less than complete information about patients and their situations, but to wait until the information is complete drastically limits necessary care. Nurses, with the patient and any others involved, therefore should make a decision for action weighing the probability of risk against the probability of benefit. An excellent description of the decision-making process can be found in Bower's *The Process of Planning Nursing Care*.[106a]

Cooperation among workers and consistency in treatment and care are fostered by patient conferences and by the use of written plans of care kept with the patient's record. Written plans of care seem to provide the surest means of making the schedule known to all concerned. Planning treatment and care on an individual basis means that those who plan it must acquire a certain amount of information about the patient in order that they may analyze his or her problems and needs. Such data make up the *patient studies* in medicine, nursing, and social work. All professional workers in attendance on the patient share the responsibility for continuously assessing the patient's needs; therefore, a record system that makes the findings or observations of each available to all should be used. All categories of health workers should have a clear understanding of their functions in relation to planning and executing the care of the patient. If they are not defined, there are apt to be overlapping and omissions.

Collecting all pertinent information about a patient is known as *a patient study*. William Osler and great doctors in all ages have stressed the present practice of teaching medicine through the study of individual cases. It seems self-evident that nurses cannot make effective plans for care of the patient without preparing such studies. The study need not necessarily take written form. If nurses are to discuss the patient's care in a conference, however, they may find it valuable to make notes on the salient facts and the way in which they affect nursing care; or, if they are preparing a study of a patient to be published or read by others, they may give this information in a narrative form. The following is a longer narrative type used as a basis for planning nursing care.

Patient Study of a Young Boy with Cavernous Hemangioma

Michael Gonzales is a 10-year-old boy, born in the United States of Mexican parentage. His father left the family shortly after Michael's birth and his whereabouts is unknown. Michael had two brothers, both of whom died in an apartment house fire when Michael was an infant. Michael and his mother recently moved to _____ (state), and Michael came to the attention of the plastic surgical service at _____ (hospital) upon referral from his school nurse. Michael and his mother presently live in a three-room apartment and are supported entirely by state welfare. Michael speaks Spanish and English, and his mother speaks only Spanish.

Michael was born with a cavernous hemangioma of his left face. It extends from the lower half of his left cheek to his upper neck and includes part of his lips. A cavernous hemangioma is a subcutaneous collection of blood vessels with normal, but bluish overlying skin. The large and irregular vessels, filled with blood, do not regress spontaneously and surgical incisions is the preferred treatment.[106b] Michael had undergone 11 surgical procedures to remove the hemangioma, but after each procedure it grew back. The right side of Michael's face is that of an attractive child, but the left is markedly disfigured. The surgeons planned to excise the hemangioma, using a more radical procedure than was carried out at the previous operations. In this way they hoped to prevent its further growth. Recognizing that such a radical excision would require skin grafting to close the wound, they explained to Michael and his mother that Michael would have more than one hospitalization before the surgery would be successfully completed. The wound would finally be closed and the face reconstructed with pedicle and split thickness skin grafts. These procedures continued for five hospitalizations for the next 2 years. This report will describe Michael's care during the first admission in which the hemangioma was excised.

Dr. Roberts, who examined Michael on admission to the children's unit, made the following notes on his condition:

Patient was born with a purplish mass on left cheek. This grew with him and he had several operations and hospitalizations in _____ (city) in an attempt to remove this hemangioma. The last surgery was about 1 year ago in _____ (city). The mass has recurred with each attempt at excision. He has only bled recently, about 2 or 3 months ago, when he bit the inside of his lip. He has never bled spontaneously. There has been no recent change in the character of the mass and no history of other cutaneous vascular malformations.

His height and weight are in the 50th percentile for his age. His heart rate is 94, respiratory rate 22, and blood pressure 110/60. His vision and hearing are normal. In the mouth dilated loops of vessels are visible. The mass over the left face is not tender and measures about 16 × 4 cm. The remainder of the physical examination is completely normal. Michael is well developed for his age, and his face is obviously deformed by the mass extending from the angle of the jaw to the midline of the left face and to just below the left eye.

After this examination, the diagnosis of cavernous hemangioma was made and the plan of treatment was surgical incision. Laboratory examinations of blood and urine and radiographic examination of the chest were carried out in preparation for the surgery. (See Chapter 47 on preoperative preparation.) Michael's general health was excellent and surgery was to be carried out two days after admission.

A conference was held by the nurses who would be caring for Michael to plan for instruction and emotional preparation for Michael and his mother (see Figs. 8-10 and 8-11). The staff regretted that the time for Michael's preparation was so short. The nature and timing of preparation for hospitalization and surgery for children are determined by several factors, some of which are the type of surgery and anticipated length of stay in the hospital, the age of the child, emotional and intellectual development, past experiences with hospitalization and surgery, the nature of relationship with mother, father, and other adults. (See Chapter 47 for a general discussion of preoperative preparation.) A child cannot be helped apart from his or her parents, and the parent is the greatest resource in planning the preparation. Preparation is carried out successfully when all persons who will be involved in the patient's care know what kind of preparation has been offered to the parent and child and their response to the preparation. The physician, nurse, and other workers in pediatric units (such as the child life worker) usually decide together the responsibility each will have in the preparation. The nurse, in turn, plans with all other nursing staff who will be caring for the patient and how the preparation will be implemented and changed based on the child's and parent's response. The report at the end of an 8-hour shift and the nursing team conference are times when preparation for the child and family can be planned and evaluated.

Background information on Michael's emotional response to past hospitalizations was not available. Neither Michael nor his mother could put into words their impressions of these events. Michael did enjoy drawing with the nurse who carried out the initial interview, and it was noted that all his drawings were of normal children. He refused to draw a picture of himself, his mother, or the hospital. Michael drew pictures with the nurse with obvious pleasure, and it was the first indication of how much Michael could trust helping adults. This trust was his major resource over subsequent weeks marked by physical pain, isolation, and temporary loss of speech.

A simple explanation was given of the anesthesia and the kind of dressings Michael would have on his face when he awakened. The mother met with the plastic surgeon who discussed the entire operation with her with the help of a Spanish-speaking interpreter. A narrative note in Michael's record written preoperatively describes Michael's reaction to the stress of hospitalization and pending surgery.

Preparation for surgery: Report of Nursing Staff Meeting. Michael has expressed fears primarily of "the mask" during anesthesia. He has said that on Friday he will hide so that he cannot be found for surgery. He is afraid "they are going to brain me." He is able to remember the intensive care unit and is afraid to be there. Michael's behavior is that of clinging to adults, and testing limits which staff set for him. He goes to the playroom somewhat reluctantly and plays alone. He knows he will have a bandage over the left side of his face when he awakens. Impression: Michael's intense activity, clinging, and somewhat demanding behavior are confusing. They seem to indicate that he is poorly defended for this experience. His strengths are his ability to become attached to helping adults and to follow directions and participate in games.

Plans are to have Michael visit the intensive care unit before surgery to become acquainted with the staff and with the appearance of the room. He will start an activity with the child life worker which will require that it be continued after the operation. He will "pack" his favorite things to have with him in intensive care, especially books for his mother to read to him. We hope to give him the sense that we expect him to "continue" as before the operation and let him know that we expect him to take responsibility for helping himself when possible.

Michael's operation lasted approximately 6 hours and the major complication was blood loss, requiring transfusions of 23 units of blood. The indications of the adequacy of the blood-clotting mechanisms were followed closely postoperatively. When massive transfusions of stored blood are given, a complex disturbance of homeostasis may ensue, due to the loss of platelets and decreasing activity of labile coagulation factors, such as factor VIII.[106c]

Nursing care in the intensive care unit consisted of careful monitoring of Michael's vital signs and level of consciousness, precise calculation of fluid balance, and maintenance of body temperature in the lower ranges of normal by a cooling mattress.*

The dressing at the site of the excised hemangioma was changed daily using sterile technique and the site of the incision was observed for signs of separation of wound edges or infection. (Techniques of wound care are discussed in Chapter 43.) The wound was drained of accumulated fluid by the insertion of drainage tube attached to a plastic container, compressed to create a vacuum (Hemovac). Michael's mother was encouraged to stay with him for long periods. An interpreter came regularly to the intensive care unit to keep the mother informed of Michael's progress and to explain the treatments to her. The interpreter also spoke to Michael in Spanish and answered his questions. Although Michael spoke English very well before surgery, he was comforted in the postoperative period by hearing and speaking Spanish. This was a normal and temporary return to an earlier stage of development; a means of coping with severe physical or emotional stress helpful to persons of all ages. Figure 8-12 shows the hourly plan of care for Michael as recorded on a nursing care "Kardex." The staff nurse made notes from the plan of care in a form convenient for use while at the bedside (see Fig. 8-13).

The nursing measures used to give Michael comfort and rest were the judicious use of medications by injection to control pain and helping Michael to turn, cough, and take deep breaths to prevent poor aeration of the alveoli of the lung and subsequent collapse of alveoli (atelectasis) and increased susceptibility to infection. The nurse touched Michael with her whole hands and moved them slowly over his body when giving a back rub or bath. This enabled Michael to maintain his orientation to his own body and prevented the anxiety that often results postoperatively from inability to perceive familiar body sensations and the sense that the body is still intact. All procedures happening to Michael were explained quietly and in simple terms. Eye contact with the nurse giving care was encouraged. The nearly constant presence of mother and nurse at the bedside prevented Michael from becoming frightened or disoriented during his stay in the intensive care unit. On the third postoperative day,

Michael returned to his own room. The central venous catheter, the intravenous catheter, and catheter in the bladder were removed prior to the transfer. Michael could void in adequate amounts without difficulty (over 30 ml per hour) and could retain liquid feedings by mouth.

An initial complex problem in Michael's care was nutrition and the experience of putting food in the mouth, tasting, chewing, and swallowing. Since the vessels of the hemangioma extended from the cheek into the mucous membranes inside the mouth, the resection of the mass extended to the mouth. Therefore, the area had to be protected and kept at rest as much as possible. A tube for liquid feedings was passed through the nose and into the stomach, and a formula containing adequate amounts of nutrients was fed to him through the tube every 2 hours. Thus he was denied the sight, smell, and taste of accustomed food and could not experience normal chewing or swallowing. The moisture and tactile sensation of mouth care were especially important in addition to its cleaning action.

Before nursing approaches could be designed to relieve any of these problems of care, Michael suffered a hemorrhage from the operative site. The left common carotid artery had been slowly eroded by the drainage tube, and Michael was close to death in minutes. He returned to the operating room for an emergency ligation of the left common carotid artery to stop the bleeding. This procedure saved his life, but required that the sutures of the wound be removed and that the wound closure occur by slow granulation of tissue. A tracheostomy had to be carried out for breathing. A volume-limited ventilator was required for 3 days postoperatively to maintain adequate respirations.* Within days it was evident that Michael was developing pneumonia. His body temperature rose to 39° to 40°C (102.2° to 104°F). Respirations were 30 to 40 per minute, and secretions suctioned from the tracheostomy were purulent. Breath sounds were diminished in both the right and left lungs, and a radiographic examination of the chest showed infiltrates in both lungs. The white blood count was elevated (18,000 cubic mm), and *Staphylococcus aureus* was cultured from the blood. *Klebsiella* was also cultured from the urine. Michael then had to undergo a prolonged course of treatment with intravenous antibiotics and was kept in a private room for 4 weeks, where adequate isolation technique could be carried out. (See Chapter 44 for discussion of infection control.) Chest physiotherapy, including intermittent positive pressure breathing, chest percussion, and postural drainage, was instituted every 4 hours to maintain adequate ventilation and promote expectoration of secretions from the trachea and bronchi. Feeding by nasogastric tube was continued for the next 3 weeks, and Michael was confined to bed. This determined the manner in which his needs for personal hygiene and elim-

---

* See Chapters 6 and 42 for a complete explanation of the temperature-regulating mechanism of the body and the rationale for and means of lowering body temperature.

* The indications for and maintenance of the tracheostomy and volume-limited ventilator are discussed in Chapter 20.

DATE (MO., DY., YR.)	LOCATION	SERVICE		

10 yrs.

AGE   **DOCTOR** *Roberts*   IF NO PLATE, PRINT NAME, SEX, AND HISTORY NO.

DATE & TIME	NURSING PROGRESS RECORD (SIGN ALL ENTRIES WITH NAME AND TITLE)	DATE & TIME	NURSING PROGRESS RECORD (SIGN ALL ENTRIES WITH NAME AND TITLE)
	ADMISSION NOTE		VALUABLES BROUGHT TO UNIT/DISPOSITION
	TIME: *1 pm* DATE:		*None*
	METHOD OF ADMISSION: (walking) wheelchair stretcher, other		ASSISTIVE DEVICES: (none) dentures eyeglasses; contact lens, hearing
	ACCOMPANIED BY: (specify relationship) *Mother*		aid, other.
	IDENTIBAND PRESENT: (yes) no		
	PATIENT'S STATED REASON FOR ADMISSION: *Mother states "tumor" is to be removed surgically.*		CUSTOMARY DIET: *Regular*
			BOWEL HABITS: *Normal for age.*
	PATIENT'S MAJOR PROBLEM: *Cavernous hemangioma left face*		BLADDER FUNCTION: *Normal for age*
			SLEEPING PATTERN: *10-12 hours per night, no naps.*
	PRIOR HOSPITALIZATIONS/REASONS *11 previous surgical procedures in an attempt to remove hemangioma. Continues to grow.*		SOCIAL HISTORY: Family Unit: *Mother and Michael* Dwelling: *Apartment, adeq. heat* Occupation: *Unemployed* Language: *Spanish-English*
	OTHER ILLNESSES *None*		Other: *Father unknown, 2. brothers died in fire.* IDENTIFY LIMITATIONS: (mental, sensory motor, communication) *None*
	ALLERGIES: *None*		
	MEDICATIONS: Regularly taken: *None*		T *98⁶* P *94* R *22* HGT. *54in.* WT. *68 lbs.*
			DOCTOR NOTIFIED: *Dr. Roberts*
	Taken today: *None*		Name Time: *2pm*
	Brought to hospital/disposition of *None*		Title

(8-75)

43458   THE NEW YORK HOSPITAL   SIGN ALL ENTRIES WITH NAME AND TITLE   (OVER)

Figure 8-10. The nursing assessment provides information on which to base the patient's plan of care. (Courtesy of Nursing Service, Cornell University–New York Hospital, New York, N.Y.)

ination were met. He presented several complex physical and emotional problems of care.

All of his activities of daily living had to be carried out for him. These included bathing, dressing, feeding, elimination, and exercise. Ways were sought in which he could assist, give directions, and help plan the timing of these care activities, in order to move him to an appropriate level of independence for a 10-year-old child as his condition improved.

Adequate dosage of antibiotics to overcome the infection could be maintained only by intravenous

DATE & TIME	NURSING PROGRESS RECORD (SIGN ALL ENTRIES WITH NAME AND TITLE)	DATE & TIME	NURSING PROGRESS RECORD (SIGN ALL ENTRIES WITH NAME AND TITLE)
	NURSING ASSESSMENT		
	10 yr. old boy, born in United States of Mexican-American parents, with nontender purplish mass over left face, extending from angle of jaw to midline of face, including part of lips, extending to just below eye.		
	Speaks English well. Mother speaks limited English. Attends ___ school, fourth grade, says he likes school.		
	Constant activity during interview, inability to recall events of previous hospitalizations, indicate that he uses denial predominately to defend himself for this experience. Willingness to play, approach other children indicate capacity to form a relationship with other adults and children. This could be developed to aid in pre-operative preparation. Plan to use drawings as means of preparation and visit to intensive care unit.		
	Mother will require an interpreter for instruction and informed consent for surgery.		
	_____ R.N.		

SIGN ALL ENTRIES WITH NAME AND TITLE

Figure 8-10. (continued)

route. Therefore, intravenous therapy was initiated and continuously monitored for the hazards and complications subsequent to having a needle placed in a vein: such as trauma, pain, infiltration of the medication into the subcutaneous tissues, and blockage of the needle.

Exposure of the wound with complete breakdown of the suture line required a treatment regimen to prevent infection and to promote granulation of tissue in preparation for skin grafting. Sterile normal saline soaks were maintained on the wound and changed every 2 hours through-

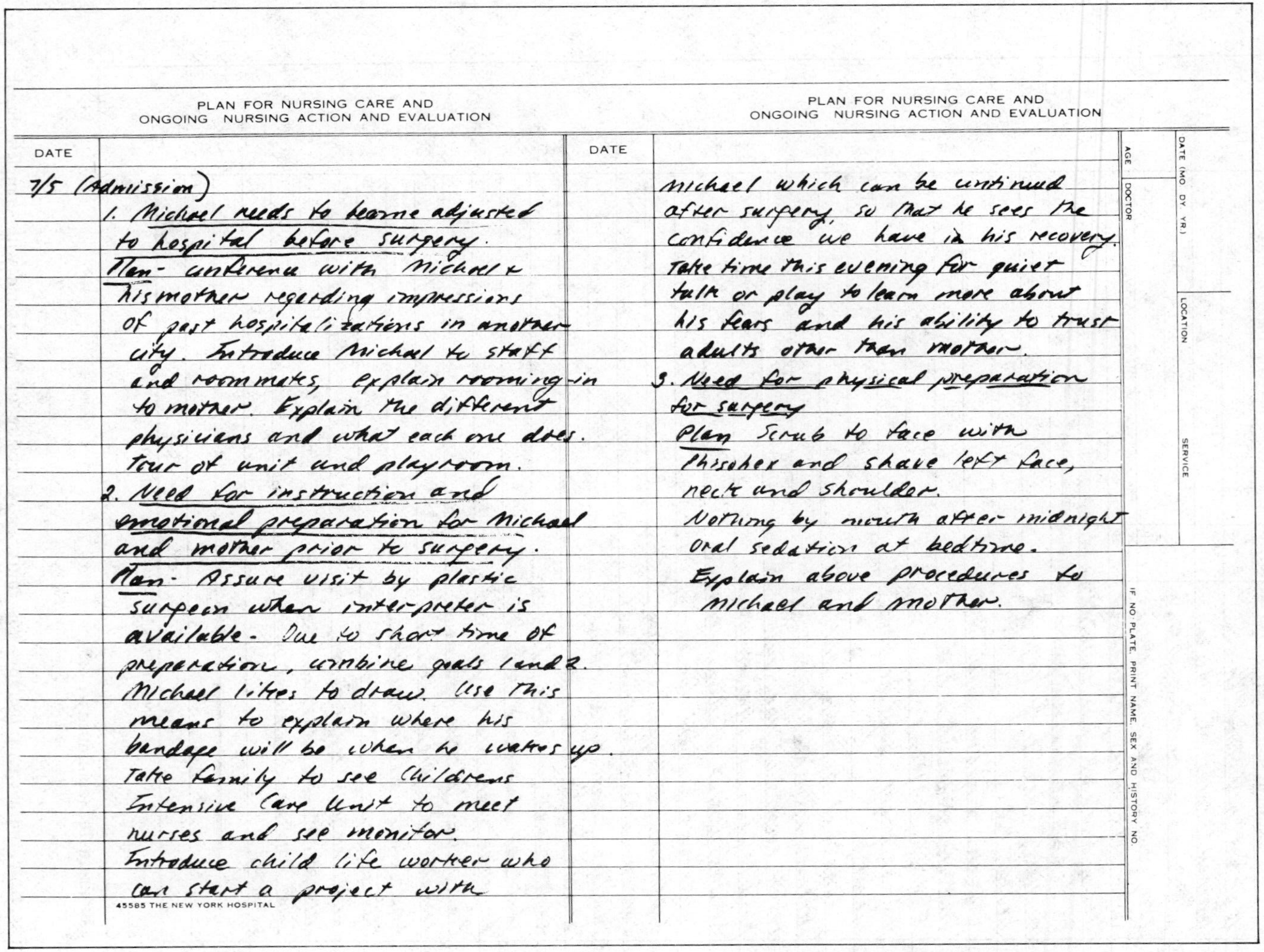

PLAN FOR NURSING CARE AND ONGOING NURSING ACTION AND EVALUATION

DATE	PLAN FOR NURSING CARE AND ONGOING NURSING ACTION AND EVALUATION	DATE	PLAN FOR NURSING CARE AND ONGOING NURSING ACTION AND EVALUATION
7/5	(Admission)		Michael which can be continued
	1. Michael needs to become adjusted		after surgery, so that he sees the
	to hospital before surgery.		confidence we have in his recovery.
	Plan- conference with Michael &		Take time this evening for quiet
	his mother regarding impressions		talk or play to learn more about
	of past hospitalizations in another		his fears and his ability to trust
	city. Introduce Michael to staff		adults other than mother.
	and roommates, explain rooming-in		3. Need for physical preparation
	to mother. Explain the different		for surgery
	physicians and what each one does.		Plan Scrub to face with
	Tour of unit and playroom.		Phisohex and shave left face,
	2. Need for instruction and		neck and shoulder.
	emotional preparation for Michael		Nothing by mouth after midnight
	and mother prior to surgery.		Oral sedation at bedtime.
	Plan- Assure visit by plastic		Explain above procedures to
	surgeon when interpreter is		Michael and mother.
	available. Due to short time of		
	preparation, combine goals 1 and 2.		
	Michael likes to draw. Use this		
	means to explain where his		
	bandage will be when he wakes up.		
	Take family to see Childrens		
	Intensive Care Unit to meet		
	nurses and see monitor.		
	Introduce child life worker who		
	can start a project with		

AGE | DOCTOR | DATE (MO. DY. YR.) | LOCATION | SERVICE

IF NO PLATE, PRINT NAME, SEX AND HISTORY NO.

45585 THE NEW YORK HOSPITAL

Figure 8-11. A plan for nursing care is usually designed without restrictive headings in order to allow development for a wide range of patients. A common method of writing the plan is to state the problems, goals, nursing action, including teaching, and evaluation and future planning. (Courtesy of Nursing Service, Cornell University–New York Hospital, New York, N.Y.)

out the day. Creative methods of supporting a bulky wet dressing at the side of the face were devised for protection of the wound and comfort for Michael.

Maintaining adequate respiration required meticulous care of the airway. The dangers of trauma and infection with a tracheostomy are well known and sterile technique must be used in suctioning secretions from the tracheostomy. Constant observation is required to prevent blockage of the airway, inspissated secretions, and trauma to the mucous membranes of the trachea. Radiography of the chest is used to confirm the correct placement of the tube in the trachea above the bifurcation of the right and left main bronchi and is also used to monitor the effect of chest physiotherapy and antibiotics on the course of the pneumonia.

Nutrition and fluid balance were first completely maintained by intravenous feeding. Tube feedings of a nutritionally balanced formula were instituted by the fifth day post ligation of the left carotid artery. Michael progressed to oral fluids by the end of the third postoperative week. Careful records were kept to assure adequate intake and output of fluids, and Michael was weighed on the bed scale once a week. Blood was drawn periodically to monitor the electrolyte concentration, another measure of the adequacy of hydration.

The maintenance of isolation for protection of other patients and staff from *Staphylococcus aureus* and *Klebsiella* must be planned with the needs of the child for his mother and other comforting adults, for play and for social stimulation provided by television, radio, and phonograph. The child life workers were responsible for providing toys and crafts for both recreation and learning. Since this hospitalization occurred in the summer, the school program was not in session. Simple procedures for the staff to follow in moving in and out of the room are described in Chapters 15 and 44, as is the cleaning of the equipment used in isolation.

Michael could not communicate verbally for 3 weeks. The meaning of being unable to communicate verbally is discussed in Chapter 46. Aids used to communicate were pointing, shaking the head, or moving other parts of the body. When he was particularly distressed and knew that his request was not clear to others, he would kick his feet against the bed in anger. A "magic slate" was used for writing messages when one of his hands was free from an intravenous line. Sharing a game with him or a drawing project brought his nurse closer both physically and emotionally. Touch, smiling, and crying all helped in maintaining his orientation to his environment, human contact, and a sense of caring and love throughout a markedly stressful period.

Growth and development do not stop when a child is hospitalized. The environment of the pediatric unit and the interaction among health workers, child, and parent should reflect understanding of the child's emotional and intellectual level of development. Michael was 10 years old.

He was inquisitive and enjoyed a challenge, such as solving a puzzle or following the directions of a new game or craft project. He was more at ease with adults and would initiate projects he and a nurse or child life worker could do together. He did not initiate conversation or games with children his own age as often as he did with adults while in the hospital. This may be because he had to be isolated most of his hospitalization from the other children. In subsequent hospitalizations he showed increasing interest in participating in group play and the school program. A plan of care was written following a nursing conference which was held as Michael was recovering from his second surgical procedure. It reflects the nursing staff's understanding of developmental needs of school-age children in general and of Michael's special needs for some control and mastery over his situation and an opportunity to express his feelings when he could not put these feelings into words.

Have him help with self care, dressing changes and IPPB * treatments.

Give choices when possible, i.e., where to sit, holding mask himself. Give information regarding medical plan of care, course of healing, why he coughs, has fever, needs medication, what is happening to the incision.

Anticipate what he wants and bring it to him without his having to use crying to keep someone with him. Ignore crying and kicking at time of IPPB treatment, carry it out promptly.

Anger seems to be Michael's primary feeling. When he kicks and cries say to him "You're angry," to convey it's an acceptable feeling that you recognize. Promote the expression of anger in play.

A child of 10 years of age will be dependent on his or her parents, but the quality of the dependency is quite different when compared, for example, to that of the 2-year-old child. School-age children will enjoy being with children their own age, and playing both cooperatively and competitively within the group. The parent is expected to help the child toward independence by encouraging his or her participation in activities outside the home. At the same time the parent is available "to come home to" for the periods of warmth and closeness reminiscent of an earlier age period. Michael was able to trust adults other than mother. He understood when his mother would be staying with him and when she would be away from the hospital. Michael could play games with the nurses happily if his mother was not there. At times of severe stress, his mother stayed continually in the hospital and helped to give care. At those times, Michael watched constantly for her presence as would a much younger child. Both the mother and the other helping adults accepted this behavior, and by this acceptance Michael was better able to move from

* Intermittent positive pressure breathing (see Chapter 20).

PLAN OF NURSING CARE

Name _Gonzales, Michael_ Division _Pediatrics_ History Number _629731_

Hour	Date Treatments and Nursing Care	Notes to Assist in Giving Care
AM 7:00	Offer urinal, measure and record output. Temp, pulse, respiration, blood pressure. Total intake and output	Record response to treatment and behavior last 8 hours. Tell Michael who his nurse will be
7:30	Report to on-coming nurse Check IV - Naso-gastric tube feeding.	during day.
8:00	Temp, pulse, respiration, blood pressure. Bath, mouth care, range of motion exercises.	Let him help with hygiene. Remember suture line in left mucus membrane of mouth.
8:30	IPPB, deep breathing, cough, postural	Likes to hold mask for IPPB.
9:00	drainage, percussion, check IV. Temp, pulse, respiration, blood pressure	May move to all positions for postural drainage.
9:30	Naso Gastric Tube feeding, check IV	
10:00	Temp, pulse, respiration, blood pressure	Involve mother in Michael's care when possible. Talk to both about reasons for treatments.
10:30	Dressing change if damp. Temp, pulse, respiration, blood pressure Check IV	
11:00	Offer urinal	
11:30	Oxacillin Gm I I.V. Naso Gastric tube feeding	Dilute in 30cc fluid, slow drip. Check IV after medication
12:00 PM	Temp, pulse, respiration, blood pressure	completed.
12:30		
1:00	Temp, pulse, respiration, blood pressure. Check IV	Provide for quiet in room for nap.
1:30		
2:00	Naso Gastric Tube feeding. Check IV Temp, pulse, respiration, blood pressure	If not coughing productively,
2:30	IPPB, deep breathing, cough, postural drainage, percussion	stimulate by placing suction catheter at glottis.
3:00	Temp, pulse, respiration, blood pressure Check IV	
3:30	Dressing change if damp. Total intake and output for 8 hours	Record response to treatment and behavior last 8 hours.
4:00	Naso Gastric tube feeding. Check IV Temp, pulse, respiration, blood pressure	
4:30	Report to on-coming nurse	Tell Michael who his nurse will be during evening.
5:00	Temp, pulse, respiration, blood pressure. Check IV	Interpreter will visit. Notify
5:30	IPPB, deep breathe, cough, postural drainage, percussion.	Dr. Roberts
6:00	Naso Gastric tube feeding Temp, pulse, respiration, blood pressure.	
6:30	Oxacillin Gm I IV	Dilute in 30cc fluid, slow drip Check IV after medication completed.

Figure 8-12. An hourly plan of nursing care is often written by a nurse to use while with a patient. These plans vary with the needs of the patient, the nurse's experience, and the accessibility of the Kardex or patient record to the nurse giving care.

complete dependency on his mother's presence to more independent ways of behaving such as sleeping comfortably without her at night and leaving mother to go to the playroom.

In teaching Michael about his care, the staff took advantage of his ability to reason, to make generalizations, and to understand the concept of time. Michael, like other 10-year-old children, was curious, familiar with the names of parts of the body, and interested in pictures, teaching dolls,

Hour	Date	Treatments and Nursing Care	Notes to Assist in Giving Care
PM 7:00		Temp, pulse, respiration, blood pressure. Mouth care. Check I.V.	Remember suture line left mucus membrane of mouth.
7:30		Range of motion exercises	
8:00		Naso Gastric tube feeding. Temp, pulse, respiration, blood pressure check IV	Promote enjoyment of touch and bodily movement.
8:30		Dressing change if damp.	Ask Michael and Mother about how they think things
9:00		Temp, pulse, respiration and blood pressure. Check I.V.	are going for them. Learn their perceptions of care.
*9:30		IPPB, Deep breathing, cough, postural drainage, percussion.	
10:00		Temp, pulse, respiration, blood pressure. Check I.V.	Likes back rub.
10:30		Naso-Gastric tube feeding. Offer urinal. Prepare for sleep.	Mother staying over night.
**11:00		Temp, pulse, respiration, blood pressure. Check I.V.	
11:30		Total Intake and output. Report to on coming nurse.	Record child's response to treatment and behavior past 8 hours.
12:00 AM		Oxacillin Gm I I.V. Naso-gastric tube feeding	Dilute in 30cc IV fluid. Slow drip. Check IV after medication completed.
12:30		Check IV	
1:00		Observe condition of dressing.	
1:30			
2:00		Pulse, respiration Check I.V. Naso gastric tube feeding.	Observe pattern of sleep. Observe position for comfort.
2:30			
3:00		Check I.V.	Talk to Michael if he awakens.
3:30			
4:00		Pulse, respiration Check I.V. Naso gastric tube feeding.	
4:30			
5:00		Check I.V.	
5:30		IPPB, Deep breathing, cough, postural drainage, percussion.	
6:00		Temp, pulse respiration, blood pressure Oxacillin Gm I I.V. Naso-gastric tube feeding	Dilute in 30cc IV fluid, slow drip. Check IV after medication completed.
6:30		Dressing change if damp.	

*IPPB and postural drainage treatments during night are dependent on the chest X-Ray and type of secretions in the past 24 hours. Treatments are deferred between 12 midnight and 6am if pneumonia clearing.

**Temperature and blood pressure are deferred to promote sleep, if vital signs are stable in previous 8 hours and other observations do not indicate a change in vital signs.

Figure 8-12. (continued)

and other visual aids which are used in preoperative instruction. The effect of the instruction was clearly demonstrated on one occasion when Michael was recuperating. He carefully arranged a bed and bedside table in the playroom into a hospital unit and supplied it with articles commonly found in the hospital. Then he took persons to see "his room" and explain all its features.

His mother was encouraged to work with the nurses throughout Michael's hospitalization. She watched the care of the wound from the beginning and was able to change the dressing and clean the area of granulation tissue without help by the time Michael was ready to return home.

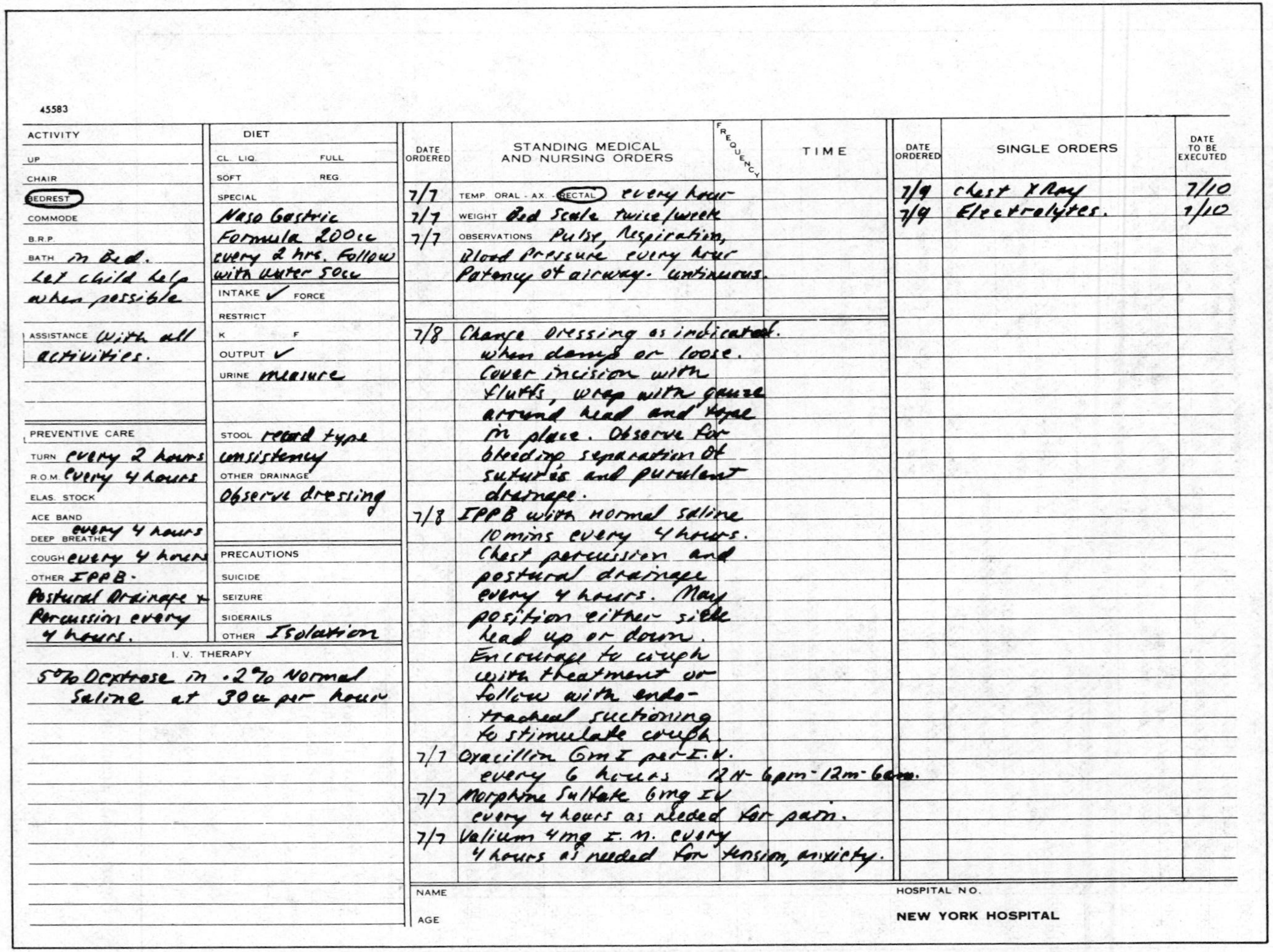

45583

HOSPITAL NO.

Figure 8-13. Medical and nursing directives for patient care are transcribed on a worksheet, which may be discarded after final use. (Courtesy of Nursing Service, Cornell University–New York Hospital, New York, N.Y.)

Two months following the surgery to remove the hemangioma, the following notes were made on Michael's condition:

This 10-year-old Mexican-American male is an unfortunate youngster plagued by a massively invasive cavernous hemangioma of the left cheek and face. He has undergone ablative and excisional surgeries in _____ (city) and most recently at _____ (this hospital) on _____ (date). Massive excisional surgery was on _____ (date), subsequently developed *Klebsiella* in urine, *Staphylococcus aureus* septicemia and pneumonia postoperatively. He also had postoperative problems secondary to treatment with 23 units of blood during surgery. Tracheostomy and volume-limited respirator were also used postoperatively, after the patient underwent emergency ligation of his left common carotid artery, secondary to its rupture and a massive bleed. Neurologic deficit almost miraculously has not been noted subsequently.

In the past month the following progress has been made by the patient. Nasogastric tube feedings with Sustagen * have progressed to a regular diet by mouth. The orocutaneous fistula through the left lower cheek is slowly closing and healing well. Staphylococcal pneumonia changes on chest x-ray are slowly clearing. The patient is now able to speak again; his tracheostomy is closed. The progress of this patient from isolation with nasogastric feeding and intravenous fluids to the present state of free oral intake and ambulation on the unit is truly remarkable.

Plan: 1. Check culture of orocutaneous fistula site.
2. Recheck x-ray for progressive clearing.
3. Talk with Mrs. Gonzales via an interpreter. She is especially concerned to know the time of future procedures for correction of Michael's left face and lip with secondary closure of the orocutaneous fistula.
4. Visiting nurse referral for daily dressing change in the home (see Fig. 8-14).
5. Possibility of home teacher. This should be looked into with Miss _____ (teacher for children's in-patient unit).
6. A great deal of compassion for this family, once numbering five and now only two. This little boy has undergone a lot of medical treatment and is still not at the end of his therapeutic course.

Two days later, Michael returned home. His first return appointment to the clinic was 1 week later. As is evident from the above progress note, several plans were made to assure that Michael and his mother were ready for the responsibilities of going home and for resuming normal activities, such as attending school (see Fig. 8-14). These

* Complete therapeutic nutriment. Provides a complete diet or extranutritional support. Mead Johnson Laboratories.

goals were not immediately realized, and there was a major role to be played in discharge planning and home care by the nurse in the clinic, who saw Michael weekly for 1 month, then monthly for 6 months. At the first return visit, this note was written by the nurse:

Nursing problems and plans:
1. VNA has not been visiting regularly or helping mother as planned. New referral written and telephone call to be made to Mrs. _____ (visiting nurse) for specific instructions on wound care.
2. Not going to school and wants to go. States he is not worried about the other children seeing his dressing. School nurse will be called to explain Michael's needs in school and that he can attend school.
3. Form completed for welfare so that family can be adequately supplied with dressings. The clinic will supply these until the Department of Welfare will approve the cost of dressings.
4. Michael's attitude and behavior at home: Has been eating soft food, gained 2 lb in one week. Is helping mother at home. Has seen his wound in the mirror and thinks this procedure has made him uglier; before he felt he looked all right. Positive aspects are his drawings, which reflect his interest in personal appearance and show his home as a cozy place with family. He talks readily about himself, is interested in helping with his dressing, explains what he needs, and keeps up his personal appearance with the help of his mother.
5. Will follow and will see Michael at each clinic visit to give him the opportunity to talk about his feelings, his treatment, and adjustment to school and peers. The medium of drawing is very helpful in getting a conversation started with Michael. It is of interest to see his willingness to draw pictures of his home and the hospital, whereas in the hospital he never drew anything that was affecting him personally.

The visiting nurse responded to the request for more information about their program of home care. Their letter also clarified the unfortunate misinterpretation by the school authorities of Michael's condition and their need for more complete information.

_____ (visiting nurse) visits the Gonzales family two times a week. Mrs. Gonzales manages Michael's care well and has a good understanding regarding the child's dietary needs.
1. The greatest problem is in the obtaining of dressings, because the Welfare Department has not approved the request as yet.
2. Transportation to _____ (hospital) is difficult and may be cause for Michael to miss appointments.
3. The school nurse has refused Michael's readmission to school. Fears that an infection might ensue. In the meantime, the child is being tutored on a home basis. It is a feeling of the agency, however, that Michael

| DATE (MO., DY., YR.) | LOCATION | SERVICE | |
| AGE | DOCTOR | | IF NO PLATE, PRINT NAME, SEX, AND HISTORY NO. |

1. What does the patient/family understand about the —

a. Medical diagnoses? *Consider hemangioma to be a "tumor." Understand that chance of regrowth slight due to radical excision.*

b. Prognosis? *Know that Michael will have more hospitalizations for skin grafting.*

c. Resumption of physical activities? *Know that full activity can be resumed, including school.*

d. Needs for continuing health care? *Know that frequent visits to clinic will be required.*

2. Significant emotional, social and family factors:
   (e.g. living arrangements, economics, transportation considerations, etc.)

Housing adequate, lives near relatives who can help with transportation. Income provided by welfare.

3. Profile of Activities	NEEDS NO HELP	NEEDS HELP	Identify Difficulties & Required Assistance
a. Mobility	☑	☐	*Progress to all foods as chewing and*
b. Eating	☐	☑	*swallowing improve. Voice is hoarse,*
c. Communication	☐	☑	*need to be patient listening to him.*
d. Hygiene	☐	☑	*Mother will help with teeth brushing.*
e. Sleeping	☑	☐	
f. Elimination	☑	☐	
g. Vision	☑	☐	

4. Equipment/Supplies Provided: *Gauze for face dressing. Silver Nitrate applicators; apply twice a day to promote granulation of wound.*

To be obtained:

5. MEDICATIONS to be taken at home	DOSE	FREQ. & MODE	Indicate what patient/family **understands** about Desired Action; **important** Side Effects and Contraindications.
None			

REV. 2-74
43465

6. Name of person(s) instructed about drugs:................................ Relationship:................................

THE NEW YORK HOSPITAL   **NURSING PROGRESS AND DISCHARGE SUMMARY**   (over)

Figure 8-14. The nursing discharge or transfer summary provides a tool for concise communication among nurses in many care settings. The summary includes current care information, reference to past planning and results, and predictive ideas which may influence future care. (Courtesy of Nursing Service, Cornell University–New York Hospital, New York, N.Y.)

7. PATIENT/FAMILY EDUCATION   Indicate name(s) of person(s) instructed:

Subjects taught	TAUGHT BY NAME, DEPT.	METHOD	OUTCOMES OF TEACHING (Include evidence of learning)
Wound Care Dressing Change every four hours except at night, dependent on drainage. As this lessens, change only as necessary. Place dry fluffs in wound and wrap gauze around head to hold in place.	R.N. Nursing	Demonstration - Return Demonstration	Mother changes dressing daily in hospital. Stays in place and is comfortable for patient for several hours.

8. Recommendations for additional teaching: Check if Michael is being advanced to regular diet.

9. REFERRALS: List specific clinic names, revisit dates, other appropriate names.

		Private Physician	☐
Home Care	☐		
Visiting Nurse	☑ Ms. ___ PHN, Town of ___	Clinics	☑ Dr. ___ Plastic, Date ___
Social Worker	☐	Other	☐

NURSING SUMMARY OF PATIENT'S PROGRESS

10 yr. old Mexican-American boy who underwent surgical excision of cavernous hemangioma, left face, followed by difficult post-operative recovery. Now mother performs wound care well. Child needs to begin to see himself as recovering and able to return to school. Becomes discouraged easily but is able to do everything for self, except care for wound. Voice is hoarse from tracheostomy. Be patient when he is trying to speak. Prepare regular diet in small amounts. May need frequent meals and liquids. As fistula closes, eating will become easier. A visiting nurse will follow in home and support mother. Dressing materials and silver nitrate sticks, used to promote granulation of tissue will be supplied to family through the clinic until Welfare approves purchase through local surgical supply store.

NURSE'S SIGNATURE: DATE:

Figure 8-14. (continued)

return to school as quickly as possible in order to make the peer contact which he needs.

signed,

＿＿＿, R.N.

The problem of transportation to the clinic was quickly resolved through help of social service, which arranged for a volunteer driver from the Red Cross to bring Michael and his mother to clinic. On occasion a family relative also drove the family to the clinic, and Michael never missed an appointment in 6 months. The problem of attendance at school was solved by the following letter written to the school nurse by the physician and nurse. Rather than waiting for mail delivery, the letter was taken directly to the school nurse and personally delivered by the Red Cross volunteer who drove Michael and his mother to clinic. The volunteer requested to do this, and her personal interest probably shortened the time that Michael was out of school by at least a week.

Dear ＿＿＿

This letter is written to explain the medical care of Michael Gonzales and to aid in helping him return to school and to the company of other children his age.

Michael was hospitalized at ＿＿＿ (hospital) from July 5 to September 12 for plastic surgical repair of a cavernous hemangioma of the left face. The incision is healing well. Other surgical procedures will be done in the coming years to improve the appearance of his face, but it was not necessary to prolong this hospitalization at this time for surgical procedures. It was our wish to have Michael at home and to learn to see for himself as a well child who can do the same things as other children his age. His dressing changes are minor procedures which his mother can do with ease. He has a slight difficulty in chewing which is continually improving. His mother will change his dressings at noontime at school and bring him the kind of food he can easily eat.

The mother and Michael are happy to have the home teacher, but Michael wants very much to return to the company of other children. The mother finds it difficult to motivate him to study at home, and thinks the competition of the other children will help this.

In summary, there is no medical reason why Michael cannot be in school. It is unlikely that he will become infected nor is he infectious to anyone else. The school will need a little patience as Michael's swallowing becomes easier and his voice becomes more distinct. This will happen. There has been major improvement since his discharge. The mother has the time and is willing to help in any way while Michael is at school. We sincerely hope you will give him the opportunity to demonstrate his ability to adjust to his problem and to grow up as normally as possible.

Sincerely,

＿＿＿＿, M.D.

＿＿＿＿, R.N.

After readmission to school, Michael's mother went daily to change the dressings as the school nurse was not able to spend the entire day at Michael's school. Thus she could not take responsibility for helping Michael with his dressing. In approximately 2 months, new granulation tissue completely closed the orocutaneous fistula and the dressing was changed only in the morning before Michael left for school. After about 3 months Michael slept without his dressing, which promoted further healing. He kept the dressing over his wound until it was permanently closed by a pedicle skin graft, which was accomplished by surgical procedure 6 months following the excision of the hemangioma.

His subsequent hospital admissions were not easy, but the relationships which were established at the initial hospitalization, the assessment of the family's needs, and the plans for care sustained Michael, his mother, and the professional staff through the difficult periods that occur when skin grafting is taking place.

Data-Processing and Plans of Care. The use of data-processing equipment requires that nurses consistently use a systematic approach to gathering and reporting information about patients, identifying their needs and problems, defining health goals, and listing appropriate nursing action. A computer is a tool that "facilitates" nursing care rather than one that "determines" nursing care. Current uses of the computer include taking over many time-consuming activities of the nurse such as delivering messages and requests for service to various hospital departments; printing laboratory findings directly on the patient's chart; recording and processing the physician's "orders" without the necessity of writing requisitions for the services of other departments; storing significant clinical information about the patient; and many clerical tasks of preparing work sheets and census lists that are necessary for the on-going activities of a hospital. [107-108b] For an example of a computerized patient record, see Chapter 4.

Computers have the potential capability of describing necessary nursing action for a given patient at a given time; however, this requires that nurses develop a program that takes into account many of the factors about the patient that are described earlier in this chapter, as well as the nursing action appropriate to each factor. For example, work is in progress at the Texas Institute of Rehabilitation and Research to develop computer programs for each of the aspects of daily living.* In the case of the one activity of "positioning," 16 different ob-

---

* Personal communication to first author from S. A. Cornell, Coordinator, Nursing Research and Education, Texas Institute of Rehabilitation and Research, Houston.

jectives have already been described, each of these has a set of appropriate nursing actions, each nursing action has a set of factors that can modify the nursing action, and each objective has an evaluation check.

4. REHABILITATING THE SICK AND DISABLED

Rehabilitation as an Essential Aspect of All Health Care. Helping a person regain independence or become rehabilitated during and after his hospitalization is considered by the authors to be an integral part of nursing care, although the most effective rehabilitation may involve the coordinated help of physicians, nurses, physical therapists, social workers, occupational counselors, and others. The point was made earlier that comprehensive care that restores *each* individual to his or her optimum physical, mental, social, vocational, and economic usefulness should be available to everyone. When Ambrose Paré operated on a French nobleman in the sixteenth century he sometimes stayed with him until the patient could resume his normal life. Paré provided medical attention, nursing care, occupation, and entertainment in various forms. Although he didn't use this term he was *rehabilitating* his patient. It seems strange that an idea, demonstrated throughout the ages by great practitioners, should be considered new. As far as we know, however, the modern concept of rehabilitation has only recently been clearly stated and generally accepted.

About rehabilitation there are two prevailing viewpoints: the first, that it is the restoration of *certain categories* of handicapped persons to their optimum physical, mental, social, vocational, and economic usefulness; the second, that this restorative process is a part of the comprehensive care which should be available to everyone.

We believe the first persons in this country to make the concept of rehabilitation crystal-clear were Mary E. Brown, George G. Deaver, and John N. Smith, Jr. They accomplished this by developing a record for an adult, based on one designed for child care by Marjorie P. Shelton, that listed the essential daily activities of an independent person.[109] Using this as a guide, they evaluated the degree of disability of those who applied to the Institute for the Crippled and Disabled in New York City, which has been in operation since 1917 when it was organized as a vocational training center. Observing individuals in such functions as walking, getting in and out of a chair, eating a meal, or dressing themselves, they discovered which of the daily activities they could perform unaided, those with which they needed assistance, and those which were beyond them. The program from then on was designed to develop independence. The person might have had sufficient motor power and coordination, but might lack confidence. Assessment included the latter as it did the client's insight into his or her condition. As its name implies, this institute was devoted to the rehabilitation of those with neuromotor disabilities. The activity record, therefore, stresses motor function, but it includes the essential daily activities, and, in a modified form, the record can be used for anyone: the person who has a loss of vision, a colostomy, or a metabolic disorder. At first glance it may not seem to apply to the psychotic patient whose major problem is a breakdown in human relationships; however, on the psychiatric service, as on the orthopedic, the person who independently performs the daily activities listed on this record is rehabilitated. In other words the mentally ill demonstrate emotional stability through physical acts.

To plan care that takes into account both the present and future health condition of the patient is difficult, and it is essential that the nurse be a member of a team composed of the kinds of professional workers described on pages 573–76. The nurse's role in rehabilitation varies greatly according to the number of specialists available in the situation. She or he may have to substitute for a variety of therapists, or, when they are not present, the nurse helps the patient continue the program that therapists have instigated. Too often a program of rehabilitation taught in a special unit fails because it is not understood by those persons with whom patients spend most of their time. In private duty nursing, in homes, in doctors' offices, in industrial nursing, and in some visiting nurse agencies, the nurse is the only person at all prepared to work with doctors in their efforts at rehabilitation. This will continue to be so until there are sufficient physical, occupational, recreational, and speech therapists, psychiatric social workers, clinical psychologists, teachers of the blind, and so on to staff health services.

The term "rehabilitation" came into use following World War I when it replaced such terms as "physical reconstruction" and "reclaiming the cripple." World War II, the Korean and Vietnam hostilities, industrial accidents, increasing numbers of injuries from automobile accidents, and the saving of infants with severe congenital handicaps have expanded the requirement for special measures and encouraged the application of new technologies in rehabilitation. Unfortunately, this has reinforced the notion that it is a "third stage" in the healing process that calls only on the skills of a certain kind of health worker who begins treatment after other therapy is completed.

Recently, social scientists, public health officials, and others concerned about gaps and inadequacies in health care for people in the United States have suggested that illness be defined as the disruption of an individual's ability to carry out effectively his social roles and tasks rather than a disease process.[110,111a] This definition seems to be particularly helpful to the rehabilitative point of view proposed in this text. If nurses consistently approach all patients with the thought that hospitalization is only a portion of their lives, that they come with past experiences and responsibilities for family and community, which will continue when they leave the hospital, then they will plan their programs of care with more comprehensiveness and continuity than if they unconsciously assume their lives begin and end with hospitalization.

Rehabilitation as the Last Phase of Care. Some health workers look upon rehabilitation as "the third phase of treatment," considering it a process to be carried out for selected patients in a special service, or rehabilitation center. Others believe that it is inherent in good health care, that it should be practiced by every health worker in every situation, and that every patient should be rehabilitated to the extent demanded by his condition. In other words, the disabling effects of illness should be assessed with each patient and his or her program of therapy designed to minimize, and eliminate when possible, every crippling effect, early or late, mild or severe, physical or emotional. This means that throughout the time the patient, or client, is under treatment, consideration is given to the part he or she should play in every therapeutic and hygienic activity. The patient should never be a passive recipient of care when he or she would ultimately benefit by participating in, or even assuming responsibility for, the activity.

When rehabilitation is looked upon as a separate program to be carried out by experts after ordinary health personnel have done what they could for the patient, it too often happens that the work of these experts is doubled or tripled and the patient has to be brought to independence by slow stages of unlearning a dependence that need never have developed. Every patient could be so nursed and so treated by physicians and special therapists that he or she would be able on discharge to carry out all of the daily activities that give us what we call independence, or as many as are consistent with an irreversible disability, if there is one.

Figure 8-15 is a list of daily activities that embody our concept of independence. Anyone who can do all of these things unaided is physically "rehabilitated." It is apparent that the independence of a patient undergoing an appendectomy is threatened for only a few hours or days, whereas that of the person who is blinded or paralyzed in all extremities is permanently curtailed. In between these two extremes lie all those with moderate to severe handicaps of short or long duration.

Rehabilitation Units in Hospitals. Special units have been established in hospitals to help persons with physical disabilities that keep them from moving freely in their environments; they admit both inpatients and outpatients, in some cases. Furnishings and their arrangement is such that independence of the individual is facilitated. A detailed description of these is given in the following section, but the furnishings will vary from institution to institution depending on its commitment to this type of service and its economic status.

The basic health team usually includes the doctor, nurse, patient, and family. Frequently physical and occupational therapists are a part of the team and in some units a psychologist and social worker are included. The role and function of all members of the health team in rehabilitation are discussed in the following section as well as various types of programs that are part of an increasing number of rehabilitation units in hospitals in the United States.

Rehabilitation Centers (Independent or "Free Standing"). Rehabilitation has, in the sense of a "third stage" of treatment, become a specialty and as such focuses on disabilities that keep individuals from moving freely in their environments; on social-emotional or mental disabilities that interfere with constructive human relations; and on defective sight, speech, and hearing. Special rehabilitation centers have been established to help clients with these problems, and while many of the centers are independent agencies others are a part of the hospital and serve both inpatients and outpatients. Such centers may be organized to give 24-hour service to patients or function as day centers only.

The design and furnishings of rehabilitation units are usually different from those of most traditional hospital divisions. However, some hospitals are trying to do some of the following things. Efforts are made to dispel the "sickroom" atmosphere. Sleeping rooms are sometimes furnished to look like sitting rooms. Day-

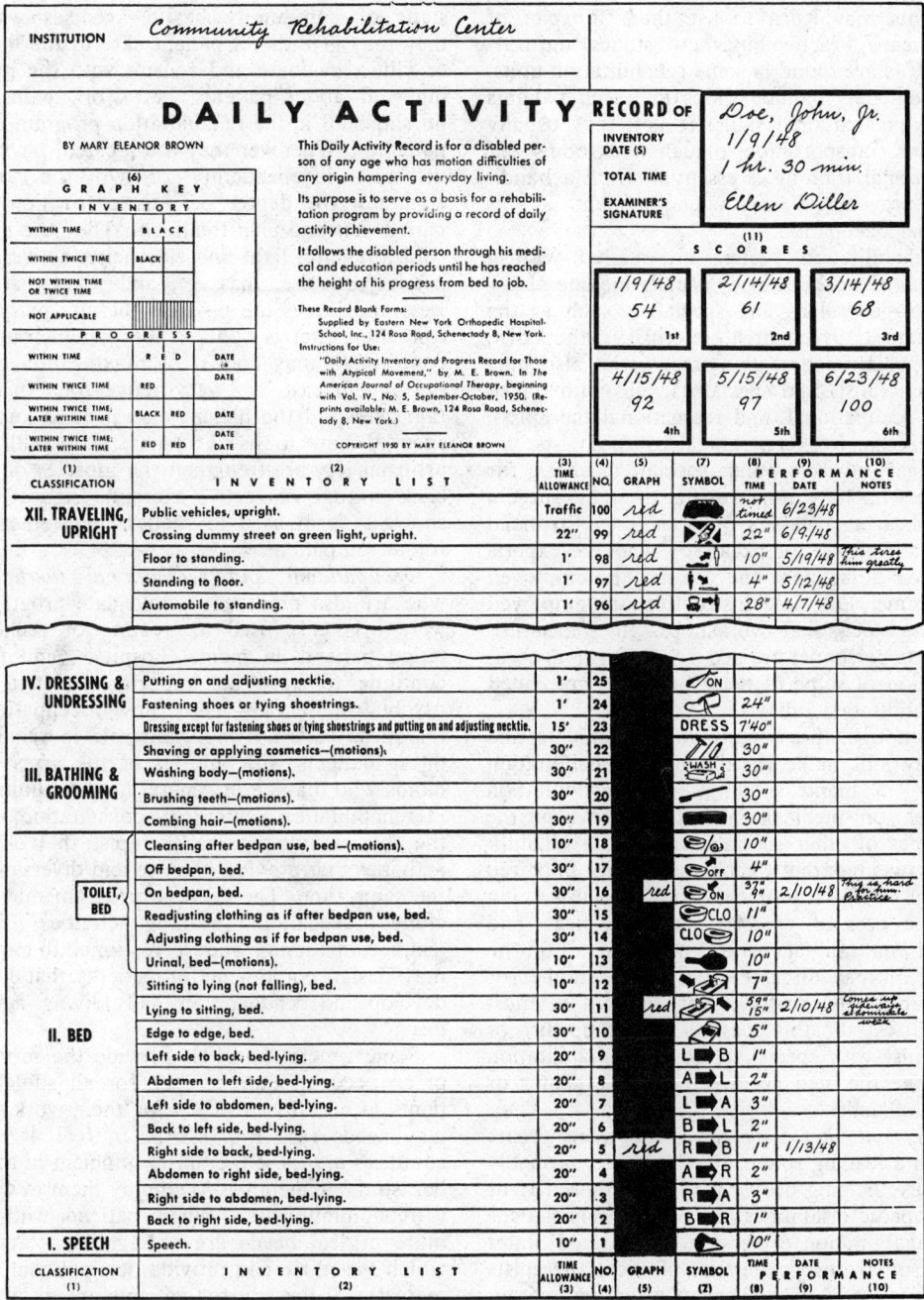

Figure 8-15. Record of daily activities, prepared for handicapped persons during the period of rehabilitation. (Brown, Mary E.: "Daily Activity Inventory and Progress Record for Those with Atypical Movement," *Am. J. Occup. Therap.*, 4:195, [Sept.] 1950.)

rooms are provided with books, games, radios, televisions, and whatever might stimulate normal interests and activities. People of both sexes and children and adults may be treated in the same area. Communal dining is encouraged for all who can feed themselves, or who need minimum help. Workrooms offer patients an opportunity for sewing and laundering. All kinds of household equipment such as stoves, refrigerators, and vacuum cleaners are provided so that patients may learn to use them in spite of handicaps. Practice buses, curbstones, and traffic lights are found in some rehabilitation units. Centers may include shops in which patients learn occupational skills. If not, they usually furnish transportation to such workrooms, for vocational training is essential when a handicap prevents a man's employment in his former occupation.

Rehabilitation centers are staffed with a variety of workers. They usually include physicians—generalists and specialists such as the physiatrist, psychiatrist, internist, orthopedist, and pediatrician; with nurses—who also may be generalists and specialists; and with physical, occupational, and recreational therapists; with social workers, clinical psychologists, vocational advisers, and special teachers for those who have impairments of sight, speech, and hearing. Makers of prostheses (artificial legs and arms, for example) who are experts in their adjustment and use may be employed part-time. Full-time instructors are employed in the vocational workshops. In some programs, personnel trained to perform a combination of some of these functions are called "rehabilitation officers."

Although the doctor, nurse, patient, and family still make up the basic rehabilitation team, in many situations the rehabilitation center or medical institution provides the services of other specialists. In those rehabilitation centers that treat patients with impaired motor ability, a physician with special training in the uses of exercise, massage, heat, and other "natural" agents (a *physiatrist*) is on the staff, or may direct the unit. The number of prepared physiatrists is very limited in most countries; for this reason, an orthopedist or internist with special interest in rehabilitation may be the medical director of the center or hospital unit.

Physical therapists have for many years taken a leading role in rehabilitation, probably because helping people with neuromuscular or orthopedic disabilities has been a major focus in rehabilitation centers. In the United States and some other countries, physical therapists are prepared in collegiate programs within medical schools and can participate effectively in plans for comprehensive medical care.[112] These therapists are usually assigned to specific patients and treat them day after day. Occasionally they act as independent professional workers and give treatments in the home to patients referred to them by physicians. Actually they *aren't* "independent" until they can practice without medical prescription. Only when a patient can come to them without referral by the physician will they be independent. Some physical therapists are now on the staffs of community health agencies where they may give direct patient care in the home or clinic, evaluate and consult with the nursing staff about patients, and work with the nursing staff in the rehabilitation program of a patient.[113] Wherever they are located, physical therapists independently, or with the physician, test the degree of muscle function the patient has and plan treatment. They use heat, cold, pressure, light and electricity, active and passive exercise, massage, and manipulation. Less and less is the physical therapy program something that is done *to* the patient; on the contrary, it may consist of re-education with the patient cast in a very active role. In certain cases, all the patient may need is knowledge of how to use crutches, walk with an artificial leg, or strengthen the muscles of the back through corrective exercise. Figure 8-16 shows a form used to request physiotherapy for an outpatient.

Occupational and recreational therapists, who are also prepared in collegiate programs, were originally used in treating or rehabilitating patients in mental hospitals, and they continue to have an important role in all psychiatric services. But now occupational therapists have an important role in rehabilitating patients with injuries of the arms and hands who may be in general hospital units or in rehabilitation centers. In consultation with the physician or physical therapist, they devise activities that provide exercise and diversion at the same time. The exercise program may include prevocational training activities. Physical, occupational, and recreational therapists may design equipment for patients that helps develop independence in daily living activities.[114]

Some general hospitals provide the services of an occupational therapist for all adult patients in an effort to care for their work and play needs (see Fig. 8-17). In few, if any, countries are these therapists sufficient in number, so the tendency is to employ them to work in rehabilitation units where patients with the more critical needs are segregated. Ways in which the nurse can provide occupational and recreational therapy for patients are discussed in Chapter 17.

Some rehabilitation centers have *vocational guidance counselors* who help patients find or train for occupations where they can be productive in spite of their disabilities. For instance, individuals who have motor disabilities of the legs or who are blind can be productive workers in industries where they assemble solid-state circuits for electronic equipment. The vocational guidance officer usually consults with other professional workers about the patient and gives the patient a battery of tests

University Hospital

OUT-PATIENT REQUEST FOR PHYSIOTHERAPY

Patient's Residential Telephone No. ____________

Place of Employment ____________

Business Telephone No. ____________

WCB ____________ Other ____________

PRIMARY DIAGNOSIS ____________

☐ Confirmed ☐ Suspected Date of Onset ____________

SECONDARY DIAGNOSIS ____________

OPERATIVE PROCEDURES ____________ DATE(S) ____________

RELEVANT FINDINGS & PRECAUTIONS ____________

PHYSICIAN'S OBJECTIVES ____________

TREAT ☐ As follows ____________

☐ As recommended above - change and progress at discretion of physiotherapist.

☐ At discretion of physiotherapist.

For co-ordination purposes please indicate relevant services involved:

☐ Inhalation Therapy ☐ Occupational Therapy ☐ Other

☐ Speech Therapy ☐ Social Services

PHYSICIAN'S SIGNATURE ____________ DATE ____________

84-687-0220

Figure 8-16. Out-patient request for physiotherapy. (Courtesy of University Hospital, University of Western Ontario, London, Ont.)

to determine how he or she can be helped. They may include aptitude tests, psychologic tests, and educational achievement tests.

Social workers, psychiatrists, and *psychologists* are often on the staff of a rehabilitation center. The kind of restorative care discussed here is very costly, and one function of the social worker is to help families get financial aid or community agencies that can help with a particular aspect of rehabilitation. All of these workers are prepared to help the patient and the family meet the psychologic and social stresses accompanying illness or injury requiring prolonged treatment.

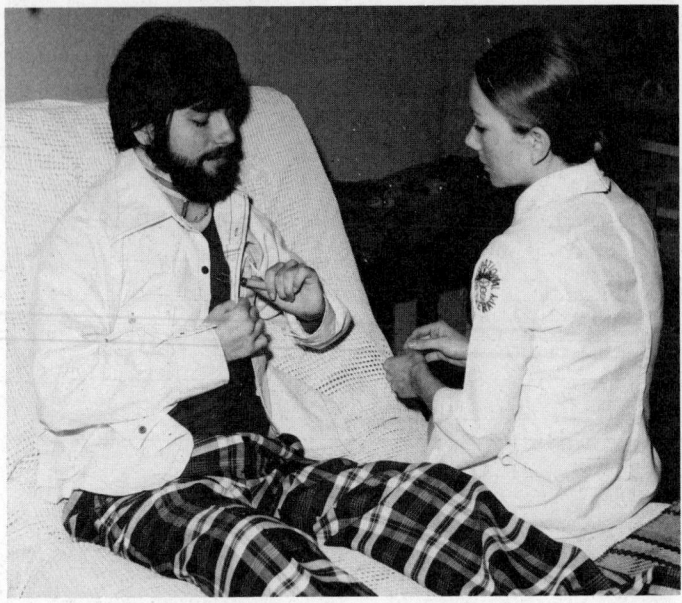

Figure 8-17. Patient with a spinal cord injury (C6–7) learns, with the aid of an occupational therapist, to button his jacket by using a buttonhook. (Courtesy of Veterans Administration Hospital, Houston, Tex.)

Rehabilitation Centers for the Mentally Retarded and for Those With Cerebral Palsy or Other Handicaps. There are rehabilitation or habilitation centers for the mentally retarded; also centers for children with cerebral palsy. Both types may use many of the therapists just described. In addition, they have teachers who are especially prepared to help children with learning problems and to teach youths work skills whether their handicaps are intellectual or physical. There are also centers that help patients who have defective sight, hearing, or speech. These centers have teachers of Braille, or a speech therapist, or a worker who is especially prepared to help a blind person use a "seeing-eye" dog. Psychiatrists, other physicians, nurses, physical therapists, social workers, and others may be employed full-time or part-time. Judging by the literature, nurses have not contributed conspicuously to the development of such programs, although they seem to have been more effective in some countries than others.

All rehabilitation units or centers, whether for children or adults, have as a major purpose helping patients to be as independent as possible in their daily activities—moving from place to place, eating, getting to bed, eliminating, keeping clean and well-groomed, working, playing, and worshipping (see Fig. 8-18). Nurses may or may not be full-time staff members but are often in a position to give information that will help the rehabilitation staff plan more effectively with the patients. If patients are hospitalized when rehabilitation therapy is started, nurses are re-

sponsible for promoting throughout the patient's day what he or she learned during the daily session of special therapy. To ensure this, some institutions have the policy of sending the staff nurse assigned to the patient to stay with him or her during the session in the rehabilitation unit. Nurses are also responsible for getting information from therapists about treatment that should be continued if a patient is rehospitalized.

Specialized Rehabilitation Programs. Although rehabilitation focuses on the restoring of function, preventing and maintaining function are the first phase—for example, preventing the contracture of a knee, shoulder, or hand; or maintaining the strength of an arm or leg whether or not this seems threatened by the diagnosis. A well arm or shoulder or a painful one can be ankylosed. Joseph J. Panzarella, discussing rehabilitation units for motor disabilities, says: "Many authorities have reported that approximately 80 per cent of the patients . . . referred to the rehabilitation centers . . . would never have had a need for referral if the concept of early total rehabilitation had been understood and practiced at the general hospital level." *

If throughout the care of all patients nurses bear in mind the goal of helping them retain or regain independence in breathing, eating, eliminating, sleeping, moving, dressing, communicating, and establishing satisfactory human relationships—in other words, carrying

* Panzarella, Joseph J., Jr.: "Rehabilitation," *Hosp. Prog.,* **45**:85, (Nov.) 1964.

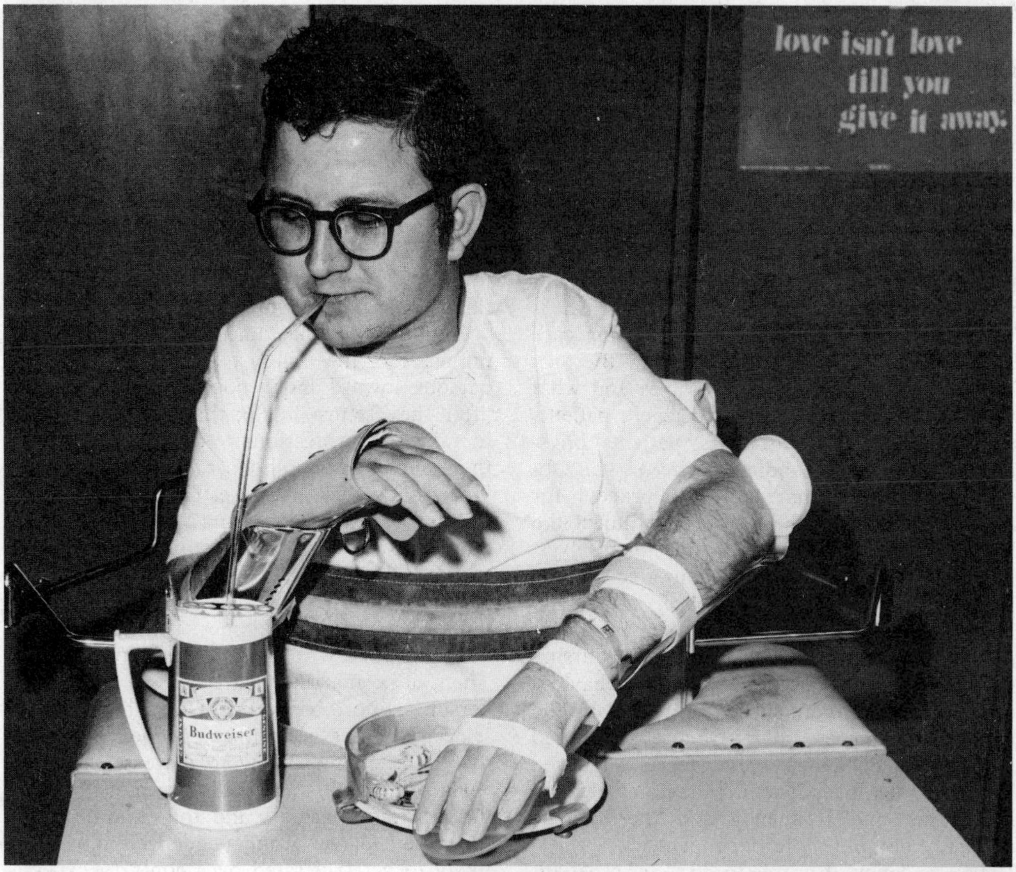

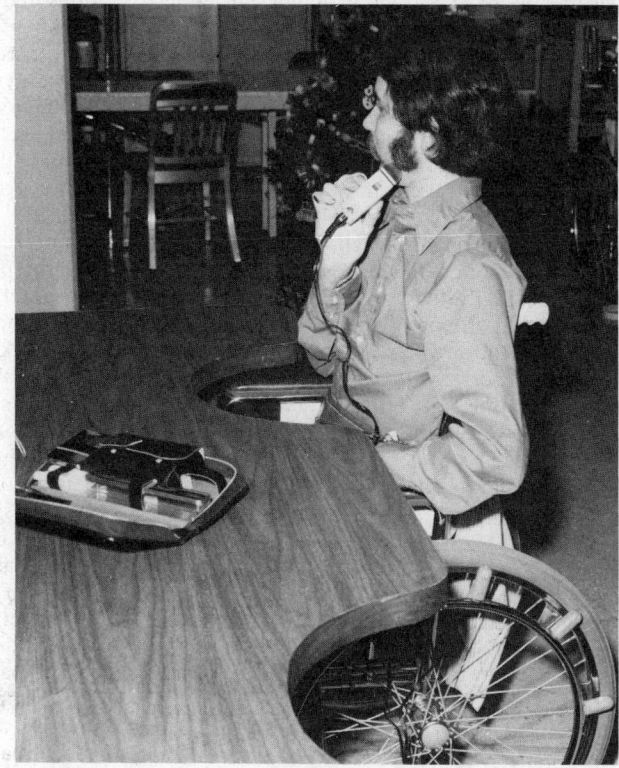

Figure 8-18. Patients with physical disabilities learning independent self-care activities. (Courtesy of Veterans Administration Hospital, Houston, Tex.)

on daily activities—then nurses are taking a leading role in rehabilitation. This process of assessing, teaching, and encouraging is not to be confused with the all too prevalent practice of allowing prostrated patients to take their own baths, of letting patients, unaided, grope their way toward an effective use of crutches, or insisting that overprotected children dress themselves. Nor does it mean turning over physical care to the untrained worker. It is rather an attempt throughout all nursing care and treatment to decide what part of the procedure nurses should do themselves and what part they should encourage, or teach, patients to perform. Nurses must assess patients' physical strength, understanding, desire or will. Obviously this is a more difficult process for nurses than to give the entire bath, inject the hypodermic, or irrigate wounds themselves. Nurses are traditionally ones who give service. Patients may enjoy dependence, and, who knows how often, nurses may revel in "being needed." * A study of patients in a nursing home showed that as the dependent behaviors of these patients were subtly reinforced by the unconscious approval of nurse attendants, and independent behaviors were generally ignored by them, the independent behaviors lessened in number and frequency and the patients gradually became more dependent.[115]

The tendency of nurses to do "for" a patient whether he or she needs it or not can be lessened if during the nursing interview information is solicited about the patient's self-care status, and this information is incorporated into the plan of care. In some institutions, codes are used to indicate the extent of a patient's independent abilities. For instance, one institution uses the code "Do For," "Help," "Watch," and "Self" indicating the patient is dependent, needs assistance, needs supervision, or is independent.[116] When each activity of daily living is judged and recorded as occurring on one of these levels, all nursing personnel know when and where the patient needs the most assistance or needs no assistance. Since the status of a patient may change hourly, however, the evaluative process must be continued.

Nurses should never lose sight of the very

important part the family of the patient plays in rehabilitation. Family members should know what patients can do and how they can help. In one rehabilitation center, Polaroid pictures are taken of patients in various positions in bed and are attached to the nearby wall. Relatives can then use these pictures as guides to help the patient change position, pillows, and other supports so the patient maintains good body alignment.

Studies show that during hospitalization the influence of the family to "motivate" disabled persons toward independence is weaker than after they return home; that is, patients tend to take the professional worker's estimate of their dependent or independent level as more "true" than the family's estimate. However, if family ties are close and patients are encouraged by their families to be independent, they are likely to make good progress. Once disabled persons have left an institution, the influence of their families (particularly the husband or wife) increases considerably. Then, if a marriage partner sees a disabled person as more independent than he sees himself or she sees herself, independence in daily living activities is likely to increase, and vice versa. Finally, if there is disagreement between the marriage partners and the children about the patient's level of independence, he or she is likely to get frustrated over contrary expectations and demands. In this case, he or she may simply give up making an effort.[117,118]

Nurses who see all nursing as rehabilitative find ways to help patients with chronic disabilities such as myocardial infarcts, strokes, diabetes, emphysema, cystic fibrosis, colostomies, ileal conduits, or ulcerative colitis, to name a few conditions where help is greatly needed.[119-126a] The nurse's aim is always to minimize disability as much as possible by helping patients learn new ways of performing those activities of daily living affected by the illness; or by showing patients adaptive devices that make activities possible and acceptable. Nurses also help patients plan and make adjustments to the environment.[127,127a] To be an effective member of a rehabilitation team, the nurse must be able to promote patients' full participation in their daily regimens. This may involve simple procedures but it may also include skills that are quite foreign to normal living—and for the nurse may involve hundreds of procedures with almost as many modifications.

Rehabilitation in psychiatry assumes different patterns according to the psychiatrists' school of thought. For instance, R. D. Laing and his associates see mental illness as a person's reaction to a way of life imposed on

---

* While it may not be necessary to make this comment, let no one suppose that the positive aspect of dependence is overlooked. It is appropriate and desirable under some circumstances to do things for patients that they are entirely able to do themselves. This is a normal expression of interest and feeling for others. At certain stages of illness, patients may need the assurance that they are liked by nurses, doctors, or therapists, more than they need physical independence. As was mentioned earlier, interdependence is characteristic of healthy human relationships.

him or her that is inconsistent with his or her instinctive desires and potential for accomplishment and human happiness. Rehabilitation, they seem to say, lies in allowing people to regress and withdraw from "life," as most persons know it, until they can find their way to a new and more satisfying existence. Rehabilitation consists of physical and emotional support throughout this period.[128-130] Alan W. Watts[131] suggests that Eastern therapies seek relief for men's loneliness and fear of death by helping them feel a part of the universe and continuing life. Increasingly, however, mental illness is looked upon as a failure to establish or maintain satisfying relationships with others in the society of which the person is a part. The corollary is that rehabilitating patients means helping them accomplish this. If the last sentence is a simple statement, the process referred to is not, and putting it so simply may be misleading. Dorothy Mereness[132] and others discuss the important role of nurses in creating a therapeutic environment which is consistent, rational, safe, and as homelike as possible, and where the patient is encouraged to function as independently as possible.

Rehabilitative nursing care of a psychiatric patient who had psychosurgery and a left leg amputation is described by Elizabeth W. Palmieri. For 15 years this man had been confined to a wheelchair, had never been away from the psychiatric ward, and had become increasingly rage-ridden and unkempt. Following surgery, nursing focused on supplying the patient's basic psychologic needs. At the end of a year of such care, the patient was a "well-groomed man who apparently cared about his appearance, socialized to some extent with others, walked, attended group therapy, had a limited grounds pass, and even went home for an occasional weekend." *

The development of therapeutic communication skills, necessary for all nurses, is discussed in Chapter 16. Related skills of helping patients meet their needs for work and play are described in Chapter 17.

Since children are more obviously in the process of "becoming" than are adults, it may be helpful to think of their care as "habilitative" rather than "re-habilitative." (This statement can be challenged since, ideally, all life can be a process of growth—physical, intellectual, emotional, or spiritual.) Habilitative nursing should include plans for helping a child learn many behaviors that are usually

learned in the home, such as drinking from a cup, using a spoon, being continent, walking, and riding a tricycle. Children with handicaps require more consistent and persistent help in learning these activities than will nonhandicapped children, but nursing care for all children should include planning to initiate these behaviors at appropriate times.[133] Care should be planned also to help children who have acquired these skills to continue their use. For instance, the 18-month-old child who has recently learned to drink from a cup should be encouraged in this behavior and not given a bottle because it is easier and because during illness there is a tendency to regress. A 5-year-old who is toilet trained should be shown the bathroom or taught to use a bedpan, not put into diapers again because it may seem easier to nursing personnel. A teenager, groping for independence and self-identity, should be consulted about and have explanations for his or her care rather than be treated as a child.[134,135]

Every child, every day, needs play activities that are appropriate to his or her age, sex, physical and mental development, and former experience. Some persons think it helpful for all children to have opportunities to express their feelings about their illness through play. If they are hospitalized, they can also show the knowledgeable health worker their reactions to this experience. Finally, all children deserve concrete explanations of things and people around them rather than symbolic verbal explanations only[136,137] (see Chapter 17).

The serious effects of separating young children from their mothers during a crisis, such as hospitalization, are widely recognized, and various kinds of arrangements for mothers to stay with their children are made by different institutions. Many mothers do stay with their children. To keep these women from feeling like "captive mothers," nurses should plan the child's care with them. In effect, the pediatric nurse should consider the mother and child as a unit (a dyad).[138-140] Mothers not only want to care for their children as much as they can, but also want to understand what is happening to them. While most emphasis has been placed on the mother-child relationship when the child is 5 years or younger, school-age children and their mothers also need consideration and planning to maintain their relationships.

In *The Growth and Development of Mothers,*[141] Angela McBride pleads that fathers be allowed and encouraged to share the parental role more evenly with the mothers. It might be appropriate here to suggest that institutions consider the possibility of having a father instead of a mother live in an institution and

---

* Palmieri, Elizabeth W.: "Recognition of Basic Human Needs and Reeducation: The Keys to the Resocialization of a Lobotomy Patient," in *ANA Clinical Sessions, 1970.* Appleton-Century-Crofts, New York, 1971, p. 219.

participate in the care of his child when this is conducive to the child's and family's welfare.

Special centers have been established for children who have congenital neuromuscular handicaps, severe and extensive burns, residual disabilities from disease such as poliomyelitis, who are blind, or who are mentally retarded. Each of these centers has some, if not all, of the therapists mentioned earlier. A child who has never walked, never been able to hear or see, requires different approaches to therapy than does an adult with any of these same disabilities. Frequently, toys are used to help the child learn ways of meeting his or her disability. A child with cerebral palsy, for example, is helped to learn about the relationship of the body to space by being bounced on a trampoline or rolled about on a large inflated ball.

Finally, in all rehabilitation efforts the importance of self-help cannot be overstressed. In Chapter 5 attention was called to Andrew Malleson's emphasis on self-help in the arrest of alcoholism and obesity which he thinks has in each case been demonstrated by studies. Francine Sobey's title, *Nonprofessional Revolution in Mental Health* (Columbia University Press, New York, 1970), is in itself a testimonial to this concept. Judith A. Bumbalo and Delores E. Young, writing on "The Self-Help Phenomenon," say:

Although the effectiveness or success of self-help may not be supported by research data, there can be little argument that this approach has been helpful to many.

. . .

People who have lived with a problem for many years may well acquire first-hand knowledge not readily accessible to or comprehended by those not directly involved.*

They go on to give an "unqualified yes" in answer to questions as to whether nurses should identify those who would benefit from participating in self-help groups and whether professionals could learn to be more effective by incorporating some self-help methods in their practice. In discussing alcoholism in Chapter 21, the three organizations designed to help alcoholics, their families and friends, and Synanon, the organization to help other drug abusers, are discussed. The Appendix lists these and other groups that offer unique services. Nurses and others engaged in rehabilitative efforts should familiarize themselves with the programs of these self-help groups.

* Bumbalo, Judith A., and Young, Delores E.: "The Self-Help Phenomenon," *Am. J. Nurs.,* **73:**1588, (Sept.) 1973.

5. TERMINATING CARE ("DISCHARGING" PATIENTS)

Discharge from Hospitals or Other Health Agencies. Discharge from the hospital or other health agency should never come unexpectedly to patients or to any of those attending them. The aim of the health team, patient, and the family, throughout the illness, is to make him or her independent. From the first, everyone should look forward to the day when the person can leave the hospital. Except in illnesses that leave no temporary or permanent disability, discharge from the hospital should be preceded by a planned program of health guidance or teaching that extends over a large part, or the entire period, of therapy. Too often the patient is given explanation or instruction about treatments, diets, formulas, exercises, or medications just before he or she leaves the institution. This is no longer thought adequate. Patients should not be discharged until they have had a chance to demonstrate and practice independence, if this is expected of them after they leave the institution. Directions for home care should be written. Illustrated and diagrammed directions often further the understanding of patients and their families.[142-143a] Dates and hours for return visits to clinics should be put in writing. It cannot be said too often that all such plans should be made *with* patients and families in an unhurried and cooperative atmosphere. Figure 8-19 is an example of a form for discharge medical prescriptions and home care instructions used with children.

Learning new habits for daily living is a complex and often slow process. Because health teaching on a "one patient to one nurse" basis is thought to be too time consuming, many institutions and agencies are organizing groups of patients with the same health problem to teach them about their health and self-care. Some group sessions are conducted during the patients' hospital stay, as, for instance, learning and using bed exercises; others are conducted after the patient leaves the hospital, for example, a six-session "course" for patients with coronary disease; and others are conducted over a period of weeks for patients who attend a clinic but do not need hospitalization, such as diabetic patients or those with arthritis.[144,145] Group teaching (rather group learning) is less time consuming than individual teaching, but it can be more effective if it is so conducted that patients can learn from each other. Psychiatric institutions conduct group sessions over a year, or even years, for outpatients. The meetings of Alcoholics Anonymous are one example of ongoing group therapy sessions that may extend indefinitely for those who need continued help.

The American Hospital Association's *Patient's Bill of Rights* includes the following statements about the patient's moral and legal rights:

The patient has the right to obtain from his physician complete current information concerning his diagnosis, treatment, and prognosis in terms the patient can be reasonably expected to understand. When it is not medically advisable to give such information to the patient, the information should be made available to an appropriate person in his behalf. . . .

The patient has the right to receive from his physician information necessary to give *informed consent* prior to the start of any procedure and/or treatment. Except in emergencies, such information for informed consent should include but not necessarily be limited to the specific procedures and/or treatment, the medically significant risks involved, and the probable duration of incapacitation. Where medically significant alternatives for care or treatment exist, or when the patient requests information concerning medical alternatives, the patient has the right to such information. The patient has the right to know the name of the person responsible for the procedures and/or treatment.

The patient has the right to expect reasonable continuity of care. He has the right to know in advance what appointment times and physicians are available and where. The patient has the right to expect that the hospital will provide a mechanism whereby he is informed by his physician or a delegate of the physician of the patient's continuing health care requirements following discharge.*

A number of persons (including nurses) who have been patients appeal to all health workers to tell patients that they have such "rights" as stated above.[146-148] It is encouraging that some hospitals give a copy of *A Patient's Bill of Rights* to all patients.

Referrals and Insuring Continuity of Care. In some cases, persons are discharged from one health agency to another better suited to their needs or economic resources. In all cases, the best results are seen when those concerned agree upon the date and are ready for the discharge. In some institutions, the doctor, nurse, and social worker meet weekly, or more often, to discuss plans for the discharge of patients or for continuing care. Ideally the patient and family concerned and representatives of all major departments contributing to the program of therapy should participate in such conferences. It is obvious that plans should be made far enough in advance to enable the staff

of another agency, the family, and the patient to arrange things so that his or her needs will be met. In some cases, a person leaves the hospital cured and rehabilitated, ready to take up his or her former way of life; very often he or she faces a period of convalescence or training for a more limited existence. Frequently the elderly, who need a longer convalescent and rehabilitative period than do younger persons, enter a nursing home. Most of these homes offer a sheltered environment with custodial rather than therapeutic care.[149] In any case, patients and their families should be prepared for the new environment and what can be expected from it. Because the elderly require some time to adjust to new surroundings and people, it is helpful for them to meet the nursing home personnel and to at least see pictures of it before they are discharged from the hospital.

Another type of social agency that helps people return to normal life is the "halfway house." Most of them are designed to help psychiatric patients and particularly drug abusers. Some are for youths and adults leaving penal institutions who are greatly in need of rehabilitation.

Hospitals and other health agencies differ greatly in the responsibility they assume for continuity of care; however, an increasing number are employing a nurse (or nurses) called the "liaison nurse" to provide for continuity. Liaison nurses assess family and patient needs on the basis of a home visit, a visit with the institutionalized person, and a review of his or her records. They are responsible for preparing referral forms and home instruction forms and are available to either the institutional nurse or the community health nurse for consultation or additional patient care planning.[150] If a liaison nurse is not available and the patient needs help from a second agency, the professional personnel of the first agency can promote the patient's welfare by communication with the personnel of the second. This is usually accomplished through "referral forms" (see Fig. 8-20 *A* and *B*). On the form the physician can make a note on treatment, the nurse, on nursing care, the social worker, on social problems, the physical therapist, on such treatment as he or she has been giving, the nutritionist, on nutritional problems, and so on. In special cases it is desirable that workers in the second agency visit the patient before he or she is admitted so that they will know something about his or her problems on admission, and so that the patient will not feel entirely strange when he or she gets there. This exchange of information can be accomplished by letters, or telephone communica-

* American Hospital Association: *A Patient's Bill of Rights*. The Association, Chicago, Nov. 17, 1972.

HOME CARE

CHILDRENS HOSPITAL OF LOS ANGELES

**DISCHARGE ORDERS AND
HOME CARE INSTRUCTIONS**

Page 1.

1. Date _____ Time _____   Referring Doctor _____
2. Discharge _____   Address _____
3. Summary _____ Dictated _____ Not Dictated   _____
4. Record diagnosis on face sheet   Phone _____

PHYSICIAN'S ORDERS (Cont.)	NURSE'S INSTRUCTIONS

1. Diet: _____ Regular _____ Special   1. Diet: _____

2. ACTIVITIES:

____ NO RESTRICTIONS   2. ACTIVITIES:

   ____ Full Play Activity and/or

   ____ Return to school

____ RESTRICTIONS

   ____ Complete Bed rest

   ____ Up for meals and bathroom   Type bath:

   ____ Frequent Rest   Shower _____ Sponge _____ Tub _____

   ____ May not return to school

   ____ Indoor play only   Shampoo: _____ Yes _____ No

3. MEDICATIONS: 3. MEDICATIONS: (First dose, etc.)

_____ M.D.   _____ R.N.

WHITE—CHART
CANARY—PARENT/GUARDIAN
PINK—PHARMACY
CAT. 46-1100 REV. 8/75

Figure 8-19. Form for discharge orders and home care instructions. Copy 2 goes to the parents, copy 3 to pharmacy, and copy 1 remains a permanent part of the chart. (Courtesy of Children's Hospital of Los Angeles.)

tion, or interagency conferences.[151] In any event, systematic use should be made of written referral forms similar to those shown in Figure 8-20 A and B.

Some institutions are providing for con-tinuity of care in homes by sending members of the hospital staff to see patients discharged from the hospital. Patients in some "home care programs" are still registered with the hos-pital.[152-154] Other institutions are providing a

H.O.M.E.C.A.R.E

CHILDRENS HOSPITAL OF LOS ANGELES

DISCHARGE ORDERS AND
HOME CARE INSTRUCTIONS

Page 2.

PHYSICIAN'S ORDERS	NURSING INSTRUCTIONS
4. TREATMENTS/PROCEDURES: (include equipment)	4. TREATMENTS/PROCEDURES: (Equipment/Supplies)

5. TINE TEST (Check one): Pos. ☐ Neg. ☐
_____ To be read _____ Was not ordered.

_____ M.D.   _____ R.N.

5. FOLLOW-UP

__ a. Dr. _____ would like to see your child in about _____ .
Please call for an appointment.

__ b. Out Patient Department Childrens Hospital _____ .
Please bring clinic card and appointment slip. _____ .

__ c. Public Health Nurse. She will contact you about home care.

__ d. Other _____ .

6. DISCHARGE COMPLETION:

I have reviewed the above instructions with the physician and nurse and release my child from Childrens Hospital.

NAME _____ ADDRESS _____

RELATION _____ _____

DATE: _____ TIME _____ PHONE _____

SCHOOL: The following may be detached and used for Return to School

To whom it may concern:

_____ has been a patient in Childrens Hospital of
Los Angeles and under my care from _____ to _____ .
Permission is hereby granted to return to school on _____ .
Special Instructions: _____

_____ M.D.

WHITE – CHART
CANARY – PARENT/GUARDIAN

CAT. 46-1100 REV. 8/75

Figure 8-19. (continued)

"hot line," originally started for drug users and persons who were potentially suicidal, that gives mothers of new infants access to competent advice over the telephone at any time.

When those concerned have agreed on the time that a patient should leave a health agency for home, or another institution, the doctor in charge of treatment writes a discharge note on the chart and signs it. The person (usually the head nurse) responsible for the general management of the clinical unit notifies the financial office in advance, and arrangements are made for the payment of the patient's bill. The medical record is brought up to date, and as the patient leaves, the hour of departure and the mode of locomotion, whether on foot, in a chair, or on a stretcher, are noted by the nurse. A medical summary is prepared by the physician, and the completed data are sent to the medical records department to be filed.

In preparation for the patient's departure, his or her belongings are assembled, checked, and packed. It is customary for the patient to sign a record indicating that the articles listed have been returned to him or her. Nurses give patients whatever help is needed in dressing. They make every effort through cooperation with families or the social service department to see that patients have suitable garments for the journey to the next destination. The nurse is usually the person who, like a good hostess, speeds the parting guests and makes them feel that those they leave behind wish them well

and will be interested in seeing them again. The nurse, or some other member of the staff, goes with them and their families to the front door, seeing that what baggage they have is delivered to them and that they have the necessary mode of conveyance. Their welcome and farewell are major factors in the total impression made on patients by the institution. The nurse plays an important role on both occasions, and, if it is possible, should allow time to make these first and last services thorough, effective, and graceful. The attitude the patient acquires toward the institution may determine his or her willingness to return to the clinic, to keep up the suggested program, or to continue treatment in another agency.

Throughout the chapters of this text, the importance of helping patients regain independence is stressed; however, nurses should be continually aware that hospitalization often allows or even encourages a person to become dependent on others. This feeling of depend-

---

**REQUEST FOR PUBLIC HEALTH AND
VISITING NURSE SERVICE**

•

Washtenaw County Health Department
and Affiliated Agencies

•

(Address)	(Office)	(Phone)
720 E. Catherine	Ann Arbor	2-5581
1761 Stamford Rd.	Willow Run	2892
26 S. Prospect St.	Ypsilanti	1525

Date_____

Name_____ Approx. Age_____

Address _____

Diagnosis _____

ORDERS:

Dr._____

Figure 8-20. *A*. Referral form used to request visiting nurse service. (Courtesy of Washtenaw County Health Department and Affiliated Agencies, Ypsilanti and Ann Arbor, Mich.)

White Copy—Patient Record
Blue Copy—Billing
Yellow Copy—Physician
Pink Copy—Initiator

DHHA/CHS Form 21-ICTP
© 1973 National League for Nursing

INTERAGENCY CARE AND TREATMENT PLAN
(Physician's Certification)

TO _____   FROM _____

_____   _____

_____   _____

AGENCY PROVIDER No. _____

☐ REFERRAL   ☐ REPORT   ☐ REQUEST FOR ORDERS   EFFECTIVE DATES: From _____ To_____

PATIENT NAME _____

ADDRESS _____

Birth Date	Soc. Sec. No.
Medicare No.	Medicaid No.
Other Insurance	No.

REPORT OF AGENCY PERSONNEL

PROBLEMS	PROGRESS, PLANS, RECOMMENDATIONS

PHYSICIAN'S ORDERS

DIAGNOSES (current, complete, date of onset—use ICDA codes)   PROGNOSIS_____

_____   FUNCTIONAL LIMITATIONS (motor or sensory deficits): _____

_____

CURRENT ORDERS — INCLUDE FREQUENCY AND DURATION, MEDICATIONS, SUPPLIES, ETC.

DIET:_____

☐ NURSING

☐ H.H. AIDE

☐ P.T.

☐ O.T.

☐ S.T.

☐ M.S.W.

☐ OTHER (Specify)

Last seen by physician___Date:_____

Recertification due____Date:_____

Sent to physician____Date:_____

Received by Agency___Date:_____

RECERTIFICATION STATEMENT: I certify that the above-named patient (1) is under my care, (2) is homebound except when receiving outpatient services, (3) requires skilled nursing care on an intermittent basis or physical or speech therapy as specified in the original orders with the modifications listed above.
Is Recertification Statement pertinent to this patient? ☐ Yes ☐ No

FORM 21-ICTP

_____
(Physician's Signature)   (Date)

Figure 8-20. *B*. Interagency referral form. (Courtesy of National League for Nursing, New York, N.Y.)

White Copy—Patient Record
Blue Copy—Billing
Yellow Copy—Physician
Pink Copy—Initiator

DHHA/CHS Form 21-SICT
©1973 National League for Nursing

SUPPLEMENT TO INTERAGENCY CARE AND TREATMENT PLAN

PATIENT NAME _____

PATIENT I.D. No. _____

All entries must be signed with name, title, and date.

☐REFERRAL   ☐REPORT   ☐REQUEST FOR ORDERS   EFFECTIVE DATES: From _____ To _____

FORM 21-SICT   Sign and date entry

Figure 8-20. *C.* Supplement to interagency care and treatment plan. (Courtesy of National League for Nursing, New York, N.Y.)

ence and the patient's (or nurse's) past experiences with separation may give one or both a sense of loss when the patient leaves. If nurses understand that this may happen, they will consistently reinforce indications of a healthy independence, stressing the positive aspects of the life to which the patient is returning.[155]

Once in a while patients or their families are dissatisfied with the treatment given in the hospital, and leave against the advice of the physician. In such cases, the patient or guardian and a member of the family are asked to sign a statement before he or she leaves. This is a protection to the hospital authorities, who may be sued if the patient is convinced that he or she was maltreated or if it can be proved that the patient was detained for treatment against his or her will. Unless they are committed psychiatric patients, have a communicable disease that limits their freedom, or are prisoners of the law, patients are free to leave the hospital at their discretion. Every effort is made to resolve any difficulty between patients and those responsible for their care and to prevent a premature termination of treatment.

Some hospital administrations attempt to improve their service by systematically soliciting criticism from patients. Administrative officers may visit patients and get such comments conversationally, or they may ask them to fill in questionnaires as they leave. Nurses could learn a great deal about the subjective aspect of illness if they kept a card file of significant comments made to them by patients. Periodically such comments could be summarized and valuable generalizations made.

Terminal Care. It must also be mentioned that some people never leave the hospital alive, death being inevitable. The care of the dying and the dead is discussed in Chapter 50.

6. EVALUATING CARE—INCLUDING REHABILITATION

General Considerations. Evaluating patient care and its effectiveness focuses on patient evidence or "outcomes," that is, the end results of the care. Avedis Donabedian says, "It is extraordinarily difficult to define what quality is. Very probably quality is not a homogenous property but a larger bundle of characteristics." * Other major problems in developing adequate criteria for evaluating quality care

are that nursing care is a very complex function and patient responses are equally complex. As nurses, patients, physicians, and other health workers may be looking at different characteristics as indicators of quality of care, it is helpful to have some agreement on what aspects of care are to be assessed.[156] If the goal of care is the attainment of healthy independence, then emotional, social, and physical characteristics that describe such a state must be agreed on and stated so that patient evidence may be collected to determine the degree of effectiveness of care.

The effectiveness of the plan of care and of the way in which it is carried out is demonstrated in various ways. Nurses may measure their success in preventive nursing by patient evidence that health is maintained. In nursing those who are sick, the recovery and rehabilitation of the individual in the shortest possible time are what nurses, in cooperation with other health workers, hope to accomplish. Another way of expressing this is to say that the patients' health problems are solved or they learn to cope with them. In nursing those who have an incurable and painful disease, success is judged largely by relief of the patients' discomfort. Success in nursing is evidenced by a spirit of friendliness and cooperation among nurses, patients, families, and friends, and between nurses and other health workers. Any manifestations of effective nursing in the behavior of others and their own consciousness of having solved problems in a situation that comes within their province give nurses increased professional confidence. It is difficult to imagine anything that offers more satisfaction than a well-conceived and skillfully executed plan of care.

Maintenance of Health. In any nursing program for healthy individuals, there is no better indication of successful care than their vigor and freedom from disease. Nurses are always cooperating with others in health programs; it is difficult to measure their success and to determine to whom it is due. In this country where nurses are the largest single health group and consequently give the most service to the patient, in point of time, they can assume that the success of a community project is some indication that they are working effectively. Nurses, working with doctors in schools, expect to see, as a result of their combined efforts, a reduction in the occurrence of colds, local infections, digestive troubles, headaches, poor posture, and other minor ills and defects. Successful nursing in schools, then, would be evidenced by the practice of good hygiene by the students.

Districts in which hospitals and community

* Donabedian, Avedis: "Part II—Some Issues in Evaluating the Quality of Nursing Care," *Am. J. Public Health,* **59**:1834, (Oct.) 1969.

nursing services are well organized should show not only lower morbidity and mortality rates but also general improvement in health practices. While the results of preventive nursing are more convincingly demonstrated by statistics on a large group of persons, *it is nevertheless what the nurse accomplishes with the individual that is measured.*

Patient's Recovery and Return to Health. In the case of a sick person, the success of the program of care is strikingly demonstrated by his or her recovery. This is clearly demonstrated in intensive care units, especially in patients with a diagnosis of acute myocardial infarction during the first few days of their illness. The mortality rate of these patients has been greatly reduced during the past decade.

Nurses are often heard to express their preference for taking care of critically ill patients. Their recovery gives them satisfaction and leaves them with a sense of achievement. There is more drama in nursing those who are acutely ill than those who are chronically ill or mildly ill. The changes during an acute illness are more obvious. While the patients are struggling against the forces of disease, the skilled nurse thinks for them, anticipates their needs, and supplies their wants, thereby making the individuals very *dependent.* Nurses and doctors sometimes give patients and their families the impression that they take more interest in getting patients over the critical stage of illness than in helping them to become *independent* during convalescence and in giving them the guidance that prevents a recurrence. Nurses or doctors who make the patient rely upon them unduly may be as mistaken as the mother who discourages self-reliance in her child. Nursing sick persons is not completely successful unless the patient is helped to maintain and acquire optimum independence throughout all stages of illness. Normal habits of living should be reestablished as rapidly as the condition of the patient permits rehabilitation.

Although healthy independence is a complex criterion, it is most important in evaluating quality of care. Another very important criterion is the patient's ability to *"cope"* with his disability or to *adjust* to some loss. Evidence of "coping" or adjusting is usually found in psychological and social behavior.

Relief of Symptoms, Including Pain and Discomfort. In Part V (Chapters 35 to 50) symptoms (or problems) of individuals are discussed; disturbances of health and its maintenance are described in Part III (Chapters 9 to 18). It is obvious, therefore, that a detailed discussion here of *symptoms* as criteria for evaluating patient care in detail is impracticable. The nature (causes and manifestations) of the symptom

and effective methods of prevention and treatment as well as evidence of its resolution give some indication of the degree of responsibility of the various health workers in the patient's care. For example, insomnia (a disturbance of normal sleep) may be viewed as a symptom or a problem. Nurses probably carry the greatest responsibility for its treatment except for prescribing tranquilizers and sedatives. When patients reestablish their normal sleep patterns without sedatives, the nursing activities are effective because insomnia (the symptom or problem) is not present. In Chapter 41 the management of insomnia, which we think can be relieved in large part by nursing care, is discussed.

Other signs of successful nursing care are the relief of pain and discomfort in the severely ill,[157-159] the establishment of confidence between the nurse and the patient and his or her family, and increased cooperation with other health workers. The control of pain and discomfort is the joint responsibility of the patient's health attendants, but of this group the nurse probably carries the largest share. The doctor prescribes narcotics and with surgery and other forms of therapy may remove the cause of pain, but the main purpose of many nursing activities is to make the patient comfortable. Well-planned nursing care, skillfully executed, makes patients actually *look* comfortable; for example, they look relaxed, in an easy position; the bedclothes, pillows, and clothing are so arranged that there is no pull or strain on any part of the body; the skin, hair, and nails look well cared for. There is order in the room; it is free from glare; there are no disagreeable odors; and the temperature is within the range of comfort. Whenever the nurse gives a treatment, a capable one avoids causing unnecessary pain or discomfort. If the daily nursing care makes the patient uncomfortable, there is usually something wrong with its plan or the way it is carried out unless the patient has "intractable" or uncontrollable pain. When the patient's disease is self-limited and there is hope of recovery, a plan of care that effects a cure is the main consideration. On the other hand, when the person has an incurable and painful disease, the chief aim of the doctor and nurse may be simply to make him or her comfortable. In such a case, the estimate of the success of the nursing plan is measured almost entirely by the relief given the patient. Chapters 49 and 50 discuss the management of pain, which, even though severe, can always be controlled, we believe.

A sign of successful nursing is the establishment of mutual confidence and respect between the nurse and the patient, family, and friends. In community health work, cooperation with the family is stressed because the nurse must frequently depend on help from members of the patient's household; but in the hospital the family and friends are likely to be given less consideration because the need for their cooperation, while it exists, is less evident. The patient's peace of mind, and consequently his or her physical condition, is affected by the feeling of confidence the family shows in the health attendants. The respect and liking of the patient and members of the household are an important indicator of successful nursing in any setting, and without it almost any plan, no matter how technically correct, is likely to fail.

It has been pointed out repeatedly that the most successful service is given when all those associated with the care of the patient are working together to accomplish a common purpose. A nursing plan that furthers this ideal and stimulates effective working relationships among the doctor, the nurse, the dietitian, the social worker, and special therapists has accomplished a good deal. The satisfaction of their associates in the care nurses give their patients is one of the signal marks of sucessful nursing. While professional loyalties should never take precedence over the welfare of the patient, in the writers' opinion, mutual respect and confidence among health workers are essential elements of the highest type of service. Plans for nursing should be made with consideration for those concerned with giving the care as well as for the patient. In hospitals the welfare of one patient must not be sacrificed for that of another. This means that the hours of service available to patients and the available supplies must be distributed with consideration for the demands of each individual. Nurses who take unfair means of benefiting their patients at the expense of others are likely to lose the support of the persons with whom they work. Intelligent patients sense the attitude of those around them and are favorably affected by the harmony that exists. The nurse who works well with others not only gets greatest personal satisfaction but also gives better patient care than one who doesn't.

The Nursing Audit. The term *audit* is most frequently associated with an official examination of business records to see whether reputable business practices have been followed, and to account for monies coming into and going out of that business. The "nursing audit" has a similar meaning—an official examination of nursing care records—but is not related to fees and payments for nursing services.[160-166] When the problem-oriented record system is used, the nursing audit is part of the audit of the entire patient's record. The focus is on the quality of patient data, the analysis of these data, and the performance of all health workers in solving the patient's problems.

Agencies or institutions that audit nursing differ in the methods they use. Frequently a clerical worker or a medical records librarian checks to see whether certain information is in the record; whether all necessary forms have complete information; and whether a minimal amount of medical and nursing information is present. The nursing auditor or audit committee then reviews the record to see whether the nursing history has sufficient pertinent data about the patient; whether health problems and nursing needs are identified, objectives defined, and nursing actions described; and whether there is evidence that outcome criteria have been met.[167-169] In most instances, only a few records are reviewed at any one time, but audits are planned for specific dates and a specific number of reviews over a period of time. The nursing audit may then be used during a nursing conference on a particular unit or for an inservice educational program for several units.

The purpose of the nursing audit and the nursing process is to help nurses attain and maintain standards of excellence in nursing care. John W. Gardiner says, "excellence implies more than competence. It implies a striving for the highest standards in every phase of life. We need excellence in all its forms—in every kind of creative endeavor, in political life, in education, in industry—in short, universally." *

Increased Nursing Ability. With the care of each patient, nurses should feel that they have added something to their store of knowledge and have increased their professional skill. If they do not have this satisfaction of having worked out problems successfully, it is very likely there was something wrong with the care they gave patients and they should try to find out in what respect they failed. Nothing could be more helpful to nurses than collecting and studying clinical nursing plans used for their patients. With each plan, notes could be kept on the condition of the patient and the reasons for, and the degree of success or failure of, the nursing measures employed.

REFERENCES

1. Garfield, Sidney R.: "The Delivery of Medical Care," *Sci. Am.*, **222**:15, (Apr.) 1970.
2. Slater, Reda R.: "Triage Nurse in the Emergency Department," *Am. J. Nurs.*, **70**: 127, (Jan.) 1970.

* Gardiner, John W.: *Excellence.* Harper & Row, New York, 1961, p. 160.

3. O'Boyle, Catherine: "A New Era in Emergency Services," *Am. J. Nurs.*, **72**:1392, (Aug.) 1972.

3a. Quinn, Joan L.: "Triage: Coordinated Home Care for the Elderly," *Nurs. Outlook*, **23**:570, (Sept.) 1975.

4. American Hospital Association: *Principles and Recommended Procedure As a Guide for the Identification of the Newborn in Hospitals.* The Association, Chicago, 1957.

5. American Academy of Pediatrics: *Standards and Recommendations for Hospital Care of Newborn Infants.* The Academy, Evanston, Ill., 1964, p. 46.

6. Hoover, J. Edgar: "The Newborn's Footprints," *Hospitals*, **33**:38, (Nov. 16) 1959.

7. Hellman, Louis M., and Pritchard, Jack A.: *Williams Obstetrics*, 14th ed. Appleton-Century-Crofts, New York, 1971, p. 487.

8. Abbott, Nancy C., et al.: "Dress Rehearsal for the Hospital," *Am. J. Nurs.*, **70**:2360, (Nov.) 1970.

9. Hunnisett, Frank W., and Knowles, David J.: "Orienting Prospective Patients," *Hospitals*, **44**:51, (Apr. 16) 1970.

9a. Rhymes, Julina: "The Prehospitalization Visit to Help a Child Cope with Stress," in Anderson, Edith H., et al. (eds.): *Current Concepts in Clinical Nursing*, Vol. IV. C. V. Mosby Co., St. Louis, 1973.

10. Auer, Edward T.: "The Invisible Patient," in Schwartz, Lawrence H., and Schwartz, Jane L.: *The Psychodynamics of Patient Care.* Prentice-Hall, Inc., Englewood Cliffs, N.J., 1972, p. 36.

11. Tagliacozzo, Daisy L., and Mauksch, Hans O.: "The Patient's View of the Patient's Role," in Jaco, E. Gartley (ed.): *Patients, Physicians, and Illness*, 2nd ed. Free Press, New York, 1972, p. 172.

12. Smith, Gary M.: "Experiencing Dehumanization in the Role of a Patient," *Ment. Hyg.*, **56**:75, (Winter) 1972.

12a. American Hospital Association: *A Patient's Bill of Rights.* The Association, Chicago, Nov. 17, 1972.

13. Belmont, Herman S.: "Hospitalization and Its Effects upon the Total Child," *Clin. Pediatr.*, **9**:472, (Aug.) 1970.

14. Conway, Barbara: "The Effect of Hospitalization on Adolescence," *Adolescence*, **6**:77, (Spring) 1971.

15. Kosa, John, et al.: *Poverty and Health.* Harvard University Press, Cambridge, Mass., 1969.

16. Clark, Margaret: *Health in the Mexican-American Culture*, 2nd ed. University of California Press, Berkeley, 1970.

17. Stone, Virginia: "Give the Older Person Time," *Am. J. Nurs.*, **69**:2124, (Oct.) 1969.

17a. Burnside, Irene Mortenson: "Listen to the Aged," *Am. J. Nurs.*, **75**:1801, (Oct.) 1975.

18. Anderson, Barbara J., et al.: "Two Experimental Tests of a Patient-Centered Admission Process," *Nurs. Res.*, **14**:151, (Spring) 1965.

19. Elms, Roslyn R., and Leonard, Robert C.: "Effects of Nursing Approaches During Admission," *Nurs. Res.*, **15**:39, (Winter) 1966.

20. Johnson, Dorothy M.: *The Stress of Children upon Admission to the Hospital.* Unpublished Master's thesis, Texas Woman's University College of Nursing, Houston Center, 1972.

20a. Robinson, G. Canby: *The Patient As a Person.* Commonwealth Fund, New York, 1939.

20b. Duff, R. S., and Hollingshead, A. B.: *Sickness and Society.* Harper & Row, New York, 1968.

20c. Bettelheim, Bruno: *A Home for the Heart.* Alfred Knopf, New York, 1974.

20d. Maguire, J., and McNalley, A. J. "Head Infestations in School Children: Extent of the Problem and Treatment," *Community Med.*, **128**:374, (Aug. 4) 1972.

20e. Wigley, Blodwen: "Patient Community Organization," in Barnes, Elizabeth (ed.): *Psychosocial Nursing.* Tavistock Publications, London, 1968, p. 78.

21. Veninga, Robert: "Communications: A Patient's Eye View," *Am. J. Nurs.*, **73**:320, (Feb.) 1973.

22. Weed, Lawrence L.: *Medical Records, Medical Education, and Patient Care.* Press of Case-Western Reserve University, Cleveland, 1970.

22a. Beeby, Nell: "Where and What Shall We Teach?" *Am. J. Nurs.*, **37**:64, (Jan.) 1937.

22b. Abdellah, Faye G., et al.: *Patient-Centered Approaches to Nursing.* Macmillan Publishing Co., Inc., New York, 1960.

22c. Nite, Gladys, and Willis, Frank N., Jr.: *The Coronary Patient; Hospital Care and Rehabilitation.* Macmillan Publishing Co., Inc., New York, 1964.

23. Mayers, Marlene G.: *A Systematic Approach to the Nursing Care Plan.* Appleton-Century-Crofts, New York, 1972, p. 228.

24. Little, Dolores E., and Carnevali, Doris L.: *Nursing Care Planning.* J. B. Lippincott Co., Philadelphia, 1969, p. 66.

25. Hamilton, Constance B., et al.: "The Nurse's Active Role in Assessment," *Nurs. Clin. North Am.*, **4**:249, (June) 1969.

25a. Aspinall, Mary Jo: "Development of a Patient—Completed Admission Questionnaire and Its Comparison with the Nursing Interview," *Nurs. Res.*, **24**:377, (Sept.–Oct.) 1975.

26. Rothberg, June S.: "Why Nursing Diagnosis?" *Am. J. Nurs.*, **67**:1040, (May) 1967.

26a. Nursing Development Conference Group: *Concept Formalization in Nursing. Process and Product.* Little, Brown & Co., Boston, 1973.

26b. Schwab, Sister Marilyn: "Nursing Care in Nursing Homes," *Am. J. Nurs.*, **75**:1812, (Oct.) 1975.

26c. Horn, Mildred: "Hospital-Based Home Care," *Am. J. Nurs.*, **75**:1811, (Oct.) 1975.

27. Noonan, Barbara R.: "Eight Years in a

Medical Nurse Clinic," *Am. J. Nurs.,* **72:** 1128, (June) 1972.

28. O'Boyle, Catherine: *op. cit.*

29. Cipolla, Josephine A., and Collings, Gilbeart H., Jr.: "Nurse Clinicians in Industry," *Am. J. Nurs.,* **71:**1530, (Aug.) 1971.

30. Biggs, Bee: "Nurse-Clinician-Practitioner-Assistant-Associate," *Am. J. Nurs.,* **71:**1936, (Oct.) 1971.

31. Stearly, Susan, et al.: "Pediatric Nurse Practitioner," *Am. J. Nurs.,* **67:**2083, (Oct.) 1967.

32. Kaku, Kanae, et al.: "Comparison of Health Appraisals by Nurses and Physicians," *Public Health Rep.,* **85:**1042, (Dec.) 1970.

33. Smith, Dorothy W.: "Patienthood and Its Threat to Privacy," *Am. J. Nurs.,* **69:**509, (Mar.) 1969.

33a. Thorndike, E. I.: *Human Nature and the Social Order.* Macmillan Publishing Co., Inc., New York, 1940.

33b. Maslow, Abraham H.: "The Influence of Familiarization on Preference," *J. Exp. Psychol.,* **21:**162, 1937.

33c. Hoffer, Eric: *The Ordeal of Change.* Harper & Row, New York, 1963.

33d. Kogan, Benjamin A.: *Health: Man in a Changing Environment.* Harcourt, Brace & World, New York, 1970.

33e. Dubos, René: *So Human an Animal.* Charles Scribner's Sons, New York, 1968.

34. Bowlby, John: *Attachment and Loss,* Vol. 1. Basic Books, Inc., New York, 1969.

35. Yarrow, Leon J.: "Separation from Parents During Early Childhood," in Hoffman, Martin L., and Hoffman, Lois W. (eds.): *Review of Child Development Research,* Vol. 1. Russell Sage Foundation, New York, 1964, p. 89.

36. Bullard, Dexter M., et al.: "Failure to Thrive in the 'Neglected' Child," in Chess, Stella, and Thomas, Alexander (eds.): *Annual Progress in Child Psychiatry and Child Development.* Brunner/Mazel Publishers, New York, 1968, p. 540.

37. Nash, John: *Developmental Psychology— A Psychobiological Approach.* Prentice-Hall, Inc., Englewood Cliffs, N.J., 1970, p. 315.

38. Hoggart, R.: *The Uses of Literacy.* Beacon Press, Boston, 1961.

39. Ardrey, R.: *The Territorial Imperative.* Atheneum, Inc., New York, 1966.

40. McClelland, D.: *The Roots of Consciousness.* Van Nostrand Reinhold, New York, 1964.

41. Krause, Marie V., and Hunscher, Martha A.: *Food, Nutrition and Diet Therapy,* 5th ed. W. B. Saunders Co., Philadelphia, 1972, pp. 34, 107.

42. Cooke, Robert E. (ed.): *The Biologic Basis of Pediatric Practice.* McGraw-Hill Book Co., New York, 1968, p. 996.

43. *Ibid.,* p. 442.

44. Haller, J. Alex: *The Hospitalized Child and His Family.* Johns Hopkins Press, Baltimore, 1967.

45. Millar, T. P.: "The Hospital and the Pre-School Child," *Children,* **17:**171, (Sept.–Oct.) 1970.

46. Adams, Martha L., and Berman, Dorothy C.: "The Hospital Through a Child's Eyes," *Children,* **12:**102, (May–June) 1965.

47. Blom, Gaston E.: "The Reactions of Hospitalized Children to Illness," *Pediatrics,* **22:** 590, (Sept.) 1958.

48. Mason, Edward A.: "The Hospitalized Child—His Emotional Needs," *N. Engl. J. Med.,* **272:**406, (Feb. 25) 1965.

49. Dombro, Robert H.: "The Surgically Ill Child and His Family," *Surg. Clin. North Am.,* **50:**759, (Aug.) 1970.

50. Mahaffy, Perry R., Jr.: "The Effects of Hospitalization on Children Admitted for Tonsillectomy and Adenoidectomy," *Nurs. Res.,* **14:**12, (Winter) 1965.

51. Cautela, Joseph R.: "A Classical Conditioning Approach to the Development and Modification of Behavior in the Aged," *Gerontologist,* **9:**109, (Summer) 1969.

52. Tallmer, Margot, and Kutner, Bernard: "Disengagement and the Stresses of Aging," *J. Gerontol.,* **24:**70, 1969.

53. Weinberg, Jack: "Environment, Its Language and the Aging," *J. Am. Geriatr. Soc.,* **18:**681, (Sept.) 1970.

54. Bischof, Ledford J.: *Adult Psychology.* Harper & Row, New York, 1969, p. 3.

55. Caudill, William, and Weinstein, Helen: Maternal Care and Infant Behavior in Japan and America," in Lavatelli, Celia, and Stendler, Faith (eds.): *Readings in Child Behavior and Development,* 3rd ed. Harcourt Brace Jovanovich, New York, 1972, p. 78.

56. Clark, Margaret: *op. cit.*

57. Leininger, Madeleine M.: "Nursing Care of a Patient from Another Culture—A Japanese-American Patient," *Nurs. Clin. North Am.,* **2:**747, (Dec.) 1967.

58. Opler, Marvin K.: "Cultural Induction of Stress," in Appley, Mortimer, and Trumbull, Richard (eds.): *Psychological Stress.* Appleton-Century-Crofts, New York, 1967, p. 209.

59. Chilman, Catherine S.: *Growing Up Poor.* US Department of Health, Education, and Welfare, Washington, D.C., 1966 (Welfare Administration Pub. No. 13).

60. Marans, Allen E., and Lourie, Reginald: "Hypotheses Regarding the Effects of Child-Rearing Patterns on the Disadvantaged Child," in Hellmuth, Jerome (ed.): *Disadvantaged Child,* Vol. I. Brunner/Mazel Publishers, New York, 1967, p. 19.

61. Gurin, Gerald, et al.: *Americans View Their Mental Health.* Basic Books, Inc., New York, 1960.

62. Pratt, Lois: "The Relationship of Socioeconomic Status to Health," *Am. J. Public Health,* **61:**281, (Feb.) 1971.

63. Fredrickson, Donald T.: *How To Stop Smoking!* American Heart Association, New York, 1969.

64. Duval, Evelyn Willis: *Family Development,* 4th ed. J. B. Lippincott Co., Philadelphia, 1971, p. 116.

65. Jackson, Don D.: "The Question of Family Homeostasis," *Psychiatr. Q. (Suppl.),* **31:** 79, 1957.

65a. Goldwyn, W. M.: "Disease Is a Family Affair," *Arch. Surg.,* **106:**610, (Apr.) 1973.

66. Anthony, E. James, and Koupernik, Cyrille (eds.): *The Child in His Family.* John Wiley & Sons, New York, 1970, p. 143.

67. Merrow, Dorothy L., and Johnson, Betty Sue: "Perceptions of the Mother's Role with Her Hospitalized Child," *Nurs. Res.,* **17:** 155, (Mar.–Apr.) 1968.

68. Freiberg, Karen H.: "How Parents React When Their Child Is Hospitalized," *Am. J. Nurs.,* **72:**1270, (July) 1972.

69. Baumgart, Alice J., and Smith, Ethel M.: "Day Care for Young Children Undergoing Surgery," *Nurs. Clin. North Am.,* **6:**531, (Sept.) 1971.

70. Condon, Sherrilyn R.: "Day-Time Hospital for Children," *Am. J. Nurs.,* **72:**1431, (Aug.) 1972.

71. Hargreaves, Anne, et al.: "A Day Hospital for Psychiatric Patients," in Mereness, Dorothy: *Psychiatric Nursing,* Vol. I, 2nd ed. Wm. C. Brown Co., Dubuque, Iowa, 1971, p. 200.

72. Libow, L. S., et al.: "The Extended Care Facility at Mount Sinai City Hospital Center, Elmhurst, New York: Three-Year Experience," *J. Am. Geriatr. Soc.,* **16:**1164, (Oct.) 1968.

73. Henderson, Myrtle: "ICU, CCU, and Now a PCU," *Am. J. Nurs.,* **71:**1557, (Aug.) 1971.

74. Pearse, Innes, and Crocker, Lucy H.: *The Peckham Experiment. A Study of the Living Structure of Society.* Yale University Press, New Haven, Conn., 1944.

75. Shetland, Margaret L.: *Family Health Service: A Study of the Department of Educational Nursing of the Community Service Society.* Institute of Welfare Research in cooperation with the Department, New York, 1953.

76. Richardson, Henry B.: *Patients Have Families.* Commonwealth Fund, New York, 1945.

77. Jaco, E. Gartley (ed.): *Patients, Physicians, and Illness,* 2nd ed. Free Press, New York, 1972, p. 1.

78. Seidenfeld, Morton A.: *Psychological Aspects of Medical Care.* Charles C Thomas, Publisher, Springfield, Ill., 1949, p. 17.

79. Joint Commission on Accreditation of Hospitals: *Standards for Accreditation of Hospitals.* The Joint Commission, Chicago, 1969, p. 33.

80. US Social Security Administration: *Conditions of Participation for Hospitals: Federal Health Insurance for the Aged.* (Code of Federal Regulations, Title 20, Chapter 3, Part 405, Section 1024-g.) US Government Printing Office, Washington, D.C., June 1967.

81. Ciuca, Rudy L.: "Over the Years with the Nursing Care Plan," *Nurs. Outlook,* **20:**706, (Nov.) 1972.

82. Alman, Beatrice: "Patients Participate in Nursing Care Conferences," *Am. J. Nurs.,* **67:**2331, (Nov.) 1967.

83. Unangst, Carol: "The Clinician's Use of Nursing Rounds," *Am. J. Nurs.,* **71:**1566, (Aug.) 1971.

84. McPhetridge, L. Mae: "Nursing History: One Means to Personalize Care," *Am. J. Nurs.,* **68:**68, (Jan.) 1968.

85. Sweet, Philothea R., and Stark, Irmagene: "The Circle Care Nursing Plan," *Am. J. Nurs.,* **70:**1300 (June) 1970.

85a. Nursing Development Conference Group: *op. cit.*

86. Mauksch, Ingeborg G., and David, Miriam L.: "Prescription for Survival," *Am. J. Nurs.,* **72:**2189, (Dec.) 1972.

87. Carrieri, Virginia K., and Sitzman, Judith: "Components of the Nursing Process," *Nurs. Clin. North Am.,* **6:**115, (Mar.) 1971.

88. Hurst, J. Willis, and Walker, H. Kenneth (eds.): *The Problem-Oriented System.* Medcom, Inc., New York, 1972.

89. Bloom, Judith T., et al.: "Problem-Oriented Charting," *Am. J. Nurs.,* **71:**2144, (Nov.) 1971.

90. Schell, Pamela L., and Campbell, Alla T.: "POMR—Not Just Another Way to Chart," *Nurs. Outlook,* **20:**510, (Aug.) 1972.

91. Bonkowsky, Marilyn L.: "Adapting the POMR to Community Child Health Care," *Nurs. Outlook,* **20:**515, (Aug.) 1972.

92. Field, Frances W.: "Communication Between Community, Nurse, and Physician," *Nurs. Outlook,* **19:**722, (Nov.) 1971.

93. Aiken, Linda H.: "Patient Problems Are Problems in Learning," *Am. J. Nurs.,* **70:** 1916, (Sept.) 1970.

94. Pierce, Lillian M.: "A Patient-Care Model," *Am. J. Nurs.,* **69:**1700, (Aug.) 1969.

95. Nadler, Gerald, and Sahney, Vinod: "A Descriptive Model of Nursing Care," *Am. J. Nurs.,* **69:**336, (Feb.) 1969.

96. Tayrien, Dorothy, and Lipchak, Amelia: "The Single-Problem Approach," *Am. J. Nurs.,* **67:**2523, (Dec.) 1967.

97. Kraegel, Janet M., et al.: "A System of Patient Care Based on Patient Needs," *Nurs. Outlook,* **20:**257, (Apr.) 1972.

98. Smith, Dorothy M.: "Writing Objectives as a Nursing Practice Skill," *Am. J. Nurs.,* **71:**319, (Feb.) 1971.

98a. Vitale, Barbara, et al.: *A Problem Solving Approach to Nursing Care Plans.* C. V. Mosby Co., St. Louis, 1974.

98b. Hefferin, Elizabeth A., and Hunter, Ruth E.: "Nursing Assessment and Care Plan Statements," *Nurs. Res.,* **24:**360, (Sept.–Oct.) 1975.

98c. Schaefer, Jeanette: "The Interrelatedness of Decision Making and the Nursing Process," *Am. J. Nurs.,* **74:**1852, (Oct.) 1974.

98d. Gebbie, Kristine, and Lavin, Mary Ann (eds.): *Classification of Nursing Diagnoses. Proceedings of First National Conference, Oct. 1–5, 1973.* C. V. Mosby, Co., St. Louis, 1975.

99. Wagner, Berniece M.: "Care Plans—Right, Reasonable, and Reachable," *Am. J. Nurs.,* **69:**986, (May) 1969.

100. Mayers, Marlene G.: *op. cit.*

101. Little, Dolores E., and Carnevali, Doris L.: *op. cit.,* p. 164.

102. Baumeister, Alfred A. (ed.): *Mental Retardation.* Aldine Publishing Co., Chicago, 1967, p. 196.

103. Bower, Fay L.: *The Process of Planning Nursing Care.* C. V. Mosby Co., St. Louis, 1972, p. 14.

104. White, Marguerite B.: "Importance of Selected Nursing Activities," *Nurs. Res.,* **21:**4, (Jan.–Feb.) 1972.

105. Kaufmann, Margaret A.: "Autonomic Responses as Related to Nursing Comfort Measures," *Nurs. Res.,* **13:**45, (Winter) 1964.

106. Hallstrom, Betty J.: "Contact Comfort: Its Application to Immunization Injections," *Nurs. Res.,* **17:**130, (Mar.–Apr.) 1968.

106a. Bower, Fay L.: *op. cit.*

106b. Nelson, Waldo E. (ed.): *Textbook of Pediatrics,* 9th ed. W. B. Saunders Co., Philadelphia, 1969, p. 1382.

106c. *Ibid.,* p. 1070.

107. Cornell, Sudie A., and Brush, Frances: "Systems Approach to Nursing Care Plans," *Am. J. Nurs.,* **71:**1376, (July) 1971.

108. Taylor, Deane B.: "A Clinical Information System: A Tool for Improving Nurses' Decisions in Planning Patient Care," in *ANA Clinical Sessions, 1970.* Appleton-Century-Crofts, New York, 1971, p. 159.

108a. Reiften, B., et al.: "The Use of Computers in Ambulatory Care. Lessons from 3000 Computers," *Comput. Biol. Med.,* **3:**101, (Sept.) 1973.

108b. Goodwin, Judy Ozbolt, and Edwards, Bernadine Symons: "Developing a Computer Program to Assist the Nursing Process: Phase I—From Systems Analysis to an Expandable Program," *Nurs. Res.,* **24:**299, (July–Aug.) 1975.

109. Brown, Mary E.: "Daily Activity Inventory and Progress Record for Those with Atypical Movement," *Am. J. Occup. Ther.,* **4:**195, (Sept.–Oct.) 1950; **4:**261, (Nov.–Dec.) 1950; **4:**23, (Jan.–Feb.) 1951.

110. Parsons, Talcott: "Definitions of Health and Illness in the Light of American Values and Social Structure," in Jaco, E. Gartley (ed.): *Patients, Physicians, and Illness,* 2nd ed. Free Press, New York, 1972, p. 117.

111. Blum, Henrik L., et al.: *Health Planning 1969.* American Public Health Association, Washington, D.C., 1969, p. 308.

111a. Riffle, Kathren L.: "Rehabilitation: The Evolution of a Social Concept," *Nurs. Clin. North Am.,* **8:**665, (Dec.) 1973.

112. Holley, Lydia: "The Physical Therapist—Who, What, and How," *Am. J. Nurs.,* **70:**1521, (July) 1970.

113. Holmes, Jean E.: "The Physical Therapist and Team Care," *Nurs. Outlook,* **20:**182, (Mar.) 1972.

114. West, Wilma L.: "Occupational Therapy—Philosophy and Perspective," *Am. J. Nurs.,* **68:**1708, (Aug.) 1968.

115. Mikulic, Mary Ann: "Reinforcement of Independent and Dependent Patient Behaviors by Nursing Personnel: An Exploratory Study," *Nurs. Res.,* **20:**162, (Mar.–Apr.) 1971.

116. Cornell, Sudie A., and Brush, Frances: *op. cit.*

117. Littman, Theodore: "The Family and Physical Rehabilitation," *J. Chronic Dis.,* **19:**211, (Feb.) 1966.

118. New, Peter, et al.: "The Support Structure of Heart and Stroke Patients," *Soc. Sci. Med.,* **2:**185, (June) 1968.

119. Dahlin, Bernice: "Rehabilitation and the Assessment of Patient Need," *Nurs. Clin. North Am.,* **1:**375, (Sept.) 1966.

120. Murray, Ruth L. E.: "Principles of Nursing Intervention for the Adult Patient with Body Image Changes," *Nurs. Clin. North Am.,* **7:**697, (Dec.) 1972.

121. Germain, Carol P.: "Exercise Makes the Heart Grow Stronger," *Am. J. Nurs.,* **72:**2169, (Dec.) 1972.

122. Barry, Ethel M., et al.: "Hospital Program for Cardiac Rehabilitation," *Am. J. Nurs.,* **72:**2174, (Dec.) 1972.

123. Guerrieri, Belga O.: "Survey of the Knowledge of the Nurse in Direct-Care Services Concerning Proper Bed Positioning of the Patient with Hemiplegia," *Nurs. Res.,* **17:**157, (Mar.–Apr.) 1968.

124. Stuart, Sarah: "Day-to-Day Living with Diabetes," *Am. J. Nurs.,* **71:**1548, (Aug.) 1971.

125. Murray, Barbara S., et al.: "The Patient Has an Ileal Conduit," *Am. J. Nurs.,* **71:**1560, (Aug.) 1971.

126. Reif, Laura: "Managing a Life with Chronic Disease," *Am. J. Nurs.,* **73:**261, (Feb.) 1973.

126a. Waltrous, W. B.: "Rehabilitation Nurse: Counselor and Coordinator," *Occup. Health Nurs.,* **21:**16, (Dec.) 1973.

127. Stryker, Ruth P.: *Rehabilitative Aspects of Acute and Chronic Nursing Care.* W. B. Saunders Co., Philadelphia, 1972, p. 17.

127a. Christopherson, V. A., et al.: *Rehabilitation Nursing; Perspectives and Applications.* McGraw-Hill Book Co., New York, 1974.

128. Laing, R. D.: *Self and Others.* Pantheon Books, Division of Random House, New York, 1969.

129. Cooper, David: *Psychiatry and Anti-Psychiatry.* Ballantine Books, New York, 1967.

130. Laing, R. D.: *The Politics of Experience.* Ballantine Books, New York, 1967.

131. Watts, Alan W.: *Psychotherapy, East and West.* Ballantine Books, New York, 1961.

132. Mereness, Dorothy: *Psychiatric Nursing,* Vol. I, 2nd ed. Wm. C. Brown Co., Dubuque, Iowa, 1971, p. viii.

133. Waechter, Eugenia H.: "Developmental Correlates of Physical Disability," *Nurs. Forum,* 9:91, (No. 1) 1970.

134. Erickson, Florence: "Nurse: Viewpoints on Children in Hospitals," *Hospitals,* 37: 47, (May 16) 1963.

135. Meyer, Herbert L.: "Predictable Problems of Hospitalized Adolescents," *Am. J. Nurs.,* 69:525, (Mar.) 1969.

136. Langford, William S.: "Physical Illness and Convalescence: Their Meaning to the Child," *J. Pediatr.,* 33:242, (Aug.) 1948.

137. Morgenstern, F. S.: "Facilities for Children's Play in Hospitals," *Dev. Med. Child Neurol.,* 10:111, (Feb.) 1968.

138. Grant, Wilson W.: "The Child Plus the Parent Equal 1 Patient: An Important Lesson," *Clin. Pediatr.,* 11:433, (Aug.) 1972.

139. Meadow, S. R.: "The Captive Mother," *Arch. Dis. Child.,* 44:362, (June) 1969.

140. Moran, Patricia A.: "Parents in Pediatrics," *Nurs. Forum,* 2:25, (No. 3) 1963.

141. McBride, Angela Barron: *The Growth and Development of Mothers.* Harper & Row, New York, 1973.

142. Kekich, Edna B.: "Illustrated HELP for Diabetic Patients," in *ANA Clinical Sessions, 1970.* Appleton-Century-Crofts, New York, 1971, p. 30.

143. Moss, Fay T.: "Select-A-Meal: An Aid for Teaching Diabetic Diet," in *ANA Clinical Sessions, 1970.* Appleton-Century-Crofts, New York, 1971, p. 37.

143a. Moreland, Helen J., and Schmitt, Virginia C.: "Making Referrals Is Everybody's Business," *Am. J. Nurs.,* 74:96, (Jan.) 1974.

144. Valentine, Lois R.: "Self-Care Through Group Learning," *Am. J. Nurs.,* 70:2140, (Oct.) 1970.

145. Baden, Catherine A.: "Teaching the Coronary Patient and His Family," *Nurs. Clin. North Am.,* 7:563, (Sept.) 1972.

146. Casoly, Rose Marie: "Give the Patient His Due," *Am. J. Nurs.,* 72:1101, (June) 1972.

147. Bergeron, Janet H.: "A Patient's Plea: Tell Me, I Need to Know," *Am. J. Nurs.,* 71: 1572, (Aug.) 1971.

148. Dodge, Joan S.: "What Patients Should Be Told: Patients' and Nurses' Beliefs," *Am. J. Nurs.,* 72:1852, (Oct.) 1972.

149. Ornstein, Sheldon: "A Nursing Home Is Not a Hospital," *Nurs. Outlook,* 21:28, (Jan.) 1973.

150. Deakers, Lynne P.: "Continuity of Family-Centered Nursing Care Between the Hospital and the Home," *Nurs. Clin. North Am.,* 7:83, (Mar.) 1972.

151. Peabody, Sylvia R.: "Assessment and Planning for Continuity of Care from Hospital to Home," *Nurs. Clin. North Am.,* 4:303, (June) 1969.

152. Calleia, Patricia, and Boswick, John A., Jr.: "A Home Care Nursing Program for Patients with Burns," *Am. J. Nurs.,* 72: 1442, (Aug.) 1972.

153. Nielsen, Sharon: "Home Visiting for Patients Receiving Special Care," *Nurs. Clin. North Am.,* 7:383, (June) 1972.

154. Taylor, Sharon: "The Initiation and Development of a Hospital-Based Home Health Agency," in *ANA Clinical Conferences, 1969.* Appleton-Century-Crofts, New York, 1970, p. 113.

155. Nehren, Jeanette, and Gilliam, Naomi R.: "Separation Anxiety," in Mereness, Dorothy (ed.): *Psychiatric Nursing,* Vol. I, 2nd ed. Wm. C. Brown Co., Dubuque, Iowa, 1971, p. 121.

156. Donabedian, Avedis: "Part II—Some Issues in Evaluating the Quality of Nursing Care," *Am. J. Public Health,* 59:1833, (Oct.) 1969.

157. Billars, Karen S.: "You Have Pain? I Think This Will Help," *Am. J. Nurs.,* 70: 2143, (Oct.) 1970.

158. Chambers, Wilda G., and Price, Geraldine G.: "Influence of Nurse Upon Effects of Analgesics Administered," *Nurs. Res.,* 16: 228, (Summer) 1967.

159. Moss, Fay T.: "The Effect of a Nursing Intervention on Pain Relief," in *ANA Regional Clinical Conferences, 1967.* Appleton-Century-Crofts, New York, 1968.

160. Rubin, Charlene F., et al.: "Nursing Audit —Nurses Evaluating Nursing," *Am. J. Nurs.,* 72:916, (May) 1972.

161. Dann, H. W., and Morgan, I. M.: *The Nursing Audit.* National League for Nursing, New York, 1968 (League Exchange No. 84).

162. Pardee, Geraldine, et al.: "Patient Care Evaluation Is Every Nurse's Job," *Am. J. Nurs.,* 71:1958, (Oct.) 1971.

163. Freeman, Ruth B., and Lowe, Marie: "A Method for Appraising Family Public Health Nursing Needs," *Am. J. Public Health,* 53:47, (Jan.) 1963.

164. Schwartz, Doris R.: "Toward More Precise Evaluation of Patients' Needs," *Nurs. Outlook,* 13:42, (May) 1965.

165. Phaneuf, Maria: *Nursing Audit: Profile for Excellence.* Appleton-Century-Crofts, New York, 1972.

166. Rinaldi, Leena Alto, and Rubin, Charlene F.: "Adding Retrospective Audit," *Am. J. Nurs.,* 75:256, (Feb.) 1975.

167. Block, Doris: "Evaluation of Nursing Care in Terms of Process and Outcomes: Issues in Research and Quality Assurance," *Nurs. Res.,* 24:256, (July–Aug.) 1975.

168. Johnson, Marion: "Outcome Criteria to Evaluate Postoperative Respiratory Status," *Am. J. Nurs.,* 75:1474, (Sept.) 1975.

169. Moore, Dianne A., and Cook-Hubbard,

Karen: "Comparison of Methods for Evaluating Patient Response to Nursing Care," *Nurs. Res.*, **24**:202, (May–June) 1975.

Additional Suggested Reading

Alexander, Edythe L.: "Symposium on Management and Supervision of Patient Care," *Nurs. Clin. North Am.*, **8**:203, (June) 1973.

Alfano, Genrose J.: "There Are No Routine Patients," *Am. J. Nurs.*, **75**:1804, (Oct.) 1975.

Anderson, Nancy: "Rehabilitative Nursing Practice," *Nurs. Clin. North Am.*, **6**:303, (June) 1971.

Apgar, Virginia, and Beck, Joan: *Is My Baby All Right.* Trident Press, New York, 1973.

Aradine, Carolyn R., and Guthneck, Margaret: "The Problem-Oriented Record in a Family Health Service," *Am. J. Nurs.*, **74**:1108, (June) 1974.

Ayrault, Evelyn West: *Helping the Handicapped Teenager Mature.* Association Press, New York, 1971.

Ballantyne, Donna J.: "CCTV for Patients," *Am. J. Nurs.*, **74**:263, (Feb.) 1974.

Bayer, Mary: "Easing Mental Patients' Return to Their Communities," *Am. J. Nurs.*, **76**:406, (Mar.) 1976.

Bielski, Mary T.: "Continuity of Care for the Patient with Coronary Heart Disease," *Nurs. Clin. North Am.*, **7**:413, (Sept.) 1972.

Brady, Eugenia: "Grief and Amputation," in *ANA Clinical Sessions, 1968.* Appleton-Century-Crofts, New York, 1969.

Brink, Pamela: "Natural Triad in Health Care," *Am. J. Nurs.*, **72**:897, (May) 1972.

Carlson, Sylvia: "A Practical Approach to the Nursing Process," *Am. J. Nurs.*, **72**:1589, (Sept.) 1972.

Chamberlin, Robert W.: "Social Data in Evaluation of the Pediatric Patient; Deficits in Outpatient Records," *J. Pediatr.*, **78**:111, (Jan.) 1971.

Chastko, Helen E., et al.: "Patients' Posthospital Evaluations of Psychiatric Nursing Treatment," *Nurs. Res.*, **20**:333, (July–Aug.) 1971.

Culbert, Pamela A., and Kos, Barbara A.: "Aging: Considerations for Health Teaching," *Nurs. Clin. North Am.*, **6**:605, (Dec.) 1971.

Davitz, Lois J., and Davitz, Joel R.: "How Do Nurses Feel When Patients Suffer?" *Am. J. Nurs.*, **75**:1505, (Sept.) 1975.

Eyres, Patricia J.: "The Role of the Nurse in Family-Centered Nursing Care," *Nurs. Clin. North Am.*, **7**:27, (Mar.) 1972.

Falknor, H. M., et al.: "Resocializing: Through a Stroke Club," *Nurs. Outlook*, **21**:776, (Dec.) 1973.

Feller, I., et al.: "The Team Approach to Total Rehabilitation of the Severely Burned Patient," *Heart Lung*, **2**:701, (Sept.–Oct.) 1973.

Fuller, Dorothy, and Rosenaur, Janet Allan: "A Patient Assessment Guide," *Nurs. Outlook*, **22**:460, (July) 1974.

Garant, Carol: "A Basis for Care," *Am. J. Nurs.*, **72**:699, (Apr.) 1972.

Geddes, Dolores: *Physical Activities for Individuals with Handicapping Conditions.* C. V. Mosby Co., St. Louis, 1974.

Gowan, Naomi M., and Morris, Miriam: "Nurses' Responses to Expressed Patient Needs," *Nurs. Res.*, **13**:68, (Winter) 1963.

Gozzi, Ethel K., et al.: "Gaps in Doctor-Patient Communication," *Am. J. Nurs.*, **69**:529, (Mar.) 1969.

Hassett, Marjorie: "Teaching Hemodialysis to the Family Unit," *Nurs. Clin. North Am.*, **7**:349, (June) 1972.

Hayes, Evelyn R.: "Clinic Waiting Room Experience: An Exploratory Study," *Nurs. Res.*, **17**:361, (July–Aug.) 1968.

Henderson, Gloria M.: "Teaching-Learning for Rehabilitation of the Spinal Cord-Disabled Individual," *Nurs. Clin. North Am.*, **6**:655, (Dec.) 1971.

Henderson, Virginia: *ICN Basic Principles of Nursing Care,* 4th ed. International Council of Nurses, Geneva, 1968.

Holdaway, David: "Educating the Handicapped Child and His Parents," *Clin. Pediatr.*, **11**:63, (Feb.) 1972.

Johnson, Dorothy E.: "Powerlessness," *J. Nurs. Educ.*, **6**:39, (Apr.) 1967.

Kalisch, B. J.: "Summer Theater: Another Way to Learn," *Nurs. Outlook*, **22**:31, (Jan.) 1974.

Katona, Elizabeth A.: "A Patient-Centered, Living-Oriented Approach to the Patient with an Artificial Anus or Bladder," *Nurs. Clin. North Am.*, **2**:623, (Dec.) 1967.

Korsch, Barbara, et al.: "How Comprehensive Are Well Child Visits?" *Am. J. Dis. Child.*, **122**:483, (Dec.) 1971.

LaFargue, Jane P.: "Role of Prejudice in Rejection of Health Care," *Nurs. Res.*, **21**:53, (Jan.–Feb.) 1972.

Lederer, Henry D.: "How the Sick View Their World," in Skipper, James K., and Leonard, Robert C. (eds.): *Social Interaction and Patient Care.* J. B. Lippincott Co., Philadelphia, 1965, p. 155.

Leonard, Beverly J.: "Body Image Changes in Chronic Illness," *Nurs. Clin. North Am.*, **7**:687, (Dec.) 1972.

Lewis, Edith P.: "Everybody's Patient Is Nobody's Patient," *Nurs. Outlook*, **23**:551, (Sept.) 1975.

Little, Dolores E., and Carnevali, Doris L.: "The Nursing Care Planning System," *Nurs. Outlook*, **19**:164, (Mar.) 1971.

Lunt, J.: "Bridging the Gap in Continuity of Care," *Nurs. Times*, **66**:372, (Mar. 19) 1970.

McCain, R. Faye: "Nursing by Assessment—Not Intuition," *Am. J. Nurs.*, **65**:82, (Apr.) 1965.

McCloskey, Joanne Connie: "The Problem-Oriented Record vs. the Nursing Care Plan: A Proposal," *Nurs. Outlook*, **23**:492, (Aug.) 1975.

McWhinney, Ian R.: "Beyond Diagnosis: An Approach to the Integration of Behavioral Science and Clinical Medicine," *N. Engl. J. Med.*, **287**:384, (Aug. 24) 1972.

Malecki, Madge A.: "What's the Name of the

Game?" in *ANA Clinical Sessions, 1968.* Appleton-Century-Crofts, New York, 1969.

Manthey, Marie: "A Guide for Interviewing," *Am. J. Nurs.,* **67:**2088, (Oct.) 1967.

Marshall, Jon C., and Feeney, Sally: "Structured Versus Intuitive Intake Interview," *Nurs. Res.,* **21:**269, (May–June) 1972.

Mayers, Marlene: "A Search for Assessment Criteria," *Nurs. Outlook,* **20:**323, (May) 1972.

Mezzanotte, Elizabeth J.: "Group Instruction in Preparation for Surgery," *Am. J. Nurs.,* **70:**89, (Jan.) 1970.

Millsap, Mary: "Occupational Health Nursing in an Alcohol Addiction Program," *Nurs. Clin. North Am.,* **7:**121, (Mar.) 1972.

Molde, Donald, and Wiens, Arthur: "Interview Interaction Behavior of Nurses with Task Versus Person Orientation," *Nurs. Res.,* **17:**45, (Jan.–Feb.) 1968.

Moore, Bernice M.: "Education for Family Living—What Is It?" *Nurs. Clin. North Am.,* **4:**359, (June) 1969.

Moses, Dorothy V.: "The Older Patient in the General Hospital," *Nurs. Clin. North Am.,* **2:**705, (Dec.) 1967.

Neely, Elizabeth, and Patrick, Maxine L.: "Problems of Aged Persons Taking Medications at Home," *Nurs. Res.,* **17:**52, (Jan.–Feb.) 1968.

Neuman, Betty M., and Young, Rae Jeanne: "A Model for Teaching Total Person Approach to Patient Problems," *Nurs. Res.,* **21:**264, (May–June) 1972.

Nicholls, Marion E.: "Quality Control in Patient Care," *Am. J. Nurs.,* **74:**456, (Mar.) 1974.

Ohno, Mary I.: "The Eye-Patched Patient," *Am. J. Nurs.,* **71:**271, (Feb.) 1971.

O'Neill, Mary: "Guidelines for Teaching Home Dialysis," *Nurs. Clin. North Am.,* **6:**641, (Dec.) 1971.

Orme, June Y., and Lindbeck, Rosemary S.: "Nurse Participation in Medical Peer Review," *Nurs. Outlook,* **22:**27, (Jan.) 1974.

Owens, Margaret L.: "Special Care for the Patient Who Has a Breast Biopsy or Mastectomy," *Nurs. Clin. North Am.,* **7:**373, (June) 1972.

Palm, Mary L.: "Recognizing Opportunities for Informal Patient Teaching," *Nurs. Clin. North Am.,* **6:**669, (Dec.) 1971.

Palmer, Irene S. (ed.): "Symposium on Nursing in Long-Term Illness," *Nurs. Clin. North Am.,* **5:**1, (Mar.) 1970.

Peplau, Hildegard E.: "Talking with Patients," *Am. J. Nurs.,* **60:**964, (July) 1960.

Quinn, Nancy, and Somers, Anne R.: "The Patient's Bill of Rights, a Significant Aspect of the Consumer Revolution," *Nurs. Outlook,* **22:**240, (Apr.) 1974.

Ramphal, Marjorie: "Peer Review," *Am. J. Nurs.,* **74:**63, (Jan.) 1974.

Reid, Margaret F., and Waddicor, Pamela E.: "Continuity of Patient Care," *Nurs. Times,* **66:**798, (June 8) 1970.

Rossman, Isadore: "The Montefiore Hospital After-Care Program," *Nurs. Outlook,* **22:**325, (May) 1974.

Rothberg, June S. (ed.): "Symposium on Chronic Disease and Rehabilitation," *Nurs. Clin. North Am.,* **1:**352, (Sept.) 1966.

Safilios-Rothschild, Constantina: *The Sociology and Social Psychology of Disability and Rehabilitation.* Random House, New York, 1970.

Scahill, Mary: "Preparing Children for Procedures and Operations," *Nurs. Outlook,* **17:**36, (June) 1969.

Scanlon, Mary E.: "An Industrial Visiting Nurse," *Nurs. Clin. North Am.,* **7:**143, (Mar.) 1972.

Schmidt, Joan: "Availability: A Concept of Nursing Practice," *Am. J. Nurs.,* **72:**1086, (June) 1972.

Schulman, Jerome L.: et al.: "Videotape Sampling of the Child's Day in the Hospital," *J. Pediatr.,* **76:**728, (May) 1970.

Schultz, Nancy: "How Children Perceive Pain," *Nurs. Outlook,* **19:**670, (Oct.) 1971.

Severyn, Betty Rose: "Nursing Implications with a Loss of Body Function," in *ANA Clinical Conferences, 1969.* Appleton-Century-Crofts, New York, 1970.

Shields, Mary: "An Evaluation Model for Service Programs," *Nurs. Outlook,* **22:**448, (July) 1974.

Shope, Joanne: "Parental Involvement Program," *Nurs. Outlook,* **18:**32, (Apr.) 1970.

Skipper, James K., and Leonard, Robert C.: "Children, Stress and Hospitalization: A Field Experiment," *J. Health Soc. Behav.,* **9:**275, (Dec.) 1968.

Smith, Dorothy M.: "A Clinical Nursing Tool," *Am. J. Nurs.,* **68:**2384 (Nov.) 1968.

Spock, Benjamin, and Lerrigo, Marion O.: *Caring for Your Disabled Child.* Macmillan Publishing Co., Inc., New York, 1968.

Steen, Joyce: "Liaison Nurse: Ombudsman for the Chronically Ill," *Am. J. Nurs.,* **73:**2102, (Dec.) 1973.

Stohl, Dora J.: "Preserving Home Life for the Disabled," *Am. J. Nurs.,* **72:**1645, (Sept.) 1972.

Struempler, Lorraine: "A Mother of a Child with Facial and Other Visible Anomalies," in Anderson, Edith H., et al. (eds.): *Current Concepts in Clinical Nursing,* Vol. IV. C. V. Mosby Co., St. Louis, 1973.

Tapia, Jayne A.: "The Nursing Process in Family Health," *Nurs. Outlook,* **20:**267, (Apr.) 1972.

Tryon, Phyllis A.: "Patient Participation vs. Patient Passivity," *Nurs. Forum,* **2:**48, (No. 2) 1963.

————, and Leonard, Robert C.: "The Effect of the Patient's Participation on the Outcome of a Nursing Procedure," *Nurs. Forum,* **3:**79, (No. 2) 1964.

Tyzenttouse, Phyllis: "Care Plans for Nursing Home Patients," *Nurs. Outlook,* **20:**169, (Mar.) 1972.

Vincent, Pauline: "Factors Influencing Patient Noncompliance: A Theoretical Approach," *Nurs. Res.,* **20:**509, (Nov.–Dec.) 1971.

Volicer, Beverly J., and Bohannon, Mary Wynne: "A Hospital Stress Rating Scale," *Nurs. Res.,* **24:**352, (Sept.–Oct.) 1975.

Wagner, Mary M.: "Assessment of Patients with Multiple Injuries," *Am. J. Nurs.,* **72:**1822, (Oct.) 1972.

Weinberg, S. L.: "Patient Education as a Part of Critical Care," *Heart Lung,* **3:**47, (Jan.–Feb.) 1974.

Weiner, Florence: *Help for the Handicapped Child.* McGraw-Hill Book Co., New York, 1973.

Williams, Barbara P.: "Life Styles of Severely Burned Men," in *ANA Clinical Conferences, 1969.* Appleton-Century-Crofts, New York, 1970.

———: "The Burned Patient's Need for Teaching," *Nurs. Clin. North Am.,* **6:**615, (Dec.) 1971.

Williams, Mary E.: "The Patient Profile," *Nurs. Res.,* **9:**122, (Summer) 1960.

Wu, Ruth: *Behavior and Illness.* Prentice-Hall, Inc., Englewood Cliffs, N.J., 1973.

Zimmerman, Donna, and Gohrke, Carol: "The Goal-Directed Nursing Approach: It Does Work," *Am. J. Nurs.,* **70:**306, (Feb.) 1970.

Gladys Nite
Catherine Temple
Virginia Henderson

The authors acknowledge the help of Roberta O'Grady who prepared the patient study.

PART III

Fundamentals of Nursing Care—Helping Others Provide for Their Basic Needs

CHAPTER 9

Respiration

1. RESPIRATION, A REVIEW OF CONCEPTS

The development of respiratory physiology is a fascinating subject showing the evolution of an advanced science from folklore. "The breath of life" is an expression found in early records. The mechanisms of this mystical function were not understood by primitive man, but the process of breathing was appreciated as a necessity for the maintenance of life and the power to breathe was attributed to a supernatural spirit.

Hippocrates (460–377 B.C.) introduced the idea that the main purpose of breathing was to cool the heart, a theory accepted by the Greeks for over five centuries. Galen (A.D. 130–201) advanced man's understanding of respiration with his teaching on circulation, diaphragmatic contractions, and movements of the chest wall. These insights antedated the scientific developments of the seventeenth century. Discovery of the closed system of peripheral and pulmonary circulation by William Harvey (1578–1657) provided a basis for research in respiration. Yet, Harvey himself remained uncertain as to the function of respiration and could not discard the idea of refrigeration of the heart. Antoine Laurent Lavoisier's discovery of oxygen as the vital ingredient of the air marked the beginning of a new era in respiratory chemistry and helped establish the dependence of medical progress on the basic sciences. By the nineteenth century, "laws" explaining the behavior of gases had been established that helped explain respiratory function. During the twentieth century, great advances have been made in the understanding of this function. The present concept of respiration evolved from mysticism, religion, philosophy, and speculative medicine into a scientific theory.[1-3]

Respiration is defined as the exchange of gases between an organism and its environment, specifically, for animals, the transport of oxygen from the atmosphere to the cells and the transport of carbon dioxide from the cells to the atmosphere. Respiration is common to all living things because it is essential to metabolism, on which life depends. The human body can survive for weeks without food, except that from its own tissues, but only for a matter of minutes without oxygen. However, animal tissues can be kept alive outside the body if they are perfused with oxygen and nutrients just as the fetus is kept alive in the uterus without pulmonary respiration.

Normal respiration involves pulmonary ventilation, diffusion and transport of gases, and regulation of respiration.

2. PULMONARY VENTILATION [4-6]

Definition. Pulmonary ventilation refers to the actual flow of air between the atmosphere and the alveoli, that is, the movement of air into the lungs with inspiration, followed by expulsion of the gases with expiration.

The Respiratory System. The upper respiratory system filters, humidifies, and warms the air as it passes to the lungs. The bronchi divide into the terminal bronchioles, the respiratory bronchioles, the alveolar ducts, atria, and the alveoli (see Fig. 9-1).

Air containing roughly 20 per cent oxygen and 0.04 per cent carbon dioxide is drawn into the lungs, where the lining of approximately 750 million air sacs provides a very large "surface" where the blood in its capillaries can rapidly pick up oxygen and give up carbon dioxide. The expired air contains approximately 16 per cent oxygen and 4 per cent carbon dioxide. In addition to providing for the exchange of gases, the respiratory system functions in sneezing, coughing, phonation (speaking), yawning, and sighing.

Mechanics of Breathing. Air is moved into and out of the lungs by movements of the diaphragm and associated muscles of respiration

623

(see Fig. 9-2). Inspiration is the active phase of breathing and involves contraction of the diaphragm, the external intercostal muscles, and the *small* neck muscles. On inspiration, the thoracic cavity elongates as the diaphragm descends. Contraction of the external intercostal muscles lifts the rib cage and increases the volume of the chest cavity. On expiration, the diaphragm ascends, the rib cage falls, and, because of elasticity, the lungs recoil. The abdominal muscles can be recruited for active expiration but are normally relaxed during quiet expiration.[7,8] Muscular work is required during labored breathing and forced expiration such as coughing, straining, or whistling. It is obvious that the strength of all of these muscles influences the effectiveness of breathing and the amount of work necessary to carry out this vital function.

Mechanics of Air Flow. Ventilation is accomplished by alternating compression and distention of the lungs. During inspiration, the intrapulmonary pressure is slightly negative (−3 mm Hg) and air flows into the respiratory passage and inflates the lungs; on expiration, the intrapulmonary pressure rises to +3 mm Hg, and air is forced out of the passage. The maximum intrathoracic pressure, achieved

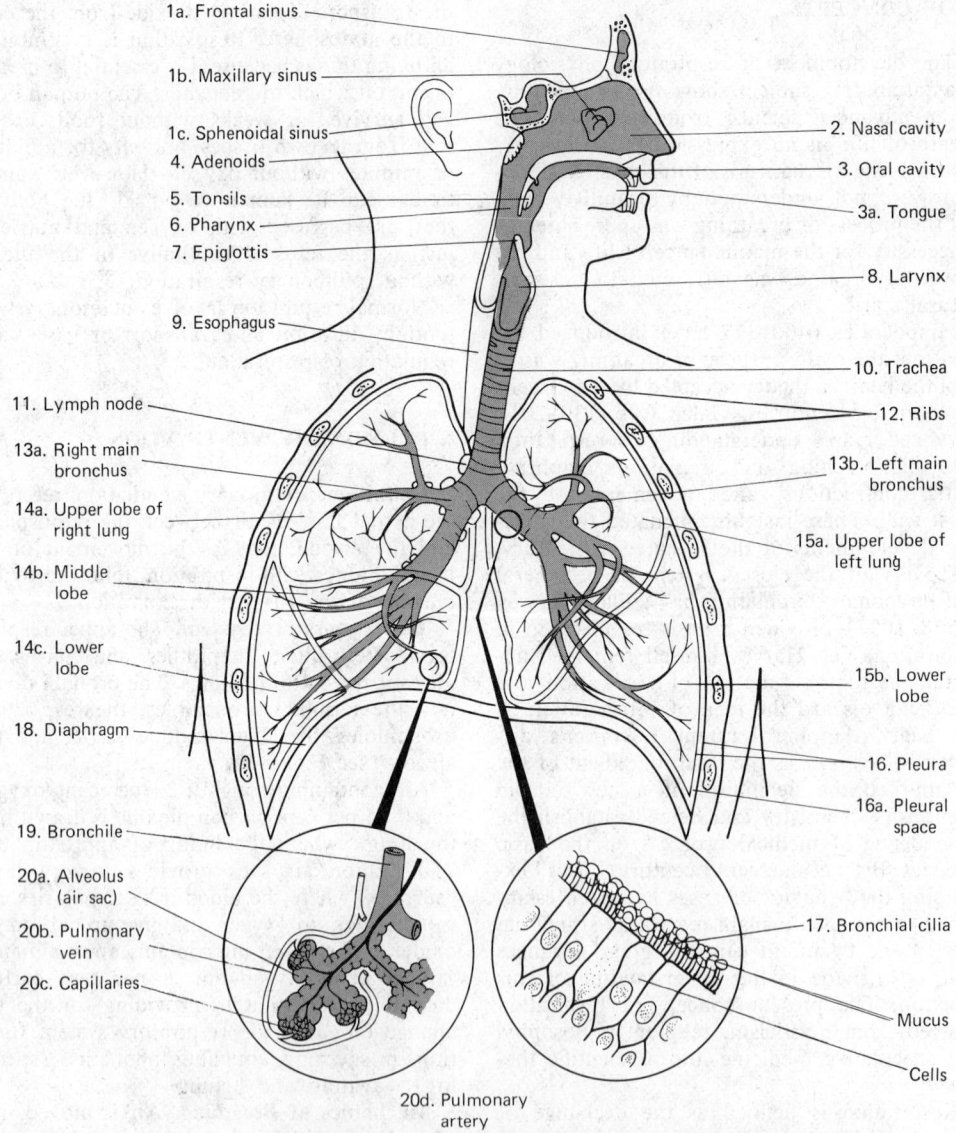

1a. Frontal sinus
1b. Maxillary sinus
1c. Sphenoidal sinus
4. Adenoids
5. Tonsils
6. Pharynx
7. Epiglottis
9. Esophagus
11. Lymph node
13a. Right main bronchus
14a. Upper lobe of right lung
14b. Middle lobe
14c. Lower lobe
18. Diaphragm
19. Bronchile
20a. Alveolus (air sac)
20b. Pulmonary vein
20c. Capillaries
20d. Pulmonary artery

2. Nasal cavity
3. Oral cavity
3a. Tongue
8. Larynx
10. Trachea
12. Ribs
13b. Left main bronchus
15a. Upper lobe of left lung
15b. Lower lobe
16. Pleura
16a. Pleural space
17. Bronchial cilia
Mucus
Cells

Figure 9-1. A detailed diagram of the respiratory system. (Courtesy of American Lung Association, New York, N.Y.)

by forced expiration against a closed glottis (Valsalva maneuver), may exceed 100 mm Hg and may occur during daily activities such as lifting heavy objects or straining at stool.* Excessive intrathoracic pressure can be dangerous for those persons with an impaired cardiac function. Inspiration against a closed glottis (Mueller's maneuver) can decrease the intrathoracic pressure to −80 mm Hg.

The intrapleural pressure, that pressure between the lung and chest wall, is normally negative to atmospheric pressure (see Fig. 9-3). This negative pressure keeps the lungs expanded or prevents their collapse. As the intrapleural pressure decreases during inspiration, the intrapulmonary volume increases, the pressure of the gases in the lungs decreases, and air moves from the area of higher pressure in the atmosphere to the area of lower pressure in the lungs until equilibrium is reached.[9,10]

The lungs are normally expanded, but tend to collapse when exposed to atmospheric pressure; this tendency to collapse is influenced by two factors, the surface tension of the layer of fluid lining the alveoli and the elasticity of the lung.

Surfactant is a phospholipid product of alveolar tissue metabolism which prevents collapse of the alveoli by decreasing the surface tension of the fluid lining the alveoli and the respiratory passages as they contract. All alveoli are not the same size, yet the pressure in the lungs is reasonably uniform. By altering the surface tension of the fluid in the alveoli, surfactant maintains the integrity of the respiratory system and prevents overinflation of the larger alveoli and the collapse of the smaller ones. On expiration, the size of each alveolus is decreased; the surfactant molecules become concentrated and decrease the surface tension. During inspiration, the size of each alveolus is increased; the molecules of the surfactant disperse, become less concentrated, and the surface tension is increased.

The surfactant may be altered by disease or by mechanical procedures; for example, hyaline membrane disease in the newborn is due to inadequate production of surfactant. Surfactant is also reduced following cardiopulmonary bypass, shock, trauma, aspiration, and smoke and chemical inhalation. Increased surface tension makes it difficult for the alveoli to expand. Oxygen, administered at several atmospheres of pressure, can decrease the level of surfactant and be a great hazard to children and adults.[11]

Compliance is the expansibility of the lungs and thorax and may be defined as the volume change in the lungs for each unit of intraalveolar pressure change. Considerable energy must be exerted by the muscles of inspiration to expand the thoracic cage as well as the lungs; the lungs removed from the chest are

* It is often remarked that strokes and heart attacks occur during expulsion of a hard stool.

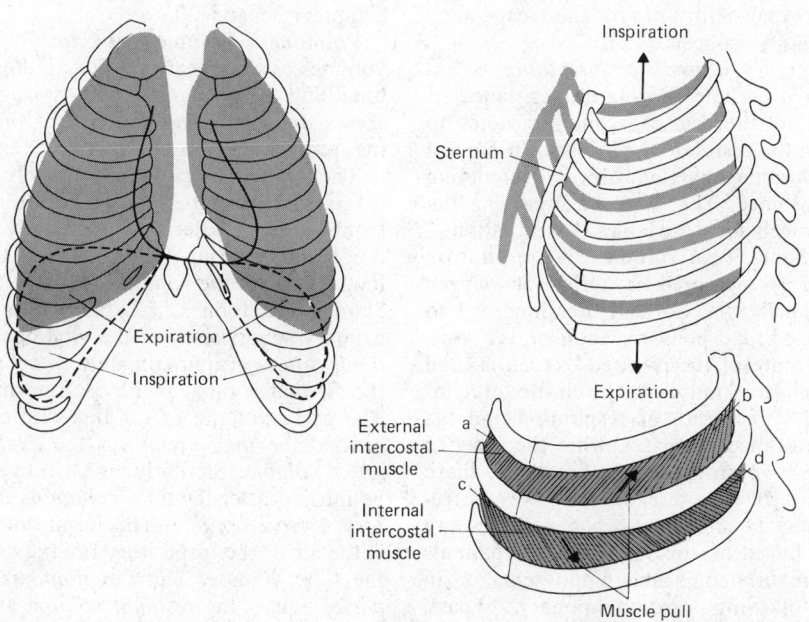

Figure 9-2. Diagram showing position of lungs, ribs, and sternum during inspiration and expiration. (From Tuttle, W. W., and Schottelius, Byron A.: *Textbook of Physiology,* 16th ed. C. V. Mosby Co., St. Louis, 1969, p. 309.)

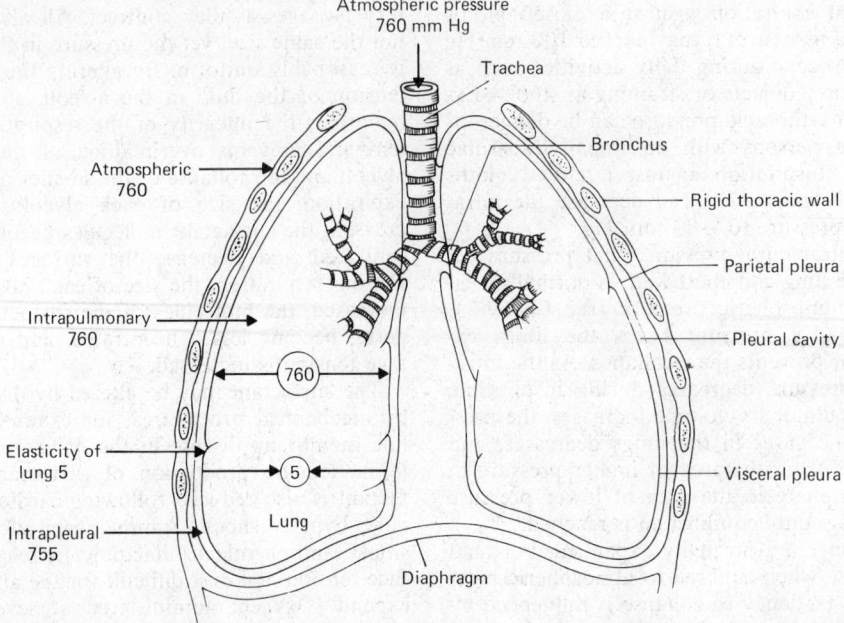

Figure 9-3. Illustration of thoracic cavity structures showing intrapulmonary and intrapleural pressures with chest wall in resting position. (From Tuttle, W. W., and Schottelius, Byron A.: *Textbook of Physiology,* 16th ed. C. V. Mosby Co., St. Louis, 1969, p. 310.)

almost twice as distensible as the lungs enclosed by the thorax.[12]

Abnormal compliance may be the result of disease or damage of lung tissue, fibrosis, edema, blocked alveoli, or abnormality that reduces the expansibility of the chest cage such as kyphosis or scoliosis.

The *energy required for breathing* is expended to overcome the elastic resistance of the lungs and thoracic cage and resistance to gas flow in the respiratory passages. In normal lungs, the primary part of work is overcoming elastic resistance. The work of breathing depends on mechanical variables of ventilation—respiratory rate, tidal volume, and respiratory level—and is measured in terms of oxygen costs. Normally, the work of breathing is 1 to 3 per cent of total body metabolism. As work increases, more of the inspired oxygen is used by the respiratory muscles. The elastic force increases with the depth of respiration and the airway resistance increases with the rate of respiration.[13] In normal, quiet breathing, there is minimal airway resistance; however, resistance may be increased when passages are narrowed by edema or secretions. In patients with severe bronchitis and emphysema or in patients following cardiopulmonary bypass, there may be an increase of the energy expenditure in the work of breathing. The work

of breathing and alveolar ventilation may be decreased by using bronchiolators, expectorants, or glucocorticoids, or by giving mechanical respiratory assistance.[13a] These conditions and methods of treatment are discussed in Chapters 35 and 20.

Pulmonary Volume and Capacity. The lung volumes can be measured during the phases of breathing. (See Fig. 9-4 for a "spirogram" that shows the fluctuating capacity of the lungs as the respiratory muscles contract and relax.)

The *vital capacity* (approximately 21 cc per lb) is the amount of air a person can expel from his lungs after first maximally filling his lungs and expiring fully. The gas left in the lungs is called the *residual volume.* N. Balfour Slonim and John L. Chapin[14] describe three primary subdivisions of the vital capacity. The *tidal volume* (approximately 3 cc per lb) is the air that is moved with each normal breath. The extra volume of air that one can exhale beyond the *tidal volume* is the *expiratory reserve volume.* Similarly, the volume that can be inhaled after the *tidal volume* is the *inspiratory reserve volume.* The inspiratory capacity is the air of the inspiratory reserve volume and the tidal volume. The *functional residual capacity* equals the *residual volume* and the *expiratory reserve volume.* The *total lung capacity* (approximately 30 cc per lb or 10

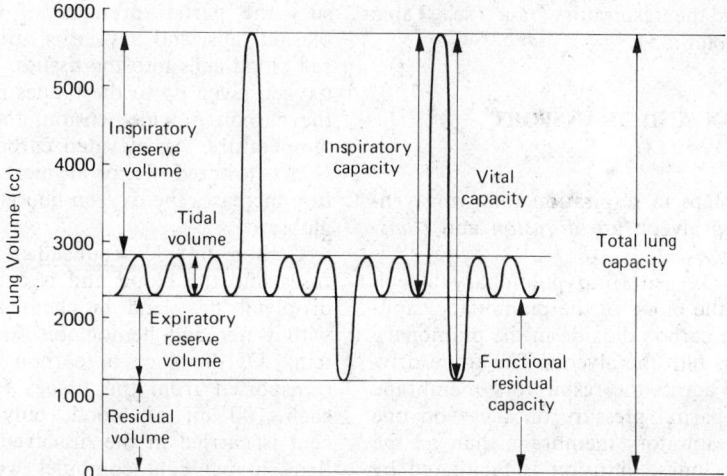

Figure 9-4. A spirogram, showing the divisions of the respiratory air. (From Guyton, Arthur C.: *Functions of the Human Body,* 2nd ed. W. B. Saunders Co., Philadelphia, 1964, p. 182.)

times the tidal volume) is the *vital capacity* and the *residual volume* combined.

The pulmonary volumes and capacities vary with the individual and with each person according to his or her physical condition. Volumes are generally less in women by 20 to 25 per cent. Athletes and large people usually have a greater volume and capacity. Lying down decreases both tidal volume and vital capacity because it increases the intrathoracic blood volume and the abdominal contents press upward on the diaphragm. The vital capacity is an important clinical measurement in the assessment of some types of pulmonary problems but by itself is a limited diagnostic tool. It is more effective to consider vital capacity in conjunction with other pulmonary measurements and estimates of arterial blood gases.

Alterations in the lung volumes and the subdivisions are most commonly associated with cardiopulmonary diseases. Pleural adhesions, bronchitic emphysema, bronchiogenic tumors, and anything that decreases the compliance of the lungs will decrease the vital capacity. Conditions producing fibrosis, such as tuberculosis and certain viral pneumonias, reduce the total lung capacity, but cause an increase in the residual volume because of the shrinkage and stiffness. An increase in the residual volume indicates that the lungs are hyperinflated and signifies changes in the thoracic cage, in the respiratory muscles, or in the pulmonary tissue. Thoracic deformities, whether congenital, developmental, or acquired, will cause a reduction in the total lung capacity and the vital capacity.[15,16]

The purposes of pulmonary function tests are to show any impairment in pulmonary ventilation, to determine whether the person has difficulty in getting the air in or out of the lungs, and to measure the extent of the impairment. All pulmonary volumes and capacities except residual volume, and hence total lung capacity, can be measured by a process called spirometry. This test, described in Chapter 7, should be used to record only a few breaths at a time because there is a buildup of carbon dioxide and loss of oxygen in the air chamber that can be hazardous to the patient. For continuous readings, a respirometer is used because this instrument removes the carbon dioxide as it forms. The following measurements cannot be made by spirometry: residual volume, the functional residual capacity, and the total lung capacity. Plethsmography, or indirect gas dilution methods, are used in making these determinations.[17]

Finally, pulmonary ventilation is influenced by the *dead space* in the lungs. This is described as that part of the respiratory system where there is no gaseous exchange. The amount of air that a person is able to move in and out of the respiratory passages each minute is the *minute respiratory volume*. This volume is equal to the tidal volume multiplied by the respiratory rate, or about 6 liters per minute. However, this volume of air is not entering the alveoli each minute because approximately one third of each breath goes into the *dead space*. The amount of air that enters the alveoli each minute for renewal is equal to the tidal volume minus the dead space volume times the respiratory rate (see Table 35-1 in Chapter 35).

3. DIFFUSION AND TRANSPORT OF GASES

The next steps in respiration following ventilation of the alveoli are *diffusion* and *transport* of the gases.

Diffusion. Oxygen from pulmonary alveoli diffuses into the blood of the pulmonary capillaries and the carbon dioxide in the pulmonary blood diffuses into the alveoli. The force driving the gases across the respiratory membrane is a greater partial pressure of a gas on one side of the respiratory membrane than on the other. In the lungs, diffusion is facilitated by the thinness of the respiratory epithelium, the large surface area, the pressure gradient across the membrane, and the solubility of the gases.[18,19]

In the tissues, oxygen moves from the plasma into tissue fluid and then into cells. As cells metabolize various foodstuffs and consume oxygen, carbon dioxide is formed. The carbon dioxide in the cells increases, diffuses into the blood, and is transported back to the lungs. Each minute the metabolizing cells of the human body consume about 250 cc of oxygen and produce about 200 cc of carbon dioxide. The amount of oxygen released to the tissues and the extent of diffusion of carbon dioxide from the tissues into the blood are governed primarily by the partial pressure of these gases and the activity of the body's tissues.

Transport. Oxygen is carried in the blood in physical solution and in chemical combination with hemoglobin; it attaches to the hemoglobin in the red blood cells. Each hemoglobin molecule can transport four oxygen molecules and each oxygen molecule that attaches to the hemoglobin increases the affinity of the hemoglobin for the next oxygen molecule. The amount of oxygen actually combined with hemoglobin is determined by the partial pressure of oxygen in the blood. In normal arterial blood with 15 gm per cent hemoglobin, fully saturated hemoglobin carries 1.34 cc of oxygen per gm (20 vol per cent). Arterial blood is normally 97 to 98 per cent saturated, venous blood 75 per cent saturated. Anemic persons suffer from insufficient capacity to carry oxygen to maintain normal metabolic processes as well as normal daily activities. They seem tired and, if the anemia is severe, listless.

The oxygen most immediately available to the tissues is that in physical solution in the plasma. As this oxygen is taken up by the tissues the partial pressure of oxygen in the plasma falls, and oxygen is liberated from the red blood cells into the tissues. The amount of oxygen given up to the tissues is influenced by the carbon dioxide tension, the pH, and the temperature. An elevated carbon dioxide tension, a lowered pH, or an increase in temperature increases the oxygen liberated from hemoglobin.[20]

Carbon dioxide produced in the tissues diffuses into the blood and is carried both in a dissolved state and in chemical combination with water and hemoglobin and plasma proteins. Of the 4 cc of carbon dioxide that is transported from the tissues to the lungs in each 100 ml of blood, only about 7 per cent is carried in the dissolved state and less than 30 per cent combines with hemoglobin and the plasma proteins. The largest proportion of carbon dioxide is transported in the form of bicarbonate.[21]

In the lungs, carbon dioxide diffuses from the blood into the alveoli because of the lower pressure in the alveoli. As long as the integrity of the respiratory system is maintained, diffusion and transport of gases is easily and efficiently accomplished in the so-called normal, healthy individual.[22]

4. REGULATION OF RESPIRATION [23,24]

Respiration is regulated by neural and humoral mechanisms; however, sensory stimuli, as well as the acid–base balance of the body, also affect the regulation of respiration.

Neural Regulation. Flourens, who discovered it, called the respiratory center "the vital knot." It is in the medulla and the pons, and has three areas of influence: the medullary respiratory area, the apneustic area, and the pneumotaxic area. The basic rhythm of respiration is not maintained by any single one of these areas but by the integrated action of all three. Signals enter the medullary respiratory center from the spinal cord, from the cerebral cortex and the midbrain, from the pneumotaxic area in the upper pons, and from the apneustic area in the lower pons, and modify the rhythm of respiration and contribute to the normal smooth pattern of respiration. The inflation reflex (*Hering-Breuer*) and the pneumotaxic reflexes are important in maintaining the rhythm of respiration and controlling inflation and deflation of the lungs. There are receptors in the lungs and thorax that detect the expansion of the lungs and send impulses to the respiratory center via the vagus nerve; inspiration is inhibited and expiration occurs. In passive expiration, there is deflation of the lungs to a certain extent, then automatic activity of the inspiratory center discharges impulses for the next inspiration. If it were not for the Hering-Breuer reflex, respiration would be much deeper.

Humoral Regulation. Chemoreceptors are located centrally on the surface of the medulla and peripherally in the carotid and aortic bodies. These receptors respond to a change in the levels of carbon dioxide and oxygen and the hydrogen ion concentration in the blood.

An increase in the blood tension of carbon dioxide is the most potent respiratory stimulus of the respiratory center. Inspiration and expiration are speeded up and there is an increase in the rate and depth of respiration. A change in the hydrogen ion concentration of the blood (pH) directly affects the respiratory center and only to a lesser degree the peripheral chemoreceptors. Ventilation increases as blood pH decreases and vice versa.

Although oxygen is vital for life, a change in the oxygen level of the blood has almost no direct effect on the respiratory center. However, when the oxygen tension is decreased, the chemoreceptors of the carotid bodies and the aortic arch become strongly stimulated; impulses are transmitted to the respiratory center and alveolar ventilation is increased.

Sensory and Temperature Stimuli. Respiration may be influenced by impulses from sensory surfaces and higher brain centers. Pulmonary ventilation increases if the ambient temperature rises beyond 27° to 29° C (80.6° to 84.3° F). In animals that pant, the temperature-regulating center has access to the respiratory center and panting is a form of hyperventilation.

Stimulation of almost any afferent nerve can influence respiration. A cold shower or plunge into cold water produces a gasp followed by an increase in respiratory rate. A pin-prick or digital manipulation of the anal canal may stimulate respiration.

Consciousness has extraordinary effects on ventilation. Man can voluntarily increase his ventilation twentyfold for short periods or may produce apnea for many minutes. Breathing patterns can be altered at will, yet involuntary control is of primary importance, such as straining (when lifting an object) and Valsalva maneuvers. Cerebral activity (for example, concentrating before hitting a golf ball) may depress the respiratory center, causing shallow and slow breathing. The accumulation of carbon dioxide overrides inhibiting impulses from the cerebrum and the result is a sigh—a deep inspiration followed by a deep expiration.[25] It is essential that breathing be involuntary. If persons try to control their respiratory rate

they will soon find themselves very uncomfortable, for it is impossible to consciously determine the oxygen need or to maintain an appropriate rhythm for long. Strong emotion can alter the depth and rate of respiration so markedly that it can produce unconsciousness. Hearing a marauder in the house can momentarily paralyze respiration. Because thinking about how we are breathing disturbs the rate of respiration, the nurse should, if possible, count the respiratory rate when the person is unaware of its being done. (See page 454 for the suggested method.)

Acid–Base Balance. The biochemical processes of the body are dependent on homeostasis of the internal environment. Acids are formed in the body as a result of metabolic activity and base radicals are ingested in foods. A quantitative index of the balance of acid and base is the hydrogen ion concentration of the blood (pH). The normal pH is 7.4 with a range of 7.35 to 7.45. A decrease in pH indicates acidosis and an increase in pH indicates alkalosis (see Chapter 35 for a more detailed discussion). Acid–base balance is maintained by the chemical buffer systems, the respiratory system, and the kidneys.

Acid–base imbalances are classified as respiratory or metabolic. Alterations in gas exchange leading to alveolar hyper- or hypoventilation affect the arterial pH and lead to compensatory measures by the kidney. Metabolic disturbances altering the carbon dioxide and bicarbonate levels are compensated for by the respiratory system.

Increased alveolar ventilation with the loss of a large volume of carbon dioxide from the blood causes an increase in pH. The result is alkalosis. There is lack of stimulation for respiration and apnea can occur. A pH of 7.8 may produce tetany. Respiratory regulation is dependent on the relationship between alveolar ventilation and the concentration of carbon dioxide, bicarbonate, and hydrogen ions.

A rise in the level of carbon dioxide causes a decrease in the pH, producing acidosis. The respiratory center is stimulated and ventilation is increased. There is an increased acidity of the urine and increased excretion of ammonium salts by the kidney. A high degree of acidosis will produce coma and a pH below 6.9 is often fatal.

The acid–base balance of the blood may be upset by renal failure, diabetes mellitus, depression of the respiratory center, altered metabolic states (fever, vomiting, ketosis), excessive exercise, and any condition producing either hyperventilation or hypoventilation. Arterial blood gases, serum bicarbonate levels, and pH provide the most quantitative index of the level of adequacy of ventilation and of acid–base balance.[26]

5. FACTORS AFFECTING NORMAL RESPIRATION

Smoking. In the past few years, cigarette smoking has been implicated as a causative factor in cancer, bronchitis, emphysema, and coronary heart disease. It is generally known that coughing (excessive or abnormal), sputum, wheezing, breathlessness, and respiratory symptoms occur more often in individuals who smoke than in those who do not (see Fig. 9-5).

It has been suggested that the parts of the lungs initially damaged by inhaled cigarette smoke are the terminal bronchioles. Other changes reported by David V. Bates [27] are loss of surfactant (discussed earlier), metaplasia of cells, and inflammation and destruction of the alveoli (see Fig. 9-6). Oscar Auerbach and associates [28] report that examinations of lung specimens have shown the following conditions that account for the symptoms seen in patients: (1) fibrosis of the alveolar septa, (2) rupture of the alveolar septa, and (3) thick-

ening of the walls of the arteries and arterioles. These histologic changes increased with age and were greater in smokers than in nonsmokers.

In a recent study of 289 young adult (men) cigarette smokers, an increased susceptibility to epidemic influenza and other acute respiratory infections was noted. Smokers had fewer residual antibodies against influenza antigens than nonsmokers, the indication being that cigarette smoking alters the persistence of humoral antibody.[29]

According to the National Health Survey, there is remarkable diminution or disappearance of symptoms of bronchopulmonary disease following the cessation of smoking. Pulmonary function improves, and forced expiratory volume and expiratory flow rate increases. On autopsy, the lung changes in ex-smokers were more like those of nonsmokers. There also were less pulmonary fibrosis, less rupture of the alveolar septa, and less thickening of the wall of the arterioles in the parenchyma of individuals who had stopped smoking cigarettes for 5 years or more as compared with smokers. There is also good evidence to document reversal of bronchitic changes.[30]

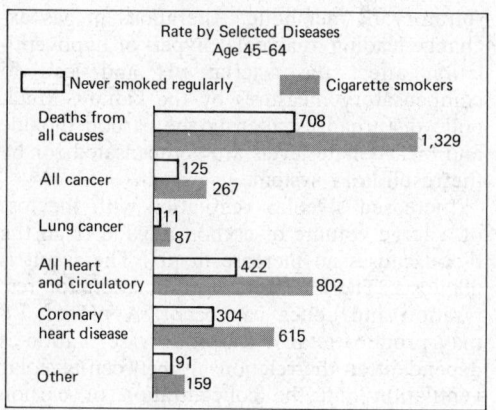

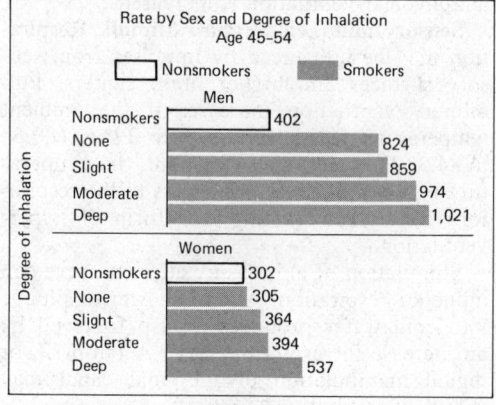

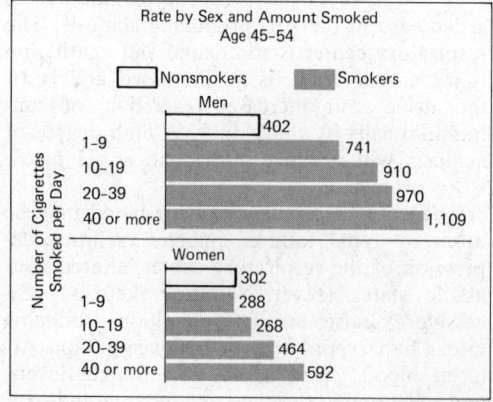

Figure 9-5. Death rates (per 100,000 person-years) of smokers compared to nonsmokers. (From Hammond, E. C.: *Smoking in Relation to Death Rates of One Million Men and Women,* 1966).

There are active programs by the American Heart Association, the American Cancer Society, and the American Lung Association to influence the public to stop smoking. Many nurses participate in these programs. (They can be most persuasive through example.) Literature on ways to stop smoking is available through these organizations to individuals and groups. Man has the ability to preserve the integrity of the respiratory system and reduce his risk of disabling pulmonary disease. To these benefits must be added the increased comfort, the feeling of well-being, and positive health. However, it should be added that many persons stop smoking, or resist the temptation to smoke, only to be poisoned by the contaminated air they breathe. Environmental pollution, close kin to the danger of smoking, is discussed on page 632.

Age. Old age distinguishes itself by both physiologic and anatomic changes of the respiratory and circulatory systems. The elderly person usually experiences dyspnea on exertion, shortness of breath, and decreased tolerance for physical activity, such as walking, that are not necessarily associated with pulmonary disease.*

One of the most common changes in the aged is muscular atrophy and increased thickness of the alveolar and capillary membranes, which results in impaired ventilation and diffusion. There is loss of lung elasticity, an increase in lung compliance, and a reduction of vital capacity. The residual lung volume is increased and ventilation distribution becomes uneven. The ratio of dead space ventilation to alveolar ventilation is increased, thereby decreasing the diffusing capacity of the lung.[31] The work of breathing is increased, yet the efficiency of gas exchange and distribution is decreased. L. Tlusty [32] says that the decrease in aerobic capacity * demonstrated in elderly individuals is not due solely to physiologic changes, but that social and psychologic factors that accompany aging also intensify the physiologic changes. Almost certainly the commonest cause of decreased lung capacity is the loss of an erect posture in old age. Ways of combatting spinal curvatures are discussed in Chapter 12. Part of the program is physical, part is emotional or psychologic.

Whether changes in normal respiration associated with aging are purely physiologic or psychophysiologic, the nurse can do a great deal to help the person maintain his optimum respiratory function. The changes associated with aging may be prevented or diminished through physical activities and training. Deep breathing and isometric exercises can help maintain the tone and efficiency of the respiratory muscles. Good posture, standing, walking, sitting, and lying make optimum ventilatory exchange possible. Emotional support and reassurance can help the elderly individual become more secure.

Obesity. It has been demonstrated that normal pulmonary function is impaired in obese

---

* It is still a question how much age should affect the capacity of the individual for activity. A man said to be 105 who is employed as a waiter at the St. Francis Hotel in San Francisco is said (in the summer of 1973) to be running 5 miles daily. He appears periodically on television shows and young men attest to his ability to outrun them.

* Aerobic capacity is a measure of an individual's physical fitness. The amount of oxygen (measured in cubic centimeters per kilogram of total body weight per minute) the body utilizes during exhausting work marks a person's aerobic capacity. See Chapter 12.

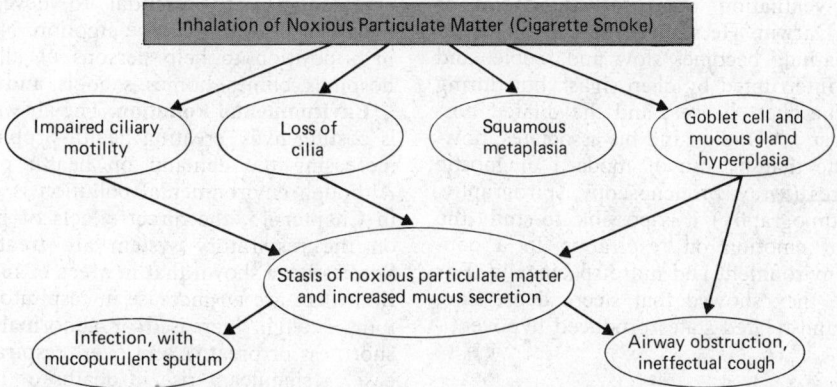

Figure 9-6. Pathophysiology of chronic bronchitis. (From Rodman, Theodore: "Management of Tracheobronchial Secretions," *Am. J. Nurs.,* **66:**24–75, [Nov.] 1966.)

people. James K. Alexander and associates [33] report that studies of obese persons have shown that ventilatory demand is greater than in normal subjects—as one would expect, for they are literally carrying a heavy load with every step they take. Their most common symptoms are exertional dyspnea and a reduced vital capacity. These findings are explained by several physiologic changes accompanying obesity: (1) in the overweight individuals, there is an alteration in the center of gravity, with resultant thoracic kyphosis which grossly limits respiratory excursions; (2) the increased size of the abdomen elevates the sternum and the chest becomes relatively fixed in a position of moderate inspiration; and (3) changes in the lung volume have to be brought about almost entirely by the action of the diaphragm.

The work of breathing is increased in obese persons and the oxygen cost of breathing is three times as great as in healthy persons of normal weight.[34] The reduction in lung capacity and alveolar ventilation, as well as the increase in oxygen consumption, ventilation, and work of breathing, may lead to cardiac and respiratory failure, hypoxemia, and hypercapnia. Serious impairment of pulmonary function can be produced even in the absence of a respiratory disease.[35]

There is convincing evidence that the abnormalities of mechanics of breathing and respiratory gas exchange may be significantly improved or removed following weight loss. The nurse has both the opportunity to teach and responsibility for teaching the overweight population the desirable effects of weight loss, which include preserving normal respiratory function. The reader should consult Chapters 10 and 36 for a more detailed discussion of this subject.

Emotions. Donald L. Dudley and associates, discussing the effects of emotions on pulmonary ventilation, refer to the studies of Charles Darwin. He showed that during grief "the breathing becomes slow and feeble, and is often interrupted by deep sighs" but during anger "the chest heaves, and the dilated nostrils quiver." * Dudley and his associates, however, note that by use of modern diagnostic procedures (x-ray, bronchoscopy, spirography, and pneumography) it is possible to study the effects of emotion on respiration in a controlled environment and more specifically. For example, they showed that sleep, depression, apathy, and related states produced hypoventi-

lation; whereas anger, exercise, and anxiety resulted in hyperventilation. In another study,[36] they found that the initiation of a hypnotic state had minimal or no effect on respiration. Following anger, anxiety, or exercise, there was respiratory hyperfunction with an increase in alveolar ventilation, oxygen uptake, and a decrease in carbon dioxide concentration. When there were deep relaxation and depression, respiratory hypofunction was noted with a decrease in alveolar ventilation, oxygen uptake, and an increase in the concentration of carbon dioxide.

Martin A. Jacobs and associates [37] discuss "life stress and respiratory illness." They report that in a group of 179 (men) college students, respiratory illness and symptoms were associated with "situations" characterized by failure, unresolved role crisis, and social isolation.

Normally, a person is unaware of his breathing unless he consciously thinks about it. In emotional states, however, there is an increased awareness of breathing and the person may complain of difficulty in breathing (dyspnea) even though there is no organic cause. This is a subjective complaint and may be perceived only by the individual experiencing it. However, a very observant nurse can often see that the person feels smothered, out of breath, or wants more air, or is breathing rapidly or slowly. The respiration may be shallow, regular, or irregular. Dyspnea may be produced by fear, excitement, anger, or any associated emotional state.[38-40a] Dyspnea as a common symptom of respiratory insufficiency and organic disease is discussed in Chapter 35.

Normal respiration may be restored by alleviating fear, reassuring the person, and dealing with the emotional problem or condition. Getting the person to express his fear, excitement, or anger is the first step; listening carefully and helping to understand what he is experiencing are essential to developing a means of dealing with the emotion. Nurses are in a position to help persons of all ages in hospitals, clinics, homes, schools, and industry.

Environmental Pollution. The air we breathe is costing lives, creating health problems, and increasing the demand on health personnel. Although environmental pollution is discussed in Chapter 15, the direct effects of pollutants on the respiratory system are treated here. Studies have shown that in areas of high pollution there are an increase in respiratory symptoms (cough, increased or abnormal sputum, shortness of breath) and overt respiratory disease, a significant rise in deaths of men over age 55, and an increase in morbidity and mortality from respiratory disease.[41,42]

---

* Dudley, Donald L., et al.: "Psychophysiologic Studies of Pulmonary Ventilation," *Psychosom. Med.*, **26:**645, (Nov.–Dec.) 1964.

Irritants in the environment act on different parts of the respiratory system and produce varying symptoms. In the bronchi, these pollutants cause paralysis of the cilia, which removes one of the body's foremost barriers against infection. Ultimately, there is destruction of the cilia, with replacement by squamous cells that may degenerate into cancerous lesions. With continuous irritation, mucous glands increase secretion of a soothing liquid to bathe the inflamed air passages. The hypertrophy of the mucous glands lining the respiratory passages and their increased secretions may close some of the smaller air passages. The inflamed passages swell, increasing the airway resistance, decreasing the air circulation, and preventing adequate drainage of secretions. All these changes in the major bronchi increase susceptibility to infection.[43] In the terminal bronchioles, irritants destroy normal defenses. With the loss of surfactant, there is impaired collateral ventilation and gas exchange within the lung. Inflammation obliterates some passages and prematurely closes small airways. In the alveoli, there is an increase in the cells and macrophages of the lungs which leads to infection and release of certain enzymes that may destroy alveoli.[44]

Miners, stonemasons, chemical workers, and textile workers face pollution from inorganic dusts. Asbestos is a common pollutant which causes pneumoconiosis, a progressive fibrotic condition in the lung, and mesothelioma. Studies of persons in these occupations have shown a decrease in pulmonary function, especially vital capacity, and a prevalence of pulmonary fibrosis.[45-47b]

The automobile contaminates the air with carbon monoxide, nitrogen oxides, and various hydrocarbons. When the exhaust meets sunlight, chemical reactions occur, producing smog. The photochemical smog and nitrogen dioxide can damage the nose, throat, and lungs. Even a low level of oxidants irritates the upper airways, causing dry throat and watery eyes. Nitrogen oxides are unique in that they produce a disease like human emphysema in animals. The acute pulmonary insufficiency found in farmers is attributed to the nitrogen dioxide found in hay.[48]

Carbon monoxide does not irritate the lung, but rather insidiously deprives the body of oxygen. Carbon monoxide combines with hemoglobin, thereby interfering with the transport of oxygen. Small children and small animals are more quickly overcome than adults and large animals. Recovery from carbon monoxide poisoning may still leave the nervous system damaged from the resultant hypoxia.[49]

In a study of 3485 persons in Tucson, Arizona, Michael D. Lebowitz [49a] reports that use of aerosol appears to be related to respiratory symptoms. Aerosols are commonly used for personal and household care, but there are current efforts to ban or control their use.

The magnitude of the pollution problem is overwhelming and ecologists are predicting that we will eventually destroy ourselves with environmental pollution. The federal government has established commissions to control disposal of wastes and to regulate the needless pollution of the environment.[49b]

Public education is emphasized by most who write about pollution. Nurses are qualified to know about the health hazards of pollution and to help make people aware of its dangers and their present and eventual consequences. They are in strategic positions throughout the world to arouse public awareness of environmental health problems and to stimulate the public to action.[50] The American Heart Association and the American Lung Association (formerly the National Tuberculosis and Respiratory Disease Association) have programs and materials for educating health professionals and laymen. Such materials and others should be used by nurses as they work with persons (sick or well) on an individual basis or with groups in all settings—industries, schools, clinics, hospitals, private homes, nursing homes, outpatient departments, and penal institutions.

There are certain measures most persons can control that affect the environment. Temperature and humidity, for example, can increase or reduce pollution. High humidity is dangerous because it increases chemical interaction of the water vapor with the irritant gases. Low humidity can be equally harmful because it dries the air passages which predispose the trachea and bronchi to irritation. "Postnasal drip" and early morning cough are often attributed to low humidity in steam-heated buildings. Benjamin Kogan [50a] gives a list of things to do when there is a warning of dangerous pollution: for example, remain indoors when the pollution index is high and keep the windows closed. Those with known respiratory disease should be advised to take antibiotics as a prophylactic protective measure, according to Stephen M. Ayres.[51]

Anesthesia and Surgery. There are multiple effects that general anesthesia and surgery, even under the most ideal conditions, may have on the respiratory system and respiration. Sedatives, narcotics, and anesthetic agents depress the respiratory center, suppress the cough reflex, and may weaken and paralyze the muscles of respiration. Preoperative restriction of fluids and administration of anticholinergic drugs thicken mucus and increase the difficulty of eliminating it. The trauma of the surgical procedure which sometimes causes the syndrome "shock" may damage the lung or intensify existing problems. Following surgery, there may be loss of surfactant and an increase in surface tension that decreases lung compliance. This happens particularly with patients who have cardiovascular surgery with a cardiopulmonary bypass. Severe loss of surfactant may result in alveolar collapse and atelectasis. Vital capacity may be reduced by decreased compliance, by incisional pain that makes the person unwilling to breathe deeply, or by abdominal distention. Underventilation during the operative procedure may cause more severe problems of respiratory insufficiency, hypoxia, and acidosis. Mouth breathing and drugs may dry secretions and induce bronchospasm and airway obstruction.

Nurses can provide preoperative and postoperative care that will include the use of expectorants, bronchodilators, postural drainage, breathing exercises, coughing, or the use of positive pressure devices (see Chapters 47 and 48). Their observations are important in the over-all assessment of the patient's ability to sustain a good ventilatory effort. They should be alert to conditions that predispose patients to respiratory problems, for example, the habit of smoking, infancy or old age, occupational hazards, or obesity. All of these affect a patient's maximal breathing capacity and may be the origin of complications following surgery and anesthesia that demand special care.

REFERENCES

1. Gottlieb, Leon S.: *A History of Respiration.* Charles C Thomas, Publisher, Springfield, Ill., 1964, p. 54.
2. Dudley, Donald L.: *Psychophysiology of Respiratory Physiology,* 2nd ed. C. V. Mosby Corp., New York, 1969, p. 1.
3. Slonim, N. Balfour, and Chapin, John L.: *Respiratory Physiology,* 2nd ed. C. V. Mosby Co., St. Louis, 1971, p. 2.
4. Haas, Albert: *Essentials of Living with Pulmonary Emphysema.* New York University Medical Center, New York, 1963, p. 3.
5. Slonim, N. Balfour, and Chapin, John L.: *op. cit.,* p. 26.
6. Proctor, Donald F.: "Physiology of the Air Passages," in Safar, Peter (ed.): *Respiratory Therapy.* F. A. Davis Co., Philadelphia, 1965, p. 20.
7. Tuttle, W. W., and Schottelius, Byron A.: *Textbook of Physiology,* 17th ed. C. V. Mosby Co., St. Louis, 1973, p. 325.
8. Secor, Jane: *Patient Care in Respiratory Problems.* W. B. Saunders Co., Philadelphia, 1971, p. 3.
9. Slonim, N. Balfour, and Chapin, John L.: *op. cit.,* p. 41.
10. Tuttle, W. W., and Schottelius, Byron A.: *op. cit.,* p. 327.
11. Guyton, Arthur C.: *Textbook of Medical Physiology,* 5th ed. W. B. Saunders Co., Philadelphia, 1976, p. 518.
12. *Ibid.,* p. 519.
13. Slonim, N. Balfour, and Chapin, John L.: *op. cit.,* p. 43.
13a. Traver, Gayle A.: "Living with Chronic Respiratory Disease," *Am. J. Nurs.,* **75:**1777, (Oct.) 1975.
14. Slonim, N. Balfour, and Chapin, John L.: *op. cit.,* p. 22.
15. Foley, Mary F.: "Pulmonary Function Testing," *Am. J. Nurs.,* **71:**1136, (June) 1971.
16. Tuttle, W. W., and Schottelius, Byron A.: *op. cit.,* p. 330.
17. Guyton, Arthur C.: *op. cit.,* p. 522.
18. Tuttle, W. W., and Schottelius, Byron A.: *op. cit.,* p. 332.
19. Green, J. H.: *Basic Clinical Physiology,* 2nd ed. Oxford University Press, London, 1973, p. 50.
20. Cherniack, Reuben M., et al.: *Respiration in Health and Disease,* 2nd ed. W. B. Saunders Co., Philadelphia, 1972, p. 75.
21. Guyton, Arthur C.: *op. cit.,* p. 553.
22. Zuck, David: "Life, Metabolism and Hypoxia I," *Nurs. Times.,* **64:**1680, (Dec. 13) 1968.
23. Slonim, N. Balfour, and Chapin, John L.: *op. cit.,* p. 109.
24. Guyton, Arthur C.: *op. cit.,* p. 557.
25. Tuttle, W. W., and Schottelius, Byron A.: *op. cit.,* p. 345.
26. Lyons, Harold A.: "Respiratory Acidosis: Diagnosis and Management," *Med. Clin. North Am.,* **51:**293, (Mar.) 1967.
27. Bates, David V.: "Air Pollutants and the Human Lung," *Am. Rev. Resp. Dis.,* **105:**1, (Jan.) 1972.
28. Auerbach, Oscar, et al.: "Smoking Habits and Age in Relation to Pulmonary Changes," *N. Engl. J. Med.,* **269:**1045, (Nov. 14) 1963.
29. Finklea, J. F., et al.: "Cigarette Smoking and Hemagglutination Inhibition Response to Influenza After Natural Disease and Immunization," *Am. Rev. Resp. Dis.,* **104:**368, (Sept.) 1971.
30. Schumann, Leonard M.: "The Benefits of Cessation of Smoking," *Chest,* **59:**421, (Apr.) 1971.
31. Jennings, Muriel, et al.: "Physiologic Functioning in the Elderly," *Nurs. Clin. North Am.,* **7:**237, (June) 1972.
32. Tlusty, L.: "Physical Fitness in Old Age. I. Aerobic Capacity and the Other Parameters of Physical Fitness Followed by Means of Graded Exercise in Ergometric Examination of Elderly Individuals," *Respiration,* **26:**163, 1969.
33. Alexander, James K., et al.: "Observations on Some Clinical Features of Extreme Obesity, with Particular Reference to Cardio-

respiratory Effects," *Am. J. Med.*, **32:**512, (Apr.) 1962.

34. Addington, W. W., et al.: "Obesity and Alveolar Hypoventilation," *Respiration,* **26:** 214, 1969.
35. Cherniack, Reuben M., et al.: *op. cit.*, p. 409.
36. Dudley, Donald L., et al.: "Changes in Respiration Associated with Hypnotically Induced Emotion, Pain, and Exercise," *Psychosom. Med.*, **26:**46, (Jan.–Feb.) 1964.
37. Jacobs, Martin A., et al.: "Life Stress and Respiratory Illness," *Psychosom. Med.*, **32:** 233, (May–June) 1970.
38. Cherniack, Reuben M., et al.: *op. cit.*, p. 180.
39. Olsen, Arthur M.: "What Is Dyspnea," in Banyai, Andrew L., and Levine Edwin Rayner (eds.): *Dyspnea: Diagnosis and Treatment.* F. A. Davis Co., Philadelphia, 1963, p. 3.
40. Dudley, Donald L., et al.: "Dyspnea: Psychologic and Physiologic Observations," *J. Psychosom. Res.*, **11:**325, 1968.
40a. Chrisman, Marilyn: "Dyspnea," *Am. J. Nurs.*, **74:**643, (Apr.) 1974.
41. Bates, David V.: *op. cit.*
42. Carnow, Bertram W.: "Air Pollution Invites Disease," *Natl. Tuberc. Resp. Dis. Assoc. Bull.*, **57:**7 (Sept.) 1971.
43. Bates, David V.: *op. cit.*
44. *Ibid.*
45. Worth, G., et al.: "Lung Function in Iron Workers," *Respiration,* **26:**225, (Suppl) 1969.
46. Weiss, William: "Cigarette Smoking, Asbestos, and Pulmonary Fibrosis," *Am. Rev. Resp. Dis.*, **104:**223, (Aug.) 1971.
47. Gunn, A. D. G.: "Abuse of the Air," *Nurs. Times,* (Feb. 18), 1971, p. 197.
47a. Kleinfeld, M., et al.: "Mortality Experiences Among Talc Workers: A Follow-up Study," *J. Occup. Med.*, **16:**345, (May) 1974.
47b. Merchant, J. A., et al.: "Dose Response Studies in Cotton Textile Workers," *J. Occup. Med.*, **15:**222, (Mar.) 1973.
48. Ayres, Stephen M.: "The Automobile— What a Way to Go," *Natl. Tuberc. Resp. Dis. Assoc. Bull.*, **68:**4, (June) 1972.
49. Tuttle, W. W., and Schottelius, Byron A.: *op. cit.*, p. 351.
49a. Lebowitz, Michael D.: "Aerosol Usage and Respiratory Symptoms," *Arch. Environ. Health,* **31:**83, (Mar.–Apr.) 1976.
49b. Kogan, Benjamin A.: *Health: Man in a Changing Environment.* Harcourt, Brace & World, New York, 1970.
50. Diekema, Anthony J.: "The Changing Environment: Some Implications for Health," *Occup. Health Nurs.*, **18:**20, (July) 1970.
50a. Kogan, Benjamin A.: *op. cit.*, p. 78.
51. Ayres, Stephen M.: "Patient Advice During Acute Air Pollution Episode," *Arch. Environ. Health,* **22:**591, (May) 1971.

Additional Suggested Reading

Anderson, William H.: "Acute Exposure to Cigarette Smoke as a Cause of Hypoxia," *Chest,* **59:**33, (May) 1971.

Brewer, George J., et al.: "Cigarette Smoking as a Cause of Hypoxemia in Man at Altitude," *Chest,* **59:**30, (May) 1971.

Cahill, John M.: "Respiratory Problems in Surgical Patients," *Am. J. Surg.*, **116:**362, (Sept.) 1968.

Cotton, Raymond D.: "Environmental Quality— 1971," *Arch. Environ. Health,* **24:**288, (Apr.) 1972.

Cullen, James H., and Formel, Paul F.: "The Respiratory Defects in Extreme Obesity," *Am. J. Med.*, **32:**525, (Apr.) 1962.

Fletcher, C. M.: "A Paper—Cigarettes and Respiratory Disease," in *Summary, World Conference on Smoking and Health, 1967.* American Cancer Society, New York, 1967.

Foss, Georgia: "Postural Drainage," *Am. J. Nurs.*, **73:**666, (Apr.) 1973.

Gelperin, A.: "Sudden Death in an Elderly Population from Aspiration of Food," *J. Am. Geriatr. Soc.*, **22:**135, (Mar.) 1974.

Gordon, I.: "A Paper—Smoking Education: When, Where and How," in *Summary, World Conference on Smoking and Health, 1967.* American Cancer Society, New York, 1967.

Hamilton, William K.: "Postoperative Respiratory Complications," in Safar, Peter (ed.): *Respiratory Therapy.* F. A. Davis Co., Philadelphia, 1965.

Heim, Edgar, et al.: "Dyspnea: Psychophysiologic Relationships," *Psychosom. Med.*, **35:**405, (Sept.–Oct.) 1972.

Higgins, L. T. T., et al.: "Smoking and Chronic Respiratory Disease: Findings in Surveys Carried Out in 1957 and 1966 in Staveley in Derbyshire, England," *Chest,* **59:**34, (May) 1971.

James, Ralph H.: "Prior Smoking as a Determinant of the Distribution of Pulmonary Ventilation," *Am. Rev. Resp. Dis.*, **101:**105, (May) 1970.

Keough, Gertrude: "Providing the Patient with Proper Humidification," in *ANA Clinical Conferences, 1970.* Appleton-Century-Crofts, New York, 1971.

Kilburn, Kaye H., et al.: "Byssinosis: Matter from Lint to Lungs," *Am. J. Nurs.*, **73:**1953, (Nov.) 1973.

Kurihara, Marie: "Assessment and Maintenance of Adequate Respiration," *Nurs. Clin. North Am.*, **3:**65, (Jan.) 1968.

Lask, Aaron: *Asthma: Altitude and Milieu.* J. B. Lippincott Co., Philadelphia, 1967.

Merchant, J. A.: "An Industrial Study of the Biological Effects of Cotton Dust and Cigarette Smoke Exposure," *J. Occup. Med.*, **15:**212, (Mar.) 1973.

Modrak, Marion, et al.: *Better Living and Breathing; A Manual for Patients.* C. V. Mosby Co., St. Louis, 1975.

Orwin, A.: "Respiratory Relief: A New and

Rapid Method for the Treatment of Phobic States," *Br. J. Psychiatry,* **119:**635, (Dec.) 1971.

US Public Health Service: *Report of Advisory Committee to Surgeon General, USPHS. Smoking and Health.* US Government Printing Office, Washington, D.C., 1966 (Pamphlet #2019).

———: *The Health Consequences of Smoking. A Report of the Surgeon General, 1971.* US Government Printing Office, Washington, D.C., 1971.

Wade, J. F.: *Respiratory Nursing Care; Physiology and Technique.* C. V. Mosby Co., St. Louis, 1973.

Yoder, Franklin D.: "Implications of the Changing Environment to Occupational Health," *Occup. Health Nurs.,* **18:**23, (July) 1970.

Gladys Nite

The author acknowledges the assistance of Dorothy Cumby, R.N., M.S., Instructor of Medical-Surgical Nursing, College of Nursing, Medical University of South Carolina, Charleston, in the preparation of this chapter.

CHAPTER 10

Nutrition

1. NUTRITION AND THE QUALITY OF LIFE

Although devastating wars have overshadowed this century, and the development of laborsaving machines and man's flight in space are its most obvious achievements, history may attach more importance to twentieth-century discoveries on the nature and needs of man himself. Of these none is more tangible nor more far reaching in effect than those of the physiologic chemist in the field of nutrition. We know that human beings, like animals, can instinctively select edible materials from the environment. By and large, superior individuals have always eaten more wisely than inferior men, their parents' wise choice of foods being largely responsible for their superiority. In previous centuries, however, man had little help in food selection except his cravings and the empiric wisdom of his elders.* Civilized man has lost much of this ability to recognize "hidden hungers," or food cravings, but a literate society can, if economically able, select a diet that will increase height, motor power, and capacity for intellectual achievement. Such a diet will at the same time eliminate scurvy, beriberi, pellagra, rickets, and a host of diseases not so generally recognized as nutritional deficiencies, which scourged peoples of the past and still take heavy tolls. The food chemist of today can provide us with proof, lacking in the past, because he has watched the effect of controlled diets on hundreds of generations of small mammals whose

behavior is in many respects comparable to that of humans. Scientific feeding of livestock and dietary studies made on human volunteers have added to our store of knowledge.

With increased communication between nations and literacy within, there is a growing realization that a large majority of the human race is underfed in quantity and quality. For example, the Eighth International Congress of Nutrition, held in Prague in 1969 with almost 1800 participants, passed the following resolutions:

Recognizing that malnutrition at present seriously affects a large proportion of the preschool children and adults as well—

Recognizing that early malnutrition causes not only retarded physical growth but also may impair the learning and behavior of children upon whom social and economic development must depend—

Recognizing the problem to be primarily social, economic and moral, since the application of present scientific and technical knowledge to agricultural, food, health and population problems of developing countries could eliminate most malnutrition—

Strongly urges all governments to reexamine their allocation of resources in order to provide needed support for the prevention of malnutrition in developing countries directly and through the United Nations Family of organizations through the application of scientific and technical knowledge to food production, storage, processing and consumption together with disease control, health promotion, nutrition education and training, and family planning.*

Because most hungry people now see and read about the more fortunate, they are not so willing to accept hunger philosophically as

---

* Josué de Castro contends that hunger is a "man-made plague," that it is the cause, not the result, of overpopulation and that many societies considered "primitive" have selected a varied and complete diet, producing a healthy people living in a balanced economy. (*The Geography of Hunger*, Little, Brown and Co., Boston, 1952.)

* Masek, J.: "Preliminary Report on the Eighth International Congress of Nutrition," *Nutr. Rev.*, **28**:60, (Mar.) 1970.

those who in the past lived unaware of the well-fed. Present even more than past governments will prosper or fall according to their ability to improve the national diet. Many students of the international scene maintain that peace depends on recognition of this fact, the distribution of food and the dissemination of knowledge of how to produce and use it to optimum advantage. Texts such as Josué de Castro's The Geography of Hunger [1] and Stringfellow Barr's Citizens of the World [2] develop this theme. Julian S. Huxley's On Living in a Revolution [3] discusses the changing emphasis from the era of "economic man" to the future era of "social man." In Our Plundered Planet [4] Fairfield Osborn shows the necessity of conserving the land while raising the standard of living. If enough good food is to be produced, there must be what has been referred to as "a marriage of agriculture and health." Some might say there must be also a "marriage of nutrition and politics"—national and international. In an editorial, "Nutrition, Agriculture, Foreign Aid and the Population Problem," Charles S. Davison says:

With proper agriculture, conservation of land and other biological resources, and free exchange between the nations, man could now feed himself. Current knowledge of nutrition indicates that he could probably feed himself well, if such knowledge were applied. . . . . If sufficient food and water were available for all, the banning of war would have some chance of success. With men, cities and nations crowded together and underfed, war seems inevitable. . . . . The opportunity for each individual to develop his capabilities to the utmost is impossible if he is hungry, underclothed and crowded.*

Experiments with laboratory animals and livestock suggest that improvement of diet offers unlimited possibility for increasing the average life span and, more important, the quality of human life.† More and more studies

showing the effect of nutrition on growth and development of children appear in the literature. According to statistics on over 8 million Japanese children reported by the Ministry of Education, the stature of these children has increased: boys at 14 years showed an increase of 7.6 cm, girls at 11 years an increase of 6.6 cm. These changes in stature are evident in children born since World War II and, therefore, not subjected to a limited diet during their preschool years.[5] Figure 10-1 shows the increased height of children during the last half century. Titles such as We Are What We Eat,[6] Eat Well and Stay Well,[7] and Climate Makes the Man [8] (because climate affects his food) are attempts to popularize the findings of scientists. National governments through their Ministries of Health have extensive educational programs in nutrition. Many countries have improved the average diet by requiring food producers to enrich certain staples and by better methods of preserving and distributing foods. In the United States, the Department of Agriculture and the Public Health Service through its various bureaus give educational and consultant services to state health departments. Nutritionists are regular members of such departments and are more and more consistently found in public and private agencies offering generalized health services. The Nutrition Foundation and other agencies are engaged in nutrition research, education, or service. Schools and hospitals of any standing in this country must provide specialists in nutrition who can plan and teach optimum dietaries. The effect of public education is seen in the improved use of the food dollar as reported in studies of the US Department of Agriculture over the last 70 years. We are slowly learning to buy the essentials first. For example, in 1942 we spent more than in the first quarter of the century on the following items: milk and cheese, fruits and vegetables. Less was spent on sweets, grains (bread), meat, fish, poultry, and eggs.[9]

* Davison, Charles S.: "Nutrition, Agriculture, Foreign Aid and the Population Problem" (editorial), Am. J. Clin. Nutr., 13:66, (Aug.) 1963.
† Josué de Castro says: "There is no doubt whatever that the low stature of tropical peoples is not a racial characteristic, but is the result of defective diet that is insufficient in protein. The average Chinese weighs 121 pounds and the average European 139, a difference due to hunger rather than to race. . . .
"On the Shetland Islands . . . grew the smallest horses in the world, hardly more than toys for children. It used to be thought that these Shetland ponies constituted a separate race of horses, stabilized by inbreeding. . . . The fact is, there are no separate races of ponies. Shetland ponies are descendants of English horses . . . ; the extreme poverty of the northern soil in certain minerals, and the consequent poverty of the pastures, led to a progressive deterioration of the species. Even after hundreds of generations, when the

ponies were taken to areas with richer soils they regained the characteristics of their ancestors.
"Exactly the same sort of phenomenon takes place with certain human groups. The Chinese and Japanese may be considered 'human ponies,' their height and weight reduced by chronic malnutrition; . . . individuals of these races, emigrating to the United States, take only two generations to produce descendants with a significant increase of several inches in height. . . . The Pygmies of Equatorial Africa lose their Pygmy characteristics when transplanted to the plain's regions where agriculture and cattle raising provide much more varied alimentary resources than their . . . limited diet of wild products of the rain forest. Thus the so-called 'inferior races' turn out to be starved races; properly nourished, they are in all respects equal to the would-be superior races." (Op. cit., pp. 38, 64, 65.)

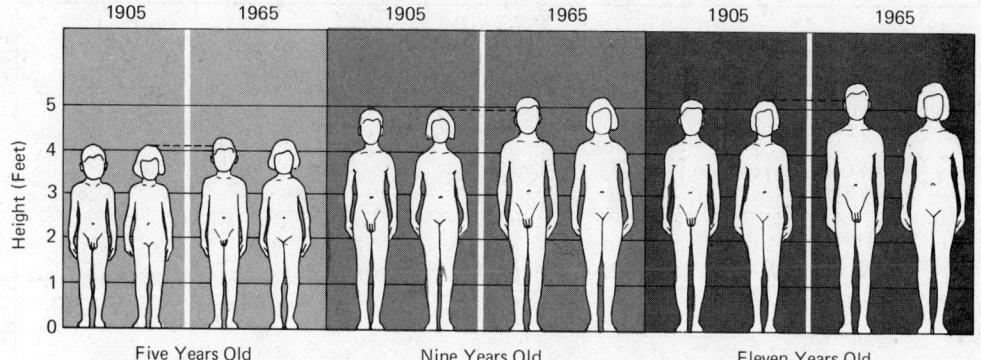

Figure 10-1. Increased size of children stems mainly from earlier maturation. A boy and girl aged five in 1965, and of average economic circumstances, were taller by about two inches than their counterparts of a half-century ago; nine-year-olds of 1965 averaged some three inches taller and 11-year-olds nearly four inches taller. The figures are based on measurements made in the United States and Europe. (From Tanner, James: "Early Maturation in Man," *Scientific American* **218:**21, [Jan.] 1968. Copyright © 1968 by Scientific American, Inc. All rights reserved.)

In 1965–66, the Agricultural Research and Marketing Service of the Department of Agriculture conducted the most comprehensive survey to date, involving 15,000 households. Their findings include the following: (1) 20 per cent of the diets were poor; (2) though families spent more money for food than in 1955, the dietary levels were similar; (3) the three nutrients most frequently provided at less than recommended levels were vitamin A, calcium, and ascorbic acid; and (4) thiamine, riboflavin, protein, iron, and niacin were provided at less than recommended levels in about 5 to 10 per cent of the households.[10] During 1963–1966, we spent more money on meat, poultry and fish, and fruits and vegetables; less money on dairy products and cereals and bakery products.[11] We are still a long way from Henry C. Sherman's and Caroline S. Lanford's recommendation (of 1951) that whatever the level of expenditure:

(1) At least as much should be spent for milk (including cream and cheese if used) as for meats, poultry, and fish; and

(2) At least as much should be spent for fruits and vegetables as for meats, poultry, and fish.*

Present-day food planners and providers have scientific and convenient guides for feeding families and large groups. Examples are *Family Fare: Food Management and Recipes,*[12] *Food: For Families with School Children,*[13] both published by the Department of Agricul-

ture; *Food for Peace Around the World,*[14] published by the Department of State; *Balance Food Values and Cents,*[15] *Saving Ways in Food Buying,*[16] both published by the University of California Agricultural Extension Service; *Health Foods: Facts and Fakes,* published by Public Affairs Committee, Inc.[16a]; *Normal and Therapeutic Nutrition*[17] by Corinne H. Robinson; *Introductory Nutrition*[18] by Helen Andrews Guthrie; and such specialized publications as *Nutrition and Family Health Service*[19] by Linnea Anderson and John H. Browe, and *Maternal Nutrition and the Course of Pregnancy,*[20] published by the National Academy of Sciences. Articles in the *Journal of the American Dietetic Association, Nutrition Review, Journal of Nutrition, Nutrition Abstracts Review,* and many other scientific journals provide the most up-to-date and accurate reports on current questions. Much of this information is simplified for general reading and published in popular magazines and texts. These are often reliable guides, but nurses, if they suggest such sources to patients, should use them critically.

Nurses especially should be prepared to help those they serve choose foods according to their needs. Much of the improvement in dietary habits in this and other countries is the result of the work of nurses, particularly "public health nurses." While community nursing services employ nutritionists as consultants, nurses carry the major part of the teaching program.[21-23] Nurses, being one of the most informed classes of health workers, and the most numerous, are in a position to promote legislation influencing nutrition and related questions such as protection of the public from contami-

* Sherman, Henry C., and Lanford, Caroline S.: *Essentials of Nutrition,* 3rd ed. Macmillan Publishing Co., Inc., New York, 1951, p. 352.

uh University Hospital

Dietary Continuing Care
Dietary Services

Diet prescription

Calories ————————————————

Protein (gm) ——————————————

Fat (gm) ————————————————

Cho (gm) ————————————————

Cho distribution ——————————————

Meal Pattern	Breakfast	10 A.M.	Lunch	3 P.M.	Dinner	H.S.
Meat exchange						
Vegetable A exchange						
Vegetable B exchange						
Bread exchange						
Fat exchange						
Fruit exchange						
Milk exchange						

Comments

————————————————————
Dietitian's Signature

Figure 10-2. A diet prescription form to be completed by a dietitian. (Courtesy of University Hospital, University of Western Ontario, London, Ont.)

nated foods. In working with families and other social groups they can help influence the psychologic climate of meals as well as the provision of appealing and nutritious food. Both are fundamental aspects of good human relations and physical health. The fact that families move oftener in this than in other decades, that the mothers are more often employed, and that other conditions threaten the stability of family life have changed the pattern of family meals—for the worse. On the other hand, there have never been so many young persons informed about and interested in nutrition. Health-food shops * are on the increase and television programs on food prep-

* Prices in such shops are higher for the same items than in regular markets and probably unjustified since at present there are inadequate guarantees of superior quality.

aration are among the most popular. Nurses, dietitians, and others might well expect a more highly motivated public, with respect to nutrition, in this age than in any former one —certainly a more informed public.

The psychologic effects of inadequate diets can scarcely be measured. Eating clay (pica) and paint, which produces lead poisoning if the paint has a lead base, are two conditions all too commonly found in the United States among those who cannot afford a good diet.[23a] Some pregnant women, who can afford an adequate diet, choose to buy starch (Argo) for eating. Some also eat clay.

The importance of clean, as well as balanced, diets cannot be overstated. Reduction in the death rate, with the increased average life span in this country during this century, discussed in Chapter 15, is due largely to cleaner food and drink than was available in the last.

The Food and Drug Administration and the Department of Agriculture largely control wholesome food—processing, packaging, and distribution in interstate commerce. Food sanitation programs are also under local and state control. They include service, preparation, processing, sale, and distribution of food on a local level. Other aspects of the subject, such as sterilization of dishes and food poisoning, are discussed in Chapters 15 and 36, respectively.

In hospitals, where diet is a vital part of the therapeutic plan for each patient, the physician usually prescribes the general nature of the diet, but depends on the nurses and dietitians to see that the patient is well fed—in fact, some physicians have, in the writer's opinion, taken too little responsibility for nutrition in health and sickness. Many persons under treatment for vague complaints are simply malnourished; many patients who seem to be making slow progress toward recovery in severe illness are suffering from weeks of incomplete dietaries. A nurse, who may be a student of nutrition, should be guided by the patient's needs, as he or she sees them, in suggesting diets or methods of feeding no matter what the setting. The patient, the family, and health workers (see Fig. 10-2) may all be involved in dietary plans and procedures.[23b, 23c]

In a review of nutritional requirements of the young, infants, and children, Robert L. Jackson and his associates say:

Frequency, severity and manifestations of malnutrition vary considerably in degree and kind in different areas of the world, between different sections of a country, at different ages, and in different social groups. Advances in nutrition and their application have almost eliminated nutritional deficiency diseases in our country. Nevertheless, despite our abundance of high quality foods, many Americans are malnourished. Malnutrition includes overnutrition as well as undernutrition, and we have to concern ourselves with inadequacies, imbalances and excesses.*

Eugene F. DuBois [21] demonstrated many years ago that a typhoid patient with a dietary requirement greater than that of the normal person could, if adequately fed, be brought through a 6-weeks' illness with no loss of weight. He admits, however, that feeding a sick man 3000 calories daily requires great nursing skill.

The "good mother" and the "good nurse" must know how to provide for the nutritional needs of those in their care. This includes ensuring appetizing food and providing such assistance in eating as these persons require, and helping individuals gain a better understanding of their nutritional needs in health and in illness. Sherman and Lanford, summing up the "nutritional improvement of life," say:

Thus we are now in a new era of nutritional knowledge, in which this knowledge serves the improvement of life in two ways: (1) correctively, in the cure and prevention of deficiency diseases and of the less well recognized states of nutritional shortage or subnormality; and (2) constructively, in the improvement of already-normal health.*

2. DIETARY ESSENTIALS AND THEIR FUNCTIONS

Essentials of Adequate and Optimum Dietaries. Diets are measured quantitatively in calories (see page 444) and qualitatively according to how well they supply the following elements: protein, carbohydrate, fat, minerals, and vitamins. Water is of course a most necessary element, but in health its availability is usually taken for granted. The role of each of the nutrients may be discussed separately, but the reader should realize that all are combined in most natural foods. A complete diet is one that provides (1) food fuel, the oxidation of which supplies energy for the varied, unceasing body activities; (2) what is needed for tissue building and upkeep; and (3) materials that regulate body processes or the components from which these regulators are formed. All of these processes are essential to life, so nature has combined in our foods carbohydrates and fats, which are chiefly fuels; proteins, essential to tissue building and repair; and minerals, vitamins, and water, usually classified as regulators of body processes. Since none of these elements can act independently, such a statement may be a misleading simplification of a complex subject. The four food groups (milk-cheese group, meat group, vegetable-fruit group, and bread-cereals group) are used as a guide in planning an adequate daily diet.

Carbohydrates. Sugar and starches are the chief *source* of carbohydrates. They are composed of carbon, hydrogen, and oxygen, the latter elements in the same relationship to each other quantitatively as in water; hence, the name. According to their molecular structure they are classified chemically as monosaccharides, disaccharides, and polysaccharides. All carbohydrates are hydrolyzed in digestion into the monosaccharides or simple sugars and absorbed rapidly in the small intestine, and, when oxidized within the cells, their end products are carbon dioxide and water. Glucose, fructose, and galactose are simple sugars that are

---

* Jackson, Robert L., et al.: "Nutritional Requirements of Infants and Children," *Pediatr. Clin. North Am.,* **9:**879, (Nov.) 1962.

* Sherman, Henry C., and Lanford, Caroline S.: *op. cit.,* p. 7.

important nutritionally; sucrose, lactose, and maltose are disaccharides in common use; and starch, glycogen, cellulose, and dextrine are polysaccharides that must be hydrolyzed into many simple sugar molecules before they can be utilized by the tissues. Of all foods the simple sugars are most readily utilized; glucose infused into the tissues is available immediately for cell metabolism. Carbohydrate is stored largely in the liver but also in the muscles as the polysaccharide glycogen and is converted by the liver into glucose as needed.

The physiologic *function* of carbohydrate is the production of energy. After its conversion by the digestive process into simple sugars, it is oxidized at once within the cells or carried to the liver, converted to glycogen, and stored there, in the muscles, or in traces throughout the body for future use. The liver cells can store up to 8 per cent of their weight and muscle cells up to 1 per cent. Some physiologists believe that glycogen is stored in two forms: *free* glycogen, which is readily released, and *fixed* glycogen, which is released only slowly.[25] When carbohydrate intake exceeds the immediate needs of the body and its capacity or need for glycogen storage, it is converted into fat—a much more concentrated fuel that the body can accommodate in large quantity. Those who understand and accept these fundamental principles of carbohydrate metabolism can make two obvious applications to everyday living and health practice: (1) simple sugars yield an immediate return in energy, and (2) a diet with carbohydrate in excess of actual needs inevitably fattens the body.

Because sugars, starchy roots, and grains are palatable and relatively cheap, there is rarely a question of meeting the *need* for carbohydrate. Proteins and fats are, on the other hand, relatively costly. Ordinarily, diets should be planned to supply the necessary proteins and fats, leaving the remaining caloric needs to be met by carbohydrate. It is possible to reduce the carbohydrate intake too much. Irving L. Schwartz and Martin Fein [26] say it has been clearly demonstrated by numerous experiments that carbohydrates act as a protector of body protein; carbohydrates are burned in preference to fat or protein. Studies have demonstrated that a diet deficient in carbohydrates can result in urinary loss of sodium, excessive nitrogen loss, and progressive loss of weight for at least three days as well as marked fatigue. Ketosis also occurs. These findings suggest that some carbohydrates should be retained in the diet of persons wishing to lose weight.[27] The fact that most natural foods combine fats and proteins and carbohydrates indicates that the metabolism of each is enhanced by the presence of the others; investi-

gators continue to study the metabolic interaction between these nutrients.[28] Some studies show that the interchange of potassium between the cells and the intercellular fluid is dependent (to some extent) on the presence of glucose and that the oxidation of glucose depends upon the presence of potassium. Both sodium and potassium must be present for optimum absorption of glucose. As more is learned about nutrition, a greater number of such dependencies will undoubtedly be established.[29-32]

When carbohydrate and fat intake is insufficient to supply the body's energy needs, protein foods, and if necessary the tissue proteins, must be drawn upon. This results in wasting, or emaciation. Even when the process does not proceed this far, the utilization of protein as a major source of energy is uneconomical. When enough protein is eaten, the body actually meets the energy needs and stores fat. Carbohydrate can be synthesized from protein, and fats from the resultant carbohydrate. Most authorities agree that when an individual is on an almost exclusively protein diet, the fat formed is similar in composition to that synthesized from dietary carbohydrates.

Many persons (diabetics and those trying to lose weight) are using artificial sweeteners. It should be noted that a number of studies indicate that some of these persons develop dermatitis.[33] Cyclamates are off the general market, and Britain, Canada, and Sweden, as well as this country, have banned the chemical from foods, according to *Consumer Reports, 1970*. Studies have shown that rats develop bladder cancer when given massive doses of cyclamates. Saccharin, a popular noncaloric sugar substitute used by many people, is also undergoing study to determine whether or not it is harmful to humans.

Fats and Lipids. Cream, butter, fatty meats and fish, and oils from vegetables and nuts are the chief *sources* of food fats and lipids. Fats and lipids are sometimes called lipins and lipoids. A true fat is in chemical nature a triglyceride, almost all of which during digestion is broken down into glycerol and three fatty acids: oleic acid, stearic acid, and palmitic acid. According to most authorities, there are several theories of fat absorption, a complex process. Arthur C. Guyton [34] says that fats are believed to be absorbed through the intestinal membrane in the form of fatty acids and monoglycerides, although triglycerides and diglycerides are also absorbed. As they pass through the epithelial cell, they are resynthesized to triglycerides and "wend their way into the lacteals of the villi and from here are pumped by the lymphatic pump upward through the thoracic duct to be emptied into the great veins of the neck." * Between 80 and 90 per cent of fat is absorbed as described and transported to the blood through the thoracic lymph. About 10 to 20 per cent of fatty acids are absorbed directly into the portal blood. Bile salts increase the rate of absorption of fatty acids and glycerides. Protein seems to be necessary in the transfer of lipids from the cells to the lymph or blood. In the fasting state, the lipid components of plasma (expressed in mean values in mg per 100 ml) are as follows: total lipid 530 mg, total fatty acids 316 mg, neutral fat 142 mg, phospholipid 165 mg, total cholesterol 152 mg, free cholesterol 46 mg, and cholesterol esters 178 mg.[35] Physiological chemists believe that more knowledge of fat metabolism may enable us to control hypertension and other diseases in which unusual blood lipid values are observed. Charles H. Best and Norman B. Taylor say:

Serum cholesterol levels can be reduced, in man, through control of the diet in three ways (a) by reducing excess caloric intake, (b) by reducing the intake of animal fats and (c) by increasing the intake of vegetable oils. These oils are rich in unsaturated fatty acids.[†]

Fat metabolism is dependent on secretions of the liver and pancreas, as well as on those of the small intestine.[35a]

Fats are ultimately oxidized to form carbon dioxide and water. During the process, intermediary compounds are formed that are collectively named "ketone bodies." The blood normally contains minute amounts (1 to 3 mg in 100 ml blood or 0.001 to 0.003 per cent). When this value is markedly increased, as it may be in diseases of the pancreas or thyroid, or when fever or starvation upsets metabolic balance, "ketosis" or "acidosis" occurs. The blood does not actually become acid because if the pH of arterial blood, which remains remarkably constant around 7.4, rises above 7.8 or drops to 6.8, death occurs. However, the push toward the acid side given by these intermediate products of fat oxidation is dangerous and greatly dreaded.[36]

Lipids are fatlike substances that accompany fats. They are soluble in fat solvents or in fats themselves. Best and Taylor classify them as (1) phospholipids, examples of which are lecithin, cephalin, and sphingomyelin; (2) cerebrosides or glycolipids, to which group belong phrenosin and kerasin; and (3) waxes, important examples of which are the choles-

terol esters. Helen S. Mitchell *et al.* classify sterols as lipids, but Best and Taylor list them separately, mentioning free cholesterol and ergosterol as examples. They also put the fatty hydrocarbons, such as squalene and carotene, into a separate category. In discussion of metabolism studies, blood chemistry, and special diets, nurses will hear reference made to these fatlike substances. Diets are planned in some conditions to control the cholesterol and lecithin content.

Fats vary in character and food value according to their component fatty acids and vitamins. Like carbohydrates, fats are derived from carbon, hydrogen, and oxygen, but there is proportionately less oxygen in the molecule. The oxidation of glucose ($C_6H_{12}O_6$) is accomplished readily, while the oxidation of stearic acid ($C_{18}H_{36}O_2$), derived from the digestion of certain facts, is a far slower and more complex process.

Fats *function* chiefly as a source of energy. Like carbohydrates, they are stored for future use as adipose tissue. As fuel, these two dietary elements are largely interchangeable, but some investigators have shown that a fat-free diet retards growth.[37] The term *essential fatty acids* (EFA) appears frequently in the literature, although authors do not always say which they consider essential. Linoleic acid, a polyunsaturated acid, is usually referred to as the main essential fatty acid. Since it is not synthesized by the body, it must be included in the diet. Following an extensive survey of the literature (354 references) on essential fatty acids, E. Aaes-Jørgensen concludes:

Thirty years of intensive work in many laboratories have significantly improved our knowledge and understanding of the role of different dietary fats. However, many problems still remain to be solved and many apparent controversies in the interpretation of experimental data have yet to be cleared up.

. . . EFA are necessary for infants. A probable figure for an adequate daily supply of EFA for infants is of the order of about 4% of the dietary calories as linoleic acid. The possible requirement of adults needs clarification. From the dietary standpoint the essential fatty acids occur in abundant amounts in most vegetable oils, and, to a lesser extent, in most animal fats. There it is generally agreed that a reasonable variation in the diet will supply man with the necessary amounts of EFA under normal conditions.[*]

Studies continue to be reported showing the importance of linoleic acid for infants' nutrition in promoting growth and preventing dry scaly skin with thickening.[38]

Culturally, diets vary greatly in fat content.

* Guyton, Arthur C.: *Textbook of Medical Physiology,* 5th ed. W. B. Saunders Co., Philadelphia, 1976, p. 891.
† Best, Charles H., and Taylor, Norman B.: *The Physiological Basis of Medical Practice,* 8th ed. Williams & Wilkins Co., Baltimore, 1966, p. 1402.

* Aaes-Jørgensen, E.: "Essential Fatty Acids," *Physiol. Rev.,* **41:**46, (Jan.) 1961.

Americans consider a diet low in fats unpalatable. Mitchell and associates [39] say that during the past 50 years statistics for the entire country show an increased per capita use of fats. These authorities say that while there is no physiological proof that the human body needs as much fat as Americans eat neither is there proof that such amounts are harmful—however, some experts recommend that 25 to 30 per cent of the total calories in the diet be in the form of fat. Most authorities mention the importance of supplying special vitamin-carrying fats for infants and adults. Discussing the function of fats, Robinson says:

In addition to providing energy, fats serve as (1) padding around the organs, holding them in place and absorbing the shocks to which they might otherwise be subjected; (2) protection for the nerves; (3) insulators for the body, thus avoiding rapid changes of body temperature by excessive heat loss from its surface; (4) spares of body proteins, since a sufficient amount of carbohydrates and fats furnishes the energy needed to carry on the work of the body; (5) carriers of the fat-soluble vitamins; (6) lubricants of the gastrointestinal tract; and (7) depressors of gastric secretion, thus delaying the emptying of the stomach and retarding the appearance of hunger.*

Hundreds of references (opinions and investigations) may be found in the literature on cholesterol and its relationship to coronary vascular disease and atherosclerosis. The average layman knows about the role of cholesterol in health and sickness and ways of decreasing it in his diet. However, it should never be considered an abnormal substance in the body as it has vital functions to perform. It is, for example, a precursor of vitamin D; it is closely related to several hormones in the body; and it is an essential constituent of many cells, especially nerve and glandular cells.[40] There is question about the interrelationships of fats, proteins, carbohydrates, and cholesterol.[41-43a] The relationship of cholesterol and atherosclerosis is far from settled.

Because fats are the least easily digested of the food elements and because animal fats, which are more digestible than the vegetable, are costly, many old people, particularly, reduce their fat intake below the optimum point. Lessened activity and a falling metabolic rate reduce the caloric need, and therefore the intake of carbohydrates and fats should be reduced proportionately, but if the reduction is made largely through fats, the diet is dangerously low in fat-soluble vitamins.[44,45]

* Robinson, Corinne H.: *Normal and Therapeutic Nutrition*, 13th ed. Macmillan Publishing Co., Inc., New York, 1967, p. 89.

Dietaries for the very ill are made up of foods quickly and easily digested, which are usually low in fats. Care is taken, however, during this limited period of illness to give vitamin supplements as indicated. The coating of foods by fats, as in frying, is believed to retard contact of the food with digestive secretions. Many dietary items well tolerated in other forms cause distress if so cooked. Some physicians maintain that hydrochloric acid excretion in the stomach is diminished in the aged and that this and inactivity may account largely for the "indigestion" that is such a common complaint of the elderly. Such physicians prescribe hydrochloric acid to combat this condition and warn against the common practice of taking sodium bicarbonate for "heartburn" as this discomfort is often called.

Proteins. That element in the diet essential to tissue growth and repair is called protein from the Greek verb *prōteios,* to take first rank. The protein molecule is complex in nature. It contains nitrogen and sulfur in addition to carbon, hydrogen, and oxygen and is constructed of building units known as amino acids. According to Best and Taylor, 21 amino acids have been identified, and it is believed that some proteins contain almost all of these, making a very large molecule that can stretch or fold up. Protein is the basis of all living things, animal and vegetable; muscle is almost entirely protein. Some authorities believe that all protein molecules are essentially fibrous but that they vary enormously according to the number and arrangement of the building units, the molecular weight and shape, and chemical behavior.

Animals and plants are the chief *sources* of protein foods, as has been implied. Each animal or plant species is thought to have its chemically distinct protein. The possible arrangements of the amino acids, or building units, is infinite since a protein molecule may contain a few or most of those known and there may be hundreds of links within the molecular structure. Plants can synthesize or build their characteristic proteins from materials in the soil and air. Animals are dependent upon their food for material with which to build proteins. They can synthesize some amino acids within their bodies, but others they cannot and are therefore dependent upon protein foods containing the amino acids they must have but cannot synthesize or perhaps cannot synthesize in sufficient quantities. Nutrients containing such tissue-building units are said to contain the nutritionally essential amino acids.

Mitchell and associates [46] point out that as the physiologic significance of proteins came to be understood and as it was realized that the specific amino acids they contain determines the nutritive value of proteins, many investigations were conducted to learn which of the amino acids were essential in the diet. They list nine amino acids that are essential to normal growth and body function: (1) lysine, (2) tryptophan, (3) valine, (4) phenylalanine, (5) leucine, (6) isoleucine, (7) threonine, (8) methionine, and (9) histidine. To maintain nitrogen balance (loss of nitrogen in the excreta is approximately equal to the nitrogen in the protein intake) within the body, the adult's diet should contain all these amino acids except the last one, histidine. In infancy, histidine is required for normal growth, and withdrawal is associated with eczematoid dermatitis.[47] Several authors suggest that arginine, as well as histidine, should be included in the diets of infants and children as they may affect growth. Nonessential amino acids are those the body can synthesize in sufficient amounts to meet its needs if the total intake of protein is sufficient in quantity and quality. Mitchell and associates[48] classify proteins according to their nutritive value as follows: (1) "complete" proteins are those that maintain and support growth—an example, casein, a milk protein; (2) "partially incomplete" proteins are those that maintain life but do not support growth—gliadin (wheat protein) is representative of this group; and (3) "incomplete" proteins are those that do not maintain life as they are lacking in one or more of the essential amino acids—zein (corn protein) belongs to this group.

Fortunately, almost all foods except gelatin contain more than one kind of protein. Animal protein is generally superior to vegetable. Whole milk and eggs take first place; animal tissues are next in importance, liver and kidneys being even more valuable than muscles. Whole grains provide important protein, particularly if fed with a diet containing milk. In the diets of children, pregnant or lactating women, or of emaciated invalids it is especially important to include abundant milk and eggs as sources of body-building proteins.[49,50]

The *function* of protein is implied in its source. If protein is the chief component of protoplasm, it follows that its function is to build and repair living tissues. Both cells and intercellular substances contain protein; it is found in the complex molecular structure of hormones and other regulators of body activity. A diet that does not supply the protein need affects every aspect of the body economy. It is such a threat to the future of a race or species that, according to some experts, nature responds to inadequate diets, but particularly

to those deficient in protein, by increasing fertility. This is not just a theory. It is explained physiologically by studies showing that protein deficiency makes the liver less able to inactivate estrogens; excess estrogen raises the level of fertility in women. De Castro thinks that, while the scientific explanation is only partially available and the information even less widely known and accepted, the relationship between poverty and fecundity has been apparent for centuries. He cites the Latin expression, "The table is meagre, but fertile is the bed of misery," and the meaning of the Roman word for the poor and undernourished—"proletarian," he who has many *proles* or offspring. He goes on to say, "Cattle raisers have long known that animals which get too fat may become sterile and that reduced rations will reestablish fertility." * James R. Slonaker[51] studied six generations of rats and found that diets containing more than 18 per cent of the total calories in protein retarded the epoch of fertilization of the females, reduced the number of offspring in the litters and the number of litters. At the same time, the progeny, although fewer in number, showed a higher survival rate and a greater resistance to disease.

While substandard diets, particularly protein hunger, may increase the birth rate, starvation diets would not. The life of the starving individual rather than the continuation of the race is then at stake. He is actually ill, and his energy is concentrated on survival. Sex interest and, in fact, every aspect of the libido wane.[52-54] Anemia and decreased hormonal activities (sexual hormones and thyroid activity) have been demonstrated.[55,56] Numerous studies during the last decades have demonstrated that a diet deficient in protein interferes with physical growth and development, and a number suggest that it also influences the mental capacity in children. It has been reported that little cell division occurs in the human brain after 5 months of age and that further growth occurs by increase in protein, RNA, and lipid content of cells. Fewer brain cells have been found in malnourished children (less than 1 year of age) as compared to those who were well-nourished. It is not known, however, how severe the nutritional deprivation must be to show these events or if this represents irreversible change.[56a,56b]

Nevin S. Scrimshaw says:

The world-wide importance of protein malnutrition lies in the high frequency with which malnutrition and infection act synergistically in young children in technically underdeveloped

* De Castro, Josué: *op. cit.,* p. 70.

areas from the time breast milk is no longer an adequate source of protein until approximately five years of age. By the age of five years those children who do survive will have acquired resistance to many of the common infectious diseases, will have been allowed to share fully in the diet of the family, and will have a somewhat lower requirement for protein per kilo of body weight. Because of the synergism between malnutrition and infection, mortality is from 10 to 60 times higher in children one to five years of age in technically underdeveloped areas than in the well-nourished populations of the developed countries. Moreover, surviving children experience some permanent retardation in physical growth as well as in psychomotor development.*

The African name kwashiorkor is given to a protein deficiency disease of young children whose diet contains little or no protein, and children with this condition may be found in all parts of the world.[57] According to J. S. Garrow,[58] disturbance of function in children with this condition includes poor cardiac function, impaired renal function, deficiency of intestinal lactose and all pancreatic enzymes, numerous endocrine abnormalities, and diarrhea; in fact, there is evidence that the function of almost every organ is impaired.

In summary, the studies cited suggest the possibility of reducing to some extent the quantity of animal or human life and markedly improving the quality by feeding optimum diets, particularly with respect to protein.

The protein need in sickness is likely to be higher than in health, contrary to general opinion in the not so distant past. Whenever there is a breakdown in tissue, as with ulcers or abscesses, when there is hemorrhage or seepage from wounds and burns, or when fever raises the metabolic rate, dietary protein should exceed the individual's normal intake. Gone for good, we hope, is the once classic invalid's diet of toast and tea, baked potato, and rice with an occasional custard and a little beef extract. Such feeding inevitably led to protein hunger with all its ills and the avitaminoses and mineral deficiencies that almost routinely accompanied protracted illness. There is abundant evidence that healing takes place more rapidly with a high-protein rather than with a low-protein diet. This is so generally accepted that even in the critical stage of a self-limited illness, when it may be necessary to feed the patient through the veins, solutions of predigested proteins, whole blood, and plasma are given in sufficient quantities to meet the requirement. Liquid diets include milk, eggs,

finely ground meats, poultry, fish or predigested animal protein, and even vegetable proteins according to the special demands of each patient. Protein supplements are used in all sorts of diets. Protenol is an example of such a preparation; sodium-free Lanolac is used in sodium-poor diets. These supplements can be given in orange juice, tomato juice, soup, or milk. (Chocolate-flavored Protenol is more palatable than the plain variety.) Vegetable protein mixtures such as INCAP and CMS (mixture of corn, soy, and milk) have been developed and are used successfully in treating Kwashiorkor in technically underdeveloped countries. And some infants in the United States are being fed on such milk substitutes. Of the many studies published on this subject, some are included in the references.[59-64]

The amount and kind of protein required depend on the immediate tissue needs for growth and repair. Protein need is greater in periods of growth, during pregnancy and lactation, and following periods of malnutrition or diseases characterized by tissue destruction as in carcinoma, infectious diseases, exophthalmic goiter, and pernicious anemia, in which the cells are always poorly nourished. The amount required *by the adult* for tissue repair is relatively small and constant. The Food and Nutrition Board of the National Research Council recommends the following: 65 gm of protein per day for a healthy man weighing 70 kg or 0.09 gm of protein for each kilogram of body weight; 55 gm of protein per day for a woman weighing 58 kg, or 0.09 gm of protein for each kilogram of body weight; for boys of 15 to 18 years of age, approximately 1⅓ gm of protein per kilogram of body weight; for girls of the same age, slightly more than 1 gm of protein to each kilogram of body weight; and for a child from 1 to 3 years, slightly more than 2½ gm of protein per kilogram of body weight.[65] The recommended amount of protein for infants varies, and most authors state that it is a complex problem with many questions yet unanswered. However, when using body weight in determining requirements of the infant for essential amino acids, they are far higher than those of the adult.[66] When cow's milk makes up the bulk of the diet, 3.5 gm of protein per kilogram of body weight is advocated.[67] For premature infants, 4 to 6 gm protein per kilogram of body weight is recommended.[68] For the adult, youth, and children, some authorities recommend less, others, more, than those given above.

In order that about two thirds of the daily allowance be complete proteins, an adult's daily diet should include one moderate serving of meat, one egg, and two glasses of milk; the

* Scrimshaw, Nevin S.: "World-Wide Importance of Protein Malnutrition and Progress Toward Its Prevention," *Am. J. Public Health*, **53**:1787, (Nov.) 1963.

remainder may be furnished by cereals and vegetables. For *children* a relatively higher proportion of protein is required (about 15 per cent of the total calories), and at least two thirds of this allowance should be complete (animal) proteins. Two or three glasses of milk and an egg daily are advisable, with other foods such as beef (stew meat) providing the proper amount and kind of protein.

Physiologists have demonstrated that storage of large quantities of amino acids in the cell does not occur; however, some are stored as protein that can be decomposed into amino acids. Tissues that have high metabolic rates, such as the liver, kidney, and intestinal mucosa, store some protein but each type of cell has a limit on the amount it can store.[69]

The body maintains a nitrogen balance by increasing nitrogenous wastes when protein foods are eaten in excess of body needs. When the daily nitrogen intake equals the daily nitrogen output, the body is said to be in *nitrogen balance,* or equilibrium. Because the kidneys bear the brunt of excreting nitrogenous waste, a high-protein diet is believed by some physicians to injure them. The fact that Eskimos, who live almost entirely on meat, do not show a high incidence of renal disease has cast doubt on this theory. While 20 gm of protein may keep an adult male weighing 70 kg in nitrogen balance, the consensus is that the quality of life is improved by a higher intake.[70,71,71a]

An idiosyncrasy to certain proteins is not unusual. For instance, some persons are allergic to eggs; others, to shellfish. Allergy is the term used for this sensitiveness to a food or an inhaled protein. The irritating factor in an article of diet, a pollen, feathers, or hair is believed to be a protein. Diets are restricted when idiosyncrasies are known or suspected, and attempts are usually made to desensitize the victim. Persons with severe food allergies are sometimes fed protein hydrolysates because the hydrolyzing process destroys the specificity of the protein to which the person is susceptible.

Mineral Elements. Most authorities separate mineral elements into two groups: principal minerals, those that occur in the body in relatively large amounts, and trace elements, those that occur in foods in traces and are needed in only minute amounts. Table 10-1 lists the principal minerals, important sources, daily requirements, and effects of deficiencies. Mitchell and associates [72] say the body requires the following *principal minerals:* calcium, phosphorus, potassium, chlorine, sodium, sulfur, magnesium, iron, and iodine. Our knowledge of the functions of these elements in the

body and in foods is incomplete, and it is not known whether all of them are physiologically significant. It has been established, however, that certain minerals present in minute amounts, such as iodine, are nevertheless essential dietary components. A varied diet of plants and animals grown in most habitable areas yields all the mineral elements. A monotonous diet or one taken from the products of depleted soil can fail to provide many of these minerals in sufficient quantity for optimum health. Pure carbohydrates and fats furnish no minerals, but man is dependent upon the sulfur that enters into the composition of proteins. Proteins also yield phosphorus, iron, and calcium. Most authorities say that an adequate supply of all minerals except sulfur can be supplied by foods other than protein, though it is a better source.

All components of the body are widely distributed in natural foods with the exception of sodium. De Castro says that although there are 13 metalloids and 16 metals always present in living matter, and "man may suffer sporadically from shortages of any or all of the mineral elements that go to make up his tissues, there are only a few whose deficiency may ordinarily be considered of social significance. They are iron, calcium, sodium, and iodine." * Diets should, therefore, be planned to include an adequate supply of these elements. Where the drinking water contains a sufficient concentration of iodine its provision is no problem.

Minerals *function* as constituents of rigid and soft tissues, and mineral salts in the body fluids act as regulators. A few of these functions are discussed briefly in the following pages. Nurses should, however, make a far more detailed study of the subject in such texts as those suggested at the end of this chapter.

Calcium is the most abundant mineral in the body; *phosphorus* is an element of every known cell. These two minerals are often considered together. Both function as constituents of hard and soft tissues and as regulators. Combined as calcium phosphate, they are preponderant in bone and tooth structure.

They are both widely distributed in plants; calcium is concentrated in the leaves and phosphorus in the seeds, while they are present in equal amounts in roots and stems. Calcium deficiencies are therefore common in animals when leafy foods are eliminated, and phosphorus deficiencies when grains are omitted. Animal foods, including milk, are a rich source of both these minerals, but the meat of grazing livestock may be relatively poor in phosphorus.

---

* De Castro, Josué: *op cit.,* p. 41.

There may be a slight loss of calcium and phosphorus in cooking vegetables, especially if the water is discarded; therefore, to provide a margin of safety, foods should be chosen that supply a liberal amount of these minerals.[73] If diets are planned to include sufficient calcium, the need for phosphorus will be met as the foods rich in calcium are rich in phosphorus,

but the reverse is not true.[74] Since phosphorus enters into the composition of all body tissues, any attempt to list its functions is obviously absurd. Because approximately 90 per cent of the body's phosphorus is in the skeleton, its deficiency, like that of calcium, is most apparent in abnormal bone structure.

Calcium deficiency is often said to be the

Table 10-1.   Principal Minerals, Sources, Daily Requirements, and Effects of Deficiencies *

Mineral	Major Sources	Daily Requirements	Effects of Deficiency

Calcium (Ca)	Animal:
	  Oysters, shrimp, clams, salmon
	  Milk
	  Cheese
	  Egg yolk
	Plant:
	  Whole grains
	  Legumes, nuts
	  Turnip, collards, kale, and other leafy green vegetables
	  Broccoli
		Children
		  1–10 yr, 1.2–1.4 gm
		Teenagers
		  Boys
		  10–18 yr, 1.2–1.4 gm
		  Girls
		  10–18 yr, 1.2–1.3 gm
		Adults 0.8 gm
		Pregnancy 1.2 gm
		Lactation 1.3 gm
			Stunted growth
			Malformation of bones and teeth
			Rickets
			Osteoporosis
			Tetany
			Renal calculi

Phosphorus (P)	Animal:
	  Meat, fish, fowl
	  Milk
	  Cheese
	  Egg yolk
	Plant:
	  Whole grains
	  Legumes, nuts
		Infants 0.2–0.5 mg
		Children 0.7–1.4 mg
		Adults 0.8 mg
		Pregnancy 1.3 mg
		Lactation 1.3 mg
			Poor mineralization
			Poor growth
			Rickets

Potassium (K)	Animal:
	  Meat, fish, fowl
	
	Plant:
	  Cereals
	  Fruits and vegetables
		Approximately 2–4 gm
		Diet adequate in protein, calcium and iron contains adequate potassium
			Muscle weakness
			Loss of appetite
			Nausea
			Vomiting
			Irritability
			Apathy
			Drowsiness
			Irregular heart rhythm

Chlorine (Cl)	Animal:
	  Meat
	  Milk
	  Eggs
	  Table salt
		Approximately 0.5 gm
		
		Diet contains
		  about 2–9 gm
			Disturbances in acid-base balance
			Hypochloremic alkalosis in a prolonged diarrhea and tube drainage

Sodium (Na)	Animal:
	  Meat, fish, fowl
	  Milk
	  Eggs
	
	Plant:
	  Carrots, beets, celery, spinach
	
	Table salt
		Approximately 0.5 gm
		
		Diet contains
		  about 2.6 gm
			Impaired osmotic pressure and water balance
			Nausea and nerve irritability
			Extreme losses by:
			  Sweating
			  Vomiting
			  Diarrhea
			Large intakes may be related to high blood pressure

Table 10-1 (continued)*

Mineral	Major Sources	Daily Requirements		Effects of Deficiency
Sulfur (S)	Animal: Meat Milk Cheese Eggs Plant: Legumes, nuts	Diet adequate in protein contains adequate sulfur		Impaired process of detoxification of toxic materials
Magnesium (Mg)	Animal: Meat Seafoods Milk Plant: Whole grains Cereals Legumes, nuts Dark green vegetables Fruits	Children 100–300 mg Adults 300–400 mg Pregnancy 450 mg Lactation 450 mg		Rare in humans Can cause neuromuscular irritability, cardiovascular calcification, and renal damage
Iron (Fe)	Animal: Liver and other meats Egg yolks Plant: Whole grains, enriched bread and cereals Legumes, nuts Peaches, apricots, prunes, raisins Potatoes Kale Dark green vegetables	Infants 0.3 mo 3–6 mo 6–12 mo Children 1–3 yr 3–10 yr Teenagers Men Women (under 55) Older women	6 mg 10 mg 15 mg 15 mg 10 mg 18 mg 10 mg 18 mg 10 mg	Reduced hemoglobin resulting in anemia
Iodine (I)	Animal: Seafoods Plant: Seafoods Iodized salt	Infants Children Men Women	25–45 mcg 55–140 mcg 140 mcg 100 mcg	Goiter Cretinism Thryotoxicosis

* Adapted from tables in Robinson, Corinne H.: *Normal and Therapeutic Nutrition,* 14th ed. Macmillan Publishing Co., Inc., New York, 1972, pp. 140–43; and Williams, Sue Rodwell: *Nutrition and Diet Therapy,* C. V. Mosby Co., St. Louis, 1969, pp. 134–35, with information on minerals taken from various sources.

most frequent and widespread dietary inadequacy. Because it is irregularly distributed in the soil and because its chief sources—milk, egg yolk, and certain vegetables—are limited in supply and therefore expensive, calcium hunger is one of the "hidden hungers." V. H. Mottran says:

Of all the elements included under the term "mineral elements," calcium is the most "weighty," and for a number of reasons.
(1) The body contains more of it than any other mineral element. All this must have come from the food.
(2) It is essential for the structures of bones and teeth.
(3) It catalyses reactions which result in con-

traction of muscles and conduction of nervous impulses.
(4) There are many parts of the world, and the whole strata in society, in which the calcium intake is deficient.*

Infants are born "calcium poor" so that they will be flexible during the process of birth. Small wonder that the infant deprived of calcium, or having a condition such as a deficiency in vitamin D that promotes its assimilation, develops a misshapen body. The daily recommended allowance of the National Research Council is as follows: 0.7 to 1.0 gm

* Mottran, V. H.: *Human Nutrition.* Edward Arnold (Publishers) Ltd., London, 1963, p. 71.

of calcium from 1 to 10 years; 1.2 to 1.4 gm for boys during the years of 10 to 18; 1.2 to 1.3 gm for girls during this age span; for adults (men and women) 0.8 gm and for women during pregnancy 1.2 gm and during lactation 1.3 gm. According to Philip L. White, Secretary of the Council on Foods and Nutrition of the American Medical Association, there is disagreement about the daily minimum requirements for dietary calcium for humans. He says:

It is generally agreed that there is no convincing evidence of harm at intakes of slightly less than 300 mg/day or as high as 2,000 mg/day in normal individuals. There is disagreement, however, about minimum dietary requirements for calcium for all age groups. Some believe the Recommended Dietary Allowances of the National Research Council are too high; others believe they should be increased for certain individuals.*

The views of six authorities are presented in a symposium on calcium requirements. The interested reader will find these helpful.[75] Diets meeting such standards will go a long way toward increasing man's vitality and life span and toward preventing rickets in the young and fractures in the elderly. We may come to look upon the bowed legs of infancy and old age as a sign of the same dietary deficiency, although at present we tend to stress the needs of the young and ignore those of the aging.

Iron has such vital functions in the human body that, while the amount needed is small, the provision of an adequate quantity in the diet is essential to health. It enters into the composition of oxygen-carrying hemoglobin and into the chromatin in the nucleus of every cell. It is therefore necessary for cell respiration, and deficiencies produce anemias with their widespread effects of oxygen want and other depletions. *Copper* enters into the composition of the hemoglobin molecule, but it is thought that most diets provide adequate amounts without special planning.[76] Iron-deficiency anemia is recognized as a problem in millions of people in the world today as it was in the past; this is especially true of women of childbearing age and infants. The 1965 food consumption surveys conducted by the US Department of Agriculture showed that dietary iron intake of the female population (10 to 55 years of age) averaged 11 mg per day, yet the recommended dietary allowance is 18 mg per day.[77,78] Lean meats are the chief source of iron in the adult diet of most Americans, Europeans, and others. Bread and cereals, enriched with iron, are another important source of this mineral. In addition, potatoes, certain vegetables such as kale, and fruits (especially prunes and raisins) may be selected to meet the present recommended daily allowance of 18 mg per day for females between the age of 10 and 55 years, including those who are pregnant or lactating; for men 18 to 75 years, 10 mg, with an increase of 8 mg (total 18 mg) for boys 10 to 18 years; children 1 to 3 years, 15 mg and between 3 and 10 years, 10 mg; for infants, birth to 3 months, 6 mg, 3 months to 6 months, 10 mg, and 6 months to 1 year, 15 mg. Irving Schulman[79] believes diets of all premature infants should include iron supplementation. Egg yolks, vegetable purées, and fortified cereals are valuable sources of iron for the infant.

Iodine is essential in human physiology even though the entire body may contain as little as 25 mg. Traces are present in natural waters and plants, but the quantity varies markedly in different geographic areas. The iodine-poor lands are most often inland and mountainous. It is well known that goiter is endemic in such regions. Iodine deficiency decreases the amount of thyroxin secreted by the thyroid gland, and the gland enlarges in an effort to fulfill its function. Since all vertebrates depend on a balanced endocrine activity for their normal development and emotional stability, a dietary deficiency that decreases the thyroid secretion has a profound effect. Most readers will have some knowledge of cretinism and myxedema and the results of treatment with thyroxin. Even more important is the prevention of these deficiency diseases. In "goiter" regions there are public health requirements on the reinforcement of table salt (sodium chloride) with one part of sodium or potassium iodide to 5000 or even 200,000 parts of sodium chloride. This is harmful to no one and should be considered a replacement of an element that is normally in the dietary.[80] Robinson says, "Many nations of the world have adopted laws that require the iodization of all salt used. In the United States, iodization is voluntary, but many people use salt without added iodine. The Food and Nutrition Board has recommended that federal legislation be enacted to make the iodization of salt mandatory."*

Sodium and *chlorine* in the form of sodium chloride are the chief mineral constituents of the extracellular fluids, including the blood and

---

* American Medical Association, Council on Foods and Nutrition: "Symposium on Human Calcium Requirements," *J.A.M.A.*, **185**:588, (Aug. 17) 1963.

* Robinson, Corinne H.: *Normal and Therapeutic Nutrition,* 14th ed., Macmillan Publishing Co., Inc., New York, 1972, p. 117.

lymph. Although both sodium and chlorine are widely distributed in foods and drink, man and some other vertebrates have developed an apparent need for more sodium chloride than is furnished by natural foods and water. The craving for what we call salt is so great that the people of India recovered it from sea water when, as a political protest against the English, they stopped buying taxed and manufactured products. A porcupine will gnaw through the thickest beams of a house, and buffaloes will travel miles, to lick salt.

In tropical countries where sweating is profuse and an excess of sodium chloride is lost in sweat, an adequate supply of salt is a serious economic and social problem as pointed out in Chapter 11. Because less salt is lost in sweat from the unclothed than the clothed body, natives of hot countries have learned to conserve sodium chloride by baring large skin areas. Fair-skinned Europeans living in the tropics cannot compete with native laborers because they don't want to conform to this custom and could not tolerate the exposure. Colonizers tend to manage rather than labor manually. De Castro says:

. . . the unavoidable deficiency of one mineral —sodium—played an extremely important role in the exploitation of a large part of the world's surface. There can be no doubt that this specific hunger, ever since the first colonization of tropical areas, has constituted a terrible handicap to these peoples' economic and social progress.*

According to Robinson,[81] the daily intake of 6 to 15 gm or more of sodium in the diet is far in excess of physiologic requirements. During acclimatization to very hot weather additional sodium may be necessary. Sodium deficiency may also occur in the presence of excessive diarrhea or vomiting. The average person in this country probably eats more salt than is needed under ordinary circumstances and neglects to increase his or her intake to compensate for losses in sweating. Recent studies show that sodium intake may account for some of the differences in blood pressure even at the age of 20 years.[82] Physicians who believe that a high salt intake contributes toward hypertension would encourage us to salt our foods lightly, or not at all, as we grow older. Sodium–potassium chloride mixtures, as a substitute for table salt, have been developed for use in processing as well as in seasoning foods. The addition of potassium makes the mixture palatable and "similar in saltiness to equal weights of sodium chloride." [83]

Potassium salts predominate in the fluid inside the cell as sodium salts do in the inter-

cellular fluids. Magnesium is found chiefly inside the cells, while the calcium in solution is largely in the intercellular fluid. The constancy of these salts must be maintained to preserve the equalizing osmotic pressures inside and outside the cell wall that preserve the integrity of the cell. This is discussed more fully on page 662. Health depends upon a constancy of these minerals for other reasons. Acting as buffer substances, they preserve the neutrality of body fluids and maintain a normal state of muscle tone and irritability of nerves. Louis S. Goodman and Alfred Gilman have stated that both a deficiency and an excess of calcium ions alter the function of cardiac muscle.[84] The presence of sodium is essential to muscle contraction, and the normal function of all tissues seems to depend upon the antagonistic action between the substances that stimulate and those that inhibit activity.

Vegetable foods are rich in potassium, and most diets contain an adequate amount. It is now realized that persons fed parenterally must be given potassium as well as sodium salts. It is probably unfortunate that a solution of sodium chloride was ever called "normal" or "physiological" saline. Great advances are to be expected in parenteral therapy as the nutritional value of food elements is established.[85-87]

Magnesium, one of the four "bulk" metals in man (the others—calcium, potassium, and sodium), has been recognized as an essential nutrient since 1932. It is concerned with regulating cardiac and skeletal muscle and nerves. Studies of deficiency states show neuromuscular irritability, cardiovascular calcification, and renal damage. There is no evidence, however, of widespread dietary magnesium deficiency except in conditions of excessive excretion and malabsorption.[88] The recommended daily allowance for adults is 300 to 400 mg, with 450 mg for women during pregnancy and lactation. Nuts, cereals and whole grains, seafoods, meats, and legumes are the chief sources of magnesium. Fruits, dairy products, and green vegetables are other sources. Vegetables lose magnesium in cooking; therefore, any liquid resulting should be used in soups, vegetable drinks, and sauces.

Less is known about the functions of *manganese, cobalt,* and *zinc.* Although they are accepted as dietary essentials, so little has been reported about their functions that discussion of them is unprofitable here. *Fluoride* is not considered essential for life but it has been proved beneficial to teeth, especially in the young. In fact, tooth decay diminishes when fluoride occurs naturally in or is added to drinking water or foods.[89]

* De Castro, Josué: *op. cit.,* p. 49.

Table 10-2. Vitamin Nomenclature, Sources, Daily Requirements, and Effects of Deficiencies *

Vitamin Group	Terminology	Water-Soluble Vitamins — Major Sources	Daily Requirements	Effects of Deficiency
Vitamin B group	Water-soluble vitamin B B-complex vitamins	Animal: Liver, kidney, and other organ meats Pork Lean meats Poultry Fish		Lack of appetite Nervous instability Depression Sleepiness Fatigue Gastrointestinal atony and constipation
Vitamin B complex	The B vitamins	Milk, liquid and powdered Eggs Cheese Plant: Brewer's yeast Wheat germ Whole grain cereals and breads Soybeans, legumes, peanuts, powdered whey Green, leafy vegetables Dried yeast, enriched foods Corn Potatoes Tomatoes Molasses Fruits		Nausea, vomiting, and other symptoms specific to each particular vitamin
Vitamin B₁	* Thiamine Antiberiberi vitamin Antineuritic vitamin		Birth to 1 yr—0.2 to 0.5 mg 1 to 8 years—0.6 to 1.1 mg Females, 10 to 55 yr—1.0 to 1.1 mg with increase to 1.2 mg at ages 12 to 18 yr Pregnant and lactating women —0.5 mg Males, 10 to 55 yr—1.2 to 1.3 mg	Beriberi, polyneuritis Muscle weakness, cardiac failure, edema
Vitamin B₂	*Riboflavin (formerly lactoflavin, vitamin G)		1.3 to 2 mg	Cracks at corner of mouth (cheilosis) Inflammation of lips and tongue Burning, itching of eyes Photophobia, blurred vision

Nicotinic acid	**Niacin** Niacinamide Antipellagra vitamin (originally called P-P [pellagra-preventing vitamin]) Coenzyme I Coenzyme II	Children and youth—8 to 25 mg Women—17 to 20 mg (maximum for those pregnant and lactating) Men—15 to 19 mg	Pellagra: gastrointestinal, skin and neurological changes
Vitamin B_6 group	**Pyridoxin** Pyridoxal Pyridoxamine	Infants and children—0.5 to 1.2 mg Adults—2 mg	Hypochromicanemia, convulsions in infants, impaired growth, seborrheic dermatitis, soreness of lips and tongue, conjunctivitis, peripheral neuritis
Vitamin B_{12} group	**Vitamin B_{12}**, **Cobalamin**, cyanocobalamine, antipernicious anemia factor; Castile's extrinsic factor	5 mg.	Pernicious anemia, macrocytic anemia, and degenerative change in nervous system
Pantothenic acid	**Pantothenic acid**	Diet that includes plant and animal foods will supply about 10 mg per day	Not observed with natural diet. Feeding antagonist produces loss of appetite, nausea, indigestion, abdominal pain, sullenness, mental depression, peripheral neuritis, repeated infections, fainting sensations, rapid pulse, lowered blood pressure, disturbed fluid balance
Biotin	**Biotin** Vitamin H Coenzyme R Anti-egg white injury factor		Deficiency unlikely in man but experimental deficiency produced in man by use of high egg white intake results in dermatitis, nervousness, anorexia, anemia, ashen pallor
Folic acid group	**Folic acid**, folacin, or pteroylglutamic acid (PGA); tri- and hepta-pteroylglutamates; folinic acid; citrovorum factor; leucovorin		Deficiency unlikely in man from dietary defects but may occur secondarily to disease such as sprue, or megaloblastic anemia or pregnancy. Symptoms include macrocytic anemia, glossitis, diarrhea, malabsorption

Table 10-2. (continued)

Water-Soluble Vitamins

Vitamin Group	Terminology	Major Sources	Daily Requirements	Effects of Deficiency
Choline	*Choline			Deficiency unknown in man
Inositol	*Inositol			Not reported in man
Para-aminobenzoic acid	*Para-aminobenzoic acid (PABA)			Not observed in man
Vitamin C	*Vitamin C Ascorbic acid Antiscorbutic vitamin	Citrus fruits Tomatoes Strawberries Cantaloupe Cabbage Broccoli Kale Potatoes	Birth to 10 yr—35 to 40 mg (depending on age and/or weight) Over 10 yr—40 to 50 mg (depending on age, weight, and sex) Pregnant and lactating women—60 mg Other women—55 mg Men—60 mg	Cutaneous hemorrhages Improper bone development, weakened cartilages, muscle degeneration, anemia, stunted growth, susceptibility to infection, scurvy

Fat-Soluble Vitamins

Vitamin Group	Terminology	Major Sources	Daily Requirements	Effects of Deficiency
Vitamin A group	*Vitamin A Provitamin A, alpha-, beta-, gamma-carotene, crytoxanthine, retinol, retinal, and retinoic acid	Animal: Fish-liver oils Liver Butter, cream Whole milk Whole-milk cheese Egg yolks Plant: Dark green leafy vegetables Yellow vegetables Yellow fruits Fortified margarine	Under 1 yr—1500 units (I.U.) 1 to 3 yr—2000 units (I.U.) 4 to 6 yr—2500 units (I.U.) 6 to 10 yr—3500 units (I.U.) 10 to 12 yr—4500 units (I.U.) 13 to 20 yr—5000 units (I.U.) Adults—5000 units (I.U.) Pregnant women—6000 units (I.U.) Lactating women—8000 units (I.U.) (USP Unit = 0.6 microgram of an internationally standardized preparation of pure beta-carotene)	Faulty bone and tooth development Night blindness Keratinization of epithelium and mucous membranes, especially xerophthalmia

654

Vitamin D group	**Vitamin D** Vitamin D_2 Calciferol, viosterol, activated ergasterol Vitamin D_3 Activated 7-dehydro-cholesterol Antirachitic factor	Fish-liver oils Fortified milk Activated sterols Exposure to sunlight Very small amounts in butter, liver, egg yolk, salmon, sardines	All ages—400 units (I.U.)	Rickets in children, soft fragile bones, enlarged joints, bowed legs, chest, spinal and pelvic bone deformities Delayed dentition Tetanic convulsions in infants Osteomalacia in adults
Vitamin E group	**Vitamin E** Alpha-, beta-, gamma-, delta-tocopherol Antisterility vitamin	Plant tissues, oils of wheat germ, rice germ, cottonseed, green leafy vegetables, nuts, legumes Possibility of intestinal synthesis	Under 1 yr—5 units 1 to 6 yr—10 units 6 to 10 yr—15 units 10 to 14 yr—20 units 14 to 18 yr—25 units Women over 18 yr—25 units Pregnant and lactating women—30 units Men over 18 yr—30 units	In humans, hemolysis of red blood cells, mild anemia; in animals, sterility in male rat, resorption of fetus in female rat, muscular dystrophy, creatinuria, macrocytic anemia
Vitamin K group	**Vitamin K** Antihemorrhagic vitamin Coagulation vitamin K_1—Phylloquinone or phytanadione K_2—Farnoquinone K_3—Menadione	Green leaves, such as alfalfa, spinach, cabbage Liver Synthesis in intestine	Not now included in dietary planning because widely distributed in natural foods	Prolonged clotting time Hemorrhagic disease in newborn infants Bleeding tendencies in biliary or surgical procedures

* Adapted from tables in Robinson, Corinne H.: *Normal and Therapeutic Nutrition*, 14th ed. Macmillan Publishing Co., Inc., New York, 1972, pp. 158 and 186–88; and Williams, Sue Rodwell: *Nutrition and Diet Therapy*. C. V. Mosby Co., St. Louis, 1969, pp. 106–107. Information on vitamins is taken from various sources. (Asterisks within table indicate official name; boldface type, common name.)

It is not possible even to mention all the important known functions of minerals or to list the conditions attributed to their deficiencies. Perhaps enough has been said to suggest the importance of a varied diet and the danger of investing many calories in pure carbohydrates and pure fats, neither of which supply the essential minerals. Diets containing abundant vegetables, fruit, meat, eggs, and dairy products, unless grown on impoverished land, provide the needed minerals.

Vitamins. Through health education and commercial exploitation, the importance of the so-called vitamins is familiar to most of us. Before the chemical nature of any of them was established, it was recognized that there were highly specialized substances in food, the lack of which produced specific disease. Some were believed to be soluble in fatty foods; others, soluble in water; and as knowledge of these increased, they were so designated. By 1920, vitamins A, B, and C were recognized in the science of nutrition. Because they were believed vital to health and in order to unify the rapidly expanding literature, it was proposed that they be called *vitamins*. The name was adopted, and they were divided into *fat-soluble* and *water-soluble* vitamins. Texts usually classify and discuss them under these headings rather than in alphabetical order. (This distinction will disappear as manufacturers convert fat-soluble to water-soluble preparations.)

The term *vitamins* is so entrenched that the nutritionists now, 50 years later, find it difficult to get the public to adopt names that suggest their chemical nature. British and American terminology differ. Standardization of terminology and dosage is now in progress. Table 10-2 gives the present nomenclature, important sources, and daily requirements for some of the vitamins and conditions resulting from their deficiencies. If the chemical nature of the vitamin is known, it is now possible to discover its concentration in the blood. Physical examination may include such estimates. The blood level, in some cases also, may be computed from the amount excreted in the urine.[90] Only those vitamins whose function is best understood are discussed in this book. Again, nurses are urged to study nutrition in more specialized works.

Ascorbic acid (vitamin C) affects the body profoundly by entering into oxidation–reduction reactions and the formation and maintenance of intercellular material that keeps the cells in normal relationship to each other. Following its chemical identification in 1932 by Charles G. King and his co-workers, the isolation and synthesis of ascorbic acid were accomplished by a number of laboratories. A deficiency of ascorbic acid is associated in the mind of the public with scurvy, and its name is designed to perpetuate this association. It is now thought, however, that a wide range of pathology may result from a very low vitamin C intake. To it one author attributes the following: structural changes in gums, teeth, bones, and cartilage, with displacement of bones, due to weakness of supporting cartilage; anemia, caused by interference with cell-forming bone marrow; degeneration of muscles, including the heart muscle; and even damage of the sex organs. This is not hard to accept when one sees the acute suffering of the person with scurvy and its fatal effect if unchecked. Mitchell and associates say:

During the 1960's an increased number of cases of infantile scurvy had been reported in the medical literature from such areas as Canada, Newfoundland, and Australia. A survey in Canada during 1961–1963 found 87 cases of infantile scurvy. These cases occurred mostly in small communities where there was ignorance, poverty, and poor health supervision.*

In 1969, a survey in Great Britain showed that the average daily vitamin C intake during the winter months was 37 mg, with more than half the individuals receiving less than 31 mg per day.[91] Ascorbic acid deficiency does occur in adults, but it is difficult to recognize as a deficiency syndrome. King[92] lists among the symptoms of a vitamin C deficiency the decreased capacity to combat infections and heal wounds. The adrenal cortex contains a high concentration of ascorbic acid which is depleted when stimulated by hormones or certain toxins; some authorities believe that ascorbic acid may play an important role in the body's reaction to stress.[93]

Vitamin C is widely distributed in foods, but is concentrated in many fruits and vegetables. It is easily destroyed by oxidation, which is accelerated by heat. Ascorbic acid is also destroyed more rapidly in the presence of alkalies. It is recommended that exposure of foods to air and heat be reduced to a minimum, and that no soda be added in cooking or processing. Most of the ascorbic acid in the American diet is provided by fruits and vegetables. The following foods known to be rich in ascorbic acid are included in most dietaries: tomatoes, citrus fruits, and cabbage. Young and sprouting vegetables are particularly valuable sources. Canned, frozen, dried, and stored fruits and vegetables have some of their ascorbic acid destroyed, but they are protective

---

* Mitchell, Helen S., *et al.: Nutrition in Health and Disease*, 16th ed. J. B. Lippincott Co., Philadelphia, 1976, p. 298.

if taken in sufficient quantity to compensate for the loss through oxidation. Estimates of the antiscorbutic value of foods are based on the processes to which they have been exposed.

There have been some changes in the recommended allowances for ascorbic acid in the past few years. Those given by the Food and Nutrition Board of the National Research Council in 1968 are as follows: daily intake for children from birth to 10 years, 35 to 40 mg depending on their age and/or weight; for children over 10 years, 40 to 50 mg depending on age, weight, and sex; for pregnant and lactating women, 60 mg, other women 55 mg per day; and for men, 60 mg per day.

Vitamin B, accepted as an entity in 1920, has since been broken down into many vitamins with much more specific functions than those attributed to the original. The chemical composition of some but not all members of the B group, or B complex, is known. The isolation of all reported members has not been generally accepted. At the present time, 12 fractions of the vitamin B complex are generally recognized, while others are postulated.[94] Some are thought to be more important than others in good nutrition. Norman Jolliffe says:

Because my associates and I are very much interested in human nutrition in general and not in hematology alone, we have shown again and again that folic acid, like thiamine, niacin, riboflavin, pyridoxine, pantothenic acid, and vitamin B_{12}, is an important constituent of the vitamin B group. Our concept is that each of these vitamins is an indispensable part of living matter and functions in living cells whether of plant or animal origin. Their importance, even their necessity for life, has now become self-evident.*

Only those members of the B group now thought to be most important are discussed in this book.

Thiamine, thiamine chloride or *hydrochloride* (vitamin B_1), was identified as the factor whose deficiency caused beriberi before it was isolated chemically in 1936 in the laboratory of Dr. R. R. Williams. It was first called vitamin B; it has been known as *aneurin,* a name that suggests its therapeutic claim; and it is referred to as the antineuritic factor. While a marked deficiency of thiamine results in a multiple neuritis with cardiac symptoms and edema, its lack is manifested much earlier in a loss of appetite and, in the young, by retarded growth. It is believed to enter into carbohydrate metabolism, which explains the generalized symptoms of a deficiency. Studies with animals and humans

have shown that the capacity for learning and the actual performance in a wide range of skills is improved on an optimum thiamine intake. With a thiamine deficiency there is an abnormal accumulation of lactic and pyruvic acid in the brain. In such conditions the tissue is restored to normal by the administration of vitamin B_1. To what extent psychoses can be attributed to this and other vitamin deficiencies is debatable, but some psychiatric units are studying the primary relationship of metabolism to so-called mental illness. Some psychiatrists are reporting successful treatment of persons diagnosed as schizophrenic with massive doses of vitamins. Malnourished alcoholics and patients with other types of inanition show depression, irritability, insomnia, and hallucinations associated with the more typical neuritis.[95] Most authors note that the peripheral nervous system, the gastrointestinal tract, and the cardiovascular system are predominantly affected by thiamine deficiency.

As thiamine cannot be stored in the body, it is important that it be supplied regularly in the diet. Thiamine is widely distributed in animal and vegetable foods but minimally in most foods. Of the meat and egg group, pork contains an abundance of thiamine. Organs such as liver, heart, and kidney are especially good sources. Fruits are considered to be a poor source; vegetables slightly better. Because it is difficult to meet the daily requirements of thiamine, the enrichment of bread and cereals was instigated, making it easier economically for the average person to meet his or her needs. It has been established that as much as 40 per cent of the daily thiamine requirement is now being supplied by these foods in the United States. The layman and health worker alike should know that some cereals contain considerably more thiamine than others. Before making a purchase everyone should read the labels on cereal boxes that give the minimum amount of vitamins in the product.

Like ascorbic acid, but not to the same extent, thiamine is thermolabile and is more rapidly destroyed in an alkaline medium. Roasting is said to destroy from 25 to 50 per cent of the thiamine present in meats.[96] Both vitamins are water soluble and are therefore partially lost when water in which they are cooked is discarded. Nurses as health teachers should encourage housekeepers to conserve the full value of foods by using cooking water for soups or vegetable "cocktails." In bakery products, vitamins are lost through oxidation in mixing and baking. When refined flours and/or soda is used, the loss is enormous. Public health regulations for the enrichment of

* Jolliffe, Norman, *et al.* (eds.): *Clinical Nutrition,* 2nd ed. Paul B. Hoeber, New York, 1962, p. 636.

flour by the addition of synthesized thiamine have to some extent offset these losses. Authorities, nevertheless, encourage the use of whole-grain products and discourage the use of soda. The recommended daily allowances of thiamine as given by the Food and Nutrition Board are as follows: for infants birth to 1 year, 0.2 to 0.5 mg; children 1 to 8 years, 0.6 to 1.1 mg; males 10 to 55 years, 1.2 to 1.3 mg, with an increase to 1.5 mg at age 14; females of the same age (10 to 55 years), 1.0 to 1.1 mg, with an increase to 1.2 mg at ages 12 to 18 years. During pregnancy and lactation it is recommended that thiamine intake be increased by 0.1 to 0.5 mg. It is now possible to determine the amount of thiamine utilized and requiring replacement by measuring urinary excretion of thiamine metabolites.[97]

Riboflavin (B₂) and *niacin, niacinamide* or *nicotinic acid,* are here considered together because their deficiencies are associated with pellagra and its related symptoms. Riboflavin was synthesized by Kuhn and his co-workers in 1935.

Riboflavin is a heat-stable substance widely distributed in plants and animals. It is believed to be essential to growth and normal nutrition, and for this reason nature concentrates it in eggs and milk to ensure the health of the young. Riboflavin deficiency produces widespread tissue changes, including general weakness, dermatitis, fissures of the lips, and reddened eyes. A long-term deficiency shortens life, decreases the vitality of the people, and lowers resistance to disease. It is doubtful whether present knowledge of this vitamin enables the nutritionist to assess its values or to provide reliable human requirements. Its deficiency is widespread even in this economically favored country, but particularly among families with low incomes because their consumption of animal protein tends to be low. Some writers suggest that the health improvement noticeable after an increase of animal protein in the diet is due in large part to its riboflavin content. A quart of milk a day or a serving of liver will meet the daily requirement of 1.3 to 2 mg. Other meats, eggs, cheese, and wheat germ are valuable sources. Weight by weight, some leafy green vegetables, such as broccoli, kale, and spinach, have about one tenth as much riboflavin as liver and the same concentration as milk. Being economically available to many, they are important sources. Enriched bread must contain specified amounts of riboflavin as well as thiamine, niacin, and iron.[98]

Niacin, or niacinamide (improperly termed nicotinic acid), is a heat-stable substance whose distribution in natural foods somewhat parallels that of riboflavin. While it is highly concentrated in yeast, dietary improvement results from emphasis on palatable and ordinary food in which it is abundant.

Severe niacin deficiency causes pellagra, the disease characterized by the three D's—dermatitis, diarrhea, and dementia. Some writers say four D's and add death. This disease occurs in areas where the land is given over to "cash crops," cotton and tobacco, for example. It is rare among peoples who raise their own food and who can therefore afford variety. Pellagra is cured by including milk, eggs, lean meats, fish, tomatoes, peas, and leafy vegetables in the diet. In addition to these foods, niacin and riboflavin are usually given to hasten recovery. Niacin is produced within the body by some bacteria. Milk probably encourages the growth of niacin-producing organisms, for pellagra is not found among those children who live largely on milk. Tryptophan, an amino acid, is a precursor from which niacin may be synthesized in the body; total niacin equivalents therefore equal the preformed niacin plus the niacin equivalents available from protein.[99] The Food and Nutrition Board recommends in "niacin equivalents" a daily range of 15 to 19 mg for men; 17 to 20 mg for women, the maximum for those who are pregnant and lactating; 8 to 25 mg for children and youth. Niacin requirements, like those for thiamine, may vary with energy expenditure. An optimum diet, as has been said, will usually provide an ample supply of this vitamin.

Vitamin B₆ consists of three related chemical compounds: *pyridoxine, pyridoxal,* and *pyridoxamine.* The need for this vitamin in both adults and infants has been proven conclusively. It helps the body utilize proteins and convert tryptophan to niacin, and it is involved in some way with the synthesis of highly unsaturated fatty acids.[100] A deficiency of vitamin B₆ may result in nervous disorders, irritability, depression, muscular weakness, and dermatitis around the eyes and angles of the mouth, with soreness of the tongue and lips. Infants have been known to develop nervous irritability and convulsive seizures when given a proprietary milk diet in which vitamin B₆ was accidentally destroyed. The daily recommended amount of 2 mg for adults may be provided by a varied diet including those foods rich in other B vitamins—meats, whole grain cereals, and vegetables.[101] The requirement for infants and children is 0.5 to 1.2 mg.

Another of the vitamin B complex group is *pantothenic acid,* also considered essential in human nutrition. It is concerned with the synthesis of amino acids, fatty acids, sterols, and steroid hormones. Pantothenic acid is widely distributed in plant and animal foods; a diet that includes both will supply about 10 mg per day. This is another example of the importance of eating a varied diet.[102,103]

Vitamin B_{12} is a cobalt-containing substance whose active principle has been named *cobalamin;* the term *cyanocobalamine* is also used. This vitamin has been broken down into several forms, but the effectiveness of all of them in treating pernicious anemia is due to the cobalamin content, and this refined substance is now used instead of the crude-liver extracts formerly given for their B_{12} content. It is effective taken orally or parenterally. Successful treatment with high oral doses of B_{12} in pernicious anemia and other states of B_{12} deficiency is extensively used in Sweden and is an acceptable alternative to the conventional method of injections.[104] Innumerable studies have been made on this nutritional element, and much has been written because it so effectively controls a once fatal and fairly prevalent disease. The level of absorption (which occurs in the ileum) depends on the presence of Castile's *intrinsic factor,* a mucoprotein enzyme secreted in the stomach. Liver is a rich source of vitamin B_{12}, and many years ago patients with pernicious anemia had to eat it in large quantities before concentrates were developed. While this vitamin is found chiefly in animal protein, it is also present in milk, cheese, and eggs. It is practically absent in plants. The recommended daily allowance is 5 mg.[105-107]

Folic acid, a water-soluble vitamin, is a member of the B complex group. Its chemical name is folacin or pteroylglutamic acid. This vitamin is found in a wide variety of foods— green leafy vegetables, cauliflower, and organ meats have a high content; beef, veal, and wheat and its products contain a medium amount of folic acid. In a summary statement, Jolliffe says:

Clinically, folic acid is the most effective therapy for nutritional macrocytic anemia, sprue, pernicious anemia of pregnancy, and megaloblastic anemia of infancy. A dominant feature of these conditions is a macrocytic anemia, and certainly nutritional deficiency is related to its development. Dietary studies have indicated the presence of a chronic deficiency of protein as well as folic acid. The occurrence of this type of anemia is more frequent in areas in which various nutritional deficiencies have long been endemic and their incidence in these areas has decreased during the last 15 to 20 years in parallel with that of other nutritional deficiencies.*

* Jolliffe, Norman, et al. (eds.): *op. cit.,* p. 644.

Breast-fed infants receive more folic acid than do those who are formula fed, as heat destroys some of the folates.[108]

Water-soluble vitamins, other than the ascorbic acid (C) and the B group, are biotin, para-aminobenzoic acid (PABA), inositol, choline, and betaine—all B complex factors. Knowledge of these is incomplete. Para-aminobenzoic acid is no longer considered a vitamin and it is thought that the body can synthesize the inositol that it needs. Because choline and betaine are structural components of the body cell (and not catalysts), their classification as vitamins is questioned by some. A deficiency in choline is unlikely since it is widely distributed in plants and animals. Betaine is formed by oxidation of choline. Biotin is synthesized in the intestines and widely distributed in foods, and a deficiency of it is unlikely.[109]

The first fat-soluble vitamin was A, but since 1920 the specificity of *fat-soluble vitamins D, E, and K* has been established. These may be further broken down, and the list might be still further enlarged in a full report of vitamin research, which is expanding so rapidly that any account of it is out of date before it can be published.

Vitamin A, found so abundantly in the liver oils of fresh- and salt-water fish, is also found in milk, eggs, and other animal fats. It has not been found in plants, but the dark green and yellow vegetables contain precursors, for convenience referred to as "the carotenes," that give rise to Vitamin A in the body.

Deficiencies in vitamin A, even though slightly below the optimum intake, are believed to limit growth. The development and maintenance of normal eyes are also closely associated with this vitamin. When a deficiency is present, adjustment to dull light is slowed; this is especially obvious when driving at night as the lights of an approaching automobile will tend to "blind" the driver—this is referred to as "night blindness" or "glare blindness." Another function of vitamin A is helping to maintain normal epithelial membranes and stimulating mucous secretions; consequently, a deficiency results in changes of the lining of the air passages, alimentary canal, and genitourinary tract, which is known as keratinization. Of course, dermatitis may also occur. The ultimate function of vitamin A is to help protect the body against infections that enter it through the respiratory, gastrointestinal, or urinary systems. Animal experiments have demonstrated that this vitamin is essential to normal reproduction in rats and other animals.[110]

Vitamin A is absorbed in the intestinal wall

and absorption is facilitated by the presence of bile. Any factor that limits fat absorption is likely to decrease absorption of vitamin A. Mineral oil should never be taken immediately before or after a meal as it coats the mucosa and interferes with the absorption of carotene. Unlike many nutritional elements, vitamin A can be stored for future use. It has been estimated that as much as 95 per cent of vitamin A in the entire body may be stored in the liver. Other storage spaces are adipose tissue, lungs, and kidneys. This reserve is important in meeting increased requirements or temporary shortages.[111]

The indiscriminate use of vitamin A supplements by the layman has resulted in serious physiologic signs and symptoms such as increased intracranial pressure, gastrointestinal distress (anorexia and vomiting), and desquamation. Ida G. Braun says:

At a time when lack of Vitamin A is responsible for wide-spread disease and blindness in many parts of the world, medical literature of Western countries contains more articles concerning the effects of Vitamin A excess. . . .

Because the body can store or break down relatively large amounts of Vitamin A, normal dietary sources do not provide quantities sufficient to cause symptoms of intoxication. It is only since Vitamin concentrates have become available to physicians and patients alike that hypervitaminosis A has become more common. The manifestation of acute and chronic poisoning differ, and both have been described in patients of all age groups.*

Nurses should caution people about the use of additional vitamins, especially the fat-soluble vitamins, as they are stored in the body. Space does not permit an elaborate discussion of vitamin A intoxication, but a few of the articles found in the literature are included in the references at the end of this chapter.[112-114]

The recommended daily allowances of the National Research Council are as follows: for children under 1 year, 1500 units; children from 1 to 3, 2000 units; children from 4 to 6, 2500 units; children from 6 to 10, 3500 units; children from 10 to 12, 4500 units; young people 13 to 20, 5000 units; adults, 5000 units except during pregnancy, when the allowance should be 6000 units, and lactation, when it advances to 8000 units. Both the International Unit (I.U.) and the United States Pharmacopeia Unit (U.S.P.) of vitamin A have a value equal to that of 0.6 microgram of an internationally standardized preparation of pure beta-carotene.

* Braun, Ida G.: "Vitamin A Excess, Deficiency, Requirements, Metabolism and Misuse," *Pediatr. Clin. North Am.,* **9:**935, (Nov.) 1962.

Vitamin D (now known to occur in several forms) is another of the fat-soluble groups whose function in human nutrition is well established. It is essential to the utilization of calcium and phosphorus, and its deficiency produces faulty bone and tooth structure. When calcification of growing bones is slowed up by insufficient minerals or vitamin D, the strain of supporting the body deforms the bones, and results in bowlegs or knock-knees, enlarged joints, the beady processes at the cartilaginous junctions of the ribs, and the pigeon breast of rickets. Vitamin D is known as the "antirachitic factor," although a diet adequate in minerals and exposure of the body to sunlight are also antirachitic factors.

The activating effect of ultraviolet light, or direct sunlight, on the utilization of nutrients was recognized in ancient times although knowledge of its functions was less specific. Modern medicine has confirmed the theory that in the presence of direct sunlight the body can synthesize vitamin D from sterols found in plants and animals. In our culture and particularly in cold climates it is difficult to expose the body to a sufficient quantity of sunlight or artificial ultraviolet light to produce adequate amounts of vitamin D from its precursors. The only safe alternative is a diet that includes a liberal allowance of vitamin D in the form of activated sterols. This is generally accepted as essential in feeding infants and children. Emphasis in the past has been on development of normal bone structure in the young, but there is a growing tendency to stress the dietary prevention of bone disease in the aging. Irradiation of foods has not proved effective in the same way as has irradiation of the body. The emphasis is, at present, on exposure of the body to a reasonable amount of direct sunlight, use of foods reinforced with vitamin D, and the administration of fish oils. The latter is particularly important in infancy, childhood, and youth. There is good evidence that vitamin D is needed throughout life, from birth through old age; 400 units (I.U.) are recommended for all ages.[115,116]

The role of *vitamin E* is not thoroughly established, although its deficiency in animal experimentation is characterized by sterility in male and female. Other manifestations of the deficiency are muscular dystrophy, stunted growth, and degeneration of the renal tubular cells. One of its main functions is thought to be prevention of oxidation of the unsaturated fatty acids. For the first time a recommended daily allowance has been given by the National Research Council because recent evidence indicates that vitamin E deficiency affects infants. The recommended daily allowances are as follows: for children under 1 year, 5 units; children from 1 to 6, 10 units; children from 6 to 10, 15 units; children from 10 to 14, 20 units; young people from 14 to 18, 25 units; all men over 18, 30 units; and all adult women, 25 units except during pregnancy and lactation when it should be increased to 30 units. Major sources of vitamin E include the oils of wheat germ, cottonseed, rice germ and germs of other seeds. It is also present in dark green leafy vegetables, legumes, and nuts. [117,118]

The *K vitamins,* the last of the fat-soluble vitamins to be mentioned, are not now included in dietary planning because they are widely distributed in natural foods and little progress has been made in clarifying how they act in higher animals. Vitamin K was demonstrated by Dr. Dam of Copenhagen about 1935. It is synthesized by bacteria in the intestinal tract and is supplied by the diet. The main function of vitamin K is to maintain normal plasma levels of prothrombin, and it has been called the "Koagulation Vitamin." Clinically, vitamin K may be given to newborns to raise the prothrombin level, and to adults with conditions that interfere with the synthesis of the vitamin in the intestines, as well as in biliary and liver disease. It is used in the control of hemorrhage.[119,120]

Should vitamins be taken without the doctor's advice? This question often confronts the nurse. It is not easy to give an answer that would meet with general approval. Most physicians would probably say they should not; on the other hand, many nutritionists might say that under certain circumstances they should. Health experts agree that if we could get an optimum diet, animal and vegetable, from lands that had not been depleted, made up of foods neither stored, dried, frozen, nor canned, and if we could spend a reasonable time out of doors, we would need no additional vitamins for health maintenance. Because, however, many of us lead indoor, sedentary lives and eat many stale and processed foods, our health often demands vitamin supplements. Because they are foods and because it is doubtful whether quantities in excess of body needs (with the exception of vitamin A) can have harmful effects, their sale to the public is not regulated. Undoubtedly, we should work to make the use of vitamins outside food items unnecessary for the healthy individual.

3. FLUID BALANCE

Critical Nature of Fluid Balance. Water is necessary for all the chemical and physical activity on which life depends. It is a constituent of all protoplasm. In it are suspended the circulating cells and the colloids, and in it are dissolved organic and mineral nutrients and wastes. Throughout this book there has been repeated reference to Claude Bernard's dictum that health depends on the constancy of the fluids that make the "internal environment," or, in other words, the extracellular fluids. Their constancy depends on the nature of the intracellular fluids, and since there is a continuous interchange of water between the cells and their environment, the fluids of each must be studied together. The water need is in direct relation to the concentration of solids dissolved in the body fluids. If their intake does not keep pace with the water ingested and eliminated, the cells drown—they are waterlogged. When the water intake does not keep pace with the intake and output of solids, the cells shrivel—they are dehydrated. Excretory organs, particularly the kidneys but also the sweat glands, the intestines, and the lungs, maintain this balance between water and solids as long as they can. When the tissues hold water in excess of their needs (edema), a positive water balance is said to exist; dehydration is referred to as a negative balance. Figure 10–3 shows the ways that body fluids are gained and lost.

Total Body Fluid, Compartments, and Composition. Various investigators estimate that approximately 55 to 65 per cent of body weight is water. Total body water in a man of average weight (70 kg) is about 40 liters, 25 of which is intracellular fluid while 15 liters is extracellular fluid. While intracellular fluid is found within the most basic unit of the body, the cell, extracellular fluid is found around the cell. Extracellular fluids include interstitial fluid, plasma, cerebrospinal fluid, intraocular fluid, and fluids of the gastrointestinal tract. The interstitial fluid lies between the cells and, by the process of diffusion, dissolved substances can move freely through it. Plasma is that part lying within the blood vessels and surrounding the blood cells.[121]

It has been established that the composition of plasma and interstitial and intracellular fluid varies. The most prevalent cation (positive ion) in plasma and interstitial fluid is sodium, while the major anions (negative ions) are chloride and bicarbonate; in addition, there are small amounts of potassium, calcium, magnesium, phosphate, sulfate, and organic acids. Intracellular fluid electrolytes are chiefly potassium and magnesium cations and phosphate, bicarbonate, and sulfate anions. Protein is present within the cell and plasma but is absent in the interstitial fluid (see Fig. 10–4).

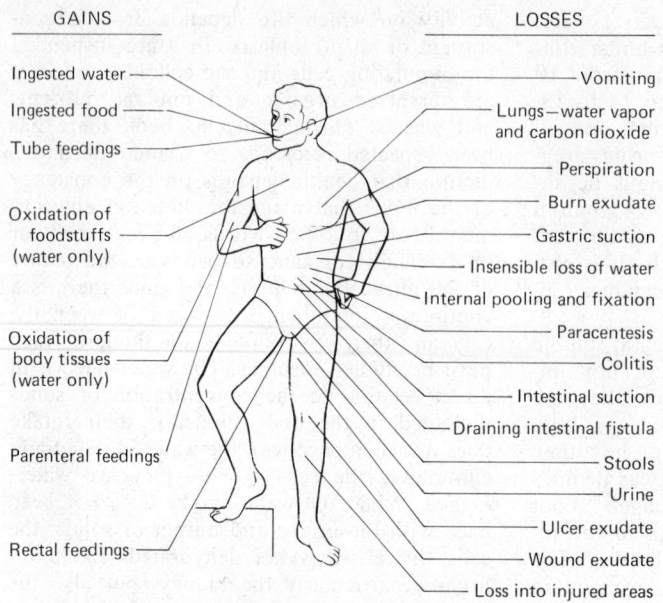

Figure 10-3. Gains and losses of body fluids. (From Snively, W. D., Jr., and Beshear, Donna R.: "Water and Electrolytes in Health and Disease," in Kintzel, Kay Corman (ed.): *Advanced Concepts in Clinical Nursing.* J. B. Lippincott Co., Philadelphia, 1971, p. 247.)

Regulation of Fluid Balance. To understand how fluid balance is regulated within the different fluid compartments, some basic concepts relating to osmotic pressure must be examined. It is the osmotic pressure of intracellular and extracellular areas that maintains fluid within each compartment. Osmosis, a process by which water molecules diffuse through a semipermeable membrane, is caused by a concentration gradient. When the concentration of a nondiffusible solute is greater on one side of the membrane than on the other, water will diffuse to the side of the greater concentration. Therefore, osmotic pressure is determined by the *numbers* of particles (be they nonionizable molecules or ions) per unit volume of fluid. The "osmol" is the basic unit of measurement of osmotic pressure. According to Guyton, *"One gram mol of dissolved nondiffusible and nonionizable substance is equal to 1 osmol."* * However, if two ions result from one gram molecular weight of substance when dissolved, such as sodium and chloride ions from sodium chloride, one ion is equal to 1 osmol. To facilitate expressing osmolality in relation to the body, the term *milliosmol* (1/1000 of 1 osmol) is used. Total osmolality of each fluid compartment has been determined by investigators to be approximately 300 milliosmols; however, the osmolality of plasma is slightly higher than interstitial fluid because of the presence of plasma proteins.[122]

The presence of protein within plasma is important because of the colloid osmotic pressure (oncotic) which it exerts. Albumin and globulin comprise most of the protein in plasma. Because the capillary membrane is relatively permeable to all substances in the blood except the large protein molecules, they remain within the capillary, exerting an oncotic pressure which draws interstitial fluid into the vascular area, thus maintaining blood volume.

The cell, too, has a relatively high protein content. Partially because of the presence of protein, osmotic pressure draws extracellular fluid into the cell. To offset this pressure, sodium is necessarily found outside the cell. Sodium is kept in its extracellular position, not because the cell membrane is impermeable to it, but because of what is thought to be an "active sodium extrusion mechanism," a "pump" located in the outer plasma membrane of all cells which continuously ejects sodium from the cell as quickly as it enters. In addition to other consequences, this results in a high intracellular concentration of potassium and an exclusion of small, negatively charged ions such as chloride from the cell interior. This high concentration of potassium within the cell offsets the negatively charged ions and allows for electric equilibrium. The extracellular position of sodium depends on a continuous supply of energy to eject this ion. Cell volume, in turn, is maintained by a "dynamic steady state" rather than a static condition. When the metabolic energy that "pumps" sodium out of the cell is inhibited, sodium can be accumulated within the cell. Chloride and water then follow the sodium into the cell and consequently the potassium leaves, and the

* Guyton, Arthur C.: *op. cit.,* p. 387.

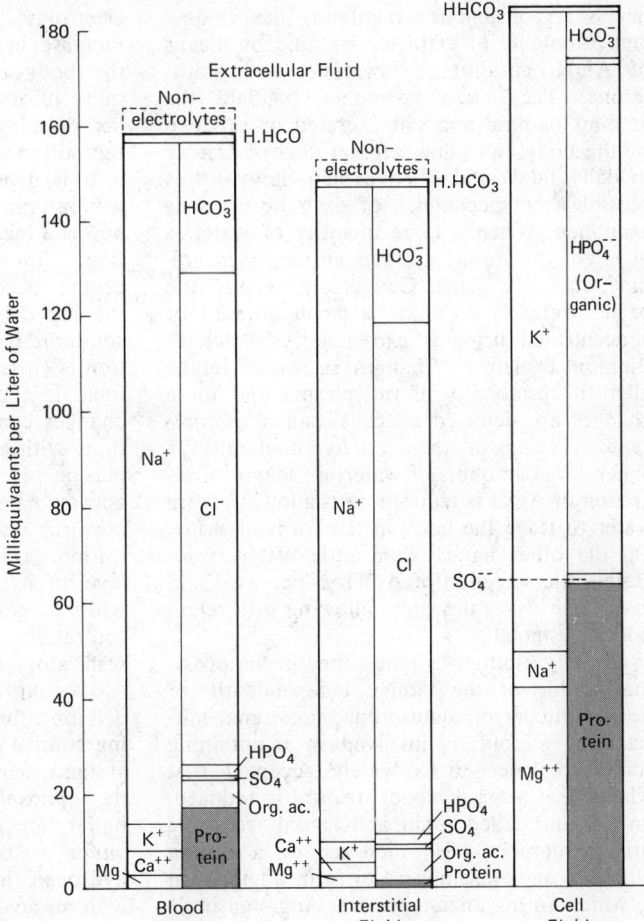

Figure 10-4. The composition of plasma, interstitial fluid and intracellular fluid. (From Guyton, Arthur C.: *Textbook of Medical Physiology*, 4th ed. W. B. Saunders Co., Philadelphia, 1971, p. 385.)

cell becomes water logged. This process is reversible as long as the cell is again supplied with metabolic energy to "pump" out the sodium. Regulation of intracellular fluid volume is obviously a function of each cell.[123]

Guyton [124] says that the osmolalities of extra- and intracellular fluid remain exactly the same except during the first few minutes after a change in one of the fluid compartments. In addition, the number of osmotically active substances remains the same in each compartment unless one of these substances moves, is added to, or is taken away. It is therefore important to note what happens to the cell when changes occur in the extracellular compartment. Isotonic solutions, such as normal saline, do not alter the osmolality of the respective fluid compartments and no water exchange occurs even though there is an increase in extracellular fluid. However, when plain water or hypotonic solutions are added, the extracellular fluid becomes hypotonic in relation to intracellular fluid. A pressure gradient results in water entering the cell

where the concentrate of solute is greatest, and the cell is distended. On the other hand, when water is removed from, or a hypertonic solution is added to, the extracellular fluid, water leaves the intracellular compartment and the cell shrivels, resulting in dehydration. The intracellular volume therefore is a function of the quantity of solute within the cell, whereas water moves back and forth across the cell membrane as necessary to equalize its activity in intracellular and extracellular compartments.

According to Sue Rodwell Williams,[125] the average adult metabolizes 2½ to 3 liters of water per day. The body is able to maintain a state of fluid balance by regular fluid intake and through normal renal and extrarenal excretion. Water enters the body not only through fluids and foods ingested but by oxidation of nutrients in the body. Water is lost from the body insensibly through the skin and lungs, as well as through urine, perspiration, and feces. Total daily water intake averages from 2100 to 2800 ml for the adult.

Among other important functions, the kidney is responsible for regulating the volume and osmolality of extracellular fluid by means of ADH, antidiuretic hormone, and aldosterone. These two hormones regulate the amount of fluid and salt excreted or retained by the body and allow a great deal of leeway in daily fluid intake. To explain how this is possible, the mechanism of each hormone is examined. When a large quantity of water is ingested, the kidney excretes an increased volume of dilute urine. Conversely, when little or no water is taken in, a small amount of concentrated urine is excreted. As Peter F. Binnion explains, "Changes in water intake alter the osmolality of the plasma and these changes are detected by cells, called osmoreceptors, lying in the . . . hypothalamus." * When large amounts of water are taken in, secretion of ADH is reduced, thus allowing more water to leave the body in the form of urine. On the other hand, when little water is ingested, the secretion of ADH is increased and less water leaves the body, allowing it to retain normal osmolality.[126]

Although sodium is reabsorbed in the proximal tubule of the kidney independently of hormonal control, aldosterone, an adrenal salt-retaining steroid, is involved in maintaining sodium balance. It is widely accepted that when renal arterial blood pressure is reduced, an enzyme called renin is released from the juxtaglomerular cells which acts on a plasma globulin, angiotensinogen, to form angiotensin I, which forms angiotensin II. Angiotensin II is a powerful vasoconstrictor which stimulates the release of aldosterone from the adrenal cortex. Aldosterone, in turn, causes retention of sodium (and water) by the renal tubular cells which results in an increase in extracellular fluid and renal blood flow. Once renal blood pressure has been raised, the stimulus disappears. By means of these two hormones, sodium and water excretion are regulated by the kidney.[127]

The colon, too, has the capacity to conserve electrolytes. Ghislain J. Devroede and Sidney F. Phillips [128] have shown that the colon absorbs sodium and chlorides against large concentration gradients. Although it effectively absorbs over 3000 ml of water per day, this process is probably a result of osmosis, that is, water follows the sodium ion. It is therefore apparent that many mechanisms are at work in the body that help to establish and maintain fluid and electrolyte balance.

Acid–base balance depends on the constancy of body fluids and their dissolved electrolytes. It has long been known that an increase in bicarbonate, for example, pushes the body toward alkalosis. However, much more information has accumulated within the last decades which should shed more light on this still incompletely understood subject.

It is generally accepted that an acid is a proton donor; that is it provides hydrogen ions and can increase the hydrogen (H^+) of a solution. It lowers the pH. Conversely, a base is a proton acceptor. It accepts hydrogen ions, thereby decreasing the hydrogen (H^+) of a solution. It raises the pH. Acid–base regulation is closely related to the level of hydrogen ions in body fluids. Because even slight changes can alter the rates of chemical reactions within the cell, it is important that the plasma pH be maintained at its normal level, approximately 7.4. The terms *acidosis* and *alkalosis* denote changes in hydrogen concentration. *Acidosis* means there is an increased level of hydrogen ion within the body fluids, while *alkalosis* indicates a low hydrogen concentration. Both disorders may result from respiratory or metabolic disturbances.

To counteract an excess or deficit in hydrogen ions, the body is equipped with the following control systems: (1) The acid-base buffer systems, which include the bicarbonate buffer, the phosphate buffer, and the protein buffer, are supplied to all body fluids. These buffer systems prevent excessive changes in hydrogen ion concentrations by combining with an acid or alkali. The bicarbonate buffer system (a mixture of carbonic acid and sodium bicarbonate) is probably the most important because the respiratory systems can regulate the carbon dioxide, and the kidney, the bicarbonate ion. The pH of the blood can be increased or decreased by the respiratory or renal systems. (2) The respiratory system regulates acid–base balance by eliminating carbon dioxide from body fluids. If the rate of carbon dioxide production is increased, the lungs compensate by increasing the rate of respiration. On the other hand, if respiration is somehow decreased or inhibited, a buildup of carbon dioxide results in respiratory acidosis due to an increase in carbonic acid and hydrogen ions. If respiration is greatly increased, respiratory alkalosis may result due to excessive removal of carbon dioxide and hence, carbonic acid. (3) The kidney is the third regulator of acid–base balance, and is also the principal regulator of the internal environment. In addition to controlling, in part, the hydrogen ion concentration by excreting either an acid or alkaline urine, it is responsible for regulating the volume and osmolality of the extracellular fluid and the excretion of nitrogenous waste products.[129]

---

* Binnion, Peter F.: "Modern Views of Physiology: IX. Control of Body Salt and Water," *Practitioner,* **203:**375, (Sept.) 1969.

Maintaining acid–base equilibrium in body fluids becomes very important when the effects of acidosis and alkalosis are realized. Acidosis results in depression of the central nervous system and, if uncorrected, leads to death. Alkalosis causes an over-excitability of the central nervous system and, if uncorrected, tetany of the respiratory muscles will develop, which may be fatal.[130] With the rapid development in physiologic chemistry within the last decades, there has been a shifting emphasis in fluid and electrolyte therapy.

In health, thirst and appetite regulate the fluid, electrolyte, and acid–base balance, if the individual has access to adequate food and drink. The balance is upset whenever shock, anesthetics, drugs, or incapacitating illness dulls normal desires in eating and drinking or makes their satisfaction impossible. Infants and children are especially susceptible to upsets in fluid and acid–base balance because they have less freedom in satisfying their appetites and because the body chemistry is less stable. Now with the increased use of surgery and its accompanying anesthesia, loss of blood, interruption of diet, narcosis, and general incapacity, the problem of maintaining balance in body chemistry assumes major proportions. Effective medicine is dependent upon successful nutrition; modern medicine must often rely on extraoral methods of feeding, and the medical workers must assume responsibility for accomplishing what the appetites so effortlessly dictate in health.

As physicians learned to introduce fluid into veins and subcutaneous tissues, they learned that the aims of fluid therapy must be to replace previous losses, provide maintenance requirements, and meet concurrent losses. According to William W. Pfaff, the "principle of fluid therapy is to maintain optimum volume and concentration of body fluid constituents so as to place the patient in the midpoint of normal range. . . ." *

Determination of electrolyte imbalance is usually based on laboratory analyses that show the level of serum sodium, potassium, chlorides, and carbon dioxide or its equivalent. Electrolyte studies are among the most frequently requested laboratory tests. Although serum sodium values do not indicate whether there is an excess or deficit in total body sodium, they do indicate the relation of salt to water, and thus the tonicity of body fluids.[131] Table 10–3 indicates the normal values for serum electrolytes.

Although it is now possible to measure electrolyte blood levels, it is still difficult to

Table 10-3.   Normal Values for Serum Electrolytes *

Cations	
Sodium	135–147 mEq/liter
Potassium	3.5–5.5 mEq/liter
Calcium	4.5–5.5 mEq/liter
Magnesium	1.5–3.0 mEq/liter
Anions	
Chloride	98–106 mEq/liter
Bicarbonate	26–30 mEq/liter
Phosphate and sulfate	2–5 mEq/liter
Organic acids	3–6 mEq/liter
Proteins	15–19 mEq/liter

* Dutcher, Isabel E., and Fielo, Sandra B.: *Water and Electrolytes.* Macmillan Publishing Co., Inc., New York, 1967, p. 19.

determine the volume of fluid that should be replaced. The physician must therefore rely on the history and physical examination of the patient, the nature of his disease, quantity and quality of the urinary output, and, if necessary, monitoring of central venous pressure. Although the best fluid replacement method is drinking, this may not always be possible. In such cases other methods, such as gastrointestinal or intravenous feedings, may be instituted.

According to D. A. K. Black,[132] the maintenance of fluid balance for short periods involves mainly water and he thinks that 2 liters per day is adequate for most patients unless there is fever or polyuria, in which case more fluids are needed. C. H. Wyndham and N. B. Strydom [133] have shown the necessity for replacing fluid during marathon running to prevent excessive temperature rise and heat stroke. A large fluid deficit (2½ to 7 pints) was created in marathon runners through excessive perspiration which resulted in body temperatures of 39.44°C (103°F) and above. Heavy persons were at a disadvantage because perspiration and heat were produced at much higher rates. Large fluid deficits were found to be preventable simply by drinking small amounts of water throughout the race. Healthy individuals may lose excessive fluids in very hot weather even when they are not engaged in such unusual activity as marathon running.

Fluid loss is often accompanied by electrolyte imbalance. In the event of decreased serum sodium (hyponatremia) which may result from excessive intravenous feeding or inappropriate release of ADH, a decreased plasma volume occurs. When sodium is lost, water follows. If 5 per cent dextrose in water is used to replace the fluid loss, glucose will metabolize, leaving hypotonic water. When this occurs, water moves into the cell until

* Pfaff, William W.: "Electrolyte Disorders," *Int. Anesthesiol. Clin.,* **6:**151, (Spring) 1968.

Intake	Vol.	Na$^+$	Cl$^-$	K$^+$	HCO$^-$	N		Output	Vol.	Na$^+$	Cl$^-$	K$^+$	HCO$^-$	N	Cal.
Oral								Urine							
Intra-venous								Insen-sible							
Total								Total							

Name _____ Service of _____

Period from _____ to: _____ Equals _____ Hrs. _____ Day: _____

Estimated Balances at Start: Water _____ Na$^+$ _____ Cl$^-$ _____ K$^+$ _____ Nit. _____

Day of Study: _____ Weight in kilograms _____

Daily water balance ....
Daily Na$^+$ balance ....
Daily K$^+$ balance ....
Daily Cl$^-$ balance ....
Daily nitrogen balance..................................

Cumulative water balance ....
Cumulative Na$^+$ balance ....
Cumulative K$^+$ balance ....
Cumulative Cl$^-$ balance ....
Cumulative nitrogen balance ....

Na$^+$, Cl$^-$, HCO$_3^-$, K$^+$, pH, BUN, HKT, Eos., Sugar, Protein, Other

Lab. Studies:

Day of Study:

Period from: _____ to _____ = _____ hrs. _____ Weight in kilograms _____

Intake	Vol.	Na$^+$	Cl$^-$	K$^+$	HCO$^-$	N	Cal.	Output	Vol.	Na$^+$	Cl$^-$	K$^+$	HCO$^-$	N	Cal.
Oral								Urine							
Intra-venous								Insen-sible							
Total								Total							

Daily water balance ....
Daily Na$^+$ balance ....
Daily K$^+$ balance..................................
Daily Cl$^-$ balance ....
Daily nitrogen balance..................................

Cumulative water balance ....
Cumulative Na$^+$ balance ....
Cumulative K$^+$ balance ....
Cumulative Cl$^-$ balance ....
Cumulative nitrogen balance ....

Na$^+$, Cl$^-$, HCO$_3^-$, K$^+$, pH, BUN, HKT, Eos., Sugar, Protein, Other

Lab. Studies:

Figure 10-5. Water, electrolyte, calorie, and nitrogen balance sheet. (From Bland, John: *Clinical Metabolism of Body Water and Electrolytes.* W. B. Saunders Co., Philadelphia, 1963, p. 213.)

osmotic pressure equalizes and extracellular fluid remains decreased. However, if Ringer's lactate solution is given, there is no change in osmolality nor a rush of fluid into the intracellular space. Correction of hyponatremia must be carried out with cautious monitoring of results over a period of hours or days. Because of an upset in the pressure gradient at the arteriole end of the capillary, hypernatremia results in edema, excess fluid in the interstitial compartment. Treatment must include correcting the predisposing cause, followed by restricted sodium and fluid intake and diuretics.[134]

Increased serum potassium (hyperkalemia) depresses conduction of nerve and muscle impulses along membranes which may lead to cardiac weakness and eventually cardiac arrest. Because of these serious consequences, serum potassium should be carefully checked following surgery, injury, or during renal insufficiency. Infusion of potassium solutions should be avoided until adequate renal function is ascertained. To correct hyperkalemia, Pfaff[135] recommends administering glucose and insulin to increase glycogen deposition, thereby increasing intracellular potassium, or by giving ion exchange resins over a period of several hours. If all else fails, hemodialysis or peritoneal dialysis may be instituted to correct increased serum potassium. Decreased serum potassium (hypokalemia) may cause muscular paralysis due to increased membrane potentials in the motor nerves which inhibits transmission of impulses to muscles. This can be corrected by infusion of potassium solutions or oral replacement.

Medicine has for many years been aware of the importance of maintaining accurate records of intake and output. An awareness of the pathologic consequences of fluid imbalance has stimulated a search for developing more accurate fluid records. Various approaches have been devised to fill this need. The traditional method of recording intake and output is still used in most hospitals. However, it has often proved inadequate or unsuccessful, making it difficult to construct a fluid profile which will be helpful in treating the patient. Edward F. Patula[136] recommends improving the traditional method by using a multiple part form to prepare intravenous solutions for administration which can be entered in a patient fluid profile summary form. This form places emphasis on detail in relation to output. Another method to improve intake and output monitoring has been attempted by Ted T. Huang and Roger D. Williams.[137] It involves a mechanical measurement of fluid intake and output with a central printout at the nursing station, which eliminates a chance for error. The method is quite costly at present but it may represent the direction in which automation may be used in nursing. Figure 10–5 illustrates a work sheet of a running balance study which shows water, electrolyte, calorie, and nitrogen balance. Such an arrangement gives one a true picture of the patient's clinical status.

Nurses render invaluable service by observing and reporting the signs of plus-and-minus fluid balances as just listed. In many cases this balance depends on their skill in feeding patients. Nurses' records of intake and output of fluids and solids are essential to the doctor's estimate of the patient's needs. This topic is discussed further in Chapter 36.

Water is so essential to body economy and the demand for it is so insistent that drinking water should always be within the patient's reach unless the physician has restricted his intake. While there are no hard and fast rules for the amount to be drunk in a 24-hour period, it should be sufficient in the case of adults to ensure the elimination of at least 1000 to 1500 ml (1 to 1½ qt) of urine.

4. FOOD SELECTION AND THE OPTIMUM DIET

Factors Affecting the Caloric Requirement. The amount of food required per unit of body weight depends on the rate at which the body utilizes nutrients. Theodore C. Ruch and Harry D. Patton[138] list the following factors as affecting the metabolic rate: age, sex, size, activity, temperature, diet, race, climate, pregnancy, and endocrine hormones, specifically epinephrine and thyroxin. Temperament or glandular makeup—and the psychic state—affects the metabolic rate. For example, the hyperthyroid person may have a metabolic rate of +30 which will fall within the normal range (+15 to −15) after a thyroidectomy. In 1929 George W. Henry[139] called attention to the difference between the caloric needs of the same individual in the hyper- and the hypoactive phases of a manic-depressive psychosis.

To estimate scientifically the caloric requirement of a subject it is necessary to measure the metabolic rate and then to take into account the factors just listed. Such estimates are complicated and impracticable for everyday use, but the average caloric needs of persons of all ages with typical builds and in various occupations, usually shown in tabular form, are arrived at by such exact calculations made on hundreds of subjects. A study of such data shows that the caloric need per unit of body weight gradually diminishes from youth to old age. Activity and the rate of growth decrease with the years, and hence we need less food as we grow older. Those who fail to change their habits of eating as they pass from young adulthood to old age get fat.

For young adults the caloric need per kilogram of body weight varies from 33 calories per day for a sedentary woman to 66 calories for a laborer who needs strong muscles.[140] The caloric needs of all other adults fall between the two extremes.

Maintenance of Normal Weight. It is not possible to determine the *normal weight* for anyone. Averages for normal males and females of all ages and body builds have been adopted as "norms." (See Table 36-3, Chapter 36.) Mortality statistics prepared by life insurance companies have influenced medical opinion to set the normal weights at lower figures than were used in past decades. The findings of animal experimentation have been popularized in such articles as "The Thin Rats Bury the Fat Rats." [141] Thorstein Veblen, however, in his *Theory of the Leisure Class* [142] shows the relationship between the cultural pattern and what we consider normal weight. In societies, for example, where "the ideal woman" can labor all day and bear many children without much interruption of her work, normal weights in relation to heights are higher than those in cultures where the "ideal woman" does little with her hands and is cherished as an ornament to the man's household. Height-weight tables should therefore be used with reference to a specific people, their body build, and the kind of life they lead. Following an analysis and comparison of height-weight tables used in various countries, Ancel Keys and Francisco Grande say:

All the foregoing discussion leads to the conclusion that the specification of "optimal" or "ideal" weights is hazardous business. For body weight and relative obesity, at least, the only point on which there will be full agreement is that major departures from the population averages should be avoided.*

Undernourishment and malnutrition are the great plague of mankind. Hunger with its far-reaching effects has been discussed in the introduction to this chapter. Its prevalence in all countries, even the economically favored, is

recognized by the experts. One of the basic principles of the charter of the Food and Agriculture Organization (FAO) of the United Nations is to "free the world from starvation." [143] Wendell H. Griffith,[144] in the Geiger Memorial Lecture, noted that subnutrition and malnutrition are prevalent in the world today in spite of the advancement in knowledge during the past 50 years; and there is evidence of faulty food practices in the United States which suggest that we have not been successful in educating people about good nutritional practices or motivating them to act on what knowledge they have.

Many of us eat a diet adequate in calories but suffer from "hidden hungers" because our food is unwisely chosen or disease may interfere with its assimilation. Fashion often dictates a figure, and some cults influence their followers to adopt a diet incompatible with good nutrition. The weakness, irritability, inability to concentrate on given tasks, and the general inertia characteristic of underfeeding are such universal experiences that the ills of malnutrition would seem self-evident, needing no emphasis in a text for health workers. It may, however, be necessary to keep reminding ourselves that what we eat is conditioned more by habits and custom passed from one generation to another than by intelligence. Some one has said, "We like what we eat," rather than eat what we like. Nutritionists find repeatedly that the diet of most persons in certain large geographical areas is inadequate in kind, quantity, and quality. Anyone can become so habituated to a low-vitamin, low-calorie diet that appetite loses its protective function.

A healthy, normal person suddenly deprived of food may be crazed by hunger. To get food, crimes are committed by the starving, even murder and cannibalism. This acute state differs, however, from that of the chronically and habitually undernourished. The latter assume that their incapacity for sustained effort is normal. It is not easy to change the eating habits of such persons or, in fact, to stimulate them in any way. The beneficial effects of vitamins as a means of increasing desire for food has been mentioned. Insulin, which speeds up the metabolism of carbohydrates, and produces acute hunger, has been used as an artifiical whip to the appetite in extreme cases. Adoption of adult diets that include the basic four food groups would eliminate gross malnutrition.

The quantities and proportions of nutrients should be adjusted to the individual according to age, sex, and genes, and to other relevant variables such as emotional strain, environmental stress, physical activity, and presence of

---

* Keys, Ancel, and Grande, Francisco: "Body Weight, Body Composition and Calorie Status," in Goodhart, Robert S., and Shils, Maurice E. (eds.): *Modern Nutrition in Health and Disease,* 5th ed. Lea & Febiger, Philadelphia, 1973, p. 8.

Table 10-4. The Energy Requirement of Adults *

Estimate of Energy Requirement for 1 Day

I Activity	II Time (hr)	III Factor (cal per kg per hr)	IV Cal per kg II × III
Lying still, awake	0.50	0.1	0.05
Sitting	1.25	0.4	0.50
Standing relaxed	0.75	0.5	0.38
Sitting, writing, or eating	8.00	0.4	3.20
Standing at attention	0.25	0.6	0.15
Dressing and undressing	1.75	0.7	1.23
Light exercise	1.00	1.4	1.40
Walking (3 miles per hr)	1.00	2.0	2.00
Dancing	1.00	3.8	3.80
Skating	1.00	3.5	3.50
Walking up stairs (4 flights)		0.036	0.14
Walking down stairs (4 flights)		0.012	0.05
	16.50		16.40

Body weight, 56 kg
Total calories for activities per kg (sum of column IV), 16.40 cal
Total cost of activities (56 × 16.40 cal), 918 cal
Saving in sleeping 7.5 hr (0.1 × 56 × 7.5), 42 cal

Total for Day	Calories
Basal metabolism for 24 hr	1297
Saving in sleep, to be deducted	42
Corrected basal metabolism	1255
Cost of day's activities	918
Total cost of metabolism	2173
"Tax" for influence of food (10 per cent)	217
Day's requirement	2390

Daily Energy Requirement According to Occupation *

Type of Occupation	Total Calories per Day Men	Women	Cal per kg per day
At rest but sitting most of day	2000–2200	1600–1800	30–33
Work chiefly done sitting	2200–2700	1900–2200	34–37
Work chiefly done standing or walking	2800–3000	2300–2500	38–42
Work developing muscular strength	3100–3500	2600–3000	43–50
Work requiring very strong muscles	4000–6000	—	55–70

* MacLeod, Grace, and Taylor, Clara M.: *Rose's Foundations of Nutrition*, 5th ed. Macmillan Publishing Co., Inc., New York, 1956, pp. 54, 55, 59.

disease. In this way the more elusive forms of underfeeding would be eliminated.[145]

Malnutrition, where the person's food supply is adequate, often has its origin in an emotional disturbance. Indigestion and aversion to food frequently accompany stress, although many neurotics seek comfort in food and get fat. Malnutrition in children is a common symptom of unhappy family relationships. For all these and other reasons, nurses soon find how difficult it is to change eating patterns.

Overeating and the resulting *obesity* is a common nutritional disorder in the economically favored countries. It is considered to be one of the major health problems of western civilization.[146] The danger of excess weight is now generally accepted but in the past it was viewed as a "reserve" to be drawn upon during illness.

Most persons in this country must change their eating habits after young adulthood or suffer a weight increase. This may not be necessary for future generations who have learned to follow the dictum, "No calories without vitamins." This automatically eliminates most concentrated fats and carbohydrates or processed foods, in contrast with natural foods.

Authorities are in agreement that overeating is the primary cause of obesity. Michael G. Wohl, however, notes several other factors that may be involved. He says:

Obesity is of multiple etiology. The principal general cause of the condition, however, is an imbalance between energy intake and energy output resulting in a positive caloric balance. The factors influencing the energy imbalance may be environmental (excessive food intake, physical activity), hereditary, psychological, endocrine or metabolic aberrations.*

In a study of 1600 adults living in New York City, Mary E. Moore and associates [147] report the following findings: (1) obesity is more prevalent (7 times greater) among women of the lowest socioeconomic level than among those of the highest level; (2) the same relationship exists for men though to a lesser degree; (3) the prevalence of obesity increases with increasing age; (4) obese persons, regardless of age and socioeconomic level, show more evidence of immaturity, suspiciousness, and rigidity than those of normal weight.

Wohl outlines reduction diets and exchange lists of foods. They are similar to those prepared in nutrition clinics of hospitals, schools, and industries. Life insurance companies distribute lists of *weight control materials*.[148] They, convinced that excess fat taxes vital organs such as the heart, interferes with body mechanics, and in various ways undermines health, find it profitable to give away pamphlets, charts, and diagrams that spread the facts of weight control. Noting that it is better to eat no more than 80 per cent of one's capacity, Philip Kapleau says:

A Japanese proverb has it that eight parts of a full stomach sustain the man; the other two sustain the doctor. The *Zazen Yojinki* (Precautions to Observe in Zazen), compiled about 650 years ago, says you should eat two-thirds of your capacity. It further says that you should choose nourishing vegetables (of course meat-eating is not in the tradition of Buddhism and it was taboo when the *Yojinki* was written) such as mountain potatoes, sesame, sour plums, black beans, mushrooms, and the root of the lotus; and it also recommends various kinds of seaweed, which are highly nutritious and leave an alkaline residue in the body. . . . . Eat more vegetables of the kind

mentioned, which are alkalinic in their effect. In ancient days there was a *yang-yin* diet. The *yang* was the alkaline and the *yin* the acid, and the old books cautioned that a diet ought not be either too *yang* or too *yin*.*

The problems of obesity and starvation are discussed in Chapter 36.

The Optimum Diet. The best diet is one that provides all the food elements a person needs in that quantity and in those proportions that will keep him or her in optimum health. Obviously, our concept of the optimum diet must be influenced by each major discovery in the field of nutrition. People complain because what health workers tell them one year they refute in the next. This will continue until man loses his capacity to learn. There is, then, no such thing as the optimum diet, but nutritionists have given us general rules epitomizing present-day knowledge.

It isn't possible in a book of this sort to discuss all considerations in feeding an individual. Many have been suggested in the pages on dietary elements: carbohydrates, fats, proteins, minerals, vitamins, and water. For the reader's convenience, however, and because these topics are so important, some major questions on the feeding of infants and the aged are given special treatment.

Infant Feeding. The first question the young mother will want answered about infant feeding is the relative value of breast and bottle feeding.[148a,b] During the first half of this century, as sanitation made clean milk available to babies, there was a tendency, even among medical workers, to think that artificial feeding was a good substitute for the baby's natural food—breast milk. There were always some physicians who disagreed, who did all they could to promote breast feeding, but in recent years obstetricians, pediatricians, and psychiatrists have combined to bring the value of nursing the baby to the attention of mothers. Custom so far prevails, however, that many women are convinced that bottle feeding is as good, if not better, for the child and more convenient for them. Benjamin Spock [149] takes the reasonable stand that at least two persons are concerned and that the woman should not be made to feel that she is a failure as a mother if she cannot or will not nurse her infant. He, of course, advocates *breast feeding* because he thinks it (1) makes the mother feel close to the baby emotionally, (2) gives the baby a sense of security or oneness with the mother, (3) saves the mother's time in preparing a formula, (4) saves money, (5)

* Wohl, Michael G.: "Obesity," in Wohl, Michael G., and Goodhart, Robert S. (eds.): *Modern Nutrition in Health and Disease*, 4th ed. Lea & Febiger, Philadelphia, 1968, p. 974.

* Kapleau, Philip: *The Three Pillars of Zen.* Beacon Press, Boston, 1965, p. 37.

protects the child from intestinal upsets because breast milk is sterile, and (6) the mother's nipple satisfies the sucking reflex more adequately than the artificial nipple, and the infant is less likely to be a thumb sucker. To these advantages should be added the protection offered the baby in the antibodies of breast milk.

According to Harold H. Williams, the milk of all species contains the same nutrients but in different proportions, and the quantitative differences of these nutrients seem to be adapted to the requirements of the young of each species. Pediatricians are credited with the successful modification of cow's milk for use by the human infant but the "ideal substitute for human milk is not available." Comparing the two types of milk, he says:

Although the two types of milk are comparable in total caloric value and percentage of calories derived from fat, human milk provides only 10% of the calories as protein and 40% as lactose. Cow's milk furnishes the latter two nutrients in equicaloric amounts. Striking differences in the pattern of minerals, fatty acids, vitamins, and several amino acids are evident. Some of these differences may be significant in the interrelated biochemical and nutritional roles of certain constituents of milk. Consequently, they also may be significant in the utilization of milk from one animal species by another.*

Nurses who are convinced of its value can greatly encourage breast feeding. Without this conviction it is hard to help mothers keep trying until the flow of milk is established. The nurse who does not make this effort for the mother wishing to nurse her baby has a great deal to answer for, as has the doctor who discourages or is neutral to breast feeding.

Generally speaking, artificial feeding and the preparation of formulas have been simplified. Whole milk, condensed milk, and dried-milk preparations are commonly used. The pasteurization or boiling of mixtures made of fresh milk was formerly advocated to protect infants from bovine tuberculosis, dysentery, and other communicable diseases. However, the necessity of this is questioned now where the water supply is "pure" and the ingredients free from contamination. Establishment of human milk bureaus in which breast milk is collected under aseptic conditions, packed in ice, or frozen, has made this food available for many sick or premature infants.

Formulas for infants. sick or well, are usually prepared in a central laboratory or kitchen, from which the bottles, labeled with names of the babies for whom they are intended, are sent to the clinical services. The formula is usually given at room temperature. If nipples have been put on in the laboratory, they are covered with a paper cap. If nipples are applied by the clinical nursing staff, they are so handled as to keep the whole nipple as clean as possible and the part coming in contact with the baby's mouth uncontaminated. Individual feedings are now prepared in disposable sacks designed to simulate the breast and the mother's nipple. See Figure 10-6 for a variety of nipples for premature and term infants.

With both breast- and bottle-fed babies, other foods are added to the milk diet within the first few months of life. Orange juice and cereals are usually the first additions, but by the sixth month many infants are getting puréed fruits, vegetables, and meats. Vitamin supplements (particularly the fat-soluble A and D vitamins) are also added to the diet soon after birth. This is thought to be particularly important for infants in cold climates.

Regularity has been especially stressed in the feeding of infants. One reason is that their stomachs are small and the baby's total needs will not be met unless he is fed frequently. Feedings are usually spaced at 3- or 4-hour intervals, being less frequent at night. A typical schedule is 6-9-12-3-6-10-2. After the child is a few months old, he or she will usually sleep through the two o'clock feeding and will demand food at longer intervals. A few physicians may have hard and fast rules for the spacing of feedings, but most now believe that each child should establish his or her own rhythm. Even this, however, implies regularity. The writings of Spock for health workers and laymen have revolutionized the feeding of children. Some psychiatrists believe that rigidity in feeding infants builds up hostility and insecurity since the baby may interpret the withholding of food he craves as an expression of dislike or rejection by the mother; or "the big person." Actually, if babies are fed on their demand—which means those signs of hunger they make—they usually establish regular habits of nursing every 3 or 4 hours.[150,151]

Infants show that they are hungry by putting their hands to their mouths and by "rooting" movements. Finally they will cry. Mothers soon learn to recognize a hungry cry but almost any crying infant should be offered food since hunger is the most common cause of discomfort.

Authorities generally agree that infants should be held in a comfortable position when fed by bottle or breast (Fig. 10-7*A*). Contact

* Williams, Harold H.: "Differences Between Cow's and Human Milk," *J.A.M.A.,* **175:**107, (Jan. 14) 1961.

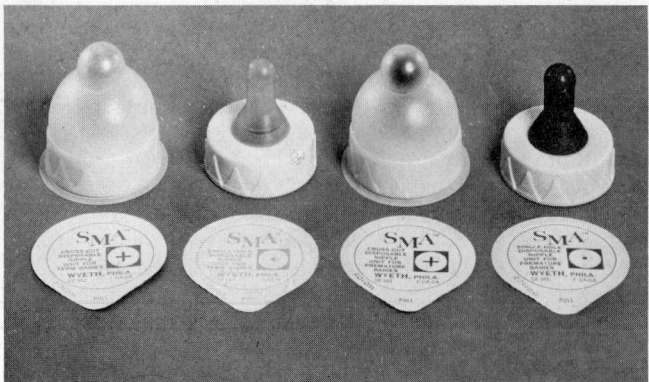

Figure 10-6. A variety of nipples for premature and term infants. The choice of a nipple may make the difference between successful and unsuccessful feeding in the newborn period. The strength of the infant's sucking and swallowing ability must be evaluated before the infant is discharged from the hospital. (Courtesy of SMA, Wyeth Laboratories, Philadelphia, Pa.)

with the mother's body or the nurse's body when they are fed by bottle gives infants the reassurance their nature demands as does the sight of her smiling face and the comforting sounds she makes. Propping the bottle, even with the so-called safe holder, should be avoided. Strangulation and death have resulted from such practices. Holes in the nipple should be such as to allow the food to pass through neither too rapidly nor too slowly. The feeding of an infant should take from 10 to 20 minutes.

Air swallowed with the food from the bottle or the breast may fill the stomach before the child has had enough. In order to prevent this the infant should be held with the head higher than the abdomen while nursing, a position said to make the gas rise toward the cardiac opening of the stomach. Some physicians recommend that at least once during the feeding period and at the end the infant be held over the shoulder for several minutes. Gentle pressure exerted by patting the baby while he is in this position helps to produce eructations (see Fig. 10-7B).[152,152a]

Premature infants, because of their extreme delicacy and sensitiveness to chilling and infection, are not usually removed from their warm surroundings for feeding periods. Lula O. Lubchenco[153] notes that it is difficult to supply premature infants with adequate foodstuffs because of the small capacity of the stomach, slow emptying time of the stomach during illness, and the danger of regurgitation with overfeeding. If premature infants have a strong enough sucking response to a nipple and a coordinated swallowing reflex they should be fed with a bottle. It is important for their development that this sucking reflex be stimulated. When it is not possible to feed infants by mouth, they are fed through a tube inserted into the stomach through the nostril, introduced intermittently or left in position (see Chapter 23 for suggested gavage procedure). However, this method of feeding

should be replaced with bottle feeding just as soon as possible. Infants weighing 1500 gm or more can usually be fed with a bottle. Roberta O'Grady[153a] gives seven signs to indicate when bottle feeding should replace gavage.

Eileen Hasselmeyer and Edward H. Hon[153b] have reported cardiorespiratory changes associated with a catheter in the back of the pharynx, when it passes the cardiac sphincter and when the stomach is rapidly extended with the formula. O'Grady describes and illustrates with photographs the signs of hunger and the normal behavior before, during, and after feeding. The relief of tension usually brings sleep when the experience is satisfying to the infant. O'Grady also discusses what the nurse can do for the mother so that she and the baby can develop a healthy feeding pattern.

There are a number of devices designed to facilitate feeding infants. The infant feeding bottle can be used effectively whenever the sucking reflex is present. A *Breck feeder* is a glass cylinder with a nipple on one end and a bulb on the other that can be squeezed to exert pressure on the contents. This feeder is used for infants with cleft palates. It is easy to strangle the baby by giving him more milk than he can swallow; an eye dropper with the tip protected by rubber is perhaps a safer instrument.

Mothers and guardians of infants and children are often in need of guidance in preparing and serving their foods. Community nurses all over the country are giving such help. In some hospitals it is customary for the nursing staff to teach the parents whatever is necessary about the preparation and administration of feedings before the infant or child is discharged. Conferences, demonstrations, moving pictures, and written directions are used as teaching methods. Frances Y. Henthorn[154] describes an interesting and successful teaching program for children in the Cleveland schools conducted by nurses who were rightfully con-

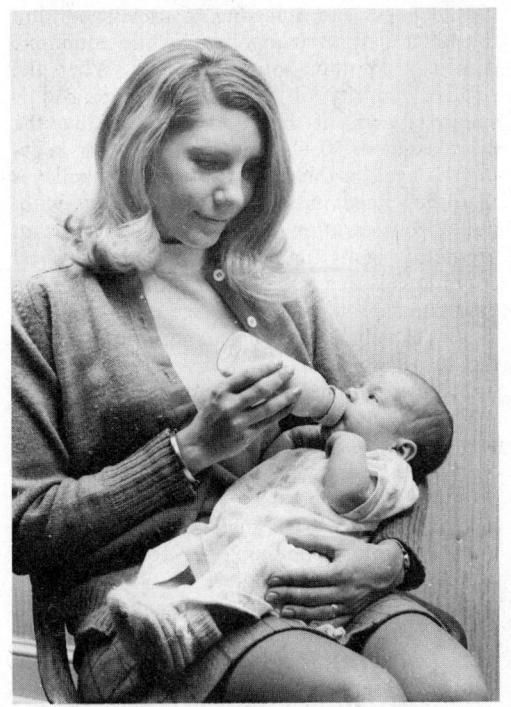

A

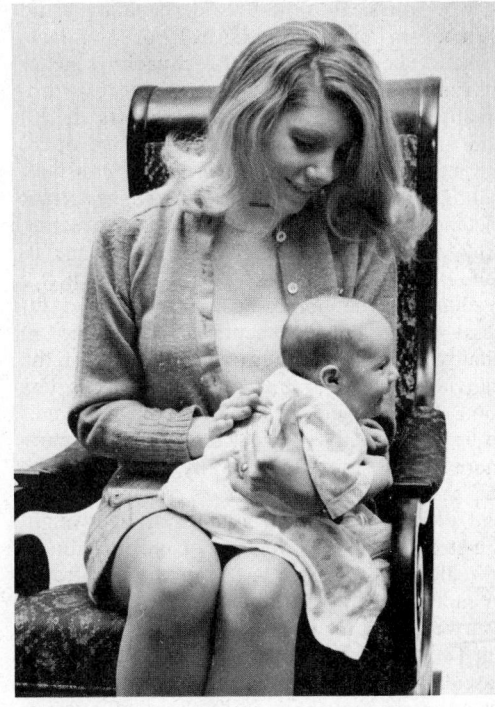

B

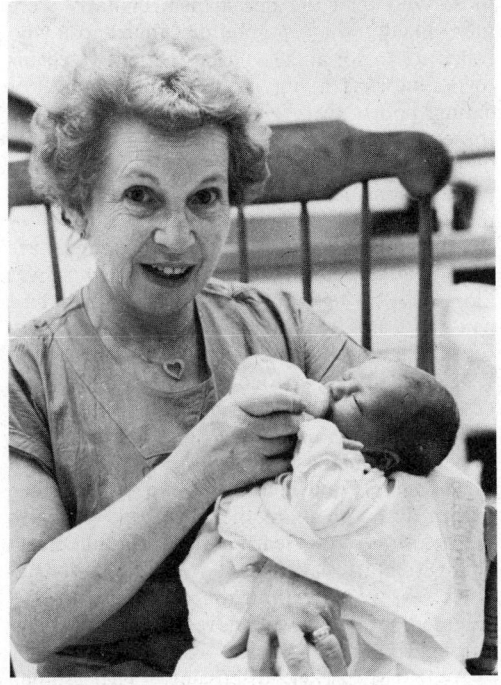

C

Figure 10-7. *A.* Whether breast or bottle feeding, the mother makes herself comfortable before starting and holds her baby close to impart a feeling of warmth and security. *B.* The mother burps the baby during and after feeding to relieve him of the discomfort caused by air sucked in with his milk. She can hold him against her shoulder, with a diaper or towel protecting the clothing, or lean him forward in her lap and pat his back gently. (Courtesy of SMA Wyeth Laboratories, Philadelphia, Pa.) *C.* Nurse in charge of a nursery in the Loyola University Medical Center, Maywood, Ill., sits in a rocking chair as she holds an infant during bottle feeding. (Photograph by Bev Montgomery.)

cerned about the inadequate breakfast that most children were eating; teachers as well as parents became active participants. Many helpful suggestions are offered in the literature for nutritional counseling of the child in and out of the hospital; a few references are included at the end of this chapter.[155-157d] This subject is referred to in Chapter 5, The Health Examination.

Feeding the Aged. People differ so greatly in the rate at which they age that it is hard to generalize about their nutritional needs. A. L. Vischer[158] shows a chart on which are graphed the curves of mental capacity, procreative power, physical fitness and capacity, and metabolism of a hypothetical, or standard, person. The curve of mental capacity reaches maximum height around the age of 60; procreative power at 30; physical fitness at 20; and metabolism at birth. After the age of 20 the metabolic rate remains nearly constant, falling less than 5 per cent. This suggests that metabolic needs, at least in quantity, are not, after adulthood, materially altered by age itself. Between the ages of 20 and 90 there is a gradual decline in physical capacity and fitness—about 20 per cent. This decline in vitality usually too reduces the activity of the individual, and for this reason he needs less food. If, however, the older person continues to be a very active person, he may need many more calories than is generally believed to be the case. The maintenance of normal weight and particularly the avoidance of overweight are stressed. The prevention of chronic illness by caloric restriction has been demonstrated by morbidity and mortality statistics among the overweight.[159] Diabetes mellitus is said to occur two and a half times as often, and cardiovascular-renal disease one and one-half times as often, in the obese as in those of average weight.[160]

No authorities have been found advocating a diet for the aged differing materially from the optimum diet in younger adulthood. Geriatrists repeatedly say that the protein, mineral, and vitamin needs are little altered by age. Occasional reference is made to the diminished secretion of the digestive enzymes and the difficulty some elderly persons find in digesting fats in particular. While no one advocates trying to force on the elderly a diet better than the one they are eating, it must be recognized that a fixed and unwholesome habit of eating can be the cause of the poor appetite and the inability to take care of the meager fare that is eaten.*

Authorities generally agree that caloric intake should be reduced so that there is no appreciable gain in weight and a generous intake of fluids should be maintained.

The faulty teeth and poor posture so often seen in the aged contribute to poor nutrition. Marked improvement may be impossible until these conditions are corrected. Food should be of a texture that the person can masticate until the dental problems are solved. The constipation that accompanies faulty body mechanics must be treated until the cause can be removed, because a poor appetite is one of the effects of constipation.[161,162]

Loneliness and a feeling of uselessness dull the latter part of many lives, while economic want is a common source of stress. When the relative security of a home for the aged is sought, years of boredom are usually the price exacted. Vischer makes a plea for keeping the aged in the current of life. He believes that they need its stimulation and that without a consideration of the psychic causes of premature aging the correction of the physical conditions is to a large extent futile. Discussing nutritional problems of the aged, Joyce Grant says: "Loneliness, eating alone, poor cooking facilities, and financial worry lead to depression, apathy, and lack of initiative." *

Depression in elderly patients in a geriatric unit of a general hospital has been shown to be associated with subnutrition.[163] Doris Schwartz and associates [164] studied 182 elderly chronically ill patients under care of a general medical clinic, concluding the following: (1) 29 per cent reported diets that were inadequate; (2) patients with no formal education reported the highest proportion of poor or inadequate diets; (3) those patients living with two or more persons had a better diet than those living alone or with only one person; (4) those who read the newspaper regularly were more likely to have a good diet than those who failed to do so; and (5) if a "patient rated his own illness as a big problem, his chance of eating poorly was greater than one out of three; and he was a 'high-risk' candidate for dietary problems." These findings are important considerations in helping elderly people to maintain good nutrition.

Fortunately, food services and resources are now available to the aged person who lives alone or who has limited assistance so that he can enjoy hot, nutritious meals. Some of these services include Home Help Service, Meals on Wheels,† and Luncheon Clubs.[165] Day-care centers also make it possible for some elderly persons who cannot shop and prepare meals to keep a home base.

Changing Food Habits. Young nurses, filled with a desire to share their enlarged concepts of nutrition, soon learn that it is difficult to change dietary patterns. If we are honest with ourselves, we will admit that we apply a small fragment of what we know about health, including food needs, in our own life.

Agnes M. Erkel, discussing "The Human

---

* An eminent physician, in discussing the ills of one of his elderly patients, explained some of them by saying "You see she's a tea and toaster."

* Grant, Joyce: "The Feeding of the Elderly in Their Own Homes: Defining the Need," *Proc. Nutr. Soc.,* **27:**35, 1968.

† These services have come to be so helpful that the federal government has produced a directory—US Public Health Service: *Home Delivered Meals. A National Directory.* US Government Printing Office, Washington, D.C., 1971, (127 pp).

Side of Eating," quotes a bulletin prepared by Margaret Mead for the United Nations:

First of all, we eat that which is available within the confines of the community; how it is prepared is dependent upon the equipment available for cooking. The ultimate result in any home, in any society, is a set pattern of food habits. . . .

Erkel goes on to say:

In every community there are patients, young and old, whose dietary habits we are trying to change. It does take time to individualize one's teaching, . . . progress will be slow . . . until we recognize the fact that eating habits are an expression of a pattern of living and . . . change must be built upon . . . the patient's economic and social background.*

Anderson and Browe [166] suggest that if we are going to be successful in helping people to develop good nutritional habits, the following is necessary: knowledge of normal nutrition, skills in guidance and counseling, an understanding of the cultural behavior of the family, and information about the composition of the family, including age categories (infancy through aging).

These authors sound a warning and give advice which, in the writers' opinion, most inexperienced health workers need. Successful nutritionists, including the nurse when she or he can qualify under this title, must be students of their subject and of society as well. They must be able to help individuals plan normal diets and follow diets prescribed by the physician; they must be prepared to help housewives plan meals for healthy families and invalids, and all of this within the cultures and economic resources of those they serve.[166a-e] The tables on pages 648–49, 652–55 in this text are helpful in the solution of such problems, but the more specialized sources listed at the end of this chapter should be consulted.

5. CONDITIONS THAT FAVOR DIGESTION AND ASSIMILATION

Sight and Smell of Savory Food. Walter B. Cannon [167] cites his experiments and those of Pavlov, Richet, and others showing that the smell and sight of appetizing food stimulates digestive juices and muscular movement of the alimentary tract. P. Teitelbaum and A. N. Epstein report their experiments on normal animals and those with hypothalamic damage. They conclude:

Normal regulation depends on adequate motivation. Taste and smell are powerful motivating stimuli. They are psychic energizers that contribute to the animal's hunger drive. However, in the normal animal, retaining intact all other sources of the urge to eat, they are dispensable. But when the drive is diminished by central neural damage, the importance of taste and smell is magnified, and they may become the dominant motives to eat. Therefore, whenever motivation is impaired, taste and smell are essential for regulation.*

This knowledge should be applied in health and sickness. A person may not be hungry, or if questioned may say that he does not want anything to eat, and yet have his appetite aroused by seeing and smelling a tempting dish. Bed patients who are too ill to feed themselves should see the food that is fed them for the psychic effect on digestion, if for no other reason. Some agencies use frozen prepared meals and microwave ovens so that patients receive a truly hot meal.†

Food Preferences. Discussing the role of food preferences, Henry W. Brosin says:

We learn to like and dislike foods from our earliest days, and often these patterns are thoroughly fixed in adult life. The nature of the memories associated with the early ingestion of food will determine preferences in a manner independent of logical considerations, and hence will be puzzling to the physician who is attempting a rational therapy for a patient with nutritional problems. If we remember the old adage about there being no disputing matters of taste, or the wide variations in diet among the various nations of the earth, it will be easier to tolerate the food vagaries of our patients.‡

It is often surprising to see the ill unable to tolerate simple bland foods and yet able to eat without discomfort some dish ordinarily considered indigestible but which they especially relish. Health workers learn to study the likes and dislikes of patients and to provide them with foods meeting their needs but also appealing to their palates.

Freedom from Pain, Stress, and Fatigue. It is well known that strong emotions, even though pleasurable, interfere with digestion.

---

* Erkel, Agnes M.: "The Human Side of Eating," *Pub. Health Nursing,* **42:**606, (Nov.) 1950.

* Teitelbaum, P., and Epstein, A. N.: "The Role of Taste and Smell in the Regulation of Food and Water Intake," in Zotterman, Y. (ed.): *Olfaction and Taste,* Vol. I. Macmillan Publishing Co., Inc., New York, 1963, p. 359.

† This comment must not be interpreted as a recommendation for wholesale, mechanized food preparation. Nutritional values and flavor suffer when food is exposed to extremes of temperature and storage.

‡ Brosin, Henry W.: "The Psychology of Appetite," in Wohl, Michael G., and Goodhart, Robert S.: *Modern Nutrition in Health and Disease,* 4th ed. Lea & Febiger, Philadelphia, 1968, p. 63.

Experiments have shown that pain, excitement, worry, fear, anger, passion, depression, irritability, nervousness, homesickness, or distress of any kind inhibits the flow of saliva, gastric juice, intestinal and pancreatic juice, and also the motor activity of the alimentary tract. Pain or violent emotion involves the autonomic nervous system which also controls alimentation.

Eating should be postponed, if possible, until excitement of any sort has abated. Infants and children should not be excited even by play immediately before or after a meal. Pleasurable emotions and sensations, however, if not too exciting, aid digestion, and so one hears such expressions as "Laugh and grow fat," and "Joy never kills." The beneficial effect of pleasure and laughter on the digestion was recognized in the custom of having a jester present at the evening meal or in our own day by soft music with meals.

Excessive fatigue is close kin to pain. Insofar as possible everyone, sick or well, should avoid eating when very tired or hurried. Physical exhaustion can usually be relieved by resting before the meal, and mental fatigue overcome by substituting a pleasant train of thought for exciting or disturbing ideas. Hurried eating is likely to inhibit digestion because the food is neither adequately ground by the teeth nor throughly mixed with the saliva.

A Pleasant Environment. Attractive surroundings and a cheerful atmosphere add greatly to the enjoyment and hence the digestion of a meal. The environment should be free from anything offensive to the senses, such as noise, disorder, confusion, dirt, unpleasant odors, excessive heat or cold, or anything to arouse unpleasant associations. Those with whom one shares a meal, who serve the meal, or even the company in the room can contribute much to creating an atmosphere conducive to digestion. Visitors who demand attention from the patient should be excluded tactfully while a sick person is eating, but an agreeable and understanding companion should be encouraged. The mildly sick and, in fact, most ambulatory patients should eat in groups rather than in solitude except under special circumstances. Many hospitals are now designed to foster communal meals.

Regularity in Eating. Periodic recurrences of hunger demand that human beings and animals eat at regular intervals. Hunger is associated with rhythmic contractions of the stomach. It is under the control of the hypothalamus where the feeding center is located and as the nutrient stores in the body fall below normal, the feeding center becomes active.

When the gastrointestinal tract, especially the stomach, is distended, the desire for food decreases. Chewing, swallowing, taste, habit, and other factors affect the rhythm so that individuals feel the need of food at different intervals. Regularity is probably desirable for everyone, sick or well, since meals too close together may overload the stomach and too far apart decrease effective effort in work and play.

Rigid feeding schedules versus self-demand feeding for infants are discussed under "Infant Feeding" on page 671. Because their stomachs hold so little, it is obvious that they must be fed frequently and with some degree of regularity.

The elderly are often psychologically dependent upon regularity. Since their activities and interests tend to be curtailed, they have a keener anticipation of their food than do busy young adults. Their habits, also, are more fixed, and a delayed dinner can be a serious annoyance. With the decreased vitality of age they may also feel a more acute need of refueling.

Meal Spacing. Through a study of variations in muscle power, believed by Howard N. Haggard and Leon A. Greenberg [168] to be an index of the individual's efficiency, they have shown that meal spacing affects efficiency. They believed the American custom of three meals a day to be the result of an industrial system that allowed one rest period during the working day, rather than consideration of body needs. They demonstrated that motor power is lowest in the morning before breakfast in spite of the long preceding rest, and that feeding individuals five meals a day instead of three resulted in a more uniform state of efficiency. Prevention of fatigue is highly important in health and even more so when the body is fighting disease.

It is customary to feed the very ill at frequent intervals, and in some cases nutrients are injected continuously into the veins. In most hospitals midmorning and midafternoon nourishments are served to patients, and in many cases are available to the staff. Meal spacing is of great interest to nurses, for, while the physician usually prescribes the diet, he or she may leave it to their judgment and its administration is the responsibility of nurses. Institutions, especially psychiatric hospitals, are developing food services that enable patients to participate in food selection and preparation at times. Some hospitals make "snacks" available to patients as they want them, and the opportunity to choose diets is more and more common. Actually it constitutes an opporunity for nutrition education.

6. DIET IN SICKNESS

Special Feeding Problems in Illness. All forms of illness affect digestion and assimilation, either directly as a result of organic disease or indirectly from poor circulation, lack of exercise, or the worry and depression that often accompany illness. Lack of exercise lessens muscle tone and reduces the metabolic rate, so diminishing the food requirement. As less food is needed, and eaten, bulk is decreased unless the diet is wisely chosen. This diminishes the stimulation of the muscular walls of the intestines brought about through distention. Constipation is the natural result, and sensations evoked by it retard appetite. Muscle tension characteristic of emotional states is favorable to action but unfavorable to the process of digestion. Bacteria and other toxins act directly on digestive glands and muscles as chemical poisons and in this way alter digestion; or they may produce nausea and vomiting or diarrhea. A dry mouth, a bad taste, and even more distressing symptoms may accompany fever and discourage eating.

Illness limits variety in persons' lives and turns their thoughts inward. With too much time to think about details they exaggerate the importance of what they eat. The limitation of their diet, due to the nature of their illness, may be a source of irritation and make it difficult to plan their meals. Acute illness and conditions that limit motion may make feeding themselves or even eating an effort. They must in many cases be fed, and unless this is very skillfully done, it detracts greatly from the pleasure of the meals.

These are only a few of the many problems involved in feeding the sick. Their solution may be the main factor in the patient's recovery. No one can live for many days without water. The omission of food for the same length of time is much less harmful, but even short periods of starvation produce discomfort and lessen the powers of resistance. D. M. Dunlop in an article, "Modern Trends in Therapeutic Diets," decries the old methods that rarely included all dietary essentials. Referring to the surreptitious drinks from flower vases and hot-water bottles, he says patients deprived of food and water were often "wiser" than the doctor. He advocates complete diets individually planned and says: "There can be few instances in dietetic out-patient departments in which the giving out of printed diet sheets is justifiable. Advice on diet should be individual. . . ." *

* Dunlop, D. M.: "Modern Trends in Therapeutic Diets," *Br. J. Nutrition,* **4:**225, (Feb.) 1950.

In spite of Dunlop's recommendation, it is common practice for physicians to prescribe the patient's diet on admission in some such terms as the following: General diet, high-caloric, low-caloric, soft, low-fat, low-cholesterol, high-vitamin, low-protein, high-protein, liquid, or other diet. If there is a good working relationship among the physician, dietitian, nurse, patient, and the family, modifications are made consistent with Dunlop's recommendations. Too often these diets are rigidly planned and administered and far too often deprive the patient of basic food needs either because they don't include them or because the diet, being unpalatable, is only partially eaten.

Responsibility of the Nurse. Although the physician in this country usually prescribes the diet and it may be prepared and served by a dietary staff, there is still much expected of nurses in the matter of feeding the patient. They may be expected in many cases to suggest the nature and content of the diet, and, it may be repeated, they are responsible for the patient's being served the prescribed diets. They observe likes and dislikes. This observation will guide them if they are preparing and serving the food themselves, or they may report it to the dietary department if the patient is in the hospital. It is essential that the physician know whether the sick person is eating the food served. The nurse, who is with the patient almost constantly, is in the best position to estimate and report what the patient eats. The nurse should be given and should accept the responsibility for the patient's getting concentrated dietary supplements through some channel when his or her needs are not met by what he or she eats at meals. In some cases where the amount consumed must be accurately determined, as in metabolic disorders such as diabetes, food left on the tray is often weighed and measured. The nurse is responsible, as far as possible, for making the patient comfortable and the surroundings pleasant at meal times. In some situations where there is no one else who can do it so well, the nurse must plan, prepare, and serve the food. The nurse may even have to select and purchase food supplies. Often the spacing of feedings is left to the nurse. In many cases the nurse is the person most able and best qualified to guide the planning of diets consistent with the doctor's orders, general health needs, and the family budget. The nurse may also be the most experienced in selecting, buying, preparing, and serving foods and in modifying habits of eating. When the patient is helpless or acutely ill, it is the nurse's responsibility to feed him or her or to teach some member of the family, volunteer, or other worker to do so.

The nurse can do a great deal in preparing the patients to go home, helping them to make changes in their diets within the framework of the usual family meals. The nurse can also be of assistance to those outside the hospital walls with *their particular* nutritional problems. Moore [169] describes how one can help a family of four plan a variety of appetizing nutritious meals for only $15.00 per week, even in 1966—a year of high prices. Such competence is greatly needed by nurses in many settings.

7. NURSING MEASURES IN ORAL FEEDING

Preparation of the Environment. The *room* should be well ventilated, quiet, and in order during meals and the patient undisturbed by treatments, dressings, visitors, or doctors' rounds. Also, in homes the atmosphere should be conducive to enjoyment of the meal. All disturbing sights should be removed, insofar as possible. In a ward, for example, disturbing

patients are screened. In most institutions bedpans are offered at regular intervals between or half an hour before meals.

The patient's *bed* should be comfortable and orderly. All unappetizing objects (for example, a sputum container) should be out of sight, and the bedside stand made as attractive as possible.

The *table holding the tray of food* should be cleared except for flowers, which, if not overpowering, add to the pleasure of the meal. In every case the food should be in front of the patient, who is in a comfortable position. When overbed tables are available (see Figs. 10-8 and 10-9), bedside stands should not be used, because the patient has to turn on one side, support himself or herself with one elbow, and eat with one hand. A sick person will often give up the struggle before having eaten as much as he or she would relish if more comfortable.

A return to normal habits should be encouraged; therefore, as soon as the patient is able to be up for part of the day, it is a good thing to draw a suitable table up to his or her chair to eat one or more meals sitting up. Patients are encouraged to eat in groups

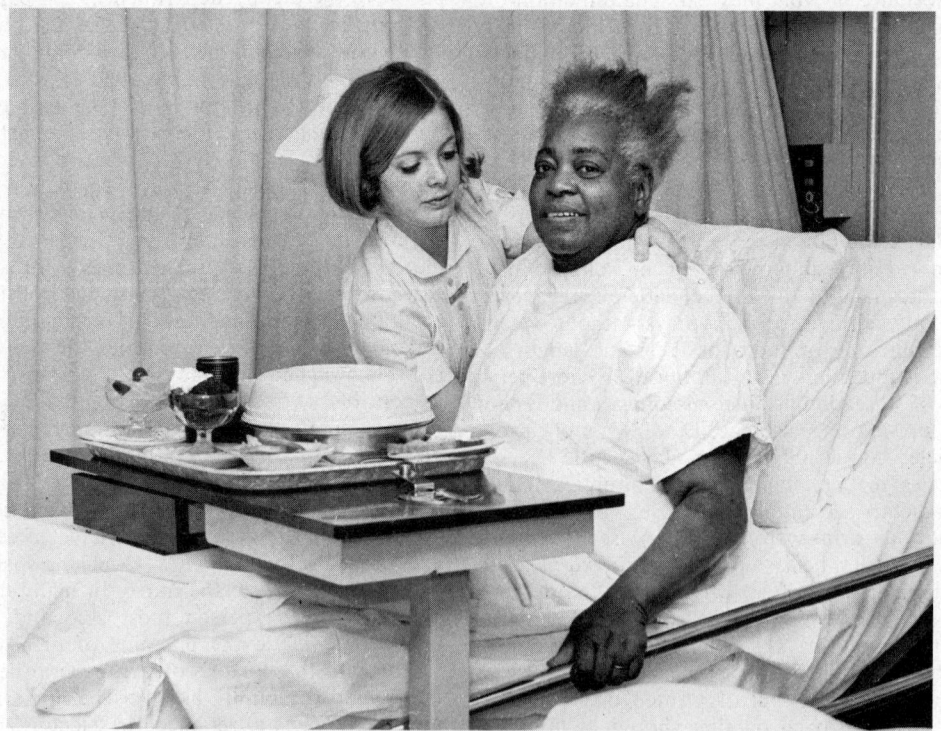

Figure 10-8. An adjustable table that fits over the bed is ideal for holding food trays. (From Robinson, C., and Lawler, M.: *Normal and Therapeutic Nutrition,* 15th ed. Macmillan Publishing Co., Inc., New York, 1977. Photo courtesy of School of Nursing, Thomas Jefferson University, Philadelphia, Pa.)

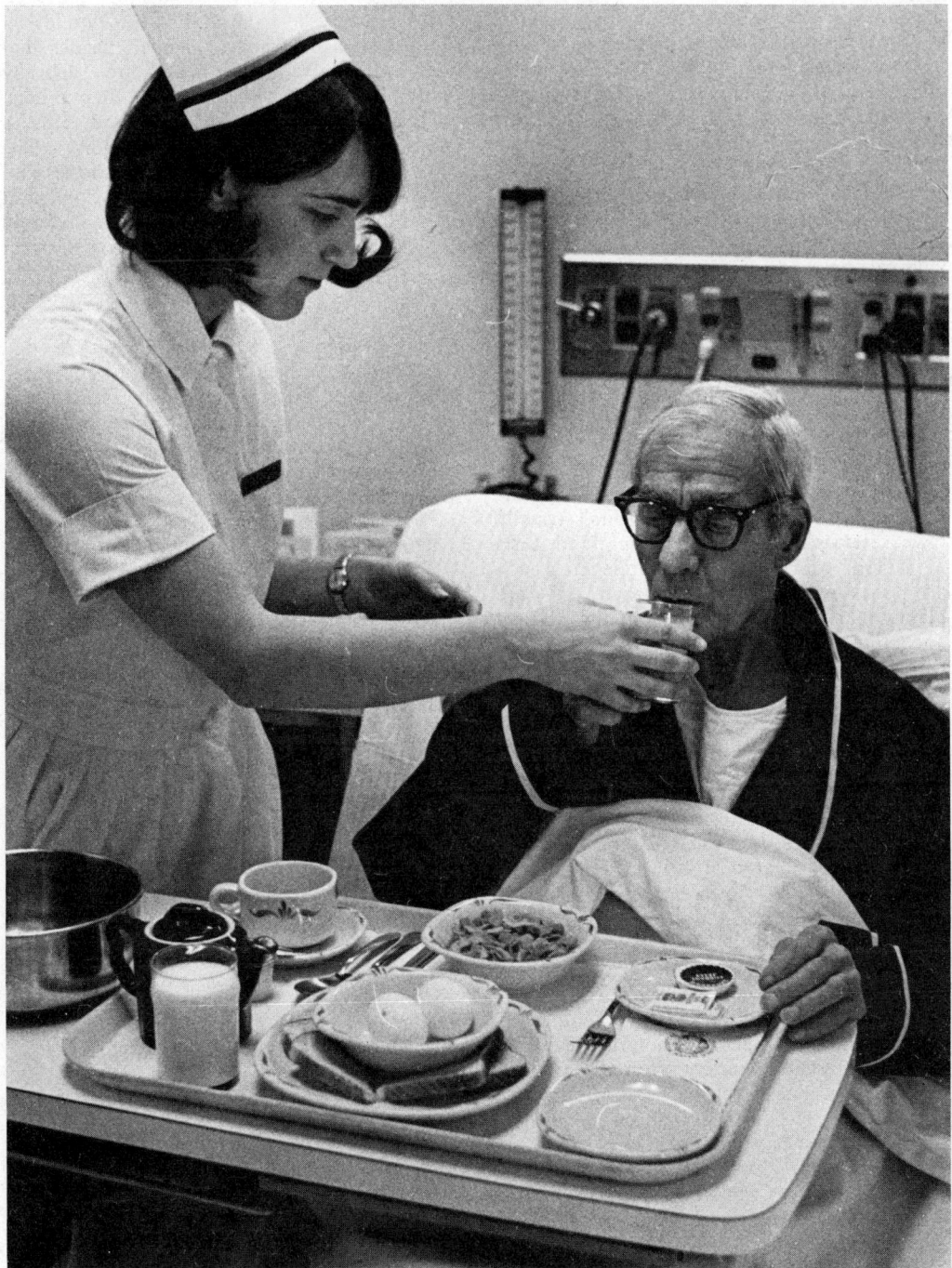

Figure 10-9. Another type of overbed table that allows the tray to be placed in a position that is convenient for the patient. (Photo courtesy of Yale–New Haven Medical Center, New Haven, Conn.)

around a table when facilities are available.

Many very sick patients prefer not to have *visitors* during meals. While it is pleasant to share a meal with another, it is tiring to have to attend to a meal and a visitor at the same time. A member of the patient's family or an intimate friend may in some cases be a pleasure and, moreover, improve the appetite. Friends and volunteer workers are often asked to help nurses feed patients. No hard and fast rule can be made for all situations. Because hospital regulations are made in the interests of the majority, however, in wards, visiting sometimes is restricted during meal hours. In private rooms and homes the visiting periods should be regulated according to the special demands of the patient.

The Patient's Diet. Since in many cases the patient's recovery depends largely on getting the prescribed diet, and errors may have far-reaching and serious results, hospitals usually have a rigid schedule about serving food. Lists of patients with the diets prescribed for each are posted in the divisional kitchen; trays are plainly marked with the names of the patients and often with the type of diet. Some terms used for diets are *regular* or *full, high-caloric, soft, clear* or *full liquid, strict* or *moderate low sodium, nonconstipating,* and numerous others. The general nature of some of these is suggested by the foods of which they are composed. For more information on diets, see Appendix with suggested references. Often colored cards are used to differentiate diets.

There is a great deal to learn about the successful feeding of persons on liquid diets. The inexperienced nurse thinks that any liquid may be given. Actually, this may not be intended, and he or she should determine, for example, whether milk is included in the liquids to be given a particular patient. C. J. Speas,[170] decrying the common tendency to omit some essential nutrients from liquid diets, has published one which he, with Milla Newland, has worked out. An analysis of this diet shows that it met what was then the recommended daily requirements for fats, carbohydrates, proteins, minerals, and vitamins. When milk is eliminated from the diet, other nourishing fluids must be substituted. Eggs are an item in most high-caloric liquid diets. Sugars, such as lactose, and preparations, such as Cerelose, which are not as sweet as cane sugar may be used in fairly large quantities. On the basis of personal experience, Sir Stanley Davidson and R. Passmore[171] recommend the use of Complan (milk proteins including carbohydrates, fat, minerals, and vitamins), Casilan (milk proteins), Prosparol (fat emulsion), and Lonalac (milk protein). These supplements may be incorporated into liquids by the use of a mechanical blender. Drinks that are neither sweet nor heavy are generally more easily tolerated in nausea than others. Ginger ale, although it has little food value, is often refreshing. (See the Appendix.) The surgical liquid diet supplies a few calories and small amounts of sodium and potassium chloride; its greatest contribution is probably relief of thirst. In the United States, Sustacal (see Fig. 10-10), a product of Mead Johnson Laboratories, is frequently used to augment the diet of an individual who is unable to take sufficient nutrients. Each serving contains one third the recommended daily allowances for protein, vitamins, and minerals (see Figure 10-11; also see Appendix for more on diets).

Preferences of the patient should be considered insofar as possible, and there are various ways of making them known to the person in charge of planning and serving diets. There is considerable disagreement as to whether patients should be asked what they want to eat, since this robs the meal of the pleasant element of surprise, pleasant to everyone, sick or well. The selection of dishes is often a bore and persons will name the first thing they think of, whereas there may be many they would enjoy more. To avoid both difficulties, hospitals have adopted the practice of printing advance menus. Patients choose

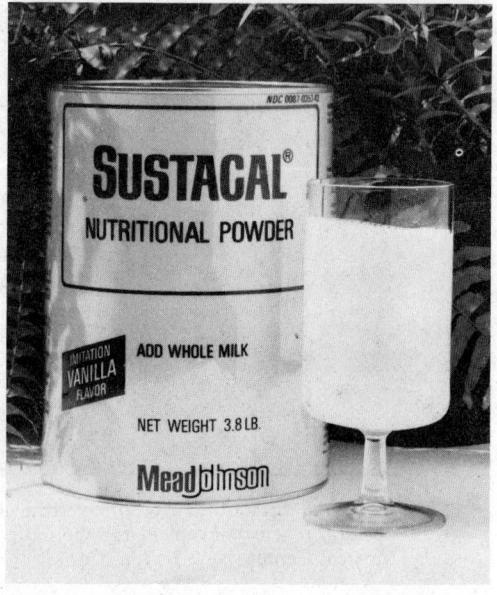

Figure 10-10. SUSTACAL is a pleasant-tasting nutritional drink that is well tolerated by patients with a wide variety of nutritional needs. The 3.8 lb. can is economical. (Courtesy of Mead Johnson Laboratories, Evansville, Ind.)

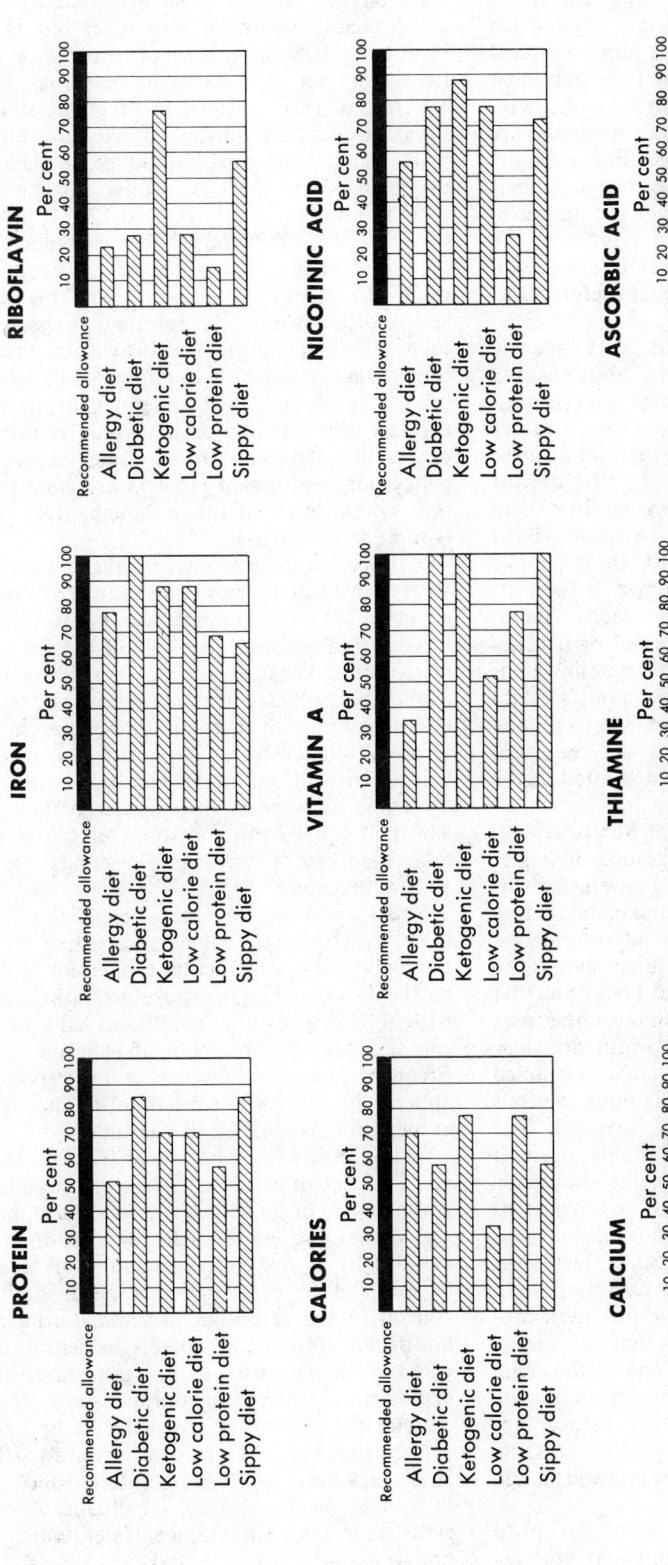

Figure 10-11. Comparison of nutrients in special therapeutic diets with recommended allowances. (From Spies, Tom D.: *The Birmingham Study, Rehabilitation Through Better Nutrition.* W. B. Saunders Co., Philadelphia, 1947.)

from a variety of dishes on Tuesday, for example, what they would like for dinner on Thursday and Friday. Checking a printed list requires little effort, and by the time the meal is served, patients have usually forgotten what they selected. This system is expensive; therefore, simpler, if less effective, methods are ordinarily used in ward service. For example, dietitians on visits to patients may ask their likes, dislikes, and idiosyncrasies; or the nurse may make such notes and send them to the dietary department. Forms may be used indicating the beverage, or the cereal preferred, or how to cook eggs.

All health workers should have specific knowledge of *racial, religious,* and *national habits of eating.* Having learned general customs, such as that Italians use olive oil rather than lard or butter in cooking, that the Chinese have rice and tea with all meals, that the orthodox Jew does not eat dairy products and meat in the same meal, nurses have some basis on which to help plan meals for these people. In helping patients in their homes in food selection and when discussing specific therapeutic diets, the nurse will find her or his suggestions much more likely to be followed if they do not run counter to the family's established dietary habits. It isn't possible to discuss here the characteristic diets of different peoples, but books on the subject are listed at the end of this chapter.

Preparation of the Patient for Meals. Analysis of conditions favoring digestion indicates that in preparing anyone, sick or well, for eating, a calm frame of mind and a body free from pain and discomfort are important. Not even the most accomplished nurse can make every patient easy in mind and body, but that should be the aim. The means the nurse uses will vary with the situation. Painful dressings or any upsetting event should be so scheduled as not to occur near the meal hour. Serious or upsetting topics should be avoided. The patient should be in a comfortable position and helped to feel fresh by having the hands washed and the mouth cleaned, or other steps taken according to the demands of the case and his or her own wishes. Some fastidious persons will demand more preparation than the distribution of nursing time provides; others will not realize until shown that cleanliness adds to the pleasure of meals and at the same time helps to control communicable diseases. Children, especially, require help in the practice of hygienic habits of eating. Infants should be changed, if necessary, and made comfortable before feedings.

Serving Diets. The service has much to do with making a meal appetizing—or the reverse. Trays should be large enough to hold the contents without crowding. Linen covers are probably the most attractive, but if the family or institution cannot provide a sufficient number, it is better to substitute paper covers that can be fresh for each meal. The same observation applies to napkins. Silverware, glass, and china should be spotless, its arrangement on the tray similar to that used on the dining table (see Fig. 10-12). If the patient is left-handed, he or she will appreciate the thoughtful attendant who reverses the order. In homes an attractive and matching set of dishes should be selected; in hospitals there is a tendency to get away from institutional types of china. Gaily flowered dishes are often seen. A child will sometimes drink from a pretty cup when he or she would refuse the nourishment from an ordinary one. Chromium coffee pots and cream pitchers are good looking and easily cared for, although silver plate is still commonly used.

A nurse caring for one patient can usually serve a meal in courses. This is likely to make it more appetizing, since hot foods can be served from the stove and cold dishes from the refrigerator. When this is not possible, covers should be provided for hot dishes and every effort made to see that cold dishes are chilled. Hospital kitchens often serve trays on moving belts so that all food items can be put on them by a line of workers in a matter of seconds. The belt moves the tray onto elevators that take them in a few more seconds to the clinical division.

Small servings are more appetizing than large. A heaped-up plate is appalling to the sick, who are in many cases indifferent to their meals, if not actively averse to eating. It is wise to serve dainty meals and add to the caloric intake by nourishment between meals. Frequent feedings, however, if they spoil the appetite for the more substantial foods offered at mealtimes, should be discontinued.

A liquid diet *must* be fed at frequent intervals in order to get an adequate caloric intake. If the choice of fluids is left to the nurse, he or she should use some such guide as that developed by Speas and Newland. This should be adapted to each patient's needs and, of course, to the resources at hand. Ordinarily, hot drinks are most acceptable in the morning when the patient wakes up; warm, nourishing drinks are given to encourage sleep. If the patient has a fever, it is usually at its height in the afternoon; then cold drinks are particularly appealing. In feeding infants and very ill persons on liquid diets, punctuality is especially important. Since concentrated foods cannot so easily be used to make up the 24-hour

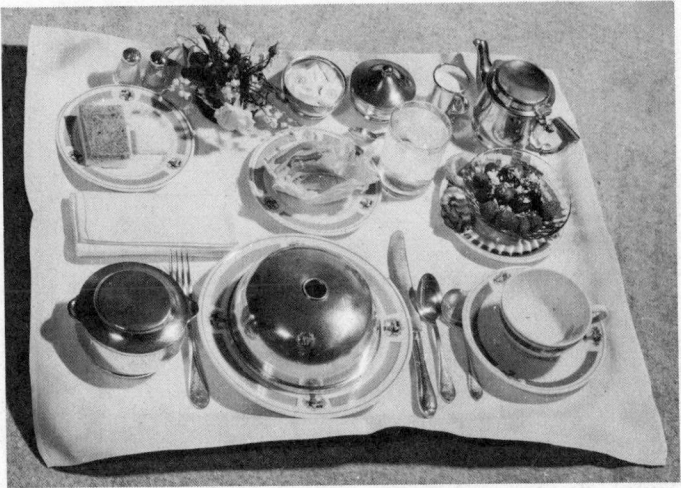

Figure 10-12. Dinner tray showing proper arrangement of dishes and silverware. (Courtesy of St. Luke's Hospital, New York, N.Y.)

food requirement, the loss of even one feeding is serious. Infant feedings are largely liquid, but the major aspects of this highly specialized subject are brought together for brief treatment on pages 670–73.

Assistance in Eating and Rehabilitation of the Handicapped. All normal persons prefer to feed themselves. Illness or disability may, however, reduce people to the helplessness of infancy. The need for assistance in getting food to the mouth is usually temporary; in rare cases it is a permanent handicap. It should be the aim of the nurse in every case to establish independence as soon as possible.

Brief and temporary help is usually needed when severe illness prostrates or weakens the patient or when burns and wounds make it impossible to use the hands or when the patient is in a respirator. Permanent help is required by anyone who loses the use of the arms and hands and who cannot be fitted with a functioning prosthesis. Some form of assistance is needed by many patients until they can adjust to their handicap and learn new techniques of eating.

The following are *general recommendations:* Help the patient into a comfortable position. Unless contraindicated by the nature of the disease, the head should be elevated and supported by pillows or a back rest. The tray of food should be within the range of vision; the sight of it whets the appetite and gives him or her the opportunity to suggest the rotation in which he or she wishes the food. The nurse should see that clothing and bedding are well protected so that the patient will not be afraid of soiling them.

If the nurse is seated, the patient loses the sense of hurry and some of the embarrassment over "causing so much trouble." A high stool

that brings the nurse on a level with the patient is illustrated in Figure 10-13. Liquids are most easily taken through tubes. Glass tubes are seldom used, because expendable tubes of waxed paper, cellophane, or plastic are more satisfactory. Irrational patients and young children who may break glass tubes might possibly swallow a piece. Nurses who see themselves as the patient are usually more successful at feeding. The patient may occasionally suggest what he or she would like next, but if this must be done often, it is tiring. No hard and fast rule can be made as to whether or not the nurse should talk during the meal. In some way the nurse should convey the impression that he or she is glad to give this service and above all is not feeling hurried or bored. Friendly remarks every now and then certainly contribute to a pleasant atmosphere, while stories to which the patient must give close attention are likely to be a bore.

The patient will prefer to wipe his or her own mouth if possible. If not, the nurse keeps the patient "neat." If the regular napkin is spread over the chest, an extra, small napkin that can be held in the hand should be provided. Sometimes the patient cannot manipulate utensils but can hold bread and butter or celery in the hand. The patient should be encouraged to help himself or herself up to the point of fatigue or frustration. An attempt should be made to judge the size of the mouthful to which he or she is accustomed. The nurse should avoid imposing on the patient his or her own eating habits. Any health teaching at mealtimes must be done skillfully; otherwise, it may irritate the patient and set up a psychologic state inhibiting appetite and retarding digestion.

Sick or weak persons can often feed them-

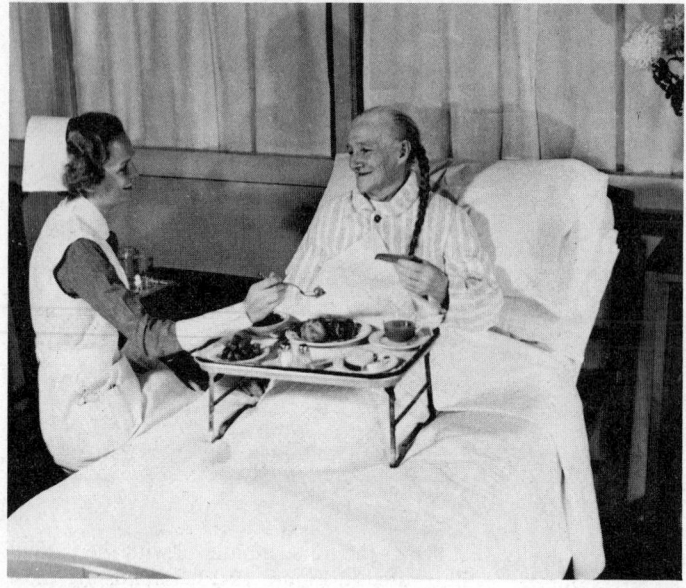

Figure 10-13. Nurse feeding a cardiac patient who is not allowed to feed herself. Note the comfortable position of the patient and the nurse. (Courtesy of the Yale University School of Nursing, New Haven, Conn.)

selves if everything is within reach, bread buttered, and other foods cut into bits. Some sensitive individuals will leave food untasted rather than ask for help.

The *blind* need special help in eating. Juliet Bindt,[172] blind herself, makes these suggestions: Help the person to use ordinary table appointments so that he or she acquires increasing independence. Place utensils in conventional positions, for this is where the blind person expects to find them. Help the newly blinded to acquire the technique of locating what is before them with careful movements of the hand. It should be held half closed, palm down, and the little finger used as a feeler. Tell the patient in a low tone what foods are served and give their location by imagining that the plate is a clock. For example, "The beef is at one o'clock, the potato at five, and the spinach at nine; celery and pickles are beside the plate at ten, and coffee at two o'clock." If there are shells, artichoke leaves, or bones to be discarded, provide an empty plate to separate waste from foods to be eaten. Try to treat him or her in every possible respect like a normal person, giving help inconspicuously rather than solicitously. Other special needs of the blind are discussed in Chapter 46.

Persons with motor disabilities can usually feed themselves if they have devices and utensils suited to their handicap. Use of special devices and foods of special textures, however, should be reduced to a minimum because dependence on them is itself a handicap in visiting or traveling. The child with cerebral palsy,

the adult with an injury to the motor area of the brain, or with a disease such as paralysis agitans or muscular dystrophy that affects motor power, coordination, or both, needs special help. Everything possible should be done to enable these patients to feed themselves (see Fig. 10-14), but rehabilitation should be so gradual that they are never discouraged by failure. When a meal becomes a physical struggle it ceases to be a pleasure, and the patient is likely to eat less than he or she needs. Marjorie Abel[173] points out that a 12-year-old child with cerebral palsy may require 6000 calories daily because tension and muscle spasm set energy expenditure at such a high point. The child and the mother must be helped to relax and enjoy mealtime; otherwise, it is difficult to get the child to meet his or her nutritional needs. Foods are selected primarily to meet nutritional requirements, but they should be chosen also for the ease with which the patient can eat them. Those with motor handicaps may be able, for example, to grasp a banana, a hard-boiled egg, or celery. Food textures must be considered, especially when the muscles used in swallowing are affected.

The child should sit in a chair that gives him or her the optimum support at a table of the right height. Edward W. Lowman and Howard A. Rusk,[174] and Alice B. Morrissey[175] show a number of mechanical aids for those with motor disabilities. These include a table with depressions into which dishes can be set to keep them from sliding out of place; utensils with cylindrical or built-up handles, designed to give maximum contact when grasped;

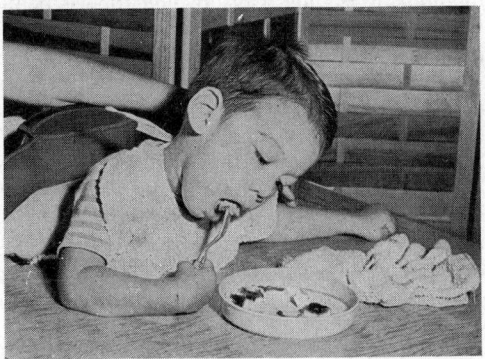

Figure 10-14. Children with cerebral palsy can learn to feed themselves with help and encouragement from nurses and parents. (From Abel, Marjorie: "Feeding the Child with Cerebral Palsy," *Am. J. Nurs.,* **50:**558, [July] 1950.)

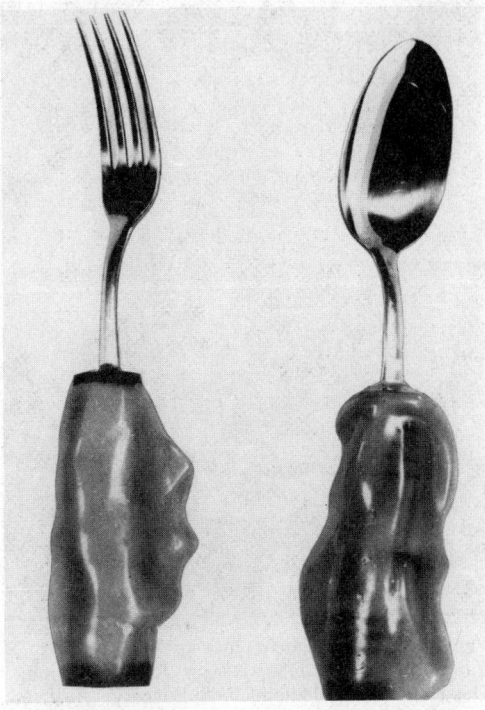

Figure 10-15. Plastic handles on fork and spoon molded to fit hands with limited grip. (From US Veterans Administration, Department of Medicine and Surgery: *Bulletin of Prosthetics Research. Prosthetic Aids and Service.* [BPR 10–15.] US Government Printing Office, Washington, D.C., 1971, p. 166.)

forks and spoons with short handles to help those with poor coordination; others with lengthened or bent handles to serve those whose motion is limited; cups with handles; drinking tubes in cartons and glasses with crocheted jackets to help prevent spilling liquids; bands, into which a fork or spoon can be fixed for those who lack the muscle power to hold one; plates with rims to prevent food from being pushed onto the table by the hand with limited control; and lastly, the rocker splint that supports the arm in an elevated flexed position while allowing a range of motion that enables the patient to get food to the mouth. Frank H. Krusen and Frederic J. Kottke,[176] discussing devices that may be used by persons with limited mobility or coordination of the upper extremity, mention the Warm Springs feeder, a balanced deltoid aid, as well as a rocker feeder. See Figures 10-15 and 10-16 for two devices used by the US Veterans Administration to help the handicapped with eating problems.

While in some cases it may be easier to teach the handicapped more independence in eating when alone with the health worker, communal eating should be the goal in most cases. Patients can sit at the table in wheelchairs and can come on crutches. A sufficient number of trained persons should be present to give them whatever help they may need. Music is conducive to a relaxed atmosphere for most, but it must be unobtrusive; otherwise, it will distract or irritate.

Whenever there is poor control of table utensils, the clothing should be protected. The bib or napkin should be fixed in place. It should have a top absorbent layer and a water-proof lining. Disposable protectors are best, economically and esthetically.

Feeding the Moribund and Unconscious. Although it is more and more common in hospitals to nourish the very ill extraorally with intravenous infusions and with intubations, these methods may be impossible in homes, and most people can be successfully fed orally if their attendants have sufficient time and patience. The touch of a spoon on the lips or the presence of food in the mouth elicits the swallowing reflex even when all cerebral activity seems to have ceased, as in severe illness. In such cases food must be given very slowly, very frequently, and in small amounts. Eye droppers, cups with spouts, and tubes of various kinds are used in the care of both children and adults, according to their condition and the particular demands of the case. Food put into the mouth of a deeply unconscious patient may, however, be sucked into the lungs instead of the esophagus. Paralysis or dystrophy of the muscles of swallowing makes oral feeding hazardous, and food must be put into the

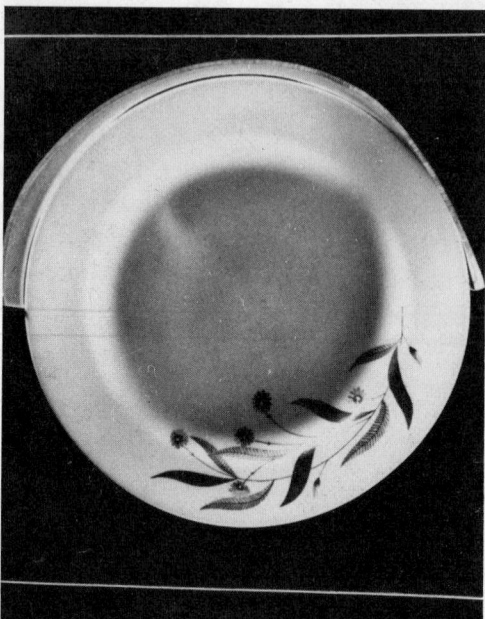

Figure 10-16. A plate holder to keep plate stationary. (From US Veterans Administration, Department of Medicine and Surgery: *Bulletin of Prosthetics Research. Prosthetic Aids and Service.* [BPR 10-15.] US Government Printing Office, Washington, D.C., 1971, p. 167.)

patient's mouth with extreme care. Many unconscious patients die from lung infections as a result of oral feeding or of the drippings from tube feedings. A weak cough reflex and inactivity contribute to the development of pneumonitis and lung abscess. When a patient with weakened reflexes is fed by mouth, a suctioning device should be at hand if possible. Motor-driven suctioning machines may, in some situations, be rented from hospital supply houses for home use. Unless it is contraindicated, the head should be elevated so that gravity favors the passage of food from the mouth to the stomach.

Records and Charting in Oral Feeding. All health workers rely upon the nurse's reports on the amount the patient eats, his or her appetite, likes and dislikes, and any resultant discomfort from feeding. The nature of these reports varies according to the patient's condition and the importance of diet in the treatment. Detailed reports are made, for example, on the feeding of babies and young children because so much depends on their getting the proper amount and kind of food and because they are unable to describe their needs and difficulties. In acute illness careful reports must be made because the physician prescribes other

methods of feeding if insufficient food is being taken by mouth. In diabetes and other metabolic diseases it is sometimes necessary to weigh and measure and record the food left on the patient's tray in order to make a sufficiently accurate estimate of the food intake to serve as a basis for the prescribed therapy.

Written reports on diet and feeding may be incorporated in the nurse's notes, as these daily running comments are usually called, or special forms may be provided. See Figure 10-2, page 640, which includes caloric intake as well as each of the nutrients.

REFERENCES

1. De Castro, Josué: *The Geography of Hunger.* Little, Brown & Co., Boston, 1952.
2. Barr, Stringfellow: *Citizens of the World.* Doubleday & Co., New York, 1952.
3. Huxley, Julian S.: *On Living in a Revolution.* Harper & Row, New York, 1944.
4. Osborn, Fairfield: *Our Plundered Planet.* Little, Brown & Co., Boston, 1948.
5. Mitchell, Helen S.: "Nutrition in Relation to Stature," *J. Am. Diet. Assoc.,* **40:**521, (June) 1962.
6. Tranter, G. A.: *We Are What We Eat.* Currawong Publishing Co., Ltd., Sydney, Australia, 1945.
7. Keys, Ancel, and Keys, Margaret: *Eat Well and Stay Well.* Doubleday & Co., New York, 1959.
8. Mills, Clarence A.: *Climate Makes The Man.* Harper & Row, New York, 1942.
9. Sherman, Henry C., and Lanford, Caroline S.: *Essentials of Nutrition,* 3rd ed. Macmillan Publishing Co., Inc., New York, 1951, pp. 318, 351, 353.
10. Robinson, Corinne H.: *Normal and Therapeutic Nutrition,* 14th ed. Macmillan Publishing Co., Inc., New York, 1972, p. 8.
11. Williams, Sue Rodwell: *Nutrition and Diet Therapy,* 2nd ed. C. V. Mosby Co., St. Louis, 1973, p. 309.
12. US Bureau of Human Nutrition and Home Economics: *Family Fare, Food Management and Recipes.* US Department of Agriculture, Home and Garden Bull. No. 1. US Government Printing Office, Washington, D.C., 1966.
13. US Bureau of Human Nutrition and Home Economics: *Food for Families with School Children.* US Department of Agriculture, Home and Garden Bull. No. 13. US Government Printing Office, Washington, D.C., 1962.
14. *Food for Peace Around the World.* US Department of State Agency for International Development. US Government Printing Office, Washington, D.C., 1962.
15. Cook, F., and Groppe, C. C.: *Balance Food Values and Cents.* University of Cali-

fornia Agricultural Extension Service, Berkeley, 1967, HXT-42.

16. ———: *Saving Ways in Food Buying.* University of California Agricultural Extension Service, Berkeley, 1967, HXT-64.

16a. Margolius, Sidney: *Health Foods: Facts and Fakes* (No. 498). Public Affairs Committee, Inc., New York, 1973.

17. Robinson, Corinne H.: *op. cit.*

18. Guthrie, Helen Andrews: *Introductory Nutrition.* C. V. Mosby Co., St. Louis, 1967.

19. Anderson, Linnea, and Browe, John H.: *Nutrition and Family Health Service.* W. B. Saunders Co., Philadelphia, 1960.

20. Food and Nutrition Board, Committee on Maternal Nutrition: *Maternal Nutrition and the Course of Pregnancy.* National Academy of Sciences, Washington, D.C., 1970.

21. Parran, Thomas: "Nutrition in Public Health Programs," *Nutr. Rev.,* **4:**129, (May) 1946.

22. Downes, Jean, and Baranovsky, Anne: "An Experiment in Nutrition Teaching by Public Health Nurses," *Milbank Mem. Fund Q.,* **23:**227, (July) 1945.

23. Moore, Mary Lou: "When Families Must Eat More For Less," *Nurs. Outlook,* **14:**66, (Apr.) 1966.

23a. Robischon, Paulette: "Pica Practice and Other Hand-Mouth Behavior and Children's Development Level," in Downs, Florence S., and Newman, Margaret A.: *A Source Book of Nursing Research,* F. A. Davis Co., Philadelphia, 1973, p. 85.

23b. Nelson, Alice H.: "Self-Recorded Diet Histories," *Am. J. Nurs.,* **72:**1601, (Sept.) 1972.

23c. Canada. Department of National Health and Welfare, Health Protection Branch Educational Services: *Selected Teaching Nutrition Aids for Public Health Nurses.* Information Canada, Ottawa, 1973.

24. DuBois, Eugene F.: *Fever and the Regulation of Body Temperature.* Charles C Thomas, Publisher, Springfield, Ill., 1948.

25. Guyton, Arthur C.: *Textbook of Medical Physiology,* 5th ed. W. B. Saunders Co., Philadelphia, 1976, p. 905.

26. Schwartz, Irving L., and Fein, Martin: "Amino Acids and Proteins: The Molecular Framework and Machinery of Living Systems," in Brobeck, John R., et al. (eds.): *Best and Taylor's Physiological Basis of Medical Practice,* 9th ed. Williams & Wilkins Co., Baltimore, 1973, pp. 1–130.

27. "The Role of Carbohydrates in the Diet," *Nutr. Rev.,* **20:**102, (Apr.) 1964.

28. "Interactions Between Carbohydrate, Protein, and Fat Metabolism in Starvation," *Nutr. Rev.,* **27:**256, (Sept.) 1969.

29. Weller, John M., and Taylor, Isaac M.: "Some Problems of Potassium Metabolism," *Ann. Intern. Med.,* **33:**607, 1950.

30. Retterbush, William C.: "Potassium Me-

tabolism," *Med. Arts Sci.,* **4:**9, (First Quarter) 1950.

31. Bland, John H.: *Clinical Metabolism of Body Water and Electrolytes.* W. B. Saunders Co., Philadelphia, 1963, p. 572.

32. Hightower, N. C., Jr., and Janowitz, Henry D.: "Secretion and Absorption in the Intestines," in Brobeck, John R., et al. (eds.): *op. cit.,* pp. 2–87.

33. "Artificial Sweeteners—Possible Photosensitizers," *Nutr. Rev.,* **28:**122, (May) 1970.

34. Guyton, Arthur C.: *op. cit.,* p. 890.

35. Neely, James R., and Oram, James F.: "Control of Fatty Acid Metabolism in Adipose Tissue," in Brobeck, John R., et al. (eds.): *op. cit.,* pp. 7–123.

35a. Mansback, Charles M.: "Conditions Affecting the Biosynthesis of Lipids in the Small Intestines," *Am. J. Clin. Nutr.,* **29:**295, (Mar.) 1976.

36. Neely, James R., and Oram, James F.: *op. cit.*

37. McAmis, Avor J., et al.: "Growth of Rats on Fat-Free Diets," *J. Biol. Chem.,* **82:**247, (May), 1929.

38. "Linoleic Acid in Infant Nutrition," *Nutr. Rev.,* **22:**45, (Feb.) 1964.

39. Mitchell, Helen S., et al.: *Nutrition in Health and Disease,* 16th ed. J. B. Lippincott Co., Philadelphia, 1976, p. 32.

40. *Ibid.,* p. 135.

41. "Further Studies of Cholesterol, Fats and Fatty Acids," *Nutr. Rev.,* **18:**146, (May) 1960.

42. Cohen, A. M.: "Fats and Carbohydrates as Factors in Atherosclerosis and Diabetes in Yemenite Jews," *Am. Heart J.,* **65:**291, (Mar.) 1963.

43. Keys, Ancel: "A Practical, Palatable Way of Eating," *Minn. Med.,* **52:**1259, (Aug.) 1969.

43a. AMA Council on Foods and Nutrition, and Food and Nutrition Board, National Academy of Science-National Research Council: "Diet and Coronary Heart Disease," *J.A.M.A.,* **222:**1647, (Dec. 25) 1972.

44. Vinther-Paulsen, N.: "Investigations of the Actual Food Intake of Elderly Chronically Hospitalized Patients," *J. Gerontol.,* **5:**331, (Oct.) 1950.

45. Community Service Society, Nutrition Service: *Foods for Health—As We Grow Older.* The Society, New York, 1949.

46. Mitchell, Helen S., et al.: *op. cit.,* p. 36.

47. "Histidine Requirement in Infancy," *Nutr. Rev.,* **22:**114, (Apr.) 1964.

48. Mitchell, Helen S., et al.: *op. cit.,* p. 39.

49. Lewis, Howard B.: "Problems in Nutrition," *J.A.M.A.,* **138:**207, (Sept 18) 1948.

50. Ohlson, Margaret A., et al.: "Studies of the Protein Requirements of Women," *J. Am. Diet. Assoc.,* **24:**744, (Sept.) 1948.

51. Slonaker, James R.: "The Effect of Different Per Cents of Protein in the Diet in

Successive Generations," *Am. J. Physiol.*, **123**:526, (Aug.) 1938.

52. Jacobs, Eugene C.: "Effects of Starvation on Sex Hormones in the Male," *J. Clin. Endocrinol. Metab.*, **8**:227, (Mar.) 1947.

53. Keys, Ancel: "Human Starvation and Its Consequences," *J. Am. Diet. Assoc.*, **22**:582, (July) 1946.

54. "Recovery Rates of Children Following Protein-Calorie Malnutrition," *Nutr. Rev.*, **28**:118, (May) 1970.

55. Cravioto, Joaquin: "Application of Newer Knowledge of Nutrition on Physical and Mental Growth and Development," *Am. J. Public Health*, **53**:1803, (Nov.) 1963.

56. Yoshimura, Hisato: "Adult Protein Requirement," *Fed. Proc.*, **20**:103, (Mar.) 1961.

56a. Winick, Myron: "Changes in Nucleic Acid and Protein Content of the Human Brain During Growth," *Pediatr. Res.*, **2**:352, 1968.

56b. Dayton, Delbert H.: "Early Malnutrition and Human Development," *Children*, **16**:211, (Nov.–Dec.) 1969.

57. "Hunger: Disease of Millions. 3. The Hungry and the Sick," *Indian J. Med. Sci.*, **17**:691, (Aug.) 1963.

58. Garrow, J. S.: "The Effects of Severe Protein Deficiency on the Human Infant," in Bianchi, C. Paul, and Hilf, Russell: *Protein Metabolism and Biological Function*. Rutgers University Press, New Brunswick, N.J., 1970, p. 36.

59. Schaeffer, Alexander J.: "Effect of Certain Amino Acids on Healing of Experimental Wounds of the Cornea," *Proc. Soc. Exp. Biol. Med.*, **61**:165, (Feb.) 1946.

60. Elman, Robert: *Parenteral Alimentation in Surgery with Special Reference to Proteins and Amino Acids*. Paul B. Hoeber, New York, 1947.

61. Lund, Charles C., and Levenson, Stanley M.: "Protein in Surgery," *J.A.M.A.*, **128**:95, (May 12) 1945.

62. Scrimshaw, N. S., and Bressani, R.: "Vegetable Protein Mixtures for Human Consumption," *Fed. Proc.*, **29**:80, (Mar.) 1961.

63. Vilter, Richard W.: "Nutritional Problems in Surgical Patients," *Postgrad. Med.*, **36**:34, (July) 1964.

64. "Corn-Soy-Milk, a Nutritional Supplement," *Nutr. Rev.*, **27**:156, (May) 1969.

65. Sebrell, W. H.: "Recommended Dietary Allowances—1968 Revision," *J. Am. Diet. Assoc.*, **54**:104, (Feb.) 1969.

66. Holt, L. Emmett, and Snyderman, Selma E.: "The Amino Acid Requirements of Infants," *J.A.M.A.*, **174**:100, (Jan. 14) 1961.

67. Woodruff, Calvin W.: "Protein Requirements of Full-Term Infants," *J.A.M.A.*, **174**:114, (Jan. 14) 1961.

68. Gordon, Harry H.: "Protein Allowances for Premature Infants," *J.A.M.A.*, **174**:107, (Jan. 14) 1961.

69. Guyton, Arthur C.: *op. cit.*, p. 931.

70. Cuthbertson, D. P.: "Quality and Quantity of Protein in Relation to Human Health and Nutrition," *Nutr. Abstr. Rev.*, **10**:1, (July) 1940.

71. Holt, L. Emmett, et al.: "The Concept of Protein Stores and Its Implications in Diet," *J.A.M.A.*, **181**:699, (Aug. 25) 1964.

71a. Garza, C., et al.: "Human Protein Requirements; The Effect of Variations in Energy Intake Within the Maintenance Range," *Am. J. Clin. Nutr.*, **29**:280, (Mar.) 1976.

72. Mitchell, Helen S., et al.: *op. cit.*, p. 51.

73. *Ibid.*, p. 52.

74. Mottram, V. H.: *Human Nutrition*. Edward Arnold (Publishers) Ltd., London, 1963, p. 72.

75. American Medical Association, Council on Foods and Nutrition: "Symposium on Human Calcium Requirements," *J.A.M.A.*, **185**:588, (Aug. 17) 1963.

76. Davidson, Sir Stanley, and Passmore, R.: *Human Nutrition and Dietetics*, 5th ed. Williams & Wilkins Co., Baltimore, 1972, p. 115.

77. "Recommendation for Increased Iron Levels in the American Diet," *Nutr. Rev.*, **28**:108, (Apr.) 1970.

78. Finch, C. A.: "Iron-Deficiency Anemia," *Am. J. Clin. Nutr.*, **22**:512, (Apr.) 1969.

79. Schulman, Irving: "Iron Requirements in Infancy," *J.A.M.A.*, **175**:118, (Jan. 14) 1961.

80. Kimball, O. P.: "Endemic Goiter—a Food Deficiency Disease," *J. Am. Diet Assoc.*, **25**:112, (Feb.) 1949.

81. Robinson, Corinne H.: *op. cit.*, p. 129.

82. "Sodium Intake and Blood Pressure," *Nutr. Rev.*, **27**:280, (Oct.) 1969.

83. Frank, Robert L., and Mickelsen, Olaf: "Sodium-Potassium Chloride Mixtures as Table Salt," *Am. J. Clin. Nutr.*, **22**:464, (Apr.) 1969.

84. Goodman, Louis S., and Gilman, Alfred: *The Pharmacological Basis of Therapeutics*, 5th ed. Macmillan Publishing Co., Inc., New York, 1975, p. 784.

85. Smith, Francis H.: "Potassium Deficiency in Gastrointestinal Disease," *Gastroenterology*, **16**:73, (Sept.) 1950.

86. Randall, H. T., et al.: "Potassium Deficiency in Surgical Patients," *Surgery*, **26**:341, (Mar.) 1949.

87. Bland, John H.: *op. cit.*, p. 217.

88. Schroeder, Henry A., et al.: "Essential Metals in Man, Magnesium," *J. Chronic Dis.*, **21**:815, (11/12) 1969.

89. Hodge, Harold C.: "Metabolism of Fluorides," *J.A.M.A.*, **177**:313, (Aug. 5) 1961.

90. Pearson, William N.: "Biochemical Appraisal of the Vitamin Nutritional Status in Man," *J.A.M.A.*, **180**:50, (Apr. 7) 1962.

91. "Vitamin C Intake in Great Britain," *Nutr. Rev.*, **27**:139, (May) 1969.

92. King, Charles G.: "Vitamin C," *J.A.M.A.*, **142:**563, (Feb. 25) 1950.

93. Mitchell, Helen S., et al.: *op. cit.*, p. 94.

94. *Ibid.*, p. 96.

95. Neal, Robert A., and Sauberlich, Howerde E.: "Thiamin," in Goodhart, Robert S., and Shils, Maurice E.: *Nutrition in Health and Disease*, 5th ed. Lea & Febiger, Philadelphia, 1973, p. 186.

96. Mitchell, Helen S., et al.: *op. cit.*, p. 101.

97. Ziporin, Z. Z., et al.: "Thiamine Requirement in the Adult Human as Measured by Urinary Excretion of Thiamine Metabolites," *J. Nutr.*, **85:**297, (Mar.) 1965.

98. Jolliffe, Norman, et al. (eds.): *Clinical Nutrition*, 2nd ed. Paul B. Hoeber, New York, 1962, pp. 606, 616.

99. Mitchell, Helen S., et al.: *op. cit.*, p. 102.

100. Shue, G. M., and Hove, E. L.: "Interrelation of Vitamin B₆ and Sex on Response of Rats to Hypercholesterolemic Diets," *J. Nutr.*, **85:**247, (Mar.) 1965.

101. Martin, Ethel Austin: *Nutrition in Action.* Holt, Rinehart & Winston, New York, 1963, p. 151.

102. Sauberlich, Howerde E.: "Pantothenic Acid," in Goodhart, Robert S., and Shils, Maurice E.: *Nutrition in Health and Disease*, 5th ed. Lea & Febiger, Philadelphia, 1973, p. 203.

103. Mitchell, Helen S., et al.: *op. cit.*, p. 108.

104. Berlin, Hans, et al.: "Oral Treatment of Pernicious Anemia with High Doses of Vitamin B₁₂ Without Intrinsic Factor," *Acta Med. Scand.* **184:**247, 1968.

105. Bethell, Frank H., et al.: "Cobalamin (Vitamin B₁₂) and the Intrinsic Factor of Castile," *Ann. Intern. Med.*, **35:**518, 1951.

106. Yamamoto, R., et al.: "Further Studies on the Absorption of Vitamin B₁₂ Following Oral and Parenteral Administration," *J. Nutr.*, **45:**507, (Aug.) 1951.

107. Hall, Charles A.: "Transport of Vitamin B₁₂ in Man," *Br. J. Haematol.*, **16:**429, 1969.

108. Matoth, Y., et al.: "Studies on Folic Acid in Infancy. III. Folates in Breast Fed Infants and Their Mothers," *Am. J. Clin. Nutr.*, **16:**359, (Apr.) 1965.

109. Mitchell, Helen S., et al.: *op. cit.*, p. 108.

110. De Luca, H. F., and Suttie, J. W. (eds.): *The Fat-Soluble Vitamins.* University of Wisconsin Press, Madison, 1970, p. 257.

111. Robinson, Corinne H.: *op. cit.*, p. 146.

112. Pease, Charles N.: "Retardation and Arrestment of Growth of Bones Due to Vitamin A Intoxication," *J.A.M.A.*, **182:**110, (Dec. 8) 1962.

113. Smith, Barbara M., and Malthus, Eileen: "Vitamin A Content of Human Liver from Autopsies in New Zealand," *Br. J. Nutr.*, **16:**213, 1962.

114. "Toxic Reactions of Vitamin A," *Nutr. Rev.*, **22:**109, (Apr.) 1964.

115. De Luca, H. F.: "Metabolism and Function of Vitamin D," in De Luca, H. F., and Suttie, J. W. (eds.): *The Fat-Soluble Vitamins.* University of Wisconsin Press, Madison, 1970, p. 3.

116. Jolliffe, Norman, et al. (eds.): *op. cit.*, p. 506.

117. Robinson, Corinne H.: *op. cit.*, p. 156.

118. Guyton, Arthur C.: *op. cit.*, p. 984.

119. "Dietary Factors and Vitamin K," *Nutr. Rev.*, **22:**225, (Aug.) 1964.

120. Suttie, J. W.: "Mechanisms of Action of Vitamin K," in De Luca, H. F., and Suttie, J. W.: *The Fat-Soluble Vitamins.* University of Wisconsin Press, Madison, 1970, p. 447.

121. Guyton, Arthur C.: *op. cit.*, p. 390.

122. *Ibid.*, p. 431.

123. Leaf, Alexander: "Regulation of Intracellular Fluid Volume and Disease," *Am. J. Med.*, **49:**291, (Sept.) 1970.

124. Guyton, Arthur C.: *op. cit.*, p. 439.

125. Williams, Sue Rodwell: *op. cit.*, p. 158.

126. Binnion, Peter F.: "Modern Views on Physiology. IX. Control of Body Salt and Water," *Practitioner,* **203:**375, (Sept.) 1969.

127. *Ibid.*,

128. Devroede, Ghislain J., and Phillips, Sidney F.: "Conservation of Sodium, Chloride, and Water by the Human Colon," *Gastroenterology,* **56:**101, (Jan.) 1969.

129. Guyton, Arthur C.: *op. cit.*, p. 485.

130. Black, D. A. K.: *Essentials of Fluid Balance*, 4th ed. Blackwell Scientific Publications, Oxford, 1967, p. 26.

131. Thompson, W. T., Jr.: "Salt and Water" (editorial), *Va. Med. Mon.*, **95:**587, (Sept.) 1968.

132. Black. D. A. K.: *op. cit.*, p. 145.

133. Wyndham, C. H., and Strydom, N. B.: "The Danger of an Inadequate Water Intake During Marathon Running," *S. Afr. Med. J.*, **43:**893, (July 19) 1969.

134. Pfaff, William W.: "Electrolyte Disorders," *Int. Anesthesiol. Clin.*, **6:**151, (Spring) 1968.

135. *Ibid.*

136. Patula, Edward F.: "Upgrading of the Quality of Patient Fluid Profiles," *Am. J. Hosp. Pharm.*, **25:**370, (July) 1968.

137. Huang, Ted T., and Williams, Roger D.: "Mechanical Monitoring of Fluid Intake and Output in Surgical Patients," *Am. J. Surg.*, **117:**687, (May) 1969.

138. Ruch, Theodore C., and Patton, Harry D.: *Howell-Fulton, Physiology and Biophysics*, 19th ed. W. B. Saunders Co., Philadelphia, 1965, p. 1043.

139. Henry, George W.: "Basal Metabolism and Emotional States," *J. Nerv. Ment. Dis.*, **70:**598, (Dec.) 1929.

140. MacLeod, Grace, and Taylor, Clara M.: *Rose's Foundation of Nutrition*, 5th ed. Macmillan Publishing Co., Inc., New York, 1956, p. 57.

141. Rorty, James: "The Thin Rats Bury the Fat Rats," *Harper's Magazine*, **198:**28, (May) 1949.

142. Veblen, Thorstein: *The Theory of the Leisure Class.* Modern Library, New York, 1923.

143. Autret, M.: "Applied Nutrition," *Isr. J. Med. Sci.,* **4**:443, (May–June) 1968.

144. Griffith, Wendell H.: "Food as a Regulator of Metabolism," *Am. J. Clin. Nutr.,* **17**:392, (Dec.) 1965.

145. *Ibid.*

146. Chrestakis, George: "Obesity and Nutrition Education," *Minn. Med.,* **52**:1279, (Aug.) 1969.

147. Moore, Mary E., et al.: "Obesity Social Class and Mental Illness," *J.A.M.A.,* **181**:966, (Sept. 15) 1962.

148. Metropolitan Life Insurance Company: *Weight Control Materials.* The Company, New York, 1970.

148a. Knafl, Kathleen: "Conflicting Perspectives on Breast Feeding," *Am. J. Nurs.,* **74**:1848, (Oct.) 1974.

148b. Brack, Datha Clapper: "Social Forces, Feminism, and Breastfeeding," *Nurs. Outlook,* **23**:556, (Sept.) 1975.

149. Spock, Benjamin: *Baby and Child Care.* Cardinal Edition, Pocket Books, Inc., New York, 1968, p. 72.

150. Senn, Milton J. E. (ed.): *Problems of Infancy and Childhood. Transactions of the Fourth Conference, New York, March, 1950.* Josiah Macy, Jr. Foundation, New York, 1951.

151. Lubchenco, Lula O.: "Formulas and Nutrition," *Am. J. Nurs.,* **61**:73, (May) 1961.

152. Vaughan, Victor C., III, and McKay, James R.: *Nelson's Textbook of Pediatrics,* 10th ed. W. B. Saunders Co., Philadelphia, 1975, p. 162.

152a. Murdough, Sister Angela, and Miller, L. Ellen: "Helping the Breast-Feeding Mother," *Am. J. Nurs.,* **72**:1420, (Aug.) 1972.

153. Lubchenco, Lula O.: *op. cit.*

153a. O'Grady, Robert S.: "Feeding Behavior in Infants," *Am. J. Nurs.,* **71**:736, (Apr.) 1971.

153b. Hasselmeyer, Eileen G., and Hon, Edward H.: "Effects of Gavage Feeding of Premature Infants Upon Cardiospiratory Patterns," *Milit. Med.,* **136**:252, (Mar.) 1971.

154. Henthorn, Frances Y.: "Better Breakfasts," *Am. J. Nurs.,* **63**:98, (Aug.) 1963.

155. Younathan, Margaret T.: "Nutritional Counseling of the Pediatric Patient," *Lancet,* **1**:81, (Mar.) 1966.

156. Zindwer, Renee, et al.: "Pediatric Dietary Practices: Scurvy Promotes Ideas for Improvement," *Hospitals,* **38**:62, (May) 1964.

157. Cherry, Robert K.: "School Lunch Program," *Ill. Med. J.,* **136**:301, (Sept.) 1969.

157a. US Public Health Service: *Screening Children for Nutritional Status; Suggestions for Child Health Programs.* US Government Printing Office, Washington, D.C., 1971 (Pub. No. 2158).

157b. McFarlane, Judith, and Hames, Carolyn C.: "Children with Diabetes Learning Self-Care in Camps," *Am. J. Nurs.,* **73**:1362, (Aug.) 1973.

157c. Schorr, Bernice, C., et al.: "Teenage Food Habits," *J. Am. Diet. Assoc.,* **61**:415, (Oct.) 1972.

157d. US Department of Health, Education, and Welfare: *Practice of Low-Income Families in Feeding Infants and Small Children with Particular Attention to Cultural Subgroups.* US Government Printing Office, Washington, D.C., 1972 (Pub. No. [HSM] 72–5605).

158. Vischer, A. L.: *Old Age: Its Compensations and Rewards.* Macmillan Publishing Co., Inc., New York, 1947, p. 31.

159. Watkins, Donald M.: "Nutrition for the Aging and the Aged," in Goodhart, Robert S., and Shils, Maurice E.: *Nutrition in Health and Disease,* 5th ed. Lea & Febiger, Philadelphia, 1973, p. 681.

160. Vilter, Richard W., and Thompson, Carl: "Nutrition and Control of Chronic Disease," *Public Health Rep.,* **66**:630, (May) 1951.

161. Weinsaft, P.: "The Management of Constipation in Geriatric Patients," *J. Am. Geriatr. Soc.,* **12**:295, (Mar.) 1964.

162. Stafford, Nora Harris: "Bowel Hygiene of Aged Patients," *Am. J. Nurs.,* **63**:102, (Sept.) 1963.

163. Fowlie, H. C., et al.: "Depression in Elderly Patients with Subnutrition," *Gerontol. Clin.,* **5**:215, 1963.

164. Schwartz, Doris, et al.: *The Elderly Ambulatory Patient: Nursing and Psychosocial Needs.* Macmillan Publishing Co., Inc., New York, 1964, pp. 145, 146.

165. Pearson, R. C. M.: "Feeding the Elderly in Their Own Homes: Meeting the Needs," *Proc. Nutr. Soc.,* **27**:37, 1968.

166. Anderson, Linnea, and Browe, John H: *op. cit.,* p. 1.

166a. Dwyer, Lois S., and Fralin, Florence G.: "Simplified Meal Planning for Hard-to-Teach Patients," *Am. J. Nurs.,* **74**:664, (Apr.) 1974.

166b. Caghan, Susan B.: "The Adolescent Process and the Problem of Nutrition," *Am. J. Nurs.,* **75**:1728, (Oct.) 1975.

166c. Fleshman, Ruth P.: "Eating Rituals and Realities," *Nurs. Clin. North Am.,* **8**:91, (Mar.) 1973.

167. Cannon, Walter B.: *The Wisdom of the Body.* W. W. Norton & Co., New York, 1939.

168. Haggard, Howard N., and Greenberg, Leon A.: *Diet and Physical Efficiency.* Yale University Press, New Haven, Conn., 1935.

169. Moore, Mary Lou: *op. cit.*

170. Speas, C. J.: "The Liquid Therapeutic Diet," *J. Tenn. Med. Assoc.,* **43**:321, (Sept.) 1950.

171. Davidson, Sir Stanley, and Passmore, R.: *op. cit.,* p. 451.

172. Bindt, Juliet: *A Handbook for the Blind.* Macmillan Publishing Co., Inc., New York, 1952.

173. Abel, Marjorie: "Feeding the Child with Cerebral Palsy," *Am. J. Nurs., 50*:558, (Sept.) 1950.

174. Lowman, Edward W., and Rusk, Howard A.: *Self-Help Devices, Part I.* Institute of Physical Medicine and Rehabilitation, New York University Medical Center, New York, 1962, p. 3.

175. Morrissey, Alice B.: *Rehabilitation Nursing.* G. P. Putnam's Sons, New York, 1951, p. 70.

176. Krusen, Frank H., and Kottke, Frederic J.: *Handbook of Physical Medicine and Rehabilitation,* 2nd ed. W. B. Saunders Co., Philadelphia, 1971, p. 492.

Additional Suggested Reading

Abernathy, Josephine Miller, et al.: "Metabolic Patterns in Preadolescent Children. XII. Effects of Amount and Source of Dietary Protein on Absorption of Iron," *J. Nutr., 85*:265, 1965.

Allison, James B.: "The Ideal Aminogram," *Fed. Proc., 20*:66, 1961.

American Academy of Pediatrics, Committee on Nutrition: "Should Milk Drinking Be Discouraged," *Pediatrics, 53*:576, (Apr.) 1974.

Avioli, Louis V.: "Absorption and Metabolism of Vitamin D_3 in Man," *Am. J. Clin. Nutr., 22*: 437, (Apr.) 1969.

Berg, Alan: "Priority of Nutrition in National Development," *Nutr. Rev., 28*:199, (Aug.) 1970.

Brink, M. F., et al.: "Nutritional Value of Milk Compared with Filled and Imitation Milk," *Am. J. Clin. Nutr., 22*:168, (Feb.) 1969.

Campbell, Teresa, and Chang, Betty: "Health Care of the Chinese in America," *Nurs. Outlook, 21*:245 (Apr.), 1973.

Cohn, Clarence, et al.: "Feed Frequency: A Factor in Dietary Protein Utilization," *Proc. Soc. Exp. Biol. Med., 115*:1057, (Apr.) 1964.

Correa, Hector, and Cummins, Gaylord: "Contribution of Nutrition to Economic Growth," *Am. J. Clin. Nutr., 23*:560, (May) 1970.

"Council Report on Dietary Fat Regulation," *Nutr. Rev., 21*:36, (Feb.) 1963.

Culley, William J.: "Caloric Requirements of Mentally Retarded Children with and without Motor Dysfunction," *J. Pediatr., 75*:380, (Sept.) 1969.

Darby, William J.: "Research Developments in International Nutrition," *Am. J. Public Health, 53*:1789, (Nov.) 1963.

Davenport, Horace W.: "Why the Stomach Does Not Digest Itself," *Sci. Am., 226*:87, (Jan.) 1972.

Davis, Thomas R. A.: "The Influence of Climate on Nutritional Requirements," *Am. J. Public Health, 54*:2051, (Dec.) 1964.

Dickens, Margaret L.: *Fluid and Electrolyte Balance.* F. A. Davis Co., Philadelphia, 1974.

Dowdy, Richard P.: "Copper Metabolism," *Am. J. Clin. Nutr., 22*:887, (July) 1969.

Eichenwald, Heinz, and Fry, Peggy Crooke: "Nutrition and Learning," *Science, 163*:644, (Feb.) 1968.

Elwood, P. C.: "Some Epidemiological Problems of Iron Deficiency Anemia," *Proc. Nutr. Soc., 27*:14, 1968.

Exton-Smith, A. N., et al.: *Nutrition of Housebound Old People.* King Edward's Hospital Fund for London, London, 1972.

"Feeding Premature Infants," *Nutr. Rev., 22*:108, (Apr.) 1964.

"Galactose Ingestion and Urinary Excretion of Calcium and Magnesium," *Nutr. Rev., 18*:147 (May), 1960.

Ganguly, Jagannath: "Absorption of Vitamin A," *Am. J. Clin. Nutr., 22*:923, (July) 1969.

"The Green Revolution," *Nutr. Rev., 27*:133, (May) 1969.

Guthrie, Diana W., and Guthrie, Richard A.: "Diabetes in Adolescence," *Am. J. Nurs., 75*: 1740, (Oct.) 1975.

Hollifield, Guy, and Parson, William: "Metabolic Adaptations to a 'Stuff and Starve' Feeding Program. I. Studies of Adipose Tissue and Liver Glycogen in Rats Limited to a Short Daily Feeding Period," *J. Clin. Invest., 41*:245, (Feb.) 1962.

Johansen, Erling: "Nutrition, Diet, and Calcium Metabolism in Dental Health," *Am. J. Public Health, 50*:1089, (Aug.) 1960.

Johnson, Ogden: "A Conference on Nutritional Teaching in Medical Schools," *Nutr. Rev., 21*: 33, (Feb.) 1963.

Kermode, G. O.: "Food Additives," *Sci. Am., 226*:15, (Mar.) 1972.

Keys, Ancel, et al.: *The Biology of Human Starvation.* University of Minnesota Press, Minneapolis, 1950.

Kretchmer, Norman: "Lactose and Lactase," *Sci. Am., 227*:71, (Oct.) 1972.

Lake, Dolores Mae. "Nursing Implications From an Investigation of Mothering, Diet, and Development in Two Groups of Children with Phenylketonuria," in *ANA Clinical Sessions, 1968.* Appleton-Century-Crofts, New York, 1968.

Lang, Virginia M., et al.: "Manganese Metabolism in College Men Consuming Vegetarian Diets," *J. Nutr., 85*:132, 1965.

Latham, Michael C.: "Starvation of Politics, or Politics of Starvation," *Lancet, 2*:999, (Nov. 8) 1969.

"Malnutrition and Physical and Mental Development," *Nutr. Rev., 28*:176, (July) 1970.

Matrin, P. E.: "Human Nutrition; the Information Requirements of a Government Department," *Proc. Nutr. Soc., 27*:116, 1968.

Mills, C. F., et al.: "Metabolic Role of Zinc," *Am. J. Clin. Nutr., 22*:1240, (Sept.) 1969.

Monckeberg, Fernando B.: "Malnutrition and Human Behavior," *Nutr. Rev., 27*:191, (July) 1969.

"Nutritional Status—U.S.A.," *Nutr. Rev., 27*:196, (July) 1969.

Olson, James Allen: "Metabolism and Function of Vitamin A," *Fed. Proc.,* **28**:1670 (Sept.–Oct.) 1969.

Picciano, Mary Frances, and Guthrie, Helen A.: "Copper, Iron, and Zinc Contents of Mature Human Milk," *Am. J. Clin. Nutr.,* **29**:242, (Mar.) 1976.

"Potassium Supplementations During Fasting for Obesity," *Nutr. Rev.,* **28**:177, (July) 1970.

Prasad, Amanda D.: "Role of Zinc in Nutrition," *Med. Times,* **97**:132, (Mar.) 1969.

Pyke, Magnus: "Food Technology and Society," *Nutr. Rev.,* **28**:31, (Feb.) 1970.

Rasch, Philip J., and Pierson, William R.: "Effect of a Protein Dietary Supplement on Muscular Strength and Hypertrophy," *Am. J. Clin. Nutr.,* **11**:530, (Nov.) 1962.

"Riboflavin Coenzymes and Congenital Malformations," *Nutr. Rev.,* **21**:24, (Jan.) 1963.

Robertson, Barbara R.: "Homemaking Classes for Low Income Families," *Can. J. Public Health,* **59**:479, (Dec.) 1968.

Robischon, Paulette: "Pica Practice in Childhood," in Anderson, Edith H., et al. (eds.): *Current Concepts in Clinical Nursing,* Vol. 4. C. V. Mosby Co., St. Louis, 1973.

Robson, J. R. K., et al.: "Zen Macrobiotic Dietary Problems in Infancy," *Pediatrics,* **53**:326, (Mar.) 1974.

Roels, Oswald A.: "The Fifth Decade of Vitamin A Research," *Am. J. Clin. Nutr.,* **22**:903, (July) 1969.

Sanpitak, N., and Chayutimonkul, L.: "Oral Contraceptives and Riboflavine Nutrition," *Lancet,* **1**:836, (May 4) 1974.

Seelig, Mildred S.: "The Requirement of Magnesium by the Normal Adult," *Am. J. Clin. Nutr.,* **14**:342, (June) 1964.

Shephard, R. J., et al.: "Factors Affecting Body Density and Thickness of Subcutaneous Fat," *Am. J. Clin. Nutr.,* **22**:1175, (Sept.) 1969.

Smith, Victor E.: "Agricultural Planning and Nutrient Availability," *Nutr. Rev.,* **28**:143, (June) 1970.

Snell, Barbara, and Mclellan, Connie: "Whetting Hospitalized Preschoolers' Appetites," *Am. J. Nurs.,* **76**:413, (Mar.) 1976.

Sukhatme, P. V.: "Size and Nature of the Protein Gap," *Nutr. Rev.,* **28**:223, (Sept.) 1970.

Taylor, Andrew: "Botulism and Its Control," *Am. J. Nurs.,* **73**:1380, (Aug.) 1973.

Umbarger, Barbara Jean: "Phenylketonuria, Dietary Treatment," *Am. J. Nurs.,* **64**:96, (Jan.) 1964.

"Utilization of Fructose by Working Muscle," *Nutr. Rev.,* **18**:296, (Oct.) 1960.

Virtanen, Artturi S.: "Some Central Nutritional Problems of the Present Time," *Fed. Proc.,* **27**:1374, (Nov.–Dec.) 1968.

Vitamin Manual. The Upjohn Company, Kalamazoo, Mich., 1961.

Walike, Barbara C., et al.: "Studies of Eating Behavior," in Downs, Florence S., and Newman, Margaret A.: *A Source Book of Nursing Research.* F. A. Davis Co., Philadelphia, 1973.

Watson, G.: *Nutrition and Your Mind.* Harper & Row, New York, 1972.

Weston, Agnes B.: "A New Approach to Meet Nutritional Needs of Older People," *Can. J. Public Health,* **60**:180, (Apr.) 1969.

Youmans, John B.: "The Changing Face of Nutritional Disease in America," *J.A.M.A.,* **189**:672 (Aug. 31) 1964.

Gladys Nite
Virginia Henderson

The authors acknowledge the assistance of Elvira Kuhn, R.N., M.S., St. Joseph Hospital, Houston, Texas, in the preparation of the section on fluid balance.

CHAPTER 11

Elimination

1. IMPORTANCE OF ELIMINATION

Elimination in Health and in Disease. As seen in the previous chapter, the quality of life depends on diet, digestion, and assimilation; but equally important is elimination of metabolic waste products.

The excretory organs are the kidneys, bowels, skin, and lungs. So important is elimination that urinalysis is included in all physical examinations, the patient is always questioned on bowel habits, the feces are often examined, and the vital capacity of the lungs is measured.*

If, during illness, the kidneys and bowels can be kept active so that waste is eliminated as fast as it is formed, the patient will have a good chance of recovery. There is always great danger, however, that excessive wastes of metabolism or bacterial or chemical toxins may be so irritating to the organs of elimination (especially the kidneys) that they cease to function. Constipation can cause discomfort and even injury, but when the kidneys "shut down," death occurs within a matter of hours or a few days. Elimination of water and dissolved substances in the form of sweat is physiological, but when this function is partly destroyed, as with burned patients, the kidneys can often compensate. Although the lungs do excrete some water, their major function is to eliminate carbon dioxide from the cells (internal respiration) and finally (during external respiration) from the lungs. We all know that death follows respiratory failure within a few minutes, although resuscitation is possible if instituted soon enough.

Elimination presents for every society a serious ecologic and epidemiologic problem. These questions are dealt with in Chapter 15 to some extent. The fact that excreta have characteristic odors, sometimes very foul ones,

makes elimination an esthetic problem, and this undoubtedly contributes toward the overall sociopsychic problems of elimination and the importance of providing for it adequately. The esthetics of the environment, including the control of odors, is discussed in Chapter 15, but some specific suggestions in relation to elimination are included here.

While elimination within a normal range is largely dependent on a healthy organic structure and the food we eat and the air we breathe, the effect on function of psychosocial conditions can hardly be overemphasized. In fact, the psychic and physical aspects of elimination are so interrelated that it is difficult to separate them.

References have been made repeatedly in this book to the stages of human development as described by Erik H. Erikson (see page 568). Many psychiatrists and clinical psychologists refer to the first years of infancy and early childhood as the oral, the anal, and the genital-locomotor ages or stages. If children are allowed to develop normal and healthy habits of elimination unassociated with embarrassment or guilt, they are likely to outgrow the anal phase with its overemphasis on bowel activity especially. If, however, children are made to feel that there is something to be ashamed of in urinating or defecating, they may never outgrow their preoccupation with these functions. Again, if, during the genital-muscular age (the third age of man, according to Erikson), children are made to feel ashamed of their genitals or the sensations associated with them, it is believed that they may never have a healthy attitude toward genital sexuality.

Since the principal organs of reproduction are in the same body area as the openings of the bladder and the rectum, the functions of elimination and reproduction tend to be confused, and the embarrassments, inhibitions, and taboos that a culture develops tend to embrace the excretory and the sexual functions

* This test is discussed on page 456.

even in the minds of many adults. The inappropriate names given to these organs and their functions and their common and often grotesque application in "vulgar parlance" to almost any subject suggest the extent to which human development has been arrested—the extent to which many persons are overly concerned with elimination and genital sexuality. This connection between elimination and sexuality suggests the complexity of helping people of all ages, sick and well, to eliminate normally and to adapt at all ages to the facilities provided for elimination in the various settings where people live and work.

Health personnel in schools, prisons, industrial settings, and particularly mental hospitals know the extent to which the use made of toilets demonstrates the asocial (unhealthy) development of persons of all ages and the close relationship that exists in the minds of many persons between elimination and sexuality.

These are special problems that cannot be dealt with adequately in a work of this kind but they are mentioned to suggest the range of competences nurses must develop if they are to practice effectively in all situations and serve those thought of as healthy and those considered sick. Common disorders of elimination are discussed in Chapter 37.

Responsibility of the Nurse. As a member of a health service in an agency, institution, camp, or home, a nurse should work with other types of health personnel in providing optimum facilities and conditions for elimination. In general, these include accessibility of toilets, privacy, cleanliness, freedom from odors, and immediate disposal of excreta in such a way that they do not menace human, animal, or plant life. During sickness or in preventive medicine, the facilities and conditions may include those for collection, preservation, measurement, examination, and reporting relevant data on excreta and the process of elimination. In many places, provision must be made for accessibility to toilets of patients in wheelchairs, and for the very sick or elderly there must be call systems to summon help. For the critically ill provision must be made for the conservation of the patient's energy and even the constant attendance of nursing personnel.

In their capacity as *health counselors,* nurses have many opportunities to teach good habits of elimination, and to prevent disease by encouraging periodic health examinations.

In their *care of infants,* and all those too sick to assume the responsibility for themselves, the nurses note the number, quantity, and character of eliminations from the bowels and kidneys or help members of a family caring for the sick to do this. In answer to a critic of present-day nursing, who thought giving and emptying bedpans a waste of a "professional" nurse's time, Sally Johnson, teacher and leader of nurses, said that the macroscopic examination of excretions by the nurse is just as "professional" a function as the microscopic or chemical examination by the physician or pathologist. In a contemporary medical textbook, Maurice M. Rathman and Albert B. Katz say this about the importance of observation of feces by the physician:

In the diagnosis of gastrointestinal complaints too little attention is paid to the examination of stools. No gastrointestinal survey is complete until the feces have been analyzed. The gross and microscopic examination are routinely practiced by most gastroenterologic internists whereas the bacteriologic examinations and chemical analyses are reserved for special cases. However, the information obtained from a report is only as reliable as the technician who performs the test. . . .

In the hospital and in the office the gross specimen is seldom observed by the clinician, who usually only reads a report. A finger cot specimen of stool can be obtained for the study of gross appearance and occult blood, which can be performed at the patient's bedside.*

Nurses should cultivate the habit of noting the appearance and odor of body discharges as indices of the patient's condition. Before emptying a bedpan or urinal, the nurse, or any other attendant, should see whether the urine is to be measured and charted, whether it is to be sent for examination, whether all the urine voided is to be saved for examination, and whether a specimen of the stool is to be saved for examination. The diagnosis, treatment, and recovery of the patient may depend on these precautions. Metabolic studies are based principally on dietary measurements and analysis of excretions.

It is largely the responsibility of the nurse to provide patients with the proper facilities and the privacy people want during urination and defecation. At the same time, when a person is critically ill, defecating may increase the work load of the heart, and it is important for the nurse to stay with the patient.

For those unable to judge the adequacy of elimination and to get needed help, it is the responsibility of nurses to make estimates of the patient's needs based on a thorough assessment and to get medical advice if necessary.

* Rathman, Maurice M., and Katz, Albert B.: "Analysis of Feces," in Bockus, Henry L.: *Gastroenterology,* Vol. II, 2nd ed. W. B. Saunders Co., Philadelphia, 1964, p. 694.

They observe and report pain or discomfort associated with urination or defecation. Both should be painless—actually pleasurable as a relief from the tension that acts as a stimulus.

Nurses work with the physician in rehabilitating those, such as paralytics, whose loss of bladder and bowel control represents their major social handicap. A discussion of this may be found in Chapter 37, page 1541.

2. ELIMINATION OF WASTE FROM THE INTESTINES

Physiology of the Intestines As It Affects Elimination. "The length and complexity" of the alimentary tract of vertebrates are affected by the nature of their diets, according to Walter C. Alvarez.[1] When it consists chiefly of meats, the tract is relatively short, especially the distal portion, the colon; and digestion is nearly completed within the small intestine. When the diet is composed of plant foods, the tract is longer, particularly the distal portion, and digestion is continued in the large intestine by the fermentive action of resident bacteria. Alvarez thinks that the usual estimates of the length of the tract are misleading because they are made on cadavers. Having lost their tone, the organs from the dead body may stretch to many times their length in the living body. Alvarez cites the work of R. J. Noer and C. G. Johnson, who concluded that the tract from mouth to anus might be about 2.4 to 3 meters (8 to 10 ft). They had healthy adult subjects swallow strings in order to make their estimates. It is possible, however that the intestine may have been pleated on these strings. Meyer O. Cantor[2] reports that the swallowed end of intubation tubes approximately 130 cm (52 inches) in length have repeatedly worked their way through the anus within 48 hours. This means, of course, that the small intestine was gathered on them as the casing of a curtain is on a rod. William S. Haubrick[3] also states that the length of the tract in animals depends, to some degree, on their dietary habits—in the herbivora it may be 25 times the length of the body while in carnivora it rarely exceeds 8 times its length. Although he says it is recognized that man is an omnivore, he thinks "his colon resembles more that of the herbivora." For an individual with an extremely long colon, who limits his or her diet to meats and starches, constipation may be expected but can be overcome by a high-residue diet, according to Haubrick. When discussing the intubation studies in living humans conducted by Blankenharn, Hirsch, and Adhrens, he points out that the length of

the intestine varies according to body size and individually among normal persons of the same size.

Joel E. Goldthwait and his associates point out structural and physiologic differences in the slender, intermediate, and stocky types of men and women. They say:

Not only are the mechanics of the body and the potentialities of strain different in the various types of body structure, but the physiologic processes differ also.

Probably the greatest variation lies in the functioning of the gastro-intestinal tract. In the slender type it is short, as in carnivorous animals; here, a more concentrated kind of diet is indicated, since the ingested food passes quickly through the tract, and therefore assimilation must be rapid. In the stocky type there is a long intestinal tract, as in the herbivora; here, a less concentrated type of diet is indicated, since the passage of food is slower, and assimilation can be carried on for a longer time. The result of this differentiation in the length of the tract is shown by the protest of the digestive system of slender children to a high-caloric, high-fat diet in large amount when this is given in an attempt to obtain the weight specified in height-weight tables.*

In man the small intestine is the essential organ of digestion and absorption; the colon's function is chiefly that of absorbing water and eliminating waste from the alimentary canal. Man can live for years deprived of the stomach or colon, but he could not exist for long without the small intestine.

Secretions of the gastrointestinal tract, from the mouth to the distal end of the ileum, and to some degree in the colon, are vital in the ultimate digestion of food and absorption of its end product. In addition to these digestive enzymes, mucus is also secreted throughout the tract, lubricating and protecting it.[4,5]

Digestion, started in the mouth and carried a little further in the stomach, is virtually completed by the time the contents of the tract reach the cecum. This is particularly true if the diet is a mixed one or composed of largely animal foods. The breakdown of cellulose is thought to depend on the action of bacteria in the large intestine; therefore, when diets high in cellulose enter the colon, they are not so completely digested.

Absorption of end products of digestion takes place almost entirely in the small intestine because food is not digested sufficiently in the stomach nor is the stomach's mucous membrane adapted to absorption, as is that of the small intestine. The stomach absorbs in-

* Goldthwait, Joel E., et al.: *Essentials of Body Mechanics in Health and Disease,* 5th ed. J. B. Lippincott Co., Philadelphia, 1952, p. 26.

significant amounts of water, glucose, and alcohol. Many authorities say the colon absorbs most of the water and significant amounts of salts. Iron is an exception for it is said to be absorbed from the stomach.

Discussing water absorption in the various areas of the gastrointestinal tract, N. C. Hightower and Henry D. Janowitz [6] say that most studies to date are of little value because it is so hard to distinguish between water secreted into the intestine and water leaving the intestine by absorption. However, they cite the studies of Scholer and Code showing the following: (1) water is absorbed rapidly from the intestine and (2) there is an appreciable amount of water absorbed from the stomach, which is contradictory to the usual statements found in the literature—that little water is absorbed from the stomach. In 1954, J. F. Scholer and C. F. Code [7] attempted to determine the rate of absorption of water from the stomach and small intestine in humans by administering deuterium oxide and sampling arterial blood. They found that the rate of absorption was much more rapid from the small intestine (26.1 per cent per minute) than from the stomach (2.5 per cent per minute) and the small intestine absorbed 95 per cent of the administered water in 10 minutes, whereas it took the stomach 54.2 minutes to accomplish the same task.

The liquid content of the small intestine is held in the colon until, under normal circumstances in the human being, it is dejected in a soft formed mass, although in some vertebrates, the rabbit, for example, the feces are so dry it will float on water.

Movements of the alimentary tract churn and break up the contents and keep them moving from the mouth to the anus. A number of authorities say that several or all of the following conditions affect the rate at which a meal passes through the tract: (1) the character of the food; (2) the individual's intestinal motility and rate of absorption, affecting the consistency of the contents; (3) the "fullness" of the bowel; (4) concurrent muscular exercise; and (5) emotional states.[8,9] It is well known that emotion can cause nausea and vomiting, diarrhea, and other profound changes in the usual alimentary activity.[9a] This question is discussed at some length in Chapter 36.

In health, an ordinary mixed meal leaves the stomach in 3 to 4½ hours. Its progress through the small intestine is rapid in the duodenum and jejunum but slows considerably in the ileum. It passes in spurts into the large intestine anywhere from 4 to 8 hours after it leaves the stomach and may stay in the colon from a few hours to days according to individual differences in the irritability of the colon and habits of elimination and other conditions. Because most estimates cited are made from barium test meals, colored beads, and tubes (with or without balloons), which are foreign objects, they do not show the normal progress of food through the alimentary canal. In a study of 51 patients, Alan A. Bloom and associates [10] found that ingesta was passed in the stool within 48 hours in 72 per cent of the subjects; the shortest time was 6 hours and longest was 5 days.

Apparently, the small intestine empties only part of its contents into the cecum daily, and a certain proportion may be held back as much as a week. The gross appearance of stools after certain foods, like cranberries, are eaten is evidence of this, but controlled experiments have demonstrated it even more convincingly. Tiny colored beads were mixed with a normal diet and fed to healthy young men. Using different colored beads on different days, the experimenters found that the average subject eliminates only 75 percent of a given color bead in 4 days.[11]

Food is propelled from the mouth through the anus by (1) the voluntary muscles used in swallowing and defecating, (2) by the involuntary muscles of the alimentary canal, and (3) by waving movements of the villi (microscopic fingerlike projections on the surface of the intestine). The movements of the walls of the tract vary according to the structure of its component organs and according to the function of each. The movements are not described by all authorities in the same terms, but the following are commonly used: (1) *peristalsis,* a band of contraction beside a band of relaxation in a muscular organ which pushes the contents forward toward the anus; (2) *antiperistalsis,* a band of relaxation followed by a band of contraction forcing the contents backward toward the mouth; (3) *segmenting movements,* described by Walter B. Cannon as simultaneous restrictions spaced regularly along a bowel; (4) *pendular movements,* described by Arthur C. Guyton as small constrictive waves that sweep forward and then backward over a few centimeters of the small intestine; and (5) *mass peristalsis,* pushing the contents of the bowel for considerable distances. This last peristaltic rush is the movement that sweeps segments of fecal matter into the rectum, compared by Alvarez to pushing cars off a siding.

Authorities agree that our knowledge of colonic physiology, in health and disease, is incomplete, and conclusions on the mechanism of propulsion in the small intestine cannot be made.[12,13]

Whatever the nature of the movements, food

is normally propelled from the mouth to the anus but held in each part until that organ has performed its functions. The sphincters of the stomach, the ileocecal valve, and to some extent the transverse constrictions throughout the colon slow the progress of the contents through the digestive tract. There is evidence that in health the colon, particularly, reverses the movement of its contents. If feces deposited in the rectum are not expelled, they are in some cases carried back to the transverse colon. This is called *retrotransport*. Movements of the colon are reported to be powerful enough to break a steel clamp. Vomiting, a reverse peristalsis, or spasm, can be so forceful that the contents of the stomach are shot across a room.

It is difficult to find a definite answer to the question, "Is the rectum normally empty?" There is considerable evidence to support the theory that the presence of feces in the rectum usually gives rise to the *defecation impulse* and that this act empties it. There is also some reason to believe that if the person does not obey the impulse, the stool in the rectum ceases to act as an irritant, and so the stool may stay in the rectum. There it gets smaller, drier and harder, and therefore more difficult to expel. In some cases, as has been noted, it may be "retrotransported" into the upper parts of the colon.[14,15]

The bulk of evidence supports the view that mass movements that push segments of the contents of the colon into the rectum occur, usually after eating, once, twice, or oftener during a 24-hour period. When this happens the person has an urge to defecate. This more or less automatic rhythmic activity of the colon is apparent in paralyzed animals and human beings, who establish regular habits of defecating once or twice a day. When the voluntary control of the anus is lost, it apparently relaxes to empty the rectum whenever feces is deposited there.

The psyche can stimulate mass peristalsis just as eating and drinking do. Alvarez tells about a patient with an incompetent anal sphincter who had a bowel movement after each meal. Between times he did not dare think of eating or even pass a restaurant because the thought or sight of food caused an involuntary bowel movement. Pleasurable excitement, such as that accompanying the purchase of a desired object, acts as a cathartic on a woman known to the second writer. Persons with a colostomy (an artificial anus, but lacking a sphincter, made by surgery into the abdominal wall) who have a regular daily evacuation under ordinary circumstances may have their routine completely upset by any unusual or exciting event. The nerve supply is too complex and controversial to be included in this brief discussion, but the severance of sensory pathways is said to affect the rectum more than injury to the motor nerves.

It is common knowledge that diet affects the rate at which food progresses through the alimentary canal. Foods that are completely absorbed, or nearly so, leave no residue, and therefore do not distend and stimulate the walls of the intestine to contract and force its contents onward. Low-residue diets are used to control diarrhea; and high-residue diets, to combat constipation. Alvarez says there is reason to believe that diets with a high-cellulose content are laxative not because they make bulk in the colon but because in their breakdown through bacterial action an irritating substance is released. Bacterial action also produces gas and a bolus of gas may act like a balloon, dilating and stimulating the colon to expel it.

Regular and Adequate Bowel Elimination. The defecation act involves both involuntary and voluntary processes. As the fecal mass is transported from the sigmoid into the rectum (by mass peristaltic movements as the gastrocolic reflex), the rectal walls are distended, causing tension which results in the urge to defecate. The internal and external anal sphincters are relaxed, the abdominal muscles contracted. Voluntary intraabdominal pressure is accomplished by contracting the diaphragm and the muscles of the abdominal wall and by spinal flexion which presses the abdomen on the thighs.[16-18]

Healthy persons tend to have a soft, formed stool at approximately the same time daily. Equally healthy individuals empty the rectum twice a day, or every other day. When evacuations are regular and the stool is soft and formed, we say that bowel elimination is *normal*. When the stools are frequent and liquid the person has *diarrhea,* and this means that the contents of the colon are ejected before the usual percentage of water has been absorbed from it. Premature defecations are the result of "an irritable colon." When the stools are irregular and excessively dry, or hard, the patient is *constipated*. Formed stools with very small diameters may indicate a rectal growth which narrows its lumen.

For those who have no serious psychologic or structural handicap, normal bowel movements can usually be effected by: (1) reasonable freedom from stress; (2) making an effort to empty the rectum at the same time or times every day, and *responding to the defecation urge when it occurs;* (3) sufficient exercise to maintain normal tone of the muscles used in defecation; (4) a squatting posture or the one that makes pressure on the bowel contents possible; (5) a diet containing foods that leave sufficient residue in the bowel; and (6) a sufficient fluid intake.

Regularity in defecation is clearly important as shown by the fact that the person who has lost voluntary control eliminates rhythmically. Moreover, if the feces are not ejected as they are deposited in the rectum by movements of the colon, they shrink, dry, and harden, making the act of defecation painful and even injurious to the mucous membrane of the anus. Children, fearing this discomfort, often postpone defecation. A simple explanation may help them to realize that this will only increase their difficulty. Everyone must learn that ignoring the stimulus finally weakens it, so that the rectum becomes habituated to the presence of feces.

Since the powerful intestinal contractions that push small masses into the rectum usually occur after meals, it is logical to select the hour after breakfast for having the daily bowel movement. This may not be desirable for the person hurrying to get to school or work, since stress interferes with relaxation of the anal sphincter and with normal vegetative functions in general. The contractions elicited by breakfast may be induced by drinking several glasses of water. Many people accomplish a daily evacuation before breakfast in this way.

That the emotions affect visceral activity has long been recognized by the observant health worker as well as the layman. The gastrointestinal tract is especially responsive to the emotions. Rathman and Katz say:

I believe that there are few people who may not occasionally experience symptoms of the irritable colon if the stimulus, usually emotional tension of some type, is sufficiently great. However, symptoms responsible for visits to the physician are more common in susceptible persons.*

Following a discussion of some of the major studies made on the subject of emotions, they consider that motor hyperactivity is caused by feelings of anger, resentment, hostility, anxiety, and apprehension—behaviors of the fighting attitude; whereas hypomotility is attributed to feelings of fear, fright, despondency, and dejection—behaviors of the running-away attitude.

Most psychiatrists, pediatrists, psychologists, and anthropologists believe that bowel function and mental health have a very close relationship. George P. Mardock and John W. M. Whiting, studying forms of marriage and parental behavior, arranged their data around a very few activities. During the child's infancy they studied the behavior of parents in relation to (1) nursing and (2) dependency; subsequently, they studied the parents' behavior toward (1) weaning, (2) toilet training, (3) independence training, (4) aggressive training, and (5) sex training.[19] These studies were made in the hope that they would lead to a clearer understanding of the effect of early training on adult behavior. It is significant that the parents' treatment of the infant and child in relation to his bowel and bladder evacuations was included. About 30 social scientists from numerous professions, discussing these studies at a conference, accepted the thesis that adult personality is profoundly affected by childhood experiences connected with elimination. Too early or too rigid bowel training with punishment for lack of control or excessive approval for control changes a normal, natural function into something that involves an emotional upheaval. This association between elimination and the individual's relationships with those he loves or hates becomes a part of him and is expressed in ways that are now only partially understood. Dorothy Baruch tries to show some of this in the story of One Little Boy.[20] Thomas P. Almy, reporting experiments on "the irritable colon," in which he contrasted the behavior of 50 healthy persons with 100 persons having some form of colitis, concluded that:

When under stress induced by experimental stimuli, both healthy persons and patients with irritable colon may show disturbances. . . . Two patterns of altered, sigmoid motility have been recognized: the one an increase in tone and/or wave-like contractions associated with overt moods of hostility and aggression; the other a decrease in tone and/or contractions associated with overt behavior symbolizing hopelessness and defeat.

. . . We therefore conclude that in most instances irritable colon is a bodily change accompanying emotional conflict in response to environmental stress.*

William J. Grace and his associates offer visible proof of this theory in their monograph. They were able to observe the response to stress in the colonic mucous membrane of four patients, parts of whose large intestines had herniated through abdominal fistulas (openings from the abdominal cavity). Their thesis that the "threatened" individual responds with the ejection-riddance reaction (vomiting and diarrhea) or the "holding fast" reaction (constipation) is so convincingly presented that

---

* Rathman, Maurice M., and Katz, Albert B.: *op. cit.*, p. 731.

* Almy, Thomas P.: "Experimental Studies on the Irritable Colon," *Am. J. Med.,* **10:**60, (Jan.) 1951.

Allen Gregg, in the Foreword, suggests that this almost irrefutable demonstration of the relationship between the psyche and the soma may influence the whole field of preventive medicine and therapy. He and the authors believe that stress may affect other organs as it is shown here to affect the colon. All health workers would find a study of this report profitable. The following summary of material in Grace's book gives the reader an idea of its value.

The ejection-riddance reaction, Grace and associates believe, is a protective pattern of defense that involves the stomach, duodenum, and large bowel. The reaction varies in intensity and pattern with the age and temperament of the individual. A feverish, fretful child who is teething may try to protect himself by the bodily reaction of vomiting and diarrhea, even though the gastrointestinal tract is not primarily involved. As the child approaches adolescence, he usually abandons this nonspecific reaction to "assault," unless there are noxious agents actually present in the gastrointestinal tract. Some adults in stressful situations in which they feel inadequate and thwarted may experience a similar body reaction. "Thus, a person who has 'taken on more than he can handle' or feels inadequate to the demands of his life situation, or a thwarted and passive person filled with hatred, defiance, contempt, and the unconscious aim to eject a threatening or overwhelming situation may have diarrhea. However, the riddance pattern being integrated through unconscious processes, the subject exhibiting violent diarrhea may be calm, sweet mannered, and seem serene."

The "holding fast" reaction, also a protective pattern of defense, involves the skeletal muscles and the large bowel. Various body postures of alertness or abjection associated with states of tension or despair are examples of sustained skeletal-muscle patterns that give rise to complaints. Such skeletal-muscle and pressor cardiovascular responses are often associated with constipation. During bodily preparation for violent exercise or competitive sports, the urge to defecate does not occur. In addition to prolonged periods of active exercise, situations evoking sadness, dejection, or cheerless striving may inhibit the gastrocolic reflex, induce nonpropulsive phasic contractions in the sigmoid, and interfere with the mass reflex. It is as though the person facing an immediate "assault" reacts by "holding on." *

Constipation continues to be found in all age groups, male and female, and in all types and stages of illness as well as in the person enjoying good health. Causes of simple constipation, in many instances, can be attributed to poor individual health practices. A detailed discussion of this problem is included in Chapter 37.

Persons, sick or well, should be encouraged to feel that they are primarily responsible for maintaining regular elimination. Even during hospitalization they are able to go to the bathroom, to exercise, and to use discretion in food selection.

The most modern hospital construction makes it possible for patients who cannot walk to wheel themselves or be wheeled to toilets. Movable commodes are now available (see Fig. 11-1). Bedside units have been constructed to make the patient confined to bed independent of his attendant and the usual bedpan; the high cost and the present emphasis on ambulation have delayed its adoption. With the assistance of the hospital engineer, bedside commodes can be adjusted to meet the needs of many bed patients.* Figure 11-2 shows an adjustable toilet seat with safety frame.

In order to retain or develop regular elimination in bed patients, bedpans must be given at regular intervals. As we have said, the impulse to defecate is, with most persons, felt immediately or shortly after breakfast. The bedpan, if patients *must* use one, should therefore be given at this time unless they have the habit of defecating at another hour, in which case it should be given to them then. The impulse to urinate is felt at more frequent intervals. For this purpose, the bedpan or urinal should be given before bedtime, on waking in the morning, and before each meal. Except when the patient has had a cathartic or has diarrhea or some disease of the urinary tract which makes frequent voiding a necessity, the irregular use of bedpans should be discouraged. Every consideration, however, should be shown the patient who cannot conform to this regimen. If regularity is observed, it not only benefits the patient but also eliminates the use of the bedpan during mealtime, visiting hours, doctors' rounds, and at other undesirable moments.

Esthetics. Because most persons prefer that the acts of defecating and urinating be performed in privacy, every effort must be made to maintain an environment free of odors from and the sight of utensils used in performing these functions. *Urinals and bedpans should be kept out of sight,* in the bedside table or some enclosed cabinet. The control of odors

---

* Grace, William J., et al.: *The Human Colon; An Experimental Study Based on Direct Observation of Four Fistulous Subjects.* Paul B. Hoeber, New York, 1951, pp. 209*ff.*

* A bedside commode was modified by the hospital engineer in one hospital and used with a group of coronary patients. (Nite, Gladys, and Willis, Frank N.: *The Coronary Patient; Hospital Care and Rehabilitation.* Macmillan Publishing Co., Inc., New York, 1964, p. 89.)

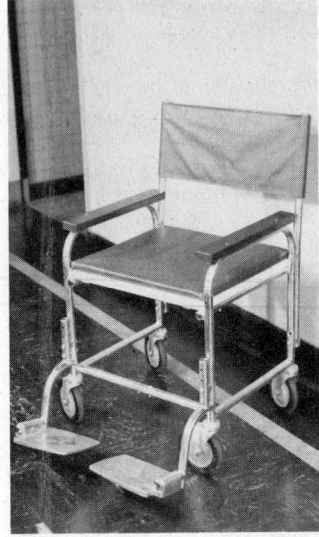
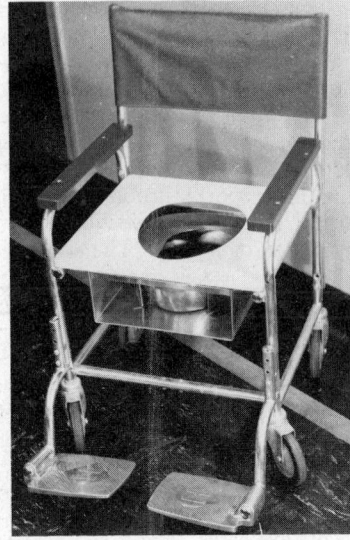
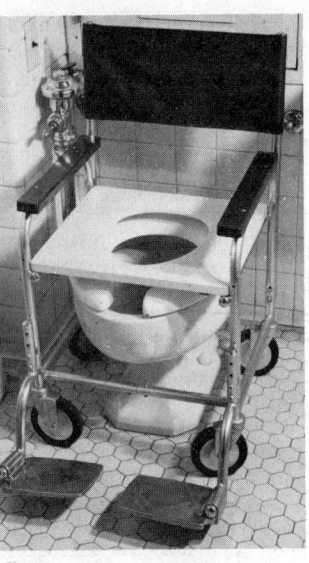

A   B   C

Figure 11-1. A commode that has many uses. *A.* In this view it is used as an ordinary wheelchair with a solid top over fenestrated seat. *B.* A stainless steel tray containing a bedpan has been suspended on runners under the seat. *C.* Tray and bedpan have been removed, and the commode is in place over the toilet. The toilet seat should always be raised to prevent soiling. (Courtesy of Columbia-Presbyterian Medical Center, New York, N.Y., and Clay-Adams Co., New York, N.Y.)

associated with excreta is important and can be accomplished by emptying the containers *immediately,* washing thoroughly under running water, and using a brush and cleaning agent. Special deodorants * are available. A small amount may be placed directly in the bedpan or urinal to control odors, but if the odors are noticeable in the room, the wick of the bottle should be pulled slightly above the rim. An environment free of unpleasant sights and odors is important to all persons, sick or well.

Method of Giving a Bedpan to a Patient. A bedpan should always be completely covered and carried to and from the patient as unobtrusively as possible, although false modesty should never be allowed to interfere with its use. The bed should be screened, the bedpan warmed and placed gently under the patient in the proper position. Bedpans are usually made of Monel metal, and while they may not look or feel as nice as an enameled pan they are more durable. Avoid use of a bedpan with chipped enamel, or if it is chipped, cover the seat with a pad, because of the danger of injuring the skin. A pad should always be used over an unyielding surface when the skin is

* Re-Odit, available from Fuller Laboratories, Eden Prairie, Minn.

tender. Cushions made of sponge rubber with a smooth outer covering are now available for this purpose and are very satisfactory. Molded nylon bedpans are now available that withstand the heat of sterilizers. They have the advantage of feeling warm to the touch. Figure 11-3 shows a disposable bedpan.

Voiding or defecating in a horizontal position is unnatural and those whose treatment (for example, a body cast) makes this necessary must learn to do so. Ordinarily the person should be put in a sitting position on the bedpan.

If patients need help in getting on the bedpan, direct them to roll on the side away from you. After covering the bed with a waterproof pad or protector, place the bedpan over the buttocks, asking the patient to roll over on the pan. Elevate the head of the bed, place a pillow covered with waterproof material under each knee for support if the patient is weak, and place a protective guard in front of the bedpan to keep urine and feces from soiling the sheets. If the bedpan is placed properly over the buttocks when the patients are on their sides, they will be in a comfortable position for defecating after they roll on their backs. The use of this technique requires little effort on the part of the patient or nurse. When the bedpan is in use, place the cover on the bar

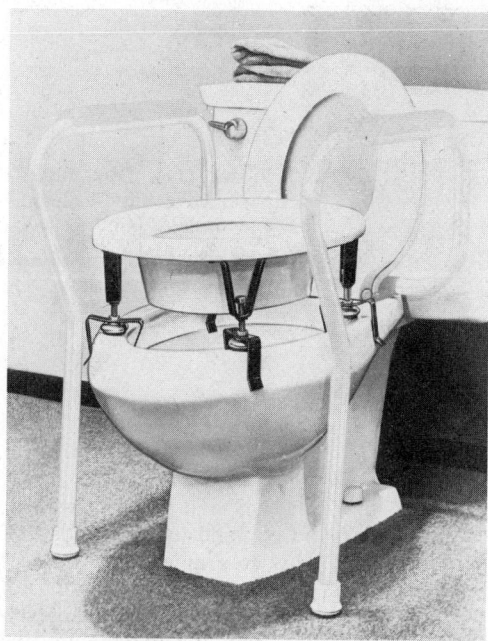

Figure 11-2. Adjustable toilet safety frame and adjustable toilet seat that fits most toilets. (Courtesy of Lumex, Inc., Bay Shore, N.Y.)

of the bed out of sight, so that the patient need not be embarrassed should someone come in the room or behind the screen. Leave the patients alone unless they are very ill or weak and likely to faint or get very tired. Give them plenty of time, but do not leave any patient longer than necessary on the bedpan. The importance of staying with certain patients, such as those who are fearful during defecation, has been emphasized.

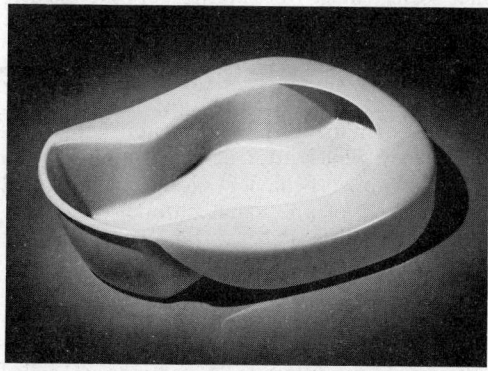

Figure 11-3. A disposable bedpan that performs the same function as metal bedpans. It may be used repeatedly by the same patient and taken home for use, when indicated. (Courtesy of Premium Plastics, Inc., Chicago, Ill.)

In removing the bedpan use the same procedure as before, asking the patients to roll on their side. Cover the bedpan immediately (see Fig. 11-4). If patients are able to clean the pubic region and buttocks, see that toilet paper, basin of water, and washcloth or sponges are within reach. If they are unable to do this satisfactorily and without fatigue, the nurse must do it for them. In hospitals there are generally a sufficient number of orderlies to give men any assistance they need in the use of the urinal and bedpan, but when there aren't, women nursing personnel must give men the help they need. Perineal bathing (sometimes referred to as "crotch care") is discussed in Chapter 25. The bedpan should be removed from the bedside as soon as possible and washed first with cold running water, then cleaned with a brush, a detergent, and hot water. When automatic bedpan washers are available, as they are in most hospitals, the pan is put directly in this apparatus. (Sterilization of bedpans is discussed in Chapter 32.) In some hospitals all equipment is processed in a central supply service. While the inclusion of bedpans and urinals in such a service might save equipment and personnel, it will make observations of excreta by the attendants concerned very difficult.

Women nurses should not attempt to put helpless adults on the bedpan, for they may injure themselves and hurt the patient. A trapeze makes it possible for many disabled persons to lift themselves. A turning sheet should be used when patients cannot help themselves or when their condition makes it important that they maintain all segments of the body in the same plane. Figure 11-5 *A* and *B* show the use of the turning sheet for this purpose. Figure 11-6 shows a patient learning to move from the chair to the toilet without assistance.

Remember that the use of a bedpan is embarrassing to the average person, is esthetically distasteful, and is physiologically undesirable. It should never be used if it is possible to substitute a mobile commode or a toilet. Leaving bedpans and urinals on tables, chairs, or the floor, or anywhere they can be seen by visitors is a practice to be condemned, but those who use them should have the assurance that bedpans and urinals are within reach or that their call for help from a nurse will be answered immediately.

Toilet Training and Changing the Infant's Diaper. In the Conference on Problems of Infancy and Childhood, where the discussion centered on the mid-century White House Conference theme, "How Can We Rear an Emotionally Healthy Generation?" there was

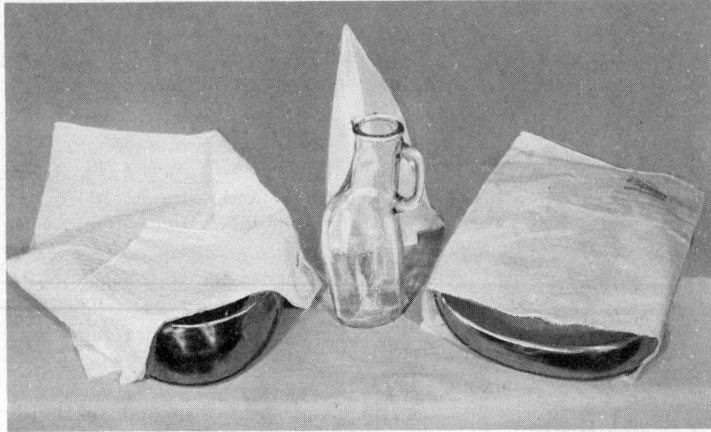

Figure 11-4. Disposable paper covers for bedpans and urinals. (Courtesy of Clay-Adams Co., New York, N.Y.)

a consensus that toilet training is one of the main areas affecting personality development (see pages 697–704). Children whose mothers expressed disgust when they soiled their clothes or who punished them for it will have associations with defecating that make it difficult to develop normal habits of elimination. Worse still, their self-confidence will be shaken and they will learn to fear the person they love best. On the other hand, children whose mothers show undue concern over their eliminations may learn that they can please or punish her with them, and so an emotional association is set up that, operating on the unconscious level, can lead to psychosomatic disease in later life when they may punish themselves or others with alimentary disorders.* Psychologists working with animals have demonstrated that for reward or punishment they can control functions thought of as autonomous, such as intestinal mobility or the rate of the heartbeat. Psychiatrists and clinical psychologists believe that this has been amply demonstrated by the behavior of humans.

In the cultures described by the anthropologists of the Child-Care Conferences, parental behavior toward the child's elimination varies from no effort to train the child in adult habits to the rigid chamber training in our culture as described in pediatrics texts 35 years ago. Most peoples wait until the baby can walk and talk. John W. M. Whiting reported only the Madagascan, Japanese, and American middle class as training in bowel habits before this time. The Knoma people did not understand what toilet training meant. One parent said "What do you mean, toilet training? I don't understand. I don't see any problem. We wait

until the child can walk and talk and we say, 'This is where you go,' and the child does it." Whiting adds "This was indeed the case." *

Even though we recognize the limitations of our knowledge and understanding, it is nevertheless agreed that emptying the rectum and the bladder are physical satisfactions in the same class as eating or giving and receiving expressions of love. Tension is the result of unsatisfied hunger, or drives, and pleasure should accompany relief of this tension. While all training or education consists of a discipline of native drives, a discipline which is beyond the capacity of the individual substitutes frustration and failure for the satisfaction or pleasure that comes with normal tension-relief activity.

It is doubtful whether a healthy, loving mother would ever have forced a rigid toilet training on her baby had she not been taught to do so by her elders. There is general acceptance of Lawrence K. Frank's insistence that society must trust and respect the dictates of maternal (and paternal) affection. As applied in this instance no rule should be set for toilet training at a chronological age. Milton J. Senn thinks that toilet training, like weaning, should be influenced by the child's total development. Since rates of maturation vary, a range of toilet behavior should be accepted for children of the same chronological age. Some pediatrists believe, however, that the child is more easily "trained" between the ages of 8 and 12 months than either earlier or later.[21,22] Ronald S. Illingworth [23] emphasizes the importance of recognizing the difference between "conditioning," commonly called

* It has been suggested by some social scientists that patients of any age may punish their attendants by incontinence.

* Senn, Milton J. (ed.): *Problems of Infancy and Childhood: Transactions of the Fourth Conference, New York, March, 1950.* Josiah Macy, Jr. Foundation, New York, 1951, p. 16.

A

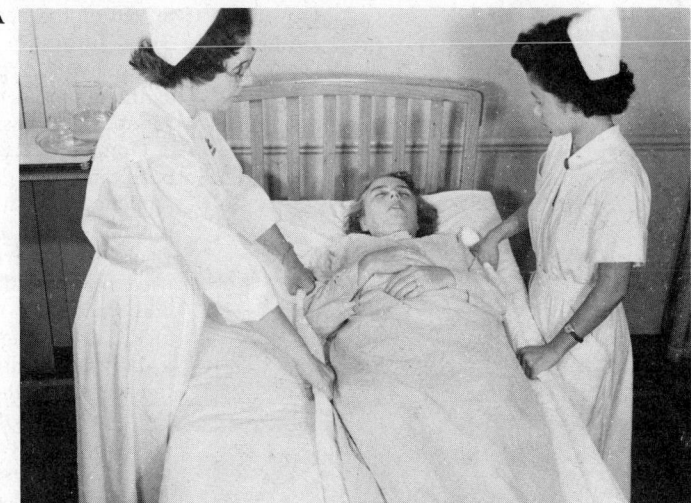

Figure 11-5. *A.* Moving a help-less patient is facilitated by the use of a turning sheet that extends from the occiput to the knees.
  B. Holding the patient on her side with the turning sheet. In this position a patient can be supported by one nurse, while the second nurse straightens the bottom sheet. Effort is reduced if additional personnel are available for this maneuver. A turning sheet is also used to help a patient on a bedpan. (Courtesy of Columbia-Presbyterian Medical Center, New York, N.Y., and Clay-Adams Co., New York, N.Y.)

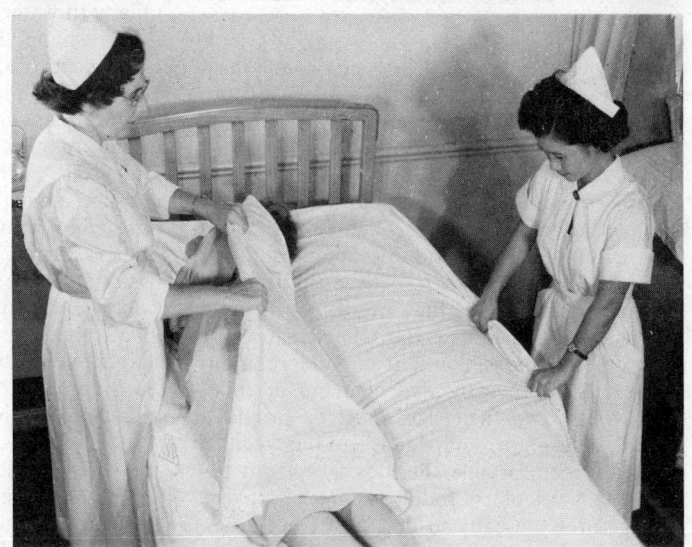

B

"training," and voluntary sphincter control, which most children do not begin to learn until 15 to 18 months of age. Waldo E. Nelson thinks that most children acquire control of anal and bladder sphincters during the second or third year of life. In discussing toilet training he says:

He [the child] is not ready to use the toilet until he is old enough to understand what it is for and to let his mother know of his needs, until his bowel movements come at fairly regular times, and until he is willing to sit on the toilet.*

Benjamin Spock and Mabel Huschka more than thirty years ago made the following rec-

ommendation to parents on training in cleanliness:

Premature and drastic toilet training are often important contributing factors in the development of emotional difficulties . . . training should not be started until the child spontaneously begins making his toilet wants known, for this means he is psychologically ready to accept training. This he will do by grunting, wriggling, putting his hands to his genitals, or by such signs as . . . a slight tension in the legs. He may begin making his wants known as early as eight months; more often he will do so after fifteen months. . . .
  In the long run the mother benefits . . . as well as the child.*

* From Spock, B., and Huschka, M.: The Psychological Aspects of Pediatric Practice, in Blumer, G. L.: *Practitioners Library of Medicine and Surgery,* Vol. 13. Appleton-Century-Crofts, New York, 1938, p. 757.

* Nelson, Waldo E., et al.: *Textbook of Pediatrics,* 9th ed. W. B. Saunders Co., Philadelphia, 1969, p. 195.

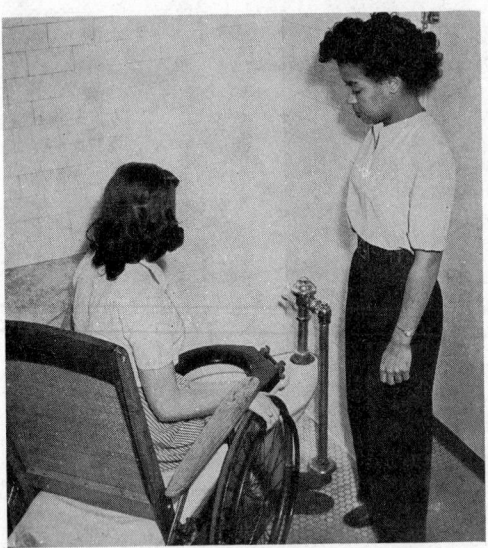

Figure 11-6. Instruction and supervision of a wheelchair patient so that she can move from the chair to the toilet without assistance. (Courtesy of National Foundation.)

Parents and nurses will find conflicting opinions to confuse them, but few persons now recommend rigid training or punishment. Most experts in child care believe that normal and happy children as they begin to walk and talk will want to imitate the toilet customs of their parents and siblings, if a good relationship exists between them. Chambers or toilet seats, adapted to their size, must be provided so that defecation, and, later, voiding will be physically comfortable. Periods free from excitement, particularly following meals, may be arranged for the baby so that his or her attention is not diverted from the stimulus provided by intestinal movements likely to follow eating. Many babies, even at 6 months, have a single daily bowel movement after their first feeding; many continue to defecate more frequently. Regularity and normal consistency are the more important criteria for judging whether or not the infant's elimination is healthy.

Discomfort from soiled diapers differs in infancy with the age and, of course, with the individual. Urine, however, is irritating to the skin, and stools, particularly liquid stools, are likely to be excoriating. To prevent chafing, rashes, or frank skin lesions, it is necessary to change a baby's diapers frequently. The practice of "waterproofing" babies so that adults are protected from their soiled diapers should be discouraged. The skin in such cases is not only macerated by the wet cloth but is also de-

prived of the healing and drying power of air. Beds, furniture, and clothing should be protected by waterproof fabrics, but pants made of them should not be put on the baby except for special occasions.

Opinions vary greatly on skin care of newborn and older infants. There is a growing tendency to reduce handling and treatment of the skin to the absolute minimum for the first week. In some hospitals, however, oil is still used for skin cleaning; in others, plain water and water with detergents. Nelson and associates,[24] discussing physical hygiene, recommend a daily bath with more frequent sponges during warm weather. The importance of rinsing the genitalia with clear water after soap has been used is stressed. Oil, powder, or lotion is usually unnecessary except when the skin is dry or irritated in the diaper area. Collections of secretion should be removed from the genitalia with water or oil on cotton applicators.

A rash on the buttocks may be the result of neglect or improperly laundered diapers. The latter should be thoroughly washed with a mild soap and boiled to kill bacteria that might reinfect the skin. Rinses (such as Diaparene *) have been developed that discourage urea-splitting and therefore ammonia-producing bacteria. Soft and loosely woven diapers dry quickly. Many layers should be used. The most satisfactory type are more bulky toward the center, or can be folded to give this effect. Rectangular or kite-shaped diapers are thought to make less pressure over the genitalia, to be less restricting, and to provide better protection than triangles.

If cleanliness and proper diapers do not prevent irritation, it may be necessary to use a bland ointment or to expose the buttocks to the warmth and light of the sun or an electric light suspended from a cradle over the bed. Chemicals that retard bacterial action may also decrease the irritating alkaline ammonia. Cleanliness, however, has the same effect, and when there is time for this, drugs of any sort are rarely necessary.

Soft expendable paper diapers are a convenience in traveling or whenever laundering service is unavailable. Institutions may find disposable materials an economy when labor is costly. The ecologic problem of waste disposal suggests, however, that they should be adopted cautiously.

What to Observe About the Feces. The principal points to be observed are the number of movements in 24 hours and any accompanying pain or straining; the consistency, shape,

* Pharmaceutical Division, Homemakers Products Corp., New York, N.Y.

color, and odor of the stool, and the presence of unusual matter. The expulsion of gas, or flatus, should be noted.

Although the *number of movements* varies in adult life, there should usually be one satisfactory daily movement; with some, two daily movements are normal unless cathartics have induced a large stool, in which case the intestinal tract may be so completely emptied that it will require 48 hours or more for the deposit of sufficient feces in the colon to stimulate contraction. As Alvarez says, the empty colon will not contract.

The stool should be formed, but not hard, and molded to the shape and size of the rectum. Henry L. Bockus [25] says the usual amount of feces is from 75 to 170 gm a day. The significance of small, dark, hard stools has been discussed as has the more common explanation of diarrhea, or frequent fluid stools. Often, but not always, fluid stools contain a substance that irritates the anus and that makes their elimination uncomfortable, or even painful. Nurses must note and record this if they observe signs of it, or if the patient complains of it. Changes in bowel habits, even of short duration, are said to be one of the early signs of cancer. Specialists are constantly urging people, particularly as they grow older, to have x-rays of the colon after a few weeks of diarrhea or constipation. Earl F. Wolfman, Jr., and C. Thomas Flatte [26] report that in a periodic physical examination offered to faculty members at the University of Michigan, one or more polyps have been detected in 33 out of a total of 400 asymptomatic individuals. For this and other reasons some internists include proctoscopy in health examinations.

The *color* of feces is normally a greenish brown, due chiefly to the bile they contain. Pale or clay-colored stools indicate its absence. This usually means either that the liver is not secreting bile or that there is some obstruction to its passage into the intestines. In the latter case bile passes into the bloodstream, and the patient is jaundiced. Light-colored stools may also be due to undigested fat. When the stool is dark and of a tarry consistency, one suspects the presence of partly digested blood. Red cells, when broken up, free hematin. A dark, tarry stool therefore indicates that a hemorrhage into the intestines occurred sometime previously, probably high up in the intestines or in the stomach. Bright red undigested blood is a sign of either a very recent hemorrhage or one from the colon. Blood from the rectum appears on the surface of the stool, while blood from the stomach or small intestines is mixed throughout. Every person who passes a bloody stool should have a careful examination. Wendell G. Scott concludes an article on rectal bleeding with the following:

(1) Cancer of the colon is common. (2) The best protection . . . is the complete periodic health check-up. (3) The surgical treatment of cancer of the colon has progressed ahead of consistent ability to diagnose it in the early stages. (4) The most urgent phase in the problem . . . is the education of people over 35 to seek medical attention for minor changes in their bowel habits and the elimination of self-medication. (5) The most important step is the education of physicians to institute examinations of the colon for suggestive symptoms and not to wait for the appearance of the advanced signs of cancer.*

D. Berkowitz,[27] reporting on a careful analysis of 200 deaths from gastrointestinal hemorrhage, concludes that diagnostic error could be attributed to (1) failure to consider acute stress ulcers as a cause of bleeding; (2) failure to consider extrahepatic causes of bleeding in patients with known liver disease; (3) failure to consider additional causes for bleeding in patients with known ulcers or varices; and (4) assumption that bleeding in elderly patients is due to malignancy.

Any bloody discharge from the body should be treated as a grave symptom. Bloody stools may be the result of rectal fissures or fistulas, of varicosities of the rectum or intestines, of ulcers or malignancies in any part of the tract, and of hemorrhage from other causes. The nurse should describe the appearance of the stool exactly, indicating whether the bright red color is on the outside of the stool or whether it is distributed throughout; whether the entire mass is of a dark, tarry consistency or whether only a part of it has this appearance, and so on. When the patient is menstruating it should be noted, since this may be the source of bright red blood on the surface of the stool.

When the presence of blood is suggested by the appearance of the stool, laboratory tests are made. These are described briefly in Chapter 7. Color and odor vary with foods eaten and with some drugs. For instance, a green color may be due to the chlorophyll from vegetables, and black stools to iron and bismuth preparations. Stools discolored by beets may suggest the presence of fresh blood.

Although the *odor* of the stool, as a rule, has no particular significance, any unusual odor should be noted. It may be caused by food or drugs, but is usually the result of bacterial action producing odoriferous gases,

* Scott, Wendell G.: "Significance of Rectal Bleeding and the Importance of Diagnosing Early Cancer of the Colon," *J. Natl. Med. Assoc.*, **42:**352, (Nov.) 1952.

such as hydrogen sulfide. Alvarez thinks excessive gas formation, especially if associated with reverse peristalsis, may account for the foul breath characteristic of intestinal stasis.

The *presence of any other unusual matter* such as pus, mucus, and worms should of course be reported.

Irritation of mucous membrane causes increased secretion of mucus. Excessive *mucus* gives the stool a *slimy* appearance. With inflammation, as in dysentery, the stool may consist of nothing but mucus and blood and defecation is accompanied by pain and tenesmus (an urge to evacuate the bowels or the bladder, without result).

Pus in the stool is the result of suppuration in the intestines, liver, or pancreas, or an abscess in the intestinal tract. Pus is hard to see in any but a fluid stool.

Intestinal parasites most commonly found in the stools are the pinworm or threadworm (*Enterobius vermicularis* or *Oxyuris vermicularis*); the roundworm (*Ascaris lumbricoides*); the whipworm (*Trichuris trichiura*); the hookworm (*Ancylostoma duodenale* and *Necator americanus*); the various tapeworms of pork and fish (*Taenia solium, Taenia saginata,* and *Diphyllobothrium latum*); and in another classification, the protozoan amebae. (See Fig. 11-7.) Worm infestation is far more prevalent than most people realize as is pointed out in Chapter 15. In people sufficiently well nourished to feed themselves and the parasites, some may produce no disease symptoms, but worms are a serious menace to the undernourished. Control lies chiefly in sanitation, and in thorough cooking of foods through which certain parasites are transmitted. The person whose intestinal tract is infested is given a drug to kill or paralyze the parasite. Such drugs are usually accompanied by a cathartic so that the worms will be removed and so that the absorption of the drug, usually toxic to the patient as well as the parasite, is reduced to a minimum. In *Diddie, Dumps and Tot*, a story of plantation life, there is a vivid description of dosing the children with "vermifuge" each spring, a necessary precaution in the last century. Some modern vermifuges or anthelmintics are piperazine hexahydrate (Antepar) and pyrvinium pamoate (Povan) for pinworm; piperazine bephenium hydroxynaphthoate (Alcopar) or hexylresorcinol for roundworm; dithiazanine iodide, tetrachlorethylene, hexylresorcinol, thiabendazole, or stilbazium iodide for whipworm; tetrachlorethylene, bephenium hydroxynaphthoate (Alcopara), hexylresorcinol, or dithiazine iodide (Delnex, Telmid) for hookworm; quinacrine hydrochloride (Atabrine) or oleoresin of aspidium for beef, pork, or fish tapeworm. The patient, family, laboratory technicians, nurses, and others will have to examine stools to determine the effectiveness of treatment.[28,29]

The *pinworm* or *threadworm* occurs quite frequently in the rectum and colon. Its presence causes itching, irritation, restlessness, insomnia, anorexia, and, finally, anemia. It appears in the stools as fine threads, usually moving actively.

Roundworms and *whipworms* are very common parasites occurring chiefly in children. They cause restlessness, irritability, twitchings, and convulsions. They are easily recognized in the stool.

When pinworms, roundworms, or whipworms are found in the stools, the greatest precaution must be taken to prevent spreading the infection to others and also to prevent patients (usually children) from reinfecting themselves by contaminating their hands. These parasites enter through the mouth. The anus and surrounding parts must be carefully washed and also the hands of both patient and nurse. Infected persons should never be allowed to handle foods.

The *ameba* is the cause of amebic, or tropical, dysentery, which is characterized by inflammation and ulceration of the intestines and abscesses in the liver. Since stools contain amebae, strict precautions must be taken to prevent the spread of the infection (see Chapter 15). The ameba is a one-celled organism that can be seen only under the microscope.

Tapeworms are taken into the alimentary tract usually in infected pork, beef, and fish which have not been thoroughly cooked. They lodge in the intestines and cause pain, nausea, diarrhea, and anemia. Infected with worms in the larval stages, cysts may form in the nervous system with such serious effects as epilepsy. These worms may be from 5 to 20 ft or more in length. Segments may be passed frequently in the stool, but until the head is removed the worm will continue to grow. When treatments are given, therefore, to expel the tapeworm, the minute head, about the size of a pinhead, with a very fine neck like a thread must be found, difficult as it is.

A stool to be examined for a tapeworm should be received in a bedpan containing water at body temperature and every bit examined. Toilet paper in the bedpan interferes with the search for the head of the tapeworm. All segments should be burned, never thrown into the toilet.

When a stool has an unusual appearance, indicating the presence of mucus, blood, pus, or worms, it should be saved, undisturbed, for inspection by the doctor, who will decide

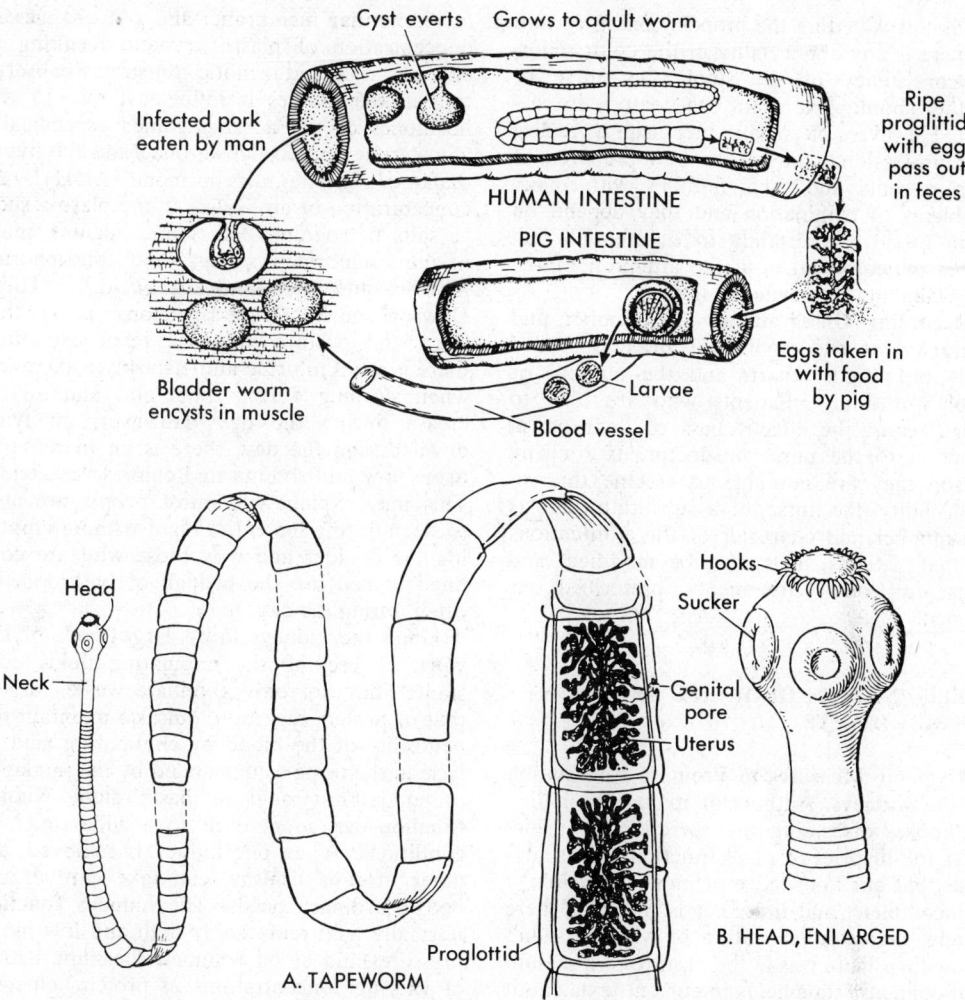

Cyst everts   Grows to adult worm

Infected pork eaten by man

HUMAN INTESTINE

PIG INTESTINE

Ripe proglittids with eggs pass out in feces

Bladder worm encysts in muscle

Larvae

Blood vessel

Eggs taken in with food by pig

Head

Neck

Hooks

Sucker

Genital pore

Uterus

Proglottid

A. TAPEWORM

B. HEAD, ENLARGED

Figure 11-7. The pork tapeworm, *Taenia solium.* (Top) Diagram of life cycle of *Taenia solium.* (From Storer, Tracy I.: *General Zoology,* 2nd ed. (After Bucksbaum.) McGraw-Hill Book Co., New York, 1951.) (*Left*) Specimen about 8 ft. long, consisting of about 900 proglottids, with four sections omitted. The uterus filled with eggs is shown in the last two proglottids. The worm is shown about four times natural size. (*Right*) Head, enlarged about 40 times. (From Hegner, Robert W., and Stiles, Karl A.: *College Zoology,* 6th ed., Macmillan Publishing Co., Inc., New York, 1951.)

whether a specimen should be sent to the laboratory for further examination. In any case, when it is suspected that the stool contains any abnormal substance, and an examination will help in diagnosis, a specimen is required for examination. Usually, a small amount is adequate, but sometimes it is necessary to save the whole undisturbed.

The character and number of the stools of an infant differ in some respects from those of adults. A normal breast-fed infant ordinarily has two or three stools daily during the first week. It is important for the nurse to watch the number and character of the stools during this period. An absence of bowel movement may be caused by some congenital malformation of the anus, rectum, or colon, which should have the immediate attention of a surgeon. After the first month, there are usually two stools each day; there should be at least one daily bowel movement.

The stool of a breast-fed infant is orange yellow in color, soft, smooth, mealy, or stringy in consistency, having a pungent odor and acid reaction. The stool of an artificially fed infant changes in appearance with the food given.

The character of the stool indicates whether

the infant is getting the proper feeding or not. If there is any abnormality in the color, odor, or consistency of the stool, the nurse or mother should save it for the doctor's inspection. However, physicians increasingly realize that professional nurses are well prepared to help patients and their families with many problems of elimination and they depend on them to do so; certainly to differentiate between patients who need the attention of the physician and those who do not.

Recording Observations. The number and character of the stools are often recorded daily on infants' charts and the number of stools for adults. Patients who are able to judge report the effectiveness of their bowel function to the nurse or doctor. If for any reason they are not able to assume this responsibility, the nurse, or a substitute, reports the number and character of the eliminations so that patients' diets may be modified, and drugs or other treatments prescribed, as needed.

3. ELIMINATION OF WASTE BY THE KIDNEYS

Hygienic Measures to Promote Elimination by the Kidneys. Authors of major physiology textbooks, discussing the secretion of urine, refer to "theories of renal function." This suggests that our knowledge of kidney physiology is incomplete, and indeed it is. Perhaps there is now a greater realization of what we don't know than there was in the past, for we seldom find dogmatic statements in current texts about diet and fluid intake in relation to kidney functions.

It is believed that urine is manufactured by the kidney through a filtration of the blood in the glomeruli with a selective reabsorption in the tubules of substances from the filtrate. The glomerular filtrate with the exception of protein, of which there is less than 0.03 per cent, is the same as plasma. Approximately 180 liters of glomerular filtrate is formed each day. Ninety-nine per cent of this is usually reabsorbed by the tubules; the remainder is passed into the urine.[30] The conditions under which the kidney functions normally are not entirely understood, but it is known that anything increasing the rate of filtration or reducing the rate of reabsorption increases the volume of urine. The reverse actively decreases the urine volume.

The rate of glomerular filtration is influenced by (1) changes in arterial pressure and the general circulation; (2) changes in arterial construction; (3) pore size and permeability of glomerular membrane; and (4) changes in concentration of plasma protein resulting in changes in colloid osmotic pressure. Reabsorption in the tubules is influenced by (1) the hormones of the adrenal glands (specifically aldosterone and corticosterone) and the hypothalamus (antidiuretic hormone, ADH); (2) concentration of any solids in the plasma such as salts of sodium, potassium, calcium, magnesium, chloride, sulfur, and phosphorus, glucose, and urea and uric acid.[31,32] Hugh Dawson and M. Grace Eggleton[33] report that sleep and posture influence renal excretion; there is a fall in urine and electrolyte excretion when sleeping during the night, and an increase during the day. However, on lying down during the day, there is an increase in urine flow and sodium and chloride excretion. This may explain why most people are able to sleep during the entire night without emptying the bladder and why those who are confined to bed use the bedpan or bathroom so often during the day.

Upon the kidneys fall a large share of the work of keeping the circulating fluids constant. They not only eliminate waste, largely that of protein digestion, but also maintain the neutrality of the blood by eliminating acid or base in the urine as demanded by the intake of preponderantly acid or basic diets. Kidney function can adapt itself to a wide range of conditions. When one kidney is removed, the other, if it is healthy, can take care of the body's ordinary needs. The kidneys function normally with remarkably high and low blood pressures and blood volumes; the same is true of varying concentrations of protein, glucose, electrolytes, hormones, and nitrogenous wastes. We must realize, however, that when any one of these conditions exceeds the limits tolerated by the kidneys, they break down; when this happens, the acid–base balance is disrupted, nitrogenous wastes and water accumulate in the tissues, and death follows rapidly.

Normal kidney function is encouraged by living a sane life with respect to food and drink, exercise, rest, and sleep. Since the emotions affect blood pressure, digestion, and in fact the entire body economy, mental health is part of this sane life. It is no longer believed that simple rules for drinking water and avoiding protein, or any other dietary element, are the answer. Avoidance of irritating chemicals, particularly those eliminated by the kidneys, and freedom from bacterial poisons, of course, help to maintain the kidneys in a normal state.

What to Observe About Urine. A nurse should note the amount of urine voided in 24 hours and the amount at each voiding; the frequency, and any urgency, effort, discomfort, or pain that accompanies voiding; also the transparency, color, and odor of the urine. According to standard texts on physiology, the *amount of urine* voided by the average adult in a 24-hour period varies from 1000 to 2000 ml (1 to 2 qt). Most authorities, however, comment on the very wide range in health according to the intake of fluids, the diet, and the amount of water through "insensible loss" (skin and lungs), sweat, or feces. Guyton reports the amount of daily water loss by each avenue for the average person during normal temperature, hot weather, and prolonged heavy exercise (see Table 11-1). It is important to recognize that water loss through the skin is *not* necessarily limited to that excreted by the sweat glands as sweat. The cornified layer of the skin acts as a protector against loss of water normally but when it is destroyed, as by a burn, the patient may lose as much as 3 to 5 liters from the body surface in 1 day.

Average daily excretion of urine for healthy children as given by Nelson is shown in Table 11-2. The amount, either in children or adults, may be greatly increased by disease, or temporarily by physiologic conditions. In acute nephritis, the amount may be only 200 to 500 ml, while it has been reported that in diabetes insipidus (caused by a lesion in the midbrain) 43 liters or quarts of urine was passed in 24 hours.[34] The voiding of a large amount of urine is called *polyuria;* when the amount voided is scanty, the condition is called *oliguria;* when there is a total absence or marked deficiency, *anuria.*

Failure to void the normal amount of urine should be reported immediately. In diseases marked by either an increase or decrease in urine, it must be carefully measured and the amount recorded.

When a person's sleep is disturbed so that he or she wakes to empty the bladder, this is

Table 11-1. Loss of Water Each Day (in Milliliters) *

	Normal Tempera-ture	Hot Weather	Prolonged Heavy Exercise
Insensible Loss:			
Skin	350	350	350
Lungs	350	250	650
Urine	1400	1200	500
Sweat	100	1400	5000
Feces	200	200	200
Total	2400	3400	6700

* Guyton, Arthur C.: *Textbook of Medical Physiology,* 5th ed. W. B. Saunders Co., Philadelphia, 1976, p. 425.

Table 11-2. Average Daily Excretion of Urine in Childhood *

Age	Cubic Centimeters
First and second day	30–60
Third to tenth day	100–300
Tenth day to 2 months	250–450
2 months to 1 year	400–500
1–3 years	500–600
3–5 years	600–700
5–8 years	650–1000
8–14 years	800–1400

* Nelson, Waldo E. (ed.): *Nelson's Textbook of Pediatrics,* 9th ed. W. B. Saunders Co., Philadelphia, 1969, p. 1106.

called *nocturia,* whereas an involuntary or unconscious voiding during sleep is *enuresis,* considered normal in children under 5 years of age. *Nocturia* and *frequency* are usually associated with bladder infection and/or obstruction. Other terms indicating urinary dysfunction include: *paradoxical* or *overflow incontinence,* a continuous dribble of urine; *stress incontinence,* intermittent leaking of urine caused by physical or emotional strain; *total incontinence,* bladder unable to retain any urine; *urgency,* sudden, almost uncontrollable, desire to urinate; and *pneumaturia,* the passing of gas with urine.[35]

Transparency is a characteristic of most normal urine. Cloudy urine or the deposit of a sediment may indicate disease or may be due to such simple causes as a change in the reaction of the urine on standing or to protein derived from the epithelial lining of the bladder and urinary passages. Normal urine is acid in reaction and always contains phosphates, which are held in solution in an acid medium. Under certain conditions, such as the ingestion of large quantities of vegetables, administration of alkalies (e.g., sodium bicarbonate) by mouth, or by prolonged forced breathing, the phosphates are no longer held in solution but are precipitated out.[36] This makes the urine cloudy, and when it stands, a sediment is formed. Even acid urine will turn alkaline and cloudy in a few hours because normal waste products in it, urea, for example, are decomposed by bacteria, setting free ammonia, which is highly alkaline. This will again precipitate the phosphates. People are sometimes needlessly alarmed by cloudy urine thinking they have "kidney trouble." Adding a little acid to the urine will determine whether the cloudiness is caused by phosphates. If it is, the cloud will disappear. Sometimes, also, people may be needlessly alarmed by a brick-red sediment in urine that has been in a specimen bottle for some time. This sediment consists of normal waste products, urates and uric acid crystals. Urine when voided is warm, and this heat keeps the urates, etc., in solution; when cooled, particularly if concentrated, they are precipitated. To test the urine, heat it; if the cloud of sediment is caused by urates, it will disappear.

When a cloud or sediment cannot be removed but is increased by adding acid or by heating, it is always due to abnormal substances—albumin, pus, blood, epithelial cells, or casts. (Urine tests are described briefly in Chapter 7).

The *color* of urine depends on the amount and kind of pigment, concentration of the urine, the amount and kind of solids, decomposition of the solids, the presence of abnormal constituents, and the action of drugs. In most cases (except those whose kidneys are unable to concentrate urine), *the color of urine is not of any great importance in diagnosis of disease, but it is an important guide for the nurse. A pale urine is a dilute, low specific gravity urine and shows that the patient is drinking enough water; amber-colored urine is concentrated, and of high specific gravity, indicating that the patient is not getting sufficient water.* Some clinicians think the color and specific gravity of the urine a more helpful guide than the record of intake and output.

The *odor* of newly voided urine is characteristic. It is caused by volatile, aromatic components. When urine stands it smells of ammonia, liberated on the decomposition of urea by bacteria. When freshly voided urine has this odor, it shows that decomposition has taken place in the bladder and this suggests cystitis. In diabetes the urine may have a sweetish odor, due to the presence of acetone. The odor of ammonia or of acetone should therefore always be reported, as either one indicates disease. Drugs and foods may also alter the odor of urine.

Some Causes of Increased Urine. A marked increase in the amount of urine voided may be caused temporarily by drinking a large amount of fluids, by excitement, cold baths, by food, and by diuretic drugs. In winter, urine is voided more frequently because less water is eliminated by perspiration. Because, however, less water is drunk in cold weather, this may not follow.

The amount is usually increased in conditions such as hysteria, chronic nephritis, diabetes mellitus, and diabetes insipidus. In chronic nephritis without edema, the diseased kidneys have difficulty eliminating solid wastes so they eliminate a small amount of solids and, to dilute them, they at the same time eliminate a large amount of water. In such cases the urine is pale and of a low specific gravity. In uncontrolled diabetes mellitus, the blood sugar rises, and this makes patients thirsty, just as eating candy does. They drink quantities of water in order to dilute the sugar and eliminate it through the kidneys.

Some Causes of Decreased Urine. A marked decrease in the amount voided may be caused *temporarily* by drinking small amounts of fluid, by the loss of body fluids by perspiration, by vomiting, diarrhea, and by the action of drugs, such as opium, that check the secretion of urine; by *suppression* of urine, failure of the kidneys to secrete urine; and by *retention* of urine, failure of the bladder to expel urine contained in it.

It is very important to know whether failure to void urine (anuria) is caused by *suppression* or *retention,* as the effect of the body and the treatment required differ greatly.

Suppression of urine, or anuria, is a very grave condition, indicating that renal function is severely impaired. Waste products in the blood, normally eliminated through the kidneys, are held in the body, and it must find another means of getting rid of them. Part will be eliminated by the bowels and the skin, but they cannot do the work of the kidneys; some of the waste products will of necessity accumulate, and give rise to serious symptoms. The symptoms of *retention* are largely local—that is, discomfort confined to the region of the bladder, but those of *suppression* are general.

Retention means that urine secreted by the kidneys is retained in the bladder. *Retention with overflow* sometimes occurs; that is, some urine is voided but the bladder is not emptied. The distended bladder can often be felt through the abdominal wall.

The symptoms of retention are failure to void; fullness and discomfort, sometimes severe pain; and a distended bladder. Any of these symptoms should be reported immediately. If voiding cannot be induced by nursing measures, catheterization must be resorted to. This is accompanied by some risk to the patient, and should be avoided if possible. It is discussed in Chapter 24.

Symptoms of suppression are dizziness, nausea, vomiting, headache, drowsiness, forgetfulness, and generalized edema which may be pronounced under the eyes. In suppression, no urine flows from a catheter inserted into the bladder, because there is none; whereas in retention the urine immediately flows from the instrument. Every nurse should be alert to the preceding symptoms and realize the importance of reporting them at once. In treatment, emphasis is placed on establishing the diagnosis—determining the primary cause. Anuria and its treatment are discussed in Chapter 37.

Nursing Measures to Stimulate Micturition. Nurses can most effectively relieve retention if to some extent they understand bladder physiology. While there is much more to learn about it than is now known, a great deal of data have been accumulated through cystometry (estimates of intervesicular pressure) in recent years.

Micturition, urination or voiding, is initiated by the stretching of the bladder walls, or by the pressure of urine. The stretching, or the pressure required to elicit the desire to empty the bladder, varies with the person and with his condition. Under stress a very small amount can give rise to an urgent desire to urinate, while the same person, under other circumstances, can store a large volume of urine without discomfort. Physical and psychic factors affect bladder function, which is, for normal children and adults, a reflex act under voluntary control. Guyton says:

The micturition reflex is a completely automatic cord reflex, but it can be inhibited or facilitated by centers in the brain. . . .

The micturition reflex is the basic cause of micturition, but the higher centers normally exert final control of micturition by the following means:
1. The higher centers keep the micturition reflex partially inhibited all the time except when it is desired to micturate.
2. The higher centers prevent micturition by continual tonic contraction of the external urinary sphincter until a convenient time presents itself.
3. When the time to urinate arrives, the cortical centers can (a) facilitate the sacral micturition centers to initiate a micturition reflex and (b) inhibit the external urinary sphincter so that urination can occur.*

By cystometry (described in Chapter 24) it has been learned that in the average adult the bladder adapts itself, by periods of contraction and relaxation, to its contents until 400 to 600 ml of urine has accumulated. Up to this point it maintains its tone; when it is distended beyond the physiologic point, it tends to lose its muscular character and behave more or less like an elastic bag. While there are great individual differences in bladder function, it empties most normally at that point when it is, physiologically speaking, full—rather than partially filled or distended. Voiding occurs most easily when nothing interferes with the removal of the voluntary inhibition. Reflex

* Guyton, Arthur C.: *Textbook of Medical Physiology,* 5th ed. W. B. Saunders Co., Philadelphia, 1976, p. 503.

acts are dependent on the sensitivity of the nerves and muscles involved; therefore, anesthetics, narcotics, hypnotics, or anything that depresses neuromuscular mechanisms may interfere with micturition. Some such drugs retard the formation of urine; some delay

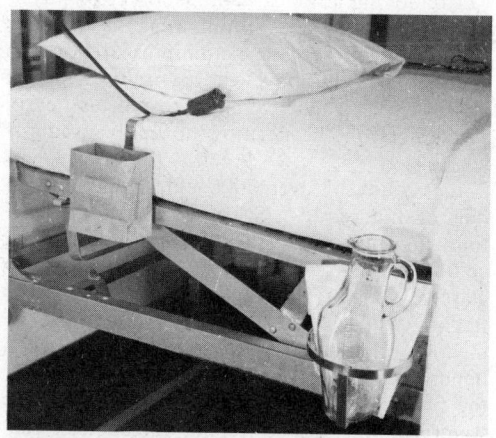

A

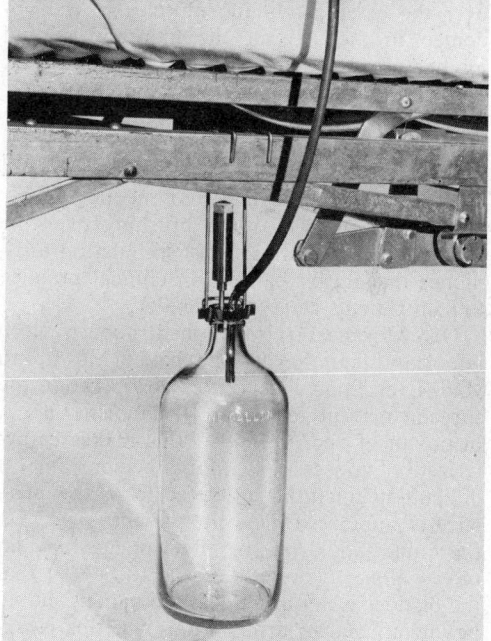

B

Figure 11-8. *A.* In many cases it is necessary to leave a urinal within reach of the patient. A metal holder, as illustrated, is a desirable type. A disposable paper cover is placed over, or beside, the urinal. (Courtesy of Columbia-Presbyterian Medical Center, New York, N.Y., and Clay-Adams Co. New York, N.Y.)

B. Tomac deodorizing drainage bottle. (Courtesy of American Hospital Supply Corp., Evanston, Ill.)

emptying of the bladder; while large doses may remove the voluntary control and cause incontinence.

When patients are not voiding and there is reason to believe that they are storing urine, nurses may encourage micturition by (1) promoting mental and physical relaxation through such measures as the particular case demands; (2) removing any distracting sources of physical discomfort; (3) stimulating the bladder walls by gentle massage and pressure on the abdominal wall above the *symphysis pubis;* and (4) seeing that patients are put, as nearly as possible, in the position normally used for voiding.

In a study of over 3000 elderly patients in nursing homes, Jean Saxon [37] reports that the following nursing measures were helpful in getting patients to urinate: (1) drinking a glass of water; (2) "slight digital pressure or tickling with cotton over or to the side of the meatus" (in women); (3) placing the patient's hands in warm water; (4) pouring water over the perineum; or (5) letting the patient hear water running. Sister Regina Elizabeth [38] recommends light brushing and application of ice over the external oblique muscles in the abdomen in the area of the first and second lumbar nerves to effect voiding. In a study of 12 postoperative women, Nancy I. Bergstrom [39] reports that eight were successful in voiding after rubbing of ice from the crest of the ilium to the groin (endings of eleventh and twelfth thoracic and first and second lumbar nerves) followed by rapid brushing over the same area. These are sensory stimulation techniques that nurses can use in clinical practice to help patients empty the bladder.

Of every measure mentioned, none is more important than having the patient sit up to void. Even immediately after an operation the surgeon may prefer having the patient sit up, in or out of bed, to void if this makes catheterization unnecessary. Many persons find it difficult to micturate or defecate in the presence of another. Unless the patient is very ill, the nurse should try the effect of leaving him or her alone. If there is reason to believe that the bladder is not distended, the patient should be encouraged to drink water, but this is unsuccessful when the bladder walls are already stretched beyond the point where they function effectively. Some physicians ask that patients be catheterized rather than to allow them to suffer from retention for any length of time. Thinning of the walls, with its effect of decreasing the blood supply, is believed by some authorities to predispose the bladder to infection and to be as much of a hazard as the introduction of a catheter. With skillful nursing these dangers can be minimized, but a catheter always introduces some bacteria into the bladder. It nearly always produces a cystitis—mild or severe.

4. ELIMINATION OF WASTE BY THE SKIN AND LUNGS

Excretory Function of the Skin. Water and electrolytes are lost through the skin by *insensible perspiration* and *sweat.* Insensible perspiration is water, lost by diffusion through the skin. The person is unaware of its presence; it is invisible and is not produced by the sweat glands. The average person loses about 350 to 450 ml water daily through insensible perspiration. Sweat, a product of the sweat glands, consists of water and electrolytes; it can be seen. It is a hypotonic solution containing sodium, chloride, potassium, and other excretory products such as urea. The amount of water lost by sweat varies. Most authors give 100 ml as the daily amount lost by the average adult under normal room temperature. However, Dixon M. Woodbury [40] notes that as much as 11 to 15 liters (25 per cent of total body water) has been lost in 24 hours during maximal sweating.

Heat is lost primarily from the skin by radiation, conduction, convection, and the evaporation of sweat and insensible perspiration. When the humidity is low, sweat evaporates and the body is cooled by the process; when the humidity is high, sweat does not evaporate and this process no longer cools the body.[41] The concepts of heat loss are discussed in Chapters 28 and 29. Sweat also helps to keep the skin supple, protecting it from mechanical influences, and it plays a role in protecting the skin from ultraviolet rays and infectious diseases.[42]

Anhidrosis and *hyperhidrosis* are two terms often found in the literature when sweating is discussed and are worth explanation. *Anhidrosis* can be defined as "the inability of the body to produce and/or deliver sweat onto the skin surface." * It may be caused by congenital ectodermal dysplasia, extensive scar tissue such as in burns, and damage to the thermal sweating center by some disease condition. Yas Kuno describes a young man (18 years of age) with the last condition as spending his summer days repeatedly taking cold baths because of his great suffering. *Hyperhidrosis* is the production of an excess of sweat over the whole body surface, as may be seen in some diseases, or it may be limited to a particular area such as the palms and soles, the axillae, and face.

---

* Kuno, Yas: *Human Perspiration.* Charles C Thomas, Publisher, Springfield, Ill., 1956, p. 347.

The terms *"mental sweating"* and *"stress sweating,"* used synonymously in the literature, are self-explanatory. Some, perhaps most, persons sweat freely when they are worried, fearful, anxious, or in other emotional states. Such sweating may occur over the entire body or on the palms, soles, and axillae in low, normal, and high temperatures and persists until the particular stimulus no longer exists.[43] Kuno describes the prevalence of sweating among Japanese students:

The sweating may be so copious occasionally that sweat drops are scattered about on the floor when the hands are waved. . . . Their mental trouble is great, much greater than others suspect; and to make matters worse, they are usually nervous in nature. There is a tendency not only with this hyperhidrosis but with all other hyperhidrosis for the sweating rate to increase in intensity as time passes. This is probably so because the reflex arc and the sweat glands concerned are trained by repetition of sweating.*

Some Conditions Affecting Loss of Heat, Water, and Electrolytes. Of the authors consulted, all list several of the following as causing the body to excrete heat, water, and electrolytes: (1) high environmental temperatures; (2) exercise; (3) strong emotions; and (4) certain bodily conditions such as fever, extensive abrasions or burns of the skin, debilitating diseases, as tuberculosis, and injury to the sweat production mechanism.

According to John H. Bland, insensible water loss is increased 10 per cent for each degree Fahrenheit during fever. He says: "Because of their hyperpnea, patients with metabolic acidosis are likely to have high rates of insensible water loss. As the nature of the respiration changes, one may anticipate prompt and large changes in rate of insensible water loss." † It has been known for some time that the denuded skin, such as in burned persons, loses large quantities of water. Richard H. Fallon and Carl A. Moyer[44] report that the dry burn eschar (6 days following the burn) transmits water vapor to the air 75 times faster than the normal skin. (See Chapter 42 for a discussion of this problem.) The badly burned person therefore needs large amounts of fluids and electrolytes. Age also influences the rate of insensible water loss. Infants lose proportionately more water than do adults because of their relatively high caloric expenditure, and the aged lose less water and heat because of atrophic changes and circulatory deficiency.[45] Sweat increases during sleep, especially when the room temperature is 29°C (84°F).

* *Ibid.,* p. 351.
† Bland, John H.: *Clinical Metabolism of Body Water and Electrolytes.* W. B. Saunders Co., Philadelphia, 1963, p. 267.

Heat, water, and electrolyte loss by the skin can be controlled to some extent by cooling the atmosphere, wearing thin and light color clothing, increasing the evaporation of sweat by using fans that circulate air, and decreasing the amount of food eaten, especially protein and fat.[46]

When large amounts of fluid and electrolytes are lost, they must be replaced. The methods used will depend on the condition of the person, but if a sufficient amount can be taken by mouth, this is the avenue of choice. Fluid loss can be estimated by weight loss, assuming the caloric intake is consistent. Weighing the person each day at the same time on the same scale will give a fairly accurate picture of fluid loss.

Chloride that is lost in sweat can be replaced by adding more salt in the diet than is ordinarily used and by taking salt in tablet form. John R. Brobeck[47] believes that after the individual becomes accustomed to a new climate, sodium chloride tablets daily for an adult may be required to maintain sodium balance.

Accurate observations on excessive loss and replacement of body fluid must be made and recorded. The patient and family will usually help collect and record this important information if they are encouraged to participate in the therapeutic program and believe that they can make an important contribution. A form kept at the bedside, available for all, increases the probability that the collected data are accurate.

Excretory Function of the Lungs. The principal function of the lung as an excretory organ is the elimination of carbon dioxide which is a waste product of all metabolism. Elimination of carbon dioxide, produced at the cell level, depends on diffusion across the alveolocapillary membrane and an adequate volume and distribution of pulmonary capillary blood flow. Factors that influence the rate of diffusion are the thickness of the membrane, the surface area of the membrane, and the pressure gradient between two sides of the membrane.[48,49] Any condition that changes the "normal" of one or more of these will interfere with the excretion of carbon dioxide. Any condition that interferes with capillary blood flow, such as occlusion (partial or complete) of one pulmonary artery or arterioles, destruction of lung tissue, emboli, or thrombosis, will also affect excretion of carbon dioxide. The subject of exchange of gases (oxygen and carbon dioxide) is discussed in Chapter 9 and should be consulted for a thorough understanding of carbon dioxide elimination.

Water is eliminated by the lungs through the process of breathing since the inspired air contains less water vapor than the expired air.

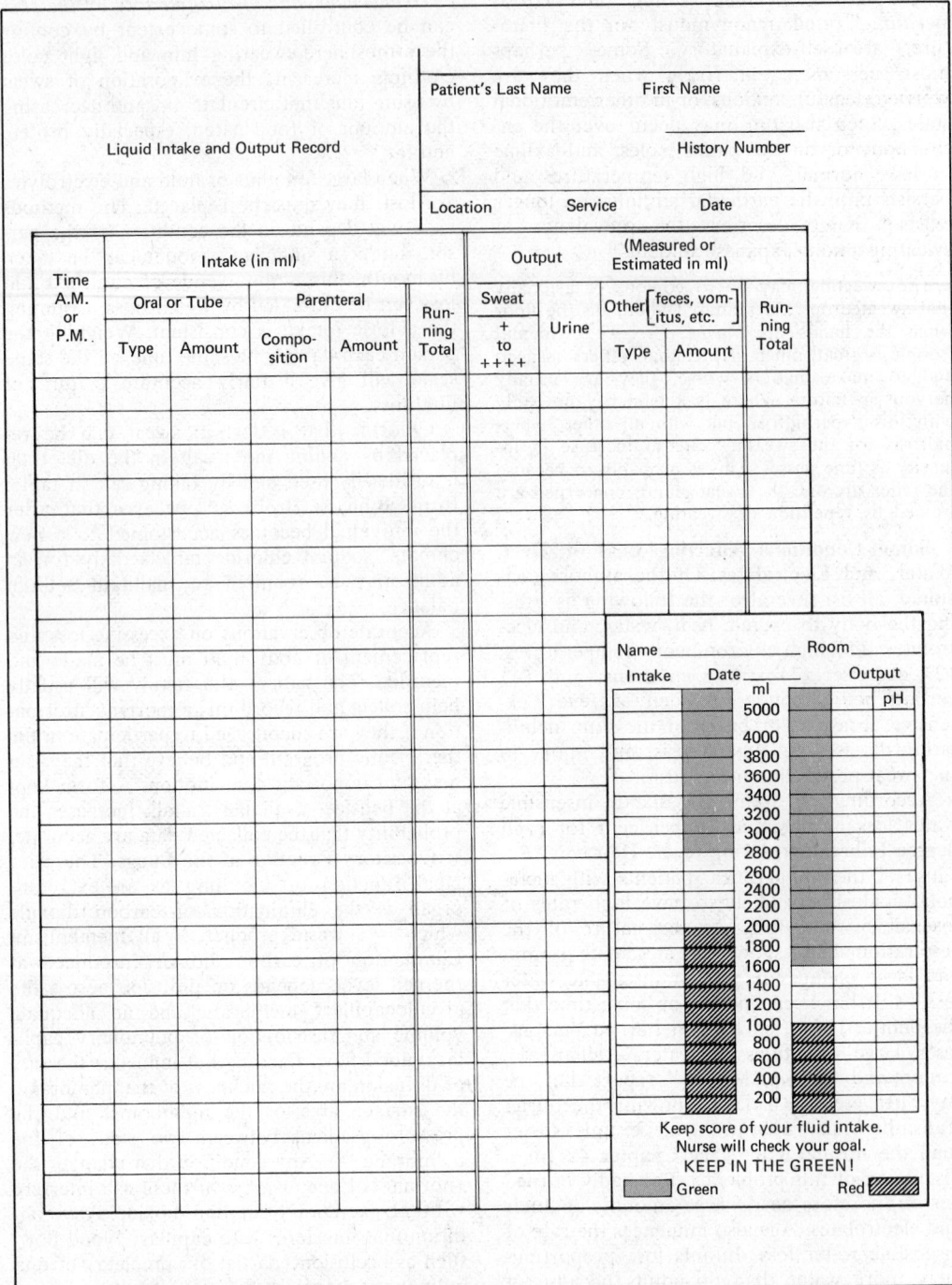

Figure 11-9. Liquid intake and output records, designed by Dr. George A. Schumacher. (From Bland, John H.: *Clinical Metabolism of Body Water and Electrolytes.* W. B. Saunders Co., Philadelphia, 1963, p. 215.) *Inset at right:* Fluid intake and output record which the patient fills in with the help of the nurse. (Copyright 1944 by American Hospital Supply Corporation, Evanston, Ill.)

Water loss is increased, especially in elderly persons, in centrally heated buildings and dehydration can occur unless fluid intake is increased. When respiration is increased, as in hyperventilation, the loss of water can be quite high, particularly in a dry atmosphere. With increased respiratory rates, more carbon dioxide is eliminated. Finally, altitudes also affect the loss of water vapor and carbon dioxide. In mountain climbing, for example, the loss of water vapor and carbon dioxide increases.[50]

Prevention and early detection of conditions that interfere with the elimination of waste products of respiration are important. Persons noting changes in their respiration should, of course, consult a phsyician. For a detailed discussion of this subject, see Chapter 35.

5. MEASURING AND RECORDING ELIMINATION

The elimination of metabolic waste products is the function of the intestines, kidneys, skin, and lungs. A daily record of defecation is a regular item of every patient's record. The nature of the stool (and any discomfort experienced) should be recorded.

When one considers the critical nature of kidney function, it is not surprising to find great emphasis put on accurately recording urinary output of most hospital patients or those sick elsewhere. Judgments on the fluid–electrolyte and acid–base balance in the body are based on these records. In many illnesses single specimens of urine and/or samplings of the 24-hour output are sent to the laboratory daily for analysis. The persons most concerned —the patients—are encouraged to keep their own record to the extent that this is possible. Figure 11-9 shows a daily form that patients and family members may be taught to keep.

To estimate the amount of fluid loss by the skin, patients should be weighed each day and their weight recorded. Observation and recording of any change in the nature of respiration should also be a part of the patient's record. Fluid–electrolyte, acid–base, and nitrogen balance is discussed in Chapter 10. Nutrition and elimination cannot be completely separated. These two chapters should be studied as a unit.

REFERENCES

1. Alvarez, Walter C.: *An Introduction to Gastro-enterology.* Paul B. Hoeber, New York, 1948, p. 607.
2. Cantor, Meyer O.: *Intestinal Intubation.* Charles C Thomas, Publisher, Springfield, Ill., 1949, pp. 112, 133.
3. Haubrick, William S.: "Anatomy of the Colon," in Bockus, Henry L.: *Gastroenterology,* Vol. II, 2nd ed. W. B. Saunders Co., Philadelphia, 1964, p. 505.
4. Hightower, N. C., Jr., and Janowitz, Henry D.: "Secretion and Absorption in the Intestines," in Brobeck, John R., et al. (eds.): *Best and Taylor's Physiological Basis of Medical Practice,* 9th ed. Williams & Wilkins Co., Baltimore, 1973, p. 2–79.
5. Guyton, Arthur C.: *Textbook of Medical Physiology,* 5th ed. W. B. Saunders Co., Philadelphia, 1976, p. 869.
6. Hightower, N. C., Jr., and Janowitz, Henry D.: *op. cit.,* p. 2–84.
7. Scholer, J. F., and Code, C. F.: "Rate of Absorption of Water from the Stomach and Small Bowel of Human Beings," *Gastroenterology,* **27:**568, (Nov.) 1954.
8. Guyton, Arthur C.: *op. cit.,* p. 858.
9. Bockus, Henry L.: *Gastroenterology,* Vol. II, 2nd ed. W. B. Saunders Co., Philadelphia, 1964, p. 626.
9a. Willacker, Jean: "Bowel Sounds," *Am. J. Nurs.,* **73:**2100, (Dec.) 1973.
10. Bloom, Alan A., et al.: "Motility of the Intact Human Colon," *Gastroenterology,* **54:** 232, (Feb.) 1968.
11. Burnett, F. L.: "The Intestinal Rate and the Form of Feces," *Am. J. Roentgenol. Radium Ther. Nucl. Med.,* **10:**599, (Aug.) 1923.
12. Chandhary, N. A., and Truelove, S. C.: "Colonic Motility: A Critical Review of Methods and Results," *Am. J. Med.,* **31:**86, (July) 1961.
13. Farrar, John T., and Zfass, Alvin M.: "Small Intestinal Motility," *Gastroenterology,* **52:** 1028, (June) 1956.
14. Texter, E. Clinton, et al.: *Physiology of the Gastrointestinal Tract.* C. V. Mosby Co., St. Louis, 1968, p. 137.
15. MacBride, Cyril Mitchell, and Blacklow, Robert Stanley: *Signs and Symptoms: Applied Pathologic Physiology and Clinical Interpretations,* 5th ed. J. B. Lippincott Co., Philadelphia, 1970, p. 384.
16. Haubrick, William S.: "Physiology of the Colon," in Bockus, Henry L.: *Gastroenterology,* Vol. II, 2nd ed. W. B. Saunders Co., Philadelphia, 1964, p. 627.
17. Welsh, Jack D.: "Physiology of Bowel Evacuation," *Nebr. State Med. J.,* **50:**52, (Feb.) 1965.
18. Duthie, H. L.: "Anal Continence," *Gut,* **12:** 851, (Oct.) 1971.
19. Senn, Milton J. E. (ed.): *Problems of Infancy and Childhood; Transactions of the Fourth Conference, New York, March, 1950.* Josiah Macy, Jr. Foundation, New York, 1951, p. 22.
20. Baruch, Dorothy: *One Little Boy.* Julian Press, New York, 1952.
21. Senn, Milton J. E. (ed.): *op. cit.,* pp. 57, 59.
22. Fries, Margaret E.: "The Child's Ego De-

velopment and Training of Adults in His Environment," *Psychoanal. Study Child II*, 1946, p. 85.

23. Illingworth, R. S.: *The Normal Child*, 5th ed. J. & A. Churchill, Ltd., London, 1972.

24. Nelson, Waldo E., et al.: *Textbook of Pediatrics*, 9th ed. W. B. Saunders Co., Philadelphia, 1969, p. 196.

25. Bockus, Henry L.: *op. cit.*, p. 695.

26. Wolfman, Jr., Earl F., and Flatte, C. Thomas: "Carcinoma of the Colon and Rectum," *Am. J. Nurs.*, **61**:60, (Mar.) 1961.

27. Berkowitz, D.: "Fatal Gastrointestinal Hemorrhage: Diagnostic Implications from a Study of 200 Cases," *Am. J. Gastroenterol.*, **40**:372, (Oct.) 1963.

28. Brown, H. W.: *Basic Clinical Parasitology*, 3rd ed. Appleton-Century-Crofts, New York, 1969, p. 112.

29. Faust, Ernest C., et al.: *Animal Agents and Vectors of Human Disease*, 3rd ed. Lea & Febiger, Philadelphia, 1968, p. 225.

30. Guyton, Arthur C.: *Basic Human Physiology: Normal Function and Mechanisms of Disease*. W. B. Saunders Co., Philadelphia, 1971, p. 274.

31. Berliner, Robert W.: "Urine Formation," in Brobeck, John R., et al. (eds.): *Best and Taylor's Physiological Basis of Medical Practice*, 9th ed. Williams & Wilkins Co., Baltimore, 1973, p. 5–17.

32. Guyton, Arthur C.: *Textbook of Medical Physiology, op. cit.*, p. 396.

33. Dawson, Hugh, and Eggleton, M. Grace: *Starling's Human Physiology*, 13th ed. Lea & Febiger, Philadelphia, 1962, p. 700.

34. Houssay, Bernardo A., et al.: *Human Physiology*. McGraw-Hill Book Co., New York, 1955, p. 569.

35. Leader, Abel J., and Carlton, C. Eugene: "Urologic Diagnosis and the Urologic Examination," in Campbell, Merredith W.: *Urology*, 3rd ed. W. B. Saunders Co., Philadelphia, 1970, p. 207.

36. Dawson, Hugh, and Eggleton, M. Grace: *op. cit.*, p. 690.

37. Saxon, Jean: "Techniques for Bowel and Bladder Training," *Am. J. Nurs.*, **62**:69, (Sept.) 1962.

38. Regina Elizabeth, Sister: "Sensory Stimulation Techniques," *Am. J. Nurs.*, **66**:285, (Feb.) 1966.

39. Bergstrom, Nancy I.: "Ice Application to Induce Voiding," *Am. J. Nurs.*, **69**:283, (Feb.) 1969.

40. Woodbury, Dixon M.: "Physiology of Body Fluids," in Ruch, Theodore C., and Patton, Harry D.: *Physiology and Biophysics*, 19th ed. W. B. Saunders Co., Philadelphia, 1965, p. 893.

41. Brobeck, John R.: "Control Systems That Establish Regulations," in Brobeck, John R., et al. (eds.): *Best and Taylor's Physiological Basis of Medical Practice*, 9th ed. Williams & Wilkins Co., Baltimore, 1973, p. 9–129.

42. Kral, Jiri A., et al.: "Sweat and Exercise," *J. Sports Med. Phys. Fitness*, **3**:110, (June–Sept.) 1963.

43. Kuno, Yas: *Human Perspiration*. Charles C Thomas, Publisher, Springfield, Ill., 1956, p. 104.

44. Fallon, Richard H., and Moyer, Carl A.: "Rates of Insensible Perspiration Through Normal, Burned, Tape Stripped, and Epidermally Denuded Living Human Skin," *Ann. Surg.*, **158**:915, (Dec.) 1963.

45. Bland, John H.: *Clinical Metabolism of Body Water and Electrolytes*. W. B. Saunders Co., Philadelphia, 1963, p. 321.

46. Houssay, Bernardo A., et al.: *Human Physiology*. McGraw-Hill Book Co., New York, 1955, p. 522.

47. Brobeck, John R.: *op. cit.*, p. 9–131.

48. Guyton, Arthur C.: *Textbook of Medical Physiology, op. cit.*, p. 539.

49. Comroe, Julius H., et al.: *The Lungs; Clinical Physiology and Pulmonary Function Tests*, 2nd ed. Year Book Medical Publishers, Chicago, 1962, p. 114.

50. Green, J. H.: *Basic Clinical Physiology*, 2nd ed. Oxford University Press, London, 1973, p. 89.

Additional Suggested Reading

Brooks, Frank P.: *Control of Gastrointestinal Function: An Introduction to the Physiology of the Gastrointestinal Tract*. Macmillan Publishing Co., Inc., New York, 1970.

Brundage, Dorothy J.: *Nursing Management of Renal Problems*. C. V. Mosby Co., St. Louis, 1976.

Caldwell, K. P.: "Sphincter Stimulators to Prevent Incontinence," *Nurs. Times*, **69**:1524, (Nov. 15) 1973.

Costill, D. L., et al.: "Water and Electrolyte Replacement During Repeated Days of Work in the Heat," *Aviat. Space Environ. Med.*, **46**:795, (June) 1975.

Dickens, Margaret L.: *Fluid and Electrolyte Balance*. F. A. Davis Co., Philadelphia, 1974.

Given, Barbara A., and Simmons, Sandra J.: *Gastroenterology in Clinical Nursing*, 2nd ed. C. V. Mosby Co., St. Louis, 1975.

Herxheimer, H.: *A Guide to Bronchial Asthma*. Academic Press, New York, 1975.

Jay, Arthur N.: "Is It Indigestion," *Am. J. Nurs.*, **58**:1552, (Nov.) 1958.

Mehbod, H.: "Bongo Drum Hematuria," *Ohio State Med. J.*, **70**:169, (Mar.) 1974.

Ryder, Henry W., et al.: "Future Performance in Footracing," *Sci. Am.*, **234**:109, (June) 1976.

Stanescu, Dan C.: *Early Detection of Chronic Bronchitis and Pulmonary Emphysema*. J. B. Lippincott Co., Philadelphia, 1976.

Young, Jimmy Albert: *Principles and Practice of Respiratory Therapy*, 2nd ed. Year Book Medical Publishers, Chicago, 1976.

Gladys Nite
Virginia Henderson

CHAPTER 12

Body Mechanics—Transportation and Prevention of Pressure Sores

1. BODY MECHANICS AND ITS RELATION TO DISEASE
2. GOOD POSTURE—STANDING, SITTING, AND LYING
3. EXERCISE IN HEALTH AND SICKNESS
4. HELPING THE SICK AND HANDICAPPED TO MOVE
5. TRANSPORTATION IN ILLNESS AND TRAVELING WITH PATIENTS
6. PREVENTION AND TREATMENT OF PRESSURE SORES (BEDSORES OR DECUBITUS ULCERS)

1. BODY MECHANICS AND ITS RELATION TO DISEASE

Body mechanics is an over-all term defined by the White House Conference on Child Health and Protection as "the mechanical correlation of the various systems of the body with special reference to the skeletal, muscular and visceral systems and their neurological associations. Normal body mechanics may be said to obtain when this mechanic correlation is most favorable to the function of these systems." * Far too many health workers, including nurses, are likely to think of body mechanics as including posture and the use of the body in moving and lifting, but it encompasses more than this. Joel E. Goldthwait and his associates [1] in 1952 attributed many chronic ailments to poor body mechanics. They pointed out that posture affects the size and shape of the thoracic, abdominal, and pelvic cavities and that this in turn affects the position of, and pressure on, the viscera. Posture also determines the distribution of weight and pull on the joints. Lack of balance or poise may create tension throughout the body, affecting the vascular, nervous, and muscular systems. Discussing many chronic conditions, they reported marked improvement or complete relief of symptoms chiefly by correction of defective body mechanics. Pictures of patients showing postural changes over many years are convincing evidence of the success of these orthopedists. John G. Kuhns (1962) in his article, "Diseases of Posture," says:

While we cannot say that any disease results from posture alone, faulty alignment produces in various parts of the body many deformities and disabilities that encourage the development of disease. When disease is already present, its symptoms are made worse by the disalignments in the body and often are improved by correction of the faulty posture.

In the chronically ill patient one is given one helpful point of attack in combating the disease. Faulty posture is a condition that is found in the majority of individuals, not only in childhood but also in adult life. In adult life symptoms [of] disease frequently are found with exaggeration of the faulty adjustment of the parts of the body. With each decade, one can expect less efficient use of the body and more evidence of malfunction of the organs.*

Most authorities say that mankind can be divided into structural types; they include the slender, the intermediate, and stocky figures. The intermediate is probably nearest to normal, while the slender and stocky figures have characteristic temperaments, and each group seems subject to characteristic disorders. That these disorders might be explained on a structural basis is not too farfetched since the viscera of the slender and stocky figures differ in size and shape and in the position they assume in the body cavity. Goldthwait et al. make this comforting statement, however:

. . . while the type of the body cannot be changed, the manner in which it is used can be modified greatly. The health of the individual depends largely on this, as well as whether or not he will succumb to one of the diseases of which he is a potential victim. Good health is possible

---

* White House Conference: *Body Mechanics*. Appleton-Century-Crofts, New York, 1932, p. 5.

* Kuhns, John G.: "Diseases of Posture," *Clin. Orthop.*, **25**:69, 1962.

in all the variations from the so-called normal, or intermediate, body type*

Many authorities believe that had man continued to walk on all fours, he would not be subjected to so much pathology involving the spine and its supporting muscles and nerves. However, some students of the subject maintain that the upright body is an efficient mechanism, that its difficulties are the result of misuse, and that if good posture is once established little effort is required to maintain it. They think that postural faults originate in the misuse of our capacities rather than in the structure of the body.[2,3] Adults often suffer from mistakes made in infancy. For example, they may have been forced to sit, stand, or walk before they were developmentally ready. It is believed that an infant will spontaneously do all these things when the structures involved are strong enough. If he or she does them earlier, faulty relationships in body segments are started that tend to be exaggerated in later life unless a great effort is made to overcome them. Joseph H. Kite [4] says the infant who is allowed to sleep consistently on the stomach, knees doubled under with feet turned under, is likely to develop a "bowing" of the entire leg. This position—"Moslem at prayer" or "knee-chest"—is often one of choice as it is similar to the fetal position, aids in the expulsion of flatus, and prevents strangling on regurgitation. There is no harm in the child assuming this position occasionally. Another faulty position that the child may assume is sitting on one foot. This can result in knock-knees or bowlegs. Almost any position in infancy if too prolonged can be harmful. Play pens that condemn crawlers to relative inactivity are harmful. Overweight infants who sit too much of the day are said by some authorities to develop short necks and exaggerated lumbar curves.

Obstetricians, midwives, and obstetric nurses place considerable emphasis on posture for a woman with child. They advocate especially correcting lordosis with its accompanying backache. Such correction should increase circulation, lessen physical strain, minimize fatigue, and reduce the bulge of the expectant mother, making her look less pregnant.[5]

Hans Kraus [6] contends that back pain is frequently precipitated by tensions, sometimes of occupational origin, other emotional problems, and unaccustomed work; also strain from sports or other physical activity. Backache is defined as a "disease of civilization," a lack of

adaptation to changes which have recently been more dramatic than the mechanical changes experienced by man over hundreds of thousands of years. Discussing tension syndrome, he writes:

In our civilized cities we lead the lives of caged animals, with little opportunity to respond, without inhibition, to outside irritations. There is often the added burden of emotional problems, which increase need for release. Since our civilization does not permit the natural response through fight or flight, and since we do not have vicarious outlets through heavy exercise, tension is stored up in our muscles. This constant tension shortens muscles and deprives them of elasticity. Once the muscle tightness has reached a sufficiently high level, and lack of physical activity has weakened the tense muscles, the stage is set for the first episode of back pain.*

Figure 12-1, based on research by Kraus and by others, demonstrates how underexercise combined with overstimulation (which is inherent in our way of life and elicits fight and flight responses) may result in physical and emotional pathology.

The spine is the fundamental basis of sup-

* Kraus, Hans: *Clinical Treatment of Back and Neck Pain.* McGraw-Hill Book Co., New York, 1970, p. 5.

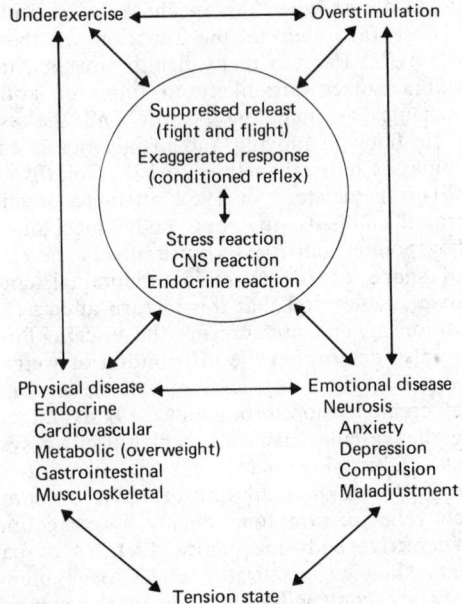

Figure 12-1. Diagram of forces acting on the typical urban person, who is overrested, overfed, overstressed, underexercised, and underreleased. (From Kraus, Hans: *Clinical Treatment of Back and Neck Pain.* McGraw-Hill Book Co., New York, 1970, p. 12.)

* Goldthwait, Joel E., et al.: *Essentials of Body Mechanics—In Health and Disease,* 5th ed. J. B. Lippincott Co., Philadelphia, 1952, p. 8.

port and movement in vertebrates, so abnormal spinal curves profoundly affect the entire body. Nutritional status affects the body's mechanical efficiency. A starved child with protruding abdomen maintains balance by increasing the lumbar curve. Less severe stages of malnutrition at any age are characterized by a musculature too weakened to hold the body erect. We are born in a bow and if we live long enough, most of us will return to it. We learn to stand erect, but the maturing process brings changes in cartilage and bone that make the maintenance of this carriage difficult. David E. Morton found by dissection of the cadavers of persons past middle age that 28 showed "brown degeneration of intervertebral discs that resulted in exaggeration or decrease in normal vertebral curvatures." [*] He considered degeneration sufficiently marked to have produced considerable discomfort as well as poor posture. The point here, however, is that without being facetious we might say that our life represents an effort to stay erect—at least physically.

That bodily attitudes reflect our innermost feelings is commonly accepted. Rene Cailliet says:

There is no doubt that posture can be considered a somatization of the psyche. We stand and move as we feel. Our stance and our movements mirror clearly to the observer our psychologic inner drives or their absence. Consciously or unconsciously we assume a pose to portray our inner feelings, and we move in a manner that depicts our attitudes toward ourselves, our fellow man, and our environment. Our posture is "organ language," a feeling-expression, in fact a postural exteriorization of our inner feelings.[†]

Some Eastern philosophies reflect the position taken in this chapter that posture and movement are influenced by the mood, emotion, or spirit. This body language is clearly shown by. Da Liu,[‡] a teacher of T'ai Chi Ch'uan, which he calls "a choreography of body and mind." The movements he teaches are based on *The I Ching or Book of Changes* [§] which in one form or another has influenced China for 3000 years. First translated into French and German, it is now available in English and it is influencing Western thought. It embodies the wisdom of Tao, Confucius, and other leaders of Eastern thought. Da Liu says this in the Introduction to his illustrated text on this system of exercise:

Although its roots are in ancient China, T'ai Chi Ch'uan is very suitable for tense Westerners. It has the advantages of regular exercise combined with a definite emphasis on the gracefulness and slowness of pace that Western society so conspicuously lacks. T'ai Chi Ch'uan can give those who live in industrialized fast-paced cities a compensating factor in their lives. It relaxes the mind as well as the body. It helps digestion, quiets the nervous system, benefits the heart and blood circulation, makes joints loose, and refreshes the skin.

Any age group can practice T'ai Chi. Liu Shoting, a contemporary T'ai Chi master, at eighty-four years of age still teaches it to students. He began to practice after he had a heart attack at the age of sixty. In three years, he was out of danger with a stronger and more vigorous body than before.

Throughout the world T'ai Chi is performed for a variety of reasons. Dance and theater schools in America use it as part of their training routines. Medical institutions in China use it to aid in restoring health. In New York it is even taught in old-age homes. For daily exercise and for maintaining health it is an ideal regimen.

T'ai Chi is taught the military as a means of defense but Da Liu says "Personally, I agree with the great master Chang San-feng when he said, 'This exercise will lead many practitioners to health, happiness, and longevity. The defense is secondary.' I don't like to emphasize competition or pushing hands in my classes. Still, in its proper place, T'ai Chi Ch'uan is an effective defense form and I teach it when I am sure sufficient forms have been mastered." [*]

The idea of defending oneself without injuring the other person is appealing and reflects a state of mind. There are other such forms of self-defense taught now, Karate for example, but as Da Liu says the idea of grace of movement, or enhancement of life generally, is the best reason for acquiring this total discipline.

By the development and maintenance of good body mechanics we may hope to make possible our optimum physical effectiveness and prevent many chronic ailments, but we can expect with equal assurance that the mental and emotional aspects of life, if they can be said to be separated from the physical, will likewise be affected. Goldthwait and his as-

[*] Morton, David E.: "An Anatomical Study in the Human Spinal Column with Emphasis on Degenerative Changes in the Cervical Region," *Yale J. Biol. Med.*, **23**:126, (Feb.) 1950.

[†] Cailliet, Rene: *Low Back Pain Syndrome*, 2nd ed. F. A. Davis Co., Philadelphia, 1968, p. 16.

[‡] Da Liu: *T'ai Chi Ch'uan and I Ching*. Harper & Row, New York, 1972.

[§] *The I Ching or Book of Changes*, 3rd ed. The Richard Wilhelm Translation rendered into English by Cary F. Baynes. Foreword by C. G. Jung. Princeton University Press, Princeton, N.J., 1967.

[*] Da Liu: *op. cit.*, p. 2.

sociates believe that efforts to develop good posture should begin at birth and that children should be universally taught the right way to stand, walk, run, lift, and so on. With their methods of reeducation they are able to help the cooperative patient of almost any age. Henry O. Kendall and associates assume that nature takes a more aggressive role in developing good posture. They say:

Most postural deviations in the growing individual fall in the category of developmental deviations; when patterns become habitual they may result in postural faults. . . . A young child is not very likely to have habitual faults and can be harmed by corrective measures that are not needed. Over-correction may lead to atypical faults more harmful and difficult to deal with than the ones which caused original concern. . . .*

W. Harry Fahrni believes that much of our postural difficulties can be attributed to postural training which is often based on military connotations. Following a comparative study of postures of a primitive society (Bhil tribe of India), he concludes:

An analysis of the postures of these primitive people suggests that they, in a spontaneous and untutored manner, practice methods of rest and locomotion that closely approach the mechanical ideal. If such is the case, the resulting improvement in function should result in demonstrable reduction in their susceptibility to the back troubles that our civilization knows so well. . . . The symptoms of back pain, sciatica, and back strain, so common in our part of the world, are completely lacking in the jungle. The women recognize no back pain except that occurring with labor pains, and the men associate it with no less an episode than a fall from the top of a palm tree.†

While there may be points of disagreement among orthopedists, most would agree that with an adequate diet and minimum help from experts almost everyone in this country could avoid the now-prevalent structural defects with their threat of concomitant ailments. It is hard to think of a preventive program more far reaching in its effects. Nurses should learn as much as they can about body mechanics in order to practice what they learn for their own benefit; they will soon realize, however, that not only are they able to influence others by their example but also that almost every activity of patient care offers an opportunity to foster good habits in their patients or improve poor ones. As far as this topic is concerned, we are all trainees subject to stress and strain,

and should be constantly alert to danger. Nurses will often leave their patients beautifully "postured" to promote rest and sleep and then themselves lie down to rest in an atrocious position; or they will lift prostrated patients to spare them effort, not considering that they may incapacitate themselves for further service.[6a] Barbara W. Narrow [7] found that 81 per cent of 173 nurses did not use a lifter in moving patients as it did not "save time." Obviously, these nurses did not recognize the purpose of the lifter—to protect both the patient and worker from injury. The writers suggest that nurses study this chapter for its value to them as individuals and workers. In many cases no effort will be made to differentiate these values since it is assumed that a principle of body mechanics is as applicable to one person as another. School and industrial nurses are in a particularly good position to contribute to the prevention of structural defects and so-called orthopedic illness.[7a] They can help to select and design chairs, stools, ladders, tables, and desks that make good body mechanics for students and workers possible.* Clothing and particularly shoes affect posture; their choice is especially important during infancy and childhood, and in pregnancy. Many industries present special orthopedic hazards as, for example, those that require workers to maintain one posture or that necessitate wearing heavy equipment. It may take the combined efforts of the industrial physician, the nurse, the industrial engineer, and the workers themselves to control fatigue and prevent disease in the occupations concerned.

No attempt has been made to cover the treatment of orthopedic conditions. Nurses should develop the habit of consulting articles and texts in the fields of body mechanics, neurology, and pediatrics as they are faced with complex orthopedic problems in patient care.

Readers interested in various methods for assessing mobility and functional status of patients should consult additional references at the end of this chapter.[7b-d]

2. GOOD POSTURE—STANDING, SITTING, AND LYING

Standing Posture. "Ideal," "normal," and "standard" postures as described usually refer

---

* Kendall, Henry O., et al.: *Posture and Pain.* Williams & Wilkins Co., Baltimore, 1952, p. 167.
† Fahrni, W. Harry: *Backache Relieved Through New Concepts of Posture.* Charles C Thomas, Publisher, Springfield, Ill., 1966, p. 50.

* The second writer is forcibly reminded of this obvious need at the moment. Working in a beautiful *medical* library where the only seats are the traditional Windsor chairs, whose arms keep them at a respectful distance from the table on which she writes, she must use a pad in the seat to keep from being thrown backward and a footstool made from her materials to keep her feet from dangling.

to the standing position. The terms are often used interchangeably and refer to skeletal alignment. The ideal posture may be seen only occasionally among young people at the university track field but is rarely seen in the middle-aged, according to Fahrni.[8] Because of the body's continual motility, the calculation of its center of gravity is difficult. The body cannot be held immobile long as it undergoes unconscious muscular contractions. An examination of frozen cadavers has shown that the center of body gravity is toward the superior part of the third sacral vertebra. However, this is an arbitrary localization because the person who even raises an arm without shifting the position of the feet changes the center of gravity 7 cm above that shown with cadavers.[9] J. V. Basmajian, on the basis of his research and that of others, concludes:

The idealized normal erect posture is one in which the line of gravity drops in the midline between the following bilateral points: (1) the mastoid processes, (2) a point just in front of the shoulder joints, (3) the hip joints (or just behind), (4) a point just in front of the center of the knee joints, and (5) a point just in front of the ankle joints. Muscular activity is called upon to approximate this posture or, if the body is pulled out of the line of gravity, to bring it back into line.*

Usually there is no awareness of this muscular activity or of the mechanical forces involved, as these responses occur in a graded fashion and are associated with all voluntary movements and postural adjustments of the body as a whole to maintain equilibrium.[10] Based on their studies of boys and adults, Erling Asmussen and Klaus Klausen [11] report that the back muscles are most frequently used to counteract the force of gravity but the abdominal muscles are used in about 20 to 25 per cent of the cases.

A good standing posture is characterized by poise or balance without tension or rigidity. It is maintained by the coordinated activity of the muscles which is largely automatic.[12] Nila Kirkpatrick Covalt gives a more complete description of the requirements for the standing (vertical) position or lying (horizontal) position:

The head is aligned on the neck, and the entire spine is in a vertical straight line. The two normal curves in the cervical and lumbar areas are in accordance with this alignment. Both legs are straight, being supported from the pelvis. The feet are at right angles and pointing straight ahead.†

She describes standard alignment essentially as that given by Basmajian (above) and says the neutrality of this position has been documented by electromyography (a study of muscle contractions induced by electric stimulation).

The effects of good posture and body mechanics include a proper relationship between the various segments of the body with minimum energy expended in balancing the segments as well as in the ease and grace of movement.[13]

In the past, emphasis was placed on "throw the shoulders back"; present emphasis is on "stand tall" and pulling in the abdomen. It is now believed that the older method of maintaining "good" posture was detrimental because the person generally assumed a position of extreme lordosis—this prevented correct use of the lower abdominal muscles. To maintain correct trunk alignment which is the basis of good posture, it is important that the lower abdomen is pulled in and up, the buttocks tucked in, the back flat, the head up and the chin in, and that the weight is thrown well forward on the outer borders of the feet. The body is then stretched tall but without rigidity. Only with such a posture can correct weight-bearing lines be maintained. When the lower abdominal muscles only are pulled in, there is no interference with normal breathing.

No posture is a good one if it is taut. Directions to "hold" any position is not only wrong but impossible to follow for any length of time. When it is necessary to stand for long periods it helps to separate the feet and thus to broaden the base supporting the body. This is done instinctively when standing in a moving vehicle. If the weight is shifted from one leg to the other by flexing one knee, the transverse axis of the pelvis should be kept horizontal with the floor to prevent lateral spinal curvatures. Because it is almost impossible to stand correctly in the wrong shoes it is advisable, before describing sitting and lying posture, to discuss their selection and emphasize the position the feet should assume.

Foot Posture and Selection of Shoes. A well-balanced body is only possible if the feet are in the relationship to it described in the preceding paragraphs and shown in Figure 12-2. Likewise, the most normal feet are those of persons whose bodies are in good alignment. Orthopedists warn against treating the back, for example, without considering the feet or trying to correct a foot disability without attempting to modify an accompanying spinal curvature. Minor structural foot defects often disappear when body mechanics in other parts of the body is improved, although many conditions require local treatment.

* Basmajian, J. V.: "Man's Posture," *Arch. Phys. Med. Rehabil.,* **46:**26, (Jan.) 1965.
† Covalt, Nila Kirkpatrick: *Bed Exercises for Convalescent Patients.* Charles C Thomas, Publisher, Springfield, Ill., 1968, p. 42.

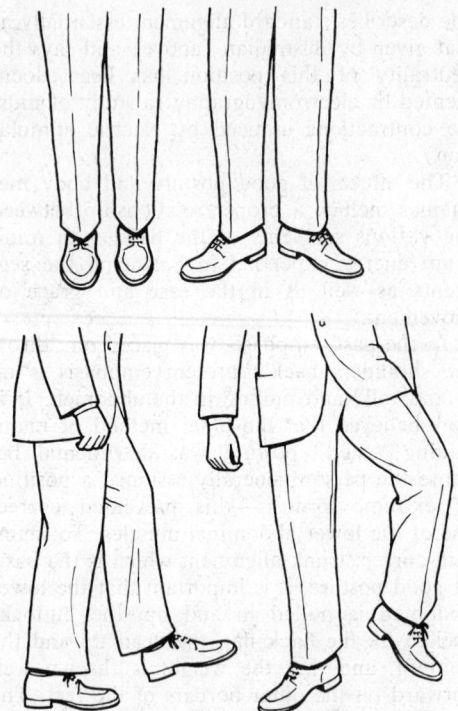

Figure 12-2. (*Top left*) Correct standing position; (*top right*) incorrect standing position. (*Bottom left*) Correct walking posture; (*bottom right*) incorrect walking posture. (Based on Krusen, Frank H.: *Physical Medicine.* W. B. Saunders Co., Philadephia, 1941.)

Most persons are born with potentially efficient feet; a few have congenital defects such as flatfoot or clubfoot, missing or extra toes. In flatfoot the connective tissues holding the bones together (ligaments and fascia) are too relaxed to preserve the arched arrangement of the tarsals and metatarsals seen in the average foot. The condition appears in both feet, whereas it is rare to find more than one clubfoot—a condition of inversion and rotation with abnormally short tendons, or contracted fascia, in parts of the foot producing and maintaining this abnormal position. Normal feet in a normal standing posture are parallel with each other; inverted feet are called *talipes varus,* while feet turned outward, or everted, are called *talipes valgus.* Inversion is more likely to be a congenital defect; eversion is more likely to be acquired as a result of faulty posture of the entire body. A short Achilles tendon is sometimes present at birth but is usually found in those who habitually wear high heels. Other acquired foot deformities associated with poor body mechanics are pronation of the foot (eversion of the heel with depression of the longitudinal arch) and the

changes that result from wearing high-heeled shoes over a long period of time. Besides shortening the tendon of Achilles (the tendon of the gastrocnemius muscle) this practice thickens the muscles above the ankle and spreads the forefoot which bears the weight of the body. Wearing shoes with high heels also interferes with the development of the tissues of the heel and increases the risk of lateral tilting and ankle sprain, as in the tilted foot the heel bears no weight, being used merely as a "feeler" in walking.[14] Donald K. Mathews and Edna P. Wooten [15] report that more oxygen was consumed per minute by women when walking in high-heeled shoes on a horizontal plane and on a 6 per cent grade plane than when they were wearing "saddle and loafer" shoes or when walking barefoot. Short shoes, especially if pointed and coupled with high heels, turn the big toe away from the midline of the body and enlarge the metatarsophalangeal joint (*hallux valgus*). Over this joint a protective cushion soon forms which we call a bunion. When the weight of the body is thrust on the point of the foot the second toe is often elongated (a "hammer toe") and calluses form on it. Calluses (corns) form on any area of the foot where irritation is constant. Nature develops them, like bunions, to protect underlying tissues.

It seems quite obvious that training in body mechanics, including selection of proper shoes, will prevent many difficulties. The effects of foot defects on the general health and motility, including work and leisure, are far-reaching. They are costly to the person, sometimes in treatment, but frequently in the purchase of many pairs of shoes that must be discarded long before they are worn out. People with a foot defect suffer discomfort or pain locally or in other parts of the body; they are tired and their gait is abnormal. They are robbed of much of the joy of life.[16] The child with a well-balanced body will stand and walk with the feet parallel. Stressing this position of the feet helps to promote good posture throughout the body but correcting only this aspect of posture is rarely enough. Shoes should be chosen with utmost care, and the child helped to understand why certain features of their construction are important. Charles LeRoy Lowman and Carl Haven Young say:

. . . if a child's feet are not properly shod before 7 years of age, during the formative period, they are likely to be more seriously injured than they would be later in life during the same length of time.*

---

* Lowman, Charles LeRoy, and Young, Carl Haven: *Postural Fitness, Significance and Variance.* Lea & Febiger, Philadelphia, 1960, p. 67.

They also emphasize the importance of wearing proper shoes during adolescence. Laurence Jones [17] says there are three types of shoes on the market: flexible, semiflexible, and rigid, and, of the three types, only the rigid can satisfactorily hold up under the weight-bearing stress to which they are subjected. He describes a technique that can be used in recognizing a suitable shoe (see Fig. 12-3). All health workers will find his description helpful. It is too long to cite here but he emphasizes a well-fitted heel, reinforcement with a steel shank, and plastic counter and room for the toes, enabling each in turn to bear weight in walking. The points stressed by most orthopedists are shown in Figure 12-4: (1) a straight inside line, (2) adequate space for the forefoot without undue spreading, (3) sufficient length to prevent pressure on the end of toes, and (4) a low heel as broad as the foot itself.

Persons who suffer from foot defects should seek the advice of an orthopedist who may correct the posture, the gait, and the selection of shoes. Occasionally surgery is indicated.

Sitting Posture. The same objectives should be kept in mind for sitting that have just been implied in the discussion of standing. Spinal curves should not be exaggerated, but the trunk held or supported in an upright position with the lower abdomen in, the back flat, and the chin in. To "sit tall" is just as important as to "stand tall." The chair seat should be deep enough to support the buttocks and most of the thighs and the chair low enough to allow the feet to rest on the floor. There should be no lateral curvature from leaning to one side.

Reclining chairs should be constructed with a straight back that supports the entire trunk and head. Mechanical chairs that can be operated by the occupant are very desirable, especially if they permit slight changes of posture so that the pressure on the supporting body surfaces can be modified at frequent intervals. A concave back rest results in a spinal flexion that crowds the thoracic viscera, relaxes the abdomen, and displaces its contents. Everyone should observe these rules for the sake of health; nurses who make provisions for, and help patients into sitting postures should see that these conditions are met. In some situations improvisation will be necessary; with well-chosen hospital equipment it is merely a matter of using it correctly.

For the average patient who is confined to bed, flexion of the knees is essential for comfort, and to prevent sliding down. But the angle of the knee bend should be less than 15 degrees to prevent pressure on blood vessels which interferes with circulation and may contribute to the development of blood clots. However, those with a motor disability, such as paraplegia and hemiplegia, should have their extremities extended so that contractures may not develop. No patient, in fact, should be kept in the same position for long periods.[17a] The back should be straight from the

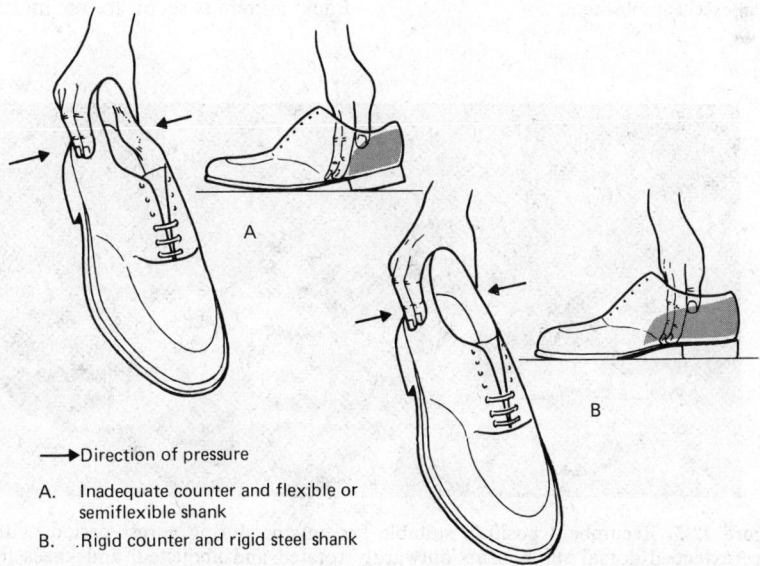

→ Direction of pressure

A. Inadequate counter and flexible or semiflexible shank

B. Rigid counter and rigid steel shank

Figure 12-3. Tests for structural weakness in shoes. *A*. A structurally weak shoe. *B*. An adequately strong shoe. (From Jones, Laurence: *The Postural Complex: Observation as to Causes, Diagnosis and Treatment.* Charles C Thomas, Publisher, Springfield, Ill., 1955, p. 80.)

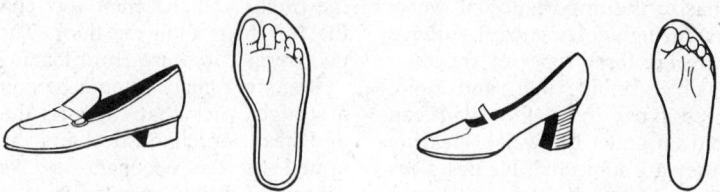

Figure 12-4. (*Left*) Correct style of shoe, and toes in natural position; (*right*) incorrect style of shoe, and toes cramped. (Based on Krusen, Frank H.: *Physical Medicine.* W. B. Saunders Co., Philadelphia, 1941.)

coccyx to the occiput. A small pillow to fill in the cervical curvature adds to comfort.* If the arms are supported with pillows, as in an armchair, it is easier to maintain the elevation of the ribs that prevents pressure on the thoracic organs. A footboard in bed takes the place of the floor when sitting in a chair. It helps the patient to maintain erectness of the spine and it prevents "foot drop."

Most authorities consulted make the point that there are many ways of sitting correctly and incorrectly. A good sitting posture is one that prevents crowding of the viscera, exaggeration of normal vertebral curves, contractures, or fatigue from lack of support. Kraus, discussing tension and associated pain in various parts of the body, emphasizes the importance of good posture in sitting, properly

* The second author finds a folded bath towel extremely comfortable under the head. During hot weather when perspiration often wets a pillow, a towel that can be easily replaced when damp and that has a clean odor is an excellent substitute.

constructed seats, and frequent changes of position. No matter how comfortable it is at first, any position is tiring if maintained for long. On the basis of many studies, F. Gaynor Evans [18] says the body weight is supported primarily by the ischial tuberosities and the soft tissues beneath them. It is not surprising to see people of all ages changing their position frequently.

Lying Posture. A firm bed is essential to good alignment of body segments in a horizontal position. Too often springs and mattresses allow the heaviest part of the body (the hips usually) to sink far below the level of the head and shoulders, which results in a marked lateral, posterior, or anterior spinal curvature according to whether the person is lying on the back, side, or abdomen. Orthopedists are discouraging the use of inner-spring mattresses, and there is such a general demand for firm beds that some hotels will supply patrons with "bed boards" on request. Back ailments seem to be increasing. Inner-

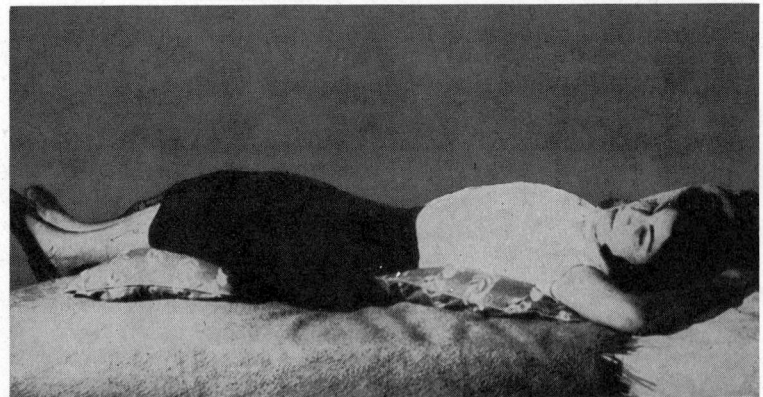

Figure 12-5. Recumbent position suitable for anyone during a rest period, with hyperextended dorsal spine, arms outwardly rotated and abducted, and knees flexed to relax abdominal muscles and flatten lower back. This position is healthy for the prenatal patient, arthritic, or person with round shoulders. It elevates the chest, brings the diaphragm higher, and makes more room for abdominal organs. (Courtesy of Joint Orthopedic Nursing Advisory Service, New York, N.Y.)

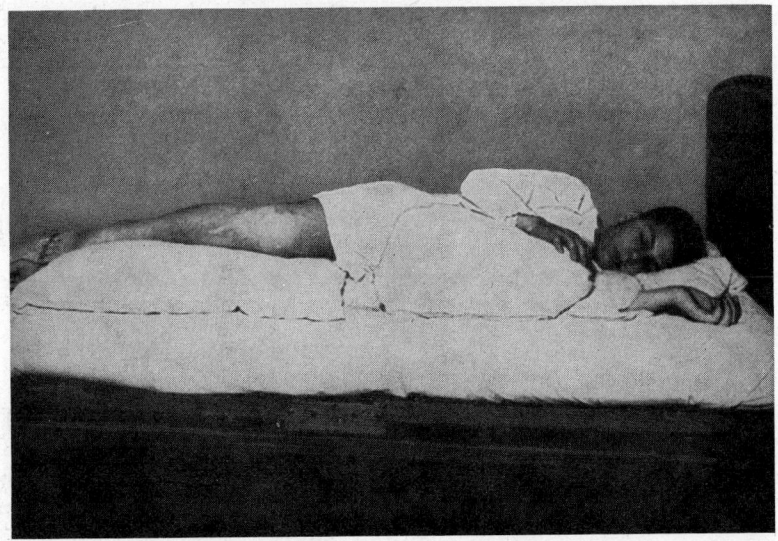

Figure 12-6. Correct side-lying position. A small pillow or pad under the head preserves alignment of cervical spine. Pillows to support upper arm and thigh prevent strain on ligaments and on joint capsules of shoulder and hip. (Courtesy of Joint Orthopedic Nursing Advisory Service, New York, N.Y.)

spring mattresses, automobiles that discourage walking, and all the laborsaving mechanisms that replace muscular activity are contributing factors.

Figures 12-5, 12-6, and 12-7 show what is believed to be correct *supine, side-lying* (lateral), and *prone* positions. In each, the following principles are observed: (1) the back is straight, or its normal curves unexaggerated, from the coccyx to the occiput; (2) the legs are flexed to relieve the strain on the lumbar

spine, the abdomen, and the legs; (3) the ribs are elevated and the "rib cage" enlarged, or constriction prevented; (4) the legs are supported so that the weight of one does not fall on the other; and (5) excessive ankle extension is prevented.

Many modifications of these positions are used according to patients' special needs. See Figure 12-8 for positioning of infants with myelomeningocele. For example, weak or paralyzed muscles require more extensive support

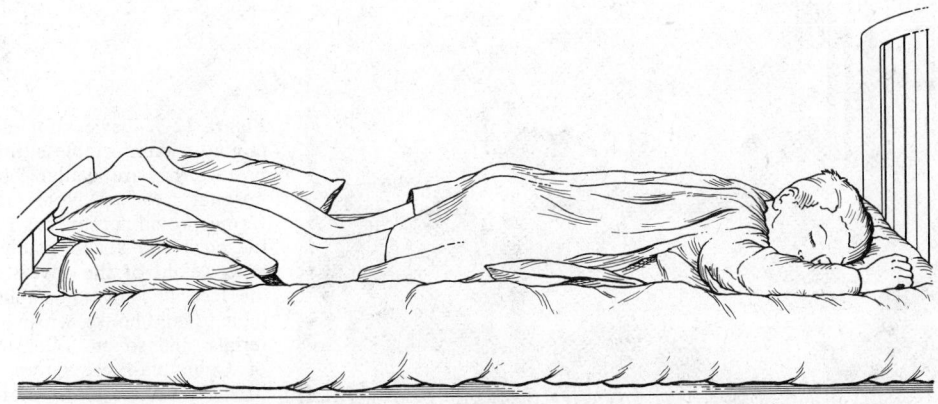

Figure 12-7. Diagram to illustrate prone position. Pillow under abdomen preserves alignment of spine. Pillows permit knee flexion, prevent pressure on toes, and allow good position of feet. If knees are straight, feet should hang over end of mattress at right angles and a small pad should be placed under ankles. Small roll under shoulders maintains shoulder girdle in correct alignment. (Courtesy of Joint Orthopedic Nursing Advisory Service, New York, N.Y.)

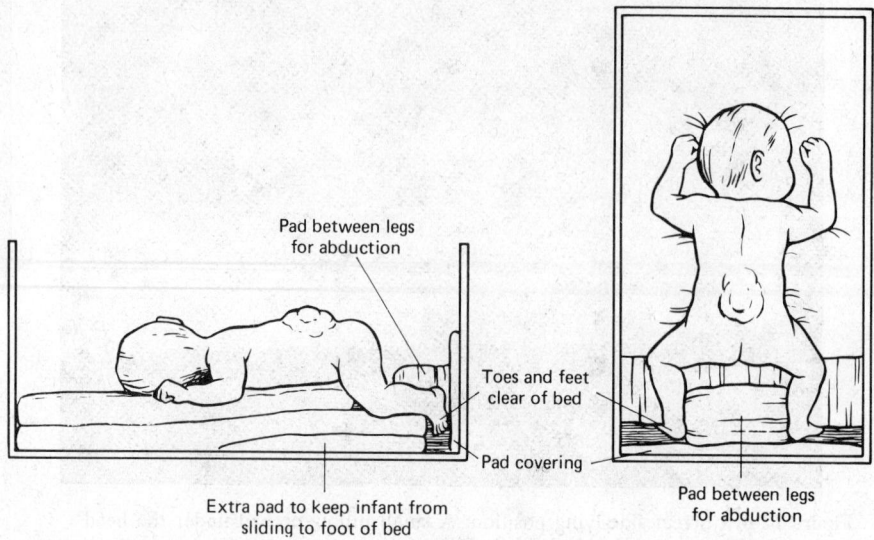

Pad between legs
for abduction

Toes and feet
clear of bed

Pad covering

Extra pad to keep infant from
sliding to foot of bed

Pad between legs
for abduction

Figure 12-8. An infant with myelomeningocele can be maintained in this position either in an incubator or an open crib. The position is used before repair of the defect, and afterward until sutures are removed and the skin is well healed. (From Passo, Sherrilyn DeJean: "Positioning Infants with Myelomeningocele," *Am. J. Nurs.*, **74:**1658, [Sept.] 1974.)

from pillows, rolled towels, sandbags, and other devices; pain in the back or the abdomen may call for increased flexion of the legs, and in spastic conditions contractures are prevented with splints, trochanter rolls, and other devices. An effective bed positioning program helps prevent decubiti and deformities.[19] Norman L. Browse [20] notes that damage to the intima of the blood vessel may be caused by an improper lying position (on side) with the upper leg resting on the lower leg which makes the upper knee press on the lower popliteal vein. Those who are conscious will usually move, finding a more comfortable position, but the totally unconscious patient will not. (Note that in Figure 12-6, the upper leg has been brought forward and is supported with a pillow.) Nurses will find Browse's book, *The*

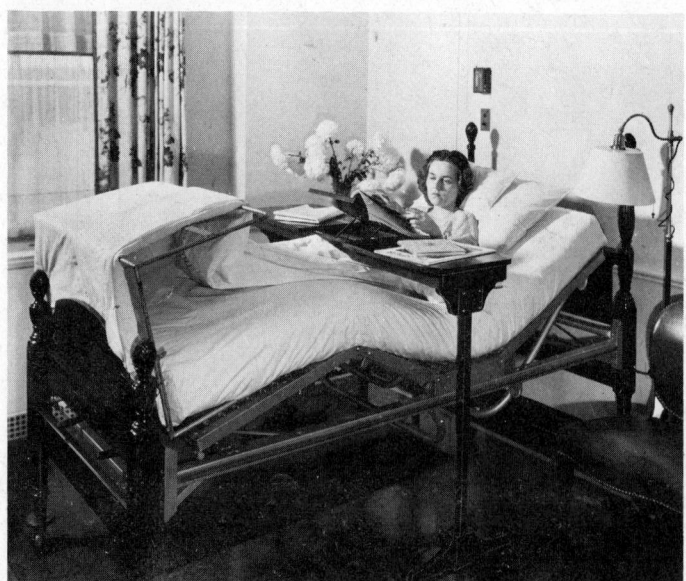

Figure 12-9. Devices for maintaining a comfortable sitting posture that are available to hospital patients. Note Gatch frame providing support for the back and knees, cradle to take weight of the covers off the feet, and an adjustable table to hold books, writing materials, and so on. (Courtesy of Columbia-Presbyterian Medical Center, New York City.)

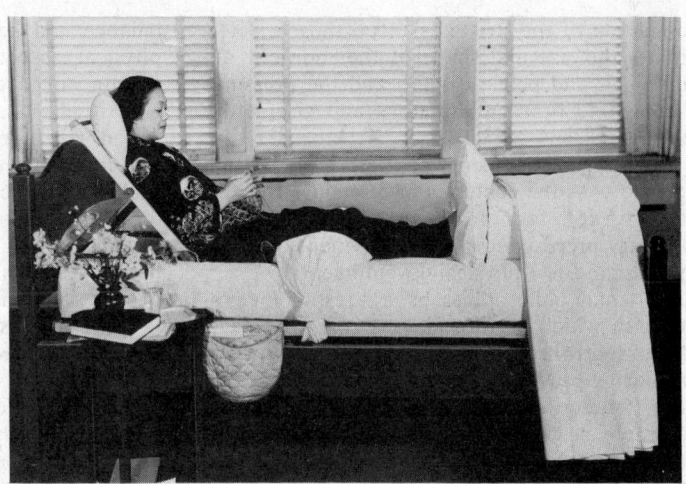

Figure 12-10. Devices for maintaining comfortable sitting posture in bed that are available in most homes. Note inexpensive removable back rest, pillow wrapped in a sheet and tied to bedsprings for knee support, a wooden box weighted by bricks to support the feet, prevent foot drop, and keep the weight of the covers off the toes.

Physiology and Pathology of Bed Rest, informative and provocative. Texts on orthopedic and neurologic nursing should be consulted, also, for amplification of the subject.

Foot Boards and Cradles. The weight of the bedclothes may often cause pain or distort posture. In such cases a board is placed between the mattress and foot of the bed to keep the feet in dorsal flexion and to support the covers, or a cradle is put on the bed over the feet to support the covers. Of the two, the foot board is by far the best. If used properly, it supports the feet in dorsal flexion, and foot-drop will not occur in most patients regardless of the length of time they are confined to bed. A great variety of cradles are available.

Equipment used in hospitals should be light so that it can be transported easily, and collapsible so that it can be stored in a small space. It should be possible to use a cradle on any part of the bed and to fix it in position. Figure 12-9 shows an aluminum cradle made in two parts and having these qualifications. It can also be equipped with a removable, thermostatically controlled light bulb to warm the air under the cradle or furnish heat prescribed for therapy. Cradles may be improvised in homes from a variety of materials. In Figure 12-10 the box used as an improvised foot rest also keeps the weight of the covers off the toes. A suitably shaped carton or wooden box with the bottom and one side removed makes an excellent cradle over a leg or arm.

Terms Used in Faulty Postures. The orthopedist uses the following terms in describing common postural faults or deviations: An anterior, posterior, or lateral *tilt* of the pelvis or *rotation* of the pelvis or thorax; *lordosis,* a forward curve of the spine used with reference to an increase in the lumbar curve; *kyphosis,* a backward curve of the spine most commonly

seen in the thorax; *round shoulders,* abduction of the scapula associated with a forward position of the shoulders; "bowlegs," lateral outward curvature of the legs from postural or structural causes; *knock-knees,* touching of the knees when the feet are separated; *pronation,* weight-bearing on the inside of the sole; and *supination,* weight-bearing on the outer side of the foot.

3. EXERCISE IN HEALTH AND SICKNESS

Life is a series of actions and reactions. Living cells have rhythms of increased and decreased activity. Contraction followed by relaxation, the "specialty" of muscle cells, is the most conspicuous cell activity. The muscles of the body, of which there are more than 600, constitute almost one-half of the body weight. Their contraction and relaxation give the face its expression, produce voice sounds and movements of the body characteristic of species and individuals. There is some form of movement in every part of the body. When we speak of exercise we usually refer to activity of voluntary or striated muscle. We are likely to forget that life is far more dependent on the smooth muscles of the viscera. Because they are involuntary, not under the control of the cerebral cortex, we are likely to forget that normal visceral activity depends indirectly on the tone of the voluntary musculature.* The

* While visceral muscles are not ordinarily controlled consciously, the mind can control them. Experiments with laboratory animals have shown that with a system of rewards and punishment they can be made to increase or decrease their heart rate and intestinal motility. Psychologists and psychiatrists have pointed out that children can learn how to induce nausea and
(Continued)

condition of the striated skeletal muscle determines the size and shape of the thoracic, abdominal, and pelvic cavities and the pressures brought to bear on excretory and circulatory organs.

A study of the history of exercise shows that people over the centuries have engaged in this activity for four reasons: (1) health; (2) military preparedness; (3) enjoyment or social values; and (4) physical development.

Oriental philosophies have stressed meditation, in which posture plays a role, and carefully controlled body activity as a means of achieving peace of mind and a sound body. Da Liu [20a] describes and shows in a series of photographs a system of slow-flowing movements that are based on *The I Ching or Book of Changes,* in which Confucianism and Taoism have common roots.[20b] Its content is derived from 64 hexagrams that existed before 1150 B.C., at about which time commentaries were added by King Wen and the Duke of Chou.[20c] The English version of this book is now in its ninth printing. The ideas in it have meaning for our time. Body control based on Zen, Karate, Yoga, and other Oriental thought appeals to many Western peoples. Among their uses is self-defense with minimum violence. A small person who has learned balance and maximum use of motor power can ward off a blow, or even toss a person twice his or her size half-way across the room. Such methods of self-defense have been part of military training in armies of the East.

Among the Western peoples the Greeks are thought to be the first advocates of exercise as promoting health. The idea that people can recover from illness and weaknesses through exercises was promoted by Galen, a Greek physician born in A.D. 130. The Greeks were also concerned with fitness for military service, which was considered a citizen's responsibility, and they were intrigued with the symmetry and beauty of the body. Emphasis was placed on

balance and harmony in the intellectual and physical aspects of life. In the late 1800s, Britain advanced the concept of good health consisting of exercise, general hygiene, and sound nutrition. Richard T. Mackey [20d] says that it was not until Catherine Beecher (1856) published her book, *Physiology and Calisthenics for Schools and Families,* that Americans began to think of exercise as influencing their health. Women's clothing and the concepts of proper feminine behavior made exercise difficult. The musical *Bloomer Girl* was a commentary on the women's liberation of the nineteenth century that included freedom to dress appropriately for sports. Physical training programs were instituted but the enjoyment of exercise or sports has continued to be important for both sexes from that time to the present.

Eugene S. Ferguson [21] writes that as machines began to replace the muscles of man as a source of power, serious investigators began to find out how much physical labor a man could be expected to do in a day. He notes that the effort continued into the present century. Because our way of life has changed so drastically, Egill Snorrason thinks that planned physical exercise is now necessary for all. He says:

Machines have taken over the heavy work of daily life, and motorization eases the burden of mankind in industry, on the farm, in the office, and in the home. But even mechanization demands physical fitness to manage and coordinate the ever-increasing mastery of machines, for without it the fate of the "Sorcerer's Apprentice" shall be that of man. Physical fitness is necessary to meet the exigencies of the moment. As the relentless demands of the times are a drain on health, it must be maintained by exercise, for health is not a permanent gift. Daily exercise will maintain physical fitness in young and old; it has become a necessity of life just as it was once necessary in making a living.*

Da Liu, commenting on the system of exercises derived from *The Book of Changes,* says they are especially useful for those who live in an industrialized urban setting with its ever-present stress.

During the past two decades, numerous studies, with as many as 10,000 subjects, have been conducted on the physical fitness of North American children as compared with those of other countries including Great Britain, Italy, Sweden, Austria, Japan, and Pakistan; the findings of these studies consistently

---

vomiting, produce abdominal cramps or a headache, if they find them useful ways of being excused from distasteful work or going to an uncongenial school, although they may not realize that they are using a symptom as a means of manipulating others. The effect of thought, or the recall of former experience, on visceral activity is the explanation of so-called psychosomatic illness. There is still much to learn about the effect of "the unconscious" on involuntary muscles. Sidney M. Jourard takes the extreme position that all illness is rebellion against frustration. He says "People inevitably *sicken* as they live in the ways their society seems to demand. I have come to see sickness of all kinds, whether 'physical' or 'mental' *as a form of protest against a way of life that is not fit for the person who is living it.*" (Jourard, Sidney M.: *Disclosing Man To Himself.* Van Nostrand Reinhold Co., New York, 1968, p. 38.)

* Snorrason, Egill: "Exercise for Healthy Persons," in Licht, Sidney (ed.): *Therapeutic Exercise,* 2nd ed. rev. Elizabeth Licht, Publisher, New Haven, Conn., 1965, p. 896.

Table 12-1. Physical Fitness of Austrian and American Males *

Fitness Category	Per Cent
1157 Austrian Males—Initial Testing (18 to 20 years of age)	
I. Very poor	0.6
II. Poor	3.6
III. Fair	20.5
IV. Good	44.5
V. Excellent	30.8
1370 American Males—Initial Testing (18 to 20 years of age)	
I. Very poor	3.0
II. Poor	6.7
III. Fair	31.2
IV. Good	52.8
V. Excellent	6.3

* Cooper, Kenneth H.: *The New Aerobics.* Bantam Books, Inc., New York, 1970, p. 33.

show that American children are less physically fit than those of other countries, and therefore are likely to develop a variety of physical problems in later life.* Lack of exercise because too much time is spent on the school bus, or in an automobile, in the play pen, or watching television or movies is thought to be responsible for the lack of physical fitness of American children.[22-24] Poor physical fitness, begun in childhood, extends into adulthood as would be expected. Kenneth H. Cooper[25] cites the work of Zechner (1969), a captain in the Austrian army, who used the 12-minute and 1.5-mile test (developed by Cooper) to determine the physical fitness of young Austrian males whose average age was 19 years. A comparison of his findings with those of Cooper (who used the same test) on a comparable group of Americans is shown in Table 12-1. It is obvious that the Austrian male is better off than his counterpart in the United States. Walking and cycling are common means of transportation in Austria and country hikes are a favorite Sunday activity, whereas in the United States the automobile is our chief mode of transportation and we have what may be called fancier entertainment.

* The "play pen" in which so many North American infants are confined while the mother goes about her business is particularly harmful. It discourages crawling, which is the natural means of developing muscles that will enable the baby to stand, walk, and run, and the pen prevents exploration of the environment from which he or she learns the shape, texture, temperature, and use of everything in it.

Studies have shown that lack of activity correlates very closely with neck and back pain.[26]

Cooper, who developed and tested a simple exercise program used by members of the US Air Force, as well as many persons of all ages in our society, and who continues to study the effects of exercise on physical fitness, believes that Europe (especially Scandinavia) is years ahead of North America in the study, promotion, and practice of exercise as a means of developing and maintaining physical fitness. He says:

In Sweden alone, there are more than five hundred bicycle ergometers (stationary bicycles on which the subject pumps against a work load fed into the machine) distributed around the country. And they are not buried in research laboratories, but are available for public use in schools, clinics and factories.*

He contends that the results of a workout for a few minutes on such a machine will tell the person what his or her physical condition is at the moment. There is no such machine available to the average person in the United States; the closest public facility to a health indicator is the weight scale which gives a superficial indication of the person's health.

As a result of the physical fitness program instituted by the late President John F. Kennedy, the President's Council on Physical Fitness has published (1964) a series of pamphlets for all ages: (1) *Adult Physical Fitness* (a home exercise plan for men and women); (2) *Youth Physical Fitness* (suggestions for school programs); (3) *Physical Fitness Elements in Recreation* (suggestions for community programs); (4) *Vim* (a complete exercise plan for girls 12 to 18); and (5) *Vigor: A Complete Exercise Plan for Boys 12 to 18.* Each of these pamphlets emphasizes the importance of regular exercise and its positive effects on a healthy and productive life. *The New Aerobics*[27] and *Aerobics*[28] include a planned exercise program for persons of different ages, how much exercise each person needs, and how to measure the benefits; they are informative, easy to read, and entertaining —a rare combination. Nurses will find all of these publications useful for themselves and as references for their patients in any setting.

Robert C. Darling,[29] writing in Sidney Licht's text, discusses the following physiologic effects of active exercise: (1) increased respiratory rate and oxygen consumption; (2) liberation of heat with increase of body temperature; (3) increase in the number of active

* Cooper, Kenneth H.: *Aerobics.* M. Evans & Co., New York, 1968, p. 44.

capillaries; (4) increased venous return to the heart resulting in (5) larger output of blood with each stroke; (6) rise in blood pressure; and (7) pulse rate and increased production, distribution, and elimination of lactic acid and carbon dioxide. Any increase in metabolism is attributed to circulatory stimulation and is therefore an indirect effect. Rodolfo Margaria [29a] says the immediate source of muscular energy is adenosine triphosphate (ATP), while the ultimate sources are the combustion of food and the breakdown of glycogen.

Analysis of these reactions suggests that exercise has a beneficial effect as long as it is moderate and does not overtax the compensatory mechanisms. With exercise the oxygen need may increase from 250 to 4000 cc, and the pulse rate may rise from 20 to 40 beats or more per minute. An abnormal heart or lungs cannot adjust to such excessive demands, nor can hypertensive arterioles adjust to an increased blood volume that raises the systolic blood pressure 60 to 70 mm of mercury. For these reasons exercise in health and sickness should be adapted to the body needs of all ages and under varying conditions. Recent studies suggest that exercises before and after surgery shorten the convalescence period.[29b] These are discussed in Chapter 30. Regular and appropriate activity results in physiologic development and in improvement of every function, including thought. It stimulates the brain by increasing its supply of oxygen and food and by removing metabolic wastes; movement also increases messages received through the sense organs. Just as the mobility of man has enabled him to control his environment to a greater degree than any other creature, the exposure of the individual to a variety of stimuli enlarges his outlook. Bodily motion is in itself a satisfaction. This engagement of rhythmic movement through suitable occupations and diversion is among the most beneficial effects of exercise. Dr. Paul Dudley White,[30] the late internationally known cardiologist, discusses five benefits of exercise, applicable to all ages: (1) establishing and maintaining the muscle tone throughout the body, especially the heart and diaphragm; (2) producing positive effects on the psyche ("antidote for nervous tension and strains, anxiety, and mental concentration"); (3) reducing nervous tension, resulting in more effective gastrointestinal function; (4) helping to control obesity; and (5) increasing the function of the lungs in gaseous exchange by deepening respiration. Several authorities say that exercise delays the aging process.

The type and amount of exercise for healthy persons as well as those who are ill or recovering from an illness are questions that continue to be discussed. White believes the type of exercise in health is not so significant, but emphasizes the importance of selecting exercises that are in accord with the strength, aptitude, and liking of the person who is using them. Based on studies of more than 5000 subjects, Cooper found that the best exercises are running, swimming, cycling, walking, stationary running, handball, basketball, and squash—and in the order given. He describes a program of exercises for persons (by age group) that includes the first four activities listed above as well as a simple method of determining physical fitness (see Table 12-2). With a group of medical consultants, Cooper [31]

Table 12-2 12-Minute Test *
(Distances in Miles Covered in 12 minutes)

Fitness Category	Age (Yr)			
	Under 30	30–39	40–49	50+
I. Very poor	<1.0	<0.95	<0.85	<0.80
	<.95	<0.85	<0.75	<0.65
II. Poor	1.0–1.24	0.95–1.14	0.85–1.04	0.80–0.99
	.95–1.14	0.85–1.04	0.75–0.94	0.65–0.84
III. Fair	1.25–1.49	1.15–1.39	1.05–1.29	1.0–1.24
	1.15–1.34	1.05–1.24	0.95–1.14	0.85–1.04
IV. Good	1.50–1.74	1.40–1.64	1.30–1.54	1.25–1.49
	1.35–1.64	1.25–1.54	1.15–1.44	1.05–1.34
V. Excellent	1.75+	1.65+	1.55+	1.50+
	1.65+	1.55+	1.45+	1.35+

(The second requirement in each case is for women.)
< Means less than.
* Cooper, Kenneth H.: *The New Aerobics.* Bantam Books, Inc., New York, 1970, p. 47.

has published a useful article titled "Guidelines in the Management of the Exercising Patient" that includes the type of initial medical examination, physical fitness testing, contraindications and abnormal responses to exercise, and restrictions on older exercising patients. Nurses will find this article useful in advising others on the hazards associated with exercise as well as the use of exercise as therapy. F. J. Kottke [32] notes that a person puts all parts of the body, "including joint capsules, muscles, subcutaneous tissue and ligaments, through full range of motion many times each day." If for any reason these activities are prevented, tightness of the muscles results, with restricted motion. Nurses should be aware of this fact for their own sakes and for the sake of their patients; obviously it is much easier and less costly to prevent tightness than it is to correct the difficulty after it has developed. Janet Travell, personal physician of the late President John F. Kennedy, who suffered from an old back injury, discusses six helpful guidelines in avoiding the abuse of muscles in housework:

Scramble your tasks. Don't insist on finishing one which drains a set of muscles. . . . Develop rhythm of movement and the gift of short periods of relaxation. . . . Avoid hurrying—it puts too great a strain on the whole body. . . . Take short rest periods once an hour. These need not be longer than two minutes. . . . Don't overload your muscles. Each individual's strength varies. . . . Don't sit too long in one position.*

Regardless of the kind of activity (work or planned exercise), these guidelines will be useful.

In health we take for granted the free movement in all parts of our anatomy and the freedom of our person. Table 2-4, page 126, shows that 13.6 per cent of personal expenditures in the United States goes for transportation. Active games are included in recreation, which takes 6.5 per cent of personal expenditures. Health workers, usually active persons, should continually remind themselves of the psychologic and physical handicap of illness that limits free movement—either of a part or of the whole person. Emphasis has shifted within the last two decades from advocating rest—bed rest—as a panacea for all ills to advocating ambulation when it is possible and can be tolerated. Browse devotes the last chapter of his book, *The Physiology and Pathology of Bed Rest,* to a discussion of "The Dangers of Rest in Bed." Some of the complications attributed to bed rest (directly or indirectly) are (1) deep

vein thrombosis and pulmonary thromboembolism; (2) pneumonia; (3) pressure ulcers; (4) constipation; (5) difficulty with micturition; (6) development of renal calculi; (7) vasomotor instability; (8) musculoskeletal disorders; and (9) psyche disturbances. He says:

In general one can say that good attentive nursing care will prevent many of the complications of bed rest and the contribution of modern nursing to the success of modern medicine and surgery must never be forgotten.*

The adverse effects of immobilization, including bed rest, are discussed in considerable detail in Chapter 38, which the reader should consult for a thorough understanding of the problem.

During illness, the physician often takes the initiative in planning the patient's activity. In many situations he leaves this question up to the nurse and/or patient. In most cases, however, the physician's directions are limited and stated in general terms. For example, he says that the patient may go to work, use stairs, be up a whole or part of the day, sit in a chair, or stay in bed. Very often he prescribes a certain amount of walking or specifies passive movements, massage, or pressure devices as substitutes for exercise. But there are many other ways in which the patient's energy may be expended or conserved, and these must be regulated by the nurse, who is with the patient constantly. It may be highly desirable for the patient to have the exercise of turning, moving about freely, of feeding himself or herself, or assisting with the bath; in rare cases is it harmful. Exercises to help maintain full range of joint motion are carried out routinely by nurses in some hospitals, whereas in others the physician prescribes them. In addition many patients have other prescribed exercises to be repeated every few hours or every day. They may be the most important part of therapy. When the patient cannot have *active* exercise, *passive* exercise in the form of massage may be given to supply the benefits of exercise.

When exercises are the chief means of reestablishing normal function, as in the treatment of skeletal deformities and diseases, the patient is usually under the supervision of a physical therapist. Nurses who specialize in orthopedic nursing also may be prepared to give massage, special types of manipulation, and expert assistance in carrying out prescribed exercises. (See Figs. 12-11*A* and *B*.) Physical therapists and orthopedic nurses

---

* Travell, Janet: "Use and Abuse of Muscles in Housework," *J.A.M.W.A.,* **18:**159, (Feb.) 1963.

* Browse, Norman L.: *The Physiology and Pathology of Bed Rest.* Charles C Thomas, Publisher, Springfield, Ill., 1965, p. 160.

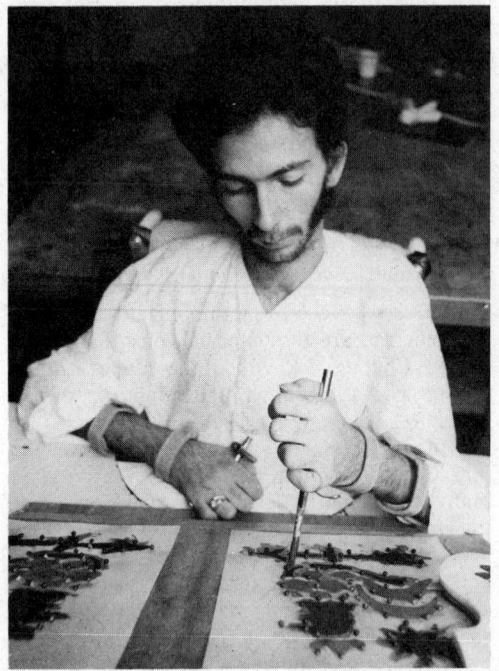
A

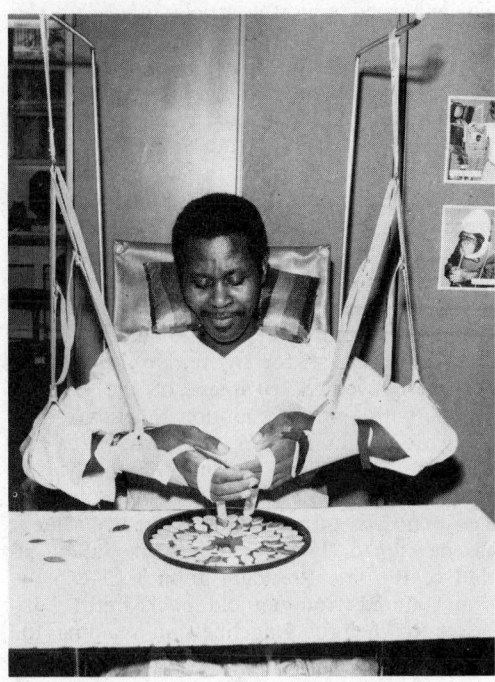
B

Figure 12-11. *A*. Patient with a spinal cord injury (C4–5) increases range of motion and coordination by using ADL (activities of daily living) hand splints to support and hold utensils. *B*. Patient with similar injury learns to develop upper extremities by picking up mosaic tiles with tongue blades. With treatment this patient's shoulder strength gradually improved so that he no longer required sling supports. (Both photos courtesy of Veterans Administration Hospital, Houston, Tex.)

should, however, be available for consultation on the problem of body mechanics presented by any patient. Chapter 30 deals briefly with the techniques of range of joint motion, massage, pressure mechanisms, and therapeutic exercises. Its contents may be studied in conjunction with this chapter. Postoperative ambulation and exercise are discussed in Chapters 47 and 48.

4. HELPING THE SICK AND HANDICAPPED TO MOVE

Importance of Moving Frequently. A healthy person has an almost unlimited choice of posture, and most of us change it every few minutes. Repose is said to be a charming quality but this does not mean immobility. Nothing is more foreign to average behavior than the stillness imposed, for example, during photography, or the fitting of clothes. Yet helpless patients are thought to be adequately nursed if a major change is made in their positions every hour. This is probably the maximum inactivity a person can tolerate. The chronically ill who are unable to move themselves and those who have nothing more than custodial care may be suffering very largely from the baleful effect of far fewer than hourly changes of posture. The first writer has seen patients lying in the same position for a period of 8 hours except when turned for bedmaking and bathing. Such practices are generally condemned.

Everything possible should be done to make patients independent in moving. Any mechanical device that is always within reach is preferable to human help that must be summoned —that is not constantly available. The services of men workers should always be used in moving adult patients if possible. One nurse alone should never try to lift an adult because of the danger and strain on both nurse and patient. Few patients have confidence in the strength of a woman nurse; and while they may laugh during the effort, they may really be excited and alarmed. At least two women nurses are required to lift a small person. To spare medical personnel, institutions should supply hoists. Home care may be possible for the permanently helpless person if such devices are provided. The purpose of an invalid lifter is to help the attendant lift and move the patient with as little effort or strain as possible on the part of the patient and the helper. Erbert F. Cicenia and associates, noting that many hydraulic lifters are available on the market, suggest useful criteria in their selection; they should be safe and easy to use and easily transported and stored. In the severely disabled, the hydraulic lifter is a multipurpose device used in transferring the patient to and from the bed, wheelchair, toilet, bathtub, and car. It is a boon to taking the severely disabled person out of a one-room existence. The importance of teaching all persons—health workers and families—who share in the care of the patient cannot be overemphasized.[32a] They say:

The family should be afforded the opportunity to observe a therapist setting up the lifter, placing the slings or harness straps on the patient, and maneuvering the lifter and patient through various daily activities. At the New York State Rehabilitation Hospital those who must look after the severely disabled patient are taught how to assist and handle the patient. If a lifter has been recommended, the instructions include assembly, operation, and maintenance of the lifter. After definite sling or harness positions have been determined and after successful methods and skills have been worked out by the therapist, the family is taught, under the supervision of a therapist, how to handle the patient and maneuver the lifter.*

In an attempt to learn why nurses do not use the hydraulic lifter as often as its use is indicated, Narrow,[33] in a survey of 173 nurses in six hospitals in Syracuse, New York, found that only 19 per cent said they used the lifter regularly or frequently, even though 85 per cent had received some instruction in its use and a lifter was available. The reasons they do not use the lifter, according to statements on the questionnaire, are that they are afraid to use it and that it does not save time or require fewer workers. Narrow believes the nurses questioned missed the point entirely as they ignored the purpose of the lifter, which is to protect the person or persons doing the lifting [and the person lifted] from injury. When this type of equipment is not available, as in some homes where it is not economically feasible, nurses must depend on the help of families and neighbors, the use of lifting sheets, and their knowledge of body mechanics.

Nurses should bend their efforts toward developing independence of patients and should move them "log fashion" only when patient participation is prohibited. A nurse may be able to move a small helpless child; two to four persons may be required to move such an adult. Margaret C. Winters[34] suggests that the weight of objects to be lifted not exceed 35 lb and that when several persons lift a heavy object together each person's share not exceed this amount. Heavy patients and objects should be transported on carriers equipped with casters or wheels.

Jesse T. Littleton[35] describes an "all-purpose stretcher," inexpensive and easily constructed, which has been shown to reduce the number of transfers of the acutely injured from 11 to only 2. The device is a slab of ¾-inch plywood, 2 by 6½ ft, with ball casters attached on the underside of the slab to facilitate rolling from place to place. The undercarriage of this device is an old x-ray table with a hydraulic lift so that the level of the carriage may be raised or lowered to any table or bed height. A radiolucent foam plastic mattress may be added for the comfort of the patient. This device has been successfully used to take the injured from the site of the accident through all outside-hospital and in-hospital moves, and ultimately to the patient's hospital bed.

Patients are likely to lie on their backs much of the time because in this position they can eat their meals, read, and talk to visitors. While the strain on the muscles of the legs, abdomen, and back can be relieved with pillows and pads, contractures of the knees result if the patient is in this position too constantly. Pressure on the calf muscle is thought also to promote the development of thrombi and phlebitis. Change of position is most important in all cases, but especially so when the position is one of marked flexion. Jessie L. Stevenson[36] (in 1942) shows how necessary it is for those doing general nursing to be alert in noticing symptoms that indicate skeletal disease and deformity. She describes the serious plight of a patient who recovered from typhoid fever, but who had contractures of both hips and knees because the legs had been kept flexed throughout the illness. Kottke[37] (1965) describes a patient in the standing position after being bedfast for 2 years following a stroke. He had contractures of the hips and knees and thoracic kyphosis. A variety of pads and pillows can be used to maintain the body in the alignment, discussed on page 726. In each position the patient must be studied to see that the weight of the arms is not dragging the shoulders forward, that the straight line of the back is maintained, and that no muscles are stretched or strained. Pillows at the back or against the abdomen give a comforting sense of warmth and support.

When patients can turn themselves without injury, and they can in almost all cases, the

---

* Cicenia, Erbert F., et al.: "Use of the Invalid Lifter in the Care of the Severely Disabled Patient," *Arch. Phys. Med. Rehabil.*, **38:**101, (Feb.) 1957.

nurse encourages them to do so. For instance, when movement causes pain, as after an abdominal operation, patients can turn themselves with greater ease and comfort than can the nurse. They will turn very slowly, first one part of the body, then another, instinctively making those adjustments that cause the least pain. Nurses may get useful hints if they watch patients.

Winters, in her discussion of lifting and moving heavy objects in *Protective Body Mechanics in Daily Living and in Nursing: A Manual for Nurses and Their Co-workers,* discusses ways to conserve effort. The writers' summary of her material includes a number of Winters' suggestions.

1. Roll or slide rather than lift an object whenever possible.
2. Remove all causes of friction (such as a wrinkled sheet) before rolling or sliding the object.
3. Roll or slide a heavy patient on a level rather than a sloping surface if possible (keep the patient who requires help on a firm bed).
4. Keep the weight to be moved as near the worker's hip level as possible (elevate a low bed or stand on a fixed platform in moving a patient).
5. Stand near the weight to be moved in order to maintain balance and use the large muscles.
6. Separate the legs to get a broad base and to enable the worker to shift the weight of her body as the object is moved.
7. Move an object toward rather than away from the worker.
8. Keep the back as straight as possible, flexing the hips or the knees rather than bending the back to get on the proper level to move an object. In this way the large muscles of the trunk and thigh are used in lifting rather than those of the arm.

These recommendations are based on the principles of simple machines or leverage. Their application to nursing is discussed in the manuals by Winters and Bernice Flash,[38] and in articles by the Royal Committee on Working Conditions of Sweden,[39] by Roberta F. Works,[40] and by others.[41] Such sources should be studied for a more thorough treatment of moving and lifting than can be given in the following suggested procedures.

Moving a Patient to the Side of the Bed and Helping Him to Turn on His Side. When one nurse moves the patient, she or he puts the forearms under the body, sliding first the head and shoulders, next the hips, and then the legs across the bed. This requires more effort than rolling the patient over, log fashion. A turning sheet as shown in Figure 12-12 *A–F* requires the least effort.

When patients have effective arm and trunk muscles and are encouraged to use them, they are taught to turn on the side. Patients with completely paralyzed lower extremities learn to do this with ease.

Turning the Patient into a Prone Position. Turning from the supine to the prone position is accomplished with three steps if persons are in a single bed. They move or are moved to one side of the bed while supine; they then turn on the side or are turned; and in the third stage they tip over on their face by a slow rotation of the hips and shoulders. In this process, it is important to adjust the arms and legs so that they will not be pinned under the body and so that their weight is used to help rather than hinder the movement of the body in the desired direction. The person with paralyzed legs learns to turn over without assistance by manual placement of the legs in the proper position for each phase of the move.

Approved prone posture and the use of supports are shown in Figure 12-7. For patients who must spend a major part of their time in a prone position the Stryker frame (see page 1468) is a boon because it is mobile and its structure makes occupation in the prone position more possible.

Moving the Mattress and the Patient Up in Bed. There is a tendency for the mattress and the patient to slide toward the footboard with any elevation of the head of the bed. To correct this condition begin, if possible, by making the mattress level; it is wasted effort to pull or push a weight uphill. If patients' condition permits, they can help bring the mattress up by grasping the headboard and pulling upward as the nurse moves the mattress into position. They can often push themselves up in bed by flexing the knees and pushing on the mattress with both feet. Grasping the head of the bed or overhead trapeze attached to the head of the bed also helps. If the patient is allowed to stand up or sit in a chair, the mattress should be adjusted while the bed is unoccupied. If a mechanical hoist is unavailable, it is often desirable to move a patient who must remain horizontal to a stretcher while the bed is remade.

Helping the Patient into a Semireclining or Sitting Position. Before elevating the upper part of the body, the patient must be far enough up in bed so that the back is straight from the coccyx to the occiput when the head of the bed, or backrest, is raised. This upward movement must be made while the patient and the mattress are horizontal.

With a Gatch bed, sitting postures are ac-

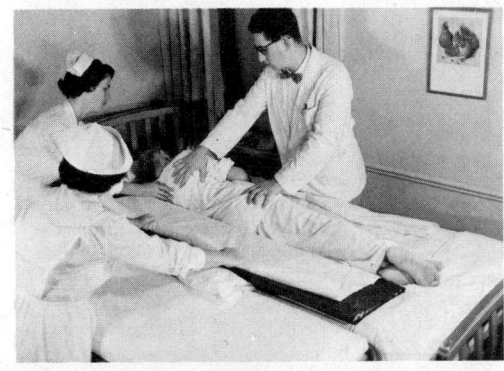

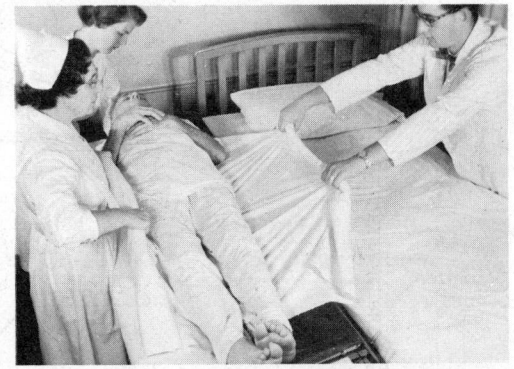

A

E

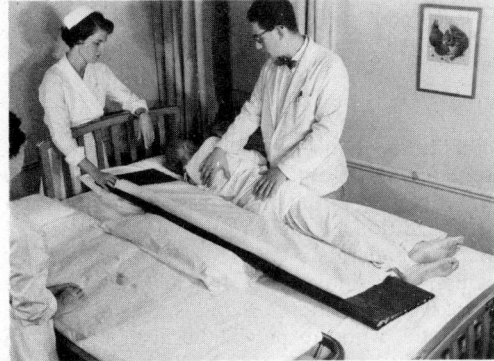

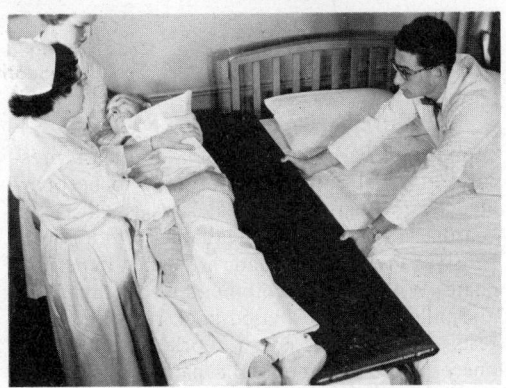

B

F

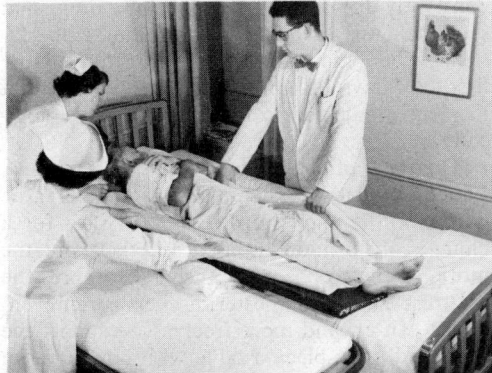

C

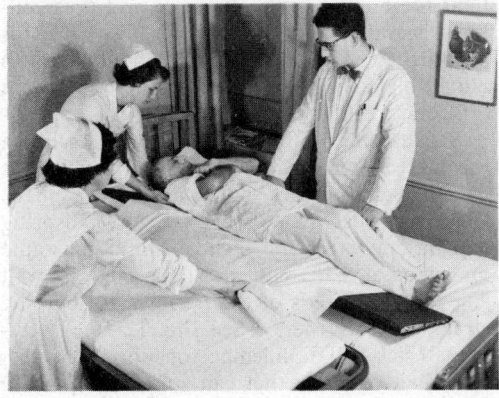

D

Figure 12-12. *A.* A roller is used to move a patient, who is unable to cooperate, from bed to stretcher. Roller in place on bed with the lifting sheet over it and under the patient. Note the pillow placed so that the roller cannot get wedged in the crack between the bed and the stretcher. *B.* Workers are easing the patient over onto the roller. *C.* One nurse is pulling the lifting sheet, the second nurse is supporting the head, and the aide is elevating his rolled edge of the lifting sheet. *D.* Another phase of the passage from bed to stretcher. *E.* The shift has been completed. *F.* The aide is removing the roller while the nurses steady the patient who has been rolled on his side with the lifting sheet. (Courtesy of Columbia-Presbyterian Medical Center, New York, N.Y., and Clay-Adams Co., New York, N.Y.)

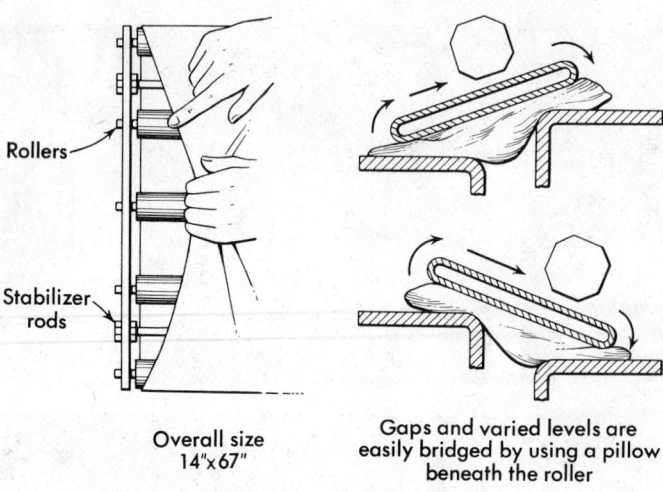

Rollers

Stabilizer rods

Figure 12-13. Diagram to show construction of the Davis patient roller. (Courtesy of Gilbert Hyde Chick Co., Oakland, Calif.)

Overall size 14"x67"

Gaps and varied levels are easily bridged by using a pillow beneath the roller

complished with the turn of a crank or pressure on a button; many are made to be operated by the patient. Special beds, such as the "cardiac bed," are also available, although expensive; they can be made into the shape of a chair. When such equipment is not available and pillows or improvised back rests and knee rests must be used, several workers are needed; one or more to support the patient in a sitting position while another worker adjusts the back rest. Most patients can lift themselves with an overhead trapeze (Fig. 12-14*B*), which should always be provided for those who are partially helpless for any length of time. Patients may lift themselves, using the nurse as a fixture as shown in Figure 12-15, but weak and heavy persons are likely to put too much weight pulling on the woman nurse in this maneuver. Too often she attempts to support patients in this way and at the same time to reach over them to adjust the pillows. This is likely to unbalance her, with disastrous results to the nurse and patient. It is far better in most cases to call a second worker. When adjustment of pillows is attempted by one nurse, she can remember that she is less likely to be unbalanced if she draws a pillow toward her than if she pushes it away from the central axis of her body. Figures 12-9 and 12-10 show patients in semireclining and sitting positions with modern hospital and improvised equipment. The principles emphasized on page 725 have been observed, and the arms and shoulders protected.

With the present emphasis on bed exercises and walking as soon as the patient's condition permits, change of position rarely causes the circulatory symptoms so much dreaded in the past when complete bed rest and virtual immobility were advocated as treatment for many

conditions. Nurses should, however, be observant and forestall accidents by noting the pulse before and after the assumption of each new exertion of the person who has been ill or has undergone surgery. Faintness and/or nausea are indications for a return to the horizontal position. Patients, such as the paralytic, who are put in the upright position with a tilt board (to reduce the cardiovascular deconditioning process) should be observed constantly for signs of nausea, sweating, and syncope. An attendant should stay with patients when they are up, at least during the first few days or until there is evidence that they have adjusted to this position physiologically.[42]

The Use of a Bedside Table in Dyspnea. Patients obliged to sit up in order to breathe with comfort may want to lean forward for a change of position. Sometimes they breathe more easily so, because the pressure of the mattress against the posterior chest is removed, and it can expand more freely. To support the head and arms place a table with one or more pillows on it over the bed in front of the patient for him or her to lean on, and press pillows against the lower part of the back for support. Protect the back and shoulders with a light blanket or jacket, according to the room temperature.

Because it is difficult to eliminate strain on the legs and loin muscles sitting in bed, it is usually better to get the patient into a chair. "Cardiac beds" are so made that the bedspring can be converted mechanically into the same angles as a chair. An adjustable chair is well suited to the needs of the person with chronic circulatory disorders. (See Fig. 12-16.) Actually all sick and disabled persons should be provided with a chair that can support the entire

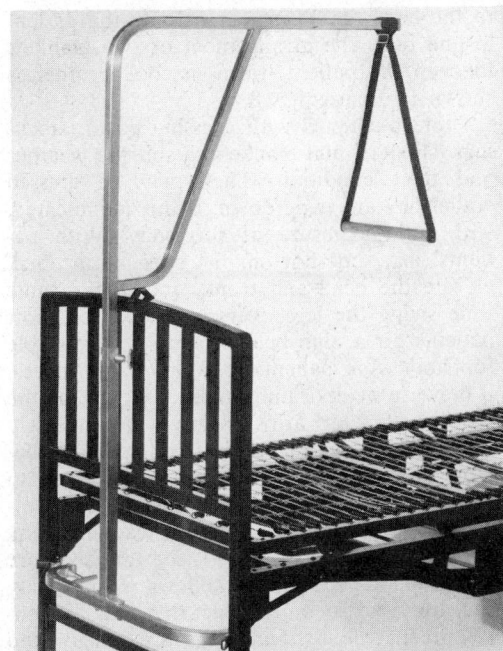

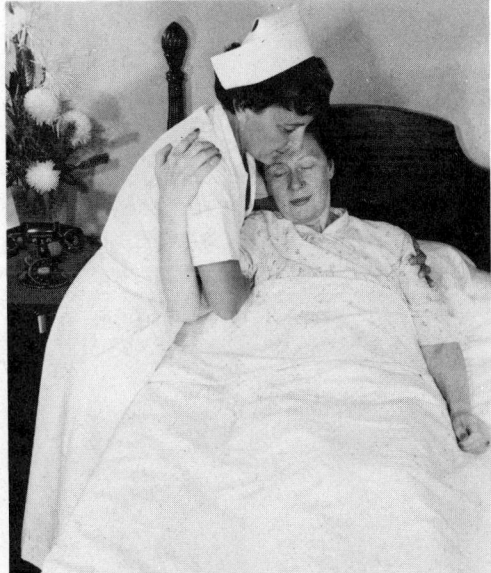

Figure 12-15. A nurse helping a patient to sit up. Note that the patient is cooperating by pulling herself up, using the nurse's shoulder as a fixed point. The nurse is cradling the patient's head with her left arm. (Courtesy of Columbia-Presbyterian Medical Center, New York, N.Y. and Clay-Adams Co., New York, N.Y.)

body and that can be mechanically manipulated to enable the occupant to change the position of the trunk and extremities—even to lie flat in the chair. If the chair is on wheels that can be both used and immobilized there will be few patients who must be confined to a bed in one room—a fate that is so likely to induce withdrawal, regression, and other personality changes.

Helping the Patient into a Chair from the Bed. Placing a patient in a wrong-size wheelchair usually results in a slumped posture, compression of the vessels under the knee if the distance to the footrests is too long, kinking of the vessels in the hip if the distance is too short, and overexertion if the chair is too wide making the armrests too far apart.[43] Consequently, selection of an appropriate wheelchair for a patient needs considerable thought. P. M. Ellwood says:

> . . . wheelchairs are fitted to patients, not patients to wheelchairs. . . . Experience has shown that certain wheelchair features are virtually standard requirements. They include high degree of durability, ease of folding, easy propulsion, brakes, removable footrests and 8 inch front casters.*

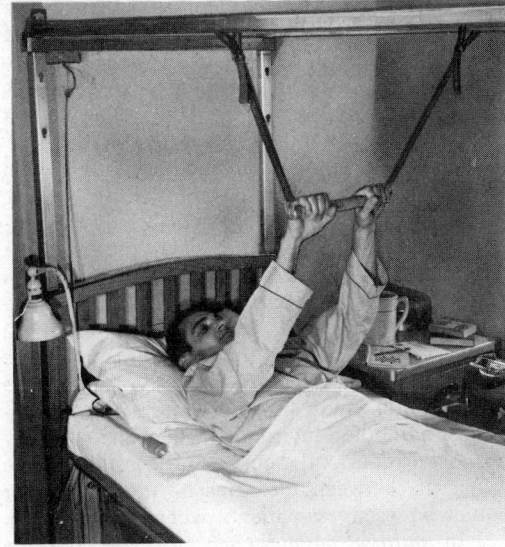

Figure 12-14. *A.* An exercise bar is a desirable attachment for the bed in almost any long-term illness. The patient can lift himself when indicated during nursing care and treatments. This gives the patient needed exercise and reduces moving and lifting by the staff. A sponge-rubber grip for the cross bar is available, if its use is indicated. (Courtesy of Simmons Co., New York, N.Y.) *B.* Another type of exercise bar. Such equipment should be provided for any patient on a Balkan frame. Its use strengthens the patient's muscles and gives needed exercise. (Courtesy of Columbia-Presbyterian Medical Center New York, N.Y., and Clay-Adams Co., New York, N.Y.)

* Ellwood, P. M.: "Prescription of Wheelchairs," in Krusen, F. H., et al.: *Handbook of Physical Medicine and Rehabilitation,* 2nd ed. W. B. Saunders Co., Philadelphia, 1971, pp. 431, 433.

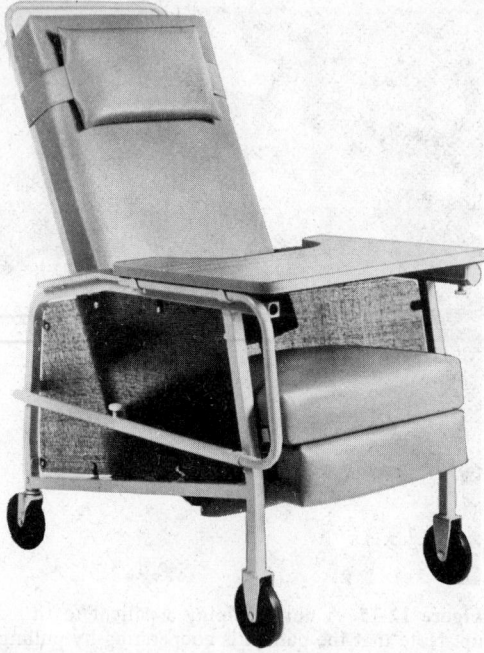

Figure 12-16. Recliner chair-table with extra-wide and extra-long armrests. Two side-mounted folding tables can be attached to provide ample and convenient surfaces for treatment utensils and materials for both the patient and attendant. This equipment is ideal for dialysis units, blood collection, and general use for the patient with eight-hour comfort capability. (Courtesy of Lumex, Inc., Bay Shore, N.Y.)

Herman L. Kamenetz,[44] in *The Wheelchair Book: Mobility for the Disabled*, says the British Ministry of Health lists four sizes: *Child*—up to 4 ft tall and 70 lb, *Junior*—up to 62 inches (5 ft, 2 inches) and about 112 to 126 lb, *Standard*—for taller persons weighing up to 196 lb, and *Outsize*—for those up to 224 lb. In the United States he says five sizes are available: *Small Child, Large Child, Junior, Adult,* and *Oversize*. Nurses who are working with disabled persons should consult this source. When selecting a wheelchair by size, consideration should be given to the following: (1) the width and depth of the seat; (2) height of the armrests (they should allow for comfort of the patient without excessive shoulder abduction or pull of the arms on the shoulder); and (3) adjustable footrest which may be set for support of the lower extremity in good alignment. Figure 12-17 shows a wheelchair prescription form. If movement of the patient is desirable (which it nearly always is) a mobile chair must be selected.[45] See that it is in good repair, protected with cushions or pillows, and placed conveniently (at right angle to the bed) for lifting, or helping the patient in and out. The arrangement of two blankets to keep the patient warm in cool weather is shown in Figure 12-18.

Protect patients with dressing gown, stockings, slippers, and blankets to suit the weather and their condition. They may be dressed while they are lying down, if this is indicated, with little exposure of the body. With patients near, but not on, the edge of the bed, elevate the head and trunk, and at the same time swing the legs over the edge. For short patients on a high bed, provide a very stable footstool. Ask patients to support themselves, if they are weak or unbalanced, by grasping the nurse's arm, or arms, firmly. Move slowly until the seat of the chair is immediately behind the patients' thighs, and direct them to grasp the arms of the chair as they lower themselves into it with the nurse's steadying help. When they are in the chair, see that they are well supported, with no hollows in the back; that the head is comfortable; that in a cool environment the feet and legs are snugly and neatly wrapped in the blanket; that a footrest keeps the feet from the floor; and that even a hot-water bottle is provided for the feet if necessary. The arms should be free and supported with armrests. If the legs are edematous or ulcerated, or the joints painful, keep them elevated.

Watch for signs of fatigue and don't wait until patients are exhausted before putting them back to bed. Patients who have been bedfast are seldom allowed to sit up the first time for more than half an hour. While they are in the chair, the mattress may be turned and the bed aired and remade. If patients are in a wheelchair, an effort should be made to give them a change of scene by rolling them outdoors, into a sun porch, solarium, or into almost any other environment than the one they must so constantly occupy. A portable table that fits between the arms of the wheelchair may be used by patients when they are up.

In *putting patients back to bed,* observe the same care as when lifting them into the chair, reversing the steps taken in getting them up. Undress them without exposure; make them comfortable and let them rest. Chart the rate and character of the pulse, the time allowed in the chair, and the effect on the patient.

Wheelchairs are made stationary by locking the wheels, but if this device is not part of the chair, a worker must hold it still or a sandbag or heavy piece of furniture must be used to brace it as the patient gets in and out.

If this is the patient's first change from a reclining or semireclining position, there is some danger that the stimulation of the circulation

Date _____

Name _____ Age _____ Address _____

Clinical diagnosis _____ Weight _____

Disability diagnosis _____

Size { Adult / Junior / "Tiny Tot" }   Type { Universal / Traveler / Amputee }

Driving mechanism: Manual < One-wheel < Right / Left / Two-wheel

Electric
Other, specify _____

Wheels: Large, 20-inch, 24-inch, 26-inch   Casters: 5-inch, 8-inch

Tires: Regular   Pneumatic < Semi / Full

Brakes: Regular   Extension < Bilateral / Unilateral

Handrims: Regular   Rubber-covered   Other _____

Seat: Hard   Soft   Cushion   inches _____

Back: Standard   Reclining < Semi / Full   Raised   Detachable

Arms: Regular   Headrest   Detachable   Desk   Wooden / Upholstered

Legrest: Standard   Elevating / Swinging   Fabric legrest panel

Footrest: Fixed   Removable   Parallel   Toe loops   Heel loops
         Heel straps

Special accessories: Arm supports and slings
                     Utility tray
                     Commode

Remarks _____

_____ M.D.

Encircle the desired specifications.

Figure 12-17. Wheelchair prescription. (From Rusk, Howard: *Rehabilitation Medicine,* 3rd ed. C. V. Mosby Co., St. Louis, 1971, p. 311.)

may dislodge a clot that has formed in a blood vessel (*a thrombus*), setting it in motion (*an embolus*), and causing death if the clot obstructs a vital artery in the heart, lungs, or brain. For this reason nurses have been cautioned to move the patient with great gentleness and to count the pulse before and after getting the patient into the chair. With bed exercises and early ambulation this accident is increasingly rare.

Teaching the Patient to Move from the Bed to a Chair and from One Chair to Another. One of the activities in the rehabilitation of the person with motor paralysis of the legs is moving from the bed to a chair without assistance. Health workers help the patient to

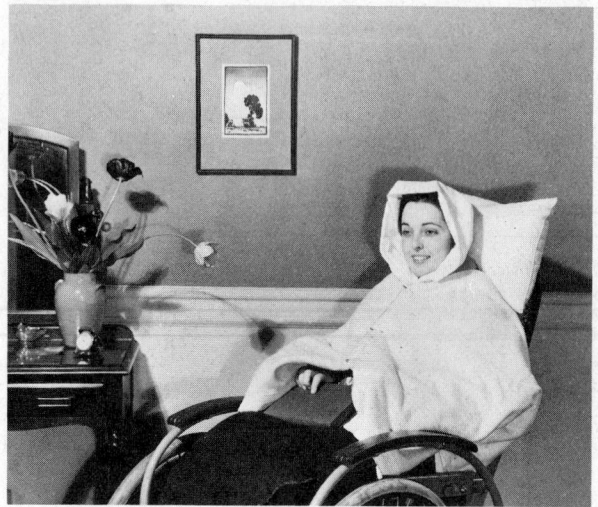

Figure 12-18. Patient prepared to go out of doors. Note the warm blanket around the patient, hood for protection of head and neck, and folded blanket pinned around shoulders leaving the hands free.

progress to complete independence as rapidly as possible. Patients eventually learn to adjust their brace lying in bed and to move freely from bed to wheelchair and from wheelchair to another chair or a toilet seat.

The bed must be the right height or the move is too difficult. In one method the seat of the chair is placed against and at right angles to the mattress at the level of the buttocks. (Patients learn to leave the chair at this spot with the brake on or with the wheels stopped by sandbags.) In a sitting position, patients push themselves off the bed with the arms and swing the legs around until they are across the bed with the buttocks hanging slightly over the seat of the chair. They reach behind, one hand at a time and grasp the arms of the chair; they can then pull themselves into the chair seat. Releasing the chair brake, they wheel it backward until the ankles are resting on the mattress; they then lower each flaccid leg to the footrest, holding it with both hands around the calf.

In the second method the chair seat is placed parallel with the length of the bed and slightly above its center. Patients hitch to the side of the bed, reach over the chair, and grasp the far armrest. Then, pushing on the bed with the other hand, they slide the buttocks over the near chair arm and into the seat. The legs are then grasped with the hands and one after the other swung from the bed into position. Getting from the chair into the bed is accomplished by reversing these processes.

A patient can be taught to move from a wheelchair to the toilet seat, from a wheelchair to a bed, (see Fig. 12-19), and from a wheelchair to the car.

In all these moves it is essential that the patient have strong arm and trunk muscles

with confidence in their powers. It is essential that the bed and chair brakes be locked. (In the home where these pieces of furniture have no brakes, they must be braced securely.) If either rolls out from under its occupant, he or she may be badly injured, and it will almost certainly destroy their self-confidence.

Teaching the Patient to Move from a Wheelchair into a Tub and Back to the Chair. The seat of the chair is covered with a waterproof square and a large turkish towel. Patients, dressed in a bathrobe, are told to bring the chair as close as possible to the tub, facing it. After braking the chair, they lift each foot into the tub. Pushing up on the arms of the chair, they move toward the tub so that the buttocks are partly on the edge of the chair and partly on the rim of the tub. Leaning forward and grasping the tub on each side, or a handle on one side of certain tubs, they can lower the buttocks into the water. A paralyzed leg can be lifted and flexed so that the foot and lower part can be bathed. Bracing the foot against one end of the tub or resting against the back steadies the body.

To get out the process is reversed. With the body braced against the back of the tub, it is brought out of the water by pushing up on the rim. The buttocks rest first on the edge of the tub and with another push are moved over on the seat of the chair. After unlocking the brakes, the chair is moved out about 6 inches, and the legs are removed singly from the tub. The body is dried and the gown replaced.

Teaching the Patient to Move from a Wheelchair to the Automobile. The method suggested in the following description is based on the ideas of Kamenetz.[45a] So that the person can regain as much independence as possible, it is important that he or she is taught

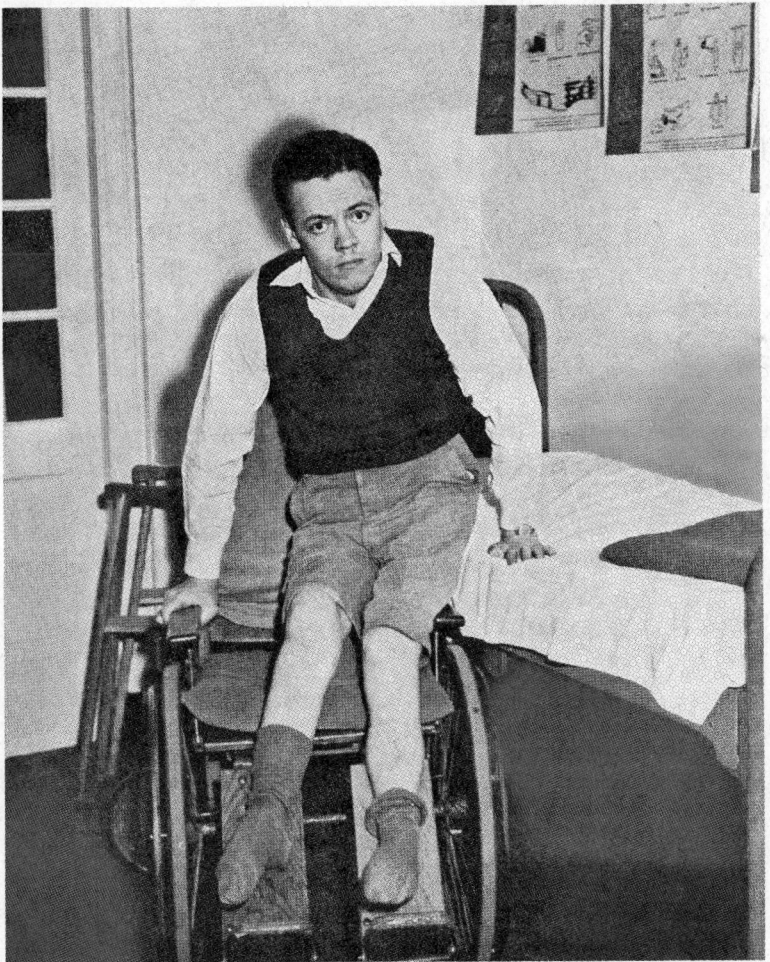

Figure 12-19. Patient moving from wheelchair to bed. (Courtesy of National Foundation, New York, N.Y.)

to move from the wheelchair to an automobile.

The automobile of choice for the wheelchair user is the one with two doors. When in the street, it must be standing against the curb (preferably right curb) and the brakes must be locked so that it will not roll, regardless of where it is parked. With the window down, the right door should be open in such a way that it does not move by itself.

One person aligns the wheelchair to the open door, puts the footrests up, locks the brakes, and removes the left armrest. Both left wheels of the chair must be against the right side of the car. If the wheelchair does not have removable armrests, the patient puts the wheelchair in an oblique position with its left front wheel against the car.

After sliding on the wheelchair seat to its front edge, patients use the right hand for support by grasping the right wheelchair arm, wheelchair seat, or car door (if they can reach it) and the left hand by grasping the doorframe or car seat; then they push themselves up, carrying themselves over to the car seat. The legs are brought into the car.

When transferring from the left door, all sides of the above description must be changed. Figure 12-20 shows a different method—placing the feet into the car first which might allow the person to bring the chair closer to the car than the above method.

Persons with physical disabilities are given instructions in driving an automobile with special assistive devices (see Fig. 12-21).

Turning the Mattress with the Patient in Bed. When the patient is in bed for a long time, the mattress may become uneven or uncomfortable, so that it is necessary to turn it, to change it, or to move the patient to another bed. The mattress may be easily

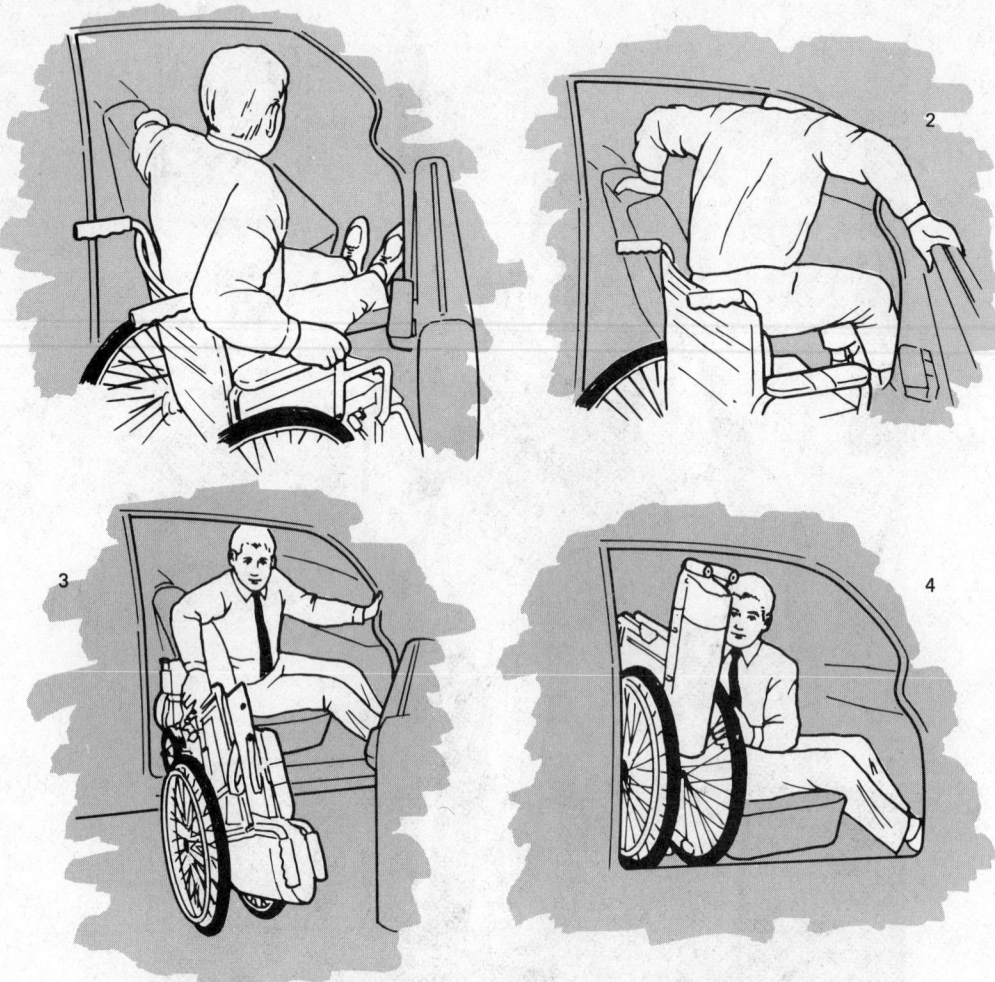

Figure 12-20. Paraplegic moving from wheelchair to car. *1.* The feet are placed into the car. *2.* Pushup and carry-over to car seat. *3* and *4.* After unlocking the brakes, the folded chair is lifted by its front posts and rolled on its large wheels over the edge and onto the car floor. (Adapted from Kamenetz, Herman L.: *The Wheelchair Book.* Charles C Thomas, Publisher, Springfield, Ill., 1969, p. 185.)

turned or changed with no discomfort to the patient. *One method* is to remove the pillows and all the top bedclothes except the sheet and blanket, which are folded back neatly over the patient. The under linen is rolled toward the patient, making a firm roll on either side. The patient is lifted to one side of the mattress, which is drawn from the side partly off the springs. Pillows are placed on the springs, the patient is moved on to the pillows, and then the mattress turned (from the head toward the foot), after which the patient is lifted on to the mattress, the pillows are removed, and the mattress placed in position. The bed is then remade. If the mattress is to be changed, the procedure is essentially the same. A *second*

and far simpler method used in the hospital is putting the patient on a stretcher or another bed while the mattress is turned. Most often the patient can be put into a chair while the mattress is turned.

Moving the Patient from One Bed to Another. Put a lifting sheet under the patient. Place the beds (if of equal height) close together, and draw the patient to the fresh bed by pulling him on the lifting sheet. When the beds cannot be put side by side, the upper sheet and blanket may be rolled snugly around the patient, who may then be lifted and carried to the fresh bed. All those who lift the patient stand on the same side, one supporting the head, shoulders, and back; the other, the back,

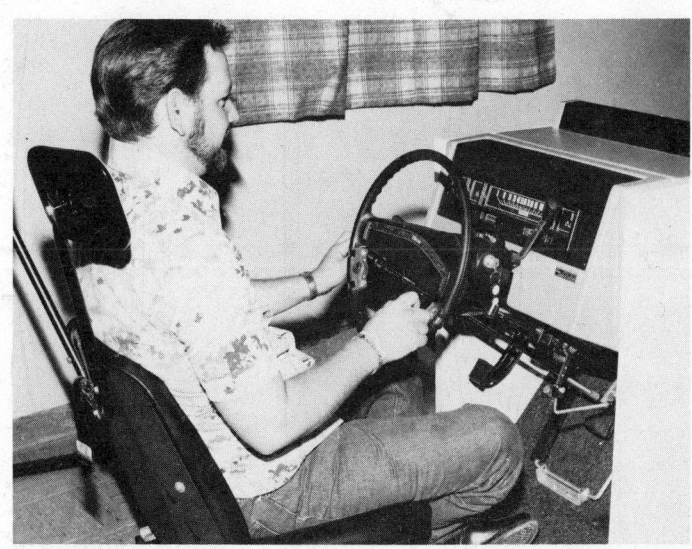

Figure 12-21. Driver education and training program for individuals with physical disabilities. A patient (with paraplegia) learns preception, proper driving procedures, and use of assistive devices in the simulator. (Courtesy of Veterans Administration Hospital, Houston, Tex.)

thighs, and feet. First draw the patient to the edge of the bed, and together lift gently, the patient holding himself or herself stiff.

Crutches. During recovery from skeletal injuries and, in some cases, as compensation for useless or partially useless legs, a patient must use crutches. Many types are available, several of which are shown in Figures 12-22, 12-23, and 12-24. Tripod crutches are sometimes used when the maintenance of balance is especially difficult. Springs have been introduced, rockers and wheels tried, and a variety of hand grips used. Adjustable crutches are especially desirable when they are rented or to be sold after short usage. Tips should be fitted with rubber caps. Sponge-rubber covers or pads are also available for axillary bars and hand bars. While the axillary bar should es-

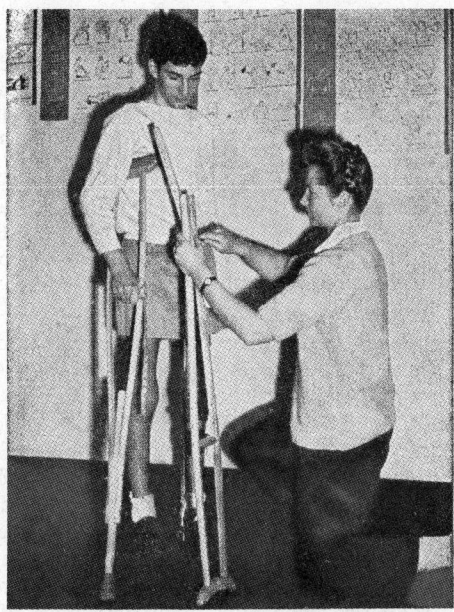

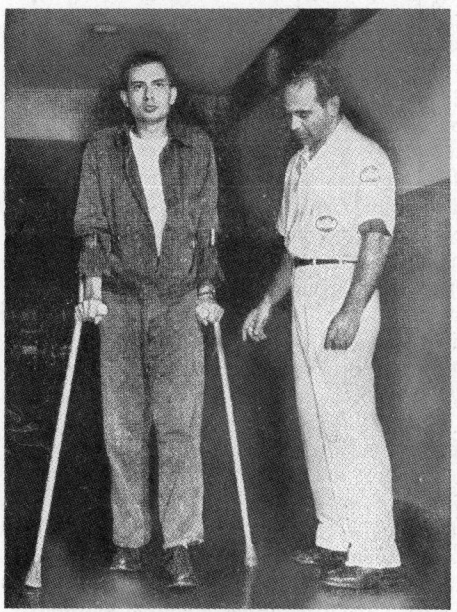

A

B

Figure 12-22. *A*. Therapist adjusting crutches to correct length. (Courtesy of National Foundation, New York, N.Y.) *B*. When a patient can walk unassisted, greater attention is paid to the development of a proper gait. (Courtesy of Veterans Administration, Washington, D.C.)

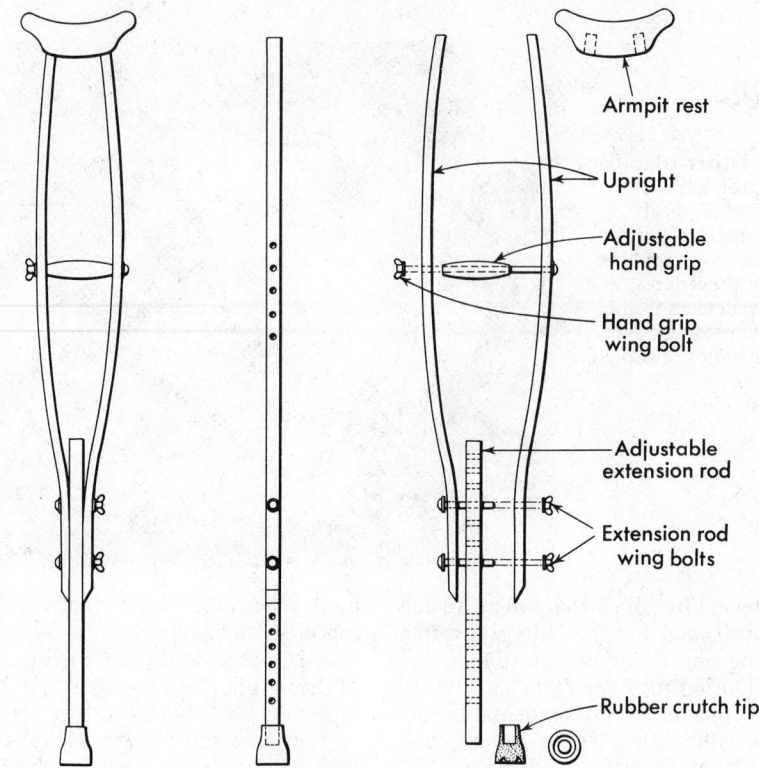

Armpit rest

Upright

Adjustable hand grip

Hand grip wing bolt

Adjustable extension rod

Extension rod wing bolts

Rubber crutch tip

Figure 12-23. Wooden adjustable crutch.

cape the axilla when the crutch is in use, many patients prefer to have it padded or made of a soft leather sling. White pads bandaged on are soon soiled and unsightly, and a heavy pad is likely to extend the crutch too much. The sponge-rubber cover is probably the most satisfactory type.

It is essential that crutches be exactly the right length. Crutches that are too long cause pressure in the armpit and elevation of the shoulder girdle. Pressure on the radial nerve as it passes through the armpit may injure it and impair the function of the hands. If the weight is borne on the top of the crutch constantly it can cause a "crutch" (arm) paralysis.[46] When crutches are too short the user has to crouch and cannot get adequate leverage. The person should always wear well-fitted shoes with rubber heels and avoid wearing ill-fitting and loose garments as they may get caught in the crutches.[47] Several methods for *measuring for crutches* (some more elaborate than others) are described by various authorities. Covalt describes a simple method:

If the patient can stand in parallel bars, the hand grips will already have been measured. A crutch is put under the arm and adjusted so that the person doing the measurement can easily get

three fingers between the top of the crutch and the axilla. Once the length is adjusted the hand-piece is then set at the proper level.

If the measurement must be made in bed, the most commonly used method, with the patient lying flat and without a pillow, is to measure from the anterior axillary fold to a point 6 inches from the side of the foot. Another method is to measure from the axillary fold to the side of the foot and add 2 inches. (In either of these methods the length will include the length with the crutch tip on.) The angle of the elbow is approximated and all the measurements rechecked when the patient stands.*

Patients should be thoroughly prepared for the use of crutches. In some instances they may be given practice before orthopedic surgery that will necessitate their use later. In all cases exercises should be taught that will strengthen the hands and arms and shoulder girdle (see Fig. 30-6, Chapter 30). Bed patients can strengthen these muscles by the use of the trapeze and by pushing themselves up with their hands, and by resistive exercises (exercises made difficult by resistance of the

---

* Covalt, Nila Kirkpatrick: *Bed Exercises for Convalescent Patients.* Charles C Thomas, Publisher, Springfield, Ill., 1968, p. 209.

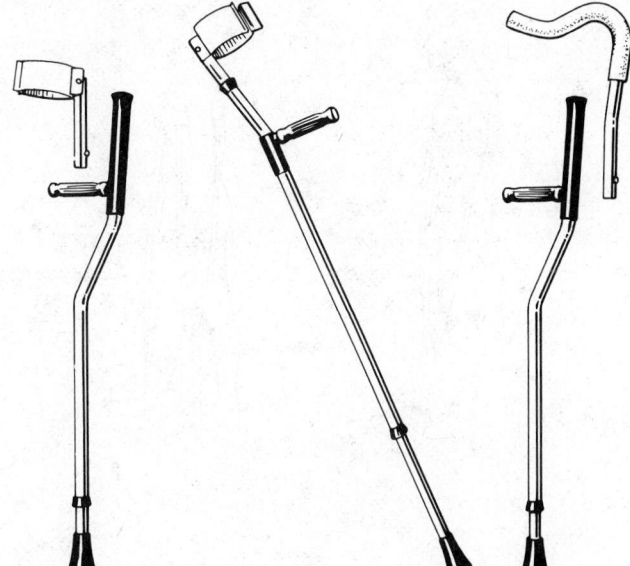

Figure 12-24. A variety of crutches from which suitable ones may be selected. Ortho-crutches are convertible from underarm to forearm crutches; top sections may be purchased separately.

operator or by other means such as gravity) described in Chapter 30.

Unless patients have had an opportunity to learn the proper use of crutches, considerable instruction is necessary. They must be taught to bear their weight on the hand bar rather than on the top of the crutch that fits under the arm. If the weight of the body is borne on the top of the crutch, making pressure on nerves over any length of time, the arms may be seriously injured. Some of the gaits used include: "the four point," "three point," "two point," "swing to," "swing through," "rocking chair," and "tripod." [48] The health team should help the patient adopt the gait, or several gaits, best suited to his or her needs. In cases where the injured leg is not to be used at all in walking, the weight is borne on the normal foot while both crutches are brought forward at once; then the normal foot is drawn in line with the crutches while the body is supported on the hand bars of the crutches. If the physician wishes the person to make some use of the injured leg, the crutches, like the feet, are put forward alternately, the sequence being (1) the left crutch, (2) the right foot, (3) the right crutch, (4) the left foot, and so on (see Fig. 12-25). Cane walking is shown in Figure 12-26. Orthopedic and rehabilitation texts should be consulted for further details on crutch walking.

When crutches are used for a child over any appreciable length of time, they must be replaced frequently as the child grows taller; otherwise, he or she will develop postural defects that may be difficult to correct.

Mechanical devices that support the patient more completely than crutches are available for use in teaching patients to walk with an artificial leg or in other conditions that interfere with normal locomotion. These so-called *walkers* are a framework on large casters or wheels, that have an adjustable seat, crutches, hand rests, and foot supports (see Fig. 12-27). This type of apparatus gives patients a feeling of greater security, because they know that they can stop and rest at any time. However, most authorities warn against the continued use of these and say a patient should not be sent home with a walker. Figure 12-28 *A-B* shows two patients at various stages of ambulation following amputation of a lower extremity.

5. TRANSPORTATION IN ILLNESS AND TRAVELING WITH PATIENTS

Moving the Patient from One Room to Another. In hospitals patients can be transferred from one room to another simply by moving them on the bed, on a stretcher, or, if their condition allows it, in a wheelchair. In homes it may be necessary to improvise a stretcher or litter from a table top or a stoutly woven cloth with poles through hems on each side. If three strong persons are available, they can move the patient log fashion; or strong individuals who make a packsaddle of their hands can carry a person who is able to sit up. Patients may be carried in an armchair if it is

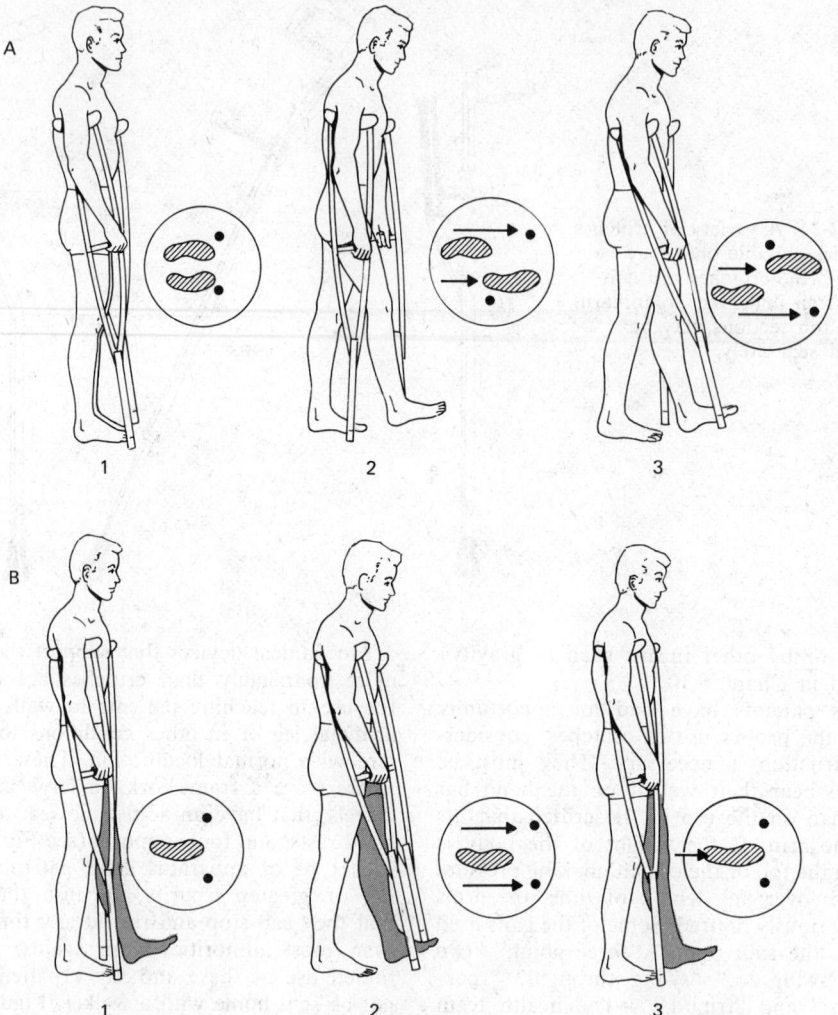

Figure 12-25. Crutch walking. *A*. Two-point gait: 1, position of rest; 2, the left crutch and the right foot are advanced simultaneously; 3, the right crutch and the left foot are advanced simultaneously. *B*. Three-point gait: 1, weight is on the uninvolved extremity; 2, with the weight on the uninvolved extremity, the crutches and the involved extremity are advanced; 3, the uninvolved extremity is advanced. *C*. Four-point gait: 1, position of rest; 2, right crutch is advanced; 3, left foot is advanced; 4, left crutch is advanced; 5, right foot is advanced. (From Dison, Norma Greenler: *An Atlas of Nursing Techniques.* C. V. Mosby Co., St. Louis, 1971, pp. 68–69.)

well built and can be firmly grasped on each side by the rungs. No matter how patients are to be moved, the method should not be discussed before them, because they themselves are likely to be fearful and even uncooperative if those moving them fail to proceed with confidence.

Moving the Patient from House to House. If ambulances are available, the transportation from one house to another is easy. When such facilities are lacking, moving patients may

present so many hazards as to be contraindicated while they are acutely ill. Children and small adults may be made comfortable if stretched out on the seat of an automobile and supported with pillows. The greatest difficulty is to get the patient in and out of the conveyance. In every case the services of a strong man are needed, and he should be shown how to lift and carry the patient so that there will be as little jarring as possible.

Collapsible wheelchairs are very useful if

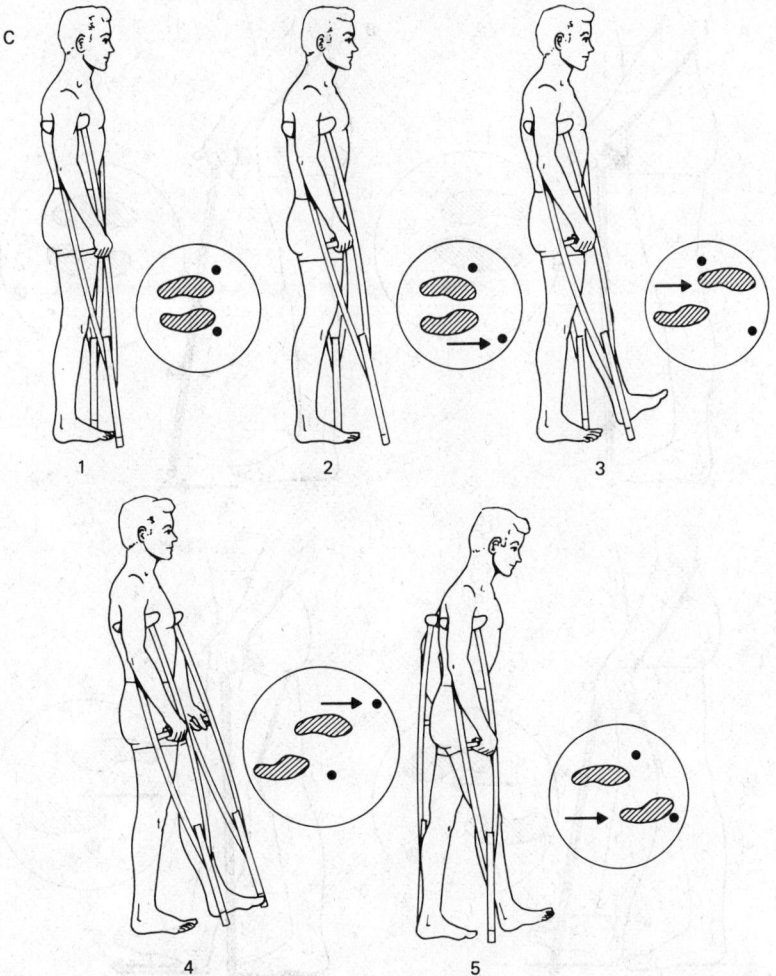

the person has a serious motor disability. Such chairs can be folded and put in an automobile or stored on a train. Patients may be wheeled from their room to an automobile, taken to their destination, and when there wheeled into the house. This saves effort on the part of those helping them and makes them feel less dependent and more comfortable. In all large cities and many other communities, wheelchairs may be rented, and welfare organizations are often prepared to lend them to persons unable to pay. The Red Cross in many communities offers transportation as does such agencies as FISH. Figure 12-30 shows a specially designed vehicle used to transport patients from their homes to the hospital.

Modes of transportation used for emotionally disturbed persons are the same as those used in other illnesses. To be able to anticipate problems that may occur in transit, knowledge of the patient's pattern of behavior and mental state is essential. It is wise to avoid deception about the destination as this is likely to produce hostility and lack of confidence on the part of the patient in future relationships with those deceiving him.* If restraints are used, of course, the patient should be told, as well as the reason for their application. An attitude of calmness and patience should prevail.[49] E. Beadle and associates [50] in England describe camping tours abroad (including Belgium, Holland, France, and Switzerland) for long-stay psychiatric patients as a means of stimulating interest in life. Two nurses and one physician accompanied a group of eight patients, men and women, between the ages of 35 and 68. The only contraindications for travel in this group were inability to dress and eat without full assistance, greatly impaired health, and incontinence.

* Someone has said that the price of lying is not being believed—as great a price as one can pay.

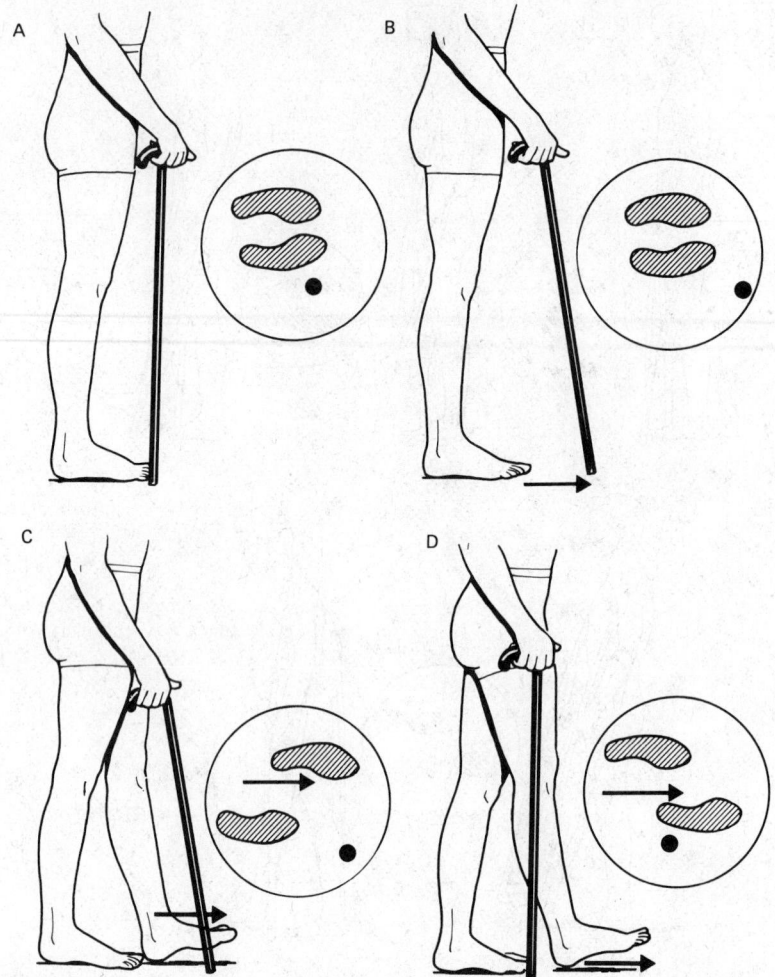

Figure 12-26. Cane walking. *A.* The cane is positioned about 4 to 6 inches away from the toe of the uninvolved extremity. *B.* The cane is moved forward about the length of the patient's foot. *C.* The involved leg is moved forward until the toe is parallel to the cane. *D.* The uninvolved leg is moved forward until its heel is parallel to the cane. (From Dison, Norma Greenler: *An Atlas of Nursing Techniques.* C. V. Mosby Co., St. Louis, 1971, p. 67.)

Traveling with Patients. The responsibility of nurses when they travel with a patient varies with the nature and severity of the illness.[50a] Their preparation for the trip will be modified accordingly, but in any event they should be well informed and prepared for emergencies. An attempt should be made to relieve patients of all anxiety; they should feel that the nurse is capable of solving the problems connected with the journey, and, unless they will benefit by helping, nothing that will tax them is expected of them.

A suitable means of taking patients to the railroad station, dock, or airport should be provided. This depends upon their condition.

Wheelchairs and elevators are available in most large stations. The nurse should learn by telephone well in advance of starting the journey what facilities are available and to what entrance the sick person should be taken. The patient is often sensitive and nervous, and will be grateful to the nurse for providing as much privacy as possible. The average person dislikes undue notice in public, and the nurse should try to see that the sick person is not made conspicuous during his or her travels.

The acceptance of the incapacitated passenger, according to Otis B. Schreuder,[51] is a common occurrence in regularly scheduled flights of the world's major airlines. Patients

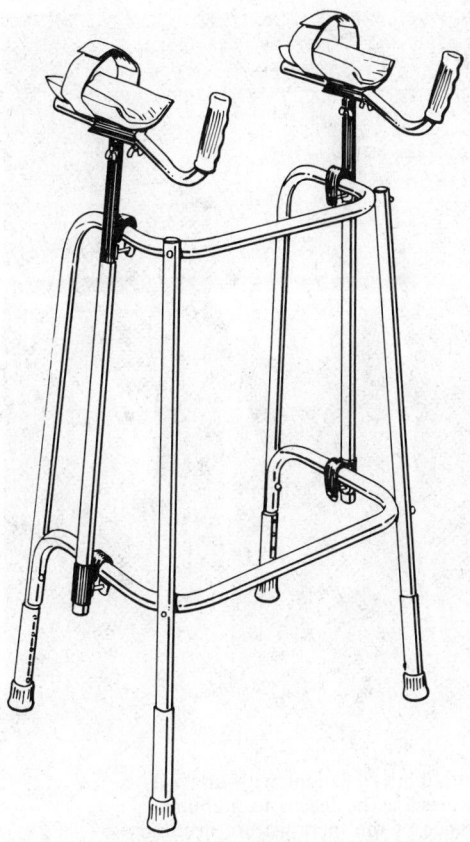

Figure 12-27. Walker with forearm attachments provides a comfortable support and added safety for the patient with weak or arthritic hands and wrists. Walker may be used without attachments. (Courtesy of Lumex, Inc., Bay Shore, N.Y.)

may be transported long distances for special medical care not available in a particular community or city, "for example from Bangkok or Buenos Aires to New York." Medical criteria have been developed that are useful to the physician in approval of air travel for a patient; some knowledge of the characteristics of the plane is also important. He says, "the pressurization in the turbo-jet aircraft (Boeing 707, Douglas DC-8, and Convair 880) is far superior to that of the piston-engined aircraft (DC-7). A relatively low cabin altitude is important to the comfort of all passengers and particularly so to the patient being transported by air." * Contraindications to air travel in commercial planes, according to A. B. Barbour,[52] include very severe and critical heart conditions, conditions with entrapped gas in the body such as pneumothorax or ventric-

ulography (air introduced into ventricles), severe cases of otitis media, acute or communicable disease, pregnancy beyond the thirty-second week, poliomyelitis of less than one month's duration, recent surgical patients without healing of the wound, unattended psychiatric patients in need of heavy sedation, contagious or repulsive skin conditions, fractures of the skull, cranial diseases involving increased pressure, intestinal obstruction, mediastinal tumors, and extremely large unsupported hernias. It is obvious that commercial airlines are attempting to protect both patients and other passengers. Discussing the facilities available, Barbour says:

These facilities range from the free loan of portable oxygen sets for those passengers with limited cardiac, respiratory, or similar conditions, to the provision of a special airborne stretcher-bed, supporting gear, safety restraining harness (for use during take-off and landing, or at times when lap-straps are worn by normal passengers), privacy curtains, essential bed nursing equipment, etc., for the transfer by air of a seriously ill person in what virtually amounts to a private air cabin.*

Medical personnel are rarely found on any but hospital planes. Commercial airplane and railroad companies have medical services prepared to advise passengers and to give medical attention at large terminals, although the latter is usually confined to first aid. The physician in charge of the patient should furnish the nurse with careful instructions about drugs to be used in an emergency. If the journey is to be a long one and the patient's own doctor therefore not available, the nurse should ask him or her to supply the names of physicians or hospitals en route should the patient need medical attention.

There are customs in relation to tipping, making reservations, protection of luggage, and similar matters with which nurses should familiarize themselves if they hope to avoid difficulties and embarrassment in traveling.

The art of companionship plays an important part in traveling with convalescents and those who are mildly ill. When a trip is part of a plan for rehabilitation, the nurse's problem may be largely that of tactfully limiting activity or suggesting diversions and occupations that will help to bring about a return to health.

Whether the journey is long or short, the patients acutely or mildly ill, it is the function of the nurse to see that they are as comfortable as circumstances permit, that hygienic care and

---

* Schreuder, Otis B.: "General Medical Problems in Passenger Flying," *Conn. Med.,* **27**:390, (July) 1963.

* Barbour, A. B.: " 'Special Delivery' Invalid Air Passengers. Some Medical Considerations," *The Medical Annual,* 1965, p. 10.

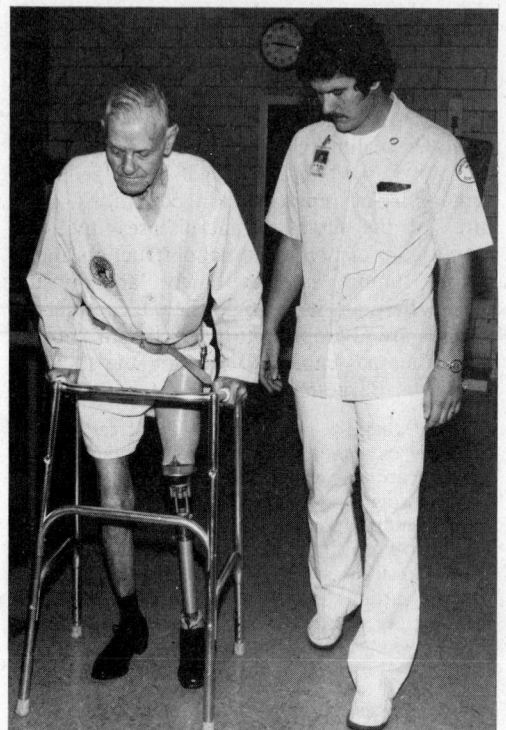

A

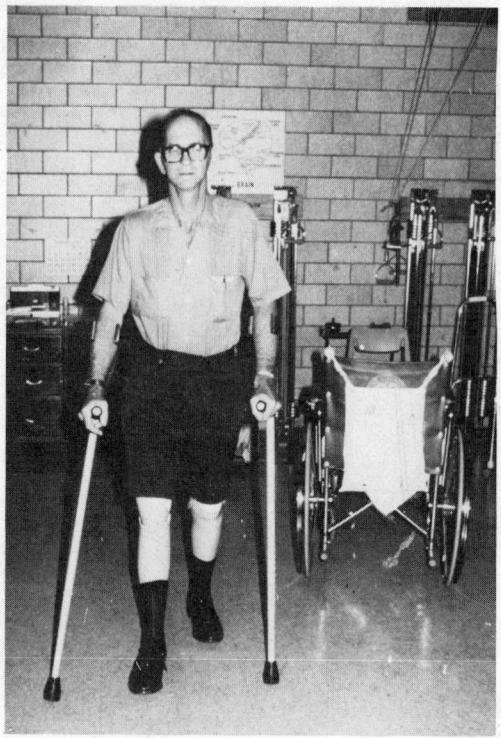

B

Figure 12-28. Patients learn to walk after amputation. *A.* Patient with above knee (AK) left amputation wears a preparatory prosthesis as he learns to ambulate, using a four-point walker. Instruction and assistance of the therapist are necessary during the early stages. *B.* Patient with bilateral amputation, above knee (AK) right and below knee (BK) left, uses a two-point gait with forearm crutches in independent ambulation. (Courtesy of Veterans Administration Hospital, Houston, Tex.)

diet are disrupted as little as possible, and that they get an adequate amount of exercise, rest, and sleep.

6. PREVENTION AND TREATMENT OF PRESSURE SORES (BEDSORES OR DECUBITUS ULCERS)

Nature of a Decubitus Ulcer. A decubitus ulcer, pressure sore, or bedsore may be defined as a localized area of cellular necrosis. Since normal cell metabolism is dependent on receiving nutrients and eliminating wastes (metabolites), any condition that interferes with this exchange will affect the function of the cell. Any alteration in the circulation leads to cellular changes. Pressure on the skin, transmitted through the subcutaneous tissues and muscles to the bone, can interfere with the circulation to such an extent that the tissue, deprived of nourishment, literally dies and becomes gangrenous, or necrotic. Skin areas lying between bony prominences and the bed are most subject to pressure sores. An area of discoloration (reddened, bluish, or mottled appearance of the skin) is an incipient pressure sore. When the process develops to the point where the skin breaks, a true pressure sore results and the wound is soon infected with *Staphylococcus aureus,* hemolytic streptococci, colon bacilli, procyaneus bacilli, diphtheroids, and others.

Predisposing and Direct Causes of Pressure Sores. Although a number of factors are associated with the development of pressure sores, authorities agree that *pressure* is the major cause.[53] Phyllis J. Verhonick and associates report a method for investigating the relationship between pressure and temperature in the development of pressure areas in humans. Data on the problem of pressure sores have been collected on 100 persons and will be examined in relation to the following factors: "pathophysiology, mobility, general nutrition, body build, laboratory findings (blood and urine), nursing and medical regi-

Figure 12-29. A means of transporting infants and children that seems more familiar to them and less formidable than the usual hospital stretcher. (Courtesy of Children's Memorial Hospital, Chicago, Ill.)

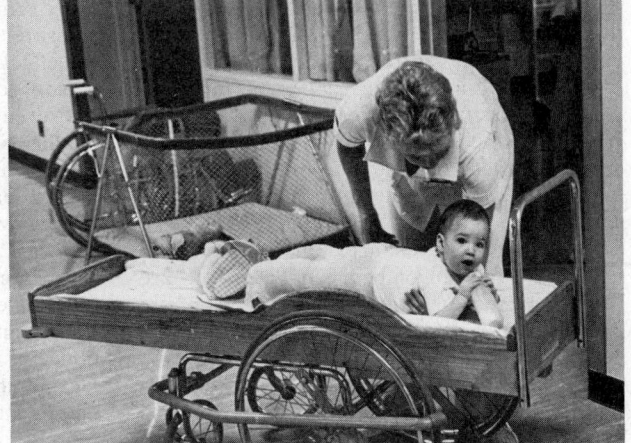

mens, and skin conditions." * In addition, a comparison between high-risk and nonhigh-risk decubitus ulcer patients will be made and reported at a later date. In a study of 26 subjects, Anne Williams [53a] found that thin people (subjected to more *pressure* over bony prominences) who have a higher than normal body temperature (fever) and are receiving corticosteroids are likely to develop decubitus ulcers. Animal experiments have been conducted over a period of years in an attempt to determine the amount and duration of pressure that tissue (cells) can tolerate without damage. T. Housain [54] (1953) reported that when pressure as low as 100 mm Hg was applied for as little as 2 hours to rats, cellular infiltration, interstitial capillary hemorrhage, and cellular degeneration was evident on microscopic

examination 24 hours after application; however, no gross changes were noted. More severe changes occurred when the duration of the pressure was extended to 6 hours. After application of only 60 mm Hg pressure for one hour, Michael Kosiak [55] found microscopic evidence of cellular infiltration, extravasation, and hyaline degeneration, but when the amount and duration of pressure were increased, muscular necrosis and venous thrombosis, as well as cellular infiltration and extravasation occurred. In a later study involving 80 experiments on 40 albino rats, he concludes that the "critical time interval at which pathologic change occurs in both normal and denervated skeletal muscle following application of pressure . . . was between one and two hours." * Some studies suggest that low pressures main-

* Verhonick, Phyllis J., et al.: "Thermography in the Study of Decubitus Ulcers," *Nurs. Res.*, **21**:237, (May–June) 1972.

* Kosiak, Michael: "Etiology of Decubitus Ulcers," *Arch. Phys. Med. Rehabil.*, **42**:19, (Jan.) 1961.

Figure 12-30. A specially designed vehicle transports patients from their homes to the hospital. The patients can be left in a wheelchair or placed on the bench seat. (From Rossman, Isadore: "The Montefiore Hospital After-Care Program," *Nurs. Outlook*, **22**:325, [May] 1974.)

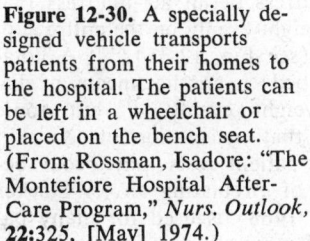
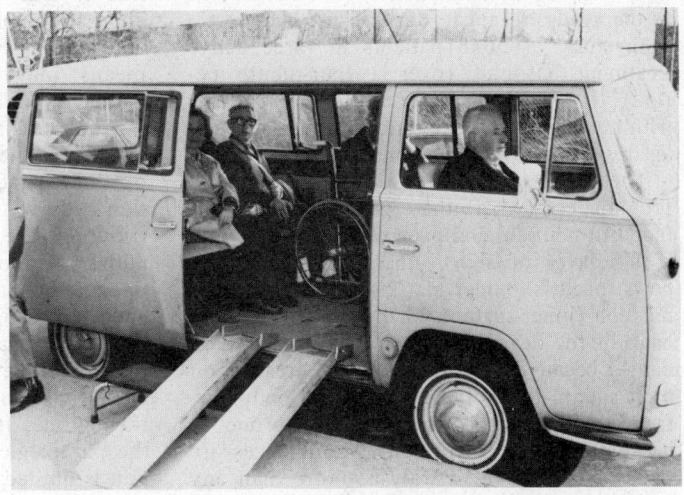

tained for long periods are more damaging to the tissues than high pressures for short periods.[56] Patients in the usual hospital bed or chair with a 2-inch foam rubber pad are subjected to pressure of at least 100 to 150 mm Hg, but as much as 300 to 700 mm Hg have been recorded on the sacrum and ischial tuberosities when sitting on a hard, unpadded surface.[57,58]

Fortunately we change our position frequently in and out of bed, but those who are unable to move freely for any reason are prone to the development of pressure sores.

Another form of pressure is "shearing force," a lag in the subcutaneous tissues behind the bony prominences that move forward when a patient slides down in bed or chair. The "shearing force" is reversed when a patient is pulled up in bed rather than lifted. Small blood vessels are damaged or destroyed in such instances.[59]

Pressure may result from the body lying too long in one position, or from splints, casts, bandages, or bedclothes. The effect of pressure is frequently aggravated by heat, moisture, and decomposing and irritating substances on the skin, such as perspiration, urine, feces, or vaginal discharge. Wrinkles in the undersheet, crumbs, friction from restlessness, rubbing of the bedclothes or of two surfaces of the skin in contact, all predispose to bedsores.

Anything that interferes with the circulation or nutrition of a part, especially if the nerve supply is deficient (as in paralysis, in some fracture cases, and after operations in which nerves have been severed), is likely to result in a pressure sore. Anemia, hypoproteinemia (whatever the cause), and vitamin deficiency play a larger role than is generally thought.[60] Great emphasis is now placed on high-vitamin and high-protein diets for patients in danger of developing decubiti. The debilitated, as well as the aged, are apt to develop pressure sores. In a study of 5648 patients in three active treatment hospitals (over a four-month period), L. W. Gerson [60a] reports that patients with neoplastic and circulatory disease and the aged were predisposed to pressure sores.

The *danger points* on the body are the bony prominences (where there is a poor supply of blood to nourish, and over which there is only a thin layer of skin)—the coccyx, hips, elbows, heels, shoulder blades, knees, and inner malleoli (inner surfaces of the ankles), and the back of the head in infants. The obese are in danger because they exert so much pressure on each square inch of the supporting body surface; the emaciated are especially prone to bedsores because their bony prominences are uncushioned by fat. Paralysis, more than any

other condition, predisposes the subject to pressure sores because he or she cannot feel the effect of pressure or respond as the normal person does with a change of position.

Preventive Measures and the Responsibility of the Nurse. Prevention of bedsores is the responsibility of nurses. As students they should learn how to take care of a patient in such a way as to prevent bedsores, for with sufficient nursing care they can be prevented. The carelessness, neglect, and ignorance of one nurse may in a few hours undo the most skilled and painstaking care of another. "An ounce of prevention is worth a pound of cure." Development of a pressure sore is a reflection on the nursing care the patient has received. Hospital nursing staffs make such an effort to prevent their occurrence that student nurses may have little if any opportunity in some situations to see the treatment of a well-developed lesion unless patients come to the hospital with this condition from homes where skilled care was not available.

Pressure sores are dreaded by the patient and medical attendants because they are painful and very difficult to heal. After the skin is broken, the area almost inevitably becomes infected. Considerable difference of opinion and variability in practice exist in the prevention of bedsores; everyone agrees, however, that the most important measure is the relief of pressure on bony prominences.

It is important to identify those patients who are likely to develop pressure areas so that preventive measures may be instituted before they occur.[60b] Following a review of the literature (including 90 references) Mary R. Bliss [61] concludes that the mechanical methods used in preventing decubiti are based on three principles: (1) distributing body weight over a wide area; (2) tipping or turning the patient from side to side by mechanical means; and (3) alternating pressure. When patients are in danger of developing pressure sores, various means may be used to implement these principles.[61a] They may be kept on an alternating pressure mattress or an air mattress that distributes the weight evenly on the entire supporting surface (see Fig. 12-31).[62,63] A flotation bed (water bed) is another means of distributing the weight evenly,[64–66] but some authorities note that maceration of the skin upon which the patient rests may occur because of a lack of circulating air. A Stryker frame (see page 1468) is used for many patients and is even more effective in distributing the weight since the patient is first supine and then prone. It is recommended especially for the paraplegic whose range of voluntary motion is limited at best.

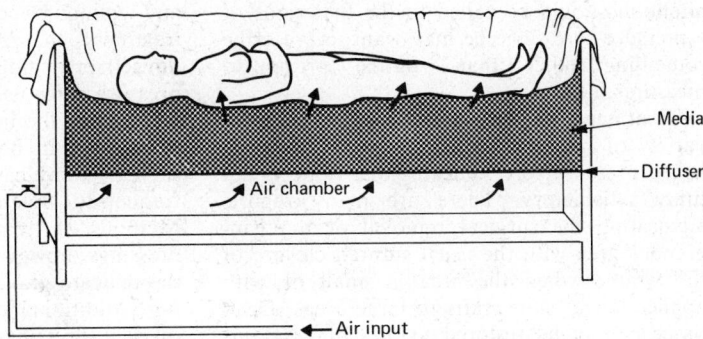

Figure 12-31. Diagram of the air bed. (From Harvin, J. Shand, and Hargest, Thomas S.: "The Air-Fluidized Bed: A New Concept in the Treatment of Decubitus Ulcers," *Nurs. Clin. North Am.* **5:**182, [Mar.] 1970.)

Silastic flotation pads (composed of silastic gel the consistency of human fat) placed into a previously cut-out square (16 inches) of a covered soft sponge rubber mattress may be used. The pad also may be placed in the chair when the patient is up.[67] When such equipment is not available, support the weight of the body and protect all bony prominences by the use of pillows and padding and bandaging joints. Rubber rings and "doughnuts" made of cotton and bandages should not be used as they only transfer pressure from one point to another. Self-adhering material made from polyether urethane foam may be applied to the heels to relieve pressure [68] and sheepskin may be put directly under the patient.

Turn the patient frequently—the position may have to be changed every hour or oftener. Avoid careless use of the bedpan, such as using a chipped pan or leaving the patient on it too long; cover the pan with a pad when there is danger of a pressure sore. When a person has involuntary passages of feces or urine, protect the bed as described in Chapter 37. When there is vaginal discharge, watch the back carefully as the discharge is likely to moisten the back under the dressing or pad and excoriate the skin. Next to an adequate diet and the relief of pressure, absolute cleanliness is the most important preventive measure. Bathe the pubic area and buttocks frequently to remove decomposing urine and other discharges; apply olive oil or cocoa butter to prevent the urine from coming in contact with and irritating the skin. A neutral detergent should be used. Ordinary soap changes the pH of the skin, which is believed to be a protection against bacterial growth (see page 783). See that the patient's gown, bed linen, and coverings of pillows are clean, dry, and free from wrinkles or crumbs. It is customary in most nursing services to rub the skin and surrounding tissue frequently with alcohol—morning and evening, three times a day, every four or two hours, or every hour, as the case demands. The alcohol cools, refreshes, and is believed to harden and dry the skin. There is great question, however, as to whether this is desirable. The writers believe that drying increases the tendency of the skin to break or crack, and recommend an emollient such as "Lubriderm" and a protective waxy coating such as "Keradex" (see Chapter 11). An ointment containing vitamins A and D is also recommended. Whatever lotion is used, however, there is benefit from the rubbing accompanying its application. When the skin is broken, rub only around the lesion and with a circular motion away from the part so as to stimulate the outflow of venous blood and the inflow of arterial blood. Exposure of the reddened area to electric light and radiant heat from a metal reflector is an effective means of improving the circulation and preventing further tissue damage. Keep the skin dry and prevent friction by the use of powder, but do not use enough to cake or roll into hard particles.

Symptoms of a Bedsore. The first symptoms are heat, redness, tenderness, discomfort, and smarting. Heat and redness show that nature has come to the rescue with an increased supply of arterial blood to nourish and revive the injured tissue. At this point it is damaged and congested but still living, and the chances of recovery are good with immediate and constant care. Studies by Kosiak and Housain (discussed earlier) suggest that visual evidence of a pressure sore may not be apparent before 2 to 9 days after the underlying tissues are damaged—all the more reason why prevention is so important.

If pressure is not relieved, the tissues become more congested. The superficial veins first feel the pressure so that the outflow of blood is reduced and the veins engorge, which mechanically prevents an inflow of arterial blood. This congestion makes the part blue, purple, or mottled, like a bruise; it is also cold and insensitive. If the pressure is not immediately relieved and normal circulation restored, true gangrene results. The physician's attention should be called to the first signs of a pressure sore since he may want to prescribe something other than routine preventive measures.

Treatment of Pressure Sores. The great variety of methods used in treating an established pressure sore indicates that none is entirely satisfactory. There are many reports advocating the surgical removal of the gangrenous area with the usual sutured closure of the wound when the area is small or with application of skin grafts to large areas. Dead tissue cannot be restored to life, but remains as a slough (dead flesh in living flesh) that must either be absorbed and carried away by the circulation or removed externally before healing can take place. Ferments or enzymes liberated from the dead and dying cells gradually decompose or soften it so that it may more easily slough away, or be absorbed by the blood and later eliminated. When the slough is removed, an open raw surface or ulcer remains. Only the physician should attempt to separate the dead from the living tissue because of the danger of hemorrhage.

When surgery is not used, a "bedsore" may be treated by sealing it off under a waterproof dressing. Theoretically, the exudates from the lesion form a water cushion that protects the granulating surface. Cellulose film and waterproof adhesive dressings have been used with some degree of success. A great variety of ointments has been advocated as wet or dry dressings, including zinc oxide, boric acid, vitamins A and D, balsam of Peru, and ichthyol; antiseptic powders and liquids including sulfonamides, antibiotics, horse serum, sodium hypochlorate (Carrell-Dakins solution), and Aveeno (a colloid) paste. Some clinicians recommend leaving the ulcer uncovered and exposed to sunlight, if available, or more practically to light bulbs suspended from a cradle over the pressure area. It has been reported that keeping patients in sawdust beds prevents bedsores, and relieving pressure by suspending the body by Kirschner wires through the shoulder and hip girdle has been reported as successful, but it seems heroic treatment. Patients threatened with pressure sores are often placed on Stryker frames (see Chapter 34). Any management of decubiti is successful if at the same time pressure is relieved and a high nutritional status is maintained by having the patient eat a diet high in protein and vitamins B and C. All measures suggested in prevention are used in treatment. Any therapy fails if the underlying causes are not removed.

A pressure sore must be cleaned and the dressing applied with the same care as with any wound. Depending upon the nature of the treatment, the physician may do the dressing himself or at times delegate it to others. Since pressure sores usually occur on the supporting surfaces of the body, their dressings are likely to be soiled by body excretions, and it is necessary, in many cases, to change these dressings frequently unless they are well protected. Methods of treatment that demand frequent dressings, however, tend to remove and injure the delicate granulating tissue formed in healing. Additional data on care of wounds and surgical dressings are found in Chapters 33 and 43.

REFERENCES

1. Goldthwait, Joel E., et al.: *Essentials of Body Mechanics—In Health and Disease,* 5th ed. J. B. Lippincott Co., Philadelphia, 1952.
2. Kendall, Henry O., and Kendall, Florence P.: *Muscles, Testing and Function.* Williams & Wilkins Co., Baltimore, 1949.
3. Kraus, Hans: *Clinical Treatment of Back and Neck Pain.* McGraw-Hill Book Co., New York, 1970.
4. Kite, Joseph H.: "Exercise in Foot Disabilities," in Licht, Sidney (ed.): *Therapeutic Exercise,* 2nd ed. Elizabeth Licht, Publisher, New Haven, Conn., 1965, p. 672.
5. Fitzhugh, Mabel Lum, and Newton, Michael: "Posture in Pregnancy," *Am. J. Obstet. Gynecol.,* **85:**1091, (Apr. 15) 1963.
6. Kraus, Hans: *op. cit.,* p. 10.
6a. Hoover, Sally A.: "Job-Related Back Injuries in a Hospital," *Am. J. Nurs.,* **73:**2078, (Dec.) 1973.
7. Narrow, Barbara A.: "An Hydraulic Patient Lifter," *Am. J. Nurs.,* **60:**1273, (Sept.) 1960.
7a. Sells, Clifford J. and May, Eleanor A.: "Scoliosis Screening in Public Schools," *Am. J. Nurs.,* **74:**60, (Jan.) 1974.
7b. Snyder, Mariah, and Baum, Rebecca: "Assessing Station and Gait," *Am. J. Nurs.,* **74:** 1256, (July) 1974.
7c. Mikulic, Mary Ann, et al.: "Clinical Applications of a Standardized Mobility Test," *Arch. Phys. Med. Rehabil.,* **57:**143, (Mar.) 1976.
7d. Granger, Carl V., and Greer, David S.: "Functional Status Measurements and Medical Rehabilitation Outcomes," *Arch. Phys. Med. Rehabil.,* **57:**103, (Mar.) 1976.
8. Fahrni, W. Harry: *Backache Relieved Through New Concepts of Posture.* Charles C Thomas, Publisher, Springfield, Ill., 1966, p. 5.
9. Saussez, Marcel: *Walking and Limping, A Study of Normal and Pathological Walking.* J. B. Lippincott Co., Philadelphia, 1968, p. 20.
10. Hurwitz, L. J.: "Modern Views on Physi-

ology. XIII. The Control of Posture in Adult Man," *Practitioner*, **204:**188, (Jan.) 1970.

11. Asmussen, Erling, and Klausen, Klaus: "Form and Function of the Erect Human Spine," *Clin. Orthop.*, **25:**55, 1962.

12. Roberts, T. D. M.: "The Mechanics of the Upright Posture," *Physiotherapy*, **55:**398, (Oct.) 1969.

13. Rusk, Howard A.: *Rehabilitation Medicine, A Textbook on Physical Medicine and Rehabilitation*, 3rd ed. C. V. Mosby Co., St. Louis, 1971, p. 88.

14. Kummer, B.: "Gait and Posture Under Normal Conditions, with Special Reference to the Lower Limbs," *Clin. Orthop.*, **25:**39, 1962.

15. Mathews, Donald K., and Wooten, Edna P.: "Analysis of Oxygen Consumption of Women While Walking in Different Styles of Shoes," *Arch. Phys. Med. Rehabil.*, **44:**569, (Oct.) 1963.

16. Gorrie, Mary G.: "Preventing Foot Deformities," *Nurs. Times*, **58:**1250, (Oct. 5) 1962.

17. Jones, Laurence: *The Postural Complex: Observations as to Causes, Diagnosis and Treatment*. Charles C Thomas, Publisher, Springfield, Ill., 1955, p. 79.

17a. Ellis, Rosemary: "After Stroke Sitting Problems," *Am. J. Nurs.*, **73:**1898, (Nov.) 1973.

18. Evans, F. Gaynor: "Stress and Strain of Posture, Expressed in the Construction of Man's Weight-Bearing Skeletal Structures," *Clin. Orthop.*, **25:**53, 1962.

19. Ellwood, Paul M., Jr.: "Bed Positioning," in Krusen, F. H., et al.: *Handbook of Physical Medicine and Rehabilitation*, 2nd ed. W. B. Saunders Co., Philadelphia, 1971, p. 463.

20. Browse, Norman L.: *The Physiology and Pathology of Bed Rest*. Charles C Thomas, Publisher, Springfield, Ill., 1965, p. 163.

20a. Da Liu: *T'ai Chi Ch'uan and I Ching*. Harper & Row, New York, 1972.

20b. *The I Ching or Book of Changes*, 3rd ed. The Richard Wilhelm Translation Rendered into English by Cary F. Baynes. Foreword by C. G. Jung. Princeton University Press, Princeton, N.J., 1967, p. xlvii.

20c. *The I Ching or Book of Changes*, 3rd ed. *op. cit.*, p. liii.

20d. Mackey, Richard T.: *Exercise, Rest and Relaxation*. Wm. C. Brown Co., Publishers, Dubuque, Iowa, 1970, p. 4.

21. Ferguson, Eugene S.: "The Measurement of the Man-Day," *Sci. Am.*, **225:**96, (Oct.) 1971.

22. Kraus, Hans, et al.: "Minimum Muscular Fitness Tests in School Children," *Res. Q. Am. Assoc. Health Phys. Educ.* **25:**178, (May) 1954.

23. ———, et al.: "Role of Exercise in the Prevention of Disease," *G.P.*, **20:**121, (Sept.) 1959.

24. ———: *Clinical Treatment of Back and Neck Pain*. McGraw-Hill Book Co., New York, 1970, p. 7.

25. Cooper, Kenneth H.: *The New Aerobics*. Bantam Books, Inc., New York, 1970, p. 33.

26. Kraus, Hans, and Weber, Sonya: "Back Pain and Tension Syndromes in a Sedentary Profession," *Arch. Environ. Health*, **4:**408, (Apr.) 1962.

27. Cooper, Kenneth H.: *op. cit.*

28. ———: *Aerobics*. M. Evans & Co., New York, 1968.

29. Darling, Robert C.: "Physiology of Exercise and Fatigue," in Licht, Sidney (ed.): *Therapeutic Exercise*, 2nd ed. rev. Elizabeth Licht, Publisher, New Haven, Conn., 1965, p. 34.

29a. Margaria, Rodolfo: "The Sources of Muscular Energy," *Sci. Am.*, **226:**84, (Mar.) 1972.

29b. Adolfson, Göran: "Rehabilitation and Convalescence After Surgery," *Scand. J. Rehabil. Med.*, **1:**14, (No. 1) 1969.

30. White, Paul D.: "The Role of Exercise in the Aging," *J.A.M.A.*, **165:**70, (Sept. 7) 1957.

31. Cooper, Kenneth H.: "Guidelines in the Management of the Exercising Patient," *J.A.M.A.*, **211:**1663, (Mar. 9) 1970.

32. Kottke, F. J.: "Therapeutic Exercise," in Krusen, F. H., et al.: *Handbook of Physical Medicine and Rehabilitation*, 2nd ed. W. B. Saunders Co., Philadelphia, 1971, p. 389.

32a. Shepard, Katherine F., and Barsotti, Louise M.: "Family Focus—Transitional Health Care," *Nurs. Outlook*, **23:**574, (Sept.) 1975.

33. Narrow, Barbara V.: *op. cit.*

34. Winters, Margaret C.: *Protective Body Mechanics in Daily Life and Nursing: A Manual for Nurses and Their Co-Workers*. W. B. Saunders Co., Philadelphia, 1952.

35. Littleton, Jesse T.: "All-Purpose Stretcher Reduces Transfers of Acutely Injured," *Hospitals*, **38:**46, (Aug. 1) 1964.

36. Stevenson, Jessie L.: *Posture and Nursing*. The Joint Orthopedic Nursing Service of the National Organization for Public Health Nursing and the National League of Nursing Education, New York, 1942.

37. Kottke, Frederic J.: "Deterioration of the Bedfast Patient, Causes and Effects," *Public Health Rep.*, **80:**439, (May) 1965.

38. Flash, Bernice: *Kinesiology in Nursing*. McGraw-Hill Book Co., New York, 1952.

39. Royal Committee on Working Conditions: "The Right Way to Lift and Carry," *Phys. Ther. Rev.*, **38:**99, (No. 2) 1958.

40. Works, Roberta F.: "Hints on Lifting and Pulling," *Am. J. Nurs.*, **72:**260, (Feb.) 1972.

41. "Seven Basic Rules for Proper Lifting Procedure," *Hosp. Manage.*, **100:**54, (Nov.) 1965.

42. Morrissey, Alice B., and Sherman, Nadine: "The Tilt Board . . . An Aid to Rehabilitation," *Am. J. Nurs.*, **56:**1146, (Sept.) 1956.

43. Kamenetz, Herman L.: "Selecting a Wheelchair," *Am. J. Nurs.*, **72:**100, (Jan.) 1972.

44. ———: *The Wheelchair Book; Mobility for the Disabled.* Charles C Thomas, Publisher, Springfield, Ill., 1969, p. 128.

45. Ellwood, P. M.: "Prescription of Wheelchairs," in Krusen, F. H., et al.: *Handbook of Physical Medicine and Rehabilitation,* 2nd ed. W. B. Saunders Co., Philadelphia, 1971, p. 452.

45a. Kamenetz, Herman L.: *op. cit.,* p. 128.

46. Covalt, Nila Kirkpatrick: *Bed Exercises for Convalescent Patients.* Charles C Thomas, Publisher, Springfield, Ill., 1968, p. 209.

47. Moskowitz, Eugene: *Rehabilitation in Extremity Fractures.* Charles C Thomas, Publisher, Springfield, Ill., 1968, p. 24.

48. Sorenson, Lois, et al.: *Ambulation; A Manual for Nurses.* American Rehabilitation Foundation, Minneapolis, 1966, p. 20.

49. Rogers, Jack M.: "Transportation of the Emotionally Disturbed Patient," *Bull. Am. Coll. Surg.,* **48:**227, (Sept.–Oct.) 1963.

50. Beadle, E., et al.: "Travelling Abroad with Long-Stay Psychiatric Patients," *Lancet,* **1:**322, (Feb. 8) 1964.

50a. Sherwood, C.: "Transportation Is a Problem: The Nurse Finds the Way," *Front. Nurs. Serv. Q. Bull.,* **48:**19, (Spring) 1973.

51. Schreuder, Otis B.: "General Medical Problems in Passenger Flying," *Conn. Med.,* **27:**390, (July) 1963.

52. Barbour, A. B.: " 'Special Delivery' Invalid Air-Passengers—Some Medical Considerations," *Medical Annual,* 1965, p. 9.

53. Exton-Smith, A. N.: "The Prevention of Pressure Sores," *Gerontol. Clin.,* **3:**65, (No. 2) 1961.

53a. Williams, Anne: "A Study of Factors Contributing to Skin Breakdown," *Nurs. Res.,* **21:**238, (May–June) 1972.

54. Housain, T.: "Experimental Study of Pressure Effects on the Tissues," *J. Pathol.,* **66:**347, (Oct.) 1953.

55. Kosiak, M.: "Etiology and Pathology of Ischemic Ulcers," *Arch. Phys. Med. Rehabil.,* **40:**62, (Feb.) 1959.

56. Exton-Smith, A. N., et al.: "The Prevention of Pressure Sores; Significance of Spontaneous Bodily Movements," *Lancet,* **2:**1124, (Nov. 18) 1961.

57. Kosiak, Michael, et al.: "Evaluation of Pressure as a Factor in the Production of Ischial Ulcers," *Arch. Phys. Med. Rehabil.,* **39:**623, (Oct.) 1958.

58. Kosiak, Michael: "Etiology of Decubitus Ulcers," *Arch. Phys. Med. Rehabil.,* **42:**19, (Jan.) 1961.

59. Clay, Elizabeth C.: "Operation Pressure Sore, I," *Nurs. Times,* **64:**394, (Mar. 22) 1968.

60. Hicks, Dorothy J.: "An Incidence Study of Pressure Sores Following Surgery," in *ANA Clinical Sessions, 1970.* Appleton-Century-Crofts, New York, 1971, p. 49.

60a. Gerson, L. W.: "The Incidence of Pressure Sores in Active Treatment Hospitals," *Int. J. Nurs. Stud.,* **12:**201, (No. 4) 1975.

60b. Rubin, Charlene F., et al.: "Auditing the Decubitus Ulcer Problem, *Am. J. Nurs.,* **74:**1820, (Oct.) 1974.

61. Bliss, Mary R.: "A Consideration of Mechanical Methods of Preventing Bedsores in Elderly Patients," *Gerontol. Clin.,* **6:**10, (No. 1) 1964.

61a. Lang, Christine, and McGrath, Anne: "Gelfoam for Decubitus Ulcers," *Am. J. Nurs.,* **74:**460, (Mar.) 1974.

62. Bliss, Mary R., and McLaren, Rhoda: "Preventing Pressure Sores in Geriatric Patients," *Nurs. Mirror,* **123:**379, (Jan. 27) 1967.

63. Harvin, J. Shand, and Hargest, Thomas S.: "The Air-Fluidized Bed: A New Concept in the Treatment of Decubitus Ulcers," *Nurs. Clin. North Am.,* **5:**181, (Mar.) 1970.

64. Weinstein, J. D., and Davidson, B. A.: "A Fluid Support Mattress and Seat for the Prevention and Treatment of Decubitus Ulcers," *Lancet,* **2:**625, (Sept. 25) 1965.

65. Pfaudler, Marjorie: "Flotation, Displacement, and Decubitus Ulcers," *Am. J. Nurs.,* **68:**2351, (Nov.) 1968.

66. Noonan, Joan, and Noonan, Lawrence: "Two Burned Patients on Flotation Therapy," *Am. J. Nurs.,* **68:**319, (Feb.) 1968.

67. Walden, Richard H., et al.: "Inoperable Pressure Sores, Prevention and Management," *NY State J. Med.,* **71:**657, (Mar. 15) 1971.

68. Kosiak, Michael: "An Effective Method of Preventing Decubital Ulcers," *Arch. Phys. Med. Rehabil.,* **67:**724, (Nov.) 1966.

Additional Suggested Reading

Abelson, L. C., et al.: "Twenty Years of Medical Support in Aircraft Disasters at Kennedy Airport," *Aerosp. Med.,* **44:**560, (May) 1973.

"Air Support Bed," *Am. J. Nurs.,* **75:**1863, (Oct.) 1975.

Astrand, Per-Olof, and Rodahl, Kaare: *Textbook of Work Physiology.* McGraw-Hill Book Co., New York, 1970.

Bedford, P. D., et al.: "The Alternating Pressure Mattress," *Gerontol. Clin.,* **3:**69, (No. 2) 1961.

Berecek, Kathleen H.: "Etiology [and Treatment] of Decubitus Ulcers," *Nurs. Clin. North Am.,* **10:**157, (Mar.) 1975.

Blass, Rosemary A.: "Improved Cushions," *Am. J. Nurs.,* **70:**2605, (Dec.) 1970.

Boyer, John L., and Kasch, Fred W.: "Exercise Therapy in Hypertensive Men," *J.A.M.A.,* **211:**1668, (Mar. 9) 1970.

Brownlow, Miriam A., et al.: "New Washable Woolskins," *Am. J. Nurs.,* **70:**2368, (Nov.) 1970.

Carter, Earl T.: "Clinico-Physiologic Aspects of Passenger Flight," *Conn. Med.,* **27:**385, (July) 1963.

Chesley, Leon C., and Sloan, Donald M.: "The Effect of Posture on Renal Function in Late Pregnancy," *Am. J. Obstet. Gynecol.,* **89:**754, (July) 1964.

Cobey, James C., and Cobey, Janet H.: "Chronic

Leg Ulcers," *Am. J. Nurs.*, **74:**258, (Feb.) 1974.

Cotes, J. E.: "Exercise Limitation in Health and Disease," *Br. Med. Bull.*, **19:**31, (Jan.) 1963.

Downs, Florence S.: "Bed Rest and Sensory Disturbances," *Am. J. Nurs.*, **74:**434, (Mar.) 1974.

Frankel, Victor H., and Burnstein, Albert H.: *Orthopedic Biomechanics*. Lea & Febiger, Philadelphia, 1970.

Griffin, Winnie, et al.: "Group Exercise for Patients with Limited Motion," *Am. J. Nurs.*, **71:** 1742, (Sept.) 1971.

Hogsett, Stanley G.: *Airline Transportation for the Handicapped and Disabled*. National Easter Seal Society for Crippled Children and Adults, Chicago, 1971.

Jebsen, Robert H.: "Use and Abuse of Ambulation Aids," *J.A.M.A.*, **199:**63, (Jan. 2) 1967.

Johnson, Philip C., et al.: "Vascular and Extravascular Fluid Changes During Six Days of Bedrest," *Aerosp. Med.*, **42:**875, (Aug.) 1971.

Jose, Anthony D., et al.: "The Effects of Exercise and Changes in Body Temperature on the Intrinsic Heart Rate in Man," *Am. Heart J.*, **79:**488, (Apr.) 1970.

Langworthy, Orthello R.: *The Sensory Control of Posture and Movement*. Williams & Wilkins Co., Baltimore, 1970.

Line, Rose E.: "Polyether Urethane Foam," *Nurs. Clin. North Am.*, **1:**417, (Sept.) 1966.

Mann, George V., et al.: "The Amount of Exercise Necessary to Achieve and Maintain Fitness in Adult Persons," *South. Med. J.*, **64:**549, (May) 1971.

Marcus, Daniel F., et al.: "The Effect of Exercise on Intraocular Pressure. I. Human Beings," *Invest. Ophthalmol.*, **9:**749, (Oct.) 1970.

Morehouse, Laurence E., and Miller, Augustus T.: *Physiology of Exercise*. C. V. Mosby Co., St. Louis, 1967.

Olson, Sharon C., and Meredith, Diane K.: *Wheelchair Interiors*. National Easter Seal Society for Crippled Children and Adults, Chicago, 1974.

Passo, Sherrilyn DeJean: "Positioning Infants with Myelomeningocele," *Am. J. Nurs.*, **74:** 1658, (Sept.) 1974.

Poller, L., et al.: "Platelet Aggregation and Strenuous Exercise," *J. Physiol.*, **213:**525, (Mar. 1971.

Roat, Darlan D., and Van Tyn, Robert A.: "A Device and Method for the Atraumatic Transportation of the Injured Patient," *Surgery*, **58:** 327, (Aug.) 1965.

Robertson, Caroline E.: "Gel Pillow Helps Prevent Pressure Sores," *Can. Nurse*, **67:**44, (Oct.) 1971.

Rosenthal, Arow M., and Schurman, Alan: "Hyperbaric Treatment of Pressure Sores," *Arch. Phys. Med. Rehabil.*, **52:**413, (Sept.) 1971.

Rowan, Noel M.: "New System for Supporting the Patient in the Management of Decubitus Ulcer: Preliminary Report," *J. Am. Geriatr. Soc.*, **18:**421, (Nov. 5) 1970.

Scales, John T., and Hopkins, L. A.: "Patient-Support System Using Low-Pressure Air," *Lancet*, **2:**730, (Oct. 23) 1971.

Settel, Edward: "Decubitus Ulcer, A Double Blind Study of an Old Problem," *Med. Times*, **97:**220, (Apr.) 1969.

Siegel, Irwin M., and Turner, Myrna: "Postural Training for the Blind," *Phys. Ther.*, **45:**683, (July) 1965.

Simonson, Ernst (ed.): *Physiology of Work Capacity and Fatigue*. Charles C Thomas, Publisher, Springfield, Ill., 1971.

Sorenson, Lois, and Ulrich, P. G.: *Ambulation Guide for Nurses*. Sister Kenny Foundation, Minneapolis, 1974.

Trigiano, L. L.: "Independence Is Possible in Quadriplegia," *Am. J. Nurs.*, **70:**2610, (Dec.) 1970.

Wallace, Gladys, and Hayter, Jean: "Karaya for Chronic Skin Ulcers," *Am. J. Nurs.*, **74:**1094, (June) 1974.

Waller, Julian A.: "The Dangers of the Bicycle," *N. Engl. J. Med.*, **285:**747, (Sept. 23) 1971.

Warren, H. J.: "Air-Sea Rescue," *Nurs. Mirror*, **135:**34, (Nov. 24) 1972.

Gladys Nite
Virginia Henderson

CHAPTER 13

Rest and Sleep

1. GENERAL VALUE OF REST IN HEALTH AND ILLNESS

Rest, mental and physical, is a physiologic necessity, as everyone knows. Even a few minutes of complete relaxation, here and there throughout the day, will go a long way toward conserving mental and physical energy, relieving tenseness, and preventing fatigue. During recent decades a great body of literature has grown up around the effects of "stress," which is defined by Hans Selye as *"essentially the rate of wear and tear in the body."* * Any condition or situation that disturbs the physiologic or psychologic equilibrium of the body is stressful. Selye urges us to follow the ancient Greek admonition to "know thyself" so that we can intelligently cope with the many psychologic and physical stresses that are present in health and illness.

Henry O. Kendall and associates [1] in their classic text, *Posture and Pain,* define stress as "any force that tends to distort a body"; "tension" as a force that lengthens a body; and "strain" as injurious tension in contrast to tautness, which they use for tone or noninjurious tension. Physical and mental fatigue produce strain and would be eliminated in an ideal state. Actually, few people succeed in regulating their lives so as to avoid fatigue. Industrial health programs are aimed very largely at reduction of fatigue. Workers' tools and their environment are studied for their effect on fatigue; work schedules are tried out for the duration and spacing of work periods. For example, telephone operators are found to make more mistakes and machine workers have more accidents if their concentrated service is not interrupted by frequent and regularly spaced rest periods. More accidents are said to occur during the latter part of the afternoon when workers are tired and fewest in the early morning when they are rested. When a person habitually wakes rested after a night's sleep, his or her occupation cannot be said to cause "stress."

All too frequently it is assumed that when a person is lying in bed he is resting. This is not necessarily so. For example, to lie motionless in bed all day is not relaxing for an active man or woman. Adequate rest depends on the degree of muscular relaxation that is present, as well as freedom from mental stress. Insufficient muscular relaxation is reflected in body movements such as frowning and wrinkling of the forehead, tapping the fingers on the bed or armchair, fidgeting, tossing and turning in the bed, or shifting position frequently when sitting in a chair. Samuel W. Gutwirth [2] recommends periodic rest periods during the day for those persons whose work is demanding; short periods are more effective than long periods, especially following the completion of an activity. In addition, he suggests resting after the noon meal and before the evening meal (in a reclining position, if possible) for middle-aged and elderly business or professional men and women. We all know that in many countries it is customary to rest after the noon meal.

Since some muscular contraction accompanies mental activity, one would expect "the worrier" to have difficulty in achieving rest, or freedom from stress. Gutwirth,[2a] in his book on sleep, says that a person who has the habit of worrying must be taught to recognize the accompanying tension patterns if he or she is to achieve peace of mind. It is futile to tell these persons "don't worry" or "forget it"; in fact, such statements only increase the frustration and hostility of the individual.

In a series of lectures given between 1860 and 1862 by John Hilton, a surgeon at Guy's

---

* Selye, Hans: *The Stress of Life.* McGraw-Hill Book Co., New York, 1956, p. 3.

Hospital, London, the concept of rest as a therapeutic measure was introduced to the medical world. Unfortunately, according to Norman L. Browse,[3] the words of Hilton were misinterpreted, and bed rest was viewed as a cure for every illness. In Browse's book, *The Physiology and Pathology of Bed Rest,* based on an analysis of current research, he says the advantages of rest in bed include the following: (1) increases cardiac output and venous return; (2) eliminates the effect of gravity; and (3) promotes relaxation of muscles and relieves weight-bearing strain from bones and joints. These advantages are limited when one considers the variety of conditions that are treated by rest in bed. The effects of hypoactivity are discussed in Chapter 38 and of hyperactivity in Chapter 39; both states threaten health.

Sleep is recognized as rest par excellence. The ability to fall asleep and stay asleep for an unbroken period is a measure of mental and physical health. The psychotic and psychoneurotic suffer as acutely from want of sleep as from any other aspect of their condition. Some psychiatrists ask that graphic records be kept showing the pattern of sleep because this helps them to assess therapeutic progress. Some experts believe that the sleep pattern of the frightened or anxious patient is different from that of the depressed. As depression or anxiety lessens, for example, subjects sleep for longer periods, and instead of waking at 2 or 3 in the morning they will sleep until 4 or 5, or until finally they reestablish their normal pattern. "Neural vigilance," as one writer terms consciousness,[4] is so exaggerated in these disturbed patients that hypnotics may not overcome the wakefulness for any length of time. Those who have attempted suicide will often say that they could not face any more sleepless nights and the accompanying physical symptoms. Herbert Hendin, studying 600 cases of attempted suicide, says:

A number of patients, particularly those with neurotic depression, gave sleeplessness as a major cause and precipitating event in their suicidal attempts. While the dynamics of the individual personality are responsible for the insomnia, once sleeplessness becomes a symptom, it in turn would then act to lower the "threshold" with regard to suicide.*

Nurses must face the fact that broken sleep from which the person wakes fatigued is a disorder, and must realize that unless patients have natural and relatively unbroken and restful sleep, their rehabilitation is incomplete.

The health team should consider their work unfinished when they discharge a patient who has very abnormal habits of sleeping, or who is dependent on drugs. It can be said unequivocally that no hypnotic has been discovered that is not habit forming, that does not have harmful side effects, and that does not require larger and larger doses to be effective. Doctors and nurses should hesitate to induce an unnatural loss of consciousness except for acute pain whose cause cannot be removed by any other means. Continued use of hypnotics and narcotics with the associated reduction of muscle tone results in depression of the respiration, circulation, digestion, and elimination; appetite and thirst are often so inhibited that the acid-base balance is seriously upset. The normal stimulation of all these processes that comes from mental and physical activity is also lessened by the sluggish consciousness of the "doped" individual. Henry K. Beecher,[4a] discussing the resuscitation of wounded military personnel, emphasizes the harmful effects of morphine even in emergencies where its need is believed most urgent. Paul Barringer, writing his memoirs at the end of a long and distinguished medical career, says:

. . . none of us [medical students] appreciated for a moment the profound change in medicine that an accurate thermometric record [thermometer] would bring any more than we foresaw the evils that could follow the foolish and indiscriminate use of the hypodermic as a "pain reliever." *

The use and abuse of drugs, including sedatives, tranquilizers, alcohol, and more recently LSD, to promote relaxation and induce sleep are major problems in the United States and many other countries. Stimulants, commonly referred to as "pep pills," are used by some to keep awake during stressful periods, followed by sedatives or tranquilizers for sleep—setting in operation a vicious circle. The magnitude of the problem was vividly described in 1966 by Gay Gaer Luce and Samuel Segal; they say:

Doctors administer barbiturates to some twenty million patients each year, and stimulants such as dexedrine to about ten million. The upward surge of demand for and dependence upon such drugs has been noticed in England and in other European countries as well. Americans pay about $100 million for prescription sedatives each year—about $350 million if over-the-counter drugs and hospital purchases are included. About $250 million are spent on tranquilizers, and the yearly

---

* Hendin, Herbert: "Attempted Suicide; a Psychotic and Statistical Study," *Psychiatr. Q.,* **24:**39, 1950.

* Barringer, Paul: *The Natural Bent.* University of North Carolina Press, Chapel Hill, 1949, p. 226.

purchase of Americans' foremost psychotoxic drug—alcohol—amounts to nearly $13 billion.

These figures barely suggest the extent to which these drugs have been used to substitute for a well-balanced nervous system. The U.S. Food and Drug Administration has estimated that about half of our barbiturates and amphetamines are diverted from the legal market. We produce about 6 to 10 billion barbiturate capsules and 8 billion amphetamine capsules a year. Illegal traffic in "pep pills" alone amounts to something between $200 million and $400 million a year.*

A few sedatives and tranquilizers are sold without prescription; some of these, by trade name, are Nytol, Sominex, Sleep Eze, and Dormin.[5] Surely, all health workers must view the indiscriminate use of these drugs as a serious health problem and do everything possible to help individuals avoid their unnecessary use in all health agencies, as well as in the home. Drug dependence is discussed in greater detail in Chapter 41, dealing with anxiety, depression, and insomnia, and in Chapter 49, which is on persistent or intractable pain; drug abuse is discussed in Chapter 21.

One of the major aims of nursing care, and one of the measures of its success, is the induction of normal sleep and the reestablishment of what is for each individual a normal pattern of sleeping. Closely allied to this is the acceptance of a regimen that eliminates fatigue, or certainly the exhaustion unrelieved by a night's rest.

Ian Oswald[6] says that we are kept awake by stimuli, which, on reaching the thalamus (by way of the reticular formation), are relayed to the cerebrum. If this is true, it follows that the way to induce sleep is to reduce such stimuli to a minimum. Edmund Jacobson,[7] (in 1948) in his classic text *You Must Relax,* developed the thesis that it is largely the stimuli from contracted muscles that keep us awake. This concept continues to be accepted today by many experts. Hans Kraus, discussing therapeutic exercises in 1963, says:

Since the mind's only outlet is the striated muscle, whatever disturbs a person is reflected in muscle action. If irritations, be they emotional or extrinsic, recur daily and establish similar patterns of response, it can be readily understood that an habitual pattern of muscular reaction is formed.
        . . .
Once the state of tension has reached the borderline of physiology, it can become either more localized, . . . or generalized, as evidenced by sleeplessness, hyper-irritability or poor general health. These symptoms may add up to what used to be called "nervousness" and more recently "tension syndrome"—its main cause the constantly suppressed fight and flight response. . . . It has been shown that by teaching a person how to relax, this complex can be immensely relieved, and that muscular relaxation may in addition help to relieve muscular tension.*,†

2. THE NATURE OF SLEEP AND THEORIES OF SLEEP INDUCTION

Sleep is a variable function of a circadian (rhythmic repetition of certain phenomena in living organisms at about the same time each day) life cycle alternating periodically with wakefulness; it is believed to serve a restorative, recuperative function as it is necessary for the preservation of life and it markedly reduces interaction with the environment.[8,8a] The functions of sleep as outlined by Ernest L. Hartmann are shown in Figure 13-1. Wilse B. Webb, recognizing that we are unable to specify the particular effects of sleep, goes so far as to say:

I believe that sleeping is required for the fulfillment of a complex of very basic needs analogous to the fulfillment of nutritional needs by eating. The strength of sleep as a need is evidenced by the ravages which result from sleep starvation. Further, sleeping places the animal in a very vulnerable condition in relation to its environment. His sensitivity to that environment is considerably reduced. In spite of this danger, the presence of sleep in all vertebrates studied suggests a vital role of sleep for the survival of the organism.‡

The work of many investigators using thousands of EEG "sleep graphs" has shown that the persons studied shift from light to deep sleep (and back again) many times during the night, probably awaking several times without remembering that they have done so (see Fig. 13-2). In uninterrupted sleep, there are two major classes (or parts) of sleep: rapid eye movement (REM), and nonrapid eye movement (NREM), which is divided into stages 1, 2, 3, and 4. Stage 1, entered on going to sleep, is light sleep, and each succeeding stage

---

* Luce, Gay Gaer, and Segal, Samuel: *Sleep.* Coward-McCann, New York, 1966, p. 141.

* Kraus, Hans: *Therapeutic Exercise,* 2nd ed. Charles C Thomas, Publisher, Springfield, Ill., 1963, pp. 236, 237, 238.
† The work of Neal Miller and others[7a,b] shows that the "mind" or "thought" affects unstriated muscle *as well as striated muscle.* For reward or punishment, animals and humans will increase or inhibit intestinal movements. Children can induce vomiting to persuade parents they are too sick to go to school. We therefore question the statement above that "the mind's *only* outlet is the striated muscle."
‡ Webb, Wilse B.: *Sleep: An Experimental Approach.* Macmillan Publishing Co., Inc., New York, 1968, p. 51.

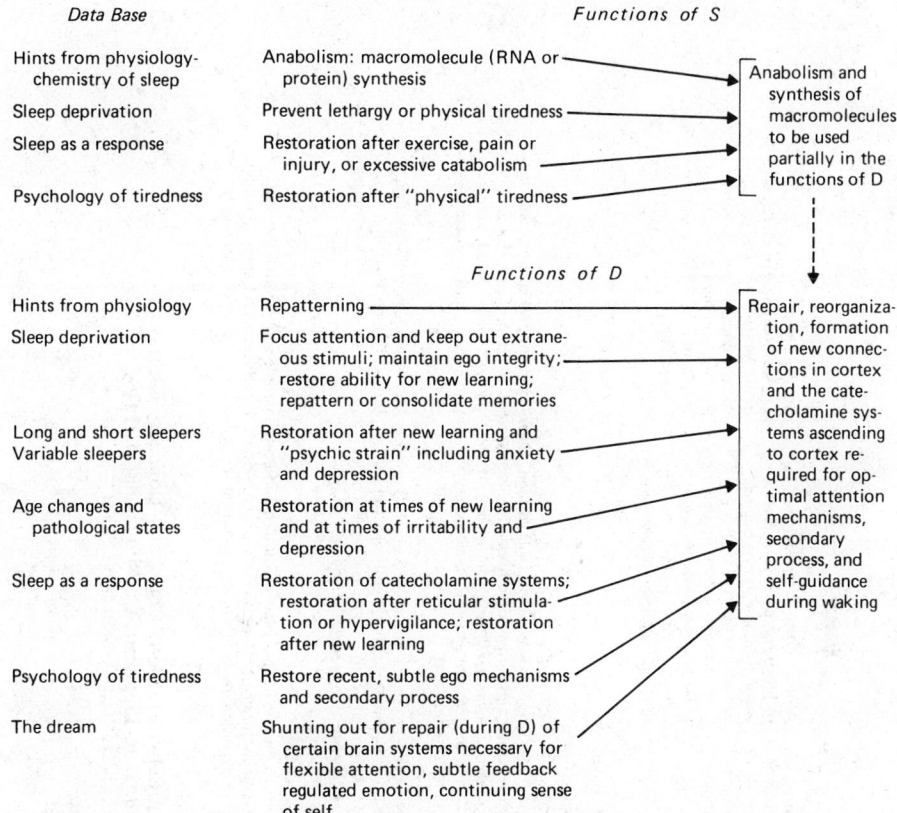

Figure 13-1. The function of sleep. (From Hartmann, Ernest L.: *The Functions of Sleep.* Yale University Press, New Haven, Conn., 1973, p. 146.)

(2 and 3) is deeper than the other until stage 4, which is deepest sleep. Having arrived at this deepest sleep stage, subjects swing back to one of the lighter sleep stages and begin the cycle again. The first "REM sleep" (which has been shown to be the stage most regularly associated with dream recall) occurs 70 to 100 minutes after onset of sleep.[9-11] Figure 13-2 shows patterns and stages of sleep. It is interesting to note that the brain waves of high voltage occur during deepest sleep and low voltage during light sleep; this is explained by the theory that during light sleep the brain cells are alert, scanning activities within the environment.[12] Webb [13] reports that the average number of sleep stage shifts for his subjects was 34 during the first 6 hours of sleep. He thinks this gives one the "impelling impression" of the sleeper being "pulled" between two vital forces: "The need to monitor, and maintain contact with the environment and the need to sleep deeply and profoundly."

During stages 1 and 2, the sleeper is sensitive to *relevant* stimuli in the environment. A mother, for example, will wake from these stages of sleep to a cry from her baby when much louder sounds fail to disturb her. A city dweller will sleep through the roar of traffic but will wake to the click of an opening door. In contrast, as sleep deepens, this capacity to discriminate between sounds is sharply reduced. Even though the sleeper seems to be "pulled" into deep sleep, he or she is able to maintain it for a short time only. Throughout the night there seems to be a continuous struggle between two forces—one demanding deep sleep and the other preventing it.

Joost A. M. Meerloo [14] goes so far as to say that there is no sharp division between being asleep or being awake. While many people sleep full of inner alert (called the sleep of hares), others who call themselves awake live automatically without wakefulness or awareness. The study of the unconscious, the study of dreams, and the relationship of both to man's overt behavior is receiving more and more attention. It is, however, too complex a subject to be treated here in any detail.

The amount of sleep time for each stage in the normal young adult varies considerably:

Waking State
EEG: Brain waves pinched and irregular scrawl; rapid irregular brain charges—low voltage.

Two major classes of sleep:
REM (rapid eye movement) class of sleep—activated sleep state
non-REM (non-rapid eye movement) class of sleep is found in 4 stages

Relaxation
Respiration grows regular—pulse even, temperature declines, aimless thoughts.

Border of Waking/Sleeping
EEG: Scrawl not so pinched, bursts at an even rhythm 9-13 per second, alpha rhythm relaxed and serene, drifting of mind like raft on water.

Stage I Sleep
Light state of sleep: increase in moderate brain waves; voltage and frequency interspersed, and bursts resembling wire spindles; REM appears here in stage I.

Stage II Sleep
Enters this stage with images and fragmentary dreams; brain waves grow longer and slower, medium depth sleep.

Stage III Sleep
EEG: Large, slow waves 1 per second; may be reached about 20 minutes after falling asleep; brain waves slower but with increasing voltage.

Alpha rhythm changes, eyes begin to roll slowly. Images or vague thoughts as one begins to traverse gates of consciousness. Sudden spasm, myoclonic jerk—may awaken one momentarily. Normal sign of movement to sleep—sleeper easily awakened.

Stage IV Sleep
EEG: Large slow waves at high voltage. Deep sleep follows stage III in a few minutes; sinks into bottomless oblivion (lasting 10-20 minutes). Exceedingly hard to awaken (sleep of the weary); if awakened will be confused, remember nothing. When bedwetting, sleep walking, nightmares, or screams occur—restorative sleep.

REM (rapid eye movement) periods in sleep occur periodically throughout the sleep cycle at regular intervals of 85–110 minutes (average of every 90 minutes). This would equal approximately 4-5 episodes of dream activity (when breath and pulse become irregular, penile erections occur, but body feels flaccid; if awakened before muscle tone returns will feel paralyzed). Character of sleep changes throughout the night; as sleep becomes lighter by morning, REM epsodes are longer, more bizarre. Each person, however, has his own REM pattern which changes throughout the life cycle.

Sleep needs change with the life cycle
REM normally decreases markedly from birth to the age of five years. Children and young people spend much more of the early portion of night in deep sleep (when growth hormones reach peak in the blood). Depth of sleep begins to vanish after age 30. Longer periods of lighter sleep in declining years. Extra REM during early years may be related to mental growth.

REM sleep is not a unity but a conjunction of physiologic rhythms and experiences essential to one's well-being.

Figure 13-2. Sleep patterns and stages. (From Sutterley, Doris Cook, and Donnelly, Gloria Ferraro: *Perspectives in Human Development.* J. B. Lippincott Co., Philadelphia, 1973, p. 214.)

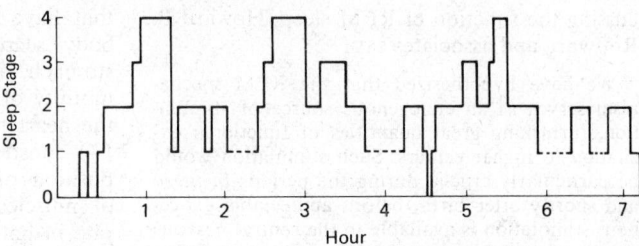

Figure 13-3. Stages of sleep across a night. Dotted lines identify periods of stage 1—REM. (From Webb, Wilse B.: *Sleep: An Experimental Approach.* Macmillan Publishing Co., Inc., New York, 1968, p. 53.)

REM sleep comprises about 20 to 25 per cent of the time; stage 1, 5 per cent; stage 2, 50 to 55 per cent; stage 3, 10 per cent; and stage 4, 10 per cent (see Fig. 13-3). Studies have shown that REM and stage 4 sleep are greatly reduced with age although the nightly percentage of REM sleep varies only slightly (with the exception of the infant) within the various age groups—children, young adults, and the elderly [15] (see Fig. 13-4). During REM sleep,

called the activated stage of sleep and in which vivid dreams may be experienced, the central nervous system functions at intensities as great as, or greater than, during wakefulness. Current evidence suggests that the REM mechanism is located in the pons and that impulses are sent to the motor as well as to sensory areas of the brain. The impulses, after reaching the thalamus from the pons, appear to follow the usual pathways to the cortex.[16] Dis-

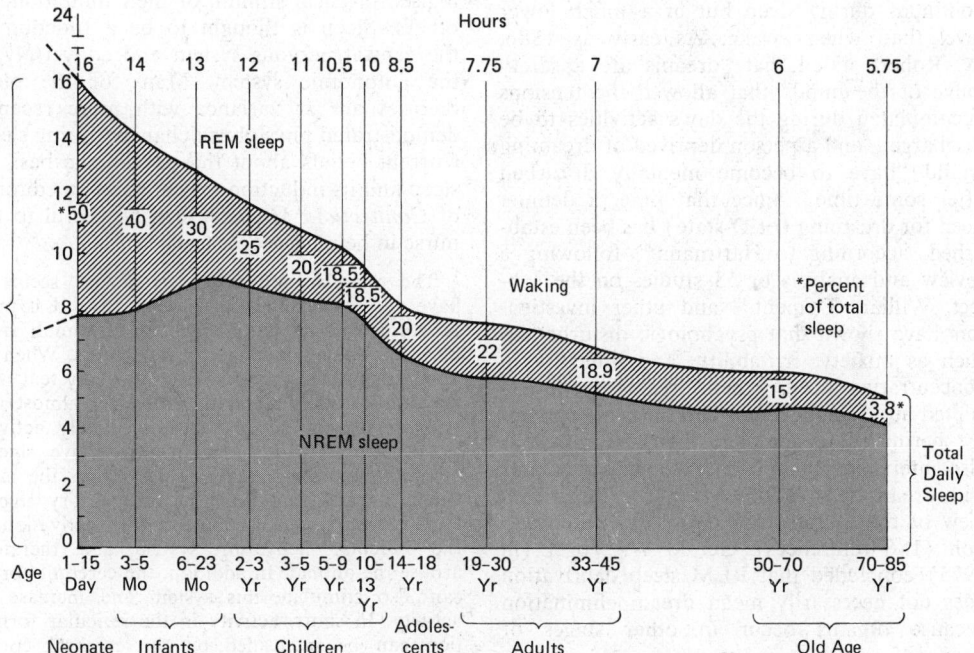

Figure 13-4. Graph showing changes (with age) in total amounts of daily sleep and daily REM sleep, and in percentage of REM sleep. Note sharp diminution of REM sleep in the early years. REM sleep falls from 8 hours at birth to less than 1 hour in old age. The amount of NREM sleep throughout life remains more constant, falling from 8 hours to 5 hours. In contrast to the steep decline of REM sleep, the quantity of NREM sleep is undiminished for many years. Although total daily REM sleep falls steadily during life, the percentage rises slightly in adolescence and early adulthood. This rise does not reflect an increase in amount; it is due to the fact that REM sleep does not diminish as quickly as total sleep. Work in progress in several laboratories indicates that the percentage of REM sleep in the 50- to 85-year group may be somewhat higher than represented here. (From Webb, Wilse B.: *Sleep: An Experimental Approach.* Macmillan Publishing Co., Inc., New York, 1968, p. 140.)

cussing the function of REM sleep, Howard P. Roffwarg and associates say:

We have hypothesized that the REM mechanism serves as an endogenous source of stimulation, furnishing great quantities of functional excitation to higher centers. Such stimulation would be particularly crucial during the periods *in utero* and shortly after birth, before appreciable exogenous stimulation is available to the central nervous system. It might assist in structural maturation and differentiation of key sensory and motor areas within the central nervous system, partially preparing them to handle enormous rush of stimulation provided by the postnatal milieu, as well as contributing to their further growth after birth. The sharp diminution of REM sleep with development may signify that the mature brain has less need for endogenous stimulation.*

We may or may not remember dreams but it is generally thought that most people do dream during REM sleep. However, Nathaniel Kleitman [17] says "there is no proof that dreaming does not occur continuously during the entire night's sleep. . . ." Cortical activity continues during sleep but at a much lower level than when awake. As early as 1886, W. Robert stated that "dreams are a safety valve of the mind" that allowed the tensions accumulated during the day's activities to be discharged, and a person deprived of dreaming would "have to become mentally disturbed after some time." Since that time, a definite need for dreaming (or D-state) has been established, according to Hartmann [18] following a review and analysis of 53 studies on the subject. William Dement [19] and other investigators have shown that psychologic disturbances such as anxiety, irritability, and difficulty in concentrating occur when dreams are interrupted but do not occur when the same persons are permitted to complete their dreams. It is also interesting to note that appetite increases with dream deprivation. After an extensive review of the literature on REM sleep deprivation (186 references) Gerald W. Vogel (in 1975) concluded that REM sleep deprivation does not necessarily mean dream elimination because dreams occur in other stages of sleep. [19a]

Most authorities say that sleep is the most common variant of consciousness, but in spite of the fact that a third of human life is spent in sleep, and it is much discussed by poets, essayists, and scientists, very little is known about its nature. Oswald [20] discusses the following physiologic changes during NREM sleep

that have been established: (1) lessening of body secretions—mouth, nose, throat, eyes, stomach, and bilary system; (2) reduction of motility of the small intestine; (3) slowing of the heart rate with a fall in systolic pressure; (4) constriction of the pupils with no definite position of the eyes; (5) general relaxation of muscles; (6) decrease in basal metabolic rate in both normal and anxious persons; (7) little change if any in the blood glucose level except in persons with diabetes, who have marked variations that cannot be attributed to their last meal; (8) fall in body temperature associated with variations in body metabolism and increased heat loss caused by peripheral vasodilation; and (9) slower and shallower respirations. In REM sleep, however, respiratory rate, heart rate, blood pressure levels, and oxygen consumption levels are higher than in NREM sleep. [21-23]

Some investigators believe sleep is an active, others, a passive, process; chemical change is believed to be a major factor by certain physiologists, physical stimuli, or their inhibition, by others. Sleep is thought to be a function of the central nervous system and conversely of the autonomic system. Many of the older theories are at variance with more recently demonstrated physiologic changes during sleep. Current beliefs about the physiologic basis of sleep and its induction presented in an editorial of *Connecticut Medicine* can be useful to the nurse in helping people to sleep:

The reticular activating system . . . seems to have very little intrinsic activity. Instead it must be stimulated to action by sensory stimuli from both the body and higher brain centers. When an animal is asleep, the reticular activity system is in an almost totally dormant state. Yet almost any type of sensory signal can immediately activate the system. For instance proprioceptive signals from the muscles, pain impulses from the skin, visual signals from the eyes or auditory signals from the ears, can all cause sudden activation of the reticular activating system and therefore arouse the animal. In addition, the cerebral cortex can also stimulate this system and increase its activity. In short, activity in the reticular formation can be intensified by the cerebral cortex from above and by bodily stimulation from below. The highest degree of arousal activity seems to be derived from muscle signals and brain signals.*

Werner P. Koella [24] views sleep as a reflex mechanism and makes the assumption that the "manifold changes in body functions which constitute sleep occur in response to adequate stimuli." Recognizing that our knowledge

---

* Roffwarg, Howard P., et al.: "Otogenetic Development of the Human Sleep-Dream Cycle," in Webb, Wilse B.: *Sleep: An Experimental Approach.* Macmillan Publishing Co., Inc., New York, 1968, p. 164.

* "Physiology of Sleep" (editorial), *Conn. Med.*, **28:** 245, (Apr.) 1964.

about these hypnogenic factors is not very advanced, he says there is enough known about a multitude of such factors operating in the induction of sleep to provide a basis for classifying them into the following four groups: (1) endogenous factors, which may be related to tiredness; (2) endogenous rhythmic factors (internal clocks) that alter in a cyclic fashion the stimulation of the sleep control apparatus; (3) unconditioned factors (such as darkness, quietness, reclining position, and sensory monotony) that influence sleep apparatus via the sensory afferent systems; and (4) conditioned factors (such as getting used to going to bed at a certain time or other presleep rituals) that influence sleep onset.

3. INDUCING SLEEP

Since the state of relaxation parallels the soundness of sleep, nurses may well approach sleep promotion primarily through inducing relaxation. Jacobson [25,25a] and Gerhard B. Haugen and associates [26] (psychiatrists) describe methods of relaxing practically every muscle of the body (and the body as a whole). Nurses might study and teach their patients these methods. Jacobson includes a manual for the patient. All people could profit by the neuromuscular control that enables them to make their body feel heavy, loose, and relaxed as if it were melting into the bed. Even without this special technique, however, the nurse can see that the body is in postures favoring relaxation, such as those illustrated in Figures 12-5, 12-6, and 12-7, Chapter 12, or in the special positions demanded by the patient's peculiar needs. It seems obvious that the relief of emotional disturbance, insofar as this can be accomplished by the nurse, will eliminate one source of tension. Consequently, nurses should help patients explore their fears and anxieties so that they may gain some understanding of their situation. Exercise during the day, health permitting, is suggested by several authorities as inducing sleep. Frederick Baekeland and Richard Lasky [27] found that exercises in the afternoon increased the amount of stage 4 sleep, whereas exercise and complex mental activity before bedtime has a stress effect on the sleeper, producing a disturbed type of sleep.*

Diverting occupation during the day promotes sleep, but exciting activities of all sorts should be avoided at bedtime. The accumulation of lactic acid from muscular exercise is possibly a chemical state conducive to the normal state of semiconsciousness; a marked acidosis results in coma. Reducing the stimuli or message from the eyes, ears, nose, and tactile sense organs induces sleep. A dark, quiet, cool room, free from disturbing odors, a smooth bed, and soft, loose sleeping garments all invite sleep. A neutral bath is a classic treatment for psychotic excitement. Hyperactive patients will nearly always sleep if supported in a tub of water that is kept at body temperature.

Limitation of movement, which is conducive to relaxation, has been shown to induce sleep in animals and children. Persons asked to "lie quietly" in preparation for a test of basal metabolism rate (BMR) will often fall asleep. Kleitman says:

The simple procedure of rocking the cradle, sometimes accompanied by the singing of a lullaby, has long been a favorite way of inducing sleep in infants. Holding a baby in one's arms, quietly restraining its movements, has also stood the test of time as a physical specific.*

The amount of coffee drunk 30 minutes before bedtime has been shown to affect sleep. While one cup of coffee had no effect on sleep of 18 healthy male subjects (20 to 30 years), two and four cups reduced total sleep time, stage 4, and latencies to first REM period and first awakening.[27a] Persons who drink several cups of coffee before bedtime frequently say that when they first go to sleep they dream when "half asleep." Because decaffeinated coffee does not affect sleep, it may be drunk prior to going to sleep.

When planning the patients' presleep activities, it is important to learn their usual regiments, their usual bedtime and routine, measures they take (if any) to induce sleep, and any problems they have had with sleep. Whenever possible, patients should be prepared for sleep at their regular bedtimes and provisions made so that they may go through their regular "presleep ritual," as Meerloo [28] calls it. Following individual patterns is difficult unless a patient is in a private room, but every effort should be made to respect this principle. Serious illness that necessitates treatment during the night interrupts the normal regimen, but this should be reduced to a minimum. Conditions likely to interfere with sleep, if noted early, can often be corrected before bedtime. Sometimes the nurse can relieve them; in many cases medical help is necessary.

---

* It has been my experience that corrective exercises taken before bedtime are very conducive to sleep. V. H.

* Kleitman, Nathaniel: *Sleep and Wakefulness*, rev. ed. University of Chicago Press, Chicago, 1963, p. 195.

Studies at the Cassel Hospital in London, England, for psychoneurotic patients suggest that the hospital atmosphere may itself promote insomnia. Nurses are "on duty" all night, lights are on in the corridors, and there may be conversations at the nurses' station. Doctors tend to readily prescribe and nurses to readily give drugs to induce sleep as if the fact of being hospitalized prohibits sleep. Nurses making the study in the Cassel Hospital concluded that drugs were often given to relieve the nurse's frustration over a wakeful patient rather than to help the patient. In this hospital, where patient government as well as the analytic approach to problems plays a dominant role, the following changes were made: Nurses were no longer "on duty" but one nurse slept in the hospital and was on call. An "orderly" was "on duty" in each unit. Lights were put out at an hour set by the patients. Doreen Weddell, "the matron," reports in 1968 that "Nowadays it is quite rare for anything to happen after 11 P.M. When we first began this system the nurse stayed up until 1 A.M. and then went to bed, but we found the same phenomenon—patients stayed up too. Now the whole hospital is pretty well bedded down by 11 P.M. without any administrative action at all, just as a family sets its own night-time routine and people go to bed when ready." * The nursing staff came to the conclusion that drugs and times . . . were more or less interchangeable. Patients asked for drugs as a means of "achieving extra nursing contact." Weddell says that in general hospitals "the sedative may be the token of being cared for and protected." The use of sedatives was recognized as an expression of a state of mind for the patient and the nurse. At the Cassel Hospital "sedatives are no longer given as a routine." Weddell says "It must be emphasized that the very real intra-psychic pain experienced by the patient is fully recognized with sympathy and understanding, but experience has shown that sedatives as such do not usually help the situation, particularly when given over a period of time." With the changed atmosphere on the patient units and the elimination of drugs given at the nurse's discretion, patients tend to sleep all night.

Massage is a form of passive exercise and if skillful is very soporific. Stroking motions should predominate when massage is used to induce sleep. The patient must be in a relaxed position. The back, neck, arms, and legs may

be rubbed, although for patients who have had recent surgery massage of the legs is contraindicated, particularly if they complain of leg pain. Following operations blood clots may lodge in the vessels, and in the past the leg was a common site for a thrombus. With the emphasis on postoperative exercise and ambulation, blood clots and inflamed vessels are infrequent accidents, but nurses must be alert to this danger.

While the room air should be cool, body warmth induces sleep. Muscles respond to cold by contracting, and this bombards the central nervous system with messages from the proprioceptive sense organs. A hot-water bottle or an electric pad to the feet or abdomen is often more conducive to relaxation and sleep than a hypnotic drug.

Methods of inducing sleep must, like most aspects of care, be individualized to be effective.[28a] Treatment that is relaxing and soothing to one person may be disturbing and exciting to another. The very young and the very old require more warmth than the vigorous person as a rule. Both are very sensitive to the effect of narcotics and hypnotics. Most hypnotics produce a marked decrease in REM sleep with a rebound increase in this sleep following drug withdrawal which may be accompanied by unpleasant dreams, nightmares, anxiety, and fatigue. It should be noted, however, that absence of REM rebound after barbiturate withdrawal has been reported.[28b] Altered sleep patterns by these drugs may be a major factor in drug dependency, according to Anthony Kales and associates.[29] The type and quantity of sleep medication for each patient must be carefully evaluated by the nurse and physician. Such drugs must be given with great caution, and nurses should ask elderly people whether they have ever noticed untoward reactions to drugs of this sort. Doctors often leave very general orders for hypnotics and narcotics. The nurse must often rely on her own judgment and discretion in following these orders. All preparation for the night should be finished before sedatives are given so that the patient will derive the full benefit. Drugs are given to induce sleep when other measures fail. Nurses, and doctors too, should avoid this too easy solution for one problem that creates others more difficult to solve.

4. AMOUNT OF SLEEP NEEDED

Sleep requirements of individuals vary widely and they vary with age (see Table 13-1). For many years it has been thought that older people required less sleep than other

---

* Barnes, Elizabeth (ed.): *Psychosocial Nursing. Studies from the Cassel Hospital, London.* Tavistock Publications, Ltd., London, 1968, p. 66. (Distributed in the United States by Barnes & Noble.)

Table 13-1. Total Number of Sleep Hours by Age *

Age Group	Number of Hours in 24
Newborn infants	10.5–23
Infants to 6 months	12–16+
Preschool children	12–13
Growing children	8.5–7
Youths (13 to 21)	8.75–7
Adults	6–9 (average 7.5)

* Kleitman, Nathaniel: *Sleep and Wakefulness,* rev. ed. University of Chicago Press, Chicago, 1963, p. 114.

adults; the research of Philip Tiller,[30] however, casts doubt on this. In a group of 83 patients over the age of 60, he found that those who slept 8 hours or more had less discomfort, such as tension, fatigue, apprehension, dizziness, feeling of confusion, gastrointestinal symptoms, musculoskeletal pain, and headache, than those who slept fewer than 7 hours. He says:

It is concluded that this study does not support the idea that either the amount of sleep or the need for sleep decreased with age.*

Findings of a later study by Webb and Heather Swinburne [30] support Tiller's conclusions. They also found that sleep in men varied considerably between subjects. If individuals want to learn the amount of sleep they need, they could do so by merely, for a few days, going to bed and sleeping until they wake in the morning without an alarm clock or any other help. Because it is believed that the average individual requires 20 minutes to fall asleep after going to bed, that time should be subtracted from the time spent in bed before waking.

There have been many investigations of man's tolerance for sleeplessness, but the lethal dose has never been established. D. B. Tyler [31] worked with 600 subjects, some of whom went without sleep for 112 days. He found no significant effect on blood chemistry, hemoglobin, red or white cells, body temperature, or weight, and only slight changes in the respiratory rate, pulse rate, and blood pressure. There were, however, marked psychologic changes; notably, irritability, hallucinations or illusions, inattention, and loss of memory. The behavior of some subjects suggested mild schizophrenia. After a review and analysis of studies dealing with sleep deprivation, Kleitman concludes:

* Tiller, Philip: "Bed Rest, Sleep, and Symptoms: Study of Older Persons," *Ann. Intern. Med.,* **61**:98, (July) 1964.

Exhaustion and unconquerable sleeplessness in man are always accompanied by extreme muscular weakness. The failure to find specific predictable changes in the visceral activities points to the absence of an effect on these activities from lack of sleep. Mental and muscular performance in various tests can be maintained at normal levels if the tests are of short duration, but sustained effort is impossible. The increased sensitivity to pain, impairment of the disposition, tendency to hallucinations, and other signs of this character are the outstanding and significant findings in all studies on lack of sleep. They suggest a fatigue of the higher levels of the cerebral cortex—the levels that are responsible for the critical analysis of incoming impulses and the elaboration of adequate responses in the light of one's previous experience.*

According to Luce and Segal,[32] "noticeable changes in brain tissue" have occurred in animals when they have been kept awake for long periods. There are hundreds of publications on sleep deprivation in the literature; a few are included at the end of this chapter.

It has been repeatedly noted that the young suffer most acutely from loss of sleep. Nature protects them by making them sleep long and soundly. Infants, if they are moved gently, will scarcely wake when the mother turns them. Although infants are not very sensitive to their surroundings, sudden noises, a bright light, and any physical discomfort that might wake them should be avoided. Good sleeping habits should be formed early. Infants should be put to bed at a regular time each day and night. (Putting to bed should not be used as a punishment.) Mental excitement, nervousness, and fear of the dark should be prevented. Children should not be told bedtime stories or watch television programs that excite them; in fact, anything should be avoided that may cause sleeplessness or a dislike of going to bed.

The quality as well as the quantity of sleep determines its value. Human beings acquire a daily sleep rhythm; infants and some animals have frequent periods of sleep within the cycle of night and day. Adults tend to get all their sleep in one stretch but this is probably to meet cultural rather than physiologic needs. The soundness of sleep varies from hour to hour. Deep sleep is dreamless and restful. Dreaming precedes waking during light sleep. The deeper the sleep, the more complete the relaxation. This partly explains why a short period of sound sleep can be more restful than a long period of fitful slumber. Another explanation lies in the fact that many somatic functions are greatly affected by the quality of sleep. For example, while the volume of urine

* Kleitman, Nathanial: *op. cit.,* p. 229.

is decreased in sleep, the excretion of urinary phosphate is increased, as is the secretion of sweat and gastric juice. A person's general appearance and outlook on life are in some cases dramatically improved by an uninterrupted period of deep, natural sleep. Studies have shown that poor sleepers are less well-adjusted and have more symptomatic complaints than good sleepers.[33] Patients and nurses do not always agree on how well the patient sleeps; however, the patient's views should always be considered in planning sleep and rest periods.[34] (Insomnia is discussed in detail in Chapter 41.)

5. PREPARATION OF THE PATIENT FOR THE NIGHT

The *purpose* of the preparation is to refresh patients after the discomforts of the day and to remove or minimize causes of restlessness and sleeplessness. Ward patients are in many hospitals wakened early; the day is long, it may have been monotonous and dreary, or patients may have passed through ordeals and be exhausted by pain, discomfort, and the long hours in bed with hot, aching, cramped limbs; they may have been tired by visitors, by worry or excitement, and by the active and sometimes trying scenes around them. Actually, the kind of preparation for the night needed by patients varies so much that any description suggests a routine that disregards individual needs. The following procedure should always be modified by the patient's condition and wishes.

The Evening Toilet. If the patient is in bed, get ready by screening him or her and bring the necessary articles—a basin of water, rubbing lotion, powder, comb and brush, and requisites for cleaning the mouth, clean linen, if necessary, and whatever may be required for their special needs.

The bedpan should first be offered to those who cannot go to the toilet. If the upper bedclothes are loosened and turned back at the foot (without exposing the feet), the clothing will be aired and cooled, and the feet given more freedom. A cotton blanket is of course used to replace the upper bedclothes if a bath or partial bath is given. If the patient can sit in a chair, the unoccupied bed can be more easily made.

Clean the mouth, face, hands, and back. To dabble the hands in water is refreshing, soothing, and restful to the patient; a full bath may be indicated in some cases. Rub the back with lubricant or lotion and powder, giving particular attention to parts that are red or in danger of becoming a bedsore. Patients should be in a relaxed, prone position, if their conditions permit. If a person is wearing a binder, loosen it when washing or rubbing the back. Inspect dressings for bleeding or discharge and see that they are changed or reinforced if necessary. Replace a soiled gown or binder with a clean one. Remove all crumbs from the gown or bed linen. Loosen the drawsheet if one is used and pull it through to give the patient a cool place to lie on. Tighten and smooth the bottom bed sheet. Remove, shake, turn, and rearrange the pillows. Brush and comb the hair. Straighten the upper bedding. If the patient has a hot-water bottle, an icecap, or a water pitcher, see that it is refilled. Give any special attention he or she may require and attend to all requests. While giving this physical care, show an equal consideration for the patient's psychic or emotional needs. Indications of interest or sympathy cannot be formalized or stereotyped. Patients sense them, however, and if the interest and sympathy are genuine, they will talk to the nurse about fears that she or he may be able to dissipate or problems that may solve themselves in the telling.

Report and record significant changes in the condition of the patient, any problems identified, and measures used by the nurse in dealing with them. Note any physical change or any expressions of anxiety or disturbing emotion. The night nurse should be informed about the patient's condition and possible developments. The day nurse should see also that all supplies that may be required for the patient during the night are on hand.

6. SELECTING AND MAKING BEDS

Importance of a Comfortable Bed. As comfort, rest, and sleep are all important in maintaining health and in promoting recovery from disease, special attention, both in homes and hospitals, should be given to providing healthful beds and bedding. In addition, means of signaling attendants must always be available to the patient. Figure 13-5 illustrates devices that hold a signal cord.

Skill in making a bed so as to ensure comfort is one of the first accomplishments of the housekeeper. Non-nursing personnel make empty beds in many hospitals, but nurses should be skillful in making all sorts since in many situations they will prefer to prepare the patients' beds, or they may have to teach bedmaking to others.

Selection of Beds and Bedding. Beds suitable for care of the sick, whether in the home or hospital, differ in certain important respects

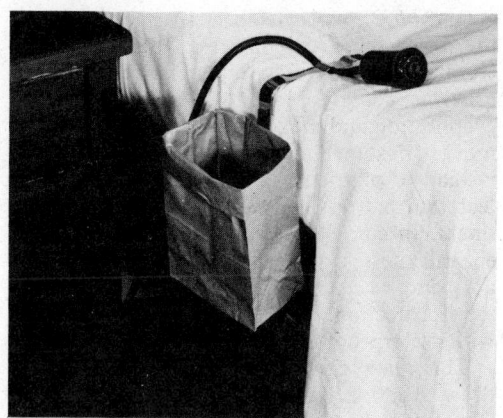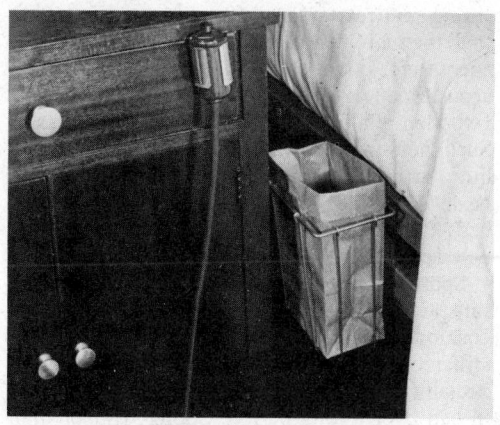

A   B

Figure 13-5. *A.* A device that holds a bell cord and push button in place on the bed and provides attachment for a paper bag. *B.* Two separate devices for these two purposes. (Courtesy of Columbia-Presbyterian Medical Center, New York, N.Y., and Clay-Adams Co., New York, N.Y.)

from those for the well. The sick person not only rests and sleeps but may have meals, recreation, occupation, and exercise in it, and here all the bodily functions must be attended to in some cases. Hospital beds should be adapted also to the needs of those who care for the sick so that their time and energy are conserved.

In psychiatric hospitals or other institutions where patients are ambulatory, patients' rooms can be made into sitting rooms. This gets rid of some of the hospital atmosphere and promotes more normal living. In such cases beds can be designed to look like couches.

The standard hospital bed is single, 6 ft 6 inches long, 3 ft wide, and 26 inches from the floor. Because a lower bed is desirable for ambulatory patients, many hospitals have beds that can be raised and lowered from the floor so that patients can get in and out of bed by themselves. It is simple in design; light; easily moved; easy to handle, clean, and disinfect; and is strong and durable. Hard-rubber casters or hard-rubber tires make it possible to move the bed without jarring the patient. The springs are usually woven wire, but box springs are also used. Adjustable beds, such as the Gatch bed, are now common, and many hospitals have some electrically operated beds which can be placed in a variety of positions and at various heights from the floor by simply punching a button. The motorized rocking bed, mounted on a frame rather than the bedstead, moves slowly and constantly like a seesaw; it is used in circulatory disorders. Beds longer than standard and those with head- and footboards that can be lowered to mattress level should be available for special cases.

There is considerable economy in having the bed furnished with rubber bumpers that keep it clear of walls, door frames, and furniture; this also reduces jarring the patient when the bed strikes an object. Paints used on babies' beds should always be free of lead, as babies frequently bite the frame with the resulting danger of lead poisoning. Some states have laws protecting infants and children from lead paint.

The *bed in the home* is usually much lower and broader, and the linen and blankets are often shorter and narrower in proportion, all of which will require special adjustments when caring for the sick in the home. For instance, blocks may be used to raise the bed to the height that makes lifting and turning the person easier, and linen may be tied to the mattress to make it tight, smooth, and secure, or permanently mitered corners may be made if contour sheets are not available. A piece of cloth sewed to the end of a short blanket at the foot makes tucking possible.

Mattresses for the hospital are generally made of stout, blue-and-white linen ticking (cotton ticking is not so cool or durable), stuffed with horsehair, felt, silk floss, cotton, or kapok. Horsehair mattresses are firm, cool, light, and, because they are nonabsorbent, easy to clean. Curled hair is the best type. Both cotton and kapok mattresses are hard and likely to be lumpy. Mattresses should be even, smooth, and firm to give a sense of support. Innerspring mattresses are widely used in hospitals. They are the most acceptable type to many patients, and maintain their shape and resiliency over a long period. Many authorities in body mechanics condemn the use of innerspring mattresses for sick or well, maintaining that they allow the body to sag and thereby encourage poor posture. Many persons are accustomed to sleeping on a "bed board" (wooden platform the size of the mattress). Such persons are uncomfortable on anything but a straight firm surface. Bed boards should be available to those who want them but all beds that fail to provide firm support should be discarded.

Sponge-rubber mattresses are proving very satisfactory in some situations. They have air cushions on the under surface, being constructed somewhat like a waffle, and are especially valuable for patients who must remain in bed over a long period. Sponge-rubber mattresses are inflammable and when burning give off a noxious gas. Unless properly protected with a fireproof cover, they are a hazard. Compartmentalized air mattresses attached to a motor that progressively empties and fills the rubber compartments with air are available. They are called "alternating pressure" mattresses (see Fig. 12-31, Chapter 12). All mattresses should be protected with washable covers or made with waterproof surfaces. *Water beds* are used in some cases where it is desirable to lower body temperature with cool water or where equalization of pressure is indicated.

There are usually *two pillows* for each bed —one hard pillow stuffed with hair and one soft pillow stuffed with feathers (2½ to 3 lb). Foam- or sponge-rubber pillows are especially useful for individuals with allergies. Because they tend to absorb body heat and do not mold to the head as other pillows do, many persons find them uncomfortable. The hard pillow is used under the feather or rubber pillow for support to the head and shoulders and sometimes without the soft pillow for coolness. It is used for various other purposes, such as to support a limb or to hold it in a fixed position. Smaller pillows also are used for special support or comfort. A very light rubberized silk or plastic cover with zipper fastening may be used successfully to protect the allergic patient; and such covering should be used when a patient has a respiratory infection.

When patients sweat profusely, pillows get wet, soiled, and odoriferous. Folded turkish towels that are replaced at frequent intervals, used in place of a pillow or over the pillow, help to deal with this problem. Keeping pillows free from odors is very difficult in institutions.

Many mattresses have a two-piece zippered covering that is waterproof and fire resistant and can be laundered or sterilized. Such coverings are very important in controlling infection.

A *rubber or plastic* sheet is used to protect the lower sheet and mattress. It must be free from thin places or wrinkles. Because plastic prevents access of air to the skin, it delays evaporation and makes the patient feel hot and moist. In some hospitals quilted cotton pads instead of plastic draw sheets are used to protect the mattress, unless the patient is incontinent. In emergencies at home, pads made of six thicknesses of newspapers inside a removable and washable cotton cover give satisfactory protection to the bed. Mattresses made with waterproof surfaces need less protection.

The *linen* consists of two large sheets, a draw sheet, a spread, and two pillow cases. The large sheets should be strong enough to stand pulling tightly and large enough to tuck in well under the mattress all around (72 by 108 inches is a good size). "The contour sheet" is a desirable substitute for the ordinary undersheet, for it stays tight indefinitely and saves the worker's time. The *draw sheet,* which may be made of single or double cotton, must be wide enough and stout enough to pull tightly and tuck well under the mattress. It is called a draw sheet because it is easily withdrawn, and formerly was made wide enough to be partly withdrawn in order to give the patient a cool place on which to lie. The *spread* should be light and easily laundered; dimity washes and wears well. *Pillow slips* should fit the pillows but not so tightly that they distort the shape.

Blankets should be light and warm. They are lighter in proportion to the warmth, depending upon the amount of wool present. A blanket with 60 to 80 per cent wool is generally used because a blanket with a cotton warp is durable and shrinks less in washing. The usual weight is from 4½ to 7 lb per pair. "Thermal" blankets (a spongy basket weave) are used frequently in hospitals and homes because they are light and warm. Electrically heated blankets are popular in cold climates but they are impractical for institutions, and in countries where there is a power shortage their use may be discouraged.

The Art of Bedmaking. The chief *objectives* in making a bed are comfort for the occupant and economy of materials, time, and energy. Finished appearance is also important. Figures 13–6*A–F* illustrate various aspects of making an unoccupied bed.

The *method* of achieving these ends varies in hospitals and homes, but the following principles apply in all situations. To economize time and effort, everything necessary for bedmaking should be on hand before beginning. To ensure comfort the under sheet must be tight and smooth. "The contour sheet" with

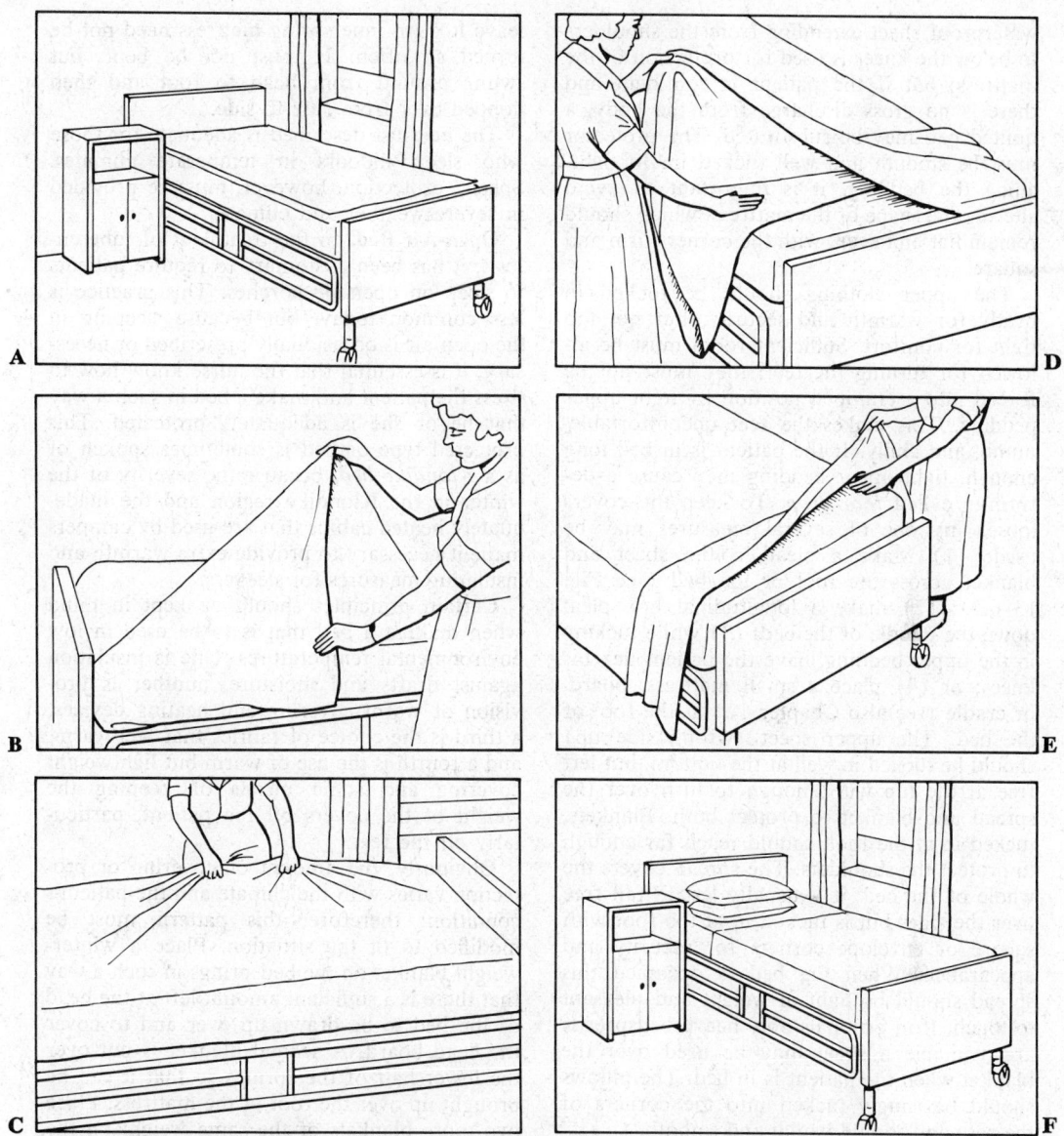

Figure 13-6. Making the unoccupied bed. *A*. The mattress is covered with a plastic, waterproof, insectproof cover. *B*. To maintain the mitered corner the worker is holding the sheet against the mattress with the left hand as she drops the edge to be tucked with the right. *C*. Pulling the bottom sheet taut. This tautness is maintained because the worker tucks the sheet far under the mattress. (The edge of the sheet should almost reach the middle of the mattress.) *D*. The next step is making the horizontal pleat. Note that the pleat is made in the upper sheet and blanket simultaneously. *E*. Bring the pleat to the edge of the mattress. *F*. The finished bed. Note that the spread comes to the head of the bed and that the corners at the foot are square rather than mitered.

manufactured mitered corners eliminates the problem of getting a lastingly smooth lower sheet. If the ordinary kind of sheet is used, it should be placed perfectly straight on the bed; otherwise it will be impossible to make it tight. The top of the mattress should be covered for

protection and the linen tucked far enough under the mattress to keep it fixed, tight, and smooth. It is tucked in on one side and tightened as it is tucked in on the opposite side. Each article of bedclothing is placed on the bed and tightened separately. In the hospital a waterproof sheet extending from the shoulders to below the knees is used for protection of the mattress; but if the patient is continent and there is no gross discharge from the body, a quilted pad may be substituted. The protector must be smooth and well tucked in. In tightening the bedding, it is important to avoid altering the shape of the mattress, which should remain flat and even, with the corners firm and square.

The upper clothing should be tucked in neatly for warmth and security, but not too tight for comfort. Sufficient room must be allowed for turning the feet; they must not be forced into a cramped position by tight upper bedding. This makes the feet uncomfortable, numb, and chilly. If the patient is in bed long enough, tight upper bedding may cause a deformity called *foot drop*. To keep the covers loose, any one of several measures may be used: (1) Make a pleat in the sheet and blanket across the foot of the bed (see Fig. 13–6D); (2) make a longitudinal box pleat down the middle of the bed; (3) while tucking in the upper bedding, have the patient flex his knees; or (4) place a small mattress, board, or cradle (see also Chapter 12) at the foot of the bed. The upper sheet (wrong side up) should be tucked in well at the bottom, but left free at the top with enough to turn over the spread and blanket to protect both. Blankets, tucked in at the foot, should reach far enough to protect the shoulders. The spread covers the whole of the bed; it is usually left to fall free over the sides but is tucked in at the foot with square or envelope corners for security and appearance. When the bed is occupied this spread should be light in weight and pleasant to touch. If in hospitals only heavy bedspreads are available a sheet may be used over the blanket when the patient is in bed. The pillows should be snugly tucked into the corners of the case and should be flat and smooth.

When *stripping an empty bed to remake it,* put beside the bed one or two chairs in position to receive the bedclothes as they are removed. Pillows are taken off first, then the bedding loosened all around and removed one article at a time, each article being folded in quarters and spread over the chairs to air. Caution is used to prevent them from touching the floor. Care should be taken not to throw into the soiled linen container objects such as dentures, jewelry, instruments, and equipment such as a hot-water bag, all of which may be left in the bed through error. They may be lost or injured, and they damage laundry machinery. To avoid unevenness from constant pressure in one place, the mattress should be turned daily from head to foot when the patient can

leave it.* An innerspring mattress need not be turned so often. It must not be bent, but swung around from head to foot and then flopped over from side to side.

The bed just described is adequate for those who sleep indoors in temperate climates. Special protection, however, must be provided in severe weather and climates.

Open-Air Bed. In the treatment of tuberculosis, it has been customary to require patients to sleep on open-air porches. This practice is less common today, but because sleeping in the open air is occasionally prescribed or necessary, it is essential that the nurse know how to dress the patient and make a bed in such a way that he or she is adequately protected. This protected type of bed is sometimes spoken of as a *Klondike bed,* because the severity of the winter in the Klondike region and the inadequately heated cabins that are used by campers make it necessary to provide extra warmth and insulating measures for sleepers.

Certain principles should be kept in mind when making a bed that is to be used in low environmental temperatures. One is insulation against drafts and moisture, another is provision of warm covering and heating devices, a third is the choice of fabrics that feel warm, and a fourth is the use of warm but lightweight covering and some means of keeping the weight of the covers off the patient, particularly off the feet.

Obviously, the amount of covering or protection varies with the climate and the patient's condition; therefore, this pattern must be modified to fit the situation. Place a winter-weight blanket on the bedsprings in such a way that there is a sufficient amount left at the head of the bed to be drawn up over and to cover the head board. A second blanket is put over the lower half of the springs so that it can be brought up over the foot of the mattress. Place two more blankets of the same weight on the springs, leaving enough on each side to come over the mattress and cover it. The selvage of these blankets should be placed at the upper edge of the springs. Before placing the mattress on the springs, cover the area under the mattress with a piece of rubber sheeting or oilcloth. If this is not available, five or six thicknesses of newspapers provide good insulation. The bed is now made like any ordinary bed except that cotton blankets replace sheets. Use

---

* To some this is very important. A strong-minded acquaintance of the second author, up for the first time after a major abdominal operation, asked the person making her bed in the hospital to turn the mattress. Her request was refused. She replied, "Step aside," and turned the mattress herself.

a footboard, a bolster, or large sandbags to keep the weight of the bedclothes off the patient's feet. A cradle is not suitable because the large air pocket that it makes is too difficult to heat.

Before the patient gets into bed, a hot-water bottle or a heating pad is used to warm the bed and is left at the feet. Bags of heated sand are available in the country and are an effective means of providing warmth. If it is possible to roll the bed on to a porch it is desirable to make the bed in a warm room and have the patient get into it there. For baths, meals, and treatment, the patient is brought indoors.

As soon as patients are in bed, tuck the top bedding in snugly but not so tightly that their movements are restricted. The blanket at the foot of the bed is then brought up like an envelope over the bottom of the mattress. Next bring the excess blanket hanging from each side of the springs over the pillows, folding the corners so that the blankets come under the chin and lap over the midline of the bed. The first blanket, which has been pinned in place over the head of the bed, is used to make a triangular-shaped windbreak on either side of the head of the bed. A sleeping bag is a good substitute for this bed.

The patient should wear outing-flannel night clothes, preferably pajamas. Sleeping socks, mittens, and a warm jacket with a hood (sometimes called a *parka*) are usually necessary. Occasionally a shoulder blanket that can be brought over the face is a necessity in very cold climates.

Patients who are on porches need especially careful supervision. They must be provided with a means of signaling attendants, and since there is always a good deal of danger that they may be chilled, there should be no possibility that their call will go unanswered for any appreciable time.

Care of Beds and Bedding. *Equipment* for beds (mattresses, pillows, blankets, linen) and its repair and renewal are among the heaviest items of expense in the hospital. Rigid economy and scrupulous care are important. The need for clean linen depends upon the amount of time patients spend in bed. If they are up during the day, it is obvious that they do not need as frequent change of bed linen as they do when they are in bed day and night and eat their meals in bed. Other considerations are unavoidable odors due, for example, to drainage from wounds and incontinence. Hospitals should provide for the specific needs of each patient rather than make changing bed linen routine. Squares of plastic and soft paper should be used freely to prevent soiling sheets and blankets while treatments are given or when the patient uses the bedpan.

Special precautions should be taken in the care of blankets. Stains should be sponged off at once or the blankets sent to the laundry to have the stain removed. Cotton blankets should be used during treatments or when soiling is likely. The supply, use, and provision for cleaning or washing blankets varies in different hospitals. Some hospitals have established modern laundries equipped with special machinery that makes it possible to wash blankets as frequently as desirable without shrinking or spoiling their appearance or making them harsh or uneven. Some modern laundries now clean blankets by steam, a method that is said not to shrink but to keep them soft and fluffy. In other hospitals not so equipped, blankets are sent to the cleaners to be dry-cleaned, or, if badly soiled, to the laundry.

After the discharge of a patient, in addition to the daily dusting of the bed and care of bedding, a more thorough cleaning is given than is possible when the patient is in bed. The danger of infection in communal living is discussed in Chapter 15, as is concurrent and terminal disinfection in homes and hospitals. All furniture and equipment should be examined to see whether it is in need of repair. Special attention should be given the mattress in some situations to see that there are no bedbugs in the tufts. Waterproof sheets and pillow cases should be scrubbed with warm water and soap, dried, and aired. When not in use, they should be rolled on or suspended over wooden rollers. Folding is likely to crack rubber or plastic. (Making the bed with a patient in it is discussed in Chapter 14, and changing and turning the mattress for a bed patient are discussed in Chapter 12.)

REFERENCES

1. Kendall, Henry O., et al.: *Posture and Pain.* Williams & Wilkins Co., Baltimore, 1952.
2. Gutwirth, Samuel W.: *How to Sleep Well: The Cultivation of Natural Sleep.* Vantage Press, New York, 1959, p. 84.
2a. *Ibid.,* p. 89.
3. Browse, Norman L.: *The Physiology and Pathology of Bed Rest.* Charles C Thomas, Publisher, Springfield, Ill., 1965, p. 148.
4. Head, H.: "The Conception of Nervous and Mental Energy," *Br. J. Psychol.,* **14:**126, 1923.
4a. Beecher, Henry K.: *Resuscitation and Anesthesia for Wounded Men.* Charles C Thomas, Publisher, Springfield, Ill., 1949, p. 115.
5. Luce, Gay Gaer, and Segal, Samuel: *Sleep.* Coward-McCann, New York, 1966, p. 147.

6. Oswald, Ian: "The Experimental Study of Sleep," *Br. Med. Bull.,* **20:**60, (Jan.) 1964.

7. Jacobson, Edmund: *You Must Relax,* 3rd ed. McGraw-Hill Book Co., New York, 1948.

7a. Miller, Neal E.: "Learning of Glandular and Visceral Responses," in Shapiro, David et al. (eds.): *Biofeedback and Self-Control.* Aldine Publishing Co., Chicago, 1973.

7b. Jonas, Gerald: *Visceral Learning. Toward a Science of Self Control.* Viking Press, New York, 1973.

8. Lindsley, Donald B.: "Summary and Concluding Remarks," in Clemente, Carmine D., et al.: *Sleep and the Maturing Nervous System.* Academic Press, New York, 1972.

8a. Hartmann, Ernest L.: *The Functions of Sleep.* Yale University Press, New Haven, 1973.

9. Kales, Anthony, and Kales, Joyce: "Evaluation, Diagnosis, and Treatment of Clinical Conditions Related to Sleep," *J.A.M.A.,* **213:**2229, (Sept. 28) 1970.

10. Kales, Anthony: *Sleep: Physiology and Pathology.* J. B. Lippincott Co., Philadelphia, 1969.

11. Oswald, Ian: *Sleeping and Waking: Physiology and Psychology.* Elsevier Press, New York, 1962.

12. Roche Laboratories: *The Anatomy of Sleep.* Hoffmann-LaRoche, Nutley, N.J., 1966, p. 11.

13. Webb, Wilse B.: *Sleep: An Experimental Approach.* Macmillan Publishing Co., Inc., New York, 1968, p. 53.

14. Meerloo, Joost A. M.: "To Sleep or Not to Sleep," *Med. Times,* **93:**727, (July) 1965.

15. Hartmann, Ernest L.: "The D-State; A Review and Discussion of Studies on the Physiologic State Concomitant with Dreaming," *N. Engl. J. Med.,* **273:**30, (July 1) 1965.

16. Roffwarg, Howard P., et al.: "Ontogenetic Development of the Human Sleep-Dream Cycle," in Webb, Wilse B.: *Sleep: An Experimental Approach.* Macmillan Publishing Co., Inc., New York, 1968, p. 144.

17. Kleitman, Nathanial: "The Nature of Dreaming," in Wolstenholme, G. E. W., and O'Connor, Maeve: *Ciba Foundation Symposium on the Nature of Sleep.* Little, Brown & Co., Boston, 1960, p. 354.

18. Hartmann, Ernest L.: *op. cit.*

19. Dement, William: "The Effect of Dream Deprivation," *Science,* **131:**1705, (June 10) 1960.

19a. Vogel, Gerald W.: "A Review of REM Sleep Deprivation," *Arch. Gen. Psychiatry,* **32:**749, (June) 1975.

20. Oswald, Ian: *op. cit.,* p. 168.

21. Snyder, Frederick, et al.: "Changes in Respiration, Heart Rate and Systolic Blood Pressure in Human Sleep," *J. Appl. Physiol.,* **19:**417, (May) 1964.

22. ————: "Blood Pressure Changes During Human Sleep," *Science,* **142:**1313, (Dec. 6) 1963.

23. Brebbia, D. R., and Altshuler, K. Z.: "Oxygen Consumption Rates and Electroencephalographic Stage of Sleep," *Science,* **150:**1621, (Dec. 17) 1965.

24. Koella, Werner P.: *Sleep: Its Nature and Physiological Organization.* Charles C Thomas, Publisher, Springfield, Ill., 1967, p. 132.

25. Jacobson, Edmund: *Anxiety and Tension Control: A Physiological Approach.* J. B. Lippincott Co., Philadelphia, 1964.

25a. Jacobson, Edmund: *Modern Treatment of Tense Patients.* Charles C Thomas, Publisher, Springfield, Ill., 1970.

26. Haugen, Gerhard B., et al.: *A Therapy for Anxiety Tension Reaction.* Macmillan Publishing Co., Inc., New York, 1963.

27. Baekeland, Frederick, and Lasky, Richard: "Exercise and Sleep Patterns in College Athletes," *Percept. Mot. Skills,* **23:**1203, (Dec.) 1966.

27a. Karacan, Ismet, et al.: "Dose-Response Effects of Coffee on Objective (EEG) and Subjective Measures of Sleep," in Levin, P., and Koella, W. P. (eds.): *Sleep 1974. Proceedings of the Second European Congress on Sleep Research, Rome, April 8–11, 1974.* S. Karger, New York, 1975, p. 504.

28. Meerloo, Joost A. M.: *op. cit.*

28a. Sheerin, E.: "A Programme Which Led to Reduction in Night Sedation in a Major Hospital," *Med. J. Aust.,* **2:**678, (Oct. 6) 1973.

28b. Feinberg, I., et al.: "Absence of REM Rebound After Barbiturate Withdrawal," *Science,* **185:**534, (Aug. 9) 1974.

29. Kales, Anthony, et al.: "Effect of Hypnotics on Sleep Patterns, Dreaming, and Mood State: Laboratory and Home Studies," *Biol. Psychiatry,* **1:**235, (July) 1969.

30. Tiller, Philip: "Bed Rest, Sleep, and Symptoms: Study of Older Persons," *Ann. Intern. Med.,* **61:**98, (July) 1964.

30a. Webb, Wilse, B., and Swinburne, Heather: "An Observational Study of Sleep of the Aged," *Percept. Mot. Skills,* **32:**895, (June) 1971.

31. Tyler, D. B., et al.: "Effects of Experimental Insomnia on Rate of Potential Changes in the Brain," *Am. J. Physiol.,* **149:**185, (Apr.) 1947.

32. Luce, Gay Gaer, and Segal, Samuel: *op. cit.,* p. 94.

33. Monroe, Lawrence J.: "Psychological and Physiological Differences Between Good and Poor Sleepers," *J. Abnorm. Psychol.,* **72:**255, (June) 1967.

34. Fass, Grace: "Sleep, Drugs, and Dreams," *Am. J. Nurs.,* **71:**2316, (Dec.) 1971.

Additional Suggested Reading

"Age and Sleep" (editorial), *Lancet,* **2:**1053, (Nov. 14) 1964.

Agnew, H. W. et al.: "Comparison of Stage Four

and 1-Rem Sleep Deprivation," *Percept. Mot. Skills,* **24:**851, (May) 1967.

Akert, K.: "The Anatomical Substrata of Sleep," *Prog. Brain Res.,* **18:**9, 1965.

Allison, Sarah E.: "The Meaning of Rest. An Exploratory Study," in *ANA Clinical Sessions, 1970.* Appleton-Century-Crofts, New York, 1971.

———: *The Meaning of Rest: Some Views and Behaviors Characterizing Rest as a State and a Process, An Exploratory Nursing Study.* Unpublished doctoral (Ed.D.) dissertation. Teachers College, Columbia University, New York, 1968.

Baker, D. R., et al.: "Evaluation of an Electric Sleep Device," *Minn. Med.,* **47:**1341, (Nov.) 1964.

Bennett, Donald R.: "Sleep Deprivation and Major Motor Convulsions," *Neurology,* **13:**953, (Nov.) 1963.

Dowd, Kathleen M.: *An Exploratory Study of Sleep and Rest in Postoperative Cardiovascular Patients.* Term paper, Yale University School of Nursing, New Haven, 1967.

Downs, Florence S.: "Bed Rest and Sensory Disturbances," *Am. J. Nurs.,* **74:**434, (Mar.) 1974.

Felton, Geraldine: "Effects of Time Cycle Change on Blood Pressure and Temperature in Young Women," in Downs, Florence S., and Newman, Margaret A. (eds.): *A Source Book of Nursing Research.* F. A. Davis Co., Philadelphia, 1973.

Hamilton, Lyle H., et al.: "Effect of a Bedtime Snack on Sleep," *J. Am. Diet. Assoc.,* **48:**395, (May) 1966.

Hartmann, Ernest: "The 90-Minute Sleep-Dream Cycle," *Arch. Gen. Psychiatry,* **18:**280, (Mar.) 1968.

———, et al.: "Psychological Differences Between Long and Short Sleepers," *Arch. Gen. Psychiatry,* **26:**463, (May) 1972.

———: "Sleep and Depression," *N. Engl. J. Med.,* **286:**269, (Feb. 3) 1972.

Hauri, Peter: "The Influence of Evening Activity on the Onset of Sleep," *Psychophysiology,* **5:**426, (Jan.) 1969.

Hess, W. R.: "Sleep as a Phenomenon of the Integral Organism," *Prog. Brain Res.,* **18:**3, 1965.

Johnson, J., and Kitching, R.: "A Simple Sleep Recorder for Clinical Situations," *Br. J. Psychiatry,* **120:**569, (Apr.) 1972.

Karacan, Ismet, et al.: "The Effects of Naps on Nocturnal Sleep: Influence on the Need for Stage-I REM and Stage 4 Sleep," *Biol. Psychiatry,* **2:**391, (Oct.) 1970.

———: "Longitudinal Sleep Patterns During Pubertal Growth: Four-Year Follow-up," *Pediatr. Res.,* **9:**842, 1975.

———: "The Effect of Acute Fasting on Sleep and the Sleep-Growth Hormone Response," *Psychosomatics,* **14:**33, (Jan.–Feb.) 1973.

———: "Sleep-Related Penile Tumescence as a Function of Age," *Am. J. Psychiatry,* **132:**9, (Sept.) 1975.

——— (ed.): "Proceedings of Sleep Symposium Held at 19th Annual Academy Meeting," *Psychosomatics,* **14:**71, (Mar.–Apr.) 1973.

Khatri, Ibrahim M., and Freis, Edward D.: "Hemodynamic Changes During Sleep," *J. Appl. Physiol.,* **22:**867, (May) 1967.

Kollar, Edward J., et al.: "Psychological, Psychophysiological, and Biochemical Correlates of Prolonged Sleep Deprivation," *Am. J. Psychiatry,* **126:**488, (Oct.) 1969.

Long, B.: "Sleep," *Am. J. Nurs.* **69:**1898, (Sept.) 1969.

Mandell, A. J., et al.: "The Stress Responsive Indole Substance in Sleep Deprivation," *Arch. Gen. Psychiatry,* **10:**299, (Mar.) 1964.

Miller, C. H.: "Dreams and Dreaming: The Current State of the Art," *Am. J. Psychoanal.,* **35:** 135, (Summer) 1975.

Oswald, Ian: "Some Psychological Features of Human Sleep," *Prog. Brain Res.,* **18:**160, 1965.

Rechtschaffen, Allen: "Hypersomnia With Sleep Drunkenness," *Arch. Gen. Psychiatry,* **26:**456, (May) 1972.

US Department of Health, Education, and Welfare: *Current Research on Sleep and Dreams.* US Government Printing Office, Washington, D.C., 1966.

Williams, Donald H.: "Sleep and Disease," *Am. J. Nurs.,* **71:**2321, (Dec.) 1971.

Williams, Robert L., and Webb, Wilse B.: *Sleep Therapy.* Charles C Thomas, Publisher, Springfield, Ill., 1966.

Williams, R. L., et al.: "The Encephalogram Sleep Patterns of Middle-Aged Males," *J. Nerv. Ment. Dis.,* **154:**22, (Jan.) 1972.

Gladys Nite
Virginia Henderson

Keeping Clean and Well Groomed, Dressing and Undressing, Protecting the Integument

1. THE MORNING TOILET

Importance of Personal Cleanliness. Habits of personal cleanliness are among the first requisites of hygienic living, and they include daily care of the skin, nails, mouth, hair, clothing, and, under some conditions, the eyes and nose. Good grooming contributes to a sense of well-being, and the absence of it, in most cultures, suggests a low morale. This is even true in the animal world, where healthy creatures are seen to keep themselves clean by various means. The first record found of the importance of personal appearance, both psychologic and physiologic, goes back more than 3500 years when Egyptian scribes recorded on papyrus remedies for skin conditions and detailed descriptions of cosmetics and their uses. Emphasis on maintaining an attractive skin and well-groomed hair has continued throughout recorded history.[1] It is interesting to note, however, that soap, which we consider essential to cleanliness, was first manufactured in England in 1641. Even then its use was discouraged by the government which controlled the amount produced and imposed a high excise tax.[2]

Theodore Rosenthal, discussing personal cleanliness in relation to public health says: "No single article can compare with soap in respect to the amount of sickness and death prevented by its use." * He thinks that basic health truths are often treated so casually by

doctors that patients overlook their advice on hygienic measures. Because hands are the tools that bring food to the mouth, clean body orifices, or rub an itching part, it is particularly important that they are washed many times a day, but especially after contamination with feces. Staphylococcal infections have become a major problem in many of our health institutions and agencies. Communal living anywhere increases exposure of individuals to microorganisms for which they have developed no immunity. Emphasis must be placed on prevention, as many of these infections are serious health hazards.[2a,2b] (Controlling communicable conditions, including worm infestations and staphylococcal infections, is discussed in Chapters 15 and 44.)

Cleanliness is essential to a normal physical and mental state, as this is interpreted in our society, although "normal" persons vary greatly in their standards.

All that can be said about the physiologic and psychologic value of cleanliness in health has added significance in illness. The sick must be fortified with every weapon that will overcome disease and promote the zest for life. Many diseases inhibit physiologic functions, such as lacrimation, salivation, or sweating, that, in a sense, clean the body. Therefore, cleansing processes, adequate in health, may require modification in sickness. The beneficial effects of hygienic measures on the appearance, emotions, and general condition of the patient contribute substantially to diagnosis and treatment. Florence Nightingale[3] wisely observed that persons, whose hygienic care had been

---

* Rosenthal, Theodore: "Personal Cleanliness: A Basic Problem in Hygiene and Public Health," *Med. Times*, 78:497, (Nov.) 1950.

neglected, might seem very ill when they are only hungry and uncomfortable. Such discomforts she thought often misleading to the doctor in diagnosis and therapy. In many cases the restless and sleepless need food and drink or a good bath rather than a sedative or narcotic. Personal appearance, cleanliness, and attractiveness in dress are some of the indices used in assessing improvement of persons under treatment for mental or emotional illness. But, regardless of diagnosis, those in general hospitals as well as in psychiatric hospitals are now encouraged to be well-groomed and to wear their own clothes and, insofar as it is possible, preserve their distinct personalities.

Beginning a New Day. Healthy people usually begin the day refreshed by a night's rest; sick people, although relieved to see the dawn, may be anything but refreshed. They may have had a sleepless night; they may dread what lies in store for them—a feared diagnosis, a painful dressing, an operation, or just another period of boredom. If nurses do not irritate them by thrusting their morning cheerfulness in their face, so to speak, they will unconsciously absorb some of the strength and *joie de vivre*. While wakeful hospital patients often say the sound of the day staff coming "on duty" is music to the ears, there is nothing about which there is more general complaint than noisy personnel beginning, only too early, the day's brisk round of activities. Hospital economy often demands that the patient's day begin early. There are seldom enough nurses to give highly individualized care, and it is thought desirable to have patients bathed and ready to see their physicians during the morning visiting hours. If reasonable hospital routines are explained to patients and there is a genuine effort to reduce regimentation, such routines may be resented less. An increasing number of nurses are planning patients' daily activities with them, varying these according to their likes and dislikes as well as considering their particular needs. Such planning is obviously constructive. Hospitals for the psychoneurotic or for long-term care are developing a form of patient government that allows residents to set their own hours for getting up, going to bed, and for meals. In one such hospital patients help staff the hospital also.[3a]

At the beginning of the usual hospital day, the nurses who have a number of persons assigned to their care should try to determine who requires their attention first, which patients would like to sleep longer, and what, in general, are the needs of each. This analysis depends largely on nurses' powers of observation and sympathy.

In homes, where the nurse is freed from hospital routine, sick persons should under most circumstances be surrounded by quiet until they wake naturally. If they must be waked, the hour should be determined by what is best for them, although in some cases the welfare of the household must also be considered. While a daily regimen is desirable in health, in sickness rest is usually more important than regularity.

Most persons, sick or well, are conscious of their appearance. Even the very ill may be favorably or unfavorably affected by it and dislike being seen at their worst. Most patients like to have their morning toilet completed before they have visitors, or even before they see their doctor.

Morning care usually includes "taking" the temperature, pulse, and respiration, then helping patients with their morning toilets, changing beds, and serving breakfast. It is wise in many cases to give the bath and make the bed after breakfast. If this is done, patients should be prepared for the meal by having their teeth brushed, face and hands bathed, and hair combed.

The help patients need from nurses depends on their condition. They may be so ill or so weak that nurses must care for them as they would infants, or they may need little if any help. The "good" nurse will prevent harmful exertion on the part of the sick but will also encourage children and invalids to develop independence. Hospital nurses who send convalescents home unnecessarily helpless have, to that extent, failed.

2. CARE OF THE SKIN AND NAILS

Hygienic Care of the Skin. The appearance of the skin is not an accurate index of *general health,* but it often reflects the condition of the body as a whole. Figure 14-1 shows a diagram of the skin. A clear complexion and good color go a long way toward making a person look healthy. Assessment of the skin for color and temperature is important for some patients.[3b] Skin, like all other tissues, is affected by its supply of the circulating body fluids and their quality. Changes in the caliber and condition of the vessels affect the quantity and quality of the blood and lymph they carry. Food and fluid intake affect available nutrients, whereas drugs, bacterial toxins, irritating proteins, and endotoxins may contaminate the fluids supplying the skin. Systemic diseases are reflected in the skin. Dermatitis is one of the pathognomonic signs of pellagra, a nutritional deficiency; papules on the back are a common sign of continued use of bromides; fairly typical eruptions are the most prominent symptom of such systemic infections as scarlet fever,

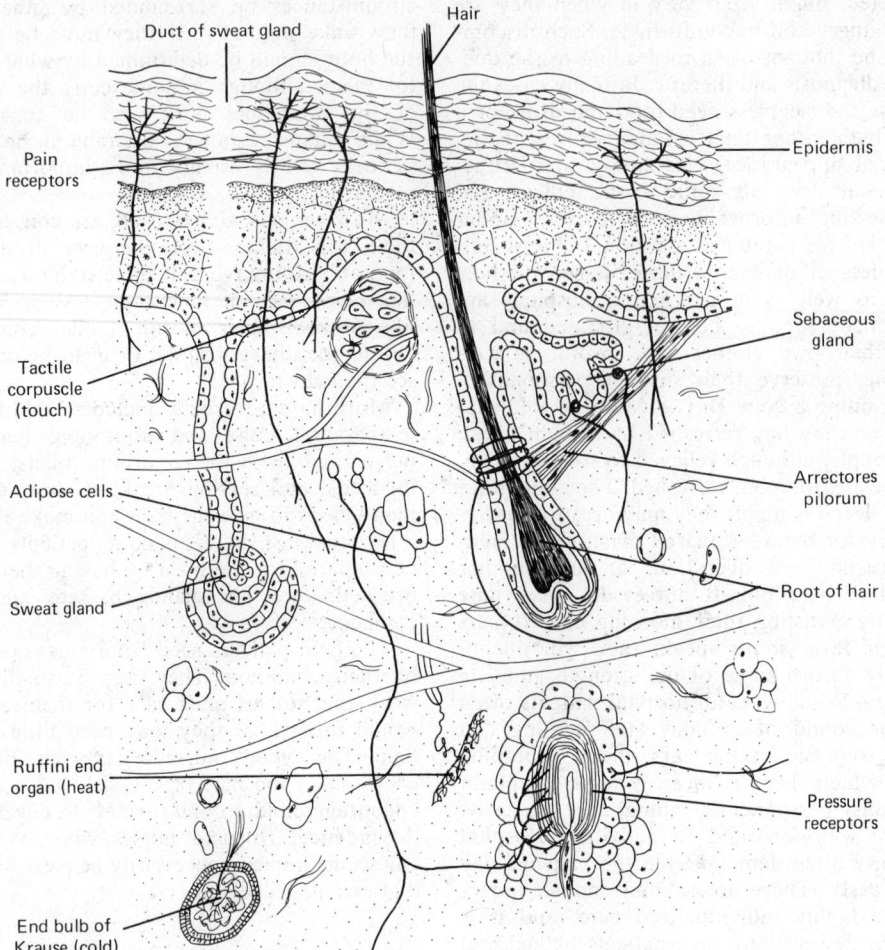

Figure 14-1. Diagram of skin showing receptors for pain, pressure, touch, heat, and cold.

measles, and shingles (herpes zoster); "hives" are a common response to foreign protein in foods or to antibiotic drugs, and the discharge of bile into the skin gives the familiar discoloration and the itching so characteristic of jaundice. This selective list of systemic conditions that may affect the quantity or quality of the skin's circulating fluids omits one of the most important. It is now generally accepted that intense or prolonged emotional stress, with the parallel effect on the endocrine system, may produce such marked changes in the caliber of the blood vessels and in the colloids of the skin that eruptions result; for example, research findings now suggest that exacerbations of acne can follow emotional stress.[4]

Because the skin reflects the condition of the body as a whole (including what is called "the mind"), its hygiene involves a wholesome daily regimen in all its aspects. Obviously, the skin must also be protected from environmental dangers: harmful temperatures, mechanical or chemical irritants, and parasites and microorganisms that may gain access to the skin's deeper layers. Age affects the kind and amount of attention given the skin. Infants have very delicate skin, easily injured mechanically and with relatively low resistance to infection. The newborn's skin should have minimum handling, and all infants and children should be gently bathed, massaged, and protected from harsh and soiled clothing. After the first few weeks all babies and children should be bathed daily. In hot weather several baths are desirable.

After puberty and up to middle age special care is needed to control odors from the secretions of skin glands that are particularly active during the childbearing period. During the teens, eruptions are most likely to appear on the face; therefore, it should be kept especially clean and free from irritation. During the active, hardworking span of life, the skin of the hands and feet need a great deal of attention. The necessity for repeated handwashing may require daily replacement of oils. In a study of 200 cases of "housewives' eczema," Sven Gösta Blohm and Anders Lodin [5] (in Sweden) suggest that the hands should be protected against chemical substances used in water by wearing cotton gloves covered by synthetic rubber gloves. The cotton gloves should be washed frequently and rinsed in boiling water. The amount of detergent used, whether or not gloves are worn, should never exceed that recommended by the manufacturer.

The aged need a different regimen from the young. With age the skin gets less moist and supple, and may lose some of the underlying fat which cushions it against injury. As glandular activity slows, the skin is less moistened by sweat and less lubricated by sebum. Moreover, the lowering of water content is said to be characteristic of aging cells, and the circulatory system may be less efficient in bringing nutrients and removing wastes. The elderly, sensing these changes, tend to bathe less often and may even use vegetable oil, cocoa butter, or lanolin to counteract dryness. The habit of oiling the finger nails and toenails daily is especially desirable as they tend to get brittle. If neglected, the toenails may grow so thick and hard that it is impossible or unsafe for persons themselves to cut them. Soaking the feet or applying pads saturated with warm oil softens the nails. Visits to podiatrists are a boon to the elderly, especially those with dim vision or those who cannot reach their feet. Areas such as heels, toes, and elbows should be rubbed with oil. Because alcoholic lotions are drying, they are not good for the aging skin. Massage is beneficial but should be gentle, and an oil or fat should be used to lubricate the hands of the operator.

Neutral detergents are recommended in place of soaps that change the pH of the skin. Daily baths should not be forced on the elderly. Any compulsion is damaging to the spirit, and frequent bathing still further dries the already dry skin. Incontinence of the bladder or rectum, discussed in Chapter 37, constitutes a special problem that may demand repeated baths.

Skin Diseases and Importance of Medical Treatment. Real skin pathology should be treated by physicians. No one should postpone medical help since the longer the duration of the disease, the more difficult the cure, and the greater likelihood of scarring, and, if the condition is communicable, the greater the danger of transmitting it.[5a,b] The physician always tries to remove the cause, but the etiology of some of the most familiar skin diseases is not established. Acne, for example, is being treated as an allergy by eliminating foods such as chocolate from the diet; as a vitamin deficiency by giving large doses of vitamin A or mixed vitamins; as an unbalanced glandular condition by giving cortisone or estrogens; and as a bacterial disease by chemotherapy or administering antibiotics.[6-11] Where systemic treatment fails in this, as in all skin diseases, the eruption is treated locally with preparations to clean, retard secondary infection, or relieve itching and burning. E. J. Moynahan [12] points out the danger of applying locally the chemotherapeutic and antibiotic agents which, themselves, may produce an "allergic sensitization dermatitis." He thinks there is less danger in oral medication and believes great strides have been made in controlling skin conditions with these two classes of therapeutic agents, with vitamins, the fungicide undecylenic acid, with antihistamines, and with cortisone and ACTH. Gordon C. Sauer,[13] Arthur Bobroff,[14] and other physicians recommend early treatment, with active participation of patients, who assume special responsibilities for their diet, cleanliness of skin and hair, and other general health habits. Bobroff says, "I am shocked at the enormous disfigurement, scarring, and facial destruction among young people. Acne is, in most cases, an easily curable disorder. What is more, it can be controlled before it disfigures." * Donald M. Ruch believes that treatment must be multiphasic, directed toward alleviating "(1) follicular plugging, (2) secondary infection, (3) correction of acnegenic dietary and hormonal stimuli, and (4) prevention of scarring." †

While the value of sunlight and of its substitutes is recognized in psoriasis and some other skin conditions, the medical profession is increasingly wary of any generalized application of radiation. The public should be educated to fear unlimited exposure to sunlight and "sun lamps" and even more the application of repeated doses of x-ray to large skin areas. Excessive exposure to sun contributes to the early development of the "aged skin" which is similar to that of "farmer's skin" or "sailor's skin." It is not uncommon to see young persons with this type of skin. The value of the various vitamin and hormone creams is questionable and disappointing, according to

---

* Bobroff, Arthur: *Acne.* Charles C Thomas, Publisher, Springfield, Ill., 1964, p. vii.

† Ruch, Donald M.: "Acne Vulgaris: Review of One Hundred Cases," *Med. Times,* **93:**1287, (Nov.) 1965.

Hymen Rogachefsky.[14a] A defect (or error) in the metabolism of the tryptophan → niacin pathway, which is present in some people, is brought on by sunlight and artificial light and, in fact, may be provoked or aggravated by both. In persons with pellagra there is a reduction of niacin synthesis, according to recent findings reported by Maurizio Binazzi and Paolo Calandra.[15]

Age seems to affect the type of skin disorders to which the human being is susceptible. Infants and small children are most likely to contract diseases caused by microorganisms, like impetigo, and the so-called children's diseases, characterized by rashes. Adolescents and young adults who have not acquired an immunity during childhood may, of course, have all of these infections, but they seem peculiarly prone to acne and to dermatoses that are thought to have an emotional causation.* In the aged, eczemas, seborrhea, keratoses, and other skin tumors are common.[16-18] Faulty diet is believed to be one of the chief causes of skin diseases in this group. Lessened activity of the glands of internal secretion and of the sweat and sebaceous glands and a low water content —all contribute to the wrinkled, dry, and sometimes scaly skin of the aged. J. R. Owen[19] (in 1951) said that this aging process, as it is often regarded, could be mitigated and the frank skin diseases of old people cured by improved diets, regular application of lubricants such as lanolin, and the administration of estrogens. Neurodermatitis, while not so common in the aged, does occur. Correction of the emotional disturbance is then, as always in this condition, more important than local treatment. Perry A. Sperber[20] (in 1965), discussing the various theories of aging, is in general agreement with Owen; he emphasizes, however, the contribution of plastic surgery. "Face-lifting" is commonplace among actors and actresses and others whose appearance affects their occupational status. There is disagreement about the effectiveness of hormone creams in the care of the aging skin. As was mentioned above, Rogachefsky questions their value, but Richard K. Brown, following a study of 145 women age 30 to 73 years, comes to the following conclusion:

In the majority of subjects there was a moderate improvement in the over-all appearance of the facial skin area where creams containing hormones were used as compared with the facial skin treated with placebo creams.*

He goes on to note other effects such as improvement in the "emolliency" and "feel" of the skin and a decrease in folds of the skin around the eyes and corners of the lips of many of the women.

Itching and burning should be relieved by removing the cause, but temporary relief is often necessary. David T. Graham and associates define two aspects of itching: "(a) first pain: a sharp superficial, well-localized pain of short latency, and (b) second pain: slower, diffuse, burning." †

Medical authorities generally agree that itching is a modified form of pain, transmitted on the slow afferent fibers; there is disagreement, however, on the neurologic basis of the itch sensation. Itching is markedly affected by psychologic and emotional factors and appears to be under cerebral control to some extent.[21] Lotions that paralyze or reduce stimulation of cutaneous nerves relieve itching. When skin or mucous membrane is irritated by acid secretions of the body, a neutralizing lotion may be prescribed.

"Chapping" of the skin is an abnormal condition that plagues many, particularly workers who must wash their hands frequently. A serious and stubborn dermatitis is often the result of continued exposure to soap and water, disinfectants, and irritating chemicals, such as surgeons or hairdressers use. The outermost layer of the skin is composed of practically dead cells, whose protoplasm has changed to a protein called keratin, acting as a waterproof covering for the body. This *stratum corneum*, as it is called, is acid in reaction and is damaged by alkalis. The oil secretion (sebum) of the sebaceous glands lubricates the corneum; and sweat, which is acid, tends to neutralize materials that might injure it and also prevents drying of the waxy keratin. Because of a low water content of the stratum corneum and a low skin surface temperature during the winter, "chapped hands," with their characteristic dry, cracked, and reddened appearance, are most common in cold weather.[21a] Persons in various industries are cautioned against excessive exposure to alkalis, acids, strong soaps, detergents, solvents, wetting agents, and moisture as they interfere with the intactness and hydration of the keratin layer as well as its

---

* Irving Shapiro notes that acne usually makes its appearance at puberty and that it is not found in eunuchs. He says it is much commoner in males than females. (Shapiro, Irving: "Estrogens and Local Applications in the Treatment of Acne Vulgaris," *Arch. Dermatol. Syph.*, **63**:224, [Feb.] 1951.)

* Brown, Richard K.: "Evaluation of Dermatologic Creams Containing Female Hormones," *J.A.M.W.A.*, **21**:493, (June) 1966.
† Graham, David T., et al.: "Itch Sensation in the Skin; Experimental Observations on the Neural Mechanisms Involved," *Trans. Am. Neurol. Assoc.*, p. 135, 1950.

surface pH.[22,22a] Contact dermatitis continues to be the most common occupational dermatosis, according to C. L. Meneghini [23] following an analysis of 1000 cases. In any occupation where the worker handles fabrics, the hands are chapped by constant removal of secretions from the skin.

To prevent "chapping," cleansing agents should be neutral in reaction or should have the pH of the skin. Gerd K. Steigleder and Wolfgang P. Raab,[24] in an investigation of eight ointments (including those containing silicone), concluded that white petrolatum showed the best protective effect of the skin surface against contact with water; they say, however, that the effectiveness of an ointment should not interfere with the performance of the work to be done. Donald J. Birmingham, noting that no one cream will serve all purposes in industry, says:

There is a lack of information regarding the tested protective capacity of barrier creams. Some manufacturers develop baseline data on the protective qualities of their products; however, the lack of uniform testing procedures probably accounts for this deficiency.*

A condition called "warm-water-immersion foot" was common among soldiers who were forced to go days without changing their socks or drying their feet in the rain-soaked coastal lowlands of Vietnam. Their feet became wrinkled, white, and so painful that it was difficult even to walk. Silicone-treated socks have proved to be effective in reducing the incidence of this condition in an experimental group of marines living under similar conditions in the North Carolina swamps.[25]

It is possible that when the hands are washed very frequently, the fat-soluble vitamins are removed from the skin. At any rate, the writers have seen stubborn occupational dermatoses successfully treated with local application of vitamin A and D ointment and large oral doses of vitamin A. Some doctors and nurses regularly apply such ointments to the hands at the first signs of irritation.

Bathing and the Control of Skin Odors. While the skin reflects the condition of the body as a whole, external cleanliness is important. Physiologically speaking, the skin is bathed by sweat and oil from its glands, but even animals, fur-bearing and otherwise, contrive to help nature with this cleaning process. For persons, as for animals, there are many ways of doing this. Peoples with low hygienic standards, according to our customs, do not

necessarily have a high incidence of skin disease; however, those with skin lesions and low hygienic standards tend to have pathogenic organisms (as shown by cultures made from skin swabs) twice as often as those whose skin hygiene is satisfactory. It is safe to assume that, other things being equal, clean skin is less subject to disease than dirty skin.[26] The protective mechanism of the skin has been compared to the surgeon's glove; theoretically, a normal hand with skin intact (no scratches, cuts, or bruises) can be immersed in a media containing virulent organisms without danger, but if there are any cuts, nicks, scratches, or bruises, the organisms will find their way through these to various internal organs.[27] It is doubtful that anyone is aware of the many small nicks or scratches on the skin; people tend to notice only those that cause discomfort. Acidity of sweat discourages bacterial life. If skin bacteria are heavily coated with the oil of unwashed skin, they are protected from the action of sweat and are therefore more likely to cause trouble when the integrity of the skin is destroyed.

Besides its cleansing value, a bath stimulates the circulation, and for the sedentary is particularly important since it is to some extent a substitute for exercise. Richard May,[28] discussing "The [many] Medical Hazards of [public] Bathing," enumerates infection of the skin, respiratory tract, sinuses, eyes, ears, and the intestinal tract; he includes the danger of allergy in pools, where some persons are sensitive to chlorine, loss of life from muscular cramps, and mechanical injury. Even so, he concludes that the advantages of bathing outweigh its dangers and thinks that if the hazards are known, they can usually be avoided.

Daily bathing for the normal person up to middle or old age should be stressed as an *esthetic* necessity rather than a health essential. Secretions of the skin, while they may clean it physiologically, contain waste products such as creatine, uric acid, ammonia, amino acids, glucose, and lactic acid that, particularly on decomposition by bacterial action, have ammoniacal and fetid odors distasteful to people of our culture.[29] Comparison of the chemical composition of sweat, the secretion of the eccrine glands, and dilute urine reveals their similarity.

Natural factors that affect the development and activity of the apocrine glands, according to Harry J. Hurley and Walter B. Shelley,[30] are age, sex, and race. The apocrine secretions begin at puberty, reaching the peak of activity during sexual life of adulthood and diminishing in amount in later years; these glands appear somewhat smaller in women than in men

* Birmingham, Donald J.: "Skin Hygiene and Dermatitis in Industry," *Arch. Environ. Health,* **10:**653, (Apr.) 1965.

and the difference in secretions is minimal. However, there is a great difference among racial groups, the Caucasian having significantly smaller apocrine glands with less secretions than the Negro, and the Orientals, especially the Japanese, having little or no body odor, which indicates that the glands are smaller and less active than in the other two (Negro and Caucasian). They go on to say there are conflicting reports in the literature about activity of the glands during pregnancy and the menstrual cycle, some writers stating there is an increase in sweat production while others hold the opposite view. Nevertheless, secretions of the apocrine glands in the hairy body areas, such as the axillae and pubis, have a particularly strong odor which even daily bathing may not counteract. Young people should be prepared for this physiologic change and helped to develop a regimen that controls body odors. Girls, particularly, should be taught that the apocrine glands are subject to stubborn infections and that the axillae and pubes should be kept very clean; this is even more important during the menses as some authors say that the glands do enlarge and become more active just before and during this time. For all these reasons cleanliness of the female pudenda is not a simple matter. Manufacturers exploit this fact to promote devices and preparations designed to absorb, control, and deodorize excretions and discharges. Some are useful, others useless, others harmful, and some even dangerous. Uncleanliness combined with the use of irritating drugs that attempt to stop or deodorize perspiration is particularly dangerous and should be avoided (see Chapter 25). There is no substitute for soap and water to clean the pubic area and the wearing of clean clothing, both of which will go a long way in eliminating offensive body odor.

Application of deodorants to control odor and antiperspirants (astringents) to control perspiration in the axillae is widely practiced. Most products on the market include several chemicals—some having a deodorizing effect and others an astringent effect, or a combination of both. These substances are usually harmless unless the individual is sensitive to the chemicals they contain or uses them excessively. There are, however, exceptions. Zirconium, a chemical alleged to be of value as a deodorant and antiperspirant and included in many brands, has been found to cause dermal granulomas. Eight years after it was introduced in the United States, a total of 70 cases were reported in the literature, according to Shelley and Hurley.[31] They say this condition is characterized by a chronic papular eruption in the axillae which may persist for months or years,

pruritus and acute inflammation are occasionally present, and major changes occur in the dermis. Although numerous therapies have been tried—such as topical steroids, Grenz-rays, x-rays, and "dry ice"—none has been especially beneficial. On the basis of an analysis of the literature and their own clinical and experimental studies, Shelley and Hurley conclude that "deodorant granulomas result from a specific acquired allergic hypersensitivity to zirconium."

Flow of perspiration is diminished by the action of astringents in coagulating the proteins of the skin, and swelling of the openings of the sweat glands blocks and reduces the flow of sweat, according to Napier Thorne.[32] He says aluminum, zinc, chromium, iron, lead, mercury, as well as zirconium salts, all possess the property of protein precipitation, but because of undesirable side effects of some of these, zinc and aluminum salts are the astringent bases most often found in commercial preparations. Tannic acid may also be used. People should develop the habit of reading labels to find out what is in a product before buying it.

Manufacturers have claimed that chlorophyll taken by mouth will deodorize virtually all body secretions. In 1951, 8 million dollars was spent on advertising chlorophyll, according to Joseph J. Seldin.[33] Some studies supported the claim that water-soluble chlorophyll promotes healing, controls bacterial growth, and has deodorizing properties.[34,35] However, the Council on Pharmacy and Chemistry of the American Medical Association (in 1951) said: "it does not exert a significant disinfectant action, and the mechanism of its deodorant effect on foul-smelling chronic lesions is not clear." *

John C. Brocklehurst [36] (1953), in a thorough investigation, found that chlorophyll mixed with strong-smelling solutions did not remove the smell from these solutions even after 1 month or more. These findings have been supported by other investigations.[37] It seems obvious that no one can depend on a sufficient intake of chlorophyll outside their food to affect body odors.

Many chemicals control odors by oxidizing odoriferous materials or by inhibiting bacterial growth and delaying putrefaction. Sodium borate (borax), zinc peroxide, aluminum, and anion-cation exchange resins are the active agents in many skin deodorants. Borax is a cheap, harmless powder that may be dusted on the skin after a bath. Some authorities

---

* American Medical Association, Council on Pharmacy and Chemistry: *New and Nonofficial Remedies.* J. B. Lippincott Co., Philadelphia, 1951, p. 420.

recommend a mixture of zinc peroxide and cold cream in proportions of about 1 to 8 as a skin deodorant. Medicinal odors in such preparations are undesirable; to some persons they may be as unpleasant as those the deodorant is designed to destroy.

It seems natural that antibiotics in cosmetics would be tried as good results were achieved with antiseptics. A number of studies support their effectiveness in suppression of bacterial growth with no adverse reactions.[38] Their use, however, has not found much commercial favor because of the danger of sensitization and emergence of antibiotic-resistant strains. In 1959, the Committee on Cosmetics of the American Medical Association authorized publication of a report by Carl T. Nelson and Marion B. Sulzberger on the inclusion of antibiotics in products intended for nontherapeutic purposes. They make the following statement:

There seems to be essential agreement that antibiotics generally useful in the treatment of systemic infections should not be used in cosmetics. The risk of sensitization of cosmetic users to such antibiotics could be dangerous. Moreover, and perhaps even more important, the widespread use of cosmetics containing these antibiotics would be unwise because of the possible increased incidence of acquired microbial resistance to such drugs. Therefore, under no circumstances should the antibiotics used in cosmetics include agents of this type.
. . . Evidence has already been presented to show that the widespread topical use of neomycin may increase the number of patients who develop moniliasis as a complication of their therapy. Those who would include such antibiotics as bacitracin, tyrothricin, neomycin, and polymyxin in cosmetics should be prepared to show that their widespread use would not result in an increased incidence of infections due to micro-organisms that are resistant to these agents.*

Publications sponsored by the American Medical Association and the Consumers' Research Annual Bulletin expose false claims of manufacturers and give reliable advice on selection of cosmetics.

The skin may be cleaned by water and soap or soap substitutes. Reports of numerous studies including those by A. L. Hudson [39] and a discussion of many others by F. Ray Bettley [40] and Napier Thorne [41] have shown that soaps, having an alkaline reaction, destroy the protective acidity of the skin's secretions. For this reason, they question the habitual use of soap and would substitute a sulfonated oil detergent, which has a neutral reaction of a pH similar to that of the skin. While allergic reactions to some soaps are fairly common, Richard B. Stoughton,[42] discussing the "controversy" of the relationship of soap to eczematous dermatitis, says soap used routinely has "no detectable adverse influence on the course of eczematous dermatitis." Noting that the results of his controlled studies are in agreement with those of other authors, Stoughton says:

The disproportionate amount of attention focused on soaps and detergents has turned our attention away from other factors which are probably more important in the etiology and aggravation of this common and frustrating disease.*

All writers and researchers do not agree; for example, J. S. Pegum [43] suggests the use of a detergent, "Sevana," while Milton Reisch and Mark R. Marciano [44] recommend "Tridenhex," an "olive-oil-surfactant hexachlorophene mixture" as a cleanser and bath additive for persons with dry, sensitive skin; they do *not* recommend its use for everyone.

Numerous studies [45,46] have been reported on the bacteriostatic effect of hexachlorophene. It is claimed that addition of it in liquid form to the bath water and application to the skin as a powder destroys many bacteria, including the staphylococci. Some writers say it is helpful in controlling cross-infections. A recent study of the effectiveness of antibacterial soaps, containing 1.5 per cent of a mixture of hexachlorophene and triclocarban, on a sample of over 1000 healthy persons showed a significant decrease in superficial cutaneous bacterial infections as compared with those using soap that did not contain the antibacterial ingredients. In addition, no irritation or photosensitivity was noted.[47] Jay P. Sanford [47a] emphasizes that hexachlorophene is *not* a germicide but has limited antimicrobial activity against gram-negative bacilli (*Pseudomonas aeruginosa,* other species of *Pseudomonas, Klebsiella-Enterobacter* species, *Alcaligenes fecalis,* and *Serratia marcescens*) of the type with which nurses and physicians are now concerned. Antimicrobial agents that have been used extensively in detergents, soaps, and creams include hexachlorophene, bithionol, and tribromosalicylanilide. Photoallergic contact dermatitis, however, has been associated with the latter two. In fact, in 1961, a British report warned that "epidemic proportions" had been reached in contact and photocontact dermatitis caused by soaps containing tetrachlorosalicylanilide.[48] In 1972, the US Food and Drug

---

* Nelson, Carl T., and Sulzberger, Marion B.: "Inclusion of Antibiotics in Cosmetic Preparations," *J.A.M.A.,* **169:**1626, (Apr. 4) 1959.

* Stoughton, Richard B.: "The Influence of Soap on Eczematous Dermatitis," *Arch. Dermatol.,* **92:**281, (Sept.) 1965.

Administration banned the use of hexachlorophene in products such as soaps, detergents, and cosmetics sold to the general public and warned doctors and other health professionals to discontinue use of products such as *pHiso-Hex* in routine body bathing in infants and adults because of deaths of some infants and demonstrated brain lesions in baby monkeys. Currently *pHisoHex* (a trade term for hexachlorophene) is used for selected patients *on prescription by the physician only.*[48a,48b]

Because the face and hands are more exposed to soiling and drying, fats such as lanolin, the base of cold creams, and vegetable oils are often used as a substitute for, or in addition to, other agents. Eskimos use oil and sun baths in place of soap and water, and physicians may prescribe oil baths for persons with excessively dry skins.

The consciousness of being clean and of wearing fresh clothing raises the self-respect. A person once accustomed to a morning bath is vaguely uncomfortable all day if deprived of it. It may be of interest to note that in recent prison riots one of the major complaints of inmates has been their limited opportunities for bathing. No one should be more scrupulously clean than nurses; they are in close proximity to others, who are often hypersensitive to odors, and they teach hygiene by example. Besides daily bathing nurses should control axillary perspiration with an approved nonperspirant; if a hypersensitive skin prohibits controlling the secretion of sweat, a harmless deodorant should be substituted.

Removal of Superfluous Hair. Most of the body is covered with hair, although, particularly in women, it is unnoticeable on large areas. Glandular activity influences hair growth; therefore, the location and quality of body hair is loosely associated with masculinity and femininity. Few persons have accurate knowledge of this relationship, but in each country custom dictates that noticeable hair on some parts of man or woman is superfluous. Those sensitive to public opinion, and few are not, should adopt a safe method of removing superfluous hair; its presence inevitably affects self-respect. Hair may be pulled out with tweezers, cut off with scissors, shaved with a razor, removed with wax stripping or depilatories, or the roots destroyed with an electric needle or radiation. According to Earle W. Brauer[49] *electrolysis* in the hands of a specialist is safe and effective. The process is, however, lengthy and expensive. *Radiation* is unequivocally condemned.

Shaving is universally practiced by men and is recommended for both men and women. H. H. Hazen notes that a woman who shaves

the legs or armpits shrinks from shaving the face. He believes this is because it increases her "feeling of masculinity." He thinks that if woman can work and play as man does, she might as well "shave" and says, "Possibly she will come to it." *

A popular misconception that it coarsens hair probably keeps many women from shaving. The stubble that appears a few days after shaving feels like coarser hair but actually isn't. The quality of a man's beard usually remains unchanged from maturity to old age even though he shaves daily or oftener.

Shaving should be preceded by skin cleaning. The skin may be cut by the razor, allowing access of bacteria to the readily infected deeper layers. Thorne[50] describes three types of shaving soaps and creams: lather creams, brushless creams, and aerosols. He suggests that lather creams are more effective, as it is the lathering qualities of a soap or cream that help soften the hair shaft. As the brushless creams cannot do this, it is necessary to first wash the face thoroughly with soap and hot water. Softening the hair makes for a more effective shave and moreover, the razor is not so likely to injure the skin. Stretching the skin lessens the danger of nicking and gives a cleaner shave because it eliminates wrinkles and pits. The angle at which the razor should be held depends upon the make. Lester Hollander and E. T. Casselman[51] say that it should be at least 28 to 30 degrees. Dull razor blades pull but are not so likely to cut the skin. It is economical to get cheap safety razor blades and discard them often. Electric razors, used by so many persons, do not nick the skin and therefore are not considered a hazard.

Cutting superfluous hair with scissors leaves a stubble. Hair *extracted with tweezers* is replaced by a new growth in about six weeks. Paste *depilatories* may soften and partially destroy the hair shaft or may harden around the hair and mechanically remove it when the dried paste is removed. Hazen says most depilatories consist of barium or sodium sulfide. He thinks their action identical with shaving except that the skin is more likely to be irritated.

After the climacteric, body hair gets straighter, finer, and sparse, while the eyebrows often coarsen, and superfluous hair appears on the face. The aged may need more encouragement and help than younger people in controlling undesirable hair growth. Hairs should never be pulled from moles, and, if they are cut, care should be taken not to

---

* Hazen, H. H.: "Cosmetics," *Am. J. Nurs.*, **38**:791, (July) 1938.

prick the mole. Such disfiguring growths should be surgically removed.

Care of the Skin in Sickness. Bathing and its stimulating effect on the circulation are even more important in illness than in health. The sick, especially those confined to bed, are deprived of exercise, particularly in the open, where air currents and changes in temperature may stimulate perspiration but also evaporate it and keep clothing dry. Bed patients of necessity live in garments and between sheets that, as the day goes on, get increasingly permeated with body excretions. In some cases they are sweating excessively; in others the skin is dry and failing to eliminate body wastes normally. In illnesses of any duration skin care is of prime importance. The skin should be stimulated by massage, heat, light, and air motion; the body, kept clean and comfortably dry. Odors should be controlled with nonirritating preparations. Some are so cheap that any hospital could supply them. Frequent change of clothing and bedding is essential.

Very sick persons should, in most cases, have at least one complete bath daily. Exception to this generalization includes the acutely ill patient suffering from a myocardial infarction whose activity, in some cases, should be very limited. Even a bath by a skilled nurse may be too much effort for a damaged, overworked heart. With the exception of the elderly and such patients as the acutely ill cardiac, most patients would enjoy and benefit from a daily bath. Unfortunately, few hospitals are equipped and staffed for this. When baths are limited, there are usually "routines." Lists are kept so that all patients get at least two baths a week and partial baths on other days.

Ideally, baths would be given to each patient at the hour habitual to him or her. Actually, they are usually given when there is adequate personnel and when they don't interfere with treatments, meals, and visiting hours. Rigidity should be avoided here, as in all dealings with people. Kathleen Newton and Helen C. Anderson say:

How many aged patients have been made miserable in the hospital by such trivial rules as having to take showers instead of tub baths, and to take them in the morning instead of at night. Perhaps for fifty years the patient's routine has been to take a tub bath just before retiring. Such unimportant rulings often make the patient unhappy and resistive to important hospital procedures. Evidence of such inflexibility on the part of nurses is fortunately quite rare today.[*]

[*] Newton, Kathleen, and Anderson, Helen C.: *Geriatric Nursing,* 4th ed. C. V. Mosby Co., St. Louis, 1966, p. 50.

In hospitals the usual times for baths are early morning and at bedtime. It is believed that a bath should not immediately follow a meal because it increases the volume of blood in the skin and thereby decreases the supply to the digestive organs.

Any doubts about the value of bathing are dispelled by seeing the effects on the very sick. Patients who in the morning after a sleepless night look hopelessly ill may fall into a natural restful slumber after a warm bath, a massage, and a change of linen. Their whole appearance is altered, and pulse and respiration rates are nearer normal. If the doctor does not see patients before they are so refreshed, the appraisal of nurses who see them at their worst should be shared with physicians.

The Cleansing Tub and Shower Bath. If the patient's condition permits (when the pulse is of good quality and there is no exhaustion or other contraindication), a tub bath or shower is usually preferred by the patient. A bed bath is at best a poor substitute for an immersion bath or shower. While nurses, who are with patients most constantly, are best able to judge whether patients are able to take tub baths or showers, physicians in some countries prefer to make this decision, even putting it into the "doctor's orders." When patients need help with tub baths or showers, a nurse or some attendant should see that the bathroom is warm, that the bath is prepared at the right temperature, generally 37.8° to 40.6°C (100° to 105°F), and that everything necessary is available. This includes soap, wash cloth, towel, nail brush, comb, nightgown or pajamas, bathrobe, slippers, and stockings in some cases. If the patients have no toothbrush or other requisite, it should be provided by those responsible for their care. Patients should be given any necessary assistance. With sufficient help, and in tubs such as those shown in Figure 14-2, a tub bath can be taken with little fatigue. In hospitals in the United States, attendants of the same sex as the patient help with tub baths, and most persons' sense of modesty would suffer if this were not so; on the other hand, health workers consider unwillingness to give any patient needed help of this sort a form of prudery. In countries such as Japan where both sexes habitually bathe together, such unwillingness would seem absurd.

Patients should not be allowed to remain in the bathroom alone for any length of time if sick and never alone with the door locked. The attendant can keep busy close by, and, although not in the room with the patient, should be fully aware of his or her condition while bathing. The patient may become chilled or faint, may be burned or fall and injure him-

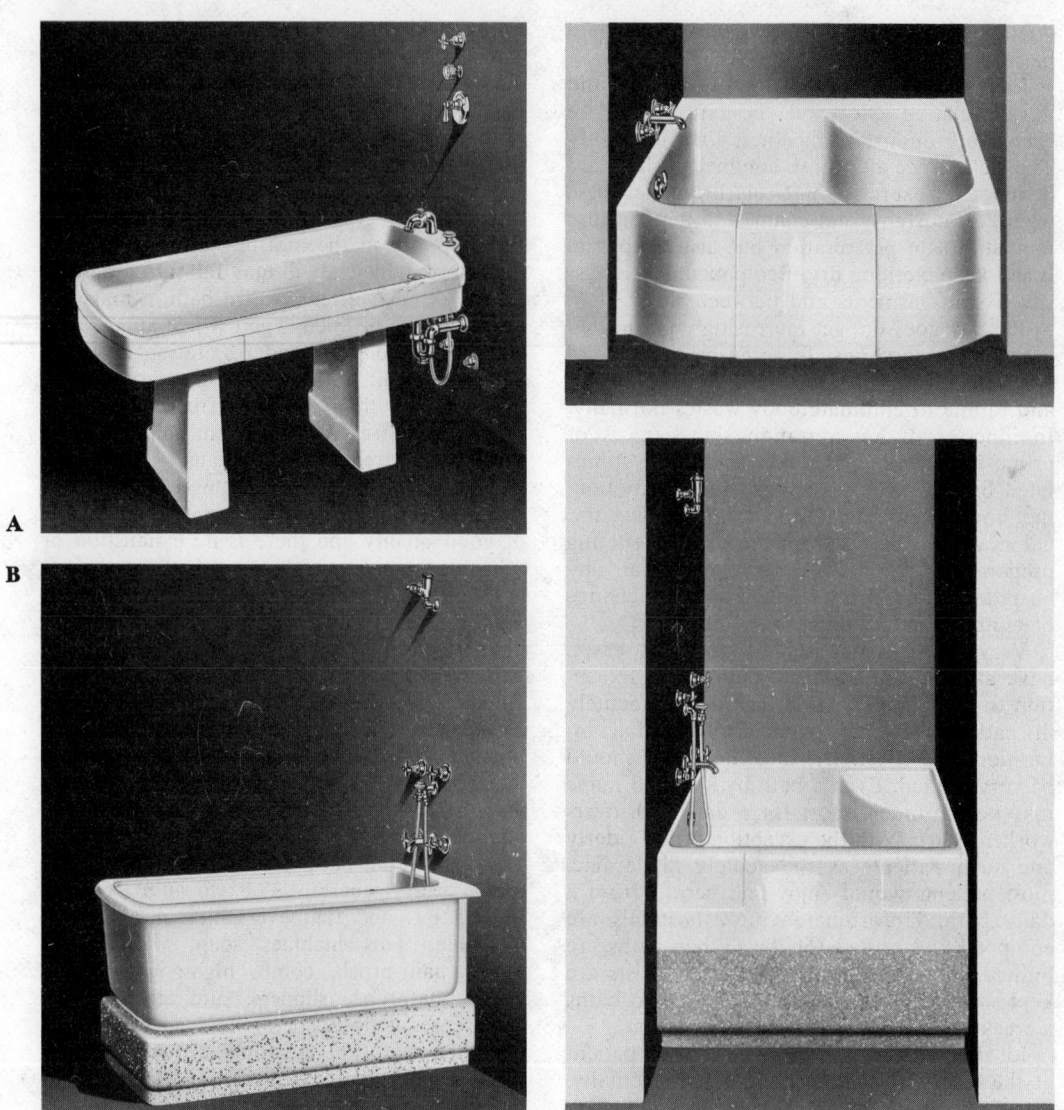

Figure 14-2. *A*. A bed patient may be put into a free-standing tub of stretcher height. *B*. A free-standing tub of this height makes it possible to give ambulatory patients assistance from both sides. *C*. A tub with a seat should be provided when chest or abdominal dressings prohibit immersion baths. *D*. A child's tub that prevents unnecessary stooping by the person giving assistance. (Courtesy of Crane Co., Chicago, Ill.)

self or herself. Since patients have both purposely and accidentally drowned in bath tubs, nurses who are responsible must take every precaution to prevent this. Patients often resent supervision, and feel that their privacy is invaded. The amount of supervision needed varies considerably, and although hospitals must protect themselves by rules to prevent accidents, the individual should not be treated in a routine fashion. After the bath, the patient should be warmly clothed and covered, ac-

cording to the environmental temperature, to prevent chilling.

If a person's comfort is dependent on a tub bath or shower, they can usually be given one. There are mechanical hoists that lift patients from the bed and lower them into a tub; many types are available. In homes, a seat or stool may be put on or into the tub or under a shower to reduce the effort of bathing to a minimum (see Fig. 14-3). Wide doors to bathrooms that admit wheelchairs, stretchers,

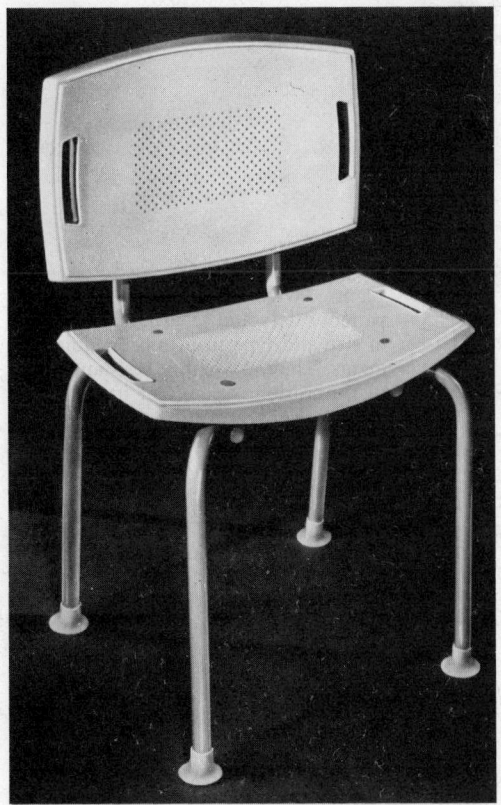 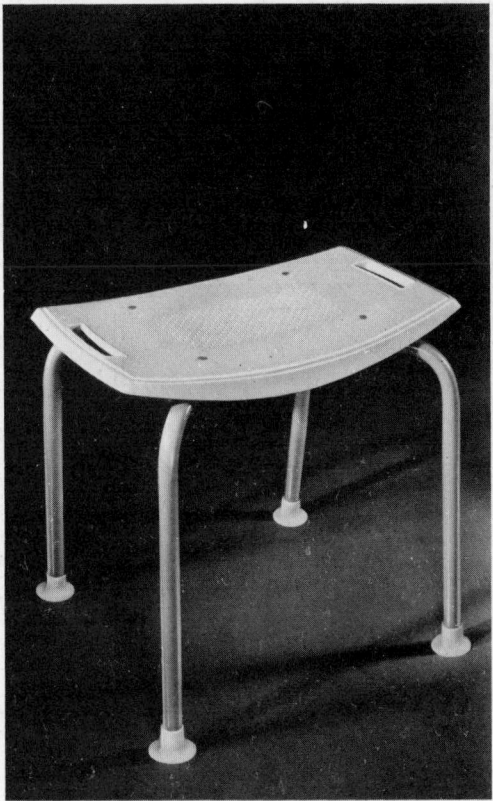

Figure 14-3. Rustproof bath seat made of reinforced polypropylene plastic. The detachable back rest and bottom have nonslide textured surface with water drainage holes. Legs have suction tips for stability. (Courtesy of Lumex, Inc., Bay Shore, N.Y.)

and hoists in hospitals and nursing homes facilitate tub baths and showers. Grab bars attached to the wall will ensure the safety and security of the patient (see Fig. 14-4).

Children should never be left alone while taking a bath. Tub baths and showers for infants and children are given at temperatures ranging between 32.2° and 37.8°C (90° and 100°F). (This temperature is one that feels comfortably warm to the elbow, which, because of its sensitivity, is used for testing temperatures when a bath thermometer is not available.) Well infants are given tub baths when cared for in homes. However, the difficulty of controlling infection in hospital or any institution makes the use of tubs and showers for bathing infants especially difficult. Decontamination of communal tubs and slabs on which babies lie for table shower baths is almost impossible. Babies and children are so much more likely than adults to contract skin diseases from contaminated tubs and showers that it makes such baths for them impractical.

Bed baths involve an exposure of the body

to which many persons are unaccustomed. Exposure of the genitalia is probably the chief cause of discomfort. When patients' conditions permit, they bathe the genital-anal region themselves, but nurses must be prepared and willing to give this service. Because in almost all cultures the genitalia are covered, exposure of the pudenda is embarrassing to most persons. The extent to which so-called modesty is innate or acquired is the subject of endless discussion. Health practices should be based on the assumption that, whether innate or acquired, the exposure of the genitalia is distasteful to many if not most persons. Having the genitalia touched is an even greater infringement of privacy and it may elicit an erotic response. In the boy or man there may be an erection of the penis. But in spite of these consequences it is obvious that help must be given some persons in keeping the genitalia clean in order to eliminate odors and to reduce the danger of infections. Unconscious patients cannot bathe themselves, nor should prostrated persons. Those with injured or burned hands

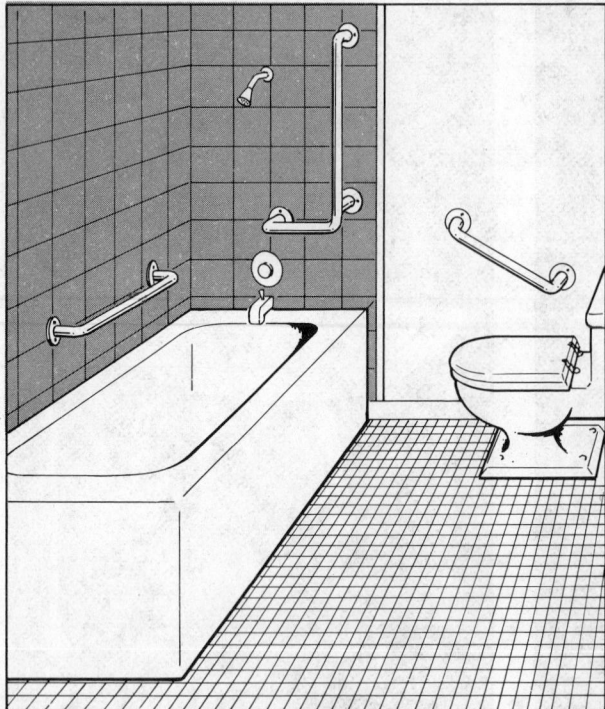

Figure 14-4. Grab-bars for greatest patient safety and security are available in size and type to fit most requirements. They are highly resistant to rust, abrasion, wear, and impact damage, yet warm to the touch.

cannot keep the genitalia clean and other circumstances give the patient a "self-care deficit" of this sort.

In many health institutions and agencies, an effort is made to provide workers of the same sex to give what is sometimes called "crotch care." But, since this is not always possible both men and women nurses should learn to feel comfortable in providing this necessary service. The "crotch" offers conditions that favor bacterial growth—warmth, darkness, and moisture. The excretions and secretions of this area have strong odors, as has been noted, so for many reasons the patient's comfort and health are dependent on cleanliness of this area. Smegma is a thick lubricating secretion of the sebaceous glands of the clitoris and labia minora in the female and of the sebaceous glands of the inner aspect of the prepuce in the male. If the genitalia are not bathed properly, collection of smegma cannot only be odoriferous but irritating. A connection between this condition and penile carcinoma has been suggested.[51a] The prepuce in the uncircumcised male covers the flaccid penis. Normally the prepuce can be retracted to expose the corona and glans penis. When the prepuce is so tight, or the opening so small, that it cannot be retracted over the glans, the condition is called phimosis. If this condition exists or if the prepuce has not been retracted and the corona and glans cleaned, both may be so coated with smegma that all of the secretion should not be removed in one bath because the process would be too irritating.

In females, even infants, secretions may collect between labial folds until the area is inflamed. Therefore, in both males and females thorough cleaning of the genitalia is important.

The genitalia of both sexes are very sensitive to touch. Touching the clitoris of the female and the penis of the male may evoke an erotic sensation but the male testicle is very tender and pressure is painful. Eroticism is partly a reflex and partly a conscious response; sexual stimulation is therefore influenced by the reaction of nurses to giving "crotch care." If the patient senses that nurses have a mature attitude toward sex, if they can give this service without embarrassment in a matter-of-fact way, they are less likely to feel sexually stimulated. W. B. Obermeyer,[51b] a man nurse, thinks it helpful to talk to patients on some diverting topic while giving this care. Both Obermeyer and Gertrude E. Gibbs,[51c] another nurse, suggest wearing gloves to reduce skin contact. Obermeyer recommends the use of a small towel for handling the genitalia when this is possible (see Fig. 14-5A–D).

Flushing the crotch with soapy and then plain warm water while the patient lies on a bedpan or douche pan (as described in Chapter 11) or using a disposable sitz bath, if he or she is able, are substitutes for showers or tub baths. When such equipment is not at hand the person can be made comfortable by bathing

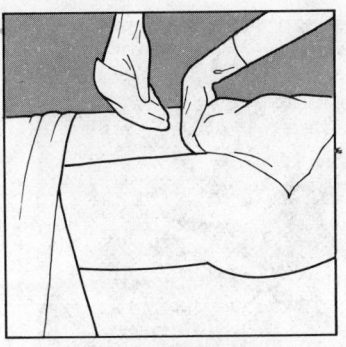

A

In cleansing the perineum, the area is exposed by lifting the genitalia up and back toward the pubes.

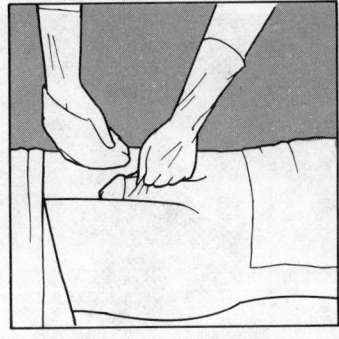

B

The prepuce must be retracted so that its inner surface and the glans penis can be cleansed.

Figure 14-5. Procedures for cleansing the genitalia. (From Obermeyer, William B.: "Crotch Care," *Am. J. Nurs.,* **57:**618, [May] 1957.)

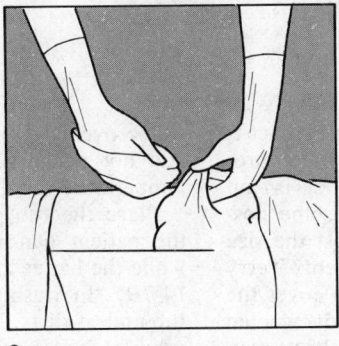

C

With the penis placed up toward the pubes, the scrotum is washed gently. Because the testicles are extremely sensitive, minimum pressure is used.

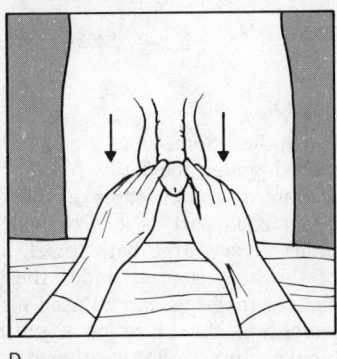

D

When the prepuce and glans penis have been cleaned and dried, the prepuce is drawn downward over the glans into its normal position.

with a wash cloth or disposable sponges. Bathing the anal region last reduces the risk of infecting the urethra and bladder with microorganisms of the rectum. The more extensive the surgery in the area or breaks in the skin from other causes, the greater the risk and the more meticulous the procedure should be from the standpoint of infection control. Intrusive treatments, such as indwelling catheters, increase the risk and make careful perineal cleaning more than ordinarily important. If nurses give patients complete baths it enables them to see, or otherwise detect, pathology over the entire exterior of the body. This is a distinct asset in trying to identify patients' problems and give them the help nurses are qualified to give or report to physicians (and others) such problems as demand their attention.

Cleansing Bed Bath. The purposes of the bath are to clean the skin and refresh the patient. The nurse should see that the room is warm, that the windows are closed and the patient protected from drafts, that the bed is

screened, and that everything necessary is at hand. The *technique* will vary in different hospitals and homes according to the facilities, but certain principles are the same for all bed baths.

A unit similar to that found in modern railroad trains during recent decades is now available for hospital use. Without such a unit the articles needed include a large basin or foot tub of water at 43.3° to 46.1°C (110° to 115°F), a bath towel and face towel, wash cloths, soap, nail brush, comb and brush, rubbing lotion, talcum powder, protection for the bed, and covering for the patient. Each should have his or her own basin, or basins in general use should be disinfected by boiling (see Fig. 14-6). Encourage patients to clean the mouth and teeth and to take as much of the bath as their condition permits, but the nurse is responsible for their preparation and for seeing that patients do not tire themselves and that the bath is adequate.

Preparation of patients includes covering them with a blanket and removing the upper

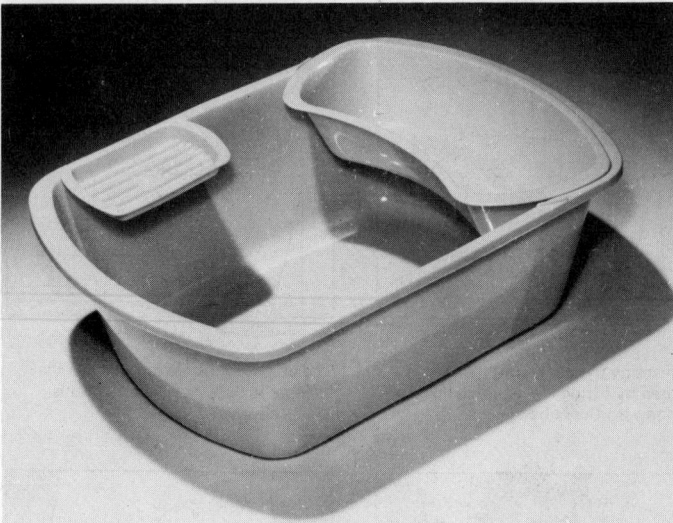

Figure 14-6. A single-patient personal care combination consisting of wash basin, soap dish, and graduated emesis basin. The three pieces fit together as one unit or can be used individually. The non-porous polyethylene wash basin has a 7-quart capacity. The soap dish can be attached or lifted from the basin without tilting. The emesis basin is graduated to 700 ml in 50 ml increments and to 24 oz. in 1 oz. increments. (Courtesy of Sherwood Medical Industries, Inc., St. Louis, Mo.)

bedclothes. Sometimes a cotton bath blanket is placed under the body for warmth and protection; in other cases a bath towel is put under each part as it is bathed. In some hospitals a very large bath towel, almost the size of the bed, is used under the patient. Terry cloth bath sheets can be used also to cover the patient in the place of a cotton or woolen blanket. In very hot weather cotton sheets may be substituted for blankets. Leave one pillow under the head, unless this position is uncomfortable or contraindicated by the patient's condition. If necessary, put a hot-water bottle at the patient's feet for warmth; in most cases, except during warm weather, this is comforting. With the patient prepared in this way, clean the mouth, and remove the gown.

In *bathing patients,* proceed in the following order—face, ears, neck, chest, arms and hands, abdomen, back, thighs, legs, feet, and pubic region. Give special attention to the ears, the skin between the fingers and toes, axillae, umbilicus, and pubic region. Work quickly, quietly, smoothly, and wash with firm but *gentle* pressure. It is almost necessary to have a compassionate feeling to get a sufficiently gentle touch for the very sick person who "hurts all over." Avoid the appearance of hurry, but if the bath is given slowly, the water becomes cold and the patient exhausted.

Make a mitten of the washcloth, holding the ends in the palm of the hand with the thumb (see Fig. 14-7*A*). If the ends dangle, they feel cold and uncomfortable. Washcloths made like thumbless mittens are very satisfactory. Expose, wash, and dry each part separately and thoroughly, covering the area immediately (see Fig. 14-7*C*). Do not drip

water over the patient. Change the water or add hot water sufficiently often to keep the temperature comfortably warm.

Place the tub or basin on the bed so that the patient can put the hands in the water while the hands and arms are bathed (see Fig. 14-7*B*). In washing the feet, put them in the tub and, if dirty, let them soak. The illusion of a tub bath is created somewhat by bathing the flexed leg and thigh while the foot is in the tub, letting the water flow over the parts from the cloth or sponge (see Fig. 14-7*D*). While the feet are soaking, the fingernails may be cleaned and trimmed. Remove the feet from the tub and dry them carefully, particularly between the toes. Clean and trim the toenails.

After bathing and drying the back, massage or rub it thoroughly to stimulate the circulation. To rub the back, help the patient, if necessary, to turn on the abdomen or on the side with the back toward the nurse and the body near the edge of the bed to be as close to the operator as possible. If the prone position is used and the patient is a woman, a pillow under the abdomen and hips removes pressure on the breasts and favors relaxation (see Fig. 14-7*E*).

In rubbing, use firm long strokes and kneading motions. (The amount of pressure to exert depends upon the patient's condition and preference.) Massage with both hands and work with a stronger upward than downward stroke. Give particular attention to pressure areas in rubbing. Most patients are especially grateful for massage of the neck and the lower part of the back, but some object to massage of these parts of the body; consequently, it is wise to ask the patient before taking this step.

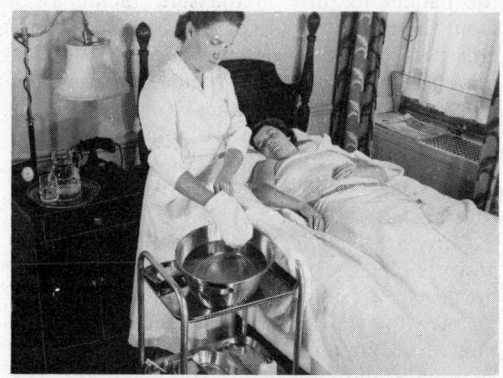

A

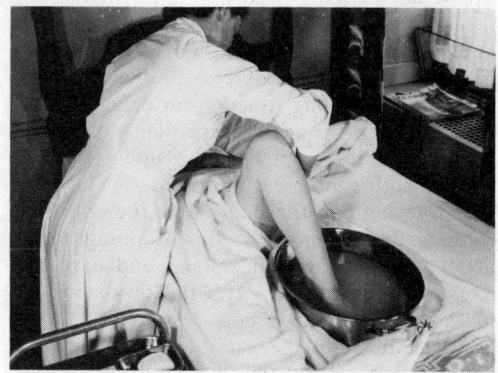

D

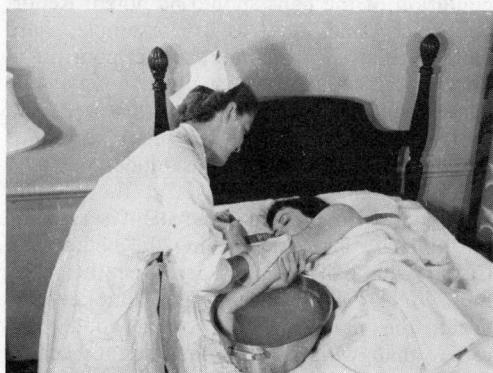

B

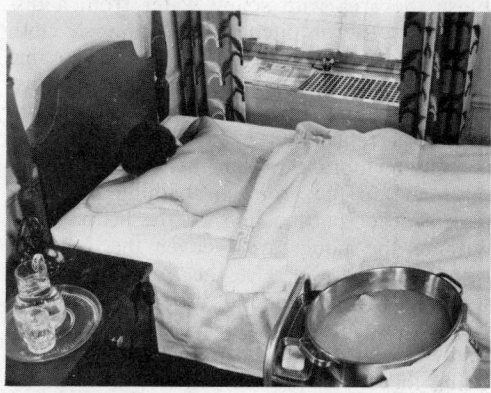

E

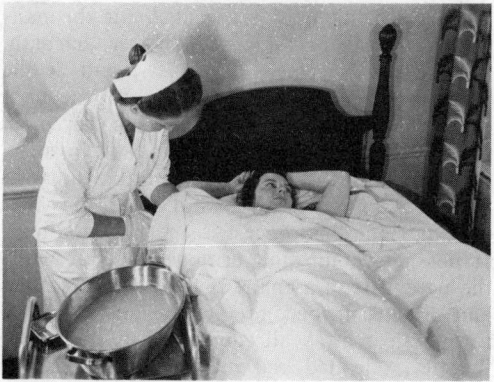

C

Figure 14-7. *A.* Giving a bed bath. Note the thumbless mitten washcloth that reduces dripping. *B.* The arm is supported and bathed while the hand rests in the water. *C.* The axilla, breast, and abdomen can be bathed with little exposure of the patient. Note the bath towel lining the bath blanket to prevent wetting the latter. *D.* The foot is soaking while the leg and thigh are bathed. Note care in draping to prevent exposure of the pubic area. *E.* The patient should be in a relaxed position while the back is bathed, rubbed, and powdered. Note the large pillow under abdomen and hips and the small pillow under the head. (Courtesy of Columbia-Presbyterian Medical Center, New York, N.Y., and Clay-Adams Co., New York, N.Y.)

Lubricating the operator's hands with cocoa butter or talcum increases the comfort of massage. Alcohol is more generally used for its refreshing effect, but it is not a good lubricant for rubbing and it tends to dry the skin.* Powder the area at the completion of the process, which should consume from 3 to 5 minutes, or more.

* "Lubriderm" is a commercial skin lubricant containing vegetable oils that is very effective in skin care. (It is made by Ayerst Laboratories, Inc., New York City.)

Throughout the bath encourage people to do as much of it as they can without tiring. Most persons prefer to wash the face, neck, and ears. Unless they are very ill or disabled, they also prefer to bathe the genitalia. Fold a bath towel and put it under the buttocks, placing an empty bedpan under the patient so that plenty of water can be used without wetting the bed. Place what patients will need where they can reach it and leave them in privacy for a few minutes. It is routine in some hospitals to flush the genital area daily with warm water in a plastic bottle that has a dispensing tip. When patients need assistance in bathing this area, they usually like to have a nurse or attendant of the same sex; no false modesty, however, should interfere with the performance of any nursing function on which the patient's comfort and welfare depend. When nurses bathe the genitalia, it is important that they be both gentle and thorough.

Before bathing the pubic area, be sure that patients understand that this is going to be done and that they understand and accept it as a necessary part of care. Put on disposable plastic gloves if this seems desirable and they are available. Put the patient on a bedpan or douche pan. Have the legs well separated. Flush the area with soapy water from a dispensing bottle or pitcher. With a wash cloth used only for this purpose, or with disposable sponges, clean the genitalia thoroughly, rinsing off the soap with plain water. If the patient is a female, clean, rinse, and dry the mucous membrane or skin between the labial folds and in the groin. In bathing the male patient, after putting him on the bedpan and flushing the pubic area, cover the genitalia with a small towel. Use the towel to lift the scrotum, then clean and dry the perineum. Next expose and clean the scrotum, being very gentle since the testicles are extremely tender. Using the towel, lift the penis so that all aspects of the scrotum can be cleaned. Pull the skin tight to eliminate folds in the scrotal covering if the area is badly soiled. Next clean the penis using long strokes from the base to the tip with special attention to the folds at the base. In uncircumcised patients, retract the prepuce with gentle pressure of thumb and forefinger on top of the penis until the prepuce is entirely retracted, exposing the corona and glans. Clean quickly and very gently with warm soapy water, removing any accumulated smegma. Rinse with clear water and dry all exposed areas, including the inner aspect of the prepuce. Next draw down the prepuce over the corona and glans. Grasping the prepuce on each side draw it down over the glans (as shown in Fig. 14-5D) restoring it to its original position.*

After cleaning and drying the genitalia, remove the bedpan, if one was used, and ask the patient to turn on the side, facing away from the nurse. (If the patient is helpless, several persons are needed for turning and lifting.) To clean the anal region, separate the buttocks, bathe, rinse, and dry the area. If powder is used to make the patient feel thoroughly dry or for its deodorizing property, avoid using an excess that forms irritating rolls in skin folds.

Care of the nails is usually left until the gown is replaced. Cutting is said to make them brittle; so a fastidious patient usually prefers to have the fingernails filed. A daily application of an emollient like cold cream helps to keep nails and cuticles in good condition. The condition of the nails should be noted. Report abnormal conditions, as for example, hard nails in children, which may reflect poor nutritional status;[52] brown nail-bed pigmented bands, which may indicate renal disease,[53] and dystrophies of the nails, which may be caused by cosmetics, especially if base-undercoats and "stick-on nails" are used.[54] Cut the toenails rather close to prevent the patient scratching the opposite leg and catching the bedclothes. Cutting the nails straight across, rather than in a curve, helps prevent ingrowing toenails. Clean the nails with an orangewood stick rather than with a metal instrument because the latter roughens the nail and makes it harbor dirt. Soaking in water and a detergent or in warm oil may be necessary if the nails are very dirty or thickened.* After the bath, remake the bed (see page 770), and at the same time remove bath blankets. Whenever it can be done without tiring patients, get them into a chair, on a stretcher, or on an "Invalift" while making the bed. It is desirable to postpone combing the hair until after the bedmaking since this process disarranges the hair. If possible, comb and arrange the hair while the patient is in a chair. If the hair is combed and brushed in bed, protect the pillow with a towel. Clear away all equipment used and see that it is cleaned and returned to its proper place. Put the patients' unit in order, and attend to their immediate wants, such as a drink or a hot-water bottle, so that they can at once get the benefit of rest that naturally follows a bath.

Bathing Infants and Children. Bed baths for infants and children are essentially the same as those for adults. Until infants' temperature-

---

* Obermeyer makes the following observation: "If the patient's prepuce is extremely redundant, it may best be retracted by enveloping the penis in the towel and encircling it with the left hand at a point just below the glans. Grasp it gently and draw the prepuce back until the entire interior is exposed, without folds, and accessible to cleaning. Occasionally it is necessary to hold the prepuce in this position to prevent its immediate return to the redundant position." (Obermeyer, William B.: "Crotch Care," Am. J. Nurs., 57: 618, [May] 1957.)

* Special care must be taken in caring for the feet of the aged and debilitated patient and the diabetic, all of whom are prone to infection. When there are difficult problems of foot care and patients cannot go to podiatrists, the latter may come to the hospital, bringing their specialized instruments, as, for example, those that cut thickened nails.

regulating mechanism is well established, they are particularly susceptible to chilling; therefore, the room should be kept warm and only small body areas exposed.

Practices for bathing the newborn may vary from institution to institution. While in some hospitals the vernix caseosa (sebaceous material covering the baby at birth) as well as excess blood and meconium is removed by dry or moist cotton balls, in others a daily sponge bath is given after the baby's temperature has stabilized. The Committee on Fetus and Newborn of the American Academy of Pediatrics (1972) says "use of hexachlorophene for total body bathing of newborn infants in hospital nurseries or at home is contraindicated." * They recommend dry skin care for the newborn infant (those born premature and at term) and washing with tap water only or with plain nonmedicated soap when needed. Because premature infants are prone to develop infection, some authorities recommend daily dilute hexachlorophene baths to prevent colonization of staphylococcus on the skin and nasal passages. Scrupulous hand washing by nurses and physicians before entering the nursery and before and after handling each infant is important in controlling infections in the nursery. The buttocks and genitalia are cleaned daily and as needed with cotton balls moistened in warm water; consequently some cleaning of the baby occurs daily. When the mother goes home she is told to bathe her baby with a wet wash cloth and a small amount of mild soap and to remove the soap with a fresh wash cloth rinsed in clear warm water. Oil is generally *not* accepted in infant care today, and as powder tends to cake in body creases it is *not* routinely used. Most authorities recommend a minimum handling of the skin of the newborn, especially the premature infant. Equipment used for the care of the skin is kept in the infants' unit, the nurses' hands are clean, and they are often gowned and masked.[55,56] In this way, it is thought, skin and respiratory infections are reduced to a minimum.

The US Food and Drug Administration and USPHS Center for Disease Control in 1972 jointly recommend that nurseries maintain the following infection control practices:

1. Adequate numbers and placement of hand-washing facilities,
2. Ability to isolate and treat neonatal disease promptly.
3. Reliability of systems for surveillance of neonatal disease,

4. Adequate number and type of personnel involved in patient care,
5. Avoid relative crowding of facilities, and
6. Ability to practice infant cohorting routinely *

By adhering to these practices it is thought that staphylococcal infections can be controlled and that hexachlorophene bathing should not be used as a substitute for these infection control practices.

Baths for young preschool children differ slightly from the adult in that they should be given the opportunity to play in the bath water, essentially to add to their sensory experiences. A tub bath is preferred; however, when this is not possible, the children play in the water with their hands.

The Partial Bath. When a partial bath is substituted for a complete one, the face, hands, arms, and pubes are bathed. Morning care for bed patients should always include cleaning the mouth, rubbing the back, combing and brushing the hair, and making the bed. The most scrupulous attention should be given the mouth and pressure areas on the skin of the bedfast even though their condition or lack of nursing personnel prohibits a full daily bath.

3. SHAVING THE MAN PATIENT

Men accustomed to shaving daily are uncomfortable when illness interrupts the habit. An unshaven face makes a sick man look sicker. This lowers his morale and distresses those who love him. Hospital barbers, orderlies, and men nurses usually shave men unable to shave themselves. A woman nurse in the hospital often helps the bed patient by putting the necessary articles within his reach; in home nursing she may be more skillful in shaving a patient than anyone else available. Because a man, who practices daily, is likely to be more adept than a woman, the nurse may ask a man in the family to shave the very ill patient if a barber is not available.

If the patient is able to shave himself, he needs light and mirror, a basin of warm water, towel, squares of soft paper, waste receptacle, razor, special soap and shaving brush or a cream not requiring the use of a brush. An electric razor eliminates the use of shaving soap and brush. All these articles should be left within reach, and the patient put in a comfortable position for shaving. He will usually

* "Hexachlorophene and 'Skin Protection' in the Newborn," *Clin. Pediatr.*, **11:**254, (May) 1972.

* US Public Health Service, Center for Disease Control: "Follow-up on Nursery Staphylococcal Disease and Its Relationship to the Use of Hexachlorophene— United States," *Morbidity and Mortality Weekly Report,* **21:**253, (No. 30) July 29, 1972.

prefer to be left alone during the procedure if he needs no assistance.

To shave a helpless patient, collect the articles just enumerated and put them on a table near the operator's hand. See that the patient is in a position comfortable for him and convenient for the worker. Protect the bedding and clothing with a towel. Wash the face thoroughly before starting the process. A towel soaked in hot water may be put on the face for a few minutes to soften the beard, which helps prevent scratching and nicking the skin. Make a thin lather on the face with soap, warm water, and shaving brush or shaving cream. Allow a few minutes for the lather to soften the beard. Keep the razor and the skin wet while shaving. Hold the skin taut, use short strokes, and keep the razor at an angle of about 30 degrees. In most areas shave against the direction taken by the hairs for a close shave. Shave very carefully around sensitive areas, such as the nose and lips. If able, the patient prefers to shave these parts himself. The razor should be kept clean by frequently rinsing. Wash the soap off the face after the shave and apply a soothing lotion if the patient has one and likes it.

An electric razor is preferred by many men. Because it cannot be sterilized, it is not suitable for communal use in hospitals.

4. CARE OF THE MOUTH, TEETH, AND DENTURES

Importance of Mouth Care in Health and Illness. Because the mouth is the portal of entry for food, and digestion is started here, its condition directly affects health. The mouth is molded to some extent by the person's character, and it can lend charm to the face or spoil its appeal. For physical and psychologic reasons a healthy mouth is highly prized. In his text, *Patients Have Families,* Henry B. Richardson [57] attributes a series of family misfortunes to the father's failure to preserve his teeth and prevent halitosis (bad breath)!

Decayed teeth and sensitive gums cause such discomfort in eating that food is likely to be swallowed before it is thoroughly chewed and mixed with saliva, which contains the digestive enzyme ptyalin. Infected teeth, gums, and tonsils can infect other parts of the digestive and respiratory systems by direct extension; by contaminating the bloodstream, they can cause joint or heart disease. An unpleasant breath can be attributed to the condition of the tonsils or the stomach, but it is often caused by diseased teeth, gums, or bony sockets.

The knowledge that one is offensive in appearance or odor is damaging to the self-respect. From this brief list of the dangers and disadvantages of neglecting the mouth, it can be seen that a person's general welfare is seriously affected by its condition.

Oral Hygiene. The development and maintenance of healthy teeth and gums are dependent on the constitutional factor, or the inherited quality of teeth and surrounding structures, and the environmental factor, or the condition of the tissues and fluids surrounding the teeth throughout life. The text of Joseph L. Bernier and Joseph M. Muhler [58] and their collaborators gives an excellent review of dental research. There seems to be general agreement that primitive peoples, whose diets have not been influenced by others, have better teeth than civilized peoples. It has been suggested that in mixed races individuals may inherit a racially characteristic narrow arch from one parent and large teeth that do not fit into it from the other. The pure race and their unrefined and varied diet probably account for the relatively normal mouths of primitive people.

A person may have teeth of poor quality at birth because the mother had an inadequate prenatal diet. After birth, while the teeth are developing, the diet and general health of the individual are thought to affect teeth. The relationship between healthy mouths and the minerals and vitamins in the diet is not well established, nor is the relationship between dental health and general health entirely clear. Most authorities would agree, however, that an optimum diet and good general health are conducive to development and maintenance of a normal condition of the mouth and teeth. Since caries (the chief disease of the tooth itself) is a disease of civilization, refined and often monotonous diet is thought to be the chief predisposing factor.

Dentistry is a comparatively new science, and until very recently it has dealt with treatment rather than prevention of disease. The most striking advances in this field of knowledge mark recent decades. Old theories have been disproved, and a new era of therapy and oral hygiene is dawning. Even the latest published opinions are likely to be out of date before they reach the public. There is a rapidly extending program of public health dentistry, including research. With the passage of the Social Security Act in 1935, dental departments were established in public health agencies. The Dental Research Act of 1948 has enabled the United States Public Health Service to enlarge its program. Federal dental programs are administered through the United

States Public Health Service, the Children's Bureau, the Office of Indian Affairs, the Veterans Administration, the Army, and the Navy. State and local health departments offer dental services of varying types. At present, public health programs concentrate on services to school children, health education, consultation service, and demonstrations of preventive methods. All types of services in the federal program are available to certain government charges and employees.

It is not possible with the existing number of dentists to offer adequate dental service to the entire population. In an effort to make dental care more universally available, Alfred C. Fones organized a school for dental hygienists. Prepared originally to give oral prophylaxis and to supplement the technical services of dentists in the schools, they are now employed to clean teeth, to serve as technicians wherever dental care is given, and to provide preventive and educational services in many settings, including clinics and schools.[59] Markedly improved methods of disease prevention and control and the extension of dental services to all segments of the population are possible developments within the near future. Bernier and Muhler say, "The day is in sight when the handpiece and the forceps will be no more than incidental symbols of the profession" [of dentistry].* In other words, caries will be controlled and the necessity for filling and extracting of teeth eliminated. They think in the future far more attention will be put on prevention.

Diseases of the mouth fall into two main groups: diseases of the teeth themselves (the main one being caries), and diseases of the bony structures and soft tissues of the mouth, called periodontal disease.

Discovery of the means of preventing and controlling dental *caries* is one of the most dramatic medical accomplishments of this century. W. D. Miller is credited with laying the foundation on which modern treatment is based. He demonstrated the existence of a substance in saliva that converts carbohydrates to lactic acid and showed that this acid dissolves tooth enamel, permitting bacterial invasion and the development of caries. Since he found that sterile (or boiled) saliva will not convert carbohydrate, he concluded that the converting principle was a bacterial enzyme. This theory is now generally accepted, and the conditions essential to the development of caries are believed to be the presence in the

mouth of the enzyme-producing bacteria (loosely referred to as the lactic acid bacilli group) + saliva in which the bacteria can function + carbohydrates (particularly sugars) + tooth enamel susceptible to caries. Alter any of these factors, and the chain of events known as caries formation is broken. Individuals who can eat sweets freely and remain immune to caries have been shown to be free from the lactic acid bacilli. It is thought that their saliva contains a substance that discourages growth of the microorganisms although the exact mechanism is not established. There is evidence that persons whose intake of fluorine is high (as in areas where the water contains relatively more fluorine) have few lactic acid bacilli in their mouths. It is also thought that fluorine has entered into the composition of the teeth during the formative period (during the prenatal period and the first 8 years of life) and that the resulting enamel is more resistant to caries.

Other substances including chlorophyll, ammonia-liberating compounds, certain antibiotics, and enzymes have been studied to determine if they discourage the growth of lactic acid bacilli, either directly or by encouraging organisms antagonistic to the lactic acid bacillus; these substances have *not* been shown to be effective in preventing caries, according to Bernier and Muhler.[60] *The positive relationship between the intake of refined carbohydrates and the incidence of caries has been amply demonstrated.* Gullorm Toverad,[61] (in 1949), reporting on caries during World War II in Norway, concluded that the low intake of refined carbohydrates accounted for the lowered incidence of caries in that country. He said that similar reports came from England and Italy. Later studies [62-64] conducted in the United States and other countries support the findings of Toverad. Carbohydrates also affect the amount and type of bacteria in plaques of man and animals.[65] It is conceded, therefore, that caries can be successfully controlled by two methods: (1) by diet, and (2) by the use of fluorine compounds (or some other inhibitor) to discourage the growth of lactic acid bacilli and/or to make enamel resistant to the action of the bacterial enzyme.

Philip Jay [66] says that good results may be expected with the reduction of carbohydrates to 100 gm daily for 2 weeks with the elimination of sugar, bread, potatoes, and other foods rich in carbohydrate. During the next two weeks sugar only is eliminated, and if the mouth is relatively free from lactic acid bacilli, no further dietary restriction may be necessary for months or, possibly, years. The dentist is guided by the bacterial mouth count. Ob-

---

* Bernier, Joseph L., and Muhler, Joseph C. (eds.): *Improving Dental Practice Through Preventive Measures,* 3rd ed. C. V. Mosby Co., St. Louis, 1975, p. 2.

viously, this treatment is more successful if pursued with adults than with children, whose food intake is regulated with difficulty, but any treatment consistently adhered to yields richer rewards in the young than in the adult who has already suffered tooth damage.

Treatment based on inhibiting the growth of lactic acid bacilli by means other than diet has been most successfully demonstrated with fluorine. The low incidence of caries in certain areas of this country where drinking water is relatively high in fluorine content has led the health departments of Grand Rapids, Evanston, and other cities to experiment in treating the drinking water with sodium fluoride. Caries in the permanent teeth were reduced 60 per cent on an average, after 10 years of fluoridation in Newburgh, N.Y., and Grand Rapids, Mich.[67] It is estimated that the yearly cost per person is 5 to 15 cents in communities with over 1000 inhabitants while in smaller communities of less than 1000 persons it may be $1.22 if installation devices and supervision of addition of fluoride is economically oriented.[68] About 23 per cent of the people in the United States do not have the benefit of drinking water with fluorine naturally present or the addition of a fluoride supplement. One part of fluorine in one million parts of water is thought to be effective without causing noticeable mottling of the tooth enamel. The nature of the caries-inhibiting properties of fluoride water is not established, according to a number of authorities, but it is believed that children exposed to this treatment for the first 8 years of life enjoy a high degree of immunity. Another method of control with fluorine is to apply sodium or stannous fluoride solutions directly to the teeth of children. In many states, mobile units continue to demonstrate this simple process, and dentists throughout the United States include the procedure in their practice. The fluoride solutions are used in varying strengths (depending on the age of the individual, the type of solution used, and the particular beliefs of the dentist). They are applied after prophylaxis. Most authorities note that stannous fluoride is more effective than sodium fluoride and some studies have found that it is effective with adults.[69-71] Following an analysis and comparison of studies (276) dealing with the problem of caries and their prevention with a fluoride, George K. Stookey comes to the following conclusion:

It has been shown that . . . no substitute for the use of a water supply containing the optimal amount of fluoride may be recommended at this time . . . means of providing topical fluoride therapy to the erupted dentition indicates that (1) sodium fluoride is of value as a caries preventive agent, but only in children reared in the absence of communal fluoride, (2) stannous fluoride provides significant benefits to all aspects of our populations, (3) certain other fluorides, including fluoride-phosphate systems, presently indicate promise as anticariogenic agents . . . and (4) by far the greatest contribution toward the complete control of dental caries may be obtained through a multiple treatment stannous fluoride program that includes the use of stannous fluoride in a compatible prophylactic paste, a solution for topical application, and a calcium pyrophosphate dentrifice for home use in an area with optimal fluoride in the communal water supply.*

Signs of disease in the tissues surrounding the teeth include inflammation, swelling and tumors (hyperplasia or hypertrophy), lesions of various sorts, necrosis, and atrophy. The loss of teeth is more often due to disease of the periodontal, or surrounding, tissue than to disease of the tooth itself, William Boyd[72] states. Anything that traumatizes tissue predisposes it to disease; anything that interferes with normal metabolism is an indirect cause. The conditions mentioned above are given names with which the nurse should be familiar. Inflammation of the gums is called *gingivitis;* inflammation of the deeper tissues surrounding the roots of the teeth (an extension of gingivitis) is called *periodontitis* or *periodontoclasia,* although many persons still use the term *pyorrhea.* Degeneration of the periodontal tissues, *periodontosis* (a rare condition), is a result of systemic disease. Atrophy of the tissues in which the teeth are embedded is common in the aged, although the fact that marked atrophic changes are not universally found in old age makes it doubtful whether this is a necessary accompaniment of the aging process. Inflammation that extends over the entire mouth, lips, tongue, and gums is called *stomatitis.* A gingivitis that progresses to a necrotic stage and is associated with the presence of fusospirochetal organisms is known as *Vincent's infection* or *trench mouth.*

Irving Glickman,[73] in his text *Clinical Periodontology,* emphasizes food impaction, improperly used toothbrushes and toothpicks, and chemical irritation as causative agents in periodontal inflammation. Gingivitis, however, is most often initiated by trauma from deposits, or calculi, at the gum margins. He considers *neglect* to be the primary reason for dental problems and makes the following statement:

Neglect is to blame for most if not all gingival and periodontal disease—neglect of the healthy mouth that permits disease to occur, neglect of

---

* Stookey, George K.: "Fluoride Therapy," in Bernier, Joseph L., and Muhler, Joseph C. (eds.): *Improving Dental Practice Through Preventive Measures,* 2nd ed. C. V. Mosby Co., St. Louis, 1970, p. 145.

early disease that permits it to destroy the tooth-supporting tissues, and neglect of the untreated mouth that permits disease to recur. Poor oral hygiene which permits plaque, calculus, and materia alba to accumulate overshadows all other local factors responsible for gingival disease. The status of the individual oral hygiene determines the prevalence and severity of gingivitis.*

In normal occlusion, the force exerted by the bite is distributed over all the teeth, but with malocclusion this very powerful pressure of the jaw action falls on those teeth that hit; likewise, the teeth that have no contact with those of the opposing jaw lack the normal stimulation of the bite. Healthy periodontal tissue is therefore dependent on the alignment of teeth, jaw structure, the inherited quality of the tissues themselves, diet and general health, and freedom from trauma by agents put into the mouth and from accretions on the teeth, either food or calculi, particularly at or near the gingival crevice or sulcus (the space between the gum and the tooth surface). Healthy gums are also dependent on effective oral hygiene carried out day after day, year after year.

Admittedly, there is much to be learned about the prevention of periodontal disease, but what has been said about its cause suggests the means of preventing and curing it. Leaving out the question of eugenics, or controlling structural factors through the genes, the mother can contribute something through the selection of an optimum prenatal diet; likewise, an optimum diet for the child throughout her guardianship. Dental supervision from early childhood prevents defective occlusion in many cases. Regular and frequent prophylaxis removes the traumatic tooth deposits and, if dentists are teachers they will help the individual reduce the hazards of food left between the teeth and calculi formation, while caring for the mouth without traumatizing tissues. It is now recognized that some persons most zealous in the care of their mouths have, by incorrect or too frequent brushing pushed the protecting gums away from the teeth, exposing an area of dentin that should remain covered. Improper habits of brushing may also wear away the enamel. It has been shown that primitive peoples have effective methods of cleaning the mouth and teeth, and the action of chewing their relatively rougher diet has a cleansing effect.

It cannot be urged too strongly that all persons from early childhood through old age visit the dentist at least twice a year. Figure

14-8 shows a form used to request dental consultation. In the elderly, cancer of the mouth is not uncommon.[74] Early signs of it and immediate treatment can be instituted if there are visits to the dentist at short intervals. Dental prophylaxis, in its broadest sense, includes removal of all injurious deposits and stains on the teeth, reduction of bacterial action, repair of carious teeth, the correction of defective occlusion and misfitting dentures, smoothing of roughened surfaces, and instruction in oral hygiene.

There is sufficient evidence that certain vitamins are important in the prevention of periodontal disease. The role of vitamins is discussed more fully in Chapter 10, but it might be indicated here that those contributing most to healthy bone and mucous membrane elsewhere in the body and to bacterial resistance are of special significance. Animal research has shown that nutritional deficiencies of vitamins A, B complex, C, and D, protein, tryptophan, magnesium, phosphorus, and calcium *adversely* influence the integrity of the periodontal tissues. Authorities differ to some degree on the effectiveness of supplemental vitamins and protein in the treatment of periodontal disease but there is agreement on the importance of optimal nutrition in such conditions.[75,76] Gingivitis and its extension, periodontitis, are late accompaniments of many long-drawn-out illnesses, if diets used are not varied and are high in refined carbohydrates and low in the vitamin-rich foods.

Daily care of the teeth includes use of a toothbrush, a dentifrice or cleansing agent, dental floss, and, recommended by some authorities, interdental stimulators. A mouthwash is not thought necessary, although a number of writers mention its value in the control of *halitosis* (foul breath).* It is, of course, desirable to remove all causes of bad breath. Hydrogen peroxide (used in the strength of about 1 per cent) removes decaying food by its bubbling action and may reduce

---

* Glickman, Irving: "Preventive Periodontics," in Bernier, Joseph L., and Muhler, Joseph C. (eds.): *Improving Dental Practice Through Preventive Measures*, 2nd ed. C. V. Mosby Co., St. Louis, 1970, p. 209.

* Discussing a study of halitosis, P. P. Morris and R. R. Read report that saliva "putrefies rapidly," giving rise to objectionable odors. According to them, dilution with water does not materially affect putrefaction. They add: "Dentifrice helps materially up to 2 hours. Antiseptic rinse (a saturated 27% aqueous alcohol solution of thymol, menthol, eucalyptol, and methyl salicylate with benzoic acid and boric acid) helps three hours, also tobacco odors are reduced by the antiseptic rinse. . . . There are certain resistant types of odors, such as garlic, that are systemic in origin, and are not affected by water or antiseptic rinse." They also report that complete dental prophylaxis reduces mouth and breath odors, as one would expect. (Morris, P. P., and Read, R. R.: "Halitosis: Variations in Mouth and Total Breath Odor Intensity Resulting from Prophylaxis and Antisepsis," *J. Dent. Res.* 28:324, [June] 1949.)

uh University Hospital

DENTISTRY CONSULTATION REQUEST AND REPORT

DESCRIPTION OF PATIENT'S CONDITION AND REASON FOR CONSULTATION (INCLUDE LABORATORY FINDINGS IF AVAILABLE)

NAME OF CONSULTANT _____

___ CONSULTATION ONLY ___   ___ CONSULTATION AND CONCURRENT SUPPORTIVE CARE ___   ___ CONSULTATION AND TOTAL TRANSFER OF FOLLOW-UP CARE

DATE

DAY   MO.   YR.   ATTENDING PHYSICIAN   M.D.

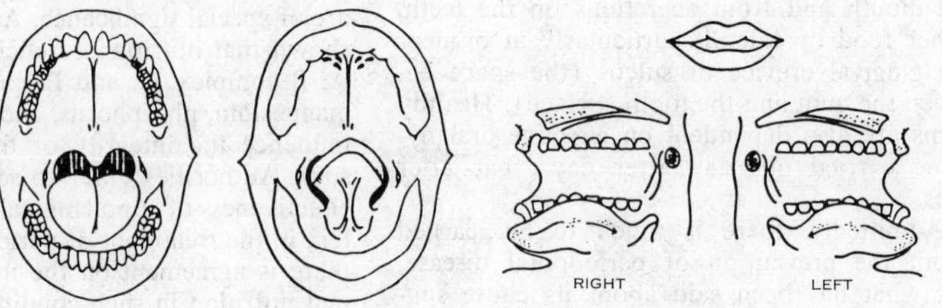

RIGHT   LEFT

CONSULTANT'S FINDINGS AND RECOMMENDATIONS

DATE

DAY   MO.   YR.   ATTENDING DENTIST   D.D.S.

TREATMENT REPORT

DATE

DAY   MO.   YR.   ATTENDING DENTIST   D.D.S.

FINAL DISPOSITION

84-696-0117 (03/73)

CHART

Figure 14-8. Dentistry consultation request and report used by physicians and nurses. (Courtesy of University Hospital, University of Western Ontario, London, Ont.)

bacterial activity thereby, striking at a common factor in halitosis. Hydrogen peroxide can injure the gums. It should be used only on the advice of the dentist. The claims by some manufacturers, in the past decade or two, on the deodorizing effect of chlorophyll denti-frices is reported less often in the literature. In 1952, the American Dental Association[77] noted that there was no scientific evidence to support their use; currently, most dental experts agree with this statement. There is no one toothbrush best suited to everyone because actual and potential dental problems vary from individual to individual; in general, a toothbrush should be small enough to reach all aspects of the teeth; a soft or medium-hard bristle brush is preferred to the hard bristle brush if the subgingival spaces are cleaned; a straight-handle brush is usually preferred to a curved handle; and two or three rows of bristles should be set in tufts spaced well apart and in equal lengths, according to most writers. Esther M. Wilkins [78] gives these specifics: the length of the brush should be about 6 inches; the head, 1 to 1¼ inches long; the bristles, 7/16 inch long.

The use of the electric toothbrush has increased greatly in the past few years. Many persons brush more frequently, especially after making the initial purchase. Some authorities believe that those persons who do not have good toothbrushing habits may benefit by using the electric brush as it does a large part of the work for them. Many investigations have been conducted on the comparative effectiveness of the mechanical (electric) and manual toothbrushes; some studies suggest that a mechanical toothbrush is superior to a manual toothbrush in removing dental plaques,[78a-79] preventing and removing calculus deposits,[80] and promoting gingival health,[81,82] but other reports fail to confirm these findings.[83-86] If an electric toothbrush is used, the following precautions should be taken: select a brand that is approved (a list of brands and their ratings may be found in *Consumers' Research*); avoid brands that operate on the 115-volt supply; do not permit children to use or play with any powerline-operated toothbrush; check the cord for breaks or other defects; and, if the toothbrush falls into the water or if there is any evidence of electrical failure or defect, *be sure to pull the plug* before touching the appliance or the water. Brushes should be rotated so that the bristles may dry (and stiffen) and bacterial action may be inhibited by the drying process. Brushes recommended for children have the same characteristics, but should be proportionally smaller. Some dentists recommend cleaning the teeth with a thin turkish toweling washcloth, as well as a brush, to remove dental plaques.

Dentifrices may take the form of a powder or a paste. Most authorities agree that, while they are not absolutely necessary to a thorough cleaning, they make the process easier and pleasanter. The stannous fluoride–calcium pyrophosphate dentifrice is the only product that is effective in children and adults, especially when the child's teeth developed in an optimal fluoride area. Most pastes, powders, and liquids for cleaning the teeth contain one or more of the following: an abrasive, a soap, and a flavoring. Pastes seem to have no advantage over powders except that they are controlled more easily. Powders may be insufflated by anybody but particularly by small children and irrational persons. Dentifrices that claim to remove stains may be injurious and are not recommended; those that are strongly abrasive should not be used. Water only is preferred for persons who use electric toothbrushes and should certainly be used for all those with exposed root surfaces. The advantage of using water alone is that there is less wearing away of teeth than when it is used with paste or powder. A homemade preparation of equal parts of sodium chloride, sodium bicarbonate, and prepared chalk, seasoned with oil of peppermint, is acceptable. The American Dental Association does not give ratings on dentifrices; *Consumer Reports* continues to serve as a reliable, readily available reference on the subject.

Flat dental floss is preferred to round, and some dentists advocate the unwaxed variety. Interdental stimulants are pointed wooden or rubber instruments made to fit between the teeth. The rubber tip fastened to the handle of the toothbrush is used on the inner and posterior interdental spaces.

The motion used in brushing is important. The main object is to clean the surfaces of the teeth. Some authorities believe that a second object is to stimulate and harden the gingiva as fibrous food is thought to harden the gums of primitive peoples. This value is questioned by some students, who claim that the chewing of coarse foods, rather than their contact with the gums, is responsible for their beneficial effect. There is agreement that the motions used should be such as to produce no traumatic effect. Horizontal and rotary motions are discouraged, the former failing to remove material from between the teeth and both inclined to push the gums away from the teeth. A dental health manual recommends that teeth be brushed in the direction in which they grow.[86a] Dorothy Hard, writing in Russell W. Bunting's text, recommends for general use a downward stroke for the upper teeth and an upward stroke for the lower teeth, each process carried out in two parts. She makes the following suggestion:

Instead of simply sweeping the bristles over the teeth, the stroke is done in two parts. First, the side of the toothbrush bristles is pressed against the gingival mucosa with sufficient force to blanch the tissues momentarily. Second, by rolling the wrist, the tips of the bristles are moved slowly and firmly lengthwise over the tooth surfaces.*

* Hard, Dorothy: "Oral Prophylaxis," in Bunting, Russell W., et al.: *A Textbook of Oral Hygiene.* Lea & Febiger, Philadelphia, 1959, p. 281.

Hard suggests establishing a pattern and looking in a mirror to see that all surfaces are covered. The motion described does not reach the occlusal surface of the teeth; therefore, an additional motion across the grinding, or cutting, surfaces is used (see Fig. 14-9). Dental tape, or floss, should be slipped carefully between the teeth, avoiding any injury to the interdental gingiva (see Fig. 14-10). Friction with wooden or rubber stimulators between the teeth discourages the formation of tartar, or calculi, and promotes healthy gums. It is advocated that this thorough cleaning be car-

ried out three times daily, and it is obvious that it is most effective if it follows eating. For many people, however, brushing the teeth before breakfast is esthetically important. The Water Pik, developed in recent years, is used by many. It ejects a thin stream of water which is directed between the teeth to forcefully remove particles of food. It should be used only on the advice of a dentist.

To summarize, the essentials of oral hygiene include the following: (1) an adequate diet containing enough coarse food to necessitate considerable chewing, (2) effective use of

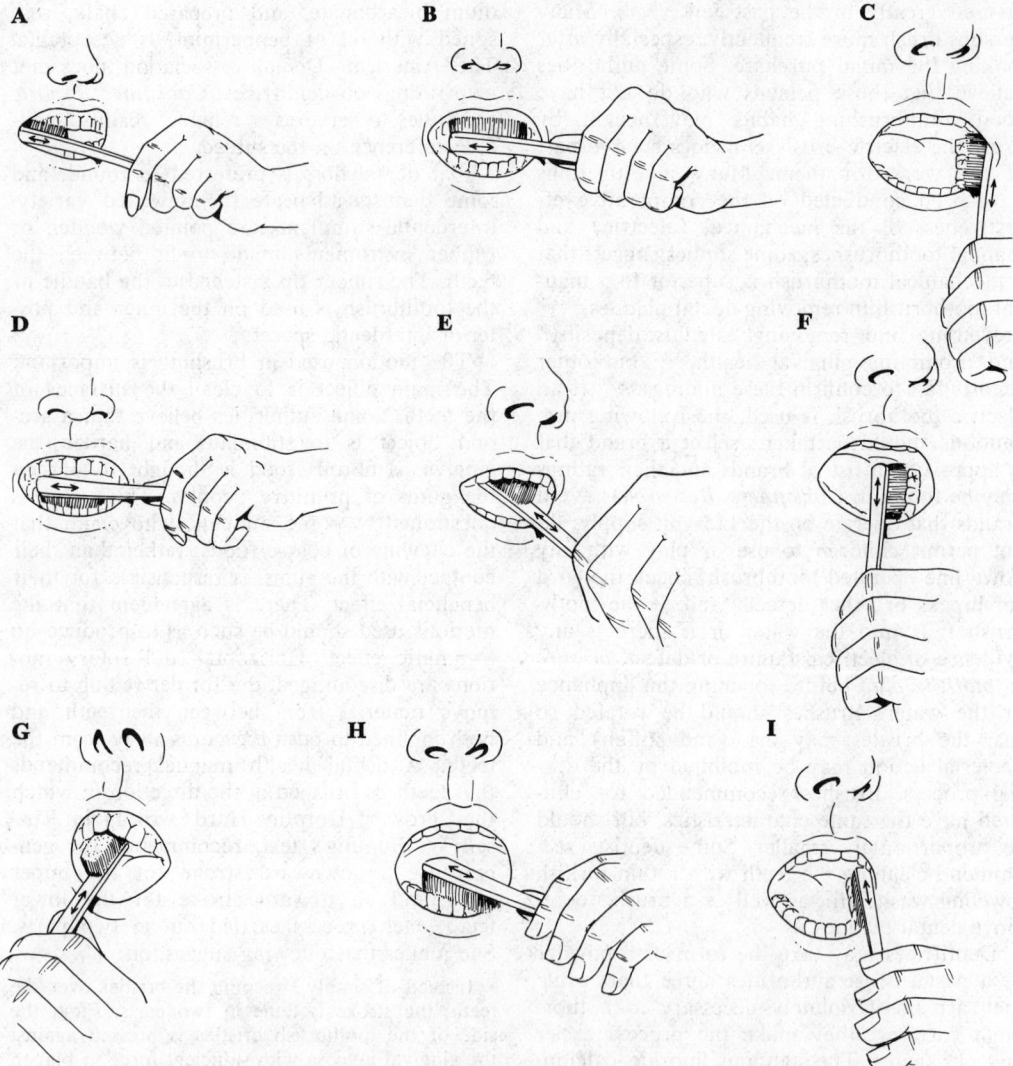

Figure 14-9. Brushing of teeth. *A*. Position the brush with bristles at junction of teeth and gums for brushing outside surfaces of all teeth as well as the inside surfaces of back teeth. *B–F*. Brush briskly back and forth with short strokes several times. *G*. and *H*. Hold the brush vertically when brushing the inside surfaces of the upper and lower front teeth. *I*. Brush back and forth to clean the biting surfaces. Study each figure carefully.

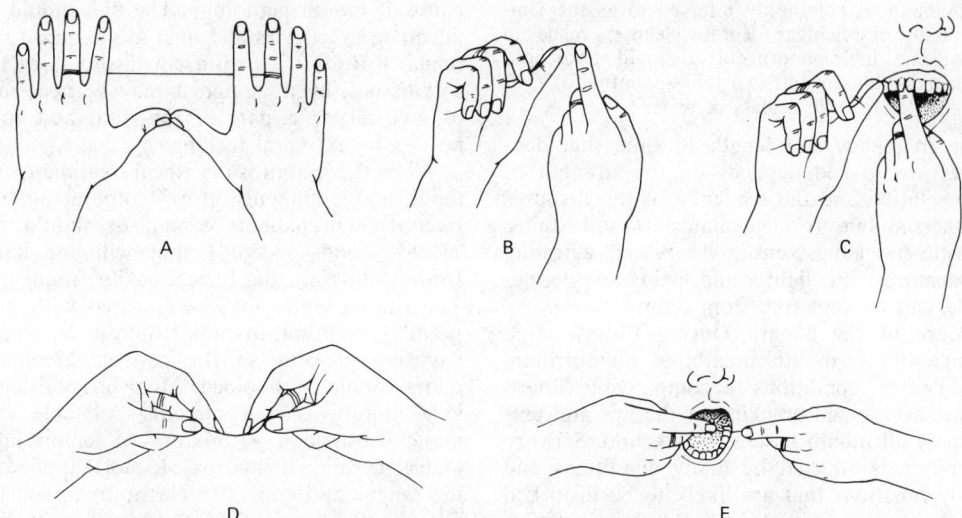

Figure 14-10. Flossing techniques. *A*. Wrap floss on middle fingers. *B*. Place thumb to outside for upper teeth. *C*. Floss between upper back teeth. *D*. Hold floss for lower teeth. *E*. Floss between lower back teeth.

toothbrush, dental tape, dental "stimulators," and dentifrice two to four times a day, preferably after meals and at bedtime; and, if prescribed, (3) effective use of the Water Pik after meals, especially for those persons who have ulcerative gums. Dental supervision is essential for the removal of irritating deposits, the early treatment of caries, and correction of malocclusion and other structural defects. Most dentists urge their patients to have a dental examination and prophylaxis at least twice a year. These visits should begin at the age of 2½ to 3 years and extend through the life span.

Care of Dentures. Since most persons having artificial teeth are sensitive about it, nurses should be especially thoughtful in helping those who wear them. Ambulatory patients will usually prefer to clean their mouths, plates, or bridges in the bathroom with running water; bed patients must have water, a dentifrice, brush, and a waste receptacle brought to them. If they are too ill to make the effort required, nurses must help them rinse their mouths and must clean their dentures.

For the sake of morale, the sick should be encouraged to wear their dentures unless their condition contraindicates it. Many persons sleep with false teeth in place. When not worn, plates and bridges made of plastic or vulcanite should be kept moist in a covered container of water to keep them from warping or getting brittle. A few drops of peppermint essence in the water give them a pleasant odor. Wet dentures are more easily inserted than dry ones. Transparent containers should

not be used for storage; false teeth exposed in a glass are grotesque and usually embarrass their owner. Plates are breakable; they must be kept in a safe place.

Plates and bridges should be cleaned when they are removed from the mouth for any purpose and after eating. The patient usually has a special powder recommended by the dentist, but any mildly abrasive tooth powder or ordinary soap may be used and applied with a brush. When nurses give this service to patients they should take the dentures to a source of running water, because they can be more satisfactorily cleaned if there is an abundant water supply. Water should be warm, never hot, since heat can distort the plastic or vulcanite. If patients clean the dentures, they should be given an ample amount of water and a large waste basin. They will ordinarily prefer to be unobserved.

Vulcanite is porous and absorbs food debris that, on deterioration, gives plates a sour odor unless properly cleaned and treated. Stains and foreign material tend to accumulate on dentures even though they have been cared for meticulously; use of immersion cleaners are, therefore, recommended. Commercial immersion cleaners are effective, but for the persons who may wish to prepare their own cleaner, Frank E. Jerbi recommends one of the following:

1. A solution of one teaspoonful of 28 per cent ammonia in a glass of water.
2. A solution of one tablespoonful of white vinegar in a glass of water (effective in removing films of hard deposits).

3. A mixture, commonly referred to as the University of Michigan denture cleanser, made up of one tablespoonful of a liquid household laundry bleach and two tablespoonfuls of Calgon detergent in a glass of water.*

The frequency and length of time that dentures are soaked depends on the strength of the solution and the tendency of the dentures to accumulate foreign materials and stains. Plastic has almost entirely replaced vulcanite in dentures. It is lighter and, being less permeable, can be kept free from odor.

Care of the Mouth During Illness. High temperatures, mouth breathing, malnutrition, and other conditions accompanying illness cause drying and cracking of the lips and predispose all mouth tissues to infection. Salivary secretion is affected by many conditions and body functions that are likely to be disturbed in illness. For example, salivary flow is diminished in fever, with profuse sweating, diuresis, diarrhea, and hemorrhage from loss of fluid and lack of fluid intake. When there is a negative fluid balance (loss of fluid) in the tissues, the secretions of the salivary glands are diminished. We all know that emotional factors have definite effects on salivary secretions (the dry mouth when frightened) and that during sleep the flow is depressed. The flow of mouth secretions is stimulated by appetizing sights and odors, by the presence of food in the mouth, by chewing, and by talking. Excessive flow may occur during pregnancy and is associated with lesions or irritation of the mouth, esophagus, stomach, and even the small intestines.

If patients are too sick to brush their teeth and clean their mouth or they do not know how to do it properly, someone must supply the needed energy and skill. In prolonged illness the examination and prophylactic treatment by the dentist, usually sought by the patient, should be provided by a dental service within the hospital or other health facility, and at more frequent intervals in sickness than in health. Dental consultation should be available to the physician and nurse when the patient has bleeding gums or other pathology. While gingivitis and pyorrhea during illness are often the direct result of an inadequate diet, they may be aggravated by the presence of tartar or other remediable conditions and by poor oral hygiene. The patient's food and fluid intake should be checked. Inadequate fluids or a deficient dietary essential can be the chief cause of mouth pathology. The diet should be adequate in calories and high in vitamins, particularly B and C, to prevent disorders of the soft tissues, even though it may be necessary to give all or a part of the fluid and food needed by extraoral feeding.

When the mouth is dry, local treatment with fluids and emollients gives temporary relief. Even though patients cannot or should not swallow foods or fluids, they will find it refreshing to rinse the buccal cavity frequently. The rinsing water may be flavored with peppermint, menthol, thymol, lemon juice, or any flavoring pleasing to the patient. Medicinal odors should be avoided. Most hospitals provide mouthwashes containing palatable aromatic substances. A mixture of lemon juice and glycerin (a trihydroxyalcohol) applied to the tongue and gums is a classic treatment for dry mouth. Louis S. Goodman and Alfred Gilman say: "Glycerin absorbs water and, therefore, in high concentration it is somewhat dehydrating and irritating to exposed tissue. Concentrated solutions, for this reason, are slowly bactericidal." *

The effectiveness of lemon juice and glycerin and their mode of action is debatable. Both are foods and harmless if swallowed, the lemon juice containing the much needed vitamin C and the glycerin having a sweet taste especially appealing to children. Lemon juice stimulates secretion of saliva and so may be of definite value. Glycerin, being hydroscopic, attracts moisture and therefore softens dry tissue, but if too concentrated it is dehydrating and irritating. In a study of 136 geriatric patients who were in a nursing home but *not* acutely ill, Jennie VanDrimmelen and Helen F. Rollins found that a mixture of lemon juice and glycerin (in a one to one proportion) had a more drying effect on the oral tissues than saline when both agents were used over a 5-day period. In conclusion, they say "If these results occur with well patients, it can be predicted that equal or more pronounced effects could occur with ill patients." † The continued use of this mixture is questionable.

Carbonated drinks such as ginger ale, give comfort as a mouthwash. It is possible that the bubbles of gas break up tenacious mucus and make its expectoration easier. Plain or flavored oils are often applied with applicators or an atomizer to the inside of the mouth. The latter method is more effective. This treatment is

---

* Jerbi, Frank E.: "Preventive Prosthodontics (Complete Dentures)," in Bernier, Joseph L., and Muhler, Joseph C. (eds.): *Improving Dental Practice Through Preventive Measures*, 2nd ed. C. V. Mosby Co., St. Louis, 1970, p. 291.

* Goodman, Louis S., and Gilman, Alfred: *The Pharmacological Basis of Therapeutics*, 5th ed. Macmillan Publishing Co., Inc., New York, 1975, p. 947.
† VanDrimmelen, Jennie, and Rollins, Helen F.: "Evaluation of a Commonly Used Oral Hygiene Agent," *Nurs. Res.*, **18**:327, (July–Aug.) 1969.

not always acceptable to the patient, and there is the ever-present danger that the oil may run down into the lungs. If the oil is not absorbed, it acts as an irritant, or foreign body, and may cause a pneumonitis or an abscess.[87] Mineral oils are the most dangerous, and vegetable oils the least; P. H. Rossier and A. Bühlman [88] say that animal oils cause necrosis or abscess formation. Lanolin and cocoa butter salves applied to the lips are of definite value. Petroleum jelly is effective, but is distasteful to most persons. In a study of 31 groups (10 each) of guinea pigs with x-irradiated induced ulcers of the mucous membrane of the mouth, Miriam K. Ginsberg and Ann E. Yoder [89] used glycerin, ascorbic acid, alkaline mouth wash, normal saline and hydrogen peroxide (applied locally), and systemic treatment (streptomycin with ascorbic acid, streptomycin alone, and ascorbic acid alone) in an attempt to test the effectiveness of some of the local treatments commonly used by nurses in the care of patients with stomatitis. They conclude that, regardless of the form of treatment, there was no difference in the day of onset of the lesion or the length of its duration. They note in an earlier study of patients with acute renal failure no mouthwash was shown to be superior to another; however, Joyce Y. Passos and Lucy M. Brand [90] report improvement in the oral cavity of 22 patients when hydrogen peroxide or milk of magnesia was used as opposed to an alkaline aromatic mouthwash. They state that hydrogen peroxide was more effective in patients over 50 years, whereas milk of magnesia was best for those under 50 years.

If the mouth is coated and lesions have developed and as a result the mouth is in a serious condition, the physician may prescribe some special application, such as sodium perborate, in addition to the general treatment suggested above, or may combat the infection with systemic antibiotics.

In sickness teeth should be brushed at least as often as in health. Because many illnesses lower resistance of oral tissues, it is desirable to clean the mouth after each meal or feeding. *Hospitals should provide toothbrushes to patients who need them. Cotton applicators are no substitute; their inadequacy as cleansing agents accounts for the poor condition of many mouths during illness when they were substituted for the toothbrush.* Cotton when wet is slippery and doesn't clean teeth or a coated tongue. As a substitute for a toothbrush some nurses use gauze strips wrapped around the finger or a tongue blade. The sensation of gauze catching on the teeth is disagreeable, and if it is used, care should be taken to reduce this to a minimum. It is not an effective procedure. Ginsberg suggests that the following principles serve as a guide in giving oral hygiene to those persons who are seriously ill:

1. The mucous membranes of the mouth, nose, and lips must be kept clean and moist at all times. . . .
2. The airway must be kept patent. . . .
3. The frequency of administration of oral hygiene nursing care is determined by the condition of the patient.*

She goes on to say that, although these principles may be simple, by scrupulously following them stomatitis was prevented in a group of patients with acute renal failure.

It is more difficult to brush someone else's teeth than one's own, and nurses often practice on each other until they are skillful. Figure 14-11*A–E* illustrates some of the major aspects in cleaning the mouth that are suggested in the following procedure.

Suggested Procedure in Cleaning the Mouth of the Bed Patient. *If patients are able to brush their own teeth,* support them in a sitting position with a waste basin before them, if possible on a table, and protect the chest with a towel. If they cannot assume a sitting position, have them turn on the side with the face extending over the edge of the pillow. (Put a right-handed person on the left side and vice versa.) In this case, protect the bedding under the head with a towel and place the waste basin on the towel beside the cheek. Obviously, people will need more assistance if they are recumbent than if they are sitting up.

Provide a cup of cool rather than hot water because the latter softens bristles and is not so refreshing. Patients will need toothbrush, dentifrice, dental tape, possibly dental stimulators, and a mouthwash. "Celluwipes" should be at hand. If the patient is lying down, a drinking tube is needed.

If the patient is unable to manipulate the toothbrush and the nurse is going to do it, place the person in the side-lying position as described above. Wet (and rinse) the brush by pouring water over it, *not* by dipping it in the cup; this soils the water and makes it repellent as a rinse. Brush the central incisors first. Ask the patient to open the mouth; then while the mouth is open, insert the brush and bring it out against the cheek in position to brush the outer aspect of the right molars as the patient approximates the teeth. Repeat this process on the left side; then, while the patient holds the mouth open, brush the inner aspects of the teeth. Use a dentifrice of the patient's choice, or select the most appropriate one available. Let the patient rinse the mouth frequently, using the drinking tube and allowing the water to flow from the mouth into the emesis basin. When the patient is unconscious or likely to insufflate fluids that are in the mouth, use a

* Ginsberg, Miriam K.: "A Study of Oral Hygiene Nursing Care," *Am. J. Nurs.,* **61**:67, (Oct.) 1961.

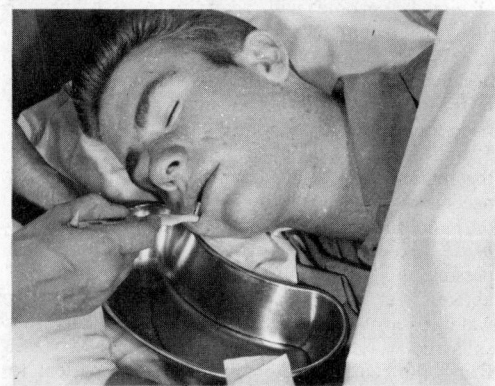

Figure 14-11. *A*. Mouth care of the conscious patient who is unable to hold a toothbrush. The nurse is introducing the toothbrush into the open mouth. *B*. The toothbrush is drawn out against cheek. *C*. The brush is in position for brushing the outer surface of the upper and lower right molars. *D*. With the water and tube held in the proper position, the patient does not have to raise his head to rinse his mouth or to drink. *E*. Rinsing water will flow from the mouth if the head is in the right position. The bed will not be wet if the basin is placed at the edge of the pillow and the patient's face hangs over the basin. (Courtesy of Columbia-Presbyterian Medical Center, New York, N.Y., and Clay-Adams Co., New York, N.Y.)

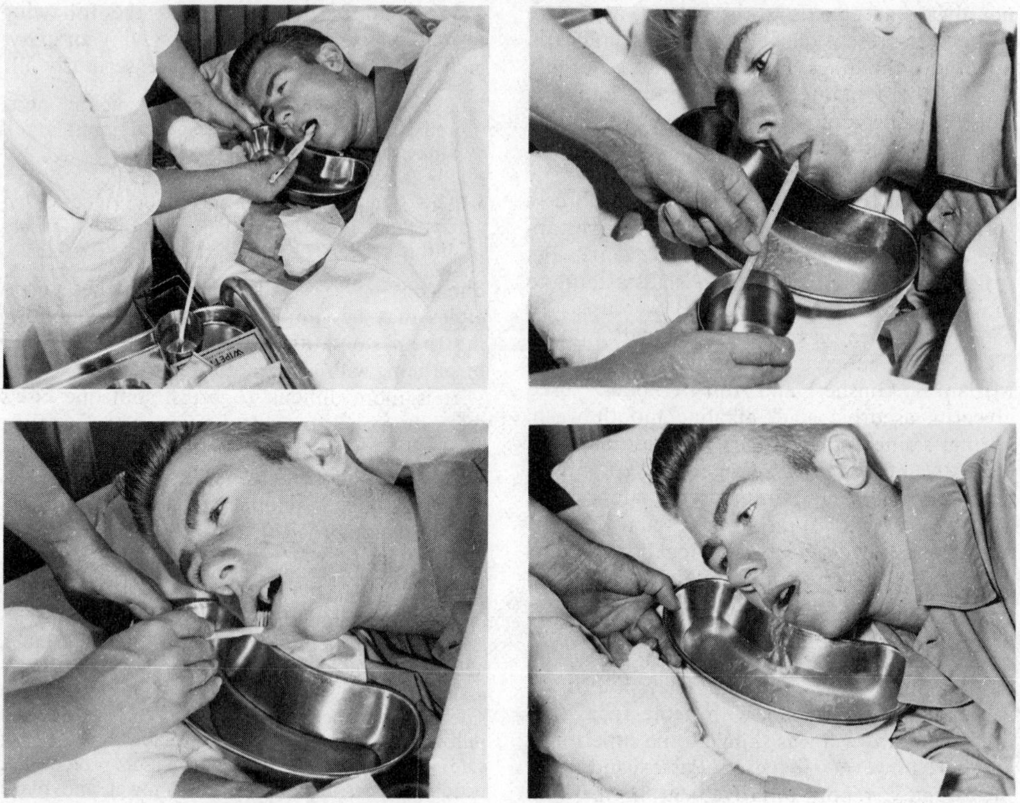

suction machine throughout the cleaning process, if one is available. An asepto syringe can be used to draw the fluid from the mouth but it is not very satisfactory. If the nurse places his or her finger over one end of a drinking tube, it may serve as a small siphon that makes it possible to put water in the mouth of the irrational patient who cannot, or will not, suck on the tube.

When cotton applicators saturated with mouthwash are used to clean the mouth, they are discarded into a paper bag as used.

Throughout the procedure, try to observe the wishes of the patients, at the same time using this as an opportunity, if the need is indicated and

interest can be aroused, to teach patients the fundamentals of mouth care. Methods used by the nurse in either home or hospital serve as a model to the patient. Teaching a method of correct toothbrushing has been shown to reduce plaques on teeth of hospitalized patients.[91] Instruction in oral hygiene is thought so important in some hospitals that specialists are employed to teach patients and to give them prophylactic treatment. There are dental clinics in hospital outpatient departments, and dental internes are found in a number of large institutions.

If the patient is unconscious, vary the procedure as illustrated in Figure 14-12*A–C*.

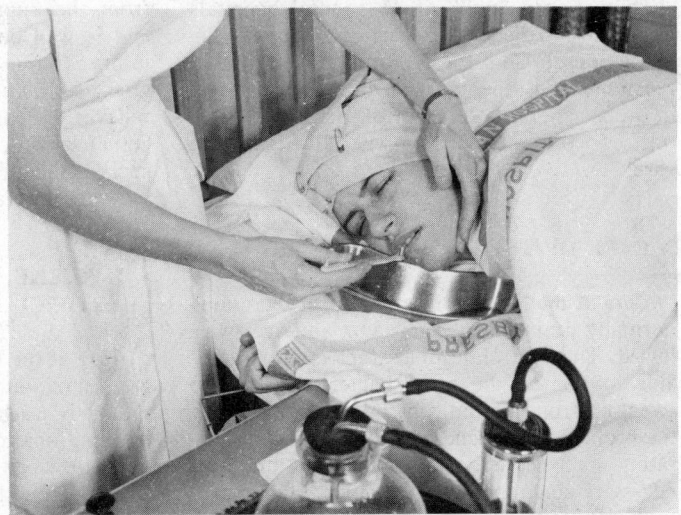

Figure 14-12. *A.* Mouth care of the unconscious patient. The nurse is brushing the teeth with the same motions advocated for the person in health. *B.* Water is introduced with an Asepto Syringe and suction is maintained at the same time. (Note that tip is protected with a piece of rubber tubing.) *C.* Excess fluid is carefully suctioned from the mouth at the termination of the cleansing process. (Courtesy of Columbia-Presbyterian Medical Center, New York, N.Y., and Clay-Adams Co., New York, N.Y.)

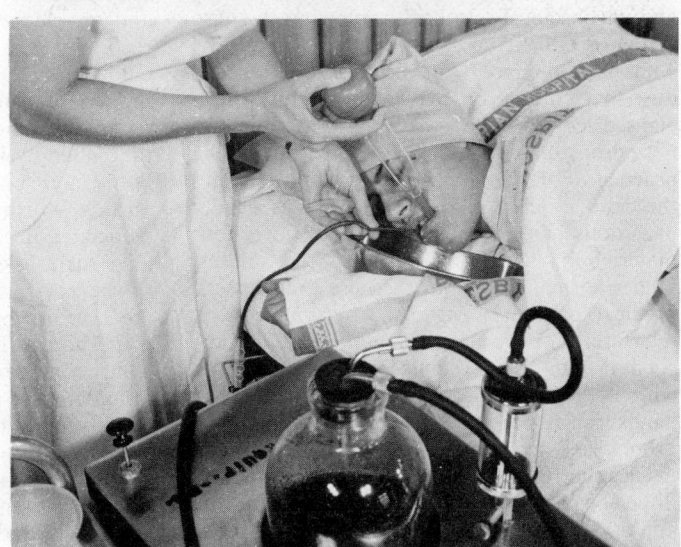

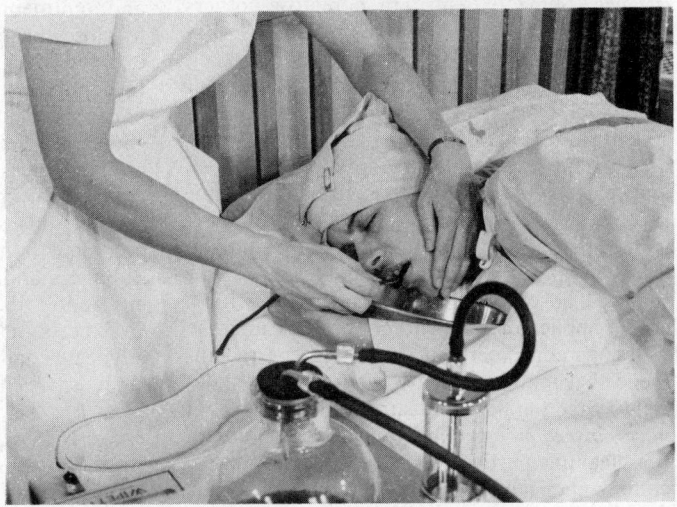

Discussing a "poll" of 41 general hospitals and their experience in a particular one, J. Orton Goodsell and R. E. Roper [92] (in 1951) recommended a dental department, or service, in every general hospital of 300 or more beds, this service to offer preventive and therapeutic care.

5. CARE OF THE NOSE

Care of the Nose in Health. Nasal secretions normally drain into the pharynx and are swallowed. The gastrointestinal tract is apparently able to destroy the nasal bacteria and those swept up from the lungs by ciliary motion into the bronchi and trachea. The habit of expectorating such secretions is unpleasant and unnecessary since they are of the same character as those that the individual swallows constantly and unconsciously. In health, blowing the nose gently is all that is necessary to keep the anterior nares free from dried secretions and dust that collects on the nasal mucus. Physicians discourage the use of nasal sprays and nose drops unless prescribed as treatment. The practice of snuffing water or salt solution into the nose to clean it is considered especially hazardous, the danger being that infectious material may be drawn up into the sinuses. Under normal conditions the nose drains itself. Medical opinion is against any unnecessary interference. Even blowing the nose is discouraged; if practiced, it should be done gently and with both nostrils open and the used paper handkerchief collected in a plastic (or waterproof) sack and later burned.

Cleaning the Nose in Sickness. Infants and ill persons are likely to have crusts form in the anterior nares. Being more or less helpless, they are unable to remove these without assistance. Some patients are comatose, others may be too weak to use a handkerchief. Patients who have nasal infections may also need instruction in cleaning the anterior nares. Paper handkerchiefs that are destroyed as soon as soiled are recommended in health and disease as a means of preventing infection of others and reinfection of the person using the handkerchief. A vegetable oil, such as cottonseed, is recommended for softening and removing dried nasal secretions, although water may suffice. The cleansing agent is applied with a cotton applicator. The end of the stick must be well covered. Experts in infant hygiene recommend that mothers use a wet soft cotton material to wipe the nose and surrounding areas but *never insert any foreign object in the nostril* for cleaning purposes. Nurses, when using a cotton applicator, should remove the stick

from the applicator because, even when the end is well covered, there is some danger of injury. If the skin around the nose is excoriated, petroleum jelly or cold cream usually relieves the condition. In cases where there are actual lesions, the physician may order some such medication as a mild mercurial, sulfur, or vitamin ointment.

6. HYGIENE OF THE EYES AND ARTIFICIAL EYES

Care of the Eyes. When the lachrymal glands are functioning normally, the eyes are continuously washed with their secretion and need no additional cleaning; in some diseases of the eyes, or when the neuromuscular mechanism that protects them by blinking is not functioning adequately, the nurse may have to protect and/or clean the eye. Francis H. Adler [93] recommends a 1.5 per cent solution of sodium chloride as a cleansing agent because it approximates normal tears. Commercially prepared eye lotions for daily use are foisted on the public by high-pressure advertising. A pint bottle may contain nothing more than water and 5¢ worth of boric acid powder, a drug associated in the public mind with eyes. Boric acid has a low saturation point, and so undissolved crystals, that act as foreign bodies in the eye, are not uncommon. Clement Brooke and Thomas Boggs, reporting the death of a child from boric acid poisoning and a review of previously reported cases, comment on its toxicity and the readiness with which it is absorbed from injured surfaces. They say: "The therapeutic value of boric acid is doubtful and its antiseptic quality minimal. There are better and safer substances available for uses as antiseptics, irrigations, wet dressings, and ointments." * When a person is unable to close the eyelids adequately, the cornea is exposed. This condition is serious and is found in conditions such as coma, unconsciousness, paralysis of the facial nerves, and lethargy caused by sedatives or anesthesia. Under such circumstances the nurse should put liberal amounts of sterile petroleum jelly in the eyes and the lids should be carefully closed. Such treatment is important in sight conservation. [94] Blindness and sight conservation are discussed in Chapter 46.

Experts in the care of the newborn do not advocate daily bathing of the eyes, except when silver nitrate has been instilled. In this

* Brooke, Clement, and Boggs, Thomas: "Boric Acid Poisoning: Report of a Case and Review of the Literature," *Am. J. Dis. Child.*, **82**:465, (Oct.) 1951.

case, they recommend irrigating the eyes with saline, using an eyedropper; otherwise, they recommend removing any crust that may form on the lids with a sterile eye cotton sponge wet with sterile water. This method may be used for everyone, or eyes may be flushed with an eyedropper or small syringe. If the latter is used and it is made of glass or plastic it is a wise precaution to cover its tip with a short piece of rubber tubing. Eye irrigations and removal of foreign bodies are discussed in Chapter 27.

During the past decade or so, rigid or flexible contact lenses as a replacement or supplement for ordinary glasses have become increasingly popular, especially among young women who are myopic and dislike wearing glasses, particularly at social functions. According to Jeffrey Baker,[95] the greatest advantage of contact lenses for about 90 per cent of the wearers is their cosmetic effect. Some of the disadvantages discussed include the following: (1) when lenses are not well fitted or kept clean, the wearer may experience "fogging" or flare, or visual symptoms of edema, lessening visual acuity; (2) the wearer's range of vision is limited to straight ahead unless the head is turned; (3) the cost of contact lenses is $150 to $300—a major disadvantage, and they are easily lost and broken; and (4) corneal abrasions occur frequently in some wearers. The conventional lens case (moist) in which lenses may be stored has been found to provide conditions for bacterial survival and, in fact, contains a significantly greater number of colonies of organisms, "predominantly Gram-negative rods, including *Pseudomonas* and *Aerobacter*" than the ventilated container (dry),* according to Charles H. Winkler and Joseph M. Dixon.[96] Obviously the cases must be kept scrupulously clean and the wetting agent changed each day. Most authorities agree that persons who wear contact lenses should be under the supervision of an ophthalmologist and should always carry an identification card (see Fig. 14-13). The ophthalmologist should recommend a reliable ophthalmic technician to fit the lenses and teach the wearer how to insert and remove them. Because the eye and eyelid structure differs considerably from person to person, methods of insertion and removal will, of necessity, vary.[97] One suggested method for removal of lenses is shown in Figure 14-14*A–C*. In addition, directions for removing lenses in various positions are shown in Figure 14-15*A–C*. Unskilled handling or fitting of lenses has been attributed to serious impairment of vision. According to *Consumers' Research Annual Bulletin*,[98] in 1966, 14 cases of blindness have been reported and 700 persons with temporarily impaired vision. Contact lenses should *not* be worn under the following conditions: (1) in industrial work where dust or dirt particles are in the air; (2) in the presence of chemicals; (3) in strenuous sports, especially those involving bodily contact; (4) while swimming; (5) in eye irritation, corneal edema, or any infection in any part of the body; and (6) when any member of the family has conjunctivitis or a bacterial infection. Figure 14-16 lists steps to follow if the wearer becomes helpless. To prevent eye infection and enhance good vision, the lenses, of course, must be kept scrupulously clean; prior to insertion, the hands should be washed well with soap and water, the lenses cleaned with the fingers using a few drops of an antiseptic wetting solution on both surfaces and edges, and then dipped in clean tap water. Some authorities say that contact lenses should not be worn longer than six consecutive hours. Flexible (soft) plastic contact lenses are currently available. Since these are less irritating than those developed earlier, they need to be taken out only two times weekly.[98a] Wearers are advised to keep their regular glasses, avoid depending on contact lenses when traveling, especially in foreign countries or other places where a qualified ophthalmologist is not readily available, and always to carry a copy of the prescription for contact lenses when traveling.

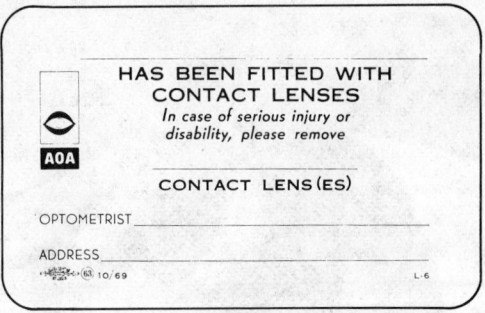

Figure 14-13. A card carried by a contact lens wearer. (Courtesy of American Optometric Association, St. Louis, Mo.)

Care of Artificial Eyes. Ocular prostheses vary greatly. They may be spherical, the size and shape of the normal eye, they may be a shell worn over a socket built up by plastic surgery, or they may fit into an implant. An implant is a spherical, nearly eye-shaped frame of polymethyl methacrylate or some other material that the tissues will tolerate. It is so

* Ventilated cases are flat plastic type with perforations on each side. (Mueller-West Co., Chicago, Ill.)

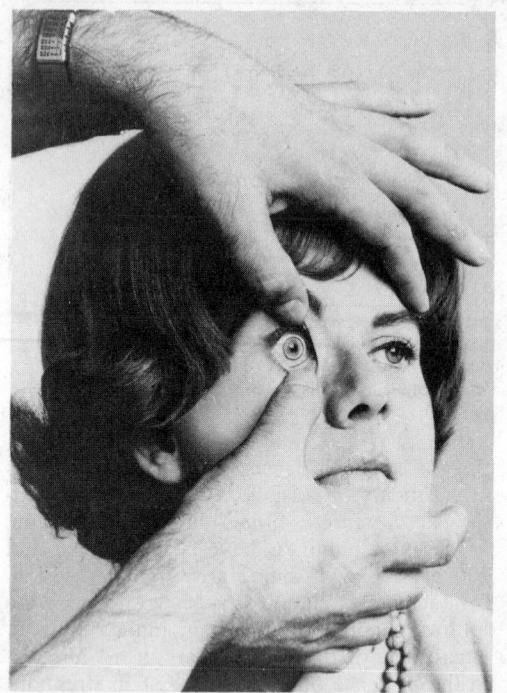

A

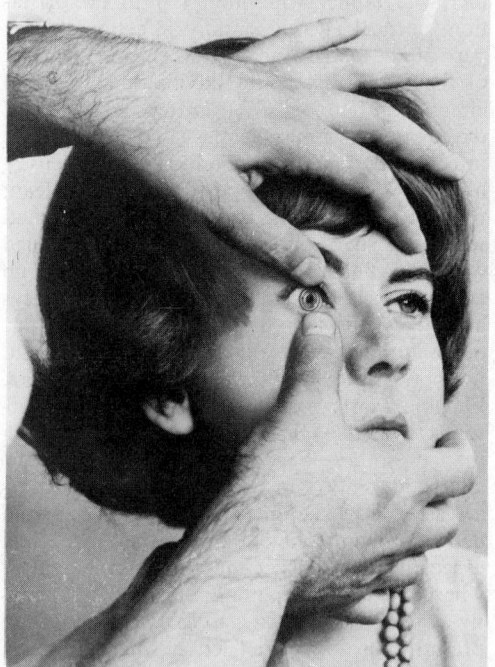

B

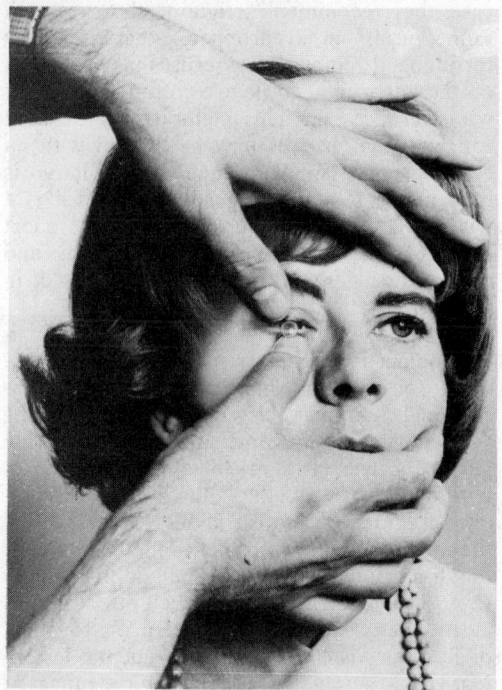

C

Figure 14-14. How to remove contact lenses. *A*. After the eyelids have been separated and the corneal contact lens has been correctly positioned over the cornea, widen the eyelid margins beyond the top and bottom edges of lens (as shown). *B*. After the lower eyelid margin has been moved near the bottom lens edge and then the upper eyelid margin has been moved near the top lens edge, move under the bottom edge of the lens as shown by pressing slightly harder on the lower eyelid while moving it upward. *C*. After the lens has tipped slightly, move the eyelids toward one another and thereby cause the lens to clide out between the eyelids. (Courtesy of American Optometric Association, St. Louis, Mo.)

constructed that the surrounding tissues and the muscles moving the eye may be attached to it permanently. The anterior visible portion, or the artificial eye, is held on the implant by some device that makes its removal possible. Newer artificial eyes are made so that the entire conjunctiva is in contact with the eye. This makes for greater mobility and comfort.

According to William Stone,[99] writing in 1965, the secretions of the socket roughen the surface of the glass prosthesis, and when this occurs surface polishing may help, but the

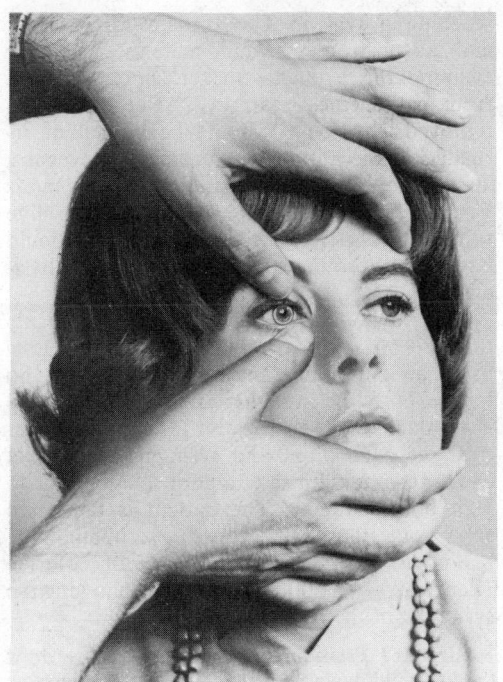

A

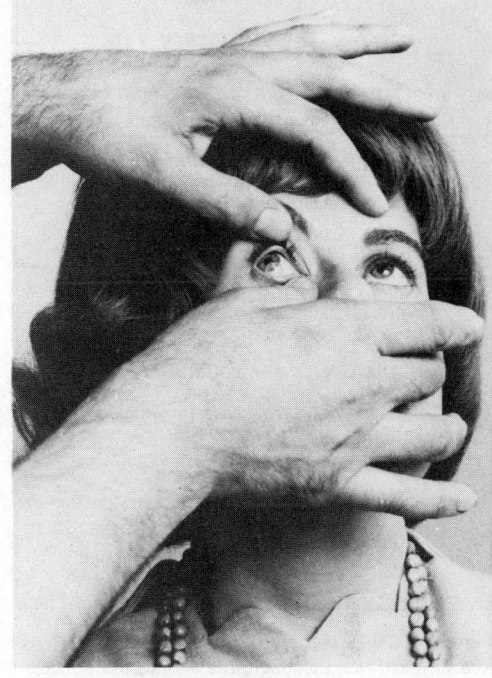

C

B

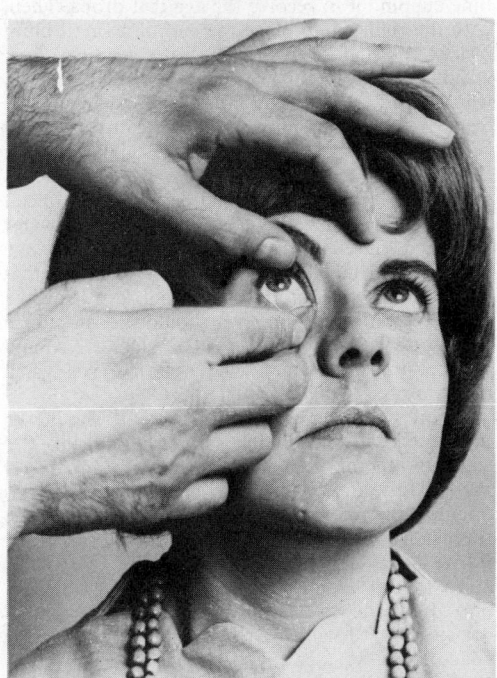

Figure 14-15. Various positions of contact lenses and directions for removal. *A.* Directly over the cornea. This normal wearing position of a corneal contact lens is also the correct position for removing it. If the lens cannot be removed, however, slide it onto the sclera. *B.* On the sclera only. Here the lens can remain with relative safety until experienced help is available; other white areas of the eye to the side or above the cornea might also be used. If the lens is to be removed, however, slide it to a position directly over the cornea. *C.* On both the cornea and sclera. A lens in this position—or a similar one anywhere around the periphery of the cornea— should be moved as soon as possible. If the lens is to be removed, slide it to a position directly over the cornea; if the lens cannot be removed immediately, slide it onto the sclera. (Courtesy of American Optometric Association, St. Louis, Mo.)

glass eye usually must be replaced; the plastic eye may also be roughened by infection of the socket and deposition of concretions on the surface and by drying of the prosthesis from incomplete closure of the lids. Treatment includes eliminating the cause, if possible, and irrigating the eye socket with an antiseptic solution. Sir Stewart Duke-Elder [100] said in 1970 that the glass eye must be replaced each year. Both authors recognize the advantages of the plastic over the glass prostheses.

Beliefs and practices in the care of the prosthesis and the eye socket vary. Irving P. Filderman and Paul F. White,[101] writing in

CONTACT LENS EMERGENCY CARE

1. DETERMINE IF PATIENT IS WEARING CONTACT LENSES:

a. Ask
b. Check I.D. Card
c. Check Medic Alert Medallion
d. Look for contact lenses

2. IF YOU SUSPECT THE LENSES ARE STILL ON THE EYE:

a. Apply adhesive tape strip to patient's forehead or adjacent area and label "Contact Lenses"
b. Consult emergency aid file when time permits

3. IF THE LENSES ARE FOUND:

a. Place in a case or bottle and label with patient's name (Mark "right" or "left," if known)
b. Record on emergency tag

Provided as a public service
by the
AMERICAN OPTOMETRIC ASSOCIATION

Figure 14-16. Steps to follow if the contact lens wearer becomes incapacitated by accident, sickness, or other cause. Contact lenses are designed to be worn only while awake and fully conscious. (Courtesy of American Optometric Association, St. Louis, Mo.)

1969, say a reformed eye should be removed every 2 to 3 weeks, cleaned with warm soapy water, and rinsed, followed by polishing with a soft cloth; whereas, a shell eye should be removed every night, cleaned, and stored in a contact lens-soaking solution. Duke-Elder said a plastic eye should be removed and washed only once a week. Stone notes that prior to World War II wearers were advised to remove the prosthesis each night, but improved methods now make it unnecessary for the patient to remove the artificial eye at any time. In fact, he says the person "is cautioned never to remove the prosthesis from the socket."

The socket may be infected by the following routes: (1) the hands of the patient by ever-present *Staphylococcus aureus* and with *Escherichia coli* when improper toilet habits are used; (2) the hands and the instruments of the eye-fitter following work on other patients with infected sockets; and (3) nasal and sinus infections of the patient, in retrograde fashion, through the nasolacrimal duct to the socket.[102]

Those persons who are fitted with an artificial eye that must be removed will prefer to care for the eye and socket themselves when in the hospital, but nurses must know how to do it for the very sick or handicapped; and they may also have to reinforce the doctor's

teaching in hygiene. The hands of the operator and all instruments and material used for cleaning the eye and socket should be free from pathogenic organisms. After the eye is removed, the socket should be bathed or irrigated. Some authorities recommend eyecups, an undine, or a glass syringe with an emesis basin to receive the waste. A physiologic saline solution (0.9 per cent sodium chloride) should be used if no other is prescribed by the physician.

Stone, who uses the newer motility implants that are not removed by the subject, suggests using an antibiotic ointment (one that is no longer used for systemic treatment, so there is no danger of sensitization) in the conjunctival sac each night and syringing the socket each morning with salt solution (¼ tsp salt to 1 qt boiled water). The patient is taught to carry out these procedures, scrubbing the hands first. Aqueous benzalkonium chloride (Zephiran)—1:3000—is instilled following the syringing of the eye.*

Suggested Procedure. *To remove the eye* draw the lower lid down with the left hand, at the same time cupping it to receive the eye if it drops. Then, with the right hand, place the end of a small blunt instrument under the edge of the artificial eye, which is made to slip forward over the lower lid, when it will readily drop out. This maneuver must be carried out with care, as the eye can very easily be destroyed by dropping on a hard surface. *Clean the eye* before putting it away or returning it to the socket. Filderman and White say the artificial eye should be washed with a mild soap and water and then rinsed with clear water, as does one maker of artificial eyes who also cautions that alcohol dims the luster of a plastic eye. For the same reason a plastic eye should be stored in water rather than left dry, while a glass eye should be kept in a box lined with soft material when not in use.†

Before inserting an artificial eye it should be moistened with physiologic saline. J. H. Prince [102a] suggests dipping it in "pure castor oil." *To insert the eye* raise the upper lid with the tips of the two middle fingers, holding the hand flat against the forehead. Push the artificial eye beneath the upper lid with the right hand, and as it slips into place, allow the lid to fall over it. The eye must be supported by the left hand while the lower lid is drawn forward with the right hand over the lower edge of the eye (see Fig. 14-17).

If the eye is not to be removed, equipment and materials necessary for eye care in the morning must be provided. They include sterile saline or salt solution (¼ tsp salt to 1 qt boiled water), a

---

* Recent work on Zephiran (see Chapter 15) has led many persons to doubt its current usefulness. If writing currently, Stone might recommend a different antiseptic.

† *Facts on the Care of an Artificial Eye.* Mager and Gougleman, Inc., New York.

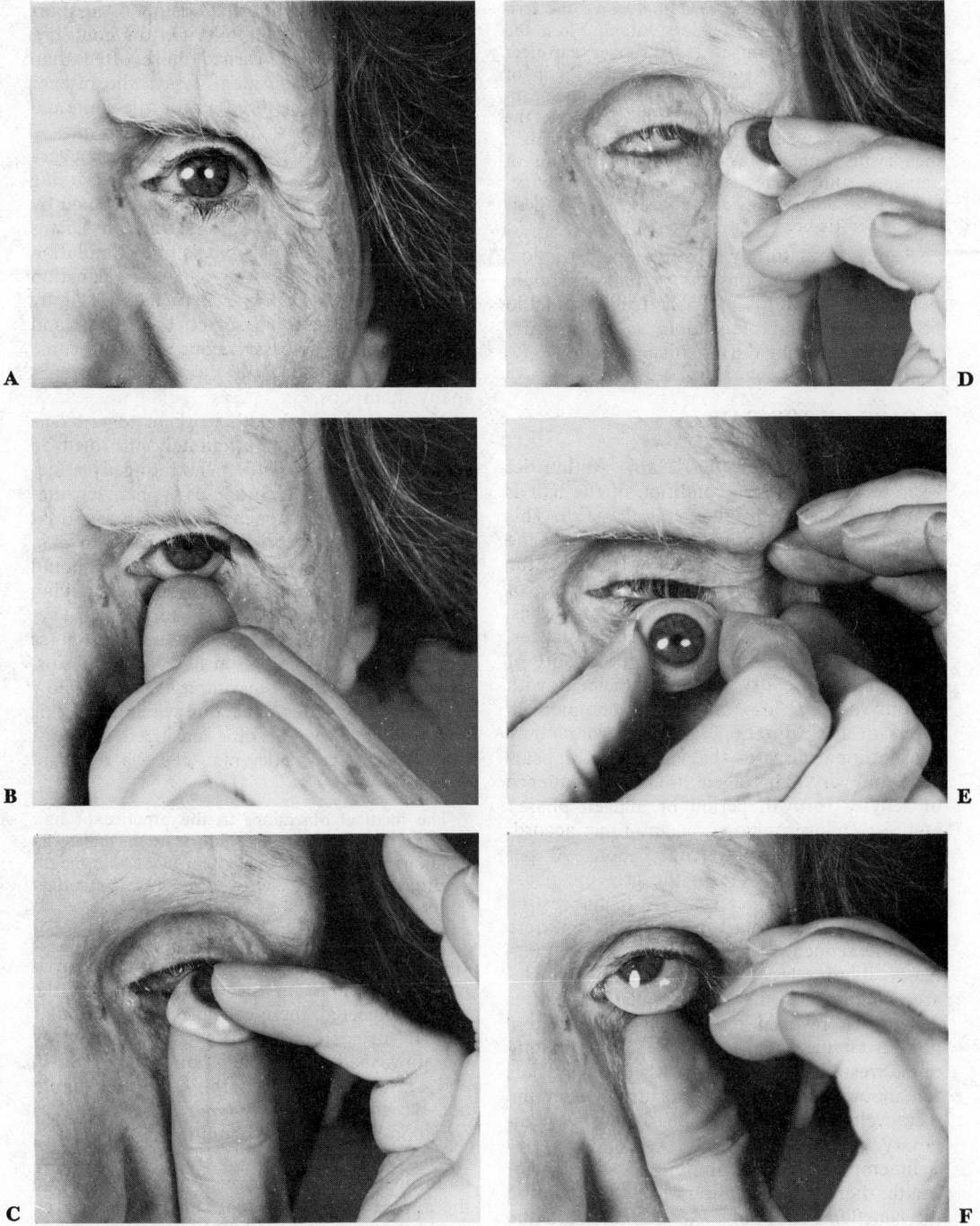

Figure 14-17. Removal and insertion of an artificial eye by a patient. *A*. Artificial eye in the socket. *B*. With the thumb, patient dislodges eye slightly, prior to removal. *C*. As eye is removed, patient holds it firmly between the thumb and forefinger. *D*. Patient holds eye alongside the empty socket; note shell form of artificial eye. *E*. For insertion, patient places left hand on forehead to left of socket and exerts slight pressure to raise upper eyelid; artificial eye is held between thumb and forefinger prior to insertion. *F*. Final step in insertion of artificial eye; patient gently pushes eye in place with thumb. (Courtesy of Alfred Spitzer.)

sterile rubber syringe, a bowl to receive the irrigating solution and antiseptic solution. Flush the eye with several syringes (soft rubber ear-ulcer syringe) full of salt solution, placing the tip of the nozzle behind the prosthesis at the inner canthus while using the other hand to keep the prosthesis from being pushed out of the socket; then instill with an eye-dropper about 4 ml of antiseptic solution in the eye, and afterward (according to Stone's advice) polish the prosthesis with paper tissue.

People are naturally sensitive about the loss of an eye and anxious that attention should not be attracted to it. Their feelings should be respected, and precautions taken to safeguard their privacy during this procedure.

7. CARE OF THE HAIR

Hygienic Care of the Hair. Authorities seem to agree that the condition of the hair is materially affected by the *general health*. This is easily understood when one realizes that the visible portion, or shaft, is nourished by the root embedded in the scalp. The supply of nutrients to the root, the removal of wastes, and the lack of certain physiologic substances, such as thyroxin, seem to affect the quality of the hair. Coarse dry hair is associated with hypothyroidism, loss of hair is common in fevers of long duration, and there are many constitutional diseases that change its appearance. In every hair follicle, there is a sequence of activity (growth period or anagen phase) and rest (telogen phase); at any time, according to Norman Orentreich,[103] about 90 per cent of the follicles are in the growing phase while the other 10 per cent are in the resting phase. Certain factors can, however, interfere with the sequence; for example, during pregnancy, there is less loss of hair as the follicles are maintained in the growing phase, but after delivery, a reversal may occur with a large number of the follicles going into the resting phase, resulting in a profuse shedding of hair for about 3 months. This disturbance in the hair cycle, fortunately, is nearly always temporary.

In emphasizing the importance of general health, there is no intention of underestimating the beneficial effect of *local treatment* on the scalp and hair shaft. Stimulating the circulation of the scalp by massage and brushing is conceded to be desirable. Brushing the hair vigorously not only stimulates the circulation, but also, if the brush is clean, removes dirt particles and dead cells from the scalp.

Washing the hair every week or two is advocated by most authorities consulted. There seems to be no adequate basis for the commonly expressed belief that shampoos at short intervals make the hair oily. On the contrary, oily hair should be washed more often than dry. Howard T. Behrman [104] says the oftener it is washed the better it is for the hair and scalp. He thinks a shampoo every five days is a good general rule; every two days, or every day, in very oily conditions of the scalp. Drying alcoholic lotions for oily hair are advocated by proprietors of beauty parlors, but physicians usually recommend cleanliness and stimulation of the scalp to make the oil glands function more normally. Dry hair may be treated by applying small amounts of oil to the hair and scalp. With age the sebaceous glands become less active, and the hair does not require as many shampoos.

No matter how health workers regard *hair dyeing,* they should be accurately informed on its hazards. The basis of penetrating dyes, according to A. J. Reiches,[105] is *p*-phenylenediamine, "a potent skin sensitizer." He says that while there are surprisingly few cases of skin irritation due to hair dye reported, dye should be used with caution. He recommends making a patch test behind the ear 24 to 48 hours before each dyeing. G. W. G. Jackman notes that persons suffering from hay fever, rhinitis, dermatitis, or other idiosyncrasies should know that they may suffer a reaction when using hair dyes and once they become sensitized, the most innocuous of cosmetics may cause a reaction. He says:

The medical objections to the practice of hair dyeing are three-fold: (1) injury to the hair; (2) insidious poisoning of the system by certain metals or drugs included in the dye; and (3) the danger of local dermatitis.*

The body surface, including the scalp, is constantly shedding dead cells. Exfoliation is rarely noticeable on the body, but when the hair is neglected, these cells produce a granular "scurf," or scale, which is caught and held by the unwashed, unbrushed hair. Agnes Savill and Clara Warren [106] say this condition should not be confused with *dandruff,* which is a common but abnormal condition.

Pityriasis capitis is the medical term for dandruff. There are various types according to the appearance of the scale and scalp, as well as the organisms found. Pityriasis may occur alone or in conjunction with other scalp and skin diseases. It is often confused with other scaly eruptions.

Pityriasis simplex is believed to be caused by the *Pityrosporum.* This has been described as

* Jackman, G. W. G.: "Hair Dyes," in Savill, Agnes, and Warren, Clara: *The Hair and Scalp,* 5th ed. Williams & Wilkins Co., Baltimore, 1962, p. 286.

a bottle-shaped bacillus, but Savill and Warren say it is now classed under the group of *Monilia* or yeast organisms. This condition, which rarely occurs before puberty, responds readily to treatment but tends to recur. Behrman thinks it is highly transmissible, but Savill and Warren disagree, saying that many persons are immune to attack by the bottle bacillus. If this disease is neglected, a more stubborn form of infection follows in which the sebaceous glands appear irritated and hyperactive. This is known as *pityriasis steatoides,* sometimes less correctly called seborrheic dermatitis, of the simple type. A second organism, the *Micrococcus cutis communis,* or *morococcus,* is associated with the *Pityrosporum* in this oily dandruff. Severer forms of pityriasis may be associated with staphylococcal or streptococcal infections, or with an "eczematized form of seborrheic dermatitis."

All authorities consulted believe that good hygiene plays an important role in the prevention and cure of any pityriasis. When treated early a complete cure can be effected; in many cases persons susceptible to dandruff must maintain a vigilant hygienic program and use antiseptic lotions or salves at regular intervals. Behrman puts more emphasis on the etiologic part played by the endocrines than do Savill and Warren, but all three recognize their relationship to this and other scalp disorders. Some dermatologists believe that the causative organisms are residents of the normal scalp and only cause trouble when conditions are especially favorable to their growth; Savill and Warren question this theory. Behrman says that with visits to barber shops and beauty parlors, where disinfecting methods are almost never lethal to causative organisms, infection is almost inescapable.

Pityriasis is a disease that should be treated by a physician. Massage and thorough brushing several times a day are generally advocated. Shampoos every two or three days may be prescribed.

Savill and Warren make the following observation:

Innumerable are the combinations of drugs and the forms of spirit [alcohol] which have been recommended for pityriases. . . . The majority of these formulae are based on sulphur, tar and mercury, or phenol and salicylic acid, with spirit and water, together with an amount of oil or glycerine which has to be varied for the individual case. Only experience can teach the correct proportion of oil and spirits suitable for the individual scalp.*

They give several formulas, and suggest frequency and method of application. The value of adequate diet, daily massage, brushing, and exposure of the scalp to air and sunlight are stressed. Hats and caps, which exclude light and air, should be worn as seldom as possible, until the condition is controlled; sunlight is beneficial.

Three factors are thought to be important in the development of typical male baldness (alopecia): (1) heredity, (2) age, and (3) male hormones.[107,108] Susceptibility to baldness may be inherited from either parent and, in fact, it may skip one or more generations. Most individuals lose a certain amount of hair with advancing age but those (men) who develop baldness usually begin to lose their hair in their late teens or early twenties, a gradual process extending over a period of years. Men, who are far more susceptible to baldness than women, should follow the established methods of promoting healthy hair, and before using any "tonic" or "cure" for baldness should investigate its claims. Orentreich believes that "the great majority of past and present 'hair restorers,' by and large directed toward 'nourishing,' 'stimulating,' or 'revitalizing' bald areas are totally worthless, as is the concept that vigorous or frequent brushing to stimulate the scalp will do anything except groom the remaining hair." * Other factors involved in hair loss, which may be temporary, include the following: (1) physical injury to the hair, as from excessively tight braids, pony tails, upsweeps, curlers, and teasing the hair; (2) chemicals in cosmetics that cause dermatitis; (3) x-rays and atomic radiation; (4) infection of the scalp by fungi, bacteria, or viruses, and systemic infections that produce a high fever; (5) a variety of drugs and poisons and even vitamin A in high doses; and (6) internal factors including many hormonal disorders.[109] The psychologic importance of hair loss should certainly not be underestimated; fortunately, hairpieces are available and worn by many women and men who have scalp and hair problems. Many wigs are made of human hair or synthetic material that is similar to the color and texture of the wearer's. They are cleaned in the same way as regular hair and scalp. Some people have several wigs so they may be "dressed" by the beautician.

Shampoo preparations are usually liquid because such detergents are more easily rinsed from the hair than pastes or solids. Neutral detergents, such as the sulfonated ethers, are largely replacing liquid soaps. Potassium oleates (liquid soaps) are more expensive than sodium oleates (solid soaps), and where cost is important, soap jellies and solutions can easily be made from flakes of sodium soap. Household synthetic detergents should *not* be used as they tend to leave the scalp dry and the hair unmanageable and some are also harmful to the skin. Use of an acid, such as vinegar or lemon juice, in one of the rinsings helps to remove soap and possibly to improve the texture of hair.

During the past decade or so aerosol sprays have become increasingly popular. They were originally a solution of shellac in alcohol, which is still available, but polyvinylpyrrolidone (PVP) and polyvinyl acetate (PVA) are now the major constituents of hair sprays. Whether hair sprays cause disease in man has been debated in the recent medical literature, according to Michael A. Nevins and associates.[110] They describe two cases of pulmonary granulomatosis—one, a compulsive user of spray deodorants and the other, a hairdresser who had a heavy exposure to hair sprays. Reports have been found of 16 patients with pulmonary conditions thought to be caused by use of hair sprays. Some researchers have been unable to reproduce the disease in animal experiments. Although the F.D.A. (Federal Food and Drug Administration) has taken the position that hair sprays containing PVP-PVA, PVP, DMHF, lanolin, methacrylate, and shellac are nonhazardous, since no major illness can be attributed beyond doubt to hair sprays, this does not mean that such sprays can be used excessively and indiscriminately.[111] Sprays can best be applied by a second person, using a sweeping motion, with the nozzle held about 14 inches from the head. The room should be well ventilated and both the sprayer and the sprayed should avoid inhaling the spray. E. Suskin and A. Boutys,[111a] following experimental studies of three hair sprays on 12 subjects, concluded that hair sprays can cause acute reversible narrowing of small airways; manufacturers are urged to test these "potentially harmful products" before marketing them.

Stiff bristles are recommended for *hairbrushes*. Nylon bristles are stiff, durable, and cheap; hair from the Australian boar makes excellent but costly brushes. Wire brushes are unyielding and tend to scratch the scalp. If tufts of bristles are set far apart, the brush is more readily cleaned. Public health regulations require manufacturers to sterilize all brushes to control transmission of disease, particularly anthrax from infected natural bristles.

Combs are usually made from plastics, hard rubber, or tortoise shell; occasionally from metal and pressed paper. Teeth should be dull so as not to scratch the scalp. Metal combs are likely to be injurious, and their use is discouraged in spite of their being unbreakable and resistant to sterilizing temperatures. Pressed-paper combs are very inexpensive and fairly satisfactory for brief use.

When more than one person uses a comb or brush, sterilization is essential to prevent possible spread of disease. In some hospitals, when patients have failed to provide themselves with toilet articles, the institution supplies them and puts the cost on expense accounts; in others the comb or brush remains the property of the institution, and is cleaned and sterilized after the patient is discharged. This process usually consists of washing in soapsuds containing a small amount of sodium borate (borax) or ammonium hydroxide and soaking for several hours in an odorless disinfectant, such as diphenyl or mercuric oxycyanide.

Care of the Hair in Sickness. Some illnesses demand such complete rest that a certain amount of neglect of the hair is inevitable, but in most cases it is possible to keep it in good condition. Generally, hair and scalp should receive the same treatment in sickness as in health. The hair should be brushed and combed twice a day and washed every few weeks or even weekly. A shampoo can be given to bed patients with almost no exertion on their part, and the consequent improvement in appearance is cheering to a man, woman, or child.

In rare cases a regular shampoo requires too much exertion on the part of the patient; in such cases a "dry shampoo" may not. Dry shampoos are actually liquid dry cleaners but because they have alcohol or carbon tetrachloride instead of water as their solvent, they evaporate rapidly and leave the hair and scalp dry in no time. The shampoo is applied to the scalp and hair with a large piece of cotton or gauze sponge. Hair oil, dissolved in the shampoo, is then removed with towels following the sponging. The scalp and hair should be treated in sections.

Combing and brushing short hair present no special difficulties, but during an illness that confines the patient to bed, care of long, heavy hair requires time and skill. Hair must be kept free from snarls, combed and brushed without hurting or irritating the patient, and should be arranged in a comfortable but becoming fashion. Appearance should always be considered; even when patients seem indifferent to their looks, they affect the spirits of family and friends.

Long hair is ordinarily parted down the middle of the scalp and plaited in two braids. They should not be very tight and should be

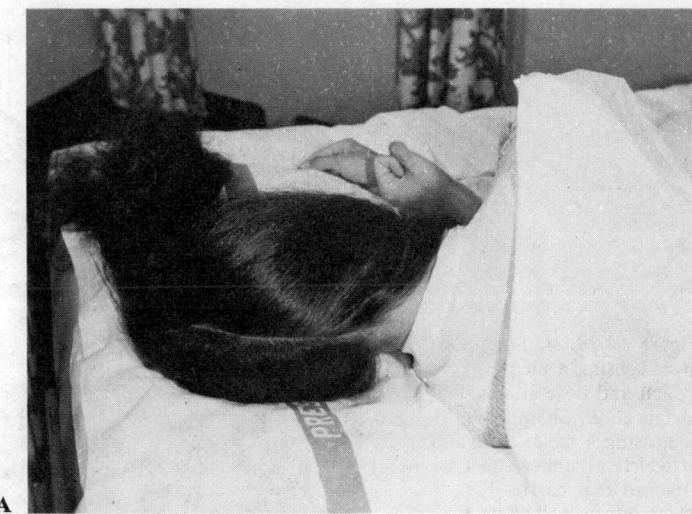

Figure 14-18. *A.* To comb long hair. The head is turned so that the hair can be parted down the back, and access of the brush and comb to the entire scalp made possible. *B.* The nurse has wrapped a strand of hair around her forefinger and is holding it slack between her hand and the scalp so that she can remove tangles without discomfort to the patient. *C.* The plaits are crossed and tied in front of the ears with ribbons. This is a becoming and comfortable way to dress the long hair of the bed patient. (Courtesy of Columbia-Presbyterian Medical Center, New York, N.Y., and Clay-Adams Co., New York, N.Y.)

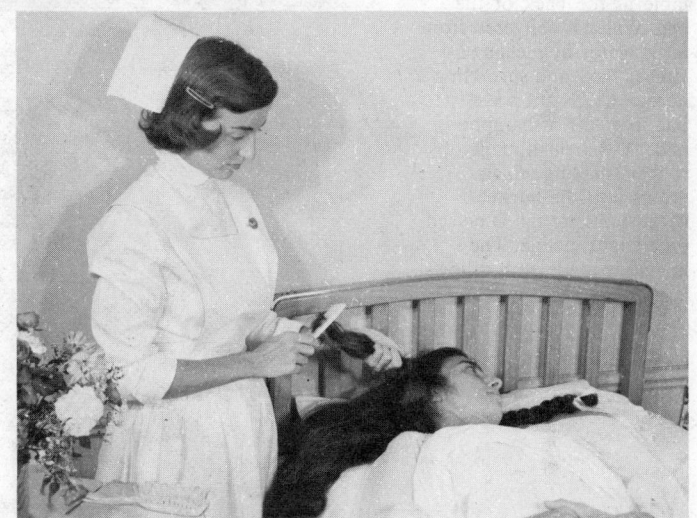

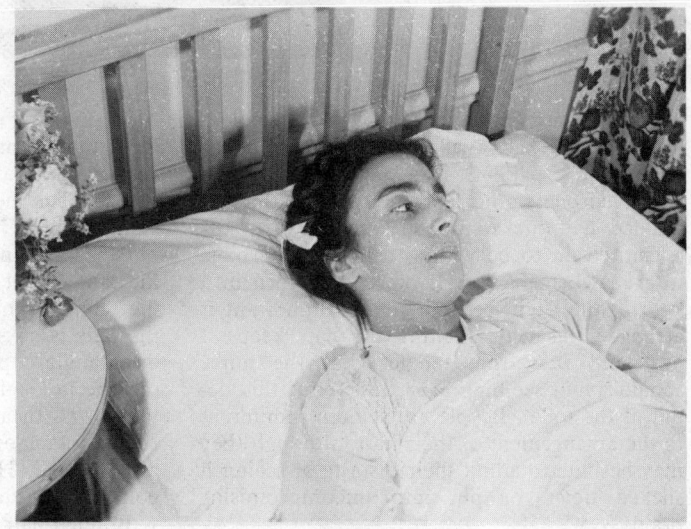

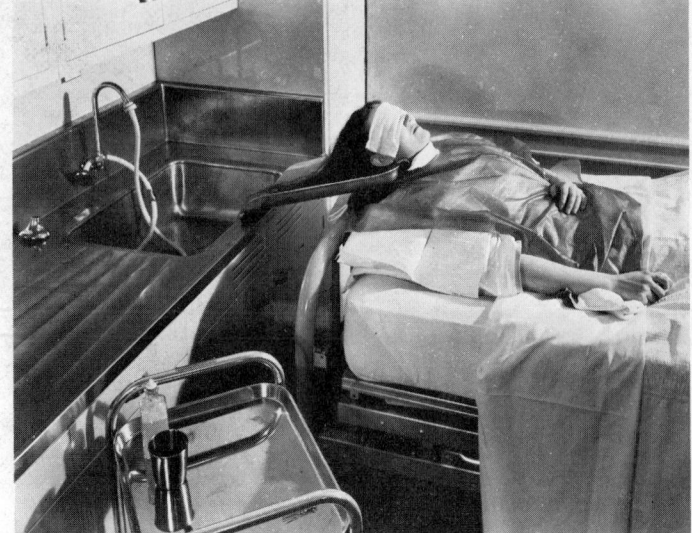

Figure 14-19. *A.* Shampoo in bed, using a metal trough and hose attached to faucet. *B.* Shampoo in bed, using a metal trough to which a rubber sheet is attached that carries the water into a bucket on a table at the back of the bed. Water is delivered from an irrigator by means of a rubber hose and sprinkling nozzle. *C.* Use of a Kelly pad in giving a shampoo in bed. *D.* A trough made of rubber sheeting which drains into the bucket because the trough is placed on a slight incline. The incline is made with pillows.

A

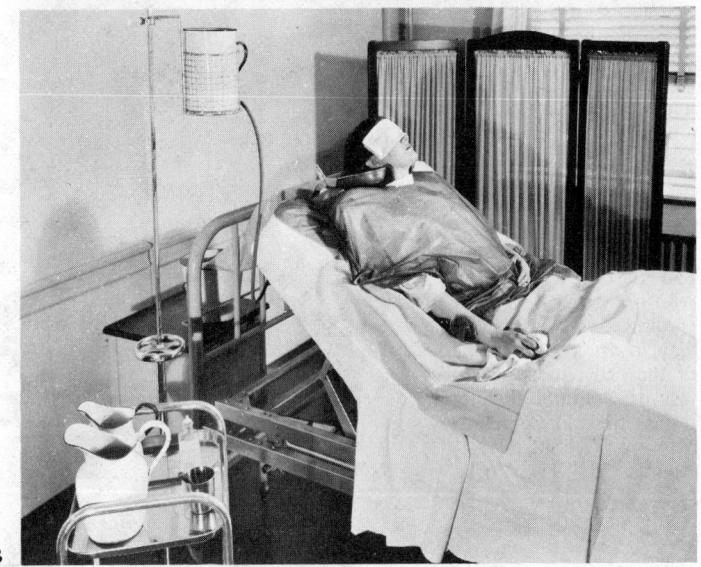

B

started toward the front so that a patient lying on the back will not be conscious of them. Some patients like the braids pinned into a coronet; others prefer to have the unbraided hair tucked up on top; few are sufficiently vain to be willing to lie on hairpins; so even when the hair is ordinarily worn in a knot at the back, bed patients seldom want it arranged this way. Plaiting the hair keeps it neat and free from tangles, but the nurse should avoid seeming arbitrary about this detail of the toilet. People are seldom indifferent to the arrangement of their hair, although they may hesitate to admit their distaste at seeing it slicked down or put into uncompromising braids.

In combing or brushing matted hair tackle it in small strands (see Fig. 14-18*B*). To prevent pulling and further tangling, hold the strand slack between the scalp and the part being combed so that the pull comes on the nurse's hand, not on the hair roots, and comb the tangles out progressively from the ends to the scalp. Comb gently but thoroughly. When the hair is so snarled, that it is impossible to disentangle it painlessly, it may be best to cut out the tangled parts. Applying oil or wetting the hair with alcohol as it is combed helps to remove tangles, but time and patience are also needed. Hair never mats when properly combed each day.

Braided hair should be held at the ends with

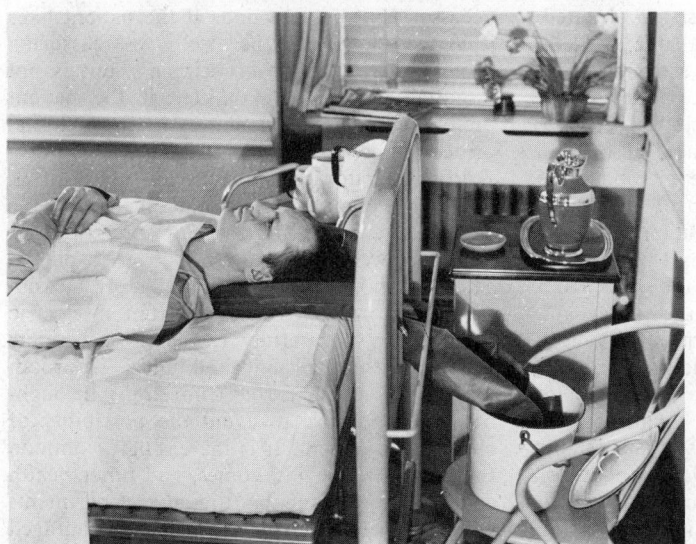

C

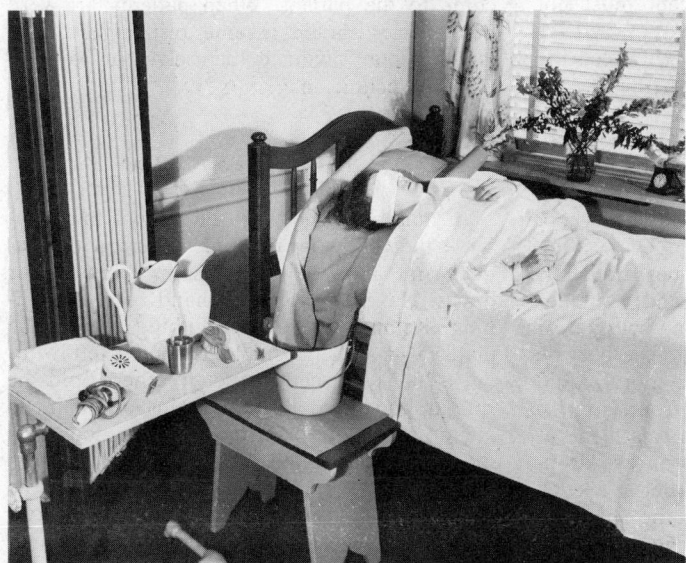

D

ribbon, or if this is not available, with tape or rubber bands. Use of hair combings for this purpose is obviously unpleasant and would not be mentioned but that the practice is sometimes seen.

Washing the Hair of a Patient in Bed. A shampoo may be given with the patient either sitting or recumbent if the proper equipment is available. Figures 14-19A–D illustrate how the hair may be washed in these positions and the use of three kinds of troughs for carrying off the cleaning agents.

The metal trough is the type seen in hairdressing parlors. It has a metal rod to hold it in position. In Figure 14-19A the rod is inserted between the end of the mattress and the footboard; in Figure 14-19B the rod is placed between the mattress and the patient's pillow. The pressure of the body against the rod holds it in place.

In Figure 14-19A the shampoo is being given in a treatment room. The patient has been placed so that the head is at the foot of the bed and the trough drains into a sink. The hose is attached to the water supply controlled by a pedal. If there is running water in the patient's unit, the shampoo may be given there, using this method. Of the two positions the recumbent is probably more comfortable, but there are some patients, for example, those suffering from certain types of heart disease or asthma, whose breathing is embarrassed except when the head and chest are elevated.

If a metal trough is not available, a Kelly pad may be used, or better still a trough made by rolling bath towels in the two edges of a rubber sheet or piece of oilcloth (see Fig. 14-19C and D). The rubber sheet or oilcloth is more easily cleaned, and the method more adaptable to home nursing, since Kelly pads are not available except in institutions.

No matter what the trough is made of, it must be so arranged as to carry the water from the head. If this is done and the pillow and shoulders covered with a waterproof material, the patient's clothing and bedding need not even be dampened. To make the rubber trough drain properly, a very gradual incline should be built at the head of the bed so that it slants toward one side. It is well to place a board or ordinary tray under the top pillow on which the head rests in order to keep it from sinking into the pillows. While the trough should slope toward the edge, the patient must not have the sensation of falling out of bed. A small pillow under the shoulders will keep the body more or less straight while the head is on an incline.

An ample supply of water must be provided; otherwise the soap will not be entirely rinsed away. It is convenient to have the water flow from a nozzle, attached to a faucet where there is running water or to a large irrigating can. If pitchers are used, large ones should be provided for the general supply and a smaller one from which to pour. The soap solution or its substitute should be brought to the bedside in a convenient container. Any pure liquid soap may be used in strengths from 2 to 10 per cent. Liquids prescribed for treatment of the scalp should be applied with an eye dropper or a small syringe. All articles needed should be at the bedside before the shampoo is started so that it will consume no more time than necessary. A movable table or cart facilitates the nurse's work.

To get the hair clean, it is necessary to produce a good lather and rinse it off two or three times. If the oil of the hair is not thoroughly emulsified, it tends to hold the soap in the hair and makes its removal difficult. An unsatisfactory shampoo is in most cases the result of using too little soap. Massaging the scalp thoroughly with the balls of the fingers adds to the comfort and effectiveness of the shampoo.

If the juice of a lemon or an ounce of vinegar is used as a rinse, it should be applied in about 1000 ml (1 qt) of water before the last clear rinsing. The water used throughout should be comfortably warm. Rinsing with cool water at the end of the procedure is not necessary but may be done if the patient likes it. A wet cloth over the eyes gives reassuring protection from soap or drippings but is not essential and may be omitted if the patient prefers. Nonabsorbent cotton in the external orifice of the ear protects it from water, but a skillful operator can prevent the need for it.

At the completion of the shampoo, the trough is removed and the hair spread out on a bath towel over a rubber-covered pillow. The hair should be dried immediately by rubbing with towels, by warm air from an electric drier, or by a carefully regulated Thermolite (a lamp with a high-powered bulb). The room should be warm and free from drafts throughout the procedure to avoid the possibility of chilling the patient. It is increasingly common for hospitals, nursing homes, and other health agencies to provide hairdressing departments with expert operators. Patients are encouraged to use them or employ the personnel who will come to the patient. When patients are very sick, nurses should assume responsibility for the shampoo, giving it themselves or working with the technician.

8. MAKING THE PATIENT'S BED

In making a bed with the patient in it, observe the following principles: Screen the patient and allow no unnecessary exposure or drafts. Have everything at hand before beginning. Remove the upper clothing except one blanket—a patient should never be left without a blanket except in hot weather. Fold the spread, and place all the clothing on chairs to air; do not allow them to touch the floor. Remove the pillows also unless this is uncomfortable for the patient. One pillow may be left. Their removal provides a change of position, usually restful to the patient; it allows the pillows to cool and makes it easier for the patient to turn and the nurse to work. Loosen the lower bed linen. Shake out all crumbs from the patient's gown or change it if damp or soiled. Remove the rubber sheet and muslin drawsheet and allow them to air. Brush all crumbs from the lower sheet or change if necessary. Move the patient from one side of the bed to the other as occasion demands and his or her condition permits. Straighten the mattress and tighten or replace the under-sheet. Replace the rubber sheet and muslin drawsheet or substitute a clean one. See that they are tight and smooth and in the proper position. Shake, turn, and replace pillows and upper bedclothes; be sure the latter are loose over the feet. This can be accomplished by having the patient keep the knees flexed while the sheet and blankets are tucked at the foot or by making a horizontal or vertical pleat over the toes (see Fig. 13-6D, Chapter 13). Remove all articles used in the toilet, and see that the bed, table, and other furnishings of the unit are in order and that the whole has a finished appearance.

In Chapter 3, the opinion was expressed that facilities for long-term ambulatory patients should provide beds that look more like a couch. Patients' rooms should look like sitting rooms rather than bedrooms and should, by their appearance, stimulate normal daily activities.

9. PROVIDING THE PATIENT WITH SUITABLE CLOTHING

Types of Clothing. Institutions must supply clothing for patients when articles brought by them are inadequate in supply, uncomfortable or inconvenient in cut, torn, soiled, or otherwise unsuitable for use in the hospital. Many patients are unable to provide themselves with private laundry service, and the administrative difficulty of getting clothing returned from the hospital laundry to patient-owners makes it impossible for the institution to provide this service for everyone. In some hospitals private patients wear their own clothing, and a laundry service is provided; or the family or friends see that fresh clothing is available as required.

In most hospitals the newly admitted patient is automatically undressed and put to bed in a nightgown. While this is often convenient for the examining physician, the practice is open to criticism unless the reason is explained and unless persons are encouraged to get up and dress if there is no longer any necessity for them to stay in bed. The value of maintaining as normal a regimen as possible during sickness and the danger of sensory deprivation of all sorts is generally accepted, as is the danger of continuous bed rest. For its physiologic effect normal daytime activity should be encouraged; for its emotional value normal clothing and good grooming should be stimulated. Recovery is most rapidly promoted in hospitals that provide patients with an opportunity to lead as vigorous and regular a life as their condition permits.

The clothing needed by the patient depends upon age, condition, the nature of the treatment, and the climate. The choice of clothing is particularly affected by the patient's status, whether bedfast or ambulatory. General and specialized hospitals may supply nightgowns, pajamas, dressing gowns, shoulder wraps, leggings, caps, underclothes, dresses, coats, trousers, slippers, shoes, and even outdoor wraps. The economic resources of institutions vary; therefore the quantity and quality of the clothing supplied to patients must also vary.

Clothes have a more marked relationship to mental and physical health than most persons realize. Marston Bates [112] discusses the disastrous effects of forcing on a people, in the name of morals, customs of dress unsuited to their climate and mores. There are certain clothing needs, typical of each culture, that a health agency should attempt to supply, if the patient, or client, lacks them. In this country each hospital bed patient should have an adequate supply of clean, comfortable sleeping garments, and a shoulder wrap of some kind. He or she should be provided with a dressing gown or wrapper, socks or stockings, and slippers. Ambulatory patients who have their meals in dining rooms and mix with other patients should have underclothes and proper outer garments and shoes. Those who go outdoors need wraps suited to the weather. Bed patients who are given fresh-air treatment in cold climates must have special outing-flannel gowns or pajamas, woolen jackets, mittens, sleeping socks, and caps. For pelvic examinations and operative procedures, patients are dressed in special garments, and in some cases leggings are used.

While institutional clothing can perhaps never have the charm of that bought especially for the individual, there is a noticeable trend toward the choice of becoming and cheerful garments. Colorfast dyes make it possible to use colors in all types of garments. State hospitals that formerly provided uniforms for ambulatory patients are now providing dresses of many colors, patterns, and styles. The choice of a dress, a gown, or a jacket provides diversion for all persons, young and old. Interest in the appearance is almost universal in healthy normal individuals. Individual dress provided by patients and their families is increasingly encouraged.

Nurses in homes, convalescent homes, and hospitals often have opportunities to select clothing for the sick or to make recommendations for its selection. The following are some suggestions in relation to specific articles.

Nightgowns should be loose in cut, allowing the patient to move without restriction. A full-length opening simplifies nursing care. A back opening facilitates the use of the bedpan; a front opening is convenient for pelvic dressings, examinations, and, in the care of obstetrical patients, for nursing infants. Figure 14-20 shows a gown with a wide lap, tucks at

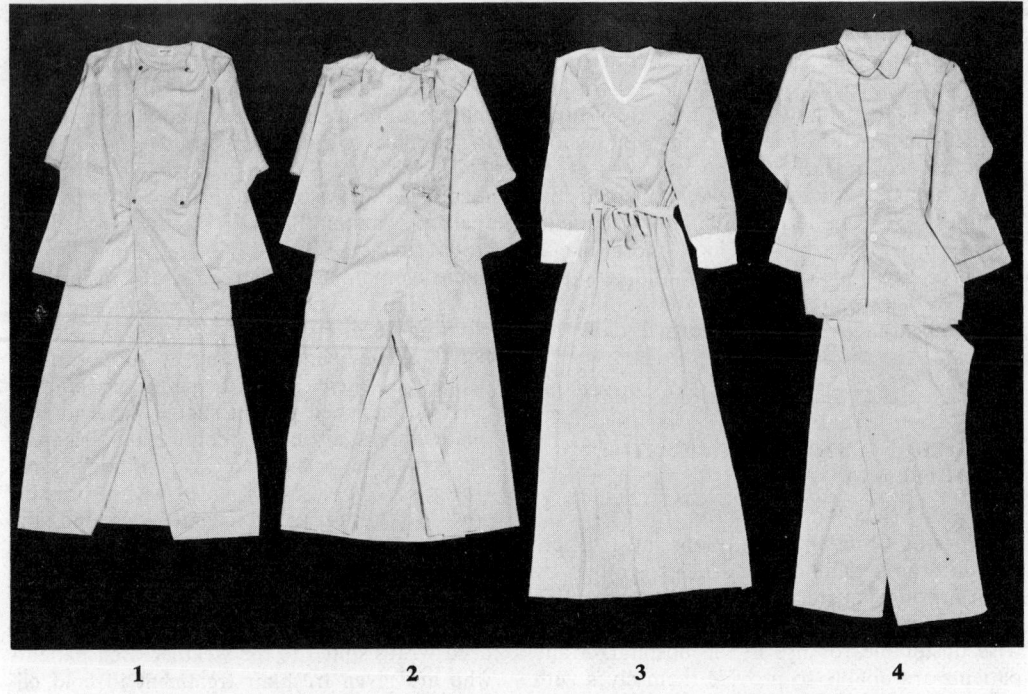

1   2   3   4

Figure 14-20. Gowns and pajamas: (*1*) a soft, gingham gown with lapping front suitable for a man or woman; (*2*) the same gown fastened with tapes instead of snaps and made so that it can be worn open in the front or back; (*3*) a jersey gown that is soft, absorbent, and easily laundered; and (*4*) pajamas, preferred by most men and a few women, and desirable for all patients who are sleeping on porches.

the shoulders, and a special neck line that makes the gown equally comfortable with the opening in the back or in the front.

Gowns should be made of a soft, absorbent, durable material. It is economically desirable that the material be one that does not require ironing. In Figure 14-20 a jersey or balbriggan gown is shown. Seersucker also is a satisfactory material for gowns if a good soft quality is selected. Knitted fabrics and Canton flannel are most comfortable when the patient perspires a great deal. A material that does not show the figure underneath is convenient because it makes it possible in hot weather to appear modestly dressed without a second garment.

It has been traditional to make hospital gowns short, or knee length, for the convenience of the nurse, or the surgeon, in caring for the patient. Since many persons wear sleeping garments to the ankles, they are more likely to prefer this length when they are in a hospital. Long gowns are also preferred by some patients who must get in and out of bed and who dislike the exposure likely with short gowns. Certain operative procedures, dressings, and examinations may call for knee-length garments, but there seems to be *no good reason for the general use of short hospital gowns* unless the person prefers them. If the same gown is worn in the winter and summer, it is probably desirable to have it made with long, loose sleeves that can be rolled above the elbow in hot weather. The sleeve should be loose enough to allow for differences in the size of arms and to permit venipunctures and other procedures requiring exposure of the arm.

White sleeping clothes are generally acceptable, but many individuals enjoy wearing colors. Hospital gowns might well be available in white, blue, and pink. This is not uncommon in children's departments at the present time.

Pajamas should be available for men patients who prefer them and who are not too sick to be exhausted by the effort required to put them on and take them off. Women patients on sleeping porches may also be more comfortable in pajamas.

Dressing gowns or wrappers should be available in different weights for hot and cold weather (see Fig. 14-21). Since cotton is less likely than wool, rayon, or other synthetic material to change its texture in laundering, it

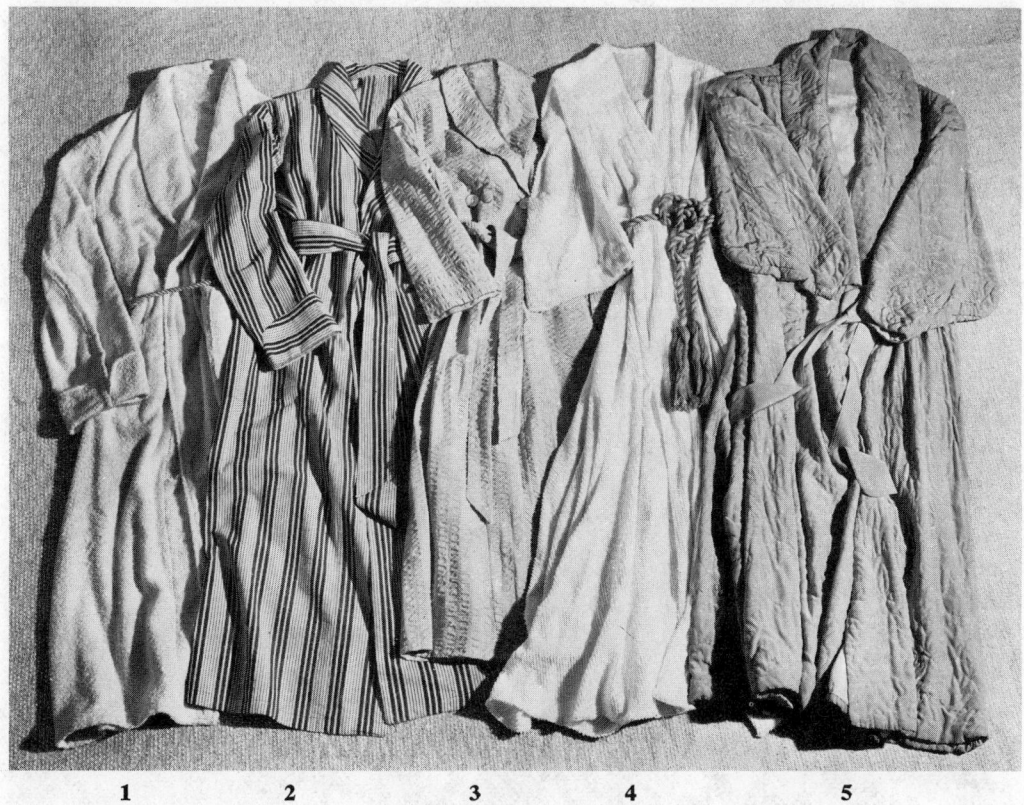

1   2   3   4   5

Figure 14-21. Dressing gowns or wrappers: (*1*) a man's robe made of toweling; (*2*)
a man's robe made of seersucker; (*3*) a woman's seersucker robe; and (*4*)
a woman's robe made of toweling. All of these garments are inexpensive and
launder satisfactorily. (*5*) A silk-and-wool quilted robe that is very warm and light.

is the preferred material. Terry cloth (bath toweling) is a satisfactory fabric for winter dressing gowns since it holds air in its meshes and is therefore warm; it does not require ironing, and has a pleasant, soft texture. In cold climates heavy outing flannel also is used for dressing gowns. Quilted robes are very warm, but are practical only for private use, since they should be dry-cleaned rather than washed. For summer weather, dressing gowns made of seersucker are comfortable, and, as they do not require ironing, are especially practical.

Like sleeping garments, institutional dressing gowns, which must fit many shapes, should be loose in cut. They should have an ample lap in front and should come in several sizes. A variety of colors adds to the patients' pleasure in wearing them.

Shoulder wraps have been called *nightingales,* after Florence Nightingale, who advocated them. It seems obvious that a person who is temporarily living in bed needs more protection for the arms while he or she is eating or reading than is afforded by the sleeves of gowns or pajamas. Many hospitals provide strips of outing flannel or small blankets to put over the shoulders. Many patients provide themselves with bed jackets, which need not be discussed here except to say that they should be soft, loosely cut, and easily washed or cleaned.

Caps must be adjustable, or made so that they will fit heads of varying sizes. They are used following brain surgery, or while treating scalp diseases or injuries. They must be designed so that they do not cut or bind at the edge and so that they can be brought well down over the head and held in position. Stockinet is a soft elastic fabric woven in tubes of different sizes. Caps made of this material are comfortable, adjustable, inexpensive, and if made with a chin strap or a draw string at the edge, are easily kept in place. A cap of this material is shown in Figure 14-22. Unless the patient is desperately ill, his or her morale will be raised by camouflaging caps used for therapeutic purposes. For women artificial bangs

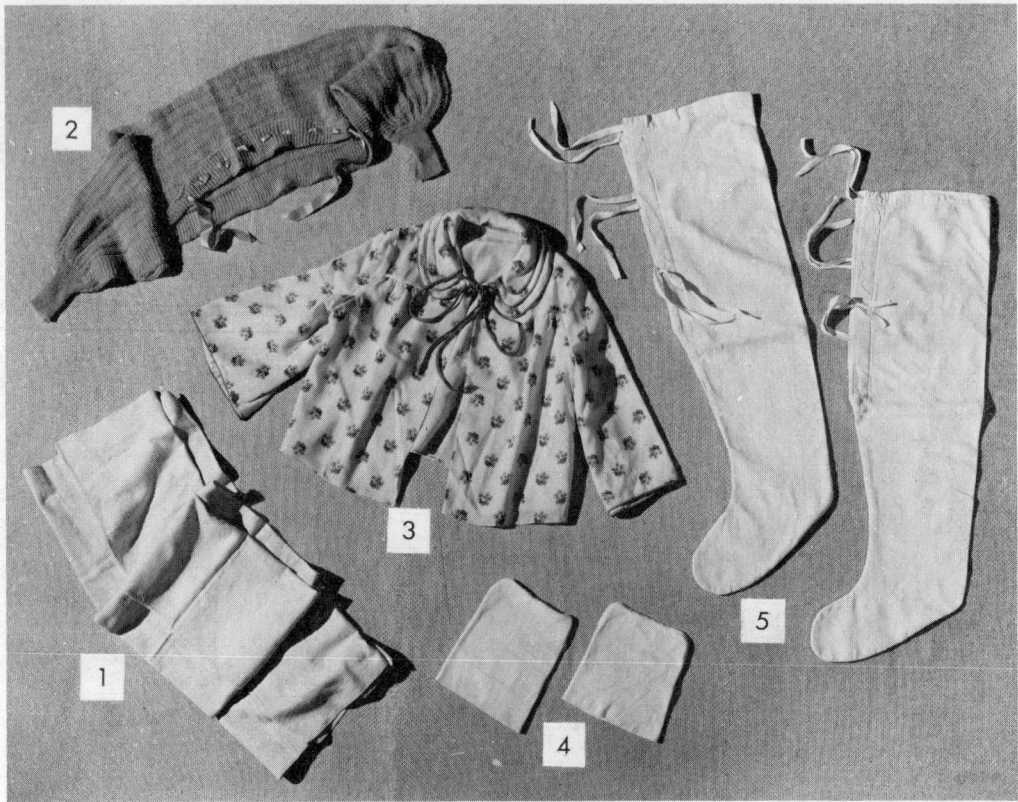

Figure 14-22. Jackets, leggings, and caps: (*1*) a strip of flannelet serves the same purpose as the jackets (*2* and *3*), although they are more attractive; (*4*) knitted caps in two sizes; and (*5*) flannelet leggings often used to protect patients during operations.

may be attached to silk kerchiefs or other suitable headgear. For men berets and skull caps of velvet, silk, or wool are appropriate. While in certain cultures and in different eras caps were worn more frequently than they are today in the United States, many older people (especially women) wear some type of head covering because they say their heads get cold when sleeping. The writers know a number of older and younger women who regularly use a towel or cotton scarf to cover the head at night.

Slippers should provide support and protection if worn by ambulatory patients. The quilted silk slipper shown in Figure 14-23 is suitable for the patient who gets up in a chair but does not walk about very much. Leather slippers are more practical for ambulatory patients. Silk and leather slippers are so expensive that few institutions can provide them, and in many cases the patient is unable to purchase slippers. The canvas slipper lined with Canton flannel illustrated in Figure 14-23

is an appropriate type for the hospital to provide. It costs very little, launders well, and is relatively durable. The crepe-paper slipper, shown next to the canvas slipper, is useful in examining rooms and departments where it is desirable to give protection for a short time only; these slippers are worn by only one person and are discarded after use. A canvas shoe with a composition sole is shown in Chapter 34. It is supplied by some institutions to patients wearing a "walking cast" or having a bulky foot dressing.

In the admission of a patient one of the nurse's duties is to see that he or she is comfortably clothed, adequately protected from chilling, and conveniently dressed for the physician's examination. Before clothing some patients, however, a cleansing bath and special care of the nails may be indicated. In order to determine the need for this, certain tactful questions may be asked and certain observations can always be made as the nurse helps the patient to undress.

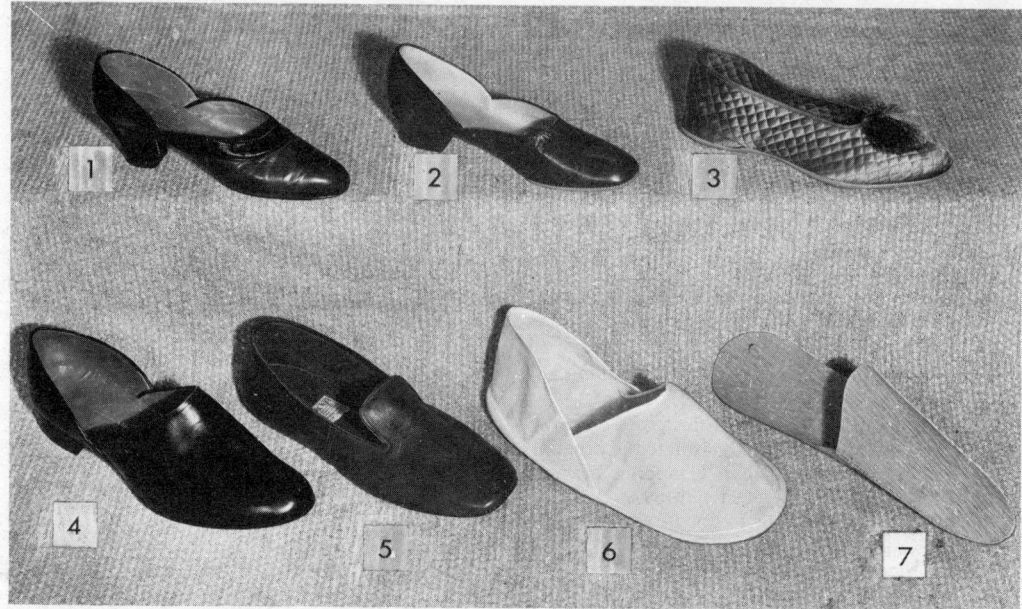

Figure 14-23. Slippers suited to the needs of the sick: (*1, 2, 4,* and *5*) for ambulatory patients; (*3*) comfortable for a patient sitting in a chair; (*6*) a washable canvas slipper which the hospital may provide; and (*7*) a paper slipper, which can be worn only once and is suitable for use in examination rooms.

REFERENCES

1. Sperber, Perry A.: *The Treatment of the Aging Skin and Dermal Defects.* Charles C Thomas, Publisher, Springfield, Ill., 1965, p. 3.
2. Thorne, Napier: "Cosmetics and the Dermatologist: Soaps," *Br. J. Clin. Pract.,* **19:** 111, (Feb.) 1965.
2a. Fox, Marian K., et al.: "How Good Are Handwashing Practices," *Am. J. Nurs.,* **74:** 1676, (Sept.) 1974.
2b. Dineen, P., and Drusine, L.: "Epidemics of Post-operative Wound Infections Associated with Hair Carriers," *Lancet,* **2:**1157, (Nov. 24) 1973.
3. Nightingale, Florence: *Notes on Nursing: What It Is and What It Is Not.* (Facsimile of 1859 ed.) J. B. Lippincott Co., Philadelphia, 1946, p. 6.
3a. Barnes, Elizabeth: *Psychosocial Nursing.* Tavistock Publications, London, 1968.
3b. Roberts, Sharon L.: "Skin Assessment for Color and Temperature," *Am. J. Nurs.,* **75:** 610, (Apr.) 1975.
4. Kenyon, F. E.: "Psychosomatic Aspects of Acne," *Br. J. Dermatol.,* **78:**344, (June) 1966.
5. Blohm, Sven Gösta, and Lodin, Anders: "Eczema of the Hands in Women—'Housewives' Eczema," *Acta. Derm. Venereol.,* **48:**7, (Jan.) 1968.
5a. Rice, Alice K.: "Common Skin Infection

in School Children," *Am. J. Nurs.,* **73:**1905, (Nov.) 1973.
5b. North, Carolyn, and Weinstein, Gerald D.: "Treatment of Psoriasis," *Am. J. Nurs.,* **76:**410 (Mar.) 1976.
6. Savitt, Leonard E., and Obermayer, Maximilian E.: "Treatment of Acne Vulgaris and Senile Keratoses with Vitamin A: Results of a Clinical Experiment," *J. Invest. Dermatol.,* **14:**283, (Feb.) 1950.
7. Kline, Paul R.: "Role of Parenteral Multivitamin Therapy in Treatment of Acne," *Arch. Dermatol.,* **62:**661, (Nov.) 1950.
8. Shapiro, Irving: "Estrogens and Local Application in the Treatment of Acne Vulgaris," *Arch. Dermatol.,* **63:**224, (Feb.) 1951.
9. Bobroff, Arthur: *Acne.* Charles C Thomas, Publisher, Springfield, Ill., 1965.
10. Sauer, Gordon C.: *Teen Skin.* Charles C Thomas, Publisher, Springfield, Ill., 1965.
11. Ruch, Donald M.: "Acne Vulgaris, Review of One Hundred Cases," *Med. Times,* **93:** 1287, (Nov.) 1965.
12. Moynahan, E. J.: "Some Recent Advances in the Treatment of Skin Diseases," *Med. Press,* **225:**187, (Feb.) 1951.
13. Sauer, Gordon C.: *op. cit.*
14. Bobroff, Arthur: *op. cit.,* p. vii.
14a. Rogachefsky, Hymen: "Care of the Aging Skin," *NY State J. Med.,* **64:**2988, (Dec. 15) 1964.
15. Binazzi, Maurizio, and Calandra, Paolo: "Identification of an Error in the Trypto-

phan Niacin → Pathway in Carriers of Some Dermatoses Conditioned or Aggravated by Sunlight," *Arch. Klin. Exp. Dermatol.*, **239**:368, (Jan.) 1971.

16. Stoughton, R. B.: "Physiological Changes from Maturity Through Senescence," *J.A.M.A.*, **179**:636, (Feb. 24) 1962.

17. Knox, J. M., et al.: "Etiological Factors and Premature Aging," *J.A.M.A.*, **179**:630, (Feb. 24) 1962.

18. Rogachefsky, Hymen: *op. cit.*

19. Owen, J. R.: "Skin Diseases of the Aged," *Med. Press*, **225**:178, (Feb.) 1951.

20. Sperber, Perry A.: *op. cit.*, p. 94.

21. Cormia, Frank E.: "The Basis of Itching," *J. Pediatr.*, **66**:207, (Jan.) 1965.

21a. Middleton, J. D.: "The Effect of Temperature on Extensibility of Isolated Corneum and Its Relation to Skin Chapping," *Br. J. Dermatol.*, **81**:717, (Oct.) 1969.

22. Birmingham, Donald J.: "Skin Hygiene and Dermatitis in Industry," *Arch. Environ. Health*, **10**:653, (Apr.) 1965.

22a. Harmon, Vera M., and Steele, Shirley M.: *Nursing Care of the Skin; A Developmental Approach*. Appleton-Century-Crofts, New York, 1975.

23. Meneghini, C. L.: "Evolution of Etiological Factors and Clinical Patterns in Occupation Noneczematous Dermatoses," in Flarer, F., et. al. (eds.): *XIV International Congress of Dermatology*. Excerpta Medica Foundation, Amsterdam, 1972, p. 16.

24. Steigleder, Gerd K., and Raab, Wolfgang P.: "Skin Protection Afforded by Ointments," *J. Invest. Dermatol.*, **38**:129, (Mar.) 1962.

25. Buckels, Larry J., et al.: "Prophylaxis of Warm-Water-Immersion Foot," *J.A.M.A.*, **200**:681, (May 22) 1967.

26. Selwyn, S., et al.: "Factors in the Bacterial Colonization and Infection of the Human Skin," *Indian J. Med. Res.*, **55**:652, (June) 1967.

27. Reisch, Milton, and Marciano, Mark R.: "A Bacteriostatic Emollient: Its Use as a Cleanser and Bath Additive," *Indust. Med. Surg.*, **32**:430, (Oct.) 1963.

28. May, Richard: "The Medical Hazards of Bathing," *Practitioner*, **164**:545, (June) 1950.

29. Grollman, Sigmund: *The Human Body, Its Structure and Physiology*, 3rd ed. Macmillan Publishing Co., Inc., New York, 1974, p. 173.

30. Hurley, Harry J., and Shelley, Walter B.: *The Human Apocrine Sweat Gland in Health and Disease*. Charles C Thomas, Publisher, Springfield, Ill., 1960, p. 62.

31. Shelley, Walter B., and Hurley, Harry J.: "The Allergic Origin of Zirconium Deodorant Granulomas," *Br. J. Dermatol.*, **70**:75, (Mar.) 1958.

32. Thorne, Napier: "Cosmetics and the Dermatologist: Deodorants and Antiperspirants," *Br. J. Clin. Pract.*, **17**:747, (Dec.) 1963.

33. Seldin, Joseph J.: "Chlorophyll: Fact or Fraud," *The Nation*, **175**:11, (July) 1952.

34. Combes, Frank C.: "Chlorophyll in Topical Therapy," *NY State J. Med.*, **52**:1025, (Apr.) 1952.

35. Westcott, F. H.: "Oral Chlorophyll Fractions for Body and Health Deodorization," *NY State J. Med.*, **50**:698, (Mar.) 1950.

36. Brocklehurst, John C.: "An Assessment of Chlorophyll as a Deodorant," *Br. Med. J.*, **1**:541, (Mar. 7) 1953.

37. Hurley, Harry J., and Shelley, Walter B.: *op. cit.*, p. 96.

38. Tenenbaum, Saul, and Allen, Emma G.: "The Safety and Efficacy of Neomycin-Containing Deodorants," *Curr. Ther. Res.*, **6**:646, (Oct.) 1964.

39. Hudson, A. L.: "The H-ion Concentration of Normal and Diseased Skin," *Can. Med. Assoc. J.*, **64**:19, (June) 1951.

40. Bettley, F. Ray: "Some Effects of Soap on the Skin," *Br. Med. J.*, **1**:1675, (June 4) 1960.

41. Thorne, Napier: "Cosmetics and the Dermatologist: Soaps," *Br. J. Clin. Pract.*, **19**:111, (Feb.) 1965.

42. Stoughton, Richard B.: "The Influence of Soap on Eczematous Dermatitis," *Arch. Dermatol.*, **92**:281, (Sept.) 1965.

43. Pegum, J. S.: "Clinical Trial of a 'Soapless Soap' in Skin Diseases," *Practitioner*, **195**:78, (July) 1965.

44. Reisch, Milton, and Marciano, Mark R.: *op. cit.*

45. Ayliffe, G. A. J., et al.: "The Disinfection of Bath Water with Hexachlorophene," *Lancet*, **2**:456, (Sept. 26) 1959.

46. Simpson, K., and Tozer, Rosemary C.: "Prevention of Staphylococcal Sepsis in a Maternity Hospital by Means of Hexachlorophane," *Br. Med. J.*, **1**:315, (Jan. 30) 1960.

47. MacKenzie, Albert R.: "Effectiveness of Antibacterial Soaps in a Healthy Population," *J.A.M.A.*, **211**:973, (Feb. 9) 1970.

47a. Sanford, Jay P.: "Disinfectants That Don't," *Ann. Intern. Med.*, **72**:282, (Feb.) 1970.

48. "The Bane of Body Odor" (editorial), *J.A.M.A.*, **197**:50, (July 4) 1966.

48a. Wade, Nicholas: "Hexachlorophene: FDA Temporizes on Brain-Damaging Chemical," *Science*, **174**:805, (Nov. 19) 1971.

48b. "Hexachlorophene Drama: Where Are Those Drug Regulations?" *Sci. News*, **102**:212, (Sept. 30) 1972.

49. Brauer, Earle W.: "Cosmetic Management of Selected Skin Changes of the Legs," *South. Med. J.*, **63**:1190, (Oct.) 1970.

50. Thorne, Napier: "Shaving Soaps and Creams," *Br. J. Clin. Pract.*, **19**:423, (July) 1965.

51. Hollander, Lester, and Casselman, E. T.: "Factors Involved in Good Shaving," *J.A.M.A.*, **109**:95, (July) 1937.

51a. Bleich, A. R.: "Prophylaxis of Penile Carcinoma," *J.A.M.A.*, **143**:1054, (July 22) 1950.

51b. Obermeyer, W. B.: "Crotch Care," *Am. J. Nurs.*, **57**:618, (May) 1957.

51c. Gibbs, Gertrude E.: "Perineal Care of the Incapacitated Patient," *Am. J. Nurs.*, **69**:124, (Jan.) 1969.

52. Robson, J. R. K., and El-Tahaw, H. D.: "Hardness of Human Nail as An Index of Nutritional Status: A Preliminary Communication," *Br. J. Nutr.*, **26**:233, (Sept.) 1971.

53. Stewart, W. K., and Raffle, E. J.: "Brown Nail-bed Arcs and Chronic Renal Disease," *Br. Med. J.*, **1**:784, (Mar. 25) 1972.

54. Bentley-Phillips, B.: "Dystrophies Due to Nail Cosmetics," *S. Afr. Med. J.*, **44**:1293, (Nov. 14) 1970.

55. Hellman, Louis M., and Pritchard, Jack A.: *Williams Obstetrics*, 14th ed. Appleton-Century-Crofts, New York, 1971, p. 487.

56. Fitzpatrick, Elise, et al.: *Maternity Nursing*, 12th ed. J. B. Lippincott Co., Philadelphia, 1971, pp. 367, 415.

57. Richardson, Henry B.: *Patients Have Families*. Commonwealth Fund, New York, 1945, p. 30.

58. Bernier, Joseph L., and Muhler, Joseph C. (eds.): *Improving Dental Practice Through Preventive Measures*, 3rd ed. C. V. Mosby Co., St. Louis, 1975.

59. Peterson, Shailer: *Clinical Dental Hygiene*, 4th ed. C. V. Mosby Co., St. Louis, 1972.

60. Bernier, Joseph L., and Muhler, Joseph C. (eds.): *op. cit.*, p. 170.

61. Toverad, Gullorm: "Diseases in Caries Reported by England, Norway, and Italy," *J. Am. Dent. Assoc.*, **39**:127, (Aug.) 1949.

62. Horsenell, A. M.: "Nutrition and Dental Disease," *Aust. Dent. J.*, **7**:48, (Feb.) 1962.

63. Gustaffsson, B. E., and Lank, L. S.: "The Effect of Different Levels of Carbohydrate Intake on Caries in 436 Individuals Observed Over Five Years," *Acta Odontol. Scand.*, **11**:232, 1953.

64. Fadich, L. S.: "The Reduction of the Incidence of Dental Caries," *J. Am. Dent. Assoc.*, **40**:133, (Feb.) 1956.

65. Bowen, William H.: "Effects of Food on Oral Bacterial Populations in Man and Animals," *J. Dent. Res.*, **49**:1276, (Nov.–Dec.) 1970.

66. Jay, Philip: "Dental Caries: Prevention and Immunology," in Hunting, Russel W. (ed.): *Oral Hygiene*, 3rd ed. Lea & Febiger, Philadelphia, 1957.

67. *Ibid.*, p. 168.

68. Stookey, George K.: "Fluoride Therapy," in Bernier, Joseph L., and Muhler, Joseph C. (eds.): *Improving Dental Practice Through Preventive Measures*, 2nd ed. C. V. Mosby Co., St. Louis, 1970, p. 95.

69. Shannon, I. L.: "Water Free Solutions of Stannous Fluoride and Their Incorporation into a Gel for Topical Application," *Caries Res.*, **3**:339, (Oct.–Dec.) 1969.

70. ———: "Preventive Dental Services in Veterans Administration Hospitals," *J. Public Health Dent.*, **30**:156, (Oct.) 1970.

71. ———: "A Pumice Zirconium Silicate Prophylaxis Paste Containing 2% Stannous Fluoride in Water Free Solution," *J. Pharmacol. Ther. Dent.*, **1**:24, (Jan.) 1970.

72. Boyd, William: *A Textbook of Pathology*, 8th ed. Lea & Febiger, Philadelphia, 1970, p. 1436.

73. Glickman, Irving: *Clinical Periodontology*, 4th ed. W. B. Saunders Co., Philadelphia, 1972.

74. Kaplan, Herman: "The Oral Cavity in Geriatrics," *Geriatrics*, **26**:96, (Dec.) 1971.

75. Parfitt, Gilbert J., and Hand, Cletis D.: "Reduced Plasma Ascorbic Acid Levels and Gingival Health," *J. Periodontol.*, **34**:347, (July) 1963.

76. Glickman, Irving: "Nutrition in the Prevention and Treatment of Gingival and Periodontal Disease," *J. Dent. Med.*, **19**:179, (Oct.) 1964.

77. Bolton, William: "That's a Good Question," *Today's Health*, **30**:2, (May) 1952.

78. Wilkins, Esther M.: *Clinical Practice of the Dental Hygienist*, 3rd ed. Lea & Febiger, Philadelphia, 1971, p. 282.

78a. Cross, W. G., et al.: "A Comparative Study of Tooth Cleansing Using Conventional and Electrically Operated Toothbrushes," *Br. Dent. J.*, **113**:19, (July 3) 1962.

78b. Parfitt, Gilbert J.: "Cleansing the Subgingival Space," *J. Periodontol.*, **34**:133, (Mar.) 1963.

79. Ritsert, E. F., et al.: "Adolescents Brush Better with An Electric Toothbrush," *J. Dent. Child.*, **34**:354, (Sept.) 1967.

80. Manhold, J. H., Jr.: "Gingival Tissue Health with Hand and Power Brushing: A Retrospective with Corroborative Studies," *J. Periodontol.*, **38**:23, (Jan.–Feb.) 1967.

81. Lobene, R. R.: "Evaluation of Altered Gingival Health from Permissive Powered Toothbrushing," *J. Am. Dent. Assoc.*, **69**:585, (Nov.) 1964.

82. Fraleigh, C. M.: "Tissue Changes with Manual and Electric Brushes," *J. Am. Dent. Assoc.*, **70**:380, (Feb.) 1965.

83. Glickman, Irving, et al.: "The Effect of Powered Toothbrushing and Interdental Stimulation Upon Microscopic Inflammation and Surface Keratinization of the Interdental Gingiva," *J. Periodontol.*, **36**:18, (May–Apr.) 1965.

84. Elliott, J. Roy: "A Comparison of the Effectiveness of a Standard and an Electric

Toothbrush," *J. Periodontol.*, **34:**375, (July) 1963.

85. Ash, M., Jr., et al.: "Evaluation of Manual and Motor-Driven Toothbrushes," *J. Am. Dent. Assoc.*, **69:**67, (Sept.) 1964.

86. Glass, Robert L.: "A Clinical Study of Hand and Electric Toothbrushing," *J. Periodontol.*, **36:**322, (July–Aug.) 1965.

86a. Canada. Department of National Health and Welfare: *Dental Health Manual.* [Ottawa, the Department, 1969,] p. 26.

87. Schneider, Louis: "Pulmonary Hazard of the Ingestion of Mineral Oil in the Apparently Healthy Adult," *N. Engl. J. Med.*, **240:**284, (Feb.) 1949.

88. Rossier, P. H., and Bühlman, A.: "Oil Pneumonia After Use of Liquid Paraffin as Nose Drops Over a Period of Years" (trans.), *Schweiz. Med. Wochenschr.*, **79:** 685, (July) 1949.

89. Ginsberg, Miriam K., and Yoder, Ann E.: "The Effectiveness of Some Traditional Methods in Oral Hygiene Nursing Care," *J. Periodontol.*, **35:**513, (Dec.) 1964.

90. Passos, Joyce Y., and Brand, Lucy M.: "Effects of Agents Used for Oral Hygiene," *Nurs. Res.*, **15:**196, (Summer) 1966.

91. Klocke, Joleen M., and Sudduth, Ardith G.: "Oral Hygiene Instruction and Plaque Formation During Hospitalization," *Nurs. Res.*, **18:**124, (Mar.–Apr.) 1969.

92. Goodsell, J. Orton, and Roper, R. E.: "The Place of Dental Care in the General Hospital," *Hospitals*, **25:**62, (Jan.) 1951.

93. Adler, Francis H.: *Textbook of Ophthalmology*, 7th ed. W. B. Saunders Co., Philadelphia, 1962, p. 523.

94. Brueggen, Stella L.: "Nurses' Opportunities To Conserve Sight," *Nurs. Outlook*, **10:**658, (Oct.) 1962.

95. Baker, Jeffrey: *The Truth About Contact Lenses: Everything the Wearer, or Potential Wearer, Should Know.* G. P. Putnam's Sons, New York, 1970, p. 79.

96. Winkler, Charles H., Jr., and Dixon, Joseph M.: "Bacteriology of the Eye. III. A. Effect of Contact Lenses on the Normal Flora. B. Flora of the Contact Lens Case," *Arch. Ophthalmol.*, **72:**817, (Dec.) 1964.

97. Chambers, Wilda G.: "Learning to Wear Contact Lenses," *Am. J. Nurs.*, **61:**82, (June) 1961.

98. "Contact Lenses," *Consumers' Research Annual Bull.*, **40:**121, 1966.

98a. Wilson, M. et al.: "Therapeutic Use of Soft Contact Lenses," *Proc. R. Soc. Med.*, **68:**55, (Jan.) 1975.

99. Stone, William: "Complications of Evisceration and Enucleation," in Fasanella, R. M. (ed.): *Complications in Eye Surgery*, 2nd ed. W. B. Saunders Co., Philadelphia, 1965, p. 420.

100. Duke-Elder, Sir Stewart: *Parsons' Diseases of the Eye*, 15th ed. Little, Brown & Co., Boston, 1970, p. 438.

101. Filderman, Irving P., and White, Paul F.: *Contact Lens Practice and Patient Management.* Chilton Book Co., Philadelphia, 1969, p. 298.

102. Stone, William: *op. cit.*, p. 394.

102a. Prince, J. H.: *Recent Advances in Ocular Prostheses.* Williams & Wilkins Co., Baltimore, 1950.

103. Orentreich, Norman: "Hair Problems," *J.A.M.W.A.*, **21:**481, (June) 1966.

104. Behrman, Howard T.: *The Scalp in Health and Disease.* C. V. Mosby Co., St. Louis, 1952, p. 125.

105. Reiches, A. J.: "Skin Reactions to Hair Dyes," *Arch. Dermatol.*, **65:**619, (May) 1952.

106. Savill, Agnes, and Warren, Clara: *The Hair and Scalp*, 5th ed. Williams & Wilkins Co., Baltimore, 1962, p. 164.

107. Orentreich, Norman: *op. cit.*

108. Mercantini, Edward S.: "Hair and Physiological Baldness," *Can. Med. Assoc. J.*, **92:** 1345, (June 26) 1965.

109. Orentreich, Norman: *op. cit.*

110. Nevins, Michael A., et al.: "Pulmonary Granulomatosis," *J.A.M.A.*, **193:**266, (July 26) 1965.

111. "Cosmetics and Toilet Sundries," *Consumers' Research Annual Bull.*, **40:**108, 1966.

111a. Suskin, E., and Boutys, A.: "Acute Airway Responses to Hairspray Preparations," *N. Engl. J. Med.*, **290:**660, (Mar.) 1974.

112. Bates, Marston: *Where Winter Never Comes.* Charles Scribner's Sons, New York, 1952.

Additional Suggested Reading

Abrahamson, Ira A.: *Know Your Eyes.* Medcom Press, New York, 1972.

Aronson, Samuel B., and Elliott, James H.: *Ocular Inflammation.* C. V. Mosby Co., St. Louis, 1972.

Belin, L., et al.: "Enzyme Sensitisation in Consumers of Enzyme-Containing Washing Powder," *Lancet.*, **2:**1153, (Dec. 5) 1970.

Cetin, E. T., et al.: "Study of Oral, Nasal and Skin Flora in an Investigation on Hospital Infection," *Pathol. Microbiol.*, **37:**324, (May) 1971.

Christie, R. M.: "Improving Mouth Care for the Incapacitated," *Nurs. Times*, **19:**22, (Dec.) 1970.

Comaish, Stanley: "Metabolic Disorders and Hair Growth," *Br. J. Dermatol.*, **84:**83, (Jan.) 1971.

Crane, G.: "New Bath System Saves Man-Hours," *Nurs. Times*, **68:**618, (May 18) 1972.

Cranin, A. Norman, and Dennison, Thomas A.: "Implants in Modern Dentistry," *Am. J. Nurs.*, **73:**1595, (Sept.) 1973.

Crounse, R. G., et al.: "Quantitative Tissue of Human Malnutrition Using Scalp Hair Roots," *Nature*, **228:**465, (Oct. 31) 1970.

Davies, D. M.: *The Influence of Teeth, Diet, and Habits on the Human Face*. William Heinemann Medical Books, Ltd., London, 1972.

DeLa Ruguera, I. Gonzalez, et al.: "The Importance of Food Sensitization in Atopia Dermatitis," *Dermatologica*, **143**:288, (No. 4) 1971.

DeWalt, Evelyn M., and Haines, Sister Ann Kathleen: "The Effects of Specified Stressors on Health and Oral Mucosa," in Downs, Florence S., and Newman, Margaret A. (eds.): *A Source Book of Nursing Research*. F. A. Davis Co., Philadelphia, 1973.

Dowling, G. B., and Naylor, P. F. D.: "The Source of Free Amino Acids in Keratin Scrapings," *Br. J. Dermatol.*, **72**:57, (Jan.) 1960.

Dunkin, R. T.: "A New Approach to Oral Physiotherapy with a New Index of Evaluation," *J. Periodontol.*, **36**:315, (July–Aug.) 1965.

Eller, Joseph J., and Silver, Stephen: "Psychosomatic Diseases of the Skin," *Behav. Neuropsychiatry*, **1**:25, (Feb.–Mar.) 1970.

Englander, H. R.: "A Perspective on Prophylaxis of Dental Caries by Topical Fluoride," *Dent. Clin. North Am.*, **16**:673, (Oct.) 1972.

Epstein, E., and Orkin, M.: "Could That 'Maddening Itch' Be Lice or Mites?" *Patient Care*, **7**:94, (Nov. 1) 1973.

Ferriman, David: *Human Hair Growth in Health and Disease*. Charles C Thomas, Publisher, Springfield, Ill., 1971.

Finn, Sidney B., et al.: *The Year Book of Dentistry 1972*. Year Book Medical Publishers, Chicago, 1972.

Flindt, M. L. H.: "Pulmonary Disease Due to Inhalation of Derivatives of *Bacillus subtilis* Containing Proteolytic Enzyme," *Lancet*, **1**:1177, (June 14) 1969.

Fraleigh, Claud M.: "Gingival Health as Related to the Electric Toothbrush," *J. Dent. Med.*, **20**:147, (Oct.) 1965.

Harrison, Jos. W. E., et al.: "Effect of Enzyme-Toothpastes upon Oral Hygiene," *J. Periodontol.*, **34**:337, (July) 1963.

Hoover, Donald R., and Lefkowitz, William: "Reduction of Gingivitis by Toothbrushing," *J. Periodontol.*, **36**:21, (May–June) 1965.

Hull, D. S., et al.: "Clinical Experience with the Therapeutic Hydrophilic Contact Lens," *Ann. Ophthalmol.*, **75**:555, (Apr.) 1975.

Jelinek, J. E.: "Cutaneous Side Effects of Oral Contraceptives," *Arch. Dermatol.*, **101**:181, (Feb.) 1970.

Kass, G. S.: "Recent Developments in Hair Preparations," *J.A.M.W.A.*, **21**:487, (June) 1966.

Leopold, Irving H.: "Anti-Inflammatory Agents in Ophthalmology," *Am. J. Nurs.*, **63**:84, (Mar.) 1963.

Löe, Harold, and Schiott, C. Rindom: "The Effect of Mouthrinses and Topical Application of Chlorhexidine on the Development of Dental Plaque and Gingivitis in Man," *J. Periodont. Res.*, **5**:79, 1970.

Mandel, Irwin D.: "New Approaches to Plaque Prevention," *Dent. Clin. North Am.*, **16**:661, (Oct.) 1972.

McCord, Carey P.: "Artificial Eyes, The Early History of Ocular Prostheses," *J. Occup. Med.*, **7**:61, (Feb.) 1965.

McNamara, Thomas F., et al.: "The Role of Microorganisms in the Production of Oral Malodor," *Oral Surg.*, **34**:41, (July) 1972.

Moore-Robinson, Miram: "Cutaneous Responses to Aspirin and Its Derivatives," *Br. J. Dermatol.*, **82**:319, (Mar.) 1970.

Muller, Sigfrid A.: "Viral Infections of the Skin and Mouth: A Selected Review," *Oral. Surg.*, **32**:752, (Mar.) 1970.

Parran, John J., and Brinkman, Richard E.: "The Effect of Human Skin Surface Lipids upon the Activity of Antimicrobial Agents," *J. Invest. Dermatol.*, **45**:89, (Aug.) 1965.

Pickett, Hal G., et al.: "Changes in the Denture Supporting Tissues Associated with the Aging Process," *J. Prosthet. Dent.* **27**:257, (Mar.) 1972.

Potten, Christopher S.: "Some Observations on the Post-Plucking Depression in Tritiated Thymidine Utilization in Mouse Skin and Some Tentative Cell Kinetic Determinations," *J. Invest. Dermatol.*, **58**:180, (Apr.) 1972.

Ralph, J. P., and Stenhouse, D.: "Denture-Induced Hyperplasia of the Oral Soft Tissues," *Br. Dent. J.*, **132**:68, (Jan. 18) 1972.

Roberts, Marguerite, and Comaish, Stanley: "Notable Advances in Dermatological Treatment Over the Past Twenty-five Years," *Br. J. Clin. Pract.*, **25**:341, (Aug.) 1971.

Rook, Arthur: "Some Chemical Influences on Hair Growth and Pigmentation," *Br. J. Dermatol.*, **77**:115, (Mar.) 1965.

Seropian, Richard, and Reynolds, Benedict M.: "Wound Infections After Preoperative Depilatory Versus Razor Preparation," *Am. J. Surg.*, **121**:251, (Mar.) 1971.

Shaw, James H.: "Nutritional Guidance in the Prevention of Oral Disease," *Dent. Clin. North Am.*, **16**:733, (Oct.) 1972.

Smith, J. Graham, and Kiem, Iris M.: "Allergic Contact Sensitivity in the Aged," *J. Gerontol.*, **16**:118, (Apr.) 1961.

Snyder, Fred H., et al.: "Safety Evaluation of Zinc 2-Pyridimethiol 1-Oxide in a Shampoo Formulation," *Toxicol. Appl. Pharmacol.*, **7**:425, (May) 1965.

Stafford, G. D., and Russell, C.: "Efficiency of Denture Adhesives and Their Possible Influence on Oral Microorganisms," *J. Dent. Res.*, **50**:832, (Aug.) 1972.

Summers, Margaret M., et al.: "Hair as a Reservoir of Staphylococci," *J. Clin. Pathol.*, **18**:13, (Jan.) 1965.

Thorne, Napier: "Hair Grooming," *Br. J. Clin. Pract.*, **18**:627, (Oct.) 1964.

Tindall, John P., and Smith, Graham J., Jr.: "Skin Lesions of the Aged and Their Association with Internal Changes," *J.A.M.A.*, **186**:1039, (Dec. 21) 1963.

Trowbridge, Janet E., and Carl, William: "Oral

Care of the Patient Having Head and Neck Irradiation," *Am. J. Nurs.,* **75:**2146, (Dec.) 1975.

Vellar, Odd D.: "Composition of Human Nail Substance," *Am. J. Clin. Nutr.,* **23:**1272, (Oct.) 1970.

Wexler, Lewis: "Gamma Benzene Hexachloride in Treatment of Pediculosis and Scabies," *Am. J. Nurs.,* **69:**565, (Mar.) 1969.

Whitner, Willamay, and Thompson, Margaret C.: "The Influence of Bathing on the Newborn Infant's Body Temperature," *Nurs. Res.,* **19:**30, (Jan.–Feb.) 1970.

Zuenick, Martha: "Care of an Artificial Eye," *Am. J .Nurs.,* **75:**835 (Mar.) 1975.

Gladys Nite
Virginia Henderson

The authors acknowledge the assistance of Carol Adamson, R.N., Ph.D., Assistant Professor, School of Nursing, St. Thomas University, Houston, Tex., in review of literature of selected topics in this chapter.

CHAPTER 15

Controlling the Environment for Maintenance of Optimal Atmospheric Conditions, Sanitation, Esthetics, and Protection from Infection and Other Dangers

1. ENVIRONMENTAL HEALTH ESSENTIALS

Environmental Components. Broadly speaking, environment is "the aggregate of all the external conditions and influences affecting the life and development of an organism".* Environment has a biologic component, consisting of all living things: plants, animals, microorganisms—the whole realm of animate nature—and a physical component, in which all living things operate. The physical sphere consists of sunlight, water, oxygen, carbon dioxide, organic compounds, and other nutrients used by plants for growth. Biologic and physical components together form an ecosystem, which is the sum total of all living and nonliving parts that support a chain of life within a given area.[1] There is a delicate balance, a precarious interdependent relationship, between living organisms and their surroundings; if one

part is substantially changed, all other parts are affected. There is a third behavioral component, which for human beings includes social interactions, customs, and economic, legal, political, and religious systems. All of these bear on human health. In addition, all animate and inanimate activity takes place within the dimensions of *time* and *space,* each of which has an important impact on human behavior and well-being.

Human Ecology and Environmental Pollution. In recent years there has been a growing recognition of man's influence on his environment. Most people are now keenly aware that extraordinary technologic advances, with the depletion and misuse of natural resources and "the population explosion," have upset the ecologic balance. This turn of events has serious consequences for health and well-being, and, if the trend is not reversed, the survival of mankind is at stake.

Environmental pollution has become a personal experience for young and old. Air pollution, mainly from combustion processes, is

* *Webster's New Collegiate Dictionary.* G. & C. Merriam Co., Springfield, Mass., 1961.

increasingly harmful to humans, plants, animals, and property. Water pollution, from improper disposal of excreta and radioactive and other chemical wastes, is depleting the usable water supply, spoiling lakes and streams, and killing fish in coastal waters. Food is polluted by insecticides, chemical additives, hormones, and antibiotics. Soil is polluted by chemical fertilizers, weed killers, and pesticides, which in turn destroy beneficial wildlife. Then, when land is cleared for construction projects, trees and plants that hold the soil in place are removed and erosion results. Land, a limited resource, is being depleted and more and more of the remaining wilderness destroyed. Noise in urban areas is a health hazard. The production of solid wastes is increasing at a prodigious rate and their disposal is more and more difficult. Plastics, for instance, stay in their original state almost indefinitely. Most methods used to dispose of solid wastes do some damage to the environment. Land for dumping is running out, and land dumps are breeding places for disease-carrying animals and insects. Burning wastes increases air pollution, while dumping wastes into rivers and oceans contributes to water pollution. "Man's pollutions are now literally out of this world," states Benjamin A. Kogan, as litter from space ships orbits the earth, and human litter invades the moon.* Care of the environment is a worldwide problem. All forms of life on earth are affected. As one writer states, "We live on a finite planet with limited resources and a limited capacity to support life. Expanding technology, industrialization, and exploding population growth are putting ever increasing pressure upon a vanishing resource base." †

This chapter examines ways in which the environment affects health and the quality of human life, as well as ways of controlling the surroundings to promote and maintain health and well-being. The emphasis is mainly on the physical, or nonhuman, environment in which nursing care takes place, as differentiated from the interpersonal environment, which is discussed in Chapter 16. It is hoped that nurses working with individuals or with groups of patients will not lose sight of conditions in the larger community that have an impact on health and disease. Attention must be paid to the issues of war, poverty, environmental pollution, population density, inadequate housing, racial discrimination, and unequal opportunities for work and education.

The Nurse's Role in Controlling the Environment. Nurses as citizens can combat these problems. They can, for example, help conserve natural resources and prevent pollution by using public transportation, sharing rides, walking, or using bicycles. They can support efforts to provide proper sewage disposal and recycling of waste water; they can use non-polluting detergents, avoid open-air burning, and select clean burning fuels. If nurses have gardens, they can avoid using harmful pesticides and chemical fertilizers, and instead build up, and use, compost, which returns nutrients to the soil. They can use containers that can be recycled, avoiding plastic and other materials that do not readily decompose. All health workers can participate in conservation activities and use their influence as consumers to bring about constructive change. Finally, they can support family planning programs and share opinions on issues such as war, poverty, discrimination, education, and prison and welfare reform with legislators, newspapers, television and radio stations, and educators. What each citizen does to help create a world in which life, and health as a quality of life, is valued, is perhaps more important than the narrower task each person sets for himself or herself as a member of a profession or occupation.[2]

As the nurse's role and function expands, nurses move into increasingly varied settings or environments. Each presents a unique challenge. Whether nursing in a home, a hospice, a prison, a parent-child center, a rural health agency, or a modern city hospital, the following essentials of environmental health must be considered: (1) optimal organization of time and space; (2) access of light during the day and adequate artificial lighting when there is insufficient daylight; (3) an atmospheric temperature and humidity that promote normal body functions; (4) air movement sufficient to evaporate sweat and favor vascular changes within the skin and to remove appreciable quantities of dust, injurious chemicals, and pathogenic bacteria from the air; (5) atmospheric or gas pressures within man's tolerance; (6) pure, wholesome food and water, and provision for disposal of excreta and waste; and (7) reasonable cleanliness of all surfaces and furnishings that the individual is likely to handle.

Order, freedom from disagreeable odors and noise, harmony of color and design in the immediate surroundings, and the opportunity for privacy affect the mental state and indirectly the physical welfare. Individuals vary, however,

---

* Kogan, Benjamin A.: *Health: Man in a Changing Environment.* Harcourt, Brace & World, New York, 1970, p. 56.

† Nelson, Gaylord: "The Common Roots of Poverty and Pollution," *The Progressive,* (Feb.) 1973, p. 33.

according to temperament and training in their desire for quiet, beauty, and privacy, whereas the conditions listed above are truly essential to well-being. It goes without saying that a healthful environment provides facilities for all the physiologic functions, such as eating, sleeping, and evacuation, and that the dwelling is reasonably free from fire hazards, faulty construction, and insect and animal pests.

Those accustomed to living surrounded by every convenience and comfort lose sight of the fact that these things are not essential to health or happiness. Nurses who find the organization of the patient's surroundings one of their functions must not be discouraged if only the necessities can be provided, for the patient who has proper medical treatment and nursing care usually recovers as rapidly in simple surroundings as in luxurious ones. For the patient's benefit, however, it is often necessary to modify his or her surroundings.

Nurses should work closely with others on environmental questions. Nurses, acting alone, cannot ensure that the persons under their care have adequate space, light, pure air, and other health essentials; they can, however, take part in planning hospitals, schools, clinics, and other domiciles, and health services in schools, industries, and penal institutions. In homes, nurses may help the family select the room for an infant or an invalid. In every situation nurses who know physiologic and psychologic reactions to temperature and humidity, light and color, gas pressures, odors, noise, chemical impurities, and microorganisms can organize and make the best use of the facilities available. Sanitation, architecture, and housekeeping, per se, are not nursing, but nurses must know something about all these and, if the welfare of the patient demands it, they may be obliged to function in any of these fields.

During epidemics of contagious diseases or in the event of disasters such as earthquakes and floods, nurses must, in addition to improvising temporary shelters and engaging in a host of other activities,[3,4] teach and practice methods of sanitation, such as decontaminating drinking water. When the patient is very ill, nurses may clean the room or prepare the food if they believe they can perform these services in such a way that the patient will be benefited. In home nursing, the professional nurse may find it necessary to clean, wash, and cook, until a suitable person can be found to take over these tasks. Although housekeeping is not what the nurse is best qualified for, and is misdirection of the energy that should go into nursing the patient, it is nevertheless a false idea of dignity to think that anything contributing to the total welfare of the patient is "unprofes-sional" or degrading. Sickness upsets a home, and if nurses can help restore peace and order, they are giving a high type of service. When sickness disrupts the management of the house, a housekeeper should be employed to supply the domestic service that has sometimes, in the past, been confused with nursing care; or Homemaking Services, which go beyond housekeeping, may be indicated in some cases.

In the hospital and other treatment centers the nurse is the "first line of defense" in the control of hospital-associated (nosocomial) infection. This will be discussed later in the chapter as well as ventilation, lighting, fire control, and other aspects of environmental control. For further study of these topics the reader is referred to texts and articles listed at the end of the chapter.

A Comparison of Environmental Needs in Health and Sickness. Almost everything that contributes to a wholesome environment of persons in health may at one time or another require modification during sickness; for example, atmospheric temperatures normally desirable are too low for the burned patient; higher humidities than those ordinarily found indoors may be indicated for the person with bronchitis; atmospheres filtered free of pollens, foreign proteins, or microorganisms are prescribed for the asthmatic patient, or one with heightened susceptibility to infectious disease; air containing a much higher concentration of oxygen than is found in nature is used in the treatment of many conditions characterized by lowered blood oxygen; and airtight chambers with regulated atmospheric pressures are used to recompress and slowly decompress the patient with caisson disease, "the bends," or "diver's palsy." It is possible to mention here only a few examples of ways in which special conditions within patients' surroundings are used to treat disease.

As more is learned about the effect of environment on health and disease, hospitals, homes, and other structures are planned and constructed to provide optimal environmental conditions. Because nosocomial (hospital acquired) infections are increasingly common and hard to control, hospitals today are designed and arranged to decrease microbial contamination. To minimize air-borne contamination, for example, air barriers are created by controlling the direction, pressure, and rate of flow of air in "critical areas" such as operating rooms, nurseries, isolation rooms, and laundry-sorting rooms. Space is arranged to reduce the flow of traffic through and near these critical areas, which in turn reduces microbial dissemination. As more is learned about the function of space, hospital planners and architects take into account its psychologic aspects as well. When discussing hospital design, they speak of "personal-space," "mind-space," "body-buffer zones," and "territoriality."

2. TIME AND SPACE IN RELATION TO THE ENVIRONMENT

Optimal Organization of Space. Although we tend to take space for granted, it has, in recent years, become a subject of increasing interest to a wide range of professions. Space (in the form of land), like water and air, is regarded by many environmentalists as one of the most neglected and endangered of earth's limited resources. It is widely believed that better planning for the use of existing land is essential for its preservation. In another context, man's movement in and organization of space and time are referred to as the fifth dimension. Architectural or environmental design psychology is a field of study. Anthropologists have shown how space, which is arranged differently in different cultures, affects behavior. According to anthropologist Edward T. Hall, "Space speaks." [5,6] He has coined the term *proxemics* to refer to the currently burgeoning theories and observations dealing with man's use and structuring of space as a specialized elaboration of culture, particularly the unconscious patterns that deeply influence life. Hall believes that everything that man is and does is associated with the experience of space, "that nothing occurs, real or imagined, without spatial context, because space (along with time) is one of the principal organizing systems for living organisms." [7] He and others postulate that, in addition to the physical boundary that separates each living thing from its environment (skin, in the case of humans), each organism has another kind of outer boundary known as the organism's territory. Most animals, including man, lay claim to territories as a division of the space in which each exists. Hall believes that the human need to lay claim to and organize territory, and to maintain discrete distances from others, is a basic human need, along with the need for food, sex, affirmation, and so on. This does not necessarily mean ownership of property. Each person has a way of finding some kind of space for his or her use. In a family, for example, even in crowded quarters, father may have "his chair," and each person "his place" at the table; Billy may have a tree house or other area that is off limits to all but a chosen

few; Susie may have her special place under the stairs where she goes to be alone when she is anxious or unhappy. Each creates a space no one else invades. The term *body-buffer zones* refers to the distances human beings keep between themselves and others. These distances vary with the individual and are affected by circumstances such as mood and social setting. Body-buffer zones are related to the need for privacy as well as to the need to interact with others. To a large extent they are culturally determined.

The way space is arranged and organized largely determines and controls the kinds of activities and behavior that takes place within it. Certain activities are unlikely when the arrangement of space is not optimal. This is an important consideration in planning learning environments for children. By varying the arrangement of space in the classroom (or playroom in the case of a day-care center, nursery school, or pediatric ward), the teacher or nurse can introduce variety and interest to a space which is otherwise static and uninteresting. For example, activity in an auditorium where the seats are bolted to the floor is limited to sitting, whereas use of the same space equipped with folding chairs is limited only by the imagination of the occupants.

In *What Do I Do Monday?* John Holt quotes the following passages from a descriptive bulletin printed by The Tree House, a company that manufactures vertical panels used to create smaller learning spaces in large rooms:

The Tree House Learning Environment (the vertical panels) provides educators with an opportunity . . . *to use space as a medium of communication.* [Italics ours.]

The appropriateness of special enclosures as a teaching medium can be readily appreciated by observing the way children play. Give a child a large box and soon he will be inside it. Should a friend be near, he will invite him inside too. Children playing in the yard where there is lawn furniture will soon use the furniture to create a special, spatially arranged world. A bench will mark off the wall of a house, the hose will serve as the highway to the shopping center indicated by the patio table. In this activity the children are arranging space—in order to create a world in which they can relate to each other. The furniture marks off spaces in which their imaginations can make present an adult world that they can control and adjust to through play.*

Some innovative teachers use the space between floor and ceiling to allow climbing and provide privacy. In the same book, Holt de-

---

* Holt, John: *What Do I Do Monday?* Dell Publishing Co., New York, 1970, p. 284.

scribes a school setting that has balconies which "go around and about, and in and out," and "retreats to get away from everything and everybody." One retreat was described as a "box-thing soundproofed with egg cartons that seemed to hang in mid air" †—a lovely temporary hideaway from pressures of group activity.

In homes, hospitals, and other institutions, as well as in schools, the organization of space is important. Many hospitals for children now include playrooms, schoolrooms, and space for parents to "live-in." A study of overcrowding in homes that shared common socioeconomic conditions showed twice as many physical and social disorders in families where space was less than 8 to 10 square meters per person as in larger homes; children in the smaller homes were reportedly much more susceptible to the influence of crowding than adults.[8]

Two studies dealing with the effect of spatial arrangement on social interaction show that army recruits living in long, open barracks know the names of more people than recruits living in partitioned barracks, but those in the partitioned areas have more friends, or "buddies." The same phenomenon has been noted in offices; open offices lead to a greater number of acquaintances but fewer friends than partitioned offices.[9]

Importance of Time in Patient Care. An individual's perception of time is affected by many variables. It is partially determined by culture, as well as by past experiences. It varies for each individual from one situation to another depending on his or her age, level of anxiety, and role in a given situation. The measure of time is not the same for patient, family member, nurse, and doctor, but it is important for each. Small children without a well-developed concept of time may feel that they have been abandoned when their mother leaves them for only a short period. An hour may seem interminable to a wife waiting for her husband to return from the operating room. Time is a valuable commodity for those who dispense health care, and their use of it in relation to the patient may be beneficial or detrimental. Time and the passage of time may be distorted in any illness, especially when patients are forced to give up their usual activities. When hospitalization is necessary, the artificiality of the hospital routine accentuates distortion. Health workers in many countries have noted that the longer patients stay in the hospital, the fewer and less frequent are their visitors, and the more important become

the ward, its people, and its activities, until even mundane happenings assume inordinate significance. Mealtimes, visiting hours, distribution of mail, and doctors' visits are finally the highlights in a patient's day.[10]

A situation in which there is no differentiation between night and day, such as an intensive care unit where there is continuous activity carried out under artificial light, may distort the patient's sense of reality. An outside window where daylight can be seen and nighttime hours designated for sleeping help to orient a person to time and space. Clocks, calendars, and current periodicals the patient can see may help prevent distortion in the sense of time. For a small child, a window with a view of the road can be an intangible link with home. Irene M. Burnside,[11] writing about nursing care of the aged, points to the unfortunate lack of clocks and calendars in patients' rooms in most hospitals and nursing homes. She believes the elderly should be helped to "maintain the rhythm of their lives" and suggests having chimes announce the hours over the intercom, as well as having the "most cheery-voiced" staff member begin each morning by announcing the date and day of the week.*

The consideration of time, as well as the organization of space, is particularly important in care and treatment of patients in mental hospitals. Otto A. Will, Jr.,[12] a physician, has eloquently described the importance of these and other aspects of the physical environment in the treatment of a chronically ill, schizophrenic girl. When Will took over the management of her treatment, she had been ill for 12 years and was markedly regressed and beset by growing social isolation, despair, and a chronic state of low morale, which was shared by the caretaking staff. Although her subsequent treatment included an enormous amount of personal input on the part of the staff, changes in the hospital's physical environment were an important part of the psychotherapeutic approach which led to her recovery. In Will's words:

The ward on which Miss X lived was dismal. The walls were dark and without decoration, lighting was dim, the windows were heavily screened, furniture was durable but uncomfortable and unattractive, there were no movable lamps and no pictures, and the floors were bare. . . . As the ward was on the 4th floor, access to the out-of-doors was difficult and, for many patients, infrequent. The restlessness and sudden explosive outbursts of some patients intensified the feeling of being crowded. Privacy

* *Ibid.*, p. 282.

* We add that it would be nice also to give the weather forecast.

was an unavailable luxury. The physical surroundings conveyed to both staff and patients a message of unchanging hopelessness. For the patients the timeless quality was emphasized by the absence of clocks, calendars, current literature, and by their isolation from the daily routines of the outside world. Miss X had no personal possessions on the ward to remind her of a happier past or suggest a more promising future. There was nothing to confirm her identity as a woman and a person of sensitivity. Her own low self-esteem was reflected in her environment.

Although we could not at this time modify the entire ward, we did redecorate Miss X's room. The walls were repainted and the worn flooring replaced. More attractive clothing was provided, and she was given her violin and typewriter to keep in her room, and a calendar and watch despite her protestations that time did not exist. . . . She was [subsequently] removed to another section of the hospital where she had a private room and bath, and special nursing. Furniture, radio, pictures, books, potted plants, and so on, were provided, and although there were days when she moved everything out of her room insisting that she wanted no thing or person near her, she did not destroy these possessions.

. . . [As treatment progressed], Miss X lived in a single room in a small cottage with about six other patients. The room was provided with furnishing from her home—her bed, rugs, pictures, lamps, chairs, and books. In the last year of our work she lived in a small apartment near the hospital. At first this was sparsely furnished, but slowly she was able to admit more color and life, until the surroundings reflected no longer despair but her increasing hope and confidence.*

Although interpersonal communication is the basis of most care and treatment in mental illness, as discussed in Chapter 16, the quality of the physical environment is important. Will favors the following environmental features in a therapeutic program:

1. Space in which patients can move about without unavoidably violating the territories of others.
2. A place in which one can be alone and find quiet.
3. A distribution of space permitting a patient to move, as he feels the need, from privacy, to contact with a small group (of two or three), and to a larger group (of eight to ten), having some freedom to choose his associates.
4. Privacy in toilet and bathing facilities.
5. Ready availability of personal possessions and items from home to reinforce a sense of identity apart from the institution.
6. Clocks, calendars, and current publications to help correct distortions of time.
7. Furnishings of varied colors and textures—

attention being given to auditory, tactile, and visual input.*

Infants and young children, in order to learn and develop, also need auditory, tactile, and visual stimulation. Hospitalization for a child can be made more tolerable when he or she is permitted to bring something from home, particularly a treasured object like a "security blanket." In this case, the personal belonging bridges the gap between hospital and home, helping to relieve the distress of separation.

Effects of Time and Space on Hospitalized Children. Time and space are both important considerations in planning care for children in hospitals. The age and phase in the child's development during which illness occurs must be taken into account if the kind of care needed to meet each child's emotional and developmental needs is to be provided. This must be done if the potential trauma of hospitalization and illness is to be reduced. To assure a physical and social hospital environment appropriate for each child's age and phase of development, Helen H. Glaser,[13] a physician, suggests that, since children of different ages have varying environmental needs, the architectural design of children's hospitals should be determined by concepts of the children's growth and development. She advocates grouping children with others of their own age, as this is more conducive to meeting their social and emotional needs than segregating them by diagnosis, sex, or socioeconomic status, as is sometimes done.

Hospital Environment for Infants. Newborns should, if possible, be in rooms with their mothers. Developmental needs of hospitalized infants (other than the newborn) under 6 months of age are best met if alcoves or other spaces are provided for mothers or nurses to feed them in comfortable rocking chairs. To meet their needs for physical care and sensory and emotional stimulation, infants under 6 months need less space than older infants and toddlers, who should have room to move about. Small, self-contained subunits for three or four infants within larger nursing units enable one nurse to give total care to one small group, thus ensuring each child maximum contact with either a parent or one nurse.†

---

* Will, Otto A., Jr.: "Schizophrenia and the Psychotherapeutic Field," *Contemp. Psychoanal.* **1:**11, (Fall) 1964.

* *Ibid.*
† Apart from its purpose of providing emotionally sound care, this method is used in the cohort plan of infant care in large newborn nurseries in order to minimize the hazard of cross-infection. Under this system, three or four infants born at approximately the same time (within a time span of a few hours) are segregated and cared for by one nurse on each shift, using barrier technique. Additional infants are

Hospitalized infants over 6 months old need space for their mothers to "live-in" with them. They also need surroundings that provide visual, tactile, and auditory stimulation, as well as experiences that promote development of motor skills. There should be a safe space in which they can crawl, pull themselves up, and walk with support; they also need a variety of toys to manipulate and moving musical mobiles to hear and watch. Glaser suggests that they also need to be able to see the world outside, to watch the changes of light and shadow as the sun moves across the room, and to see other children at play and nurses at work.

Hospital Environment for Young Children. Toddlers and preschool children need an environment that promotes independence in self-care and provides opportunities to explore the nonhuman and human worlds. They need equipment that helps them develop motor skills and physical coordination and promotes imaginative activity. Since development in children of this age proceeds through play, outdoor and indoor play areas are important. The hospital play area is not basically different from that used by healthy children, but it must be designed to accommodate children on stretchers or push-carts, in wheelchairs, and children wearing casts. If space permits, beds with attached traction frames can be wheeled into playrooms and on to porches or patios. Most play materials and equipment used in playrooms outside the hospital can be utilized, as, for example, the following: water, clay, sand, play dough, paint, blocks, beads, boards, and boxes. Clothing and surgical supplies and equipment that allow children to imitate doctors and nurses are useful in encouraging expression of feelings engendered by medical treatment.

Hospital Environment for School-Age Children. Children between 6 and 12 need facilities for continuing school work. They also benefit from music, painting, and crafts, as well as from indoor and outdoor play. During these years a child's social development includes learning the skills of working and living with others. Multipurpose space and multiple-bed rooms are appropriate for school-age pediatric patients.

Hospital Environment for Adolescents. Glaser, in discussing needs of adolescents, suggests that the hospital environment be designed to help them develop their sense of identity. Teen-agers need personal space—a clearly defined territory in which the boy or girl can keep his or her possessions and which can reflect his or her personality. They need a sanctuary where each person can function independently, away from other patients some of the time. They also need an opportunity to associate with visiting friends, or with friends made in the hospital. A day room including a kitchenette where patients and visitors can get together to play or eat is important, as is access to a telephone. In addition, adolescents, like school-age children, need an opportunity to continue schooling while in the hospital.[14]

Environment of Health Institutions for Adults. It is hard to generalize about the needs for young, middle-aged, and aged adults. Segregation according to age, sex, socioeconomic status, or race may impoverish rather than enrich life for adults. Some segregation is inevitable, however. For example, girls and women who are bearing children should be put in one area to protect them and their infants from infection. Most often adults are housed in units according to the amount of care they need. For example, there are intensive care units with the maximum life-saving equipment and self-care units where patients live as independently and with as much privacy as they might in a hotel.

Many hospitals have rehabilitation units that provide special services and special furnishings and equipment that enable patients to practice activities of daily living so that the sick and handicapped can be relatively independent when they leave the institution. When all health workers are prepared to foster independence in patients there may be less need for these specialized services.

Hospital or nursing home units, or separate institutions for the terminally ill, are discussed in Chapter 50. It is rare to find children in them but some admit adolescents.

In all services for children and adults, the environment should promote the goal of making residence within them a learning, or constructive, experience.

Hospital Space for Parents and Staff. Parents, particularly those of young children, need space in the hospital if they are to participate in their children's care. Because efficiency and occupational satisfaction depend to a great extent on the physical environment, hospital personnel need adequate space, not only for work but for interaction and relaxation as well. Glaser[15] advocates a special "territory" where

excluded from the group. When all three or four infants go home, the area is meticulously cleaned and disinfected before the next group is admitted. This system limits the transfer of potential infection to only one generation of infants. Very often the presence of infection is not recognized in nurseries, as symptoms do not appear until days, or even weeks, after the infant has been discharged. The cohort plan of infant care tends to confine the potential spread of unrecognized (inapparent) infection to small rather than large groups of infants.

the nurse can spend brief periods away from patients and the "nurses' station." For the physician, Glaser advocates office space, lounging areas, and overnight accommodations near the patient unit. Physicians need a place to talk with patients and families in private. Examination and treatment rooms, as well as consultation offices near the patient unit, encourage the use of these areas, rather than the bedside, for such procedures.

3. NATURAL AND ARTIFICIAL LIGHTING

Natural Lighting. Light and heat from the sun as solar energy reach the earth by radiation. Sunlight contains all of the wavelengths of light visible in the rainbow or in a prism. The solar spectrum also contains wavelengths outside of the portion that can be seen. Beyond the red end of the spectrum are infrared rays that produce heat when absorbed by the body. Beyond the violet end of the spectrum are ultraviolet rays that tan the skin. Sunlight is not always equally potent; some ultraviolet rays are screened out by clouds, rain, dust, and smoke in the air and by ordinary window glass, and the rays are stronger in the summer than in the winter.[16] The life-sustaining, health-promoting effects of sunlight are well known. Ultraviolet radiation on the skin is necessary for the body's production of vitamin D, and sunlight in suitable amounts enhances the healing of wounds. Nevertheless, excessive exposure to sunlight can cause severe burns, and ultraviolet light radiation from the sun is responsible for most skin cancers.[17] Exposure of the eyes to snow or to radiation from the sand on beach or desert may be intensely irritating and, if of long duration, harmful. Glasses that filter out ultraviolet, infrared, or excessive visible radiation should be worn under such circumstances.

While we can live without sight, it is hard to conceive a healthful life, in fact life at all, without sunlight. Physiologically and psychologically it is so important to us that as a general rule buildings should be designed to admit adequate natural light to every room. Northern exposures are desirable in southern countries, and windows that face the south in northern latitudes. A room well lighted by natural light has a window area equal to at least one fifth of the floor space, and to admit maximum light, windows should reach nearly to the ceiling. A room is poorly lighted if it is very much brighter in one part than another. Windows, however, should be so placed that it is not necessary to face the light when working. Provision should be made for controlling

glare. Contrasts in brightness are uncomfortable. Most eyes can tolerate outdoor sunlight because it is of uniform brightness. Visual acuity is cut down as one passes from a brightly lighted area to a darker one; therefore, passages and storage spaces should be well lighted to prevent accidents. Rooms with pale walls and white ceilings are most easily lighted; dark, dull walls absorb much of the sunlight. Shining surfaces, however, contribute to glare. Windows should be planned to fit the purpose of the room. Tall windows give greater penetration of light; broad windows give a greater diffusion. The usefulness of windows is reduced by covering them unnecessarily with curtains and shades.

Because exceedingly efficient artificial lighting and ventilation are now available, some buildings are constructed without windows, for example, factories, libraries, and art galleries. Windows are unnecessary in modern operating rooms, as all surgery is performed by artificial light.* Too much daylight can be distracting and cannot be controlled easily. Eliminating windows in operating rooms permits better control of heating and ventilation and makes a dark room possible during endoscopy. The artificial lighting system in the operating room should be backed up by a fully automatic emergency lighting system for use in case of power failure.[18] In homes and most buildings, however, windows are a necessity. Aside from the sunlight and warmth they afford, they are esthetic, and they provide the change from daylight to night that helps orient occupants to time. Sunlight discourages the growth of microorganisms and helps control infection.

Artificial Lighting. Adequate light is essential for efficient sight. When natural light does not suffice, artificial lighting is necessary both indoors and out. Most communities have building codes that prescribe standards for artificial lighting, as well as other health essentials. The US Public Health Service publishes proposed housing standards for local adoption.[19] In the United States the foot-candle † is the unit commonly used to measure the intensity of illumination. A photometer is used to assess the amount of light in an area. The amount of light is affected by the spacing of light sources, the amount of shadow and glare, the extent to which control of outside light is possible, and the brightness of the room's surfaces. Lighting standards vary, depending on the

* Some surgeons object to windowless operating rooms in spite of this.
† A foot-candle is the unit of intensity of illumination at a point of 1 ft from a standard candle. One candlepower is about equal to 1 watt consumption in a tungsten lamp.

kind of activity taking place in a given area. In work areas, proper lighting is essential for cleanliness, accident prevention, and reduction of fatigue.[20] Illumination of 50 to 70 foot-candles is recommended for prolonged reading. As much as 100 foot-candles is recommended for office work, while as little as 10 foot-candles is the illumination suggested for residential hallways, living rooms, and dining rooms.[21]

The human eye has remarkable power to adjust to conditions varying from bright daylight to semidarkness, but flickering light, which makes the eyes attempt rapid change, causes eye strain, fatigue, and nervousness. Glare and sharp contrast of light in the work area have the same effect. Fluorescent lighting, which provides a large surface of diffused light, is effective because it eliminates some of these difficulties. It is used extensively in work areas in industry. Properly placed fluorescent lighting provides steady, even illumination, free from deep shadows. It is also bright and cheerful and uses less power per lumen. Indirect lighting, which provides a source of light not visible to the eye, is also effective. If lamps are used at a desk to supplement room lighting, the whole work area should be illuminated.[22]

Much less light is needed to read a page of black print on very white paper than to read the same print on gray paper. A person sewing on black cloth needs far more light than is needed for either white or gray. Dust on light bulbs and in the atmosphere cuts down illumination. Nurses must bear in mind, too, that as persons grow older, they require more light. The middle-aged man or woman requires ten times as much light for clear vision as the young child. Persons with defective vision need more light, generally speaking, than those who see well, and, according to Sidney A. Fox,[23] the light blue eye requires less light than the dark. Health workers should be ever alert to special needs of patients and personnel.

Artificial Lighting of Patients' Rooms. On the basis of a series of studies, the US Public Health Service has provided the following guidelines for lighting patients' rooms in hospitals: lighting should be based on each patient's physical and psychologic needs, specific care and treatment needs, and considerations of safety and accident prevention. Sufficient light should be provided for all activities performed in the room, including those of nurses, physicians, technicians, therapists, housekeeping and maintenance personnel, and visitors. Various functions, particularly in a multibed room, require different illumination levels, ranging from a fraction of a foot-candle for night lighting to 100 foot-candles or more for examinations and treatments. Several steps of lighting levels within this range are needed. Glare from light sources and reflecting surfaces should be kept low enough to prevent discomfort for any person in the room. The degree of discomfort caused by glare is related to a person's physical well-being; nurses and doctors are not discomforted by brightness to the same degree as most patients. The goal of the staff should be to get enough light at the right locations to perform their tasks efficiently without subjecting the patient to uncomfortable brightness.

General lighting should be indirect, and excessive spottiness minimized. Controls for dimming lights are desirable. Fluorescent lamps should be the deluxe (warm- or cool-white) type. Reading lights should provide a reasonable degree of uniformity of lighting over an area of 3 sq ft for an adjustable light source, and 6 sq ft for a nonadjustable unit. Extension cords to connect portable lamps should be avoided; they are an electrical hazard, collect dust, and may cause accidents.

Local lighting for the purpose of observation should be provided or installed where needed and should be positioned to light the necessary equipment and the bed area; if this light remains on all night, provision should be made to shield the light from other patients. Lights for examination of patients should also be shielded or adjusted to confine the illumination to the bed area. Shadows on the lighted area should be minimized as much as possible.

Nightlights should provide a low level of illumination. They are not intended to supply enough light to see the patient's expression or to give nursing care but rather to detect conditions demanding additional light. The preferred location is near the floor, at the room entrance. A control switch mounted at the door, to switch the nightlight to a higher level, is useful.

Permanently installed light fixtures as well as movable or extendable lamps that can be attached to beds, other pieces of furniture, and the wall are useful in patients' rooms. Some types of lighting systems can be used for both examinations and for reading, but in most instances it is impractical to combine these lighting features. Permanently installed units have the advantage that they do not interfere with the staff members' use of both hands or with the free movement of doctors and nurses.[24] It is highly important that rational bed patients have within their reach a light that they can control.

Color of walls and furnishings is an important consideration in the selection and design of lighting systems. A study of the effect of color on light has shown that, with the same light source, brightness (measured by foot-lamberts) * varied with different colored walls and ceilings from 170 foot-lamberts with white walls to 20 with black, with a wide variation inbetween with different colors and shades.[25]

Lighting in the newborn nursery should permit easy detection of jaundice and cyanosis. This requires shadow-free illumination of at least 100 foot-candles intensity at the infants' level. Fluorescent tubes, deluxe cool-white, are recommended. A portable lamp containing two 15-watt fluorescent bulbs held 12 in. away from the infant will produce a light intensity of about 100 foot-candles.[26]

Chapter 46 includes a discussion of the special needs of those with defective vision.

Psychologic Aspects of Light in Illness. Everyone is susceptible to the cheering effect of sunlight, and, while sickness occasionally makes an individual hypersensitive to light, it is usually a mistake to darken "the sickroom."

Alfred W. Worcester,[27] a physician of long experience, commented on the tendency of the dying to turn toward light as vision waned. Nurses should help patients and their families to recognize the value of light and should use their influence in providing well-lighted dwellings for the sick and well. In hospitals, beds should be placed so that occupants do not face the window when lying on their back but are able to see the outdoors by turning. Since the patient's condition determines positions that can be assumed, it may be desirable in hospital rooms to have signal and electric light connections on two walls, so that several arrangements of the furniture can be made. It should be possible to regulate light with window shades. In rare cases it is necessary to shut out daylight almost entirely, although in most cases the eyes rather than the windows should be shielded.

The sick person's day is usually planned so that there are periods morning and afternoon when the room is kept light, not only for the beneficial effect of light but to facilitate medical and nursing care and to make it possible for the patient to read, to see friends, or to be occupied in some way. There should likewise be rest hours, especially after meals, when the shades are drawn and the patient is encouraged to relax or sleep. Changes such as this in the environment help to give some variety to the day and make the time pass more quickly. Good lighting, both natural and artificial, is important wherever human beings live because of its effect on mind and spirit as well as body.

* A foot-lambert is a unit of photometric brightness (luminance).

4. REGULATING ATMOSPHERIC CONDITIONS

Conditions Affecting Health. Temperature, air movement, humidity, radiation, atmospheric pressure, and the relative purity of air affect comfort and health. Man alone in the animal kingdom has been able to adapt to and control his environment to the extent that he can survive for long periods under atmospheric conditions ordinarily incompatible with human life—in polar regions, under the sea, and in outer space. He has also adapted meteorologic atmospheres for utilization in treatment of disease.

Temperature and Relative Humidity. Tolerance of heat and cold depends on the amount of moisture in the air; for this reason the two are considered together.

Tolerance for high environmental temperatures has been studied rather extensively with young men; less is known about the tolerance of older and younger persons. The ability of man to adjust to high temperature depends largely upon his condition. The following factors lower his tolerance: heavy physical work, lack of acclimatization, extensive dehydration, improper clothing, old age, lack of physical fitness, and excessive adipose tissue. Man can tolerate air temperatures as high as 115.5°C (240°F) with low humidity for short periods, whereas, for long periods under some conditions, he cannot tolerate even 31.1°C (88°F).

When thermal strain raises the pulse rate to 140 beats per minute when sitting or 180 beats per minute when exercising, the person is on the borderline of collapse. When loss of body fluid through sweating exceeds 1800 ml per hour, an individual at rest cannot sustain the fluid loss; when exercising, loss of 3900 ml is fatal. The loss of so much water or sodium chloride, which is present in concentrations of 0.06 to 0.6 per cent in sweat, is dangerous. During periods of excessive sweating, lost body fluid must be replaced, but drinking water alone does not restore the blood volume; salt must be taken at the same time (see Chapter 42 for amounts). During hot weather, people have to make a voluntary effort to drink more water periodically throughout the day, as the sensation of thirst alone does not in most cases ensure replacement of water.[28] (Chapter 10 discusses fluid balance in detail.)

In hot weather, clothing of light color should be worn because it reflects infrared rays. Fabric should also be light in weight, dry quickly, and hold a little air in its meshes. Wet garments should be exchanged for dry before the wearer goes into a cool temperature. During excessive heat, in the absence of air conditioning, hospital workers should be given frequent rest periods. Patients who can leave their beds periodically should be encouraged to sit in chairs; this allows more air movement around the body surface. Cold baths reduce body temperature to a slight degree, as do cold drinks. Exposure to excessive heat may result in heat exhaustion, heat cramps, and heat stroke. These conditions are discussed in Chapter 42.

The physiological response to cold does not seem to result in great *tolerance for cold environmental temperatures*. The inactive human body can endure less than 6 hours of exposure to air at −12.2°C (+10°F); about 4 hours at −23.3°C (−10°F); 1½ hours at −40°C (−40°F); and 25 minutes at −56.6°C (−70°F). Even shorter periods of exposure to cold water at these temperatures can be tolerated. Age, amount of fatty tissues, physical fitness, physical exercise, and clothing—all affect adjustment to cold. Ordinarily, human beings prevent a drop of more than a few degrees of body temperature by muscular exercise and the use of protective clothing. If the body temperature falls to 27°C (80.6°F), the pulse rate and blood pressure drop, and numbness, weakness, and coma set in. Under these circumstances an individual is unable to do any of the things that would raise his temperature, and death occurs when the heart is no longer able to circulate the thickened (viscous) blood.

Hypothermia is an abnormally low body temperature resulting from an imbalance between body heat production and heat loss. Seriously low temperature levels are rarely caused by diminished production of body heat, except in debilitating states such as fatigue and metabolic disorders. Hypothermia resulting from accelerated loss of heat to the environment is more serious. An inadequately protected person immersed in water 0°C (32°F) will lose consciousness in about 5 to 15 minutes and die in 30 to 60 minutes.[29]

In the last decade, attention has been drawn by British clinicians to spontaneous hypothermia, a serious condition, among elderly people who live alone in unheated houses. When the body temperatures go as low as 32°C (89.6°F) to 25°C (77°F), pulse, respiration, and blood pressure are depressed, consciousness is impaired, shivering ceases, and subcutaneous edema may occur. This condition is sometimes wrongly diagnosed as cardiovascular accident. Rapid rewarming is contraindicated; it could cause sudden peripheral vasodilation and circulatory failure. Treatment consists of wrapping the person in blankets or warm clothing to allow gradual accumulation of body heat. If body temperatures stay above 32°C (89.6°F), the person usually recovers quickly when put in a comfortable environment. It has been estimated that as many as 2000 deaths from accidental hypothermia may occur each year in Great Britain.[30] Treatment of other conditions caused by excessive cold, such as frostbite, are discussed in Chapter 42.

Hypothermia is sometimes induced in preparation for cardiovascular surgery and neurosurgery because it depresses body processes. This is discussed briefly in Chapter 42.

Humidity. Because water is a better conductor of heat and cold than air, a person suffers from extremes of temperature more intensely as the amount of moisture in the atmosphere increases. A high moisture content intensifies the sensations of heat and cold, not only on account of the physical principle that water is a good conductor, but also because evaporation of sweat from the skin is retarded. Very dry air, on the other hand, speeds up evaporation of sweat, a process that uses body heat, so this may also produce the sensation of chilliness under some conditions.

Instruments—psychrometers and hygrometers—indicate the proportion of moisture in the air. When a given quantity at a given temperature contains as much water vapor as it can hold without precipitation as rain or snow, the humidity is said to be 100 per cent; if it contains half this amount of water vapor, the humidity is said to be 50 per cent, and so on. The reading of a hygrometer, calibrated in percentages, should therefore be taken to mean the relative amount of moisture in the air and not the actual water content.

Anna M. Baetjer[31] says that relative humidity plays only a small role in comfort except at very low and very high temperatures. The normal skin temperature exceeds the air temperature except in very hot weather; therefore, vaporization of sweat is, according to this authority, relatively constant in relative humidities of 15 to 75 per cent. The body compensates by increasing sweat production. When, however, the limit of compensation is reached and the entire body is covered with sweat, the relative humidity is the controlling factor in heat loss, and high humidities cause great discomfort.

Although outdoor humidity cannot be controlled by man, the water content of indoor air can be very accurately regulated. The relationship of humidity to health, however, is not as well established as its relationship to comfort. When temperature and humidity are properly regulated, room air feels soft and warm.

Thermal Standards for Heated Buildings. There is no point on the temperature scale that is the ideal indoor temperature for everyone. Individuals differ in their reactions to atmospheric conditions, and each person has periods of increased and decreased sensitivity to heat and cold. The ideal indoor temperature may be defined as one that does not make the person sitting in the room feel chilly, but is at the same time not warm enough to enervate or cause perceptible perspiration. Optimal conditions depend on the individual, his or her sensations, health, sex, age, and activity at a given time. Recommended temperature and humidity ranges vary from temperatures of 20° to 25°C (68° to 77°F) with relative humidities of 10 to 60 per cent.* Indoor humidity of 60 per cent or higher, however, would cause condensation and the possibility of mildew, corrosion, and decay.[32]

Relative humidity of 50 per cent is believed by some researchers to provide maximum comfort for most individuals and is most effective for removing microorganisms from the hospital atmosphere when a mechanical air-control system is in use. The relative humidity should be above 50 per cent in operating rooms, however, to reduce the hazard of anesthesia gas explosion.[33] This hazard is also reduced by a ventilation system that exchanges air frequently, which prevents accumulation of anesthesia gas.

"Cold steam" humidifiers that disseminate mist, are often used to combat dryness in overheated homes. They should not be used in hospitals, however, because they may harbor and spread gram-negative microorganisms. When hospitalized patients require higher humidity, it is usually provided by inhalation devices or, in the case of infants, by incubators, rather than by increasing the humidity in the room. (See Chapter 20.)

Temperature Control and Ventilation in Nurseries for the Newborn. Newborn and high-risk infants who have immature heat-regulating mechanisms need protection from radiant heat exchange with the environment. Special conditions are necessary to prevent excessive heat loss (or gain). At the time of birth the air temperature in the delivery room should be 22° to 24°C (71.6° to 75.2°F), with a relative humidity of approximately 50 per cent for the comfort of the working personnel. A source of radiant heat (heat lamp, heated bed, or warmed incubator) should be available for the infant immediately after birth, and later when the infant is undressed or out of a warm environment for special procedures.

Air temperature in the nursery should be

28° to 30°C (82.4° to 86°F), with a relative humidity less than 50 per cent, again for comfort of the staff. Ideally, the nursery should be air-conditioned, with ventilation and heat units separate from the main hospital system so that they may be turned off in an emergency. The intake of fresh, uncontaminated air should be near the ceiling and the output near the floor, with the air pressure inside the room slightly greater than in adjacent areas. There should be at least 12 changes of room air every hour, and the room should be free of drafts. Neither chemical air disinfectants nor ultraviolet lamps should be used to decontaminate the air in nurseries.

Small or premature infants may require a relatively high environmental temperature—34°C (93.2°F) or even higher to prevent a drop in body temperature; larger infants need less supplemental heat—30°C (86°F). In order to determine the correct environmental temperature, the temperature of the infant and of the immediate environment should be taken simultaneously. A body temperature of 36.5° to 37°C (97.7° to 98.6°F) is considered normal, but the precise optimal body temperature for low birth weight infants has not been determined. Relative humidity should be 50 to 65 per cent in incubators. Higher humidities may be necessary to reduce heat loss in infants weighing less than 1500 gm (3 lb, 5 oz) who cannot otherwise be kept warm. High humidities are not necessary to maintain body temperature when supplemental heat is provided by radiant sources rather than warmed air in the incubator.[34]

Oxygen Therapy for Infants. Oxygen, when necessary, must be administered to newborn infants with caution because of the risk of causing blindness due to abnormal growth of fibrous tissue behind the crystalline lens (retrolental fibroplasia). Arterial blood gas should be measured when possible, in order to determine safe oxygen concentration levels. A normal newborn has an oxygen tension in arterial blood of 60 to 100 mm Hg. Oxygen-enriched mixtures should be regulated to keep the oxygen tension close to this range. Mixtures of oxygen and room air may be delivered to the infant by endotracheal tubes, masks, funnels, hoods, or incubators. Mixtures should be warmed and humidified regardless of method of delivery. Incubators should be thoroughly cleaned and decontaminated after each use. (See also Chapter 20.)

Air Movement and Variability. Warm air weighs less than cold and therefore tends to rise. Air currents of different temperatures have a refreshing effect on the body. They induce circulatory changes and lower the skin

---

* People from Europe generally find North American buildings overheated. Many authorities have commented on this as a health hazard.

temperature by increasing evaporation of sweat and also by carrying the air heated by the body away from it. High indoor and outdoor temperatures can be tolerated if there is sufficient air movement. On the other hand, discomfort from low temperatures is increased when there is marked air movement, because rapid evaporation of sweat, with its accompanying heat loss, chills the body. Since outdoor air usually has the virtue of variability, it is much more refreshing than indoor air. Good ventilation requires that the air contain a suitable amount of moisture, and that it be in gentle motion, free from offensive odors, poisonous fumes, and large amounts of dust, and that it be of a comfortable temperature. When the outdoor air is clean, the temperature neither too hot nor too cool, the humidity consistent with human comfort, and the atmospheric pressure within tolerable limits, dwellings can be adequately ventilated with doors, windows, and chimneys. This is called natural ventilation. An enclosed space is said to be *air-conditioned* when the contained air is circulated, impurities removed, and the temperature and humidity regulated. With air conditioning, it is now possible to approximate indoors the desirable features of outdoor air. When natural ventilation by means of windows, doors, and fireplaces is not sufficient, as in public buildings, air movement and variability can be effected by one of three types of mechanical ventilation: (1) the vacuum system, which withdraws air from the room by exhaust or suction fans; (2) the plenum system, which forces air into the room by fans; and (3) a combination of both. Efficient air-conditioning systems, particularly in areas where air is polluted, filter and exchange, or recirculate, air to keep it as free as possible from contaminants. In hospitals, ventilation is a factor in control of infection. An adequate ventilation system, well maintained, helps keep airborne microbial contamination of the environment at a low level. Microorganisms attached to particles of dust, lint, and respiratory droplets should not be permitted to move from one area of the hospital to another in uncontrolled airstreams. Such movement is particularly serious if contaminated air is allowed to enter areas housing susceptible patients or sterile equipment and supplies. By regulating the amount of air blown into and drawn out of a room it is possible to dilute the air, thereby removing almost all airborne contamination. This does not prevent microbial shedding from people in the room, however— a constant occurrence—nor does it protect against contamination by direct contact with contaminated hands, a far more serious and

more frequent cause of microbial transfer than air transmission.

It is generally agreed that sensitive areas of a hospital such as operating rooms, delivery rooms, and nurseries should be provided with air as nearly bacteria-free as possible. To accomplish this, all outdoor inlets should be located as high above ground level as possible. Inlets should not be near ventilation discharge outlets, incinerators, or boiler stacks. High efficiency filters should be used in systems serving these and other high-risk areas. Departmental zoning of air systems helps confine the air to a single department, reducing the possibility that air from one unit mixes with air from other parts of the hospital. Finally, air pressure in specific areas should be controlled so that it is greater inside the room than out, thus preventing contaminated air from entering through doorways to adjacent areas.[35] In critical areas, however, doors should be kept closed, even when air pressure is regulated.

The aerospace industry has developed a method of filtering and controlling air movement to exclude or remove virtually all airborne particulate matter, even that shed by room occupants. With the method of controlling air known as laminar flow, a large volume of highly filtered air is moved uniformly to a confined or enclosed area. The air circulating in the room is self-cleaning, as it carries particulate matter away from critical work areas. It is forced into the room through high-efficiency filters in the ceiling and out of the room through gratings in the floor, or it is forced from wall to wall with filters on one side of the room and grates in the opposite wall. The laminar flow principle is used in a variety of areas, ranging from small hood-type enclosures to full size rooms.[36] Laminar flow has been used in operating rooms and in rooms for patients with severe burns. Even though it is expensive to install and is not widely used in health care facilities at this time, laminar flow systems may eventually help control contamination in many critical areas of the hospital such as nurseries, isolation areas, intensive care units, central supply work areas for the processing of sterile supplies, autopsy rooms, and microbiologic laboratories.[37]

Air Conditioning. Today, many homes in the United States and most public buildings, as well as public vehicles, are air-conditioned. Over the past 25 years air conditioning has brought many changes in life styles and has become a valuable adjunct in patient care and treatment—in operating rooms, nurseries, maternity and delivery rooms, x-ray rooms, and wards for control of allergic disorders. It has affected people's mobility by allowing them to choose where to live or work without being restricted by considerations of comfort. It has brought about changes in building codes and building design by permitting use of space away from windows, which was formerly considered submarginal. By permitting the closing out of street noise and dust, it has made lower floors as acceptable as upper. It permits higher occupancy per square foot of floor space and less expensive floor plans by eliminating the need for narrow wings or light and ventilation courts. By permitting higher lighting intensities, air conditioning has improved work efficiency.[38] In hot areas, air conditioning of homes, office buildings, and industrial plants has markedly decreased the lethargy attributed to those who live in the debilitating climate. Perhaps one of the most important benefits of air conditioning is the removal of noxious agents from the air.*

In private dwellings, activated charcoal filters, which remove most irritating pollutants, can be added to standard air-conditioning equipment. Such filters, along with well-ventilated cooking stoves and heating equipment, make it possible for people living in polluted areas to have purer air inside than out. Electrostatic air-cleaning units are also available, but they produce ozone gas and do not remove chemical smoke from the air.[39] The best air-cleaning units combine an absolute filter with the activated carbon unit and the air conditioner.

Purity of Air. Absolutely pure air is rarely if ever found; the air over the ocean and on mountain summits is most free of contaminants. Today, air pollution, particularly over congested areas, is a major health hazard. Smog caused by air inversion can be lethal to people already suffering from chronic respiratory or cardiovascular diseases. Air pollution has been responsible for a number of disasters. In London in 1952, one incidence of smog took the lives of 4000 persons. In 1956, during an 18-hour period, 1000 persons died when heavy smog settled over New York City. In December 1930, 60 persons died in the Meuse River Valley in Belgium when a fog polluted by oxides of sulfur lay over the area. In October 1948, in Donora, Pennsylvania, there were 17 deaths and hundreds were ill during a similar episode. In 1950, in the oil-refining town of Poza Rica, Mexico, over 300 people were ill and 22 died when hydrogen sulfide gas was accidentally spilled. All of these episodes

occurred under extraordinary meteorologic conditions that reduced the volume of the air in which the pollutants were diluted.[40] Aside from these and other dramatic episodes, the particulate and gaseous irritants in polluted air exert a continuous, insidious, cumulative effect. One 6-year study showed that the over-all death rates for people living in heavily polluted areas were twice as high as the death rates in less polluted areas, while the death rates from tuberculosis and stomach cancer were three times as high. Other diseases associated with air pollution are bronchial asthma, chronic bronchitis, lung cancer, and conjunctivitis.[41]

In addition to being harmful to health, pollutants in the air damage property, equipment, and facilities. Pollution makes more frequent cleaning and use of air-filtering equipment necessary and intercepts part of the light from the sun, increasing the use of electricity in the daytime. Damage done by air pollution to plants, trees, livestock, and food crops is estimated at $500 million a year in the United States. Carbon monoxide is the principal pollutant by weight, and the motor vehicle, which also discharges lead from gasoline, is the major contributor, followed by industry and power plants. Other sources of air pollution are agricultural spraying of pesticides, orchard heating devices, exhausts from various commercial processes, rubber from tires, asbestos dust from brakes, mist from spray-type cooling towers, the use of cleaning solvents and household chemicals, various aerosols, and, last on this list but by no means least, tobacco smoke. Stack pollution from processing nuclear fuel and nuclear reactors, and nuclear explosions are also potential sources of pollution.[42]

Not all pollution is man-made, however. Natural pollutants, consisting of spores and pollen given off by plants, and fungi are a menace to persons who are allergic to them. Dust disseminated by wind, earthquakes, volcanic eruptions, and traffic is a potential hazard to respiration.[43]

Air stagnation is a contributing factor. In the Los Angeles area, mountain ranges prevent unobstructed horizontal flow of the surrounding air, while frequent temperature inversion conditions limit vertical movement. Pollutants trapped under the inversion layer move back and forth under alternating sea and land winds. This meteorologic condition is not limited to the west coast of the United States; it is a frequent occurrence over the whole country wherever air inversion results from a cold layer of air remaining close to the ground.[44]

Prevention and Treatment of Air Pollution. Although it is possible to exclude some pollutants from indoor air by air conditioning and

---

* The disadvantages of "climate control" should be mentioned. All air conditioning requires electric or other forms of energy, thus depleting even further our limited energy resources.

filtering systems, there are no methods for improving the quality of outdoor air. Control measures must therefore combat the sources of pollution. Federal and local governments, industry, and concerned citizens' groups are working toward that goal. Air pollution in London has, for example, been significantly reduced in recent years through such cooperation. There are a few measures that may be taken to combat some of the ill effects anywhere. In Los Angeles, the County Medical Association has advised residents to stay indoors from mid-morning to mid-afternoon when smog is heavy and to keep doors and windows closed and use air conditioners that filter and recirculate inside air without drawing outside air in. People are advised to avoid strenuous physical activity, to get extra rest, to avoid stimulating foods, drinks, and medicines that increase metabolism, and to reduce to a minimum major cooking, cleaning, and shopping activities. They are advised not to smoke, to avoid dusts, fumes, sprays, or aerosols, and to avoid congested or dangerous freeway traffic. Those with respiratory diseases are advised that, prior to any emergency, they should seek treatment and instruction in the use of oxygen and bronchodilator drugs; they should also learn techniques of respiratory assistance with intermittent positive pressure breathing devices.[45] (See Chapter 20.)

Air Pressure. When man invades the ocean's depths or the stratosphere, or even climbs very high mountains, the effect on health of atmospheric pressure must be considered.

At sea level the atmosphere exerts a pressure of 14.7 lb per square inch on any object, including the body. This pressure decreases progressively with the altitude. At sea level the atmosphere supports a column of mercury 760 mm in height; at 50,000 feet above sea level, only 87 mm. (This mercury instrument is called a barometer, and atmospheric pressure is often called barometric pressure.) Atmospheric pressure of 14.7 lb per square inch is spoken of as 1 atm (atmosphere); the pressure under water at 300 ft below sea level is equal to 10 atmospheres or 147 lb per square inch. Because the atmosphere and the ocean exert an equal pressure over all parts of the living organism, the body is not destroyed by this enormous force. On the other hand, all animals are sensitive to marked changes in the pressures of gases, particularly oxygen, in air and water. The proportion of gases in the air is constant at all altitudes (nitrogen 79 per cent, oxygen 20.96 per cent, carbon dioxide 0.04 per cent, and traces of other gases), but at high altitudes, where the air pressure is low, the number of molecules of each gas in a given quantity of air is actually smaller and therefore the "partial pressure" of each gas is low. Under these circumstances the inhaled air is relatively poorer in oxygen, nitrogen, and carbon dioxide. At low altitudes the air in any given volume contains more molecules of each gas than that same amount of air at sea level. Since the concentration of oxygen and nitrogen in the blood is directly related to their partial pressures in the inhaled air, reactions to high and low altitudes are the result of lowered or raised concentrations of these gases in the tissues.

Man's body economy with relation to exchange of gases is apparently geared to the partial gas pressures near the earth's surface. Rachel L. Carson [46] says that marine animals who live near the surface of the ocean cannot sustain life in the ocean depths and that deepsea fish are thought to be destroyed when upheavals of the sea bring them to the surface. When human beings travel great distances into the air or the depths of the sea, they must surround themselves with airtight chambers in which gas pressures can be regulated or oxygen fed to them, just as in some diseases affecting the amount of oxygen available to victims, they must be provided with an environment in which the contained gases are regulated to the patient's needs. (See Chapter 20.) When persons exposed to high altitudes for a long time descend rapidly to sea level, when miners go down a mine shaft, or when a deepsea diver descends into the ocean, they may, on their return to sea level, suffer the *toxic effect of high gas pressure,* or of compression, unless ascent is gradual, or made in stages.

The symptoms experienced as they are *decompressed* occur from 30 minutes to 12 hours after rapidly ascending from a low altitude and are believed to be caused by bubbles of nitrogen that, in the higher altitude, can no longer be held in solution in the blood. This condition is variously called decompression sickness, caisson disease, the "bends" (because pain makes the victim double up), the "chokes" (because of nausea, vomiting, and coughing), the "staggers" (because of dizziness), and the "itches." Death can and does result if the person is not again compressed and then gradually decompressed. This requires a decompression chamber.

Hazards Associated with Diving. Diving, either with or without scuba equipment, involves certain hazards. Mechanical injuries to lungs may result from pressure changes. If the breath is held while diving, the thoracic cage is compressed to the position of maximal expiration. On further descent, air within the lungs can no longer be compressed to counter the increasing external pressure, resulting in a condition known as thoracic squeeze, which is characterized by pulmonary congestion, edema, and hemorrhage. Breathing denser air delivered by scuba equipment while under water or through a long snorkel tube may also create a relatively negative pressure within the lungs, with similar consequences. After breathing the denser air while under water it must be released from the lungs during ascent. Otherwise, expanding air in the lungs builds up sufficient pressure to rupture lung tissue, resulting in pneumothorax, mediastinal emphysema, or air embolism. Air embolism has reportedly been caused by dives into water as shallow as 9 ft.[47]

In addition to the danger of air embolism, scuba (self-contained underwater breathing apparatus) * diving to depths greater than 30 ft may result in decompression sickness. Today, scuba diving is one of the fastest growing sports in the United States. Millions of people who lack basic understanding of the effects of increased underwater pressure are making hazardous dives with scuba gear. Learning to breathe underwater with this equipment is deceptively simple, and anyone may buy and use it without demonstrating proficiency in its use. Consequently, decompression sickness is an increasingly common occurrence. A high percentage of patients treated in US Navy recompression chambers are civilian recreational scuba divers.[48]

Scuba equipment requires the diver to breathe through a mouthpiece without protection of a helmet. Low air supply, or any mishap, forces the relatively unprotected diver to ascend rapidly to the surface without adequate decompression, which is normally achieved by ascending in stages.[49] Rapidity of ascent should be governed by the depth of the dive and the amount of time spent at that depth. Inadequate decompression can produce nitrogen bubbles in tissues and bloodstream, asphyxia, or paralytic injury to the spinal cord. Either air embolism or serious decompression sickness requires treatment in a recompression chamber at the earliest possible moment. Meanwhile, mouth-to-mouth artificial respiration should be carried out if necessary.[50]

Albert Behnke,[51] a physician, suggests that all diving groups should have a small, one-man portable chamber pressurized with oxygen to 3 atmospheres. A device of that kind could prevent injury and possible death. The same type of portable pressurized chamber can be used for emergency oxygen treatment in carbon monoxide asphyxia, coronary thrombosis, asphyxia of the newborn, and for vitalization of damaged tissues resulting from injury.

The Hyperbaric Environment. Hyperbaric oxygenation is achieved by increasing atmospheric pressure within sealed chambers to levels varying from two to four atmospheres. In addition to treating acute asphyxia and decompression sickness, hyperbaric therapy is used to treat fulminating gas gangrene infection and to provide increased tissue oxygenation in cardiac surgery and x-ray therapy. Hypothermia and hyperbaric oxygen have a synergistic effect. In deep hypothermia, oxygen is not released adequately from red blood cells. This can be corrected to some extent by the pressure of oxygen in physical solution brought about by the hyperbaric atmosphere. Under conditions of deep hypothermia combined with hyperbaric oxygen, the heart and brain have recovered their function following deprivation of blood for 30 minutes or more. This has opened the way for the preservation of living tissue for subsequent transplantation at a later time.[52]

Inhalation Therapy. A different kind of remedial atmosphere is provided by oxygen inhalation and aerosol therapy, which makes possible the dispersion of vasodilators and other medications as submicroscopic particles (in concentrations of 20 million particles per cubic centimeter of air) throughout the entire lung system. The amount of drug thus employed can be small enough to have no systemic effect. Wetting agents and detergents are utilized to loosen secretions in cystic fibrosis. There are disadvantages associated with respiratory therapy, however. Antibiotics such as penicillin should not be administered as aerosols because of the hazard of sensitization, and nebulizers and respirators can harbor gram-negative organisms such as *Pseudomonas* and are therefore a potential source of serious infection unless scrupulously cleaned and sterilized.[53] (See page 1426 and also Chapters 20 and 32.)

High Altitudes. Effects of high altitude differ with the person's ability to adjust to it, the rapidity of ascent, and the duration of exposure to it. Given time, the body can accommodate itself, but sudden ascents produce the *toxic symptoms of low gas pressures*. These are as follows: changes in pulse and respiratory rates and in blood pressure; headache; nausea and vomiting; fatigue; psychologic symptoms of depression or euphoria, or loss of memory; and, if the ascent is great enough, loss of voluntary muscle control, impairment

---

* A portable compressed-air reservoir that automatically delivers air to the diver on demand, at the same atmospheric pressure as that surrounding the diver.

of the special senses, coma, and death. These symptoms are associated with hypoxia, a term that refers to reduced partial pressure of oxygen at high altitudes. At 5000 ft, night vision is impaired. At about 10,000 ft, dyspnea may appear, and in some persons mental concentration is difficult. Above 15,000 ft, impaired judgment threatens the safety of fliers and mountain climbers. Between altitudes of 18,000 and 25,000 ft, unconsciousness occurs. Rapid descent or administration of oxygen is necessary to prevent death.

Acute mountain sickness is a clinical syndrome seen in some persons within a few hours after rapid exposure to high altitude, in some instances at only 8000 ft. Symptoms are incapacitating headache, dyspnea on exertion, malaise, weakness, insomnia, anorexia, nausea, vomiting, and diarrhea. Symptoms usually subside gradually in a few days. They are relieved by oxygen or by returning to a lower altitude.

Chronic mountain sickness is a loss of tolerance to hypoxia occurring in residents previously acclimatized to high altitudes. This condition is common at altitudes over 14,000 ft and is manifested by marked cyanosis, dyspnea, palpitations, headache, giddiness, muscular weakness, pain in the extremities, and episodic stupor. It can be cured only by descending to a lower altitude.[54]

Problems Associated with Air Travel. For the healthy person and for most ill patients (often transported by air) air travel is not hazardous. Before transporting patients, however, there are a few factors to be considered. In high-flying jet airplanes, cabin pressure is maintained at higher than ground level altitude, or about 75 per cent of sea level pressure. It is often equivalent to altitudes as high as 7000 to 9000 ft. At these altitudes, a bubble of gas trapped within the body will expand, causing pressure on surrounding tissues. This may interfere with blood supply and rupture tissue walls. Persons with unreduced hernia, or with perforating wounds of the eyeball or skull, should not fly, nor should patients with pneumothorax, lung cavities, lung abscesses, or recent pneumoencephalography. Similar precautions should be taken for 2 weeks following abdominal surgery. Persons with acute upper respiratory tract disease, chronic sinusitis, or allergic rhinitis may have discomfort in the sinuses or middle ear, which may be modified by use of decongestant nose drops or inhalers before flight. Because of other hazards associated with reduced oxygen, advance arrangements should be made to have supplemental oxygen continuously available during flight for patients with myocardial infarction,

angina pectoris, anemia when hemoglobin is less than 50 per cent, sickle-cell disease, developing gangrene, carbon monoxide poisoning, or any pulmonary disease severe enough to cause cyanosis at ground level.

Healthy infants tolerate air travel well, but they should be given something to suck during descent, as swallowing helps to equalize the pressure in the middle ear. Adults may find that chewing gum reduces discomfort, even pain, in the ears. Old age and pregnancy are not contraindications to flight, nor is hypertension.

There are other problems associated with flight that are not a consequence of altitude. Some of these are impaired circulation in the legs due to prolonged sitting and inactivity, and motion sickness, which is due to labyrinthine stimulation resulting from repetitive movement in space. Air travelers should move about frequently during long flights to promote circulation. Motion sickness may sometimes be prevented by the use of drugs such as Dramamine taken 30 minutes before takeoff and every 4 to 6 hours during long flights. Symptoms usually disappear soon after the journey ends. Of course, everyone who flies is subjected to the potential hazard of hypoxia from rapid decompression should cabin pressure fail. For this reason, emergency oxygen is available at every seat on high flying planes. Finally, everyone who flies across time zones is subject to disturbances in natural body rhythms.[55]

The Effect of Air Travel on Circadian Rhythms. The tie between biologic functioning and environmental or cosmic forces over which we have no control is an intriguing phenomenon. Just as certain celestial and natural events occur at periodic intervals—night following day, the ebb and flow of tide, and the rhythmic change of seasons—our life processes, too, are repetitive, periodic, and follow predictable time patterns. The biologic functioning of all living things, plant and animal alike, is governed by an inner biologic clock, which is synchronized and in harmony with the outer cosmic clock. Among our biologic rhythms are those of a beating heart, of breathing, and of waking and sleeping. Rhythm characterizes menstruation and the onset of labor and birth. Everyone has customary sleep-awake and rest-work cycles that are resistant to change. Every form of life has an inborn timetable that determines its rate of growth, maturation, and decline. Some of our biologic functions have a 24-hour cycle and are affected by light and dark—by the cycles of sunrise and sunset. The term circadian refers to the rhythmic biologic cycles that recur at approximately 24-hour intervals. It means approximately the same thing as diurnal, which means "daily." [56] Rapid, long-distance air travel across several time zones disrupts circadian rhythms, posing a stress for the air traveler. This disruption is referred to as circadian-rhythm desynchronization or, more simply, "jet-lag." It is characterized by changes in physiologic and psychologic functioning. After flights through seven to 12 time zones, fatigue and insomnia frequently occur; reaction time and decision-making may be adversely affected, and there are changes in body temperature, heart rate, water and electrolyte excretion, and other body functions. Because of potentially dangerous transitory impairment of performance, airplane crew members are required to take specified rest periods between flights. The length of the rest periods is determined by the length of travel time, and the number of time zones crossed. Out-of-phase functioning is more easily restored to normal after east-to-west flights than west-to-east. It is apparently easier to delay circadian rhythms than to advance them. Persons can delay going to sleep for a few hours with greater ease, for example, than forcing sleep when they are not ready for it. Flights from north to south and south to north that do not involve the crossing of time zones do not have the same effect. Symptoms as well as the time required to get "on schedule" at destination, are affected by times of departure and arrival, length and direction of flight, travel experience, stress, age, physical condition, and food, liquor, and other drugs consumed during the flight. Sleep during flight and changes in climate and in the new social environment also affect a traveler's reaction. Adjusting sleep habits and overcoming fatigue during the period of rephasing may take from one to several days, while the deeper physiologic cycles require longer periods—from 4 to 8 days. Travelers are advised to plan for sufficient rest before and after long flights, to avoid additional stress, including heavy eating and drinking, and to delay making important decisions in the first 24 hours after deplaning. [57-59]

5. WATER SUPPLY AND WASTE DISPOSAL

Water Supply. An adequate supply of clear, palatable, sanitary water is essential for good health.

About two thirds of the world's people are without a safe supply of water for bathing and drinking. In underdeveloped countries there is a high prevalence of waterborne disease. Even though water supplies in the United States are among the purest in the world, there are wide differences in the relative purity of water in both urban and rural communities. Sources of city water, if they are small lakes and reservoirs, are usually protected from pollution by restricting habitation around their borders. Where the water comes from large lakes or rivers, however, it is impossible to prevent pollution. In such cases the water is made relatively pure by physical processes, or by natural means of purification, such as aeration, exposure to sunlight, sedimentation, oxidation, and storage in lakes with controlled animal and vegetable life. When these measures are unavailable, or inadequate if used alone, water is treated with a chemical, such as chlorine.

Source of Water. The source of water is rainfall. It falls directly into ponds, streams, or lakes, or soaks into the ground and becomes *ground water,* which is made available at a later time through springs and wells. Water taken from rivers, lakes, and ponds is referred to as *surface water*. Today, surface water, which is the source of water for most cities, is not safe for drinking without purification. If ground water passes through sand or gravel for a considerable distance (around 100 ft), microorganisms and particles of dirt will be strained out, making the water safe to drink even though it may contain a high content of dissolved minerals. There is always danger of ground water becoming polluted, however. Water from springs or wells may be clear and cold but not necessarily safe to drink. It is possible for pollution to reach the source of ground water by a rivulet if ground is broken by limestone or rock. During heavy rains the ground may become saturated with polluted surface water. If water from a well or spring becomes turbid or colored after a rainstorm, it may possibly be polluted. To avoid contamination by sewage, a privy or septic field should be located at least 100 ft from a well, and drainage from the source of pollution should be away from the water supply, not toward it. Water from deep wells is usually more reliable than that from shallow wells, as it is less subject to pollution from surface water. About 19 per cent of the population in the United States depend on private supplies of ground water, and many small towns and cities also use ground water for drinking. It is easily protected and leaves surface water for other purposes. [60]

The US Public Health Service has outlined standards for drinking water purity. [61] Water supply systems used by ships, planes, and buses crossing state lines must conform to these standards, but thousands of small community and privately owned water supply systems are not subject to surveillance and control.

A government survey completed in 1970 showed that 16 per cent of 969 public water supply systems investigated did not comply with suggested standards. This survey covered only a small percentage of the 19,236 public water supplies known to be in operation at that time and did not include private water sources, on which millions of people were, and still are, dependent.[62]

Safety and purity of private water sources are the responsibility of the property owners. If there is doubt about water from privately owned wells or cisterns, samples may be taken to local health authorities for analysis. Many people are exposed to questionable water supplies when traveling or camping. When there is doubt about the purity of any water, it should be purified before drinking. During epidemics or disasters, when a water emergency exists, local or state health departments should be consulted, but it may become necessary to decontaminate drinking water without waiting for directions. The simplest and most reliable method of purifying small quantities of water when fuel is available is to boil it for one minute. Chlorination (adding chlorine) is a satisfactory method for purifying water not grossly polluted—water from a

relatively clean lake, stream, or well, for example. Chlorine, used as a household bleach, is readily available in powder, liquid, and tablet forms from drugstores and grocery stores. The powder is calcium hypochlorite, and the liquid, sodium hypochlorite. The strength, expressed as percentage of available chlorine, is printed on the container label.

To decontaminate water, prepare a concentrated stock solution to be added to the desired amount of water to be purified. See Table 15-1 for the quantity of chlorine needed to prepare a stock solution, and for the quantity of stock solution needed to disinfect 1 gal and 1000 gal of water. When using powder to make a stock solution, make a paste with a small amount of water and dissolve it in 1 qt of water. Allow it to settle, and use the clear liquid only. Chlorine preparations deteriorate with age and exposure to light; solutions should be stored in the dark, and stock solutions should be made up every week. After treating the water let it stand for at least 30 minutes before using.

Water-purifying tablets containing chlorine, suitable for use on camping trips, are available in drugstores. Because they are slow-acting, water treated with them should stand for 60 minutes before using. The tablets, like other forms of chlorine, also deteriorate with age. If chlorine is not available, 8 drops of 2

Table 15-1. Emergency Disinfection of Small Volumes of Water * †

Product	Available Chlorine, %	Stock Solution ‡	Quantity of Stock Solution to Treat 1 gal of Water §	Quantity of Stock Solution to Treat 1000 gal of Water †
Zonite	1	Use full strength	30 drops	2 qt
S.K., 101 solution	2½	Use full strength	12 drops	1 qt
Clorox, White Sail, Dazzle, Rainbow, Rose-X	5¼	Use full strength	6 drops	1 pt
Sodium hypochlorite	10	Use full strength	3 drops	½ pt
Sodium hypochlorite	15	Use full strength	2 drops	¼ pt
Calcium hypochlorite, "bleaching powder," or chlorinated lime	25	6 heaping table-spoonfuls (3 oz) to 1 qt of water	1 teaspoonful or 75 drops	1 qt
Calcium hypochlorite	33	4 heaping table-spoonfuls to 1 qt of water	1 teaspoonful	1 qt
HTH, Perchloron, Pittchlor	70	2 heaping table-spoonfuls (1 oz) to 1 qt of water	1 teaspoonful	1 qt

* Salvato, Joseph, Jr.: *Environmental Engineering and Sanitation,* 2nd ed. Wiley-Interscience, New York, 1972, p. 253.
† Quantity of chlorine needed to prepare a stock solution, and quantity of stock solution needed to disinfect 1 gal and 1000 gal of water.
‡ One quart contains 135 ordinary teaspoonfuls of water.
§ Let stand 30 min before using. To dechlorinate, use sodium thiosulfate in same proportion as chlorine.

per cent tincture of iodine may be used to disinfect 1 qt of water. Allow it to stand for at least 30 minutes before using.[63]

Use of Water. Although water, like air and land, is a limited resource, the total amount of the earth's water is not diminished by our use. It is eventually converted by natural processes into rain again, but is unevenly distributed, and the world population is rapidly increasing. In the last 100 years the amount of rainfall has not increased, but our population has increased fivefold from 40 to more than 200 million.

The people of the United States, even in arid sections, use water lavishly. It is used in private swimming pools and lawn sprinklers and for numerous other purposes in addition to bathing and drinking. It is estimated that the average man uses 5 gal a day to shave, wash, and brush his teeth. A running shower uses 5 gal, while another 5 to 7 gal is used every time a toilet is flushed, and almost 30 gal in one load of home laundry. Agriculture and industry, too, consume vast amounts of water, and most industries demand water of high purity. Moreover, for years industry has been discharging huge amounts of pollutants into our water supply. City water, once used, becomes a waste carrier. In some areas it is collected by sewage pipes and carried, without being exposed to treatment, into the nearest river. That practice is condemned, however, and measures are being taken to stop it.

Management of Water Pollution. Waste water is being treated and recycled for continuing use by some communities. In Santee in Southern California, for example, reclaimed sewage water is salvaged and used for irrigation, as well as for supplying a large man-made lake used by residents for boating, swimming, and fishing. Many industries are restudying their waste disposal processes. Some wastes that were formerly dumped into rivers are now being used in the manufacture of pet foods, and in some areas treated sewage is being converted into fertilizer.[64]

Increasing the Water Supply. Converting sea water to fresh water is possible, but the process is expensive. A desalination plant in Freeport, Texas, which has been in operation since 1961, distills 1 million gal of water a day at a cost of $1.00 per 1000 gal. The average cost of supplying fresh water by other methods is $0.30 to $0.40 per 1000 gal. Methods of desalination, other than distillation, are being studied, including freezing and harvesting water crystals. It is expected that salt water conversion will eventually be possible at a fraction of the present cost.[65]

Disposal of Human Excreta. Sanitary disposal of excreta is of primary importance, for upon this depends the purity of drinking water, the cleanliness of vegetables eaten raw, and the safety with which children and adults can work and play in the soil. A large part of the inhabited earth is polluted with excreta because so many persons are ignorant of, or indifferent to, the danger. The people of some overpopulated areas are dependent on human excreta ("night soil") for fertilizer, and, when used, untreated excreta pollute the land. Under such conditions the practice of storing the excreta for 2 to 6 weeks would reduce the serious danger that exists when fresh urine and feces are used. There are many sections of the United States where modern sewage disposal systems are not available. In these areas septic tanks and many types of privies and latrines are in use. If properly located, constructed, and maintained, they can be adequate sanitary devices for the disposal of human excreta. In some areas, however, human dejecta are deposited on the ground, and outdoor toilets and privies are badly constructed and improperly tended. At some camp sites excreta are deposited in trenches or pits. The deeper the pit the less danger there is of infecting flies, roaches, and animals; the more danger there may be, however, of contaminating the water supply.

Nurses serving communities without modern sanitation may cooperate with other health workers, to encourage provision of adequate toilets, as well as education of the community in sanitary practices. Proper disposal of excreta, however, without control of vermin and infected animals, and particularly without the habitual washing of hands contaminated with excreta, will not eliminate infectious conditions of the intestinal tract.

Some of the major diseases spread by the ingestion of excreta are caused by (1) the virus causing infectious hepatitis, (2) bacilli—the salmonellae, causing typhoid, paratyphoid, and related focal infections, and the shigellae causing dysenteries; (3) the vibrio of cholera; (4) protozoa—chief of which is the *Endamoeba histolytica,* causing amebic dysentery; and (5) the worms or helminths—*Ancylostoma duodenale* and *Necator americanus* (hookworms), *Ascaris lumbricoides* (roundworm), *Trichuris trichiura* (whipworm), and *Strongyloides stercoralis* and *Enterobius vermicularis* (pinworm or seat worm). The extent to which these microorganisms and worms can be found in the intestinal tracts of a populace is an index of its sanitary practice. It has been supposed that hot weather favored the growth of these organisms and for this reason diseases caused by them were more prevalent in the tropical zones. It is now recognized, however, that the shigellae, for example, live longer in cold waters than in warm and that the salmonellae survive freezing temperatures.

Safe disposal of excreta means preventing its contact with human beings, insects, animals, foods eaten raw, such as shellfish or lettuce, and with water until the disease-producing components have been destroyed by chemical action or by the forces of nature. The latter include storage, drying, fermentation, filtration, sedimentation, the action of light and oxidation, and dilution. In the United States, because raw sewage has been a major contributor to our present problems of water pollution, community sewage disposal systems that treat sewage in various ways to render it harmless are now expected to subject all sewage to at least a minimum of secondary treatment before discharge into a water source.[66]

Disposal of urine, feces, vomitus, dressings, and contaminated wastes in hospitals are discussed in the section of this chapter on control of hospital infection.

6. ESTHETIC ASPECTS OF ENVIRONMENTAL CONTROL

Appeal to the Senses. Surroundings are attractive to people if they appeal to their senses; that is, if they enjoy looking at them, if they touch them with pleasure, and if the atmosphere is fragrant or free from disagreeable odors, and free from attention-getting noise. Closely akin to these sensations is the innate desire for privacy during certain aspects of the toilet, whenever treatments require exposure of the body, or when the individual feels that his or her illness necessitates behavior of any kind that would be socially disadvantageous. There seems to be a universal desire to be alone at certain times and a definite irritation when this privacy is invaded, especially without warning.

Beauty and Order in the Surroundings. Whether people are conscious of it or not, the *design* or arrangement of a room contributes to its harmony. Balance or symmetry is a cardinal principle, and furniture can often be rearranged so that large or dark pieces are placed on opposite walls or on either side of a door, window, or mantelpiece. Balance is sometimes achieved through the use of contrasting colors in curtains, screens, and furniture.

Through skillful use of *color* almost any room can be made attractive. With advances in industrial chemistry, colorfast dyes of every hue have been brought within the reach of all, but an appreciation of colors and the art of combining them are not universal. Certain principles may be learned that may help the average person with no special talent along these lines. For example, experts say that there should be a symmetrical use of dark, medium, and light tones in a room. Most persons respond favorably to rooms in which the dark tones are kept on or near the floor. Plain, light-colored walls make rooms look larger. The amount of sunlight and kind of artificial light available affect the selection of colors. Brightly lighted rooms, especially those with extensive window space, may be painted rich, even dark, colors; and paper or paint with a good deal of white should be used to reflect the light when this is meager. Warm colors, such as yellow and pink, are usually advocated for northern exposures; cool greens, blues, and grays are more suitable for sunny rooms.

Color preferences vary with the culture, fashion, race, age, and sex, although there are strong individual likes and dislikes. Black is often associated with death and mourning, but red is also worn as a symbol of bereavement by some peoples. Today, interesting combinations and patterns of vivid colors are used increasingly in a variety of settings, health institutions being no exception. Carpets, too, are installed in hospitals, clinics, nursing homes, and other treatment centers. They are most often found in waiting areas but sometimes in patients' rooms, also. They add an aura of softness, comfort, and luxuriousness to what is sometimes an austere setting, and they reduce noise. Although the use of carpets in hospitals is controversial, no evidence has been found by the writers that they are related to disease, even though they obviously get contaminated. If used, they should not be installed in high-risk areas such as intensive care units. Carpets are not as easily cleaned as hard-surfaced floors and, if not meticulously cared for, may present a shabby, unclean appearance.

Illness may or may not affect reaction to color; some authorities think that color can be used as a therapeutic agent. Yellow, for example, is said to be exciting or stimulating and may be used for the depressed patient; lavender, gray and gray blues are quieting and therefore indicated in rooms where sedative treatments are given; pink and rose are cheering, and, because disease is likely to be depressing, free use should be made of such shades. It seems to be generally agreed that walls and floors should be colored rather than drab, but that soft shades should be used. Raymond P. Sloan [67] in 1944 recommended colored ceilings, particularly for bed patients. His text has a helpful section on mixing paints. Vivid colors in small objects should be used for contrast. Flowers and pictures, if well chosen and properly placed, give charm to a room. Pictures may be changed for variety.

The Care and Arrangement of Flowers. In some countries, such as certain South American states, flowers are so closely associated with death that they are not sent to the sick. In the United States the well-to-do err on the other side and so completely fill the sickroom with bouquets that its appearance is marred because there is seldom space enough for more than one arrangement of flowers on any piece of furniture.

Most florists now deliver flower arrangements in containers that may be kept by the recipient, but occasionally patients receive cut flowers, which must be put into containers on arrival. Volunteer workers often take care of patients' flowers. It is no longer thought that cut flowers in patients' rooms absorb oxygen. There is no necessity for removing them from the room at night except to get them out of a temperature that tends to wilt them. Flowers such as lilies that have a heavy fragrance, are often distasteful or even nauseating to the sick at any time but may be especially noticeable at night.

Patients attach great importance to the attention given their flowers. To them flowers are a symbol of the affection of their family or friends, and if the nurse takes no interest in them, it may seem to patients to be indifference to their pleasure.

The Patient's Outlook. So far very little has been said about anything but the immediate surroundings of the patient. Nothing is more refreshing to the spirit of persons who are housed for any length of time than a lovely *outlook* from their windows. This the nurse cannot manufacture, but the furniture can be so arranged that the inmates will have the best possible view. Sometimes when sick persons must lie in one position and have little variety of scene, they will enjoy having a mirror placed so that they can see any moving objects that may be reflected. With suitable equipment most sick persons can and should be moved from one room to another or into the outdoors for variety of scene. It is very rarely necessary to keep even a very ill person confined in one room.

Esthetic considerations should include *freedom from unpleasant sights*. Vessels of excreta, soiled dressings, and used linen should be covered and disposed of immediately. Trays of instruments and utensils that suggest painful treatments should be removed immediately when not in use. Special passageways and service elevators should be used in hospitals for the transportation of waste or any objects that would repel patients and visitors.

Patients who are very ill, who are vomiting, or who for any reason present a painful appearance to other patients should be in private rooms or screened if they must be cared for in multiple-bed units.

Concepts of beauty vary greatly with the individual, but pleasing proportions, balance, symmetry, order, harmonious coloring, and variety deserve universal consideration. It is particularly important that persons who are confused in mind and dispirited by illness should be surrounded by order and, if possible, by beauty.

Esthetic Sensations of Touch. Metals, wooden surfaces, and fabrics may be attractive to look at, yet unpleasant to *touch*. The choice of clothing and household equipment is influenced by this consideration, and very properly so. Sufferers from certain types of diseases, particularly those affecting the nerves of the skin, such as herpes or shingles, are particularly susceptible to irritation from rough fabrics and heavy clothing.

In both health and sickness there is a tendency to like smooth surfaces unless they are greasy, and to enjoy touching soft fabrics. Materials with curly fibers that have a nap hold air in their meshes and impart a grateful warmth in winter but are unpleasant in hot weather. Few like the feeling of blankets or woolen material next to the skin except in severe climates, and even then the sensation may be disagreeable. Warmth without weight is generally desired in blankets and bedclothes. The lightest covering may be so uncomfortable that it is necessary to support it on a framework or cradle (for further suggestions, see Chapter 12).

Woolen blankets are not recommended for use in hospitals. Any type of blanket is capable of disseminating lint and dust particles —and with them, microorganisms—into the air when handled, but cotton or synthetic blankets are preferred as they are less likely to harbor microorganisms and are easier to launder and disinfect. For hygienic as well as esthetic reasons, only clean blankets should be issued to patients; they should never be passed from one patient to another or stored in a linen closet until they have been properly laundered and disinfected.

Provision for Privacy. Eleanor A. Schuster,[68] reporting a study of privacy (or interpersonal distancing) and hospitalization, observes that the idea of privacy is "elusive" and evades the attempt to "capture it in a precise manner." She thinks it is "a comfortable condition—a desired degree of social retreat"; an "informational mode" in which the person is free "to disclose only that information about himself consistent with his circumstances and desires"; and privacy frequently connotes "propriety."

A part of the discomfort of hospital experiences for the average person is the necessity for exposing the body during physical examinations and treatments and for assistance during such physical acts as defecation, voiding, or vomiting. Added to this, in the case of the ward patient, is the necessity for staying in a room with strangers. Modesty is said by psychologists to be an acquired trait, which means that individuals differ markedly with respect to what embarrasses them. Although some patients give the impression that they have no modesty, hospital methods should be designed to protect the feelings of the most sensitive persons. Ward units should be provided with curtains that may be drawn around the bed when desirable, or screens used if curtains are not provided. In private rooms a screen may be placed between the patient and the open door. Revolving signs on doors that notify visitors when the patient is not to be disturbed give the patient a feeling of security and privacy. The practice of knocking, or otherwise announcing one's presence, is so generally observed that it seems almost unnecessary to say that the entire hospital staff is expected to follow this custom. Patients should be given as much privacy as possible; some are so sensitive that they dislike dressing, getting in and out of bed, or trying their strength by walking under observation. Nurses will often be surprised to find these acts performed during their absence, and may wonder why patients did not wait for their help. People need privacy for reflection, or meditation, and opportunities to be alone with members of their families and with friends.

Providing an environment that does not offend the senses of the patient is not an easy matter but a task for imaginative, resourceful workers. There are numerous and varied possibilities for running counter to the prejudices and preferences of patients, and in hospitals and nursing homes it is only by setting high standards of institutional management that difficulties can be avoided.

Freedom from Strong and Disagreeable Odors in the Surroundings. Some odors, such as the fetid and the acrid, are so universally objectionable that there is no question as to whether they should be eliminated from the environment. Fetid odors in hospitals have their origin in body excretions, discharges from wounds, and necrotic areas. Sweat has an acrid odor, and so do formalin and other chemicals commonly used where there is sickness. Odors that are ordinarily pleasant may on occasion be objectionable. Nausea turns any one against favorite perfumes; unhappy associations can make the smell of a fruit or flower a disagreeable experience. The use of odors as a means of giving pleasure, or the opposite, is a highly subjective matter, differing with individuals and their moods. The safest practice is to keep the atmosphere as odorless as possible in public places, and particularly in hospitals. Health workers should never use perfume and should avoid foods, such as onions, that make the breath malodorous. Many patients suffer from the smell of tobacco on the breath and hands of doctors and nurses. Soaps, detergents, and skin disinfectants as nearly odorless as possible should be selected.

Odor control in the hospital, like contamination control, depends on the cooperation of several departments. It is better to prevent than combat odors. Prevention requires frequent inspection of areas usually associated with odor formation, and application of appropriate sanitary measures. Odors commonly occur in storage areas, morgues, locker rooms, soiled linen areas, utility closets, bathrooms, and kitchens. Odors build up if there is a lack of outside air. Ventilation, with a proper air supply and air movement, is effective in preventing odors.

Deodorizing Agents. Some disinfectants deodorize by removing odors formed by bacteria, molds, and fungi. Ultraviolet lights are sometimes used in storerooms to reduce bacterial growth. Alkalies, such as borax and lime, neutralize unpleasant odors caused by acid.

Various kinds of space deodorants are available commercially. They usually work in one of the following ways: (1) By masking the disagreeable odor. An example of this is the use of perfumed deodorants in washrooms, which is not a practical method of deodorizing, as neither the source nor the composition of the preexisting odor is affected. (2) By anesthetization of the sense of smell, usually accomplished by the addition of formaldehyde to the deodorant, which is not recommended as formaldehyde is poisonous and irritating to the eyes, nose, and throat. (3) By odor-pairing, or cancelling out one odor by another. When this process is effective it results in the neutralization of both odors. Since one odor cannot neutralize all other odors, there are numerous deodorants on the market containing a variety of ingredients intended to counteract many different offensive odors. The odor-pairing deodorants are effective as a temporary measure only. (4) By the use of porous materials like charcoal and silica gel that collect vapors on their surface by adsorption. The fourth method is more effective than the first three mentioned, particularly when used in conjunction with individual or central air-conditioning systems. Deodorants usually come in pressurized dispensers (aerosol cans), wick-in-liquid form, and solid preparations in dispensers.

Odors are sometimes controlled by forcing air through filters or through a liquid such as water, alcohol, glycerin, or mineral oil; this is known as "scrubbing" the air. There are a number of electrostatic air-cleaning devices on the market termed "ion-generators" or "air-chargers" which produce ozone gas and are therefore not recommended for use in hospitals. In any case, deodorant devices should not be used as a substitute for good sanitary practice. The extent to which a hospital controls odors is to many persons an index of the quality of its total maintenance.

The Effect and Control of Noise. Noise is unwanted sound. The word *noise* is derived from the Latin words for nausea, which means sick, and noxia, which means harm.[69]

The characteristics of noise are pitch, quality, and intensity; or the number of double vibrations per second that strike the ear, the form of the sound waves, the amplitude of the vibrations set up in the vibrating body, and the nearness of the person to the vibrating object. Sound intensity is measured by the sensation produced by sound on the human ear. The *bel* or *decibel* (1/10 of a bel) is the name given this unit and is a measurement made with reference to the minimum audible sound. A low whisper 3 ft away has a noise intensity of 20 decibels; a jet engine, an intensity as high as 140 decibels. Noise from heavy traffic measures 90 decibels.

Excessive noise in the environment today is often referred to as "noise pollution." Increasingly it constitutes an environmental health problem. Human hearing begins to be damaged by prolonged exposure to more than 85 decibels. Intensities of 120 to 150 decibels sometimes cause temporary loss of hearing and may, if prolonged, cause permanent deafness. Some of the known effects of loud noise are paling of the skin, constriction of blood vessels, tensing of muscles, increased secretion of adrenal hormones, nervous tension, and increased blood pressure. Sudden loud noises produce the physical changes typical of fear.

Noise comes from a variety of sources: traffic, construction, sirens, fans, air conditioners, furnaces, television sets, radios, and other sound systems—particularly those with amplifiers *—aircraft, automobiles and numerous other mechanical items. Animals and humans

can be noisy but this "hum" of life usually goes unnoticed.

There is no way of escaping from many of these noises, but numbers of them can be controlled. Acoustic engineers have the technology to accomplish this. Many communities are passing laws to prohibit the use of equipment that emits noise above a given number of decibels (see Table 15-2 for a decibel scale of loudness).

Sick persons at home should be placed, if possible, in the quietest room in the house while they are acutely ill, and it is perfectly proper for the nurse to suggest door silencers and other reasonable devices to reduce noise. Dead silence, however, with no sign of activity may be frightening or depressing to a sick person and is particularly bad for patients who need diversion. Quiet, like every other therapeutic measure, must be used with discretion and with consideration for the individual's needs.

Hospital designers and hospital staffs are

Table 15-2.   A Decibel Scale of Loudness *

Decibels (approximate)	
160	Cannon (at close range)
150	Shotgun blast
140	Jet plane (100 ft away)
130	PAIN THRESHOLD Riveter
120	Loud discotheque
110	Loud motorcycle —Power mower
100	Noisy kitchen —Inside subway
90	—Inside auto (city traffic)
80	Day-by-day industrial noise able to cause some hearing loss
70	—Average traffic (100 ft away)
60	Ordinary conversation
50	Noisy office —Average home
40	—Quiet office
30	Whisper
20	
10	
0	THRESHOLD OF HEARING

---

* Research has shown that loud rock-and-roll music damages the hair cells in the cochlea of guinea pigs and other laboratory animals. (Kogan, Benjamin A.: *Health: Man in a Changing Environment.* Harcourt, Brace & World, New York, 1970, p. 102.)

* Kogan, Benjamin A.: *Health: Man in a Changing Environment.* Harcourt, Brace & World, New York, 1970, p. 102.

making efforts to reduce sounds of operation to a minimum. Walls and especially ceilings of workrooms and corridors can be covered with materials that deaden sound. Unfortunately, some of the materials that deaden sound also create a fire hazard and harbor and disseminate microorganisms—some of them, such as asbestos, are known to be harmful when inhaled over long periods—while hard, polished, nonporous surfaces that increase noise do not harbor microorganisms and are easier to clean and disinfect.

Workrooms in clinical divisions should be segregated and, like elevators, separated from patients' rooms by corridors. Lights or bleepers should replace bells, buzzers, or voices in call and alarm systems.

All portable equipment should be furnished with rubber-tired wheels or casters, and all parts kept tight to prevent rattling. Rubber bumpers on beds, wheelchairs, and carts of all kinds reduce noise and protect walls and door jambs. Racks for bedpans and similar objects may be coated with rubber; edges of hoppers, buckets, and such articles may be protected with rubber. Tops for metal pitchers and cans are available in rubber, and mats of similar composition can be used on floor, table, sink, or shelves to deaden workroom noises. Rubber or plastic coverings on siderails of electrically operated beds afford added protection, by insulating against electrical current.

Health personnel should be taught the importance of cultivating quiet, pleasing speech. Whispering is irritating to both sick and well. It is particularly undesirable around the apprehensive, who may fear it means that their condition is serious. Both whispering and tiptoeing are objectionable because to most persons they suggest an anxious, fearful mood. Nurses, doctors, and visitors should avoid talking with one another within the hearing of patients, if they are not interested or too sick to make the effort to attend to what is said. The positive use of sound or music as a therapeutic agent is discussed in Chapters 8 and 16. (See Table 15-3 for list of sounds that are most annoying to hospitalized patients.)

7. CONTROLLING PESTS—INSECTS AND RODENTS

The Problem of Pests. Insects (arthropods) and rodents in dwellings and institutions are not only a nuisance, destructive to food supplies, textiles, books, and other equipment, but also carry filth and can transmit disease.

Insects are the most numerous and varied living things in our environment. Some are helpful; others are of no use to humans, and some, by serving as vectors, or carriers of disease, are dangerous enemies. Many persons are afraid of insects and repelled by many species.

Biting and sucking insects such as ticks introduce microorganisms by direct contact through their mouth parts, or by depositing infectious feces on the puncture wounds they make as they feed on their human hosts. Houseflies and other insects carry microorganisms from a contaminated source on their feet, wings, or bodies. In this instance, the microorganisms are conveyed to food or people by *mechanical transmission,* while *biologic transmission* is the term used to describe the process when a disease agent multiplies or undergoes some developmental change in the arthropod host. The plague bacilli multiplying in fleas that infest rats, and the malarial parasite multiplying in the mosquito are examples of biologic transmission.

Most insects that are a menace to human beings can and do live on animals. Lice, ticks, bedbugs, and fleas can all adapt themselves to human or animal hosts although each species has its favorite victim. Until the fact that fleas travel from house to house on infected rats to spread the plague among people was understood, control of the disease was impossible. To protect the population from insect-borne disease it is essential to know something of the habits and characteristics of the insect in relation to man, animals, and the environment. Domestic and wild animals may spread disease mechanically by harboring insects, and by their bite. Even when insects do not transmit disease, they interfere with sleep. Unquestionably, all human parasites lower the health status and to a greater or lesser extent menace man.

Pest control is extremely complex; no single method of control exists. In general, the control of arthropods, rodents, and weeds (which

Table 15-3. Most Prevalent Kinds of Noise in Hospitals, Arranged in Order of Annoyance to Patients *

Rank Position	Sound
1	Radio or television sets
2	Staff talk in corridors
3	Other patients in distress and recovery-room sounds
4	Voice paging
5	Talk in other rooms
6	Babies or children crying
7	Telephones
8	Pantry, kitchen, utility room

* Bond, Richard G., et al. (eds.): *Environmental Health and Safety in Health-Care Facilities.* Macmillan Publishing Co., Inc., New York, 1974, p. 134.

are pests of another sort but mentioned here because of certain characteristics of the agents used to control them) should take into consideration the life cycle of each and the conditions favorable to its growth. Joseph A. Salvato [70] has said that pest control should be achieved by using the combination of biologic, physical, chemical, and educational measures that will give the best results with the least amount of selective chemical poison and that will pose a minimum hazard to man and wildlife.

Ideally, pest control is a community affair. It cannot be achieved unless widespread measures of sanitation are instituted and carried out. The National Sanitation Foundation in the United States defines sanitation as a way of life, as "the quality of living that is expressed in the clean home, the clean farm, the clean business, the clean neighborhood, and the clean community. Being a way of life it must come from within the people; it is nourished by knowledge and grows as an obligation and an ideal in human relations." *

High standards of sanitation are particularly important where there is illness. The sick person is especially susceptible to infection, often irritable, and capricious in appetite. One small crawling object on the breakfast tray may turn him or her against all the food that is offered, and the presence of one bedbug may disturb the patient's sleep for many nights, even after the condition has been corrected.

All health workers—and, indeed, everyone —should have some knowledge of principles and methods involved in pest control. Conditions found in homes by nurses, may be reported to the local bureau of sanitation, but in some situations such expert service is not readily available, and the nurse, to give the family adequate help, must be well informed or know where to get necessary information. Certain problems, such as the delousing of persons and the control of bedbugs, mosquitoes, and flies, are ever present in some homes, hospitals, and schools and must be dealt with by the health service staff, either alone or in cooperation with exterminating experts. Nurses should have a thorough knowledge of insecticides and repellents used for these pests.

Insecticides, Pesticides, and Repellents. Insecticides are substances used to kill insects. The word pesticide is a general term that includes insecticides, fungicides, rodenticides, herbicides, disinfectants, repellents, and other chemicals used to control pests and weeds. The control of arthropodborne disease is considered

one of the great triumphs of the twentieth century. Insecticides developed within the past 25 years have been instrumental in helping to control malaria, plague, typhus, and other diseases transmitted by insects. There are thousands of formulations of pesticides and insecticides, including repellents, attractants, and impregnants, and they are all harmful to man in varying degrees.

Insecticides are classified into the following groups: (1) contact poisons, which kill insects on contact (for example, DDT); (2) stomach poisons, which cause death when ingested (for example Paris green and sodium fluoride); and (3) fumigants, which give off lethal vapors (sulphur dioxide, for example). Notable among the newer pesticides are numerous synthetic preparations. Among the most widely used of these are the chlorinated hydrocarbons, which include DDT, BHC, and dieldrin. All three are contact poisons having the characteristic of residual or prolonged action. Some have the ability to kill or repel insects by contact for months after their application. Of these, DDT has been the most widely used because it is the least toxic to people. These insecticides that offered so much promise when first introduced have their disadvantages. The principal danger of many of them is that they are persistent; that is, they are not readily decomposed by bacterial action and tend to accumulate in plants and animals. The indiscriminate use of these pesticides, notably DDT, has upset the ecologic balance between insects and other forms of life, with undesirable side effects on fish, birds, and other wildlife, as well as on man, domestic animals, and food crops. Moreover, widespread use has given rise to resistant strains of the insects the pesticides were intended to eradicate and has enabled certain other pests to flourish by destroying their natural enemies. Use of pesticides has also harmed useful insects such as the honey bee. In addition, pesticides have been a direct hazard to the workers involved in their broad-scale application. As a consequence, the use of persistent pesticides and weed killers in some countries has been restricted to disease control measures. The distribution and use of pesticides in the United States is now controlled by federal and state laws, which are enforced by the US Food and Drug Administration and the US Department of Agriculture. Spraying crops with DDT is no longer permitted. Many of the older pesticides that were replaced by the resistant synthetics are being used again. *Pyrethrum* and the oil-soluble *pyrethrin,* in use before World War II, are very effective—highly poisonous to insects and only mildly toxic to man. They are made from a species of chrysanthemum. *Rotenone,* also

---

* Park, J. E.: *Textbook of Preventive and Social Medicine.* Banarsidas Bhanot, Publishers, Napier Town, Jabalpur, India, 1970, p. 143.

extracted from plants, is in the same category.

Pyrethrum is volatile, "knocks down," or acts immediately on flies, for example, and will kill them if used in sufficient quantities. Effective repellents for use on skin and clothing are *Rutgers 612, indalone, dimethylphthalate,* and *diethyltoluamide.*

Insecticides, repellents, and poisons for animal pests are used as fumigants (gases) or in the form of sprays, dusts, or pastes. They may be added to foods that attract the insect or animal, but in such cases great care must be taken to see that human beings (especially children) and animal pets do not eat the poisoned food.

Insecticides depending for their effectiveness on contact with the pest should contain a chemical that will enable the lethal element to penetrate the insect's protective (waxy) coat. Sesame oil is an example of a substance used for this purpose. When insecticides are prepared as sprays, they are often carried in a volatile liquid, such as kerosene oil, which evaporates, leaving no trace of itself, but deposits fine particles of the lethal agent on surfaces in the environment and on the pests themselves.

Geographic location determines to some extent the varieties of insects and animals to be found in a particular area, but free travel increases the possibility that certain types of pests will become universally prevalent. In North America the common domestic pests are flies, mosquitoes, moths, bedbugs, pediculi, fleas, ticks and mites, cockroaches, rats and mice. There are poisonous spiders and other insects that have not been enumerated, but at the present time these are not commonly found inside dwellings.

Flies. Flies are probably the most common of the insect pests. Excreta from animals or people is the medium in which flies breed most prolifically. They lay eggs in any putrefying or fermenting organic matter; hence, garbage and many foods become breeding places if left exposed. The fly has a hairy body and sticky, padded feet. In feeding on filthy material, the fly covers its legs, body, and wings with microorganisms, which it transmits mechanically. One fly may carry as many as 6.5 million microorganisms.[71]

Diseases most often spread by flies are those contracted by eating contaminated food. Known to fall in this group are the intestinal diseases, such as typhoid, dysentery, and cholera. Flies may contaminate food and drinking vessels with microorganisms that cause sore throat and may deposit anthrax, tetanus, or gas gangrene organisms in a wound. Unprotected ulcers may be infected with larvae deposited by flies.

In the United States "flies," unless otherwise indicated, refer to the domestic insect that, as a rule, does not bite and that spreads disease mechanically. It is believed, however, that the deer fly, horsefly, or biting fly, so often encountered outdoors, transmits tularemia from infected animals to man or other animals. In tropical countries, where the disease yaws is prevalent, flies are believed to be carriers; kala-azar is spread by sand flies, and African sleeping sickness by the tsetse fly.

Fly control, in addition to destruction of adult flies, requires the elimination of the breeding places and food supply of the flies and the destruction of larvae. This is accomplished primarily by environmental sanitation, secondarily by the proper use of insecticides, poisoned baits, and electric grids and traps. Cleanliness, good housekeeping, and the application of sanitary control measures are mandatory in the control of flies. Garbage should be wrapped or bagged and placed in clean, covered, washable containers. Garbage grinders in homes and institutions are highly recommended when local conditions permit. Privies must be constructed so that flies and rodents cannot gain access to the pit. Sewage and waste water should be discharged into a sewage system, so that exposure of inadequately treated sewage is prevented. Barnyard excreta and incompletely digested sludge from septic tanks or cesspools should be buried in trenches with 2 ft of earth cover, at least 200 to 500 ft from any water source. Spraying with kerosene, fuel oil, or other larvicide, or dusting with borax before and while covering the trenches, will make the breeding of flies less likely.

When flies are prevalent, screening is important, particularly in kitchens, nurseries, infirmaries, and places where food is prepared and served. Fans that repel flies may be used in place of screening, although the latter is more effective. Screen doors should open outward to avoid driving flies into a room when the door is opened. Doors may be covered with wire netting carrying an electric charge strong enough to kill insects, but harmless to people. This method is used in some dairies where the use of pesticides is contraindicated. When screening is not possible, patients with communicable diseases should have their beds covered with a canopy of netting.

Spraying an approved residual insecticide * on walls and screens just before fly season is helpful, but the spray must not be applied near food, utensils, pets, stoves, or open fires. Com-

---

* State or local regulations impose certain restrictions on the use of some insecticides. Consult local health authorities for information.

plete dependence for killing flies cannot be placed on insecticides alone, as strains of houseflies that are resistant to insecticides are developing.[72]

Mosquitoes. The more important diseases transmitted by mosquitoes are dengue, or breakbone fever, encephalitis, filariasis, malaria, Rift Valley fever, and yellow fever. Of these, only malaria and the encephalitis diseases are found in the United States.

Anopheles quadrimaclatus is the principal malaria vector in the United States. The disease is spread when the female mosquito bites a person infected with malaria parasites. The parasite picked up by the mosquito goes through changes in the body of the mosquito until its cycle is completed. If the mosquito then bites a susceptible well person, the parasites are transmitted by injection and that individual may develop the disease, at the same time becoming another reservoir of infection.

Mosquitoes breed in water and are harbored by tall grass and shrubbery. This knowledge is the key to *mosquito control*. Eliminating breeding places by the draining of swamps and stagnant pools is one method of control, but is not easy to accomplish, since mosquitoes also breed on the edges of ponds, in streams, in salt marshes, in holes in stumps of trees, and in open cesspools, open septic tanks, overflowing sewage, water barrels, empty tin cans and jars, old rubber tires, or any place where water collects. Unlike flies, mosquitoes do not feed on decaying organic matter. The female mosquito feeds only on the blood of man and animals; the male mosquito feeds on the nectar from flowers. Removal of stagnant water controls them, not by eliminating their food supply, but by preventing them from reproducing.

When breeding places cannot be eliminated, biologic and naturalistic measures should be attempted before resorting to chemical control. Biologic measures include stocking ponds with fish that feed on larvae. Naturalistic measures include rendering the water unsuitable for mosquito breeding by changing its chemical or physical characteristics. Changing the salinity of water, adding acid, muddying it, changing the water level, and agitating the water's surface are all measures that discourage the growth of mosquito larvae. When chemical control is resorted to, the area may be sprayed with pesticides, and larvicides may be sprayed on the surface of the water. Nonpersistent larvicides include No. 2 fuel oil, Paris green, borax, and emulsions of pyrethrum extract in kerosene. Paris green is especially suited for control of malaria-carrying species.

Around human habitation, areas of water that cannot be drained or filled can be treated by weekly spraying with fuel oil, kerosene, or other larvicides. The spraying of shrubbery or tall grass in the early morning or evening will give temporary relief from adult mosquitoes for a week or more. A pyrethrin or dichlorvos spray around lawn furniture will help for several hours. Dichlorvos plastic strips and pyrethrin space sprays are useful for indoor control.

Temporary relief from mosquito biting can be effected by applying repellents to clothing and exposed skin. Common repellents are diethyltoluamide, indalone, dimethylphthalate, and repellent 612.[73]

Fleas. Fleas have played a dramatic role in history. As parasites on rats and human beings, both subject to bubonic plague, fleas have laid waste vast cities as they traveled between rodents and men, sick and well. Hans Zinnser, among others, tells the story in *Rats, Lice and History*.[74]

Over a thousand species of fleas have been described, but only a few are of medical importance. Fleas associated with human dwellings fall mainly into the following categories:

1. Human fleas (*Pulex irritans*), which are primarily human parasites, but can adapt to other hosts; they are not an important transmitter of disease.
2. Cat and dog fleas (*Cetenocephalides canis* and *C. felis*), which readily pass from one host to another; when animals are not around, they use humans as a source of nourishment.
3. Rat and mice fleas (*Xenopsylla cheopis*), which also live on ground squirrels and other rodents. As accidental parasites of man, they spread plague and endemic typhus.

In the United States, fleas are mainly associated with house pets. Cat and dog fleas are intermediate hosts of the dog tapeworm (*Dipylidium caninum*) which can be transmitted to humans, particularly to children. Fleas attach themselves to the animals and feed on their blood. They breed in the animal fur where the larvae hatch. They live in dust and carpets, and in cat and dog bedding.[75]

The bite of an uninfected flea is not dangerous except that when scratching it, a person may introduce microorganisms under the skin. The process of feeding, with many insects, stimulates defecation, so that as the animal sucks the blood of his host, his excrement is deposited on the skin. When this excrement contains organisms pathogenic to man, the insect bite is a serious threat. Infected insects, such as fleas or lice, produce disease when the host crushes them against the skin, if the skin is not intact. Even when fleas do not spread disease, they disturb sleep, rest, and waking comfort.

Elimination of rats is essential in *flea control*. Where rats are present, a 5 per cent DDT dust may be applied to rat runs and areas harboring them. For soil and house infestation by dog and cat fleas, sprays of 0.5 per cent diazinon, 1 per cent lindane, 2 per cent malathion, and 1 per cent ronnel are effective. Dusts of malathion, lindane, and carbaryl can also be used outdoors. Oil solutions must not be applied to domestic animals lest they be absorbed, but infested animals can safely be dusted with 1 per cent pyrethrum, 1 per cent rotenone, or 5 per cent malathion.[76]

Ticks. Ticks rank next to mosquitoes in spreading disease among men and are the greatest menace to animals of all the insects. Ticks may take many forms as they adapt themselves to different hosts and environments. Many species live outdoors on tame and wild animals, but some live in houses, as do bedbugs. The species sometimes found in houses is a bat tick. Ticks, when not engorged, resemble bedbugs in shape. Their bodies are leathery and very elastic and are about the size of an adult bedbug. When full of the host's blood, they may be half an inch long and look more like a light gray-brown bean than an insect. The *ornithodorous* and *dermacentor* species are important in North America.

Ticks attach at any point on the body, causing an inflammatory reaction. The bite is not painful and persons rarely know that they have acquired a tick, which may remain attached and suck blood for several days. If this occurs, tick paralysis may develop due to toxic substances released in the tick's saliva; this is particularly likely in children when the tick attaches itself near the child's head and neck. Pathogenic organisms carried by ticks are transferred to humans by the bite of the tick or by contact contamination of the tick's blood or feces which may be deposited on the host's skin. Infected wood ticks and dog ticks transmit Q fever, relapsing fever, Rocky Mountain spotted fever, and tularemia to human beings, although the latter is often contracted from handling infected rabbits.

When ticks are found attached to human beings or animals, it is best to cover the insect with an oil, lard, petroleum jelly, or a hydrocarbon, such as kerosene. Oil deprives the insect of oxygen and so it releases its hold on the victim. An anesthetic, such as ether or chloroform, has the same effect of making the insect let go. If the ticks are found in the ear, a bland oil may be dropped into the ear. If the tick is torn from its attachment, the sucking portion is often left in the skin and infection results. For this reason ticks should be removed with fine-pointed tweezers, applying gentle but firm pressure on the tick. Force should not be used; a slow, steady pull is required. It is a wise precaution to apply a skin antiseptic to the bite. Since bodies of ticks may contain infectious material, they should never be crushed, but burned or dropped into kerosene oil.

Wood ticks appear during spring and early summer in the northwestern United States. Dog ticks are present throughout the summer months in the eastern and southern states. Rabbits, squirrels, woodchucks, horses, sheep, and cattle, as well as dogs, may be infested with ticks.

If it is not possible to avoid tick-infested areas during tick season, one should wear clothing to protect legs, arms, and hands, and inspect the body and clothing for ticks at frequent intervals. The use of repellents on skin and clothing is a protective measure. *Ticks can be controlled* in outdoor areas by spraying with chlordane or toxaphene. Indoor areas can be treated by dusting cracks around windows, baseboards, and floors with carbaryl dust, diazinon, malathion, or lindane. Infested dogs and kennels may be dusted with lindane, carbaryl, coumaphos, or malathion. Cats should be treated with 1 per cent rotenone.[77]

Mites. Mites and ticks are similar, but mites are smaller; some are almost microscopic. *Sarcoptes scabie,* commonly known as the itch mite, causes scabies, which is also referred to as human mange or the seven-year-itch. The impregnated female mite invades the human body by burrowing into the skin. As she burrows, she lays her eggs and defecates. The eggs hatch in the tunnels, and the nymphs start new tunnels, causing skin sensitization and intense itching. Scratching the area spreads the mites and makes secondary infection likely. Scabies is treated by applying benzine hydrochloride (lindane ointment) or benzylbenzoate lotion to the entire body after a hot, soapy bath. Two applications may be necessary. Cuprex and Kwell body lotions and shampoos, available in drugstores in the United States, are also effective.

The hair follicle mite, *Demodex folliculorum,* lives in hair follicles and sebaceous glands around the face, causing blackheads, acne, or localized keratitis. These conditions are cleared up with lindane ointment.

Red bugs, or "chiggers," are picked up out-of-doors in grass or weeds. They invade the skin, not by burrowing into it, but by attaching to the outside, where they feed on tissue fluids, causing severe itching and dermatitis.

Alcohol helps allay the itching, and topical sulphur ointment is effective in eliminating the mite.[78-80] *Mites can be controlled* in outdoor areas by spraying with chlordane or toxaphene.

Bedbugs. Many people associate bedbugs with uncleanliness for the reason that this animal parasite is generally found in badly kept homes, hotels, and hospitals. Bedbugs usually infest a house by living and breeding in the cracks and crevices of beds, from which they emerge at night to feed on the blood of the occupants. They may hibernate in a house for as long as a year. They are very skillful in finding their prey. Young bedbugs are so small and light in color that they are difficult to see; a full-grown bedbug, when not swollen with blood, resembles a tick. The body is wingless, of a dark reddish brown color, and appears to be smooth and hard, but under the microscope it is seen to be covered with fine hairs at the junction of each segment; the shape and size depend upon whether or not the body is distended with blood. There is a nauseating odor about these insects that may account in part for the extreme revulsion that is felt for them.

In order to prevent infestation by bedbugs, buildings should be made as nearly insectproof as possible. The substitution of metals, concrete, and glass for wood construction helps to discourage these vermin. Constant vigilance is necessary in hospitals, however, to prevent patients and their visitors from bringing bedbugs into the buildings on their clothes or other belongings. The bugs cling to the clothing even while they are feeding on their host. The admitting division should be especially careful when storing patients' possessions.

Bedbugs hide during the day and come out at night; they generally inflict multiple bites, raising three or four small hard white elevations in a row. The sleeper is usually restless and anxious. If these signs occur, a search should be made in the cracks of the bed and in the tufts of the mattress. It is sometimes difficult to find these insects.

If constantly exposed to bedbugs, human beings seem to develop an immunity to the irritation caused by their bite. A fresh victim, however, may be very sick from the bites of a small army of bugs, and most people suffer from irritability and lassitude due to the interference with sleep. The itching is intense, the bite not actually painful, but burning. Bedbugs have never been proved to be disease carriers.

Bedbugs are controlled by determining their source and destroying their eggs, larvae, and any adult bedbugs that can be found. Habitual hiding places are usually made evident by black or brown irregular spots near the victim's sleeping quarters. Bedbugs live and lay their eggs in crevices and cracks of floors and walls, in the seams and folds of bedclothes, and in cracks in bed frames and bedsteads. Some of the insecticides effective in killing bedbugs are malathion, dichlorvos, ronnel, and lindane sprays. Pyrethrin sprays help drive bedbugs out from cracks and crevices. It may be necessary to repeat the application two or three times to kill eggs which hatch after the initial spraying. Clothing and bedding that have been sprayed should be aired 4 to 8 hours before using and should be exposed daily, if possible, to fresh air and sunlight. Hand picking, brushing with a stiff-bristled brush, and shaking blankets is also recommended. Steam, scalding hot water, and the use of a blow torch are effective when they can be applied to objects with safety.[81]

Lice. There are hundreds of varieties of lice that are parasites on human beings, animals, fowls, birds, and plants. The three following types, belonging to two genera, infest human beings: (1) *Pediculus,* from which come the human head louse, *P. humanus var. capitus,* and the body louse, *P. humanus var. corporis* or *vestimenti,* and (2) *Phthirius,* from which comes the crab louse, *P. pubis.* The latter lives in those parts of the body covered with short hairs: the pubes, the axillae, the eyebrows, and the eyelashes.

While head lice and crab lice tend to stay on the host hidden by hairs, body lice cling to the clothing, and if a "lousy" person undresses, not one may be seen on the skin. They cling to the clothing by their hind legs while they suck the blood of their host and lay their eggs on the clothing. The head and pubic lice lay eggs on the hairs, gluing them to the hairs with a waxy coating. The eggs hatch in 8 to 10 days if they are not destroyed by excessive drying or moisture.

The presence of body lice is indicated by scratches on the skin and hemorrhagic specks on the body and by the person's habit of scratching. Occasionally they may be seen on the bedding. Clusters of nits (eggs), that look like oval particles of dandruff clinging to the hair, are usually found near the ears. Bites, or pustular eruptions, are seen near the hair line behind the ears. The louse is very small, grayish white, and hard to see; the crab louse has reddish legs. The fresh victim is highly sensitive to the bite and shows what is thought to be an allergic reaction. The veteran acquires an immunity, and often an indifference. Along with resistance to the irritating chemical excretions of the louse, the human host also develops immunity to the diseases transmitted by the louse. In sections of the population where lice and typhus, for example, are present, such diseases tend to be endemic, low-grade infections in the native population. The disease may change to an epidemic and virulent form when the causative organism finds new hosts unprotected by long exposure to the disease. Epidemics occur when "lousy" and "nonlousy" groups are thrown together, as in ships and army quarters.

Lice share with other bloodsuckers the ability to transfer typhus fever, trench fever, and relapsing fever. The first two are spread by the introduction of the feces of the infected louse into the puncture it makes as it sucks blood, while relapsing fever is thought not to be transferred through the bite but from body fluids of the louse, inoculating the host as he crushes the body of the louse against his skin. Crushing lice between the teeth, as is seen in some countries, may spread intestinal diseases. Rats, mice, and other animals may act as intermediary hosts and contribute to typhus epidemics, as they have to those of plague.

The *control of lice* has many aspects. It is obvious that a high standard of personal cleanliness tends to prevent infestation, but the most fastidious person may pick up head lice from cloak rooms, from trying on hats, or from chairs in public conveyances. Crab lice may be transferred from toilet seats and through sexual intercourse.

DDT kills the adult louse and nymph, and while it does not destroy the egg, its effect on the hair or clothing remains lethal to the louse until the eggs hatch. The widespread use of DDT, however, has rendered it ineffective against resistant strains of lice and other insects. During World War II, before resistant strains made their appearance, DDT dusting was effective in delousing prisoners of war, displaced persons, and others, but resistant strains soon made their appearance. Benzine hexachloride (BHC) has also been effective, but strains resistant to it have also been observed. For most strains, BHC as a spray, powder, or ointment is recommended. As a practical, specific measure benzine benzoate emulsion is also reported to be effective. Chlordane is recommended by Ernest C. Faust and his associates as the most effective, safe alternative to DDT.[82] Haig H. Najarian [83] recommends lindane ointment. Most of the insecticide louse powders contain DDT or 1 per cent lindane or malathion as the active ingredient. Abate dust is also reported to be very effective.[84] Cuprex and Kwell body lotions and shampoos, available in drugstores in the United States, are also effective.

Before any treatment agent or pesticide is applied to the body, the hair should be shaved from the infected area and it should be bathed with hot, soapy water. Shampooing the hair using Kwell shampoo and applying Cuprex or Kwell lotion to the entire body are effective in combating head and body lice. Infested clothing and bedding should be boiled or autoclaved. In the hospital, infested linen should be bagged separately and labeled, and the bed and floor should be vacuumed before cleaning and disinfecting.

Cockroaches. The cockroach family has numerous branches that differ markedly in size and shape. The largest variety looks like a winged beetle and is 2 inches in length; the smallest type is less than an eighth that size. They are especially prevalent in crowded apartment houses, schools, stores, and similar places where they find food and moisture. Cockroaches are so dependent on water that they remain near plumbing fixtures and inhabit damp cellars. Any food or cellulose product left uncovered attracts and fosters cockroaches; some species even eat fabrics. Absolute cleanliness and the use of tightly covered containers for foods are the most effective measures in keeping them out of houses. If roaches are a problem, paper should not be used on kitchen and pantry shelves, leaking pipes should be repaired immediately, and all holes around pipes and in floors, walls, or ceilings should be closed. When trying to eliminate cockroaches, temporarily remove all food and equipment from the area. Scrub it clean, including shelves, windowsills, tops and bottoms of tables, corners, and floors under refrigerators, vegetable bins, iceboxes, sinks, and other equipment before applying pesticides. Salvato [85] recommends for *cockroach control* dust or sprays of 1 per cent baygon, 0.5 per cent dichlorvos, or 5 per cent malathion. A pyrethrum spray applied before the residual treatment will drive roaches out of cracks and crevices.

Moths. Moths are a serious menace to owners of woolen fabrics and furs. The flying moth lays eggs that hatch into the destructive larvae or worms. *Moth control* depends on eliminating breeding conditions and on the use of insecticides. These insects flourish in warm, dark places and are more abundant in the spring. They are more likely to eat soiled than clean fabrics; they avoid strong odors and are killed by fumes of some chemicals.

To prevent loss from moths, keep materials they will eat clean, well aired, and, if possible, stored in light closets. After the winter season is over, furs, woolen clothes, and household goods should be cleaned and put away with flakes of camphor or paradichlorobenzene or stored in tar bags. Moth-repellant cakes, placed in a perforated container and hung in a closet, afford adequate protection. Packing clean clothes in tightly closed boxes or cedar chests to which the moths cannot gain access is effective. Cold storage, available in large institutions, cleaning establishments, and stores, is satisfactory protection.

Rodents. Of all household pests, rats and mice are the most prevalent. They live in almost every climate and feed on a great variety of foods. Because they gain access to ships by ropes and gangplanks, they have in some cases carried disease from one continent to another. Certain laws require shipowners to use methods to prevent rats and mice from entering and leaving vessels. These animals are dangerous not only because they carry disease but also because they may bite human beings, especially infants, and gnaw matches, causing fires.

To control these pests, all buildings should be ratproof; food should be inaccessible to them. Rats and mice may be trapped or poisoned. Mice are frightened and killed by cats and dogs; ferrets kill both rats and mice.

Rats are carriers of disease germs, fleas, lice, mites, and intestinal parasites. They destroy food and cause an estimated $900 million yearly damage in the United States alone. They breed prolifically and are spreaders of filth. A rat drops 25 to 150 pellets of feces, 10 to 20 ml of urine, and several hundred hairs per day.

Rodent control depends on starving and poisoning them. Poisoning is not a substitute for basic environmental sanitation, only a supplement. Poisoning alone will only provide a temporary reduction in rat population. Other specific rat control measures include starving them by eliminating their supply of food and water, and keeping them out by ratproofing buildings and by removing their shelters.

When poison is used, it can be mixed with fish cereal, grains, or meat. Care should be taken to keep poisoned bait away from people and domestic animals. Some common agents are Red Squill and anticoagulant rodenticides such as Warfarin, Pival, Fumarin, or ANTU. Other poisons, such as arsenious oxide, yellow phosphorus, which is hazardous because of its flammability, and calcium cyanide, which releases hydrocyanic acid on exposure to moist air, should be used only by experienced exterminators and should never be used in populated areas. ANTU, Red Squill, and the anticoagulants are less hazardous to use, but are not effective against roof rats or house mice.

Anticoagulants, which cause capillaries to break down, resulting in internal bleeding, are the preferred rat poisons for most purposes. It should be recognized, however, that mouse and rat resistance to anticoagulant bait has been reported in Scotland, Denmark, England, and Wales, and there is evidence that it may be developing in North Carolina and New York State.

Various antifertility agents have been proposed to prevent the reproduction of rats. This technique has promise if used as an adjunct to basic environmental sanitation and control of rats by poisoning, particularly in areas where it is not practical to remove food, water, and shelter. A combination of methods must be used in ridding the community of rats. They must be controlled in sewers, in open areas, in rundown houses, on city dumps, and in any place where sanitation is poor. Such a program requires community action, with education through schools, the news media, posters, and the use of other methods to encourage public participation.

Mice are controlled by trapping unless the infestation is heavy. House mice populations may increase as rat populations are reduced. As with rat control, poisons should be used when other methods are not effective, and sanitary measures should be utilized to eliminate conditions that permit rodents to exist.[86]

Helminths. Parasitic worms constitute a distinct hazard in man's environment, the species depending upon the geographical area. Hookworm is a threat in warm countries where people go barefooted and unprotected from human excreta containing the worms. Obviously, *methods of control* depend on providing proper sanitary facilities and wearing shoes. Roundworms, pinworms, tapeworms, and trichinella are taken in through the mouth. Their control is effected by cleanliness of everything that goes into the mouth, including food, and by good nutrition. Since it is difficult to make sure that meats do not contain disease-producing agents, thorough cooking of all meats, particularly pork which harbors trichinella, is important.

Vermin Control in Hospitals and Other Health Care Institutions. The prevention of vermin infestation is part of a good institutional management program. The disease most commonly transmitted by vectors in the hospital is salmonellosis because domestic rodents are common reservoirs for salmonella organisms. Disease organisms can also be transmitted mechanically by filth-breeding insects such as houseflies and cockroaches. Sanitary methods of food preparation are important, as salmonella organisms are often found in eggs, and uncooked meat and poultry (see page 879).

Vermin control begins with hospital construction. Hospitals should be planned with a minimum of suitable hiding places for rodents and insects—dark, warm areas such as hollow walls, false ceilings, and dead spaces behind equipment. Screens on doors and windows and air barriers on doors frequently opened are a protection against flying insects. House-keeping measures should include strict cleanliness and the proper storage of food and disposal of garbage, using garbage grinders if possible. Chemical insecticides and rodenticides should be used as sparingly as possible in hospitals, and professional exterminators should be called in to administer these poisons when it becomes necessary to use them. Certain insecticides such as DDT are generally forbidden in food-handling areas. Good sanitation is the only permanent solution to most vermin infestations in hospitals.[87]

8. PREVENTING MECHANICAL INJURY, BURNS, POISONING, AND ELECTRIC SHOCK

Common Dangers in Health and Sickness. Possibilities of mechanical injury, electrical mishaps, burns, poisoning, and infection are ever present in our surroundings. According to the National Safety Council, as cited by Kogan,[87a] in 1968, 115,000 people in the United States died as a result of accidents. Of these, 55,200 died in automobile accidents, which also accounted for about 2 million disabling injuries. Accidents in the home caused the death of 28,500 people. Falls were responsible for 40 per cent of these deaths, and fires and burns for 20 per cent. Falls are most common among the elderly. Stair railings, nightlights, and luminous paint around light switches are suggested as safety measures.

Childhood Accidents. Accidents are the leading cause of death of persons between the ages of 1 month and 24 years, excluding sudden infant death, which occurs more frequently than accidents during the first 6 months of life. Age-associated activity is a factor in the cause of accidents in children. Accidental poisoning occurs primarily in pre-school children; drowning and firearms accidents beset school-age children; while hanging, either accidental or suicidal, occurs among older children and adolescents. Tricycle, bicycle, and motorcycle accidents are also age-associated. Suffocation is a common cause of death in infants and toddlers. Plastic bags and small objects that could occlude air passages should be kept away from young children, who use their mouths as one means of exploring their world. Measures to prevent childhood accidents include education, particularly for parents and school children. An important function of the nurse is giving anticipatory

guidance or counseling parents in advance on the types of accidents likely to happen to their children at different ages.

Burns. Every year more than 150,000 people suffer burns from clothing that has caught fire. Some fabrics are particularly hazardous. Cotton combined with acrylic is highly combustible. Some synthetic fabrics when ignited melt into sticky substances that cause severe burns. Flimsy, ruffled clothing is a potential hazard, particularly around gas stoves and other open flames. Wool is the most naturally fire-resistant of all fabrics. Denim is a good fabric for children's clothing, as it burns slowly.[88] Care of burned patients is discussed in Chapter 42.

Protection from Poisons. National and state legislative bodies have passed laws and formulated public health regulations to protect the public from the unwitting use of poisons. Druggists are not permitted to sell highly toxic and potent drugs without a prescription from a physician; labels must show the ingredients of patent medicines, and pharmacists are required to label highly toxic drugs as poison. The use of injurious chemicals as food preservatives and the employment of toxic sprays are regulated very carefully. Like all other health workers, nurses should keep themselves informed about health legislation of this type and give their support to measures that provide thorough public protection. In hospitals, drugs of a highly poisonous nature are always kept under lock and key. Some toxic antiseptic solutions, however, are usually found on open shelves in workrooms. Because it is difficult to recognize suicidal intentions, the use of *all* toxic chemicals should be reduced to a minimum and made as inaccessible to patients as possible. Pesticides, in addition to being toxic, may be flammable; their use and storage should be carefully controlled. They should not be stored in a food preparation or serving area.

Poison ingestion is a major cause of accidental death in young children, the principal poisons being aspirin, cleansing agents, and pesticides. Mothers of young children should be urged to keep poisonous substances out of reach and, when taking a child who has ingested poison to a physician, to take along the poison container. Most large cities have poison control centers that supply information about antidotes. After a child has ingested poison, the poisonous substance must be eliminated from the body as quickly as possible or be inactivated. Gastric lavage to remove the contents of the stomach is not as effective as induced vomiting because not all stomach content is small enough to be drawn through a lavage tube. The most effective way to induce vomiting in the child between 1 and 4 years of age is to administer a large dose of syrup of ipecac, 15 ml followed by another 10 to 15 ml if no vomiting occurs within 20 minutes. Many physicians prescribe a 1-oz bottle of ipecac for all children at the age of 1 year in order that parents will have it on hand in case of need. Vomiting should not be induced, however, in children who have swallowed caustics such as lye or acid, as this would cause burning of the esophagus twice. If syrup of ipecac is not available, mothers can be advised to try to induce vomiting mechanically by pressing the blunt edge of a spoon against the back of the tongue.[89]

Lead poisoning, a common occurrence in young children, is a serious environmental disease which is theoretically preventable. Lead in paint and pipes in older buildings is readily accessible to children, especially those in slum areas. The ingestion of paint chips containing lead is closely associated with the propensity of many children to eat inedible materials—a predisposition known as pica, which is itself an environmentally associated phenomenon. Factors contributing to pica are parental supervision inadequate to recognize and stop the practice, a paucity of appropriate toys and facilities for normal toddler play activities, and dilapidated walls, window sills, and furniture which provide a source of lead.

Control measures include anticipatory counseling of parents, as well as removal of lead from the environment of young children by scraping all painted surfaces and repainting them with lead-free paint, or covering surfaces with plywood or linoleum; other control measures include removal of children from the environment containing lead to newer housing.[90] The manufacture of paint containing lead is now prohibited by law in the United States.

Poisoning is also discussed in Chapter 21.

Preventing Institutional Accidents. In health care institutions, as in the larger environment, rapid advances in science and technology have imposed new hazards and risks, not only for patients but for visitors and personnel as well. Prevention must be aimed at safeguarding everyone who enters the institution.

Advances such as organ transplants, renal dialysis, lasers, cryogenics, radiation, and monitoring devices in treatment centers all require complex instruments, machines, and techniques that demand sophisticated knowledge and skills on the part of many persons. Each department within a treatment institution has hazards specific to that area. The pathology laboratory is a particularly high-risk area for personnel, as are radiation therapy departments, the kitchen, laundry, and maintenance and storage rooms. This chapter will deal mostly with accident prevention in relation to patient care. For a more comprehensive discussion of institutional safety the reader is referred to *Safety Guide for Health Care Institutions,* published by the American Hospital Association and the National Safety Council, 1972. This guide includes valuable information on the safety of patients, visitors, and employees. It also covers all types of hazards, and presents a wide spectrum of precautions, recommendations, and safety checklists, as well as a special section on fires and proper contents and location of fire extinguishers. Portions of the material presented here are adapted from that Guide. Hazards associated with use of radioactive materials are discussed in Chapter 31 of this volume.

In the United States, safety codes and regulations for health care institutions, particularly hospitals, have been established by local and federal government and other regulatory agencies. Among these are the codes and regulations of the Joint Commission on Accreditation of Hospitals, the Federal Social Security Safety Law, and the Occupational Safety and Health Act of 1970. In addition, many private agencies and business organizations are a useful source of information about institutional safety.

Accidents Among Employees of Health Care Institutions. Studies of accidents to hospital employees indicate that falls and improper lifting of heavy objects (including patients) cause two thirds of the serious disabling injuries. The remaining one third are caused by moving machinery, transportation (of patients, supplies, and equipment), incorrect use of tools, and improper handling of equipment including explosive gases. The greatest cause of disability to nurses is handling and lifting patients. In addition, nurses are frequent victims of cuts and punctures from broken glass, sharp instruments, and needles.

Patient Safety. In addition to a safe environment, the safety and security of the patient depends on proper nursing care, and safe, accurate administration of medications and treatments, as well as correct identification of the patient by means of an information-bearing tag attached to each patient's wrist; this is particularly important in the newborn.

Three major types of accidents suffered by patients are *falls, electric shock,* and *explosions* due to ignition of gas mixtures used during anesthesia, with falls being the predominant cause of injuries, especially to elderly patients.

Preventing Mechanical Injury. Normal adults can, if they try, substantially reduce the chance of having an accident or meeting accidental death. Sickness, however, often distorts judgment and weakens, and in some cases destroys, the will to live. Some sick persons must be protected from accidental injury, as must children or the unconscious, but a more aggressive type of guardianship is necessary for the patient who has suicidal compulsions. In order to keep patients from accidentally falling or intentionally throwing themselves from a window, the windows should be made in such a way that they cannot be opened wide enough to admit a human form. (Suicide and its prevention are discussed at some length in Chapter 41.)

Smooth, even floors, fixed floor coverings, and well-lighted rooms help prevent falls which cause most mechanical injuries. Hospital personnel and visitors must be warned when floors are wet, and movable objects kept out of passageways. Falls are not limited to those on their feet; it is not uncommon for children and sick people to tumble out of bed. In hospitals, beds are put on casters so that they may be easily moved, but this in itself constitutes a danger. Patients must be warned that in turning on their side and reaching for something from the bedside table there is a risk of falling; this is particularly true when inner spring mattresses are used. It is very desirable to have a brake on at least one wheel or caster of any bed or similar piece of equipment.

To minimize leaning over the edge of the bed, the bedside stand should be at the head and side of the bed. When the patient is raised to a sitting position, the stand should be moved a foot or so down from the head of the bed; frequently used items should be placed on the stand close enough so the patient can reach them without leaning over. Falls frequently occur when patients are getting out of, or into, bed. Patients who need it should be urged to ask for assistance. Prompt, cheerful answering of calls will encourage their cooperation. Electric beds should be lowered before the patient attempts to stand. If a footstool is used, it should be covered with slip-proof material, and its legs should have rubber tips. The stool should be kept within the patient's reach, not under the bed. Proper positioning of patients, while sitting in bed, wheelchair, or chair, and sufficient support to maintain their position, is necessary for elderly or weak patients. Side rails on beds should always be used if there is a possibility of a patient's rolling out of bed. Side rails are mandatory for infants, young children, and elderly, weak, seriously ill, disoriented, or unconscious patients, and whenever drainage tubes, intravenous solutions, or

catheters are used. When it is necessary to use side rails patients should be helped to understand that they are there to protect, not restrain, them.

As a measure of general patient safety, the hospital staff should keep the patients' rooms clean and tidy at all times, making sure that drawers are closed after use, and that bed crank handles are folded under. Instruments and needles should not be kept on the bedside stand.

Areas in which the patient may walk should be dry and free of obstacles and slipping hazards. Night lighting should be provided in the patients' rooms and corridors. Crutches issued to patients should be of the correct height and weight. They must have suction cup tips, free of wax and small particles. Corridor handrails should be provided, especially in geriatric areas.

All toilet, bath, and shower facilities should be equipped with grab bars to provide assistance for ambulatory patients. The latch on stall doors should be operable from both sides, and every lavatory area should have a call button connected to the nurses' station.

Proper use of wheelchairs should be demonstrated to patients; their locking devices should be checked. When patients are being transported from their room to another area of the hospital on a stretcher, they should be secured with a restraining belt and cautioned to keep their feet, hands, and arms under the covering blanket and on the stretcher. They should be positioned so that the head is on the end nearest the attendant, and should be moved feet forward. At doorways, stretchers (and carts) should be pulled through rather than pushed in, blindly. When two persons are handling a stretcher, both should face forward. When going down a ramp, one person should brace the stretcher from the front. Irrigation standards should be anchored securely, and packages, trays, or other objects should not be permitted to hang over the patient or rest on the stretcher or cart. All patient conveyances should be wheeled down the center of the corridor to prevent collision with persons emerging from doorways.

Preventing Burns. To prevent burns and shock from electric pads, the pads must be kept dry. Pins must not be put through them, and they must not be used at high temperature. Hot water bottles should be tested for temperature and covered before application. A hot water bottle or heating pad should not be placed directly against an unconscious patient, or on a hot compress. The patient's skin should be checked frequently for redness. Electric light cradles should be inspected daily for loose wiring and connections. Only 25-watt bulbs should be used, and the bulb should be protected and placed at least 18 inches from the patient's body. While in use, the cradle should be firmly secured. Infrared lamps should have guards, and should not be used without constant supervision.

Institutional safety is the responsibility of all employees and staff members. Everyone should report any unsafe condition or act that he or she observes. Damaged equipment should be removed from use until it is repaired. Everyone should be familiar with relevant work procedures and safe work practices. The provision of safety in an environment fraught with hazards requires concerted vigilance and strict observance of safety regulations.

Fire Protection in Health Care Institutions. Fire resulting in injury or death is always tragic, especially in hospitals and nursing homes, where many of the occupants are helpless and unable to save themselves. Solomon Garb and Evelyn Eng [91] report that there are approximately four fatal hospital fires each year in the United States and about four non-fatal fires every day. The National Fire Protection Association (NFPA) puts the daily number of hospital fires at around 15. A survey by NFPA of 381 hospital fires and explosions found that the two leading causes of hospital fires are smoking and electricity. The greatest number of fires are started in patients' rooms, mostly in oxygen tents and bedding. Employees' quarters and heating and power plants are also frequent sites of origin.

Fire prevention, rather than fire control, should always be stressed. Most fires are a result of carelessness. Early detection, prevention of spread, and prompt extinguishing of the fire, and, when necessary, safe evacuation of people are also of importance. Fire protection requires diligent planning, instruction in use of equipment, frequent fire drills and inspections, and strict adherence to regulations.

Design and construction of health care buildings and choice of furnishings are important in prevention.* A so-called fireproof building can be a death trap if it contains combustible materials. A hospital fire that took sixteen lives in Hartford, Connecticut, in 1961 occurred in a new, supposedly fireproof building. It was fatal largely because a

* Nursing homes should have the same requirements as hospitals. Because they are often private residences adapted to public use, patients in them are subjected to greater risks than those in hospitals. The fact that most of the inmates are old and infirm adds to the difficulty of evacuating a burning building.

combustible acoustic ceiling caught fire. Vertical passages such as stairs, laundry chutes, and shafts should be made of fireproof material and enclosed to prevent the spread of flames and asphyxiating smoke and gases. Fire doors should be installed to ensure isolation of areas of greater than normal hazard and to permit each floor to be divided into subareas. This kind of compartmentalization of the building, in addition to preventing the spread of flames and smoke, permits emergency evacuation of patients in fire-resistant buildings from one section of a floor to another when removal to another floor would be difficult and time-consuming.

Fire doors should swing to open in the direction of the exits. Equipment must not be stored in corridors, as unobstructed passageways with well marked and properly placed hand extinguishers and hose cabinets are basic to fire safety, as are well marked exits.

Proper facilities for handling disposal of linen and trash are important. Refuse should be discarded promptly so that it will not stay in the building overnight.

Papers and rugs may reach the kindling point if allowed to collect in closets, attics, or any warm place. Oil on paper or fabrics lowers the kindling point and thus increases the danger. Waste should be collected in metal containers; oiled mops and dustcloths are not to be used in health care institutions; they spread microorganisms, in addition to posing a fire hazard. The clothing of workers should be stored in ventilated fireproof lockers. Chemicals should not be discarded into refuse cans, and flammable liquids, such as ether, should be stored in refrigerators that are free of potential sparks from electric wiring on inside lights and thermostats. Smoking in institutions is increasingly restricted for health reasons other than fire, but it should never be permitted near explosive gases or in other hazardous areas. Safe ash receptacles should be provided in areas where smoking is permitted.

Early detection, when prevention has not been effective, is of utmost importance. In areas where someone is "on duty" around the clock, an outbreak of fire is likely to be discovered early, in which case immediate action should be taken to alert those responsible for fire control. Other areas, those not under constant supervision or considered to be of greater than normal risk (storage rooms, maintenance shops, trash collection rooms, etc.), should have automatic detection and alarm systems. Many experts have suggested that the most important single step in preventing fatal hospital fires is the installation of automatic sprinkler and alarm systems.

Restricting the spread of an initial outbreak

of fire may sometimes be accomplished by closing the door, thus confining the fire to its point of origin for a while at least. This also prevents passage of smoke and gases from one room to another. Fires discovered at an early stage can be held in check by proper use of fire extinguishers.

Water should be available in every part of the building for the use of fire hoses. Attempts to extinguish fire with water, however, are ineffective in some cases and often destructive to equipment and injurious to patients; other measures must also be provided.

All extinguishers operate on the same principle—the exclusion of oxygen from burning objects. Many devices contain chemicals, such as a soda solution and sulfuric acid, which, when combined, form carbon dioxide gas. When this gas surrounds the fire, it excludes oxygen as effectively as a water bath. The chemicals are usually mixed by inverting the container. Another type of extinguisher sprays the burning objects with a soap solution. Soapsuds spread rapidly over surfaces and in so doing exclude oxygen. Wool blankets or rugs thrown on a fire also exclude oxygen and extinguish flames.

Even though it is important to try to extinguish a small fire before it gets out of control, it should be understood that a fire extinguisher is a stopgap remedy to be used only while awaiting the arrival of professional fire fighters. Moreover, not all extinguishers are equally effective on different kinds of fires. Fires are classified by the type of fuel feeding the fire:

A *class A* fire is one in which ordinary combustible materials like wood, paper, and fabric are burning. They can be quenched with water or with any other type of extinguisher.

A *class B* fire is one in which flammable liquids, grease, oil, gasoline, paint, etc., are burning. Water and soda acid extinguishers cannot be used effectively since they tend to spread the fire. Class B fires are best handled by a blanketing technique.

A *class C* fire is one in which live electric equipment is involved. Water, soda acid, and foam cannot be used because they cause electric short circuits and make the fire worse. A nonconducting dry chemical extinguisher should be used. It is possible to use dry chemical extinguishers for all classes of fires.

Local fire departments can provide assistance in selecting and positioning extinguishers and can assist in training institutional personnel in appropriate use of the equipment. Fire fighting equipment is useless if no one knows how to use it.

All fire extinguishers should be inspected at least once a year by the local fire department or a qualified extinguisher service agency. In addition, a monthly inspection by a designated institutional employee should be made to ensure that extinguishers have not been removed or tampered with. An inspection tag, initialed and dated on each inspection, should be attached.

The entire institutional staff should be familiar with measures of fire prevention and control, but one individual should be responsible for the program. Each worker should know the procedures to follow in case of fire: how to turn in an alarm, use fire extinguishers, and remove a patient to a place of safety, and how to protect the nose and throat from smoke in leaving a burning building. Some engineering staffs are so well prepared to deal with a fire that all health workers are asked to turn in an alarm immediately, and then to stay on the services to which they are assigned and to maintain the usual order while the fire is extinguished by those most expert in this task.

James Feerick,[92] a professional fire fighter, answers a question asked by many nurses— "What is the first thing to do in the event of fire in a health care institution?"—by saying that we must each use our own initiative and judgment—it depends on the situation. Ordinarily, sounding the alarm would be the appropriate first action, but, if the fire is spotted in an empty room some distance from the telephone or alarm box, closing the door to confine the flames would be more appropriate. If a nurse finds a patient in bed with the clothing on fire, he or she might first extinguish the fire with a blanket, or with water from the bedside stand. The first action of an inhalation therapist might be to turn off the oxygen. Fire regulations, including designation of the person to whom fire should be reported, vary with different institutions.

Most deaths from fire occur from inhalation of smoke and toxic vapors. Patients and personnel trapped in a burning building can often survive by following procedures to keep smoke and flames out of the room they are in. Doors, transoms, and vents should be kept closed. Cracks should be plugged with wet cloths. Windows may be opened from time to time for ventilation if smoke and hot air are not drawn into the room. Procedures for removal of patients from a burning building * should be

* For suggested procedures, see National Safety Council and American Hospital Association: *Emergency Removal of Patients and First-Aid Fire Fighting in Hospitals,* The Council, Chicago, 1972. Local fire departments are also a valuable source of information about fire prevention and control. Other sources are: National Fire Protection Association; Underwriters Laboratories, Inc.; US Department of Interior, Bureau of Mines; and Factory Mutual Engineering Corporation.

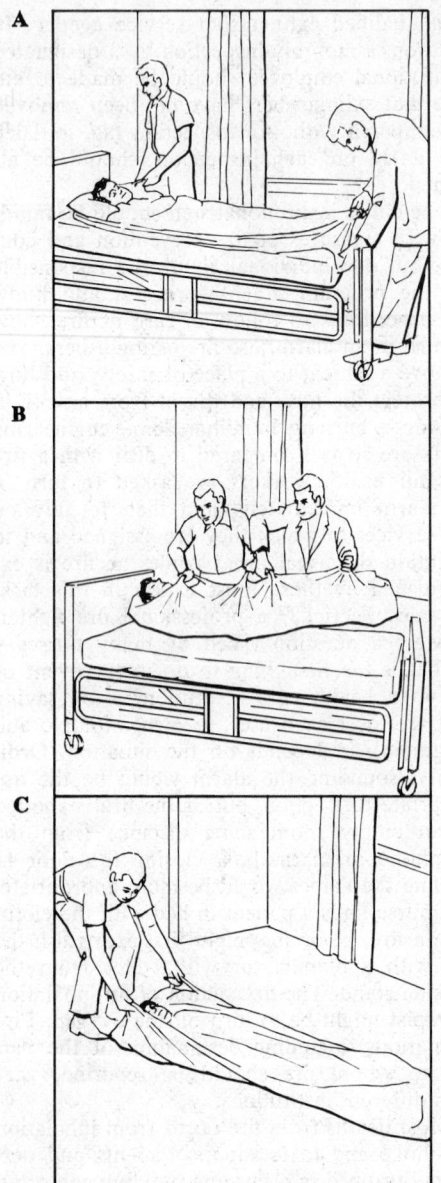

Figure 15-1. *A.* Washable fabric patient-carrier that fits over mattress if folded around patient. *B.* Lifting patient from bed. *C.* Method by which one man can evacuate a nonambulatory patient regardless of patient's size. (Adapted from Black, James B.: "Fire and Disaster," in *Environmental Aspects of the Hospital.* Vol. III, *Safety Fundamentals* [PHS Pub. No. 930-C-17]. US Government Printing Office, Washington, D.C., 1967, p. 7).

devised and rehearsed before a fire occurs [93-95] (see Fig. 15-1).

Protection from Flammable Gas. The three following types of flammable gases are commonly used in health care institutions: natural gas, for heating, cooking, and incineration; acetylene gas, for welding in institutional maintenance; and medical gases, for anesthesia and for diagnostic and treatment procedures. The hazard associated with *natural gas* is related to gas leakage either from joints in pipes or from extinguished pilot lights. It can cause death by asphyxiation, and if ignited, an explosion. Gas leaks should be reported immediately and flames and sparks kept out of the area until the leak is stopped and the gas dissipated. *Acetylene gas,* used for welding, has the greatest flammability of any commercial gas. Safety regulations require that this gas be stored in a fire-resistant storage room separated from oxygen or nitrous oxide, which are reducing agents. All gas tanks are dangerous and should be treated with respect. The pressure regulators on the tanks, particularly those of oxygen, should never be regulated by unauthorized personnel. Dangerous fires have occurred in hospitals because the regulators on oxygen tanks have been tampered with. Because of the danger of spontaneous ignition, oil or grease should never be used on oxygen or nitrous oxide equipment. Clothing or linens should not be hung on cylinders, as fabrics saturated with oxygen or nitrous oxide ignite easily. *Medical gases* administered to the patient should be used only when nonflammable materials give unsatisfactory results. For example, an inert gas like helium is preferable to hydrogen for use in tests to measure blood circulation rates. Hydrogen, because of its flammability, should never be piped through a hospital building.

Safe Use of Oxygen in Tents and Piped-in Lines. Oxygen is widely used throughout the hospital. When it is in use in a patient area the following precautions are recommended.[96]

1. Post "No Smoking" signs conspicuously. Take smoking materials and matches away from patients. Warn visitors about smoking lest they light a cigarette from force of habit.
2. Do not use alcohol, ether, or other flammable liquids, wool, silk, rayon, or nylon within the tent hood; they create flammable mixtures and static electricity sparks. Use water or noncombustible rubbing liquids. Tuck blankets over the skirt of the tent hood to prevent escape of oxygen. Do not use arcing or sparking electric equipment within or next to the tent, lest the bedclothes ignite.
3. Check the oxygen supply periodically to guard against unnoticed exhaustion.
4. Do not permit any source of ignition such as sparking toys in the area.

Ethylene and cyclopropane used in anesthesia are both flammable gases. Nitrous oxide, another anesthetic gas, is capable of supporting combustion, but is not flammable. Ethyl ether, used extensively in the past as an anesthetic, is also flammable. In 1961, a nonexplosive anesthetic gas, halothane, was introduced. Although widely used, it has not replaced explosive anesthetics entirely. Flammable anesthetic gases are given the patient in combination with oxygen, making them explosive when ignited. Anesthesia explosions can be prevented or reduced by removal of ignition sources. Cautery, endothermy, or other electric equipment employing an open spark during surgery should only be used in the presence of a nonflammable anesthetic. If this is not possible, the patient should be draped so that a barrier is provided against any escape of the flammable gas to the area in which the cautery or endothermy is applied. Other sources of ignition include electric arcs and sparks which may emanate from electric equipment, plugs, sockets, or light switches, and the insidious, often unseen, sparks of static electricity. The electric safety code requires that electric wiring be explosion-proof in the operating room and in areas where gas cylinders are stored. Mechanical ventilation at the rate of at least eight air changes an hour is recommended to prevent accumulation of explosive gas mixtures.

Protection Against Static Spark Ignitions. Static electricity is generated by friction between dissimilar substances. When the surfaces are rapidly separated, the surface of one material or object becomes positively charged and the other negatively charged. Tremendously high voltages can be produced in this fashion, but the quantity of the electricity is generally low. In nature, clouds are charged relative to each other and to the earth by the friction produced by the wind. Lightning strokes are often the result. Man-made friction machines generate millions of volts for lightning simulation and other high voltage experimentation. In dry weather, a person walking on a carpet or other good insulating surface can generate many thousands of volts of charge sufficient to cause a spark and a quite perceptible momentary shock on contact with another person or an electric conductor such as a metal doorknob.* Static charges are frequently released, causing a spark so tiny that it is unnoticed; nevertheless, such a small spark can ignite explosive gases. The act of "whipping off" a blanket from a rubber pad or rubber sheet can produce such a charge.

Some materials are more inclined to form static electricity than others. High on this list are wool, silk, rayon, nylon, and most plastics. These materials should not be brought into the operating room. On the other hand, cotton, linen, and viscose rayon are ideal for operating room clothing, towels, surgical "drapes," and blankets. They are not as likely to generate electricity, and in addition, readily absorb moisture which diminishes static sparks.

Conductive floors and shoes are required for operating rooms. A conductive floor serves the purpose of electrically connecting persons and objects. This prevents accumulation of electrostatic charges by enabling electricity to drain off to ground * before high voltages are built up. Rubber should not be used in the operating room as it is highly insulating and will prevent static electricity from draining off to ground, increasing the danger of its being discharged as sparks. If, during the manufacture of rubber, carbon black is finely disbursed through it, the rubber will lose its insulating property and become conductive. This conductive or antistatic rubber, as it is sometimes called, will allow electrostatic sparks to dissipate as rapidly as formed. Only conductive rubber should be used in the operating room. Because a highly humid atmosphere is a deterrent to the formation of static electricity, the relative humidity in the operating room should be maintained between 50 per cent and 65 per cent. All personnel must wear conductive footwear, which should be tested for conductivity before entering the operating room, and all equipment must be fitted with a grounding device to maintain a constant conductive path to the floor.[97-99]

Protection from Hazards of Electrosurgery. High-frequency electrosurgical devices, also known as Bovie equipment, are used in surgery to cut and coagulate living tissue. Although these units are among the most potentially dangerous equipment in the hospital, they are used because they save operation time, and do away with the need for conventional suturing, or tying-off, of blood vessels. In addition, high-frequency current does not cause muscular contraction during surgery. While open sparks produced by these units could cause gas explosion if used near flammable anesthetics, the most common injuries associated with electrosurgical equipment are accidental high-frequency burns.

High-frequency currents, unlike regular 60-cycle alternating current (ordinary household current), can be transferred from one con-

---

* The authors are indebted to John W. Gray, electronic engineer of Guilford, Conn., for this and other assistance in preparation of the material on electric safety.

* "Drain off to ground" refers to the propensity of electricity to find the most accessible conductive pathway to the earth.

ductor or electric cord or power line to another without direct electric connection, even when the two are separated by an insulator. Burns have been reported where electric power cords connected to machines have been draped over the patient's body. Burns have also occurred where high-frequency current makes contact with electrocardiograph and electroencephalograph electrodes attached to the patient. Rectal burns at the site of endoscopic equipment and temperature monitoring probes have been reported. Surgeons using electrosurgical equipment have been burned when the current has returned to ground through the surgeon. Fires have started when surgical "drapes" have ignited as a result of heat and arcing at an unintended ground point. Fires have also occurred when flammable skin preparation solutions such as ether, alcohol, or acetone have pooled under the patient on mattresses and "drapes." Because high-frequency current sometimes flows from one conductor to another, such fires have occurred even when the flammable solutions are some distance from the surgical site. An electrically powered proctoscope used for cutting into the bowels has reportedly ignited explosive bowel gases such as methane, hydrogen, and hydrogen sulfide. The bladder has ruptured during transurethral resections from explosion of gases within the bladder.

Another common problem associated with electrosurgery is electromagnetic interference. Radiofrequency energy (high frequency) can disrupt cardiac pacemaker circuits, and interfere with monitoring equipment in the operating room. In addition, interference can be broadcasted through hospital power lines to disrupt equipment at other locations in the hospital, affecting physiologic signals, monitoring displays, computing equipment, and equipment control circuits. Indiscriminate use of electrosurgery, or poor technique, may increase the probability of infection by prolonging healing of wounds and by causing an excess of charred and devitalized tissue at the operating site.

Burns resulting from the use of *laparoscopy* equipment have been reported. Laparoscopy is a diagnostic procedure for viewing the internal organs of the abdomen. It is often used in conjunction with electrosurgical equipment for laparoscopic tubal ligations (lap-tubals), an increasingly popular technique for female sterilization. The procedure involves inflating the abdomen with carbon dioxide through a needle inserted through the abdominal wall. The puncture site, sometimes in conjunction with a second incision, is then enlarged to permit insertion of the laparoscope (also called peritoneoscope) and electrosurgical device.

Using this equipment, a surgeon can locate, grasp, coagulate, and cut the fallopian tubes. Although electrosurgical burns to patients and surgeons are a potential hazard, this procedure is used because it is brief (about 15 minutes) and the incisions are small (about 1 cm).[100]

Protection from Other Electric Hazards. The hazards associated with careless use of electricity, in addition to fire and explosion discussed earlier in the chapter, are electric shock (both macroshock and microshock), and power failure which could result in malfunctioning of life-sustaining equipment. Malfunction or unsafe handling of electric equipment could electrocute a patient, or death could result from failure of life-sustaining devices. Recording errors from improperly functioning monitoring equipment is another hazard. Nurses are legally responsible for recognizing malfunctioning equipment and for alerting the engineering staff so that it can be repaired. Nurses are also responsible for proper use of the equipment and for observing and accurately recording all of the patient's symptoms and reactions.[101] Considering the proliferation of electronic equipment used in hospitals, and the hazards associated with its use, this is indeed a grave responsibility.

Perhaps one of the greatest challenges in nursing is care of the electrically susceptible patient, and prevention of *electric shock* which can and does electrocute patients—sometimes in very subtle ways. There are two kinds of electric shock: (1) *macroshock,* the type of shock received when electric current from an external contact enters through unbroken skin and flows through the body; and (2) *microshock,* the kind of shock in which small amounts of current bypass the protective covering of the skin by traveling through an externalized conductor directly to an electrode implanted in the heart muscle, or through a catheter leading into or near the heart. In this latter type, minute electric currents (as little as 20 microamperes) too small to be felt by sensitive fingers can cause ventricular fibrillation. Unless fibrillation is stopped and normal heart function is reestablished immediately, death results.

Until recently, macroshock was the only electric hazard requiring precautions. Now, since the introduction of electronic diagnosis and treatment devices, microshock is a serious hazard which must be scrupulously guarded against. The hazard of macroshock is present wherever and whenever electricity is used. It can usually be controlled by traditionally effective safety measures. Microshock, on the other hand, occurs only in the electrically sensitive patient, and its prevention is more difficult. It requires "a carefully designed and controlled electrical environment for the patient, and the discipline to keep him there." *

A patient who has an electric conductor connected to the heart with terminals exposed outside the body is referred to as an *"electrically sensitive"* or *"electrically susceptible"* patient (ESP). The areas in which these patients are treated, such as the cardiac catheterization laboratory, or the coronary care unit, are designated as "electrically susceptible patient locations" (ESPL). The electric environment in these locations can be controlled to some extent by installation of a carefully engineered electric power distribution network of one kind or another. Of course, it is not possible to make an area where electricity is used absolutely "electrically safe." Careful, intelligent use of electric equipment is required to reduce the hazard of microshock. The danger can be lessened somewhat by using only properly grounded equipment which will permit all leakage current to seek ground through a safe conductive pathway, preferably with an alarm or warning system which will warn hospital personnel wherever leakage current develops. Another important safety measure is periodic inspection of equipment by hospital engineering services.

The human body, like a bird perched on a high-tension wire, is immune to electric shock so long as it is not part of an electric circuit.[102] Becoming part of a circuit is a possibility whenever electric equipment is used. In order for electricity to work, it must flow in a complete circuit from the power source, through the device it is intended to energize, and from there back to the power source which is in contact with the earth through a ground wire and grounding plug. If electric current "escapes" or flows out of its intended pathway, by way of a frayed extension cord, for example, it seeks the path of least resistance to ground through the most available conductive pathway. This may be through a grounded object (anything that is attached directly or indirectly to earth, such as plumbing fixtures) or through a human body if a person touches live current and a grounded object at the same time. In that case, the person, by serving as an accidental link in the current's pathway to ground, becomes part of an electric circuit, and a victim of electric shock. Whether or not the shock will be fatal depends on the amount of current (measured in amperes) flowing through the body, the location of the current as it flows through the body, and the amount

of time the current continues to flow. These factors are highly variable, but the voltage (or pressure behind the current) is constant. The path of the current through the body depends on the points of contact. Usually this is through one or both hands and out both feet. The amount of current that will flow through the body depends on the resistance of the tissues, chiefly the intact skin. Skin resistance increases with thickness, and is diminished by moisture. For this reason, perspiration, or a break in the skin at the site of contact, significantly reduces electric resistance, permitting more current to flow. In the gross shock situation, that is, in the case of macroshock, electric current diffuses through the body from the point of entrance to the point of exit. Once the skin barrier is penetrated, the body offers little resistance to the passage of current. Blood and body fluids are excellent conductors, and the blood vessels and intravascular spaces provide an excellent conduction system.[103]

The amount of time spent in contact with alternating current is of vital importance. If sufficient current flows long enough (more than a second or two) muscular contractions may make it impossible to release contact. In general, men can free themselves from currents of 9 or less milliamperes, whereas the top "let go" value for women is 6 milliamperes.[104] At 100 milliamperes, muscular contractions can be so rapid and forceful that the victim may be involuntarily jerked away from contact with the electrical source. For this reason, high currents are often not as lethal as moderate currents. Failure to let go may result in a reduction of skin resistance due to secondary perspiration, or blistering at the side of contact, with a consequent increase in flow of current through the body.

Electricity may damage the body four ways: (1) Its effect on the nervous system may briefly stun the victim, producing reversible loss of consciousness, or it may cause cessation of respiration that could result in death. (2) Electricity affects the heart by causing ventricular fibrillation. Macroshock current affects the heart only when the heart is in the pathway between the entrance and the exit of current, that is, when the current flows through the chest area. Ventricular fibrillation caused by macrocurrent usually results when a current of about 100 milliamperes flows from arm to arm across the thorax for one second or longer.[105] This differs from microshock which can electrocute a person with current levels of only millionths of amperes if current flows directly into an implanted electrode in the heart. (3) Heat from electric current in contact with the skin may scorch and coagulate tissue. Severe burns can occur deep inside the

* Friedlander, Gordon D.: "Electricity in Hospitals," *IEEE Spectrum*, (Sept.) 1971, p. 41. (Published by the Institute of Electrical and Electronics Engineers, Inc.)

body as well as on the surface, destroying nerves and muscle tissue, or burns may be caused by flaming clothing. (4) Electricity causes muscles to contract, causing intense pain. Powerful muscular contractions may result in injury of bones or soft tissue. Contraction of the chest muscles also contributes to cessation of respiration. Even when electric shock is not severe enough to be lethal or to adversely affect the body, it may cause secondary accidents. Involuntary movements from reacting to the current may make someone spill a pan of hot liquid, or fall from a ladder, for example.

The *hazard of macroshock* in health care institutions is like the hazard in home bathrooms, kitchens, gardens, and basements. It is the normal hazard associated with the general use of electricity, and its control is covered by the national electric code. In the hospital, or anywhere, electric shock can occur whenever electric devices are used in the vicinity of grounded metal objects. A floor polisher, for example, can be an electric hazard when used near a grounded electric device such as a television set, or near a grounding point such as the radiator, a metal window frame, an overbed light, a drinking fountain, or an oxygen or vacuum outlet in the wall. In the event of a defect in the equipment being used, the person using the equipment could make contact with live voltage from the defective machine and a grounded object at the same time, thus becoming part of an electric circuit. The ensuing shock could be mild, serious enough to cause a short circuit that could blow a fuse or trip a circuit breaker, or severe enough to kill. Macroshock could also be caused by a grounded electrically operated bed and a defective electric device such as a bedside lamp, particularly if there is spillage of water, urine, blood, vomitus, or other liquid into the bed. A defective electrocardiograph machine in operation after well-moistened electrodes are applied to the outside of the patient's body could result in macroshock.[106,107]

The easiest way *to prevent macroshock,* or avoid danger from electric shock, is to keep one's body from becoming part of an electric circuit, that is, from becoming an accidental link in the current's path to ground. Certain safety measures apply wherever electricity is used: Keep electric equipment in good condition and handle with care. The cord and plug are among the most hazardous parts of any electric equipment because they are so easily damaged. Do not use electric-powered appliances or tools while standing in water or on a wet floor, as water is an excellent conductor of electricity. Remember, wet hands

and electric fixtures are a dangerous combination. Keep electrically operated devices away from bathtubs and swimming pools. Wear insulated shoes and gloves when using electrically powered garden tools. Do not grasp powered equipment and grounded objects at the same time. Never plug in or unplug equipment, turn on a light, or touch operating equipment while your other hand, or other part of your body, is in contact with a grounded fixture. Do not drape or rest electric power cords on water pipes, radiators, or other fixtures in contact with the ground. Avoid using separate ground wires to connect equipment to a pipe or radiator; have proper 3-prong grounded plugs and cords installed on the equipment. The 3-prong plug has a "built-in" grounding provision; the longer, or rounded third pin, connects the frame or chassis of the equipment to the building power system ground. The 2-blade plug does not have this feature (see Fig. 15-2). Bear in mind that plugs alone do not guarantee safety; a 3-prong grounded plug may have a hidden break in the grounding wire, or the wall receptacle into which it is plugged may not, in fact, provide a good connection to the building ground. Special equipment known as testing equipment is available in hospitals to locate these kinds of defects. Never break off the third pin of a 3-prong grounded plug to make it fit into a 2-prong wall receptacle, and, remember, a device is not grounded if an extension cord without a grounding plug is used, or if a "cheater" adaptor is used to convert a 3-prong plug to a 2-prong plug. Extension cords should be avoided. If their use is necessary, they should be as short as possible and as heavy or as large in diameter as the power line (electric cord) on the equipment.

If a person should receive a severe electric shock of macroshock intensity, breathing is likely to stop but life may be saved by prompt use of artificial respiration or *resuscitation.* When such an accident occurs, do not touch the victim, or you may become part of the electric circuit. Shut off the current if possible, or, using a dry, nonconductive implement such as rubber gloves, a dry wooden stick or rope, release the victim from the current. As soon as the person is free, if spontaneous respiration has ceased, begin mouth-to-mouth respiration, and, if possible, cardiac massage. Both artificial respiration and artificial circulation should be maintained simultaneously if possible until spontaneous breathing starts and cardiac function returns.[108]

Microshock is a hazard for persons under diagnosis and treatment with electrical devices. All seriously ill patients are more vulnerable

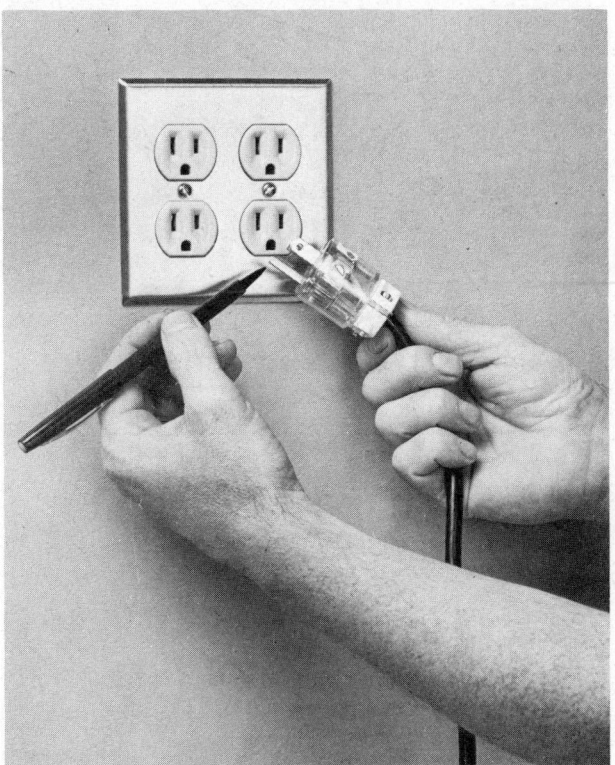

Figure 15-2. A three-prong grounding plug. The longer, round pin is grounding connection. Through a third wire in the power cord, it is connected to metal frame, chassis, or case of equipment. When plugged into a properly grounded receptacle, it connects the hospital ground to the equipment. Never break off third pin of a three-prong plug, or use a "cheater" adaptor to fit three-prong plug into wall receptacle having only two slots. Change the wall receptacle. (From Hewlett Packard Co.: *Using Electrically Operated Equipment Safely with the Monitored Cardiac Patient*. Waltham, Mass., 1971, p. 12.)

to electric shock than healthy persons; their nervous systems are more susceptible to electric current, and they are likely to perspire more and have other physiologic changes that lower resistance to electricity, but electrically susceptible patients with catheters, probes, or wires leading from within the heart to terminals outside are in double jeopardy. Their unprotected hearts are exposed to the electric environment around them, and that environment is apt to contain an array of potentially lethal electronic devices. The intracardiac catheters or electrodes they are bearing provide a low resistance path directly to the heart for small amounts of leakage current continuously emanate from ungrounded, or improperly grounded equipment. Leakage current is unwanted current which flows in the frame or chassis of all electric equipment. It serves no useful purpose, and when diverted to ground through a grounding wire, is of no consequence. Leakage current is hazardous only when allowed to pass through internal catheters or lead-wires in, or near, the vicinity of the heart. Leakage current is in the microampere range and is too weak to be perceptible to the touch of those taking care of the patient. It can only be detected with sensitive instruments, and is therefore a hidden danger as far as the nurse is concerned. *Small amounts*

of leakage current, as little as 20 millionths of 1 ampere, if directed into the patient's heart through electrodes implanted there, can electrocute the patient by causing fatal ventricular fibrillation. The density of the electric current plays a role in causing fibrillation. Each implanted electrode has only a small area of contact with the heart, but through this small area, all of the available leakage current is channeled. Although the total current may be very small, density, or concentration, is high.

Because saline and blood both conduct electricity, a fluid-filled catheter can serve as an electrode. For this reason, indwelling venous and arterial catheters used for measurement of flow and pressure, or even a fluid-filled nasogastric tube ending in close proximity to the heart, can be a means of carrying fatal current.

Some situations are especially hazardous. Since patients bearing a pressure catheter, pacing catheter, or intracardiac electrocardiograph electrodes have "electrically exposed" hearts, people taking care of them are considered part of the electric environment surrounding the patient. Under certain circumstances, a nurse simultaneously touching a current-carrying device (a lamp, or bedrail of an electrically operated bed) with one hand, and the patient with the other, may electrically

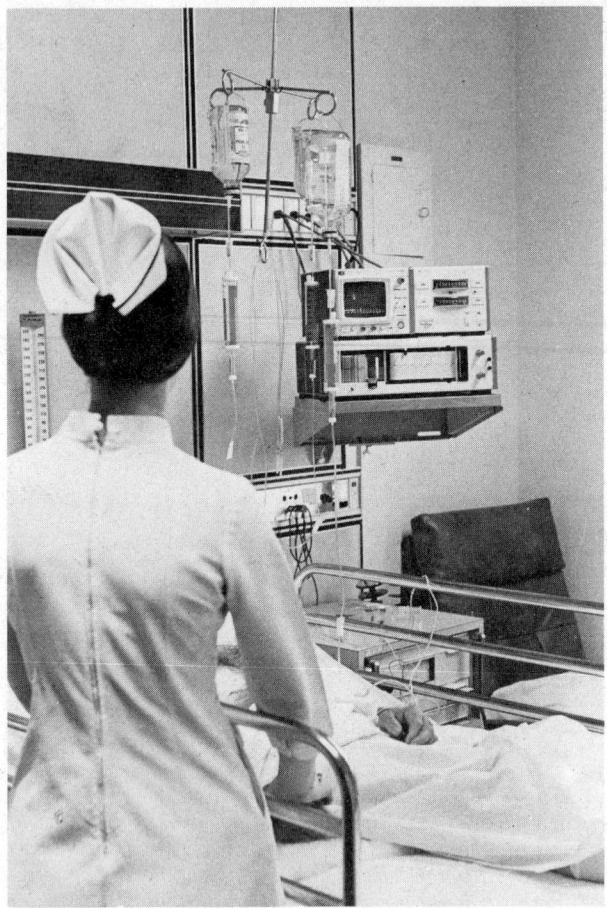

Figure 15-3. The patient being monitored by electronic equipment is highly vulnerable to microshock. The nurse in attendance is part of the "electrical environment" surrounding the patient. When several pieces of electrically operated equipment are being used, great care should be exercised to keep one device from acting as a "current source" and another as a "ground" with the patient as a current path between the two. (From Hewlett Packard Co.: *Using Electrically Operated Equipment Safely with the Monitored Cardiac Patient.* Waltham, Mass., 1971, p. 8.)

connect the two by serving as an accidental path for electric current[109] (see Fig. 15-3).

Consider the following hypothetical, but possible, situation: A patient equipped with a transvenous pacing catheter connected to a small battery-operated pacemaker is lying in an electrically operated bed which has a faulty ground connection in the power cord near the wall plug. The patient is also connected to a grounded electrocardiograph monitor. The right leg electrocardiograph electrode is connected to the hospital grounding system through the monitor. The faulty ground connection on the electric bed allows current to flow through the bed frame. Normally this current would be harmlessly conducted to ground, but the broken ground wire has permitted the current to follow another path. Assume that the nurse, or someone else in attendance, comes to the bedside to adjust the pacing catheter connections and, without thinking, touches the pacemaker terminals and the bed rail at the same time. The nurse's body, in this instance, completes the path between the power line and ground with the current going through the nurse, into the pacemaker's wire, and through the patient's heart. An assumed 100 microamperes would not be noticed by the nurse as it is below the threshold of perception of most adults. It would, however, be strong enough to cause the patient's heart to fibrillate (see Fig. 15-4).

The nurse in this situation might have suspected earlier that something was wrong if he or she had noticed a possible increase in the amount of line frequency interference on the electrocardiograph trace on the monitor, but since the electric bed would have been operating satisfactorily, the fault in the ground wire would probably not have been suspected. It could only have been discovered by careful testing with special testing equipment. *This example illustrates the importance of proper handling of equipment, vigilant observation, and meticulous checking and testing of equipment.**

* The authors thank the Medical Electronics Division of the Hewlett Packard Company, Waltham, Mass., for permission to reproduce Figures 15-3 and

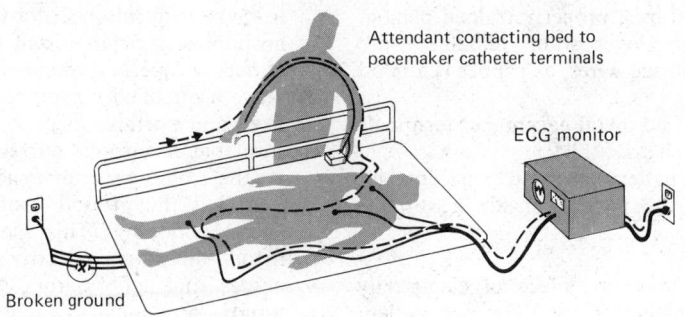

Attendant contacting bed to
pacemaker catheter terminals

ECG monitor

Broken ground

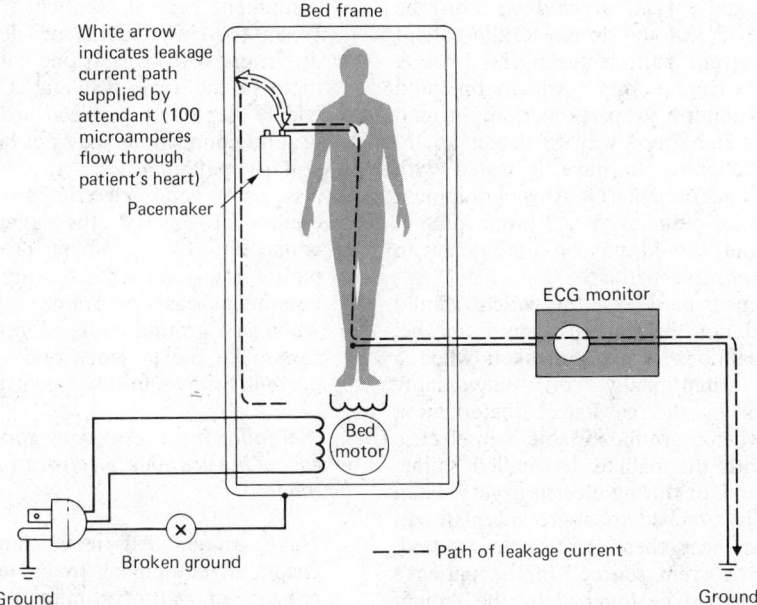

Bed frame

White arrow
indicates leakage
current path
supplied by
attendant (100
microamperes
flow through
patient's heart)

Pacemaker

ECG monitor

Bed
motor

Broken ground

- - - - Path of leakage current

Ground

Ground

Figure 15-4. Diagram of an unwitting electrocution. *Above,* the faulty ground connection on the electric bed allows a voltage to exist on the bed frame. Here, the attendant supplies the completion of the current path (from the source, through the pacemaker's wire, to the patient, to ground) when he touches the bed, thereby permitting the leakage current to flow through his body and that of the patient. *Below,* analysis of the mishap is shown in the block diagram of the leakage current's path. (From Hewlett Packard Co.: *Patient Safety.* Waltham, Mass., 1971, p. 10.)

The following are recommendations for safe care of electrically susceptible patients, *being constantly aware that the person at the bedside is part of the patient's electric environment.*[*]

15-4 and the description of the illustrations taken from the Hewlett Packard brochure, *Patient Safety,* 1971.

[*] These recommendations for anyone who works with electrically susceptible patients were summarized and adapted from the booklet, *Using Electrically-Operated Equipment Safely with the Monitored Cardiac Patient.* This is one of two booklets on care of the electrically susceptible patient printed by the Hewlett Packard Company, Waltham, Mass.

1. When adjusting instrument controls, checking electrode attachments, handling the patient, adjusting the bed, and so forth, do not touch electric devices with the other hand.
2. Keep in mind that moisture increases electric conductivity and lowers resistance of the skin, allowing more current to flow than if dry.
3. Watch for dangling power or patient cables, kinks in wires, loose plugs in wall outlets, loose electrocardiograph electrodes, or worn or frayed electric cords, and report anything suspicious immediately. Take faulty equipment out of service until it is checked

and corrected by a properly trained person.

4. Wear rubber gloves when handling bare catheter electrode wires, as rubber is a good insulator.
5. Insulate exposed metal pacemaker terminals with rubber sleeves.
6. Place a battery-operated pacemaker, strapped to the patient, inside a surgical glove.

When more than one piece of electrically operated equipment are used for one patient at the same time, it is possible for one device to serve as a "current source" and another as a "ground" and *special precautions* must be observed. Be careful and do not let the patient become a current path between the two. A current source can be any electrically operated equipment without a properly working ground connection. (The surest way to detect an inactive connection is to have it tested with appropriate instruments.) Any equipment plugged into an outlet with a 2-prong plug is dangerous and should not be used near an electrically sensitive patient.

All equipment used near the patient should be grounded but the patient should *not* be. Special precautions should be taken when a patient is intentionally or unavoidably grounded as in the cardiac catheterization laboratory when a grounded table is in electric "contact" with the patient by spilled saline, blood, or urine, or during electrosurgery when the patient is attached to a ground plate. In such circumstances, there must be no exposed, ungrounded "current source" in the patient's vicinity that could be touched by the patient or an intermediary. This could cause the patient to become a conductive path to ground. Periodic checks of all electrically operated equipment in these locations is mandatory. Do not depend on equipment failure as a warning of the presence of hazardous currents.

Keep in mind that current flowing through the exposed metal parts of the bed frame or the case of an electric device with a defective or missing ground connection may be too small to be felt by the nurse, and may not prevent the equipment from working properly, but it could cause fibrillation if permitted to flow through the nurse's body to the patient's heart. With this in mind, observe the *following precautions:*

1. Be certain all equipment is effectively grounded through 3-wire power cords, and 3-prong grounding plugs connected to grounded wall outlets.
2. Never use "cheater" adaptors or break off the round grounding pin on a 3-prong plug

to make it fit into a 2-slot wall outlet. Have hospital electrician install new 3-wire wall outlets, properly grounded.

3. Have a qualified person regularly check all fixed and portable electric equipment to be sure that hazardous current is not present on the frame, case, or exposed metal parts, and that the ground connection is intact and functioning. This includes *all* equipment—monitors, electrocardiograph machines, and defibrillators, as well as lamps, radios, nurse call switches, electric fans, television sets and their remote control units, suction machines, and other electric equipment near the patient.*
4. When two instruments or electric devices are in use with or near one patient, connect them to the same wall outlet. If different, widely separated outlets are used, their ground connections may not be at the same voltage potential.
5. Associate good electric grounding with equipment, not with the patient. A ground connection to equipment provides a safe path for any currents flowing through the equipment case or frame to "drain off," whereas a ground connection to the patient can make the patient's body the path the current follows in flowing to ground.†

The *following precautions should be taken when an intracardiac electrocardiograph is to be made:*

1. Have a qualified technician thoroughly check all equipment to be used near the patient for faulty or missing ground connections, and hazardous voltages, before it is used.
2. Connect electrode catheters to the V-lead of the electrocardiograph. (This circuit has a high electric resistance in relation to the ground.)
3. Do not connect such catheters to the indifferent or grounded electrode (usually the right leg).
4. Do not let anyone or anything that is electrically grounded touch the V-lead electrode terminals.

Potential hazards can exist and not be readily apparent. Do not rely on a possible hazard

* It is unwise to permit extraneous or unnecessary electric equipment such as radios or television sets to be brought into the area with an electrically sensitive patient. Electric fans, as well as creating an electric hazard, may disseminate pathogenic microorganisms.
† Household electric appliances such as stoves have their metal frames grounded through a third wire in the power cord and a third prong on the power plug for the same reason.

to always give a clear advance warning. The best defense against hazards is enough knowledge to enable the nurse to recognize warnings, combined with regular maintenance procedures to prevent them. The following are some *warning signals* that should alert the nurse to possible hazards:

1. If A.C. "noise" or power line interference in displayed or recorded electrocardiograph wave forms makes interpretation difficult, check for and correct loose or dried-out electrodes, or defects in the patient cable. If that does not stop the interference, it may mean potentially hazardous current is flowing in the patient leads. Investigate thoroughly, and correct the situation as soon as possible.
2. Tingling sensations which can be felt when touching or brushing against a piece of electrically operated equipment demand immediate attention.* If the equipment is not necessary to support the patient's life, it should be removed from use for repair, and labeled to warn others. If it is necessary for the patient's life support, the problem should be investigated by an electronics technician if necessary and corrected immediately.

All of the earlier suggestions on the use of 3-prong plugs, and precautions to observe while working around grounded installations discussed under the prevention of macroshock, are equally valid as *preventive measures against microshock*.

Ideally, to minimize electric mishaps, a hospital should have an electrical safety program with an equipment control officer to oversee the purchase, inspection, maintenance, and proper use of electric equipment. There should be an adequate on-going training program for personnel who use the equipment. Doctors and nurses should know how to operate it correctly and how to recognize defects. Frequent inspection of all equipment by authorized personnel is essential. In addition, each piece of equipment used with the electrically susceptible patient should be tested immediately before it is put into use. Critical testing instruments have been designed specifically for use by technicians, nurses, and physicians. The hospital should make this testing equipment available. Intelligent use of equipment, careful testing, and preventive mainte-

nance are the best safeguards against electric accidents.

9. PROVIDING AND MAINTAINING A SANITARY ENVIRONMENT

Importance of Cleanliness. The common expression "Cleanliness is next to godliness" expresses a public recognition of its importance. A sanitary environment goes a long way toward controlling disease. The development of the public health movement was based on sanitary science and many of its leaders were classed as "sanitarians." Elements of a sanitary environment are so widely known and accepted in developed countries that they may seem to need little emphasis. The fact is, however, that sanitary standards vary greatly among the developed nations and practices vary even more. "Sanitary codes," published by national, state, provincial, county, and metropolitan health departments, are far from standardized. Since problems of sanitation vary from one area to another some differences are understandable. Generally speaking, the more crowded an area the greater the risk of disease from poor sanitation; the more stable the population, and the healthier it is, the more resistance it has to poor sanitary conditions. Standards of cleanliness that might not cause disease in a home would be dangerous in a hospital.

Comparative Danger of Home and Institutional Living. Invasion of the bodies of man and animals by other living organisms is a hazard in every environment. But man and animals are also dependent on other living organisms. Coexistence is an element of every biologic system. Health and life depend on a balance between systems and on the exercise, by each organism, of its protective mechanisms.

Humans and animals build up resistance to the organisms that reside in the bodies of their associates; they have less resistance to the bacterial flora of strangers. Protective mechanisms of humans and animals are weakened by malnutrition, by polluted atmospheres, and by almost any disease process. Protective mechanisms are threatened by traveling to strange places, by living with strangers, and living under crowded conditions. Almost any institutional life, even a hotel, exposes its inmates to a greater risk of infection than family life.* An institution for the sick is especially hazardous, and large ones, particularly teaching and

---

* A tingling sensation is induced by about one-thousandth of an ampere of 50- or 60-cycle alternating current, under ordinary circumstances harmless, but nearly 50 times the current which can cause ventricular fibrillation if it flows through the patient's heart.

* A home can, of course, be so poorly maintained and crowded that living in it can be hazardous just as a hotel may be so well maintained that staying in it offers little danger of infection.

research centers, especially so, although this may be offset by the effective efforts the staff often makes—and can afford to make—to reduce risks.

Because hospital environments carry a greater risk of infection than any other, this chapter concentrates on how to protect people in them. The emphasis is also on big "modern" institutions that can provide the most highly developed facilities, equipment, and supplies. Nurses working in isolated and underdeveloped areas, in some schools, industries, corrective institutions, and homes may think the way the subject is handled offers them little help. It should be stressed, however, that the practices recommended for the most dangerous situations are those that people should strive for in all treatment centers. Practices may safely be less rigid in home nursing and in institutions where certain hazards characteristic of the general hospital do not exist; but it is desirable anywhere to use genuinely aseptic, commercially sterilized, and disposable equipment and supplies rather than those treated by boiling, by dry heat in an oven, or by ironing with a hot iron. All these "makeshift" practices are better than no effort to achieve asepsis and should be used in emergencies where reliable practices are impossible.

Visiting nurse services provide workers with manuals in which disease control measures are spelled out. In general they are adaptations of the methods discussed here. While patients in homes are exposed to fewer hazards, it is of the utmost importance that the equipment carried in the nurse's bag be kept free from disease-producing microorganisms.

Other parts of this text reinforce or supplement what is said in this chapter. In Chapter 14 there was some discussion of how people protect the body—the integument, or tissues exposed to danger; in chapters that describe particular treatments, or procedures, such as injections or intubations, special aseptic precautions are discussed; in Chapter 32 processing sterile supplies and equipment is discussed; in Chapters 33 and 43 wounds and wound dressings are discussed; in Chapter 44 systemic infections, or communicable diseases, are discussed.

Maintaining a sanitary hospital environment requires the coordinated efforts of several departments and the carrying out of a number of activities, among which are cleaning and disinfection of the inanimate environment, sterilization of certain materials, insect and rodent control, effective ventilation and laundering, sanitary handling and disposal of waste, and provision for safe water, ice, and food.

Adequate cleaning and decontamination of the physical surroundings is essential not only to help prevent the spread of infection but for esthetic reasons as well.

Psychologic Effect of Cleanliness and Order. There are many standards of cleanliness even in economically favored countries. What one person considers necessary in this respect may seem fastidious to the neighbor on the right and careless to the neighbor on the left. Generally speaking, however, most people respond favorably to symmetry and clarity of design in the arrangement of a room and cleanliness of walls, floors, and furnishings.

If the outlook of a person in good health is affected by his or her environment, that outlook is even more likely to be influenced during sickness. Those who are habitually orderly and clean are likely to be most sensitive to their surroundings, but even persons who seem unable to keep themselves and their belongings in order when well are very critical of disorder in the treatment setting. Teaching the value of cleanliness and order may be one of the nurse's most important services.

Institutional management and housekeeping is no longer the responsibility of the nurses, who are rarely experts in this field, and it is a waste of their special preparation for nursing to divert their energies to housekeeping; nevertheless, for the sake of the patient, they must be prepared to act in this role as they must often act for the physician, the nutritionist, or the social worker when they are unavailable. Because cleaning, laundering, and the care of furnishings are specialties, only the most fundamental principles can be set down in a text of this kind. More detailed information can be found in textbooks devoted to household arts and institutional management.

Scientific housekeeping is now a specialized occupation and field of study. Hotel management, including housekeeping, is a worldwide specialty. Training programs for hospital housekeepers have been established in several universities of the United States, among them Washington State, Michigan State, and Cornell. Sound hospital housekeeping practices are based on scientific principles. Cleaning procedures should be continually evaluated and modified to fit rapidly changing conditions. Cleaning and disinfection require knowledge of microbiology, chemistry, and the principles of vermin and rodent control. Housekeeping staffs must be carefully trained to assume responsibility for specific functions in various areas of the hospital. Critical patient care areas such as operating rooms, nurseries, and intensive care and isolation units require meticulous cleaning and disinfecting. Work areas such as central supply, laboratories, and kitchen and laundry areas also require specialized cleaning techniques. All hospital housekeeping personnel should know the fundamentals of infection control as well as something about general aseptic and isolation techniques. These concepts must be taught in a way suited to each group of learners. The nurse may be called on to function formally or informally as a teacher in such programs.

General Cleaning Procedures. The American Hospital Association's book, *Infection Control in the Hospital*,[110] recommends that hospitals have written directives, reviewed by the infection control committee, for the cleaning of walls, floors, windows, window frames and sills, curtains, bedside screens, fixtures, and furniture throughout the hospital. In general, it is recommended that waste receptacles should have disposable liners, and that both liners and waste are to be incinerated, that delivery of clean linen and collection of soiled linen, using special precautions for linen from infected patients, should be scheduled, and because most dust and lint settles on horizontal surfaces, all horizontal areas in patients' rooms (except for ceilings) should be wet- or damp-cleaned at least daily, with thorough terminal cleaning of rooms between patients. Walls need not be routinely cleaned except for visible soil. Fogging with disinfectants is an unsatisfactory method of decontaminating air or surfaces, and, with mechanical ventilation, airing-out periods are not necessary (see page 901). However, in most places, and to most persons, outside air brought into a room is psychologically refreshing.

Central cleaning and disinfection of supplies such as bedpans and basins is preferable to decontamination on the nursing unit. In cleaning a room in which a person has been isolated, housekeeping personnel should use the same precautions as recommended for hospital staff (immunizations, protective clothing, and aseptic measures). Double bagging (see page 896) and labeling should be used for contaminated equipment and linen, and special precautions for handling should be observed by both housekeeping and central supply personnel. (See page 900 for more about terminal cleaning of isolation areas.)

Cleaning Agents and Methods of Cleaning. The method of cleaning and choice of agents depends on the surfaces to be cleaned, the kind and amount of soil, and the condition of the soil—whether it is fresh, or dry and hardened. Some kinds of soil are soluble in water, others are not. Fatty substances must be removed with fat solvents or emulsifying agents; rust is soluble in acid, and blood and urine are soluble in alkalies. Mineral oil is soluble in organic solvents, while complex soil such as milk and dust are insoluble but can be suspended in a solution. Dust must be reduced to a minimum as dust particles may carry microorganisms to distant parts of the hospital by drafts, and through laundry and rubbish chutes, elevator shafts, and stairwells. A bag of refuse or laundry falling down a chute may create a piston effect, forcing airborne particles through openings on a succession of floors. Regardless of the kind of soil, principles of cleaning are the same in all cases. Dirt or stain is removed mechanically by brushes or mops, by suction with a vacuum cleaner, or by an abrasive of some kind. Cleaning agents are acid, alkaline, or neutral. It is important to know this property in selecting a detergent or a solvent and to consider its action on the article to be cleaned as well as its action on the disinfectant it is to be used with, as some disinfectants are inactivated by detergents. It is also important to select the most economical of the available agents, providing quality is not sacrificed. It is estimated that 90 per cent of housekeeping costs are for labor.* Relative to over-all expense, the cost of good quality disinfectants and detergents is small.

Detergents and Soaps. A *detergent* is an agent that helps remove unwanted material from a surface. All cleaning agents, including soaps, are, according to the dictionary's definition, detergents, but they may or may not be disinfectants. (In common usage *detergent* often means an agent that is not a soap.) Bacteria, if not killed, are usually removed whenever detergents are used. A *soap* is a compound of fatty acids and a soluble alkali. Used alone, they do not disinfect. When mixed with water, they remove dirt and surface bacteria that are loosely attached. The process of cleaning with a detergent is really the exchange of a soiled surface for a clean surface plus a soiled detergent. Soaps and detergents are used in hospitals for laundry, dishwashing, cleaning hard surfaces (walls, floors, furniture), handwashing, and for cleaning equipment and utensils.[111]

Disinfecting Agents. A *disinfectant* is a chemical agent used to kill vegetative forms of microorganisms on inanimate surfaces. Specific disinfectants should be chosen according to their effect on various organisms. Phenolic compounds are most active against gram-negative bacteria. Quaternary ammonium compounds, which are no longer recommended

---

* Mallison, George, in a lecture on Hospital Sanitation, US Public Health Service, Center for Disease Control, Atlanta, Ga., March 1973.

for use in the hospital outside of the kitchen, are effective only against gram-positive organisms, specifically staphylococci and streptococci. Iodophors are effective against many organisms and have a bactericidal effect on tubercle bacilli. Activated glutaraldehyde and formaldehyde kill all microorganisms including spores.

The housekeeping staff should be taught the potential danger in using disinfecting agents, as well as which materials weaken or neutralize the compounds. Cotton, soap, and hard water will inactivate quaternary compounds such as Zephiran, iodine may react with some metals, and phenols may be inactivated by protein. (See page 882 for more information about disinfectants.) Table 15-4 on page 885 lists disinfecting agents for types of objects to be disinfected as well as for specific contaminating organisms. It cannot be overemphasized that all objects or surfaces must be thoroughly cleaned before disinfectants are used in order to remove materials, particularly feces, blood, pus, or mucus that are not penetrated by disinfectants.

Care of Cleaning Equipment. Cleaning equipment should be made of noncorrosive materials and should be easy to clean. Mop heads and dusters must be laundered daily, or disposable materials used. Wet mop heads, cloths, brushes, or sponges should never be stored in a janitor's closet, nor should water be allowed to stand in containers, as any moist surface provides a medium for growth of gram-negative bacteria. Wet pick-up and dry vacuums must have efficient filters to prevent bacteria from passing through on small dust particles or in aerosol droplets. Cleaning methods should be simplified as much as possible in order to keep cleaning equipment relatively free of bacteria.[112]

Cleaning Procedures for Specific Areas. *Floors* in a hospital are always considered contaminated. Dust and soil picked up by people's feet is carried from contaminated to (relatively) cleaner areas. Hard-surfaced floors such as marble, tile, terrazzo, and some of the synthetic tiles are nonporous, nonresilient and easily maintained. Softer surfaces such as wood, linoleum, and cork tiles are porous dust collectors but are often used because they are resilient and cause less fatigue to those who tread them or stand on them.

There are differing opinions about the advisability of *carpets* in hospitals. Some studies have shown that buildup of bacteria occurs rapidly in carpets, that bacteria can survive for several months in carpeting material, and that cleaning and walking on carpets disseminates bacteria into the air.[113] Other studies have shown that proper vacuuming keeps carpets as

free of bacteria as hard-surfaced floors.[114] Even though carpets *do* get contaminated, there is little evidence that they are related to outbreaks of infection. If they are used in hospitals, however, they should not be installed in high-risk areas, such as intensive care units, or work areas where they are subjected to heavy soiling.

The most effective method of cleaning floors, while preventing dissemination of microorganisms, is a combination of scrubbing with a detergent-disinfectant and the use of a filtered wet vacuum pick-up machine (a vacuum cleaner that picks up liquids).[115,116] Carpeted floors should be vacuumed daily, and uncarpeted floors and other open areas should be flushed and scrubbed once a day with a fresh detergent-disinfectant solution using a wet vacuum pick-up machine to remove the solution from the floor following flushing and scrubbing. Vacuum cleaning of surfaces (for removal of dust) is recommended prior to wet cleaning. Vacuuming should not be substituted for wet cleaning, however. Vacuums should have effective filters to avoid dissemination of bacteria from vacuum exhaust. Dry sweeping or buffing of floors is not recommended as it may increase the microbial count in the air. New synthetic floor finishes eliminate the need for routine buffing. If a wet vacuum pick-up machine is not available, the double bucket or double mop technique may be utilized using clean mops, buckets, and solutions.* Mop heads and cleaning cloths, if not disposable, should be laundered every day. Poor housekeeping techniques can contribute to contamination. Mopping with a treated dust mop or dry dusting of any surface is condemned.

A definite regimen should be established for cleaning patients' *bathrooms* with a detergent-disinfectant twice a day, or oftener if necessary. Bathtubs, shower stalls, sinks, and toilet bowls and seats should all be cleaned and disinfected. Powdered cleaners containing chlorine can be used for scouring sinks, providing that they are not abrasive enough to roughen the surface. Phenolic-type solutions are generally recommended for bathroom disinfectants, although iodophors are also used. Quaternary ammonium compounds such as Zephiran are not recommended as they are inactivated by hard water and traces of soap and are ineffec-

---

* Continuous rinsing of the mop in a single bucket of solution contaminates the solution and spreads contamination from one part of the floor to another. The double bucket technique of floor cleaning utilizes separate buckets for the detergent-disinfectant solution and the rinse water. The mop is rinsed prior to dipping into the detergent bucket to minimize contamination of the solution and to extend its useful life.

tive against gram-negative organisms. Showers, with use of disposable, impervious shower mats for each patient, are preferred to bathtubs in order to reduce the chance of cross-contamination.

The proper care of *sinks, toilets, hoppers,* and *bedpans* is very important. Nothing should be emptied into waste pipes that will not break up into small particles. It stands to reason that the larger the drainage pipe the less likely it is to clog; however, even very large openings will be obstructed if hair, matches, cotton fibers, and grease are emptied into them in appreciable quantities. Any indications that fixtures are out of order should be immediately reported.

In many hospitals, particularly where bathrooms adjoin patients' rooms, bedpans are emptied into the toilet and cleaned with a spray. It is thought that so-called bedpan sterilizers are ineffective and may disseminate airborne microorganisms, and that bedpans should be emptied into the nearest toilet rather than carried any distance. Moreover, if bedpans are put into the bedpan flusher, they must be disinfected before being used again, even by the same patient. If possible, all patients should have their own bedpans, to be emptied and cleaned in adjoining bathrooms and replaced in their bedside stands after each use, or if the patient has his or her own bathroom, the bedpan can be kept there.*

Toilets should be vigorously brushed with a germicidal bowl cleaner both inside and out, using a disposable brush, if possible. It has been found that dysentery organisms are capable of survival on toilet seats for more than 2 weeks.[117] The practice of letting toilet brushes stand in a solution is to be discouraged. If disposable brushes are not available, the brush should stand in a phenolic solution, *not* Zephiran which may become inactivated and provide a medium for propagation of gram-negative organisms.

Providing a sanitary environment involves more than cleaning; it may involve killing disease-producing microbes or all microbial life. The following sections deal with this subject and the processes involved.

10. PROVIDING AND MAINTAINING A SANITARY FOOD SERVICE

General Principles of Sanitary Food Handling. The first step in sound food sanitation

* The practice of keeping bedpans and urinals within sight as well as within the patient's reach is highly unesthetic and offensive to many patients and visitors and is condemned by the writers.

is the purchase of good quality food, followed by safe handling and storage after delivery. Foods most likely to be contaminated at time of purchase are dairy products, cream-filled pastries, poultry, and fresh meat and fish. Only pasteurized dairy products should be purchased, and if frozen eggs are bought they should be pasteurized. Cracked eggs should be avoided because of the likelihood of salmonella contamination.[118] Stored food must be protected from rodent and insect infestation in clean, dry, well-ventilated storage rooms large enough to prevent overcrowding.

Written directions for procedures and cleaning schedules for food service workers are essential, as is good direction and an adequate training program. The program should emphasize employees' personal hygiene, and the importance of reporting all infections. Employees with upper respiratory infections, skin lesions, or diarrhea should not be allowed to handle food. An employee health program for dietary personnel should include periodic medical examinations. Stool cultures should be made before food handlers are hired to screen out carriers of salmonella and shigella.

Clean toilets and handwashing facilities should be provided near food preparation areas, preferably with the handwashing sink outside the toilet area in an easily seen location. Kitchen sinks should not be used for washing hands. All food workers should wash their hands thoroughly and frequently, especially after using the toilet.[119,120]

All work areas and equipment must be kept clean on a regular, daily cleaning schedule. Utensils and work surfaces should never be used for food preparation unless they have been cleaned and sanitized. Meat slicers, grinders, and other equipment that may harbor food particles should be dismantled and cleaned every day. Chopping blocks should be used *only* for raw meat, so that the same block used for cutting raw meat will not be used for chopping other foods. Salmonella, commonly found in raw meat and poultry, may get embedded in a wooden chopping block. Cooking meat destroys the salmonella organisms, rendering the meat safe, but the microorganisms remaining on the block may be transferred to other foods such as precooked meats or salads that are served without further cooking. For the same reason, hands should be washed after handling raw meat, before touching other foods or utensils. Salmonella is also commonly found on egg shells. Outbreaks of food poisoning have resulted from the ingestion of eggnog containing raw, salmonella-contaminated eggs. Eggs should be cooked before serving. Meringue made with raw egg whites should be thoroughly baked, not just superficially browned. Pasteurized frozen or powdered eggs should be used only in dishes requiring prolonged cooking such as baked goods.

Handling food with the fingers should be reduced to a minimum. Clean, sanitized utensils, not hands, should be used to mix food. Plastic gloves should be worn when hands are used (see Fig. 15-5). Persons having infected cuts should not work with food. One reported outbreak of food poisoning was caused by contaminated macaroni salad that had been prepared several hours before the meal. The cooked pimentos, boiled eggs, mayonnaise, and mustard used in the salad were hand-mixed by a cook who had several minor cuts on two fingers. On investigation, *Staphylococcus aureus* from the cuts were found in the salad.[121]

Foods should be served as soon as possible after preparation, and should be kept covered between the time of preparation and serving. Potentially hazardous foods (perishable foods containing milk, eggs, meat, poultry, or fish, chopped cooked foods, or other foods capable of supporting rapid growth of microorganisms) should be kept *hot* at 65.5°C (150°F) or above, or *cold* at 4.4°C (40°F) or below when not being prepared or served. Using leftover cooked food is risky and should be avoided whenever possible. In a reported outbreak of food poisoning, 150 persons had severe diarrhea and abdominal pains after eating roast beef and gravy that had been prepared the day before and allowed to cool on open trays for 24 hours without refrigeration. *Colostridium perfringens* organisms were found in the gravy. Leftovers and partially prepared foods, when used, require immediate refrigeration, stored in shallow pans to permit uniform and rapid cooling. Frozen foods should be thawed in water, or in the refrigerator; they should not be permitted to thaw slowly at room temperature.

Pork should never be eaten unless it is cooked sufficiently to reach an internal temperature of at least 65.5°C (150°F) in order to destroy *Trichinella spiralis,* organisms commonly found in pork, which cause trichinosis.

Food containers made with metal such as zinc, cadmium, and lead have been sources of foodborne illness. Utensils containing toxic materials should not be used in the preparation or storage of food. Organic acids present in fruit juice, jellies, and candies can react with metals of some containers such as tarnished copper. Walter Jopke [122] reported an incident in which 14 people became ill after drinking punch prepared and stored in a galvanized iron container. Investigation showed that acid in the punch had dissolved a considerable amount of zinc from the lining of the container.

Pesticides, detergents, and other cleaning compounds should be stored in a room separate from food to avoid mistaking them for food. Detergents have been mistaken for paprika, liquid cleaning compounds have been mistaken for cooking oils, and sodium fluoride has been confused with baking powder.[123]

Sanitary Handling of Ice in Institutions. Water from an approved source should be used in the manufacture of ice. Storage chests and ice machines should be located in "clean" areas of the hospital or other health care facility. Ice should be transported in clean, covered containers or plastic bags. Storage containers and ice machines should be washed and disinfected with a hypochlorite (chlorine) solution regularly.

Ice should never be handled with bare hands. A scoop or tongs should be used and left on a clean tray, not in the ice chest. The

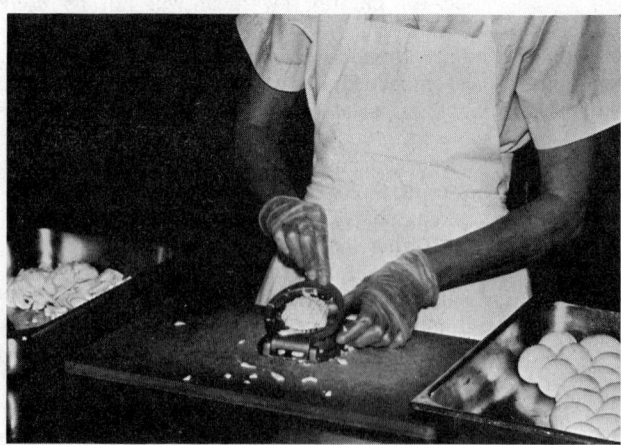

Figure 15-5. Single-service plastic gloves worn during food preparation reduce the possibility of contamination from the hands. (From Bond, Richard G., et al. [eds.]: *Environmental Health and Safety in Health Care Facilities.* Macmillan Publishing Co., Inc., New York, 1974, p. 244.)

utensils and the tray should be washed, preferably in a mechanical dishwasher, every day. Unused ice should not be returned to the storage container.

Care of Water Carafes in Institutions. Drinking water should be supplied to the patient in containers that can be effectively sanitized. Since carafes provide an excellent medium for the growth of gram-negative organisms,[124] they should be collected, washed, and sanitized every day. Carafes should never be flushed out in the wash basin of the patient's bathroom.

Environmental sampling (taking bacterial counts of the inanimate environment) will determine the effectiveness of cleaning procedures. It should be remembered, however, that bacterial sampling is a means of quality control, but it is *not* infection control. Hospital-prepared infant formula should be cultured once a week. Ice should be sampled occasionally.

Dishwashing. Dishes should be machine washed in water at a temperature of 60°C (140°F) for 20 seconds and rinsed at a temperature of 82.2°C (180°F) for 10 seconds. If dishes are washed by hand in an institution they require soaking for at least 30 seconds in an effective sanitizing solution. Dishes should never be dried by hand in treatment centers. Even in homes it is desirable to leave dishes on a clean rack to drain and dry.

Special measures used in food services for patients isolated with a communicable disease are discussed later in this chapter and also in Chapter 44.

11. MAINTAINING A SANITARY LAUNDRY SERVICE

Handling Soiled Materials. The laundry of an institution, especially a hospital, is considered an area where the risk to workers is high. Soiled linen is a significant source of microbial contamination. There is a risk for all personnel in contact with *soiled linen* and they should be taught how to protect themselves and others. Soiled linen should not be sorted in patient areas, nor should it be allowed to accumulate there. Handling linen of infectious patients is discussed on page 897.

All soiled linen should be *bagged* and transported in *covered carts* used exclusively for that purpose. If *chutes* are used they should be cleaned regularly, and should terminate in separate, well-ventilated fireproof rooms, not corridors. Rooms for sorting linen should be separate from other rooms in the hospital laundry. They should have at least ten air changes an hour, with no recirculation within the hospital. The soiled linen areas should be cleaned and disinfected daily.[125]

Clean Materials. *Clean linen* should be processed in rooms separated from sorting and washing areas. The laundry should have a soiled linen storage and sorting room, a processing room, and a clean linen area. Clean linen should be handled as little as possible and stored covered or wrapped. Enclosed linen carts used to transport and store linen in patient areas minimize contamination. Shelves of carts or linen closets must be cleaned routinely.

There are a number of advantages to treatment of linens with textile softeners and bacteriostatic agents during the washing process. Softeners make linen easier to wash and handle, softer for the patient, and less productive of lint.[126]

Some small health agencies contract for service from community laundries but the same steps should be taken to protect workers there as in a hospital laundry.

12. DISINFECTION AND STERILIZATION

Definition of Terms. *Sterilization* is the complete destruction of all forms of microbial life, including spores, viruses, parasites, and fungi. In the hospital this is usually accomplished by steam under pressure as in the autoclave.

Disinfection is the process of destroying only certain disease-producing microorganisms, usually vegetative forms of bacteria, but not resistant spores. The term *disinfection* implies chemical treatment of an inanimate surface to rid it of harmful microorganisms.

A *germicide* is a chemical agent that kills microorganisms. A *sporicide* kills spores, and a *fungicide* kills fungi. When a germicide is used on an inanimate object or surface it is referred to as a *disinfectant;* when applied to skin or mucous membranes, an *antiseptic.* This is the customary term for an agent used on living tissue to oppose sepsis, putrefaction, or decay.

Tissue cells and microbes are both living protoplasm; therefore, a physical or chemical agent that is destructive to one is likely to be destructive to both, and because tissue cells are devoid of a thick cell wall that protects bacteria and fungi from biologic effects of chemicals, it is they, not the bacteria, that are more susceptible to injury. Because only relatively weak concentrations of most chemicals can be applied safely to body surfaces, even intact skin, most antiseptics have limited bactericidal action; some are essentially bacteriostatic.[127]

A *bacteriostat* prevents organisms from multiplying; it arrests growth without killing the organisms. A *sanitizer* is a term used in the dairy industry to denote an agent that reduces microbial contamination to safe limits.

Disinfection with Chemicals or Germicides. Disinfection is practiced in every health care institution and agency and often in homes. When properly used, disinfectants are capable of very rapid destruction of microbes. Available commercial germicides (and there are hundreds) vary greatly in their capacity to kill microorganisms, and conversely, microorganisms possess a wide range of resistance to chemicals. There is no *one* all-purpose disinfectant. The type of disinfectant to be used is often not as important as the way it is used. The efficacy of any germicide is influenced by its concentration, its temperature, the amount of time it is in contact with the organisms, the chemical compatibility of the germicide and its solvents, the age, numbers, and types of microorganisms, and the cleanliness of the surface to be disinfected.

Cleanliness of the surface to be disinfected is essential. If the germicide cannot penetrate to the wall of the microorganism, it will not destroy it. Organic matter such as serum, blood, pus, or other protein substances, in addition to preventing penetration, may render the disinfectant chemically ineffective.

The higher the concentration of the germicide the greater the killing potential, but not always—70 per cent alcohol, for example, is more effective than higher or lower concentrations.

The temperature of the disinfectant solution may affect its efficacy. In general, the higher the temperature, the more rapid the action. Iodophors are an exception to this, but in general, the use of warm or hot water is preferred for disinfecting and cleaning purposes.

No chemical germicide disinfects a surface instantly. The time required for different disinfectants to kill microorganisms varies from seconds to hours. In each case, sufficient time must be allowed.

Some types of organisms are more easily killed than others. Vegetative bacteria, such as staphylococci, are more easily killed than capsule formers such as the tubercle bacilli. The spore form of an organism is most resistant while the relative resistance of viruses is not fully understood at this time. In addition, as has been pointed out, disinfectants are not equally effective for all types of organisms. The specific action of the chemical agent on the organism to be killed must be known.

When a chemical disinfectant is used in conjunction with another substance, it is necessary to consider the compatibility of the two substances. Alkalinity, acidity, oxidation, or reducing properties may adversely affect the action of a disinfectant. Hard water will neutralize some germicides, and many are inactivated by soap and detergents. The halogens (iodine and chlorine) are more effective in the acid range, whereas other disinfectants such as quaternary ammonium compounds, work better in the alkali range.[128,129]

Types of Chemical Disinfectants. The most important chemical germicides used in hospitals include the following: (1) alcohol; (2) the halogens, iodine and chlorine; (3) phenol; (4) quaternary ammonium compounds; (5) activated glutaraldehyde; (6) formaldehyde; and (7) chlorhexidine. Other chemicals used in the past include mercury compounds, pineoils, silver compounds, and dyes. Of these, only silver is still extensively used—in the form of silver nitrate, used in the eyes of newborn babies, and in the treatment of burns.

The alcohols, particularly ethyl, 70 per cent, and isopropyl, 50 to 90 per cent, are very good disinfectants. They readily kill vegetative organisms and tubercle bacilli, but are not completely effective against spores. They are safe, relatively inexpensive, have a cleaning action, act quickly, evaporate readily, and leave no residue. The addition of iodine to alcohol increases the effectiveness of both. Alcohol can also be combined with formaldehyde and certain phenolics to enhance bactericidal action. Alcohol is used for skin disinfection, cleaning thermometers, and for disinfection of instruments and needles (recommended only when a reliable method of sterilization is not available).

The halogens, of which chlorine is one example and iodine another, are good disinfectants that kill both gram-negative and grampositive bacteria, and also viruses. Chlorine is effective against spores only if the solution is neutral or slightly acid. It is not effective against acid-fast bacteria such as the tubercle bacillus. It has the disadvantage of being irritating to tissue, corrosive to metals, and injurious to rubber, and it does not combine well with detergents. Chlorine is widely used for disinfection of toilets, lavatories, and bathtubs, and as a bleach for fabrics as well as a sanitizer for dishwashing, swimming pools, and hydrotherapy tanks.

Iodine is an excellent all-around disinfectant. It is effective against spores, viruses, fungi, and bacteria, including tubercle bacilli. Iodine tincture refers to a preparation containing 2 per cent iodine and 2.4 per cent sodium iodide in diluted alcohol. Iodine solution refers to an aqueous (water) solution, and the term *iodophor* refers to a compound containing iodine and a solutizing agent, or carrier, for the iodine. In this form, the iodine is slowly liberated when diluted with water. The iodophors are stable, nonstaining, nontoxic, and odor-free. Some of these are now general purpose disinfectants. Iodine tincture is used for preparation of the skin before surgery and before inserting a needle. Iodophors are used for application to mucous membranes and for disinfection of hands. Other iodine preparations are used for disinfection of instruments and equipment such as suture materials, thermometers, dishes, and eating utensils.

Phenols are among the oldest germicides. Lister's phenol compounds and other early germicides in the nineteenth century were coal tar derivatives that had a strong, disagreeable odor and were highly caustic. Today, odorless, nontoxic phenol derivatives and synthetic phenols are available.* In correct concentrations they are effective against a wide spectrum of vegetative forms of bacteria, but are less effective against spore forms. Combined with detergents, they are widely used in hospital housekeeping as detergent-germicides on walls, floors, and furnishings, and to a lesser extent on instruments and glassware. They have been used as a laundry rinse, but recent reports indicate that diapers rinsed with phenolic compounds have been toxic to infants.[130]

Bacterial contamination of phenolic disinfectants has been reported.[131] Contamination may be facilitated by the persistence of bacteria in the space behind plastic liners in the screw-on caps of containers, or by inactivation of the disinfectant by the organic matter it is meant to disinfect, or by materials in cleaning equipment, as, for example, polyurethane floor mops.[123]

Hexachlorophene is a bisphenol that retains its bactericidal potency when combined with soap and detergents. Until recently it has been widely used as an antiseptic for handwashing and for bathing babies in newborn nurseries. Its "degerming" action is attributed to a film deposited on the skin. It is soluble in alcohol and acetone. Hexachlorophene is actually not a germicide; it is bacteriostatic rather than bactericidal, and has limited antimicrobial activity against gram-negative bacilli. It is most effective against gram-positive organisms. Solutions containing hexachlorophene have been shown to be contaminated with gram-negative organisms such as *Pseudomonas aeruginosa, Serratia marcescens,* and *Alcaligenes fecalis.*[133]

Moreover, because of its toxicity when absorbed by the skin, hexachlorophene is no longer routinely used to bathe babies. A US Food and Drug Administration (F.D.A.) ruling, December 8, 1971, restricts hexachlorophene to prescribed usage.

Quaternary ammonium compounds (the "Quats") are surface-active compounds that lower the surface tension of solutions. They are nonirritating to the skin, and are effective against gram-positive, but not gram-negative, organisms, or tubercle bacilli. In recent years, benzalkonium chloride preparations such as Zephiran, Detergex, and Detergicide have been among the most commonly used disinfectants in the hospitals. It is now known that aqueous solutions of benzalkonium chloride lose most of their antibacterial properties on contact with soap, cotton fibers such as gauze sponges, and protein, leaving a standing body of water in which gram-negative organisms may thrive. Serious infections including fatal bacteremia have been linked to mistaken dependence on these compounds.[134,135] At the present time, aqueous solutions of quaternary ammonium compounds are discouraged for hospital use outside of the kitchen.*

Activated glutaraldehyde is an alkylating agent similar to ethylene oxide or formaldehyde. Because it kills spore forms of bacteria in 3 to 10 hours, a relatively shorter time than other chemicals, it is used for "cold sterilization" of delicate lensed instruments, anesthesia equipment, and other heat-sensitive materials. It is available in a 2 per cent aqueous solution under the trade name Cidex. It is relatively costly, and its stability is limited to about 2 weeks. A buffer is commonly used with glutaraldehyde to help regulate the pH of the solution. It is irritating to the skin, and any item disinfected by it must be rinsed in sterile water before being applied to a patient.[136]

Formaldehyde gas when in solution is known as formalin. Because it is effective against spore forms of bacteria and does not corrode metal or affect cutting edges, it is sometimes used in the hospital to disinfect instruments. It has an objectionable odor, and is irritating to tissues. Instruments soaked in formalin must be rinsed before use on the patient. The most common use of formalin is in Bard-Parker Solution (20 per cent formalin, 70 per cent ethanol, and 10 per cent methanol).[137]

Chlorhexidine is a guanidine derivative that is used very little in the United States, but widely used in Great Britain. It is effective against gram-positive organisms, and in more concentrated solutions, against gram-negative

---

* Among numerous commercial disinfectant detergents on the market are Staphene and One-Stroke Vesphene made by Vestal Laboratories, St. Louis, Mo.

* US Public Health Service, Center for Disease Control, Atlanta, Ga.

bacteria. It is used mainly as an antiseptic in urology and gynecology, and as a bacteriostatic agent in ophthalmology.[138]

Sterilization. In practice, sterilization, the destruction of all microorganisms, is achieved by exposing materials to dry or moist heat, to the action of various chemical agents including some gases, or to various types of radiation. The three basic methods of sterilization in hospitals are (1) *wet heat* (pressurized steam), (2) *dry heat,* and (3) *ethylene oxide gas.* Boiling in water is *not* an effective means of sterilization as it does not kill spore forms but it may be the only process available in emergencies and in undeveloped areas.

Flowing steam sterilizers are not recommended for use in hospitals because they have the same limitations as boiling water. Liquid chemical preparations are usually considered to be disinfectants, not sterilizing agents, with the exception of glutaraldehyde and formaldehyde which, because they kill spores, are sometimes used for "cold sterilization," usually on lensed and cutting edge instruments. This is not as satisfactory a method of sterilization as moist heat, however, as it takes a long exposure time (up to 24 hours) and equipment so treated must be rinsed before using. Moreover, since equipment is not wrapped while soaking, it does not remain sterile after removal from the solution. Sterilization by radiation is currently limited to commercial processing of medical supplies, as it is not economically feasible for use in hospitals at this time.

Sunlight discourages bacterial growth and is one of nature's ways of controlling infection. Water in the middle of a lake has, for example, a very low bacterial count, and on city reservoirs and water purification plants sunlight is used as a sanitizing agent. Sunlight is not, however, relied on for sanitizing surfaces and objects in health care institutions since there are other quicker and more reliable agents. In homes, soap and water and sunlight go a long way in controlling infection.

Moist Heat Sterilization. Steam under pressure, or saturated steam in an autoclave, is the most rapid and reliable method of sterilization used in the hospital, other institutions, and health agencies. When correctly used, it destroys all forms of microbial life, even dry, resistant spores, in a relatively short time. It leaves no toxic residue, it is easily controlled, and the results can be measured. However, it has the following disadvantages: moist heat damages some materials such as plastics, laryngoscopes, and bronchoscopes; steam does not penetrate certain anhydrous materials such as oil, grease, and powder; sharp-edged instruments may be dulled by the process; and

autoclaving requires well-engineered, well-maintained, correctly used equipment.

Sterilization will not take place unless objects are packaged and loaded to permit exclusion of air and free access of steam. All air must be expelled from the chamber and correct pressure and temperature maintained. Materials to be sterilized must be clean, as soil may harbor microorganisms and may prevent steam from penetrating. An adequate drying cycle is essential, as moist packages will not remain sterile.

Four types of autoclaves are currently in use: (1) The downward displacement, or gravity discharge, type. In this older-type autoclave, air is evacuated downward and outward as steam is admitted. This method requires a longer period than some of the newer types. The complete cycle, including come-up time and exhaust and dry time, takes approximately 75 minutes. (2) The prevacuum, high-temperature steam sterilizer (prevac). This is a newer type of autoclave in which air is removed by a vacuum pump, enabling steam to be introduced into a vacuum. It is much faster than the downward displacement type. The total cycle takes about 20 minutes. It is inefficient with small loads because of difficulty in evacuating all of the air in a partially loaded chamber. (3) The high-speed pressure instrument sterilizer. This sterilizer is used primarily for high-speed emergency sterilization of surgical instruments. It incorporates very rapid air evacuation and steam penetration. Instruments, which in this case are not wrapped, can be sterilized and dried in about 10 minutes. (4) The instrument washer sterilizer. This is another speed type autoclave used for emergency sterilization of surgical instruments. It incorporates steam and an agitated high-temperature detergent bath. It can wash and sterilize a load of unwrapped instruments in about 20 minutes.[139]

Dry Heat Sterilization. Circulating hot air ovens are most commonly used for hot air sterilization. Dry heat requires higher temperatures for longer periods than steam under pressure. It is mainly used to sterilize anhydrous oils, greases, and powders not penetrated by steam, as well as materials damaged by moisture such as sharp instruments. Hot air ovens are commonly used in laboratories for glassware sterilization. In homes some objects can be sterilized in ovens; fabrics may be ironed.

Gas Sterilization. Ethylene oxide, glycol, formaldehyde, and beta-propiolactone vapor are all gases that can be used for sterilization. Of these, ethylene oxide is the most commonly used in the hospital.

Table 15-4. Disinfecting Agents for Various Types of Objects and Specific Contaminating Organisms* †

Objects	Vegetative Bacteria and Fungi Influenza Viruses Disinfection	Tubercle Bacilli Enteroviruses Except Hepatitis Viruses Vegetative Bacteria and Fungi Influenza Viruses Disinfection	Bacterial and Fungal Spores Hepatitis Viruses Tubercle Bacilli Enteroviruses Vegetative Bacteria and Fungi Influenza Viruses Sterilization
Smooth, hard-surface objects	A—10 min D— 5 min F—10 min H—10 min L— 5 min M— 5 min	B—10 min D—10 min G—10 min H—10 min L—10 min M—10 min	D—18 hr J K L— 9 hr M—10 hr
Rubber tubing, rubber catheters	F—10 min H—10 min	G—10 min H—10 min	J § K
Polyethylene tubing, polyethylene catheters	A—10 min F—10 min H—10 min	B—10 min G—10 min H—10 min	D—18 hr J § K L— 9 hr M—10 hr
Lensed instruments	F—10 min H—10 min K M—10 min	K M—10 min	K
Hypodermic needles	Sterilization only	Sterilization only	J
Thermometers ‖	C—10 min K	C—10 min K	D—18 hr L— 9 hr M—10 hr
Hinged instruments	A—20 min D—10 min F—20 min H—20 min L—10 min M—10 min	B—30 min D—20 min G—30 min H—30 min L—20 min M—20 min	J K L— 9 hr M—10 hr
Floors, furniture, other appropriate room surfaces	F— 5 min H— 5 min I— 5 min	G— 5 min H— 5 min	Not necessary or practical

* Adapted from US Public Health Service: *Isolation Techniques for Use in Hospitals.* US Government Printing Office, Washington, D.C. 1970, p. 98 (PHS Pub. No. 2054).

§ Investigate thermostability when indicated.

‖ Must be thoroughly wiped, preferably with tincture of soap, before disinfection or sterilization. Alcohol-iodine solution will remove markings on poor-grade thermometers.

† **Key:**
A. isopropyl alcohol (70–90%) plus 0.2% sodium nitrite to prevent corrosion
B. ethyl alcohol (70–90%)
C. isopropyl or ethyl alcohol plus 0.2% iodine
D. formaldehyde (8%)—alcohol solution plus 0.2% sodium nitrite to prevent corrosion
F. iodophor—75 ppm available iodine plus 0.2% sodium nitrite to prevent corrosion
G. iodophor—450 ppm available plus 0.2% sodium nitrite to prevent corrosion
H. phenolic solutions (2% aq.) plus 0.5% sodium bicarbonate to prevent corrosion
I. sodium hypochlorite (1:500 aq.—approx. 100 ppm)
J. heat sterilization   } see manufacturers recommendations
K. ethylene oxide gas   } or technical literature
L. aqueous formalin (40%)
M. activated glutaraldehyde (2% aq.)

Ethylene oxide is a colorless, pleasant-smelling, highly penetrating gas introduced to hospitals in the 1950s. It kills all microorganisms including spore forms. Ethylene oxide is used to sterilize the following materials that are damaged by moisture and heat: plastic and rubber goods, delicate surgical instruments, needles, syringes and thermometers, electric equipment, lensed instruments, blankets, mattresses and pillows, anesthesia equipment, nebulizers, infant incubators, and heart-lung oxygenators. Ethylene oxide has disadvantages, however. It is highly combustible. The vapors which become explosive when mixed with air are made safe by the addition of an inactive gas such as carbon dioxide, Freon, or nitrogen. The process of ethylene oxide sterilization is lengthy, and because it is toxic, both through inhalation and when applied to the skin, materials sterilized by ethylene oxide gas must be held ("quarantined") in a well-ventilated area for a minimum of 24 hours. Aeration of absorbent materials such as rubber and plastics may take as long as 7 days. An alternative to this long period is the use of a specially designed aeration chamber which can reduce the time to 12 to 18 hours, regardless of the material being sterilized.

The efficacy of ethylene oxide sterilization depends on the length of time of exposure which, in turn, depends on concentration and temperature. Maintenance of correct temperature during sterilization is important because at temperatures above 60°C (140°F) no ethylene oxide gas will be introduced into the sterilizer, leaving only the carrier gas (usually Freon). Humidity should be maintained in the range of 25 to 50 per cent for the greatest effectiveness, as microorganisms are resistant when dry or desiccated. Instructions on all sterilizing equipment must be followed carefully.

Items that have been previously sterilized by gamma radiation (as some commercially packaged supplies) should never be resterilized with ethylene oxide as this forms a highly toxic compound, *ethylene chlorhydrin*. Disposable items are not meant to be resterilized; they should be discarded after use.

Formaldehyde and beta-propiolactone vapor are sometimes used to disinfect whole rooms, although this practice is no longer recommended for terminal disinfection (see page 901). Formaldehyde has an irritating odor, and beta-propiolactone can produce tumors in mice, which suggests that it might be dangerous for humans. Glycols, usually triethylene or propylene, are used as vapors or aerosols in an enclosed area. They are not toxic and have no odor.[140,141] (See Table 15-4 for list of disinfecting and sterilizing agents for various types of objects and specific contaminating organisms.)

13. PREVENTING AND CONTROLLING INFECTION *

A *nosocomial* † infection is a hospital-associated infection acquired after admission to the hospital, often following surgery or other intrusive procedures that violate the body's natural barriers. Actually any treatment setting (not just hospitals) offers the risk of infection, as do all institutions. However, the sicker and more debilitated the inmates, the more "intrusive" the therapy, the greater the extent to which the therapy lessens the body's natural resistance, and the more entrenched and resistant the environment organisms, the greater the risk.

The exact number of infections acquired in hospitals is unknown, but it has been conservatively estimated that 5 per cent of all patients admitted to hospitals in the United States develop an infection that was not present or incubating at the time of admission.[142]

A recent report on surveillance of nosocomial infections in community hospitals named the urinary tract as the most frequently reported site of infection (43 per cent), followed by surgical wound infection (34 per cent), respiratory tract (16 per cent), and skin (4 per cent).[143] In recent years, nosocomial infection has become a major problem, not only in the United States, but in hospitals around the world.

Conditions Influencing the Development of Infection. Hospital-associated infection is a complex phenomenon that defies a simple cause-and-effect explanation. In the hospital, as in the world outside, scientific and technologic progress (so-called) has upset the ecologic balance or interaction between people, disease-producing microorganisms, and the hospital or treatment environment. Although infection has always been present in hospitals, the problem in the current form is often said to have started with the introduction of anti-

---

* The first author thanks Claire Coppage, R.N., M.P.H., Assistant to Chief for Infection Control Training, US Public Health Service, Center for Disease Control, Atlanta, Ga., for enabling her to attend a course on Surveillance, Prevention, and Control of Hospital-Associated Infection, March 1973.

† The word *nosocomial* is derived from the Greek words *nosos* = disease, and *komeion* = to take care of. A nosocomial infection is a disease associated with an institution intended to take care of diseases.

biotics, particularly penicillin, in the 1940s. Although chemotherapy had an upsurge with the development of the arsenicals and sulfur compounds, the antibiotics made available for the first time effective treatment for most infectious disease. This was soon followed by a false sense of security and a lowering of standards of aseptic technique which have never been fully reestablished. The subsequent use and misuse of antibiotic treatment over the years has resulted in the emergence of strains of bacteria that are highly resistant to antibiotics, making treatment ineffective in many instances. Resistant strains of microorganisms develop through genetic selection over many millions of generations in the hospital environment. Bacteria multiply about every 30 minutes as long as conditions are favorable to growth. So it is possible for one sturdy, resistant organism to give rise to a population of over 1 million in 10 hours, and in 15 hours, to more than 1 billion.[144] Moreover, antibiotics, by changing the natural bacterial flora in patients, open the way for endogenous infection (arising from within) by organisms which ordinarily are not pathogenic—organisms which, under ordinary circumstances, live in peaceful coexistence in and on the bodies of their human hosts.

Fifteen years ago staphylococcal (a gram-positive organism) infection was the most significant infection problem in hospitals. Although gram-positive infections occur today, the danger from gram-negative organisms is as great or greater than that from the gram-positive cocci. Gram-negative organisms, which include *Pseudomonas, Proteus, Escherichia coli, Serratia,* and *Klebsiella,* thrive and reproduce in water, or even in humid atmospheres. They require a minimum of "food" to sustain life, and are able to live in supposedly sterile distilled water, feeding on minute traces of phosphorus and sulfur. Many are more resistant to the effects of germicides and antibiotics than are gram-positive pathogens. In addition to being called "water bugs," [145] the gram-negative organisms are commonly referred to as "emerging pathogens" or "opportunists," as they were formerly considered to be nonpathogenic and are quick to seize the opportunity to "move in" on a compromised host (a person whose natural defenses against infection have been reduced).

Another condition that enters into the occurrence of nosocomial infection is the virulence of hospital organisms. Virulence, an important determinant as to whether infection will or will not develop when pathogens make contact with a host, is increased by rapid passage from one host to another. Many organisms commonly found in the hospital are not only more resistant to antibiotics, but are more virulent than similar pathogenic organisms found outside the hospital. As bacterial virulence and resistance to antibiotics increase, and formerly benign organisms become pathogenic, hospital personnel adopt the microbial flora of the hospital. As a result, the microorganisms that have become associated with hospital-acquired infection are permanent inhabitants of the hospital environment, existing in and on patients and staff, as well as throughout the structure, furnishings, and materials used in the hospital. Moreover, spread of these organisms within the hospital seems almost unavoidable.[146]

Another factor in considering the cause of hospital-associated infection is the particular or unique character of the hospital host, or the person invaded by disease-producing organisms. The hospital constitutes a unique community comprised of staff and visitors of varying ages and susceptibility, as well as patients who, for the most part, either have communicable diseases on admission or are highly susceptible to invasion by infectious organisms. Among them are elderly people, many of whom are suffering from chronic debilitating diseases, and infants with minimal resistance to infection. Infants of low birth weight, who in the past would not have survived very long after birth, now live to be subjected to the hazards of mists, aerosolizers, and other sources of moisture which may harbor gram-negative organisms such as *Serratia, Herellea, Achromobacter, Proteus,* and *Pseudomonas.* All of these organisms have been incriminated in outbreaks of fatal infection in hospital nurseries.[147,148] Patients with severe burns are often found in hospitals. These patients are not only highly susceptible to infection by hospital organisms, but because virtually all severe burns inevitably become infected, are a potential source of cross-infection as well. Additionally, an increasing number of seriously ill patients are kept alive on therapy that reduces the body's defenses. Among these are deep x-ray and antimetabolite, immunosuppressive, or adrenocorticosteroid drug therapy. Patients whose defenses are lowered or absent are referred to as compromised hosts.

The picture is further complicated by today's complex diagnostic and therapeutic procedures. Among these are extensive and prolonged operations such as cardiac surgery and organ transplants that expose large raw surfaces to possible infections for many hours, and other procedures that penetrate the skin, enabling microorganisms to invade the body's natural barriers. These procedures include cardiac catheterization, biopsy of bone marrow and internal organs, arteriography, continuous intravenous therapy with indwelling catheters, tracheostomies, and central venous pressure systems used during shock. All of these procedures have been associated with life-threatening or fatal infections such as gangrenous pneumonitis, enterocolitis, peritonitis, and septicemia.[149-152]

Procedures requiring insertion of instruments into body cavities, as well as those penetrating the skin, are known to be hazardous. For example, urinary catheterization and other types of urinary tract instrumentation, anesthesia, and respiratory assistance procedures during the postoperative period, as well as inhalation therapy, have all been linked to outbreaks of infection which are particularly severe and often fatal. In regard to this, Vernon Knight has written: "The growing problem of instrumentation infection is a modern dilemma created by the sheer efficiency of new drugs, vaccines, and operations that maintain life. Our modern therapies can make people into more-or-less defenseless tissue cultures, into collections of living cells devoid of natural resistance to armies of pathogens." *

In addition, increased use of large amounts of blood has become commonplace in hospitals, and transfusion always carries the risk of introduction of infective organisms, notably the virus causing hepatitis. Staff members who handle blood in the hospital are at risk in this respect, as well as patients receiving the blood. Positive pressure respirators and muscle relaxants for patients with pulmonary or central nervous system disease alter the elasticity of the body, favoring invasion by pathogenic organisms. Hypothermia, used in certain central nervous system diseases, such as encephalitis, results in metabolic changes which increase the risk of pulmonary infection by endogenous organisms.[153] Current changes in hospital practice, such as early ambulation and greater mobility of pediatric patients, increase many patients' chances of exposure to infection.

Hospital equipment and supplies have been a source of hospital-induced infection. Objects incriminated as having introduced organisms causing urinary tract infection include catheters, cystoscopes, syringes, drainage bottles, urinals, bedpans, rectal thermometers, and resectoscopes. Anesthesia apparatus found to have been grossly contaminated includes endotracheal tubes, rebreathing bags, face masks, and inspiratory and expiratory tubing. High-

humidity environments and apparatus used to promote high humidity including incubators, inhalation equipment, reservoir nebulizers, and humidification units, as well as equipment used for aspiration and suction, have all been linked to severe outbreaks of infection. Indwelling plastic intravenous catheters have been known to introduce infective organisms. Outbreaks of infection have been traced to contaminated cellulose wadding used as padding under casts, and improperly sterilized lumbar-puncture and catheterization sets. Blankets, diapers, antiseptics, medications, intravenous fluids, blood used for transfusions, pharmaceuticals and cosmetics such as hand and body lotions, detergents, and soaps, including some preparations containing quaternary ammonium compounds (Zephiran) and hexachlorophene, have all been associated with outbreaks of infection, as have hospital plumbing and air-conditioning systems.[154]

Control Measures. The prevention and control of nosocomial infection are the responsibility of almost everyone who works in the hospital. It requires a wide variety of activities, carried out on several fronts. Presently, every hospital in the United States, in order to be accredited by the Joint Commission on Accreditation of Hospitals, must have a multidisciplinary infection control committee responsible for "instituting, directing, reviewing and changing as appropriate, effective measures for control of infection." Although there is wide variation in the way hospitals conduct infection control programs, each infection control committee is charged by the Joint Commission to, at the very least, define infection for the purpose of surveillance as well as to indicate the need for (and the procedures to be used in) isolating patients; to develop, evaluate, and revise procedures and techniques for maintaining sanitation and asepsis standards; to develop a system for reporting, evaluating, and keeping records of infection among patients and personnel; to periodically review the use of antibiotics; and to assist in the development of an employee health program.*

Nurses have a major function in controlling and preventing the development and spread of communicable disease in the hospital. They are widely regarded as being "the first line of defense." By being in intimate and continuous

---

* Knight, Vernon: "Instruments and Infection," *Hosp. Practice*, **2:**95, (Sept.) 1967.

* These and other standards are published in the Joint Commission on Accreditation of Hospitals' *Accreditation Manual for Hospitals*, Chicago, the Commission, 1971. In addition, administrators of all institutional members of the American Hospital Association receive on-going recommendations and revisions of the Joint Commission's requirements.

24-hour-a-day contact with patients, and by being responsible for coordinating all aspects of patient care, nurses are in a unique position to not only protect the patient from cross-infection, but to strengthen the patient's natural defenses by carrying out health-promoting nursing measures.[155,156]

A key position in an increasing number of hospitals is that of Infection Control Nurse, sometimes called Nurse Surveillance Officer, or Nurse Epidemiologist. According to Philip Brachman of the Center for Disease Control in Atlanta, Ga., the Infection Control Nurse "has more to do with day-to-day control and prevention of hospital infection than any other person on the hospital staff." * Infection control as a separate phase of nursing is said to have begun in England in 1960 with the appointment of the first Infection Control Sister.[157] The role and function of an Infection Control Nurse in the United States have been delineated by Kathryn Wenzel,[158] one of the pioneers in this new cadre of infection fighters.

Preparation for the position of Infection Control Nurse varies. Wide experience in hospital nursing is helpful, as is public health training and epidemiology. Not all hospital infection control specialists are nurses. Many epidemiologists and health workers from other fields have joined the ranks. In the United States, the US Public Health Service, Center for Disease Control, Atlanta, Ga., offers training courses for nurses and others. The CDC training staff also supplies educational materials and recommendations for hospital practice.

The rapid increase in numbers of those engaged in infection control has given rise to an international organization—the Association for Practitioners in Infection Control (APIC), as well as regional groups.

Infections acquired in the hospital may prolong hospitalization by days, weeks, or months and may involve the institution in litigation.

Epidemiology of Infectious Disease in the Hospital. In order for an infection to spread, three elements must be present—a *source* of the infecting organism, a *means of transmission* for the organism, and a *susceptible host.* Microorganisms are everywhere in the environment. The majority are harmless to humans and many are beneficial—those used to brew beer, ripen cheese, raise bread, produce antibiotics, and keep the soil fertile. A large part of the feces is bacteria but they ordinarily do us no harm. Moreover, human contact with the relatively few organisms that are pathogenic

does not always result in disease. Development of infection depends on the organism's virulence and ability to multiply in the human body, on the resistance of the host, on the part of the body, or tissue, invaded, and on the number of organisms that gain entry. Bacteria normally present in the intestinal tract, in the nose and throat, and on the skin are harmless only as long as the barriers that separate them from critical tissues are intact. When the protective barriers such as skin or mucous membrane are broken, allowing organisms to gain entry to a part of the body where they do not belong, the entering organisms can become deadly, particularly if the body has little resistance or if there are enough of them to overwhelm the normal body defenses.[159]

The spread of infection has been likened to a chain of three interlocking links, the first link representing a source, or reservoir, of the infecting organism, the second link a means of transmission for the organism, and the third link, a susceptible host. Representationally, the spread of infection can be controlled if the chain is interrupted by breaking any one of the three links. Some diseases, such as diphtheria and smallpox, can be controlled by increasing the resistance of the host by vaccination. Other diseases are best controlled by isolating the reservoir of infective organisms (see Chapters 2 and 44). Still others are controlled by destroying the infective agent through the use of antibiotics or chemotherapy, for example, or by treating a water source to prevent the spread of a waterborne disease such as typhoid. In hospitals, since *agent* and *host* factors are more difficult to control, efforts to interrupt, or break, the chain of infection are directed primarily at *transmission*. This is done mainly by creating barriers of one kind or another between microorganisms and potential hosts. The barriers can be physical in the form of doors, gowns, masks and gloves, or air barriers such as positive pressure ventilation, or laminar flow. Barriers may also be spatial, such as restriction of visitors and segregation of infected patients in certain areas.

Source of Infection. The source of an infective agent can be a patient, a visitor, or a hospital employee who either has a disease, or is incubating a disease, or someone who is colonized by the infectious agent, but has no clinical manifestation of the disease (a carrier). Other potential sources include contaminated objects (fomites) in the environment, as well as food, water, blood, and drugs.

Means of Transmission. The four main routes for the transmission of microorganisms are *contact, vehicle, airborne,* and *vector-borne.* The contact route can be further di-

* Brachman, Philip S.: "Foreword," Symposium on Infection and the Nurse, *Nurs. Clin. North Am.,* **5**:86, (Mar.) 1970.

vided into three subgroups—(1) direct contact, that is, the transfer of organisms from one person to another, or through an intermediary. A nurse who uses poor technique may transfer organisms from one baby to another in a nursery; (2) indirect contact, that is, contact with contaminated articles such as improperly decontaminated and disinfected thermometers or bedpans; or (3) by droplet spread which is the passing of infectious organisms in the form of droplets by coughing, sneezing, or talking while in relatively close face-to-face contact. Droplets usually spread no more than 3 ft. The vehicle route applies in diseases transmitted through food, as in salmonellosis, through water, as in shigellosis, through drugs, as in *Pseudomonas* infections from use of contaminated ophthalmologic ointment, and through blood, as in hepatitis.[160]

Combatting Communicable Disease by Controlling the Source: Medical and Surgical Asepsis Measures in Patient Care. The practice of *aseptic technique* is the chief means of preventing the spread of communicable disease in the hospital. Aseptic technique refers to numerous and varied measures carried out by hospital staff and employees to protect themselves and their patients from contact with disease-producing organisms. A basic principle underlying the use of aseptic technique is "The fewer the pathogenic organisms available to the host, the less his chance of contracting infection; if organisms in numbers sufficient to overcome defense mechanisms can be prevented from reaching the host, infection probably will not occur." * This, of course, does not apply to organisms already present in the patient's body which, when resistance is lowered, may give rise to endogenous infection.

Asepsis literally means without sepsis, or without infection. *Medical asepsis* is the practice of reducing direct or indirect transfer of organisms by proper handwashing techniques, the use of barriers such as gowns, gloves and masks, safe handling of contaminated articles, body wastes, blood, food and drink, and so forth. *Surgical asepsis* is the practice of keeping an area free from all possible organisms by using sterile techniques.

Aseptic technique in the broadest sense as outlined by Margaret Benson [161] includes both patient care, and environmental control. Adapted herein, it consists of

1. Screening patients on admission, for infectious diseases or dangerously lowered

* Vandermade, Jean: From a lecture on Aseptic Technique, US Public Health Service, Center for Disease Control, Atlanta, Ga., March 1973.

resistance, with subsequent isolation as needed.
2. The use of appropriate medical and surgical asepsis in patient care.
3. The use of clean, freshly issued supplies and equipment for each patient.
4. Care in distribution of supplies with segregation of "clean" and "dirty" procedures and equipment.
5. Proper personal hygiene for patients and staff.
6. Delivery of patient care by personnel who themselves are free from infection.
7. Maintenance of a sanitary environment through effective housekeeping, proper decontamination, disinfection, and sterilization of materials, controlling traffic through critical areas, appropriate handling and disposal of wastes, insect and rodent control, efficient ventilation and laundering, and safe handling of food, water, and ice.

Skin Cleaning. Frequent cleaning of the skin of both patient and attendants is important in the control of infectious disease. In spite of the self-disinfecting powers of the skin, it is normal to find as many as 10,000 organisms to a square centimeter. The count is lower on the smooth surfaces and higher in the folds and under the fingernails. Each person harbors his or her own particular flora. The majority of the organisms are not disease-producing, but there are always pathogens present that will attack injured tissue. Skin organisms are divided into two classes—the *resident* and *transient*. The resident bacteria penetrate the hair follicles and sebaceous glands and, in contrast to the transient organisms, cannot be removed by any practical method of scrubbing. Although it would be impossible to completely sterilize the skin without destroying it, no technique for preventing the spread of disease is so important as *handwashing*. Almost one hundred years ago Ignaz Semmelweis dramatically reduced puerperal fever in a Viennese hospital by merely insisting that physicians wash their hands before touching a patient. *Handwashing* is still considered to be the cornerstone of aseptic practices, and *the single most important measure in the prevention of cross-infection.*

Handwashing. Appropriate hand cleaning consists of mechanical removal of dirt and microorganisms by sudsing, friction, flushing with running water, and the use of a detergent or germicidal preparation.

If handwashing is to be optimally carried out by hospital staff and personnel, it must be easily accomplished. Sinks for handwashing should be conveniently located near every patient. A coat rack near every sink might lessen the psychologic deterrent to handwashing caused by lack of a place to put a jacket, lab coat, or other outer clothing. There should also be an adequate supply of uncontaminated antimicrobial soap or solution, nail cleaners, and paper towels. An inappropriate requirement for lengthy washing or scrubbing may discourage handwashing. A sudsy, grease-removing scrub for even 15 or 20 seconds will remove nearly all transient bacteria from the hands. Studies have shown that hand scrubbing with a povidone-iodine preparation (Betadine Surgical Scrub) will lower bacterial counts on the hands whether scrubbed for 3, 5, or 10 minutes.[162]

Until recently, hexachlorophene-containing detergents, such as pHisoHex, have been the most widely used *handwashing agents*. At the present time, povidone-iodine preparations, such as Betadine Surgical Scrub and Betadine Antiseptic Solution have widely replaced hexachlorophene as a skin antiseptic. Hexachlorophene 3 per cent (pHisoHex) is not a germicide; it is a bacteriostatic agent that leaves a protective film on the skin when used regularly, but subsequent application of alcohol removes the protective coating of pHisoHex. It is effective against gram-positive microorganisms, especially skin-resident staphylococci, but is ineffective against gram-negative organisms and fungi. Hexachlorophene-containing detergent solutions have been found to be contaminated with *Pseudomonas* and other gram-negative organisms.[163] Moreover, because of toxicity when absorbed by the skin of infants, hexachlorophene is no longer routinely used to bathe babies; in fact, it is no longer dispensed without a prescription. Povidone-iodine preparations, on the other hand, are effective against a relatively broad spectrum of organisms; they do not require repeated use over a period of time in order to become effective; they are not inactivated by alcohol nor do they serve as a growth medium for gram-negative organisms. Betadine Surgical Scrub, one povidone-iodine preparation, is an antiseptic microbicidal sudsing cleaner that is effective against all gram-positive and some gram-negative organisms as well as yeasts, fungi, viruses, and protozoa. Numerous clinical studies have demonstrated its efficiency in degerming the hands of hospital personnel. It has been shown to be superior to hexachlorophene, benzalkonium chloride 1:1000, liquid soap, and liquid soap followed by 70 per cent ethyl alcohol.[164]

There is some disagreement about the length of time of scrubbing and handwashing. Each hospital must devise procedures appropriate to a given situation, but in general hands should be washed (1) when coming to work on a treatment unit; (2) when the hands are obviously soiled; (3) before and after giving patient care, even when gloves are used; (4) while administering to a patient, after any contact with the patient's infectious excretions or secretions before touching the patient again; (5) before touching face and mouth of patient, and before touching one's own face, hair, or mouth; (6) after using the toilet; (7) after blowing or wiping the nose; (8) after handling any contaminated material; (9) after leaving an isolation area; (10) before eating; * and (11) before leaving a treatment unit.

Soap dispensers, which can easily be contaminated, should be routinely emptied, cleaned, and disinfected. Faucet aerators can also be contaminated.[165] If they must be used to prevent splashing, they should be removed and sterilized frequently. Soap should not be left on sponges. In fact, sponges are condemned for use in hospitals unless used only once and thrown away. Disposable skin-cleaning brushes, and sponges impregnated with iodophor preparations, are available commercially. The use of brushes for hand scrubbing is thought by many to be undesirable because bristles irritate the skin, and are difficult to decontaminate.

Handwashing techniques vary with the situation. One suggested procedure, using an iodophor preparation, is as follows: Wet hands with water. Apply a single squirt of solution and, without adding more water, rub vigorously using friction on all surfaces, including areas between fingers. Clean underneath the fingernails. Wash 3 to 5 minutes when starting to work on a unit, and 30 seconds between patients. Add enough water to develop suds, and rinse thoroughly under running water. Dry completely with paper towel and use it for turning off hand-controlled faucets. Foot- or knee-controlled soap dispensers and faucets are preferred. No jewelry other than a plain wedding band should be worn.

Preoperative Skin Preparation at Operative Site. Cleaning that penetrates the skin lessens the hazard of introducing microorganisms into a surgical wound. Procedures for skin preparation vary with clinical situations and personal preference, but in general skin should be cleaned with a mechanical scrub using soap or detergent to remove dirt and oily substances,

---

* In general, personnel should not eat in patient areas. Every patient in the hospital should be considered a potential source of communicable disease. Serum hepatitis, which is now known to be spread by the oral route, is an example of a disease that may be contracted. It has a 3- to 6-month incubation period, which means that any patient in the hospital could be infectious without symptoms. Eating while "on duty" is especially dangerous in dialysis units.

followed by application of a bactericidal antiseptic. Friction is important in the cleaning process, and applying pressure enhances the use of the antiseptic. Semirough materials, such as gauze, increase friction and are more suitable as applicators than cotton. There is some disagreement about the advisability of shaving the area, as scratches on the skin provide an incubating media for bacterial growth. Shaving obstetric patients is no longer universally recommended. If the operative site is shaved, it should be done as near the time of surgery as possible, preferably the same day, using wet lather technique. The former practice of doing a sterile "prep" and wrapping the area with towels is bacteriologically unsound.

Bactericidal antiseptics for preoperative skin preparation recommended by the Center for Disease Control of the US Public Health Service are either 70 per cent alcohol, alcohol-iodine combinations, or iodophors. Alcohol in concentrations of 60 to 95 per cent is an effective nonirritating, bactericidal agent on the skin. Alcohol does not have residual activity. One per cent tincture of iodine (iodine and alcohol) rapidly kills both gram-negative and gram-positive bacteria, as well as fungi, tubercle bacilli, and viruses. It has no residual activity. Iodophors such as Virac, Io-prep, and Betadine are bactericidal complexes of iodine and organic molecules that release iodine slowly, providing prolonged bactericidal activity or residual activity. The iodophors are water soluble and are neutralized by small amounts of blood and serum. Iodophor preparations are now so widely used for a variety of purposes including handwashing and skin and mucous membrane antisepsis that there is danger of people becoming sensitized, and widespread use increases the possibility of the appearance of resistant strains of microorganisms.

Some skin antiseptics commonly used in the recent past are now believed unsuitable: organic mercurials such as metaphen, mercurochrome, and merthiolate are bacteriostatic and not able to kill bacteria on contact. Quaternary ammonium compounds such as Zephiran are not recommended as they are inactivated by traces of soap, by gauze, hard water, and organic matter, and are not effective against gram-negative organisms. Moreover, they have been linked to outbreaks of infection.[166-168] Hexachlorophene is suitable as a skin-cleaning agent, but not as an antiseptic.

Use of Gowns. Gowns are worn for protection of staff when in contact with a patient who has a disease that may be transmitted by way of clothing, or when giving care to a patient who is sneezing, coughing, or vomiting persistently. Gowns are also worn when working in hazardous areas such as the morgue, laboratory, or laundry-sorting rooms. Clean gowns are worn while in contact with infants and sterile gowns are worn to protect patients in reverse isolation, and those undergoing surgery. The protection provided by sterile gowns is from microorganisms on the clothing and bodies of attendants. Gowns should be worn once, and then discarded. Unless the patient is on strict, or protective, isolation, a gown need not be worn when entering the room to talk to a patient, or to deliver articles.

Suggested Gowning Procedure. Select a gown large enough to entirely cover the wearer's clothing. Wash hands, put gown on, fold or lap one side of the back opening over the other, and tie at waist and neck. To remove gown, untie at neck and waist, withdraw arms from sleeves, and fold gown inside out without touching uniform. Discard into laundry hamper in room. Wash hands before leaving room. In protective isolation, gowns should be removed and discarded outside the patient's room.

Use of Gloves. Gloves are worn to prevent contamination of the patient by microorganisms on the hands of the attendant, or to protect the attendant's hands from blood, infectious discharges, and contaminated articles. Gloves also protect against harsh disinfecting agents, and should be worn when cleaning and disinfecting contaminated equipment.*

The use of gloves is not intended to replace handwashing. Hands should be washed before donning the gloves, and after removal. Gloves should be worn only once, and then discarded in an appropriate receptacle. Sterile gloves are worn when carrying out procedures requiring surgical asepsis, or when caring for the patient in protective isolation.

Suggested Procedure for Donning Clean But Nonsterile Gloves. Wash hands before putting on gloves. (Hands should be washed before any procedure, even when gloves are worn.) If gown is worn, gloves should cover cuff of gown. Remove gloves by grasping edge of cuff and pulling inside out over hands. Discard into waste receptacle in room. When gloves, gown, and mask are worn, remove gloves first, then gown, then mask, using prescribed techniques for each. When wearing gloves while giving patient care and the gloved hands become soiled with the patient's infectious excretions or secretions, change to clean gloves even if care has not been completed.

Suggested Procedure for Donning Sterile Gloves. Open the outer wrapping of the package

---

* Rubber gloves are worn by the attendant to protect the electrically susceptible patient from microshock when the attendant handles lead wires connected to implanted electrodes in the patient's heart (see page 869).

leaving exposed the inner sterile glove container. Then wash the hands as directed on page 891. Remove the gloves from the package being careful to avoid touching the "contaminated" outside surface of the package. The first glove is drawn on by grasping and pulling the inside of the glove cuff; the second, by placing the gloved hand under the untouched portion of the cuff. The cuffs are turned up by manipulating only the sterile surface of the glove and not that which has come in contact with the hand. If a sterile gown is worn, it should be put on before the gloves, in order that the glove cuffs may be drawn up over its sleeves.

Use of Masks. Research on the effectiveness of various types of masks has shown that gauze or thin muslin masks have little ability to trap bacteria, especially if worn longer than 10 minutes, and plastic or cardboard masks simply serve as bouncing boards, with exhaled air pouring out, over, and around the sides of masks.[169] Fiberglass and high-efficiency filter type masks provide effective filtration for long periods. Peter Dineen,[170,171] in a study of 11 types of masks currently marketed, found that the filtration efficiency was still good up to 8 hours in the four best types: Bardic #1795, Bard Vigilon #1796, Deseret Filter Masks #505, and Johnson & Johnson Surgine #4239.

There is some disagreement about the efficacy of wearing masks, as they are useless if not properly applied. In general, masks are recommended while caring for a patient with an infection that may be communicated by droplet route, if face-to-face communication is to take place (droplets do not usually spread more than 3 ft), and when strict aseptic technique is necessary, such as during surgical procedures, or when taking care of a patient in reverse isolation. Masks are sometimes worn by infectious patients if they are unwilling or unable to control or cover their coughs and sneezes. Masks are also worn for protection of staff in hazardous areas such as laboratories, morgues, and laundry-sorting rooms. Masks should be used only once, and discarded when leaving the area or whenever they become moist. Masks should cover the nose and mouth completely and should not be lowered around the neck and reworn, nor should they be touched with contaminated hands.

Suggested Procedure for Donning Mask. Apply before entering the area, completely covering the nose and mouth. To remove mask, wash hands and untie, grasping only the ties. Discard in appropriate receptacle before leaving the area. If the patient is in protective isolation, remove mask after leaving the room.

The high-filtration type mask, made of a fiber and weave that prevents inhalation of droplet nuclei, is effective when caring for pa-

tients with infections that spread by droplet transmission. The molded fiberglass mask traps large droplets at the source, and is effective when worn by staff caring for patients in protective isolation, or when worn by patients in respiratory isolation for active pulmonary tuberculosis whenever anyone else is inside the isolation room, or whenever the patient is outside his or her room.

Dispensing and Handling Supplies and Equipment Used in Care of Institutionalized Patients. A central medical and surgical supply service for processing, storing, and dispensing supplies is an important safeguard against the hazard of contaminated equipment. In addition, a *central supply service* with a well-trained staff ensures standardization of processing and economical, efficient use of personnel. For more information, see Chapter 32.

Ideally, clean supplies and equipment, to be kept at the bedside for each patient's exclusive use, should be in the patient's unit on admission. They should include blankets, bath and emesis basin, soap and toothbrush container, a covered water pitcher, drinking glass (or paper cup) and tray, thermometer and holder, bottle of rubbing lotion, container of powder, paper handkerchiefs and a paper bag in which to discard them, bedpan, urinal, and toilet paper. While in daily use, equipment should be cleaned and disinfected or sterilized as often as necessary. When the equipment is no longer in use, it should be returned to the central processing area for cleaning, decontamination, and storage. Equipment such as heating pads or nebulizers used by a number of patients should be decontaminated after use by each patient.

Instruments and equipment should not be cleaned or decontaminated on the patient-care unit, except for such necessary measures as rinsing blood out of a reusable syringe. Used equipment from infectious patients should be placed in designated containers, bagged, and labeled "contaminated" for return to central supply. Such handling will prevent contamination of the environment on the unit and in transit, and identify contents as hazardous to personnel.

Separating Clean and Used ("Dirty") Equipment and Procedures. If equipment must be cleaned and decontaminated on the patient-care unit, there should be some provision for separation of "clean" and "dirty" equipment and procedures: separate rooms, or one room divided by a pass-through area should be provided if possible. At the very least, there should be a clearly designated service counter or table for "clean" equipment and procedures and another for "dirty" equipment and procedures. These areas should be used consistently so that everyone can rely on one surface being clean, and the other contaminated. In the same vein, there should be clearly designated "clean" and "dirty" work areas in the pharmacy, kitchen, and laundry, and supplies should be transported to and from these areas in "clean" and "dirty" receptacles.

Separation of Clean and Soiled Items Under the Friesen Concept. Today, many new hospitals utilize the Friesen concept of hospital design which minimizes the opportunity of cross-contamination by arranging patient areas so that "clean" and "soiled" activities are separated. Traffic is directed to cut down on airborne contamination. In addition, by efficient design and planning, all work effort is minimized, reducing the over-all numbers of employees needed to take care of the patient. One feature of the design is the "Nurserver" (see Fig. 15-6) consisting of a cabinet built into the wall of the patient room's nursing alcove. The cabinet has two sections, one for clean and the other for soiled supplies. The soiled section is under negative ventilation and pressure to prevent contamination of the clean side and to contain odors. The Nurserver may or may not have a pass-through door opening into the corridor, but in either case the patient is not disturbed by, and does not come into contact with, the personnel who stock the Nurserver. Because all supplies, including the patient's chart, are contained in the Nurserver, the patient's room is a self-sufficient treatment environment rather than just a bedroom. The Friesen system provides a Supply Processing and Distribution Department (SPD) which corresponds to the central supply service, but is more than that, in that all functions relative to supplies are organized under one control system. This includes not only the purchase of all supplies and equipment, but also all reprocessing and distribution, regardless of use. As a master control point in the receiving, processing, sorting, issuing, reprocessing, or disposal of all hospital supplies, the SPD is an extension of every department in the hospital. Centralization of all materials means greater control, fewer losses, and more efficient handling of equipment and supplies, as well as optimal utilization of many items that could otherwise lay dormant for long periods of time while not being used by a specific department. On each patient floor there is one Clean Holding Room where clean supplies are kept on carts temporarily until delivered to the Nurserver. Adjacent to this room is the Soiled Holding Room, where soiled items, collected from the Nurserver, are kept until scheduled to be returned to SPD for reprocessing. The

traditional utility room serving both "dirty" and "clean" needs has been eliminated. All such processing activities are within the domain of the SPD; none occurs anywhere else in the hospital. In Friesen-designed hospitals, chutes and dumbwaiters are not used. The hospital incorporates some type of automated materials-handling system instead. In a hospital using the Friesen concepts of design, the nurse is freed from duties that are not associated with patient care, providing greater opportunity for patient-centered nursing care.

Distributing and Storing Supplies. In hospitals that do not have a distribution service that separates clean and dirty supplies, clean supplies such as freshly laundered linen, and packaged sterile supplies such as dressing trays, should be transported in covered or enclosed carts and stored in enclosed cupboards. Patients' supplies should not be stored on open shelves or on an open stand in the hallway outside an isolation room. If an anteroom is not available for that purpose, an enclosed cabinet should be used. When dumbwaiters or carts are used for transporting supplies to and from Central Supply Service, some should be designated for return of used equipment, and others for distributing clean and sterile equipment. Conveyors should be cleaned at least once a day.

The use of dressing carts with trays of instruments in solution, canisters of flats, and transfer forceps is no longer recommended. Only sterile dressing trays and individually packaged sterile supplies should be used. Some hospitals have dressing teams and catheter-care teams to ensure consistent, high-quality technique in the use of sterile procedures and equipment. If instrument trays and forceps jars are used, glutaraldehyde (Cidex) or alcohol and formaldehyde (Bard Parker Solution) are preferred bactericidal solutions, and they should be changed every 48 hours. Aqueous quaternary ammonium solutions (benzalkonium chloride) such as Zephiran should not be used for they lose most of their antibacterial properties on contact with soap, organic matter, or cotton fibers such as gauze sponges, leaving residual water which is amenable to the growth of gram-negative bacteria.[172] Fatal septicemia has resulted after the use of equipment "cold sterilized" with benzalkonium chloride.[173,174]

If dressing carts must be used, they should not be taken into patients' rooms, nor should they include a container for disposal of soiled dressings. Soiled dressings should be discarded into a moisture-proof bag at the site where the dressing is removed, and the bag should be securely closed before discarding into a lined waste receptacle for transfer to the incinerator.

Protecting Stock Solutions and Pharmaceutical Preparations from Contaminaton. Single-use vials and bottles of sterile solutions and medications are preferable to multiple-use containers. If stock preparations must be used, stock containers should not be taken into the patient's room; small amounts of the material to be dispensed should be taken to the room in a paper cup or other disposable container.

A variety of antiseptics and skin cleaners are packaged commercially in single-use ampules, each with a self-contained applicator tip. Among the solutions available are 70 per cent isopropyl alcohol, PVP iodine, 70 per cent isopropyl alcohol with 10 per cent acetone, iodine 2 per cent, and green soap.

Handling and Disposal of Needles and Syringes. All used needles and syringes should be handled with utmost care as they are potentially contaminated with hepatitis virus or other microorganisms. Disposable syringes should be purposely damaged to prevent their reuse. Disposable needles should be reinserted in the original plastic sheaths and discarded in a special container provided for that purpose. Nondisposable needles and syringes should be rinsed in cold water, wrapped, using double bag technique if necessary, and returned to central supply in a rigid container to avoid injury to personnel.

Diabetics who use syringes and needles daily at home and can't afford disposable equipment can achieve considerable protection from infection by boiling the syringes and needles for 10 minutes. If these instruments are put in a strainer they can be lifted out of the water in it, the water discarded, and the syringes and needles left to drain in the strainer until cool enough to handle. If boiling is not possible in the home, chemical disinfection is probably best accomplished with 70 per cent to 90 per cent alcohol.

Cleaning and Disinfecting Thermometers. Ideally, every patient should have an individual thermometer throughout institutionalization. After each use the thermometer should be "scrubbed" clean with an alcohol sponge, or if grossly soiled it should be vigorously cleaned with soap under running (cool) water, before wiping with alcohol. Individual thermometers treated in this manner may be stored dry in a thermometer rack at the bedside or in a container of alcohol and iodine disinfectant solution (70 per cent alcohol with 2 per cent iodine). The solution should be changed and the container washed and dried every 3 days. Before use, thermometers should be rinsed in cold water. Upon discharge of the patient, the thermometer can be wrapped and sent to central supply for processing. Some hospitals discard thermometers used by isolated patients. Other hospitals let noninfectious patients take thermometers home. Still other hospitals provide a supply of sterile, singly packaged thermometers to each division every day. Each thermometer is used once, then inserted in its paper envelope to be returned to central supply service for processing. Several electronic thermometers are available. One disposable electronic thermometer records both oral and axillary temperatures in one minute, and rectal temperatures in 30 seconds. Another, battery-operated thermometer probe has disposable plastic sheaths that fit over the probe and prevent its contamination.[175] (See Chapter 6 for further discussion of this subject.)

Visiting nurses use the patient's thermometer, cleaning and storing it as described above. If the patient doesn't own a thermometer, they use one carried in their bag of equipment. It should be cleaned with soap solution, wiped with alcohol, and stored in a small vial of alcohol and iodine disinfectant, as noted above. Many agencies in the United States use plain alcohol 70 per cent. Some agencies use disposable waterproof sheaths that keep thermometers clean, but do not interfere with temperature registration.*

Disposal of Contaminated Waste and Equipment. Nurses are responsible for disposal of waste at the bedside, housekeeping personnel are responsible for removal of waste from the patient-care unit; and, in most hospitals, the final collection and disposal of waste are functions of the engineering department. Because it would make the handling more complicated to separate "clean" and "contaminated" waste, it is all handled as if it were "contaminated," although the special precaution by "double bagging" (see page 899) is used only for waste from infectious patients.

It is estimated that 300 to 400 gal of liquid waste and 6 to 9 lb of solid waste a day accumulates from the care of one patient. In addition, hospitals generate enormous quantities of single-use disposable items, as well as microbial and tissue waste from laboratory and autopsy. Hospital wastes are highly infectious and a potential hazard to everyone in the hospital and community.[176] Disposable equipment from infected patients, laboratory specimens, and autopsy wastes, if not incinerated, should be put into the autoclave before being sent to the community landfill. All con-

* Made by Johnson & Johnson, New Brunswick, N.J.

taminated wastes and equipment should be handled with caution, particularly needles and cutting-edge instruments, to reduce the danger of accidental inoculation and infection of personnel.

Two good general principles of disposal are (1) a contaminated article should be immediately placed in a special container, and (2) containers should be disposed of in the same way as their contents. Burnable bags are for things to be burned, canvas or soluble bags for materials to be laundered, and metal containers for items to be autoclaved. This eliminates the transfer of dirty articles from one container to another and provides for decontamination or disposal of contaminated containers.[177]

The double bagging technique should be used when removing contaminated articles from a contaminated area. This provides a "clean" outside surface for further handling. The double bag technique consists of securely enclosing contaminated items in a bag, then placing that bag in a second bag for disposal. In the isolation room, contaminated items are bagged, then transferred at the door to a clean (noncontaminated) bag being held by a person standing outside of the room. Care should be taken not to contaminate the outside of the clean bag during transfer.

Disposal of Discharges from the Nose and Throat. Even healthy individuals should be careful to protect others from their nasal and oral discharges. Paper handkerchiefs deposited in waste receptacles and burned are most desirable.

If patients have diseases that can be transmitted by oral and nasal discharges, contaminated paper handkerchiefs should be deposited immediately in a paper bag and the bag and its contents burned. Water used in cleaning the mouth may be emptied into hoppers and toilets. In case the patient is coughing and expectorating, a sputum cup of some kind must be provided. A tightly covered paper carton is probably the best type because it can be burned with the contents. Sawdust in the cup absorbs the water in the sputum and helps to mask any disagreeable odor that may be present. To estimate the quantity of sputum, the container may be weighed when it is given to the patient and again before it is discarded; the difference in weight is the amount of sputum.

Disposal of Soiled Dressings and Similar Refuse. Dressings removed from the patient are considered infectious whether or not clinical evidence of infection is present. They should be handled carefully, as agitation of contaminated textiles, such as dressings, can build up a level of airborne bacteria. Soiled dressings and other equipment contaminated by excretions or secretions, such as swabs, tongue blades, and disposable tubing, should be carefully disposed of in waterproof bags, and burned.

Disposal of Garbage. There is no aspect of cleaning, either in homes or institutions, that is of more importance than the efficient disposal of waste. If this is properly done, one of the greatest sources of disagreeable odors is eliminated, repellent objects are immediately removed from sight, and attraction of insects is reduced. In hospitals, solid food wastes from patients who are not in isolation are returned to the kitchen on their trays. Most urban hospitals have mechanical garbage grinders that permit disposal through the sewage system. If the patient is isolated with a communicable disease, liquid waste is discarded in the toilet on the patient unit, while leftover food is bagged and discarded in a container with an impervious liner. The liner is closed, sealed, and put into a second bag upon leaving the patient's room. It is finally burned.

Isolation. Caring for a patient in isolation is sometimes referred to as barrier nursing, or barrier technique. It is a means of preventing the spread of infection by establishing an aseptic barrier around the patient.[178] The specific method of isolating a given patient is determined by answering the question "Who is to be protected from what?" *Infected patients* are isolated to protect other people from microorganisms causing their diseases, while *unusually susceptible patients* are isolated to protect them from pathogenic organisms in the environment. This is known as *protective* or *reverse isolation*. It should be noted that this type of isolation does not protect the patient from endogenous infections caused by the patient's own bacteria, nor does it protect against violations of aseptic technique. "Germ-free" rooms cannot prevent direct contact with contaminated hands.

Requirements for isolation of the infected patient vary somewhat with the way the disease is spread. The object is to isolate the disease, not the patient, according to the mode of transmission. Since isolation is expensive in staff time, space and equipment, and because it can be psychologically hard on patients,[179] it is important that it be specifically suited to the patient being isolated, and to the disease to be controlled. Chapter 44 lists the communicable diseases which should be isolated, and recommended isolation precautions for each. For more detailed information see the US Public Health Service Manual, *Isolation Techniques for Use in Hospitals*.[180]

Ordinarily, the decision for isolating a patient rests with the attending physician. In some hospitals, however, a charge nurse may put a patient in isolation if a physician is not available. When strict isolation is necessary, the isolation room should have a private bathroom and an anteroom or entry cubicle for storing clean supplies. If this is not available, an ample supply of clean masks, gowns, gloves, and linen should be stored in an enclosed cabinet outside the patient's room. Open storage shelves and basins of antiseptic solution for decontaminating hands are condemned. A sink for handwashing is mandatory. Those in contact with the patient should wash their hands before entering, and after leaving the isolation room, and should wear gowns, masks, and gloves when appropriate. Aseptic handling of infectious wastes and of all equipment coming in contact with the patient is essential. The door to the isolation room should be kept closed even if there is a differential in air pressure. Specific isolation procedures should be posted on the corridor side of the door, and patients should be told the reasons for their isolation and given information about their part in protecting others. Needed equipment should be anticipated and put in the room for the duration of isolation, which is generally limited to the period of communicability of the disease. This may be determined by consulting the American Public Health Association's 1970 manual, *Control of Communicable Diseases in Man*.[181]

To control airborne microorganisms, the isolation room should have minimum ventilation of six air changes per hour and there should be no cross-circulation or recirculation of air between the isolation room and other sections of the hospital. Older buildings may not have mechanical air-conditioning equipment for filtering, diluting, and directing the flow of air. When modern air conditioning is not available, high-efficiency face masks should be worn when caring for a patient in strict, or respiratory, isolation, and care should be taken to avoid creating aerosols by avoiding vigorous shaking or handling of linens and other equipment that could disseminate airborne contaminants. The use of window fans that exhaust air from the room should be considered if proper air conditioning is lacking, particularly when patients are isolated with diseases spread by the airborne route, such as staphylococcal pneumonia, chickenpox, or active pulmonary tuberculosis.[182]

Isolation of the Susceptible Patient—Protective or Reverse Isolation. Protective, or reverse, isolation is commonly used to lessen the chances of infection in premature and newborn infants, in patients with hypo- or agammaglobulinemia, leukemia, or severe burns, and in patients treated with large doses of radiation, steroids, or other immunosuppressive agents.

The objective in protective isolation is to maintain the patient at a level of asepsis comparable to that in the operating room. This requires a single room with toilet, bath, and lavatory. The patient and family must be told the reasons for the isolation, and if necessary taught the principles of personal hygiene. The door should be kept closed, and all persons with definite or suspected infection excluded. All personnel and authorized visitors should wear caps, sterile gowns, and masks when in the room, and sterile gloves when in direct contact with the patient. In some hospitals, foot covering is required.[183]

Various kinds of protective environments have been devised for the infection-prone patient, ranging from individual plastic enclosures known as "life-island" units, and regulated environments for safety (RES) [184-186] to elaborately designed "bacteria-free" nursing units large enough to accommodate several patients. [187,188] (See Fig. 15-6.)

Special Measures in Caring for Isolated Patients Who Have a Diagnosed Communicable Disease. When a patient is diagnosed as having an infectious or communicable disease and is isolated in a room or cubicle, the following special precautions are taken. (Chapter 44 discusses systemic infections and includes a good deal on measures for control of communicable diseases. What is said there is built on and reinforces the material in this chapter.)

Visitors to isolated patients should be kept to a minimum and should be taught handwashing, the use of masks, gowns, and gloves, and other precautions as necessary. Because patients with communicable diseases are often children or young people with whom a parent, or parent substitute, stays during the admission procedure, or longer, it may be necessary to teach precautionary measures at once.

Transportation within the hospital of patients who have communicable diseases should be reduced to a minimum. The area to which the patient is taken should be notified of his or her arrival, and of techniques that must be used to prevent spread of infection. Patients, too, should be shown how they can help maintain a barrier against transmission of infection while they are out of their rooms.

Bed linen of isolated patients should be changed daily, and handled without vigorous shaking so as to prevent dissemination of lint harboring microorganisms. To remove contaminated sheets from the bed, loosen all around, gather corners together, gently crum-

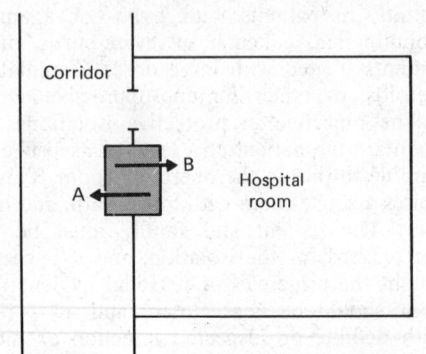

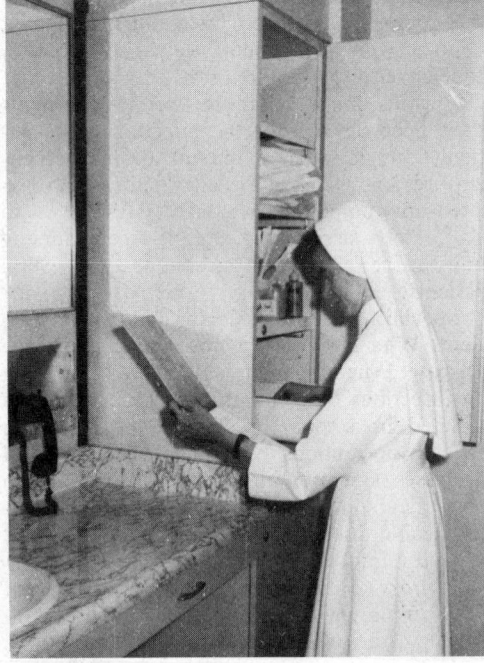

Figure 15-6. The Friesen Concept "Nurserver" is a two-way cabinet that may be supplied from the corridor and utilized by nursing personnel from the bedside. The upper half of the cabinet contains incoming, "clean" supplies and the lower half is reserved for outgoing or "dirty" items. The photograph shows the patient's room side of the unit. (Courtesy of Gordon A. Friesen International, Inc., Washington, D.C.)

ple, and place each item into the hamper inside the patient's room. Some hospitals use soluble plastic bags which may be put directly into the washing machine. Water-soluble laundry bags minimize the amount of handling necessary in the laundry. If water-soluble bags are not used, linen should be carefully put into the washing machine unsorted. Some hospitals use disposable sheets, pillowcases, and towels for patients in isolation. Bedclothes and tow-

els, regardless of the type of bag used, should be removed from the room of an infectious patient using the double bag technique. The articles, tightly closed in a bag in the contaminated area, are put in a second "clean" bag, preferably of a different color, which is held by a second person or supported by a clean hamper outside the patient's room (see Fig. 15-7). The second bag is tightly closed, taking care not to contaminate the outside, and labeled "contaminated." Sterile linen may be used for patients in protective isolation, and disposed of without special handling.

Food, ice, and drinking water must be handled differently for the patient in isolation. The food tray may be carried into the room unless the patient is on strict, or protective, isolation, in which case it is carried to the patient's door. Fresh drinking water should be kept in the patient's room in a disposable pitcher and cup. Ice should be brought into the room in a plastic or paper bag, or supplied by a second person who passes it through the doorway but does not enter the room. These same principles apply in homes. Families of patients isolated at home may prefer to supply a china, glass, or pottery pitcher which can be decontaminated by boiling in terminal cleaning of the patient's room.

Disposable *dishes* are preferred for patients on hemodialysis and for isolated patients, except for those on wound precautions and in protective isolation. If nondisposable dishes are used, they should be removed with double bag technique from the room in a moisture-proof bag clearly labeled "contaminated" (see Fig. 15-8). Dishes used by an infectious patient at home may be boiled before washing if an efficient mechanical dishwasher is not available.

Disposal of excreta varies according to the sewage system involved. Urine, feces, and vomitus of an institutionalized patient who has an infectious disease transmitted by the enteric route should be flushed down the toilet, not emptied into the bedpan flusher. Bedpan-cleaning equipment does not sterilize bedpans and spray may escape from the flusher, causing bacterial or viral aerosols. (Any bedpan placed in the bedpan flusher must be disinfected before being used again —even by the same patient.) Some health care institutions use disposable bedpans and urinals for patients in isolation. When the patient is discharged, the disposable utensils are disposed of by the double bag technique the same as for dressings and tissues. Nondisposable bedpans and urinals should be issued to each isolated patient to be used only by that patient throughout hospitalization to avoid the neces-

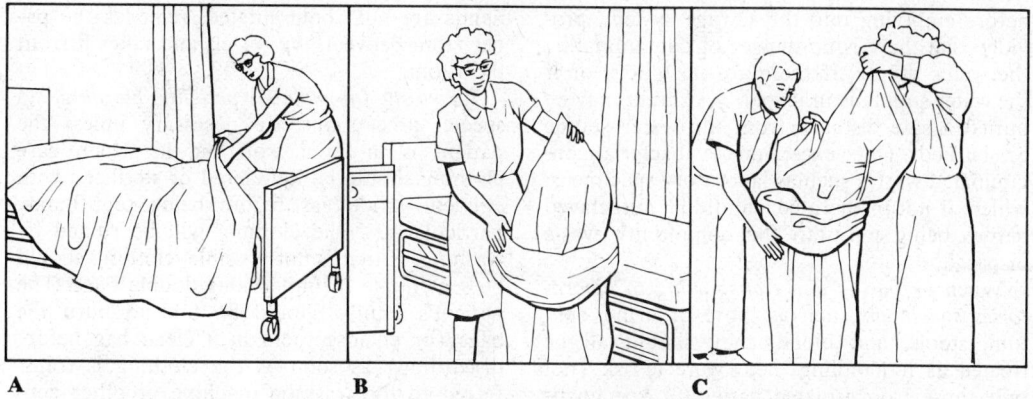

A   B   C

Figure 15-7. Procedure for removing bedding with minimum aerosol generation. *A.* Sheet is carefully loosened and gathered from corners to center of bed. *B.* Bedding is placed into color-coded laundry bag. *C.* Double-bagging is done by placing "room bag" into color-coded outer bag for isolation linen. (Adapted from Benson, Margaret: "Infection Control," in *Environmental Aspects of the Hospital.* Vol. I, *Infection Control* [PHS Pub. No. 930-C-15]. US Government Printing Office, Washington, D.C., 1970, p. 38.)

sity of concurrent sterilization. At the time of discharge, the equipment should be bagged and returned to central supply for decontamination and sterilization, preferably by autoclaving. Pus and other contents of suction bottles can be disposed of by emptying into the toilet or the clinical sink in the operating room, taking care to avoid splashing.

Soaking excreta in disinfectant solutions is no longer recommended. In view of the wide-spread distribution of disease-producing organisms in the intestinal tracts of well persons, sporadic efforts to treat feces, urine, and vomitus from sick persons are relatively useless, and penetration of organic matter by disinfectant agents is questionable. Natural decay of excreta is believed to be as effective without, as with, disinfection. Even when modern bathroom and sewage disposal facilities are not available, excreta need not be disinfected

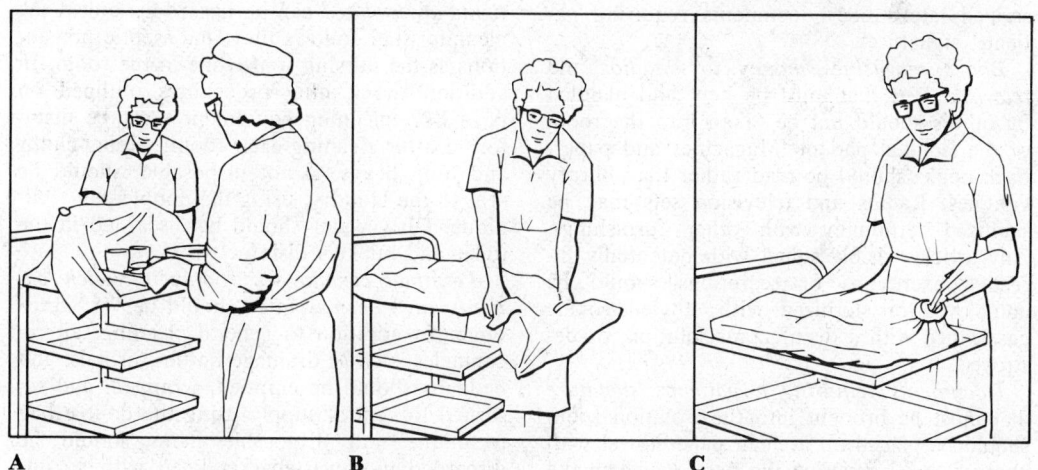

A   B   C

Figure 15-8. Removing dishes from room of patient in "strict" isolation. *A.* Diet tray is placed in a plastic bag without contaminating outside of bag. *B.* Tray bag is sealed. *C.* Tied bag ready to be labeled CONTAMINATED for return to dishwashing area. (Adapted from Benson, Margaret: "Infection Control," in *Environmental Aspects of the Hospital.* Vol. I, *Infection Control* [PHS Pub. No. 930-C-15]. US Government Printing Office, Washington, D.C., 1970, p. 38.)

before emptying into the sewage system, provided that there is no danger of contaminating the water supply. If there are no toilets, or if the water supply is in jeopardy, excreta may be buried a safe distance from the water source or burned. One exception is bacterial-contaminated wastes such as laboratory specimens, which, if not incinerated, should be autoclaved before being put into the community waste disposal.*

When *preparing and transporting to laboratories specimens* such as those of urine, sputum, stools, and blood, they should all be treated as if handling them were a risk (not only those from isolated patients). Specimens should be put into sterile labeled containers, being careful not to contaminate the outside. The lids should be securely closed. Specimens from patients on strict isolation precautions are placed in a transparent bag, using the double bag technique, and clearly labeled "contaminated" to warn laboratory personnel.

The *sphygmomanometer and stethoscope* should be kept in the isolated patient's room throughout hospitalization if possible. After discharge, the equipment should be disinfected in the manner appropriate to the microorganism causing the patient's disease. Cloth cuffs may be placed with the soiled linen and the remaining pieces wiped with a germicidal solution. Velco cuffs can be sent to central supply for sterilization by ethylene oxide gas.

Patients' charts and other hospital records should ordinarily not be taken into a room where a patient is isolated. If records must be made there, they may be protected as described later under documents requiring patients' signatures.

Books, magazines, money, toys, radios, and *television sets* that must be kept and handled by others should not be taken into the room of the isolated patient. Magazines and paperback books should be read rather than library volumes. Radios and television sets may be sanitized terminally with other furnishings. Any articles visibly soiled with potentially infective excretions or secretions should be autoclaved or sterilized with ethylene oxide gas, wiped with a disinfectant solution, or destroyed.

Documents requiring a patient's signature that must be brought into the isolation room should be placed on a clean paper towel with another towel covering the part on which the patient's hand will rest (see Fig. 15-9). After the signature is affixed, the nurse, whose

hands are not contaminated, removes the paper from between the towels and takes it from the room.

In *caring for isolated patients' clothing,* no special precautions are necessary unless the patient is in strict isolation, in which case clothing should be laundered or sterilized with ethylene oxide gas before being sent home, particularly if the clothing will be ruined by washing. If that is not possible, clothing should be sent home in impervious double bags. The patient's family should be told to burn the bags (or enclose them in a clean bag before discarding) as soon as the clothing is transferred to the washing machine or other container used for terminal disinfection. Hands should be thoroughly washed after handling contaminated clothing. All colorfast fabrics, except for silk or wool, should be washed in *hot* water in a washing machine with 1 cup of chlorine bleach (5.25 per cent sodium hypochlorite) added to the wash water along with laundry detergent. If washed by hand, the clothing should be soaked for at least 10 minutes in hot water to which laundry detergent and 1 oz (2 tbsp) of household bleach per gallon of water has been added. Silk, wool, unfast colors, or any other fabric that is damaged by chlorine bleach and hot water should be washed in warm water to which 1 cup of Lysol or other phenolic household disinfectant has been added. Add 1 cup to each washing machine load. The clothing should be washed and rinsed a second time without phenols to remove toxic residue.

Concurrent cleaning of rooms in which patients are isolated can be hazardous unless the cleaning staff follows the same aseptic precautions as the nursing staff while in the room. In addition to cleaning procedures outlined on page 877, cleaning equipment must be disinfected after cleaning each room; wiping-cloths and mop heads, if not disposable, should be sent to the laundry, using the double bag technique. Dirty water should be discarded in the toilet and buckets disinfected.

Terminal cleaning of rooms in which patients have been isolated should be very thorough. In addition to general cleaning, all receptacles such as drainage bottles, urinals, and bedpans should be emptied, wrapped, and returned to central supply using the double bag technique. All disposable items should be discarded in a wastebasket lined with an impervious plastic bag. All equipment that cannot be handled by central supply or discarded should be washed with a germicidal solution. All furniture, and mattress covers, should be washed with germicidal detergent solution. Plastic mattress and pillow covers may be sent

---

* Recommendation of Training Staff, Center for Disease Control, US Public Health Service, Atlanta, Ga., March 1973.

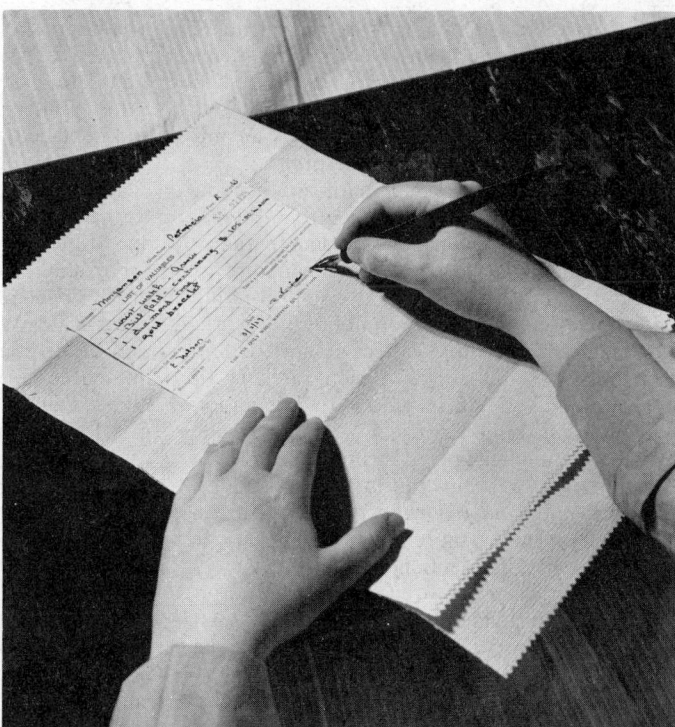

Figure 15-9. Patient signing a paper in medical asepsis. Contact between the paper and the patient, who has a communicable disease, is prevented by the use of paper towels.

to the laundry with contaminated linen. All floors should be wet-vacuumed (or mopped using the double bucket method if wet vacuuming is not available) with a germicidal detergent solution. All curtains should be sent to the laundry.

Disinfectant fogging (filling a sealed room with disinfectant mist, using a fog generator) is not an effective method of terminal disinfection of hospital rooms since mist does not penetrate contaminated surfaces. Decontamination of hospital air is best achieved by ventilation. Two air changes an hour will remove at least 90 per cent of airborne particles. Moreover, the safety of repeated exposure of humans to disinfectant fog has not been established. Finally, fogging may engender a sense of security among patients and personnel that could lead to abandonment of more effective sanitation and infection control measures.[189] Airing the room is not as effective as mechanical ventilation but if the room does not have a mechanical ventilation system a 30-minute airing period with windows open and doors closed may be indicated before terminal cleaning, particularly if the patient was in respiratory isolation. With the energy crisis we may have to go back to natural measures.

Some Infection Control Measures Other Than Those Involving Aseptic Technique. An *employee health program* is essential to infec-

tion control if patients are to be cared for by personnel who are free of infection. The American Hospital Association's book *Infection Control in the Hospital*[190] recommends the implementation of an employee health service that will detect, evaluate, prevent, and treat infection in personnel. This includes an initial examination of all applicants and an ongoing immunization program. Personnel who have direct or indirect contact with patients, including food handlers and technicians, should be excused from work when having fever, diarrhea, draining lesions of any kind, or any apparent infection. Institutional workers who develop infection in the course of their work should be transferred to tasks not involving patients or should be given leave with pay until they are no longer regarded as hazardous to others. Adoption of this practice would help to ensure adequate reporting of illness. Prophylactic treatment for workers following unusual exposure to diseases such as hepatitis should be available. For more specific recommendations on employee health, see AHA's *Infection Control in the Hospital*.

Teaching patients and families is also an important part of caring for the infectious patient. For example, patients should be taught good practices in bathing, handwashing, and use of paper handkerchiefs when coughing, sneezing, or spitting. Families must be taught how to care for patients who are sick at home without endangering themselves or other members of the family. Since parents are urged to keep infants and small children with infectious disease at home, this aspect of care is an important part of the visiting nurse program.

Teaching all health personnel is another important aspect of infection control. Educational programs should be provided to familiarize *all* hospital workers with the nature of nosocomial infections and ways of preventing and controlling them. As not all hospital workers require the same degree of instruction, programs must be suited to each category of personnel and should include both orientation and on-going inservice training sessions. The nurse epidemiologist plays an important role in designing and participating in such programs.

Surveillance and reporting programs are essential, and one of the chief functions of the epidemiologist or infection control nurse is to methodically detect and record nosocomial infection. This provides basic information about the usual endemic rate of infection in a given institution and evidence of a potential epidemic, or increase in rate. Surveillance also identifies areas in need of more specific control measures. Additionally, information gathered in this way can be useful in educational and research programs within the institution and community.[191]

Control of antibiotic use is an important part of a hospital infection control program. Most treatment centers have now adopted and enforce a policy designed to prevent the misuse of antibiotics. This is essential in order to combat the increase of resistant strains of microorganisms, and to decrease the occurrence of compromised hosts resulting from antibiotic-induced changes in microbial flora.

Controlling hospital traffic influences the spread of infection. Since microorganisms are spread by people, the chance of acquiring an infection increases wherever people congregate. Hospital design can reduce the flow of traffic from "dirty" to "clean" areas. A surgical area, for example, can be situated so that everyone who enters must pass through the dressing and gowning rooms. In general, no one but authorized personnel should be permitted to enter high-risk areas such as operating and delivery rooms, and nurseries.

Institutional ventilation and air conditioning can be designed to help control airborne microorganisms and provide a comfortable environment. This is achieved most effectively with a system that filters the air and controls the temperature, humidity, and air movement throughout the plant. To accomplish this, air is mechanically drawn into the building, where it is filtered, circulated throughout, and forced through exhausts, or outlets, to the outside. Ventilating systems require routine maintenance. Filters must be checked on schedule and replaced when damaged or clogged. Desirable ventilation rates, expressed in air changes per hour, vary with the functions performed in a given area. The sensitive areas—operating rooms, delivery rooms, and nurseries, for example—should be provided with air as nearly bacteria-free as possible without the necessity for reuse or recirculation. The location of air inlets and exhaust outlets in a room influences air movement within that room. High wall or ceiling air inlets are recommended for sensitive areas, as well as for areas of high contamination, such as autopsy and isolation rooms. High vent locations move the clean air downward toward the low exhaust outlets. Air pressure can be controlled by supplying more ventilating air into a given area than is being removed by the exhaust system. This produces an outflow around openings and lessens infiltration of air from adjacent areas. A negative air pressure is recommended for contaminated areas, while positive pressure is recommended for sensitive areas.[192]

Finally attention is called to the following *high-risk procedures and patient-care situations.* These six procedures carry above-average risk of infection and therefore require special precautions and techniques: (1) care of surgical wounds; (2) care of tracheostomies and tracheal suctioning; (3) intravenous and hyperalimentation therapy; (4) procedures requiring the use of anesthesia and respiratory therapy equipment; (5) urinary tract catheterization; and (6) renal dialysis.

Some hospitals have special wound-dressing and catheter-care teams consisting of staff members who are aware of the problems involved and skilled in meticulous sterile technique. Correct techniques for the procedures listed above are discussed in chapters dealing with these procedures. Since control and prevention of infection associated with the use of anesthesia and respiratory therapy equipment are dependent on proper cleaning, the correct processing of that equipment will be discussed here.

Inhalation therapy equipment, using reservoir nebulizers, is capable of generating aerosols containing large numbers of microorganisms. The source of contamination may be the jet of the nebulizer, improper cleaning and sterilization of the reservoir, or contaminated solutions, or medications, used in the nebulizer. Proper care requires that all contaminated components be removed and thoroughly cleaned, dried, and sterilized by steam or ethylene oxide gas, every 8 to 12 hours, and always between patients. Detachable equipment that cannot be autoclaved or sterilized with ethylene oxide should be thoroughly cleaned with hot water and a detergent and soaked in an effective germicide, then rinsed and dried. Activated glutaraldehyde (Cidex) is the recommended agent of choice. If that is not available, 70 to 90 per cent isopropyl alcohol or phenolic or iodophor germicides may be used. Disinfecting solutions must be changed frequently—at least every other week for activated glutaraldehyde, and as often as every day for some products. After soaking, the equipment should be rinsed in sterile water, dried thoroughly, and wrapped and stored, using sterile technique.*

Operating rooms, delivery rooms, nurseries, and infant-formula rooms are considered *high-risk hazardous areas* as far as patients are concerned, while laboratories, autopsy rooms, and laundry-sorting rooms are high-risk areas for personnel.

Renal dialysis units are hazardous for both patients and personnel. In the dialysis unit patients are exposed to the dangers of hepatitis, shunt sepsis, pyrogenic reactions to contaminated dialysis fluid, and severe systemic infections—peritonitis and bloodborne infection resulting from the use of an indwelling catheter or an artificial kidney, or from an infected urinary tract.[193]

Anybody in a hospital who requires transfusions of blood or a blood product, or anybody who handles blood or blood-contaminated equipment, runs a risk of acquiring hepatitis. Recent studies have shown that, among hospital personnel, surgeons have the highest rate of serum hepatitis, apparently from needle punctures and minor knife nicks. The serum hepatitis virus is so potent that only 0.001 to 0.01 ml is needed to transmit an infection. Moreover, it is now known that serum hepatitis can be transmitted by the oral, as well as the parenteral, route.

Blood should be handled so there is minimum risk of spillage and skin contact. Gloves should be worn and specimens enclosed in plastic bags for transfer to laboratories. Staff should refrain from eating, drinking, or smoking while on the clinical unit, and should carry out meticulous measures of personal hygiene. Segregation of infected patients with separation of dialysis equipment for their exclusive use is preferred to using the equipment interchangeably with patients who do not have hepatitis. Safe handling and disposal of urine, feces, and dialysis fluid and blood-contaminated equipment should be employed.[194]

Summary. The foregoing discussion of the environment as it relates to health care has dealt mainly with the inanimate, physical environment, with emphasis on ways to regulate certain aspects of it in order to make it conducive to health. Health essentials of the environment have been identified as the following: optimal organization of time and space, optimal natural and artificial lighting, and regulation of atmospheric conditions to provide healthful temperatures, humidity, and circulation of pollution-free air. This section also has included a brief discussion of some of the ways atmospheric conditions are adapted for use in the treatment of disease. Other health essentials are identified as the following: an adequate supply of fresh, safe water, safe waste disposal, at least a minimum of beauty and order in the surroundings including freedom from disagreeable odors, noise, and harmful insects and rodents, safe living and working conditions, sanitary surroundings and pure food, and the provision for preventing infection both in and out of health care institutions. A section of infection control in the hospital has included a brief discussion of the factors that contribute to hospital-associated (nosocomial) infection, as well as ways of preventing and controlling it. Included here is mention of aseptic technique, and disinfection and sterilization, certain aspects of which are covered in a number of other chapters.

That part of the nonhuman, animate environment comprised of plants and animals and the beneficial effects of our natural surroundings have not been discussed in this chapter, but the authors recognize, and wish it were possible to stress, their importance in the promotion and maintenance of health and well-being. The human environment, or its psychosocial aspect as it relates to health and well-being, is covered in Chapter 16.

---

* Recommendation of the Center for Disease Control, US Public Health Service, Atlanta, Ga.

REFERENCES

1. Henkel, Barbara O., et al.: *Foundations of Health Science,* 2nd ed. Allyn and Bacon, Boston, 1971, p. 432.
2. Henderson, Virginia A.: "Health Is Everybody's Business," *Can. Nurse,* **67:**1, (Mar.) 1971.
3. "Symposium on Disaster Nursing," *Nurs. Clin. North Am.,* **11:**285, (June) 1967.
4. Garb, Solomon, and Eng, Evelyn: *Disaster Handbook,* 2nd ed. Springer Publishing Co., New York, 1969.
5. Hall, Edward T.: *The Silent Language.* Fawcett Publications, Greenwich, Conn., 1959, p. 146.

6. ———: *The Hidden Dimension.* Doubleday & Co., Garden City, N.Y., 1966.

7. ———: "Communication and Design," a paper presented at the American Anthropological Association meeting, New York, 1971.

8. Griffin, William V., et al.: "The Psychological Aspects of the Architectural Environment: A Review," *Am. J. Psychiatry,* **125:**1057, (Feb.) 1969.

9. *Ibid.*

10. Barnes, Elizabeth: *People in Hospital.* Macmillan & Co., London, 1961, p. 90.

11. Burnside, Irene M.: "Clocks and Calendars," *Am. J. Nurs.,* **70:**117, (Jan.) 1970.

12. Will, Otto A., Jr.: "Schizophrenia and the Psychotherapeutic Field," *Contemp. Psychoanal.,* **1:**11, (Fall) 1964.

13. Glaser, Helen H.: "The Hospital as an Environment for Children and Their Families," *Pediatr. Ann.,* (Dec.) 1972, p. 10.

14. *Ibid.*

15. *Ibid.*

16. Turner, C. E.: *Personal and Community Health,* 14th ed. C. V. Mosby Co., St. Louis, 1971, p. 281.

17. Kogan, Benjamin A.: *Health: Man in a Changing Environment.* Harcourt, Brace & World, New York, 1970, p. 37.

18. Brigden, Raymond J.: *Operating Theatre Technique,* 2nd ed. E & S. Livingstone, Ltd., London, 1969, p. 11.

19. *Recommended Housing Maintenance and Occupancy Ordinance.* US Government Printing Office, Washington, D.C., 1969 (PHS Pub. No. 1953).

20. Salvato, Joseph A., Jr.: *Environmental Engineering and Sanitation,* 2nd ed. Wiley-Interscience, New York, 1972, p. 593.

21. Turner, C. E.: *op. cit.,* p. 435.

22. *Ibid.,* p. 434.

23. Fox, Sidney A.: *Your Eyes.* Alfred A. Knopf, New York, 1944, p. 94.

24. *Lighting for Hospital Patients' Rooms.* US Government Printing Office, Washington, D.C., 1967, p. 1 (PHS Pub. No. 930-D-3).

25. *Ibid.,* p. 27.

26. American Academy of Pediatrics: *Hospital Care of Newborn Infants,* 5th ed. The Academy, Evanston, Ill., 1972, p. 56.

27. Worcester, Alfred W.: *Care of the Aged, the Dying and the Dead.* Charles C Thomas, Publisher, Springfield, Ill., 1935, p. 19.

28. Baetjer, Anna M.: "Environmental and Occupational Health," in Sartwell, Philip E. (ed.): *Maxcy-Rosenau Preventive Medicine and Public Health,* Appleton-Century-Crofts, New York, 1956, p. 713.

29. Quashnock, Joseph M.: "Heat and Cold," in Beeson, Paul B., and McDermott, Walsh (eds.): *Cecil-Loeb Textbook of Medicine,* 13th ed. W. B. Saunders Co., Philadelphia, 1971, p. 32.

30. *Ibid.,* p. 32.

31. Baetjer, Anna M.: *op. cit.,* p. 729.

32. Salvato, Joseph A., Jr.: *op. cit.,* p. 817.

33. Uyeda, Charles T.: "Environmental Sanitation," *Hospitals,* **40:**57, (Apr. 1) 1966.

34. American Academy of Pediatrics: *op. cit.,* pp. 57, 89.

35. American Hospital Association: *Infection Control in the Hospital.* The Association, Chicago, 1970, p. 70.

36. Whitfield, W. J.: "Use of Laminar Flow for Environmental Control," in Conference on Environmental Sanitation, Dec. 15–16, 1966, Chicago: *Environmental Sanitation.* American Hospital Association, Chicago, 1968, p. 27.

37. Whitcomb, John C.: "Surgical Experience with Laminar Flow," in Conference on Environmental Sanitation, Dec. 15–16, 1966, Chicago: *Environmental Sanitation.* American Hospital Association, Chicago, 1968, p. 30.

38. Gordon, P. B.: "Man and His Environment: Where Are We? Where Are We Going?" in Jennings, Burgess H., and Murphy, John E. (eds.): *Interactions of Man and His Environment.* Plenum Press, New York, 1966, p. 152.

39. Garr, Doug: "Electronic Air Cleaners: What Can They Do for You?" *Popular Sci.,* (Sept.) 1972, p. 58.

40. Stern, Arthur C. (ed.): *Air Pollution,* Vol. I, 2nd ed. Academic Press, New York, 1968, p. 554.

41. Salvato, Joseph A., Jr.: *op. cit.,* pp. 39, 44.

42. *Ibid.,* p. 450.

43. Phillips, John, Jr.: *Environmental Health.* Wm. C. Brown Co., Dubuque, Iowa, 1971, p. 21.

44. Haagen-Smit, Arie J.: "The Troubled Outdoors," in Jennings, Burgess H., and Murphy, John E. (eds.): *Interactions of Man and His Environment.* Plenum Press, New York, 1966, p. 45.

45. Kogan, Benjamin A.: *op. cit.,* p. 78.

46. Carson, Rachel L.: *The Sea Around Us.* Oxford University Press, New York, 1951, p. 46.

47. Johnson, Robert L.: "Alterations in Atmospheric Pressure," in Beeson, Paul B., and McDermott, Walsh (eds.): *Cecil-Loeb Textbook of Medicine,* 13th ed. W. B. Saunders Co., Philadelphia, 1971, p. 33.

48. Dewey, A. Warner: "Decompression Sickness, an Emerging Recreational Hazard," *N. Engl. J. Med.,* **267:**759, (Oct. 11) 1962.

49. Behnke, Albert R.: "Remedial Atmospheres," in Jennings, Burgess H., and Murphy, John E. (eds.): *Interactions of Man and His Environment.* Plenum Press, New York, 1966, p. 66.

50. Johnson, Robert L.: *op. cit.,* p. 34.

51. Behnke, Albert R.: *op. cit.,* p. 67.

52. *Ibid.,* p. 65.

53. *Ibid.,* p. 64.

54. Johnson, Robert L.: *op. cit.,* p. 36.

55. Ellingson, Harold V.: "Motion Sickness and Problems of Air Travel," in Beeson, Paul B., and McDermott, Walsh (eds.): *Cecil-Loeb*

Textbook of Medicine, 13th ed. W. B. Saunders Co., Philadelphia, 1971, p. 41.

56. Siegel, Peter V., et al.: "Time-Zone Effects," *Science,* **164:**1249, (June 13) 1966.
57. Kogan, Benjamin A.: *op. cit.,* p. 9.
58. Siegel, Peter V., et al.: *op. cit.*
59. Ellingson, Harold V.: *op. cit.,* p. 41.
60. Turner, C. E.: *op. cit.,* p. 410.
61. *Public Health Service Drinking Water Standards.* US Government Printing Office, Washington, D.C., 1972 (PHS Pub. No. 956).
62. Salvato, Joseph A., Jr.: *op. cit.,* p. 104.
63. *Ibid.,* p. 252.
64. Kogan, Benjamin A.: *op. cit.,* p. 62.
65. Turner, C. E.: *op. cit.,* p. 413.
66. Salvato, Joseph A., Jr.: *op. cit.,* p. 345.
67. Sloan, Raymond P.: *Hospital Color and Decoration.* Physicians Record Co., Chicago, 1944, pp. 77, 107.
68. Schuster, Eleanor A.: "Privacy and Hospitalization Subject of Nurses Investigation," *Nurs. Res. Rep.,* **8:**1, (Oct.) 1973.
69. Phillips, John, Jr.: *op. cit.,* p. 38.
70. Salvato, Joseph A., Jr.: *op. cit.,* p. 700.
71. *Ibid.,* p. 707.
72. *Ibid.,* p. 707.
73. *Ibid.,* p. 712.
74. Zinnser, Hans: *Rats, Lice and History, Being a Study in Biography . . . With the Life History of Typhus Fever.* Little, Brown & Co., Boston, 1953.
75. Beck, J. Walter, and Barrett-Connor, Elizabeth: *Medical Parasitology.* C. V. Mosby Co., St. Louis, 1971, p. 182.
76. Salvato, Joseph A., Jr.: *op. cit.,* p. 727.
77. *Ibid.,* p. 723.
78. Beck, J. Walter, and Barrett-Connor, Elizabeth: *op. cit.,* p. 175.
79. Faust, Ernest C., et al.: *Animal Agents and Vectors of Human Disease,* 3rd ed. Lea & Febiger, Philadelphia, 1968, p. 330.
80. Najarian, Haig H.: *Textbook of Medical Parasitology.* Williams & Wilkins Co., Baltimore, 1967, p. 13.
81. Salvato, Joseph A., Jr.: *op. cit.,* p. 722.
82. Faust, Ernest C., et al.: *op. cit.,* p. 347.
83. Najarian, Haig H.: *op. cit.,* p. 15.
84. Salvato, Joseph A., Jr.: *op. cit.,* p. 727.
85. *Ibid.,* p. 728.
86. *Ibid.,* p. 732.
87. Greene, V. W.: "Part IV, Role of Housekeeping," in *Microbiological Contamination in Hospitals.* American Hospital Association, Chicago, 1970 (reprinted from *Hospitals*).
87a. Kogan, Benjamin A.: *op. cit.,* p. 108.
88. *Ibid.,* p. 117.
89. Haggerty, Robert J.: "Accidental Poisoning," in Green, Morris, and Haggerty, Robert J. (eds.): *Ambulatory Pediatrics.* W. B. Saunders Co., Philadelphia, 1968, p. 823.
90. Smith, Hugo D.: "Lead Poisoning and Pica," in Green, Morris, and Haggerty, Robert J. (eds.): *Ambulatory Pediatrics.* W. B. Saunders Co., Philadelphia, 1968, p. 825.

91. Garb, Solomon, and Eng, Evelyn: *op. cit.,* p. 185.
92. Feerick, James: "Fire! What Do You Do First?" *Am. J. Nurs.,* **70:**2579, (Dec.) 1970.
93. American Hospital Association; National Safety Council: *Safety Guide for Health Care Institutions.* The Association, Chicago, 1972, p. 185.
94. Black, James B.: "Fire and Disaster," in *Environmental Aspects of the Hospital,* Vol. III, *Safety Fundamentals.* US Government Printing Office, Washington, D.C., 1967, p. 1 (PHS Pub. No. 930-C-17).
95. Smariga, Julian: *Fire Prevention in Hospitals.* US Government Printing Office, Washington, D.C., 1965 (PHS Pub. No. 930-D-21).
96. American Hospital Association; National Safety Council: *op. cit.,* p. 66.
97. Moore, A. D.: "Electrostatics," *Sci. Am.,* **226:**47, (Mar.) 1972.
98. Brigden, Raymond J.: *op. cit.,* p. 52.
99. Hudenburg, Roy: "Flammable Gases," in *Environmental Aspects of the Hospital,* Vol. III, *Safety Fundamentals.* US Government Printing Office, Washington, D.C., 1967, p. 37 (PHS Pub. No. 930-C-17).
100. *Health Devices,* **2:**218, (June–July) 1973.
101. Creighton, Helen: "Your Legal Risks in Nursing Coronary Patients," *Am. J. Nurs.,* **71:**25, (Dec.) 1971.
102. Dalziel, Charles F.: "Electric Shock Hazard," *IEEE Spectrum,* (Feb.) 1972, p. 41.
103. Goldstein, David H.: "Electric Shock," in Beeson, Paul B., and McDermott, Walsh (eds.): *Cecil-Loeb Textbook of Medicine,* 13th ed. W. B. Saunders Co., Philadelphia, 1971, p. 44.
104. Dalziel, Charles F.: *op. cit.*
105. Stanley, Paul E.: "Electrical Shock Hazards, Part I," *Hospitals,* **45:**58, (Jan. 1) 1971.
106. Dalziel, Charles F.: *op. cit.*
107. Lubin, David: "Electrical Safety," *Hospitals,* **43:**57, (Dec. 1) 1969.
108. Goldstein, David H.: *op. cit.,* p. 44.
109. Hewlett Packard Company: *Using Electrically-Operated Equipment Safely with the Monitored Cardiac Patient.* The Company, Waltham, Mass., 1971, p. 6.
110. American Hospital Association: *op. cit.,* p. 55.
111. California Department of Public Health: *Cleaning, Disinfection and Sterilization, A Guide for Hospitals and Related Facilities.* The Department, Berkeley, 1965, p. 22.
112. American Hospital Association: *op. cit.,* p. 55.
113. Litsky, Bertha Y.: "Scientific Housekeeping and the Professional Nurse," *Nurs. Clin. North Am.,* **5:**108, (Mar.) 1970.
114. Davis, R. N.: "Carpet in the Hospital," *Hospitals,* **39:**44, (Sept. 16) 1965.
115. Gable, Tom S.: "Bactericidal Effectiveness of Floor Cleaning Methods," *Hospitals,* **40:**107, (Feb. 16) 1966.
116. Litsky, Bertha Y.: *op. cit.*

117. Hospital Bureau, Inc.: *Control of Cross Infection.* The Bureau, New York, 1966, p. 6.
118. American Hospital Association: *op. cit.,* p. 50.
119. *Ibid.,* p. 48.
120. Stauffer, Lee, and Decker, Winston: "Dietary Services," in *Environmental Aspects of the Hospital,* Vol. II, *Supportive Departments.* US Government Printing Office, Washington, D.C., 1971, p. 36 (HEW Pub. [HSM] No. 72–4003).
121. Jopke, Walter H.: "Food Hygiene," in Bond, Richard, et al. (eds.): *Environmental Health and Safety in Health Care Facilities.* Macmillan Publishing Co., Inc., New York, 1973, p. 239.
122. *Ibid.,* p. 243.
123. *Ibid.,* p. 243.
124. Walter, C. W., et al.: "Bacteriology of the Bedside Carafe," *N. Engl J. Med.,* **259:**1198, (Dec. 19) 1958.
125. American Hospital Association: *op. cit.,* p. 53.
126. Mallison, George F.: "Environmental Control in Hospitals," in *Methods of Microbiology.* American Society for Microbiology, Washington, D.C., 1970, p. 618.
127. Spaulding, E. H.: "Role of Chemical Disinfection in Prevention of Nosocomial Infection," in *Proceedings of the 1970 International Conference on Nosocomial Infections.* American Hospital Association, Chicago, 1971, p. 247.
128. Vesley, Donald, and Greene, Velvl W.: "Sterilization, Disinfection and Cleaning Techniques," in Bond, Richard, et al. (eds.): *Environmental Health and Safety in Health Care Facilities.* Macmillan Publishing Co., Inc., New York, 1973, p. 48.
129. California Department of Public Health: *op. cit.,* p. 19.
130. Vesley, Donald, and Greene, Velvl W.: *op. cit.,* p. 56.
131. Simmons, N. R., and Gardner, D.: "Bacterial Contamination of a Phenolic Disinfectant," *Br. Med. J.,* **2:**668, (June 14) 1969.
132. Leigh, D. R., and Whittaker, C.: "Disinfectants and Plastic Mop Heads," *Br. Med. J.,* **3:**435, (Aug. 12) 1967.
133. Sanford, Jay P.: "Disinfectants That Don't," *Ann. Intern. Med.,* **72:**282, (Feb.) 1970.
134. *Ibid.*
135. Plotkin, S. A., and Austrian, R.: "Bacteremia Caused by *Pseudomonas* sp. following the Use of Materials Stored in Solutions of a Catatonic Surface Active Agent," *Am. J. Med. Sci.,* **235:**621, (June) 1958.
136. Vesley, Donald, and Greene, Velvl W.: *op. cit.,* p. 56.
137. *Ibid.,* p. 56.
138. *Ibid.,* p. 56.
139. *Ibid.,* p. 48.
140. *Ibid.,* p. 51.
141. California Department of Public Health: *op. cit.,* p. 23.
142. Brachman, Philip S.: "Foreword, Symposium

on Infection and the Nurse," *Nurs. Clin. North Am.,* **5:**85, (Mar.) 1970.
143. US Public Health Service, Center for Disease Control: *National Nosocomial Infections Study Quarterly Report, Second Quarter 1972.* The Center, Atlanta, Ga., May 1973.
144. Spaulding, Earle H.: "Principles of Microbiology as Applied to Operating Room Nursing," from a paper presented at Annual Congress of Association of Operating Room Nurses, Washington, D.C., Feb. 19, 1963, modified from a version published in *AORN J.,* **1:**49, (Jan.) 1963.
145. "Water Bugs in the Bassinet" (editorial), *Am. J. Dis. Child.,* **101:**273, (Mar.) 1961.
146. Gibson, G. L.: *Infection in Hospital.* E. & S. Livingstone, London, 1971, p. 35.
147. Kresky, B.: "Control of Gram-Negative Bacilli in a Hospital Nursery," *Am. J. Dis. Child.,* **107:**363, (Apr.) 1964.
148. Foley, John, et al.: "Achromobacter Septicemia Fatalities in Prematures," *Am. J. Dis. Child.,* **101:**279, (Mar.) 1961.
149. Langmuir, Alexander D.: "A View of the Issues," in *Environmental Sanitation.* American Hospital Association, Chicago, 1968, p. 1.
150. Brachman, Philip S.: *op. cit.*
151. Gregg, Michael B.: "Communicable Disease Trends in the U.S.," *Am. J. Nurs.,* **68:**5, (Jan.) 1968.
152. Altemeier, W. A.: "Current Infection Problems in Surgery," in *Proceedings of the 1970 International Conference on Nosocomial Infections.* American Hospital Association, Chicago, 1971, p. 86.
153. Top, Frankin H. (ed.): *Control of Infectious Diseases in General Hospitals.* American Public Health Association, Washington, D.C., 1968, p. 5.
154. Mallison, George F.: "Introduction to Microbiology of the Institutional Environment," paper presented at National Communicable Disease Center, Fourth Annual Technical Meeting and Exhibit, Miami Beach, Fla., May 1965 (HEW Report No. 58). US Government Printing Office, Washington, D.C., [1965].
155. Anderson, Louise, and Himmelsbach, Clifton: "The Nurse: First Line of Defense Against Infections," *Hospitals,* **41:**84, (Oct. 1) 1967.
156. Streeter, Shirley, et al.: "Hospital Infection —A Necessary Risk?" *Am. J. Nurs.,* **67:**526, (Mar.) 1967.
157. Williams, R. E. O., and Shooter, R. A. (eds.): *Infections in Hospitals.* F. A. Davis Co., Philadelphia, 1963.
158. Wenzel, Kathryn: "The Role of the Infection Control Nurse," *Nurs. Clin. North Am.,* **5:**89, (Mar.) 1970.
159. Greene, V. W.: "Microbiological Contamination Control in Hospitals, Part I. Prospectives," *Hospitals,* **43:**82, (Oct. 16) 1969.
160. US Public Health Service: *Isolation Tech-*

niques for Use in Hospitals. US Government Printing Office, Washington, D.C., 1970 (PHS Pub. No. 2054).

161. Benson, Margaret: "Infection Control," in *Environmental Aspects of the Hospital,* Vol. I, *Infection Control.* US Government Printing Office, Washington, D.C., 1970, p. 35 (PHS Pub. No. 930-C-15).

162. Bernard, Harvey R.: "The Effect of Scrub Time on Hand Antisepsis Using Povidone-Iodine Surgical Scrub for 3–5–10 Minute Scrubs," in Polk, H. C., and Ehrenkranz, N. J. (eds.): *Medical and Surgical Antisepsis with Betadine Microbicides.* Proceedings of Symposium co-sponsored by Departments of Surgery, Epidemiology, and Public Health, University of Miami School of Medicine. Purdue Frederick Co., New York, 1972.

163. Sanford, Jay P.: *op. cit.*

164. Joress, S. M.: "A Study of Disinfection of the Skin: A Comparison of Povidone—Iodine with Other Agents Used for Surgical Scrubs," *Ann. Surg.,* **155**:296, (Feb.) 1962.

165. Wilson, M. G., et al.: "A New Source of *Pseudomonas aeruginosa* in a Nursery," *J.A.M.A.,* **175**:146, (Apr. 1) 1961.

166. Maliza, W. F., et al.: "Benzalkonium Chloride as a Source of Infection," *N. Engl. J. Med.,* **263**:800, (Oct. 20) 1960.

167. Lowbury, E. S. L.: "Contamination of Cetrimide and Other Fliuds with *Pseudomonas pyocyanea,*" *Br. J. Ind. Med.,* **8**:22, (Jan.) 1951.

168. Lee, J. C., and Fiakow, P. J.: "Benzalkonium Chloride—Source of Hospital Infection with Gram-Negative Bacteria," *J.A.M.A.,* **177**:708, (Sept. 9) 1961.

169. Adams, Ralph, et al.: "New Fashions in Surgical Attire," *Am. J. Nurs.,* **59**:1103, (Aug.) 1959.

170. Dineen, Peter: "Microbial Filtration by Surgical Masks," *Surg. Gynecol. Obstet.,* **133**:812, (Nov.) 1971.

171. Dineen, Peter: "Clinical Research in Skin Disinfection," *AORN J.,* **14**:77, (July) 1971.

172. Sanford, Jay P.: *op. cit.*

173. Plotkin, S. A., and Austrian, R.: *op. cit.*

174. Keown, K., et al.: "Open Heart Surgery, Anesthesia and Surgical Experiences," *J.A.M.A.,* **165**:781, (Oct. 19) 1957.

175. "Equipment," *Am. J. Nurs.,* **73**:1962, (Nov.) 1973.

176. Greene, V. W.: "Part 2—Role of the Engineer," in *Microbiological Contamination in Hospitals.* American Hospital Association, Chicago, 1970 (reprinted from *Hospitals*).

177. Hospital Bureau, Inc.: *op. cit.,* p. 18.

178. American Hospital Association: *op. cit.,* p. 74.

179. Goldberger, Leo: "Experimental Isolation: An Overview," *Am. J. Psychiatry,* **122**:774, (Jan.) 1966.

180. US Public Health Service: *Isolation Techniques for Use in Hospitals.* US Government Printing Office, Washington, D.C., 1970.

181. Benenson, Abram S. (ed.): *Control of Communicable Diseases in Man,* 11th ed. American Public Health Association, Washington, D.C., 1970.

182. US Public Health Service: *Isolation Techniques for Use in Hospitals.* US Government Printing Office, Washington, D.C., 1970, p. 8.

183. American Hospital Association: *op. cit.,* p. 80.

184. Seidler, Florence M.: "Adapting Nursing Procedures for Reverse Isolation," *Am. J. Nurs.,* **65**:108, (June) 1965.

185. Michaelson, George S.: "Experimental Approaches to Controlling the Environment," in *Environmental Sanitation.* American Hospital Association, Chicago, 1967, p. 33.

186. Glor, Beverly, et al.: "The RES System—A Concept of Reverse Isolation," *Milit. Med.,* **131**:421, (May) 1966.

187. McDermott, Nancy K.: "The Nursing Role in a Specialized Infection Control Unit," *Nurs. Clin. North Am.,* **5**:113, (Mar.) 1970.

188. Margolius, Francine: "Burned Children, Infection, and Nursing Care," *Nurs. Clin. North Am.,* **5**:131, (Mar.) 1970.

189. US Public Health Service, Center for Disease Control: *National Nosocomial Infections Study Quarterly Report, Third Quarter 1971.* The Center, Atlanta, Ga., May 1972.

190. American Hospital Association: *op. cit.,* p. 23.

191. US Public Health Service: *Outline for Surveillance and Control of Nosocomial Infections.* Center for Disease Control, Atlanta, Ga., 1970.

192. American Hospital Association: *op. cit.,* p. 70.

193. Gibson, G. L.: *op. cit.,* p. 43.

194. *Ibid.,* p. 43.

Additional Suggested Reading

Abelson, Philip H.: "Man Made Environmental Hazards: How Man Shapes His Environment," *Am. J. Public Health,* **58**:2043, (Nov.) 1968.

American Hospital Association: "Guidelines to Hospital Fire Safety," *Hospitals,* Special Issue, (June 1) 1962.

———: *Housekeeping Manual for Health Care Facilities.* The Association, Chicago, 1969.

———, and National Safety Council: *Safety Guide for Health Care Institutions.* The Association, Chicago, 1972.

American Insurance Association: *Safe Hospitals,* 2nd ed. The Association, Chicago, 1969.

American Sterilizer Company: "Prevacuum High Temperature Steam Sterilization," *J. Hosp. Res.,* Vol. 1, (July) 1963.

———: "Operating Room Lighting," *J. Hosp. Res.,* Vol. 2, (April) 1964.

———: "Safety from Fires and Explosions from Flammable Anesthetics in Hospitals," *J. Hosp. Res.,* Vol. 4, (July) 1966.

———: "Surgical Scrubs and Preoperative Skin Disinfection," *J. Hosp. Res.,* Vol. 5, (Dec.) 1967.

———: "The Hospital Environment and Infection," *J. Hosp. Res.,* Vol. 6, (July) 1968.

———: "Ethylene Oxide Sterilization," *J. Hosp. Res.,* Vol. 7, (Nov.) 1971.

———: "Chemical Disinfection and Antisepsis in the Hospital," *J. Hosp. Res.,* Vol. 9, Rev., (Feb.) 1972.

Aronow, S., et al.: "Ventricular Fibrillation Associated with an Electrically Operated Bed," *N. Engl. J. Med.,* **281:**31, (July 3) 1969.

Baker, Paul H.: "Human Adaptation to High Altitudes," *Science,* **163:**1149, (Mar. 14) 1969.

Baron, Robert Alex: "Noise and Urban Man," *Am. J. Public Health,* **58:**2060, (Nov.) 1968.

Basic Housekeeping Procedure Manual, 5th ed., prepared by Vestal Laboratories, Division of W. R. Grace & Co., St. Louis, 1970.

Bates, Marston: *Man in Nature,* 2nd ed. Prentice-Hall, Englewood Cliffs, N.J., 1964.

Bentley, D., and Lepper, M.: "Septicemia Related to Indwelling Venous Catheter," *J.A.M.A.,* **206:** 1749, (Nov. 18) 1968.

Bhatia, C. K.: "Hospital Acquired Infections," *N. Engl. J. Med.,* **284:**338, (Feb. 11) 1971.

Bjornson, Bayard F., et al.: *Control of Domestic Rats and Mice.* US Public Health Service Center for Disease Control, Atlanta, Ga., 1973 (DHEW Pub. No. [HSM] 72–8141).

Bocock, J., and Parker, M.: *Microbiology for Nurses,* 4th ed., rev. Williams & Wilkins Co., Baltimore, 1972.

Boettcher, E. N.: "Fire Safety Begins in the Patient's Room," *Mod. Hosp.,* **101:**98, (July) 1963.

———: "How to Make a Fire-Safe Hospital Safer," *Mod. Hosp.,* **101:**83, (Aug.) 1963.

Brennan, M. F., et al.: "The Growth of *Candida albicans* in Nutritive Solutions Given Parenterally," *Arch. Surg.,* **101:**705, (Dec.) 1971.

Bruner, J. A.: "Hazards of Electrical Apparatus," *Anesthesiology,* **28:**396, (Mar.–Apr.) 1967.

Carson, Rachel: *Silent Spring.* Houghton Mifflin Co., New York, 1962.

Chernick, V., and Raber, M. B.: "Electrical Hazards in the Newborn Nursery," *J. Pediatr.,* **77:** 143, (July) 1970.

Collins, R. N., et al.: "Risk of Local and Systemic Infection with Polyethylene Intravenous Catheters," *N. Engl. J. Med.,* **279:**340, (Aug. 15) 1968.

Commoner, Barry: *Science and Survival.* Viking Press, New York, 1967.

Corrigan, Marjorie J., and Corcoran, Lucille E.: *Epidemiology in Nursing.* Catholic University Press, Washington, D.C., 1971.

DeBell, Garrett (ed.): *The Environmental Handbook.* Ballantine Books, New York, 1970.

DeRoos, Roger L., and Michaelsen, George S.: "Solid Wastes: Handling and Disposal," in Bond, Richard, et al. (eds.): *Environmental Health and Safety in Health Care Facilities.* Macmillan Publishing Co., Inc., New York, 1973.

DeWitt, Jon S.: "These Measures Are Needed to Protect the Electrically Susceptible Patient," *Mod. Hosp.,* **116:**79, (Jan.) 1971.

Dubos, René: *Mirage of Health.* Harper & Row, New York, 1959.

———: *Man Adapting.* Yale University Press, New Haven, Conn., 1965.

———: *So Human an Animal.* Charles Scribners' Sons, New York, 1968.

Ehrlich, Paul R.: *The Population Bomb.* Ballantine Books, New York, 1965.

———, and Ehrlich, Anne H.: *Population, Resources, Environment; Issues in Human Ecology.* W. H. Freeman & Co., San Francisco, 1972.

Electrical Safety in the Hospital. Medical Economics Co., Book Division, Oradell, N.J., 1976.

Finland, M.: "Changing Ecology of Bacterial Infections as Related to Antibacterial Therapy," *J. Infect. Dis.,* **122:**419, (Nov.) 1970.

Foley, Mary E.: "Air Travel for Patients," *Am. J. Nurs.,* **73:**1020, (June) 1973.

Gilbert, G.: "Electrical Hazards in the Use of Monitors and Defibrillators," *Nurs. Clin. North Am.,* **4:**615, (Dec.) 1969.

Ginsberg, F.: "How to Decontaminate Anesthesia Circuits," *Mod. Hosp.,* **115:**88, (Dec.) 1970.

Gomez, Ann, and Bellows, Donald R.: "Formulating and Implementing an Infection Surveillance Program," *Hospitals,* **43:**91, (Mar. 16) 1969.

Grahm, Frank, Jr.: *Disaster by Default: Politics and Water Pollution.* M. Evans & Co., New York, 1966.

———: *Since Silent Spring.* Houghton Mifflin Co., New York, 1970.

Green, Henry L., et al.: "Electronic Equipment in Critical Care Areas: Status of Devices Currently in Use," *Circulation,* **43:**A101, (Jan.) 1971.

Greenberg, B.: *Flies and Disease.* Princeton University Press, Princeton, N.J., 1971.

Griffin, Noyce L.: *Electronics for Hospital Patient Care.* US Government Printing Office, Washington, D.C., 1969 (PHS Pub. No. 930-D-25).

"Guidelines for the General Hospital in the Admission and Care of Tuberculous Patients." Ad Hoc Committee on the Treatment of Tuberculous Patients in General Hospitals. *Am. Rev. Resp. Dis.,* **99:**631, 1969.

Hardin, Garrett (ed.): *Population, Evolution and Birth Control.* W. H. Freeman & Co., San Francisco, 1969.

Hayt, E.: "Legal Considerations in Control of Hospital Infections," *Hospitals,* **40:**75, (Oct. 16) 1966.

"Hepatitis in Hospitals," *Hospitals,* **44:**83, (Sept. 16) 1970.

Hochberg, Howard M.: "Effects of Electrical Current on Heart Rhythm," *Am. J. Nurs.,* **71:**1390, (July) 1971.

How to Clean Everything: An Encyclopedia of What to Use and How to Use It, 3rd ed. Simon & Schuster, New York, 1968.

Infection Control Manual. Medical Economics Co., Book Division, Oradell, N.J., 1975.

Jodais, Janet, and Rothenberg, Herbert: "An

Isolation Unit in a General Hospital," *Hosp. Manage.,* **109**:25, (Mar.) 1970.

Johnson, Cecil E. (ed.): *Social and Natural Biology.* D. Van Nostrand Co., Inc., Princeton, N.J., 1968.

Kilbourne, Edwin D. (ed.): *Human Ecology and Public Health.* Macmillan Publishing Co., Inc., New York, 1969.

Kummer, S. B., and Kummer, J. M.: "Pointers to Preventing Accidents," *Am. J. Nurs.,* **63**:118, (Feb.) 1963.

Larson, Elaine: "Bacterial Colonization of Tracheal Tubes of Patients in a Surgical Intensive Care Unit," *Nurs. Res.,* **19**:122, (Mar.–Apr.) 1970.

Lawrence, C. A., and Block, S. S. (eds.): *Disinfection, Sterilization and Preservation.* Lea & Febiger, Philadelphia, 1968.

Lipscomb, David M.: "High Intensity Sounds in the Recreational Environment: Hazard to Young Ears," *Clin. Pediatr.,* **8**:63, (Feb.) 1969.

Litsky, Bertha Y.: *Hospital Sanitation.* Clissold Publishing Co., Chicago, 1966.

Lubin, David: "Stringent Grounding Control: Last-Minute Checks Needed for Electrical Safety," *Mod. Hosp.,* **113**:86, (July) 1969.

———: "Coating Metal Surfaces Reduced Electrical Risk," *Mod. Hosp.,* **117**:68, (July) 1971.

Maki, D. G., et al.: "Prevention of Catheter-Associated Urinary Tract Infection," *J.A.M.A.,* **221**:1270, (Sept. 11) 1972.

Martin, L. W.: "Infections in Pediatric Surgery," *Pediatr. Clin. North Am.,* **16**:735, (Aug.) 1969.

McGee, Z. A., et al.: "Superinfection in Lymphoreticular Diseases," *Annu. Rev. Med.,* **22**:25, 1971.

McInnes, Betty: *Controlling the Spread of Infection, A Programmed Presentation.* C. V. Mosby Co., St. Louis, 1973.

Menzies, D. W., and McLaughlin, J. H.: "Cross-Infection Control: The Human Element. A Survey of 44 Saskatchewan Hospitals Reveals Three Approaches to This Crucial Problem," *Hosp. Adm. Can.,* **11**:32, (Nov.) 1969.

Merigan, T. C., and Stephens, D. A.: "Viral Infections in Man Associated with Acquired Immunological Deficiency States," *Fed. Proc.,* **30**:1858, 1971.

Michigan State Health Department: *A Guide to Chemical Disinfection and Sterilization for Hospitals and Related Care Facilities.* The Department, Lansing, 1963.

Morrison, Robert P., and Oviatt, Vinson R.: "Environmental Control Programs in Health Care Facilities," *Hosp. Prog.,* **52**:96, (Aug.) 1971.

National Academy of Sciences: *Electrical Hazards in Hospitals.* The Academy, Washington, D.C., 1970.

National Fire Protection Association: *The Safe Use of Electricity in Hospitals.* The Association, Boston, 1971 (Manual #76 BM).

———: *Hospital Emergency Preparedness.* The Association, Boston, 1970.

National Tuberculosis and Respiratory Disease Association: *Air Pollution Primer.* The Association, New York, 1969.

Neiburger, Morris, et al.: *Understanding Our Atmospheric Environment.* W. H. Freeman & Co., San Francisco, 1970.

O'Neill, J. A., Jr., et al.: "Suppurative Thrombophlebitis—A Lethal Complication of Intravenous Therapy," *J. Trauma,* **8**:256, (Mar.) 1968.

Perkins, J. J.: *Principles and Methods of Sterilization in Health Sciences,* 2nd ed. Charles C Thomas, Publisher, Springfield, Ill., 1969.

Read, Donald H., and Greene, Walter H.: *Health and Modern Man,* Macmillan Publishing Co., Inc., New York, 1973.

Reddish, G. F. (ed.): *Antiseptics, Disinfectants, Fungicides and Sterilization,* 2nd ed. Lea & Febiger, Philadelphia, 1957.

Remington, J. S.: "The Compromised Host," *Calif. Med.,* **117**:59, (Jan.) 1972.

Riley, H. D.: "Hospital Associated Infections," *Pediatr. Clin. North Am.,* **16**:701, (Aug.) 1969.

Rockwell, Susan: "Electricity: It Doesn't Need to Be a Problem," *R.N.,* **35**:35, (June) 1972.

Sachs, A., and Watson, J.: "Four Years' Experience at a Specialized Burns Centre," *Lancet,* **1**:718, (Apr. 5) 1969.

Santora, Delores: "Preventing Hospital-Acquired Urinary Infection," *Am. J. Nurs.,* **66**:5, (Apr.) 1966.

Sarg, Thomas J., and Hickman, Lanier H.: *Sanitary Landfill Facts.* US Government Printing Office, Washington, D.C., 1970 (PHS No. 1792).

Scheffler, G. L.: "The Nurse's Role in Hospital Safety," *Nurs. Outlook,* **10**:680, (Oct.) 1962.

Scott, Harold George: *Household and Stored-Food Insects of Public Health Importance and Their Control.* Health Services and Mental Health Administration, Center for Disease Control, Atlanta, Ga., 1972 (DHEW Pub. No. [HSM] 72–8122).

Seedor, Marie M.: *Introduction to Asepsis: A Programmed Unit in Fundamentals of Nursing,* 2nd rev. ed. Teachers College, Columbia University, New York, 1963.

Seton Hall College of Medicine and Dentistry: *The Becton, Dickinson Lectures on Sterilization.* The College, Jersey City, N.J., 1959.

Skaliy, Peter: "Ethylene Oxide as a Hospital Sterilizing Agent," *Hospitals,* **41**:100, (Nov. 16) 1967.

Stanley, Paul E.: "Electrical Shock Hazards, Part 2," *Hospitals,* **45**:73, (Jan. 16) 1971.

Starmer, Frank C., et al.: "Electrical Hazards and Cardiovascular Function," *N. Engl. J. Med.,* **284**:181, (Jan. 28) 1971.

———: "Hazards of Electric Shock in Cardiology," *Am. J. Cardiol.,* **14**:537, (Oct.) 1964.

Stead, Frank M.: "What Can Man Do Technologically to Restore His Environment," *Am. J. Public Health,* **58**:2050, (Nov.) 1968.

Still, Henry: *The Dirty Animal.* Hawthorn Books, Inc., New York, 1967.

Sykes, G.: *Disinfection and Sterilization,* 2nd ed. J. B. Lippincott Co., Philadelphia, 1965.

Travenol Laboratories, Inc.: *Hospital Sepsis, A*

New Medicom Learning System. The Laboratories, Deerfield, Ill., 1972.

Trought, Elizabeth A.: "Equipment Hazards," *Am. J. Nurs.,* **73:**858, (May) 1973.

US Public Health Service: *Dishwashing.* US Government Printing Office, Washington, D.C., 1971.

———: *The Hospital Laundry.* US Government Printing Office, Washington, D.C., 1971 (PHS Pub. No. 930-D-24).

———: *Noise in Hospitals.* US Government Printing Office, Washington, D.C., 1963 (PHS Pub. No. 930-D-11).

———: *Principles of Infection Control in Health Facilities; A Programmed Course for Housekeeping Personnel.* US Government Printing Office, Washington, D.C., 1971.

———: *Public Health Pesticides.* US Government Printing Office, Washington, D.C., 1970.

———: *Safe Practices for Health Services and Mental Health Administration Hospitals and Clinics.* US Government Printing Office, Washington, D.C., 1971.

Venhulst, Henry L., and Crotty, John J.: "Childhood Poisoning Accidents," *J.A.M.A.,* **203:**1049, (Mar. 18) 1968.

Ward, Barbara, and Dubos, René: *Only One Earth.* W. W. Norton Co., New York, 1972.

Washington State Department of Health: *A Guide to the Use of Disinfectants and Detergents.* The Department, Olympia, 1966.

Westaby, J. R., et al.: "Integrating Accident Prevention in Total Patient Care," *Nurs. Outlook,* **11:**600, (Aug.) 1963.

Westwood, J. C. N.: "Hospital Infection Control, A New Philosophy and a New Approach. Part I. The Need," *Can. Hosp.,* **47:**39, (July) 1970.

———: "Hospital Infection Control, A New Philosophy and a New Approach. Part II. The Background of Failure," *Can. Hosp.,* **47:**60, (Aug.) 1970.

———: "Hospital Infection Control, A New Philosophy and a New Approach. Part III. The Reasons for Failure," *Can. Hosp.,* **47:**62, (Sept.) 1970.

Whalen, R. E., et al.: "Electrical Hazards Associated with Cardiac Pacing," *Ann. NY Acad. Sci.,* **111:**922, (Mar.) 1964.

Whyte, William H.: *The Last Landscape.* Doubleday & Co., Garden City, N.Y., 1968.

Wilmore, D. W., and Dudrick, S. J.: "Safe Long-Term Hyperalimentation," *Arch. Surg.,* **98:**256, (Jan.) 1969.

Wolman, Abel: "Air Pollution: Time for Appraisal," *Science,* **159:**1437, (Mar. 29) 1968.

———: *Water, Wealth and Society.* Indiana University Press, Bloomington, 1969.

World Health Organization: *Vector Control in International Health.* The Organization, Geneva, 1972.

Young, Louise B. (ed.): *Population in Perspective.* Oxford University Press, New York, 1968.

Julina Rhymes
Virginia Henderson

CHAPTER 16

Communication, Human Relations, Learning, Health Goals and Guidance

1. INTRODUCTION

Communication and learning are basic, pervasive parts of our existence. John R. Pierce says:

Without external communication we might live, but we would be ignorant, lonely individuals. We would have neither the inspiration of accumulated skill and knowledge nor the support of a society. That society, which communication makes possible, supplies us with necessities we would otherwise have to obtain for ourselves. Moreover, communication with others conveys rewards far beyond the basic necessities of life.*

Colin Cherry [1] believes that communication is essentially a social affair—social in the sense of self-awareness, social responsibility, ethics, and laws; and Ray L. Birdwhistle sees communication as "that system through which humans establish a predictable continuity in life" † which, in turn, is the essence, the *sine qua non,* of sanity and humanity.

The skillful use of communication by nurses and other health workers is indispensable for recognizing and dealing with emotional aspects of illness, as well as for promoting a "helping" relationship with patients.[1a-1d] These relationships, in turn, can "affect the outcomes of all medical and nursing procedures and ultimately contribute to the physical well-being of the patient." ‡ Learning and its companion—teaching—are also indispensable and almost un-

avoidable parts of the nurse-patient or physician-patient relationship. Health workers must be constantly aware that while they are "communicating," either verbally or nonverbally, they also are "teaching," and patients are "learning." Since the triad of communication, interpersonal relationships, and learning-teaching are all but inseparable, they are discussed in a single chapter. Although it is impossible here to even summarize the enormous amount of information about communication, human relations, and learning that is available, it is hoped that the scope of these topics is indicated, and that the chapter references and suggested readings will enable the interested reader to pursue these subjects.

Study of Animal and Insect Communication. Man has complex faculties for learning, remembering, reasoning, and creating, as well as an enormous capacity for forming communication systems of diversity and purpose. Interest in the origin and evolution of these commonplace, but truly extraordinary, human abilities has led to the study of both communication and learning in animals at all levels of the evolutionary scale.

Observation of animal communication systems suggests that they are "languages" in principle like human languages, but simpler in vocabulary, in the number and complexity of combinations, and that they are not necessarily vocalized. For instance, army ants, which periodically move their nesting sites as a group and forage for food in groups, communicate the direction and route by continuously depositing a chemical trail as they run along the ground.[2] The "waggle" dance of honeybees, first decoded by Karl von Frisch, communicates to other members of the colony the direction and distance of a recently discovered pollen source. While the rules of this dance are

* Pierce, John R.: "Communication," *Sci. Am.,* **227**:31, (Sept.) 1972.

† Birdwhistle, Ray L.: *Kinesics and Context.* University of Pennsylvania Press, Philadelphia, 1970, p. 14.

‡ Bernstein, Lewis, et al.: *Interviewing: A Guide for Health Professionals.* Appleton-Century-Crofts, New York, 1974, p. x.

genetically fixed and always designate a certain direction and distance, the dance seems to have some characteristics associated with human language. That is, the dance is a symbolic representation of the messenger bee's past experience, rather than direct communication of immediate experience, and a new message is originated each time the location of the food source changes.[3] Howard R. Topoff, studying "essentially blind" army ants, notes their highly organized social behavior. He says ". . . their means of communication . . . is based mainly on chemical and tactual stimuli" although he thinks the surface has "hardly been scratched" in studying the regulatory mechanisms of this species.*

Studies of the male white-crowned sparrow show that maturation level, heredity, and learning play parts in the development of its distinctive song. If a young male is placed in isolation between 5 and 50 days of age with no opportunity to hear other sparrows, an abnormal song is developed; but, if during this period recordings of its species song and another species song are heard, the male learns the song of his own species and rejects the other.[4]

Research in communication and learning among the large water and land mammals has been most extensive with dolphins. Their ability to learn has been amply demonstrated in marine centers and by the US Navy in retrieval missions.[5] Although the sounds dolphins produce have been studied for at least 20 years, scientists are still divided in their opinions about the complexity of meaning in these sounds. Some think that dolphins may have their own language that conveys information about the past, present, and future, and that it also expresses something about the communicator, his plans, and problems. They tend to believe this "language" can be learned by humans and that communication between dolphins and man is possible. Others think that human language can be taught to dolphins if their enormous acoustic power and natural habitat are used to good advantage.[6,7]

Some scientists are studying and working with chimpanzees in hopes of determining the evolution of human language or, as in the case of Ann James Premack and David Premack,[8] to better define the fundamental nature of language, and to identify those aspects that are peculiarly human. Although chimpanzees in their natural environment have an extensive vocal call system, scientists generally believe they lack sufficient tongue mobility and a suf-

ficiently flexible vocal mechanism to produce the variety of sounds used by humans. Researchers who have been most successful in teaching words and simple concepts to chimpanzees have used the primate's natural ability to gesture (use sign language), and have taught them to communicate by manipulating objects, plastic symbols, or a computer.[9,10] It is hoped that the same techniques used with chimpanzees can be used with humans having a language difficulty caused by brain damage, with autistic children, and with mentally retarded children who cannot talk.[11]

Definitions of Communication. In spite of the fact that humans communicate with so-called lower forms of life and that these lower forms communicate within and between species, definitions of communication are nearly always confined to communication between humans. Virginia Satir says, "I see communication as a huge umbrella that covers and affects all that goes on between human beings" *; however, many people continue to think of communication only as the transfer of information, ideas, or opinions. This definition seems to focus on the content or "message," and implies the use of speech or language. Everybody is aware, however, that a smile, a frown, a clenched hand, or an arm around the shoulders in some situations "communicates" emotion just as surely, and probably more surely, than words. Doris C. Sutterley and Gloria F. Donnelly propose a definition of communication that includes nonverbal as well as verbal behavior. They say that communication "is the sum total of all behavioral events, both conscious and unconscious, that occur when people come together." † A more abstract definition of communication is suggested by George A. Miller. He says, "Communication occurs when events in one place or at one time are closely related to events in another place or at another time." ‡ In this sense, communication can be thought of as a process in addition to behavior and a message, and as occurring between persons (including the communication of genetic traits and various diseases), as well as between other living organisms, and even machines.

Miller's definition also indicates that communication spans both time and space. For

---

* Satir, Virginia: *Peoplemaking.* Science & Behavior Books, Inc., Palo Alto, Calif., 1972, p. 30.
  † Sutterley, Doris C., and Donnelly, Gloria F.: *Perspectives in Human Development. Nursing Throughout the Life Cycle.* J. B. Lippincott Co., Philadelphia, 1973, p. 106.
  ‡ Miller, George A.: "Psychology and Communication," in Miller, George A. (ed.): *Communication, Language, and Meaning.* Basic Books, Inc., New York, 1973, p. 3.

---

* Topoff, Howard R.: "The Social Behavior of Army Ants," *Sci. Am.,* **227:**71, (Nov.) 1972.

example, the work of great painters and great composers completed hundreds of years ago continues to communicate ideas and emotions today. Through current technology, such as radio and television, events occurring in almost any part of the world can be heard and seen almost immediately in any part of the world.

Because communication sounds technical rather than a term to describe a biologic function, some writers avoid it. Benjamin A. Kogan, for instance, in his remarkable text, *Health: Man in a Changing Environment*,[11a] has a chapter on "The Emotional Life," which is devoted to human relations and communication, but the word "communication" cannot be found in it or even in the index of this comprehensive text. It should, perhaps, be said here that the intent of the writers of this chapter is to stress the human need for expression in all aspects of life, regardless of the way in which communication is defined; also to stress the important role that communication plays in nursing. Current criticism of nurses by patients is not nearly so often aimed at technical incompetence as at a lack of understanding, a lack of compassion and consideration, and the inability to relate constructively to others.

Communication Theory and Cybernetics. Claude E. Shannon and Warren Weaver's [12] theory of communication, and Norbert Wiener's [13] work with servomechanisms and cybernetics have been major forces in the development of communication technology and the broadening of our definitions of communication. Communication theory describes a "system" (an interrelated combination of things or parts that make up a whole) that consists of an information source, a transmitter, a communication channel, a noise (interference) source, a receiver, and a message destination. Although the theory was originally related to technical communication engineering, such as teletypewriters and telephones, it has since been applied to many other scientific and social fields. Both Birdwhistle and Cherry believe that human communication is far more complex than this model, and is not confined to the audioacoustic channel. Birdwhistle [14] suggests that since all the sensory systems are channels for communication, they are used in overlapping ways and for various lengths of time in any one interaction. Cherry says:

. . . the human body is not to be thought of as a unit possessing a number of receptor organs, into which separate signals are received, like the wires entering a telephone exchange. A man is an organism, and the various stimuli bring into action physiological functions which set the whole organism into adjustment. Response to a stimulus of one organ may be influenced by the states of others and by the whole environment.*

Cybernetics is a word coined by Wiener to describe the concept of machines that can handle information, make decisions, and control the operation of themselves and other machines. A major proposition in the field of cybernetics is "feedback." That is, information is "fed back" to the behavior or message source about the way in which the receiver is reacting to the original behavior or message. Some common examples of feedback are thermostats for electric irons and central heating systems, the float and valve device that controls the height of water in a toilet tank, and the automatic pilot for airplanes. Examples in humans are the maintenance of a fairly even body temperature in spite of variations in environmental temperature, the opening or closing of the pupil of the eye depending on the amount of light present, learning to use a typewriter with the "touch system," or playing the piano without looking at the keyboard.

As Wiener worked with the mathematical theory of computers and automatic control devices, he noticed similarities between the way computers operate and the way the human nervous system handles information. The human system has input organs (eyes, ears, nose, etc.) and output organs (muscles, glands, etc.), short- and long-term memory, information processing, feedback, and over-all control. Generalization of the theory of communication and the concept of feedback has led to various "models" for communication that combine these ideas. A model used in this sense is a simplified abstraction about still another abstraction—the communication process. However, it helps a person visualize the elements of the complex activity of communication between two or more persons. Models, themselves, can be more or less complicated as indicated in Figure 16-1.

2. WAYS OF COMMUNICATING

Being as Communication. Every person, every living thing, every object, communicates in some way with the person who sees, hears, touches, or smells it. Even the shape and arrangement of spaces, best exemplified in Japanese garden designs and flower arrangements, communicates to those who see them.

Harold Saxton Burr [15] and others have hypothesized that any *biological system*, includ-

---

* Cherry, Colin: *On Human Communication*, 2nd ed. M.I.T. Press, Cambridge, Mass., 1966, p. 16.

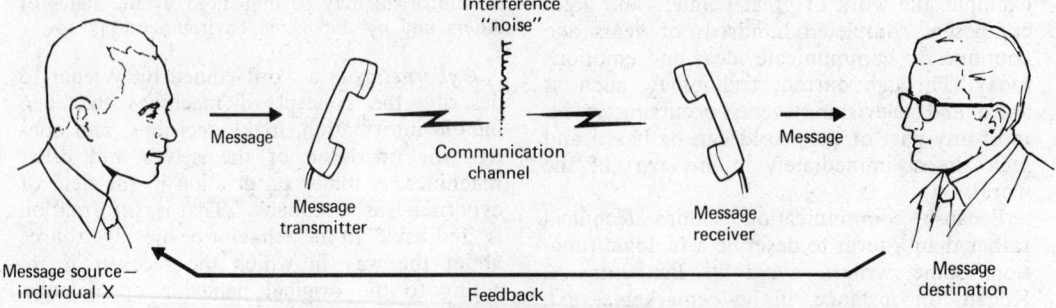

Figure 16-1. This basic model of communication is useful in that it shows the essentials of any communication system, and permits an analysis and, perhaps, modification of any one part. The model can be applied to human face-to-face communication and expanded to include all the perceptions and influences affecting individuals X and Y as message source and destination. It can also be applied to the selection of words, sounds, gestures, and uses of space as message transmitters, as well as external elements such as poor light, background sounds, or various kinds of interruptions as "noise" or interference. Feedback occurs between the individuals and/or between any of the other parts of the model.

ing man, is an *electrodynamic field* continually exchanging energy with surrounding electrodynamic fields. Dorothy Harrison, a nurse and anthropologist, is currently studying ways in which to use new electronic devices to determine such energy exchanges. Her purpose is to provide evaluative tools that will help nurses assess patients' needs, as well as the effectiveness of nursing care. (See Chapter 19.)

The extent to which thought is transmitted has been studied in every age. Researchers in *extrasensory perception* (ESP), which may be a manifestation of electrical energy exchange, believe that thoughts are communicated between persons who are emotionally close, and that dreams are often the vehicles for this communication.[16] While transmission of thought is a fascinating subject, it cannot be explored in a work of this kind. Few, however, would question the statement that to some degree the conscious and unconscious thoughts of nurses or other health workers are sensed by those with whom they are associated. The extent to which this occurs may determine their usefulness to others.

J. Samuel Bois [17] writes that while some persons seem to acquire the *"art of awareness"* without effort, others must cultivate that kind of sensitivity, and many have noted that *silence,* whether between persons or between a person and the environment may be as eloquent as speech.[18]

Although we ordinarily think of communication as occurring between living things or persons, there are several ways that communication occurs within an individual. *Remembering* is essentially communication with one's past.* It may be "pure" remembering in the sense that past events, behavior, people, or places are recalled and enjoyed again, or not enjoyed, as the case may be. Remembering also occurs with *thinking* when past information or experiences are applied to the solution of a problem or plans for the present and future.

Dreams during sleep have, since the time of Freud, had some respectability as symbolic representations of unexpressed feelings and wishes. *Daydreams,* however, have been considered at best a trivial use of time and at worst a mechanism by which individuals isolate themselves from society. For the most part, daydreaming has been ignored by researchers, but since the early 1960s Jerome L. Singer [19] has been studying daydreams to determine their functional roles in the emotional and creative processes, and he concludes that

The practiced daydreamer has . . . developed a resource that gives him some control over his future through elaborate planning, some ability to amuse himself during dull train-rides or routine work, and some sources of stimulation to change his mood through fanciful inner play.†

Meditation is another form of self-communication. The mystical East has a body of literature on thought, thought control, communication, and human relations of which the West tends to be ignorant. Many of the East-

---

* Marcel Proust, the French novelist, heightened awareness of this aspect of communication through his social study, *Remembrance of Things Past.*

† Singer, Jerome L.: "The Importance of Daydreaming," *Psychology Today,* **1:**19, (Apr.) 1968.

ern philosophies are currently of intense interest, as evidenced by the fact that the third edition of *The I Ching* (*or Book of Changes*) [20] has gone into its ninth printing. Researchers are now studying how meditation can be taught and used to enhance conscious control of vital body processes and increase the human potential. Few subjects are of more interest currently than Transcendental Meditation, commonly referred to as T.M.[21-24] (See also Chapter 18.) Meditation can result in therapeutic communication initiated by one's self, called biofeedback. (See biofeedback used in controlling blood pressure, Chapter 6.) The technology developed to study cerebral mechanisms has shown that a variety of physical and psychologic phenomena may be induced, inhibited, or modified by electrical stimulation of specific cerebral areas. José M. R. Delgado makes the following statement:

If we could modify mental mechanisms intelligently, the consequences would be far more important than the consequences of extending man's life span or limiting his birth rate, because to influence mental processes is to influence the source of all human activities.*

Use of the Senses in Communication. Although sight and hearing are often thought of as the senses primarily used for communication, all the senses—sight, hearing, taste, smell, and touch—are involved. Reports about the external world are constantly pouring into the central nervous system to be recognized, organized, and interpreted. At the same time this "external" communication is going on, muscle sense, the sense of balance, communicates "internally," evaluating where each movable part of the body is at any given time and keeping it oriented in space (usually as related to the ground). The more fully all these senses can be used for communication and learning, the better man and the environment can be known, understood, and enjoyed. (Although the senses are discussed as separate systems, this is not meant to imply that they operate alone during any kind of communication behavior.)

The *sense of smell* is thought to be man's most primitive sense [25] although it is frequently ignored except as it affects taste when someone has a cold, or as it differentiates pleasant from unpleasant odors. Since odors can be detected in extremely small concentrations, it is likely that olfaction enabled primitive man to distinguish friend from enemy, to locate food, and to help stragglers find their group. Per-

haps this need of primitive man accounts for the remarkably elaborate olfactory tract which now plays only a minor role in human life. Edward T. Hall says:

In the use of the olfactory apparatus Americans are culturally underdeveloped. The extensive use of deodorants and the suppression of odor in public places results in a land of olfactory blandness and sameness that would be difficult to duplicate anywhere else in the world. This blandness makes for undifferentiated spaces and deprives us of richness and variety in our life. It also obscures memories, because smell evokes much deeper memories than either vision or sound.*

Trygg Engen [26] and his colleagues found that infants as young as 32 to 68 hours of age reacted to irritating and unpleasant odors. They reported that with successive presentations of these substances the reactions of the 20 infants studied changed from a total, if mild, body response to a simple turning of the head away from the odor. This early "learning" may be a partial explanation of the memory arousal effect of odors.

In spite of Hall's contention about the blandness of the American olfactory environment, it can supply people with many olfactory sensations if awareness is cultivated. A few examples include the odor of bread near a bakery, of coffee brewing for breakfast, and the odor of disinfectants and cleaning compounds in hospitals, although these are faint in well-managed institutions. If such clues are ignored, people can be olfactorily deprived and can reduce the kind and number of messages they receive and, consequently, those to which they respond.

In animal populations, odors not only differentiate individuals but identify the emotional state of other organisms as well. Kathleen Smith and Jacob O. Sines [27] report that, in an experimental study, rats were adversely affected by odors from the sweat of schizophrenic patients, but not from that of non-schizophrenic patients. A few persons claim they can detect others' emotions by smell. Nurses who work with the emotionally disturbed often say a schizophrenic patient has a characteristic odor, and at least one psychotherapist is said to be able to distinguish the smell of anger in patients 6 or more feet away.[28] Among the Arabs, Hall reports, a relationship between odor and temperament is apparently recognized to such a point that marriage intermediaries may ask to smell the girl. They may even reject her "if she 'does not smell nice,' not so much on esthetic

---

* Delgado, José M. R.: *Physical Control of the Mind.* Harper & Row, New York, 1969, p. 259.

* Hall, Edward T.: *The Hidden Dimension.* Doubleday & Co., Garden City, N.Y., 1966, p. 43.

grounds, but possibly because of a residual smell of anger or discontent." *

The ability to detect odors in any one environment seems to decrease quickly through the process of adaptation. While this adaptation is a generally recognized fact of human life, the explanation for it lies in future research. It is now known, however, from electrophysiologic studies of rabbit nasal mucosa that neural olfactory adaptation is not as rapid as experience seems to indicate. Nurses should be aware that many odors in the hospital environment to which they have adapted and of which they are unconscious are very noticeable to patients and visitors. Since many hospital odors are unpleasant, every effort should be made to eliminate them by keeping the environment clean and well ventilated.

The *sense of taste* is very limited in the kind and amount of communication it supplies. Frank A. Geldard says:

We are constantly ascribing to taste those sensations that really belong to smell. . . . The sense of taste, unassisted, is able to detect the sourness of acid, the sweetness of sugar, the bitterness of quinine, and the salt taste of sodium chloride. It fails utterly to encompass the full flavor of meats, fruits, butter, and coffee. . . . Were there no sense of smell there would be no gourmets, only consumers of nutriments.†

The enjoyment of food, whether due to taste or smell, plays a large part in most cultures, and has many emotional meanings. To be only a "consumer of nutriments" because there is no sense of taste (hypogeusia), or the sense of taste is badly distorted (dysgeusia) is, therefore, depressing. In fact, some persons with these problems are said to have contemplated suicide.[29] The anorexia and refusal of food by sick persons because of hypogeusia or dysgeusia are of great concern to nurses since poor nutrition retards recovery. Until recently the cause of this distressing condition was thought to be temporary or psychosomatic. Now researchers report that in patients with thermal burns, viral hepatitis, various types of malabsorption pathology, growth retardation, and idiopathic hypogeusia, the blood level of some trace metals, particularly zinc, is very low. The oral administration of zinc ion corrects the lack of taste and the sense of smell; it improves appetite, and hastens recovery.[30-33]

The sense of taste is not only interwoven with the sense of smell, but with cutaneous sensations of astringency, texture, and temperature. In infants and young children, all these sensory receptors are liberally scattered over the tongue, palate, pharynx, tonsils, and epiglottis. Children's responses to foods are, therefore, more intense than are adult responses. This may account for the young child's tendency to eat the peas on the plate before starting the hamburger, or to separate the various foods in a casserole and eat each separately rather than as a mixture.

A phenomenon of the taste sense that is so far unexplained is the detection by "taste" of some substances given intravenously in the arm. One of these, sodium dehydrocholate (Decholin Sodium) causes a bitter taste just a few seconds after it has been given, and patients should be forewarned of this body response.

Physiologically, the *sense of touch* (tactile sense) includes sensations of touch, temperature, pressure, and vibration. The interpretation of much of the information received through this sense requires the cooperation of muscle proprioceptors and sight. For instance, when the eyes are closed a fingertip placed on the rim of a cup, and then on the edge of a ruler, cannot differentiate the two. If, however, the finger is moved around the rim or along the ruler edge, the difference is apparent. Both of these movements require the use of wrist and arm muscles which give more identifying information, but sight has to be added to be able to say, "this is a cup and this, a ruler."

Because the skin, with its many nerve endings, is a major source of tactile information, researchers have given considerable time and thought to the possibility of using the skin with an artificial receptor (eye or ear) to convey visual or auditory signals to the brain. Carter C. Collins and Paul Bach-y-Rita[34] report there is experimental evidence to show that with electrical stimulation of the abdominal skin, visual images can be transmitted to sight areas of the brain. At this time the ability to transmit small details of the object (the image resolution) depends on the equipment available, and not on the capacity of the skin to receive optical information, or the capacity of the central nervous system to process it. Prototype equipment has been successfully used to help the blind "see" through the skin. There has also been some research on using the skin to convey auditory signals. With practice, patients have "heard" various test signals, including sentences. Much more research is needed, however, before equipment that transmits ordinary speech through the skin is practical.[35]

While the direct transmission of audible speech by way of the skin is not possible at this time, spoken language can be understood

---

* Hall, Edward T.: *op. cit.,* p. 47.

† Geldard, Frank A.: *The Human Senses,* 2nd ed. John Wiley & Sons, New York, 1972, p. 438.

by the deaf-blind through vibratory tactile stimuli. This method (Tadoma) requires that the "listening" person place his or her hands on the speaker's face with the thumbs on the lips, the index fingers on the sides of the nose, little fingers on the throat, and the other fingers on the cheeks. Speech is communicated through the kinesthetic movements of finger joints and muscles as well as the stimulation of the skin surface. Helen Keller is perhaps the best-known person who used this method for communication.

Touch and the Braille code (see Fig. 16-2) have been used for over 100 years to communicate written language. Recently a device called the Optacon has been developed that optically scans ordinary reading material and sends tactile images of alphabetic shapes to the fingertips. Alphabetic codes, other than Braille, have been developed also in recent years, but seem to be no easier or faster to use than Braille. (The average speed of Braille reading is 35 words per minute while the average speed of sighted reading is 300 words per minute.) [36]

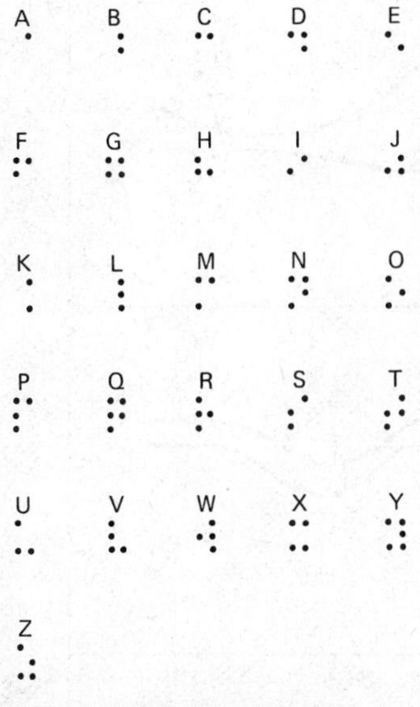

Figure 16-2. An alphabet of raised dots developed by a Frenchman, Louis Braille, in the first half of the nineteenth century, enables the blind to read. In the Braille system, various combinations of from one to six dots are used to represent letters and short words. By running his fingers over the raised points, an experienced blind person can read at the rate of 50 words per minute. Braille, who was blinded in an accident at age three, developed the reading system when he was teaching at the Institution for the Young Blind in Paris. (From *Light and Vision*. Life Science Library. Time, Inc., New York, 1966, p. 14.)

Some authorities believe that persons who can sense colors through their fingertips are demonstrating the human potential for detecting differences in reflected infrared (heat) and other wave lengths of the electromagnetic spectrum, perhaps even visible light wave lengths.[37-39] This may be somewhat analogous to the perception of light through nonretinal body structures that has been studied in fish, amphibians, reptiles, and some birds in order to understand circadian rhythms and reproductive cycles. Michael Menaker writes that while it may be difficult to accept the fact that visible light does penetrate body structures thought of as opaque, holding a turned-on flashlight cupped in the hand in a dark room can dispel this doubt. "In effect the human hand, although it is almost an inch thick, is a moderately transparent red filter." *

Touch accompanied by movement is the only sense that both receives and sends messages. Manfred Clynes, a musician, engineer, and physiologist, describes in the following incident the use of touch to send a message:

In 1967 I took part, as pianist, in Pablo Casals' master classes in San Juan, Porto Rico. One day when Casals was teaching Haydn's *Cello Concerto*, he asked a participant, a young master in his own right, to play the theme from the third movement. His playing was expert, sure and graceful. But for Casals something was missing.

The master stopped the performance. "No, no!" he said, waving his hands. "That must be graceful!"

He took up his own cello and played the same passage. And it was graceful, a hundred times more graceful than we had just heard. Yes—it seemed as though we had never heard grace before. We had experienced one of the least understood forms of human communication—a powerful and clear transmittal of feeling without words, a feeling that penetrated our defenses and transformed our states of mind.

Casals played the same notes, and at similar speed. But the muscles of his hands and arms acted precisely together with his cello according to his very clear idea of grace.†

Clynes [40] later conducted experiments to show that a single finger can express various fantasized emotions. He found that each emotion had a different pattern of minute muscle movements that occurred again and again in the same person, that different individuals in the same culture, as well as in different cultures, showed a highly similar finger tracing

* Menaker, Michael: "Nonvisual Light Perception," *Sci. Am.,* **226:**22, (Mar.) 1972.
† Clynes, Manfred: "Sentic Cycles: The Seven Passions at Your Fingertips," *Psychology Today,* **5:**59, (May) 1972.

for the same emotion. He found, furthermore, that if pattern tracings differed very much between two persons, it was because they were fantasizing the designated emotion in different ways. Anger, for instance, might have been fantasized as an irritable, ready-to-strike out kind in one person, while the other was fantasizing a slow, burning type. Figure 16-3 shows finger tracings of three different persons when fantasizing "love" and "anger." If the touch of one finger transmits a message of emotion, it is reasonable to suppose that the message is multiplied many times when the whole hand, or hand and arm, are used to express a feeling for which words are inadequate.

That touch can express thoughts and emotions seems self-evident. The blind and those with sight in the dark can often tell immediately who is touching them. The touch of a beloved person evokes a pleasurable response but the touch of a hated individual evokes an unpleasant sensation. To shrink from this touch is automatic. Reactions are especially strong if touching suggests sexual involvement. Persons who are especially fearful of this may avoid all forms of body contact, even the perfunctory forms, such as handshaking.

All interpersonal communication can be described as a reciprocal process in which there is an ebb and flow of action and reaction. The use of touch with infants is one example. The infant's "rooting" behavior and its weight in her arms gives the mother tactile signals that she responds to with caresses, patting, rocking, and voice sounds, and these are messages for the infant.

Supplying infants with many sensory experiences is known to play an important part in their development. Early tactile stimulation has a particularly important role because its sensory area in the brain is better developed at birth than is either the auditory or visual area.[41] In the first few months of life, therefore, it is likely that tactile stimuli are the major source of sensory input. John Bowlby[42] believes that a newborn's anticipatory head

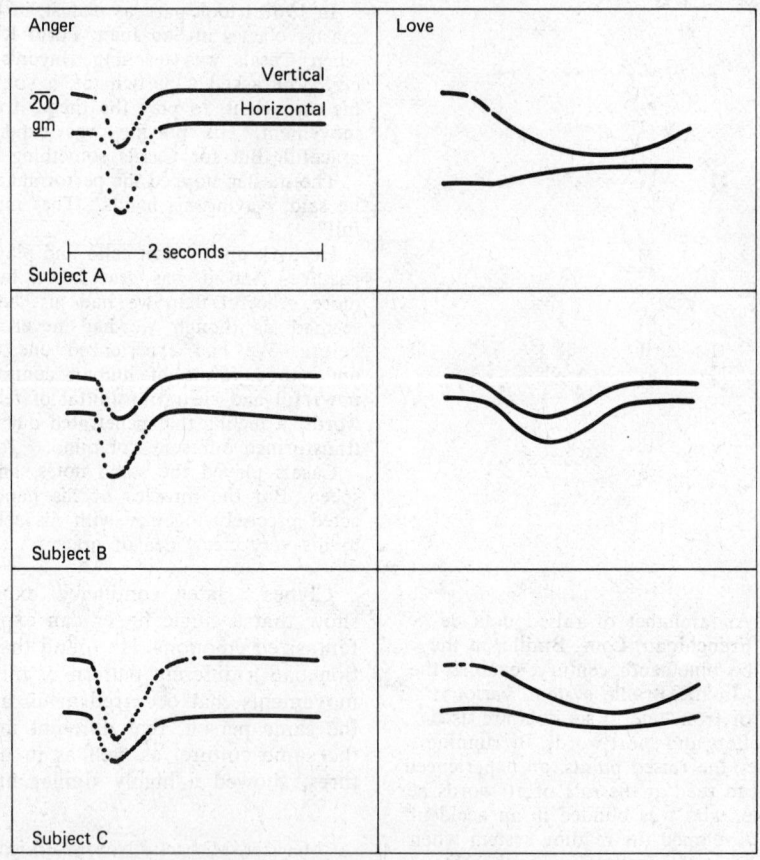

Figure 16-3. Finger tracings of three persons fantasizing anger and love. (From Clynes, Manfred: "Sentic Cycles: The Seven Passions at Your Fingertips," *Psychology Today,* 5:58, [May] 1972.)

and mouth movements toward the mother's breast at the beginning of a feeding (and on other occasions) are due to the tactile stimulation he or she receives when placed in the nursing position. Since the effect of this behavior is to turn the baby toward the mother, Bowlby says it is one important aspect of "attachment" behavior that, in turn, is vital for healthy personality development. Tactile contact with a mother, or a mother substitute, is now thought so important that holding and caressing is a part of the program of care for all infants and young children, sick or well, premature or full-term.

The newborn infant is believed by some physicians, psychologists, and others to be traumatized by birth, and regression as "return to the womb" has been discussed in psychiatric circles throughout this century. The unborn infant lies in a warm, dark, and cushioned environment and is catapulted by birth into a cool, often noisy, brightly lighted, and sometimes harsh world. It is recommended by Frederick Leboyer [42a] that the separation of the infant from the prenatal environment be made as gradually as possible. Leboyer, in his book *Birth Without Violence,* shows how he puts the infant on the mother's abdomen as soon as it is born; how he covers the body of the infant with the hands, stroking it gently, soothingly, and encouraging the mother to keep the baby close to her.* (See Fig. 16-4.) Noise is kept at a minimum in the delivery room and the newborn is put into a warm bath for the same purpose of imitating intrauterine conditions. Stroking continues to be throughout life a soothing kind of communication. Leboyer considers traditional practices in the delivery of babies seriously traumatic as, for example, slapping the baby to make it breathe. He leaves the baby attached to the mother through the umbilical cord until respiration is established. During this period the baby lies on the mother's abdomen partially covered by the hands of the doctor or midwife. Leboyer believes that this soothing treatment of the newborn is probably the most important step in developing healthy human relations.

The dependence on body contact for healthy development is seen in animals as well as humans. The degree of dependence on touch varies with the animal species, while the degree of acceptable human touching varies with each culture. Even those cultures that are the least demonstrative, however, have customs such as shaking hands with strangers. Embracing and kissing in public are more and more common in the West, and a couple holds hands, now, as freely as they walked arm in arm in the Victorian era. Sexual intercourse is, of course, recognized as the most intimate form of body contact and, in its most satisfying form, is likely to be the profoundest emotional experience that can be shared by two persons.

Although it is hard to generalize, most people believe that throughout the life span it is normal for a human being to want, or take comfort in, touching and being touched by others. By means of group therapy sessions, "sensitivity training," and sex education programs, people of all ages are learning to communicate or express their thoughts and feelings with touch and other forms of nonverbal communication. Healing by the "laying on of hands" is discussed later in this chapter under the topic Therapeutic Communication, Relationships, and Environments.

For most animals the *sense of sight* is a means of survival only, but for man it is also a means of enriching life, a channel for communicating information and ideas through written words, and a means of understanding a concept so abstract that it requires a concrete visual model for its comprehension. Man's eyes are very precise and adaptable, and with the organizing and interpreting parts (association centers) of the brain, are capable of estimating distance, size, and direction of movement, of distinguishing colors, of adapting to bright or dim light, of instantly shifting focus, and of moving with great rapidity.

The anatomic and physiologic eye is usually likened to a camera; however, vision consists of more than the simple receiving and recording of an image. It requires maturation of the visual sensory area and association centers of the brain, as well as multiple, varied, and early visual experiences.[43] Experiments conducted with infant monkeys kept in darkness from 1 to 11 weeks resulted in temporarily "blind" animals. The monkeys in darkness the longest time, when brought into the light, bumped into things, fell off tables, and were unable to locate objects by sight. It sometimes took weeks for them to "learn to see." Monkeys kept a short time (1 to 2 weeks) in darkness showed good spatial orientation in a few hours or days after being brought into the light.[44] While the number of reports about congenitally blind persons who were able to see following surgery in their adult years is very limited, it appears that these visually deprived persons had to spend

* Animal husbandmen and veterinarians habitually put a newborn animal beside the mother's nipples immediately after birth. Not only is it desirable for the young animal's survival to be close to the mother, but also the effect of nursing seems to reduce postpartal bleeding.

Figure 16-4. *A.* Communication between mother and infant immediately after birth. Frederick Leboyer says, "She (the mother) is ready to hold and touch her baby . . . a woman will simply place her hands on its body . . . hands of peace. Through such hands flow the waves of love which will assuage her baby's anguish." *B.* The face of a baby who is not yet 24 hours old who was "born without violence." Frederick Leboyer says, "The newborn baby is a mirror reflecting our image. It is for us to make its entrance into the world a joy." (From Leboyer, Frederick: *Birth Without Violence*. Alfred A. Knopf, New York, 1975, pp. 66, 113.) *C.* The touching of mother and child during the early development period continues to be an important kind of communication. (From Leboyer, Frederick: *Loving Hands. The Traditional Indian Art of Baby Massage.* Alfred A. Knopf, New York, 1976, p. 30.)

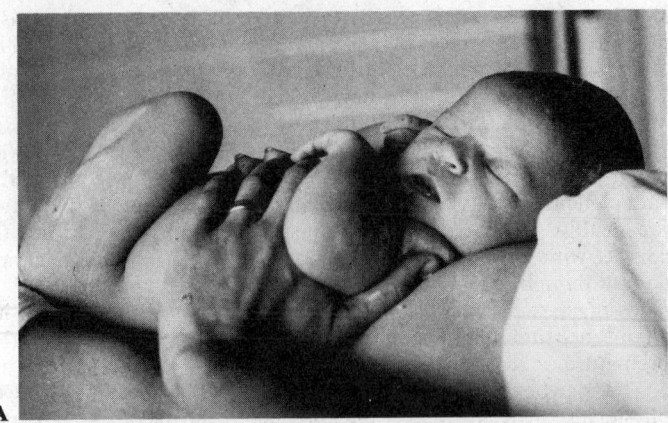

A

B

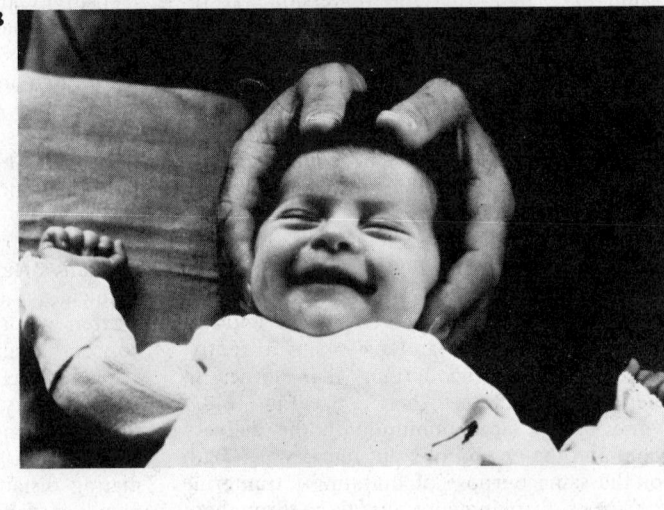

C

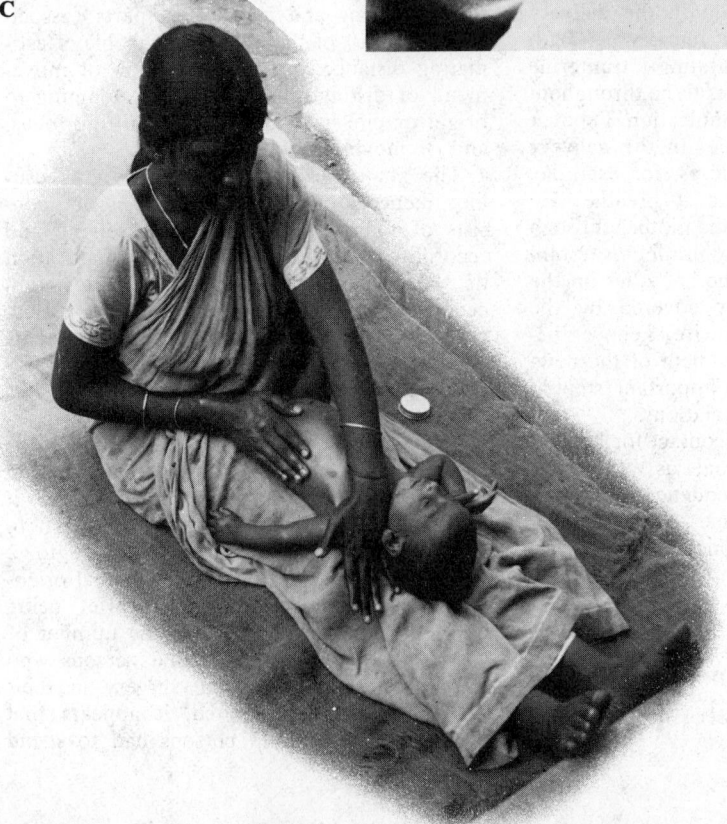

many months learning to use sight to find their way about.

Visual perception has been studied in relation to the following: the ability to perceive form; to judge depth, distance, and movement; to maintain constancy for shape, size and color of an object (no matter the angle it is viewed from); to recognize persons; to eliminate visual cues irrelevant to the moment; to "fill in" visual gaps; and to react to limited visual information. No two people draw the same conclusions from the same images produced on the retina (see Fig. 16-5). Whatever conclusions are drawn are based on past experiences and processes of identification and classification that depend on memory, learning, attention, reasoning, and language.[45] Differing eyewitness testimony about an accident or crime is a common example of the various conclusions drawn from the same visual stimuli. In one study involving a staged purse-snatching incident, only 7 of 52 "witnesses" selected the "culprit" from two lineups of five men each.[46]

Pictures, or a pattern of lines and shaded areas on a flat surface, have been drawn since the caveman era, and it might be supposed that pictorial representations constitute a universal language. Studies have shown, however, that people of various cultures persistently interpret pictorial information in different ways. Although research on these differences is in its early stages, Jan B. Deregowski[47] reports that William Hudson has established that both children and adults from various African tribes have difficulty perceiving depth in pictures. When asked to make a choice between a picture of an elephant seen from above, and a picture of an elephant seen from above but with the legs split to the sides, the African children consistently chose the split-type drawing as more representative of an elephant (see Fig. 16-6).

Communication through language is compared with visual images by E. H. Gombrich.[48] He says the functions of language as proposed by Karl Buhler are expressive, arousing, and descriptive. The expressive function gives information about the speaker's state of mind; the arousal function's purpose is to create a feeling or emotion; and the descriptive function informs of past, present, or future affairs, those that are near at hand, observable and actual, or those that are distant or conditional.

Visual imagery "is supreme" in its capacity to create moods and arouse emotions. While some persons may disclaim interest in, or disclaim being affected by, drawings, pictures, and three-dimensional art forms, they do respond to them. A room hung with El Grecos

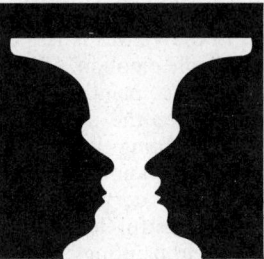

Figure 16-5. The drawing above is among many designed by Gestalt psychologists to demonstrate that the individual organizes visual sensations into perceptions. The simple black and white pattern can be organized in two ways, and the viewer does both, alternately perceiving a white goblet against a black ground or two silhouettes against a white ground.

creates a very different mood from one hung with Renoirs. Color alone has been shown to affect various emotions and physiologic drives, such as appetite. It is no accident, therefore, that many restaurants in Western cultures use shades of red in their furnishings. Florence Nightingale,[49] in a chapter on variety, notes that "little as we know about the way in which the effect is produced" form, color, and light affect people physically. She marvels that nurses, "educated people," will leave a bedridden patient to stare at a dead wall without a "change of object to vary his thought." While Florence Nightingale emphasizes variety here she also is emphasizing the visual esthetics of the environment.

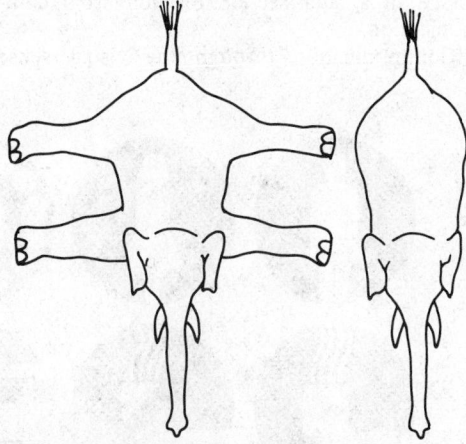

Figure 16-6. Split-elephant drawing (*left*) was generally preferred by African children and adults to the top-view perspective drawing (*right*). (From Deregowski, Jan B.: "Pictorial Perception and Culture," *Scientific American,* **227**:82, [Nov.] 1972.)

The ability of artists to communicate their state of mind to the viewer is less certain than their ability to kindle emotion. Gombrich [50] discusses Van Gogh's painting "Bedroom at Arles" and describes the sense of calm and tranquility this painting had for the artist. Persons who do not know the artist's meaning, however, usually do not perceive the pictured room as a restful haven. Some artists refuse to title their paintings or sculpture because they believe viewers should be allowed to find their own meanings in particular works of art. A few museums of art have special galleries for children where art objects can be touched, handled, and manipulated. Art can then be appreciated by way of the many sensory messages it contains, and the viewer, especially of sculpture, may come closer to understanding the artist's message.

There are many kinds of visual images that serve a descriptive function of communication —maps, graphs, charts, and highway signs, to name a few. Each of these conveys a limited amount of information that is often increased with a "key" or some verbal explanation. One of the most successful uses of informative signs was at the 1968 Olympic Games in Mexico. Because the meaning in each sign was restricted and there was enough similar past experience among the participants to make the context clear, the signs overcame some of the problems of communicating in many different languages (see Fig. 16-7).

Dance and pantomime theatricals are other forms of visual communication that add to men's enrichment and an understanding of their world. Both of these art forms are discussed in a later section on nonverbal communication.

Communication through the visual sense and the printed word has been a revolutionizing force throughout the world. As soon as information, ideas, and opinions could be transmitted without the physical presence of the message sender, knowledge spread widely and rapidly. Persons in this day and age who do not read with ease are at a distinct disadvantage.

How people learn to read, that is, to "receive" understandable messages from patterned marks on a page, is still debated. Studies show that a paragraph in which the words are printed backwards is almost as easy to read, once the pattern of the symbols is found, as is a normally printed paragraph (see Fig. 16-8). Paul A. Kohlers [51] believes the assumption is incorrect that a person's eyes move along a line of print, seeing each letter, and mentally forming each word. As a result of his experimental work he concluded that readers use an internal process of "generating" messages based on clues in the printed text rather than from seeing each word specifically. For instance, bilingual (French and English) readers would often substitute French words for English when reading aloud, but would not stop to correct themselves because the meaning of the sentence remained clear to them with either word.

For some persons, reading a message is more effective than hearing it. For those who are mute or deaf, reading and writing are important and necessary channels of communication. There are famous love affairs in which an exchange of letters between the lovers was a relatively satisfying substitute for other forms of lovemaking and communication. Eric Hoffer, the longshoreman-philosopher who was partially blind until the age of 15, exemplifies the effectiveness of wide reading as a sub-

Figure 16-7. Signs for the 1968 Olympic Games in Mexico are self-explanatory because the number of possible meanings is restricted. The use of pictorial images in international events overcomes the problem of communicating to people who speak diverse languages. (From Gombrich, E. H.: "The Visual Image," *Scientific American* **227**:82, [Sept.] 1972.)

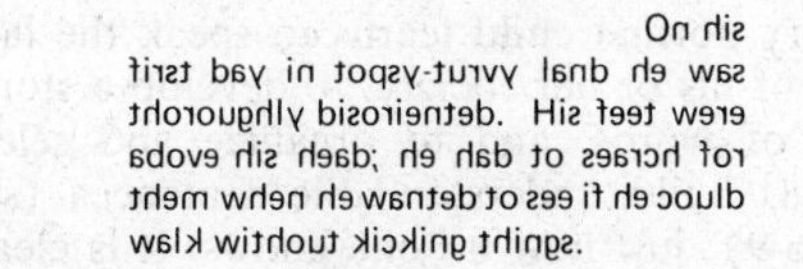

On sih
saw eh dnal yvrut-yspot ni yad tsrit
erew teet siH .detneirosid ylhguoroht
rot hcraes ot dab eh ;daeh sih evoba
dluoc eh ti ees ot detnaw eh nehw melht
stnirq quickly kriock truohtiw klaw

Figure 16-8. Reading this "backward" paragraph is probably easy because meaning rather than letters or words is important in reading. (From Kolers, Paul A.: "Experiments in Reading," *Scientific American* **227**:84, [July] 1972.)

stitute for a more formal education. Many long illnesses and prison terms have been converted into constructive experiences by reading, and many a "bookworm" has reveled in the opportunity both afforded for reading.

The value of the *sense of hearing* is not often appreciated until the plight of an infant born deaf is considered. The sounds of life, early steps to development, are beyond his or her reach. (See Chapter 46 for ways to identify and teach congenitally deaf children.) Many authorities believe that it is hearing, and its offspring speech, that has given man the extraordinary capacity to communicate and "master" the world. Working together, the anatomic and neurologic structures of the ear can discriminate among some 400,000 sounds. A person with normal hearing can locate the source of a sound by hearing alone. Blind persons can often use hearing to find their way by listening to the echoes that bounce off buildings or other large objects.

Throughout the waking hours man's ears receive an almost uninterrupted stream of messages that must be screened, sorted, filed, or acted on. Even during sleep the ears function with great efficiency. In combination with the limbic system of the brain, sound signals can be selected and interpreted so that an alarm clock buzz wakes the sleeper but noisy traffic throughout the night does not.

Depending on the brain's interpretation, sounds may be judged as "noise," harsh and dissonant, or "music," harmonious and pleasing. They may produce a quickening heartbeat, laughter, or tears; they may trigger memory, or bring forth speech or movement. Music,* like paintings, communicates most effectively in arousing emotion or mood. Clara Schuman wrote to Johannes Brahms after getting and playing one of his compositions, "Oh, Johannes, do you really feel this way?"

Many persons, particularly the younger generation, are so accustomed to having the radio

or television turned on that they say they cannot concentrate in a quiet environment. Others say they can't go to sleep in one. Institutional regulations that prohibit music and noise at certain hours may pose a real problem for such persons. Until they can form other patterns of living, it may be important to provide them with earphones for radios or television sets.

Not all sounds heard by the human ear are man-made. For example, bird song is not only expressive to birds, but to humans. We speak of something being as cheerful as the sparrow's chirp, or as mournful as the song of the dove. While few may be aware of nature's separate sounds or meanings, animals, birds, and insects provide the background music for life outdoors.

Speech is, of course, the most important of sounds for communication, learning, and thought. Because it is so vital to the human condition it is discussed separately.

Speech and Language. Of all the ways that humans use to send messages to others, language is the most extraordinary, flexible, and productive. It is used to talk about what has happened, what is happening, or what can or will happen. William G. Moulton makes the following statement about language:

We can use it to convey wishes and commands, to tell truths and to tell lies, to influence our hearers and to vent our emotions, and to formulate ideas which could probably never arise if we had no language in which to embody them.*

Every *language* consists of many *styles,* that is, different ways of speaking (or writing) that are used more appropriately in one situation than in another. For instance, most persons have one style in speaking with close friends, and vary the style if it is a woman-to-woman, woman-to-man, man-to-woman, or a man-to-man conversation. Another style is used when speaking with a person older or younger; another, if being interviewed by a prospective employer. Some health workers have different styles when speaking with patients, and still other styles if speaking with patients' families or with physicians.† Subtle differences in styles of address are apparently learned at a very

---

* While making and writing music are important ways for sending messages, the emphasis in this discussion is on hearing or receiving a message from music.

* Moulton, William G.: "The Nature of Language," *Daedalus,* **120**:17, (Summer) 1973.

† The extent to which a person treats all human beings with equal courtesy, simplicity, and understanding is believed by some to be a measure of integrity. The different "styles" of language used in hospitals led one patient to say to the second author of this chapter, "The doctors and nurses seem to be having very interesting conversations but as for me I feel as if I'm in a secret society and don't know the passwords." Making patients feel excluded is, of course, most undesirable.

early age, and Susan H. Houston believes that the current notion that disadvantaged children (especially black children) speak a "quasi-foreign" English is based on their use of a particular language style in school settings, with authority figures, or in any formal, constrained circumstances. She found that in contrast to the nonfluency and strange language used by these children in restrictive situations, when playing, they "engaged in constant language games, verbal contests, and narrative improvisations far removed from linguistic disability." * In addition, during these play times they used all the grammatic patterns characteristic of their age group.

* Houston, Susan H.: "A Reexamination of Some Assumptions About the Language of the Disadvantaged Child," in Chess, Stella, and Thomas, Alexander (eds.): *Annual Progress in Child Psychiatry and Child Development, 1971.* Brunner/Mazel Publishers, New York, 1971, p. 240.

Every normal child learns to speak the language of his or her society, to develop a storehouse of words, and to organize and select them to build understandable sentences (see Fig. 16-9); just how no one knows. It is clear, however, that language is connected with human experience—and with the audible sound of speech. Linguists, psychologists, neurobiologists, and other scientists continue to examine the languages of the world to hunt for clues that will explain what is unknown about speech.

The study of patterns of *language development* in children is not new, but the conclusions drawn from more recent observations and experiments have thrown a new light on the question. At one time it was assumed that the sounds used in adult speech were the same as those used by the babbling infant. It is now known that many of these infant sounds are acoustically different from adult sounds, some

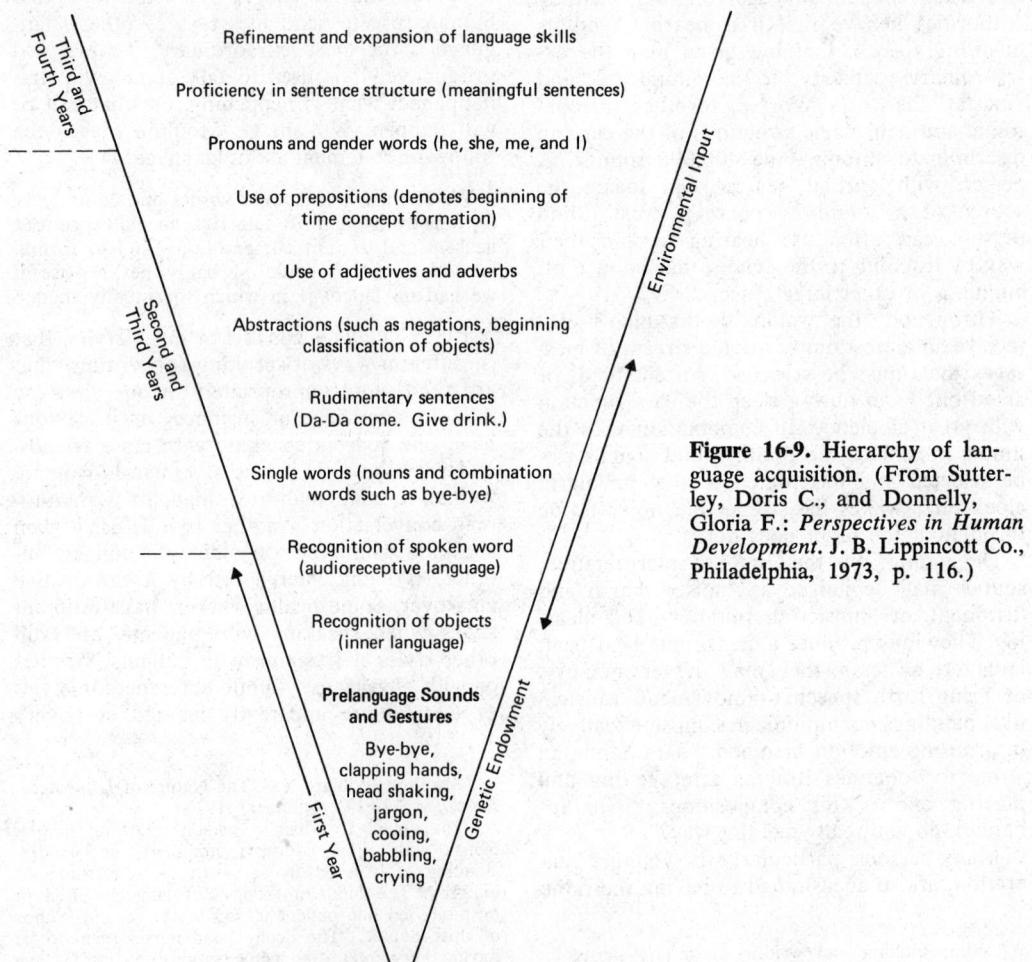

Figure 16-9. Hierarchy of language acquisition. (From Sutterley, Doris C., and Donnelly, Gloria F.: *Perspectives in Human Development.* J. B. Lippincott Co., Philadelphia, 1973, p. 116.)

of which are rarely heard in babbling, and that an adult is unable to imitate most babbling sounds.[52]

Eric H. Lenneberg,[53] a psychologist and neurobiologist, contends that language has an innate biologic basis. He points out that language is present in every culture, that children everywhere start talking at approximately the same age, and that various stages of speech development occur in a fixed sequence and at a fairly constant age. This is not to say that the rate of language development is absolutely uniform, because it often varies as the child's rate of motor development varies.

From observing hearing infants of deaf parents, Lenneberg found that early speech development differed very little from that of hearing infants with hearing parents. He also found in follow-up studies that children of deaf parents eventually learned to communicate in two languages. One was used with their parents and the other with the rest of the community.

Noam Chomsky[54] and other linguists believe that the language of young children is not just a poor copy of the adult's, but is, in fact, a different language. While the child's vocabulary is for the most part borrowed from adults, the grammar follows its own rules and is the same in all the cultures and localities studied up to this time. It would seem that families with very young children are, in a sense, bilingual—both children and adults understand one another, but produce speech with totally different grammars.[55-58] The ability to correctly use grammar in a sentence and to express the same idea in various ways—linguistic competence—is usually apparent in the conversation of 3½- to 4-year-old children; by 10 to 11 years, their competence is that of an adult.[59] While social aspects of speech—communication competence—is acquired at 10 or 11 years, it usually improves into adolescence and beyond.

Benjamin Lee Whorf, a chemical engineer and linguist, believes that all higher levels of *thinking* are *dependent on language,* and that distinct styles of thinking arise from the characteristics of the language in which thought is carried.* [60] While some investigators [61,62] disagree with this point of view, Janellen Huttenlocher says:

Certain philosophers claim that men over the ages have concerned themselves with many vacuous questions because their natural language was so poorly formulated that it tricked them into generating pseudoproblems. The argument suggests that natural language is so centrally implicated in the thought process that people may end up thinking about nothing at all if their language permits it.

From a different vantage point, cultural anthropologists have also suggested that language exerts a molding and constraining influence on thought. They have proposed that the variations in the way different languages represent people's experience is closely tied to the variations in social customs and world view in different societies.*

While the origins of spoken language are lost in prehistoric uncertainty, the earliest *written communication* is thought to be Sumerian.[63] Sumerian cuneiform writing dates back 5000 years, but is no longer used by any peoples of the modern world. Chinese writing, on the other hand, dates back 3500 years, and while there have been many stylistic changes, about half the characters found on ancient Chinese artifacts can be deciphered today.[64] Communication through writing has advantages over speech. One is that the written or printed page can be referred to again and again for its message, while the spoken word, once uttered (unless tape recorded), is gone. And, who has not been aware of some dissatisfaction when the written thoughts and feelings of a character, well described in a novel, are not as fully portrayed in a spoken radio, movie, or television drama?

The written word is a coded symbol of yet another symbolic form of human experience—the spoken word. Both of these, in turn, have other symbolic languages devised for specific communication purposes. Shorthand, mathematical equations, computer languages, Braille, and hand signs are some examples of symbolic languages that facilitate communication in the business world, in the scientific world, and in the worlds of the blind and the deaf. Cherry says, "Of all living creatures he [man] has the most complex and adaptable systems of language; he is the most widely observant of his physical environment, and the most responsive in his adjustment to it." †

Nonlanguage Communication. Perhaps facetiously, Albert Mehrabian[65] says that in human interactions 7 per cent of the impact of any one statement is due to the verbal content, 38 per cent to voice intonations, and 55 per cent to facial expression. There is no proof of such ratios, but most persons are aware that

---

* In a recent television program on teaching a chimpanzee to use the sign language, the subject elected to use two signs, one for "water" and one for "bird" instead of the sign for "duck." This certainly suggests a fairly high level of thinking. [V. H.]

* Huttenlocher, Janellen: "Language and Thought," in Miller, George A. (ed.): *Communication, Language, and Meaning.* Basic Books, Inc., New York, 1973, p. 176.

† Cherry, Colin: *op. cit.,* p. 30.

what is said is often not what is meant. Sarcasm, where the tone of voice contradicts the verbal message, is one example. Nonlanguage communication is far more limited in the kind of information that can be given than is language, but it frequently has a more powerful effect. Some examples are vocal intonations, speech hesitations, yawning, laughing, or grunting (paralanguages); facial expressions, eye movements, gestures, posture, or touch (kinesics); physical closeness or distance, or the use of space (proxemics); and variations from the generally accepted standards of clothing. In general, nonlanguage communication sends messages of emotion, liking or disliking, preferences or nonpreferences.

Mehrabian describes the work of other researchers in *paralanguage communication* and says that when the speaker's discomfort and anxiety increase, speech errors increase. There are more unnecessary word repetitions, omissions of parts of words, incomplete sentences, "ums," and "ahs." Speech habits such as very long or clipped sentences, frequent interruptions, and silent periods tell something about the speaker's feeling toward his or her companion, as well as the status of each. If the higher-status person changes his or her speech patterns, using either longer or shorter sentences, the lower-status person does the same. If the higher-status person interrupts frequently or allows long silences to develop, the lower-status person becomes quite uncomfortable.

Studies show that *body movements and positions,* as well as facial expressions, act as visual cues helping to determine the nature and intensity of the speaker's moods and emotions.[66] Frieda Fromm-Reichman, a psychoanalyst, was said to imitate the posture of her client in order to experience something of what he or she was feeling, and so come to a better understanding of what was being said in a therapeutic session. Allan T. Dittman and his colleagues [67] asked psychotherapists and professional dancers to look at silent films of a patient and then decide when the patient's mood was a positive one. When the face of the patient was masked the dancers made more correct judgments than the psychotherapists, but both groups made equally accurate judgments when the entire person was shown.

Mehrabian [68] reports that liking and status are both expressed and interpreted through sitting body postures. His findings suggest that speakers sit in either a very relaxed or very tense position when companions are disliked and a moderately relaxed position when companions are liked. As far as status is concerned, Mehrabian concludes that higher-status persons use the most relaxed position when speaking to lower-status persons who, in turn, have a less relaxed position.

Many authorities believe that *facial expression* showing interest, joy, surprise, fear, anger, shame, and other emotions are socially learned and, therefore, cannot be used or interpreted with any accuracy by persons of different cultures. However, Paul Ekman and his associates [69] report that persons in three literate cultures (Brazilian, Japanese, and American) were in high agreement when naming the emotions shown in photographed faces, and persons from preliterate cultures in New Guinea and Borneo were generally in agreement when the emotions portrayed were happiness, sadness, or anger. Ekman contends that facial expressions of emotion are similar among all peoples because of their evolutionary origin, but that a society's "rules" controlling when and where emotions are displayed, or the behavioral consequences of displaying emotion, are learned and they differ in various cultures.

Actors and dancers use nonlanguage communication in a controlled, conscious way in pantomimes, ballet, and drama. In pantomimes, the actors tell their story through gestures only. In ballet and other dance forms, such as the Japanese Kabuki dance, music is added to enhance the communication between dancer and audience. And in drama—whether film, television, or "live" productions—actors use all the nonlanguage forms of communication plus a verbal script to convey emotions and a story.

Birdwhistle [70] believes that body motion, as one kind of nonlanguage communication, has an internal structure similar to the linguistic structure of language, and he has devoted much research to identifying small muscle changes he calls "kinemes." At this time kinemes are thought to be analogous to linguistic phonemes—the smallest distinctive group of speech sounds found in any language. For example, he has isolated, among Americans, four kinemes of eyebrow movements: lifted brows, lowered brows, knit brow, and single brow movement. Ewan C. Grant [71] has devised a check list composed of 100 such units of muscle change associated with facial expression. Both of these researchers are less interested in the psychic processes and personalities indicated by nonverbal behavior than they are in the structure of the communication behavior itself.

Much of the *early learning* of children about themselves, their families, and their culture is the result of nonlanguage communication. Voice quality, touch, and facial expression all convey information to the infant. In addition, on what appears to be a very primitive level of communication, Lee Salk [72] reports that a general sense of well-being is apparently communicated to a newborn by the adult heartbeat. In an experimental study covering the first 4 postnatal days of 214 infants, Salk found there was half as much crying in nurseries playing a tape with the sound of a normal heartbeat as in nurseries without this sound. Babies in the experimental group (hearing the heartbeat) showed a median weight gain over the 4 days of 40 gm. Those in the control group showed a median loss of 20 gm although there was no significant difference in the amount of food that was taken. Salk speculates that weight gain in the heartbeat group was due to reduced crying which conserved energy.

Part of children's learning about their own cultures comes from the nonverbal language of *clothing, hair styles,* and the use of *cosmetics* and *jewelry.*[73] All children at some time in their preschool years "try-on" adult roles such as mothers, fathers, astronauts, policemen, firemen, doctors, and nurses by using clothing generally associated with these roles. As the children grow older they come to use the accepted and normal ways of dressing in their culture:

By adopting those conventions for dressing himself, a person communicates to the world that he wants to be treated according to the standards of the culture for which they are appropriate. . . . On the surface, dressing up in unusual costumes would seem to be one of the more innocent forms of dissent that a person could express, but in fact it is deeply resented by many people who still feel bound by the traditional conventions of their culture and who become fearful or angry when those norms are violated. The nonverbal message that such a costume communicates is, "I reject your culture and your values," and those who resent this message can be violent in their response.*

Undoubtedly the so-called generation gap is widened by marked differences in standards of dress and grooming. It is hard for older persons to give unprejudiced attention to a young person who has to them a bizarre appearance. However, prejudices against the opposite sex, against other races, creeds, and colors, also affect communication throughout life.

Man's *use of space* as a nonlanguage communication system has been studied extensively by Hall. He coined the term "proxemics" to describe "interrelated observations and theories of man's use of space as a specialized elabora-

tion of culture." * Hall believes, as does Whorf, that people of different cultures, not only speak different languages, but live in different sensory worlds. They, therefore, use space and their senses in quite different ways. The Japanese, for instance, erect visual screens of various kinds in their buildings, but are oblivious to the poor acoustic qualities of paper walls. The German and Dutch, on the other hand, feel that sound is an intrusion and erect buildings with thick walls and double doors. Americans are taught not to breathe in the face of another (unless a particular brand of mouthwash has been used) while Arabs commonly "bathe" one another in their breath.

Because of these culturally different ways of using their senses, the Japanese, the German, the Dutch, the American, or the Arab uses space in unconscious ways that are often at cross purposes. Although the study of the cultural uses of space is a fascinating one, it is impossible to go into great detail here. Interested readers can find additional information through the references and suggested readings at the end of the chapter.[74-77]

Animal behaviorists have determined that birds and mammals not only establish territories they occupy and defend, but that within these territories they maintain a series of uniform distances from one another. Robert Sommer and Robert Dewar [78] distinguish between the concepts of human territoriality and distance, or personal space. They say the differences are that (1) territory is a relatively stationary area, while personal space is carried around with the individual; (2) the boundaries of a man's territory are usually marked and visible to others, while the boundaries of personal space are invisible; and (3) the defense of territory may arouse aggressive action, while the defense of personal space usually brings about withdrawal.

Hall,[79] from interviews with and observations of healthy adults living along the United States northeast coastline, has tentatively described four zones of distance as a possible starting point for the study of the use of space by Americans. Each of these zones—intimate distance, personal distance, social distance, and public distance—is subdivided into a close and far phase. Figure 16-10 is a summarization of the number of feet at which each zone begins, the sensory stimuli most involved in each zone, and behavioral characteristics of each zone. If nurses can conceive of each person (including themselves) as being surrounded by a series of invisible "bubbles," their own communicative

* Miller, George A.: "Nonverbal Communication," in Miller, George A. (ed.): *Communication, Language, and Meaning.* Basic Books, Inc., New York, 1973, p. 233.

* Hall, Edward T.: *op. cit.,* p. 1.

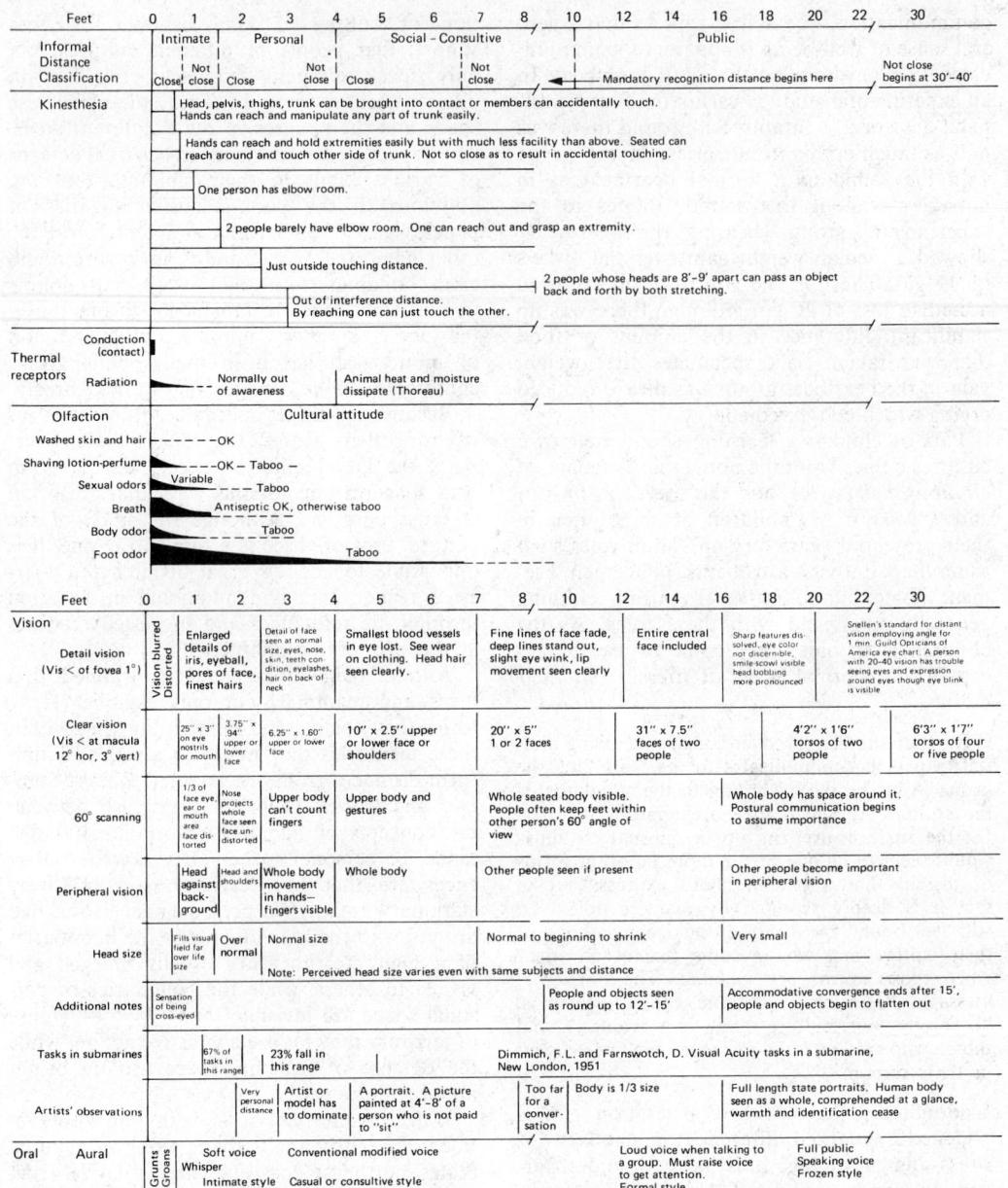

Figure 16-10. Chart showing interplay of the distant and immediate receptors in proxemic perception. (From Hall, Edward T.: *The Hidden Dimension.* Doubleday & Co., Inc., Garden City, N.Y., 1966.)

behavior, that of patients, and families may be more understandable.

The concept of space as communication includes not only our individual "bubbles" and their effects on ourselves and others, but the effect on us of architecture and objects in our surroundings. One study asked students to judge photographs of people for "energy and well-being" placed in three kinds of surroundings that ranged from attractive and elegant to dingy and ugly. The researchers found that pictures in the most unattractive room were rated as lacking energy or a sense of well-being. The research assistants when working in the dingy room complained of monotony, fatigue, headache, discontent, and irritability while they felt pleasure, enjoyment, importance, and energy when working in the attractive rooms. When questioned after the experiment only one-fourth of the students had some conscious awareness that the surroundings influenced their judgments and behavior.[80]

The design, colors, furniture, art objects, plants, flowers, and fountains used at the hospital entrance or within the hospital affect the public's feeling about it. If beauty and serenity as well as an understanding of territoriality and personal space extend to the living and treatment units, a mood of well-being is sustained. If they do not, there is more than a suggestion that beauty has no function for "persons" who become "patients," and that whatever beauty was viewed at the hospital entrance was largely for "show."

Communication Technology. The invention of the printing press is often cited as the beginning of communication technology. Later inventions such as the telegraph, telephone, radio, recorders, records and tapes, sound-color movies, television, computers, and communication satellites have increased man's capacity to send and receive messages ever faster and further. Marshall McLuhan[81] believes that any extension of ourselves, whether clothing or television (all of which he calls media), introduces into our affairs a new scale of "sense ratios or patterns of perception." George Gerbner[82] says that communication technology has not only extended human ability to exchange messages, but also has transformed the symbolic environment of human consciousness. He sees the symbolic environment as having the same relationship to the brain that air has to the lungs.

Authorities from many fields believe that the kinds of communication systems available to a society both facilitate and determine its social changes. The generation and culture gaps of this age, discussed so fully in Alvin Toffler's[83] *Future Shock* and Herman Kahn and B. Bruce-Briggs'[84] *Things to Come*, can be attributed in part to differences in the ease with which the old and the young use existing communication media. There are men and women alive today who remember the first telephone in their community and there are young people who take for granted the necessity of getting information from computers. Communication in a stable, primitive culture was largely spoken, and history passed from generation to generation by word-of-mouth. Today's highly mobile society, however, increasingly depends on all the electric means mentioned earlier for sending and receiving information.[84a-84c]

Unquestionably, the *telephone* has played an enormous part in the growth of the business and industrial world. Less apparent or less noticed is its role in helping teenagers in some aspects of adolescent growth, in helping the lonely aged to maintain some contact with the outside world, in helping those contemplating suicide to find a sympathetic, knowledgeable listener, in helping runaway youngsters send a message home, and in furthering medical care. Warren B. Miller[85] says there are several "properties" of the telephone that make it important and powerful in communication. In addition to speed, these are spatial, mechanical, and temporal properties, and the use of a single sensory channel. The telephone alters the spatial relations of persons using it and allows them to be both separated and symbolically close. McLuhan[86] comments that the telephone with the mouthpiece and earphone in a single instrument (the "French" phone) brings the voice and the ear together in an especially intimate way. Communication by way of the telephone is limited to the hearing sense * and the many visual cues of nonverbal communication cannot, of course, be utilized. Miller notes, however, that telephone conversations tend to be more sequential and logical than face-to-face conversations. For the psychiatrist or physician the telephone's temporal aspect is often of importance because the patient is not limited to a particular time or day in seeking advice as is necessary with an office appointment.

Any family with one or more teenagers is well aware of the constant, never-ending, telephone conversations of its adolescent son or daughter. (Some families surrender to the inevitable and have a separate telephone listed in the children's name.) What has escaped the attention of many adults is that the telephone, along with adolescent language, dancing, clothing, hair styles, letter writing, and poetry writing, constitutes an adolescent "culture" that is essentially an effort to find a middle course on the rocky road to adulthood. The use of the telephone is one way adolescents express the following needs:

. . . to love but to avoid excessive stimulation; to separate and differentiate from the parents but to find adequate controls; to regard themselves as unique but to be enveloped by the peer group; to express and show themselves to the world but

---

* A daily newspaper recently reported that a scientist at Bell Laboratories has patented a special light-sensitive pen with a "plasma panel" kind of writing pad with which it is possible to exchange two-way written messages over regular telephone lines. Picturephones have already been developed, but their cost is prohibitive for widespread use at this time.

to keep a secret and personal "inner space" in-violate.*

Telephone crisis "hotlines" such as those in suicide prevention centers, in centers for inter-vening with drug users, for acutely violent persons, or any who have an overwhelming problem and need a responsive listener have been developed recently. The telephone is a link between young people who have run away from home and their families. They may call Operation Peace of Mind and relay any mes-sage they wish to send. For many elderly per-sons who live alone a telephone reassurance program that uses volunteers to call them at an agreed-upon time each day does much to as-sure them that someone cares and that should they need help someone will be aware of it.

For many years pediatricians have been giv-ing reassurance and advice over the telephone to mothers caring for infants or young chil-dren.[87] Surgi-centers in which patients stay 12 hours or less make use of the telephone to follow patients' progress for a few postopera-tive days, and patients discharged from the hospital following major surgery or a serious illness find having a telephone number to call in case of an emergency or unexpected ques-tion is a great help. During hospitalization the telephone provides a special kind of communi-cation with family and friends. In addition to all the above uses, the telephone has been used for long-distance hypnosis, for international psychiatric consultation on Peace Corps vol-unteers, and, increasingly, in psychiatric and psychologic therapy. Warren B. Miller[88] re-ports that in a survey of 59 San Francisco psychiatrists 97 per cent were found to use the telephone for emergencies in the course of treatment, 45 per cent to use it with some patients as a planned adjunct to face-to-face therapy session, and 19 per cent to use it with some patients as the primary means of treat-ment.

Tapes and *tape recorders* as a medium for sending and receiving messages are so preva-lent that many cartoonists are using them for subject matter. Perhaps the best known cartoon shows an empty classroom with chairs in or-derly rows. On the teacher's desk is a large tape recorder, and on every student chair—a small tape recorder.

The comedian Fred Allen is said to have quipped that *television* is a "medium" because nothing on it is ever well done. Whether this is true or not, the influence of television on increasing vocabulary, general information, and trivial knowledge is well recognized. In fact, it has been suggested that schools stop teaching "information" but teach children to handle the flood of information that television supplies. The influence of television on the social behavior and attitudes of children is well documented. Most of the attention has been directed toward evaluating programs that show interpersonal violence. Researchers re-port that children from the preschool years through adolescence are more aggressive after viewing programs of violence. Studies also show, however, that television can encourage children to change attitudes toward people and activities in a positive direction and it can promote socially valued behavior.[89] Television has been used in behavior modification therapy with good results. When children were shown 10-minute films by means of a rear-screen film projector that looked like a television set, un-reasonable fears about dogs and dentists were reduced in eight out of nine children.[90,91]

The "instant replay" quality of video tape is being used to advantage in schools of nursing and in medical and other educational pro-grams. Small television cameras allow teachers to make their own "shows" and cassette type television monitors allow students to view the tapes without a classroom and as often as they wish.[92,93]

Television is being used more and more in medical diagnosis and consultation, and as a part of psychotherapy.[93a-93e] Televised x-rays, electrocardiograms, electroencephalograms, even close-up views of various parts of the body for detailed inspection can be transmitted over telephone lines from physicians in remote areas to physicians in medical centers. Tele-vision in combination with radio, and com-puterized telemetry is also used by emergency ambulance services. At the scene of the acci-dent attendants can communicate with an emergency room and transmit blood pressure levels, pulse, and respiration rates, as well as electrocardiograms. Immediate treatment can then be worked out by physicians in the medical center and directions transmitted to the health workers at the scene of the accident.

Computers represent for many persons the epitome of the threatening aspects of our tech-nological age. Science-fiction writers[94,95] and scientists specializing in computer technology have speculated about future uses of computers and have described both intriguing and fright-ening possibilities. Philip Handler[96] says that predicting the future role of computers in the life sciences is very difficult. While the in-creased speed and decreasing cost of com-puter-time use "guarantees that revolutionary developments will take place," our current in-ability to write appropriate instructions for some projected computer programs "makes it

---

* Group for the Advancement of Psychiatry, Com-mittee on Adolescence: *Normal Adolescence*. Charles Scribner's Sons, New York, 1968, p. 70.

almost impossible to predict which of many paths it [the computer] will take."

Computers are essentially symbol manipulators or general information processors, and as such are used in most large hospitals for the business and institutional management aspects of hospitalizaton. In addition, some hospitals and clinics are beginning to use computers for patient diagnosis, treatment, and record-keeping. These latter uses of computers are discussed in Chapters 4, 5, and 7 and are not considered further here.

The value of computer-based or computer-assisted learning has been promoted for some time. Until recently, however, it has not been economically feasible to introduce this kind of instruction in schools on a very broad base. Advances in computer technology (the "hardware" of such systems) and the development of improved programs of teaching strategies (the "software") now seem to indicate that the cost of computer-based education can be reduced.

Although few schools have been able to afford computer-based instruction, the earliest use of the computer was for elementary mathematics drill and reading vocabulary development. Since then, programs have been prepared to develop logical and critical thinking, as well as to take into account nonspecified solutions a student might give in response to a task to be completed.[97,98] Where computer-based instruction has been used, students and teachers are most enthusiastic, and in one evaluative study of 20 students in a semester-length medical science course it was found that those using computer instruction scored as well on a nationally administered test as students in a traditionally taught control group. The computer instructed group showed greater retention of the course material over a 26-week period, although they had used only one-third to one-half as many instructional hours as the conventionally taught classroom students.[99]

Charles E. Silberman argues, however, that computer-based instruction has not lived up to the promise that small-scale use of it has implied. He believes that thus far the programs developed tend to force students into an educational mold because the behaviorist approach to education and computer programming implies there is only one right answer to a problem and only one way to find it. He makes the following observation:

Our most pressing educational problem . . . is not how to increase the efficiency of the schools; it is how to create and maintain a humane society. A society whose schools are inhumane is not likely to be humane itself.*

* Silberman, Charles E.: *Crisis in the Classroom.* Random House, New York, 1970, p. 203.

There is little doubt that in the future electronic storage and retrieval of information, as well as all kinds of electronic communication, will be increasingly important. Picturephones, now in limited use, may make it possible for public health or district nurses to check accurately on patients without actually visiting them. Two-way television is also being explored, and at some time a viewer may be able to communicate directly with a teacher, consultant, therapist, or government official in a television studio by pressing a button. The uses of computers seem to be almost endless. Many telephone instruments already have a provision for future connections with computers that will order groceries, do banking, or pay bills. John McCarthy regards the computer as the "contemporary counterpart of the steam engine that brought on the industrial revolution," and he says, "Taking advantage of this opportunity may present the most urgent engineering, social and political questions of the next generation." *

3. COMMUNICATION BONDS AND BARRIERS

Strengthening Bonds and Reducing Barriers. Every health worker is concerned with strengthening bonds in, or gateways to, communication, and reducing barriers. These bonds and barriers are, in many instances, opposite sides of the same coin. Having the same language, culture, ethnic background, interests (work or leisure), age, sex, and even health problems often helps establish communication bonds, or helps people communicate more comfortably with one another.† Obviously, wide differences in these characteristics may hinder communication, and so act as barriers.

Mental States as Barriers. Communication disorders and, therefore, barriers, are reported as occurring more frequently among the *mentally retarded* than among the rest of the population, and many authorities believe that *mentally ill* persons have such different patterns of communication that they both send and receive distorted messages. Neither the special care of the mentally retarded nor the care of persons treated in psychiatric units or

* McCarthy, John: "Information," in Scientific American: *A Comprehensive Review of the Extraordinary New Technology of Information.* W. H. Freeman & Co., San Francisco, 1966, p. 1.

† An unusually frank woman once said to one of the writers, "I never enjoyed a novel in which the heroine didn't remind me of myself." Another said, "I often hear myself telling my family when I come back from a visit to friends, 'They are awfully nice people. Very much like ourselves!' "

hospitals is discussed in this book. Chapter 41, however, deals with anxiety and depression because both are found in all health services and both affect communication. Communication with *disoriented persons* is discussed in Chapters 40 and 46. It therefore seems unnecessary to pursue these subjects here.

Sensory Defects as Barriers. Some sensory defects make communication so difficult that Chapter 46 is devoted to a discussion of ways in which nurses and others can help persons with such handicaps to cope with them. Defective hearing or vision, or an inability to comprehend spoken language (auditory aphasia) interferes mainly with the handicapped person's reception of messages. Other sensory defects, such as the inability to use speech intelligibly (expressive aphasia), interfere with sending messages. The degree to which sensory defects limit communication depends to some extent on the severity of the defect, but perhaps more importantly on the intelligence and perseverance of the learner and teacher who are trying to compensate for the handicap. Van Wyck Brooks, writing about Helen Keller, said that when she was in a room everyone else seemed handicapped.

Language as Bond and Barrier. In earlier sections of this chapter it was pointed out that the transfer of many kinds of information can be accomplished without language; however, *language* is clearly the "great facilitator." Visitors to countries where the language is different often greet fellow countrymen with great delight, whether or not they are acquainted, simply because communication becomes so much easier when the same language is spoken. It takes little imagination to understand the troublesome situation a foreign-speaking patient has when language difficulties are compounded by illness.[100]

In order to create language bonds, nurses and all health workers should adopt standard speech and eliminate jargon, especially when talking with persons who have no health science education. They should also take every opportunity to be linguists of sorts. If they cannot learn to speak the principal language used in their work settings, they can, at least, learn appropriate forms of addressing persons, and some common phrases in other languages. The following are some suggestions for reducing language barriers: (1) find persons who will act as paid or volunteer translators, or interpreters, for patients in clinics and hospitals; (2) ask patients to translate for one another; (3) organize teaching and therapy groups around the language of the participants if the number of patients from a particular language group is large; and (4) give information booklets and directions for diagnostic tests and treatments which many health services translate into several languages. Since nurses are in most places the coordinators of patient care, they are almost certainly in the best position to recognize language barriers between the givers and receivers of health care, and to institute appropriate measures to lower or eliminate these barriers.[100a]

Culture as Bond and Barrier. Cultural differences and their effects on communication are just beginning to be understood and described. Only since the 1950s has the US Department of State asked anthropologists to work with foreign service personnel to help them understand the cultures of other countries so that international understanding can be improved. The anthropologist's goal is primarily to help interpret the "unconscious aspects of a culture—the things people do automatically without being aware of the full implications of what they have done," * as well as to point out the cultural taboos of a particular society.

Often the term "culture" is taken to mean a knowledge and appreciation of the fine arts or the ability to use certain forms of social behavior at the proper time, but culture, as it is used here, is defined as a society's way of life. The term includes all the material objects and tools of a society, as well as all of that society's learned behavior patterns and attitudes. Madeleine M. Leininger gives "culture" the following meaning:

Culture may be viewed as a blueprint for living which guides a particular group's thoughts, actions, and sentiments. . . . Culture includes all the accumulated ways a group of people solve problems, which are reflected in the people's language, dress, food, and a number of accumulated traditions and customs. It also includes material items, and the many social institutions which embody and sustain all these elements.†

Cultural differences appear not only between peoples of various nations, but also between people within a single society. For instance, there are a number of subgroups within the American society that have their own cultural values, beliefs, and practices. Some of these subgroups are based on age, others on economic level, others on religious beliefs, others on the national origin of parents or grandparents, and still others on professional work

---

* Hall, Edward T.: "The Anthropology of Manners," in Scientific American: *Science, Conflict, and Society.* W. H. Freeman & Co., San Francisco, 1969, p. 65.

† Leininger, Madeleine M.: *Nursing and Anthropology. Two Worlds to Blend.* John Wiley & Sons, New York, 1970, p. 49.

disciplines. Because health services are generally nondiscriminatory, and any that accept United States federal funds must have open admission policies, it is apparent that health workers are constantly obliged to communicate with persons whose backgrounds are different from their own. Table 16-1 describes the different meanings given to abstract concepts such as authority, education, and society by two subgroups of American culture, and Table 16-2 describes variations in professional values of the cultural subgroups "nurses" and "physicians."

Cultural barriers to communication are often not recognized because cultural attitudes, values and behaviors are learned from infancy and become such a part of the person that they rarely enter conscious thought. It may be that patients who are termed "difficult" or "uncooperative" are actually encountering cultural "shock" and are, therefore, unaware of the reasons for their behavior. For instance, in the lower Yakima Valley of eastern Washington State, Mexican-American men at one clinic refused to leave the examining room when their wives were having an obstetric or urogenital examination because an important part of the husband's cultural role is to protect the modesty of his wife. When a health worker with the same cultural heritage explained the patient's actions to the physician and the physician's actions to the patient, the problem was eased.[101]

It is essential that health workers understand themselves and their prejudices. While their training tends to develop objectivity, some black nurses may never thoroughly like or understand white patients and vice versa; a gentile may be prejudiced against Jews, or the other way around; the individual who has suffered persecution at the hands of nationalists from another country may never acquire objectivity in dealing with "the enemy." Cultural prejudice is obviously a barrier to communication.

All too often nurses and other health workers in the United States are unaware of their own American cultural values and the ways they influence thinking and acting. For example, the middle-class American values of activity and achievement often make nurses uncomfortable when they are encouraged to think about and plan for nursing care that is largely listening and counseling. Many believe they are "good nurses" only when they are physically active or doing something concrete for others. Cleanliness is another American cultural value, and nurses often give more emphasis to making sure that patients are neat and tidy than to their rehabilitative, emotional, or social needs. Foreign visitors are frequently amazed at Americans' stress on cleanliness, and some cultural groups contend that being somewhat unclean or even being directly exposed to dirt has a positive value.[102] A third example of the unconscious influence of culture is the American concern with time as a precious commodity which is not to be squandered. Often nurses and other health workers are so regulated by the clock that to sit by the patient's bedside in silence or even in more active communication is considered a "waste of time," and only under unusual circumstances to be condoned. There are, of course, many other American cultural behavior patterns and attitudes that might profitably be explored by nurses. A few, of varying importance, that are or could be studied are the uses of social, personal, and intimate space; [102a] voice quality under excitement or stress; and the circumstances that determine when it is desirable to call another by his or her first name.

Unless health workers maintain an open attitude in examining their personal prejudices, attitudes, and stereotyped perceptions, they cannot learn about their own cultural patterns nor those of others. Leininger suggests that the best way to learn about another culture or subculture is to follow the example of the anthropologists and "become active participants in the life ways of a particular culture . . . seeing and hearing through the eyes and ears of the people." * Since this is rarely practicable for nurses, she suggests they should be active listeners, observers, and good questioners of the people they want to learn about. There are, of course, other possibilities for learning about different cultures. Many schools of nursing have a cosmopolitan student body where students of varied backgrounds can provide one another opportunities for understanding and appreciating cultural norms and practices. Most of the cities in which these schools are located provide rich community resources for learning about cultural and subcultural groups. Visits can be made to different places of worship, to intercultural group meetings, to restaurants serving ethnic foods, to concerts of ethnic music, and to traditional ethnic festivals. Nursing education programs are putting more and more emphasis on courses such as anthropology, sociology, and psychology (see Chapter 1) that are aimed at helping nurses gain an intellectual understanding of the commonalities and differences in human behavior. Such courses, wide and thoughtful reading on these subjects, plus listening to and observing

* Leininger, Madeleine M.: *op. cit.*, p. 112.

Table 16-1.   The Cultural Chasm Reconsidered (by R. Segalman): The Ideals Espoused, the Middle Class Realities, and the View from Beneath *

The Concept of:	The Ideal Meant:	The Middle-Class Reality Meaning:	The Lower-Class Reality Meaning:
Authority (courts, police, school principal	Someone we helped choose and whose activities we are responsible for	Security—to be taken for granted, wooed, and used for personal benefit	Something to be hated and avoided
Education	A means of learning more about the world God gave us	The road to better things for one's children and one's self	An obstacle course to be surmounted until children can go to work
Joining a church	To recharge our spiritual and ethical batteries and motivations	Affiliation for social acceptance and activity	An emotional release
Ideal goal	To be a better person	Money, property; to be accepted by the successful	"Coolness"; to make out without attracting the attention of the authorities
Society	Something we all are responsible for and from which we cannot stand idly by	The pattern one conforms to in the interests of security and being "popular"	"The Man"—an enemy to be resisted and suspected
Delinquency	An act of injustice to someone or one's self	An evil originating outside the middle class home	One of life's inevitable events to be ignored unless the police get into the act
The future	Something which we make for ourselves (subject to supernatural cancellation)	A rosy horizon	Nonexistent, so live each moment fully
"The street"	A road for which we are responsible and which we need to use responsibly	A path for the auto—somewhere to throw our used beer cans and cigarette wrappers	A meeting place; an escape from a crowded home; the place where the "action" is
Liquor	Something to be used with caution and for fulfillment	Sociability; cocktail parties, etc.	A means to welcome oblivion
Violence	Something to be abhorred as destructive to humans	A last resort of authorities for protecting the law-abiding; is acceptable when used	A tool for living and getting on; a way of getting attention of those who won't listen
Sex	Only a part (but important part) of a deeper mutual intertwining of two lives	An adventure and a binding force for the family—creating problems of birth control	One of life's few remaining free pleasures
Money	Something to be used for personal growth and participation in further support and improvement of society	A resource to be cautiously spent and saved for the future	Something to be used quickly before it disappears

* Sutterley, Doris C., and Donnelly, Gloria F.: *Perspectives in Human Development.* J. B. Lippincott Co., Philadelphia, 1973, pp. 119, 120.

Table 16-2.   Phrases That Indicate Different Professional Orientations *

	Nursing	*Medicine*
Central questions of the profession	What are the patient's problems, how is he coping with them and what help does he need?	What is the patient's diagnosis and what treatment does he need?
Phenomena dealt with	Discomfort	Symptom
	Patient concern	Disease
	Vision	Eyes
	Hearing	Ears
	Mobility	Musculoskeletal and neurologic systems
	Elimination	Diseases of the colon and rectum
	The patient with tuberculosis	Diseases due to mycobacteria
	The patient with disease of bones and joints	Diseases of joints
Professional specialty areas	Maternal and Child Health	Obstretrics and Pediatrics
Process of improving the patient's future health	Promotion of health and well-being, health care supervision	Preventive medicine
Expressing esteem for the physician	He really knows his patients	He really knows his medicine
People served	Patients	Clinical material, teaching material, cases †
People served who are especially valued	Good patients, nice patients, cooperative patients, patients really need help	Fascinating patients, good clinical material, great cases

* Lynaugh, Joan E., and Bates, Barbara: "The Two Languages of Nursing and Medicine," *Am. J. Nurs.*, 73:67, (Jan.) 1973.
† Medical center dialect.

others are all ways that if consciously and consistently used help nurses develop the ability to create cultural communication bonds.*

Although information about the health care practices and beliefs of different cultures and subcultures is not extensive, it is increasing.[103-109a] There has been, in the last several years, a dramatic increase in the general literature describing cultural similarities and differences, only a few of which are listed in the references.[110-116]

Age-Related Communication Bonds and Barriers. As a person progresses through the life cycle there are various developmental stages, roughly age-related, when communication seems to be easier with peers than with either younger or older persons.[116a] Sometimes common psychologic changes facilitate communication, as with the late school-age child (9 to 10 years) or the adolescent, whose lengthy telephone conversations with peers have been mentioned. Sometimes communica-

tion is facilitated by being in similar family developmental stages, as with newly married couples, those having preschool children, or those whose children are leaving "the nest." Sometimes communication is easier with peers as in the case of older adults when retirement problems and pleasures are of central concern and striving for success is no longer important. Perhaps the only age groups that do not find it easier to communicate with peers are the toddlers, preschoolers, and early school-age children.

Health workers, particularly nurses, cannot confine their communication effort to their own peer group. While some seem able almost instinctively to penetrate all age barriers, there is little doubt that those who do not have this "innate talent" can improve their communication skills. To do this, it is important to know the capabilities, "normal" interests, values, emotional and physical needs, and motives of persons in various stages of the life cycle. Erik Erikson's psychosexual stages of human development (see page 570) and Abraham Maslow's hierarchy of human needs (see page 566) have been stressed throughout this book, and both indicate requirements for "healthy" development. According to Eric Berne,[116b] each

* Since the International Council of Nurses as well as nursing organizations of the United States and most other countries have for many years barred discriminatory membership practices, nursing meetings can also provide a forum for intercultural communication.

person communicates from three aspects of his or her personality. At one time it may be from the Child ego state, at another time from the Parent ego state, or at still another time from the Adult ego state. In the Child state people respond as they did when a child and reproduce the behaviors and feelings of a particular moment or period in their development. When people react in the Parent ego state, Berne says, they borrow the responses, attitudes, feelings, and behaviors observed in the past in their parents. And when responding in the Adult state people use behaviors commonly called problem-solving. While it is impossible to discuss Berne's theory of transactional analysis in any detail here, the interested reader can find a nontechnical description in Thomas A. Harris's [116c] book *I'm OK—You're OK*. Harris points out that communication is likely to be unsatisfactory when an adult remark elicits a childish response, or when any two persons are responding to each other on different levels, or states, particularly when they are doing so without realizing what is happening.

In addition to knowledge about human development, health workers should make use of all their senses when receiving information and should be especially aware of the nonlanguage communication (either sent or received) that may contradict what is said. And finally, nurses and other health workers should keep in mind that effective communication is also dependent on recognizing individual differences and respecting the uniqueness of each person.[117]

Communication during *infancy and the preschool years* depends in large part on the health worker's ability to interpret and use nonlanguage channels in sending and receiving messages. Young children understand more of what is said to them than they can put into language themselves; however, because their life experiences are still very limited, much of what is said continues to be beyond real comprehension. For instance, young children in the hospital or entering nursery school should be constantly reassured that their mother will return. Until they have many experiences of mother's return, coupled with verbal reinforcement, they are not likely to believe or understand.* Children require much more nonlanguage communication when they are in stressful situations than do adults. Cuddling, caressing, singing, and rocking are often far more effective than soothing words (see Fig. 16-11). Because young children learn through

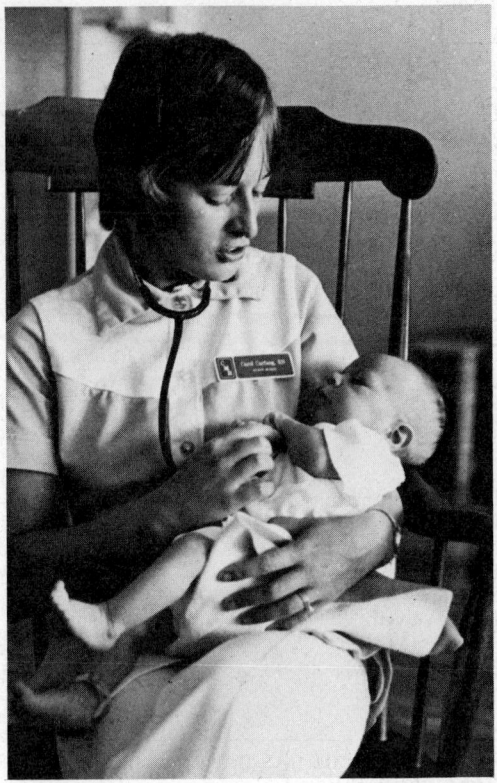

Figure 16-11. A nurse taking time to rock and talk to a baby. (Courtesy of Children's Memorial Hospital, Chicago, Ill.)

all their senses but haven't the ability to use language in abstract ways, they need concrete experiences of holding, manipulating, smelling, and tasting many kinds of objects rather than just seeing or being told about them. Play is, of course, children's major medium for communication. During play they not only receive information from objects and people, but send information to those who observe with discrimination and understanding. Chapter 17 has further discussion about the uses of play for both children and adults.

Communication and understanding between parents or other authority figures and *adolescents* has always been difficult. In 800 B.C., Hesiod, a Greek poet, said:

I see no hope for the future of our people if they are dependent on the frivolous youth of today, for certainly all youth are reckless beyond words. . . . When I was a boy, we were taught to be discreet and respectful of elders, but the present youth are exceedingly wise and impatient of restraint.*

* Because a young child cannot differentiate between temporary and permanent loss of a parent (or a substitute), hospitals now encourage parents to stay with children as much as is possible, even sleeping in the child's room.

* Quoted in Group for the Advancement of Psychiatry, Committee on Adolescence: *Normal Adolescence.* Charles Scribner's Sons, New York, 1968, p. 7.

Although cultural influences for resolving the developmental tasks of adolescence differ, the tasks themselves are the same: to learn how to work for economic and social reasons, how to love another outside the family of origin, how to separate from the family of origin, and how to nurture others instead of being nurtured.[118] As one adolescent boy said, "Growing up is sure hard work!" Parents, too, think that helping an adolescent grow up is "hard work," since fine judgments are often needed to decide when appropriate controls are necessary and wanted, or even what are appropriate controls.

Many authorities believe that current adolescent problems, at least in the American culture, are due in large part to a lack of satisfying communication with parents or other adults who might be able to provide needed help. Jack C. Westman [119] believes that the lack of communication results in part from the differing views that adults and adolescents have about the adolescent years. He says that too often adults see adolescence only as a preparatory period for something later in life. Adolescents, on the other hand, although they can intellectually and idealistically contemplate the past and future, are actually most concerned with living fully in the present. He makes the following observation:

One of the pitfalls for adults in approaching younger people is the hope that it is possible to really completely understand adolescents and convert them to adult ways. . . . The parent who talks about establishing a close relationship with an adolescent is fighting the growth process. He runs counter to the burgeoning independence of the teenager. From birth onward, children grow away from adults at a rate that accelerates during the adolescent years. We often are inclined to overlook the necessary and useful distance between generations.*

Westman also contends that much adolescent behavior is a bid for recognition as well as a challenge to adults to define their own positions. The current problem of adolescent and adult drug abuse, which includes alcoholism, may be an example of this point. Charles A. Ramsey,[120] in his controversial book *The Greening of America: The Coming of a New Consciousness and Rebirth of a Future,* states his belief that a better world is evolving from this generation's protest, and that adults should listen to and learn from young people as well as advise them.

Talking freely with competent health advisers about human relations, particularly sexual relations, contraception, abortion, the dangers

of venereal disease, and the misuse of drugs has never been more important for teenagers than it is today. But one of the communication difficulties they face is the fact that these concerns are often seen as "taboo" subjects by adults. School nurses, or nurses in homes, hospitals, and corrective institutions, must have current, accurate knowledge about these problems, and the ability to discuss them without embarrassment or a judgmental attitude toward the questioner. Nurses' understanding of their own beliefs and feelings are absolutely essential for reducing communication barriers with adolescents on these subjects. There is further discussion of this subject under other headings in this chapter.

There is a saying attributed to Confucius that the first part of life is for oneself, the second for one's family, the third for the community, and the last for meditation. Although most of us spend the greater part of our lives as adults, psychologists and others have devoted their efforts mainly to the study of childhood, adolescence, and old age. Ledford J. Bischof [121] suggests that studying adults may be worthwhile if for no other reason than to relieve the frustration of not knowing how the children in child studies turned out. He also suggests that since so little attention has been paid to the healthy development of the years between 25 and 65 we may need "well-adult clinics" in addition to "well-baby" clinics.

Most health workers, being themselves young adults or middle-aged, can easily identify and communicate with those who are neither very young nor very old. Among *young adults,* the problems of choosing occupations, achieving success in them, achieving a satisfying sexual relationship, having a child or children, establishing a home, and developing constructive family relationships with their children as well as with their own parents are principal subjects of communication. In addition, in today's world many young adults are deeply concerned about population control and having a family of healthy children who can be adequately provided for. Since young couples are frequently unable or unwilling to seek parental advice about family planning, health workers are often asked for help. The effectiveness of nurses' communication depends in very large part on their beliefs about family planning and their willingness to respect the beliefs of others.

The years between 45 and 65 are often called *middle age,* and this period has its own special problems. The end of the childbearing period is especially difficult for many women; however, some men's fear of impotence is perhaps even more troublesome because it is so

---

* Westman, Jack C.: "Understanding Teenagers," *Minn. Med.,* **56:**94, (Feb.) 1973.

seldom discussed. Sexual maladjustment is, in its broadest sense, a problem of all ages, but it is particularly acute in middle age. Nurses who are familiar with studies such as those of Alfred C. Kinsey and his associates [122,123] and of William H. Masters and Virginia E. Johnson [124-126] can understand and discuss patients' problems more effectively than the uninformed. Perhaps more important, however, is the necessity for health workers to be aware that their social values and emotional reactions to the discussion of sex also affect their ability to help others. Those who consider expression of sexuality inappropriate in middle and later life will be unable to help these age groups. While the following point has been made elsewhere, it bears repeating for emphasis: Effective health care for all ages should encourage rather than discourage healthy sex expression. Institutions and agencies offering care and treatment should not separate patients, or clients, from their mates unless this is a desirable aspect of the plan of care and treatment.

Another common preoccupation of the middle-aged is the loss of children from the home as the latter marry or leave to make their own way in life. This alters the parental role completely, and whether the relationship is more or less satisfying, the parent or parents find their lives greatly changed.

The extent to which nurses, and all health workers, have lived fully or have for themselves made constructive decisions in their own lives influences the degree of success they are likely to have in communicating with their own and other age groups. Let it also be said, however, that vicarious experience through listening, observing, and reading about the reactions of others add enormously to nurses' ability to create communication bonds. The warm reception of Angela Barron McBride's [127] book, *The Growth and Development of Mothers,* lies in her honest (and entertaining) subjective analysis of the maternal experience. As a psychiatric nurse, she can discuss the psychologic foundation for her anxieties, her envy, her frustrations, and resentment. Primarily, however, the subject of this autobiographic communication comes through as a normal, healthy, successful mother.

While some adolescents and adults find it hard to communicate with infants and children, an even greater number find it difficult to communicate with the *elderly.* People can, with more or less effort, recall their childhood, but until their time comes they cannot know firsthand how the aged feel.

The position of elders in a society varies with the culture and with the times. In some stable cultures the memory of ancestors is kept alive; the oldest living man or woman is revered and cherished by an extended family, a tribe, or a community; the counsel of the elders is sought and their advice taken. In rapidly changing societies, however, the culture a person of 65 was born into no longer exists, and the elderly are not thought wise so often as out-of-date, incompetent, or even a liability. There is, however, wide variation in the vigor and mental capability of aged persons. While some are content to sit and remember, others are as energetic and alive as they were at an earlier age. Simone de Beauvoir with great feeling says:

If old people show the same desires, the same feelings and the same requirements as the young, the world looks upon them with disgust: in them love and jealousy seem revolting or absurd, sexuality repulsive and violence ludicrous.*

In spite of the increasing number of studies about aging and the aged, little is actually known about the process of aging. The results of aging are apparent, however, and it is known that the amount of information taken in by the sensory processes is quite reduced. Sight, adaptation to darkness, hearing, and olfactory sensitivity are all decreased. Loss of memory and inadequate processing of information has been thought to be a hallmark of aging; however, evidence seems to be accumulating that when older persons are given enough time to learn specified material, they are able to recall it as effectively as a younger person. [128-128b]

Some authorities believe that as people grow older there is a purposeful withdrawal from social obligations and contact (disengagement). James E. Birren [129] says that disengagement includes four elements: less involvement with other people; a reduction in the variety of social roles played; more use of mental ability and less physical or social activity; and a recognition of less physical strength for sustained activity. Some investigators suggest that disengagement is a developmental stage that is triggered by retirement, while others believe it is a phenomenon beginning in the middle-age years. [130]

Retirement for some elderly means a "desirable unharried, unhurried, and dignified closure to life," but for others it is "hollow survival, feeling useless, unneeded and burdensome." [131] In the latter instance, severe depression is a common reaction. Jacques Choron,[132] in a study of suicide, which accounts

---

* de Beauvoir, Simone: *The Coming of Age.* G. P. Putnam's Sons, New York, 1972, p. 3. Translated by Patrick O'Brian.

for 1 per cent of all yearly deaths, says the rates are highest in the 60 to 65 age group. Depression and suicide are discussed in Chapter 41, where the point is made that they both represent profound disruptions of communication. Those who can help people identify and talk about the cause or causes of their depression make it possible for them to cope with it by changing conditions that can be changed, or accepting those that cannot.

Erikson calls the last developmental crisis of man "ego integrity versus despair" and believes that the following is a healthy resolution of this stage:

. . . acceptance of one's one and only life cycle and of the people who have become significant to it as something that had to be and that, by necessity, permitted of no substitutions. It thus means a new and different love of one's parents, free of the wish that they should have been different, and an acceptance of the fact that one's life is one's own responsibility. It is a sense of comradeship with men and women of distant times and of different pursuits who have created orders and objects and sayings conveying human dignity and love.*

The frequently observed tendency of the elderly to reminisce about the past may be in effect a "life review" so that past experiences and unresolved conflicts can be surveyed, reintegrated, and placed in perspective.[133]

The majority of aging and aged adults in the United States do not live in institutions, and even those with some physical impairment are able to manage their own lives. Nurses, however, usually have their most frequent contact with those elderly who are more incapacitated, and, consequently, they draw on this experience to provide clues to creating communication bonds. In general, when health workers speak clearly, and not too rapidly, and then give the older person time to comprehend what was said as well as time to respond, communication is eased.[134,135] Irene M. Burnside,[136] in a description of group work with disabled aged persons, points out that these patients often are unaware of the nonlanguage communication that takes place because of sight and hearing deficits. Nurses must take care, however, that they do not assume that all persons over 65 years have sensory impairments and routinely treat them as if they were deaf, blind, or childish.

When communicating with patients, but particularly the elderly, the health worker's manner of addressing the person should show consideration and respect regardless of his or her physical condition or social status. A friend of one of the writers came back from a hospital stay indignant because nurses had addressed her by her first name. While no rules can ever be made for interpersonal relations, the careless use of endearments may be resented by any adult. Warmth of feeling can be shown in other ways: listening with interest, taking time, and using to advantage the many opportunities for appropriate and comforting physical contacts that nursing offers (see Fig. 16-12).

Most aged adults have health problems, and the relatively new health specialties of geriatrics and geriatric nursing are helping to combat them. Nursing and medical literature on the aged is growing rapidly. Psychologists, sociologists, ecologists, architects, economists, urban planners, and others are contributing a wide variety of studies on aging and the many elements that isolate or help integrate the elderly in today's society.[137-149]

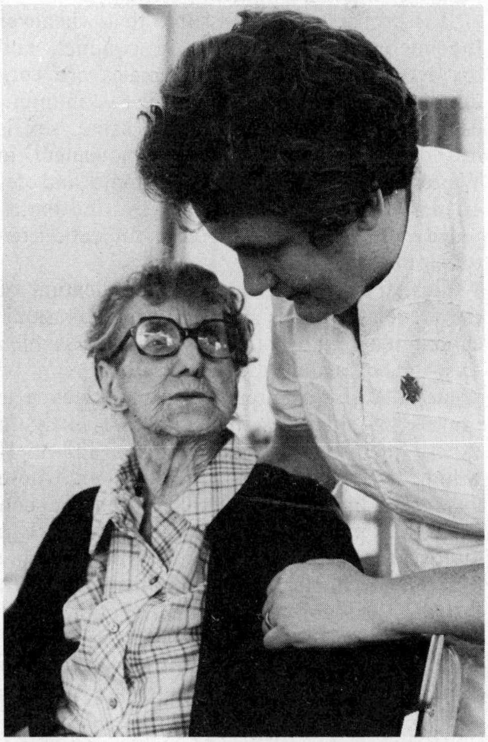

Figure 16-12. Registered nurse at Bestview Lodge (Toronto area senior citizen's nursing home) comforts expressed anxieties of a patient who is receiving long-term care and physical rehabilitation. (Photograph by Dugal Bichan in Handbury, Eric: *Nurse.* McClelland & Stewart, Ltd., Toronto, Ont., 1975. Sponsored by the Registered Nurses Association of Ontario for the celebration of its 50th Anniversary.)

* Erikson, Erik H.: *Identity: Youth and Crisis.* W. W. Norton & Co., New York, 1968, p. 139.

Sex-Related Communication Bonds and Barriers. In some cultures the roles of males and females are well-defined and totally different. Volumes have been written on the differences in the upbringing of girls and boys in various societies, a few of which are listed among the references.[149a-149d] Anthropologists stress the inescapable effect of early training on the roles in a society of adult men and women.

Where the male and female roles are very different, the effect of sex on communication is most marked. If girls are not supposed to take part or be interested in sports or politics they are not very likely to be able to participate or be interested in them as women. If boys are not supposed to play with dolls, help care for younger children, or participate in household tasks they are not likely to share the parental and homemaking roles as men. If sexual freedom is permitted, or even advocated, for boys but frowned on, or even punished, when practiced by girls, these conflicting standards will be reflected in the sexual behavior of men and women.

It is probably fair to assume that whenever the interests, the standards of conduct, and the activities of males and females are very different, sex constitutes a barrier to communication, and where they are the same, sex is less of a barrier. The unisex movement in Western society, applauded by some and decried by others, may have, at least, the undisputed virtue of facilitating communication between the sexes.

This is, of course, an oversimplification of the sex-related bonds and barriers in communication. There are other angles from which this subject should be discussed. It can be argued that, for example, when society expects bravery of all males they are least likely to expose their fears to other males and most willing to expose them to a female of whose love and admiration they are assured. In such cases the opposite sex encourages rather than discourages communication. It is not possible in a single chapter of a comprehensive work to treat this subject adequately, but it might be worthwhile to stress the importance of having male and female health workers on services for both male and female patients and for, in fact, avoiding the segregation of the latter.

Hospitalization and Illness as They Affect Communication. In general, adults who are ill, but not critically so, come to the hospital with the expectation of being cured and, in the American culture, according to Talcott Parsons,[150] the obligation to get well. Before they can fulfill these conditions, however, they require information that helps them plan co-operatively with health personnel the measures essential to their welfare and survival.* James V. Skipper and his colleagues [151] describe communication that serves this function as "instrumental," that is, helps promote action toward a future goal. At the same time patients are emotionally dependent in varying degrees on hospital personnel and look to them for acceptance, understanding and support. The satisfaction of these needs has been called the "expressive" function of communication.

Skipper found in a study of 86 men and women between the ages of 40 and 60 that 65 per cent wanted good explanations of their illness, what was going to happen, and when. Communication of this kind increased their understanding, their ability to cooperate, their trust, and their ability to assess their "rights." ("Rights" in this instance were based on a judgment of the degree of their illnesses, that is, the sicker the patient, the better the "right" to more care and attention.)

Patients were concerned about their safety and thought that the more they knew about what was happening, the better able they were to protect themselves from possible errors. In addition, they wanted to know the regulations and customs of the hospital so they could judge how they were expected to behave. Finally, Skipper concluded in the following terms that when health workers used communication that helped relieve patients' loneliness, helped pass the time, showed kindness and emotional support:

Patients used this type of communication as a sign that not only were their nurses and physicians dedicated and interested in their care and cure and would not reject them, but also that these persons were technically qualified, possessing the knowledge and skill to get them well.†

Seriously ill patients often show characteristics that act as barriers to communication. For instance, they may be totally self-centered and want every need gratified immediately. They may be so emotionally dependent that every act of a health worker is seen as an acceptance or rejection of them, or they may be preoccupied with bodily functions to the exclusion of everything but the present moment. Their senses are dulled by their physical state and, frequently, medications they are taking.

---

* It is repeatedly stressed in this book that health workers should plan *with,* not *for,* patients and that health workers should cooperate with patients rather than the other way around.

† Skipper, James V., et al.: "What Communication Means to Patients," *Am. J. Nurs.,* **64:**101, (Apr.) 1964.

For these reasons, plus the total newness of the experience, their ability to interpret what is heard and seen is usually disrupted. And, to compound these difficulties, some very ill patients have tubes in the respiratory tract so they cannot speak and let others know about their fears and misinterpretations.[152]

Robert Senescu,[153] writing about communication with the seriously ill, says there are four fundamental goals: (1) seeing that patients do not cause themselves more distress than is already present from their condition; (2) helping them to take advantage of medical and nursing plans; (3) seeing to it that patients do not give up usual sources of pleasure; and (4) helping them to maintain sociocultural and familial functions as much as possible. The last two goals Senescu believes apply particularly with patients who have diagnoses of disease thought to lead inevitably to death. Since Chapter 50 discusses specific ways to help patients die as they wish to die there seems little need to discuss them further here.

4. THERAPEUTIC COMMUNICATION, RELATIONSHIPS, AND ENVIRONMENTS

Therapeutic Communication and Relationships. The goals of all health workers are to promote health, to prevent and cure disease, to help people cope with disease or health problems that can't be corrected, and to help people die well when death is inescapable. To reach these goals physicians and nurses in their daily work use communication of some kind with patients, families, and co-workers, in developing interpersonal relationships that are helpful rather than merely neutral or damaging. Although the idea that communication can and should be used in a therapeutic way by all health workers is increasingly stressed, psychotherapists and psychiatric nurses have used communication as treatment with the emotionally disturbed for some time. Now there is growing recognition that every person with a physical illness has emotional problems that are most effectively managed when there is a constructive communicating relationship between the health worker and patient.[153a]

Jurgen Ruesch says that *therapeutic communication* during any interpersonal encounter helps "people overcome temporary stress, [helps them] to get along with other people, to adjust to the unalterable, and to overcome psychological blocks which stand in the path of self-realization." * He believes that com-

municating with therapeutic effect is not limited to psychotherapists, but takes place during many ordinary conversations. He says, "At times this process is referred to as therapy; at other times as education; some call it counselling; others simply friendship." *

Carl R. Rogers[154] and Abraham H. Maslow[155] both discuss psychotherapy as *therapeutic relationships,* and both believe that the relationship between a therapist and client is only a special instance of helping relationships in general. Rogers describes a helping relationship as one that intentionally promotes growth and development, and improves people's use of latent inner resources they possess. Maslow calls this goal "self-actualization" and believes that it can be reached best through interpersonal relationships that satisfy fundamental human needs of safety, belongingness, love, feelings of worth, and self-esteem. Rogers and Maslow both contend that this "basic therapeutic medicine" is, or can be, present in any good relationship such as the relationship between husbands and wives, parents and children, teachers and students, or nurses and patients.

It is undoubtedly true, as Ruesch points out, that many persons are able to use communication in a therapeutic way without recognizing that they have done so. However, it is a part of the professional health workers' responsibility to consciously try to make all their communication efforts with client-patients, or co-workers, as "therapeutic" as possible.

Nurses who see themselves as assisting patients when they lack the will, knowledge, or strength to perform activities contributing to health will make efforts to know the patients, understand them, and, in effect, "get inside their skins." This process of putting oneself in another's place is always difficult and only relatively successful. It requires a listening ear and constant observation and interpretation of both verbal and nonverbal behavior. It also demands of nurses self-understanding and the recognition that their own emotions may block their concentration on the patients' needs and interfere with helpful responses to these needs. And, finally, it calls for a willingness on the part of nurses to selectively express what they are feeling and thinking so that a *mutual* understanding may develop between nurse and patient.

Analytic Approaches to Nurse-Patient Interaction. Hildegard E. Peplau[156] and Gwen E. Tudor (Wills),[157] both psychiatric nurses, were the first to point out in the early 1950s the necessity of nurses' analyzing their relation-

---

* Ruesch, Jurgen: *Therapeutic Communication.* W. W. Norton & Co., New York, 1973, p. 7.

* Ruesch, Jurgen: *op. cit.,* p. 31.

ships with patients; of recognizing and analyzing the hospital ward as a network of reciprocal, communicating interpersonal relationships; and of helping patients identify and analyze emotions they were experiencing, as well as the situations that aroused them, and the behavior patterns that relieved them. Since those early descriptions of analytic nurse-patient relationships, Ida Jean Orlando (Pelletier) [158] and Ernestine Wiedenbach [159] have discussed a "deliberative" nursing approach. They describe specific instances of patients' behavior as observed by nurses, what the nurses thought or felt at that time, and what they said or did in response to these thoughts or feelings. In addition, the nurse authors describe and discuss the ways patients responded to the nurses' interpretations of their behavior, and finally, they discuss ways nurses can evaluate their "deliberative" nursing efforts. Others have used this approach to communication with patients and there are many reports of it.[160-165]

The Communication Theory Model to Describe Nurse-Patient Interaction. Earlier in this chapter, communication was described as a system having a message source, a transmitter, a channel for transmitting messages, a message receiver, and a destination. While human communication cannot be totally explained by this model, it is useful as a framework for giving some order to complex human interaction. Either nurses or patients may be message sources and encoders converting knowledge, ideas, and feelings into signs and symbols that are transmitted through actions and words. Communication channels may be conceived of as light and sound waves, or, more concretely, for example, as oral speech, the printed page, a painting, or a musical composition. The human counterpart of the model's message receiver may be viewed as the sensory organs, and the destination or decoder as the remembering, thinking, evaluating, decision-making brain cells of the patient or nurse.

Since our purpose here is to emphasize that professionally responsible nurses consciously use communication to inform, comfort, support, reassure, and help patients bear the seemingly unbearable, the focus here is on the nurse as the message source and destination, or message sender and receiver. Much of what is said in the following paragraphs about the *nurse as a communicator* is applicable to communicating with a single patient, a group of patients, patients' families, or colleagues. It applies to nurses working in hospitals, public health agencies, clinics, industrial dispensaries, schools, penal institutions, homes, or in any setting.

Margaret Colliton and associates [165a] have

shown in a "Symposium on the Use of Self in Clinical Practice" the way in which psychiatric nurses make communication therapeutic with their patients. Actually, such methods are applicable to nursing anywhere. Because psychiatric nurses have special preparation in communication they may be used as consultants for staff and patients in nonpsychiatric services.[165b] They may be called liaison nurses and sometimes ombudsmen for patients.[165c] Ability to communicate with patients is considered so essential to effective nursing that measuring this competence is suggested as a way of evaluating nurse practitioners.[165d] The National League for Nursing has distributed the pamphlet *Communicate or Else*,[165e] psychiatric nursing texts deal with this subject in great detail, and Maureen J. O'Brien [165f] has a full-length work, *Communications and Relationships in Nursing*.

It goes without saying that nurses who are able to inform patients must have a broad *knowledge* about the factors that can influence the maintenance of health or recovery from illness. Environmental conditions, economic level, sociocultural factors, physiologic functioning, and methods to correct dysfunction are only a few of the areas of knowledge necessary for nurses in order to communicate with therapeutic intent.

It has been pointed out repeatedly that *self-understanding* is basic to understanding others, and this is particularly important for the development of therapeutic communication. Nurses, as unique individuals, have values, feelings, and opinions that affect the ways they initiate communication or react to others. Because values, feelings, and opinions (facets of personality) may not be consciously recognized, and may emerge at inappropriate times or in ways that distort or disrupt communication, nurses are responsible for a continuous self-assessment.[166,167]

To examine one's own attitudes and values is a difficult task, since new and unwelcome feelings may be aroused when we begin to question our own personalities, our motives, our actions. Past experiences have instilled in us judgments of "right" and "wrong" behavior as well as descriptions of feelings that we "should" or "should not" have. However, Ann C. Burgess and Aaron Lazare [168] point out that it is important to remember when making a self-assessment that establishing blame or finding excuses is not its purpose. Its purpose is to understand.

Self-assessment involves becoming aware of qualities and skills that can be developed further, and, just as importantly, talents and assets that the nurse already has. Herbert A.

Otto, describing a human potentialities research project, makes the following statements:

A recurrent finding, based on 18 experimental groups, was that healthy or "normal" people of all ages, including members of diverse professions, have a clearer perception of their problems or weaknesses than of their strengths and assets. Less than one-tenth of 1 percent of all the participants had ever taken inventory of their personality assets or strengths, but approximately 20 times that number (2 percent) had at some time in their lives made a list of their problem areas.

Another finding was that the process of taking inventory of one's strengths is in itself strengthening. This can be done periodically and can result in one's developing a more well-rounded self-concept and a healthier self-image.*

Otto says that the process of taking an inventory of their strengths and personality resources led one nursing student to exclaim, "I am beginning to see strengths or the 'good side' of people I never thought had any."

There are many ways that self-assessment can be undertaken and self-understanding developed. For instance, nurses may decide to spend a quiet and private half-hour each day taking "stock" of their personal strengths and weaknesses.† Some nurses may decide to participate in sensitivity groups,[169] while others may choose to examine feelings, attitudes, and behavior with a friend, classmate, or instructor. Whatever approach is used, patience and persistence are as necessary with one's self as they are with patients or others.

The ability to see positive aspects in all patients, no matter how demanding or unattractive, leads to an *attitude of respect* for others that is crucial to all helping relationships. Nurses communicate respect and their appreciation of the worth and dignity of others by taking them seriously, by listening carefully, by being honest and dependable, and by seeing them as persons—not objects. Burgess and Lazare say, "Interest and caring about an individual are not technical skills; they are the basic arts of psychic healing." ‡

Therapeutic communication requires that nurses continually strive to become *nonjudgmental* in their encounters with others. Judith D. Goldsborough [170] suggests there are at least four steps that are helpful in becoming nonjudgmental: (1) recognition and acknowledgment that each person, including one's self, has judgmental attitudes; (2) acceptance of one's own judgmental attitudes; (3) attempts to find the origins of such attitudes; and (4) the realization that each new interpersonal experience requires the first three steps to be repeated.

It is inevitable that the behavior of patients and that of co-workers will call forth various *feelings* in the nurse. These may be feelings of pleasure, surprise, confusion, anxiety, or anger, to name a few. Henry T. Close [171] maintains that since emotions are just as much a part of an internal state as is being hungry, thirsty, or tired, there is little point in pretending a feeling does not exist. He says that the greater the strength of the feeling the more we are moved to *do something,* that is, to take some kind of action. That being the case, Close suggests that when extreme feelings are aroused there are four possible courses of action a person may take: (1) to conceal the feelings; (2) to communicate them; (3) to exhibit them; or (4) to act them out on other people. Each of these choices may be appropriate in some circumstances and inappropriate in others.

Nurses who have some self-understanding are free to attend to *decoding, or interpreting, messages* from other persons and from the environment. Decoding makes careful observation of facial expression, gestures, posture, and other nonlanguage behavior a necessity, and also requires nurses to listen with care to the verbal message.

Although both *listening and hearing* [172-174] involve an awareness of sound, they are not the same. Hearing is essentially a passive and often subconscious process. We may hear a siren or train horn in the distance, or the radio or television playing close at hand without attaching any meaning to these sounds and, in fact, without thinking about them at all. Almost the same kind of "hearing" can be observed during conversations between two or more persons. Frequently, the persons being spoken to are almost visibly forming replies that will stun the speaker even though his or her comments have not yet been completed. Many nurses are guilty of "hearing" patients in this same way. They, consequently, make stereotyped responses such as, "Don't worry. Your doctor knows what he's doing," or they introduce unrelated topics of conversation, or even interrupt while patients are speaking.[175] This, of course, tends to prevent communication rather than encourage it.

Listening, on the other hand, is an active,

---

* Otto, Herbert A.: "The Human Potentialities of Nurses and Patients," *Nurs. Outlook,* **13:**32, (Aug.) 1965.

† This is an effective part of the Alcoholics Anonymous and Al-Anon programs, and is recommended to both the alcoholic and his or her relatives.

‡ Burgess, Ann C., and Lazare, Aaron: *Psychiatric Nursing in the Hospital and Community.* Prentice-Hall, Inc., Englewood Cliffs, N.J., 1973, p. 36.

conscious process. S. I. Hayakawa says, "Listening requires entering actively and imaginatively into the other fellow's situation and trying to understand a frame of reference different from your own.* Deliberative nursing, described earlier, is one way of actively listening to patients. When nurses put into their own words their reactions to, or interpretation of, what patients have said or the way they look, they let patients know they have really been heard or, at least, someone is trying to understand the meaning of their communication. Orlando describes as follows a nurse-patient relationship during which the patient told the same story to the nurse ten different times:

The next time the patient repeated the story, the nurse explored her reaction by saying, "I don't want to sound impolite, but I can't help wonder why you keep telling the same story over and over again." The patient replied, "Well, that's a relief. You looked as if you were listening, but I wasn't really sure. I just wanted to be sure you knew how miserable that woman made my life." †

This approach to listening and decoding a patient's message focuses on the here-and-now, and is not an attempt to make a profound interpretation of the psychologic meanings that may be attached to the patient's behavior.

In the recent past, nurses have been encouraged to decode the messages of patients by simply repeating their last statements, that is, "reflecting" their verbal communication. This technique is a rather poor imitation of the nondirective counseling school of thought originated by Rogers during the 1940s and 1950s. Rogers' idea was that the counselor *should reflect in his or her own words the feeling state of the patient* and not, in most cases, the last words spoken. Nurses who use the first procedure often find they have completely missed the point of the patient's communication and the interaction generally comes to a standstill.[176]

One final concept of decoding patients' behavior should be commented on here, that is, *covert behavior*. Most persons have learned that it is unmannerly to question a friend's behavior in social situations, and we accept it at face value—as a description of his or her thoughts or feelings of the moment. We tend to respond the same way in the work situation,

although patients do not always act in ways that directly reveal their feelings nor do they always mean what they say. Of course, not all behavior has a hidden meaning. Some patients, however, find that illness and hospitalization arouse extremely painful feelings, and these can be so difficult to face that they deny them and behave in ways that refute their existence. When patients' behavior is surprising, because of its inappropriateness, nurses should be alerted that they may require considerable help in expressing what they are really experiencing.[177]

Throughout their association with clients, or patients, health workers are continually *encoding, or converting into a code, and sending messages* to others. The largest share of these are informational, and the importance of information to patients has already been described. While it seems fairly obvious that the words used to convey information must be understood by the persons to whom they are directed, nurses and physicians often use medical jargon that is incomprehensible to laymen.[177a] Few persons are willing to expose their ignorance of a subject they are assumed to understand, and many patients and families do not ask for clarification. On the other hand, more and more medical information is appearing in newspapers, popular periodicals, and on television so that a very elementary definition of many medical terms is not desirable either. Nurses must determine what the patient understands and use words that fit this understanding.

Silence, in combination with other nonlanguage behavior such as a frown or touch, can be as important a way to send a message as any use of words. Silence may convey sympathy, composure, tranquility, reservation, or temporary speechlessness. Because many persons find silence something to be avoided, they fill it with sound, and often are talking when they should be silent and listening. Dominick A. Barbara[178] believes that when we use silence constructively we can develop stronger ties and deeper feelings than words can possibly achieve.

Nurses, through their *sense of humor,* can convey important messages while promoting the harmony of their relationships with patients, families, and colleagues. Vera M. Robinson[178a] says that humor and laughter are healthy when they deal with immediate issues and ease the way for individuals to meet reality. Nurses who can see what is absurd in their own behavior as well as that of others also have a sense of what is tragic. Like the best of the comedians, they are often realists as opposed to romanticists, and can use humor

* Hayakawa, S. I.: "How to Attend a Conference," quoted in Lewis, Garland K.: *Nurse-Patient Communication.* Wm. C. Brown Co., Dubuque, Iowa, 1969, p. 32.

† Orlando, Ida Jean: *The Dynamic Nurse-Patient Relationship.* G. P. Putnam's Sons, New York, 1961, p. 57.

as an antidote for false or cheap sentimentality.

Laughter and humor between patients and health workers can be as good as, or better than, a medication. It can create a warm "climate," promote good interpersonal relationships, and relieve feelings of frustration, anxiety, or hostility. As Konrad Z. Lorenz points out, "Barking dogs may occasionally bite, but laughing men hardly ever shoot." *

A number of articles and books have been written that suggest some "do's and don't's" that health workers may wish to take note of in improving their communication skills. These suggestions are often helpful, but nurses who adhere to them too rigidly may find they interfere with their ability to pay close attention to what patients are saying. Rules too rigidly followed may destroy all vestiges of spontaneity in conversation.[179-186]

Therapeutic Communication Through Touch, Music, Other Art Forms, Role-Playing, Reading, and Writing. Popular literature and that of various health disciplines, including nursing, abounds in books and articles on the behavioral expression of "tender loving care" (T.L.C.), and the therapeutic effect of *touching* others.[187-194e] Sidney M. Jourard makes the following observation on touching:

The touch is an action which bridges the gulf many people develop between themselves and others, and between their "self" and their body. When I touch someone, I experience his body and my own simultaneously. To be touched is an almost infallible way of having one's attention seized and diverted from anything it was occupied with. . . . Touching another person is the last stage in reducing distance between people. Each person lives as if with an invisible fence around his body, a fence that keeps others at that distance which one feels most safe and comfortable. Let another person approach nearer than the boundary, and the one approached will step back, to keep the distance optimum—even if it means successively stepping back until considerable distance has been covered, with one approaching, the other retreating. To actually touch a person who is thus walled behind an invisible fence is often to invite violence or panic . . . we know little about the conditions under which a person will permit another to touch him, the meanings people attach to touching and being touched, the loci of acceptable touch, and little of the consequences of body contact.†

Nursing is the one helping profession that is permitted, and, in fact, expected, to use touch to provide its services. Nevertheless, nurses

must continually bear in mind that each person is unique in responding to being touched and touching others. The same behavior of one nurse may seem reserved to one patient and warm to another. A pat on the shoulder from a nurse may be welcomed by one person and resented by another. In spite of these differences, Marion S. Lesser and Vera Keane,[195] studying nurse-patient relationships in a hospital maternity service, found that the mothers they studied valued most the nursing personnel who served them with their hands as well as their heads. Lesser and Keane concluded that, as far as the public is concerned, the nurse is the person who makes physical contact with the patient.

In order to provide a "compassionate use of hands" and to appreciate the extent that it is needed or wanted by patients of all ages, nurses and other health workers must have some understanding of themselves.[196] Through methods of self-assessment already described, they can learn to recognize their own cultural taboos, as well as their personal inhibitions and capabilities in the physical expression of

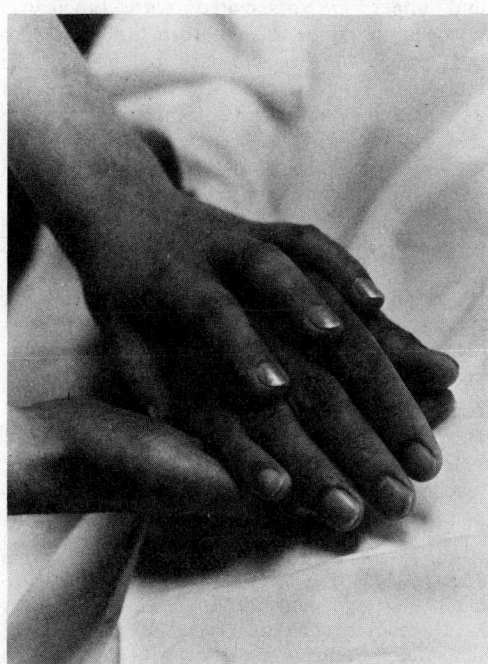

Figure 16-13. The comforting touch of a hand is but one of many different ways in which the "caring quality" of nursing is expressed. (Photograph by Dugal Bichan in Handbury, Eric: *Nurse*. McClelland & Stewart, Ltd., Toronto, Ont., 1975. Sponsored by the Registered Nurses Association of Ontario for the celebration of its 50th Anniversary.)

* Lorenz, Konrad Z.: *On Aggression.* Harcourt, Brace & World, New York, 1966, p. 294.

† Jourard, Sidney M.: *Disclosing Man to Himself.* Van Nostrand Reinhold Co., New York, 1968, p. 136.

thoughts and feelings. Whether they realize it or not, they have a philosophy, or point of view, on what is a "normal" or "healthy" range of behavior in the demonstration of affection, love, and sexual attraction. Their philosophy affects how and how much they use touch in their relations with patients and their professional associates. It also affects, in a less direct way, policies about visiting hours in institutions, for allowing parents, spouses, and others to have "rooming-in" privileges, about patient day-care and night-care services; it affects policies about week-end leaves for persons in extended care facilities, psychiatric hospitals, and correctional institutions.

Healing by the "laying on of hands" has been described in various cultures over the centuries. Expressing sympathy, compassion, or a desire to help by touching the person who is troubled or in pain seems to be instinctive. Little experimentation on the extent to which touch can be healing has been found by the authors.

Attention is called in Chapters 5 and 31 to Harold Saxton Burr's study of the bioelectric fields of life. He and his associates demonstrated that emotional states such as depression and anger are associated with bioelectric changes and since they in turn are related to disturbance in the acid-base balance of the body it is not farfetched to think that contact of one living body with another can produce measurable results. Albert Szent-Gyorgyi's [196a] study of *The Living State* is as much concerned with physics and chemistry as with the physiology of cell structure. In applying his findings to cancer, he points out that the problem is to find out how to arrest "senseless proliferation." The answer may lie in the use of agents that restore the bioelectric balance. To the extent that pathology is a disturbance of the electromagnetic fields of the body, healing can result from anything that reestablishes the balance of negative and positive elements.

Dolores Krieger, a nurse who is practicing, teaching, and studying the subject of therapeutic touch, makes the following observation:

An extensive search of the literature from Western countries . . . did not yield a clue to the modus operandi of this healing process. I have a considerable background in the study of comparative religions, particularly the Eastern religions, so I reread material I had come upon several years ago for clues that might guide my search.

The East holds different assumptions about man and a different view of the dynamics of human relationships than the West, particularly about the personal interaction that occurs during the laying-on of hands. The basis for this interaction between healer and subject is thought to be a state of matter for which we in the West have neither a word nor a concept. In Sanskrit it is called *prana*. Our nearest translation would be vitality or vigor. Eastern literature states that the healthy person has an overabundance of prana and that the ill person has a deficit. Indeed, the deficit is the illness. . . . Prana can be activated by will and can be transferred to another person if one has the intent to do so. The literature also states that prana is intrinsic in what we would call the oxygen molecule.*

Krieger goes on to discuss the possibilities of chemical changes in the cells in response to touch.† She calls "therapeutic touch" the "imprimatur of nursing" and her studies and those of Dorothy Harrison (see page 1385) may help produce results that will convince skeptics that the healing power of touch has a "scientific" explanation.[196b-196e]

Shirley Farrah,[196f] a psychiatric nurse presenting a survey of the literature and the results of her own experience, lists inappropriate and appropriate situations for using touch, which are given, in part, as follows:

Inappropriate situations. When it is sexually suggestive, or when a person has an aversion to sex or to touch; when it doesn't convey a "genuine" message; when a person has an extreme fear of dependency; when a person sees physical contact as a form of communication reserved for children or the handicapped; when a person is angry or suspicious; when the health worker feels "unnatural" or embarrassed in touching the patient.

Appropriate situations. When a person is depressed or anxious and fails to respond to verbal communication; when the person needs encouragement to take a difficult step; when a person is fearful; when health workers want to show that they share another's joy or that they sympathize with another's sorrow or grief; when a person needs "mothering"; when they "reach out" in periods of stress or need assurance of their acceptability; when a person is disoriented, unconscious, terminally ill, or dying; when they are in pain, rejected, lonely or sensorily deprived.

In concluding, Farrah makes the following generalization about touch:

There is no intention on the part of the author to suggest that touch be used indiscriminately as a way of relating to patients. It is the author's belief, however, that the judicious use of touch can be a valuable asset in nursing care. The avoidance of touch should not be taken for granted as taboo by the nurse, rather, it should be recognized, discussed, clarified, and evaluated

---

* Krieger, Dolores: "Therapeutic Touch: The Imprimatur of Nursing," *Am. J. Nurs.,* 75:784, (May) 1975.

† The profound and pervasive physical response to the emotion aroused during lovemaking suggests that the psychic phenomenon of faith could have as profound and pervasive a physical response.

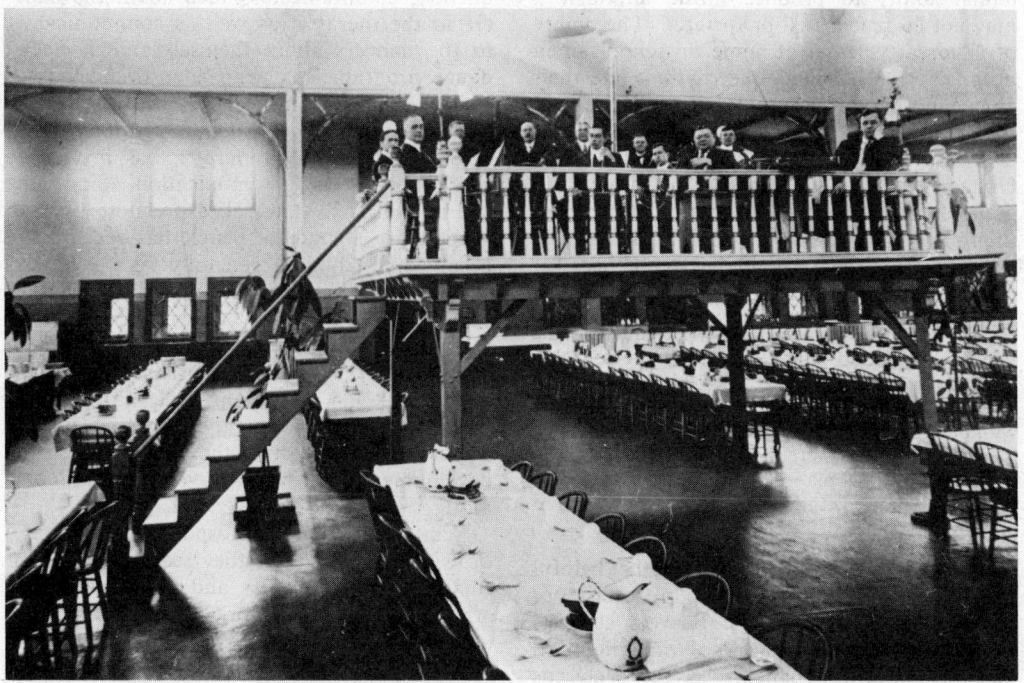

Figure 16-14. Dining room of the Connecticut Valley Hospital (formerly General Hospital for the Insane of the State of Connecticut) about 1900, showing orchestra that played for patients during the evening meal. (Carini, Esta, et al.: *The Mentally Ill in Connecticut: Changing Patterns of Care and the Evolution of Psychiatric Nursing, 1936–1972.* Connecticut Department of Mental Health, Hartford, 1974, p. 28.)

within the general framework of the nurse-patient relationship. The use of touch should be determined according to each patient's individual needs and wishes and not by the nurse's predetermined bias.*

Music has the ability to communicate the composer's ideas and feelings or to help the hearer call to mind his or her own images and feelings. The often misquoted lines by William Congreve—"Music hath charms to soothe a savage beast/To soften rocks, or bend a knotted oak"—describe beautifully and concisely the effects that music can have. In fact, it was so taken to heart by building managers and administrators that for a time music was heard throughout the majority of public buildings. Figure 16-14 shows the dining room of a mental hospital in 1900 with an orchestra of twelve pieces which must have materially affected the atmosphere during meals. Since David played his harp to soothe Saul, the quieting effect of music has been recognized, but

health workers may not have given the subject as much attention as it deserves.*

Age, experience, and cultural background affect the kind of music people enjoy. Some reject much of the contemporary music while others prefer it and have little interest in the classics. Occidentals find it hard to understand or enjoy oriental music and vice versa. In any case, different patterns, harmonies, and rhythms that are strange may make a person inhospitable to a particular kind of music. Mark Twain is credited with the comment, "Wagner's music is better than it sounds." While there is certainly no requirement that people like all the music they may hear, it is one thing to refuse to listen to the new and another to listen but still prefer what they have grown to love. Obviously, when music is to be used in a therapeutic way, the preferences of patients are of great importance, and the freedom to make choices is vital.

Emma D. Sheehy says everyone has a po-

---

* Farrah, Shirley: "The Nurse—the Patient—and Touch," in Duffey, Margery, et al. (eds.): *Current Concepts in Clinical Nursing,* Vol. III. C. V. Mosby Co., St. Louis, 1971, p. 258.

* A woman of middle age, describing the "routine" she and her husband had established in their home after he was told that he had inoperable cancer, said "we keep beautiful music on the stereo all the time."

tential ability to produce music although it may not be recognized or fostered. The ability of children, whether at home, in school, or in hospitals, to beat out simple rhythms and their enjoyment of it substantiates her statement as does the popularity of choral groups, orchestras and bands in schools throughout the United States. As an example of pleasure in a simple music-making activity, Sheehy gives the following description of one of her experiences in tuning one hundred water glasses for a college dinner party:

All of the glasses at a table were tuned to the same interval and numbered. Each person was given a "score" indicating when his number was to be played. The entire group sang the song first with only the piano accompaniment; the next time the tuned glasses were added. *Jingle Bells,* the favorite song, was played four times: I will never forget this music time in which one hundred players participated.*

Kathryn J. Ammon [197] studied the helpful effect music has on children in respiratory distress and Stacie Virginia Beavers suggests the therapeutic advantages of studying and making music for patients at the Veterans Administration Hospital in Topeka, Kan.:

Active patient participation in music study and practice offers the challenge of expansion of knowledge, provides the discipline of orderly activity, and promotes improvement in concentration, attention span, and memory. Pride of achievement is another healthy result. Patients are sometimes able to solve some of their personal problems after they have developed the ability to solve problems in the musical setting. Music therapists hope that through changes effected by music therapy, a patient will experience greater understanding of himself and the world about him and achieve a more satisfactory adjustment to society.†

Courses in music therapy are relatively new. In Finland, with its advanced health care system, the first course of this kind was offered in 1973, for instance.[197a]

Dance, as therapeutic communication, requires active participation and is, therefore, limited to patients who are physically able. With children or adults it may be used to help develop coordination, to give them a sense of freedom or a sense of their physical relationship to space, and to allow them to show feelings through unrestricted body movements. Dance therapy used in this way is not bound by patterns of accepted social dances, and, consequently, communicates much about the dancers to the therapist as well as communicating to the dancers about themselves.[198-200] Social dance programs may engender friendships as well as promote physical well-being.*

Art in other forms, such as *painting, sculpture,* and various *handicrafts,* has been used for centuries as communication. Since the 1930s the idea that self-expression through graphic art is good for people has been widely accepted.[201] Children generally take every opportunity available to use graphic materials, and since the discovery that children's drawings and paintings develop in predictable sequence, there has been less insistence that their works look like something real.[202,203] According to Edith Kramer, art therapy † is primarily a means of "supporting the ego, fostering the development of a sense of identity, and promoting maturation in general." ‡

School children in a hospital frequently use drawings to show how they see it. Feelings of smallness, powerlessness, and abandonment are often shown. Health workers and parents can use these productions to help children tolerate their hospitalization and even make it a constructive experience.[204,205]

The value of art therapy with psychotic adults is debatable, according to George Serban,[206] although it has been widely used as a diagnostic tool for many years. Some therapists claim that the course of a psychotic episode can be traced in the drawings and paintings of a manic-depressive patient, for example. Serban concluded from a study made of 32 patients that art therapy with other rehabilitative measures was of some use in the treatment of psychiatric patients, but not a significant factor in their improvement. In Serban's study, no art therapists were used and it may be that while the freedom to show dreams and subconscious ideas overcame the inhibitions of the patients, there was no person sufficiently knowledgeable to help the "artists" turn their fantasies into constructive imagina-

---

* Experimental programs for geriatric patients have included dancing sessions and one physician told the second author that he considered them the most effective aspect of the program he was directing.

† As an interesting sidelight, the Navajo and other southwestern Indian tribes use art as therapy in a unique way. Their sand paintings are a part of "curing" ceremonies in which traditional designs are "painted" on the ground. The ill person sits on the colored sand while more sand is sprinkled over him by the medicine man. "The supernatural powers intrinsic in the sand supposedly enter the patient's body and the evil spirits return to the sand. The sand painting is then destroyed before sunset." (*Newsweek,* Apr. 14, 1975, p. 76.)

‡ Kramer, Edith: *Art as Therapy with Children.* Schocken Books, New York, 1971, p. xiii.

---

* Sheehy, Emma D.: *Children Discover Music and Dance.* Henry Holt & Co., New York, 1959, p. 33.
† Beavers, Stacie Virginia: "Music Therapy," *Am. J. Nurs.,* **69:**89, (Jan.) 1969.

tive forms or to help them develop the ability to see their surroundings and themselves more accurately.

Role-playing as psychodrama is a form of group psychotherapy. It provides a structure for the *spontaneous* dramatization of a patient's personal and emotional problems or the problem of a group operating with some direction from a professional worker trained in this form of therapy.[207,208] For instance, an adolescent may be directed to play himself or herself or the part of a parent while others in the group take complementary roles. Since the goal of this kind of therapeutic communication is self-realization, it requires a highly skilled therapist-director.

Modifications of this technique are used in studying group dynamics, training for leadership, and to help students develop understanding of human behavior in some schools of nursing. For example, students studying rehabilitation nursing were asked to live for 24 hours as severely handicapped persons with classmates to act as their caretakers. After this experience all the students developed a greater appreciation of the frustrations and problems faced by the handicapped.

Role-playing can be seen often in children's play. Children "try on" the roles "Mommy," "Daddy," the "plumber," or "baby" to see how it feels to be powerful, or helpful, or helpless. In general, this is a part of growing up, but if a child insists on playing only one role, parents, teachers, and nurses should make special efforts to decode this communication.

Taking part in amateur theatricals does not have the same purpose as role-playing in an educational setting or group therapy. However, many persons derive great satisfaction in playing a part that is unlike their role in everyday life.[208a]

Reading provides hours of enjoyment for many persons. Information can be communicated, new ideas triggered, or feelings which are largely unverbalized by the reader can be beautifully expressed by a poet or author. If nurses are sufficiently well read, they can give patients very specific help with reading material, and help them to use bookmobiles and libraries. Since many adults need help identifying and getting reading materials, some health services employ librarians full- or part-time. While nurses cannot be librarians they can be aware of and use such references as *The Reader's Advisor*,[209] "A layman's guide to the best in print in the categories of General Biography, History, Bibles, World Religions, Philosophy, Psychology, the Sciences, Folklore, the Living Arts, Communications, and Travel."

Reading in a group, with or without discussion of what was read, has been found helpful to psychiatric patients and to the elderly.[210,211] Reading to a small group of hospitalized children is a fascinating activity to experience or observe. Children who have books read to them from a very early age develop reading skills with relative ease and usually maintain a lifelong interest in books.

Although *writing* themes, essays, reports, critiques, poetry, and short stories is a part of every child's educational program in the United States and in some other countries, many people cannot or do not use writing skills in later years. Letter-writing, for instance, once used by most literate persons to carry on conversations with distant friends is, in this age, often replaced by telephone calls or taped letters.

Roger Lauer[212] has described the use of creative writing with a group of ten psychiatric patients. He reported that nearly all the patients found they could write productively, and that it gave them enjoyment, satisfaction, pride, and a sense of accomplishment. The writing seemed to release some creative force so that these patients began to use music, painting, ceramics, and film-making in creative ways. And, finally, patients found that writing helped them deal in new and positive ways with problems such as unemployment, drug abuse, and loneliness. Encouraging persons to write creatively need not be limited to psychiatric patients. However, it seems easier to use this therapeutic communication tool with those in long-term care programs than with patients in short-term programs.

Communicating with Families and Groups in Varied Settings. Whether nurses are communicating with patients, their families, or with a group, they should be aware of all the elements that enter into the decoding and encoding of verbal or nonverbal messages. When three or more persons are communicating the messages are, of course, multiplied proportionately. It takes understanding, effort, and practice to develop communication that is constructive and, at the same time, seems natural, unstilted, unforced.

Unless nurses are on a psychiatric unit the groups they are likely to be working with are teaching-learning groups. Some of the skills and methods for use in these kinds of groups are discussed in a later section, but it should be said here that when communication "flows" from the nurse to group members, between group members, and back to the nurse (not necessarily in this order) in a reciprocal process, good communication results. How to help the too-talkative person, the too-silent person, or the person who continually introduces extraneous ideas into a group discussion cannot be treated here, but there are references on this subject that can be consulted by the reader.[213-215]

The settings in which nurses communicate with families and groups are, of course, varied. The setting should be as free from distractions as possible. Studies show that with groups of 15 or fewer persons, a circle arrangement is most conducive to interaction. Where the nurse is communicating with one family member, sitting at a corner of a table is helpful. How people arrange themselves within a group depends, in part, on their personalities and their cultural backgrounds. Knowledge about the interpersonal spatial behavior of people in groups is still limited, but it is a subject of current research.[216-221]

Nurses who make home visits, particularly the first few times, often comment on the difficulty of communicating with the patient or family. This may be related to the anthropologic concepts of territoriality and personal space. In the home, patients and families are in their own "territory" and can control the use of space, whereas in the hospital, school, clinic, or penal institution, the opposite is true. If nurses feel uncomfortable during home visits they are likely to listen less, observe less, and misinterpret whatever they observe or hear. A study of 48 home visits made by 12 nurses showed that nurses who asked many questions but gave little information about social-emotional problems generally made short visits and were dissatisfied with 50 per cent of them. Patients, however, usually reported that they were pleased with the visits and wanted more of them.[222] Once again, self-understanding and self-analysis of the nurse's communication can lead to improvement of interaction skills.

Requirements for a Therapeutic Environment. An environment may be described, for our purposes, as the sum of the conditions, influences, things, and their attributes that surround people in space and time. Authorities in systems-thinking conceive of an environment as a system made up of other systems. In either case, when one of the elements or systems of an environment changes, this brings about changes in the remaining elements or systems and changes the total environment, which, in turn, affects the systems or elements. The changed element may be as tangible as a piece of furniture, or as intangible as the "atmosphere" created by a smile or a frown.

The ideal health care environment in which those served can communicate freely with those who serve them, and where there is free communication within each of these two groups, assumes the presence of a favorable organizational structure, constructive administrative practices, pleasing age-appropriate surroundings, a sense of "team" work in decision-making, and the effective use of all learning situations for all members.[223-226a]

The terms *therapeutic environment* and *therapeutic community* came into use in the middle 1940s and early 1950s to describe a treatment approach to psychiatric patients, and, although somewhat different in meaning, the terms are often used interchangeably. While initially used with psychiatric patients, over the years a therapeutic environment has come to mean the deliberate establishment and use of physical and interpersonal elements in a given situation to further the health goals of any classification of patient. A therapeutic community, according to T. F. Main of the Cassel Hospital in England, is as follows:

. . . an attempt to use a hospital . . . as a community with the immediate aim of full participation of all its members in its daily life and the eventual aim of the resocialization of the neurotic individual for life in ordinary society. Ideally, it has been conceived as a therapeutic setting with a spontaneous and emotionally structured (rather than medically dictated) organization in which all staff and patients engage.*

Further ideas of a therapeutic community were described by Maxwell Jones [227,228] and its characteristics are summarized by Marvin I. Herz as follows:

Treatment responsibility is distributed among patients and staff. The patient is expected to participate actively and responsibly not only in his own treatment but in that of his fellow patients as well.
Traditional staff roles and status are changed. The social distance between echelons of staff and between staff and patients is reduced so that the behavior of both patients and staff may be freely discussed.
A democratic and permissive atmosphere is assiduously cultivated.
A high value is placed on sharing feelings and information in order to improve the quality and quantity of communication. To that end, communalism is practiced, with no privileged communications.
Social learning takes place and acting-out behavior is controlled through the medium of patient-staff meetings.†

Herz believes that while these concepts have opened channels of communication, promoted

* Main, T. F.: "The Hospital as a Therapeutic Institution," in Barnes, Elizabeth (ed.): *Psychosocial Nursing.* Tavistock Publications, London, 1968, p. 6.
† Herz, Marvin I.: "The Therapeutic Community: A Critique," *Hosp. Community Psychiatry,* **23:**69, (Mar.) 1972.

active patient participation in ward management and decision-making, and decreased the dehumanizing effect of institutionalization, they are not totally applicable to all psychiatric patients. He says, "It seems obvious that a milieu should be tailored to the needs of a particular population and that there must be many different types of therapeutic communities."

A series of papers about the Cassel Hospital —*Psychosocial Nursing*,[229] edited by Elizabeth Barnes,—gives a fairly concrete description of an institution that seems to have achieved a therapeutic environment. The final chapter of this book is called "Change as a Learning Situation," and this title may be the clue to a therapeutic environment. Perhaps such an environment is one that permits people to grow and change as a member of a family and a community.

Many persons will say that the accomplishments in psychiatric settings cannot be transferred to health services in general hospitals, schools, industry, corrective institutions, and homes. It is the opinion of the writers, however, that generalists can profit by the work of specialists in human relations and that many aspects of programs such as that at the Cassel Hospital can be adapted to any health program. A dominant role like that allowed patients there could result in a level of patient education and an acceleration of rehabilitation that might revolutionize health services.

During the last decade an effort has been made in the United States to allow for the *participation of consumers* on various policy-making bodies of health services. Public funding of some health services carries with it the proviso that there be consumer representation at several organizational levels, and even some form of community control. Community mental health services in the United States might be cited as typical of those giving the consumer a prominent organizational role.* Although few steps have been taken toward providing structures through which all groups of health care providers, as well as consumers, could be heard, the necessity exists if open communication and a therapeutic environment are to be developed. Sociologists Basil S. Georgopoulous and Floyd C. Mann, in the following statement, suggest that hospitals, considered generally, are not therapeutic communities as characterized by Herz:

The hospital is a formal, quasi-bureaucratic, and quasi-authoritarian organization which, like most organizations of this kind, relies greatly on conventional hierarchical work arrangements and on rather rigid impersonal rules, regulations and procedures. But, more importantly, it is a highly departmentalized, highly professionalized, and highly specialized organization that could not possibly function effectively without relying heavily for its internal coordination on the motivations, actions, self-discipline, and voluntary, informal adjustments of its many members.*

Both the organizational structure and administrative practices of today's large health service institutions are too complex to be adequately treated in a general discussion of communication. This complexity, plus economic factors and an increased technology in health care, may partially explain the many articles and books in which the theme is the health care consumers' feelings of helplessness, the lack of opportunity to express their needs, dissatisfaction with the help they are getting, and their inability to meet health care costs.[230-232]

Reporting the conclusions of an international study about common human problems in general hospitals, Barnes says:

General hospitals today give many satisfactions to patients and to staff. But the almost exclusively physical approach to disease, both in the care of patients and the training of staff, the stratified administrative structure and the increasing pressure and fragmentation of clinical work have produced a social climate which makes it difficult for people to consider the emotional impact of their work on either the patients or themselves—much less the therapeutic or non-therapeutic aspects of that impact.†

All of the 18 study groups in the project reported by Barnes agreed that an *overriding problem* in hospitals is communication among health workers as well as health workers and patients. Albert F. Wessen [233] found, after observing and interviewing all levels of personnel in the work setting at one hospital, that 75 per cent of the communication of doctors was with other doctors, and that 62 per cent of the nurses' and other health workers' communication was with members of their own groups. He contends that patients have little part in this communication system, and only act as a reference group toward which health workers orient their action and attitudes.

Wessen noted also that while physicians initiated and directed 23 per cent of their communications toward nurses, nurses initiated and directed only 9 per cent of their messages toward the physician. He suggests this as an

---

* The role of the consumer is of special importance in creating laws affecting the care of psychiatric patients because their human freedom and dignity have frequently been threatened or denied.

* Georgopoulous, Basil S., and Mann, Floyd C.: "The Hospital as an Organization," in Jaco, E. Gartley (ed.): *Patients, Physicians, and Illness*, 2nd ed. Free Press, New York, 1972, p. 311.

† Barnes, Elizabeth: *People in Hospital*. Macmillan & Co., Ltd., London, 1961, p. ix.

example of other sociologic findings, as does Jean L. J. Lum,[234] that persons of higher rank originate interaction toward lower rank persons more often than the latter originate interaction upward. Barnes [235] comments that the relationship of communication and the status of various persons or groups in hospitals was often a theme of discussion during the international study mentioned earlier. One group thought that the idea "the patient comes first" developed because health workers were uncertain or nonaccepting of the work status assigned to them. The study group concluded that even though the facts show that all facets of hospitalized patients' lives are directed and managed by someone else (indicating very low status), hospital staff accords them lip service of "coming first" in order to avoid facing the issue of their own status.

The American Hospital Association [236] has recently felt it necessary to develop and distribute *A Patient's Bill of Rights* (see Chapter 3, page 198) in which is made plain the patient's right to all kinds of information about his or her illness, treatment, and rehabilitation; the right to be informed of hospital rules and regulations that affect his or her conduct; the right to privacy and confidentiality; and the right to refuse to participate in research projects or to refuse treatment to the extent permitted by various laws. This document, if completely implemented, would make certain "the patient comes first" in fact as well as fancy. States are enacting laws to protect the *rights of mental patients* which may include the protection of fundamental civil rights and the provision of professional services. They may include the right to register and vote in elections; to practice religion; to be outdoors at regular intervals; to refuse medication (if patients have committed themselves), never to have it "administered as punishment"; to be "free from excessive medication"; to be given medication only as prescribed by a physician; to be protected from "experimental research, shock treatment, psychosurgery, or sterilization" without informed consent, following consultation with counsel or "an interested party of the patient's choice." Experimental research not directly related to the specific goals of treatment may be prohibited and treatment centers required to post a list of the rights of patients in a prominent place and given to each patient.[236a] With health legislation that provides for the inclusion of consumers on health planning and regulating bodies, protective laws will undoubtedly be more inclusive and specific in this and other countries.

Obviously, once a therapeutic environment is established, it must be maintained, and *nurse-to-nurse communication* is one important

aspect. The hospital change of shift report has been a time-honored mechanism for nurses to tell each other relevant facts about patients that are necessary for the continuity of the patient's care, and, in effect, the maintenance of the therapeutic environment. Linda L. Clair and Patricia M. Trussell [237] found, however, in a study of ten nurses and their reports that very little information the nurses believed should be reported actually was reported. For instance, they all believed that for noncritical as well as critically ill patients information about the nature of patients' nursing care problems, the solutions attempted, and their results should be given. In spite of these beliefs, the nurses almost never gave this information. Perhaps hospital nursing personnel should collaborate on guidelines so that nurses know what goes into a change of shift report and how to evaluate the results of reporting.

Margaret Treat and Marlene Kramer found in a study of 201 nurses that the questions supervisory personnel ask of persons on the next lower administrative level establish the "climate" of patient care in any work setting. Nurses in the study were encouraged through these questions to focus on the completion of nursing tasks and tasks that kept the organization running. Nurse-patient interactions and patient reactions to medications, treatments, diet, and so forth were infrequently questioned. Treat and Kramer say:

The way in which nurses begin to perceive what activities are important and the ones for which they receive rewards is analogous to throwing a rock in a quiet pond. As the director of nursing service, at the center of the organization, *evidences concern* and questions her administrative staff about the allocation of personnel and materials, they in turn question the head nurses, the head nurses question the staff nurses and they, also evidencing concern, question auxiliary personnel. As this wave reaches the shore of the pond, the patient also perceives that he is rewarded by conforming to the task-oriented expectations of nursing personnel.*

Other studies about the effectiveness of supervisory personnel's communication have shown that communicative behaviors directly affect the morale and performance of subordinate workers, patients' recovery rates, and the evaluation others place on supervisors' performances.[238-240] †

* Treat, Margaret, and Kramer, Marlene: "The Question Behind the Question," *J. Nurs. Admin.,* **2:**20, (Jan.–Feb.) 1972.
† In Chapter 3 the role of a nursing "supervisor" is discussed. The point is made there that the work of professional workers is rarely "supervised." The work of registered nurses may be more satisfying as and when they are held responsible and accountable for their actions.

Hospitals, as well as the practice of medicine and nursing, have historical roots in religious and military organizations. It is, therefore, not surprising that the *communication and interpersonal relationships of physicians and nurses* have been characterized for the most part by medical authoritarianism and nursing dependence.[241-244] Some authorities believe that the need for an "omnipotent" leader in an anxiety-producing situation, the system of rewards and punishment for interaction patterns, and the fact that most physicians are male, and nurses, female, also play important parts in these interpersonal relationships. Leonard I. Stein and Pamela Levin and Eric Berne [245] say that doctor-nurse communications (and some nurse-patient communications) have a special quality that fit a "game" model of interaction. According to Stein, the "game" objective is for the nurse to show initiative and make responsible, significant recommendations about patients' care to the physician, but at the same time to let the suggestions appear to be initiated by the physician. He says, "The major disadvantage of a doctor-nurse-like game is its inhibitory effect on open dialogue, which is stifling and anti-intellectual." * Sutterley and Donnelly [246] point out that when nurses and physicians share a common view of their roles, communication is smooth, but when physicians see nurses as dependent and nurses see themselves as independent, communication is difficult. According to the reports of observers such as Victor W. and Ruth Sidel [246a] and Felix Greene,† hierarchies in medical personnel have been reduced to a minimum in the People's Republic of China. This may partially account for the remarkable improvement in the health status of its people. In Chapter 3, an effort was made to show that under the reorganized National Health Service in Great Britain nurses and doctors are more likely to work as colleagues. It is possible that when the fee-for-service system of health care is abandoned by all health workers it is easier to establish colleague relationships and common goals than when some of them operate under this system and others do not.

Since physicians have traditionally made decisions about diagnosis, prognosis, and treatment, and mistakes in any one of these areas subject them to criticism or charges of malpractice, they carry a heavy burden. Many doctors have said, "We are the end of the road—we can't afford to be wrong." This may result in their making ambiguous statements, failing to commit themselves, or being unwilling to share their doubts and fears with nurses or patients. Some critics of health care believe that physicians must accept the concept of teamwork where all (including the patient) have the same interests and goals, and to the extent it is possible, the same information.[247] Michael Crichton,[248] in his study *Five Patients. The Hospital Explained,* comments that when the medical world taught diabetics the nature of the disease, how to assess its status, and how to control it, they opened up a new era of medicine in which the patient plays the most active role in treatment.

Communication, as earlier portions of this chapter indicate, uses many avenues. For instance, *the clothing worn by health workers or patients* may affect the give-and-take of communication. In many mental health facilities the personnel wear street clothes, and find they feel better about themselves, are less likely to be viewed by patients as "the authority," and are more likely to be seen as helping persons.[249,250] In general hospitals, on the other hand, patients use the distinctiveness of health workers' clothing to identify them and to determine what to communicate. For example, patients communicate different concerns to an intern than to a staff physician, or they communicate differently with a professional nurse than with a nursing aide. It must be said, however, that no matter what the current "fashion" for clothing in any one health care setting, the patients' experiences and values will determine whether they view the health workers' appearance and grooming as an invitation or deterrent to communication.

The way that patients are clothed also affects the free exchange of ideas and feelings. In mental hospitals, pediatric units, and nursing homes when patients are allowed to wear their own clothes and encouraged to look their best, the result has been more self-respect, better interpersonal relationships, and more interest in the world about them.

Physical surroundings make up an important part of any environment, and color, harmony of design, variety, and pleasing textures all contribute to the therapeutic environment, as do order and cleanliness. While some might argue the point, everyone, consciously or subconsciously, responds to beauty in their surroundings. Of course, the culture from which persons come and the experiences they have had affect their taste, so what is beautiful or familiar to one may not be to another.

Bruno Bettelheim describes the arrangement and uses of various furnishings in the first room that children and their parents see at the Orthogenic School in Chicago, Ill. There is an

---

* Stein, Leonard I.: "The Doctor-Nurse Game," *Arch. Gen. Psychiatry,* **16:**699, (June) 1967.

† Felix Greene has shown over television during the summer of 1975 a series on life in the People's Republic of China that confirms many of the Sidel's observations.

antique carved wood throne, a large antique rocking crib, a Victorian doll house, a comfortable sofa and chairs, open bowls of candy on low tables, and there are pictures on the walls and books on the shelves. Explaining why the room is so furnished, he says:

We wanted it [the living room] to express our therapeutic convictions, as well as our human concern for the feelings of a patient just arriving at the School, and we wanted it to be in accord with both. As with so much else in our work— from the way we arranged the building and its details, to how we treat the patient—we started out on the basis of our theoretical convictions of what we thought might feel good to him, and did in fact feel good to us. Afterward, if it did indeed appeal to the patients, we tried to understand how and why; if not, on this basis we changed things around.*

Nurses in *pediatric units and clinics* have found that when child-size tables, chairs, commodes, lavatories, creative toys, creative materials (paint, paper, clay), and toys that can be used to express anger and hostility are available to children, the children communicate and can be communicated with more easily than if there are no such furnishings.

As concern about human ecology and environment has increased, so have the studies of human territoriality and usage of space. Sommer and DeWar [251] report that in mental hospitals overcrowding increases disturbed behavior of patients. Other studies show that certain patients are happier in multibed accommodations than private rooms because they are less lonesome and bored.[252] In Chapter 50, on Death and Dying, the value of four-bed units for many terminally ill patients is emphasized.

Alton J. De Long discusses a desirable *spatial environment for elderly persons* and says it should be planned in light of the kind of sensory information the elderly depend on for communication. For instance, the aged use peripheral vision more than younger people do, and rely heavily on their tactile, olfactory, and thermal senses. They, therefore, prefer a small cluttered space to a spacious, roomy area. De Long describes an arrangement of rooms in one nursing home composed of six private rooms with a shared social area, says the use of these rooms by the patients can be compared to the use of a house (private room), porch (small social area), and street (corridor), and makes the following comments:

. . . when there were no private spaces, residents established personal domains in the corridor.

When there was a private space but no semi-private:semi-public space, residents used the corridor as a social space. And when both private and semiprivate:semi-public spaces were available, the corridor became a characteristically public space for the first time.*

Because it is so difficult to make an institutional environment "homelike" in feeling and appearance (and because institutional care is so costly) there is general agreement that more people, especially the chronically ill and elderly, should have health care provided in their own homes. If they must be institutionalized for extended periods, the environment is more likely to be "therapeutic" when they are allowed to partially or entirely furnish their room with familiar belongings.

In order for an environment to be "therapeutic" it should contain some novelty and variety, as well as allow for activity and exploration. When stimuli for the latter are not present, there is *sensory deprivation* with resulting boredom, monotony, inactivity, regression, and distorted thinking. The term "sensory deprivation" is in actuality a misnomer since sensory experience is never totally absent (see Chapters 34 and 38). Studies of stimuli in depleted environments have shown that when stimuli such as diffuse, unchanging light and a monotonous humming sound were present the aftereffects on most of the subjects were more severe and prolonged than when the environment was completely dark and silent. Although both situations affected the experimental volunteers in adverse ways, the researchers concluded that the environment that prevented people from finding meaning in the stimuli present was the most detrimental. In other words, perceptual deprivation was more dangerous than sensory deprivation, per se.[253-256]

5. LEARNING

Learning is a function of all animals. That is, all animals have the capacity to use experience as the basis for modifying behavior— the ability to learn.† Learning in humans, like

---

* Bettelheim, Bruno: *A Home for the Heart.* Alfred A. Knopf, New York, 1974, p. 133.

* De Long, Alton J.: "The Micro-Spatial Structure of the Older Person: Some Implications of Planning the Social and Spatial Environment," in Pastalan, Leon A., and Carson, Daniel H. (eds.): *Spatial Behavior of Older People.* University of Michigan, Ann Arbor, 1970, p. 85.
† This characteristic may be present in all forms of matter. Père Teilhard De Chardin [256a] has been cited elsewhere as believing that matter is in constant motion, always seeking a higher, or better, configuration of its elements. Change and adaptation may be interpreted as learning processes.

communication, is both a complex behavior and a process. It has a commonly understood and used meaning—the act or process of acquiring knowledge and skill—that only partially describes what learning is or when it occurs. Ernest R. Hilgard and Gordon H. Bower say:

There are many activities which everyone will agree count as illustrations of learning: acquiring a vocabulary, memorizing a poem, learning to operate a typewriter. There are other activities, not quite as obviously learned, which are easily classified as learned once you have reflected upon them. Among these are the acquiring of prejudices and preferences and other social attitudes and ideals, including the many skills involved in the social interplay with other people. Finally, there are a number of activities whose acquisition is not usually classifiable as a gain or improvement because their utility . . . is not readily demonstrable. Among these are tics, mannerisms, and autistic gestures.*

They go on to say that any formal definition of learning must distinguish between behavioral changes that result from maturation, native response tendencies (such as imprinting † in ducklings), or a temporary state of the learner (such as habituation). Robert M. Gagné says, "Learning is a change in human disposition or capability, which can be retained, and which is not simply ascribable to the process of growth." ‡ Since learning may be a change in attitudes, interests, or values in addition to behavior, most educators and educational psychologists say that learning cannot be measured directly, but can only be inferred.

For many years psychologists have been studying learning in animals with the expectation that whatever was discovered could be applied to man. As information has accumulated, however, some question the assumption. It now seems obvious that the animal species studied, as well as the stage of human development to which the results are being applied, must be considered when making generalizations from animal learning to human learning. Researchers have concluded from animal laboratory experiments that (1) simple stimulus-response learning is acquired as easily by lower animal species as by higher species; (2) mature higher animal species can learn more complex relationships than can mature lower animal species; and (3) the higher the animal on the phylogenetic scale the longer learning takes and the longer the period of immaturity.[257]

Some authorities believe that these studies and a few comparative animal-human studies indicate that the nature of learning in humans is of two kinds. They propose that one type, related to learning in lower animal species, occurs in early childhood, and the second more complex type occurs later, so that learning during human development changes both in degree and kind.[258] Jean Piaget, a Swiss biologist, philosopher, and child psychologist, who has spent more than 40 years uncovering the nature and direction of human intellectual development by closely watching and recording the behavior of his own infants and children (later a larger sample), appears to agree with this notion. One of the many important ideas he has proposed is that in all areas of human behavior, including the intellectual, there are distinct organizational differences between childhood and adult behavior.[259,260]

Learning and Perception. Only that which is perceived through sensory receptors can be learned, and in the maturing human what is learned depends in part on the unique ways sensations are attended to. William James made the following observation decades ago:

Millions of items of the outward order are present to my senses which never properly enter into my experience. Why? Because they have no interest for me. My experience is what I agree to attend to. Only those items which I notice shape my mind—without selective interest, experience is an utter chaos.*

He pointed out that the focus of a person's attention was like the small area of a huge dark room lighted by a candle. The room is the mind in which the unlighted contents are just as real but of which the owner may be unconscious. Study of the effect of the unconscious, or the unlighted content of the mind, is in its infancy.

Perception is described by child development authorities on the one hand as sensation (the change that occurs in the central nervous system after a sensory receptor has been stimulated), and on the other hand as the organization and interpretation of sensation so that

---

* Hilgard, Ernest R., and Bower, Gordon H.: *Theories of Learning*, 3rd ed. Appleton-Century-Crofts, New York, 1966, p. 2.

† Imprinting is defined as an innate tendency birds and animals have for developing attachments to their parents. Lorenz used the term to describe the commonly observed "following" behavior of ducklings and goslings. (Lorenz, Konrad Z.: *King Solomon's Ring.* Thomas Y. Crowell Co., New York, 1952.) Some psychologists believe that an infant's recognition of his or her mother is based on this same tendency.

‡ Gagné, Robert M.: *Conditions of Learning.* Holt, Rinehart & Winston, New York, 1965, p. 5.

* James, William: *The Principles of Psychology,* Vol. I. [reprint] Dover Publications, New York, 1950. p. 402.

meaning is derived from what is seen, heard, touched, smelled, or tasted. In the adult it is impossible to differentiate one kind of perception from the other. In young children, however, the assumption is made that perception is largely sensation alone. This assumption is based on the known immaturity of the child's central nervous system, as well as his or her lack of experience. Studies of the visual ability of week-old infants show what seems to be an innate "preference" for looking at certain forms—mainly those resembling the human face, but researchers believe that the ability of 2-month-old infants to give selective visual attention to various forms and movement represents the early stage of perceptual-intellectual development and perception as interpretation. [261,262] By the time infants are 3 or 4 months old some perceptual organization has taken place since it is apparent they have learned to differentiate their mothers' faces and voices from other faces and voices. The infant's innate temperament,[263] the family's educational and economic status, the language and culture of the community and of the nation will all affect what sensations the growing infant gives meaning and importance to. The tendency of different people to give different meanings to the same visual experience has already been discussed in relation to communication. If one scene communicates different ideas to different persons, each one is obviously learning something different at that time.

Learning Through the Life Cycle. To observers or parents of *young children* it is obvious that early learning does not and cannot depend on verbal communication as much as it does on touch, physical closeness, the opportunity to observe people and the environment, the manipulation of objects, participation in many kinds of sensorimotor activities, and imitation of the behavior of parents and others.[264-267] The need of children and young animals for an age-appropriate, stimulating environment has been extensively studied. Unfortunately many conclusions about infants and preschoolers were largely drawn from studies of institutionalized children in sensory deficient environments rather than from experimental studies. One of the reasons that Piaget's theories are so widely accepted is the fact that he bases them on minute observation of his own children and other children in normal environments.

Piaget's research has shown that intellectual development occurs when children are encouraged to explore their environments in play, and to discover for themselves the physical attributes of objects as well as the logical relations between them. Because all learning takes time and tends to both influence and build on earlier learning, it is essential that children are not forced into too early a development of concepts and ideas about their worlds. According to students of Piaget's theories, he believes that cognitive development has a biologic basis and points out that learning occurs in progressive stages that are somewhat related to age. He says that later stages in cognitive development are not entered until earlier stages have been passed through. It is only in adolescence that the use of abstract concepts and adult logic is possible.[268,269] Table 16-3 is a brief summary of Piaget's concept of cognitive development.

The increasing ability of *adolescents* to deal with abstractions contributes to new interests and learning activities in the arts, sciences, humanities, and philosophy.[270] At the same time adolescents' concern for, and interest in, their physiologic changes makes them ready to learn about health practices, especially those related to their immediate and intense concerns. Language is increasingly important as a mediator in learning, and allows more rapid learning; it eliminates the necessity for rediscovering through individual effort many important facts about the universe.

Evidence about learning and intellectual capacity in *adults* indicates that the greatest intellectual creativeness occurs before the age of 30, while the greatest intellectual productiveness appears in the middle 30s and early 40s.[271] This is not to say, however, that intellectual creativity and production do not occur in younger or older persons since numerous examples of such early or late productivity can be found.

Many studies have been made of the intellectual capacity and learning ability of middle-aged and elderly persons (50 years and older). The conclusions are contradictory. This may be due to the kinds of testing instruments used (most are designed for testing children); the settings for testing (laboratory experiments rather than real-life settings); and to the fact that some studies have failed to test subjects for minimal but important brain damage.[272] Bischof, after reviewing a number of studies of intelligence, memory, and learning ability in older adults, says:

And so we come to the general conclusion [that] the old dog can learn new tricks but [that] the answer is not a direct and simple one. It appears that the old dog is reluctant to learn new tricks. He is less likely to gamble on the results, particularly when he is not convinced that the new trick is any better than the old tricks, which served him so well in the past. He may not learn the new trick as rapidly as he did in the past, but learn it he does. Further, the best evidence seems to indicate that if he starts out as a clever young pup, he is very likely to end up as a wise old hound.*

It seems obvious that in order to live a full and productive life it is important and necessary to continue to learn and to be able to change at every age. Today's rapid accumulation of scientific knowledge makes it impera-

* Bischof, Ledford J.: *Adult Psychology*. Harper & Row, New York, 1969, p. 224.

tive that professional workers are constantly involved in *continuing education*. It has been said that 50 per cent of the information an engineer now graduating from college has acquired will be obsolete in 7 years. Nurses are aware that they, too, cannot consider their learning as complete when they have received a diploma, but must continue throughout their working life to learn and change. (Continuing education for nurses and some others is discussed in Chapter 1.)

Learning Theory. Although learning has been studied by psychologists for the past 100

Table 16-3.   A Summary of Jean Piaget's Stages of Cognitive Development *

Stage I: Sensorimotor (Birth to 2 Years)	Stage II: Preoperational Thought (Ages 2 to 7 Years)	Stage III: Concrete Operations (Ages 7 to 11 Years)	Stage IV: Formal Operations (Ages 12 to 15 Years)
During this period the child learns to coordinate his actions with what he perceives. He learns to utilize the elementary behaviors in his repertoire in relation to many different objects (e.g., he can follow an object with his eyes, grasp it, shake it, rattle it, suck it, etc.). During this time he learns that objects exist even out of sight and he achieves a rudimentary understanding of some relationships in space, causality and time. The key words are *assimilation* and *accommodation* for this period which is concerned with evolution of the abilities necessary to construct and reconstruct objects. This is the period of experimentation and exploration through incorporation. Reasoning is by means of mental image.	Experimentation continues through this period with language, and thought and active learning to manipulate the world through action. This is the stage where he establishes the relationship between experience and action. During this stage the child begins to develop and use language. He learns to represent the world through images and words. Through his imaginative play, questioning and talking, listening and experimenting, he constantly reorganizes his picture of the world. What is primarily lacking at this stage is the concept of reversibility, that is, for every action or operation, there is one that cancels it (e.g., the child cannot grasp the idea that when the shape of a ball of clay is changed it can be brought back to its original shape).	An "operation" is a way of organizing facts about the real world so that one can use them selectively in problem-solving. During this period the child can perform *concrete operations*, that is, he can deal with properties of the *immediately present* world in solving new problems but he cannot yet *deduce* or reason hypothetically. Reasoning at this level can only be *inductive*. During the earlier part of this stage he is gradually building up the ideas of the conservation of matter, and length, and weight, and volume later on.	During this stage the child develops the capacity to make free use of hypothetical reasoning, of *deductive* reasoning. He learns to attack problems from the angle of all possible combinations of relations, systematic isolation of variables, and deductive hypotheses—testing. This would be true formal thought, the culmination of the development of logical thought and the last stage enumerated by Piaget.

Era I (0–2)—sensory motor intelligence—use of imagery

Era II (2–5)—transition to abstract—reflective thought, pre-logical, symbolic, intuitive (without logical relations.)

Era III (6–10)—logical processes, formation of stable categorical classes—quantitative and numerical relations of invariance

Era IV (11 to adulthood)—inferences through logical operations upon propositions or "operations upon operations"—reasoning about reasoning—true formal thought

* Sutterley, Doris C., and Donnelly, Gloria F.: *Perspectives in Human Development*. J. B. Lippincott Co., Philadelphia, 1973, p. 159.

years, and by physiologists, biochemists, and neurologists for a shorter time, a single, workable theory of learning has not yet been described. Most of the theories found so far relate to single aspects of learning and were developed from laboratory experiments with young adults or animals. They are, therefore, only partially applicable to many situations in which humans of various ages learn.[273-275]

Hilgard and Bower [276] have summarized and grouped into three categories statements about learning from various psychologic schools of thought: stimulus-response theory, cognitive theory, and motivation and personality theory. They note that these generalizations are too imprecise to be considered "laws" of learning (at least from the researcher's point of view), but that both unstructured experience and experiments (structured experience) tend to confirm their general applicability. The following statements, adapted from Hilgard and Bower, may therefore be useful to nurses as they plan learning experiences either with patients or for themselves:

Principles emphasized within stimulus-response theory are: (1) The learner should be active, rather than a passive listener or viewer; (2) Frequent repetition is important in acquiring skill and in bringing enough overlearning to guarantee retention; (3) Reinforcement is important. Positive reinforcements (rewards, successes) for correct responses are better than negative reinforcements (punishment, failure) for incorrect responses; (4) New behavior can be increased and refined through the use and imitation of models.

Principles emphasized within cognitive theory are: (1) The organization of information to be learned should be from simple to complex, not from arbitrary meaningless parts to meaningful wholes, but from simplified wholes to more complex wholes; (2) Learning with understanding is more permanent and more transferable than rote learning or learning by formula; (3) Goal-setting by the learner is important as motivation for learning, and his or her success or failure in reaching initial goals determines how he or she sets future goals; (4) Divergent thinking which leads to inventive solutions of problems or to the creation of novel and valued products is to be nurtured along with convergent thinking which leads to logically correct answers. Such divergent thinking requires the learner to perceive himself or herself as potentially creative through appropriate support from the teacher for his or her tentative efforts at originality.

Principles emphasized within motivation and personality theory are: (1) The learner must be understood in terms of the postnatal influences that have shaped his or her development, as well as the possible hereditary determiners of his or her ability and interests; (2) Learning is culturally relative, and both the wider culture and the subculture to which the learner belongs affect learning; (3) The learner's abilities are important, and provision has to be made for slow and rapid learners, as well as for those with special abilities; (4) The anxiety level of the individual learner may determine the beneficial or detrimental effects of certain kinds of encouragement to learn. With some tasks high-anxiety learners perform better if not reminded of how well (or poorly) they are doing, while low-anxiety learners do better if they are interrupted with comments on their progress; (5) The individual's organization of motives and values is important. Since long-range goals often affect short-range activities, some college students, for instance, may do better in courses seen as relevant to their majors than in those seen as irrelevant; (6) The same objective learning situation may tap appropriate motives for one learner and not for another. For example, some learners are motivated by relationships within a group, while others are motivated by their own achievement; (7) The group atmosphere of learning (competition vs. cooperation, authoritarianism vs. democracy, individual isolation vs. group identification) affects satisfaction in learning as well as the products of learning.

One of the most widely discussed and used of the stimulus-response or conditioning theories of learning is based on B. F. Skinner's experimental work with animals and pigeons.[277] The terms *operant conditioning, reinforcement therapy, behavior modification,* and *programmed learning* are all used to describe the application of this theory to cognitive learning, visceral learning, and some forms of psychotherapy. It is impossible to go into the details of Skinner's theory here, but it can be described in an oversimplified way as the learning of new behavior patterns by systematically applying rewards. The rewards may be as concrete as giving candy every time a child is able to put his or her shoes on the correct feet, or as fleeting as a smile or nod to indicate approval.

Operant conditioning is used in everyday activities, often without thinking about it. William S. Verplanck [278] was interested in applying operant conditioning to ordinary conversations between two persons, and asked a number of his college students to report on their conversations with one other person. The students were told to smile, nod, express agreement, or paraphrase any statement made to them that begin with "I think," "I believe," "I feel," or "it seems to me." Later in the 30-minute conversation they were to disagree or remain silent when such statements were made. When the students agreed or reinforced the speakers' opinions, all increased the rate at which they expressed those opinions, but when the students disagreed or were silent the speakers markedly decreased their rate of stating opinions. To name a few of its applications, operant conditioning has been used to teach the mentally retarded daily tasks of living, to modify the behavior of psychiatric patients, to help a speech-deficient child learn to speak, and to correct incontinence in neuropsychiatric geriatric patients.[279-285a]

"Programmed learning" is another application of operant conditioning that has been used in textbooks, workbooks, and computers. An adaptation of B. R. Bugelski's description of some of the requirements of an effective "program" follows:

(1) Learning proceeds in small steps. Not only are the steps in the program small, but they incorporate considerable repetition, review, and self-testing.
(2) Reinforcement is immediate. As soon as the learner writes down his or her answer he or she can confirm it by glancing at the supplied answer.
(3) The student is called upon to formulate, produce, "compose," or "create" the answer and to write it down. Programmers consider that this practice involves activity.
(4) There is no time limit. Every learner can proceed at his or her own rate. This is sometimes referred to as "self-pacing."
(5) The answers called for provide a record. Such records can be checked to determine whether or not any specific item is too difficult or unnecessary.[285b]

While the over-all effectiveness of programmed learning is questioned by many educators because it does not allow for creative problem-solving, other educators believe it is of value when the material to be learned can be presented in a logical way.

Neurologic and biochemical studies and theories of learning are in their early phases, but they indicate that learning occurs in different structures and locations of the brain, and that memory, as one aspect of learning, goes through various stages. Researchers speculate that a learning experience may (1) set in motion electrical circuits among the neurons; (2) physiologically change nerve synapses so that previously ineffective connections become effective; (3) anatomically change the synapses with additional "sprouts" at the connecting neuron terminals; (4) change the biochemicals that mediate the transmission of memory across synapses; and/or (5) change the coding of information in nerve cell macromolecules such as RNA.[286]

Learning, which is an aspect of communication (and vice versa), involves use of all the senses, and what is learned affects not only the intellect, but the personality as a whole. People not only learn to communicate, but communicate to learn, and the ways in which both are accomplished may determine the effectiveness of professional health workers.

6. HEALTH GOALS AND HEALTH GUIDANCE

International and National Health Goals. The definition of learning as change in behavior, interest, or capability assumes that a definite goal for change is in view. Many nations and individuals are beginning to set, or already have set, goals for health that require new values, attitudes, and behavior. In 1973, an international symposium, organized by the Ciba Foundation, focused on Human Rights in Health and discussed the "four fundamental human rights in health as the minimum at which mankind should aim." The conclusions of the symposium are as follows:

. . . safe water to drink, [implying good general sanitation] sufficient food, protection against communicable disease, and access to the means of controlling fertility. All are interlinked, and they lead to a fifth—the right to have within reach at least some form of health care—which could, if interpreted in a wide sense, cover all the others.*

There are, of course, many nations that have already adopted and provided for these minimum health "rights" either through governmental or private resources. These and other factors that contribute to health, good housing, adequate income, and education, for instance, are being improved for some disadvantaged areas and groups within the United States and in other populations. However, as industrialization, urbanization, and levels of prosperity increase, other health problems develop: pollution of the environment, overeating, lack of physical exercise, excessive smoking, abuse of drugs and alcohols, a long list

* Wolstenholme, G. E. W., and Elliott, Katherine: "Introduction," in Ciba Foundation Symposium 23 (New Series): *Human Rights in Health*. American Elsevier Publishing Co., New York, 1974, p. 2.

of chronic diseases, "the constant bombardment of stimuli, [and] the inescapable estrangement of civilized life from the natural biological rhythms . . ." * More and more scientists are coming to realize that many factors influence health in simultaneous, and often unrecognized, ways. They are also aware that changes in any part of the ecology may affect other parts in ways they had not foreseen.[287] National, as well as individual, health goals differ, therefore, and depend in part on the resources, economics, development, and industrialization of a society. Margrethe Kruse, as president of the International Council of Nurses, made a plea for "a world of unity" and showed the influence the ICN has had since its inception on the creation of international standards in nursing care and the development of international health goals.[287a]

Individual Health Goals. Health workers in many countries tend to view individual good health in the limited sense of an absence of illness even though they give lip service to the World Health Organization's definition and goal of health as "a state of complete physical, mental, and social well-being . . ." † About this Halbert L. Dunn says:

Perhaps this is because their training has been oriented toward disease rather than toward positive wellness; and they therefore find disease more *interesting* than wellness. Also, it's easier to fight *against* sickness than to fight *for* a condition of greater wellness.‡

According to a study of health practices and opinions conducted for the US Food and Drug Administration, however, many health service consumers see their health goals not as an absence of illness, but as a state of well-being that consists of a feeling of unlimited energy, freedom from anxiety and depression, and the presence of contentment and happiness ("super health" in the words of the report). Those who wrote the report of the study say that trying to achieve this goal leads large numbers of individuals to use questionable health practices and to place greater value on their own judgment of health products than on the physician's judgment. Some of these questionable health practices are (1) the excessive use of vitamins without medical guidance; (2) an overemphasis on nutrition and "health foods" as the method for reaching health goals; (3) the unnecessary use of laxatives; and (4) an almost unquestioning acceptance of advertising claims for nonprescription health products.* [288] The authors speculate that, among other reasons, health courses taken in school "with their stress upon general well-being rather than specific diseases and disorders, may also contribute to the super health orientation." † The results of this study seem to indicate that consumers of health services know the goals toward which they are striving, but have little accurate knowledge about how to reach them.‡

* A recent study of 208 fifth and sixth grade children shows that 70 per cent of 781 television health commercials were believed; in addition, *all* the health commercials were believed by 47 per cent of the children. (Lewis, Charles E., and Lewis, Mary Ann: "The Impact of Television Commercials on Health-Related Beliefs and Behavior of Children," *Pediatrics,* **53:**431, [Mar.] 1974.)

† National Analysts, Inc.: *A Study of Health Practices and Opinions.* National Technical Information Service, Springfield, Va., 1972, p. xviii.

‡ Some social scientists believe that the major health improvements in developed countries have been the result of governmental regulations and laws rather than enlightened choice by health service consumers. For example, they think the dramatic decrease in many communicable diseases followed legal requirements that all children entering public schools must have certain immunizations; other examples they cite are the effects of sewage treatment plants and water purification systems on health.

This age has seen in both the Union of Soviet Socialist Republics and the People's Republic of China a most dramatic demonstration of how the level of health in a population can be raised rapidly through health legislation and through the provision of universal health education and health service. Health has actually been politicized in China. The Red Liberation Army, since the 1965 revolution, activates the policies of the central government. Medical workers as part of this army work with the population in the community where the medical unit is stationed. In fact, the army is constantly engaged in helping citizens with road building, agriculture, health care, and other activities essential to the welfare of the community. Citizens, in turn, help the military if they need training in certain skills or other services, but the maintenance of a high level of health is a political goal.

There have been (over a longer period) less rapid, but still impressive, gains in health in New Zealand, Australia, Scandinavia, Great Britain, and other European countries where health legislation assures the provision of health care for all citizens. As pointed out in Chapter 2, since Canada has achieved in all its provinces a health service available to all citizens, the United States is the only remaining developed country that lacks such a service and that leaves the achievement of health goals so largely to individual initiative.

The provision of health care is actually a political question in every country. Preventive medicine and health education are likely to be neglected when public funds aren't available for the payment of providers. Lucie Young Kelly, a nurse directing a program of consumer education, says:

. . . only a few insurance plans and some aspects of Medicaid provide any reimbursement to anyone for

* Dubos, René: *So Human an Animal.* Charles Scribner's Sons, New York, 1968, p. 155.

† World Health Organization: "Constitution of the World Health Organization," *Chron. World Health Org.,* **1:**29, (Nos. 1–2) 1947.

‡ Dunn, Halbert L.: *High-Level Wellness.* R. W. Beatty, Ltd., Arlington, Va., 1961, p. 3.

Health Education for Promotion of Health and Prevention of Illness. With growing recognition that treatment of disease is costlier than prevention, in terms of money and human suffering, more and more attention is given to the dissemination of health knowledge. As in most aspects of education, it seems wise to begin with the child in order to prevent the formation of habits and prejudices that interfere with learning later on. Better health could be promoted and the incidence of disease could be reduced enormously if health education in schools were as thorough as it might be.

Health education is believed by many to be one of the major functions of the school.[289] The fact that health, education, and welfare are combined into one large division of the United States Government suggests how closely related they are thought to be. A recent nationwide survey of health education in the United States indicated that 37 of the 44 states responding to the questionnaire have health education guidelines in use in their public schools. However, only 31 of the responding states have requirements for some kind of health instruction for all students.[290]

Health educators in the United States tend to believe that health education is a discipline that requires specialized preparation.[291] However, as shown in Chapter 3, school nurses see themselves as health educators. In fact, some nurses in all specialties claim this function. Pam Arnold,[291a] describing the work of one of the 174 "teacher-nurses" in the Chicago schools, notes that all have degrees, more than half advanced degrees, and they must have "18 hours of college credit in education."

---

patient teaching, much less community health education, but there is a gradual trend in this direction. . . . It is logical that reimbursement will call for organized plans, documentation of teaching, and evaluation of results. (Kelly, Lucie Young: "Nurse-Teacher Role Overlaps" [editorial], *The American Nurse*, 7:4, [Sept.] 1975.)

Rosamund C. Gabrielson, as president of the American Nurses' Association, is quoted as testifying against certain current bills before the American Congress that failed to recognize adequately the role of nurses as health educators and that teaching is inherent in nursing. In testifying, she noted that recently:

. . . definitions in licensure laws have specified client teaching as a nursing function—a legal commitment to a traditional responsibility. ("Bills Must Recognize Health Education Roles," *The American Nurse*, 7:15, [Sept.] 1975.)

The salaries of city and county public health nurses (some of the latter claim to be public health nurses who happen to be working in schools) are paid from public funds. Their preventive work and health teaching is therefore a part of the public health service provided in the United States. But, generally speaking, monies for curative health care have exceeded those for preventive health care in the United States.

In most elementary and middle (junior high) schools of the United States, the classroom teacher is largely responsible for health education, while in the majority of senior high schools, physical education instructors are responsible. A survey made of 357 teachers from kindergarten through grade 12 in one city in New York State found many misconceptions of current health, first aid, and safety knowledge. Among the erroneous beliefs are the following and some figures on the number of teachers who held them:

64% Were unaware that a severe head injury is usually accompanied by a change in consciousness.

76% Did not believe that knowledge lessens anxiety. They felt that panic was unaffected by knowing the facts.

92% Believed barefoot contact with floor surfaces will cause "athlete's foot."

44% Continue to believe alcohol is a stimulant while less than half correctly labeled alcohol a depressant.

65% Answered that *everyone* needs a quart of milk daily.

66% Felt that "health foods" were useful additions to most diets.

32% Responded that *added* vitamins to the diet were always needed.

53% Of the teachers believed bowel movements on schedule were essential for health.

60% Did not know barbiturate and aspirin were two of the leading accidental poisoning substances in the U.S.A.

72% Believed that general character traits and conduct patterns could not be significantly altered even with adequate therapy.*

Nutrition is taught in most schools at every grade level, and if most teachers hold the same beliefs as those of teachers in the study cited, there can be little argument with the view that school health courses are responsible for much misinformation.[292] Furthermore, studies of the nutritional knowledge of high school students indicate that the majority have 50 per cent or less of the information considered essential to good nutrition.[293,294] While the increase in height in many national groups during the last decades is usually ascribed to improved nutrition, the individual's nutritional knowledge, per se, is not the only factor involved.[295-297] It may be that some of the important factors are beyond the control of the individual. For instance, Eugene B. Hayden,[298] president of the Cereal Institute, Inc., points out that cereal manufacturers in the 1940s began to add various nutrients to cereals to restore those removed in processing the grains,

---

* Keeve, J. Philip, and Specter, Gerald J.: "Responses to a Teacher Health-Knowledge Inventory," *J. Sch. Health*, 37:384, (Oct.) 1967.

and that since 1955 they have increased the vitamin and iron content to higher than the natural levels of the unprocessed grains. Ruth P. Fleshman,[298a] who is directing a commune health education project in the Haight-Asbury Medical Clinic, San Francisco, Calif., discusses the attitude of young people toward food—its meanings for them. She urges health educators to take a human rather than a technical approach to teaching nutrition.*

Nurses who work in schools have responsibility for improving both teachers' and students' knowledge of nutrition, while those who work in other institutions or agencies have frequent opportunities to discuss nutrition with patients and their families. Chapter 10 has a detailed discussion of nutrition as well as the nutritional needs of people of various ages, and Chapter 36 discusses malnutrition and obesity. (In Chapter 3 the function of nurses in all settings is discussed.)

A number of studies have been conducted to determine the *health needs and interests* of students, teachers, counselors, and parents so that planning for health education in the schools could be improved. In West Virginia, investigators found that topics of highest interest and need were family health, mental health, drugs and narcotics, and safety education.[299] In South Carolina, the community's health interests focused on illegitimacy, venereal disease, drug abuse, accidents, alcoholism, heart disease and cancer.[300] The results of a Connecticut study,[301] shown in Figure 16-15*A, B*, indicate not only the subject matter of interest, but the grades at which students have the highest interest in the subjects. It must be kept in mind, of course, that while all these studies show commonalities, the interests are not necessarily universal nor permanent. The specific needs and interests of the groups or individuals being taught must continually be determined by teachers and nurses in health education.

The so-called "sex revolution" has brought to the attention of the schools, nurses, physicians, and other professional workers, as well as the general public, the need for *sex education* of all age groups. Studies repeatedly show that approximately 40 per cent of the young people get their first sex information from peers; literature is the second primary source; mothers are the third; and schools are the fourth. Professional persons, who might be supposed to have the most accurate and complete knowledge, supply little information.[302-304] Part of the difficulty has been that health professionals have indeed little more information than those who seek guidance. Fortunately, seminars, workshops, and courses on sexuality and sexual counseling are offered more and more frequently to nurses and physicians.[305-307] Churches and other organizations are sponsoring marriage encounter groups; there are groups that focus on the human potential; and there is an increase in the number of articles in popular, as well as professional, literature calling attention to the fact that human beings are sexual beings throughout the life cycle.[308-309] Anna Freud has enunciated the concept of sexuality that we believe is generally accepted today:

The sexual instincts of man do not suddenly awaken between the thirteenth and fifteenth year, i.e., at puberty, but operate from the outset of the child's development, change gradually from one form to another, progress from one state to another, until at last adult sexual life is achieved as the final result from this long series of developments.*

Sex can be thought of as an appetite gratified only by the coupling of two bodies, or it can be considered a pervasive element in personality development from birth to death. Jeanne D. Fonseca [309a] titles an article "Sexuality—A Quality of Being Human." The latter view is vindicated by the results of sex-modifying glandular therapy and surgery that can completely alter the appearance and behavior of individuals, especially when the treatment is begun at an early age. Changes include attitudes toward both sexes and ways of communicating with all ages. (See Chapters 5 and 47 for further discussion of this subject.)

Sexual drives may be expressed in many ways—not only, or necessarily, by consummation through physical intercourse. On the other hand, sexual attraction without the gratification of intercourse can, of course, be a source of frustration and the underlying cause of unhappiness in human relations. In discussing alcoholism, the impotence of the alcoholic was instanced as one of the underlying causes of divorce and deteriorating family relationships. Health workers who have the broadest knowledge of acceptable and unacceptable sex expression for all ages in different cultures are obviously best prepared to help patients give satisfying expression to sexual

---

* Food can mean love, a sensation, a status symbol, poison, therapy, and health maximizer. To help patients, nurses must know the meaning food has for them.

* Quoted in Sex Information and Education Council of the United States (comps. and eds.): *Sexuality and Man.* Charles Scribner's Sons, New York, 1970, p. 3.

A

Topics*	K	1	2	3	4	5	6	7	8	9	10	11	12
General health	*	*	*										
Health habits				*	*	*	*						
The body													
Structure					*	*	*						
Functions							*	*					
Growth and development							*	*	*	*			
Food and nutrition							*	*					
Weight control							*	*	*				
Exercise and physical education													
Body build						*	*	*	*	*	*	*	*
Skills													
Recreational activities							*	*	*	*	*	*	*
First aid				*	*	*							
Safety													
Mental health													
Self and others							*		*		*		
Fears					*	*	*						
Social-emotional development													
Peers							*	*	*				*
Parents and family							*	*	*	*			
Sex education							*	*	*				*
Reproduction							*	*	*	*			

*From evidence in the data, the above topics seem to be desired at all levels with emphasis where the asterisks are placed.

B

Topics*	K	1	2	3	4	5	6	7	8	9	10	11	12
Babies	*	*	*	*	*	*	*	*					
Puberty							*	*	*				
Personal sex problems							*	*	*		*	*	*
Social problems							*	*	*		*	*	*
Diseases					*			*			*		
Alcohol													
Individual problem						*	*						
Social problem											*		
Drugs													
Individual problem								*					
Social problem											*		
Smoking													
Individual problem					*		*						
Social problem											*		

*These topics seem to be desired, with major emphasis, in the grades indicated.

Figure 16-15. *A.* Health topics of interest to Connecticut school children in every grade with emphasis in particular grades where the need is greatest. *B.* Health interests of Connecticut school children to be taught about in specific grades. (From Byler, Ruth et al.: *Teach Us What We Want to Know.* Mental Health Materials Center, New York, 1969, p. 170.)

drives.* Unless health workers are knowledgeable and comfortable in discussing sexuality, in all forms of its expression, they are very limited in their ability to help patients.

The Sex Information and Education Council of the United States (SIECUS) suggests

that as knowledge and understanding of sex and gender roles increase through research, the term "sexuality" instead of the term "sex" may better indicate "that sex expression is a deep and pervasive aspect of total personality —the sum total of one's feelings and behavior not only as a sexual being, but as a male or a female." * They cite a number of criteria now

* An experienced internist who was asked what explained the great differences in the aging process said, "I don't know but there is one thing that I'm sure keeps people young—interest in the opposite sex."

* Sex Information and Education Council of the United States (comps. and eds.): *op. cit.,* p. 4.

in use to classify individuals as male or female: chromosomal, gonadal, and hormonal sex, internal accessory reproductive structures, external genital structures, sex of assignment and rearing, and gender roles and sexual orientations established while growing up. These criteria may operate independently of one another and create personality conflicts that result in unwanted teenage pregnancies, promiscuity, and marital discord, or in special problems such as transsexualism, homosexuality, rape, and child molestation.

Although it is impossible to discuss here in any detail the various stages or the many elements involved in sexual development, references helpful to the reader are listed at the end of this chapter.[310-316] Nurses, as health teachers, must learn to be comfortable with their own sexuality and aware of the sex information needs and concerns of *adolescents, parents of young children, young adults, the middle-aged,* and *the elderly,* whether they are well or ill.[316a-316e]

The need for sexual activity and sexual gratification in the elderly is often ignored or considered "depraved."[317] However, many older persons believe as a current automobile bumper sticker proclaims, "I'm not a dirty old man, I'm just a sexy senior citizen!" It is, of course, true that sexual deprivation may be experienced more frequently by the elderly than by younger persons since it may result from organic impairment of sexual function, from the loss or absence of a sexually fulfilling personal relationship, or from environmental constraints, such as separation in a nursing home or other institution.[318] However, the presence of any of these circumstances does not negate the importance of the role of sex in old age, and sex counseling is considered as necessary for the aging as for the adolescent. Stanley T. Dean says:

In the final analysis, aging is regarded as a demon that heralds approaching death, whereas sex is equated with life. That is why sexuality is especially significant for an older person's morale; it is an affirmation of life, a denial of death. Even when short of complete fulfillment, there is enough beauty in it to make the journey as well as the destination full of rapture and delight.*

Sexual deprivation is not only a possible problem for the elderly, but may present a problem to the young or middle-aged person. Imprisonment and its effects on sexuality and sexual gratification have only recently been discussed with any openness, and the possibilities of outside visiting privileges for some prisoners explored. Long-term hospitalization, frequent or long separations of married couples because of military or work-related responsibilities, inadequacy of the sexual responses of one or both partners, or severe injury, surgery, or illness may also result in sexual deprivation.[319]

All health workers should know about the various ways in which sexuality is expressed which include *heterosexual* and *homosexual* activities, *masturbation,* and other forms of erotic stimulation. Many expressions of sexuality once thought to be *perversions,* or abnormal manifestations of sex, are now believed by some experts to be universal practices and to represent stages of sexual development.

The literature on sexuality has been extensive for many years and there are volumes on erotic art. Articles in nursing journals on this subject appear with increasing frequence. In 1973, Mary H. Browning and Edith P. Lewis compiled such articles appearing in publications of the American Journal of Nursing Company in a volume titled *Human Sexuality: Nursing Implications.*[319a] The articles are grouped under human sexuality (including "mind-body continuum," masturbation, homosexuality, transsexualism); sex education (emphasizing the role of the nurse, education of young persons); fertility regulation (including family planning, contraceptives, sterilization); abortion (stressing attitudes toward it, legal aspects, administration of abortion services, counseling, methods, preparation of personnel in abortion clinics); and venereal disease (including incidence, types, tests, treatment). In 1975, *The Nursing Clinics of North America* published a "Symposium on Human Sexuality,"[319b] which included articles on education and counseling, human response patterns, "myths" in sexuality, trauma of children and adolescents, sexuality in later life, dysfunction (temporary or permanent) in reversible and irreversible health limitations. These two series provide nurses with a fairly comprehensive review of the topics that can be treated only superficially in a general work such as this.

As health workers and the public learn more about sexuality and sexual expression they will be in a strong position to promote healthy attitudes and activities. They will also be able to give specific help to patients with illnesses or physical handicaps that affect sexual attitudes and activities. Far more research is needed, however, before optimum help can be offered most persons with sexual problems. It is only within the past decade or two, for instance, that the sexual activity potential of spinal cord–injured patients has been given much at-

---

* Stanley T. Dean, quoted in "Those 'Dirty Old Men'—Just Sexy Senior Citizens," *Geriatric Focus,* **12:**1, (July–Aug.) 1973.

tention, and the paraplegic or quadriplegic patient and his or her partner offered help in adjusting to their sexual roles.[320] Before guidance can be given to these couples and specific measures recommended, a basic neurologic examination of the injured person must be made, and the attitudes and beliefs of the couple determined. It hardly seems necessary to say that any guidance must be given to the couple and not to just one partner.

Sexual gratification is a "very delicate problem and one of central importance" for a large number of persons with colostomies or ileostomies, according to Barney M. Dlin and Abraham Perlman.[321] While many physicians and patients assume that such surgery disturbs sexual potency, a 1958 study by LeRoy H. Stahlgren and F. Kraeer Fergusson [322] found that of 25 men studied, 20 considered themselves equally or more sexually capable after their surgery, and 24 of the 26 women in the study felt they were as competent or more competent after surgery. Dlin and Perlman found that the understanding and support given by the spouse of the patient becomes a major factor in the patient's favorable recovery. Masters and Johnson say:

. . . fear of inadequacy is the greatest known deterrent to effective sexual functioning, simply because it so completely distracts the fearful individual from his or her natural responsivity by blocking reception of sexual stimuli either created by or reflected from the sexual partner.*

Nurses in their care and health guidance of ostomy patients must, therefore, give particular attention to helping the marriage partner as well as the patient.

Although patients and their physicians believe that sexual behavior affects and can be affected by medical disorders, there is little factual information about the degree to which or the circumstances under which this is true.[323,324] Charles A. Pinderhughes and his colleagues,[325] in a review of literature on this subject, found general agreement that various aspects of patients' lives, including sexual activity, are affected by nearly all physical or emotional alterations in their being. They also found that if physicians (and presumably nurses) were more fully aware of the known relationships between medical problems and sexual functioning, some patients could be relieved of their self-imposed, medically unnecessary restrictions and others could be helped to adjust to situations where sexual functioning was likely to be adversely affected. It can be

argued, then, that most patients need some sexual counseling, and nurses should develop the ability to create a nurse-patient relationship conducive to a discussion of sex. Development of this ability presupposes, of course, that nurses have a broad and current knowledge of sexual psychology, physiology, and functioning.

Surveys and articles in the literature report an increase in the number of never-married teenagers who have sexual intercourse, an enormous increase in the number of teenage cases of venereal diseases, and a two- to threefold increase in the number of unwanted pregnancies in teenage girls.[326-329] The serious negative consequences of pregnancy to teenage mothers and their infants include (1) higher maternal mortality rates; (2) a higher incidence of the complications of pregnancy; (3) greater risk their infants will be stillborn, die shortly after birth, be premature, or have serious physical or mental handicaps; and (4) greater possibilities that the adolescent mother will develop postpartum psychiatric symptoms. In addition, studies indicate that children born to teenage mothers perform less well on measures of intelligence, while the teenage parents appear to be less effective as parents.[330,331]

Although knowledge about contraception is not the only factor necessary to prevent or avoid pregnancy, it is basic. Howard J. Osofsky and Joy D. Osofsky say:

All too often, professionals have discovered that teenagers of both sexes, who claim to have understanding of their bodies, have information which, if utilized, would result in certain pregnancy unless one or both of the sexual partners were sterile. Many teenagers believe that the safe period occurs halfway between the menses; Saran Wrap condoms and Pepsi Cola douches are commonly used as contraceptives. Their parents, unfortunately, may be no more enlightened.*

Teenagers, themselves, want sex education that is explicit and answers their questions.[332] While few answers to such questions can be given here, some books helpful to adolescents and their parents are listed in the references.[333-335] Parents need help in understanding that sex education in the schools is education concerning bodily functions, and not an attempt to remove responsible social and psychologic restrictions or to proscribe a particular kind of morality.

Some authorities believe that *venereal diseases* are now pandemic in the United States. Increased incidence is attributed to a number

---

* Masters, William H., and Johnson, Virginia E.: *Human Sexual Inadequacy*. Little, Brown & Co., Boston, 1970, p. 12.

* Osofsky, Howard J., and Osofsky, Joy D.: "Let's Be Sensible About Sex Education," *Am. J. Nurs.*, 71:532, (Mar.) 1971.

of causes, among them the following: sexual intimacies, romantic notions of the desirability of spontaneous intercourse, the widespread use of oral contraceptives instead of condoms, a false sense of security about the efficiency of antibiotics for treatment, breakdown of the family unit, and increased mobility.[336] Surprisingly, surveys of high school students show that although information gaps exist, their knowledge of venereal disease is much better than their knowledge of sex in general.[337,338] It has been suggested that greater emphasis on venereal diseases as communicable rather than social diseases may be helpful in encouraging infected persons of any age to have early treatment. Nurses in public health agencies, schools, college health centers, in industries, doctor's offices, and in penal institutions should take advantage of the many opportunities they

have to teach and counsel any patient, his or her contacts, and the families about venereal disease.[339-341] (See also Chapter 44.)

Recently, health education that encourages greater *participation of the public in health care* has been stressed. For example, Robert R. Huntley and Keith W. Sehnert of the Georgetown University Community Health Plan describe to reporters Arlene and Howard Eisenberg [342] a patient education program in which adults are being taught to use stethoscopes, sphygmomanometers, and otoscopes; to take vital signs; what to do in emergencies; the symptoms of minor illnesses and what to do for them (see Fig. 16-16A–B). Harvey P. Katz and Robert R. Clancy [343] describe a successful program in which mothers learn to take cultures from their children's sore throats so that streptococcal infections can be diagnosed early,

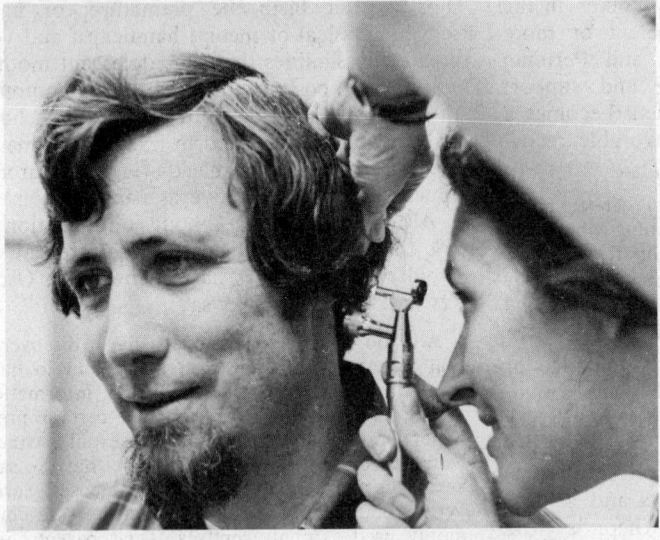

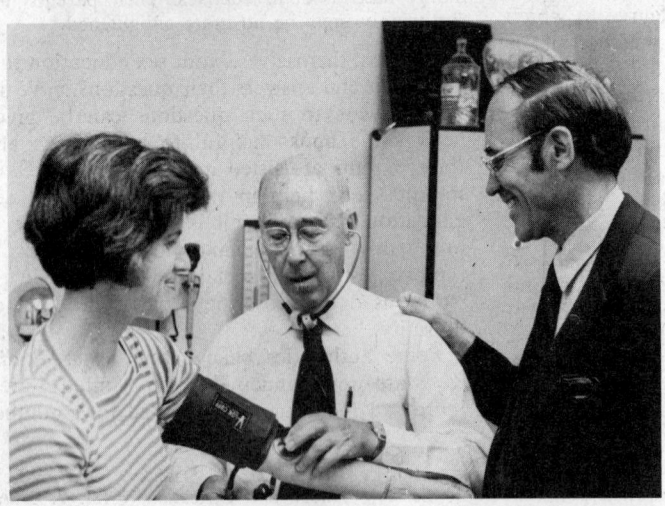

Figure 16-16. *A*. Husband and wife learning to use an otoscope in self-help preventive medical care. *B*. Learning to take the blood pressure for self-help preventive medical care. (Courtesy of Georgetown University Community Health Plan, Washington, D.C.)

and Louis H. Black and Donald D. Brown [344] report a study in which an intensive educational effort by nurses and physicians was made for one year to inform citizens of the early symptoms of myocardial infarction. Attention was called in Chapters 2 and 3 to the high level of citizen participation in health care in the U.S.S.R. and the People's Republic of China.

Other professional health workers are studying more intensively the characteristics of adults who seek out health information, as well as the characteristics of the communication media that convey the information. For instance, one study found that white women college graduates, as a group, are more likely to read health information than to listen to it, and have more information about major diseases than do other groups.[345]

Responsibility of Nurses for Health Guidance. Nurse leaders throughout the life of professional nursing have emphasized teaching, or health guidance, as an inherent aspect of nurses' work. Although many social institutions with their specific professionally skilled workers help others change and move toward Maslow's concept of "self-actualization," nurses are in a particularly advantageous position to do so. They have frequent chances to teach persons who are healthy, those called by some the "worried well," and those whose health has been impaired or depleted. Unfortunately, recent reports indicate that many nurses do not take the responsibility, nor recognize their opportunities, for giving health guidance. In addition, much of the health guidance by nurses is inadequate.[346-348] Jan Robinson [349] found that only 46 per cent of a group of 300 new mothers had been given advice about feeding their new infants before they were discharged from the hospital, and when teaching was done only 40 per cent of the essential information about feeding was included. Vivian Vreeland Clark [350] reported that 52 patients with coronary occlusions were given only 44 per cent of the information they needed about their illness and self-care, and almost all of that was given by the physician. In Chapter 21 attention is called to the studies of Doris Schwartz [350a] showing the woeful inadequacy of guidance in the use of drugs. Teaching is undoubtedly a complex, difficult task, but it appears that nurses must increase the time, effort, and thought they devote to it.[351-358]

To define the nurse's responsibility for health teaching is difficult. Attention has frequently been called to the overlapping of the functions of health workers. There is as much confusion about their teaching activities as there is in distinguishing between nursing procedures, medical treatments, and the appropriate activities of social workers, physical therapists, and health educators.

The hygienic care of patients and the home care of the sick are the particular responsibility of nurses, although a disability may make any ordinary daily activity so difficult that patients will need the combined efforts of a rehabilitation team to solve the problem. Nurses through their teaching may help patients to organize and maintain a healthful environment when it is obvious that they need and want such help. Nurses should be able to give such patients accurate information about matters of personal cleanliness and habits of elimination; they may help others to select and prepare normal diets; still others with habits of sleep, rest, and exercise and problems of mental hygiene related to these questions. They should also be able to give advice in getting competent medical care and in making use of the health services in the community. Nurses should be able to recognize and give some guidance to the psychologic or emotional aspects of all these questions. They must be able to differentiate between a deep-seated and serious disturbance that is interfering with appetite or sleep, for example, and one less serious that the patient may be easily helped to recognize. In psychotherapy the nurse is one member of a team with a common plan for the patient.

Because the science of healthful living is developing so rapidly, there is rarely a final answer to any problem. Nurses are of greatest service to patients when they help to arouse their interest, guide their study, and then develop health practices based on the knowledge and insight they have acquired.

During their care of patients questions such as the following will come up which nurses should refer to the physician: questions related to the physician's reasons for employing the prescribed therapeutic measures; the significance of symptoms; and the probability of recovery. Physicians usually prefer to explain the purpose of the prescribed treatment to their patients. They are certainly the best interpreters of this as they are best fitted to discuss the causes of pain and other symptoms of disease. However, under some circumstances, physicians may ask nurses to interpret the prescribed treatment or to amplify their directions. Whenever they act as the agent of a particular physician, nurses should be certain that they comply with his or her wishes and that their interpretation is similar to the physician's. If nurses believe that physicians are dangerously misinformed or incompetent, they cannot conscientiously assume the responsibility of carrying out their wishes, and will not be willing to act for them.

Rules, however, must never take the place of reason or common sense, and although these general principles may be used to help nurses in the practice of health guidance, occasions will undoubtedly arise when, as in emergencies, they may find it necessary to assume some of the functions of the physician or other medical specialist. As pointed out in many parts of this book and most specifically in Chapters 1, 3, and 5, nurses and other health workers are now assuming more and more diagnostic and therapeutic responsibilities for individual patients and groups of patients in many countries.

Student nurses need a great deal of help in dealing with patients' questions. They must learn which they should be able to discuss, which should be referred to an experienced nurse, and which should be referred to a physician. Student nurses should be encouraged to talk about these problems with instructors capable of making constructive criticism of the way in which a teaching opportunity is handled. Students profit by listening to conferences between patients and graduate nurses who can teach effectively. Afterward, students and graduates should discuss the experience. Throughout their period of preparation for nursing, students need as much help with the health guidance they give as with the manual skills they use in the care of the sick.

Nurse Qualifications for Health Guidance. Nurses who offer effective health guidance or counseling are constantly aware that the *relationships between teacher and learner* are very important. Just as in communicating therapeutically, teaching effectively requires that nurses recognize and understand their own attitudes, values, and perceptions. It requires them to see patients and their families as persons worthy of respect, with the right to know what is being done to and for them, with the ability to learn and change, and with the desire to make the best possible use of their capabilities and potentialities. It seems self-evident that helping others to learn about health and disease also means that nurses must have a thorough knowledge of the health sciences, an understanding of the patient's goals and the plans made with the patient by all health workers concerned. All those giving health guidance should have an understanding of the environment in which the patient and family live. Nurses should know as much as they can about motivation and the ways that people of all ages learn; they should know where to find and make use of the many learning aids that are available; and constantly look for and use opportunities for teaching health. In countries that have most successfully raised the level of health knowledge, health practice, and population stabilization, there has been a coordinated program in which health workers collaborated with economists, legislators, educators, and consumers, or representatives of the community.

Although nurses often think of teaching as just giving information or as a well-organized, logical (at least to the teacher), formal exposition of a subject, in actuality, *nurses are almost constantly teaching.* It may be through their verbal responses to the questions, comments, or actions of patients, or through nonverbal communication. What patients, coworkers, or students learn from nurses is often quite different from what the latter intended. But whether or not nurses feel qualified or like teaching it is *inherent in nursing* and makes health guidance an obligation.

Settings and Opportunities for Health Guidance. Because health teaching is such an integral part of health care, wherever and whenever it is offered patients should be learning. However, the purpose of the agency or institution, the commitment of the administration to health promotion, and the space available for individual or group teaching will influence what nurses teach and how they accomplish it.[359-361] Chapter 3 discusses the settings in which nurses work. It is impossible to describe every setting or every teaching opportunity nurses have, but the following are some examples.

Public health agencies and visiting or district nurse associations maintain clinics and give home nursing advice or care to persons who are not acutely or critically ill. Since these patients are, as a rule, assuming responsibility for managing their own health problems, their need for guidance is apparent. There are some well-established *clinics* focusing on the maternity cycle, the care of infants, and the problems of parenthood; other clinics of this nature are of recent origin.

In classes for expectant parents, the process of reproduction is explained and problems of mental and physical hygiene during pregnancy and the care of the newborn are discussed. Where natural childbirth is stressed, the teaching program is especially thorough and includes explanation of the process, special exercises designed to help the woman and her husband prepare for labor and delivery. Many husbands are learning to help their wives during labor and to play a helping role during the delivery.[361a] Findings of studies indicate that this "family" involvement leads to more combined decision-making and less uncertainty about the process of childbearing.[362]

Individual instruction is given patients according to their particular needs. Opportunities are made for conferences with health workers at regular intervals. Advisers try to uncover the fears so common during pregnancy. Often these fears are groundless and disappear if given expression or if shown to be without basis. Even when there is some cause for anxiety, the patient is relieved by knowing the best way to face it and by realizing that the health workers recognize that the danger exists and are prepared to give the assistance required. Many patients have physical difficulties, such as varicose veins, and need instruction in relation to treatment by posture and the elimination of tight clothing; others have abdominal discomfort, and benefit from advice on the selection and adjustment of supports. Nutrition, rest, exercise, elimination, personal hygiene, sexual intercourse during pregnancy, and other problems are also discussed.[363,364] The incidence of eclampsia and other complications of pregnancy is greatly reduced by teaching women the danger signs and symptoms and the importance of early treatment.

Pregnant teenagers, whether married or unmarried, present a special challenge for health teaching.[365-367] Most of them have not yet completed their own physical (to say nothing of the psychologic) growth and development, but must, nevertheless, be concerned about the growth of another. Physicians, nurses, social workers, and other health personnel in clinics and schools often work with teachers and counselors in helping these young mothers. Lucille Davis and Helen Grace put the goals in helping them in the following terms:

. . . enhance the girl's physical and emotional development during this time of stress, increase her understanding of her own body and that of the baby, and prepare her emotionally, physically, and pragmatically for the motherhood role.*

Unfortunately we have found no evidence that help is available for the teenage expectant father or that his physical and emotional needs in the role of married or unmarried fatherhood have been studied.[368,369]

During prenatal classes, in clinics or elsewhere, in the hospital postpartum units, or in the home, nurses teach mothers how to prepare the baby's formula, including handling of the food, bottles, and nipples. When the mother is able to nurse the infant, the nurse shows her how to keep the breasts clean; discusses the value of breast feeding from the emotional and physical standpoints; and helps her to overcome any difficulties in nursing (see Fig. 16-17). Later, if there are problems in the child's eating habits, the nurse may be called upon to help the parents identify the causes, help them to understand their own or the child's difficulties, and to overcome them. Some feeding difficulties, however, are the result of such deep emotional disturbance in the mother that the psychiatrist's help may be needed. Infants' baths are often demonstrated to the parents in the hospital and home, and they practice this procedure with the nurse present to help them if necessary. The equipment for the care of the baby may be selected and the room in which the baby sleeps arranged after consultation with the nurse.

Other health guidance that is offered by nurses in *well-child clinics* concerns the value of and schedule for immunizations against various communicable diseases*; anticipatory guidance in normal growth and development; and counseling and guidance for problems encountered on a daily basis by families of growing children. Such clinics should offer new mothers the kind of help that gives them a growing confidence and a feeling that their needs as well as those of the child are recognized and respected.

The apparently high incidence of *neglected, sexually or otherwise abused children* should be of concern to all nurses, and particularly to those who work with mothers and children.[370-373] There are multiple factors involved in this problem, such as family emotional and financial stresses related to unemployment or poverty, and a cultural pattern of "an ample measure of physical violence inflicted upon children in their homes, in schools, in child care facilities, and in various children's institutions." †

---

* Childhood communicable diseases as major health problems in highly developed countries are no longer as life-threatening as they once were. Programs for prevention, research into the development of new vaccines, and an informed population have decreased the incidence of these diseases. The role of community health nurses still involves casefinding and education, but is almost completely focused on prevention. In many underdeveloped countries lacking health care resources, or where the culture or understanding of the people places little value on preventive immunization, however, communicable diseases are still major problems. Obviously, nurses working in such countries need a different orientation to nursing and its health teaching responsibilities than they do when working in developed countries.

† Gil, David G.: "Violence Against Children," *J. Marr. Fam.*, 33:637, (Nov.) 1971.

* Davis, Lucille, and Grace, Helen: "Anticipatory Counseling of Unwed Pregnant Adolescents," *Nurs. Clin. North Am.*, 6:581, (Dec.) 1971.

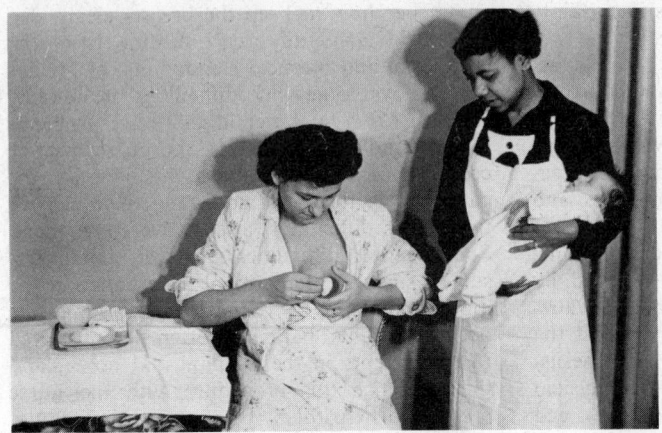

Figure 16-17. Nurse teaching mother breast care. (Courtesy of Visiting Nurse Association of Brooklyn, Brooklyn, N.Y. and Clay-Adams Co., New York, N.Y.

Researchers might, however, agree with John J. Spinetta and David Rigler who make the following statement:

. . . abusing parents lack appropriate knowledge of child rearing, and . . . their attitudes, expectations, and child rearing techniques set them apart from nonabusive parents. The abusing parents implement culturally accepted norms for raising children with an exaggerated intensity and at an inappropriately early age.*

School nurses and maternity and well-baby clinic nurses all have responsibility for teaching teenagers and parents about child and family development and helping them to understand the continuing effort and attention-giving that parenthood requires.[374,375] Parents who are violent with their children are often addicted to alcohol or other drugs (alcohol is sometimes called a "family disease"). Child abusers are emotionally disturbed to some degree and need help. There are special programs for such persons and self-help organizations for abusive parents are listed in the Appendix.

It is only within the recent past that *family planning clinics* have been available to a majority of women in the United States and other developed nations. Health teaching and guidance is a major emphasis of the nursing care offered in these clinics. Since many of the neglected and abused children come from large families, nurses who work with family planning can make a significant impact on this problem through health teaching.[376,376a] Overpopulation is so serious a problem worldwide that many countries, through health programs, are trying to reduce or stabilize their birth rates. Nurses give guidance to women and teenage girls about various contraceptive methods such as using the rhythm method, the "pill," intrauterine devices (IUDs), the diaphragm, and gels and foams. They may counsel men and their wives about the advantages and disadvantages of vasectomies.* Nurses in family planning clinics may also teach teenagers and others about venereal disease. They, as well as other informed nurses, should be able to advise marital partners so they will find greater sexual fulfillment in their marriage. These are sensitive and difficult matters for most persons to discuss and the attitude of nurses toward them and a broad and up-to-date store of knowledge are of prime importance.[377-381]

Genetic counseling clinics are of fairly recent origin although at least one was established in England as early as 1946.[382] There are approximately 300 such clinics in the United States and most are associated with large medical centers where genetic research is in progress. Many parents coming to these clinics are facing severe emotional problems that may interfere with understanding what the physician tells them. It may be the responsibility of nurses to make certain that the parents understand the information given about the risks of subsequent pregnancies and that they have the information they need and want about contraception.[383-386]

Health workers in *medical, surgical, and psychiatric clinics*, whether the clinic's primary purpose is supervisory, diagnostic, or therapeutic, usually realize that the weekly or monthly service they give patients will not affect their health nearly so much as the daily

* Spinetta, John J., and Rigler, David: "The Child Abusing Parent: A Psychological Review," *Psychol. Bull.,* 77:296, (Apr.) 1972.

* Tying the fallopian tubes in women is rarely recommended as a method of contraception. This is a major operation with all its dangers and there are many safer methods for women to use.

care they give themselves. Health workers in clinics understand that their chief service to patients is the help they give them in working out a regimen that they can carry out. The continued well-being of diabetic patients, for example, depends almost entirely on the understanding they have of their condition and the steps they must take to control it. Physicians, nurses, dietitians, and social workers may all participate in teaching individuals, or groups of diabetics. The physician ordinarily explains the physiology, the significance of the symptoms, and the prescribed treatment, which may be diet alone or a combination of diet and insulin. The dietitian may show patients how to calculate, plan, and prepare their diets,[387] and the social worker may help patients get financial assistance for needed insulin or foods. Nurses often must clarify patients' and families' understanding of the information given them. They must often teach patients and families how to test urine for the presence of sugar, to administer insulin when it is a part of the treatment, to give proper attention to the care of skin, nails, and feet, to be aware that exercise may change their insulin needs, and to recognize the symptoms of insulin shock. Nurses often recommend steps that should be taken to prevent colds or other illnesses. Teenage diabetic patients present a particular challenge to nurses for they must help them resolve the problems of normal adolescent rebellion while developing a good, consistent diabetic regimen. The teaching of any diabetic patient should always involve the family since their understanding of what the diabetic faces from this time forward is essential to his or her daily regimen.[388-392]

It is unusual to find any patient attending a therapeutic clinic who does not need or would not profit by some sort of instruction. There are few if any cases in which a patient should be kept in ignorance of his or her condition. Patients, including health workers when they are sick, are more and more insistent that they be told exactly what is wrong and that they be given some choice, if there is a possible choice, in treatment. Although much of this teaching is done by the physician, the cooperation of the nurse is usually essential. When nurses are aware of and make use of the opportunities a clinic affords for teaching, this is their most important service.

When patients are in a hospital or nursing home, however, they assume less responsibility for their own care since the care they require is provided by the staff. Unfortunately, nurses and doctors may lose sight of what will happen to patients after they leave. This failure to recognize the patients' need of assistance in the period following their discharge from the hospital or nursing home results in many incomplete cures and unnecessary complications during convalescence. There is a growing recognition of the importance of discovering how much and what kind of assistance the person should have, and of providing as much of this as possible while the patient is in the institution where doctors and nurses are available to teach the fundamentals of nursing and medical care needed in each case. Although it is possible for patients to learn a good deal simply by being in a health care institution, observing its operation, and asking questions, planned programs of guidance for each patient should be more highly developed. The necessity for cooperation among health workers is as important here as in any other part of the patient's program of care.

Some hospitals, nursing homes, and hospices have community liaison nurses who may refer discharged patients to visiting or district nurse agencies for follow-up health teaching, or who may, themselves, extend the institutionally initiated teaching to the home. For orthopedic or neurologic conditions, nurses may show the patient and the family how to maintain prescribed postures in lying, standing, or sitting; they may be asked by the physician to teach the mother of a sick child corrective manipulation and massage; they can often help in the arrangement of the room and in the provision of facilities for moving the patients about so that their lives will be more nearly normal. Unless there is a physical therapist and an occupational therapist in attendance, nurses must to some extent fulfill the functions of both of these specialists. Most health agencies employ such specialists who advise nurses.

Nurses who visit in the home often help cardiac patients work out a plan for regulating the daily regimen in accordance with their condition. They are taught the importance of limiting exercise, of resting at well-spaced intervals, and of eating frequent simple and light meals. In some cases they are encouraged to cultivate occupations that do not make too great a demand on their strength.

Patients with chronic respiratory disease, whether an adult with emphysema or a child with cystic fibrosis, usually need assistance finding, using, and perhaps adapting to the home special equipment to relieve respiratory distress. In addition, they may need advice on effective ways of alternating exercise and rest.

Patients with colostomies, ileostomies, or indwelling catheters are often taught while in the hospital how to care for themselves at home. However, they may need considerable guidance from a visiting nurse in adapting what they learned to the home setting. No matter how vivid the patient's description is of his or her home conditions, nurses in the hospital cannot visualize them very well, and usually are unable to incorporate these variations into their teaching.*

Besides the problems involved in the physical care of patients, there are the many and varied mental adjustments to be made by the person who is sick and by members of the family. The depression, the sense of futility, the nervousness or irritability that often accompany illness may be more difficult to deal with than the physical limitations imposed by disease. Nurses may be able to do nothing more than listen sympathetically, but in many cases, if they are skillful, they can relieve the patient's discouragement or irritation by helping him or her to understand the source of it and to substitute constructive for destructive ideas.

Few personnel are as well prepared to give psychiatric guidance as they are to help those with physical problems. The great need for a general knowledge of the emotional components of health and illness has been stressed throughout this text. It has been pointed out that mind and body cannot be separated and that in every illness there are psychic problems. Attention has been called to a number of studies showing that approximately half the persons who apply to medical clinics have conditions caused by emotional stress.

Nurses of *occupational health services* who interpret their functions broadly are health counselors to management and labor. Occupational health services function as clinics, but since the physician is rarely present full time, the nurse carries a particularly heavy burden of responsibility. In the United States, since the passage of the Occupational Safety and Health Act of 1970,[383] nurses in industry are taking on new health guidance responsibilities. Some have instituted home visiting for employees who have been hospitalized or who request a home visit for any one of a variety of reasons; others have instituted programs to help the alcoholic worker; while still others have developed programs to increase the flow of information from employer/employee to referral agencies back to employer/employee.[394-396] (See also Chapters 3 and 21.) Although many occupational health nurses concern themselves only with the sick or injured employees of the company for which they work, they have the opportunity to offer preventive health guidance and, perhaps, to help establish well-adult clinic programs. In some countries occupational health has been upgraded with different systems. (See Chapter 3 for some discussion of the roles of feldshers in the U.S.S.R. and indigenous workers in the People's Republic of China.)

In *school health services* the nurses work with the physician, helping with periodic examination and inspection; they give first aid and teach the protection of wounds from infection, and the importance of treatment of colds and other mild diseases. Since they are usually responsible for testing the students' vision and hearing at regular intervals, and for notifying the parents when abnormalities are found, school nurses have many opportunities for health guidance (see Fig. 16-18). Some school nurses make home visits to children who have a school-discovered health problem or children who are frequently absent from school because of illness. In some school systems nurses teach health courses, in others they are responsible for "rap" sessions about drug abuse or other subjects, and in still others they take part in programs for pregnant teenagers.[397-402]

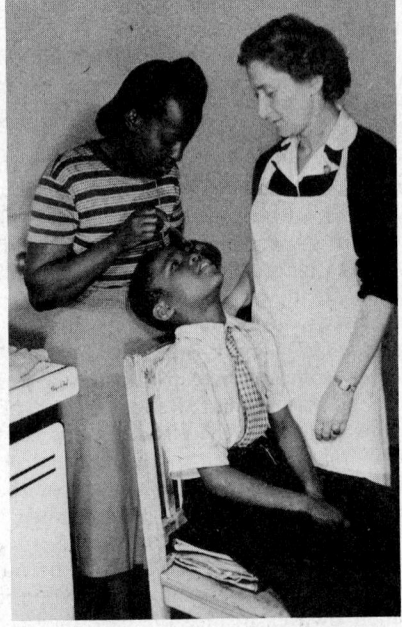

Figure 16-18. Instruction in eye care of a school child. (Courtesy of Visiting Nurse Association of Brooklyn, Brooklyn, N.Y., and Clay-Adams Co., New York, N.Y.)

---

* Some hospitals have such effective home care programs that health personnel in hospitals can make home visits. In some hospitals there are branch offices of visiting nurse agencies that facilitate continuity of care for ostomy patients and many others for whom it is so important.

In *college health services* nurses do not always take advantage of the opportunities they have to give health guidance. In one survey it was found that 50 per cent of the students preferred to rely on self-diagnosis and self-treatment and one-third of the students never used the health service.[403] Studies have also shown that college students have faulty and inadequate information about sexuality, birth control, pregnancy, and appropriate ways of managing emotional tensions. The need for health guidance for college students is apparent.[404-406]

In Chapter 3 *health services in correctional institutions* are discussed briefly. It was pointed out that from all accounts found they are woefully inadequate. If it is assumed that criminal conduct is a form of sick, or warped, behavior, the need is for reeducation rather than incarceration of those exhibiting antisocial behavior. Nurses, especially pediatric and psychiatric nurses, could play an important teaching role in prison health services if and when they are based on the assumption that people can learn to be law-abiding—to want to be law-abiding. And since the populations of correctional institutions have as many, if not more, physical problems than the general population, nurses in their health services have as many opportunities for general health teaching as do nurses in schools and colleges, hospitals, and other settings.

Planning for Health Guidance. Planning is as much a requirement for the incidental health teaching that goes with answering a patient's questions as it is for more formalized teaching such as demonstrating infant care to new mothers. All patients should have health learning needs thoughtfully provided for in their nursing care plans so that they are not overlooked. Learning needs of critically ill patients may have a low priority in the early phases of hospitalization but are increasingly important as they assume more responsibility for self-care.[406a] On the other hand, the learning needs of mothers attending well-baby clinics are usually the most important aspect of their care and have the highest priority from the beginning.

The *nurse's over-all objectives* for health teaching may be described as helping patients find the information they need, helping them to think through steps in solving a particular health problem, or helping them to be aware of alternative courses of action.[407-409] In the final analysis it is the patient who must make the decision to use any health worker's guidance and to change his or her health practices.

In order for nurses to prepare a plan to help patients learn, they must have *informa-tion about the patients:* their prior knowledge, their age and educational level, their cultural background, their occupation, their place in the family group, the language they speak, are among the essential kinds of information. With these basic facts as a starting point, nurses and patients together can determine what help they need; what skills may have to be learned; what, if any, changes in the home environment should be made; and how these can be achieved. In other words, patients and health workers together decide what *the patient's unique learning goals or objectives* should be.

Communication between a patient and nurse or any health worker is difficult when they have different goals. Raymond S. Duff and August B. Hollingshead,[409a] in a study of patient care on the medical and surgical units of a medical center in the eastern United States, noted how common it was for a patient to be treated for something that did not concern him or her, while the health problem that did worry them was ignored. Patients who resist regimens planned for them by others are often said to be "uncooperative," sometimes "unpopular" or "difficult."[409b] While, from the patient's standpoint, caretakers may seem all these things, the expression "an uncooperative doctor" or "an uncooperative nurse" would have a strange ring in most countries and would undoubtedly arouse resentment.

Some generalizations can be made about the kinds of information patients want. Joan S. Dodge[410] found from an analysis of 116 interviews with medical and surgical patients that sex, age, education, and the nature of the illness, whether short- or long-term, affected the information they sought. Patients most wanted information that would let them plan realistically for their immediate and long-range living arrangements, but were also concerned about the cause and possibility of recurrence of illness—in order to prevent it, if possible, Dodge suggests.

Men wanted information that enabled them to judge how their condition and post-hospital need for care would affect their ability to earn a living, while women wanted information that allowed them to maintain their role of family health protector. Young patients were most interested in their day-to-day progress and the time when "subgoals" of improvement would be reached; middle-aged patients wanted information about the extent or complexity of their illness and the ways that their daily living habits might be modified by it; and older patients were interested in many of the details of their care, but showed little concern about the total time that would be involved.

Dodge also found that poorly educated patients wanted information that was relatively nontechnical and that stressed the personal, emotional aspects of their illness. High school graduates were concerned with knowing the details of their care; and the patients with the most education sought information that could be integrated with their own knowledge and used in reaching their own conclusions.

Once the patient and health workers have identified goals to be reached, nurses are responsible for *determining the methods* and finding the resources that they can use in helping patients learn what they need to know or to learn the skills they will need. The most common, but not necessarily the best, method of teaching is through speech. Nurses often assume if they *tell* patients what they are to do, the kind of diet that is most nutritious, the dangers of smoking, or the consequences of not having their children immunized, that learning occurs, and that, subsequently, patients eat a good diet, stop smoking, and have their children immunized. As Catherine M. Norris [411] points out, however, knowledge about good health practice does not necessarily translate into appropriate behavior. (Readers may be able to give examples from their own behavior where they "know better" but find it hard to "do better.") This is not to say that patients should not be given health information, but only that giving or having information does not mean that health practices improve accordingly.

If nurses view the "telling" aspects of health teaching and guidance as *persuasion,* it may help them see their patient-teaching function in a somewhat different light. Television advertisers and politicians are famous (or infamous) for their persuasive techniques. Psychologists, as well as other social scientists, frequently study persuasion in an effort to understand why people behave the way they do, and why they change their behavior. William J. McGuire [412] says there are six steps a person must go through before he or she is persuaded to adopt some new attitude or action: (1) the information must be presented; (2) the persons being persuaded must pay attention to the message; (3) they must understand it; (4) agree with it, at least verbally; (5) retain it for future use; and finally (6) they must act on it.

In health teaching, fear is a common condition played on in gaining people's attention and persuading them to adopt a particular health goal. Studies indicate that it sometimes accomplishes this goal, but when too much fear is aroused, anxiety, hostility, and noncompliance are the frequent reactions.[413] Observations on the health behavior of United States citizens leads to the suspicion that fear-arousing messages have a short-term effect, but are relatively useless in the long run. Although regular physical examinations and self-performed breast examinations have been advocated by health professionals for decades, it was only after breast cancer was found in the wives of both the President and Vice-President of the United States that physicians, clinics, and hospitals in this country were inundated with women seeking breast examinations. Nurses, then, who are trying to encourage certain health regimens should be cautious in using fear-arousing tactics to persuade others.

It seems obvious that in order for a message to be persuasive it must be understood. However, physicians and nurses are often hurried and unaware that the language they use is incomprehensible to patients or that they are giving too much information at one time. The following statements made by a number of investigators may be useful to nurses who are trying to increase patients' understanding.[414-418] (1) The more medical knowledge a patient has, the better he or she understands and remembers the information being given. (2) The number of facts or instructions given at one time should be limited. (3) The information is understood and remembered better if arranged in categories, such as "this is how you take the medicine," and "this is how the medication will act." (4) The most important information should be given first because early statements of a series are the best remembered. (5) Important instructions or information should be repeated since anxiety levels may interfere with both hearing and remembering them. (6) Written materials that patients may take or keep with them act as reminders about the information given; however, nurses should bear in mind that many patients cannot profit from written health materials because they have little or no reading ability. (7) There is some evidence that learning is increased when nurses tell patients they are going to "teach" and ask the patients to be temporary "students." (8) Patients are more likely to understand, accept, and follow through on suggestions given by health personnel they like, and with whom they have good relationships. For this reason the use of indigenous health workers is advocated for some patient populations. The assumptions are that similarity of background and experience allows workers to relate more easily with those who are essentially their neighbors, and that workers can perceive the problems of patients most accurately under such conditions. While studies have shown that indigenous workers do perceive local problems and predict their neighbors' attitudes and perceptions better than do the workers from another culture. they were less effective in actually changing their neighbors' attitudes or behavior than was expected. [419-421]

Demonstrations of skills patients may need for self-help of any kind are another frequently used teaching method. Since learning is sounder and more lasting when as many of the senses as possible are used along with active mental work, demonstrations followed with practice by patients are especially effective. While nurses usually have a particular way of doing a procedure, there may be many safe and effective methods. If they encourage patients to suggest procedure modifications that fit their own circumstances and still meet the necessary physiologic and hygienic or sterility requirements, patients become mentally involved and are likely to learn with more ease. Supervised practice not only lets the patient try out the skill, but provides a kinesthetic "memory" of the muscle movements needed to carry it out.*

Most of the nurse's teaching is done with individuals and their families; however, there are many instances when patients receive minimal instruction because health workers cannot or do not find time for teaching individually; under these circumstances *group instruction* may be used. Prenatal classes and infant care classes have been given for many years, but group teaching is now used for many categories of hospitalized patients. Actually there are a number of advantages in group teaching—for instance, participation in group discussion, going to meetings at a designated time and place, and having, usually, a well-prepared teacher with a consistent presentation of the material to be learned. [422-426] In some cases, groups of patients meet without professionals and learn through helping each other. The *self-help* movement is thought by some students of the health scene to be the most significant development of this era. In the Appendix is a list of names and addresses of self-help organizations.

A third frequently used method in health teaching for persons in or out of hospitals is the *lecture-discussion* method. Group meetings for persons with the same or a similar health problem may be arranged with a lecture in the first meeting to give some basic information and later meetings used to ask and answer questions, exchange ideas about solving common problems, and to offer emotional support to one another. Of course, group meetings that do not have a lecture included are also a frequent teaching method.

Nurses may decide to use audiovisual aids such as *movies, filmstrips, or videotapes as resources* for helping a group of patients learn. Other resources for either a group or an individual patient are former patients who have made successful recoveries and lives after a colostomy, ileostomy, mastectomy, amputation, a heart attack, or a stroke. [427] Health literature is an excellent source of information for many persons, and nurses should be able to help any who ask them to find libraries to use and appropriate *books, articles, films, recordings,* or other learning materials in health science libraries. [428]

Communication technology is being used increasingly by health care agencies to improve health teaching [429] (see Fig. 16-19). Many agencies and institutions are using commercially prepared slides and tapes to teach patients. In some cases institutions prepare their own. [430,431] For example, the Texas Institute for Rehabilitation and Research in Houston has developed a learning packet for patients who require frequent catheterizations because of paralysis. The packet consists of a filmstrip and tape cassette that visually and aurally explains the equipment and procedure. The packet also contains a programmed learning booklet and samples of the equipment to be used. Patients and families can use this learning material together as often as they wish after the initial demonstration by nurses. In the same institution, Polaroid pictures are taken of patients in various positions, on their sides, back, and abdomen. These snapshots are attached to the wall near the patient's bed so that family members or other health workers can use them as guides when changing the patient's position. They can also be taken home as continual references when the patient is discharged.*

Closed circuit television systems are used in some hospitals not only for in-service education, but for patient education. Programs are developed and videotaped to help patients learn about their care in the hospital and at home, and also to explain Medicare, hospitalization insurance, billing procedures, and the operation of various hospital departments, such as housekeeping and dietary. [432-432b] Marjorie H. Bartlett and her associates describe a program in Madison, Wisc., hospitals where

---

* There is a saying all teachers should take to heart: "We forget what we hear, we understand what we see, we know what we do,"—in other words, experience is the best teacher.

* Personal communication from Sudie A. Cornell, Texas Institute for Rehabilitation and Research, Houston.

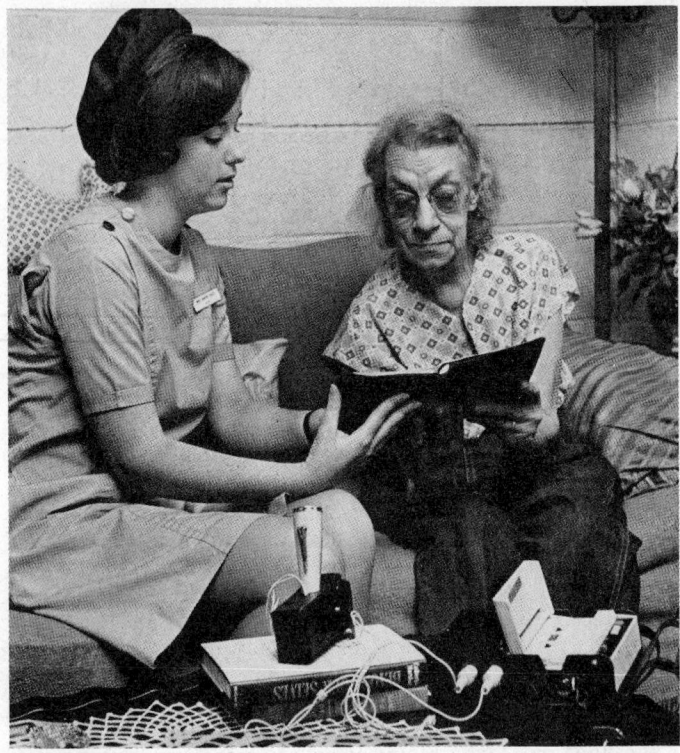

Figure 16-19. Student nurse using tape recorder during a patient interview as a means of reviewing and improving her communication skill. (From Smith, Virginia Whitmore: "I Can't Believe I Said That!" *Nurs. Outlook,* **18:**50, [May] 1970.)

patients may use hospital telephones to get information they need through a "Dial Access Library." [433]

Television is being used on a broad scale to disseminate health information. Although we cannot cite studies that have tested the effectiveness of this kind of health teaching, many believe it to be effective. The Children's Television Workshop has produced for adults a series of programs, called *Feeling Good,* that cover a variety of topics, as, for example, mental health, dental hygiene, nutrition, alcoholism, and hypertension. The increasing sophistication of patients is attributed by many to the public's exposure to health education over television.

In summary, it can be said there is an increasing tendency to put more responsibility for the practice of health upon health-care consumers, to encourage them to participate in planning for health practices, and to make them independent through health instruction. Because nurses and physicians are health advisers, teaching is unavoidable for them. Patients constantly ask questions, and the nurse as well as the physician should strive to give accurate information and adequate help. One of the commonest criticisms of members of the health professions is that they so often give equivocal answers or vague and incomplete explanations and fail to take the responsibility

for the patient's rehabilitation through adequate instruction. And far too often they fail to give written instructions.

Nurses must learn to distinguish between matters on which they can advise patients and those that they must refer to other health workers, to sense situations in which their help is needed and welcome. Nurses can do harm by injudicious teaching, just as they can fail to do good by neglecting legitimate opportunities. Wherever they practice nursing— in the home, hospitals, clinics, schools, industrial plants, correctional institutions—nurses are teaching directly or indirectly, consciously or unconsciously. When nurses recognize teaching as one of their major functions, they will be more concerned about preparing themselves to teach effectively.

REFERENCES

1. Cherry, Colin: *On Human Communication,* 2nd ed. M.I.T. Press, Cambridge, Mass., 1966, p. 3.
1a. Gould, Grace Thersa: "Symposium on Compassion and Communication in Nursing," *Nurs. Clin. North Am.,* **4:**651, (Dec.) 1969.
1b. Wu, Ruth: *Behavior and Illness.* Prentice-Hall, Inc., Englewood Cliffs, N.J., 1973.
1c. Kogan, Benjamin A.: *Health: Man in a*

Changing Environment. Harcourt, Brace & World, New York, 1970.

1d. Rohan, V.: "Be a Human Being to Those You Deal With," *Austr. Nurses J.,* **2**:11, (Aug.) 1973.

2. Topoff, Howard R.: "The Social Behavior of Army Ants," *Sci. Am.,* **227**:71, (Nov.) 1972.

3. Wilson, Edward O.: "Animal Communication," *Sci. Am.,* **227**:53, (Sept.) 1972.

4. Marler, Peter: "Speech Development and Bird Song: Are There Any Parallels?" in Miller, George A. (ed.): *Communication, Language, and Meaning.* Basic Books, New York, 1973, p. 73.

5. Wood, Forrest G.: *Marine Mammals and Man.* Robert B. Luce, Inc., New York, 1973.

6. Lilly, John Cunningham: *The Mind of the Dolphin.* Avon Books, New York, 1967.

7. Fichtelius, Karl-Erik, and Sjölander, Sverre: *Smarter Than Man? Intelligence in Whales, Dolphins, and Humans.* Pantheon Books, New York, 1972.

8. Premack, Ann James, and Premack, David: "Teaching Language to an Ape," *Sci. Am.,* **227**:92, (Oct.) 1972.

9. *Ibid.*

10. Rumbaugh, Duane M., et al.: "Reading and Sentence Completion by a Chimpanzee," *Science,* **182**:731, (Nov. 16) 1973.

11. Colby, Kenneth Mark, and Smith, David Canfield: "Computers in the Treatment of Nonspeaking Autistic Children," *Curr. Psychiatr. Ther.,* **11**:1, 1971.

11a. Kogan, Benjamin A.: *op. cit.,* p. 318.

12. Shannon, Claude E., and Weaver, Warren: *The Mathematical Theory of Communication.* University of Illinois Press, Urbana, 1959.

13. Wiener, Norbert: *Cybernetics or Control and Communication.* M.I.T. Press, Cambridge, Mass., 1961.

14. Birdwhistle, Ray L.: *Kinesics and Context.* University of Pennsylvania Press, Philadelphia, 1970, p. 70.

15. Burr, Harold Saxton: *The Fields of Life.* Ballantine Books, New York, 1973.

16. Ullman, Montague, et al.: *Dream Telepathy: An Experimental Odyssey.* Macmillan Publishing Co., Inc., New York, 1973.

17. Bois, J. Samuel: *The Art of Awareness,* 2nd ed. Wm. C. Brown Co., Dubuque, Iowa, 1973.

18. Cage, John: *Silence.* Wesleyan University Press, Middletown, Conn., 1961.

19. Singer, Jerome L.: "Daydreaming and the Stress of Thought," *Am. Sci.,* **62**:417, (July–Aug.) 1974.

20. Wilhelm, Richard, and Baynes, Cary F. (trans.): *The I Ching or Book of Changes.* Bollinger Series xix. Princeton University Press, Princeton, N.J., 1967.

21. Nideffer, Robert M.: "Alpha and the Development of Human Potential," in Shapiro, David, et al. (eds.): *Biofeedback and Self-Control, 1972.* Aldine Publishing Co., Chicago, 1973, p. 167.

22. Orme-Johnson, David W.: "Autonomic Stability and Transcendental Meditation," in Miller, Neal E., et al. (eds.): *Biofeedback and Self-Control, 1973.* Aldine Publishing Co., Chicago, 1974, p. 476.

23. Gellhorn, Ernst, and Kiely, William F.: "Mystical States of Consciousness: Neurophysiological and Clinical Aspects," in Miller, Neal E., et al. (eds.): *Biofeedback and Self-Control, 1973.* Aldine Publishing Co., Chicago, 1974, p. 484.

24. Weil, Andrew: *The Natural Mind.* Houghton Mifflin Co., Boston, 1972.

25. Geldard, Frank A.: *The Human Senses,* 2nd ed. John Wiley & Sons, New York, 1972, p. 445.

26. Engen, Trygg, et al.: "Olfactory Responses and Adaptation in the Human Neonate," *J. Comp. Physiol. Psychol.,* **56**:73, (No. 1) 1963.

27. Smith, Kathleen, and Sines, Jacob O.: "Demonstration of a Peculiar Odor in the Sweat of Schizophrenic Patients," *Arch. Gen. Psychiatry,* **2**:184, (Feb.) 1960.

28. Hall, Edward T.: *The Hidden Dimension.* Doubleday & Co., Garden City, N.Y., 1966, p. 46.

29. Sutterley, Doris C., and Donnelly, Gloria F.: *Perspectives in Human Development. Nursing Throughout the Life Cycle.* J. B. Lippincott Co., Philadelphia, 1973, p. 111.

30. Hambridge, K. Michael, et al.: "Taste Acuity, Appetite, Stature, and Hair Zinc Concentrations in 'Normal' Children," *Clin. Res.,* **20**:256, (Feb.) 1972.

31. Henkin, Robert I., et al.: "Idiopathic Hypogeusia with Dysgeusia, Hyposomia, and Dysomia," *J.A.M.A.,* **217**:434, (July 26) 1971.

32. ———, and Smith, Frank R.: "Hyposomia in Acute Viral Hepatitis," *Lancet,* **1**:823, (Apr. 24) 1971.

33. Cohen, I. Kelman, et al.: "Hypogeusia, Anorexia, and Altered Zinc Metabolism Following Thermal Burn," *J.A.M.A.,* **223**:914, (Feb. 19) 1973.

34. Collins, Carter C., and Bach-y-Rita, Paul: "Transmission of Pictorial Information Through the Skin," *Adv. Biol. Med. Phys.,* **14**:285, 1973.

35. Kirman, Jacob H.: "Tactile Communication of Speech: A Review and an Analysis," *Psychol. Bull.,* **80**:54, (July) 1973.

36. *Ibid.*

37. Steinberg, Danny D.: "Light Sensed Through Receptors in the Skin," *Am. J. Psychol.,* **79**:324, (June) 1966.

38. Youtz, Richard P.: "Dermo-optical Perception," *Science,* **152**:1108, (May 20) 1966.

39. Makous, W. L.: "Cutaneous Color Sensitivity: Explanation and Demonstration," *Psychol. Rev.,* **73**:280, (July) 1966.

40. Clynes, Manfred: "Biocybernetics of the

Dynamic Communication of Emotions and Qualities," *Science,* **170:**764, (Nov. 13) 1970.

41. Nash, John: *Developmental Psychology. A Psychobiological Approach.* Prentice-Hall, Inc., Englewood Cliffs, N.J., 1970, p. 98.

42. Bowlby, John: *Attachment and Loss, Vol. I: Attachment.* Basic Books, Inc., New York, 1969, p. 277.

42a. Leboyer, Frederick: *Birth Without Violence.* Alfred A. Knopf, New York, 1975.

43. Fantz, Robert L., and Nevis, Sonia: "Pattern Preferences and Perceptual-Cognitive Development in Early Infancy," in Chess, Stella, and Thomas, Alexander (eds.): *Annual Progress in Child Psychiatry and Child Development, 1968.* Brunner/Mazel Publishers, New York, 1968, p. 22.

44. Fantz, Robert L.: "The Origin of Form Perception," in Scientific American: *The Nature and Nurture of Behavior.* W. H. Freeman & Co., San Francisco, 1972, p. 66.

45. Vernon, M. D.: *Perception Through Experience.* Barnes & Noble, New York, 1970, p. 1.

46. Buckout, Robert: "Eyewitness Testimony," *Sci. Am.,* **231:**23, (Dec.) 1974.

47. Deregowski, Jan B.: "Pictorial Perception and Culture," *Sci. Am.,* **227:**82, (Nov.) 1972.

48. Gombrich, E. H.: "The Visual Image," *Sci. Am.,* **227:**82, (Sept.) 1972.

49. Nightingale, Florence: *Notes on Nursing. What It Is and What It Is Not.* Appleton-Century-Crofts, New York, 1946. (Facsimile of 1859 edition.)

50. Gombrich, E. H.: *op. cit.*

51. Kohlers, Paul A.: "Experiments in Reading," *Sci. Am.,* **227:**84, (July) 1972.

52. Ervin-Tripp, Susan: "Language Development," in Hoffman, Lois Wladis, and Hoffman, Martin L. (eds.): *Review of Child Development Research,* Vol. II. Russell Sage Foundation, New York, 1966, p. 55.

53. Lenneberg, Eric H.: "On Explaining Language," in Chess, Stella, and Thomas, Alexander (eds.): *Annual Progress in Child Psychiatry and Child Development, 1970.* Brunner/Mazel Publishers, New York, 1970, p. 104.

54. Chomsky, Noam: *Aspects of the Theory of Syntax.* M.I.T. Press, Cambridge, Mass., 1965.

55. McNeill, David: *The Acquisition of Language: The Study of Developmental Psycholinguistics.* Harper & Row, New York, 1970.

56. Slobin, Dan I.: "Children and Language: They Learn the Same Way All Around the World," *Psychology Today,* **6:**71, (July) 1972.

57. Moore, Terence: "Language and Intelligence: A Longitudinal Study of the First 8 Years," *Hum. Dev.,* **10:**88, 1967.

58. Herriot, Peter: "The Comprehension of Tense by Young Children," *Child Dev.* **40:** 103, (Mar.) 1969.

59. Nash, John: *op. cit.,* p. 332.

60. Carroll, John B. (ed.): *Language, Thought, and Reality. Selected Writings of Benjamin Lee Whorf.* M.I.T. Press, Cambridge, Mass., 1956, p. 65.

61. Furth, Hans G.: "Linguistic Deficiency and Thinking. Research with Deaf Subjects 1964–1969," in Chess, Stella, and Thomas, Alexander (eds.): *Annual Progress in Child Psychiatry and Child Development, 1972.* Brunner/Mazel Publishers, New York, 1972, p. 191.

62. Bonvillian, John D., et al.: "Psycholinguistic and Educational Implications of Deafness," *Hum. Dev.,* **16:**321, (No. 5) 1973.

63. Pei, Mario: *The Story of Language,* rev. ed. J. B. Lippincott Co., Philadelphia, 1965.

64. Wang, William S.-Y.: "The Chinese Language," *Sci. Am.,* **228:**51, (Feb.) 1973.

65. Mehrabian, Albert: "Communication Without Words," in *Readings in Psychology Today.* Communications/Research/Machines, Inc., Del Mar, Calif., 1969, p. 276.

66. Ekman, Paul, and Friesen, Wallace V.: "Head and Body Cues in the Judgment of Emotion: A Reformulation," *Percep. Mot. Skills,* **24:**711, 1967.

67. Dittman, Allen T., et al.: "Facial and Bodily Expression: A Study of Receptivity of Emotional Cues," *Psychiatry,* **28:**239, (Aug.) 1965.

68. Mehrabian, Albert: "Significance of Posture and Position in the Communication of Attitudes and Status Relationships," *Psychol. Bull.,* **71:**359, (No. 5) 1969.

69. Ekman, Paul, et al.: "Pan-Cultural Elements in Facial Displays of Emotion," *Science,* **164:**86, (Apr. 4) 1969.

70. Birdwhistle, Ray L.: *op. cit.,* p. 101.

71. Grant, Ewan C.: "Facial Expressions and Gesture," *J. Psychosom. Res.,* **15:**391, (Dec.) 1971.

72. Salk, Lee: "The Role of the Heartbeat in the Relations Between Mother and Infant," *Sci. Am.,* **228:**24, (May) 1973.

73. McLuhan, Marshall: *Understanding Media: The Extension of Man.* McGraw-Hill Book Co., New York, 1964, p. 119.

74. Esser, Aristide H. (ed.): *Behavior and Environment.* Plenum Press, New York, 1971.

75. Ball, Donald W.: *Micro-ecology: Social Situations and Intimate Space.* Bobbs-Merrill Co., Indianapolis, 1973.

76. Watson, O. Michael: *Proxemic Behavior: A Cross-Cultural Study.* Humanities Press, Atlantic Highlands, N.J., 1970.

77. Sommer, Robert: *Tight Spaces. Hard Architecture and How to Humanize It.* Prentice-Hall, Inc., Englewood Cliffs, N.J., 1974.

78. ———, and Dewar, Robert: "The Physical Environment of the Ward," in Freidson, Eliot (ed.): *The Hospital in Modern Society.* Free Press of Glencoe, New York, 1963, p. 319.

79. Hall, Edward T.: *op. cit.*, p. 110.
80. Sommer, Robert, and Dewar, Robert: *op. cit.*, p. 325.
81. McLuhan, Marshall: *op. cit.*, p. 18:
82. Gerbner, George: "Communication and Social Environment," *Sci. Am.*, **227**:153, (Sept.) 1972.
83. Toffler, Alvin: *Future Shock*. Bantam Books, New York, 1970.
84. Kahn, Herman, and Bruce-Briggs, B.: *Things to Come. Thinking About the 70's and 80's*. Macmillan Publishing Co., Inc., New York, 1972.
84a. Fowkes, R. L., et al.: "Communications and Mass Media," *Lamp*, **30**:21, (Feb.) 1973.
84b. Althafer, C., et al.: "Now It's Health Information by Phone. Tel-Med," *Am. Lung Assoc. Bull.*, (Jan.–Feb.) 1974.
84c. Sullivan, Richard A., et al.: "Telephone Services for the Disabled: Patient and Equipment Evaluation," *Nurs. Clin. North Am.*, **4**:555, (Sept.) 1969.
85. Miller, Warren B.: "The Telephone in Outpatient Psychotherapy," *Am. J. Psychother.*, **27**:15, (Jan.) 1973.
86. McLuhan, Marshall: *op. cit.*, p. 266.
87. Tripp, Sally: "Telephone Techniques in Pediatric Practice," *Am. J. Nurs.*, **71**:1722, (Sept.) 1971.
88. Miller, Warren B.: *op. cit.*
89. Leifer, Aimee Dorr, et al.: "Children's Television. More Than Mere Entertainment," *Harvard Educ. Rev.*, **44**:213, (May) 1974.
90. Hill, Jae H., et al.: "Vicarious Extinction of Avoidance Behavior Through Films: An Initial Test," *Psychol. Rep.*, **22**:192, (No. 1) 1968.
91. Herskovitz, Antol, et al.: "A Motion Picture as a Substitute for Experience in a Health Delivery Environment," *J. Biol. Photogr. Assoc.*, **38**:193, (Oct.) 1971.
92. Wittkopf, Berniece: "Self-Instruction for Student Learning," *Am. J. Nurs.*, **72**:2032, (Nov.) 1972.
93. Barlow, Donna Jean, and Bruhn, John G.: "Role-Plays on Television," *Nurs. Outlook*, **21**:242, (Apr.) 1973.
93a. Niles, A. M.: "Nursing Dial Access—Audiotapes by Telephone," *Superv. Nurse*, **4**:12, (Oct.) 1973.
93b. Ricks, M. C.: "Maritimers Have a T. V. Nurse," *Can. Nurse*, **66**:33, (Sept.) 1970.
93c. Murphy, R. R., Jr., et al.: "Telediagnosis; A New Community Health Resource. Observations on the Feasibility of Telediagnosis Based on 1,000 Patient Transactions," *Am. J. Public Health*, **64**:113, (Feb.) 1974.
93d. Hudson, H. E., et al.: "Medical Communication in Alaska by Satellite," *N. Engl. J. Med.*, **289**:1351, (Dec. 20) 1973.
93e. Anderson, C. J., et al.: "Use of Videotape Feedback as a Psychotherapeutic Nursing Approach with Long-Term Psychiatric Patients. A Pilot Study," *Nurs. Res.*, **22**:507, (Nov.–Dec.) 1973.
94. Levine, Ira: *The Stepford Wives*. Random House, New York, 1972.
95. Crichton, Michael: *The Terminal Man*. Alfred A. Knopf, New York, 1972.
96. Handler, Philip (ed.): *Biology and the Future of Man*. Oxford University Press, London, 1970, p. 532.
97. Reed, Fay Carol, et al.: "Computer Assisted Instruction for Continued Learning," *Am. J. Nurs.*, **72**:2035, (Nov.) 1972.
98. Collart, Marie E.: "Computer Assisted Instruction and the Teacher-Learning Process," *Nurs. Outlook*, **21**:527, (Aug.) 1973.
99. Alpert, D., and Bitzer, D. L.: "Advances in Computer-Based Education," *Science*, **167**:1582, (Mar. 20) 1970.
100. Mueck, Marjorie A.: "Overcoming the Language Barrier," *Nurs. Outlook*, **81**:53, (Apr.) 1970.
100a. Samora, Julian, et al.: "Medical Vocabulary Knowledge Among Hospital Patients," in Skipper, James K., Jr., and Leonard, Robert C. (eds.): *Social Interaction and Patient Care*. J. B. Lippincott Co., Philadelphia, 1965.
101. Lurie, Hugh James, and Lawrence, George L.: "Communication Problems Between Rural Mexican-American Patients and Their Physicians," *Am. J. Orthopsychiatry*, **42**:777, (Oct.) 1972.
102. Leininger, Madeleine M.: *Nursing and Anthropology. Two Worlds to Blend*. John Wiley & Sons, New York, 1970, p. 58.
102a. Rodgers, Janet A.: "Relationship Between Sociability and Personal Space Preference at Two Different Times of Day," in Downs, Florence S., and Newman, Margaret A. (eds.): *A Source Book of Nursing Research*. F. A. Davis Co., Philadelphia, 1973.
103. Milio, Nancy: "Project in a Negro Ghetto," *Am. J. Nurs.*, **67**:1006, (May) 1967.
104. Clark, Margaret: *Health in the Mexican-American Culture*, 2nd ed. University of California Press, Berkeley, 1970.
105. Lego, Suzanne M.: "Competing Sets of Appraisal in White Nurse-Negro Patient Relationships," in *ANA Clinical Sessions, 1966*. Appleton-Century-Crofts, New York, 1967, p. 1.
106. Gregg, Elinor D.: *The Indians and the Nurse*. University of Oklahoma Press, Norman, 1965.
107. Campbell, Teresa, and Chang, Betty: "Health Care of the Chinese in America," *Nurs. Outlook*, **21**:245, (Apr.) 1973.
108. Madson, William: *Mexican-Americans of South Texas*, 2nd ed. Holt, Rinehart & Winston, New York, 1973.
109. Anderson, Gwen, and Tighe, Bridget: "Gypsy Culture and Health Care," *Am. J. Nurs.*, **73**:282, (Feb.) 1973.
109a. Redmann, Ruth E.: "Black Child—White Nurse: A Nursing Challenge and Privilege," in Duffey, Margery, et al. (eds.): *Current*

Concepts in Clinical Nursing, Vol. III. C. V. Mosby Co., St. Louis, 1971.

110. Goldstein, Bernice, and Tamura, Kyoko: *Japanese and American English Language, Culture, and Personality.* C. E. Tuttle Co., Rutland, Vt., 1973.

111. Lester, Anthony, and Bindman, Geoffrey: *Race and Law in Great Britain.* Harvard University Press, Cambridge, Mass., 1972.

112. Lewis, Oscar: *Anthropological Essays.* Random House, New York, 1970.

113. Lewit, David W., and Abner, Edward V.: "Black-White Semantic Differences and Interracial Communication," *J. Appl. Soc. Psychol.,* **1:**263, (July–Sept.) 1971.

114. Minuchin, Salvador, et al.: *Families of the Slums.* Basic Books, Inc., New York, 1967.

115. Bullough, Bonnie, and Bullough, Vern L.: *Poverty, Ethnic Identity, and Health Care.* Appleton-Century-Crofts, New York, 1972.

116. Kosa, John, et al. (eds.): *Poverty and Health.* Harvard University Press, Cambridge, Mass., 1969.

116a. Will, Gwen T.: "Developmental Concepts Relating to Psychiatric Nursing Practice," in Anderson, Edith H., et al. (eds.): *Current Concepts in Clinical Nursing,* Vol. IV. C. V. Mosby Co., St. Louis, 1973.

116b. Berne, Eric: *Principles in Group Treatment.* Oxford University Press, New York, 1966, p. 220.

116c. Harris, Thomas A.: *I'm OK—You're OK.* Avon Books, New York, 1969.

117. Veninga, Robert: "Communications: A Patient's Eye View," *Am. J. Nurs.,* **73:**320, (Feb.) 1973.

118. Group for the Advancement of Psychiatry, Committee on Adolescence: *Normal Adolescence.* Charles Scribner's Sons, New York, 1968, p. 34.

119. Westman, Jack C.: "Understanding Teenagers," *Minn. Med.,* **56:**94, (Feb.) 1973.

120. Ramsey, Charles A.: *The Greening of America: The Coming of a New Consciousness and Rebirth of a Future.* Random House, New York, 1970.

121. Bischof, Ledford J.: *Adult Psychology.* Harper & Row, New York, 1969, p. 1.

122. Kinsey, Alfred C., et al.: *Sexual Behavior in the Human Male.* W. B. Saunders Co., Philadelphia, 1948.

123. ———: *Sexual Behavior in the Human Female.* W. B. Saunders Co., Philadelphia, 1953.

124. Masters, William H., and Johnson, Virginia E.: *The Human Sexual Response.* Little, Brown & Co., Boston, 1966.

125. ———: *Human Sexual Inadequacy.* Little, Brown & Co., Boston, 1970.

126. ———: *The Pleasure Bond.* Little, Brown & Co., Boston, 1975.

127. McBride, Angela Barron: *The Growth and Development of Mothers.* Harper & Row, New York, 1973.

128. Moenster, Phyllis A.: "Learning and Memory in Relation to Age," *J. Gerontol.,* **27:** 361, (July) 1972.

128a. Greenberg, B.: "Caring for the Aged: Reaction Time in the Elderly," *Am. J. Nurs.,* **73:**2056, (Dec.) 1973.

128b. Rossi, A. O., et al.: "Treating Old People Like Children Can Bring on Mental Breakdown," *Mod. Nurs. Home,* **29:**62, (Sept.) 1972.

129. Birren, James E.: *The Psychology of Aging.* Prentice-Hall, Inc., Englewood Cliffs, N.J., 1964.

130. Bischof, Ledford J.: *op. cit.,* p. 8.

131. Lidz, Theodore: *The Person.* Basic Books, Inc., New York, 1968, p. 476.

132. Choron, Jacques: *Suicide.* Charles Scribner's Sons, New York, 1972.

133. Butler, Robert N.: "The Life Review, an Interpretation of Reminiscence in the Aged," in Kastenbaum, Robert (ed.): *New Thoughts on Old Age.* Springer Publishing Co., New York, 1964, p. 265.

134. Panicucci, Carol L., et al.: "Expanded Speech and Self-Pacing in Communication with the Aged," in *ANA Clinical Sessions, 1968.* Appleton-Century-Crofts, New York, 1969, p. 95.

135. Stone, Virginia: "Give the Older Person Time," *Am. J. Nurs.,* **69:**2124, (Oct.) 1969.

136. Burnside, Irene M.: "Communication Problems in Group Work with the Disabled Aged," in *ANA Clinical Conferences, 1969.* Appleton-Century-Crofts, New York, 1970, p. 125.

137. Rossman, Isadore (ed.): *Clinical Geriatrics.* J. B. Lippincott Co., Philadelphia, 1971.

138. Jaeger, Dorothea, and Simmons, Leo W.: *The Aged Ill—Coping with Problems in Geriatric Care.* Meredith Publishing Co., New York, 1970.

139. Chinn, Austin B. (ed.): *Working with Older People—A Guide to Practice.* Vol. IV: Clinical Aspects of Aging. US Government Printing Office, Washington, D.C., 1971.

140. Burnside, Irene M.: *Psychosocial Nursing: Care of the Aged.* McGraw-Hill Book Co., New York, 1973.

141. Brantt, Virginia M., and Brown, Sister Marie Raymond: *Readings in Gerontology.* C. V. Mosby Co., St. Louis, 1973.

142. Birchenall, Joan, and Streight, Mary E.: *Care of the Older Adult.* J. B. Lippincott Co., Philadelphia, 1973.

143. Anderson, Helen C.: *Newton's Geriatric Nursing,* 5th ed. C. V. Mosby Co., St. Louis, 1971.

144. Anderson, Catherine J.: "Alienation in the Aged: Implications for Psychiatric Geriatric Nursing," in *ANA Regional Clinical Conferences, 1967.* Appleton-Century-Crofts, New York, 1968, p. 115.

145. American Nurses' Association: *Standards for Geriatric Nursing Practice.* The Association, New York, 1973.

146. "ANA Asks Stepped-Up Research on Aged

and Aging," *Am. J. Nurs.,* **72:**1368, (Aug.) 1972.

147. Butler, Robert N., and Lewis, Myrna I.: *Aging and Mental Health—Positive Psychosocial Approaches.* C. V. Mosby Co., St. Louis, 1973.

148. Eisdorfer, Carl, and Lawton, M. Powell (eds.): *The Psychology of Adult Development and Aging.* American Psychological Association, Washington, D.C., 1973.

149. Riley, Matilda W., et al.: *Aging and Society,* Vols. I, II, III. Russell Sage Foundation, New York, 1968–1972.

149a. McBride, Angela Barron: "Can Family Life Survive?" *Am. J. Nurs.,* **75:**1648 (Oct.) 1975.

149b. Mead, Margaret: *Male and Female.* William Morrow & Co., New York, 1949.

149c. Janeway, Elizabeth: *Man's World, Woman's Place.* William Morrow & Co., New York, 1971.

149d. Steinberg, David: "Redefining Fatherhood: Notes After Six Months," in House, L. K. (ed.): *The Future of the Family.* Simon & Schuster, New York, 1972.

150. Parsons, Talcott: "Definitions of Health and Illness in the Light of American Values and Social Structure," in Jaco, E. Gartley (ed.): *Patients, Physicians, and Illness,* 2nd ed. Free Press, New York, 1972, p. 117.

151. Skipper, James V., et al.: "What Communication Means to Patients," *Am. J. Nurs.,* **64:**101, (Apr.) 1964.

152. Reichle, Marian J.: "Psychologic Aspects of the Acutely Stressed in an Intensive Care Unit," in Bushnell, Sharon S. (comp.): *Respiratory Intensive Care Nursing.* Little, Brown & Co., Boston, 1973, p. 219.

153. Senescu, Robert: "The Problem of Establishing Communication with the Seriously Ill Patient," *Ann. NY Acad. Sci.,* **164:**696, 1969.

153a. Anderson, Evelyn R.: "The Role of the Nurse in Communications and Interpersonal Relations," in Anderson, Evelyn R.: *The Role of the Nurse.* Royal College of Nursing, London, 1973.

154. Rogers, Carl R.: "The Characteristics of a Helping Relationship," in Bennis, Warren G., et al. (eds.): *The Planning of Change,* 2nd ed. Holt, Rinehart & Winston, New York, 1969, p. 153.

155. Maslow, Abraham H.: *Motivation and Personality,* 2nd ed. Harper & Row, New York, 1970, p. 248.

156. Peplau, Hildegard E.: "Interpersonal Techniques. The Crux of Psychiatric Nursing," in Mereness, Dorothy (ed.): *Psychiatric Nursing,* Vol. 1, 2nd ed. Wm. C. Brown Co., Dubuque, Iowa, 1971, p. 127.

157. Tudor, Gwen E.: "A Sociopsychiatric Nursing Approach to Intervention in a Problem of Mutual Withdrawal on a Mental Hospital Ward," *Psychiatry,* **15:**193, (May) 1952.

158. Orlando, Ida Jean: *The Dynamic Nurse-Patient Relationship.* G. P. Putnam's Sons, New York, 1961.

159. Wiedenbach, Ernestine: *Clinical Nursing. A Helping Art.* Springer Publishing Co., New York, 1964.

160. Dumas, Rhetaugh G., and Leonard, Robert C.: "The Effect of Nursing on Postoperative Vomiting," *Nurs. Res.,* **12:**12, (Winter) 1963.

161. Anderson, Barbara J., et al.: "Two Experimental Tests of a Patient-Centered Admission Process," *Nurs. Res.,* **14:**151, (Spring) 1965.

162. Elms, Roslyn E., and Leonard, Robert C.: "Effects of Nursing Approaches During Admission," *Nurs. Res.,* **15:**39, (Winter) 1966.

163. Schmidt, Joan: "Availability: A Concept of Nursing Practice," *Am. J. Nurs.,* **72:**1086, (June) 1972.

164. Dumas, Rhetaugh G., and Johnson, Barbara A.: "Research in Nursing Practice: A Review of Five Clinical Experiments," *Int. J. Nurs. Stud.,* **9:**137, (Aug.) 1972.

165. Diers, Donna, et al.: "The Effect of Nursing Interaction on Patients in Pain," *Nurs. Res.,* **21:**419, (Sept.–Oct.) 1972.

165a. Colliton, Margaret, et al.: "Symposium on the Use of Self in Clinical Practice," *Nurs. Clin. North Am.,* **6:**691, (Dec.) 1971.

165b. Clark, C.: "The Clinical Specialist as Communication Consultant," *Superv. Nurse,* **4:**20, (Apr.) 1973.

165c. Robinson, Lisa: *Liaison Nursing—Psychological Approach to Patient Care.* F. A. Davis Co., Philadelphia, 1974.

165d. Richards, S. J., et al.: "Communication with Patients: A Parameter in Evaluating Nurse Practitioners," *Mo. Med.,* **70:**719, (Oct.) 1973.

165e. Gallagher, M.: *Communicate or Else.* National League for Nursing, New York, 1973.

165f. O'Brien, Maureen J.: *Communications and Relationships in Nursing.* C. V. Mosby Co., St. Louis, 1974.

166. Callaghan, Perquilla: "Development of Awareness of Self for the Professional Nursing Student," in Carlson, Carolyn E. (coordin.): *Behavioral Concepts and Nursing Intervention.* J. B. Lippincott Co., Philadelphia, 1970, p. 283.

167. "Developing Self-Understanding," in Mereness, Dorothy (ed.): *Psychiatric Nursing,* Vol. I, 2nd ed. Wm. C. Brown Co., Dubuque, Iowa, 1971, p. 2.

168. Burgess, Ann C., and Lazare, Aaron: *Psychiatric Nursing in the Hospital and Community.* Prentice-Hall, Inc., Englewood Cliffs, N.J., 1973.

169. Coleman, Margaret, and Glofka, Peter T.: "The Effect of Group Therapy on Self-Concept of Senior Nursing Students," *Nurs. Res.,* **18:**274, (May–June) 1969.

170. Goldsborough, Judith D.: "On Becoming

Nonjudgmental," *Am. J. Nurs.,* **70:**2340, (Nov.) 1970.

171. Close, Henry T.: "Expressing One's Feelings," *Voices: Art, Sci., Psychother.,* **8:**54, (Summer) 1972.

172. Blum, Lucille H.: *Reading Between the Lines. Doctor-Patient Communication.* International Universities Press, New York, 1972, p. 160.

173. Suhrie, Eleanor Brady: "The Importance of Listening," in Stewart, Dorothy M., and Vincent, Pauline (eds.): *Public Health Nursing.* Wm. C. Brown Co., Dubuque, Iowa, 1968, p. 96.

174. Wilson, Lucille M.: "Listening," in Carlson, Carolyn E. (coordin.): *Behavioral Concepts and Nursing Intervention.* J. B. Lippincott Co., Philadelphia, 1970, p. 153.

175. Hays, Joyce S.: "Analysis of Nurse-Patient Communications," *Nurs. Outlook,* **14:**32, (Sept.) 1966.

176. Ujhely, Gertrud B.: "The Uses and Abuses of the So-Called 'Nondirective Technique' in Nursing," in *ANA Regional Clinical Conferences, 1967.* Appleton-Century-Crofts, New York, 1968, p. 299.

177. Bliss, Rachel: "Covert Behaviors: Recognition and Intervention," in *ANA Clinical Sessions, 1968.* Appleton-Century-Crofts, New York, 1969, p. 309.

177a. Baziak, Anna Teresa, and Dentan, Robert Knox: "The Language of the Hospital and Its Effect on the Patient," in Skipper, James K., Jr., and Leonard, Robert C.: *Social Interaction and Patient Care.* J. B. Lippincott Co., Philadelphia, 1965.

178. Barbara, Dominick A.: *The Art of Listening.* Charles C Thomas, Publisher, Springfield, Ill., 1958, p. 179.

178a. Robinson, Vera M.: "Humor in Nursing," in Carlson, Carolyn E. (coordin.): *Behavioral Concepts and Nursing Intervention.* J. B. Lippincott Co., Philadelphia, 1970, p. 129.

179. Thomas, Mary Durand: "Trust in the Nurse-Patient Relationship," in Carlson, Carolyn E. (coordin.): *Behavioral Concepts and Nursing Intervention.* J. B. Lippincott Co., Philadelphia, 1970, p. 117.

180. Peplau, Hildegard E.: "Talking with Patients," in Mereness, Dorothy (ed.): *Psychiatric Nursing,* Vol. I, 2nd ed. Wm. C. Brown Co., Dubuque, Iowa, 1971, p. 76.

181. Peitchinis, Jacquelyn A.: "Therapeutic Effectiveness of Counseling by Nursing Personnel," *Nurs. Res.,* **21:**138, (Mar.–Apr.) 1972.

182. Owens, Charlotte: "Concepts of Interviewing," in Stewart, Dorothy M., and Vincent, Pauline (eds.): *Public Health Nursing.* Wm. C. Brown Co., Dubuque, Iowa, 1968, p. 71.

183. Harper, Mary W., et al.: "Do Attitudes of Nursing Personnel Affect the Patient's Perception of Care." *Nurs. Res.,* **21:**327, (July–Aug.) 1972.

184. Francis, Gloria M., and Munjas, Barbara: *Promoting Psychological Comfort.* Wm. C. Brown Co., Dubuque, Iowa, 1968, p. 55.

185. Kron, Thora: *Communication in Nursing,* 2nd ed. W. B. Saunders Co., Philadelphia, 1972.

186. Gardner, Kathryn: "Patient Groups in a Therapeutic Community," *Am. J. Nurs.,* **71:**528, (Mar.) 1971.

187. Barnett, Kathryn: "A Theoretical Construct of the Concepts of Touch as They Relate to Nursing," *Nurs. Res.,* **21:**102, (Mar.–Apr.) 1972.

188. Hallstrom, Betty J.: "Contact Comfort: Its Application to Immunization Injections," *Nurs. Res.,* **17:**130, (Mar.–Apr.) 1968.

189. McCorkle, Ruth: "Effects of Touch on Seriously Ill Patients," *Nurs. Res.,* **23:**125, (Mar.–Apr.) 1974.

190. Durr, Carol A.: "Hands That Help . . . But How?" *Nurs. Forum,* **10:**392, (No. 4) 1971.

191. Howard, Jane: *Please Touch.* McGraw-Hill Book Co., New York, 1970.

192. Davis, Ellen D.: "Give a Bath?" *Am. J. Nurs.,* **70:**2365, (Nov.) 1970.

193. Amacher, Nancy Jean: "Touch Is a Way of Caring," *Am. J. Nurs.,* **73:**852, (May) 1973.

194. Johnson, Betty Sue: "The Meaning of Touch in Nursing," *Nurs. Outlook,* **13:**59, (Feb.) 1965.

194a. Preston, T.: "Caring for the Aged: When Words Fail," *Am. J. Nurs.,* **73:**2064, (Dec.) 1973.

194b. Burnside, J. M.: "Caring for the Aged: Touching Is Talking," *Am. J. Nurs.,* **73:**2060, (Dec.) 1973.

194c. Day, F. Ann: "The Patient's Perception of Touch," in Anderson, Edith H., et al. (eds.): *Current Concepts in Clinical Nursing,* Vol. IV. C. V. Mosby Co., St. Louis, 1973, p. 206.

195. Lesser, Marion S., and Keane, Vera: *Nurse-Patient Relationships in a Hospital Maternity Service.* C. V. Mosby Co., St. Louis, 1956.

196. Mereness, Dorothy: "Your Self-Image and Your Practice," *Am. J. Nurs.,* **66:**96, (Jan.) 1966.

196a. Szent-Gyorgyi, Albert: *The Living State. With Observations on Cancer.* Academic Press, New York, 1972, p. 107.

196b. Krieger, Dolores: "The Response of In-vivo Human Hemoglobin to an Active Healing Therapy by Direct Laying-on of Hands," *Hum. Dimensions,* **1:**12, (Autumn) 1972.

196c. ———: "Healing by the Laying-on of Hands as a Facilitator of Bioenergetic Change: The Response of In-vivo Human Hemoglobin," *Psychoenergetic Systems,* **3:** (No. 3) 1974.

196d. Schlotfeld, R. M., and Krieger, Dolores: "The Relationship of Touch with Intent to Help or Heal to Subjects' In-vivo Hemoglobin Values: A Study in Personalized Interaction," in *Ninth Nursing Research Conference*. American Nurses' Association, New York, 1973.

196e. Krieger, Dolores: "Therapeutic Touch: The Imprimatur of Nursing," *Am. J. Nurs.*, **75**:784, (May) 1975.

196f. Farrah, Shirley: "The Nurse—the Patient —and Touch," in Duffey, Margery, et al. (eds.): *Current Concepts in Clinical Nursing*, Vol. III. C. V. Mosby Co., St. Louis, 1971, p. 256.

197. Ammon, Kathryn J.: "The Effects of Music on Children in Respiratory Distress," in *ANA Clinical Sessions, 1968*. Appleton-Century-Crofts, New York, 1969, p. 127.

197a. "First Music Therapy Course," *Sairaanheitaga*, **49**:10, (Sept. 25) 1973.

198. Riess, Bernard F.: "Developments in Dance Therapy," *Curr. Psychiatr. Ther.*, **9**:195, 1969.

199. Gunning, Susan V., and Holmes, Thomas H.: "Dance Therapy with Psychotic Children," *Arch. Gen. Psychiatry*, **28**:707, (May) 1973.

200. Puttock, Denise: "Dance Therapy," *Nurs. Times*, **68**:960, (Aug. 3) 1972.

201. Shifman, Audrey F.: "The Value of Art Therapy in Psychotherapy," *Voices: Art, Sci., Psychother.*, **8**:37, (Summer) 1972.

202. Kellogg, Rhoda, and O'Dell, Scott: *The Psychology of Children's Art*. Random House, New York, 1967.

203. Di Leo, Joseph H.: *Young Children and Their Drawings*. Brunner/Mazel Publishers, New York, 1970.

204. "Viewpoints on Children in Hospitals," *Hospitals*, **37**:43, (May 16) 1963.

205. Fleming, Juanita W.: "Understanding Children Through Drawings," in *Eighth Nursing Research Conference*. American Nurses' Association, New York, 1972, p. 133.

206. Serban, George: "A Critical Study of Art Therapy in Treating Psychotic Patients," *Behav. Neuropsychiatry*, **4**:2, (Apr.–May) 1972.

207. Freedman, Alfred M., et al.: *Modern Synopsis of Comprehensive Textbook of Psychiatry*. Williams & Wilkins Co., Baltimore, 1972, p. 535.

208. Underwood, Patricia R.: "Communication Through Role-Playing," *Am. J. Nurs.*, **71**: 1184, (June) 1971.

208a. Kalisch, B. J.: "Summer Theater: Another Way to Learn," *Nurs. Outlook*, **22**:31, (Jan.) 1974.

209. Courtney, Winifred F. (ed.): *The Reader's Advisor*, Vol. II. R. R. Bowker Co., New York, 1969.

210. Johnston, Nina: "Group Reading as a Treatment Tool with Geriatrics," *Am. J. Occup. Ther.*, **19**:192, (July–Aug.) 1965.

211. Kirshenbaum, Elaine, and Glasgow, Douglas: "Group Work Method in Psychiatric Nursing Practice," in Mereness, Dorothy (ed.): *Psychiatric Nursing*, Vol. I, 2nd ed.

Wm. C. Brown Co., Dubuque, Iowa, 1971, p. 224.

212. Lauer, Roger: "Creative Writing as a Therapeutic Tool," *Hosp. Community Psychiatry*, **23**:55, (Feb.) 1972.

213. Auerbach, Aline B.: *Parents Learn Through Discussion*. John Wiley & Sons, New York, 1968.

214. Mills, Theodore M.: *The Sociology of Small Groups*. Prentice-Hall, Inc., Englewood Cliffs, N.J., 1967, p. 119.

215. Sommer, Robert: "Working Effectively with Groups," in Mereness, Dorothy (ed.): *Psychiatric Nursing*, Vol. II, 2nd ed. Wm. C. Brown Co., Dubuque, Iowa, 1971, p. 331.

216. Abercrombie, M. L. J.: "Face to Face— Proximity and Distance," *J. Psychosom. Res.*, **15**:395, 1971.

217. Batchelor, James P., and Goethals, George R.: "Spatial Arrangements in Freely Formed Groups," *Sociometry*, **35**:270, (No. 2) 1972.

218. Baxter, James C.: "Interpersonal Spacing in Natural Settings," *Sociometry*, **33**:444, (No. 4) 1970.

219. Mehrabian, Albert, and Diamond, Shirley G.: "Seating Arrangement and Conversation," *Sociometry*, **34**:281, (No. 2) 1971.

220. ————: "Effects of Furniture Arrangement, Props, and Personality on Social Interaction," *J. Pers. Soc. Psychol.*, **20**:18, (No. 1) 1971.

221. Sommer, Robert: "Small Group Ecology," *Psychol. Bull.*, **67**:145, (Feb.) 1967.

222. Conant, Lucy H.: "Give-and-Take in Home Visits," in Stewart, Dorothy M., and Vincent, Pauline (eds.): *Public Health Nursing*. Wm. C. Brown Co., Dubuque, Iowa, 1968, p. 51.

223. Bennis, Warren G.: "Post-Bureaucratic Leadership," *Trans-Action*, **6**:44, (July) 1969.

224. Graves, Helen Hope: "Can Nursing Shed Bureaucracy?" *Am. J. Nurs.*, **71**:491, (Mar.) 1971.

225. Russell, Charles H.: "Survey Shows How Doctors, Nurses and Hospitals Agree and Disagree on Health Care Issues and Outlook," *Mod. Hosp.*, **115**:88, (Nov.) 1970.

226. Kramer, Marlene: "The Consumer's Influence on Health Care," *Nurs. Outlook*, **20**:574, (Sept.) 1972.

226a. Kavaler, F., et al.: "Nursing Home Residents' Council; a 'New Wrinkle' in Consumer Participation," *Nurs. Homes*, **21**:8, (Oct.) 1972.

227. Jones, Maxwell: *The Therapeutic Community*. Basic Books, Inc., Inc., New York, 1953.

228. ————, et al.: *Beyond the Therapeutic Community*. Yale University Press, New Haven, Conn., 1968.

229. Barnes, Elizabeth (ed.): *Psychosocial Nursing*. Tavistock Publications, London, 1968.

230. Cook, Fred, Jr.: *The Plot Against the Pa-*

tient. Prentice-Hall, Inc., Englewood Cliffs, N.J., 1967.

231. van Velde, Jacoba: *The Big Ward.* Simon & Schuster, New York, 1960.

232. "The Plight of the U.S. Patient," *Time,* Feb. 21, 1969, p. 53.

233. Wessen, Albert F.: "Hospital Ideology and Communication Between Ward Personnel," in Jaco, E. Gartley (ed.): *Patients, Physicians, and Illness,* 2nd ed. Free Press, New York, 1972, p. 325.

234. Lum, Jean L. J.: "Interaction Patterns of Nursing Personnel," *Nurs. Res.,* **19:**324, (July–Aug.) 1970.

235. Barnes, Elizabeth: *People in Hospital.* Macmillan & Co., Ltd., London, 1961, p. 59.

236. American Hospital Association: *A Patient's Bill of Rights.* The Association, Chicago, 1972.

236a. "Mental Patients' Rights Guaranteed in Jersey Under New Law," *Am. J. Nurs.,* **75:** 1210, (July) 1975.

237. Clair, Linda L., and Trussell, Patricia M.: "The Change of Shift Report," *Hospitals,* **43:**91, (Oct.) 1969.

238. Dyer, Elaine, et al.: "Can Job Performance Be Predicted from Biographical, Personality, and Administrative Climate Inventories?" *Nurs. Res.,* **21:**294, (July–Aug.) 1972.

239. Jain, Harish C.: "Supervisory Communication Effectiveness and Performance in Two Urban Hospitals," *Personnel J.,* **50:** 392, (May) 1971.

240. Slocum, John W., et al.: "An Analysis of Need Satisfaction and Job Performance among Professional and Paraprofessional Hospital Personnel," *Nurs. Res.,* **21:**338, (July–Aug.) 1972.

241. Bates, Barbara: "Doctor and Nurse: Changing Roles and Relations," *N. Engl. J. Med.,* **283:**129, (July 16) 1970.

242. Christman, Luther: "Nurse-Physician Communication in the Hospital," *J.A.M.A.,* **194:** 539, (Nov. 1) 1965.

243. Dodge, Joan: "Nurse-Doctor Relations and Attitudes Toward Patients," *Nurs. Res.,* **11:** 32, (Winter) 1960.

244. Peplau, Hildegard E.: "Nurse-Doctor Relationships," *Nurs. Forum,* **5:**60, (Jan.) 1966.

245. Levin, Pamela, and Berne, Eric: "Games Nurses Play," *Am. J. Nurs.,* **72:**483, (Mar.) 1972.

246. Sutterley, Doris C., and Donnelly, Gloria F.: *op. cit.,* p. 123.

246a. Sidel, Victor W., and Sidel, Ruth: *Serve the People. Observations on Medicine in the People's Republic of China.* Beacon Press, Boston, 1973, p. 96.

247. Korsch, Barbara M., and Negrete, Vida F.: "Doctor-Patient Communication," *Sci. Am.,* **227:**66, (Aug.) 1972.

248. Crichton, Michael: *Five Patients. The Hospital Explained.* Alfred A. Knopf, New York, 1970.

249. Klein, Robert H., et al.: "Psychiatric Staff: Uniforms or Street Clothes?" *Arch. Gen. Psychiatry,* **26:**19, (Jan.) 1972.

250. Petrovich, Donald V., et al.: "Nursing Apparel and Psychiatric Patients: A Comparison of Uniforms and Street Clothes," *J. Psychiatric Nurs.,* **6:**344, (Nov.–Dec.) 1968.

251. Sommer, Robert, and Dewar, Robert: *op. cit.,* p. 327.

252. Angell, M. Faith, and Spaeth, G. L.: "Multibed Rooms Improve Morale, Patient Survey Shows," *Hospitals,* **42:**57, (Nov. 1) 1968.

253. Vernon, M. D.: *op. cit.,* p. 109.

254. Chodil, Judith, and Williams, Barbara: "The Concept of Sensory Deprivation," *Nurs. Clin. North Am.,* **5:**453, (Sept.) 1970.

255. Jackson, C. Wesley, Jr., and Ellis, Rosemary: "Sensory Deprivation as a Field of Study," *Nurs. Res.,* **20:**46, (Jan.–Feb.) 1971.

256. Shore, Herbert: "Total Environment vs. Creative Living," *Geriatric Nurs.,* **4:**18, (Aug.) 1968.

256a. De Chardin, Père Teilhard: *The Phenomenon of Man.* (English Translation.) Harper & Row, New York, 1959.

257. Nash, John: *op. cit.,* p. 234.

258. *Ibid.,* p. 238.

259. Piaget, Jean: *Six Psychological Studies.* (Translated by Anita Tenzer.) Random House, New York, 1967.

260. Siegal, Linda: "The Development of the Ability to Process Information," *J. Exp. Child Psychol.,* **6:**368, (Sept.) 1968.

261. Fantz, Robert L.: "Pattern Vision in New-Born Infants," *Science,* **140:**296, (Apr. 19) 1963.

262. ———, and Nevis, Sonia: *op. cit.,* p. 22.

263. Thomas, Alexander, et al.: "The Origin of Personality," *Sci. Am.,* **223:**102, (Aug.) 1970.

264. Korner, Anneliese F., and Thoman, Evelyn B.: "The Relative Efficacy of Contact and Vestibular-Proprioceptive Stimulation in Soothing Neonates," in Chess, Stella, and Thomas, Alexander (eds.): *Annual Progress in Child Psychiatry and Child Development, 1973.* Brunner/Mazel Publishers, New York, 1974, p. 30.

265. Montagu, Ashley: *Touching. The Human Significance of the Skin.* Columbia University Press, New York, 1971.

266. White, Sheldon H.: "The Learning Theory Tradition and Child Psychology," in Mussen, Paul H. (ed.): *Carmichael's Manual of Child Psychology,* 3rd ed. Vol. I, John Wiley & Sons, New York, 1970, p. 657.

267. Brooks, Marion R.: "A Stimulation Program for Young Children Performed by a Public Health Nurse as Part of Well Baby Care," in *ANA Clinical Sessions, 1970.* Appleton-Century-Crofts, New York, 1971, p. 128.

268. Maier, Henry W.: *Three Theories of Child Development.* Harper & Row, New York, 1965, p. 75.

269. Kohlberg, Lawrence: "Early Education: A Cognitive Developmental View," in Chess, Stella, and Thomas, Alexander (eds.): *Annual Progress in Child Psychiatry and Child Development, 1969.* Brunner/Mazel Publishers, New York, 1969.

270. Group for the Advancement of Psychiatry, Committee on Adolescence: *op. cit.,* p. 76.

271. Horn, John L.: "Intelligence—Why It Grows, Why It Declines," *Trans-Action,* **5:**23, (Nov.) 1967.

272. Bischof, Ledford J.: *op. cit.,* p. 150.

273. Hilgard, Ernest R., and Bower, Gordon H.: *Theories of Learning,* 3rd ed. Appleton-Century-Crofts, New York, 1966.

274. Handley, Philip (ed.): *Biology and the Future of Man.* Oxford University Press, New York, 1970.

275. Bugelski, B. R.: *The Psychology of Learning Applied to Teaching,* 2nd ed. Bobbs-Merrill Co., New York, 1971.

276. Hilgard, Ernest R., and Bower, Gordon H.: *op. cit.,* p. 562.

277. Skinner, B. F.: *The Behavior of Organisms: An Experimental Analysis.* Appleton-Century-Crofts, New York, 1938.

278. Verplanck, William S.: "The Control of the Content of Conversation: Reinforcement of Statements of Opinion," *J. Abn. Soc. Psychol.,* **51:**668, (Nov.) 1955.

279. Bensberg, Gerald J., et al.: "Teaching the Profoundly Retarded Self-Help Activities by Behavior Shaping Techniques," *Am. J. Ment. Def.,* **69:**674, 1965.

280. Baker, Roger: "The Chronic Psychiatric Patient—A New Hope for Treatment?" Part I, *Nurs. Times,* **68:**1161, (Sept. 14) 1972.

281. Rosenthal, G., et al.: "The Chronic Psychiatric Patient—A New Hope for Treatment?" Part II, *Nurs. Times,* **68:**1182, (Sept. 21) 1972.

282. Hoffey, Virginia A.: "Behavior Modification Utilizing a Token Economy Program," *J. Psychiatric Nurs.,* **8:**31, (Mar.–Apr.) 1970.

283. Wheeler, Andrew J., and Sulzer, Beth: "Operant Training and Generalization of a Verbal Response Form in a Speech-Deficient Child," *J. Appl. Behav. Anal.,* **3:**139, (Summer) 1970.

284. Grosicki, Jeanette P.: "Effect of Operant Conditioning on Modification of Incontinence in Neuropsychiatric Geriatric Patients," *Nurs. Res.,* **17:**304, (July–Aug.) 1968.

285. Wagner, Bernard R., and Paul, Gordon L.: "Reduction of Incontinence in Chronic Mental Patients: A Pilot Project," *J. Behav. Ther. Exp. Psychiat.,* **1:**29, (Mar.) 1970.

285a. Berni, Rosemarian, et al.: *Behavior Modification and the Nursing Process.* C. V. Mosby Co., St. Louis, 1973.

285b. Bugelski, B. R.: *op. cit.,* p. 240.

286. Handler, Philip (ed.): *op. cit.,* p. 415.

287. Jamann, Joann S.: "Health Is a Function of Ecology," *Am. J. Nurs.,* **71:**970, (May) 1971.

287a. Kruse, Margrethe: "A World of Unity. From Nationalism to Internationalism," *Imprint,* **20:**14, (Apr.) 1973.

288. National Analysts, Inc.: *A Study of Health Practices and Opinions.* National Technical Information Service, Springfield, Va., 1972, p. xviii.

289. Van Dorn, Mark: *The Meaning of a Liberal Education.* Henry Holt & Co., New York, 1943.

290. Leigh, T. M.: "Nationwide Profile of Health Instruction," *Sch. Health Rev.,* **4:**35, (May–June) 1973.

291. Eiseman, Seymour, and Marshall, Larry: "The Status of Professional Preparation of Health Educators in Selected California Community Colleges," *J. Am. Coll. Health Assoc.,* **20:**280, (Apr.) 1972.

291a. Arnold, Pam: "Chicago Teacher-Nurses," *The American Nurse,* **7:**8, (Sept.) 1975.

292. National Analysts, Inc.: *op. cit.*

293. Dwyer, Johanna T., et al.: "Nutritional Literacy of High School Students," *J. Nutr. Educ.,* **2:**59, (Fall) 1970.

294. Tifft, Margaret, and Stanton, J. B.: "Nutrition Misconceptions of Secondary School Youth," *Sch. Health Rev.,* **3:**12, (Nov.–Dec.) 1972.

295. Mitchell, Helen S.: "Nutrition in Relation to Stature," *J. Am. Diet. Assoc.,* **40:**521, (June) 1962.

296. Greulich, William W.: "Growth of Children of the Same Race Under Different Environmental Conditions," *Science,* **127:**515, (Mar. 7) 1958.

297. Abramowicz, Mark: "Heights of 12-Year Old Puerto Rico Boys in New York City: Origins of Differences," *Pediatrics,* **43:**427, (Mar.) 1969.

298. Hayden, Eugene B.: "Breakfast and Today's Lifestyles," *J. Sch. Health,* **45:**83, (Feb.) 1975.

298a. Fleshman, Ruth P.: "Eating Rituals and Realities," *Nurs. Clin. North Am.,* **8:**91, (Mar.) 1973.

299. Ramsdell, Les C.: "An Analysis of the Health Interests and Needs of West Virginia High School Students," *J. Sch. Health,* **42:**477, (Oct.) 1972.

300. Newman, Ian M., and Mayshark, Cyrus: "Health Education Planning and Community Perceptions of Local Health Problems," *J. Sch. Health,* **43:**438, (Sept.) 1973.

301. Byer, Ruth, et al.: *Teach Us What We Want to Know.* Mental Health Materials Center, New York, 1969.

302. Thornburg, Hershel D.: "A Comparative Study of Sex Information Sources," *J. Sch. Health,* **42:**88, (Feb.) 1972.

303. Warren, Carrie Lee, and St. Pierre, Richard: "Sources and Accuracy of College

Students' Sex Knowledge," *J. Sch. Health,* **43:**588, (Nov.) 1973.

304. Pauly, Ira B., and Goldstein, Steven G.: "Physicians' Ability to Treat Sexual Problems," *Med. Aspects Hum. Sex.,* **4:**24, (Oct.) 1970.

305. Mandetta, Anne F., and Woods, Nancy Fugate: "Learning About Human Sexuality —A Course Model," *Nurs. Outlook,* **22:** 525, (Aug.) 1974.

306. Mims, Fern, et al.: "Effectiveness of an Interdisciplinary Course in Human Sexuality," *Nurs. Res.,* **23:**248, (May–June) 1974.

307. Malo-Juvera, Dolores: "Seeing Is Believing," *Nurs. Outlook,* **21:**583, (Sept.) 1973.

308. Moore, Bernice Milburn: "Education for Family Living—What Is It?" *Nurs. Clin. North Am.,* **4:**359, (June) 1969.

309. Krizinofski, Marian T.: "Human Sexuality and Nursing Practice," *Nurs. Clin. North Am.,* **8:**673, (Dec.) 1973.

309a. Fonseca, Jeanne D.: "Sexuality—A Quality of Being Human," in Browning, Mary H., and Lewis, Edith P. (comps.): *Human Sexuality: Nursing Implications.* American Journal of Nursing Co., New York, 1973.

310. Sutterley, Doris C., and Donnelly, Gloria F.: *op. cit.,* p. 127.

311. Sex Information and Education Council of the United States (comps. and eds.): *Sexuality and Man.* Charles Scribner's Sons, New York, 1970.

312. Lidz, Theodore: *op. cit.*

313. Benedek, Therese: "Parenthood During the Life Cycle," in Anthony, E. James, and Benedek, Therese (eds.): *Parenthood. Its Psychology and Psychopathology.* Little, Brown & Co., Boston, 1970, p. 185.

314. Kagan, Jerome: "Acquisition and Significance of Sex Typing and Sex Role Identity," in Hoffman, Martin L., and Hoffman, Lois Wladis (eds.): *Review of Child Development Research,* Vol. I. Russell Sage Foundation, New York, 1964, p. 137.

315. Simon, William, and Gagnon, John: "Psychosexual Development," *Trans-Action,* **6:**9, (Mar.) 1969.

316. Stephens, Gwen J.: "Mind-Body Continuum in Human Sexuality," *Am. J. Nurs.,* **70:** 1468, (July) 1970.

316a. Juhasz, Anne McCreary (ed.): *Sexual Development and Behavior.* Dorsey Press, Homewood, Ill., 1973.

316b. Burt, John J., and Meeks, L.: *Toward a Healthy Sexuality.* W. B. Saunders Co., Philadelphia, 1973.

316c. Krizinofski, Marian T.: *op. cit.*

316d. Oksisabor, J. A.: "Assessment of Masculinity and Femininity," *Niger. Nurse,* **5:**30, (Jan.–Mar.) 1973.

316e. Schlesinger, Arthur, Jr.: "An Informal History of Love, U.S.A.," *Med. Aspects Hum. Sex.,* **4:**64, (June) 1970.

317. "Sexual Attitudes and Behavior in the Elderly," *Geriatric Focus,* **12:**1, (May) 1973.

318. Barton, David: "Sexually Deprived Individuals," *Med. Aspects Hum. Sex.,* **6:**88, (Feb.) 1972.

319. *Ibid.*

319a. Browning, Mary H., and Lewis, Edith P. (comps.): *Human Sexuality: Nursing Implications.* American Journal of Nursing Co., New York, 1973.

319b. Mims, Fern H. (ed.): "Symposium on Human Sexuality," *Nurs. Clin. North Am.,* **10:**517, (Sept.) 1975.

320. Comarr, A. Estin, and Gunderson, Bernice B.: "Sexual Function in Traumatic Paraplegia and Quadriplegia," *Am. J. Nurs.,* **75:**250, (Feb.) 1975.

321. Dlin, Barney M., and Perlman, Abraham: "Sex After Ileostomy or Colostomy," *Med. Aspects Hum. Sex.,* **6:**32, (July) 1972.

322. Stahlgran, LeRoy H., and Fergusson, F. Kraeer: "Influence on Sexual Function of Abdominoperineal Resection for Ulcerative Colitis," *N. Engl. J. Med.,* **259:**873, (Oct. 30) 1958.

323. Pinderhughes, Charles A., et al.: "Interrelationships Between Sexual Functioning and Medical Conditions," *Med. Aspects Hum. Sex.,* **6:**52, (Oct.) 1972.

324. Oaks, Wilbur W., and Moyer, John H.: "Sex and Hypertension," *Med. Aspects Hum. Sex.,* **6:**128, (Nov.) 1972.

325. Pinderhughes, Charles A., et al.: *op. cit.*

326. Reichelt, Paul A., and Werley, Harriet H.: "A Sex Information Program for Sexually Active Teenagers," *J. Sch. Health,* **45:**100, (Feb.) 1975.

327. Kantner, John F., and Zelnik, Melvin: "Sexual Experience of Young Unmarried Women in the United States," *Fam. Plann. Perspect.,* **4:**9, (Oct.) 1972.

328. US Public Health Service, Center for Disease Control: *VD Fact Sheet, 1973.* US Government Printing Office, Washington, D.C., 1974.

329. ———: *Abortion Surveillance Summary in the United States, 1972.* US Government Printing Office, Washington, D.C., 1974.

330. Osofsky, Howard J., and Osofsky, Joy D.: "Adolescents as Mothers," in Chess, Stella, and Thomas, Alexander (eds.): *Annual Progress in Child Psychiatry and Child Development, 1971.* Brunner/Mazel Publishers, New York, 1971, p. 556.

331. De Lissovoy, Vladimir: "Child Care by Adolescent Parents," *Children Today,* **2:**22, (July–Aug.) 1973.

332. Gordon, Sol: "What Adolescents Want to Know," *Am. J. Nurs.,* **71:**534, (Mar.) 1971.

333. Hastings, Donald W.: *A Doctor Speaks on Sexual Expression in Marriage,* 2nd ed. Little, Brown & Co., Boston, 1971.

334. Pierson, Elaine C.: *Sex Is Never an Emergency,* 3rd ed. J. B. Lippincott Co., Philadelphia, 1973.

335. Yale University, Student Committee on Human Sexuality: *The Student Guide to Sex on Campus.* New American Library, New York, 1971.

336. Brown, Mary Agnes: "Adolescents and VD," *Nurs. Outlook,* **21:**99, (Feb.) 1973.

337. Reichelt, Paul A., and Werley, Harriet H.: *op. cit.*

338. Yacenda, John A.: "Survey of VD Knowledge Among Young People," *Health Serv. Rep.,* **87:**394, (May) 1972.

339. Vandermeer, Daniel C.: "Meet the VD Epidemiologist," *Am. J. Nurs.,* **71:**722, (Apr.) 1971.

340. Brown, William J.: "Acquired Syphilis—Drugs and Blood Tests," *Am. J. Nurs.,* **71:**713, (Apr.) 1971.

341. Brown, Mary Agnes: *op. cit.*

342. Eisenberg, Arlene, and Eisenberg, Howard: "A New Teaching Program. How To Be Your Own Doctor—Sometimes," *Parade, New Haven Register,* Feb. 24, 1974, p. 11.

343. Katz, Harvey P., and Clancy, Robert R.: "Accuracy of a Home Throat Culture Program: A Study of Parent Participation in Health Care," *Pediatrics,* **53:**687, (May) 1974.

344. Black, Louis A., and Brown, Donald D.: "Public Information and Heart Attack. Report of an Educational Program," *Ohio State Med. J.,* **69:**369, (May) 1973.

345. Swinehart, James W.: "Voluntary Exposure to Health Communications," *Am. J. Public Health,* **58:**1265, (July) 1968.

346. Pearman, Eleanor C.: *Historical Study of the Emotionally-Supportive and Patient-Teaching Roles of the General Duty Nurse from 1900–1970.* Doctoral Dissertation, Boston University, Boston, 1971.

347. Pender, Nola J.: "Patient Identification of Health Information Received During Hospitalization," *Nurs. Res.,* **23:**262, (May–June) 1974.

348. Boosinger, Jeannene C. K.: *Nurses Perception of Responsibility for Health Education of Patients.* Doctoral Dissertation, University of Nebraska, Lincoln, 1971.

349. Robinson, Jan: "Do Nurses Tell Mothers Enough About Feeding Problems?" *Lamp,* **29:**7, (Aug.) 1972.

350. Clark, Vivian Vreeland: *Learnings of the Patient with Coronary Occlusion About His Illness and Self-Care.* Doctoral Dissertation, Columbia University, New York, 1967.

350a. Schwartz, Doris: "Medication Errors Made by Elderly, Chronically Ill Patients," *Am. J. Public Health,* **52:**2018, (Dec.) 1962.

351. Aiken, Linda Harman: "Patient Problems Are Problems in Learning," *Am. J. Nurs.,* **70:**1916, (Sept.) 1970.

352. Culbert, Pamela A., and Kos, Barbara A.: "Aging: Considerations for Health Teaching," *Nurs. Clin. North Am.,* **6:**605, (Dec.) 1971.

353. Grout, Ruth E., and Watkins, Julia D.: "The Nurse and Health Education," *Int. Nurs. Rev.,* **18:**248, (No. 3) 1971.

354. Hallburg, Jeanne C.: "Teaching Patients Self-Care," *Nurs. Clin. North Am.,* **5:**223, (June) 1970.

355. Healy, Kathryn M.: "Does Preoperative Instruction Make a Difference?" *Am. J. Nurs.,* **68:**62, (Jan.) 1968.

356. Jason, Hilliard: "The Health-Care Practitioner as Instructor," in *Fostering the Growing Need to Learn,* Part I. Regional Medical Programs Service, Syracuse University, Syracuse, N.Y., 1973, p. 225.

357. Redman, Barbara K.: "Patient Education as a Function of Nursing Practice," *Nurs. Clin. North Am.,* **6:**573, (Dec.) 1971.

358. Storlie, Frances: "A Philosophy of Patient Teaching," *Nurs. Outlook,* **19:**387, (June) 1971.

359. Bird, Ida Stanley: "Breast-Feeding Classes on the Postpartum Unit," *Am. J. Nurs.,* **75:**456, (Mar.) 1975.

360. Copp, Laurel A.: "The Waiting Room—A Health Teaching Site," *Nurs. Outlook,* **19:**481, (July) 1971.

361. Hayes, Evelyn R.: "Clinic Waiting Room Experience: An Exploratory Study," *Nurs. Res.,* **17:**361, (July–Aug.) 1968.

361a. Wonnell, Edith B.: "The Education of the Expectant Father for Childbirth," *Nurs. Clin. North Am.,* **6:**591, (Dec.) 1971.

362. Steiner, Joseph Ray: *The Effects of Family-Centered versus Wife-Centered Obstetrical Care Upon Family Life.* Doctoral Dissertation, Ohio State University, Columbus, 1972.

363. Quirk, Barbara, and Hassenein, Ruth: "The Nurse's Role in Advising Patients on Coitus During Pregnancy," *Nurs. Clin. North Am.,* **8:**501, (Sept.) 1973.

364. Otte, Mary Jane: "Correcting Inverted Nipples," *Am. J. Nurs.,* **75:**454, (Mar.) 1975.

365. Barnard, Janice E.: "Peer Group Instruction for Primigravida Adolescents," *Nurs. Outlook,* **18:**42, (Aug.) 1970.

366. Curtis, Frances L.: "Observations of Unwed Pregnant Adolescents," *Am. J. Nurs.,* **74:**100, (Jan.) 1974.

367. Minder, Laurie: "Sex Education on a Psychiatric Unit," *Am. J. Nurs.,* **74:**1865, (Oct.) 1974.

368. Burgess, Linda C.: "The Unmarried Father in Adoption Planning," *Children,* **15:**71, (Mar.–Apr.) 1968.

369. Pannor, Reuben: "Casework Services for Unmarried Fathers," *Children,* **10:**65, (Mar.–Apr.) 1963.

370. Light, Richard J.: "Abused and Neglected Children in America: A Study of Alternative Policies," *Harvard Educational Rev.,* **43:**556, (Nov.) 1973.

371. Giovannoni, Jeanne M.: "Parental Mistreatment: Perpetrators and Victims," *J. Marr. Fam.,* **33:**649, (Nov.) 1971.

372. Goode, William J.: "Force and Violence

in the Family," *J. Marr. Fam.,* **33:**624, (Nov.) 1971.

373. Barnard, Martha Underwood, and Wolfe, Lorraine: "Psychosocial Failure to Thrive," *Nurs. Clin. North Am.,* **8:**557, (Sept.) 1973.

374. Kyle, Jean R., and Savino, Anne B.: "Teaching Parents Behavior Modification," *Nurs. Outlook,* **21:**717, (Nov.) 1973.

375. "Education for Parenthood," *Children Today,* **2:**3, (Mar.–Apr.) 1973 (Special Issue).

376. Light, Richard J.: *op. cit.*

376a. Hubbard, Charles William: *Family Planning Education. Parenthood and Social Disease Control.* C. V. Mosby Co., St. Louis, 1973.

377. Arnold, Elizabeth: "Individualized Nursing Care in Family Planning," in Browning, Mary H., and Lewis, Edith P. (comps.): *Human Sexuality: Nursing Implications.* American Journal of Nursing Co., New York, 1973, p. 75.

378. Connell, Elizabeth B.: "The Pill and the Problems," in Browning, Mary H., and Lewis, Edith P. (comps.): *Human Sexuality: Nursing Implications.* American Journal of Nursing Co., New York, 1973, p. 120.

379. Davis, Joseph E.: "Vasectomy," in Browning, Mary H., and Lewis, Edith P. (comps.): *Human Sexuality: Nursing Implications.* American Journal of Nursing Co., New York, 1973, p. 141.

380. Gonzales, Betty: "Voluntary Sterilization," in Browning, Mary H., and Lewis, Edith P.: *Human Sexuality: Nursing Implications.* American Journal of Nursing Co., New York, 1973, p. 134.

381. Wiedenbach, Ernestine: "The Nurse's Role in Family Planning," *Nurs. Clin. North Am.,* **3:**355, (June) 1968.

382. Carter, C. O., et al.: "Genetic Clinic: A Follow-Up," *Lancet,* **1:**281, (Feb. 6) 1971.

383. Arehart, Joan L.: "Prenatal Diagnosis: How Fast, How Far?" *Sci. News,* **100:**44, (July 17) 1971.

384. Finley, Sara C.: "Genetic Counseling," *South. Med. J.,* **64:**(Suppl. #1) 101, (Feb.) 1971.

385. Friedmann, Theodore: "Prenatal Diagnosis of Genetic Disease," *Sci. Am.,* **225:**34, (Nov.) 1971.

386. "Perspectives in Genetic Counseling," *Pediatric Curr.,* **20:**9, (Feb.) 1971.

387. Tani, Gwen S., and Hankin, Jean H.: "A Self-Learning Unit for Patients with Diabetes," *J. Am. Diet. Assoc.,* **58:**33, (Apr.) 1971.

388. Collier, Boy N., Jr., and Etzwiler, Donnell D.: "Comparative Study of Diabetes Knowledge Among Juvenile Diabetics and Their Parents," *Diabetes,* **20:**51, (Jan.) 1971.

389. Leifson, June: "Glycosuria Testing and the Nurse," in *ANA Clinical Conferences, 1969.* Appleton-Century-Crofts, New York, 1970, p. 94.

390. Martin, Elizabeth Jean: "Diabetic Foot Care: Knowledge and Practice," in *ANA Clinical Conferences, 1969.* Appleton-Century-Crofts, New York, 1970, p. 143.

391. Nickerson, Donna: "Teaching the Hospitalized Diabetic," *Am. J. Nurs.,* **72:**935, (May) 1972.

392. Skelton, Judith M.: "A Diabetic Teaching Tool," *Can. Nurse,* **69:**35, (Dec.) 1973.

393. Goldstein, David H.: "The Occupational Safety and Health Act in 1970," *Am. J. Nurs.,* **71:**1535, (Aug.) 1971.

394. Millsap, Mary: "Occupational Health Nursing in an Alcohol Addiction Program," *Nurs. Clin. North Am.,* **7:**121, (Mar.) 1972.

395. Scanlon, Mary E.: "An Industrial Visiting Nurse," *Nurs. Clin. North Am.,* **7:**143, (Mar.) 1972.

396. Tinkham, Catherine W.: "The Plant as the Patient of the Occupational Health Nurse," *Nurs. Clin. North Am.,* **7:**99, (Mar.) 1972.

397. Chinn, Peggy: "Relationship Between Health and School Problems: A Nursing Assessment," *J. Sch. Health,* **43:**85, (Feb.) 1973.

398. Hilmar, Norman A., and McAtee, Patricia A.: "The School Nurse Practitioner and Her Practice: A Study of Traditional and Expanded Health Care Responsibilities for Nurses in Elementary Schools," *J. Sch. Health,* **43:**431, (Sept.) 1973.

399. Lowis, Evelyn M.: "An Appraisal of the Amount of Time Spent on Functions by Los Angeles City School Nurses," *J. Sch. Health,* **39:**254, (Apr.) 1969.

400. Pelizza, John J.: "A Comparative Study of How Parents from Different Social Classes Perceive School Health Services," *J. Sch. Health,* **43:**176, (Mar.) 1973.

401. Simon, Helen M.: "A Look at Secondary School Health Services," *Nurs. Outlook,* **16:**42, (Aug.) 1968.

402. Van Arsdell, William R., et al.: "Visits to an Elementary School Nurse," *J. Sch. Health,* **42:**142, (Mar.) 1972.

403. Storrs, Rosa Tolbert: "A Survey of Attitudes of Students Toward Utilization of the University Health Center," *J. Am. Coll. Health Assoc.,* **20:**204, (Feb.) 1972.

404. Amdur, Shiela B., and Oreschnick, Robert W.: "A Descriptive Study of a Pregnancy Counseling Service in a University Health Service," *J. Am. Coll. Health Assoc.,* **21:**149, (Dec.) 1972.

405. Lopater, David, and Hursh, Lawrence M.: "Report on Student Views of the Illinois Health Service," *J. Am. Coll. Health Assoc.,* **20:**299, (Apr.) 1972.

406. Sidhu, Satwant, and Klotz, Addie L.: "Student Awareness and Utilization of a College Student Health Service," *J. Am. Coll. Health Assoc.,* **19:**298, (June) 1971.

406a. Weinberg, S. L.: "Patient Education as a Part of Critical Care," *Heart-Lung,* **3:**47, (Jan.–Feb.) 1974.

407. Grout, Ruth E., and Watkins, Julia D.: *op. cit.*

408. Levine, Myra E.: "The Intransigent Patient," *Am. J. Nurs.,* **70:**2106, (Oct.) 1970.

409. Collins, Rosella Denison: "Problem Solving. A Tool for Patients, Too," *Am. J. Nurs.,* **68:**1483, (July) 1968.

409a. Duff, Raymond S., and Hollingshead, August B.: *Sickness and Society.* Harper & Row, New York, 1968.

409b. Stockwell, Felicity: *The Unpopular Patient.* Royal College of Nursing, London, 1972.

410. Dodge, Joan S.: "Factors Related to Patients' Perceptions of Their Cognitive Needs," *Nurs. Res.,* **18:**502, (Nov.–Dec.) 1969.

411. Norris, Catherine M.: "Delusions that Trap Nurses . . . into Dead End Alleys Away from Growth, Relevance, and Impact on Health Care," *Nurs. Outlook,* **21:**18, (Jan.) 1973.

412. McGuire, William J.: "Persuasion," in Miller, George A. (ed.): *Communication, Language, and Meaning.* Basic Books, Inc., New York, 1973, p. 248.

413. Holder, Lee: "Effects of Source, Message, Audience Characteristics on Health Behavior Compliance," *Health Serv. Rep.,* **87:**343, (Apr.) 1972.

414. Kramer, Charles H.: "Communicating with the Patient," *Geriatric Nurs.,* **4:**15, (Sept.) 1968.

415. Ley, P., et al.: "A Method for Increasing Patients' Recall of Information Presented by Doctors," *Psychol. Med.,* **3:**217, (May) 1973.

416. Marks, Janet, and Clarke, Margaret: "The Hospital Patient and His Knowledge of the Drugs He Is Receiving," *Int. Nurs. Rev.,* **19:**39, (No. 1) 1972.

417. Mohammed, Mary F. Bucklin: "Patients' Understanding of Written Health Information," *Nurs. Res.,* **13:**100, (Spring) 1964.

418. Packard, Rose B., and Van Ess, Harriet: "A Comparison of Informal and Role-Delineated Patient-Teaching Situations," *Nurs. Res.,* **18:**443, (Sept.–Oct.) 1969.

419. Holder, Lee: *op. cit.*

420. Roberts, Beryl J., et al.: "An Experimental Study of Two Approaches to Communication," *Am. J. Public Health,* **53:**1361, (Sept.) 1963.

421. Grossen, Charles F.: "Local Residents as Mediators Between Middle-Class Professional Workers and Lower-Class Clients," *Soc. Serv. Rev.,* **40:**56, (Mar.) 1966.

422. Carroll, Bettie: "Fingers to Toes," *Am. J. Nurs.,* **71:**550, (Mar.) 1971.

423. Griffin, Winnie, et al.: "Group Exercise for Patients with Limited Motion," *Am. J. Nurs.,* **71:**1742, (Sept.) 1971.

424. Lindeman, Carol A.: "Nursing Intervention with the Presurgical Patient. Effectiveness and Efficiency of Group and Individual Preoperative Teaching. Phase II," *Nurs. Res.,* **21:**196, (May–June) 1972.

425. Mezzanotte, Elizabeth Jane: "Group Instruction in Preparation for Surgery," *Am. J. Nurs.,* **70:**89, (Jan.) 1970.

426. Valentine, Lois R.: "Self-Care Through Group Learning," *Am. J. Nurs.,* **70:**2140, (Oct.) 1970.

427. Mullen, Patricia Dolan: "Health Education for Heart Patients in Crisis," *Health Serv. Rep.,* **88:**669, (Aug.–Sept.) 1973.

428. Horkheimer, Foley A. (comp. and ed.): *Educators Guide to Free Health, Physical Education, and Recreational Materials,* 5th ed. Educators Progress Service, Randolph, Wisc., 1972.

429. Ambrosino, R. J., and Anzola, Anne M.: "Keeping Healthy After 60 by 2-Way Radio," *Health Serv. Rep.,* **87:**583, (Aug.–Sept.) 1972.

430. Brylski, Eleanor, and Gillen, Janet: "Audiovisuals Made to Order," *Nurs. Outlook,* **20:**385, (June) 1972.

431. Langhoff, Howard F.: "Audiovisual Equipment," *Am. J. Nurs.,* **72:**2032, (Nov.) 1972.

432. Catania, James J.: "Closed-Circuit TV Helps Patients Understand and Adjust to Environment," *Mod. Hosp.,* **109:**66, (July) 1967.

432a. Ballantyne, D. J.: "CCTV for Patients," *Am. J. Nurs.,* **74:**263, (Feb.) 1974.

432b. Lovrien, J.: "Utilize Closed Circuit Television in an Inservice Program," *J. Contin. Educ.,* **4:**13, (July–Aug.) 1974.

433. Bartlett, Marjorie H., et al.: "Dial Access Library–Patient Information Service," *N. Engl. J. Med.,* **288:**994, (May 10) 1973.

Additional Suggested Reading

Alfano, Genrose: "Whom Do You Care For?" in *ANA Clinical Conferences, 1969.* Appleton-Century-Crofts, New York, 1970.

Bates, Barbara, and Chamberlin, Robert W.: "Physician Leadership as Perceived by Nurses," *Nurs. Res.,* **19:**534, (Nov.–Dec.) 1970.

Bedard, Evelyn M.: "Unmet Needs Versus Perceived Needs—The Effect of Inadequate Communication," in *ANA Clinical Conferences, 1967.* Appleton-Century-Crofts, New York, 1968.

Bellugi, Ursula: "Learning the Language," *Psychol. Today,* **4:**32, (Dec.) 1970.

Bird, Brian: *Talking with Patients,* 2nd ed. J. B. Lippincott Co., Philadelphia, 1973.

Bower, T. G. R.: "The Object in the World of the Infant," *Sci. Am.,* **225:**30, (Oct.) 1971.

Breed, George, and Porter, Maynard: "Eye Contact, Attitudes, and Attitude Change Among Males," *J. Genet. Psychol.,* **120:**211, (June) 1972.

Brink, Pamela J.: "Role Distance: A Maneuver in Nursing," *Nurs. Forum,* **11:**323, (No. 3) 1972.

Brooks, Patricia A.: "Masturbation," in Browning, Mary H., and Lewis, Edith P. (comps.): *Human Sexuality: Nursing Implications.* American Journal of Nursing Co., New York, 1973.

Brown, Roger: *Psycholinguistics: Selected Papers.* Free Press, New York, 1970.

Brunswick, Ann F.: "Health Needs of Adolescents: How the Adolescent Sees Them," *Am. J. Public Health,* 59:1730, (Sept.) 1969.

Chapanis, Alphonse: "Interactive Human Communication," *Sci. Am.,* 232:36, (Mar.) 1975.

Charlip, Remy, et al.: *Handtalk, An ABC of Finger Spelling and Sign Language.* Parents Magazine Press, New York, 1974.

Chomsky, Carol: "Stages in Language Development and Reading Exposure," *Harvard Educational Rev.,* 42:1, (Feb.) 1972.

Couture, Nancy A.: *Communicating with Patients. Approach and Content Used by Nurses.* Doctoral Dissertation, St. Louis University, St. Louis, 1967.

Crayton, Josephine K.: "Talking with Persons Who Have Cancer," *Am. J. Nurs.,* 69:744, (Apr.) 1969.

Cronenwett, Linda R., and Newmark, Lucy L.: "Fathers' Responses to Childbirth," *Nurs. Res.,* 23:210, (May–June) 1974.

Davis, Milton S.: "Variations in Patients' Compliance with Doctors' Advice: An Empirical Analysis of Patterns of Communication," *Am. J. Public Health,* 58:274, (Feb.) 1968.

Douglas-Wilson, I., and McLachlan, Gordon (eds.): *Health Service Prospects. An International Survey.* Little, Brown & Co., Boston, 1973.

Ellsworth, Phoebe, et al.: "The Stare or a Stimulus to Flight in Human Subjects," *J. Pers. Soc. Psychol.,* 21:302, (No. 3) 1972.

Engen, Trygg: "The Sense of Smell," *Ann. Rev. Psychol.,* 24:187, 1973.

Fast, Julius: *Body Language.* Pocket Books, New York, 1971.

Flanagan, James L.: "The Synthesis of Speech," *Sci. Am.,* 226:48, (Feb.) 1972.

Fleming, Joyce D.: "Field Report: The State of the Apes," *Psychol. Today,* 7:31, (Jan.) 1974.

Gardner, Richard A.: *Therapeutic Communication with Children: The Mutual Storytelling Technique.* Science House, New York, 1971.

Gerbner, George: "Cultural Indicators: The Case of Violence in Television Drama," *Ann. Am. Acad. Pol. Soc. Sci.,* 388:69, (Mar.) 1970.

Geschwind, Warren H.: "Language and the Brain," *Sci. Am.,* 226:76, (Apr.) 1972.

Hadley, Betty Jo: "Current Concepts of Wellness and Illness: Their Relevance for Nursing," *Image,* 6:21, (No. 2) 1974.

Hall, Edward T.: "Environmental Communication," in Esser, Aristide H. (ed.): *Behavior and Environment. The Use of Space by Animals and Men.* Plenum Press, New York, 1971.

Horowitz, Mardi J.: "Spatial Behavior and Psychopathology," *J. Nerv. Ment. Dis.,* 146:24, (No. 1) 1968.

Huey, Florence L.: "In a Therapeutic Community," *Am. J. Nurs.,* 71:926, (May) 1971.

Hutcheson, Hazel Ann, and Wright, Nicholas H.: "Georgia's Family Planning Program," in Browning, Mary H., and Lewis, Edith P. (comps.): *Human Sexuality: Nursing Implica-*

tions. American Journal of Nursing Co., New York, 1973.

Kelly, Holly Skodol: "The Meaning of Current Dance Forms to Adolescent Girls: An Exploratory Study," *Nurs. Res.,* 17:513, (Nov.–Dec.) 1968.

Kelly, Marge: "Birthright—Alternative to Abortion," *Am. J. Nurs.,* 75:76, (Jan.) 1975.

Koch, Sigmund: "The Image of Man in Encounter Groups," *Am. Scholar,* 42:636, (Autumn) 1973.

Lada, Alice Kahn: "Information and Social Support as Factors in the Outcome of Breast Feeding," *J. Appl. Behav. Sci.,* 8:110, (Jan.–Feb.) 1972.

Lennenberg, Eric H.: "The Neurology of Language," *Daedalus,* 102:115 (Summer) 1973.

MacNamara, John: "Cognitive Basis of Language Learning in Infants," in Chess, Stella, and Thomas, Alexander (eds.): *Annual Progress in Child Psychiatry and Child Development, 1973.* Brunner/Mazel Publishers, New York, 1973.

Malo-Juvera, Dolores: "What Pregnant Teenagers Know About Sex," in Browning, Mary H., and Lewis, Edith P. (comps.): *Human Sexuality: Nursing Implications.* American Journal of Nursing Co., New York, 1973.

Marshall, Jon C., and Feeney, Sally: "Structured Versus Intuitive Intake Interview," *Nurs. Res.,* 21:269, (May–June) 1972.

Meadows, Kathryn P.: "Early Manual Communication in Relation to the Deaf Child's Intellectual, Social, and Communicative Functioning," *Am. Ann. Deaf,* 113:29, 1968.

Minckley, Barbara B.: "Space and Place in Patient Care," *Am. J. Nurs.,* 68:511, (Mar.) 1968.

Morimoto, Kiyo, et al.: "Notes on the Context for Learning," *Harvard Educational Rev.,* 43:245, (May) 1973.

Nash, Helen: "Perception of Vocal Expression of Emotions by Hospital Staff and Patients," *Genet. Psychol. Monogr.,* 89:25, (Feb.) 1974.

Oettinger, Anthony G., and Zapol, Nikki: "Will Information Technologies Help Learning?" *Teachers Coll. Rec.,* 74:5, (Sept.) 1972.

Parker, Ross D., et al.: "Hostile and Helpful Verbalizations as Regulators of Nonverbal Aggression," *J. Pers. Soc. Psychol.,* 23:243, (Aug.) 1972.

Pastalan, Leon A.: "Privacy as an Expression of Human Territoriality," in Pastalan, Leon A., and Carson, Daniel (eds.): *Spatial Behavior in Older People.* University of Michigan, Ann Arbor, 1970.

Pattullo, Ann W., and Barnard, Kathryn E.: "Teaching Menstrual Hygiene to the Mentally Retarded," *Am. J. Nurs.,* 68:2572, (Dec.) 1968.

Pluckham, Margaret L.: "Territoriality: A Problem Affecting the Delivery of Health Care," *Nurs. Forum,* 11:300, (No. 3) 1972.

Porter, Carol S.: "Grade School Children's Perceptions of Their Internal Body Parts," *Nurs. Res.,* 23:384, (Sept.–Oct.) 1974.

Riekehof, Lottie: *Talk to the Deaf.* Gospel Publishing House, Springfield, Mo., 1968.

Spaulding, Margaret R.: "The Effectiveness of

Tape Recordings with Primiparas of the Lower Socioeconomic Group in Coping with Mothering Tasks," in Batey, Marjorie V. (ed.): *Communicating Nursing Research*. Western Interstate Commission for Higher Education, Boulder, Colo., 1969.

Thompson, Richard F., et al.: "The Neurophysiology of Learning," *Ann. Rev. Psychol.*, 23:73, 1972.

Tillich, Paul: "The Meaning of Health," *Perspect. Biol. Med.*, 5:92, (Autumn) 1961.

Ujhely, Gertrud: *Determinants of the Nurse-Patient Relationship*. Springer Publishing Co., New York, 1968.

Wilkins, R. H.: "The Health Visitor and the Alcoholic," *Health Visit.*, 46:366, (Nov.) 1973.

Zaenglein, Mary Margaret, and Smith, Clagett: "An Analysis of Individual Communication Patterns and Perceptions in Hospital Organizations," *Hum. Rel.*, 25:493, (Dec.) 1972.

Zuger, Bernard: "Understanding Human Freedom: A Necessary Ingredient in Treating Adolescents," *Am. J. Psychother.*, 26:263, (Apr.) 1972.

Catherine Temple
Virginia Henderson

The authors acknowledge the assistance of Margaret Colliton (formerly Associate Professor, Psychiatric Nursing, Yale University School of Nursing, and Clinical Specialist in Psychiatric Nursing, Connecticut Mental Health Center, New Haven, Conn.) in the preparation of this chapter.

CHAPTER 17

Work—Occupation; Play—Recreation

1. WORK
2. PLAY
3. THE NURSE'S ROLE IN PROVIDING OPPORTUNITY FOR WORK AND PLAY

1. WORK

The Nature and Meaning of Work. Mark Twain has said, "Work consists of whatever a body is *obliged* to do, and Play consists of whatever a body is not obliged to do." The term *occupation* is applied to an activity yielding tangible results, or products, and is usually done with serious intent and for material gain.

In health, a normal infant spends few, but steadily increasing, hours in play (which is undistinguishable from work) because he or she sleeps so many hours and eats at frequent intervals. Preschool children spend most of their waking hours in some form of work-play, according to the culture in which they grow up. At school, learning—or work—comes to be differentiated from play and gradually the pattern of the young person's life assumes more and more of the characteristics of adulthood in which work may fill the major part of the waking hours until "retirement" when, in Western cultures, there is an abrupt reversal of this pattern.

While health personnel do not ordinarily think of themselves as being responsible for providing conditions under which constructive work and play activities are available to well persons of all ages, it is quite clear that normal human development depends upon them. A healthy regimen must include them, just as a health history must include information on how the subject spends his or her time in work and play.

During illness or recovery from injury, at any age, the daily rhythms of work are suddenly, in some cases gradually, interrupted. The interruption may be necessary; often it is not. The chasm that exists between the sick and the well is probably brought about by the change in the way persons spend their day more than by the pain or discomfort they suffer. As long as they can go about their business, or keep in "the stream of life" they don't feel separated from the well even though they may actually be quite sick. If this is true, health personnel should see that there is minimum interruption of work and play patterns. These questions are seriously considered in rehabilitation services; they are often neglected in other services.[1] Rehabilitation is discussed in Chapter 8 and referred to in many others. The point is made here that opportunities for, and the value of, work and play should be considered *for every person served by the nurse and should be thought of as a part of every daily regimen.*

In helping patients in these aspects of their life, nurses can be guided by what they know about universal human needs, the hierarchy or importance of these needs in human development, and the effects of sensory and kinesthetic deprivation. In Chapter 8, theories of Maslow, Erikson, and others were discussed. The material on pages 564–70 might be reviewed and the points they are designed to make applied to the discussion of work and play in this chapter. Both are as directly related to human development, as are the persons' endowment at birth, the air they breathe, and the food they eat. During work and play individuals are—or are not—satisfying their psychologic needs, their need for safety, love—or sense of belonging—, esteem, fulfillment ("self actualization"), their desire to know, and their thirst for beauty. Deprived of constructive play and work, the individuals develop some negative qualities identified by Erikson as mistrust, shame or doubt, guilt, inferiority, isolation, stagnation, and despair.

Throughout man's history various meanings have been attached to the concept of work. The ways in which men have made their living have been some of the chief factors that determined the form and organization of human societies. We can infer from the little information we have about earliest man that simply to exist required continuous labor and the participation of all group members. It is likely that he lived in small bands for protection and mobility in his unending hunt for sufficient wild game and other naturally occurring foods.

It is also probable that at this time work and leisure had no separate or distinct meanings.

As man and his social organizations became more complex, a division of labor occurred, with status, position, and roles attached to certain occupations. For instance, when societies based on the herding of animals developed, the breeding and care of these successfully domesticated animals constituted the only acceptable occupation of the adult male; at about the same time, the development of agricultural societies resulted in farming and land-holding, so *it* was a status occupation, with the amount of land determining to a large extent his position in society. Western culture has been most influenced by the history of the countries bordering the Mediterranean Sea—most particularly that of Greece. In its classical period, immediately preceding the Christian era, all useful work in the city-states was performed by slaves, serfs, or noncitizens, while the Greeks regarded work for themselves as degrading and servile, and looked for ways to make wise use of their leisure.* This negative attitude toward work continued to exist into the early Middle Ages in the form of agrarian feudalism, but began to change when monastic brotherhoods developed. In these communities, work was valued as a way "to discipline the soul," and as an instrument of expiation and charity. The Protestant Reformation is credited by some historians with the spread, rather than the initiation, of this new meaning of work. Work acquired a moral dignity in its own right, and what had once been a way of life for monks acquired religious sanction for the laity. In Colonial America, particularly Calvinistic New England, this ethical concept of work, together with an abundance of land, a scarcity of labor, a preoccupation with manufacturing and trade, and a general anti-aristocratic opinion, combined to make hard work the path to success and security.[1a] Some individuals, however, in every country, cling to the concept, as suggested by Mark Twain, that work is something they must do rather than something they want to do.

Terence Carroll[2] suggests that while work is a necessary activity and must be performed by many people, work has no inherent virtue in and of itself. He believes that whatever virtue work is currently seen as having has developed through learned attitudes. Eugene Friedmann and Robert Havighurst[3] believe

there are certain functions and characteristics found in all situations defined by society as "a job." They describe these characteristics as (1) providing income; (2) regulating the worker's pattern of time and energy expenditure; (3) providing identification and status; (4) fixing patterns of associations; and (5) offering the worker meaningful life experiences. Although they were able to describe this limited number of the functions of work as applicable to all workers, they found there were many meanings of work, and these were not the same for all workers. In general, they reported the meanings of work fell into two large categories: (1) the individual's recognition of the part the job played in his or her life, and (2) the kind of affective response he or she made to it. They concluded that persons who see work as primarily a way of making a living want to retire at 65 (or the normal retirement age), while those who stress the values of work do not look upon this as desirable. Table 17-1 presents the relationships between the functions and meanings of work as reported by Friedmann and Havighurst.

A number of researchers have concluded that for various reasons the Protestant work ethic has declined in America and that work is no longer a central life interest.[3a,3b] Others believe that the importance of work to Americans has shown no sign of disappearance, and that habits of work and its prestige continue to persist.[3c,3d] Sigmund Nosow and William Form say:

The separation of work from other realms of life has been erroneously interpreted by some as indicating that work is no longer a central life interest of modern man. The available evidence does not confirm this, for work continues to be the driving force giving direction and meaning to contemporary living. While it is true that work satisfaction tends to decrease with level of occupational skill, work still occupies a central role in the lives of most people. The primary reason for this is that there is no other activity which provides as much social continuity to life as does work. Certainly leisure has not yet replaced work as a central organizing principle of life. It is work, not leisure, that gives status to the individual and his family.*

James E. Birren goes so far as to suggest that work is such a pervasive force that although many young people are attending school beyond the required twelve years (delaying their formal entry into the labor force) and theoretically at leisure, "the frequent use of schol-

---

* The Greek term for work, *ponos,* has the same root as that of *poena* which in Latin means sorrow. This concept is echoed in the story of the Garden of Eden where Adam and Eve lived in "innocence," idleness, and abundance and from which they were banished to live and work in the world.

* Nosow, Sigmund, and Form, William (eds.): *Man, Work and Society.* Basic Books, Inc., New York, 1962, p. 11.

Table 17-1.   The Relation Between the Functions and Meanings of Work*

Work Function	Work Meaning
1. Income	(a) Maintaining a minimum sustenance level of existence (b) Achieving some higher level or group standard
2. Expenditure of time and energy	(a) Something to do (b) A way of filling the day or passing time
3. Identification and status	(a) Source of self-respect (b) Way of achieving recognition or respect from others (c) Definition of role
4. Association	(a) Friendship relations (b) Peer-group relations (c) Subordinate-superordinate relations
5. Source of meaningful life experience	(a) Gives purpose to life (b) Creativity; self-expression (c) New experience (d) Service to others

* Friedmann, Eugene, and Havighurst, Robert: *The Meaning of Work and Retirement.* University of Chicago Press, Chicago, 1954, p. 7.

arships implies that many students are in truth employed by society to study." * Gladys Nite and Frank N. Willis,[4] when reporting their findings on the nursing care of patients with myocardial infarctions, noted the frequency with which patients in the experimental group showed concern about their future work. Few, if any, seemed pleased with the possibility of reorganizing their post-recovery lives about leisure-time activities rather than work-time activities.

The Meaning and Nature of Leisure. Alexander Reid Martin[5] believes that a capacity for leisure as well as a capacity for work is a necessity for health and creative development.† He also believes that the health profession (particularly medicine) has a major interest in understanding the work-leisure cultural changes that affect health and disease, and that it has a major responsibility for helping individuals adapt to them.

Havighurst and his associates,[6] in a series of studies, investigated the nature and values of leisure-time activity. They found that most of the values attached to leisure-time activities were the same as those attached to work (see Table 17-1). The two exceptions were "just for the pleasure of it" and "a welcome change from work." They suggested that because the value-meanings of work and leisure are similar, many persons can find the same satisfactions in leisure they find in work. For instance, if patterns of associations have a high work-life value for the individual, he or she will get similar satisfaction from leisure-time group activity rather than from leisure-time solitary activity. They also suggest that the meanings of work and play may be complementary; that is, if creative activities are not available in the work situation, they may be sought and found in the recreational situation.

As the average life span of modern man has increased, and as technologic science, with its accompanying economy of abundance, has developed, there is an apparent increase in leisure time. The length of time before entering employment has lengthened through additional years of schooling; the daily number of hours of free time available to individuals in the labor force has almost doubled since 1900 (see Fig. 17-1); and the average number of years in retirement has increased by 50 per cent. This would all seem to indicate that people are more and more able to enjoy the "fruits of their labor" in the satisfying use of leisure time. Because of this increased leisure time, a number of sociologists and social commentators believe that the use of so much free time may become a social problem. However, Martin[7] and Sebastian de Grazia[8] think that while many persons consciously want leisure time, they are uneasy when they have it, are too busy to plan for it, or continue to work to avoid it. A Twentieth Century Fund study of work and leisure conducted in the early 1960s indicated that with increased "over-time" work, paid or unpaid, "moonlighting," other forms of multiple employment, increased travel time to and from work, and more "do-it-yourself" home repairs, the time available for

* Birren, James E.: *The Psychology of Aging.* Prentice-Hall, Englewood Cliffs, N.J., 1964, p. 205.
† Genius has been described as the recapture of childhood which includes the zest for all of life which, in fact, makes work of play and vice versa. For those who work compulsively and who seem to use work as an escape, the term "workaholics" is sometimes used facetiously.

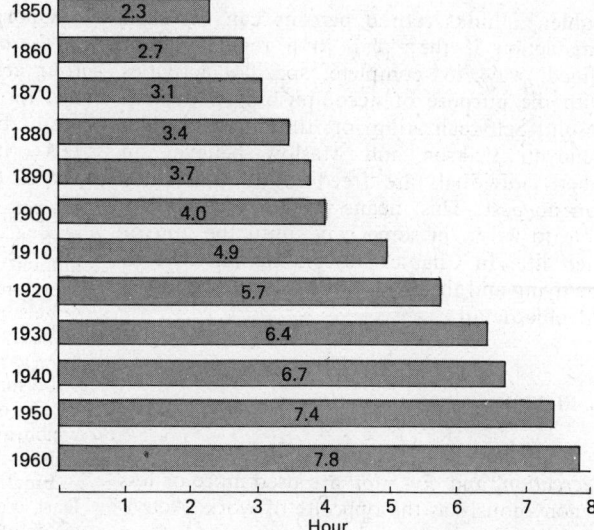

Figure 17-1. Hours free after work, eating, and necessities, 1850–1960. Projected on a six-day work week. Includes seven hours' sleep, one hour for eating, two hours of miscellaneous activity. (From Kaplan, M.: *Leisure in America.* John Wiley & Sons, Inc., New York, 1960.)

free-choice activities was only slightly more than was available to a worker in 1900.

A recent study by Eric Pfeiffer and Glenn Davis [9] indicated that in the 46- to 71-year-old middle and upper income group they investigated, the majority of subjects took greater satisfaction in their work than in their leisure, and that those who were working had "fun" more recently than the nonworking subjects. They concluded that "individuals now in their middle age will arrive in old age essentially unprepared for the meaningful utilization of large amounts of free time." * They suggested that in order to help individuals to a more satisfying old age, our society should distribute work and leisure more evenly over the life span; or provide preparation for using leisure, particularly in middle age; or create more opportunity for continual employment in old age.

Retirement and Leisure Time. Because of the importance of work in the lives of Americans, and the obvious lack of it among most retired persons, a number of studies have investigated the activities of those in the postretirement period with its wanted or unwanted increase in leisure time. These studies,[10-13] indicate that if the retired individual has (1) good health, (2) adequate financial resources, (3) a prior hobby or other interest, and (4) lives in a retirement community, he or she is likely to have a "good" retirement. However, in 1965, approximately one-third of the 11.5 million families living in poverty were headed by persons of retirement age or older,[14] and

studies [15,16] among this economic group have indicated that they are frequently in poor health, have inadequate transportation facilities, and have economic problems that prevent the use of leisure time in the diverse ways these persons might like. It is often this group that feels shunted aside once they have left their jobs.

Ronald Chen [17] believes that the social and emotional impact of the retirement process is similar to "anxiety separation" in a much younger population. He thinks there is some evidence that anticipation of retirement may be a problem before actual retirement occurs. He points out that there are definite signs and symptoms which, if not recognized, may lead to profound psychologic problems. Among these signs and symptoms he lists the development by persons nearing retirement of critical attitudes toward themselves, irrational anger toward others, and mood swings from depression to elation in an apparent effort to minimize the loss of work and its many meanings.

A study of healthy elderly men conducted by Birren and others [18] at the National Institute of Mental Health showed that men who had undergone physical or psychologic environmental losses such as retirement brings tended to show poor performances on cognitive and psychomotor tests. This was thought to indicate that current life circumstances of the older individual rather than central nervous system degeneration are of considerable significance in governing the individual's emotional state and social productivity.

Many students of our current social problems are suggesting that modern men (and women) need an alternate rhythm of work and leisure to feel content, and Charlotte

* Pfeiffer, Eric, and Davis, Glenn: "The Use of Leisure Time in Middle Life," *Gerontologist,* **11:**192, (Autumn, Part 1) 1971.

Buhler[19] thinks retired persons can get such satisfaction if they plan in a regular, disciplined way to complete specific activities with the purpose of accomplishing a definite result. Self-realization or fulfillment is dependent, Erikson and Maslow believe, on when individuals are freed to do what they can do best. This means that they should be able to work, in some way, until the end of their life. In Chapter 50, on nursing care of the dying and the dead, this subject is discussed in some detail.

2. PLAY

Adult Play and Recreation. The terms *play, recreation,* and *diversion* are used more or less synonymously as the opposite of work. Activities that have no serious motive and from which there is no material gain are usually thought of as play or diversion. Recreation, or an activity that "re-creates" the individual, has a slightly deeper meaning. The distinction between work and play, however, lies in the mental attitude. Baseball can be the work by which the professional ball player makes his living or it can be play, diversion, or recreation.

The history of play is a long one. Aristotle, for instance, spoke of the value of play in releasing pent-up emotions. Most play theories developed from observing children in their daily play. Schiller explained play as an expression of surplus energy; Groos and Bower explained play as rehearsal for adult activities; Freud and Erikson pointed out the many symbolic meanings found and used in play; and Piaget developed theories of cognition (the act of knowing) based on observation of children's play.[20]

Jacqueline Hott[21] cites Davis, who suggests that for adults play and recreation may emphasize the attitudes involved in an activity, the aim of the activity, or the mechanics of the activity (see Fig. 17-2). Play and recreation may be thought of as an art, a science, a discipline, or a point of view. Allen V. Sapora and Elmer D. Mitchell[22] believe that entertainment-seeking and escapism are currently the most pervasive elements in adult play and recreation. They point out that these elements are in contrast to earlier historical patterns, where play was an integral and alternating part of all life's activities.*

George Lundberg, in what is considered one of the classic studies of leisure, has developed four criteria for the use of leisure in which the terminology "recreation or play" might easily be substituted for the word "leisure." His criteria with the substitutions described are as follows:

Leisure [recreation or play] has, in a relatively high degree, both its original incentive and its fulfillment in the individual himself rather than in coercions of the social and economic order.

Leisure [recreation or play] must possess the capacity of being relatively permanently interesting (variety).

Leisure [recreation or play] should involve activities or states as different as possible from those which are consciously forced upon us by our station in life.

Finally, leisure [recreation or play] should be at least compatible with, if not conducive to, physical, mental and social well-being.*

Although most people would likely agree with Lundberg's criteria, studies and surveys indicate that the recreational activities most frequently reported by people of all age groups tend to be passive. For example, a 1957 survey of a national sample of 5021 people, 15 years of age and older, and living in private households showed that the four most common recreational activities were watching television, visiting with friends and relatives, working around the yard and garden, and reading magazines.[23] A 1970 survey of 502 men and women in the middle and upper income groups, aged 46 to 71 years, 13 years later, duplicated these findings.[24] Surveys of this nature do not, of course, indicate the pleasure other recreational activities such as games, arts and crafts, traveling, or participation in music and dancing hold for large numbers of people of varying ages; however, they would seem to indicate, as mentioned earlier in this chapter, that some kind of training for many individuals in leisure-time activities is necessary.

Children's Play. The meaning of children's play is like that of the adult's only in one respect—that the activity is not carried out for material gain. Where the adult frequently plays for the purpose of "re-creation" and a renewal of life, the child plays to promote physical growth and to learn about life. Child psychologists and experts in human development have pointed out that when children play, in addition to expressing their current interests, abilities, and feelings, more significantly they are finding out about themselves

---

* We all know persons who prescribe recreation for themselves as if it were medicine and their reaction to it is correspondingly devoid of spontaneous enjoyment.

* Lundberg, George, as quoted in Kaplan, Max: *Leisure in America: A Social Inquiry.* John Wiley & Sons, New York, 1960, p. 28.

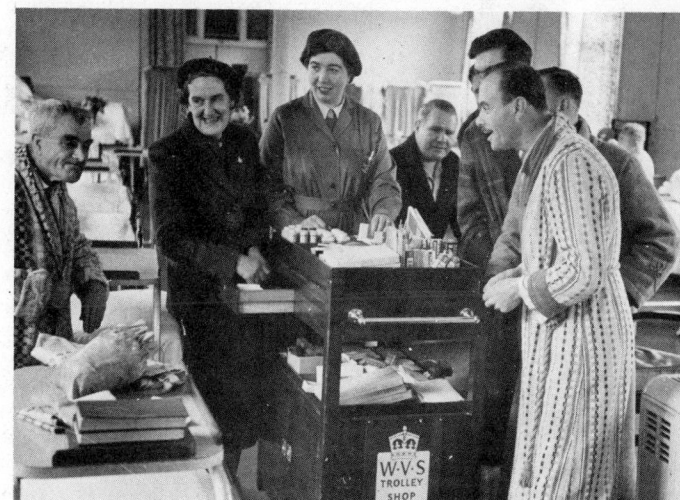

A

B

Figure 17-2. Selected social activities for groups of adults. *A*. Hospital volunteers in Great Britain. (Photo by Radio Times Hulton Picture Library.) *B*. Stockholm's Karolinska Hospital. (W.H.O. Photo by Jean Mohr.)

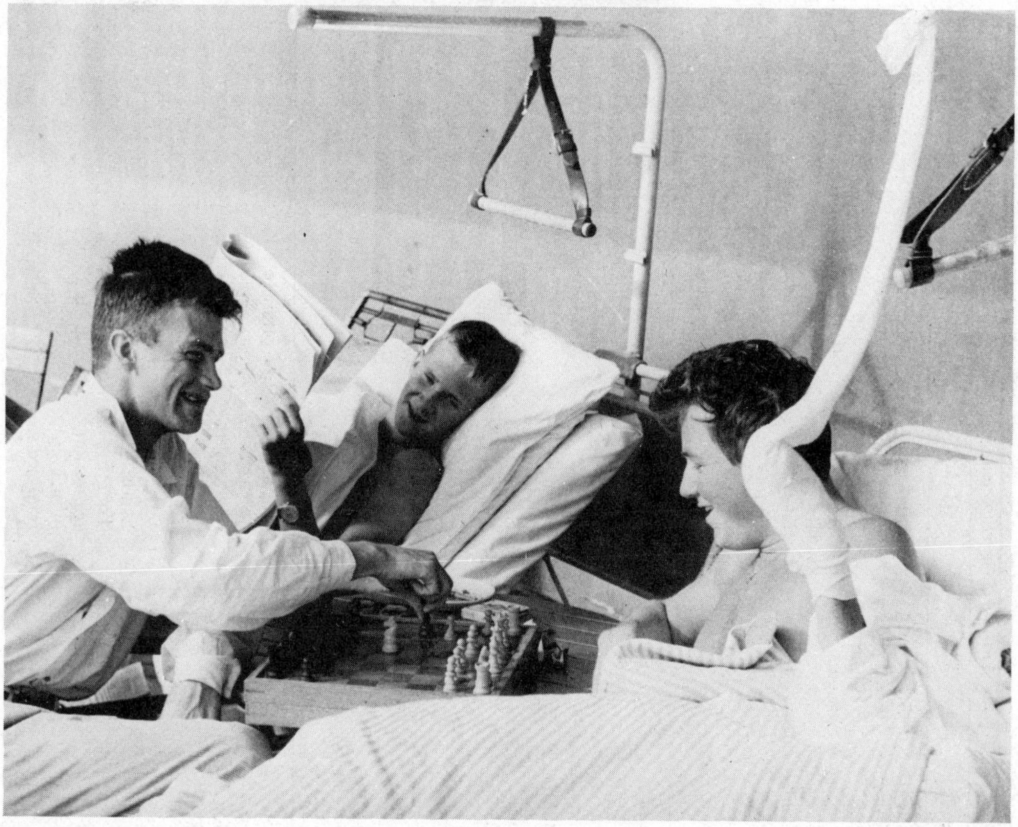

and the world in which they live.[25-27] This aspect of children's play is a most serious one and has brought about the use of the hyphenated term "work-play" to describe much of their activity.

The Time Children Spend in Play. There are other differences between the play of adults and that of children. Perhaps the most obvious one is the proportion of time children spend in play. Infants, before they are able to get around independently, have their play limited by their physical needs that demand so much of their time and by their limited ability to move. However, when they are not eating or

Table 17-2. Toys for Infants *

Age	Physical Development					Social Development	Appropriate Toys
	Eyes	Ears	Hands	Torso	Standing		
Birth–3 months	Searches with eyes; follows an object. Focuses on an object.	Stops activity on hearing sound.	Random defensive movements; hand is still fisted but will grasp object placed near hand.	Head and shoulders droop in sitting position. Turns from side to back. Raises head longer and higher.		Enjoys cuddling and motion. Responds to presence of people.	Nursery mobiles: hanging, unbreakable mirrors Crib dangle bells; see-through crib bumpers Music boxes with moving figures Balloons
3–5 months	Capable of most complicated eye movements—horizontal, vertical, and circular. Sees in color.	Turns head toward voice.	Awkward grasping. Thumb apposition begins. Grasping more coordinated. Can reach-grasp-release.	Turns from back to side. Rests on forearms with head high. Can pull up to sitting position.		Usually pursues moving person. Knows mother, stares at strangers. May smile at mirror image. Shows interest in father and siblings.	Rattles; crib exerciser Cradle gym Small rattling or squeeze-squeak toy that will fit into palm of baby's hand Small plastic blocks; rubber squeeze blocks; weighted toy (i.e., clown)
5–7 months	Can show consistent regard for person or object.	Turns head toward bell. Listens to own sounds and those of others.	Can accept one object when given to him. Corrals with both hands. Thumb apposition in picking up objects.	Complete turn from stomach to stomach. Hitching (backward locomotion while sitting). Can sit alone unsupported with body erect. Crawling.		Fear of strangers developing. Shows affection for family group.	Grip balls Soft blocks and squeeze-squeak toys Soft animals Teething toys

Age						
7–9 months	Visual pursuit of dropped object.	Listens to conversations and singing tones. May respond to name and word like "no."	Can accept 2 objects. Starts to grasp with thumb and first two fingers.	Sits unsupported, usually for 10 or more minutes. Draws up on knees.	Supports entire weight.	Waves hands. Initiates play. Chooses toy deliberately.	Activity boxes in crib or tub. Soft blocks for stacking. Sturdy cloth or cardboard picture books. Nesting cups. Bath toys—boats, rubber and plastic or foam animals
10 months	Sees individual objects as separate from others. Searches for hidden object if he sees it hidden.	Listens with interest to familiar words. Understands commands—"give it to me."	Can accept 3 objects. Begins to hold drinking cup; reaches for spoon.	Crawls, trunk still dragging. Creeps.	Stands on toes with support.	Initiates sounds and actions. Shows moods—happy, sad. Begins sexual identity.	Colorful, sturdy cars and trucks. Musical toys—cymbals, tambourine, maracas, drum. Baby drinking cup. Stacking squares or rings
11–12 months	Reaches accurately for something as he turns away.	Produces more sounds and babbles short sentences.	Throws or rolls ball. Builds tower of blocks. Points with index finger.	Climbs up and down stairs.	Pulls up to a standing position. Walks, using support.	May release object on request. Solicits attention. Offers object to a familiar adult. Talks to mirror.	Unbreakable mirror which child can hold and manipulate. First push-and-pull toys (e.g., dog, turtle). Shape and/or color matching toys

Reprinted from *American Baby Magazine*, April 1974.
* Feldman, Marie: "Cluster Visits," *Am. J. Nurs*, **74**:1485, (Aug.) 1974.

NAME:

(Check O, observed and/or D, discussed, Mother)
(Check CO, observed and/or CD, discussed, Caretaker)

	1 mo	2 mo	3 mo	4 mo	5 mo	7 mo	9 mo	11 mo
I. Visual								
A. Magazine cutouts								
B. Picture books								
C. Designs and beauty								
II. Auditory								
A. Talk to child, distinctly								
B. Describe activities to child								
C. Encourage new words								
D. Name objects								
E. Listen to child talk								
F. Encourage to tell experiences								
G. Sing to child								
H. Soft music, radio								
III. Tactile								
A. Cuddling, kissing								
B. Bath, pouring water, permit playing								
C. Play while dressing								
D. Various textures								
E. Permit mud pies								
F. Finger paint								
G. Allow to hold cup								
spoon								
food								
IV. Motor								
A. Allow jumping, climbing								
B. Use of large muscles								
C. Permit some noisy play								
D. Large blocks, balls								
E. Use of parks								
F. Use pencil and crayons								
G. Help with home toys								
V. Encourage exploration								
Looking								
Touching								
Encourage questions								
Answer all questions								
VI. Miscellaneous								
A. Company other children								
B. Place for own toys								
C. Rewards for pleasing behavior								
D. Encourage independence								
E. Alleviate superstition								
F. What landmark to look for next								
G. Enjoy child								
H. Accident prevention								
VII. Overstimulation (and what kinds)								

A

NAME:

(Check O, observed and/or D, discussed, Mother)
(Check CO, observed and/or CD, discussed, Caretaker)

	1 mo	2 mo	3 mo	4 mo	5 mo	7 mo	9 mo	11 mo
I. Visual								
A. Magazine cutouts, puzzles								
B. Picture and alphabet books								
C. Designs and beauty, nature								
II. Auditory								
A. Talk distinctly to child, say his words back								
B. Encourage new words								
C. Describe activities to child								
D. Name objects, parts of body								
E. Listen to child talk								
F. Encourage to tell experiences								
G. Sing to child								
H. Music, radio, rhythm								
III. Tactile								
A. Cuddling, kissing								
B. Bath, pouring water, allow playing								
C. Play while dressing								
D. Various textures								
E. Play-do, sand								
F. Finger paint (in bathroom)								
G. Mirror play								
IV. Motor								
A. Allow jumping, climbing, rhythm								
B. Use of large muscles								
C. Permit noisy play								
D. Large blocks, balls, cartons								
E. Parks, zoo, free programs								
F. Use crayons and lots of paper								
G. Homemade toys								
H. Musical toys								
I. Imitative play-sweeping, cooking, etc.								
V. Exploration and Curiosity								
A. Looking, touching								
B. Answer all questions								
VI. Miscellaneous								
A. Play with own age group								
B. Need for possessions, a safe place								
C. Reward frequently, praise								
D. Admire results of efforts								
E. Encourage independence								
F. Alleviate fears								
G. What progress to look for								
H. Enjoy child								
I. Accident prevention								
VII. Overstimulation (and what kinds)								

B

Figure 17-3. *A*. Stimulation check list (1 to 2 years). *B*. Stimulation check list (2 to 3 years). (From Brooks, Marion R.: "A Stimulation Program for Young Children Performed by a Public Health Nurse as Part of Well Baby Care," in *ANA Clinical Sessions, 1970.* Appleton-Century-Crofts, New York, 1971, pp. 135, 136.)

sleeping they explore their hands and feet, their mother's eyes, ears, and nose, and the objects they can see or touch within their limited range of vision or their arm's reach. As their ability to get from one place to another increases, as they become more skilled in controlling both the large and small muscles of the body, more able to communicate with words, and increasingly adept in the understanding and use of symbols, the time they spend in play increases and finally consumes the largest number of their waking hours. Later, as they take on the tasks and the responsibilities of being a student, the time they spend in play is reduced. When they reach the point of being a productive worker, they use play as adults commonly use play.*

The Changing Character of Children's Play. Another difference between the play of adults and children is the developmental and changing character of children's play activity. As children grow, their play activities pass from simple motor activities to socialized play, to creative, dramatic, constructive play, and, finally, to team and competitive play. (These activities vary culturally. The observations in this chapter most accurately describe child activity in the Western world.)

Initially, much of young children's play is exploratory, that is, finding out about this "thing" (including people) outside themselves. Then they begin experimenting—experimenting for its own sake—for example, does the object move, bend, or break? Because they find so many things interesting and their attention span is so short, during this developmental period, they need many materials to satisfy them. They are experimenting and learning to trust others and objects in their environment. During play time infants should be fondled. In hospitals, mother figures hold, rock, and caress infants. Erikson calls this the oral-sensory age of man. Infants will put almost anything into their mouth. They "play" with their bottle, their fingers, or a pacifier. As they grow, infants are interested in other children as objects, and sometimes seem to explore them in the same way. They may play side by side with another child, but there is little if any interaction except the unabashed appropriation of a wanted toy.† The expression "the terrible

two's" is based on some of these propensities (see Table 17-2).

At about 3 or 4 years of age, having grown more adept physically, children seem to have time and energy available to participate in small group play but mainly they are learning to be autonomous, to use their muscles. Later, they begin to dramatize the events in their life that have impressed them, as they think they happened, or possibly, as they think they should happen (see Fig. 17-4). During this period of growing they continue to improve their fine muscle abilities. Their skill in manipulating constructive "raw" material changes and seems more purposeful. When they are about 5 years old their fine muscle coordination is such that they can use scissors, manipulate paste, draw firm lines, and construct a fairly elaborate block structure. One play activity will now occupy them for a much longer period and they want to finish a project, or leave it to be completed, or leave it to be used again at a later time. During this period their initiative should be encouraged. During the early school years or middle years of childhood (7 to 10) they play more in groups for dramatizations or cooperative competition and seem dedicated to the improvement of physical skills requiring fine muscle control.[28,29] Children up to the age of puberty are normally so active or "industrious" that an adult harnessed to them would soon drop with fatigue.

The Changing Use of Play Materials. As children grow and develop, the changing character of their play parallels the changing character of the kind of objects or materials they find interesting, and the changing way in which they use the "raw" materials. As infants the materials they use are entirely determined by the adult, and are simple in purpose, that is, to look at, to listen to, to bite, to shake, or to drop. Between the ages of 1 and 2 years when they are learning to walk, talk, and reach out to the world just beyond their crib and play pen, anything and everything within their exploring, experimenting reach is an object for play. They need objects as toys that they can explore with their mouth without injury, that they can pull, push, sit on, fit together or take apart, pile up and knock down, pound, and throw. At first they are not inter-

---

* In Chapter 12 on body mechanics the importance of crawling and exploring in infancy is stressed. An infant who spends many hours in cribs or "play pens" is deprived of the muscular and intellectual stimulation he or she gets from free movement and exploration of the environment.

† Marion R. Brooks reports on a 5-year project in Washington, D.C., which included a "stimulation program"—visual, auditory, tactile and motor—for

underprivileged infants. The "preliminary results" show higher developmental status for the 23 stimulated infants than for the 22 "well" infants not exposed to this program. (Brooks, Marion R.: "A Stimulation Program for Young Children Performed by a Public Health Nurse as Part of Well Baby Care," in *ANA Clinical Sessions, 1970.* Appleton-Century-Crofts, New York, 1971.) See Fig. 17-3 *A-B* for stimulation check list [of activities] for 1 to 2 and 2 to 3 years.

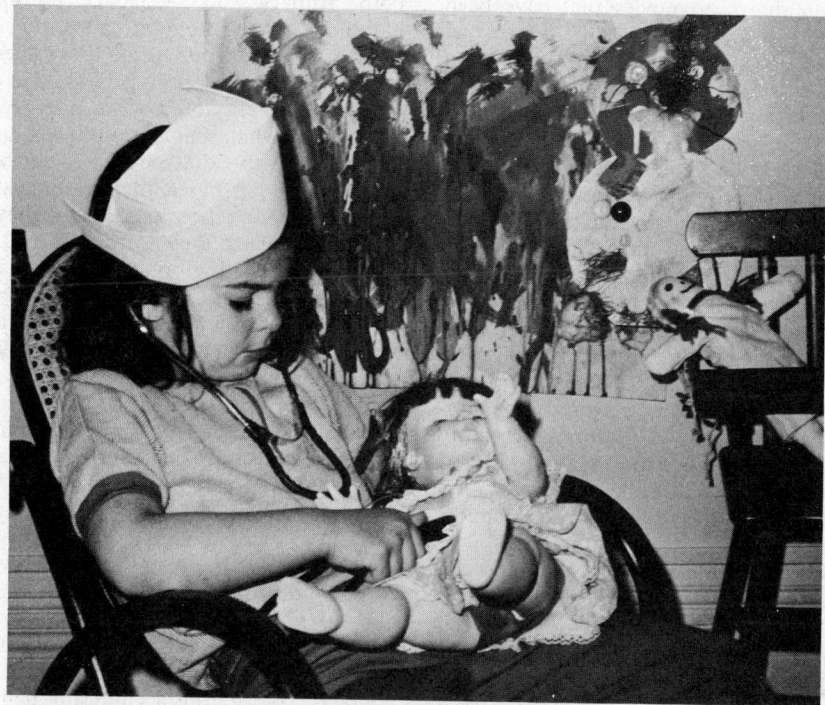

Figure 17-4. This child casually incorporates new experiences in her play. (Photo by Sirgay Sanger, from Petrillo, Madeline, and Sanger, Sirgay: *Emotional Care of Hospitalized Children*. J. B. Lippincott Co., Philadelphia, 1972.)

ested in materials that will later help in their play of imitating grownups, nor are they interested in crayons, paint, paint brushes, or clay.

In the next stage (between 3 and 4) children use many things that help their play which is imitation of adults. This is not the cooperative dramatic play of the 5- to 6-year-old, although the same materials are used. In some cultures children's play things are objects used in adult life and, in fact, children at very early ages participate in the activities of their elders. Some anthropologists believe that maturity is delayed in many Western countries because children are not included in homemaking activities, in caring for the sick, and in ceremonies such as weddings and funerals.

Dramatic play in the preschool period is usually simple and of short duration—a kind of experimentation with specific objects and roles. Children in this period also are beginning to use smaller objects such as peg boards, pounding boards, hammer and large nails, long-handled paint brushes, clay, and large crayons—all of which they may have explored a little as a younger child, but did not put to use. They are not yet interested in a product from their activity but, simply, in the activity.

As adults we often place a burden on these young children when we insist that they tell us the nature or meaning of their product. Since it has no meaning and represents nothing to which they can attach a name, they feel an inadequacy which is not really there and tend to avoid interesting and creative materials and a repetition of this frustrating experience.

When children are nearly 6 they will use all but their very early play materials in new ways, and add games of simple physical prowess and mental skill. For example, they want to learn to jump rope, to roller skate, to throw and catch a ball, and to swim. Boys and girls begin to show marked differences in the kinds of materials they use for play, and the kinds of activities they carry on with these materials.* Dramatization continues to be used, but now includes stories that have been heard or read,

* To what extent this differentiation is innate or learned is a moot question. If it weren't for social disapproval many more small boys might play with dolls and many more small girls with bats and balls. Not long ago when a bee flew into the car I said to a boy of 17, "Bill, you're the only man here, it's your job to get rid of the bee." His answer was "I don't believe in sex roles." [V. H.]

or television shows or movies that have been seen.

From the age of 8 years competitive card games and other table games engage children and they can and will follow rules. (At the age of 6, game rules are seen as quite elastic, and changed as the game progresses because it is so important for the 6-year-old to win.) Collections and hobbies become important to the child from 8 to 11, but they change frequently as the child's interests and learning broaden.[30,31]

With puberty and young adulthood, the individual is trying to find his or her place in an adult world. He or she needs forms of play that teach him or her the arts of companionship outside the family group. A healthy young adult forms intimate relationships or suffers from a feeling of isolation. Play should include group activities with increasing opportunity for developing adult relationships.

Purposes of Children's Play. Perhaps the major purpose of children's play involves learning—about themselves and their world; in other words, to grow up. Other purposes of their play are (1) to translate ideas into forms, that is, a house of blocks must have a roof, a door, and a window; (2) to translate concepts into shapes, as for example, a bridge of blocks must go up, and over; (3) to turn impressions into products, such as a picture of the hospital as a big bed with a tiny person in it, and a huge syringe and needle nearby; and (4) to transform feeling into action or a product. Anger and frustration, for example, are pounded onto a large inflated plastic clown, or a painting is splashed with strokes of bright color. A wish to be powerful is transformed into giving an injection to a doll, or applying a dressing like a surgeon, or "performing" an operation. Children will take any material, shape, or form and breathe something of themselves into it. The more unstructured the material, the better it serves them to project feelings and ideas.

Nurses should utilize their understanding of the changing characteristics and purposes of children's play in order to help mothers promote healthy growth in childhood which leads into a balanced rhythm of adult work and play. Nurses can also utilize this knowledge in constructing a totally "therapeutic milieu" for the hospitalized child.

3. THE NURSE'S ROLE IN PROVIDING OPPORTUNITY FOR WORK AND PLAY

The Adult Nonhospitalized Client. With nurses taking an increasingly active part in both primary and secondary prevention of pathologic states, the importance of each nurse having an understanding of the values, meaning, and activities comprising the complementary concepts of work-leisure seems self-evident. In whatever circumstances nurses are associated with adults of any age, but especially retired persons in the community, clinics, nursing and/or retirement homes, they can include as a part of their assessment of the client his or her needs for leisure-time activities. Sickness dislocates life in most cases. Many clients might use counseling and encouragement to keep their daily lives as full and as normal as possible.[31a-c]

Edward L. Bortz [32] warns that the inactivity, aimless living, and separation from fellow workers and responsibility that retirement brings may precipitate discontent, unhappiness, and illness. These, in turn, may set the stage for neurosis and depression, and complete the vicious circle for the individual by causing disturbed appetite, bowel function, and all kinds of circulatory disturbances. It has been reported that retired persons need a routine of activity, opportunity for personal contacts, status from a culturally defined role, opportunities to help others, and an intrinsic satisfaction in the activity itself.[33] The nurse can find community resources such as sheltered workshops, senior citizen groups, and community volunteer bureaus and suggest their use to clients. When encouraging volunteer community service, the nurse must be aware of the importance to the individual of payment for services given. In a study conducted by Frances M. Carp,[34] the time-filling, time-scheduling, and social contact aspects of volunteer service were not enough to keep all retired workers content. Many saw payment as a value placed by society on their contribution. The nurse must also be aware that people age in ways that are consistent with their earlier life-histories and when offered choices of activities will select that combination that fits best with their established values and self-concepts.[35] Maslow described the fulfilled or "self-actualized" person who is not concerned with status, but he makes it clear that the fully matured adult is a rarity.

Since available evidence indicates many people approach retirement with little knowledge of the satisfying use of leisure-time, the nurse can encourage family members to help plan, with the older person, for the use of his or her free time. In this way the nurse may involve younger family members so that all can learn about rewarding leisure-time activities—the development of interests that can be pursued throughout life.

The Adult Hospitalized Client. When the nurse is responsible for assessing the needs and planning for a patient's play or recreation at the time the patient is hospitalized, she or he should be aware that during the acute stage of an organic disease, instinct seems to dictate to patients that they concentrate their energy on self-preservation. It has often been remarked that physically ill or starving men, women, and children seem to lose interest in family and friends; they are indifferent to everything but the bodily processes concerned with survival. At such times occupations, diversions, and recreation, as we understand them, are usually suspended, although some rare persons manage to maintain their interests in people and their environment even when they are acutely ill and suffering. Except in periods when life itself is threatened, occupation and diversion are essential aspects of an effective therapeutic program.[35a]

Hospitalization can be a constructive experience instead of a morbid period overloaded with idleness and boredom, introspection and anxiety. Health care can be based on a recognition of the universal needs of man, and the patient can learn in the hospital to lead a fuller richer life. Special institutions for the care of the psychotic, the retarded, and the physically handicapped have made a science of recreational and occupational therapy; the general hospitals are less well prepared to give this service, and many doctors seem to overlook these therapies. Health services in schools, camps, and prisons, or in any situation where education or rehabilitation is important, should make a special study of the work and play programs.

Before prescribing a drug or a diet it is necessary to study the individual. It may be just as important in some cases to assess his or her need for occupation and diversion. For example, in planning occupations and recreation with and for the patient, the following are taken into account: age (chronologic and intellectual), sex, tastes, interests, experience, cultural prejudices, the physical condition, and the mood, emotional slant, attitude, or maturity (see Fig. 17-5).

With the growing emphasis in occupational therapy on developing interests and skills that will persist beyond hospitalization, many of the handicrafts that yielded a product of doubtful beauty or value have disappeared. It is likely that with the tendency for women to enter more and more occupations there will be less and less differentiation in the occupational therapy offered the sexes. In recreational therapy the same general trends are apparent. Perhaps the most interesting change is that

of encouraging men and women patients to work and play together in health institutions. This alone will help to develop a greater mutuality of tastes and interests although this is only one of the desirable outcomes. Emotional maturity is thought by many persons to include good heterosexual relationships.

A person's interests are, of course, affected by experience, and this should be taken into account. While novelty has its charm, new skills, games, exercises etc., should be introduced gradually. Many persons are self-conscious in a learning situation and until they feel at home with the therapist or the nurse, they will prefer a familiar activity. A knowledge of national customs and mores is of great value to all health workers.

The physical status, of course, limits the choice of occupation and recreation, as does the patient's mood. During a prostrating physical illness, exertion and emotional tax are contraindicated, and only the thoughtless or ignorant try to amuse or occupy the patient. Gradually as strength increases and interest returns, diversional and occupational activities are introduced. Nothing requires more sensitivity and imagination on the part of nurses than the management of this phase of illness. They can do a great deal to prevent the dependence, depression, or anxiety that often accompanies convalescence (see Fig. 17-6).

Nite and Willis [36] found in their study of patients with coronary disease that the patients groped with the problem of how to fill time during their convalescence and rehabilitation. When assistance with this problem was not forthcoming from the staff, the patient lost interest in pursuing a solution and was frequently seen moving aimlessly in bed, staring idly at the ceiling, and unable to express interest in any topic other than his or her own illness. On the other hand, when the nurse suggested and supplied materials for activities within the physical limitations of the patient (such as reading materials, radio, television, record players and records, games, pictures for the walls, and nonmedical conversation), the frequency with which patients seemed bored was significantly lower than it was among patients who did not have these materials made available to them.

A report on one patient demonstrated the effectiveness of the nurse's imaginative use of recreational activity:

A 60-year-old retired city fireman, whose major interests were city politics, his family, his one-half acre garden, and building birdhouses, displayed a picture of complete boredom with life in the hospital and continually rebelled against the "new way of life." Though he had no interest in art,

A

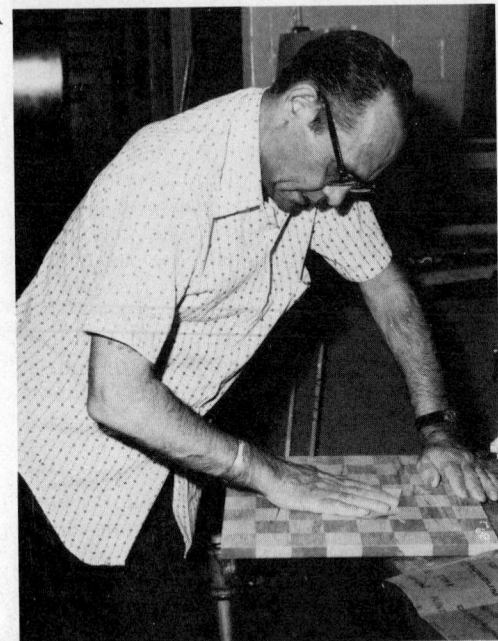

B

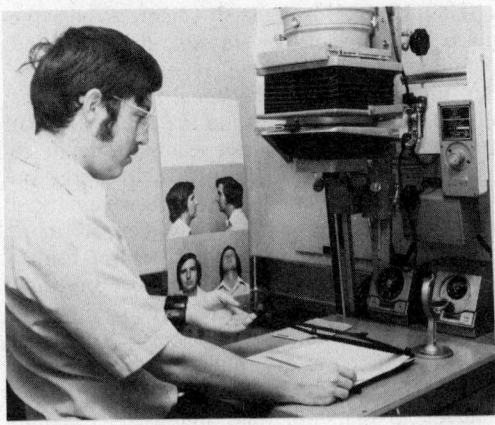

Figure 17-5. Patients learn new skills or improve old ones. (Courtesy of Veterans Administration Hospital, Houston, Tex.)

C

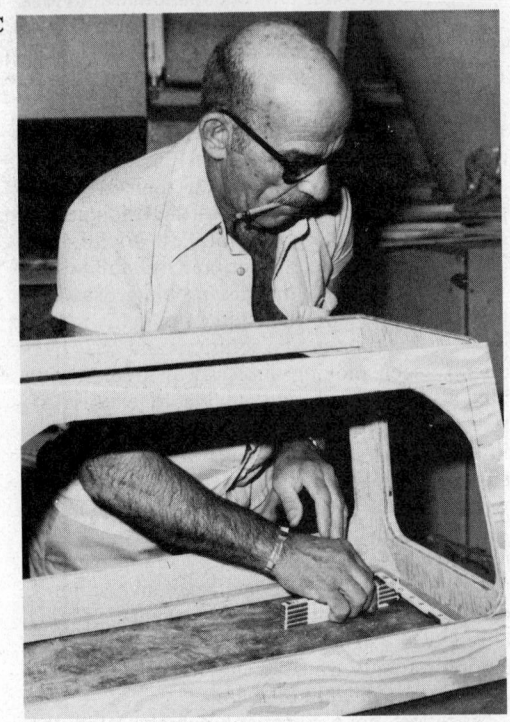

D

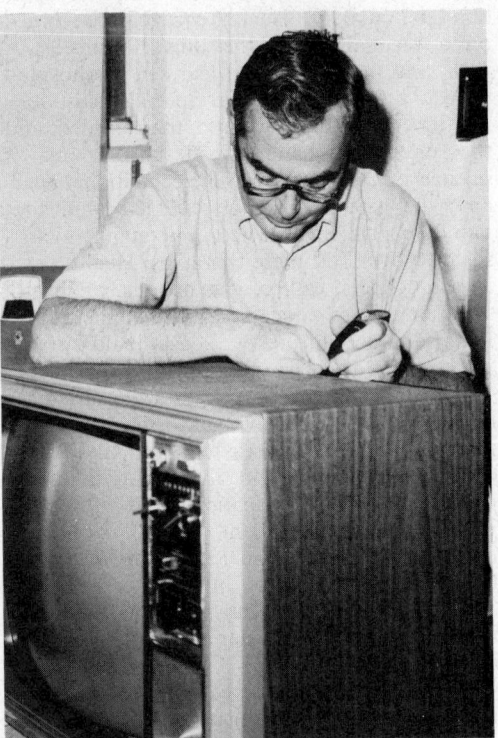

when the nurse enthusiastically presented him with a large assortment of reprints of paintings from which he was asked to select those of his choice and to supervise her in the hanging of these on the walls, his entire attitude changed. With obvious delight and studied care, he selected prints and had the nurse cover every conceivable spot on the wall. His choices were predominantly outdoor scenes, including some by Van Gogh. These pictures proved to be a great source of joy to the patient, and he would discuss them with his physicians, nurses, and visitors. A later visit to his home revealed two pictures on the wall, which probably came from the "dime store." *

* Nite, Gladys, and Willis, Frank N.: *The Coronary Patient; Hospital Care and Rehabilitation.* Macmillan Publishing Co., Inc., New York, 1964, p. 71.

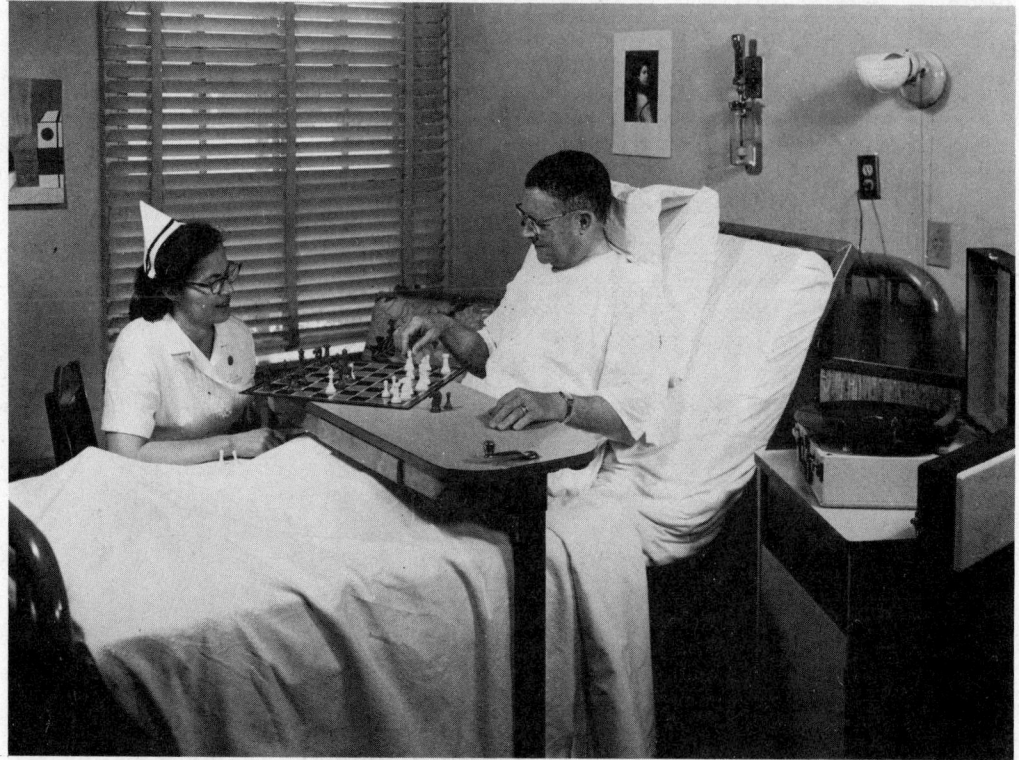

Figure 17-6. Recreation is an important part of the nursing program. The patient and nurse play a game of chess, his choice. The record player with a variety of records is also available and the patient makes his own selection. (From Nite, Gladys, and Willis, Frank N.: *The Coronary Patient; Hospital Care and Rehabilitation.* Macmillan Publishing Co., Inc., New York, 1964, p. 148. Photo courtesy of Independence Hospital, Independence, Mo.)

In well-organized and adequately staffed psychiatric services, patients frequently have prescribed programs of physical, recreational, and occupational therapy. They go to these departments daily, and specialists may work with them on the clinical services. Patients also have access to psychologists, psychiatric social workers, and others prepared to give special help. If, however, a therapeutic community is to exist throughout the hospital, or wherever we find patients, nurses must be able to participate in most aspects of the program. The nurse in psychiatry has greatest need for psychologic knowledge and skill, although the same art can be used in preventive psychiatry elsewhere. Musical, dramatic, and other social talents are assets. It is difficult for a person to enter enthusiastically into any social activity if she or he is inept.* For this reason, as well as for their own sake, nurses should cultivate a wide variety of interests.

The development of the concept of "milieu therapy" for psychiatric patients has enhanced the need for nurses to develop broad interests, their own talents, and greater social adeptness since a significant goal of this therapy is the resocialization of the patient through activities usually found in normal living. Frequently the nurse is responsible for planning bowling parties, pool parties, trips to parks and museums, organized classes in cooking, dancing, or current events, or other group activities. Figure 17-7 shows examples of some of these recreational activities. Otto von Mering believes there is a danger in *requiring* patients to participate in occupational and recreational activities simply because "treatment is assumed to occur through a variety of environmental pressures that require the patient to be con-

* Francoise R. Morimoto,[37] who made a study in the Boston Psychiatric Hospital under an American Nurses' Association grant, concluded that most of the nurses' social skill can be used in patient activity, that nurses tend to let patients initiate activity, and that they gravitate to patients who share their own interests and skills. If typical, this study suggests the importance of a catholicity of tastes on the part of the nurse.

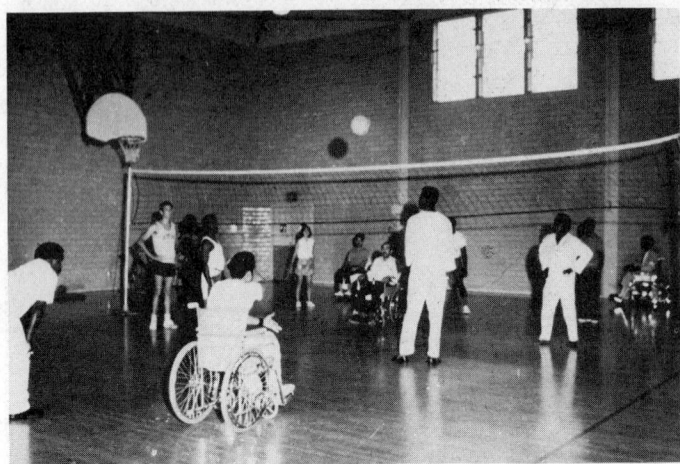

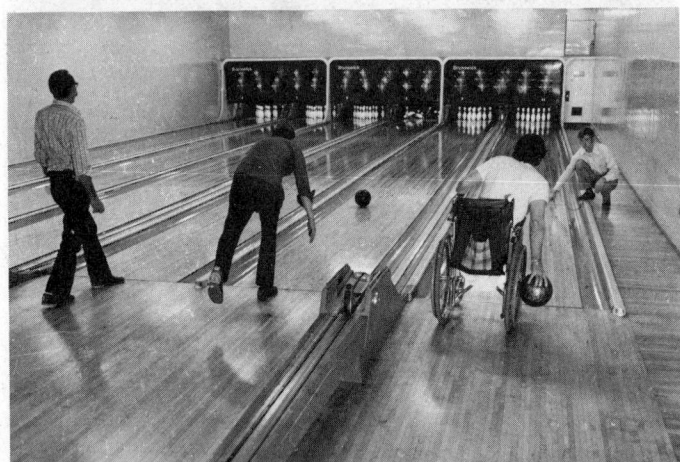

Figure 17-7. Examples of recreational activities available to individuals with a variety of physical disabilities. (All photos courtesy of the Veterans Administration Hospital, Houston, Tex.)

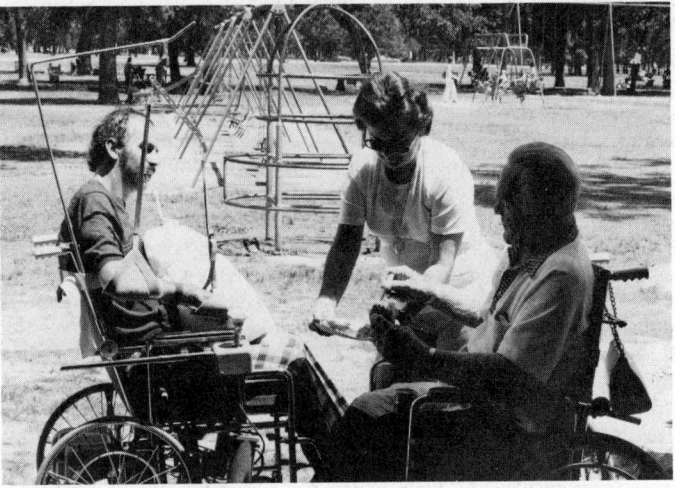

tinuously exposed to an activity wheel of planned recreational activity or 'canned joy' programs." *

While we have been speaking particularly of the psychiatric patient in the paragraphs above we are all "emotionally disturbed" during illness. Some of us manage to hide it more successfully than others; some of us express this disturbance in socially acceptable behavior, others do not. The mood or attitude of the patient is to be considered in planning the program of every patient. This does not imply that there is a specific activity for a given diagnosis; each prescription must be suited to the particular needs of the patient. It goes without saying that the patient should be encouraged and invited to participate rather than forced into the activity, as remarked by von Mering, above.

The patient who is hospitalized and immobilized because of neurologic or orthopedic pathology is especially in need of recreational activity. Studies [37a] of kinesthetic deprivation indicate that a number of negative behavior changes occur that are due largely to the restriction of movement. The nurse caring for the patient with these kinds of problems must be particularly innovative. At least one study showed that even though various kinds of auditory stimulation and some visual stimulation through the use of pictures projected overhead were used, undesirable behavior changes developed. Sensory deprivation is one of the major causes of illness in and outside the hospital. Sidney M. Jourard in his various writings states repeatedly that, in his opinion, all illness is rebellion against the environment.† While his views seem extreme, they have received a good deal of attention.

Diversions and Occupations Available in Most Situations. In making the daily plan of care for most patients the nurse should realize that rehabilitation is fostered by providing the variety that people in a culture expect in a "normal day." Most of us in the Western world like to spend part of the day alone with some interesting occupation, but the average person seeks company for many of his or her activities. We look upon reading as a daily diversion, or duty, and music in some form enters into the daily pattern of many lives. Games are a standard form of recreation, and, to creative individuals the day is lost if they

don't make something—or work on some productive task.

Congenial companionship is of course a source of recreation and the one most lacking in the sick man's day. The potential therapeutic value of the health worker's personality is often discussed. Whereas we have just come through a "scientific" era in which nurses were taught that it was "unprofessional" to sit and talk with patients, we now realize that the provision of a listening, interested companion is one of the most important forms of therapy. The patient may be in greater need of the nurse's unhurried attention than of any aspect of physical care.

Most patients have *visitors* to provide company and affection. Ideally the amount of visiting should be determined by the effect upon the patient. Because there is limited visiting on many ward services it should not be assumed that the underprivileged person has less need for family and friends than the person in the private room. "Visiting hours" are an administrative device to regulate activity in treatment areas. Some hospitals have instituted unlimited visiting, and, according to some observers, the increased well-being of the patients more than compensates for the extra demands made on the staff. Indeed, some people believe that the visitors help with the care of the patient and incidentally are prepared to promote the patient's rehabilitation at home in proportion to their opportunity to serve and participate in the hospital. Occasionally visitors have an unwholesome effect; in such cases it is the responsibility of the doctor and the nurse to control their visits or at least to help the patient solve this problem.

Visitors should be made comfortable and welcome. They should be within the patient's sight and hearing. They should not sit on or jar the bed. It often tires the patient less to have two visitors who talk to each other than to have one demanding his or her full attention. If a visitor can enjoy an occupation or a meal with an institutionalized patient so much the better, but few rules can be made about such individual matters.

Letters, flowers, and other gifts are means of preserving personal relationships. For patients who can't write, the services of a nurse or a volunteer worker should be provided if possible.

The satisfaction of making purchases to supply daily needs and desires is taken for granted until one is deprived of it; therefore, carts containing such items as magazines, bouquets, soaps, edibles, tooth paste, writing paper, stamps, and other things are a pleasure to bed patients who have no access to shops

---

* von Mering, Otto: "Beyond the Legend of Chronicity," in Mereness, Dorothy: *Psychiatric Nursing, A Book of Readings*, Vol. II, 2nd ed. Wm. C. Brown Co., Dubuque, Iowa, 1970, p. 74.

† Jourard, Sidney M.: *The Transparent Self*, rev. ed. Van Nostrand Reinhold Co., New York, 1971.

within the hospital. With ambulation encouraged for most persons who aren't physically incapacitated or suffering from a communicable disease, such provisions are needed less and less often. Eventually we may learn to provide minimum institutionalization. Some persons need help at night, others during the day only. Self-care units that give residents the privilege of signing in and out during the day or night are revolutionizing care.

Reading is an unending source of diversion and learning for well and sick clients. Patients may visit a library in the hospital or books may be brought to them on carts. Bibliotherapy is often discussed as a means of altering a mood or an attitude. The use of specific books as therapy is, to the writers' knowledge, rare, but reading as recreation and for educational rehabilitation is well established.* Nurses should be able to read aloud so that it gives pleasure since volunteer workers, who might do this, are rarely available. Also, mechanical aids may be available for patients unable to hold a book (see Fig. 17-8). The American Library Association, the Child Study Association, and other agencies can provide lists to those who need help in selecting books according to age and interest.

---

* The present trend is toward making medical libraries "health science libraries" that all health workers use. Some persons believe that patients, or clients, of health services should have free access to what has been published in any communication media. The knowledge patients have of their needs, their illness or disability, is more likely to influence their behavior than any advice given them by medical workers.

Radio and television have put music and drama within the reach of the sick population (see Fig. 17-9), also some very effective health teaching. Music therapy has been discussed since David soothed Saul with his harp and his songs and probably long before that. Recently there have been some experiments with the use of music in psychiatry.

Music for and by the sick is certainly receiving an increasing amount of attention. Active participation in concerts and theatrical entertainment undoubtedly helps to reestablish the patient's self-confidence and enables him or her to have a normal group interest, for diversion is most satisfactory in a form that allows the patient a choice.[37b]

Variety in dress and provision of suitable clothing is a part of every rehabilitation program. Children and adults enjoy deciding what they will wear. Even in otherwise poor state hospitals, uniforms have been discarded because of their depressing effect. More than a hundred years ago Florence Nightingale suggested that nurses wear different colored uniforms and that pictures be changed in "the sick room" from time to time to combat monotony. Normal dress is encouraged in a rehabilitation program, and patients may be taught how to make suitable attractive clothing.

Meals can be pleasurable events if appetite is present. Enjoyment depends upon a combination of good food, attractive service, and companionship. Communal dining is encouraged for patients who can feed themselves and who will not be tired by company. The psychologic effect of eating alone is admittedly

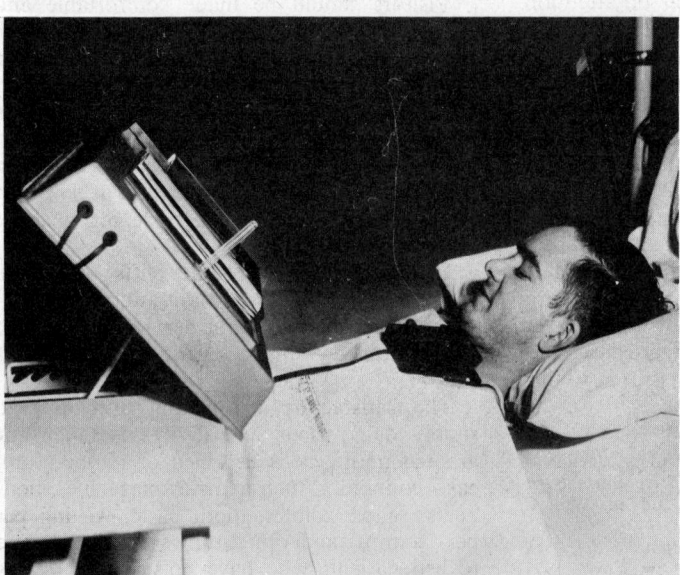

Figure 17-8. An electromechanical page turner, molded from laminated plastics, light in weight but strong and durable. Thin metal clips tied by a series of knots on a thread are slipped on the edges of successive pages of a book. When a switch adjusted under the chin is depressed by the patient, a motor-driven rotating cylinder automatically pulls the metal clips and a page is turned. (Courtesy of General Textile Mills, Inc., New York, N.Y.)

bad, and it should be avoided in institutions and homes unless the patient's condition indicates it. In these circumstances the nurse and the dietary service should use every means at their disposal to make the solitary event a pleasurable one. This is discussed in Chapter 10 as well as the desirability of giving institutionalized persons a chance to get a "snack" for themselves or even prepare a meal.

A change of scene is possible for all patients who aren't critically ill. Beds and their occupants can be wheeled to roofs or porches. Helpless persons can be lifted into wheelchairs, and taken almost anywhere. Motorized wheelchairs have been available for years. As soon as patients are ambulatory they may be moved to parts of the hospital where normal living is the order of the day. Some military and civil hospitals are classifying patients according to their independence, or the type of service they need. As the acute stage of the illness passes the patient is moved to a unit operated more like a club or a hotel and equipped and staffed differently from the acute service. Properly managed, this will certainly promote rehabilitation. More and more hospitals are adopting the practice—always common in certain countries—of admitting family members with patients. The average hospital could adopt certain aspects of such programs.

Most of the facilities mentioned in this section are generally available. The use made of them depends on the interest, imagination, and talents of health workers. For many patients, no other activities are needed for their rehabilitation; for others, organized programs of games, entertainment, and handicrafts are indicated. Some of these are discussed in Chapter 8.

Play for the Nonhospitalized Child. Recent child development research has not only pointed out the ways in which spontaneous learning develops in the infant and young child, but also the importance of supplying the child with a wide variety of toys and activities for physical, intellectual, and emotional growth.[38-39a] Many mothers are unaware of very simple and inexpensive materials that can be used as toys for children, but nurses in clinics, community settings, and the hospital can help them by showing examples and demonstrating ways in which the materials might be used (see Fig. 17-10). Student nurses are learning in their educational programs to help both mothers and children develop healthfully through play; however, the reader might like to consult an article by Mary M. Alexander[40] and various publications of the Play Schools Association, Inc.,[41] for additional ideas about interesting and inexpensive toys.

The waiting areas of pediatric outpatient clinics are often places of boredom and anxiety for children. As a consequence there may be crying and misbehavior. However, some clinics[42,43] are recognizing the benefits play has for the relief of feelings, and are providing play areas staffed with volunteers and sometimes qualified nursery school teachers. In addition to providing relief for the child (and parent), it permits the boy or girl to develop positive feelings about clinics and medical personnel. Such programs can teach the mother ways to help her child through play, and they present many opportunities for professional students from several disciplines to learn about children. Where space is insufficient for a permanent play area, "magic carts" and "magic carpets" (a play area de-

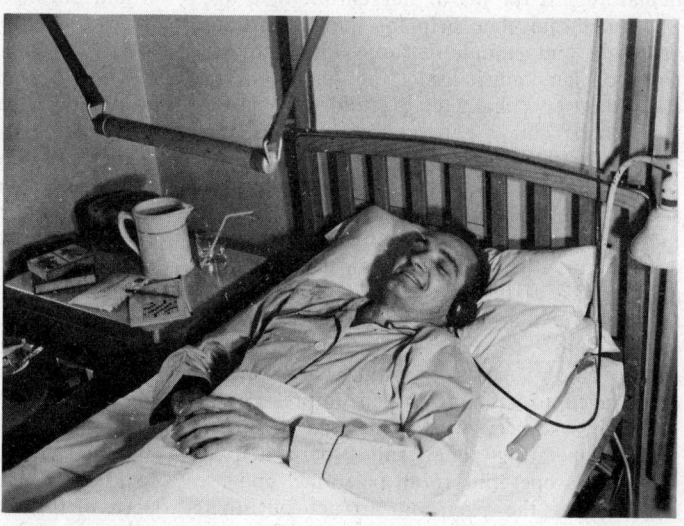

Figure 17-9. Patient with earphones listening to one of six programs available in the hospital. A pull on the black cord changes the station. (Courtesy of Columbia-Presbyterian Medical Center, New York, N.Y. and Clay-Adams, Co., New York, N.Y.)

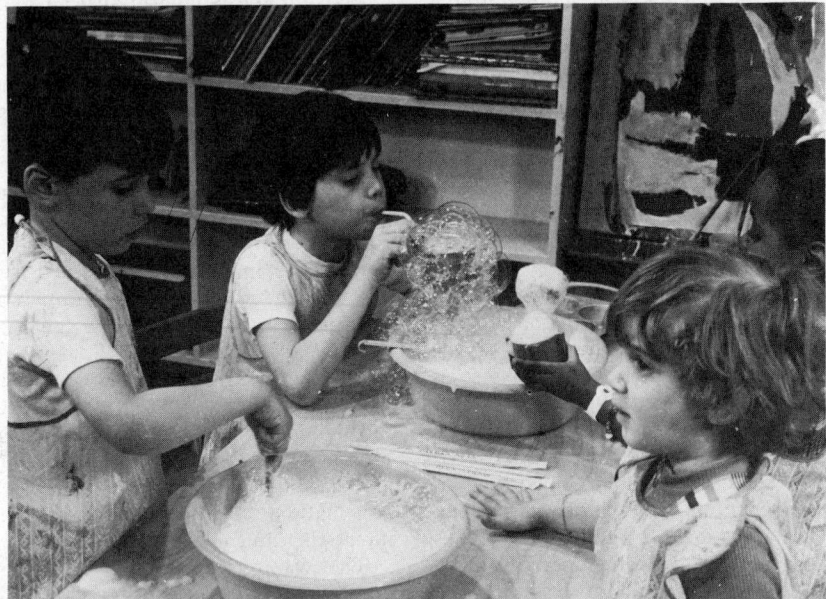

Figure 17-10. Group play consists of both imaginary and real stimuli. A child who can only allow one or the other is quickly revealed. (Reproduced with permission from Petrillo, Madeline, and Sanger, Sirgay: *Emotional Care of Hospitalized Children.* J. B. Lippincott Co., Philadelphia, 1972. Photo taken from the film "Play in the Hospital," Play School Association, Campus Films.)

fined by the size of a fairly large carpet) can be used to promote play and its values for children.[44]

According to Benjamin Spock,[45] parents of well children rarely ask for advice about toys and playing, while parents of retarded or handicapped children frequently ask such questions. Since the child is first a child, and then a child with a disability, the nurse should evaluate the developmental level without particular regard for his or her chronologic age. The nurse may then help the mother find appropriate and stimulating toys and activities based on her knowledge of the developmental continuum and character of children's play as well as the child's capabilities.

Play for the Hospitalized Child. Many hospitals use play to prepare children for surgical and other medical procedures.[46-49] Children may be brought to the hospital as much as a week before their admission or the program may be part of their surgical experience after admission. Children may be taken on a tour, usually before or sometimes after surgery, to see an empty operating room. They can be encouraged to dramatize their impression of impending surgery with dolls and a miniaturized operating room suite; permitted to dress up as operating room personnel and use a corner of the playroom to act out their

impressions of an operation; or they may be permitted and even encouraged to explore such equipment as stethoscopes, sphygmomanometers, thermometers, tongue blades, and needles and syringes. Unfortunately, what is not so frequently found in hospitals is a well-equipped and staffed play area which can be used by and for children as an ordinary part of their hospital day, or equipment and staff to arrange for play activities for children who would not be able to come to a play area, as, for example, the sandbox brought to the child's bed.[50-52a]

There are many opportunities for play with children in the course of their regular care. Story-telling, nursery rhymes, finger plays, snatches of songs, water play, and even simple games like "peek-a-boo" can be carried out while bathing a child, making his or her bed, or irrigating a catheter.[53-55] These activities are not only pleasurable to the child, but stimulate varied aspects of his or her development, as stressed earlier.

When children must be hospitalized at a distance from their homes, parents are often unable to be with them all the time. For such children, the time just prior to bedtime is very difficult. A group of nursing students elected to take as a project the alleviation, through play, of this crisis time for one group of children. They found that sharing the evening mealtime (students brought sack lunches), providing a period for active release of pent-up feeling, followed by quieting stories and simple games, plus cuddling or conversation prior to "tucking the child in," enhanced the child's ability to go quickly to sleep and to sleep well all night. The regular staff nurses were pleased with the children's response to this regime, but, regrettably, felt they could not continue with the project because of the pressure of the prescribed treatment plans and other ward duties.* The value of volunteer foster parents has been mentioned. It should be stressed that this is therapeutic for both those giving and receiving "T.L.C." (tender loving care).

A recent publication by Madeline Petrillo and Sirgay Sanger[56] might be consulted by the nurse responsible for or interested in the care of children for its many suggestions about play for the hospitalized child.

* Personal communication, Catherine Temple.

Donna Juenker[57] suggests that a play profile be used as an assessment tool at periodic intervals throughout a child's illness. While the initial information for such a profile may be a recounting of the child's play behavior by the parents, later information should be derived from the pooled observations of nursing staff who are responsible for the care of the children on that particular unit, and the nursing care modified in relation to this information.

A recent study by Veronica B. Tisza and associates indicates that for most children between the ages of 3 and 8, the threats inherent in illness and hospitalization create so much anxiety that the children "either regress or struggle against regression with resultant primitivization or even absence of play activity." * They also concluded from this study that the continuity of relationships with the

* Tisza, Veronica B., et al.: "The Use of a Play Program by Hospitalized Children," *J. Am. Acad. Child Psychiatry,* **9:**515, (July) 1970.

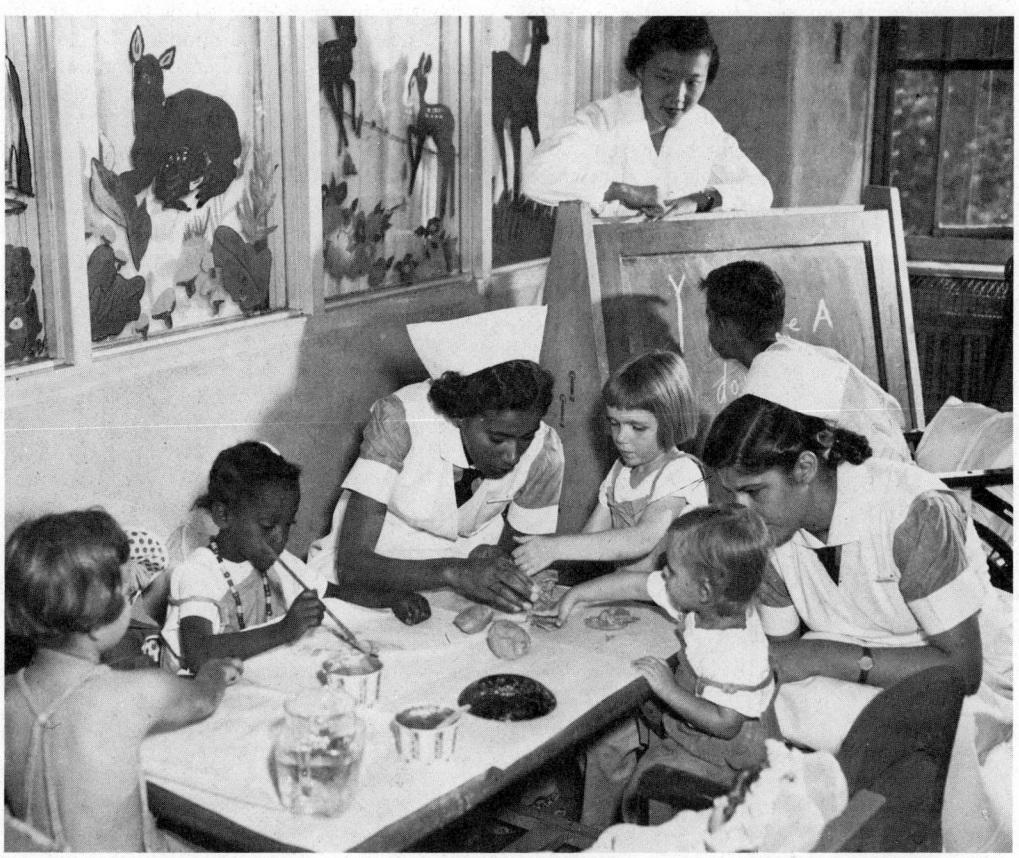

Figure 17-11. Play teacher and two student nurses supervising recreational activities of hospital patients. (Courtesy of Yale University School of Nursing, New Haven, Conn.)

playroom teacher, for children from 3 to 6 years (and to a lesser extent for children up to 8 years), lessened the "separation anxiety" so prevalent in the young hospitalized child, and permitted the child to regain the use of play for mastery purposes before the 3-day observational period of the study ended. Lawrence K. Frank [58] believes that children need the participation of adults in their "pretending" play in order to reassure them of the validity of their play and to encourage them, through participative approval, to continue to strive for mastery in the play situation. This implies that a truly effective pediatric nurse is one who not only provides for but participates in the hospitalized child's play as knowledgeably and conscientiously as she or he provides for the patient's personal hygiene and prescribed medical treatment (see Fig. 17-11).

Most pediatric hospitals or pediatric departments allow extended visiting hours for the parents of hospitalized children, and an increasing number are planning for and permitting parental rooming-in. This gives the nurse an excellent opportunity, not only to obtain information about the child, but to help the mother anticipate future developmental characteristics and the play needs of children.

Play therapy has a slightly different connotation from the kind of play program we have been discussing.[59] Virginia M. Axline [60] says play therapy is based upon the assumption that children have a growth impulse which makes mature behavior more satisfying to them than immature behavior, and that they have within themselves the ability to solve these problems when they are given some help. She describes play therapy as the opportunity given to the child to "play out his accumulated feelings of tension, frustration, insecurity, aggression, fear, bewilderment, [and] confusion" * (see Fig. 17-12). The therapist reflects these attitudes and feelings expressed in play back to the children verbally in such a way as to help them understand themselves a little better, but continually conveys to them the feeling that she is understanding and accepting them at all times, regardless of what they say or do. Play therapy is defined by Axline as not an appropriate therapeutic measure for children who are too young to have developed language skills; however, a therapeutic effect results when a preverbal child's play behavior is accepted and approved of by the adult with the only limitations placed on the child those of preventing injury to himself or herself or others, or destroying valued nonplay objects. Erik Erikson in *Childhood and Society* describes many instances in which his analysis of the

* Axline, Virginia M.: *Play Therapy*. Ballantine *Books,* Inc., New York, 1969, p. 16.

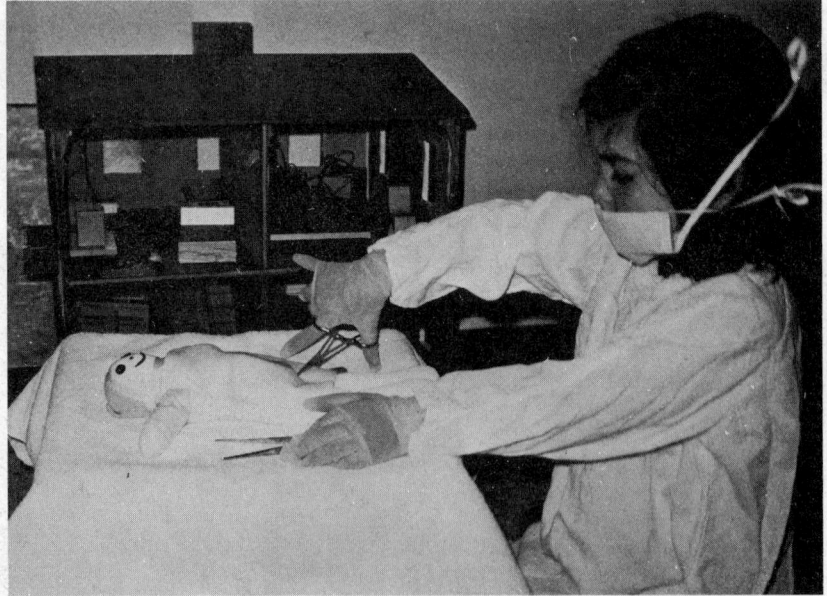

Figure 17-12. Each child uses supplies in her own way to reenact events that are stressful. (Photo by Sirgay Sanger from Petrillo, Madeline, and Sanger, Sirgay: *Emotional Care of Hospitalized Children.* J. B. Lippincott Co., Philadelphia, 1972.)

child's (and the parent's) problems are based on his observation of the child at play.

With an understanding about play characteristics and needs of children at various ages, a knowledgeable nurse can help mothers, nurses, and other hospital personnel plan and carry out play activities that provide outlets for children's emotions, for their socialization, for physical activity, for intellectual stimulation, for positive sensory stimulation of all kinds, and for growth and well-being.

REFERENCES

1. Riffle, Kathryn L.: "Rehabilitation: The Evolution of a Social Concept," *Nurs. Clin. North Am.*, **8:**665, (Dec.) 1973.
1a. Neff, Walter S.: *Work and Human Behavior.* Atherton Press, New York, 1968.
2. Carroll, Terence: "The Ideology of Work," *J. Rehabil.*, **31:**26, (July–Aug.) 1965.
3. Friedmann, Eugene, and Havighurst, Robert: *The Meaning of Work and Retirement.* University of Chicago Press, Chicago, 1954.
3a. Kaplan, Max: *Leisure in America.* John Wiley & Sons, New York, 1960.
3b. Loether, Herman: "The Meaning of Work and Adjustment to Retirement," in Shostak, Arthur, and Gomberg, William (eds.): *Blue Collar World.* Prentice-Hall, Inc., Englewood Cliffs, N.J., 1964.
3c. Berger, Peter: *The Human Shape of Work.* Macmillan Publishing Co., Inc., New York, 1964.
3d. Blauner, Robert: "Work Satisfaction in Modern Society," in Galnson, Walter, and Lipset, Seymour (eds.): *Labor and Trade Unionism.* John Wiley & Sons, New York, 1960.
4. Nite, Gladys, and Willis, Frank N.: *The Coronary Patient; Hospital Care and Rehabilitation.* Macmillan Publishing Co., Inc., New York, 1964.
5. Martin, Alexander Reid: "Man's Leisure and His Health," *Bull. NY Acad. Med.*, **40:**21, (Jan.) 1964.
6. Havighurst, Robert: "The Nature and Values of Meaningful Free-Time Activity," in Kleemeier, Robert (ed.): *Aging and Leisure.* Oxford University Press, New York, 1961.
7. Martin, Alexander Reid: "Urgent Need for a Philosophy of Leisure in an Aging Population," *J. Am. Geriatr. Soc.*, **10:**215, (Mar.) 1962.
8. de Grazia, Sebastian: *Of Time, Work, and Leisure.* Twentieth Century Fund, New York, 1962.
9. Pfeiffer, Eric, and Davis, Glenn: "The Use of Leisure Time in Middle Life," *Gerontologist*, **11:**187, (Autumn, Part 1) 1971.
10. Pfeiffer, Eric.: "Survival in Old Age: Physical, Psychological and Social Correlates of Longevity," *J. Am. Geriatr. Soc.*, **18:**273, (Apr.) 1970.
11. Ryser, Carol, and Sheldon, Alan: "Retirement and Health," *J. Am. Geriatr. Soc.*, **17:**180, (Feb.) 1969.
12. Beckman, R. O.: "Acceptance of Congregate Life in a Retirement Village," *Gerontologist*, **9:**281, (Winter) 1969.
13. Bultena, Gordon L., and Wood, Vivian: "The American Retirement Community: Bane or Blessing?" *J. Gerontol.*, **24:**209, (July) 1969.
14. Wendel, Richard S.: "The Economic Status of the Aged," *Gerontologist*, **8:**32, (Spring) 1968.
15. Sheets, Alfred W., et al.: "The Aged: Satisfied or Dissatisfied?" *J. Am. Geriatr. Soc.*, **16:**314, (Mar.) 1968.
16. Vogel, Bruce S., and Schell, Robert E.: "Vocational Interest Patterns in Late Maturity and Retirement," *J. Gerontol.*, **23:**66, (Jan.) 1968.
17. Chen, Ronald: "The Emotional Problems of Retirement," *J. Am. Geriatr. Soc.*, **16:**290, (Mar.) 1968.
18. Birren, James E.: *The Psychology of Aging.* Prentice-Hall, Inc., Englewood Cliffs, N.J., 1964.
19. Buhler, Charlotte: "Meaningful Living in the Mature Years," in Kleemeier, Robert (ed.): *Aging and Leisure.* Oxford University Press, New York, 1961, p. 370.
20. Sapora, Allen V., and Mitchell, Elmer D.: *The Theory of Play and Recreation*, 3rd ed Ronald Press, New York, 1961.
21. Hott, Jacqueline: "Play PRN in Pediatric Nursing," *Nurs. Forum*, **9:**288, (No. 3) 1970.
22. Sapora, Allen V., and Mitchell, Elmer D.: *op. cit.*
23. de Grazia, Sebastian: *op. cit.*, p. 460.
24. Pfeiffer, Eric, and Davis, Glenn: *op. cit.*
25. Erikson, Erik H.: *Childhood and Society*, 2nd ed. W. W. Norton & Co., New York, 1963.
26. Hartley, Ruth E., et al.: *Understanding Children's Play.* Columbia University Press, New York, 1952.
27. Murphy, Lois Barclay: *The Widening World of Childhood.* Basic Books, Inc., New York, 1962.
28. Gesell, Arnold, et al.: *The Child from Five to Ten.* Harper & Row, New York, 1946.
29. Ilg, Frances, and Ames, Louise: *Child Behavior.* Harper & Row, New York, 1955.
30. Hartley, Ruth E., and Goldenson, Robert M.: *The Complete Book of Children's Play.* Thomas Y. Crowell Co., New York, 1963.
31. Hawkes, Glenn, and Pease, Damaris: *Behavior and Development from 5 to 12.* Harper & Row, New York, 1962.
31a. Robison, Sandy: "Home Visits to the Elderly," *Am. J. Nurs.*, **74:**908, (May) 1974.
31b. Langrehr, Audry A.: "Social Stimulation," *Am. J. Nurs.*, **74:**1300, (July) 1974.
31c. Hargreaves, Anne G.: "Making the Most of the Middle Years," *Am. J. Nurs.*, **75:**1772, (Oct.) 1975.
32. Bortz, Edward L.: "Retirement and the In-

dividual," *J. Am. Geriatr. Soc.,* **16:**1, (Jan.) 1968.

33. Sherman, E. David: "Retirement," *J. Am. Geriatr. Soc.,* **18:**780, (Oct.) 1970.

34. Carp, Frances M.: "Differences Among Older Workers, Volunteers, and Persons Who Are Neither," *J. Gerontol.,* **23:**497, (Oct.) 1968.

35. Neugarten, Bernice L.: "Personality and the Aging Process," *Gerontologist,* **12:**9, (Spring) 1972.

35a. McLellan, E. I.: "Patients' Recreation Program," *Can. Nurse,* **69:**37, (Mar.) 1973.

36. Nite, Gladys, and Willis, Frank N.: *op. cit.*

37. Morimoto, Francoise R.: "The Socializing Role of Psychiatric Ward Personnel," *Am. J. Nurs.,* **54:**53, (Jan.) 1954.

37a. Zubek, John P.: "Sensory and Perceptual-Motor Effects," in Zubek, John P. (ed.): *Sensory Deprivation: Fifteen Years of Research.* Appleton-Century-Crofts, New York, 1969, p. 248.

37b. Gaston, E. Thayer (ed.): *Music in Therapy.* Macmillan Publishing Co., Inc., New York, 1968.

38. Brooks, Marion R.: "A Stimulation Program for Young Children Performed by a Public Health Nurse as Part of Well Baby Care," in *ANA Clinical Sessions, 1970.* Appleton-Century-Crofts, New York, 1971.

39. Murphy, Lois B.: "Spontaneous Ways of Learning in Young Children," *Children,* **14:**211, (Nov.–Dec.) 1967.

39a. Brooks, Marion R.: *op. cit.*

40. Alexander, Mary M.: "Homemade Fun for Infants," *Am. J. Nurs.,* **70:**2557, (Dec.) 1970.

41. Shoemaker, Rowena: *All in Play.* Play Schools Association, Inc., New York, 1958.

42. Azarnoff, Pat: "A Play Program in a Pediatric Clinic," *Children,* **17:**218, (Nov.–Dec.) 1970.

43. Wootton, M., et al.: "Shaping Preschoolers' Play Behavior in the Child Health Conference Waiting Area," *Can. J. Public Health,* **61:**10, (Jan.–Feb.) 1970.

44. Wheeler, Ann C.: "The Magic Cart," *Am. J. Nurs.,* **71:**2172, (Nov.) 1971.

45. Spock, Benjamin: *On Being the Parent of a Handicapped Child.* National Society for Crippled Children and Adults, Chicago, 1961.

46. Erickson, Florence: "Reactions of Children to Hospital Experience," *Nurs. Outlook,* **6:**501, (Sept.) 1958.

47. Webb, Carolyn: "Tactics to Reduce a Child's Fear of Pain," *Am. J. Nurs.,* **66:**2698, (Dec.) 1966.

48. Petrillo, Madeline: "Preventing Hospital Trauma in Pediatric Patients," *Am. J. Nurs.,* **68:**1469, (July) 1968.

49. Cassell, Sylvia, and Paul, Milton H.: "The Role of Puppet Therapy on the Emotional Responses of Children Hospitalized for Cardiac Catheterization," *J. Pediatr.,* **71:**233, (Aug.) 1967.

50. Brooks, Mary M.: "Why Play in the Hospital?" *Nurs. Clin. North Am.,* **5:**431, (Sept.) 1970.

51. Hott, Jacqueline: *op. cit.*

52. "Clever Chaos," *Hospitals,* **43:**51, (Oct. 1) 1969.

52a. Dittemore, I.: "Play Utilized by a Burned Child," *Matern. Child Nurs. J.,* **2:**203, (Fall) 1973.

53. Reese, E. M.: "The Story-Lady Nurse," *Nurs. World,* **132:**16, (Oct.) 1958.

54. Pierce, June: *Finger Plays and Action Rhymes.* Wonder Books, New York, 1955.

55. Call, Justin: "Games Babies Play," *Psychol. Today,* **3:**34, (Jan.) 1970.

56. Petrillo, Madeline, and Sanger, Sirgay: *Emotional Care of Hospitalized Children.* J. B. Lippincott Co., Philadelphia, 1972.

57. Juenker, Donna: "Play as a Tool of the Nurse," in Steele, Shirley (ed.): *Nursing Care of the Child with Long-Term Illness.* Appleton-Century-Crofts, New York, 1971, p. 76.

58. Frank, Lawrence K.: "Play in Personality Development," in Seidman, Jerome M. (ed.): *The Child, A Book of Readings.* Holt, Rinehart & Winston, New York, 1963.

59. Hyde, Naida D.: "Play Therapy: The Troubled Child's Self-Encounter," *Am. J. Nurs.,* **71:**1366, (July) 1971.

60. Axline, Virginia M.: *Play Therapy.* Ballantine Books, Inc., New York, 1969, p. 16.

Additional Suggested Reading

Abbott, Nancy, et al.: "Dress Rehearsal for the Hospital," *Am. J. Nurs.,* **70:**2360, (Nov.) 1970.

Carlson, Bernice, and Ginglend, David: *Play Activities for the Retarded Child.* Abingdon Press, New York, 1961.

Diamond, Florence: "A Play Center for Developmentally Handicapped Infants," *Children,* **18:**174, (Sept.–Oct.) 1971.

Dolan, Patricia O'Connor, and Flumere, Judith A.: "Patients' Coffee Hour," *Am. J. Nurs.,* **74:**479, (Mar.) 1974.

Galligan, Ann Costello: "Books for the Hospitalized Child," *Am. J. Nurs.,* **75:**2164, (Dec.) 1975.

Hoke, Bob: "The Game of Work," *Arch. Environ. Health,* **19:**232, (Aug.) 1969.

Honig, Alice: "The Role of the Nurse in Stimulating Early Learning," *J. Nurs. Educ.,* **9:**11, (Jan.) 1970.

Hopkins, Helen L.: "Occupational Therapy Management of Cerebrovascular Accident and Hemiplegia," in Willard, Helen S., and Spackman, Clare S. (eds.): *Occupational Therapy,* 4th ed., J. B. Lippincott Co., Philadelphia, 1971.

Johnson, June: *838 Ways to Amuse a Child.* Harper & Row, New York, 1960.

Kellogg, Rhoda, and O'Dell, Scott: *The Psychology of Children's Art.* Random House, New York, 1967.

Kleeman, James A.: "The Peek-A-Boo Game,

Part I," in Eissler, Ruth, et al. (eds.): *The Psychoanalytic Study of the Child,* Vol. XXII. International University Press, New York, 1967.

Langrehr, Audrey A.: "Social Stimulation," *Am. J. Nurs.,* **74:**1300, (July) 1974.

Larson, David, and Spreitzer, Elmer: "The Disabled Role, Affluence, and the Meaning of Work," *J. Rehabil.,* **36:**29, (July–Aug.) 1970.

Lemkau, Paul: "The Importance of Play for the Child in the Hospital," in Haller, J. Alex (ed.): *The Hospitalized Child and His Family.* Johns Hopkins Press, Baltimore, 1967.

Lewis, C. E., and Lewis, M. A.: "The Impact of Television Commercials on Health-Related Beliefs and Behavior of Children," *Pediatrics,* **53:**431, (Mar.) 1974.

Lloyd, Susan: "Playing the Health Game," *Nurs. Outlook,* **18:**36, (Oct.) 1970.

Martin, Alexander: "Idle Hands and Giddy Minds," *Am. J. Psychoanal.,* **29:**147, 1969.

McBride, Angela Barron: "Can Family Life Survive?" *Am. J. Nurs.,* **75:**1648, (Oct.) 1975.

Nixon, C.: "The Work of the Occupational Therapist Today," *Health Visit.,* **46:**221, (July) 1973.

Plank, Emma: "Drawings Help Children Express Their Anxieties," *Hosp. Topics,* **43:**93, (Oct.) 1965.

Shannon, Phillip D.: "Work Adjustment and the Adolescent Soldier," *Am. J. Occup. Ther.,* **24:**111, (Mar.) 1970.

Gladys Nite
Catherine Temple
Virginia Henderson

CHAPTER 18

Worship

1. THE SEARCH FOR MEANING IN LIFE

It seems to be a human characteristic to believe, or want to believe, that there is a beneficent purpose in life and that there is a divine spark in man. The search for "the good," "the beautiful," "the perfect," or "the divine" is what most distinguishes man from animals. However, for some, even this differentiation of man from other aspects of the universe is unsatisfying. For instance, Pierre Teilhard de Chardin,[1] who was a scientist and Jesuit priest, believed that the atoms of all matter, animate and inanimate, are in constant motion, attempting an alignment of their component parts that more nearly approaches what is good, beautiful, or perfect. This striving for perfection he saw as a universal quality of matter. This concept is so appealing to those who search for unity that students of his life and writings have formed a society in his name. Since his death in 1955, many books have been written about him and his theories.[2-6] His attempt to reconcile science and theology has helped many who have worried over this difficult issue.

Ours is considered an age of doubt or even godlessness by some persons. Arthur Koestler[7] refers to this as "The Spiritual Ice Age." Titles such as *God in Exile*,[8] *Can Faith Survive?*,[9] *Religion and the Rise of Skepticism*,[10] *Nihilism*,[11] and *Varieties of Unbelief*[12] are not uncommon in the literature of today. Others believe that there is also a revulsion against materialism and technology, a new emphasis on spiritual values. Mahatma Gandhi, Albert Schweitzer, Martin Luther King, and Mother Teresa are leaders of our times who, like Teilhard de Chardin, have spiritually influenced and are influencing millions on every continent. Albert Einstein influenced science more profoundly than any other person of this century, but his ethical interpretation of life has also had a striking effect on those who have studied his work. Some historians who take the long view see man as continuously striving for life that is better for all mankind. Jacob Bronowski, a physician, biologist, and historian, called this historical record *The Ascent of Man*. Bronowski thought the intellectual leadership of the twentieth century "rested with scientists," but he said that this posed "a grave problem" because science is a source of power that "walks close to government" and "the state wants to harness this power." He thought that if science allowed itself to be "harnessed," the beliefs of the twentieth century would "fall to pieces in cynicism." Bronowski reached the following conclusion: "It is not the business of science to inherit the earth, but to inherit the moral imagination; because without that man and beliefs and science will perish together." *

Although this is generally thought to be an age of scientific discovery and technological advance, some see life or nature as an infinitude of unanswered questions, essentially a mystery. In 1974, Lewis Thomas, a physician, said we hadn't a "complete set of information concerning at least one living thing." He doubted whether, with the help of the most sophisticated computer, we could learn in a decade all there is to know about even a simple form of life such as *Myxotricha paradoxa* "which inhabits the inner reaches of the digestive tract of Australian termites." †

Kenneth Boulding,[13] an economist and a Quaker, sees hope in "an invisible college" of people who (worldwide) are recognizing the dangers in economic development, are analyz-

---

* Bronowski, Jacob: *The Ascent of Man*. Little, Brown & Co., Boston, 1973, p. 432.

† Thomas, Lewis: *The Lives of a Cell. Notes of a Biology Watcher*. Viking Press, New York, 1974, p. 27.

ing ideologies, and are changing their lives from "unexamined" to "examined" ones.

Even as some writers stress the revolutionary changes brought about by technology, others stress revolutionary changes stemming from the data that are accumulating on the behavior of man. James Hillman[14] thinks the discovery of the unconscious (the soul?) sets the twentieth century apart from the past; Joseph Fletcher,[15] a theologian, writes about "the new morality" which is based on love and individual decision-making ("situation ethics") rather than on dogma; Gene Outka,[16] a theologian, presents an "ethical analysis" of "agapé," the love commandment and interfaith groups are celebrating feasts of brotherly love under this title—agapé. Faith rather than doctrine, nonviolent political resistance, sensitivity training, group therapy, and the emphasis on open and friendly communication are characteristic of this age.[17-19] Ashley Montagu's[20] book *Touching* has had a wide audience.

Whether or not history will stress the technical achievements of this age more or less than its efforts to understand human nature, the guiding beliefs of people are products of what Bronowski calls "the moral imagination." Before discussing these beliefs, it might be interesting to see the various meanings attached to the words "religion," "worship," "faith," and "mysticism."

Religion is the belief in a divine or superhuman power or powers to be obeyed and worshipped; expression of a belief in conduct and ritual; any specific system of belief, worship, conduct—often involving an ethical code and a philosophy; a state of mind, a way of living that expresses love for and trust in God and an effort to act according to God's will; any object of conscientious regard and pursuit; and the practice of religious observances or rites.

Worship is prayer, church service, or other rite showing reverence for or devotion to a deity—religious homage or veneration; and extreme devotion or intense love and admiration.*

Faith is unquestioning belief; unquestioning belief in God, in religion, or a system of religious belief. Faith can be applied to anything believed, complete trust, confidence, reliance, loyalty or allegiance to a person or thing.

Mysticism is the doctrine that it is possible to achieve communion with God through con-

templation and love without the medium of human reason.

In every era of recorded history, men and women have tried to understand life's meaning, to put their beliefs into words, and to evolve from their beliefs a guide to conduct. Paul Hutchinson, a theologian, says:

Endless are the forms man's religion has taken. . . . His irresistible urge to worship has been explained by a leading American anthropologist who says that man, unlike other animals, is "the creature who comprehends things he cannot see and believes in things he cannot comprehend." *

People feel so strongly about their religious beliefs that, sadly enough, they wage war in their names.† As Hutchinson says:

There is a tendency, a product of the egotism in all of us, to mock the unfamiliar in other men's faith and worship. Such words as "heathen," "idolatry," "superstition," are used more often as smear words or in derision than in their legitimate meanings. They are the words we hurl at others; seldom do we apply them to ourselves. Yet every man should command respect in the moment when he bows before his God. We may believe that his conception of the Divine lacks valuable, even essential elements. His forms of worship may appear to us bizarre, sometimes even repellent. But in that moment of prayer every man is at his best; if we are as wise as we like to think ourselves, it is then that we will attempt to understand him.‡

While religion has separated nations or been used as an excuse for wars, the works of anthropologists, such as James Frazer's *The Golden Bough*,[21] and those of historians, such as Arnold Toynbee's *An Historian's Approach to Religion*[22] point to common origins and parallel customs or festivals in all religions.§ Today, as practiced, the same religion seems different from country to country because as the people of any land adopt a new faith they keep certain elements of the one they gave up, combining the old and new beliefs, customs, and practices. The writer heard a Hindu Swami (leader or priest) say that there are as many religions as there are people in the world. He was expressing the opinion that,

---

* "Worship" is used as a title in England or as a form of address, "Your Worship," signifying a high office.

* Hutchinson, Paul: "Introduction. How Mankind Worships," in *Life*, Editorial Staff: *The World's Great Religions*. Time, Inc., New York, 1955, p. 9, Vol. 1.

† Many so-called religious wars have been political power struggles, with leaders using the strong feelings excited by religious beliefs to further the military success that would enable them to retain or acquire political power.

‡ Hutchinson, Paul: *op. cit.,* pp. 9–10.

§ A good example is the use of fire or light which is current today. Frazer traces the use of light to sun worship, to purification through fire, burning of effigies—witches, harmful spirits—and burnt offerings or sacrifices.

since each person is unique, he or she develops a particular combination of beliefs, hopes, and fears derived from intuition (the id or ego), what has been taught by parents and authority figures (the superego), and what has been learned from experience. Obviously, no two persons can have exactly the same combination of all these influences. It is hard to question the statement that even the most devout or orthodox subscribers to a religious faith make their own interpretations or adaptations. Even professed atheists (those who deny or disbelieve the existence of a god or gods) hold some beliefs that have a religious origin—beliefs that hark back to the early teaching of authority figures; agnostics (those who hold that the ultimate cause, God, and the essential nature of things are unknown or unknowable, or that human knowledge is limited to experience) are simply those in whom doubt is stronger than their faith and their hope. Archbishop Anthony Bloom,[23] a physician and theologian, in *God and Man* discusses "belief, doubt and unbelief" that lie at the center of man's experience. He thinks that doubt is always ready to disturb the most devout.

The search for unifying forces in all religions goes on; the ecumenical movement within religions, and the efforts of young people, especially, to identify common ideas and to disregard dogma and practices that tend to separate people is characteristic of this age.[24-30] The ease with which man can travel from one continent to another fosters the concept of unity—of worldwide acceptance of ideas, beliefs, and practices. However, conditions must change radically if religious wars are to be avoided and divisive forces within religious groups mitigated. *Peace and Nonviolence*[31] is a collection of essays on this theme by writers representing the major religions of the world. It emphasizes the common beliefs and hopes underlying all religions and asks for tolerance of the differences. It is a hopeful sign to see the clergy writing tracts that explain their religions to those outside the faith, for example, Rabbi Stuart E. Rosenberg's[32] *Bridge to Brotherhood, Judaism's Dialogue with Christianity,* René Laurentin's and S. J. Neuner's[33] "Declaration on the Relation of the Church to Non-Christian Religions," or J. Edgar Bruns's[34] *The Christian Buddhism of St. John.*

There are many current efforts by Occidentals to understand Oriental mysticism and to make the benefits of meditation available to peoples of all religions.[35-39] Transcendental Meditation (T.M.), so widely used on all continents, is associated in most person's minds with Eastern religions, with Yoga and other such disciplines, but the search for peace of mind through meditation has been practiced by Christians from the beginning of the Christian era.[40,40a]

There are people whose religion seems compartmentalized and as not affecting their actions; there are others whose every action seems dictated by their religious beliefs. It is the second category of persons who have had worldwide influence; Buddha, Moses, Muhammad, St. Francis of Assisi, and Mother Teresa are some examples. It seems wrong, however, to single out individuals of any age who have lived their religions since there are so many who might be mentioned. Communities or communes have been formed in every age by those who hoped they could create a society where they could achieve their spiritual ideal of living. George R. Fitzgerald[41] discusses this movement in the United States. Jean Vanier[42] in *Be Not Afraid* calls on followers of Jesus to "live his message." Sue Mosteller[43] in *My Brother, My Sister* describes the Mother Teresa Foundations in India that serve the indigent, and particularly the lepers, and the Jean Vanier houses for retarded adults that are practical expressions of Christianity. Malcolm Muggeridge[44] titles his book about Mother Teresa's work *Something Beautiful for God.* Dom Helder Camara and his associates[45] in *The Church and Colonialism* calls for just treatment of the poor; Anthony Padovano[46] in *American Culture and the Quest for Christ* uses striking photographs to show parallels between the life of Jesus and present-day Christian lives.

Even in affluent North America, material poverty exists, and poverty of the spirit invades all classes. Ethical leaders and health workers alike call for the development of a social system that abolishes hunger and inadequate shelter and clothing.[47-49] Mohandas K. Gandhi,[50] who reduced his material wants to a minimum, said that it was almost futile to try to interest the hungry in anything but food. Abraham H. Maslow, so often quoted in this book, discussed the hierarchy of needs; he believed that if the lower basic physical needs are not satisfied, the (higher) spiritual needs will not develop. In other words, the development of the highest form of human behavior cannot be realized.

While some persons would separate religion and ethics, others look upon them as two sides of a coin. While some persons believe in separation of religion and politics, few would separate ethics and politics. While some look upon science as the antithesis of religion, even of morality, others reconcile it with both, as did Teilhard de Chardin.

Maslow made the observation that the ruthless man of today is more dangerous than in any other age because "neutral" science has put such devastating weapons in his hands. He said:

. . . the classical philosophy of science as morally neutral, value free, value neutral is not only wrong, but is extremely dangerous as well. It is not only amoral; it may be antimoral as well. It may put us into great jeopardy. Therefore I would stress again that science itself comes out of human beings and human passions and interests, as Polanyi . . . has so brilliantly set forth. Science itself must be a code of ethics as Bronowski . . . has so convincingly shown, since if one grants the intrinsic worth of truth, then all sorts of consequences are generated by placing ourselves in the service of this one intrinsic value. I would add . . . that science can *seek* values, and can uncover them within human nature itself. As a matter of fact, I would claim it has already done so, at least to a level that would make this statement plausible, even though not adequately and finally proven. Techniques are now available for finding out what is good for the human species, that is, what the intrinsic values of human beings are. . . . what makes man healthier, wiser, more virtuous, happier, more fulfilled.*

Young people in every era have included idealists. Medical and nursing students are no exception. In groups, with other health workers, they are trying to bring health services to underprivileged communities, in their way, making religious, moral, or spiritual values come alive.

Edmund D. Pellegrino, discussing medicine as "the most humane science," said:

Medical students in the last three or four years have initiated a third and quite imaginative method for remedying some of the insensitivity to humane values in contemporary medicine, education, and practice. They have plunged into early and direct clinical experiences and roles of advocacy for medically disenfranchised patients and communities. These efforts have effectively revolutionized certain aspects of the medical curriculum. In the process, even faculties and deans have become more responsive to the importance of "involvement" in the major social medical issues of our day.†

Pellegrino advocated (as partial solutions to the educational deficiencies created by the present state of the humanities) three approaches: (1) behavioral science, (2) religion, and (3) direct clinical experience.

It would seem that if people are to be viewed whole, by any health worker, their moral, ethical, spiritual, and religious values cannot be ignored, nor should the practice of health workers violate their own moral, ethical, spiritual, and religious values. Nurses, physicians, and others should therefore be educated in a way that enables them to see patients as unique persons. Pellegrino called for "the truly educated person in the liberal tradition"; his three approaches he calls "partial solutions to the educational deficiencies created by the present state of the humanities." * Pellegrino, with many other physicians, is calling for a renewed emphasis on the *art* of medicine as opposed to the *science* of medicine. The art of medicine demands an understanding of broad human needs, not only the disease or diseases identified by the physicians. However, Pellegrino said that

. . . the movement *toward man* which the young so rightly and earnestly press upon . . . must not be synonymous with a flight *from reason*. We applaud those who feel deeply the responsibilities of medicine as an instrument of social purpose. Their purposes, too, will be immeasurably advanced, if heart and head are in the closest possible dialogue.†

Hundreds of books, journal articles, and other learning media addressed to health workers might be cited that stress the importance of understanding the human beings they serve. The position is taken throughout this text that the ability of nurses to help others depends on their competence in identifying clients' problems or assessing their "self-help deficits." These problems or deficits, or the reasons why one person needs help from another, are influenced by everything that creates disruption in a person's life. Religious beliefs, ethical concepts, moral values, or the meaning of life lie at the roots of each personality. The achievement of health is to some extent dependent on harmony between belief and behavior. David Belgum [51] and Orval H. Mowrer,[52,53] theologians, and Sidney M. Jourard,[54,55] a psychologist, press this point, and Karl Menninger,[56] a psychiatrist, would seem to question eliminating "sin" as an underlying cause of mental illness. The relationship between guilt and mental illness is accepted by many, as is the relationship between emotional upheaval and physical disease.

Health workers who have a broad knowledge of other cultures, including their reli-

* Maslow, Abraham H.: *The Farther Reaches of Human Nature.* Viking Press, New York, 1971, p. 2.
† Pellegrino, Edmund D.: "The Most Humane Science: Some Notes on Liberal Education in Medicine and the University," *Sixth Sanger Lecture,* Medical College of Virginia, *Bull. Med. Coll. Va.,* (Summer) 1970, p. 11.

* *Ibid.*
† Pellegrino, Edmund D.: "Humanism in Medicine. A Version for Today," *The Pharos of Alpha Omega Alpha,* **32:6,** (Jan.) 1969.

gions, will find it easier to understand human problems. Such health workers are also more likely to design and operate health services that meet people's needs regardless of their religious affiliations or lack of them.

In countries where there is a separation of church and state, public (tax-supported) agencies and institutions are prohibited from forcing any religious practice on those they serve and are supposed to give all people the same opportunity to live within the tenets of their faiths. Representatives of the dominant religion of a country often overlook these principles and impose on those of other religions some practices that run counter to their belief in what is "good" or "right." For example, prohibited foods are served with no alternate choices, only one form of religious service is made available to staff and patients in health agencies, and the only holidays recognized are those of the dominant religion.

Some persons who are socially experienced, either through travel or through reading and other ways of learning, know the history of the world's principal religions, their sacraments and holy days; however, most persons have little knowledge of religions other than their own or the faiths their parents professed. Because so many health workers, including nurses, find themselves hampered by ignorance in their efforts to help persons with different religious beliefs, this chapter gives some basic information on the world's living religions and suggests some books and articles that enable readers to pursue this subject. The principal living religions are discussed in chronological order. Their central beliefs are given, their customs and sacraments are identified, their religious holidays and rites are listed. The role of their religious leaders on the health team is discussed in general terms and some ways in which workers can foster religious practices by clients or patients are suggested.

To summarize what has been said about man's search for meaning in life, everyone believes in *something*. Even hedonists believe in "the pleasure principle." They think that what is enjoyable is good or desirable. Language is full of common expressions showing the human tendency to recognize a higher power. Strong language in emotion evokes the name of God (or gods), and, in great stress, men seem to pray, whether or not they are "religious." Common expressions suggest that most people recognize a god-like quality in other humans. A child is said to worship his father, a man to worship his wife or a woman her husband. Of a man, it might be said that "money is his God" or "he worships power," suggesting that a man must worship something. Piaget, the great student of childhood, is said to believe that all children are religious.

Most people believe that there is order in the universe; few persons who have studied nature in any of its myriad manifestations can think that its balance, harmony, or interdependence is the result of chance. The mystery of life is so awe inspiring and the plan of nature is so complex as to defy human comprehension. Whatever force lies behind this mystery, this plan of nature is "worshipped" by most, if not all, human beings. Whatever form this worship takes, it is an essential activity in the lives of children and adults. Health services should enable healthy clients and sick patients to continue the forms of worship that bring them satisfaction or comfort and that can provide opportunities for developing more mature expressions of their faiths.

2. MAJOR LIVING RELIGIONS

Membership in the Nine Major Living Religions. *The World Almanac and Book of Facts 1977* [57] gives nine religions under which the religious population of the world is categorized (see Table 18-1). Of the total world population of 3,953,125,000, it is reported that 2,550,249,665 belong to one of the nine major living religions: Christian, Islam or Muslim, Hindu, Buddhist, Confucian, Shinto, Taoist, Jewish, or Zoroastrian—in this order of magnitude. The proportionate membership of the principal religions in North America differs greatly from the world membership. For example, there are more Christians in North America than all other religions put together. Over one third of the Jews in the world are in North America, making Judaism the second largest religion. In 1976, there were 235,000 Muslims, 148,000 Buddhists, 96,000 Confucians, 70,000 Hindus, 55,000 Shintos, 16,000 Taoists, and 250 Zoroastrians.

Some of the nine religions listed above may have branches or subdivisions with such differences in their beliefs and practices as to be considered by some persons to be separate religious bodies. In 1974, a committee of physicians and chaplains in Rochester, Minnesota, compiled a guide, *Religious Aspects of Medical Care,* [58] to which they gave the subtitle *A Handbook of Religious Practices of All Faiths.* The committee listed 37 "religious groupings." Thirty-four are based on the teachings of Jesus and, liberally interpreted, might be considered denominations of the Christian faith. They include Quakers, Christian Scientists, Unitarians, and the Salvation Army. Besides these bodies, the committee listed only three non-Christian

Table 18-1. **Religious Population of the World by Continents in Nine Major Living Religions***

Religion	N. America [1]	S. America	Europe [2]	Asia	Africa	Oceania [3]	Total
Total Christian	225,504,750	161,583,500	352,597,100	86,811,000	100,465,100	17,104,000	944,065,450
Roman Catholic	128,884,000	151,600,000	171,748,500	45,122,000	32,039,500	3,188,000	532,582,000
Eastern Orthodox	4,115,000	54,000	65,534,600	1,835,000	17,410,000	353,000	89,301,600
Protestant [4]	92,505,750	9,929,500	115,314,000	39,854,000	51,015,000	13,563,000	322,181,850
Jewish	6,346,525	678,700	3,960,700	3,026,150	299,465	75,000	14,386,540
Muslim	235,000	191,200	8,730,000	422,208,000	97,678,500	66,000	529,108,700
Zorastrian [Zoroastrian]	250	—	—	224,650	475	—	225,375
Shinto	55,000	90,000	—	62,004,000	—	—	62,149,000
Taoist [5]	16,000	12,000	—	31,360,700	—	—	31,388,700
Confucian [5]	96,000	83,000	30,000	205,725,700	500	41,500	205,976,700
Buddhist	148,000	180,300	220,000	247,951,500	2,000	15,000	248,516,800
Hindu	70,000	502,000	350,000	512,418,000	463,400	629,000	514,432,400
Totals	232,471,525	163,320,700	365,887,800	1,571,729,700	198,909,440	17,930,500	2,550,249,665

Source: The 1975 Encyclopaedia Britannica Book of the Year.
[1] Includes Central America and the West Indies.
[2] Includes the USSR where it is difficult to determine religious affiliation.
[3] Includes Australia. New Zealand. and islands of the South Pacific.
[4] Protestant figures include "full members" rather than that all baptized persons and are not comparable to those of ethnic religions or churches counting all adherents.
[5] Statistics for Confucianism and Taoism are underterminable in China since the Cultural Revolution.

faiths: "Buddhist Churches of America," "the Islamic Society," and "Judaism." In a country that is predominantly Hindu instead of Christian, a handbook of religious practices might show a listing of the various branches of the Hindu religion that would equal or exceed in number the branches of the Christian religion shown in this handbook.

The nine principal living religions of the world, as listed in the *World Almanac* in an order from the oldest to the newest, are described briefly in the following pages. However, something should be said first about the religions of the less developed peoples of the world that are sometimes called "primitive" religions.

Religions of "Primitive" Cultures. Anything approaching a history of religion in a book such as this would be the height of pretension; however, it seems necessary to remind nurse readers that the earliest known forms of religion exist in certain parts of the world today. John B. Noss,[59] in *Man's Religions,* called attention to the following characteristic features of religions in existing primitive cultures: (1) *awe before the sacred* (belief that impious handling of the sacred may cause suffering, even death); (2) *expression of anxiety in ritual* (rituals include those for purification or expiation); (3) *ritual and expectancy* (rites performed to bring health, offspring, or other blessings, and "rites of passage" such as in birth, marriage, and death); (4) *myth and ritual* (belief in stories told by the authority figure that directs the tribe to behave in a certain way or that explains creation and great events); (5) *use of magic* of various kinds for various purposes (the imitation of rain by throwing rocks down a hill, for example, to end a drought, "black magic" such as sticking pins in the effigy of an enemy, or the use of fetishes—objects with presumed powers—or shamanism—the conjuring out of a spirit or disease in another through the intervention of the shaman who is himself or herself spirit-possessed—a witch-doctor); (6) *divination* (recourse to the shaman or other prophetic figure who is thought to have communion with holy spirits or gods, and who can read signs or omens); (7) *mana* (belief in a force thought transmissible from an object in nature to man, from person to person, or from person to things); (8) *animism* (the belief that motionless objects as well as living creatures have a soul and that souls leave the body during dreams and finally at death; (9) *veneration and worship of spirits* (worship of the object itself, which may be anything between heaven and earth or in the heavens, including stones, plants, trees, animals, and the elements—earth,

air, fire, and water); (10) *recognition of high gods* (belief in beings or spirits sometimes thought to have lived on the earth and retired to the heavens, sometimes thought to have created the world, established rituals, "fathered all things"); (11) *taboo* (acceptance of "hands-off," warnings applied to things, persons, and actions based on fear of "mana"— a spirit—loss of health, power, or luck); (12) *purification rites* (the use of cleansing ceremonies, sometimes to break a taboo); (13) *sacrifice* (giving up or destroying—usually by burning—an inanimate object or a living creature to please the spirit, spirits, or gods; (14) *wariness in treating the dead body* (for example, putting fences around graves, making propitiatory offerings, or providing the dead with their worldly needs *); (15) *totemism* (believing that a more or less intimate relationship exists between groups of humans and classes or species of animals, plants, or inanimate objects. Tribes may have one or more totems).

A list of characteristics of primitive religions such as the one just given can do little more than encourage readers to study sources such as Frazer's [60] *Golden Bough,* the works of Mircea Eliade,[61-64] William James's [65] *Varieties of Religious Experience,* and Carl Clemen's [66] *Religions of the World: Their Nature and History,* or anthropologic tracts on the peoples in which the readers are particularly interested. Articles by nurses, physicians, and others who have lived and worked with North and South American Indians (Native Americans), African tribes, or Australian Aborigines can give many interesting examples of behavior based on these primitive religions. Most health workers in cultures foreign to their own find it necessary to study the religion and the history of the people. It must be obvious, however, to any thoughtful reader that peoples in undeveloped countries have much in common, from the standpoint of religion, with the more sophisticated cultures. Eliade is especially helpful in identifying the universal religious themes.

In Chapter 1, attention was called to currently effective health experiments in undeveloped areas where care has been taken to build a program around the fundamental beliefs of the people, or to use folk medicine

---

* Noss says that, within living memory, the deaths of kings in Africa have "been an occasion of 'sending along' hundreds of men and women" (Noss, John B.: *Man's Religions,* 4th ed. Macmillan Publishing Co., Inc., New York, 1969, p. 21). Kings in some cultures were sacred and no sacrifice could be too great. See also Frankfort, Henri: *Kingship and the Gods.* University of Chicago Press, Chicago, 1948.

(which always involves religion) as well as so-called scientific medicine.[67-69]

No effort will be made to discuss in any detail the major living religions historically or geographically, but most readers should find both approaches rewarding. It is hard to understand present-day India, for example, without knowing a good deal about the history of Hindus and Buddhists, or to understand the influence of Chairman Mao's socialist philosophy on the people of Mainland China without studying Confucius's teaching. He was another leader who was more of a philosopher than a *religieuse*. While Mao emphasized national loyalty, Confucius emphasized family loyalty.[70] This has led to a conflict between the State and "religion."

About India, Noss makes the following observation:

The religions of India are inexhaustively fertile in the suggestions they offer for meeting the need man feels for rational and mystical adjustment to life and the world. This suggestiveness is both a present and a past fact. The religions of India can be said to have offered almost every answer to religious need that can be thought of, and to have discarded none; all the answers made in the past are preserved, like bees in amber, along with those offered in the present. One feels, in studying the development of Indian religions, like an archeologist digging down through the layers of Near East civilizations and finding the old forever preserved beneath the new.*

Hinduism and Buddhism are discussed next but in so abbreviated a fashion that the reader cannot possibly acquire any understanding of the diversified forms they have taken over the centuries in the various countries where they are practiced. Hinduism, especially, is an inclusive rather than an exclusive religion. Robert C. Zaehner[71] says Hinduism is free from any "dogmatic affirmations about god." Gandhi, who was a devout Hindu, included in his daily devotional services both Christian and Muslim prayers and excerpts from the Bible and the Koran.[72]

Hinduism. According to Noss,[73] modern Hindus use the ancient word *dharma* (meaning "way of life") for Hinduism unless they are speaking to, or writing for, Westerners. The origin of Hinduism goes back beyond recorded history. It is thought that the people of India in 2500 B.C., practiced an "advanced religion" that contained "the germ" of ideas expressed in the Law of Karma and reincarnation. The early expression of Hinduism in Pre-Aryan India (before 1500 B.C.) is distinguished by some writers from later Hinduism. Noss calls early Hinduism the passage from ritual sacrifice to mystical union; later Hinduism, he says, is religion as the basis of social behavior.

Knowledge of ancient Hinduism is an interpretation of the Vedic literature or the *Rig-Veda, Sama-Veda, Yajur-Veda,* and *Atharva-Veda* (*Veda* means "sacred knowledge"). These sacred writings were followed by later collections known as the *Brahmanas,* the *Aranyakas,* and the *Upanishads.* Some Hindus refer to all these works, which come in several versions, as "the Vedas." All the older writings are seen as *shruti* ("heard" revelations and sacred writ); later writings as *smriti* ("remembered" or composed by human authors). The latter include *sutras, shastras, epics,* or the *Mahabharata* and *Ramayana* and the *Puranas* (ancient stories) and *Tantras* (threads, basic teaching). The *Mahabharata* contains the *Bhagavad Gita,* or Song of the Blessed Lord, which interweaves all three ways of religious expression, *knowledge, works,* and *devotion.*

The Hindu looks upon this life as an opportunity to seek the ultimate good, to comprehend the eternal, to reject the immediate and the material reward and accept the spiritual. Joseph M. Kitagawa[74] refers to the Hindu's sacramental view of the universe—the concept that all work is sacrifice. Reincarnation, rebirth, or the transmigration of souls (which is not peculiar to Hinduism) enables a soul to exist on different planes. According to the Law of Karma, which is part of Indian Hinduism, a person's thoughts, words, and deeds determine whether the soul will enter a lower or higher form of life in rebirth. This process of repeated rebirth is known as "The Wheel." Hindus believe that there is a realm of being where one is released from "The Wheel." This realm of being—free from suffering and striving—where human imperfection is transcended is *Nirvana.* There, the soul's essence is united with the absolute. The state of Nirvana represents true and real, or Brahman, freedom and is only attained by the holy man. *Yoga* is a general term for any ascetic technique and any method of meditation. For those studying forms of Yoga in India, Eliade's[75] *Yoga: Immortality and Freedom* is a valuable source. In earlier forms of Hinduism, the devout sought Nirvana in solitude—withdrawing from the world; modern Hindus seek it in good works, trying to better the lot of mankind.

Noss says:

In the more universal forms of Hinduism a triad of great gods appears. These beings—Brahma the Creator, Shiva the Destroyer, and Vishnu the Preserver—are recognized by the Brahmins as un-

* Noss, John B.: *op. cit.,* p. 86.

doubtedly standing for realities within the frame of the universe. In any event, they command the believing trust and devotion of millions of the common people of India.*

With their different characteristics, these gods now variously influence their followers, and rival loyalties have developed, with separate temples and forms of devotion. However, these personal gods of the Hindus are all seen as manifestations of the spiritual absolute. Many students of the subject believe these god-figures are essential to the majority of people and are a means of holding them in Hinduism when they might otherwise be attracted to other faiths, such as the Buddhist, that offer devotional objects.† A. L. Basham [76] describes the Hindu cyclic concept of the world and the characteristics of its principal gods.

Since there are so many branches of Hinduism, it is not easy to list the customs or practices of its members. Most abstain from meat, even eggs, and also from alcohol. Life is held sacred and animals may roam unharmed among the people. India is famous for its sacred cows. Gandhi [77] called this reverence for life the central fact of Hinduism and considered the cow symbolic of the whole subhuman world. Most leaders practice and teach some form of bodily discipline, such as Yoga (a Sanscrit word meaning "yoking," or "union"), which is believed to free the spirit from domination by the body. The holy men or leaders are called gurus and addressed as Swami. Many of them have come to the United States and have built up large followings. Ralph Waldo Emerson and other intellectuals of his day were influenced by Hindu philosophy. Swami Vivekananda's statements at the 1893 World Parliament of Religions in Chicago made a lasting impression. His Vedanta Hinduism was revived by the mystic, Ramakrishna, who also won converts in the West. Most recently, Swami Bhaktivedenti in the 1960s established the Krishna Consciousness movement. Its chanting monks in saffron robes are seen on the streets of numerous large cities today. Basham [78] credits Vivekananda with restoring the faith of educated Hindus which the earlier reformers had not succeeded in doing.

Various meditative disciplines have evolved within Hinduism. Transcendental meditation is a form of nonreligious self therapy; it was made popular in this country largely through the teaching of Maharishi Mahesh Yogi.

The Yogi system of disciplining mind and body is, according to Noss, first mentioned in the Upanishads. It was refined by Patanjali in the second century A.D. There are eight steps in the Raja Yoga of Pantanjali but two are other forms of Yoga. Sri Aurobindo Ghose, a Bengali Brahmin who died in 1950, taught "integral Yoga" and, like Teilhard de Chardin, hoped for an evolution of mankind. Aurobindo Ghose's teaching is said to fill 30 volumes in English and is being studied in ten centers within the United States as well as in the Aurobindo Ashram in Pondichérry, India. He and Sarvepalli Radhakrishnan [79] have sought a reconciliation of Eastern and Western thought about religion.

Hindus worship at home or in temples as they feel the need. A priest or family member (who may be a man or woman) conducts domestic rites before an image of the household god, and he or she and all of the community may attend ceremonies performed several times a day by local priests in temples. Many descriptions of Hinduism note that Hindus get their greatest religious satisfaction in being in the presence of holy men (gurus) and in pilgrimages to holy places.[80-83]

Hindus practice cremation of the dead. This may take the form of a public ceremony, with the funeral pyre floating on a river as the body burns. Gandhi's pyre floating on the holy river, the Ganges, with his body surrounded by offerings of marigolds, expressing the love of hundreds of people, was seen over television by millions of viewers of this era.

Jainism. Like Hinduism, Jainism originated in India. It is an outgrowth of or a "reform" movement within Hinduism. Its founder is Mahavira (meaning Great Man, or Hero), whose real name was Nataputta Vardhamana. He is believed to have been a prince who lived from 599 to 527 B.C. He renounced his princely life when he was 30 and joined a body of monks. He neglected his body and is said to have wandered completely naked in his "quest of release from the cycle of birth, death and rebirth." According to Noss:

His two convictions were (1) that saving one's soul from evil (that is, purging contaminating matter from the soul) is impossible without practicing the severest asceticism, and (2) that maintaining the purity and integrity of one's own soul involves practicing ahimsa, or noninjury, to any and all living beings. Neither of these convictions was new, for Mahavira took them from his predecessors in the tradition of thought with which his name is now associated, but the faithfulness and sincerity with which he lived by them were remarkable.*

---

* *Ibid.*, p. 207.
† Noss says: "The common man of India is uncritically and perhaps limitlessly polytheistic, . . . their deities numbering 330 millions. They may go from shrine to shrine, making innumerable pilgrimages." (*Ibid.*, p. 217.)

* *Ibid.*, p. 113.

Finally, after 13 years of a stringently ascetic life, it is recorded that Mahavira reached Nirvana. After this, until his death at 72, he was called Jina (the Conqueror) and his followers were called Jains. Of the five vows taken by Jainist monks, the first is Ahimsa—to kill no living things; other vows are to renounce "all vices of lying speech," to renounce taking anything that is not given, to renounce sexual pleasures and all attachments. For lay members of the Jainist faith, the code is a modification of these stringent practices and, according to Noss, there is no sharp distinction between monks and laymen. Both observe the "recurring events" of their religious calendar. About the end of August, there is a period of fasting and repentance (Purushana) followed by rejoicing, the Jain's New Year's Day. The Jains believe that the world is in a period of decline or degeneration, but that the "golden age" will return. It is estimated that there are about 2,000,000 Jains. Their temples in Calcutta and Bombay are among the most beautiful in India. Basham [84] thinks that, while Jains are few, they have been influential. He thinks that Gandhi's philosophy owes much to the strict *ahimsa* (non-violence) of Jainism.

Buddhism.* Like Jainism, Buddhism is an outgrowth of or "reform" within Hinduism. Buddha, its founder, like Mahavira, was a rich man. He was a member of a prominent Kshatriya family who left his wife and child to lead the homeless life of a mendicant. His name was Siddharta (Pali, Siddharta) Gautama (Pali, Gotama) who lived from 643 to 563 B.C. After achieving Nirvana, he became the Buddha (the Enlightened One).

Written records of Buddha's life are said by some to date from the third century B.C. Noss † remarks, "The relative lateness of written transmission [or oral accounts] obviously magnified the uncertainties of textual criticism also."

While biographies of the Buddha differ, they agree in the main. Siddharta Gautama lived in luxury and was shielded from sights of poverty and sickness until after his marriage when, leaving home against his father's wishes, he saw the sick, the old, the suffering, and the dead. He is said to have shaved his head, put on a monk's yellow robe, and sought, through solitude, meditation, and association with other ascetics, to achieve enlightenment, or Nirvana. He is often represented in sculpture as sitting, sometimes under a bo-tree, unmoved by temptation. After his enlightenment, he preached for 45 years and made many converts in India. His first sermon is said to have contained the germ of the Four Noble Truths and the Noble Eightfold Path and the Five Precepts which are the basis of Buddhism as practiced worldwide. The following is a brief version of the "truths" of the path:

The Four Noble Truths are the following (1) Suffering is universal; (2) The cause of suffering is craving, or selfish desire: (3) The cure of suffering is the elimination of craving; (4) The way to eliminate craving is to follow the Middle Way, a technique which embodies the Noble Eightfold Path.

The Path consists of (1) right knowledge, (2) right intention, (3) right speech, (4) right conduct, (5) right means of livelihood, (6) right effort, (7) right mindfulness, (8) right concentration.*

Through a purifying life of ethical thinking and behaving (good deeds), the Buddhist achieves an impersonal ultimate reality. Buddhists are said to believe in reincarnation but not, like Hindus, in the transmigration of souls through various forms of life. Buddhism is essentially monastic, requiring withdrawal from life and relinquishing the eating of meat and owning of personal property. Most Buddhist boys and men spend a part of their lives as monks, but most return to the life of laymen. Even four-year-olds may be initiated into a monastic order and spend a night in a monastery. The initiation ceremony is said to be more important to Burmese Buddhists than weddings or funerals. A few Buddhist sects permit monks to marry. Most Buddhists are essentially compassionate, avoid killing animals, and may be vegetarians. Asoka, the great emperor of India who ruled from 269 to 237 B.C., became a Buddhist and was so impressed with its pacifist principles that, after years of conquest, he foreswore killing and made Buddhism the state religion of India. During this time, Buddhism dominated Hinduism, but today Buddhism has largely disappeared from India. It is said to be the gentlest of religions. The Buddhist saint, Sariputta, is quoted as saying, "Shame on him that strikes, greater shame on him who, stricken strikes back." †

Buddhism has been taken to all continents and it is the dominant religion in many coun-

---

* Noss says: "Like the Hindus, the Buddhists, when referring to what the West calls 'Buddhism' or the 'Buddhist religion,' use the term *Dharma* (*Pali Dharma*). Their only difference from the Hindus in this respect lies in their linking of this term with the teaching and moral injunctions of one man, Gautama Buddha. An alternative term is *Sasana* which means the whole body of beliefs and practices of the Buddhist faith, broadly, the Buddhist 'dispensation' or 'system.'" (*Ibid.*, p. 123.)

† *Ibid.*, p. 124.

* *Life*, Editorial Staff: op. cit., p. 54, Vol. 1.

† *Ibid.*, pp. 54, 62, 65.

tries. It has encouraged tolerance, nonviolence, respect for the individual, love of nature, and the spiritual equality of human beings.

The religion of Buddhism has dominated Japan, Manchuria, Mongolia, China, Tibet, Burma, Thailand, and Cambodia. In some form, it exists on every continent. In the United States, there are more Buddhists and Buddhist communities than members of any other Eastern faith.

For Westerners who find the Buddhist religion hard to understand, Jane Hamilton-Merritt's book, *A Meditator's Diary*,[85] is useful. She studied meditation (which she says is "central to Buddhism") with the abbots and monks in two Thai Wats, or Theravada Buddhist communities. A journalist who had had assignments in Vietnam, Cambodia, Laos, and Thailand, she understood and spoke the Thai language. Quoting from her journal, she carries the reader through her experience in studying Theravada Buddhism. She explains the way of life of the Buddhist, the eight "precepts" to which she adhered while living in the Chiang Mai Wat. She describes her sensations and the effect of meditation, including its effect on pain, and the "shedding of desires," they, according to Buddhist teaching, being the source of all suffering. The following is excerpted from Hamilton-Merritt's summation.

Meditation . . . is learning to still the mind, to control it, to centre the mind's potential energy. In this quietness or condensation of the mind's energy, the mind expands and is capable of producing more accurate realizations. . . .

The process of meditation seems to involve a shedding of desires, of the need for unnecessary possessions, of a demanding ego, of the importance of the trite, superfluous, loud or ostentacious. When these fall away—as they will in meditation—it becomes possible to know something of the true self. . . .

Inherent in Theravada Buddhist meditation is self analysis—a willingness to examine oneself. The Buddhist concept of being *Awake* is the realization that all of us can save ourselves from our own suffering. All of us have within us the potential to win our own freedom.*

As often happens with a religion, the teachings of the founder are differently interpreted. The Buddhists of China, Japan, and Tibet follow a later interpretation—the new doctrine being known as Mahayana or "The Greater

Vehicle"; the orthodox Theravada Buddhism of Ceylon, Thailand, and Burma as Hinayana or "The Lesser Vehicle." In the later version, the austere Gutama Buddha is replaced by the Amitabha Buddha, or "Buddha of Infinite Light." His virtue is not so much in philosophical detachment as in compassion.[86]

Buddhists have various "holy" days in eight of the twelve months of the year.* It is suggested in *Religious Aspects of Medical Care* [87] that, since some "could be quite emotional," surgical treatment on one of them might be unwise, according to the patient's convictions. Buddhists have no sacraments in the sense used by Christians but some equate with Baptism the expression of faith in the Three Treasures (Buddha, Dharma, and Sangha) which is the symbolic act of becoming a Buddhist.

Cremation is common among the Buddhists, but the body may also be buried after a service at a temple or at the graveside. Since the aim of the devout Buddhist is enlightenment and spiritual peace, prolongation of life until this end is achieved is desirable, but after enlightenment, euthanasia might be accepted.

Buddhism has undergone so many variations in China and Japan that, according to Noss,[88] attempting to trace the differences among the schools and sects in the two countries would be as tedious and difficult as to trace the differences between Protestant (Christian) sects in Europe and America. He thinks, however, the following five main trends among the Buddhist schools are distinguishable:

1. *The Pure Land School.* In China, the Ching-t'u School looks upon salvation as the gift of Amitabha Buddha if there is unquestioning faith in him. In Japan, the Jodo and Jodo-Shin sect believe in redemption by humility and faith in Anitabha Buddhi. Their "Hail Amida Buddha," or "Namu Amida Butsu," is abbreviated to "Nembutsu."

2. *The Intuitive School.* In China, this is the Ch'an School, pronounced Zen in Japan. In both schools, the emphasis is on enlightenment and salvation through meditation rather than on study or good deeds. The inward search for the essential is reflected even in art, architecture, flower arranging,

---

* Hamilton-Merritt, Jane: *A Meditator's Diary. A Western Woman's Unique Experience in Thailand Temples.* Harper & Row, New York, 1976, pp. 143, 145. The concluding chapter contains specific directions for meditation practice.

* Holy days of Buddhists are said to be January 1st and 16th, February 15th, March 21st, April 8th, May 21st, July 15th, September 1st and 23rd, and December 8th and 31st. (Medicine and Religion Committee, Zumbro Valley Medical Society, Rochester, Minn. (compilers): *Religious Aspects of Medical Care; A Handbook of Religious Practices of All Faiths.* Catholic Hospital Association, St. Louis, 1975, p. 5.)

and social intercourse which makes for simplicity and restraint. Ch'an and Zen Buddhism deserve far more attention than can be given them here.

3. *The Rationalist School.* In China, this school is represented by the T'ien-T'ai sects. Followers of this school believe that the Gutama Buddha saw three levels of truth: one for those who believe in the reality and value of the material world, another for those who seek spiritual peace living in this world, and a third for those who seek redemption through meditation. The followers of this school see Buddha as having reconciled the three. In Japan, this school is known as Tendai.

4. *The Mystery or True World School.* In China, the Chen Yen or Mystery School puts emphasis on the supernatural, on a long list of gods and formulas, gestures, invocations, and rites. In Japan, the Mystery School formed the Shingon sect that worship the Dhyanni Buddha. They have a doctrine and ritual that is a synthesis of Buddhism and Shinto which is very appealing to the Japanese.

5. *The Socio-political School* is an expression of Japanese Buddhism founded by Nichiren ("Sun-Lotus") which is described in his *Lotus of the Good Law*—an attempt to restore original and true Buddhism. This sect is strongly nationalistic and maintains a headquarters including the largest temple in the world at the foot of the Sacred Mount Fuji:

Tibetan Buddhism is of a special character with an admixture of Trantrism which is a devotion to natural energy, or *shakti*—the concept that everything in nature is a union of male and female elements. Studying Tibetan art, it is noticeable that Buddhas and Bodhisattvas have spouses. There is a strong element of magic in this religion. The prayer wheel or mill is believed to protect the devout who carry it from a variety of evils. The clergy are called *lamas,* which means superior. They are encouraged to marry. The Grand Lama at Lhasa acquired the name Dalai Lama in the sixteenth century. Before communism, one fifth of the population lived in lamaseries which were centers of political influence and learning. Changes wrought by communism are too complex for discussion here.

Writings on Buddhism are extensive. Sir Edwin Arnold's [89] narrative poem, *The Light of Asia* first published in 1884, introduced many English readers to the character of "Lord Buddha—Prince Siddartha styled on earth" (as the poem began) and his teachings.

Students of this religion will find additional sources among suggested readings at the end of this chapter.

The Confucian Philosophy and Chinese Religions. Although Confucianism is often considered a religion, the authorities consulted by the writer seem to agree that the teachings of Confucius represent a philosophy more than a religion. Fêng Yu-lan,[90] in *The Spirit of Chinese Philosophy,* includes Confucius, Mencius, Lao Tzu, and the Inner Light School of Buddhism. However, a religious cult has been formed around the teachings of Confucius. In 195 B.C., Emperor Kao Tsu of the Han Dynasty is said for the first time to have offered official sacrifices at Confucius' tomb. Subsequent emperors added honors, and in A.D. 59 it was ordered that there be sacrifices in his name in urban schools. Since the seventh century, the Chinese have built Confucian temples. In 1906, the last Manchu emperor elevated Confucius to the highest position of worship, along with Heaven and Earth.

The people of China from primitive times have tried to understand nature, seeing in it a sublime beauty and order. Man was believed to be happy living in harmony with nature rather than dominating it and using it to his ends.[91-95] Heaven, Earth, and man were believed to have an indivisible unity governed by Tao (cosmic law). Tao literally means "a way" or "a road," or "the way to go." Noss gives the following explanation:

The Tao is emphatically a way of harmony, integration, and cooperation. Its natural tendency is toward peace, prosperity, and health. If it were not for the perverse men and demonic beings that refuse to adjust themselves to it, this would quickly become evident. In fact, if the Tao were ever to be followed everywhere, heaven, mankind, and earth would form a single, harmonious unit, in every part cooperating toward universal well-being.*

This state of perfection was thought to have existed in the Golden Age when Tao and Shun, the good emperors, ruled according to Tao. As early as 1000 B.C. perhaps, the Chinese sought to understand matter and the opposing forces, or energy modes. They believed that Yang (male) and Yin (female) forces existed in the same object, and that object might be Yang (or male) at one time and Yin (or female) at another. For example, a dried log appears to be a Yin object but, when burning, it has the Yang qualities of warmth and brightness. This ancient Chinese concept —that all matter is in a changing dynamic state and that harmony depends on balance

* Noss, John B.: *op. cit.,* p. 251.

between the positive and negative elements—seems strangely modern.*

About the *I Ching,* Jung said:

The *I Ching* does not offer itself with proofs and results; it does not vaunt itself, nor is it easy to approach. Like a part of nature, its waits until it is discovered. It offers neither facts nor power, but for lovers of self-knowledge, of wisdom—if there be such—it seems to be the right book. To one person its spirit appears as clear as day; to another, shadowy as twilight; to a third, dark as night. He who is not pleased by it does not have to use it, and he who is against it is not obliged to find it true. Let it go forth into the world for the benefit of those who can discern its meaning.†

Earth worship is characteristic of ancient China. A mound of earth called the *she* was made in each village and, according to Noss,[96] ceremonies around it, resembling the European Maypole festival, continue into modern times. Worship of heaven comes down from ancient times. Tien (heaven) meant the abode of the Great Spirits; Chou and subsequent emperors were Tien Tzu, or "Son of Heaven." The Chinese believed spirits inhabited heaven and earth and that not all were beneficent. Spirits were finally categorized into the *Shen* (good) and the *Kwei* (bad or unpredictable). The good were associated with daylight, the sun, and flowering plants; the bad were everywhere and made night or the dark dangerous. This danger could be mitigated by carrying a lantern. These beliefs are expressed in modern-day customs. For example, the Chinese New Year is celebrated by fires, torches, candles, lanterns, and fire crackers to scare the evil spirits away for the coming year. Spring is celebrated with branches of peach blossoms and red paper in imitation of them, and sayings of wise men are tacked to the houses.

Ancestor worship was, and still is, practiced by the Chinese who thought of themselves as surrounded by the living and powerful spirits of members of the family who had died. These spirits promoted the welfare of the family. Living members made sacrifices of food and drink to the ancestors who were supposed to have inhaled the essence of the sacrifice.‡

Homes contained, as many do today, an ancestral shrine, where ceremonies such as marriage might take place or where the head of the family might announce an important business venture. Loyalty and duty to the family were considered preeminently virtuous. Confucius taught, for instance, that a father should conceal the crimes of a son, or vice versa.*

Until recent times China was not a united country but a group of feudal states. This feudal system was preserved by a rigid code of behavior for emperors, nobles, officials, and common people. This behavior included religious practices. It was considered improper for the common man to worship the hills and streams that belonged to the feudal lords. Only the emperor could address the sublime spirit, or Tien, at the Altar of Heaven outside the capitol of the empire. Common men could, with propriety, only worship their ancestors, the spirits guarding their dwellings, their health, and their "luck." Confucian precepts tended to preserve the status quo, to encourage a code of behavior or custom based on a rigid social hierarchy.

Confucianism can be said to have been preceded by Taoism since Confucius is believed by some to have been a pupil of Lao-tzu whose treatise is the basis of Taoism. Wing-tsit Chan [97] says, "No one can understand China or be an intelligent citizen of the world without some knowledge of Tao-te Ching (the Classic of the Way and Its Virtue). . . ." In Chan's monograph, dates for Lao-tzu range from the eighth to the fifth centuries B.C. Noss [98] says there is some confusion between Lao Tan, a legendary person, and Li Erh of the fourth century B.C., presumably nicknamed Lao-tzu.

Volumes have been devoted by Chinese scholars to defining Taoism, so it seem presumptuous to try to reduce it to a few paragraphs here. The early Taoists were said to think the secret of a good life was following the inevitable, being indifferent to things, paying no attention to the past or future—allowing things to take their natural course or not interfering with the Tao (the eternal Way of the Universe—the cosmic mode of action).

Next to Lao-tzu, Chuang-tzu of the fourth century is said to be the most famous of the Taoist philosophers.[99] His essays, like the brief writings attributed to Lao-tzu, are basic to understanding Taoism. In A.D. 165, the Emperor Huan of the second Han Dynasty had

---

* C. G. Jung in the foreword to Richard Wilhelm's translation of The *I Ching, or Book of Changes* said: "The ancient Chinese mind contemplates the cosmos in a way comparable to that of the modern physicist who cannot deny that his model of the world is a decidedly psycho-physical structure."

† *The I Ching or Book of Changes,* 3rd ed. The Richard Wilhelm translation rendered into English by Cary F. Baynes. Princeton University Press, Princeton, N.J., 1950, pp. xxiv, xxxix (Bollingen Series XIX).

‡ After a proper interval, the priests or sacrificers ate the food.

* Communism considers this teaching of Confucius absolutely wrong and a crime against the state.

a temple built to Lao-tzu, but Taoism was not recognized as an organized religion until the seventh century A.D. when, to stop the inroads of Buddhism, it is said, Taoism was endowed with some comparable characteristics to make it more appealing to the common man. As a religion, Taoism is in decline, but the influence of its philosophy is hard to estimate or separate from that of Confucius. *The I Ching or Book of Changes,*[100] which is thought to be the common source for both philosophies, is widely read both inside and outside China. Hellmut Wilhelm, in the preface to the third edition of the translation, makes the following statement that shows the importance of this book and the role of Confucian philosophy in the Republic of China:

Reference has been made to recent Chinese scholarship regarding the Book of Changes. This renewed interest in the Book is fundamentally different, of course, from the one that produced the abundance of I Ching studies during Imperial times. The Book is no longer considered part of Holy Writ but is submitted to the same type of analysis as any other ancient text would be. The results have been highly rewarding. There is, however, evidence of a continued strain of reverence which has by now overcome—or more cautiously: is about to overcome—the fashion of the earlier republican times to see in the Book only a conglomerate of superstition or, at the least, murk. Everybody knows, of course, that a host of problems still remains unsolved; but sober scholarship gradually recognizes again that what has been dealt with in the Book is a unique manifestation of the human mind. The more emotionally inclined have proceeded to regard the Book again as one of the most treasured parts of the Chinese tradition. To the extent that opinions can be expressed, this is true even in the context of Communist China. Kuo Mo-jo, who until his recent purge was the foremost cultural official of Communist China, devoted himself to the Book extensively, particularly in his earlier years. And when, in the early 1960's the ideological reins were somewhat relaxed and it was possible for a time to deal with matters of intellectual concern, the two issues which engendered nationwide discussions were the ethical system of Confucius and the Book of Changes. By now these discussions have been curtailed, but the phenomenon persists: whenever the rare chance of expression is given, the Book emerges as one of the foremost concerns of Chinese intellectuals even under the specific set of circumstances prevailing on mainland China.*

The Confucian philosophy might be termed elitist, and it is easy to see why these teachings run counter to the egalitarian philosophy of the late Chairman Mao and other Communist leaders. However, it is easier to understand the influence of a poet and a philosopher such as Mao when one considers that the majority of the Chinese have been followers of the sage Confucius rather than the religious mystics whose teachings have dominated other Eastern countries.

The Maoist regime, with its emphasis on loyalty to the nation, discouraged the family loyalty that under Confucianism took precedence over all others. Those who want to understand modern-day China must study the opposing philosophers of the past and the present.[101,102]

Judaism. The first strictly monotheistic religion is said by many writers to be that of Judaism, a characteristic shared by the later religions of Christianity and Islam. Judaism is the oldest of the living religions of the West. While the Jewish people trace their ancestry to Abraham and God's covenant * with him, the issuance of the Commandments to Moses around 1400 B.C. is the beginning of Judaism—particularly the Commandment, "Thou shalt have no other gods before [or but] me." Arthur Hertzberg [103] says that "to this day" the convert to Judaism is adopted as "a child of Abraham" (one of the family of his descendants) as well as a member of the Judaic faith. The Israelite monarchy was founded by Saul in the eleventh century B.C., and was divided under David and his son Solomon (who built the great temple) into the kingdom of Israel in the north and Judah in the south.

Judaism has been called "a kingdom of priests," the greatest being Moses. The prophets of the eighth and seventh centuries B.C. influenced the character of Judaism, and much of its literature is the various interpretations of their prophecies.

The kingdom of Israel was destroyed by the Assyrians in 722 B.C. and Solomon's Temple was razed during this war. Many of its people (afterward referred to as "the ten lost tribes") disappeared; others were carried captive into Babylonia. When Babylonia was conquered by the Persians, the Jews were free to reestablish a Jewish state. The Temple was rebuilt around 515 B.C., only to be destroyed again in A.D. 70 when the Romans, under Titus, took Jerusalem. Jews were allowed after that to enter the city only to mourn on the anniversary of the Temple's destruction. The "wailing wall" in Jerusalem remains today a symbol of the irreparable losses the Jewish people have suffered.

After the Roman Conquest the Jews were dispersed (dispersed Jews are still called the Diaspora) and, according to the country in

---

* *The I Ching or Book of Changes: op. cit.,* p. xvi.

* See Genesis 15.

which they lived, Judaism took on slightly different characteristics, although it has remained a remarkably unified faith. Dispersed among nations though they were and are (as are the peoples of other religions), their priests, leaders, teachers, or rabbis have interpreted the Laws of Judaism with more uniformity than is found in most religions.[104]

The Jews attempt to determine God's will as expressed in the Torah,* which is called "the heart of the Jewish religion." Torah (which comes from *Yarah* having to do with shooting an arrow) means law and teaching. It includes the five books of Moses—Genesis, Exodus, Leviticus, Numbers, and Deuteronomy. Interpretations of the Mosaic books resulted in a large body of oral law known as *Mishna* (from *Shanah* meaning repeat), and commentary on the Mishna which is called *Gemara*. When both of the latter were written (about the sixth century A.D.), the result was, and is, known as the *Talmud*. This publication, in a sense, held the Jewish people together after they were scattered throughout the Near East and Europe. In the persecution of the Jews, the Talmud was burned repeatedly since it seemed to be what preserved them as a people. Jews fared best during the Middle Ages in Spain when this country was under Moslem rule. As pointed out in Chapter 1, Jewish physicians of Spain practiced the most enlightened medicine of medieval times.[105-107]

Jews are noted for their scholarship and their great admiration for learning. Their priests are the rabbis who are their teachers, or interpreters of the law. As long as Jews were persecuted and confined to a narrow life within a ghetto, the interpretation of Judaic law tended to be restricted. With elimination of the ghettos and especially with the migration of almost half of Jewry to America during the eighteenth, nineteenth, and twentieth centuries, the interpretation of the law was liberalized and diversified. The literature on Judaism is so extensive that Morton M. Applebaum's [105] small book *What Everyone Should Know About Judaism* is especially useful.

In a series of essays edited by Judah Goldin under the title *The Jewish Expression* (Yale University Press, New Haven, Conn., 1976), the student of Judaism can get some idea of the wide range of beliefs held by individuals

who call themselves "Jews" and by members of Jewish congregations.*

The heart of Judaism is belief in one God, Jehovah, a personal God, though not in the sense of being a person with a body. God deals with man through justice, anger, and love, and God created the world for a purpose. While Jews may or may not believe in life after death, as they practice their religion, their emphasis is on ethical use of life on earth. They look upon the Torah as an ethical guide. Man is thought to have a divine spark; he is faced every moment with a choice of good or evil and is free to choose one or the other. Because of his human weakness, he cannot escape sin, but, to the extent that he loves God and hence man, he will choose the good or right way.†

It is believed by Conservative and Reform Jews that ethical and spiritual values of Judaism remain unchanged, but that practices expressing these values should change according to the needs or customs of the persons they serve. Reform Jews look upon the Torah as a source of ethical ideals but they do not necessarily accept it as divine revelation. Orthodox congregations do not rule out adaptation of the law to modern needs but they rule out changes that are believed to be for convenience only.

While Jews worship as "congregations" in "temples" or synagogues, the home is also a place of worship, and for devout Jews it is dominated by religious practices. For instance, there may be a small box at the door called a *mezuzah* (meaning doorpost) holding 15 verses from scriptures.‡ Meals are governed by die-

---

* The Torah is a sacred scroll of the law which is kept in the ark (cabinet) in the temple. On it are handwritten the first five books of the Bible. These sacred scrolls are on parchment and may not be destroyed. If worn, they are repaired or kept reverently in an appropriate place. The word Torah is also used for all scriptures—not just the books of Moses—on which the Judaic law is based. A religious school may be called a Talmud Torah. (*Life*, Editorial Staff: *op. cit.*, p. 147, Vol. 2.)

* It is not easy to define Jewry. Is it a race, a religion, or a nation? Mordecai M. Kaplan is quoted as defining Judaism as "a civilization and the Jews as a people linked by a common history, a common language or prayer, a common and vast literature and a sense of common destiny." "The Law of Judaism," in *Life*, Editorial Staff: *op. cit.*, p. 147, Vol. 2.)

Judah Goldin says in the Introduction to *The Jewish Expression* (Yale University Press, New Haven, Conn., 1976) ". . . it is impossible to say that the Jewish people were perpetually dominated by this or that single idea from the beginnings to now. The complexity of Jewish reaction is itself one of the most noteworthy lessons to be learned from a reading of Jewish literature or from a study of the different chapters of Jewish history; the essays in the present volume are themselves reports—analyses and descriptions—of that complexity."

† According to Applebaum, Jews welcome but do not seek converts. He maintains that ". . . based on rabbinical teachings, Judaism claims no monopoly on salvation . . . [but] reasons that whatever the rewards of the future world may be, all God-revering people will share therein." (Applebaum, Morton M.: *What Everyone Should Know About Judaism.* Philosophical Library, New York, 1959, p. 7.)

‡ These verses are Deuteronomy 6:4–9 and 11:13–21. (*Ibid.*, p. 22.)

tary laws derived from prohibitions against foods thought unclean, such as pork and shell-fish. Meat must be from animals slaughtered quickly to reduce the blood left in it; dishes and utensils used for meat are kept separate from those used for milk. The Sabbath (from dusk on Friday to sundown on Saturday) is strictly observed. Candles are lit and wine is sipped as the family gathers for the evening meal on Friday. The annual "holy days" are said to have held the Jewish people together regardless of the differences in their beliefs. The following are the most important: *Rosh Hashanah* is the Jewish New Year, the Day of Memorial, the Day of Blowing the Alarm (in September or October), and *Yom Kippur* (the Day of Atonement). The two comprise a 10-day period of repentance including a 24-hour fast. *Passover* or *pesoch* is a festival celebrating the liberation from Egyptian bondage or the anniversary of Israel's natal day (March or April). The ceremonial meal is called the *Seder* feast. Prescribed dishes are served that have special meaning and the *Kiddush* cup is passed and a glass of wine is set for the prophet Elijah who some Jews believe will arrive on a Passover to announce the coming of

the Messiah. There is a ritual reading of scripture known as the Haggadah in the form of questions and answers to teach the children the meaning of Passover.

Other festivals are *Simchath Torah,* or Rejoicing in the Law (September or October), which ends the yearly cycle of Torah readings; *Purim,* a holiday on which masquerades are used to teach children the Jewish aspect of history as related in the book of Esther; *Shabuot,* or Feast of the First Fruits (May or June), which recognizes the handing down of the Ten Commandments (children in Reform families are confirmed then); *Succoth,* an 8-day autumn thanksgiving; and *Hanukkah* (Chanukah), or the Feast of Lights (November or December), an 8-day celebration of the victory of the Maccabees over the Syrians and the rededication of the temple by Judas Maccabee in 165 B.C. There is a ceremonial lighting of the Hanukkah menorah or seven-branch candelabra, and the last day there are presents for the children.

Weddings are performed with great ceremony and, although divorce is permitted, marriage is sacred. Circumcision of male children is performed on the eighth day after birth. It

Table 18-2. Jewish Holidays, Festivals and Fasts Showing Hebrew Date and Date on the Gregorian Calendar. *

Festivals and Fasts	Hebrew Date		1976–1977 (5737)	1977–1978 (5738)	1978–1979 (5739)
Rosh Hashana (New Year) †	Tishri	1	Sept. 25 Sa	Sept. 13 Tu	Oct. 2 Mo
Fast of Gedalia	Tishri	3	Sept. 27 Mo	Sept. 15 Th	Oct. 4 We
Fast of Gedalia	Tishri	4	... .	... .	... .
Yom Kippur (Day of Atonement)	Tishri	10	Oct. 4 Mo	Sept. 22 Th	Oct. 11 We
Sukkoth (Feast of Tabernacles). 1st Day †	Tishri	15	Oct. 9 Sa	Sept. 27 Tu	Oct. 16 Mo
Sukkoth. 8th Day (Shemim Atzereth)	Tishri	22	Oct. 16 Sa	Oct. 4 Tu	Oct. 23 Mo
Simchat Torah (Rejoicing of the Law)	Tishri	23	Oct. 17 Su	Oct. 5 We	Oct. 24 Tu
Chanukah (Feast of Lights)	Kislev	25	Dec. 17 Fr	Dec. 5 Mo	Dec. 25 Mo
Fast of Tebet ‡	Tebet	10	Dec. 31 Fr	Dec. 20 Tu	Jan. 9 Tu
Fast of Esther‡	Adar	13	Mar. 3 Th	... .	Mar. 12 Mo
Fast of Esther ‡	Adar II	13	... .	Mar. 22 We	... .
Purim (Feast of Lots)	Adar	14	Mar. 4 Fr	... .	Mar. 13 Tu
Purim	Adar II	14	... .	Mar. 23 Tu	... .
Pesach (Passover) 1st Day †	Nisan	15	Apr. 3 Su	Apr. 22 Sa	Apr. 12 Th
Pesach. 7th day †	Nisan	21	Apr. 9 Sa	Apr. 28 Fr	Apr. 18 We
Lag B'Omer	Iyar	18	May 6 Fr	May 25 Th	May 15 Tu
Shavuoth (Feast of Weeks) †	Sivan	6	May 23 Mo	Jun. 11 Su	Jun. 1 Fr
Fast of Tammuz ‡	Tammuz 17		Jul. 3 Su	Jul. 23 Su	Jul. 12 Th
Tisha B'Av (Fast of Av) ‡	Av	9	Jul. 24 Su	Aug. 13 Su	Aug. 2 Th

All Jewish holidays, etc., begin at sunset on the day previous.

The months of the Jewish year are: 1 Tishri; 2 Chesvan (also Marchesvan); 3 Kislev; 4 Tebet (also Tebeth); 5 Sebat (also Shebhat); 6 Adar; 6a. added month some years. Adar Sheni (II); 7 Nisban, 8 Iyar; 9 Sivan; 10 Tammuz. 11 Av (also Abh); 12 Elul.

Source: Synagogue Council of America.
* Adapted from *The World Almanac Book of Facts 1977.* Newspaper Enterprise Association, Inc., New York, 1977, p. 357.
† Also observed the following day.
‡ Hebrew date varies to avoid conflict with Sabbath.

commemorates God's covenant with Abraham. At 13, a boy becomes a son of the commandment (*bar mitzvah*) and assumes adult religious duties. At this time, following a religious service, there is a feast and a gathering of relatives and friends. *Mitzvah* means commandment, and devout Jews live by a series of *mitzvot;* every aspect of life is governed by them. The creed of Moses ben Maimon, usually called Moses Maimonides (a medieval Jewish scholar), is said to be the best-known expression of Orthodox Jewish concepts. He reduced the Mishnah to 13 cardinal principles.

The varieties of "Jewish expression" have been emphasized, so it may be unnecessary to remind the reader that the observances of the rituals, festivals, and customs as just described differ among Jewish families. Only by reading many authorities or talking with many Jews can those outside the faith have any idea of the range of "expression" of Judaism. Regardless of the differences, Jacob Neuser concludes his 1972 study of American Judaism with a comment on "the astonishing continuity of Judaism." [108-114]

Jewish scholars, or rabbis, put different emphases on a knowledge of history, on knowledge of the laws and their observance, and on mysticism. Mysticism and emotionalism as expressed in the Hasidic doctrine of joyous communion with God has been interpreted by Martin Buber in a number of his books. [115,116] *Hasidim* (pious ones) dates from the middle of the eighteenth century in Poland. Hasidic Jews are recognizable by their black archaic garb, their hats, their beards, and their side curls.

In spite of the freedom of Jews in many countries in this and the last century, some have thought that security lies in the creation of a Jewish state. Noss [117] says this viewpoint was expressed by Theodor Herzl in *The Jewish State* published in 1896. A movement known as Zionism supported and promoted this view; some Reform Jews opposed it.* The Balfour Declaration of 1918 established Palestine as a national home for Jewish people. In 1947, the United Nations Assembly voted the partition of Palestine, making the Zionist State of Israel a fact.

It might bear repeating for emphasis that Jewish viewpoints range widely, including

those of the Orthodox, the Zionists, the Hasidists, the Conservative, the Reform, and the Reconstructionists. Most religious scholars speak of the Judaic-Christian faith since the Old Testament is part of the bible of each faith. All Jews and Christians have much in common from a religious standpoint. Archeological and historical studies of today and ecumenical efforts by representatives of both faiths are fostering mutual understanding and acceptance.

The Messianic question has been studied by Jewish and Christian scholars—the question as to whether there has been or will be a Messiah. A few sources are listed among the references, but the different Hebraic points of view are too numerous to be discussed, including the assumption that Jesus was the Messiah.*[118-120]

R. J. Zwi Werblowsky [121] said in 1959 that Jewry has polarized into two centers—Israel and America, which represent the Judaism of the homeland and the Judaism of the Diaspora (Jews living outside Israel). They live side by side in time and will probably lead to a "reformulation" of Judaism.

Shinto. The name of the native Japanese religion, Shinto, is derived from the Chinese Shen-tao, "The way of the higher spirits or gods." Its Japanese equivalent is *Kami-no-michi* or the *Kamis'* way. Kami can refer to gods or, more inclusively, to beings of higher potency who are not necessarily divine.

To understand any religion, it is necessary to know something about the history of the country in which it originated and of the country or countries in which it developed. This is particularly true of Shinto.[122] It is inextricably intertwined with the history of the Japanese people, who are partly Korean, partly Mongolian, and partly Malaysian. The Japanese islands were inhabited largely by primitive peoples in the first century B.C., with only small centers of "culture" at Izumo and Yamato on the island of Kyushu. These primitive clans or tribes inhabiting the islands worshipped gods of the sea, the storm, or the heavens. According to Noss, the Yamato clans, possibly in the fourth century

---

* Alfred M. Lilienthal, author of *What Price Israel?* (Henry Regnery Co., Chicago, 1953), in his Foreword said: "The resulting confusion [from the creation of the State of Israel in 1948] has seriously affected the position of the free world in the Middle East, has dangerously complicated the lives of Jews everywhere, and now endangers Judaism, the oldest monotheistic faith in the world."

* Arthur Katz, writing with Jaime Buckingham, in *Ben Israel. Odyssey of a Modern Jew* (Logos International, Plainfield, N.J., 1970), tells the story of his acceptance of Jesus as the Messiah foretold by the Hebrew prophets of the Old Testament. A group of Jews who believe as he does published a New Testament that includes related prophesies throughout. It begins with the following prayer in English and in Hebrew: "O God of Abraham, Isaac, and Jacob, show me the Truth as I read this Book; and help me to follow the Light that is given me by Thee. Amen." (*New Testament; Old Testament Prophecy Edition*). [no publisher, no date.]

A.D., declared their chieftain an emperor descended from the Sun. Some other groups were ruled by matriarchs credited with special powers.[123]

Because Japan was for so long a collection of feudal states, often at war with each other, successful warriors were revered and patriotism was the highest virtue. Religion was mixed with magic, as in primitive societies. The ancient Shinto religion is spoken of as formless until the fifth century A.D. when Japanese nationalism was challenged by Buddhist and Confucian ideas from Korea and China. These ideas were effecting what is referred to as the "first transformation" in the national life and outlook of the Japanese. Noss makes the following comment:

Almost at a bound the people passed from a primitive to a relatively advanced type of national culture. . . . Confucian ideas brought about permanent changes of emphasis in morals. There followed in particular a powerful re-enforcement of the ideal of filial piety. Old Shinto had been mainly a haphazard cult of nature-worship, loosely tied in with ancestor-worship. It now took on the aspect of history's most comprehensive ancestor-cult. Not only did the emperor's descent from the sun-goddess receive stress, but the higher officials began to trace their own descent from the deities most closely related to the sun-goddess, and the common people were supposed to be descendants of the more distantly related deities. In this way the mythological basis was laid for the claim (so greatly emphasized during the last decades of the nineteenth century and the beginning of this) that the people were organically related to the emperor by a divine family relationship.

But an even greater impact was made upon the Japanese by Buddhism, coming first by way of Korea and then from China. When this religion came to Japan in the sixth century, it brought with it an exciting literature, a new, rich art, an emotionally satisfying ritual, and fresh insights in every field of human thought and action, including logic, medicine, and social service. Buddhism broke down Japanese provincialism by bringing the overseas world into the religious picture, for in the eyes of the Buddhist priests, the seat of religious reality and authority lay not in Japan, but in India and China.*

There were efforts in the seventh century A.D. and later to preserve the Shinto myths and traditions by putting them in writing. The *Kujiki* or Chronicle of Old Events appeared in A.D. 620, the *Kojiki,* Chronicle of Ancient Events in A.D. 712, the *Nihongi,* Chronicles of Japan, in A.D. 720, the *Kogoshui,* Gleanings from Ancient Stories, and in the tenth-century the *Engi-shiki,* a compendium of Shinto tradi-

tions in 50 parts—the first ten including Shinto prayers and rituals called *norito*.[124]

According to the Shinto myth,* the Japanese islands are a special divine creation. The myth explains how the primal male *Izanagi* and the primal female *Izanami* made the islands and how they created the Japanese deities, the most revered being *Amaterasu,* goddess of the sun.

Japan, according to the myth, was peopled by divine beings; it was called "the Land of the Gods." The emperor was believed to be descended from Amaterasu, whose temple at Isé remains today the most revered of Japan's thousands of shrines.†

While the emperor was descended from the sun-goddess, all the Japanese were descended from greater or lesser deities called, collectively, *Karmi.*

By the eighth century A.D., Buddhism was a dominant influence in Japan but, as happens in transplanting religions from one country to another, it and Confucianism were interwoven with Shinto, or reconciled with certain Shinto beliefs. (The genius of the Japanese for taking from other cultures and making what they take their own is generally recognized.) The Shinto *Kami* came to be the protectors of Buddha's Law, and some were given the title *bosatsu* (bodhisattra). By the ninth century A.D., the Kami of Shinto were equated with Buddhas. Amaterasu was said to be the manifestation of the Buddha Maha-Vairocana; Hachiman, the war-god, was the Bodhissattva Kshitigarbha in Japanese guise, and so forth. Such beliefs led to *Ryobu* or Mixed Shinto (the Twofold Way of the Gods). Some authorities speak of Japan as a Buddhist nation during this period.[125,126]

From the fourteenth to the end of the sixteenth century, any national unity stemming from the power of the emperor was threatened by powerful feudal nobles and dictators (*shoguns*) who tried to control the nobles and the military (*samurai*). This period ended when three strong dictators successively took national leadership, encouraged native customs and beliefs, and tried to reduce or eliminate non-Japanese influences. Japan was said to have been closed to outsiders from the end of the sixteenth until the middle of the nineteenth century; to have become a "hermit nation" with ports closed to all but a few Chinese and Dutch traders. During this period,

---

* Noss, John B.: *op. cit.,* p. 318.

---

* As used here, myth means a tale that explains, validates, or justifies the origin of a belief or custom.

† According to Noss, the state shrines under the Home Ministry numbered about 110,000 within the last century. (Noss, John B.: *op. cit.,* p. 328.)

Japanese scholars tried to disentangle Shinto beliefs from Buddhism and Confucianism. Christians, who had brought their religion to Japan, were persecuted and encouraged to leave the country.

The "second transformation" of Japan is said to have occurred under the Emperor Meiji who established Shinto as the state religion, abolishing Buddhist elements from Shinto shrines.* Until 1945, Shinto shrines were put under the control of the state. Because it proved impractical to eliminate Buddhism, it was granted autonomy by the government in 1877, and in 1889 religious liberty was guaranteed to all citizens. The government retained a Department of Shrines, later divided into a bureau for the control of Shinto shrines under the Department of Home Affairs and a bureau of religions under the Department of Education.[127-130]

The treaty between Japan and the United States effected by President Millard Fillmore with the help of Admiral Matthew C. Perry in 1854 opened Japan to Western influence. The emperor was restored to sovereignty over the nation in 1868 and a strong central government encouraged a study of the past, respect for "imperial ancestors," and a reverence for religious shrines. Citizens were encouraged to make at least one pilgrimage within a lifetime to the Grand Imperial Shrine of Isé which is sacred to the goddess Amaterasu. Shinto shrines are usually unpainted structures with an entrance guarded by two uprights held together by a horizontal bar (the *torii*). The inner sanctuary houses a treasured object which is reverently protected or surrounded by two fences or barriers, with no one but the priests having access to the sanctuary.† During festivals, sacred objects (*shintai*) may be borne, sometimes in treasure chests, through the streets in a religious procession. The *torii* of a Shinto shrine is said to have the same meaning to a devout person that a temple has to the Chinese or the minaret has to the Muslim.

The emperor was directly concerned with state ceremonies at the Grand Imperial Shrine of Isé. The *O'Harai* or Grand Purification, the most important Shinto ceremony, occurred twice a year (June and December). Purification wands were waved over the people who brought offerings to the Shrine.[131]

The Shinto religion has been closely associated with the military. During the feudal period, the *Bushido* code (the warrior–knight way) evolved. It has been compared with the European code of chivalry closely associated with Christianity and the Crusades.

The *Bushido* code is an unwritten law expressing ideal behavior through eight attitudes: loyalty (to the emperor and the nobles under which the individual serves), gratitude, courage, justice, truthfulness, politeness, reserve, and honor—death being preferable to disgrace.

The last attitude is the one for which the Japanese warrior or soldier of today is best known, for he prefers death to capture and suicide to disgrace. Wives of defeated warriors may commit hari-kari (disembowelment) with their husbands. For this and other reasons that have been mentioned, the Shinto religion and the nationalism of Japan are closely related.

The attitude of the Japanese toward death has affected the people in various ways. From earliest times, the Japanese have emphasized cleanliness. Their fear of pollution from the dead resulted in immediate burials. After a 10-day period of mourning, the whole family went into the water to bathe and the structure in which death occurred might be abandoned. Noss says:

This practice imposed a peculiar difficulty upon the early emperors. Each new emperor perforce abandoned the old capital and built a new palace in another part of the country, and this meant that with each accession to the throne the government was temporarily disorganized. . . .*

Industrialization and other aspects of modernization have greatly changed most aspects of Japanese life. It is said that disbelief in the native religion, and in fact all religions, is widespread. Joseph M. Kitagawa [132] speaks of the present "rootlessness" of the Japanese people. However, recent visitors comment on the inability of even the most "westernized" Japanese to think of living permanently away from their country.[133] In 1945, the Shinto shrines (110,000 of them) once under the control of the Home Ministry were cut off from state funds and supervision. According to Noss, some are kept in repair by local shrine associations and 86,000 are now maintained by a private nationwide shrine association.

The present government of Japan has withdrawn from control of religions. It is said that hundreds of sects have formed and by 1969

---

* According to Daniel C. Holtom, state Shinto was disestablished December 15, 1945, and Shinto has since been a privately supported sect. (Holtom, Daniel Clarence: *Modern Japan and Shinto Nationalism; A Study of Present-day Trends in Japanese Religions,* rev. ed. University of Chicago Press, Chicago, 1947.)

† If the *shintai* is a natural object such as a rock or a tree, it may be left visible to the shrine pilgrim.

* Noss, John B.: *op. cit.,* p. 317.

about 60 had registered with the government as sectarian Shinto denominations. Some include faith healing, and one, the *Tenri Kyo,* is said to be the Christian Science of Japan.[134,135]

The festivals of Japan, in which all participate, are said to support Shrine Shinto. Five festivals are grouped as the *go-sekku:* the New Year; the First Moons Festival with national holidays; the Peach Festival, also called the Girls Festival in March; the Boys Festival, which coincides with the Iris Festival in May; the Festival of the Star Vega in summer; and the Chrysanthemum or Indian Summer Festival. There is also the Cherry Blossom Festival in spring. The emperor's birthday is celebrated, as are dates in the imperial history throughout the year and the harvest festival in the fall.

In Shinto homes there is a *kami-dana* or god-shelf. Memorial tablets with names of ancestors or the name of a patron deity may be on it. Talismans of pilgrimages or any object associated with family history or a significant event may be added to the shelf. As in most countries, customs persist long after their origins are known or underlying beliefs held. Some recently formed semireligious groups are not Shintoist but hold a synthesis of beliefs and principles drawn from many religions and social sciences.[136,137]

Zoroastrianism. The religion of Zoroaster is thought to have the same origin as Hinduism. The Indo-European people who settled in India many centuries before Christ and those who settled in ancient Persia (now Iran) are of the same stock. Noss [138] suggests that the nature of the land affected the temperament of these peoples, making the Persians "more aggressive and realistic" and the Indians more romantic and philosophical.

Zoroaster (which is a Greek version of Zarathustra) was born to a well-to-do family around 660 B.C. or earlier and lived in what is now Persian Khorasan or possibly the Turkman Republic of the Union of Soviet Socialist Republics. According to Noss,[139] he is referred to in Greek sources. Ruhi Muhsen Afnan [139a] has made a study of Zoroaster's influence on Greek thought. Cyrus the Great, Darius, and Xerxes are said to have been Zoroastrians and Plato wanted to go to Persia to study Zoroaster's teaching but was prevented by the Persian–Spartan War in 396 B.C. According to W. B. Henning,[140] Zoroaster held the hereditary office of witch doctor or medicine man for his tribe. Henning pays tribute to him as an original thinker.

About this time, writers such as Euripides were questioning the gods of the ancient Greek Pantheon. In a number of countries, people were ready for a monotheistic religion and this was the characteristic of Zoroastrianism that most differentiated it from Hinduism.

Zoroaster had a vision in which the archangel *Voho Manah* (meaning Good Thought) told his spirit to ascend to the presence of *Ahura Mazda* (the wise Lord or Supreme Being). In this celestial realm, he was taught what he, as a prophet, was to teach to mortals.* This experience was followed by subsequent revelations with the six principal archangels.†

Noss and Afnan compare Zoroaster to Moses, for both were great originals who taught unique ethical monotheism "based solidly on inherited beliefs"; both wanted to stamp out the worship of daevas, deities, or evil spirits who were represented by all manner of "idols." [141,142] Zoroastrians of today consider Jesus, as well as Zoroaster, a prophet.

Robert C. Zaehner says:

Zoroaster himself is a prophet and no more than a prophet. Like Muhammad he is simply the vehicle through which the divine Word is transmitted to man. The "Good Religion," however, of which he was the vehicle, is not quite identical with the Avesta: it is not so much a book, it is rather a principle. It can be summed up in the following words—order, righteousness or justice, and the Mean. [the Aristotelian mean].‡

Zoroaster's concepts, greatly abbreviated, were embodied in the following eight statements: (1) the one true religion is that revealed by *Ahura Mazda* and he is its prophet; (2) *Ahura Mazda* is the one supreme deity who causes everything to exist and who will finally destroy evil and establish right; (3) *Ahura Mazda* works his will through *Spenta Mainyu* (Holy Spirit) and "Immortal Holy Ones" or forms of ethical behavior as *Vohu Manah* (Good Thought or Good Sense), *Asha* (Right), *Kshathra* (Power or Dominion), *Hauvatat* (Prosperity), *Armaiti* (Piety), and *Ameretat* (Immortality); (4) while *Ahura Mazda* is supreme, he is opposed by evil forces; there is the lie as well as the truth, death as well as life, there is the false as well as the true religion and man has freedom of choice; (5) good and bad are at war within each man's soul; (6) since good and evil are

---

* Noss says that Zoroaster did not invent the concept of a wise lord who was a supreme being. *Ahura Mazda* was, there is little doubt, no other than the god of the moral and natural order whom the Aryans of India worshipped under the name of *Varuna.* (*Ibid.,* p. 347.)

† The idea of angels is often attributed to Zoroastrianism but adopted by Christianity.

‡ Zaehner, Robert C.: *The Teachings of the Magi; A Compendium of Zoroastrian Beliefs.* G. Allen and Unwin, London; Macmillan Publishing Co., Inc., New York, 1956, p. 83.

not clearly defined, each man must decide for himself, using the *Gathas* (devotional hymns of Zoroaster) to guide him; (7) animal sacrifice, magic, idolatry, and drinking intoxicating haoma juice to enhance religious ecstasy must be eliminated—the sacred fire must not be worshipped but used as a symbol of *Ahura Mazda;* and (8) good will outlast evil and, in a final judgment, good men will be separated from the bad, the former dwelling in "The House of Song" where the sun shines forever and the latter in "The House of the Lie," which is dark and foul smelling.[143]

Zoroastrianism seems to have spread rapidly and to have been adopted by the prince and the nobles as well as the common man of Persia. A Zoroastrian group in Media were known as "the Magi," but there is some mystery about them. In the spread of this religion, Zoroaster's teachings were modified by its priests and the princes who supported the faith. The official creed came to be known as *Avesta. Ahura Mazda* was still the supreme deity but, according to Noss: "The old Aryan nature gods whom Zoroaster condemned and fought, crept back into the faith and provided powerful figures around *Ahura Mazda* to share his powers. . . . But these Holy Immortal Ones . . . seemed much less important than the *Yazatas,* or angels, of whom forty are named." *

Mithra, one of these Holy Immortal Ones, assumed great importance in later Zoroastrianism. The sacred intoxicant, haoma, was brought back and animal sacrifices, both of which Zoroaster had denounced. Another development was the *Fravashis,* who were first spirits or angels guarding each person, and the ideal person, or the soul, within each man. Noss makes the following observation about developments with Zoroastrianism:

In all this we see monotheism relapsing into polytheism, a not uncommon fact in the history of religions. In all faiths there is a joyful acceptance of prophetic utterances and ideals in difficult and degenerate days, but reform is generally succeeded by relapse, a falling away from "thoughts that are high and deeds that are noble" to a more comfortable accommodation of doctrine and practice to the easy going ways of the masses of men "who like not thinking better than to follow habit." †

Other changes were the struggle against the demonic powers of impurity with the use of powerful *mantras*—passages from the *Gathas* of Zoroaster—repeated without flaw and used as incantations. Libations of haoma juice were used. Zoroastrians of this age use libations made from twigs of a sacred plant which are drunk in part by officiating priests.

Dead bodies were thought polluting and even Zoroastrians of today attempt to prevent contamination of the earth and streams by the dead. Any portion of a body is defiling, including nail parings and even exhaled air. Horror of contaminating the earth or the streams with dead bodies led to the exposure of the dead in the *dakhmas,* or "Towers of Silence." A circular stone floor in three sections or levels with a pit in the center is surrounded by a wall. The highest section is for men, the middle for women, and the lowest for children. Dead bodies are borne to the Tower by six bearers followed by white-clad mourners. The body is laid in a shallow pit and partially exposed by slitting the clothing. As the mourners depart, vultures swoop down from the wall and soon the skeleton is laid bare. Within days after the bones are dry, mourners return to place them in the pit where they are allowed to crumble and disappear, anonymously. In small communities where there are no *dakhmas,* the dead may be buried in stone or lead coffins. People of this faith came to believe in an elaborate doctrine of life after death. The fate of good and bad souls is described in a *Pahlevi* text, the *Bundahishn.*

Zoroastrians were driven out of Persia during the Muslim Conquest, many going to India where they were called *Parsis* (Persians). Those who continued to live in Persia were called Gabars (which means infidels) by Muslims. While present-day Zoroastrians are divided into two sects using different yearly calendars, both worship according to the *Avesta,* which is a faith quite different from that of the founder Zarathustra.

A Zoroastrian Mountain Fire-Temple may look like an ordinary building, or it may be a room in a dwelling. According to Noss, these temples in India are devoted to the fire-keeping ceremonies. The temples are of varying degrees of holiness—some fires purified by longer and more complicated rituals, compounded of many fires and originating from various sources—from a bolt of lightning or from flints, for instance.

The sacred fire is in the center of the temple or room and is fed with sandalwood by attendants who wear masks over their mouths to keep from polluting the holy fire. Worshipers come singly at any time they wish. Inside the Temple, they wash the uncovered parts of the body, say a prayer, and go barefooted to the threshold of the inner room containing the fire. They give money or sandalwood to the priest who, in return, gives them

* Noss, John B.: *op. cit.,* p. 357.
† *Ibid.,* p. 355.

ashes from the sacred fire which worshipers rub on the forehead or eyelids.

On the Parsi New Year, worshippers put on new clothes to worship at the temple and, after giving alms to the poor, spend the remainder of the day visiting friends and feasting. One Parsi festival honors *Mithra*, another *Farvadin*, the deity who presides over spirit ancestors. During the 10-day festival, the celebrants visit ancestral homes and attend special ceremonies at *dakhmas*. Another festival honors *Voho Manah*, the guardian of cattle, and for a week worshippers are especially kind to animals. There are other Zoroastrian festivals or feasts commemorating six phases of creation—heaven, water, earth, trees, animals, and man. According to Noss, there were in the last decade more than 100,000 Parsis in India, most around Bombay and Calcutta.[144-147]

Christianity. Of all religions, Christianity is the most widespread and its followers are the most numerous. It is based on the teachings of Jesus as expressed in the New Testament. Jesus questioned some of the beliefs of Judaism as recorded in the Old Testament; nevertheless, the "Old" and the "New" testaments constitute the Bible which is, in different versions, the foundation of all Christian faiths.

The prophets of the Old Testament foretold the coming of a Messiah, an idea that is found also in Hinduism and Zoroastrianism.[148-150] Some parties or divisions within Judaism did not believe in the Messianic doctrine, and even those that did had varying concepts. One concept, however, involved the salvation of the righteous, the destruction of the wicked, a reign of justice, the resurrection of the dead, and "the last judgment." For his disciples or followers, Jesus became the Messiah, or Christ,* as he is for some Jews even today.[151] In the Gospel of Mark (13:30–33), Jesus refers to "the reign of God," in Matthew (8:11–13) to "the Kingdom of Heaven." Some interpret these and other sayings of Jesus as an acceptance of the Messianic doctrine, certainly as an indication that he believed he was sent to establish God's Kingdom.[152]

Noss maintains that there have been more books written about the first Christian centuries than any other comparable period of history and that it is difficult to tell the story of the Christian religion "briefly and clearly." He says:

Historical criticism has been particularly busy with them [the Gospels and Epistles of the New Testament] during the last seventy-five years and has reached the verdict that in the New Testament the early Christian religion *about* Jesus has overlaid and modified the record of the religion *of* Jesus himself, but there is no unanimity about the degree of modification. It is known that Jesus himself did not write down his teachings but relied upon his disciples to go about preaching what he taught, from memory. It is generally assumed by historians that after his death some of them did write down his sayings, with occasional notes of the historical setting, before they should be forgotten, and that thus a document, or group of documents, came into being that scholars call "Q" (from the German word Quelle or "source")*

Any history of Christianity distinguishes between the record of Jesus's life and teaching and the history of the Christian Church. As with all religions, it is impossible to understand them in depth without knowing a good deal about the setting in which they developed. The following facts are those most often given by historians:

Jesus was born in Nazareth into a Jewish community of Galilee, which was part of Palestine.† Jews, Greeks, Phoenicians, and others who lived there were all under the domination of the Roman Empire. The Jews themselves were divided into sects or groups; for example, the Pharisees, the Sadducees, the Zealots, and the Essenes. Jesus grew up in a period when there was controversy between the various nationalities living in the region and also among the Jews who professed a common faith. It is thought that Jesus belonged to a strictly religious family who, unlike the stern Pharisees, believed more in the spirit of the Jewish faith than in the laws governing it. Some groups believe that Jesus was the oldest of at least seven children. The names of the sisters are unknown; those of the brothers are James, Joses, Simon, and Jude. Jesus was a carpenter and, except for the fact that he seems to have been very religious and at home in the temple even as a child, not very much is known about his early life. Jesus was baptized when he was almost 30 years of age by John, who became known as John the Baptist. John thought that the end of the world was at hand and that the appearance of the Messiah was imminent. In Mark's

---

* Noss, John B.: *op. cit.*, p. 426.

† According to Noss (*op. cit.*, p. 431), the Christian church in the middle of the sixth century A.D. began to reckon time from the date of Jesus's birth. The monks who made the first calculations on which B.C. (Before Christ) and A.D. (Year of Our Lord) are based made an error of four to six years, for the best historical evidence shows that Jesus was born in 4 B.C. or earlier.

---

* Christ comes from the Greek *Christos*, anointed, which is a translation of the Hebraic Māshīah, anointed, or Messiah. (Stein, Jess, and Urdang, Laurence [eds.]: *Dictionary of the English Language.* Random House, New York, 1973.) It would therefore be more correct to say Jesus, the Christ than Jesus Christ.

Gospel (1:9–11), the baptism of Jesus is described and his mystic experience of hearing a voice from heaven saying "You are my Son, my Beloved! You are my Chosen!" [153–157]

After this experience, Jesus went into the wilderness for, it is believed, forty days to consider how he would carry out his mission.* After this, he ceased to work as a carpenter and spent his time carrying his message, as described in the Gospels, throughout the area known now by Christians as the Holy Land. Jesus immediately made four disciples, Simon Peter and his brother Andrew, and James and his brother John, all of whom were fishermen.† Jesus preached in the synagogue or temple, in the streets, beside the sea, or, when the multitudes on the shore got unmanageable, he taught from a boat a little offshore (Mark 4:1).

There are so many books on the teaching of Jesus that it is hard to single out the most cited. Stephen Neill's [158] *Jesus Through Many Eyes: Introduction to the Theology of the New Testament* (1976) will guide the reader to what may be considered the most significant. Volumes have been written interpreting the Gospels and it would be presumptuous to attempt anything more here than to suggest some of the more important points on which scholars seem to agree.‡ One point is that Jesus pictured a righteous and just God but also a merciful and forgiving God who never ceases to love man no matter how low he falls, and to offer redemption at any stage of his life. Jesus taught his followers to question the outward manifestations of correct behavior and examine people's motives. He questioned the morality of some of the Jewish laws, saying that they didn't go far enough. Murder, for example, was outlawed, but Jesus taught that a man should not get angry with or curse his brother (Matthew 5:33); violence was justified under the Jewish law in righteous retaliation—"An eye for an eye, a tooth for a tooth"—but Jesus taught that if a man sued for your shirt you should "let him have your coat too" (Matthew 5:38–40). In other words, a person should return good for evil.

The ethical code embodied in Jesus's teaching is found throughout the Gospels but the Sermon on the Mount (Matthew 5–7) embodies the principles underlying the Christian religion. Although Jesus taught a demanding moral code, he also brought the comforting concept of a living and forgiving God—the idea that faith could make a man whole; he put emphasis on the importance of each personality; his teaching was understandable and the prayer (The Lord's Prayer) he taught his disciples has come to have the widest usage of any.

Jesus questioned the laws of Judaism as, for instance, those on observance of the Sabbath. "The Sabbath was made for man, not man for the Sabbath" (Matthew 2:27). This antagonized the Pharisees; his advocacy of nonviolence alienated the Zealots. He taught that those who took to the sword would perish by it. Other groups found his teachings a threat to their beliefs and way of life, and his large following began to dwindle. The rumor was spread that Jesus was "possessed" of an evil spirit and leading the people astray (Mark 6:4). His family was alarmed and tried to put an end to his ministry.

Knowing what awaited him, that the opposing forces within the Jewish community would connive with the rulers to bring about his death, Jesus went to Jerusalem at the annual Jewish festival of the Passover. He is often pictured riding down the Mount of Olives on a colt or donkey, accompanied by his disciples. His followers threw palm branches in his way.* With bread and wine, Jesus's disciples celebrated the Passover with him in "an upper room" in Jerusalem, and he foretold his betrayal by one of them (Mark 14:22–24). This simple ceremonial meal is the sacrament of Communion which is celebrated in most Christian churches. During illness, when the sick cannot go to church, it may be celebrated in a hospital or a private home.

In the Garden of Gethsemane, Jesus's identity was made known to armed men, who were sent out by the high priest of the Sanhedrin, by a kiss from Judas Iscariat (one of the disciples). A "Judas kiss" remains to this day the symbol of betrayal. The Sanhedrin passed judgment on Jesus as a political criminal and handed him over to Pilate, who found no fault with him and turned him over to Herod Antipas, Governor of Galilee. Herod returned

---

* This is the reason why many Christians observe Lent, a 40-day period before Easter in which they make certain dietary or other sacrifices and attend special religious services.

† The fish has ever since been symbolic of the early Christians and it is said to have been used by them as a symbol.

‡ Edith Hamilton's *Witness to the Truth, Christ and His Interpreters*, (W. W. Norton and Co., Inc., New York, 1948) is a group of helpful essays on the Gospels. It includes an essay on Socrates, whose moral code she compares with that taught by Jesus.

* Christians celebrate the Sunday before Easter as Palm Sunday. Some groups bring home from church a piece of palm, which they may cherish throughout the year.

Jesus to Pilate who tried to get the crowd to accept him as the prisoner of the year to be released. Instead, the crowd demanded the release of Barabbas, a Zealot insurrectionist, which resulted in the crucifixion of Jesus. This has made the cross the symbol of Christianity throughout the world.[159-161]

According to Noss,[162] the events following the death of Jesus were more important to first-century Christians than those that preceded it. Jesus was buried in a tomb belonging to Joseph of Arimathaea. On the third day following his crucifixion and burial, his Galilean followers found the tomb empty. An angel appeared who told them Christ had risen. Later, Peter and other disciples saw and talked with Jesus and this convinced them that he was the promised Son of Man who would judge the nations. When Jesus's disciples living in Jerusalem met at the Harvest Festival (the Jewish festival of Pentecost), tongues of flame settled on the heads of the leaders (called the Apostles) and the Holy Spirit entered into them, enabling them to speak in foreign languages.* This is said to be the beginning of the efforts of the Apostles to preach in the name of Jesus.

The early church in Jerusalem was split into two parties. One was composed of those who believed that Christians should follow the law of Moses (including circumcision) as well as Jesus's teaching. They were called Judaizers, later Ebionites or Nazarenes. The other party, led by Peter, approved of the baptism of the uncircumcised, and its members were more liberal in their outlook. To this group belonged Paul (or Saul) of Tarsus, who never saw Jesus except as a "spiritual body" after his crucifixion.

Noss says[163] that Paul is frequently called the "second founder of Christianity." † He was a great leader but had to depend on the disciples for his knowledge of Jesus's teaching. A non-Palestinian Jew with the legal status of a free-born Roman, he had, as a Pharisee, participated in the persecution of Jesus's followers. He himself said he was "fanatically devoted" to what his forefathers had "handed down." On his way to Damascus (to further punish those who believed in Jesus) he was converted to Christianity by hearing a voice

saying, "Saul! Saul! why persecutest thou me?" (Acts 9:2). He wrote that Jesus appeared in a bright light which blinded him for 3 days during which he neither ate nor drank.

Paul's role in establishing the Christian church can hardly be overstated. He went to most of the countries on the Mediterranean Sea—Italy, Greece, Asia, Lycia, Galatia, Cilicia (Turkey), Cyprus, and Syria. Paul accepted Jesus as the Messiah but also as a divine being—as the Lord who has the nature of God. "He is the likeness of the unseen God, born before any creature, for it was through him that everything was created in heaven and earth, the seen and the unseen, angelic thrones, dominions, principalities, authorities,—all things were created through and for him" (Colossians 1:15).

All through the Mediterranean countries, the Apostles, Paul, and other early Christians carried the teaching of Jesus, in spite of opposition and persecution. According to Noss,[164] the Christian communities developed self-contained units. The services were of two kinds: (1) services modeled on those of the synagogue, which were open to inquirers as well as believers, and (2) the agapé or "love feast," an evening meal commemorating the Last Supper. This ceremony was in the form of a thanksgiving which the Greeks named Eucharist ("the giving of thanks").*

The earliest part of the New Testament is the Epistles of Paul; the earliest and briefest Gospel (of Mark) was probably written in Antioch about A.D. 65 to 70. It is believed to be the recollections of Peter as recorded by John Mark who lived in Jerusalem before coming to Antioch. The virgin birth is not in the Gospel of Mark, but is in the Gospels of Matthew and Luke. The fourth Gospel, that of John, follows most closely the belief held by Paul, reconciling the living Lord experienced by Paul in his conversion with the Jesus of the first three Gospels. In this Gospel, it is claimed that God's Word (the Logos) "became flesh and blood and lived among us" (John 1:1-14). Jesus is the Son of God. The difference in the four Gospels has given rise to endless interpretations of Christianity and to so-called "heresies." Just when the Gospels were written and by whom is a subject of endless debate. John A. T. Robinson, at one time Bishop of Woolwich, whose 1963 book *Honest to God* provoked wide comment, has devoted years of study to historical sources. He has concluded all four Gospels may have

---

* This is the origin of the Apostolic Succession, with Peter considered by many Roman Catholics to be the first Pope.

† Paul Hutchinson and Wilfred E. Garrison, writing in 1959, expressed the opinion that there were more "objections" to the obscuring of Jesus's teaching by Paul "a few years ago" than at the time they were writing (*20 Centuries of Christianity*, Harcourt Brace Jovanovich, Inc., New York, N.Y., 1959, p. 15).

* To this day, some Christians think that the Eucharist, or the taking of Communion, should be part of every church service.

been written before A.D. 70; some historians give later dates for the Gospels of Matthew, Luke, and John.[165-169]

In an effort to unify the Christian churches, Irenaeus, Bishop of Lyon, in Gaul (now France), issued a book *Against the Heresies* (especially the Gnostic and Marcionite doctrines). Based on his insistence that the apostles were the authentic source of knowledge, the Church of Rome (about A.D. 150 to 175) framed the Apostles' Creed. It is used in almost the same form in some Christian churches today.

Despite the persecution of the early Christians, their faith spread rapidly throughout the countries bordering the Mediterranean. By A.D. 287, Christianity was the state religion of Armenia. The Roman Emperor Constantine, in the edict of Milan, A.D. 313, legally sanctioned Christianity. He was baptized on his deathbed and was considered the patron of the church. Under Theodosius, made emperor in A.D. 379, Christianity became the official religion of the Empire.

The Epistles of Peter and Paul show some of the basic disagreements among the early Christians. Constantine, who saw Christianity as a unifying force in the Roman Empire, called and presided over a council of 300 bishops at Nicaea, in A.D. 325, to settle the dispute over the question of whether Jesus, the Christ, was of the *same* substance as God, the Father, or, as the Bishop Arius of Alexandria believed, of *like* substance. Out of this council came the Nicene Creed which espouses the belief of Athanasius, who came to be the chief opponent of Arius.*

The authority of the Church, as time went on, centered in Rome where the patriarch claimed to be the successor of Peter and the ranking officer of the Church. The term Catholic was first used in the sense of the universal Church. There was, however, very soon a schism between the western church of Rome and the eastern Church of Constantinople which has persisted to this day. There is still the Roman Catholic Church and the Eastern Orthodox Church.

The Popes, or heads of the Western Church, have been secular as well as religious leaders. At one time, three bishops claimed to be the true Pope, and each hurled scandalous charges at the others. The abuses of the Papacy that led to the Reformation under John Calvin

and Martin Luther are known to have ultimately divided Christian churches into Roman Catholic, Eastern Orthodox, Anglican, and Protestant.[170-175] The emphasis and interpretation of events in the history of the church vary, as is true with all history. In Zaehner's [176] *Concise Encyclopedia of Living Faiths,* the Early Church, the Eastern Orthodox, the St. Thomas and Medieval Theology, Protestantism, and the Catholic Church since the Reformation are treated separately by five different authorities.

It is one of the precepts of Christianity to bring the message of Jesus to all parts of the world. Roman Catholic missions are in every country. Christopher Dawson's the *Formation of Christendom* (Sheed and Ward, New York, 1967) describes the "uniqueness and universality" of the [Roman] Catholic Church. Protestant churches also send missionaries worldwide. In 1946, the Federal Council of Churches, the Foreign Missions Conference, and the American Committee of the World Council of Churches jointly established an organization called the Church World Service as a Division of Overseas Ministries. In 1976, it listed 20 "participating denominations and related organizations." * The editors of *Life* reported that there were 225 recognized Protestant sects in 1963.[177]

While in 1963 110 million of 185 million inhabitants of the United States are reported to be Christians, the First Amendment to the Constitution says, "Congress shall make no law respecting an establishment of religion." This legally separates church and state, but the Christian holidays (Christmas, celebrating the birth of Jesus, the Christ, and Easter, celebrating the resurrection) are generally recognized and celebrated by Christians and non-Christians alike. Table 18-3 shows the calendars of religious observances in Protestant, Greek Orthodox, and Roman Catholic bodies.†

This is an age that seems to be characterized by religious tolerance, with interfaith meetings held all over the world. Edward J. Jurgi has edited the report of a symposium entitled *The Ecumenical Era* in Church and Society.[177a] All branches of the Christian faith are participating in an ecumenical movement. In an effort to make the teaching of the church understandable to more people, the liturgy is

---

* The *Ecclesiastical History* of Eusebius is said to be the best source of information on the history of the first Christian centuries. (Wilken, Robert L.: *The Myth of Christian Beginnings; History's Impact on Belief.* Doubleday and Co., Inc., Garden City, N.Y., 1971, p. 52.)

* Church World Service. Division of Overseas Ministries: *Church World Service—Thirtieth Anniversary,* 1946-1976, New York, 1976.

† The church calendar shows saints' days throughout the year, but the only one generally celebrated is St. Patrick's Day in March. Other events, such as Pentecost and Ash Wednesday, the beginning of Lent, are observed by some Christians.

Table 18-3. Calendar of Religious Observances in Protestant, Greek Orthodox, and Roman Catholic Religious Bodies.*

	1977	1978
Christmas (Birth of Jesus)	Dec. 25	Dec. 25
Festival of the Christening of Jesus (New Year's Day)	Jan. 1	Jan. 1
Twelfth Night (Epiphany Eve)	Jan. 5	Jan. 5
Epiphany (Baptism of Jesus)	Jan. 6	Jan. 6
Week of Prayer for Christian Unity	Jan. 18 to 25	Jan. 18 to 25
Brotherhood Week	Feb. 20 to 27	Feb. 19 to 26
Ash Wednesday (Beginning of Lent)	Feb. 23	Feb. 8
St. Patrick's Day	Mar. 17	Mar. 17
The Annunciation of the Virgin Mary	Mar. 25	Mar. 25
Holy Week	Apr. 3 to 9	Mar. 19 to 25
Palm Sunday	Apr. 3	Mar. 19
Good Friday (Burial of Jesus)	Apr. 8	Mar. 24
Easter (Latin) Sunday	Apr. 10	Mar. 26
Easter (Orthodox) Sunday	Apr. 10	Apr. 30
Festival of the Christian Home (Mother's Day)	May 8	May 14
Ascension Day	May 19	May 4
Whitsunday (Pentecost)	May 29	May 14
Children's Sunday	June 12	June 11
Father's Day	June 19	June 18
The Transfiguration (also last Sunday after Epiphany)	Aug. 6	Aug. 6
Labor Day	Sept. 5	Sept. 4
World Communion Sunday	Oct. 2	Oct. 1
Thanksgiving Day (Canada)	Oct. 10	Oct. 9
All Saints' Day	Nov. 1	Nov. 1
Thanksgiving Sunday (U.S.)	Nov. 20	Nov. 19
Thanksgiving Day (U.S.)	Nov. 24	Nov. 23

* Adapted from "A Calendar for Church Use," in Jacquet, Constant H., Jr. (ed.): *Yearbook of American and Canadian Churches.* Abingdon Press, Nashville and New York, 1975, pp. 1–3.
(The Greek Orthodox Church Calendar for earlier years shows slightly different dates for some of these events. The Greek Church in 1923 adopted the Gregorian Calendar.)

couched in the vernacular of the day in some Roman Catholic and Protestant Churches, and versions of the Bible in current English are used by many instead of the standard King James version or the Roman Catholic Vulgate, St. Jerome's version.[178,179,179a] Evangelists attract millions, and among some in the younger generation, there is an effort to follow the teachings of Jesus literally.*

* Those unfamiliar with the Bible who want to select one must choose from a bewildering number. The best known are the *Roman Catholic Latin Vulgate* (and its later translations) and the *King James Ver-*

Among churchmen and churchgoers, there is what Robinson refers to as a "reluctant revolution" comparable to the religious upheavals of the past. A characteristic of this age is the willingness of representatives of all religions to discuss the nature of God, the relation between God and man, religious pluralism, the nature of faith, and other questions of fundamental importance to all religions. Changes in the Roman Catholic Church under Pope John have had a profound effect worldwide.[181-183]

Roman Catholics, Protestants, and distinguished representatives of all other living religions have been on an editorial board of *Religious Perspectives,* a group that between 1960 and 1972 published 22 volumes dealing with fundamental ethical, moral, and religious matters. A study of these volumes gives an impressive record of the progress made in ecumenical understanding. Zaehner calls it "concordant discord." [184] Ruth Nanda Ashen, editor of the series, makes the following statement:

Religious Perspectives represents a quest for the rediscovery of man. It constitutes an effort to define man's search for the essence of being in order that he may have a knowledge of goals. It is an endeavor to show that there is no possibility of achieving an understanding of man's total nature on the basis of phenomena known by the analytical method alone. It hopes to point to the false antinomy between revelation and reason, faith and knowledge, grace and nature, courage and anxiety. Mathematics, physics, philosophy, biology and religion, in spite of their almost complete independence, have begun to sense their interrelatedness and to become aware of that mode of cognition which teaches that "the light is not without but within me and I myself am the light." *

sion, the English translation prepared from various sources between 1604 and 1611. There have been so many translations under the title *The King James Version* that Frederick Fyvie Bruce has written a short history, *The King James Version; the First 350 Years 1611–1961* (Oxford University Press, 1960). The effort to make the Bible increasingly authentic and intelligible to readers goes on into this era with biblical scholars working singly or in groups. Recent archeological discoveries have made this work especially significant. The following are some of the titles found today in a theological library: *The Student's Bible, King James Version* (1907); *The Holy Bible, An Exact Reprint . . .* of the 1611 Version (1911); *The Companion Bible* (1932); *The Bible for Today* (1941); *The Readers Bible* (1951); *The Oxford Self-Pronouncing Bible* (1956); *The Interpreters' Bible* (1951 and 1957); *The Westminster Study Edition of the Holy Bible* (1965); *The Jerusalem Bible* (1966); *The Geneva Bible, a Facsimile of the 1560 edition* (1969); *The Bible in Living English* (1972).
* Ashen, Ruth Nanda [Editor of the Series], from Preface in Zaehner, Robert C.: *Matter and Spirit, Their Convergence in Eastern Religions.* In Vol. 8, of *Religious Perspectives,* Harper and Row, New York, 1963.

While this account of Christianity may seem to have emphasized the differences within it, the teachings of Jesus, as recorded in the Gospels, remain as always the unifying force. Its sacraments also help to unify Christendom.

There are seven sacraments in the Christian Church, all observed by Roman Catholics and only certain ones by other faiths: (1) Baptism (the first act of faith by the individual or, in the case of infants, their sponsors; (2) Confirmation, the assumption of spiritual responsibility by the child, youth, or adult; (3) Communion or Holy Eucharist, the taking of bread and wine commemorating the Last Supper; (4) Marriage, recognizing the union of man and woman and sanctifying human love and procreation of children; (5) Penance or Confession and the granting of forgiveness of sins; (6) Unction, or annointing the sick with oil and the saying of a prayer over them; and (7) Ordination of ministers or priests by bishops or higher prelates within the church.[185,186]

Islam. The word *Islam* means "peaceful submission to God's will." The term can refer to the faith of Muslims,* which is based on the teachings of Muhammad (or Mohammed) as recorded in the Qur'an (or Koran); Islam can also refer to the whole body of Muslims, their civilization, and the countries in which their religion is dominant.[187,188] The *Cambridge History of Islam*[189] is not predominantly a history of the religion but of its synthesizing effect in different eras and different countries.

Islam is the newest of the great living religions. Its founder, Muhammad, is said to have been born in Mecca in A.D. 570; Arthur Jeffery[190] says in the year of the elephant.† Muhammad's father was a Quraysh of the Hashimite clan. At the age of six, Muhammad was an orphan. He grew up in poverty as a ward of his grandfather and later of an uncle. His family, the Quraysh, held the office of trustee of the Ka'ba, meaning a cube. The Ka'ba is a holy shrine in Mecca that contained, in Muhammad's youth, images of local and distant gods and the Black Stone.‡

---

* Muslims do not like to be called Muhammadans since they dislike the implication that they look upon Muhammad as divine. He is the greatest of the prophets (Morgan, Kenneth W. [ed.]: *Islam. The Straight Path Interpreted by Muslims.* Ronald Press, New York, 1958. p. viii.)

† The Muslim calendar is different from the Gregorian calendar. According to the *Columbia Encyclopedia,* 3d ed. (Columbia University, New York, 1963, p. 317.), it is the only purely lunar calendar, its year varying from 354 to 355 days. For the names of the months, see Table 18-4.

‡ The Black Stone is said to be an outcropping of limestone measuring 58 by 44 feet. It is a meteorite referred to by Diodorus Siculus (a Roman historian) about 60 B.C. Arabians worshipped it as falling from heaven in the days of Adam. The Ka'ba was built

Table 18-4. Lunar Calendar Used by Islam Showing Relationship of Dates to the Gregorian Calendar Used Throughout Countries That Are Predominantly Christian.*

The Islamic calendar, often referred to as Mohammedan, is a lunar reckoning from the year of the hegira, A.D. 622 when Mohammed moved to Medina from Mecca. It runs in cycles of 30 years, of which the second, 5th, 7th, 10th, 13th, 16th, 18th, 21st, 24th, 26th, and 29th are leap years. Common years have 354 days, leap years 355, the extra day being added to the last month, Zu'lhijjah. Except for this case, the 12 months beginning with Muharram have alternately 30 and 29 days. The month begins at sunset on the day before that given in the tables.

Year	Name of Month	Month Begins
1396	Muharram (New Year)	Jan. 3, 1976
1396	Safar	Feb. 2, 1976
1396	Rabia I	Mar. 2, 1976
1396	Rabia II	Apr. 1, 1976
1396	Jumada I	Apr. 29, 1976
1396	Jumada II	May 30, 1976
1396	Rajab	Jun. 28, 1976
1396	Shaban	Jul. 28, 1976
1396	Ramadan	Aug. 26, 1976
1396	Shawwai	Sept. 25, 1976
1396	Zu'lkadah	Oct. 24, 1976
1396	Zu'lhijjah	Nov. 23, 1976
1397	Muharram (New Year)	Dec. 23, 1976
1397	Safar	Jan. 22, 1977
1397	Rabia I	Feb. 20, 1977
1397	Rabia II	Mar. 22, 1977
1397	Jumada I	Apr. 20, 1977
1397	Jumada II	May 20, 1977
1397	Rajab	Jun. 18, 1977
1397	Shaban	Jul. 18, 1977
1397	Ramadan	Aug. 16, 1977
1397	Shawwai	Sept. 15, 1977
1397	Zu'lkadah	Oct. 14, 1977
1397	Zu'lhijjah	Nov. 13, 1977

* From *The World Almanac Book of Facts 1976.* Newspaper Enterprise Association, Inc., New York, 1976, p. 498.

The principal Meccan gods were Habal and Al-Uzza. The Meccans also believed in jinn, demons, or Satan, and in good and bad omens.[191]

Muhammad grew up in the religious tradition of the community, but he is said to have been disturbed by its polytheism, the immorality at religious gatherings, the burial of live, unwanted female infants, the intertribal anarchy, and the bloodshed of ensuing wars.

over it. Nearby is the holy well, Zamzam. After Hagar was expelled from Abraham's tent, she is supposed to have brought Ishmael, her son, to the site of Mecca. Ishmael, a sick child, is believed to have created the well by kicking the earth in a tantrum. The Ka'ba and the well are the chief objectives of Muslim pilgrims. (Noss, John B.: *op. cit.,* p. 519.)

Muhammad was employed by Khadija (or Khadeejie), a rich widow, whom he later married. He is thought while in her employ to have learned about the Jewish and Christian religions. The monotheism of Judaism appealed to him, while the Trinity of Christianity is said to have suggested polytheism and hence to have been rejected by him; he accepted the idea of a last judgment and the destruction of idolators by fire. He seems also to have been impressed by the Zoroastrian belief and to have adopted its concept of angels.

When Muhammad was about 40 years old, he went to a cave at the base of Mount Hira, near Mecca, to brood over the change in his religious beliefs. One night (called by Muslims "The Night of Power and Excellence"), the vision of an angel appeared to him who, as the Messenger of God, said:

Recite: In the Name of the Lord, who Created Man of a blood clot.
Recite: And thy Lord is the Most Generous who taught by the Pen, taught Man that he knew not. . . .*

Beset by doubts after this meeting with the angel (said to be Gabriel by some, but not all, Muslims), he nevertheless before long assumed the role of a prophet and began to recite in verse form revelations of the Lord. His followers wrote down his sayings which eventually formed the Qur'an. He came to believe that the Lord was giving (through him) a scripture that was more authentic than that of Judaism or Christianity. Muhammad accepted the prophesies of the Jews, and of Jesus as the greatest of the prophets, but not as a divinity.[192,193]

Sura II (Chapter II) of the Qur'an includes the following lines:

Say you: "We believe in God, and in that which has been sent down on us and sent down on Abraham, Ishmael, Isaac and Jacob, and the Tribes and that which was given to Moses and Jesus and the Prophets, of their Lord; we make no division between any of them, and to Him we surrender." †

Within four years, Muhammad is said to have won forty converts to his beliefs, which can be organized under the headings as follows: 1. *Iman, or articles of faith.* Belief in God, Allah, who stands alone and is omniscient and omnipotent who, on the day of judgment will save believers and place them in paradise. There are various interpretations on the extent to which man is free or controlled by God's will which is revealed to him by Mu-

hammad his prophet, by the Qur'an and by the angels. 2. *Ihsan or right conduct* to achieve salvation. Such conduct includes believing in God, the Last Day, the angels, the Book and the Prophets; giving to kinsmen, orphans, the needy, the travelers, beggars, and to ransom the slave. Good conduct includes praying and paying alms, fulfilling covenants; enduring with fortitude misfortune, hardship, and peril; being kind to parents; not slaying children for fear of poverty; never exchanging the corrupt for what is good; never approaching fornication. Good conduct includes marriage: "marrying women as seems good to you, two, three or four; but if you fear you will not be equitable then only one." Good conduct includes giving orphans their property ("Those who devour the property of orphans unjustly, devour Fire in their bellies and shall assuredly roast in a Blaze"); it involves retaining a divorced woman until she "can be set free honorably"; "fighting in the way of God with those who fight with you, but aggress not; God loves not aggressors. . . . Fight them, till there is no persecution and the religion is God's; then if they give over, there shall be no enmity save for the evil doers." Right conduct involves dietary laws: carrion, blood, and flesh of swine are prohibited. Gambling is prohibited, as are the use of "divining arrows" and the worship of idols.* 3. *Ibadat or religious duty,* this includes "Five Pillars" (*al-Arkan*). (1) Repetition of the creed (*Shahada*) "La ilāha, illa Allāh; Muhammad rasūl Allāh" ("There is no God but Allah, and Muhammad is the prophet of Allāh"). (2) Prayer (*Salat*) five acts a day—at dawn, noon, midafternoon, sunset, and fall of darkness, the devout bowing low toward Mecca and repeating the Fatiha, the Arabian Lord's Prayer: "Praise belongs to God, the Lord of all Being, the All-merciful, the All-compassionate, the master of the day of Doom. Thee only we serve; to Thee alone we pray for succour. Guide us in the straight path, the path of those whom Thou hast blessed, not to those against whom Thou art wrathful, nor of those who are astray." (3) Almsgiving (Zakăt). Originally exacted by religious officials as a "loan to Allah," it is now mostly voluntary. (4) Fast during the sacred month of *Ramadan,* no food taken from the time a white thread can be differentiated from a black, at dawn, until sundown when the difference is no longer perceptible to the eye. (5) Pilgrimage (*Hajj*)

---

* The last has influenced Islamic art, which never includes sacred figures. The remarkable mosaics of Islamic mosques are geometric in design, with symbolic leaves, flowers, and calligraphy. This is also true of the design of rugs that cover the floors of mosques.

---

* Arberry, Arthur T.: *The Koran Interpreted.* George Allen and Unwin, Ltd., London, 1955, p. 344, Vol. II.
† *Ibid.,* 1955, p. 344, Vol. I.

once during a lifetime to Mecca during the sacred month of *Dhu-al-Hijja* for the sacred circumambulation of the Ka'ba at Mecca; the Lesser and Greater pilgrimages, and the Great Feast. The devout wear seamless white garments, abstain from sexual acts, and by day from food and drink, and do no harm to the living—animal or vegetable.[194]

When Muhammad began his teaching, there was, of course, opposition to it, as there always is to change, especially if it affects religious beliefs. The Quraysh especially objected to Muhammad's claim that he was God's prophet, which gave him dominance over the community. His wife Khadija accepted his mission, as did his adopted sons Zaid and 'Ali, the son of Abu Talib; also a kinsman, Abu Bakr, who was his first successor or Caliph, and Uthman, his third successor, or third Caliph. When Muhammad's wife and Abu Talib died, his position in Mecca was weakened and he decided to go to another area. After an unsuccessful attempt to establish himself in Ta'if, he went to Yathrib, whose name was later changed to Medina (*Madinat an nabi*, the City of the Prophet). In Medina, Muhammad established himself as a prophet, built the first mosque, and evolved what Noss [195] calls "a new cultus," with weekly services on Friday and prostration during prayers. Prayers were first directed toward Jerusalem but later toward Mecca.*

In A.D. 630, Muhammad marched against and took control of Mecca, becoming the greatest chief in Arabia as well as Allah's prophet. He removed the idols from the Ka'ba and even removed the paintings of Abraham and the angels from the walls. He treated the Black Stone reverently and sanctioned the use of the well Zamzam. He tried to unify the factions in Arabia under Allah, the one and only God, but he died in 632 before this was accomplished.

Joseph Schacht, writing on Islamic law, said that Muhammad's aim was

. . . to teach men how to act, what to do, and what to avoid in order to pass the reckoning on the Day of Judgment and to enter Paradise. This is why Islam in general, and Islamic law in particular is a system of duties comprising ritual, legal, and moral obligations on the same footing, and bringing them all under the authority of the same religious command.†

Khan [196] calls Muhammad "a law bearing prophet," and John A. Williams [197] maintains there is no sharp distinction between religion and law in Islam.

Muhammad's faith and teachings did spread rapidly, but Islam has been beset by the questions of who should succeed to Muhammad's leadership role and how the teaching in the Qur'an should be interpreted. Muhammad died suddenly in A.D. 632 and had not specified his successor. Three political parties, the Companions, the *Muhajirin* or Emigrants, and the *Ansar* or Supporters, had different interpretations. The leaders, or Caliphs, that followed Muhammad sometimes died a natural death, but in a number of cases they were assassinated by rival factions.* It is not within the scope of this book to give, even in summary form, the story of these factions, or of the spread of Islam. Noss † describes the Muslim conquest of country after country and the creation of the various Islamic Empires, one of which was the Ottoman Empire, stretching from Palestine into Egypt, which "endured to World War I."

The Islamic religion seems to have sanctioned conquest but not persecution of the vanquished. The treaty of Damascus in A.D. 635 makes the point "in the name of Allah, the compassionate, the merciful" that as long as the inhabitants of the city pay the poll tax "nothing but good shall befall them." [198]

Many conquered countries adopted the Islamic religion. M. Naseem,[199] a Muslim, argues that the Islamic religion is characterized by tolerance. However, it is a mistake to assume complete consistency throughout Islam. Schools of Islamic Law developed that interpreted differently the teachings of the Qur'an and that put more or less emphasis on the *Hadith,* or Tradition. The Hadith consisted largely of recollections of Muhammad's sayings and doings traced back through attestors or authorities to Muhammad himself or to a companion in Medina. The Traditions, or Hadiths, ran into the thousands, and their authenticity was often challenged. The controversy over the meaning of the Qur'an and the value of the

---

* Strangers to Islam will find helpful Constance Padwick's *Muslim Devotions* (Society for Promoting Christian Knowledge, London, 1961), which is a study of the prayer manuals in common use around 1960.

† Schacht, Joseph: *Introduction to Islamic Law.* Oxford University Press, London, 1966. p. 11.

---

* Muhammad and Khadija had two sons who died in infancy. Four daughters survived. Those claiming descent from their daughter Fatima were called Fatimads and successfully ruled Islam from A.D., 909 to 1171. At that time, Islam stretched from India to Spain. (Muhammad also had two adopted sons.)

† Noss says, "On the whole, then, the Muslim conquests represent one more of a long succession of Semitic migrations from the Arabian desert—the last and the greatest." (The Semites are said to have outnumbered non-Semitic peoples in Arabia whose people included Sumerians, Babylonians, Persians, and Hamitic Egyptians.) (Noss, John B.: *op. cit.,* p. 535.)

Hadith has persisted among Muslim scholars. Some of the divisions within Islam mentioned by Noss include the Mu'tazilites, characterized by reason and argument in defense of the faith of Islam; the Sunnis, or Traditionists, led by Ash'ari, the four schools of law, and the mystics who include the Sufis, which means wool-wearers. According to Noss:

Islam had no priests, then or now, ordained and set apart for a life dedicated to the worship of God and the pursuit of holiness, and yet everyone knew that Muhammad had been a true man of God, wholly dedicated to his mission, who in the period before the revelations came had retired at times from the world to meditate in a cave. It was thus that he had become an instrument of God's truth.*

The yearning for unworldly lives and union with God in life led some Muslims to adopt an ascetic life which they tried, against opposition, to reconcile with Muhammad's teaching. The *iman* or leader of worship in the Friday service is a layman who may give part-time or full-time to God's work, but the "monkish" life of the mystics and the religious ecstasies of the Sufis as dervishes or fakirs was believed by many to be contrary to the teachings of the Qur'an.

The famous *iman* Ash'ari, a Persian of the eleventh century, is believed to have revivified Islam by reconciling or synthesizing divergent groups. But Noss said "Islam is not and never has been a monolithic faith." He described the Great Dissent that divided the Muslim world. The *Shi'ites* believe that Muhammad and his descendants are the divinely appointed and supernaturally guided leaders of the faith; that the role of Muhammad could only be filled by his cousin and son-in-law 'Ali.† They believe that the appointment of Abu Bakr, Umar, and Uthman as Caliphs after Muhammad's death was usurpation of 'Ali's leadership. The murder of 'Ali and the death of his two sons "has haunted the lives of the party (Shi'a) of 'Ali." ‡ Noss discusses the Shi'ite sects that have formed and that represent divisions within Islam today. He mentions, for example, the Zaidites, the Ishmaelites or Seveners, and their offshoots, which include the Assassins. The Nizarites of Pakistan, India, Persia, and Syria were said to number 250,000 in 1969 and to have as their head Agha Khan IV.[200]

The religion of Islam has continued to change, with its leaders calling for reforms that may result in, according to Noss, "purification, secularism, conservatism, reformation or syncretism." Mustapha Kemel, for instance, in 1924 overthrew the Ottoman Caliphate and introduced Western ideas into Turkey and separated church and state. This affected marriage, divorce, the status of women (including their dress), and education. In Egypt, the Young Men's Muslim Association and the Muslim Brotherhood have had great influence. Jamal Abdal-Nasir ("Nasser"), by establishing the United Arab Republic, tried to achieve the unity of Islam. The creation of Pakistan as a Muslim state should be mentioned as evidence of the current strength of Islam, as should the creation of *Bahai.* The latter is an independent pacifist faith which has a Shi'ite background, has its headquarters in Palestine, and is active in the United States.

It is apparent from the most superficial study of the literature that there are widespread efforts at mutual understanding between representatives of Islam and other religions. Readers who want to follow this line of study will find some books cited among the references for this Chapter.[201-205] H. A. R. Gibbs,[206] writing in Zaehner's *Concise Encyclopedia of Living Faiths,* said in 1959 that the question for the future is whether Islam will remain a "comprehensive culture" based on a religion or become a "church" accepted by smaller or larger bodies of followers within a secular civilization.

Islam has its own calendar, as mentioned earlier (the Muslim Year). Its religious festivals are as follows, although they may be differently observed by the various divisions within Islam: There are two feasts (1) *'Id al-Fitr,* or "little feast," on the first day of the month Shawwal, and (2) *'Id al-Adha,* or the "great feast," on the tenth day of the month Dhu-al-Hijja. The latter represents the ritual offering of allowed animals when pilgrims outside Mecca have returned half way from their Great Pilgrimage. There are three festivals: (1) *Muharram,* or New Year, observed during the first day of the first month—observed by Shi'ites with lamentation over the death of 'Ali and his sons; (2) *Mawlid an-Nabi,* festival of the Prophet's birthday on the twelfth day of the month Rabi al-awwal; and (3) *Lailat al-Mir'aj,* the festival of the Prophet's Night Journey,* observed usually on the night

---

* *Ibid.,* p. 545.

† Noss compares this with the Christian doctrine that Jesus bestowed supernatural powers on Peter, with the resulting concept of the Apostolic succession.

‡ The population of Iran is Shi'ite (Twelver Sect), Islam is the state religion, and the Shah was at one time its representative.

---

* Muhammad is believed to have been taken into the presence of Allah one night. Jeffery says there are "many versions of the story." (Jeffery, Arthur [ed.]: *Islam; Muhammad and His Religion,* Liberal Arts Press, New York, 1958.)

before the twenty-seventh of the month of Rajab. Mosques and minarets are lighted and accounts of the journey are read.[207-209]

While Muslims have no priests or sacraments, they do have the ritualistic practices known as the Five Pillars of Islam, as outlined on page 1045, and the moral and legal ordinances. As mentioned, Muslims may not eat blood, the flesh of animals that have died of themselves, or pork; they may not drink fermented liquor, practice usury, or make idols.[210]

While the Qu'ran does not mention it, Muslims practice circumcision and, as in Judaism, a joyous ceremony accompanies it, with music and feasting. In *Islam, Its Meaning for Modern Man,* Khan [211] says that a Muslim with any faith at all believes in life after death. He says that life on earth is not a perfect whole. "Too often it comes to an end like a snapped ribbon." After death, the body is bathed, the hands placed as in prayer, the body enshrouded. Before the head is covered, relatives say farewell and a catechism may be whispered: "Who is thy God? Allah. What is this Religion? Islam. Who is thy prophet? Muhammad." This is said to prepare the dead for questioning by the angels. The body may be buried without a coffin so it can "sit up for the angels." [212]

3. RELIGIOUS LEADERS AS MEMBERS OF HEALTH TEAMS

Students of the health sciences in the industrialized cultures of the West tend to think of all health care as initiated by the physician, and as based on "science" rather than on a philosophy or a religious belief. The following statement by Henry S. Sigerist is worth pondering:

There are people who consider medicine whatever the physician does. He who is not a physician is a layman and what he does cannot be medicine. This is a very narrow viewpoint and one that certainly does not hold true in historical studies.
. . . The great majority of all cases of illness, moreover, even today [1951] are never seen by a physician. They are treated by the patient himself or by his relatives.*

In another context, Sigerist observes:

Ancient traditions are still alive today in many countries. In India the overwhelming majority of close to 400 million people receive medical services from indigenous practitioners who treat their patients either according to the principles of Ayurvedic or ancient Hindu medicine, or according to the teaching of Unani or Graeco-Arabic medicine, or some other ancient or medieval system. . . . The classics of Arabic Medicine are still read and followed in Mohammedan countries of North Africa and the Near East.*

In all of the systems of health care that retain ancient or medieval practice, religious and philosophical elements are present. Anyone who uses these systems should recognize the latter and understand their significance.

The role of religion in health care in the United States is so established that the American Medical Association has a Committee on Chaplaincy, the Catholic Hospital Association has a Department of Pastoral Care Services, the American Protestant Hospital Association sponsors a College of Chaplains, and the New York Board of Rabbis has a Liaison Committee on Jewish Chaplaincy.[213] Those who want to learn more about this subject might ask for publications from such organizations. As with all professions, there are many journals for religious advisors, for example, *The Journal of Pastoral Care* or *The Journal of Religion and Health.*

Ministry to the terminally ill has had a phenomenal amount of attention in this decade, as has the ethical question of extending human life with technical support. Both are discussed fully in Chapter 50, but it might be worth noting here that in 1954 the Institute of Religion and Human Development was founded in the Texas Medical Center at Houston to "provide a graduate center for education, service and research in religious ministry and health." †

William A. Bean, a physician, speaking of "doctors and priests" in the Foreword to *Religion and Medicine,* tried to show their interdependence. He said there were three "intertwining elements" that give unity to human life—the mind, or *psyche;* the body or *soma;* and the spirit, or *pneuma.* He thinks the medical scientist "had better know all he can" about the psyche and the pneuma, as well as the soma, dismissing what he believes to be a mistaken conflict between science and religion. He harks back to antiquity when the "physician-priest" tried to give patients "an inner glow" by making them "feel good the way friends make friends feel good." He

---

* Sigerist, Henry S.: *A History of Medicine,* Vol. I: *Primitive and Archaic Medicine.* Oxford University Press, New York, 1951, p. 7.

* Ibid., p. 25.
† McCarthy, Donald G. (ed.): *Responsible Stewardship of Human Life. Inquiries into Medical Ethics II.* The Catholic Hospital Association, St. Louis, 1976, p. iii.

thinks "the wise and kind" physician does this today, helped *by those who minister to the religious needs of the patient"* (italics ours).[214] If this statement implies separate components it should be stated that I, the writer, disclaim this concept and agree with Paul Tillich in the following: "Man should not be considered as a composite of several levels, such as body, soul, spirit, but as a multidimensional unity." *

In the volume *Religion and Medicine,* ten theologians, seven physicians, four psychologists, and a health educator discuss the relationship of spiritual, emotional, and physical well-being and the role of the minister, priest, or spiritual advisor in therapy. The extent to which people believe health dependent on peace of mind or emotional balance determines their willingness to assign the priest a place in health agencies. Some people believe that disease in human beings is primarily a protest against the way in which they are forced to live by their social circumstances; many attribute mental illness to guilt or wrongdoing and the anxiety or stress arising from knowledge of it by the subject. Medical and theological libraries abound in books and journals dealing directly or indirectly with this subject. The psychiatrist Carl G. Jung [215] has said that among his patients over 35 there hasn't been one whose problem "in the last resort" was not finding "a religious outlook on life."

Gordon W. Allport, student of personality and social relations, discussing mental health, asks, "How, in the helping . . . can we recover some of the common sense that we seem to have lost along the way?" † He says the conviction that "man's psyche is secondary to his soma became set"; he thinks that "when scientific dogma alone rules the roost a curious caste system develops with the patient at the bottom"; he questions the ultimate effectiveness and the wide use of drug therapy [in mental illness] and recalls Philippe Pinel's revolutionary success with what he called "moral treatment," which Allport thinks might be more accurately described as "morale treatment." He thinks Pinel's concepts are again gaining favor and cites the work of H. B. Adams, I. S. Bockovern, and Carl R. Rogers that point to the importance of self-understanding in the recovery of the mentally ill and the rehabilitation of juvenile delinquents.

In his research on religion and mental health, Allport differentiates between extrinsic and intrinsic religion. The first is something to use but not to live; the second is not instrumental —it does not exist to serve the person, but rather the person serves it. Intrinsic religion is integrating and healing, extrinsic religion tends to be "a matter of convenience." He thinks the task of the religious counselor is to help the person move from an extrinsic to an intrinsic religion; he thinks the principle of "discovering and holding fast to one direction the first law of mental health." Allport cites a psychiatrist's statement that "a sense of sin" is the "chief lesion" in mental illness. He agrees with William James that the confessional is healing and that the minister has a "more balanced wisdom" in dealing with "private sacramental penance under the seal of secrecy [than others]."

Victor E. Frankl,[216] in his compelling book *Man's Search for Meaning,* shows the human capacity for enduring and surviving extreme suffering when there is a reason for survival. While he, a psychiatrist, believes that it is within the realm of his practice to help others identify a purpose and value in life, this is admittedly a major concern for the priest, minister, rabbi, or any spiritual advisor.

James B. Ashbrook,[217] a professor of pastoral theology, thinks that "as long as life runs smoothly we can avoid facing the depths of experience." Illness may make ordinary concerns seem "strangely irrelevant." Face to face with the possibility of death or the inability to continue living as they had before their illness, sick men or women may, almost for the first time, begin to search for the meaning of life. The sick must work through this problem before they can be whole again, achieve harmony, salvation, a state of grace, or peace of mind.

Gotthard Booth,[218] a psychiatrist, says, "mankind has known intuitively since early times that the body speaks a very basic and honest language through the healthy and unhealthy functioning of its organs" and he thinks religions have "at all times and in all places expressed an intuitive insight into the meaning of illness and death." He thinks modern medicine has ". . . flagrantly sidestepped the insight which was so evident to religious ages, that man is [his] own executioner." * Booth obviously believes that the health worker should cultivate insight into the meaning of illness but he also sees a place on

---

* Tillich, Paul: "The Meaning of Health," in Belgum, David (ed.): *Religion and Medicine.* Iowa State University Press, Ames, 1967, p. 6.

† Allport, Gordon W.: "Mental Health: A Generic Attitude," in Belgum, David (ed.): *Religion and Health.* Iowa State University Press, Ames, 1967, p. 47.

* Booth is quoting John Donne in *Devotion XII.* Donne was a seventeenth-century theologian and poet. (Hayward, John [ed.]: *Complete Poetry and Selected Prose.* Nonesuch Press, 1929, p. 529.)

health teams for religious advisors who, by the nature of their calling, see meaning in sickness and death and consider it a part of their work to discuss this meaning with patients and their families.

Orville S. Walters, a psychiatrist, discussing "religion and psychopathology," comments on the importance of understanding religious symptoms, emphasizing the religious obsessions in schizophrenia, but he thinks collaboration between medicine and theology has not gone far enough. He says:

Increasing collaboration between psychiatry and religion has brought the clergyman and the psychiatrist closer together. Programs of clinical training have made the minister better acquainted with mental illness in its various forms. But there has not been any comparable movement to acquaint psychiatry with religious experience in its healthy expressions.*

Gordon E. Jackson,[219] a theologian, discusses "the problem of guilt" as seen by Sigmund Freud, Erik Erikson, Emil Brunner, Reinhold Niebuhr, Lewis Joseph Sherrill, Alfred North Whitehead, Paul Tillich, and others. Russell J. Becker,[220] another theologian, discusses "Sin, Illness and Guilt," with special emphasis on the concept of "original sin" and the Judaic-Christian ethic. Gunter Elsässer,[221] a psychiatrist writing on "objective guilt and neurosis," notes that the concept of guilt, in even more pervasive forms, dominates other religions. He cites the 18th Canto of the Bhagavad Gita: "Whatever man touches is loaded with guilt, as fire is with smoke." Elsässer says, "Just as the neurotic patient first has to learn how properly to sleep, eat, drink, love, work, defend himself, and so on, so he has to learn on psychotherapeutic treatment how to get along with his fragmentary human nature and the guilt entanglements that spring from it." He refers to man's conscience as his "shadow," an inescapable companion.

So far, the emphasis may seem to have been on people who might be classified as psychotic, neurotic, or emotionally disturbed. While it is true that among physicians, nurses, and social workers those associated with the mentally ill have more often collaborated with religious counselors than have those associated with the physically ill, hospitals of all kinds have resident or visiting chaplains, and there are chaplains associated with military medical services, with prison health services, and, of course, with institutions and agencies

giving terminal care. Gerald R. Niklas, a Roman Catholic priest, and Charlotte Stefanics, a psychiatric nurse, in their monograph *Ministry to the Hospitalized*,[222] estimated that unfortunately, less than one third of the hospitals in the United States had salaried chaplains (in 1975). They said that visitation of the sick was "the duty of all Christians." They discussed the special needs of obstetrical and gynecological patients, those who have suffered disfigurement, the critically ill, the old, the dying, and their families. Robert D. Wheelock, director of pastoral care services of the Catholic Hospital Association, has prepared a guide to organization management and evaluation of health care ministries. He suggested that if only one salaried chaplain could be employed, a clergyman should be chosen whose faith represented that of the majority of the patients. He says:

Increasingly today Catholic health facilities are hiring full time Protestant and Jewish religious health care professionals to minister as full members of the pastoral care team. Ecumenism has been very functional in the hospital ministry. Pastoral care personnel visit, counsel, and minister to all people in need regardless of their religious affiliation; yet there are times when only a clergyman of one's own faith can fulfill the needs of the patient or family.*

Wheelock outlines the certification requirements for Roman Catholic chaplaincy and the nature of programs to prepare priests for ministry to the sick.

The position is taken in this book that *all* illness has emotional and physical components; that there is no health service that does not have a spiritual aspect. There are many centers where the clergy are prepared to function in health services. Some have a very broad base. There is, for instance, the Institute of Religion and Human Development at the Texas Medical Center in Houston, founded to "provide a graduate center for education, service, and research in religion, ministry, and health." † In a recent workshop that clergymen sponsored, physicians, a nurse, and several lawyers spoke to the question of "responsible stewardship of human life." In the last analysis, all patients are "terminal cases," since dying is part of every life. To put it negatively, most illness is threatening; to put it positively, all illness can be a learning experience. The presence of the spiritual advisor on the health team should help to reduce the fear and anxi-

* Walters, Orville S.: "Religion and Psychopathology," in Belgum, David (ed.): *Religion and Medicine.* Iowa State University Press, Ames, 1967, p. 133.

* Wheelock, Robert D.: *Health Ministries; A Guide to Organization, Management, Evaluation.* Catholic Hospital Association, St. Louis, 1975, p. 51.
† McCarthy, Donald G. (ed.): *op. cit.,* p. iii.

ety associated with illness and increase opportunities for developing self-understanding.

4. SOME WAYS IN WHICH NURSES AND OTHERS HELP THOSE THEY SERVE MEET THEIR SPIRITUAL NEEDS

There can be no real distinction between what physicians, nurses, social workers, psychologists, and others do to help patients attain or maintain the peace of mind that is one of the aims, if not the principal aim, of spiritual ministry, of worship, or of religious practice. Any health worker can establish a relationship with clients or patients that enables them to express their fears, their need for help, and the conditions of their illness that have created emotional and spiritual problems —that have interrupted their habits of worship, shaken their faith, or that have created new needs. Actually, the help given by workers to healthy clients and sick patients may be no different from that given by relatives and friends; however, until people express their fears, their hopes, or their conflicts, or until they confide in others, it is almost impossible to give the needed help.

Sickness often precipitates frustration, with an overflow of grief that takes the form of sobbing. David Sobel,[223] a psychiatrist, noted that this release from an effort to control the hurt is often followed by the ability to express tenderness or the ability to confide in others. Therefore, allowing a person to cry and accepting subsequent confidences is a form of therapy many persons can offer. Nathaniel Hawthorne, a nineteenth-century writer, makes the following observation on the relation of doctors and patients. (In the writer's opinion it applies equally to the nurse, the clinical psychologist, the family counselor, or the social worker.)

If . . . [the doctor] possess[es] native sagacity and a nameless something more, . . . if he have the power, which must be born with him, to bring his mind into such affinity with his patients' that this last shall unawares have spoken what he imagines himself only to have thought: if such revelations be acknowledged not so often by an uttered sympathy as by silence, an inarticulate breath, and here and there a nod, to indicate that all is understood; if to these qualifications of a confidant be added the advantages afforded by his recognized character as a physician;—then, at some inevitable moment, will the soul of the sufferer be dissolved, and flow forth in a dark, but transparent stream, bringing all its mysteries to light.*

* Hawthorne, Nathaniel: *The Scarlet Letter.* Random House, Modern Library Edition, New York, 1950, p. 140.

William W. Zeller,[223a] a psychiatrist, who cited Hawthorne's observations, discusses "values" in sickness and health. He defines value as a personal estimate of what is desirable and discusses the way these values change as a person matures, or how childish values may persist or be challenged by sickness.* Sickness may paralyze the value system, he says, just as it may paralyze the motor system. He thinks, as so many do, that, if treated constructively, illness may offer an opportunity for growth—an opportunity to recover or acquire integrity, wholeness, holiness, or health—all words with related origins. This recovery depends upon the understanding of those associated with the sick, their ability to refrain from passing moral judgment, but also their ability to help the sick achieve self-understanding. Alcoholism is instanced as an illness for which sufferers may feel socially condemned. Zeller thinks that if they can be helped to understand that the use of alcohol is "but the symptom of turbulent emotions, of anxiety, of severe depression, and not infrequently of overwhelming guilt," they may recover and lead a happier life than before.†

Mack Lipkin, writing for medical students in *The Care of Patients,* emphasizes the art as well as the science of medical practice. He has this to say about the mystery of faith-healing:

Religion has played an important role in the treatment of countless people throughout history. Faith having brought more comfort to more people than physicians in any age, priests, ministers, and rabbis are today becoming more involved in psychiatry, and many schools of theology offer instruction in pastoral psychiatry. For those patients who have religious faith, hospital chaplains afford great solace. The equanimity based on faith in God's care that is shown by some patients facing death can be impressive. Many doctors who think of themselves as medical scientists are inclined to scoff at faith healers, but the fact that they often bring great comfort cannot be denied. Our inability to explain such relief in physico-chemical terms is reason for humility rather than for scorn.‡

Since nurses are with patients more than any other health workers, they have the greatest opportunity to listen—to be the patient's confidante. The more spirituality nurses have, the more comfortable they are in discussing

* J. B. Phillips thinks many people retain a childish concept of God that fails to support them in life's crises. Written for Christians, his book, *Your God Is Too Small* (Macmillan Publishing Co., Inc., New York, 1961), has been widely used.

† The feeling of being "reborn" is often described by members of Alcoholics Anonymous, and corresponding behavior may be noted by their friends and families.

‡ Lipkin, Mack: *Care of Patients. Concepts and Tactics.* Oxford University Press, New York, 1974, p. 231.

spiritual questions, the more likely it is that people—patients and their families—will confide in them.

Jean Stallwood and Ruth Stoll,[224] writing in Irene L. Beland and Joyce Y. Passos's comprehensive text, *Clinical Nursing,* discuss "spiritual dimensions of nursing practice." They discuss a conceptual model of personality, assessing spiritual resources and needs, the counseling function of the nurse, and the use of religious literature; they review a range of opinion which provides the nursing student with sources (chiefly Judaic-Christian) for further study. Stallwood and Stoll illustrate three types of nursing intervention—for comfort, for its catalytic effect, or to challenge the patient. They give specific responses the nurse might make to patient's expressed needs in various stages of illness that suggest denial by the patient, anger, bargaining, depression, or acceptance. Lucie Young Kelly,[225] in *Dimensions of Professional Nursing,* has a helpful section on "Religion and the Nurse" in which she discusses the nurse's role in meeting spiritual needs of patients. She makes specific suggestions for Jewish and Christian patients and for how nurses may help clergymen. Kelly describes Judaism and Christianity and, under "Other Organized Religions," discusses very briefly Christian Science, Jehovah's Witnesses, Society of Friends (Quakers), Mormons, the Unitarian Universalist Association, Seventh Day Adventists, and, under "Other Major World Religions," Islam, "the second largest religion in the world." Kelly's explanation of the Sacraments in Roman Catholicism is especially helpful.

By their ethical codes, nurses worldwide are committed to serving all peoples the same way without regard to their religion, and they are committed to holding in confidence what they learn about people while they nurse them.

The International Council of Nurses' 1973 Code of Ethics includes the following statement:

The need for nursing is universal. Inherent in nursing is respect for life, dignity and rights of man. It is unrestricted by considerations of nationality, race, creed, colour, age, sex, politics or social status. . . .

The nurse, in providing care, respects the beliefs, values and customs of the individual.

The nurse holds in confidence personal information and uses judgment in sharing this information.*

The American Nurses' Association Code for Nurses (1968) includes similar statements:

1. The nurse provides services with respect for the dignity of man, unrestricted by considerations of nationality, race, creed, color, or status.
2. The nurse safeguards the individual's right to privacy by judiciously protecting information of a confidential nature, sharing only that information relevant to his care.*

In current books and articles, nurses are urging other nurses to care for people in their entirety.[226-231] This always includes a spiritual aspect and always or sometimes, according to the way in which the terms are used, includes a religious aspect. Sister Madeleine Clémence Vaillot interprets the term "spiritual" as ". . . the essential principle influencing us. Spiritual, although it might, does not necessarily mean religious: it also includes the psychological. The spiritual is opposed to the biological and mechanical, whose laws it may modify." †

If nurses believe that personality is unique and that all behavior is the result of physical structure and function, emotion, thought, and the person's motivation or spiritual values, it is not possible to ignore any of the inseparable aspects of the personality. If they (nurses) are trying to help a person maintain or develop healthy behavior, they must be prepared to work with the whole person, not with one facet of his or her life. Motivation, spiritual values, and aspirations are rooted in religious beliefs of the culture in which the personality is formed, although, since each person's experience is unique, the beliefs or cultural values are uniquely modified by the individual's experience. In order to understand a person's motivations, it is necessary to know something about the religious climate in which he or she grew up and the way in which life has affected the person's values or aspirations.

Most health histories include a statement on religious affiliation. Just as nurses note other aspects of the history, they note this fact or the fact that the person disclaims any connection with an established faith. Depending upon the duration and quality of the nurse-patient relationship, there will be few or many opportunities for nurses to learn more than is in patients' histories about their beliefs and the place that religion has in their lives.

The extent to which nurses are informed about the religions to which their patients subscribe influences the patients' tendencies to talk to them about religious needs or questions.

* International Council of Nurses: *1973 Code for Nurses.* The Council, Geneva, 1974.

* American Nurses' Association: *The Code for Nurses (1968).* The Association, Kansas City, Mo., 1969.
† Vaillot, Sister Madeleine Clémence: "The Spiritual Factors in Nursing," *J. Pract. Nurs.,* **20**:30, (Sept.) 1970.

The extent to which nurses can see the commonalities in religions and recognize the differences in them determines to a large extent their ability to meet patients on their own grounds, to accept people of all faiths and help them with problems that involve religion or spiritual values.

The knowledge nurses have, their own spiritual strength and experience and the catholicity of their sympathies, affects their usefulness to their clients or patients, but the situation also determines what they can do and what they may be willing to do. Missionary nurses, for instance, may think conversion a part of their work; generally speaking, health workers do not try to influence the religious beliefs of those they serve, nor is religious counseling or the performance of religious rites among their functions. However, many persons facing death or crises in their lives may turn to institutions or agencies staffed by health personnel who are also members of religious orders. In effect, such patients or clients may be asking for the support that the religious nurse's faith can bring them. Emotionally disturbed patients for whom the nurse is the principal therapist may ask for help with problems that pose ethical and religious questions. In medical centers and in many settings, religious advisors (minister, priest, rabbi, swami, or other) are available to patients, but in many circumstances they are not. The nurse may be the only worker available to the person and his or her family in need of help that involves a spiritual problem or a religious practice. If religion, faith, or spiritual values are seen as woven into the fabric of life, it is an inescapable function of nurses to recognize them.* Having done this, a nurse may deal with them negatively, rejecting any responsibility for helping people with problems of this nature, or they may accept responsi-

bility for giving such help as they may be prepared to give.

Young nurses may have had little experience with illness, death, and bereavement. It may be especially helpful for them to join groups made up of psychiatrists, psychologists, chaplains, nurses, social workers, and others who meet to discuss these questions. It is especially desirable that they have some experience in group discussions that include patients and their families. Discussions of the health problems of almost any client or patient might involve spiritual counselors; many books and articles, however, emphasize their role in mental illness, ethical decisions about prolonging life, the care of the dying, bereavement, experimenting with human subjects, transplanting organs, genetic counseling, sexual behavior, and family life.[232-241]

For the benefit of those who find specific suggestions helpful, and with apologies to those who are put off by a simplistic concept of the nurse's role, I offer the following list of steps nurses might take in helping people meet their spiritual needs:

1. Try to identify their own (the nurses') values, spiritual needs, religious beliefs.
2. Learn as much as possible about living religions—their fundamental beliefs, practices, sacraments, and holidays—by reading, by talking with others, and by attending religious services. It is particularly important to learn how religions, rituals, and values affect the meaning of illness, the concept of therapy, and hence the treatment the patient may be willing to follow.
3. When caring for well clients or sick patients, note their religious affiliation on charts or records.
4. Listen with interest to anything patients or families say about their ethical values, spiritual needs, or religious beliefs, noting any aspect of treatment or care that runs counter to these values or makes it impossible for them to meet their spiritual needs or act consistently with their religious beliefs. Accept their statements nonjudgmentally; avoid questions that suggest idle curiosity, but invite confidence by genuine interest and informed understanding. Above all, be honest and natural.
5. When people express the wish to see a spiritual advisor, communicate this need to an appropriate person or persons; this may or may not include speaking directly to the priest, minister, rabbi, or other religious representative.

---

* Margaret Read, an anthropologist, discussing "values underlying ritual and religious ceremonies," says that it is difficult, but not impossible for people of one culture to understand the values of another. She makes the following suggestion: "try to discover the occasions on which cultural values are stressed and made articulate. . . . Religious ceremonies emphasize, to those who participate in them, their concepts about the nature of the universe, how the supernatural elements in the universe impinge on man in his life on earth and how this concept in turn affects the relation of man to his fellowmen. . . ." She notes that among the Navaho [Native Americans] health is a central objective in religious behavior and is believed to represent the correct balance between man and his physical, social and supernatural environment. (Read, Margaret: *Culture, Health, and Disease. Social and Cultural Influences on Health Programmes in Developing Countries.* Tavistock Publications, London; J. B. Lippincott Co., Philadelphia, 1966, p. 79.)

6. When religious advisors visit patients, see that as much privacy as possible is provided; see that the patient and the surroundings are ready for the visit. See that clergymen have the articles they need for any sacraments to be administered. Answer the clergyman's questions about the patient's condition and offer additional information that, in your judgment, the clergyman may need in order to help the patient.

7. Learn to administer sacraments that it is appropriate for lay persons to administer in emergencies when religious representatives are not available and when receiving the sacrament is of importance to the patient and/or the family.

8. Read prayers or other religious literature at the request of patients or their families.

9. Work with others in health agenices to see that there are suitable resources (space, furnishings, objects, and services) for religious observances by patients and staff. The resources include written guides, or information on this subject for staff and clients, or patients.

10. Respect the property of patients that has religious significance and, to the extent consistent with the welfare of others, allow patients to keep such articles with them, or nearby.

11. To the extent that it is possible, enable patients to continue religious practices whether this involves bringing a service to them or taking them to the service.

12. Participate in interdisciplinary conferences that deal with managerial problems such as offering health workers and patients religious freedom and an opportunity to serve and be served "without regard to creed."

5. SUMMARY

The intuitive belief in a higher power is accompanied by reverence for and devotion to this power—or God. When expressed in prayer or ritual, this reverence and devotion are known as worship. Anthropologists say that human beings, unlike animals, comprehend things they cannot see and believe in things they cannot comprehend. Humans endow the object of worship with the qualities they most admire. Religions are expressions of human values. People's values determine their purposes in life. Good health seems to be dependent upon the belief that life has meaning or a "good" purpose and upon behavior that is consistent with this meaning, this purpose, or

value system; upon behavior that brings people nearer their goal in life.

More than half of the world's inhabitants belong to nine major living religions; others belong to primitive religions or have no religious affiliation; but all have value systems that lie at the roots of their being. Sickness should ideally be an opportunity to strengthen, rather than weaken, the personality; to clarify goals and to establish more satisfying or valid goals. Opportunity to worship according to one's faith is important to many in maintaining their integrity, strengthening their faith, and raising their aspirations. Health workers should know enough about living religions to enable them to foster habits of worship, to help clients and patients use the spiritual resources within a community, and to promote conditions within health agencies and institutions that encourage rather than discourage forms of worship.

This chapter describes nine major living religions in chronological order, from the oldest, which is the Hindu religion, to the youngest, which is the Islamic, or Muslim, religion. Recurrent themes in these religions are noted and even their kinship with primitive religions. Although some refer to this age as "Godless," others look upon this century as characterized by a "new morality" with an ecumenical movement aimed ultimately at a worldwide acceptance of basic religious or ethical beliefs.

Health organizations, institutions, and agencies in the United States and other countries promote or foster the participation of the clergy in health services. Many members of the clergy have special preparation for such work. The knowledge health workers have of religions and their ability to serve people of any faith with understanding determine the range and quality of their usefulness. Men and women in nursing who have faced honestly the serious questions in life, who have developed their inherent spirituality, will be more effective and more comfortable than those who haven't when they work with people in crises. This chapter suggests some steps nurses might take to help well clients and sick patients with the ethical, moral, spiritual, and religious aspects of health and illness.

REFERENCES

1. Teilhard de Chardin, Pierre: *The Phenomenon of Man.* Harper and Brothers, New York, 1959, p. 318.
2. Birx, James H.: *Pierre Teilhard de Chardin's Philosophy of Evolution.* Charles C Thomas, Pubisher, Springfield, Ill., 1972.
3. Braybrooke, Neville: *Teilhard de Chardin:*

Pilgrim of the Future. Seabury Press, New York, 1964.

4. Gray, Donald P.: *The One and the Many; Teilhard de Chardin's Vision of Unity.* Herder & Herder, New York, 1969.

5. Lubac, Henri de: *Teilhard de Chardin: The Man and His Meaning.* (Translated by René Hague.) Hawthorne Books, New York, 1965.

6. Kessler, Marvin, and Brown, Bernard (eds.): *Dimensions of the Future; The Spirituality of Teilhard de Chardin.* Corpus Books, Washington, D.C., 1968.

7. Koestler, Arthur: *The Trail of the Dinosaur and Other Essays.* Macmillan Publishing Co., Inc., New York, 1955, p. 257.

8. Fabro, Cornelio: *God in Exile: Modern Atheism; A Study of the Internal Dynamics of Modern Atheism from Its Roots in the Cartesian Cogito to the Present Day.* (Translated and edited by Arthur Gibson.) Newman Press, Westminster, Md., 1968.

9. Eisendrath, Maurice N.: *Can Faith Survive?* McGraw-Hill Book Co., New York, 1965.

10. Baumer, Franklin L.: *Religion and the Rise of Skepticism.* Harcourt Brace & Co., New York, 1960.

11. Thielicke, Helmut: *Nihilism.* Harper & Row, New York, 1961 (Religious Perspectives Series Vol. 4).

12. Marty, Martin E.: *Varieties of Unbelief.* Holt, Rinehart & Winston, New York, 1964.

13. Boulding, Kenneth: *The Meaning of the 20th Century. The Great Transition.* Harper & Row, New York, 1965, p. 2.

14. Hillman, James (ed.): *The Myth of Analysis: Three Essays in Archetypal Psychology.* Northwestern University Press, Evanston, Ill., 1972.

15. Fletcher, Joseph: *Situation Ethics—The New Morality.* Westminster Press, Philadelphia, 1966.

16. Outka, Gene: *Agape. An Ethical Analysis.* Yale University Press, New Haven, Conn., 1972.

17. Mellert, Robert B.: *What Is Process Theology?* Paulist-Newman Press, Paramus, N.J., 1976.

18. Gandhi, Mohandas Karamchand: *Gandhi on Non-violence.* (With introduction by Thomas Merton.) New Directions Publishing Co., New York, 1965 (paperback).

19. Mowrer, Orval H. (ed.): *Morality and Mental Health.* Rand McNally, Chicago, 1967 (Rand McNally Psychology Series).

20. Montagu, Ashley: *Touching: The Human Significance of the Skin.* Columbia University Press, New York, 1971.

21. Frazer, James: *The Golden Bough. A Study in Magic and Religion.* (Abridged ed.) Macmillan Publishing Co., Inc., New York, 1926.

22. Toynbee, Arnold J.: *An Historian's Approach to Religion.* Oxford University Press, London, 1956.

23. Bloom, Anthony: *God and Man.* Paulist-Newman Press, Paramus, N.J., 1976.

24. Baum, Gregory: *Ecumenical Theology No. 2.* Paulist-Newman Press, Paramus, N.J., 1967.

25. Grant, John Webster: *The Canadian Experience with Church Union.* Butterworth, London, 1967 (Ecumenical Studies in History No. 8). Also John Knox Press, Richmond, Va.

26. Jurji, Edward J.: *The Ecumenical Era in Church and Society; A Symposium in Honor of John A. Mackey* [by] Hugh T. Kerr [and others]. Macmillan Publishing Co., Inc., New York, 1959.

27. McNeill, John Thomas, and Nichols, James Hastings: *Ecumenical Testimony; The Concern for Christian Unity Within the Reformed and Presbyterian Churches.* Westminster Press, Philadelphia, 1974.

28. Rouse, Ruth, and Neill, Charles (eds.): *A History of the Ecumenical Movement,* 2nd ed. Westminster Press, Philadelphia, 1967–1970.

29. Sheerin, John B.: *Christian Reunion; The Ecumenical Movement and American Catholics.* Hawthorne Books, New York, 1966.

30. Vatican Council, 2nd, 1962–1965: *The Decree on Ecumenism of the Second Vatican Council.* (New translation by Secretariat for Promoting Christian Unity with commentary by Thomas F. Stransky.) Paulist-Newman Press, Paramus, N.J., 1965.

31. Guinan, Edward (comp.): *Peace and Non-Violence; Basic Writings.* Paulist-Newman Press, Paramus, N.J., 1973.

32. Rosenberg, Stuart E.: *Bridge to Brotherhood; Judaism's Dialogue with Christianity.* Abelard-Schuman, New York, 1961.

33. Laurentin, René, and Neuner, S. J. (eds.): "Declaration on the Relation of the Church to Non-Christian Religions," in *Vatican Council Two—Constitution of the Sacred Liturgy.* Paulist-Newman Press, Paramus, N.J., 1966.

34. Bruns, J. Edgar: *The Christian Buddhism of St. John; New Insights into the Fourth Gospel.* Paulist-Newman Press, Paramus, N.J., 1971.

35. Conza, Edward: *Buddhist Meditation.* George Allen & Unwin, London, 1956.

36. Hamilton-Merritt, Jane: *A Meditator's Diary. A Western Woman's Unique Experience in Thailand Temples.* Harper & Row, New York, 1976.

37. Bright, D., et al.: "What School Physicians, Nurses and Health Educators Should know About Transcendental Meditation," *J. Sch. Health,* **43:**192, (Mar.) 1973.

38. Byles, Marie Beuzeville: *Journey into Burmese Silence.* George Allen & Unwin, London, 1962.

39. Deffner, Donald Louis: *Christ on Campus; Meditation for College Life.* Concordia Publishing House, St. Louis, 1965.

39a. Merton, Thomas: *Contemplative Prayer.* Herder & Herder, New York, 1969.

40. Lunn, Henry Simpson: *The Secret of the Saints; Studies in Prayer, Meditation and Self-Discipline.* Macmillan Publishing Co., Inc., New York, 1933.

40a. Kelsey, Morton T.: *The Other Side of Silence. A Guide to Christian Meditation.* Paulist-Newman Press, Paramus, N.J., 1976.

41. Fitzgerald, George R.: *Communes, Their Goals, Hopes, Problems.* Paulist-Newman Press, Paramus, N.J., 1971.

42. Vanier, Jean: *Be Not Afraid.* Griffin House, Toronto, 1975.

43. Mosteller, Sue: *My Brother, My Sister.* Story of the Mother Teresa Foundations in India and Jean Vanier Houses for Retarded Adults. Paulist-Newman Press, Paramus, N.J., 1973.

44. Muggeridge, Malcom: *Something Beautiful for God. Mother Teresa of Calcutta.* Collins-Fontana Books, London, 1973.

45. Camara, Helder, et al.: *The Church and Colonialism. The Betrayal of the Third World.* Dimension Books, Denville, N.J., 1969.

46. Padovano, Anthony T.: *American Culture and the Quest for Christ.* Sheed & Ward, New York, 1970.

47. Perella, Frederick J., and Procopio, Mariellen: *Poverty Profile USA.* Paulist-Newman Press, Paramus, N.J., 1976.

48. Milio, Nancy: *The Care of Health in Communities; Access for Outcasts.* Macmillan Publishing Co., Inc., New York, 1975.

49. Storlie, Frances: *Nursing and the Social Conscience.* Appleton-Century-Crofts, New York, 1970.

50. Gandhi, Mohandas Karamchand: *My Religion.* (Compiled and edited by Bharatan Kumarappa.) Navajivan Publishing House, Ahmedabad, 1958.

51. Belgum, David: *Guilt: Where Religion and Psychology Meet.* Prentice-Hall, Inc., Englewood Cliffs, N.J., 1963.

52. Mowrer, Orval H.: "The Neurosis Confession and Recovery of a Protestant Minister," in Belgium, David (ed.): *Religion and Medicine.* Iowa State University Press, Ames, 1967.

53. Mowrer, Orval H.: *The Crisis in Psychiatry and Religion.* Van Nostrand Co., Princeton, N.J., 1961.

54. Jourard, Sidney M.: *The Transparent Self,* rev. ed. Van Nostrand Reinhold Co., New York, 1971.

55. Jourard, Sidney M.: *Disclosing Man to Himself.* Van Nostrand Reinhold Co., New York, 1968.

56. Menninger, Karl: *Whatever Became of Sin?* Hawthorne Books, Inc., New York, 1973.

57. *The World Almanac and Book of Facts 1976.* Newspaper Enterprise Association, New York, p. 488.

58. Medicine and Religion Committee, Zumbro Valley Medical Society, Rochester, Minn.: *Religious Aspects of Medical Care. A Handbook of Religious Practices of All Faiths.* Catholic Hospital Association, St. Louis, 1975, p. vii.

59. Noss, John B.: *Man's Religions,* 4th ed. Macmillan Publishing Co., Inc., New York, 1969, p. 10.

60. Frazer, James: *op. cit.*

61. Eliade, Mircea: *Myths, Dreams and Mysteries, the Encounter Between Contemporary Faiths and Archaic Realities.* Harvill Press, London, 1960.

62. ———: *Patterns in Comparative Religion.* Sheed and Ward, New York, 1958.

63. ———: *The Quest; History and Meaning in Religion.* University of Chicago Press, Chicago, 1969.

64. ———: *From Primitive to Zen; a Thematic Sourcebook of the History of Religions.* Harper & Row, New York, 1967.

65. James, William: *Varieties of Religious Experience.* Longmans Green Co., New York, 1902.

66. Clemen, Carl (ed.): *Religions of the World: Their Nature and History.* George G. Harrap & Co., London, 1931.

67. Djukanovic, V., and Mach, E. P. (eds.): *Alternative Approaches to Meeting Basic Health Needs in Developing Countries.* World Health Organization, Geneva, 1975.

68. Read, Margaret: *Culture, Health and Disease; The Social and Cultural Influence on Health Programmes in Developing Countries.* Tavistock Publications, London, 1966. (J. B. Lippincott Co., Philadelphia, distributors in USA and Canada.)

69. Udupa, K. N.: "The Ayurvedic System of Medicine in India," in Newell, Kenneth W. (ed.): *Health by the People.* World Health Organization, Geneva, 1975.

70. Kitagawa, Joseph M.: *Religions of the East* (enlarged edition). Westminster Press, Philadelphia, 1968, p. 96.

71. Zaehner, Robert Charles: *Hinduism.* Oxford University Press, New York, 1962.

72. Gandhi, Mohandas Karamchand: *An Autobiography. The Story of My Experiments with Truth.* Beacon Press, Boston, 1940.

73. Noss, John B.: *op. cit.,* p. 89.

74. Kitagawa, Joseph M.: *op. cit.,* p. 153.

75. Eliade, Mircea: *Yoga: Immortality and Freedom.* Pantheon Books, New York, 1958.

76. Basham, A. L.: "Hinduism," in Zaehner, R. C. (ed.): *The Concise Encyclopedia of Living Faiths.* Hawthorne Books, New York, 1959, p. 225.

77. Gandhi, Mohandas Karamchand: *An Autobiography. The Story of My Experiments with Truth.* Beacon Press, Boston, 1940.

78. Basham, A. L.: *op. cit.,* p. 257.

79. Radhakrishnan, Sarvepalli: *Eastern Religions and Western Thought.* Oxford University Press, New York, 1940.

80. Morgan, Kenneth William: *The Religion of*

the Hindus (with contributors). Ronald Press, New York, 1953.

81. Noss, John B.: *op. cit.*

82. Renou, Louis (ed.): *Hinduism.* George Braziller, New York, 1961.

83. Zaehner, Robert Charles: *op. cit.*

84. Basham, A. L.: "Jainism," in Zaehner, R. C. (ed.): *The Concise Encyclopedia of Living Faiths.* Hawthorne Books, New York, 1959, p. 266.

85. Hamilton-Merritt, Jane: *op. cit.*

86. *Life,* Editorial Staff: *The World's Great Religions.* Vol. I: *Religions of the East.* Time Inc., New York, 1963 p. 64.

87. Catholic Hospital Association: *Religious Aspects of Medical Care. A Handbook of Religious Practices of All Faiths.* The Association, St. Louis, 1974, p. 5.

88. Noss, John B.: *op. cit.,* p. 178.

89. Arnold, Sir Edwin: *The Light of Asia,* 65th ed. K. Paul, Trench, Truber, London, 1925.

90. Fêng, Yu-lan: *The Spirit of Chinese Philosophy.* Routledge & K. Paul, London, 1962.

91. Hughes, E. R., and Hughes, K.: *The Religion of China.* Hutchinson's University Library, London, 1950.

92. Lao-Tzu: *The Way of Lao Tzu (Tao-tê Ching).* Bobbs-Merrill, Indianapolis, 1963.

93. Lin Yutang: *The Wisdom of China and India.* Random House, New York, 1942.

94. Yang, C. K.: *Religion in Chinese Society.* University of California Press, Berkeley, 1961.

95. Shryock, John K.: *The Origin and Development of the State Cult of Confucius.* Century Company, New York, 1932. (Reprinted by permission of Appleton-Century-Crofts.)

96. Noss, John B.: *op. cit.,* p. 257.

97. Chan, Wing-tsit: *Religious Trends in Modern China.* Columbia University Press, New York, 1953.

98. Noss, John B.: *op. cit.,* p. 259.

99. *Ibid.,* p. 246.

100. *The I Ching or Book of Changes.* The Richard Wilhelm Translation rendered into English by Cary F. Baynes. Princeton University Press, Princeton, N.J., 1950 (Bollingen Series XIX).

101. Kitagawa, Joseph M. (ed.): *Understanding Modern China.* Quadrangle Books, Chicago, 1969.

102. Chan, Wing-Tsit: *op. cit.*

103. Hertzberg, Arthur (ed.): *Judaism.* George Braziller, New York, 1961, p. 21.

104. *Life,* Editorial Staff: *op. cit.,* pp. 147–57.

105. Applebaum, Morton M.: *What Everyone Should Know About Judaism.* Philosophical Library, New York, [1959].

106. Hertzberg, Arthur (ed.): *op. cit.*

107. *Life,* Editorial Staff: *op. cit.,* p. 158, Vol. 2.

108. Applebaum, Morton M.: *op. cit.*

109. Blau, Joseph L.: *Modern Varieties of Judaism.* Columbia University Press, New York, 1966.

110. Gordis, Robert: *Judaism in a Christian World.* McGraw-Hill Book Co., New York, 1966.

111. Hertzberg, Arthur (ed.): *op. cit.*

112. *Life,* Editorial Staff: *op. cit.,* Vol. 2.

113. Neuser, Jacob: *American Judaism: Adventure in Modernity.* Prentice-Hall, Inc., Englewood Cliffs, N.J., 1972, p. 156.

114. Noss, John B.: *op. cit.,* pp. 363–425.

115. Buber, Martin: *Hasidism.* Philosophical Library, New York, 1948.

116. Sholem, Gershorn G.: "Martin Buber's Interpretation of Hasidism," in Goldin, Judah (ed.): *The Jewish Expression.* Yale University Press, New Haven, Conn., 1976.

117. Noss, John B.: *op. cit.,* p. 422.

118. Katz, Arthur (with Jaime Buckingham): *Ben Israel. Odyssey of a Modern Jew.* Logos International, Plainfield, N.J., 1970.

119. Klausner, Joseph: *The Messianic Idea in Israel, From Its Beginning to the Completion of the Mishnah.* Macmillan Publishing Co., Inc., New York, 1955.

120. Sholem, Gershorn G.: *The Messianic Idea in Judaism and Other Essays on Jewish Spirituality.* Schocken Books, New York, 1971.

121. Werblowsky, R. J. Zwi: "Judaism or the Religion of Israel," in Zaehner, Robert Charles (ed.): *The Concise Encyclopedia of Living Faiths.* Hawthorne Books, New York, 1959, p. 49.

122. Ballou, Robert Oleson: *Shinto, the Unconquered Enemy; Japan's Doctrine of Racial Superiority and World Conquest with Selections from Japanese Texts.* Viking Press, New York, 1945.

123. Noss, John B.: *op. cit.,* pp. 316–40.

124. Wheeler, Post (ed. and translator): *The Sacred Scriptures of the Japanese.* H. Schuman, New York, 1952.

125. Ballou, Robert Oleson: *op. cit.*

126. Noss, John B.: *op. cit.,* p. 322.

127. Herbert, Jean: *Shinto; at the Fountainhead of Japan; with a Preface by Marguis Yukitada Sasaki.* George Allen & Unwin, London, 1967.

128. Muraoka, Tsunetsugu: *Studies in Shinto Thought.* (Translated by Delmer M. Brown and James T. Araki.) Japanese National Commission for UNESCO, Tokyo, 1964.

129. Ross, Floyd Hiatt: *Shinto, the Way of Japan.* Beacon Press, Boston, 1965.

130. Noss, John B.: *op. cit.,* pp. 123–26.

131. *Ibid.,* pp. 325–31.

132. Kitagawa, Joseph M.: *Religion in Japanese History.* Columbia University Press, New York, 1966.

133. Keith, Agnes Newton: *Before the Blossoms Fall. Life and Death in Japan.* (An Atlantic Monthly Press book.) Little, Brown & Co., Boston, 1975, p. 307.

134. Noss, John B.: *op. cit.,* p. 340.

135. Thomsen, Harry: *The New Religions of Japan.* Tuttle, Rutland, Vt., 1963.

136. Noss, John B.: *op. cit.,* p. 337.

137. *Life,* Editorial Staff: *op. cit.,* p. 15, Vol. 1.

138. Noss, John B.: *op. cit.,* p. 343.

139. *Ibid.,* p. 346.

139a. Afnán, Ruhi Muhsen: *Zoroaster's Influence on Greek Thought.* Philosophical Library, New York, 1965.

140. Henning, W. B.: *Zoroaster, Politician or Witch Doctor?* Oxford University Press, New York, 1951.

141. Noss, John B.: *op. cit.,* pp. 345–48.

142. Afnán, Ruhi Muhsen: *op. cit.*

143. *Songs of Zarathustra.* The Gathas Translated from the Avesta by Dastar Framroze, Ardeshir Dade and Piloo Nanavulty. George Allen & Unwin, London, 1952.

144. Duchesne-Guillemin, Jacques: *Symbols and Values in Zoroastrianism, Their Survival and Renewal.* Harper & Row, New York, 1966.

145. Modi, J. J.: *Religious Ceremonies and Customs of the Parsis,* 2nd ed. J. B. Karani's Sons, Bombay, 1937.

146. Noss, John B.: *op. cit.,* pp. 345–52.

147. Zaehner, Robert Charles: "Zoroastrianism," in Zaehner, Robert Charles (ed.): *The Concise Encyclopedia of Living Faiths.* Hawthorne Books, New York, 1959, p. 209.

148. Hutchinson, Paul, and Garrison, Winfred E.: *20 Centuries of Christianity.* Harcourt Brace, New York, 1959, pp. 7, 14.

149. Walker, Williston: *A History of the Christian Church,* 3rd ed. Charles Scribner's Sons, New York, 1970.

150. Noss, John B.: *op. cit.,* pp. 215, 352–58, 402–405.

151. Katz, Arthur (with Jaime Buckingham): *op. cit.*

152. Noss, John B.: *op. cit.,* p. 434.

153. Burke, J. Bruce: *Foundations of Christianity.* Ronald Press, New York, 1970.

154. Hutchinson, Paul, and Garrison, Winfred E.: *op. cit.,* pp. 1–8.

155. Noss, John B.: *op. cit.,* pp. 430–33.

156. Riggin, George A.: *Messianic Theology and Christian Faith.* Westminster Press, Philadelphia, 1967.

157. Robinson, James M.: *A New Quest of the Historical Jesus.* Studies in Biblical Theology. Student Christian Movement Press, London, 1959.

158. Neill, Stephen: *Jesus Through Many Eyes. Introduction to the Theology of the New Testament.* Fortress Press, Philadelphia, 1976.

159. Noss, John B.: *op. cit.,* pp. 459, 213.

160. Walker, Williston: *A History of the Christian Church,* 3rd ed. Scribners, New York, 1970.

161. *Life,* Editorial Staff: *op. cit.,* p. 215.

162. Noss, John B.: *op. cit.,* pp. 443–46.

163. *Ibid.,* p. 449.

164. *Ibid.,* p. 454.

165. Neill, Stephen: *op. cit.*

166. Noss, John B.: *op. cit.,* p. 455.

167. Robinson, John A. T.: *Honest to God.* Westminster Press, Philadelphia, 1963.

168. Robinson, John A. T.: *In the End, God.* Religious Perspectives Vol. 20. Harper & Row, New York, 1968.

169. Robinson, John A. T.: *The Human Face of God.* Westminster Press, Philadelphia, 1973.

170. Biggs, Wilfred W.: *Introduction to the History of the Christian Church.* E. Arnold, London, 1965.

171. Dawson, Christopher: *The Formation of Christendom.* Sheed & Ward, New York, 1967.

172. Hutchinson, Paul, and Garrison, Winfred E.: *op. cit.*

173. *Life,* Editorial Staff: *op. cit.,* pp. 215–39, Vol. 2.

174. Meyer, Carl S., and Tjernagel, Neelak S.: *A History of Western Civilization.* Concordia Publishing House, St. Louis, 1971.

175. Noss, John B.: *op. cit.,* pp. 481–83, 487–92.

176. Zaehner, Robert Charles: *op. cit.*

177. *Life,* Editorial Staff: *op. cit.,* p. 220, Vol. 2.

177a. Jurgi, Edward Jabra: *The Ecumenical Era in Church and Society. A Symposium in Honor of John A. Mackey.* Macmillan Publishing Co., Inc., New York, 1959.

178. *The New English Bible with the Apocrypha.* Oxford University Press, New York, 1971. (Prepared under the direction of representatives of 13 Protestant and Roman Catholic Organizations.)

179. *Good News Bible. The Bible in Today's English Version.* American Bible Society, New York, 1976. (Prepared under the direction of the American Bible Society and the British and Foreign Bible Society.)

179a. *The Way. The Living Bible Illustrated.* Tyndale House Publishers, Wheaton, Ill., 1971.

180. Robinson, John A. T.: *Honest to God, op. cit.*

181. Cullman, Oscar: *Vatican Council II; The New Direction.* Essays Selected and Arranged by James D. Hester. (Religious Perspectives). Harper & Row, New York, 1968.

182. Falconi, Carlo: *The Popes in the Twentieth Century. From Pius X to John XXIII.* Little, Brown & Co., Boston, 1967.

183. Pope John XXIII: *Pacem in Terres. Encyclical of Pope John XXIII.* Paulist-Newman Press, Paramus, N.J., 1975.

184. Zaehner, Robert Charles: *Concordant Discord: The Interdependence of Faiths.* Oxford University Press, New York, 1970.

185. Connell, Francis J.: *The Seven Sacraments.* Paulist-Newman Press, Paramus, N.J., 1966.

186. *Life,* Editorial Staff: *op. cit.,* pp. 308–19, Vol. 2.

187. Noss, John B.: *op. cit.*

188. Morgan, Kenneth Williams: *Islam, The Straight Path; Islam Interpreted by Muslims.* Ronald Press, New York, 1958.

189. Holt, P. M., et al. (eds): *The Cambridge History of Islam.* Cambridge University Press, Cambridge, Eng., 1970, 2 vol.

190. Jeffery, Arthur (ed.): *Islam: Muhammad*

and His Religion. Liberal Arts Press, New York, 1958.

191. Khan, Muhammad Zafrulla: *Islam; Its Meaning for Modern Man.* (Religious Perspectives Vol. 7.) Harper & Row, New York, 1962, p. 20.

192. Watt, W. Montgomery: *Muhammad: Prophet and Statesman.* Oxford University Press, New York, 1961.

193. Noss, John B.: *op. cit.,* p. 524.

194. *Ibid.,* p. 534.

195. *Ibid.,* p. 526.

196. Khan, Muhammad Zafrulla: *op. cit.,* p. 66.

197. Williams, John A. (ed.): *Islam.* George Braziller, New York, 1961.

198. Noss, John B.: *op. cit.,* p. 536.

199. Naseem, M.: *Religious Toleration in Islam.* London Mosque, London, 1965.

200. Noss, John B.: *op. cit.,* p. 554.

201. Hitti, Philip Khuri: *Islam, A Way of Life.* Henry Regnery Co., Chicago, 1970.

202. Sidjabat, Walter Bonar: *Religious Tolerance and the Christian Faith.* (Dissertation submitted to Princeton University.) Penerbit Kristen Day Missions, Badan.

203. Spencer, H.: *Islam and the Gospel of God; A Comparison of the Central Doctrines of Christianity and Islam Prepared for the Use of Christian Workers Among Muslims.* S.P.C.K., Delhi, 1956.

204. Watt, William Montgomery: *Islamic Revelation in the Modern World.* Edinburgh University Press, Edinburgh, 1969.

205. Jaehner, Robert Charles: *Christianity and Other Religions.* Hawthorne Books, New York, [1964].

206. Zaehner, Robert Charles: *The Concise Encyclopedia of Living Faiths.* Hawthorne Books, New York, 1959.

207. Noss, John B.: *op. cit.,* p. 557.

208. Khan, Muhammad Zafrulla: *op. cit.,* pp. 112–116.

209. Noss, John B.: *op. cit.,* p. 557.

210. Khan, Muhammad Zafrulla: *op. cit.,* p. 112.

211. *Ibid.,* p. 184.

212. *Life,* Editorial Staff: *op. cit.,* p. 127, Vol. 2.

213. Wheelock, Robert D.: *Health Care Ministries. A Guide to Organization, Management, Evaluation.* Catholic Hospital Association, St. Louis, 1975, p. 112.

214. Bean, William A.: "Of Doctors and Priests," in Belgum, David (ed.): *Religion and Medicine.* Iowa State University Press, Ames, 1967, p. V.

215. Jung, Carl: *Modern Man in Search of a Soul.* Harcourt, Brace & Co., New York, 1934, p. 264.

216. Frankl, Victor E.: *Man's Search for Meaning.* Beacon Press, Boston, 1963.

217. Ashbrook, James B.: "The Impact of the Hospital Situation in Our Understanding of God and Man," in Belgum, David (ed.): *Religion and Medicine.* Iowa State University Press, Ames, 1967, p. 61.

218. Booth, Gotthard: "The Voice of the Body," in Belgum, David (ed.): *Religion and Medicine.* Iowa State University Press, Ames, 1967, p. 96.

219. Jackson, Gordon E.: "The Problem of Guilt," in Belgum, David (ed.): *Religion and Medicine.* Iowa State University Press, Ames, 1967, p. 216.

220. Becker, Russell J.: "Sin, Illness and Guilt," in Belgum, David (ed.): *Religion and Medicine.* Iowa State University Press, Ames, 1967, p. 236.

221. Elsässer, Gunter: "Objective Guilt and Neurosis," in Belgum, David (ed.): *Religion and Medicine.* Iowa State University Press, Ames, 1967, p. 245.

222. Niklas, Gerald R., and Stefanics, Charlotte: *Ministry to the Hospitalized.* Paulist-Newman Press, Paramus, N.J., 1975.

223. Sobel, David: "Love and Pain," *Am. J. Nurs.,* **72:**910, (May) 1972.

223a. Zeller, William W.: "Values in Sickness and Health," in Belgum, David (ed.): *Religion and Medicine.* Iowa State University Press, Ames, 1967, p. 256.

224. Stallwood, Jean, and Stoll, Ruth: "Spiritual Dimensions of Nursing Practice," in Beland, Irene L., and Passos, Joyce Y.: *Clinical Nursing: Pathophysiological and Psychosocial Approaches,* 3rd ed. Macmillan Publishing Co., Inc., New York, 1975, p. 1086.

225. Kelly, Lucie Young: *Dimensions of Professional Nursing,* 3rd ed. Macmillan Publishing Co., Inc., New York, 1975, pp. 222–40.

226. Dickinson, Sister Corita: "The Search for Spiritual Meaning," *Am. J. Nurs.,* **75:**1789, (Oct.) 1975.

227. Piepgras, Ruth: "The Other Dimension: Spiritual Help," *Am. J. Nurs.,* **68:**2610, (Dec.) 1968.

228. Rogers, Martha E.: *Nursing Science I. An Introduction to Theoretical Basis of Nursing.* F. A. Davis Co., Philadelphia, 1970.

229. Travelbee, Joyce: *Interpersonal Aspects of Nursing.* F. A. Davis Co., Philadelphia, 1966.

230. Ujhely, Gertrud B.: "What Is Realistic Emotional Support?" *Am. J. Nurs.,* **68:**762, (Apr.) 1968.

231. Vaillot, Sister Madeleine Clémence: "Existentialism: A Philosophy of Commitment," *Am. J. Nurs.,* **66:**504, (Mar.) 1966.

232. Carkhaff, Robert: *Helping and Human Relations.* Holt, Rinehart & Winston, New York, 1969, 2 vols.

233. Elkington, J. R.: "The Experimental Use of Human Beings" (editorial), *Ann. Int. Med.,* **65:**371, (Aug.) 1966.

234. Fletcher, G. P.: "Legal Aspects of the Decision Not to Prolong Life," *J.A.M.A.,* **203:** 65, (Jan. 1) 1968.

235. Freund, P. A.: "Ethical Problems in Human Experimentation," *N. Engl. J. Med.,* **273:** 687, (Sept. 23) 1965.

236. Graubard, S. R. (ed.): "Ethical Aspects of Experimentation with Human Subjects," *Daedalus,* Spring 1969.

237. Calderone, Mary S.: "Sex, Religion and Mental Health," *J. Religion Health,* (July) 1967.
238. Johnson, Eric W.: *Love and Sex in Plain Language.* J. B. Lippincott Co., Philadelphia, 1965.
239. Wynn, John Charles (ed.): *Sex, Family, and Society in Theological Focus.* Association Press, New York, 1966.
240. World Health Organization, Expert Committee on Human Genetics: *Genetic Counselling; Third Report of the Expert Committee. . . .* The Organization, Geneva, 1969 (Tech. Rep. Series No. 416).
241. Wolstenholme, G. E. W., and O'Connor, M. (ed.): *Ethics in Medical Progress with Special Reference to Transplantation.* A Ciba Foundation Symposium. Little, Brown, & Co., Boston, 1966.

Additional Suggested Reading

Bane, J. Donald, et al.: *Death and the Ministry. Pastoral Care of Dying and Bereaved.* Schocken Books, New York, 1975.
Berkowitz, P., et al.: "The Jewish Patient in the Hospital," *Am. J. Nurs.,* **67:**2335, (Nov.) 1967.
Catholic Hospital Association: *The Updated Chaplaincy. Workshop Proceedings.* The Association, St. Louis, [1975].
Cousins, Ewert H. (ed.): *Process Theology: Basic Writings.* Newman Press, New York, 1971.
Dickinson, Sister Corita: "The Search for Spiritual Meaning," *Am. J. Nurs.,* **75:**1789, (Oct.) 1975.
Feldman, David M.: *Birth Control and Jewish Law; Marital Relations, Contraception, and Abortion as Set Forth in the Classic Texts of Jewish Law.* New York University Press, New York, 1968.
Frazier, Claude A.: *Healing and Religious Faith.* United Church Press, Philadelphia, 1974.
Jakobovits, Immanual: *Jewish Medical Ethics. A Comparative and Historical Study of the Jewish Religious Attitude to Medicine and Its Practice.* Bloch Publishing Co., New York, 1975.
Kelsey, Morton T.: *Healing and Christianity; In Ancient Thought and Modern Times.* Harper & Row, New York, 1973.
Laurentin, René: *Liberation, Development and Salvation.* Translated by Charles Underhill Quinn. Orbis Books, Maryknoll, N.Y., 1972.
Marty, Martin E.: *The Pro and Con of Religious America. A Bicentennial Argument.* Word Books, Waco, Tex., 1975.
Morris, Karen, and Foerster, John: "Team Work: Nurse and Chaplain," *Am. J. Nurs.,* **72:**2197, (Dec.) 1972.
O'Rourke, Kevin D. (ed.): *Mission of Healing.* Catholic Hospital Association, St. Louis, 1974.
Tillich, Paul: *The Courage To Be.* Yale University Press, New Haven, Conn., 1952.
Tournier, Paul: *The Healing of Persons.* Harper & Row, New York, 1965.
Whitman, Helen H., and Lukes, Shelby J.: "Behavior Modification for Terminally Ill Patients," *Am. J. Nurs.,* **75:**98, (Jan.) 1975.
Wilson, C. R. M.: "The Public Health Nurse and the Parish Minister," *Can. J. Public Health,* **61:**112, (Mar.–Apr.) 1970.

Virginia Henderson

Therapeutic Measures, Procedures, or Techniques that Nurses Perform or Help Patients, Their Families, and Medical Workers (Other Than Nurses) Perform

CHAPTER 19

Basis for the Selection of Method. Research as a Means of Improving Nursing Practice

1. BASIS FOR THE SELECTION OF METHOD

Part IV, which this chapter introduces, is devoted to therapeutic measures, procedures, or techniques. Every profession embodies method as well as theory, and the competence of its practitioners can be measured by their mastery of method as well as their knowledge of underlying principles. Creativity, a quality characteristic of those who practice, not only competently but imaginatively, is hard to measure but is perhaps the most important quality in a rapidly changing environment.*

The position is taken by the authors of this text that nursing is both a science and an art. Those who practice it are urged to be scientists, which means a lifetime of study, for without it they may be implementing discredited data †; but they are also urged to be

---

* Benjamin A. Kogan, in his work *Health: Man in a Changing Environment* (Harcourt, Brace & World, New York, 1970), says the central and recurring theme of his book is how people can achieve harmony between their "slowly changing inner environment and their rapidly changing outer environment" (p. IX).

† *Truth*
For what is truth?
Since it is found to be,
Later, no more than sooth-
sayer's early fantasy
So often! But may you
Guard what your conscience tells
Or mind thinks to be true;
For he who conscience sells;
That sale will rue!

Evelyn Princeps

creative in their practice. Painters respond to an inner prompting that says this is "true" or "beautiful," but without a knowledge of technique they cannot make their inner vision a reality or paint a picture whose colors remain unchanged; architects may design a beautiful house, but if it is to withstand the elements they must know the science of building.

The science of nursing is ultimately as useful as it is effective in helping people achieve a higher standard of health. Since each person is unique, his or her plan of care and the way it is implemented must be unique to some extent; therefore, the methods in Part IV are "suggested procedures," modifiable as the situation demands.

The suggested procedures are based on all that the writers have learned. People learn in various ways and base their conclusions, or judgments, on intuition, authority, tradition, inductive and deductive reasoning, random and planned experience, and on scientific investigation, or research. These processes range from the most inborn, or universal, to the most learned, selective, or sophisticated. They include the chief bases for action among primitive peoples, the Socratic method of reasoning —which put the Classical Greek intellectually ahead of his contemporaries—and the process of research, which is modern man's approach to solving problems of education, industry, government, and all professional practice, including that in the field of health.

Before presenting a suggested procedure in Chapters 20 through 34, pertinent research or the conflicting views of experts in the field found in the literature are cited. In discussing preparation for nursing in Chapter 1, we showed that basic nursing curricula in the universities of the United States included the widest range of physical, biologic, and social sciences. The position was taken that all health workers are dependent on the knowledge developed in these fields and that "medical science" and "nursing science" are questionable entities since the boundaries between them and between each with other sciences are constantly shifting. So it will not surprise readers to find that the research cited in Part IV is drawn from many fields; it may or may not surprise them to see that a small proportion of the investigations cited were conducted by nurses. The fact that there is comparatively little research on nursing practice is explained in the following pages.

2. THE DEVELOPMENT OF NURSING RESEARCH

Nursing, which as someone has said, was born in the church and bred in the military, has relied heavily on authority and tradition, not to mention intuition. There is evidence, however, that some "professional" nurses in every decade since 1860 have used the approach of a researcher in seeking solutions to problems. In Chapter 1, we noted that Florence Nightingale spent many more years in research on health problems than in administering nursing services—the work for which she is famous. She was an expert statistician who persuaded the British Government to make changes in the military and colonial health services because she collected, reported, and interpreted the facts about current practices so thoroughly and effectively that she could show the advantage of change over the status quo.[1]

The system of nursing in our Western culture derives from the practices Florence Nightingale advocated in *Notes on Nursing* and other publications on nursing education written before 1900. These works and the Nightingale pattern of nursing have been widely acclaimed; few people seem to have recognized and emulated Miss Nightingale's ability to conduct investigations and use the findings as leverage for social action or as a basis for nursing practice. While certain British nurses, such as Ethel Gordon Fenwick, may have appreciated the full range of Florence Nightingale's accomplishments, M. Adelaide Nutting and Isabel M. Stewart in the United States were certainly aware of the importance of her research as well as her revolutionary concepts

about health promotion and the care of the sick. They showed this awareness in their writings and they followed her example to some extent.

In 1907, Nutting [2] conducted a survey of nursing schools addressed to the US Office of Education. It is often referred to as the first full-scale investigation in nursing. Stewart and other outstanding nurses of that period, as, for example, Annie W. Goodrich, continued to use surveys and statistical reports to demonstrate the need for change in nursing education and administration. In 1909 a national survey of public health nursing showed the wide variety of practice and administrative policy.[3] It introduced a new era in this type of nursing which soon attracted independent and well-prepared nurses who continued to rely on surveys of practice.

During the twenties and thirties there was a movement toward standardization in industry, education, and health agencies.* Frank Taylor and Frank Galbraith conducted many highly publicized industrial studies and Lillian M. Galbraith (wife of Frank) continued this work after his death up until recent times.[4]

The American Hospital Association, seeing in the operation of hospitals many parallels with industry and education, set up a Simplification and Standardization Committee whose recommendations soon influenced working conditions, hospital structure, furnishings and supplies.[5] The committee worked closely with the US Bureau of Standards and nongovernmental agencies set up to protect and inform consumers. In this era, industries created research units that resulted in standardized products and processes. Labor shortage in World War I (and later in World War II) intensified the search for uniform and reliable machine-made products. Supplies that were once made by nurses, as, for example, dressings and solutions, were replaced by commercially prepared supplies. Time, motion, and cost studies were instituted in this period. Ralph M. Barnes [6] gives the history of these processes and the related aspects of industrial management. Blanche Pfefferkorn and Marion Rottman's *Clinical Education in Nursing* [7] was actually an activity analysis and time study.

---

* William Bagley, an educator at Teachers College, Columbia University, discussing standardization in education during the 1920s, used to say that the French Minister of Education claimed that, on looking at his watch during a school day, he could say what every child in every grade of the French schools was doing at that moment. It is small wonder that the first national curriculum in nursing, published by the National League of Nursing Education in 1917, was called *The Standard Curriculum*.

But even earlier, Stewart realized the applicability of time, motion, and cost studies to nursing. She also sensed the limitation and possible danger of the standardization movement. She pointed out the difference between industry, where the goal is a uniform product, and a health service, where the product must not be standardized because the needs of each person served are unique. In an article titled "Possibilities of Standardization in Nursing Technique," [8] she emphasized the importance of using what she believed were "flexible" standards. She said, in effect, that the reliability of each procedure should be judged on the following basis:

1. Does it provide maximal *safety* for the patient, the nurse and other persons involved?
2. Is it *therapeutically effective?*
3. Does it provide the greatest degree of *comfort and happiness (or least amount of pain) for the patient* that is consistent with accomplishing the therapeutic aim?
4. Is it as *economical* of time, effort, and materials as it can be made without sacrificing the first three factors?
5. Does the equipment present a pleasing appearance and [does] the performance give an impression of finished workmanship?
6. Is the procedure as *simple* as it can be made without destroying its therapeutic effectiveness, safety, and comfort, and is it *adaptable* to hospital and home nursing?

Had she added the questions Does it take into consideration the patient's wishes? and Does it provide for optimum patient independence, participation, and learning? the Stewart criteria would be as acceptable today as they were in 1919. Her article was the cornerstone for a course initiated at Teachers College, Columbia University, about 1930 that was later called "Comparative Nursing Practice." It introduced students to the research process. Nursing procedures or techniques were evaluated for their safety, therapeutic effectiveness, comfort, economy, and esthetic appeal. Each student, either alone or with others, conducted a library investigation, an interview or questionnaire survey, and a laboratory experiment or some other kind of study.*

Stewart and her associates, appreciating the importance of research, proposed in 1930 the establishment of an institute for nursing research within the Department of Nursing Education at Teachers College.[9,10] Jean Broadhurst, a bacteriologist there, strongly supported this position. Her support is evidenced by the number of bacteriologic studies made by graduate nurse students under her direction in the 1920s and 1930s.* With Martha Ruth Smith of the Nursing Faculty, Broadhurst edited a text on the principles of nursing care [11] which dealt with the science underlying nursing rather than its techniques. During the publication of the *Nursing Education Bulletin* at Teachers College, it carried very little except the reports of studies by students and faculty. An Institute of Research and Service in Nursing Education was finally established at the College in 1953 (and was the first such institute in a university), but the studies conducted under its sponsorship since have rarely been directly related to nursing practice.† In fact, until this decade, nursing research has focused on educational or occupational problems (see Table 19-1). Leo W. Simmons and Virginia Henderson showed this clearly in their 1964 report, *Nursing Research—A Survey and Assessment.*[12] ‡ Because so many studies were focused on the nurse rather than nursing, the second author, while making this survey, was moved to write an editorial in *Nursing Research,* the journal initiated in 1952, "Research in Nursing—When?" [13]

For the first three or four decades of the twentieth century, studies focused on practice were designed chiefly to make a nursing procedure, or specific activity, more valid; just as most medical research was designed to make a laboratory test more reliable, an operation or a drug safer and more effective. Research in the health field was more likely to be technical

* The following are examples of studies made by students: (1) the effect of smoking just before measuring body temperature by mouth; (2) the sedative effect of a cold wet sheet pack as compared with a warm wet sheet pack; (3) the optimum temperature for a perineal cleansing solution, an eye or ear irrigation; (4) the amounts of fluid held, or the distention of the colon tolerated, by persons while having a cleansing enema; (5) the fears and discomforts of a person in a body cast; and (6) the safety

and comfort factors with different types of lubricants for urinary, nasal, or rectal intubations. A number of such studies were published in nursing journals of this era.

* In this era, before the development of the sulfa drugs and antibiotics and many of the vaccines, infectious diseases were man's chief enemies. Medical research focused on them very largely and it is not surprising that nursing studies of this period did likewise.

† Because of the emphasis on education research, Harriet Werley and Fredericka P. Shea describe the Center for Nursing Research at Wayne State University, Detroit, Mich., as "The First Center for Research in Nursing," (*Nurs. Res.,* **22:**217, [May–June] 1973.)

‡ The history of research in nursing is traced in this report during the period of development [of nursing] 1870–1900; period of expansion 1900–1930; period of stock-taking and upswing in research 1930–

Table 19-1. Table Showing 1464 Master's Theses and Papers Written During the Late 1940s and 1950s Showing the Preponderant Emphasis on Study of Educational Problems.*

Classification	Number	Per Cent of Total
A. History, culture, philosophy	186	12.70
B. Occupation (general)	71	4.85
C. Occupation (special fields)	94	6.42
D. Nursing organizations	2	.10
E. Nursing service administration	158	10.79
F. Nursing care	211	14.47
G. Patients' reactions to identifiable variables	35	2.39
H. Human relations—interaction	27	1.84
I. Education	680	46.44
Total	1464	100.00

* Simmons, Leo W., and Henderson, Virginia: *Nursing Research: A Survey and Assessment,* Appleton-Century-Crofts, New York, 1964, p. 119.

rather than philosophic. The virtue of the health system had not come under such a barrage of criticism as it has in this era. It was generally assumed that if the parts of which it was composed were each more reliable, the system as a whole might meet the needs of man. However, some persons in every decade *were* doubtful about the health care system. Some nurses, and others too, questioned the way students were selected for nursing, the way they were prepared, the conditions under which they worked, and in general, the utilization of the services they were prepared to give. In the survey of research reported by Simmons and Henderson in 1964, the most persistent question asked by approximately 500 persons interviewed was, "What is the [proper] function of the nurse?"

In 1950, the American Nurses' Association instituted a 5-year program to study the function of the nurse. By 1957, $400,000 had been spent on 21 separate studies conducted in 17 states and reported in 1958 by Everett C. Hughes et al. in *Twenty Thousand Nurses Tell Their Story.*[14] While this momentous nationwide effort failed, apparently, to give a final and satisfactory answer to the question, "What is the function of the nurse?" it provided an enormous amount of information about nursing. One study, for example, showed the wide range of nursing activities (more than 400) for hospital nurses in one statewide investigation and other studies threw considerable light on the concepts held about nurses and nursing and on many occupational problems.[15] As noted earlier in this text, this investigation is one of six or more nationwide studies that, made periodically during the twentieth century, have identified and focused attention on occupational problems. Some of the data collected in such studies is now kept current in

the United States by the ANA's annual publication, *Facts About Nursing.*[16] The Canadian Nurses' Association publishes a comparable annual publication titled *Countdown.*[17] National nursing organizations around the world are committed to occupational research but they are also beginning to promote research on nursing practice.

In 1953, the major national nursing organizations in the United States implemented the recommendations of their Structure Study begun in 1948 and research units were created in each.* In 1956, the American Nurses' Foundation was established as an independent agency to accept funds, make grants for, and conduct research. It maintains a directory of nurses with earned doctoral degrees.[18] Generally speaking, most graduate programs now offer or require clinically oriented research experience. Educational programs for graduate nurses were first nothing more than post-basic experience in hospitals. However, a midwifery program based at Teachers College was developed during the 1930s, and in the next decade, programs in pediatric, psychiatric, and medical-surgical nursing were developed. Other programs in general public health, school nursing, or industrial nursing at Teachers College offered field experience with emphasis on practice. After World War II the national nursing organizations began to emphasize the importance of post-basic, collegiate study of clinical nursing. Presently, this is the emphasis in most graduate programs rather than the functions

* The ANA now has a Commission on Nursing Research and a Council of Nurse Researchers responsible to the Commission, who are nurses with earned doctor's or master's degrees who are engaged in research. (Notter, Lucile E.: "The New Council of Nurse Researchers," *Nurs. Res.,* 21:293, [July–Aug.] 1972.)

of teaching, supervision, and administration. The fact, however, that so many degree-holding nurses were then and still are fully occupied in teaching, supervision, and administration has undoubtedly led graduate students to investigate nonclinical questions. The current preoccupations with recognizing, legalizing, and preparing the nurse for an expanding clinical role, eliminating nonnursing functions, and reducing the administrative superstructure in health service, have created an insistent demand for research centered on nursing practice.

Many of the national nursing investigations, as, for example, that directed by Esther Lucile Brown,[19] reported in 1948 under the title, *Nursing for the Future*, stressed the importance of research. The latest study by the National Commission for the Study of Nursing and Nursing Education, reported as *An Abstract for Action*,[20] gives the most persuasive argument for the research approach in dealing with all aspects of nursing—practice, administration, and education.

Nurses employed in the national, state, provincial, and local governments of many countries, most particularly in the United States, have made signal contributions to the development of nursing research. For example, Marion Ferguson and Pearl McIver of the US Public Health Service began, even before World War II, to foster nursing investigations. During World War II, with the creation of the Cadet Nurse Corps in 1943 and the Division of Nursing of the USPHS in 1949, nursing research was seen as essential to the development of nursing. Faye G. Abdellah, Margaret Arnstein, Ava Dilworth, Lucile Petry Leone, Jessie Scott, and Ellwynne Vreeland are among those who have fully appreciated the importance of research. Studies conducted or sponsored by the Division were, at first, surveys of nursing needs and resources. In 1954, Abdellah reported that since 1947, "37 states, the District of Columbia, and the Territory of Hawaii have used the nursing survey as a tool for identifying the most important community nursing problems which demand action and about which something can be done." * During the last and the current decade the national nursing agencies and health agencies of which nursing is a part in the United States tend to encourage other types of studies and particularly clinical investigations.

Since the creation of the Division of Nursing in the USPHS, grants totaling approximately $39 million (fiscal years 1956–June 1976)[21] have been made for all kinds of nursing studies. Figure 19-1 shows total federal outlays for health research in 1969 and 1974. Nurses in these agencies have worked with the ANA's Research and Statistics Unit and have played important roles in the creation of the Journal *Nursing Research* and in international, regional, state, and local conferences devoted to discussing and promoting nursing research. The National Center for Health Services Research and Development, established in 1968, and reorganized as the Bureau of Research and Evaluation in 1973, is said by Faye G. Abdellah, the former Deputy Director, to have as one of its primary goals the evaluation of new types of health manpower vital to the improved delivery of health services." * Rita K. Chow, a former member of the Bureau's staff, has reported a method for identifying and categorizing nursing action in the care of patients with cardiac surgery that has general application. Reviewing current proposals for reducing the roadblocks in the delivery of health care, she says, "There is urgent need for increased efforts by all health professionals to analyze and synthesize more efficient modes of organizing and delivering health services research." † She presents a diagram suggesting the needed (interdisciplinary) research methodology.

While it is not possible to discuss even the high points in the development of nursing research around the world, we might mention that the Canadian Nurses' Association publishes an annual list of nursing studies, *Index of Canadian Nursing Studies*[22]; the Finnish Foundation for Nursing Education's *Yearbook of Nursing* is a collection of study reports[23]; there is an international journal devoted to research, the *International Journal of Nursing Studies*.

Professional nurses have always been involved in the physician's clinical research but they have, for the most part, played a passive and relatively uninformed role. Stanhope Bayne-Jones,[24] a physician writing in 1950, said that the role of a laboratory technician was more likely to be recognized in written reports of research in medical journals than that of the nurse. However, today, interdisciplinary research (but with the nurse as full partner) is more likely, in some quarters, to find a sponsor than research devoted to the concern of one discipline. Research-conscious and often knowledgeable nurses are working closely with physicians, statisticians, physical, biologic, and

---

* Abdellah, Faye G.: "Surveys Stimulate Community Action," *Nurs. Outlook,* **2:**268, (May) 1954.

* Abdellah, Faye G.: "Evolution of Nursing as a Profession. Perspective on Manpower Development," *Int. Nurs. Rev.,* **19:**319, (No. 3) 1972.
† Chow, Rita K.: "Research + Primex = Improved Health Services," *Int. Nurs. Rev.,* **19:**319, (No. 4) 1972. (Primex is a family nurse practitioner or a "primary care extender.")

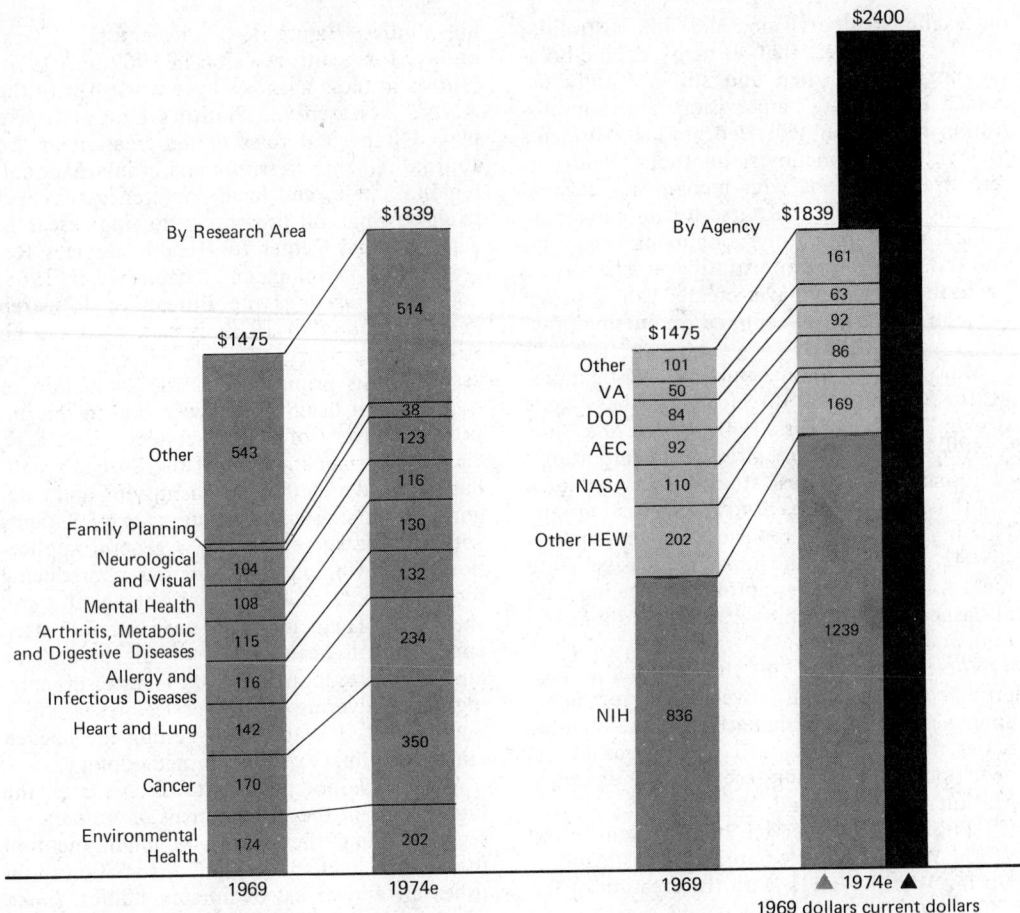

Figure 19-1. Graph showing federal outlay for research in 1974 as compared with 1969. (Center for Health Policy Studies, National Planning Association: *Chartbook of Federal Health Spending, 1969–74*. The Association, Washington, D.C., 1974, p. 9.)

social scientists in such agencies in the United States as the National Center for Health Services Research and Development, and the National Institutes of Health, as well as in many health organizations and foundations. Nurses in some states have, with physicians, social scientists, and others, designed and carried out interdisciplinary studies under the sponsorship of regional medical programs.

Vernon W. Lippard, in *A Half Century of American Medical Education: 1920–1970* (Josiah Macy, Jr. Foundation, New York, 1974, p. 73), showed the expansion of federal funds for medical research. He noted that 1930 legislation changed the name of the Hygienic Laboratory, established in 1887, to the National Institute of Health. Its appropriation in 1931 was $43,000. The National Cancer Institute was created in 1937. The establishment of the Office of Scientific Research

and Development in the 1940s led to large-scale appropriations. The National Science Foundation was established in 1950. The P.H.S. Omnibus Act this same year empowered the Surgeon General to establish separate institutes to support research in neurologic diseases and blindness, arthritis, and metabolic disease, allergy, and infectious diseases. Within 20 years the total dollars for medical research increased 24 times.

While physicians may have been slow to collaborate with nurses as full partners in clinical research, many social scientists seem to have embraced the opportunity. These circumstances and the current and growing emphasis on the psychosocial aspects of health and disease may account for the fact that most of the clinical nursing research lies within this area.

Since 1958, a number of volumes devoted to

nursing research have been published. Some are surveys, others are source books, and others are on method; some serve many purposes.[25-31] The authors of these works are nurses and social scientists. A 1970 publication by three sociologists (all of whom are members of the faculties in university schools of nursing) is titled *Behavioral Science, Social Practice, and the Nursing Profession.*[32] The authors accept the position (which they seem to think is held by most nurses) that the physician's goal is cure or "the more or less permanent correction of the patient's diagnosed pathology" and "The goals of nursing treatment [meeting the patient's 'situationally derived needs,' including his response to the biophysical treatment] are usually short term and palliative rather than curative." The writers say that the boundaries of research in any profession are set by the limits of its responsibility for prescribing action and they suggest that it is only within the realm of social science (or human interaction) that the nurse is free to prescribe. Hence the supposition that finding the rational bases for nursing practice through research is largely a task for nurses in collaboration with social scientists. Robert Leonard, the third author of this monograph, with Florence Wald [33] published an often-cited article "Toward Development of Nursing Practice Theory" in which they follow this same line of reasoning—that nursing contribution is largely one of interaction. The authors suggest that research methods used in the physical and biologic sciences aren't appropriate for the study of nursing practice.

In discussing the term "nursing science" in Chapter 1, we took the position that it was not different from medical, or health, science; nor were these independent or different from the biologic sciences. In other words, a rational practice for any health practitioner depends on research that may take the researcher into the field of the physicist, the chemist, the microbiologist, the physiologist, the psychologist, the anthropologist, the sociologist, the lawyer, or the economist. We believe that the nurse is presently, and within the legal meaning of nursing as defined by nurse practice acts (and statements of official nursing organizations), initiating or prescribing treatments or protective measures that relate to all these fields. Nurses, for example, decide how to keep the mouth of an unconscious patient clean, how to prevent pressure sores, or when the comatose are sufficiently recovered to be safely fed by mouth, just as they initiate measures to persuade the mute to talk or the agitated and anxious to express their fears. Even though a treatment, such as an enema, may be pre-

scribed by physicians, nurses select the equipment, often the injected liquid, and they help the patient take the treatment so that the therapeutic purpose is accomplished. While physicians prescribe and sometimes (but not always) start an intravenous feeding or medication, its safe and effective administration is largely dependent on nurses. Some procedures, as for example lumbar punctures, are prescribed and carried out by physicians but nurses work with them in preparing patients, giving the treatment, and giving aftercare. Whether or not nurses play a major or minor role in prescribing, initiating, and carrying out a treatment, they have a professional responsibility for validating, or rationalizing through research, what they do and how they do it.

Tracing the development of nursing research from the time of Florence Nightingale to the present, we find an uneven progression with changing emphases. First we note in the nineteenth century Nightingale's studies using such data as morbidity and mortality statistics to persuade a national government to alter health services; in the first decades and throughout the succeeding decades of the twentieth century, periodic nationwide educational and socioeconomic surveys; in the third and fourth decades, a number of studies designed to make specific procedures more valid, especially as related to medical and surgical asepsis or the control of infection; in the fourth and fifth decades, surveys of nursing needs and resources and studies of the role and function of the nurse; in the sixth and seventh decades, the emphasis on interaction between nurse and patient—or client—and on studies aimed at the validation or improvement of nursing practice. There is at present a high priority on research and especially on evaluation of nursing care, either alone or as an aspect of health service. In some cases the research attempts to relate the value of care to the type of preparation for nursing. Presently, as pointed out in Chapter 1, there is considerable preoccupation with the development of nursing theory, with assessing the quality of nursing care, and particularly the care given by nurses with special preparation for assuming more than the usual responsibility for clinical management.

3. CRITERIA FOR EVALUATING METHOD OR ASSESSING THE QUALITY OF CARE

The difficulty of measuring the effect of nursing as distinct from the effect of care by other health workers, most notably treatment by the physician, is obvious. Louis I. Dublin,[34] in 1932, evaluated frontier nursing and midwifery services in the Kentucky mountains and was able to show that their first 1000 deliveries were almost totally free from morbidity or mortality. This compared most favorably with mortality rates in the United States or any other country. Nurse-midwifery is, however, atypically independent of medicine in its practice.

The survey and assessment of nursing research by Simmons and Henderson,[35] in the chapter on studies of nursing care, attempts to identify types of evaluative studies through 1963, to give outstanding examples, and to list the research methods or techniques used in making judgment about, or measuring, quality.*

Quality assessment is believed by many persons to be essential in substantiating the claims of professions (including nursing) that the kind (length, content, and methods) of learning in the educational process affect the kind of care graduates give. While patient opinion polls, such as that by Abdellah and Eugene Levine [36] in 1957, indicate that patients rate the services of better-prepared nursing personnel higher than those of less well-prepared ones, the issue is still alive and the search for criteria in measing quality goes on.

Since the roles of nurses, physicians, physical therapists, social workers, and others often overlap, and since what each health worker does affects the total outcome of care, evaluation of any system of care is really a joint responsibility. Paul J. Sanazaro and his associates [37] note that all medical and health care professions and the federal government are involved. Professional Standards Review Organizations (PSRO) composed of physicians have been established in many states and in two states (Utah and Hawaii) include nurses. In 1970, legislation was introduced in the US

Congress to establish such organizations in each state for the purpose of monitoring all medical services reimbursed under provisions of the Social Security Act (P.L. 92–603).*

Effective nursing has always been dependent on the nurse's knowledge of the treatment plan. As nurses assume more responsibility for therapeutic management and as the patient-problem-oriented system of health care spreads, it will be increasingly necessary to make interdisciplinary evaluations.†

Avedis Donabedian,[38-41] discussing the evaluation of medical care between 1966 and 1969, distinguished between assessing the process of care, the organizational structure under which it is given, and the outcome. The Donabedian model provides a basis for an assessment of total quality of care.‡

John W. Williamson [42,43] in 1968 and 1971 discussed priorities and a strategy for relating outcome and process in assessing quality of patient care. This is akin to the Donabedian model.

Another investigator, Beverly C. Payne,[44] developed in 1966 an extensive set of process criteria by which care for in-hospital patients could be assessed.§

---

* These methods or techniques are:

1. Opinionnaires or questionnaires answered in writing or verbally by patients, nurses, doctors, and others; accompanied, or unaccompanied by pictures showing persons or situations—comparing what someone thinks the patient needs with what he gets.

2. Analysis of critical incidents showing effective and noneffective, or even destructive, nursing.

3. Interviews, with or without written schedules, "Q-sorts" or pictures, and other descriptive materials, such as case studies.

4. Observation and analysis of patient-nurse (or other) interaction and changes in the behavior or appearance of patients.

5. Clinical tests for changes in physical status such as measurement of blood pressure, body temperature, or gain of weight.

6. Study of patients' records to find evidence of certain services to the patient or of physical changes, psychosocial behavior and the status of patients with relation to independence or rehabilitation.

---

* Monitoring would answer the questions, Were the services medically necessary and of an acceptable professional standard. This would include hospitalization.

† This system, usually called "the Weed System," is discussed in Chapters 4 and 8 and is referred to repeatedly throughout this text. (See also Weed, Lawrence L.: *Medical Records, Medical Education and Patient Care: The Problem-Oriented Record as a Basic Tool.* Case-Western Reserve University Press, Cleveland, 1969.)

‡ I. *Physician Behavior*—A. Technical management of health and illness, 1. adequacy of diagnosis, 2. adequacy of therapy, 3. parsimony or minimum redundancy in diagnostic and therapeutic procedures, 4. full exploitation of medical technology, 5. full exploitation of professional and functional differentiation; B. Socioeconomic management of health and illness, 1. attention to social and environmental factors, 2. use of larger social units as the units of care wherever appropriate, 3. use of community resources on behalf of the patient, 4. attention to broader community interests; C. Psychological management of health and illness; D. Integrated management of health and illness; E. Continuity and coordination in the management of health and illness. II. *Client-Provider Relationship*—A. Some formal attributes of the client-provider relationship; B. Some attributes of the content of the client-provider relationship.

§ Assessment of quality care was accomplished by three techniques: (1) review of the medical record alone, (2) review of the medical record with the criteria presented in the *Hospital Utilization Review Manual*, and (3) a combination of the medical record, the criterion list, and a case abstract prepared by a nonprofessional. If readers are interested in the specifics they will find a list of criteria for evaluating the care of a patient with pneumonia in the hospital in the monograph by Payne titled *Quality Assurance of Medical Care*, Regional Medical Programs Service, US Department of Health, Education, and Welfare,

At best, assessment of the quality of care given by physicians is complex; it may be equally so for all health professions.

Measuring the Quality of Nursing. Attempts to answer the question "What is good nursing care?" are as old as professional nursing. The remarkable reduction in the death rate among British soldiers in the Crimean hospitals after the arrival of Florence Nightingale and the nurses associated with her gave some sort of measurement because she described the nursing care given and provided before-and-after statistics.[45] Jane E. Hitchcock's [46] report in 1902 of 500 cases of pneumonia was not so much a report on this disease as a comparison between the effectiveness of nursing care given in hospitals and by Henry Street visiting nurses. Dublin's report on the first 1000 deliveries of the Frontier Nursing Service, mentioned earlier, was a form of measurement. The Stewart "yardstick," also cited earlier in this chapter, was an attempt to provide specific criteria for measuring the reliability of a single activity. In reviewing the literature it is clear that these attempts have steadily increased. In 1950, Frances Reiter and Marguerite E. Kakosh [47] identified the following 12 components of nursing care: control of environment; mental adjustment; condition of skin and mucous membranes; elimination; posture, position, and exercise; rest and sleep; nutrition; observation of signs and symptoms; administration of laboratory tests; administration of medicines; administration of treatments; and teaching health. Each component was defined in operational terms. An observational guide was developed. The six following qualitative categories were defined as criteria that might be quantitatively scaled: *Dangerous:* The patient's health or welfare is endangered by the nursing care he received; *Safe:* No harm comes to the patient for having had nursing care; patient's life and values protected; *Adequate:* To the extent that it is possible, the patient's standards and customary way of living are kept as normal as possible; that he recovers to the greatest extent his former state of health at his own rate of recovery; *Optimum:* The patient's integrity is respected and he is helped to improve his state of health and is better able to care for himself; *Maximum:* The design of patient care is based on the best known scientific advances to date; *Ideal:* Patient care is examined and evaluated for the purpose of improvement through controlled research in nursing.

February 1973, pp. 252–254. Payne is now extending his research to include the development of criteria for ambulatory care.

Kakosh,[48] in a doctoral dissertation that took the form of a film script, tried to show the "differentiating characteristics of professional nursing care." In 1955, Myrtle Kitchell Aydelotte and her associates [49] initiated a long-range study using skin condition, mental attitude, and mobility of patients as criteria. In 1964, Gladys Nite and Frank Willis [50] reported a 4-year study of hospitalized patients with myocardial infarction, identifying "measuring rods" that could be used in evaluating care given to such patients. They concluded that nursing practice is therapeutic when in each case patients' problems are correctly identified and nursing care is directed toward resolution of these problems (a very close parallel with the Weed approach). Nite and Willis identified specific criteria to measure the progress of cardiac patients. Some examples are the following: patients will gradually show less apprehension toward pain as they gain an understanding of the physiologic process causing pain; patients permit the nurse to perform necessary activities for them; patients will tend to sleep during the day after major activities and during the entire night without medication.

A number of attempts have been made to compare the effect on patients of a traditional (less analytic) type of nursing with a deliberate (more analytic) process as described in Ida Jean Orlando's *The Dynamic Nurse-Patient Relationship*.[51] One such study, discussed in Chapters 47 and 48, was conducted by Rhetaugh G. Dumas and Robert C. Leonard,[52] its aim being to observe the effect of an experimental nursing process on the incidence of vomiting during recovery from anesthesia.

A research team at Rush-Presbyterian–St. Luke's Medical Center and the MEDICUS Systems Corporation have developed a methodology for monitoring quality of nursing care. Emphasis is placed upon an outcome assessment, and the researchers suggest that the relationship between process and outcome may be different for different types of patients. Many factors affect nursing quality, one of which is hospital management control. The quality-monitoring methodology has merit for nursing management in controlling nursing performance at the unit level. Nursing management must know and understand both process and outcomes to make decisions regarding quality of nursing care.[52a]

A significant breakthrough has been achieved by the American Nurses' Association, as a result of a contract with the Department of Health, Education, and Welfare in the development of model sets for criteria for screening quality, appropriateness, and necessity of nursing care in settings for which Professional Standard Review Organizations (PSROs) have responsibility. The manual *Guidelines for Review of Nursing Care at the Local Level* describes the development and organization of PSROs, a model for quality assurance in nursing, and explains the process for identifying outcome criteria.[52b]

Discussing the difficulty of evaluating nursing, Dorothy M. Smith[53] proposes that practice be measured more indirectly than directly. She thinks measurement of the nursing care of a "patient as a whole" may not be possible. She suggests that measurement of quality nursing (as Nite and Willis have also suggested) might be made on the basis of the "scientific rightness" of the assessment of the patient's nursing problems and the nurse's management of them. Smith proposed that "we need a system—an organized framework wherein we can see plainly and definitely what is to be done and what we must do to accomplish it." * She proposed that the nursing problems that professional nurses are called upon to assess and manage daily might form the basis for evaluating quality nursing care. Quality nursing might be measured indirectly by examining the system or organization provided for dealing with these nursing problems. For example, the degree to which communications are systematized might be one of the most important criteria that can be used in assessing quality nursing practice.

The identification of criteria of nursing practice poses many problems. Measurement of quality care will have to be both direct and indirect before a complete assessment of the effects of nursing practice upon patient welfare can be made.

Eleanor C. Lambertsen identifies six criteria for evaluating nursing care related to the plan of nursing care. These are as follows: is coordinated with the over-all plan of medical care, based on scientific principles, is therapeutically effective, ensures minimum physical and emotional safety and security for the patient, reflects immediate and long-range planning for regaining or maintaining maximum degree of health attainable for the patient, meets the psychosocial needs of the patient, and provides for patient-family participation.†

Dorothy Harrison, a nurse and anthropologist, is designing a study that will use electronic devices in measuring patient status which will also evaluate the effect of nursing. She says:

Inasmuch as technology today is advancing at an ever more rapid pace, I believe that nursing as a profession should make use of technological tools to meet its particular needs. Nursing is a discipline that demands not only an understanding of internal physiology and disease processes, but understanding of the whole person in an environment—physical and social. Medicine and most other helping and healing disciplines have tended to see and study separate parts and operations. It is especially important in nursing to see and integrate the whole. In the past, nurses have had to put the pieces that go to make the whole together on a more or less intuitive basis. Ability to do this varies with the particular nurse's alertness, power of observation, knowledge, and skill. An objective analysis and evaluation of this process of integration is needed. It is now possible to make this analysis and evaluation electronically, using electromagnetic field theory. All forms of matter, including living systems, possess constantly interacting electromagnetic properties. Electronics today can be called upon to do things that were heretofore undreamed of, to sense and measure minute electrical activity. I shall therefore attempt to use electronic devices to detect, measure, and study integration of the person, including interaction with some major environmental factors, which will provide nursing with the assessment tools it needs.*

Her work will be based on that of Harold S. Burr whose book for laymen, *The Electric Fields of Life* (Ballantine Books, New York, 1972), has been cited in various chapters of this text.

Standards for Nursing Practice. Definitions of nursing and standards based on them were discussed in Chapter 1 but it might be pointed out here that both are related to assessing the quality of nursing practice. Standards should derive from, or be consistent with, an accepted definition of nursing. They should also be sufficiently specific to describe effective practice. Standards may be so inclusive that they describe practice in any setting, or separate standards may be set up for nursing practice in hospitals, homes, schools, industry, penal institutions, and so on. Some of these standards have been given in earlier chapters but the point was also made there that this process is on-going—never completed. Definitions and standards appropriate for one era may need revision in the next.

Jean K. McFarlane,[54] engaged in 1970 in a 2-year study of nursing care, comments on the difficulty of establishing criteria (standards) of quality nursing care. She comments that health care professions lack precise goals and the goals of one profession may conflict with the goals of another. Standards for motor skills can be spelled out but the skills of observa-

---

* Smith, Dorothy M.: "Myth and Method in Nursing Practice," *Am. J. Nurs.,* **64:**68, (Feb.) 1964.
† Lambertsen, Eleanor C.: "Evaluating the Quality of Nursing Care," *Hospitals,* **39:**61, (Nov.) 1965.

* Personal communication.

tion, judgment, and applying the results to individuals cannot be spelled out, nor can human relation skills be defined. For these latter it is especially hard to establish criteria of performance.

Grace Fivars and Doris Gosnell,[55] also discussing the problems of evaluation, say it is recognized that in any activity where performance must be evaluated acceptable minimum standards are needed. Establishing standards of performance requires a thorough knowledge of what should be done to complete an assignment and the kinds of behavior it requires.

There seems to be a consensus among nurse educators that a program that prepares nurse practitioners is performance-based if

1. Competencies (knowledge, skills, behaviors) to be demonstrated by graduates are derived from explicit conceptions of roles stated in measurable terms.
2. Criteria (standards) for assessing competencies make explicit expected levels of mastery under specified conditions.
3. Assessment of the nurse practitioner is based on performance, and evidence of knowledge relevant to planning for, analyzing, interpreting, or evaluating situations or behavior.

Determining Standards of Performance.
Having agreed upon a definition of nursing and the scope of nursing functions, the next step would be to identify the components of performance that determine the desired level of proficiency. For example, when a patient's blood pressure is taken, the nurse should be able to complete the activity within a specified period of time, get an accurate reading, and handle the equipment with dexterity. So there are minimum requirements for each performance that, when they occur together, represent adequate performance.

David J. Klaus and his associates [56] say that on developing standards of performance for various nursing behaviors, attention is usually given to absolute (criterion referenced) standards rather than to normative standards. By *normative* is meant the performance of many individuals with the same training and experience when it is ordered along a continuum and an arbitrary point along this continuum is selected as the standard of acceptable performance. Most standards are stated in terms of measured performance, or the adequacy of performance in a test situation.

The following are some recent efforts to produce "instruments" for measuring nursing performance:

Charles M. Bidwell and Doris J. Froebe [57]

have developed an instrument for evaluating hospital nursing performance for "clinical nurse practitioners" in patient care and administrative "tasks," teaching, and formulation of objectives.

Margaret A. Dunn [58] constructed an instrument to measure the performance of professional nurse practitioners and she reports that it was found to be reliable in describing and evaluating clinical performance. The PETO System *[59] indexes nursing care needs and is a useful management tool for measuring nursing workload and resource planning. It is particularly useful when correlated with a nursing audit. The critical criteria, or seven areas in which evaluations are made, are diet, toileting, vital signs and measurements, respiratory aids, suction, cleanliness, and turning and/or assisted activity. These criteria are derived partly from the work of R. White et al.[60] R. Wilda Routhier [61] developed a tool to evaluate patient care. The tool is a 79-item questionnaire that includes direct and indirect elements of patient care and involves auditing the patient's record. The tool builds upon Irene L. Beland's [62] guide for assessing patients' needs.

Joy E. Gelder [63] describes a *Flow Process Chart* as a simple way of looking at a procedure in a systematic way. The procedure to be analyzed is described in detail. Each step is coded as to whether it is an operation, transportation, storage or waiting, and inspection. Specific questions are asked such as: What is its purpose? Why is it necessary? What should be done? Where should it be done and why? When should it be done and why? Who should do it and how is the best way to do it?

Lawrence L. Weed's [64] *Problem-Oriented Record* system of medical care with its revolutionary computerization provides a logical basis for planning, giving, and evaluating and/or auditing care. It allows health workers (physician, nurse, others) to define and follow clinical problems one by one and organize them for solution. This system has been described in some detail in Chapters 4 and 8. Attention was called there to the problem approach embodied in an article by Nell Beeby in 1937;[65] also the suggestion in Chapter 34 of the 1955 edition of this text that nursing care be taught and organized around nursing problems; and the development by Abdellah and associates [66] of 21 "nursing problems," published in 1960 under the title *Patient-Centered Approaches to Nursing*.

---

* PETO is an acronym of the surnames of the pediatrics team that developed the system: Marilyn Poland, Nellie English, Nancy Thorton, and Donna Owens, Medical College of Georgia, Augusta.

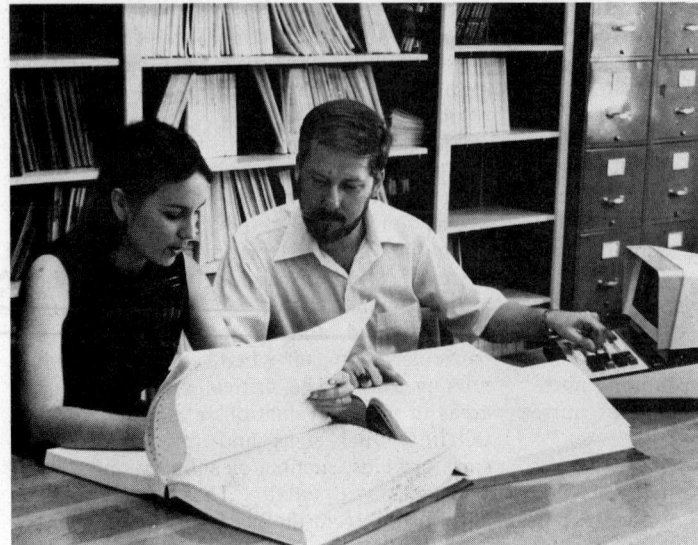

Figure 19-2. The use of the computer in analyzing patient care information allows health researchers to study large numbers of clinical situations. (Courtesy of Yale University School of Nursing, New Haven, Conn. Photo by Knollmueller.)

Mabel A. Wandelt and Maria C. Phaneuf [67,68,69] have described three instruments for measuring the quality of nursing care: the *Slater Nursing Competences Rating Scale,* the *Quality Patient Care Scale,* and the *Nursing Audit.* The Slater Scale, with 84 items, measures the nurse's competence in giving care in any setting, over a period of 2 weeks to 1 year. The Quality Patient Care Scale, with 68 items, is derived from the Slater Scale but has a slightly different emphasis. The Nursing Audit, developed by Phaneuf, has 50 items and measures the care received by the patient in his or her own home, a nursing home, or a hospital. It provides a basis for written appraisal of nursing care after discharge of the patient through analysis of patient care records.* The Nursing Audit is a useful tool in evaluating the quality of the care provided in any program and setting in which a record is an integral part of providing comprehensive and continuing nursing care.

4. THE NURSE'S ROLE IN RESEARCH RELATED TO IMPROVEMENT OF CARE

Nursing is a health science profession to the extent that its practice is based on science and that its research is practice-oriented. Nurses who participate in research can enrich their own practice and validate, rationalize, and improve their methods. Research challenges nurses to find answers to problems or questions. Research should be a part of every nurse's practice. All practitioners should be able to read and apply findings of research reports and take part in research. Speaking to this point, Dorothy Mereness says:

Research is not a set of skills which can be added to an individual's educational equipment at will. Rather, it is a way of seeking solutions to problems, a way of thinking and working, a way of collecting data and treating it once it has been collected, a way of making use of the results of a study once these results have been identified— in short, it is a way of life.*

As the authors have pointed out, the idea that all who practice nursing should be aware of and participate in research is relatively new. Abdellah and Levine [70] emphasize this in their 1965 publication *Better Patient Care Through Nursing Research.* In 1962, the American Nurses' Association Committee on Research and Studies [71] presented what it called a "Blueprint for Research in Nursing." It is a guide in outline form giving areas in which research is needed. Ten years later, Werley,[72] who is directing the Center for Health Research, Wayne State University College of Nursing, comments on the paucity of clinical nursing research but also on some encouraging signs, as, for example, the existence, since the 1950s, of a nursing research department in the Walter

---

* Quality of care with relation to the following functions is judged: (1) application and execution of physician's legal orders; (2) observation of symptoms and reactions; (3) supervision of the patient; (4) supervision of those participating in care; (5) reporting and recording; (6) application of nursing procedures and techniques; (7) promotion of health by direction and teaching.

* Mereness, Dorothy: "Preparing the Nurse Researcher," *Am. J. Nurs.,* **64:**78, (Sept.) 1964.

Reed Army Institute of Research, the support given by the US Department of Health, Education, and Welfare of clinical nursing research, and its support in universities. Werley identifies 18 reasons for the "paucity" of clinical research. They include "not enough clinical researchers . . , lack of research role models . . , instruction often not based on research . . , students do not gain . . . research awareness . . , textbooks not based on research-documented content," and "In the last analysis, one might wonder if there is not a lack of meaningful commitment to research on the part of both the profession and the many individuals who profess commitment." * There is no doubt that nursing has in the past depended on other disciplines rather than developing its own body of scientific knowledge. Leonard, discussing the development of research in the practice-oriented discipline of nursing, observes that "Nurses are pressed to act, act often, and act swiftly. In the face of the urgent and constant demand for nursing services, a body of nursing practice which incorporates many untested assumptions has become imbedded in hospital policies and textbooks for nursing students. Such principles [assumptions] are likely to be rationalizations for existing practices rather than scientifically based propositions that have been rigorously tested by our best research methods." †

While nursing research can be defined as "a systematic, detailed attempt to discover or confirm facts that relate to a . . . problem or problems in the field of nursing . . ." the research is referred to as "clinical" when "the ultimate goal is . . . to improve nursing practice." ‡

In Chapter 1 the expanding role of nursing was discussed at some length and reference made to the report of the Committee of the (former) Secretary of the US Department of Health, Education, and Welfare, *Extending the Scope of Nursing Practice* [73] as one of the publications that have fostered this development. Clinical research as a basis for determining the value of an extended role for nurses is the subject of many commentaries. [74-76] In *Better Patient Care Through Nursing Research*, Chapter 5 outlines the major steps in the research process: (1) formulate the problem; (2) review the literature; (3) formulate

the framework of theory; (4) formulate hypotheses; (5) define the variables; (6) determine how variables will be quantified; (7) determine the research design; (8) delineate the target population; (9) select and develop method for collecting data; (10) formulate method of analyzing the data; (11) determine how results will be interpreted (generalized); and (12) determine method of communicating results.*

"Clinical research" can be conducted in any clinical setting in which the nurse and patient are together, as, for example, a hospital unit, a nursing home, a school or industrial or penal health service, a clinic, or in a patient's home. The investigator (nurse researcher and/or practitioner) collects data through direct observation of the patient. Phyllis J. Verhonick says, "All too frequently the changes that have been made in nursing practice have been the result of the application of expedient measures rather than systematic investigation." †

It is the responsibility of every nurse to appraise his or her practice and identify ways of improving it. Leonard F. Stevens [77] describes a program at the Veterans Administration Hospital, St. Cloud, Minn., which created a climate that encouraged nurses to evaluate their practices and to make use of studies in doing this more effectively. Research was considered a means of improving nursing practice rather than an end in itself.

Lucille E. Notter [78] comments on the time lag that always exists between research and its implementation despite the increasing opportunities for publication and dissemination of research reports through reviews and source books.

In the 1970s nurse investigators are placing increased emphasis upon clinical research. Some excellent examples are provided in the ANA publication, *Research in Nursing: Toward a Science of Health Care*, 1976.

Examples of research in clinical nursing will be found in many chapters of this text. In discussing procedures such as enemata or taking temperatures, studies by nurses are cited; in discussing pain, preparing the patient for surgery, or caring for the dying, numerous studies by nurses are also used as a basis for suggesting methods or ways of helping patients. It is hoped that those who use this text will come to look upon the conduct, use, and interpretation of research as an essential element of nursing practice. Every nurse should

---

* Werley, Harriet H.: "This I Believe—About Clinical Nursing Research," *Nurs. Outlook*, **20**:718, (Nov.) 1972.

† Leonard, Robert C.: "Developing Research in a Practice-Oriented Discipline," *Am. J. Nurs.*, **67**:1472, (July) 1967.

‡ Abdellah, Faye G.: "Overview of Nursing Research 1955–1968, Part I," *Nurs. Res.*, **19**:6, (Jan.–Feb.) 1970.

---

* Abdellah, Faye G., and Levine, Eugene: *Better Patient Care Through Nursing Research*. Macmillan Publishing Co., Inc., New York, 1965, p. 91.

† Verhonick, Phyllis J.: "Clinical Investigations in Nursing," *Nurs. Forum*, **10**:81, (Summer) 1971.

at the very least know where to find published research.

The analytical aspects of the nursing literature published in English between 1900 and 1959 is indexed and annotated in the *Nursing Studies Index*.[79] Henderson [80] in 1957 and Abdellah [81] in 1970 published reviews of nursing research, which included clinical studies. Simmons and Henderson in 1964 published *Nursing Research—A Survey and Assessment*,[82] Chapter 13 of which is devoted to Studies of Nursing Care. Abdellah with Levine in 1965 published *Better Patient Care Through Nursing Research* [83] which dealt with "how some of the important methodological tools can be applied to problems that are uniquely nursing," giving throughout examples of how these methods have been used and citing hundreds of studies. The bimonthly journal *Nursing Research*, besides publishing full-length reports of major studies, gives abstracts of many others. Abstracts under the heading "Nursing Practice and Related Care" in the May–June 1973 issue outnumber those in any other category. This same trend is noticeable in the *International Journal of Nursing Studies*. It is tempting to mention certain investigations that might be considered "milestones" in the development of clinical nursing research but this is coming to be as difficult as it would be to select outstanding studies in any other health field.

More and more often nurses are working with other health workers on problems of common concern. A good example is the work of the US Department of Health, Education, and Welfare's Center for Disease Control, an agency of the Public Health Service. There, bacteriologists, epidemiologists, nurses, and physicians are studying ways of preventing the spread of infection. An example is the [abortive] nationwide swine flu program directed by the Public Health Service. The Center is discussed in Chapter 15 and specific studies emanating from there are cited throughout this text. In some cases nurses studying in this Center are afterwards employed in hospitals as epidemiologists. Most health institutions and agencies realize that practice must change and that it should be under constant surveillance. Nurses are assuming more and more responsibility for this work.

5. ORGANIZATION WITHIN PRACTICE SETTINGS THAT FOSTERS THE IMPROVEMENT OF CARE

An analysis of practice settings in which nurses work indicates the need for establishing a formal mechanism for the study of procedures, practices, and method in the care of patients. Figure 19-3 illustrates one organizational approach developed by Henderson that might be used in a hospital.

At Case-Western Reserve University, Jannetta MacPhail directed *An Experiment in Nursing: Planning, Implementing, and Assessing Planned Change* [84] that resulted in an effective approach. A Committee on Nursing Practice Guidelines was established as a counterpart of the Procedures Committee of the Medical Council. The purposes of the Committee on Nursing Practice Guidelines were defined as follows: (1) to review existing policies and procedures, identifying those which pertain to nursing practice, and to recommend the need for policy revisions or the development of policies where none now exist; and (2) to submit policy statements to the Nursing Council for review and preparation of guidelines for the implementation of the policy. This Committee had six representatives from medical-surgical nursing, a centralized staff development group faculty appointee, and related clinical specialty representatives.

In any agency, the Research Review Committee usually studies research proposals from all angles but its most important function is to protect human subjects. (This will be discussed in the next section of this chapter.)

In most hospitals the Committee on Research in Central Storage and Processing of Supplies, including equipment, is an important one. Representation on this committee must include one or more persons in this field as well as knowledgeable workers in clinical services who can interpret the needs of these services. This committee is responsible for reviewing requests for change in supplies or equipment, getting needed information, and collecting data or testing supplies and equipment and recommending selection. The effectiveness of such committees will depend upon the opportunities they provide for continuing education. This is stressed by Marjorie Cantor [85] and Abdellah.[86]

6. ETHICAL ASPECTS OF CLINICAL RESEARCH

Advances made in biomedical science and technology have raised perplexing problems and increased professional and public interest in ethical issues and moral decisions. James Carmody [87] discusses this in a report that includes a bibliography on this subject. The revision of practices based on experiments involving human subjects—the prolongation of

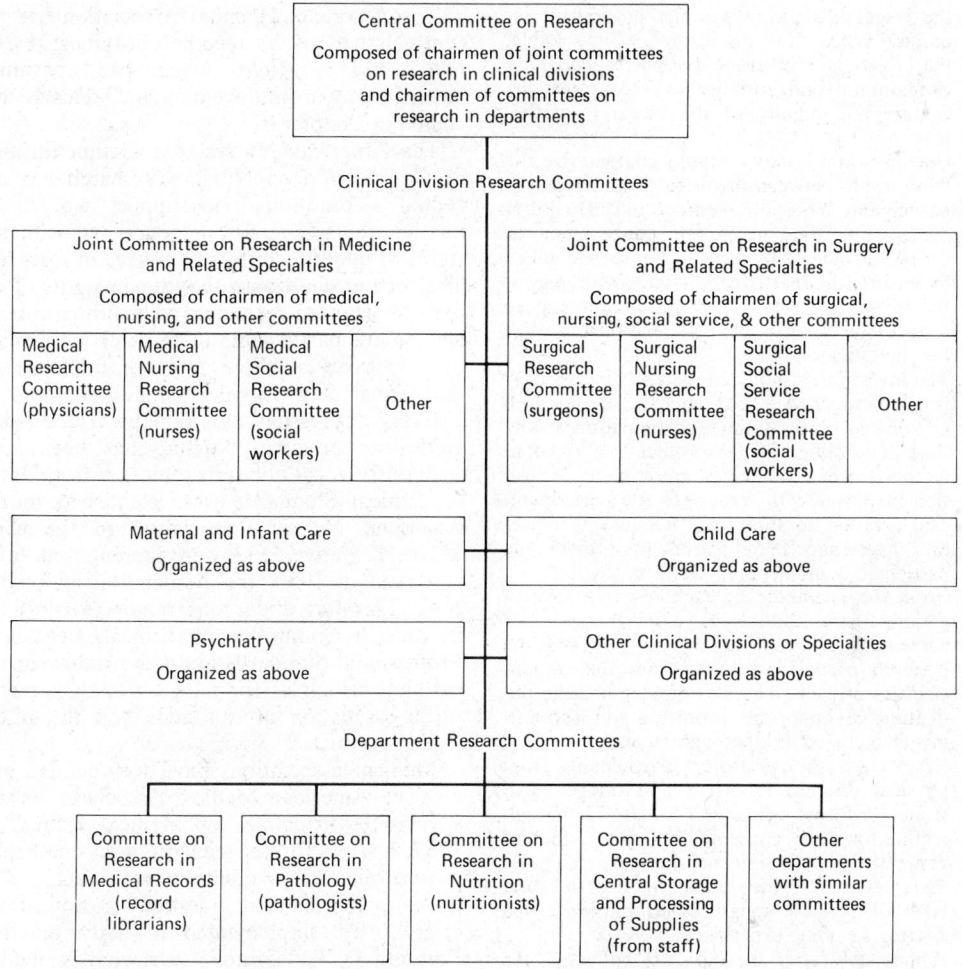

Figure 19-3. Suggested organization within a hospital to promote study of method in patient care. (Prepared by Virginia Henderson for meeting of Connecticut League for Nursing, Sept. 29, 1961.)

life, the survival of malformed neonates, organ transplantation, the control of population—all necessitate ethical decisions. As nursing research moves more and more in the direction of clinical research the legal and ethical aspects of using human subjects for experimentation must be continuously examined. Abdellah discussed this question at some length in a 1967 article.[88]

The most far-reaching study of ethical standards for research with human subjects has been undertaken by the American Psychological Association. It proposes the following ethical principles:

1. It is the personal responsibility of the investigator to make a careful evaluation of the ethical acceptability of each study he plans to undertake, taking into account the following guidelines for research with human beings. To

the extent that this appraisal, weighing scientific and humane values, leads the investigator to consider a deviation from any principle, the investigator incurs a correspondingly greater obligation to seek ethical advice and to observe more stringent safeguards to protect the rights of the human research participant.

2. The final responsibility for the establishment and maintenance of acceptable ethical practice in research always remains with the individual investigator. The investigator is also responsible for the ethical treatment of research participants by collaborators, assistants, students and employees, all of whom, however, incur parallel obligations.

3. The investigator should inform the participant of all features of the research that reasonably might be expected to influence willingness to participate. In addition, the investigator should explain all other aspects of

the research about which the participant inquires. When full disclosure is impossible, the investigator incurs increased responsibility to maintain confidentiality, and to protect the welfare and dignity of the research participant.

4. Openness and honesty should characterize the relationship between investigator and research participant. When the methodological requirements of a study necessitate concealment or deception, adequate measures must be taken to ensure the participant's understanding of the scientific grounds for this action and to restore the quality of the relationship with the investigator.

5. The investigator should respect the individual's freedom to choose to participate in research or not and to discontinue participation at any time. The obligation to protect this freedom increases when the investigator is in a position of power with respect to the participant. The decision to limit this freedom increases the investigator's obligation to protect the participant's dignity and welfare.

6. From the beginning of each research investigation, there should be a clear and fair agreement between the investigator and the research participant that defines the responsibilities of each. The investigator has the obligation to honor all promises and commitments included in that agreement.

7. Researchers should protect participants from physical discomfort, harm and danger, and from all forms of mental stress. If the potential for such consequences exists, the investigator should inform the participant of that fact, secure his consent to proceed, and take all possible measures to minimize the distress he may experience.

8. Immediately after the data are collected, the investigator should provide the participant with a full clarification of the nature of the study and remove any misconceptions that may have arisen. Where scientific or humane values justify withholding information, every effort must be made to assure that this has no damaging consequences for the participant.

9. Where research procedures may result in undesirable consequences for the participant, the investigator has the responsibility for employing appropriate measures to detect and remove or correct these consequences, including, where relevant, long-term after-effects.

10. The investigator should keep in confidence all information obtained about research participants. When any known possibility exists that others may obtain access to such information, this possibility, together with the plans for protecting confidentiality, should be explained to the participants as a part of the procedure for obtaining informed consent.*

* American Psychological Association: "Ethical Standards for Research With Human Subjects," The Association, Draft document (May) 1972.

The American Hospital Association has recently issued to its member hospitals *A Patient's Bill of Rights* which had consumer participation in its development.[89] This is discussed in Chapter 8.

The American Nurses' Association through its Commission on Nursing Research has accepted a commitment to support two sets of human rights. The first is concerned with the rights of qualified nurses to engage in research. The second deals with the human rights of all persons who are recipients of health care services or are participants in research performed by investigators whose research impinges on the patient care provided by nurses.[89a]

Every profession has an ethical code that guides its practice. Nursing has been conspicuously vocal about its ethics. A Committee on Ethical Standards was established in the American Nurses' Association in the early 1920s. Tentative codes were presented at intervals, and in 1950, the Association adopted a code. This has undergone major revisions by its present Committee on Ethical, Legal and Professional Standards and has resulted in ten cardinal principles for nurses.[90] See Chapter 1 for a discussion of this code and the ICN's Code of Ethics.

Medical associations have well-defined ethics. The American Medical Association issued a revised "Principles of Medical Ethics" in 1957.[91] While formal recognition by the health professions that patients have rights is important, the critical question is how these "rights" are implemented in daily practice. Edmund D. Pellegrino[92] says what is notably lacking is the critical reassessment of traditional professional roles and functions that will permit the fullest exploitation of new scientific knowledge while protecting the patients' rights.

Experimentation with new procedures, practices, and/or methods should be encouraged. Any changes in procedures or reassignment of tasks that involves two or more types of personnel must be decided by a joint practice committee or a research committee (discussed previously) where ethical principles that protect the rights of the patients and workers are operative.

REFERENCES

1. Nutting, M. Adelaide: "Florence Nightingale as a Statistician," *Public Health Nurse,* **19:** 207, (May) 1927.
2. ———: *The Education and Professional Position of Nurses.* US Government Printing Office, Washington, D.C., 1907. (Reissued as *Educational Status of Nursing,* Bull. No. 7 of US Office of Education.)
3. Waters, Yssabella: *Visiting Nursing in the*

United States. Charities Publication Committee, [New York], 1909.

4. Galbraith, Lillian M.: "Management Engineering and Nursing," *Am. J. Nurs.,* **50:**780, (Dec.) 1950.

5. American Hospital Association: "Report of Simplification and Standardization Committee," in *Transactions, American Hospital Association Meeting, Detroit, 1932.* The Association, Chicago, 1933.

6. Barnes, Ralph M.: *Motion and Time Study,* 3rd ed. John Wiley & Sons, New York, 1949.

7. Pfefferkorn, Blanche, and Rottman, Marion: *Clinical Education in Nursing.* Macmillan Publishing Co., Inc., New York, 1932.

8. Stewart, Isabel M.: "Possibilities of Standardization in Nursing Technique," *Mod. Hosp.,* **44:**46, (Oct.) 1919.

9. ————: "An Opportunity to Cooperate in a Plan for Improving Nursing Practice," *Nurs. Ed. Bull.,* n. s. **1:**4, 1930.

10. ————: "A Search for More Exact Measures of Reliability and Efficiency in Nursing Procedures," *Nurs. Ed. Bull.,* n. s. **1:**4, 1930.

11. Smith, Martha Ruth, and Broadhurst, Jean (eds.): *An Introduction to the Principles of Nursing Care.* J. B. Lippincott Co., Philadelphia, 1937.

12. Simmons, Leo W., and Henderson, Virginia: *Nursing Research—A Survey and Assessment.* Appleton-Century-Crofts, New York, 1964.

13. Henderson, Virginia: "Research in Nursing —When?" (editorial), *Nurs. Res.,* **4:**99, (Feb.) 1956.

14. Hughes, Everett C., et al.: *Twenty Thousand Nurses Tell Their Story.* J. B. Lippincott Co., Philadelphia, 1958.

15. Kroeger, Louis J., et al.: *Nursing Practice in California Hospitals.* California State Nurses Association, San Francisco, 1953.

16. American Nurses' Association: *Facts About Nursing 74–75.* The Association, Kansas City, Mo., 1976.

17. Canadian Nurses' Association: *Countdown 1973. Canadian Nursing Statistics.* The Association, Ottawa, 1974.

18. American Nurses' Foundation: "Directory of Nurses with Earned Doctoral Degrees," *Nurs. Res.,* **18:**465, (Sept.–Oct.) 1969.

19. Brown, Esther Lucile: *Nursing for the Future.* Russell Sage Foundation, New York, 1948.

20. National Commission for the Study of Nursing and Nursing Education: *An Abstract for Action.* McGraw-Hill Book Co., New York, 1970.

21. Abdellah, Faye G.: "Overview of Nursing Research, 1955–1968, Part III," *Nurs. Res.,* **19:**239, (May–June) 1970. (Financial data updated by author Oct. 1976.)

22. Canadian Nurses' Association: *Index of Canadian Nursing Studies.* The Association, Ottawa, 1973.

23. [Finnish] Foundation for Nursing Education: *Sairaanhoidon Vuosikirja X.* The Foundation, Helsinki, 1973.

24. Bayne-Jones, Stanhope: "The Role of the Nurse in Medical Progress," *Am. J. Nurs.,* **50:**601, (Oct.) 1950.

25. Brown, Amy Francis: *Research in Nursing.* W. B. Saunders Co., Philadelphia, 1958.

26. Meyer, Burton, and Heidgerken, Loretta E.: *Introduction to Research in Nursing.* J. B. Lippincott Co., Philadelphia, 1962.

27. Simmons, Leo W., and Henderson, Virginia: *op. cit.*

28. Skipper, James K., and Leonard, Robert C. (eds.): *Social Interaction and Patient Care.* J. B. Lippincott Co., Philadelphia, 1965.

29. Abdellah, Faye G., and Levine, Eugene: *Better Patient Care Through Nursing Research.* Macmillan Publishing Co., Inc., New York, 1965.

30. Fox, David J.: *Fundamentals of Research in Nursing.* Appleton-Century-Crofts, New York, 1966.

31. Wandelt, Mabel T.: *Guide for the Beginning Researcher.* Appleton-Century-Crofts, New York, 1970.

32. Woolridge, Powhatan J., et al.: *Behavioral Science, Social Practice, and the Nursing Profession.* Press of Case-Western Reserve University, Cleveland, 1968.

33. Wald, Florence, and Leonard, Robert: "Toward Development of Nursing Practice Theory," *Nurs. Res.,* **13:**309, (Fall) 1964.

34. Dublin, Louis I.: "First 1,000 Midwifery Cases of the Frontier Nursing Service in Kentucky," *Public Health Nurse,* **24:**582, (Oct.) 1932.

35. Simmons, Leo W., and Henderson, Virginia: *op. cit.*

36. Abdellah, Faye G., and Levine, Eugene: *Patients and Personnel Speak. A Method of Studying Patient Care in Hospitals.* US Department of Health, Education, and Welfare, Division of Nursing, Washington, D.C., 1957. (USPHS Pub. No. 527.)

37. Sanazaro, Paul J., et al.: "Research and Development in Quality Assurance. The Experimental Medical Care Review Organization Program," *N. Engl. J. Med.,* **287:**1125, (Nov. 30) 1972.

38. Donabedian Avedis: "Evaluating the Quality of Medical Care," *Milbank Mem. Fund Q.,* **44:**166, Part 2, 1966.

39. ————: *A Guide to Medical Care Administration,* Vol. II; *Medical Care Appraisal— Quality and Utilization.* American Public Health Association, New York, 1969.

40. ————: *Evaluating the Quality of Medical Care, Program Evaluation in the Health Fields.* (Edited by H. C. Schulberg *et al.*) Behavioral Publications, New York, 1969, p. 186.

41. ————: "Promoting Quality Through Evaluating the Process of Patient Care," *Med. Care,* **6:**181, 1968.

42. Williamson, John W.: "Evaluating Quality of Patient Care—A Strategy Relating to Outcome and Process Assessment," *J.A.M.A.,* **218:**564, (Oct. 25) 1971.

43. ————, et al.: "Priorities in Patient-Care Re-

search and Continuing Medical Education," *J.A.M.A.*, **204:**303, (Apr. 22) 1968.

44. Payne, Beverly C.: *Hospital Utilization Review Manual*. University of Michigan Press, Ann Arbor, 1966.

45. Woodham-Smith, Cecil: *Florence Nightingale 1820–1910*. Constable, London, 1950.

46. Hitchcock, Jane E.: "Five Hundred Cases of Pneumonia," *Am. J. Nurs.*, **3:**169, (Dec.) 1902.

47. Reiter, Frances, and Kakosh, Marguerite E.: *Quality of Nursing Care*. A Report of a Field Study to Establish Criteria 1950–1954. Institute of Research and Studies in Nursing Education, Division of Nursing Education, Teachers College, Columbia University, New York, 1963.

48. Kakosh, Marguerite E.: *Differentiating Characteristics of Professional Nursing Care*. Ed. D. Dissertation, Teachers College, Columbia University, New York, 1954.

49. Aydelotte, Myrtle Kitchell, and Tener, Marie E.: *An Investigation of the Relation Between Nursing Activity and Patient Welfare*. State University of Iowa, Utilization Project, Iowa City, 1960.

50. Nite, Gladys, and Willis, Frank: *The Coronary Patient; Hospital Care and Rehabilitation*. Macmillan Publishing Co., Inc., New York, 1964.

51. Orlando, Ida Jean: *The Dynamic Nurse-Patient Relationship. Function, Process and Principles*. G. P. Putnam's Sons, New York, 1961.

52. Dumas, Rhetaugh G., and Leonard, Robert C.: "The Effect of Nursing on the Incidence of Postoperative Vomiting," *Nurs. Res.*, **12:**12, (Winter) 1963.

52a. Haussman, R. K. Dieter, et al.: *Monitoring Quality of Nursing. Part II. Assessment and Study of Correlates*. US Department of Health, Education, and Welfare, Public Health Service, Bethesda, Md., July 1976 (Pub. No. [HRA] 76–7).

52b. American Nurses' Association: *Guidelines for Review of Nursing Care at the Local Level*. The Association, Kansas City, Mo., 1976 (Pub. No. NP-54).

53. Smith, Dorothy M.: "Myth and Method in Nursing Practice," *Am. J. Nurs.*, **64:**68, (Feb.) 1964.

54. McFarlane, Jean K.: "Study of Nursing Care —The First Two Years of a Research Project," *Int. Nurs. Rev.*, **17:**102 (No. 2) 1970.

55. Fivars, Grace, and Gosnell, Doris: *Nursing Education: The Problem and the Process*. Macmillan Publishing Co., Inc., New York, 1966, p. 47.

56. Klaus, David J., et al.: *Controlling Experience to Improve Nursing Proficiency*. Background and Study Plan, Report No. 1. American Institutes for Research, Pittsburgh, 1966, p. 40.

57. Bidwell, Charles M., and Froebe, Doris J.: "Development of an Instrument for Evaluating Hospital Nursing Performance," *J. Nurs. Admin.*, **1:**10, (Sept.–Oct.) 1971.

58. Dunn, Margaret A.: "Development of an Instrument to Measure Nursing Performance," *Nurs. Res.*, **19:**502, (Nov.–Dec.) 1970.

59. Clark, E. Louise, and Diggs, Walter W.: "The PETO System Offers a New Method of Matching Patient Needs with Available Nursing Care," *Hospitals*, **45:**96, (Sept. 16) 1971.

60. White, R., et al.: *Patient Care Classification: Methods and Application*. Johns Hopkins University, Baltimore, 1967.

61. Routhier, R. Wilda: "Tool for Evaluation of Patient Care," *Supervisor Nurse*, **3:**15, (Jan.) 1972.

62. Beland, Irene L.: *Clinical Nursing*, 2nd ed. Macmillan Publishing Co., Inc., New York, 1970.

63. Gelder, Joy E.: "The 'Flow Chart' Assists Nursing," *Can. Hosp.*, **48:**81, (Oct.) 1971.

64. Weed, Lawrence L.: *Medical Records, Medical Education, and Patient Care: The Problem-Oriented Record as a Basic Tool*. Case-Western Reserve University Press, Cleveland, 1969.

65. Beeby, Nell: "Where and What Shall We Teach?" *Am. J. Nurs.*, **37:**64, (Jan.) 1937.

66. Abdellah, Faye G., et al.: *Patient-Centered Approaches to Nursing*. Macmillan Publishing Co., Inc., New York, 1960.

67. Wandelt, Mabel A., and Phaneuf, Maria C.: "Three Instruments for Measuring the Quality of Nursing Care," *Hosp. Topics*, **150:**20, (Aug.) 1972.

68. Phaneuf, Maria C.: "Quality of Care: Problems of Measurement Part I—How One Public Health Nursing Agency Is Using the Nursing Audit," *Am. J. Public Health*, **59:**1827, (Oct.) 1969.

69. ———: *The Nursing Audit. Profile for Excellence*. Appleton-Century-Crofts, New York, 1972.

70. Abdellah, Faye G., and Levine, Eugene: *Better Patient Care Through Nursing Research*. Macmillan Publishing Co., Inc., New York, 1965.

71. American Nurses' Association: "ANA Blueprint for Research in Nursing," *Am. J. Nurs.*, **62:**69, (Aug.) 1962.

72. Werley, Harriet H.: "This I Believe . . . About Clinical Nursing Research," *Nurs. Outlook*, **20:**718, (Nov.) 1972.

73. US Department of Health, Education, and Welfare: *Extending the Scope of Nursing Practice*. A Report of the Secretary's Committee to Study Extended Roles for Nurses. US Government Printing Office, Washington, D.C., (Nov.) 1971.

74. Diers, Donna: "Application of Research to Nursing Practice," *Image*, **5:**7, (No. 2) 1972.

75. Notter, Lucille E.: "The Vital Significance of Clinical Nursing Research," *Cardio-Vasc. Nurs.*, **8:**19, (Sept.–Oct.) 1972.

76. Verhonick, Phyllis J.: "Clinical Investigations in Nursing," *Nurs. Forum*, **10:**81, (Summer) 1971.

77. Stevens, Leonard F.: "Look at Your Own Practice," *Am. J. Nurs.*, **65:**106, (June) 1965.

78. Notter, Lucille E.: "The Editor's Report—

January 1973," *Nurs. Res.,* **22:**3, (Jan–Feb.) 1973.

79. Henderson, Virginia (ed.): *Nursing Studies Index. An Annotated Guide to Reported Studies, Research Methods, and Historical and Biographical Materials in Periodicals, Books, and Pamphlets Published in English* (1900–1959). J. B. Lippincott Co., Philadelphia, 1964–1972, 4 vols.

80. Henderson, Virginia: "An Overview of Nursing Research," *Nurs. Res.,* **6:**61, (Oct.) 1957.

81. Abdellah, Faye G.: "Overview of Nursing Research, 1955–1968," Parts I, II, III. *Nurs. Res.,* **19:**6, (Jan.–Feb.) 1970; **19:**151, (Mar.–Apr.) 1970; **19:**239, (May–June) 1970.

82. Simmons, Leo W., and Henderson, Virginia: *op. cit.*

83. Abdellah, Faye G., and Levine, Eugene: *Better Patient Care Through Nursing Research.* Macmillan Publishing Co., Inc., New York, 1965.

84. MacPhail, Jannetta: *An Experiment in Nursing: Planning, Implementing, and Assessing Planned Change.* Case-Western Reserve University, Frances Payne Bolton School of Nursing, Cleveland, 1972, p. 8.

85. Cantor, Marjorie: "Standard 5—Education for Quality Care," *J. Nurs. Admin.,* **3:**49, (Jan.–Feb.) 1973.

86. Abdellah, Faye G., et al.: *New Directions in Patient-Centered Nursing,* Macmillan Publishing Co., Inc., New York, 1973.

87. Carmody, James: *Ethical Issues in Health Services. A Report and Annotated Bibliography.* US Department of Health, Education, and Welfare, National Center for Health Services Research and Development, Report HSRD #70–32, (Nov.) 1970.

88. Abdellah, Faye G.: "Approaches to Protecting the Rights of Human Subjects," *Nurs. Res.,* **16:**316, (Fall) 1967.

89. American Hospital Association: *A Patient's Bill of Rights.* The Association, Chicago, 1972.

89a. American Nurses' Association: *Human Rights Guidelines for Nurses in Clinical and Other Research.* The Association, Kansas City, Mo., 1975 (Pub. No. D-46).

90. American Nurses' Association: "Code for Nurses," *Am. J. Nurs.,* **68:**2581, (Dec.) 1968.

91. American Medical Association: "Principles of Medical Ethics," *J.A.M.A.,* **164:**1484, (July 27) 1957.

92. Pellegrino, Edmund D.: "Ethical Implications in Changing Practice," *Am. J. Nurs.,* **64:**110, (Sept.) 1964.

Additional Suggested Reading

American Nurses' Association: *Quality Assurance for Nursing Care Institute, Oct. 29–31, 1973. Proceedings.* The Association, Kansas City, Mo., 1974.

Barber, Bernard, et al.: *Research on Human Subjects; Problems of Social Control in Medical Experimentation.* Russell Sage Foundation, New York, 1974.

Batey, Marjorie V. (ed.): *Communicating Nursing Research; Critical Issues in Access to Data.* Western Interstate Commission for Higher Education, Boulder, Colo., 1975.

———: *Communicating Nursing Research. Is the Gap Being Bridged?* Western Interstate Commission for Higher Education, Boulder, Colo., 1971.

———: *Communicating Nursing Research. Problem Identification and the Research Design.* Western Interstate Commission for Higher Education, Boulder, Colo., 1969.

———: "Some Methodological Issues in Research," *Nurs. Res.,* **19:**511, (Nov.–Dec.) 1970.

British Columbia, University of, School of Nursing: *First National Conference on Research in Nursing Practice.* Canadian Nurses' Association, Ottawa, 1971.

Chater, Shirley: *Understanding Research in Nursing.* World Health Organization, Geneva, 1975.

Chow, Rita K.: "Significant Research and Future Needs for Improving Patient Care," *Milit. Med.,* **139:**302, (Apr.) 1974.

Chung, Hsin Hsin: "An Exploratory Study of Clinical Nursing Activities as a Preliminary Step for Planning Changes in Care Delivery System," *Int. Nurs. Rev.,* **18:**291, (No. 4) 1971.

Collins, Rosella D.: "Problem Solving a Tool for Patients, Too," *Am. J. Nurs.,* **68:**1483, (July) 1968.

Diers, Donna: "Research for Nursing," *J. Nurs. Admin.,* **3:**8, (Jan.–Feb.) 1973.

Downs, F. S., and Newman, M. A.: *A Source Book of Nursing Research.* F. A. Davis Co., Philadelphia, 1973.

Drew, Jacqueline: "Determining Quality of Nursing Care," *Am. J. Nurs.,* **64:**82, (Oct.) 1964.

"Ethics of Nursing Research," *Can. Nurse,* **68:**23, (Sept.) 1972.

Greenberg, B. G.: "Introduction to Research," in *International Conference on the Planning of Nursing Studies, Sevres, France, Nov. 12–14, 1956.* International Council of Nurses, London, 1957.

Hamburger, Jean, and Crosnier, Jean: "Moral and Ethical Problems in Transplantation," in Rapaport, Felix T., and Dausset, Jean: *Human Transplantation.* Grune & Stratton, New York, 1968.

Hulicka, Irene M., and Hulicka, Karel: "To Design Experimental Research," *Am. J. Nurs.,* **62:**100, (Jan.) 1962.

Malone, Mary: "From Practitioner to Researcher," *Am. J. Nurs.,* **62:**65, (Aug.) 1962.

Marram, G. D.: "Patients' Evaluation of Their Care: Importance to the Nurse," *Nurs. Outlook,* **21:**322, (May) 1974.

Michigan Department of Public Health: *Kidney Transplantation Services. Minimal Criteria and Guidelines.* The Department, Lansing, 1972.

"Moral Problems in the Use of Borrowed Organs, Artificial and Transplanted" (editorial), *Ann. Intern. Med.,* **60:**309, 1964.

Notter, Lucille E.: *Essentials of Nursing Research.* Springer Publishing Company, New York, 1974.

———: "Research in Nursing—A Critical Need"

(editorial), *Nurs. Res.,* **20:**195, (May–June) 1971.

Notter, Lucille E., and Spector, Audrey F.: *Nursing Research in the South.* Southern Regional Education Board, Atlanta, Ga., 1974.

Platt, Lord: "Human Guinea-Pigs," in Clow, Archie (ed.): *Morals and Medicine.* Oxford University Press, New York, 1971.

Ponton, T. R.: "Measuring the Work of the Physician," *Bull. Am. Coll. Surgeons,* **13:**11, (June) 1929.

Roy, Sister Callista: "Adaptation: A Basis for Nursing Practice," *Nurs. Outlook,* **19:**254, (Apr.) 1971.

Royal College of Physicians, Committee on the Supervision of the Ethics of Clinical Research Investigations in Institutions: *Supervision of the Ethics of Clinical Research Investigations in Institutions.* The College, London, 1973.

Schlotfeldt, Rozella M.: "Reflections on Nursing Research," *Am. J. Nurs.,* **60:**492, (Apr.) 1960.

Stone, R. S.: "The Rights of Human Beings Participating as Subjects in Biochemical Research" (editorial), *J. Lab. Clin. Med.,* **85:**184, (Feb.) 1975.

Treece, Eleanor Walters, and Treece, James William: *Elements of Research in Nursing.* C. V. Mosby Co., St. Louis, 1973.

"Utah University Creates Nursing Research Center" (news), *Nurs. Outlook,* **24:**141, (Mar.) 1976.

Verhonick, Phyllis J.: "Research Awareness at the Undergraduate Level," *Nurs. Res.,* **20:**26, (May–June) 1971.

———: (ed.): *Nursing Research 1.* Little, Brown & Co., Boston, 1975.

Vreeland, Ellwynne M.: "Nursing Research Programs of the Public Health Service," *Nurs. Res.,* **13:**148, (Spring) 1964.

Werley, Harriet H.: "Different Research Roles in Army Nursing," *Nurs. Outlook,* **11:**134, (Feb.) 1963.

———: "Promoting the Research Dimension in the Practice of Nursing Through the Establishment and Development of a Department of Nursing in an Institute of Research," *Milit. Med.,* **127:**219, (Mar.) 1962.

Western Interstate Commission for Higher Education: *Newly Initiated and Completed Research in the Western Region,* Vol. II. The Commission, Boulder, Colo., 1975.

Williams, Carolyn A.: "Nurse Practitioner Research: Some Neglected Issues," *Nurs. Outlook,* **23:**172, (Mar.) 1975.

Woodruff, M. F. A.: "Ethical Problems in Organ Transplantation," *Br. Med. J.,* **1:**1457, (June) 1964.

Faye G. Abdellah
Virginia Henderson

CHAPTER 20

Administration of Oxygen and Other Gases and the Use of Ventilators (Respirators)

1. INTRODUCTION TO THE ADMINISTRATION OF OXYGEN AND OTHER GASES

Oxygen in excess of that in the atmosphere is administered in a number of conditions, and under these circumstances the gas that is normally inhaled is considered a therapeutic agent. Oxygen therapy is used in conditions in which there is a direct or indirect interference with normal oxygenation of tissues. Some of these *conditions* include respiratory diseases, heart disease, shock, infections with fever, industrial asphyxia,† to mention only a few. Oxygen may be used instead of air in diagnostic treatments such as a pneumoencephalogram (see page 1311). Since oxygen is absorbed more rapidly than air, the excruciating headache which is a frequent sequela of the test disappears more rapidly and the patient's discomfort is greatly eased; occasionally oxygen may be prescribed by the physician and is then administered by means of a face mask following the pneumoencephalogram.‡

Besides oxygen, other *gases* are used in inhalation therapy. These gases and vapors have little in common except that they are absorbed chiefly by the respiratory tract; on a pharmacologic basis, they have been classified into three main groups—therapeutic, noxious, and inert. In the therapeutic group are the anesthetic gases and vapors, oxygen and carbon dioxide, as well as helium. Helium, even though it is an inert gas, is included among the therapeutic gases since it has valuable therapeutic actions because of its physical properties.[1] Of the therapeutic gases, only oxygen, helium, and carbon dioxide are discussed in this chapter. The *method of administration* is chosen according to the patient's condition or needs, and is, of course, dependent on the facilities and equipment available. An inhalation therapy record is maintained for each patient (see Fig. 20-1).

2. ADMINISTRATION OF OXYGEN

Nature of the Gas and Definition of Oxygen Therapy. Oxygen, which comprises 20.93 per cent of normal air, is a colorless, odorless, and tasteless gas that is heavier than air. It is a constituent of air, water, crust of the globe, and all plant and animal life. It supports combustion and must be kept away from inflammable materials.

Tissue cells must be constantly supplied with oxygen by the circulation since they have no reserve store; oxygen inhalation in humans is

---

* Mechanical devices which help a person in respiratory failure to breathe were first called respirators. This term has been replaced by what is thought to be the more accurate term "ventilator". The public and some members of the health professions may still use the term "respirator."

† Several simple industrial asphyxiants include nitrogen, hydrogen, and acetylene. When such gases are used, there may be insufficient oxygen present; thus they can act as asphyxiants. Examples of chemical asphyxiants include carbon monoxide and cyanide. Because carbon monoxide has the property of combining with the hemoglobin of the blood, thus excluding oxygen, it is called a chemical asphyxiant. Cyanide may be a chemical asphyxiant since it acts upon the tissues and temporarily deprives them of the capacity to use the oxygen in the blood.

‡ This therapy supplements other more general measures such as urging the patient to lie flat in bed,

keeping the room darkened and adequately ventilated, and offering the patient fluids at frequent intervals and in small amounts—all of which will help the patient obtain needed rest and sleep until the headache has subsided.

INHALATION THERAPY RECORD

| Family Name | First Name | Attending Physician | Room No. | Hosp. No. |

Diagnosis:

Date Ordered	Date Discontinued	PHYSICIAN'S ORDERS	Physician

| | APPARATUS | DETAILS | USE OF O_2 | REMARKS | Nurse or Therapist |

Date | Time | Aerosol | Catheter | Croupette | Incubator | IPPB | Mask | Tent | Continuous | Intermittent | Stand By | Liters/Min. | Time of Analysis | O_2 Concentration | Time Catheter Changed | Time On | Time Off | Total Hours | REMARKS | Nurse or Therapist

12 M-8 AM | 4 PM-12 M | 8 AM-4 PM

Daily Total (Hours) O_2 Administered →

12 M-8 AM | 4 PM-12 M | 8 AM-4 PM

Daily Total (Hours) O_2 Administered →

12 M-8 AM | 4 PM-12 M | 8 AM-4 PM

Daily Total (Hours) O_2 Administered →

FORM D-1051   PHYSICIANS RECORD CO., BERWYN, ILLINOIS · PRINTED IN U.S.A.   INHALATION THERAPY RECORD (OVER)

Figure 20-1. Inhalation therapy record. (Courtesy of Physicians' Record Co., Berwyn, Ill.)

therefore essential for life. However, there is a wide difference in the critical need of oxygen by the various body cells. Cells in the cerebrum must have oxygen constantly; if the supply of oxygen to the cerebral cells is cut off for from 5 to 7 minutes, irreversible changes occur in the cells. In the heart, however, Andrew C. Ivy [2] says that the myocardial cells would have to be completely deprived of blood (and the oxygen the blood contains) for 30 to 40 minutes before irreversible changes occur.

Oxygen may be administered by tent, face mask, or intranasal catheter. Oxygen adminis-

INHALATION THERAPY RECORD

Family Name		First Name	Attending Physician		Room No.	Hosp. No.

Diagnosis:

Date Ordered	Date Discontinued	PHYSICIAN'S ORDERS	Physician

Date	Time	APPARATUS							DETAILS							USE OF O₂			REMARKS	Nurse or Therapist
		Aerosol	Catheter	Croupette	Incubator	IPPB	Mask	Tent	Continuous	Intermittent	Stand By	Liters/Min.	Time of Analysis	O₂ Concentration	Time Catheter Changed	Time On	Time Off	Total Hours		

(Columns: Date; Time [12M-8AM, 8AM-4PM, 4PM-12M]; Apparatus: Aerosol, Catheter, Croupette, Incubator, IPPB, Mask, Tent; Details: Continuous, Intermittent, Stand By, Liters/Min., Time of Analysis, O₂ Concentration, Time Catheter Changed; Use of O₂: Time On, Time Off, Total Hours; Remarks; Nurse or Therapist)

Daily Total (Hours) O₂ Administered →

Daily Total (Hours) O₂ Administered →

Daily Total (Hours) O₂ Administered →

Figure 20-1. (continued).

tration through an endotracheal tube or tracheostomy tube in conjunction with mechanical ventilation is often used for the critically ill.

Since World War I the therapeutic value of oxygen has been scientifically investigated, and oxygen is now recognized as a valuable therapeutic agent.[3]

Physiologic Basis of Therapeutic Use. Oxygen is used principally to relieve *hypoxia,* or oxygen want, which occurs in diseases of the respiratory and cardiovascular systems, as well as in conditions secondarily affecting these systems.

It is not the purpose of this chapter to give in detail the physiology of respiration. For this the reader should refer to Chapters 9 and 35. However, to understand oxygen therapy it is essential to know that the lungs and the circulatory system supply oxygen to the tissues and remove carbon dioxide in a continuous cycle which consists of four phases: (1) *ventilation,* or the movement of air into and out of the lungs, (2) *absorption,* or passage of oxygen from the alveoli of the lungs into the blood hemoglobin, (3) *transportation,* or movement of the oxygenated blood through the cardiovascular system from the lungs to the tissues, and (4) *tissue absorption,* or passage of the oxygen into the cells of the body from the blood. A failure of any one phase of the respiratory cycle will cause a deficiency in the oxygen supply available to the cells of the body (in part or completely). The hypoxia which results may be classified according to the type of disturbance of the oxygen-supplying mechanism by which it is caused.[4]

Types of Hypoxia, or Oxygen Want. Lack of oxygen to breathe or disturbance of the phase of ventilation may produce *hypoxic hypoxia.* This type of hypoxia is characterized by a low arterial oxygen tension with the result that the exchange of oxygen in the lungs is interfered with. When such conditions as pulmonary edema, atelectasis, or bronchospasm are present, they act as a mechanical hindrance in the lungs and prevent the free diffusion of gases from the alveoli into the lungs. There is sufficient concentration of oxygen in the lungs, but the amount in the arterial blood is below normal because it does not diffuse readily.

Disturbance of the *absorption phase* may result in *anemic hypoxia.* This condition occurs when the hemoglobin in the blood is reduced in quantity with a consequent reduction in the capacity of the blood to carry oxygen. Causes of this condition include hemorrhage and anemia. The tissues, therefore, fail to receive an adequate supply of oxygen.

Disturbance of the *transportation phase* of the oxygenated blood from the lungs to the tissues may result in *stagnant hypoxia.* The tissues receive insufficient oxygen because their circulation is inadequate in conditions such as the following: low cardiac output or congestive heart failure, reduction of blood volume (dehydration), lowered arterial blood pressure (shock, hemorrhage), and local circulatory insufficiency from constricted or diseased blood vessels.

Disturbance of the *phase of tissue absorption* may result in *histotoxic hypoxia,* which is caused by an interference in the ability of the cells to utilize oxygen. Alcohol, narcotics, and certain other poisons can cause such interference.

Because several varieties of hypoxia can exist at the same time, there is a fifth type, referred to as the *combined form.* For example, the patient with shock from hemorrhage has both the anemic and stagnant forms of hypoxia.

When an oxygen want exists, the basic cause or type of hypoxia must be determined so that effective therapy can be instituted. In anemic hypoxia, the basic condition—anemia—must be treated; in histotoxic hypoxia, the cause of the diminished ability of the cells to utilize oxygen must be determined and corrected if possible. In general, it may be stated that oxygen therapy is most effective in hypoxic conditions when the hypoxia arises from inadequate oxygenation of the blood passing through the lungs (that is, hypoxic hypoxia). Unless shock is preceded or accompanied by hemorrhage, oxygen therapy does little to relieve stagnant hypoxia because blood, even though its circulation has been slowed down, is being saturated with oxygen to a normal degree.

Indications for Oxygen Therapy. The first essential in oxygen therapy is early recognition of the developing hypoxia. The nurse is the person most often in a position to see the signs of oxygen want, and he or she should be alert to report them promptly. The signs of hypoxia include one or more of the following: an *increased pulse rate, rapid and shallow breathing or deep and labored breathing,* occasionally *cyanosis,* and an increasing *agitation* or *confusion.* Sometimes symptoms such as *headache, cardiac pain,* and *muscle twitching* develop.[5] H. H. Bendixen and associates [6] include in the clinical signs of hypoxia a *fall in blood pressure* (hypotension) or a *rise in blood pressure* (hypertension) in addition to rapid shallow breathing and cyanosis. They believe that hypotension should be assumed to be secondary to cyanosis until another explanation has been found. Hypotension results in tissue hypoxia regardless of its cause and therefore oxygen administration is always indicated. Hypertension, especially when occurring suddenly, may be an early compensatory response to hypoxia. Hypoxia is a powerful stimulus of sympathetic activity that results in selective vasoconstriction (vasoconstriction in tissues less vital to maintaining life), thus raising peripheral resistance and resulting in a moderate rise in blood pressure.[7] Bendixen and associates state further that cyanosis is a late sign of hypoxia and that it is unreliable as an index of arterial oxygenation:

In general . . . cyanosis will appear particularly late in those patients who are capable of increasing their blood flow in the presence of hypoxia. If the hemoglobin content is only 10 grams, such a patient could suffer a degree of hypoxia that is inconsistent with survival, without any signs of cyanosis.*

Although the absence of cyanosis does not mean that tissues are well oxygenated, some hypoxic states are characterized by cyanosis. In these cases it is helpful to recall four factors that modify the appearance of cyanosis described by Arthur E. Guedel.[8] These include color of the skin, thickness of the epidermis, density of the capillary network, and lighting and color effects in the patient's unit or in the operating room. In fair-skinned persons the threshold value for the appearance of cyanosis is lower than in persons with a darker skin. Because there are no blood vessels in the epidermis, it acts as a screen through which the cyanosis must be observed; cyanosis in areas of thick epidermis is not as readily apparent as when the epidermis is thin. When capillaries are abundant and the epidermis thin (as in an ear lobe), cyanosis can be observed more quickly and accurately. The evaluation of cyanosis is influenced by the character of the light in which it is observed; cyanosis can be observed more accurately and promptly in bright daylight than in artifical light.

For patients who are critically ill, the determination of hypoxia may be made more precisely by monitoring equipment available in hospitals. In this setting, the nurse notes the usual signs of hypoxia and is also able to draw and prepare arterial blood samples for blood gas analysis.†

The signs of hypoxia are compensatory efforts of the body.[9] The body attempts to increase the rate of oxygen transport by increasing cardiac output, so the heart beats more rapidly (tachycardia). A person with a weakened heart muscle (myocardium), such as would occur following occlusion of one of the coronary arteries, would not be able to increase his or her cardiac output in response to hypoxia. In fact, hypoxia might precipitate or worsen existing heart failure.

Another way to increase the rate of oxygen transport is to breathe more rapidly to increase ventilation in the alveoli. An individual who

has a depressed respiratory center (for example, an overdose of a narcotic) or insufficient muscular strength cannot respond to hypoxia by increasing the rate of respiration. The astute clinician does not simply keep in mind a fixed set of signs that represent hypoxia, but evaluates hypoxia in the individual patient by the signs he or she may be capable of demonstrating.

Therapeutic Uses. The factors upon which a normal supply of oxygen to the tissues depends are: (1) an adequate oxygen pressure in the atmosphere; (2) an unobstructed passageway from the nose or mouth to the lungs; (3) an adequate lung capacity; (4) an adequate supply of blood to the lungs; and (5) blood characterized by a red blood cell count, a hemoglobin content, and a buffer salt content, all within physiologic limits. Any atmospheric condition or disease that interferes with these requirements produces *a state of oxygen want or hypoxia*. The administration of air rich in oxygen is of at least temporary benefit whenever the body tissues are receiving an inadequate supply no matter what the cause, but only in marked oxygen want and under certain conditions is it prescribed.

The obstacles to oxygen and carbon dioxide transport are best understood by describing the basic physiologic disturbance, not by describing a particular disease state (such as asthma). If the physiologic disturbance is identified, it can explain why the effect of oxygen therapy is temporary. Only hypoxia due to a decreased arterial oxygen concentration in the blood will respond dramatically to oxygen therapy.[10]

The following are the chief *causes of respiratory failure.* (1) *Increased physiologic shunting* is a condition in which a part of the blood leaving the heart does not participate in pulmonary blood-gas exchange and returns to the left side of the heart unoxygenated. This can occur when there is no oxygen available in part of the lung from, for example, atelectasis or collapse of alveoli. Defects in the ventricular septal wall can cause blood to go from the right to the left ventricle, completely bypassing the lung.[11,12] (2) *Increased wasted ventilation* is another cause of respiratory failure. Only the air that exchanges with pulmonary blood has any physiologic significance. This volume of air is called alveolar ventilation, or effective ventilation. The portion of the total ventilation that does not exchange with blood is wasted ventilation (dead space). If an alveolus is being ventilated, but the pulmonary capillary is not being perfused, the air in that alveolus is wasted ventilation. A pulmonary embolus is an example of a condition that leads to increased dead space because a ven-

---

* Bendixen, H. H., et al.: *Respiratory Care.* C. V. Mosby Co., St. Louis, 1965, p. 129.

† The measurement of dissolved oxygen pressures in the blood in relation to dissolved carbon dioxide pressure, hydrogen ion concentration, and oxyhemoglobin saturation give a much more precise picture of the state of hypoxia and its effect on the body. Modern ventilatory care, oxygen therapy, and respiratory therapy are based upon the immediate availability and accuracy of the blood gas laboratory. For a complete description of the blood gas machine and how it operates to measure gases dissolved in the blood, see Shapiro, Barry A.: *Clinical Application of Blood Gases,* Year Book Medical Publishers, Inc., Chicago, 1973.

tilated lung is not being perfused. There is also an increase in dead space following hemorrhage or a drop in blood pressure.[13] (3) *Increased work of breathing* demanded by resistance is a third cause of respiratory failure. The work of breathing is performed to overcome airway resistance as well as the elastic and viscous (or tissue) resistance against inflation offered by the lungs and chest wall.[14] Pulmonary emphysema, chronic bronchitis, and bronchial asthma are always associated with increased airway and tissue resistance. Passing a suction catheter through an endotracheal or tracheostomy tube increases airway resistance. For this reason, 100 per cent oxygen is insufflated into the breathing passages before suctioning takes place and intermittently throughout the procedure. The common causes of increased resistance (compliance or distensibility of lungs and chest wall) are atelectasis, pneumonia, and the respiratory distress syndrome of the newborn. Increased tissue resistance may also occur following prolonged use of extracorporeal circulation (heart-lung bypass). The respiratory frequency decreases with increased airway resistance and increases with increased tissue resistance. When there is a substantial increase in the work of breathing the expiratory muscles begin to use a critical portion of the total oxygen consumption. Therefore, ventilator support is usually indicated to reduce the work of breathing and rest respiratory muscles. (4) *Decreased hemoglobin content of blood* and inadequacies in the volume and distribution of cardiac output will decrease oxygen transport in blood and contribute to respiratory failure. An increase in the inspired oxygen concentration increases the amount of dissolved oxygen carried by the blood and makes oxygen available to the tissues where oxygen reserves are, for practical purposes, nonexistent.

To summarize, hypoxia may result from problems of absent or uneven perfusion of the alveoli by the blood, problems that inhibit movement of air into the lungs or its even distribution, problems that increase the work of breathing, and problems of oxygen transport by the blood to the tissues. The person may show signs of oxygen want in all these cases, but oxygen alone may not be therapeutic. For example, in cases of airway obstruction, the obstruction must be removed. Valuable time is lost in trying to give oxygen. When the work of breathing is exhausting the patient, oxygen is administered with the assistance of the mechanical ventilator. Normal blood volume must be restored in hemorrhagic shock, although the administration of oxygen is of temporary benefit.

Dosage and Means of Controlling It. Atmospheric air contains 20.93 per cent oxygen, 0.03 per cent carbon dioxide, and 79.04 per cent nitrogen. To be effective therapeutically, the inspired mixture of gases must contain considerably more oxygen than ordinary air.

Oxygen should be ordered and administered in specific dosages as are other therapeutic agents. Accurate recordings are made by the nurse of the duration of the therapy and the patient's physical and mental reactions. Dosage in oxygen inhalation therapy is expressed in *fractions of inspired oxygen content of air or per cent of inspired oxygen*. The symbol for the fraction is F_IO_2. An example of a prescription for oxygen is: "F_IO_2 0.4" (0.4 atmosphere) or simply "inspired oxygen concentration—40%." Because *liter flow per minute is not an accurate guide*, the only way to determine the percentage of oxygen in the inspired air is to analyze a sample of the mixture that the patient is breathing. In oxygen therapy this should be done every few hours and following any treatment that has necessitated a loss of oxygen from a tent or room. The technique of making this analysis is discussed on page 1104.

It is difficult to predict the inspired oxygen fractions required for patients with various respiratory patterns, and it is even more difficult to estimate alveolar oxygen tensions in diseased states.[15,16] This makes it necessary to use both clinical observations and blood gas measurements to assess the adequacy of oxygen therapy, rather than computing the amount of oxygen being given.[17]

In all cases where supplemental oxygen is needed, the oxygen-carrying capacity of the blood must be optimal. A blood transfusion may be indicated to raise the hemoglobin to the normal range of 12 to 14 gm per 100 ml of cells (adult) and 10.5 to 12 gm (infant). If oxygen therapy is required in the newborn period (for example in the treatment of respiratory distress syndrome), it is suggested that oxygen tension in the arterial blood be kept in the range of 60 to 100 mm Hg (millimeters of mercury).[18] In cases of obstructive pulmonary disease, an arterial oxygen tension of approximately 60 to 70 mm Hg is desired, as these patients are dependent on lower concentrations of oxygen as a stimulus to breathe (see Chapter 35).

Precautions in the use of oxygen and hazards of oxygen therapy are reviewed by Louis S. Goodman and Alfred Gilman, Barry A. Shapiro, H. H. Bendixen and associates, H. Pontoppidan and associates, N. Balfour Slonim and Lyle Hamilton, and Donald F. Egan.[19-24] In spontaneously breathing patients with neurologic injuries involving the respiratory centers or who have had prolonged hypercarbia or hypoxia, as in chronic pulmonary disease, the administration of oxygen may cause apnea. Apnea occurs because the response of the respiratory centers of the medulla to carbon dioxide is depressed. Respiratory drive must be maintained by aortic and carotid chemoreceptors (specialized nerve cells in the angle of the bifurcation of the common carotid arteries and at the level of the aortic arch). These arterial chemoreceptors differentiate between concentrations of hydrogen ions and oxygen ions in the blood perfusing them and stimulate the medullary centers to increase ventilation when there is a drop in oxygen tension. Therefore, the administration of oxygen and consequent rise in arterial pressure of oxygen may cause apnea by removing the chemoreceptor drive to respiration. In these cases the patient's need for oxygen may be met with controlled mechanical ventilation rather than breathing spontaneously, but inadequately, to an hypoxic drive from the chemoreceptor mechanism.

Another hazard of oxygen administration is the collapse of alveoli resulting from inhalation of high concentrations of oxygen. Breathing 100 per cent oxygen depletes nitrogen, the gas in highest concentration in the alveoli. Nitrogen, normally coming from inspired air, keeps the alveoli expanded. If it is depleted or "washed out," the alveoli tend to collapse.

Pontoppidan and associates make the following statement:

Current clinical practice is based on the assumption that an F_1O_2 of 50 per cent (0.5 atmosphere) or higher is likely to produce serious changes when used for more than two days. The higher the F_1O_2, the more rapid the onset of damage. Except in patients with chronic hypoxemia, one should select an F_1O_2 that will result in a P_aO_2 (partial pressure of oxygen in arterial blood) in the normal range.*

Symptoms of oxygen toxicity in the conscious patient are irritation of the mucous membranes, substernal pain, paresthesia of the arms and legs, and nausea and vomiting. A serious consequence of giving high concentrations of oxygen (80 to 100 per cent) over long periods is the formation of a membrane on the alveolar walls, similar to the hyaline membrane of the alveoli found in premature infants with respiratory distress syndrome. The child or adult subjected to prolonged treatment with high concentrations of oxygen may

develop noncompliant lungs due to the presence of this membrane and the loss of pulmonary surfactant.

A vascular proliferative disease of the retina (retrolental fibroplasia), causing blindness, is an example of the toxic effect of high levels of oxygen in the retinal capillaries of the premature infant.[25] This complication of oxygen therapy can be avoided by careful monitoring of the partial pressure of oxygen in arterial blood (P_aO_2) during the administration of oxygen to premature infants. The best practice is to administer the smallest amount of excess oxygen for the shortest possible time, and, in general, maintain the P_aO_2 between 50 and 100 mm Hg. Sheldon B. Korones[26] says there is no documented level of oxygen that is invariably toxic to the retinal vessels, nor are there data to indicate the length of time a high level of oxygen in arterial blood is tolerated.

Oxygen administration is contraindicated for newborn infants who depend on an open or patent ductus arteriosus to perfuse either the pulmonary circulation or the systemic circulation. The ductus arteriosus must be patent in order for the blood to bypass either obstructive valvular and vascular lesions of the right side of the heart (such as tetrology of Fallot or pulmonic stenosis) or those of the left side of the heart (hypoplastic left heart syndrome).[27] In order to understand why the administration of oxygen to these infants may be life-threatening, the reader must recall the changes in the heart and circulation occurring at birth. Following the infant's first breath, systemic arterial oxygen saturation begins to rise, and the ductus begins to constrict due to its particular susceptibility to the increase in partial pressure of oxygen in arterial blood. The hypoxia resulting from cyanotic congenital heart disease prevents the ductus arteriosus from closing. It is the usual practice to offer oxygen for a brief period to a cyanotic infant and to observe his or her response. The infant who is dependent on the open ductus arteriosus for pulmonary or systemic perfusion will respond to the administration of oxygen with increasing signs of cardiac failure.

In summary, considering the present state of knowledge of oxygen toxicity, clinicians do not withhold oxygen from an hypoxic patient because of the danger of oxygen toxicity but when giving oxygen they watch the patient closely to see whether it is helpful or harmful. Inspired oxygen concentrations, blood gases, lung volumes, circulatory status, and level of consciousness are continually monitored. When patients have had oxygen therapy over a brief period it must be discontinued gradually. The higher the concentration of the oxygen ther-

---

* Pontoppidan, H., et al.: "Acute Respiratory Failure in the Adult," (Second of Three Parts), N. Engl. J. Med., **287**:748, (Oct. 12) 1972.

apy, the more gradual should be its concentration reduction. A careful watch should be maintained and the pulse and respiratory rate observed closely. The partial pressure of oxygen in arterial blood may also be measured, but when facilities and equipment for this measurement are unavailable, the respiratory and pulse rates and rhythm are reliable guides to the patient's condition. If there are no arrhythmias, marked change in pulse rate, or respiratory rate, nor significant fall of P_aO_2, it may be assumed that the patient's general condition is satisfactory, and additional decreases can be carried out over a period of hours.

Regulation of Carbon Dioxide Content in the Inspired Air. Atmospheric air contains 0.03 per cent carbon dioxide; expired air, 4 per cent. The concentration of this gas in the inspired air can be increased markedly without any appreciable effect; however, the effect of too great concentrations is injurious since carbon dioxide in the blood stream stimulates the respiratory center in the medulla. According to Goodman and Gilman, as little as 2.0 volumes per cent of carbon dioxide in the inspired air increases its alveolar concentration.[27a] Concentrations above 2.0 volumes per cent for patients receiving oxygen therapy are undesirable, because the deep respirations produced may be exhausting.

Since the expired air contains such a high concentration of carbon dioxide, there is some danger of the air inside an oxygen tent or other chamber (such as an oxygen hood for infants) containing too large a proportion of this gas. However, it has been found that with a fairly high concentration of oxygen (approximately 50 per cent), the circulation of air produced in a tent by the inrush of oxygen (maintenance flow, 8 to 10 liters per minute) is sufficient to blow the carbon dioxide out and keep its concentration down below 2.0 volumes per cent. When the plastic oxygen hood is used for infants, the circulation of air can be maintained by a warmed moist flow of compressed air so that the oxygen can be delivered at exactly the per cent required for normal arterial oxygenation. Bendixen and associates [27b] explain the technique for measuring expired carbon dioxide concentrations. The infrared analyzer used for this purpose is more difficult to calibrate than an oxygen analyzer and, in the presence of an enlarged dead space, underestimates the actual arterial carbon dioxide tension. At the time of this writing it is thought to have limited value in patient care.

Control of Humidity. It is very important in both health and disease to provide a sufficient amount of moisture in the inspired air. A discussion of this subject may be found in Chapter 9. For patients receiving oxygen therapy, the regulation of the humidity is especially important.

Compressed gases are dry and, even when the upper airway is not bypassed, oxygen must never be administered without humidification for more than brief periods.[28] The humidifying capacity of a standard bubble humidifier is suitable for use with a nasal catheter or face mask, as the mouth and pharynx can supply additional warming and humidification. Ventilation through an endotracheal or tracheostomy tube bypasses the normal humidifying and warming action of the upper airway, and cools and dries the lower airway.[29] Therefore, humidifiers and nebulizers are used to add more moisture to the air for endotracheal and tracheostomy intubation. The addition of heat improves the absolute humidity (water vapor content) of humidifier output. The water in the humidifier is usually heated to a higher temperature than that of the body as it begins to cool as soon as it leaves the humidifying apparatus. However, the patient still has to provide body heat to vaporize the droplets once in the lung. If the tubing from the humidifier to the patient is allowed to fall in dependent loops, it can become obstructed by water. This water acts as a trap which removes the nebulized water droplets, and it must be drained periodically.

All mechanical ventilators must be used with at least one humidification device, either a heated humidifier or a particle generator (nebulizer). The humidity reservoirs of all ventilators are filled with sterile distilled water. See Chapter 15 for a discussion of the infection hazards associated with humidification equipment.

Oxygen tents and chambers are so constructed that the temperature of the atmosphere may be controlled. Ice chambers or refrigerating coils are used to cool the gas mixture in the tent. Condensation of water vapor in the expired air will remove excess moisture from the environment, but at least 50 per cent relative humidity is generally desirable. When 100 per cent humidity is required, humidifiers and nebulizers are used to supply the necessary moisture.

Methods of Administering Oxygen. Oxygen may be administered in the following ways: (1) by introducing a *catheter into the oropharynx;* (2) through *hollow tubes that fit into the nose* (nasal cannula); (3) by *face masks* of various types; (4) by an *oxygen tent or chamber;* and (5) by *mechanical ventilator.* Whatever method is selected, the means of administering oxygen is connected with a supply of oxygen (either individual tank or an outlet from the oxygen piping system) to which an oxygen regulator has been attached.

The *choice of method* depends on the patient's condition, the concentration desired, the facilities available, and the patient's and the doctor's preference. Should a patient be more comfortable with a face mask than with a nasal catheter in place, the former method would then be the preferred one, providing the prescribed concentration can be maintained. Less oxygen is usually required to maintain therapeutic concentrations using a catheter, nasal cannula, or mask than to operate a tent or ventilator. Nursing care varies widely depending upon the severity of illness and the means of delivering oxygen—from simple bedside measures of comfort and hygiene, to instruction in effective breathing and coughing, clearance of secretions by utilization of gravity and chest percussion (postural drainage), physiologic monitoring, and evaluation of mental status.

Responsibility for the operation of oxygen-therapy apparatus varies from one institution to another, as well as in homes. In large hospitals there are usually respiratory therapists who make the initial adjustment of the apparatus, inspect it at frequent intervals, test the inspired air for oxygen and carbon dioxide concentrations, and repair the equipment as necessary. In such cases the physician, nurse, and respiratory therapist together plan, implement, and evaluate the complex therapies available to help patients in any stage of respiratory impairment. Nurses are usually the persons most constantly at the bedside and, therefore, in the best position to anticipate the changing requirements of patients, and to prevent errors of dosage and other untoward incidents. They should understand the manipulation of cylinders, regulators, humidifiers, catheters, inhalers, face masks, tents, and ventilators; they should be able to make analyses of the air for concentrations of oxygen and carbon dioxide, draw and prepare venous or arterial blood samples for blood gas analysis, measure lung volumes, and adjust gas concentrations and ventilator volume and pressure in accordance with therapeutic requirements. Nurses should know how to clean and sterilize equipment and to store it so that deterioration is reduced to a minimum. It is their particular responsibility to study and devise ways of giving nursing care so that there is no interruption in the administration of oxygen or in other means of ventilatory support.

Nurses in leadership positions in respiratory and critical care units should keep informed on the latest developments in oxygen and ventilatory equipment by attendance at professional meetings and clinical symposia and consultation with physicians and respiratory therapists. They are then able to advise on the purchase of safe and economical equipment, prepare adequate budgets for purchase of equipment, and teach their staffs how to use it when the equipment is made available.

An important factor in successful oxygen therapy is the cooperation of patients. Unless the treatment has been adequately explained, they will be fearful, anxious, and tense. Explanation is also given to members of the patient's family who may otherwise be apprehensive; they must also be told of the great danger of smoking in the patient's room—signs on the tent and the door are not sufficient warnings.

No matter what technique is used, an *adequate supply of oxygen* must be maintained. Most hospitals now have a liquid oxygen supply with distribution to patient care areas (see Fig. 20-2). Standard line pressure is 50 lb psi (pounds per square inch). Oxygen may also be purchased in large cylinders at a pressure of 2000 lb psi. If cylinders are used as the oxygen supply, the following methods of handling oxygen in cylinders and other precautions must be kept in mind. The tanks may be taken directly to the patient's bedside or the oxygen delivered to the clinical division through an outlet from a manifold, or group of oxygen tanks, kept in a special oxygen supply room. On account of the danger of fire and explosion, installation of an oxygen manifold in a hospital is very desirable since the weight of tanks makes transportation difficult and since there is a possibility of errors in marking tanks "full" and "empty." Oxygen cylinders (or tanks) should be stored in a cool temperature away from inflammable material and where they are not likely to be knocked over. High temperatures cause expansion of the gas with consequent loss through the safety valve. While in use, an oxygen cylinder should be strapped to the tent, bed, or wall. In some types of oxygen tents there is space for the tank in which it is secured by a metal door.

The supply of oxygen must always be equipped with a regulator. A regulator changes the pressure at which the oxygen escapes from the tank to that needed for oxygen administration and keeps it flowing evenly. The flow gauge is usually calibrated in liters of oxygen per minute. The operator sets the gauge for the prescribed flow, and the regulator automatically controls it.

Before attaching a cylinder to a regulator it is important to do what is known as "cracking the valve." This means opening the valve

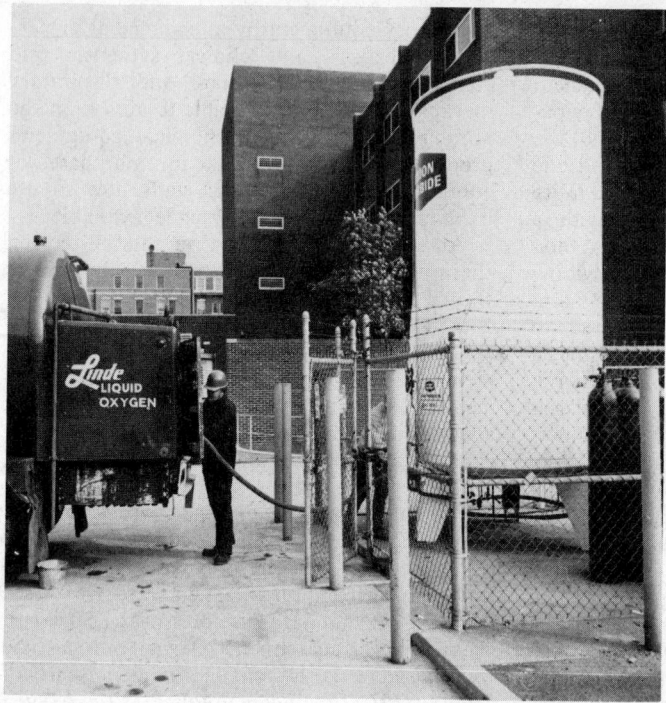

Figure 20-2. Liquid oxygen storage facility in a hospital setting. (Courtesy of Union Carbide Corporation, Linde Division, New York, N.Y.)

at the top of the cylinder slightly until a hissing sound is heard and then closing the valve quickly. Dust particles that may have lodged in the opening are thus removed. A failure to take this precaution may result in an injury to the regulator and possibly to the person operating the apparatus. The person cracking the valve should stand at the side, rather than the front, of the outlet.

An absolute rule in using any oxygen regulator is to avoid the use of oils. In the presence of high oxygen concentration, oils are likely to ignite and explosions have occurred as a result. A set of directions is supplied with each piece of oxygen equipment, and every operator should study and follow them carefully.

No rule can be given for regulating oxygen flow. To maintain a concentration of 50 per cent oxygen in the inspired air, Peter Safar[30] says a minimum flow of from 6 to 10 liters per minute is required according to the method of administration and the construction of the equipment; if no oxygen analyzer is available, flows of 10 to 14 liters per minute are indicated. As previously stated, the only sure method of maintaining the prescribed dosage is to make frequent analyses of samples of air as close to the patient's airway as possible.

A cylinder should not be replaced until it is entirely empty. A special gauge on the regulator shows the pressure of oxygen in the tank at any given time. When the amount of oxygen

is low (about 300 lb) as indicated on the regulator, another cylinder is ordered from the oxygen therapy unit so that it can be connected when the tank in use registers "empty." This will ensure continuous treatment. (At 8 liters per minute, the 300 lb remaining in the cylinder should last nearly 2 hours).*

Every doctor, nurse, technician, patient and his or her visitors should be aware of the *danger of fire and explosion* in oxygen therapy. Warning signs should be placed outside and inside oxygen tents and on ventilators. With the catheter and mask, the signs should be put where anyone near the bed can see them. As far as the writers have been able to discover, all fires that have been reported in connection with oxygen therapy have been caused by the lighting of a cigarette or pipe in a tent or in the vicinity of the oxygen supply. The hazard of using oil or grease on oxygen apparatus has been mentioned. Ungrounded electric devices and open flames should be banned. While the danger of accidents must be stressed in order to avoid them, there is no reason to be afraid

* Andrews' formula to determine duration of flow from oxygen cylinders is useful. He says: (1) multiply the pressure by 3, and (2) divide by flow in liters per minute. E.g.: $300 \times 3 = 900 \div 6 = 150$ minutes (or about 2 hours and 30 minutes). (Andrews, Albert H., Jr.: *Manual of Oxygen Therapy Techniques,* 2nd ed. Year Book Medical Publishers, Chicago, 1947, p. 23.)

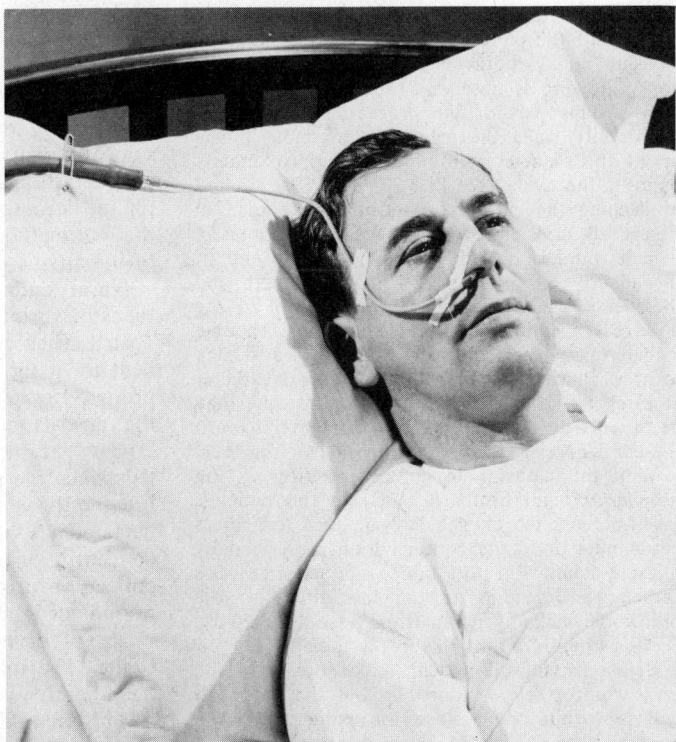

Figure 20-3. Oropharyngeal catheter in place and fastened to the patient's face with adhesive tape. Note how tubing is securely fastened to pillow with safety pin. There must be sufficient slack to permit free movement of the patient's head. (Courtesy of Union Carbide Corporation, Linde Division, New York, N.Y.)

of using oxygen apparatus if proper precautions are taken. Fires are usually the result of carelessness and need never occur. The same is true of explosions. See Chapter 15 for a discussion of electric safety.

Oropharyngeal Catheter Technique. Administration of oxygen by oropharyngeal catheter makes it less difficult to examine the body, give nursing care, or any sort of treatment. One of the great advantages of this method is that the patient is able to move about freely in bed; on the other hand, administration of oxygen by catheter is likely to irritate the mucous membrane. It is the combined responsibility of the physician, nurse, and respiratory therapist to help patients accept the treatment willingly and then to reduce the irritation of the nose and throat by the use of the humidifier and by changing the catheter at least every 8 hours or more often when indicated. This is the most common and inexpensive method of oxygen administration. It is recommended for short-term use, as in the immediate postoperative period. Prolonged use may lead to irritation of the nasal mucosa [31] (see Fig. 20-3).

Suggested Procedure. Fill humidifier jar half full or to indicated water level with distilled water and be sure it is working properly. Plug humidifier into outlet from the oxygen manifold or onto the cylinder of oxygen. Attach approximately 9 ft of oxygen tubing (usually plastic disposable) to humidifier. Attach the plastic, disposable nasal oxygen catheter (size #8 to #10 French for children and size #12 to #14 for adults, perforated with fine holes in its terminal 2½ cm) to the oxygen tubing. If a rubber oxygen catheter is used, a metal adapter is needed to make the attachment. Adjust flow rate to 2 to 3 liters.

To insert the catheter: Measure the distance from the tip of the nose (external nares) to the lobe of the ear (tragus), and mark this point on the catheter with a small piece of tape (to indicate the approximate distance the catheter is to be inserted).

Lubricate the catheter sparingly while the oxygen is flowing; then hold the tip of the catheter in a glass of water to make sure the terminal holes are not plugged with the lubricant.*

Determine the direction of the natural "droop" of the catheter: (1) hold the taped part with the thumb and forefinger, and (2) slowly rotate the catheter until its tip hangs at the lowest level. Elevate the tip of the nose, and pass the end of the catheter (in the position of its greatest "droop") gently along the floor of the nasal cavity into the oropharynx, *with the oxygen flowing.* Observe the position of the catheter through the patient's open mouth.

To make certain the catheter is in the correct

_____
* A lubricant that is not soluble in water (e.g., petroleum jelly) is satisfactory.

position, insert it slowly beyond the measured depth until the patient has swallowed a bolus of oxygen; then withdraw it back to a point where no swallowing is observed (about ⅔ cm or ¼ inch). (This part of the procedure can be followed only when the patient is conscious.) The tip of the catheter will now rest approximately opposite the uvula (see Fig. 20-4A–B). A method of keeping the catheter in position is shown in Figure 20-3. A piece of adhesive, approximately 1 inch wide, is placed on the nose. One end of the adhesive is split about 1 inch in length and these ends are left hanging from the tip of the nose. Place catheter between split ends; encircle catheter with each end, bringing both ends back to nose. Place small piece of tape across catheter at forehead. If the patient prefers, the tube may be fastened to the cheek and brought over toward the ear where it is taped to the side of the face.

With the catheter in correct position in the *oropharynx* and firmly fastened to the patient's face, increase the oxygen flow up to 4 to 6 liters per minute or to the concentration prescribed by the physician. Pin the tubing—attached to the catheter and leading to the humidifier—to the pillow or back of the mattress (see Fig. 20-3). See that there are no kinks in the tubing.

Before leaving the patient, make sure he or she is as comfortable as possible and that the call bell is within reach since the patient may be apprehensive. At stated intervals check the humidifier and add water as indicated.* Also check the catheter to be sure it does not adhere to the inside of the nose. Change the catheter every 8 hours as previously described, using the other

---

* When water is to be added to the humidifier, turn off the oxygen before adding water and fill quickly so that the patient is without oxygen for a minimal period.

nostril and a new lubricated catheter. If the disposable catheters are not available, the rubber type is washed and sterilized before it is used again.

In giving oxygen by this method there is some difficulty in accurately determining the concentration of oxygen in the inspired atmosphere, because it is not possible, as it is with the tent method, to test a representative sample of the air the patient is breathing.

Nasal Cannula. Plastic nasal cannulas are tubes of various sizes with tips that fit into the nostrils. The prongs are malleable and can be bent to fit the facial contour; the ends of the prongs are lubricated and then inserted into the nostrils about ¼ to ½ inch (see Fig. 20-5). The prongs must not occlude the nostrils since the patient would then be forced to breathe through the mouth, negating the beneficial effects of the treatment by diluting the concentration of oxygen. Because the vapor collects in drops of water in the nosepiece, a humidifier is not used unless the patient complains of dryness of the nasal mucous membrane. The inhaler is held in position with a head band.

This method may be valuable in tapering off oxygen therapy; also it is easily adapted for self-administration.

Oxygen Face Mask—Types. Face masks are used to administer oxygen in varying concentrations, as prescribed by the physician (see Fig. 20-6). They are available in the following four types: the simple face mask, the partial rebreather mask, the nonrebreathing mask, and the concentration mask. Bendixen and asso-

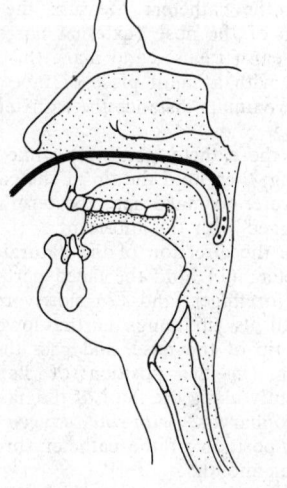

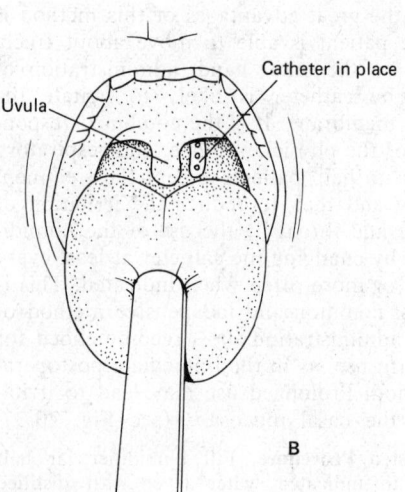

Figure 20-4. *A.* Sagittal section of the head to show depth to which oropharyngeal catheter is inserted. *B.* Tip of the catheter shown in relation to the uvula.

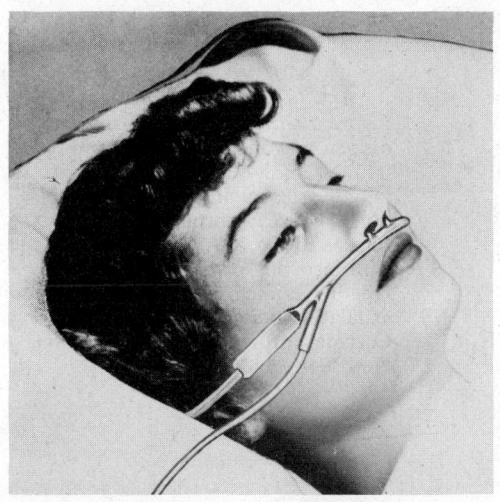

Figure 20-5. Administration of oxygen by nasal oxygen cannula. (Courtesy of Union Carbide Corporation, Linde Division, New York, N.Y.)

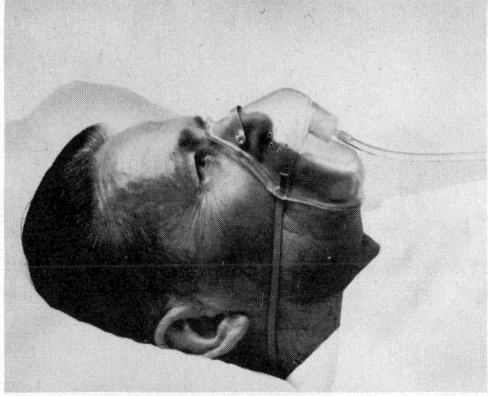

Figure 20-6. Administration of oxygen by simple plastic mask with oxygen inlet and exhalation holes. (Courtesy of Union Carbide Corporation, Linde Division, New York, N.Y.)

ciates [32] describe a face hood, a plastic device (not disposable) which may be strapped to the head, providing a snug fit underneath the chin, but leaving a wide opening at the top. It is used with a wide bore tube that connects to the hood at the level of the patient's mouth. The hood is used for administration of high humidity in the form of a mist. They state that this therapy is often effective in short-term treatment of laryngeal edema or in cases of very thick tracheobronchial secretions.[33]

Face masks are used for short-term oxygen therapy. Safar makes the following statement:

> The disadvantages of masks are that they are uncomfortable for the ill patient; there may be difficulty in obtaining a leak free seal, particularly in the unattended patient; and in opaque masks, mouth and nose are obscured from view.*

The mask must fit the patient's face, and careful adjustment of the head band is essential. The conscious patient can tell the nurse whether the head band should be placed above or below the ears for greater comfort. The nurse must be meticulous in the placement of the band so that there is no pressure on the top of the ear. A piece of gauze or sponge rubber over the bridge of the nose prevents irritation when a rubber face mask must be in position for a long time.

When oxygen therapy by means of a face mask is instituted, the nurse must spend sufficient time with the patient to be certain that he or she understands and will tolerate this

treatment. When the nurse leaves, she or he makes sure the call bell is close at hand.

Partial rebreathing bag-mask units are masks that contain reservoir bags enabling the patient to partially rebreathe exhaled gases. Exhaled gases are eliminated through ports or holes, utilizing high flows of oxygen into the mask (see Fig. 20-7). In order for the carbon dioxide accumulation to be minimized, Safer says the oxygen flow must be greater than the volume of gas breathed by the patient in one minute (minute volume).[34] The oxygen flow is adjusted so that during inhalation the reservoir bag does not deflate by more than half its capacity. The "B.L.B." unit,* a rubber mask with a latex bag and sponge rubber ports for overflow and emergency air inlet, is a type of partial rebreathing bag-mask unit. Others are plastic disposable bag-mask units. The per cent of inspired oxygen is dependent on the fit of the mask. Concentration of 80 to 100 per cent will be provided when the oxygen is on high flow (12 to 15 liters per minute).

Suggested Procedure. After the approximate size has been determined by the patient's facial contour, connect the tubing from the mask by an adapter to a 9 ft length of plastic tubing that is attached to the humidifier, which is, in turn, attached to the outlet of the oxygen regulator. The flow of oxygen is usually set at 6 to 8 liters per minute. Apply the mask to the patient's face as he or she exhales into the mask. Oxygen enters the mask through perforated rubber tubing that opens directly under the external nares. Most patients breathe more deeply or more rapidly

---

* Safar, Peter (ed.): *Respiratory Therapy.* F. A. Davis Co., Philadelphia, 1965, p. 154.

* The name *B.L.B. mask* is taken from the first letters of the surnames of the men who devised it: W. M. Boothby, W. R. Lovelace, and A. H. Bulbulian.

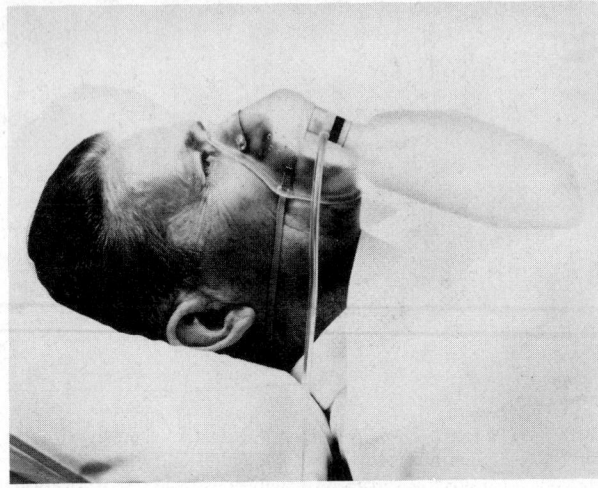

Figure 20-7. In the partial rebreathing oxygen mask the oxygen flows directly into the mask during inspiration and into the reservoir bag during exhalation. The early portion of exhaled air returns to the bag to be rebreathed with incoming oxygen in the next breath. Terminal air escapes from the exhalation ports. (Courtesy of Union Carbide Corporation, Linde Division, New York, N.Y.)

when a mask is first applied. For this reason, it is advisable to increase the flow up to from 10 to 12 liters per minute. As soon as the initial abnormal breathing has subsided, reduce the flow to from 6 to 8 liters per minute; the breathing bag should almost, but not quite, collapse during inspiration. Usually the mask is removed at stated intervals (every 2 hours) so that the patient's face may be washed, dried, and powdered lightly before the mask is reapplied.

A disadvantage of the oronasal face mask is that oxygen administration must be discontinued when the patient eats and drinks. It is used, however, because the equipment is inexpensive, because it simplifies nursing care, and because some patients with a tendency to claustrophobia prefer a mask to a tent. It does not have the disadvantage of irritating the oronasal mucous membranes as does the catheter technique.

Nonrebreathing masks prevent the inhalation of exhaled gas. Inhaled gas comes from a bag by way of the inhalation valve, and all exhaled gas is eliminated through the exhalation valve. Oxygen must be supplied at a flow to satisfy the minute volume of the patient; that is, to keep the reservoir bag full at the beginning of each inhalation. Should the bag collapse completely during inhalation, a safety air inlet valve opens.[35,35a] Oxygen flow is regulated by an attached concentration meter, and not by the liter flow per minute as with the partial rebreathing mask.

When the oxygen concentration is changed by resetting the meter disk, the liter flow must be either raised or lowered. The plug in the meter mask can be removed if suction is indicated. If the plug is removed inadvertently and not replaced, there will be a loss of oxygen by leakage.

The meter mask comes equipped with specially designed large-diameter tubing. It is important to use this tubing; if a smaller diameter tubing is substituted, the percentage of oxygen actually administered will vary from that shown on the meter. There must be no kinks in the tubing.

The meter mask is available in both nasal and oronasal styles. The meter that mixes air with oxygen and on which the required concentration of oxygen is indicated is attached to the outlet of the oxygen regulator after the hose nipple and nut have been removed. (It is important to store these two items carefully to prevent loss.) The large-diameter tubing from the mask is attached to the outlet at the back of the meter. This type of mask is now rarely used since the development of the disposable concentration masks which deliver controlled low concentrations of oxygen.

Suggested Procedure. Check the inlet connection of the mask to make sure the large-diameter tubing has been attached so that the inlet connection is pointing downward at a slight angle. Then turn the meter disk to the prescribed oxygen percentage by rotating the disk so that the number corresponding to the desired percentage is at the top. Have the meter disk set at approximately 10 liters when applying the mask. After the patient has been breathing normally for several minutes, turn the flow of oxygen down to from 6 to 8 liters per minute. Apply the mask as the patient exhales. Adjust the head band above the ears so that it fits snugly; be sure that there is no pressure on the ears. The breathing bag which must not collapse completely during inhalation indicates correct flow of oxygen.

Should the patient complain of dryness of the mouth, nose, and throat, increase the moisture of the inhaled oxygen by injecting 15 to 20 ml of water into the meter, either through the large hole in the meter disk or through the hose connection on the back of the meter. Remove the meter mask at stated intervals (usually every 2 hours) so that the patient's face can be washed, dried, and powdered.

Concentration masks (sometimes referred to as venturi masks) deliver a relatively low but predictable and constant oxygen concentration of 24 to 40 per cent, along with a high total gas flow. No exhaled gases are rebreathed due to the high flow and the exhalation ports on the mask. The mask is designed to draw in or "entrain" room air to mix with oxygen. Oxygen passes through a precisely sized oxygen inlet and pulls in room air through ports in the surrounding cylinder.* The high flow exceeds the patient's minute volume so that the mask need not be fitted tightly to the face. The cooling action of the high flow is often a comfort to the patient even when heated humidity is used.

Suggested Procedure. After the approximate mask size has been determined by the patient's facial contour, connect the large bore tubing from the mask to the oxygen inlet attachment containing the venturi and air entrainment orifice. At the time of this writing, the oxygen inlet attachments presently available are four sizes to deliver 24, 28, 35, and 40 per cent oxygen concentration. Then connect the oxygen inlet attachment to the plastic tubing which, in turn, is attached to a humidifier and to the outlet of the oxygen regulator. Set the oxygen flow at 4 liters for the 24 and 28 per cent oxygen inlet and 8 liters per minute for the 35 and 40 per cent oxygen inlet. The procedure of applying an oxygen mask to the face and adjusting it for comfort has been previously described under Oxygen Face Mask—Types, page 1094.

Safar[36] states that oxygen therapy masks cannot be used for positive pressure artificial ventilation because of their structurally loose design, poor mask fit, and leaks during inflation attempts. Bendixen and associates and Safar agree that the expiratory positive pressure provided by these masks is of value in treating patients with mild pulmonary edema,

and sometimes in emphysematous patients who require positive and expiratory pressure to prevent collapse of small bronchi.[37,38]

Oxygen Tent. An oxygen tent consists of a cabinet that may be connected to a supply of oxygen and a canopy to cover the patient and the whole or part of the bed (see Fig. 20-8). There are various tents on the market and they may be grouped under the classification of motor-driven and motorless tents. In the first type, oxygen is forced into the tent by a motor-driven rotary blower. The oxygen is temperature controlled in the cabinet before it enters the canopy. In the second type, oxygen is forced into an air-conditioning chamber by pressure from the oxygen cylinder only. Because cold air is heavier than warm air, currents form inside the canopy and cabinet, cold air falling as hot air rises. If the outlets in the cabinet are properly placed and the whole mechanism well constructed, therapeutic concentrations of oxygen can be maintained in a motorless tent with a very much lower oxygen consumption than in the motor-driven tents. To prevent gradual accumulation of carbon dioxide, a flow of oxygen exceeding the minute volume of the patient must be provided, usually 12 to 14 liters or more, of oxygen per minute.[39] Motor-driven tents require a flow of from 6 to 12 liters to maintain oxygen concentrations around 50 per cent, while some

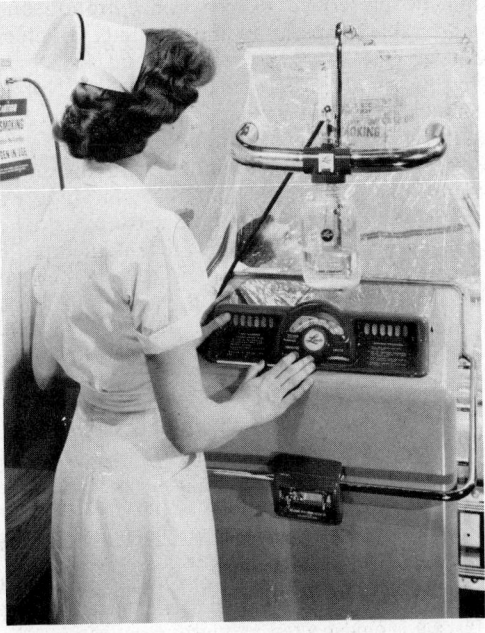

Figure 20-8. The oxygen tent. (Courtesy of Union Carbide Corporation, Linde Division, New York, N.Y.)

---

* The principle of operation is based on the "Bernoulli effect" (Daniel Bernoulli, 1700–1782). The principle states that pressure exerted by a steady flow of fluid through a tube varies inversely as the velocity of the fluid. When there is an abrupt narrowing of the tube, there will be a presure drop distal to the restriction. A modification of the Bernoulli effect is found in a venturi (Giovanni Venturi, 1742–1822). The "Venturi principle" states that the pressure drop distal to the restriction may be restored closely to the pre-obstruction pressure if the tube is dilated immediately after the narrowing, with an angle of divergence not to exceed 15 degrees. (Walker, Charles G.: *Mix-O-Mask, Low Concentration Oxygen Mask,* O.E.M. Medical Inc., Edison, N.J.)

motorless tents maintain the same concentrations with a flow of from 6 to 10 liters. When an oxygen analyzer is not available, an oxygen flow of from 10 to 14 liters per minute is recommended to maintain a 40 per cent concentration. In addition, after the tent has been opened, it should be generously flooded with oxygen to reestablish the desired concentration.

The temperature of the air can be satisfactorily regulated with either type. A desirable temperature is thought to range around 21°C (69.8°F) although higher temperatures may be indicated for infants and the aged. A relative humidity of 40 to 60 per cent should be maintained.

In older oxygen tent cabinets the circulation of air occurred in the main unit. These models have to be stripped and mechanically cleaned. In newer models the circulation of air is through a separate refrigerated coil inside the canopy, thus permitting sterilization of all parts of the unit that come in contact with the patient.[40]

Canopies are made of various plastics. The larger the transparent area, the better the patient likes it and the more easily the nurse can observe the patient. From the occupant's standpoint, canopies that cover the entire bed are preferable, but they require a higher oxygen consumption than the smaller canopies and make nursing care more difficult.

While taking care of a patient in an oxygen tent, a nurse is often responsible for maintaining the prescribed oxygen concentration and a desirable temperature and humidity. In older models, ice has to be renewed and soda lime for absorbing carbon dioxide changed. Nurses should feel that it is their responsibility to give nursing care in such a way that the patient's needs are adequately fulfilled with the minimum loss of oxygen from the tent. It is essential that each institution set up its own nursing procedure for oxygen tent therapy in accordance with the type of tent in current use at that institution, even though the basic principles in effective tent therapy are applicable to any type of tent. The following method summarizes the steps in starting tent therapy:

Suggested Procedure. Check the tent and its accessories outside the patient's room to make sure the unit is complete. With the canopy over the top of the frame, wheel the tent into the patient's room, having first talked with him or her and explained the advantages of the treatment and having tried to discover and minimize anxiety. Place a shoulder wrap around the patient.

Plug unit into electrical outlet and adjust temperature setting to 21.1°C (70°F) or −11.1°C (12°F) below room temperature, if room temperature is over 26.7°C (80°F). Turn on the oxygen flow. Adjust the tent canopy over the patient, being careful that the edges of the canopy do not touch the patient's face. Then tuck the canopy under the mattress as far as it will go at the head and sides of the bed. With a sheet or cotton flannel bath blanket, fasten the front of the canopy by making a wide double cuff; tuck the ends firmly under the mattress. Flood the tent with oxygen either with the flush valve for at least 2 minutes or by raising the oxygen flow to 15 liters per minute and maintaining this flow for approximately 15 minutes. At the end of this period, analyze the atmosphere within the tent to make certain the patient is receiving the prescribed oxygen concentration (usually 40 per cent). Check the temperature gauge on the unit to make sure the temperature is not too low for the patient's comfort. (In older models, the thermometer may be placed inside the tent.) If the patient feels cold, give him or her an extra shoulder wrap and/or raise the temperature control to medium or warm. *No electric appliances* (such as an electric heating pad, signal cord, or device of any kind) *are to be used within the tent.*

Check the oxygen concentration approximately every 3 to 4 hours or as necessary prior to opening the tent to give care. Before leaving the room make sure the patient has a hand bell.

If the patient has accepted the tent therapy without undue apprehension and seems relaxed and comfortable, it is wise for the nurse to explain again briefly and calmly why no electrical appliances are to be used within the tent as well as emphasizing that visitors are not to smoke in the room while the treatment is in progress. The nurse must check to make sure there are no matches and cigarettes in the patient's bedside stand. It is also the nurse's responsibility to give the family adequate and frequent reminders of these hazards. Signs on the tent canopy and door of the patient's room need reinforcement through repeated verbal warnings to the patient and his or her visitors, just as the warning has been repeated within this chapter.

To conserve oxygen, the following precautions should be taken: (1) examine the canopy frequently for cracks and tears; (2) keep the canopy well tucked under the mattress, sealing the free edge with a folded sheet or cotton bath blanket if the canopy does not entirely cover the bed; (3) when using the sleeve or zippered opening to hand the patient food or drink, bathe the face, or clean the mouth, draw the sleeve tightly around the arm; (4) in bathing the patient's body or making the bed, slide the canopy up around the neck of the patient and tuck it under the pillow (see Fig. 20-9). In some hospitals, patients are removed from the tent and given oxygen by catheter or mask while they are bathed.

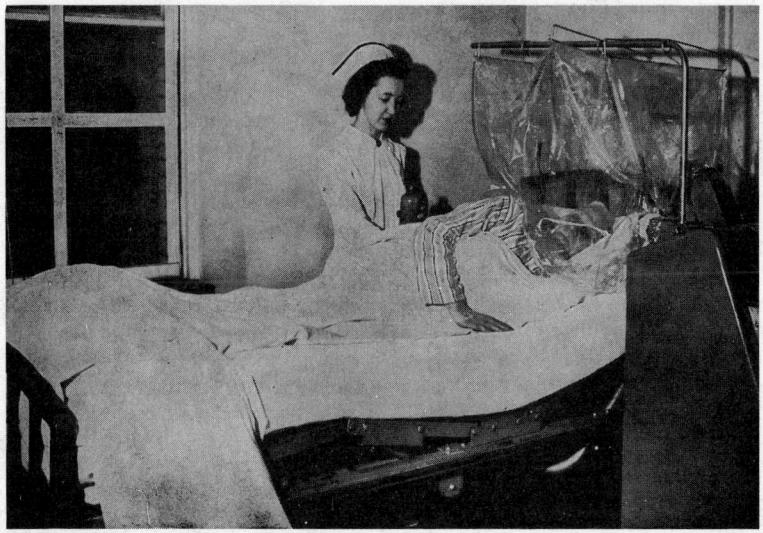

Figure 20-9. Patient being cared for in an oxygen tent. The canopy is tucked under the pillow, above the shoulders, so that patient receives continuous oxygen. (Courtesy of New York Hospital, New York, N.Y., and West, John P., Keller, Manelva W., and Harmon, Elizabeth: *Nursing Care of the Surgical Patient,* 6th ed. Macmillan Publishing Co., Inc., New York, N.Y.

For the febrile patient, low temperatures inside an oxygen tent are usually comfortable. It is wise, however, to provide a head and shoulder wrap, for the air entering the tent on the side with the cabinet is very cool and the unprotected neck and shoulders are likely to be chilled. If the tent has louvers, they are adjusted so that the incoming atmosphere is not blown directly on the patient.

Analyses of the air inside the canopy should be made at regular intervals (every 3 or 4 hours) and whenever examinations or treatments necessitate opening the canopy. Either the liter flow per minute is increased to 15 for a 15-minute period, or if the tent is equipped with a flush valve, the tent may be flooded rapidly with extra oxygen for 2 minutes. However, when the latter method is used, the patient must be warned of the rushing sound this makes. Even though the flow of oxygen is always increased following treatments, there is no certainty that the prescribed concentration has been reestablished until an oxygen analysis of the atmosphere in the tent has been made.

When oxygen therapy is to be discontinued, it may be advisable to taper off the treatment. This may be done by loosening the canopy to create leakage; however, this is an expensive method. As an alternative, the patient may be removed from the tent for short intervals of 15 to 20 minutes. If the pulse rate does not

increase, such intervals can be lengthened. A third method would be to give the patient oxygen either by catheter or face mask, with a slower rate of liter flow per minute. A very slow rate of oxygen flow cannot be utilized in a tent because of the possibility of carbon dioxide build-up within the tent should the flow of oxygen be so reduced that there is insufficient force to blow out the excess carbon dioxide.

Modern canopies are disposable. If the reusable canopy is used, the tent should be thoroughly washed with soap and water, and aired before it is stored. Soaking in a chemical disinfectant such as activated gluteraldehyde is recommended by some authorities. Great care should be taken in storage to prevent tearing or cracking tents. If space is available, it is best not to fold them at all.

Administration of Oxygen to Infants and Children. The five main factors that influence the administration of oxygen to infants and children are (1) the patient's size; (2) his or her ability to comply with the treatment; (3) the nature of respiratory conditions in the pediatric age group; (4) the influence of drugs, trauma, and foreign bodies in the child's ventilation; and (5) in some cases the equipment available. The professional worker who gives oxygen therapy or other forms of respiratory therapy to children must be familiar with the child's developmental needs and his or her response to stress, in addition to possessing adequate technical knowledge about respiratory therapy equipment for children.

Masks of various types may be used for children provided the size is correct and the configuration is suitable to fit the child.[41] Disposable plastic masks and reusable masks are available in pediatric sizes. Because very young children are naturally active, it is difficult to keep a mask tightly applied to the face, and other types of equipment for the delivery of oxygen are easier to use. The canopy tent designed for pediatric use ("croup" tent) is of great benefit for children when high concentrations of oxygen and mist are desired (see Fig. 20-10).*

The "croup" tent is essentially a small oxygen tent. It can be improvised in the home, but in most hospitals today a device is available called a "Croupette." † In its current form, cooling is accomplished by the use of ice in a container at the back of the unit. The "Croupette" has a self-contained nebulizer. The entire unit can be cleaned with a chemical disinfectant, and disposable canopies are available. The small size of these units is reported to make the control of oxygen concentration, humidity, and temperature a much simpler task than in adult oxygen tents.[42] Avery and her associates present the following and differing point of view on the efficacy of the treatment using the "Croupette":

The distressing habit of ordering mist by writing the trade name of a commercial tent has pervaded many services, leaving [unspecified] the crucial decision of the rate of gas flow, use of air or oxygen and temperature regulation. . . . If ice cubes are added to cool one surface of the tent, the internal temperature may fall to levels which require of the patient shivering, vasocon-

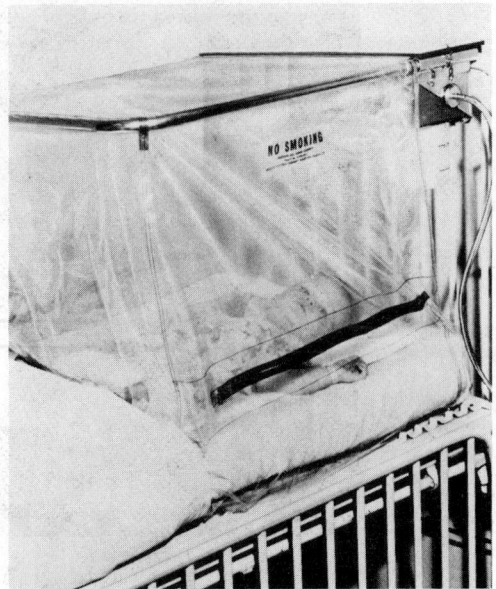

Figure 20-10. "Croupette" or canopy tent for children. The side rails of the crib have been lowered for the photograph. (Courtesy of Union Carbide Corporation, Linde Division, New York, N.Y.)

striction, and increased oxygen consumption. Droplets of water on the skin or wet clothes aggravate heat loss . . . failure to watch the tent temperature may lead to overheating.*

Suggested Procedure. Check the "Croupette" and its accessories outside the patient's room to make sure the unit is complete. Fill the jar with distilled water and see that it is working properly. It is usually recommended that ice be added to the chamber before bringing the unit to the patient's bedside. Practical experience shows that it is often easier to fill the chamber after the unit is in place on the bed or crib, as it is heavier with the ice added and difficult to maneuver.

Open the canopy frame and place the unit over the patient with the ice chamber at the head of the bed. It is helpful to have the assistance of another person (parent or nurse) to hold the child out of the bed or otherwise be alert for his or her safety, while the equipment is being moved into place.

Plug the flow meter into the oxygen outlet and adjust to 8 liters per minute. Attach tubing from flow meter to "Croupette." Check pressure gauge on the "Croupette" to make sure it is operating correctly. The indicator moves into the green area on the dial. If air compressor is used (for mist therapy without added oxygen) adjust air flow so that pressure gauge needle is in the green area. Make sure damper is in "open" position.

* Mary E. Avery and her associates express the following views in relation to the pediatric age group:

At present, technical advances in the generation of mists and the knowledge of the deposition of particles *exceeds* knowledge of the role of mist in the treatment of respiratory disorders. Some evidence exists that viscous secretions can be thinned by mist; upper airway cooling and drying can be decreased by added humidity. . . . No evidence exists that lower airway obstructive disease or bronchopneumonia in the absence of much sputum is improved by mist. Humidified oxygen can be given without mist. . . . It would be useful practice for the physician to consider whether the aim is to provide oxygen or air, humidity or mist and to weigh the hazards of a wet, uneven thermal environment versus uncertain gain from mist in the treatment of respiratory disease. (Avery, Mary E., et al.: "Mist Therapy," *Pediatrics*, **39**:160, [Feb.] 1967.)

† "Croupette" is a name used by Air Shields Co., Hatboro, Pa., National Cylinder Gas Co., Chicago, Ill., and Union Carbide Corp., Linde Division, New York, N.Y., to describe the canopy tent for pediatric use that they manufacture.

* Avery, Mary E., et al.: *op. cit.*

This enables the tent to be flushed with air or oxygen.

Place the child in the tent. Place canopy over frame and tuck it under frame and mattress. Attach tubing to the condensate drain and place the end in a receptacle. This prevents moisture from soaking the child's bed. Move damper to "closed" position. This provides for adequate flow of oxygen or air and for fine particles of mist to flow without forming droplets of water vapor, which only serve to wet the child and the bed.

The temperature inside the "Croupette" should be checked frequently, also the oxygen concentration. G. E. Burch reports that a tent temperature of 23° to 25°C (73.4° to 77°F) for the clothed infant is optimal from the aspect of cardiac work.[43] The oxygen concentration for the ill child should be adjusted according to his or her blood gas analysis. If blood gases are not being monitored, skin color, pulse, and respirations measure the effect of the oxygen concentration. It is difficult to get concentrations of oxygen greater than 50 per cent inside the "Croupette" due to leakage.

The unit must be checked to see that it is fogging properly and that the pressure gauge is operating in the green area. The nebulizing jar should be filled with distilled water. Excess water should be drained from the ice chamber and fresh ice brought to refill it as needed. The child may keep toys or any other comforting object from home inside the tent. The reader is referred to textbooks on pediatric nursing for suggestions on feeding, bathing, and providing emotional comfort for the child who requires oxygen and mist therapy by "Croupette."

The *infant incubator* * is a unit designed primarily to maintain a constant temperature in the environment of the infant. In addition to a built-in heating unit, it has provision for humidification and oxygen delivery (see Fig. 20-11). Concentration of oxygen in an incubator cannot generally be raised beyond 60 to 70 per cent. An imperfectly fitting plastic lid and the opening of portholes to gain access to the infant deplete ambient oxygen concentrations rapidly (see Fig. 20-12).[44] The incubator is not the method of choice for the administration of oxygen because the concentration

---

* The use of the infant incubator or "Isolette" is discussed here only from the standpoint of the administration of oxygen. The reader is referred to textbooks on the care of the newborn and seriously ill infant for a complete discussion of the use of the infant incubator in the management of the environment of the seriously ill newborn.

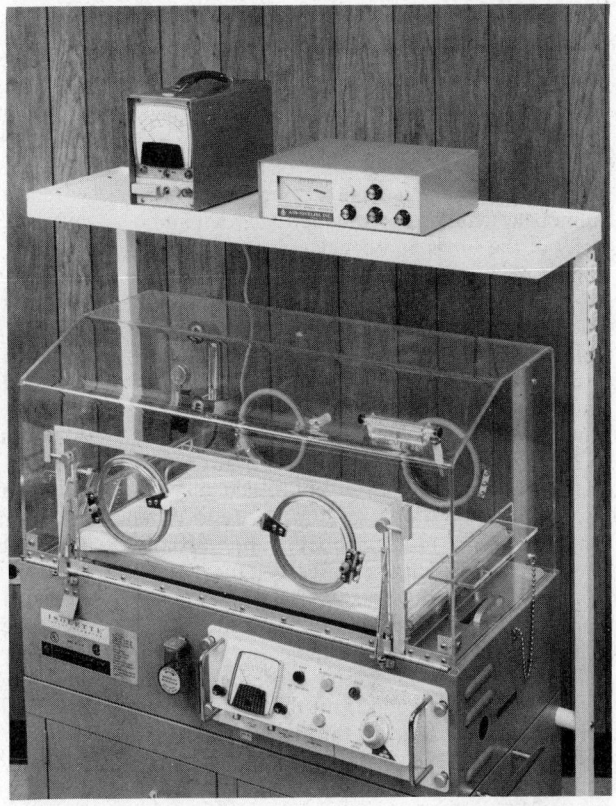

Figure 20-11. Incubator to provide an infant with an environment of controlled oxygen concentration, temperature, and humidity. An accessory shelf provides space above the hood for placement of monitoring, respiration, or other adjunct equipment. (Courtesy of Air-Shields, Inc., A Narco Health Company, Hatboro, Pa.)

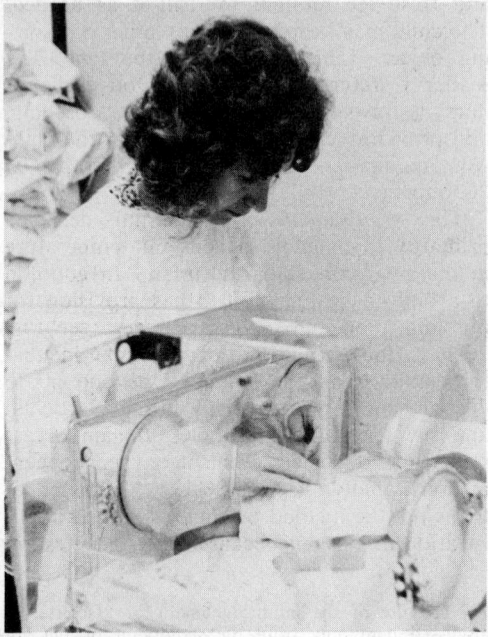

Figure 20-12. When giving care to an infant in an incubator, the nurse or parent inserts her hands through plastic, washable cuffs. This minimizes the loss of heat and humidity and helps maintain a constant temperature in the infant's environment. (Courtesy of Yale University School of Nursing, New Haven, Conn.)

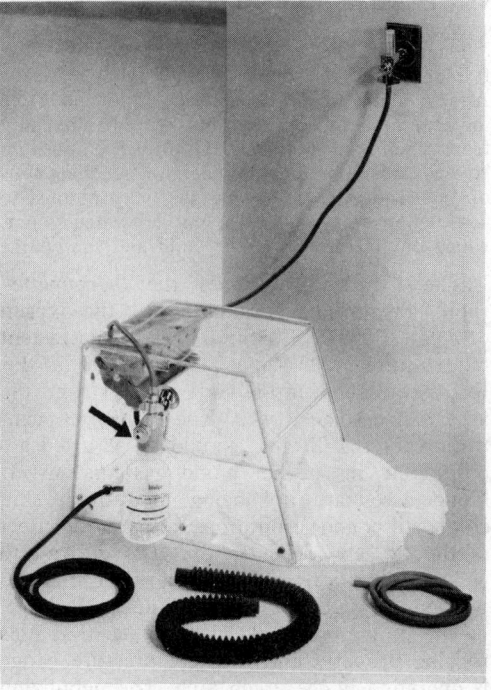

Figure 20-13. One type of plastic head hood for oxygen administration. (Courtesy of Union Carbide Corporation, Linde Division, New York, N.Y.)

is so variable, but also because the hypoxic infant usually needs administration of oxygen under positive pressure. The infant is hypoxic because of the increased work of breathing (or decreasing compliance of the lungs) and intrapulmonary shunting subsequent to the immaturity of the lungs and deficiency of surfactant. The primary problem, therefore, is to enable air to move into the lungs with the least amount of effort on the part of the infant. This is usually accomplished by mechanical positive pressure ventilation rather than by simply adding oxygen to the air that the infant is struggling to inhale.

The *plastic head hood* is a useful alternative method for maintaining a controlled elevated oxygen concentration (see Fig. 20-13). When a hood is in use in an incubator, the portholes may be opened without affecting the oxygen concentration in the hood.[45] The hood is especially helpful for an hypoxic infant who is being treated on an open table supplied with radiant heat from an overhead source. Oxygen is delivered to the hood from the wall or cylinder source after passing through a heated humidifying unit. The recommended temperature is 31° to 34°C (87.8° to 93.2°F). The use of cold, unhumidified air-oxygen mixture by way

of a face mask or head hood results in large increases in oxygen consumption despite an apparently adequate thermal environment surrounding the infant. This occurs because the temperature-sensitive zones of the face and forehead are stimulated.[46] A flow of oxygen or air mixed with oxygen of at least 6 liters per minute is essential to "wash out" exhaled carbon dioxide from the hood. Sufficient flow of air is provided by a compressor or cylinder of compressed air when oxygen concentrations are being decreased.

Administration of Oxygen in the Home. Oxygen may be prescribed for therapy at home for patients suffering from chronic respiratory disease. These patients, usually in the stable phase of their disease, require an organized approach to home care with ready access to instruction in self-care and assistance in getting the proper equipment and medications. Thomas L. Petty[47] and Joanne Lagerson[48] describe home care programs designed to increase patients' comfort, their ability to work and to enjoy more normal daily activities, in spite of having a progressively debilitating disease. These programs may be directed by a nurse with special preparation in care of patients with respiratory diseases. They may be located in hospitals and clinics, visiting nurse associations, respiratory disease associations, or public health agencies. The patient's physician, nurse, respiratory therapist, and social worker usually consult together in planning a home care program. They provide for patient education in all measures used to clear the airways of secretions (bronchial hygiene), breathing retraining, and physical reconditioning. Oxygen is reserved for patients with hypoxia and marked disability.

Oxygen therapy is provided most efficiently with a portable liquid oxygen reservoir that contains about a 3-day supply of oxygen. The portable 7-lb canister, containing approximately a 3-hour supply of oxygen, is filled from the reservoir and worn by patients strapped to the back or carried with them about the house or out-of-doors during work or recreation. The patient receives the oxygen through a nasal oxygen cannula connected to plastic oxygen tubing. The mucous membranes of the nose humidifies the gas so that bubbling the oxygen through water is not necessary. Petty and Louise M. Nett [49] report that oxygen by mouth is more drying, and they recommend the nasal cannula.

Oxygen can also be stored in the home in cylinders (tanks). When this method of administration is used the patient is confined to the area where the tank is. Oxygen cylinders are available in all sizes for the home from the "A" cylinder, 3 inches in diameter and 10 inches in height, to the "H & K" cylinder, 9 inches in diameter and 55 inches in height.[50] The smallest cylinder contains sufficient oxygen for 20 minutes and may be carried in a car or brief case. The larger cylinders will provide oxygen for 4 to 6 hours, depending on the gauge pressure (pounds per square inch or "psi") and flow rate (liters per minute). Because these cylinders are large and hard to move and store they are rarely used in the home. Douglas R. Gracey [51] reports on a newer development in home oxygen therapy for patients who require a stationary oxygen source. This is the molecular sieve system * which removes nitrogen, carbon monoxide and hydrocarbons from room air and leaves an enriched oxygen supply (see Fig. 20-14). The units are small and provide any concentration of oxygen from 22 to 90 per cent. These devices should fill an important need in remote areas where tank and reservoir replacement calls are difficult.

Precise instruction to the patient and his or her family must be given on the safety precau-

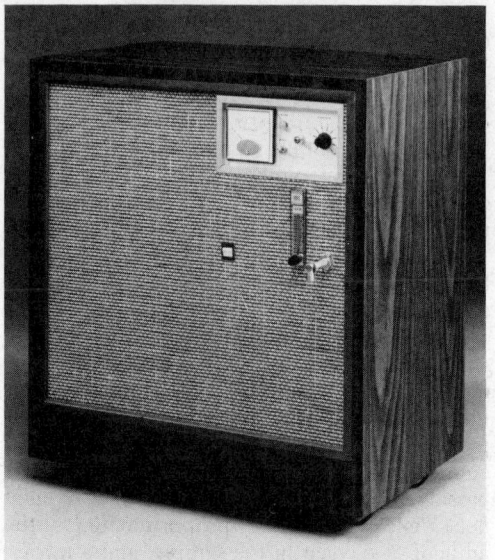

Figure 20-14. A system with molecular sieves which remove nitrogen, carbon monoxide, and hydrocarbon from room air, providing an enriched oxygen supply for the patient who needs oxygen therapy in the home. (Courtesy of Marx Medical Incorporated, La Jolla, Calif.)

tions while using oxygen. The nurse should make a home visit before discharge of the patient to plan with the family the location of an oxygen cylinder and how to secure it so that it can't fall. The nurse should be in the home at the time the oxygen is delivered to give further instructions on opening the cylinder and regulating the flow. The companies that bring oxygen to the home also provide instruction in its use and explain safety precautions to the patient and family. Spencer H. Robley,[52] a patient with emphysema, has written a helpful guide to self-care for other victims of emphysema. He tells how to get oxygen delivered, how to operate the cylinders in the home, and describes safety precautions. He notes that oxygen is much less expensive when gotten from a welding supply company. The oxygen cylinders carried by these companies are labeled usable as medical oxygen.

The nurse consulting with patients who require oxygen at home should seek help from the local or state respiratory disease association. They can advise on availability and cost of equipment in the patient's area and sources of financial support for rental or purchase of equipment. Financial support can come from private medical insurance, federal medical insurance ("Medicare" under Social Security), state medical benefits ("Medicaid" and other welfare programs), state crippled children's services, and various voluntary groups and

---

* Marx Oxygen System, Marx Medical Incorporated, LaJolla, Calif., and Bendix Respiratory Support System, Bendix Corp., Health Care Products, Davenport, Iowa.

parents' associations, such as associations for the care of children with cystic fibrosis.

Analysis of Air for Oxygen Content. Oxygen analyzers can be divided into two basic *types:* units that require manual aspiration of a quantity of gas into a sampling chamber, and devices that monitor oxygen concentration continuously by means of an attached or remote sensor [53] (see Figs. 20-15 and 20-16). The first permits only intermittent analysis, but the second permits either intermittent or continuous analysis.

The units that require manual aspiration of gas into a sampling chamber operate on one of two basic principles: paramagnetism or thermal conductivity. In the former, the sample of gas is drawn into the instrument by compression of a rubber bulb and dried by passing through desiccant crystals. The magnetic field is distorted proportionate to the amount of oxygen in the sample, and a mirror moves in the field. A beam of battery-powered light is reflected onto a translucent scale calibrated to translate the magnetic force into per cent of oxygen in the air sample. The other intermittent oxygen analyzers operate on the principle of thermal conductivity or the fact that heat conductivity of oxygen is different from that of nitrogen. The rate at which a temperature-sensitive thermistor is cooled in the sampling chamber depends on the oxygen concentration in the chamber. The rate of cooling of this thermistor is compared with the rate of cooling of a similar control thermistor,

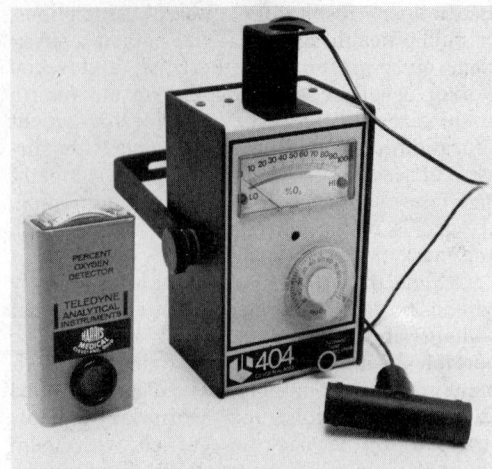

Figure 20-16. An oxygen analyzer that monitors oxygen continuously by means of an attached sensor. (Courtesy of Union Carbide Corporation, Linde Division, New York, N.Y.)

and the difference is displayed as a meter reading of oxygen concentration.[54]

All of the continuous oxygen analyzers operate on electrochemical principles, using either polarographic sensors or galvanic cells.[55] In the polarographic technique, oxygen diffuses through a membrane and electrolyte solution to a bipolar electrode across which a polarizing potential is applied. To compensate for temperature changes, a thermistor is incorporated into the sensor, allowing it to respond only to the changing *partial* pressure of oxygen. An electric current is generated proportionate to the diffusion of oxygen. The flow of current is amplified and indicated on a meter in per cent concentration of oxygen. Polarographic sensors require periodic replacement of the electrolyte solution and an external power source.

In a galvanic cell, the polarizing potential is internally generated, and periodic replacement of electrolyte solution is not required. The galvanic cell has a limited life span and must be replaced after 6 months to 1 year.[56] Once exposed to room air, the limited life of the sensor begins.

Nurses, respiratory therapists, and physicians must have precise understanding of the *operation of the analyzer* used in the patient care area. For example, the paramagnetic, intermittent sampling analyzers can test only dry gas. They are equipped with a cartridge containing desiccant crystals which must be replaced when there is a color change (this occurs when the crystals cannot absorb anymore moisture from samples of gas). One of the intermittent sampling analyzers that op-

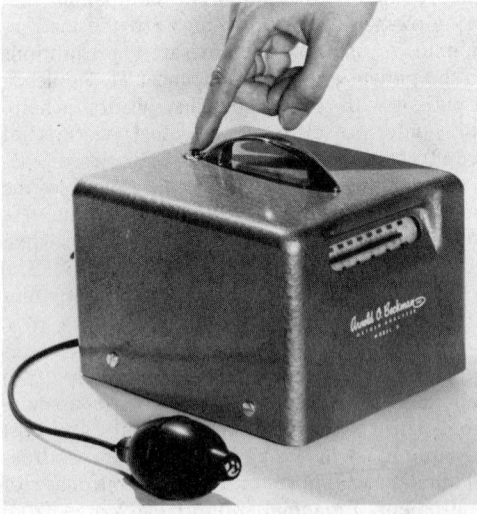

Figure 20-15. An oxygen analyzer that requires manual aspiration of a quantity of gas into a sampling chamber. (Courtesy of Union Carbide Corporation, Linde Division, New York, N.Y.)

erates on the principle of thermal conductivity analyzes wet gas and contains a silica gel which adds moisture to the dry gas. A carbon dioxide absorbing agent is also required when an intermittent analyzer is used to measure gas samples in the expiratory line of ventilators. Carbon dioxide will alter the thermal conductivity of oxygen.[57] Some analyzers are accurate only when placed on a flat surface and give inaccurate readings when hand held.

The electrochemical analyzers are very susceptible to condensation on their sensors, which could easily occur when used in a mist tent or in the inspiratory lines of ventilators. The oxygen concentration readings will be erroneously low because the film of water retards the diffusion of oxygen into the sensor. Wiping the sensor clean of accumulated moisture is a simple but easily forgotten procedure. It has already been noted that the polarographic sensor may be cleaned and reused. The recharging process must be understood in order to get accurate readings of oxygen percentage in the sample. Disposable sensors may be purchased for some units.

Calibration is the crucial part of the maintenance of all oxygen analyzers. Nurses and respiratory therapists should know the particular method prescribed for the analyzer that they are using. Most analyzers are calibrated first in room air (21 per cent oxygen) and then at 100 per cent dry oxygen. For the latter step, the sensor is placed in the bottom of a small container and 100 per cent dry oxygen is allowed to flow around the sensor at 2 to 3 liters per minute. Oxygen is heavier than air and will settle in the bottom of the container. It is important to note that any calibration error made in room air increases proportionately when the sensor is placed in oxygen. Some devices require battery replacement and this should be known at the time of purchase.[58]

The process of making the analysis of oxygen is very simple, but *most important* to help ensure adequate and safe oxygen therapy.

3. ADMINISTRATION OF HELIUM

Nature of the Gas. In 1866, J. Norman Lockyer observed the chromosphere of the sun through a special telescope that he had designed, and saw a yellow line in the solar spectrum that could not be identified as sodium. This bright yellow line was later identified as the gas, helium (*helios* = sun). However, it was not until 1895 that its existence on earth was determined and confirmed by Sir William Ramsey, a London professor. Its therapeutic use was reported by Alvan L. Barach

in 1934. "Helium is an inert gas which owes its pharmacologic actions exclusively to its physical properties." *

Helium is an odorless, colorless, and tasteless gas. It is found in the atmosphere, in minerals, and in natural gases, the latter being the commercial source. Helium is an extremely light gas, and a mixture of 80 per cent helium and 20 per cent oxygen is only one third as heavy as air. Other physical properties include its low coefficient of solubility and high rate of diffusion.

Therapeutic Uses. The act of inspiration requires an expenditure of energy which, as Slonim and Hamilton [59] point out, is influenced by the weight of the volume of air that is moved in the respiratory act. When gas moves slowly and steadily through a straight, smooth, rigid, large caliber, cylindrical tube, it flows in a laminar pattern. This is another way of saying that the gas flows in layers. Resistance to laminar flow is dependent on viscosity of the gas, and helium is relatively more viscous than oxygen. When gas flow reaches a certain critical velocity, the flow changes from laminar to turbulent, which is a chaotic movement of air currents running contrary to the main current. Resistance to turbulent flow varies with gas density, and helium has one-eighth the density of oxygen. Since the tracheobronchial tree is an irregularly branching system of tubes, gas must move in a turbulent manner, slowed by projections and changing directions. The significance in respiration of these two patterns of gas flow is that it requires greater pressure to move gases flowing in a turbulent pattern than it does to move gases flowing in a laminar pattern. If gas flow becomes turbulent in the normal tracheobronchial tree, it is easy to understand that secretions, mucosal edema, and constriction of bronchial tubes will increase turbulent flow, thus increasing the resistance to breathing.

Since turbulent gas flow is, to a certain extent, proportional to the weight or density of the volume of gas inspired, it is reasonable to assume that given conditions of increased, turbulent flow in respiratory disease, a gas that is lighter than air will be easier to breathe. This is the rationale for having patients breathe a gas mixture of 20 per cent oxygen and 80 per cent helium. When flow is turbulent the force required for drawing 80 per cent helium with 20 per cent oxygen into the lungs is only one-half that necessary for air, which is 20 per cent oxygen and 79.7 nitrogen.

---

* Goodman, Louis S., and Gilman, Alfred: *The Pharmacological Basis of Therapeutics,* 5th ed. Macmillan Publishing Co., Inc., New York, 1975, p. 897.

Goodman and Gilman [60] state that the use of a helium-oxygen mixture may be helpful in cases of obstruction of the respiratory tract of an acute and self-limiting nature, but that it does not replace specific therapy. In status asthmaticus, the patient is often refractory to drug therapy and in great need of oxygen since only a limited amount of air can reach the alveoli of the lungs through constricted bronchioles; Goodman and Gilman also state that the administration of helium-oxygen mixture leads to partial relief at once and that helium may be valuable in the treatment of inflammatory obstructions in the air passages. They report that when helium is used as a diluent in anesthetic mixtures containing cyclopropane and oxygen, it decreases flammability; however, it is not widely used for this purpose. Helium is not superior to 100 per cent oxygen, oxygen diluted with nitrous oxide, or nitrogen for insufflation into the lung during cardiopulmonary bypass when ventilation of the lung has been discontinued.[61]

Because of its physical properties, helium is effective in shortening the decompression period of divers and other persons who have breathed compressed air under high pressure. Since nitrogen has a high solubility and relatively low rate of diffusion, a long period of time is required to rid the body of excess nitrogen. When a helium-oxygen mixture is used, the period of decompression is much shorter. This is due to the low solubility of helium and its poor affinity for lipids which limit the amount of helium dissolved in body fluids. The rapid escape of helium is further increased by its high rate of diffusion. Substitution of helium for nitrogen in the breathing mixture of divers also prevents the intoxicated condition called nitrogen narcosis, thought to be caused by inhaling nitrogen under high pressure.[62] Knowledge of the physical properties of helium is essential in determining its effective use in untoward respiratory conditions.

Method of Administration. Because of its low molecular weight and density, helium-oxygen escapes more easily than nitrogen-oxygen (air). It is better to give helium-oxygen by *face mask* (partial rebreathing or concentration) than by tent or oropharyngeal catheter. Helium-oxygen can be given in a nonrebreathing system, but this is expensive.[63] When it is administered in a closed system, provision must be made for the absorption of carbon dioxide. Helium-oxygen may also be used with mechanical ventilators.

Helium mixed with oxygen in the desired proportions is available in large cylinders. Special regulators calculated for helium should be used. A regulator that has been used for helium, or for carbon dioxide, or for mixtures of either gas with oxygen, must not be used on an oxygen cylinder. Some helium and carbon dioxide cylinders are compressed with oil-lubricated compressors, and may contain very fine particles of oil. If any of these particles lodge in the regulator, it is hazardous to use the regulator on a cylinder of oxygen. Oil coming in contact with oxygen under high pressure can ignite violently.

4. ADMINISTRATION OF CARBON DIOXIDE

Nature of the Gas. Carbon dioxide was discovered by J. B. van Helmont (1577–1644) in the products of combustion and fermentation. It is a colorless gas, with a faint pungent odor and a slightly acid taste. It occurs in the atmosphere, is a product of metabolism in animal life, and can be made commercially in various ways. In pure form it is highly toxic and can cause death. According to A. S. Blumgarten,[64] carbon dioxide snow ("dry ice") destroys living tissue by freezing. For medicinal purposes, carbon dioxide is usually given in combination with oxygen, and cylinders (both large and small tanks) containing the two gases in varying proportions (carbon dioxide 5 to 10 per cent and oxygen 90 to 95 per cent)[65] are available. The pressure and volume during carbon dioxide administration are regulated by a gauge.

Therapeutic Uses. In normal physiology, carbon dioxide is a gas of paramount importance in the control of both the respiration and circulation.[66] It stimulates the respiratory center located in the medulla oblongata, increasing the rate and depth of respiration. Respiratory integration areas in the brain stem are also acted upon by impulses from arterial chemoreceptors.[67] The intensity of this action is affected by concentration of carbon dioxide in the blood (which is determined by the composition of the alveolar air inhaled) and the responsiveness of the respiratory center. If the center has been depressed by morphine, the response to carbon dioxide is minimal.[68]

The circulatory effects of carbon dioxide are the result of its direct local effects and its centrally mediated effects on the autonomic nervous system.[69] Carbon dioxide has a direct effect on the heart, resulting in diminished contractile force and a slowed rate of contraction. It also acts directly on blood vessels, producing vascular dilation. The autonomic actions of carbon dioxide result in activation of the sympathetic nervous system with an increase in plasma levels of epinephrine and norepinephrine. The results of sympathetic nervous system activity are, in general, opposite to the local effects of carbon dioxide. They are an increase in the force and rate of cardiac contractions and the constriction of many vascular beds. Therefore, the total circulatory response to carbon dioxide is determined by the balance of the opposing local and sympathetic nervous system effects. The local vasodilating effects exert more of an influence than the sympathetically mediated vasoconstrictive effects. Carbon dioxide is a potent cerebral vascular dilator and must be used with caution as it may elevate intracranial pressure.

Carbon dioxide has been used therapeutically as a respiratory stimulant and in the drowned and drug-poisoned person, but Goodman and Gilman discourage its use in the following terms:

In all types of respiratory depression, asphyxia, and coma, reliance should be placed on mechanical support of the respiration plus the administration of oxygen.*

Intermittent carbon dioxide inhalation has been used postoperatively to increase ventilation, but intermittent positive pressure breathing, tracheal suctioning, coughing, and voluntary deep breathing can produce the same or better results. Egan [70] states that one of the most specific indications for carbon dioxide therapy is in the treatment of hiccups (singulation or hiccough). The customary means of treating hiccups, such as forced inspiratory breath holding, taking long drinks of water, and breathing into a paper bag, produce some degree of hypercapnia. The effect of hypercapnia on the respiratory center is to initiate impulses which overcome the spasmodic contractions of the diaphragm. In the hospital, low concentrations of carbon dioxide may be administered to stop a severe attack of hiccups.

Contraindications. According to Goodman and Gilman, the contraindications are relative rather than absolute. Whenever concentrations of 5 per cent carbon dioxide are administered for a period of 30 minutes or more, the patient should be observed carefully for *signs of toxicity*. These include the following: unbearable dyspnea, vomiting, disorientation, and a markedly elevated systolic blood pressure.[71] A rise in arterial pCO_2 above 80 to 100 mm Hg may cause carbon dioxide narcosis. When such symptoms appear, administration of the gas must be discontinued at once. In general, it seems best to discontinue its use as soon as the desired effect on respiration is observed.

* *Ibid.,* p. 896.

Methods of Administration. Carbon dioxide may be administered with the type of *mask* used in anesthesia that delivers a mixture of oxygen and carbon dioxide in prescribed percentages (5 to 10 per cent carbon dioxide in oxygen, but usually 5 per cent). One hundred per cent carbon dioxide may be given from a cylinder through a tube held a few inches above the patient's face. Since carbon dioxide is heavier than air, it falls over the patient's face, is diluted with room air, and inhaled. When this method is used there is no way to know the inhaled concentration of carbon dioxide.[72] Safar [73] describes the use of the *rebreathing tube* to increase respiratory dead space. The supply of carbon dioxide comes from the patient's exhaled gases which are rebreathed. Oxygen must be added to prevent hypoxia from the rebreathing of gases, and is delivered in a 4-liter flow to the distal end of the rebreathing tube. This method of increasing respiratory dead space is rarely used.

Carbon dioxide may be added to the inspired gas mixture delivered by a *ventilator* when the required minute volume lowers the arterial carbon dioxide tension. This state, if left untreated, would result in respiratory alkalosis and occasionally tetany. Adding carbon dioxide to the gas mixture is an alternative to adding mechanical dead space (extra tubing between the exhalation port and the patient, enabling the patient to rebreathe expired gas containing carbon dioxide).

During the administration of carbon dioxide the patient requires constant attention to prevent overstimulation of the respiratory center in the medulla with subsequent hyperventilation. The effectiveness of the treatment is determined by a satisfactory increase in rate and/or depth of respiration or arterial pCO_2 within the normal range. The professional person in attendance must be skilled in techniques of respiratory therapy and knowledgeable about the effects of carbon dioxide inhalation. The nurse or respiratory therapist can be prepared to administer the treatment and evaluate its effects. Nurses may often plan the treatment in accordance with the on-going plan of care for patients and they instruct patients so that they will benefit from the plan.

5. USE OF VENTILATORS (RESPIRATORS)

General Indications. Ventilatory assistance is indicated in patients whose respiratory system cannot provide adequate oxygenation, carbon dioxide excretion, and removal of secretions, or pulmonary expansion.[74] The methods for evaluating the adequacy of ventilation presented in the first section of this chapter should be reviewed. The clinician who provides care for persons in need of ventilatory assistance must have clearly in mind the signs and symptoms of hypoxia and hypercarbia, the meaning of static and functional lung volumes and how these are measured, the significance and techniques of blood gas measurement, and the pathologic processes of the respiratory, circulatory, and nervous systems causing inadequate ventilation. The following discussion is an introduction to the use of ventilators in patient care, and the reader is referred to comprehensive works on the subject listed in the references and additional suggested readings at the end of this chapter.

Intermittent Positive Pressure Ventilation. Examples of short-term ventilatory assistance are positive pressure ventilation with the operator's exhaled air, manually-assisted ventilation with a self-inflating bag and mask, and mechanically-assisted ventilation. All these methods exert a positive pressure at the upper airway to effect the necessary pressure gradient needed to move a volume of air into a patient's lungs.[75] Positive pressure ventilation with the operator's exhaled air (mouth-to-mouth resuscitation) is described in Chapter 35. It is the basis for ventilation in cardiopulmonary resuscitation. This technique is studied and practiced by all who are giving care to persons who risk accidents, asphyxia, and cardiopulmonary failure. The professional nurse frequently plans and conducts courses in this technique for policemen, ambulance attendants, and firemen.

Manually Assisted Ventilation—Bag and Mask. The use of a self-inflating breathing bag and mask may be indicated in an effort to avoid ventilation using an endotracheal tube (see Fig. 20-17).[76] Bag and mask ventilation does not depend on a supply of oxygen for positive pressure breathing, but oxygen is usually added to the bag inlet. There are several self-inflating bag and mask units available in adult and pediatric sizes, and the clinician should investigate certain features of the bag and mask unit before recommending purchase. The nonrebreathing valve should have no forward or backward leak. It should have low resistance, small dead space, and minimal opening pressure without sticking. It should resist clogging by secretions or vomitus and be lightweight. The valve should also be transparent and easy to clean and sterilize. The bag itself should be soft, easily sterilized, and capable of rapid refilling.[77] The tubing leading from the oxygen source is attached to the "intake" valve. Information from the manufacturer about the concentration of oxygen which can be de-

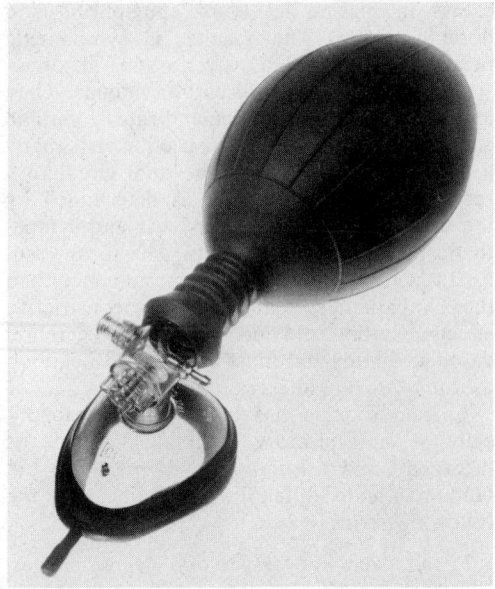

Figure 20-17. An example of a self-inflating breathing bag and mask. (Courtesy of Union Carbide Corporation, Linde Division, New York, N.Y.)

livered by the bag must be available to those who use the equipment. Some bags cannot deliver a concentration over 40 per cent.[78] Lloyd F. Reddick and others[79] report on the delivered oxygen concentration in six currently available self-inflating breathing bags when they are used with supplemental oxygen. Oxygen percentages are approximately 35 per cent when the flow rate of added oxygen is 5 liters per minute. The bags vary greatly in their capacity to increase the percentage of oxygen delivered at flow rates of 10 and 15 liters per minute. None of the bags tested delivered more than 88 per cent oxygen at 15 liters per minute.

Suggested Procedure. Place the mask firmly with one hand over the patient's mouth and nose with the operator's thumb at the part of the mask closest to the nose and the index finger on the part of the mask closest to the chin. With the third, fourth, and fifth fingers pull the patient's chin upward and backward. With the operator's other hand, compress the bag until the chest moves and release the bag for exhalation. Bag release should be quick to permit proper nonrebreathing valve action (see Fig. 20-18).

The number of compressions per minute (rate) is dependent on the size of the patient, the heart rate, and the partial pressure of carbon dioxide in the blood. The normal adult respiratory rate is 16 to 20 breaths per minute. The rate for the newborn infant is 40 to 60. It may be necessary

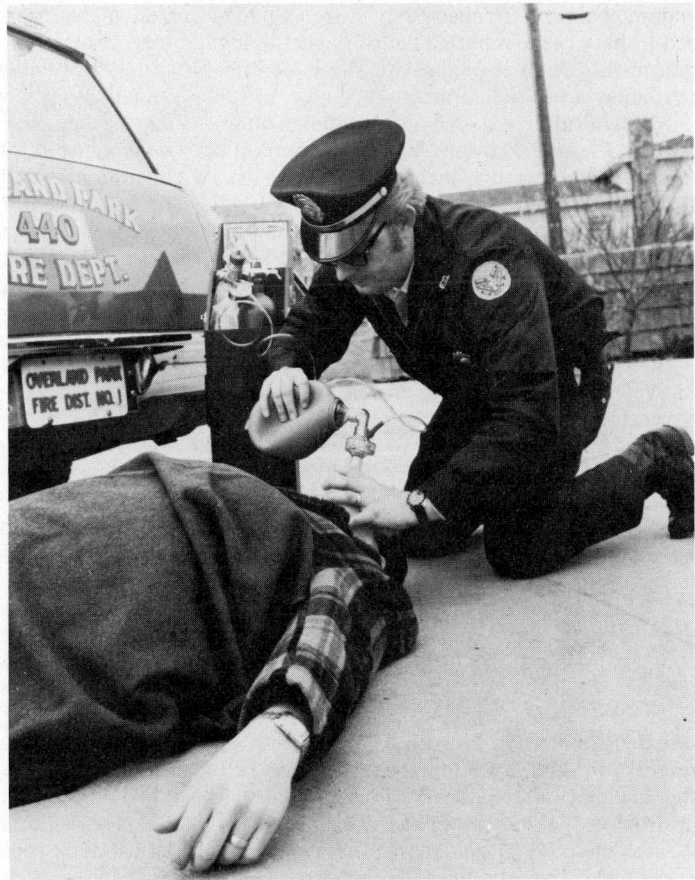

Figure 20-18. Resuscitation using self-inflating breathing bag and mask. Note the position of the operator in relation to the patient and the position of the operator's hands. (Courtesy of Puritan-Bennett Corporation, Kansas City, Mo.)

to increase the respiratory rate above what is normal for the patient to stimulate a more rapid heart beat and prevent bradycardia. Increasing the respiratory rate enables the patient to eliminate carbon dioxide in arterial blood and correct a state of respiratory acidosis (pCO_2 greater than 50 mm Hg). Conversely, a slower rate may be necessary to enable the patient to retain carbon dioxide and correct a state of respiratory alkalosis (pCO_2 less than 35 mm Hg).

Effective use of the bag requires training and practice. Reddick[80] and others provide data on the volumes of gas delivered by a bag when a trained and an untrained person is the operator.

Rapid gastric distention can be a problem when using bag and mask ventilation technique on an infant. If the operator passes an orogastric tube with the free end left open, the gas passing into the stomach can be released. Infants are never ventilated with bag and mask if they have a feeding remaining in their stomach. If they should vomit during compression of the bag, the gastric contents would be forced into their lungs. Because of this problem of gastric dilation and regurgitation with aspiration, infant resuscitation more often calls for endotracheal intubation. Resuscitation by bag and mask is also contraindicated when there is bleeding in the oropharynx. An

endotracheal tube is passed before resuscitation is attempted.

The bag and mask or bag with adaptor for endotracheal or tracheostomy tube must *always* be available in a patient care setting and there should be one at the bedside of every critically ill patient. *At any time* hand support of ventilation may be required.

Even when a mechanical ventilator is available, the patient must be ventilated by hand during the time it takes to set up a mechanical ventilator or correct a malfunction. Often bag and mask ventilation is used to provide the patient on a mechanical ventilator with hyperexpansion (a deep breath or sigh) which prevents alveolar and small airway collapse, thus preventing or reversing intrapulmonary shunting. It is also used to insufflate 100 per cent oxygen * to the lung prior to suctioning of the

---

* As previously described, it is questionable whether a resuscitation bag can deliver 100 per cent oxygen. However, the technique is to attach oxygen tubing from an oxygen source to the bag and insufflate the oxygen at the highest per cent which the bag can provide.

endotracheal or tracheostomy tube. Sudden death has been reported during suctioning, presumably from hypoxia with subsequent arrhythmias and cardiac arrest.[81,82]

Mechanically Assisted Ventilation: Intermittent Positive Pressure Breathing. Intermittent positive pressure breathing (IPPB) is a form of assistance to ventilation carried out mechanically by means of a mask or mouthpiece and a pressure-powered device that blows air or oxygen-enriched air with or without aerosolized medication or water into the airway.[83]

Intermittent positive pressure breathing therapy attempts to (1) prevent or correct atelectasis by deep lung inflations; (2) produce mechanical bronchodilation; (3) improve distribution and deposition of aerosols; (4) promote clearing of bronchial secretions; (5) counteract pulmonary congestion or edema; (6) decrease the work of breathing; and (7) regulate inspiratory and expiratory gas flow patterns.[84] It has been shown to be useful in the prevention of postoperative respiratory complications, and in the treatment of asthma, pulmonary edema, and atelectasis. In contrast, evidence of its beneficial effects in chronic lung disease is limited.[85,86] Terring W. Hieronimus [87] reports on investigations that showed IPPB therapy injurious to patients with severe chronic obstructive pulmonary disease because it decreased the pCO_2 and increased the physiologic dead space. These findings led the investigators to the conclusion that the more severely diseased the airways, the more harmful the effects of IPPB. Safar [88] also supports these findings and notes that European anesthesiologists and chest physicians seem reluctant to adopt this mode of therapy, relying more upon breathing exercises and spontaneous inhalation of aerosols.

The clinician can expect to see changes in the use of intermittent positive pressure breathing therapy as investigation of it continues. Where the technique is shown to be helpful, the benefits will be realized only when intelligent use is made of the equipment.

The IPPB ventilator has the following *features,* regardless of the model purchased (see Fig. 20-19): (1) The machine moves air by exerting an increasing pressure, the limit chosen and set by the operator (pressure limited). The volume of air is secondarily determined by the mechanical characteristics of the system into which the pressure is directed.[89] (2) It will initiate an inspiration when the patient makes an effort to inspire, allowing patients to set their own respiratory rate and assisting each respiratory cycle. This mechanism of operation is called "assist mode," and the machine is said to be "sensitive" to the patient's inspiratory effort. Many IPPB machines can be adjusted to ventilate the lungs at a rate determined by the operator. In other words, they can be adjusted to be "insensitive" to the patient's inspiratory effort. This mechanism of operation is called "control mode" and is not used for IPPB therapy. (3) The pattern of gas flow is characterized as a square wave or a sine wave. The square wave is a diagrammatic representation of flow, rising immediately to a determined maximum rate and remaining at this rate until limiting pressure is reached. The sine wave is a diagrammatic representation of flow that rises more slowly to a peak and then to zero before expiration begins. Theoretically, the sine wave flow pattern should improve intrapulmonary distribution toward the end of inspiration.[90] (4) An air dilution valve assures that oxygen-enriched air will be delivered to the patient, but the inspired oxygen concentrations are completely unpredictable, varying from 40 to 90 per cent. Delivered oxygen concentration varies with cycling pressure and flow rate. The only way to know what oxygen concentration is being delivered is to analyze the gas at the patient's mouth.[91,92] (5) Tidal volume is influenced primarily by pressure and is in turn dependent upon patient cooperation, airway resistance, and compliance of lungs and thorax. (6) A variable "sensitivity" adjustment permits minimal effort to initiate or trigger cycling by the patient. (7) The length of the inspiratory phase is determined by the patient. Inspiration is prolonged by increasing cycling pressure or decreasing inspiratory flow. (8) Retarding exhalation is possible by using a variable orifice retardation adaptor, attached to the exhalation valve. This has the same effect as if the patient exhaled through pursed lips. It helps prevent bronchial collapse and air trapping in the alveoli. (9) There is provision for nebulization and humidification of inhaled gases. (10) All parts of the ventilator which come into contact with the patient's gases are easily taken apart and cleaned and sterilized.

Safar makes the following statement:

Effective administration of IPPB to a conscious patient is an art. It depends upon the degree of cooperation of the patient and the skill and understanding of the therapist. IPPB should be "taught" to the patient, not "given." *

Suggested Procedure. Prior to starting an IPPB treatment, know the desired oxygen concentration, the time and length of administration, type and dosage of nebulized solutions, and if expiratory retardation is to be used. Desired pressure

---

* Safar, Peter (ed.): *op. cit.,* p. 225.

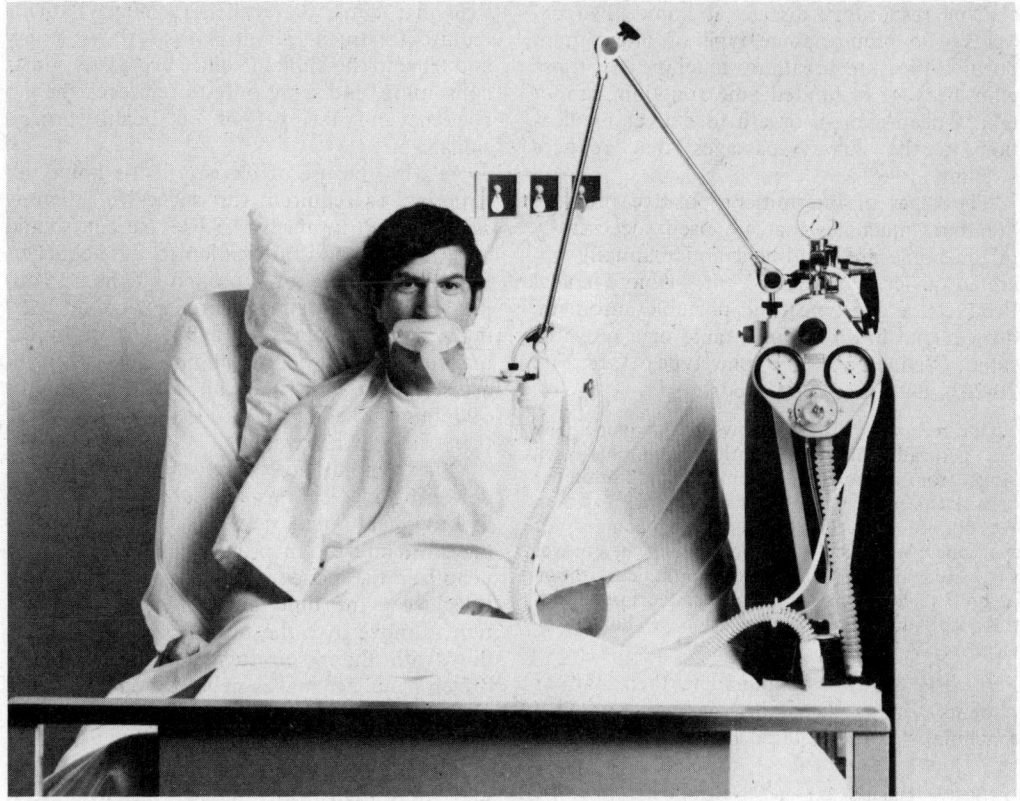

Figure 20-19. A patient receiving intermittent positive pressure breathing therapy. Note that the patient is sitting and using a mouthpiece without a nose clip. In this example, the ventilator is powered by oxygen compressed in a cylinder. The source gas may also be oxygen from a wall outlet, compressed air, or a mixture of compressed air and oxygen. (Courtesy of Puritan-Bennett Corporation, Kansas City, Mo.)

or volume may be indicated, but the flow rate and cycling pressures, which determine pressure and volume in the patient's airway, should be determined when therapy is instituted. They vary with each patient and cannot be prescribed in advance. The air dilution valve is set for air dilution. The automatic cycling mechanism (control mode) is turned off. Set peak pressure initially for 15 ml of water and change according to the patient's needs. Fill the nebulizer with an appropriate solution and check for "fog" production before the patient begins treatment and during treatment.

The same therapist should administer treatments to the same patient if possible, to maintain continuity and personal rapport. Explain the treatment to the patient and demonstrate how the machine works by using a balloon on the end of the breathing tube. (Some companies make a small bag called a "test lung" for demonstration and teaching.) Adjust the sensitivity by using a balloon or test lung and adjust during the treatment if indicated. Have the patient in the sitting position. Young children are comfortably supported in the therapist's or parent's lap. Use a

mask or mouthpiece according to the patient's preference. Nasal leaking is avoided with the mouthpiece if a nose clip is used. Experienced patients learn not to inhale or exhale through the nose when using a mouthpiece and do not require the nose clip. Never leave the patient alone. If he or she should not be able to trigger the ventilator, immediate intervention by the therapist is necessary.

The treatment is evaluated by observation of color, breathing pattern, and pulse rate. Tidal volume is measured during and after the treatment by a bedside spirometry device. (The Wright Respirometer is usually used.) Portable equipment is now available to measure peak inspiratory flow rate, forced expiratory capacity, and timed forced expiratory capacity. The physician, nurse, respiratory therapist, and personnel of the pulmonary function laboratory should collaborate in evaluating the effect of the treatment on each patient.

The Administration of Intermittent Positive Pressure Breathing in the Home. Intermittent positive pressure breathing (IPPB) machines are available for patients suffering from chronic respiratory disease at home. The patients who require some type of intermittent positive pressure breathing machine are those who, because of limited lung function, cannot take a deep enough breath to deliver medication to the airway passages that reduces swelling.

The types of intermittent positive pressure breathing machines that are used successfully in the home are hand-held and manually operated devices ("Hand-E-Vent," Ohio Medical Products, is one type) and portable automatic devices that fit on top of a table or a movable stand (Bennett AP-5 is one type) (see Fig. 20-20). Petty and Nett report:

Our recent experience shows that anyone who can naturally draw medications into his own lungs from a powered nebulizer or humidifier does not need something to do this work for him. We do not prescribe home IPPB machines for everyone. We select the individual who moves very little air and who needs good nebulization of both medications and steam in the home. For this individual we do prescribe a home device. . . .*

Petty and Nett [93] recommend further that for patients who do need therapy with an IPPB machine, it is best offered in the home, rather

* Petty, Thomas L., and Nett, Louise M.: *For Those Who Live and Breathe: A Manual for Patients with Emphysema and Chronic Bronchitis,* 2nd ed. Charles C Thomas, Publisher, Springfield, Ill., 1972, p. 54.

than in a clinic or physician's office. Patients require treatment about 3 to 4 times a day and trips to the clinic or office are costly, time-consuming, and serve only to reinforce the dependency of the patient on health professionals.

As with the use of oxygen in the home, instruction is required for successful therapy with the IPPB machine. The patient should know how to add medication to the nebulizer, how the machine turns on and off, how to adjust the inspiratory pressure to take increasingly deeper breaths, and how to clean the machine after use. The tubing and nebulizer are scrubbed with soap and water, soaked for 10 minutes in a bleach solution such as Clorox, then rinsed with water.[94]

Other simple and less expensive methods of delivering medications to the airway passages are the hand bulb nebulizer and the pump-driven nebulizer. In order to use a hand-held nebulizer the patient must have the strength to squeeze the bulb and sufficient coordination to move it to the mouth and regulate the flow with the respiratory cycle. The pump-driven nebulizer makes nebulization of inhaled air more convenient. The initial cost is greater, but if used over years, as is expected in cases of chronic respiratory disease, the convenience may more than justify its cost. As with IPPB equipment, the nebulizer should be cleaned frequently to prevent contamination. The cleaning procedure is similar to that described for IPPB

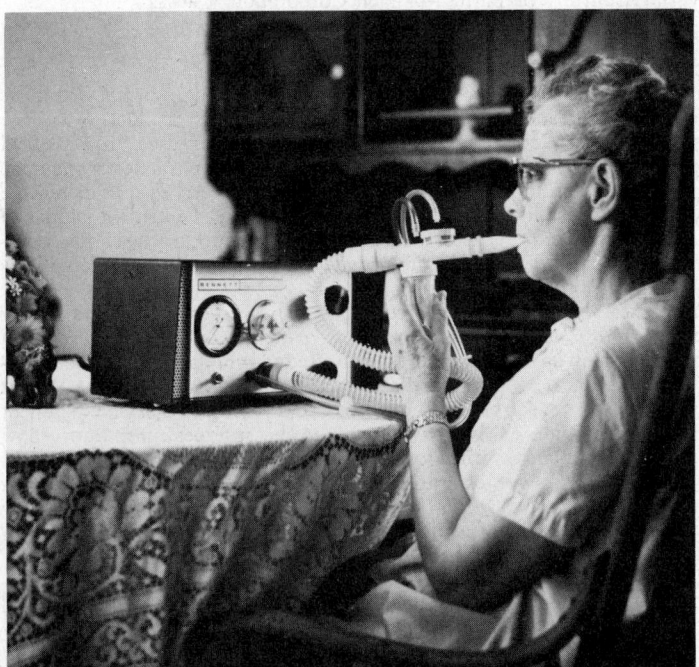

Figure 20-20. Patient using a portable, automated breathing machine at home (Bennett AP-5). (Courtesy of Puritan-Bennett Corporation, Kansas City, Mo.)

machines. Soaking the glass part of the nebulizer twice a week in a 1:6 solution of vinegar (white) and water is recommended to destroy organisms commonly found in inhalation equipment.[95]

In addition to nebulization of drugs into the airway, the home care program includes the delivery of moisture into the lungs to loosen and thin secretions. Encouraging the patient to take fluids is a good method of maintaining hydration in the lungs and loosening secretions. The ability of the commercially available humidifiers to deposit either water or medication into the lungs has been questioned, and the efficiency of these humidifiers has been tested primarily with children suffering from cystic fibrosis, who were required to sleep in mist tents. The consensus of recent studies[96-99] is that exposure to mist has no advantage in the delivery of water to peripheral airways, to liquefy tracheobronchial secretions and improve pulmonary function. Children with cystic fibrosis now use the hand nebulizer or pump-driven nebulizer only for the administration of medications.

Prolonged Mechanical Artificial Ventilation. The following are *conditions* that can occur singly or in combination, in which *prolonged mechanical artificial ventilation proves beneficial*[100-102]: (1) Inadequate ventilation (air movement in and out of lungs that makes possible exchange of gas molecules within pulmonary blood). Paralysis, trauma, and overdose of sedative and narcotic drugs are conditions that cause inadequate ventilation. Neurologic or muscular pathology interferes with the transportation of air into and out of alveoli. (2) Inadequate oxygenation. Illness or disease that causes shunting (passage of blood from artery to vein without undergoing gas exchange) such as atelectasis, hypoventilation, and diffusion defects leading to inadequate oxygenation. (3) Inadequate removal of carbon dioxide. Inadequate tidal volume caused by low respiratory rate or rapid, shallow breathing, acute pulmonary embolus, or uneven distribution of blood flow to the lungs, or ventilation in excess of perfusion (for example, the septal alveolar wall degeneration of emphysema) or bronchoconstriction with air trapping, leading to inadequate removal of carbon dioxide. (4) Secretion removal. Excessive and tenacious secretions, which are difficult to remove, accompany many of the disease states previously described and occur frequently in the immediate postoperative period. Intubation for continuous ventilation and meticulous suctioning, combined with humidification and chest physiotherapy can prevent or reverse infection and airway obstruction

caused by retained or inspissated secretions. (5) Inadequate expansion of lungs and thorax for mechanical reasons. The defect in ventilation associated with crushed chest is due to the instability of the chest wall which moves in a paradoxical manner during spontaneous ventilation; that is, contracting on inspiration and expanding on expiration. This results in decreased compliance and increased work of breathing, all of which can be corrected by the proper application of mechanical artificial ventilation. Another type of restriction that limits ventilation by reducing lung-thorax compliance is the respiratory distress syndrome of the infant and the adult. (6) Overwhelming metabolic needs. Mechanical artificial ventilation is increasingly part of the treatment of hypoxia, and decreased pulmonary compliance that may accompany overwhelming infection and metabolic acidosis, with marked increase in the work of respiration. Other hypermetabolic states are hyperthermia and early shock caused by gram-negative sepsis.

The prophylactic use of ventilators has been brought about by the development of special patient care units, the increasing knowledge and technical skill of nurses and other supportive medical personnel in respiratory therapy, and the increasing safety and effectiveness of ventilators. They are used to prevent complications that might follow extensive abdominal and thoracic surgery or in the treatment of severe trauma and shock.

The ventilator helps the critically ill patient or those subjected to physical stress by reducing the work of breathing and reducing oxygen consumption. The effect is to return arterial oxygen, carbon dioxide, and pH values to normal or near normal.[104] It accomplishes this by initiating inspiration when the patient makes an effort to inspire ("assist mode") or it can ventilate the lungs at a rate determined by the operator ("control mode"). The responsible physician makes the decision on when to start artificial ventilation. The absolute indications are controversial, but with the increasing use of more precise tools of diagnosis, such as blood gas measurements, spirometric measurements, estimation of alveolar and arterial oxygen tension gradients, shunt fractions, and dead space-tidal volume ratios, the decision can be reached more reliably for the benefit of the patient.[105]

Indications for respiratory support differ depending on the age of the patient and the acuteness or chronicity of the ventilatory problem. Philosophical questions may also enter into the decision to initiate controlled mechanical artificial ventilation—for example, is the patient capable of survival? If he or she survives, will life have some meaning? Will the patient be aware of and able to maintain or develop satisfying relationships with others? Should a vegetative existence be prolonged by the use of mechanical respiration?

Hieronimus [106] and Korones [107] give the following physiologic indications for intubation and mechanical artificial ventilation which would apply to the child and adult: (1) respiratory rate in the adult greater than 35 (acceptable range 12 to 25), in the child greater than 50, and in the infant greater than 80 to 100; (2) vital capacity less than 15 ml per kg (acceptable range 20 to 30); (3) inspiratory force less than 25 ml of water (acceptable range 100 to 50); (4) alveolar-arterial oxygen tension difference $(A - aDO_2)$ greater than 350 mm Hg (acceptable range 50 to 200 mm Hg) after breathing 100 per cent oxygen for 15 minutes; (5) arterial oxygen tension less than 70 on mask oxygen (acceptable range 100 to 75 in room air); for the infant less than 50 after breathing 100 per cent oxygen for 20 minutes; (6) ratio of dead space ventilation to tidal volume (V_D/V_T) greater than 0.5 (acceptable range 0.3 to 0.4); (7) arterial carbon dioxide tension greater than 60 mm Hg or rising rapidly, except in chronic hypercapnia (acceptable range 35 to 45 mm Hg).

When the decision has been reached to start mechanical artificial ventilation, *intubation* may be thought desirable or necessary. The patient is usually intubated with an orotracheal or nasotracheal tube or tracheostomy. In contrast to a mask, the tube prevents gastric inflation and variable air leaks and facilitates tracheobronchial suctioning. Prolonged artificial ventilation by mask has been found feasible, but the risk of injury to the skin, leakage, gastric insufflation, and hypoventilation is said by Safar [108] to be great. The *choice* of orotracheal, nasotracheal, or tracheostomy tube is made after consideration of several factors. Some of these instanced by Hieronimus [109] are the following: (1) The oro- or nasotracheal tube is the airway of choice for the infant, as the removal of a tracheostomy is often delayed for months or years, due to the tendency of the infant's trachea to stenose after a tracheostomy tube has been in place. (2) Skill of the clinician; in some centers, physicians or their associates have more practice in one method of intubation than another. The competence of nurses in caring for patients with different types of airways may also be a determining factor in the success of the procedure. It is the responsibility of nurses in critical care units to develop competence in the management of *any type* of airway. (3) Anticipated duration of mechanical artificial venti-

lation affects the choice of method. Safar [110] reports that some authorities say tracheostomy is indicated when the need for an endotracheal airway of several days' duration is anticipated. Hieronimus [111] gives an example of preference for an oro- or nasotracheal tube over the tracheostomy tube, even during prolonged periods of mechanical artificial ventilation. In general he thinks the oro- or nasotracheal tube should be used until the patient's condition has sufficiently stabilized to allow a tracheostomy.

An inflatable cuff should be used on the endotracheal or tracheostomy tube to prevent air leakage. This provides a constant tidal volume, and prevents aspiration of foreign material. However, the cuff requires meticulous management to prevent trauma to the tracheal mucosa in the form of compression necrosis, ulceration, cartilaginous erosion, and infection. Since infants and children are more susceptible to these problems than adults, uncuffed tubes are used for them. The uncuffed tubes fit more tightly than in the adult and leakage is a minor problem. Before endotracheal and tracheostomy tubes were designed with bonded inflatable cuffs, there was the hazard that the cuff would slip off the tube and occlude the airway; with bonded cuffs this hazard has been eliminated.

Suggested Procedure—Nasal Endotracheal Intubation.* (See Chapter 35 for a description of the technique of orotracheal intubation. An oral endotracheal tube is frequently used first to establish an airway before nasal intubation is attempted.)

Select an endotracheal tube of appropriate size depending on the patient's size. The average adult will accommodate a tube with an internal diameter of 8 to 9 mm.[112] Tubes with an internal diameter of 3 mm are appropriate for the infant. Check the cuff for leaks by inflating it with air.

Elevate the patient's occiput and tilt the head backward. Insert the laryngoscope from the right corner of the patient's mouth and push the tongue to the left. Lift the epiglottis (directly with a straight blade and indirectly with a curved blade) for visualization of the arytenoid cartilages, glottis, and vocal cords. An assistant can facilitate exposure by pressing the patient's larynx backward.

Insert a well-lubricated tube through the patient's nostril (nasal topical anesthesia is used in some instances) and pass it beyond the nasopharyngeal angle. Curved forceps (Magill type) are used to direct the tube. The use of a stylet may be necessary. Immediately after the tube is

---

* Only in an emergency, to save a life, would nurses carry out these procedures. They are described here because nurses should understand them to be able to help physicians as needed and to be able to discuss the procedure with patients and their families.

passed check its location by auscultation of each lung, particularly the upper lobes, for breath sounds. A chest x-ray is required to indicate precisely the position of the tube.

Inflate the cuff just enough to prevent an air leak or to allow a minimal leak at 25 to 30 cm water pressure.

Suggested Procedure—Tracheostomy.* Discuss the need for a tracheostomy with the patient and family and get an informed consent to the procedure and a local or general anesthetic. Although the equipment to perform an emergency tracheostomy is kept in all critical care areas, the procedure is usually carried out in the operating room. Usually children are intubated with an oral or nasal endotracheal tube to use as a guide prior to performing a tracheostomy. Remove the endotracheal tube after the tracheostomy tube is secure.

Select the largest size tracheostomy tube that can be accommodated by the trachea. Small cannulae increase resistance to ventilation and are occluded more easily with secretions. Check the cuff for air leak. The cuff should be pre-softened or hyperexpanded to soften before use.

Following the placement of the tube, secure it by a ribbon around the neck, knotted on the side for easy visibility and access. Do not put a dressing under the tube. Particles of cotton dressings can be aspirated into the lungs and gauze dressings can dislodge the tube, particularly in infants and children.

Suggested Procedure for Care of the Patient with an Artificial Airway. Successful management of artificial airways requires a well-defined and comprehensive program which everyone understands and follows precisely.†

Use sterile technique with sterile gloves and sterile catheters; use them only once.

Hyperoxygenate and hyperinflate the patient's lungs with the self-inflating breathing bag. Aspirate the pharynx before deflating the cuff so that oral secretions are not aspirated when the cuff is deflated. Deflate the cuff. Instill a minimum of 0.5 ml to a maximum of 5 ml sterile normal saline by syringe, with needle removed, directly into the endotracheal or tracheostomy tube to thin secretions. The amount of normal saline instilled in the tracheostomy is dependent on the size of the tube.

---

* Only in an emergency, to save a life, would nurses carry out these procedures. They are described here because nurses should understand them to be able to help physicians as needed and to be able to discuss the procedure with patients and their families.

† The procedure described is generally appropriate for the critically ill patient who is being ventilated by machine through an artificial airway. The technique of aspirating through a tracheostomy tube will be modified for the child or adult who has a tracheostomy for months or years. These persons learn to manage their own tracheostomy care. Deep bronchial suctioning is not necessary and may even be harmful to the tracheal mucosa. With the help of postural drainage techniques, adequate exercise, and fluid intake, they cough up secretions and prevent pneumonia and atelectasis without bronchial suctioning.

Administer by bag and adaptor (which fits snugly into the endotracheal or tracheostomy) 100 per cent oxygen for a few inspirations. Provide for effective ventilation. Aspirate secretions by passing a catheter small enough to fit comfortably into the airway, but large enough for adequate suctioning power. Moisten the catheter with sterile water, attach to a Y tube, and insert *without applying suction*. Insert just past the tip of the tube. Turning the patient on the right side and then on the left facilitates passage of the suction catheter into first the right and then left bronchus (see Fig. 20-21). Apply suction by putting thumb intermittently over the Y tube and slowly withdrawing the catheter with rotation. *Never* prolong a period of aspiration beyond 10 seconds. If suction is repeated, reinflate the lungs by bag and adaptor with 100 per cent oxygen.

Cardiac arrest sometimes occurs during prolonged aspiration. Bendixen and associates[113] say that it is probably caused by massive removal of oxygen from the airway and massive reduction in lung volume, with subsequent hypoxia. Therefore, the patient should be ventilated and oxygenated before each passage of the aspirating catheter.

Reinflate cuff until audible leakage is faintly

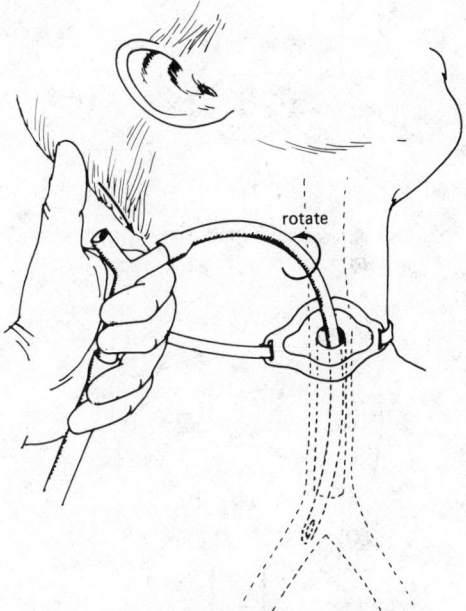

1. Patient is turned on to right side with head to the left. Catheter is moistened with sterile water and inserted just past the tip of the tube.

2. Suction is applied by intermittently putting thumb over opening in Y tube, while at the same time slowly withdrawing and rotating catheter.

3. Sterile water may be aspirated through the catheter to clean it; the patient may then be turned, and the procedure repeated to suction the left bronchus.

Figure 20-21. Steps in suctioning a tracheostomy.

heard (minimal leak technique) or just stopped, but no further. If a tracheostomy tube with an inner cannula is used, remove the inner cannula and clean it as necessary every 4 hours (see Fig. 20-22).

Heated humidification should be continuous, to avoid thickening (inspissation) of secretions.

The prevention and treatment of infection require scrupulous attention to aseptic technique and proper removal of secretions. Bendixen and associates[114] recommend sending deep tracheal aspirate, collected in a sterile sputum collector, to the laboratory for culture and sensitivity determination every other day. Safar and Hieronimus

recommend that endotracheal and tracheostomy tubes be changed every 24 to 48 hours.[115,116] Bendixen and associates[117] state that the tube should be changed only when there is mechanical failure, such as a leaking cuff or a cannula with excessive secretions.

The *types of ventilators* used in prolonged mechanical artificial ventilation are the pressure-limited and volume-limited ventilators. The pressure-limited ventilator was described in the section of this chapter on intermittent positive pressure breathing. When this type of ventilator is used for continuous artificial ventilation, the expired minute volume and the tidal volume must be monitored frequently to ensure that the pressure setting of the ventilator and inspiratory flow rate result in adequate alveolar ventilation. The tidal volume produced by the pre-set pressure-limited ventilator is a function of elastic and airway resistance of the patient's lungs and the inspiratory flow rate. The pressure-limited ventilator, which can vary the speed at which air flows into the lungs (flow variable), is preferred in continuous ventilation to those pressure-limited ventilators in which the speed of air flow varies directly with the cycling pressure. Intrapulmonary air distribution is more adequate when the ventilator has a variable flow rate.[118,119]

Suggested Procedure for Pressure-Limited Ventilator Used for Continuous Ventilation.* Attach tubing to power source. In the pressure-cycled ventilator, this is always compressed gas. Attach a balloon or "test lung" to the main breathing tube to regulate the ventilator before attaching it to the patient. Set the pressure limit control at a pressure considered adequate to ventilate the patient. Set the inspiratory flow rate control to govern the length of the inspiratory phase. Set the expiratory timer to control the length of expiration, which then determines the respiratory rate.

Pull the air mix control out to produce oxygen-enriched air. The control may be pushed in to provide 100 per cent oxygen, but the flow variable feature of this ventilator is lost when this is done. Oxygen concentration may be increased by adding oxygen to the ambient air chamber of the ventilator. Air mix does not supply a uniform, predictable oxygen concentration. The actual inspired concentration must be measured with each new adjustment of the ventilator. The sensitivity control is off during controlled ventilation and regulated as previously described for intermittent positive pressure therapy, when the ventilator is on "assist mode."

Provide humidification in prolonged ventilation

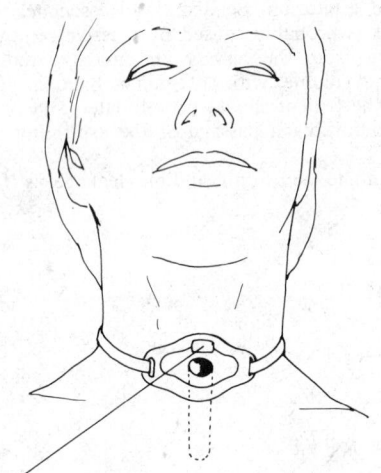

1. Patient's head is tilted upward and back.

2. Locking key is turned to release inner cannula.

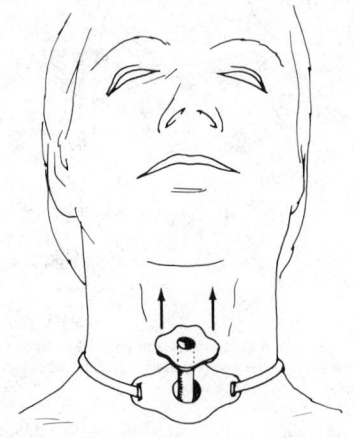

3. Inner cannula is lifted out, cleaned with the appropriate agent, *rinsed in sterile water*, and replaced by reversing these steps. Care must be taken to relock the key.

Figure 20-22. Steps in cleaning the inner cannula of a tracheostomy tube.

* The Bird Mark 7 is described as it is a typical pressure-limited ventilator. The study of its operation is made easier by its clear plastic construction, in which the major parts can be visualized during ventilation. (Bird Corp., Palm Springs, Calif.)

by a large mainstream nebulizer that can be heated. The small nebulizer located at the nonrebreathing valve is inadequate for continuous humidification.

When all controls are synchronized, using the "test lung," attach the ventilator to the patient. Adjust settings to the patient's needs with adequate monitoring of ventilation. Monitoring is accomplished by blood gas measurement, spirometric measurements, observation of the patient's color, heart rate and respiratory rate, chest expansion, intra-arterial or cuff measurements of arterial blood pressure, inspired oxygen concentration, and auscultation by stethoscope for breath sounds.

Periodic hyperinflation of the lungs (sigh) is accomplished by increasing the pressure and lengthening the inspiratory time for two to three deep breaths, about every 30 minutes. Care must be taken to return all the controls to their previous settings, following hyperinflation.

Exhalation may be retarded as described on page 1110 under the description of intermittent positive pressure ventilation.

The volume-cycled ventilators move a volume of air which is determined either by the operator or by the patient (see Fig. 20-23A–D). The pressure exerted in moving the volume is determined by the following physical characteristics of the system into which the volume is moved: mechanical connectors and tubes, airways, and the patient's lungs and their condition.[120] In other words, the ventilator exerts a higher airway pressure in a "stiff" lung (as found in pneumonia) than in a "compliant" lung (as seen in narcotic poisoning) when a constant volume is generated.* The Emerson, Bennett MA 1, and Bourns Adult Volume Ventilator (Bear 1) are representative of this type of machine. The Bourns Infant Ventilator is a volume-limited ventilator, designed for use on infants. Small tidal volumes of less than 150 cc can be delivered by this ventilator.

Suggested Procedure—Volume-Limited Ventilator Used for Continuous Ventilation.† Plug electric cord of the ventilator into a power source.

Connect the oxygen tubing to the oxygen source. Room air is forced into the breathing tubing by means of an electric blower. Set directly and independently, by the clearly labeled dials on the control panel, the tidal volume, inspiratory flow rate, ratio of inspiration to expiration, peak pressure limit, inspired oxygen concentration, and cycling rate per minute (respiratory rate).

Set directly, by dials on the control panel, the hyperinflation control and hyperinflation volume (sigh control, number of sighs per minute and tidal volume during the sigh).

Place the ventilator on assist or control mode by separate controls.

Provide humidification by a heated humidifier. The temperature of the inspired gases is registered in the inspiratory breathing line near the attachment to the patient's airway. An adjustable control introduces expiratory resistance or exerts a negative pressure on expiration.*

A built-in alarm system indicates accidental disconnection of the breathing tube from the patient's airway (registered on the pressure gauge as a sudden drop in pressure) or other failures, such as an oxygen concentration that falls below the pre-set concentration.

Set and check all controls by use of a "test lung" or balloon before attaching the breathing tube to the patient. Adjust settings to the patient's needs by using the same measurements described in the suggested procedure for the pressure-limited ventilator.

Bendixen and associates [121] say that any ventilator used for a patient must have the following features: dependability—that is, the ventilator must operate for days or weeks with minimal service; the basic controls of pressure, flow, phase, and volume should be clearly marked and calibrated in the accustomed units of measurement; the inspired oxygen concentration should be variable from 21 per cent to 100 per cent; the humidification system must provide for the delivery of gas saturated with water vapor at or near body temperature (provision for warming the water by a thermostatically controlled heating element in the humidifier is necessary); the expiratory valve should be designed to allow easy connection of ventilation meters for measurement of expired gas volume and for collection of inspired gas; the ventilator should operate on both "assist" and "control mode"; the duration of inspiration and expiration should be set independently and be calibrated in seconds or fractions of seconds; all parts of the ventilator exposed to moisture (humidifier, tubing, and valves), should be easily detachable for sterilization; the system should incorporate a one-way valve open to the atmosphere in order to permit the patient to inspire freely during any phase of the respiratory cycle. There should be an alarm system to warn of mechanical failure, but this does not negate the need for continu-

---

* The volume-cycled ventilator becomes pressure-cycled when the pressure required to maintain a preset volume reaches the pressure limit of the ventilator (usually about 60 cm of water).

† The Bennett MA 1 is described as it is a typical volume-limited ventilator.

* Indications for the use of expiratory resistance have already been discussed. Negative pressure at the end of exhalation was originally thought to promote exchange of gas in the alveoli and improve venous return to the heart. This mode of ventilation is no longer used as its hazards (airway collapse and air trapping) are believed to outweigh its benefits.

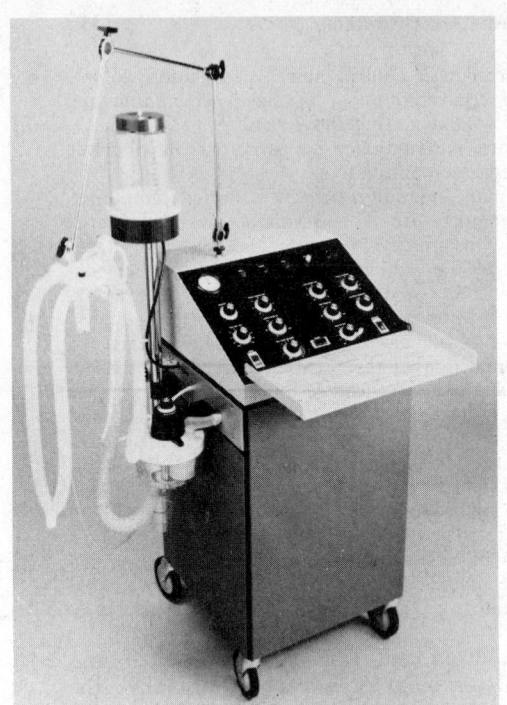

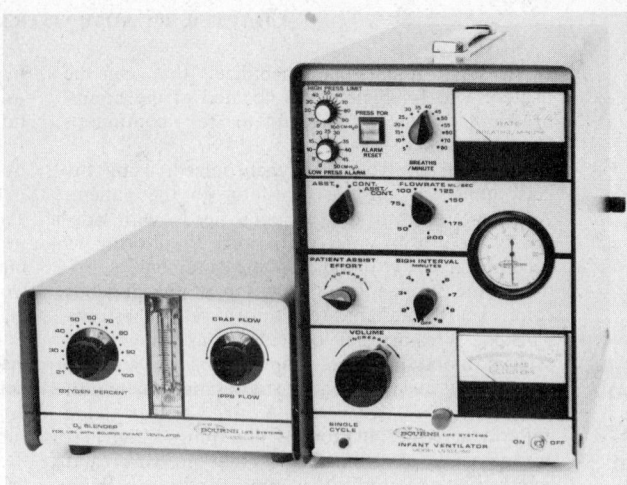

C

D

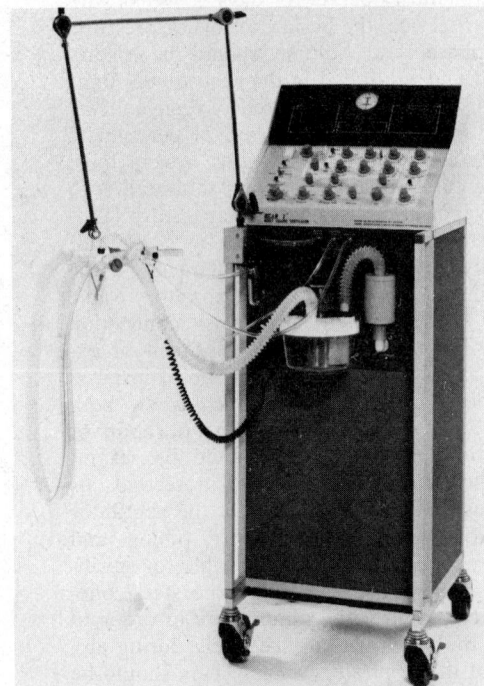

A

B

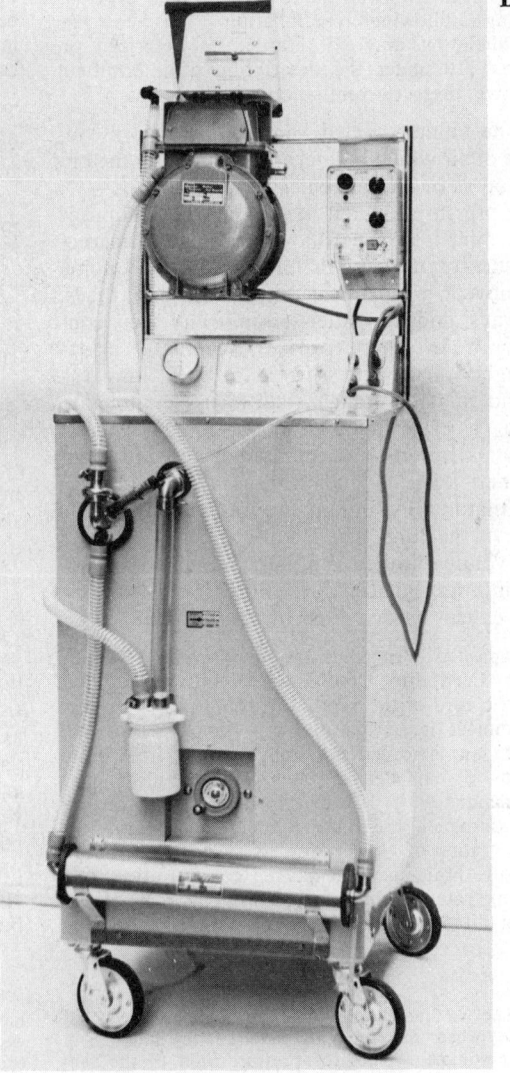

Figure 20-23. Ventilators that move a volume of air determined either by the operator or by the patient. *A*. The Bennett MA-1, a volume-cycled ventilator. (Courtesy of Puritan-Bennett Corp., Kansas City, Mo.) *B*. Bourns adult volume ventilator (Bear 1). (Courtesy of Bourns Life Systems Division, Riverside, Calif.) *C*. Bourns ventilator, only for the premature or term infant. The maximum tidal volume the machine is able to deliver is 150 cc. (Courtesy of Bourns Life Systems Division, Riverside, Calif.) *D*. Emerson ventilator. (Courtesy of J. H. Emerson Company, Cambridge, Mass.)

ous care of the patient and supervision of ventilator therapy.

Other Positive Pressure Techniques of Mechanical Ventilation. Intermittent inflation of lungs with negative pressure around the body, with the airway exposed to atmospheric pressure, is the principle of the "tank" respirator described by Safar.[122] The Drinker/Emerson Body Respirator, Monoghan Chest, or Cuirass Respirator, also described by Safar,[123] and the Air Shields Incubator Respirator for infants described by V. Chernick [124] are examples of tank or body respirators. Positive pressure is the correct term to use for these respirators because in each peak lung inflation the intrapulmonary pressure is higher than the pressure surrounding the patient.[125,126] In the United States, prior to 1961, prolonged artificial ventilation was provided by tank respirators, but at present the authorities consulted say that their advantages or usefulness for the occasional patient who is not intubated is outweighed by their disadvantages, although Chernick [127] in 1973 advocated chest wall pressure therapy for the newborn infant with hyaline membrane disease. Safar [128] gives their disadvantages as inadequate ventilatory reserve power in conditions of decreased lung-thorax compliance and increased airway resistance; leaks at the collar around the patient's neck; difficulty in providing care to a person enclosed in an airtight compartment; and bulkiness of the equipment. The tank respirator may be used for intubated patients who have normal lung-thorax compliance, provided that heated, humidified gas is supplied to the endotracheal tube.

Positive End Expiratory Pressure. Positive end expiratory pressure (PEEP) means that pressure is maintained throughout expiration.* This method of mechanical ventilation is considered the major advance in the treatment of the respiratory distress syndrome of the adult †

and the respiratory distress syndrome of the infant (hyaline membrane disease).[129-131] To understand what positive end expiratory pressure can accomplish for a patient with respiratory distress syndrome, it is helpful to consider the infant's way of compensating for alveoli that tend to collapse. When the infant is immature or has an impaired ability to generate surfactant (see Chapter 9 for an explanation of surfactant), the alveoli do not stay expanded following the first breath. In other words, air is not left behind in the aveoli, and they collapse to the tubular conformation characteristic of the lung before birth. Thus the work of breathing is the same for every subsequent breath as it is for the first. The infant has two ways to compensate for this inadequate function of the lungs. He or she can breathe more rapidly and can grunt. This grunt is an expiratory effort against a partially closed glottis, and it creates a positive pressure in the airway which helps to keep alveoli from collapsing. The same effect can be achieved by a variety of adaptations of mechanical ventilators or simply having the patient exhale into a system of tubing that is immersed to a specified depth in a cylinder of water or attached to an anesthesia bag and manometer. The positive pressure exerted during expiration usually begins at about 5 cm of water and may be increased to as much as 20 cm of water, depending on the patient's condition and response to the treatment.

Harvey J. Sugarman and his associates [132] report that positive end expiratory pressure was first introduced in 1938 for the treatment of pulmonary edema, secondary to heart failure, and it was studied in the 1940s in relation to the problems of high-altitude flying. Indications for institution of positive end expiratory pressure are similar to indications for mechanical artificial ventilation. These indications are inability to maintain arterial oxygen tension above 70 mm Hg, with inspired oxygen concentration of 50 per cent, respiratory rate greater than 35 per minute, vital capacity less than 10 to 15 cc per kg of body weight, and arterial carbon dioxide tension greater than 50 mm Hg (see page 1090 for the value of these parameters in the infant).

Korones and Chernick [133,134] report that continuous positive airway pressure breathing

* Other terms used to describe pressure maintained throughout expiration are continuous positive pressure breathing (CPPB), continuous positive pressure ventilation (CPPV), and continuous positive airway pressure (CPAP). At the time of this writing, positive end expiratory pressure is the preferred term and refers specifically to the application of pressure throughout expiration when the patient is intubated and breathing is completely controlled by a mechanical ventilator. Continuous positive airway pressure (CPAP) is the preferred term for exactly the same maneuver when it is applied to a patient who may or may not be intubated, but is breathing spontaneously against a pressure.

† Synonyms for the adult form of respiratory distress syndrome are adult hyaline membrane disease, shock lung, pump or respirator lung, and post-traumatic pulmonary insufficiency. The latter terms have been used because the syndrome often follows a

critical surgical or medical illness in which cardiopulmonary bypass or the mechanical artificial ventilator is used. F. William Blaisdell and Richard M. Schlobohm in their article "The Respiratory Distress Syndrome; A Review," (*Surgery,* **74**:251, [Aug.] 1973), list a total of 27 synonyms for this condition and review the pathologic changes, etiology, prevention and treatment of the condition.

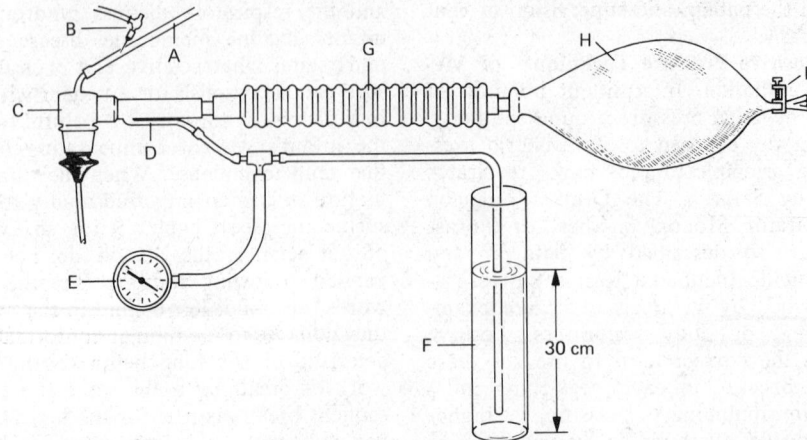

Figure 20-24. Equipment for one type of continuous positive airway pressure (CPAP) system used for the infant. The infant breathes spontaneously through an endotracheal tube. *A.* Line through which the mixture of oxygen and air enters the system at a flow rate of twice the minute volume of respiration. *B.* Sampling site for measuring oxygen concentration. The gas passes through a heated humidifier (not shown) before it reaches the patient. The expired gas and excess gas entering the system leave the unit through *C* and *D,* the Norman elbow and Sommers T piece, and *G,* corrugated tubing, into *H,* the reservoir bag, and out through the terminal exit port. *E.* Aneroid manometer for measuring airway pressure. *I.* Stopcock at the terminal exit port of the system; setting of the screw clamp determines the airway pressure. *F* "Pop-off" safety valve to assure that the airway pressure never exceeds 30 cm of water. If respiratory assistance is needed, the infant can be ventilated manually using the reservoir bag. There are no valves within the system. Rebreathing is prevented by using a flow rate of gas into the system which exceeds two times the respiratory minute volume of the infant. (Adapted from Barratt-Boyes, Brian G., et al. [eds.]: *Heart Disease in Infancy.* Williams & Wilkins Co., Baltimore, 1973, p. 311.)

may reduce the need for mechanical respirators in the infant suffering from respiratory distress syndrome. The atelectatic characteristics (imperfect lung expansion) of this syndrome is overcome by maintaining pressures above zero at the end of expiration. A further advantage is that the arterial oxygen is increased at relatively low concentrations of inspired oxygen. Thus the hazard of lung toxicity from high oxygen concentrations is minimized.

M. Brooke Nicotra and associates[135] have reported on a series of 36 adult patients treated with positive end expiratory pressure. They found that the measure increased oxygen tension in patients with hypoxemia and required lower concentrations of inspired oxygen than are ordinarily used with ventilatory support not using positive end expiratory pressure.

Blaisdell and Schlobohm[136] describe the untoward side effects of positive end expiratory pressure. There is a possibility of tension pneumothorax and lung rupture. They recommend constant evaluation of the patient and

daily assessment of the need for positive end expiratory pressure. Petty[137] reports that the efficacy of positive end expiratory pressure has not been established in conditions of chronic airway obstruction, status asthmaticus, and pneumonia. He considers it to be a treatment for impaired oxygen transport associated with the respiratory distress sydrome.

The suggested procedure for instituting positive end expiratory pressure or continuous positive airway pressure varies according to the type of mechanical ventilation equipment used, whether or not the patient is intubated, and if he or she is being ventilated on the "control" or "assist mode." Any of the presently available mechanical volume-limited ventilators can be modified to add positive end expiratory pressure.

Suggested Procedure. Intubate by endotracheal or tracheostomy tube, as previously described. (Orotracheal or nasotracheal intubation is preferred over tracheostomy for infants.)

Set up the ventilator as previously described if the mechanical ventilator is being used with the modification for positive end expiratory pressure.

If the water seal or anesthesia bag is used, measured concentrations of warmed humidified oxygen are delivered to the patient's airway and expired gas is conducted through an outflow system that maintains end expiratory pressures above zero (see Fig. 20-24). Pressure within the system is displayed continuously on a gauge.

Monitor blood gas exchange and suction periodically. Hyperventilation and other measures to maintain normal exchange of gases are effected by a mechanical ventilator.

General Principles of Care for Patients Who Require Prolonged Mechanical Artificial Ventilation. The patient who requires prolonged artificial ventilation is critically ill. Bendixen and associates make the following statement:

These patients are cared for best in a special unit where there can be assembled both a wide variety of diagnostic and therapeutic equipment and also the accumulated experience of nursing staff and physicians. These patients can never be left unattended.*

Many surgical patients know well in advance that a ventilator will be used to help them through a part of their illness, usually postoperatively. Explanation of the therapy is crucial in helping patients maintain a sense of control over their bodies and the immediate environment and in promoting trust in the professional staff. Instruction in the purpose of the ventilator, how it operates, and how the experience may be perceived and felt by the patient is an important part of a preoperative teaching program. (See Chapter 47 for further explanation of preoperative teaching.) The postoperative patient may require other support equipment as well (see Fig. 20-25). Children benefit from hearing the sound of a ventilator, touching the tubing, and trying on the mask or mouthpiece (in the case of intermittent positive pressure breathing therapy). The ventilator can be placed beside their bed a day or two before surgery so that they and their parents become accustomed to what it looks like and how it operates.

Patients who must be placed on the ventilator without prior preparation, such as the victims of an automobile accident, present a somewhat different problem in support and instruction. They may be conscious prior to intubation, but some awaken from surgery with an endotracheal or tracheostomy tube and the ventilator in operation. This is a time for accurate and simple explanations given to the patient and the family in a calm and confident manner. The procedures intended to help the patient to take a deep breath, to loosen secretions from the alveoli and bronchi, to promote drainage of secretions from the lungs, and to suction these secretions from the airway may cause much apprehension for patients. They will fear that they will not be able to breathe. The feeling of suffocation experienced during tracheobronchial aspiration or change of the endotracheal or tracheostomy tube is alleviated by pre-oxygenation (insufflation of 100 per cent oxygen by self-inflating bag and adaptor) and limiting the aspiration to 10 seconds. At the same time, the nurse must use sight, touch, and voice to reassure patients who are helpless and totally dependent on their nurses to maintain their sense of self, their body integrity, and their ability to communicate. Patients suffer especially from the difficulty of communicating. Some will be able to speak if the cuff on the tube is deflated. The patients who have a hand free from intravenous or intra-arterial catheters are provided with a pad and pencil on which to write their requests. Small children and others who cannot write are not able to express themselves and suffer most from a feeling of isolation.

Constant care interrupts sleep and contributes to the patient's anxiety and depression. It is difficult to strike a balance between optimal respiratory care and sufficient rest. Thoughtful planning of treatments and grouping of nursing care activities help promote rest and sleep.

The patient on the ventilator may be anxious, depressed, and afraid of many things, including death, and the inability to express these emotions to family and staff makes them all the more unbearable. It is helpful to study the content of Chapters 41, 46, 47, 48, and 50 on nursing intervention for the anxious, frightened, and depressed patient, and on the approach to the patient who fears that he or she is dying, before accepting responsibility for the care of the patient on the ventilator. Touching the patient in a comforting way with the whole hand, holding his or her hands, giving considerable time to the bath and passive range-of-motion exercises, and rubbing the back keep the patient from losing a sense of his or her own body and feeling depersonalized. Maintaining eye contact and speaking directly to the patient are other helpful measures. The family can be taught these and other ways of maintaining contact with the patient. Linda R. Thomson,[138] a registered nurse, has written a very moving account of her personal experience as a patient in a critical care unit which focuses particularly on the aspect of loneliness and sensory deprivation that she experienced. Everyone around the patient must be particularly vigilant to avoid talking across the bed to each other about the patient or about ir-

* Bendixen, H. H., et al.: *op. cit.,* p. 137.

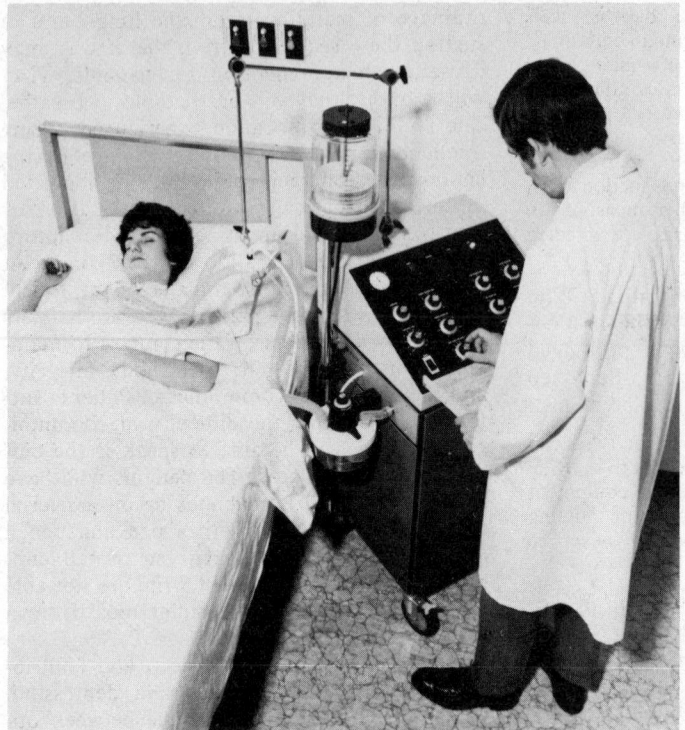

Figure 20-25. A model demonstrates the position of the ventilator and tubing in relation to the patient who has a tracheostomy. The patient who requires a ventilator to maintain respirations would also have an intra-arterial catheter for monitoring arterial blood pressure and blood gases; a venous catheter for measurement of central venous pressure; a peripheral catheter for maintenance of fluids; and other support equipment as required. (Courtesy of Puritan-Bennett Corporation, Kansas City, Mo.)

relevant topics. The nurses of one pediatric intensive care unit are careful to post signs on the children's beds that say things like "My name is Nancy. Please talk *to* me, not *about* me." The best health workers abide by this injunction with all patients. Many nurses in critical care units consult with hospital administration on the design of the units, in order to make the environment itself less a source of anxiety to patients and their families. In some hospitals this collaboration has resulted in comfortable waiting rooms for families, chairs at the bedside, rockers for holding small children, windows (so that the cycle of night and day is not lost), clocks and calendars to maintain the patient's orientation to time, and radios and television for familiar sights and sounds.

A common reaction of the patient on the ventilator is to breathe in an asynchronous pattern to that set by the operator. This may be caused by inadequate alveolar ventilation with hypercarbia, by hypoxemia, inadequate expansion, or by low cardiac output, leading to hypoxemia.[139] The psychologic causes have yet to be studied systematically, but the preparation of patients for this form of therapy undoubtedly plays an important role in the ability of the patient to adapt to the pattern set by the operator. Tranquilizing and analgesic medications help the patient to gain the needed physical and emotional rest but they must be skillfully used to be effective and prevent ad-

diction. (See Chapters 13, 23, 49, and 50). Manually controlled ventilation with 100 per cent oxygen may help the patient breathe with the ventilator. If this is not successful within 5 to 10 minutes, Bendixen and associates[140] recommend giving morphine intravenously in small doses (2 mg to the average adult) every 5 minutes until the patient can breathe with the ventilator. They say that in some cases the patient must be paralyzed with a long-acting relaxant to allow controlled ventilation.[141] The helplessness that is experienced by the paralyzed conscious patient is overwhelming. The quality of the nurse-patient-family relationship as previously described takes on even greater importance. The patient who is no longer using a ventilator may benefit from psychotherapy during his or her rehabilitation.

Termination of Prolonged Mechanical Ventilation. It is the goal of all ventilatory therapy to discontinue it as soon as possible. At the same time, the patient must be as carefully prepared for this step as for its initiation. Safar describes the following two physiologic problems that must be taken into account:

These patients may have "reset" their respiratory center to the lower $PaCO_2$ (tension of carbon dioxide in arterial blood) maintained during artificial ventilation. They . . . become dyspneic at $PaCO_2$ levels below 40 mm Hg. . . . These patients may crave deep lung inflations, presumably because pulmonary or chest wall stretch receptor reflexes became addicted to the sensation of deep inflations.*

The termination of mechanical ventilation is called "weaning." It cannot be started before the patient can maintain a tidal volume of 5 to 7 cc/kg and a vital capacity of 10 cc/kg. Vital capacities less than this are usually inadequate to provide the necessary deep inhalations, and progressive atelectasis results.[142] Weaning is also guided by serial determinations of the arterial tensions of carbon dioxide and oxygen and pH (the blood gases). Patients must be able to maintain normal pCO_2 and pH and pO_2 of 80 mm Hg on inspired oxygen concentrations of 40 per cent, or a pO_2 of 60 mm Hg on room air.

Patients may be prepared for the weaning process from the time artificial ventilation is initiated by explaining that this is a temporary measure. Other opportunities to help patients to be emotionally ready for the experience are at the times of suctioning when the ventilator tubing is removed. Efforts to move the chest are noted as a good sign, and patients should be encouraged to breathe with the ventilator turned off. The staff can discuss with the alert patient the progress made in acquiring independence from the ventilator. It is helpful to remember that the endotracheal or tracheostomy tube takes away the sensation of movement of gases into the lungs, and the patient may lose the sense of chest movement. After short-term ventilation the patient may have reduced tidal volume or vital capacity. The patient tends to take shallow breaths since deep breathing with the tube in place is uncomfortable.

Weaning from the ventilator is begun during the day, with the staff in constant attendance. It is obvious that patients must be refreshed and alert to cope with their feelings of dependence on the ventilator and fear of being unable to breathe. They must also feel the security of the familiar persons who have been supportive throughout the experience of using the ventilator.

The patient should breathe a humidified oxygen-enriched atmosphere when the ventilator is discontinued. This may be provided by a tracheostomy mask, an oxygen hood (in the case of infants), or a device that blows humidified oxygen over the endotracheal tube or tracheostomy tube ("blow-by"). The cuff is deflated. The first time "off the ventilator" is short, depending on the patient's tolerance, and may be from 1 to 15 minutes. Rather than lengthening the time the ventilator is turned off, the time the ventilator is turned on is gradually shortened.

* Safar, Peter (ed.): *op. cit.,* p. 126.

The ventilator may be used at night for several days after weaning has started. It can be set to initiate an inspiration when the patient makes an effort to inspire ("assist mode"), or it can be set to initiate inspiration without the patient's effort ("control mode"). Another technique in this highly individualized procedure is to progress the patient first to "assist mode" and then to breathing on his or her own in the oxygen-enriched atmosphere.

Intermittent mandatory ventilation is another system of weaning a patient from prolonged mechanical artificial ventilation. The ventilator is not disconnected from the patient as in the conventional weaning procedure. However, the patient breathes spontaneously, at his or her own rate, and at intermittent, preset intervals, a mechanical hyperinflation is delivered to the airway. This is a supportive, automatic "sigh," and it can be gradually reduced in frequency until weaning is complete.

The intermittent mandatory ventilation function can be adapted to any mechanical ventilator breathing circuit. Michael J. Banner and James R. Clark [143] show diagrams of the breathing circuit and commonly used adult and infant ventilators equipped with the circuit. They present their own and other clinical observations on weaning using an intermittent, pre-set hyperinflation and consider it psychologically superior to conventional weaning techniques. The patient who is apprehensive and lacking in confidence in his or her ability to resume spontaneous breathing has some mechanical ventilatory support.

The chest respirator and the rocking bed have been used in the past during the weaning period for patients treated in the body (tank) respirator. Safar [144] reports that the chest respirator and rocking bed cannot be relied upon to provide adequate tidal volumes in apneic or comatose patients or in the presence of "non-compliant" lungs and bronchial secretions.

Removing the tracheostomy tube follows the termination of ventilatory support and is dependent on the patient's ability to cough effectively, swallow, and maintain normal blood gases over several days. Egan [145] observes that the same considerations enter into the decision to remove an endotracheal tube. The risk of early removal of these tubes may be lessened as, in the hands of a skilled physician, they are easier to replace. A common practice in the past was to deflate the cuff of the tracheostomy tube and plug before removing it. This method was used primarily for patients with laryngeal edema and neuromuscular causes of respiratory failure. They usually had normal lungs and normal air passages distal to the trachea. Their tubes were plugged to evaluate the degree of return of neuromuscular ventilatory function before extubation. If a tube is plugged for a patient with pulmonary disease, it only impedes airflow, which was the reason why the artificial airway and ventilatory assistance was originally required.

REFERENCES

1. Goodman, Louis S., and Gilman, Alfred (eds.): *The Pharmacological Basis of Therapeutics,* 5th ed. Macmillan Publishing Co., Inc., New York, 1975, p. 881.
2. Ivy, Andrew C.: "The Physiology of Respiratory Diseases," *W. Va. Med. J.,* **43**:71, (Feb.) 1947.
3. Barach, Alvan L., et al.: *Physiology of Anoxia.* Linde Air Products Co., New York, 1943, p. 24.
4. Goodman, Louis S., and Gilman, Alfred (eds.): *op. cit.* p. 882.
5. Livingstone, Huberta M.: "Oxygen as Therapy," *Am. J. Nurs.,* **48**:17, (Jan.) 1948.
6. Bendixen, H. H., et al.: *Respiratory Care.* C. V. Mosby Co., St. Louis, 1965, p. 127.
7. *Ibid.,* p. 28.
8. Guedel, Arthur E.: *Inhalation Anesthesia,* 2nd ed. Macmillan Publishing Co., Inc., New York, p. 113.
9. Bendixen, H. H., et al.: *op. cit.*
10. Shapiro, Barry A.: *Clinical Application of Blood Gases.* Year Book Medical Publishers, Chicago, 1973, p. 112.
11. *Ibid.,* p. 41.
12. Bendixen, H. H., et al.: *op. cit.,* p. 12.
13. *Ibid.,* p. 21.
14. *Ibid.,* p. 22.
15. *Ibid.,* p. 130.
16. Shapiro, Barry A.: *op. cit.,* p. 106.
17. *Ibid.*
18. Bendixen, H. H., et al.: *op. cit.,* p. 130.
19. Goodman, Louis S., and Gilman, Alfred (eds.): *op. cit.,* p. 887.
20. Shapiro, Barry A.: *op. cit.,* p. 121.
21. Bendixen, H. H., et al.: *op. cit.,* p. 132.
22. Pontoppidan, H., et al.: "Acute Respiratory Failure in the Adult," (Second of Three Parts), *N. Engl. J. Med.,* **287**:748, (Oct. 12) 1972.
23. Slonim, N. Balfour, and Hamilton, Lyle: *Respiratory Physiology,* 3rd ed. C. V. Mosby Co., St. Louis, 1976, p. 165.
24. Egan, Donald F.: *Fundamentals of Respiratory Therapy,* 2nd ed. C. V. Mosby Co., St. Louis, 1973, p. 272.
25. Korones, Sheldon B.: *High Risk Newborn Infants,* 2nd ed. C. V. Mosby Co., St. Louis, 1976, p. 96.
26. *Ibid.,* p. 153.
27. Talner, Norman S.: "Congestive Heart Failure in the Infant," *Pediatr. Clin. North Am.,* **18**:1011, (Nov.) 1971.
27a. Goodman, Louis S., and Gilman, Alfred (eds.): *op. cit.,* p. 894.
27b. Bendixen, H. H., et al.: *op. cit.,* p. 70.
28. *Ibid.,* p. 105.
29. Hieronimus, Terring W.: *Mechanical Artificial Ventilation,* 2nd ed. Charles C Thomas, Publisher, Springfield, Ill., 1971, p. 117.
30. Safar, Peter (ed.): *Respiratory Therapy.* F. A. Davis Co., Philadelphia, 1965, p. 154.
31. Bendixen, H. H., et al.: *op. cit.,* p. 133.
32. *Ibid.,* p. 134.
33. *Ibid.,* p. 135.
34. Safar, Peter (ed.): *op. cit.,* p. 154.
35. *Ibid.,* p. 156.
35a. Egan, Donald F.: *op. cit.,* p. 283.
36. Safar, Peter (ed.): *op. cit.,* p. 154.
37. *Ibid.,* p. 157.
38. Bendixen, H. H., et al.: *op. cit.,* p. 135.
39. *Ibid.*
40. Safar, Peter (ed.): *op. cit.,* p. 158.
41. *Ibid.,* p. 161.
42. *Ibid.*
43. Burch, G. E., et al.: "Influence of Temperature and Oxygen Concentrations in Oxygen Tents," *J.A.M.A.,* **176**:1017, (June 24) 1961.
44. Korones, Sheldon B.: *op. cit.,* p. 154.
45. *Ibid.,* p. 154.
46. Stern, Leo: "The Use and Misuse of Oxygen in the Newborn Infant," *Pediatr. Clin. North Am.,* **20**:447, (May) 1973.
47. Petty, Thomas L.: *Intensive and Rehabilitative Respiratory Care,* 2nd ed. Lea & Febiger, Philadelphia, 1974, p. 301.
48. Lagerson, Joanne: "Nursing Care of Patients with Chronic Pulmonary Insufficiency," *Nurs. Clin. North Am.,* **9**:165, (Mar.) 1974.
49. Petty, Thomas L., and Nett, Louise M.: *For Those Who Live and Breathe: A Manual for Patients with Emphysema and Chronic Bronchitis,* 2nd ed. Charles C Thomas, Publisher, Springfield, Ill., 1972, p. 69.
50. Egan, Donald F.: *op. cit.,* p. 250.
51. Gracey, Donald R.: "Home Oxygen Therapy for the COPD Patient," *Heart & Lung,* **4**:792, (Sept.–Oct.) 1975.
52. Robley, Spencer H.: *Emphysema and Common Sense.* Parker Publishing Co., West Nyack, N.Y., 1968, p. 73.
53. "Portable Oxygen Analyzers," *Health Devices,* A Test Evaluation and Advisory Service of The Emergency Care Research Institute, Philadelphia, **1**:203, (May) 1972.
54. *Ibid.*
55. *Ibid.*
56. *Ibid.*
57. *Ibid.*
58. *Ibid.*
59. Slonim, H. Balfour, and Hamilton, Lyle: *op. cit.,* p. 62.
60. Goodman, Louis S., and Gilman, Alfred (eds.): *op. cit.,* p. 898.
61. *Ibid.,* p. 927.
62. Slonim, H. Balfour, and Hamilton, Lyle: *op. cit.,* p. 164.
63. Goodman, Louis S., and Gilman, Alfred (eds.): *op. cit.,* p. 898.
64. Blumgarten, A. S.: *Textbook of Materia Medica, Pharmacology and Therapeutics,* 7th

ed. Macmillan Publishing Co., Inc., New York, 1937, p. 297.
65. Goodman, Louis S., and Gilman, Alfred (eds.): *op. cit.*, p. 896.
66. *Ibid.*, p. 894.
67. *Ibid.*, p. 894.
68. *Ibid.*
69. *Ibid.*
70. Egan, Donald F.: *op. cit.*, p. 300.
71. Goodman, Louis S., and Gilman, Alfred (eds.): *op. cit.*, p. 895.
72. *Ibid.*, p. 896.
73. Safar, Peter (ed.): *op. cit.*, p. 163.
74. Hieronimus, Terring W.: *op. cit.*, p. 5.
75. *Ibid.*, p. 11.
76. Korones, Sheldon B.: *op. cit.*, p. 57.
77. Reddick, Lloyd F., et al.: "An Evaluation of Hand Operated Self-Inflating Resuscitation Equipment," *Anesth. Analg.*, **49**:28, (Jan.–Feb.) 1970.
78. Korones, Sheldon B.: *op. cit.*, p. 134.
79. Reddick, Lloyd F., et al.: *op. cit.*
80. *Ibid.*
81. Hieronimus, Terring W.: *op. cit.*, p. 129.
82. Selecky, Paul A.: "Tracheostomy: A Review of Present Day Indications, Complications and Care," *Heart Lung*, **3**:272, (Mar.–Apr.) 1974.
83. Hieronimus, Terring W.: *op. cit.*, p. 111.
84. Safar, Peter (ed.): *op. cit.*, p. 220.
85. *Ibid.*
86. Hieronimus, Terring W.: *op. cit.*, p. 111.
87. *Ibid.*
88. Safar, Peter (ed.): *op. cit.*
89. Hieronimus, Terring W.: *op. cit.*, p. 11.
90. *Ibid.*, p. 14.
91. *Ibid.*, p. 20.
92. Safar, Peter (ed.): *op. cit.*
93. Petty, Thomas L., and Nett, Louise M.: *op. cit.*, p. 55.
94. *Ibid.*, p. 57.
95. *Ibid.*, p. 43.
96. Chang, N., et al.: "An Evaluation of Nightly Mist Tent Therapy for Patients with Cystic Fibrosis," *Am. Rev. Resp. Dis.*, **107**:672, (Apr.) 1973.
97. Chang, N., and Levinson, H.: "The Effect of Nebulized Bronchodilator Administered with or without Intermittent Positive Pressure Breathing on Ventilatory Function in Children with Cystic Fibrosis and Asthma," *Am. Rev. Resp. Dis.*, **106**:817, (Dec.) 1972.
98. Barker, R., and Levinson, H.: "Effects of Ultrasonic Nebulized Distilled Water on Airway Dynamics in Children with Cystic Fibrosis and Asthma," *J. Pediatr.*, **80**:396, (Mar.) 1972.
99. Motoyama, E. K., et al.: "Evaluation of Mist Tent Therapy in Cystic Fibrosis Using Maximum Expiratory Flow Volume Curve," *Pediatrics*, **50**:299, (Aug.) 1972.
100. Safar, Peter (ed.): *op. cit.*, p. 94.
101. Hieronimus, Terring W.: *op. cit.*, p. 44.
102. Egan, Donald F.: *op. cit.*, p. 396.
103. Safar, Peter (ed.): *op. cit.*, p. 95.
104. *Ibid.*, p. 94.

105. Shapiro, Barry A.: *op. cit.*, p. 45.
106. Hieronimus, Terring W.: *op. cit.*, p. 7.
107. Korones, Sheldon B.: *op. cit.*, p. 158.
108. Safar, Peter (ed.): *op. cit.*, p. 97.
109. Hieronimus, Terring W.: *op. cit.*, p. 124.
110. Safar, Peter (ed.): *op. cit.*
111. Hieronimus, Terring W.: *op. cit.*
112. Bendixen, H. H., et al.: *op. cit.*, p. 111.
113. *Ibid.*, p. 117.
114. *Ibid.*
115. Safar, Peter (ed.): *op. cit.*, p. 57.
116. Hieronimus, Terring W.: *op. cit.*, p. 128.
117. Bendixen, H. H., et al.: *op. cit.*, p. 118.
118. *Ibid.*, p. 153.
119. Hieronimus, Terring W.: *op. cit.*, p. 16.
120. *Ibid.*, p. 12.
121. Bendixen, H. H., et al.: *op. cit.*
122. Safar, Peter (ed.): *op. cit.*, p. 101.
123. *Ibid.*
124. Chernick, V.: "Continuous Negative Chest Wall Pressure Therapy for Hyaline Membrane Disease," *Pediatr. Clin. North Am.*, **20**:407, (May) 1973.
125. Safar, Peter (ed.): *op. cit.*
126. Hieronimus, Terring W.: *op. cit.*, p. 95.
127. Chernik, V.: *op. cit.*
128. Safar, Peter (ed.): *op. cit.*, p. 102.
129. Blaisdell, F. William, and Schlobohm, Richard M.: "The Respiratory Distress Syndrome: A Review," *Surgery*, **74**:251, (Aug.) 1973.
130. Korones, Sheldon B.: *op. cit.*, p. 155.
131. Chernick, V.: *op. cit.*
132. Sugarman, Harvey J., et al.: "Positive End Expiratory Pressure (PEEP); Indications and Physiologic Considerations," *Chest*, **62**:865, (Nov.) 1972 (Suppl. Part II).
133. Korones, Sheldon B.: *op. cit.*, p. 155.
134. Chernick, V.: *op. cit.*
135. Nicotra, M. Brooke, et al.: "Physiologic Evaluation of Positive End Expiratory Pressure Ventilation," *Chest*, **64**:10, (July) 1973.
136. Blaisdell, F. William, and Schlobohm, Richard M.: *op. cit.*
137. Petty, Thomas L.: "PEEP" (editorial), *Chest*, **61**:309, (Apr.) 1972.
138. Thomson, Linda R.: "Sensory Deprivation: A Personal Experience," *Am. J. Nurs.*, **73**:266, (Feb.) 1973.
139. Bendixen, H. H., et al.: *op. cit.*, p. 140.
140. *Ibid.*
141. *Ibid.*
142. Safar, Peter (ed.): *op. cit.*, p. 127.
143. Banner, Michael J., and Clarke, James R.: "IMV: Innovation in Long-Term Ventilation," *Respiratory Ther.*, **2**:83, (Mar.–Apr.) 1973.
144. Safar, Peter (ed.): *op. cit.*, p. 128.
145. Egan, Donald F.: *op. cit.*, p. 429.

Additional Suggested Reading

Avery, Mary Ellen, and Fletcher, Barry D.: *The Lung and Its Disorders in the Newborn Infant*, 3rd ed. W. B. Saunders Co., Philadelphia, 1974.
Bates, David V., et al.: *Respiratory Function in*

Disease, 2nd ed. W. B. Saunders Co., Philadelphia, 1971.

Corden, E., and Hughes, T.: "An Evaluation of Manually Operated Self Inflating Resuscitation Bags," *Anesth. Analg. (Cleve.),* **54**:133, (Jan.–Feb.) 1975.

Crozier, D. N.: "Cystic Fibrosis," *Pediatr. Clin. North Am.,* **21**:935, (Nov.) 1974.

Downs, John B., et al.: "Intermittent Mandatory Ventilation: A New Approach to Weaning Patients from Mechanical Ventilators," *Chest,* **64**:331, (Sept.) 1973.

Fagerhaugh, Shizuko Y.: "Getting Around with Emphysema," *Am. J. Nurs.,* **73**:94, (Jan.) 1973.

Feeley, Thomas W., and Hedley-Whyte, John: "Weaning from Controlled Ventilation and Supplemental Oxygen," *N. Engl. J. Med.,* **292**:903, (Apr. 24) 1975.

Gold, Martin: "The Current Status of IPPB Therapy," *Chest,* **67**:469, (Apr.) 1975.

Graff, Thomas: "Humidification: Indications and Hazards in Respiratory Therapy," *Anesth. Analg. (Cleve.),* **54**:444, (July–Aug.) 1975.

Greenberg, Mark, and Edmonds, John: "Chronic Respiratory Problems in Neuromyopathic Disorders," *Pediatr. Clin. North Am.,* **21**:927, (Nov.) 1974.

Hadley, Florence, and Bordicks, Katherine J.: "Respiratory Difficulty—Causes and Care," *Am. J. Nurs.,* **62**:64, (Oct.) 1962.

Helming, Mary G. (ed.): "Nursing in Respiratory Disease—A Symposium," *Nurs. Clin. North Am.,* **3**:381, (Sept.) 1968.

Kirkpatrick, Barry V., et al.: "Complications of Ventilator Therapy in Respiratory Distress Syndrome: Recognition and Management of Acute Air Leaks," *Am. J. Dis. Child.,* **128**:496, (Oct.) 1974.

Kurihara, M.: "Postural Drainage, Clapping, and Vibrating," *Am. J. Nurs.,* **65**:76, (Nov.) 1965.

Nett, Louise M., and Petty, Thomas L.: "Acute Respiratory Failure," *Am. J. Nurs.,* **67**:1847, (Sept.) 1967.

Rodman, Theodore: "Management of Tracheobronchial Secretions," *Am. J. Nurs.,* **66**:2474, (Nov.) 1966.

Traver, Gayle A. (ed.): "Care in Respiratory Disease," *Nurs. Clin. North Am.,* **9**:97, (Mar.) 1974.

Yanda, Roman L.: "Quality Control of Inhalation Therapy," *Chest,* **66**:61, (July) 1974.

Roberta O'Grady
Virginia Henderson

CHAPTER 21

Oral Administration of Drugs

1. THE USE OF DRUGS

While such a chapter in most books on nursing deals with the use of drugs prescribed as therapeutic agents by physicians, or by those to whom this responsibility has been delegated, almost equal attention here is devoted to self-medication. Far more money is spent by most societies on self-prescribed than medically-prescribed drugs. In the first place, alcohol is a drug and so are tobacco, marijuana, hashish (cannabis or Indian hemp) and other plants that are widely distributed and widely used on the public's initiative.* These specified drugs are first taken for their "pleasurable" effects or to conform to custom and later because their use becomes a habit or creates a craving. But apart from drugs used for their social or euphoric effects (in most cases because they remove inhibitions), drugs are commonly self-prescribed to produce forgetfulness, relaxation and sleep; to relieve pain or discomforts such as burning or itching; to "kill germs"; to stimulate bowel activity; or to cure a lesion, a growth, or some other manifestation of disease. (Needless to say the effects of drugs taken for these various reasons are not in many cases those anticipated.)

Erwin DiCyan, a pharmacist, and Lawrence Hessman, a physician, have written a book titled *Without Prescription* which they say is "a guide to the selection and use of medicines you can get over the counter without prescription for safe self medication." [1] They list 562 products under the following headings: The Common Cold; Drugs for Children; Stomach and Abdominal Discomfort; Pain;

Eye, Ear, Nose, Throat and Mouth; Feminine Hygiene; Insomnia and Fatigue; Allergy; and Skin. Before listing the proprietary, or "over-the-counter" drugs (as opposed to "legend drugs," or those available only on prescription), DiCyan and Hessman tell enough about the products in each category to enable people to make, as they think, an "informed choice." There is now in every sort of health service an emphasis on health education, prevention, and self-help. The informed use of drugs and management by individuals of their medicines is timely.

The use and misuse of drugs are, and probably always have been, among the most serious problems humans face. Health workers should be leaders in programs designed to help people use drugs wisely and to establish the causes of drug abuse—or misuse. They should be leaders in programs to educate the public; to promote legislation protecting people from dangerous drugs and from persons who promote ("push") the illicit sale of drugs for profit; and leaders in programs that offer treatment for addicts.

Nurses, in their daily practice, by example and by using every opportunity to help patients make a constructive use and informed choice of all kinds of drugs, can affect the so-called drug problem. Drugs, as opposed to foods, are potent substances that are to be feared as well as valued.* In our judgment, health workers should feel as obligated to teach patients about the drug the patient is taking as to prescribe

---

* While alcohol is an ingredient of many beverages, the National Institute of Mental Health titles a 1972 publication *Alcohol Is a Drug* (US Government Printing Office, Washington, D.C.).

* Differentiation between food and drugs is not as simple as it may seem. Webster says a drug is "any substance used as a medicine"; therefore if prune juice is used in place of a pill to stimulate bowel activity, it might be defined as a drug, while vitamins added to breads to increase their nutritive value are consumed daily as food rather than as therapeutic agents.

and administer the most appropriate drug in the appropriate dosage. The economic waste in harmful or useless drug consumption is almost incalculable—as are the illnesses attributable to it. Health workers who use drugs unwisely and who fail to teach their patients, or clients, the dangers of drugs must share the blame for the accusation that ours is "a drugged society."

2. THE ABUSE OF DRUGS

Definitions. Kenneth L. Jones and his associates[2] define *drug addiction* * as a state of periodic or chronic intoxication caused by repeatedly taking a natural or synthetic drug. Addiction is characterized by an overpowering compulsion to take the drug, to get it by any means, and to gradually increase the dosage because there is a developing tolerance. It is also characterized by a psychologic and physical dependence on the drug that results in a personal, family, and community problem. *Drug dependency,* a less serious state, is defined as one that results from repeated use of a drug. Its characteristics are a desire (but not an overwhelming compulsion) to continue taking the drug, little or no tendency to increase the dosage, and a psychologic rather than a physiologic dependency that results in a personal problem but not necessarily a family or community problem. While "alcoholism" includes alcohol addiction and dependency and is one form of drug abuse, it is often considered separately.

In 1952, the World Health Organization gave the following *definition of alcoholics:*

Alcoholics are those excessive drinkers whose dependence on alcohol has attained such a degree that they show a noticeable mental disturbance or an interference with their mental and bodily health, their interpersonal relations and their smooth social and economic functioning; or who show the prodromal signs of such developments. They therefore need treatment.†

While this statement would probably go unchallenged in most discussions of alcoholism, there are many public views on it, and even in the professional literature, definitions vary.[3]

One emphasizes the extent of the drinking—if drinking goes beyond dietary and social custom, it is considered alcoholism. Another emphasizes the effects of drinking—when drinking interferes with the physical, personal, and social aspects of life, it is alcoholism. A third definition emphasizes the similarity between alcoholism and other forms of drug addiction or the compulsive nature of the drinking, the increasing tolerance, the obsessive efforts to get alcohol, the physical deterioration, the personality change, and the resulting social problems.

Incidence and Causes of Drug Abuse. Throughout man's history consciousness-altering drugs have been used and abused. They are as old and familiar as alcohol or as new and unfamiliar as methaqualone. Many primitive peoples use the "mood modifiers" found in native plants in their tribal rituals. According to Andrew Weil,[4] the Indians of the Amazon Basin today use more drugs of plant origin than any other peoples. In technologic societies, drugs are nearly always highly refined and often synthesized chemicals that are extremely potent, in comparison with those used in the form of plants where the concentration is in most cases low. When used wisely, under competent medical direction, many of the refined potent drugs are helpful and may be essential to the cure or control of diseases of body and mind—if the latter can be considered separately. When drugs of any kind are abused, however, they are threats to individuals and societies. The most commonly abused drugs today are alcohol, marijuana, morphine, codeine, amphetamines, the various chemical compounds called tranquilizers, and the barbiturates.

National commissions have been appointed in recent years to study drug dependency and addiction. The incidences reported have been alarming. Many persons believe drug abuse (and associated crime) is the major problem of this era. But drug abuse takes many forms and it is not necessarily associated with crime. As knowledge about drug abuse increases, some distinctions can be made among the people who abuse drugs. For instance, Leon Wurmser[5] says the majority of drug users are *experimenters* who should be differentiated from *compulsive users* whose behavior indicates that they have psychologic problems. However, it is dangerous to experiment with consciousness-altering drugs, for it can always lead to compulsive use. Each person is a unique combination of physical and emotional forces, and the effects of any drug differ with the individual and they even vary with the individual from one day to the next.

---

* Frequently abused chemicals and their specific action on the central nervous system and other body systems are discussed in most textbooks of therapeutic pharmacology. Interested readers should consult such texts.

† World Health Organization, Expert Committee on Mental Health: *Alcohol Subcommittee Second Report.* The Organization, Geneva, 1952 (Tech. Report Series No. 48).

Jerome H. Jaffe * thinks that in addition to distinguishing between the experimental and compulsive drug users, more should be known about why particular groups use particular drugs—especially if these groups are to be treated effectively. Teenagers, for example, may be rebelling against authority, testing themselves in a dangerous situation, and searching for their identities. They are in an ambivalent age. By using drugs of which the grown-ups disapprove, adolescents can express independence; at the same time, by using drugs, they can render themselves helpless and so remain children. The need that young people have for group approval and support is thought by some authorities to account for the current epidemic of youthful drug experimentation. Jaffe says that although the parental use of cigarettes, alcohol, tranquilizers, and barbiturates gives a "set" to an adolescent's attitude toward drugs, friends of the same age group have the most influence.[6]

While the preceding statements apply chiefly to young people who use drugs (including alcohol) for the first time, or on rare occasions, many authorities believe that compulsive drug users are emotionally troubled individuals. Wurmser[7] says the patients he has treated have a general unwillingness to accept limitations, commitments, or responsibilities. Their prevailing feelings on a deep emotional level are rage, boredom, and a vague tension; on a still deeper level they seem to be profoundly demanding. While they would like to be omnipotent they have a sense of helplessness. Other authorities describe the young drug abuser as a person who is apathetic, passive, unable to tolerate frustration, and unable to communicate effectively. Frequently, these young people take drugs to relieve anxiety, depression, pressure, and tension.

Andrew Malleson[8] thinks the publicity given young drug users by the press obscures what he believes to be the much more common use by the middle-aged of the "nice drugs" like the slimming pills, the barbiturates, the antidepressant and antianxiety drugs. He calls this "the pot and kettle story" because he thinks the very people who take these drugs which he calls "brain poisons" condemn the young addicts. Malleson is highly critical of physicians who too readily prescribe addictive drugs and even more critical of the drug industry that spends millions on high-pressure advertising of addictive drugs. He, and many others, think the depression, hypoactivity, and

* Former director of the Special Action Office for Drug Abuse Prevention activated by the United States Government, June 1971.

apathy so common among the elderly, and especially the institutionalized elderly, is attributable in part to the injudicious use of tranquilizers. In nursing homes and mental hospitals, chemical restraint has been substituted for physical restraint, and it is hard to say which is more destructive.

As other addictive drugs become less available, alcohol, which is legalized and readily available in a wide range of beverages, is more often used by the young as well as those who have reached their majority. While some youthful drinkers may escape addiction, an alarming number are becoming alcoholics.

There are many theories on the cause of alcoholism and no single theory prevails. Suggested physiologic causes of alcoholism are allergic reactions, metabolic defects, nutritional deficiencies, and abnormal levels of body hormones. Proposed psychologic causes include oral cravings, pleasure fixation, unconscious urges to destroy oneself or dominate others, and feelings of inferiority or insecurity. Sociologic studies indicate that alcoholism is, certainly to some extent, cultural. The incidence of alcoholism varies with the country, with ethnic and religious groups, and from one era to another. The economic level and educational status also influence the incidence of alcoholism, although the abuse of alcohol is worldwide and few groups escape entirely.

Most students of alcoholism differentiate between a high consumption of alcohol by a class, or people, and a high incidence of alcoholism. Selden D. Bacon,[9] writing on the social aspects of alcohol addiction, notes that drinking is very common among Jewish-Americans and Italian-Americans, but the incidence of alcoholism is very low. Malleson says France reportedly has the highest consumption of alcohol per person and 10 per cent of the deaths are from cirrhosis of the liver. Yet no one thinks of "the drink" as typically French. Malleson cited another study showing that 2 per cent (or 350,000 persons) in the population of Great Britain were alcoholics. He said, however, that "Americans drink the British under the table," 4 per cent being alcoholic and $300 million being spent each year in advertising booze. Figures reported on alcoholism in Russia are comparable to those for the U.S.A.[10] Programs to reduce drug abuse in mainland China are reportedly very effective.

Because many people can drink large quantities of alcohol without becoming so-called alcoholics, the concept of alcoholism as a disease is widely accepted today, and is the basis for the "treatment" approach used by Alcoholics Anonymous. The successful use of disulfiram (Antabuse) as a therapeutic method in alcoholism and research in the use of lithium for treating alcoholics are also based on the concept of disease or illness. Clearly, alcoholism is a complex problem that does not have a simple cause or cure.[11-12a]

The epidemiology of all types of drug abuse is a subject that might fill volumes. Whether the drug is alcohol or an opiate, the incidence varies with sex, age, race, religion, culture, and economic status. Its prevalence in this era is attributed to so many different conditions that any statement made in this brief discussion of the subject seems an oversimplification. The safest position may be that of the person who stresses the universality of the problem; the fact that both sexes, all ages, all races, religious cultures and classes are affected. While some psychiatrists believe drug abuse indicative of emotional instability, others note that persons thought most stable by their associates fall victim to drugs, and most particularly alcohol, if conditions in their lives foster dependence and addiction.[13-20] Because there is no stigma attached to social drinking in many cultures, the prevalence of alcoholism is easily understood.

Sociologists tend to stress environmental conditions as causative factors in drug dependency and addiction, psychiatrists see personality structure as the major explanation, but a few doctors [21] say, like Thomas Szasz,[22] "Bad Habits Are Not Diseases." His article on the subject is subtitled "A Refutation of the Claim That Alcoholism Is a Disease." Malleson [23] seems inclined to think that those who seek refuge in drugs have failed to "learn life's lessons" and those who prescribe addictive drugs are practicing "unhealthy doctoring." He says "proper behavior does not come in bottles."

Nurses in most, if not all countries, in every clinical specialty, and every occupational field encounter drug abuse, although they may fail to recognize it if they are uninformed. Midwives and obstetric nurses should be alert to the dangers to mothers and their unborn babies if the mother is drug dependent or addicted;[24,25] they should also realize that the mother needs special help if the husband or any member of the household is abusing drugs. Pediatric nurses, particularly those in school health, should know the incidence and the signs of drug abuse in pupils or students. School nurses are also in a position to help young people who live with addicted parents. The neglected child often has one or both parents addicted to drugs.[26-34]

Many industries have drug dependency and addiction programs.[35] This is also true for military health services and even for those in prison where health care is probably of the lowest order. National legislation of the 1970s has made funds available in federal prisons for drug abuse programs and also to state and local agencies that sponsor such programs in prisons as well as mental health centers, clinics, hospitals, and rehabilitation units.[36] States have councils on drug abuse and often separate councils on alcoholism.

Health personnel employed in institutions where programs are in operation are usually made aware of the incidence of drug abuse, its manifestations, and at least the treatment approach used in the particular institution.

Many persons admitted to general hospitals for surgery and for medical treatment are also drug-dependent or addicted. Patients may themselves be in the denial phase and families are often too proud to admit that their relative is addicted. Unless it is known and withdrawal reactions modified by treatment, these reactions may greatly affect the patient's prognosis. Nurses who are aware of this danger, who know the signs of addiction, and nurses whose nonjudgmental attitude invites confidence may be the means of forestalling withdrawal crises. Knowledgeable nurses are essential to effective crisis intervention.[37-41a]

Nurses in hospitals, or in fact any health institution or agency, should realize that employees may be addicted. LeClair Bissell and his associates, writing about alcoholism ("the lonely illness") in hospital employees, comment on the lack of help available to them as compared with employees in "other industries." They make the following observations: "Studies in private business and industry (including hospitals), as well as in government, indicate that between 5 and 10 percent of the employees on an organization's payroll are alcoholics." * Speaking of the widespread and effective programs in most industries, Bissell and his associates ask the following questions:

Where, within a major hospital, is an alcoholism program for the physician, nurse, social worker or technician? Are we any less valuable than the worker on the assembly line, the army officer, the executive? Are we any more difficult to reach because we are used to treating others rather than ourselves? †

Parenthetically, these questions are answered in part by the authors' description of the alcoholism program at the Roosevelt Hospital in New York City, under the joint auspices of medicine and psychiatry, that is offering hospital employees the same consideration shown patients. The same principles that apply to

---

* Bissell, LeClair, et al.: "The Alcoholic Hospital Employee," *Nurs. Outlook,* **21:**708, (Nov.) 1973.
† Bissell, LeClair, et al.: *op. cit.*

alcoholism apply to other types of addiction; help should be available in all cases.[42-47]

There are countless studies of the incidence of drug abuse but they are all rough estimates. It is generally conceded that there are more persons addicted to alcohol than to any other drug because it is a legalized, socially acceptable, easily available drug. Of those who drink alcoholic beverages, it is estimated that at least 1 in 14 is an alcoholic. The total figure for the United States is put at 9 to 10 million persons; the figure for heroin users is around 500 to 600 thousand.[48,49] Alcoholics and all drug abusers tend to hide their addiction as long as possible and this makes estimates of incidence subject to question.

Addicts rarely seek help in early stages, and even in the late stages of addiction denial is common, since they fear treatment, fear life without the drug on which they are dependent, and, of course, fear the social disapproval that may make them lose their place in the family, in school, or wherever they are employed. **Recognizing Drug Addiction by its Symptoms.** Since addictive drugs differ in their effects and individuals differ in their response to the same drug, there is no easy answer to the question "How can a drug dependent or drug addict be identified?" Bonnie L. Long and Donna Sammarco Krepick[50] list the following categories of drugs that are abused and their immediate and long-term effects which differ from one category to another: *hallucinogens* (marijuana, alcoholic extract of marijuana, hashish, LSD, Psilocybin, mescaline or peyote, STP, Phenyclidine, or Sernyl); *sedative-hypnotics* (barbiturates, organic solvents such as glue, plastics, gasoline, or cleaning fluid, ethyl alcohol, Librium, Valium, Miltown, methaqualone; *stimulants* (amphetamines, cocaine); *opiates* (heroin, morphine sulfate, methadone, codeine).

While it isn't possible in a general discussion of drug abuse to give all its symptoms, there are some that are common to a number of categories listed above: The following are *immediate effects:* relaxation and relief from anxiety; euphoria, followed by sedation depression, and, in some cases, loss of consciousness; slowed reflexes and impaired coordination with slurred speech; loss of inhibitions and emotional control; impaired judgment and memory. Among the *long-term* effects are craving for the drug with a need for increased dosage; restlessness and insomnia; decreased appetite, malnutrition, weight loss, and excessive fa-

Table 21-1. Phases and Symptoms of Alcoholism

First Phase

1. First blank period or amnesia
2. Sneaking drinks
3. Preoccupation with drinking
4. Gulping drinks
5. Becoming evasive about drinking
6. Second blank period or amnesia

Second (or Crucial) Phase

7. Loss of control of drinking
8. Manufacturing alibis
9. Extravagant and grandiose behavior
10. Aggressive behavior
11. Persistent remorse
12. Periods of total abstinence ("going on water wagon")
13. Tries changing pattern of drinking
14. Begins dropping friends
15. Leaves or loses jobs
16. Becomes *more* preoccupied with alcohol
17. Loses outside interests
18. Indulges in orgies of self-pity
19. Impulse to escape from environment (actual or contemplated)
20. Experiences unreasonable resentments
21. Protects his supply of alcohol (hides bottles)
22. Malnutrition (the alcoholic neglects to take food)
23. Hospitalization
24. Decrease or loss of sexual desire
25. Alcoholic jealousy
26. The morning drink (needs a "bracer" to start the day)

The Final (or Chronic) Phase

27. First prolonged intoxication
28. Ethical deterioration
29. Impairment of thinking
30. Drinking with social inferiors
31. Debasement of taste—if necessary drinks methylated spirit, bay rum, or surgical spirit in toilet preparations
32. Loss of tolerance for alcohol
33. Vague, indefinable fears
34. Persistent tremors
35. Cannot perform simple muscular tasks without alcohol
36. Drinking becomes obsessive
37. Vague religious desires develop
38. Alibis and rationalizations fail, and the patient admits defeat

* Kogan, Benjamin A. *Health: Man in a Changing Environment.* Harcourt, Brace & World, New York, 1970, p. 401.

tigue; sweating; constipation; decreased sexual desire and impotency; social alienation.

Marty Mann,[51] a recovered alcoholic, in her *New Primer on Alcoholism,* lists and discusses the early, middle, and late symptoms, most of which are the same as for other sedative-hypnotics. In 1973, the National Council on Alcoholism published an extract of her Primer in a pamphlet titled *How to Know an Alcoholic.*[52] Her description is too long to cite but interested readers can get this pamphlet on request from the Council (address: 2 Park Avenue, New York, N.Y.). Table 21-1 lists the phases and symptoms of alcoholism.

Mary Millsap, discussing her role as an occupational nurse in an alcohol addiction program, says that employees suspected of alcoholism are handed the following questionnaire to answer:

	YES	NO
1. Have you lost time from work due to drinking?	( )	( )
2. Has drinking made your home life unhappy?	( )	( )
3. Do you drink because you are shy with people?	( )	( )
4. Has drinking affected your reputation?	( )	( )
5. Have you gotten into financial difficulties because of your drinking?	( )	( )
6. Do you turn to lower companions and an inferior environment when drinking?	( )	( )
7. Does your drinking make you careless of your family's welfare?	( )	( )
8. Has your drinking decreased your ambition?	( )	( )
9. Do you want a drink "the morning after"?	( )	( )
10. Does your drinking cause you to have difficulty sleeping?	( )	( )
11. Has your efficiency decreased since drinking?	( )	( )
12. Has drinking ever jeopardized your job or business?	( )	( )
13. Do you drink to escape from worries or troubles?	( )	( )
14. Do you drink alone?	( )	( )
15. Have you ever had a complete loss of memory as a result of drinking?	( )	( )
16. Has your physician ever treated you for drinking?	( )	( )
17. Do you drink to build up self-confidence?	( )	( )
18. Have you ever been in an institution or hospital on account of drinking?	( )	( )
19. Have you ever felt remorse after drinking?	( )	( )
20. Do you crave a drink at a definite time daily?	( )	( )

These questions were developed by the late Dr. Robert V. Seliger. It has been the experience of the membership of Alcoholics Anonymous that if a man answers "yes" to as few as three questions, he can be reasonably certain that alcohol has become, or is becoming, a problem for him. Although it has inherent weaknesses because it is a self-appraisal tool, it has become a widely accepted method of getting the patient to look at himself.*

The above questionnaire is often cited and we think it could be used by nurses in settings other than industry to identify persons who need help with alcoholism.

It should be remembered that drug abuse affects the addicts' families. It is anxiety-provoking for anyone close to them; disturbed family relationships are therefore symptomatic. Alcoholism is often called "a family disease."[53] It is not unusual for the wife of an alcoholic to land in a mental hospital before the extent of the husband's addiction is generally known; husbands of alcoholic wives frequently seek divorce.† Parents of drug-addicted sons and daughters are often so alienated that the young people leave home. When drug addiction is suspected, it should be treated as a family problem.

Because the abuse of alcohol is so common, because "social drinking" is so universal, most people find it hard to accept the fact that alcohol, no matter what the amount, is a depressant, not a stimulant. The apparent stimulation results from the depression of cortical centers that control judgment; therefore, persons who are normally inhibited and self-controlled may seem stimulated or happy because they lose their inhibitions or their self-control. The ability, under the influence of alcohol, to express emotion that is ordinarily repressed is part of the relief sought by certain alcoholics.

While some people survive years of alcohol abuse, it is, nevertheless, a poisonous substance. As noted earlier, Malleson calls it a "brain poison." According to Laurence A. Senseman,[54] microscopic examination of nerve cells in acute alcohol poisoning shows little

* Millsap, Mary: "Occupational Health Nursing in an Alcohol Addiction Program," *Nurs. Clin. North Am.,* 7:121, (Mar.) 1972.

† Husbands and wives who tell their story at joint meetings of Alcoholics Anonymous, Al-Anon, and Alateen sometimes say that the drinking partner often thinks the nondrinking partner "crazy" and that the relationship between the children and the drinking parent may be better than that between the children and the sober parent. A nondrinking wife is likely to be so disturbed that friends and relatives often exclaim "I don't blame her husband for staying drunk!" There is a saying among wives of alcoholics that the wife "stands alone."

difference from cells in other kinds of poisoning, such as lead or arsenic. While such cell changes are at first reversible, they accumulate and are more marked as "addiction" to alcohol develops.

Alcoholism, in contrast to other drug addictions, has a slow rate of progress and may take from 5 to 15 years to develop. According to reports of E. M. Jellinek's now classic study, most alcoholics pass through definite progressive stages with characteristic symptoms.[55] Figure 21-1 presents a modified version of these stages and their associated behaviors. As can be noted in the figure, rehabilitation of alcoholics cannot begin until they admit they are alcoholics, that they need and honestly want help. Actually, effective treatment of any addict is dependent on their readiness to stop using the addictive drug.

Treatment of Drug Abuse. At no time in history has treatment for drug abuse been so widely discussed or so widely available. There is universal emphasis on traffic in drugs and on drug abuse. The World Health Organization has an Expert Committee on Drug Dependence that has published about 20 reports.[56] National commissions have been appointed in many countries.* State and provincial commissions and councils are working on the problem with, usually, separate councils on alcoholism, and there is a wealth of literature addressed to the public and professionals.[57-64]

Addiction to opiates—cocaine and other such habit-forming drugs—has been treated as a disease throughout this century. There are, and have been for decades, federal and state laws in the United States designed to control the illicit use of such drugs and to enforce treatment. Comparative studies of drug abuse in various countries are designed to measure the effectiveness of differing legal approaches to the problem. While the United States Prohibition Law of 1918 (the 18th Amendment to the Constitution or the Volstead Act which was ratified in January 1919 and repealed in December 1933) was an attempt to control the production and sale of alcoholic beverages, alcoholism has only recently been considered a disease. "Drunks" have been laughed at, or if a public nuisance, sent to jail rather than to the hospital. Until very recently, general hospitals refused to admit alcoholics. Current federal legislation making funds available for

treatment has helped change this, but the generally accepted concept of alcoholism as a disease has had the more pronounced effect on treatment.

The public's attitude toward drug abuse seems to be changing. Artists often sense social change before average persons. Eugene O'Neill's *Long Day's Journey into Night*,[65] written in 1956, showed the effect on a family of opiate addiction; *The Iceman Cometh*[66] in 1946 gave a vivid picture of alcoholism. Both plays drew on O'Neill's personal experience and he is only one of many artists—writers, actors, and painters—who have helped people understand the causes and the effects of addiction. *The Story of Mrs. Murphy*[67] and *Lost Weekend*[68] were popular books, and many television programs, with prominent actors who have had personal experience with addiction, have encouraged families to bring the problem into the open, to seek help, and to consider the addict a sick human being rather than a "disgrace."

Passage of the Comprehensive Alcohol Abuse and Alcoholism Prevention, Treatment and Rehabilitation Act of 1970 (Public Law 91–616) established the National Institute on Alcohol Abuse and Alcoholism within the National Institute of Mental Health. This has had a marked effect on the treatment of alcoholism in the United States and has put addiction to alcohol in the same class with addiction to other drugs. It has established alcoholism as a disease and made funds available for research, training, development of services, and public education. The report of the first national symposium in 1970, edited by Nancy Mello and Jack H. Mendelson,[69] is a guide to the most significant lines of research on alcoholism. In 1971, the US Public Health Service published a descriptive pamphlet, *Developing Community Services for Alcoholics, Some Beginning Principles*,[70] and in 1972, *A Guide to Drug Abuse Education and Information Materials*.[71] The treatment of persons addicted to alcohol runs parallel with the treatment of those addicted to other drugs.

However, while the "recovery" of many prominent persons (actors, writers, and politicians) is a matter of public record, at this time there is no treatment for drug abuse that can be applied successfully to all persons. The following approaches, all controversial, are in current use: (1) methadone maintenance; (2) narcotic antagonists; (3) detoxification centers; and (4) therapeutic communities with emphasis on self-help, health education, or character rebuilding.

Methadone maintenance treatments (many of them given through outpatient programs)

---

* In December, 1974, the American Nurses' Association Division of Psychiatric and Mental Health Nursing, as a member of the Congress on Alcohol and Drug Problems, was one of the 40 sponsoring agencies for the most comprehensive international forum ever held on alcoholism and other forms of drug abuse.

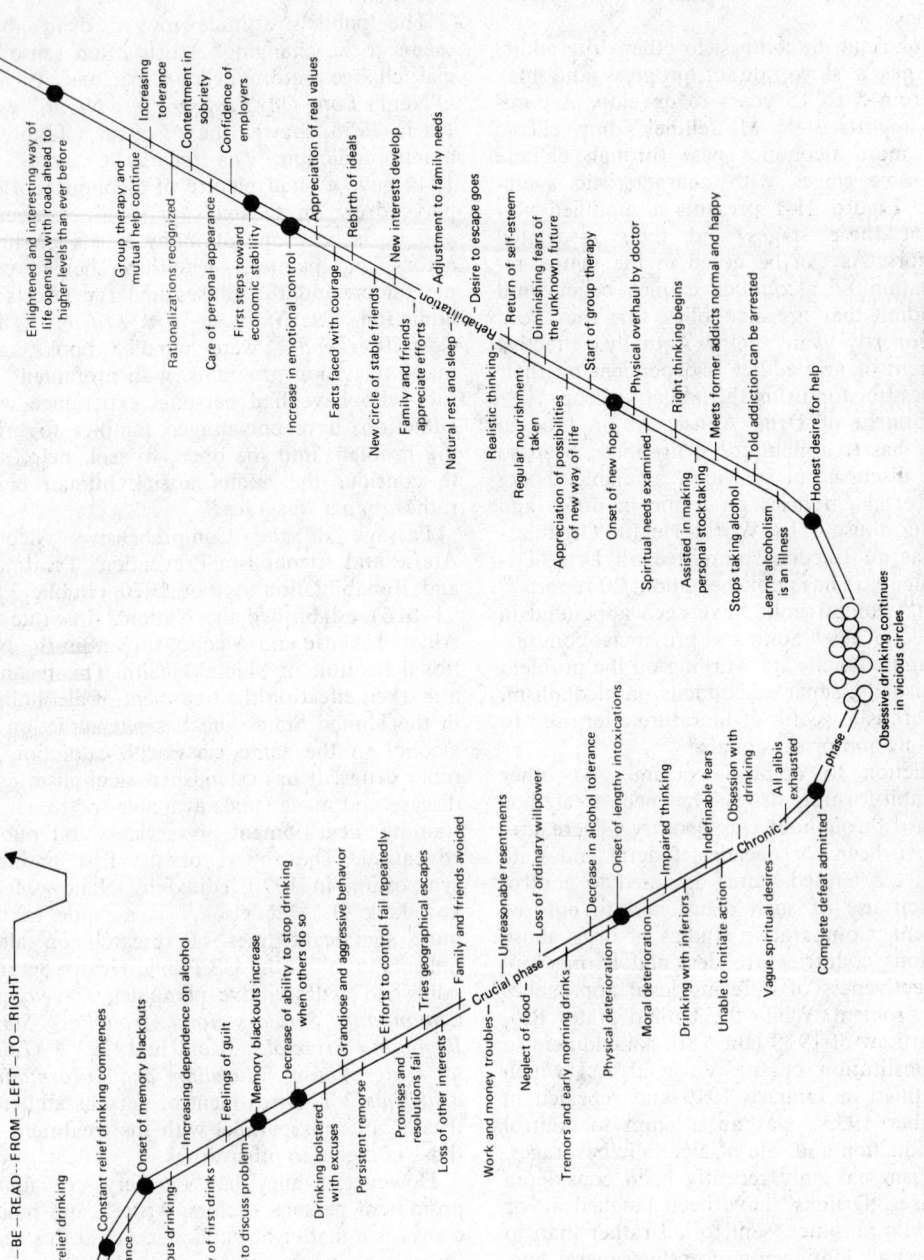

Figure 21-1. A chart of alcohol addiction and recovery. (From Millsap, Mary: "Occupational Health Nursing in an Alcohol Addiction Program," Nurs. Clin. N. Am., 7:121, [Mar.] 1972.)

TO—BE—READ—FROM—LEFT—TO—RIGHT

Occasional relief drinking
Constant relief drinking commences
Increase in alcohol tolerance
Onset of memory blackouts
Surreptitious drinking
Increasing dependence on alcohol
Urgency of first drinks
Feelings of guilt
Unable to discuss problem
Memory blackouts increase
Decrease of ability to stop drinking when others do so
Drinking bolstered with excuses
Grandiose and aggressive behavior
Persistent remorse
Efforts to control fail repeatedly
Promises and resolutions fail
Tries geographical escapes
Loss of other interests
Family and friends avoided
Work and money troubles
Unreasonable resentments
Neglect of food
Loss of ordinary willpower
Decrease in alcohol tolerance
Onset of lengthy intoxications
Physical deterioration
Impaired thinking
Moral deterioration
Drinking with inferiors
Indefinable fears
Unable to initiate action
Obsession with drinking
Vague spiritual desires
All alibis exhausted
Complete defeat admitted

Crucial phase
Chronic phase

Obsessive drinking continues in vicious circles

Honest desire for help
Learns alcoholism is an illness
Stops taking alcohol
Told addiction can be arrested
Meets former addicts normal and happy
Right thinking begins
Physical overhaul by doctor
Assisted in making personal stocktaking
Spiritual needs examined
Onset of new hope
Start of group therapy
Appreciation of possibilities of new way of life
Diminishing fears of the unknown future
Regular nourishment taken
Return of self-esteem
Realistic thinking
Natural rest and sleep
Desire to escape goes
Adjustment to family needs
Facts faced with courage
New interests develop
New circle of stable friends
Rebirth of ideals
Family and friends appreciate efforts
Appreciation of real values
Increase in emotional control
Confidence of employers
First steps toward economic stability
Care of personal appearance
Contentment in sobriety
Rationalizations recognized
Increasing tolerance
Group therapy and mutual help continue
Enlightened and interesting way of life opens up with road ahead to higher levels than ever before

Rehabilitation

use methadone, a synthetic narcotic, to satisfy the drug "hunger" created by addiction to an opiate. Methadone is also an addictive drug and there are two common views on how it should be used to interrupt the chronic use of a narcotic.* One is that, if necessary, the narcotic users be given methadone for the rest of their lives; the other, that once the cycle of the original addiction is broken, methadone be withdrawn. In either case, when patients have reached their individual maintenance level (acquired over 3 to 6 weeks), they are given counseling and rehabilitative services for at least a year—and often much longer—to help them acquire new goals, new activities, and new friends. [72-76]

In the search for solutions to the problem of drug abuse, *narcotic antagonists* (cyclazocine and naloxone) are on trial. These drugs come from the poppy seed, as do heroin, morphine, and codeine. However, the antagonist drugs have had the nitrogen atom of the alkaloid modified, while the narcotic drugs have the alkaloid's hydroxyl groups modified. Giving a narcotic antagonist is based on the theory that drug abuse is learned (conditioned) behavior. According to Thomas J. Crowley,[77] reports from drug abusers "leave little doubt" that certain drugs give intense physical pleasure with the first use, and so are used repeatedly. To explain the hold that some drugs have on some persons, even after one experience, the intense physical pleasure (the "rush") is compared by some experts with sexual gratification. The pleasurable effect "conditions" the user to respond to certain unpleasant stimuli by taking a drug which either removes or changes the stimuli to something pleasanter. Narcotic antagonists interfere with the pleasurable sensations produced by the opiates and, therefore, "negatively reinforce" the drug-taking habit. The first antagonists used were short-acting and had many undesirable effects; however, additional chemicals are being tested with the hope that more effective antagonists will be found.[78]

When "negative reinforcers" are given to alcoholics, it is called *aversion therapy*. Patients are advised to take Antabuse, which causes very unpleasant physiologic reactions (such as chills, tremors, and vomiting) with the first alcoholic drink. Antabuse must be taken daily in order to produce these effects.

Another kind of aversion therapy is to give the alcoholic a drink of liquor along with a nausea-producing drug. This method is based on the principle that two different responses (pleasure and vomiting) to one stimulus (alcohol) cannot take place at the same time, so one will inhibit the other. Alcohol, that once gave a pleasurable reaction, now causes a distasteful reaction, vomiting. Other operant conditioning techniques, relaxation techniques, and group sessions focused on the practical problems of living with alcohol addiction are often used in conjunction with aversion therapy.[79,80]

Psychiatrists and clinical psychologists are treating alcoholics and other addicts both individually and in family counseling. They may or may not prescribe drugs used to combat insomnia, depression, anxiety, and other common symptoms of addiction; they may or may not combine psychotherapy with aversion therapy and/or association with a therapeutic community. While some persons seem to have profited from prolonged and deep psychotherapy, great skepticism about its value and justification for the expense to the addict is expressed in some circles. Stirring up buried fears and resentments can be dangerous unless the problems they raise can be resolved. The sick addict is rarely well enough physically or can afford sufficiently prolonged psychotherapy to solve such problems. Malleson, a psychiatrist, makes the following observation on psychiatric treatment of alcoholics, which in his book is carefully documented:

Psychiatrists are also singularly unsuccessful at stopping people drinking. The World Health Organization expert committee on mental health defines the criterion for cure of an alcoholic as two years of total abstinence. . . . Only 18 per cent of fifty alcoholics treated at the Mecca of English psychiatry, the Maudsley Hospital, fulfilled this criterion of success. . . . The alcoholic unit at Warlingham Park Hospital has an international reputation for success. This unit, quite properly, carefully selects alcoholics who are most likely to benefit by treatment, and it keeps them in hospital for three months. Nevertheless, its cure rate is only 33 per cent. . . . Most hospitals have much less success. Since many doctors themselves believe that problems can be cured by chemicals, it may be that doctors, just like the proverbial alcoholic's wife, are not good for boozers. So far, doctors have been more successful at causing addiction than at curing it.

Going on to discuss self-help for alcoholism and obesity, he says:

Self-Help is Best Help
  If: *the overweight ate less*
     drinkers drank less
     smokers stopped smoking
     and everyone took a little more exercise

---

* The idea of substituting one addiction for another is not new. Malleson notes that in 1885 the German doctors "confirmed the value of cocaine in the cure of the morphine habit . . ." (Malleson, Andrew: *Need Your Doctor Be So Useless?* George Allen & Unwin, Ltd., London, 1973, p. 57.) Some critics of the methadone program applaud such analogies.

then we would save more life years and eradicate more disease than we could possibly do by supplying even the best and the most expensive of modern treatments for the cure of already established diseases.*

The American Psychiatric Association and the National Association for Mental Health have a Joint Information Service. Speaking for it, Raymond M. Glasscote and associates [81] reported in 1972 on *The Treatment of Drug Abuse: Programs, Problems, Prospects.* For those interested in the more official psychiatric viewpoint, this review is helpful.

Physiologists, psychiatrists, and psychologists are studying the biochemical basis of drug addiction; family behavior patterns; the addicts' self-image; the effect of drugs on sleep, on memory ("black-outs"), on liver and adrenal functions, and on genetics.[82-91] The variety of approaches suggests the lack of consensus on the effect and treatment of drug abuse by professional health workers.

Legal aspects of drug abuse are under study. In some states persons who break the law because they are under the influence of drugs may have compulsory treatment. People arrested for drunken driving may, for example, be required to go to AA meetings. Special AA meetings for such persons are called the Honor Court in Connecticut. Some industries deal with alcoholism by requiring attendance at AA meetings.[92-99]

Detoxification centers are used for all types of drug abusers. Addicts work up to crises during which they are helpless and often critically ill. They are physically unable to get and take the drug on which they are dependent and at the same time are in danger from the symptoms of withdrawal. Patients in drug withdrawal crises are not infrequently seen in emergency rooms where they may be given immediate treatment.[100]

The hallucinations and convulsions of sudden alcohol withdrawal are well known; withdrawal from heroin has been publicized in current films and television programs. Withdrawal reactions are frightening to those who experience them and to those who watch them.

Detoxification centers withdraw the drug gradually, using sedatives, vitamins, and parenteral fluids to support and build up a person who is toxic, dehydrated, and malnourished. Antibiotics may be given if there is a local or systemic infection. S. C. Kaim and associates,[101,102] discussing the treatment of alcohol withdrawal syndrome, recommend drugs to suppress the symptoms, advocating chlordiazepoxide as an anticonvulsant, used effec-

tively in studies reported by the Veterans Administration. (See Figure 21-2 showing withdrawal symptoms and time of appearance after withdrawal.) Sidney M. Wolfe and Maurice Victor [103] found a respiratory alkalosis and lowered blood magnesium. They suggest the administration of carbon dioxide or some other agent to mitigate symptoms of alcohol withdrawal.

Patients are usually kept in detoxification centers from 10 days to 2 weeks but are helped to find long-term postdetoxification programs where they may learn to change and improve their lives. Some general hospitals now have detoxification centers and some offer long-term inpatient and outpatient rehabilitation programs.[103a-113] As mentioned earlier, the role of general hospitals in preventing, controlling, or arresting drug abuse is changing radically.

Nurses watching a person with acute withdrawal symptoms may be frightened; some have a judgmental attitude and intentionally or unintentionally show disgust for the addict. Ethel H. Russaw, a nurse who helped plan a narcotic detoxification unit in one of Chicago's general hospitals, expresses the following opinion:

The nurse must be firm, consistent, orderly, and giving, responding with attentive interest and concern to the patient's feelings and behavior. All addicts need understanding and acceptance as sick persons.

. . .

I see the role of the nurse with the addict as . . . supportive. . . . Her willingness to help as evidenced by her presence meets an important need of addicts withdrawing from drugs.*

Among the *therapeutic communities* helping drug abusers are Synanon, Daytop, Narcotics Anonymous, Phoenix House, and communities for alcoholics.[114-116] In 1971, Florence L. Huey [117] gave a vivid illustrated report of visits to Phoenix House and Daytop Village in New York. Most of these communities are administered by ex-addicts, including "recovered" alcoholics.

Complete abstinence from drugs is the community's major focus. In some of these communities the addict is allowed to suffer withdrawal symptoms without suppressant drugs, but experienced residents (ex-addicts) support them through this ordeal, called in the addict's slang, "cold turkey." Residents in Synanon, for example, *can* remain as long as they think they need help and are drug-free ("clean"). The use of any addictive drugs—antidepressants or antianxiety drugs—is not

---

* Malleson, Andrew: *op. cit.,* pp. 36, 37.

* Russaw, Ethel H.: Nursing in a Narcotic-Detoxification Unit," *Am. J. Nurs.,* **70:**1720, (Aug.) 1970.

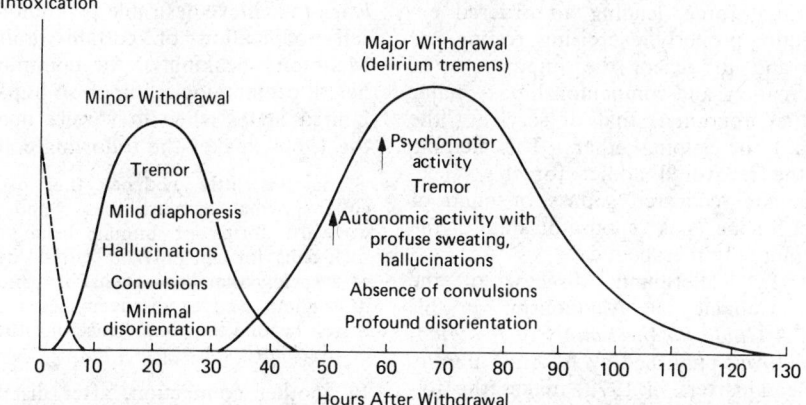

Figure 21-2. Clinical findings during the minor (early) alcohol withdrawal syndrome and the major withdrawal syndrome (delirium tremens). (From Wolfe, Sidney M., and Victor, Maurice: "The Physiological Basis of the Alcohol Withdrawal Syndrome," in Mello, Nancy, and Mendelson, Jack H. [eds.]: *Recent Advances in Studies of Alcoholism.* National Institute on Alcohol Abuse and Alcoholism, Rockville, Md., 1971, p. 189.)

allowed. One slip disqualifies the person for residence in some instances. Group psychotherapy, encounter groups, and individual psychotherapy are used to help community members, who must be highly motivated, to remain drug-free.[118] Work and recreation, or keeping occupied, is also stressed. Residents and volunteers maintain many of these centers.

While these self-help communities accept the idea of addiction as a disease, they also stress the concept of self-cure. The addict, or the alcoholic, can only recover if he or she stays "clean," or, in the case of the alcoholic, sober.

Members of Alcoholics Anonymous never use the term "cure." They maintain that alcoholics are always alcoholics; that they may recover their sobriety but that they must guard this zealously as long as they live. They always say they are sober for *today*. Those who have had experience with addiction seem most able to help addicts. The ex-addict cannot be fooled by the addict and can speak convincingly on abstinence, and, above all, the happy recovered addict gives the unrecovered addict hope. Few persons who have not been addicted have the knowledge, the understanding, the patience, the ability to get through to the addict that most recovered addicts demonstrate.

The program conducted by Alcoholics Anonymous is the best known and most effective program for helping alcoholics. Started in 1935 by two men, a former stockbroker and a doctor, the name Alcoholics Anonymous was adopted in 1939 when a book with this title was written by and about some of the group members. The book is affectionately

called by members "The Big Book" or "The Black Book." It contains the now famous 12 steps, the traditions, slogans, and concepts that guide its members. At first wives, husbands, parents, children, and other relatives and friends went with the alcoholics to AA meetings. The nonalcoholics, recognizing their need for help in living with an alcoholic, often met separately and discussed their common problem. So "Family Groups" were organized and at first listed in the directory of Alcoholics Anonymous. In 1954, the Al-Anon Family Group Headquarters, Inc., was established in New York City; Alateen, an organization for teenage children, still later.* All three organizations have spread worldwide and all have a common base—recovery through "the 12 steps," group unity through the "traditions," and service through the concepts.[119–121]

Therapeutic communities offer what might be termed in psychiatric circles "behavior therapy." Neurotic, and even psychotic, behavior can be thought of as learned bad habits. Habits that are learned can be unlearned and replaced by new healthy learned habits. Addicts who have "recovered" in the AA, Al-Anon, or Alateen programs seem more effective than professional medical workers in helping "newcomers" accept addiction as a disease, accept the necessity of giving up the drug, making an honest self-appraisal, relying on a higher power

* Telephone directories in most large communities list numbers for all these groups. See the Appendix for headquarters' addresses of all self-help groups mentioned in this book. Headquarters staff offer counsel to visitors and usually free literature on request.

or a spiritual force, leading an ordered existence, eating properly, exercising, resting and relaxing; and to accept the importance of work, recreation, and companionship. A major part of the program is that of service ("the 12th step"), or helping others. This helping role of the recovered addict for the "sick" addict, or the recovered spouse or child of the addict for the "sick" spouse or child of the addict is mutually therapeutic.

Joseph L. Kellermann, director of the Charlotte Council on Alcoholism, in his pamphlet *A Guide for the Family of the Alcoholic,* which was published by Al-Anon Family Group Headquarters in 1972, makes the following statement:

The "next of kin" or person most responsible for the alcoholic may need more assistance and counseling than the alcoholic if an effective recovery program is to be launched. Alcoholism is an illness, but one which has tremendous emotional impact upon the immediate family. Those most affected by the alcoholic are the spouse, parent, sister, brother and child. The more distorted the emotions of these persons become the less adequate their help will be. The interaction may and often does become destructive rather than helpful.*

Most, if not all, alcoholics are dependent, yet they develop a strong hostility toward those on whom they must depend. In *Alcoholism, A Merry-Go-Round Named Denial,*[122] Kellermann shows how families can perpetuate and intensify this dependency, never allowing the alcoholics to suffer the consequences of addiction so that they are never persuaded that they must conquer it if they are to avoid death or insanity.

Methods for preventing and treating drug abuse other than those discussed in this section are being explored. For instance, there are reports that long-time drug users have given up drugs after learning to use "transcendental meditation" or yoga to alter consciousness. Weil says empirical evidence indicates that "the highs obtained by meditation are better than the highs obtainable through drugs . . . ." † In addition, the use of meditation has been shown to change a number of autonomic system responses. This information, together with application of the work of Neal E. Miller [123] and other researchers in the voluntary control of selected visceral responses in animals, leads some authorities on drug abuse to suggest that in the future individuals can learn to achieve desirable psychologic states by self-modification of certain brain waves.[124] Malleson, speaking of the community mental health centers, looked upon so hopefully in the United States when they were opened during the 1960s, makes the following comment:

There is little evidence that psychiatry can either prevent or cure these "undesirable" and wayward forms of human behavior. Probably such behavior can only be "cured" by the vitality of a society that knows what it wants and where it is going, and to discover these cultural goals is well beyond the competence of either psychiatry or psychiatrists.*

In another connection, after discussing some medical gains, he emphasizes the inability of any health providers to prevent, control, or cure disease. He says:

How then can our good health be further improved? The answer is simple, though discomforting. We can do it ourselves. Ordinary citizens are now in the best position to make effective advances in the prevention of disease. The ball is in our court.†

When it comes to preventing and controlling drug abuse, the ball is certainly in the court of the ordinary citizen. However, the attitude of nurses toward addiction, their knowledge of its symptoms and treatment is of utmost importance. Because nurses are more numerous than any other health workers and their relationship with the public often invites confidence, they have a unique opportunity to help. Addiction is so widespread that most nurses have opportunities to work with persons who are directly or indirectly affected. Nurses in detoxification programs can with skillful nursing greatly affect the physiologic recovery of the patient. After withdrawal is completed, nurses may play an important role in the counseling program. In many of the methadone and aversion therapy clinics nurses are important members of the staff.

Marjorie B. Rykken makes the following observations on counseling alcoholic patients:

An accepting, nonjudgmental, firm but kind attitude on the part of the nurse can help remove some of the barriers to the alcoholic's motivation to get well. As the nurse demonstrates such an attitude and ministers to the physical needs of the patient in his acute phase of alcoholism, she establishes rapport and sets the stage for the counseling role. The patient will come to devaluate himself less and feel some hope for his problem.

The nurse's positive attitude toward the members of the patient's family can also help them to

---

* Kellermann, Joseph L.: *A Guide for the Family of the Alcoholic.* Al-Anon Family Group Headquarters, New York, 1972, p. 3.
† Weil, Andrew: *The Natural Mind.* Houghton Mifflin Co., Boston, 1972, p. 68.

* Malleson, Andrew: *op. cit.,* p. 221.
† *Ibid.,* p. 34.

accept and understand the patient more easily. The family's acceptance and understanding, in turn, can give the patient some of the support he needs to give up alcohol. . . . The nurse can help the family to understand the "up's and down's" of the patient on the road to recovery and the length of time it may take before sobriety and wellness are achieved. Accepting, nonjudgmental, and sincere attitudes will eventually help to produce positive results in a number of alcoholic patients.*

The same attitudes on the part of nurses are necessary when they are working with patients and families with any drug problem. Carol Distasio and Marcia Nawrot,[125] discussing the use of methaqualone, say that nursing is just beginning to assume an "active dynamic posture toward the problem of drug abuse." They suggest in-service seminars on drug abuse and the participation by nurses in drug abuse research.

Nurses who know the local and state resources have countless opportunities for helping drug abusers, their families, and friends to get the help they need. This includes telling addicts and their families about the self-help programs that are meeting with such undisputed success.

In 1971, the US Public Health Service awarded a grant of $40,000 to the American Nurses' Association to develop a curriculum on drug abuse for nursing education programs throughout the United States.[126] While many physicians refuse to treat drug addicts, saying, frankly, that they know nothing about it, medical schools are beginning to stress drug abuse in the medical curriculum.[127] We believe that all students and practicing nurses and all health workers should know the major approaches to treatment, have sufficient experience in each type of program mentioned in this section to give them an informed opinion on its value, an ability to make judicious referrals, and the ability to participate effectively in programs of their choice. Readers will find listed references to books and articles ranging from those written for experts to those addressed to the average citizen.[127a-143] An indifferent or moralistic attitude toward drug addiction can hardly be justified in this era.

3. DRUGS USED TO PREVENT DISEASE

"Medicines" are sometimes used to promote health and prevent disease. Vaccines and sera,

* Rykken, Marjorie B.: "Counseling Patients Who Are Dependent on Alcohol," in *ANA Clinical Conferences, 1969.* Appleton-Century-Crofts, New York, 1970, p. 107.

for example, are given to protect people and animals from communicable diseases; quinacrine (Atabrine) is taken regularly as a preventive by susceptible persons living where malaria is rife; drinking water is reinforced with iodine in certain regions to prevent goiter, and in some places with fluorine to control dental caries; insulin is occasionally used to promote appetite; and vitamins are given in the form of a medication when the diet is substandard in quantity or quality or minerals are added to food to improve their nutritive value. Health workers, however, tend to think of drugs as substances prescribed by physicians. While a more realistic view of how drugs are used by society might result in revision of laws governing their prescription and sale, this chapter deals with drugs given to cure or control a disease or to allay the accompanying pain and discomfort, and the abuse of drugs used at first to give pleasure and eventually to satisfy a craving.

4. DRUG THERAPY

Responsibilities of the Nurse. Giving drugs and observing their effects are among the nurse's most demanding functions. Persons who are under treatment but who do not need nursing care may prepare and take their own medication. They can, in most cases, learn enough about the drug and their condition to do this with safety, and they should be helped to gain this independence even while they are hospitalized. Nurses, in contrast, have a more difficult task because they must know about many drugs and in giving these must be able to follow any physician's plan of therapy for any patient. To get the best results, drugs should be given exactly as prescribed in relation to route, time of administration, preparation, and dosage. The person who is giving, or taking, the drug must know enough to carry out the doctor's directions but also to recognize and report reactions that would make the physician want to change the prescription. It is important that the nurse (as an administrator of drugs) and the patient (as the recipient), or the parents of a child, know the nature of the drug; its local and systemic action and the underlying physiology; also why the drug is prescribed and the result the physician hopes to get; the signs of the intended effect; and the signs of an overdose or of a cumulative toxic effect, or indications that the patient has an idiosyncrasy to the drug. The nurse must know how to use the apothecaries' and metric systems of measurement and how to convert one to the other (see the Appendix for tables of equivalents). While most countries, including the United States, have "gone metric," it is not possible to complete this conversion overnight.[144,145] All those who take part in drug therapy should know the minimum and maximum dosage of any drug they use. Nurses should know how age, sex, body weight, and time of administration affect the dose. They should know how drugs are excreted for the excretory organ is the first to show signs of toxicity. For example, the kidneys are irritated by mercury, arsenic, and the sulfa drugs. The nurse should understand that drugs cannot change the functions of body cells but they can stimulate or depress these functions and eventually destroy the cells if either of these effects is carried beyond physiologic limits. A knowledge of the selectivity of drugs will help the nurse to understand the wide variety of reactions to medication. The person giving or taking the drug should know when it is to be pushed to its physiologic limit—which means until symptoms of toxicity occur. A classic example is digitalis which is often given until the pulse is slowed to 60 beats per minute.

While the physician is primarily responsible for ordering the medication in the correct dosage he or she, being human and often overworked, is subject to error.* Lives have been saved by nurses who have recognized mistakes in written orders for drugs, and lives have been lost because similar mistakes were not detected. Moreover, nurses can be successfully prosecuted for carrying out a doctor's order for the wrong drug, or a toxic dose, if the court is persuaded that the preparation of the nurses qualified them to recognize the danger of the drug or the dosage. Irene A. Murchison and Thomas S. Nichols, in discussing the legal duty of the nurse to execute the physician's orders, say:

When a nurse encounters an illegible or incomplete order, her duty is obvious; she must contact the physician who wrote the order and find out what was intended, for such an order does not constitute precise instructions and therefore is not an order at all. If the nurse were to give what she thought the doctor intended and the patient suffered harm because the wrong drug or dosage was given, she would bear full legal responsibility.

Another source of danger is when the nurse is given what appears to be an erroneous order. It

would indeed be a misconception for a nurse to lull herself into a false sense of security and to believe that to follow a doctor's order would obviate all legal responsibility for her part of the act. She is a person of substantial preparation in the use of medications and has a responsibility to use that knowledge. To request confirmation of a doctor's order is simply a part of intelligent nursing practice. It is not only accepted, but is encouraged by the medical practitioner who is aware of the dual responsibility of the doctor and the nurse. Indeed, in circumstances where injury is foreseeable, the nurse has not merely the privilege but the obligation to question the order, for by failing to do so she compounds the negligent giving of an erroneous order, and implicates herself in the resulting harm to the patient, should it occur.

. . .

Another area in which the legal duty of the nurse is clear is when she is confronted with an order for a mode of administration that she does not feel competent to carry out. Her duty to her patient, derived from her ability to foresee the harm she might do if the procedure were not carried out with safety, would lead her to withhold administration and report to her supervisor, if she were in a hospital setting. If she were working alone, in a public health or industrial area, she should advise the doctor. At times, to withhold action or refuse to act, if it is done in the best interest of the patient, is in itself a good legal defense.*

In school and industrial nursing, and other situations where the physician is often unavailable, the nurse gives, or advises patients to take, certain drugs for which "standing orders" have been set up by the physicians of the service. The shortage of physicians in this country has forced them increasingly to delegate to others responsibility for prescribing medication—a function that has in the past been uniquely theirs. Other health workers in assuming this responsibility may be technically protected by working "under the supervision of the physician." This is the term used in some recent medical practice acts to justify changing practice. A number of sociologists have called the corner druggist "the poor man's doctor" and there is no doubt that he often advises the inquiring customer or sick person. At any rate, more nonprescription drugs are sold than those ordered by physicians. Until the ratio of physicians to the population changes radically, interdisciplinary health commissions (national, state, and local) must develop ways of using such knowledge as all health workers have in relation to drugs to the

* The term "doctor's order" suggests that the patient is compelled to take the drug and the nurse to give it. We (the authors) object to this term but because it is in such common usage in discussing drugs it has not been changed to "doctor's prescription" which we believe more appropriate. Any patient may refuse to take a drug and the nurse should recognize his or her right to do so.

* Murchison, Irene A., and Nichols, Thomas S.: *Legal Foundations of Nursing Practice.* Macmillan Publishing Co., Inc., New York, 1970, pp. 125, 126.

best advantage of the people they serve. Ways must be devised for safeguarding those who give and receive drugs, for they are all potentially dangerous. In the opinion of the authors, all professional health workers should be legally responsible for their acts. Therefore, if in any state physicians and nurses agree that the latter will assume responsibility for prescribing medication, the nurse's preparation must include enough pharmacology and therapeutics to prepare her or him to do this safely, and nursing and medical practice laws must be changed to protect the public, the nurse, and the physician. The latter are in such short supply that they cannot begin to meet the needs of the public for medical care and certainly they cannot, even if it were desirable, direct, or "supervise," the work of other health professionals.

In any case, it is obvious that in order to protect the patients and themselves nurses should know the therapeutic and maximum doses of the drugs they give no matter who prescribes them. Nurses should be informed on their legal status in drug therapy wherever they practice. It is a protection to know the federal laws and regulations restricting the use of drugs, the most important law being the Federal Food, Drug and Cosmetic Act that in 1940 replaced the Pure Food Law of 1906 and the (Federal) Harrison Anti-Narcotic Act of 1914 (revised many times since) with the related (state) Uniform Narcotic Drug Acts.[146-148]

This competence is acquired in "courses," but it is also built up gradually through a study of each patient and the medication used for him or her. Nurses must have considerable knowledge of chemistry, physiology, and general principles of therapy in order to read medical reports with understanding and administer drugs safely. They should be familiar with the indexes to current medical periodicals; they should know that "U.S.P." indicates that a drug is made according to the standards published in the *Pharmacopoeia of the United States of America,*[149] that the *National Formulary*[150] ("N.F.") supplements that publication, and that virtually all therapeutic agents listed in these two are also in *AMA Drug Evaluations*[151] prepared by the Council on Drugs of the American Medical Association. In addition, this publication, which is published annually, includes new drugs not included in official publications; it replaces *New and Nonofficial Remedies, New and Nonofficial Drugs and New Drugs* previously prepared by the Council. Nurses will, also, find the *Physicians' Desk Reference*[152] (usually called PDR), an annual publication, a useful reference; it

should be kept on each patient unit. Most agencies require physicians to use official nomenclature in writing drug orders.

Nurses should develop the habit of looking up every unfamiliar drug they give.* Drugs should be thought of as potentially dangerous, and no nurse should dare to be ignorant, uninterested, or mechanical in the administration of them.

Daniel A. Hussar, a pharmacist, comments on the complexity of the drug scene in an article entitled "Drug Interactions by the Hundreds! How Can You Possibly Remember Them All?" He believes there are nine "basic mechanisms" that nurses can learn which will enable them to anticipate drug "interactions," the beneficial and harmful ones.[153]

Patients ask nurses many questions about drugs prescribed for them and drugs they use on their own. Increasingly, doctors like their patients to be partners in the therapeutic plan and usually they are very frank about the nature and purpose of the drugs they prescribe. The nurse, physician, and in some cases the pharmacist, should develop a plan for teaching patients to avoid duplication of effort, omissions, and misunderstandings. In the treatment of diabetes, pernicious anemia, hypothyroidism, and many long-term diseases, control is only possible if the patient and the family understand the use of therapeutic agents.

Discussing the reasons why prescription drugs should be labeled with their names and strength, the Council on Drugs of the American Medical Association says, "The patient has a right to be informed about his illness and the medications prescribed." † In addition, it believes that patients with allergies should know what drugs they are taking. It would seem that these beliefs apply equally to the patient in the hospital. Nurses should listen with interest to anything patients may ask or tell them about medication, their mental attitude toward the treatment, the experiences the patients have had with drugs, and particularly any idiosyncrasies to drugs. The latter should be reported at once, but at all times nurses should take every opportunity to learn from patients themselves and should report what they know promptly and accurately. On the basis of the nurse's observations drugs are often discontinued and dosage changed.

---

* When a physician is prescribing a new, and especially an experimental, drug, he or she should supply the workers giving the drug with some literature on it. More and more patients also may expect this help from the doctor.

† AMA Council on Drugs: *AMA Drug Evaluations,* 1st ed. American Medical Association, Chicago, 1971, p. xxvii.

In general, nurses should reinforce the doctor's information to patients by teaching them how to prepare and take drugs, by explaining that certain results, as, for example, a dry mouth from belladonna, or dark stools from bismuth, or diarrhea from oxytetracycline (Terramycin), are to be expected, while warning them to watch closely for toxic signs such as a reduction in urine with sulfa drugs or headache and skin eruptions from bromides. Nurses should impress patients with the danger of self-medication (using drugs without a physician's knowledge and approval). They should also teach them to look for evidence of high standards of quality in drugs. Instruction must often include demonstrations and super-

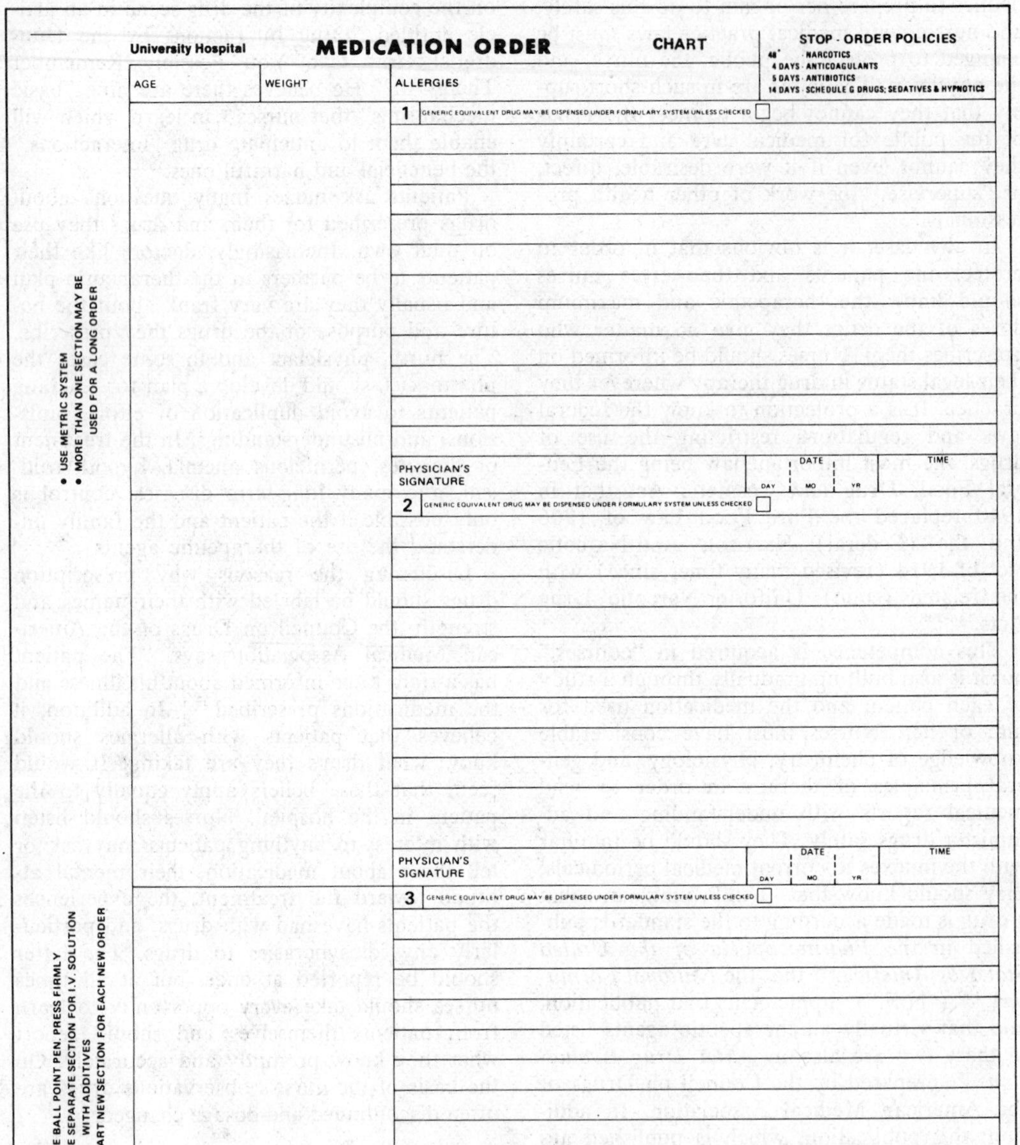
University Hospital MEDICATION ORDER CHART

STOP - ORDER POLICIES
48" - NARCOTICS
4 DAYS - ANTICOAGULANTS
5 DAYS - ANTIBIOTICS
14 DAYS - SCHEDULE G DRUGS; SEDATIVES & HYPNOTICS

AGE | WEIGHT | ALLERGIES

• USE METRIC SYSTEM
• MORE THAN ONE SECTION MAY BE USED FOR A LONG ORDER

1 GENERIC EQUIVALENT DRUG MAY BE DISPENSED UNDER FORMULARY SYSTEM UNLESS CHECKED ☐

PHYSICIAN'S SIGNATURE | DATE (DAY MO YR) | TIME

2 GENERIC EQUIVALENT DRUG MAY BE DISPENSED UNDER FORMULARY SYSTEM UNLESS CHECKED ☐

PHYSICIAN'S SIGNATURE | DATE (DAY MO YR) | TIME

• USE BALL POINT PEN. PRESS FIRMLY
• USE SEPARATE SECTION FOR I.V. SOLUTION WITH ADDITIVES
• START NEW SECTION FOR EACH NEW ORDER

3 GENERIC EQUIVALENT DRUG MAY BE DISPENSED UNDER FORMULARY SYSTEM UNLESS CHECKED ☐

84-680-0024 (09/73)

PHYSICIAN'S SIGNATURE | DATE (DAY MO YR) | TIME

Figure 21-3. Doctor's medication order. (Courtesy of University Hospital, University of Western Ontario, London, Ont.)

vised practice in the measurement and administration of drugs. It is as much the nurses's function to teach the patient how to take medications as to give them to him or her. For this reason it is desirable that patients handle their medication while nurses are avaliable to help them learn to do it correctly.

The importance of teaching patients, sick or well, about prescribed drugs cannot be overemphasized. Doris Schwartz and her associates, studying the care of ambulatory and elderly patients, reported specifically on the shocking numbers and kinds of errors they made at home in taking medications prescribed for them by hospital physicians.[154,155] Two British nurses (Janet Marks and Margaret Clarke) report a study of inpatients' knowledge of the drugs they are receiving and they find it is usually inadequate, although it is especially so in the case of the elderly.[156] Ignorance of the underlying sciences, poor memory, poor hearing and sight, are all handicaps in learning that are more common in the old than in the young.

Because it is apparently difficult to ensure accurate use of prescribed drugs, teaching must be individualized and there must be a clear understanding of the physician's, nurse's, pharmacist's, and, possibly, the social worker's role. It seems very desirable to have patients manage their own medication in the hospital where they have the help of a professional staff while they are learning to do this. Reading matter designed for different levels of comprehension should be available. When patients go home it may be helpful in some cases to use colored cards and correspondingly colored labeled bottles to differentiate the "heart medicine" from the "digestion medicine" or the "asthma pills." Too often all the drugs persons are taking are capsules or tablets that look alike to them and very often the containers look alike. For the blind patient, it may be necessary to set up a system based on differentiation by touch. In all cases written directions should be given patients. Either patients or those who are nursing them should know the composition and action of the drugs they are taking. The name alone is insufficient.

Accuracy, Punctuality, and Efficiency. To ensure that the right patient is given the right medicine at the right time, each hospital has developed or adopted a system for the administration of medicines, which usually includes the following steps.

On each ward there is a *doctor's order book* or file in which the doctor's orders are written (see Fig. 21-3). In an increasing number of hospitals, orders are written on the patient's chart. Except in emergencies, no medicine should be given a patient unless the doctor

writes the order and signs it.* When an emergency prevents this, the order should be dictated and signed later. All orders must be clearly written. (A nurse should never give a medicine if in doubt as to the drug or dosage.) Sometimes there is a separate order book for day and night, but, in any case, the date and hour should be clearly indicated. Nurses should look at this book (or the charts if orders are written on them) frequently, because a doctor may write an order without calling the attention of a nurse to it and the patient may be suffering from want of the medication. In some hospitals, the doctor puts a red tag or some other identifying marker on the front of the patient's chart, or he or she may leave the chart open to show that an order has just been written. When the medicine ordered is not be be repeated, the order should be marked off with red ink as soon as the drug is given, and the time of administration indicated, or some other method may be used which is understood by all workers. If the original order was not written on the doctor's order sheet, which is a permanent record, but in a book (called doctor's order book), the order and time are copied on the chart. If such an order is not marked off, the drug may be given a second time and endanger the life of the patient. Those orders for drugs that are to be repeated are marked off when transferred to the medication tickets, or cards. White "tickets," or cards, (usually 2 inches square) are commonly used; however, colored "tickets," or cards, continue to be used in some hospitals. Each color indicates the time of administration as in the following:

Color of Ticket	Time of Administration
Plain yellow	Every 4 hours
Yellow with corners cut	Four times a day
Plain pink	Three times a day
Pink with corners cut	Every 3 hours
Orange	Before meals
Orange, ½ ticket	Every night
Blue	After meals
Pale orange	Twice a day
Red	Every 6 hours
Red, ½ ticket	Every morning
White	Every 2 hours
Green	When required

* Drugs are often given under "standing orders." This means that the medical staff or a specific physician of an institution or agency has authorized the administration of a particular drug in a given dosage to a patient under given circumstances. An example is a sleep-inducing drug the night before surgery. In such cases the nurse does not have to get a written order each time the drug is given.

Commercial cardboard covers for medicine glasses are available that have space for writing all the information given on the ticket. If they have different colored borders they serve the same purpose as medicine tickets and also provide covers for the glasses (see Fig. 21-4.) An increasing number of workers prefer to have all cards the same color, depending entirely on what is written on the card.

In a hospital or nursing home it is necessary to give the following information on each card: (1) the patient's full name, (2) the room and bed number, (3) the drug, (4) the dosage, and (5) the hour and frequency. It is convenient to give the date the drug was ordered and the date on which it is to be discontinued, if this is known. In some places it is assumed that drugs are to be given by mouth unless otherwise indicated on the card.

When the card system is used, the doctor's orders are transferred from the order book to cards, usually by one person, such as the ward clerk or head nurse. In any event it must be clearly understood who is responsible for this. The cards should be kept near the medicine closet in a convenient holder; this may be an oblong box with slots designated according to hour for each patient or one for all patients according to hour. These should be clearly marked.

There should be a record by which the number of medications to be given at different hours can be checked daily. This should be tallied with the medication cards and the patients' charts. When an order for a drug is altered or discontinued the ticket is often put on the desk of the head nurse, or of the person assigned the responsibility for seeing that drugs are accurately given, who then destroys it.

When nurses administer the medications they place the tickets of the drugs to be given at that hour in a row. As they prepare each dose they attach the corresponding ticket to the glass and do not remove the ticket until they give the medication to the patient.

The following rules, or precautions, in giving drugs make for accuracy.*

1. Arrange, if possible, to be free from interruption while preparing a medication. Avoid conversation or anything that prevents concentration on the task in hand.
2. Check the doctor's order and make certain that it is signed. Read the medicine ticket and be sure that it tallies with the doctor's order; keep the ticket in sight while preparing the medication.
3. Check the order (medicine ticket) with the label on the bottle. Read the label three times—before taking the bottle from the shelf, before pouring the medication, and before returning the bottle to the shelf.
4. Measure the dose exactly, using standard weights and measures: use graduated

---

* These "rules" are observed in hospitals where nurses give medications. In some hospitals, patients are allowed to keep drugs in their rooms, and it is the function of the nurse to help them become self-reliant in measuring, preparing, and taking drugs as prescribed by the physician.[156a] This, obviously, is the objective of the nurse in schools, in industry, and in home nursing. If the patient is disoriented, the nurse works with others who care for the patient or with the parents if the patient is a child.

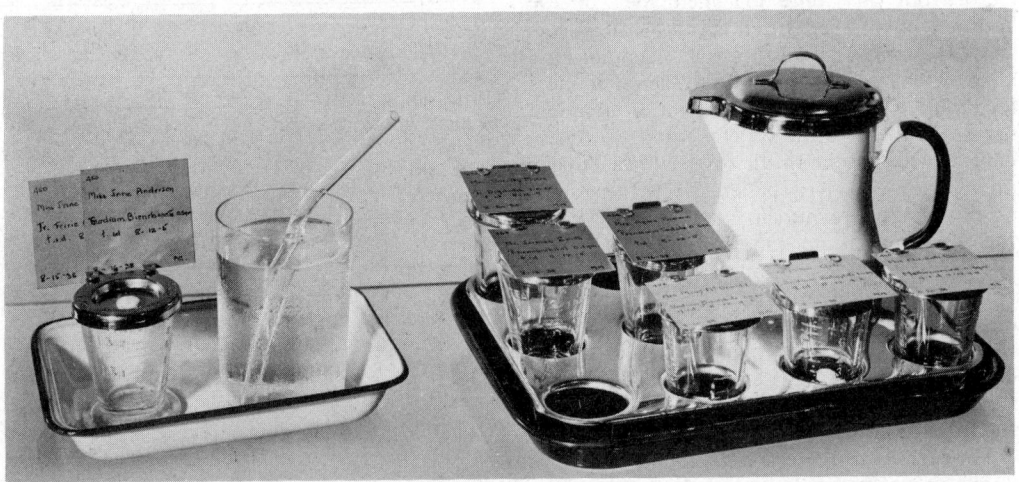

Figure 21-4. Equipment for administering medicines by mouth. *Left:* Tray to be used when medications are given individually; *right:* convenient setup for group technique in giving medicines.

glasses for measuring cubic centimeters (milliliters), ounces, and drams; a minim glass for minims, and a pipette or medicine dropper for drops. Never give minims for drops, or vice versa. (Some pipettes are calibrated for minims and drops.)

5. When measuring fluids hold the graduate so that the eye is on a level with the line indicating the desired quantity.

6. Shake fluid medications. Don't use a fluid if there is a change of color, or if there is a sediment in a preparation that does not have "shake well" on the label.

7. Give each liquid drug in a separate glass, or cup.

8. If an excess of the drug is poured do not return it to the bottle; in general this is dangerous, even with pills, tablets, and capsules.

9. Take the drug to the patient with the identifying ticket on it. (The nurse who measures the drug should give it; drugs should not be sent to a patient by another patient.) Use the person's name in handing him or her the drug to give him or her a chance to correct mistaken identity.

10. Stay with the patient while he or she takes the drug but try to avoid the impression of compulsion and haste. If circumstances make it impossible or undesirable for the person to take the medication at the time ordered, consultation with the doctor may be indicated. The drug should not be left with the patient, but a fresh dose taken to him or her if the medication is given later.

11. Be sure that the person is able to take the medication as it is prescribed. Semiconscious and irrational patients should not be given drugs in liquid form. Pills, capsules, and tablets may be held in the mouth or they may be inhaled and lodge in the trachea, occluding the air passages. (Patients whose swallowing reflex is absent should not be given anything by mouth.)

Medications should be given to patients by the nurse asigned to care for them. In this way the patients are most likely to have the maximum help from the nurse, and she or he is best able to observe the physiologic and/or emotional effect of the drug. The nurse is likely to learn most about the clinical uses of the drug and its relationship to the patient's progress under these circumstances. The graduate nurse should require no supervision of this function; for the welfare of all concerned, medications given by student nurses should be checked by the graduate staff. Many hospitals assign the giving of drugs to one nurse even though most of the nursing care of patients is individualized. Under these circumstances it is more likely to be a routinized, rather than an individualized, process.

Recording Medications. A part of every medical record is the sheet on which the doctor's orders for the patient are written. This gives the date, the drugs prescribed, their dosage and route of administration, and the date of cancellation. Another part of the record is the sheet on which nursing care is reported. On this is a record of the medications—the day, the hour, the dosage, and route of administration (see Fig. 21-5). Practice in charting medications varies in several respects. In certain hospitals nurses are asked to record every drug they give, in other hospitals they are expected to record giving only selected drugs, a list of which is posted. In some agencies nurses are required to sign their initials or their name after every medication they give but in most places after potent drugs only. Nomenclature used in all records should be official, and abbreviations, when used in records, should be taken from a standard source. (See the Appendix for a list of abbreviations with which nurses should be familiar.)

The Medicine Cupboard and Care of Drugs. All medicines should be kept in a separate room near the head nurse's station, or office. Each patient's medicines are kept in a designated place as in an oblong box (clearly marked with the patient's name), on a shelf, or compartment of the medicine cupboard. A sink with running water should be a part of the unit. It is necessary to prevent some patients, occasionally with suicidal intent, from taking hospital supplies. For this reason particularly the medicine cupboard is always locked; the keys are tagged and given to qualified personnel only. Solutions, ointments, and liniments for external use should be in a compartment that separates them from substances for internal use. Solids and liquids are separated; poisons should be in a special part of the cupboard in bottles clearly marked *poison,* differentiated by color, roughened surface, and shape. All potent drugs such as morphine and strychnine, usually given hypodermically, should be in a separate compartment. The alphabetical arrangement of drugs within the groups just mentioned saves time in finding the desired substance. Organic oils should be kept in a cool place—they are decomposed by heat and exposure to air. Sera, vaccines, and antibiotics, such as penicillin and oxytetracycline, are kept in a refrigerator. The medicine cupboard should be well supplied with all drugs likely to be required, but it should not be overstocked. Its contents should be checked fre-

NURSES' MEDICATION RECORD

Family Name	First Name	Attending Physician	Room No.	Hosp. No.

PARENTERAL DRUGS	DATE	AM	PM	AM	PM	AM	PM	AM	PM	AM	PM	AM	PM
	Time												
	Site												
	Initials												
	Time												
	Site												
	Initials												
	Time												
	Site												
	Initials												
	Time												
	Site												
	Initials												
	Time												
	Site												
	Initials												
	Time												
	Site												
	Initials												
ORAL, Suppositories and Other Drugs													
	Time												
	Initials												
	Time												
	Initials												
	Time												
	Initials												
	Time												
	Initials												
	Time												
	Initials												
	Time												
	Initials												
	Time												
	Initials												
	Time												
	Initials												
	Time												
	Initials												
	Time												
	Initials												
	Time												
	Initials												
	Time												
	Initials												

ABBREVIATIONS: L.G. (Left Gluteus Muscle)   R.G. (Right Gluteus Muscle)   L.D. (Left Deltoid Muscle)   R.D. (Right Deltoid Muscle)
L.L. (Left Leg)   R.L. (Right Leg)   L.A. (Left Arm)   R.A. (Right Arm)

FORM D-836   PHYSICIANS' RECORD CO., BERWYN, ILLINOIS - PRINTED IN U.S.A.   NURSES' MEDICATION RECORD (OVER)

Figure 21-5. Nurse's medication record. (Courtesy of Physicians' Record Co., Berwyn, Ill.)

quently. Day nurses should see that there is sufficient for the needs of the day and should be particularly watchful to see that the necessary supply is on hand for the night. Drugs should be ordered in small amounts since many deteriorate or lose their effectiveness if not fresh. Any change in color, odor, or consistency should be noted and the bottle returned to the pharmacy. Bottles should be tightly covered and labeled. Labels should be indestructible and clean. Labels should be changed by the pharmacist. In some hospitals the personnel of the pharmacy check drugs in the clinical divisions and assume responsibility for providing, storing, and maintaining supplies of drugs.

To avoid soiling the label when pouring the solution from the bottle, the label should be held uppermost. The rim of the bottle should always be cleaned afterward. Medicine should never be left in an unmarked glass or bottle. If a drug has two commonly used names it is wise to have both names on the label. The dosage of potent medicines is sometimes printed on labels. Bottles for drugs of the same group should be of a uniform size and shape, and arranged so that each label is visible. Discontinued prescriptions should be returned to the drug room. There are desirable types of bottles for powders, liquids, and tablets. When a screw cap is used, it covers the mouth of the bottle and protects it from contamination. Glass-stoppered bottles, while attractive looking, are expensive and impractical, the stoppers not being interchangeable and affording no protection to the bottle lip.

Automation. One of the major changes in some hospitals today is the method of drug distribution to patients. A number of authors suggest that in the future such change will be commonplace. Because of the increasing incidence of medication errors and the number and complexity of drugs prescribed for individual patients, some members of the health team are suggesting that the hospital pharmacist should be the controlling figure in drug administration. Anne K. Byrne,[157] in 1953, reported one of the first studies of medication errors by student nurses. Since that time, an increasing number of articles and studies of the causes of medication errors and suggestions for their elimination have appeared in the literature. A comprehensive study by Kenneth Barker [158] in 1969 showed that of 11,015 drugs administered by nurses over a 6-month period, the error rate was as high as 31.2 per cent of all drugs given. Barker [159] then studied the effect of keeping all medications in the pharmacy and dispensing them in unit doses to the nurse at the time the drug was scheduled to be given the patient; only 13.4 per cent incidence of error occurred with this method. This method was more costly but the author suggests that each hospital should assess its benefits.

Most authors agree that unit dose packages are far superior to the more common method of preparing drugs in bulk. The unit dose package contains the amount of drug ordered for a single dose and in the proper form for administration; they are properly labeled with the generic and trade name of the drug, strength of the dose, warnings or precautions to be taken, expiration date, and storage suggestions (such as store in a cool place). An increasing number of drugs, especially those in common use, are being prepared in unit dose packages by pharmaceutical companies.

The *unit-dose system* is usually described as including a number of activities: A carbon copy of the physician's medication order is sent to the pharmacy where it is interpreted by the pharmacist who prepares the individual dose, labels it, and delivers it in unit dose to the patient care unit at the appropriate time. The pharmacist and physician discuss directly all questions of interpretation of orders, and the pharmacist is always on call. The responsibility of the nurse is that of giving the proper medication at the right time to the right patient and of observing the physiologic and/or psychologic effects of the drugs. Edmund D. Pellegrino says:

The system was devised with several objectives in mind; to save precious nurse time, to reduce medication errors, and to make optimal use of the pharmacists' superior knowledge of the constantly changing field of new drugs, dosage forms, incompatibilities, and side effects.*

This system has been introduced and used in a number of hospitals for several years.[160,161] W. G. Blasingame and associates [162] describe the use of single-unit packaged drugs in five hospitals of different size and geographic location, using different drug distribution and administration systems. They conclude that the use of single-unit packages of drugs does not necessarily increase hospital medication costs and can be adapted to any type of system used.

Other than costs, there are the following advantages in using the unit dose: decrease in medication errors, greater ease in administering the drug, greater assurance for patients that they are getting the correct medication and dosage and that they are being charged for only the medication they receive.

The role and function of the pharmacist is changing. Some are stationed on large units where they work closely with the physician, nurses, and others, holding conferences on drug therapies. Their functions include delivery of all drugs to the unit in the dosage and form ordered by the physician, getting a drug history on patients, interpreting the medication order to patients and the nurse, helping the nurse observe patients for drug reactions, teaching patients about drugs to be taken at home, and preparing special medications on the unit (especially parenteral fluids including all additives in intravenous solutions). Nurses should recognize that pharmacists have special knowledge and their collaboration should be sought in all hospitals.[163,164]

---

* Pellegrino, Edmund D.: "The Unit Dose System," *J.A.M.A.,* **205:**24, (Aug. 9) 1968.

5. FACTORS MODIFYING DOSAGE AND EFFECTS OF DRUGS

As has been said, nurses are not usually responsible for the dose prescribed but it is often their function to see that the patient gets the drug in the amount intended by the physician. To help prevent errors in medication they must know, or be able to find information on, the minimum and maximum dosage and they should have some appreciation of the way in which the following factors modify dosage.

Age. Since it is impossible to memorize doses for all ages, rules have been established for computing the child's dose from the adult therapeutic dose. The dosage is usually based on age and weight. Clark's rule is suggested most frequently by authorities.[165] (Child's dose $= \dfrac{\text{weight of child in pounds}}{150} \times$ adult dose.) The AMA Council on Drugs,[166] however, thinks that the child's dose should be based on the area of body surface; it emphasizes that the detoxification and excretion of drugs in premature and newborn infants is very different from that of older children and adults.

No formulas can be applied mechanically because children respond differently to different kinds of drugs. For instance, children require small doses of narcotics, while, on the contrary, the child's dose of a cathartic approaches that of an adult. In old age the dose of weakening or depressing drugs, such as irritant cathartics or narcotics, is smaller than the usual therapeutic dose. For an elderly person who has not developed a tolerance for it, an ordinary dose of morphine (for example) may be fatal.

Sex. The adult dose is based on the average weight of a man. As women weigh less than men, the dose ordered is often smaller. Women are more susceptible to the action of certain drugs, and, during pregnancy, special precautions are taken as the fetus may also be affected by the drug. In fact, medical authorities usually say that no drugs (including aspirin and nose drops) should be taken unless the pregnant woman has specific approval from her physician.

Previous Habits or Toleration. When a patient has been in the habit of taking drugs, such as morphine or alcohol, it is often dangerous to stop the drug suddenly. For instance, following an accident, when the patient has been in the habit of drinking heavily, whisky is administered to prevent delirium tremens. In such cases large doses are necessary to produce any effect. If the patient has been in the habit of taking morphine only a large dose will relieve pain or induce sleep. Patients quickly develop a tolerance for all sedatives.

Idiosyncrasy and Susceptibility. Certain foods and drugs that may be given to most people with safety produce in others very unusual and poisonous effects. Some people are very susceptible to cocaine or derivatives of opium, for example, so that even small doses cause nausea and other toxic symptoms.

Condition of the Patient. Rate of Excretion and Cumulative Action. For intense pain, large doses of morphine may be ordered. When the patient's breathing is already difficult, smaller doses of morphine are given, and the patient is watched closely for further depression of the respiratory center. In shock or collapse, the dosage of stimulants ordered may be larger than usual. When drugs are given as antidotes for poisoning, large doses are prescribed. On the other hand, in diseases of the kidneys or in any disease with edema, smaller doses of drugs eliminated by the kidney may be ordered, and at greater intervals. Failure of the kidneys to eliminate the drug makes it accumulate in the body. When there is edema, the drug may accumulate and be dissolved in the excess fluid. In conditions that prevent the elimination of a drug through the normal avenue of excretion the nurse should be on the alert for symptoms of cumulative poisoning.

Nature and Form of Medication. Some drugs are eliminated very rapidly, as, for example, ammonia and epinephrine (Adrenalin). The effect of such drugs is fleeting, therefore, and they can be repeated in therapeutic doses without fear of toxicity; other drugs, such as digitalis and iron, are eliminated slowly and for this reason they are effective when given less frequently, but the patient must be watched for signs of cumulative poisoning.

Liquid medications, particularly drugs dissolved in water, act more rapidly than pills and powders. Powders should be dissolved or given in capsules. Absorption of powders and capsules is hastened, and swallowing made easier, if they are taken with a large quantity of liquid.

Some drugs have a *biphasic action;* that is, doses on different levels have different effects. Average doses (0.4 to 0.6 mg) of atropine slow the heart rate, probably by stimulating the medullary vagal nuclei; large doses increase the cardiac rate by blocking vagal effects on the S-A pacemaker.[167]

Time of Administration. The effect of drugs given by mouth is more marked if the stomach and upper part of the intestinal tracts are empty. For instance, the same amount of alcohol is much more intoxicating taken before than after a meal. If given after meals, larger doses of drugs are usually necessary to produce the effect desired.

Drug Combinations. When two drugs that have similar actions are given at the same time the dosage of each is smaller than if it were given alone. Drugs that act in this way are called *synergistic;* drugs whose actions oppose each other are called *antagonistic.* There are numerous drugs that cannot be given in combination with others. If there is any question about the compatibility of two drugs, the pharmacist should be consulted.[167a-b]

The Route of Administration. The dose varies according to the rapidity with which it is absorbed; for instance, when given intravenously, the dose is small because the full effect of the drug is felt immediately. When given by rectum the dose ordered may be larger than when given by mouth because the rate and amount of absorption from the rectum is slow and uncertain.

Route of Excretion. Drugs are selective in their avenues of excretion. They may be eliminated by one or all of the following: the kidneys, the alimentary tract, the lungs, the skin, and mucous membranes of the nose and throat. When the patient's disease cripples the excretory function of any of these organs the physician avoids, or gives in small dosage, drugs that must be eliminated by them.

6. ROUTES AND METHODS OF ADMINISTERING DRUGS

Medicines may be given by any of the following routes and methods depending upon the effect desired (a direct local effect, a systemic effect, or a remote local effect), the rapidity of action needed, the nature and amount of drug to be given, and the condition of the patient: (1) by needle injection—intra-arterial, intravenous, intramuscular, subcutaneous, intracardial, intraperitoneal, intraspinous, intraosseous, and intradermal; (2) by mouth—swallowed and sublingual; (3) by inhalation; (4) by application to the mucous membranes of the rectum, vagina, urethra and bladder, the eye, ear, nose and throat; and (5) application to the skin (see Table 21-2). The speed of action is more or less in the order given, from the most rapid to the least rapid. (The introduction of drugs through the skin by means of a jet of liquid under high pressure

Table 21-2.   Routes Used in Giving Medications

Routes	Methods of Administration

Directly into the tissues or serous cavities with a needle or cannula	By needle injection into the
	Artery—intra-arterial injection
	Vein—intravenous injection
	Muscle—intramuscular injection
	   (intracardial—into the heart muscle)
	Peritoneum—intraperitoneal injection
	Spinal cavity—intraspinal injection
	Bone—intraosseous injection
	Subcutaneous tissue—subcutaneous injection
	   (usually referred to as a hypodermic injection)
	Derma, or corium—intradermal injection

By the mouth to the alimentary tract	Oral medication swallowed or held under the tongue (sublingual)
By the nose to the lung	Inhalation of drugs in vapor, or steam

By the mucous membrane of
  Eye
  Ear
  Nose
  Throat
  Rectum
	Application with swab or sponge
	Irrigation of surface or cavity
	Instillation of medication held in a body of liquid
	   into a cavity

By the skin	Application with swab or sponge (Application of a drug in a jet of liquid under high pressure penetrates the skin and gives results comparable to subcutaneous needle injections)

gives results comparable to needle injections. This procedure is discussed on page 1180.)

Since the techniques of giving drugs with needles and through tubes into body cavities require detailed directions they are described in a chapter devoted to the subject; other methods of medication are described here.

By Mouth. Drugs are given by mouth in the following *forms:* (1) liquids—oils, water solutions as infusions, decoctions, or suspensions, and alcoholic solutions as extracts or tinctures; (2) solids—tablets, powders (often put in capsules), pills, and lozenges.

The person preparing an oral medication should consider the effect desired and how to get it, the nature of the drug, how to protect the mouth and teeth if the drug is injurious to them, and how to make the dose acceptable to the patient.

It is important to know why a medication is prescribed in order to decide whether it should be well diluted or given in a more concentrated form. If, for example, a systemic or a remote local effect is desired, drugs should be well diluted to promote absorption. (As water is usually the best solvent, all drugs, except oily preparations, are given with water unless otherwise ordered.) Water is given freely with all diaphoretics, diuretics, and narcotics. A hot drink following administration of such drugs is thought to hasten their action. When sweating is induced by drugs, such as the salicylates, care should be taken to keep the patient from getting chilled.

Some drugs, such as aromatic spirits of ammonia, although given for a systemic effect, owe their action to a reflex response following irritation of nerve endings in the mucous lining of the mouth or throat. Such drugs must be diluted sufficiently to prevent irritating the tissues, but not so much as to interfere with the effect on the nerve endings.

Drugs, such as syrup cough mixtures, prescribed for a local soothing or sedative effect on the mucous lining of the respiratory tract, are usually given undiluted. Drugs given for a local effect on the stomach are only slightly diluted. They may be given before meals, when the stomach is empty and at rest, to soften mucus or to stimulate the flow of gastric juice. They may be given *during* or *after* meals to supply a deficiency of hydrochloric acid or enzymes, or to counteract abnormal conditions present.

Time of administration is chosen with reference to the desired effect. Drugs given by mouth for a systemic effect usually depend upon absorption from the intestines rather than the stomach. They act most rapidly when the stomach and upper intestines are empty; they are therefore prescribed between meals.

Sodium bicarbonate, when given in acidosis, to neutralize an acid tendency in body fluids, is usually given between meals. If given after meals, more of the alkaline salt is combined with hydrochloric acid, and absorbed as sodium chloride. It should rarely be given in a capsule but should be dissolved in a glass of water and followed by more water.

In order to give a sedative or narcotic intelligently nurses must know the effect desired, and also the time required for the drug to act. The *hour* of administration and the need for the drug are often left to their judgment. Before giving the drug nurses should see that the patient's surroundings and his or her mental and physical condition are all conducive to rest. Because of the depressing effect of all sedatives and narcotics, the character of the patient's sleep should be noted. In Chapter 13, the effect of natural as against induced sleep is discussed. The use of drugs for pain is discussed in Chapter 49 on pain and also in Chapter 50 on death and dying.

The effect desired sometimes determines the *amount of drug* given. For instance, when ipecac is used to cause vomiting by a direct local effect on the stomach, a large dose is given well diluted; but when used as an expectorant, through its remote control effect on the bronchial tubes, a small dose is given undiluted in a cough mixture.

Cold water is commonly used to dilute drugs; but when a drug, such as peppermint, is given for a carminative effect, hot water should be used, as heat promotes the expulsion of gas from the stomach or intestines.

The *nature of the drug and its possibly injurious effects* should be fully considered by the nurse. Many drugs, such as dilute acids, iron, arsenic, salicylates, iodides, bromides, digitalis, and mercury, are irritating to the mucous lining of the stomach and may cause pain, nausea, and vomiting. All such drugs should be well diluted. They are usually given after meals so that they may be mixed with the stomach contents which reduces the effect on its walls. Dilute acids such as hydrochloric acid and liquid preparations of iron are destructive to the teeth. They should be given through a glass tube or a straw. Dilute hydrochloric acid is frequently added to a drinking glass of water or fruit juice, and the patient is asked to sip it during the meal, in this way approximating the normal secretion in the stomach. The mouth should receive careful attention when such drugs are given. Some doctors prescribe bicarbonate of soda with aspirin and other preparations of the salicylates to lessen the irritation in the stomach and to prevent acidosis.

Every nurse should know how to make

medicine as acceptable as possible to a patient. There are a few drugs, such as the bitter stomachics, quinine, gentian, and nux vomica, that owe their stimulating effect on the appetite to their bitter taste. These drugs are therefore given undiluted with no attempt to disguise the taste. In all other cases the taste should be made as unobjectionable as possible. Unpalatable drugs should be diluted, and cold water should be given immediately afterward from a clean glass. Ice may be held in the mouth before and after the medication in order to numb the nerve endings which include the taste buds. It is unwise to try to disguise the taste with food because this is likely to turn the person against the food.

Although a nurse's manner should not be hurried when giving a medication she or he should encourage the patient to take it promptly. Delay only prolongs the period of dread and intensifies dislike of the drug. Mouthwash should be offered persons who must take unpalatable concoctions or who are getting drugs which, like the iodides, are excreted in the saliva.

Castor oil is a heavy oil with a taste universally disliked in this country. A tasteless preparation is on the market but the consistency is still unpleasant, and memory supplies the taste to those who know it. To make this drug acceptable to most persons it should be disguised. It may be bought flavored with peppermint or its cloying consistency may be changed by mixing it thoroughly with a carbonated drink such as root beer. The following method is simple and satisfactory to many persons:

Rinse the medicine glass with lemon juice. Pour a teaspoonful of lemon juice into the glass, then the oil, and on top of that more lemon juice. Place the glass in a small saucer and surround it with small pieces of chipped ice. Chilling a substance dulls the flavor and warming intensifies it. Give the patient ice to hold in the mouth before and after taking the oil. Orange juice, Vichy or Seltzer water, or an olive given afterward will often prevent the feeling of nausea that sometimes follows a dose of castor oil.

Pills or tablets should be broken up, powdered, and dissolved when it is difficult for patients to swallow them. Powders that will not dissolve readily or that have a disagreeable taste may be given in capsules. Because compound licorice powder is not easily dissolved, it should be made into a paste with a small amount of water. Sufficient water should be added to enable the patient to swallow it; adding too much water is likely to cause nausea.

Attractive looking equipment helps to make medicines less distasteful. The articles shown in Figure 21-4 were chosen for their neat appearance, durability, and convenience. Disposable paper medicine cups and drinking tubes save labor. Medicine glasses and glass tubes must be "sanitized" as described for dishes in Chapter 15. A short drinking tube has an advantage over a long one because it is better balanced. When drugs are given to a group of patients an extra water supply is carried on the tray, but the nurse giving the medicines should see that each patient who is to receive medicine is provided with a glass and fresh drinking water.

By Inhalation. Drugs may be given by inhalation for either a *systemic* or a *local* effect. The systemic effect is produced immediately because of the large surface area of the lungs and the rich supply of blood vessels. Drugs used for *local effect* may be in the form of medicated steam and fumes, although the latter method is rarely used. Fumes from stramonium leaves (or stramonium with belladonna) may be inhaled to relax spasms of the involuntary muscles. Stramonium leaves may be made into cigarettes, or they may be burned in a fireproof vessel and the fumes inhaled through a cone fitted over the vessel.

Some drugs that are used for their *systemic effect* are: Ammonia gas (from ammonia water or smelling salts). It is inhaled as an emergency heart and respiratory stimulant in fainting or mild collapse. Amyl nitrate is inhaled to relax the coronary arteries and relieve an attack of angina pectoris or to relax spasms of the muscles of the bronchial tubes in asthma. This drug comes in small glass capsules, or pearls, which are broken in a paper or gauze handkerchief and held a short distance above the nose for a few minutes. Aminophylline, amphetamine (Benzedrine), penicillin, streptomycin, cyclopentamine hydrochloride (Clopane), and ergotamine, when introduced by aerosol spray, produce a systemic effect.[168] These are discussed in detail in Chapter 35.

The inhalation of fumes from volatile drugs, or burning drugs, is *dry inhalation;* the inhalation of plain steam or steam impregnated with a drug is *moist inhalation.*

Moist or *steam inhalations* are used chiefly for the following purposes: (1) to relieve inflammation of the mucous membrane in acute colds and in sinusitis; (2) to relieve inflammation of the larynx; (3) to soften thick, tenacious mucus and relieve coughing from many causes; and (4) to warm and moisten the air when, following operations such as a tracheotomy, room air is drawn into the trachea without being warmed and moistened by the nose and upper respiratory passages as it is in normal breathing.

Steam for moist inhalations is generated,

most often, in an electrically heated unit as shown in Figure 20-24. Antiseptics, such as tincture of benzoin, turpentine, menthol, creosote, and eucalyptol, are sometimes vaporized in the steam. Most authorities, however, believe that the virtue of an inhalation lies chiefly in the action of moist heat. Some physicians believe that the patient should stay in a very humid room rather than inhale steam intermittently. Windows and doors are kept closed, and steam is released from a special outlet on a steam radiator, from an electrically heated humidifier, or from a kettle of water boiling in the room over any source of heat. Usually, the treatment is given intermittently for a period of one-half hour every three or four hours during the day. The method depends upon the equipment available. Inhalators with incorporated electrical heating units are most convenient and safest.

A croup tent arranged around and over the head of the bed is advisable, particularly for a child with croup, and in all cases in which it is desirable to have a patient breathe warm moist air continuously or for a prolonged period (see Fig. 20-10). This prevents the discomfort, strain, and exhausting effect of keeping the face turned constantly toward the steam and overcomes the difficulty of maintaining this position during sleep. In this, and in all other methods used, the greatest precaution must be taken to protect the patient from burns or scalds. The outer covering of the tent may be a cotton sheet, but the inner layers must be a blanket or a large piece of turkish toweling to absorb the moisture; otherwise, the hot condensed steam might fall on the patient or bed. The head of the bed must be securely enclosed to prevent the escape of steam. There should be ample ventilation however, and, although there must be no drafts, the tent should not be kept so warm that both patient and nurse get a steam bath. The humidifier or kettle should be on the floor, a low table, or chair, according to the design, with the spout extending into the tent at the side or back. The spout must not extend far enough for the patient to touch it or for condensed steam to fall from it on the patient. When electric inhalators are not available other methods of generating steam may be used. Boiling water or the boiling medicated solution may be poured into a narrow-necked pitcher, and a towel, or a cone of cardboard or oiled paper, placed over it to direct the steam toward the mouth and nose of the patient. (To avoid burning the patient the pitcher must be filled only two thirds full.) An ordinary teakettle may be used in the same way. The croup kettle—a tin kettle with a long spout—is occasionally used in the hospital. An electric stove is the best and safest means of keeping the contents of the kettle steaming hot. In all methods, the patient should be in a comfortable position.

Inhalations involve a risk of scalding the person or of scorching the bedding. Every precaution should be taken to prevent such accidents, and the patient should be closely watched. During this treatment blood vessels of the skin and mucous membrane of the head are dilated. For this reason the patient is easily chilled; therefore, he or she should not go into a cold atmosphere for several hours.

Many persons suffering from chronic upper respiratory disease get considerable relief from inhaling steam. Very often the doctor prescribes this treatment to be used by patients in their home. The nurse should, in such cases, devise and teach patients a method that is adapted to the circumstances in which they live. When room air is centrally heated in houses the air is dry. Doctors may suggest that for even healthy persons the air be moistened by humidifiers that are electrically operated. They may be kept plugged in and operating constantly or only during the night in bedrooms.

Another way of medicating the respiratory passages is to *spray* the nose or throat with very finely divided liquids. If the particles are extremely small the liquid is said to be *nebulized*. Devices for mechanically dividing medications are called atomizers and nebulizers. Both operate on the principle that a column of gas forced through a liquid will collect and carry with it particles of the liquid. Air is forced through the atomizer with the hand bulb, or a stream of oxygen may be passed through the nebulizer. The latter is one way of giving antibiotics, such as penicillin, when the patient has a lung infection. Because the lungs have such an abundant blood supply, inhaled nebulized drugs, such as epinephrine, may be rapidly absorbed and show immediate systemic action.[169]

When nebulizers are used, the physician intends that the drugs reach the lungs. (The finer the particles the more likely they are to penetrate the lungs.) Patients must be taught to inhale as the bulb collapses in order to draw the vapor into the lungs and to avoid swallowing the drug. If swallowed it may be inactivated and wasted, or it may cause discomfort. The exact dose is put in the nebulizer; the mask is fitted to the patient, and oxygen allowed to flow through the nebulizer at the rate of 5 or 6 liters a minute until all the drug has been vaporized.

Gases—oxygen, helium, and carbon dioxide —are given by inhalation as therapeutic agents. Because there is so much detail to be discussed in connection with their administration, Chapter 20 is devoted to this subject.

By Mucous Membranes. There are numerous blood vessels in the mucous membrane under the tongue (sublingual vessels). Tablets and lozenges held under the tongue in the front of the mouth are rapidly dissolved and absorbed. Louis S. Goodman and Alfred Gilman [170] say that nitroglycerin is absorbed more efficiently by the sublingual than by the intestinal route. While drugs to be absorbed are most often given by mouth they can reach the circulation from the mucous lining of the oropharynx, nose, eyes, rectum, vagina, urethra, and bladder. Ordinarily those regions are medicated for a local effect, but sometimes it is convenient to give systemic medications by these routes, as, for example, general anesthesia by rectum. Topical medications and irrigations of these areas and the introduction of suppositories into these various body cavities are described in Chapters 23, 24, 25, 26, and 27.

By the Skin. In the simplest forms of life the surface of the organism is very sensitive to its environment, chemicals penetrate the outer cells, and the organism dies if it is not in a fairly stable medium. The higher forms of life, in contrast, are able to exist in more unstable surroundings because most chemicals in the creature's or the human's (outer) environment do not penetrate their skins, or hides. Drugs, therefore, are rarely applied to the skin for anything but a local effect. If the skin is clean and the drug is carried in an oil, or fat, it can penetrate the hair follicles and sebaceous glands and through them the subcutaneous tissue according to Goodman and Gilman.[171] They say also that drugs that ionize can be made to migrate through the epidermis by means of a galvanic current, a procedure called *iontophoresis.* Discussing the protective structural characteristics of the skin, Eric W. Martin and associates [172] say a number of factors increase percutaneous passage of drugs. Examples are a macerated skin caused by moist applications, injured or diseased epithelial layer of skin, and certain chemicals called "wetting agents."

With an instrument called the *Hypospray,* or *Dermo-jet,* described in Chapter 22, a jet of liquid drug can be directed at the skin with such force that it will penetrate the unbroken skin and will give a systemic effect similar to that of a hypodermic.

Drugs carried in fats or oils and applied to the skin for their systemic effects are called *inunctions.* Mercurial ointment was at one time used this way in the treatment of syphilis. A drug is absorbed most readily in regions where the skin is thin, such as the axilla, the inner surface of the arm, the thigh, and groin. The skin should be clean and the blood vessels dilated by a warm bath. The ointment or oil should be warm also. To prevent irritation the ointment is never applied to the same area on successive days. The areas just listed may be used in rotation; this is called a "course" of applications. The treatment is then omitted for a day and the parts are washed to remove any of the ointment that may remain in the pores of the skin. The "course" is then begun again in the same order. The treatment should be recorded on the chart each day. If nurses are rubbing an irritating drug on a patient's skin they should wear gloves, otherwise their hands may be affected or the drug may be absorbed and act on them systemically. Most applications to the skin are made for the purpose of cleaning, soothing, or disinfecting the skin. The concept of "feeding the skin" with fats, vitamins, and proteins has little credence in medical circles. The effectiveness of local applications to the skin of fat-soluble vitamin ointment in conditions associated with constant removal with soap and water of skin oils is evidence, however, that the skin can, in a sense, be "fed" certain food elements.

7. DRUG POISONING

Ingestion of poison by mistake and with suicidal intention is, unfortunately, a fairly common emergency. Poisoning by food and by drugs used in therapy is not uncommon * (see Fig. 21-6).

The number of drug addicts, young and old, who die from overdoses is shocking the people of many countries. A discussion of this and the problem of the depressed person who poisons himself or herself cannot be treated adequately here. However, the role of the nurse in helping the depressed patient is discussed briefly in Chapter 41. Regardless of the cause of poisoning the removal of or neutralization of the toxic substance is done in the same way for the accidentally or intentionally poisoned person. What is said in this chapter on the subject applies in both cases. The subsequent treatment of the suicidal and the non-

---

* A physician reports that in 1939, 1 per cent of the children admitted to a large city hospital were brought there for treatment of poisoning. About a fourth of them were accidentally poisoned; about one-half were poisoned from the use of substances used therapeutically. (Gold, Harry [ed.]: *Cornell Conference on Therapy,* Vol. 4. Macmillan Publishing Co., Inc., New York, 1951, p. 1.)

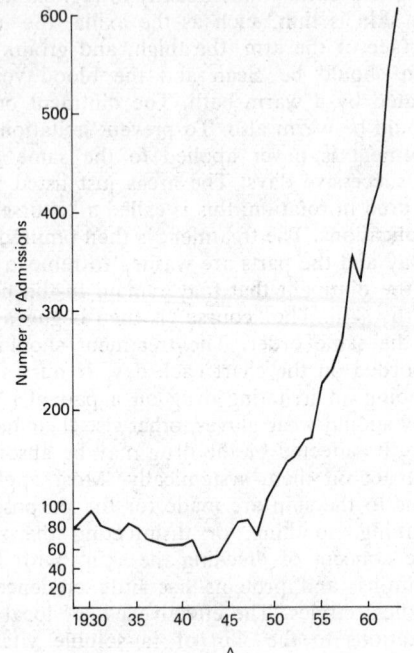

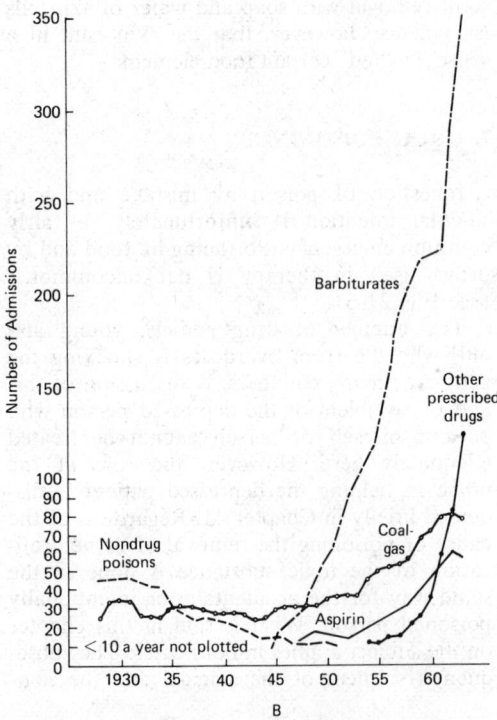

Figure 21-6. Yearly admission rates of poison patients to the Royal Infirmary at Edinburgh. *A.* Total number of patients admitted each year. *B.* Type of poison employed. (From Malleson, Andrew: *Need Your Doctor Be So Useless?* George Allen & Unwin Ltd., London, 1973, pp. 75 and 76.)

suicidal persons is different. The suicidal always needs psychiatric help.

First aid is often given at home because time is of the essence. It would be a good thing if everyone understood the underlying principles of emergency treatment. The nurse may be called on to teach these and to put them into practice. In many cases there is no way of determining the nature of the toxic agent, and, as some authorities point out, time spent in trying to discover this before starting treatment in acute poisoning may cost the patient's life.

It has been stressed throughout this chapter that nurses should be students of drug action so that they will recognize toxic symptoms in their patients. The signs of chronic drug poisoning should be part of the study of each potent drug. It is not within the scope of this volume, however, to discuss the toxicology of even the commonest drugs. All that is attempted is an outline of the principles underlying the treatment of acute poisoning when an emergency occurs.

In acute poisoning, the person giving first aid may be seeing the patient for the first time. Immediate action is demanded. Information should be solicited, but first-aid measures can be initiated while the family, the friends, or the patient himself or herself is explaining what happened. Needless to say, the services of a physician should be solicited at once.

First Aid or Immediate Treatment of Acute Poisoning. Goodman and Gilman [173] list the following steps in treatment: (1) remove the poison from the body, (2) administer antidotes, and (3) give supportive or symptomatic treatment.

Poison is removed from the stomach most effectively by gastric lavage. (See page 1224 for a discussion of this procedure.) Lavage may be contraindicated when the poison is highly corrosive for the tube might, in such cases, perforate the injured esophagus or stomach. Lavage should not be used when the poison is a convulsant drug, such as strychnine, since the procedure will induce or exaggerate convulsions. Goodman and Gilman point out that lavage not only removes the toxic agent from the stomach, but offers a means of introducing a saline cathartic into the stomach after the stomach is washed out, which promotes further elimination of the poison.

Emetics are advocated in some first-aid texts. Goodman and Gilman state that "only in rare cases are such drugs of value." They suggest that of all the emetics, apomorphine given hypodermically is most rapidly effective. Mustard water (in the proportion of one teaspoonful to a glass of tepid water) taken until vomiting occurs may be tried when a stomach tube and apomorphine are not available. Vomiting should not be induced in comatose patients for they will almost inevitably insufflate the vomitus and, with it, the poison. The danger is obvious.

If the poison has not been ingested but is in contact with the skin, repeated bathing with running water is effective unless the irritant is insoluble in water. In such cases a bland substance that will dissolve the poison should be used as, for example, vegetable oil or alcohol, according to the nature of the toxic agent.

When contact with poisonous plants is suspected, a thorough scrubbing with yellow laundry soap is advocated. (Inoculations of susceptible persons are effective in some cases as a preventive but cannot be relied upon for control of poison ivy dermatitis.)

Because many ingested poisons are eliminated by the kidneys, patients should be encouraged to drink as much water as they will take. This dilutes the toxic substance and thereby minimizes its harmful effect upon the kidneys.

Volatile substances that are eliminated by the lungs can be gotten rid of more rapidly if respiration is stimulated. Carbon dioxide as a stimulant should be administered only by specially trained personnel.

In Volume 4 of the *Cornell Conferences on Therapy* [174] there are two interesting chapters on household poisoning. A number of physicians reported cases in which the antidote used in treating the victim did more harm than good and was even a more dangerous substance than the so-called poison. One physician urged those who are unsure, or limited in the knowledge of antidotes, to resist the temptation to use them.

Goodman and Gilman point out that antidotes are of two kinds: chemical and physiologic. Chemical antidotes are those that inactivate the poison by chemical reaction; physiologic antidotes are substances that combat the harmful physiologic effect of the poison. An acid is, for example, a chemical antidote for an alkali; a drug that stimulates respiration is a physiologic antidote for a respiratory depressant.

Even if the person giving first aid knows the specific antidote for the ingested poison, it is rarely available. Goodman and Gilman suggest the following household agents as antidotes one might expect to find and that are safe to use.

Poison	Antidote
For poisoning by heavy metals	Milk and egg white
For poisoning by any irritant (starch is especially effective against iodine)	Flour and starch water
For poisoning by alkaloids	Strong tea and diluted tincture of iodine

The following is a list of antidotes for common poisons as compiled from the discussion in Volume 4 of *Cornell Conferences of Therapy:*

Poison	Antidote
For nicotine poisoning	Potassium permanganate for lavage
For arsenic poisoning (including therapeutic arsenicals such as oxophenarsine [Mapharsen] or Fowler's solution)	BAL (2,3-dimercaptopropanol)
For poisoning by mercuric compounds	BAL (2,3-dimercaptopropanol)
For effects of lead poisoning	Calcium (large amounts)
For cyanide poisoning	Sodium nitrite and sodium thiosulfate (intravenously)
For most alkaloids	Potassium permanganate for lavage
For barbiturate poisoning	Picrotoxin and amphetamine sulfate (Benzedrine sulfate)

It should be understood that antidotes are often and most effectively used as a lavage in water solutions.

Pharmacology texts include the treatment of toxic doses in the discussion of every poisonous drug. Frank poisons usually give the antidote on the label of the bottle. Poisoning of children often results from ingestion of a cleaning fluid, a poison put down for insects or animals, or some other household chemical whose container may not be available or which may fail unfortunately to provide the needed information on its label.

Supportive, or symptomatic, treatment probably needs no explanation, but the authorities emphasize that it is as important as other aspects of therapy. There may be oxygen want or excessive loss of fluids; the patient may be in shock, or, if suicidal, in a critical emotional state. These and many other symptoms, or groups of related symptoms, demand either immediate attention or consideration after neutralizing or removing as much of the drug as possible from contact with the body.

REFERENCES

1. DiCyan, Erwin, and Hessman, Lawrence: *Without Prescription.* Simon & Schuster, New York, 1972.
2. Jones, Kenneth L., et al.: *Drugs and Alcohol.* Harper & Row, New York, 1969, p. 9.
3. Ivy, Andrew C.: "Definitions of Terms Basic to the Problems Created by the Consumption of Alcohol," in Narcotics Education, Inc.: *Toward Prevention. Scientific Studies on Alcohol and Alcoholism.* University Press, Berrien Springs, Mich., 1971, p. 50.
4. Weil, Andrew: *The Natural Mind.* Houghton Mifflin Co., Boston, 1972, p. 98.
5. Wurmser, Leon: "Drug Abuse: Nemesis of Psychiatry," *Am. Scholar,* 41:393, (Summer) 1972.
6. Harris, T. George: "A Conversation About the Drug Epidemic with Jerome Jaffe," *Psychology Today,* 7:68, (Aug.) 1973.
7. Wurmser, Leon: *op. cit.*
8. Malleson, Andrew: *Need Your Doctor Be So Useless?* George Allen & Unwin, London, 1973, p. 65.
9. Bacon, Selden D.: "The Process of Addiction to Alcohol—Social Aspects," *Q. J. Stud. Alcohol,* 34:1, (Mar.) 1973.
10. Malleson, Andrew: *op. cit.,* pp. 35, 59.
11. Christopher D. Smithers Foundation, Inc.: *Understanding Alcoholism.* Charles Scribner's Sons, New York, 1968, p. 7.
12. Jellinek, E. M.: *The Disease Concept of Alcoholism.* College and University Press, New Haven, Conn., 1960 (In association with Hillhouse Press, New Brunswick, N.J., on behalf of Christopher D. Smithers Foundation).
12a. Jones, Kenneth L., et al.: *op. cit.,* p. 100.
13. "Epidemiologic Studies and Control Programs in Alcoholism," *Am. J. Public Health,* 57:955, (June) 1967.
14. Barchha, R., et al.: "The Prevalence of Alcoholism Among General Hospital Ward Patients," *Am. J. Psychiatry,* 125:681, (Nov.) 1968.
15. Cahalan, D., et al.: *A National Study of Drinking Behavior and Attitudes.* Rutgers Center of Alcohol Studies, New Brunswick, N.J., 1969 (Monograph No. 6).
16. Crowley, Thomas J.: "The Reinforcers for Drug Abuse. Why People Take Drugs," *Compr. Psychiatry,* 13:51, (Jan.) 1972.
17. Frederick, Carl: "Drug Abuse as Self-Destructive Behavior," *Drug Ther.,* 2:49, (Feb.) 1972.
18. Knupfer, G.: "The Epidemiology of Problem Drinking," *Am. J. Public Health,* 57: 973, (June) 1967.
19. Robins, Lee N., and Guze, Samuel B.: "Drinking Practices and Problems in Urban Ghetto Populations," in Mello, Nancy, and Mendelson, Jack H. (eds.): *Recent Advances in Studies of Alcoholism.* National Institute on Alcohol Abuse and Alcoholism, Rockville, Md., 1971.
20. Plaut, Thomas F. A.: *Alcohol Problems. A Report to the Nation by the Cooperative Commission on the Study of Alcoholism.* Oxford University Press, New York, 1967.
21. Johnson, Gordon F.: "Alcoholism—Disease and Irresponsibility," *Can. J. Public Health,* 60:416, (Nov.) 1969.
22. Szasz, Thomas: "Bad Habits Are Not Diseases. A Refutation of the Claim that Alcoholism Is a Disease," *Lancet,* 2:83, (July 8) 1972.
23. Malleson, Andrew: *op. cit.,* p. 44.
24. Finnegan, Loretta P., and MacNew, Bonnie A.: "Care of the Addicted Infant," *Am. J. Nurs.,* 74:685, (Apr.) 1974.
25. Ramsey, M. A.: "Drug Addicted Mother and Child," *Nursing '73,* 3:46, (Feb.) 1973.
26. Caskey, K. K., et al.: "The School Nurse and Drug Abusers," *Nurs. Outlook,* 18:27, (Dec.) 1970.
27. Fox, V.: "Alcoholism in Adolescence," *J. Sch. Health,* 43:32, (Jan.) 1973.
28. Caskey, K. K., et al.: *op. cit.*
29. Barty, Naomi, et al.: "Drug Abuse Education; A Practical Approach for Elementary School," *Educ. Can.,* 13:10, (Mar.) 1973.
30. Child Study Association of America: *You, Your Child and Drugs.* Child Study Press, New York, 1971.
31. Cockett, R.: *Drug Abuse and Personality in Young Offenders.* Appleton-Century-Crofts, New York, 1971.
32. Dambacher, Betty, and Hellwig, K.: "Nursing Strategies for Young Drug Users," *Perspect. Psychiatr. Care,* 9:201, (Sept.–Oct.) 1971.
33. Dearden, M. H., et al.: "A Pilot Program in High School Drug Education Utilizing Non-Directive Techniques and Sensitivity Training," *J. Sch. Health,* 41:118, (Mar.) 1971.
34. Finnegan, Loretta P., and MacNew, Bonnie A.: *op. cit.*
35. Millsap, Mary: "Occupational Health Nursing in an Alcohol Addiction Program," *Nurs. Clin. North Am.,* 7:121, (Mar.) 1972.
36. Miller, Donald E.: "An Emerging Federal Role," *Hospitals,* 45:15, (Aug. 1) 1971.
37. Barchha, R., et al.: *op. cit.*

38. Freeman, J. W., et al.: "Management of Patients Unconscious from Drug Overdose," *Med. J. Aust.,* **2:**1165, (Dec. 19) 1970.

39. Foreman, Nancy Jo, and Zerwekh, Joyce V.: "Drug Crisis Intervention," *Am. J. Nurs.,* **71:**1736, (Sept.) 1971.

40. Moody, P. M.: "Attitudes of Nurses and Nursing Students Toward Alcoholism Treatment," *Q. J. Stud. Alcohol,* **32:**172, (Mar.) 1971.

41. Morgan, Arthur James, and Moreno, Judith Wilson: "Attitudes Toward Addiction," *Am. J. Nurs.,* **73:**497, (Mar.) 1973.

41a. Wilkins, R. H.: "The Health Visitor and the Alcoholic," *Health Visitor,* **46:**366, (Nov.) 1973.

42. Brewster, J. T.: "Let's Diagnose Ourselves When Treating Addicts," *Can J. Ment. Health,* **20:**14, (Nov.–Dec.) 1972.

43. Ferneau, E. W., et al.: "Attitudes of Nursing Personnel Regarding Alcoholism and Alcoholics," *Nurs. Res.,* **18:**446, (Sept.–Oct.) 1968.

44. "Nurse Addicts Have Special Unit at Federal Hospital, Lexington, Ky.," *Am. J. Nurs.,* **72:**2138, (Dec.) 1972.

45. Lipp, Martin R., et al.: "Marijuana Use by Nurses and Nursing Students," *Am. J. Nurs.,* **71:**2339, (Dec.) 1971.

46. Kraus, A. S., et al.: "Non-Medical Use of Drugs by Students and Alumni of Queen's University," *Can. J. Public Health,* **63:**296, (July–Aug.) 1972.

47. DeLeon, George: "Phoenix House: Criminal Activity of Dropouts," *J.A.M.A.,* **222:**686, (Nov. 6) 1972.

48. Krepick, Donna S., and Long, Bonnie L.: "Heroin Addiction: A Treatable Disease," *Nurs. Clin. North Am.,* **8:**41, (Mar.) 1973.

49. Malleson, Andrew: *op. cit.,* p. 58.

50. Long, Bonnie L., and Krepick, Donna Sammarco: "New Perspectives on Drug Abuse," *Nurs. Clin. North Am.,* **8:**25, (Mar.) 1973.

51. Mann, Marty: *New Primer on Alcoholism.* Holt, Rinehart & Winston, New York, 1958.

52. Mann, Marty: *How to Know an Alcoholic.* National Council on Alcoholism, New York, 1973.

53. *Alcoholism, The Family Disease.* Al-Anon Family Group Headquarters, Inc., New York, 1964.

54. Senseman, Laurence A.: "Alcohol and the Nervous System," in Narcotics Education, Inc.: *Toward Prevention. Scientific Studies on Alcohol and Alcoholism.* University Press, Berrien Springs, Mich., 1971, p. 77.

55. Jellinek, E. M., *op. cit.*

56. World Health Organization: *WHO Expert Committee on Drug Dependence. 18th Report.* The Organization, Geneva, 1971.

57. Ball, J. C., and Chambers, C. D. (eds.): *The Epidemiology of Opiate Addiction in the United States.* Charles C Thomas, Publisher, Springfield, Ill., 1970.

58. Eckert, W. G.: *The Medical, Legal and Law Enforcement Aspects of Drugs and Drug Abuse. A Bibliography of Classic and Current References.* The Author, Wichita, Kan., 1972.

59. Meyers, R. E.: *Guide to Drug Rehabilitation.* Beacon Press, Boston, 1972.

60. National Council on Alcoholism: *Alcoholism Publications.* The Council, New York, 1973.

61. Philipson, Richard V. (ed.): *Modern Trends in Drug Dependence and Alcoholism.* Appleton-Century-Crofts, New York, 1970.

62. Zinberg, Norman E.: *Drugs and the Public.* Simon & Schuster, New York, 1972.

63. US National Library of Medicine, Toxicology Information Program: *Drug Interactions; An Annotated Bibliography with Selected Excerpts, 1967–1970.* The Library, Bethesda, Md., 1972.

64. US Congress: *Narcotics Research, Rehabilitation and Treatment,* Parts 1 and 2. US Government Printing Office, Washington, D.C., 1971.

65. O'Neill, Eugene G.: *Long Day's Journey Into Night* (A Play). Yale University Press, New Haven, Conn., 1956.

66. ———: *The Iceman Cometh* (A Play). Random House, New York, 1946.

67. Scott, Natalie A.: *The Story of Mrs. Murphy.* E. P. Dutton & Co., New York, 1947.

68. Jackson, Charles: *Lost Weekend.* Farrar, Straus & Giroux, New York, 1944.

69. Mello, Nancy, and Mendelson, Jack H. (eds.): *Recent Advances in Studies of Alcoholism.* National Institute on Alcohol Abuse and Alcoholism, Rockville, Md., 1971.

70. US Public Health Service: *Developing Community Services for Alcoholics, Some Beginning Principles.* US Government Printing Office, Washington, D.C., 1971.

71. US Department of Health, Education, and Welfare, National Institute of Mental Health: *A Guide to Drug Abuse Education and Information Materials.* US Government Printing Office, Washington, D.C., 1972 (Pub. No. [HSM] 71–9077).

72. "Methadone—Yes or No?" *J.A.M.A.,* **219:**1275, (Mar. 6) 1972.

73. Wolfson, Edward A.: "Alternatives to Methadone," *Hospitals,* **45:**53, (Aug. 1) 1971.

74. Harris, T. George: *op. cit.*

75. Nelson, Karin: "The Nurse in a Methadone Maintenance Program," *Am. J. Nurs.,* **73:**870, (May) 1973.

76. Pearson, Barbara: "Methadone Maintenance in Heroin Addiction," *Am. J. Nurs.,* **70:**2571, (Dec.) 1970.

77. Crowley, Thomas J.: *op. cit.*

78. Fink, Max, et al.: "Narcotic Antagonists. Another Approach to Addiction Therapy," *Am. J. Nurs.,* **71:**1359, (July) 1971.

79. Dunn, Robert B.: "A New Comprehensive, Intensive Care Program for the Treatment

of Alcoholism," *Psychosomatics,* **13**:397, (Nov.–Dec.) 1972.

80. Kimmel, Mary E.: "Antabuse in a Clinic Program," *Am. J. Nurs.,* **71**:1173, (June) 1971.

81. Glasscote, Raymond M., et al.: *The Treatment of Drug Abuse: Programs, Problems, Prospects.* Joint Information Service of the American Psychiatric Association and the National Association for Mental Health, Washington, D.C., 1972.

82. Davis, V. E., and Walsh, M. J.: "Alcohol, Amines, and Alkaloids: A Possible Biochemical Basis for Alcohol Addiction," *Science,* **167**:1005, (Feb. 13) 1970.

83. Weiner, S., et al.: "Familial Patterns in Chronic Alcoholism: A Study of Father and Son During Experimental Intoxication," *Am. J. Psychiatry,* **127**:1646, (June) 1971.

84. Nathan, P. E., et al.: "Behavioral Analysis of Chronic Alcoholism," *Arch. Gen. Psychiatry,* **22**:419, (May) 1970.

85. Johnson, L. C., et al.: "Sleep During Alcohol Intake and Withdrawal in the Chronic Alcoholic," *Arch. Gen. Psychiatry,* **22**:406, (May) 1970.

86. Gross, Milton M., et al.: "Sleep Disturbances in Alcoholic Intoxication and Withdrawal," in Mello, Nancy, and Mendelson, Jack H. (eds.): *Recent Advances in Studies of Alcoholism.* National Institute on Alcohol Abuse and Alcoholism, Rockville, Md., 1971.

87. Goodwin, D. W., et al.: "Loss of Short-Term Memory as a Predictor of the Alcoholic 'Blackout'," *Nature,* **227**:201, (July 11) 1970.

88. Rubin, E., and Lieber, C. S.: "Alcohol-Induced Hepatic Injury in Man," in Sardesia, V. M. (ed.): *Biochemical and Clinical Aspects of Alcohol Metabolism.* Charles C Thomas, Publisher, Springfield, Ill., 1969.

89. Isselbacher, Kurt J., and Carter, Edward A.: "Effect of Alcohol on Liver and Intestinal Function," in Mello, Nancy, and Mendelson, Jack H. (eds.): *Recent Advances in Studies of Alcoholism.* National Institute on Alcohol Abuse and Alcoholism, Rockville, Md., 1971.

90. Motoi, Ogata, et al.: "Adrenal Function and Alcoholism: II. Catecholamines," in Mello, Nancy, and Mendelson, Jack H. (eds.): *Recent Advances in Studies of Alcoholism.* National Institute on Alcohol Abuse and Alcoholism, Rockville, Md., 1971.

91. Epstein, S. S., et al. (eds.): *Drugs of Abuse; Their Genetic and Other Chronic Nonpsychiatric Hazards.* Massachusetts Institute of Technology Press, Cambridge, 1971.

92. "Nurses Slated for Key Role in Federal Program Against Employee Alcoholism," *Am. J. Nurs.,* **71**:2088, (Nov.) 1971.

93. Curran, William J.: "Drug Addiction and Alcohol Abuse Under Workmen's Compensation," *N. Engl. J. Med.,* **285**:559, (Sept. 2) 1971.

94. Ditman, K. S., et al.: "A Controlled Experiment on the Use of Court Probation for Drunk Arrests," *Am. J. Psychiatry,* **124**:160, (Aug.) 1967.

95. Gallant, Donald M.: "Evaluation of Compulsory Treatment of the Alcoholic Municipal Court Offender," in Mello, Nancy, and Mendelson, Jack H. (eds.): *Recent Advances in Studies of Alcoholism.* National Institute on Alcohol Abuse and Alcoholism, Rockville, Md., 1971.

96. Hughes, Margaret E.: "The Role of Law in the Control of Alcohol and Drug Use," *Addictions,* **16**:1, (Summer) 1969.

97. Orr, Michael: "Business and the Compulsive Drinker," *Addictions,* **19**:38, (Summer) 1972.

98. Pfeffer, A. Z., et al.: "A Treatment Program for the Alcoholic in Industry," *J.A.M.A.,* **161**:827, (June 30) 1956.

99. Slovenski, R. S.: "Alcoholism and Criminal Law," *Bull. Menninger Clin.* **31**:105, (Mar.) 1967.

100. Chapel, J. L.: "Emergency Room Treatment of the Drug-Abusing Patient," *Am. J. Psychiatry,* **130**:257, (Mar.) 1973.

101. Kaim, S. C.: "Drug Treatment of the Alcohol Withdrawal Syndrome," in Mello, Nancy, and Mendelson, Jack H. (eds.): *Recent Advances in Studies of Alcoholism.* National Institute on Alcohol Abuse and Alcoholism, Rockville, Md., 1971.

102. ———, et al.: "Treatment of the Acute Alcohol Withdrawal State: A Comparison of Four Drugs," *Am. J. Psychiatry,* **125**:54, (June) 1969.

103. Wolfe, Sidney M., and Victor, Maurice: "The Physiological Basis of the Alcohol Withdrawal Syndrome," in Mello, Nancy, and Mendelson, Jack H. (eds.): *Recent Advances in Studies of Alcoholism.* National Institute on Alcohol Abuse and Alcoholism, Rockville, Md., 1971.

103a. Simpson, R. K.: "Controlling Delirium Tremens and Treating the Alcoholic," *Med. Insight,* **4**:46, (Jan.) 1972.

104. American Hospital Association: *Who Cares About an Alcoholism Program in the General Hospital?* The Association, Chicago, 1972.

105. Phillips, D. F.: "Are Hospitals Too Late and Too Square? Drug Abuse Programs," *Hospitals,* **45**:55, (Jan. 16) 1971.

106. Mantle, Sister Audrey: "Hospital's Responsibility Towards Drug Users," *Catholic Hosp.,* **2**:5, (May) 1971.

107. Imhoff, John E., et al.: "The Emerging Role of the Hospital in Drug Abuse Education and Prevention," *J. Sch. Health,* **42**:472, (Oct.) 1972.

108. Hickox, R. F.: "Hospitals Open Their Doors to Alcoholics. . . . Slowly," *Hosp. World,* **1**:1, (Jan.) 1972.

109. Hacker, Carlotta: "Do You Have a Bad

Trip if You Go to the Hospital?" *Can. Nurse,* **67**:39, (June) 1971.

110. Freilich, Herbert: "Hospitals Urged to Take Active Part in Effort to Control Drug Addiction," *Hosp. Top.,* **49**:45, (Dec.) 1971.

111. "Detoxification Centres: Should They Be Inside Hospitals?" *Hosp. Admin. (Can.)* **13**:14, (Dec.) 1971.

112. Couture, J.: "National Symposium on Hospital Responsibility Towards Drug Users," *Can. Assoc. Med. Res. Librarians Bull.,* **4**:53, (Nov.) 1971.

113. Burkhalter, Pamela K.: "The Alcoholic in a General Hospital," *Superv. Nurse,* **3**:25, (Apr.) 1972.

114. Endore, G.: *Synanon.* Doubleday & Co., New York, 1968.

115. Keller, Oliver J., and Alper, Benedict S.: *Halfway Houses.* D. C. Heath Co., Boston, 1970.

116. Yablonsky, L.: *The Tunnel Back: Synanon.* Macmillan Publishing Co., Inc., New York, 1965.

117. Huey, Florence L.: "In a Therapeutic Community for the Treatment of Drug Addiction," *Am. J. Nurs.,* **71**:926, (May) 1971.

118. Hyde, Margaret O. (ed.): *Mind Drugs.* McGraw-Hill Book Co., New York, 1968, p. 90.

119. Christopher D. Smithers Foundation, Inc.: *op. cit.,* p. 5.

120. Fox, Richard P., et al.: "A Therapeutic Revolving Door," *Arch. Gen. Psychiatry,* **26**:179, (Feb.) 1972.

121. Al-Anon Family Group Headquarters, Inc.: *Living with An Alcoholic.* Al-Anon, New York, 1973.

122. Kellermann, Joseph L.: *A Merry-Go-Round Named DENIAL.* Al-Anon Family Group Headquarters, Inc., New York, 1969.

123. Miller, Neal E.: "Learning of Glandular and Visceral Responses," in Shapiro, David, et al. (eds.): *Biofeedback and Self-Control, 1972.* Aldine Publishing Co., Chicago, 1973, p. 90.

124. Wallace, Robert K., and Benson, Herbert: "The Physiology of Meditation," in Shapiro, David, et al. (eds.): *Biofeedback and Self-Control, 1972.* Aldine Publishing Co., Chicago, 1973, p. 353.

125. Distasio, Carol, and Nawrot, Marcia: "Methaqualone," *Am. J. Nurs.,* **73**:1922, (Nov.) 1973.

126. "Drug Abuse Focus of ANA Project," *ANA in Action,* **3**:1, (Fall) 1971.

127. "Medical School Education on Abuse of Alcohol and Other Psychoactive Drugs," *J.A.M.A.,* **219**:1746, (Mar. 27) 1972.

127a. Gibbons, Robert J., et al. (eds.): *Research Advances in Alcohol and Drug Problems.* John Wiley & Sons, New York, 1974.

128. American Association for Health, Physical Education and Recreation: *Resource Book for Drug Abuse Education.* The Association, Washington, D.C., 1970.

129. Blakeslee, Alton L.: *Alcoholism—A Sickness That Can Be Beaten.* Public Affairs Committee, New York, 1970 (Public Affairs Pamphlet No. 1184).

130. Brill, Leon, and Harms, Ernest (eds.): *Yearbook of Drug Abuse.* Behavioral Publications, New York, 1973.

131. ———, and Lieberman, Louis (eds.): *Major Modalities in the Treatment of Drug Abuse.* Behavioral Publications, New York, 1972.

132. Canadian Department of National Health and Welfare, Commission of Inquiry into the Non-Medical Use of Drugs: *Treatment.* Information Canada, Ottawa, 1972.

133. Canadian Medical Association: *Policy Statement; Non-Medical Use of Drugs.* The Association, Ottawa, 1972.

134. Child Study Association of America: *op. cit.*

135. Chipp, D. L.: "The Nurse's Role in the Use and Abuse of Drugs," *Aust. Nurses J.,* **1**:1, (Suppl.) June 1972.

136. DeDain, Gerald: "Drugs and Society: What Can a Public Inquiry Do?" *Addictions,* **9**:18, (Summer) 1972.

137. Kalant, Harold, and Kalant, Oriana J.: *Drugs, Society and Personal Choice.* Paper Jacks; for Addiction Research Foundation of Ontario, Don Mills, Ont., 1971.

138. McCarrick, H.: "A City That Has Controlled Heroin Addiction," *Nurs. Times,* **65**:945, (July 24) 1969.

139. Malcolm, Andrew I.: *The Pursuit of Intoxication.* Alcoholism and Drug Addiction Research Foundation, Toronto, 1971.

140. Saltman, Jules: *What We Can Do About Drug Abuse.* Public Affairs Committee, New York, 1970 (Public Affairs Pamphlet No. 390).

141. "Drug Abuse: Where to Find the Facts," *Today's Health,* **49**:57, (Mar.) 1971.

142. Wilbur, Richard S.: "How to Stamp Out a Heroin Epidemic—Army Style," *Today's Health,* **50**:9, (July) 1972.

143. World Health Organization: *Youth and Drugs; Report of a WHO Study Group.* The Organization, Geneva, 1973 (Pub. No. 516).

144. US Department of Commerce, National Bureau of Standards: *A Metric America. A Report to Congress. A Decision Whose Time Has Come.* US Government Printing Office, Washington, D.C., 1971.

145. Odone, Jeffrey V.: "Going Metric," *Am. J. Nurs.,* **74**:1078, (June) 1974.

146. DiPalma, J. R. (ed.): *Drill's Pharmacology and Medicine,* 4th ed. McGraw-Hill Book Co., New York, 1971, p. 1877.

147. Murchison, Irene A., and Nichols, Thomas S.: *Legal Foundations of Nursing Practice.* Macmillan Publishing Co., Inc., New York, 1970, p. 335.

148. Bergersen, Betty S.: *Pharmacology in Nurs-*

ing, 12th ed. C. V. Mosby Co., St. Louis, 1973, p. 16.

149. *Pharmacopoeia of the United States of America,* 18th revision, by Authority of the United States Pharmacopeial Convention. Mack Publishing Co., Easton, Pa., 1970.

150. *National Formulary,* 13th ed. Prepared by Committee on National Formulary under the supervision of Council by Authority of the American Pharmaceutical Association. The Association, Washington, D.C., 1970.

151. AMA Council on Drugs: *AMA Drug Evaluations,* 1st ed. American Medical Association, Chicago, 1971.

152. *Physicians' Desk Reference to Pharmaceutical Specialties and Biologicals* (PDR), 31st ed. Medical Economics, Oradell, N.J., 1976.

153. Hussar, Daniel A.: "Drug Interactions by the Hundreds! How Can You Possibly Remember Them All?" *Nursing '72,* **2:**7, (Jan.) 1972.

154. Schwartz, Doris, et al.: *The Elderly Ambulatory Patient.* Macmillan Publishing Co., Inc., New York, 1964.

155. Schwartz, Doris: "Medication Errors Made by Elderly, Chronically Ill Patients," *Am. J. Public Health,* **52:**2018, (Dec.) 1962.

156. Marks, Janet, and Clarke, Margaret: "The Hospital Patient and His Knowledge of the Drug He Is Receiving," *Int. Nurs. Rev.,* **19:**39, (No. 1) 1972.

156a. Schwartz, Doris: "Safe Self-Medication for Elderly Outpatients," *Am. J. Nurs.,* **75:**1808, (Oct.) 1975.

157. Byrne, Anne K.: "Errors in Giving Medications," *Am. J. Nurs.,* **53:**829, (July) 1953.

158. Barker, Kenneth: "The Effect of an Experimental Medication System on Medication Errors and Costs, Part One: Introduction and Errors Study," *Am. J. Hosp. Pharm.,* **26:**324, (June) 1969.

159. ———: "The Effect of an Experimental Medication System on Medication Errors and Costs, Part Two: The Cost Study," *Am. J. Hosp. Pharm.,* **26:**388, (July) 1969.

160. Kern, M. S.: "New Ideas About Drug Systems," *Am. J. Nurs.,* **68:**1251, (June) 1968.

161. Slater, Wallace E., and Hripko, Joseph R.: "The Unit-Dose System in a Private Hospital," *Am. J. Hosp. Pharm.,* **25:**641, (Nov.) 1968.

162. Blasingame, W. G., et al.: "Some Time and Motion Consideration with Single-Unit Packaged Drugs in Five Hospitals," *Am. J. Hosp. Pharm.,* **26:**310, (June) 1969.

163. Mehl, Bernard: "An Experiment in Clinical Pharmacy," *Am. J. Hosp. Pharm.,* **25:**631, (Nov.) 1968.

164. Levine, Myra E.: "Breaking Through the Medications Mystique," *Am. J. Nurs.,* **70:**799, (Apr.) 1970.

165. Martin, Eric W., et al. (eds.): *Techniques*

of Medication. J. B. Lippincott Co., Philadelphia, 1969, p. 31.

166. AMA Council on Drugs: *op. cit.,* back of cover.

167. Goodman, Louis S., and Gilman, Alfred: *The Pharmacological Basis of Therapeutics,* 5th ed. Macmillan Publishing Co., Inc., New York, 1975, p. 518.

167a. Tobey, Lee E., and Covington, Tim R.: "Antimicrobial Drug Interactions," *Am. J. Nurs.,* **75:**1470, (Sept.) 1975.

167b. Lambert, Martin L.: "Drug and Diet Interactions," *Am. J. Nurs.,* **75:**402, (Mar.) 1975.

168. Martin, Eric W., et al. (eds.): *op. cit.,* p. 98.

169. *Ibid.*

170. Goodman, Louis S., and Gilman, Alfred: *op. cit.,* p. 731.

171. *Ibid.,* p. 8.

172. Martin, Eric W., et al. (eds.): *op. cit.,* p. 46.

173. Goodman, Louis S., and Gilman, Alfred: *op. cit.,* p. 39.

174. Gold, Harry (ed.): *Cornell Conferences on Therapy,* Vol. 4. Macmillan Publishing Co., Inc., New York, 1951, p. 1.

Additional Suggested Reading

Al-Anon Family Groups: *Living with an Alcoholic with the Help of Al-Anon.* AFGA, Inc., New York, 1973.

Allendorf, Elaine Erickson, and Keegan, M. Honor: "Teaching Patients About Nitroglycerin," *Am. J. Nurs.,* **75:**1168 (July) 1975.

B., Elaine, et al.: "Helping the Nurse Who Misuses Drugs," *Am. J. Nurs.,* **74:**1665, (Sept.) 1974.

Bagnell, Barbara: "Heroin: A Rising Tide?" *Addictions,* **19:**44, (Summer) 1972.

Bakwin, Harry, and Bakwin, Ruth M.: *Behavior Disorders in Children,* 4th ed. W. B. Saunders Co., Philadelphia, 1972.

Beard, J. D., and Knott, D. H.: "Fluid and Electrolyte Balance During Acute Withdrawal in Chronic Alcoholic Patients," *J.A.M.A.,* **204:**133, (Apr. 8) 1968.

Bell, Billie Simmons: *A Study of Medication Errors Made by Aged Clinic Patients.* Unpublished Master's Thesis, Texas Woman's University College of Nursing, Houston Center, 1970.

Bennett, B. V.: "Drug Distribution in Nursing Homes," *Nurs. Homes,* **20:**18, (May) 1971.

Blatherwick, Carol E.: "Understanding Glue Sniffing," *Can. J. Public Health,* **63:**272, (May–June) 1972.

Boyd, H. S., and Sisney, V. V.: "Immediate Self-Image Confrontation and Changes in Self-Concept," *J. Consult. Psychol.,* **31:**291, (No. 3) 1967.

Boyer, Catherine M.: "Caring for a Young Addict with Tetanus," *Am. J. Nurs.,* **74:**265, (Feb.) 1974.

Burkhalter, Pamela K.: *Nursing Care of the Al-*

coholic and Drug Abuser. McGraw-Hill Book Co., New York 1975.

Cahn, Sidney: *The Treatment of Alcoholics. An Evaluative Study.* Oxford University Press, New York, 1970.

Campbell, Charles M.: "Information System for a Short-Term Hospital," *Hospitals,* **38:**71, (Jan. 1) 1964.

Canadian Department of National Health and Welfare: *A Parents' Guide to Drug Abuse.* The Department, Ottawa, 1972.

Conn, Howard F.: *1976 Current Therapy.* W. B. Saunders Co., Philadelphia, 1976.

Csaky, T.: *Introduction to General Pharmacology.* Appleton-Century-Crofts, New York, 1969.

Cutting, Windsor Cooper: *Handbook of Pharmacology.* Appleton-Century-Crofts, New York, 1969.

Davis, William N.: "The Treatment of Drug Addiction: Some Comparative Observations," *Br. J. Addict.,* **65:**227, 1970.

Dilenno, J.: "Medicine or Myth," *J. Albert Einstein Med. Center,* **19:**57, (Summer) 1971.

Dilling, Walter James: *Clinical Pharmacology.* Bailliere, Tindall and Cassell, London, 1969.

Drugs of Abuse. US Department of Justice, Drug Enforcement Administration, Washington, D.C., 1976.

Edwards, Lillian G., and Barker, Kenneth N.: "Pharmacy Notes for Nurses," *Am. J. Nurs.,* **62:**68, (Oct.) 1962.

Falconer, Mary W., et al.: *The Drug, The Nurse, The Patient.* W. B. Saunders Co., Philadelphia, 1974.

Frederick, Calvin J., et al.: "Self-Destructive Aspects of Hard Core Addiction," *Arch. Gen. Psychiatry,* **28:**579, (Apr.) 1973.

Freedman, A. M.: "Narcotic Addiction; New Approaches," *Compr. Psychiatry,* **12:**587, (Nov.) 1971.

Fuchs, Victor R.: *Who Shall Live? Health, Economics, and Social Choice.* Basic Books, New York, 1974.

Gallant, Donald M., et al.: "The Revolving-Door Alcoholic," *Arch. Gen. Psychiatry,* **28:**633, (May) 1973.

Gallelli, Joseph F., et al.: "Role of the Hospital Pharmacist in the Operation of a Life Island," *Am. J. Hosp. Pharm.,* **25:**354, (July) 1968.

Garb, Solomon: *Pharmacology and Patient Care.* Springer Publishing Co., New York, 1966.

————: *Clinical Guide to Undesirable Drug Interactions and Interferences.* Springer Publishing Co., New York, 1971.

Geis, Gilbert: *Not the Law's Business? An Examination of Homosexuality, Abortion, Prostitution, Narcotics and Gambling in the United States.* (Crime and Delinquency Issues, a Monograph Series.) US Government Printing Office, Washington, D.C., 1972 (Pub. No. [HSM] 72–9).

Gimble, Josephine G.: "Oral Medications and the Older Patient," in *ANA Regional Clinical Conferences, 1967.* Appleton-Century-Crofts, New York, 1968.

Glicksberg, Kolman, and Jacobson, H. M.: "Study

of Chicago Industry Drug Abuse and Alcoholism," *Occup. Health Nurs.,* **20:**16, (Sept.) 1972.

Goth, Andres: *Medical Pharmacology.* C. V. Mosby Co., St. Louis, 1970.

Griffith, John D., et al.: "Dextroamphetamine— Evaluation of Psychomimetic Properties in Man," *Arch. Gen. Psychiatry,* **26:**97, (Feb.) 1972.

Grollman, Arthur: *Pharmacology and Therapeutics,* 7th ed. Lea & Febiger, Philadelphia, 1970.

Group for the Advancement of Psychiatry, Committee on Mental Health Services: *Drug Misuse.* Charles Scribner's & Sons, New York, 1971.

Groves, Barbara Bloom: *Attitudes and Behavior: Liking for Patients and Medication Errors.* Unpublished Master's Thesis, Texas Woman's University College of Nursing, Houston Center, 1970.

Hartley, Herbert L.: "Medication Errors in Hospitals," *Northwest Med.,* **68:**239, (Mar.) 1969.

Heen, Esther: *An Exploratory Study of the Nursing Role in a Methadone Maintenance Program.* Unpublished Master's Report, Yale University School of Nursing, New Haven, 1971.

Heller, William M.: "Packaging for Centralized Unit-Dose Dispensing," *Bull. Parenter. Drug Assoc.,* **17:**17, (July–Aug.) 1963.

Hoblitzelle, Lucy F.: *Pharmacology Applied to Patient Care.* F. A. Davis Co., Philadelphia, 1969.

Kaufman, Arthur, et al.: "Tranquilizer Control," *J.A.M.A.,* **221:**1504, (Sept. 25) 1972.

Kiene, Catherine L.: *Follow-up Study of Young Drug-Users After Participation in a Day Treatment Program.* Unpublished Master's Report, Yale University School of Nursing, New Haven, 1971.

Kline, N. S.: "The Future of Drugs and Drugs of the Future," *J. Social Issues,* **27:**73, (Mar.) 1971.

Kogan, Benjamin A.: *Health: Man in a Changing Environment.* Harcourt, Brace & World, New York, 1970.

Koscal, Jessie MacDonald: "How Patients Use a Logbook," *Am. J. Nurs.,* **74:**1307, (July) 1974.

Krantz, John Christian: *The Pharmacologic Principles of Medical Practice.* Williams & Wilkins Co., Baltimore, 1969.

Kubie, L. S.: "Some Aspects of the Significance to Psychoanalysis of the Exposure of a Patient to the Televised Audiovisual Reproduction of His Activities," *J. Nerv. Ment. Dis.,* **148:**301, (Apr.) 1969.

Laurence, Desmond Roger: *Clinical Pharmacology.* Little, Brown & Co., Boston, 1966.

Lembeck, Fred: *Pharmacological Facts and Figures.* Springer Publishing Co., New York, 1967.

Levine, David G., et al.: "A Special Program for Nurse Addicts," *Am. J. Nurs.,* **74:**1672 (Sept.) 1974.

Lober, Gertrude: "Sources of Drug Information," *Am. J. Nurs.,* **63:**101, (Dec.) 1963.

Long, Edna S.: "How to Survive Hospitalization," *Am. J. Nurs.,* **74:**486, (Mar.) 1974.

Louria, D. B.: *Overcoming Drugs.* McGraw-Hill Book Co., New York, 1971.

MacIlwain, William: *A Farewell to Alcohol.* Random House, New York, 1971.

Maloney, Elizabeth M.: "Remarks on the Physiological and Psychological Factors Influencing Addiction," in Anderson, Edith H., et al. (eds.): *Current Concepts in Clinical Nursing,* Vol. 4. C. V. Mosby Co., St. Louis, 1973.

Martin, Eric W., et al.: *Hazards of Medications.* J. B. Lippincott Co., Philadelphia, 1971.

Martin, William R., et al.: "Methadone—A Reevaluation," *Arch. Gen. Psychiatry,* **28:**286, (Feb.) 1973.

Metropolitan Life Insurance Company: *To Young Teens on Druggism,* and *to Parents About Drugs.* The Company, New York, 1972 (2 pamphlets).

Modell, W. (ed.): *Drugs in Current Use.* Springer Publishing Co., New York, 1969.

————: *Drugs of Choice.* C. V. Mosby Co., St. Louis, 1970–1971.

Moser, J.: *Problems and Programs Related to Alcohol and Drug Dependence in 33 Countries.* World Health Organization, Geneva, 1974.

Musser, Ruth D.: *Pharmacology and Therapeutics.* Macmillan Publishing Co., Inc., New York, 1969.

Nowlis, Helen: *Drugs on the College Campus.* Doubleday & Co., New York, 1969.

O'Keefe, Maureen Imelda: *A Nursing Approach to the Treatment of Drug Addicts: Evaluation of an Educational Program.* Unpublished Master's Report, Yale University School of Nursing, New Haven, 1971.

Parke, Dennis V.: *The Biochemistry of Foreign Compounds.* Pergamon Press, Elmsford, N.Y., 1968.

Rauffenbart, Mary: "Drug Administration by Automation," *Nurs. Clin. North Am.,* **1:**611, (Dec.) 1966.

Reibel, Eleanor Mannino: "Study to Determine the Feasibility of a Self-Medication Program for Patients at a Rehabilitation Center," *Nurs. Res.,* **18:**65, (Jan.–Feb.) 1969.

Richards, Louise, and Carroll, Eleanor: "Illicit Drug Use and Addiction in the United States," *Public Health Rep.,* **85:**1035, (Dec.) 1970.

Robson, John Michael: *Recent Advances in Pharmacology.* J. & A. Churchill, London, 1968.

Rodman, Morton Joseph: *Pharmacology and Drug Therapy in Nursing.* J. B. Lippincott Co., Philadelphia, 1968.

Root, Walter Stanton: *Physiological Pharmacology.* Academic Press, New York, 1967.

Serrano, R. S.: "Drug Security in Hospitals," *Superv. Nurse,* **3:**65, (Oct.) 1972.

Silverman, Milton M., and Lee, P. R.: *Pills, Profits and Politics.* University of California Press, Berkeley, 1974.

Sperandio, G. J., and Belcastro, P. F.: "The Clinical Pharmacist: Adviser, Teacher, Consultant," *Mod. Hosp.,* **108:**100, (Nov.) 1968.

Steiner, Claude: *Games Alcoholics Play: The Analysis of Life Scripts.* Grove Press, New York, 1971.

Sutherland, Violette Cutter: *A Synopsis of Pharmacology.* W. B. Saunders Co., Philadelphia, 1970.

Szasz, Thomas: "The Ethics of Addiction," *Am. J. Psychiatry,* **128:**541, (Nov.) 1971.

US Department of Health, Education, and Welfare: *Alcohol and Health.* US Government Printing Office, Washington, D.C., 1972.

US National Institute of Mental Health: *Alcohol Is a Drug.* US Government Printing Office, Washington, D.C., 1972.

Walter, Paul, et al.: "Drug Use and Life-Style Among 500 College Undergraduates," *Arch. Gen. Psychiatry,* **26:**92, (Jan.) 1972.

Whitehead, Paul C.: "Drug Education, Parents and the Information Gap," *Canada's Ment. Health,* **19:**13, (Nov.–Dec.) 1971.

Zinberg, Norman E.: "Heroin Use in Vietnam and the United States," *Arch. Gen. Psychiatry,* **26:**486, (May) 1972.

Gladys Nite
Catherine Temple
Virginia Henderson

CHAPTER 22

Parenteral Administration of Food, Fluids, and Medications

1. GENERAL CONSIDERATIONS IN PARENTERAL THERAPY

Definition. Parenteral therapy is a term for the giving of therapeutic agents, including foods, outside the alimentary tract (*para* = beside; *enteron* = intestine). By definition, inhalation and insufflation of drugs might fall under parenteral therapy, but the conventional use of the term is confined to the administration of drugs by the routes with the corresponding procedures given in the table on page 1149.

Parenteral fluids might conceivably be given in any but the most unyielding tissues. Those tissues (and areas) enumerated above are injected in current practice, although some procedures are rarely used.

Choice of route depends upon whether a local or systemic action is desired, how rapid an effect is needed, the amount of fluid to be injected, the nature of the fluid, whether blood vessels are accessible and suitable for injection, the wishes of the patient and his or her family, and the skills and preferences of the physician or operator.

As long as the heart beats, the lungs can exchange gases, and the kidneys eliminate waste products, a person can be nourished and live almost indefinitely if fed parenterally. Many irreversibly ill patients who are alive only in a vegetative state, or who may be suffering intensely, have their life prolonged for days, weeks, or months by artificial feeding.

When parenteral feeding is used to prolong death rather than life, the patient or the family should, in the opinion of the authors, have the right to ask that it be discontinued. This and related questions are discussed in greater depth in Chapter 50.

Health workers tend to take parenteral injections as an essential part of the therapeutic regimen and they may fail to realize that they always elicit some degree of fear or psychic trauma. They always involve some risk and physical injury. The psychologic and physical preparation of the patient is discussed later in this chapter, but it should be stressed that food and drugs should be given parenterally only if they cannot be safely swallowed and if they cannot be effectively absorbed from the gastrointestinal tract so they are therapeutically effective.

Materials Injected. Water, electrolytes, vitamins, sugars, digested proteins, whole blood and its component parts, so-called "blood substitutes," vaccines and protective sera, and many drugs used for diagnosis and therapy are all given parenterally. Some of the fluids most often given by each route are discussed under each procedure heading.

Fat, a necessary nutrient for effective parenteral therapy, continues to be studied in an attempt to produce a product that may be administered safely to the patient. In 1964, Dr. Oscar Schuberth[1] of Sweden reported their clinical experience with 2500 infusions with fat emulsions administered principally to surgical patients. After several years of research on animals, they found INTRALIPID (a trade name) prepared from soybean oil and egg phosphatides to have the fewest side effects. In 1400 infusions of this preparation the frequency of side effects was remarkably low and complications considered to be severe were not observed. K. E. D. Shuttleworth[2] of England, writing in the same year, notes that before preparations of fat emulsions may be considered safe for general use, the fat particles must be small and remain small, the emulsion must be sterile, nontoxic, and stable, and the body must be capable of utilizing the emulsion. In a comprehensive discussion of present knowledge of intravenous fat emulsions, Dr. Richard J. Jones[3] (1966) at the University of Chicago says there are two fat emulsions that have reached the stage of commercial availability: (1) in the United States a 15 per cent cottonseed oil emulsion is available and (2) Sweden now has available a 20 per cent soybean oil emulsion. He and others discuss many problems that await solution before these products are used generally. In conclusion he writes:

. . . it must still be said that artificial fat emulsions are not yet perfected to the point where they can be recommended for general use in patients requiring temporary parenteral nutrition. On the other hand, continued improvement over the last 20 years in the purity of the oils and the emulsifiers used has reduced the incidence and intensity of side effects, so that there is reason to hope that further understanding may soon lead to their ultimate inclusion.*

Some of the fluids most often given by each route are discussed under each procedure heading.

Dangers Common to All Injections. Whenever the skin is punctured or incised there is risk of *infection*. (This risk is reduced to a minimum when the equipment is prepared as for a surgical operation.) Many of the substances injected are foreign and often toxic so that the patient may have an *allergic* or *toxic reaction* to the treatment. This is likely to be most severe with intravenous and intra-arterial injections because they are most rapidly absorbed.

Tissue trauma is the inevitable accompaniment of an injection. If the treatment is given skillfully, tissue destruction is negligible and the wound heals readily, but it is possible to inflict a lasting, or fatal, injury with a needle. For example, a nerve can be injured, causing

serious damage, especially with intramuscular injections. There are a number of reports in the literature of sciatic nerve injury in infants and children resulting in paralysis of the lower extremity following intragluteal injections.[4,5] Although the newborn infant (especially the premature infant) is more likely to have this complication, any age group may be affected and only one injection is necessary, according to Mollie A. Combes, et al.[6] The exact cause of the damage, according to Richard K. Richards,[7] has not been determined; he says faulty technique, chemical irritation by the medication, or pressure are thought to be responsible. After conducting a number of experiments on guinea pigs, using a 10 per cent aqueous solution of amobarbital sodium, which was injected along the sciatic nerve, Richards concludes that intramuscular injection of a soluble barbiturate can produce nerve damage. These studies will be discussed in more detail under the procedure of intramuscular injections. Injury may result if the needle strikes a bone or if it is broken off and left embedded in the tissues. Irritating drugs should not be given subcutaneously as they can cause necrosis of the facia and skin; when given intramuscularly, they are more readily tolerated, but seem to cause less adverse effect when administered *slowly* intravenously, according to Stanley Alstead and J. Gordon MacArthur.[8]

Needles range in size from 27 gauge (the finest) to 13 gauge (the largest). The finest gauge that can be used effectively should be chosen in each case.

Choice of Equipment. Skin-cleaning equipment is needed for all injections; in some cases this includes articles for shaving the area. It is most convenient if the equipment is sterilized separately in units such as those shown in Figure 22-1. Waterproof disposable containers can be substituted to bring to the patient sponges, or applicators, already wet with the cleaning and disinfecting solutions.

Any preparation for parenteral use (including drugs) should be put up in a sealed plastic or glass ampule, vial, flask, or bottle from which the contents can be removed without contaminating it. (The solute and solvent are put in separate containers when the drug in solution is unstable.) Commercially prepared parenteral fluids in plastic or glass containers from which they are dispensed are one of the most important developments in modern asepsis and medical economy. Sterile disposable syringes, needles, and tubing have been brought within a possible cost range for most sections of the country, and, in many cases, their purchase represents a saving. When commercially prepared sets are not used a reservoir for the

---

* Jones, Richard J.: "Present Knowledge of Intravenous Fat Emulsions," *Nutr. Rev.,* 24:225, (Aug.) 1966.

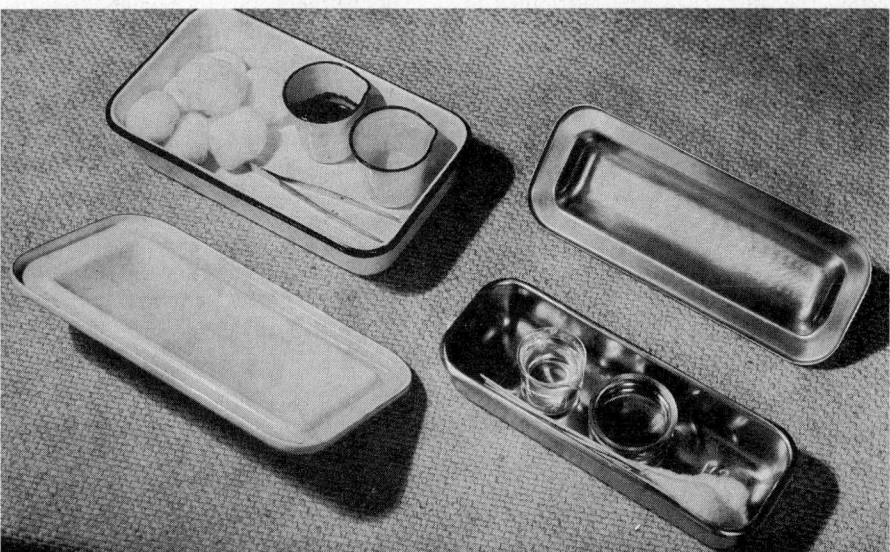

Figure 22-1. Skin-cleaning trays. Supplies are taken to the patient's unit in the amounts needed to avoid contamination of stock supplies. Trays and cups are sterilized after use and left sterile until needed when solutions, sponges, and a forceps or applicators are added.

solution must be provided. For small quantities (up to 60 ml or 2 oz) a syringe is used; for larger quantities a burette or flask. The burette (a glass cylinder from which the solution flows by gravity in an open system) is going into the discard for it necessitates transferring solutions from one container to another with the inherent danger of contamination. The Fenwal flask is a satisfactory reservoir because the solution can be both sterilized in it and dispensed from it. Varieties of flasks, tubing, and syringes are illustrated and discussed in Chapter 32. The importance of selecting equipment that will not react with the water, food, and drugs given parenterally was emphasized. When needles are used more than once it is convenient to sterilize them in glass vials or transparent envelopes so that they may be seen when selected and kept sterile if not used. Choice of needle, its length, gauge, and bevel, is discussed with each procedure.

Tubing, sufficient in length to reach without tension from the reservoir to the needle, is necessary. The transparent or semitransparent type is desirable. Disposable, presterilized plastic tubing is used increasingly. A heavy-walled pure gum rubber may be used but plastic tubing is rapidly replacing other varieties. Whatever the kind, it must be fitted with clamps to regulate the flow. The drip bulb is usually placed just below the reservoir so that the rate at which the solution flows can be regulated with exactness. The end of the tub-

ing to be attached to the needle is fitted with an "adapter."

Some operators feel more secure if the site of injection is surrounded with sterile towels and if they wear sterile rubber gloves when injecting veins, giving transfusions, or injecting the spinal canal. In most cases the operator works without gloves or from any sterile area other than that made by the inside of the covering of the sterile equipment. The patient's clothing and bedding should be protected by paper or cotton squares backed by waterproof paper, plastic, or rubber, if they are likely to be wet or soiled during the procedure.

Preparation of Equipment. Sterilization of needles, syringes, tubing, and solutions is discussed in Chapters 15 and 32. It was emphasized that such materials used for surgery should be sterilized with steam under pressure, or hot air at very high temperatures, to destroy spore forms of microorganisms. Tetanus and the gas-forming bacilli, common in nature, are particularly dangerous if they are injected into the tissues with a puncture wound. Sources of the organisms are thought to include medications, needle, syringe, personnel, and the patient. The problem is considered to be much greater in European countries than in the United States where 18 cases have been reported since 1936, according to Ronald B. Berggren and associates.[9] It is well known that the reported cases represent a small percentage of accidents that have occurred.[10-12] Epidemics of infectious hepatitis have been attributed to improperly disinfected syringes, needles, and surgical implements.[13,14] It is recognized that the many individuals who are infected by improperly sterilized equipment are not included in the reports found in the literature. Paul B. Beeson and Walsh McDermott say:

Inoculation of as little as 0.0004 ml of infected blood may transmit SH (serum hepatitis). Professional personnel (particularly those who work in chronic dialysis units) are subject to occupational exposure, and heroin addicts who share infected needles constitute a major fraction of the patients with icteric hepatitis.*

The first author has known a number of nurses who were infected by improperly sterilized needles and syringes. P. M. Inman and associates [15] report multiple abscesses in the arms of 12 patients seen over a period of 14 months; the source of infection was thought to be a batch of histamine solution which had become infected with the organism *Mycobacterium abscessus.*

For sterilizing equipment a pressure cooker may be used when an autoclave is not available. Boiling-water sterilization should not be used, even in homes, when steam under pressure is available. Sterilization with chemicals is uncertain and risky. Equipment for injections should be prepared in commercial laboratories or in hospital central supply services by technicians whenever possible. The use of sterile, assembled, disposable equipment prepared by reliable commercial firms gives maximum protection and is economical where labor costs are high. It is widely used in military medicine and in disasters. When assembled sterile disposable units are not available and it is necessary to protect a community by vaccinating thousands of persons in a short time, platinum needles that can be sterilized with a flame are used, and many injections are made with the same syringe. The need for immediate immunization may outweigh the risk of poor aseptic technique and in some cases it may be necessary to even use the same needle for many persons.

Psychologic Preparation of the Patient. Medical personnel, accustomed to seeing very painful treatments accepted by many patients with little visible protest, tend to forget man's natural fear of the unknown and the unwillingness of most persons to acknowledge this fear. The writers have seen strong men faint in anticipation of "a hypodermic." It is routine to give an infusion to any persons undergoing

major surgery, but to patients or their family it may be an indication that they are very ill. In an investigation by L. R. C. Haward of intramuscular injections administered manually and by a *mechanical injection* * on a group of 300 psychiatric patients, he concludes that the mechanical injection is superior to the manual injection as it is virtually painless and only one patient in five was aware that the injection had occurred. Haward believes this is a useful technique when injections have a strong emotional meaning for the patient; he says:

These findings have an important implication in physiological measurement other than that involving injections, mechanical or otherwise. They indicate that a carry-over effect operates so that if the patient believes a previously unpleasant situation is to be repeated, he will react relative to his preconceptions and not merely to the real situation.†

The relationship between the nurse and patient, according to Klaus W. Berblinger,[16] can influence the action of a drug. He says, for example, that his early experience with corticosteroid hormones given by "an aggressive" physician produced a rise in blood pressure but when injected by a relaxed, permissive resident caused the blood pressure to fall. The giving of a drug should be viewed as a means of communicating with a patient.

The purpose and nature of the treatment should be explained to the patient and his or her cooperation elicited. (An exception to this generalization is in times of an emergency when time is of the essence.) Physicians may prefer to do this themselves, especially with the more complex procedures, but, if not, the nurse assumes the responsibility. The explanation is given before patients are faced with the syringe or transfusion set; and even if they appear to be unconscious it is wise to assume that they can hear an explanation. Patients should understand the treatment and be willing and ready to submit to it; they should know how much discomfort they can expect. When feasible, pain may be minimized with a cooling spray (such as ethyl chloride or "Formula A" which consists of 15 per cent dichlorodifluoromethane and 85 per cent trichloromonofluoromethane [17]) or other local anesthetics. Substances like *hyaluronidase*, that

* Beeson, Paul B., and McDermott, Walsh (eds.): *Cecil-Loeb Textbook of Medicine*, 13th ed. W. B. Saunders Co., Philadelphia, 1971, p. 1390.

* Palmer Injectors Ltd., Torlundy, Fort William, Scotland.
† Haward, L. R. C.: "Some Psychological Aspects of Intra-Muscular Injections," *J. Ment. Sci.*, **108:**853, (Nov.) 1962. The mechanical injector consists of a pistol-type body carrying a syringe-loaded carriage operated by a trigger. When the trigger is released, the needle penetrates the tissues to a specified depth and the contents of the syringe is released.

reduce pain by speeding absorption, are also used. Restraint seldom is needed when this approach is used. For any treatment involving fear, discomfort, or pain, tension is reduced by keeping the patient warm and relaxed in a sitting or recumbent position.

Preparation of the Skin at the Site of Injection. Skin disinfection was discussed at length in Chapter 14 and will not be treated in detail here. An injection of a needle is a minor surgical procedure, and the area should be prepared as for surgery. A cleaning agent, such as alcohol 70 per cent, ether, or water and a detergent, should be followed by a skin disinfectant, such as tincture of iodine or benzalkonium (Zephiran). Iodine preparations are available that retain all bacterial properties of iodine but eliminate the staining and toxic properties which were formerly so troublesome. Newer preparations include Isodine, Betadine, and Wescodyne. Thomas A. Koons and George M. Boyden [18] recommend them and deplore the use of 70 per cent alcohol as it does not control spore-forming organisms; they report a case of gas gangrene following preparation of skin for an injection with 70 per cent ethyl alcohol. T. C. Dann [19] questions the usual skin preparation for a different reason. He reports that there have been no infections following over 5000 injections without preparing the skin at the Medical Center of the University College of Swansea, Singleton Park, Swansea, Wales.

Applicators or sponges and forceps, with which the disinfectant is applied, should be sterile. Disinfectants that stain clothing, such as iodine, should be removed when the treatment is over.

Restraint of the Patient. It is obviously desirable to immobilize a joint, the elbow for example, if a needle is inserted into the arm, but only irrational adults are restrained for injections. Even with infants and very small children restraints are avoided whenever possible.

Technique for Injecting the Needle. Whenever a needle is injected the object is to get the needle into the intended locale with minimum discomfort for the patient and minimum injury to body tissues. Almost everyone, brave or cowardly, is tense as they wait for an injection. A sharp needle injected skillfully *into relaxed tissue* is so unexpectedly painless, however, that the patient is often waiting for the prick when the treatment is over. There are various ways of evoking relaxation. A diverting thought, a deep breath, or a light blow or pinch near the site of injection will usually relax the patient. For subcutaneous and intramuscular injections a successful technique is

that of striking the patient sharply with the hand, then immediately inserting the needle. A similar effect results from grasping the area to be injected between the thumb and forefinger, or pinching the area. The tissues grasped in this fashion make a firm cushion, which the needle punctures easily. The second method is safer with thin patients, for it draws the muscle away from the bone and makes striking the bone less likely. Injecting the needle quickly, as one throws a dart, minimizes the discomfort.

Injecting needles between the layers of the skin, into veins, serous-lined cavities, and bones present special problems. While the nurse does not ordinarily make these injections, the techniques are discussed briefly under the procedures involved, and more and more workers are learning intravenous techniques. Soldiers are taught to give each other life-saving parenteral therapy in emergencies. Technicians in laboratories acquire great skill in finding and entering veins. For these reasons there is a tendency to overlook the potential hazards of trauma, infection, and chemical poisoning from intravenous injections.

The angle of the needle and the depth to which it should be inserted depend upon what lies between the skin at the site of injection and the spot in the tissues that the needle point should reach when the needle is in place. Knowledge of anatomy and physiology, judgment as to the amount of fat lying in the subcutaneous tissue, and experience all contribute to making successful injections.

Factors That Favor Absorption. As defined by Andres Goth,[20] absorption is a process by which a drug is made available to the body's fluids of distribution. The rate of absorption depends on solubility of the preparation and the blood flow through the area. It is obvious that fluids injected into the bloodstream will most rapidly find their way to all parts of the body. Likewise substances injected into the muscles or into red bone marrow are quickly distributed by the abundant blood supply in these tissues. When fluids are deposited in the subcutaneous tissues, they are taken up less readily because there are relatively fewer blood vessels than in the muscles. Fluids may accumulate in subcutaneous tissues to a dangerous degree. By any route, however, liquids may be given more rapidly than they can be absorbed.

Application of heat over the site of the injection or the use of warm solutions has been recommended. Microfilms have proven that heat dilates blood vessels and that the effect on the capillaries lasts for hours. August K. Krogh [21] has shown that dilated capillaries are more permeable, and it follows that their capacity for absorption is increased. Raising the temperature of the solution, therefore, within the limits of physiologic tolerance, should increase the rate of absorption. Many devices for maintaining the temperature of the solution at the desired point have been described. In some methods heat is applied around the reservoir; in others, around the tubing. Hot-water bottles, heating pads, and other devices have been used as the source of heat. Cardiac arrest has occurred following rapid massive injection of cold blood.[22] At the present time blood is most often warmed by the heat exchange coils (see Fig. 22-2) when it is thought necessary; a microwave blood warmer is under investigation.[23,24] As most intravenous fluids are stored at room temperature and few require refrigeration, the temperature of intravenous fluids (other than blood) is rarely significant.

In spite of the probability of hastening the absorption by warmth the practice of heating parenteral fluids is disappearing. With all known methods it is time consuming and with most methods uncertain. A solution that is heated in a reservoir drops from 2.3° to 9°C (5° to 20°F) according to room temperature and other conditions, as it flows through the tubing. Heating the tubing may result in dangerously hot injections.

Massage is believed to increase the local blood supply and increase the rate of absorption. Most authorities recommend massage as a factor in promoting absorption. It is usual to follow a hypodermic or an intramuscular injection with gentle massage of the area.

The rate of absorption differs with the *composition of the fluid* injected. In parenteral therapy, especially intravenous and intra-arterial therapy, it is well to bear in mind Claude Bernard's thesis that all vital mechanisms of the body have but one object—to preserve constant conditions of life in the internal environment.[25] In sections of this text dealing with nutrition, fluid and electrolyte balance, and emotional stability, it is pointed out that the aim of therapy is to maintain a balance of fluids and electrolytes (solutes) in all fluid compartments. See Chapter 10, where these concepts are discussed. Whatever interferes too greatly with the equilibrium of body fluids endangers life. When a solution with a lower content of solutes than is present in plasma and interstitial fluid is injected into the tissues, the body cells take in some of the water (solvent) and give off some of their electrolytes (solutes) to equalize the hydro-

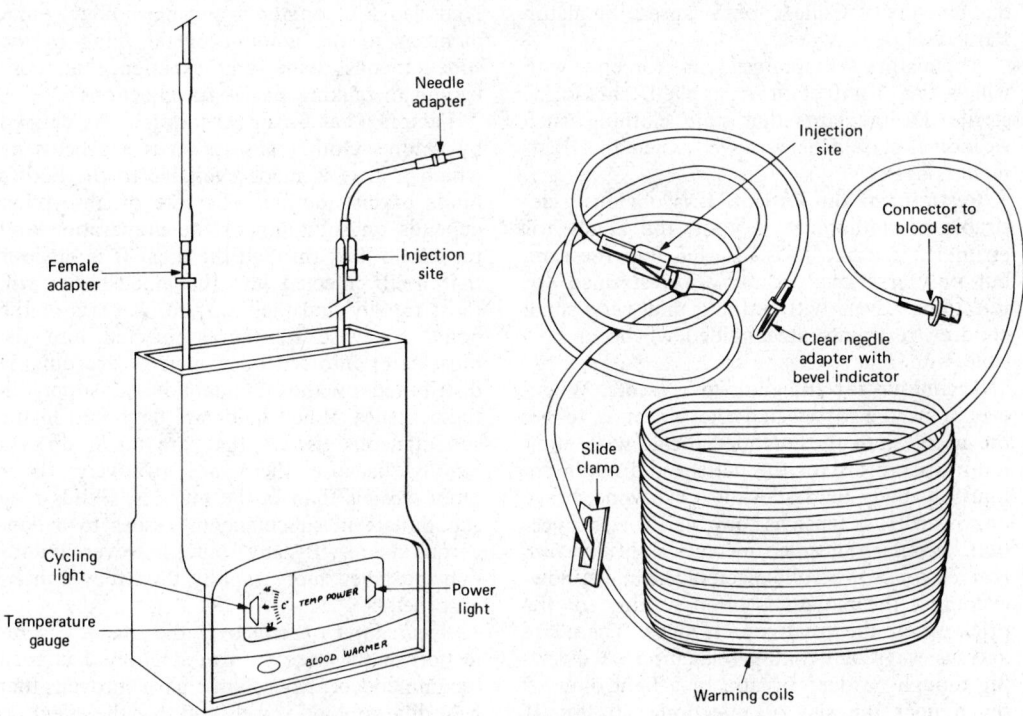

Figure 22-2. Blood warmer and blood-warming coils. The water bath is constantly cycled between 39°C and 40°C. Blood entering the coil at 2°C to 6°C will exit the coil at 35°C ± 2°. (Courtesy of McGaw Laboratories, Glendale, Calif.)

static pressure inside the cells and in the fluids surrounding them. Likewise when a solution with a higher content of solutes than is found in the plasma and interstitial tissue is injected, the cells give off some of their water content and take in some of the solutes to equalize the pressure inside the cells and in the fluids surrounding them. This process of osmosis (the passage of water molecules through a membrane) and diffusion (the passage of solid molecules through a membrane), if carried far enough, can destroy cells by shrinking them as they give off water, or by bursting them as they take in more water than the cell membrane can support. A solution is spoken of as isotonic when it exerts the same osmotic pressure as the blood; hypertonic when it exerts a greater osmotic pressure; and hypotonic when it exerts a lesser osmotic pressure. Hypertonic solutions can shrink, or crenate, cells and sclerose tissues; hypotonic solutions can hemolyze cells ("lake" the blood) and cause generalized edema. Fortunately, a cell's membrane has a selective action and will allow some molecules to pass through and not others. The exchange of solutes and water that goes on between the cell and its environment is constant and, within limits, physiologic. If given time, a cell can adjust itself to many changes in its fluid environment. Generally speaking, however, fluids that are isotonic, or nearly so, with the blood and interstitial fluid are most easily absorbed.

The passage of drugs across body membranes is a complex process; additional references are included at the end of this chapter for those who are interested in further study of the subject.[26-28]

Absorption can be markedly increased by the addition of a substance that tends to break down the natural resistance of the tissues to the injected fluid. Research of the past 40 years has established the fact that extracts of certain mammalian organs, leeches, some bacteria, and snake venom contain a "spreading factor." *Hyaluronidase* is the name given this enzyme because it breaks down, or depolymerizes, hyaluronic acid, a mucopolysaccharide which is the main component of the intercellular ground substance, or cement substance, of tissues. Karl Meyer[29] says hyaluronic acid "holds cells together in a jelly-like matrix and serves as a lubricant and shock absorber in joints." Because hyaluronidase breaks down this matrix, injections of it have proved useful as an accompaniment of hypodermoclysis solutions. It also increases the diffusion and absorption of other injected substances such as penicillin and speeds the absorption of solutions of diagnostic agents. When injected directly into local accumulations of transudates

of blood, hyaluronidase facilitates reabsorption. It has been incorporated in local anesthetic solutions to facilitate distribution of the anesthetic agent but it is little used at present because of its cost and the following disadvantages: When hyaluronidase is used there is a higher rate of systemic reactions to the anesthetic drugs and the success rate is not increased when it is used in nerve blocks in which the anesthetic is confined within a fascial plane. Hyaluronidase injected in areas that are infected or cancerous greatly increases the danger of spreading the infection or malignancy.[30]

Hyaluronidase is available for clinical use as a pyrogen-free extract of bovine testes. It is on the market as a powder or stabilized solution in ampoules containing either 150 or 1500 N.F. units. Dosage is always prescribed by the physician, and the nurse's responsibility is the same here as in other medication. Fortunately, it seems to be nontoxic. Improvement in its preparation is said to have eliminated occasional allergic reactions. When hyaluronidase is given with small quantities of another drug it may be drawn into the same syringe or injected first into the selected site; when given in hypodermoclysis it may be introduced into the tubing with a needle immediately after the fluid starts flowing into the tissues, or it may be incorporated with the solution in the reservoir. The bulk of fluid entering the tissues in hypodermoclysis exerts enough pressure to stimulate absorption; when hyaluronidase is injected into a hematoma a pressure bandage should be applied over the area.

More specific discussion of the major types of injections follows. The sequence chosen has nothing to do with the rate of absorption by the different types. It seems more reasonable to discuss first the procedures most commonly used, "the hypodermic," and the intramuscular injection. The chapter should be read as a whole because in each section there is an assumption that the reader is familiar with the preceding sections.

2. SUBCUTANEOUS MEDICATION OR HYPODERMIC INJECTION (INCLUDING INSULIN ADMINISTRATION)

Definition. *Hypodermic* is derived from *hypo* (under) and *derma* (skin). In common parlance and medical practice the term "hypodermic" is used for the introduction of a small quantity of fluid into the subcutaneous tissues with a needle.

Therapeutic Uses. A drug is given by "hypodermic" when (1) the patient cannot or will not swallow a drug or when it is dangerous for him or her to attempt it; (2) the person is vomiting or having gastric suction; (3) the action of the drug is destroyed by secretions of the gastrointestinal tract or is irritating to the tract; and (4) the drugs act more quickly or effectively if absorbed from the subcutaneous tissues.

Selection of Method. The importance of sterility for all injection equipment has already been stressed, and the best method of *sterilization* discussed. Maximum safety probably lies in the commercially prepared ready-to-use disposable unit, of which there is an increasing number available; some of these include *Tubex, Isojet, Parentopak,* and *Monojet.* Disposable injection units were first developed for military uses, for example *Ampin,* but were found to be equally suitable for civilian medicine.[31] Robert R. Cadmus [32] reports a substantial savings when commercially prepared ready-to-use disposable units were substituted for a common method of hypodermic injection in one of Cleveland's large hospitals. Most of the units in use employ the "cartridge-type" injection device such as found in the *Tubex.* Over 80 per cent of all injections of 2½ ml and under that are used in hospitals are available in prefilled *Tubex* units which consist of a glass cartridge and needle [33] (see Fig. 22-3). The cartridge is placed in a metal syringe with cut-out sides that allow full visi-

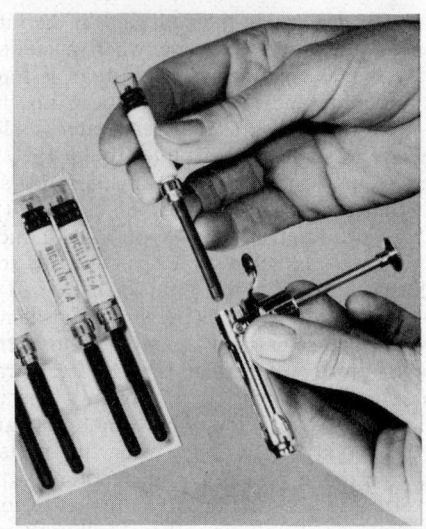

Figure 22-4. Disposable closed injection system. Sterile cartridge-needle unit contains medication which is placed in hypodermic syringe and ready for instant use. (Courtesy of Wyeth Laboratories, Philadelphia, Pa.)

bility of calibrations. By pressing the plunger after the needle is inserted the solution is made to flow into the tissue. Some companies use an all-plastic prefilled disposable syringe (see Fig. 22-4). Kenneth N. Barker and associates [34] report two studies of "nurse acceptance evaluation" of some prefilled disposable injection devices mentioned above. After determining the characteristics nurses thought were important and how they ranked currently available devices, Roehr Products Company designed an all-plastic disposable syringe which was prefilled. This device was used by 42 nurses, each giving 40 injections; important conclusions included the ease of maintaining sterility. We believe the use of the disposable units will certainly increase since their advantages far outweigh any disadvantages they may have. As this type of unit is not used in all institutional or private practice and all drugs are not available in the disposable units, nurses must be familiar with other methods of giving hypodermic injections. The jet injection technique is discussed on page 1180.

Sterilization in the central supply service of an assembled syringe and needle put up in a glass or metal tube is probably, next to the commercially prepared disposable unit, the method of choice. Drugs in multiple (or single) dosage in rubber-stoppered vials are prepared commercially and in hospital pharmacies. The difficulty of sterilizing the rubber stoppers, through which the drug is drawn

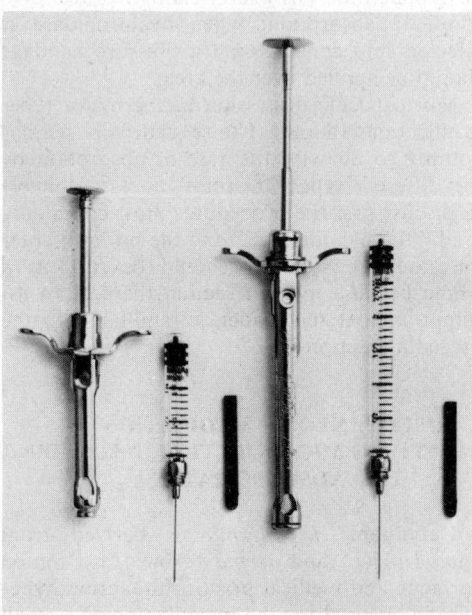

Figure 22-3. Hypodermic syringes, 1- and 2-ml size, and prefilled sterile "cartridge-needle units." (Courtesy of Wyeth Laboratories, Philadelphia, Pa.)

with the needle and syringe, makes this type of container less safe than the single-dosage sealed glass ampule. Hospital pharmacies in increasing numbers assume the responsibility for preparing the hypodermic so that it is ready for use. Sister Mary Hiltrudis Chlebik [35] describes the use of this method in an 80-bed hospital, emphasizing its accuracy and safety. When it is necessary to combine drugs in an injection, compatibility of the drugs must be considered; Jan N. Bair, a pharmacist, says:

The hospital pharmacist seems to be the only professional in the hospital environment who is in a position to provide the needed answer to the incompatibility problem.*

When vials or ampules are not used, *preparation of the solution* is a problem because the drug is in tablet form. Lack of moisture in the bottle discourages the growth of bacteria, but it can hardly be claimed that the contents of a bottle that is opened repeatedly remains sterile. Tablets must be mixed with a solvent, but the solution should not be boiled afterward because heating might alter its chemical composition. While tablets can be handled in such a way as to reduce contamination of the solution to a minimum, hypodermic injections prepared with tablets are never free from microorganisms. Sterile physiologic saline and sterile distilled water are commonly used as solvents. Arthur Grollman [36] suggests normal saline or Ringer's solution instead of plain water whenever possible; Alstead and MacArthur [37] note that sterile water or physiologic saline may be used and that isotonic solution causes little discomfort. Burdellis L. Carter,[38] in a study of 40 young healthy women, found that injections of distilled water produced more discomfort than those of normal saline; however, both types of solution caused some discomfort. When commercially prepared solutions are not available —as in the home—boiled tap water may be used. There is some question as to whether minerals in natural waters combine with the drug to make it less active or irritating. About 2 ml (30 m) of the solvent is ordinarily used.

The site of injection may be almost any of the less sensitive areas of the body where no bones or large blood vessels are near the surface. The outer aspect of the arms and thighs fulfill the requirements and are convenient sites, but muscular areas of the body wall may be used also. When a patient is getting hypodermics frequently, the sites of

the injection should be rotated and an attempt made to avoid puncturing the same spot twice.

Preparation of the skin was discussed in Chapter 14 and again on page 1167.

Insertion of the needle is described in general terms on page 1167. For subcutaneous injections the needle should be held at an angle of about 90 deg. and inserted quickly, as a dart is thrown, to the depth of 1½ cm (½ in.). If the individual is obese the needle can be inserted as much as 2 cm or more; if he or she is emaciated an injection 1 cm in depth will take the drug into the areolar tissue.

Factors affecting the rate of absorption are numerous. There is general agreement on some points but not on all. Drugs given in aqueous solution are absorbed more rapidly than those given in oil or wax suspensions. When physicians want to slow the rate of absorption so that the drug will be available to the body over a period of hours (as with penicillin or insulin), they prescribe it in an oil or wax suspension. This is an example of the principle that the rate of absorption is influenced by the solubility of the preparation. Authorities are in general agreement that the amount of blood flow through the area injected also influences the speed of absorption. For example, Goth [39] says when peripheral circulatory failure is present, absorption may be very slow from a subcutaneous site. Carl J. Wiggers [40] cites experiments demonstrating the presence of drugs in the thoracic duct two minutes after they (in aqueous solution) were injected subcutaneously. John J. R. MacLeod [41] says that methylene blue injected in the thigh appears in the urine before it is seen in the thoracic duct. While it is evident that the drug gains access immediately to the blood and lymph circulations, it is probably true that massage and heat, both of which dilate blood vessels, hasten absorption. When irritating drugs are given, gentle massage and the application of heat may reduce discomfort caused by the continued presence of the drug in the tissues.

Equipment. Because hypodermic injections are often given in an emergency, with an immediate response the prime object, it is particularly important that the equipment be ready for use. Obviously, a presterilized assembled unit, such as the *Tubex* or a disposable syringe and needle is most satisfactory. When these are not available, the syringe with needle attached that has been sterilized by steam under pressure is the best substitute. Any containers or wrapping for a needle should protect the point. Extra needles in glass tubes should be available. Ampoules, files, and sterile paper or gauze squares, to protect the hands in breaking ampoules, should be stored

* Bair, Jan N.: "A Brief Review of Drug Compatibility and Stability Literature," *Am. J. Hosp. Pharm.,* **23:**346, (July) 1966.

nearby. If tablets are used they, too, should be kept with the other articles used in giving hypodermics. Solvents should be sterilized in small flasks with a rubber cover through which the liquid can be drawn, or a cap that can be replaced without contaminating the lip of the flask. Sterile sponges, handling forceps, and a skin disinfectant complete the essential equipment unless tablets are used; then it is necessary to have a small flat-bottomed receptacle in which the tablet can be dissolved, such as tiny waxed paper cups, a birdseed dish, or a saltcellar. Small packages may be made for individual injections containing a dish, the sponges needed, and a small square of waxed paper on which the prepared "hypodermic" may be carried to the bedside. Very large cotton applicators in a waterproof paper envelope, in which they may be carried wet with the skin disinfectant, are a convenience in keeping the applicators uncontaminated and the bedside table clean and dry. The practice of embedding the needle in an alcohol sponge is undesirable because the discomfort of the injection is increased.

In some hospitals and in home nursing it may be necessary to boil the syringe and needle and even the solvent, but this practice is becoming increasingly obsolete as commercially presterilized disposable syringes and needles may be purchased at most corner drugstores. In a very few places chemical disinfection of syringes and needles is practiced, but this should be considered the last resort. When boiling a hypodermic syringe and needle or when sterilizing them in a pressure cooker, it is convenient to support them in a sieve. The point of the needle in the sieve swings free and so is protected from blunting. Attempts to sterilize a needle in a spoon over the flame from a lamp should be discouraged.

Syringes (except disposal plastic ones) should be made of heat-resistant alkaline-free glass. A small-gauge needle should be used whenever possible because it punctures the skin more easily than a large needle and causes less pain and tissue damage. Most subcutaneous needles have a moderately long bevel or cutting edge. Some operators believe that the needle with a lateral bore causes least discomfort. The length of the needle for ordinary subcutaneous injections should be about 2 cm (¾ inch) and the gauge 25 or 24. A larger gauge is necessary when oily drugs that do not readily pass through a fine needle are administered; longer needles are used when it is desirable to inject the drugs deep in the tissues. *Safety or security* needles have a bead-like construction just below the juncture of the shaft and the hub. The needle is most likely to break at this point, and the bead keeps the broken-off shaft from getting lost in the tissues.

Suggested Procedure. If a sterilized assembled disposable unit is available, take this from the cabinet in which it is stored, observing the usual precautions to see that the drug and its dosage are correct. Carry the unit on a small tray to the bedside with a waterproof paper or envelope containing sponges or applicators, one or more wet with the skin antiseptic. After cleaning the skin remove the guard over the needle, release the solution according to the directions of the manufacturer of the unit, and after striking, or grasping, the area insert the needle as a dart at an angle of about 90 deg. (The patient is less likely to feel the prick if diverted, and if he or she is not watching the process.) Inject the solution slowly. Remove the needle quickly while exerting pressure over the area with a dry sponge; maintain the pressure for a few seconds and rub the area gently.

When a sterile assembled needle and syringe are used with the drug in an ampule (see Fig. 22-5), collect these articles and the skin-cleaning equipment. Warm, but do not heat, the drug if it is a thick oil or suspension that cannot be drawn readily through the needle. Twirling the vial or ampoule between the palms of the hands both warms and mixes a suspension. Work quickly and give the injection immediately; otherwise, the drug will stiffen and "lock" the syringe. Clean the neck of the ampoule with alcohol. Collect all the drug in the bottom of the ampoule by tapping the tip until the liquid leaves it. File the neck of the ampoule and break it, protecting the fingers with a sterile gauze or paper square; then withdraw the contents, or part of the contents of the ampule, as prescribed, through the needle into the syringe. If the drug is in a rubber-stoppered vial, clean the rubber stopper. Draw into the syringe (see Fig. 22-6) as much air as drug to be withdrawn from the vial. Insert the needle into the vial cap and force the air into the liquid; the pressure of this air makes it easy to withdraw the drug from the vial. Before giving the medication see that all but a small bubble of air is expelled from the syringe. This air bubble will rise to the surface of the liquid as the hypodermic is given and, being injected last, tends to fill the channel left by the needle as it is removed. Theoretically, this prevents leakage of drugs through the skin opening, and the air is soon absorbed. In carrying the equipment to the patient, protect the needle with a sterile, dry gauze or cotton sponge.

When a tablet is to be used, the solution is prepared in the following manner: Pour a small amount of saline solution into the mixing receptacle; draw up 2 ml (30 m), or the desired amount, into the syringe and discard what remains. Drop the tablet into the vessel and discharge the saline solution from the syringe upon it; draw the solution back and forth in the syringe until the tablet is dissolved; fill the syringe and attach the needle.

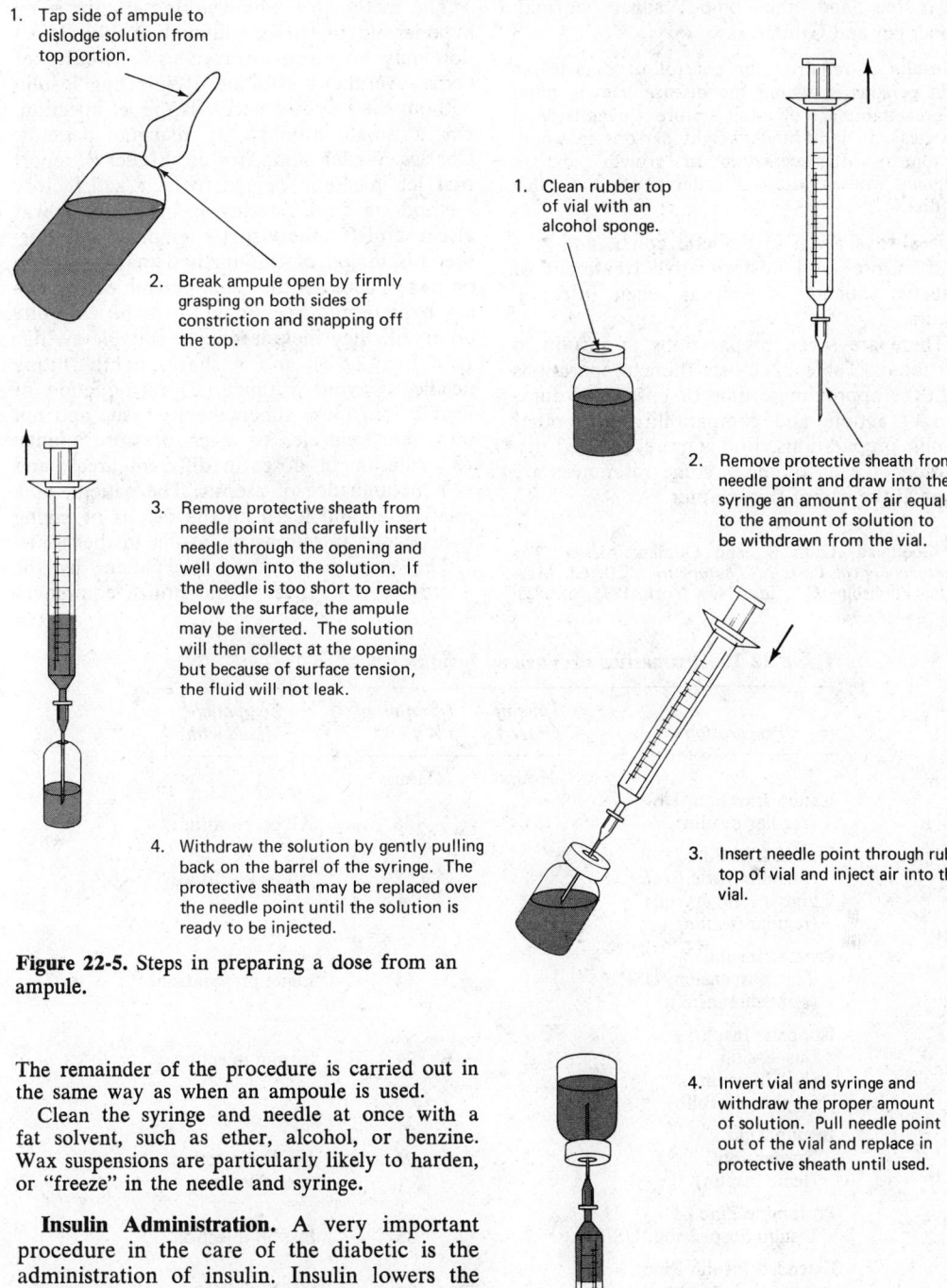

1. Tap side of ampule to dislodge solution from top portion.

2. Break ampule open by firmly grasping on both sides of constriction and snapping off the top.

1. Clean rubber top of vial with an alcohol sponge.

2. Remove protective sheath from needle point and draw into the syringe an amount of air equal to the amount of solution to be withdrawn from the vial.

3. Remove protective sheath from needle point and carefully insert needle through the opening and well down into the solution. If the needle is too short to reach below the surface, the ampule may be inverted. The solution will then collect at the opening but because of surface tension, the fluid will not leak.

3. Insert needle point through rubber top of vial and inject air into the vial.

4. Withdraw the solution by gently pulling back on the barrel of the syringe. The protective sheath may be replaced over the needle point until the solution is ready to be injected.

Figure 22-5. Steps in preparing a dose from an ampule.

The remainder of the procedure is carried out in the same way as when an ampoule is used.

Clean the syringe and needle at once with a fat solvent, such as ether, alcohol, or benzine. Wax suspensions are particularly likely to harden, or "freeze" in the needle and syringe.

Insulin Administration. A very important procedure in the care of the diabetic is the administration of insulin. Insulin lowers the blood sugar, promotes combustion of carbohydrates, and prevents acidosis. It is not a cure, or a substitute for strict regulation of the diet, but it is an aid of immeasurable value in arresting the disease, in prolonging life, and in restoring the patient to health more quickly. It is given when the patient's own insulin production is so deficient that regulation of the diet alone is not enough to keep the urine

4. Invert vial and syringe and withdraw the proper amount of solution. Pull needle point out of the vial and replace in protective sheath until used.

Figure 22-6. Steps in preparing a dose from a vial.

sugar-free and the blood sugar normal. Goodman and Gilman say:

Insulin is required for control of diabetes in most persons in whom the disease has its onset before attainment of adult stature (juvenile-onset diabetes), in most underweight persons in whom it appears after cessation of growth, and in pregnant women whose disorder is not controlled by diet.*

It is always given in diabetic coma, and it is used in pre- and postoperative treatment of diabetic patients as well as when infection occurs.

There are seven preparations of insulin in use today. Table 22-1 lists these preparations with the approximate time of onset and duration of action, and compatibility with other insulin preparations. For a more detailed discussion of each of these, some references are given at the end of this chapter.[42-44]

* Goodman, Louis S., and Gilman, Alfred: *The Pharmacological Basis of Therapeutics*, 5th ed. Macmillan Publishing Co., Inc., New York, 1975, p. 1525.

The method of administering insulin is by hypodermic injection, although insulin injection may be given intravenously in cases of coma. Another technique of injecting insulin without the use of a needle is the jet injection. On a small number of diabetic patients, Charles Weller and Morton Linder[45] report that jet injection seemed to be a satisfactory method of administering insulin and it was also useful for the visually handicapped. Further discussion of this method may be found on page 1180. All the usual precautions in giving hypodermic injections are to be carefully observed; they include: (1) a suitable syringe (see Fig. 22-7) and a sharp, tightly fitting needle to avoid trauma; (2) introduction of insulin into loose subcutaneous tissue and not into skin, muscle, or over pressure points; (3) rotation of doses in different areas; and (4) maintenance of asepsis. The patient, or a relative, should learn all the details of giving hypodermic injections of insulin in the home.

The procedure taught the patient by the doctor or the nurse should utilize equipment

Table 22-1. Properties of Various Insulins * ‡

Preparation	Time of Onset †	Duration of Action †	Compatible Mixed with
	Hours	Hours	
Insulin Injection, USP (regular insulin)	1	6	All preparations
Insulin Injection, USP "Insulin made from zinc-insulin crystals" (regular insulin)	1	8	All preparations
Prompt Insulin Zinc Suspension, USP (semilente insulin)	1	14	Lente preparations
Isophane Insulin Suspension (NPH insulin, isophane insulin)	2	24	Insulin injection
Insulin Zinc Suspension (lente insulin)	2	24	Insulin injection, semilente
Protamine Zinc Insulin Suspension, USP	7	36	Insulin injection
Extended Insulin Zinc Suspension, USP (ultralente insulin)	7	36	Insulin injection, semilente

* A 2–3:1 mixture of regular insulin and protamine zinc insulin behaves essentially like isophane insulin; a less than 2:1 mixture of regular insulin and protamine zinc insulin possess essentially the properties of protamine zinc insulin.

† These figures are not absolute; they are representative and may vary over a wide range, depending on the dose administered and the individual patient.

‡ Goodman, Louis S., and Gilman, Alfred: *The Pharmacological Basis of Therapeutics*, 5th ed. Macmillan Publishing Co., Inc., New York, 1975, p. 1517. Adaptation of Table 71-1.

Figure 22-7. Various insulin syringes. Styles and colors of marking on insulin syringes are standardized, and only one scale appears on "official" syringes approved by the American Diabetes Association. Markings are red for U-40 insulin, green for U-80, and either amber or black for U-100. These colors correspond to the colors used on commercial insulin preparations, and to avoid dangerous medication errors, the appropriate syringe should always be used. (Courtesy of Eli Lilly & Co., Indianapolis, Ind.)

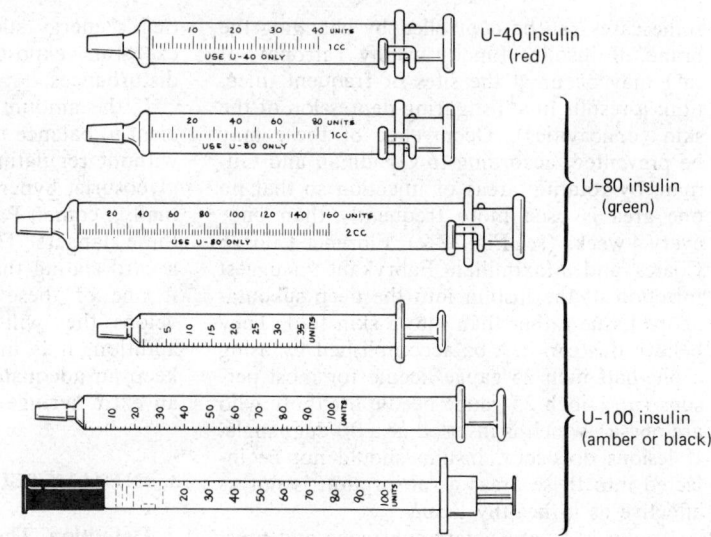

that is readily available, and the method employed should be simply and fully explained and demonstrated by the nurse. Then the patient should demonstrate that he or she can carry out the procedure accurately and safely (see Fig. 22-8). The method of preparing a hypodermic in the home that is described on page 1172 applies to the administration of insulin. Alcohol is usually advocated to clean the skin and the rubber stopper of the insulin vial.

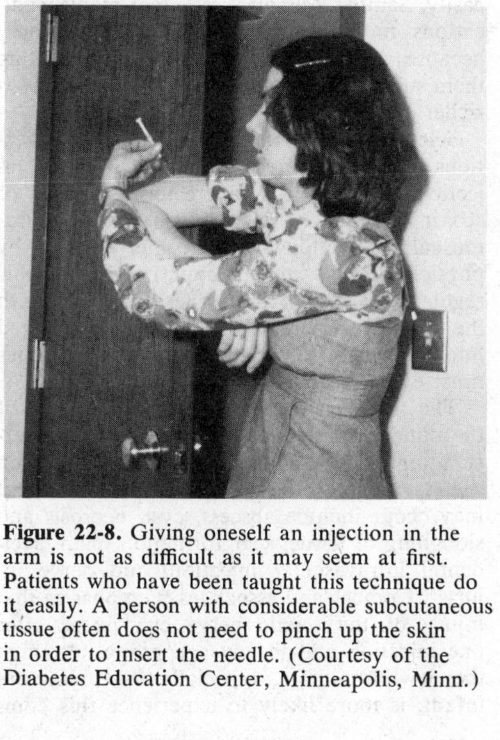

Figure 22-8. Giving oneself an injection in the arm is not as difficult as it may seem at first. Patients who have been taught this technique do it easily. A person with considerable subcutaneous tissue often does not need to pinch up the skin in order to insert the needle. (Courtesy of the Diabetes Education Center, Minneapolis, Minn.)

Medicated rubbing alcohol, 70 per cent, can be bought in any drugstore and is a satisfactory preparation. A device for holding the insulin syringe for automatically injecting the needle is available for persons who find it difficult to inject the needle into their tissues.

Because protamine zinc insulin is a suspension, the vial must be rotated gently or rolled between the hands before use to ensure an even distribution of the insulin particles and thus to ensure accurate dosage. Formation of foam on the surface should be avoided and, if present, should not be drawn into the syringe and considered part of the dose. Although protamine zinc insulin is said to be a stable compound if kept at room temperature, authorities recommend storing all insulin preparations in a cool place such as a refrigerator. However, if a diabetic is traveling and it is not possible to keep the vial of insulin in a refrigerator, there should be no anxiety, especially when the insulin is self-administered by the patient at least once daily. (This would result in emptying the vial within a matter of days.)

Goodman and Gilman say there is a low incidence of serious untoward reactions to insulin. Local reactions may occur, but these are frequently the result of poor injection technique. Allergic reactions may prove troublesome, and are indicated by swelling, erythema, and itching at the site of injection. Generalized urticaria and a severe constitutional reaction are seen occasionally. The following are other symptoms that may appear: swelling of the lips, reddening of the eyes, puffiness of the face, weakness, epigastric pain, nausea, and vomiting. If the reaction cannot be traced to poor technique, hypersensitivity in some cases can be controlled by changing the brand of insulin. Lipodystrophy (atrophy of fat) may occur at the sites of frequent injection; it results in a disfiguring depression of the skin (concavities). Occurrence of these may be prevented, according to Goodman and Gilman, by rotating areas of injection so that no one area is used more frequently than once every 4 weeks (see Fig. 22-9); Florence Cuozzo Coates and Maximilian Fabrykant [46] suggest injection of the insulin into the deep subcutaneous tissue rather than into a skin fold. They believe this can best be accomplished by using a one-half inch 25-gauge needle for most persons (a ¾-inch 25-gauge needle for those who are obese) which is inserted at a 90-deg. angle. If lesions do occur, insulin should not be injected into these areas as absorption is not as effective as in healthy tissue.

Insulin is a very potent substance and must be used with caution and exactitude. An error in dosage, time, and frequency of administration or in the diet to which it bears a direct relationship may prove serious. The following are other factors that affect the insulin requirement: interferences with the absorption of the diet such as vomiting and diarrhea; or anything that makes great demands on the pa-

tient's energy such as unusual exercise, overexertion, exposure to cold, or emotional disturbances.

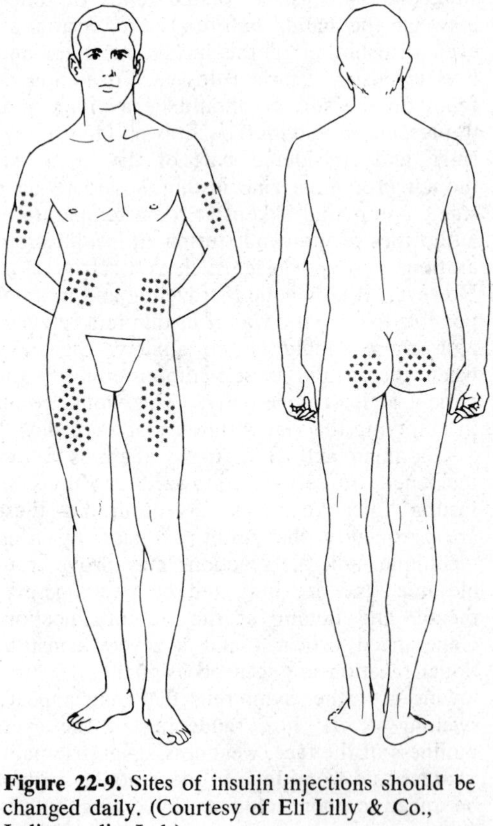

If the amount of insulin given is not sufficient to balance the diet, or if a dose is omitted without regulating the diet, the result will be glycosuria, hyperglycemia, acidosis, and, eventually, coma. Patients should be warned of these dangers. They should be urged to carry a card stating that they have diabetes so that, if one of these untoward complications develops, they will receive prompt treatment. In addition, it is important for each diabetic to keep an adequate supply of insulin as well as an extra syringe and needle on hand.

3. INTRAMUSCULAR INJECTION

Definition. The meaning of the term is self-evident. It is applied to the injection of drugs in quantities that usually range from 2 to 10 ml. Much larger doses of sera or blood are occasionally introduced into the muscles.

Therapeutic Uses. Fluids are injected into muscles for the same reasons that they are given subcutaneously. The intramuscular route is chosen in preference to the subcutaneous route when (1) the substance is irritating, (2) more rapid absorption is desired than is thought possible with the subcutaneous route, and (3) when there is a larger quantity of the fluid (as with injection of blood and some sera) than the subcutaneous tissues can absorb easily. Samuel Zelman [47] says that many medications must be given intramuscularly only because greater pain is caused by injecting them subcutaneously where the nerve supply is richer.

Selection of Method. Intramuscular injections involve more risk than subcutaneous injections since there is a greater likelihood of striking nerves and large blood vessels. Intramuscular injections were formerly given by physicians, but in this country nurses now regularly carry out this procedure, and, with the more widespread use of agents injected into the muscles, the patients and their families must often be taught the techniques.

The selection for the *site of injection* is of the utmost importance and requires an understanding of the anatomy of the area in which the injection is to be given. Complications that may occur include abscess, cyst, necrosis and sloughing of tissue, scar formation, pain, accidental intravascular injection, and nerve injury.[48] Combes and associates [49] emphasize that injury of the sciatic nerve can occur after one injection and in any age group, although the newborn infant, especially the premature infant, is more likely to experience this com-

Figure 22-9. Sites of insulin injections should be changed daily. (Courtesy of Eli Lilly & Co., Indianapolis, Ind.)

plication. They report 12 infants so affected after intragluteal injection. Foot drop, persistent paralysis, and sensory and sweating loss in the lower leg and foot were signs of nerve injury most often observed. Because the total gluteal region is small in the infant, the preferred site of injection is the mid-anterior aspect of the thigh, with the quadriceps muscle as the recipient of the injected substance. Paul H. Curtis and Howard J. Tucker [50] report a follow-up study of 10 premature infants who experienced partial sciatic palsy caused by the needle or the agent injected and they conclude that the ventrogluteal injection site is safer than the traditional dorsogluteal site. For the adult, the sites most frequently suggested are the dorsogluteal, ventrogluteal, laterofemoral (also referred to as *vastus lateralis* site), and deltoid.[51-53]

The dorsogluteal site is used most frequently for intramuscular injections in adults because the *gluteus maximus*, a big muscle, is there and it can absorb large quantities of solution, making irritating drugs less painful. Because there is danger of trauma to the sciatic nerve and the superior and inferior gluteal artery, it is necessary that the site be located anatomically so that the needle will not be misplaced. The upper outer quadrant of the gluteal area is the recommended site and may be located by drawing a line from the posterior superior iliac spine to the greater trochanter of the femur. Any injection given lateral and superior to this line will be some distance from the sciatic nerve (see Fig. 22-10). The patient should be placed in a prone position with feet internally

rotated and in plantar flexion when the site is located by palpation. This position ensures relaxation of the muscle as the injection is given. The standing or sitting position, according to Zelman,[54] should not be used because relaxation of the muscle is impossible and there is danger of a sudden jerking movement that may break the needle.

The ventrogluteal site, recommended by von Hochstetter in 1954, is considered the safest area for injections in children and is used increasingly for adults (see Fig. 22-11). There are several advantages: the gluteal muscles (medius and minus) are thicker than the maximus; there are no major nerves and vessels in the area; the patient may be in any position when the injection is given; and the area is more likely to be free from contamination of feces and urine. Barbara J. Horn describes the location of the site:

To accurately locate the site place the tip of the left index finger on the right anterior superior iliac spine of the patient; place the third finger just below the iliac crest. The index finger and the third finger form an area in the shape of a V. The area within the V constitutes the correct site for injection into the ventrogluteal area.*

The laterofemoral site or *vastus lateralis* site is located on the lateral aspect of the thigh, one hand's breadth below the greater trochanter and one hand's breadth above the knee. There are no major vessels or nerves deep in

* Horn, Barbara J.: "Intramuscular Injections: The Nurse's Responsibility," *Univ. Mich. Med. Cent. J.,* **32:**31 (Jan.–Feb.) 1966.

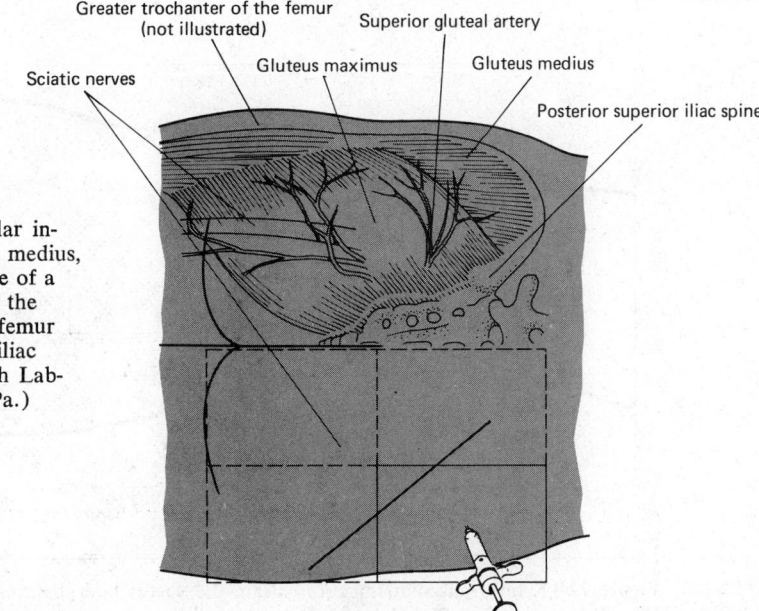

Figure 22-10. Intramuscular injection site of the gluteus medius, which is above and outside of a diagonal line drawn from the greater trochanter of the femur to the posterior superior iliac spine. (Courtesy of Wyeth Laboratories, Philadelphia, Pa.)

Greater trochanter of the femur (not illustrated)

Superior gluteal artery

Sciatic nerves

Gluteus maximus

Gluteus medius

Posterior superior iliac spine

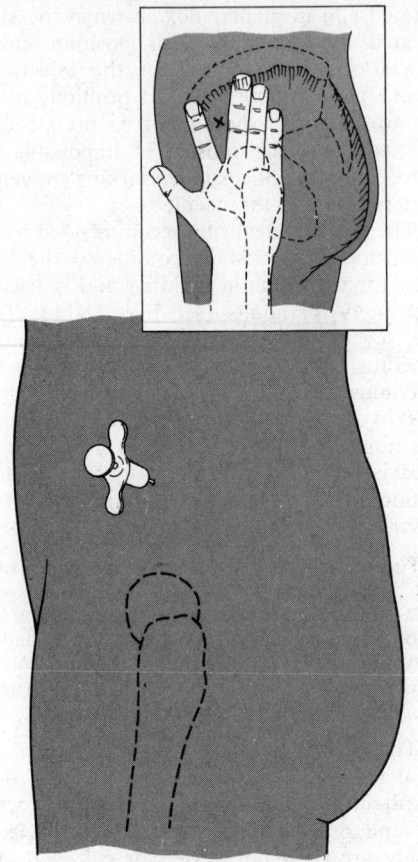

Figure 22-11. Intramuscular injection site in the ventrogluteal area within the limits of a triangle formed by the greater trochanter of the femur and the posterior and anterior edges of the iliac crest. (Courtesy of Wyeth Laboratories, Philadelphia, Pa.)

the area but the lateral femoral cutaneous nerve is superficial. Absorption is slower in this area than those described above; consequently, it should not be used for frequent injections. The area is readily accessible with the patient in the prone or supine positions and it is easily located (see Fig. 22-12).

The deltoid site, easiest to expose and most acceptable to patients, is the least desirable area because the muscle is not as large as the gluteals and the radial nerve is near the injection site. The area should not be used in adults except when the most nonirritating substance is injected, according to Daniel J. Hanson.[55] In locating the site for injection, a rectangle is drawn on the lateral arm beginning with the lower edge of the acromion (point where the scapula articulates with clavicle) on the top and ending at the point opposite the axilla on the bottom (see Fig. 22-13). This site may be used for small doses (not to exceed 1 ml) of nonirritating drugs and when other sites are not available.[56]

Sterilization of equipment, preparation of the drug, and preparation of the skin are the same as for a subcutaneous injection. To prevent the likelihood of injected materials seeping into the sinus made by the needle, it is important to retract the skin and subcutaneous tissue when injecting the needle into the skin and muscle.[57] The needle is inserted at a right angle to the skin (see Fig. 22-14).

Equipment. The articles required are practically the same as those needed in giving a subcutaneous injection, the size of the syringe varying with the amount to be given and the gauge and length of the needle with the type of drug it is intended to carry and the condi-

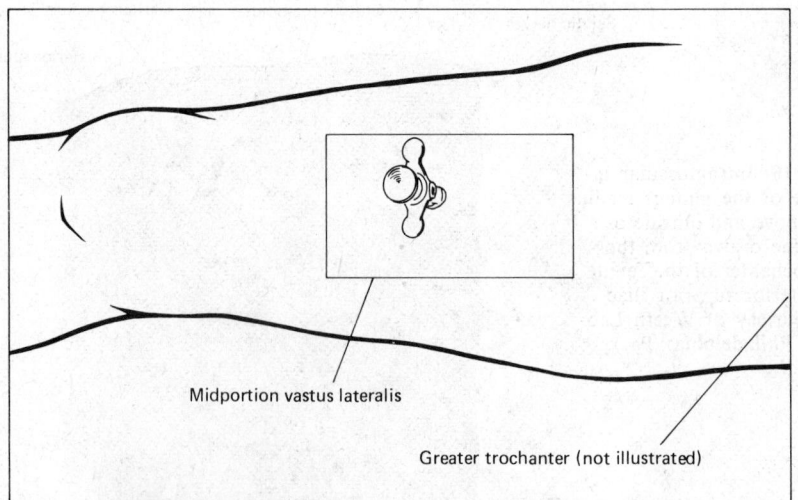

Midportion vastus lateralis

Greater trochanter (not illustrated)

Figure 22-12. Intramuscular injection site in the vastus lateralis area. (Courtesy of Wyeth Laboratories, Philadelphia, Pa.)

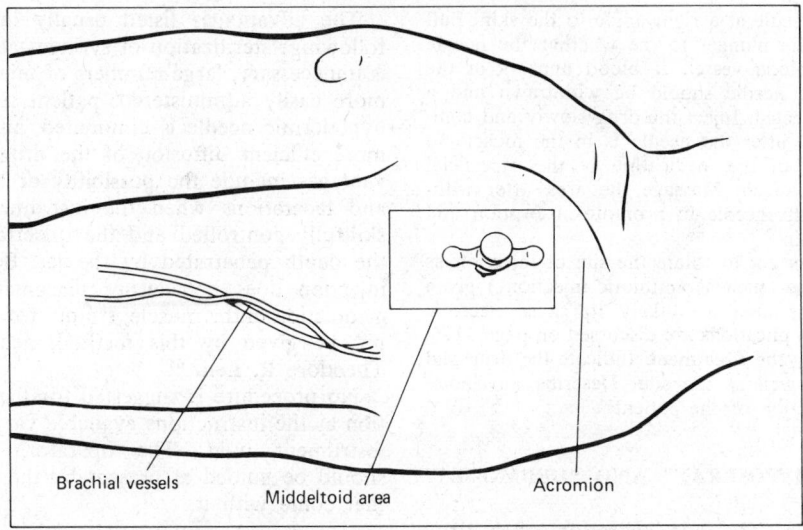

Figure 22-13. Intramuscular injection site of the middeltoid area. (Courtesy of Wyeth Laboratories, Philadelphia, Pa.)

tion of the tissues. Sizes of the latter range from 19 to 22 gauge and from 3½ to 6 cm (1½ to 2½ inches) in length. Fine needles may be used for thin liquids, heavier ones for suspensions; short needles are satisfactory when the person is thin and flabby; longer needles are necessary when the patient is obese. For injections into the arms or thighs, needles range from 2.5 to 3½ cm (1 to 1½ inches) in length. The size of the syringe depends upon the amount of liquid to be injected.

Suggested Procedure. Prepare the drug and carry the equipment to the bedside in the same way as for a subcutaneous injection, first being sure that the patient is willing to have the treat-

ment. In selecting the site of injection, consider the amount and properties of the drug to be injected and the condition of the patient, especially painful areas. Expose the area and palpate the site of injection, using anatomical landmarks. If the dorsogluteal site is selected, the patient is placed in the prone position with feet internally rotated and in plantar flexion. Clean the skin thoroughly (using a circular motion starting from the central to the peripheral zone) with an appropriate agent such as tincture of iodine, acetone, or 70 per cent alcohol. To avoid escape (tracting) of the drug in superficial tissues, which can cause necrosis, wipe the needle free of the drug or, even better, use a different needle than the one used in withdrawing the medication from the vial. After retracting the skin and subcutaneous tissue,

Figure 22-14. Intramuscular injection of the arm. Note needle held at a right angle to the skin.

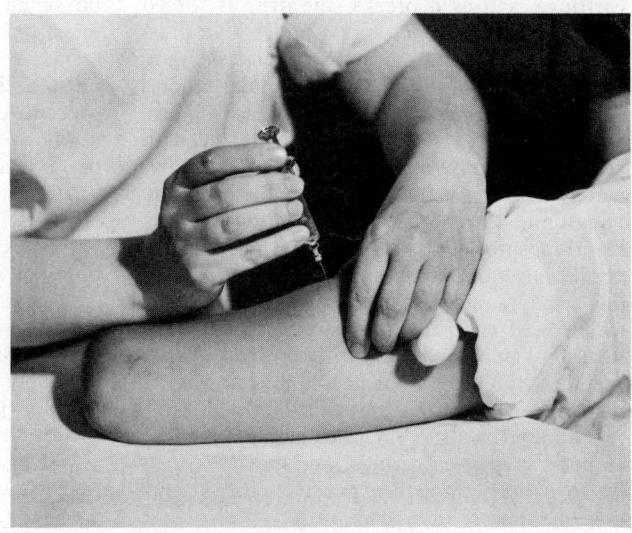

insert the needle at a right angle to the skin. Pull gently on the plunger to see whether the needle entered a blood vessel. If blood appears in the syringe, the needle should be withdrawn and a new site selected. Inject the drug slowly and completely only after the needle is in the muscle so that escape of the medication in the superficial tissues is avoided. Massage the area after withdrawal of the needle to promote absorption and diminish pain.

It is important to rotate the site of injection as certain drugs (such as antibiotic injections) given in the same area are likely to cause necrotic lesions. Complications are discussed on page 1176.

Recording the Treatment. Indicate the drug and amount as well as the site. Describe any noteworthy reaction of the patient.

4. THE "HYPOSPRAY" AND "DERMO-JET"

Definition. The administration of a drug through the skin, without a needle, in the form of a jet of fluid under high pressure is called the jet injection. The instruments used are called the *Hypospray* or the *Dermo-jet*.

Therapeutic Uses. Jet injection has been used to administer various materials since the initial development of the Hypospray in 1947. Theoretically, jet injection may be substituted for the subcutaneous and intramuscular administration of an unlimited number of therapeutic agents. It may therefore have the same uses as the "hypodermic" and intramuscular injections. Its more common use has been multiple immunizations of large groups such as school children and armed forces.[58]

Method. The Hypospray (and Dermo-jet) are metal barrels with a very small opening at the end from which the drug is discharged. They contain a plunger operated by a spring, and the drug is in a metal cartridge. Release of the spring forces the plunger against the cartridge, and as it breaks, the drug is forced out in a fine stream, or spray, under high pressure. Robert Hingson and associates[59] and W. Royce Hodges[60] report two similar studies on the Hypospray in venereal disease clinics. Approximately 150 patients were treated with penicillin given by the Hypospray and approximately 50 with penicillin by needle injection. Hingson et al. report 97.5 per cent cures using the Hypospray and 97.9 per cent cures using needle injection. Hodges' results with virtually the same number of patients in the experimental and control groups were identical. In treating "tennis elbow" with hydrocortisone acetate by Hypospray or needle injection in 50 patients, G. R. V. Hughes and H. L. F. Currey[61] found the success rates similar, but the Hypospray was less painful and more acceptable to patients, though expensive.

The advantages listed usually include the following: sterilization of syringes and needles is unnecessary, large numbers of injections are more easily administered, patient fear of the hypodermic needle is eliminated, and there is more efficient diffusion of the drug.[62] Disadvantages include the possibility of contusions and lacerations when the instrument is not skillfully controlled and the uncertainty over the depth penetrated by the jet. Because jet injection does not ensure placement of the medication in the muscle, tetanus toxoid should not be given by this method, according to Theodore R. Lenz.[63]

No procedure is suggested for the jet injection as the instructions available vary with the instrument used. The operator, therefore, should be guided at present by the directions that come with it.

5. INTRADERMIC OR INTRACUTANEOUS INJECTION

Definition. *Intradermal injection* is the term used to describe the introduction of a substance into the corium or the upper layers of the skin.

Therapeutic Uses. In allergic conditions, such as hives or hay fever, when the physician wants to see the local reaction of tissue to bacteria, their toxins, or foreign proteins, he or she introduces them under the superficial layer of the skin. Because absorption from the skin takes place more slowly than from the areolar tissue or muscle, it may be desirable to inject intradermally therapeutic doses of very potent substances that produce severe generalized body reactions.

Selection of Method. Because intradermal injections are used for diagnostic purposes and sometimes dangerous or delicate therapy, the physician generally prefers to prepare the drug, inject it, and watch the reaction. The nurse may, in some situations, prepare the equipment or she or he may carry out the entire procedure.

The *sterilization of equipment* and *preparation of the drug* are the same as for subcutaneous and intramuscular injections. Drugs given intradermally are nearly always put up in ampoules because, if used for diagnostic purposes, it is essential that they be pure.

The *site of injection* is usually the inner aspect of the forearm. Local reactions, if they occur, are most easily recognized if the skin is relatively free from hair and pigment and if the skin is thin. Disinfectants that discolor or irritate are avoided in the *preparation of the skin* because the physician does not want the reaction of the skin to the injected agent to be obscured. Alcohol 70 per cent is commonly used.

Injecting the needle so that the point goes no deeper than the first layer of the skin is very important; in order to do this the needle is held at a very slight angle to the skin with the opening of the needle up and the point of the bevel lying on the skin. The needle is injected about 2 mm or ⅛ inch, and when in position for the injection the opening of the needle should be visible through the skin.

Equipment. Materials for cleaning the skin are required as in any injection. A slender syringe that enables the operator to hold the needle at a slight angle and to measure very small doses in the syringe should be provided. The most desirable needle is one with a rounded sloping hub that allows the shaft to lie close to the skin. It should be about 1 cm (⅜ inch) in length and from 26 to 27 gauge. When injections are made for diagnostic purposes, at least two syringes and needles are necessary since a control wheal is usually made.

Suggested Procedure. Give patients a suitable explanation of the treatment if there is any doubt about their understanding it. See that patients are in a comfortable position with the forearm supported on a firm surface. They may sit or lie down, but if there is any tendency on their part to be nervous, they are less likely to feel faint or nauseated if they are recumbent. Clean an area about 7½ cm (3 inch) in diameter on the inner surface of the forearm midway between the wrist and the elbow; allow the skin to dry. Holding the needle and syringe almost parallel with the arm, introduce the needle about 2 mm (⅛ inch) with the opening upward and the bevel visible under the skin. When the needle is in place, introduce the drug, making a wheal, or circumscribed elevation of the skin. The area is not cleaned or massaged following the removal of the needle.

When foreign proteins are administered, a very minute amount is usually given and the patient observed for symptoms of allergic shock before proceeding with the administration of the total dose. In serum therapy, in which an anaphylactic reaction is likely, a preparation of epinephrine as an antidote should be available for immediate subcutaneous administration.

If injections are made for diagnostic purposes, a control injection of sterile saline solution is given on the other arm and a careful record kept to avoid possible errors in reading the tissue reaction.

6. SUBCUTANEOUS INFUSION OR HYPODERMOCLYSIS

Definition. The word *hypodermoclysis* is derived from *hypo,* meaning under, *derma,* the skin, and *clysis,* to cleanse. In medical practice the term is used to designate an injection of a large amount of fluid into the subcutaneous tissues by means of a needle, for the purpose of supplying the body with fluids, and not, as the name implies, for the purpose of cleansing the area into which the solution is injected.

Therapeutic Uses. Subcutaneous injections are given to supply the body with fluids that closely resemble the electrolyte content and tonicity of extracellular fluid when the patient is unable to take adequate amounts by mouth and by rectum and when administration of fluids into the veins is contraindicated or impractical. It is most often used when intravenous fluids are difficult to start, for example, with the infant, obese, and aged (see Fig. 22-15). But hypodermoclysis injections have been largely replaced by the intravenous injections.

Selection of Method. In some hospitals every step of this procedure is carried out by the nursing staff; in others, the physician injects the needles and starts the flow of solution; in both cases the nurse may prepare the equipment, regulate the flow of solution, and take care of the patient before, during, and after the treatment. Since the physician and the nurse share the responsibility for this procedure, the basis on which the selection of method is made is a matter of concern to both. The chief objectives in any method are the promotion of rapid absorption and the prevention of undue distention, irritation, infection, and unnecessary pain or discomfort to the patient.

There are *few solutions* that can be given by this method and they are prescribed by the physician. Those considered to be reasonably safe are: isotonic saline (0.9 per cent sodium chloride), half-isotonic saline (0.45 per cent sodium chloride) with 2½ per cent dextrose, Ringer's solution, Lactated Ringer's solution, half-strength Ringer's solution with 2½ per cent dextrose, and half-strength Lactated Ringer's with 2½ per cent dextrose. Patients require many fluids which cannot be given by the subcutaneous route. Sugar solutions that are electrolyte free are contraindicated as they may produce circulatory difficulties (hypotension and anuria, for example), especially if given to patients with a sodium deficit, a low blood volume, or renal impairment. Edema is increased in the injection area and plasma volume reduced because there is a shift of body fluid and electrolytes in an attempt to maintain equilibrium. If hypertonic solutions are not absorbed, body fluids will be drawn into the injection area which may result in reduced fluid volume with threatening circulatory collapse. Solutions containing alcohol are irritating to the tissues and may cause slough-

A

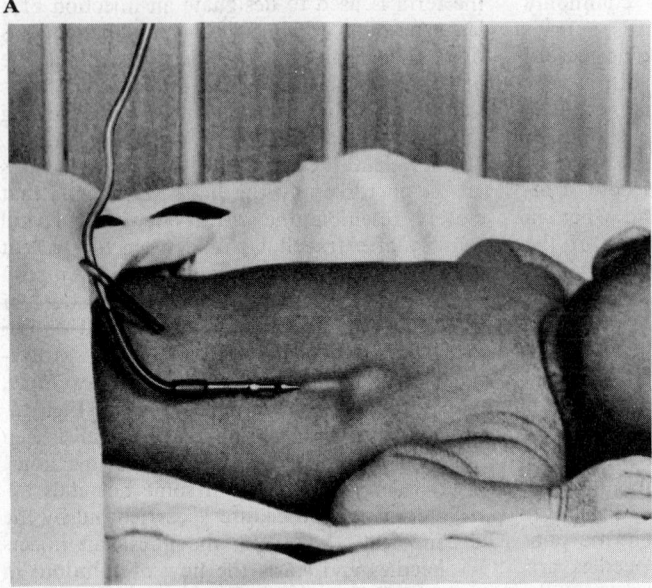

Figure 22-15. *A*. Administration of fluid by hypodermoclysis is frequently indicated in infants with poor superficial veins. The addition of hyaluronidase prevents painful swelling and speeds absorption. *B*. Note swelling of tissues following a hypodermoclysis to which hyaluronidase has not been added. (Courtesy of Wyeth Laboratories, Philadelphia, Pa.)

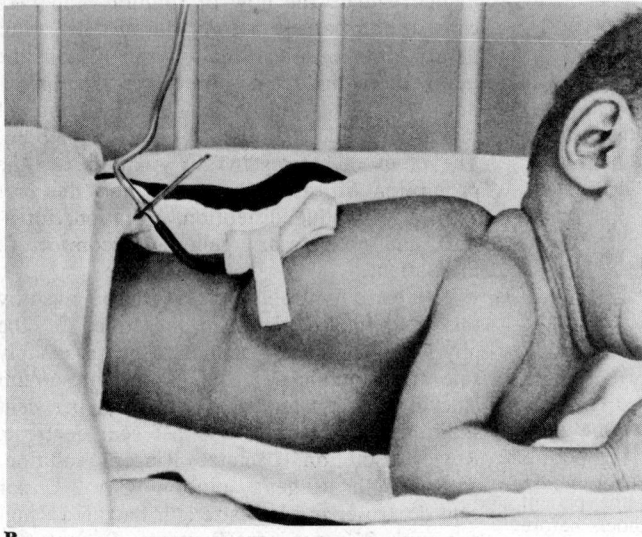

B

ing; albumin in solution is not absorbed because of its high molecular weight. Fat emulsions and any solution that differs significantly from the body pH (such as in gastric replacement solutions) are contraindicated.[64,65] Norma Milligan Metheny and William D. Snively say: "Orders for the subcutaneous administration of any of these solutions should be questioned." *

The preparation of parenteral fluids and the

* Metheny, Norma Milligan, and Snively, William D.: *Nurses' Handbook of Fluid Balance,* 2nd ed. J. B. Lippincott Co., Philadelphia, 1974, p. 128.

dangers of pyrogens are discussed in Chapter 32. Infections are not uncommon when fluids are given in the subcutaneous tissues and are related proportionately to the amount of distention and the length of time required for the treatment.

Maintaining the *temperature of the solution* at, or near, body heat was discussed on page 1168. Unless the physician requests that the fluid be warmed, subcutaneous infusions are, in most places, given at room temperature.

The *amount of solution* to be given depends on the size and condition of the patient. When large amounts of solution are needed in a hurry, this route is undependable, according to Metheny and Snively.

The *rate of administration* is determined by the individual's rate of absorption. A larger quantity may be given more rapidly if the solution is injected into two areas of the body simultaneously. Fluids are absorbed more rapidly by thin than by fat persons because the areolar tissue is not so packed with fat cells. The degree of dehydration of the tissues is also a factor in absorption. As much as 250 to 500 ml may be given at one site in one hour to an adult when the fluid is absorbed well.[66] Hyaluronidase, injected into the tissues at the injection site or added to the infusion, will increase absorption.

The nurse should check the patient frequently and regulate the rate of flow according to the rate of absorption of the fluids. When swelling (edema) of the area occurs, the infusion should be stopped completely. Discomfort and pain are caused by pressure of the fluid and the edematous sites are fertile fields for infections.

The most commonly used *sites of subcutaneous injection* are (1) the outer front of the thighs between the knee and the hip, (2) under and near the outer margin of the breast, and (3) the abdominal wall above the crest of the ileum. In choosing the area the objects are to select loose tissue; to avoid large blood vessels and nerves; and also to limit the patient's movement as little as possible.

Preparation of the skin and *sterilization of the equipment* are based on the principles discussed in Chapters 14, 15, and 32.

The *position of the patient* should be one in which he or she is relaxed and comfortable. If the fluid is given under the breast, the patient is probably most comfortable lying on the back; if it is given in the abdominal wall above the crest of the ileum, the patient should be turned on the opposite side and supported with pillows. When the needles are introduced into the thighs, the patient is placed in the dorsal recumbent position with the knees slightly flexed and supported.

The *technique of injecting the needles* varies according to the area into which the solution is given. When injecting the needles under the breast, it is important to lift the breast away from the body and insert the needle into the space between the chest wall and the mammary gland. The needle should be held almost parallel with the body wall to avoid the possibility of striking a rib, passing the needle through the intercostal muscles, or injuring the glands of the breast. When inserting the needle into the thigh, the tissue should be grasped firmly in the left hand and the needle introduced quickly, at a slight angle, for a length of approximately 3 cm (1¼ inch). If the needle is sharp and the injection made with a quick movement, it is only slightly more painful than a hypodermic injection. The fluid entering the tissues and the resulting pressure produce a burning, tingling sensation that is very uncomfortable and nerve-racking even to a well person. Some physicians inject the area first with a local anesthetic, such as procaine (Novocaine), and this appreciably reduces the discomfort. Hastening absorption with hyaluronidase eliminates most of the sensations induced by pressure of the fluid.

There would seem to be no justification for *massaging* the part while the needle is injected; the movement of the point of the needle is obliged to destroy and damage the surrounding tissue cells and to cause a good deal of pain. Robert T. Gants[67] and O. P. Humpstone[68] reported fatalities following the administration of hypodermoclysis under the breast and in the thigh, and each concludes that one of the injurious factors was the massage that accompanied the administration of the fluid.

Equipment. If small amounts of solution are administered, it may be convenient to give the treatment with a Luer or Record syringe, but in most cases a reservoir of some type is used. It is desirable that this reservoir is the flask or bottle in which the solution is sterilized in order to prevent the possibility of bacterial contamination in transferring the solution. An Erlenmeyer, a Fenwal, or a Florence flask may be used. Commercially prepared solutions are used in most hospitals and almost universally in home, office, industrial, and military medicine. A 180-cm (6-ft) length of plastic or rubber tubing about 1 cm (⅜ inch) in diameter is needed to deliver the solution; if two needles are used, a glass Y tube should be introduced into the tubing with about 35 cm (14 inches) of tubing attached to each arm of the Y tube. The end or ends of the tubing to be connected with the needle, or needles, must be provided with suitable adapters. The tubing should be equipped with a drip bulb, so that the solution may be regulated to drops per minute, if so ordered. A screw clamp is necessary above the drip bulb to control the rate of flow; and screw clamps on each arm of the Y are also important in controlling the rate of flow.

Needles used range from 22 to 19 gauge and from 3.7 cm (1½ inches) to 5 cm (2 inches) in length and have a moderately long bevel. Small needles cause less discomfort and less tissue damage. Some physicians use a very small-gauged needle as a means of slowing the rate of flow; if a sufficiently fine needle is employed, the drip bulb and screw clamp can be dispensed with. An irrigating pole, or standard, is necessary to support the reservoir. If a siphonage system is used, a syringe to start the flow of solution from the reservoir should be provided.

Materials for cleaning the skin include the disinfectant and either sponges and forceps or cotton applicators. Four or five gauze squares to be used as dressing and strips of adhesive on crinoline may be sterilized in the package with the tubing. A small basin for waste solution and a paper bag for soiled sponges are needed. A moistureproof bed protector with a soft cover to place under the puncture area is desirable; sterile towels are unnecessary, but one may be used for convenience to supply a sterile field on which to handle the tubing and needles. Sterile rubber gloves are also unnecessary because it is possible to manipulate the equipment with sterile forceps and clean hands without contaminating any surfaces that should be kept sterile. The drip bulb, the glass Y tube, and the adapters should be inserted into the tubing before they are sterilized.

Treatment blankets should be available for draping the patient. A cart on which the equipment can be wheeled to the bedside saves time and effort.

Preparation of the Patient. Hypodermoclysis may be used when patients are unconscious or too ill to want an explanation of the procedure. The importance of gaining the rational patient's understanding and cooperation has been discussed.

The room should be comfortably warm; the patient placed in a suitable position and supported to avoid strain; the bed covers turned down to expose the area in which the needles are to be injected; patient's clothing and the bedding arranged to avoid soiling; and treatment blankets properly adjusted to protect uncovered parts of the body. Only the necessary skin area should be exposed. The skin is prepared as for any surgical operation. The fold of upper bedclothes just below the site of injection may be covered with a sterile towel or a square of soft crepe paper. If the equipment is not brought into the room on a treatment wagon, a table must be cleared and placed at the bedside.

Suggested Procedure. If the puncture is made on a hairy part of the body, shave the area before starting the treatment. Clean and disinfect the skin as described and inject the local anesthetic if it is to be used. Attach the tubing and its connections to the reservoir; hang the reservoir about 90 cm (3 ft) above the level of the bed and allow the solution to fill the tubing, and, at the same time, expel the air from the tubing. Pierce the center of a square gauze dressing with the needle;

then, holding the needle at a slight angle, inject it quickly into the subcutaneous tissue at the specified site. Attach the tubing to the needle by the adapter. Fix the needle (or needles) in position with a strip of adhesive brought around the needle hub and carried over the gauze square to the skin on either side. When the needles are in position draw the bedding or treatment blanket over the patient. Adjust the flow of solution to the prescribed rate. When hyaluronidase is used inject it with a fine needle into the tubing as the solution starts to flow. In all cases the rate at which the fluid is given should be such that the tissues around the needle stay nearly normal in tension and appearance. If the rate of absorption is very low, the physician may want the treatment discontinued before the prescribed amount is given. The injection may last from 30 minutes to 6 hours or more according to the rate of flow and the amount of fluid needed by the patient.

At the end of the treatment, withdraw the needles quickly, making pressure over the puncture wound with a sterile gauze dressing. Fix a dry, sterile gauze square over the wound with adhesive. Arrange the patient's clothing and bedding.

It is important that the nurse stay nearby while the solution is flowing to prevent the occurrence of accidents and to reassure the patient. The screw clamp may loosen and allow the solution to flow in too quickly; a sudden movement of the patient may disconnect the tubing from a glass connection; or the patient may turn and displace a needle.

Recording the Treatment. Indicate the nature, amount, and temperature of the solution given; state the rate of flow and the total amount of time over which the treatment extended; report briefly the patient's reaction to the treatment.

7. INTRAVENOUS INFUSION OR INJECTION

Definition. *Infusion* comes from *infundere,* to pour into. *Intravenous infusion* is used to designate the giving of fairly large amounts of fluids into the veins. *Intravenous injection* is the term more often used if the quantity is small and if it is a drug. If blood is given, the infusion is called a *transfusion. Parenteral hyperalimentation* or *total parenteral alimentation* is used to designate the giving of large amounts of basic nutrients sufficient to achieve tissue synthesis and growth. The reader should consult references at the end of this chapter on this method of treatment. [68a-f]

Therapeutic Uses. Intravenous infusions are given (1) to correct water deficit and electrolyte imbalance; (2) to maintain daily requirements of these, (3) to supply the body with food in the form of glucose, amino acids, protein hydrolysates, or whole blood when there is hypoproteinemia from burns or other causes, or when there is a metabolic crisis, such as acidosis, with an immediate need for a food like glucose in the tissue fluids; (4) to alter vascular pressure by introducing hypertonic saline and/or glucose solutions, dextran, or albumin solutions; and (5) to supply one or more of the blood's components by injections of whole blood, cell suspensions, plasma, "plasma substitutes," or elements of plasma. Some of the indications for infusing blood, blood components, and their substitutes are discussed under *transfusion* on page 1194.

Drugs are injected into the veins when (1) a very rapid effect is needed, (2) when the drug is given for its action on the blood stream or the vessels, and (3) when the drug would be irritating or ineffective given by other routes.

Selection of Method. Because so many risks are inherent in the procedure, physicians, in the past, have preferred to give intravenous medications, or to train special technicians for this task. With the increased demand for hospital care and for intravenous therapy, and the disproportionate increase in physicians and medical technicians, many nurses are included in the personnel prepared to give intravenous infusions. Although more responsibility for administering parenteral fluids, including the venipuncture, is being allocated to the nurse, this practice is not uniform among hospitals and states. In large hospitals, parenteral teams composed of nurses may be responsible for all intravenous therapy, whereas in small hospitals a nurse on each unit is responsible. And, in some teaching centers, the intern or resident performs the venipuncture.

The legal responsibilities of the professional nurse who initiates intravenous therapy continues to be questioned. Rulings have been made by some state boards of nursing and state attorney generals, and joint policy statements have also been made by professional nursing and medical organizations in an attempt to clarify the role of the nurse in intravenous therapy. Policy statements are helpful but nurses should realize that they do not relieve them of their responsibility for their own acts.[69]

Those who give intravenous injections should know how to locate blood vessels suitable for injection; they should have sufficient knowledge of anatomy to avoid injury to nerves, bones, and glands; they should understand the nature and action of the substances they inject and the appropriate doses should be checked; they should be keenly aware of the dangers involved and complications that may occur; and, obviously, they should be skilled in the procedure itself.

Whether or not the nurses actually perform the venipuncture, they have an important role in intravenous therapy. They should participate in designing the method used for infusions, including the selection of equipment, since they are the persons who most often regulate the flow of solution and who watch and record the patient's reaction during the treatment. Throughout the procedure the nurses should work with the physician; the more thoroughly they understand the treatment, the better their service to the patient.

The *solution* is prescribed by the physician. He or she may be giving it to supply any one or several of the following: water, electrolytes, or drugs; or food in the form of glucose, amino acids, protein hydrolysates, fat emulsions, or vitamins. If the blood volume is diminished, or if there is a lessening of the cell or plasma content, the physician will order whole blood, plasma, or plasma substitutes. Infusion of blood, plasma, or the so-called substitutes is discussed in detail under the heading of *transfusion* on page 1194.

Effects of introducing *hypotonic, isotonic,* and *hypertonic* solutions were treated on page 1169. The reader is referred to that discussion since the dangers of intravenous therapy cannot be understood without some knowledge of the reaction of the blood to solutions of varying osmotic pressures.

Sodium chloride solution at approximately 0.9 per cent is considered isotonic with the human blood, and is the strength commonly used. Other saline preparations, such as Ringer's, Lactated Ringer's (Hartmann's), Fox's, and Darrow's solutions, containing a number of the plasma electrolytes beside sodium chloride, are also used. Bernard Zimmermann, discussing water and electrolyte balance in *Davis-Christopher Textbook of Surgery*,[70] says that sodium chloride in large amounts is not required for maintenance of patients unless they suffer from external losses. This is because the normal kidney has the ability to conserve sodium in the absence of intake; however, this does not hold true for potassium ion since 30 to 40 mEq of potassium may be excreted by persons who are not receiving any by mouth or parenterally. Consequently, 2 to 3 gm of this salt (such as potassium chloride) daily is necessary for maintenance after normal renal function has been established following surgery. Many of the untoward effects of infusions can be avoided when their prescription is based on blood analyses. When the blood tends toward an acid reaction (acidemia), an alkalinizing solution such as sodium lactate ⅙ M may be administered. Hypertonic solutions of sodium chloride (5 per cent sodium chloride) may be given to correct hypotonicity of the body fluids; such a concentration will draw water from all body compartments, thereby increasing tonicity. Sodium bicarbonate solutions should never be heated because heat converts this salt to the very toxic sodium carbonate solution. Fortunately, commercial solutions prepared under special conditions are available in most situations and should be used if possible. When metabolic alkalemia is severe enough to require treatment, ammonium chloride (2.14 per cent) may be given to adults and 0.9 per cent to children.[71]

Carbohydrates administered intravenously include glucose, fructose, and invert sugars; all of these are monosaccharides and readily utilized by the body cells. John H. Bland[72] says that fructose exerts a greater protein-sparing effect than glucose. Glucose is administered in 5, 10, 20, and even 50 per cent solutions, although concentrations over 5 per cent are hypertonic. To supply the necessary calories (such as 1600 daily for an adult) with 5 per cent dextrose solution would require a volume exceeding the tolerance of most patients. Alcohol and glucose mixtures are useful because of their high caloric content and limited bulk. Concentrated solutions, such as 20 or 50 per cent, should be administered slowly and intermittently so that the glucose may be utilized and diluted by a relatively large volume of blood, diminishing the possibility of damage to the vessel wall, according to Metheny and Snively.[73] They are given to supply calories for patients with renal insufficiency or to those who are unable to tolerate larger volumes of fluid. Glucose in 50 per cent solution has been used to sclerose varicose veins; but in such cases it is injected with a special technique, more rapidly than in an infusion for a systemic effect. Glucose is most often given in saline solutions, but if there is no object in administering sodium chloride, the solution may be prepared with distilled water. Glucose is administered with insulin in diabetic coma.

Amino acids prepared from enzymatic digests of complete protein are given with carbohydrate and alcohol whenever possible so that the protein will be used for tissue repair. Protein hydrolysate solutions supply the body with the same end products of protein digestion that are found in normal blood plasma. A variety of preparations are available, such as *Amigen,** a pancreatic hydrolysate of casein, *Aminosol,†* a modified fibron hydrosylate, and *Travamin,‡* a hydrolyzed bovine plasma, all available in 5 and 10 per cent solutions. These and similar preparations are said to be capable of bringing the person with hypoproteinemia into nitrogen balance. (Protein preparations

should be given with glucose. As in the metabolism of a complete diet, the body uses the glucose for energy and the protein is left for tissue growth and repair.)

Dextran,* a polydipseroid polymer of glucose with a molecular weight similar to albumin and a specific gravity between blood and plasma, like albumin, gelatin, acacia, and pectin, is given to increase the volume of circulating fluids rather than to serve as food. Two types of dextran solution are available for clinical use: (1) medium molecular weight dextran (average molecular weight of 75,000) and (2) low molecular weight dextran (average molecular weight of 40,000). The molecules of all these solutions are sufficiently large to keep them from passing through the capillary walls readily and so they hold water in the blood system. These preparations are given chiefly because whole blood and blood plasma are not available in sufficient quantity to serve the public need. Most blood substitutes have limited value and are in a developmental stage.[74]

The *temperature of the solution* is rarely of significance as few of them require refrigeration. Most solutions are stored at room temperature; those that require refrigeration include hyperalimentation solutions and blood. The custom (in the past) of warming solutions has been discontinued because many parenteral solutions include electrolytes that may be altered by heat, and it is generally thought that the solution assumes the internal heat of the body as it mixes quickly with the blood. The dangers of overheating parenteral solutions and the precautions to be observed in preventing this were discussed on page 1168.

The *amount of solution and the rate of flow,* as in hypodermoclysis, varies with the size of the body, the need for fluids, cardiac and renal status, the nature of the fluid used, the patient's age, and his or her reaction during the infusion. The size of the vein used is also a factor. The physician should prescribe the type and rate of solution. Robert Kaye and associates say:

Written orders should be explicit as to the type of solution and the rate of administration. Rate should be specified in drops per minute, by which the flow is adjusted, as well as in cubic centimeters per hour, by which progress is gauged. It is advisable to have available for ready reference a flow-rate table equating cubic centimeters per hour to drops per minute.†

---

* Mead Johnson Laboratories, Evansville, Ind.
† Abbott Laboratories, North Chicago, Ill.
‡ Baxter Laboratories, Dallas, Tex.

* Pharmacia, Stockholm, Sweden.
† Kaye, Robert, et al.: "Solutions for and Techniques of Parenteral, Oral and Rectal Administration," *Pediatr. Clin. North Am.,* **11:**1074, (Nov.) 1964.

A

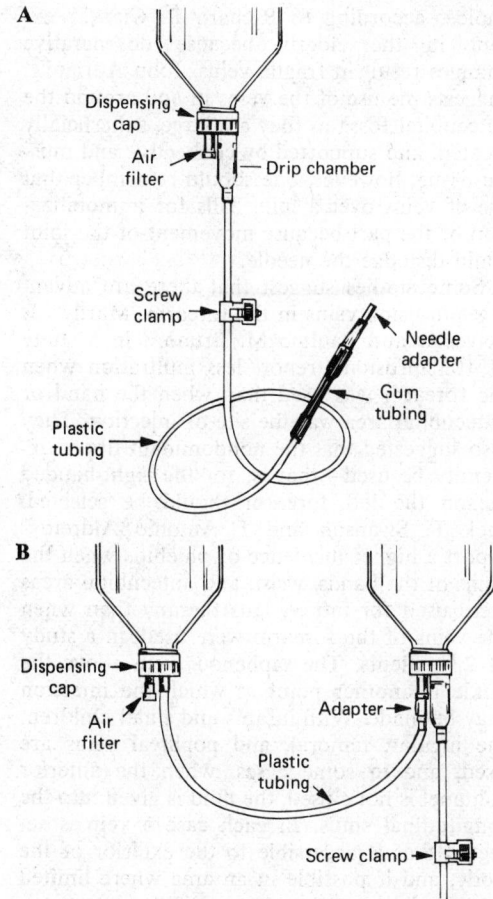

B

Figure 22-16. *A.* Simple disposable intravenous set. Additional medications may be injected in the gum rubber insert after cleaning area with an antiseptic solution and allowing to dry. *B.* Secondary hookup. A simple means of adding or changing fluids while an infusion continues by attaching the secondary bottle to the primary container. The secondary container always empties first. (Courtesy of Abbott Laboratories, North Chicago, Ill.)

The rate of the infusion should usually be slow except in emergency so that overloading the cardiovascular system is avoided. The usual infusion rate is 3 ml per square meter of body surface per minute. The larger an individual, the more nutrients and fluids he or she requires and the faster he or she can utilize these; consequently, the rate is influenced. The patient's need for fluid is another factor that influences rate, for example, an infusion is given rapidly when a patient is in hypovolemic shock. But, on the other hand, it is given at a much slower rate if there is cardiac or renal impairment. The very young and the older person should re-

ceive fluids at a slower rate as there is usually some cardiac and renal damage in the elderly and the infant and child are prone to pulmonary edema when receiving fluids at a rapid rate. The composition of the fluid is another important factor to consider in rate of infusion. In the normal adult the maximum amount of glucose that may be given is 0.5 gm per kilogram of body weight in 1 hour without producing glycosuria. Concentrated solutions of glucose, such as 20 and 50 per cent, must be administered slowly so that the glucose may be utilized by the cells. Protein hydrolysate solutions should be given slowly at the beginning of the treatment as some persons are sensitive to certain amino acids; if any untoward symptoms occur, the infusion should be stopped. Too rapid administration of these preparations may cause nausea, vomiting, flushing, abdominal pain, and mild fever; but, if the rate is decreased these symptoms will usually disappear. One liter of a 5 per cent protein hydrolysate solution may be given in 1½ to 2½ hours.[75] The patient should be checked frequently as individuals vary greatly in their rate tolerance. Suggested maximum rates of infusions of 1000 ml of carbohydrate and water solutions for adults vary from 1½ to 6 hours depending on the type of carbohydrate. Some authorities say that fructose can be given more rapidly than glucose, while the rate of infusing invert sugar lies between the two.[76] It is obvious that determining the rate of flow is complex. The rate may be gauged by counting the drops, but one must remember that the size of a drop varies. It may take as many as 10 to 25 drops or more to make one ml of fluid, depending on the nature of the fluid and the apparatus used. Fortunately, manufacturers include the rate and amount that may be given for each of their products. Also, "calculators" * are available for determining the rate of administration and the number of drops in a milliliter. If for some reason these are not available the following formula is a quick and easy method for computing flow rate in drops (gtt) per minute: Drops per minute of the given set ÷ 60 minutes × total hourly volume = number of drops per minute to be given.[77,78] Infusion pumps † that maintain the exact rate of flow are available in the United States (see Fig. 22-17). A. Baumgarten and C. C. Curtain [79] describe a small electrolytically driven infusion pump developed

* Normosol Calculator by Abbott Laboratories, North Chicago, Ill. Minislide by Baxter Laboratories, Dallas, Tex.
† The Holter pump is manufactured by Extracorporeal Medical Specialties, Inc., Mt. Laurel, N.J.

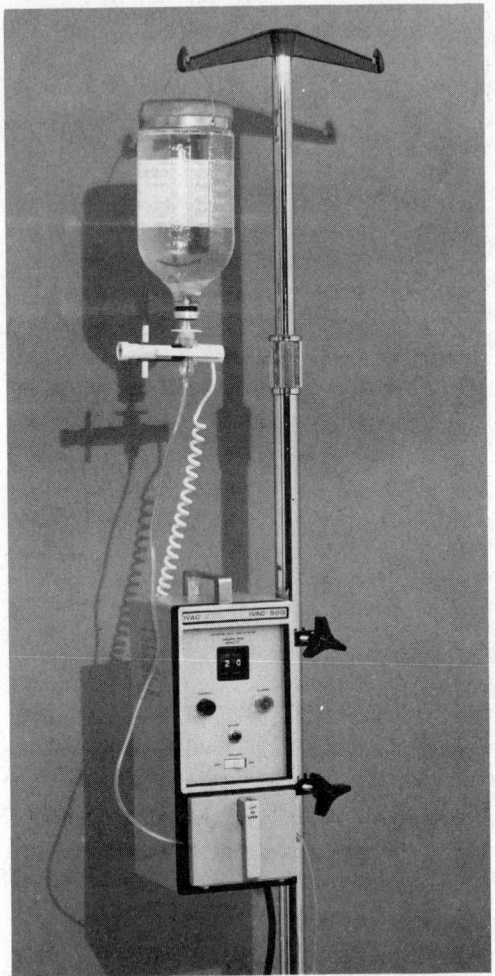

Figure 22-17. One of many types of pumps or controllers for safe and accurate administration of intravenous fluids. This pump administers fluids by peristaltic action at a rate of from 1 to 99 drops per minute, selected by switch setting. Any standard intravenous administration set may be used with this equipment. (Courtesy of Ivac Corp., San Diego, Calif.)

in Australia which can control a flow rate of 0.5 to 25 milliliters per hour.

The vein selected for the *site* of injection should be well supported by surrounding tissue and adequate in size to accommodate the needle. The veins of the forearm (especially the cephalic vein) are suggested as the most suitable for continuous intravenous therapy (see Fig. 22-18). They are less tortuous than the antecubital veins, well supported by subcutaneous tissue, and immobilization of the part is rarely needed, which allows the patient more freedom of movement. The veins located on the dorsum of the hand are a good second

choice, according to Richard B. Clark,[80] except in the elderly because degenerative changes result in fragile veins. John Adriani [81] suggests the use of the veins in and around the antecubital fossa as they are large, superficially located, and supported by connective and muscle tissue; however, one should remember that use of veins over a joint calls for immobilization of the part because movement of the joint could dislodge the needle.

Some studies suggest that there are advantages in using veins in the forearm. Marilyn J. Sylvester and Pauline M. Bruno,[82] in a study of 103 infusions, report less infiltration when the forearm was used than when the hand or antecubital area was the site of injection. They also suggested that the nondominant upper extremity be used—that is, for the right-handed person the left forearm should be selected. Jack T. Swanson and J. Antonio Aldrete [83] report a higher incidence of phlebitis when the veins of the hands, wrist, and antecubital areas were used for intravenous therapy than when the veins of the forearm were used, in a study of 23 patients. The saphenous vein above the ankle is another point at which the injection may be made. With infants and small children, the jugular, femoral, and popliteal veins are used, and in some cases, when the anterior fontanel is not closed, the fluid is given into the longitudinal sinus. In each case a vein is selected that is accessible to the exterior of the body, and if possible in an area where limited motion does not cause the patient unnecessary discomfort.

Patients who cannot eat and drink are kept alive during a protracted illness with parenteral fluids. Repeated injections of veins tend to sclerose the walls, and ultimately it is difficult to find an accessible vein that is patent. Some patients have poor veins, and under certain conditions it is hard to enter anyone's veins. These facts have led to the use of *intravenous catheters* that are "indwelling" or fixed in the vein (see Fig. 22-20). Catheters are believed by some persons to be less irritating than a needle.[84] Some operators get excellent results with the indwelling Lindemann needle. This is blunt at the end and has a sharp cannula and trochar, which are removed after the needle is in place. Michael Ladd and George E. Schreiner [85] and Lawrence Meyers [86] describe the successful use of plastic intravenous catheters. Although a catheter facilitates prolonged therapy, its use increases the risk of thrombophlebitis. Swanson and Aldrete [87] report a higher incidence of phlebitis when large catheters (15, 16, and 18 gauge) were used as compared to a 19-gauge needle. Similar findings were reported by selected staff at the Joseph Brant

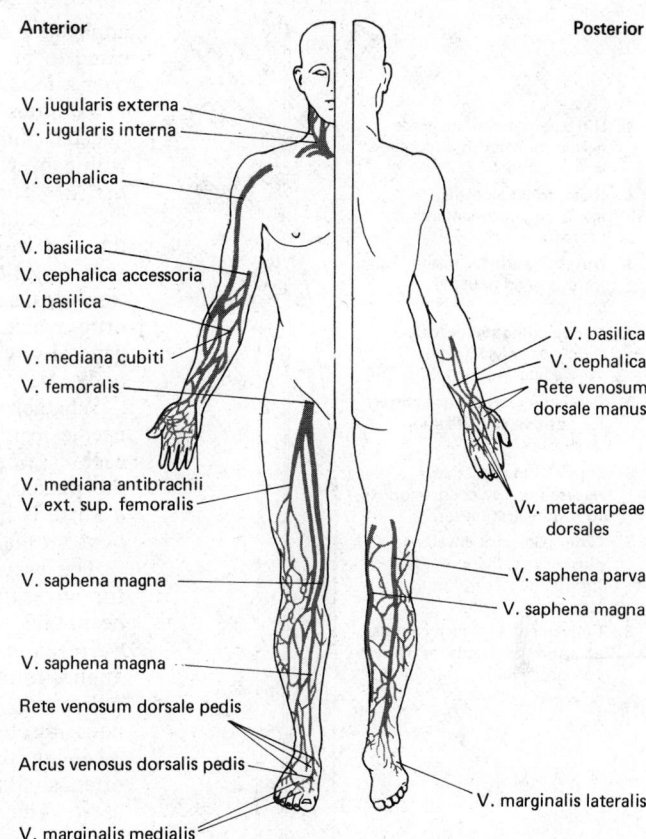

Anterior   Posterior

V. jugularis externa
V. jugularis interna

V. cephalica

V. basilica
V. cephalica accessoria
V. basilica

V. mediana cubiti
V. femoralis

V. basilica
V. cephalica
Rete venosum
dorsale manus

V. mediana antibrachii
V. ext. sup. femoralis

Vv. metacarpeae
dorsales

V. saphena magna

V. saphena parva
V. saphena magna

V. saphena magna

Rete venosum dorsale pedis

Arcus venosus dorsalis pedis

V. marginalis lateralis

V. marginalis medialis

Figure 22-18. The superficial veins used in blood transfusion or intravenous injection. (From *Proceedings Staff Meetings, Mayo Clinic,* **12:**122–25, 1937.)

Memorial Hospital, Burlington, Ontario.[88] Benedict P. Mariano and associates [89] suggest that radiopaque catheters should be used because catheters or parts of them have been lost in the circulatory system. They describe a patient in whom a catheter progressed from an injection site in the right antecubital vein to the lung. Catheters come in sizes equal to needles of 27 to 15 gauge. They can be passed

into the vein for 4 to 5 inches through a needle, which is then removed. The free end of the catheter is attached to the reservoir of solution by tubing, or to a syringe. In both cases appropriate adapters are needed. Ada Lawrence Plumer says:

If the venipuncture is unsuccessful the needle and catheter must be removed *together;* to pull

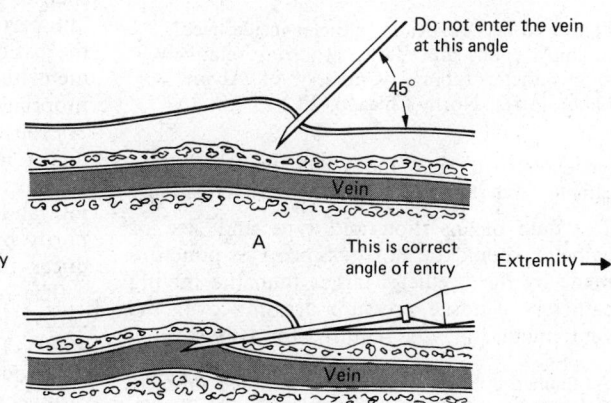

Figure 22-19. Angle of entry of needle in venipuncture of the forearm. (Courtesy of Cutter Laboratories, Berkeley, Calif.)

Do not enter the vein at this angle

45°

Vein

← Body

A

This is correct angle of entry

Extremity →

Vein

B

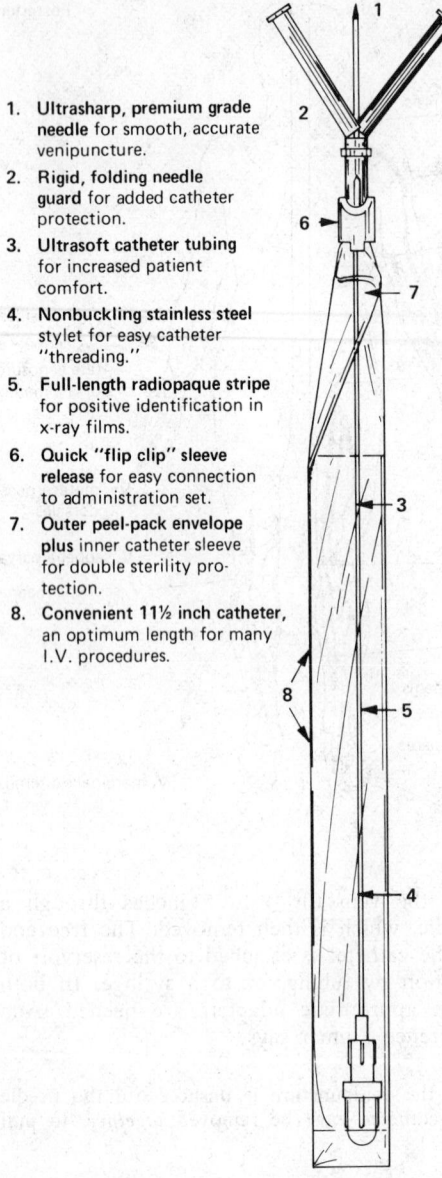

1. **Ultrasharp, premium grade needle** for smooth, accurate venipuncture.

2. **Rigid, folding needle guard** for added catheter protection.

3. **Ultrasoft catheter tubing** for increased patient comfort.

4. **Nonbuckling stainless steel stylet** for easy catheter "threading."

5. **Full-length radiopaque stripe** for positive identification in x-ray films.

6. **Quick "flip clip" sleeve release** for easy connection to administration set.

7. **Outer peel-pack envelope plus** inner catheter sleeve for double sterility protection.

8. **Convenient 11½ inch catheter,** an optimum length for many I.V. procedures.

Figure 22-20. Venocath, catheter-inside-needle for intravenous procedures, requiring relatively long catheter tubing. (Courtesy of Abbott Laboratories, North Chicago, Ill.)

the catheter through the needle may sever the catheter and result in its loss in the circulation.*

The date of insertion and type and size of catheter should be noted. Since the puncture made by the needle is larger than the inlying catheter, a sterile pressure dressing over the venipuncture may be required for a short time;

*Plumer, Ada Lawrence: *Principles and Practices of Intravenous Therapy*. Little, Brown & Co., Boston, 1970, p. 56.

application of an antibiotic may also be indicated to prevent infection. If the catheter lies over a joint, an armboard should be used.

Solutions containing some drugs may be injected into arteries, especially for patients with cancer. This method is called *arterial perfusion*. The only difference between this method and the usual intravenous method is that the drug is introduced under pressure into an artery flowing directly into the area to be treated. Consequently the full strength of the drug reaches the tumor before entering the general circulation and tissues throughout the body.

Whether to *immobilize the area* in which the needle (or catheter) is inserted depends in each case on the site of injection, condition of the patient, and duration of the treatment. If a nurse is in constant attendance, immobilization is usually unnecessary.

The *preparation of the skin* is the same as for any skin puncture or incision. What has been said about the importance of complete *sterilization of equipment* for other injections applies to infusions.

Because *unfavorable reactions* to intravenous injections continue to occur, the patient receiving this treatment should be observed often so that complications may be detected early. The nurse should check the patient's general response to the infusion, the rate of flow and amount of solution in the bottle, as well as the appearance of the injection site. Complications, as cited by Metheny and Snively, include thrombophlebitis, local infiltration, pyrogenic reactions (pyrogens in the solution or those introduced by poor technique), circulatory overload, speed shock, and air embolism. J. Hästbacka and associates[90] in Finland report a clinical study of infusion thrombophlebitis involving 1048 patients; the problem seems to be great. Incidence of phlebitis is associated with a number of factors, such as composition and duration of infusion, but particularly the latter. In the event that the patient responds unfavorably to the treatment, the infusion should be stopped and appropriate action taken.

Preparation of the solutions and tubing requires intelligent direction, well-trained technicians, and good equipment. The use of tubing and solutions prepared and tested for purity by reliable firms is widespread and reduces risk.

The *technique of injecting the needle* concerns all those who participate in the treatment. The vein should be dilated with a tourniquet or digital pressure between the site of injection and the heart, and the pressure released as soon as a flow of blood from the needle indicates that the vein has been entered. If the attempt to enter the vein is unsuccessful and the process long drawn out, the circulation is allowed to return to normal before the next attempt. In some cases it is necessary to make an incision and expose the vein. When an incision is made a local anesthetic is always used; some physicians anesthetize the area in preparation for a needle puncture. Another method of dilating a poorly filled vein is shown in Figure 22-21.

Equipment. Small amounts of solution may be given with a Luer or Record syringe, but when the quantity is sufficient to necessitate refilling the syringe, a reservoir is better. The reservoir, tubing, regulating clamps, and adapters are similar to those used for subcutaneous infusions. Commercial sets are available and used in general practice (see Figs. 22-22 and 22-23). This new equipment ensures greater accuracy in regulating the rate of flow and in controlling volume; because it is disposable, it has replaced permanent rubber tubing and consequently reduced pyrogenic reactions. An inline filter aids in preventing infections and air emboli.[91-93]

Intravenous needles range in length from 4 to 5 cm (1½ to 2 inch) and from 20 to 18 gauge. They should have a medium bevel. The Lindemann needle is often used when the infusion is to last for days. It is less likely to injure the lining of the blood vessel and to get clogged. An irrigating pole, or standard, is necessary when a reservoir is used. Materials are needed for skin disinfection as in all injections. Gauze dressings and strips of adhesive on crinoline may be sterilized with the tubing or in a separate package. Sterile towels enable the operator to handle the area surrounding the point of injection without contaminating his or her hands. Like sterile gloves they are a convenience rather than a necessity. If the physician prescribes the administration of a solution above room temperature a heating device must be provided. A tourniquet is required for dilating the vein to be injected. A moisture-proof pillow is often needed to support the part of the body in which the injection is made and a small blanket to cover the shoulders or exposed areas of the body, according to the room temperature. Containers for liquid and dry waste should be provided. As in all such treatments it is convenient to bring the equipment to the bedside on a moving table or cart. In some institutions patients are taken to treatment rooms. Splints and restraints are selected according to the requirements of each patient. A small hair pillow strapped to the arm makes a less uncomfortable elbow restraint than the rigid type.

Preparation of the Patient. Because the area of injection is different, the patient's position and the arrangement of clothing and bedding are different; in other respects the preparation of the patient is the same as for a subcutaneous infusion. The operator needs a good light on the area where the vein is to be injected, and the patient's eyes should be shielded from it.

Suggested Procedure. Attach the tubing with its connection to the reservoir. (If a syringe is used, attach the needle and fill the syringe with the solution.) Expel the air inside the tubing with solution from the reservoir before attaching the needle to it. Hang the reservoir about 90 cm (3 ft) above the bed. (If a local anesthetic is used, it is given at this point.) Apply the tourniquet above the site of the puncture; as soon as the vein is sufficiently distended inject the needle into the vein, and when the flow of blood from the needle shows that the vein has been entered, release the tourniquet.

In describing the venipuncture, Adriani says:

The puncture is made an inch or so below the contemplated point of entry of the needle into the vein. The needle is introduced with the bevel facing upward, almost parallel to the skin but inclined slightly downward toward the vein. Then, as the point enters the tissues, the shaft is shifted to a more parallel position in relation to the vein but still in a somewhat downward direction. . . .

The operator continues to advance the needle toward the vein until it is felt to pierce the vessel wall. This produces the sensation of a snap if the vein is distended. Blood immediately appears in the syringe. [This assumes that one is using a syringe attached to the needle.] . . . . The direction of the needle is then shifted so that the shaft lies parallel to the vessel wall, and the needle is advanced until it is "threaded" into the lumen for a distance of approximately ½ to ¾ inches.*

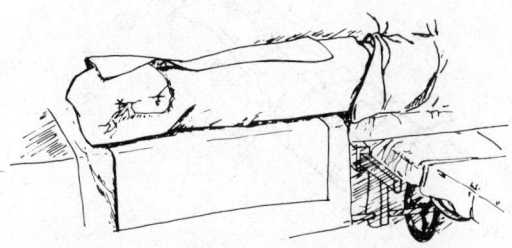

Figure 22-21. Method of applying moist heat to dilate poorly filled veins. The arm is wrapped with a Turkish towel wrung out of hot water, over which is placed a rubber sheet enclosed in turn by a dry Turkish towel. This is left in place 10 to 20 minutes. (Courtesy of Abbott Laboratories, North Chicago, Ill.)

* Adriani, John: "Venipuncture," *Am. J. Nurs.,* **62:**69, (Mar.) 1962.

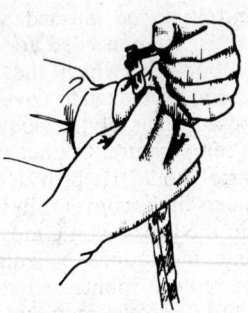

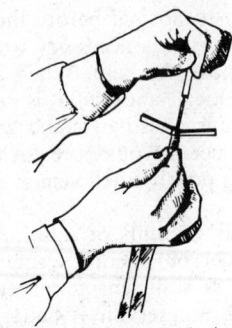

1. *To open* — Leave the sterile inner sheath intact until immediately before use. Then grasp base of blue needle guard and strip sheath down enough to expose only two thirds of guard.

2. *Expose needle* — Slide back clear plastic ring on needle guard, and open guard wings. Discard inner white cover, exposing needle.

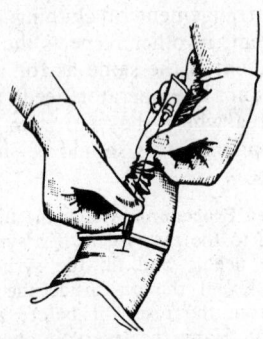

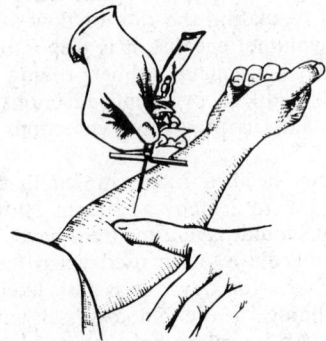

3. *Enter vein* — Make venipuncture, holding needle bevel up. Grasping catheter through its protective sheath, slowly push catheter well into vein. (If during this maneuver, it becomes necessary to withdraw catheter, always withdraw needle simultaneously; this prevents severing of catheter by needle.)

4. *Withdraw needle* — After blood fills catheter, apply finger pressure over catheter in vein. Hold it thus while withdrawing needle. Discard sheath. Snap hub of needle guard into white adapter at catheter end.

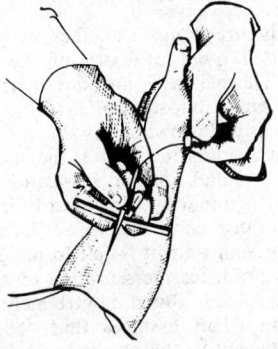

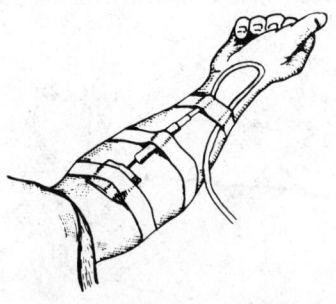

5. *Withdraw stylet* — Remove protective cap from white adapter, and withdraw wire stylet. Immediately connect administration set to adapter.

6. *Close needle guard* — Close wings of guard in place over needle, and slide ring back to distal end of wings, to lock them in place. Tape catheter, needle guard, and end of administration set for proper immobilization.

Figure 22-22. Steps in assembling and operating the Venocath. (Abbott Laboratories: *Parenteral Administration.* Abbott Laboratories, North Chicago, Ill., 1969, p. 32.)

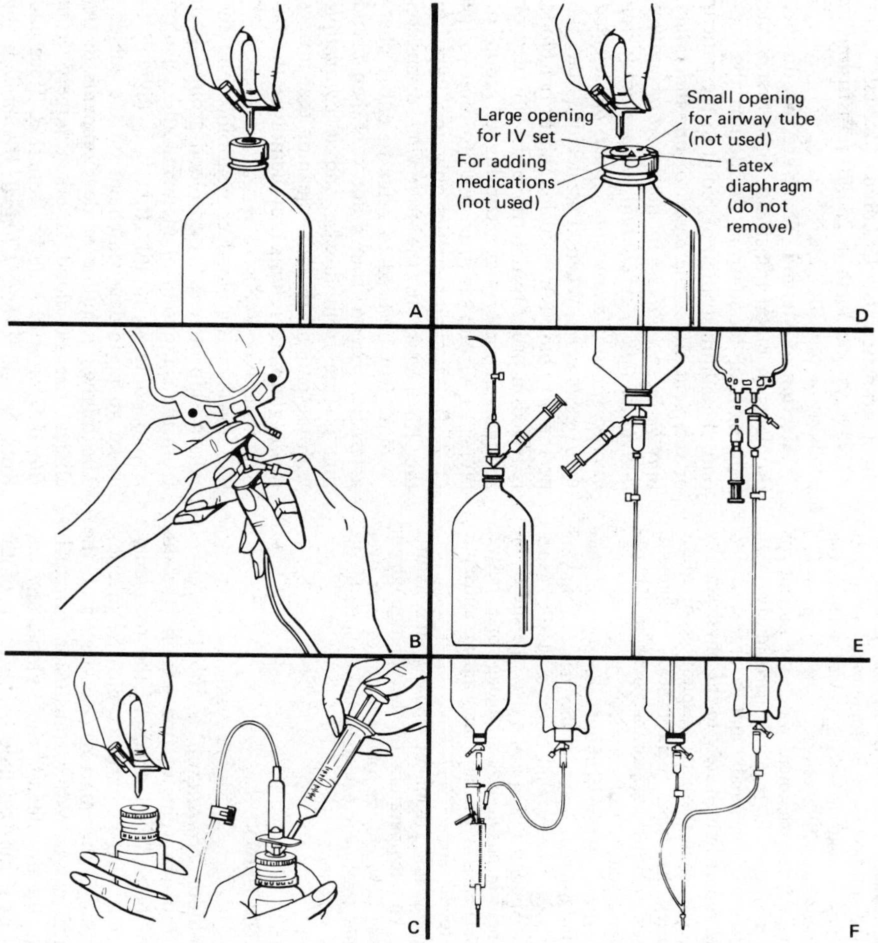

A. Venoset and vacuum bottle with solid rubber stopper

Thrust piercing pin through center of stopper. Do not twist or angle. When bottle is immediately inverted, vacuum can be checked by observing rising filtered air bubbles. Proper fluid level is established in drip chamber automatically (half full).

B. Venoset and plastic IV bag

Replace air filter with needle adapter cover. Insert piercing pin into entry port and penetrate internal plastic seal. Suspend bag and prime set by squeezing flexible drip chamber until half full.

C. Venoset and small volume drug additive containers for IV use

No need to use an air vent needle. Just insert Venoset and remove air filter. Inject diluent through air inlet, using syringe *without* needle. Replace air filter and proceed with administration.

D. Venoset and vacuum bottle with air vent tube

Do *not* remove protective rubber diaphragm under metal seal. Cleanse exposed rubber diaphragm with antiseptic. Insert Venoset piercing pin through diaphragm into largest outlet hole in stopper. IV system is now closed to unfiltered air. When bottle is immediately inverted, vacuum can be checked by observing rising bubbles. Proper fluid level is established in drip chamber automatically (half full).

E. Add compatible medications

Medications can be added to the bottle through the additive port while upright (left) or while suspended and running (center). Medication should be added to the plastic bag only through the injection site on the bag, or via "Y" or latex injection site on the Venoset.

F. To "piggyback"

Administer precision volume additives through Y injection site atop Additive Soluset (left). When it is undesirable to mix additive with primary solution, use Secondary Venoset with needle inserted into Y injection site of primary set.

Small opening for airway tube (not used)

Latex diaphragm (do not remove)

Large opening for IV set

For adding medications (not used)

Figure 22-23. The all-purpose Venoset. (Courtesy of Abbott Laboratories, North Chicago, Ill.)

If the syringe method is used, the operator remains with the patient and injects the total amount; but if the solution is delivered from a reservoir, those caring for the patient keep the apparatus adjusted so that the solution flows at the prescribed rate. Fix the needle in the vein by passing a strip of adhesive around the needle hub and applying the ends to the skin; or, the adhesive may be applied over the hub of the needle, with the ends on the skin. The latter method prevents movement of the needle which may displace it.

When the puncture is made in the bend of the elbow attach a padded splint to the arm. Other necessary restraints, as determined by the condition of the patient, the site of injection, and the amount of nursing attendance available, are applied by the physician or nurse. Stay with or observe the patient as frequently as possible while the solution is flowing and the needle is in the vein, in order to prevent accidents and reassure the patient. There is always the possibility that the clamps on the tubing may loosen and allow the solution to flow into the vein too rapidly, a sudden movement of the patient may disconnect the tubing from one of its connections, or he or she may displace the needle and injure the surrounding tissues. If for some reason the temperature of the solution is to be maintained near that of the body, provide a heating device such as the electric heating coil.

Throughout the treatment watch the patient for signs of unfavorable reaction, particularly when the solution is given rapidly and in large quantity. Note and report immediately to the physician any marked changes in the pulse, respiration, or color; also nausea, headache, nervousness, excitement, restlessness, or any unfavorable signs in the patient's condition.

When the prescribed amount of solution has been administered, remove the needle, making pressure over the wound with a sterile gauze dressing. Apply a dry dressing over the site of injection, held in position by a bandage or adhesive. The physician may or may not want an antiseptic applied to the area.

Recording the Treatment. Indicate the nature, amount, and temperature of the solution given; the rate of flow and the total amount of time over which the treatment extended; report briefly the patient's reaction.

8. TRANSFUSION

Definition. *Transfusion* is the transfer of blood from the veins of one person (the donor) to the veins of another (the recipient). Blood may also be infused into the arteries, the muscles, the marrow cavities, and the peritoneal cavity. While transfusion primarily refers to the transfer of whole blood, any discussion of it must include the infusion of the component parts—cells, plasma, and plasma derivatives.

Therapeutic Uses. Blood or its constituents are infused when (1) the circulating blood volume is suddenly reduced, as in acute hemorrhage, trauma or burns; (2) the concentration of circulating hemoglobin is at an inadequate level in those types of anemia that are not relieved by specific measures, such as Vitamin B_{12} and iron therapy; (3) certain blood substances are lacking, such as plasma protein, clotting factors, and antihemophilic globulin; and (4) there is an infection in leukopenia patients. In this last condition transfusions of white blood cells from patients with chronic myelocytic leukemia have been used with some success.[94]

In case this listing gives the impression that blood transfusion is common, it may be well to state that all authorities consulted say that even with the most up-to-date methods and skillful operators transfusion still involves serious risks. Maxwell M. Wintrobe notes that the use of blood and blood products has become so commonplace that the dangers as well as the advantages have been "multiplied manifold." In 1960 Albert Ehrlich [95] estimated that 5000 fatalities occurred due to incompatible blood transfusions; Crichton McNeil [96] (in 1967) says one death in 25,000 transfusions is probably a realistic rate.

Selection of Method. There are two distinct problems in blood transfusion: the first is the collection of blood from the donor; the second, the administration of blood to the patient or recipient. *Since the blood of one individual may be incompatible with the blood of another individual and may contain disease-producing microorganisms the donor must be selected with great care.* When it is decided that the person is to have a transfusion, his or her blood is tested in order to determine its inherited or acquired characteristics according to "group" or "type." ("Group" is often used to refer to the O, A, B, AB characteristics only and "type" to the Rh factor. In the following discussion "group" will be used to refer to either characteristic.) Blood from a donor is then found that is free from disease and is *compatible* with the patient's blood—meaning that it does not agglutinate (clump) or hemolyze the patient's red blood cells.

Knowledge of blood compatibility and the relationship of heredity to blood groups, both from the standpoint of medicine and genetics, is expanding so rapidly that it is difficult to make an up-to-date statement on the subject. The following outline of developments in the clinical use of blood is taken largely from *Blood Groups in Man* by Robert R. Race and Ruth Sanger [97] and *Clinical Hematology* by Wintrobe.[98]

There are records of attempts to transfuse blood from animals and well human beings to sick persons as far back as the seventeenth

Table 22-2.   Landsteiner Blood Groups as Defined by Anti-A and Anti-B Factors

Percentage of the Population in United States and Europe	International Nomenclature	Jansky Numbering	Moss Numbering	Agglutinogens or Antigens in Red Blood Cells	Agglutinins or Antibodies in Serum
45	O	I	IV	O	Anti-A (alpha factor) Anti-B (beta factor)
42	A	II	II	A factor	Anti-B (beta factor)
10	B	III	III	B factor	Anti-A (alpha factor)
3	AB	IV	I	A and B factors	None

century. These attempts were rare because the methods were crude; there was little understanding of blood compatibility, and the chance of surviving the treatment was about fifty-fifty.

In 1900, Landsteiner reported that red cells from one human being were agglutinated, or clumped, when mixed with the blood serum of some human beings but not others. Within two years he and his associates were able to announce that people can be divided into four groups according to the behavior of their blood cells and sera. This led to wide experimentation by scientists in various parts of the world. A conflicting nomenclature sprang up for these blood groups and the mysterious qualities, or factors, that make some blood compatible, others not. Although Landsteiner's nomenclature for the four blood groups was rivaled by those of Jansky and Moss, it is now in general use (see Table 22-2).

As can be seen when one studies Table 22-3, a person who has group O blood has red blood cells that are not agglutinated by the blood serum from any of the other groups. He or she is often (with undue confidence) called a *universal donor*. A person with group AB blood has serum with no anti-A and anti-B agglutinins to clump the cells from the A and B groups, so he or she is termed the *universal recipient*. Actually, these statements are oversimplifications. Since the discovery of these four blood groups, O, A, B, and AB, subgroups have been recognized in A and AB groups. These are

designated as subgroups A_1 and A_2, A_1B and A_2B. (Differences in the behavior of bloods of two persons belonging in the A group or the AB group are clinically significant and point to the necessity of proving the blood of the donor compatible with the blood of the recipient before each transfusion.) Next in importance to the discovery of the original blood groups was the introduction in 1914 of sodium citrate as an anticoagulant by Lewinsohn in the United States, Hustin in Belgium, and Agote in Argentina. This made "delayed transfusion," with a simple aseptic procedure, possible. The discovery of *pyrogens* by Seibert in 1923, and the development of blood banks and blood preservation from 1933 to the present have all contributed toward safer transfusions.

In 1927, Landsteiner and Levine reported that human beings could again be divided into three groups according to the way their blood cells reacted to two sera, one of which they named anti-M and the other anti-N. Bloods agglutinated by anti-M serum they designated *type M*, those agglutinated by anti-N they termed *type N;* those agglutinated by both sera, *type MN*. In 1947, Race reported an *S group* which he classifies with the MN category. Another category of blood groups Landsteiner and Levine have reported as *type P+* and *type P−*. Mourant in 1946 and Andresen in 1948 discovered the Lewis system which is closely related to the ABO system and is defined by two antigens, Le^a and Le^b and the two antibodies, anti-Le^a and anti-Le^b. Observation

Table 22-3.   Interactions of the Four Blood Groups

Cells	AB Serum No Agglutinins	B Serum (Anti-A)	A Serum (Anti-B)	O Serum (Anti-A, Anti-B)
AB	−	+	+	+
A	−	+	−	+
B	−	−	+	+
O	−	−	−	−

(+ means agglutination, or clumping; − means no agglutination.)

also strongly indicates that a substance on group O cells and in group O secretions is not a direct product of the O genes; this substance has been renamed "H." Wintrobe [99] notes that many of the confusing observations made since Landsteiner's discovery can be appreciated by the recognition of the four closely interrelated gene systems: ABO, Hh, Lele, and Sese. The five blood group specificity (A, B, H, Le^a, and Le^b) may be detected in human secretions, and combinations of the four gene systems permit recognition of six main groups of gene combinations.

A much more important discovery, from the clinical standpoint, is the *Rh facto*r (antigen or agglutinogen) reported by Landsteiner and Weiner in 1940. They described studies in which rabbits were injected with red cells of the Rhesus monkey, the rabbits developing an antiserum that was found to agglutinate the red cells of human beings in about 85 per cent of those tested, regardless of the absence, or presence, of the agglutinogens AB, MN, or P. They called the agglutinogen or antigen in the cell the *Rh factor* after the Rhesus monkey. Persons whose erythrocytes are agglutinated by the antiserum are termed *Rh positive;* those whose cells were not agglutinated are termed *Rh negative*. About 85 per cent of the Caucasians are estimated to be *Rh positive*, 15 per cent *Rh negative*. At first the *Rh factor* was thought to be a single antigen; now "almost 30 different specificities of Rh-Hr antisera" have been reported in the literature, according to Wintrobe. The Hr factor (an agglutinin) was discovered in the serum of the Rh-positive

mother of an erythroblastotic infant; this agglutinin acted upon all Rh-negative bloods as well as on certain Rh-positive bloods. J. Garrott Allen says:

Six different cell characteristics are identifiable in the Rh system. These are designated as Rh$_o$, rh', rh'', Hr$_o$, hr', and hr'', respectively; or by the British corresponding nomenclature of D, C and E, and d, c and e. However, these do not refer to the potential number of combinations of Rh groups which total 27 possibilities.

The erythrocytes of every person must contain at least one member of each of these 3 pairs of antigens. The red cells of some individuals may contain 4, 5 or even 6, so that the number of combinations possible is rather large.*

Not only has complexity been compounded by disagreement in nomenclature (Wiener vs Fisher-Race) but by differences in theories postulated by Wiener and Fisher. Table 22-4 shows Wiener's gene designations, corresponding agglutinogens, and blood factors, as well as Fisher-Race notations. Health workers must be familiar to some extent with both nomenclatures until a single system is widely accepted. A numerical coding system to fit with the schemes of the two opposing schools (Wiener and Fisher) has been proposed, such as Rh1, Rh2, and so on; hopefully, some standard terminology will soon be established.

Since the *Rh factor* was recognized and publicized as the cause of severe transfusion

* Allen, J. Garrott: "Blood Tranfusions and Related Problems," in Moyer, Carl A., et al.: *Surgery Principles and Practice*, 3rd ed. J. B. Lippincott Co., Philadelphia, 1965, p. 158.

Table 22-4.   Wiener's Gene Designations, Corresponding Agglutinogens and Blood Factors, and Fisher-Race Notations *

Genes		Frequency Among Caucasoids, %	Corresponding Agglutinogens	Blood Factors Present
Wiener	Fisher-Race			
r	*cde*	38.0	rh	hr',hr'',hr
r'	*Cde*	0.6	rh'	rh',hr''
r'^{w}	*C^{w}de*	0.005	rh'^{w}	rh',rh^w,hr''
r''	*cdE*	0.5	rh''	rh'',hr'
r^y	*CdE*	0.01	rh^y	rh',hr''
R^o	*cDe*	2.7	Rh$_o$	Rh$_o$,hr',hr'',hr
R^1	*CDe*	41.0	Rh$_1$	Rh$_o$,rh',hr''
R^{1w}	*C^{w}De*	2.0	Rh$_1$^{w}	Rh$_o$,rh',rh^w,hr''
R^2	*cDE*	15.0	Rh$_2$	Rh$_o$,rh'',hr'
R^z	*CDE*	0.2	Rh^z	Rh$_o$,rh',rh''

Wiener, in his publications, uses italics for gene symbols and for genotypes, regular type for agglutinogens and phenotypes, and boldface type for symbols for blood factors and for the corresponding antibodies used to detect the blood factors in question. Further, to distinguish the symbols for genotypes and phenotypes, the letter "h" is omitted and only superscripts are used in gene symbols.

* Wintrobe, Maxwell M.: *Clinical Hematology*, 6th ed. Lea & Febiger, Philadelphia, 1967, p. 372.

reactions and erythroblastosis foetalis (hemolytic anemia of the newborn characterized by jaundice with an increased number of nucleated red blood cells), the *Rh factor* has come to be a familiar term in this country. Many nonmedical persons know the danger in transfusing an *Rh negative* individual with *Rh positive* blood; they even know the precautions that must be taken to protect the *Rh negative* woman and her offspring if she marries an *Rh positive* man, or if she gets transfusions of *Rh positive* blood. It will be a good thing when everyone knows that *Rh positive blood should never be given to any person who is Rh negative.* This has often happened, and, as a result, many *Rh negative* persons who have received repeated transfusions of *Rh positive* blood have developed antibodies against the *Rh positive* cells, or they have been "sensitized" to *Rh positive* blood. The *Rh negative* mother carrying a fetus who has (inherited) *Rh positive* blood cells may develop antibodies against the *Rh positive* cells of the fetus, and these antibodies in the mother's blood cause erythroblastosis foetalis. This reaction, or sensitization, is more marked with each *Rh positive* fetus the mother carries. This explains why the third or fourth child is more likely to develop erythroblastosis than the first born. If the sensitized *Rh negative* mother is given a transfusion of *Rh positive* blood she is likely to have a very serious reaction, that can be fatal. According to P. L. Mollison,[100] the *maximum* incidence of hemolytic disease of the newborn due to Rh incompatibility is between one in 150 to one in 200 births; however, only 60 per cent or one in 300 of all newborn infants requires treatment. Intrauterine transfusions (red blood cells introduced into the peritoneal cavity) have been given when the fetus has reached 31 weeks' maturity. It is thought that red cell destruction is established by about the fourth month of pregnancy and is detected by testing maternal serum for antibodies. If the test is positive and there is a likelihood of disease in the offspring, plans should be made for an "exchange transfusion" as soon as the baby is born. The erythroblastotic blood of the infant is replaced with *Rh negative* blood from a female donor. The exchange transfusion is often made through the umbilical vein. (*Rh negative* persons should be urged to donate blood to blood banks so that their blood will be available in such eventualities. *Rh negative* blood should never be used for *Rh positive* recipients.) Other blood groups, recognized between the years 1946 and 1951, include the Lutheran, Kell, Duffy, and Kidd groups, named for those persons in whose blood they were first discovered. Not all of these are thought to be clinically significant. The anti-K (Kell group) is a cause of hemolytic disease of the newborn and may be the cause of transfusion reaction. This group as well as the others mentioned above are important in the study of anthropologic characteristics of man. Fourteen human blood group systems and more than 60 different blood group factors are known today.[101] It must be obvious from even so brief an account of blood groups that health workers must be alert to new progress in the study of blood physiology.

The fact has been established that blood groups are inherited through the Mendelian law of inheritance. Given the blood group characteristics of a baby, the experts in genetics can say whether it is possible or impossible for a man, on the basis of his blood characteristics, to be the father of the child. Blood grouping has therefore a very important role in *forensic* (pertaining to a law court), or legal, medicine. Blood tests may help an accused man to prove that he is not the father of a child, or they may help a man suspected of a crime by proving that the blood stains on him were not made by the blood of the victim. It has been suggested that newborn infants have their blood tested and records kept. This means of identification would be a protection for hospitals in lawsuits over the ownership of babies. All persons should carry with their identification a record of their blood type to prevent delay in giving a transfusion should they be seriously injured and need immediate replacement of lost blood.

A commercial blood donor service has on hand a number of cells to be used by laboratories in checking blood types, but it is only occasionally that some of these cells are needed.

Early in 1950, the National Institutes of Health established *minimum standards* for the safe preparation and preservation of blood for transfusions, including the selection of donors. These have been adopted by the American Association of Blood Banks and endorsed by the American College of Surgeons. Such action facilitates easy exchange of blood between blood banks and offers protection to donors and recipients as well as the physician and other health workers involved in transfusions, including the hospital.[102,103] Donors must have a normal temperature and blood pressure, be free from syphilis, malaria, and upper respiratory disease and give no history of viral hepatitis. They must not have been pregnant within the last six months, and their hemoglobin must not fall below 12.5 gm per 100 ml of blood. In addition, M. C. Crocker says: "A recent history of any illness, use of drugs, vaccinations,

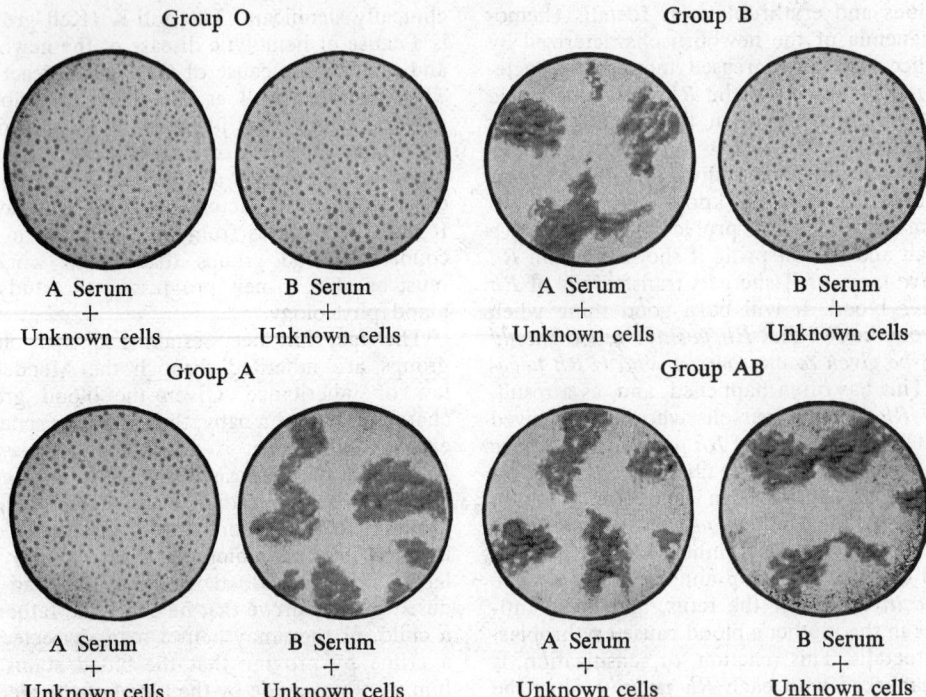

Figure 22-24. Diagrams showing the behavior of blood when compatible or incompatible blood serums are added. *Upper left:* The corpuscles of *group O* are not agglutinated by serum from groups A and B. *Lower left:* The corpuscles of *group A* are agglutinated by group B serum. *Upper right:* The corpuscles of *group B* are agglutinated by serum from group A. *Lower right:* The corpuscles of *group AB* are agglutinated by serums of groups A and B. (Courtesy of LaVerne Ruth Thompson and Clay-Adams Co., New York, N.Y.)

travel to the tropics or history of contact with communicable diseases should be obtained." * Some individuals are sensitive to certain drugs (such as salicylates and penicillin) and vaccine. Persons who suffer from allergies may transmit an allergic reaction to recipients. Most donors are between 18 and 65 years of age. When the blood is collected from the donor a sample is taken, and from this sample a serologic test for syphilis is made and the blood is "typed" or "grouped." (Blood from a syphilitic patient is either rejected or used in such a way that transmission of the disease is impossible. Actually, the spirochete causing syphilis is easily killed and, according to the National Institutes of Health will not survive in blood that is stored for 96 hours.) Crocker believes that the blood of a person known to have syphilis should be excluded. All blood is typed for O, A, B, and AB groups and for the Rh factor, using an anti-Rh$_0$ (anti-D) typing serum. Allen says that most clinicians feel more secure when

the common subgroups, as well as major groups, are identified in both the donor and recipient. For example, in testing for the Rh antigens, cells may be examined for the presence of Rh$_0$, rh', and rh", using the antisera anti-Rh$_0$ (anti-D), anti-rh' (anti-C), and anti-rh" (anti-E). The same holds true for the ABO group—A$_1$, A$_2$, A$_3$, A$_1$B, and A$_2$B (see Table 22-5). Although group O blood has been used successfully for groups A and B after being titered (strength measured) for isoagglutinins, its use is not recommended except in grave emergencies. (The prefix *iso* comes from the Greek word, *isos* = equal or same. Here this refers to the same group.) If group O blood has a high titer of isoagglutinins, "group specific substances" may be added to reduce the titer so that the blood is more compatible with other groups. Even though plasma isoagglutinins are usually absorbed by the recipient cells, due to their large surface area, the "universal donor" plasma may contain "immune" or "second order" anti-A or anti-B which may cause hemagglutination and hemolysis. In other words, the patient's own red

* Crocker, M. C.: "Blood Transfusion," *Anesthesia,* **23:**372, (July) 1968.

Table 22-5. Anti-Rh Typing Serums and Rh Factor(s) Reacting *

Anti-Rh Serum	Rh Factor(s) Reacting
Anti-Rh$_0$ (Anti-D)	Rh$_0$ (D)
Anti-rh' (Anti-C)	rh' (C)
Anti-rh" (Anti-E)	rh" (E)
Anti-Rh$_0$' (Anti-CD)	Rh$_0$ (D), rh' (C)
Anti-Rh$_0$" (Anti-DE)	Rh$_0$ (D), rh" (E)
Anti-Rh$_0$rh'rh" (Anti-CDE)	Rh$_0$ (D), rh' (C), rh" (E)
Anti-hr' (Anti-c)	hr' (c)
Anti-hr" (Anti-e)	hr" (e)

The Pharmacopeia of the United States of America, 18th rev., United States Pharmacopeia Convention, Washington, D.C., 1970, p. 841.

cells are lysed (dissolved) and serum hemoglobin rises. Several deaths have resulted from the use of "universal donor" blood.[104] Some writers say that the terms "immune sera" and "universal donors" should be discarded because they give a false impression. They point out that transfusions to other groups of group O blood, or plasma, may have cumulative effects that are at first unnoticeable but build up to marked blood changes.

The donor's blood may be used as citrated whole blood or the cells and platelets and the plasma may be used separately. Because it may be stored, transported without refrigeration, and rapidly reconstituted when dried, plasma has been used successfully in emergency military situations and in treatment of coagulation deficiencies; however, because of the availability and superiority of whole blood for treatment of hemorrhage, its use has decreased over the last two decades. In addition, investigators have shown that administration of pooled plasma (a mixture of plasma from various numbers of donors) carries with it a high incidence of serum hepatitis which varies directly with the number of donors in the pool. The possibility of transmitting hepatitis may be reduced by processing plasma from single units of blood and by storing plasma for 6 months or longer at a temperature of 31°C (87.8°F). However, the stored plasma is still not completely free of hepatitis virus. Transfusion reaction may also occur as a result of plasma infusion.[105]

In summary, the serologic test is made for syphilis on the donor's blood. It is typed for *O, A, B groups* and the *Rh (CDE) factor*. It is titered and subtyped in special cases. Before the whole blood (blood cells) from any donor is given to any recipient it must be cross-

matched. The donor's cells are mixed with the recipient's serum (plasma), and the recipient's cells are mixed with the donor's serum. All these tests must be negative for agglutination before the blood can be safely given. Ordinarily, plasma or its proteins (albumin and globulin) are given without crossmatching; some physicians, in some cases, insist on group-specific plasma. All containers of blood and plasma must be clearly marked with the information as indicated above.

The technique of collecting blood from the donor and giving it to the patient has been revolutionized in recent years. Textbooks continue to list *direct* and *indirect* methods. The direct method, though rarely used today, may involve one of the following: (1) vessel anastomosis, (2) cannula anastomosis, (3) vein-to-vein connection by tubing and valve or pump, (4) paraffined tube method, and (5) multiple syringe method.

In the *immediate* or *direct* methods the donor and recipient are placed side by side, and blood taken from one person is given directly to the other so that, theoretically, the blood has no time to clot. Actually all direct techniques are difficult and hazardous compared with indirect methods. Direct transfusion, now rarely used, is a procedure for the operating room and will not be discussed in this book.

With *delayed* or *indirect* transfusions, blood is taken from the donor and given to the recipient days or weeks later in, perhaps, another hemisphere. *Clotting is prevented* by the addition of an anticoagulant solution and the blood preserved by refrigeration. The storage of blood has been extended to as long as 28 days due to the various types of anticoagulants, which must be chemically free, pyrogen-free, and sterile. Three anticoagulant solutions are currently used: Table 22-6 gives the formulas for each of these. In ACD (acid-citrate-dextrose) solutions, sodium citrate is used as an anticoagulant because of its ability to bind calcium, while citric acid slows cellular metabolism and prolongs storage life. The addition of dextrose allows cellular metabolism and thus preserves viability of the red cells.[106] CPD (citrate-phosphate-dextrose) reduces the net loss of potassium from red blood cells and allows for longer survival.[107] Calcium-chelating agents may also be used as alternative anticoagulants to collect blood, an example is EDTA (ethylene diamine acetic acid).[108] In addition, heparin is used as a collection anticoagulant, especially in blood collected for extracorporeal circulation. Heparinized blood must be used within 48 hours due to poor red cell viability, but if it is not used within this period, it may be citrated with ACD solution

Table 22-6.   Formulas for Anticoagulant Solutions *

Solution	Contents	Amount/500 ml blood
ACD, Formula A (Acid-Citrate-Dextrose)	Trisodium citrate	1.65 gm
	Citric acid anhydrous	0.6 gm
	Hydrous dextrose	1.83 gm
	Water for injection	75 ml
ACD, Formula B	Trisodium citrate	1.58 gm
	Citric acid anhydrous	0.53 gm
	Hydrous dextrose	1.76 gm
	Water for injection	120 ml
CPD (Citrate-Phosphate-Dextrose)	Trisodium citrate	1.94 gm
	Citric acid anhydrous	0.24 gm
	Monobasic sodium phosphate	0.157 gm
	Hydrous dextrose	1.83 gm
	Water for injection	75 ml

* Graves, Constance: "Massive Transfusion," *Int. Anesthesiol. Clin.,* **5**: 928, (Winter) 1967.

within 24 hours to avoid wasting the blood.[109]

The equipment for the collection of blood from the donor and the administration of blood to the recipient is very similar. Materials for disinfecting the skin are identical. The container in which the blood is collected from the donor serves as the reservoir in which it is stored and from which blood is given to the recipient. Commercially prepared, disposable units that include polyvinyl and glass reservoirs, tubing, needles, filter, and clamps offer by far the best protection and are, in the long run, most economical in this country. In the donor set the reservoir is connected with the donor's vein by a 40-inch length of plastic tubing. The tubing for the polyvinyl bag has a 16-gauge needle on one end and is incorporated into the bag itself on the other end. The tubing for the glass bottle has a piercing cannula or needle on one end with a needle on the opposite end. The polyvinyl bag expands during collection and collapses during administration and thereby prevents foaming, hemolysis, and potential air embolism. An air vent needle should *never* be inserted into a polyvinyl bag. Multiple closed-system vinyl blood collecting units are available to transfer whole blood or (by differential centrifugation) combinations of plasma, red cells, and platelets. Abbott Laboratories states: "Since all transfers are closed, there is maximum protection of sterility and no waste of blood." Multiple plasmapheresis units are also available to permit collection of blood for plasma with immediate return of red cells to the donor.[110] Blood is drawn from the donor by gravity, or with suction by a vacuum in the reservoir.

Crocker cautions that the tourniquet should be held inflated at a pressure of 40 to 60 mm Hg while blood is being drawn to prevent air embolism. In addition, the receiving bottle or bag should always be held below the level of venipuncture, and collection tubing should be clamped prior to tourniquet release because of the increased venous and bottle pressure caused by its use.[111] A small amount of air is not thought dangerous, but a large amount may be fatal. Blood and anticoagulant solution should be mixed gently and often during collection. A blood collection balance or spring scale is recommended for accurate weighing of blood. A means of regulating the flow in collecting and giving blood should be provided; therefore, it is desirable to have the tubing fitted with a disposable clamp. But disposable clamps are *not* adequate in maintaining a vacuum in certain collection sets. In such cases, a metal clamp or hemostat should be used. During collection, the rate of flow should be adjusted so that 5 to 7 minutes are required for collection of one unit of blood.[112]

For administering blood, a longer tube (6 to 7 ft) is used. It is fitted with a cannula that is inserted into the reservoir. Incorporated in the drip chamber is a filter. *Filtration of the blood going in the patient is essential.* The National Institutes of Health say the filter must be one that removes "particular matter of a size potentially dangerous to the patient" but must not reduce the rate of blood flow unnecessarily (see Figs. 22-25 and 22-26). A dressing to cover the puncture wound is needed for the donor and recipient. Splints and restraints may be required for the recipient. While blood is

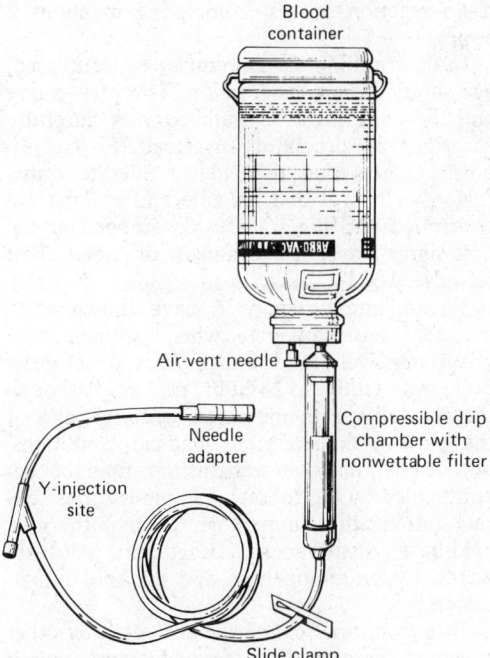

Figure 22-25. Blood administration set with filter in drip chamber. (Courtesy of Abbott Laboratories, North Chicago, Ill.)

often given in tandem with saline, or saline with glucose, the practice of mixing nutrients or drugs with blood is frowned on. For rapid infusion of blood, a blood pump or pressure unit may be used with the glass container or vinyl bag, respectively [113] (see Fig. 22-27). Because refrigeration slows decomposition of blood cells, blood is cooled rapidly after collection to a temperature of 4°C (39°F) and kept so until it is used.[114,115] However, when given in large amounts at a rapid rate (such as 500 ml per 5 minutes), in treatment of massive hemorrhage for example, the patient who is already cold can be further chilled and the state of shock deepened.[116] Instead of being a lifesaving measure, rapid transfusion of cold blood may produce cardiac or generalized hypothermia and even death. In such cases it is necessary to warm blood immediately before transfusion. Blood may be warmed by passing it through a coil of 24 ft of disposable, sterile plastic tubing submerged in a 37°C (99°F) water bath while the transfusion is carried out. The long coil, however, offers resistance to the flow of cold blood and reduces the maximal rate of transfusion, which could be a disadvantage when rapid blood replacement is necessary. (Another device, under investigation, called the microwave blood warmer, allows heating of blood within one minute.) The

vinyl blood bag is placed in a cylinder with metal shielding on both ends to produce a more uniform final temperature. Additional studies must be performed, however, to ensure that no significant changes will result from microwave warming. *Unused, warmed blood should not be returned to the blood bank for reuse.*[117]

Disinfection of the skin at site of puncture is the same as for the other procedures described in this chapter. The donor and the patient should both be prepared to cooperate through suitable explanations of what is to happen. The sites for transfusion are virtually the same as those for infusion. Blood is ordinarily collected from the median basilic or cephalic vein of the donor after an application of a tourniquet, but any good-sized patent vein may be used. Blood is given to the recipient in veins of the arm, leg, hand, foot, or neck. When for any reason the veins cannot be used, blood is injected into the peritoneal cavity and bone marrow. Occasionally when a patient is in a critical condition, blood may be given into an artery, especially if an artery is exposed as during an operation. Transfusions for infants are difficult because their veins are small. While the fontanel is still open, blood can be given into the superior saggital sinus. Because, however, the danger of a hematoma in the cranium is so serious, this site seems to be unanimously condemned.

The amount of blood taken from the donor

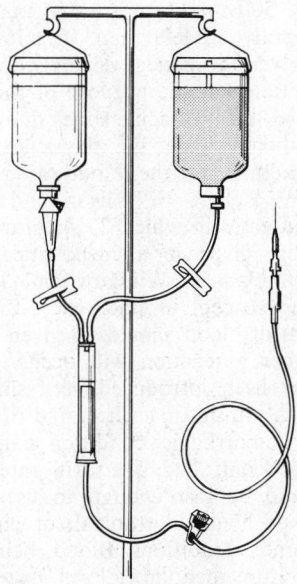

Figure 22-26. "Y" set-up for blood and solution. (Courtesy of Cutter Laboratories, Berkeley, Calif.)

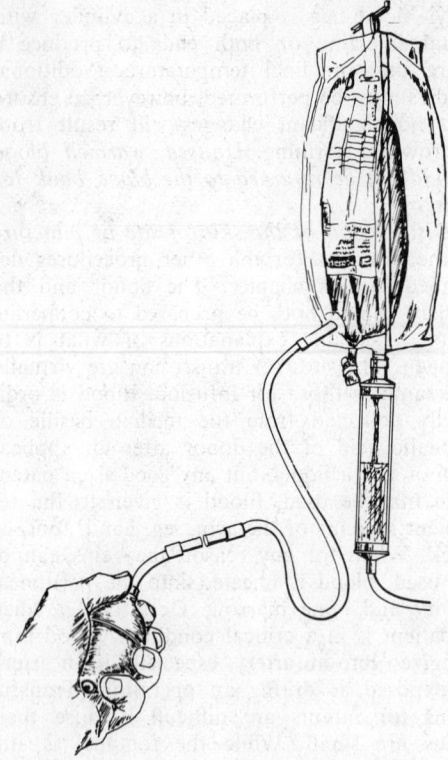

Figure 22-27. Plastic blood bag with pressure bulb. (From Abbott Laboratories: *The Uses of Blood.* Abbott Laboratories, North Chicago, Ill., 1967, p. 55.)

is usually 500 ml (1 pt) and it may be collected rapidly, in less than 10 minutes. The amount given the patient depends upon his or her condition and the purpose of the transfusion. In treatment of acute shock due to uncontrollable hemorrhage, the physician may decide to administer the blood as rapidly as possible.[118] Robert F. Wilson and others [119] have cited cases in which 25 or more units of blood were given in a 24-hour period. According to Jan T. Williams and Daniel F. Moravec,[120] except in emergency, the first 50 to 100 ml of blood should be given slowly to see whether a reaction will occur. Although blood has been introduced very slowly as a continuous infusion over a period of 24 hours when a hemorrhagic condition exists which cannot be controlled, the drip rate of each unit should be fast enough to use all of it within four hours in tropical, or eight hours in temperate, conditions. Blood, being an excellent culture medium, allows growth of organisms if the temperature is permitted to rise.[121] According to Francis D. Moore,[122] an elective transfusion should be started at 20 to 40 drops per minute and speeded as necessary

if no reaction occurs, completing in about 2 hours.

In determining the amount to be transfused, age should be a consideration. The very young and the aged must be watched very carefully for signs of circulatory overload. F. J. Gibbins [123] states that the elderly tolerate transfusion well, provided the rate and volume are controlled and the transfusion stopped at the first sign of dyspnea, cyanosis, or moist chest sounds.

Wilson and others [124,125] have shown a 45 per cent mortality rate when patients were given massive blood transfusions of at least 5000 ml within a 24-hour period. Although the mortality rate increased with the age of the patient, complicating medical conditions, and shock, massive transfusions may be accompanied by the following complications: citrate intoxication, hyperkalemia, hypothermia, acid-base disturbances, coagulation disturbances, hyperammonemia, and nitritoid intoxication.

In anemia that cannot be corrected by other types of therapy, the object of transfusion is to increase the red blood cell count until a given hemoglobin concentration is reached. This can be calculated by established formulas. Roughly, 500 ml of blood should raise the hemoglobin concentration in an adult 10 per cent. Slow (drip) administration of blood gives best results. Even at this slow rate, blood is rarely given continuously, so it may take almost four days to raise the hemoglobin concentration 30 per cent. To keep from "overloading the circulation," anemic and cardiac patients are sometimes given concentrated suspensions of erythrocytes (whole citrated blood from which some of the plasma has been removed). The term, "packed cells," is often used to refer to blood from which plasma

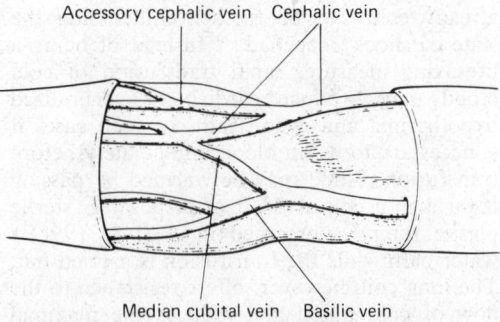

Figure 22-28. Diagram showing veins used for collection of blood from the donor and for administration of blood to the recipient. (*Guide for Venipuncture and Intravenous Therapy in Emergency Medical Services.* New York State Department of Health, Albany, N.Y., 1952.)

has been removed. James M. and Peter Vogel [126] state that packed red cells prepared from blood collected in glass reservoirs or single-unit vinyl bags must be used within 24 hours because entry increases the risk of contamination. However, packed cells collected in the multiple-pack bags may be stored for 21 days since this is a closed system. They further state that transfusion of packed cells may decrease transfusion reaction due to a plasma factor.

Most authorities say there are *no substitutes for whole blood*. When the oxygen-carrying red blood cells are needed, citrated whole blood or packed cells should be used. In some conditions the blood count is normal, but the volume of circulating fluid is low. In such cases blood plasma (fresh, frozen, or dried) is used. Albumin solutions, packed platelets, platelet-rich plasma (PRP) as well as leukocytes and fibrinogen are also given. Substitutes for plasma are discussed briefly on page 1186 under *infusion*. Even with blood banks, the collection of blood from persons who have met accidental death, and the improved methods of preserving whole blood, blood cells, plasma, and albumin, there is still an insufficient supply. Health workers should take every opportunity to make the public mindful of this need. Considerate, appreciative treatment of donors and skillful collection of blood are most effective in promoting both voluntary and paid donations.

Although the mechanism responsible for clotting is not well understood, platelets arrest bleeding from injured vessels, prevent petechial hemorrhages, and promote conversion of prothrombin to thrombin. In patients with thrombocytopenia due to leukemia, platelet transfusion has not only decreased the risk of infection and the rate of fatal hemorrhage by 50 per cent, it has also permitted intensive chemotherapy. Other conditions in which platelets may be transfused are hemorrhage resulting from massive transfusion, septicemia, aplastic anemia, or dengue hemorrhagic fever.[127,128] Platelets may be transfused in the form of whole fresh blood, platelet-rich plasma, and platelet concentrates. Because the half-life of platelets in the recipient is 1 to 2 days, platelets should be infused within 6 hours of their donation. Since fever and septicemia further decrease the half-life of platelets, the frequency of infusion depends upon their post-transfusion survival rate. Plasmapheresis (a process used for removing platelet rich plasma from the donor) has greatly increased the availability of platelets because each donor can supply more than 40 times as much platelet-rich plasma as whole blood.[129] While it has been shown in several

patients with aplastic anemia that they may become refractory to repeated platelet transfusions over a longer period of time (presumably due to antibody formation), this could be controlled by splenectomy which improves response to platelet transfusion.[130]

Even though platelet transfusion has become quite common, leukocyte transfusion has not increased as rapidly because of the difficulty of getting adequate numbers of cells from normal donors. Several investigators have used leukopharesis (a process of removing leukocytes from the blood of the donor) to get white cells from patients with chronic myelocytic leukemia to infuse into leukopenic patients. Results show that infusion of adequate numbers of leukocytes is followed by disappearance of fever and partial or complete remissions from the disease itself. However, leukocyte transfusion may result in a high incidence of fever, chills, leukocyte-antibody production, and a secondary syndrome identical to that which complicates the grafting of allogenic bone marrow in man.[131]

Two noncellular substances in blood may also be transfused. Albumin, a serum protein, is useful as a plasma expander in certain types of shock because it exerts oncotic pressure. In addition, dessicated human fibrinogen is used to treat clinical conditions associated with hypofibrinogenemia.[132]

Accidents, Reactions, and Complications. McNeil [133] lists the following types of reactions to blood transfusion: (1) allergic reaction and unexplained, transient fever, (2) plasma reaction, (3) leukocytes agglutinin reaction, (4) platelet agglutinin reaction, (5) hemolytic reaction and sensitization, (6) blood contamination—bacterial and viral hepatitis, (7) circulatory reactions due to overload, air embolism, and cold blood, and (8) potassium intoxication and citrate toxicity.

Many of these dangers are eliminated by the blood bank, or the blood collecting service, if the department furnishes the patient with compatible pyrogen-free and sterile plasma or blood, properly treated with an anticoagulant. From this point on the patient must be protected by physicians, nurses, and by all who work with him or her. Labels identifying the blood must be checked and rechecked with the patient's name by several persons who understand the danger involved. (The second author has seen the administration of the wrong blood to a sick man prevented by the vigilance of a student nurse in her early study period.)

No matter what precautions are taken, the patient must be watched closely during and after a transfusion. The most common symptom of reaction to transfusion is fever, which may be followed by other symptoms such as a chill, urticaria, pruritus, and even asthma. The cause is rarely identified, but there appears to be a correlation between allergic reaction and previous transfusion. Treatment of febrile and allergic reactions should include supportive care, and the transfusion should be discontinued if the symptoms include only chills and fever in order to determine the true cause. However, if itching and urticaria alone are present, the transfusion should rarely be stopped since these symptoms subside in 2 to 6 hours.[134] Allergic reaction, if severe, resembles anaphylactic shock, and should be controlled with antihistamine drugs such as adrenalin.[135]

Plasma reaction usually occurs after the transfusion has been completed and is characterized by severe chills, fever, and sometimes shock. This complication may be confirmed by giving 5 to 10 ml of cell-free compatible plasma and observing for a minimum of 2 degrees rise in temperature. It is often difficult, however, to determine the true cause of a reaction because fever is a symptom of different reactions. Occasionally, a rise in temperature may result from leukocyte and platelet antibody formation or bacterial contamination of blood.[136] Organisms such as pseudomonas are capable of growing even at low temperatures, and if contaminated blood is infused, septic shock may occur. Therefore, it is important not to add medications or other substances to blood that might increase the possibility of contamination.[137]

Potassium intoxication may result from transfusion because this ion is released from red cells during storage at low temperatures. Although hyperkalemia has not been noted after infusion of small amounts of blood, it may be a dangerous side effect of multiple transfusion. Therefore, symptoms of hyperkalemia should be noted.[138] Also, tetany may follow multiple transfusions, citrate toxicity, and hypocalcemia. In addition, hypothermia, acid-base disturbances, coagulation disturbances, and hyperammonemia may result from the "storage lesion" of banked blood—changes caused by addition of anticoagulants and breakdown of metabolic products that accumulate with storage.[139]

Symptoms of hemolytic *reactions* caused by blood incompatibility vary. Some reactions are severe and may result in death; others so mild that they may be unnoticed. The characteristics of an acute hemolytic reaction are: severe chills, fever, sharp lumbar pain, and dyspnea within 10 minutes of the start of transfusion, hematuria, shock with rapid blood pressure fall, gradual onset of oliguria to anuria (depending upon the amount of blood

transfused, leading to impending uremia), and hemorrhagic diathesis in mucous membranes and skin.[140] Treatment of the uremic stage is too complex to be discussed here.

Still a major problem resulting from blood transfusion is the risk of viral hepatitis. Because of the difficulty involved in detecting the virus, one cannot be sure that the blood given is free of this organism.[141] Elizabeth J. Bottcher [142] believes that the need for transfusion should be reevaluated in those patients who receive 1 to 2 units of blood. Since there is question whether patients who receive this small amount of blood really are in need of transfusion, the probability of post-transfusion complications could be greatly reduced.

Suggested Procedure. *For the removal of blood from the donor's vein* place the person in a comfortable recumbent position, the arm or leg to be injected supported and the table or bed on which it rests protected. See that the individual has a thorough understanding of what is to be done, and try in every way to relieve him or her of such anxiety he or she may feel. Keeping the person engaged in conversation helps to prevent fainting, which is thought to have a psychic origin. Disinfect the skin; apply a tourniquet but release it as soon as the needle enters the vein. Allow 500 ml (1 pt) of blood to flow into the receiving unit unless the donor is faint or nauseated, in which case terminate the procedure. Keep the blood and anticoagulant in a gentle swirling motion throughout the collection of blood. Fill a small test tube with blood to be used for laboratory tests if a bottle is used, and attach it to the receiving unit at the end of the procedure. When the needle is withdrawn cover the wound with a dressing. Provide a half hour's rest and quiet for donors. Give them a palatable drink to replace some of the body fluid they have just lost.

For the administration of blood to the recipient prepare him or her as for an infusion. Check and recheck the blood or plasma to be given. Prepare the patient as for any infusion and give the blood or plasma with the usual technique for infusions with the following exceptions: Be sure that a filter is incorporated in the tubing; give the blood very slowly at first and watch the patient carefully for an adverse reaction. If a physician is not present and the patient is extremely nervous and complains of any of the symptoms listed on page 1203, stop the blood flow and report the condition at once. Have epinephrine available for immediate injection.

Recording the Treatment. Institutions have different regulations for recording transfusions. Whether the physician or the nurse records the treatment, it is important to indicate the time and manner in which the blood was administered, by whom the treatment was performed, the amount of blood injected, and the patient's reaction. This report is normally made on the patient's chart, and a second report is often sent to the blood bank supplying the blood. (See Fig. 22-29.)

TRANSFUSION RECORD

Donor No.	Amount Drawn	Preliminary Grouping			Group
	Diluent_____	ANTI-A ◯	ANTI-B ◯		Rh

Family Name	First Name	Middle Name	Home Phone	Occupation

Address	City	Zone	State	Sex M F	Age

DONOR'S MEDICAL HISTORY

Malaria ____ Antimalaria Drugs ____ Tuberculosis ____ Fainting Spells ____ Convulsions ____ Rheumatic Fever ____ Blood Infections ____

Undulant fever ____ Epilepsy ____ Heart disease ____ Eczema ____

Glandular Swelling ____ Dyspnoea ____ Venereal Disease ____ Persistent Cough ____ Illness in past three months ____

Jaundice ____ Blood Transfusion Received ____ Recently Pregnant ____ Asthma ____ Hay Fever ____ Diabetes ____

Food last eaten ____ a.m. p.m. Date Time Food: ____

Hg. ____ B.P. ____ Pulse ____ Temp. ____ Wgt. ____ Serology ____ Icterus Index ____

Blood Group ____ Veins ____ Hematoma ____ No. punctures ____ Heart ____ / ____ Skin ____ Spleen ____

Donor Reaction ____

I hereby certify that this donor appears to be free from diseases transmissible by blood transfusion and is a suitable donor for removal of not more than ____ cc. of blood.

Date ____ Signed ____ M.D.
Examining Physician

DONOR'S AUTHORIZATION TO TAKE BLOOD

I hereby certify that I have truthfully answered the above questions concerning diseases and conditions and give permission to the Blood Bank Service of this hospital, to withdraw up to 500 cc. of blood for the use of the service, and I further release this hospital and each and all of its physicians, nurses, technicians or other members of its staff from any claims which I may have against them relative or incidental to or in consequence of such withdrawal of blood.

Date ____

Signature of Donor or Signature and Relationship of Guardian if Donor is a Minor

Witness ____ Technician ____

RECIPIENT'S RECORD

Family Name	First Name	Physician	Room No.	Hosp. No.

Cross-matching reveals patient and donor compatible:
Yes ☐ No ☐ See laboratory reports.   Technician's Signature ____ Date ____

Previous transfusions: Dates ____ Reactions: ____

Indication for this transfusion ____ Date ____ a.m. p.m.

Method: Direct ☐ Indirect ☐ Amt. blood given ____ cc. Amt. saline ____ cc. Amt. dextrose ____ cc.

Reactions: respiratory distress ____ chill ____ nausea-vomiting ____ urticaria ____ shock ____ cyanosis ____ anuria ____ hematuria ____ jaundice ____

Pulse: one hour before ____ one hour after ____ temp. one hour before ____ temp. one hour after ____

To be filled out in triplicate and when donor's blood is to be used all copies should be sent to the patient's medical record. Within 24 hrs. after transfusion, forms should be completed in triplicate sending the two carbon copies back to the Blood Bank and the original remaining on the chart.

FORM E-402   PHYSICIANS' RECORD CO., BERWYN, ILLINOIS - PRINTED IN U.S.A.   TRANSFUSION RECORD

Figure 22-29. Transfusion record. (Courtesy of Physicians' Record Co., Berwyn, Ill.)

9. INTRAPERITONEAL INFUSION OR INJECTION

Definition. The injection of fluid into the peritoneal cavity by means of a needle is an intraperitoneal infusion or injection. (If the fluid is aspirated after it is injected, the treatment is termed an irrigation.)

Therapeutic Uses. When it is difficult to give fluid by vein, as with infants and small children, the peritoneal route is used. The peritoneal cavity is sometimes irrigated for several days when renal failure is thought to be reversible. This procedure (peritoneal dialysis) allows the removal of metabolic products by dialysis through use of irrigating fluids containing certain electrolytes designed to establish the electrolyte balance of the patient. A discussion of treatment by this method may be found in Chapter 24.

Selection of Method. An intraperitoneal injection or infusion is like a subcutaneous and an intravenous infusion except that the needle is injected into the abdominal, or peritoneal, cavity. *The equipment* is the same except that a short needle with a short bevel is used. A 20-gauge needle, 3¾ cm (1½ inches) in length is suggested. Obviously the length of the needle should be chosen with relation to the thickness of the abdominal wall. A short bevel makes puncturing the intestine less likely. The needle is inserted in the midline halfway between the umbilicus and the symphysis pubis with the needle pointing upward. It is important that the bladder be emptied in preparation for the treatment. A full bladder can rise to the point of the injection and the thin wall of the distended bladder can be easily penetrated with the needle. To avoid the danger of puncturing the abdominal or pelvic organs some operators make a small incision and introduce a blunt needle, or trochar.

Preparation of the equipment and preparation of the skin at the site of injection are the same as for infusions. As is the case of any injection where a large needle must be used, a local anesthetic lessens discomfort. It is important with this, as with all treatments, to have the understanding and cooperation of the patient. Intraperitoneal injections for the administration of blood or nutrient fluids are more often given to infants and small children than to adults; for these patients restraints are usually necessary. The *solutions* are approximately the same as those given by vein. Eric W. Martin [143] says that some drugs are absorbed more slowly from the abdominal cavity than from the vein but that the effect may be more lasting. He thinks that not more than 100 ml of fluid should be given a child at one time which will necessitate frequent injections as this amount is about half the usual fluid intake at one oral feeding. O. Ransome-Kuti and associates [144] report the successful use of normal saline with 28 mEq of potassium chloride per liter; or for those babies who are hypertonically dehydrated, half strength Darrow's solution. They think that intraperitoneal injection is a simple procedure which can be carried out in situations where complex medical equipment is not available if the baby is premedicated with promazine.

10. INTRACARDIAC INJECTION

Definition. As currently used, an *intracardiac injection* refers to the introduction with a needle of a drug into the atrium or ventricle of the heart.

Therapeutic Uses. Authorities consulted agree that this treatment should be used in cardiac arrest (when the heart stops beating) regardless of cause. The patient can often be saved if given an intracardiac injection, pulmonary resuscitation, heart massage, and parenteral fluids. External electrical defibrillation is the treatment of choice if ventricular fibrillation is the cause of arrest.

Selection of Method. It is obvious that only the physician is qualified to give a cardiac injection, but a patient with cardiopulmonary arrest may be given artificial ventilation by mouth-to-mouth breathing or other appropriate means by the person present most skilled in the process. External cardiac massage may also be instituted as a first aid measure to circulate the blood oxygenated by artificial ventilation. Samuel Bellet [145] says that once effective artificial circulation and respiration have been established, epinephrine 0.5 mg diluted to 5 ml may be given every 3 to 5 minutes either directly into the heart or intravenously. Norepinephrine may also be given directly into the heart. When ventricular fibrillation is present, electrical defibrillation is the treatment of choice and must be instituted promptly along with artificial ventilation and external cardiac compression. Intracardiac norepinephrine may also be administered. Martin [146] recommends a long thin needle of 20 gauge, 4 inches in length. Any hypodermic syringe will serve the purpose. The skin should be disinfected as for a surgical operation, but the entire procedure must be carried out with the utmost speed. The area just to the left of the sternum in the fourth or fifth intercostal space is used for ventricular puncture and just to the right of the sternum in the third intercostal space for atrial puncture. (The latter is said to be the more difficult operation.) In some emergencies the surgeon may think it wiser to risk infection than to take time for aseptic precautions.

11. INTRAOSSEOUS INFUSION OR INJECTION

Definition. The introduction of fluid into the marrow cavities of bones is called an intraosseous infusion.

Therapeutic Uses. This procedure is carried out when it is difficult or impossible to give fluids intravenously, as, for example, when there are extensive burns.

Selection of Method. First described in 1941, intraosseous infusions have been used for adults and children, but chiefly for the latter. Martin says that the action of an intraosseous injection is almost as rapid as that of an intravenous injection. The puncture is always made by the physician. As in all procedures the patient's understanding and cooperation are sought. If the patient is a child the parents should have the treatment explained carefully since this is an uncommon procedure.

A thorough *preparation* of the skin is of particular importance, for the treatment is very traumatic and the injured bone is especially susceptible to infection. The skin is washed and shaved if necessary; iodine and alcohol or other suitable antiseptics are applied. The area is draped with sterile towels. The physician scrubs as for a surgical procedure and usually wears sterile gloves. *The equipment* is similar to that used for any infusion (or transfusion) except that a local anesthetic, such as procaine, is always provided and the needles used in entering the bone are quite different although a short-beveled, 18-gauge spinal puncture needle 3 to 4 cm in length with a lumen of 1 to 2 mm in diameter can be used. Wintrobe recommends an adjustable guard attached to the sternal needle so that the depth penetrated may be known. The outer guiding needle is 14 gauge, the inner trephine needle 17 gauge. The outer needle is 2 cm (¾ inch) in length and has a cutting tip and a stylet. This outer needle is left in the bone and is the tube through which the fluid flows into the bone marrow. The inner needle is a trephine. It is passed through the outer needle and used to saw and remove a plug of bone to make a pathway for the introduction of the larger outer needle. When the outer needle is in place the inner needle is removed. The outer needle is equipped with an adapter that will fit a syringe or tubing. Besides its stylet the needle has a cap that can be fitted over the hub. If repeated infusions are given through the needle, the opening or hub may be protected from gross contamination by the cap. The right-angle "observation tube" is said to make it easy to tape the tubing to the skin. The most common *site of insertion* of the needle in adults is the upper portion of the sternum between the second and third ribs because the bone is less likely to bend at this point. In children under 4 years of age the proximal end of the tibia is the site of choice as the cavity of the sternum is not large enough to use for infusion.[147]

Solutions that may be given by this route include blood and other fluids given intravenously. Advocates of this technique report that adults can tolerate a *rate of flow* of 50 ml (1⅔ oz) per minute in some cases, while admitting that too rapid flow causes discomfort and pain. H. I. Arbeiter and J. J. Greengard[148] report that infants were given plasma in the tibia with an average rate of flow 1.44 ml (22 gtt) per minute. Small quantities of fluid can be given with a syringe, but the administration of the fluid from a container, in which it has been sterilized, offers better protection from infection.

It is generally conceded that the administration of fluids by the intraosseous route presents difficulties and hazards. Infections, fat and air emboli, and varying degrees of pain may result. If the sternum is used in children, there is danger of puncturing the mediastinum as the bone is thin.[149]

REFERENCES

1. Schuberth, Oscar: "Clinical Experience with Fat Emulsions for Intravenous Use," *Acta Chir. Scand., Suppl.,* **325:**43, 1964.
2. Shuttleworth, K. E. D.: "Intravenous Fat Therapy," *Nurs. Times,* **60:**1330, (Oct. 9) 1964.
3. Jones, Richard J.: "Present Knowledge of Intravenous Fat Emulsions," *Nutr. Rev.,* **24:**225, (Aug.) 1966.
4. Scheinberg, Labe, and Allensworth, Mollie: "Sciatic Neuropathy in Infants Related to Antibiotic Injections," *Pediatrics,* **19:**261, (Feb.) 1957.
5. Curtiss, Paul H., "Sciatic Palsy in Premature Infants," *J.A.M.A.,* **174:**1586, (Nov. 19) 1960.
6. Combes, Mollie A., et al.: "Sciatic Nerve Injury in Infants," *J.A.M.A.,* **173:**1336, (July 23) 1960.
7. Richards, Richard K.: "Nerve Injury from Intramuscular Barbiturate Injection," *Clin. Pharmacol. Ther.,* **2:**262, (Feb.) 1961.
8. Alstead, Stanley, and MacArthur, J. Gordon: *Clinical Pharmacology* (*Dilling*), 22nd ed. Bailliere, Tindall & Cassell, London, 1969, p. 12.
9. Berggren, Ronald B., et al.: "Clostridial Myositis after Parenteral Injections," *J.A.M.A.,* **188:**1044, (June 22) 1964.
10. Koons, Thomas A., and Boyden, George M.: "Gas Gangrene from Parenteral Injection," *J.A.M.A.,* **175:**46, (Jan. 7) 1961.
11. "Tetanus Following Subcutaneous Injections of Saline Solutions" (editorial), *J.A.M.A.,* **81:**2210, (Dec. 29) 1923.
12. "Gas Gangrene from Injections" (editorial), *J.A.M.A.,* **87:**453, (Aug. 7) 1926.
13. Mosley, James W., and Dull, Bruce H.: "Transfusion-Associated Viral Hepatitis," *Anesthesiology,* **27:**409, (July–Aug.) 1966.
14. Mervine, Charles K., and Schechter, David C.: "The Prevention and Treatment of Blood Transfusion Reactions," *New Physician,* **11:**6, (Jan.) 1962.
15. Inman, P. M., et al.: "Outbreak of Injection Abscesses Due to *Mycobacterium abscessus,*" *Arch. Dermatol.,* **100:**141, (Aug.) 1969.
16. Berblinger, Klaus W.: "The Influence of Per-

sonalities on Drug Therapy," *Am. J. Nurs.,* **59:**1130, (Aug.) 1959.

17. Travell, Janet: "Factors Affecting Pain of Injection," *J.A.M.A.,* **158:**369, (June 4) 1955.

18. Koons, Thomas A., and Boyden, George M.: *op. cit.*

19. Dann, T. C.: "Routine Skin Preparation Before Injection: An Unnecessary Procedure," *Lancet,* **2:**96, (July 12) 1969.

20. Goth, Andres: *Medical Pharmacology,* 7th ed. C. V. Mosby Co., St. Louis, 1974, p. 17.

21. Krogh, August K.: *The Anatomy and Physiology of Capillaries.* Yale University Press, New Haven, Conn., 1922, p. 96.

22. Boyan, C. P.: "Cardiac Arrest and the Temperature of Bank Blood," *Bibl. Haemetol.,* **23:**1136, 1965.

23. Metheny, Norma M., and Snively, W. D.: *Nurses' Handbook of Fluid Balance,* 2nd ed. J. B. Lippincott Co., Philadelphia, 1974, p. 156.

24. Restall, Charles J., et al.: "A Microwave Blood Warmer: Preliminary Report," *Anesth. Analg.,* **46:**625, (Sept.–Oct.) 1967.

25. Bernard, Claude: *Introduction to the Study of Experimental Medicine* (translated by Henry C. Greene). Macmillan Publishing Co., Inc., New York, 1927.

26. Goth, Andres: *op. cit.,* p. 15.

27. DiPalma, Joseph R.: *Drills Pharmacology in Medicine,* 4th ed. McGraw-Hill Book Co., The Blackenstone Division, New York, 1971, p. 21.

28. Schanker, Lewis S.: "Passage of Drugs Across Body Membranes," *Pharmacol. Rev.,* **14:**501, (Dec.) 1962.

29. Meyer, Karl: *Conference on the Ground Substance of the Mesenchyma and Hyaluronidase,* New York Academy of Science, New York, Dec. 3–4, 1948.

30. Goodman, Louis S., and Gilman, Alfred: *The Pharmacological Basis of Therapeutics,* 5th ed. Macmillan Publishing Co., Inc., New York, 1975, p. 956.

31. Rovenstine, Emery A., and Baterman, Robert C.: "The Use of Ampin, an Automatic Ampule Injector for Routine and Emergency Hypodermic Medications," *J. Lab. Clin. Med.,* **35:**795, (May) 1950.

32. Cadmus, Robert R.: "Medications Cost Study," *Mod. Hosp.,* **75:**68, (Sept.) 1950.

33. *Administering Closed System Injection.* Wyeth Laboratories, Philadelphia, 1964, p. 3.

34. Barker, Kenneth N., et al.: "A Nurse Acceptance Evaluation of Some Prefilled Disposable Injection Devices," *Am. J. Hosp. Pharm.,* **23:**138, (Mar.) 1966.

35. Chlebik, Sister Mary Hiltrudis: "Dispensing Direct to the Patient," *Am. J. Hosp. Pharm.,* **23:**581, (Oct.) 1966.

36. Grollman, Arthur: *Pharmacology and Therapeutics,* 7th ed. Lea & Febiger, Philadelphia, 1970, p. 60.

37. Alstead, Stanley, and MacArthur, J. Gordon: *op. cit.,* p. 12.

38. Carter, Burdellis, L.: "Comparison of Individual Pain Reactions to Injections of Distilled Water and Normal Saline," in *ANA Regional Clinical Conferences, 1967.* Appleton-Century-Crofts, New York, 1968, p. 219.

39. Goth, Andres: *op. cit.,* p. 19.

40. Wiggers, Carl J.: *Physiology in Health and Disease,* 5th ed. Lea & Febiger, Philadelphia, 1949, p. 1089.

41. MacLeod, John J. R.: *Physiology and Biochemistry,* 6th ed. C. V. Mosby Co., St. Louis, 1930, p. 112.

42. Goodman, Louis S., and Gilman, Alfred: *op. cit.,* pp. 1516, 1524.

43. Beland, Irene L., and Passos, Joyce Y.: *Clinical Nursing: Pathophysiological and Psychosocial Approaches,* 3rd ed. Macmillan Publishing Co., Inc., 1975, p. 1030.

44. Beeson, Paul B., and McDermott, Walsh (eds.): *Cecil-Loeb Textbook of Medicine,* 14th ed. W. B. Saunders Co., Philadelphia, 1975, p. 1616.

45. Weller, Charles, and Linder, Morton: "Jet Injection of Insulin vs. the Syringe-and-Needle Method," *J.A.M.A.,* **195:**844, (Mar. 7) 1966.

46. Coates, Florence Cuozzo, and Fabrykant, Maximilian: "An Insulin Injection Technique for Preventing Skin Reactions," *Am. J. Nurs.,* **65:**128, (Feb.) 1965.

47. Zelman, Samuel: "Notes on Techniques of Intramuscular Injection," *Am. J. Med. Sci.,* **241:**568, (May) 1961.

48. Hanson, Daniel J.: "Intramuscular Injection Injuries and Complications," *Am. J. Nurs.,* **63:**99, (Apr.) 1963.

49. Combes, Mollie A., et al.: *op. cit.*

50. Curtiss, Paul H., and Tucker, Howard J.: *op. cit.*

51. Hanson, Daniel J.: *op. cit.*

52. Horn, Barbara J.: "Intramuscular Injections: The Nurse's Responsibility," *Univ. Mich. Med. Cent. J.,* **32:**31, (Jan.–Feb.) 1966.

53. Pitel, Martha, and Wemett, Mary: "The Intramuscular Injection," *Am. J. Nurs.,* **64:**104, (Apr.) 1964.

54. Zelman, Samuel: *op. cit.*

55. Hanson, Daniel J.: *op. cit.*

56. Horn, Barbara J.: *op. cit.*

57. Zelman, Samuel: *op. cit.*

58. Dreyer, Carl V., and Winter, Chester C.: "Use of the Dermo-jet in Urology," *Ohio State Med. J.,* **65:**254, (Mar.) 1969.

59. Hingson, Robert, et al.: "Hypospray Administration of Penicillin in the Treatment of Gonorrhea," *J. Ven. Dis. Inform.,* **29:**61, (Mar.) 1948.

60. Hodges, W. Royce: "Continued Use of Hypospray in Treatment of Syphilis and Gonorrhea," *Anesth. Analg.,* **28:**231, (July–Aug.) 1949.

61. Hughes, G. R. V., and Currey, H. L. F.: "Hypospray Treatment of Tennis Elbow," *Ann. Rheum. Dis.,* **28:**58, (Feb.) 1969.

62. Kutscher, Austin H., et al.: "A Comparative Evaluation of the Jet Injection Technique

(Hypospray) and the Hypodermic Needle for the Parenteral Administration of Drugs: A Controlled Study," *Am. J. Med. Sci.,* **244:** 418, (Oct.) 1962.

63. Lenz, Theodore R.: "Foreign Body Granuloma Caused by Jet Injection of Tetanus Toxoid," *Rocky Mt. Med. J.,* **63:**48, (Jan.) 1966.

64. Plumer, Ada Lawrence: *Principles and Practice of Intravenous Therapy.* Little, Brown & Co., Boston, 1970, p. 189.

65. Metheny, Norma Milligan, and Snively, William D.: *op. cit.,* p. 128.

66. *Ibid.,* p. 128.

67. Gants, Robert T.: "Fatal Thrombosis Following Hypodermoclysis," *J. Kans. Med. Soc.,* **33:**13, (Jan.) 1932.

68. Humpstone, O. P.: "Unusual Sequelae of a Submammary Hypodermoclysis," *Med. Rec.,* **65:**216, (Feb.) 1904.

68a. Dudrick, Stanley J., and Rhoads, Jonathan E.: "Metabolism in Surgical Patients: Protein, Carbohydrates, and Fat Utilization by Oral and Parenteral Routes," in Sabiston, David C., Jr. (ed.): *Davis-Christopher Textbook of Surgery; The Biological Basis of Modern Surgical Practice,* 10th ed. W. B. Saunders Co., Philadelphia, 1972, p. 160.

68b. Winters, Robert W., and Hasselmeyer, Eileen G.: *Intravenous Nutrition in the High Risk Infant,"* John Wiley & Sons, New York, 1975.

68c. Dudrick, Stanley J., and Duke, James H., Jr.: "Nutritional Complications in the Surgical Patients," in Artz, Curtis P., and Hardy, James D.: *Management of Surgical Complications,* 3rd ed. W. B. Saunders Co., Philadelphia, 1975, p. 264.

68d. Tsallos, G., and Bann, D. C.: "Home Care Total Parenteral Alimentation," *Am. J. Hosp. Pharm.,* **29:**840, (Oct.) 1972.

68e. Calley, Rita, and Phillips, Karen: "Helping with Hyperalimentation," *Nursing '73,* **3:**6, (July) 1973.

68f. Baker, Dorothy I.: "Hyperalimentation at Home," *Am. J. Nurs.,* **74:**1826, (Oct.) 1974.

69. Plumer, Ada Lawrence: *op. cit.,* p. 3.

70. Zimmermann, Bernard: "Fluid and Electrolyte Balance in Surgical Patients," in Sabiston, David C., Jr. (ed.): *Davis-Christopher Textbook of Surgery,* 10th ed. W. B. Saunders Co., Philadelphia, 1972, p. 101.

71. Metheny, Norma Milligan, and Snively, William D.: *op. cit.,* p. 141t.

72. Bland, John H.: *Clinical Metabolism of Body Water and Electrolytes.* W. B. Saunders Co., Philadelphia, 1963, p. 219.

73. Metheny, Norma Milligan, and Snively, William D.: *op. cit.,* p. 132.

74. Atik: "Dextrans, Their Use in Surgery and Medicine," *Anesthesiology,* **27:**425, (July–Aug.) 1966.

75. Metheny, Norma Milligan, and Snively, William D.: *op. cit.,* p. 134.

76. *Ibid.,* p. 133.

77. Plumer, Ada Lawrence: *op. cit.,* p. 68.

78. "Intravenous Technique," *Spectrum,* **9:**80, (Sept.–Oct.) 1961.

79. Baumgarten, A., and Curtain, C. C.: "A Small Electrolytically Driven Infusion Pump," *J. Appl. Physiol.,* **20:**793, (July) 1965.

80. Clark, Richard B.: "The Art of Venipuncture," *New Physician,* **13:**253, (Aug.) 1964.

81. Adriani, John: "Venipuncture," *Am. J. Nurs.,* **62:**67, (Mar.) 1962.

82. Sylvester, Marilyn J., and Bruno, Pauline M.: "Factors Associated with Infiltration During Continuous Intravenous Therapy," *Nurs. Res.,* **15:**255, (Summer) 1966.

83. Swanson, Jack T., and Aldrete, J. Antonio: "Thrombophlebitis after Intravenous Infusion," *Rocky Mt. Med. J.,* **66:**49, (Apr.) 1969.

84. Anderson, L. H.: "Venous Catheterization for Fluid Therapy: A Technique and Results," *J. Lab. Clin. Med.,* **36:**645, (Oct.) 1960.

85. Ladd, Michael, and Schreiner, George E.: "Plastic Tubing for Intravenous Alimentation," *J.A.M.A.,* **154:**642, (Mar. 3) 1951.

86. Meyers, Lawrence: "Intravenous Catheterization," *Am. J. Nurs.,* **45:**930, (Nov.) 1945.

87. Swanson, Jack T., and Aldrete, J. Antonio: *op. cit.*

88. Muir, A. P.: "Intravenous Complications," *Appl. Ther.,* **6:**1004, (Dec.) 1964.

89. Mariano, Benedict P., et al.: "Accidental Migration of an Intravenous Infusion Catheter from the Arm to the Lung," *Radiology,* **86:**736, (Apr.) 1966.

90. Hästbacka, J., et al.: "Infusion Thrombophlebitis," *Acta Anaesthesiol. Scand.,* **10:**9, 1965.

91. Wilmore, Douglas W., and Dubrick, Standly J.: "An In-Line Filter for Intravenous Solutions," *Arch. Surg.,* **99:**492, (Oct.) 1969.

92. "Innovations in I.V. Equipment," *Am. J. Nurs.,* **62:**80, (Mar.) 1962.

93. Blumberg, Mark S.: "How Electronics Can Improve I.V. Safety," *Mod. Hosp.,* **104:**54, (May) 1965.

94. Wintrobe, Maxwell M.: *Clinical Hematology,* 7th ed. Lea & Febiger, Philadelphia, 1974, p. 474.

95. Ehrlich, Albert: "Causes and Prevention of Blood Transfusion Fatalities," *Hospitals,* **36:** 60, (Sept. 16) 1962.

96. McNeil, Crichton: "Complications of Blood Transfusion," *Int. Anesthesiol. Clin.,* **5:**1023, (Winter) 1967.

97. Race, Robert R., and Sanger, Ruth: *Blood and Blood Groups in Man,* 5th ed. F. A. Davis Co., Philadelphia, 1968, p. 9.

98. Wintrobe, Maxwell M.: *op. cit.,* p. 451.

99. *Ibid.,* pp. 454, 455.

100. Mollison, P. L.: *Blood Transfusion in Clinical Medicine,* 5th ed. Blackwell Scientific Publications, Oxford and Edinburgh, 1972, p. 621.

101. Wintrobe, Maxwell M.: *op. cit.,* p. 456.

102. Allen, J. Garrott: "Blood Transfusion and

Related Problems," in Rhoads, Jonathan E., et al.: *Surgery, Principles and Practice,* 4th ed. J. B. Lippincott Co., Philadelphia, 1970, p. 164.

103. "Standards and Accreditation Programs of the American Association of Blood Banks," *Transfusion,* **5:**107, (Mar.–Apr.) 1965.
104. McNeil, Crichton: *op. cit.*
105. Vogel, James M., and Vogel, Peter: "Transfusion of Blood Components," *Anesthesiology,* **27:**368, (July–Aug.) 1966.
106. Graves, Constance: "Massive Transfusion," *Int. Anesthesiol. Clin.,* **5:**926, (Winter) 1967.
107. Wintrobe, Maxwell M.: *op. cit.,* p. 473.
108. Crocker, M. C.: "Blood Transfusion," *Anaesthesia,* **23:**372, (July) 1968.
109. Bunker, John P.: "Metabolic Effects of Blood Transfusion," *Anesthesiology,* **27:**446, (July–Aug.) 1966.
110. Abbott Laboratories: *The Use of Blood.* Abbott Laboratories, North Chicago, 1968, p. 34.
111. Crocker, M. C.: *op. cit.*
112. Abbott Laboratories: *op. cit.,* p. 47.
113. *Ibid.,* p. 54.
114. Barton, Jane: "How Safe Is Hospital Blood Service," *Mod. Hosp.,* **99:**76, (July) 1962.
115. Wintrobe, Maxwell M.: *op. cit.,* p. 472.
116. Crocker, M. C.: *op. cit.*
117. Restall, Charles J., et al.: *op. cit.*
118. Crouch, Madge L., and Gibson, Sam T.: "Blood Therapy," *Am. J. Nurs.,* **62:**71, (Mar.) 1962.
119. Wilson, Robert F., et al.: "Five Years of Experience with Massive Blood Transfusions," *J.A.M.A.,* **194:**851, (Nov. 22) 1965.
120. Williams, Jan T., and Moravec, Daniel F.: "Intravenous Therapy," *Hosp. Manage.,* **101:**66, (Feb.) 1966.
121. Crocker, M. C.: *op. cit.*
122. Moore, Francis D.: "Blood Transfusions: Rates, Routes, and Hazards," *Nurs. Clin. North Am.,* **1:**285, (June) 1966.
123. Gibbins, F. J.: "Blood Transfusion in the Elderly," *Br. J. Clin. Pract.,* **20:**22, (Jan.) 1966.
124. Wilson, Robert F., et al.: *op. cit.*
125. Graves, Constance: *op. cit.*
126. Vogel, James M., and Vogel, Peter: *op. cit.*
127. Zucker, Marjorie B., and Lundberg, Ante.: "Platelet Transfusions," *Anesthesiology,* **27:** 385, (July–Aug.) 1966.
128. Freireich, Emil J.: "Effectiveness of Platelet Transfusion in Leukemia and Aplastic Anemia," *Transfusion,* **6:**50, (Jan.–Feb.) 1966.
129. "Platelet Transfusion Procedures," *Cancer Chemother. Rep.,* **52:**3, 1968.
130. Flatow, Frederick A., and Freireich, Emil J.: "Effect of Splenectomy on the Response to Platelet Transfusion in Three Patients with Aplastic Anemia," *N. Engl. J. Med.,* **274:**242, (Feb. 3) 1966.
131. Schwarzenberg, M. D., et al.: "Study of Factors Determining the Usefulness and Complications of Leukocyte Transfusions," *Am. J. Med.,* **43:**206, (Aug.) 1967.

132. Vogel, James M., and Vogel, Peter: *op. cit.*
133. McNeil, Crichton: *op. cit.*
134. Baker, R. J., et al.: "Transfusion Reaction: A Reappraisal of Surgical Incidence and Significance," *Ann. Surg.,* **169:**687, (May) 1969.
135. McClaughry, Robert I.: "Transfusion Reactions," *Med. Clin. North Am.,* **46:**551, (Mar.) 1962.
136. McNeil, Crichton: *op. cit.*
137. Baker, R. J., et al.: *op. cit.*
138. Bunker, John P.: *op. cit.*
139. Graves, Constance: *op. cit.*
140. McNeil, Crichton: *op. cit.*
141. Mosley, James W., and Dull, Bruce H.: *op. cit.*
142. Bottcher, Elizabeth J.: "Use of Whole Blood Transfusions in a General Hospital," *NY State J. Med.,* **62:**1196, (Apr. 15) 1962.
143. Martin, Eric W.: *Techniques of Medication, A Manual on the Administration of Drug Products.* J. B. Lippincott Co., Philadelphia, 1969, p. 137.
144. Ransome-Kuti, O., et al.: "Intraperitoneal Fluid Infusion in Children with Gastroenteritis," *Br. Med. J.,* **3:**500, (Aug.) 1969.
145. Bellet, Samuel: *Clinical Disorders of the Heart Beat,* 3rd ed. Lea & Febiger, Philadelphia, 1971, p. 595.
146. Martin, Eric W.: *op. cit.,* p. 134.
147. Wintrobe, Maxwell M.: *op. cit.,* pp. 40, 41, 473.
148. Arbeiter, H. I., and Greengard, J. J.: "Tibial Bone Marrow Infusions in Children," *J. Pediatr.,* **25:**1, (July) 1944.
149. Wintrobe, Maxwell M.: *op. cit.,* p. 474.

Additional Suggested Reading

Atik, M.: "Dextran 40 and Dextran 70," *Arch. Surg.,* **94:**664, (May) 1967.

Barry, Kevin G., and Crosby, William H.: "The Prevention and Treatment of Renal Failure Following Transfusion Reactions," *Transfusion,* **3:**34, (Jan.–Feb.) 1963.

Brisman, Ronald et al.: "Anaphylactoid Reactions Associated with the Clinical Use of Dextran 70," *J.A.M.A.,* **204:**824, (May 27) 1968.

Buchman, Robert J.: "Subclavian Venipuncture," *Milit. Med.,* **134:**451, (June) 1969.

Copeland, Edward M., III, et al.: "Prevention of Microbial Catheter Contamination in Patients Receiving Parenteral Hyperalimentation," *South. Med. J.,* **67:**303, (Mar.) 1974.

Darrow, Daniel C.: "The Physiological Basis for Estimating Requirements for Parenteral Fluids," *Pediatr. Clin. North Am.,* **11:**819, (Nov.) 1964.

Dudrick, Stanley J.: "Rational Intravenous Therapy," *Am. J. Hosp. Pharm.,* **28:**82, (Feb.) 1971.

Dudrick, Stanley J., and Rhoads, Jonathan E.: "Total Intravenous Feedings," *Sci. Am.,* **226:** 73, 1972.

Erickson, Larry, et al.: "A Peculiar Cutaneous

Reaction to Repeated Injections of Insulin," *J.A.M.A.*, **209:**934, (Aug. 11) 1969.

Foukalsrud, Eric W.: "Reduction of Infusion Thrombophlebitis with Buffered Glucose Solutions," *Surgery*, **63:**280, (Feb.) 1968.

Fowler, Thomas J.: *Injectable Solutions and Additives*. Springer Publishing Co., New York, 1971.

Gallub, S., et al.: "The Bleeding Tendency Associated with Plasma Expanders," *Surg. Gynecol. Obstet.*, **124:**1203, (June) 1967.

Grant, Jo Ann Nallinger, et al.: "Parenteral Hyperalimentation," *Am. J. Nurs.*, **69:**2392, (Nov.) 1969.

Greenhill, P. J.: *Obstetrics*, 13th ed. W. B. Saunders Co., Philadelphia, 1965.

Hays, Doris: "Do It Yourself the Z-Tract Way," *Am. J. Nurs.*, **74:**1070, (June) 1974.

Hellman, Louis M., and Pritchard, Jack A.: *Williams Obstetrics*, 14th ed. Appleton-Century-Crofts, New York, 1971.

Hilkemeyer, Renilda: "Intra-Arterial Cancer Chemotherapy," *Nurs. Clin. North Am.*, **1:**295, (June) 1966.

Imperiale, Marie, and Krebs, Theodora: "The Intravenous Therapy Nurses," *Am. J. Nurs.*, **61:**53, (May) 1961.

Kernicki, Jeanette: "Needle Puncture: Health Asset or Menace," *Nurs. Clin. North Am.*, **1:**269, (June) 1966.

Kilman, Allan: "Presently Useful Plasma Volume Expanders," *Anesthesiology*, **27:**417, (July–Aug.) 1966.

Langer, B., et al.: "Prolonged Survival After Complete Small Bowel Resection Using Intravenous Alimentation at Home," *J. Surg. Res.*, **15:**226, (Sept.) 1973.

Lary, Banning G.: "Continuous Intra-Arterial Infusion Using Compressed Gas for Power," *South. Med. J.*, **59:**294, (Mar.) 1966.

Lawrence, Patricia A.: "U-100 Insulin: Let's Make the Transition Trouble Free," *Am. J. Nurs.*, **73:**1539, (Dec.) 1973.

Lenenstein, Barbara P.: "Intravenous Therapy: A Nursing Specialty," *Nurs. Clin. North Am.*, **1:**259, (June) 1966.

McCarter, Donna: "Nourishing the Solute-Sensitive Patient," *Am. J. Nurs.*, **73:**1935, (Nov.) 1973.

Merritt, John A.: "Complications Related to Blood Replacement," *Am. J. Surg.*, **116:**333, (Sept.) 1968.

Pitel, Martha: "The Subcutaneous Injection," *Am. J. Nurs.*, **71:**76, (Jan.) 1971.

Ruberg, R. L., et al.: "Progress in Parenteral Protein Nutrition," in Brown, Henry (ed.): *Protein Nutrition*. Charles C Thomas, Publisher, Springfield, Ill., 1974.

Rush, Benjamin F., and Stewart, Robert A.: "More Liberal Use of a Plasma Expander, Impact on a Hospital Blood Bank," *N. Engl. J. Med.*, **280:**1202, (May 29) 1969.

——, et al.: "Limitations of Blood Replacement with Electrolyte Solutions, A Controlled Clinical Study," *Arch. Surg.*, **98:**49, (Jan.) 1969.

Sapira, J. D., et al.: "Liver Disease in Narcotic Addicts, II. The Role of the Needle," *Clin. Pharmacol. Ther.*, **9:**725, (June) 1968.

Schmidt, Paul J.: "Erythroid Homograft Following Leukocyte Transfusion in a Patient with Acute Leukemia. II. Serologic and Immunochemical Studies," *Blood*, **26:**567, (Nov.) 1965.

Seal, Anna L.: "The Nurse's Responsibility in Anticoagulant Therapy," *Nurs. Clin. North Am.*, **1:**325, (June) 1966.

Tepe, Pauline F.: "A Physiological Approach to Pediatric Medications," *Nurs. Clin. North Am.*, **1:**111, (Mar.) 1966.

"Total Parenteral Nutrition," *Nutr. Rev.*, **28:**286, (Nov.) 1970.

Voda, Anna M.: "Body Water Dynamics, A Clinical Application," *Am. J. Nurs.*, **70:**2594, (Dec.) 1970.

Webb, John W.: "A p^H Pattern for I.V. Additives," *Am. J. Hosp. Pharm.*, **26:**31, (Jan.) 1969.

Wemple, Bertha M.: "The New and the Old Intramuscular Injection Sites," *Am. J. Nurs.*, **61:**56, (Sept.) 1961.

Williams, Jan T., and Moravec, Daniel F.: "Intravenous Therapy, Part 3—Procedures and Techniques," *Hosp. Manage.*, **101:**63, (Mar.) 1966.

Gladys Nite
Virginia Henderson

CHAPTER 23

Intubation of the Alimentary Tract for Feeding, Medication, and Drainage

1. INTUBATION OF THE STOMACH AND INTESTINES

Definition. Intubation, decompression, suction-siphonage, nasogastric suction and gastrointestinal suction are some of the terms used for the introduction of a tube through the nose into the alimentary tract to remove its contents by suction which is applied to the end of the tube outside the body. Any organ or cavity having an opening to the surface of the body may be decompressed in this way. Suction, or negative pressure, is exerted whenever a vacuum exists. "Nature abhors a vacuum," and atmospheric pressure forces into a vacuum any gas or fluid at the opening of the chamber in which the vacuum exists. Suction-siphonage, or decompression of the alimentary tract, occurs when a vacuum large enough (a negative pressure strong enough) to remove its contained fluids and gases is applied.

Therapeutic Uses. Intubation of the alimentary tract is used for four general purposes: (1) to remove gas and fluids in the prevention or treatment of distention following abdominal operations, (2) occasionally to study with x-rays the response of the alimentary tract to opaque liquids introduced through the tube, and (3) to remove the contents of the alimentary tract when its distention is caused by an obstruction. In the latter case when obstruction is the result of a mechanical condition, such as kinking, intubation alone may correct it; more often, suction-siphonage precedes surgical treatment. (4) A fourth use of

intubation is the removal of the stomach contents as preparation for, and during, general anesthesia.[1] As early as 1949, Henry K. Beecher[2] recommended intubation of the stomach of all wounded patients before surgery because distention of the stomach interfered with circulation. Gastric suction is commonly used before and after many types of surgery to reduce the stomach size, increase exposure of the operative site, and remove air swallowed by the patient.

Aspiration of gastric contents is said by George Culver and his associates to be "a common and serious complication of anesthesia and surgery." * (To determine its frequency these physicians used dyes opaque to x-rays.) In a study of 300 unselected surgical cases at the Massachusetts General Hospital they found that 79 regurgitated and 49 aspirated gastric contents before the completion of the operation, and there was "frank vomiting" in 24 instances, with 16 of these aspirating gastric contents. Another 25 patients aspirated "silently." In a review of 1000 deaths associated with anesthesia, G. Edwards and associates[3] report 18 per cent of these were due to regurgitation and vomiting. Therefore, it is apparent that the operative patient is in constant danger of developing serious pulmonary problems from aspiration of stomach contents.

---

* Culver, George, et al.: "Frequency of Aspiration of Gastric Contents by the Lungs During Anesthesia and Surgery," *Ann. Surg.*, **133**:289, (Mar.) 1951.

Gastric tubes during the operation are said to exert a protective effect. Double-lumen tubes (the D'Eloia, for example) prevent suction from drawing the mucosa into the drain lumen. Intubation is used less frequently for other purposes in selected areas; these include: (1) eradication of intestinal parasites by introducing a vermicide through the tube to the site of the area where they are; (2) gastric and small intestinal lavage in the management of reversible acute renal failure when for some reason other means of dialysis are not desirable or possible; (3) removal of intestinal contents in the ileum to prevent its entering the colon in selected cases of ulcerative colitis (called medical ileostomy); and (4) compression of esophageal varicies for the arrest of bleeding in patients with portal hypertension.[4]

Selection of Equipment and Method. Methods of intubation and the equipment used vary considerably now, as in the past. Meyer O. Cantor (in 1949) believed these differences indicated that the procedure presented difficulties to most, if not all, operators. Henry L. Bockus (1964) says:

It is not a method for the casual worker. For satisfactory results the work of passing a long intestinal tube is best assigned to individuals who will make a careful study of the procedure and devote to it the time that it requires. . . . The patient cannot afford to lose valuable time while unsuccessful attempts are made to pass a tube.*

Cantor's monograph shows very clearly that the operator should understand the anatomy and physiology of the alimentary tract, and should be familiar with the available instruments and the physical principles governing their use. In practice, nurses are often expected to carry a large share of the responsibility for intubation, especially gastric intubation. Consequently they should study the procedure just as physicians must. Although the value of intestinal intubation in the treatment of obstruction has been accepted for more than 30 years, the merits of long intestinal tubes and gastroduodenal tubes are still debated. Alexander P. Remenchik and Peter J. Talso[5] believe there has not been a properly designed study of the advantages of one tube over another.

The choice of equipment is the physicians' responsibility. They must decide how they want negative pressure or suction created and applied, and what kind of tube to use. Five *types of suction* as described by Cantor and Roland P. Reynolds[6] are used: (1) simple

* Bockus, Henry L.: *Gastroenterology,* Vol. II, 2nd ed. W. B. Saunders Co., Philadelphia, 1964, p. 369.

suction; (2) continuous hydraulic, or water-displacement suction; (3) electric, motorless pump exerting intermittent suction through expansion and contraction of air (Gomco thermotic pump); (4) a pump "activated by electromagnetic coils on the same principle as the electric meter" (Stedman pump); and (5) motor-driven pumps. "Wall" or "piped-in" suction is available in many hospitals.

Emptying the stomach with simple suction has been practiced for more than a century. Devices to induce vomiting were used in ancient times, but since the invention of the gastric tube by Hunter in 1776 it has been possible to wash out the stomach as well as feed patients by intubation.[7]

Philip Syng Physick (1800) is believed to be the first to wash out a stomach with a tube and syringe.[8] From this time on, stomach tubes have been improved, and in 1909, duodenal intubation was developed. It was found that when a tube was passed into the stomach or intestine their contents flowed out forcibly, since the liquids and gases in the alimentary tract, because of its muscular walls, are under greater than atmospheric pressure. The longer the tube and the greater the drop from the patient to the container into which the contents flows, the greater the suction. When the flow ceases, it can be reestablished with a syringe or a vacuum bottle.

Decompression with water displacement is commonly used where means of creating suction with electric power is unavailable. Hydraulic suction is based on the fact that negative pressure is created by the flow of water from a higher to a lower level. In this method a bottle, usually of 4-liter capacity, is suspended from an irrigating standard at any convenient height, but higher than the patient's bed. This bottle is connected by rubber tubing to one of similar size placed on the floor; water flowing from the upper to the lower bottle creates a vacuum in the upper that is transmitted through a tube to the patient's stomach or intestine. An airtight system is, of course, essential for the creation of a vacuum. Fluid or gas in the alimentary tract is drawn into the upper bottle, causing the water in it to flow to the bottom bottle.

According to Bockus, the Wangensteen suction apparatus creates a negative pressure of 65 to 70 cm of water when fluids are aspirated, but the pressure increases to 150 to 160 cm as gaseous inflation occurs. (Some authors describe this as mild suction.) Two or three times this amount of pressure may collapse the tube and with continuous excessive negative pressure, necrosis of the intestinal wall may occur. Following experimental tests and clinical trials, Wangensteen and Paine concluded that when continual suction was used, the optimal negative pressure was 75 to 100 cm water.

The greater the perpendicular distance between the level of the stomach and the drainage bottle, the greater the pull on the stomach, or the greater the negative pressure and the larger the tube the less amount of suction is needed to withdraw the same amount of fluid from a cavity.

A third bottle may be added to the apparatus. Then the vacuum created by the flow of water from the upper to the lower bottle is transmitted to the third bottle and in turn to the tube inserted into the stomach or duodenum. The chief advantage of this modification is that the material aspirated from the stomach or the duodenum is kept in the third bottle. The material may be observed for color and consistency and may be more easily measured if kept separate from the water in the other two bottles. In this method only one of the three bottles is contaminated by the contents of the stomach, and the cleaning of the equipment is simplified. In the three-bottle method, it is a convenience to color the water in the two bottles used to produce the vacuum, because this enables the nurse to see the level of the liquid from a greater distance. A hospital-made water-displacement suction set can be assembled; its commercial counterpart is shown in Figure 23-1.

While effective decompression can be accomplished with the suction devices just described, electrically operated units are in general use. Of these the most desirable are the motorless ones because they are noiseless. Small portable units are more convenient than the large cumbersome variety. An increasing number of hospitals, large and small, are installing "wall-suction" or "piped-in-suction" in every room with an outlet over each bed which requires the use of only one bottle, a stopgap between the source of suction and the patient. Most machines show a low, medium, and high suction mark; low or medium suction is used for decompression of the alimentary canal. One type of drainage pump is shown in Figure 23-2.

No matter how the suctioning device is constructed, it cannot be made "fool-proof." Health workers must understand the principles on which it operates. Since nurses are most constantly with patients during the days and nights when the tube is in place, successful decompression depends to a large extent on the faithfulness with which they check the mechanism and their ability to use it effectively.

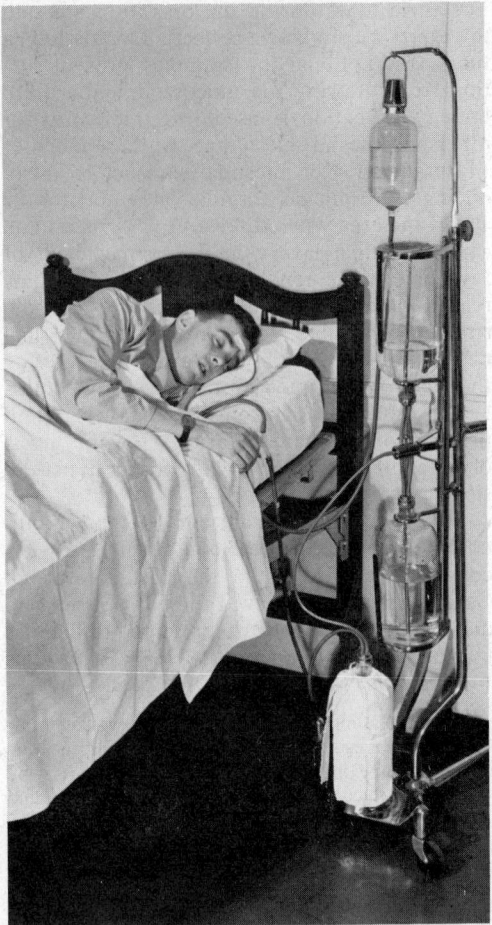

Figure 23-1. Patient having stomach drained through a tube in the nose. Three-bottle method is illustrated. Bottles that create suction are on a pivot. The upper bottle, which has no part in the suction-siphonage system, is attached to the nasal tube by a glass Y tube and contains saline solution that is used to wash out the tubing and to provide the patient with fluid as needed; the stomach contents are drawn into the lower bottle by a vacuum.

Tubes for intubation of the gastrointestinal tract are available in bewildering variety but are basically of two types—"short" tubes (gastroduodenal, such as the Levin tube for aspirating contents of the stomach) and "long" tubes (the Miller-Abbott, a prototype for all long tubes for aspirating contents of the small intestines).[9] There are *four decompression (long) tubes* in common use in this country. These are (1) the Harris; (2) the Johnston; (3) the Miller-Abbott; and (4) the Cantor tubes (see Fig. 23-3). Other tubes in use include the double-lumen tube by D'Eloia for

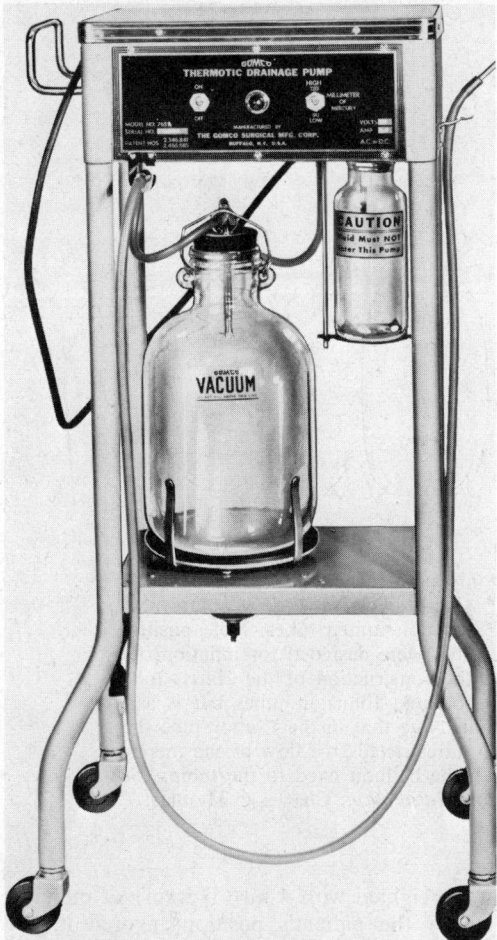

Figure 23-2. Electrically driven drainage pump; unit creates a negative pressure that can be regulated within the recommended range. (Courtesy of Gomco Surgical Manufacturing Co., Buffalo, N.Y.)

"roentgen visualization of the interior of the stomach," a tube within a tube arrangement with an air vent by Devine to prevent obstruction by suction of mucosa into holes of the tube, a polyethylene duodenal tube with a metal-weighted bucket by Matzner and associates to prevent irritation caused by rubber tubes, and a long plastic tube and flexible stylet arrangement by Smith to guide the tube into the upper part of the small intestine.[10]

Because of the difficulty in passing the tube through the pylorus, Baker developed a 40-inch #20 French double-lumen plastic tube (essentially a long Foley catheter) which is introduced into the jejunum about 12 inches below the Treitz ligament through a stab wound. Albert Behrend and Mabim C. Piezas[11]

report satisfactory results with the use of this tube in small bowel obstruction.

The Abbott-Rawson tube provides for simultaneous aspiration of the stomach and jejunal feeding. It is a double lumen tube with a single lumen extension. The double lumen portion of the tube ends in the stomach while the single lumen extension protrudes beyond the stoma of the gastroenterostomy. It is called a gastroenterostomy tube.[12] While the nurse may not encounter this tube very often, the existence of an instrument whose two parts can be passed to different sections of the intestinal tract seems worth mentioning. The Argyle Dennis tube is a three-lumen gastrointestinal sump tube, designed for decompressing the intestinal tract prior to or after gastrointestinal surgery. It allows inflation or deflation of the balloon at any point during the procedure and the sentinel line and sentinel eye permit confirmation of position of tube by x-ray or fluoroscopy (see Fig. 23-4).

The Sengstaken-Blakemore tube is used to control bleeding from esophageal or gastric varicies in patients with portal hypertension. It is a nasogastric tube with separate esophageal and gastric balloons, and a separate lumen for gastric aspiration. When the tube is in place, the two balloons are inflated, exerting pressure on the varicies in the esophagus and at the top of the stomach. Because these tubes serve a purpose different from those discussed above they are not fully described here. References listed at the end of the chapter will be helpful to the reader especially interested in this topic.[13-17]

Cantor says the Levin tube is usually discussed in connection with decompression, but it is not in the same category with the four tubes mentioned because it will decompress only the stomach and duodenum. Nevertheless, these newer tubes are modifications of the Levin tube in use since 1921. The Levin tube is a #16 French plastic (formerly rubber) tube with a closed weighted tip and opening along the side. Because this tube would often fail to pass the pylorus and because it was not long enough to drain the length of the alimentary tract, as is sometimes necessary, variations have been designed. Some medical authorities believe that sufficient drainage may be effected by the use of gastroduodenal tubes, such as the Levin tube, and that use of long tubes is not necessary. Andreas J. Høyer and Kaare Solheim,[18] discussing the therapy of 493 patients with small bowel obstruction, say that they use a duodenal tube to aspirate the stomach before and during surgery and strongly advise others to avoid using the Miller-Abbott tube. Johathan E. Rhoads and associates[19] say short

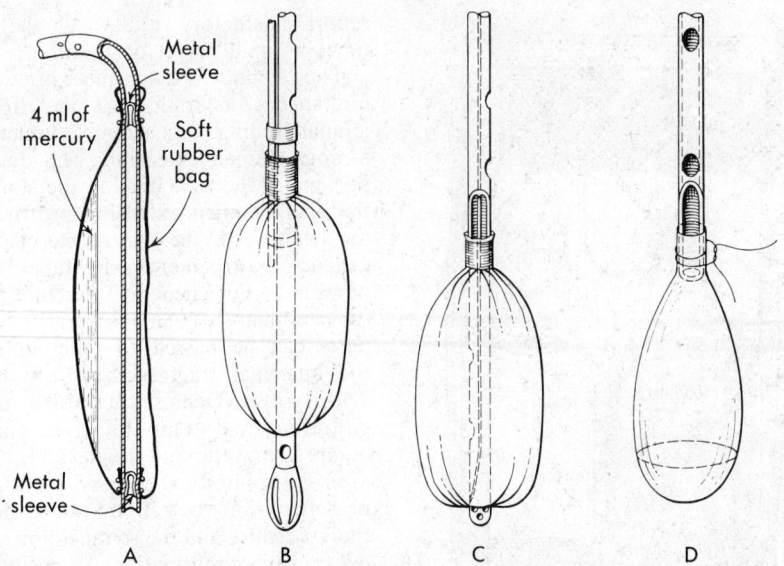

Figure 23-3. Tube heads of the most commonly used intestinal decompression tubes. *A.* Harris tube; *B,* Johnston tube; *C.* Miller-Abbott tube; *D.* Cantor tube. The Johnston tube and Miller-Abbott tube are double-lumen tubes. Note position of balloon along the shaft of the tube. These tubes were designed for inflation of the balloon with air to propel the tube. Note the construction of the Harris tube head. It is exactly the same as the Miller-Abbott and Johnston tubes but is a single-lumen tube and uses mercury as a weight. Note that in the Cantor tube the loose balloon at the tip of the tube permits an unrestricted free flow of the mercury. A later model of the Cantor tube is made with the balloon fixed to the tubing. See Figure 23-5. (From Cantor, Meyer O.: *Intestinal Intubation.* Charles C Thomas, Publisher, Springfield, Ill., 1949.)

tubes are fairly effective in preventing distention in mechanical obstruction of the small bowel.

In order to make the decompression tube pass beyond the pylorus, a number of modifications of the tip have been devised, and the decompression tubes have been lengthened and the number of holes in them increased so that negative pressure can be applied to any part of the intestinal tract. To combat the difficulty of obstruction of the tubes, their caliber has been increased.

The four decompression tubes in current use, shown in Figure 23-3, have balloons fixed to their tips, or just above them. The Miller-Abbott tube was the first. This is a single double-lumen tube with a weighted tip. The tube is passed with the balloon deflated, and it is not inflated until the tip of the tube has been carried through the pyloric valve of the stomach. The double lumen enables the operator to introduce air into, or deflate, the balloon at any point in the procedure. Because many operators had difficulty in getting the Miller-Abbott tube to go through the pyloric sphincter, this instrument has been modified.[20] Franklin I. Harris[21] found that if the balloon

was weighted with 4 ml (1 dram) of mercury and if the patient's position favored it, the tube would be carried by gravity through the alimentary tract and the inflation of the balloon with air was unnecessary. The Harris tube is a single-lumen tube, because it is not necessary to inflate the balloon. The Johnston tube is based on the same principle as the Miller-Abbott tube—that a balloon will be propelled onward by peristalsis of the alimentary tract. Charles G. Johnston[22] improved the Miller-Abbott tube by increasing the diameter of the decompression portion. The Miller-Abbott tube is a double-lumen tube enclosed in one sheath; Johnston's instrument is composed of two tubes attached to one tip and enclosed in one balloon a short distance above the tip which is an elongated fenestrated metal bulb. With Walter B. Cannon's findings in mind, that the pylorus would not open to the stimulus of a hard object, Cantor eliminated the hard tip and put the balloon containing mercury on the end of the tube (see Fig. 23-5). Because Cantor and Harris tubes depend upon the free flow of mercury to carry them by gravity through the intestinal tract, and because the balloon, with mercury in it, is passed through the nose,

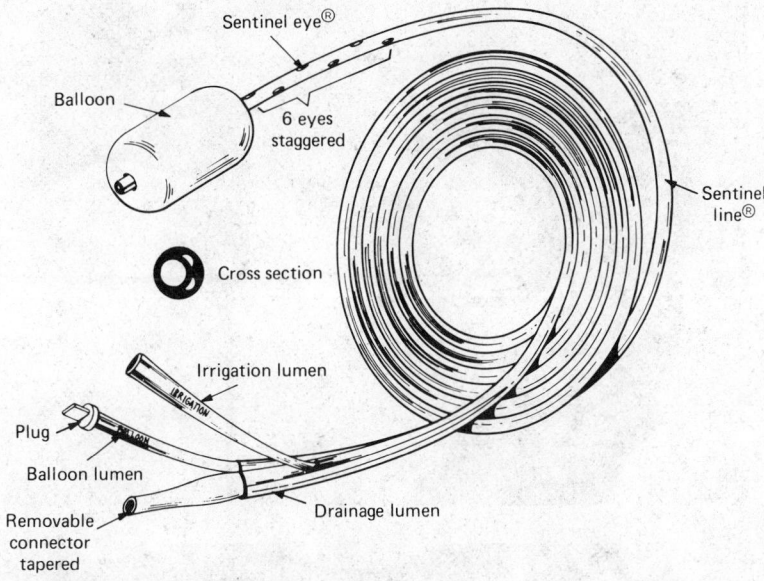

Figure 23-4. A three-lumen gastrointestinal sump tube, the Argyle Dennis tube. (Courtesy of Aloe Medical, St. Louis, Mo.)

these are single lumen tubes. The Cantor tube is #18 French with a sufficient series of large holes to provide for decompression of the intestinal tract all along its course. There is least likelihood of stoppage in a tube of this type. E. Nicholas Sargent and Harvey I. Meyers [23] describe a teflon-coated wire guide (12 ft long) that is used with a Cantor tube for rapid small bowel intubation.

The decompression tubes described are usually made of radiopaque vinyl plastic. They are less irritating than the soft rubber tubes used in the past. In modern practice surgeons depend on the help of the x-ray in determining the position of the tube. At certain stages in the passage of the tube they may work with the patient under the fluoroscope.

The *amount of mercury* used in the Harris tube is usually 4 ml (1 dram) and in the Cantor tube 1½ to 5 ml according to the age, size, and condition of the patient. When intestinal movement is normal, or nearly so, peristalsis will propel the tube onward; when the small intestine is atonic, as often happens following surgery, the weight of the tube rather than intestinal movement carries it onward. If the balloon breaks during its transit through the intestinal tract no harm will result from the presence of this small amount of mercury, according to most authorities.

Lubricants used in passing decompression tubes include water, glycerin, and vegetable and mineral oils. Cantor recommends the latter, but the danger of insufflation of mineral oil (see page 1331) should be kept in mind.[24] A vegetable oil is a safer choice. The lubricant should be applied to the tube with a cotton sponge. If the tube is dipped in the lubricant, the excess is most likely to drop into the air passages. As long as the tube is in the nose the part just outside the nares must be kept lubricated; otherwise, a crust forms which is irritating to the mucous membrane and slows the passage of the tube.

The *temperature* of the tube as it is passed has been thought important. Many texts advocate icing the tube to stiffen it; with tubes in current use this is not generally thought necessary.

Successful intubation is dependent upon getting the tip of the tube through the pylorus. *Many methods of passing the tube through the pyloric sphincter* have been advocated. Stylets to stiffen the tube have been used. Under the fluoroscope the operator can then maneuver the tube to the pylorus.[25,26] (He or she sometimes does this through the abdominal wall without a stylet.) This is uncomfortable for the patient and admittedly dangerous in any but the most skilled hands.[27] Devine, and also James, have recommended a magnetized head on the tube with a magnet used outside the body to pull the head through the pylorus.[28] Amyl nitrate has been recommended to relax the pyloric sphincter. Cantor claims that if the patient's position favors it, the tube containing free-flowing mercury will, by gravity, pass easily through the pylorus and a paralyzed ileum. The

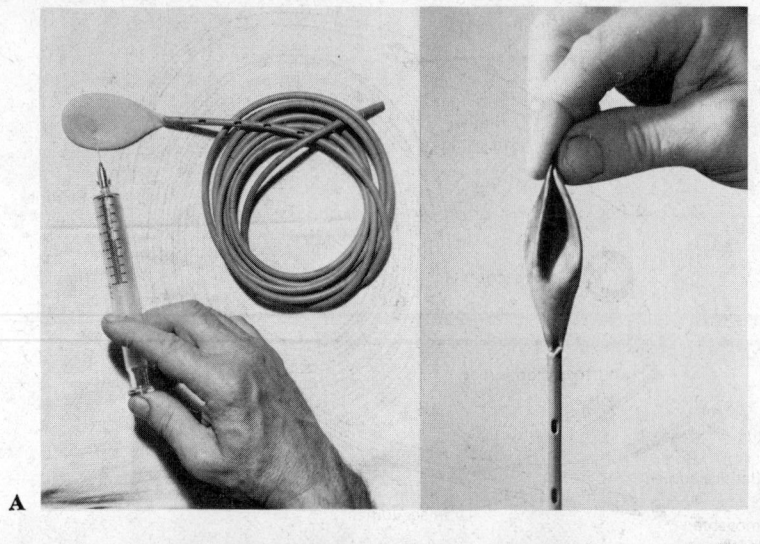

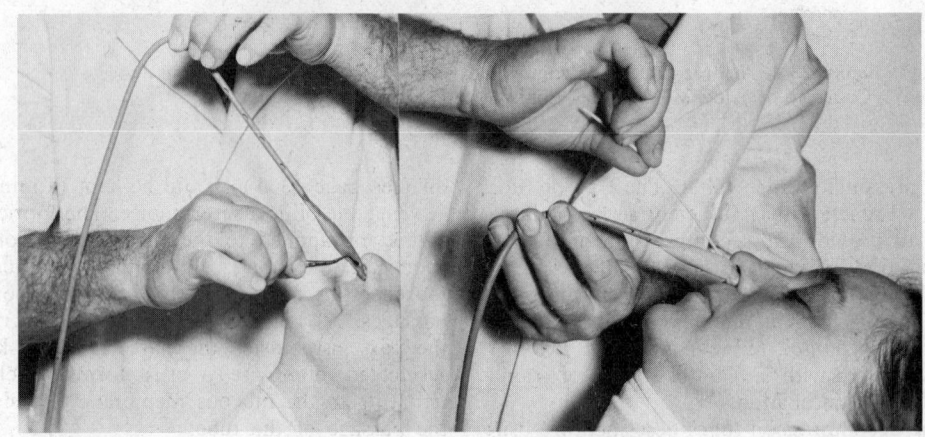

Figure 23-5. *A.* Mercury being injected into balloon of Cantor tube. *B.* End of tube held by balloon so that mercury will flow to tip by gravity. *C.* Insertion of Cantor tube started with metal forceps, and (*D*) continued with a long cotton-tipped applicator. (After Cantor, Meyer O.: *Intestinal Intubation.* Charles C Thomas, Publisher, Springfield, Ill., 1949. Courtesy of Clay-Adams Co., New York, N.Y.)

Cantor tube with the "mushy" balloon on the end most nearly approximates the consistency of the stomach contents, to which the pylorus normally opens. If, however, operators cannot visualize the tortuous course of the alimentary canal, it is difficult for them to put the patient in postures that favor a passage of the tube through the canal by gravity. If they have opaque x-rays of the patient's stomach and intestines, made previous to the intubation, to which they can refer, their problem is somewhat simplified.

After the tube is in the stomach, positioning the patient on the right side (without pillow) with the foot of bed elevated 12 inches helps the tube to pass through the pylorus, accord-

ing to some authorities. Because the head of the tube may not reach the point in the intestinal tract intended by the surgeon within 24 or even 48 hours, nurses must participate in promoting its progress unless the physician is present. They should insist upon written and specific directions for changing the patient's position, for elevating the bed, and for getting the patient on his feet. They must also know whether the tube outside the nares should be free or fixed to the face; and if the latter, how it should be fastened on the face. Most authorities say the tube should never extend over the nose and be anchored to the forehead as the pressure will cause necrosis of the nares. Nurses need equally specific directions as to when and how much of the tube is to be fed into the nose. The point is made repeatedly that the tube should not be pushed forcibly. Intestinal movement and/or the weight of the tube will carry it toward the anus with almost no help if it is not held back. Bockus thinks 6 inches of tubing should be fed every half hour. If too much is pushed in at once, it tends to coil in the tract.

Gases in the alimentary tract have been known to permeate, distend, and stop the progress of the balloon. Cantor, with associated physicists, discusses this problem in his text. They say:

It has been well established that practically all the gas found in the gastro-intestinal tract in early post-operative intestinal distension is due to swallowed air, after the anesthetic agent has been dissipated if general anesthesia was used. . . . In cases of small bowel obstruction, however, . . . the composition of intestinal gases . . . is seen to consist of the following:
   Nitrogen—70 to 80%. . . .
   Oxygen—1 to 10%. . . .
   Carbon dioxide—4 to 18%. . . .
   Hydrogen—1 to 6%. . . .
   Hydrogen sulphide—2 to 12%. . . .*

In such cases unless precautions are taken, the balloon could be dangerously distended, for natural rubber found in many of these instruments is highly permeable to carbon dioxide; and balloons of latex are permeable to hydrogen sulfide, as are Neoprene balloons to a lesser extent. Cantor says:

In a very small percentage of cases in which the intestinal tube is permitted to remain in the gastro-intestinal tract for longer than five days, it may be found that the balloon-tipped intestinal tubes take up gas into the balloon from the bowel. Because of this, check-up roentgen studies may show that the balloon is more inflated than the amount of air inserted, or the presence of air may be noted in the balloon of the Cantor tube where no air was supposed to be.†

When such accidents occur, their correction is the surgeon's problem, but the nurse can help to prevent them. The Cantor tube provides an air vent by injecting the mercury into the balloon with a hypodermic needle. The tiny hole that is left permits the escape of gas. The nurse usually participates in the preparation of equipment and can see that this precaution is taken. The air-filled balloons of the Johnston and Miller-Abbott tubes can be deflated at any time by opening the communicating lumen of the tube. While intestinal tubes are used chiefly to remove gas and fluids

from the intestinal tract, they are a means of washing it out and giving food, as tolerated. Intubated patients are usually very ill and for the first few days are ordinarily fed intravenously. Fluids are introduced during this time to keep the tube patent, to distend the tract ahead of the tube and make its passage easier, or to wash out the tract. As the distention subsides, increasing amounts of food are given as tolerated by the patient. When food is taken without nausea or distention, and the bowels move normally, the tube can be safely withdrawn. Sodium chloride solutions are commonly used to irrigate gastric and intestinal tubes. If water is used, sodium and potassium pass very rapidly into the water from the gastric and intestinal mucosa and are washed out of the body.[29] Provision must be made for returning to the patient, intravenously or by mouth, the water and salts removed by suction-siphonage; otherwise the fluid-electrolyte, acid-base balance is dangerously upset (see page 665). More than 20 years ago Rhoads mentioned fluid and electrolyte imbalance as one of the abuses of the Miller-Abbott tube. Current authorities continue to refer to the abuses which he summarized in the following terms:

Abuse has occurred mainly in cases of mechanical obstruction where it has sometimes led to delay in operation in patients who have gangrene of the bowel. . . .
Abuse consists in leaving balloon inflated and fastening tube at the anterior nares. Peristaltic action of bowel makes persistent drag on tube, resulting in skin necrosis at the nares and mucosal ulceration at the cardia. When tube has advanced far enough, balloon should be deflated when tube is fastened. Since mercury can seldom be withdrawn completely, a tube with mercury in the balloon is best avoided when it is desired to fix tube at a particular level.
Passing tube requires skill and judgment must be exercised as to how much time, how much of patient's strength, and how much x-ray exposure can be justifiably expended for this purpose.
To employ tube for suction without adequate negative pressure (usually about 5 ft of water), or without frequent irrigation, is an *abuse* in that it generally fails to function effectively.
Another abuse occurs when suction drainage is instituted without adequate replacement of water and electrolytes, including sodium, potassium, chloride and bicarbonate.*

To understand the problem of fluid and electrolyte imbalance in patients with gastro-intestinal problems, some basic information about absorption and secretions must be re-

---

* Cantor, Meyer O.: *Intestinal Intubation.* Charles C Thomas, Publisher, Springfield, Ill., 1949, p. 247.
† *Ibid.,* p. 184.

* Rhoads, Jonathan E.: "The Use and Abuse of the Miller-Abbott Tube," *Surg. Gynecol. Obstet.,* **92:** 244, (Feb.) 1951. By permission of *Surgery, Gynecology, and Obstetrics.*

Table 23-1.   Rates of Turnover of Water by Various Organs in a 70-Kilo Human Individual in Milliliters per 24 Hours *

Organs	Minimum	Liberal
Salivary glands	500	1500
Stomach	1000	2400
Intestinal wall	700	3000
Pancreas	700	1000
Liver (bile)	100	400
Lymph	700	1500
Total recovered by body	3700	9800

*From data in Wangensteen, O. H.: *Intestinal Obstructions*. 3rd ed. Charles C Thomas, Springfield, Ill.

viewed. It is estimated that the absorptive surface of the small bowel exceeds 10 square meters or about 8 times the skin area of an average adult. This large surface is made possible by the innumerable villi folds of the bowel mucosa. As is said in Chapter 11, most nutrients, electrolytes, and water are absorbed in the small intestines, although some water is absorbed in the stomach, cecum, and right half of the colon.

Most authors say approximately 8000 to 10,000 ml of secretions enter the alimentary tract in 24 hours and about 200 ml of water is excreted with the feces. This means that more than 95 per cent is reabsorbed. The amount of secretions at each level of the intestinal tract varies to some extent (see Table 23-1) whereas the electrolyte content varies significantly, depending on where the fluid is derived. Table 23-2 shows the average and range of variation in the concentration of sodium, potassium, chloride, and bicarbonate in the fluid from different levels of the intestine in patients with a variety of causes of the drainage. Of these secretions, only bile and pancreatic juice are approximately isotonic in their electrolyte content.

An examination of these tables indicates that the entire loss of any one of these fluids that normally enter the gastrointestinal tract could be fatal if it was not corrected by replacing appropriate amounts of electrolytes and fluids. If a patient with a mid-ilial obstruction loses about 2500 ml of gastrointestinal contents, Rhoads and associates [30] estimate the electrolyte losses (and the necessary replacements for these losses) would be as follows: sodium, 290 mEq; chloride, 265 mEq; potassium, 12 to 25 mEq; and bicarbonate, 50 mEq. Table 23-3 gives the average concentration of sodium, potassium, and chloride in the gastrointestinal secretions removed by indwelling tubes. This clearly shows the importance of accurately measuring and recording all fluid losses so that appropriate replacement may be made. Table 23-4 shows a list of imbalances that result from fluid loss of specific body fluid.

When fluids and electrolytes are lost by pro-

Table 23-2.   Electrolyte Concentration of Gastrointestinal Secretions * †

Source of Fluid	Na, mEq/liter	K, mEq/liter	Cl, mEq/liter	Effective HCO₃, mEq/liter
Saliva, average of 3 pt (based on 1 ml/minute)	60	20	16	50
Gastric, average	59	9.3	89	0–1
Range	30–90	4.3–12	52–155	
Upper small bowel, average	105	5.1	99	≅10
Range	72–128	3.5–6.8	69–127	
Ileum, average	117	5.0	106	15–20
Range	91–140	3.0–7.5	82–125	
Bile, average	145	5.2	100	≅50
Range	134–156	3.9–6.3	83–100	
Pancreatic fistula, average of 3 pt	141.6	4.6	76.6	≅70

† The concentration of sodium (Na), potassium (K), chloride (Cl), and bicarbonate (HCO₃), or its equivalent in organic ions, at various levels of the gastrointestinal tract. Range represents values for the middle two-thirds of a series of patients, except for gastric secretion, where a group of patients with high gastric acidity and a high CL⁻ concentration in gastric juice have been included at the upper limit.

* Modified from H. W. Davenport, "Physiology of the Digestive Tract," The Year Book Medical Publishers, Inc., Chicago, 1961, and Schwartz, Seymour I., et al., *Principles of Surgery*, Vol. I. McGraw-Hill Book Co., New York, 1969, p. 56.

longed gastric suction, the body tries to compensate by increasing renal excretion of bicarbonate, decreasing hydrogen ion and ammonia secretions in the renal tubule, and decreasing carbonic acid excretion by diminishing pulmonary ventilation. The plasma pH rises and metabolic alkalosis occurs when these compensatory adjustments are no longer effective. In this type of acid-base imbalance, serious depletion of potassum (hypokalemia) may occur, largely by way of the kidney.[31] Robert Turell says these deficits (fluids and electrolytes) can best be corrected by administration of "0.9 per cent sodium chloride solution with generous amounts of potassium chloride added to the infusion." * He recommends removal of the tube as quickly as possible, rather than prolonged use of suction and replacements by veins, so that fluid and electrolyte losses are minimized.

When the small bowel becomes distended and atonic, a considerable loss of protein may occur. In fact, as much as 20 to 30 gm of protein per liter of small bowel drainage has been reported. Plasma proteins are replaced by giving plasma in addition to electrolytes and additional fluids, depending on the needs of the patient.[32] Table 23-5 gives a semiquantitative method for replacing losses from differ-

Table 23-3. Average Concentration of Sodium, Potassium, and Chloride in the Gastrointestinal Tract Secretions Removed by Indwelling Tubes, Milliequivalents per Liter *

	Sodium	Potassium	Chloride
Through gastric tube			
Salivary ⎫ Gastric ⎭	59	9.3	89.0
Through small bowel tube			
Bowel wall ⎫ Bile ⎬ Pancreas ⎭	104.9	5.1	98.9
Through Miller-Abbott suction			
Ileum	116.7	16.2	105.8
Through ileostomy	129.5	20.6	109.7
Through cecostomy	79.6		48.2

* From Randall, H. T.: *Surg. Clin. North Am.,* **32:**2, 457, 1952.

* Turell, Robert (ed.): *Diseases of the Colon & Anorectum,* Vol. I, 2nd ed. W. B. Saunders Co., Philadelphia, 1969, p. 120.

Table 23-4. Imbalances Resulting from Fluid Loss of Specific Body Fluid *

Fluid Being Lost	Imbalances Likely to Occur
Gastric juice	Extracellular fluid volume deficit Metabolic alkalosis Sodium deficit Potassium deficit Tetany (if metabolic alkalosis is present) Ketosis of starvation Magnesium deficit
Intestinal juice	Extracellular fluid volume deficit Metabolic acidosis Sodium deficit Potassium deficit
Bile	Sodium deficit Metabolic acidosis
Pancreatic juice	Metabolic acidosis Sodium deficit Calcium deficit Extracellular fluid volume deficit
Sensible perspiration	Extracellular fluid volume deficit Sodium deficit
Insensible water loss	Water deficit (dehydration) Sodium excess
Wound exudate	Protein deficit Sodium deficit Extracellular fluid volume deficit
Ascites	Protein deficit Sodium deficit Plasma-to-interstitial fluid shift Extracellular fluid volume deficit

* Snively, W. D., Jr., and Beshear, Donna R.: "Water and Electrolytes in Health and Disease," in Kintzel, Kay Corman (ed.): *Advanced Concepts in Clinical Nursing.* J. B. Lippincott Co., Philadelphia, 1971, p. 264.

ent levels of the gastrointestinal tract. Although nurses are not responsible for prescribing these fluids, they should understand their therapeutic uses. They are the health workers who see the patient most consistently and over the longest period.

Intubation of the stomach and intestines does not always proceed smoothly. Some authorities say a common difficulty of intubation is kinking of the tube in the stomach or intestines, which interferes with aspiration of the contents; others say that vomiting frequently occurs when long tubes are used because the stomach and duodenum fill with fluids. Abdominal and duodenal distention can be corrected by inserting a Levin tube in the stomach or cutting additional holes in the long tube at the level of the stomach and duodenum. W. D. Mackay and associates [33] in a study of

Table 23-5. Semiquantitative Electrolyte Replacement for Fluids Lost from the Gastrointestinal Tract *,†

Fluid or Source of Fluid	Dextrose in H_2O, %	Dextrose in 0 . 9% NaCl Solution, %	$M/6$ $NaHCO_3$, %
Saliva	50	25	25
Gastric:			
Average	33	67	0
High acidity	0	100	0
Low acidity	50	50	0
Upper small bowel	20	70	10
Ileostomy (fresh)	15	70	15
Bile	—	67	33
Pancreatic juice	—	50	50
Diarrhea:			
Up to 1000 ml / day	50	50	0
Large volumes	30	60	10

† Based on volume-for-volume replacement of losses. These solutions are used for volume replacement of measured or, if necessary, accurately estimated losses of fluids from the gastrointestinal tract and are used in addition to base-line fluid requirements. $M/6$ $NaHCO_3$ contains 167 mEq of $NaHCO_3$/liter. $M/6$ sodium lactate may be used instead if liver function is normal. Add 20 mEq of KCl to each liter of replacement infusion unless contraindicated by dehydration or hyperkalemia. 500 ml of plasma or of 5% human albumin solution should be administered for each 2000 to 3000 ml of small intestinal content loss. Count the volume and electrolyte content as part of replacement of abnormal losses. Large volumes of diarrhea also require protein replacement.

* Schwartz, Seymour I. et al.: *Principles of Surgery,* Vol. I. McGraw-Hill Book Co., New York, 1969, p. 56.

over 50 individuals conclude that the nasogastric tube does not adversely affect pulmonary ventilation, interfere with coughing, or predispose to postoperative atelectasis—a belief held by many. They attribute respiratory complications to factors such as unwillingness to cough (or inability, as in the very ill), nasopharyngeal mucorrhea, and infection. While intubation is in some cases a life-saving measure, it has its dangers and it is always a trial for the patient.

The Psychologic and Physical Preparation of the Patient. More than in most procedures the preparation of the patient is of utmost importance. Fear and anger make successful decompression much more difficult. Before starting the procedure, patients, if not too ill, should be shown the tube, pictures, and diagrams that help them to understand its function. Surgeon, nurse, and roentgenologist need patients' cooperation, and they are more likely to gain it if they understand the procedure. An explanation from the physician in charge means most to patients usually, but this may be left to the nurse. Patients with obstruction are so sick that they often welcome something that promises relief. In all cases Cantor recommends the administration of morphine sulfate to allay nervousness and relax the stomach sphincters. (This is contraindicated for patients who are nauseated by morphine or have some other negative reaction to the drug.) It is, of course, essential that the subject be willing to swallow the tube when it passes into the oral pharynx. The *position of the patient's head* for intubation is one of the chief factors in successful passage of the tube through the nose, and the subject is most likely to maintain it if he or she visualizes the course the tube should take.[34]

Most physicians writing on this subject recommend painting or spraying the nostril to be intubated with a local anesthetic such as tetracaine (Pontocaine) 2 per cent. Shrinking the area with ephedrine 2 per cent is indicated when the passage is narrow.

Passing the tube into the stomach through the nose is the physician's responsibility, but the nurses can help him or her and the patient most effectively if they understand the technique. The patient's head should be in the hyperextended position shown in Figure 23-5D. He or she may be sitting or recumbent. Hyperextension of the head is the position in which the weighted end of the tube can be made to fall most readily into the nasopharynx. The tube should be directed downward and backward as it is passed. It should never be pushed up into the nose. The deflated balloon, with or without mercury, is folded so that the tip of the tube is pointed or small; a Levin tube, of course, requires no special manipulation. Thorough lubrication facilitates passage of the tube, and for this reason an oily lubricant is preferred to water or glycerin by most operators. Since nausea is often present a tasteless lubricant is desirable.

The patient's discomfort during intubation should be minimized as much as possible, for at best this is a traumatic experience. The tube is a foreign body, and the mucous membrane secretes excessively in order to protect itself. The patient is conscious of what feels like a noxious mass lying in the throat and, already nauseated, must constantly swallow or spit out the excess and tenacious mucus. The throat soon gets sore and if the tube falls constantly over the openings of the Eustachian tubes a middle ear infection may result. Frequent change of position helps to prevent this. The best possible oral hygiene should be practiced before and after insertion of the tube.

The teeth should be brushed three or four times daily, and a mouthwash kept in the unit for the patient. Some patients find very dilute cool lemon juice refreshing; others have used ginger ale because the bubbles of gas seem to break up the thick mucus that is so hard to spit out. Cracked ice to suck (the amount of water should be estimated and recorded, when used), chewing gum (sometimes Aspergum), and oil sprays are variously advocated to combat throat irritations and the parotitis (inflammation of the parotid gland) that sometimes accompany intubation.[35] Change of position and ambulation minimizes and equalizes the pressure of the tube on pharyngeal surfaces. If patients can tolerate it, hearing a diverting story read aloud or having the radio or television on may take their mind off their discomfort.

The patient's bedding and clothing should be protected. Nausea is often present, and intubation may precipitate vomiting. Several emesis basins and a box of paper handkerchiefs should be available. The nauseated patient usually prefers to be flat in bed, and the treatment may be started in this position with the head hyperextended over a pillow. Some operators think it easier to pass the tube through the nose when the patient is sitting.

Suggested Procedure. Having prepared the patient and gained his or her cooperation, bring the necessary equipment to the bedside. Check the suctioning apparatus to be sure it is functioning properly. With an electrical device, or pump, see that it will draw water from a bowl into the attached bottle which will later receive the contents of the stomach and intestine. Establish suction in a hydraulic system by allowing water to run from the upper to the lower bottle. As soon as suction can be felt, or otherwise demonstrated at the opening of the tube from the source of the vacuum (to be connected with the intubation tube) the tube is clamped off. Check the tube for patency as well as leaks by submerging it in a basin of water and forcing air in the lumen. If the tube has been sterilized by a solution, make sure that it has been removed by rinsing the lumen with water.* Protect the patient and the bedding with waterproof and absorbent covers and give him or her some paper handkerchiefs. See that the patient is sitting or lying with the head back, the neck hyperextended. The physician checks the condition of the tube and balloon, if one is used. He or she attaches the latter to the tube and inserts the mercury into the balloon with

a syringe and 18-gauge needle. After aspirating the air the physician ties it off as described by the designer of the particular instrument. (Cantor suggests that a nasal speculum to stretch the mouth of the balloon facilitates its fixation on the tube. He also advocates a "25 pound pull fishline of braided silk" for the tie.) The physician next swabs or sprays the nostril with a local anesthetic (tetracaine 2 per cent), lubricates the tube, and passes it through the nostril into the nasopharynx. When the tip falls into the nasopharynx, the neck is straightened, the patient, preferably, sits up, and the nurse immediately gives him or her water through a drinking tube. This swallowing carries the tube into the stomach. With the Cantor tube an "S" (stomach) appears at the nares when the tube is in the stomach. With other tubes, measures in centimeters or inches, the points at which the tube would be in different parts of the alimentary tract, are predetermined by the operator. The nature of the fluid aspirated indicates the position of the tube to some extent. From the time the tube is in the stomach Cantor advocates the following program.*

1. For the first 2 hours keep the patient turned on his right side with the face inclined downward and raise the foot of the bed.
2. For the next 2 hours have the patient in Fowler's position (a position with the back rest elevated 18 to 20 in.) and gently feed another segment of the tube until the letter "D" (duodenum) appears at the nares. If the Johnston or Miller-Abbott tube is used, the doctor will inflate the balloon. The presence of bile in the aspirated fluid is some indication that the tube is in the duodenum unless there is reverse peristalsis. This side of the tube should be marked "Balloon—doctor only" and must stay clamped firmly.
3. For the third 2-hour period turn the patient on his left side and pass another 4 inches of tubing.

(Bockus says when the Miller-Abbott tube is used about 6 inches may be fed through the nose every half hour and the balloon will usually pass through the small intestine in 3 to 6 hours. Intubation is usually carried out under fluoroscopy, but when this is not possible x-rays are taken at intervals to check the progress of the tube.)

Arrange the tube in loose coils on the bed in such a way that ample slack is allowed, and attach it to the linens. *Never fix the tube to the face or over the nose to the forehead,* for this will obviously stop its progress. This is a common mistake made by both doctors and nurses. When the Levin tube is used for gastric suction, it may be attached loosely to the side of the face so long as there is no pull on the tube.

There are several methods of determining whether or not it has passed from the stomach

---

* The death of a woman, 35 years old, was attributed to failure to remove lysol, the sterilizing solution, by those preparing the equipment and finally, those using the equipment. (Cantor, Meyer O., and Reynolds, Ronald P.: *Gastro-Intestinal Obstruction.* Williams & Wilkins Co., Baltimore, 1957, p. 498.)

* If gastric suction alone is desired, the tube (usually a Levin rather than the Cantor, Miller-Abbott, or Johnston tube) is attached to a suction device and left to drain the stomach as long as indicated. (Cantor, Meyer O., and Reynolds, Ronald P.: op. cit., p. 498.)

into the intestine. One is to have the patient drink (or inject through the tube) a colored solution; then immediately aspirate the fluid or observe the liquid that comes back into the drainage bottle. A quick return of colored fluid obviously indicates that the tube is still in the stomach. Another test, with the Johnston or Miller-Abbott tube, is to inject the amount of air required to inflate the balloon. Attach a loose-fitting empty syringe to the tube and retract it slightly. If the balloon is in the duodenum, the rhythmical movements of the intestine produce changes in pressure on the balloon that will make the plunger move back and forth in the barrel. The latter test is always made by the physician.

Proceed with intermittent or continuous suction as prescribed by the physician. It may be necessary to irrigate the tube, or flush it with a syringe at intervals. When a double-lumen tube is used, take every precaution to avoid injecting the irrigating solution into the lumen communicating with the balloon. This mistake can have very serious results. To irrigate the tube, stop the suction by shutting off the clamp on the tube leading to the vacuum. Attach a syringe to the tubing on one arm of the glass Y tube and gently force the irrigating solution through the tube. It may be aspirated with the syringe, or the suction may be turned on to remove the fluid. If a reservoir is attached to the Y tube, allow the desired amount of solution to run into the stomach and turn on the suction to aspirate the fluid. The patient may assume different positions during the progress of this treatment, but care must be taken not to dislodge the tube.

The amount and kinds of fluid to be given by mouth will be prescribed by the physician and will vary depending on the condition of the patient. Clear fluids are usually given after the tube has passed far down the gastrointestinal tract and the distention is under control. Fluids, electrolytes, vitamins, and calories in the form of predigested protein, glucose, and alcohol may be given by vein at the same time, depending on the amount of drainage and concentration of plasma electrolytes.

To prevent irritation of the nasopharynx, apply an anesthetic and shrinking spray, clean the nasal secretions and all adhesive from the tube, and always avoid pressure by the tube on the nares. Check the patient frequently for evidence of inflammation or irritation of the middle ear, pharynx, and nose.

Empty the bottle into which the drainage is aspirated as necessary. If the treatment is continued for a long period, it may be necessary to remove the tube, to give the nose and throat a rest for a few hours and introduce a clean tube. This has obvious disadvantages and is rarely considered essential.

When the treatment is to be discontinued, the physician slowly withdraws the tube through the nose. (If by accident the end has passed through the anus it is withdrawn through the rectum.) Cantor says the removal of a tube should be gradual enough to consume 20 minutes or more.

Decontaminate all equipment by suitable methods. Do not soak intubation tubes in disinfectants, such as carbolics, that might leave an odor. Discard balloons. Disposable tubing is used by some operators, especially for short intubation periods.

Recording the Treatment. Note the hour at which the treatment is begun, and record the patient's reaction. Record daily the amount of fluid the patient has received by mouth or parenterally. It is likewise important for the physician to know the amount of fluid and gas aspirated from the gastrointestinal tract. If a three-bottle method is used, the fluid in the third bottle may be easily measured and recorded. If the two-bottle apparatus with hydraulic suction is used, the siphonage is begun with a known amount of water (4000 ml) in the upper bottle and in the lower bottle (400 ml). As gas and fluid are aspirated into the top bottle, fluid will flow into the bottom bottle. The difference between the amount originally in the lower bottle (400 ml) and the amount present at the time of the reading is the amount of gas and fluid aspirated from the stomach. The gas remains in the top bottle; it may be measured by means of the calibrations on the bottle. The total amount of fluid in the lower bottle minus the original amount of water in that bottle, minus the amount of gas aspirated will give the amount of fluid aspirated. Such readings should be taken and recorded at prescribed intervals and always when changing the apparatus.[36] Record the character of the drainage, which will vary depending on the site of intubation and treatment of the patient. Following gastric surgery, it will probably be pink and scanty in amounts with a few clots of blood but will become brownish green by the first postoperative day, eventually assuming the color of normal bile drainage. With small bowel obstruction, there may be yellow or brown fecal drainage in large amounts, up to 3000 ml (3 liters or quarts).[37]

2. GASTRIC LAVAGE

Definition. Lavage is a French word derived from the Latin *lavare*, to wash out, and as used here it means the washing out of the stomach.

Therapeutic Uses. A gastric lavage is used (1) to remove undigested food and toxic substances in persistent vomiting, when the stomach may be enlarged or atrophied with lessened secretions; (2) in acute dilation of the stomach and to prepare the patient for gastric surgery; (3) to remove ingested poisons; (4) to control gastric hemorrhage; or (5) for emergency surgery as discussed on page 1212. More often in the latter case the gastric contents are removed by suction, but the stomach is not washed out.

Selection of Method. The gastric lavage is usually accomplished by means of the siphon. It is a well-known physical law that the atmosphere exerts a pressure equal to a column of water 34 feet high. If the two ends of a tube are each placed in a container of water, the fluid will run from the container that is on the higher level to the container on a lower level, because the atmospheric pressure plus the weight of the column of water in the tube forces the water into the lower container. In the lavage, one end of the stomach tube is resting under the level of the fluid in the stomach and when the funnel end of the tube is inverted and extended below the level of the distal end of the tube, the contents of the stomach will drain out. Slight suction may be used to begin the siphonage, but that is usually unnecessary. As long as the distal tip of the tube is below the level of fluid in the stomach and the funnel end of the tube inverted, the fluid will drain from the stomach. When continuous gastric drainage is indicated before, during, or after surgery, a Levin tube is passed through the nose and attached to a suctioning device, such as those described on pages 1213–14. Richard K. Hughes and D. Gareth Wootton [38] contend that a double-lumen gastric sump tube (a pit or reservoir serving as a drain) connected to a graduated water seal drainage bottle attached to a suction is more effective than drainage by a Levin tube (see Fig. 23-6).

The most commonly used solution is saline. Sodium bicarbonate or tap water may be used also. In the removal of poisons from the stomach a neutralizing solution may be used. The temperature of the solution may be from 37.8° to 41.1°C (100° to 106°F). However, to control gastric hemorrhage, the saline solution must be 0°C (32°F) to promote hemostasis [39] (see Fig. 23-7). The quantity varies from 4000 ml to 12,000 ml (1 to 3 gal). When prescribed for cleansing purposes, the treatment may be continued until the return flow is clear.

The time and frequency of treatments vary, but a lavage is usually an emergency treatment in gastric dilation, hemorrhage, or in poisoning. If repeated lavage is indicated, the intubation just described is more satisfactory. Some persons who habitually swallow more than the normal amount of air have learned to pass a stomach tube to relieve distention. This self-treatment should, of course, be discouraged, and the source of this neurosis corrected if possible.

Equipment. Articles necessary for a gastric lavage include a stomach tube, a large pitcher for the irrigating solution, and a container for the return flow. A waste basin and paper handkerchiefs and a paper bag that may be discarded are also needed. The patient's bedding and clothing should be protected. A bib of plastic, rubberized silk, or cellulose film and an absorbent cover provide satisfactory protection. Lubricants are likely to be unpleasant in taste and consistency and increase the tendency to nausea, but they reduce the irritation caused by passage of the tube.

Some operators ask that the stomach tube—a medium-sized, smooth, flexible tube about 4½ to 5 ft long—be placed on ice to prepare it for use. A stiff, cold tube is thought to be more easily passed. A funnel is attached to one end of the tube to receive the solution. Ordinarily no suction is needed to remove the

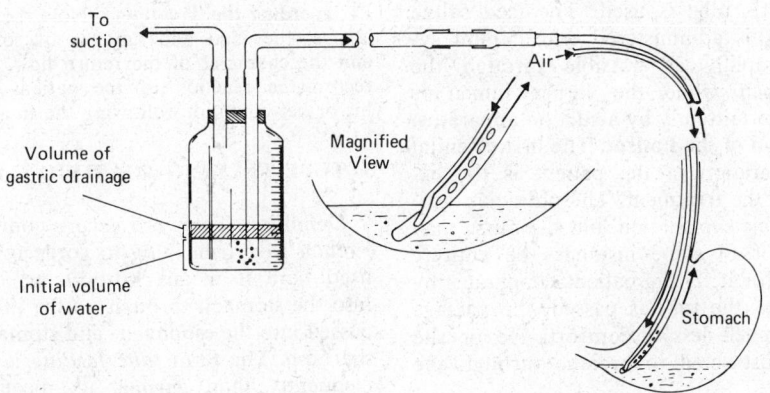

Figure 23-6. Gastric sump drainage with water seal monitor. The gastric sump tube is shown in the stomach. Room air is pulled down the smaller tube to the inside of the tip. The air and gastric fluid are pulled back through the larger tube to the water seal trap. Continuous air flow through the water seal signifies patency of the tube. (From Hughes, Richard K., and Woolton, D. Gareth: "Gastric Sump Drainage with a Water Seal Monitor," *Surgery*, **61:**193, [Feb.] 1967.)

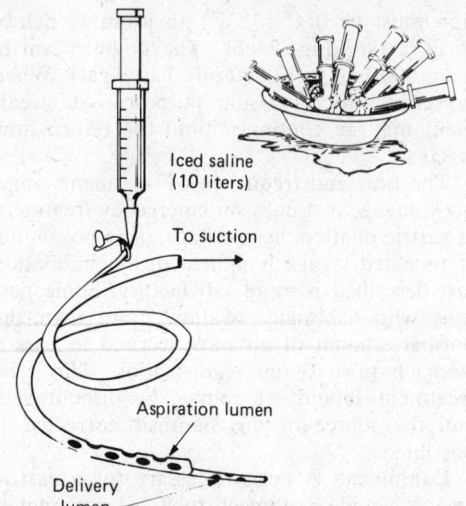

Iced saline
(10 liters)

To suction

Aspiration lumen

Delivery
lumen

Figure 23-7. Gastric lavage with iced saline using the double-lumen nasogastric tube. (Moss, Gerald: "Technique of Iced Saline Gastric Lavage in Upper Gastrointestinal Hemorrhage," *Am. J. Surg.,* **122:**569, [Oct.] 1971.)

stomach contents, but some stomach tubes are equipped with a small bulb about midway that can be used to produce mild suction. The tube is usually marked about 45 cm (18 inches) from the gastric end. If the tube is inserted this distance, it indicates, in the average adult, that the end of the tube is in the stomach. A tube is passed through the mouth to lavage a cooperative patient, but a smaller tube must be passed through the nose if an uncooperative patient bites the tube to prevent its passage.

To control hemorrhage, a double-lumen nasogastric tube * about the size of a #24 French Harris tube is used. The iced saline 0°C (32°F) is administered with 50 ml syringes as rapidly as possible through the smaller lumen while the larger lumen is aspirated intermittently by a suction apparatus.

Preparation of the Patient. The first essential in the preparation of the patient is the explanation of the treatment. The physician usually makes this explanation, but the nurse may amplify it or in some instances be entirely responsible for it. If the patient cooperates by swallowing as the tube is passed, the passage will cause much less discomfort. He or she should be instructed to breathe through the mouth.

The patient should preferably be in a sitting or horizontal recumbent position. If the head is held slightly forward, swallowing is easier

---

* United States Catheter & Instrument Corporation, Glens Falls, N.Y.

and passage of the tube is facilitated. The bedding and clothing should be well protected. The patient should have paper handkerchiefs within reach.

Suggested Procedure. The doctor passes the stomach tube, the nurse giving whatever assistance is necessary. Passage of the tube is never forced. As soon as the tube is in place, permit the stomach contents, if present, to drain into the receptacle for the return flow. Fill the funnel with the irrigating solution, allowing the fluid to run in slowly. The solution should be poured so that the funnel never completely empties because this introduces air. When 2 or 3 funnelfuls have flowed into the stomach, and before the funnel is completely empty, pinch the tube, invert the funnel over the waste receptacle, and allow the solution to siphon back. If the tube is completely empty it may be difficult, if not impossible, to establish siphonage. About 500 ml of solution should be allowed to run in before it is siphoned back. Continue the treatment by alternately introducing fluid into the stomach and permitting it to run back until the return flow is clear or until the prescribed amount of solution has been used.

To discontinue the lavage, pinch off or clamp the tube and withdraw it quickly. The patient may appreciate the use of some pleasantly flavored mouthwash after the tube is removed. Wipe the mouth and remove the rubber protector. Remove the equipment from the bedside and clean and disinfect it appropriately.

In some emergency departments in this country and in England, nurses are performing this treatment. David Wingate [40] (of England) contends this procedure "is the responsibility of doctors" and can be a hazard to the airway, especially in the unconscious patient. Nurses who perform this procedure should be fully aware of all its hazards. They should have special instructions and directed practice before carrying out the treatment without the physician.

Recording the Treatment. Note the time of the lavage, the kind and amount of solution used, and the character of the return flow. In addition, record the reaction of the patient during and his or her condition following the treatment.

3. TUBE FEEDING—GASTRIC GAVAGE

Definition. The word *gavage* comes from the French *gaver,* meaning to gorge fowls, and as used here it means introducing liquid food into the stomach through a tube that has been passed into the esophagus and stomach through the nose. The term *tube feeding* is used more frequently than *gavage;* its meaning is the same.

Therapeutic Uses. Gavage is often employed in the practice of medicine. It has an advantage over other unnatural methods of feeding in that it allows the administration of a complete diet. Its common uses are as follows:

when the patient refuses food; when conditions of the mouth or esophagus make swallowing difficult or impossible; when operations on the mouth make it desirable to keep it as clean, dry, and as inactive as possible; when the patient is unconscious, or semiconscious; when the patient is unable to retain food (anorexia nervosa and vomiting, for example); and when severe illness makes it difficult to take large amounts of nutrients and calories, as in acute and chronic infections, severe burns, terminal malignancy, and malnutrition.[41,42] Some authors list more than 20 conditions in which tube feeding has been used. The extent to which forced feeding is justified in terminal illness and other conditions in which the patient opposes it is an ethical and philosophic question too complex to discuss in this chapter. It is discussed in some detail in Chapter 50.

Selection of Method and Equipment. In tube feeding, the nasogastric tube which is inserted into the stomach is used when possible. However, it may be passed into the duodenum when a fistula or partial blockage is present. In partial obstruction and some selected conditions, Frank S. Butler and William F. Harrigan[43] say the feeding tube should be surgically inserted into the esophagus (oesophagostomy) at the cervical or thoracic level or into the stomach (gastrostomy). They believe this method of feeding is superior to nasogastric tube as the patient requires no assistance in feeding and the tube can be concealed by clothing. Shattuck W. Hartwell and Owen R. Cole[44] report the use of feeding by cervical oesophagostomy in 51 patients with cancer of the head and neck without complication. They, too, believe this method is superior to nasogastric intubation and gastrostomy for long-term gavage.

Feeding by gastrostomy and jejunostomy has been used in medical practice for years. When tumors, fistulas, or operations on the upper alimentary tract make it impossible for food to reach the intestine by the normal route, it may be necessary to bring a part of the stomach or the small intestine to the abdominal wall and make an artificial opening, or mouth, and insert a tube through which food can be passed into the part of the alimentary tract remaining. Medical authorities disagree to some extent on the advantages and disadvantages of these methods. Additional references are given at the end of the chapter for the interested reader.[45-49]

Sir Stanley Davidson and R. Passmore[50] list the following advantages of gastric feeding by tube over parenteral feeding when the patient cannot take food by mouth: (1) an adequate amount of all types of nutrients, including distasteful foods and medications, can be supplied; (2) large amounts of fluids can be given with safety, which is important with dehydrated patients; (3) the dangers of parenteral feeding (venous thrombosis, for example) are avoided; (4) nasogastric tube feeding may be continued for weeks without danger to the patient; and (5) the stomach may be aspirated at any time if it is desirable.

The *feeding* must be liquid in form, but may contain a wide variety of ingredients. Electric grinders and blenders reduce almost any foods to particles small enough to pass through a tube. Any type of feeding should contain the necessary amounts of calories, carbohydrates, fats, proteins, vitamins, and minerals. In addition, water must be supplied to meet the daily requirement. Daily requirements for dietary components are discussed in Chapter 10. A liquid diet made in a blender, which is described in the Appendix, and some commercially prepared liquid feedings listed there are suitable for gavage. Sustacal has proved to be effective in very ill patients over long periods and it is easy to use, requiring only the addition of water. However, no single formula should be taken as a standard. The diet administered by gavage should be calculated for each child or adult with even more care than that given by mouth, since the patient's appetite does not control what he or she eats. Because the liquid feeding is an ideal medium for the growth of bacteria, it must be kept refrigerated.[51] Commercial canned tube feedings are available and used in some parts of the United States. They are reported to be convenient, economical, and safe. Annette Gormican[52] says their greatest advantage is the absence of bacterial contamination.

Tube feedings are usually administered by gravity flow; however, for some patients a mechanical pump is used. Among the *articles* required for this procedure is a feeding tube, usually a thin polyethylene tube with a diameter of less than 2.5 mm. This small tube is preferred because it is well tolerated by the nasal passages and may be left in place up to 4 months, without irritating the tissues or clogging. Some operators, however, prefer a plastic Levin or a polyvinyl plastic tube. It is desirable to use a tube marked off in centimeters or inches so that it is not necessary to indicate the length of insertion with an adhesive strip. A bowl of ice to cool and stiffen the tube is usually advocated. A lubricant for the tube should be used. Oil softens the tube and may be disagreeable to taste and touch. Glycerin is believed by some authorities to be the most satisfactory substitute. An ideal lubricant for this purpose has not been found.

The lubricant should be applied to the tube with a paper square. If the tube is dipped in a liquid such as milk or glycerin, make sure that the blind end is not left filled with the fluid, because this may drop into the larynx during the passage of the tube. A drop of mineral oil, because it is not absorbed by the lung tissue, acts as a foreign body. Water-soluble lubricants dropped into the larynx can strangulate and may carry pathogenic organisms, but on the whole they are not so dangerous as the hydrocarbons. The tube should be open at the side rather than at the end.

A funnel or Asepto syringe attached to the feeding tube, with an effective clamp, is commonly used. This equipment is simple and easy to care for. In addition, patients may feed themselves as soon as their condition permits. When the feeding is given over a long period, another type of apparatus is used. A resterilized parenteral fluid bottle and disposable intravenous tubing attached directly to the nasogastric tube is economical and reduces the chance of contamination of the feeding as it is a closed system. A thin feeding mixture is necessary to prevent clogging of the tubing and ice bags applied to the bottle will diminish the possibility of bacteria growth in

the mixture. A Kelly Flask or Vitex Salvarsan tube with a Murphy drip is frequently used because the equipment is available in most hospitals and can be sterilized and used repeatedly. Unfortunately it is an open system which allows contamination of the mixture. Commercial disposable gastric feeding units,* consisting of a 1800 ml graduated polyethylene bag, drip chamber, shut-off for measurement of flow, and wide plastic tube, are available (see Fig. 23-8). The tubing is connected to the nasogastric tube or to the gastric or duodenal tube by the use of a Sims connector. The apparatus is a closed system and accommodates both thin and thick mixtures given over long periods. The equipment may be used repeatedly for the same patient if it is thoroughly cleaned after each feeding. Figure 23-9 shows equipment used in feeding premature infants.

The Barron food pump (a commercial, mechanical food pump) was developed by James Barron, of the Henry Ford Hospital, and the Engineering and Medical Departments of the Chrysler Corporation, in 1949. Barron [53] discusses his experiences with this method of tube feeding in "several hundred patients." A viscous feeding can be given constantly and

* Daval Rubber Co., Providence, R.I.

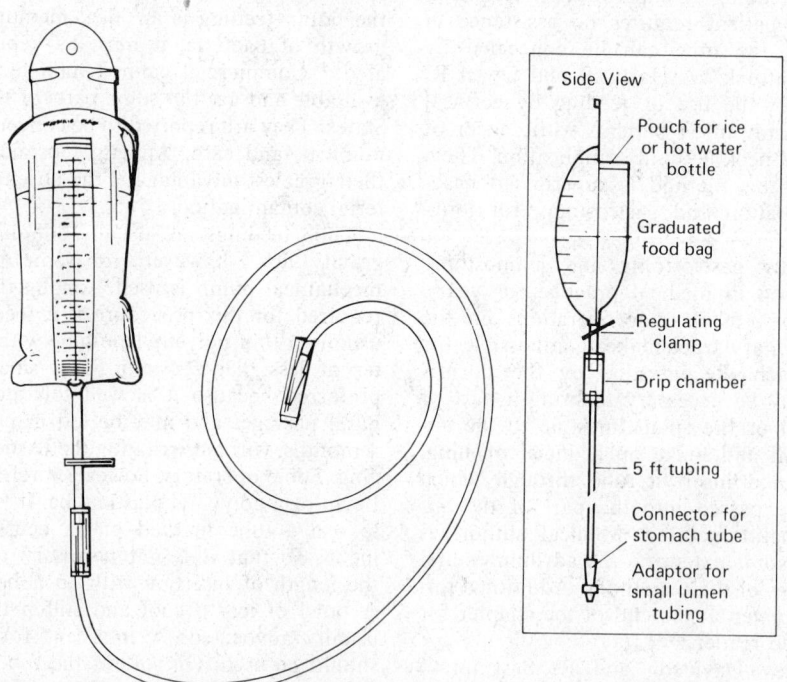

Side View

Pouch for ice or hot water bottle

Graduated food bag

Regulating clamp

Drip chamber

5 ft tubing

Connector for stomach tube

Adaptor for small lumen tubing

Figure 23-8. A tube feeding set that keeps food solution warm or cold as long as desired (note insert of side view). (Courtesy of Chesebrough-Pond's, Inc., Hospital Products Division, Greenwich, Conn.)

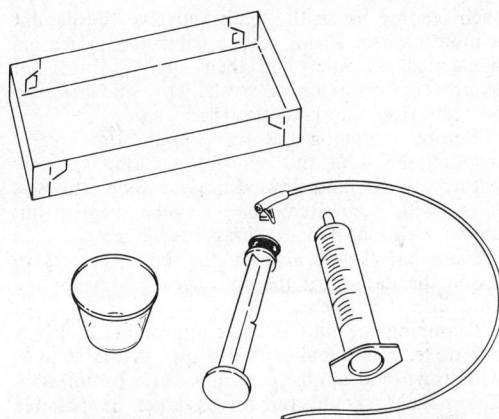

Figure 23-9. Components for feeding the premature infant. Plastic feeding tube is inserted in the proper position, then syringe is attached to the distal end. By pouring formula into the syringe, a gravity feed is obtained. No preparation is required other than measuring the formula into the graduated medicine cup provided. Transparent polyvinyl chloride feeding tube minimizes irritation to mucosa and allows the nurse to observe formula flow. The whole package is disposable. (Courtesy of Medicon, Inc., Holbrook, Mass.)

the patient is able to move freely and get out of bed without disrupting the flow of the mixture—which is not possible when the gravity drip method is used. Multiplication of bacteria in the feeding is negligible as the food bottle is kept in an insulated ice container. With this equipment it is possible to refeed gastric juice, bile, and pancreatic juice that has been removed by suction and then given with the feeding beyond the level from which they were obtained. These gastrointestinal juices contain essential electrolytes and enzymes that are difficult to replace by the intravenous route. The speed of the feeding rate is determined by the physician. The first speed delivers 42 ml of feeding in an hour; the second speed, 67 ml an hour; the third speed, 110 ml an hour; and the fourth speed, 200 ml an hour.[54] For best results, the nurse should study the instructions that accompany the pump.

Liquid medication, with the exception of oily preparations, may be given through the feeding tube by a syringe, followed by an injection of clear water to clean the tube. Tablets must be crushed, dissolved, and given by a syringe and the tube cleaned in the same manner.

The type of equipment used will depend on what is available, the viscosity of the feeding mixture, and the condition of the patient. The mechanical food pump is best when a constant slow rate of feeding is necessary—for example, with patients needing duodenal or jejunal feeding. When a thick mixture is given, tubing with a wide diameter or a mechanical food pump is necessary to prevent clogging of the apparatus.[55] Regardless of the apparatus used it must be thoroughly washed with hot, soapy water, rinsed following each feeding, and resterilized frequently. When not in use, it should be stored in such a way that it will not be contaminated.

Preparation of the Patient. When the physician prescribes tube feeding, he or she usually indicates the method for administering the mixture and explains the nature of the procedure to the patient. As in all such therapy, the nurse amplifies and reinforces the physician's original explanation and instruction. The patient's cooperation should be gained if possible, since physical and psychic resistance interferes with digestion and may even cause nausea and vomiting, greatly increasing the danger of strangulation and mechanical injury. If the feeding apparatus is brought to the bedside in a covered container on a tray with the feeding beside it in an attractive pitcher, the patient is less likely to be offended and his or her appetite inhibited by a method of feeding, unesthetic at best. Because the food is not warmed by chewing and swallowing, it should be heated to body temperature. However, when the Barron pump is used the mixture is not heated because it is given at a slow rate.

There is some question whether gavage is a medical or nursing procedure. In some institutions it is performed by the medical staff; in others by the nursing staff. Certainly, there are dangers of mechanical injury to the tract, of strangulation, and of lung infections, from allowing the tube or some part of the feeding to enter the respiratory passages. Such dangers can be prevented, and, since there are many situations in which there is no physician available to give this service, it seems important that nurses at least know how to carry out the procedure. When they must assume responsibility for gavaging the patient, nurses should insist that a physician give the first feeding in order to determine whether there is any obstruction to the passage of the tube. The patient should be *protected* by a large waterproof bib, and paper handkerchiefs are needed to wipe mucus from the mouth and to wrap the tube where the operator holds it. The operator usually wears a waterproof apron as vomiting sometimes occurs. There is also, with resistant disturbed psychotic patients, considerable danger of soiling the clothing.

Gavage is performed with the patient in either a lying or sitting position. While the passage of the tube may be facilitated by the sitting position, nausea is less likely when the patient is recumbent.

Some *restraint of the patient may be necessary* if he or she is an infant, is irrational, or is resisting gavage. If restraint is necessary, it should be limited to essentials. The operator should be calm, quiet, and reassuring. In the case of patients who have refused to eat, there should be no implication that they are being punished, although the dread of the tube feeding often acts as an incentive to eat. In such case the gavage should not be administered until patients have refused the food served to them, and they should be given to understand that the treatment will be discontinued as soon as they resume normal eating.

There are several methods of *determining whether the tube is in the alimentary or the respiratory tract*. If the tube has been passed through the larynx, it will be impossible for the patient to speak; if a few drops of normal saline are injected slowly into the tube, the patient will cough violently; and if the funnel or syringe barrel is inverted in water, bubbles of air will appear, and there will be hissing breath sounds at the open end of the tube. Gurgling noises from the stomach may be mistaken for breath sounds, however, so one of the first two means of determining the position of the tube should be used. Another method that is commonly used is syringe aspiration of the tube for gastric contents, which if obtained is assurance that the tube is in the stomach.

Suggested Procedure. After gaining the patient's cooperation, place him or her in a comfortable, relaxed position. If the patient is sitting or the head is elevated, ask him or her to tilt the head slightly forward so that the tube may pass along the floor of the nasal cavity. After applying a water-soluble lubricant to the tube, insert it into the largest nostril and ask the patient to breathe deeply as the tube is passed. This tends to relax the voluntary muscles and to divert the person from the discomfort. Tell the patient to swallow as the tube reaches the mouth of the esophagus. This tends to carry the tube into the opening and inhibits gagging. Give repeated directions to swallow and pass the tube downward immediately afterward, each time the esophagus relaxes.

After the tube is in place, tape it to the side of the face and wait for a few minutes until peristalsis has subsided before *introducing the feeding,* which should be allowed to flow in slowly. Nausea and vomiting are more likely if the food is given rapidly. At the end of the feeding, pour some water through the tube to remove food particles and thereby lessen the danger of clogging.

For tube-fed patients, frequent mouth and nostril care is necessary to reduce nausea. Before each feeding brush the teeth and give the patient a mouth wash. Clean the nostril with applicators moistened in water and then apply a lubricant to prevent formation of crusts. To avoid pressure necrosis, use alternate nostrils.[56]

Before removing the tube, pour some water through the tube and adjust the clamp securely before all the fluid flows from the tube and it is filled with air. Remove the tube gently but quickly to shorten a disagreeable process, to prevent passage of air into the stomach, and to lessen the danger of the entrance of some of the fluid into the trachea.

Clamping the tube is most important. If this is not done, the liquid will run out as the tube is withdrawn and almost certainly cause insufflation. The patient should remain as quiet as possible after the feeding in order to lessen the tendency to nausea and vomiting.

Recording the Treatment. Record the amount of feeding given as well as the amount of water added before, after, and between the feedings. Also, record the patient's reaction. Careful attention should be given to urinary output which should be about the same amount as the water taken by tube; it, too, should be recorded.

4. SELECTION OF METHOD IN COLONIC TREATMENTS

Anatomic, Physiologic, and Physical Facts Influencing Colonic Treatments. The large intestine begins at the ileocecal valve and extends to the anus. The colon surrounds, or frames, the small intestine; the transverse colon is closely associated with the liver and gallbladder, the stomach and spleen; the ascending and descending colons are in front of the kidneys (see Fig. 23-10). A hot or cold solution in the colon, therefore, acts as a local application of heat or cold to these organs. Eric W. Martin [57] says hot or cold enemas are used to raise or lower the body temperature. The average adult's colon is thought to be about 2.4 to 3.0 meters (8 to 10 ft) long. Although the amount of fluid necessary to fill the colon in healthy adults varies, Bernard P. Widman [58] believes the average is perhaps 1065 ml (approximately 1 qt). An atonic colon may hold as much as 4000 ml (4 qt). (See Chapter 11 for review of intestinal motility.)

While some person's defecating habits seem to keep the rectum empty, physicians find feces in the rectums of many patients when making examinations in the office. If an opaque enema is injected into the rectum under moderate pressure, the colon is filled within 2 to 5 minutes.[59] S. G. Flavell Matts and K. H. Gaskell [60] demonstrated that a single rectal injection of 100 ml of a 40 per cent suspension of barium in water would penetrate the ascending colon in persons with ulcerative colitis, but ascend

Figure 23-10. Semidiagrammatic view of the large intestine; the figures give in hours the average times after taking a meal that its debris reaches the various parts. This diagram shows the transverse colon in a higher position than it occupies when man is erect, and rather higher than the average even in the horizontal position. (From Haliburton, W. D., and McDowell, R. J. S.: *Handbook of Physiology.* Blakiston's Sons and Co., Philadelphia, 1934.)

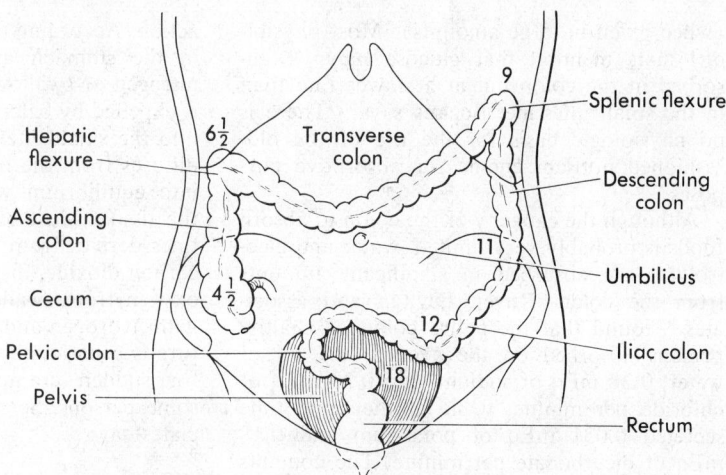

only to the splenic flexure in those persons with a relatively healthy colon. Their explanation for the difference is that the colon in ulcerative colitis lacks tone and has lost haustration contractions, offering less resistance to the upward flow of solutions injected rectally. The

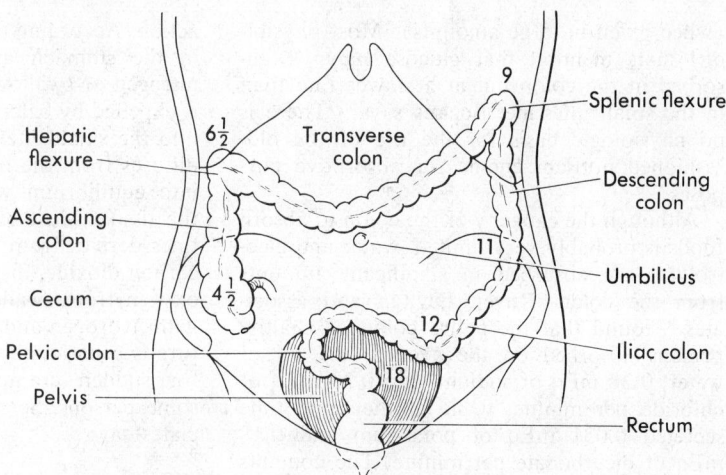

Figure 23-11. X-ray of colon immediately after the injection of a barium enema, showing that the whole length of the colon is completely filled by the liquid. (Courtesy of Columbia-Presbyterian Medical Center, New York, N.Y.)

rapid filling of the colon by large amounts of fluid may be explained on the basis of dilation and distention, that is, motility is decreased in a distended colon (see Figure 23-11).

The ileocecal valve, whose primary function is to prevent backflow of fecal content from the colon into the small intestines, can usually resist considerable reverse pressure, as much as 50 to 60 cm of water.[61] Widman[62] says the competency of the ileocecal valve may be overcome by allowing the flow of fluid to continue until the ascending colon is markedly distended; in other words if too much fluid is given it may pass the ileocecal valve into the small intestines.

In medical practice, food, drink, and drugs are administered by rectum; therefore, a consideration of *absorption* in the large intestine is important in the study of colonic treatments. This is also discussed in Chapter 11. Complete digestion of a carnivorous animal's diet takes place before it reaches the large intestine, and the absorption of most of the end products of digestion is believed to have been accomplished by the small intestine. Alvarez says that man's alimentary tract is similar to that of carnivorous types. J. C. Goligher[63] also says that the colon's role in the absorption of food is insignificant. Others imply, however, that food materials that find their way into the colon are absorbed.[64] Foods broken down into forms that are readily taken up and utilized by the cells *may* be absorbed in the large intestines. Bockus[65] says the absorption of dextrose and sucrose in the distal segment of the colon "has been demonstrated following their introduction into colonic segments distal to colostomies." Reginald A. Cutting[66] found that dogs could absorb 30 gm an hour; A. Dahlquist and D. L. Thomson[67] report that rats absorb as much as 25 per cent of lactose (when given in large amounts). Most physiology texts mention that glucose *may* be absorbed in the colon but at a slower rate than in the small intestine. Bockus says: "There is no physiologic basis for the use of the old-fashioned nutrient enema for absorptive purposes." *

Although the capacity of the colon to absorb foods is probably very limited, water and electrolytes are absorbed in significant amounts from the colon. Ruven Levitan and associates [68] found that the entire colon of healthy persons absorbed on the average 1.7 ml of water, 0.28 mEq of sodium, and 0.39 mEq of chloride per minute, while at the same time secreted 0.031 mEq of potassium and 0.18 mEq of bicarbonate per minute. The contents (approximately 500 ml of chyme per day) of the alimentary tract, as it enters the cecum, is about 90 per cent water, whereas a normal stool is a semisolid mass; this shows how much water passes from the large intestine into the tissues during its normal activity. Bockus says that a proctoclysis is only of value to the body if sodium chloride or a sugar is added to the water. Charles H. Best and Norman B. Taylor note that "more water is absorbed from hypotonic than from isotonic solutions and more from isotonic than from hypertonic solutions." †

The amount and rate of absorption of drugs depend upon the drug and how it is injected. According to Robert Turell,[69] some drugs and foreign substances are absorbed promptly from the colon, while others are not absorbed at all. Besides the physical processes of osmosis and diffusion, by which water and solid particles pass through animal membranes, there appears to be a selective activity of the cells lining the large intestine, enabling them to accept certain materials and reject others. A great deal of experimental work has been done on absorption, but the findings and opinions vary. However, there is evidence that glucose, certain electrolytes, ether, and other drugs are absorbed. Injecting the solutions in hypotonic concentrations, under low pressure and near body temperature, favors absorption in the colon. A large number of medications are available in the form of rectal suppositories that are adequately absorbed.

There is general agreement among authorities that much of the intestinal gas enters the tract through the esophagus during swallowing but some is formed by chemical and bacterial action. According to Arthur C. Guyton,[70] gases in the stomach are principally oxygen and nitrogen or swallowed air. Gas in the stomach is expelled by belching, but small amounts pass into the small intestines where carbon dioxide diffuses from the blood into the air to bring it into equilibrium with the carbon dioxide of the tissue. Most of the gas in the large intestines derives from bacterial action. It includes carbon dioxide, methane, and hydrogen. When oxygen from swallowed air is properly mixed with hydrogen and methane, an explosive mixture is occasionally formed. This may account for sudden cramping pains experienced by some persons. Seymour I. Schwartz and associates say:

Gases are absorbed from the intestines at rates that are directly related to the partial pressure of the particular gas in the intestine, in the plasma, and in the air breathed. Thus with nitrogen there is little diffusion, since the partial pressures of the gas are virtually the same in the intestine, plasma, and air. On the other hand carbon dioxide diffuses very rapidly, because the partial pressure of carbon dioxide is high in the intestine, intermediate in plasma, and very low in air. For this reason, though carbon dioxide is produced in large amounts in the intestine, it contributes little to gaseous distension because of its rapid diffusibility.*

On the average about 7 to 10 liters of gases either enter or are formed in the intestines each day while about 0.5 liter is expelled and the remainder is absorbed. However, large quantities may be expelled at times because of excessive motility of the colon.[71] Sickness or any condition that lessens muscle tone will tend to make the expulsion of gas more difficult.

It is certainly true that the passage of gas along the intestinal tract requires a greater muscular effort than the passage of food. The second writer has seen the violent contractions produced by the injection of air into a rabbit's alimentary canal whose motor function was preserved by suspending it in a tank of warm saline solution. Such contractions in the living animal may cause a pull on sensitive areas of the peritoneal attachments and so cause considerable pain. No matter what the mechanism, there is no doubt that discomfort and pain are associated with a distended abdomen, a condition known as *tympanites* or *meteorism*. Treatments, such as colonic irrigation, enemas, and proctoclysis, should be given in such a manner as to facilitate the escape of gas. How-

---

* Bockus, Henry L.: *op. cit.,* p. 620.

† Best, Charles H., and Taylor, Norman B.: *The Physiological Basis of Medical Practice, 8th ed.* Williams & Wilkins Co., Baltimore, 1966, p. 1180.

* Schwartz, Seymour I., et al. (eds.): *Principles of Surgery,* Vol. II, 2nd ed. McGraw-Hill Book Co., New York, 1974, p. 982.

ever, we believe these treatments are used infrequently for relief of distention since the advent of nasogastric suction.

Experiments with dogs have shown that enemas of physiologic salt solution, tap water, soap solution, and mixtures of ox gall, glycerin, and water did not have any effect on mobility of the small intestine but that injections of hypertonic salt solution do increase peristalsis of the small intestine and should therefore be more effective in relieving abdominal distention.

Austin Smith [72] gives the following formulas for "purgative enemas": Glycerin 30 ml, magnesium sulfate 60 gm, and water 120 ml; another larger preparation consists of warm soapsuds 0.5 liter, magnesium sulfate 60 gm, glycerin 60 ml, and oil of turpentine 15 ml emulsified in the yolk of an egg. This type of enema is rarely used today. When a fecal impaction is present an oil retention enema is given followed by gentle manipulation with the gloved finger in the rectum to break up the mass.

Physical principles *regulating* (positive) *pressure* when dilating the colon and suction (negative pressure) when draining it are of great importance. Persons administering such treatments must bear in mind that the greater the height of the column of liquid, the greater the pressure, the more rapid the dilation, and the greater the stimulation of the intestinal musculature; also, the larger the caliber of the outlet of the column of liquid, the more rapid the flow. Likewise, the greater the drop, or length of the drainage column below the level of the anus, the greater the suction and the more rapidly the colon empties. If sufficient suction were exerted on the bowel, the mucosa might be sucked into the opening of the tube, occlude it, and possibly injure the mucosa. Nice regulation of the pressure and rate of flow in filling and draining the colon is for this reason important. Although the colon can probably stand a good deal of pressure without injury to the organ, Adolph Walkling [73] has reported several cases of rupture of the rectum resulting from distention during proctoscopic examinations. According to Henry C. Frech and L. Richard Lanier,[74] 31 cases of colonic perforation caused by an improperly administered enema have been reported in the literature. They think that the two types of patients who are particularly vulnerable to perforation by enema are those over 55 years of age and pregnant women at term. Emphasis is placed on inserting the enema nozzle just past the sphincter, using small rectal tubes, and cautioning the patient to avoid sneezing, coughing, moving suddenly, or straining while the enema tip is in the rectum. The nurse must not lose sight of this danger.

Physiologic response to the *insertion* of a rectal tube or any foreign body into the anal canal is a contraction of the anal sphincter. This protective reflex makes the introduction of the tube difficult and possibly painful if the tube is forced into the canal while the body is trying to prevent its entrance. The following method should reduce the discomfort of the patient and the difficulty of the worker: Expose the anal region, keeping the patient as well covered otherwise as possible; a good light on the area is required; if he or she is able to cooperate, ask the patient to bear down as if having a stool (this opens the orifice) and to inhale deeply in order to relax the abdominal wall; then insert the tube slowly and gently. The tube should be well lubricated. Vegetable and mineral oils make effective lubricants, but the heavy hydrocarbons, such as petroleum jelly, are most effective. Since oils, and particularly hydrocarbons, are destructive to rubber, vegetable jellies, which have little if any effect on the life of rubber and are nearly as satisfactory as lubricants, are extensively used. If a small amount of solution is injected as the tube is inserted, the fluid will distend the rectum and leave a free passage for the introduction of the tube.

When introduction of the tube is painful or difficult, the nurse should remove the tube and report the condition. The patient may have hemorrhoids, a stricture of the rectum, an abscess, or some condition that would make the usual introduction of a rectal tube dangerous. The ability to determine whether an unnatural amount of discomfort is experienced by the patient is acquired through experience. Student nurses should err in being too careful rather than incautious in such cases.

5. CLEANSING, OR EVACUATING, ENEMAS

Definition. An enema given to remove fecal material from the colon is often called a *clyster*. This comes from the Greek *klysis,* meaning a washing out of stagnant or waste materials by means of injection of fluid. An enema for this purpose is given in such a way as to stimulate the defecation impulse.

Therapeutic Uses. A cleansing, or evacuating, enema may be prescribed if the number or character of the stools indicate that waste products are not being properly eliminated (as in constipation or fecal impaction); in preparation for surgery or delivery of a fetus so that the rectum and lower colon is cleaned, ensuring a clean field; in preparation for examination of the rectum by proctoscope or x-ray so that the physician can see the mucous membrane; and if the intestines are abnormally distended by gas. An enema given to stimulate the expulsion of gas is called a *carminative enema*. The purpose of the treatment is to soften hardened fecal matter and to stimulate the contraction of the colon by distending the walls or by irritating them with high or low temperatures or with chemicals. William Lieberman in "Some Historical Notes on the Enema" * says: ". . . the use of the enema recedes far into the past beyond the earliest recorded times." People are likely to resort to enemas without any medical advice whatever.

Some physicians warn against the continued use of cleansing enemas, saying that they interfere with normal bowel movements, cause gradual dilation of the colon, and wash out the mucus which is the natural lubricant of the colon as well as the bacteria that function in cellulose digestion. Morcella F. Dunning and Fred Plum [75] report an excessive loss of potassium (hypokalemia) in a patient who received repeated and prolonged enemas. Most authorities say this problem can occur when enemas are used indiscriminately.

Selection of Method. The *kind* and *amount of fluid* depend upon the age and condition of the patient, the purpose of the treatment, and the judgment of the physician. Solutions most commonly given are sodium chloride, sodium bicarbonate, and a weak solution of a neutral soap; plain water is also used. Hypertonic solutions (sodium phosphate and biphosphate, for example) in commercially prepared disposable enema units are used increasingly in hospitals and homes.† Medicated carminative enemas include solutions and mixtures containing purgative salts, glycerin, turpentine, oil, alum, ox gall, milk, molasses, asafetida, and other substances in various combinations and proportions. (Most texts list these substances but the writers think they are rarely used. Formulas for these various enemas are given in the Appendix.) There is a good deal of variation in the nomenclature and in the proportions of the drugs used for enemas. Most hospitals give directions in their procedure manuals for preparing special enemas.

When the physician orders a cleansing enema and fails to prescribe *the solution*, the nurse is probably safe in using physiologic saline solution. Attention has been called to the fact that physiologic solutions are nonirritating. Although dilute soap solutions are used, they are irritating; this is dramatically demonstrated every time that soap gets into the eyes during a shampoo. In experiments with animals, soap-solution enemas have produced hemorrhages and ulcerations of the colon. Harold H. Rosenfield and associates [76] report that 60 of 100 women complained of "griping" or "discomfort" during administration of a soapsuds enema. Excessive mucus and spasm of the mucosal lining of the colon has been observed, also.[77] Water intoxication following tap water enemas has been demonstrated in animals and several deaths of humans have been reported. Howeven, Alan Ziskind and Sidney S. Gellis [78] found that tap water enemas had no adverse effect on 11 healthy children but that five children with chronic constipation and a dilated colon showed a decrease in serum sodium concentration. The reason for the increased absorption of water was an increase in the absorptive surface area and decreased peristaltic action which permitted the hypotonic solution to come in contact with the bowel wall for long periods. In conclusion, they write:

If tap-water enemas are not administered to patients receiving intravenous hypotonic solutions, to unconscious patients, and to patients with chronic constipation, water intoxication is unlikely to develop. The judicious use of one tap-water enema in an otherwise normal patient is permissible and carries little risk of producing water intoxication.*

The commercially prepared individual enema units containing hypertonic solutions of sodium phosphate can produce harmful effects on patients with certain conditions. Following administration of one of these enemas containing 165 mEq of sodium, Edgar H. Flentie and Arthur Cherkin [79] found that on the average 35 mEq or 21 per cent of sodium was retained. They suggest that this type of enema should not be used for patients on a low-sodium regimen. Eugene Y. Berger and associates [80] demonstrated, by the use of cation exchange resins, that the colon of the edematous patient with congestive heart failure and cirrhosis of the liver retains sodium to a greater degree than does the colon of persons who are healthy. It is obvious, therefore, that solutions containing sodium should not be used with patients having these conditions. Distention and irritation of the bowels by temperatures above

---

* *Rev. Gastroenterol.*, **13:**215, (May–June) 1946.

† These small hypertonic enemas in disposable units are convenient to use but the fluid may cause more local discomfort than blander solutions given in larger quantities.

* Ziskind, Alan, and Gellis, Sidney S.: "Water Intoxication Following Tap-Water Enemas," *Am. J. Dis. Child.*, **96:**699, (Dec.) 1958.

or below that of the body are sufficient to stimulate peristalsis. Ordinarily, physicians prescribes the solution; they may indicate the strength of the drug and the proportions to be used in compounded enemas; or, if in a hospital, they may use the customary name which in that institution designates the particular solution or mixture.

Medical opinion and custom vary with respect to the *temperature* of solutions given. The practice of making the fluid about 41.7°C (107°F) so that it enters the rectum around 40.6°C (105°F) is probably most general. Temperatures above 43.3°C (110°F) should not be used, as they may injure the tissues.

Apparently no rule can be laid down for the *amount* of solution, as quantities varying from 500 ml (1 pt) to 2000 ml (2 qt) are advocated. For infants and children, proportionately smaller amounts are injected. Reports of studies and medical opinion indicate a growing disapproval of large quantities because of excessive loss of potassium, water intoxication, and decrease of muscle tone caused by abnormal distention of the bowel. In commercially prepared enema units the amount varies from 100 to 130 ml but as little as 5 ml of hypertonic solution is reported as being effective.[81,82] If additional fluid is needed, Turell suggests refilling the squeeze bottle with plain tap water.

In abdominal and pelvic surgery, if the abdomen is distended with gas and the pressure on the operative site from this distention is causing discomfort or actual pain, especial care should be exercised to avoid increasing distention any more than is necessary. If the patient is an adult, it is desirable to introduce about 240 ml (8 oz) of the enema and insert a rectal tube or allow the patient to use the bedpan before continuing to give the total amount prescribed. Usually the physician orders the enema as a means of emptying the lower bowel and is willing to have as little or as much solution used as is necessary to stimulate evacuation, depending on the condition of the patient.

Much of the discomfort patients suffer during administration of enemas is caused by rapid dilation of the colon. Attention has been called to the importance of giving fluids under low *pressure*. This precaution is repeated here for emphasis. Mention has been made also of the fact that solutions injected into the rectum with a tube inserted 7½ to 10 cm (3 to 4 inches) have been shown to reach the cecum in 5 minutes or less. Because of the possibility of injuring the rectum, most authorities say insertion of the tube should not exceed 5 cm (2 inches)—further insertion may result in coiling of the tubing or perforation of the anterior wall.[83]

Velvet-eyed catheters or rectal tubes (tubes with side rather than end openings) are preferred for all rectal injections. It is now generally agreed that the *position of the patient* makes little if any difference in the results of an enema. Abdominal relaxation decreases pressure and consequent discomfort; this is favored by having the patient in the lateral position with the knees flexed. In some cases, especially those in which there is loss of control over the anal sphincter, it is necessary to give the enema with the patient on the bedpan. As patients may get very tired in this position a rubber-covered pillow should be placed under the small of the back so that they will feel supported, and unless they can keep their knees flexed without tiring, another rubber-covered pillow should be placed under them for support. When giving an enema to infants who are unable to retain the solution, provision must be made for its immediate return. In hospitals, regular treatment tables are provided for this purpose; in homes the infant may be supported over a douche pan or a waste container of any kind. Care must be taken to protect the infant from the edges of the pan.

Equipment. Regardless of the method and equipment used, there seems to be advantages and disadvantages attached to each. The disposable unit for giving enemas which is in common use today is a labor-saving device; some disadvantages have been discussed. Turell[84] (in 1960) discusses injuries to the anorectum of 12 patients following self-administered concentrated enemas in disposable containers. Injuries included the following: laceration of the anal canal and internal hemorrhoids, bleeding, and suppuration. The extent of the injuries were thought to be caused by the chemical effect on the lacerated areas and the physical injury caused by the enema tip. In 1969, he recommended their use if there was no inflammatory disease of the distal colon. The disposable unit is a plastic bag or bottle with an attached rectal tip, containing the solution. By squeezing the flexible container, the solution is forced into the rectum. These are suited for hospital, home, and office use and are esthetically appealing to the patients.[85] The solution can be warmed by immersing the container in a water bath.

The solution may be administered from a reservoir (an irrigating can or rubber douche bag) or it may be poured from a pitcher into a funnel attached to a length of tubing. Because it is more convenient for the worker and there is less likelihood of introducing air with the solution, the reservoir method is preferable. The funnel-and-pitcher method is frequently used by nurses in homes because it is easy for them to carry this equipment in their bags. If an irrigating can is used, a standard should be provided for its support. It is necessary to have a clamp on the tubing to stop or regulate the flow of solution. Tubing attached to the can and connected to the rectal tube by a glass connecting tube should be approximately 90 cm (3 ft) in length. The rectal tube should be a #22 or #24 French, with a velvet eye; the smaller sized catheters are used in giving enemas to infants. (Hard-rubber rectal tubes are likely to irritate or injure the rectum, and their use should be discouraged.) A lubricant for the tube, such as a vegetable or petroleum jelly, is essential. Usually a small portion of the lubricant is brought to the bedside in a folded piece of toilet tissue by which means it is applied to the tube. A waste basin is needed for the used rectal tube. The bed should be protected by some means; this may be a piece of plastic sheeting with a cotton or paper cover, or a pad of cellucotton with a piece of impervious paper as a base. A pad made of newspapers and covered with old sheeting is an excellent protector to use in the home if plastic sheeting is not available. A treatment blanket covers the upper part of the body, and toilet articles must be at hand for cleaning and drying the patient after the treatment.

In order that it may enter the rectum at the proper temperature, the solution is prepared at a temperature a few degrees higher than that prescribed. If a soap-solution enema is ordered, the suds should be removed from the surface of the liquid, since, for reasons already pointed out, the injection of air into the rectum should be avoided. A tray or treatment wagon is used to convey the equipment to the bedside.

Suggested Procedure. Before taking the equipment to the bedside, explain the treatment to the patient and gain his or her cooperation. As in all such cases, the explanation must be suited to the patient. Discomfort is reduced and the effectiveness of the treatment increased if fear and resistance are eliminated. Preparation of the patient includes protection of the bottom sheet, replacing the top bedclothes with one or more treatment blankets, screening the patient, and putting a sign on the door of a private room to ensure privacy.

If an irrigating can is used, hang it so that the level of the solution is never more than 45 cm (18 inches) above the anus. Ordinarily, half this height will result in a steady, slow injection, which is desirable. Expel air in the tubing by allowing a small amount of solution to run through it into a waste basin. With the patient in the proper position and the blanket adjusted in such a way that only the anal region is exposed, insert the lubricated rectal tube slowly and gently for a distance of approximately 5 cm (2 inches) (see Fig. 23-12). *Let the solution flow into the rectum slowly.* Do not allow the can or the funnel to empty as this draws air into the rectum. If the patient complains of discomfort, the solution is probably flowing too rapidly and should be stopped to allow peristalsis to quiet down. In some cases it is desirable to remove the tube and ask the patient to use the bedpan. If a good bowel movement results, it may not be necessary to give the remainder of the solution. Irritation of the rectum is reduced to a minimum during the removal of the tube if this is done gently and quickly. Manual pressure over the rectum with a cellucotton pad inhibits defecation temporarily. In some instances it may be desirable to have the patient retain the solution for a few minutes before using the bedpan, but if a large amount of solution has been injected, he or she is seldom able to do this. The bedpan should be warm, and the diagonally folded protection sheet drawn up between the legs like a diaper to form a shield that prevents the upper bedclothes from being soiled and helps to control odor. If patients are weak or ill, they should not be left alone, since an enema is tiring and they may faint from the effort made to expel the solution. Ordinarily, patients prefer privacy, but the nurse must be near and a means of summoning him or her within their reach. If she or he is not called within a reasonable length of time, the nurse should make certain that the patient is all right.

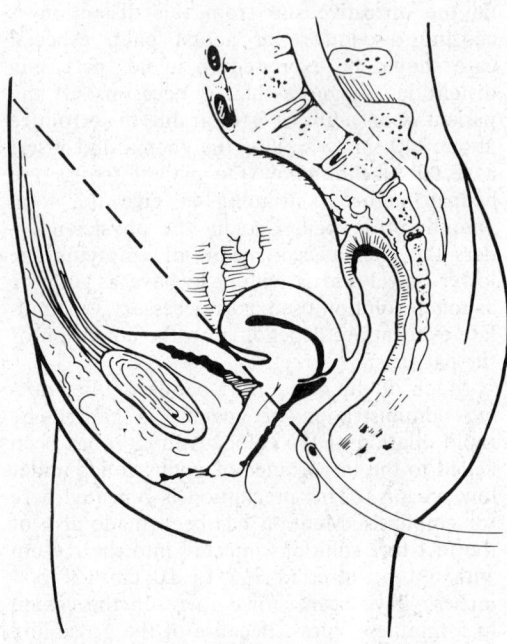

Figure 23-12. When inserting the enema tube, direct it toward the umbilicus and insert about 2 inches (5 cm).

Sometimes patients are unable to expel the enema. Retention of a cleansing enema is likely to occur if the patient is dehydrated. The solution injected is then absorbed to supply fluid which the tissues need. In cases of this kind, reinsert the rectal tube, place the end in a bed pan, and if the nurse is a student she or he should report the condition to the head nurse. Further measures will probably be prescribed.

After the enema is expelled, remove the pan, turn patients on their side, and clean the buttocks with toilet tissue and soap and water, if they are unable to do this for themselves. Remove the bed protector and readjust the clothing. The importance of sterilization of equipment used, including container, connecting tubes, and rectal tube, cannot be overemphasized. Contamination of the equipment, including the container for the solution, with transmission of bacteria has been demonstrated.[86,87,88] Sterilize all equipment that may be used again.

Recording the Treatment. Consider the purpose of the treatment and chart the results—whether retained or expelled, whether the return was satisfactory in amount, whether it was fluid or contained small, hard masses, the amount of flatus, and the presence of any abnormality. Also note the effect on the patient—whether the treatment was accompanied by pain or discomfort, or followed by signs of weakness or exhaustion.

6. COLONIC IRRIGATION, OR ENTEROCLYSIS

Definition. *Enteroclysis* is derived from two Greek words: *enteron,* meaning intestine, and *klysis,* a washing out of stagnant or waste material. There seems to be no sharp dividing line between enemas and irrigations, but their purposes are different. The ordinary enema is given to induce defecation while the irrigation is given to wash out material situated above the sigmoid colon and to lavage the wall as high as the water can be made to reach. Usually this requires that the fecal mass in the lower colon be expelled and the liquid pass into the colon gently so that the defecation reflexes are not stimulated.

Therapeutic Uses. Colonic irrigations are given for the following purposes: (1) To clean the colon and rectum when impacted with feces or when coated with a barium preparation, or in fecal incontinence and in cases of poisoning to dilute and remove any of the toxic agent that may be present in the large intestine.[89,90] (2) To supply heat to the colon, or to the pelvic and abdominal organs surrounding the large intestine for the relief of pain and to bring about circulatory changes. Cold as well as hot irrigations may be used for the thermal effect on the colon and nearby organs. Ice water enemas may be given in

sunstrokes.* In treatment of prostatitis local application of heat may be accomplished by low rectal irrigations.[91] (3) As a means of applying local remedies to the colon in the treatment of infections and other pathologic conditions. (4) To empty the colon when the patient is so weak and ill that he or she is unable to go to the toilet or use a commode or the bedpan without exhaustion.

With the development of the sulfa drugs and the antibiotics, colonic irrigations are rarely used in the treatment of infections. Several authors recommend irrigating the bowel below a tumor in the colon to avoid spreading carcinoma cells during the operation. Harry E. Bacon [92] uses two or three flushings, 1000 ml each, of chlorpactin (0.5 per cent) just before surgery is performed. The procedure is carried out in the operating room.

Selection of Method. The equipment and method depends upon the purpose for which the treatment is ordered, the condition of the patient, and the facilities available. The physician may prescribe the method or simply order a colonic irrigation and leave it to the judgment of the nurse to decide how to give it. In either case the nurse should have a thorough understanding of the basis on which the choice of method is made. He or she should determine whether the treatment is prescribed for its cleansing, thermal, or chemical action, or as a means of supplying fluid to the body; and whether the physician intends that the solution reach the entire length of the colon or only the distal portion. Having this information, the nurse administers the treatment, keeping in mind its purpose and the condition of the patient.

Variations in method most often mentioned are the use of one or two tubes. There is probably little difference in the results or in the ease with which the two methods are used. In the one-tube method, the rectal tube is attached to one prong of a glass Y tube, a drainage tube is attached to the other prong, and the tubing from the reservoir is attached to the base of the Y tube. Stopcocks on the inlet and drainage tubes enable the operator to introduce a given quantity of solution and then drain the bowel by closing the inflow tube and opening the drainage tube. In the second method an inflow and a drainage tube are inserted into the rectum at once, and the bowel may be drained constantly while the solution is being administered; or, with the use of the stopcocks on the tubing, the treatment may consist of periods of injection of the solu-

---

* Medical texts usually recommend cold baths in the treatment of sunstroke.

tion with the outflow tube closed and periods of drainage while the inflow is cut off.

The size of the rectal tube varies from #22 to #32 French. Raymond J. Jackson [93] recommends a #18 to #26 French catheter for patients with fecal incontinence. A Bardex-Foley type of rectal bag and catheter may be used instead of the regular catheter when a large anal defect is present. Another device that is helpful in retaining the fluid is a catheter threaded through a soft rubber ball which may be purchased at the dimestore. This is accomplished by drilling a hole in the ball and pulling the catheter through so that it is well anchored. This device, like the Bardex bag, produces pressure on the anal defect so that water can be retained (see Fig. 23-13). The Harris Flush Tube may be used to give an enema, rectal irrigation, or flush (see Fig. 23-14).

A colonic lavage machine, designed by Henderson at St. Mark's Hospital, London, is used to clean the bowel before radiography. It operates in such a way that fluid flows in by gravity and, when the colon is full, it automatically ceases and fluid returns under slight negative pressure. A metal nozzle serves as a rectal tube.[91] It seems that such an instrument

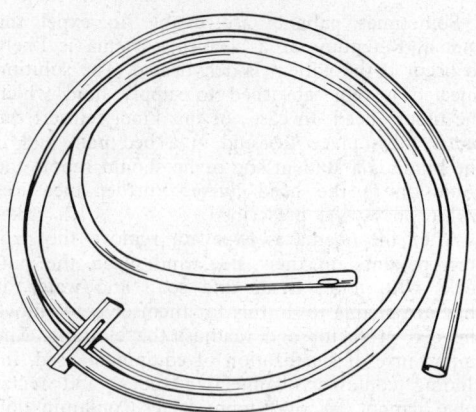

Figure 23-14. Harris flush tube for enema, rectal irrigation or flush. (Courtesy of Aloe Medical, St. Louis, Mo.)

could injure the rectum unless the operator is knowledgeable and skilled in the procedure.

Equipment. In any method the following equipment is necessary: a reservoir (an irrigating can, a large pail with a spigot at the base to which tubing may be attached, or a large glass cylinder, any of which must be calibrated so that the worker can determine the amount of solution injected into the patient), tubing for the solution, rectal tubes, and connecting tubes of suitable size. If the one-tube method is used, a #30 to #32 French with a closed end and velvet eye is generally satisfactory for an adult; if two tubes are employed, this size may be used for the outflow or drainage and a smaller size (#22 to #24 French) for the inflow. It is desirable to select tubes that are calibrated in centimeters or inches, with some indelible marking (silver nitrate may be used on rubber tubes). Clamps must be provided for both inflow and outflow tubes; a lubricant, such as a vegetable or petroleum jelly, is essential; a calibrated pail or jar for the return, which should be covered; an Asepto syringe that can be used to wash out the drainage tube if it clogs; pitchers or other containers for the total amount of solution to be used; a waterproof bed protector; an irrigating pole; and a suitable tray or treatment wagon for conveying this equipment to the patient. A bedpan should be available and toilet articles for cleaning and drying the patient after the treatment.

The *solution* used, its *temperature,* and the *amount* depend upon the purpose of the treatment, the condition of the patient, and the preference of the physician. Physiologic saline, tap water, and bicarbonate 1 to 2 per cent is usually used. The disadvantages of different solutions have been discussed on pages 1231–

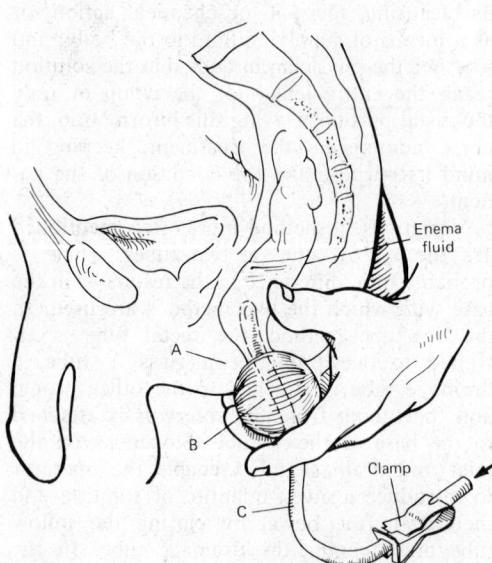

Figure 23-13. Mechanical method of retaining fluid in irrigation of lower part of intestine in patient with defective anus. *A.* Incompetent anus. *B.* Rubber ball pressed against the perineum acting as dam to assist in retaining fluid. *C.* Catheter threaded through ball. (From Jackson, Raymond J.: "Fecal Incontinence—Nonsurgical Treatment, *J.A.M.A.,* **166:**1284, [Mar. 15] 1958.)

1233 in this chapter; however, for *emphasis*, we repeat there is danger of water intoxication following extensive and prolonged use of tap water. If the nurse must make the choice, physiologic saline would be safe as this is the more normal habitat of body cells and it is reasonable to suppose that it could have little if any harmful effect. The recommended temperature is near that of the body.

Although the amount of solution used depends on the purpose of the treatment and the preference of the physician, most authors consulted warn against using large amounts of fluid over a long period and usually recommend 2000 to 3000 ml. As much as 4000 ml may be used for some patients.

When the treatment is ordered chiefly for its thermal effect, the solutions are usually those mentioned. The temperature of the solution will be prescribed by the physician. If for some reason the nurse must make the decision, temperatures above 43.3°C (110°F) should not be used. A cold irrigation is uncommon, because it is seldom desirable to reduce the temperature of the abdominal and pelvic viscera, except in sunstroke.

The type of solution used for medical purposes is prescribed by the physician. Silver nitrate 1:5000 to 1:1000, potassium permanganate 1:5000, tannic acid 1:100, thymal 1:500, and alum 1:100 are used for various conditions. In any infection, the object in selecting an antiseptic solution is to find a drug that is specifically destructive to the causative organism in such a strength as will not be injurious to the tissues.

Position and Preparation of the Patient. The room should be comfortably warm, and the bed table, floor, and furniture that might be injured by wetting suitably protected. Protection and privacy of the patient should be assured by draping, screening, and a sign on the door. Since the patient's cooperation is essential, the nurse should give an explanation suited to his or her intelligence, experience, and condition. The position of the patient is usually prescribed by the physician; the dorsal recumbent, the right and left lateral, the supine, and the knee-chest positions are variously advocated.

If the abdominal muscles are relaxed patients have less sensation of pressure as the intestine is distended; therefore, regardless of whether they are on the side or back, the knees should be flexed. They should be supported with pillows and made as comfortable as possible in whatever position they are placed. Their clothing should be folded up above the waist and they should be covered with one or more treatment blankets, according to the room temperature and their condition. A cellucotton pad with a nonabsorbent base placed directly under the anus absorbs any seepage there may be around the tube and keeps the bed dry.

An important point in preparing a patient for a colonic irrigation is determining whether the rectum is empty or filled with fecal matter. If fecal matter is present, it may be hardened from having remained in the rectum where absorption of water takes place. This hardened mass is difficult to break up or soften and drain from the rectum with the drainage tube; it is likely to clog the tubing and should therefore be evacuated before giving the irrigation. Some physicians advocate a cleansing enema before the irrigation, but if the patient has had a normal stool a few hours earlier or is having daily colonic irrigations, this should not be necessary. If an enema is given, the irrigation should not be started for 20 to 30 minutes after the enema has been expelled, because the enema will have stimulated the defecation impulse, and stimulation of this reflex interferes with successful irrigation. To reduce pressure within the abdominal and pelvic cavities, the bladder should be emptied before a colonic irrigation.

Suggested Procedure. Hang or support the reservoir so that the surface of the liquid is not more than 45 cm (18 inches) above the level of the anus; attach the large catheter (or small rectal tube) to the glass connecting tube; allow the solution to run to the tip of the tube to expel the air, and clamp off the tubing. Place the pail or jar for the return on a stool, chair, or stand, so that the top of the container is not more than 15 to 20 cm (6 to 8 inches) below the anus. To avoid splashing, see that the drainage tube reaches well into the container. Insert the tip of the smaller inflow tube into the eye of the larger drainage tube; lubricate the tubes and insert them together. When they are well in the rectum, about 5 to 7½ cm (2 to 3 inches), make traction on the smaller tube in order that the tip will be drawn out of the eye of the larger tube. Continue the insertion of the two tubes separately until the inflow tube is inserted 12½ to 15 cm (5 to 6 inches), and the outflow, or drainage tube 7½ to 10 cm (3 to 4 inches). If calibrated tubes are not available, mark with narrow strips of adhesive or on rubber tubing with a silver nitrate solution. As soon as the tubes are in place, start the inflow with the outflow tube closed. Allow the solution to run into the bowel at the rate of approximately 100 to 150 ml a minute under gentle pressure. When about 500 ml have been injected, open the drainage tube and adjust the height of the outflow column so that the bowel drains at the same rate of speed while the fluid is being injected; this keeps the bowel distended with approximately 500 ml of fluid until the end of the irrigation. Then clamp off the inflow tube and leave the drainage tube open and in the rectum as long as there is any return flow.

The outflow tube may be left in position for 10 minutes or more after the treatment, or the patient may be allowed to use the bedpan if he or she wishes.

In case the patient complains of abdominal pain during the treatment, clamp off the inflow and increase the rate of flow through the drainage tube by lowering the waste container, thereby lengthening the drop in the tubing. If the solution is given under sufficiently low pressure and not allowed to accumulate in or distend the colon too much, the patient should have no pain and very little sensation of any kind.

Should the drainage tube clog, pinch it or move it gently back and forth in the rectum to open it; if this is not effective, force some fluid through the tube with a bulb syringe or, if necessary, remove, clean, and reinsert. Note the nature of the return flow throughout the treatment and whether gas is expelled; this is indicated by bubbles seen through the plastic tubing or the glass connection in the drainage tube. As soon as the treatment is completed, clamp and remove the tubes gently and quickly; clean and dry the patient; remove the bed protection; readjust the clothing; and leave the patient in a comfortable position with the surroundings in order.

Recording the Treatment. Indicate the nature, amount, and temperature of the solution used; make a report of the fecal matter, the odor, and the presence of mucus, gas, and food particles if noted in the return. Describe briefly the patient's reaction to the treatment.

Modifications and Adaptions. A satisfactory irrigation may be given with the one-tube method, partially described under another heading.

One rectal tube is attached to a glass Y tube, to the other arm the drainage tube is attached, and the base of the Y to the tubing from the reservoir. The irrigation consists of a series of injections of approximately 500 ml each, with intervening periods of drainage through the outflow tube.

If a reservoir is not available, the colon may be lavaged just as the stomach is lavaged, with a tube and funnel. This method requires more care and skill in order to prevent the introduction of air and soiling the bedding and surroundings.

7. PROCTOCLYSIS, MURPHY DRIP, RECTAL INFUSION, OR RECTAL SEEPAGE

Definition. *Proctoclysis* comes from the Greek: *proktos,* meaning anus or rectum, and *klysis.* The treatment is sometimes called *Murphy drip,* after the noted surgeon who first used and described it. It is a form of rectal injection in which the solution is introduced drop by drop, with a device on the inflow tubing that provides for the escape of gas from the rectum. The treatment is designed to extend over a period of hours or days.

Therapeutic Uses. Rectal infusions are given in order (1) to supply fluid and sometimes food in the form of glucose during postoperative periods and acute stages of illness when the patient is unable to get sufficient water and nourishment by mouth, and intravenous and subcutaneous injections are not available or practicable; (2) to dilute toxins that may be in the intestines; (3) to administer selected medication; and (4) to provide an outlet for the escape of gas from the colon and rectum. Because chemicals, antibiotics, and intravenous therapy are now so effective in combatting most of the conditions for which proctoclysis was used, this procedure is now rarely seen in the United States.

As early as 1948, Guy W. Daugherty and associates [95] reported improvement in a patient with renal insufficiency which they attributed to continuous lavage of the colon. Even though peritoneal dialysis and hemodialysis are currently used in treating this condition, medical texts continue to mention intestinal lavage as a means of treatment.

Treatment of ulcerative colitis with local hydrocortisone administered intrarectally by a slow-drip method has been shown to be effective in several studies conducted and reported by S. C. Truelove [96-98] (in England). Using essentially the same method and medication, Geoffrey Watkinson [99] reports a similar study of patients with ulcerative colitis. In the first study (1956), Truelove used 250 mg of hydrocortisone dissolved in 50 ml of 50 per cent ethyl alcohol which was added to 500 ml of normal saline in an infusion bottle. The solution was allowed to drip into the rectum at a slow and steady rate. Patients learned to administer the treatment at home. In 1957, his second study, hydrocortisone hemisuccinate sodium (100 mg of hydrocortisone) dissolved in 120 ml of normal saline was administered by the same method—rectal infusion by slow-drip from an intravenous infusion bottle. He thinks any volume up to about 250 ml would be suitable.

Equipment. The following articles are needed: an irrigating pole and a reservoir with attached tubing to deliver the solution (the reservoir may be a calibrated irrigating can, glass cylinder, or infusion bottle); and a drip bulb, which enables the worker to regulate the flow in drops per minute, introduced into the tubing about 30 cm (12 inches) below the reservoir. A glass Y tube is attached by one prong to the delivery tube a few centimeters below the bulb. The base of the Y is attached to the tubing inserted into the rectum; the other prong is attached to a piece of tubing long enough to reach up into the reservoir; this latter piece of tubing provides a means of escape for gas from the intestinal tract. A catheter, #20 to #22 French, is used to deliver fluid to the rectum, since a small tube is less irritating. Tubing should be supplied with sufficient clamps to enable the nurse to regulate the flow and to detach and clean parts of the equipment.

The *solutions* used should be hypotonic to favor their passage from the intestines into the tissues. Those commonly used are water, sodium chloride 0.5 per cent or lower concentration, and glucose 2 to 5 per cent in water or in hypotonic sodium chloride. If the treatment is specific, as in ulcerative colitis, the physician will prescribe the dosage of the medication. The *amount* required depends upon the length of time over which the treatment is extended and the ability of the patient to absorb the fluid. Daugherty and associates used a solution containing sodium, potassium, magnesium, and calcium chloride with sodium bicarbonate, sodium acid phosphate (anhydrous), and glucose.

As it enters the rectum, the *temperature* of the solution should be near body temperature, or slightly higher, to promote absorption. If the treatment extends over a long period, a heating coil (see Chapter 22, page 1168) may be used to maintain the desired temperature. Rhoads and associates [100] (1970) say the solution should be given slowly, whereas Hamilton Bailey and associates [101] (1962) recommend no more than 60 drops per minute.

A lubricant, preferably a vegetable jelly, is necessary. Adhesive or Scotch tape is needed to strap the catheter to the buttock so that it will not be displaced when the patient moves. A perineal T binder and an especially designed tube that can be attached to the binder may be used for persons with very sensitive skin.

Waterproof protection for the bed should be provided. Since a rectal infusion is a protracted treatment, especial care should be taken to make the patient comfortable.

In order to keep accurate record of the amount of absorption, it is desirable to have paper and pencil at the bedside to chart the amount of solution added to the reservoir and the estimated absorption taking place.

The room and bed should be prepared and the treatment explained as described under colonic irrigation.

Since this treatment may be continued over a long period of time, no one position should be maintained; on the contrary, the nurse should encourage or help the patient to change position frequently and so arrange the tubing, heating devices, and reservoir that this is possible. Relaxation of the abdominal wall is desirable and encourages retention of the solution. The bladder should be emptied frequently in order to reduce abdominal pressure. At the beginning of the treatment, the bedding may be folded to the anal region and the top of the body covered with a bath blanket; the patient's clothing should be folded up above the waist to avoid soiling.

It is important before starting this treatment, as it is before irrigating the colon, to make sure that the rectum is empty. Fecal matter in the rectum interferes with the introduction of the solution and its absorption, and particles of fecal material may occlude the tube. The physician may order a cleansing enema or a colonic lavage as preparation for the proctoclysis. Since an enema stimulates the defecation reflex, the proctoclysis should not be given for 20 to 30 minutes after the enema is expelled.

Suggested Procedure. Hang or support the reservoir high enough to keep the drip bulb in an upright position well above the bed level. Attach the catheter to the glass connecting tube and allow the solution to flow through it until it warms the catheter and eliminates the air in the tubing. Lubricate and introduce the catheter 10 to 12½ cm (4 to 5 inches); when in position, attach it to the side of the buttock with adhesive or Scotch tape; care must be taken not to apply it over the pubic hair. It may be necessary to shave the area. As soon as the apparatus is adjusted and the patient comfortable, start the solution flowing at the rate prescribed by the physician; this may vary from 10 to 60 drops per minute, according to the patient's ability to absorb it. No matter what rate the physician specifies, however, he or she will expect the nurse to regulate the flow to prevent dilating the rectum and filling the tubing as far as the drip bulb. The nurse should note and report the rate at which the patient appears to be absorbing the solution. If all factors are favorable for absorption—that is, an empty rectum, a comfortable position, unoccluded tubing, a slow rate of injection, a nonirritating and hypotonic solution, and the temperature of the solution around that of the body—and yet there is little if any absorption taking place, the nurse should report the condition to the physician, who will probably stop the treatment. This treatment requires a good deal of skill, and a nurse can justifiably feel a fair measure of satisfaction if she or he is able to administer as much as 1000 to 2000 ml in 24 hours by this method. If the drainage tube gets clogged, move it back and forth in the rectum; or pinching the tube may dislodge a particle of fecal material in the eye of the catheter. If the tube is still occluded, force solution through the catheter with a bulb syringe or remove and clean the tubing.

Recording the Treatment. Throughout the treatment, note the amount of solution absorbed, the gas bubbling through the outlet tube, soiling of the solution by fecal matter, and the patient's reaction to the treatment. Make written reports at regular and frequent intervals so that the physician may be able to judge whether the treatment is effective or whether other means must be adopted to accomplish its purpose.

8. HARRIS DRIP, OR PROCTOCLYSIS BY A TIDAL-STAND METHOD

Definition. This treatment is a modification of the Murphy drip, and is likewise named after the physician who designed it. The distinctive feature of this method of proctoclysis is that the reservoir for the solution is hung about the level of the rectum, so that there tends to be a flow of solution into the rectum from the reservoir and a return of the solution, with an expulsion of gas and fecal material from the rectum into the reservoir, according to changes in pressure within this area; such movement of the solution and the contents of the rectum is encouraged by periodically raising and lowering the reservoir.[102]

Therapeutic Uses. The purposes of the Harris drip are the same as those listed under the Murphy drip. This treatment is rarely used; it was not mentioned by any of the recent sources consulted. The interested reader can find it described in the Fifth Edition of this book.

9. RECTAL FEEDING, OR NUTRITIVE ENEMAS

Definition. A nutritive enema is the injection into the rectum of a liquid food selected on the basis of the supposed ability of the colon to absorb it. Since opinions differ on absorption in the colon, practice will differ in the use of nutritive enemas. It is conceded that liquid foods must be used that are broken down to such a simple state as to be ready for absorption.

Therapeutic Uses. Nutritive enemas are resorted to as a means of feeding the patient if oral feeding is contraindicated (for example, following operations on the mouth or upper alimentary tract) and in case nutritive infusions are unavailable; also when some condition, such as hemophilia, makes injection of a vein an undesirable proceeding. Nutritive enemas are now seldom used; Bockus says the old-fashioned nutritive enema has no useful purpose.

Equipment. Articles used in giving an enema that is to be retained differ in the following respects from those required for giving a cleansing enema: A catheter is substituted for a rectal tube in order to reduce to a minimum the irritation likely to stimulate defecation; a funnel and pitcher may be used instead of an irrigating can, because the amount of solution given is so small that a proportionately large amount is lost adhering to the sides of the can and tubing, and it is cooled in passing through the can and tubing. A bedpan should be within reach, but since the object of the treatment is defeated if the patient expels the solution, it should not be within sight of the patient because it suggests defecation.

The food most commonly used is a glucose solution; whisky and brandy and predigested proteins were prescribed in the past. It has been noted that some physicians recommended that the intestinal contents recovered by intubation be reintroduced by rectum to maintain the electrolyte balance.

Although no fixed rule can be given for the *amount* of solution to be administered, 500 ml (1 pt) is probably the maximum prescribed for an adult and 240 ml (8 oz) is about the average amount given; proportionately smaller amounts are prescribed for infants and children. The *temperature* of the solution as it reaches the rectum should be near that of the body to avoid stimulating its contraction. The solution should be prepared at approximately 42°C (107.6°F) to allow for cooling while the patient is prepared, and for the drop in temperature as the solution passes through the funnel, or the reservoir and tubing.

Preparation of the Patient. The directions for preparing a patient for the administration of proctoclysis may be followed here. His or her cooperation is even more essential, and every effort should be made to gain it. Protection of the bedding is of course important. The position advocated is usually the left lateral, but the right lateral or dorsal-recumbent position, with the knees flexed, may be substituted. To reduce pressure within the abdominal cavity, the bladder and rectum should be empty. When rectal feedings are prescribed, the physician ordinarily directs that a cleansing enema be given once or twice daily and the feedings four or five times during the 24-hour period. To quiet the patient the physician may prescribe a sedative, sometimes an opium suppository, to be inserted before the feeding; or he or she may direct that a sedative be added to the enema. If the patient has hemorrhoids, or for other reasons the anal canal or rectum is very sensitive, it may be necessary to apply a local anesthetic.

Suggested Procedure. A nutritive enema is given in the same general manner as any other rectal injection to be retained. The following encourage retention and absorption: A small tube, well lubricated, inserted gently and slowly and removed gently but quickly, the height of the insertion probably not exceeding 12½ cm (5 inches); regulation of the temperature so that it is not much above or below that of the rectum, administration of the solution or mixture under low pressure, which means that the surface of the column of the liquid should not be more than 20 cm (8 inches) above the anus; and manual pressure over the rectum with a cellucotton compress, or other suitable material, after the catheter is removed. If possible the patient should refrain from using the bedpan for several hours after the treatment; otherwise the whole, or a portion, of the feeding may be expelled. Patients should be kept comfortable and quiet following the treatment, the bed protection left undisturbed to avoid moving them and to prevent soiling the bed in case the enema is expelled or there is seepage from the anus. In some cases, when patients find it difficult to retain the fluid, it is helpful to clamp the catheter but leave it inserted in the rectum for 15 to 20 minutes after the completion of the treatment.

10. MEDICATED RETENTION ENEMAS

Definition. A medicated enema is the rectal injection of a fluid drug. The drugs prescribed vary with the purposes for which the treatment is given.

Therapeutic Uses. When given for their systemic effect, or effect after absorption, the medicated enemas used are: (1) sedatives, such as paraldehyde; (2) analgesics and anesthetics, as, for example, tribromoethanol (Avertin) and ether; and (3) stimulants, such as coffee (now seldom used). Medicated enemas that are prescribed for local effects are: (1) oils to soften fecal matter and aid in its expulsion; (2) salts to draw fluid from the tissues in edema, or to stimulate peristalsis; (3) anthelmintics to kill or paralyze pinworms; (4) emollients to relieve irritation of the rectum; (5) astringents to check bleeding; and (6) corticosteroids for ulcerative colitis. For example, Matts [103] (1961) reports intrarectal treatment of 100 ulcerative colitis patients with Prednisolone-21-Phosphate enemas. A commercially prepared bag containing 20 mg of prednisolone is given to the patient who administers the solution slowly into the rectum after going to bed at night. He or she is encouraged to go to sleep as quickly as possible after the injection. F. Avery Jones and associates [104] describe the procedure they teach their patients.

Equipment and Suggested Procedure. All enemas to be retained are given in the same manner, and therefore the equipment needed for the administration of a medicated enema is the same as that for a nutritive enema. The same factors aid in retention and absorption. The physician prescribes the amount and kind of solution. When irritating drugs are given, such as anthelmintics, they are sometimes siphoned off after a stated period or removed by a cleansing enema. Sedatives and analgesics also are removed in some cases as soon as the desired sedation or analgesia is reached. Such drugs as tribromoethanol, the purpose of which is to produce a partial anesthesia, usually preceding the administration of an inhalation anesthetic, are given by an anesthetist. (Formulas for enemas are given in the Appendix. Most hospitals have nursing manuals that specify the particular mixtures and quantities used in their institutions.)

11. RECTAL SUPPOSITORIES

Definition. Rectal suppositories are concentrated food, soap, glycerin, and plain or medicated cocoa butter, prepared in the shape of a cone. They retain this shape at ordinary room temperatures, but when introduced into the rectum are dissolved by body heat. Drugs contained in them are then set free.

Therapeutic Uses.
1. Soap and glycerin suppositories are used to stimulate defecation. They are particularly valuable when the feces are in the lower bowel or rectum, but are not expelled because the anal sphincter will not relax. The presence of the suppository acts as an irritant that stimulates the rectum to expel its contents. Glycerin suppositories for adult use are naturally larger than those for infants and young children. Soap suppositories may be purchased, but may easily be made by taking a splinter of white soap and holding it in hot water until smooth and rounded to the required length and shape. It should be cone-shaped and from 2.5 to 7.5 cm (1 to 3 inches) long. Soap is very irritating to the mucous membrane and should not be used very often or without a doctor's prescription. Carbon dioxide-forming rectal suppositories are thought to be more effective, and have less adverse effects on the intestinal mucosa than those mentioned above.[105] They are also used with children.[106] For best results these suppositories are lubricated with water (*petroleum jelly is not used because it decreases the formation of carbon dioxide*).
2. Astringent suppositories of tannic acid, belladonna, and glycerin are prescribed in dysentery and diarrhea to contract the tissues, check bleeding, relieve pain, and dry up the secretions. Bismuth suppositories are

also used; these form a coating on the rectal mucosa and protect it from irritation.

3. Ice suppositories are sometimes used to check local bleeding or to relieve local inflammation. An ice suppository may be made in the same way as the soap suppository. It must be smooth and of a suitable shape and size.

4. Anodyne or local sedative suppositories are prescribed for hemorrhoids, dysentery, diarrhea, rectal abscesses, or postoperative conditions in which it is necessary to keep the rectum at rest. Drugs commonly used are cocaine, opium, and belladonna added to cocoa butter. Cocaine relieves pain and, by contracting the blood vessels, checks bleeding if it occurs. Opium and belladonna relieve pain, check peristalsis, and dry up secretions.

5. Suppositories containing opium or barbital (Veronal) are used for a general sedative effect if for any reason it is inadvisable to give medication by mouth.

6. Specific suppositories. In treating malaria, large doses of specifics may cause gastric disturbances. To prevent this, quinine has been given in the form of a suppository.

Suggested Procedure. Before inserting the suppository, it must be lubricated. Petroleum jelly is usually used; however, *only water* is used for lubricating the carbon dioxide-producing suppository. Wearing a glove, insert the suppository as far as the finger will reach and then apply pressure over the anus for a short time, until all desire to expel the suppository has passed.

Suppositories should always be kept in a cool place to prevent melting. It is necessary to keep glycerin suppositories under refrigeration.

12. IRRIGATION OF A COLOSTOMY

Nature of a Colostomy. Colostomy is performed for the purpose of making an artificial anus in the anterior abdominal wall, the location of the opening being determined by the pathology in the colon. This operation is usually necessary when there is an obstruction of the large intestine (colon, sigmoid, or rectum) that prevents the passage of fecal contents or a known lesion (as, for example, cancer) that will eventually cause an obstruction. Other reasons for a colostomy include the following: to divert the fecal contents so that healing of injuries and resolution of inflammatory process, such as diverticulosis and ulcerative colitis, may occur; to promote repair of a traumatic wound of the colon; and as the first step in resecting a part of the colon.[107]

The most common types of colostomies are transverse, descending, and sigmoid, indicating the location of the opening (stoma) along the colon. Transverse colostomies may be located on the right or left side or at the midline; most are temporary but they can be permanent. A transverse colostomy, by eliminating function of all bowel distal to it and by diverting the fecal stream, is performed to relieve or prevent an obstruction and to permit healing of a portion of the bowel. Two types of surgical procedures may be performed: (1) A *double-barreled colostomy* is one in which the transverse colon is divided and the ends are brought out at the margin of the skin; the proximal opening (right margin) is the outlet for the feces and the distal opening, or stoma, leads to the nonfunctioning bowel. (2) A *loop colostomy* may be described as a portion (or loop) of the colon that is brought through the abdominal wall and a bridge or rod placed under it. The surgeon usually opens the loop with an electric cautery one to four days after surgery. This procedure, which is painless, may be performed at the patient's bedside. Usually the right side of the opening leads to the functioning colon and the left side to the nonfunctioning colon. Descending and sigmoid colostomies are always permanent and they are located on the left side. They are usually performed in conjunction with an abdominal perineal resection for cancer of the rectum. After resecting the diseased portion of the colon, the end of the functioning colon is pulled through the abdominal wall, forming a single stoma.[107a]

The terms "wet" and "dry" colostomy are used to distinguish between the sites of the opening; that is, "dry" refers to an opening of the left side of the colon where the fecal content is usually soft or formed and "wet" refers to an opening of the right side where the fecal content is liquid.[108] In addition, the term "wet" colostomy is used following ileal diversion of the urine.[108a]

Preparation of the Patient for a Colostomy. Many persons having symptoms that suggest a growth in the intestine postpone a medical examination because they fear an operation and the possibility of a colostomy. When patients enter the hospital they are frightened about the surgery, they are afraid that the disease has progressed to such an extent that it may be inoperable, or that it may recur. They are concerned and anxious about change in the appearance of their body, being rejected by family members and others, and having unbearable pain if a colostomy is performed.[109,109a] The emotional shock of having to change a function so fundamental as defecation should not be underestimated. The person who accepts this cheerfully is usually a good actor.

It is the surgeon's responsibility to explain

the procedure to patients and help them accept the operation that may be essential for life; the nurse also plays an important role in this process. The patient will need understanding and emotional support to face and accept the many adjustments that a colostomy necessitates. If nurses are nonjudgmental and accept the patient's behavior, their attitude will encourage patients to talk about their feelings and fears and to ask questions; if, however, nurses are uncomfortable about cancer they could discourage all attempts on the patients' part to discuss their feelings.[110] It is important to answer all questions and correct misconceptions about the procedure before surgery.

If it is possible during the preoperative period for the patient to talk with someone who has a colostomy and has learned to manage elimination and overcome fears, such a conversation will be reassuring and informative.[111,111a] Preoperative instruction about the colostomy and how it will affect the patient is important. The nature of the colostomy and how it alters the anatomy of the large intestines and normal bowel function should be explained. Many patients are concerned about odors and spillage of feces; consequently, they should be reassured that odors can be controlled by using deodorants and omitting certain foods from the diet and that at first a plastic bag will be worn to collect liquid feces but they will be able to control elimination by irrigation and eventually only wear a small dressing, in most instances. All equipment and supplies used in irrigations and stomal care should be shown to the patient and his or her spouse. In addition they should know that they will be able to engage in all their usual activities with the exception of body contact sports (football, for example) and that sexual life is usually not affected. Above all, they should know that the colostomy need not alter their life but its care will become a routine part of daily activity.[112-112e] Goligher of England writes that the patient should be told:

. . . there are countless people in all walks of life who are enjoying splendid health and leading full normal lives despite the fact that they have such an opening. . . . many of the patients have been able to return to their previous occupations and activities even though these may have involved manual work. Similarly they have not been debarred from recreation and social life; those who desire it have been able to take part in meetings, dancing, golf, cricket, tennis and even swimming, in accordance of course with their age and general condition.*

In an emergency, when such psychologic preparation and instruction is not possible, the physician and nurse must give the patient such assistance in the postoperative period.

Because colostomy is often performed on patients having cancer, who are generally anemic, malnourished, and in poor physical condition, the preoperative treatment is especially important. Following a study of 880 colostomy patients, Earl F. Wolfman, Jr., and C. Thomas Flotte [113] recommend the following (physical) preoperative preparation: (1) a high carbohydrate, high protein (low residue) diet to restore the nutritional status to the best possible level before surgery; (2) vitamins, including ascorbic acid, as essential dietary supplements; (3) blood transfusions if necessary so that the circulating blood volume is normal; (4) vitamin K supplements; (5) electrolyte and fluids if there is an imbalance; and (6) "making the intestines as germ free as possible." If the patient is unable to take food and fluid by mouth, he or she may be given feedings by nasogastric tube and by intravenous infusion. To inhibit the colon flora and decrease the risk of infection, purgatives, enemas, and antibacterial (chemical) therapy are given.

A nasogastric tube (and in some cases a Miller-Abbott or Cantor tube) is usually inserted before surgery to minimize distention in the postoperative period and to facilitate surgery. A retention catheter is inserted in the bladder if the rectum is resected and sometimes when it is not.

Postoperative Care. If the rectum is not resected, the postoperative care of these patients does not differ from any other type of abdominal surgery except in the care of the colostomy itself. At operation a single loop of bowel is brought out on the abdomen.* The dressings protecting the operative site are not changed until after the colostomy has been opened (one to four days after surgery) by the surgeon. If the obstruction was complete, the surgeon will probably open the loop of bowel and insert a catheter to drain off fecal material.[114] This type of drainage helps to decompress the bowel. Most surgeons, however, leave the nasogastric or intestinal tube in place until peristalsis returns, making the insertion of a catheter into the colon unnecessary.

A perineal resection (removal of the sig-

---

* Goligher, J. C.: *Surgery of the Anus, Rectum and Colon,* 2nd ed. Bailliere, Tindall & Cassell, London, 1967, p. 729.

* When a colostomy is performed prior to a second operation, the surgeon constructs a double-barrel loop on the abdominal wall. The nurse must know that the upper, or proximal, loop is the one irrigated. The lower, or distal, loop is irrigated only when directed by the physician as a preliminary measure to the next surgical step.

moid and rectum) is performed when the tumor is in the low sigmoid or rectum. The colon is brought out through the abdominal wall—this is called a terminal (or permanent) colostomy. To prevent wound contamination, the surgeon applies a clamp or tie to the exposed colon (called the stoma). On the second or third day, the clamp or tie is removed and a disposable plastic collecting bag is applied over the stoma (see Figs. 23-15 and 23-16).

If a catheter was inserted in the bowel, it is connected to a drainage bottle when the patient returns to the nursing unit. The tube leading from the catheter to the bottle is fastened to the mattress with a safety pin to prevent undue pull on the catheter; kinking of the tube is thus avoided. The nurse notes whether there is drainage and the appearance of it; if the catheter seems to be clogged, preventing drainage, distention will result. To test its patency, the catheter may be irrigated with normal saline but the physician should leave directions for this procedure.

An accurate record of urinary output, fluid intake, and drainage (from wounds, nasogastric or intestinal tube, or catheter if it is inserted) is important in the postoperative period since these data are essential to the surgeon when he or she evaluates the fluid and electrolyte needs of patients. Fluids and electrolytes are given intravenously as indicated. Blood transfusions may be given also. Oral feedings are withheld

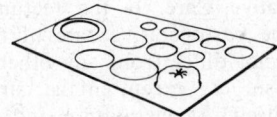

1. Measure stoma and cut hole in drain 1/8″ larger than stoma.
2. Wash skin and stoma with soap, rinse thoroughly, and pat dry.

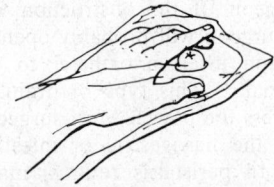

3. Peel backing from stoma drain. Place hand inside the drain and position hole over stoma. Press around stoma to form a seal. Close drain at end with rubber band. Empty as needed.
4. Rinse inside of drain daily. Under normal conditions, do not remove drain for 3 to 5 days.

Figure 23-15. Steps in applying a temporary colostomy drainage bag. A stoma measuring guide is packaged with the drain and may be used to help determine the proper size hole to be cut in drain.

until peristalsis has been established and then clear liquids are prescribed. A full liquid diet is given if there is no nausea. As soon as possible patients are given a regular or low residue diet, depending on their condition.

When the colostomy is opened, an evacuation of loose stool is likely to occur. The bed should be protected with a plastic sheet covered with a towel and an emesis basin positioned against the side of the patient to catch any fecal matter. The dressings are changed frequently to prevent disagreeable odors, excoriation of the skin, and discomfort. Because this is not a sterile procedure, the skin may be cleaned gently with soap and warm water and cotton balls or gauze squares. A light coat of talcum may be desirable.

Odors may be controlled by placing aspirin tablets *or* deodorants in the appliance, and by using "odor-proof" plastic bags, which can be discarded after a single use.[115] Derifil, a chlorophyll derivative, is highly effective when two tablets (100 mg tablet) are placed in the colostomy opening two or three times daily.[116] Bacon [117] also suggests a thorough cleaning of the upper bowel with warm potassium permanganate solution (1:10,000). He suggests giving by mouth Methylene blue (1 gr) and Kerol (3 minims), in capsule form, before breakfast, and "freshly heated charcoal" (15 to 30 gr) thrice daily to absorb gases.

Most authorities recommend cleaning the skin by washing with warm soapy water, rinsing, and patting dry. When the skin becomes irritated, as happens with diarrhea and the "wet" (right side) colostomy, creams (Desitin, for example), boiled Gelusil paste, and karaya gum paste or powder may be helpful.[118] Tenacious ointments should not be used as their removal is irritating to the skin.[119] Karaya gum powder and the karaya gum ring, which may be applied directly over an irritated skin, are probably the best products available in the care of the irritated skin.[120] For example, Robert J. McNamara and Eugene M. Farber,[121] who studied 1048 ileostomy patients in Great Britain and the United States, found that 82 per cent in Great Britain and 76 per cent in the United States who had skin problems of varying degrees reported karaya gum powder was effective in relieving skin irritation in the circumileostomy area and beneath the appliance. If a plastic collecting bag is applied over the stoma until bowel movements are regulated and if evacuations occur during irrigation thereafter, the surrounding skin should never get excoriated. When it does, however, ointments should be tried out until one is found that relieves the condition. During a bout of diarrhea, or with high colostomies or

1. Begin by sealing bottom of drainable bag with the clamp provided.

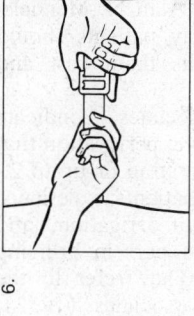

2. Thoroughly clean and dry the skin surrounding the stoma.

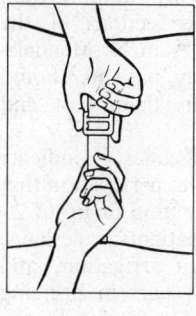

3. Peel the protective covering from the seal ring. (If using drainable bag with adhesive square, also peel paper backing from adhesive.) Seal must fit snugly around the stoma for adequate skin protection; you can adjust its shape to some degree by molding it with your fingers. Depressions in the skin or areas left exposed around an irregularly shaped stoma should be protected with a layer of colostomy paste.

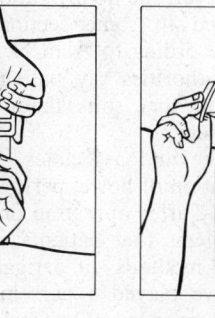

4. Fasten one end of belt to gasket of drainable bag and rotate belt into position. (Buttons on belt should point away from body.)

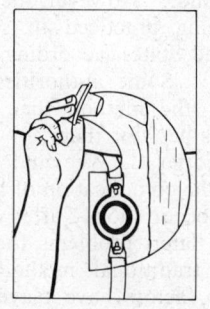

5. Holding gasket away from stoma, wrap belt around waist with soft side in contact with skin. Fasten loose end of belt to gasket and position Seal around stoma.

If using drainable bag with adhesive square, press adhesive coating firmly to the skin. Keep adhesive flat and free of puckering.

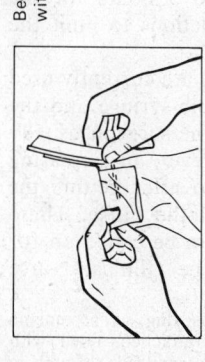

6. Adjust belt for proper fit by moving the plastic slide adjuster. Belt should be tighter when lying down than when standing. You may wish two belts, so you can keep one adjusted for each use.

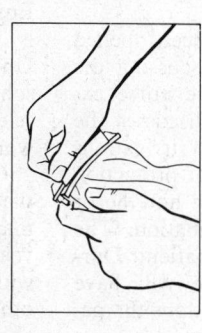

7. To empty, position bag over toilet or other receptacle. Lift bottom of bag so contents are shifted away from sealed opening.

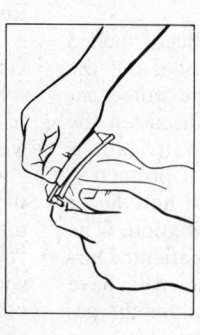

8. Remove clamp by holding bottom of bag upward with right hand, while left hand holds the bag near the clamp. Release latch with finger of left hand; hold clamp and pull bottom of bag gently, thereby opening clamp.

9. Allow bag to unfold downward and empty into receptacle. When empty, cleanse with clear water and tissue and reseal as shown in 1 and 2 above. The bag may be used several times before replacement.

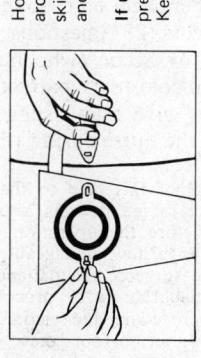

Figure 23-16. Applying and emptying a more permanent colostomy drainage. Correct size is important. The stoma should be carefully measured with the appropriate guide.

ileostomies, a plastic collecting bag should be cemented to a karaya gum ring or to the skin around the stoma *before* the skin is irritated. The digestive enzymes in the bowel contents are irritating to the skin, and it should be protected from them.

If a collecting bag is not applied when the colostomy is opened, soft absorbent dressings are used and held in place with Montgomery straps, and an abdominal binder if indicated. The dressing should be abundant and loosely applied to soak up any discharge through the stoma. This is likely to run out from under a tight or compact dressing. A waterproof cover may be applied over the dressing and arranged in such a way as to prevent soiling of the clothing and linen.

As soon as the colostomy has been opened and the patient is receptive to discussing the management of the colostomy, the nurse explains the special skin care and discusses the type of dressings, appliances, and irrigations used in the hospital and the type of protection the patient will apply at home, and how he or she will be able to control elimination. The nurse also discusses diet with the patient. During such conversations the nurse will have many opportunities to answer questions the patient will ask; the following list illustrates some of the usual queries; *

How will a colostomy change my way of living and working, and other everyday activities, such as a tub bath?
Can regularity of elimination really be established and what about odor?
What equipment will I need for self-care and where can it be bought?
What kinds of food should I eat and will my diet have to be different from that served my family?
How can I explain to the younger members of my family what a colostomy is?

Lester Breidenbach and Sophie M. Secor [122] (1956) discuss 25 questions (or problems) experienced by Secor (who has a colostomy) and over 200 colostomy patients whom she has helped. They give many suggestions that can be useful to the nurse caring for these patients.

---

* The timing of this help to the patient is an individual matter. Some persons know they will have a colostomy before the operation and it may comfort them to learn how manageable this condition is. The nurse, the surgeon, the patient—and the family, of course—collaborate in the process. A colostomy is a multilating procedure and victims must be allowed a period of grief before they can accept their fate and adjust to it. A patient who does not admit to fear or grief is almost certainly putting on an act. (Conversations with Virginia Dericks, a nurse who specializes in the care of colostomy patients.)

By study and by observing experienced workers nurses should prepare themselves to help patients with the solution of these and other problems.

When surgeons open the colostomy, they will usually do the first irrigation and then they tell the nurse which loop is to be irrigated, indicating whether there are any restrictions on the amount of irrigating solutions and whether there are any unusual deviations in the intestinal passage.

Colostomy Irrigation. In the United States, irrigations (daily or every 2 or 3 days) and diet have been used to regulate bowel movements, whereas the nonirrigation method (diet and medications) is used by most surgeons in England.[123] However, the nonirrigation method is being practiced in some sections of the United States, according to Alan N. Mendelssohn.[124] Some authorities say patients should select the method that suits them best and works best for them.

George C. Wee and associates [125] indicate that the complication of bowel perforation that may occur shortly after operation or up to 22 years later, problems that patients experience with traditional methods of irrigation, and other factors have played a part in bringing about change in practice. They refer to the work of Sutherland and associates (1952), who studied 57 patients using the Binkley * type of irrigation. The amount of water used ranged from 2 quarts to 10 gallons with half of the patients using the latter and the time required to perform the irrigation ranged from 45 minutes to 8 hours, with 16 taking more than 3½ hours. Complaints included inadequate return of fluid and evacuation of feces and spillage. Alice R. Sill [126] (1970) recommends the use of the bulb-syringe (8 oz) technique for colonic stoma irrigation because this cuts down on the fluid used. She says some of her patients were using as much as 3 or 4 quarts and spending 1½ to 3 hours for the procedure in spite of instructions to limit the fluid to 1½ pints of water.

Two methods of irrigation are currently used in the United States: the bulb-syringe and the traditional (enema) type. The surgeon usually decides on the method; however, an increasing number of physicians do so after getting the opinions of the patient and the nurse. There are resource persons who can be called on for specialized services: (1) The Clinical Nurse

---

* A system of irrigation consisting of an enema can (or bag), with a catheter attached, filled with tepid water. The catheter is introduced through a dome applied over the stoma and water enters the colon and returns through an attached sheath. The treatment is repeated every other day or every 3 days.

Specialist (called nurse clinician in some parts of the United States) with graduate preparation in clinical nursing and teaching can effect change throughout an institution or community on behalf of patients with a common problem. (2) The Enterostomal Therapist may be a lay person or nurse trained in short courses to help fill the shortage of professional personnel knowledgeable in Ostomy care. (3) Many representatives (but not all) of manufacturers or distributors of Ostomy supplies are well-informed in Ostomy care and the use of the company's products. Those who have had special training can be of great help in the selection of equipment and in its use. (4) The Ostomy Visitor, a lay person who is mature and well-adjusted to the colostomy, can be a great source for moral support and practical solutions to problems with a stoma.[126a] Hospitals have one or more of these persons to whom patients may be referred for help, which includes demonstrations by the worker and guidance of the patient as he or she carries out the procedures of skin care, irrigation if used, and cleaning the equipment.

When the colostomy is irrigated, the procedure is carried out by the nurse. (The surgeon may irrigate during a dressing to establish the patency of the opening.) The nurse begins at once to explain the steps of the procedure to patients and encourages them to participate. As soon as patients are ambulatory, the nurse helps them carry out the procedure. This hastens patient rehabilitation. A patient who chooses to remain anonymous wrote an excellent article titled "No One Knows I Have a Colostomy," * describing her inadequate preparation for self-care, her later search for understanding, and her very effective rehabilitation. She urges nurses to see that all patients are prepared before they leave the hospital to select the necessary equipment, irrigate the colostomy, and regulate bowel activity. Secor [127] says the nurse should arrange to have a member of the patient's family observe and learn the irrigating procedure so that they will know the problems of the patient and can give assistance when needed.

If the enema type irrigation is used, a 2-qt can or bag, tubing, glass connector, catheter (size #16 to #24 French are recommended by various authors, including patients), and a disposable irrigator drain or plastic sheath will be needed. To prevent backflow of enema fluid, Norman D. Nigro [128] says he uses a 1-oz rubber ear syringe with a #26 French rubber catheter inserted through a hole in its base with the tip cut off. The bulb-syringe serves as

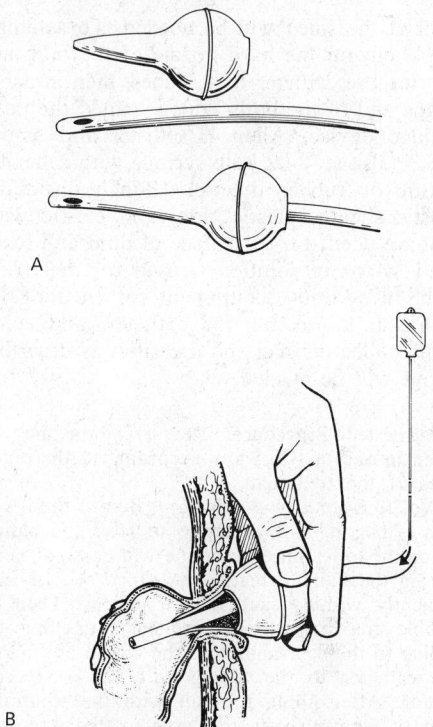

Figure 23-17. The bulb syringe method of colostomy irrigation. *A.* One-ounce ear syringe and 26 F catheter assembled. Catheter passes through syringe, which serves only as a guard. *B.* Tapered rubber syringe prevents backflow and injury is avoided because of minimal introduction of catheter. (From Nigro, Norman D.: "A Special Catheter for Colostomy Irrigation," *Dis. Colon Rectum,* **12**:61, [Jan.] 1969.)

a guard (see Fig. 23-17). Plastic reusable irrigators with a sliding stoma seal are available.* A nozzle (called the Laird tip or cone) is also available. Such devices help in preventing a perforation of the colon, *not* a rare occurrence.[128a] About 500 to 1000 ml irrigating solution (tap water or normal saline) is needed. The temperature of the fluid should be between 37.8° to 40.6° (100° to 105°F); *hot water should never be used.* A lubricant (petroleum jelly) is needed for the catheter, soft toilet tissue or cotton to clean around the opening before and after the irrigation, and a paper bag for soiled dressings. Clean dressings (soft and absorbent) are needed to apply after the irrigation or a clean plastic collecting bag for the patient who is wearing one.

For the bulb-syringe method, an 8-oz soft rubber bulb-syringe and a #24 French rubber or plastic catheter with the opening at the end (not at the side) will be needed. To assemble these, cut off the hard nozzle of the bulb and shorten the catheter to 4 inches, then attach it to the end of the bulb—this is called the bulb-syringe device. Allen H. Postel and associates [129] use an 8-oz bulb-syringe with a flexible plastic or rubber tip. An 18-inch disposable plastic sheath, plastic ring, and elastic waist belt are needed for drainage of fluid and feces. Only 24 oz of solution is used for the irrigation. In addition, equipment for cleaning the skin and lubricating the catheter, and colostomy collecting bag and dressings as described above will be needed.

Suggested Procedure. The irrigation may be given in one of two ways, according to the objectives of the treatment.

No. 1. Enema type irrigation. Before the irrigation is begun, it is desirable to have the patient sit on the toilet since he or she will do so at home during the daily irrigation. Arrange articles conveniently within reach of the patient. Then assemble the irrigation equipment, attaching the tubing to the can, and close the clamp and attach the catheter to the tubing with the glass connector. After filling the can with the solution,* hang it from an irrigating pole so that it is 4 to 4½ inches below shoulder level. At this level, the pressure of the water is kept low and only the left colon will be filled, taking about 20 minutes for the fluid to run in. (The method of holding the can 18 to 24 inches above the colostomy causes a rapid filling of the colon, loss of fluid in the transverse colon, return of the fluid in spurts from 12 to 20 hours after irrigation, and eventual delay in rehabilitation of the patient. All articles written by patients that were reviewed recommend that the can be held 4 to 4½ inches below the level of the shoulder.)

After removing the dressing or the collecting bag, clean the skin with toilet tissue, or soap and water should a more thorough cleaning be indicated. Insert the drainage sheath through the plastic ring and place over the stoma and then hook the belt clips onto the ring. Lubricate the catheter tip, allow a small amount of solution to run through the tubing to remove air. Then insert the catheter through the irrigation drain and, gently, into the colostomy opening about 7½ to 15 cm (3 to 6 inches) with full flow of water through the catheter. Allow 500 to 750 ml (½ to ¾ qt) to enter the colon; if cramps result, pinch the tube and lower the irrigating can so that the force of the flow is not so great. Tighten the clamp so that solution will return through the outlet sheath into the toilet.

The amount of solution to be used varies with each patient; however, sufficient solution must be used to prevent drainage between irrigations. If the can should be refilled, do this while waiting for the return flow of the instilled solution. The bowel may be sluggish after surgery and require a greater quantity of fluid to induce an evacuation than is later needed. The nurse and patient should experiment to determine the patient's particular needs.

After the irrigation has been completed, detach and discard the sheath, and place the collection bag over the stoma. At this point the patient should be encouraged to massage the abdomen, lean forward and from side to side, and even stand up once or twice. Activity hastens bowel movement. Let the collection bag remain in place until the patient thinks all drainage has ceased. (The nurse may suggest that the patient read a magazine or newspaper while he or she is waiting.) When reasonably sure drainage has ceased, clean the skin around the colostomy opening and dry it thoroughly. Apply a clean dressing or appliance if patient has not gained control of fecal elimination.

Clean the equipment immediately. Rinse first in cold water, then wash with soap and warm water. Store equipment when dry in a convenient place for daily use. Immediate cleaning is the best preventive against odor.

No. 2. Bulb-syringe type irrigation. Have the patient sit on the toilet, remove the colostomy dressing and clean the stoma and surrounding skin with toilet tissue and soap and water, if indicated.

After attaching the disposable sheath on the plastic ring, place the ring with the sheath over the stoma and secure with clips to the belt around the waist. Cut a small hole in the sheath above and to one side of the stoma, tuck it between the legs leading directly into the toilet bowl (see Fig. 23-18).

Fill the bulb-syringe, being sure that all air is expelled by holding the nozzle upright, compressing the bulb gently; then, place the nozzle under the water for complete filling. Lubricate the catheter tip and insert through the slit in the sheath for about 3 to 5 inches. Apply continuous and steady pressure to the bulb. When withdrawing the bulb from the stoma, it is important to maintain pressure on it so that feces is not aspirated into the nozzle.

The amount of fluid used will vary with the individual patient. Most authorities say 2 bulbsful (16 oz) is sufficient and no more than 3 (24 oz) should be used; if more fluid is used, there is likely to be retention of water in the colon which may result in spillage and accidents later in the day.

Remove the drainage sheath and discard it in a paper bag when the irrigation is completed. Clean the stoma with toilet tissue, cotton balls, or gauze and attach a temporary disposable bag to the belt to collect feces and drainage that has not been evacuated. The bag is usually left in place about 15 to 30 minutes as the patient carries out other hygienic measures (bathing, for example). After discarding the bag and thoroughly cleaning the skin with soap and water, apply a small dressing (usually two 4-inch square gauze) over the stoma. Hold the dressing in place by tape, a girdle, or a wide elasticized waist band. If the patient has not gained control of fecal elimination, apply an appliance.

---

* In the home the patient may use plain tap water or water to which is added 1 tsp of salt to every quart of solution used.

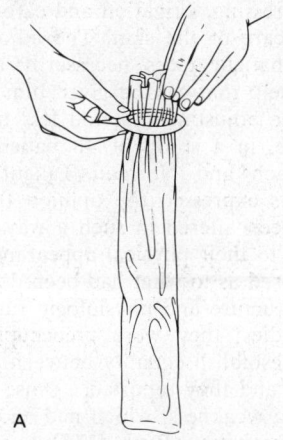

A

Insert one end of drainage sheath through the plastic ring.

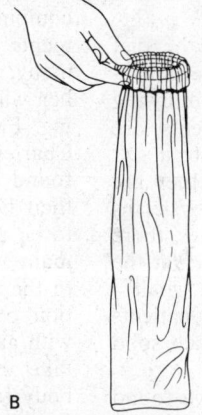

B

Fold over the edges of the sheath and roll around ring securely and evenly.

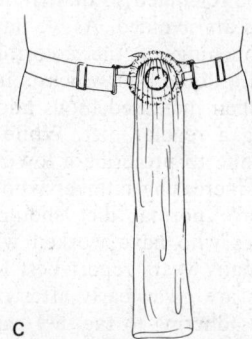

C

The ring with sheath is placed over the stoma, and the belt clips hooked onto the ring. This holds the appliance securely over the opening.

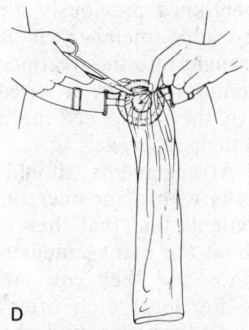

D

A small slit is cut into the sheath near the ring. The hole is made above the stoma, and to one side, to prevent leakage of the return flow.

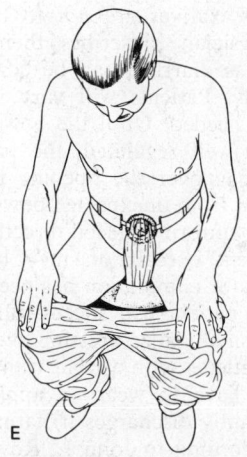

E

Tuck the sheath between the legs so that it leads directly into the toilet.

Figure 23-18. The bulb syringe method of colostomy irrigation. (Postel, Allen H., et al.: *Training the Patient in the Bulb Syringe Method of Colostomy Irrigation.* New York University Medical Center, N.Y., 1965.)

Wash the bulb-syringe and pitcher with soapy water, rinse thoroughly, and dry. Because the other items are disposable, they are discarded in a paper bag.

Charting. Note and record the time the treatment was given, the amount and kind of solution used, whether the nurse gave the treatment or whether the patient carried out the procedure and how well he or she managed self-care. Progress in rehabilitation of the patient with a colostomy should be as carefully noted as that for an amputee or a paraplegic.

Self-care and Rehabilitation. In the home, the patient may need in the bathroom a small table on which to assemble the equipment for the procedure. An orange crate may be substituted since the partition serves as a tray. After the irrigation has been completed and the equipment cleaned, the patient can store the items out of sight. With an orange crate the open side can be turned toward the wall. If the enema type irrigation is used, a hook or nail at the correct level should be inserted in the wall near the toilet on which the bag or can of solution may be suspended.

Although it may take some time, the diet can be regulated so that frequent bowel movements are avoided. As we have said, following the opening of the colostomy, patients are given a liquid diet which is increased to a soft diet then increased foods added until they are eating a regular diet. While some physicians continue to prescribe a low-residue diet, there is an increasing number who contend that the person's normal diet should be the goal.[130] Nurses who have worked with these patients for many years report best results when solid foods are given early after operation.

By adhering to the diet patients have found best for themselves, they will be able to control frequent loose stools and should be able to have a regular well-formed stool once a day. If diarrhea occurs, the patient should wear a colostomy bag, and pay special attention to the diet in an attempt to determine the food or foods that had a laxative effect. Fluid intake can be temporarily reduced at this time. If diarrhea persists, patients should consult their physician. Laxatives are *not* to be given unless the physician prescribes them. Constipation as well as diarrhea can be controlled by diet usually. Patients will vary in amounts of roughage needed. Until the bowel movements are again well regulated, the patient should wear a bag over the opening to prevent embarrassment from unexpected bowel movements. A karaya gum ring placed directly on the skin to prevent excoriation may be needed until regularity of elimination has been reestablished and the patient can successfully get along with only a small gauze dressing over the opening. Those patients with a right transverse colostomy will have to wear an appliance because it constantly discharges irritating semiliquid wastes, according to John L. Rowbotham.[130a]

Most patients wear a small dressing after bowel evacuations are established. One patient recommends a dressing of, first, a paper handkerchief, next a piece of waxed paper, and then a thin gauze dressing.

Because individuals differ, patients with a colostomy must learn what is best for them to eat and the type of dressing with which they feel most secure. Conferences with their physician to discuss problems of care and activity are needed from time to time. When a "routine" has been established, patients are much more content, since their general work and home activities can be carried on as they were before the operation.

Before leaving the hospital, the patient should clearly understand the regulation of diet, change of dressing, irrigation and care of equipment, and care of the skin. The adjustments that the patient faces necessarily are many, and any help that can be given him or her will make the adjustment period less trying. For example, in a study of 48 patients, Charles E. Orbach and Norman Tallent [131] found all subjects expressed the opinion that their body had been altered in such a way as to be destructive to their physical appearance; many were confused as to what had been done to the internal structure and physiologic function of their bodies; they were preoccupied with attempts to establish equality between intake and output; and they reported a sense of body fragility and weakness, which had an effect upon their activities. Ruth B. Dyk and Arthur M. Sutherland,[132] reporting a second study of 38 patients treated at the Memorial Center, New York City, believe that the spouse is often the key to the success or failure of patients' adaptation to their disability. In fact, the patients' adaptation to illness and the colostomy is never independent of the relationship between them and their spouse. As we have mentioned previously, the spouse or some responsible member of the family should be brought into the treatment program, as a functioning member, at an early date. To be effective, they, too, need the same instruction as the patient receives.[132a,b]

Arrangements should be made early for visits with a member of a local ostomy club. Patients find that they can learn a great deal about the management of ostomies from each other and they can attend regular meetings of the local club after leaving the hospital. They may also find the *Ostomy Quarterly,** devoted to special interests and problems of these patients, helpful. An increasing number of Stoma Rehabilitation Clinics are being established to provide a regional facility that offers service, consultation, and teaching to patients and professional persons.[133-135a]

* Published by the United Ostomy Association, Inc., 1111 Wilshire Blvd., Los Angeles, Calif.

REFERENCES

1. Bockus, Henry L.: *Gastroenterology,* Vol. II, 3rd ed. W. B. Saunders Co., Philadelphia, 1976, pp. 197, 387, 495.
2. Beecher, Henry K.: *Resuscitation and Anesthesia for Wounded Men; The Management of Traumatic Shock.* Charles C Thomas, Publisher, Springfield, Ill., 1949, p. 104.
3. Edwards, G., et al.: "Death Associated with Anesthesia, A Report on 1,000 Cases," *Anesthesia,* **2:**194, (July) 1956.

4. Bockus, Henry L.: *Gastroenterology*, Vol. II, 2nd ed. W. B. Saunders Co., Philadelphia, 1964, p. 74.

5. Remenchik, Alexander P., and Talso, Peter J.: "Medical Management of Intestinal Obstruction," *Med. Clin. North Am.*, **48**:67, (Jan.) 1964.

6. Cantor, Meyer O., and Reynolds, Roland P.: *Gastro-Intestinal Obstruction.* Williams & Wilkins Co., Baltimore, 1957, p. 347.

7. Hughes, Richard K., and Wootton, D. Gareth: "Gastric Sump Drainage with a Water Seal Monitor," *Surgery*, **61**:192, (Feb.) 1967.

8. Cantor, Meyer O.: *Intestinal Intubation.* Charles C Thomas, Publisher, Springfield, Ill., 1949, p. 20.

9. Schwartz, Seymour I., et al. (eds.): *Principles of Surgery*, Vol. II, 2nd ed. McGraw-Hill Book Co., New York, 1974, p. 986.

10. Bockus, Henry L.: *Gastroenterology*, Vol. II, 3rd ed. W. B. Saunders Co., Philadelphia, 1976, p. 198.

11. Behrend, Albert, and Piezas, Mabim C.: "Treatment of Complicated Intestinal Obstructions by Use of the Baker Tube," *Int. Surg.*, **52**:63, (July) 1969.

12. Bockus, Henry L.: *op. cit.*, p. 198.

13. Hermann, Robert E., and Traul, Don: "Experience with the Sengstaken-Blakemore Tube for Bleeding Esophageal Varices," *Surg. Gynecol. Obstet.*, **130**:879, (May) 1970.

14. Pitcher, J. Loren: "Safety and Effectiveness of the Modified Sengstaken-Blakemore Tube: A Prospective Study," *Gastroenterology*, **61**:291, (Sept.) 1971.

15. Conn, Harold O.: "Sengstaken-Blakemore Tube Revisited" (editorial), *Gastroenterology*, **61**:398, (Sept.) 1971.

16. Altshuler, Anne: "Esophageal Varices in Children," *Am. J. Nurs.*, **72**:687, (Apr.) 1972.

17. McCallister, Jean: "Nursing Care of a Patient with Bleeding Oesophageal Varices," *Nurs. Times*, **64**:621, (Nov. 29) 1968.

18. Høyer, Andreas J., and Solheim, Kaare: "The Therapy of Acute Small Bowel Obstruction," *Surg. Gynecol. Obstet.*, **109**:555, (Nov.) 1959.

19. Rhoads, Jonathan E., et al.: *Surgery; Principles and Practice*, 4th ed. J. B. Lippincott Co., Philadelphia, 1970, p. 1092.

20. Abbott, William E.: "Indications for the Use of the Miller-Abbott Tube," *N. Engl. J. Med.*, **225**:641, (Oct.) 1941.

21. Harris, Franklin I.: "A New Rapid Method of Intubation with the Miller-Abbott Tube," *J.A.M.A.*, **125**:784, (July 15) 1944.

22. Johnston, Charles G.: "Decompression in the Treatment of Intestinal Obstruction," *Surg. Gynecol. Obstet.*, **70**:365, (Feb.) 1940.

23. Sargent, E. Nicholas, and Meyers, Harvey I.: "Wire Guide and Technique for Cantor Tube Insertion," *Am. J. Roentgenol.*

Radium Ther. Nucl. Med., **107**:150, (Sept.) 1969.

24. Schneider, Louis: "Subclinical Mineral Oil Pneumonitis," *NY State J. Med.*, **51**:245, (Jan.) 1951.

25. Smith, Grafton A.: "Tube Decompression in Intestinal Obstruction," *Am. J. Surg.*, **104**:419, (Sept.) 1962.

26. Edlich, Richard F., et al.: "New Long Intestinal Tube for Rapid Nonoperative Intubation," *Arch. Surg.*, **95**:443, (Sept.) 1967.

27. Cantor, Meyer O.: *op. cit.*, p. 120.

28. Bockus, Henry L.: *op. cit.*, p. 203.

29. Rhoads, Jonathan E., et al.: *op. cit.*, p. 1091.

30. *Ibid.*, p. 1070.

31. Turell, Robert (ed.): *Diseases of the Colon and Anorectum*, Vol. I, 2nd ed., W. B. Saunders Co., Philadelphia, 1969, p. 120.

32. Schwartz, Seymour I., et al. (eds.): *Principles of Surgery*, Vol. I, McGraw-Hill Book Co., New York, 1969, p. 56.

33. Mackay, W. D., et al.: "Nasogastric Tube and Pulmonary Ventilation," *Arch. Surg.*, **87**:673, (Oct.) 1963.

34. Cantor, Meyer O.: *op. cit.*, p. 124.

35. Cleveland, Marion: *Relief of Throat Irritation During Intubation.* Unpublished Study, Nursing Education Division, Teachers College, Columbia University, New York, 1940.

36. Kehoe, Rosemary: "Recording Suction Siphonage," *Am. J. Nurs.*, **39**:126, (Feb.) 1939.

37. Drummond, Eleanor E., and Anderson, Mary L.: "Gastrointestinal Suction," *Am. J. Nurs.*, **63**:109, (Dec.) 1963.

38. Hughes, Richard K., and Wootton, D. Gareth: *op. cit.*

39. Moss, Gerald: "Technique of Ice Saline Gastric Lavage in Upper Gastrointestinal Hemorrhage," *Am. J. Surg.*, **122**:565, (Oct.) 1971.

40. Wingate, David: "Gastric Lavage in Acute Poisoning," *Nurs. Times*, **66**:648, (May 21) 1970.

41. Goodhart, Robert S. and Shils, Maurice E. (eds.): *Modern Nutrition in Health and Disease*, 5th ed. Lea & Febiger, Philadelphia, 1973, p. 832.

42. Barron, James: "Tube Feeding of Postoperative Patients," *Surg. Clin. North Am.*, **39**:1481, (Dec.) 1959.

43. Butler, Frank S., and Harrigan, William F.: "The Modern Revision of Feeding Tube Techniques," *J. Am. Geriatr. Soc.*, **14**:1107, (Nov.) 1966.

44. Hartwell, Shattuck W., and Cole, Owen R.: "The Feeding Cervical Oesophagostomy in the Management of Head and Neck Cancer," *Aust. NZ J. Surg.*, **39**:241, (Feb.) 1970.

45. Nicks, Rowan: "Combined Jejunostomy Feeding and Gastrostomy: Postoperative Management," *Med. J. Aust.*, **1**:1064, (May 24) 1969.

46. Vengusamy, Shakunthala, et al.: "A Controlled Study of Feeding Gastrostomy in Low Birth Weight Infants," *Pediatrics,* **43:**815, (May) 1969.

47. Coupland, G. A. E., and Reeve, T. S.: "Gastrostomy: A Review of Its Uses in a General Surgical Unit," *Aust. NZ J. Surg.,* **39:**150, (Nov.) 1969.

48. Heimbach, David M.: "Surgical Feeding Procedures in Patients with Neurological Disorders," *Ann. Surg.,* **177:**311, (Aug.) 1970.

49. Welch, Richard G.: "Feeding Jejunostomy," *Aust. NZ J. Surg.,* **41:**35, (Aug.) 1971.

50. Davidson, Sir Stanley, and Passmore, R.: *Human Nutrition and Dietetics,* 5th ed. Williams & Wilkins Co., Baltimore, 1972, p. 452.

51. Fason, M. Fitzpatrick: "Controlling Bacterial Growth in Tube Feedings," *Am. J. Nurs.,* **67:**1246, (June) 1967.

52. Gormican, Annette: "Prepackaged Tube Feedings," *Hospitals,* **44:**58, (Sept. 1) 1970.

53. Barron, James: *op. cit.*

54. Friedrich, Helen N.: "Oral Feeding by Food Pump," *Am. J. Nurs.,* **62:**62, (Feb.) 1962.

55. Metheney, Norma Milligan, and Snively, William: *Nurses' Handbook of Fluid Balance.* J. B. Lippincott Co., Philadelphia, 1967, p. 86.

56. Davenport, Rachel R.: "Tube Feeding for Long-Term Patients," *Am. J. Nurs.,* **64:**121, (Jan.) 1964.

57. Martin, Eric W. (ed.): *Techniques of Medication.* J. B. Lippincott Co., Philadelphia, 1969, p. 156.

58. Widman, Bernard P.: "Part I. Roentgen Examination of the Colon," in Bockus, Henry L.: *Gastroenterology,* Vol. II, 2nd ed. W. B. Saunders Co., Philadelphia, 1964, p. 677.

59. *Ibid.*

60. Matts, S. G. Flavell, and Gaskell, K. H.: "Retrograde Colonic Spread of Enemata in Ulcerative Colitis," *Br. Med. J.,* **2:**614, (Sept. 2) 1961.

61. Guyton, Arthur C.: *Textbook of Medical Physiology,* 5th ed. W. B. Saunders Co., Philadelphia, 1976, p. 863.

62. Widman, Bernard P.: *op. cit.*

63. Goligher, J. C.: *Surgery of the Anus, Rectum and Colon,* 2nd ed. Bailliere, Tindall & Cassell, London, 1967, p. 49.

64. Ruch, Theodore C., and Patton, Harry D. (eds.): *Physiology and Biophysics,* 19th ed. W. B. Saunders Co., Philadelphia, 1965, p. 974.

65. Bockus, Henry L.: *Gastroenterology,* Vol. II, 2nd ed. W. B. Saunders Co., Philadelphia, 1964, p. 620.

66. Cutting, Reginald A.: "Absorption of Dextrose and Water by the Small Intestine and the Colon," *Arch. Surg.,* **29:**643, (Oct.) 1934.

67. Dahlquist, A., and Thomson, D. L.: "The Digestion and Absorption of Lactose by the Intact Rat," *Acta Physiol. Scand.,* **61:**20, 1964.

68. Levitan, Ruven, et al.: "Water and Salt Absorption in the Human Colon," *J. Clin. Invest.,* **41:**1754, (Sept.) 1962.

69. Turell, Robert (ed.): *op. cit.,* p. 80.

70. Guyton, Arthur C.: *op. cit.,* p. 900.

71. *Ibid.*

72. Smith, Austin: *Technique of Medication.* J. B. Lippincott Co., Philadelphia, 1948, p. 131.

73. Walkling, Adolph: "Rupture of the Sigmoid by Hydrostatic Pressure," *Ann. Surg.,* **102:**471, (Sept.) 1935.

74. Frech, Henry C., and Lanier, L. Richard, Jr.: "Injuries to the Bowel as the Result of an Enema," *Am. J. Obstet. Gynecol.,* **74:**1146, (Nov.) 1957.

75. Dunning, Morcella F., and Plum, Fred: "Potassium Depletion by Enemas," *Am. J. Med.,* **20:**789, (May) 1956.

76. Rosenfield, Harold H., et al.: "Disposable Enema Unit in Obstetrics," *Obstet. Gynecol.,* **11:**222, (Feb.) 1958.

77. Page, Sidney G., Jr., et al.: "A Comparative Clinical Study of Several Enemas," *J.A.M.A.,* **157:**1208, (Apr. 2) 1955.

78. Ziskind, Alan, and Gellis, Sidney S.: "Water Intoxication Following Tap-Water Enemas," *Am. J. Dis. Child.,* **96:**699, (Dec.) 1958.

79. Flentie, Edgar H., and Cherkin, Arthur: "Electrolyte Effects of the Sodium Phosphate Enema," *Dis. Colon Rectum,* **1:**295, (July–Aug.) 1958.

80. Berger, Eugene Y., et al.: "Suppression of Sodium Excretion by the Colon in Congestive Heart Failure and Cirrhosis of the Liver Demonstrated by the Use of Cation Exchange Resins," *J. Clin. Invest.,* **31:**451, (Mar.) 1952.

81. Flentie, Edgar H., and Baptist, Victor H.: "Enema Studies: Role of Volume in the Action of Hypertonic Sodium Phosphate Enemas," *Western J. Surg. Obstet. Gynecol.,* **65:**302, (Sept.–Oct.) 1957.

82. Miller, Joseph M., and Brown, Ernest O.: "Clinical Evaluation of a Disposable Microenema," *Am. J. Proctol.,* **20:**444, (Dec.) 1969.

83. Tillery, Betty, and Bates, Barbara: "Enemas," *Am. J. Nurs.,* **66:**534, (Mar.) 1966.

84. Turell, Robert: "Laceration to Anorectum Incident to Enema," *Arch. Surg.,* **81:**953, (Dec.) 1960.

85. King, V. M., et al.: "A Miniature Disposable Enema," *Nurs. Times,* **58:**1302, (Oct. 12) 1962.

86. Steinbach, Howard L., et al.: "Transmission of Enteric Pathogens by Barium Enemas," *J.A.M.A.,* **174:**1207, (Oct. 29) 1960.

87. Meyers, Philip H., and Richards, May: "Transmission of Polio Virus Vaccine by Contaminated Barium Enema with Resultant Antibody Rise," *Am. J. Roentgenol. Radium Ther. Nucl. Med.,* **91:**864, (Apr.) 1964.

88. Meyers, Philip H.: "Contamination of Barium Enema Apparatus During Its Use," *J.A.M.A.*, **173**:1589, (Aug. 6) 1960.

89. Moeschlin, Sven: *Poisoning, Diagnosis and Treatment.* Grune & Stratton, New York, 1965, p. 15.

90. Bockus, Henry L.: *Gastroenterology,* Vol. II, 3rd ed. W. B. Saunders Co., Philadelphia, 1976, p. 951.

91. Sawyer, Janet R.: *Nursing Care of Patients with Urologic Diseases.* C. V. Mosby Co., St. Louis, 1963, p. 239.

92. Bacon, Harry E.: *Cancer of the Colon, Rectum and Anal Canal.* J. B. Lippincott Co., Philadelphia, 1964, p. 539.

93. Jackson, Raymond J.: "Fecal Incontinence—Nonsurgical Treatment," *J.A.M.A.*, **166**:1281, (Mar. 15) 1958.

94. "Colonic Lavage Machine," *Nurs. Times,* **57**:589, (May 12) 1961.

95. Daugherty, Guy W., et al.: "Continuous Lavage of the Colon as a Means of Treating Renal Insufficiency; Report of a Case," *Proc. Staff Meet., Mayo Clin.,* **23**:209, (Apr.) 1948.

96. Truelove, S. C.: "Treatment of Ulcerative Colitis with Local Hydrocortisone," *Br. Med. J.,* **2**:1267, (Dec. 1) 1956.

97. ———: "Treatment of Ulcerative Colitis with Local Hydrocortisone Hemisuccinate Sodium," *Br. Med. J.,* **1**:1437, (June 22) 1957.

98. ———: "Treatment of Ulcerative Colitis with Local Hydrocortisone Hemisuccinate Sodium," *Br. Med. J.,* **2**:1072, (Nov. 1) 1958.

99. Watkinson, Geoffrey: "Treatment of Ulcerative Colitis with Topical Hydrocortisone Hemisuccinate Sodium," *Br. Med. J.,* **2**:1077, (Nov. 1) 1958.

100. Rhoads, Jonathan E., et al.: *op. cit.,* p. 1070.

101. Bailey, Hamilton, et al.: *A Short Practice of Surgery,* 12th ed. J. B. Lippincott Co., Philadelphia, 1962, p. 110.

102. "The Harris Drip," *Am. J. Nurs.,* **28**:1212, (Dec.) 1928.

103. Matts, S. G. Flavell: "Intrarectal Treatment of 100 Cases of Ulcerative Colitis with Prednisolone-21-Phosphate Enemata," *Br. Med. J.,* **1**:165, (Jan. 21) 1961.

104. Jones, F. Avery, et al.: *Clinical Gastroenterology,* 2nd ed. Blackwell Scientific Publications, Oxford, 1968, p. 646.

105. Culp, Clyde E.: "Bowel Preparation for Proctosigmoidoscopy," *Nebr. State Med. J.,* **50**:79, (Feb.) 1965.

106. Shirkey, Harry C.: "Bowel Evacuation in Infancy and Childhood," *Nebr. State Med. J., 50:*67, (Feb.) 1965.

107. Lichtenstein, Manuel E.: "Intestinal Stomas: Colostomy and Ileostomy," in Turell, Robert (ed.): *Diseases of the Colon and Anorectum,* Vol. I, 2nd ed. W. B. Saunders Co., Philadelphia, 1969, p. 629.

107a. Jensen, Vicki: "Better Techniques for Bagging Stomas. Part 2: Colostomies," *Nursing '74,* **4**:30, (Aug.) 1974.

108. Lichtenstein, Manuel E.: *op. cit.,* p. 648.

108a. Watt, Rosemary C.: "Urinary Diversion," *Am. J. Nurs.,* **74**:1806, (Oct.) 1974.

109. Gutowski, Frances: "Ostomy Procedure: Nursing Care," *Am. J. Nurs.,* **72**:262, (Feb.) 1972.

109a. Gallagher, Ann M.: "Body Image Changes in the Patient with Colostomy," *Nurs. Clin. North Am.,* **7**:669, (Dec.) 1972.

110. Hallburg, Jeanne C.: "The Patient with Surgery of the Colon," *Am. J. Nurs.,* **61**:64, (Mar.) 1961.

111. Secor, Sophie M.: "New Hope for Colostomy Patients," *Nurs. Outlook,* **2**:642, (Dec.) 1954.

111a. Dericks, Virginia C.: "The Psychological Hurdles of New Ostomates. Helping Them Up . . . and Over," *Nursing '74,* **4**:52, (Oct.) 1974.

112. Gutowski, Frances: *op. cit.*

112a. Dlin, Barney, and Perlman, Abraham: "Sex After Ileostomy or Colostomy," *Med. Aspects Human Sexuality,* **6**:33, (July) 1972.

112b. Vukovich, Virginia, and Grubb, Reba D.: *Care of the Ostomy Patient.* C. V. Mosby Co., St. Louis, 1973.

112c. Dericks, Virginia C.: "Nursing Practices that Affect the Dynamics of Rehabilitation for Patients with an Ostomy," in *ANA 1974 Clinical Sessions.* Appleton-Century-Crofts, New York, 1975, p. 248.

113. Wolfman, Earl F., Jr., and Flotte, C. Thomas: "Carcinoma of the Colon and Rectum," *Am. J. Nurs.,* **61**:60, (Mar.) 1961.

114. Drosd, Rudolph E., and Shocket, Everett: "Effective Decompression of the Colon by Transverse Colon Tube Colostomy," *Surg. Gynecol. Obstet.,* **129**:123, (July) 1969.

115. Lenneberg, Edith, et al.: "Colostomies: A Guide for the Patient," *Dis. Colon Rectum,* **12**:201, (May–June) 1969.

116. Donaldson, Gordon A.: "Current Concepts in Therapy; Management of Ileostomy and Colostomy," *N. Engl. J. Med.,* **268**:827, (Apr. 11) 1963.

117. Bacon, Harry E.: *op. cit.,* p. 803.

118. Katona, Elizabeth A.: "Learning Colostomy Control," *Am. J. Nurs.,* **67**:534, (Mar.) 1967.

119. Dericks, Virginia C., and Robeson, Kathryn: "Problems of Colostomy Patients," *Public Health Nurs.,* **41**:16, (Jan.) 1949.

120. Gibbs, Gertrude E., and White, Marilyn: "Stomal Care," *Am. J. Nurs.,* **72**:268, (Feb.) 1972.

121. McNamara, Robert J., and Farber, Eugene M.: "Circumileostomy Skin Difficulties," *Arch. Dermatol.,* **89**:675, (May) 1964.

122. Breidenbach, Lester, and Secor, Sophie M.: "Twenty-Five Questions on Colostomy Management," *Nurs. World,* **56**:16, (Jan.) 1956.

123. Wee, George C., et al.: "Irrigation Versus Nonirrigation of Colostomy," *Mo. Med.,* **68:**622, (Aug.) 1971.

124. Mendelssohn, Alan N.: "Management of the Colonic Stoma," *Surg. Gynecol. Obstet.,* **129:**1046, (Nov.) 1969.

125. Wee, George C., et al.: *op. cit.*

126. Sill, Alice R.: "Bulb-Syringe Technique for Colonic Stoma Irrigation," *Am. J. Nurs.,* **70:**536, (Mar.) 1970.

126a. Dericks, Virginia C.: "Practical Counseling," presented at a Conference titled *Outlook of the Patient, with an Intestinal Stoma.* Sponsored by the American Cancer Society's New York City Division, New York City, New York, Oct. 24, 1972.

127. Secor, Sophie M.: "Colostomy Care— 1964," *Am. J. Nurs.,* **64:**127, (Sept.) 1964.

128. Nigro, Norman D.: "A Special Catheter for Colostomy Irrigation," *Dis. Colon Rectum,* **12:**61, (Jan.–Feb.) 1969.

128a. Lenneberg, Edith S., and Sohn, Norman: "Modern Concepts in the Management of Patients with Intestinal and Urinary Stomas," *Clin. Obstet. Gynecol.,* **15:**542, (June) 1972.

129. Postel, Allen H., et al.: *Training the Patient in the Bulb Syringe Method of Colostomy Irrigation. A Manual for Nurses.* New York University Medical Center, New York, 1965.

130. Rowbotham, John L.: "Colostomy Problems—Dietary and Colostomy Management," *Cancer,* **28:**222, (Jan.) 1971.

130a. *Ibid.,* p. 223.

131. Orbach, Charles E., and Tallent, Norman: "Modification of Perceived Body and Body Concepts," *Arch. Gen. Psychiatry,* **12:**126, (Feb.) 1965.

132. Dyk, Ruth B., and Sutherland, Arthur M.: "Adaptation of the Spouse and Other Family Members to the Colostomy Patient," *Cancer,* **9:**123, (Jan.–Feb.) 1956.

132a. Connors, Melba: "Ostomy Care: A Personal Approach," *Am. J. Nurs.,* **74:**1422, (Aug.) 1974.

132b. Gross, Linda: "Ostomy Care: A Letter to Parents," *Am. J. Nurs.,* **74:**1427, (Aug.) 1974.

133. Rowbotham, John L.: "The Stoma Rehabilitation Clinic," *Dis. Colon Rectum,* **13:**59, (Jan.–Feb.) 1970.

134. Kirsner, Joseph B.: "Stoma Therapy Clinic —University of Chicago Hospitals and Clinics" (editorial), *Int. Surg.,* **53:**6, (June) 1970.

135. Lenneberg, Edith: "Role of Enterostomal Therapists and Stoma Rehabilitation Clinics," *Cancer,* **28:**226, (July) 1971.

135a. Honesty, Henrene: *Essentials of Abdominal Ostomy Care.* Springer Publishing Co., New York, 1972.

Additional Suggested Reading

Baker, Dorothy I.: "Hyperalimentation at Home," *Am. J. Nurs.,* **74:**1826, (Oct.) 1974.

Brooks, Frank P.: *Control of Gastrointestinal Function: An Introduction to the Physiology of the Gastrointestinal Tract.* Macmillan Publishing Co., Inc., New York, 1970.

Bullock, John D.: "A Convenient Method for Inserting Small Feeding Tubes," *Gut,* **10:**599, (June) 1969.

Butler, Frank S.: "Cancer of the Esophagus: Modern Method of Maintaining Nutrition," *J. Am. Geriatr. Soc.,* **15:**462, (May) 1967.

Casten, Daniel F.: "The Use of a Triple Lumen Gastric Tube for Suction and Feeding," *Surg. Gynecol. Obstet.,* **130:**696, (Apr.) 1970.

Cobbin, Odell, et al.: "Preliminary Report of a New Intestinal Intubation Principle, with Application to the Large Bowel," *Surgery,* **55:**564, (Apr.) 1964.

Davidson, Murray, et al.: "Studies of Distal Colonic Motility in Children; I. Non-propulsive Patterns in Normal Children," *Pediatrics,* **17:**807, (June) 1956.

Davis, Larry E., and Hofmann, William: "A Long-Term Nasogastric Feeding Tube Made from Modified Penrose Tubing," *J.A.M.A.,* **209:**685, (Aug. 4) 1969.

"Dehydration with High Protein Tube Feeding," *Nutr. Rev.,* **26:**271, (Sept.) 1968.

Dennis, Clarence: "The Gastrointestinal Sump Tube," *Surgery,* **66:**309, (Aug.) 1969.

Dericks, Virginia C.: "The Controversy Over Colostomy Irrigation, A Historical Perspective," *Ostomy Q.,* (Spring) 1976, p. 32.

———: "Nursing Care of the Patient with an Ostomy," in American Cancer Society: *Proceedings of the 1973 National Conference on Cancer Nursing.* The Society, Chicago, 1974, p. 116.

French, W. Edward: "Intra-Abdominal Surgery Without Gastrointestinal Decompression," *Tenn. Med. Assn. J.,* **59:**767, (Aug.) 1966.

Gibstein, Alan, et al.: "Prevention of Postoperative Abdominal Distention and Discomfort with Simethicone," *Obstet. Gynecol.,* **38:**386, (Sept.) 1971.

Given, Barbara, and Simmons, Sandra: "Care of a Patient with a Gastric Ulcer," *Am. J. Nurs.,* **70:**1472, (July) 1970.

Given, Barbara, and Simmons, Sandra: *Gastroenterology in Clinical Nursing,* 2nd ed. C. V. Mosby Co., St. Louis, 1975.

Hamilton, Mary Sue, and Schlapper, Nancy Bryant: "Pelvic Exenteration," *Am. J. Nurs.,* **76:**266, (Feb.) 1976.

Hector, R. M.: "Improved Technique of Gastric Aspiration," *Lancet,* **1:**15, (Jan. 6) 1968.

———: "Gastric Aspiration," *Nurs. Times,* **64:**723, (May 31) 1968.

Ibach, John R.: "Tube Gastrostomy for Postoperative Decompression," *Milit. Med.* **133:**987, (Dec.) 1968.

Jay, Arthur N.: "Is it Indigestion?" *Am. J. Nurs.,* **58:**1552, (Nov.) 1958.

Langer, B., et al.: "Prolonged Survival After Complete Small Bowel Resection Using Intravenous Alimentation at Home," *J. Surg. Res.,* **15:**226, (Sept.) 1973.

Larson, Darlene: *Living Comfortably with Your Ileostomy.* Sister Kenny Institute, Minneapolis, 1974.

Nichols, Ronald L., et al.: "Alteration of Intestinal Microflora Following Preoperative Mechanical Preparation of the Colon," *Dis. Colon Rectum,* **14:**123, (Mar.–Apr.) 1971.

Paulson, Moses (ed.): *Gastroenterologic Medicine.* Lea & Febiger, Philadelphia, 1968.

Peaston, M. J. T.: "External Metabolic Balance Studies During Nasogastric Feeding in Serious Illnesses Requiring Intensive Care," *Br. Med. J.,* **2:**1367, (Dec. 3) 1966.

Ray, John E., et al.: "Postoperative Problems of Ileostomy and Colostomy," *J.A.M.A.,* **174:**48, (Dec. 24) 1960.

Reid, David H. S.: "Treatment of the Poisoned Child," *Arch. Dis. Child.,* **45:**428, (June) 1970.

Sawyer, Robert B.: "Jejunostomy for Feeding or Decompression," *Surg. Clin. North Am.,* **49:**1311, (Dec.) 1969.

Schauder, Marilyn R.: "Ostomy Care: Cone Irrigations," *Am. J. Nurs.,* **74:**1424, (Aug.) 1974.

Schulman, Norman H., et al.: "Decompression of the Colon with Complete Diversion of the Fecal Stream by an *in situ* Colonic Catheter: A Pilot Study," *Surgery,* **67:**918, (June) 1970.

Shah, N.: "Method of Fixing the Nasogastric Feeding Tube," *J. Laryngol. Otol.,* **83:**485, (May) 1969.

Smith, Grafton A.: "Long Intestinal Tubes for Operative Decompression and Postoperative Ileus," *J.A.M.A.,* **160:**266, (Jan. 28), 1956.

Spiro, Howard M.: *Clinical Gastroenterology.* Macmillan Publishing Co., Inc., New York, 1970.

Stewart, William R. C., and Samson, Ralph B.: "Rectal Tube Decompression of Left-Colon Anastomosis," *Dis. Colon Rectum,* **11:**452, (Nov.–Dec.) 1968.

Ulin, Alex W., and Ehrlich, Edward W.: "Current Views Related to Management of Large Bowel Obstruction Caused by Carcinoma of the Colon," *Am. J. Surg.,* **104:**463, (Sept.) 1962.

Walike, Joseph W.: "Tube Feeding Syndrome in Head and Neck Surgery," *Arch. Otolaryngol.,* **89:**117, (Mar.) 1969.

Gladys Nite
Virginia Henderson

CHAPTER 24

Intubation of the Urinary Tract for Medication, Irrigation and Drainage, and Dialysis

1. BASIC PRINCIPLES UNDERLYING TREATMENTS OF THE BLADDER

The bladder is a highly elastic musculo-membranous sac in the pelvic cavity behind the symphysis pubis. When distended, it reaches above the symphysis pubis and may be felt, and its outline seen except in the obese. It functions as a reservoir for the urine that is constantly secreted by the kidneys and carried from them to the bladder in very small amounts by peristaltic waves that pass over the ureters every few seconds. The tone of the bladder wall and changes in intravesical pressure as the bladder fills with urine can be estimated by use of a cystometer. According to Arthur C. Guyton,[1] when the bladder is completely empty, the intravesical pressure is zero; however, 100 ml of urine raises the pressure to about 10 cm of water but an additional 300 to 400 ml will not significantly change this pressure. Contents of the bladder that exceed this point will bring about a very rapid rise in pressure. This obviously accounts for the discomfort that may be severe at times when the bladder is distended. The bladder can be trained to increase its capacity, especially in the young. The bladder capacity is related to the size of the person.

Oswald S. Lowsley and Thomas J. Kirwin[2] say the bladder is capable of great distention without rupture. While it may be distended to hold 2000 ml (2 qt) or more, the accumulation of 240 to 300 ml (8 to 10 oz) elicits the desire to micturate or empty the bladder. This desire is a vague sensation in the penis or perineum and is thought to be initiated by rhythmic contraction of the bladder walls which is in turn initiated by stretching or distention of the bladder. After infancy the act of voiding is under the control of the will in healthy persons.[3] The mechanism of micturition is discussed in Chapter 11. This and the subject of retention should be reviewed as a basis for understanding the various treatments described in this chapter.

As is pointed out in Chapter 11, emotion may give rise to an almost constant desire to void, and this must be understood to interpret correctly the physician's directions for catheterization. Inflammation of the bladder results in this symptom of "urgency," and it is important to determine the latter's true origin. Treatment should be designed to eliminate the cause: either relief of mental stress or inflammation.

Retention, or failure to empty the bladder normally, must in some cases be relieved by catheterization, for undue *distention* of the bladder wall with consequent reduction of the blood supply is believed to predispose to infection. However, it is impossible to insert a catheter without introducing some bacteria, because the urethra opening cannot be sterilized. For this reason, some physicians avoid catheterization except in emergencies.

In catheterizing there has been some question as to whether the bladder should be emptied. Ralph A. Straffon says: "The normal bladder is completely empty at the end of micturition; the intravesical pressure is equal to the intra-abdominal pressure." [*] This suggests that the complete emptying of the bladder by catheterization is indicated. *The amount of urine to remove* by catheter has, however, been a perennial subject of discussion. When it is thought that the bladder is distended, nurses are sometimes directed to remove "half the contents" as if the abdominal and bladder walls were transparent, enabling the nurse to make such a judgment. In some hospitals it is routine to withdraw the catheter after collecting, or removing, 500 ml (1 pt.). Some physicians approve complete emptying but prescribe the instillation of 30 to 60 ml of a sterile solution to prevent a sudden change in vesicular pressure. It is believed that this sudden change may result in engorgement of the blood vessels made almost toneless by the thinning of the wall during retention. Charles D. Creevy [4] (in 1932), reporting his experience with a published record of 300 cases of urinary retention in which the bladder had been completely emptied, says that no unfavorable reaction was observed in any case. In a study of 22 patients with acute urinary retention, Theodore G. Osius and Frank Hinman, Jr.[5] (in 1963) report that because withdrawal of relatively small amounts of urine (100 ml) lowered the intravesical pressure by half, slow decompression fails in its objective. They believe that complications and death occur from infection (enhanced by slow drainage), not from hemorrhage or shock. Some urologists refer to the fractional emptying of the bladder as a moot question while others insist that it is a necessity because the bladder is less likely to bleed or set off renal reflex dysfunction than when decompressed rapidly.[6,7] Complete emptying of the bladder may be avoided by raising the drainage tube to a certain height so that the urine will flow uphill before it drains down in the collecting device. Because the urine will flow against gravity, there will always be a certain quantity in the bladder. Therefore, since it is an unsolved problem in therapy, the nurse should determine the physician's wishes in relation to this aspect of the procedure. *The amount of solution to introduce into the bladder* at a single injection during irrigations should vary with patients and their conditions and with the physician's plan of treatment. Since the objectives of the treatment are to clean, medicate, and sometimes to distend the bladder wall, the amount is usually sufficient

to get rid of the folds in the lining of the bladder and varies from 150 to 400 ml (5 to 13 oz). Larger quantities, of course, are used in the total process of the irrigation.

In describing bladder irrigations, all the urologists whose methods have been examined state that the fluid should be introduced slowly, under *gentle pressure*. Water introduced into a closed cavity exerts equal pressure in every direction, so that this force, if great enough, could carry the bladder contents up into the ureters. The total force of a liquid on a surface is equal to the area of the surface times the depth of the liquid times the density of the liquid. Applying this principle, it can readily be seen that reducing the depth of the liquid, which in this instance is the same thing as the height of the column of the irrigating fluid, reduces the force. The top of the column of the irrigating fluid should not be more than 15 to 20 cm (6 to 8 inches) above the meatus.

The cause of infections associated with catheterization has been given a great deal of attention in medical literature. *Catheter cystitis* is a term often used in the past, and this expression implies that the infection was caused by the catheter. Following an extensive analysis of relevant literature in 1955, E. H. Kass,[8] who is credited with introducing the "midstream" or "clean-catch" specimen as a substitute for the catheterized specimen, concluded that catheters and other instruments are the major carriers of organisms causing urinary infections. In 1956, he reported that 95 per cent of patients on open-catheter drainage for 96 hours developed significant bacteriuria.[9] Although indwelling catheters and instruments are more often related to bacteriuria, the likelihood of inducing bacteriuria by a single catheterization in women is 2 to 4 per cent as reflected in a sample of 2000 cases.[10] Following single urethral catheterization, Marvin Turck and associates [11] report persistent bacteriuria in only one woman of 200 physically healthy, ambulatory men and women, whereas 8 were affected in a group of 75 hospitalized bed patients (men and women). It is obvious that the sick, elderly (some were in their eighties) patients are a high-risk group; therefore, catheterization should not be performed if it can be avoided.

Pablo Morales and Anthony Y. Tsou [12] emphasize the importance of the "paraplegic" achieving urethral voiding as quickly as possible because bacteriuria was found in all 20 patients with indwelling catheters and 16 of the 20 who had achieved urethral voiding. In 100 unselected autopsies, Richard A. MacDonald and associates [13] found a substantial correlation between bacteriuria, pyelonephritis,

---

[*] Straffon, Ralph A.: "Pathological Physiology of the Kidney. Micturition," in Brobeck, John R., et al. (eds.): *Best and Taylor's Physiological Basis of Medical Practice*, 9th ed. Williams & Wilkins, Co., Baltimore, 1973, p. 5–53.

and indwelling catheters—demonstrating the seriousness of catheter-induced infection. Conversely, W. R. Cattell et al.[14] did not find any patient with "progressive renal damage" that could be attributed to catheter-induced urinary infection 10 years earlier in a group of 71 patients who had had vaginal repair.

The specific causes of infection related to the catheter or other parts of the drainage system have been investigated extensively in the past decade or so.[14a] Some authorities say infections are due to lack of an aseptic technique or lack of understanding of the mechanisms of bacterial entry into the catheter system. Robert E. Desautels[15] lists the following causes of infection associated with the catheter or a drainage system: (1) inadequate preparation of the urethra; (2) contamination of any part of the catheter; (3) trauma of the urethra or pressure necrosis of the meatus because of a large catheter or poor blood supply (as in a diabetic); (4) entry of bacteria at the junction of the catheter and the urethral meatus; (5) contamination of the connecting tube and catheter because of improper method of irrigations or disconnecting them; and (6) contamination of distal end of the drainage system. Bacteria are in large numbers on the skin and especially areas adjacent to the urethral meatus such as the vagina and rectum in the female and the foreskin in the male. A small number of bacteria are present in the urethra, only a few centimeters from the meatus.[16] Entry of bacteria by way of the urethra is discouraged by the washing effect of micturition; however, Kass and Lawrence J. Schneiderman[17] have shown that bacteria enter the urethra in patients with indwelling catheters. Sources of infection, in addition to those mentioned above, are discussed and reported by J. S. Ansell[18]: (1) bacteria from the air may contaminate urine through the open bottle (a closed system prevents this); (2) motile bacteria may migrate up the collecting tube (a urine flow rate of 50 ml per minute is thought to prevent this); and (3) contaminated hands of personnel caring for these patients may introduce bacteria into the drainage system. It is obvious from the above discussion bacteria may enter the lower urinary tract in the following ways: bacteria may be carried in by the catheter, ascend the lumen of the catheter, and enter through the space between the urethral wall and the catheter.

Most authorities place great emphasis on frequent emptying of the bladder both for the patient's comfort and the prevention of infection. With retention (residual urine), cystitis may occur. If the patient is not kept comforta-

ble by voiding, catheterization may be advised postoperatively. Indwelling catheters are sometimes inserted at time of surgery so that distention of the bladder does not occur.

In determining the frequency of catheterization several factors should be considered: the patient's description of his or her discomfort, and the normal rate of secretion. The healthy kidney secretes approximately 50 ml per hour but the amount of fluid intake actually determines the rate of urinary secretion or how frequently the bladder fills. Fortunately, less emphasis is placed now on catheterizing patients at specified time intervals, such as every 8 hours, than in the past.

There is agreement that the meatus and lower urethra contain organisms, but the normal functioning bladder flushes contaminants by voiding, thereby preventing infection. Kass says "presently available data are compatible with" the statement "that urine is normally sterile." * This implies that the bladder is also normally sterile; however, other authors indicate that the bladder is not a sterile cavity. Bacteria are taken to the bladder by the blood stream as well as by way of the urethra.

To prevent entry of bacteria by the urethra, it is helpful to know those that enter by this route. According to J. P. Sanford,[19] there is general agreement that *Escherichia coli, Klebsiella, Aerobacter, Proteus, Pseudomonas,* and enterococcus are most frequently associated with urinary tract infections. Grayson Carrol, writing in Campbell's and Harrison's text, reports the type of organisms and their frequency in 1000 patients as shown in Table 24-1. Vegetative pathogens and their spore forms may be destroyed by boiling the submerged catheter for 15 minutes, a simple and available method. Autoclaving is even more effective. Some chemical solutions, used in cold sterilization, kill most vegetative bacteria but their effects vary on the tubercle bacilli, spores, and fungi.[20] The majority of authorities consulted recommend prepackaged, disposable catheters that are sterilized commercially. Sterile catheterization kits that include all necessary equipment are also available. Some urologists believe use of this equipment helps to ensure sterility as well as standardized contents of the "packs" or "kits."[21]

Although the bacterial agent is the direct cause of infection, injury to the mucous membrane is a major predisposing factor. Urologists repeatedly state that the normal bladder and urethra with intact mucous surface can

---

* Kass, Edward H.: "Pyelonephritis and Bacteriuria, A Major Problem in Preventive Medicine," *Ann. Intern. Med.,* **56:**47, (Jan.) 1962.

Table 24-1. Frequency of Occurrence of Organisms Found in 1000 Patients with Urinary Infection *

	Percent
E. coli	24.5
Pseudomonas aeruginosa	15.9
Aero. aerogenes	12.2
Proteus vulgaris	11.7
Staphylococcus	10.0
Streptococcus	8.1
E. intermedia	5.9
Alcal. faecalis	3.8
Paracolon	3.1
Fungus	4.8

* Campbell, Meredith F., and Harrison, J. Hartwell: *Urology,* Vol. I, 3rd ed. W. B. Saunders Co., Philadelphia, 1970, p. 420.

The catheterization procedure should not be left to the novice; it takes practice to be skilled in performing this procedure without injuring the tissues.

Although the meatus cannot be sterilized and should not be irritated, an effective cleaning should always be attempted. Some authorities recommend a neutral detergent in cleaning the meatus, while others believe an antiseptic solution should be used. Irrigation of the distal urethra with an antibacterial agent (such as benzalkonium chloride 1:1000 or 1:750) with an Asepto or bulb syringe is recommended also.[22] Cotton swabs impregnated with this solution are included in some catheterization kits. This antibiotic agent is thought to inactivate the bacteria present in the urethra and the meatus. Polymixin B is reported to be effective in reducing postinstrument incidence of bacteriuria in women.[22a] Cotton sponges are

usually protect themselves from infection if no bacteria has been introduced by a contaminated catheter, but that trauma produces a vulnerable spot upon which otherwise helpless invaders can gain a foothold. The importance of maintaining the integrity of the tissues suggests that smooth, pliable, and unbreakable catheters, of the smallest effective size, should be used. It also suggests that catheters should be well lubricated and skillfully handled. Although metal, glass, and woven silk (stiffened by shellac) catheters are available, medical opinion favors a pliable catheter of rubber or plastic. Metal and glass catheters are sometimes used but only for catheterizing women. They are rigid and potentially traumatic, even to women. Glass catheters should *not* be used for children, according to most authorities. It has been reported that ten urologists (of 26 in 14 states) have known of more than one case in which a portion of a catheter was left in the bladder.*

Too much emphasis cannot be placed on the skillful handling of the catheter. It can be manipulated more sensitively if grasped by the fingers rather than by a forcep. If a stiff catheter is used, it may be held with a clean hand far enough from the tip to make its introduction bacteriologically safe, but a rubber catheter has to be held much nearer the tip and the worker should therefore wear a sterile glove. If gloves are available, they should be worn regardless of type of catheter used so that the possibility of introducing organisms is reduced.

* Studies referred to above were made in the Department of Nursing Education, Teachers College, Columbia University, New York, N.Y., 1934 and 1935. (Unpublished.)

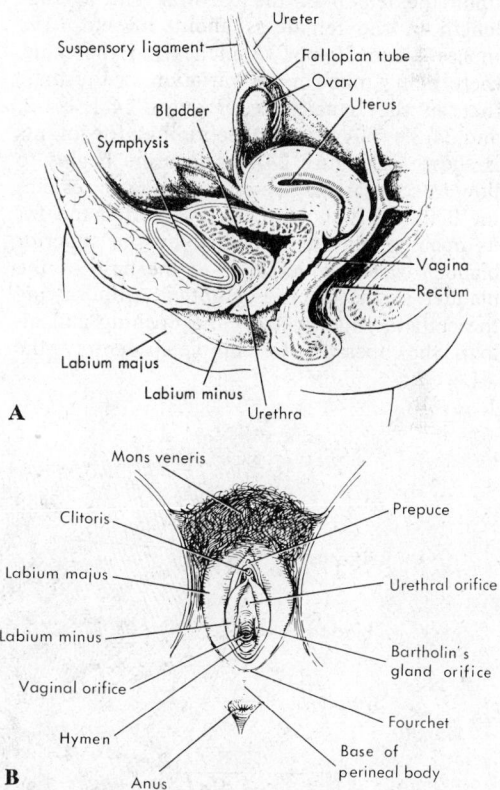

Figure 24-1. Female generative tract showing (*A*) internal and (*B*) external organs. Note normal position of urethral orifice between the clitoris and the vaginal orifice. (From Keuhnelian, J. G., and Sanders, V. E.: *Urologic Nursing,* Macmillan Publishing Co., Inc., New York, 1970; and Ziegel, E., and Van Blarcom, C. C.: *Obstetric Nursing,* 6th ed., Macmillan Publishing Co., Inc., New York, 1972.)

recommended because they are less likely to irritate than those made of gauze. To reduce the bacteria on the area as much as possible, sterile sponges are used and are manipulated with a sterile instrument.

Catheter lubricants may be one of the hydrocarbons, such as mineral oil or petroleum jelly, one of the vegetable oils, or a lubricating jelly with a water base. Although the oily substances are more effective as lubricants, the water-soluble jellies are preferred by many physicians. They are absorbed by the tissues and leave the urethra closed, whereas oils, particularly inorganic oils, tend to remain on the surface of the mucous membrane and provide a pathway over which microorganisms gain access to the bladder. Another reason for using water-soluble lubricants is that they do not destroy rubber catheters as the oils, especially the hydrocarbons, do.

The *distance to insert the catheter* depends upon the length of the urethra. The average length in the female is about 3.8 cm (1½ inches); and 20 cm (8 inches) in the male, there being much more variation in the male than in the female (see Figures 24-1, 24-2, and 24-3.) [23] A urine collection bag for infants is shown in Figure 24-4. The urine begins to flow as soon as the eye of the catheter reaches the bladder. If the catheter is inserted too far its opening may be occluded by the superior bladder wall that descends to the base of the bladder as the organ is emptied; withdrawing the catheter slightly frees the opening and allows the operator to completely empty the

cavity. The catheter should not be inserted too far, because it is possible to injure the lining of the bladder, and even to puncture the wall with a stiff catheter if enough force is exerted.

Introduction of the catheter is often made difficult by abnormalities in the meatus and urethra. The orifice varies in shape and position in the female, but is usually a sagittal slit in the center of the papilla just above the opening of the vagina and about 2½ cm (1 inch) below the clitoris. In some cases it is in the anterior vaginal wall and cannot be seen. The meatus is often difficult to find in children, or if the area is inflamed and swollen, or if the vagina is packed postoperatively. Packing in the vagina tends to displace the surrounding parts.

Since a living organism involuntarily protects itself from harmful objects, there is a natural withdrawal of the body and a contraction of the urethral orifice when an attempt is made to insert a catheter. Strong emotions and chilling, interfering with relaxation of the urethra, make the introduction of the catheter difficult. In preparing patients for catheterization, nurses should see that they are warm and, if possible, free from fear and excitement. Embarrassment over exposure and fear of being hurt are frequent causes of stress. Assurance of privacy, adequate draping, and the use of gloves or finger cots for the necessary handling of the genitalia may reduce the patient's embarrassment. A careful and truthful explanation of the procedure will relieve the patient's fear of pain if he or she has confi-

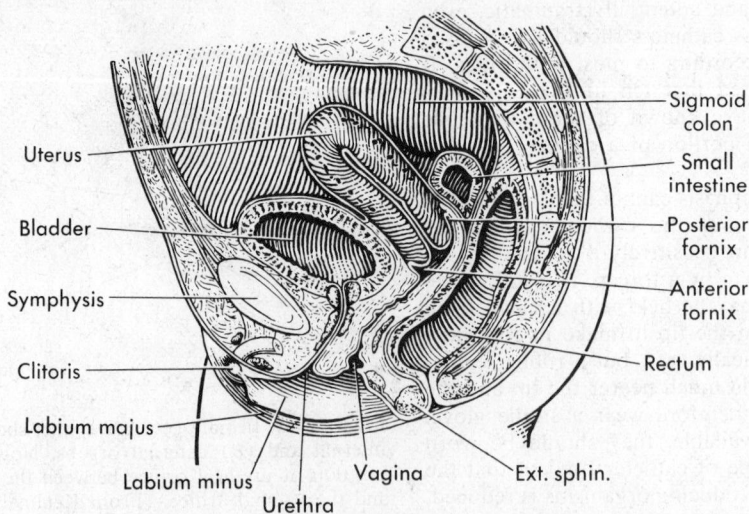

Figure 24-2. Median section of the female pelvis. Note the direction a nozzle should take to follow the normal curve of the vagina. (Miller, M. A., Leavell, L. C., and Drakontides, A. B.: *Kimber-Gray-Stackpole's Anatomy and Physiology,* 17th ed. Macmillan Publishing Co., Inc., New York, 1977.)

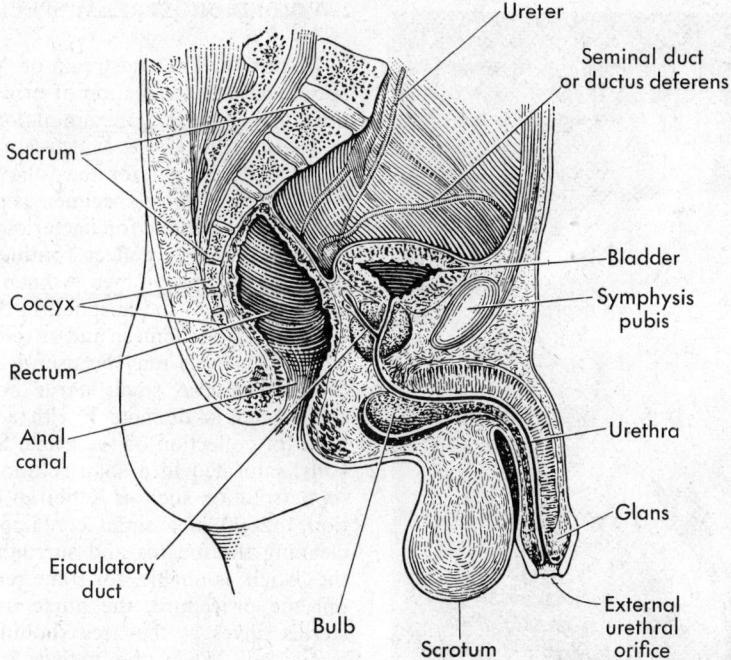

Figure 24-3. Median section of the male pelvis. Note the curve in the urethra that should be modified during the introduction of a catheter. (Miller, M. A., Leavell, L. C., and Drakontides, A. B.: *Kimber-Gray-Stackpole's Anatomy and Physiology*, 17th ed. Macmillan Publishing Co., Inc., New York, 1977.)

dence in the nurse. The treatment should be expeditious and so arranged that the patient is not left alone. The area should be well lighted so that there is no doubt as to whether the catheter is in the meatus. After the tip of the catheter is inserted, a few moments should be allowed for relaxation of the sphincter before introducing the catheter farther. If patients concentrate on deep breathing, look about the room, or do anything that takes their mind off the introduction of the catheter, relaxation is fostered. They should be discouraged from closing their eyes as this tends to increase the process of introspection, increasing tension. The catheter should be inserted by the operator in an upward and backward direction in the female; this is the course of the urethra with the patient lying in the dorsal recumbent position.

Introduction of a catheter in the male is more difficult than in the female, because the urethra is long and curving. Where it passes through the prostate gland and at various other points, there may be constriction caused by contraction of the surrounding tissue. In order to straighten the passageway as much as possible, the penis is held at an angle of 60 degrees. Ralph M. LeComte [24] says it should be drawn forward and upward from the body to stretch it slightly and in so doing straighten the anterior urethra.

Because the introduction of an instrument into the bladder is accompanied by danger of injury and infection, nurses should use all their skill and ingenuity to get the patient to void normally in cases of retention. Such measures are discussed in Chapters 11 and 37. If catheterization is unavoidable, we repeat for emphasis that the procedure must be performed in as aseptic a manner as possible and with the utmost gentleness in order to reduce the danger of trauma.

To prevent the necessity for repeated catheterization in cases where the neuromuscular mechanism is out of order, as in injuries to the lower part of the spinal cord, a retention catheter is left in the urethra. This may be opened periodically for drainage, or it may be attached to an apparatus that empties the bladder when the pressure within it approaches that which stimulates normal micturition. Periodic emptying with or without accompanying irrigation is more nearly physiologic than allowing the bladder to drain constantly.

Periodic emptying of the bladder is called tidal drainage. Closed drainage is also used, especially in the postoperative period. Both of these methods are described in this chapter.

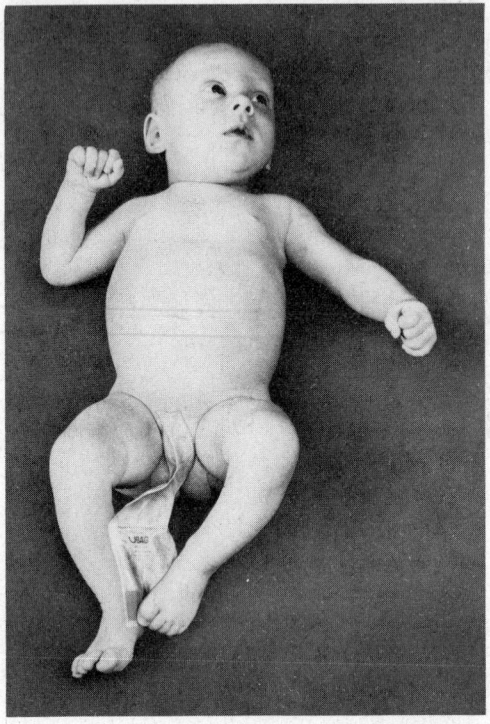

Figure 24-4. Urine collection bag for infants. The transparent patch, anatomically correct for boy or girl, has a narrow adhesive bridge that does not cover the anus, thus eliminating fecal contamination. The side-seal design lets the U-Bag collector hang tension-free between the thighs. (Courtesy of Hollister, Inc., Chicago, Ill.)

Kass introduced the voided midstream specimen as a substitute for the usual catheterized specimen. It seems logical to discuss this method before continuing the description of the catheterization.

2. VOIDED MIDSTREAM SPECIMEN

Definition. The midstream or "clean voided" specimen is the collection of urine for the purpose of bacteriologic examination.

Therapeutic Uses. Midstream urine specimens are collected for the following reasons: (1) to get as clean a specimen as possible, without catheterization, for bacteriologic examination; and (2) to collect routine urine specimens for analysis on men, women, and children on admission to the hospital, in the physician's office, nursing homes, and in other situations where urinalysis may be useful.

Equipment. A small sterile bottle (at least 1½ inches in diameter) with a screw top is used for collection of the urine. Several cotton balls, saturated in a soap solution or an antiseptic solution such as Zephiran chloride solution 1:2000 in a small container is used for cleaning the meatus and surrounding area. If the patient is unable, for some reason, to carry out the procedure, the nurse uses a pair of sterile gloves as the area should not be contaminated. When the patient is confined to bed, a sterile bedpan and waterproof pad to protect the bed is used. Mark Ridley[25] (in England) suggests that the technique (and therefore the equipment) should be simple because an elaborate technique offers more opportunity for contamination. Commercial sterilized midstream collection sets are available.

Preparation of the Patient. Of course, an explanation of the procedure is an essential first step as is an assessment of the patient's state of hydration. It is easier to void, especially in the presence of others, when the bladder is relatively full. Additional fluids may be given if they are indicated. When the patient has an urge to void, the procedure is started. If the patient is able to collect the specimen, it

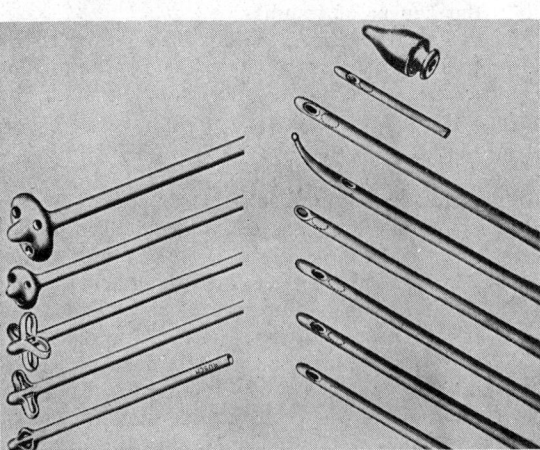

Figure 24-5. Various urologic catheters. *Left, top to bottom:* Pesser catheter, 30-mm head, three eyes, natural rubber latex with reinforced tip; Pesser catheter, smaller size, three eyes, natural rubber latex with reinforced tip; four-wing Malecot catheter, natural rubber latex with reinforced tip; and two two-wing Malecot catheters, natural rubber latex with reinforced tips. *Right, top to bottom:* Urethral tip, natural rubber; female catheter, solid tip, two eyes; Robinson catheter, hollow tip, two eyes; Tiermann catheter, coudé solid tip, olivary, one eye; whistletip catheter, one eye; Robinson catheter, red rubber, hollow tip, two eyes; Robinson catheter, amber, hollow tip, two eyes; and Nélaton catheter, red rubber, solid tip, one eye. (Courtesy of Clay-Adams Co., New York, N.Y.)

is done most easily sitting on the toilet. Following a study of 25 women, Cathryn Mainwaring[26] suggests that having the patient face the back of the toilet helps to separate the labia, provides more space, and ensures more privacy for the patient.

For the patient who is confined to bed, the specimen may best be obtained by having the patient lying on her back. The sterile bedpan should be in place and the bed protected with a waterproof pad. The top linens are folded below the hips and the chest is covered with a bath blanket. Of course, a good light is necessary.

Preparation of the man for a midstream specimen is very similar to that for catheterization. The prepuce is widely retracted and with the glans and *separated meatus* is thoroughly washed.[27] A surgical germicidal soap solution or antiseptic solution may be used. Most authorities consulted note that it is much easier to obtain an uncontaminated mid-stream specimen from men than from women. If the patient is unable to collect his own specimen, he will prefer help from a physician or male attendant but if neither is available the woman nurse will of course carry out the procedure.

Suggested Procedure. If the patient is able to collect the specimen and is a woman, accompany her to the bathroom at which time she washes her hands. If for any reason it is thought that she may contaminate herself, then gloves should be worn though this will probably not be necessary for the average person. She then sits on the toilet, facing the front or back as she prefers. Describe the technique step by step. Using the left hand, separate the labia, exposing the urethral meatus, and with the free hand, using a cotton ball saturated in a detergent or antiseptic, clean the area by making a downward stroke. Repeat this process at least twice, discarding the cotton balls in a waste container. After the meatus and surrounding area has been cleaned, hand the uncapped sterile container to the patient. Of course the left hand continues to be in place holding the labia well apart. Ask the patient to void a forceful stream, and catch a mid-stream specimen in the sterile bottle which is held away from the body—*the mouth of the bottle should never touch the body.*

For the patient who is confined to bed, the method is essentially the same. With the patient lying on her back, near the side of the bed, place the sterile bedpan and waterproof protector under the buttocks. Fold the top covers below the hips and, according to the room temperature, place the bath blanket over the upper part of the body to prevent chilling, and adjust the light. Place the equipment on the bedside table, so that it can be easily reached. After washing the hands, put on sterile plastic gloves. With the left hand, separate the labia, exposing the urethral meatus. Use the right hand to clean the area with a firm downward stroke. Discard the cotton balls in a waste

container. With the labia separated, ask the patient to void forcefully. After the stream has begun, catch at least 2 oz in the sterile bottle, never touching the labia with the container. The patient may not be able to void immediately so the nurse may have to wait awhile before the stream is begun.

In collecting a midstream specimen from a man, the same principles apply but preventing contamination of the urine is easier.

After the specimen has been collected, allow the patient to finish voiding and clean the genitalia. Remove the bedpan and bed protector. Rearrange the clothing and bedding, remove the equipment, and leave the surroundings in order.

Send the specimen to the laboratory *immediately,* labeling it with the patient's name, address (room number and patient unit in the hospital), and date and hour collected. Indicate the kind of specimen, and the type of examination desired. Note diagnosis, usually, and almost always the name of the attending physician.

Recording the Procedure. Chart the procedure, the time, and the difficulty or discomfort occasioned; also note the amount, appearance, and any unusual odor of the urine.

3. CATHETERIZATION OF THE URINARY BLADDER

Definition. The word *catheter* comes from a Greek word meaning a thing put down. Catheterization of the bladder is the introduction of a tube into the bladder, the tube being passed through the external opening or meatus. The general purpose of the treatment is to drain the bladder.

Therapeutic Uses. Catheterization is performed for the following reasons: (1) to get as clean a specimen of urine as possible for diagnostic purposes; (2) to determine whether the failure to void at all or to void a normal amount is due to inability to expel urine from the bladder (retention), or to failure of the kidneys to secrete urine (suppression); (3) to empty the bladder or remove a portion of the urine when a condition of retention is thought to exist; and (4) to prevent the patient's voiding voluntarily or involuntarily if there are surgical wounds, bedsores, or other conditions that make it important to keep the genitalia and surrounding area clean and dry.

Equipment. Commercially sterilized catheterization "kits" are available and except for the problem of disposal of waste are highly recommended. These "kits" include all necessary equipment, such as plastic forceps, several urethral catheters of different sizes, plastic gloves, specimen container, graduated plastic tray, waterproof underpad (to protect the linen and mattress), fenestrated towel, large absorbent balls, and sterilized lubricant packet.* If for some reason they are not available to the worker, then, of course, all equipment necessary to carry out the procedure effectively and safely must be assembled.

Usually several catheters are brought to the bedside in case one is accidentally contaminated, or the instrument has to be removed and reinserted (see Fig. 24-6). A pliable catheter, made of plastic or rubber, is the safest type, and should always be used for male patients, for children, for patients who are irrational and cannot be relied upon to keep still during the procedure; for obstetrical cases before delivery; for patients who have a urethral stricture or for those subject to urethral spasm; for patients who have had pelvic operations; and when the vagina is packed. Woven silk catheters are fairly pliable, but are not very satisfactory because they are destroyed by sterilization with heat. Commercially sterilized, disposable, plastic catheters are now available and highly recommended. The caliber of the catheter is determined by the size and condition of the urethra. The smallest effective catheter is preferred. Plastic and rubber catheters range in size from #10 to #22 French. If a pliable catheter is used, sterile gloves should be added to the equipment. In fact, it is always preferable to wear sterile gloves regardless of type of catheter used, otherwise the nurse must scrub the hands immediately before handling the catheter. Figure 24-7 shows the correct method for putting on sterile gloves. Unless scrubbing facilities are in the room or the nurse has an assistant, this adds to the possibility of contamination and necessitates leaving the patient, which is to be avoided if possible. If a stiff catheter is used and gloves are not available, rubber finger cots may be worn on the

* Pharmaseal Laboratories, Glendale, Calif.; Tomac, American Hospital Supply Co., Evanston, Ill.

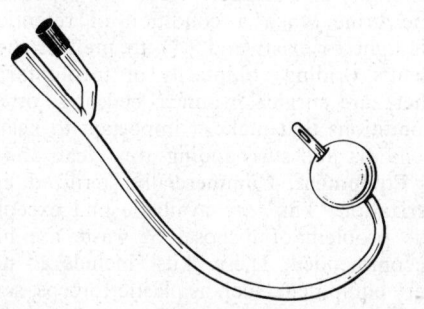

Figure 24-6. Rusch-Gold Foley catheter (made of latex impregnated with silicone) may remain in the bladder up to three weeks with proper care. (Courtesy of Rusch-Gold, Inc., New York, N.Y.)

thumb and first finger of the left hand which are used to separate the labia. A sterile lubricant is essential. An antibiotic ointment is recommended by several authorities. A small amount of warm detergent or antiseptic prescribed by the physician, such as pHisoHex or benzalkonium (Zephiran), with large cotton balls and forceps to apply it, is needed for cleaning the meatus and surrounding area. An antibacterial agent such as benzalkonium chloride 1:1000 or 1:750 prescribed by the physician, with an Asepto or bulb syringe to instill it, is needed to irrigate the distal urethra and surrounding area.

Several low, sterile-covered containers should be provided for the collection of urine. In an initial catheterization, when retention is suspected, provision should be made for the collection of 2000 ml (2 qt) of urine, as a patient may have this amount in the bladder. Since nurses cannot leave the patient to get another vessel, they are in a very awkward situation if the containers they have provided are inadequate. A paper bag or other type of receptacle should be provided for dry waste. A small rubber square with cotton or a waterproof paper pad is used to protect the bed. Sterile draping is necessary to provide a sterile field on which to work. With a male patient it is convenient to have a sterile fenestrated sheet or several sterile towels with which to surround the penis after the glans and meatus have been cleaned.

All this equipment, with the exception of the bed protector which may be kept in the patient's unit, should be brought to the bedside on a covered tray or cart, together with the catheter, lubricant, gloves, and cleansing material. Moistureproof wrappers, covered trays, or small drums are used to keep the equipment sterile.

Before preparing the equipment, the catheter should be scrutinized for defects. Only perfect instruments should be used; rubber catheters that have lost their resiliency and cracked or roughened instruments should be discarded.

Preparation of the Patient. Gain the patients' cooperation by explaining the necessity for the treatment and finding out how much or little they know about it and how they feel about having the treatment. As in all such cases, what is said to the patients depends upon their intelligence, former experience, and condition. It is most desirable that they accept the treatment; an unreceptive attitude inevitably hinders relaxation and thereby increases discomfort and possible danger.

Have the patients lying on their back near the side of the bed most convenient for the nurse. In catheterizing a female patient, the

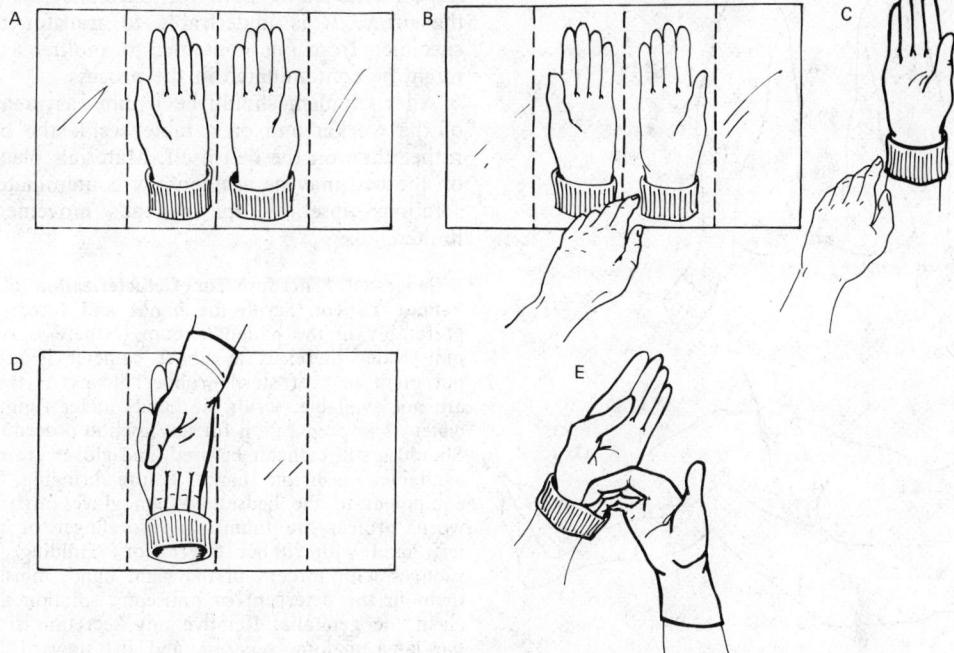

Figure 24-7. Correct method of putting on sterile gloves. Since the shaded portion of the glove is considered contaminated, it is the only part touched by the hand as the gloves are put on.

knees should be flexed, the feet flat on the bed, and the legs well separated while the meatus is cleaned and the bladder emptied (see Fig. 24-8). If the patient is weak or irrational, the flexed legs should be supported with rubber-covered pillows. In order to keep the irrational patient in the desired posture, restraining devices or several assistants may be necessary. Place the waterproof protector over the bedding between the legs and slightly under the buttocks; arrange the clothing in neat folds above the hips; replace the upper bedclothes with two treatment blankets folded in half lengthwise. Both these blankets remain over the chest and arms, but are separated over the lower abdomen so that the genitalia are exposed and each leg is wrapped or covered with one of the folded blankets. In hot weather very thin blankets or cotton sheets should be used for this draping. See that the room is warm; and, if the patient shows signs of being cold, place hot-water bottles at the feet. It is important for the patient to be warm, not only for his or her comfort and welfare but also as a means of promoting relaxation of the urethral musculature. The lateral position also may be used when catheterizing a woman. The patient may lie on either side, depending on which position is most comfortable, with the buttocks near the edge of the bed and the knees drawn toward the chest. Arrange the clothing so that the patient is kept warm and protected from unnecessary exposure. Figure 24-9 shows positions for urinary catheterization of women.

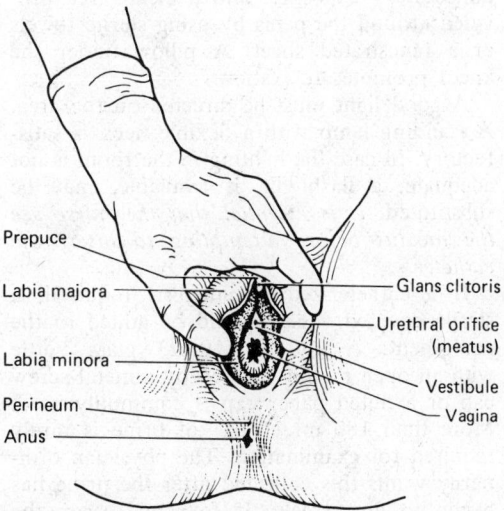

Prepuce

Labia majora

Labia minora

Perineum

Anus

Glans clitoris

Urethral orifice (meatus)

Vestibule

Vagina

Figure 24-8. With the patient in the dorsal recumbent position, separate the labia minora, clean the area, and insert the catheter.

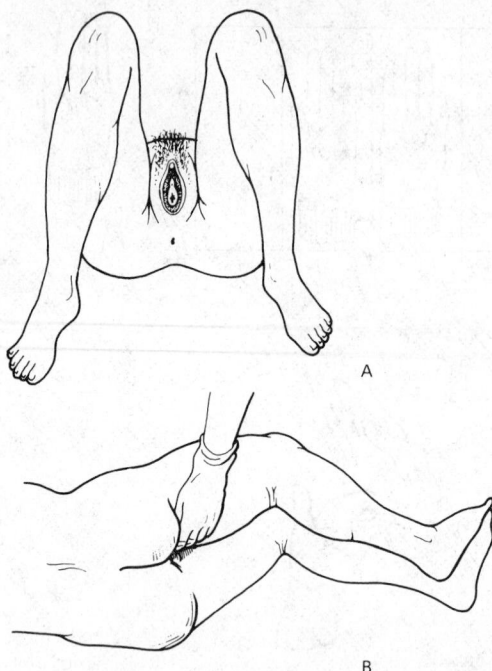

Figure 24-9. Positions for urinary catheterization of women. *A*. Dorsal recumbent position. *B*. Lateral position. Covering omitted for clarity of illustration. Use the *B* position only if *A* position is impossible.

In the preparation of a male patient, the chest may be covered with a folded treatment blanket, and the upper bedclothes turned down to the pubes and covered with a waterproof square. The patient should be protected from unnecessary exposure, and a clean area provided around the penis by using sterile towels or a fenestrated sheet. A pillow under the knees promotes relaxation.

A good light must be directed on the area. A standing lamp with a flexible neck is satisfactory. In case the lighting in the room is not adequate, a flashlight, if available, may be substituted. *It is essential that the nurse see the meatus before attempting to insert the catheter.*

If a catheterized specimen is required, a sterile covered vessel should be added to the equipment. A 300-ml (10-oz) glass bottle with an open mouth covered by a metal screw cap or a fluted paper cap is commonly used. More than 180 ml (6 oz) of urine is rarely required for examination. The physician ordinarily wants this collected after the urine has begun to flow freely. If for any reason the whole amount, or a sample from the whole amount, is required, the covered pans used to receive the urine must be kept sterile or a very

large sterile bottle used for the collection of the urine. It is undesirable to transfer the specimen from one container to another as it might be contaminated in the process.

All equipment should be within easy reach of the worker and on a table beside the bed rather than on the bed itself. Materials placed on the bed may be accidentally contaminated, solutions upset, or the patient's movements limited.

Suggested Procedure for Catheterization of a Female Patient. Scrub the hands and forearms, preferably in the patient's room if there is running water there. If a rubber catheter is used, put on a pair of sterile rubber gloves; if these are not available, scrub the hands under running water as in preparation for any aseptic procedure. Should a stiff catheter be used, and gloves are not available, wash the hands before bringing the equipment to the bedside. When gloves are not worn, protect the thumb and forefinger of the left hand with rubber finger cots. Holding the sponges with forceps in the right hand, moisten them in the detergent or antiseptic solution and clean the genitalia. Remove any secretion from the labia majora, separate and lift upward the labia minora with the thumb and forefinger of the left hand, exposing the meatus. Clean the area around the meatus with particular care. It is desirable, but not necessary, to remove the detergent with sterile water; the area should then be dried. Throughout this cleaning process, use a gentle but firm downward motion and take a fresh sponge for each stroke. The last sponge may be left in the vaginal orifice to keep any vaginal secretions from spreading upward over the meatus. (When this is done, care should be taken that the sponge is placed in the orifice and not packed in the vagina, as this would cause pressure on the urethra and interfere with the passage of the catheter.) When an antibacterial agent is used in the urethra, 5 ml may be instilled into the distal urethra with an Asepto or bulb syringe. The meatus and surrounding area is also irrigated. The area should then be dried. Without removing the fingers of the left hand from the labia, place the receptacle for the urine in position on the bed, dip the tip of the catheter into the lubricant, and insert the catheter into the urethral meatus without allowing anything to touch that portion that is to come in contact with the urethra. If a pliable catheter is used, it must be grasped near enough the tip to control its direction; if the catheter is rigid, it may be held as much as 4 inches from its eye without any loss of control by the operator. After relaxation has followed the initial contraction of the urethra, introduce the catheter about 4 cm (1½ inches), or until the urine begins to flow. Since the bladder may in some cases be empty, the rule "until the urine begins to flow" must not be followed too literally. The catheter should not be introduced much more than the supposed length of the urethra without consulting a physician. When introducing the catheter, bear in mind the upward and backward direction of the urethra. If a catheterized specimen is desired, keep the outer end of the catheter sterile until after the specimen is collected. This is received in a small sterile glass bottle after the urine begins to flow freely. If the physician wants to examine the whole amount, or a sample taken from the whole amount, collect the urine in a large sterile bottle or vessel that can be sent to the laboratory.

As soon as the urine ceases to flow freely, or drips from the end of the catheter, withdraw the instrument slightly to see whether any more urine will flow with the eye of the instrument nearer the urethral outlet. Withdraw the catheter slowly, and when the bladder appears to be empty, remove the catheter gently. If only a prescribed amount of urine is to be removed, the nurse should have some way of determining when this has been withdrawn. The procedure can be stopped at any time by removing the catheter from the bladder. After the removal of the catheter, clean the meatus of any excess lubricant. Rearrange the clothing and bedding, remove the equipment, and leave the surroundings in order. When the lateral position is used, lift the upper buttock and labia to expose the urinary meatus and carry out the procedure as described above. Sterile drapes may be used to extend the work area beyond the immediate perineal area.

Recording the Treatment. Chart the treatment, the time, and the pain or discomfort occasioned; also the amount, appearance, and any unusual odor of the urine withdrawn.

Suggested Procedure for Catheterization of a Male Patient. Wear rubber gloves or prepare the hands as for any aseptic procedure. With the left hand retract the foreskin, exposing the meatus, situated in the center of the glans. Using the forceps in the right hand to keep this hand uncontaminated, clean the area surrounding the meatus. After lubricating the catheter insert it into the meatus, gently stretching the penis with the left hand and lifting it to an angle of about 60 degrees in order to straighten the urethral canal as much as possible (see Figure 24-10). Insert the catheter approximately 17½ cm (7 in) or until the urine begins to flow. The same precaution should be taken with the male patient as with the female patient—not to insert the catheter an unreasonable distance. The bladder may be empty, and it is possible to injure its lining by forcing a catheter along its walls. Since the length and size of the penis vary in different individuals, the size of the catheter and the length of the insertion will therefore have to be determined in each case. The passage of an instrument through the male urethra is often a difficult procedure. Before attempting it, the operator should get a clear picture in his mind of the structure and position of the urethra and surrounding tissues; this is essential for an intelligent direction of the course of the catheter and for manipulation of the parts in such a way as to eliminate as far as possible the urethral folds and curvatures.

The physician usually passes the catheter in the male patient or supervises its passage. Exposure and handling of the genitalia in medical

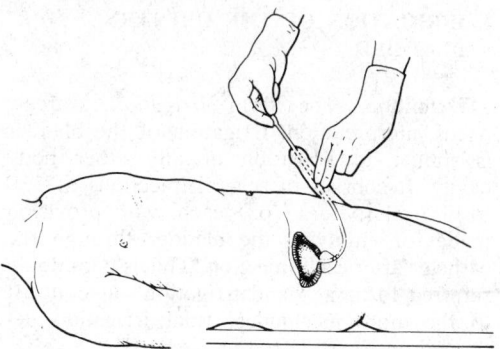

Figure 24-10. Insertion of a catheter into the male bladder. Lift the penis 60 degrees (or higher) from the body to straighten the urethral canal.

treatment and nursing care are generally less embarrassing to men and women if members of their own sex are in attendance upon them; for this reason the catheterization of a male patient is usually performed by a man physician in order to reduce the embarrassment, which is not only unpleasant for the patient but may interfere with relaxation. In some hospitals men nurses or special technicians are taught to give this treatment but any professional woman nurse should be prepared to carry out the procedure when need arises.

Self-Catheterization. A number of urologists, including Jack Lapides, who have studied the physiology of micturition, stress the importance of preventing bladder distention, which they believe predisposes the bladder to infection. In 1972 he and his associates introduced a clean self-catheterization technique so that people with neurogenic bladder dysfunction could avoid diversionary surgery, indwelling catheters, or the urine-collecting devices that are often associated with skin infection.[27a] Anne Altshuler and her associates describe a program to teach children from 8 to 17 to catheterize themselves. Parents of younger children are taught the procedure and also taught to help older children. Of the 55 children in the program of the Children's Hospital, University of Wisconsin in Madison, 37 were able to stay dry for more than 80 per cent of the time with self-catheterization. Altshuler makes the following statement:

Studies are now being conducted . . . to evaluate infection rates and long-term changes in the genitourinary tract. So far, a third of our population has been infection-free since starting CISCP [clean, intermittent self-catheterization program]; another third is on suppressive antibiotics and the rest are treated only when cultures demonstrate infection.*

* Altshuler, Anne, et al.: "Even Children Can Learn to Do Clean Self-Catheterization," *Am. J. Nurs.,* 77:97, (Jan.) 1977.

4. IRRIGATION OF THE URINARY BLADDER

Definition. The term *irrigation* scarcely needs interpretation. Irrigation of the bladder is similar to irrigation of any other body cavity. It consists of several injections of 150 to 400 ml (5 to 13 oz) each, with provision made for emptying the bladder through the catheter after each injection. This is commonly referred to as a "hand irrigation" in contrast to the more mechanical tidal irrigation described on page 1277.

Therapeutic Uses. Irrigations are given for the following reasons: (1) to clean the bladder; (2) to prevent formation of calcific deposits in and around indwelling catheters; and (3) to medicate the lining of the bladder for which usually an antiseptic, an astringent, or an anticoagulant is used. Cystitis is now more often treated with systemic drugs than with local applications. Nitrofurantoin, ampicillin, penicillin G, nalidixic acid, the tetracyclines, and the sulfa drugs are particularly effective, although methenamine (Urotropin), mandelic acid, and other drugs are often used.[27b]

Selection of Method. An irrigation of the bladder may be given with a reservoir, such as a plastic or glass container, or an irrigating can, filled with solution and attached to a two-way, or Y-shaped, catheter. The fluid flows into the bladder through one arm of the catheter and out through the other. The fluid may also be introduced through a funnel attached to the catheter, inverting the funnel to empty the bladder, and repeating these alternate steps until the prescribed amount of solution has been used or until the return is clear. A third method is injecting the solution through the catheter with a large syringe, detaching the syringe and emptying the bladder by lowering the catheter, repeating this process until the treatment is completed.

If a large amount of solution is prescribed, or if it is ordered for its thermal effect, the reservoir method is probably best, since it maintains the solution at a fairly uniform temperature. Most physicians, however, prefer the closed irrigation-drainage method which is discussed on page 1276. The funnel method is often used by nurses caring for patients in their homes because the equipment is simple and easily transported. The disadvantages of this method are that the solution cools quickly, and, unless the worker is very skilled, the instruments are contaminated, air is introduced with the liquid, and the bedding soiled. The syringe method is easy, the equipment is not difficult to procure, and it can be transported in a small space. The temperature of the solution probably remains more constant when the syringe is used rather than the funnel, and there is less risk of injecting air and soiling the bedding.

Equipment. To the articles collected for catheterization should be added a sterile calibrated container for the prescribed amount of solution and either a glass-and-rubber syringe or a funnel for injecting it. If an irrigating can is used, the solution may be carried to the bedside in it; for a female catheterization a two-way catheter, which has a short piece of rubber tubing and a clamp on the outflow arm, is needed. Clamps should be provided for the inflow tube also. In case a rubber catheter is used, a glass Y tube is inserted into the open end of the catheter to provide a passageway for the inflow and outflow.

A fairly large shallow pan, which can be placed on the bed near the meatus, must be provided for the return flow. A covered pail, large enough to hold the entire amount of fluid used in the treatment should be conveniently placed for emptying this pan each time it fills.

The *irrigating fluids* commonly used are physiologic sodium chloride solution; boric acid 2 per cent; potassium permanganate, 1:10,000; acriflavin, 1:10,000; and benzalkonium chloride, 1:20,000. These solutions are helpful in relieving vesical irritation. Silver nitrate, 1:5000, is often used following a single catheterization. Acetic acid solution (0.25 per cent) may be prescribed for severe *Pseudomonas* infection and neomycin sulfate solution (0.5 per cent) to cut down the number of bacteria. Neomycin solution must be kept in the refrigerator when not in use to prevent decomposition. Suby's solution, also known as "G" or "urologic solution," and renacidin solution (10 per cent) are prescribed when the patient has a long-term indwelling catheter. They prevent calcific precipitation which may necessitate frequent changing of the catheter. Renacidin must be kept refrigerated when not in use because the organic acids in the solution decompose rapidly at room temperature. *Any solution used must be sterile.*[28-30] Nurses are not responsible for selecting the kind of solution or the strength. They should know that high concentrations of irritating drugs are not ordinarily prescribed for the bladder, and if they should see an order for such a treatment they are justified in questioning the physician as to whether there may not have been some error in the writing of the order or misinterpretation in reading it. If, as sometimes happens, physicians prescribe a bladder irrigation without specifying the kind of solution and nurses are unable to communicate with them, he or she could safely use physiologic saline.

Unless otherwise directed, the solution

should be administered at body temperature, that is, it should be around 37.2°C (99°F) as it enters the bladder. Lowsley and Kirwin say temperatures ranging from 37.8° to 43.4°C (100° to 110°F) may be used according to the tolerance of the patient. In cystitis and urethritis the mucous membrane is highly sensitive to temperatures varying appreciably from that of the body. It is, therefore, important to regulate accurately the temperature of the solution. At room temperatures—around 25°C (77°F), 1000 ml (1 qt) of solution should be prepared at approximately 42°C (107.6°F) to allow for the cooling that takes place while the patient is catheterized and the solution injected. All equipment should be sterile, with the exception of the large covered pail used in procedure No. 1 for receiving the irrigating fluid.

Suggested Procedure. Catheterize the patient in the usual manner, keeping the outlet of the catheter uncontaminated. The irrigation may be done in any of the following ways, according to the type of equipment used:

No. 1. Using an irrigator: Hang or support the reservoir so that the surface of the liquid is not more than 15 to 20 cm (6 to 8 inches) above the level of the meatus. Attach the tubing to one arm of the two-way catheter or, if a rubber catheter is used, attach the tubing to the catheter by a glass Y-shaped tube. Expel the air from the tubing before attaching the catheter. Place the basin to receive the return under the outflow tube; clamp the outlet tube. Open the inflow tube and inject the solution in such an amount as to get the degree of distention prescribed by the physician. The amount introduced at one time varies from 30 to 500 ml (1 to 16 oz), according to the condition of the bladder and the purpose of the treatment. The physician may direct that the treatment be given so that the bladder is distended with increasingly large amounts. Between these injections of fluid, the bladder is drained by opening the outflow tube. The order for the treatment may stipulate that a definite amount of solution be used, or the physician may ask that the irrigating process be kept up until the return from the bladder is clear. At the end of the irrigation, clamp the tubing, remove the catheter gently, and complete the treatment according to the directions for catheterization on page 1268.

No. 2. Using a funnel: Attach the funnel to the catheter with the uncontaminated right hand. Place the basin for collection of the return on the bed conveniently near the meatus. Hold the funnel with one hand and with the other pour the desired amount of solution from the calibrated container down the side of the funnel. The amount of solution to be introduced at one time varies, as just stated. Physicians may want the same amount introduced at each injection, or they may request that the amount be increased with each injection. When introducing the solution, do not allow the funnel to empty. If the tubing is allowed to empty,

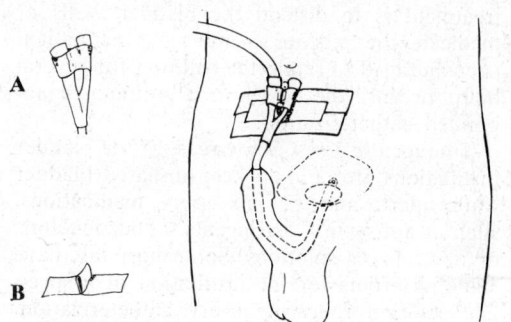

Figure 24-11. *A.* The catheter tips are taped together to prevent the tubing from turning on itself. *B.* The tape is prepared to place onto abdominal tape strips. *C.* When the catheter is taped to the abdomen a continuous "circle" is maintained, which helps prevent ulceration. (From Anderson, Edith, et al.: *Current Concepts in Clinical Nursing.* C. V. Mosby Co., St. Louis, 1973.)

air will be sucked into the bladder. To empty the bladder between injections of the irrigating solution, pinch the tubing, lower and invert the funnel over the basin for the return. The alternate processes of filling and emptying the bladder are kept up as directed above, and the treatment terminated in the same way as under method No. 1.

No. 3. Using a syringe: Clamp or pinch the catheter used to empty the bladder so that it will not drain dry, fill the Asepto syringe from the calibrated container of solution; attach the syringe tip to the catheter, being careful not to contaminate either, and inject the solution slowly into the bladder. If more than one syringeful is to be injected before emptying the bladder, pinch the tubing, detach and refill the syringe, and proceed as above. In order to empty the bladder, pinch the tubing, detach the syringe, lower the tubing over the basin for the return and remove the pressure on the tubing. Repeat these alternate processes of filling and emptying the bladder and finish the procedure as directed under method No. 1.

Recording the Treatment. Chart the treatment and the time at which it was given; any pain or discomfort experienced; the kind, concentration, and amount of solution used; the appearance of the return—whether it contained mucus, pus, bloodtinged particles, or other substances indicative of the condition of the bladder. Record the amount of urine withdrawn before the irrigation and describe its appearance.

5. INSTILLATION OF THE URINARY BLADDER

Definition. An *instillation* of the bladder is the introduction of a small amount of sterile water or some medication into the bladder through a catheter. Since the purpose of the treatment is to distend the bladder walls or medicate the mucous membrane, the patient is encouraged to retain the solution for several hours or until the next normal voiding or appointed catheterization.

Therapeutic Uses. Some reasons for bladder instillations are: (1) to keep diseased bladder walls apart; and (2) to apply medications, such as antiseptics, astringents, anticoagulants, or neutralizing solutions. Some hospitals have standing orders for the instillation of a specified solution following every catheterization. Many physicians believe that this is a necessary precaution in the prevention of infection; it is not done, however, as a substitute for aseptic technique, which is essential.

Equipment. Everything listed as necessary for catheterization is needed for bladder instillation and, in addition, a small funnel and glass and rubber connections to attach the funnel to the catheter. A glass-and-rubber syringe may be used in place of the funnel. A calibrated container, such as a measuring glass or cup, should be provided for the drug to be instilled. It is desirable to have the drug near body temperature, but chemicals whose composition is altered by heat should not be warmed. The drugs for irrigation (page 1270), as well as mild silver protein (Argyrol, 5 per cent), are used. Urinary antiseptics given systemically in many cases may be used locally. The antibiotics and sulfa drugs, for example, are sometimes instilled.

Suggested Procedure. Catheterize the patient in the usual way, completely emptying the bladder but not draining the catheter. Attach the funnel to the catheter and, holding the funnel about 12½ cm (5 inches) above the level of the meatus, pour into the side of the funnel the liquid to be instilled. Pinch the rubber attachment, or the rubber catheter if one is used, when the funnel empties; remove the catheter gently. Before giving the treatment the nurse should learn whether the physician wants the drug retained for several hours or a short period only. When irritating antiseptics are used, some physicians direct that the drug be immediately siphoned from the bladder.

Recording the Treatment. Chart the treatment, the time at which it was given, any attendant pain or discomfort, the nature, strength, and amount of the drug, and the catheterization preceding the instillation.

6. CLOSED DRAINAGE OF THE URINARY BLADDER

Definition. Drainage of the urinary bladder consists of draining its contents (urine) by way of an indwelling catheter attached to a closed system which reduces the possibility of organisms entering the lower urinary tract through the apparatus.

Therapeutic Uses. Closed drainage of the urinary bladder is used for the following purposes: (1) to empty the bladder when the patient, for a variety of reasons, is unable to void normally; and (2) to prevent bed wetting and maceration of the skin of an incontinent patient. Noting that the indwelling catheter is an essential part of medical care, Calvin M. Kunin and Regina C. McCormack say:

It is widely used to give temporary relief of anatomic or physiologic urinary obstruction, facilitate surgical repair of the urethra and surrounding structures, provide a dry environment for comatose or incontinent patients and permit accurate measurement of urinary output in severely ill patients.[*]

They describe the closed-drainage method as a way of reducing infections associated with indwelling catheters. Authorities agree that a closed drainage system should be used, but some physicians think that the danger of chronic infection following this treatment is, under any circumstances, so great that incontinence, as that following a stroke, should be tolerated until bladder control returns.

Discussing treatment of the neurogenic bladder, Donald R. Smith [31] says the use of closed drainage with irrigation three times daily is probably just as effective as tidal drainage in maintaining vesical capacity. Steve J. Misak and R. Carl Bunts [32] (in 1963) report that Veterans Administration paraplegic centers were using continuous intraurethral catheter drainage in the treatment of paraplegics. Over a 6-year period a progressive decline in urethral complications such as fistulas and diverticula was attributed to the following: (1) use of a small catheter (#16 to #18 French); (2) taping the catheter to the lower abdomen to reduce angulation at the penoscrotal junction (see Fig. 24–11); (3) using the Bunts Multiholed, 3-way catheter for long-term urethral catheter drainage; (4) irrigating the urethra and bladder 2 or 3 times a day with clorpactin (performed by technician or patient); and (5) changing the catheter weekly.

Selection of Equipment and Method. The two types most frequently used, according to John G. Keuhnelian and Virginia E. Sanders,[33] are *the straight* and *decompression* drainage. Straight drainage depends on gravity to drain the bladder. Tubing is used to connect the end of the catheter to the collecting device, which

---

[*] Kunin, Calvin M., and McCormack, Regina C.: "Prevention of Catheter-Induced Urinary-Tract Infections by Sterile Closed Drainage," *N. Engl. J. Med.*, **274:**1155, (May 26) 1966.

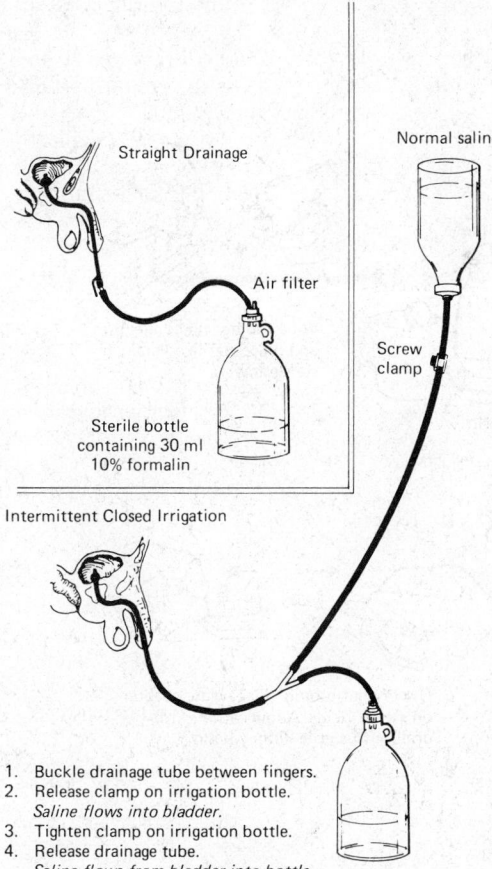

1. Buckle drainage tube between fingers.
2. Release clamp on irrigation bottle.
   Saline flows into bladder.
3. Tighten clamp on irrigation bottle.
4. Release drainage tube.
   Saline flows from bladder into bottle.

Figure 24-12. Aseptic drainage techniques. (From Ansell, J. S.: "Catheter Care," *J. Urol.*, **89**:942, [June] 1963.)

may be a bottle or plastic bag at the bedside (or attached to a wheelchair) or a bag applied to the patient's leg if he or she is up (see Fig. 37-2 and Fig. 37-4 in Chapter 37). In the latter case, the patient is able to walk about. Decompression drainage allows the bladder to empty slowly by having the urine drain uphill or against gravity. Tubing is attached to the end of the catheter and to a Y tube which has another connecting tube that extends to the collecting device. The Y tube (one end remains open) is attached to a bedside pole and is raised the necessary distance above the level of the bladder to ensure a certain quantity of urine in the bladder at all times. This method is used to slowly empty an overdistended bladder; also to control bleeding from the bladder by raising the intravesical pressure. This acts as a mild tamponade against venous bleeding.

Another method, frequently described, is the *intermittent bladder irrigation.* This allows for drainage and irrigation. The catheter is

attached to the Y connecting piece which has tubing attached to both arms, one to allow the urine to flow into the collecting device and the other (connected to a reservoir containing the irrigating solution) to allow irrigation. The bottle of solution—usually hung on a pole at the foot of the bed—is maintained for irrigating purposes [34] (see Fig. 24-15). *Frequent irrigations are discouraged by all urologists.*

The selection and use of equipment are very important in the prevention of urinary tract infection in patients with indwelling catheters. Most authors suggest a plastic, disposable, sterile drainage system. Kunin and McCormack [35] (in 1966), following a study of the effectiveness of the B-D Asepto closed drainage system, recommend it for general use. They believe it would prevent catheter-induced infection because 77 per cent of the large sample studied had sterile urine at the time the catheter was removed. Maintaining this system included the following conditions: the junction of the catheter with the drainage system was never broken; urine specimens were collected by aspirating the urine from the proximal lumen of the catheter after cleaning it with an alcohol sponge; collecting bags were never inverted but always hung on the side of the bed, chair, or stretcher; bags were drained every 8 hours; perineal care with soap and water was given twice daily; finally, catheters were irrigated only when the physician suspected an obstruction. Zachary Finkelberg and Kunin [36] (1969) contend that a multitude of mechanical devices, including closed urinary drainage systems, are being placed on the market with little or no preliminary clinical trial; consequently, they studied eight different systems manufactured by seven companies. The following problems were observed: (1) delayed urine flow which could be confused with retention; (2) cotton or other types of filters were frequently wet in systems using this device; (3) assembling the system and maintaining the proper vertical position of the bag was difficult; (4) urinary retention occurred with some systems; and (5) the outlet for drainage was difficult to clamp. The results of the study were shared with the manufacturers, and the products have been modified or withdrawn from the market; however, the authors say:

We urge each institution to conduct brief preliminary trials on those that appear most promising and select the bag which best meets the needs of patient care.*

* Finkelberg, Zachary, and Kunin, Calvin M.: "Clinical Evaluation of Closed Urinary Drainage Systems," *J.A.M.A.*, **207**:1657, (Mar. 3) 1969.

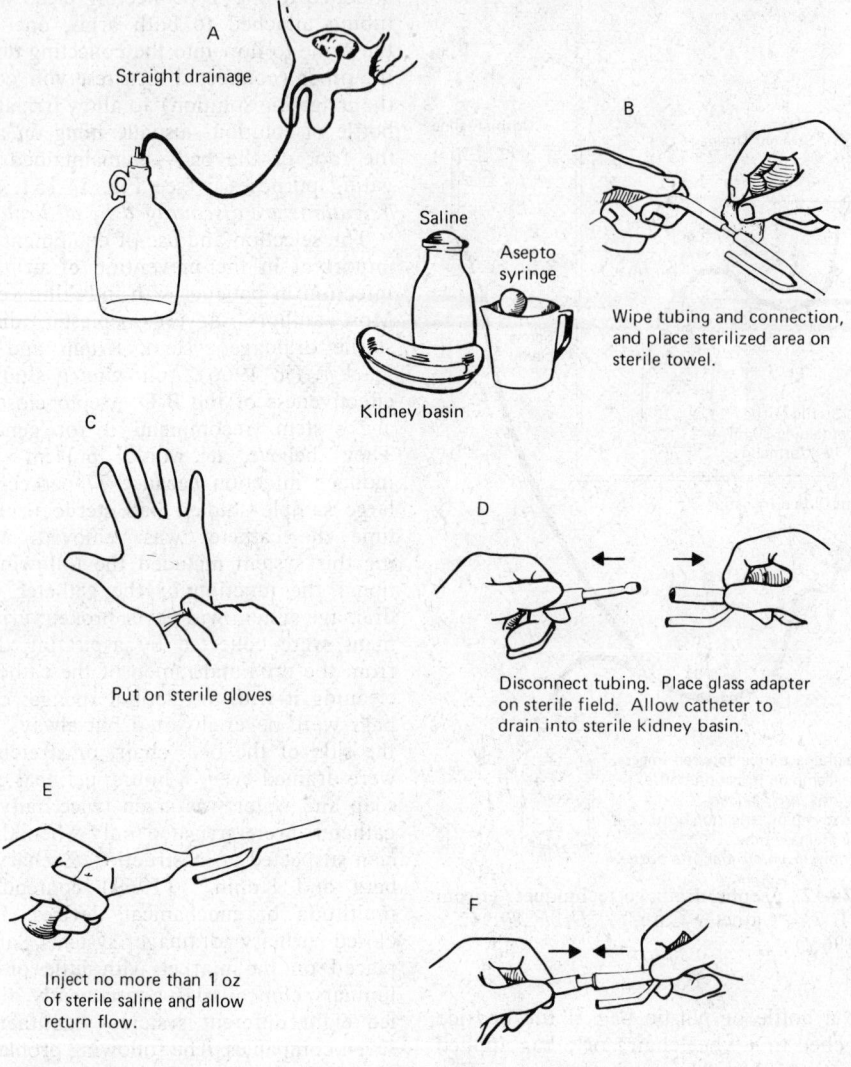

A
Straight drainage

B
Saline
Asepto syringe
Kidney basin
Wipe tubing and connection, and place sterilized area on sterile towel.

C
Put on sterile gloves

D
Disconnect tubing. Place glass adapter on sterile field. Allow catheter to drain into sterile kidney basin.

E
Inject no more than 1 oz of sterile saline and allow return flow.

F
Replace glass connector in catheter.

Figure 24-13. Technique of hand irrigation. (From Ansell, J. S.: "Catheter Care," *J. Urol.*, **89**:942, [June] 1963.)

A number of ways are recommended to prevent bacterial entry through the catheter lumen. A disinfectant such as formaldehyde (40 per cent) in the collecting bottle will control the multiplication of bacteria in the urine and air bubbles rising up the lumen of the catheter will not be a source of infection.[37] *Formaldehyde is not used in collapsible bags because of the danger of expressing the contents of the bag into the bladder.* A drip chamber in the connecting tube at the junction of the tube and the drainage bag is used in some systems, providing an air barrier between the bag and the connecting tube.[38] Virginia Cleland and associates [39] report that its use did not alter the inci-

dence of bacteriuria in a group of 184 patients; however, the products were not mechanically dependable and the staff and patients did not use them properly in all instances. When moving a patient, the drainage system should not be disconnected but goes with him or her. Urine specimens are collected by inserting a needle in the catheter after it is cleaned with an antiseptic solution. (The aspirated urine is then put in a bottle.) [40] Bacteria are less likely to ascend the lumen of the catheter when the flow of urine is greater than 25 ml per hour; therefore, patients should drink enough to ensure an adequate urinary output. Some urologists say that the patient on unrestricted fluid

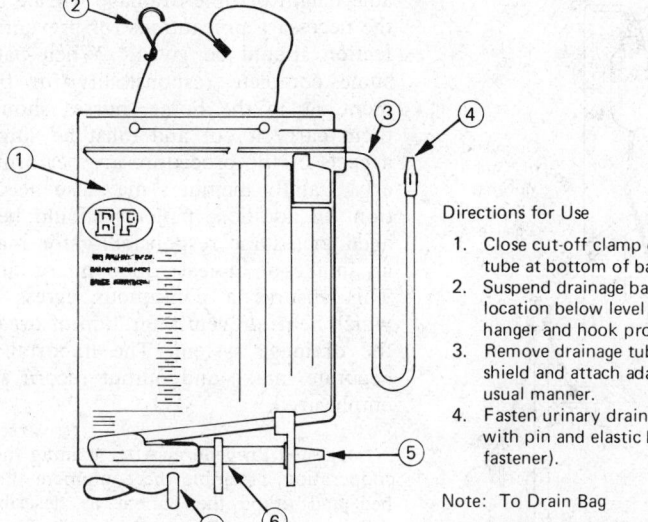

Directions for Use

1. Close cut-off clamp on the discharge tube at bottom of bag.
2. Suspend drainage bag in any desired location below level of patient, using cord hanger and hook provided on bag.
3. Remove drainage tube adaptor protector shield and attach adaptor to catheter in usual manner.
4. Fasten urinary drainage tube to bedding with pin and elastic band (drainage tube fastener).

Note: To Drain Bag

A. Remove discharge tube hanger cap.
B. Place drainage tube over collection container.
C. Open cut-off clamp and drain bag, leaving small amount of fluid in the draining tube.
D. Close cut-off clamp and pinch or milk tubing between clamp and discharge end to empty residual fluid.
E. Thoroughly clean discharge tube end and hanger cap with antiseptic solution.
F. Replace discharge tube in hanger cap.

1. 2000 ml graduated drainage bag with filtered air vent.
2. Cord hanger and hook.
3. Drainage tube.
4. Drainage tube adaptor with protector shield.
5. Discharge tube hanger cap.
6. Discharge tube with mounted cut-off clamp.
7. Drainage tube fastener.

Figure 24-14. Closed system urinary drainage set: B-P Asepto II. Left-hand column gives information about each part of bag; column on right gives directions for using and draining the bag. (Courtesy of Bard-Parker, Division of Becton, Dickinson & Co., Rutherford, N.J.)

intake with an indwelling catheter should have 3000 ml liquid daily.

Several approaches are reported as successful in preventing bacterial entry to the bladder through the space between the urethral wall and the catheter. These include use of catheters impregnated with antibacterial agents,[41] instillation of an antibacterial agent in the bladder and around the catheter,[42,43] and perineal care at least twice daily.[44,45] Cleland and associates,[46] however, found that four types of perineal care different from patient-administered self-care in a total sample of 184 female subjects had no effect on the incidence of urinary infection. Although reported studies differ in their findings on the effectiveness of perineal care in reducing urinary infection, nurses should continue to give meticulous care to the perineum with soap and water at least twice daily and more frequently if this is necessary. As we have said, Kass demonstrated conclusively that bacteria will enter the bladder through the fluid at the junction of the catheter and urethra.

The smallest size catheter that is effective is suggested by most urologists. A #16 or #18 Foley catheter is frequently used. The Gibbon catheter (developed in England) is also used but it is too small for irrigations.[47]

Solutions used to irrigate and medicate the vesical wall are similar to those listed for irrigation of the bladder "by hand." Suby's (or G) solution and renacidin (10 per cent) is recommended in long-term urinary drainage to prevent calcific deposits, usually phosphates, in the lumen of the catheter. Both of these solutions are irritating to the bladder wall and are used only when prescribed by the physician. Acetic acid 0.25 per cent solution also is used to control urinary infection in patients who have indwelling catheters for weeks or months.

All equipment should be selected before the procedure is begun. Equipment necessary for a catheterization is needed and, in addition, a sterile collecting device (bottle or calibrated plastic bag), with sterile connecting tubing, glass connector, and catheters, sizes #16 or

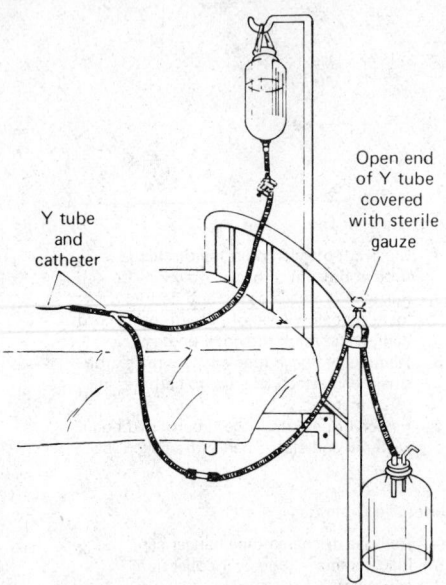

Y tube and catheter

Open end
of Y tube
covered
with sterile
gauze

Figure 24-15. Keyes intermittent bladder irrigator. (From Campbell, Meredith F., and Harrison, J. Hartwell: *Urology,* Vol. III, 3rd ed. W. B. Saunders Co., Philadelphia, 1970, p. 2502.)

#18 Foley. At least two catheters are needed in case one is contaminated during the procedure. Sterile disposable systems consisting of all equipment needed for the procedure are available and used in many hospitals, clinics, and homes in the United States. This equipment is necessary for *closed straight drainage.* When *intermittent closed irrigation and drainage* is used, additional equipment needed includes a calibrated irrigating bottle containing the irrigation solution, tubing, a screw clamp (to start and close inflow), and a Y (glass or plastic) connector. All equipment should be *sterile.* Intermittent irrigation with closed drainage is used when the lining of the bladder is inflamed, irritated, or bleeding. Irrigation of the bladder is used also with closed straight drainage and for this procedure the following equipment is needed: *sterile* towels to provide a sterile field, gloves, container with irrigating solution, aseptic syringe, and basin for receiving the returned irrigating fluid. The solutions used for irrigation are prescribed by the physician.

Preparation of the Patient. As some patients have indwelling catheters for long periods, an understanding of its function and acceptance of the importance of the treatment is necessary. In many instances the patient assumes responsibility for care of the catheter, performing the irrigations; therefore, a thorough explanation of what is to be done, the prob-

able length of time drainage will be used, and the necessary precautions for prevention of infection should be given.* When patients assume complete responsibility for this treatment, as in the home, nurses should watch them carry it out and must be sure that all aspects of the procedure are performed properly. Family members may also need instruction. In addition, patients should be encouraged to assume responsibility for maintaining an intake of at least 3000 ml of fluid daily. This ensures a continuous egress of urine which helps prevent migration of organisms up the drainage system. The importance of an accurate intake and output record should be emphasized.

Suggested Procedure. After gaining the patient's cooperation, assemble the equipment. Prepare the bed and drape the patient as described for a catheterization. After scrubbing the forearms and hands and putting on gloves, pretest the bag of the Foley catheter by inserting 5 cc of air or 5 ml sterile water. Insert the catheter and then distend the Foley catheter with 5 ml of sterile water. After the bladder is allowed to drain (the amount may be measured later), connect the drainage tube to the catheter by a glass connector with the distal end in the sterile calibrated collecting plastic bag or bottle, being sure that the end of the tube does not extend into the collected urine.

When intermittent irrigation with drainage is used, the same procedure for insertion of the catheter may be used. In addition, a calibrated sterile bottle containing the irrigating solution with tubing attached is hung on an infusion stand. After expelling the air from this tubing and filling with irrigating solution, attach it to the catheter by a Y (glass or plastic) connector which is also attached to the tubing providing the outflow. The inflow and outflow clamps are adjusted to allow a specific amount of solution to flow into the bladder and then to drain from the bladder at specified intervals. Patients may be taught to perform this part of the procedure after they have become familiar with the treatment.

The drainage tubing should be of sufficient length to reach the collecting device (bottle or plastic bag) so that the patient may move freely in the bed; yet it should not be too long because the urine will pool in the tubing, interrupting drainage from the bladder. Attach the tubing to the side of the bed (by adhesive tape or safety pins) so that no tension is placed on the catheter. The catheter is taped to the thigh of women and to the abdomen of men.

The system must be maintained as a sterile closed system at all times. If the catheter becomes disconnected, clean it with 70 per cent alcohol and attach another sterile drainage tube. When

* The risks of any treatment should be understood by patients and the wishes of those who do not want to take these risks should be respected.

patients move from their bed—sit in a chair, walk, or are transported on a stretcher—do not disconnect the drainage; move it with them.[48]

The catheter is usually changed every 1 to 3 weeks, depending on the case, and the drainage tubing daily or every 2 or 3 days. If irrigations are prescribed for those patients with closed straight drainage, one of the procedures described under the section dealing with irrigations of the urinary bladder may be used. The junction of the catheter and drainage tube must be treated as a sterile field.

Recording the Treatment. Record the time the procedure was begun, the amount and characteristics of the urine obtained, any discomfort of the patient, or any difficulties encountered. If the bladder is irrigated, the amount and composition of the solution is recorded as well as the color and odor of the drainage. If the patient has pain or discomfort, this too is recorded. An accurate intake and output must also be kept. The patient can often assume responsibility for this function; it is part of his or her rehabilitation, gaining independence.

7. TIDAL IRRIGATION (TIDAL DRAINAGE) INCLUDING CYSTOMETRY

Definition. Tidal irrigation, also called tidal drainage, is a mechanically controlled method of gradually filling the bladder with an irrigating solution, in addition to the urine, and then periodically emptying it. The apparatus enables the operator to control the pressure exerted on the bladder wall and the intervals at which the vesicle is emptied.

Therapeutic Uses. Tidal irrigation has the following uses: (1) to empty the bladder periodically when injuries of the spinal cord or surgery of the bladder interfere with normal functions; (2) to combine with periodic emptying the gradual distention of the bladder within physiologic limits to prevent retention and increase the tone in an atonic bladder and to distend and prevent continuous emptying of a hypertonic bladder; and (3) to combine with the preceding the action of antiseptic, astringent, anticoagulant, or neutralizing solutions used in periodic filling of the bladder or that used in additional flushings.[49-51]

Because of the complexity of the equipment and the need for the patient to remain in bed during the treatment, tidal drainage is used infrequently today. It has been recommended, however, as an intermediate step in rehabilitation of the patient with "a cord bladder." This term is used for a bladder that does not respond normally to pressure within because the spinal cord has been injured and nerve pathways supplying the bladder have been destroyed. If there is incontinence following such an injury

and the bladder is continually emptying itself, or if retention (usually with overflow) exists, some physicians believe that an automatic function can be more rapidly established if tidal drainage, with its gradual filling and periodic emptying of the bladder, is instituted. Edward H. Kass and Harold S. Sossen [52] (in 1959) say that tidal drainage provides a physiologic stimulus as well as a constant supply of antibacterial fluid to the bladder, but the method often will not work in persons with hypotonic or irritable bladders. In addition, it has not been well accepted by some nurses and physicians because of the complexity of equipment. An electromechanical device used to control the outflow of fluid from the bladder in a group of 100 patients with continuous urinary drainage and irrigation with 0.25 per cent acetic acid is described. They suggest this method as an alternative to tidal drainage.

Creevy [53] (in 1964) describes a simple method of bladder irrigation with closed drainage that the patient, who is in good condition and has use of his or her hands, can be taught. He believes this method is just as effective as tidal drainage. Jack Lapides [54] (in 1970) writing in Campbell's and Harrison's text, says that within 1 to 2 weeks all patients with a neurogenic bladder should have suprapubic drainage of the bladder by cutaneous vesicotomy (a nonstricturing large caliber, vesicocutaneous fistula in the suprapubic area made by surgery). By wearing an appropriate collecting device over the stoma of the fistula, the patient maintains urinary drainage and his or her clothing is protected. Lapides believes complications such as acute pyelonephritis, acute urethritis, acute cystitis, urethrocutaneous fistula, periurethral abscess, acute epididymitis, urethral stricture, and calculous disease may be avoided by performing a cutaneous vesicotomy.

Houston S. Everett and John H. Ridley [55] advocate the use of 0.25 per cent acetic acid solution in a "tidal drainage apparatus" following plastic procedures of the anterior vaginal wall in the bladder region. Those patients treated postoperatively by this method regained adequate bladder function more quickly, had fewer catheterizations, and a lower infection rate than those with straight drainage alone.

Selection of Equipment and Method. All the methods the writers have seen or seen described combine periodic emptying of the bladder by siphonage with the gradual filling of the bladder by secreted urine mixed with a sterile solution which flows by gravity from a reservoir and tubing. The rate of the solution's flow is controlled with clamps and a drip bulb.

The procedure has been criticized because the apparatus does not allow for irrigation of the bladder with the irrigating solution alone, but instead there is a mixing of the solution with considerable quantities of urine. In an attempt to solve this problem, a variety of methods have been tried over the years.

O. A. Nelson and A. W. Kretz outline the following "requirements" of a satisfactory instrument:

1. The action of the apparatus must be positive so that siphonage invariably takes place as soon as the level of the fluid reaches a certain height.
2. The bladder should be completely empty before each siphonage action ceases.
3. The apparatus must be so constructed that the intravesical pressure can be varied at will.
4. Fluid remaining in the apparatus, after the siphonage has ceased, should not be washed into the bladder.
5. As far as possible, the apparatus should be simple to operate, easy to clean and sterilize.
6. The only adjustment necessary should be the placing of the high-tide point of the apparatus at the proper height in relation to the bladder and also to regulate the rate of drip of irrigating fluid.*

These authors go on to say their instrument meets all these requirements. They describe it as consisting of:

An inverted U-shaped metal tube, placed inside a glass cylinder. Each end of the cylinder is covered by a metal cap. In the top cap are three holes. Two small ones serve as air vents and a large one admits a screw-threaded truss rod which is attached to the bottom cap. A nut on top of the rod, when tightened, draws each metal cap against the respective ends of the glass cylinder, thus holding the apparatus together.

Between the bottom end of the glass cylinder and the metal cap is a rubber gasket. Through the bottom cap is placed the tube from the bladder and also the outlet arm of the inverted U-tube or siphon. The lower end of the last-mentioned tube has three features essential to the proper function of the apparatus. First, a constriction in the tube; second, an air vent; and, third, the lower end of the tube is enlarged so as to fit a sizable rubber tube which conveys the fluid to the waste container.†

Another method commonly advocated, which the authors have seen, is the manually controlled intermittent closed drainage followed by a period of bladder training. When irrigating solutions are used, the inlet tube is opened at stated intervals (with the outlet tube clamped) and a certain amount of fluid is allowed to enter the bladder. The inlet is then closed and the outlet is opened, permitting the fluid to drain from the bladder into the drainage bottle. This process is continued until the drainage is clear. Several types of apparatus are available. Reed M. Nesbit [56] says he uses the one devised by Keyes for intermittent bladder irrigation. Nurses must learn how to operate many kinds of tidal drainage apparatus. The principles underlying all tidal drainage devices are similar.

The mechanism of tidal drainage is essentially a siphon. The fluid flows into the bladder by gravity; therefore, the reservoir must be hung above the level of the bladder. Atmospheric pressure supports the column of liquid in a siphon that empties when the pressure within the bladder exceeds the atmospheric pressure, supporting the column of fluid. The pressure exerted on its contents (urine and/or the solution from the reservoir) by the bladder wall depends upon its elasticity, the strength of its muscle contraction, and the push on the pelvic organs during abdominal contraction. The height of the siphon determines the force required to push the column of liquid through it.

It is essential that doctor and nurse understand how to operate tidal drainage apparatus; it is almost equally important in some cases that the patient and family understand it. Rehabilitation depends largely on re-establishing bladder control of which this is the first step.

The physician must always initiate tidal drainage and prescribe (1) the nature of the solution, (2) the rate of flow for the solution (drops per minute), and (3) the height of the reservoir and the siphon in relation to the symphysis pubis and the opening of the drainage or outlet arm of the tubing.

Solutions used to irrigate, medicate, and regulate pressure within the vesicle are similar to those listed for irrigation of the bladder "by hand." Since contact with the solution is protracted, irritating chemicals must be diluted. Suby's (or G) solution and renacidin (10 per cent) is recommended in long-term urinary drainage to prevent calcific deposits, usually phosphates, in the lumen of the catheter. Both of these solutions are irritating to the bladder wall and are used only when prescribed by the physician. [57]

The *rate of flow* usually varies from 40 to 60 drops per minute. At the latter rate, William F. McKenna says the average bladder will fill in about an hour, taking the secreted urine into account; at 200 drops per minute, the bladder will empty every 10 minutes. Emptying is dependent not only on the solution's rate of flow but also on the *height of the siphon—*

* Nelson, O. A., and Kretz, A. W.: "Improved Tidal Irrigator," *Northwest Med.,* **49:**374, (June) 1950.
† *Ibid.*

or the distance between the outlet to the bladder and the height of the column of liquid. The equipment is usually adjusted with the outlet to the bladder (a tubing connected to the catheter) 2 to 3 cm (about 1 inch) below the level of the anus, and the arch of the siphon about 10 cm (4 inches) above the level of the base of the bladder. With this adjustment, McKenna says: "The pressure within the bladder will not exceed that amount [10 cm]. This degree of bladder pressure is well within the limit of natural tissue elasticity of an intact bladder. . . ." *

The lower end of the drainage tube must not be too long because sufficient negative pressure may be created therein, during the drainage aspect of the cycle, to pull the bladder wall into the eye of the catheter. The drainage bottle should be suspended off the floor and *the end of the drainage tube kept above the level of fluid in the bottle.* Siphonage will not occur if the end of the drainage tube is in the fluid. A #16 to #18 Foley catheter is frequently suggested. When a balloon type is prescribed, it must be tested with 5 cc of sterile water or air before inserting it. After insertion it is inflated with 3 cc of air or sterile water to hold it in place. A balloon in poor condition can rupture and leave fragments in the bladder. Even a soft catheter makes pressure on the bladder wall, and for this and other reasons tidal drainage is discontinued periodically. To keep the balloon from pushing against the neck of the bladder, the tubing is so pinned or clipped to the bedding that it is never taut. The catheter is fixed to the leg with a narrow strip of adhesive for this same reason, or in the case of an ordinary catheter, to keep it from slipping out of the urethra. If the patient is a man, the catheter should be taped to the lower abdomen to reduce angulation at the penoscrotal junction.[58]

Even with the greatest care, organisms will be carried into the bladder and the tissues irritated by tidal drainage. *Strict asepsis* must be observed throughout. The entire apparatus is exchanged for a fresh sterile setup every 4 to 6 days or oftener.[59]

Preparation of the Patient. Since this is a step in rehabilitation, it is particularly important that patients understand and accept it. When their cooperation is gained they can assume considerable responsibility for the management of the apparatus, and the procedures may interest rather than horrify them. The nurse must realize, however, that it is difficult

for patients and family to accept so unnatural a means of performing a body function, and he or she must be sympathetic if they move slowly in this direction. As in all such therapy, the nurse amplifies and reinforces the doctor's original explanation and instruction. Eleanora A. Seidel recommends giving the patient a demonstration with a dummy setup, using a balloon for a bladder, before starting the procedure. To understand tidal drainage one must know bladder physiology. Bladder capacity was discussed in the beginning of this chapter, micturition in Chapter 11, and incontinence and retention in Chapter 37. All bladder therapy is aimed at the ultimate goal of making it possible for patients to control the emptying of the bladder, to void painlessly, and to hold comfortably in the bladder sufficient urine to enable them to carry out normal daily activities without undue interruptions. Assessment of the individual patient's capacity for storing urine, or the response of the neuromuscular elements of the bladder on filling, is made with a manometer. Since tidal drainage involves cystometry this diagnostic procedure should perhaps be discussed before continuing the description of tidal drainage. These measurements are made by the physician before prescribing the conditions of tidal drainage.

Cystometry. Measurement of pressure exerted by the bladder wall on its contents is called cystometry. The process is based on the same physical principles as those in measuring the pressure of the vessel walls on the contained blood or the pressure of the meninges on the spinal fluid. Liquids in a membranous sac behave the same way all over the body, the pressure exerted upon them depending upon the contractile elements in the walls of the sac and the pressure exerted on the outside of the sac by the surrounding structures. If a vertical tubular outlet is provided for the fluid, on which pressure is being exerted equally in all directions, the fluid will rise in the outlet to a level equivalent to the pressure exerted on the contained fluid. The level will fluctuate in the outlet with fluctuations in pressure on the fluid within the sac or cavity. Pressure on the bladder contents varies with muscular contractions of the bladder and the contractions of the diaphragm and abdominal muscles in breathing, coughing, sneezing, laughing, sighing, groaning, and, of course, defecating and voiding. The *purpose* of cystometry is to determine the following: (1) heat and cold sensations; (2) bladder capacity, including amount of urine at first desire to void; (3) type of bladder contractions; and (4) amount of residual urine.[60]

---

* McKenna, William F.: "A Simple Efficient Automatic Tidal Drainage Apparatus," *Urol. Cutan. Rev.,* **52:**18, (Jan.) 1948.

Equipment needed for cystometric measurements is that used for a bladder irrigation with the addition of a cystometer. This is nothing more than a water manometer, or a calibrated glass tube. The manometer must be supported on a fixed standard so that the heights to which the fluid rises in it above the level of the bladder can be measured. Most tidal drainage sets incorporate what is, in effect, a cystometer. Fluid used in these measurements may be normal saline or any of those listed for bladder irrigation (see p. 1270).

The *procedure* of cystometry is as follows: Ask the patient to void, and observe the time required to initiate the stream, its size, force, amount of straining, and presence (if any) of dribbling at termination. With the patient lying on the back in a comfortable position, insert the catheter in the bladder and note the amount of residual urine. Instill 60 ml of cold and then 60 ml of warm water and note if the patient has sensations of cold and warmth, respectively. (This is called testing for exteroceptive sensation.) Then attach the glass or plastic Y-tube to two lengths of rubber tubing that have been previously connected to the manometer and calibrated reservoir, respectively. Place a finger over the open end of the Y-tube (the catheter will be connected here later) so that the air may be expelled from the entire system, and open the outlet, allowing water to run from the reservoir into the manometer tube until all air is expelled. After closing the flow from the reservoir, attach the open end of the glass or plastic Y-tube to the catheter. Adjust the manometer so that the zero mark is level with the patient's pubis. Start the flow of solution at a rate of about 1 ml per second. Ask the patient to say when he or she feels the first inclination to void and again when the bladder feels full. Record the fluctuation of pressures that indicate emptying contractions. An abrupt excursion of the fluid with a slow return to a point near which it started represents a contraction of the detrusor muscles. Note the level from which the rise started and the peak. Record the first discomfort and any increase, or pain, thereafter; record at what point there is a desire to void and any leakage around the catheter. Intravesicular pressure varies in the normal bladder from 0 when it is empty to about 12 to 20 cm (water) when the bladder holds 500 ml. At this pressure, it empties. Great modifications in these figures occur in disease.

Suggested Procedure for Tidal Irrigation. Having gained the patient's cooperation, collect the equipment for the cystometric tests and tidal drainage. Prepare the bed and drape the patient as described for catheterization; then proceed with the catheterization or leave this for the physician who, with the nurse, may wish to make the cystometric measurements. The catheter inserted for emptying the bladder should serve also for cystometry and tidal drainage so it is desirable for the physician to perform all the functions that require gloved or scrubbed hands and for the nurse to be free to handle unsterile objects. Unless otherwise specified the doctor select Foley catheters (#16 to #18 for women; #18 to #22 for men.) After draining the bladder into a covered vessel or into the drainage bottle, adjust the tubing so that a measured amount of fluid can flow from a calibrated reservoir into the bladder. Tape the catheter to the thigh of women and to the lower abdomen of men. Distend the Foley catheter with 5 cc of air or sterile water injected with a sterile syringe. The inlet and drainage tubes should be closed at the start of the procedure. Adjust the height of the cystometer so that the outlet (zero point) is level with the symphysis pubis. After eliminating the air in the system of tubes, attach the inlet tube to the catheter and allow the fluid from the reservoir to flow at the specified rate and in the specified amounts. The nurse may record the findings as the cystometric tests proceed or the physician may prefer to do so. The physician, having now assessed the condition of the bladder, may immediately prescribe the rate of flow for the tidal irrigation and the height of the siphon. He or she will adjust the mechanism to the patient's condition and will test the effectiveness of the adjustment before leaving it to others.

To prevent kinking of the excess tubing, keep it coiled and fixed to the bedding with tapes or safety pins. See that it is not collapsed by the patient's leg. Leaking around the catheter (a wet bed) may be caused by an obstructed drainage tube or by blood clots or sloughing tissue in the catheter. If the tubes are unobstructed, the doctor will decrease the height of the siphon, since contractions of the bladder may be sufficient to empty it but the pressure insufficient to carry the fluid over the siphon loop.

If fluid escapes from the air vent, check the patency of the drainage tube; be sure that the end of the drainage tube is above the level of the liquid in the drainage bottle. Check all connections to prevent the introduction of air into the system. Bubbles can occlude the tubes in various places.

To control urethral irritation and prevent entry of bacteria, the perineal area should be cleaned with soap and water at least twice daily and all mucus and encrustations of dried exudate on the catheter removed. Some urologists prescribe irrigating the urethra with an antibacterial agent after cleaning the perineum.

As long as tidal irrigation is functioning, check the tubing and general operation of the apparatus. Replenish the solution when necessary, usually every 8 hours.

The catheter should not be disconnected from the drainage tubing when the patient leaves the bed; however, the irrigation may be discontinued. A *sterile closed drainage* system must be maintained at all times.

If possible, keep tidal drainage out of sight,

especially while the patient has visitors. The drainage bottle can be hung on the bed under the covers, and a screen may be placed around the standard with the irrigating fluid and the siphon.

The physician will discontinue the treatment from time to time to test the patient's ability to retain urine and void spontaneously. He or she will probably want the patient catheterized after voiding in order to know whether the bladder is emptying. It is wise to use the kind of catheter for this procedure that will be needed if it is necessary to reestablish tidal irrigation.

Recording the Treatment. Many hospitals have special forms for tidal irrigation records. Intake and output forms may be modified to include the following information: (1) the total intake of fluids, by mouth and by vein, or any other parenteral route; and (2) total output by the urinary route. Estimate this by subtracting (3) the amount of solution used from (4) the total drainage. Also record (5) the amount in the reservoir and (6) amount in the drainage bottle.

Record the initiation of the procedure and the physician who did it, the solution used, the rate of flow, and the height of the siphon in relation to the symphysis pubis. Record significant remarks of the patient showing acceptance, skepticism, or aversion to the treatment and any physiologic or mechanical difficulties encountered.

8. HEMODIALYSIS

Definition. Hemodialysis is a method of removing excessive metabolic waste products from the body and of maintaining a balance of electrolytes and water when the kidney is unable to perform this function. This process is accomplished by *diffusion,* the movement of solutes from a solvent (fluid) of higher concentration to one of a lower concentration across a semipermeable membrane. Two methods of dialysis—the artificial kidney (extracorporeal dialysis) and peritoneal dialysis—are used.

Therapeutic Uses. Hemodialysis (extracorporeal dialysis) is used in the treatment of patients with acute and chronic renal failure, exogenous poisonings (as from barbiturates), and edematous states when the object is to remove sodium and water.[61,61a] After an extensive review and analysis of literature on management of chronic renal failure, John P. Merrill[62] says that hemodialysis is used for the following: (1) sick "uremic" patients who do not respond to conservative management; (2) patients with acute renal failure, as an adjunct to good conservative management; (3) patients with chronic renal failure; and (4) critically ill patients with advanced renal failure. He notes that short-term intermittent peritoneal dialysis is well established as an adjunct to the treatment of acute renal failure where there are no contraindications, and there is considerable interest in kidney transplant for patients with chronic uremia.

The concept of external dialysis is not new, although its use in clinical medicine is relatively so. In 1913, Abel, Rowntree, and Turner used an artificial kidney made of collodion tubes enclosed in a glass cylinder containing dialysate through which dog blood was passed to remove salicylate. They recommended its use in humans as a suitable technique for removing toxins and accumulated metabolites in disease states.[63] Willem Kolff of the Netherlands built the first artificial kidney in 1943. It was successfully used for the dialysis of a patient's blood in an extracorporeal circuit with cellophane as the dialyzing membrane and heparin to prevent clotting of the blood in the extracorporeal passages.[64]

Successful treatment of patients for chronic renal failure was first reported by B. H. Scribner[65] (in 1960) who with his associates developed a Silastic-Teflon external arteriovenous fistula. This device provides a smooth surface which discourages adhesion of platelets and formation of blood clots and eliminates the need for performing a surgical cutdown for each dialysis. It is used in many centers today. Because of complications associated with the external AV shunt, Michael J. Brescia and associates[66] created a subcutaneous AV fistula by anastomosing the distal radial artery and adjacent vein side-to-side. Repeated venipunctures are possible because of the hypertrophy of the venous side of the fistula. They report successful treatment of 13 patients (without complications) in over 800 dialyses, contending that this method largely removes the clinical and psychologic problems associated with the external shunt. All authorities consulted recognize the contribution of both methods to successful treatment and rehabilitation of patients with chronic renal failure.

Following the development of various hemodialysis equipment and techniques, this method of therapy was instituted in special medical centers, community hospitals, and finally in the home. It continues to be viewed in some places as a complex medical treatment, requiring a group of specially trained physicians, nurses, and technicians; whereas, in other centers that have been in operation for a long time, it is called a nurse and technician procedure. These nurses are expert practitioners in this special area of nursing. Patient selection in chronic hemodialysis is emphasized. Following a survey of the 19 world centers, Scribner and associates in 1965 said that all investigators "stressed the fact that success of therapy depended primarily on patient cooperation with cannula care and low salt diet. Each reported success with 'cooperative' patients and endless problems with 'uncooperative' patients." * Most authorities stress potential for successful treatment and rehabilitation as well as emotional stability in selection of patients.

Successful treatment in exogenous poisoning has been reported in some community hospitals without specially trained physicians and nurses.[67] J. F. Maher and associates [68] report hemodialysis as therapeutic in barbiturate poisoning in about 200 patients in 30 different institutions; and, according to John G. Setter and associates,[69] hemodialysis was more efficient than peritoneal dialysis in 173 similar patients. Glenn D. Lubash [70] believes that peritoneal dialysis can be carried out in most community hospitals but questions the advisability of hemodialysis in these settings if specially trained personnel are not available. There are advantages and disadvantages in both methods and the one selected by the physician will depend on the particular patient and his or her condition and the available facilities.

Hemodialysis in the home was instituted because of the high cost, limited space, the need for specially trained personnel, and the large number of patients who could not travel to special centers. Shaldon in England, Scribner in Seattle, and Merrill in Boston are credited with training the first patients (and their spouses) to dialyze themselves in the home, in 1964.[71] Advantages include reduction in cost, saving of time, and flexibility in the treatment program. Patients can dialyze themselves in the evenings after work or while sleeping and dialysis may be carried out as frequently as necessary to meet the metabolic needs of the individual. Limited care dialysis facilities are used by selected patients on an outpatient basis.[71a]

William J. Johnson and associates [72] describe their experiences with chronic dialysis over a period of 5½ years with a total of 43 patients (24 men and 19 women). Thirty-three (17 men and 16 women) returned to their jobs or household responsibilities. Those on home dialysis had the lowest number of complications requiring hospitalization. In addition, annual cost of home dialysis three times a week was $3,848, whereas center dialysis twice weekly was $19,760. Some centers report annual cost of center dialysis as approximately $10,000. In 1969, of 2660 patients on chronic dialysis, 885 were on home dialysis and the remainder were in 253 dialysis facilities.[73] Since January 1967, the survival rate of those on home dialysis is better than those treated in a center.

Authorities agree that early treatment, better patient selection, and improved techniques are important in effective therapy. Jerry P. Pendras and R. V. Erickson [74] report their experience with 22 carefully selected patients in a large dialysis center; 19 were able to return to full-time work or part-time semisedentary work and only three died during the treatment period, which ranged up to 50 months. Following an analysis of data on 302 patients undergoing chronic intermittent hemodialysis in 14 centers, Edmund J. Lewis and associates [75] concluded that age was not a valid criterion in the selection of patients for treatment. There was no difference in survival rates for those under or over the age of 45. Men and women did equally well.

Selection of Equipment and Method. Artificial kidneys currently used include the Twin Coil, Mini Coil, Koff, Skeggs-Leonards, and the Modified two-layer Kiil. All dialyzers are similar in design. Richard B. Freeman and associates [76] refer to 2 types: (1) Coil dialyzers include the standard twin coil * and the modified "chronic" coil; and (2) Parallel flow dialyzers include the Skeggs-Leonards and the Kiil (four or two layer).†

Most authorities agree that the "ideal dialyzer" awaits development. Freeman and associates, therefore, conducted a 5-year study of four separate hemodialysis systems used in treating 11 patients with chronic renal failure for a period of 2 to 30 months. In conclusion, they said:

The best combination of perfusion characteristics in dialyzers currently available for chronic intermittent hemodialysis was found in the two layer Kiil dialyzer that it perfused with dialysate fluid at 1.5 to 2.4 liters/min and is not recirculated. Coil dialyzers provide an excellent reserve system for use in emergencies and may be more practical than parallel flow units in certain locations, such as those with existing coil units and those with limited technical personnel. The Skeggs-Leonards dialyzer has certain advantages for children and low flow cannulae, notably a low resistance to flow and a small priming volume. Composition of the dialysate, selection of membranes (thick, cuprophane, ultra-thin), and duration and frequency of dialysis should be adjusted to the individual needs of the patients.‡

They identified the following characteristics of the "ideal dialyzer": (1) removes nitrogenous and toxic products of metabolism efficiently; (2) is capable of removing water from the oliguric patient; (3) has a low internal vol-

---

* Scribner, B. H., et al.: "Some Therapeutic Approaches to Chronic Renal Insufficiency," *Annu. Rev. Med.,* **16:**291, 1965.

* Travenol Laboratories, Inc., Morton Grove, Ill.

† Seattle Artificial Kidney Supply Division of the Sweden Freezer Co., Seattle, Wash.

‡ Freeman, Richard B., et al.: "Hemodialysis for Chronic Renal Failure," *Ann. Intern. Med.,* **62:**519, (Mar.) 1965.

ume that would eliminate the need for priming with blood and minimize the possibility of fluid shifts during dialysis and reduce blood loss at the end of dialysis; (4) has a low internal resistance to flow if blood is to be propelled through the system by arterial pressure rather than a blood pump; (5) the dialyzer membrane and its supports, including the connecting tubing, are presterilized, disposable, and simple to assemble; (6) is reliable, safe, and requires little attention during use; and (7) is inexpensive and has low maintenance costs. Because changes in dialyzing equipment are being made almost daily, nurses working in this specialty should consult the most recent references at all times.[76a]

All dialyzers work on the same principle. Blood is circulated through layers of a semipermeable membrane (cellophane) immersed in a dialyzing solution (dialysate) similar in composition to blood plasma. By the process of *diffusion,* molecules pass through the membrane from a fluid of greater to a fluid of lesser concentration until an equilibrium is reached on both sides. It is obvious, then, that if the concentration of a waste product (urea) or an electrolyte (such as potassium) is greater in the blood than in the dialysate, both of these products will decrease in the body. If the blood level of an electrolyte is below normal, it may be added to the dialysate in concentration greater than the normal plasma level and then the level of the electrolyte in the blood will increase as dialysis proceeds. The cellophane membrane does the filtering work that is normally done by the kidney.[77]

The solution (dialysate), prescribed by the physician, is usually similar to the composition of normal plasma, containing sodium, potassium, calcium, magnesium, acetate, chloride, and glucose. For some patients the amounts of each may vary so that the solution is suited to the individual needs of the patient.[78] The addition of glucose assists in ultrafiltration. By adding lactic acid or carbon dioxide, the recommended pH of 7.4 of the bath can be maintained. The dialysate is usually prepared by the pharmacist or a specially trained technician. To maintain a steep concentration gradient from the patient's blood to the dialysate, the solution must be changed as equilibrium of substances approaches. James E. Kintzel and Elizabeth M. Cameron write:

In the older machines, the 100 liter tank dialyzers, the bath must be changed every 2 hours. In newer models, when the dialysate is passed through a separate chamber containing a coil membrane, the dialysate is discarded from the upper chamber. In this instance, enough dialysate can be mixed for an entire treatment and kept at room temperature until it is used. (This assumes that room temperature is low enough to discourage bacterial growth.) Some medical centers employ a twice-normal dialyses delivery rate and change the bath twice in order to maintain a greater concentration gradient.*

The temperature of the solution may vary from 20° to 37°C (68° to 99°F).[79-80a] The low temperature of the bath inhibits bacterial growth, preventing infection which is a great hazard to the "uremic" patient. Clotting and microbubbles are more likely to form when a solution of 20°C (68°F) is used; consequently dialysis is usually performed at 37°C (99°F). In addition, the present equipment (cellophane) is made in such a way that most bacteria are unable to enter the blood as it reenters the body.

The *site of insertion* of an arteriovenous (AV) external shunt is usually the nondominate forearm (for example in the left forearm of the right-handed person) or the lower leg. The teflon vessel tips are placed in the artery and nearby vein and joined together by a silicone rubber tubing that completes the shunt. Prior to insertion of the cannula, the area must be shaved, thoroughly cleaned with soap solution, and rinsed with an iodine preparation. The surgical procedure is carried out by the physician in the operating room, a treatment room, or in the patient's room. W. E. Quinton and associates [81] describe the development and use of the silastic-teflon cannula in a large group of patients over a 2-year period with no outright failure. They contend that with proper cannula care clotting and infection can be virtually eliminated; the life of the appliance depends on the care given it. After the initial insertion, the patient wears a forearm splint for 1 to 2 weeks. Cannula sites are washed with hexachlorophene or iodine solution (using strict aseptic technique) once or twice daily followed by redressing the area. Sterile dressings are used and a mask and cap are worn by the operator.[82] Martha Read and Mary Mallison [82a] say shunt care is similar to care given a fresh surgical wound. They describe the shunt care in their center as follows: After cleaning the entire area with hydrogen peroxide or alcohol, Betadine (an antiseptic iodine solution) is applied around the exit sites. Then an antibiotic ointment (Bacitracin or Neosporin G) is applied. A sterile applicator is used only once at one site and *not* at the other so that cross contamination of exit sites is prevented. Sterile dressings, usually

---

* Kintzel, James E., and Cameron, Elizabeth M.: "The Insulted Kidney: Medical and Nursing Intervention for Patients Undergoing Dialysis or Renal Homotransplantation," in Kintzel, Kay Corman (ed.): *Advanced Concepts in Clinical Nursing.* J. B. Lippincott Co., Philadelphia, 1971, p. 295.

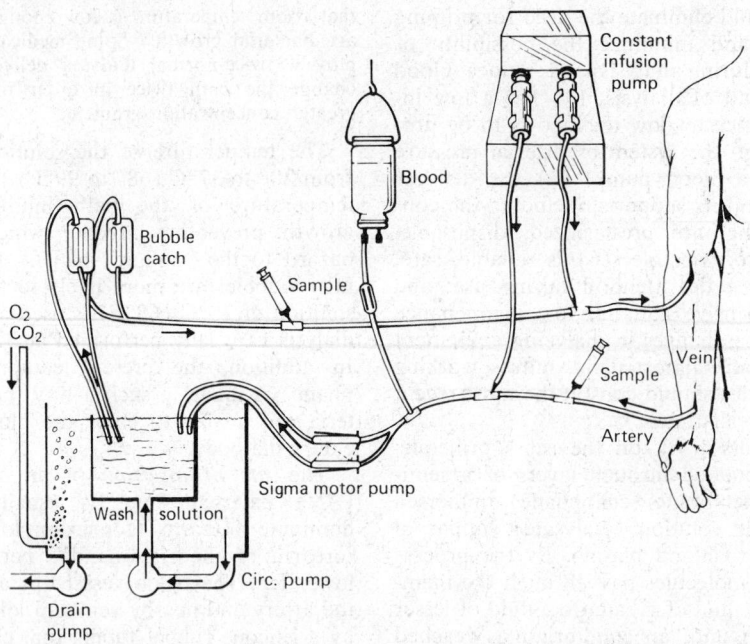

Figure 24-16. Extracorporeal blood circuit. Note heparin entering the tubing leading to the dialyzer and the protamine entering the tubing leaving the dialyzer. (From Maher, John F., et al.: "Regional Heparinization for Hemodialysis," *N. Engl. J. Med.*, **268**:454, [Feb. 28] 1963.)

two 4-inch by 4-inch sponges, are placed over each exit site and the forearm is wrapped with a sterile bandage in such a way that a small loop of the silastic tubing is visible for observing the appearance of the shunt. Patients are taught to change the dressings and check the blood flow in the shunt frequently.

The patient is heparinized, when the dialysis is begun, by intermittent systemic doses or by continuous systemic heparinization; in both methods heparin is administered intravenously. If there are sources for bleeding (for example following surgery), systemic heparinization cannot be used. Instead, regional heparinization is instituted; that is, a constant infusion pump is used to infuse heparinized, normal saline in the arterial blood as it enters the dialyzer and then before the blood returns to the patient it is infused with normal saline and protamine. (See Fig. 24-16). To maintain clotting time of the patient at approximately 10 minutes and dialyzer time more than 60 minutes, additional small amounts of heparin and protamine may be necessary.[83]

The length of time for the treatment varies. It may take as long as 24 hours but 8 hours is more common. The size of the patient and his or her rate of catabolism will influence the number of hours needed for best results. Chronic intermittent dialysis is frequently carried out at night as there are less interrup-

tions of the patient's normal living pattern.

Preparation of the Patient. Persons who are treated by hemodialysis experience many emotional problems and the period of adjustment is difficult and long. Studies show that before dialysis, patients experienced irritability, apprehension, and insomnia; during dialysis, they experienced anxiety when they were connected to or disconnected from the machine. When there were technical difficulties, patients experienced restlessness, irritability, anxiety, and often depression. After dialysis, subjects felt only relief that the procedure was over.[84,84a] It is obvious that the preparation of the patient is of utmost importance. Before starting the treatment, the patient, if not too ill, should be given detailed explanations of the procedure. The physician usually explains the purpose and nature of the treatment as well as prospects for rehabilitation. The nurse gives more detailed information about the procedure and teaches selected patients how to carry it out. The patient and family need a great deal of support and encouragement from the nurse, physician, and others who are caring for the patient. Written directions, oral explanations, and demonstrations are essential.

The *patient's discomfort* during hemodialysis should be minimized as much as possible, for at best it is traumatic. Patients are aware that their lives depend on the success of the treatment and a well-functioning machine. Those patients who are acutely ill will need a great deal of nursing care. The patients' position should be changed and they should be encouraged to cough and breathe deeply, at least every hour. Good oral hygiene and skin care are especially important.[85,86] Patients on chronic intermittent dialysis enjoy reading or watching television. If the cannula is in the lower extremity, they may do some type of handwork.

Because hemodialysis for the patient with acute renal failure is a highly specialized treatment and differs considerably from repeated dialysis in chronic renal failure, a discussion of the procedure is not included. For the same reason, home dialysis is omitted. The interested reader should consult appropriate references listed at the end of the chapter.

Suggested Procedure for Repeated Hemodialysis. After the patient has been selected for treatment by this method, the physician will explain its purposes, details of the procedure, and probable effects. The nurse supplements these explanations and answers additional questions. Every effort needs to be made to make patients as comfortable as possible and allay their fears. The attitude of the nurse is important.

So that repeated connections to the dialyzer may be made, an arteriovenous (AV) external shunt or internal (AV) fistula must be made. The internal fistula is made in the operating room by a surgeon. The insertion of the cannula for the external shunt is a surgical procedure and is performed by one or more physicians and a nurse in the operating room, a treatment room that has facilities (including sink and running water) for a surgical procedure, or the patient's room if these facilities are available. The physicians and those who assist them wear sterile gowns and gloves, masks, and caps. The patient also wears a mask. The length of time needed to insert the cannula will vary, depending on the patient and his or her condition. Before the procedure is begun, assemble all necessary equipment and wash hands as for a surgical procedure.

After scrubbing the area thoroughly with hexachlorophene, shave it and scrub again with hexachlorophene. In addition, saline and an iodine preparation may be used to clean the area after it is prepared. Place the "cutdown tray" or cannulation tray on a table near the site of operation and open it under sterile conditions. A good light over the operative field is necessary. Drape the area with sterile towels and maintain a sterile field during the procedure. A local anesthetic such as procaine or Xylocaine is used. After the procedure has been completed, the cannulas are cleaned and stabilized by taping to skin. A small, padded board may be used to immobilize the extremity. This procedure may be used in preparation for dialysis or changing a cannula that has had technical failures such as clotting of the cannula. Following the insertion of the cannula, the patient is ready for dialysis. The patient is taught to check the blood flow in the shunt frequently and to clean the area around the cannula sites and change the dressings. A member of the family may also be taught how to do these things.

Blood is sometimes needed to prime the machine before the cannulas are attached; however, this is not necessary for most stable chronic patients. Connect the arterial blood supply to the inlet of the machine and unclamp so that blood flows into the dialyzer. When the blood reaches the bubble trap, clamp the venous line and connect it to the patient's vein. After releasing the clamps, the cannulas are then opened, allowing the blood to circulate through the special cellophane panels or coils that are submerged in the dialysate.

The flow rate, prescribed by the physician, is set before the procedure is begun. Masks are worn by all personnel in the dialysis unit as the site of insertion of the cannula is a source of infection. Cover the cannula with a sterile dressing.

The patient is usually heparinized by intermittent systemic doses or continuous systemic heparinization given intravenously. When the patient needs a transfusion, packed cells are given instead of whole blood so that the amount of fluids given is decreased.

Observation of the patient is essential during dialysis. Before the procedure is begun and when it is discontinued, check the vital signs (blood pressure, temperature, pulse, and respiration) and weight. Throughout the treatment note any unfavorable signs, as for example the following: restlessness, twitching or involuntary movements, pain, leg cramps, nausea and vomiting. Check the vital signs throughout the procedure as frequently as the patient's condition may indicate.

When the dialysis is complete, drain the blood within the dialyzer into the patient by clamping the patient's outflow line and pushing the blood through the dialyzer into the patient's vein. Attach the shunt to the arterial and venous cannula and release the clamps. Clean the cannula sites and apply a sterile dressing. Many experienced patients perform this part of the procedure.

Recording the Treatment. Hospitals usually have special forms (see Fig. 24-17). In any event, record the following information: date and hour dialysis was begun and discontinued; amount and composition of the dialysate; pre- and post-dialysis body weight, temperature, pulse, respiration, and blood pressure; all medications given, including the amount and time of heparinization; all laboratory work, including the time and readings of clotting times. Record the amount and time that packed cells are given. The patient's reaction to the treatment—any discomfort, concerns, or fears—should be recorded.

9. PERITONEAL DIALYSIS

Definition. Peritoneal dialysis is a method used for the removal of toxic substances from the body by instilling a specially prepared solution (dialysate) into the peritoneal cavity and then allowing this fluid to return by gravity. The peritoneum serves as the semipermeable

University Hospital

INDIVIDUAL HEMODIALYSIS PLAN AND SUMMARY

DATE (DAY | MO. | YR.)

DIALYSIS NO. WEEK NO.

HEMODIALYSIS PLAN

1. DIALYZER ______ 2. DURATION ______
3. DIALYSATE COMPOSITION ______
   - ☐ STANDARD
   - ☐ CUSTOM
4. CIRCUIT FILLING ______
   - ☐ OWN BLOOD, SALINE DISCARDED
   - ☐ SALINE REINFUSION
5. WASHBACK (VOL. SOL'N. ± AIR) ______
6. HEPARIN — START ______
   — MAINT. ______
7. POST DIALYSIS WT. ______
8. EST'D. MEAN T.M.P. ______
9. MEDICATIONS DURING DIALYSIS ______
10. LABORATORY STUDIES ______
11. OTHERS ______

SIGNATURE ______

84-750-0260 (5/75)

HEMODIALYSIS SUMMARY

	PRE (DAY | MO. | YR.)	POST (DAY | MO. | YR.)
DATE		
HOUR		
BLOOD PRESSURE — LYING		
BLOOD PRESSURE — STANDING		
PULSE		
TEMPERATURE		
WEIGHT	PRE D. △	△ D.

ACCESS CANN. FIST. EXT. RA LA RL LL

STATUS ______

HEPARIN ____ START ____ MAINT. ____

____ TOTAL ____

C.T./D.HR. ______

DIALYZER ____ Q. DIAL ____ Q BLOOD ____

M.P. DIAL. ____ M.P. BLOOD ____ T.M.P. ____

WASHBACK (VOL. SOL'N. ± AIR) ______

MEDICATIONS GIVEN (NAME-DOSE-TIME)

1. ______ 5. ______
2. ______ 6. ______
3. ______ 7. ______
4. ______ 8. ______

CHART

Figure 24-17. Sample of hospital forms for recording hemodialysis treatment. (Courtesy of University Hospital, University of Western Ontario, London, Ont.)

membrane, permitting diffusion of excess metabolic waste, electrolytes, and water into the peritoneal cavity.

Therapeutic Uses. Peritoneal dialysis is used for (1) excessive concentration of potassium (hyperkalemia); (2) gross overhydration; (3) severe acidosis; and (4) excessive ingestion of drugs such as barbiturate, salicylate, or bromide.[87,88] Edward B. Hager and John P. Merrill[89] say it is a safe and effective adjunct to

uh University Hospital

HEMODIALYSIS WORKSHEET

PATIENT _____

DATE _____   DIALYSIS NO. _____

TIME	B.P.	PULSE A.R.	WT.	HEP.	C.T.	BLOOD FLOW RATES		PRESSURES			EST. UF	OUT-PUT	INTAKE			FLUID BAL.	COMMENTS
						Pump Set.	Flow Rate	BLD DIAL	TOT				IV	Blood	P.O.		

Predialysis Wt. _____   Blood Put Up By _____

Desired Postdialysis Wt. _____   Blood Checked By _____

84-602-0259

Figure 24-17. (continued).

the therapy of the patient with acute renal failure.

Dialysis, by use of the peritoneum, as by use of the artificial kidney, is a relatively new treatment in clinical medicine. Ganter, in 1923, performed peritoneal dialysis on anuretic rabbits and guinea pigs and in the same year introduced 1.5 liters of physiologic saline solution, intraperitoneally, into a patient with urethral obstruction. (The dialysis was followed by a slight improvement in her condition.) [90] John H. Bland [91] reports that he has had better results with peritoneal dialysis than hemodialysis in the treatment of patients with chronic renal failure. He gives the following reasons: (1) it does not require the specialized facilities and apparatus necessary in hemodialysis; and (2) after the dialysis has been started and is operating satisfactorily, the patient may be cared for by a well-prepared surgical nurse with the physician checking the physical condition of the patient and the progress of the dialysis at intervals. He believes that the complications associated with this form of treatment are few. He says peritonitis and abdominal discomfort during the procedure, especially with those patients who are apprehensive and have a "low complaint threshold," occurred infrequently. Discussing its uses and effects, he says:

Peritoneal dialysis is approximately one-fourth as efficient as hemodialysis. Nevertheless dialyses lasting twelve to twenty-four hours reduce the blood urea concentration by one-third to one-half of its initial value. Water and electrolyte equilibrium is generally attainable and systemic acidosis reversed within this time period. After dialysis the patient often feels sufficiently well to live a relatively active life. His appetite may return so that he is again able to attain a sufficiently high caloric intake to regain strength and to spare excessive protein catabolism. This improvement lasts from one to several weeks, the duration being correlated with the residual renal function and thus to the daily rate of rise of the blood urea concentration which usually is in the range of 10 to 35 mg. per 100 ml. At times dialysis must be performed at relatively frequent intervals, not because of uremia, but because of difficulties in the excretion of water and potassium. Peritoneal dialysis is an extremely efficient means of removing water and electrolytes from such patients, effective removal of as much as 1 liter per hour being easily attainable.*

S. T. Boen [92] says indications for peritoneal dialysis include the following: (1) in acute renal failure caused by lesions that are expected to be reversible; (2) occasionally, in chronic renal insufficiency when "kidney failure has been accentuated as a result of trauma, infection, vomiting, diarrhea or excessive protein intake"; and (3) in poisoning from drugs such as barbiturates, methyl alcohol, salt, boric acid, salicylates, and glutethimides. He recognizes that medical opinion varies as to the time that dialysis should be performed in acute renal failure; however, many physicians use the criterion of a blood urea concentration

above 3.5 to 4 gm/liter. Other indications are a plasma sulfate concentration above 10 mEq/liter and a chloride concentration below 85 mEq/liter. All authorities agree that dialysis is absolutely indicated in excessive concentration of plasma potassium (hyperkalemia) and extreme acidosis. Finally, Boen says that prophylactic dialysis has been advocated in more recent years, which means starting the dialysis before the patient's blood chemistry becomes grossly abnormal, as a more effective way of treating the patient.

Complications associated with this form of treatment include infection, pain, and protein loss. G. M. Berlyne and associates [93] report an additional group that affects the lungs—pneumonia, atelectasis, purulent bronchitis, and pleural effusion. They believe the lower lungs are partially collapsed by elevation of the diaphragm through distention of the peritoneal cavity with the dialysis fluid. One liter changes (rather than the customary two liters), each cycle lasting only 45 minutes and the total duration of dialysis lasting no longer than 24 hours is recommended.

Selection of Equipment and Method. The method used in peritoneal dialysis is relatively simple and the equipment needed is usually available in all hospitals, making this form of treatment accessible to more patients than hemodialysis which requires elaborate facilities and equipment (see Fig. 24-18). The method most frequently described is the infusion of the solution into the peritoneal cavity by way of two bottles (one liter each of commercially prepared solution) hung on an infusion stand, and attached to tubing and a catheter inserted into the peritoneal cavity. The outlet tubing extends into a graduated drain bottle and is connected to the inlet tubing with a glass connector. Clamps are attached to the inlet and outlet tubing so that inflow and outflow of dialysate may be regulated. The solution is allowed to flow into the peritoneal cavity as rapidly as possible (about 10 minutes is usually required), where it remains for a period determined by the physician, usually 30 to 60 minutes, during which time metabolic waste, excessive electrolytes, and water diffuse into the cavity from the body fluids through the peritoneal membrane. The fluid is then drained from the abdominal cavity by gravity or suction into a large drainage bottle connected to the closed system of drainage [94] (see Fig. 20-19). It is important to maintain a *sterile, closed system* as there is less chance of infection.

The *composition of the solution* (dialysate) is important for best results. According to Boen, it should meet the following criteria:

---

* Bland, John H.: *Clinical Metabolism of Body Water and Electrolytes.* W. B. Saunders Co., Philadelphia, 1963, p. 599.

1. It must allow maximal diffusion of retained waste products.
2. It should be able to normalize or maintain the hydration state of the patient.
3. It must be capable of correcting the abnormalities in the electrolyte composition of the plasma.*

Most authorities say the ideal solution is similar to the *electrolyte composition of plasma* so that the constituents of normal plasma are not altered but all excesses, including toxins, are removed. Glucose is added so that the solution is slightly hyperosmotic to plasma. A hypertonic (7 per cent) dialysate enhances peritoneal permeability, resulting in an increase of urea clearance.[94a] Commercially prepared solutions approach the electrolyte composition and tonicity of plasma.

If the concentration of a particular substance is increased, it may be added to only one of the bottles, as the solutions mix quickly in the cavity. Heparin is added to prevent fibrin formation on the catheter which may block its perforations, impeding the removal of the dialysate. Potassium may be added occasionally, especially if prolonged vomiting has caused a depletion of potassium. Antibiotics also may be added.

The *temperature* of the solution should be near body temperature to promote removal of waste products and excess electrolytes.[95] It is also more comfortable for the patient and prevents hypothermia. Placing the bottles in

* Boen, S. T.: *Peritoneal Dialysis in Clinical Medicine.* Charles C Thomas, Publisher, Springfield, Ill., 1964, p. 75.

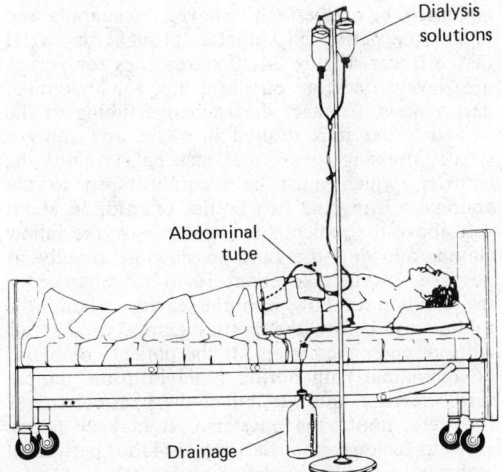

Figure 24-18. Peritoneal dialysis setup. (From Abbott Laboratories: *Impersol.* Abbott Laboratories, North Chicago, Ill., 1967, p. 16.)

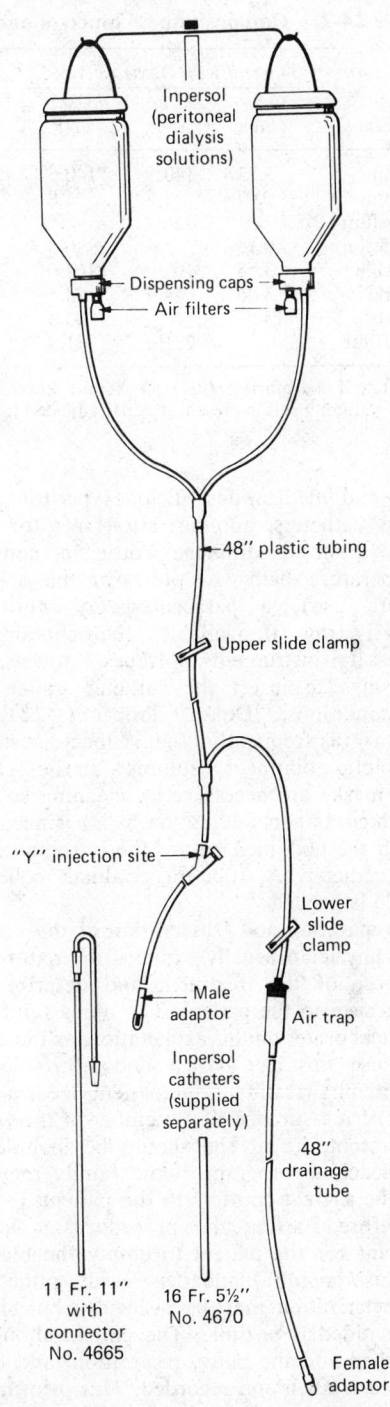

Figure 24-19. Peritoneal dialysis set, including all parts (with exception of drainage bottle) appropriately marked. (Courtesy of Abbott Laboratories, North Chicago, Ill.)

a warm bath is an effective way of warming the solution.

Equipment needed, in addition to the solu-

Table 24-2.   Composition of Inpersol and Inpersol-K Solutions *

Solute	Inpersol with Dextrose 1.5%†			Inpersol with Dextrose 7%†			Inpersol-K with Dextrose 1.5%†		
	Gm/ liter	mEq/ liter	mOsm/ liter	Gm/ liter	mEq/ liter	mOsm/ liter	Gm/ liter	mEq/ liter	mOsm/ liter
Sodium	3.23	140.5	140.5	3.23	140.5	140.5	3.23	140.5	140.5
Calcium	0.07	3.5	1.8	0.07	3.5	1.8	0.07	3.5	1.8
Potassium								0.16	4.0	4.0
Magnesium	0.18	1.5	0.8	0.18	0.8	1.5	0.18	1.5	0.8
Chloride	3.58	101.0	101.0	3.56	101.0	101.0	3.72	105.0	105.0
Lactate	3.96	44.5	44.5	3.96	44.5	44.5	3.96	44.5	44.5
Dextrose	15		83.3	70		388.8	15		83.3
Total		291.0	371.9		291.0	677.4		299.0	379.9

* Abbott Laboratories: *Inpersol*. Abbott Laboratories, North Chicago, Ill., 1967, p. 3.
† No sodium bisulfite present.   pH adjusted to 5.1 with hydrochloric acid.

tion and medications, includes peritoneal dialysis catheters, administration sets for solution, a sterile drainage bottle, a constant-temperature bath (to prewarm the solution before use), a paracentesis or peritoneal dialysis tray (if available) that contains the necessary instruments, "drapes," towels, and dressings to insert the catheter under sterile conditions. "Dukes" Trocar (#22) with side arm is frequently used. A local anesthetic, antibiotic ointment, sutures, sterile gloves, and masks are necessary. A cleaning solution (with containers and cotton balls) is needed to scrub the abdomen before the introduction of the catheter. A 1000-ml graduate collecting bottle is needed.

Preparation and Observation of the Patient.
The physician usually explains the nature and purpose of the treatment and describes the procedure to the patient. The nurse reinforces and elaborates on this explanation, as indicated. Because this can be an uncomfortable and frightening treatment, the patient needs a great deal of reassurance. If a member of the family is present, he or she should be included in the teaching program. Some family members can be a great comfort to the patient.

Before starting the procedure, it is important for the patient to empty the bladder, because a full bladder is easily punctured. Catheterization may be necessary but should be avoided if possible. The patient should be weighed and the pulse, respiration, and blood pressure taken and recorded. This information is necessary to check the fluid balance during and after the procedure.

The supine position with the head of the bed raised to about a 45-degree angle is usually the most comfortable position during treatment. However, the nurse should help the patient change position frequently, as this is a long and tiresome procedure. It may last as long as 48 hours.

Suggested Procedure. The procedure is carried out in the patient's room. After assembling all necessary equipment, the dialysis solution may be warmed to body temperature (before using) by placing the bottles in a constant-temperature bath. Be sure the bottles are well marked (a glass marking pencil can be used) and show the per cent of glucose since the labels may be loosened when wet. Before hanging the solution bottles, add the medications carefully so no contamination occurs.

Place the patient in the supine position and prepare the abdomen for a sterile operative procedure by shaving and scrubbing the abdomen with a cleaning solution (iodine may also be applied afterward), and drape the area with sterile towels or a fenestration sheet, leaving the area uncovered where the incision will be made. The physician wears sterile gloves and mask. He or she introduces the trocar and cannula, after a local anesthetic has been given and taken effect, about 1 inch below the umbilicus in the midline of the abdomen; he or she then removes the cannula and inserts the peritoneal catheter through the barrel of the trocar. Figure 24-20 shows sites for peritoneal lavage and four-quadrant taps for abdominal paracentesis. Connect the exchange tubing to the catheter after it is sutured in place, and apply a sterile dressing over the incision around the catheter, which must be securely taped to the abdomen. Hang the two bottles of solution about 4 ft above the patient's bed and release the inflow clamp, allowing the fluid to flow as rapidly as possible. It will take about 10 to 15 minutes for the solution to flow into the cavity. Clamp the tubing just before the bottles empty so that air will not enter the system. If the patient complains of abdominal pain during rapid infusion, temporarily decrease the rate, but if the pain persists or is severe, notify the physician. It may be necessary to change the location of the peritoneal catheter or to give medications for relief of pain.

To determine whether the outflow path is obstructed, drain the first infusion immediately by

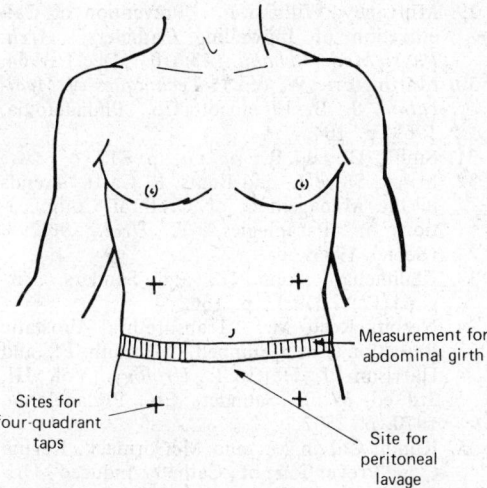

Figure 24-20. Sites for measurement of abdominal girth, for the four-quadrant taps, and for peritoneal lavage. (From Wagner, Mary M.: "Injuries to the Chest and Abdomen," *Nurs. Clin. North Am.*, 8:425, [Sept.] 1973.)

unclamping the drainage tube. The fluid should flow rapidly. The first drainage may be blood-tinged because the insertion of the trocar is traumatic. After the first drainage, the fluid is allowed to remain in the cavity for a period prescribed by the physician—usually 30 to 60 minutes. This is called the "dwell period." When the outflow phase is complete, the inflow phase is started again and the cycle continues until the dialysis, as prescribed, is completed. When the prescribed amount of dialysate has been used, remove the catheter and apply a dry, sterile dressing over the incision.

The patient may have some discomfort or pain during the procedure, especially during outflow, because the catheter may be displaced into the upper abdomen by peristalses, or the perforations of the catheter may be obstructed by fibrin. Simple measures such as changing the patient's position or applying pressure with the hands to the lower abdomen may be helpful. When these measures fail, the physician should be notified; he or she may insert another catheter. It may be necessary to give analgesics.

The amount of fluid returned should at least be equal to that infused for most patients and in many cases exceeds this amount. An accurate record of the total infusion and outflow must be maintained, showing the time and amount of each. A picture of the patient's fluid balance is reflected in this record. A "negative" fluid balance means the amount of drainage is greater than the amount of solution infused, the extra fluid being that withdrawn from the patient. In this case the patient has a fluid loss, usually considered desirable. A "positive" fluid balance means the amount of drainage is less than the amount of solution infused. In this case the patient has gained fluid by

retaining some of the infused solution. In most cases this is not desirable. The limits of negative and positive balance are set for each patient by the physician. In general, a positive balance that exceeds 500 ml or a negative balance that exceeds 1000 ml should be reported to the physician.[96]

Recording the Treatment. The importance of recording all aspects of the treatment and observations of the patient cannot be overemphasized as this information indicates the patient's reaction to the treatment. Most hospitals have special forms which include records of the amount and composition of the solution (dialysate); all medications given; vital signs (especially blood pressure and pulse), including the time they are taken; any complications that occur or discomfort experienced by the patient; and the exact time of infusion and drainages (with amounts of each). In addition, an *accurate* record of intake and output during the entire procedure should be kept and a record of the name of the physician who begins and discontinues the procedure.

REFERENCES

1. Guyton, Arthur C.: *Textbook of Medical Physiology*, 5th ed. W. B. Saunders Co., Philadelphia, 1976, p. 502.
2. Lowsley, Oswald S., and Kirwin, Thomas J.: *Clinical Urology, Vol. II*, 3rd ed. Williams & Wilkins Co., Baltimore, 1956, p. 467.
3. Straffon, Ralph A.: "Pathological Physiology of the Kidney. Micturition," in Brobeck, John R., et al. (eds.): *Best and Taylor's Physiological Basis of Medical Practice*, 9th ed. Williams & Wilkins Co., Baltimore, 1973, p. 5–54.
4. Creevy, Charles D.: "Sudden Decompression of the Chronically Distended Urinary Bladder; a Clinical and Pathologic Study," *Arch. Surg.*, **25**:356, (Aug.) 1932.
5. Osius, Theodore G., and Hinman, Frank, Jr.: "Dynamics of Acute Urinary Retention: A Manometric, Radiographic and Clinical Study," *J. Urol.*, **90**:702, (Dec.) 1963.
6. Winter, Chester C.: *Practical Urology*. C. V. Mosby Co., St. Louis, 1969, p. 169.
7. Keuhnelian, John G., and Sanders, Virginia E.: *Urologic Nursing*. Macmillan Publishing Co., Inc., New York, 1970, p. 168.
8. Kass, E. H.: "Chemotherapeutic and Antibiotic Drugs in Management of Infection of Urinary Tract," *Am. J. Med.*, **18**:764, (May) 1955.
9. ———: "Asymptomatic Infections of Urinary Tract," *Trans. Assoc. Am. Physicians*, **69**:56, 1956.
10. ———: "Bacteriuria and the Diagnosis of Infections of the Urinary Tract," *Arch. Intern. Med.*, **100**:709, (Nov.) 1957.
11. Turck, Marvin, et al.: "The Urethral Catheter and Urinary Tract Infection," *J. Urol.*, **88**:834, (Dec.) 1962.
12. Morales, Pablo, and Tsou, Anthony Y.:

"Quantitative Bacteriologic Study of Urinary Infection Among Paraplegics," *J. Urol.*, **87**: 191, (Feb.) 1962.

13. MacDonald, Richard A., et al.: "Relation Between Pyelonephritis and Bacterial Counts in the Urine," *N. Engl. J. Med.*, **256**:916, (May 16) 1957.

14. Cattell, W. R., et al.: "Catheter-Induced Urinary Infection: Follow-up Study," *Br. Med. J.*, **335**:923, (Apr. 6) 1963.

14a. Degroot, Jane, and Kunin, Calvin M.: "Indwelling Catheters," *Am. J. Nurs.*, **75**:448, (Mar.) 1975.

15. Desautels, Robert E.: "The Causes of Catheter-Induced Urinary Infections and Their Prevention," *J. Urol.*, **101**:757, (May) 1969.

16. ———: "Mismanagement of Urethral Catheterization," *Hosp. Med.*, **1**:10, (Mar.) 1965.

17. Kass, Edward H., and Schneiderman, Lawrence J.: "Entry of Bacteria into the Urinary Tracts of Patients with Inlying Catheters," *N. Engl. J. Med.*, **256**:556, (Mar. 21) 1957.

18. Ansell, J. S.: "Catheter Care," *J. Urol.*, **86**:940, (June) 1963.

19. Sanford, J. P.: "Hospital Acquired Urinary Tract Infection," in *Proceedings of National Conference on Institutionally Acquired Infection, 1963*. US Government Printing Office, Washington, D.C., 1964, p. 129 (PHS Pub. No. 1188).

20. Keuhnelian, John G., and Sanders, Virginia E., *op. cit.*, p. 129.

21. Campbell, Meredith F., and Harrison, J. Hartwell: *Urology*, Vol. I, 3rd ed. W. B. Saunders Co., Philadelphia, 1970, p. 246.

22. Desautels, Robert E.: "Mismanagement of Urethral Catheterization," *Hosp. Med.*, **1**:10, (Mar.) 1965.

22a. Chavigny, Catherine Hill: "The Use of Polymixin B as a Urethral Lubricant to Reduce the Post-instrumental Incidence of Bacteriuria in Females. An Exploratory Study," *Int. J. Nurs. Studies*, **12**:33, (June) 1975.

23. Miller, Marjorie A., and Leavell, Lutie C. (eds.): *Kimber-Gray-Stackpole's Anatomy and Physiology*, 16th ed. Macmillan Publishing Co., Inc., New York, 1972, p. 521.

24. LeComte, Ralph M.: *Manual of Urology*, 4th ed. Williams & Wilkins Co., Baltimore, 1948, p. 20.

25. Ridley, Mark: "A Bacteriologist's View," *Nurs. Times*, **59**:1501, (Nov. 29) 1963.

26. Mainwaring, Cathryn: "Clean Voided Specimens for Mass Screening," *Am. J. Nurs.*, **63**:96, (Oct.) 1963.

27. Campbell, Meredith F., and Harrison, J. Hartwell: *op. cit.*, p. 246.

27a. Lapides, Jack, et al.: "Clean, Intermittent Self-Catheterization in the Treatment of Urinary Tract Disease," *J. Urol.*, **107**:458, (Mar.) 1972.

27b. Smith, Donald R.: *General Urology*, 7th ed. Lange Medical Publications, Los Altos, Calif., 1972, p. 163.

28. Keuhnelian, John G., and Sanders, Virginia E.: *op. cit.*, p. 170.

29. Mulvaney, William P.: "Prevention of Calcification of Indwelling Catheters," *Arch. Phys. Med. Rehabil.*, **45**:610, (Dec.) 1964.

30. Martin, Eric W. (ed.): *Techniques of Medication*. J. B. Lippincott Co., Philadelphia, 1969, p. 104.

31. Smith, Donald R.: *op. cit.*, p. 317.

32. Misak, Steve J., and Bunts, R. Carl: "Trends in the Management of Urethral Complications in Paraplegics," *J. Urol.*, **90**:298, (Sept.) 1963.

33. Keuhnelian, John G., and Sanders, Virginia E.: *op. cit.*, p. 166.

34. Nesbit, Reed M.: "Transurethral Prostatic Resection," in Campbell, Meredith F., and Harrison, J. Hartwell: *Urology*, Vol. III, 3rd ed. W. B. Saunders Co., Philadelphia, 1970, p. 2502.

35. Kunin, Calvin M., and McCormack, Regina C.: "Prevention of Catheter-Induced Urinary-Tract Infections by Sterile Closed Drainage," *N. Engl. J. Med.*, **274**:1155, (May 26) 1966.

36. Finkelberg, Zachary, and Kunin, Calvin M.: "Clinical Evaluation of Closed Urinary Drainage Systems," *J.A.M.A.*, **207**:1657, (Mar. 3) 1969.

37. Roberts, J. B. M., et al.: "Long-Term Catheter Drainage in Male," *Br. J. Urol.*, **37**:63, 1965.

38. Desautels, R. E., et al.: "Technical Advances in the Prevention of Urinary Tract Infection," *J. Urol.*, **87**:487, (Mar.) 1962.

39. Cleland, Virginia, et al.: "Prevention of Bacteriuria in Female Patients with Indwelling Catheters," *Nurs. Res.*, **20**:309, (July–Aug.) 1971.

40. Miller, Ashton: "Infections of the Urinary Tract Excluding Tuberculosis," *Br. J. Urol.*, **37**:34, 1965.

41. Desautels, R. E., et al.: "Technical Advances in the Prevention of Urinary Tract Infection," *J. Urol.*, **87**:487, (Mar.) 1962.

42. Gillespie, W. A., et al.: "Prevention of Catheter Infection of Urine in Female Patients," *Br. Med. J.*, **2**:13, (July 7) 1962.

43. Roberts, J. B. M., et al.: *op. cit.*

44. Kunin, Calvin M., and McCormack, Regina C.: *op. cit.*

45. Desautels, Robert E.: "The Causes of Catheter-Induced Urinary Infections and Their Prevention," *J. Urol.*, **101**:757, (May) 1969.

46. Cleland, Virginia, et al.: *op. cit.*

47. Gibbon, Norman: "A New Type of Catheter for Urethral Drainage of the Bladder," *Br. J. Urol.*, **30**:1, 1958.

48. Santora, Delores: "Preventing Hospital-Acquired Urinary Infection," *Am. J. Nurs.*, **66**:790, (Apr.) 1966.

49. Munro, Donald: "Rehabilitation of Patients Totally Paralyzed Below the Waist, with Special Reference to Making Them Ambulatory and Capable of Earning Their Living; Tidal Drainage, Cystometry and Bladder Training," *N. Engl. J. Med.*, **236**:223, (Feb. 13) 1947.

50. Seidel, Eleanora S.: "Tidal Drainage—Its

Present Status," *Am. J. Nurs.*, **50:**702, (Nov.) 1950.

51. Everett, Houston S., and Ridley, John H.: *Female Urology.* Harper & Row, New York, 1969, p. 138.

52. Kass, Edward H., and Sossen, Harold S.: "Prevention of Infection of Urinary Tract in Presence of Indwelling Catheters," *J.A.M.A.*, **169:**1181, (Mar. 14) 1959.

53. Creevy, Charles: *Outline of Urology.* McGraw-Hill Book Co., New York, 1964, p. 313.

54. Lapides, Jack: "Neuromuscular Vesical and Ureteral Dysfunction," in Campbell, Meredith F., and Harrison, J. Hartwell: *Urology,* Vol. II, 3rd ed. W. B. Saunders Co., Philadelphia, 1970, p. 1362.

55. Everett, Houston S., and Ridley, John H.: *op. cit.*, p. 138.

56. Nesbit, Reed M., *op. cit.*, p. 2502

57. Keuhnelian, John G., and Sanders, Virginia E.: *op. cit.*, p. 170.

58. Misak, Steve J., and Bunts, R. Carl: *op. cit.*

59. Munro, Donald: *op. cit.*

60. Lapides, Jack: *op. cit.*, p. 1352.

61. Kintzel, James E., and Cameron, Elizabeth M.: "The Insulted Kidney: Medical and Nursing Intervention for Patients Undergoing Dialysis or Renal Homotransplantation," in Kintzel, Kay Corman (ed.): *Advanced Concepts in Clinical Nursing.* J. B. Lippincott Co., Philadelphia, 1971, p. 291.

61a. Gutch, C. F., and Stones, Martha H.: *Review of Hemodialysis for Nurses and Dialysis Personnel,* 2nd ed. C. V. Mosby Co., St. Louis, 1975.

62. Merrill, John P.: "Management of Chronic Renal Failure: Present and Prospective," *Am. J. Med.*, **36:**763, (May) 1964.

63. Strauss, Maurice B., and Raiz, Lawrence G.: *Clinical Management of Renal Failure.* Charles C Thomas, Publisher, Springfield, Ill., 1956, p. 50.

64. Merrill, John P.: *op. cit.*

65. Scribner, B. H., et al.: "The Technique of Continuous Hemodialysis," *Trans. Am. Soc. Artif. Intern. Organs,* **6:**88, 1960.

66. Brescia, Michael J., et al.: "Chronic Hemodialysis Using Venipuncture and a Surgically Created Arteriovenous Fistula," *N. Engl. J. Med.*, **275:**1089, (Nov. 17) 1966.

67. Smith, Warren W., et al.: "The Use of the Artificial Kidney in the Community Hospital," *Ohio State Med. J.*, **59:**1202, (Dec.) 1963.

68. Maher, J. F., et al.: "Editorial Review: The Clinical Dialysis of Poisons," *Trans. Am. Soc. Artif. Intern. Organs,* **11:**349, 1965.

69. Setter, John G., et al.: "Barbiturate Intoxication," *Arch. Intern. Med.*, **117:**224, (Feb.) 1966.

70. Lubash, Glenn D.: "Acute Renal Failure," *Hosp. Med.*, **1:**14, (Apr.) 1965.

71. Curtis, F. K., et al.: "Hemodialysis in the Home," *Trans. Am. Soc. Artif. Intern. Organs,* **11:**7, 1965.

71a. Wilkinson, Patricia Marshall: "Nursing in a Limited Care Hemodialysis Facility," *Nurs. Clin. North Am.*, **10:**491, (Sept.) 1975.

72. Johnson, William J., et al.: "Hemodialysis," *Arch. Intern. Med.*, **125:**462, (Mar.) 1970.

73. Kintzel, James E., and Cameron, Elizabeth M.: *op. cit.*, p. 294.

74. Pendras, Jerry P., and Erickson, R. V.: "Hemodialysis: A Successful Therapy for Chronic Uremia," *Ann. Intern. Med.*, **64:**293, (Feb.) 1966.

75. Lewis, Edmund J., et al.: "Survival Data for Patients Undergoing Chronic Intermittent Hemodialysis," *Ann. Intern. Med.*, **70:**311, (Feb.) 1969.

76. Freeman, Richard B., et al.: "Hemodialysis for Chronic Renal Failure," *Ann. Intern. Med.*, **62:**519, (Mar.) 1965.

76a. Smith, Linda J.: "Large Surface Area Dialysis," *Nurs. Clin. North Am.*, **10:**481, (Sept.) 1975.

77. Trusk, Carol Williams: "Hemodialysis for Acute Renal Failure," *Am. J. Nurs.*, **65:**80, (Feb.) 1965.

78. Kintzel, James E., and Cameron, Elizabeth M.: *op. cit.*

79. Freeman, Richard B., et al.: *op. cit.*

80. Cole, J. J., et al.: "The Pumpless Low Temperature Hemodialysis System," *Trans. Am. Soc. Artif. Intern. Organs,* **8:**209, 1962.

80a. Pendras, Jerry P. & Stinson, Gerald W. (eds.): *The Hemodialysis Manual,* Section VII. The Theory of Hemodialysis. Edmark Corp., Seattle, Wash., p. 5.

81. Quinton, W. E., et al.: "Eight Months' Experience with Silastic-Teflon Bypass Cannulas," *Trans. Am. Soc. Artif. Intern. Organs,* **8:**236, 1962.

82. Shaldon, Stanley, and Cook, G. C.: *Acute Renal Failure.* F. A. Davis Co., Philadelphia, 1964, p. 146.

82a. Read, Martha, and Mallison, Mary: "External Arteriovenous Shunts," *Am. J. Nurs.*, **72:**81, (Jan.) 1972.

83. Maher, John F., et al.: "Regional Heparinization for Hemodialysis—Technique and Clinical Experiences," *N. Engl. J. Med.*, **268:**451, (Feb. 28) 1963.

84. Shea, Eileen J., et al.: "Hemodialysis for Chronic Renal Failure. IV. Psychological Considerations," *Ann. Intern Med.*, **62:**558, (Mar.) 1965.

84a. Anger, Diane: "The Psychologic Stress of Chronic Renal Failure and Long-Term Hemodialysis," *Nurs. Clin. North Am.*, **10·**449, (Sept.) 1975.

85. Kintzel, James E., and Cameron, Elizabeth M.: *op. cit.*, p. 297.

86. Trusk, Carol Williams: *op. cit.*

87. Boen, S. T.: *Peritoneal Dialysis in Clinical Medicine.* Charles C Thomas, Publisher, Springfield, Ill., 1964, p. 90.

88. Twiss, Mary R., and Maxwell, Morton H.: "Peritoneal Dialysis," *Am. J. Nurs.*, **59:**1560, (Nov.) 1959.

89. Hager, Edward B., and Merrill, John P.: "Peritoneal Dialysis and Acute Renal Fail-

ure," *Surg. Clin. North Am.*, **43:**883, (June) 1963.

90. Boen, S. T.: *op. cit.*, p. 8, 10.
91. Bland, John H.: *Clinical Metabolism of Body Water and Electrolytes.* W. B. Saunders Co., Philadelphia, 1963, p. 598.
92. Boen, S. T.: *op. cit.*, p. 86.
93. Berlyne, G. M., et al.: "Pulmonary Complications of Peritoneal Dialysis," *Lancet*, **2:**75, (July 9) 1966.
94. Boen, S. T.: *op. cit.*, p. 81.
94a. Henderson, Lee W., and Nolph, Karl D.: "Altered Permeability of the Peritoneal Membrane after Using Hypertonic Peritoneal Dialysis Fluid," *J. Clin. Invest.*, **48:**992, (May) 1969.
95. Gross, Melvin, and MacDonald, Harold P., Jr.: "Effect of Dialysate Temperature and Flow Rate on Peritoneal Clearance," *J.A.M.A.*, **202:**363, (Oct. 23) 1967.
96. Kintzel, James E., and Cameron, Elizabeth M.: *op. cit.*, p. 290.

Additional Suggested Reading

Adams, Ralph: "Prevention of Infection in Hospitals," *Am. J. Nurs.*, **58:**344, (Mar.) 1958.

Ansell, J. S.: "Catheter Care," *J. Urol.*, **89:**940, (June) 1963.

Anger, Diane, and Anger, Daniel W.: "Dialysis Ambivalence: A Matter of Life and Death," *Am. J. Nurs.*, **76:**276, (Feb.) 1976.

Bengston, Edna G., and Elliot, James E.: "The Value of Water Diuresis Following Transurethral Prostatic Resection," *Nurs. Res.*, **15:**177, (Spring) 1966.

Birum, Linda Hulthen, and Zimmerman, Donna Stulgis: "Catheter Plugs as a Source of Infection," *Am. J. Nurs.*, **71:**2150, (Nov.) 1971.

Blandy, J. P.: "Catheterization," *Nurs. Mirror*, **122:**v, (Sept. 30) 1966.

Brand, Lucy, and Komorita, Nori I.: "Adapting to Long Term Hemodialysis," *Am. J. Nurs.*, **66:**1778, (Aug.) 1966.

Burton, Benjamin R., et al.: "National Registry of Long Term Dialysis Patient," *J.A.M.A.*, **288:**718, (Nov. 1) 1971.

Cameron, J. S., and Russell, Alison M. E.: *Nephrology for Nurses: A Modern Approach to the Kidney.* William Heinemann Medical Books, Ltd., London, 1970.

Chute, Ralph: "Catheters, Bacteriuria and Pyelonephritis," *J. Ky. Med. Assoc.*, **64:**403, (May) 1966.

Clark, Cheryl Lee: "Catheter Care in the Home," *Am. J. Nurs.*, **72:**922, (May) 1972.

Clifton, Janice: "Collecting 24-Hour Urine Specimens from Infants," *Am. J. Nurs.*, **69:**1660, (Aug.) 1969.

Colapinto, V., and McCallum, R. W.: "Urinary Continence After Repair of Membranous Urethral Stricture in Prostatectomized Patients," *J. Urol.*, **115:**392, (Apr.) 1976.

Corea, Anna L.: "Current Trends in Diet and Drug Therapy for the Dialysis Patient," *Nurs. Clin. North Am.*, **10:**469, (Sept.) 1975.

Cullinan, J.: "The Making and Meaning of

EDTNA (European Dialysis and Transplant Nurses Association)," *Nurs. Times*, **69:**819, (June 28) 1973.

Cummings, Jonathan W.: "Hemodialysis—Feelings, Facts, and Fantasies," *Am. J. Nurs.*, **70:**70, (Jan.) 1970.

"Dialysis, Renal Failure, and Vitamin Homeostasis," *Nutr. Rev.*, **27:**75, (Mar.) 1969.

Dobbins, Janet, and Gleit, Carol: "Experience with the Lateral Position for Catheterization," *Nurs. Clin. North Am.*, **6:**373, (June) 1971.

Downes, Ann Wright, and Cleland, Virginia S.: "Bacteriuria and Urinary Tract Infection in Infancy and Childhood, A Review," *Nurs. Res.*, **20:**131, (Mar.–Apr.) 1971.

Downing, Shirley R.: "Nursing Support in Early Renal Failure," *Am. J. Nurs.*, **69:**1212, (June) 1969.

Eschbach, J. W., et al.: "Hemodialysis in the Home," *Ann. Intern. Med.*, **67:**1149, (Dec.) 1967.

Fearing, Margery O.: "Osteodystrophy in Patients with Chronic Renal Failure," *Nurs. Clin. North Am.*, **10:**461, (Sept.) 1975.

Fellows, Barbara: "Hemodialysis at Home," *Am. J. Nurs.* **66:**1775, (Aug.) 1966.

————: "The Role of the Nurse in a Chronic Dialysis Unit," *Nurs. Clin. North Am.*, **1:**517, (Dec.) 1966.

Foy, Audrey L.: "Dreams of Patients and Staff," *Am. J. Nurs.*, **70:**80, (Jan.) 1970.

Frewen, W. K.: "Urgency Incontinence: Review of 100 Cases," *J. Obstet. Gynaecol. Br. Commonw.*, **79:**77, (Jan.) 1972.

Gombos, E. A., et al.: "One Year's Experience with an Intermittent Dialysis Program," *Ann. Intern. Med.*, **61:**467, (Sept.) 1964.

Gross, James B., and Kokkro, Juhap: "The Influence of Increased Tubular Hydrostatic Pressure of Renal Function," *J. Urol.*, **115:**424, (Apr.) 1976.

Hampers, Constantine L., and Merrill, John P.: "Hemodialysis in the Home—Thirteen Months' Experience," *Ann. Intern. Med.*, **64:**276, (Feb.) 1966.

Hampers, Constantine L., and Schupak, Eugene: *Long Term Dialysis.* Grune & Stratton, New York, 1967.

Hansen, Ginny L.: *Caring for Patients with Chronic Renal Disease.* J. B. Lippincott Co., Philadelphia, 1974.

Harrington, Joan DeLong, and Brener, Etta Rae: *Patient Care in Renal Failure.* W. B. Saunders Co., Philadelphia, 1973.

Henderson, L. W.: "Peritoneal Ultrafiltration Dialysis: Enhanced Urea Transfer Using Hypertonic Peritoneal Dialysis Fluid," *J. Clin. Invest.*, **45:**950, (June) 1966.

Henderson, L. W., et al.: "Further Experience with the Inlying Plastic Conduit for Chronic Peritoneal Dialysis," *Trans. Am. Soc. Artif. Intern. Organs*, **1:**106, 1963.

Hinckley, Bernice: "The Changing Role of the Dialysis Nurse," *Nurs. Clin. North Am.*, **4:**395, (Sept.) 1969.

Khan, Abdul J., and Pryles, Charles V.: "Urinary Tract Infection in Children," *Am. J. Nurs.,* **73**:1340, (Aug.) 1973.

Kory, Mitchell, and Waife, S. E. (eds.): *Kidney and Urinary Tract Infection.* Lilly Research Laboratories, Indianapolis, 1971.

Kossoris, Penny: "Family Therapy: An Adjunct to Hemodialysis and Transplantation," *Am. J. Nurs.,* **70**:1730, (Aug.) 1970.

Kunin, Calvin M.: "Prevention of Urinary Tract Infections in Hospitalized Patients," in *Proceedings of the International Conference on Nosocomial Infections,* Center for Disease Control, August 3–6, 1970. American Hospital Association, Chicago, 1971.

Langford, Teddy Lynn: "Nursing Problem: Bacteriuria and the Indwelling Catheter," *Am. J. Nurs.,* **72**:113, (Jan.) 1972.

Lapides, Jack: *Fundamentals of Urology.* W. B. Saunders Co., Philadelphia, 1976.

Merrill, J. P., et al.: "Hemodialysis in the Home," *J.A.M.A.,* **190**:144, (Nov. 2) 1964.

Michalov, Thelma R.: "Bowel and Bladder Management of Children with Myelomeningocele," *Nurs. Clin. North Am.,* **1**:459, (Sept.) 1966.

O'Neill, Mary: "Guidelines for Teaching Home Dialysis," *Nurs. Clin. North Am.,* **6**:641, (Dec.) 1971.

Pendras, Jerry P., and Pollard, Terrance L.: "Eight Years Experience with a Community Dialysis Center: The Northwest Kidney Center," *Trans. Am. Soc. Artif. Intern. Organs,* **16**:77, (Apr.) 1970.

Raz, Shlomo, and Smith, Robert B.: "External Sphincter Spasticity Syndrome in Female Patients," *J. Urol.,* **115**:443, (Apr.) 1976.

Reams, Gerald B., and Powell, Elma J.: "Post-operative Catheterization—Yes or No?" *Am. J. Nurs.,* **60**:371, (Mar.) 1960.

Riechers, Rogers N., and Brendler, Herbert: "Peritoneal Dialysis for Patients in Uremia Secondary to Obstructive Disease," *J. Urol.,* **107**:341, (Mar.) 1972.

Schlotter, Lowanna: "What Do You Teach the Dialysis Patient," *Am. J. Nurs., **70**:82, (Jan.) 1970.

———: "Learning to Be a Home Dialysis Patient," *Nurs. Clin. North Am.,* **4**:419, (Sept.) 1969.

Schreiner, George E., and Maher, John F.: "Hemodialysis for Chronic Renal Failure. III. Medical, Moral and Ethical, and Socio-Economic Problems," *Ann. Intern. Med.,* **62**:551, (Mar.) 1965.

Schumann, Delores: "The Renal Donor," *Am. J. Nurs.,* **74**:105, (Jan.) 1974.

Sood, Satya F.: "Prevention of Urinary Tract Infection After Gynaecological Laparotomy," *J. Obstet. Gynaecol. Br. Commonw.,* **79**:80, (Jan.) 1972

Tyler, Carl W., and Oseasohn, Robert: "The Relationship of In-lying Catheterization to Persistent Bacteriuria in Gynecologic Patients," *Am. J. Obstet. Gynecol.,* **86**:998, (Aug. 15) 1963.

Watt, Rosemary C.: "Urinary Diversion," *Am. J. Nurs.,* **74**:1806, (Oct.) 1974.

Wright, Robert G., et al.: "Psychological Stress During Hemodialysis for Chronic Renal Failure," *Ann. Intern. Med.,* **64**:611, (Mar.) 1966.

Gladys Nite
Virginia Henderson

Irrigation of the Vulva, Perineum, and Vaginal Canal for Cleaning and Medication

1. BASIC PRINCIPLES UNDERLYING THE SELECTION OF METHOD

Certain *anatomic and physiologic factors* have a definite bearing on the selection of method in cleaning and medicating the vulva and vaginal canal. For example, structural characteristics influence the length and direction of the insertion of irrigating tips or of suppositories; temperature tolerance determines, to a large extent, the heat of irrigating solutions, and resistance to bacteria determines the preparation of equipment.

Skin covers the labia majora and gradually merges into a modified mucous membrane on the labia minora. The mucous lining of the vagina is arranged in folds, which makes childbirth possible but a thorough cleaning of the canal difficult. A delicate sheet of mucous membrane, the hymen, may entirely or partially occlude the vaginal orifice in the virgin. If such an occlusion exists, the condition is referred to as an *imperforate hymen,* and an operation is indicated to allow egress of the vaginal flow. It is, of course, impossible to give a vaginal irrigation if an imperforate hymen exists. In giving this treatment for the first time, the nurse should examine the orifice carefully in order to be sure that the condition is a normal one. Physicians rarely prescribe an irrigation without having made this examination themselves.

An especially important anatomic feature of the female reproductive tract is the fact that the mucous membrane of the external genitalia is continuous with the lining of the uterus and through the fallopian tubes with the peritoneum, or the serous lining of the abdominal cavity. An infection of the vagina can therefore spread by direct extension to the peritoneum and throughout the abdomen. Since peritonitis is a highly serious condition, physicians try to prevent any possibility of its occurring and rarely irrigate the uterus. If used, *vaginal irrigations should be given under low pressure* to avoid the possibility of forcing infectious material into the uterus.

Except during menstruation and the later stages of pregnancy, the internal and external openings of the cervix (the neck of the uterus) are normally closed. This, to some extent, protects the body of the uterus from bacteria always present in the vagina. Most authorities advise against vaginal irrigations during both menstruation and pregnancy, because there is more likelihood at these times of forcing material into the uterus. Louis M. Hellman and Jack A. Pritchard [1] say several deaths in pregnancy from air embolism have occurred following use of hand bulb syringes in vaginal irrigation; consequently, their use *"must be absolutely forbidden."* The downward and outward flow of the menstrual discharge and lochia tends to wash pathogenic bacteria from the vaginal tract. Any reversal of the flow is contraindicated.

The vaginal secretions contain lactic acid that, according to Dugald Baird,[2] Lester Cohen,[3] and other authorities, discourages the growth and decreases the virulence of organisms resident in the vagina and cervix. The acidity of the vaginal secretions is due to fermentation of glycogen (which is always present in the vagina) by the Döderlein's bacillus, a large Gram-positive rod-shaped organism. The pH of vaginal secretions of healthy individuals varies according to age: the newborn infant, 4 to 5; 1-month infant, 7; adolescent (during puberty), increased acidity of secretions; adult woman during childbearing period, 4 to 5; and during the menopausal period, 6 to 7.[4] J. P. Greenhill[5] says that all uteri contain vaginal bacteria by the second day following delivery of the fetus. A number of factors, some of which may be unknown, explain why infection does not develop in all women.

There seems to be general agreement that under ordinary circumstances *the intact vaginal mucosa discourages the growth of pathogenic organisms;* however, the generative tract is peculiarly susceptible to infection during the late stages of pregnancy, at delivery, and during the post-partum period. This lowered resistance may be explained by the stretching and injury of tissues, or by the change that occurs in the chemical nature of the secretions, or to both circumstances. Undoubtedly, the introduction of foreign strains of microorganisms is especially dangerous to the obstetric or surgical patient. The low incidence of infections in home deliveries as compared to those in the hospital, when both groups receive comparable medical and nursing care, suggests the hazard of exposing a woman to a large group of attendants and to a new bacterial environment to which she has not developed immunity.

Apparently the reproductive tract is much more susceptible to infection from one type of organism than another. It is well to know that all human feces contain strains of colon bacilli and that most persons harbor welchii bacilli in the colon. Fecal organisms have easy access to the vagina, and if infections do not occur it must mean that there is natural protection. Andrew A. Marchetti[6] in 1934, in a careful study of medical literature over a long period, found only 56 cases of Welch's bacillus infections reported. Coralie Rendle-Short[7] brings this review up to 1942 and remarks on the rarity of welchii infections. Fifteen years later (1967) most authors note that infection by the welchii bacillus is, indeed, rare. James C. Caillouette[8] says the most feared intrauterine infections are those resulting from this organism. In comparison it is estimated that the streptococcus causes the majority of puerperal infections and that puerperal infections cause approximately one-fourth of the total number of maternal deaths. A large number of healthy persons are found to have streptococci in the throat. Discussing puerperal infection, Greenhill notes that there are two modes of transmitting organisms to the genital tract: exogenous and endogenous, the latter is called autoinfection. Exogenous infection (source is external) is the most common of the two. Although infection may be transferred to the genital tract from the outside in a variety of ways, special emphasis is placed on the environment, insufficiently sterilized equipment, and medical personnel. He says: "Of the many ways by which the air can become the bearer of infective particles special emphasis is laid on the streptococcus carrier who coughs, sneezes or talks the air full of germ-laden droplets of saliva and mucus." * As early as 1933, the Committee on Public Health Relations of the New York Academy of Medicine,[9] studying maternal mortality in New York City, strongly recommended that attendants giving perineal care mask the nose and mouth. J. C. Colbeck[10] (1962) believes that many of the aseptic measures introduced at that time are still of value; authorities consulted do not agree that masking the nose and mouth while giving perineal care is necessary. J. S. Tomkinson[11] (in England) says a mask should be worn, whereas Hellman and Pritchard[12] strongly recommend its use during delivery only. In the United States, masks are usually not worn when giving perineal care. A discussion of types of masks and their efficacy is included in Chapters 15 and 44. Medical personnel as well as visitors who have a respiratory infection or acute or chronic sinus infections should not come in contact with postpartal or postoperative patients.

In spite of the fact that infections by spore-forming organisms are rare, sterilization by steam under pressure is the method of choice for the preparation of sterile supplies for the postoperative or obstetric patient.

Many physicians believe that at any age and under any circumstances resistance to infection in the vagina is lowered by irrigations that wash away secretions offering a natural protection. Elaine C. Pierson[13] says that "maybe . . . most women, never douche unless required for medical reasons" and she adds that "a good percentage" of gynecologists "over the age of forty-five are absolutely against it." She herself thinks that weekly douching may control "omnipresent yeast infections associated with the pill" and that it may be beneficial under other circumstances. Robert Glynn[14] reports there was "no significant alterations in vaginal pH, as determined electronically, and no adverse effects on the vaginal mucosa as determined by Papanicolaou smears" following daily vaginal douching for 1 month with water, an alkaline powder, vinegar, or an acid powder. Larry McGowan[15] notes that some authors recommend douching as a safe procedure while others condemn it as being a hazard, even resulting in peritonitis; he reports

* Greenhill, J. P.: *DeLee's Obstetrics*, 13th ed. W. B. Saunders Co., Philadelphia, 1965, p. 1069.

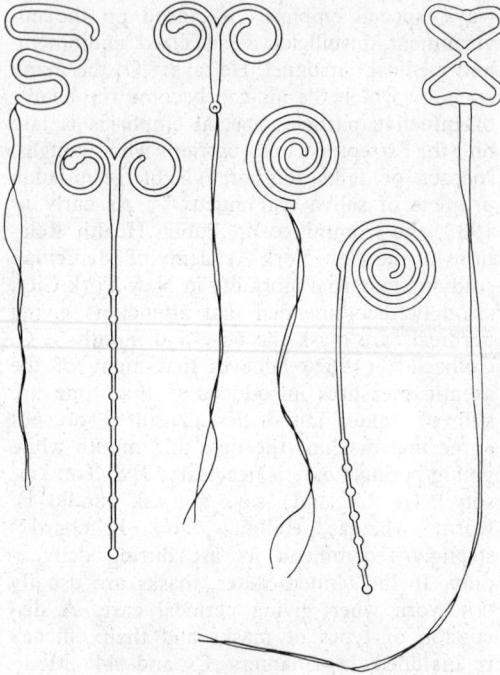

Figure 25-1. Various plastic intrauterine contraceptive devices, including (*left to right*) Lippes' loop, Saf-T-Coil with stem, Saf-T-Coil without stem, Gynecoil without stem, Gynecoil with stem, and Birnberg bow.

nine cases of pelvic peritonitis that immediately followed douching of the vaginal canal. As a result, a self-bathing technique that includes manual cleaning of the vulva and vagina with a nonirritating soap * was found to be an effective means of cleaning the areas in a group of 360 asymptomatic women. The same method employed with a group of 94 women with symptomatic *Trichomonas vaginalis* vaginitis was effective in relieving symptoms in 94.7 per cent of the women in seven days. Treatments such as these, including vaginal irrigation, should be used only when prescribed by a physician.

Many women have used douching without medical prescription as a means of avoiding pregnancy. Donald W. Hastings,[16] discussing contraception, says that douches are commonly thought to be useful but are of no value in preventing conception. He also thinks that douching following intercourse is unnecessary since "the normal vagina has an excellent ability to cleanse itself"; external bathing is therefore all that is necessary. He believes the chemicals advertised for "feminine hygiene"

* Ivory and Dial soap were used in this study.

may be irritating and may upset the delicate chemical balance of the normal vagina.

Both Hastings and Pierson discuss the following methods of contraception that are currently known: for males, vas ligation (vasectomy), condoms, and withdrawal of the penis from the vagina before ejaculation; for females, tubal ligation; "the pill" (some that depress ovulation while others bring about changes in the endometrial lining of the uterus, inhibiting implantation of the cells); injecting foams, gels, cremes (creams), and suppositories into the vagina that kill the male cell (sperm); the introduction of foreign bodies into the uterus (intrauterine devices, IUDs) that prevent implantation or the development of a fetus (see Fig. 25-1 and Table 25-1); the use of a diaphragm that closes the opening of the cervix; avoiding intercourse during the period of ovulation (rhythm method) with or without the measurement of basal body temperature; and, of course, abstinence for both male and female.

Because nurses are professional health workers, the public expects them to be informed on and able to counsel their clients or patients on sexual practice.[16a,16b,16c] A general book such as this cannot treat the subject adequately. The literature on sex goes back to Aristotle or even the first written records of human behavior. It has religious, moral or ethical, sociologic, and physiologic aspects. The extensive research of A. C. Kinsey and his associates in recent decades has thrown light on the psychosocial aspects of sex and the joint studies of

Table 25-1. Utilization of Intrauterine Contraceptive Devices *

	Approximate Cumulative Number of IUD Insertions		
Country†	Sept. 1964	Jan. 1966	Jan. 1968
South Korea	50,000	350,000	1,100,000
Taiwan	25,000	150,000	370,000
Pakistan	5,000	50,000	1,200,000
India	2,000	320,000	2,000,000

* Jordan, Clara H.: "Family Planning—A Vital Family Health Service," in Kintzel, Kay Corman (ed.): *Advanced Concepts in Clinical Nursing.* J. B. Lippincott Co., Philadelphia, 1971, p. 33. From United States Food and Drug Administration: Report on Intrauternie Devices by the Advisory Committee on Obstetrics and Gynecology. Studies in Family Planning. The Population Council, #27, 1968, p. 13.

† Accurate figures for the United States are not available. By September 1964, the major manufacturers of IUD's distributed nearly 250,000 devices. By January 1968, the total number distributed was approximately 3,000,000.

William H. Masters and Virginia E. Johnson have answered many physiologic questions and raised others in the psychosocial field. Their bibliography of 333 books and articles in their report *The Human Sexual Response* [16d] could serve as a guide to nurses who wish to study the subject in depth or who expect to specialize in counseling. Pierson has prepared a booklet, in question and answer form, entitled *Sex Is Never an Emergency. A Candid Guide for College Students.* [16e] In its first edition (1970), it was titled *A Guide for University of Pennsylvania Students.* Nurses should know the specialized counseling services in their community including those connected with the various religions. Sex behavior should not be considered apart from other aspects of life. [16f-h]

The length of the vagina varies markedly in the child, the adolescent, and in the fully developed woman. Abnormalities of the vagina occur occasionally. In the mature adult the average length of the anterior wall is 6 to 8 cm and that of the posterior wall 7 to 10 cm, according to Hellman and Pritchard. [17] In the early years of life there are numerous transverse ridges or *rugae* which form a corrugated surface of the vagina but gradually become obliterated after repeated childbirth, often resulting in a smooth vaginal wall in elderly multiparas. The intravaginal portion of the cervix projects into the vagina at such an angle that a sort of pocket is formed between the cervix and the posterior wall of the vagina. In suppurative vaginitis, or following the rupture of a pelvic abscess, pus may collect in this pocket. Irrigations to clean the vagina under such circumstances should be so administered that the solution comes in contact with this area.

The direction in which the tip or nozzle is inserted largely determines whether the solution reaches all parts of the vagina, as it should. By studying Figure 25-2, it can be seen that in the standing position the direction of the vagina is upward and backward. With the recumbent patient, the vaginal tip should be directed upward and backward at an angle of about 35 degrees. Since a reasonable amount of vaginal dilation causes no discomfort or irritation, the tip may be gently rotated without danger to the tissues.

The *position* of the patient also should favor the entrance of the irrigating solution into the upper part of the vagina. Elevating the hips and lowering the head helps to distend the vaginal walls with the irrigating fluid.

There is normally a small amount of mucous *discharge from the vagina* between the menstrual periods. A profuse or purulent discharge is an indication of pathology. Pruritus (itching) of the vulva, a distressing condition, often accompanies vaginal discharge. According to Edmund R. Novak and associates, [18] the amount of leukorrhea is not related to the degree of discomfort experienced by the person. A variety of local causes discussed include inflammatory skin diseases, ulcerative lesions of the vulva, irritating discharges from the urethra, vagina, and cervix, trichomonas and mycotic infections of the vagina, animal para-

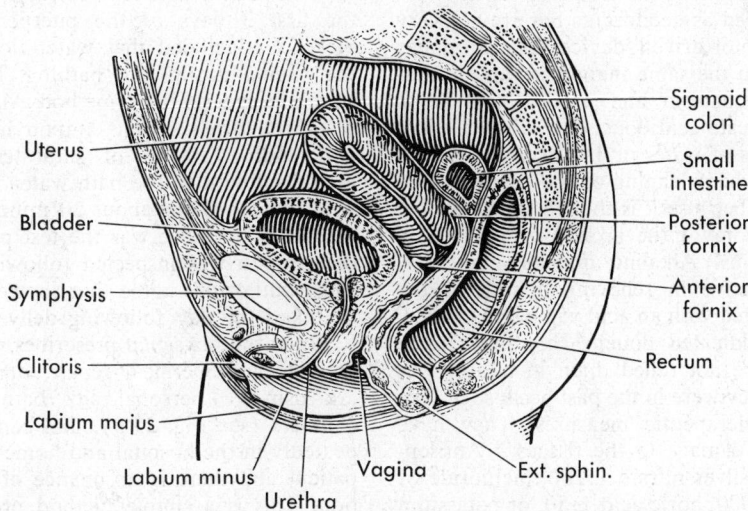

Figure 25-2. Median section of the female pelvis. Note the direction a nozzle should take to follow the normal curve of the vagina. (From Miller, M. A., Leavell, L. C., and Drakontides, A. B.: *Kimber-Gray-Stackpole's Anatomy and Physiology,* 17th ed. Macmillan Publishing Co., Inc., New York, 1977.)

sites, chemical irritation due to strong soaps, lotions, and ointments, and uncleanliness. Some of the general causes are endocrine disorders, allergy, toxic conditions, diabetes mellitus, and conditions of general physical disability. Like most body discharges, the vaginal secretions contain protein substances that on decomposition have a strong odor. Underclothing made of synthetics should not be worn; they should not be binding or too warm. Of course, the individual should be encouraged to refrain from scratching. Frequent cleaning of the vulva with a mild soap and water is esthetically essential to prevent an accumulation of these secretions in the mucous folds of all persons, including those who do not have an excessive amount of vaginal secretions. After using the bedpan, a patient should be given the necessary articles for bathing this area; or, if she is too ill to make the effort, the nurse should do it.

According to *Consumer Reports* [19] (1972), there are 30 brands of "feminine hygiene spray" on the market. These are used indiscriminately by women and men in an attempt to control genital odor. Their use is considered to be dangerous; one physician reports 30 cases of vulvitis following the use of these sprays. Authorities consulted consistently advocate soap and water as the most effective and safest hygiene.

Deodorizing powders, such as sodium borate, may be used after cleaning the vulva, but soaps or solutions having characteristic odors should never be used. The odor of the drug is itself disagreeable and comes to be associated with the odor it is intended to correct. In carcinoma of the uterus, oxidizing agents are sometimes used as deodorants but are not very effective. Motor-driven devices placed under the bed act in the same manner as an air-conditioning mechanism and are helpful. Some authors advocate acid douches (3 tbsp of vinegar to 3 liters of water or 1 tbsp of lactic acid to 2 liters) when cleaning of the vaginal canal is necessary, because it is thought that alkaline douches may favor the growth of pathogenic microorganisms. Alkaline douches, however, may be effective in relieving itching of the vulva associated with an acid vaginal discharge. Although medicated douches continue to be used, they are not relied upon in treating infections as they were in the past because of specific chemotherapeutic measures. They have caused local damage to the tissues.[20] Antiseptics, such as silver nitrate 1:200, bichloride of mercury 1:1000, boric acid 1:50, or potassium permanganate 1:2000, are used in treating vaginal infections, but must be prescribed by the doctor. Astringents such as tannic acid, acetic acid, and alum are used to check secretions.

Many irrigations are prescribed purely for the heat effect, in which case water or physiologic saline is most often used. If the physician prescribes an irrigation and fails to stipulate the kind of solution and he or she cannot be reached, it is always safe for the nurse to use water or sodium chloride 1:1000.

During postpartum, it is generally accepted that cleanliness is the primary object of so-called perineal care.[21] Many hospitals and visiting nurse organizations have given up chemical antiseptics in this procedure and substitute bathing the perineum with soap and water, using a regular washcloth or a pre-packaged disposable one that is impregnated with soap. Another method includes using a plastic (capped) bottle of warm tap water with a tube that may be attached to the bottle so that the water can be directed over the perineal area. Patients find the use of this bottle simple and effective. Authorities emphasize the importance of a simple procedure and teaching the patient to carry out the technique as soon as she is able to do so. Self care limits the number of opportunities for transmitting organisms to the genital tract by the exogenous mode.

Because of the possibility of infection by organisms from the rectum and the increased susceptibility to infection, Edward M. Davis and Reva Rubin [22] say sitz baths may be contraindicated the first week postpartum. Sister M. Juan and Reginald A. Smith,[23] however, recommend their use daily and report a morbidity rate of only 0.32 per cent in 10,000 obstetric patients. Following a study of ten women (five in the last 2 weeks of pregnancy, five in the first 3 days of the puerperium), Peter Siegel [24] concluded that water does not enter the vagina during tub bathing. He used the starch-iodine reaction method which involves placing a dried starch tampon in the vagina and adding 50 ml of saturated potassium iodide solution to the bath water in which the woman bathed for about 20 minutes. He says that in no instance was the test positive when the tampon was inspected following the bath. Most authorities agree that shower baths may be taken the day following delivery.

When the physician prescribes sitz baths for patients with perineal repair, many hospitals are using a personal sitz bath kit, called "Sitz-et" (see Fig. 25-3), that can be used repeatedly in the hospital and home by the same patient and there is no chance of cross infection. This is a simple method providing heat and cleaning the perineal area. Patients are taught to give this treatment, which consists of filling the plastic bowl half-full of warm water, placing it on the crockery of the toilet bowl

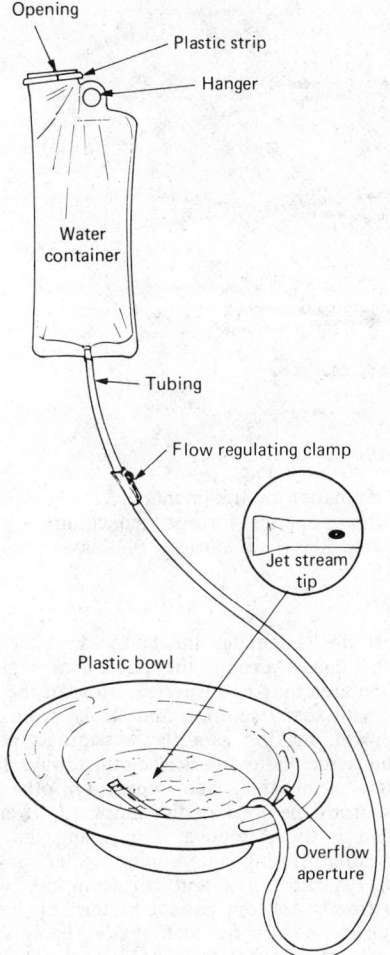

Figure 25-3. A personal sitz bath to be used in the patient's home toilet bowl.

with the overflow aperture toward the front, and then filling the water container with tap water 49°C, (120°F) and hanging it 1 or 2 feet above the bowl on an irrigating stand or wall hook. The patient sits on the bowl and puts the tubing between her legs with the jet stream top immersed in the water. The water flows in a whirlpool fashion from the container.[25,25a]

In a study of perineal care of ten patients with radical vulvectomies including bilateral groin dissection, Audrey L. Urquhart[26] reports a decrease in wound infection by 60 per cent and in wound breakdown by 40 per cent, and hospital stay decreased by an average of 22 days when the operative areas were irrigated with large amounts of normal saline and the *sitz bath was eliminated*.

Generally speaking, mucous membrane is less

sensitive to high and low temperatures than is the skin. The vaginal mucosa tolerates irrigating solutions too hot to be borne by the skin. Since any solution injected into the vagina immediately runs out over the vulva, temperatures must not be used that cause discomfort to the skin. The fact that temperatures above 46.1°C (115°F) are destructive to tissue cells must be borne in mind. The temperature of the fluid must never go above this point. Most authorities advocate a "warm solution," the temperature *not* to exceed 43.5°C (110°F). In preparing the solution allowance must be made for the cooling effect as the solution flows through the tubing. If tissues are tender or injured, a solution at body temperature causes least discomfort.

Exposure of the genitalia is embarrassing to the average person, and so the nurse should make every effort to reduce it to a minimum, to ensure privacy during the treatment, and to work expeditiously.

2. IRRIGATION OF THE VULVA AND PERINEUM (PERINEAL CARE)

Definition. An aseptic irrigation, or sponging, of the vulva and perineum given after voiding or defecation in a specified period following delivery, or an operation on the birth canal, perineum, urinary meatus, or anus is termed *perineal care*.

Therapeutic Uses. Special atttention is given to the external genitalia, perineum, and anus when any condition makes these areas susceptible to infection. The object of the treatment may be merely to clean the skin and mucous membrane under aseptic conditions or to discourage the growth of bacteria by application of antiseptics and to encourage healing with protective substances.

Equipment. The equipment necessary for cleaning the perineum following delivery includes a container of water, a bottle of soapy solution, and washcloths, or a plastic (capped) bottle of warm tap water, a tube that can be attached, and a bottle of soapy solution. The "pitcher douche" is no longer used for maternity patients "because of the feeling that pouring solution with a patient in bed will only wash into the vaginal canal any organisms which might be on the perineal area." *

A dressing is usually applied over the geni-

* Thomas, Margaret W.: *Aseptic Nursing Techniques, A Survey of Maternity Departments in Thirteen Medical Centers.* US Department of Health, Education, and Welfare. US Government Printing Office, Washington, D.C., 1960, p. 42.

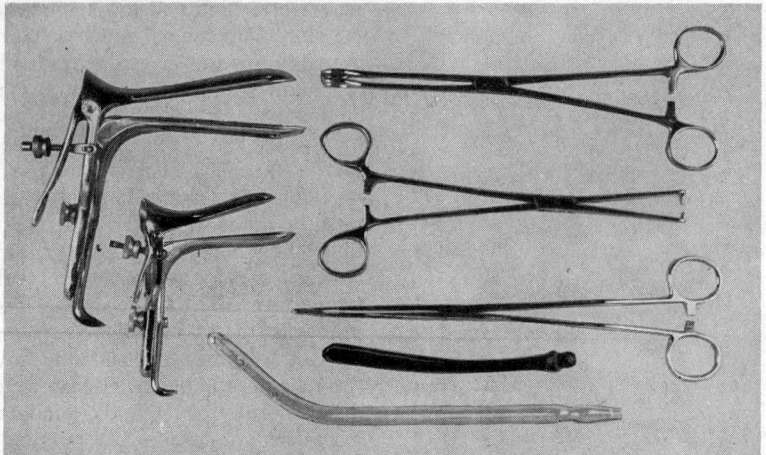

Figure 25-4. Equipment used during a vaginal examination or treatment. *Left:* Vaginal speculums, two sizes. *Right, top to bottom:* Sponge forceps, tenaculum clamp, and two douche tips (one hard rubber, one glass). (Courtesy of Clay-Adams Co., New York, N.Y.)

talia for protection and to absorb discharge. This dressing should be soft and aseptic. It should be held in place by pinning it to a belt. If possible, the belt should be elastic so that it gives with the movements of the body. If an elastic one is not available, it is essential that the belt be adjustable in size. On the theory that a perineal pad makes the discharge "back up" in the vagina, some obstetricians in the past forbade its use. In such cases the patient lies on a large absorbent pad of cellucotton that must be changed frequently as it is soon soiled. Currently most patients are out of bed the day following delivery.

The articles used in this procedure are usually kept at the bedside. When demonstrating this procedure to the patient, an impervious paper square or plastic treatment sheet covered with a piece of absorbent paper or muslin is placed under the buttocks of the patient to prevent soiling of the bed linens. The upper bedding must be folded down to expose the area to be treated and covering provided for the upper part of the body and, ideally, for draping the thighs. In most cases the upper sheet is used to drape the legs.

Suggested Procedure. Gain the cooperation of the patient by an explanation of the purpose and nature of the treatment. Before preparing the equipment, wash the hands carefully. Screen the patient or make provision for privacy, fold the upper bedding midway of the body, and cover the upper half of the body with a treatment blanket. Place the bedpan in position, remove the soiled dressing, and put it in a paper bag; allow time for the use of the bedpan before returning to the bedside, at which time remove the bedpan and

protect the bed under the buttocks. After washing the hands, expose the pubic-anal region so that the area may be inspected. Moisten the washcloth with soapy solution and stroke from above downward, making as little pressure as possible on the tissue. Fold the washcloth, always finding another clean area, and repeat on other side. Work from the median line outward. If a soap solution is used, remove it by using the washcloth after rinsing in running water or wash basin. Pat the vulva and perineum dry with a clean towel. Ask the patient to turn on her side and clean and dry the anal region, being careful not to let the washcloth come in contact with the vulva. When the bottle is used, fill it with warm tap water, attach the tubing and direct the flow of water in such a way that it does not enter the vagina. Use a washcloth with soapy solution to wash the area well and follow by rinsing. In applying the dressing, avoid touching the surface that comes in contact with the vulva and perineum; pin the compress to the belt or binder. Dispose of the soiled dressings and measure the amount of urine voided. Wash and sterilize the equipment before it is stored and used again.

In most institutions all equipment and supplies are kept in the patient's room or unit if she is in a ward, and the patient carries out this procedure in the bathroom. Most expendable supplies are packaged individually and replaced as the need arises.

In home nursing, reasonable protection is afforded the patient by using clean cotton dressings and solutions and by scrubbing the hands immediately before and after the procedure. In teaching the patient or a member of the family to give this treatment, simplify the procedure as much as possible and then stress the essentials.

The same procedure may be used for those persons with complex surgery of the perineum except all equipment must be sterile, and more solution, approximately 200 to 300 ml, is needed. A sterile Asepto bulb syringe is safe and effective in irrigating the area as the stream of solution can be directed in such a way that the solution does not enter the vagina. Sitz baths may also be used, but they are infrequently prescribed.

Recording the Treatment. Note the character and amount of discharge, the appearance of the wound and of the sutures if visible; record giving the treatment and the nature and quantity of the elimination.

3. VAGINAL IRRIGATION

Definition. A vaginal irrigation is sometimes called a *vaginal douche,* but the former term is correct, because a douche implies that a stream of water is directed against a part with force. A vaginal irrigation should be the introduction of a liquid at low pressure. It is similar to the irrigation of any open cavity, such as the external auditory canal, from which the liquid immediately returns.

Therapeutic Uses. Vaginal irrigations may be prescribed to: (1) discourage growth of bacteria by the application of an antiseptic, (2) remove a foul or irritating discharge, (3) apply heat or cold in the treatment of inflammation or possibly to control hemorrhage, and (4) clean the vagina in preparation for surgery. Vaginal douches are now less often used than in the past. The physician is able to control a large number of vaginal infections with chemotherapy and antibiotics given systemically. J. Bernard Bernstine and Abraham E. Rakoff [26a] (1953) say specifically that while the antibiotics and sulfanilamides have proved very useful in gonococcal and other infections, effective agents for the treatment of trichomoniasis and moniliasis are unknown. Novak and associates [27] (1970) note that many different methods of treatment have been tried but are not entirely satisfactory; they suggest that local and systemic antibiotic therapy has not been regularly effective. *Trichomoniasis vaginalis* vaginitis has been established as a worldwide infection; a number of other bacteria are usually present.[28] Preoperative irrigation of the vagina cannot be relied on to effectively clean the area for surgery, according to McGowan [29]; it continues to be prescribed, however, by some physicians. Heat in the form of diathermy has to some extent replaced the use of hot irrigations.

Equipment. Articles required are: a douchepan or bedpan to receive the return flow; a reservoir for the solution (an irrigating can, rubber bag, plastic or glass bottle), with a convenient length of tubing and a clamp attached; a douche tip, a small container for this tip; soft paper squares or towel for drying the patient; and a waterproof protector for the bed and a cover of muslin or paper for the protector.

Vaginal "douche tips" are made of glass, plastic, or hard rubber. Glass has the advantage of being easy to clean; hard rubber, the merit of being difficult to break. Metal tips are unsuitable, because they conduct heat too readily and would be painful to the patient if used for a hot irrigation. Tips come in various sizes suitable for children and adults. Before using a tip, it must be examined to see that it is intact and has a smooth surface.

The prescribed solution in the required amount, usually 2000 ml (2 qt), is brought to the bedside in the reservoir. The temperature must be regulated with a thermometer, according to the physician's prescription, allowing about 2°C or 5°F for cooling before the solution reaches the vagina. If neither the temperature nor the kind of solution is specified, it is safe to use water, sodium chloride 1 per cent, or sodium bicarbonate 2 per cent at 40.6°C (105°F).

The articles just listed must be *clean* or "medically aseptic" in preparation for most vaginal irrigations. Following an abortion, a delivery (contraindicated during the early part of the puerperium [30]), or a surgical operation, the treatment must be given with *sterile* equipment and must be handled with surgical asepsis. In administering a clean douche, it is convenient to bring the reservoir, tubing, tip, and treatment towel to the bedside in a clean douchepan or bedpan; if giving a sterile douche, it is more convenient to use a tray for these articles and to provide rubber gloves for manipulating the tip and cleaning and separating the labia. As in all such treatments, it is important to cover the equipment in transporting it to and from the bedside.

Suggested Procedure. Gain the cooperation of the patient by a thorough and appropriate explanation. If the treatment is given for the first time, and especially if the patient is a child or a young girl, this explanation must be made with the greatest tact. (The treatment should never be administered to a responsible patient unless she understands it and is willing to have it.) Ensure privacy with signs on the door, screen the bed, and drape the patient to avoid unnecessary exposure.

Place the patient on the bedpan or douchepan. Support the back with a pillow and cover the seat of the douchepan with a pad. It is desirable to support the flexed legs. If the irrigation is given as slowly as it should be, the patient tires in this position unless care is taken to make her comfortable.

Replace the upper bedding with two treatment blankets. Arrange these so that they separate and drape each leg, leaving the pubic region exposed. Hang the reservoir so that the base is about 30 cm (12 inches) above the vaginal meatus; this keeps the solution at low pressure, slows the rate of flow, and makes the treatment last long enough to produce a temperature effect. Allow a small amount of the solution to flow over the vulva to remove any gross discharge. If the temperature of the solution is uncomfortable and there is no therapeutic indication for giving it at this temperature, make the necessary change before continuing. Examine the nozzle carefully for cracks and nicks and, if intact, attach it to the tubing. Insert the nozzle very gently into the vagina; the patient may prefer to do this herself, and if the effort is not injurious to her, she should be helped to do so. (In cases where there is an infection such as gonorrhea, do not allow the patient to handle the tip or tubing as it is desirable to prevent contamination of a bed patient's hands. Without access to running water, it is difficult for her to get her hands clean, and there is always danger of infecting the eyes. In addition to other steps taken to maintain medical asepsis, the nurse should wear glasses to protect the eyes from accidental splashing. Gloves are not necessary for the protection of the nurse, the gonococcus being easily killed with soap and hot water, but a gown should be worn.) Directing the nozzle upward (toward the head) and backward (toward the sacrum) tends to keep the stream of water from forcing its way into the mouth of the cervix. Openings at the side and not at the end of the nozzle also help to prevent this. With the proper amount of force, the liquid should fill and distend the vagina.

After the administration of the prescribed amount of fluid, allow the patient to stay on the bedpan for a few minutes to drain the vagina. Dry the postoperative patient with sterile sponges, handled aseptically; dry other patients with toilet paper or with the folded instrument towel used to pad the seat of the douchepan.

Before emptying the douchepan, note the character of the return. Discard soiled sponges or paper squares, send used linen to the laundry, wash and return the treatment sheet to the patient's unit, and boil all other articles of equipment before returning them to storage space. In homes, or in private-hospital rooms equipped with running water, the articles required for a vaginal irrigation may be washed and kept separate for the use of the patient. This avoids the necessity for concurrent sterilization.

When douches are prescribed for women in the home, they should be instructed in the proper technique. Advise them to lie in a bathtub on a towel when taking a douche and not sit on a toilet bowl [31] since in this position the solution fails to reach the upper part of the vagina.

Recording the Treatment. Note the time the treatment was given, the kind, amount, and temperature of the solution, the character of the return flow, and the reaction of the patient. Vaginal irrigations are sometimes continued when no longer necessary if the nurse fails, for example, to state that the fluid returns clear.

4. VAGINAL SUPPOSITORIES

Definition. Vaginal suppositories are cones of cocoa butter or paraffin impregnated with a drug; they are made to approximate the length and diameter of the vaginal cavity.

Therapeutic Uses. Local applications of an astringent, an antiseptic, or other types of drugs can be made by the introduction of a suppository. Actually, this form of therapy is rarely practiced, because drugs are more easily applied in other ways. Contraceptive suppositories are used but are said to be unreliable.

Suggested Procedure. Cool and harden the suppository in a refrigerator. In hospitals, suppositories are kept stored in refrigerators. Explain the nature and the purpose of the procedure to the patient. Place the patient in the dorsal recumbent or left lateral (Sims') position. Drape the patient to expose only the vaginal orifice. Lubricate the suppository with a vegetable jelly. Gently insert the full length of the suppository into the vagina. The nurse may wear a rubber glove or finger cots on the thumb and forefinger of the hand that manipulates the suppository.

Recording the Treatment. Note the time at which the suppository was inserted, its nature, and any significant reaction, such as pain or discomfort, experienced by the patient.

REFERENCES

1. Hellman, Louis M., and Pritchard, Jack A.: *Williams' Obstetrics,* 14th ed. Appleton-Century-Crofts, New York, 1971, p. 341.
2. Baird, Dugald (ed.): *Combined Textbook of Obstetrics and Gynecology, for Students and Practitioners,* 8th ed. E. & S. Livingstone, Edinburgh, 1969, p. 844.
3. Cohen, Lester: "Influence of pH Vaginal Discharges," *Obstet. Gynecol. Survey,* **25:** 792, (Aug.) 1970.
4. Taylor, E. Stewart: *Essentials of Gynecology,* 4th ed. Lea & Febiger, Philadelphia, 1969, p. 48.
5. Greenhill, J. P.: *DeLee's Obstetrics,* 13th ed. W. B. Saunders Co., Philadelphia, 1965, p. 471.
6. Marchetti, Andrew A.: "Intrapartum Gas Bacillus Infection," *Am. J. Obstet. Gynecol.,* **26:**612, (Apr.) 1934.
7. Rendle-Short, Coralie: *"Clostridium welchii* Infection of the Uterus, Complicating Delivery," *J. Obstet. Gynaecol. Br. Commonw.,* **49:**581, (Dec.) 1942.
8. Caillouette, James C.: "Septic Abortion, Pathology and Treatment," *Am. J. Nurs.,* **66:**1045, (May) 1966.
9. New York Academy of Medicine, Committee on Public Health Relations: *Maternal Mortality in New York City, 1930–32.* Oxford University Press, New York, 1933, p. 75.
10. Colbeck, J. C.: *Control of Infections in*

Hospitals, Hospital Monograph Series No 12. American Hospital Association, Chicago, 1962, p. 53.

11. Tomkinson, J. S.: *The Queen Charlotte's Textbook of Obstetrics,* 12th ed. J. & A. Churchill, London, 1970, p. 322.

12. Hellman, Louis M., and Pritchard, Jack A.: *op. cit.,* p. 987.

13. Pierson, Elaine C.: *Sex Is Never an Emergency. A Candid Guide for College Students,* 2nd ed. J. B. Lippincott Co., Philadelphia, 1971, p. 17.

14. Glynn, Robert: "Daily Douching: Effect on Vaginal Mucosa," *Obstet. Gynecol.,* **22:**642, (Nov.) 1963.

15. McGowan, Larry: "Peritonitis Following the Vaginal Douche and a Proposed Alternative Method for Vaginal and Vulvar Care," *Am. J. Obstet. Gynecol.,* **93:**506, (Oct. 15) 1965.

16. Hastings, Donald W.: *A Doctor Speaks on Sexual Expression in Marriage,* 2nd ed. Little, Brown & Co., Boston, 1971, p. 129.

16a. Clark, Ann L., and Hale, Ralph W.: "Sex During and After Pregnancy," *Am. J. Nurs.,* **74:**1430, (Aug.) 1974.

16b. Gedan, Sharon: "Abortion Counseling with Adolescents," *Am. J. Nurs.,* **74:**1856, (Oct.) 1974.

16c. Mindek, Laurie: "Sex Education on a Psychiatric Unit," *Am. J. Nurs.,* **74:**1865, (Oct.) 1974.

16d. Masters, William H., and Johnson, Virginia E.: *The Human Sexual Response.* Little, Brown & Co., Boston, 1966.

16e. Pierson, Elaine C.: *op. cit.*

16f. Ehrman, Myra L.: "Sex Education for the Young," *Nurs. Outlook,* **23:**585, (Sept.) 1975.

16g. Manisoff, Miriam: "Family Planning Democratized," *Am. J. Nurs.,* **75:**1660, (Oct.) 1975.

16h. Arnold, Elizabeth: "Individualizing Nursing Care in Family Planning," in *Human Sexuality: Nursing Implications.* American Journal of Nursing Co., Educational Services Division, New York, 1973 (Contemporary Nursing Service).

17. Hellman, Louis M., and Pritchard, Jack A.: *op. cit.,* p. 27.

18. Novak, Edmund R., et al.: *Textbook of Gynecology,* 8th ed. Williams & Wilkins Co., Baltimore, 1970, p. 169.

19. "Should Genital Deodorants Be Used?" *Consumer Reports,* **37:**39, (Jan.) 1972.

20. Martin, Eric W. (ed.): *Techniques of Medication.* J. B. Lippincott Co., Philadelphia, 1969, p. 105.

21. Davis, Edward M., and Rubin, Neva: *DeLee's Obstetrics for Nurses,* 18th ed. W. B. Saunders Co., Philadelphia, 1966, p. 367.

22. *Ibid.,* p. 366.

23. Juan, Sister M., and Smith, Reginald A.: "Postpartum Tub Baths," *Am. J. Nurs.,* **64:**135, (Sept.) 1964.

24. Siegel, Peter: "Does Bath Water Enter the Vagina," *Obstet. Gynecol.,* **15:**660, (May) 1960.

25. "Expediting the Sitz Bath Procedure," *Nation's Hospitals,* (Fall) 1966.

25a. "Personal Sitz Baths Upgrade Hospital Efficiency, Saves Nurses' Time," *Nation's Hospitals,* (No. 2) 1969.

26. Urquhart, Audrey L.: "A Study of Nursing Care of the Vulvectomy Patient," in *ANA Regional Clinical Conferences, 1967.* Appleton-Century-Crofts, New York, 1968, p. 260.

26a. Bernstine, J. Bernard, and Rakoff, Abraham E.: *Vaginal Infections, Infestations and Discharges.* Blakiston Co., New York, 1953.

27. Novak, Edmund R., et al.: *op. cit.,* p. 186.

28. Desai, Zarin D., et al.: "A Study of 183 Cases of Leucorrhea: Incidence of Trichomonas Vaginalis, Candida Spp., and Hemophillus Vaginalis," *J. Postgrad. Med.,* **12:**91, (Apr.) 1966.

29. McGowan, Larry: "New Ideas about Patient Care Before and After Vaginal Surgery," *Am. J. Nurs.,* **64:**74, (Feb.) 1964.

30. Taylor, E. Stewart: *Beck's Obstetrical Practice,* 9th ed. Williams & Wilkins Co., Baltimore, 1971, p. 209.

31. Greenhill, J. P.: *Office Gynecology,* 9th ed. Year Book Medical Publishers, Chicago, 1971, p. 181.

Additional Suggested Reading

Allen, Andra J.: "All American Sexual Myths," *Am. J. Nurs.,* **75:**1770, (Oct.) 1975.

Avery, Wanda, et al.: "Vulvectomy," *Am. J. Nurs.,* **74:**453, (Mar.) 1974.

Barnes, Allan C., et al.: *The Social Responsibility of Gynecology and Obstetrics,* Johns Hopkins Press, Baltimore, 1965.

Behrman, Samuel J., and Gosling, John R. G.: *Fundamentals of Gynecology,* 2nd ed. Oxford University Press, London, 1966.

Benton, Barbara D. A.: "Stilbestrol and Vaginal Cancer," *Am. J. Nurs.,* **74:**900, (May) 1974.

Berkow, Sam Gordon: "A Replacement for the Vaginal Douche," *Obstet. Gynecol.,* **15:**773, (June) 1960.

Christine, Sister Marie: "Postpartum Nursing Care," *Can. Nurse,* **61:**29, (Jan.) 1965.

Danforth, David N. (ed.): *Textbook of Obstetrics and Gynecology,* 2nd ed. Harper & Row, New York, 1971.

Department of National Health and Welfare, Information Services Division: *The Application of the Principles of Medical Asepsis to Maternity and Newborn Care.* Child and Maternal Health Division, Department of National Health and Welfare, Ottawa, Ont., 1960.

Fisher, Rex R.: "Detergent Alkaline Douches," *Pac. Med. Surg.,* **73:**209, (May–June) 1965.

Fitzpatrick, Elsie, et al.: *Maternity Nursing,* 12th ed. J. B. Lippincott Co., Philadelphia, 1971.

Graber, Edward A., and Barber, Hugh R. K.: "The Case For and Against Estrogen Therapy," *Am. J. Nurs.,* **75:**1766, (Oct.) 1975.

Green, Thomas H.: *Gynecology; Essentials of*

Clinical Practice, 2nd ed. Little, Brown & Co., Boston, 1971.

Hawkins, John A., and Schulman, Harold: "Prematurity Associated with Cervicitis and Vaginitis During Pregnancy," *Am. J. Obstet. Gynecol.,* **94:**898, (Apr.) 1966.

Heald, Felix P. (ed.): *Adolescent Gynecology.* Williams & Wilkins Co., Baltimore, 1966.

Huffman, John W.: *The Gynecology of Childhood and Adolescence.* W. B. Saunders Co., Philadelphia, 1968.

"Infection Control in Maternity Unit," *Nurs. Outlook,* **12:**32, (May) 1964.

Kinsey, A. C., et al.: *Sexual Behavior in the Human Female.* W. B. Saunders Co., Philadelphia, 1953.

————: *Sexual Behavior in the Human Male.* W. B. Saunders Co., Philadelphia, 1948.

Kistner, Robert W.: *Gynecology; Principles and Practice,* 2nd ed. Year Book Medical Publishers, Chicago, 1971.

Knapp, Robert Charles, et al.: "Septic Abortion, Five Year Analysis at the New York Hospital," *Obstet. Gynecol.,* **15:**344, (Mar.) 1960.

Kroger, William S. (ed.): *Psychosomatic Obstet-*

rics, Gynecology and Endocrinology. Charles C Thomas, Publisher, Springfield, Ill., 1962.

Orley, J., et al.: "Vaginal Discharge in Puberty," *Obstet. Gynecol. Survey,* **25:**369, 1970.

Raneholt, R. T., and LaVeck, G. D.: "Staphylococcal Disease—An Obstetric, Pediatric, and Community Problem," *Am. J. Public Health,* **46:**1287, (Oct.) 1956.

Summers, Margaret M., et al.: "Hair as a Reservoir of Staphylococci," *J. Clin. Pathol.,* **18:**13, (Jan.) 1965.

University of Minnesota, School of Public Health: *National Conference on Institutionally Acquired Infections, Sept. 4, 5, 6, 1963.* US Department of Health, Education, and Welfare, Public Health Service. US Government Printing Office, Washington, D.C., 1964.

Walker, James, et al. (eds.): *Combined Textbook of Obstetrics and Gynaecology,* 9th ed. Churchill Livingston, London, 1976.

Gladys Nite
Virginia Henderson

CHAPTER 26

Incision and Puncture of Body Cavities for Drainage and Medication

1. GENERAL PRINCIPLES UNDERLYING SELECTION OF METHOD
2. THORACIC, OR CHEST, ASPIRATION
3. ARTIFICIAL PNEUMOTHORAX
4. LUMBAR PUNCTURE WITH MYELOGRAM OR ENCEPHALOGRAM
5. CISTERNAL PUNCTURE
6. ASPIRATION OF THE PERICARDIUM
7. ABDOMINAL PARACENTESIS
8. MYRINGOTOMY
9. PHLEBOTOMY OR VENESECTION

1. GENERAL PRINCIPLES UNDERLYING SELECTION OF METHOD

Conditions Requiring Aspiration and Incision: General Purpose. In certain conditions and diseases, fluid collects in body cavities and tissues. This excess fluid may result from local inflammation, trauma, or from an abnormal condition of a remote organ or organs. When a serous membrane, such as that covering the brain or the lungs or lining the abdominal cavity, is inflamed it secretes an abnormal amount. This fluid is nature's means of bathing and separating the affected tissues. It also protects the affected organs with a water cushion. When excessive fluid forms in the cranial, chest, or abdominal cavities, it exerts pressure on vital organs. This always causes discomfort or pain and menaces the function of the affected parts.

Fluid may collect in body cavities and tissues as a result of disease of the circulatory or excretory systems. For some persons with this condition, drugs, such as meralluride sodium solution (Mercuhydrin), may be prescribed and given intramuscularly to speed up elimination by the kidneys, although aspiration (removal of the fluid through a hollow needle or other instrument) may be used in conjunction with the diuretic. Aspirations not only relieve pressure caused by the fluid accumulation but also enable the physician to examine the fluid and make a more accurate diagnosis. Any aspiration, however, involves a risk of infection. Nosocomial infections (infections caused by hospital life) are discussed in Chapter 15, as well as the reasons why such infections have increased. One of these reasons is that patients in general hospitals are increasingly subject to "intrusive therapy," or the invasion of the body with tubes, needles, and other instruments. While the body has a remarkable defense system (discussed in Chapter 44), that of the hospital patient has often been weakened by the disease that brought him or her there and the "intrusive" forces, if strong enough, can overcome even normal defenses. Health workers and the public should be aware of the risks as well as the merits of "intrusive" treatment. Both should be presented to the patient, if he or she is a rational adult, or to the parent or guardian if the patient is irrational or a child, and they should be able to accept or reject the treatment.

Classification and Character of Fluid Collected in Body Cavities. For clinical purposes the fluid is classified as an *exudate* (a fluid produced by the lining of the cavity) or a *transudate* (a fluid that escapes from the blood and lymph vessels and collects in the cavity). An exudate, occurring as a result of inflammation, may be serous (watery) or it may be purulent if suppuration has developed. It usually has a high specific gravity, contains white blood cells, and, in many cases, microorganisms. The meningococcus, streptococcus, pneumococcus, staphylococcus, and tubercle bacillus are among those infecting serous cavities. An exudate may also contain fibrin or blood. In malignancies, necrotic tissue may be present. A transudate has much the same character as blood serum; it is pale yellow or greenish yellow, is alkaline in reaction, and has a low specific gravity. The amount of protein is low, and

1307

blood cells are few in comparison with those in an exudate; there are no bacteria in the fluid. Salts, glucose, and urea are found as in plasma.[1]

Methods of Drainage or Suction. Fluid may be drained through an incision if pressure on the organ or tissue is sufficient to cause drainage, or if gravity favors it. If an incision is likely to prove either ineffective or dangerous, a hollow needle or cannula is introduced, and suction applied with a syringe, vacuum bottle, or motor-driven suction pump. There are various ways of producing subatmospheric pressure (suction), but the underlying principle is the same. Air may be sucked out of a bottle or a tube, in order to create a partial vacuum, with a hand pump, a pump operated by an electric motor, or with running water.

Regulation and Measurement of Suction. As explained in Chapter 23, a vacuum is a void— theoretically, a space in which there is nothing. That "nature abhors a vacuum" is a well-known axiom of physics, and the consequence is that a complete vacuum does not exist, because an airtight chamber is hard to construct and atmospheric pressure forces air through the smallest opening. A partial vacuum is, however, easily created and occurs whenever part of the air is forced out of a bottle or cavity so that the remaining air is rarefied, expanded, or under less than atmospheric pressure. In any vacuum system it is essential that connections between tubing and needles, manometers, bottles, and syringes are tight. Admission of air at the wrong time and place destroys the vacuum. Closed systems of drainage are recommended to reduce the danger of infection since it is impossible to prevent the entrance of organisms if room air is drawn into the system (see also Chapter 15). Operation of the apparatus must be mastered before the treatment is started.[2]

In aspirating fluid from any body cavity, it is possible to measure the positive pressure the fluid is under in this cavity by attaching to the needle a perpendicular glass tube with a special adapter. The height to which the fluid rises indicates the pressure—the higher the fluid, the greater the pressure.

Importance of Asepsis. Cavities or tissues that require aspiration or incision are obviously those having no opening to the outside air. (Such cavities as open on the surface of the body may be drained through tubes inserted into these openings.) Nature has not provided closed cavities with the relative immunity to infection that exists in the mucous-lined cavities, and a more rigid asepsis is therefore required. (Actually any "intrusive therapy" carries with it the danger of trauma

and infection.) Preparation of the skin area to be punctured or incised and preparation of equipment must follow the rules for all surgical procedures as discussed in Chapters 15, 33, and 44. The skin is prepared by cleaning and by the application of an antiseptic; all dressings and instruments, including the skin-cleaning equipment, should be sterile. Commercially sterilized packs with all necessary equipment and supplies to drain fluid from the various body cavities are available and used in many hospitals and clinics; if not available, then sterilization by steam under pressure should be used. The skin-cleaning equipment may be sterilized in a separate covered tray or package so that the nurse may handle these articles without contaminating instruments prepared for the physician. The nurse is often asked to prepare the skin while the doctor is scrubbing or preparing the local anesthetic.

Reducing the Danger of Trauma. A puncture or incision inevitably injures the tissues and introduces skin bacteria since it cannot be made completely free of microorganisms. A wound is made that nature must heal. The physician and nurse should try to reduce the amount of trauma to a minimum. Voluntary and involuntary movements of the patient during the procedure usually may be prevented by a thorough and appropriate explanation; the patient should be supported in a comfortable position; the possibility of striking a bone should be reduced by selecting the proper site of injection; and, above all, needles and scalpels should be sharp and of the right size.

Preparing the Patient. To patients and their families, aspirations are minor operations, and it is not unusual to see marked anxiety or even terror expressed in word or manner. An explanation from the physician is most reassuring, but the nurse should be sure that the patient understands the nature and purpose of the procedure, the type and degree of discomfort that may occur, and the importance of remaining immobile. Terms should be used that the patient can understand, and diagrams may be helpful.* Only in rare cases should treatments such as this be given without the patients' understanding. Their cooperation is often essential to the success of an aspiration

---

* There was a case in which a patient sued a highly reputable hospital for damages. In court he testified that the nurse came in with a tray of instruments and told him he was going to have something done to him (he didn't know exactly what she said); then she turned him to the wall, tied his hands and feet, the doctor came in and hit him in the back, and he, the patient, hadn't been the same since. Any of us can recognize in this account a failure on the part of the medical worker to interpret a lumbar puncture in the patient's terms.

if they are conscious, and psychologically it is traumatic to have such an experience under duress. In some hospitals, patients are asked to sign permits; parents and guardians sign such forms for children and mental incompetents. A person's *acceptance* should be sought; or that of the parent or other family member or guardian when the person is irrational, or is a child or infant. (As the risks of these treatments are better understood the public may be less willing to submit to them.) A sedative given at the proper time may help the patient to stand the treatment much more easily. The anxiety and pain associated with these treatments should not be overlooked.

2. THORACIC, OR CHEST, ASPIRATION

Definition. A chest aspiration or thoracentesis is the withdrawal of fluid from the pleural cavity.

Therapeutic Uses. Aspiration may be prescribed if an accumulation of fluid causes pain, dyspnea, and other symptoms of pressure. A transudate may form as a result of heart, kidney, or vascular disease; an exudate may be caused by tubercular pleurisy. Pleural infections, however, can be associated with infections of the lung, or secondary infections in other parts of the body, for example, the meninges. In such cases the microorganisms found in the fluid may be the pneumococcus, streptococcus, or meningococcus. If the effusion is purulent in nature, the patient is said to have empyema, and it may be impossible to drain the cavity adequately through a needle. Fluid may collect in the pleural cavity as a result of malignant growths in the chest.[3]

Pleural fluid is often removed for diagnostic purposes; that is, to discover the causative organism in pleurisy. For this purpose it is not necessary to collect a large quantity, and no attempt is made to do so unless the fluid is causing discomfort.

Equipment. The articles required are a small plastic sheet to protect the bedding, towels or soft paper to cover the plastic, sterile draping materials (a fenestrated sheet is best); sterile cotton and skin disinfectants; a sterile hypodermic needle and syringe with ½ or 1 per cent procaine (Novocaine) for local anesthesia; sterile gloves and powder for the doctor; sterile dressings; and the aspirating set. When a motor-driven suctioning device is not available, a hand-operated apparatus is substituted. The latter consists of a calibrated glass bottle having a rubber stopper in which there is a metal tube with two branches, each provided with stopcocks. To each branch is fitted rubber tubing with metal ends or adapters. The sterile aspirating needle fits the metal end of one piece of tubing, and through the other end air may be exhausted from the bottle with an exhaust pump, leaving a vacuum in the bottle into which the chest fluid will readily flow. Such equipment is known as a *Potain aspirating set.* Harvey J. Engelsher [4] describes a small hand-operated bellows pump that is attached to the needle by one tube with an enclosed valve and to the collecting bag by another tube that also includes a valve. Commercial sets are used in most hospitals in the United States and are very satisfactory because the connections are usually airtight. If a commercial or manual set is not available, adequate negative pressure may be created in a syringe. This is troublesome and dangerous to use, however, because the amount of fluid removed is often larger than the capacity of the syringe, and air may enter the pleural cavity while detaching, emptying, and readjusting it. A suction apparatus must be used to collect fluid from the pleural cavity, because a subatmospheric pressure exists there and the fluid will not flow out by gravity. This low pressure is caused by the elasticity of the lung tissue and the resistance it offers to the elevated ribs and lung expansion. The downward pull of the elastic lung makes the atmospheric pressure greater than the pressure in the thoracic cavity, and fluid cannot run out by gravity until the external pressure in the bottle or syringe is less than the internal thoracic pressure.

When the air is exhausted from the bottle, both stopcocks must be closed. The apparatus should have been tested on starting to ensure that the chest fluid will flow into the bottle. To test the apparatus place the tubing to be attached to the aspirating needle in a container of sterile water and open the stopcock of that branch only; if the water runs into the bottle readily, the chest fluid also will run into it when the needle is inserted into the pleural cavity and attached to the tubing.

Needles of different sizes should be provided. The bevels in all cases should be short to avoid pricking the lung, but the bores should vary so that a small needle is ready in case the exudate is of a serous nature or a large one for a purulent exudate. A plastic catheter, threaded through a needle, is used by some physicians because the catheter reduces the hazard of pulmonary puncture and because it is flexible, it may be fed into a pocket of fluid. Joseph L. Kovarik [5] reports the successful use of a size 14 Angiocath (inner metal needle with outer plastic sheath or cannula) in 50 thoracenteses.

Preparation of the Patient. As in all treatments, the patient's mental and physical wel-

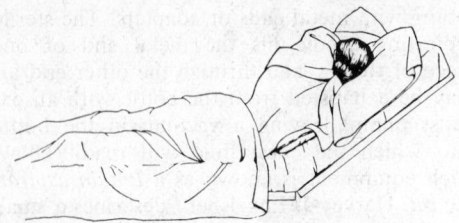

Figure 26-1. Side-lying position for a patient about to have a thoracentesis. Note small pillow under right chest wall to separate ribs where puncture will be made in opposite chest wall. (After Abbot.)

fare should be considered throughout. To lessen the danger of shock, fainting, or fatigue it is wise to have him or her lie on the side in a semirecumbent position, and on the side of the bed most convenient for the doctor (see Fig. 26-1). Some authorities believe the recumbent position is usually superior to the sitting position. William W. Stead [6] says that when a small amount of fluid is present it can be removed most easily and safely if the person lies on the affected side because the air-filled lung floats above the fluid and lessens the chance of its being punctured by the needle. When the procedure is performed with the patient lying on the affected side, the arm of that side is held above the head or forward. The position should be comfortable. The treatment may be given with the patient sitting on the side of the bed, the feet resting on a stool, and the arms on a pillow laid over the back of a chair (see Fig. 26-2). Sometimes patients lean forward on a bed tray or table. They should be warmly clad to prevent chilling and to lessen the danger of shock. There should be no more than the necessary exposure.

The lungs do not completely fill the pleural sac, so that at the anterior and inferior borders sinuses are formed. Pathologic fluids first collect in the interior or costophrenic sinus, but may collect also in the interlobular spaces. Physicians always select the site of insertion of the needle. They may clean and disinfect the skin, or the nurse may do it. In either case forceps are used to handle the sponges or other methods are used that reduce contamination to a minimum. (It is not possible to completely sterilize the skin, as has been explained repeatedly.) If sterile drapery is used, physicians usually adjust it after they have scrubbed their hands or put on sterile rubber gloves.

Suggested Procedure. The physician first anesthetizes the site of injection with ½ to 1 per cent procaine or similar drug and then inserts the needle in the skin area under which he or she believes the fluid to have collected. The site of puncture is determined by x-ray and chest sounds that indicate the location of excess serum or pus.[7] The needle is injected midway between the ribs to avoid the intercostal blood vessels and during inspiration when the spaces are wider. Either the doctor or the nurse must tell the patient not to move or cough while the needle is in the chest wall. If coughing is unavoidable, the physician may withdraw the needle temporarily. An adapter (a three-way stopcock) must be attached to the needle, so that entrance of air through the needle into the pleural cavity can be prevented by closing the stopcock. As soon as the needle is in position, the syringe or tubing from the vacuum bottle is attached. The suction produced pulls the fluid from the cavity. The stopcock to the pump remains closed after the treatment is started (unless it is necessary to renew the vacuum), and the opening to the needle should be closed until the physician asks the nurse to open it. As soon as this passageway is opened, fluid should flow into the vacuum bottle. If an uncontaminated specimen is needed for laboratory study, the physician may collect it with a syringe and transfer it to a small, wide-mouthed, covered bottle. Although the vacuum bottle is sterilized in preparation for the treatment, it is hard to get an uncontaminated specimen from this large container.

Watch the patient's condition carefully; throughout the treatment note his or her color, pulse, and respiration. Sudden withdrawal of pressure on the chest organs may cause fainting, or a hemorrhage from puncture of a blood vessel, or collapse of the lung if it is pricked.

On the withdrawal of the needle the physician applies a sterile dressing. After the treatment patients rest for a prescribed period according to their condition. Later, the sputum should be watched for the presence of blood, suggesting injury to lung tissue.

The bottle containing the fluid must be labeled with the date, patient's name, clinical division, nature of the fluid, and the purpose for which it is to be examined. If so desired by the physician,

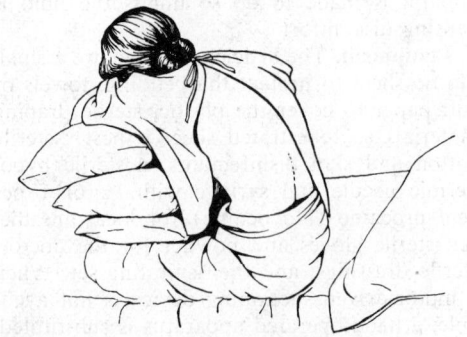

Figure 26-2. Sitting position for a patient about to have a thoracentesis. Note pillows used to support patient during treatment and covering provided. (After Abbot.)

it should be sent immediately to the laboratory to be examined for specific gravity, differential white cell count, albumin, and the specific organisms present. The amount of albumin indicates the degree of inflammation present.

Recording the Treatment. The amount, color, and type of fluid withdrawn, the time of treatment, coughing, any fatigue, syncope, or untoward symptoms either accompanying or following the procedure, as well as any beneficial effects observed, should be recorded. Note the collection of specimens and the purpose for which they were sent to the laboratory.

3. ARTIFICIAL PNEUMOTHORAX

Definition. *Pneumothorax* means air in the pleural cavity. An artificial pneumothorax is the introduction of nitrogen gas, or air, into this cavity for the purpose of creating sufficient pressure to collapse and rest the lung. This procedure was a standard form of treatment for selected patients with pulmonary tuberculosis in the 1920s, and continued to be used until about 1950, when effective antibiotic therapy was introduced. By 1955, its use was almost abandoned in North America.[8]

Studies have shown that a higher incidence of breast and lung cancer has occurred in persons treated with pneumothorax as compared to those who did not receive such therapy. Investigators suggest that frequent fluoroscopies of the chest that were necessary with the extensive use of pneumothorax collapse therapy were the cause of cancer.[9,10] Fortunately, this form of treatment is no longer used and is mentioned because readers may find reference to it in histories of older patients and may want to know its nature.

4. LUMBAR PUNCTURE WITH MYELOGRAM OR ENCEPHALOGRAM

Definition. A lumbar puncture (spinal tap) is the introduction of a hollow needle into the subarachnoid space of the spinal canal, usually in the lumbar region, for the purpose of draining the canal or injecting substances into it. When opaque substances are injected and an x-ray taken, the picture is called a myelogram; when air or oxygen is injected, the procedure is called a pneumoencephalogram.

Therapeutic Uses. The cerebral and spinal subarachnoid spaces and the fluid contained in them communicate freely with each other through the foramen magnum and with the cavity of the cerebral ventricles through the foramen of Magendie in the lower part of the roof of the fourth ventricle. The cord is suspended in cerebrospinal fluid. If the circulation of fluid is unobstructed, pressure of the fluid varies with breathing, coughing, or abdominal straining. Manual compression on large veins (jugular pressure usually) produces a rise in pressure. A stationary pressure under any of these conditions indicates a block. In a relaxed recumbent position the spinal fluid is under a pressure of 10 to 15 cm of water; 20 to 25 in a sitting position.[11] In a disease, the pressure during relaxation may rise markedly. A lumbar puncture as a diagnostic or therapeutic measure depends upon this intercommunication and interchange of fluid and the responses to varying pressures within the body, referred to as "spinal dynamics."

The subarachnoid space is entered in order to (1) withdraw cerebrospinal fluid to relieve pressure, (2) get a specimen of fluid for diagnostic purposes, (3) inject sera or drugs in the treatment of disease, (4) inject a spinal anesthetic, (5) introduce an opaque liquid before taking an x-ray for diagnosis of cord and brain lesions, and (6) measure the pressure of the spinal fluid under varying conditions. This last is referred to as the manometric test. The normal rise in spinal-fluid pressure on compression of the internal jugular veins is called "Queckenstedt's sign," because he first described it, hence "Queckenstedt's test."

Removal of excess cerebrospinal fluid is often indicated in hydrocephalus and meningitis. Meningitis caused by the meningococcus and the pneumococcus was once treated by the introduction of sera into the spinal canal. The antibotics are occasionally given in this way. Israel S. Wechsler [11a] says that the chemotherapeutic agents are irritants when injected into the spinal canal. He implies that even antibiotics are more satisfactorily given in other ways. Spinal anesthesia is administered when other types of anesthesia are contraindicated. If a tumor of the brain or spinal cord is suspected, for diagnostic purposes an opaque substance * is injected into the subarachnoid space of the spinal cord, the enlargement of this space at the base of the brain, or into one of the lateral ventricles. A cavity filled with this substance shows up on film as a dark area. A misplaced or distorted ventricle or an occluded area of the subarachnoid space indicates pressure made by a nearby tumor or lesion (see Fig. 26-3). Air is opaque to x-rays and is sometimes used instead of a drug. A lumbar puncture is contraindicated when an intracranial tumor is suspected or there is evidence of

---

* Ethyl iodophenylundecylate (Pantopaque) or iodized poppy seed oil (Lipiodol) are the drugs commonly used for this purpose.

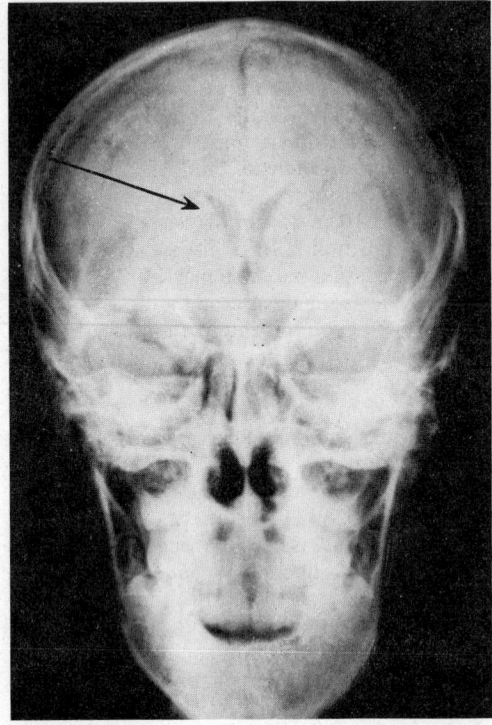

A

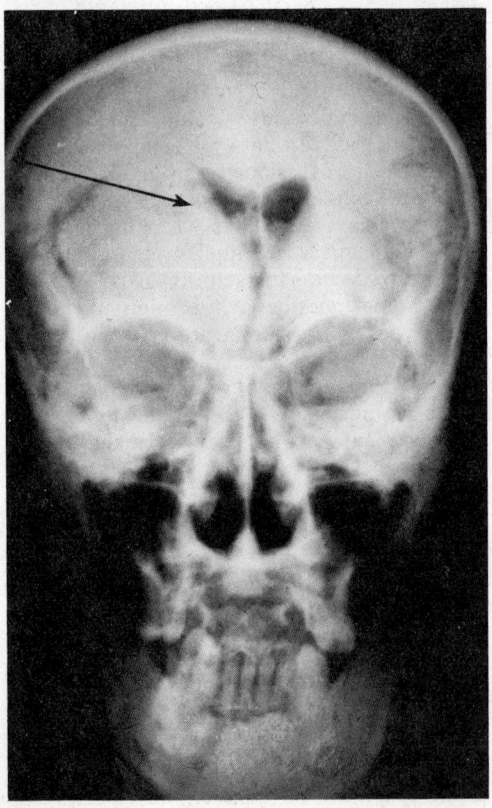

B

Figure 26-3. *A*. Anteroposterior encephalogram showing normal size lateral and third ventricles. *B*. Anteroposterior encephalogram showing moderate displacement of lateral and third ventricles to left due to a low posterior right frontal tumor. (Courtesy of Columbia-Presbyterian Medical Center, New York, N.Y.)

increased intracranial pressure (papilloedema).[12,13]

Equipment. Articles required are materials for cleaning and disinfecting the skin; sterile towels or a sterile fenestrated sheet for draping the patient; sterile rubber gloves, a mask, and gown (not universally considered essential) for the doctor; procaine (Novocaine) ½ to 1 per cent, a hypodermic syringe and two needles for administration of the anesthesia; 2 lumbar puncture needles; a water manometer for measuring the pressure of the cerebrospinal fluid; 3 small, sterile, test tubes or capped bottles marked 1, 2, and 3 to receive specimens of the fluid; and a sterile dressing to apply to the wound after the removal of the needle. In addition to these items, a plastic or rubber square and cotton or paper cover should be provided to protect the lower bedding and a treatment blanket to cover the upper part of the body, unless the room is very warm. If the bed sags, it may be necessary to place a board under the mattress. Any lateral curvature of the spine distorts the intervertebral spaces in such a way as to preclude the introduction of the needle. A pad and pencil are needed to record pressure readings. Sterile handling forceps are a convenience. Drugs to be injected must be added to the equipment as prescribed by the doctor.

In selecting needles for the introduction of the local anesthesia, choose one for the superficial tissues about 1¾ cm (¾ inch) and 25 gauge; for a deeper injection of the anesthetic, the surgeon will want a slightly longer and heavier needle. To reach the subarachnoid space, lumbar puncture needles of various sizes are used. Nicholas A. Vick[13a] recommends a fine needle (20-gauge), sharply pointed, and with a well-fitted stylet. A 22-gauge needle is preferred by some physicians. For babies, Wechsler[13b] advocates a 5-cm (2-inch) needle. It is desirable in most cases to have the needle equipped with a three-way stopcock. The needle may be attached directly to a syringe or to a manometer by an adapter, but with many types of apparatus it is connected to either of these with rubber tubing about 14 cm (5½ inches) long. This tubing should be the noncollapsible type; unless it is transparent, it should have a glass connecting tube within its length and adapters at each end to make it fit tightly to the needle and the syringe or to the needle and manometer, as the case may be.

Intraspinal medications usually come prepared in ampoules. A water bath at 40°C (104°F) is desirable to warm the liquid in the vial. The temperature of the bath must be carefully controlled because high temperatures may coagulate or change the chemical nature of a drug.

Preparation of the Patient. Explanation to the patient and family should be made and their acceptance of the procedure determined, as discussed on page 1308. Since patients must remain motionless during the treatment, their cooperation is essential (if they are older children or adults). Successful restraint of an infant or small child is possible, but it is extremely difficult to keep an adult quiet by force. If manometric readings are to be made, this aspect of the procedure must be thoroughly explained. The patient will be asked to strain (as if at stool) and to submit to manual pressure on the jugular veins or to pressure with a blood pressure cuff around the neck. Because the local anesthetic rarely reaches the meninges, pain is almost inevitable as the entrance of the needle stretches the dura and pulls on the connective tissues surrounding the vertebrae. It is wise to tell the patient that a certain amount of pain is unavoidable; otherwise he or she may not be braced for it and will move involuntarily as the needle is introduced. This move may injure the spinal nerves or cord.

While the physician is scrubbing his or her hands, draw the patient to the right side of the bed or table if the operator is right-handed; otherwise to the left. See that a stool is provided for the operator. Have the patient arch his or her back so that the head is almost touching the knees. (The patient also moves the knees up toward the chest.) If the bed sags, place a board under the mattress to correct the resulting spinal curvature. Cover the body as far as the waist with a treatment blanket, fold the upper bedding down to the separation of the buttocks, and protect the bedclothes under the lumbar region. The skin area to be cleaned and disinfected lies in a line drawn between the crests of the two ilia if a puncture is to be made in the lumbar region. The fourth lumbar interspace is most commonly used in adults, but the spinal canal can be entered at other levels. Because the spinal cord of young children extends almost to the sacral region, the site selected is usually lower than the fourth lumbar interspace.

After the skin is prepared, it is usual to surround the area with sterile towels or a fenestrated sheet (see Fig. 26-4). It is wise for

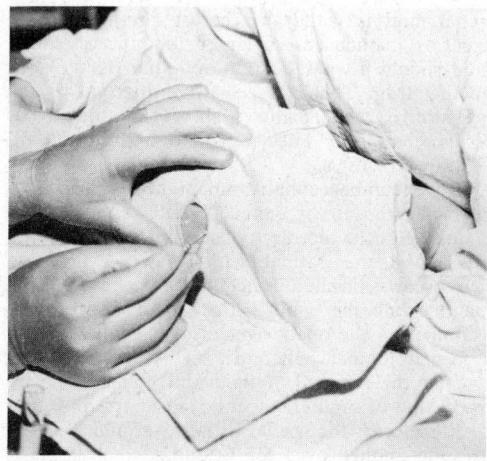

Figure 26-4. Spinal tap showing infant draped and held in position by nurse. (Courtesy of Bellevue Hospital School of Nursing, New York, N.Y., and Clay-Adams Co., New York, N.Y.)

nurses to ask physicians whether they wish them to prepare the skin area or whether they prefer to do it themselves. If the skin is hairy, it should be shaved; in any case shaving is a desirable precaution.

Wechsler says that the patient may be in a sitting position for this treatment, but in any position the back must be arched to separate the vertebrae; therefore, if a sitting posture is used, a table or chair must be provided for the patient to lean on. Any physical ordeal is more easily borne in the recumbent position; this should be used unless the physician prescribes otherwise.

Suggested Procedure. See that all sterile equipment is available and ready for the physician's use. If the patient is an infant or a child that the nurse must restrain, he or she will not be able to give other assistance during the treatment; therefore, everything must be ready for the physician, or a third member added to the team. After scrubbing the hands and putting on gloves, gown, and mask, the doctor introduces the needle. The resistance offered by the ligaments, and lastly by the dura, guides the doctor in making this puncture, which toward the last is made slowly and carefully. As soon as serum starts to drop from the needle, its position in the subarachnoid space is established. If the physician wishes to know the pressure the fluid is under, he or she attaches the manometer to the needle and then expels the air by tilting it horizontally. While the patient is in a relaxed horizontal position, the initial reading is made. Then the pressure is read during and after straining and jugular compression. Any specimens desired for laboratory analysis are collected in test tubes or small, open-mouthed bottles under aseptic conditions. In case a drug or serum is to be administered, an equal amount of spinal fluid is withdrawn before the therapeutic agent is introduced. A larger amount of spinal fluid should always be removed than is replaced by the drug. This is especially important if the pressure is abnormally high. The amount of serum commonly injected is from 20 to 30 ml (⅔ to 1 oz).

If a pneumoencephalogram or myelogram is to be made, the air or opaque liquid (about 3 ml) is injected, the needle removed, a dressing applied, and the patient with head elevated on two pillows taken at once to the x-ray department. After the x-ray picture and fluoroscopic examination the opaque material is removed with a second lumbar puncture.

After the removal of fluid and possibly the introduction of some therapeutic substance, the stopcock is closed, the needle withdrawn, and a sterile dressing applied over the wound.

Throughout the procedure the nurse should note very critically the condition of the patient. Withdrawal of fluid from around the brain may cause pressure on vital centers in the medulla. Removal of spinal fluid takes away the water cushion on which the medulla rests and allows it to fall on the uneven surface of the cranial bones. The introduction of a drug in too large amount may cause respiratory failure and other symptoms of intercranial pressure. If this occurs during the treatment, fluid is allowed to flow back through the needle. Note and call the doctor's attention to any changes in color, pulse, or respiration, and any complaint the patient makes of headache or nausea.

After the treatment keep the patient in a recumbent position for the time prescribed by the physician. Elevation of the foot of the bed may be prescribed, particularly if a drug has been administered, and the patient kept in bed for at least 24 hours in order to reestablish the circulation of the spinal fluid. It is usual for the patient to suffer from headache and backache for several days following a lumbar puncture. Quiet and good care are likely to reduce this discomfort.

Recording the Treatment. Note the amount and character of the fluid withdrawn—its color, whether cloudy or bloody—and whether withdrawn by gravity or suction. If blood is present, note whether it is in all three tubes or bottles or, as occasionally happens from trauma, merely in the first. Record the kind and amount of any drug injected and whether it was removed in whole or in part. X-rays, if taken, should be recorded. Any discomfort and any signs of the desired beneficial effects should be carefully noted. State whether specimens of fluid were sent to the laboratory for analysis. It is usual to indicate the exact time at which the treatment was given and the name of the physician who gave it.

5. CISTERNAL PUNCTURE

Definition. A cisternal puncture is the injection of a needle into the cistern magna (an enlargement of the subarachnoid space just below the cerebellum) and is like a lumbar puncture except for the area of injection. The lateral ventricle may be aspirated or injected, in which case the procedure is called a *ventricular puncture;* the x-ray picture following the injection of air, a *pneumoventriculogram;* or following the injection of an opaque drug, a *ventriculogram.* All these diagnostic measures are more thoroughly discussed in neurologic texts such as Wechsler's [13e] or neurologic nursing texts such as that by Esta Carini and Guy Owens.[13d]

Therapeutic Uses. It is desirable to enter the subarachnoid space at the cistern magna instead of the lumbar region (1) when a spinal puncture cannot be performed at the usual site (lumbar region); (2) as a means of determining subarachnoid block by performing a cisternal and lumbar puncture simultaneously; (3) to drain cerebrospinal fluid if a subarachnoid block is present or if a lumbar puncture is contraindicated, for some reason; and (4) to inject air or an opaque drug before making an encephalogram to discover the presence and location of brain lesions. (Air also may be injected directly into the lateral ventricles through the cranium. The needle can be introduced through the anterior fontanel of an infant or by way of a trephined opening through the skull of a child or an adult.)

Equipment. The only difference between the equipment for a lumbar and a cisternal puncture is the use of short-beveled spinal needles. Vick [13e] says a 20-gauge lumbar puncture needle is satisfactory, but it should be marked at 6 cm, the maximum safe depth of insertion. Since the area of insertion is always hairy, a razor is necessary to shave the site of injection. A lumbar puncture may be made at the same time, in which case it is necessary to include equipment for the two injections.

Preparation of the Patient. With exception of the position, preparation is, in general, the same as that for lumbar puncture. It is important that the spinous processes of the vertebrae and the occipital protuberance are in line; therefore the head must rest on a small hard pillow or a sand bag. The patient is told to tilt the head forward, to draw the legs up, and to fold the arms over the chest. The nurse holds the head firmly and then the physician inserts the needle between the first and second cervical vertebrae, entering the cranium through the foramen magnum.

Suggested Procedure. From the standpoint of the nurse there is no difference, after the preparation of the patient and the equipment, between this procedure and that for the lumbar puncture. In preparation for an encephalogram the physician alternately removes fluid and injects air, the amount of air depending on the size of the ventricles.

6. ASPIRATION OF THE PERICARDIUM

Definition. The term defines itself; it is the removal of fluid from the pericardial sac surrounding the heart.

Therapeutic Uses. Fluid is removed from the serous sac surrounding the heart (1) for diagnostic purposes or (2) to relieve intrapericardial pressure. Normally, only a few milliliters (about 15 to 30) of clear citron-colored fluid moisten the inner fibrous (visceral) pericardium and outer fibrous (parietal) pericardium. In acute pericardial effusion, the parietal layer may be stretched so as to allow 200 to 300 ml, producing pressure on the heart (called cardiac tamponade), while in chronic cases, where the accumulation has been gradual and the parietal layer has had time to adapt itself, as much as 2000 ml (2 qt) may collect, according to William L. Winters and Felix M. Cortes.[14] A transudate also may collect in the pericardium in heart and kidney disease.

The pericardium is pear-shaped, the base in contact with the diaphragm, the apex above. If the sac is only partly filled, the fluid may shift its position with that of the body, so that when the person is in the recumbent position, the fluid may extend into the apex, press on the bronchi, and interfere with breathing. If the person is sitting up, the fluid gravitates to the base of the sac.

If the fluid is excessive, there is pressure on the heart, lungs, bronchi, trachea, and esophagus. This causes dyspnea; a dusky, anxious countenance; a rapid weak pulse; a cough; and dysphagia. The diaphragm, liver, and stomach may be displaced downward. Removal of the fluid in such cases relieves symptoms due to pressure. Successful antibiotic therapy has reduced the necessity for pericardial aspiration. However, this procedure (called *pericardiocentesis* by some authorities) continues to be used as a therapeutic measure, especially in patients with a rapid accumulation of fluid, and in such cases it may be a life-saving measure. Pericardiocentesis is used for diagnostic as well as therapeutic purposes (see Fig. 26-5).

Equipment. Articles required for the procedure are the same as in aspiration of the pleural sac except that as the amount of fluid withdrawn is small, the aspirating set and large receptacle for the fluid are rarely required. A large, sterile syringe equipped with a three-way stopcock is ordinarily used to

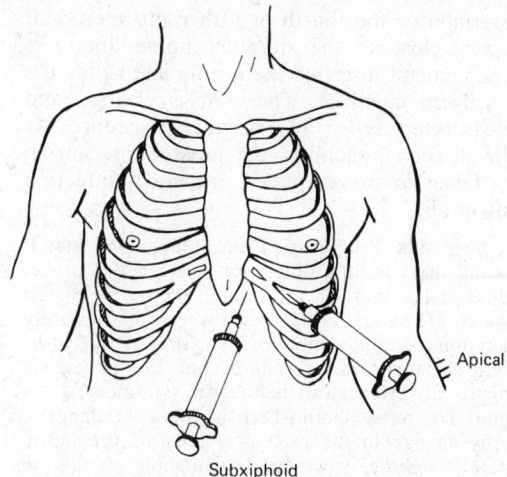

Figure 26-5. Apical and subxiphoid approaches for performing pericardiocentesis. (From Wagner, Mary M.: "Injuries to the Chest and Abdomen," *Nurs. Clin. North Am.,* **8**:425, [Sept.] 1973.)

withdraw the fluid and a sterile bottle to receive it. Usually a large short-bevel needle is used; however, the type and amount of fluid expected must be considered in the final selection of a needle. An electrocardiographic lead attached to the hub of the needle by an alligator clamp is used to determine when the needle makes contact with the pericardium which is reflected "by the instant appearance of upward ST segment displacement and/or premature ventricular contractions." * Mervyn S. Gotsman and Velva Schrire[15] (in England) describe a specially designed electrode needle used to aspirate the fluid which is attached to the electrocardiograph machine by a special wire.

Preparation of the Patient. If the patient is in a sitting or semi-upright position, the fluid tends to gravitate to the base of the lungs in the pleural sac where it can be more easily aspirated at the frontal and lower side of the chest. Pillows should be placed under the back in such a way that the spine is in marked extension. However, when patients' condition is critical and they are in great distress, they must always remain in the position in which they can breathe most easily and in which they are as free as possible from strain.

The area where the incision or puncture is usually made is the fourth, fifth, or sixth left intercostal space close to the left edge of the

---

* Winters, William L., Jr., and Cortes, Felix M.: "Pericardial Disease," in Conn, Hadley L., Jr., and Horwitz, Orville: *Cardiac and Vascular Diseases,* Vol. II. Lea & Febiger, Philadelphia, 1971, p. 1330.

sternum or the fourth or fifth right intercostal space close to the sternum. Some operators recommend inserting the needle just below the ensiform cartilage. The skin is cleaned and disinfected as for any surgical procedure. As in all such punctures, the greatest precaution is taken to prevent the entrance of infection or of air.

Suggested Procedure. From the nurse's standpoint, there is little difference between this procedure and a thoracic aspiration. She or he should watch the patient critically and report immediately any unfavorable symptoms. Not only is this in itself a dangerous procedure, but the patient is nearly always very ill before the treatment is begun. The nurse should keep in mind the dangers. Any change in the rate or quality of the pulse, pallor, sighing, yawning, or coughing should be noted and reported immediately. A stimulant is usually kept ready for instant use.

Recording the Treatment. Follow the suggestions for recording similar procedures.

7. ABDOMINAL PARACENTESIS

Definition. An abdominal paracentesis is removal of fluid from the peritoneal cavity. The condition in which a large amount of fluid has collected in the peritoneal cavity is called *ascites* from the Greek *askos,* a bag.

Therapeutic Uses. Fluid may be removed from the peritoneal cavity (1) for diagnostic purposes or (2) for drainage of an exudate in peritonitis and (3) to relieve pressure on other abdominal and chest organs if a transudate collects as a result of certain renal, cardiac, and liver diseases.

The peritoneal sac, like the pericardium, contains just enough fluid to lubricate its surface and to prevent friction between contiguous parts. The surface of the peritoneum is enormous, almost equal to that of the skin, and contains many lymph vessels. Its power of absorption is therefore great; but when "hepatic and intestinal lymph is formed in amounts that exceed the capacity of the thoracic duct to drain lymph from the abdomen," * ascitic fluid accumulates. William Boyd says the fluid may be a transudate or an exudate (inflammatory). An accumulated transudate fluid is caused by cardiac or renal disease or it may be due to obstruction of the partal vein. The condition is called *dropsical ascites.* Although the portal obstruction is usually caused by portal cirrhosis of the liver, it may be due to pressure on the vein by enlarged glands or tumors. When an exudate is present, it is caused by irritation of the peritoneum by carcinoma or tuberculosis. The exudate (inflammatory) "fluid has a higher specific gravity (above 1018) and protein content (above 3 per cent) than the dropsical" * (transudate) fluid and it may contain blood. Ascitic fluid may contain as much as 2 to 3 gm of protein per 100 ml of fluid.[16] The patient with ascites usually has a distended abdomen with weight gain and a decrease in urinary output; in addition, he or she often has great difficulty in breathing.

Because methods of treatment have improved (including low sodium intake, restriction of fluids, and oral or intramuscular injections of a diuretic drug in combination with an aldosterone blocking agent), an abdominal paracentesis, as a control measure, is used less frequently now than in the past. In fact, the procedure is avoided as long as possible so that the patient's body proteins are conserved. When it is used, not more than 3 to 5 liters of fluid is removed at any one time.

Due to the common occurrence of severe injury (see Chapter 43), diagnostic abdominal taps are frequently made.[16a] James McCoy and Fred J. Wolma say the procedure has "an accuracy rate as high as 96 per cent in determining whether significant intra-abdominal injury has occurred." † They state that fluid with "a red cell count of more than 100,000 cells, more than 500 white cells per mm, or amylase concentration of 100 units/100 ml" is considered "positive"; whereas, Theodore Drapanas and Martin S. Litwin [17] think that if one-tenth of 1 ml of fluid is obtained and especially if additional fluid can be aspirated in other puncture sites the test is "positive." Any emergency area should have peritoneal tap equipment available for immediate use.

Equipment. Articles required are similar to those needed for pleural and pericardial aspirations, except that a trocar and cannula may be substituted for a needle (see Fig. 32-9, Chapter 32). A small plastic catheter that can be threaded through the trocar and ensures very slow drainage of the fluid should be included, as some physicians prefer it. Fluid may be collected through tubing attached to the cannula or by a plastic catheter threaded through the trocar and extending to a bottle. A short and shallow preliminary incision is usually made; for this a scalpel is needed. Sometimes one or two sutures may be necessary after the treatment is finished. If so, dressing forceps,

* Jefferies, Graham H.: "Diseases of the Liver," in Beeson, Paul B., and McDermott, Walsh (eds.): *Textbook of Medicine,* Vol. II, 14th ed. W. B. Saunders Co., Philadelphia, 1975, p. 1327.

* Boyd, William: *A Textbook of Pathology, Structure and Function,* 8th ed. Lea & Febiger, Philadelphia, 1970, p. 933.

† McCoy, James, and Wolma, Fred J.: "Abdominal Tap; Indication, Technic, and Results," *Am. J. Surg.,* **122:**693, (Nov.) 1971.

needle holder, suture needles, and sutures will be required. No aspirating apparatus is needed as the fluid flows out, impelled by gravity, the pressure of the viscera, and contraction of the abdominal walls. Since this is a slow process, a seat should be provided for the doctor.

Preparation of the Patient. As in all such treatments, the patient's cooperation and understanding and acceptance of the treatment should be assured before it is begun. The bladder should be emptied, because, if full, it is easily punctured during a paracentesis.

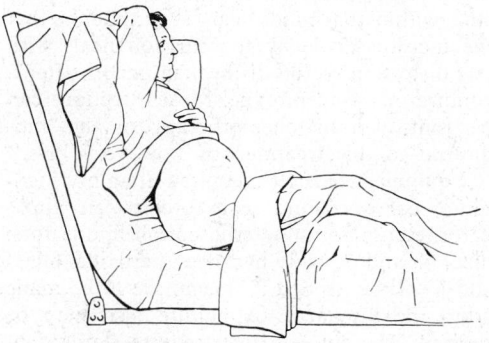

Figure 26-6. Sitting position of a patient in bed, about to have paracentesis. (After Abbot.)

Catheterization is indicated if the patient cannot void. Take the blood pressure, pulse, and respiration rate and weigh the patient as this information serves as baseline data that may be used to compare similar data during and following the procedure to determine its effect on the patient. Depending on the patients' condition, place them in one of the positions as follows: (1) bring the patient close to the side of the bed and place him or her in a sitting position, well supported (see Fig. 26-6); (2) have the patient sit on the side of the bed (or treatment table) with feet well supported on a stool or chair; or (3) ask the patient to sit in a chair that provides good back and arm support. Regardless of the position selected, be sure that the patient is warm. Nervousness is likely to produce a chilly sensation. Cover the chest with the gown, pajama top, and/or treatment blanket according to the room temperature. The lower part of the body may be protected by folding the upper bedding down to the pubic area or a treatment blanket may be used over the legs when the patient is sitting on the side of the bed or in a chair. Protect the patient and lower bedclothes with plastic, rubber, or moisture-proof paper and cover with toweling or cotton material.

Figure 26-7. The sterile specimen trap is a closed system, providing for efficient, reliable, and safe specimen analysis. Specific directions for use in a variety of situations are provided by the manufacturer. (Courtesy of Chesebrough-Pond's, Inc., Greenwich, Conn.)

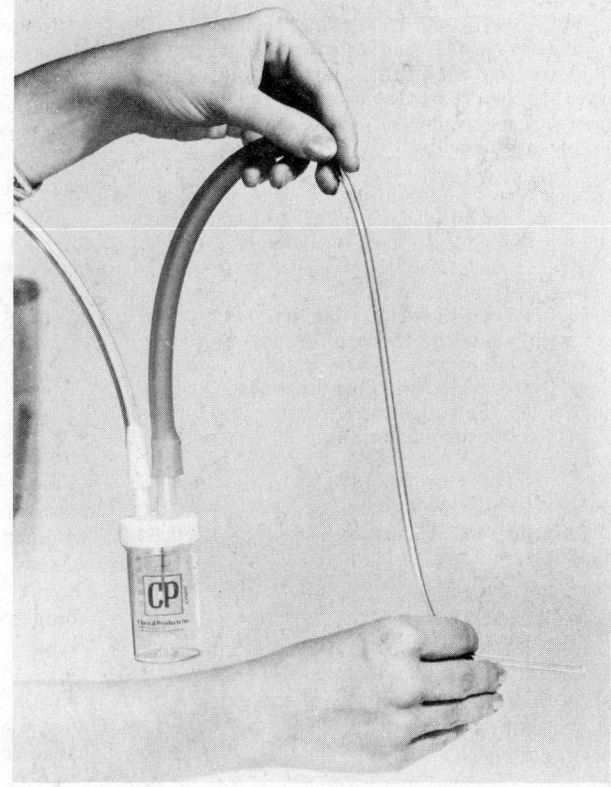

The incision is usually made in the midline of the abdomen, 2.5 to 5 cm (1 to 2 in.) below the umbilicus. The midline is chosen because an incision at the side might puncture the colon, as it is fixed in position. Clean and disinfect this area as for any surgical procedure. Shave the skin if the site of injection is hairy. When the procedure is carried out for diagnostic purposes, a puncture with a long spiral needle is made rather than a trocar and cannula which necessitates an abdominal incision.

Suggested Procedure. After the usual preparation for a surgical procedure (scrubbing, adjusting gloves, gown, and possibly a mask), the surgeon incises the skin and introduces the trocar and cannula. The trocar is removed to allow the fluid to flow through the cannula. After the collection of specimens of fluid for laboratory analysis (see Fig. 26-7), the cannula is attached to tubing that reaches from the instrument to the closed drainage bottle. This bottle is usually placed on the floor or on a low stool. The greater the vertical distance between the incision and the end of the tubing in the drainage bottle, the greater the pull on the fluid in the cavity and the more quickly the cavity is drained. Too rapid withdrawal of fluid may produce hypovolemia and shock that result from a shift of fluid from the intravascular compartment into the peritoneal cavity. Such results may be prevented by a gradual withdrawal of fluid. Usually from one-half to three-quarters of the estimated amount of fluid is removed but no more than 3 to 5 liters.

The person should be reassured, and the treatment throughout made as simple as possible. (Patients are less likely to be nervous if they have had previous treatments, as they welcome the relief that follows.) Avoid any unnecessary display of instruments, and divert the patient's attention if possible. Nurses must, however, remember the dangers involved; they should observe the patient's color, pulse, respiration, and blood pressure, and note immediately any signs of vascular collapse. A glass of ice water and a stimulant should be at hand.

The thickness of the dressing depends upon the expected amount of drainage. It should be examined for drainage, and the patient's condition checked frequently after the treatment. In addition, weigh the patient and measure the amount of fluid collected. The physician may request that samples of the fluid be sent to the laboratory for examination of its specific gravity, bacterial count, and protein concentration.

Recording the Treatment. Follow the suggestions for recording similar procedures.

8. MYRINGOTOMY

Definition. This minor operation consists of an incision, or paracentesis of the eardrum. It is performed with a special knife called a *myringotome*.

Therapeutic Uses. A myringotomy is made to provide a channel for drainage of pus or other fluid from the middle to the external ear. It is performed in otitis media when the drum is red and bulging with an accumulation of fluid or pus in the middle ear, when pain is severe, or when other symptoms, such as tenderness over the mastoid process, indicate the spread of the inflammation. Opinion among authorities consulted on the subject varies greatly as to indications for this operation. At present the tendency is to postpone the incision until there is reason to believe that the drum if not incised will burst from the pressure within the middle ear. It is thought that the incision made by the surgeon heals with less distortion of the drum than occurs after a rupture of the membrane. Most infections can be controlled by chemotherapy or the antibiotics, so this treatment is now very rare.[18]

Equipment. Articles required are a myringotome, ear speculum, ear forceps, an applicator, sterile cotton, sterile cotton applicators, alcohol, and possibly hydrogen peroxide. Glass slides will be needed if smears are to be made from the discharge. A culture also may be desired. The surgeon may require sterile rubber gloves. The myringotomy knife is usually sterilized by immersion in a chemical disinfectant or by hot air. It should be protected from any hard surface, because it is most important that its sharp edge be preserved.

Preparation and Aftercare of the Patient. Have the patient on the edge of the bed or on an operating table lying on the unaffected ear.

The surgeon performs the operation. The nurse prepares the patient and the required articles, and assists the surgeon, carries out the aftercare, and observes and reports any results of the treatments and any symptoms of complications that may develop.

A general anesthetic is nearly always given, as the incision causes agonizing pain, and local anesthetics do not desensitize the drum sufficiently. John Ballantyne and John Groves [19] say a general anesthetic should always be used. The ear is very sensitive, and even the slightest involuntary movement might cause a serious accident. Nitrous oxide gas is commonly used. (Frequently in the case of very young babies, however, no anesthetic is given; they are wrapped firmly in a sheet.) In all cases, even when a general anesthetic is used, the head should be held to prevent voluntary or involuntary motion.

As in all operations, every precaution is taken to prevent secondary infection. If possible, a short time before the operation the auricle and surrounding area are cleaned. The canal is syringed with an antiseptic solution and packed with antiseptic gauze. When the surgeon is ready, sterile towels are placed across the shoulder and around the head covering the hair. A bright light should be placed so that it will be reflected by the doctor's head mirror into the patient's ear.

The treatment following the incision varies —the necessary articles should always be in readiness. Sometimes the canal is irrigated directly after the incision in order to wash out any blood clots that might block the incision if allowed to remain. Sometimes fluid is removed by suction. Some surgeons apply a moist dressing to absorb the discharge, or a sterile gauze wick may be inserted and a dressing and bandage applied. Dressings are usually impregnated with an antibiotic. They are changed as often as necessary, depending upon the amount of discharge.

After a myringotomy the canal is sometimes irrigated until the discharge has ceased; at first every 2 or 3 hours, then as often as the amount of discharge indicates. Sterile cotton or a gauze wick may be kept in the canal between treatments. Some surgeons keep the aural canal free from all dressings, believing that anything in the canal tends to block it. In such cases a sterile cellucotton pad with an impervious paper base or a rubber or plastic sheet is placed under the draining ear as the patient lies on this side. Irrigations of an ear with an open drum are dangerous because of the possibility of forcing infectious material back into the middle ear and possibly into the mastoid cells and eustachian tubes (see Chapter 27).

9. PHLEBOTOMY OR VENESECTION

Removal of blood from a vein is a quick way to reduce blood pressure and for this purpose is occasionally used. Most often blood is withdrawn for diagnostic tests. (The technique is discussed under transfusion in Chapter 22.)

Bleeding and "leeching" were common in the past, so common that barbers did both. The striped pole in front of the barber shop represents the blood that was drawn and the white, the bandage applied to the wound. A leech (sucking worm) is said to withdraw 15 ml (½ oz) of blood before it is satiated. Another outmoded and unwarranted method of reducing blood volume is to place vacuum cups over incisions made in the tissues. The practice of bleeding patients (and giving the emetics) was so common in the seventeenth and eighteenth centuries that a person had to be strong indeed to survive "treatment." Each generation of health workers should be aware

of the possibility that current methods may be discredited because their risks outweigh their positive values.

REFERENCES

1. DeGowin, Elmer L., and DeGowin, Richard L.: *Bedside Diagnostic Examination,* 3rd ed. Macmillan Publishing Co., Inc., New York, 1976, p. 311.
2. Flitter, Hessel Howard: *An Introduction to Physics in Nursing,* 6th ed. C. V. Mosby Co., St. Louis, 1972, p. 112.
3. McClement, John H.: "Diseases of the Pleura," in Beeson, Paul B., and McDermott, Walsh (eds.): *Textbook of Medicine,* Vol. I, 14th ed. W. B. Saunders Co., Philadelphia, 1975, p. 873.
4. Engelsher, Harvey J.: "Automatic Thoracentesis," *Surg. Gynecol. Obstet.,* **122**:1320, (June) 1966.
5. Kovarik, Joseph L.: "Thoracentesis: A Modified Technic," *Postgrad. Med.,* **48**:96, (Dec.) 1960.
6. Stead, William W.: "Diseases of the Pleura," in Beeson, Paul B., and McDermott, Walsh (eds.): *Cecil-Loeb Textbook of Medicine,* 13th ed. W. B. Saunders Co., Philadelphia, 1971, p. 931.
7. Takaro, Timothy: "The Pleura and Empyema," in Sabiston, David C. (ed.): *Davis-Christopher Textbook of Surgery,* 10th ed. W. B. Saunders Co., Philadelphia, 1972, p. 1815.
8. Myrden, J. A., and Hiltz, J. E.: "Breast Cancer Following Multiple Fluoroscopies During Artificial Pneumothorax Treatment of Pulmonary Tuberculosis," *Can. Med. Assoc. J.,* **100**:1032, (June 14) 1969.
9. Gofman, John W., and Tamplin, Arthur R.: "Fluoroscopic Radiation and Risk of Primary Lung Cancer Following Pneumothorax Therapy of Tuberculosis," *Nature,* **227**:295, (July 18) 1970.
10. Myrden, J. A., and Hiltz, J. E.: *op. cit.*
11. Wechsler, Israel S.: *Clinical Neurology,* 9th ed. W. B. Saunders Co., Philadelphia, 1963, p. 76.
11a. *Ibid.*
12. Carini, Esta, and Owens, Guy: *Neurological and Neurosurgical Nursing,* 6th ed. C. V. Mosby Co., St. Louis, 1974, p. 50.
13. Vick, Nicholas A.: *Grinker's Neurology,* 7th ed. Charles C Thomas, Publisher, Springfield, Ill., 1976, p. 50.
13a. *Ibid.*
13b. Wechsler, Israel S.: *op. cit.*
13c. *Ibid.*
13d. Carini, Esta, and Owens, Guy: *op. cit.*
13e. Vick, Nicholas A.: *op. cit.*
14. Winters, William L., Jr., and Cortes, Felix M.: "Pericardial Disease," in Conn, Hadley L., Jr., and Horwitz, Orville: *Cardiac and Vascular Diseases,* Vol. II. Lea & Febiger, Philadelphia, 1971, p. 1326.

15. Gotsman, Mervyn S., and Schrire, Velva: "A Pericardiocentesis Electrode Needle," *Br. Heart J.,* **28:**566, (No. 4) 1966.

16. Fishman, Alfred P.: "Diseases of the Cardiovascular System, Heart Failure," in Beeson, Paul B., and McDermott, Walsh (eds.): *Cecil-Loeb Textbook of Medicine,* 13th ed. W. B. Saunders Co., Philadelphia, 1971, p. 958.

16a. Tucker, J. F., et al.: "Traumatic Intraperitonel Haemorrhage. Diagnosis by Paracentesis and Lavage," *Ann. R. Coll. Surg. Engl.,* **56:**33 (Jan.) 1975.

17. Drapanas, Theodore, and Litwin, Martin S.: "Trauma: Management of the Acutely Injured Patient," in Sabiston, David C. (ed.): *Davis-Christopher Textbook of Surgery,* 10th ed. W. B. Saunders Co., Philadelphia, 1972, p. 359.

18. Ballantyne, John, and Groves, John: *Scott-Brown's Diseases of the Ear, Nose, and Throat,* Vol. 2, 3rd ed. J. B. Lippincott Co., Philadelphia, 1971, p. 106.

19. *Ibid.*

Additional Suggested Reading

Bishop, L. H., Jr., et al.: "The Electrocardiogram as a Safeguard in Pericardiocentesis," *J.A.M.A.,* **162:**264, (Sept. 22) 1956.

Blount, Mary, et al.: "Obtaining and Analyzing Cerebrospinal Fluid," *Nurs. Clin. North Am.,* **9:**593, (Dec.) 1974.

Donohoe, Katherine M., et al.: "Cerebral Circulation and Cerebral Angiography," *Nurs. Clin. North Am.,* **9:**623, (Dec.) 1974.

Giacobine, J. W., and Siler, V. E.: "Evaluation of Diagnostic Abdominal Paracentesis with Experimental and Clinical Studies," *Surg. Gynecol. Obstet.,* **110:**676, (June) 1960.

Gott, P. H.: "Simplified Method for Thoracentesis and Pleural Fluid Drainage," *Am. Rev. Resp. Dis.,* **92:**295, (Aug.) 1965.

Kinney, Anna Belle, et al.: "Cerebrospinal Fluid Circulation and Encephalography," *Nurs. Clin. North Am.,* **9:**611, (Dec.) 1974.

Mandrillo, Margaret P.: "Brain Scanning," *Nurs. Clin. North Am.,* **9:**633, (Dec.) 1974.

Merritt, H. Houston: *A Textbook of Neurology,* 5th ed. Lea & Febiger, Philadelphia, 1973.

"Quick Way to Tap a Chest" (editorial), *Emerg. Med.,* **3:**31, (Jan.) 1971.

Root, H. D., et al.: "Diagnostic Peritoneal Lavage," *Surgery,* **57:**633, (May) 1965.

Tilbury, Mary S.: "The Intracranial Pressure Screw, A New Assessment Tool," *Nurs. Clin. North Am.,* **9:**641, (Dec.) 1974.

Tindal, S., and Myerowitz, B. R.: "Unusual Complications of Diagnostic Abdominal Paracentesis," *J.A.M.A.,* **193:**836, (Sept. 6) 1965.

Gladys Nite
Virginia Henderson

CHAPTER 27

Irrigation and Medication of the Eye, Ear, Nose, and Throat and Removal of Foreign Bodies

1. IRRIGATION OF THE CONJUNCTIVAL SAC

Definition. An eye irrigation is the washing out of the conjunctival sac by a stream of liquid.

Therapeutic Uses. Irrigations are given in various forms of inflammation of the conjunctiva (conjunctivitis) for cleaning, to combat infection and for temperature effects, and in chemical injury to the eyes to remove all particles of the offending agent.

Selection of Method. The conjunctiva is a continuous, thin, transparent layer of mucous membrane lining the eyelids and covering the anterior surface of the eyeball. It is exposed to bacteria, irritation from sun and wind, from smoke, dust, and other foreign bodies. It has a rich supply of blood vessels and lymphatics. It is also supplied with mucous and lacrimal glands. The conjunctiva is liable to congestion and swelling, and increased secretion when irritated or infected, the lids becoming tender, edematous, adherent, or difficult to separate. An abundant nerve supply makes the conjunctiva sensitive to minute irritation, and the resulting conjunctivitis is very painful. Secretions of the conjunctival sac drain through the lacrimal, or tear, duct into the nasal cavity.

The conjunctiva is never free from live organisms although its normal condition is not conducive to their growth. The lacrimal secretion contains lysozyme which dissolves many air bacteria. Normal tears contain comparatively few live organisms.[1] The relative immunity of the mucous membrane of the eye as compared to that in other parts of the body may be attributed to the action of lysozyme and probably other enzymes yet unrecognized, as well as the low temperature of the eye, its moderate blood supply, and the evaporation of the lacrimal fluid. It is, however, susceptible to infection by the gonococcus, staphylococcus, *Pseudomonas aeruginosa*, streptococcus, the virus of inclusion conjunctivitis of the newborn, trachoma, and the bacilli of Koch-Weeks and Morax-Axenfeld; more rarely the meningococcus and pneumococcus, the colon, diphtheria, and tubercle bacilli, and the treponema of syphilis. In 1961, Robert P. Burns and David H. Rhodes [2] reported the death of four premature infants caused by *Pseudomonas aeruginosa* infection of the eye. They say this organism, which is commonly found in hospitals, water, sewage, and soil, is a more frequent cause of conjunctivitis than gonorrheal ophthalmia and a far greater hazard. This suggests that the causes of eye infection may vary with climate, sanitary conditions, and hygienic practice. Foreign proteins, animal parasites, and growths produce hyperemia of the eye covering. Nutritional deficiencies and endocrine imbalance are contributing factors.[3]

The layman's name for any conjunctivitis, "pink eye," is dangerous because it suggests to most persons a mild condition that can be cured with home care. Now, as in the past, some individuals practice folk medicine. From 1967 to 1969, a large number of persons attending an eye clinic in Atlanta said they had used flaxseed as a home remedy at one time or another for a variety of eye problems.[4] Frederick T. Fraunfelder and F. Hampton Roy say, "Home use of topical anesthetics for ocular pain is hazardous because these agents delay normal healing and may lead to keratitis. This has been the subject of many malpractice suits." * Nurses and all health workers should be aware of the dangers of untreated eye conditions. Any conjunctivitis, therefore, suggests the need for medical care, because the treatment varies according to the etiology.

Infective agents are usually brought to the conjunctiva from the environment, that is, they are exogenous. Endogenous infection carried by the blood or lymph occurs less often. The human host, according to Burns,[5] may acquire eye infections for the following reasons: (1) a peculiar susceptibility of tissues of the eye to certain microorganisms (the virus of Newcastle disease is, for example, only pathogenic for the eye); (2) there may be a loss of the mechanical protection from the blink reflex or changes in the epithelium that permits entrance of organisms; (3) a decrease in antibacterial (lysozyme) quality of tears characteristic of some diseases of the eye; and (4) metabolic changes as in conditions such as diabetes or acidosis. Burns believes that certain organisms, however, are always pathogenic (diplobacillus Morax-Axenfeld, for example) and only require contact with the host to cause disease.

Health regulations, that enforce protective treatment for the eyes of the newborn, and the current effectiveness of antibiotics and chemotherapy have greatly reduced the incidence of conjunctivitis in most countries. Both types of agents may be given systemically or administered locally in the form of drops or ointments. Antitoxin may also be used systemically or locally. Penicillin is particularly effective in the control of eye infections. It has largely replaced silver preparations in the prevention of gonorrhea neonatorum. The sulfa drugs are very effective in trachoma and other types of conjunctivitis. Contact dermatitis of the conjunctiva and lids (sensitivity to the therapeutic agent), however, often complicates local therapy. The drugs that are the most frequent offenders are atropine, neomycin, sulfathiazole, and penicillin. Although corticosteroids are effective in therapy, they have been found "to cause or aggravate glaucoma," enhance viral and fungal disease, and promote cataract formation in rare instances. Any patient receiving these medications should be watched carefully for development of such complications.[6] *Most authorities say only an ophthalmologist should prescribe these drugs.*

When irrigations are used for any type of conjunctival infection, every precaution should be taken to control the spread of the disease. *Antiseptic solutions* for irrigations and instillations should be chosen for their effect upon the causative organisms. In a series of studies on antiseptic solutions commonly prescribed in the treatment of eye infections, Frederick Ridley [7] found a wide variation in their effectiveness on staphylococci and hemolytic streptococci. Boric acid (2 per cent) had no effect on the organisms; mercuric oxycyanide (1 per cent) and Argyrol (25 per cent) had slight effect; however, acriflavine (1 per cent) inhibited the growth of the bacteria, and silver nitrate (1 per cent) was germicidal. Sir Stewart Duke-Elder says that silver nitrate is not "strongly bactericidal" but that the organisms are caught in the coagulum that it forms and are removed with it. He says that most eye lotions cannot be used in sufficient strength to act as "efficient antiseptics." Most authorities consulted recommend isotonic saline solution for its cleansing effect. After tests of bacterial sensitivity, the appropriate drug should be given, but in the absence of such a test, a "broad spectrum antibiotic" is generally used.[8] A number of antibiotics may be instilled in the eye without causing systemic toxicity.

If irrigations are given for mechanical cleaning or for temperature effect (usually heat), it seems reasonable to use a sodium chloride solution, which is nonirritating. In a series of tests made on normal subjects the second writer found that there was less sensation of burning or smarting with a 1.0 per cent sodium chloride solution than with plain water or a 2.0 per cent boric solution. George V. Hosford and Avery M. Hicks [9] believe that the sensation when substances are instilled in the eyes is intimately associated with the hydrogen ion concentration. The pH of tears is 7.35, approximately the hydrogen ion concentration of blood and lymph. This suggests that for comfort the solutions used for eye irriga-

---

* Fraunfelder, Frederick T., and Roy, F. Hampton: "How to Treat Common External Eye Problems," *Am. Fam. Physician,* **3:**104, (Apr.) 1971.

tions should be approximately neutral in reaction.

In industries, schools, and homes, eyes are often injured; chemical burns that need immediate attention are especially common.[9a-d] The eye should be *irrigated with saline, tap water, or any other bland solution available,* regardless of the chemical—acid or alkali. Because tap water is readily available, it is used frequently. The person should be taken to the ophthalmologist as quickly as possible.[10,11] The importance of immediate and copious irrigation of the eye with water should be stressed in educational programs for workers, mothers, and children.[12] Defective vision, its many causes, and methods of prevention and treatment are discussed in Chapter 46 and care of the artificial eye and eye socket is described in Chapter 14.

Except in emergencies the irrigating solution is specified by the physician. If the physician is unavailable it would be safe in most cases for the nurse to use a physiological saline solution.

The *temperature* of the solution varies according to the effect desired, and should be prescribed by the physician. Irrigations are most comfortable if given at or near body temperature. In treatment of inflammatory conditions, they may be prescribed as hot as the patients can tolerate them. The second writer has found that solutions at a temperature of 43.3°C (110°F) are uncomfortably hot for normal subjects. Cold irrigations are rarely ordered; cold compresses, however, are common. Any increase in the rate or force of the solution intensifies the temperature sensation.

All the authorities consulted seem to agree that the *pressure* or force of the liquid should be only that required to maintain a steady flow.

The *amount* of solution also varies with the effect desired. It may range from 30 to 1000 ml (1 oz to 1 qt). When larger quantities of solution are prescribed, it is desirable to use a reservoir rather than a syringe.

Equipment. For an eye irrigation the articles required are: the prescribed solution, an irrigator, a basin for the return, eye cotton pledgets, a paper bag, a waterproof protector, and towel to cover it. The fluid may be delivered from a flask or an irrigating can, saturated absorbent cotton, an eye dropper, a soft rubber bulb, or an undine. Everything that comes in contact with the eye should be sterile. A good light is essential.

Solutions commonly used for cleaning are boric acid (2 per cent) or sodium chloride in physiologic concentration (0.9 per cent). The solution should be prepared so that it is at the prescribed temperature when it reaches the eye.[13]

Suggested Procedure. Have the patient sit comfortably or, if in bed, lie on the back with the head turned slightly to the side to be irrigated. When the patient is a small child, it may be necessary to wrap him or her firmly in a sheet in order to keep the hands away from the eyes and to prevent interference with the treatment with possible injury to the eyes from sudden, violent movements. (It may be necessary to hold, or restrain, an infant or a child whose cooperation cannot be gained.) Arrange the light in such a way that it is sufficient for the operator but does not shine in the patient's eye. Protect the patient's shoulder with a towel. Incline the head to the side being irrigated, tilted slightly backward and support it if the patient is sitting up and the nurse standing behind him or her. Show a responsive patient how to hold the basin to the side of the face to receive the return flow.

Before irrigation, carefully clean the eyelids to remove any secretions or particles of dust adhering to the lashes, which would otherwise be carried into the sac. Separate the lids very gently with the thumb and fingers of the left hand so that the fluid will reach all parts of the membrane. In separating the lids, exert pressure on the cheek and brow, never on the eyeball. Use just sufficient force in irrigating to dislodge the secretions or a foreign body if this is the purpose of the treatment. Direct the fluid from the inner angle of the eye so that it will flush the sac and discharge the secretions from the outer angle. The fluid should not flow down the lacrimal duct to the nose; this might spread the infection. Never touch the eye with the irrigator. Dry the lids as soon as the sac has been thoroughly flushed and all secretions removed. An eye pad and metal shield may be used to protect the affected eye.

In acute infections, irrigations must be given with care to prevent spread of infection to the nurse and other patients or to the nonaffected eye. Duke-Elder recommends a waterproof transparent protective dressing for the uninfected eye (called a Buller's shield). It is made with a watch crystal and adhesive, or with Scotch tape and cellophane. If by accident a drop of pus should spurt into one of the nurse's eyes, immediate steps should be taken. Only a short time is sufficient to cause serious damage, and neglect may result in loss of sight. The conjunctiva lining the upper and lower lids should be exposed and the sac thoroughly irrigated with one of the germicidal solutions previously mentioned. A few drops of mild silver protein, a 2 per cent solution of silver nitrate, or a penicillin suspension should be instilled into the eye; the other eye should be protected until all danger of infection has passed. Nurses may protect their eyes from such accidents by wearing glasses or goggles.

Recording the Treatment. Chart the type of solution used, its concentration and temperature, and the hour at which the treatment was given. Report any unusual reaction or any change in the condition of the eyes, as, for example, the relief felt if a foreign body is flushed out of the sac.

2. EYE INSTILLATIONS

Definition. An instillation means the introduction of a liquid into a cavity by drops.

Therapeutic Uses. Various drugs are instilled into the eyes for purposes of examining the eye, for the treatment of disease, and for local anesthesia. Antiseptics and astringents are frequently used; they include silver nitrate, mercury bichloride, and zinc oxide. A number of antibiotics including penicillin and corticosteroids are also used.[14,15]

Suggested Procedure. An eye dropper is generally used for the instillation of drops. In drawing up the solution from the bottle, do not draw up more than required, since excess solution must not be returned to the bottle for fear of contamination and mistaken drug identity.

To instill the drops, tilt the head of the patient slightly backward; wipe away any secretions and place the soiled cotton in a paper bag; then gently separate the lids, draw down the lower lid with the left hand, ask the patient to look up and allow the drop to fall on the center of the everted lower lid. The eye dropper should be held so that its long axis is parallel to the lid margin; if the patient suddenly moves forward, he or she is struck by the side of the eye dropper rather than the end, thereby avoiding damage to the eye [16] (see Fig. 27-1). The drops should never be allowed to fall on the sensitive cornea; that would be startling and disagreeable. The dropper should never touch the lashes, lids, or eyeball, lest this result in injury. When the lids are closed, the drops are distributed over the surface. Hold a cotton pledget over the inner angle of the eye so that the drug will not be lost down the lacrimal duct. Wipe from the lids and cheek any overflow of the drug or secretion.

The same dropper should not be used for two patients or for different solutions (see Fig. 27-2).

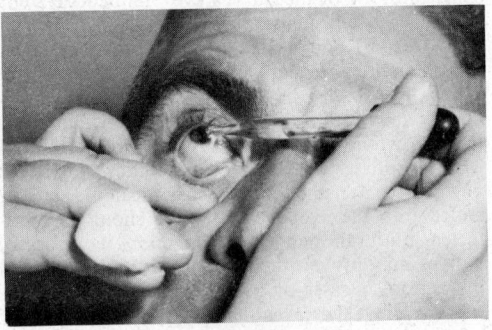

Figure 27-1. Instillation of eye drops. (Courtesy of Clay-Adams Co., New York, N.Y.)

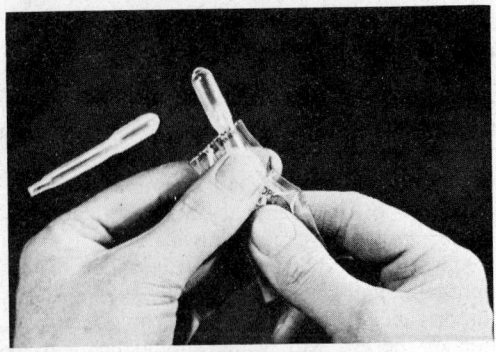

Figure 27-2. This flexible clinic dropper delivers 20 drops of solution. The plastic contains ASC-4 diaphene to prevent penetration by and growth of bacteria. (Courtesy of Medicon, Inc., Holbrook, Mass.)

Ideally, a bottle of drops should be discarded after use for one patient. (Because most medications are now available in 1- or 2-ml vials, it is not necessary to use a common bottle for all patients.) [17] All drugs to be instilled in the eyes should be inspected for changes in the color or for the formation of a sediment.

3. EVERSION OF THE EYELIDS

Skill in eversion of the eyelids is necessary in examinations, irrigations of the conjunctival sac, the removal of foreign bodies, and in the application of remedies to the conjunctiva and eyeball. Eversion of the lower lid is quite a simple matter; eversion of the upper eyelid is more difficult and requires considerable practice. In all cases precautions should be taken to avoid injury to the lids or eyeball, particularly in diseases of the eyes when the lids are likely to be tender, swollen, very sensitive, and easily injured. Chapter 5 describes methods for examining the eyes.

Suggested Procedure. *Eversion of the lower lid.* With the patient in a comfortable position and head supported, place a finger or thumb on the lower lid below the lashes and while pressing downward ask the patient to look upward. The edge of the lid will roll outward with the conjunctival sac exposed.

Eversion of the upper lid. Have the patient look downward with both eyes open. Grasp the eyelashes between the finger and thumb of one hand while, with the other, make counter pressure with the tip of an applicator, pencil, or glass rod on the skin of the lid just above the tarsal plate. Draw the lower part of the lid away from the globe, move the two hands in opposite directions which will rotate the tarsal plate above its long axis and expose the conjunctival surface of the lid (see Fig. 27-3). Tell the patient to continue looking downward. The lid can be main-

Figure 27-3. Eversion of upper lid in search for foreign body. *A.* Placing an object over which cartilage in lid can be turned. *B.* Everted upper lid. See Figure 27-4, which shows removal of a foreign body with a sterile moistened applicator. (Courtesy of Clay-Adams Co., New York, N.Y.)

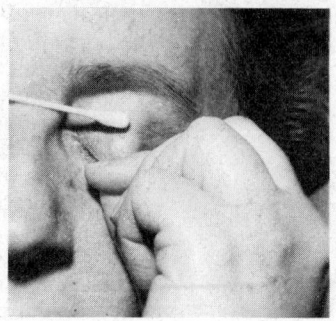
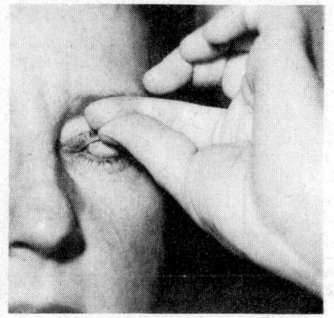

A   B

tained in this position by the pressure of a finger at its lower border.[18,19] If the patient should look upward after the lid has been everted it will return to its normal position because of the continuity of the conjunctiva over both lids and the front of the eyeball.

4. EYE MEDICATIONS

Application of Ointments. Antiseptic, irritant, or caustic ointments are frequently applied to the eyes in inflammatory diseases of the eyelids, conjunctiva, or cornea.

In *applying* the ointment, the eyelids should first be cleaned of all secretions or discharges and scales or crusts removed. A solution of borax (about half a teaspoonful in a cupful of hot water) will soften the crusts and aid in cleaning. The ointment may then be applied to the margin of the lids with a glass rod or spatula or cotton applicator. If intended for the conjunctiva or cornea, the ointment may be applied to the everted lower lid; in this way it is introduced into the conjunctival sac. Gentle massage of the lids will help to spread the ointment over the surface of the eyeball.[20] Ointments are available in tubes and, for individual use, applied directly. The ointment is dropped into the conjunctival sac from the tip of the tube, which is kept covered with a screw cap when not in use.

Application of Solutions. Antiseptic, astringent, caustic, and disinfectant solutions are painted or brushed on the everted lids in inflammatory diseases of the conjunctiva or applied directly to infected corneal ulcers. This is usually done by the physician.

5. REMOVAL OF FOREIGN BODIES FROM THE EYE

According to Harold A. Stein,[21] about 5 per cent of all injuries treated in an emergency department of a general hospital are those that involve the eye. Over half of these are foreign bodies lodged under the eyelid or on the surface of the eye. Eye injuries are common also in industries in spite of the excellent prevention programs of these agencies. When the patient is first seen, the nature and time of the injury should be determined as this will help the operator in determining the treatment.

Foreign bodies, such as glass, wood, vegetable matter, metal, dust, coal, or ashes may be carried into the conjunctival sac or may adhere to or become embedded in the cornea. Sharp particles may penetrate the chambers of the eye. When in the conjunctival sac, they often adhere to the inner surface of the upper lid. Patients can often tell the examiner where the particle is by indicating the spot where they feel greatest discomfort.

Focus a good light on the eye and ask the person to keep both eyes open while moving them from side to side and then up. If the particle is floating, it will often be found in the sac of the lower lid. The foreign body can then be removed with a moistened sterile cotton applicator. Stein believes that the home remedy of pulling the lid down and rolling the eye about to dislodge the particle can be dangerous if the particle is glass or a burr embedded under the eyelid. If the particle is not found, evert the upper lid as shown in Figure 27-3 on this page. In this maneuver the patient is asked to look down, the lashes are grasped, and the lid is everted over a match or pencil, held horizontally against the eyelid. The mucous lining of the cartilaginous lid is examined, and the moistened applicator drawn over its surface (Fig. 27-4). If these operations are ineffective, a sterile irrigation of the conjunctival sac may dislodge the mote. When all of these efforts are unsuccessful it is wise to fix a pad over the lid to keep it closed and inactive until a doctor can treat the condition. If the eye is very irritated an antibiotic may be instilled to retard infection. Strict asepsis should be maintained.

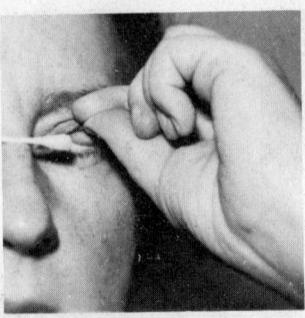

Figure 27-4. Subject about to remove a foreign body on everted upper lid with a sterile moistened applicator. See Figure 27-3 for steps in eversion of upper lid, prior to removal of a foreign body. (Courtesy of Clay-Adams Co., New York, N.Y.)

When a corneal injury or an intraocular foreign body is suspected, the eye should be put at rest with a pad strapped over it until a doctor can treat it. Corneal abrasions will show up as bright green patches after placing a strip of fluorescein-impregnated paper in the lower lid.

The removal of intraocular foreign bodies requires the skill of an ophthalmologist as well as special equipment. Stein says these include "exact localization by special x-ray techniques, foreign body locators, ultrasound, and removal by giant electromagnets or fine vitreous forceps." *

If an eye has been injured by chemicals, such as a burn, Frank J. Weinstock [22] says it should be washed out at once with tap water from a faucet for 15 minutes. Water is always available and the important thing is to remove the chemical as soon as possible. Then a standard intravenous bottle of isotonic saline or Ringer's solution (1000 ml) attached to intravenous tubing should be used for continuous irrigation for the same period (as soon as this treatment can be set up).

6. EAR IRRIGATIONS

Definition. An ear irrigation is the washing out of the external auditory canal with a stream of liquid.

Therapeutic Uses. Ear irrigations are used to combat infections of the external auditory canal or the middle ear by cleaning, antiseptic, or temperature effect, and for the removal of wax (cerumen) or some types of foreign bodies from the auditory canal.

---

* Stein, Harold A.: "Foreign Body Injuries to the Eye," *Appl. Ther.*, **11**:591, (Nov.) 1969.

Selection of Method. The difference in the structure of the auditory canal in the infant and the adult must be borne in mind when irrigating the ear.

In an *infant* the auditory canal is mostly cartilaginous and is nearly straight, but because the drum membrane at the end of the canal (separating it from the middle ear) is in an oblique position, the floor of the canal is in contact with it. When irrigating, it is necessary to draw these two surfaces apart so that the fluid can reach and clean all parts of the canal; in order to do this, the auricle of an infant is drawn gently downward and backward.

In an *adult* the canal is about 2 to 2.5 cm (¾ to 1 inch) in length; only its outer third remains cartilaginous, the inner two thirds of its walls being composed of bone. It takes a spiral course inward, forward, and upward. Lifting the ear (or pinna) upward and backward and the tragus (cartilaginous projection in front of the external meatus of the ear) forward will straighten the canal for examination, according to David D. DeWeese and William H. Saunders.[23] See Chapter 5 for methods of examining the ear. In irrigating an adult's ear the pinna is lifted upward and backward.

Other anatomic factors to keep in mind are the position and function of the tympanic membrane, the nerve supply, and the surrounding structures. The latter suggests the serious complications that may result from injury or spread of infection into the mastoid cavity or the Eustachian tube.

Irrigations were most often used in the past to remove an accumulation of discharge from the external auditory canal when there had been a rupture or a puncture of the drum, and drainage from the infected middle ear into the canal. This procedure is now rare. Lawrence R. Boies and associates [24] (1964) do not, for example, mention the use of irrigation following a myringotomy. They advocate the continued use of sulfonamide or antibiotic therapy, dry wiping of the canal with sterile cotton (the patient is taught this procedure), and lying on the affected ear to promote drainage by posture. They believe that medication (instillations of drug) is probably useless. John Ballantyne and John Groves,[25] however, do mention irrigation but say if syringing the ear is necessary, the canal must be dried afterward or a pool of water is left in the deep meatus, rendering the skin soggy and perpetuating infection. Like many other authorities they comment on the reduced incidence of otitis media since the development of sulfonamides and antibiotics. Miriam H.

Rutherford,[26] admitting the value of drug therapy for the control of the respiratory (usually streptococcal) infections, says that they may have lulled the physician into a false sense of security. Establishment of drainage is urged when the infection threatens the ear structures with resulting deafness. T. Palva and associates [26a] discuss the function of the

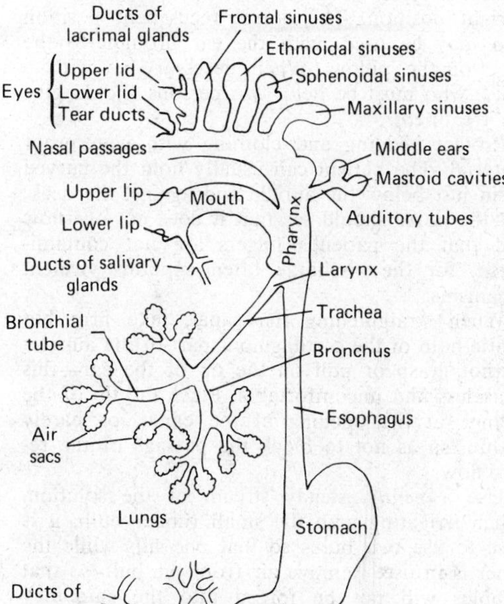

Figure 27-5. Diagram showing the continuity of the gastropulmonary mucous membrane. Note the possibilities of extending infection by improper methods of irrigating the ear, nose, and throat. (From Miller, Marjorie A., Drakontides, Anna B., and Leavell, Lutie C.: *Kimber-Gray-Stackpole's Anatomy and Physiology,* 17th ed. Macmillan Publishing Co., Inc., New York, 1977.)

middle ear mucosa in secretory otitis media.

After the drum ruptures or is incised, the infection is usually a mixed one. Since the growth of an organism may be stimulated and its virulence increased by the presence of another strain, it is important to use only sterile equipment when irrigating an ear with a punctured or incised drum. The initial infection spreads from the mouth and nose by way of the eustachian tube when the drum is intact. Figure 27-5 shows the avenues by which infection can travel from one mucous-lined cavity to the other in the head and, in fact, throughout the respiratory and intestinal tracts.

There seems to be general agreement among otologists that, if used, ear irrigations should be given with minimal *force,* unless the drum is intact. The danger of driving infectious material into the mastoid cells by forceful irrigation as well as the effectiveness of currently prescribed antibiotics has led some physicians to discontinue the use of this treatment altogether. Others advocate the irrigation and suction of the external auditory canal with an eye dropper, because they believe that it is not possible to use enough force with this device to make the solution enter the middle ear from the external auditory canal.

When a reservoir is used, the level of the solution should not be more than 15 cm (6 inches) above the level of the ear. Irrigations to remove plugs of cerumen (wax) are given with a fair amount of force, but in this case the drum is intact and there is no question of driving material from the auditory canal into the middle ear. A metal syringe is commonly used in this type of irrigation, and force is exerted by manual pressure on the piston. Physicians often remove wax with a cerumen spoon.

Irrigations are usually prescribed at 3- to 4-hour periods during the day; sometimes less frequently.

Solutions used for ear irrigations are, on the whole, similar to those prescribed for irrigations of the eye. The point is made repeatedly that the kind of solution is immaterial: the benefit to be derived from an irrigation is that, by washing the discharge from the external canal, drainage of the ear is encouraged. If irrigations are used for the removal of cerumen, a 1 per cent solution of sodium bicarbonate softens and breaks up the wax plug.* (This treatment is discussed later in this chapter.)

For the comfort of the patient the *temperature of the irrigating solution* should be near

---

* Wax in the auditory canal is a protection of the drum and the very sensitive lining of the canal. Many persons learn to prevent impaction of the canal.

that of the body. Temperatures below or above set the endolymph in motion, and this can cause vertigo (dizziness) and nausea.[27] Erik Peitersen [28] describes a 35-year-old man who periodically irrigated his ears with water, claimed to be at body temperature but not measured by a thermometer; he developed severe vertigo, nausea, vomiting, and tinnitus but these symptoms subsided in less than a week after the treatment was discontinued. In order to allow for cooling as it flows from the irrigating can or the syringe, the solution should be prepared at about 40.6°C (105°F). Cold solutions are rarely used except for diagnostic ("caloric") tests.

The *amount of solution* varies with the purpose of the treatment. In some cases the irrigation is stopped as soon as the return flow is clear, indicating that the canal has been thoroughly cleaned. Varying amounts of solution are therefore needed. If the effect of heat is desired, as much as 1000 ml (1 qt) should be used if the patient can tolerate it. An irrigating can is a satisfactory device to use for the administration of the solution because, if a syringe is used, the patient is annoyed by the repeated starting and stopping of the flow. A plastic container of a commercially prepared sterile solution is recommended.

After the irrigation is completed, the canal should be dried with sterile cotton applicators, and the patient should lie on the affected side, allowing the ear to drain on a cellucotton pad. A gauze wick, sometimes impregnated with a drug, may be inserted in the canal, but the meatus should not be plugged with cotton as this tends to hold discharges in the middle ear.

Equipment. The following articles are required: a treatment tray with the prescribed solution, an irrigator, a towel to cover the patient's shoulder, several sterile applicators, a paper bag, a curved basin for the return, a larger waste container into which the contents of the emesis basin may be emptied, and petroleum jelly if the skin is excoriated by the discharge. A good light is essential. The irrigator may be a glass or plastic bottle, a soft rubber bulb syringe, a glass syringe, or an irrigating can with tubing and glass tip; the syringe or reservoir and tubing and the glass tip should be sterile. After the treatment they should be cleaned and decontaminated.

Solutions used are similar to those listed for eye irrigations although the ear can probably tolerate a more irritating drug (see p. 1322).

The *temperature* of the solution should be such as to give a sensation of comfort; it may vary in the reservoir from 40.6° to 43.3°C (105° to 110°F). A solution that feels either cool or uncomfortably hot to the patient should never be used; it may cause mild dis-

comfort or a severe earache that lasts for hours. If the patient has a high temperature, remember that the solution of a given temperature is likely to feel cooler than when the body temperature is normal.

Suggested Procedure. Carefully explain the treatment to the patients before starting, relieve their apprehension if possible, and elicit their cooperation. If their condition permits, seat them comfortably in a chair or support them in an upright position. The dorsal recumbent position also may be used, with the ear brought to the edge of the pillow. When necessary as with a child, who must be held, two persons should give the treatment.

Protect bedding and clothing with waterproof material. The patient can usually hold the curved basin just below the auricle and against the neck, but the nurse should see that it does not overflow and that the patient's fingers are not contaminated, for the discharge often contains virulent organisms.

When straightening the canal, take firm but gentle hold of the cartilaginous part of the auricle; do not grasp or pull on the tip of the ear—this is useless and uncomfortable. Place the tip of the syringe at the opening of the canal, or barely within, so as not to block the passage of the return flow.

Use a *gentle,* steady stream of the solution. When irrigating with the small rubber bulb, it is wise to use two bulbs so that one fills while the other is in use. Remove air from the bulb so that bubbles will not be forced into the ear; they produce loud sounds and cause great discomfort. If the irrigation causes pain, dizziness, faintness, or nausea, stop it and consult the doctor.

As soon as the canal is thoroughly cleaned, dry the external area with clean cotton. Apply petroleum jelly if the skin is excoriated. The tips of applicators must be well and tightly covered with cotton. If the cotton is loose it can slip off in the ear and be difficult to remove.

Recording the Treatment. Record the amount and character of the discharge and any nausea, dizziness, or any other discomfort.

Removal of Cerumen (Ear Wax) and Epithelial Plugs. Ear wax and epithelial scales may collect in the auditory canal, obstruct the passage, and harden against the drum membrane. This condition is fostered by swimming under water and pushing a cloth into the meatus when washing and drying the ear; the wax, instead of being thrown off in the normal way, is forced inward. Impacted ears are more common in the aged because the external meatus usually flattens in later life. The symptoms of an impaction are deafness, dizziness, a sense of fullness, sometimes pain, and a reflex cough from irritation of a nerve that supplies the lungs.

The treatment of this condition is to soften the mass and remove it by syringing. Before syringing, it is desirable and sometimes necessary to instill a few drops of warm hydrogen peroxide or a vegetable oil which may soften the wax in 10 minutes, or it may be necessary to repeat the instillation at intervals. Lying on the unaffected ear encourages absorption of the "cerumen drops."

Wax is sometimes removed with a cerumen spoon; however, this method should be used only by a physician.

A 1 per cent soap, sodium bicarbonate, or normal saline solution is most often used for the irrigation. The large metal Pomeroy or Neumann ear syringe is most satisfactory, but a rubber or rubber-and-glass instrument may be substituted. Considerable practice is necessary before these metal syringes can be manipulated with safety or skill; they are heavy, difficult to handle without injury to the ear and to operate so as to get a steady stream with little force. It is a wise precaution to cover the syringe tip with a piece of rubber tubing since there would be less danger of injury if it accidentally hits the ear. In some clinics and hospitals where it is impossible for all nurses to have sufficient practice in the use of these metal syringes, nurses do not use them to give irrigations. After use they are easily cleaned and sterilized, as they can be taken apart. George Larsen [28a] says cerumen can be removed with ease by using a Water Pik at low pressure. This equipment is available at most drug stores.

Equipment used in the irrigation of an ear with an intact drum membrane should be clean (sterilized after it is used) but need not be sterile.

A good light is essential. The stream of solution must be directed between the wax and the canal at different points so as to separate it and force it outward. Care must be taken to *avoid* directing the stream of solution onto a mass of wax as this will only impact it more deeply in the canal. The canal should be inspected from time to time so that syringing will not be continued after the wax is removed.[29]

After the irrigation, the canal is dried. The physician may inject air into the middle ear through the eustachian tubes if the drum is retracted. He or she usually fills the external auditory canal very loosely with absorbent cotton and tells the patient to remove it in 12 to 24 hours.

7. REMOVAL OF FOREIGN BODIES FROM THE EAR

Foreign bodies found in the ear vary in size, shape, and substance, in their position in the canal, in their effect, and therefore in the symptoms to which they give rise. For instance, they may be small, hard, and smooth (like beads, stones, or buttons), easily inserted by a child, and pushed into the canal; they may, like peas and seeds, swell with moisture and block the meatus. They may be present for years, give rise to no symptoms, and be forgotten by the individual; or they may injure, inflame, and infect the canal and may cause deafness, dizziness, tinnitus, a reflex cough, and vomiting.[30] Live insects especially produce acute pain and anxiety.

Foreign bodies rarely cause serious trouble unless they injure the tympanic membrane, while rupture of the tympanic membrane, removal of ossicles, purulent infection of the middle ear, inner ear, and meninges have resulted from *ill-directed attempts at removal.* Death has followed clumsy and misguided first aid when no foreign body was present.

Before attempting removal of foreign bodies, therefore, the physician will first note the symptoms and history, and will inspect the ear to determine the presence, nature, and position of a foreign body, and the condition of the canal. The nurse often prepares the equipment for this examination and may give some of the treatments that follow.

Removal by irrigation, or persistent syringing with warm water, is a method commonly used. This is the best and safest method, and is the only one that should be attempted by a nurse, or by anyone who is not an expert. Even syringing may do harm, and may be contraindicated if, for instance, there is danger of forcing the object in farther. Sometimes a preliminary treatment must be given: it may be necessary to relieve inflammation and swelling of the tissues before syringing, by applying an alcoholic solution of boric acid; or, when water will cause the object to swell (as in the case of a pea or seed), it is advisable first to syringe the canal with alcohol, which will absorb the water, prevent swelling, and may possibly shrink the foreign body. The instillation of oil or glycerin also helps to remove seeds. If the foreign body is an insect, it should first be killed by the introduction of a few drops of absolute alcohol, oil, or chloroform.* When dead, it usually floats out. Syringing with water will make a living insect move, which causes great discomfort, even agony, to the patient.

When syringing the ear, incline the patient's head toward the affected side, as the force of gravity is to some extent helpful. (In the case

---

* The second author was told by a person who lives in a region where medical services are unavailable that holding a light to the ear was a common practice when an insect was believed to have crawled or flown into the ear because most insects will be attracted by the light and come out of the meatus.

of children, because the aural canal is straight, rotation in front of the ear with the finger sometimes makes a round, smooth body work its way outward.) The auricle should be held in the proper position for irrigating and the stream directed between the foreign body and the wall of the canal where the space is widest. Syringing should be continued gently until the body is removed, unless it gives rise to pain, vomiting, or other unfavorable symptoms; then it should be discontinued until further examination is made. The ear should be carefully dried and absorbent cotton left in the meatus following the treatment. Any abrasion caused by the foreign body should be treated, and precaution taken to prevent infection.

Removal by instruments is sometimes necessary, but this should be done only by a skilled otologist unless the object can be easily grasped. As a rule, instruments are used only when syringing has failed or is contraindicated by the severity of the symptoms. In the hands of an unskilled person, an instrument may push the foreign body farther into the canal, injure the tympanic membrane or the bony wall of the canal, cause severe irritation, swelling, and inflammation, and even necessitate a major operation (incision behind the ear into the canal).

8. NASAL IRRIGATIONS

Definition. A nasal irrigation is the washing out of the nasal cavity by a stream of liquid.

Therapeutic Uses. In some medical texts nasal irrigations are advocated to apply heat, to clean the nose, and to combat the disagreeable odor connected with chronic rhinitis in which there is a purulent discharge or the formation of crusts.

According to DeWeese and Saunders,[31] irrigation of the nasal passages daily with isotonic saline solution is as effective as any known medical treatment in providing symptomatic relief in atrophic rhinitis. Because there is danger of forcing infectious material into the sinuses communicating with the nose, the treatment, however, is used only when the condition fails to respond to less hazardous methods. In the experience of the writers this treatment is now rarely used. On the other hand, the partial or complete closure of the air passages of the nose by encrusted material is very uncomfortable and forces the victim to breathe through the mouth. Patients who cannot use their hands, or who are too weak to use a handkerchief, need special help; some way of softening and removing the material must be devised in each case.

Selection of Method. Because of the dangers involved, nasal irrigation must be given with great care, preferably by a physician. If administered by a nurse at the request of the physician, he or she should specify the kind of solution, its amount, temperature, and force, and the position of the patient.

The *solution* may be any one of the mild antiseptics used on the mucous membrane; physiologic saline solution is commonly advocated. Most medical authorities say the irrigating fluid should be comfortably warm; a temperature of 37.7°C (100°F) is probably best tolerated by the nasal mucosa. It is important to remember that solutions tolerated by the mucosa of the mouth and pharynx are painfully hot if applied to the nose.

The greater the *pressure* or *force* of the solution, the greater the possibility of driving material from the nose into the sinuses. E. G. Collins[32] recommends the reservoir be about 1 ft (12 inches) above the patient's head; others fail to mention this aspect of the procedure. It is generally agreed, however, that the reservoir should be so adjusted that the stream from the nozzle is a gentle steady flow when the tip of the nozzle is held at the level of the patient's head. Fluid flows from the tip into one nostril, around the posterior border of the septum and out of the other. If less force is used and if the tip does not fill the nostril, the fluid is not likely to flow through the other nostril.

The prescribed *amount* of solution varies according to the condition under treatment but usually ranges from 500 to 1000 ml (1 pt to 1 qt), because less than this does not loosen crusts or give the desired temperature effect.

Any *position* assumed by the patient must favor the return flow of the solution from the open nostril; therefore, the head must be held forward. The patient must be told to breathe through the mouth and not to speak or swallow. Changes in pressure within the nasal or aural cavity may draw material into the Eustachian tubes and sinuses. Since patients may feel impelled to speak, cough, or swallow, it is desirable to teach them how to hold the tip in the nose, how to remove it, and control the flow.

Equipment. Articles used vary with the method. The irrigation may be given with a Douglas syringe or with an irrigating bottle, rubber tubing, nasal irrigating tip, and a basin for the return. Paper handkerchiefs, a waterproof bib and a cotton cover to protect the clothing, and a receptacle for waste should be provided. The equipment need not be sterile but must be clean (sterilized after it is used and handled with clean hands).

Preparation of the Patient. Before starting the treatment it must be carefully explained to patients, and they must understand what they should do during the irrigation. Any lack of cooperation on their part increases its danger.

Suggested Procedure. Have the patient sitting in a chair or in bed and bending over a sink or basin with the head well flexed on the chest. Maintain a copious, gentle, and uniform stream of solution up one nostril, back into the nasopharynx, and around the septum, allowing it to run out the opposite nostril. Direct the patient to keep the head forward, to breathe through the mouth, and not to speak or swallow. Conversation by the nurse or doctor with the patient or with others is unwise, as the patient is tempted to say something while the irrigation is flowing.

Insert the irrigating tip or nozzle in the nostril just tightly enough to prevent the return of fluid from that nostril, unless the aim is to irrigate only this side. Support the irrigator so that the surface of the liquid in the reservoir is not more than 20 cm (8 inches) above the level of the nose, unless the physician indicates otherwise. If the patient coughs or chokes, check the flow, as coughing usually indicates that the solution, owing to some obstruction, is not returning properly. In case one nostril is more obstructed than the other, some authorities say that the stream should be directed first up the unaffected side; this washes out the discharge from the obstructed side without so much danger of forcing material into the unaffected side or into the Eustachian tubes. Other authorities advise injecting the fluid only into the narrow, obstructed side; in this method the unobstructed nostril allows free passage for the exudate. Nurses should ask physicians which method they prefer.

Patients should be warned not to blow excess fluid from the nose for several minutes after the procedure, as this may force discharges into adjoining cavities. They are also advised to stay in a warm temperature for an hour or more, since the blood vessels of the nose are dilated and more subject to chilling.

Recording the Treatment. Chart the treatment, the nature, temperature and amount of solution used, the character of the return, and any symptoms of middle-ear disturbance, such as dizziness or a feeling of fullness in the ears.

9. NASAL INSTILLATIONS

Definition. The introduction of a liquid into the nose, drop by drop, constitutes a nasal instillation.

Therapeutic Uses. Nasal instillations are used to coat the nasal mucosa with an antiseptic drug, a soothing substance, an astringent, or a local anesthetic. Roger H. Lehman and Richard I. H. Wang [33] say nasal medications should have the following characteristics of normal nasal secretions: they should be isotonic, slightly acid, and nonirritating. Although oily solutions act as lubricants and decongestants, they also impede ciliary action, which is undesirable. They may sometimes be prescribed, however, to soften and dislodge encrusted secretions.

Selection of Method and Suggested Procedure. Administer the drug from an eye dropper. The patient's head should be tilted backward—otherwise the liquid will run out of the anterior nares as soon as it is injected. If the patient is in bed, it is desirable to have him or her in the supine position with the head over the side of the bed or with the pillows removed and the head tilted backward, sometimes called the Proetz position. Insert the dropper in the nose not more than 1 to 1½ cm (about ½ to ⅔ inch). Some of the solution will run into the mouth, and since drugs used often have a disagreeable taste, provide a sputum basin, paper handkerchiefs, and a bag for waste.

If drops are put into the nose of an infant, a young child, or an irrational person who is struggling against the treatment, protect the tip with a short length of rubber tubing. Particles of mineral oil or any drug not absorbed by the tissues, passing from the nose through the larynx and trachea into the lung, may cause an abscess or pneumonitis. Health departments have warned the public against the use of such drugs. Nasal instillations should be avoided unless prescribed by the physician.

10. SPRAYING THE NOSE AND THROAT

Therapeutic Uses. Sprays are used in acute or chronic inflammation as a means of covering the mucosa with a film of antiseptic, astringent, soothing, or anesthetic drug. Estrogenic sprays are used in some diseases of the nose, according to Boies and associates.

Selection of Method. Drugs may be applied to the mucous lining of the nose or throat with a hand atomizer; the solution is forced out through the perforated tip by air pressure produced by squeezing the attached rubber bulb. The instrument should give a generous stream of droplets; a very forceful spray is injurious. There should be separate tips for watery and oily sprays, because a larger opening is necessary for heavy liquids.

Prescribed solutions vary according to the condition and results desired; if warmed to a temperature of 37.8°C (100°F) they are likely to be more comfortable. When the treatment is painful, it should be reported to the physician who may order a weaker or a different solution.

Suggested Procedure. If possible let the patient use the atomizer, but be sure that he or she carries out the treatment effectively. The end of the nose should be raised and the tip of the atomizer placed just within the nostril. Less force should be used in spraying the nose than in applying a drug to the throat. To carry the drug to the larynx, the tip should be turned downward.

11. REMOVAL OF FOREIGN BODIES FROM THE NOSE

Flying insects and objects of various kinds are often drawn into the nose during inspiration. Children frequently push peanuts, safety pins, and other small objects into the nose. Should foreign bodies lodge in the anterior nares, they may often be blown out before harm results. If they are visible, they may be removed with forceps, but great care must be taken not to force them in farther. When simple measures fail or when the object has dropped into the posterior nares, the patient should be taken to a physician who will light the cavity, discover the position of the foreign body, and remove it with special instruments. D. Dayal and A. P. Singh [34] report three rare cases of foreign bodies in the nasopharynx, one reaching this area by fracturing the ethmoids and frontal sinus and the other two through the nose.

12. THROAT IRRIGATIONS

Definition. A throat irrigation is the washing out of the oral pharynx by a stream of liquid.

Therapeutic Uses. The purposes of the irrigation are to soften the mucus and to remove accumulated secretions; to stimulate the circulation and promote absorption of inflammatory products; to relieve congestion, swelling, and pain; and to stimulate and bring to a head the inflammatory process of suppuration, so that the abscess may be incised and drained. A throat irrigation is ordered in place of a gargle if gargling is painful or if a more continuous and prolonged effect is desired. Most authorities say a gargle is of doubtful value if it does not reach beyond the tonsillar region. However, it is not easy to persuade patients to allow solutions to pass beyond this point during an irrigation.

Selection of Method. The *solution* used for a throat irrigation may be any one of those ordered as gargles and they are numerous indeed. In some cases drugs that act as a mild local anesthetic may be in the irrigating solution. The benefits are probably heat effect and mechanical cleaning; therefore, it is doubtful

whether one solution is much better than another. Since the treatment is unpleasant if a solution has a disagreeable taste, plain hot water or physiologic saline solution would seem to be the choice for cleaning and temperature effect. Nurses would be safe in using either of these if the physician failed to specify the solution and they were unable to talk with him or her.

Solutions of a *temperature* not tolerated by other parts of the body feel comfortable in the mouth. A throat irrigation is often ordered as hot as patients can stand it; however, temperatures above 49°C (120.2°F) might cause tissue damage.

If the irrigation is ordered for a temperature effect, the duration of the treatment is of some importance, and it is necessary to use from 1000 to 1500 ml (1 to 1½ qt). The *amount* of the solution may or may not be specified by the physician. In any event the treatment should not tire patients unduly, and if ill persons show signs of exhaustion before the entire amount has been used, the treatment should be stopped.

To get the desired results from a throat irrigation, a continuous stream of solution must reach the affected parts without making patients gag. If this occurs, they will probably swallow or aspirate some of the irrigating fluid. The *position* of the head must allow the solution to flow freely in and out of the mouth; the head must tilt forward so that the solution can flow over the lower lip or tilt to one side in such a way that the solution can flow from the corner of the mouth. If patients direct the stream of liquid themselves, they feel less nervous about the treatment. The purpose of the irrigation and the method of giving it should be carefully explained to patients. They are told to hold the breath while the solution is flowing, to prevent aspiration of the fluid, but they should realize that the irrigation can be stopped at any time so that they can rest or breathe. This treatment is comforting, and after patients are once taught to take a throat irrigation, the average person will cooperate fully.

If the patient is able to sit up, the return flow is received in a large basin, placed on a table under the chin. The irrigation can be even more comfortably given with the patient lying down, the head turned so that the cheek is on the edge of the pillow. In order to clean the entire throat, the patient shifts position in the middle of the procedure and lies on the other side. If the irrigation is given in this position, the return flow is received in a curved or rectangular basin placed under the cheek and mouth. The bedding must be protected with a waterproof cover.

Equipment. Articles required are an irrigating pole, irrigating can, tubing with clamp, an irrigating tip, the solution, a large pail for the return, a waste basin in which to collect the solution as it runs from the mouth, protection for the chest and shoulder of the patient, paper handkerchiefs, and a paper bag for used handkerchiefs. Equipment must be clean but need not be sterile.

Suggested Procedure. Explain the procedure to the patients. Have them in a sitting or recumbent posture, according to their condition and preference. Protect the clothing or bedding with suitable materials, such as rubber sheeting, oiled silk, or cellulose film; cover the part that goes around the patient's neck with a towel or piece of soft crepe paper. Give the patient a paper handkerchief. Place in position the basin for the collection of waste. Support the irrigating can so that the level of the solution is approximately 30 cm (12 inches) above the level of the mouth. If the treatment is new to patients allow the solution to flow for a very short time, remove the tip from the mouth and discuss any difficulties they may have had. As they acquire more confidence, they can direct the flow of solution, hold their breath for longer periods, and make the solution reach farther into the pharynx. At frequent intervals empty the waste basin into the pail to prevent spilling. If it is necessary for the nurse to look at the pharyngeal mucosa, the usual care must be taken in depressing the tongue, so as to prevent gagging and injury.

Recording the Treatment. Record the treatment, the time it was given, the kind, amount, and temperature of the solution, and the patient's reaction to it.

13. GARGLES

Gargles are used in the same conditions of the throat as those in which sprays or irrigations are used. The same solutions are used to serve the same purposes. The patient must be cautioned against swallowing the solution, although antiseptic gargles are rarely toxic if swallowed in small quantities. The editors [35] of *Consumer Reports* say that well-known gargles have little, if any, therapeutic advantage over physiologic saline solution. Gargling is likely to be fatiguing and is often painful. Its value is questioned by many doctors, who feel that the rigid control of the throat and breathing are so difficult for the already sensitive, painful, and swollen throat that the effort may be quite inadequate to bring the solution into contact with all parts of the inflamed mucous lining. For this reason, many physicians prefer sprays that may be applied directly to the diseased part, or irrigations if a temperature effect is desired.

14. REMOVAL OF FOREIGN BODIES FROM THE THROAT

The experience of having food drawn into the respiratory tract instead of being directed into the esophagus is common to everyone. The presence of a foreign body in the larynx stimulates the cough reflex, which is nature's method of getting rid of the offending object. In most cases the foreign body will be coughed up into the mouth. Lowering the head brings gravity into play and helps throw the object out of the larynx. Many a mother has saved the life of a strangling child by picking it up by its feet and shaking a bead, a marble, or a crust of bread out of the respiratory passage.

If the foreign body passes the larynx, it will lodge in the trachea or bronchi, and in case it does not occlude the air passage, it may stay in this position without causing any serious damage for a few hours or possibly a day or two; however, if it is not removed by a surgeon within a short time, infection results. In most large communities there are surgeons who specialize in removing foreign bodies from the bronchi (bronchoscopists). With highly developed skill and instruments designed for this purpose, it is now possible to extract open safety pins, fishbones, and other objects equally difficult to manipulate, from almost any part of the bronchi.[36]

REFERENCES

1. Duke-Elder, Sir Stewart: *Parson's Diseases of the Eye,* 15th ed. Little, Brown & Co., Boston, 1970, p. 149.
2. Burns, Robert P., and Rhodes, David H.: "Pseudomonas Eye Infections as a Cause of Death in Premature Infants," *Arch. Opthalmol.,* **65:**517, (Apr.) 1961.
3. Symposium, New Orleans Academy of Ophthalmology: *Infectious Diseases of the Conjunctiva and Cornea.* C. V. Mosby Co., St. Louis, 1963.
4. Humphrey, William T.: "Flaxseeds in Ophthalmic Folk Medicine," *Am. J. Ophthalmol.,* **70:**287, (Aug.) 1970.
5. Burns, Robert P.: "Characteristics of Ocular Infectious Agents that Are of Importance in the Understanding of Eye Infections," in Symposium, New Orleans Academy of Ophthalmology: *Infectious Diseases of the Conjunctiva and Cornea.* C. V. Mosby Co., St. Louis, 1963, p. 27.
6. Fraunfelder, Frederick T., and Roy, F. Hampton: "How to Treat Common External Eye Problems," *Am. Fam. Physician,* **3:**104, (Apr.) 1971.
7. Ridley, Frederick: "The Use of Antiseptics in Ophthalmology," *Proc. R. Soc. Med.,* **25:**480, (Feb.) 1932.

8. Duke-Elder, Sir Stewart: *op. cit.*, p. 154.

9. Hosford, George V., and Hicks, Avery M.: "Hydrogen Ion Concentration of Tears," *Arch. Ophthalmol.*, **13**:14, (Jan.) 1935.

9a. Blake, J.: "Eye Hazards in Rural Communities," *Practitioner*, **214**:641, (May) 1975.

9b. Moore, W. E., et al.: "Spectacle Lens Associated Eye Injuries in Louisville—1960–1974," *J. Ky. Med. Assoc.*, **73**:416, (Aug.) 1975.

9c. Havener, W. H., et al.: "Emergency Management of Ocular Injuries," *Ohio State Med. J.*, **71**:776, (Nov.) 1975.

9d. Pashby, T. J., et al.: "Eye Injuries in Canadian Hockey," *Can. Med. Assoc. J.*, **113**:663, (Oct. 4) 1975.

10. Weinstock, Frank J.: "Emergency Treatment of Eye Injuries," *Am. J. Nurs.*, **71**: 1928, (Oct.) 1971.

11. Kuhn, Hedwig S.: "How to Treat Chemical Eye Injuries," *Am. Assoc. Ind. Nurses J.*, **14**:7, (Apr.) 1966.

12. Gordon, Dan M.: "Eye Emergencies," *AORN*, **11**:78, (Jan.) 1970.

13. Dunlap, Edward A. (ed.): *Gordon's Medical Management of Ocular Disease*, 2nd ed. Hoeber Medical Division, Harper & Row, Publishers, New York, 1976, p. 273.

14. Ellis, Philip P., and Smith, Don L.: *Handbook of Ocular Therapeutics and Pharmacology*, 4th ed. C. V. Mosby Co., St. Louis, 1973, p. 64.

15. Duke-Elder, Sir Stewart: *op. cit.*, p. 155.

16. Newell, Frank W., and Ernest, J. Terry: *Ophthalmology, Principles and Concepts,* 3rd ed. C. V. Mosby Co., St. Louis, 1974, p. 95.

17. Weinstock, Frank J.: *op cit.*

18. Jackson, C. R. S.: *The Eye in General Practice,* 6th ed. E. & S. Livingstone, Ltd., London, 1972, p. 25.

19. Keeney, Arthur H.: *Ocular Examination; Basis and Technique.* C. V. Mosby Co., St. Louis, 1970, p. 36.

20. Parkinson, Roy H.: *Eye, Ear, Nose and Throat Manual for Nurses.* C. V. Mosby Co., St. Louis, 1959, p. 126.

21. Stein, Harold A.: "Foreign Body Injuries to the Eye," *Appl. Ther.*, **11**:591, (Nov.) 1969.

22. Weinstock, Frank J.: *op. cit.*

23. DeWeese, David D., and Saunders, William H.: *Textbook of Otolaryngology,* 4th ed. C. V. Mosby Co., St. Louis, 1973, p. 6.

24. Boies, Lawrence R., et al.: *Fundamentals of Otolaryngology,* 4th ed. W. B. Saunders Co., Philadelphia, 1964, p. 105.

25. Ballantyne, John, and Groves, John (eds.): *Scott-Brown's Diseases of the Ear, Nose and Throat,* Vol. II, 3rd ed. J. B. Lippincott Co., Philadelphia, 1971, p. 107.

26. Rutherford, Miriam H.: "Proper Use of Antibiotics in Treatment of Acute Otitis Media," *Calif. Med.*, **75**:98, (Aug.) 1951.

26a. Palva, T., et al.: "The Role of the Middle Ear Mucosa in Secretory Otitis Media," *J. Laryngol. Otol.*, **89**:491, (May) 1975.

27. DeWeese, David D., and Saunders, William H.: *op. cit.,* p. 303.

28. Peitersen, Erik: "Sudden Loss of Vestibular Function After Irrigation of the Ear," *J. Laryngol. Otol.*, **78**:694, (July) 1964.

28a. Larsen, George: "Removing Cerumen with a Water Pik," *Am. J. Nurs.*, **76**:264, (Feb.) 1976.

29. Sale, Charles S.: "Removal of Ear Wax," *Va. Med. Mon.*, **95**:75, (Feb.) 1968.

30. Gatley, Malcolm S.: "A Foreign Body in the Ear Mimicking Secretory Otitis Media," *Practitioner,* **207**:817, (Dec.) 1971.

31. DeWeese, David D., and Saunders, William H.: *op. cit.,* p. 237.

32. Collins, E. G.: *A Guide to Diseases of the Nose, Throat and Ear for General Practitioners and Students.* Williams & Wilkins Co., Baltimore, 1964, p. 93.

33. Lehman, Roger H., and Wang, Richard I. H.: "Topical Medication in Otolaryngology," *Wis. Med. J.*, **68**:143, (Mar.) 1969.

34. Dayal, D., and Singh, A. P.: "Foreign Body Nasopharynx," *J. Laryngol. Otol.*, **84**:1157, (Nov.) 1970.

35. Editors of *Consumer Reports: The Medicine Show,* rev. ed. Consumers Union, Mount Vernon, N.Y., 1971, p. 27.

36. Schaller, Robert, and Goff, Willard F.: "A New Mini-Corkscrew for Bronchoscopic Foreign Bodies," *Laryngoscope,* **80**:1740, (Nov.) 1970.

Additional Suggested Reading

Barsam, Paul C., et al.: "Treatment of Dry Eye and Related Problems," *Ann. Ophthalmol.*, **4**:122, (Feb.) 1972.

Bell, R. W.: "Diagnosis and Treatment of Intraocular Foreign Bodies Incurred in Vietnam," *Surg. Forum,* **24**:498, 1973.

Benda, T. J.: Perforating Foreign Body of the Esophagus," *Laryngoscope,* **79**:470, (Mar.) 1969.

Bhargava, S. K.: "Penetrating Thistle Bracts Injury," *Br. J. Ophthalmol.*, **55**:421, (June) 1971.

Cignetti, Franklin E.: "Disease of the External Eye," *J. Occup. Med.*, **12**:395, (Oct.) 1970.

Dawes, J. D. K.: "Chemotherapy in Infections of the Ear, Nose and Throat," *Practitioner,* **207**: 735, (Dec.) 1971.

Donnan, F. DeS.: "Clinical Experience of 'Xerumenex' in the Removal of Ear Wax," *Practitioner,* **200**:574, (Apr.) 1968.

Douvas, N. G.: "The Cataract Rotoextractor," *Trans. Am. Acad. Ophthalmol. Otolaryngol.*, **77**:792, (Nov.–Dec.) 1973.

Fox, Samuel L.: "The Management of External Eye Infections in Industry," *J. Occup. Med.*, **12**:390, (Oct.) 1970.

Gibb, A. G.: "Syringing the Ear," *Nurs. Times,* **66**:1246, (Oct. 1) 1970.

Gruber, Ellis: "The Red Eye and What to Do About It," *Med. Times,* **93**:1207, (Nov.) 1965.

Hardin, A. F.: "Venereal Diseases and the Eye," *Practitioner,* **214**:636, (May) 1975.

Hewitt, H. R.: "Clinical Evaluation of Choline Salicylate Ear-Drops," *Practitioner*, **204**:438, (Mar.) 1970.

Hiles, David A.: "Strabismus," *Am. J. Nurs.*, **74**:1082, (June) 1974.

Khambata, A. S.: "Ear Dressings in the Treatment of Otitis Externa," *Practitioner*, **202**:269, (Feb.) 1969.

Lawrence, Norman: "A Comparison of Analgesic Therapies for the Relief of Acute Otalgia," *Br. J. Clin. Pract.*, **24**:478, (Nov.) 1970.

Lazar, M., et al.: "Topical Hetrazan in the Treatment of Ocular Onchocerciasis," *Am. J. Ophthalmol.*, **70**:741, (Nov.) 1970.

Longridge, N. S.: "Unusual Foreign Body in the Ear," *Br. Med. J.*, **2**:728, (June 28) 1975.

Maichuk, Y. F.: "Florenal in Treatment of Herpesvirus and Adenovirus Eye Diseases," *Invest. Ophthalmol.*, **10**:408, (June) 1971.

Marks, John H.: "A Study of Otitis Externa in General Practice," *Br. Clin. Pract.*, **22**:97, (Mar.) 1968.

McDowall, G. D.: "The Management of Otitis Externa," *Practitioner*, **207**:743, (Dec.) 1971.

Newlands, William J.: "The Treatment of Ear, Nose and Throat Infections in Childhood," *Practitioner*, **204**:64, (Jan.) 1970.

Phillips, A.: "A Simple Treatment for Chronic Otitis Externa," *Practitioner*, **199**:218, (Aug.) 1967.

Polack, Frank M. (ed.): *Corneal and External Diseases of the Eye, First Inter-American Symposium.* Charles C Thomas, Publisher, Springfield, Ill., 1970.

Salomon, J. L.: "New Technique for Rapid Ear Irrigations," *J. Occup. Med.*, **9**:576, (Nov.) 1967.

Smith, Joan F., and Nachazel, Delbert P.: "Retinal Detachment," *Am. J. Nurs.*, **73**:1530, (Sept.) 1973.

Wright, P.: "The Dry Eye," *Practitioner*, **214**:631, (May) 1975.

Zetterstrom, Birgitta: "The Treatment of Contusion of the Eye," *Acta Ophthalmol.*, **47**:784, (No. 3) 1969.

Gladys Nite
Virginia Henderson

CHAPTER 28

Local Applications of Heat, Cold, and Chemicals for Circulatory Effects

1. USES AND EFFECTS OF LOCAL APPLICATIONS OF HEAT

Uses. Most authorities agree that the principal indication for therapeutic use of local heat is the relief of pain. It is used to dilate small vessels and to relax muscle tissue, both of which may be factors in the relief of pain.[1] Certainly exercises for stiff joints are less painful (and more effective) if preceded by applications of heat. When heat is used as therapy, the physician prescribes the size and mode of application, the intensity, and duration. Applications to a circumscribed part of the skin or mucous membrane are most often used in acute or chronic inflammation of the superficial tissues lying underneath or in reflexly related, deeper tissues. Another and more reliable means of getting the effect of heat in the deeper tissues and viscera is the passage of an electric current through them. The resistance offered to the current by tissues raises their temperature. Diathermy and other electrotherapeutic procedures are discussed in Chapter 31.

When heat is applied locally for comfort to warm a cold skin area, it may be instigated by the nurse unless heat is contraindicated by the patient's condition. The use of heat for comfort is instinctive for animals and humans. The danger of heat wrongly used should be part of health education.

Effect of Local Applications of Heat. The effect of heat applied locally is the same as that discussed under general hot applications except that it is more, but not entirely, circumscribed (see Chapter 29, Table 29-1). John H. Gibbon and Eugene M. Landis[2]

showed that immersion of the forearm in water of 43.3°C (110°F) raised the skin temperature of the big toe from 21.1° to 32.2°C (70° to 90°F) in about 40 minutes (Fig. 28-1). This shows that blood is an excellent media for transmitting heat and with an increase in temperature, an increase in blood flow and vasodilation occurs. The effect of a hot arm bath on the pulse and respiration cannot be compared with the systemic effect of a general hot bath. For this reason heat of greater intensity and duration can be used for applications to a circumscribed body area than to the entire body.

William Bierman[3] says the skin can tolerate high temperatures because of the presence of arteriovenous shunts that open quickly on local heating, allowing blood to bypass the capillaries. He cites the work of Williamson and Scholtz who found that temperatures of 57.8°C (136°F) applied to a small area of the forearm for 5 seconds did not cause any visible reaction; after 10 seconds, an erythematous macule occurred, and after 15 seconds, a blister was formed. With a temperature of 54.5°C (130°F) 2 minutes were required for a blister to form, whereas no blisters occurred even after 20 minutes at temperatures below 50°C (122°F). For local applications, most authorities give 43.3°C (110°F) as the upper limit to which skin temperature should be brought because temperatures hotter than this are thought to cause irreversible tissue changes.

Bierman and Sidney Licht[4] give the temperature changes in the superficial and deeper tissues with local applications of heat and cold to the leg, arm, abdomen, forehead,

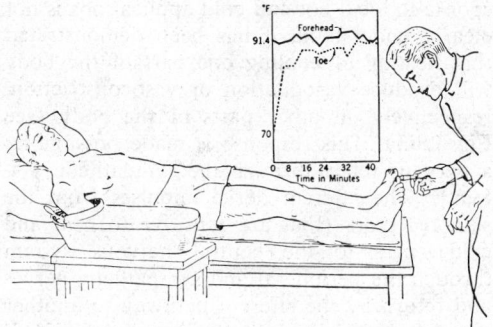

Figure 28-1. Changes in temperature of the skin surfaces of the forehead and toe when the forearm is immersed in hot water (Landis-Gibbon test). The test is useful in the diagnosis of cardiovascular disease. (From Bierman, William, and Licht, Sidney [eds.]: *Physical Medicine in General Practice,* 3rd ed. Harper & Row, New York, 1952.)

urethra (male), and vagina. Basing their judgments on their own studies and those of H. C. Bazett and L. Scribyatta,[5] Albert Kuntz,[6] Selling Brill,[7] Norman C. Lake[8] and others, they show that local hot and cold applications, respectively, raise and lower the temperature of the skin, subcutaneous tissue, and muscle lying under the hot or cold object; however, the effect is less intense in the deeper tissues, and there is a lag in its appearance. Bierman and Licht had an opportunity to observe that a cold application to the forehead reduced the temperature of the brain 1.5°F (see Fig.

28-2), but the evidence of temperature changes within the stomach from applications of heat to the abdominal wall are conflicting. On application of a hot-water bag to the human leg (calf) Bierman[9] reports the following temperature changes:

Interior of hot-water bag   133°F
Outside of towel covering hot-water bag 122°F
Cutaneous temperature rose from 90° to 110°F
Subcutaneous temperature rose from 91.2° to 105.5°F
Intramuscular temperature rose from 94.2° to 99.6°F

He says:

It requires fifty minutes for the establishment of this intramuscular temperature. Several other investigators have observed that the temperature of the skin in direct contact with the heating source rises rapidly. The subcutaneous temperature rises slower and to a lesser degree. The muscle and joint temperatures do not rise until a period of time during which body temperature may become elevated.*

Recent studies are more or less consistent with these findings and opinions of early investigators and writers.[10-12] Following a study of application of hot and cold packs to the abdominal area of dogs, Elaine D. Dyer and Howard K. Bagnell concluded that such applications on humans "could be expected to

* Bierman, William: "Physiologic Changes Produced by Heat," in Licht, Sidney (ed.): *Medical Hydrology,* Vol. 7. Elizabeth Licht, Publisher, New Haven, Conn., 1963, p. 97.

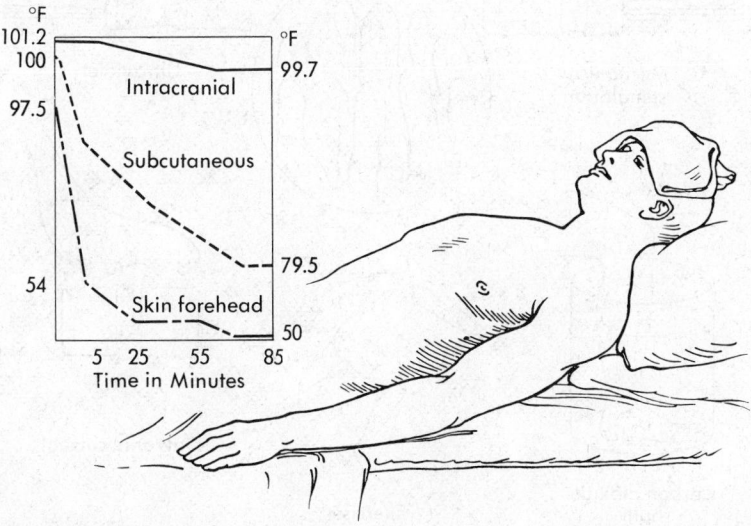

Figure 28-2. Temperature changes produced by application of ice bags to head. (From Bierman, William, and Licht, Sidney [eds.]: *Physical Medicine in General Practice,* 3rd ed. Harper & Row, New York, 1952.)

have a substantial effect on local temperatures in the skin, subcutaneous and muscle tissues" * but changes in the peritoneal cavity and body temperatures would be minimal. It is important to remember that the environmental temperature is a factor in the changes that are produced by local heating or cooling.

Although the distant or reflex thermal re-

* Dyer, Elaine D., and Bagnell, Howard K.: "Local Tissue and General Temperature Changes in Dogs Produced by Temperature Applications," *Nurs. Res.,* **19:**37, (Jan.–Feb.) 1970.

sponse to local hot and cold applications is not clearly understood, it has been demonstrated that heating or cooling one part of the body will produce vasodilation or vasoconstriction, respectively, in other parts of the body (see Fig. 28-3). This response is made possible by a nervous reflex through the sympathetic system.[12a] The afferent nerve impulses from the skin receptors (that are sensitive to heat and cold) pass to the central nervous system through the peripheral and sympathetic nerves and return by the efferent pathway to another part of the body. In addition to these local

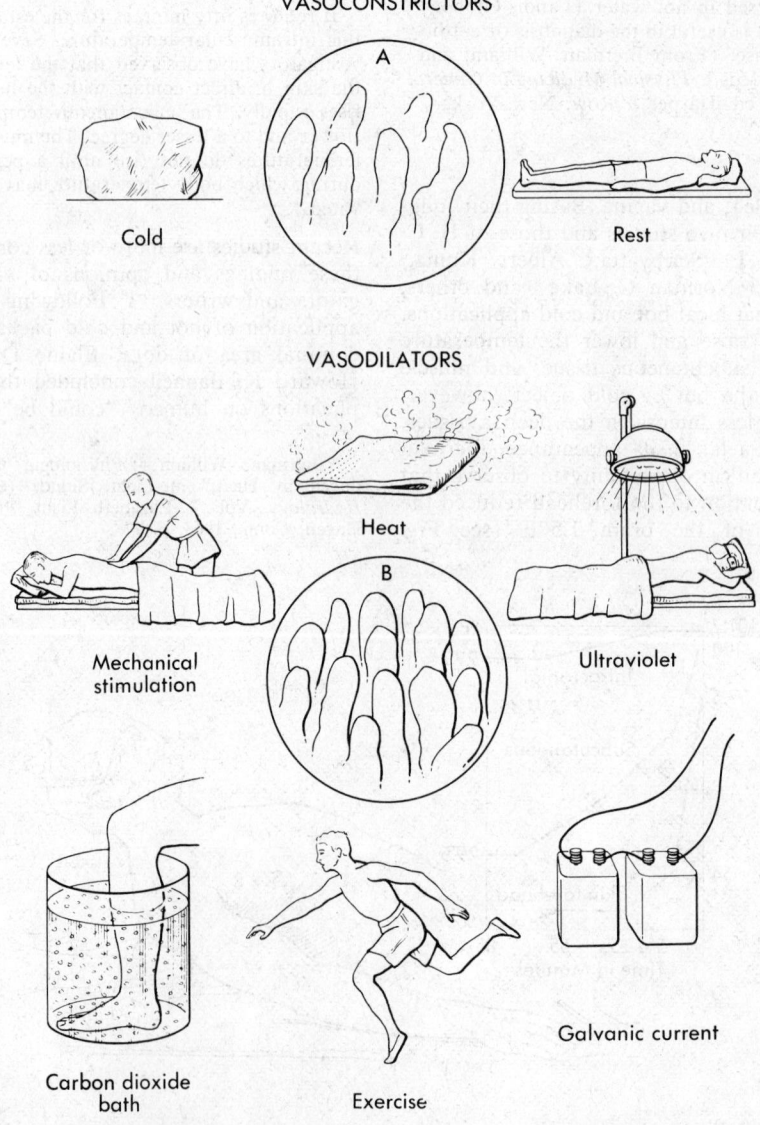

VASOCONSTRICTORS

Cold   A   Rest

VASODILATORS

Mechanical stimulation   Heat   B   Ultraviolet

Carbon dioxide bath   Exercise   Galvanic current

Figure 28-3. Physical agencies causing vasoconstriction and vasodilation. *A.* Constricted capillaries. *B.* Dilated capillaries (schematic). (From Bierman, William: *Physical Medicine in General Practice.* Harper & Row, New York, 1944.)

receptors of temperature, there is experimental evidence that deep or central receptors are present in both man and animals.[12b] John A. Downey says it is necessary to heat a large area of the body before "consensual" vasodilation will occur as a reflex to heating the skin and the "reflex blood flow increase through the forearm can be as much as 400 to 500 per cent, a change that occurs in the skin with no change or even a decrease in muscle flow." * Some doctors depend upon the application of heat to a related skin area to improve the circulation in a related deep-lying organ, such as the kidney.

Vasodilation is the principal action of heat that has been mentioned, chiefly because this is more easily measured. Other changes accompanying vasodilation—increased metabolism and relaxation of muscle and connective tissue—are discussed in Chapter 29. Heat applied to a local infection hastens the physical and chemical process of suppuration. Moist hot applications, especially, promote drainage from wounds and skin lesions; however, since the advent of antibiotic therapy, these have been supplanted by dry heat especially during the acute phase. Bierman says:

The pain occurring in acute inflammatory conditions may be aggravated by such applications, while that of subacute or chronic states may be ameliorated. The additional tissue tension due to the increased blood flow following the use of heat can account for increased discomfort in acute inflammation. Very rapid and marked temperature alterations have been shown to cause nerve excitation and contraction of skeletal muscles. . . . In subacute and chronic states, the increased circulation and the muscle-relaxing influence of heat may explain the soothing influence.†

Moist hot applications to surgical wounds have been used to reduce pain by some physicians for many years. The physiologic basis of this treatment is not clearly understood; it is thought, however, that when there is more than one form of sensory stimulation—heat plus pain, for example—the perception of either is reduced, according to Downey. In a study of 108 postoperative patients, Marilyn Halsell[13] reports that 54 patients who received hot moist packs (Hydrocollator Steam Pack) to the surgical incision three times daily consistently took fewer narcotics than those patients (54) who did not receive steam packs. Nurses working with surgical patients who are treated with hot packs for pain have repeatedly told the first writer that this is an effective method of controlling pain.

The effect of temperature depends upon the size of the area covered, whether it is intense or moderate, whether it is dry or moist, and the duration of the treatment (Chapter 29). It also depends upon the part of the body to which it is applied, the age and condition of the patient, and particularly the difference between the temperature of the hot application and the skin area involved.

Contraindications to Local Hot Applications and Their Dangers. Nurses see hot applications ordered by one physician and cold applications ordered by another in what appears to them to be similar situations. Depending upon the way in which they are used, both may increase the local blood supply; used alternately, they are very effective in doing this. Heat is usually contraindicated when vasodilation would increase pain, as in a swollen sprained ankle or when expansion of fluids or gases would intensify discomfort as in an infected tooth. In the first case cold applications are indicated, or contrasting temperatures; in the second case hot applications should be avoided. The pain in an infected tooth is caused by the pressure of gas formed by the bacteria infecting the tooth. There is less avenue for its escape in the untreated tooth, and the only relief comes from the contraction of the gas and blood vessels in the infected area. Small poultices are available at some drugstores which may give some comfort. They act by withdrawing fluid from the tissue and reducing pressure. Heat is rarely applied to the head because vasodilation of cerebral vessels makes pressure on the rigid cranium with resulting pain or discomfort.

Heat is believed to hasten a suppurative process; it is therefore contraindicated in an acute inflammatory condition as it would intensify this process and possibly result in tissue necrosis, as in appendicitis. Patients with appendicitis who are awaiting surgery, or trying to avoid it, have ice applied intermittently to the area for varying periods of time.

Heat is not used where there is a malignancy in the treatment area as increased blood flow may hasten metastases.[13a] It is contraindicated for those persons with impaired circulation or sensation. If the arterial supply is limited, the tissue will lack, to some degree, the convective action of an increased flow of blood. When heat is applied in such conditions, it should be possible to see the response to treatment. In chronic venous insufficiency, the skin has a reduced tolerance for heat; consequently, caution must be taken to prevent burning. If the patient's sensation for heat or pain is impaired for any reason, and heat is used as a form of therapy, then the greatest

* Downey, John A.: "Physiological Effects of Heat and Cold," *Phys. Ther.,* **44:**713, (Aug.) 1964.
† Bierman, William: *op. cit.,* p. 99.

Table 28-1.   Types of Local (Cold, Neutral, and Hot) Hydrotherapeutic Applications

Cold	Neutral	Hot
1. *Compresses, wet dressings,* or *packs* to induce vasoconstriction, reduce swelling, and retard the suppurative process. Alternated with hot applications to improve the tone of muscle tissue, particularly the blood vessels. Sometimes applied for reflex effect on deeper tissues and to relax muscle and connective tissue in spasticity	1. *Compresses, wet dressings,* or *packs* to soften exudates and induce drainage	1. *Compresses, wet dressings,* or *packs* to induce vasodilation and leukocytosis, to increase the metabolic rate locally, to relax muscles and connective tissue, to hasten suppuration and promote drainage. Alternated with cold applications to improve the tone of muscle tissue, particularly the blood vessels. Sometimes applied for reflex effect on deeper tissue
2. *Immersion baths* to induce vasoconstriction, etc., as above; whirlpool baths—water kept in motion giving the effect of massage to some extent (cold sitz bath for immersion of pelvic area rarely used)	2. *Immersion baths* to induce drainage and relieve pain and irritation in burns and other skin lesions. Whirlpool baths —water kept in motion giving the effect of massage to some extent	2. *Immersion baths* to induce vasodilation, etc., as above. Sitz baths for immersion of pelvic area. This is not alternated with cold bath and is used chiefly for reflex action on pelvic organs. Whirlpool baths —water kept in motion giving the effect of massage to some extent
3. *Spray baths, douches, or irrigations to body surface and communicating cavities.* Same effects as item 2.	3. *Spray baths, douches, or irrigations to body surface and communicating cavities.* Same effect as item 2.	3. *Spray baths, douches, or irrigations to body surface and communicating cavities.* Same effect as item 2.
4. *Air baths or cabinets* to induce vasoconstriction and improve the tone of all muscle tissue in the local area	4. *Air baths or cabinets* to relieve pain and irritation and promote healing of skin lesions	4. *Air baths or cabinets* to induce vasodilation and promote healing of skin lesions
5. *Cold objects*—collars, caps, and bags of various sizes filled with ice or frozen glycerin mixtures; coils and Elliot applicators containing circulating ice water have about the same effect as described under item 1		5. *Hot objects*—collars and bags of various sizes filled with hot water or chemicals that react and produce heat when water is added; electrically heated pads and bricks or stone heated in a stove produce same effect as item 1, except that it does not promote drainage to the same extent
		6. *Poultices* have same effect as item 1
		7. *Semisolids*—paraffin and mud, same effect as item 4
		8. *Counterirritant chemicals,* liniments, and plasters induce vasodilation and relaxation of muscle and connective tissues. Sometimes applied for reflex effect on deeper tissues
		9. *Diathermy* (the passage of an electric current through the tissues) heats the deeper tissues, producing in them effects similar to those listed under items 1 and 2 (it is described in Chapter 31)

care must be taken to prevent injury to the patient.[14]

Few patients other than the comatose will tolerate general applications of heat without complaint; local applications at injuriously high temperatures may go unnoticed if the person's attention has been diverted by pain or absorbing thoughts. Those who apply heat must see that the skin temperature is never raised above 43.3°C (110°F). This is the maximum temperature for wet applications since water is a good conductor of heat. Air is a poor conductor, and the skin therefore tolerates higher temperatures in air baths. Hot objects, however, and even air baths, soon induce sweating, and this may convert a dry application, for example, an electric pad, into a wet one. Some tissues, notably the mucous membrane of the mouth and pharynx, tolerate brief contact with food and drink at temperatures of 49°C (120.2°F) which could not safely be used on the skin. This should not make the nurse less cautious in applying heat.

Methods. The sources of heat by conduction (with which we are concerned in this chapter) are solids, liquids, and gases. The solids most commonly used are hot water in a bottle, electric wires embedded in a pad, heated sand, brick, and a hot poultice. Liquids used include water used as local baths or to wet compresses or packs. Melted or hot paraffin wax is another liquid used for local application of heat. Hot air or water vapor is the gas most frequently used.[15] Table 28-1 shows most of the common and some of the less common means of modifying local temperatures. Cold, neutral, and hot applications are combined to offset the disadvantages of prolonged cold and heat. For example, the vasodilation that accompanies prolonged applications of heat results in edema, and this can be avoided by alternating applications of heat and cold.

If light is used that gives off rays having chemical as well as thermal effects, there will of course be a difference between its action and that of a hot-water bottle. Many electric-light bulbs, however, produce only a heat effect. For convenience, the therapeutic use of light, both for its thermal and chemical effect, is discussed in Chapter 31, although, as a means of applying heat, it more properly belongs here.

If applying heat over a painful area, weight is to be avoided. In such cases an electric pad is preferable to a hot-water bottle, or lights suspended from a cradle placed over the area are even more desirable. When accurate regulation of temperature is important, the electric heating pad is preferable to the hot-water bottle because it maintains its temperature during use; however, because the temperature is maintained, patients are more likely to be burned by this device than hot-water bottles, especially if they lie on the heating pad.[16]

If the purpose of the treatment is to promote drainage, moist heat in the form of a local bath or compress is usually indicated. Compresses may be kept at the same temperature by putting an electric heating pad over them. The Aquamatic K-Pad * is thought to be an effective means of controlling heat of a compress for as long as 6 hours. The pad, attached to a control unit which ensures maintenance of the prescribed temperature, is placed over the compress. Hydrocollator packs (see Fig. 28-4) applied in the same way are

* Gorman-Rupp Industries, Inc., Bellville, Ohio.

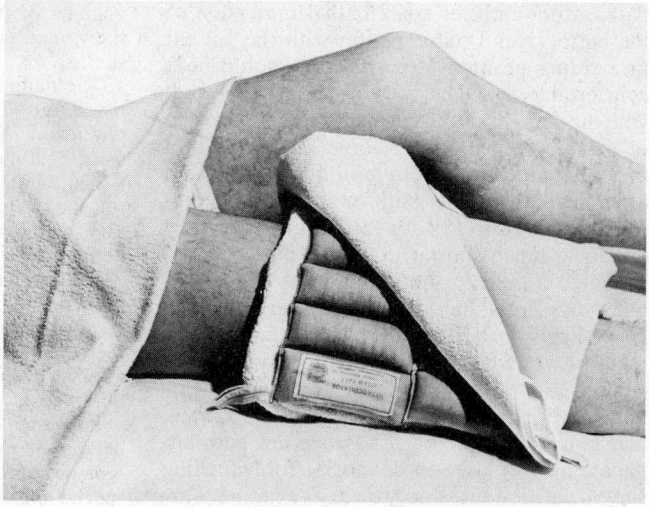

Figure 28-4. Moist heat applications with a Hydrocollator steam pack that can be applied for periods up to 30 minutes. The pack is designed so that it can be rolled along one dimension; it can also be hinged into a "V" along the other dimension. Thus, it can be adapted to practically any body contour. (Courtesy of Chattanooga Pharmacal Co., Chattanooga, Tenn.)

effective for at least 30 minutes.[17] Tub baths, containing 5 to 6 inches of warm water for postpartum patients, are reported to have been effective in relieving discomfort in the perineal or rectal area of 10,000 obstetric patients.[18] Plastic sitz baths issued individually to hospital patients reduce the danger of infecting perineal and rectal wounds. However, it is more difficult to keep the water warm and they add to the cost of care.

The following suggested procedures include the more common methods of applying heat locally, with the exception of the heated-air bath, which is discussed in Chapter 31.

2. LOCAL HOT-WATER BATHS

Selection of Method. Local baths used in the treatment of wounds and some skin eruptions should be *sterile;* if the skin is intact and the bath is prescribed for its thermal effect only, it need be nothing more than *clean*. The *temperature* of the bath depends upon the effect desired, the sensitivity of the area, and the temperature tolerance of the patient. For therapeutic baths the physician usually stipulates the temperature he or she wishes to have used. The average adult tolerates water at temperatures as high as 43.3°C (110°F); a child's skin is more sensitive and more easily injured. Generally speaking, the ventral body surface is more sensitive than the dorsal surface, and the foot and leg more sensitive than the hand and arm. Temperatures that are not bearable at first are tolerated if the bath is gradually brought to that point by adding hot water. *A thermometer should always be used to test the temperature as the skin may tolerate water hot enough to burn it.*

No matter whether the treatment is an arm bath, a foot bath, or a sitz bath (immersion of the buttocks and pubic region with the patient in a sitting position), the *posture* should be a comfortable one. The body must be supported, and the legs or arms protected from the rim of the tub with a pad of some kind. The skin must be protected from chilling during and after the bath. A foot bath or sitz bath is commonly ordered to last for 20 minutes, but may last for a much shorter or longer period.

Water is used for hot local baths ordinarily, but drugs are sometimes added and are especially likely to be used in baths for the treatment of wounds. *Solutions* commonly used for wounds are sodium chloride, sodium bicarbonate, boric acid, and magnesium sulfate, and tannic acid for burns. Potassium permanganate may be used to deodorize foul-smelling superficial lesions and to dry exuding surfaces.[19] Mustard was once added to a hot foot bath in the proportions of 1 tbsp to 1 gal of water when the bath was used to induce hyperemia of the intact skin. This treatment is rarely, if ever, prescribed, but if used, the mustard should be well dissolved in tepid water before it is added to the bath water to ensure its even distribution. Undissolved particles of mustard may burn the skin. When mustard is used, the temperature of the bath may not be more than 37.8° to 40.6°C (100° to 105°F), because the irritating quality of the mustard makes the bath seem hot to the patient.

Suggested Procedure for a Clean Foot Bath. Give the bath with the patient sitting comfortably in a chair, or in bed. When in a chair, wrap the upper part of the body in a blanket, cover the legs with a second blanket, and enclose the bath. When the patient is in bed, turn back the bedclothes, protect the bed with a rubber sheet, and cover the legs, enclosing the bath with a blanket. Before gradually immersing the feet, apply cold to the head. Support the knees with a knee rest or pillow, and pad the rim of the tub with a towel.

At the termination of the bath, (5 to 30 minutes) avoid exposure and chilling. Dry the legs and feet and leave them wrapped in the blanket for 20 to 30 minutes.

Record the time at which the treatment was given, the duration of the treatment, and the patient's reaction.

Suggested Procedure for a Sterile Foot or Arm Bath. Scrub the foot or arm as in preparation for surgery and leave the extremity wrapped in sterile towels until it is immersed in the bath, using a sterilized tub. Cover the tub with a lid made of the same material as the tub, an opening being left at the top and to one side for the arm or leg. The solution used for the bath and a thermometer for testing the temperature of the water should be sterile. At the termination of the bath apply a sterile dressing to the wound, and dry the remainder of the area with a clean towel, protecting the wound from contact with anything that is not sterile.

The nature of the solution, its temperature, and the duration of the bath are prescribed by the physician. The duration of the treatment is usually 20 to 30 minutes; however, for selected patients, the physician may prescribe such a bath for longer periods, and in such cases it is necessary to keep adding hot water to maintain the desired temperature.

Record the time the bath was given, its duration, the nature and temperature of the solution. If a wound or skin lesions are present, describe their appearance before the bath, their appearance afterward, and the amount and kind of discharge observed in the bath water.

Suggested Procedure for a Sitz Bath. This bath derives its name from the German word meaning *seat* because it is taken in a sitting position. If a special tub is available the patient may sit in the water with the feet outside. Having the patient sit in an ordinary bathtub full of water has a similar effect. This is the method commonly used. In some hospitals patients are issued individual plastic tubs that are discarded when they are no longer needed.

When the patient is in the bath, apply cold compresses to the head. An ice collar on the back of the neck is also very effective. Put a bed jacket or blanket around the shoulders of the patient, and a blanket over the thighs and legs and enclose the tub with it if possible.

Make the bath as hot as the patient can bear it. If the heat is gradually increased, a temperature of 43.3°C (110°F) may be tolerated, but it must never exceed this. The duration of the bath is about 30 minutes according to Ronald Harrison.[20] The suggested duration by other authors varies considerably, the most common being 20 to 30 minutes. Should the patient show signs of exhaustion before the end of the prescribed period, he or she is of course removed from the bath.

Record the time the bath was given, its duration, the nature and temperature of the solution, and the patient's reaction.

3. HOT WET COMPRESSES AND FOMENTATIONS (OR STUPES)

Selection of Method. Flannel and pieces of old woolen blankets are satisfactory materials for hot compresses, because a woolen fabric is light and holds a proportionately large amount of water. The pieces may be laundered afterward and used many times, but very hot water soon makes wool hard, scratchy, and unsuitable for this purpose, so that they must be replaced with new compresses at frequent intervals. In many hospitals thick gauze pads are used instead of woolen squares; expendable cellucotton and gauze pads also may be used with excellent results. The 4- by 4-inch gauze dressings are commonly used for wet sterile compresses. The gauze pads and gauze dressing type of compress is the most economical and probably the most satisfactory. A turkish towel is frequently used for large surface areas when the skin is intact and it is available in homes. The material can, of course, be sterilized and used for compresses on wounds. Whatever type of material has been selected, see that it is cut or folded to cover the area that the physician wishes to have covered. This depends upon the objective. When the fomentation is to increase the volume of blood in the skin and relieve congestion in the adjoining parts or internal organs, make it very large, so as to withdraw a large volume of blood; for instance, applications to relieve pain in the kidneys must cover the whole central and lower part of the back and come well around to the sides; to relieve inflammation of joints,

the application should be closely wrapped completely around the joint and extend several inches above and below it; to relieve pain or congestion in pelvic organs, the application must extend over the whole lower abdomen and well down over the hips and thighs; to relieve pain in abdominal organs, the application must extend from above the waistline over the hips; to relieve inflammation or congestion of the breasts, the application should be applied closely around the breasts, but the nipples must never be covered; to relieve pain and congestion in the anal area, the application must be applied between the buttocks and extend well over them; to distend vessels in preparation for a venipuncture, the application must extend well beyond the selected site; to relieve pain in surgical incisions, the compress should extend a few inches beyond the incision (a 4- by 4-inch or 4- by 8-inch compress is usually sufficient).

When applied for a purely local effect, as in the relief of an infected finger or boil, or wound, such as an infected surgical wound, the application should be no larger than necessary, to avoid dilating the artery supplying the part and thus increasing the congestion; for instance, when the object is to relieve the inflammation of the eyeball, the application should cover the eye and extend over the brow (but not over the cheek).

Suggested Procedure for Clean Compresses. Protect the patient from chilling, both during and after the treatment, by exposing no more of the body than is necessary and by covering the area of hyperemia, produced by the treatment, with a dry piece of flannel or a turkish towel after the wet compresses are removed.

To protect the skin, apply a thin coat of mineral oil over the treatment area except when a wound is present or when the treatment is used in preparation for a venipuncture.

Before applying the compresses, wring from them the prescribed solution. Test the temperature of the water or the solution with a thermometer. Keep a thermometer in the liquid, so that it can be maintained at the desired temperature; this should not exceed 55°C (131°F), for compresses wrung out of water hotter than this are likely to burn the patient unless very carefully cooled before application.

Wring the compress as dry as possible. A saturated compress is heavy, and water trickles from it over the patient. Apply one or more compresses to the area and, to maintain the desired temperature a hyperthemia pad, an electric heating pad, or a hot-water bottle may be used to cover the compress. In case the physician wants the effect of heat moderated by periodic removal of the compress, use two cloths and as the application cools renew it with a fresh hot one.

To protect the bedding and clothing, cover the wet compress with a moistureproof material such as cellophane, a processed paper, oiled silk, or plastic or rubber tissue. This also acts as insulation and helps maintain the application at the desired temperature. A turkish towel or piece of dry flannel over the waterproof material also helps to provide insulation. When an electric pad is used, take special care to prevent wetting the pad as this may cause a short circuit. Special hyperthermia pads are designed to avoid this danger. It is desirable to hold the compress in place with a loosely applied binder, so that the patient is not obliged to stay in one position throughout the treatment.

Record the treatment as given and its effect on the patient.

Suggested Procedure for Sterile Hot Wet Compresses. (Wet dressings applied directly over a wound should be sterile.) Prior to use, moisten several cotton-filled 4- by 8-inch dressings in the prescribed solution, wring as dry as possible, and place in a metal container. After autoclaving for 15 minutes at 121.11°C (250°F), they are ready for use. With sterile forceps, apply the compress to the area. If for some reason this is not possible, place the sterile compresses in the preheated sterile solution, wring them with sterile forceps or use a sterile Asepto syringe to apply the solution to the dry compresses. The latter method is less desirable.[21] Cover the wet compress with sterile abdominal pads or towels or both and then a sterile waterproof material, such as vinyl plastic sheeting. Further insulation may be effected by putting a turkish towel or a clean piece of flannel over the compress. (Other methods of maintaining the desired temperature are those described for clean compresses.)

Hot compresses to the eye are generally sterile because they are used in conditions that make the conjunctiva very susceptible to infection. Several gauze sponges, 2 by 2 inches, or a pad made of cellucotton covered with gauze may be used.* Moisten compresses by immersion in a bowl of sterile solution, then wringing them with sterile forceps; by steaming them in a sieve; or by wetting the pad with a solution applied with an Asepto syringe. Change the compresses as soon as they cool, and use a fresh compress each time. (A special forceps should be provided for handling the contaminated dressings.) The duration of the treatment is usually 20 minutes, changing the compresses every minute (because of the thickness of the compress, sufficient heat is retained for this period).[22] If only one eye is affected, protect the other eye with a clean dry dressing or shield. In addition, keep the patient's head turned slightly toward the affected side so that the solution cannot run into the unaffected eye. If both eyes are under treatment, avoid contaminating one eye with material from the other; use a separate tray for each eye.

Since the eye is very sensitive, regulate the temperature of the compress accurately within comfortable limits (it should never exceed 50°C [122°F]), and avoid putting any pressure on the eye. Place the patient in a recumbent position, the head on a pillow protected with moistureproof material, and over this an absorbent cover.

Small pads are available that will keep eye compresses hot for hours. They have waterproof covers and are filled with chemicals that, when moistened, generate heat. When available and their weight tolerated, they simplify the procedure.

4. HOT MOIST PACKS IN POLIOMYELITIS

Selection of Method. Fortunately, because of the development and widespread use of vaccine to prevent poliomyelitis, its occurrence is rare and this cumbersome treatment by hot packs is less frequently needed now than in the past. In *Cecil-Loeb Textbook of Medicine,* Louis Weinstein writes:

The preparation of formalin-inactivated virus suspensions by Salk, and later of "live virus" vaccines by Sabin, by Cox, and by Koprowski in the latter half of the 1950's, has made the greatly reduced incidence or even eradication of poliomyelitis a realistic goal.*

The value of heat in relieving the muscle spasm of anterior poliomyelitis and in relaxing muscles in preparation for reducing a fracture is generally recognized. It was popularized by Sister Kenny's methods and is still the most commonly used treatment during the acute and early convalescent stages with hot moist packs; other methods, however, are used by some physicians such as dry heat by luminous or infrared radiation, continuously or at regular intervals. Diathermy to relieve angiospasm (excessive blood vessel tone) has been found to be effective but is questioned in the treatment of acute poliomyelitis. Cold packs have been used with good results for some patients, especially those with high fever.[23] Warm baths in pools, tanks, and tubs are used in the later stages. The warmth relaxes muscles and reduces sensitivity and irritation. A body supported in water is moved with a fraction of the effort required when it is not. In the past, "polio packs" were pinned on but this required considerable movement. To reduce the patient's activity to a minimum, "lay-on" in contrast to "pin-on" packs are more often advocated now, especially during the stage of painful spasm.

---

* Specially prepared eye cotton and eye gauze pads are frequently used to prevent pieces of lint or ravelings from falling on the eyeball.

* Weinstein, Louis: "Poliomyelitis," in Beeson, Paul B., and McDermott, Walsh (eds.): *Cecil-Loeb Textbook of Medicine,* 13th ed. W. B. Saunders Co., Philadelphia, 1971, p. 406.

Sometimes pin-on and lay-on pack treatments are alternated.

"Kenny packs" are made of three layers: (1) inner moist, hot woolen (or woolen and cotton) fabric in double layers; (2) dry waterproof cover; and (3) dry outer woolen (or woolen and cotton) layer. Pin-on packs are cut in rectangles to envelop the foot, leg, back, abdomen, chest, neck, forearm and hand; triangles to envelop the thigh and shoulder. For lay-on packs the inner moist woolen layer is most often used alone. The larger rectangles, cut for pin-on packs, are suitable for this purpose. Some physicians, however, prefer all three layers for the lay-on packs. Waterproof covers may be made from cellulose film, waxed paper, oiled silk and rayon, or pliofilm. The covers should be light and flexible.

Odon F. Von Werssowetz [24] says he prefers a silicate gel pack which is heated in a special cabinet to the desired temperature and with the proper water content. It serves as the inner layer of the pack. Because the gel retains the heat for a long time, the pack is not changed unless it is used for periods longer than 30 minutes. He believes it is easy to apply, saves time, and is efficient; however, it is difficult to apply around the shoulders and hips and should not be used on an extremely sensitive patient because it is heavier than woolen packs.

The physician prescribes the number, method, frequency, and duration of the packs and the areas to be covered. The hot packs may have to be applied continuously for several hours and changed as often as every 2 or 3 minutes but as a general rule, according to Von Werssowetz, they are applied every 1 to 2 hours in severe cases, every 3 to 4 hours in moderate cases, and every 4 to 6 hours in mild cases.

Since the packs are applied as hot as can be tolerated without fear of burning, a means of heating the packs must be provided. Special portable steamers are economical of time and effort. Portable electric washing machines and wringers are the next choice. Since these treatments may be prescribed at 2-hour intervals, "polio packs" are a major economic problem in understaffed hospitals. It is important that efficient portable equipment be provided. Instrument sterilizers, tubs, stoves, and wringers of all sorts have been used, and improvisation in homes is necessary, except in centers where special electric steamers may be rented. Heating units must decontaminate packs as well as heat them unless they can be isolated.

A loin cloth should be provided for all patients, and a breast protector for older girls and women; breast and abdominal binders and pins are also needed. Thick moist cloths favor the growth of microorganisms, particularly yeasts and molds; so they must be sterilized after each use and, if possible, dried in sunlight or ultraviolet light. Washing in detergents and boiling for 20 minutes are recommended for all except woolen materials. The patient's skin must be watched closely for signs of infection, and a rash is a contraindication for "packing." Certain patients are intolerant of contact with wool, some physically, others psychologically. Turkish-toweling packs or four-layer thickness of munsingwear can be substituted, but they are heavier and will not hold heat as long as wool. A layer of gauze next to the skin makes the wool pack bearable in some cases.

Sponge baths may be indicated between packs to reduce fever and remove lint left by packing. The skin must be dried gently, for it is subject to irritation and maceration from repeated applications of packs. Oils and ointments are not recommended. There is great difficulty in preventing discoloration and odor in pack materials; heat quickly hardens woolen fibers, and this makes it necessary to replace packs frequently.

The procedure should be described to patients, and their cooperation enlisted before any equipment is brought to the bedside. A warm environment for packing is essential, for subsequent chilling would more than counteract the benefit of the packs. Speed is also important to prevent cooling the packs before they can be adjusted. At least two workers should give the treatment; more can be used with benefit in turning patients and applying the packs, especially if the equipment necessitates wringing water from the cloths.

Suggested Procedure.* Gain the patient's understanding of and cooperation in the treatment if possible. See that the room is warm. Replace the patient's gown or pajamas with a pubic binder or loin cloth and protect the breasts of adolescent girls and women. Leave the patient in the desired position and bring the pack materials to the bedside.

For lay-on packs have the patient supine if pads are to be applied to the chest; prone if to the back. Apply a rectangle of moist (not wet) woolen (or woolen and cotton) blanketing large enough to cover the prescribed area. Lay it on gently, having shaken out all wrinkles, and make sure that it is not too hot. A patient's first packs should be only moderately hot to accustom him or her to the treatment. Fear must be avoided

* This technique is based on that described in the booklet *Nursing for the Polio Patient,* prepared by the Joint Orthopedic Nursing Advisory Service of the National Organization for Public Health Nursing and the National League of Nursing Education, New York, 1948.

as it induces muscular contraction. Do not insulate the pack, but replace the cooling rectangle with a hot one every 5 minutes for the prescribed period, or until the spasm is relieved. After treating the chest, and in some cases the anterior surface of the arms and legs, put the patient in the prone position and "pack" the posterior surface. If packs are to be applied to the legs as well as the back, use one large rectangle over the neck, shoulders, arms, back, and buttocks and another over the thighs and legs. Tuck the pack at the sides to prevent air currents. If the doctor prescribes the three-layer pack, apply it in the same way as described for the single layer and leave the packs on the patient for the prescribed period, repeating the treatment as prescribed. Maintain good body alignment throughout the pack and promote relaxation with the use of pillows, pads, and sandbags as discussed in Chapter 12.

For pin-on packs the patient and the environment are prepared as described for lay-on packs except that abdominal and chest binders in addition to the three pack layers are placed under the patient ready to be drawn up over the packs after they are adjusted. Apply the inner packs, the insulating layers next, and the dry woolen layers, folding them firmly but not tightly over the inner and middle layers. Pin the binders over the packs. (In some methods binders are omitted, and the outer layer of wool is pinned over the wet and insulating layers.) Move the patient gently and support the extremities when necessary by placing the hands under the joints. Leave the packs on the patient for the prescribed period and repeat them according to the doctor's directions. Remove the packs if signs of prostration (rapid pulse and increased respiration, pallor or cyanosis, or excessive sweating) indicate an unfavorable reaction.

Record the time the pack was applied, its duration, and any systemic or local reactions.

5. POULTICES

Nature of a Poultice. A poultice is an application of moist heat in the form of a soft spongy mass that retains its heat for a varying length of time, according to the ingredient used. The effects of poultices depend upon the heat they supply.

This treatment is very rarely used. J. B. Millard [25] in 1965 says they "are used occasionally for home treatment" but there are simpler and easier ways of applying heat locally. It is doubtful that this method would be used except in situations where even a hot-water bottle is unavailable.

While any vegetable product that makes a hot mash can be used, flaxseed or linseed is a good choice if it is available. Flaxseed has mucilaginous and oily ingredients; it is soothing to the skin and may be used at high temperature without burning, and air can be readily incorporated in it, making it light in weight.

Suggested Procedure for a Flaxseed Poultice. Make the poultice large enough to cover the desired area completely. When the application is prescribed for the treatment of one lung, for example, have the patient lie on the unaffected side, and apply the poultice from the neck to the base of the lung and from beyond the midline in front to beyond the midline in the back. The poultice, flannel cover, and binder used to hold it in place should each be shaped so as to fit under the arms and at the neck.

Before beginning to make the poultice, see that everything needed is at hand. Add the flaxseed to the boiling water gradually, at the same time stirring constantly with a spatula just as in making any cereal. (The water should not stop boiling.) When the mixture will drop clean from the spatula, it is of the right consistency. Beat the mixture thoroughly, so as to introduce air and make it as light as possible. The addition of 1 tsp of sodium bicarbonate increases this effect. Spread it evenly on muslin and protect it with another piece of muslin, in each case leaving sufficient margin to turn in neatly, so that there can be no possible escape of the mixture. Then wrap it in a warm towel or piece of flannel and take it to the bedside on a hot-water bottle if available. This flannel may be left on the part after the poultice is removed, to prevent chilling.

Unnecessary weight is particularly to be avoided when a poultice is to be applied. This is particularly true if applied to the chest, as in pneumonia, when breathing is already an effort. The flaxseed mixture should be about ¼ inch thick in such cases, and when applied to the abdomen for distention or to other tender areas. Applied to the extremities, where lack of weight is not such an important factor, the poultice may be ½ inch thick or more.

The care of the skin is much the same as in the application of fomentations. Oil the skin if the applications are frequent, or if the skin is tender; apply the poultice gradually; keep raising part of it until the patient is accustomed to the heat. Avoid exposure of the part before, during, or after the treatment. Cover the poultice with flannel or oiled muslin, so as to retain the heat. Fasten it in place with the binder or bandage the part may demand. A patient who is restless, or who is in pain, should not be obliged to stay in one position or to worry about keeping a poultice in place. Fasten binders on the trunk only tightly enough to hold the poultice in place, not enough to restrict breathing.

The duration of the application in all cases should be only as long as the heat is retained (never longer than 1 hour).

After the removal of the poultice, dry the part and inspect the skin. It should have a pink glow. Oil it if tender or red, and cover with soft flannel to prevent chilling.

When a poultice is applied to relieve distention,

a rectal tube is usually inserted into the rectum (by order) to aid in the expulsion of gas.

Record giving the treatment and the patient's reaction.

6. HOT-WATER BOTTLE AND ELECTRIC PAD, AND DISPOSABLE SUBSTITUTES

Suggested Procedure. Test the temperature of the water with a thermometer. It may vary from 49° to 65°C (120.2° to 149°F), depending upon the thickness of the cover used, the area to which the application is made, and the condition of the patient and the skin. The water should not be hot enough to burn the patient should the bag

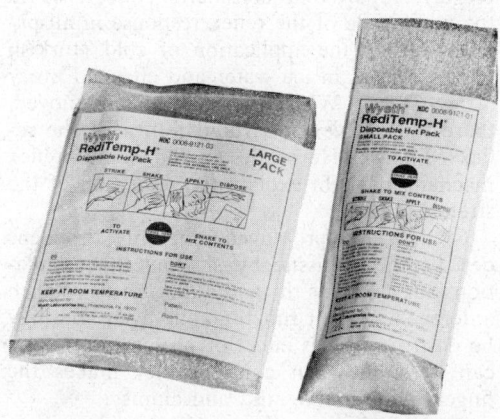

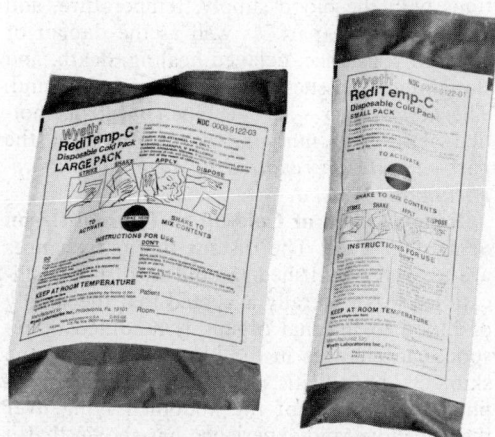

Figure 28-5. RediTemp packs are prefilled with precisely measured active ingredients to produce controlled and predictable temperatures. When a RediTemp pack is struck on the spot designated on the front of the package, a heat-producing reaction occurs between a chemical and an inner bubble of solvent. The reaction takes place inside a plastic bag, which is contained in an insulated outer wrapper. (Courtesy of Wyeth Laboratories, Philadelphia, Pa.)

leak or the rubber burst, and the bag should be completely and suitably covered.

The avoidance of unnecessary weight is important. If the patient must support the weight of the bag, as when applied to the abdomen, it should be one-third full and all the air expelled to make it pliable.

If the application is to be continued, see that the bag is regularly refilled and kept hot. Notice the position of the bag. The patient may be restless (particularly if in pain), displace the bag, roll over on it, and get burned.

Earthenware and glass bottles, if they can be tightly stoppered, are very good substitutes for rubber bags. Here the application is used to warm the feet, the chest, abdomen, or other body area. In home nursing it may be necessary to find a substitute for a rubber bag.

It is usually important to record that a hot-water bottle has been given to a patient whether for therapy or comfort and also to note the area to which it is applied.

The electric pad, an efficient substitute, is rapidly replacing the hot-water bottle. The mechanical mechanism has been improved so there is little danger of overheating or short circuits developing in the newer models, but the unit should be encased in a waterproof jacket for protection. The patient should *never* lie on the pad as pressure interferes with circulation (the system used to conduct heat throughout the body) and burns can occur.

Disposable hot packs are now available that are especially useful in emergencies and for patients who have a highly infectious condition.* The ecologic disadvantage of disposable equipment makes its excessive use questionable.

7. USES AND EFFECTS OF LOCAL APPLICATIONS OF COLD

Uses. Cold is prescribed to contract the blood vessels, thereby reducing the circulating fluids in an area and relieving pain caused by pressure. It is also used to control hemorrhage, check inflammation, and prevent suppuration, lessen abnormal muscle tone (spasticity), and relieve pain by raising the threshold of pain receptors.[26,27] A cold application may be used to affect the skin and the tissues immediately under the skin or to effect internal circulatory changes by reflex action. The latter was discussed with relation to the effect of heat (page 1338).

It is essential that those who use it understand the action of cold, because, if used improperly, it may be harmful.

---

* Wyeth Laboratories, Philadelphia, Pa., makes *RediTemp* disposable hot and cold packs in large and small sizes. Directions for their use are printed on the cover (see Fig. 28-5).

Action and Effects. The physiologic action of cold and the effects produced depend upon: the mode of application—whether in the form of moist or dry cold, for this affects the intensity; the temperature; the duration; the surface of the body covered by the application; and the condition of the tissues and the general condition of the patient.

Moist cold, like moist heat, is more penetrating in its action, because water is a better conductor of cold than air. A patient can tolerate an ice bag (a form of dry cold) for a much longer period than a local ice-cold bath.

Bierman and Licht give the following changes in skin, subcutaneous, and muscle temperature with the application of an ice bag:

With the application of cold, heat is transferred from the body to the colder substance. An ice bag placed on the calf of the leg caused the following temperature changes:

Interior of ice bag   32°F
Outside of towel covering ice bag   40°F
Cutaneous
    temperature declined from 84° to 43°F
Subcutaneous
    temperature declined from 94° to 70°F
Intramuscular
    temperature declined from 98° to 79°F

The time required for the fall in skin temperature was fifteen minutes; for the subcutaneous temperature, about one hour; for the intramuscular, about two hours.*

The effect of cold on mucous membrane is the same as that on the skin except that it is less sensitive to either heat or cold. The effect may be seen by holding ice in the mouth: the lining pales; bleeding, if present, is checked; nerves are numbed so that sensations are dulled. Ice held in the mouth before taking an obnoxious drug will make it much less distasteful. Surgeons and dentists anesthetize with a volatile liquid which, in evaporating, markedly lowers the temperature locally.

Although most authors concede that cold affects nerves, they say more research is needed before the process will be fully understood. Discussing the effects of cold in the reduction of spasticity, Licht writes:

It is most likely that suppression of the myotatic reflex is a result of (a) reduction of nerve conduction (skin afferents), (2) decrease of muscle spindle excitability by enhanced sympathetic activity and (c) increase in tissue and joint viscosity. After removal of ice packs, the skin temperature soon reaches 25°C and tends to remain at this level for at least another hour. At this time, intramuscular temperatures are lowest. Thus, discharges from the muscle spindle

which is very sensitive to cold are modified, leading to alteration of motor responses and reduction in muscle tone.

Unlike the effects of local applications, when the entire body is cooled, there is an increase of myotatic reflex activity following a decrease of the muscle spindle threshold to stretch and an increase of excitability of the motor neuron pool.*

He mentions that Hartviksen and Miglietta, working independently, agreed that early reduction in myotatic reflex activity probably resulted from blocking of skin afferents when cold was applied to the quadriceps muscle. Osvaldo E. Miglietta,[28] in another study of the effect of cold on the hyperactive stretch reflex of ten spastic patients (hemiplegic and quadriplegic), reported a considerable decrease in the magnitude of the reflex response in all patients during the application of cold (turkish towels soaked in ice water and changed every 30 seconds). When the cold was removed, there was, however, a rapid return of the reflex response. He suggested the neural reflex mechanism might explain the reduction of the stretch reflex.

Cold, if too prolonged, not only threatens destruction of tissue by slowing the circulation, but it lessens the activities of cells to such a degree that their function, and even life, may be destroyed. This effect of prolonged chilling can be seen when cold weather makes the fingers blue, numb, stiff, and clumsy.

The interference of prolonged cold applications with the blood supply, temperature, and function of the part, as well as the danger of lowered resistance, delayed healing, death, and sloughing of tissues, should be kept in mind. The *first danger signs*—a blue, purplish, mottled skin, with numbness or stiffness of the part—*should be reported at once and the applications removed.*

Reflex Action of Cold on an Internal Organ or Distant Part. The distant thermal changes are as well established in cold as in hot applications. It is generally accepted that the supply of blood to internal organs is modified in response to changes in the blood volume of the skin. In appendicitis, for example, cold is applied to the area of the abdomen lying over the appendix, and experience has shown that it allays inflammation internally. While this might result from conduction of cold through the abdominal wall, it is generally believed that cold affecting blood vessels in the skin is the first link in a chain of nerve reflexes carried

---

* Bierman, William, and Licht, Sidney (eds.): *Physical Medicine in General Practice,* 3rd ed. Paul B. Hoeber, New York, 1952, p. 5.

* Licht, Sidney: "Local Cryotherapy," in Licht, Sidney (ed.): *Therapeutic Heat and Cold,* Vol. II, 2nd ed. Elizabeth Licht, Publisher, New Haven, Conn., 1965, p. 545.

through the central nervous system that result in vasoconstriction in related organs.

Contraindications to Local Cold Applications. If signs of circulatory stasis are present, cold is contraindicated. Cold is rarely applied to injured tissue or used in any condition that suggests poor nutrition of the area. Some authorities think that a local application of cold increases the blood supply in the surrounding area, and they therefore hesitate to use cold applications when pain might be caused by congestion in the surrounding tissues.

Because warmth is associated in most minds with comfort, hot applications rather than cold are likely to be used for the relief of pain. Actually, the choice should depend upon the ultimate relief that results from correct treatment, and this is to be determined in each case by taking into consideration the cause of the pain or discomfort. It is a misconception to think that heat relieves pain and cold does not. Either can relieve pain, according to whether pain is produced by muscular contraction, a collection of pus, pockets of gas, or dilated blood vessels that cause pressure on sensory nerve endings.

In some cases, to avoid the injurious effects of too prolonged application of heat or cold, they are made alternately, as has been noted.

8. COLD WET COMPRESSES

Suggested Procedure. Cut or fold layers of gauze or turkish toweling so that they make a compress about ½ to 1 cm (⅙ to ⅓ inch) thick and shaped to fit the part. A knee compress should be large enough to completely encase the joint and surrounding area and will vary depending on the size of the person; a compress for the eye should be approximately the shape of the eye socket.

If this treatment is used repeatedly and the compress is a large one, it is wise to make it so that it will withstand laundering. Small towels are suitable for compresses to some body areas. An eye compress is discarded after one use if the eye is infected; but, if there is no infection present, an entire treatment may be given with two compresses applied alternately.

Protect the bedding and clothing from wetting by using impervious paper, cellulose film, oiled silk, or rubber tissue. See that the patient is in a comfortable posture before starting the treatment.

Cold compresses are usually wrung from water containing ice, which means that the water is only slightly above the freezing point. In a warm room the temperature of the compress changes before it can be applied; therefore, wring the compress with the hands and apply it as quickly as possible. There must be sufficient ice to maintain a very low temperature; use large pieces rather than chips, which might cling to the compress and irritate the area. Cold compresses are never sterile, because ice is not sterile, strictly speaking. If they are applied over an area that should be kept sterile, the technique of application can be made fairly safe by the use of sterile equipment, and forceps for handling the compresses.

Do not cover the compress. A cold compress that is covered soon reaches body temperature, and the effect is then that of a neutral or warm application. Physicians should stipulate the effect they wish and the duration of the treatment. If cold compresses are applied to a large area, place a hot-water bottle at the feet and take all necessary steps to prevent the sensation of chilliness.

When cold compresses or packs are used in treatment of muscle spasm, apply them over the entire length of the muscle, and after removal, massage the area lightly, which may have a sedative effect, but *avoid* vigorous massage as it may cause reflex activity and muscle spasm.[29]

The prescribed duration of cold compresses is usually 15 to 20 minutes, repeated every few hours. During the 15-minute period the compress is changed as it is warmed by the body; ordinarily this is every minute. In some cases, as, for example, when the patients have a bruised eye or an infected tooth, they may be well enough to change the compress themselves and will prefer to do so, because they know best when it loses its coldness.

If the area is infected, as in a gonorrheal conjunctivitis (which is usually treated with cold compresses), take care to protect the unaffected eye of the patient, the worker's eye, and the eyes of other persons who may come in direct contact with the infectious material. Cover the patient's unaffected eye with a clean dressing or shield (nurses should wear glasses to protect their eyes from the contaminated liquid that might be splashed into them, and the strictest medical asepsis practiced in all other respects.) Handle used compresses with forceps, discard them into a paper bag, and burn. Record the time the treatment was given and the patient's reaction.

The gonococcus is readily killed by soap and hot water, so that it is unnecessary for nurses to wear gloves. Because mucous membrane is peculiarly susceptible to infection by the gonococcus, however, every effort is made to protect nurses' eyes. If by accident their eyes or the unaffected eye of the patient is contaminated, irrigate the conjunctival sac freely with warm saline solution and instill penicillin solution (5000 units per ml) every minute for half an hour, then every 5 minutes for another half hour, and follow this with hourly instillations for at least 2 days. Watch the eye carefully for conjunctivitis.[30]

9. ICECAP AND ICE COLLAR

Icecaps are ordinarily filled with ice, but various freezing mixtures are now used with more or less success. The cap is filled with a water solution of alcohol or glycerin and then placed in an electric refrigerator until the liquid is frozen to a mushy consistency. Since the freezing point is lowered by increasing the specific gravity of the water with alcohol or glycerin, this type of ice bag is colder than one filled with ice, and it is therefore particularly important to cover it with a thick cover. The advantage of this method is that the solution may be left in the icecap, and after the outer surface has been properly cleaned and decontaminated it can be put back in the refrigerator and refrozen. In this way the nurse's time and effort are conserved. Disposable, ready-to-use cold packs in various sizes are also available as was mentioned earlier. These packs are especially useful in emergencies and highly infectious cases.

Suggested Procedure. Select an icecap or ice collar to fit the part to which the application is to be made. Fill the cap or collar approximately one-half full of pieces of ice about the size of a walnut. Expel the air before closing the cap. (Air decreases the flexibility of the bag and increases the rapidity with which the ice melts.) Test the cap for leakage. If there is leakage, a new washer may be all that is needed. Cover the cap with a soft absorbent bag, or case, made of a fabric such as Canton flannel. Water condenses on the outside of the bag; if the cap is used without a cover, bedding and clothing are likely to be wet, and the cold may be too intense.

Observe the skin carefully every hour or so. Report blueness, or mottling immediately, for the physician will probably want to stop the treatment. If an ice bag is applied over a period of days, it is usual to remove it every few hours for a short period to allow the circulation in the area to return to normal. (Gangrene may result from too prolonged applications of icecaps.)

An icecap used for its therapeutic effect must be kept cold. The rate at which the ice melts depends upon the size of the pieces of ice, the type of freezing mixture, the size of the icecap, and the temperatures of the room and the patient's body. Note the approximate length of time the bag stays cold and then establish regular hours for refilling it.

Record the application of the ice collar and any visible reaction of the patient or that which the patient describes.

10. USES AND EFFECTS OF CHEMICAL COUNTERIRRITANTS

Uses. Chemical skin irritants are used as are hot applications to induce vasodilation in the superficial tissues, or to affect the circulation or muscle tone in an underlying area or distant part by reflex action. Chemical counterirritants have been prescribed in bronchitis, pleurisy, pneumonia, joint pain, headache, abdominal distention, and many other conditions but are now seldom prescribed. Commercially prepared analgesic plasters are used by the public for "backache" and various types of rheumatic pain. In some cases their use may be justified; however, the cause of the pain should be determined, and, except in emergency, self-treatment for aches and pains should be discouraged. Since many persons still have great faith in plasters and liniments, they have a psychologic effect that is not duplicated by a hot-water bottle or pad which the writers think produces the same physiologic changes. For this reason nurses should understand the action and uses of counterirritants, the methods and dangers involved.

Action and Effects. Mustard and turpentine, camphor, menthol, and other aromatic substances found in liniments are the chemical counterirritants most often seen. (Older texts mentioned a plaster made of the powdered bodies of a fly named *Cantharis vesicatora*.) Their action is similar. When absorbed by the skin they irritate the sensory nerve endings and produce a vasodilation. Most of them blister the skin if they are left in contact with it long enough. Absorption of any drug is hastened if the drug is carried in an oil; counterirritants, called liniments, are therefore oily.[31]

Choice of Method. Application of liniments is not described here because it presents no problem other than the protection of bedding and clothing and the control of an odor which may be offensive to some persons. Their use should be avoided for this reason unless the person lives alone. The application of mustard is unusual, but nurses may find local mustard baths and mustard plasters prescribed in some situations.

In the dry form, mustard has no irritant quality; but when combined with water, a ferment or enzyme (myosin) breaks up a glucoside in powdered mustard into dextrose and volatile oil. The enzymes in the mustard flour are destroyed by a temperature of 60°C (140°F). Therefore, when the irritant effect of the volatile oil is desired, tepid water only should be added to the dry mustard.

In former years the effect of counterirritants on the skin was sometimes carried far enough to produce a blister. This practice is no longer believed beneficial; it is, on the other hand, considered dangerous, because infection of the blistered area is unavoidable. The only reason to produce a blister purposely is when the serum formed in a blister is needed in the production of an autogenous vaccine. A blister is occasionally made over a rheumatic joint, the fluid aspirated under aseptic conditions, and a vaccine prepared and administered to the same patient.

Suggested Method of Procedure. To prepare a *mustard paste* or *mustard plaster,* mix mustard and flour in the prescribed proportions (1:4 for an adult, 1:8 for a child, and 1:12 for an infant) and make into a smooth paste with tepid water. If the individual has a very sensitive skin, dilute the mustard even more with flour. The greater proportion of mustard, the less time is required for the plaster to have the desired effect and the more often the color of the skin must be checked to prevent a burn or blister. It is better to use less mustard and avoid burning the skin.

Make a paste that can be spread easily but is not runny. (The plaster should feel moist but not wet to the touch. A clammy plaster is uncomfortable, and the patient will shrink from it.) Spread the plaster on a piece of muslin large enough to cover the area, and turn up over the edges and back of the plaster. Take the plaster to the patient on a hot-water bottle, so that the application will feel warm. Turn the bedclothes down to expose the area of application. Arrange a binder in position, then apply the plaster and over it a piece of waterproof material the same size to prevent wetting or soiling the clothing. Fix the plaster in position by pinning the binder; arrange it so that observations of the skin under the plaster can be made every few minutes.

Leave the plaster in place until the skin is a deep pink. There is no stated time required for this reaction; it depends upon the individual's skin. It may redden in a few minutes, or it may be 20 minutes before a flush appears. After removing the plaster, wash the area gently with soap and water and leave it covered. If the skin shows signs of irritation, apply a vegetable oil, petroleum jelly, or cold cream. A thin coating of oil to the skin before the plaster is applied delays and decreases the intensity of the action. Ordinarily this is not necessary, but for patients who have a very tender skin it is a desirable precaution. Apply a dressing if oil is left on the skin, to avoid soiling the clothing.

Record the time at which the plaster was applied and removed, the area of application, and the reaction of the patient.

Commercially prepared plasters have directions for their use printed on them.

REFERENCES

1. Licht, Sidney (ed.): *Rehabilitation and Medicine.* Elizabeth Licht, Publisher, New Haven, Conn., 1968, p. 16.
2. Gibbon, John H., and Landis, Eugene M.: "Vasodilation in the Lower Extremities in Response to Immersing the Forearms in Warm Water," *J. Clin. Invest.,* **11:**1019, (Sept.) 1932.
3. Bierman, William: "Physiologic Changes Produced by Heat," in Licht, Sidney (ed.): *Medical Hydrology,* Vol. VII. Elizabeth Licht, Publisher, New Haven, Conn., 1963, p. 97.
4. ——, and Licht, Sidney (eds.): *Physical Medicine in General Practice,* 3rd ed. Paul B. Hoeber, New York, 1952.
5. Bazett, H. C., and Scribyatta, L.: "Effect of Local Changes in Temperature on Gas Tensions in the Tissues," *Am. J. Physiol.,* **86:**565, (Oct.) 1928.
6. Kuntz, Albert: "Relation of Automatic Nervous System to Physical Therapy," *Arch. Phys. Ther.,* **19:**24, (Jan.) 1938.
7. Brill, Selling: "Effect of Abdominal Thermal Applications on the Intraperitoneal Temperature," *Ann. Surg.,* **89:**857, (June) 1929.
8. Lake, Norman C.: "An Investigation into the Effects of Cold Upon the Body," *Lancet,* **2:**557, (Oct.) 1917.
9. Bierman, William: *op. cit.,* p. 98.
10. Abramson, D. I., et al.: "Effect of Paraffin Bath and Hot Fomentation on Local Tissue Temperatures," *Arch. Phys. Med. Rehabil.,* **45:**87, (Feb.) 1964.
11. Lehmann, Justus F., et al.: "Comparison of Deep Heating by Microwaves at Frequencies 2456 and 900 Megacycles," *Arch. Phys. Med. Rehabil.,* **46:**307, (Apr.) 1965.
12. Lehmann, Justus F.: "Temperature Distribution in the Human Thigh, Produced by Infrared, Hot Pack and Microwave Applications," *Arch. Phys. Med. Rehabil.,* **47:**291, (May) 1966.
12a. Downey, John A.: "Control of the Circulation in the Limbs," in Downey, John A., and Darling, Robert C. (eds.): *Physiological Basis of Rehabilitation Medicine.* W. B. Saunders Co., Philadelphia, 1971, p. 157.
12b. ——: "Physiological Effects of Heat and Cold," *Phys. Ther.,* **44:**713, (Aug.) 1964.
13. Halsell, Marilyn: "Moist Heat for Relief of Postoperative Pain," *Am. J. Nurs.,* **67:**767, (Apr.) 1967.
13a. Lehmann, Justus F., and DeLateur, Barbara J.: "Heat and Cold in the Treatment of Arthritis," in Licht, Sidney (ed.): *Arthritis and Physical Medicine.* Elizabeth Licht, Publisher, New Haven, Conn., 1969, p. 316.
14. Stillwell, G. Keith: "Therapeutic Heat and Cold," in Krusen, Frank H., et al.: *Handbook of Physical Medicine and Rehabilitation,* 2nd ed. W. B. Saunders Co., Philadelphia, 1971, p. 259.
15. Millard, J. B.: "Conductive Heating," in Licht, Sidney (ed.): *Medical Hydrology,* Vol. VII. Elizabeth Licht, Publisher, New Haven, Conn., 1963, p. 240.
16. Stillwell, G. Keith: *op. cit.*
17. Erdman, William J., and Stoner, Emery K.: "Comparative Heating Effects of Moisture and Hydrocollator Hot Packs," *Arch. Phys. Med. Rehabil.,* **37:**71, (Feb.) 1956.
18. Juan, Sister M., and Smith, Reginald A.: "Postpartum Tub Baths," *Am. J. Nurs.,* **64:** 135, (Sept.) 1964.
19. Shestack, Robert, and Ditto, Edward W.: *Physician's Physical Therapy Manual.*

Prentice-Hall, Englewood Cliffs, N.J., 1964, p. 53.

20. Harrison, Ronald: "Heat in Vascular Disorders," in Licht, Sidney (ed.): *Therapeutic Heat and Cold,* Vol. II, 2nd ed. Elizabeth Licht, Publisher, New Haven, Conn., 1965, p. 411.

21. Sheldon, Nola S.: "Sterile Warm Wet Compresses," *Am. J. Nurs.,* 59:982, (July) 1959.

22. Modell, Walter (ed.): *Drugs of Choice 1972–1973.* C. V. Mosby Co., St. Louis, 1973, p. 626.

23. Von Werssowetz, Odon F.: "Heat in Neuromuscular Disorders," in Licht, Sidney (ed.): *Therapeutic Heat and Cold,* Vol. II, 2nd ed. Elizabeth Licht, Publisher, New Haven, Conn., 1965, p. 436.

24. *Ibid.*

25. Millard, J. B.: "Conductive Heating," in Licht, Sidney (ed.): *Therapeutic Heat and Cold,* Vol. II, 2nd ed. Elizabeth Licht, Publisher, New Haven, Conn., 1965, p. 241.

26. Licht, Sidney (ed.): *op. cit.,* p. 18.

27. Haines, Jill: "Cold Therapy Used by Physiotherapists," *Nurs. Times,* 64:25, (July 12) 1968.

28. Miglietta, Osvaldo E.: "Evaluation of Cold in Spasticity," *Am. J. Phys. Med.,* 41:148, (Aug.) 1962.

29. Licht, Sidney: "Local Cryotherapy," in Licht, Sidney (ed.): *Therapeutic Heat and Cold,* Vol. II, 2nd ed. Elizabeth Licht, Publisher, New Haven, Conn., 1965, p. 546.

30. Duke-Elder, Sir Stewart: *Parson's Diseases of the Eye,* 15th ed. Little, Brown & Co., Boston, 1970, p. 156.

31. Shestack, Robert, and Ditto, Edward W.: *op. cit.,* p. 54.

Additional Suggested Reading

Badder, E., et al.: "Circulatory Requirements for Heat Transport," *Surg. Forum,* 24:90, 1973.

Brouda, L.: "Heat and the Older Worker," *J. Am. Geriatr. Soc.,* 10:35, (Jan.) 1962.

DonTigny, Richard L., and Sheldon, Keith W.: "Simultaneous Use of Heat and Cold in Treatment of Muscle Spasm," *Arch. Phys. Med. Rehabil.,* 43:235, (May) 1962.

Ellis, M.: "Relief of Pain by Cooling the Skin," *Br. Med. J.,* 1:250, (Jan. 28) 1961.

Gerner, E. W., et al.: "The Potential of Localized Heating as an Adjunct to Radiation Therapy," *Radiology,* 116:433, (Aug.) 1975.

Hellon, R. F.: "Local Effects of Temperature," *Br. Med. Bull.,* 19:141, (Feb.) 1963.

Hickey, M. C.: "Hypothermia," *Am. J. Nurs.,* 65:116, (Jan.) 1965.

Kamon, E.: "Ergonomics of Heat and Cold," *Tex. Rep. Biol. Med.,* 33:145, 1975.

King, C. A.: "The Effects of Ice or Heat, Comparative Study on Muscle Spasm in Cases of Low Back Pain," *J. Can. Physiother. Assoc.,* 19:208, (Apr.) 1967.

Knott, Leslie W.: "Modalities of Physical Medicine, Their Uses and Abuses," *Mod. Treat.,* 5:909, (Sept.) 1968.

Kraus, Hans: *Clinical Treatment of Back and Neck Pain.* McGraw-Hill Book Co., New York, 1970.

Licht, Sidney (ed.): *Medical Hydrology.* Elizabeth Licht, Publisher, New Haven, Conn., 1963.

Mead, Sedgwick, and Knott, Margaret: "Topical Cryotherapy, Use for Relief of Pain and Spasticity," *Calif. Med.,* 105:179, (Mar.) 1966.

Rittner, E.: "Cryotherapy as a Preparation for Exercise Treatment," *Arch. Phys. Ther.,* 19:183, (Feb.) 1967.

Wakim, Khalil G., et al.: "Therapeutic Uses of Hot and Cold Procedures," *Med. Arts Sci.,* 13:176, (May) 1959.

Waylowis, G. W.: "The Physiologic Effects of Ice Massage," *Arch. Phys. Med. Rehabil.,* 48:37, (Jan.) 1967.

Gladys Nite
Virginia Henderson

CHAPTER 29

Baths and Packs for Circulatory and Sedative Effects

1. PRINCIPLES UNDERLYING THERAPEUTIC BATHS AND PACKS

Baths and packs are used in the treatment of inflammatory conditions of the joints and nerves, such as arthritis and neuritis, or in sprains or strains of muscles, before exercising stiff joints, as well as in treatment of low back pain with associated muscle spasm; or they may be prescribed in skin diseases as, for example, scabies and urticaria, in which relief is afforded by chemicals in the baths. Baths at body temperature are used to relieve tension and induce sleep; cold packs are also sedative because they soon reach body temperature. Ice packs, cool sponges, and spray baths are prescribed for the reduction of temperature in fever. Hypothermia blankets which are used for the same purpose are discussed in Chapter 42.

None of these treatments is used now as frequently as in the past. For example, Martha M. Brown and Grace R. Fowler (in 1971) say:

Hydrotherapy was one of the earliest methods used for the symptomatic treatment of psychiatric patients, and many psychiatrists and psychiatric nurses believe that it should be available to those patients who, for some reason or other, cannot be treated with medication. Although hydrotherapy departments may no longer be considered an essential part of many psychiatric units, the use of water in various forms to facilitate relaxation and to help reduce the individual's level of tension is still as effective today as it was many years ago. . . . The use of swimming pools and various water games for patients is a fairly new innovation in hydrotherapy and can have either a relaxing or a stimulating effect as desired.*

Figure 29-1 shows a group of patients playing games in the hospital swimming pool, a common practice in some Veterans Administration hospitals.

The effect on health of exercising the blood vessels (or stimulating the circulation by contraction and dilation of blood vessel walls) was discussed in Chapter 12. There has never been a time in history when baths of all sorts were more generally available. The spreading popularity of the Finnish sauna is an example of public enthusiasm for the effects in health of hydrotherapeutic methods used also as treatment of illness or injury. A winter sun tan is the trademark of the affluent class even though it must be given from a sun lamp.

In rehabilitation units, physical therapeutic measures are more widely used than ever. Unfortunately, patients are too seldom taught to adopt these procedures so that they can be carried out at home. Still more unfortunately the nursing staffs in the clinical units of hospitals and the staffs in visiting nurse agencies

* Brown, Martha M., and Fowler, Grace R.: *Psychodynamic Nursing, a Biosocial Orientation*, 4th ed. W. B. Saunders Co., Philadelphia, 1971, p. 158.

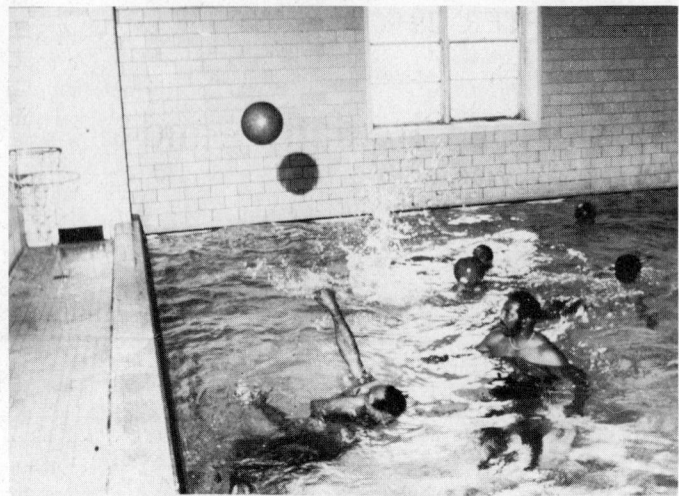

Figure 29-1. A group of patients playing volleyball in the swimming pool to promote socialization and relaxation. (Courtesy of Veterans Administration Hospital, Houston, Tex.)

often fail to help patients continue the activities taught them by experts in the physical therapy or rehabilitation unit—or make it possible for the patient to practice them. If all nursing students had some experience in such units they might be more effective in helping patients make optimum use of physical therapies—including baths and packs. As general hospitals have increased their emphasis on care of the critically ill there has been less reason and relatively less time for comforting and restorative aspects of health care, so helpful to those with long-term ailments. Nursing homes where such patients must seek care rarely have the facilities or a sufficient number of workers prepared to make the best use of them. These are some of the reasons the material in this chapter may seem "irrelevant" to many practicing nurses.

Heat can be applied in the form of hot air, steam, or vapor, and water. Heliotherapy is the use of light rays in the treatment of disease; infrared rays have a heat effect.

General applications of heat are rarely used for seriously ill patients; they have a profound effect, beneficial or harmful, according to the intelligence and skill with which they are applied. Before attempting to give these treatments, the nurse should know the patient's condition, the disease from which he or she is suffering, the action of heat, the effects desired, and how the particular procedure should be carried out to achieve the desired effect. Justus F. Lehmann and Barbara J. DeLateur, discussing effects of general applications of water, write:

. . . if the entire body is immersed, heat losses by radiation become impossible except in the area of the head, sweating becomes ineffective, and there will be interference with the systemic heat regulatory mechanisms, for only panting remains to rid the body of excess heat. With body immersion it is easy to raise the systemic temperature if the water is at or about 102°F.

Special precautions must be taken for body immersion in heated water since the artificial fever produced may be contraindicated in patients with poor heat tolerance, such as in disseminated lupus erythematosus or during cortisone withdrawal (accompanied by adrenal suppression). Water temperatures which elevate body temperatures in such patients have produced shock.*

Authorities agree that if water is applied above body temperature, a rise in the individual's temperature will occur and if the temperature of the water is below that of the body, the opposite effect will occur. Hans J. Behrend [1] says the change in body temperature may occur in less than 30 minutes.

The results depend on: (1) the water temperature itself; (2) the difference between the patient's skin temperature and that of the bath or pack; (3) the suddenness of the application; (4) the method of applying the hot or cold medium; (5) the extent of the skin surface covered by the bath or pack; (6) the duration and frequency of the treatment; and (7) the general condition, weight, and age of the patient. [2]

The effect of heat and the results of both local and general applications, but particularly the latter, depend upon the condition of the subject, the age, weight, and vitality. However, individuals respond differently to heat and cold and the reason for this is obscure. Studies

---

* Lehmann, Justus F., and DeLateur, Barbara J.: "Heat and Cold in the Treatment of Arthritis," in Licht, Sidney (ed.): *Arthritis and Physical Medicine.* Elizabeth Licht, Publisher, New Haven, Conn., 1969, p. 355.

have demonstrated that heat may have opposite effects—for example, on cardiac and kidney function—in different persons. G. Keith Stillwell [3] refers to the "idiosyncratic responses to heat" and stresses the importance of careful observation of the patient for specific effects of hydrotherapy, especially during the first treatment.

The comparative effects of hot and cold applications on the average person are listed in Table 29-1. The data are compiled from several sections of Frank H. Krusen and associates' *Handbook of Physical Medicine and Rehabilitation*,[4] Sidney Licht's *Therapeutic Heat and Cold*,[5] John A. Downey and Robert C. Darling's *Physiological Basis of Rehabilitation Medicine*,[6] and Sidney Licht's *Medical Hydrology*.[7]

Cold applications can be very injurious if they are prolonged, or if the patient hasn't sufficient vitality to carry the effects into the "reaction" phase. Elderly and debilitated subjects rarely "react" to general applications of cold; therefore, they are seldom prescribed for them or anyone with lowered vitality. In addition, they are used infrequently for the very young. Whenever cold treatments are used, temperatures should be modified to suit the condition of the patient; the more robust, the lower the temperature tolerated, as a rule.

Generalized hot applications can be so debilitating that the patient is prostrated. Hot water and steam baths are still prescribed, however, for certain conditions and in the recent past, artificial fever produced with hot-water, vapor, and light baths was used to combat infection. Other agents (the sulfonamides and antibiotics) have so nearly replaced this therapy that a discussion of it seems unnecessary.

Many hydrotherapeutic procedures include the contrasting effects of heat and cold. Hot-water or vapor baths are followed by cold showers, or extremities are immersed alternately in hot and cold water.

Hot baths are occasionally prescribed, but they are likely to be given in a hydrotherapy department under the direction of physical therapists. Patients with back injuries or with pelvic infections are sometimes advised to take hot baths at home. In such cases the nurse gives the patient some specific advice on the temperature and duration of the bath. Some persons need advice on how to get in and out of the tub and how to decontaminate it if they have a communicable disease.

Temperatures to be used in hydrotherapy and heliotherapy should be prescribed by the physician. Temperature equivalents are given in Table 29-2. All sources consulted give the same equivalents.

Several authorities comment on the high degree of discrimination that some normal subjects have for temperature of immersion baths. The difference of one degree can often be recognized. On the other hand, particularly

Table 29-1.   Comparative Effects of Cold and Hot Applications*

Effect of Brief Applications of Cold (Tonic Effect)	*Effect of Brief Applications of Heat (Atonic Effect)*
1. Peripheral vasoconstriction (pale skin)	1. Peripheral vasodilation (reddened skin)
2. Sensation of chilliness and tension	2. Sensation of warmth and general relaxation as bath progresses
3. Increase in output of blood with each heartbeat. Some authorities say the pulse rate is increased; others that it is decreased	3. Decrease in output of blood with each heartbeat is probable. The pulse rate tends to rise 10 beats with each degree Fahrenheit of body temperature
4. Increase in depth and rate of respiration	4. Increase in respiratory rate. One authority says the fall in alveolar carbon dioxide may produce alkalosis. The pH is said to rise from 0.1 to 0.3 during the hot bath
5. Rise in blood pressure	5. Fall in blood pressure, although this effect varies
6. Shivering, leading to increased heat production and the "reaction" to cold that lasts from 20 to 30 minutes	6. Decrease in heat production and profuse sweating
Reaction effect	7. Increase in number and motility of leukocytes
Peripheral vasodilation with reddened skin	8. Increase in local rate of metabolism results in increased concentration of metabolic products
Sensation of warmth and relaxation	
Decreased pulse rate with increased cardiac output	
Decreased respiratory rate	
Fall in blood pressure	

* Prepared from various sources listed above.

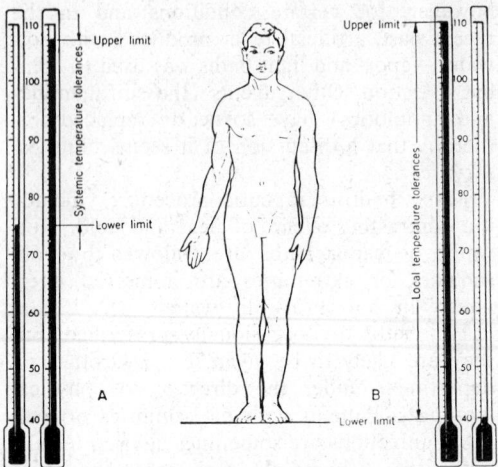

Figure 29-2. Temperatures which can be tolerated by the human body for long periods without producing irreversible damage. *A.* Systemic. *B.* Local. The indicated upper limit of systemic temperature is 107°F (41.7°C); the lower limit 75°F (23.9°C). The temperature tolerances of local tissues vary between 110°F (43.3°C) and 40°F (4.4°C). (From Bierman, William: *Physical Medicine in General Practice.* Harper & Row, New York, 1944.)

with local application of heat, the greatest care must be taken to protect the patients with fine discrimination. They may be burned. Morris B. Bender [8] found that if stimuli are applied simultaneously to two points on the body, for example, the face and the leg, the person is aware of only one stimulus. The face sensation will, in this case, take precedence over, or obliterate, that of the leg. In like manner,

Table 29-2.   Temperature Equivalents in Hydrotherapy*

Adjective Used to Describe Temperatures	Centigrade	Fahrenheit
Very cold	1° to 13°	34° to 55°
Cold	13° to 18°	55° to 65°
Cool	18° to 27°	65° to 80°
Tepid	27° to 33.5°	80° to 92°
Neutral or warm	33.5° to 35.5°	92° to 96° (neutral)
	35.5° to 36.5°	96° to 98° (warm)
Hot	36.5° to 40°	98° to 104°
Very hot	40° to 46°	104° to tolerance (115°)

* Licht, Sidney (ed.): *Medical Hydrology,* Vol. 7. Elizabeth Licht, Publisher, New Haven, Conn., 1963, p. 242.

severe pain in any body area, or a strong emotion, can obliterate the sense of discomfort from heat; therefore, the patient may be burned without his or her awareness. *Any form of heat applied to living tissue should be measured with a thermometer.*

Hydrotherapy and other means of lowering or raising the systemic or local body temperature have been used in the treatment of almost every known disease. Because water is the most universal solvent, it is used in conjunction with drugs for their chemical or physical effects. It is needless for nurses to try to memorize *all the uses* of heat and cold. Rather, they should study the physiologic action of different temperatures. This will enable them to understand why a cold, neutral, or hot application should be used; they will also be able to carry out procedures more critically. Figure 28-3 in Chapter 28 shows the response of capillaries to heat and cold. Seeing a microscopic moving film in which the vasodilation from a hot application is shown to persist for several hours usually convinces the nurse that hot dressings can promote healing of wounds. Watching a film that demonstrates the vasoconstriction of capillaries with the application of cold should explain the reduction in swelling after a sprain, for example, when cold compresses are applied. Treatment by water and sunlight has been used throughout the ages and in all cultures. It is not possible to list all the hydrotherapeutic measures the nurse is likely to encounter. Table 29-3 is an attempt to organize those most frequently mentioned in medical texts under general applications of heat and cold.

The *dangers* of excessive and prolonged cold and hot environments have been discussed in Chapters 42 and 15 and other chapters. Immersion of the body in cold and hot water and in steam has an effect similar to, but more marked than, surrounding it with cold and hot air. Prolonged local applications of intense cold and heat both paralyze the discriminatory power of the skin and interfere with the circulation.

In general applications of heat and cold there is a redistribution of the circulating fluids. Cerebral congestion can be controlled by cold applications to the forehead or back of the neck. Chilliness is mitigated by a hot application to the feet. These two practices are nearly always followed in giving sponge, spray, and hot-air baths as well as packs.

To guard against injurious effects, the pulse and respiration are taken before and after generalized hydrotherapy, and, if the therapy is prolonged, they are checked at intervals. The bath or pack is terminated if the patient

Table 29-3. Types of General Cold, Neutral, and Hot Hydrotherapeutic Applications

Cold	Neutral	Hot
1. *Immersion* (water) *bath* for tonic effect	1. *Immersion* (water) *bath* for sedative effect; if prolonged, it is called "continuous bath"	1. *Immersion* (water) *bath* to induce sweating and relaxation
2. *Shower* or *douche* for tonic effect. Often alternated with hot shower or douche	2. *Shower* or *douche* for sedative effect	2. *Shower* or *douche* to induce relaxation. Often alternated with cold shower or douche
3. *Wet sheet pack* with blanket wrapping for sedative effect	3. *Wet sheet pack* with blanket wrapping for sedative effect (used when patient cannot tolerate cold packs)	3. *Wet sheet pack* with blanket wrapping usually to induce sweating; occasionally to induce sedation
4. *Wet sheet* or *towel application* ("pack") for temperature reduction	4. *Sponge bath* for temperature reduction—water, or water and alcohol	4. *Steam bath* to induce relaxation and sweating
5. *Spray bath* or affusion for temperature reduction (patient recumbent)	5. *Spray bath* or affusion for temperature reduction (patient recumbent)	5. *Hot-air bath* or hot-air cabinet to induce relaxation and sweating
6. *Cold wet hand rub* for tonic effect	6. *Medicated baths* for sedation or for soothing or antiseptic effect on skin	
7. *Medicated baths* for tonic effect	(a) "Nauheim"—water baths charged with gas for sedation	
(a) Saline	(b) Starch, bran, or other cereal, and sodium salts for soothing effect on skin	
(b) "Nauheim"—water baths charged with gas for tonic effect	(c) Sulfur for antiseptic effect on skin	

is reacting unfavorably according to these signs or to what he or she says.

The types of general cold, neutral, and hot hydrotherapeutic applications are shown in Table 29-3. For a full description of these methods the nurse should consult such standard texts on physical medicine as those in the list of references for this chapter. The following description of some selected methods is largely based on these sources.

2. HOT TUB BATH

Selection of Method. This bath is similar to the cleansing bath with which everyone is familiar; it needs no definition. It is sometimes prescribed to induce sweating or to relieve pain and stiffness in chronic arthritic patients with multiple joint involvement and in muscle spasm, chronic myositis, fibrositis, and neuritis.[9] Some orthopedists advise a hot bath in conjunction with exercises for back and other injuries. It is prescribed for its relaxing effect, but if the water is very hot and contact with it very brief, the result is excitement and muscular contraction rather than relaxation. The temperature should rarely exceed 41.1°C (106°F). The bath should not last more than 10 minutes. Behrend says:

Its (hot water baths) widespread use taught us how rapidly the systemic temperature of some people rises when the body is immersed in water of relatively low temperature. Even in a water bath of 40°C, the temperature of a patient may rise to more than 40°C in less than 30 minutes.*

A warm or neutral rather than a hot bath should be used for a sedative effect.

Suggested Procedure. Underlying principles and precautions to be observed in giving the hot tub bath are the same as in all general applications of heat. Note the pulse, the patient's breathing, color, and expression for symptoms of excitement or signs of cerebral congestion, such as headache, nausea, and vertigo. To avert such reactions, apply cold compresses or an icecap to the head and raise the temperature of the bath slowly until perspiration begins.

Normal rate of perspiration is 1 or 1½ oz per hour or 2 pt in 24 hours, but by hot applications this may be increased to more than an ounce a minute. Remember that the loss of so much fluid has a very depressing effect on the heart, similar to that of hemorrhage. Except in edematous or dropsical conditions, encourage copious drinking of water before and during the bath.

Take every precaution to avoid burning the

* Behrend, Hans J.: "Hydrotherapy," in Licht, Sidney (ed.): *Medical Hydrology.* Elizabeth Licht, Publisher, New Haven, Conn., 1963, p. 243.

patient. The *temperature* of the water varies from 36.7° to 40°C (98° to 104°F), although sometimes, depending on the patient's condition and the effect desired, it may be increased, but never above 43.3°C (110°F). The *duration* varies from 2 to 30 minutes. After the bath the patient should lie down for at least 1 hour.

3. SEDATIVE BATH

Definition. A bath surrounding the skin with an environment free from irritation or stimuli is called a sedative bath because it favors relaxation and sleep. It is also called a neutral bath because the water is kept at about the same temperature as that of the skin, or around 33.3°C (92°F).

Therapeutic Uses. The sedative bath is used principally in insomnia to induce sleep and muscular relaxation, whenever indicated. A neutral bath is used also for its generalized vasodilation effect.

A bath at body temperature places no undue strain on the nervous or cardiovascular systems, but surrounds the body with a medium that shields it from all external stimuli or irritation of nerve endings from air, clothing, pressure, and changes in temperature. The bath is therefore soothing and quieting. If the body is supported, the patient often sleeps in a neutral bath. Until recently sedative baths were widely used in the treatment of psychiatric patients, but some current texts on therapy in the United States barely mention them or omit any reference whatever.

Hydrotherapeutic measures are at best palliative, and with the development of medication therapy and various forms of psychotherapy as well as shock therapy, less emphasis is placed on them. Some psychiatric nurses believe that this form of therapy has been used indiscriminately in the treatment of emotionally disturbed persons. Moreover, hydrotherapy demands more personnel and equipment than many of our overcrowded, understaffed psychiatric hospitals can boast. Insomnia and tension in many patients, even in general hospitals and homes, could, however, be relieved with sedative baths.

Suggested Procedure. The sedative bath is given in a full tub at a *temperature* from 33.3° to 36.1°C (92° to 97°F). Its good effects depend upon maintenance of the proper temperature. Its *duration* varies from 15 minutes to 1 hour, and the best time for it is just before bedtime. The subject then has the necessary rest following the bath with no danger from chilling.

In homes a sedative bath can be taken with ordinary bathroom facilities by simply regulating the temperature of the water. Physical therapy departments and certain bathrooms in psychiatric divisions of general hospitals are provided with special tubs for prolonged or "continuous" sedative baths. Regardless of where the bath is taken it is important that the environmental temperature be sufficiently high so that patients will not be chilled when they leave the bath.

4. CONTINUOUS BATH

Definition. When the sedative bath is continued for hours or days, it is called a continuous bath. The effect on the nervous system is the same as that of the sedative bath.

Therapeutic Uses. Continuous baths are used to quiet motor and psychic activity in diseases of the nervous system when the patient is hyperactive, excited, and unable to sleep; in certain skin diseases; in badly infected wounds; and in extensive burns and bedsores. Some physicians believe the healing process is stimulated by continuous baths; others think that it is hard for the body to form granulations and scar tissue when macerated with water. A great disadvantage of the bath lies in the fact that it cannot be made aseptic.

Suggested Procedure. Support the patient on a hammock or other device with the body immersed, the head resting comfortably on a rubber pillow. Apply cold compresses or an icecap to the brow or nape of the neck. Watch the patient very closely and take special care to see that the neutral temperature of the water is maintained. In a physical therapy department there are special tubs with provision for a constant removal of water and a fresh supply at the desired temperature. In many hospitals the water is thermostatically controlled, so that when the mechanism is set, no further adjustment is necessary. In any case, however, the thermometer should be suspended in the water so that the nurse can check the temperature.

Rub the patient's skin with petroleum jelly or oil to prevent maceration. Cover the tub with a sheet during the treatment so that there is no exposure of the patient. (Restraining devices that are buckled to the sides of the tub have been used for irrational patients.) Take care to prevent chilling by wrapping the patient warmly at the termination of the treatment (or when the patient has to leave the tub temporarily to empty the bladder or bowel); also by having him or her rest in bed after the bath for several hours.

5. COLD OR TEPID SPONGE BATHS

Therapeutic Uses. General cold baths are given in febrile conditions to relieve discomfort, to stimulate the circulation, and, where high temperatures exist, as in heatstroke, to reduce temperature. If used for temperature reduction, the treatment must be continued for some time to make it effective. Very high temperatures cause brain damage, so this treatment can be a critical factor in a person's recovery from heatstroke or from a febrile disease.

When giving general cold baths, the extremities must be massaged vigorously to overcome peripheral stagnation caused by vasoconstriction, according to Joseph M. Quashnock.[10] In a study of 130 children (ages 6 months to 5 years), Russell W. Steele and associates [11] report that sponging with ice water, 4.4° to 10°C (40° to 50°F), was just as effective as sponging with equal parts of 70 per cent isopropyl alcohol and tepid water, 29.4° to 32.2°C (85° to 90°F). Both were superior to sponging with tepid water. All children included in the study received an oral antipyretic drug (Acetaminophen) because such drugs are commonly used to reduce fever.

In the hydrotherapy department, cold spray and slush baths and cold douches are used for their tonic effect.

In the cold wet hand rub and the cold sponge bath, the water *temperature* varies from 4.4° to 24°C (40° to 75.2°F) or from 18.3° to 32.2°C (65° to 90°F), according to the age of the patients and their ability to react. The *duration* is usually about 10 minutes.

Suggested Procedure. Before starting the treatment bring everything required to the bedside. See that the room is warm. Cover the patient with a large sheet, while fanfolding the bedclothes to the foot of the bed; remove the pillows and gown. Adjust a loin cloth and place a large waterproof rectangle covered with a sheet under the patient to protect the bed. See that the body is warm before the treatment is given. Apply friction briefly to stimulate the skin, prevent chilling, and hasten the reaction. Place a hot-water bottle at the feet for comfort and to encourage the desired vascular reaction. Apply cold compresses to the head.

During the treatment the upper sheet may be removed, or it may be manipulated so that the parts under treatment are exposed in succession, then covered as reaction sets in. Vasodilation should be induced by rubbing. Two nurses may give the treatment, one applying water with the hands or with washcloths to the face, anterior surface of the trunk, and upper extremities, while the second nurse treats the lower extremities; this should last 3 minutes. The patient is then turned and the posterior surfaces treated, beginning with the neck, shoulders, chest, and so on, with special attention to the spine; this might take 7 minutes.

Watch the patients' color and pulse; if there is any indication that they are reacting unfavorably, discontinue the treatment immediately and report their condition to the physician.

When the bath is completed, pat the skin dry and cover the patient with the sheet. Remove the waterproof protector and sheet under the patient and put a warm gown on him or her. Massage the extremities to prevent venous stagnation. Arrange the pillows and bedding to make the patient comfortable. A tonic reaction to cold is promoted by hot drinks.

6. ALCOHOL SPONGE BATH

Definition. The alcohol sponge bath is a tepid or cold bath given with a 25 to 50 per cent solution of alcohol.

Therapeutic Uses. The alcohol sponge bath is prescribed for the same purposes as the tepid- or cold-water sponge—when the patient is to be disturbed as little as possible with turning or moving. Since alcohol evaporates at a lower temperature than water, the sponged parts dry more quickly, the patient's reaction is less violent, and the bedding is not so likely to be wet by the bath.

Suggested Procedure. Give the bath in the same manner as the cold sponge just described. Since, however, the alcohol solution evaporates so quickly, no rubber protectors are necessary for the bed, and, therefore, it is not necessary to turn the patient so often. Bath towels are placed at either side of the patient and under the legs. The sponge or washcloth should be only slightly wet. The back may be rubbed with the hand, moistened with alcohol, instead of with the sponge and, if advisable, without turning the patient.

7. SALINE BATH

Definition. This is an artificial sea-water bath, in which 8 lb of sea salt to 30 gal of water are used. By using 5 to 8 lb of ordinary table salt, practically the same effects may be produced. For partial baths, use 4 oz of salt to 1 qt of water.

Therapeutic Uses. Cold saline baths are used for their tonic effect. Health claims of the spas are based, rightly or wrongly, on the effect of the salts in their local waters.

Selection of Method. Sea water feels much warmer than fresh because the salt irritates or stimulates the nerves in the skin and so hastens vasodilation. The *temperature* of the bath is usually 21.1°C (70°F). The *duration* is usually 10 minutes, with friction during and after the bath. The usual precautions are taken to prevent chilling or exhaustion.

8. ALKALINE BATHS

Definition. An alkaline bath is one of natural alkaline waters or a bath prepared by the addition of an alkaline salt such as sodium bicarbonate to water.

Therapeutic Uses. Alkaline baths are most commonly used in skin diseases, to relieve itching.

Suggested Procedure. Add 4 to 12 oz of sodium bicarbonate to 30 gal of water. (For local applications ½ oz of sodium bicarbonate to 1 qt, or up to 8 oz of sodium bicarbonate to 1 gal, of water may be used.) Keep the *temperature* of the water about 36.7°C (98°F).

Encourage the patient to lie quietly in the bath for the prescribed duration. Do not apply friction during or after the bath. At its termination, wrap the patient in a sheet that has been warmed and dry by gently patting over it.

9. SULFUR BATH

Definition. A sulfur bath is a water bath (usually warm) to which potassium sulfate is added.

Therapeutic Uses. Sulfur is very toxic to lower forms of vegetable life. It is used extensively in the form of an ointment and occasionally in the form of a bath in acne and in other skin diseases such as scabies, where it is lethal to the itch mite lying within the burrows it has made in the skin. (A mixture of benzyl benzoate, DDT, benzocaine, and an emulsifier is perhaps more often used now for scabies.)

Suggested Procedure. Dissolve from ½ to 2 oz of potassium sulfate in a small amount of hot water and add this to the bath water (15 gal). The *temperature* of the bath usually varies from 32.2° to 35.6°C (90° to 96°F); the *duration,* from 10 to 30 minutes.

Metal bath tubs should be protected, as sulfur corrodes them. When the bath is given to relieve infectious skin diseases the tub must be decontaminated after use. (The writers believe this treatment is now rare.)

10. MUSTARD BATH

Definition. A mustard bath is a warm- or hot-water bath to which powdered mustard is added.

Therapeutic Uses. Mustard is an irritant, inducing vasodilation. It is sometimes used for adults with chronic arthritis or fibrositis, and in the relief of muscle spasm and pain; as mustard is irritating to the skin, it should not be used for those persons with a tender skin or skin diseases.[12,13]

Suggested Procedure. Add 1 tbsp of mustard to 1 gal of water. The mustard must be mixed into a paste with tepid water in the usual way, then further dissolved and thoroughly stirred into the bath water.

Suit the *temperature* to the patient's condition, but it may be lower than when water alone is used. It is usually 26.7° to 32.2°C (80° to 90°F), if the full effect of the mustard is desired. When the temperature is from 40.6° to 43.3°C (105° to 110°F), the mustard helps at first by hastening the desired reaction, but its effect is soon destroyed by the heat. The *duration* of the bath is prescribed by the physician, but the patient must be removed from the tub when the skin is a rosy pink.

11. EMOLLIENT OR SOOTHING BATHS

Definition. An emollient bath is a neutral tub bath to which some substance such as starch or a cereal has been added.

Therapeutic Uses. The bath is used to relieve skin irritation.

Suggested Procedure. Add 1 lb of corn starch or 4 to 6 lb of bran to 30 gal of water. The starch is boiled into a smooth paste, or the bran is boiled in a bag for 20 minutes. Either must be strained to remove large particles that would clog the plumbing. The thick liquid is then added to, and mixed thoroughly with, the bath water. The *temperature* is usually from 33.9° to 35.6°C (93° to 96°F).*

12. HOT PACK

Definition. A general hot pack is the application of blankets wrung out of water as hot as the patient can endure without pain or injury. A second wrapping of dry blankets is used to delay cooling of the hot wet pack.

Therapeutic Uses. Hot packs were at one time prescribed in diseases accompanied by suppression of urine; for example, nephritis, uremic poisoning, bichloride of mercury poisoning, and eclampsia. Modern treatments, including hemodialysis and peritoneal dialysis, are now used to control fluid and electrolyte balance; consequently, purges and sweatings are no longer mentioned in these conditions.

Jack M. Zislis [14] and William D. Robinson [15] note that the full-hot wet pack may be used for persons with extensive arthritis. Discussing treatment of the patient with rheumatoid arthritis, Robinson says:

---

* Aveeno is a patented colloid fraction of oatmeal prepared for baths and made by the Musher Foundation, Inc., New York. Its chief advantage is that it requires no boiling or straining.

Generalized heat is particularly advantageous for the patient with extensive joint involvement and has the advantage of stimulating the circulation, inducing copious perspiration and elevating the body temperature slightly.*

The *temperature* or *duration* of the pack is not mentioned by either author. Gertrude B. Finnerty and Theodore Corbitt,[16] however, suggest that the sheet or wool blanket, depending on the one used, should be soaked in water at 65.5° to 71°C (150° to 160°F) and every possible drop of moisture removed, to avoid burning the patient. The duration of the treatment may be 5 to 20 minutes. The procedure for applying the pack is essentially the same as described for the Sedative Pack, page 1362, or local hot packs used in poliomyelitis (see Chapter 28).

13. COLD AND TEPID PACKS FOR THE REDUCTION OF TEMPERATURE

Definition. A temperature-reducing pack is one in which the body is enveloped in wet sheets or towels applied at a temperature lower than that of the body.

Therapeutic Uses. So-called antipyretic packs are used to reduce dangerously high fever. They are also used as sponge baths or to make patients more comfortable and to stimulate the circulation when the body temperature goes above 39.4°C (103°F). Hypothermia is used as an anesthetic, but for other purposes within the scope of this book, the reader should consult Chapter 42.

Selection of Method. When cold is applied to the body for the reduction of temperature, care must be taken to prevent the sensation of chilliness and the consequent muscular reaction of shivering. It has already been pointed out that shivering raises the body temperature, and if the treatment is given to make the patient more comfortable, its purpose is defeated when the treatment is associated with the disagreeable sensation of being cold. This reaction is avoided by the use of friction accompanying the pack, which increases the blood supply in the skin. According to Theodore C. Ruch and Harry D. Patton[17] and other physiologists, people feel warm when the cutaneous vessels are dilated and vice versa. Bringing blood to the skin with friction not only keeps the patient from being chilly but also hastens the re-

duction of temperature by increasing the volume of blood exposed to the cooling action of the pack.

It is obvious that, when a cold pack is used for the reduction of temperature, the patient, wrapped in the cold sheet or pack, must be exposed to the air. The cooling effect of the pack is largely due to the process of evaporation. When water is changed into vapor, heat is required for the physical process, and this heat is taken from the body.

The *temperature* of the water prescribed for an antipyretic pack varies from 15.6° to 36.1°C (60° to 97°F), the higher temperatures being more commonly used than very cold ones at the present because it is believed that very low temperatures are more likely to elicit the shivering reflex and the general tonic reaction of the body to intense cold.

The *duration* of the pack varies from 15 to 30 minutes, but the treatment is discontinued at any time if any unfavorable reaction occurs.

Suggested Procedure. Prepare the patient by removing the gown and applying a protector over the pubic area, covering the lower bedding with a large waterproof rectangle, and replacing the top covers with a bath blanket. Apply a hot-water bottle to the feet, and an icecap or cold compress to the forehead.

The pack can be given with 2 or 3 small cotton sheets or 6 bath towels; the object in both methods is to keep the body covered with cool wet cloths. Encase the body with the exception of the head, feet, and hands in wet sheets or wet bath towels. Keep sheets or towels cool by having an extra sheet or towel kept in a basin of water the prescribed temperature and used as a replacement when the heat of the skin warms the covering. When sheets are used, change them about every 5 minutes; when towels are used, keep them rotating almost constantly. Apply light friction over sheets or towels. At the termination of the treatment, which usually lasts 20 minutes, dry the patient, remove the plastic and wet sheets or towels, put a dry gown on the patient and leave him or her to rest with an icecap on the head and a hot-water bottle at the feet. If there is any tendency to chilliness during the treatment, remove the pack and apply external warmth.

To see whether the treatment has reduced the fever, take the temperature and record it just before and an hour after the pack. Record the pulse at these times and at intervals during the treatment as indicated by the patient's condition.

During febrile states the physician ordinarily prescribes a high fluid intake to combat excessive water loss. While the nurse is giving an antipyretic bath or pack, she or he has an excellent opportunity to urge patients to drink such fluids as are included in their diet.

Recording the Treatment. Record the treatment, the time it was given, the duration, the temperature of the water used for the pack, the patient's temperature and pulse just before and an hour

---

* Robinson, William D.: "Diseases of Joints," in Beeson, Paul B., and McDermott, Walsh (eds.): *Cecil-Loeb Textbook of Medicine,* 13th ed. W. B. Saunders Co., Philadelphia, 1971, p. 1892.

after the pack, and any marked reaction to the pack, favorable or unfavorable.

14. SEDATIVE PACK

Definition. Sedative packs are prolonged applications of wet sheets to the body. Evaporation and cooling of the sheets, and also motor activity, are controlled by wrapping the body tightly in blankets.

Therapeutic Uses. Sleeplessness, hyperactivity, and excitement are indications for the use of a sedative pack. These symptoms occur in organic and functional diseases of the nervous system and in abnormal mental states associated with many kinds of pathology. The action of a sedative pack is similar to that of the continuous sedative tub. Although these methods were popular in the past, they are rarely used today. Of the two, the sedative pack is more likely to be used because facilities for its use are more generally available and it is a form of protective restraint for the hyperactive person.

Selection of Method. Sedating, or quieting the patient and inducing sleep, is the purpose of the pack. This is chiefly accomplished by having the sheets wet with water at the proper temperature, by insulating the wet sheets with snug wrappings, by seeing that the body is in a comfortable position, by removing stimuli from the environment, by continuing the treatment until the subject is relieved, and possibly by preventing cerebral vasodilation.

The various theories of sleep are discussed in Chapter 13. Those most often found are that sleep is induced by a reduction of sensory stimulation, by humoral or biochemicals usually produced by fatigue, and by chemicals that inhibit the activity of brain cells. Treatments used to induce sleep are usually based on the theory or theories accepted by the physician prescribing them.

Of the various factors affecting the success of a sedative pack, the *temperature* of the sheets is possibly the most important. A study made by Marguerite Kennedy et al.[18] in 1936 showed that water ranging from 8.9° to 100°C (48° to 212°F) for wetting sheets in packs was being used at that time in 24 mental hospitals. These workers experimented with temperatures of from 10° to 100°C (50°F to 212°F), using 15 young women in good health as subjects. The results of the investigation showed more complete relaxation and longer periods of sleep with cold sheets than with hot. Finnerty and Corbitt in 1960 recommended temperatures of 8.9° to 10°C (48° to 50°F) for "the active robust" patient, 15.6° to 21.1°C

(60° to 70°F) for patients of "average vitality," and 33.3° to 36.1°C (92° to 97°F) for less active patients. The less vigorous the person, the less able he or she is to stand low temperatures; several authorities say that the temperature of the pack should be determined in each case by the condition of the individual and the room temperature.

The *duration* of the treatment is 2 hours, usually, and should *not* exceed 3 hours at any one time, according to Marguerite L. Manfreda.[19] If the pack is to be continued for a longer period, the patient should be removed for at least 30 minutes, dried, and encouraged to void. When the necessity to void or defecate interrupts the prescribed time period, the pack is replaced. In cases of involuntary micturition or defecation, the patient must be removed from the pack, bathed, and re-enveloped in fresh sheets and blankets.

One of the most important points in the application of a pack is the proper adjustment of the sheets and blankets. It is important that the pack be snug, especially about the neck, so that there are no air pockets around the body; the covering must be smooth and the sheets so arranged that no skin surfaces touch. During the pack the patient perspires freely, and before sedation occurs, there may be friction from restless movements. In such cases excoriation is almost certain to result if skin surfaces are not separated. It is also important to make sure that the arms are beside the body and not caught under it. There is a difference of opinion as to whether the feet should be wrapped in the wet sheets and blankets or only in the dry blankets. It probably makes little difference in the final result, but it may be easier to keep the feet warm if they are not first encased in cold sheets. The feet should be warmed by a hot-water bottle throughout the treatment.

In all cases it is desirable to have the body firmly encased in the sheets and blankets, but this is essential if the person is resisting the treatment. Excited, irrational patients will work themselves out of this covering or, wrapped like a cocoon, will bounce themselves off the bed. Protection sheets may be placed over the chest, and sometimes over the knees as well, to prevent such accidents. Siderails are also used. Tight restraining sheets or other restraining devices should not be used for patients suffering from insomnia as they cause discomfort and fear. *The element of restraint is psychologically traumatic,* and patients are not forced to have this treatment if there are better sedative measures available.

Relaxation, which is such an important factor in promoting sleep, is induced in the dorsal recumbent position only if the knees are flexed and supported. A pillow under the knees relaxes the leg, thigh, and abdomen. Lateral and supine positions are impractical for the patient in a pack because the arms are bound to the body.

Appreciable amounts of fluid are lost in perspiration during the pack. It is therefore important to have this made up either before, during, or after the treatment. The practice of forcing fluids just before and during the pack is questionable, both because of the inconvenience of voiding and the objection to arousing a drowsy patient. A more reasonable practice is to make certain that the fluid intake is increased a few hours before and after the pack.

It is customary to place an icecap on the patient's head to relieve cerebral congestion. Some authorities suggest that the icecap be removed after the first reaction to the pack has subsided, if there is no headache, marked flushing of the face, or other indication for its use.

Sedative packs are generally said to be contraindicated in organic heart disease, in exophthalmic goiter, in advanced arteriosclerosis, certain atrophic muscular diseases, paralysis, old age, and during pregnancy and menstruation.

It is very desirable to gain the cooperation of the patient in this treatment since struggling against the pack delays its sedative effects and is psychologically traumatic. An explanation should precede the application of the pack. The nature of the explanation, as in all cases, is determined by the patient's powers of comprehension, vocabulary, and condition.

Suggested Procedure. Fanfold the top covers to the foot of the bed; protect the foundation bed, as suggested for the other packs; put a blanket crosswise on the bed so that there is an excess on one side; put a second blanket, folded crosswise, on the bed in such a way as to cover the feet on the lower third of the mattress; put a third blanket crosswise on the bed with an excess at the opposite side. The wet sheets are laid on top of the blankets. Three sheets are used, two large ones and a draw sheet in between, the latter placed crosswise on the bed approximately 10 inches below the top edge of the blankets.

One worker should arrange the bed while another prepares the patient, explains the treatment, and determines the pulse and respiratory rates. Undress the patient, drape in a sheet, and take care to see that he or she empties the bladder. Then both nurses draw the wet sheets quickly over the body, the left side of the pack sheet over the patient's left leg, under the right leg and across the body, leaving the arms free. Bring the end of the draw sheet up between the arms and the body, over the arms, fixing them to the side with the palms against the thighs. Put the third sheet over the body, covering the right leg and the feet. Wrap the blankets around the body in mummy fashion. Protect the neck and chin from contact with the blankets by a cuff made of the sheets. If protection sheets are used, place one over the chest, and if the patient is uncooperative, place another over the knees; adjust rubber-covered pillows under the head and knees; draw the top covers up and tuck a towel under the patient's chin to protect it from contact with the blankets.

Although the natural tonic reaction to the pack is a chilly sensation, this must not be prolonged. Put a hot-water bottle at the feet and use extra blankets if the patient feels cold. Apply an icecap to the forehead. Ventilate and darken the room, and disturb the patient as little as possible during the treatment. Take the temporal pulse and respiratory rates every 30 minutes until the patient is relaxed; and if there is any abnormality noted in the heart action or the respiration, as indicated by a weak, rapid pulse or cyanosis, terminate the treatment. As soon as the patient shows signs of drowsiness, remove the icecap, and adjust the top covering so that he or she is comfortable and warm.

On removal of the pack, rub the body with alcohol, rearrange the bed, put on night clothes and encourage the patient to rest for at least a half hour. The duration of the pack is prescribed by the physician. The treatment is not considered successful unless the person is relaxed or, better still, actually sleeps.

REFERENCES

1. Behrend, Hans J.: "Hydrotherapy," in Licht, Sidney (ed.): *Medical Hydrology*. Elizabeth Licht, Publisher, New Haven, Conn. 1963, p. 243.
2. Zislis, Jack M.: "Hydrotherapy," in Krusen, Frank H., et al.: *Handbook of Physical Medicine and Rehabilitation,* 2nd ed. W. B. Saunders Co., Philadelphia, 1971, p. 347.
3. Stillwell, G. Keith: "General Principles of Thermotherapy," in Licht, Sidney (ed.): *Therapeutic Heat and Cold,* 2nd ed. Elizabeth Licht, Publisher, New Haven, Conn., 1965, p. 238.
4. Krusen, Frank H., et al.: *Handbook of Physical Medicine and Rehabilitation,* 2nd ed. W. B. Saunders Co., Philadelphia, 1971.
5. Licht, Sidney (ed.): *Therapeutic Heat and Cold,* 2nd ed. Elizabeth Licht, Publisher, New Haven, Conn., 1965.
6. Downey, John A., and Darling, Robert C.: *Physiological Basis of Rehabilitation Medicine.* W. B. Saunders Co., Philadelphia, 1971.
7. Licht, Sidney (ed.): *Medical Hydrology.* Elizabeth Licht, Publisher, New Haven, Conn., 1963.
8. Bender, Morris B.: *Disorders in Perception.* Charles C Thomas, Publisher, Springfield, Ill., 1952, p. 11.
9. Zislis, Jack M.: *op. cit.,* p. 351.
10. Quashnock, Joseph M.: "Heat and Cold," in

Beeson, Paul B., and McDermott, Walsh (eds.): *Cecil-Loeb Textbook of Medicine,* 13th ed. W. B. Saunders Co., Philadelphia, 1971, p. 30.

11. Steele, Russell W., et al.: "Evaluation of Sponging and of Oral Antipyretic Therapy to Reduce Fever," *Pediatrics,* **77:**824, (Nov.) 1970.

12. Finnerty, Gertrude B., and Corbitt, Theodore: *Hydrotherapy.* Frederick Unger Publishing Co., New York, 1960, p. 157.

13. Shestack, Robert, and Ditto, Edward W.: *Physicians Physical Therapy Manual.* Prentice-Hall, Inc., Englewood Cliffs, N.J., 1964, p. 54.

14. Zislis, Jack M.: *op. cit.,* p. 350.

15. Robinson, William D.: "Diseases of Joints," in Beeson, Paul B., and McDermott, Walsh (eds.): *Cecil-Loeb Textbook of Medicine,* 13th ed. W. B. Saunders Co., Philadelphia, 1971, p. 1892.

16. Finnerty, Gertrude B., and Corbitt, Theodore: *op. cit.,* p. 117.

17. Ruch, Theodore C., and Patton, Harry D.: *Howell-Fulton Physiology and Biophysics,* 9th ed. W. B. Saunders Co., Philadelphia, 1965, p. 1056.

18. Kennedy, Marguerite, et al.: "The Sedative Wet Pack," *Am. J. Nurs.,* **36:**53, (Jan.) 1936.

19. Manfreda, Marguerite L.: *Psychiatric Nursing,* 7th ed. F. A. Davis Co., Philadelphia, 1964, p. 435.

Additional Suggested Reading

See "Additional Suggested Reading" for Chapter 28, page 1351.

Gladys Nite
Virginia Henderson

Massage, Therapeutic Exercise, and Pressure for Circulatory and Sedative Effects and Improvement of Muscle Tone

1. MASSAGE
2. THERAPEUTIC EXERCISE
3. PRESSURE AS THERAPY
4. ULTRASOUND

1. MASSAGE

Definition. Massage is scientifically designed and rhythmic manipulation of the tissues, although animals use a form of massage instinctively. Kneading, stroking, or friction may characterize the motions used.

Physiologic Effect and Therapeutic Uses. Miland E. Knapp[1] believes that many statements about the physiologic effects of massage are untrue because in the past the subject was taught by persons who had a limited understanding of physiology. He believes that through reflex effects initiated in the skin by massage, the muscles are relaxed and the arterioles are either dilated or constricted. He also mentions the "pleasurable" effects of massage. Sedation is a very important physiologic effect of massage, especially when given in a monotonously repetitive way. The return flow of blood and lymph is increased by the mechanical effects of massage. Controlled animal experimentation has failed to show that it reduces fatty tissue, and according to Gertrude Beard and Elizabeth C. Wood[2] massage will not increase muscle tone and strength or prevent atrophy. However, it will lessen the amount of fibrosis. According to the movements used, it can be a stimulant or a sedative to motor activity. General massage causes *peripheral vasodilation,* with a visible reddening of the area manipulated. With the dilation of the capillaries there is increased permeability so that the interchange of fluids and solids between the blood stream and the tissue cells is accelerated.

Massage has been considered a sedative for many years. Although it is difficult to find the scientific explanation, mothers and nurses know from experience that they can induce sleep with rhythmic stroking motions. How much of this results from the comfort of their presence and the sympathy conveyed by their touch, how much to the monotonous motion, or how much to the reflex effect is a question. Certainly an unsympathetic and rough operator can have the very opposite effect and so irritate the subject that relaxation and sleep will be delayed rather than induced.

Whether or not the effect can be shown to rest on a scientific foundation, massage is prescribed by the physician in abnormal conditions of muscles and nerves associated with disease or injury. It is used for relaxation, to relieve spasm, or to stretch contracted tissue.[3] It is also prescribed by the physician or used at the nurse's discretion as a sedative.

The physician should indicate whether massage is to be used as a stimulant or a sedative. If physical therapists are to carry out the prescription, they will know what motions to use. Since, in many cases, this type of worker is not available, both physicians and nurses should be familiar with the effect and nature of the common movements in massage so that they can prescribe them and use them effectively. If physical therapists are members of the health team serving the patient they may give a weekly or daily treatment and direct or guide nurses in supplementary massage. In conditions where long-term home care is indicated, either physical therapists or nurses may teach the families to give simple massage. Massage of the back is taught in home nursing courses and is as common as any comforting nursing measure. It is, in the last analysis, a substitute for active exercise when the patient's condition prohibits this.

Massage is contraindicated when there are skin lesions, infections, and malignancies, and

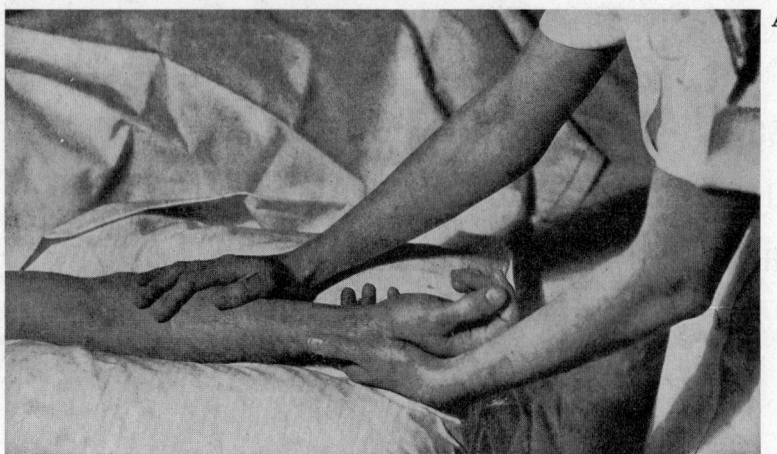

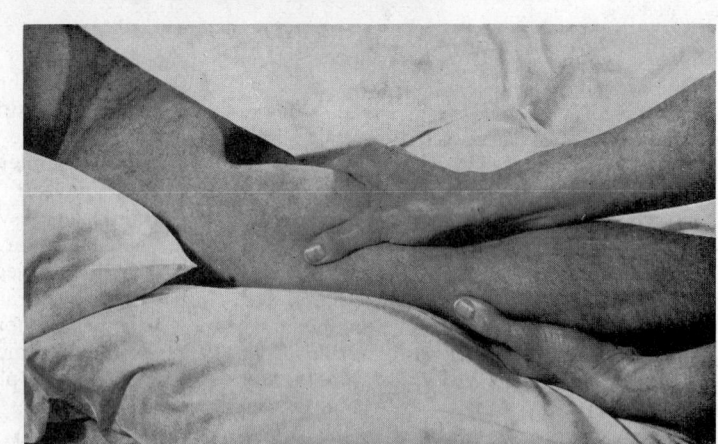

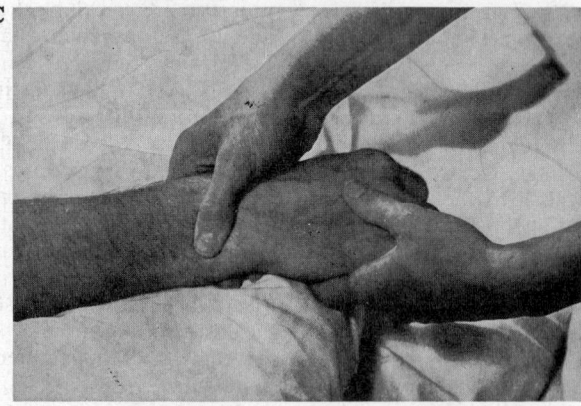

Figure 30-1. *A*. Stroking or effleurage, one of the common movements in massage. *B*. Kneading or petrissage, another common movement in massage. *C*. Friction, a third type of movement commonly used in massage. (From Krusen, Frank H. [ed.]: *Physical Medicine and Rehabilitation for the Clinician*. W. B. Saunders Co., Philadelphia, 1951.)

joints or fracture lines are avoided in giving massage. It is particularly dangerous to massage a painful extremity since the pain may be caused by a blood clot. Massage may loosen the clot and send it out into the blood stream where it may occlude a vessel supplying a vital organ, or a hemorrhage might result.[4,5]

Common Movements in Massage. Figure 30-1 *A, B,* and *C* show the three most common movements in massage: (1) *stroking* or effleurage, (2) *kneading* or petrissage, and (3) *friction.* Percussion or tapotement, which is rarely used, is not illustrated.

Suggested Procedure. See that the subject is in a relaxed (usually recumbent) position, in good alignment, and supported by pads or pillows as described in Chapter 12. Expose the area to be massaged, but make sure that the room temperature and covering will prevent chilling. (Relaxation is difficult under such circumstances.) Stand in a relaxed position facing the direction which the massage movements will take. Separate the feet to give a firm base on which the operator's weight may be shifted from the front to the back foot when long stroking movements are used. Lubricate the hands with powder, cocoa butter, mineral oil, or lanolin. Using the prescribed motions start with moderate force and rhythm; increase the force and then decrease it. Do not use the same motion on the same area more than three times but move on to another area before the subject begins to tire of the pressure or friction. Watch the patient's response and moderate the force used if he or she does not seem to enjoy the treatment.* Discourage talking by being quiet since both subject and operator should be relaxed. The following are more specific suggestions for each movement.

Stroking. Use long, slow, rhythmic movements, upward from the hand, foot, or buttocks, according to the part under treatment, and very lightly downward to begin the next stroke. Keep the entire hand or hands in contact wtih the patient's skin throughout and use firmer pressure on the upward than on the downward movement, or the return to the starting point. The force used depends on the effect desired and the tone and bulk of the muscles. It should be graduated so that the movement begins and ends gently. When stroking the back use both hands; when stroking an extremity support it under the joint with one hand while massaging with the other.

Kneading. Use a series of rhythmic, short, squeezing, wringing, or compression movements in the direction taken by the muscle kneaded. Keep as much of the hand as possible in contact with the subject's skin, but in this movement exert pressure with the thumb and the distal phalanges. Use both hands in kneading back muscles, but in treating extremities support and steady the part

---

* The interest, sympathy, or compassion of the operator is literally felt by the subject. It is impossible to massage effectively while thinking of something else.

with one hand. Pressure varies with the purpose of the massage and the patient's reaction.

Friction. With the thumb and distal phalanges exert pressure with a deep rolling or circular movement around (never over) joints or scars when the purpose of the massage is to break up adhesions.

Percussion. The nurse is rarely expected to use this type of massage, but it may be of interest to know that rapid, light, cutting, loose-wrist motions are made with the little-finger side of the operator's hand.

Aftercare. Remove excess lubricant with alcohol or soap and water if desired. This is refreshing in some cases but may tend to rouse the patient when massage is used for sedation.

2. THERAPEUTIC EXERCISE

The effect of exercise and its lack were discussed in relation to health in Chapter 12. The interrelation of thought and movement was stressed; even the philosophies based partly on body movement were touched on. The sensory deprivation from hypomobility is discussed in Chapters 12 and 38 and in other parts of this book. The intent in this chapter is to describe some of the more usual and specific exercises nurses may initiate or help patients perform after they have had specialized help from physical therapists.

If some one else will feed a human being, life can be maintained by movement of the involuntary, or visceral, muscles and those voluntary or skeletal muscles used in respiration that function reflexly and of whose action the individual is unconscious until it is interrupted. Exercise means to most people those body movements not associated with, or essential to, visceral activity. When these movements are prescribed by a physician they are termed therapeutic. Specialists in physical medicine are often more highly trained in this branch of therapy than general medical practitioners but they rarely practice independently. The patient's physician usually initiates or prescribes the treatment.

Since the services of physical therapists are not available to the majority of persons who need or would benefit from therapeutic exercise, physicians and nurses who are trained in this special branch of medicine can hasten the rehabilitation of many patients. In fact, there are few cases of illness lasting more than a few days where some form of exercise should not be used just to keep the patient from losing muscle tone. This principle has been recognized by many surgeons who make exercise a regular part of pre- and postoperative care (see Chapters 47 and 48). The same principle applies to the medical condition, as was thoroughly demonstrated by Joel E. Goldthwait and his associates [5a] a quarter of a century ago.

Nurses who expect to take a very effective part in kinesiology should make a special study of the neuromotor system in its relation to the underlying bony structure. When exercises are prescribed for their effect on a particular muscle, it is important to know its origin and insertion and its action or function. It is also important to know that all flexors are stronger than extensors, all adductors are stronger than abductors (except with the above-knee amputee), and the external rotators are stronger than internal rotators. The psychologic effect of motion was stressed in Chapter 12 but its value can hardly be overemphasized. The infant is soothed and rested by rocking as it is held in the arms or by rocking the crib; those confined to a room take comfort in rocking chairs, in beds that change the position of the occupants, or change pressure areas, and by other forms of exercise suited to their particular needs. Texts devoted to this subject describe therapeutic exercise, and anatomic monographs are available on the locomotor system that describe and illustrate every voluntary muscle that has been identified. It is not possible, however, in this book to give anything more than a bare introduction to the subject of therapeutic exercise. The student may pursue the matter by studying some of the references listed at the end of the chapter.

The purpose of therapeutic exercises is to increase or maintain mobility of joints and soft tissue.[6-6b] Such exercises may be directed toward correction of abnormalities (structural, functional) as well as toward rehabilitation (physical, social, mental). M. Dena Gardiner [7] says the aims of exercises are to minimize the effects of inactivity, correct the inefficiency of specific muscles or muscle groups, help the person maintain or regain normal range of joint motion, and perform normal functions.

After physicians evaluate the patient's general condition, physical abilities, and particular needs, they prescribe the type of exercise, its duration, and frequency.

Exercises may be *passive* (range-of-motion and massage, according to Nila Kirkpatrick Covalt) and carried out by the nurse, physical therapist, or occupational therapist without any assistance from patients (see Fig. 30-2); however, range-of-motion exercises are performed by patients when they are able. Passive movements are frequently used following removal of a cast (body, leg, or arm). They are also used for patients with a stroke, cord injury, neurologic deficit (such as multiple sclerosis, myasthenia gravis, poliomyelitis),

and for other persons who have a condition that prevents them from carrying out normal activities.

For most patients, range-of-motion exercises are used as a preventive rather than corrective therapy. Their purposes are to increase circulation, maintain joint motion, and minimize contractures. Nurses usually assume responsibility for initiating these exercises; however, in certain conditions where joints are affected (arthritis, for example) they should consult the physician.[8-10]

All joints should be put through full range-of-motion (see Fig. 30-3) five times each and repeated several times every day, depending on the patient's condition. Some authorities say these exercises should be carried out every hour depending on the patient's condition, while others suggest from two to five times daily.[11,12] Patients should be taught these exercises and encouraged to do them as their condition improves. Winnie Griffin and associates [13] describe an exercise program (including range-of-motion) for patients with orthopedic conditions.

Isometric exercises (muscle contracts against an immovable outer resistance) should be used (several times each day) by patients confined to bed rest for long periods. The exercises, also called muscle setting, are done by contracting and relaxing muscles alternately without joint movement. Mary M. Kelly says:

Setting exercises are particularly useful for maintaining the tone of the postural muscles of the buttocks, abdomen, and thighs. The patient can set the quadriceps, gluteal, and abdominal muscles separately, or he may set all of them simultaneously by lying supine with legs extended and hands at his sides, then lifting his buttocks off the bed, bearing his weight on shoulders and heels.*

E. A. Muller [14] reports that five maximal isometric contractions, each lasting 6 seconds, with a 2-minute rest period between each contraction will prevent loss of muscle strength in the immobilized person. After appropriate instruction and supervision, the average patient is able to carry out these exercises.

If patients carry out the exercise, the movement is termed *active*. O. Leonard Huddleston [15] describes the following types or levels of active exercise: (1) static, when patients contract and relax muscles alternately without joint motion; (2) assistive, when patients are helped by the operator or by other means, such as weights or pulleys, to perform the exercise (see Fig. 30-4); (3) resistive, when patients perform the exercise against resistance offered

* Kelly, Mary M.: "Exercises for Bedfast Patients," *Am. J. Nurs.*, **66:**2209, (Oct.) 1966.

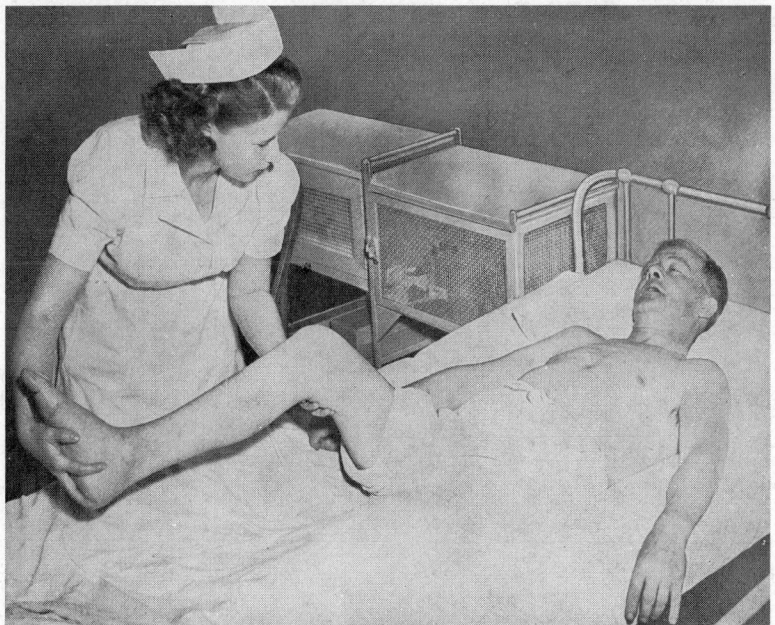

Figure 30-2. Daily passive motion of involved parts is important in the prevention of contractures. (Courtesy of Veterans Administration, Washington, D.C.)

by the operator, by gravity, or by a weight (see Fig. 30-5); (4) progressive-resistive, when weights and pulleys are used to provide a resistance load and developed in an organized system (see Fig. 30-6); (5) free, when the exercise is carried out by the patients "using minimal or optimal resistance to the motion." Figure 30-7 shows a patient engaged in exercises that strengthen muscles of upper extremities.

These local corrective exercises are selected and graduated according to the patient's needs. To be most effective they should be directed by experts. Adjustments in the scope and duration of the exercises are prescribed by the physician, but they may be instigated by requests from the patient, the family, the nurse, or the physical therapist.

In addition to exercises, the physician may prescribe immersion of a part in water. The arms or legs can be placed in a whirlpool tank, or the patient can carry out the prescribed exercise in a swimming pool. Water reduces the effect of gravity, and free movements can be carried out more easily or without tiring the patient when resistance to gravity is so minimized. Water therapy is frequently used for patients who have had poliomyelitis.

Occupations are also useful. The patient may be taught a craft such as weaving where a number of muscle groups are used and strengthened, or crafts such as knitting or blockprinting, where movements are finer.

Although nurses do not usually carry out or supervise local corrective exercises, they must be familiar with them and with the desired results. It is important that nurses know the time patients were served their meal so that they will not go to the physical therapy department for exercises until about 1 hour after they have eaten.

Nurses are responsible for noting and reporting to the physician any marked increase in the temperature, pulse, and respiration caused by the prescribed exercise or any soreness or stiffness that results from it. Nurses and physical therapists should regulate the environmental temperature so that patients are neither overheated nor chilled. Patients' records (made by nurses and physical therapists) should show the objective and subjective reactions to exercise and functional progress in the affected part. A form used to record various physical therapies and progress of a patient is shown in Figure 30-9.

In recent years, Thomas L. DeLorme and other kinesiologists have studied the effect of exercise on the size and power, or strength, of muscles. There seems to be considerable evidence that *exercise against resistance* is essential for maximum muscular development. Therefore, the physical therapist may initiate

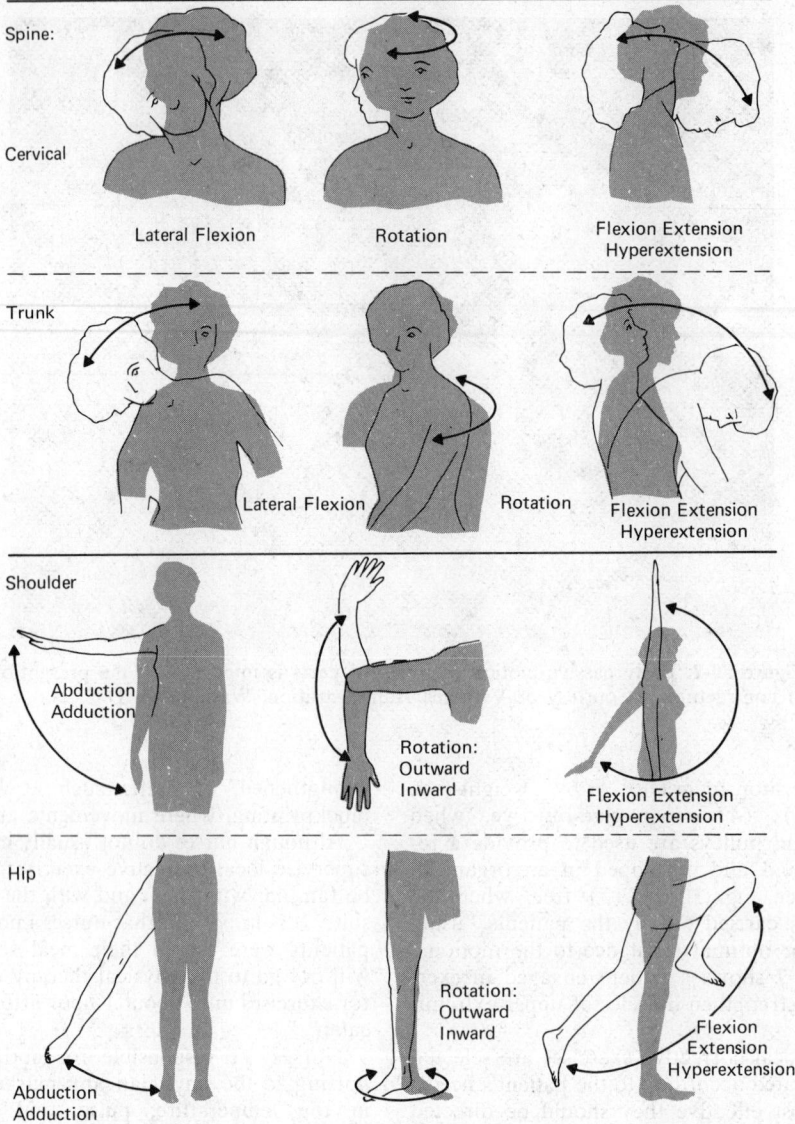

Figure 30-3. Range-of-motion exercises.

a series of exercises, prescribed by the doctor, that combine passive and active motions and include those in which the patient pushes with hand or foot against the operator's hand, or against a weight or some other object that offers resistance. Unless nurses have special preparation they cannot implement the physician's prescription without the supervision of an expert; they can, however, encourage all patients, except the most seriously ill or incapacitated, to use simple forms of exercise that will keep joints free-moving and prevent loss of muscle tone. If the complications caused by bed rest are to be prevented, all patients who

are confined to bed must be taught and encouraged to exercise. A discussion of the harmful effects of bed rest is found in Chapters 12 and 38.

All patients who are ill for long periods or unable to move themselves should have all of their joints put through full range-of-motion each day. Physicians may prescribe these exercises for specific joints of a person who has suffered a stroke, especially for the affected shoulder, hip, and thumb, several times a day. In every case the extent and frequency of exercise depends on the patient's condition, his or her physical abilities, and prognosis.

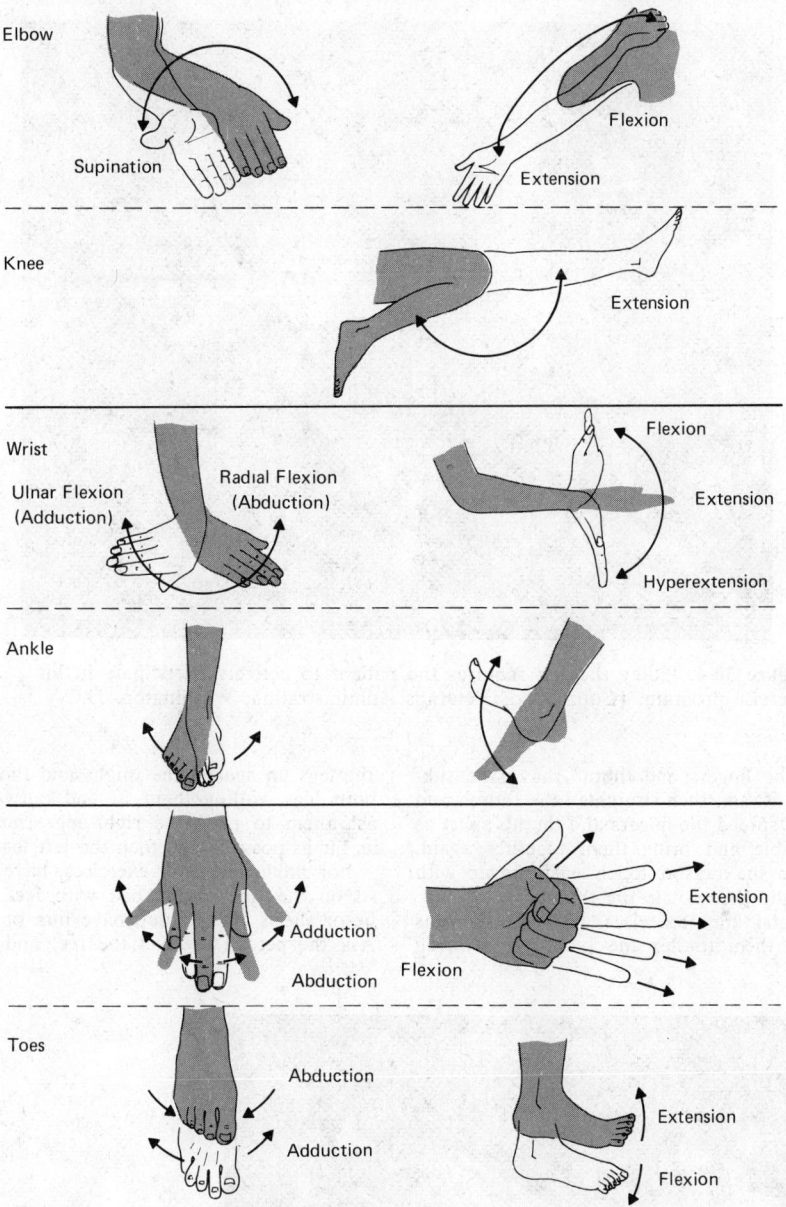

Figure 30-3. (continued).

Suggested Procedure for Range-of-Motion Exercises. Before starting the exercises, explain them thoroughly, including the benefits expected. (If patients are able to read they may be given a series of illustrated cards or a booklet to read first.) Ask subjects to indicate any pain or discomfort they have as a result of the movement. Have the person sit in a chair or in bed. Ask him or her to bend the head forward until the chin touches the chest, and then back as far as possible, turning the head to the right shoulder and then the left. When the head is in normal position, ask the subject to tilt the head toward one shoulder and then the other. For the upper extremities, ask the person to raise the arms over the head and then extend them to the side of the body and swing them in circular fashion.

To exercise the shoulder and elbow, ask the subject to raise the arm above the head and then bend the elbow, moving the palm of the hand until it rests on the back of the head. For the wrist and lower arm, have the person hold the upper part of the arm close to the body and the elbow at right angle to it and then turn the palm up, flexing the wrist, and then extend the fingers as far as possible and rotate the hand over and

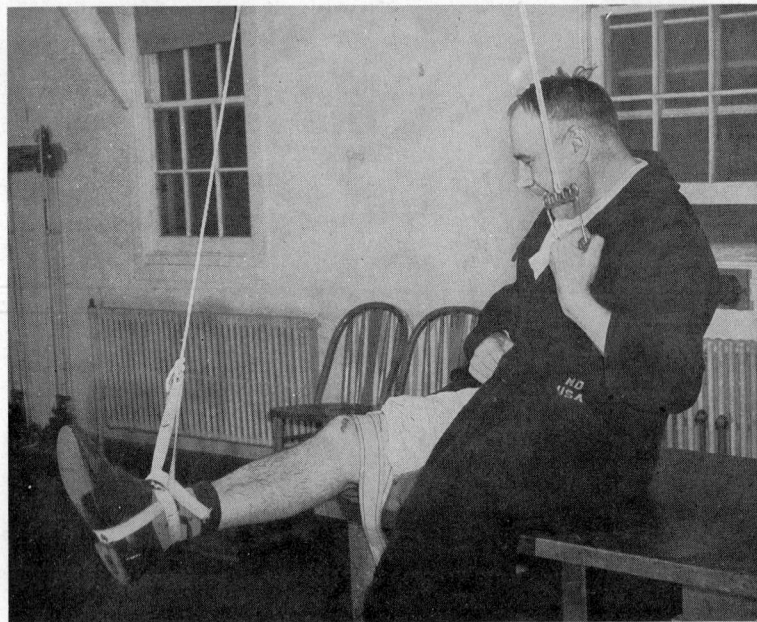

Figure 30-4. Pulley therapy requires the patient to actively participate in his exercise program. (Courtesy of Veterans Administration, Washington, D.C.)

back. For the fingers and thumb, have the subject make a fist and then straighten the thumb and fingers; next spread the fingers and thumb apart as far as possible and bring them together again. Finally have the person touch each finger with the thumb and then rotate the thumb.

For hip and knee exercises, have the subjects supine. Ask them to flex the knees by drawing the legs up against the thighs and then straighten both legs, rolling them in and outward. Finally ask them to raise the right leg straight upward as far as possible and then the left leg.

For ankle and foot exercises, have the subject sit on the side of the bed with feet dangling if he or she is able; if not, have him or her supine. Ask the person to bend the feet and toes down-

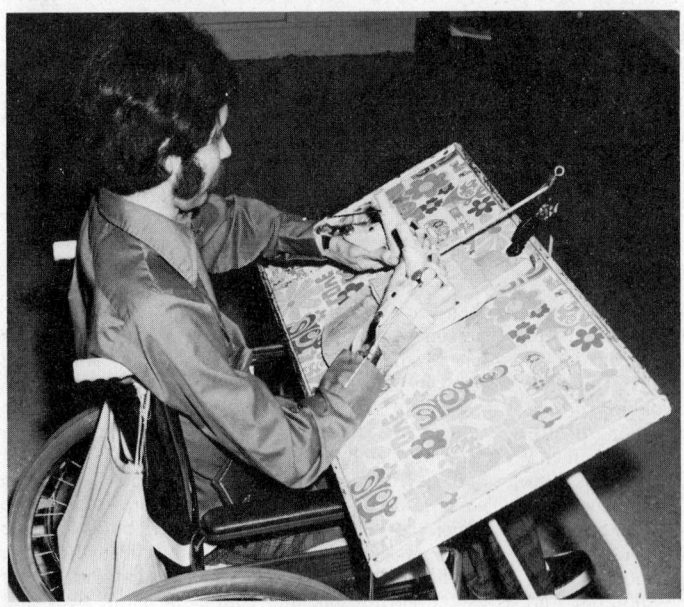

Figure 30-5. An example of progressive resistive exercise with use of a weighted sander. Note that patient uses hand splints to grasp the sander. (Courtesy of Veterans Administration Hospital, Houston, Tex.)

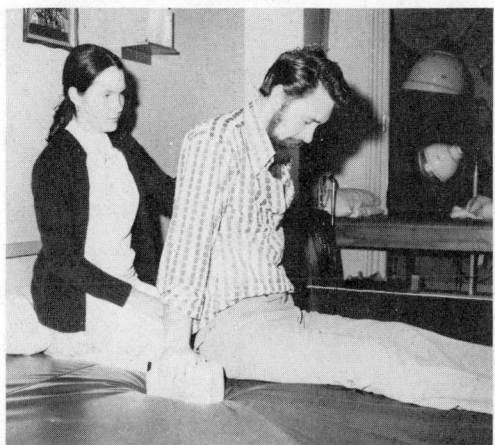

Figure 30-6. Exercises to strengthen muscles of upper extremities. (Courtesy of Veterans Administration Hospital, Houston, Tex.)

ward as far as possible and then upward, then rotate the feet outward and inward, finally circumducting the ankle.

Record the exercises and the patient's reaction.

If any of the exercises cause pain or discomfort, report this to the physician. He or she may prescribe other treatment (such as heat) to be given just before the exercises.

3. PRESSURE AS THERAPY

Uses. It has been found that circulation in an area can be stimulated by the application of pressure that is alternately more, then less, than atmospheric pressure; in other words, by alternate applications of positive and negative pressure. Some of the conditions in which this treatment is prescribed are thromboangiitis obliterans, acute peripheral stasis, as in chilblains or frozen extremities, arteriosclerosis

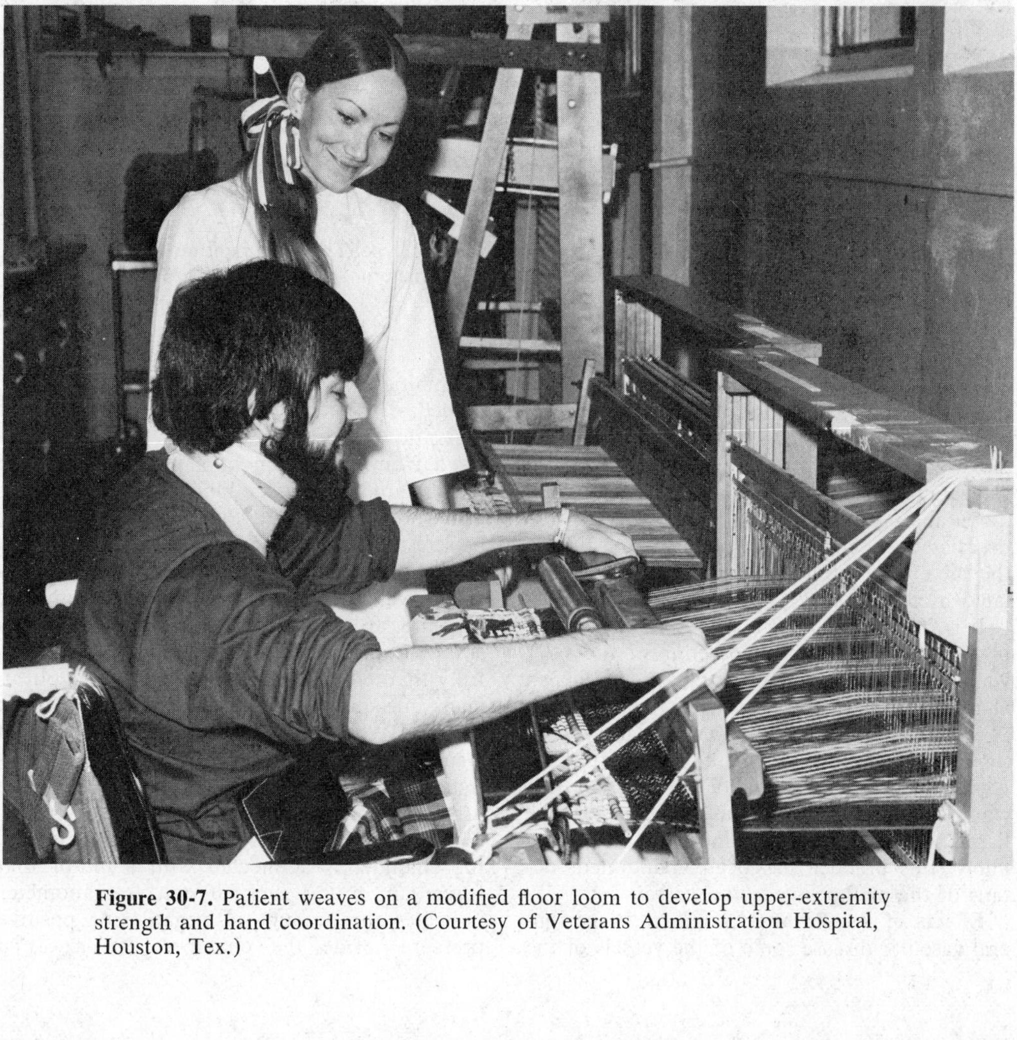

Figure 30-7. Patient weaves on a modified floor loom to develop upper-extremity strength and hand coordination. (Courtesy of Veterans Administration Hospital, Houston, Tex.)

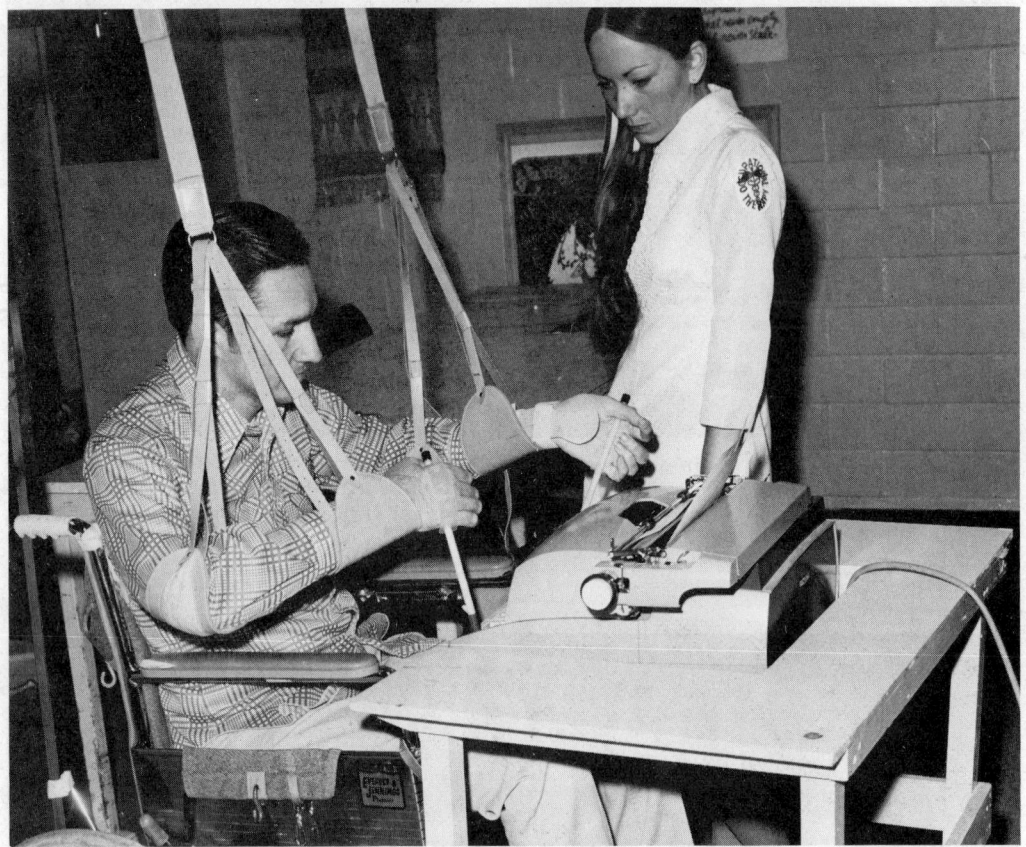

Figure 30-8. Patient with spinal cord injury learns to type. This treatment modality is also used to develop coordination. (Courtesy of Veterans Administration Hospital, Houston, Tex.)

(certain types, not all), varicose ulcers, and to reestablish the circulation following the healing of a fracture. Hadley L. Conn and Orville Horwitz [16] say the procedure is most helpful for patients who have had a recent and sudden inoperable arterial occlusion; however, it is used less frequently now than in the past since the advent of arterial surgery and the regulated oscillating bed.

It is interesting to note that "cupping," used in the past to produce hyperemia of the skin, was based on the same principle as the Pavaex chamber. It was, however, used for treatment of inflammatory rather than circulatory conditions. A negative pressure was created in glass cups by burning alcohol in them and then clapping the cups over the skin just as the flame was extinguished. Since, as far as we know, this practice has been abandoned, details of the method seem unnecessary.

Effects of the Pavaex Chamber. In peripheral vascular disease some of the vessels of the extremities may be obliterated or partially occluded. This interference may lead to areas of ulcerations and gangrene. Benefit may be derived from the action of a pressure chamber that alternately draws blood into the leg or arm and forces it out. Patency of vessels may be re-established or a nearly normal circulation established by increasing the capacity of collateral vessels. Changes in the environmental pressure are thought by some physicians to stimulate the arterial circulation more successfully than either heat or massage; other physicians question the effectiveness of the Pavaex device.[17] When used the extremity is placed in a suction-pressure chamber, which is made airtight by the use of a rubber cuff around the arm or leg at the point at which it is introduced into the chamber. The inner aspect of the chamber is connected with a motor that forces air in and sucks it out. A manometer indicates the amount of negative or positive pressure inside the chamber. *Pavaex* is a

PHYSICAL THERAPY RECORD

Date _____   Hosp. No. _____

Patient _____   Age ___ Sex ___   Clinic No. _____

Address _____   Phone _____   Attending Physician _____

Diagnosis _____

Date	PHYSICAL THERAPY MODALITIES	Technician

RECORD OF TREATMENTS

Month	1	2	3	4	5	6	7	8	9	10	11	12	13	14	15	16	17	18	19	20	21	22	23	24	25	26	27	28	29	30	31	Total

FORM L-101   PHYSICIANS' RECORD CO., BERWYN, ILLINOIS - PRINTED IN U.S.A.   PHYSICAL THERAPY (OVER)

Figure 30-9. A physical therapy record. The reverse side contains space for progress notes. (Courtesy of Physicians' Record Co., Berwyn, Ill.)

coined word from the initial syllables of the words in the phrase, *passive vascular exerciser*. The apparatus is portable, and the treatment is given to patients in their own beds. The time cycle and the pressures are ordered by the physician. Controls enable the operator to set the machine for the prescribed amount of negative and positive pressures and to time the phases.

As the pressure inside the chamber is re-

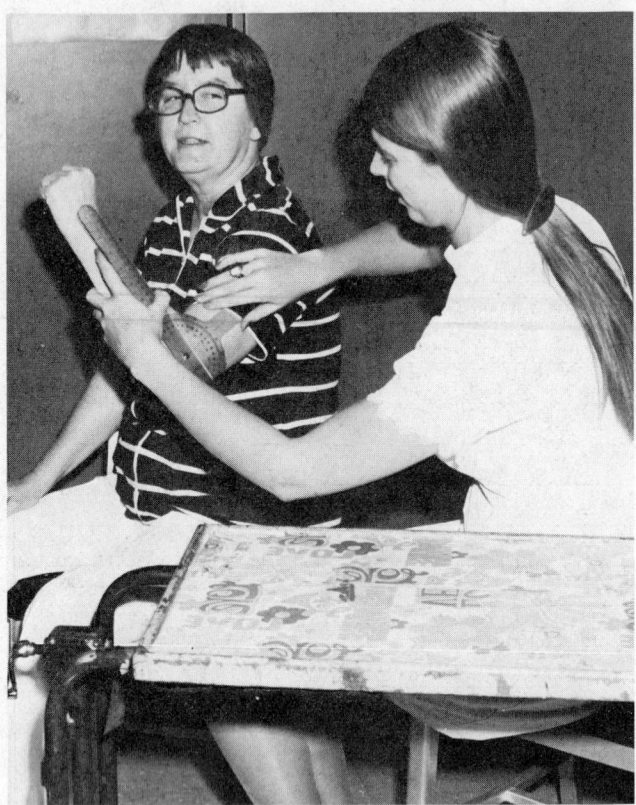

Figure 30-10. Prior to initiating a treatment program, a patient with arthritis is evaluated for range of motion. (Courtesy of Veterans Administration Hospital, Houston, Tex.)

duced below that of the atmosphere, the atmospheric pressure on the remainder of the body forces an excess amount of blood into the vessels of the extremity to fill the vacuum in the chamber. During this period, the skin flushes, the rapidity and the intensity of the reaction depending upon the extent of damage that disease has produced in the vascular system. The more intense the reaction, the less suction is needed and the shorter the time cycle. After the application of suction, air is forced into the chamber until the pressure is greater than that of the atmosphere. This phase is shorter than the suction phase, but should last long enough to force the excess blood back into the circulation. A typical cycle is one in which the period of negative pressure lasts 12 seconds and that of positive pressure lasts 3 seconds. L. Hobson [18] suggests bringing the negative pressure to 80 mm of mercury gradually and following this with a positive pressure that reaches 20 mm of mercury in the average. It is important that this change from negative to positive pressure be gradual.

In many hospitals the apparatus used for Pavaex treatment is operated by a physical therapist; in others, by a nurse. In either case it is desirable for nurses to understand the method, and if they are not responsible for the treatment, to cooperate intelligently with those who are.

The venous occlusion plethysmograph is used to measure circulation in an extremity or a part of an extremity. Its operation is like that of the Pavaex chamber. Nurses may assist the physician in this diagnostic technique.[19] The nurse's role in making this test is discussed in Chapter 7.

Suggested Procedure. Before starting the treatment, explain it thoroughly to the patient, giving some idea of the sensations he or she will have. If the person sees the apparatus before the explanation, it may be frightening; the nature of the explanation should vary, as in all such cases, with the person's physical condition and powers of comprehension.

Place the patient in a comfortable position. Since the treatment may last for as long as 5 or 6 hours, it is important that this position be one that can be maintained without strain. Elevate the extremity so that the foot or hand is slightly higher than the heart; this facilitates the return of the venous blood to the large veins.

If the leg or arm is ulcerated, remove the dressings so that the vascular changes around the ulcerated area can be seen. Protect open lesions by placing one or more sterile towels under the extremity. The leg or arm should rest on a soft pad. Since the extremity moves up and down in the chamber with the alteration of pressure, friction must be reduced to a minimum. The opening of the chamber for the admission of the leg or arm is made airtight by the use of a cuff. Powder the part where the cuff is adjusted to facilitate its application and removal. Adjust and remove the chamber carefully to avoid injuring the skin. (The conditions for which this treatment is used are ones that interfere with the healing process; therefore, any break in the skin may have serious consequences.)

Set the apparatus for the time cycle and pressure phases prescribed by the physician. Watch the skin, and if color changes are not satisfactory report it immediately, for the physician will undoubtedly change the prescription. (An effective cycle is one in which the extremity is flushed during the period of negative pressure and the flush disappears during the period of positive pressure. The desired intensity of these changes must be determined by the physician prescribing the treatment.) Having once established a satisfactory cycle, the apparatus may be left to run automatically.

The treatment causes no discomfort if properly given, and the patient often experiences great re-lief if the condition is one that responds to this type of therapy. An exaggeration of the former discomfort is an indication that the treatment should be discontinued; it is, therefore, very important to report the patient's sensations. While constant attendance is not necessary, a frequent check is, for some part of the machinery may get out of order and other untoward incidents may occur.

Record the time at which the treatment was begun and ended, skin color changes, and the subjective reaction. Also record the amount of negative and positive pressures used and the time relationship of the two phases.

The Oscillating Bed. Changes in blood volume in dependent parts may be accomplished by alternately elevating and lowering them. This treatment, combined with hot applications, is advocated in a circulatory disease described by Buerger and named after him. The exercises are also called *Buerger's exercises.* The same effect is produced by placing the patient on a bed that oscillates (see Fig. 30-11). The motorized bed, which lowers first the head and then the feet at a very slow rate, may also be used for patients who have spent

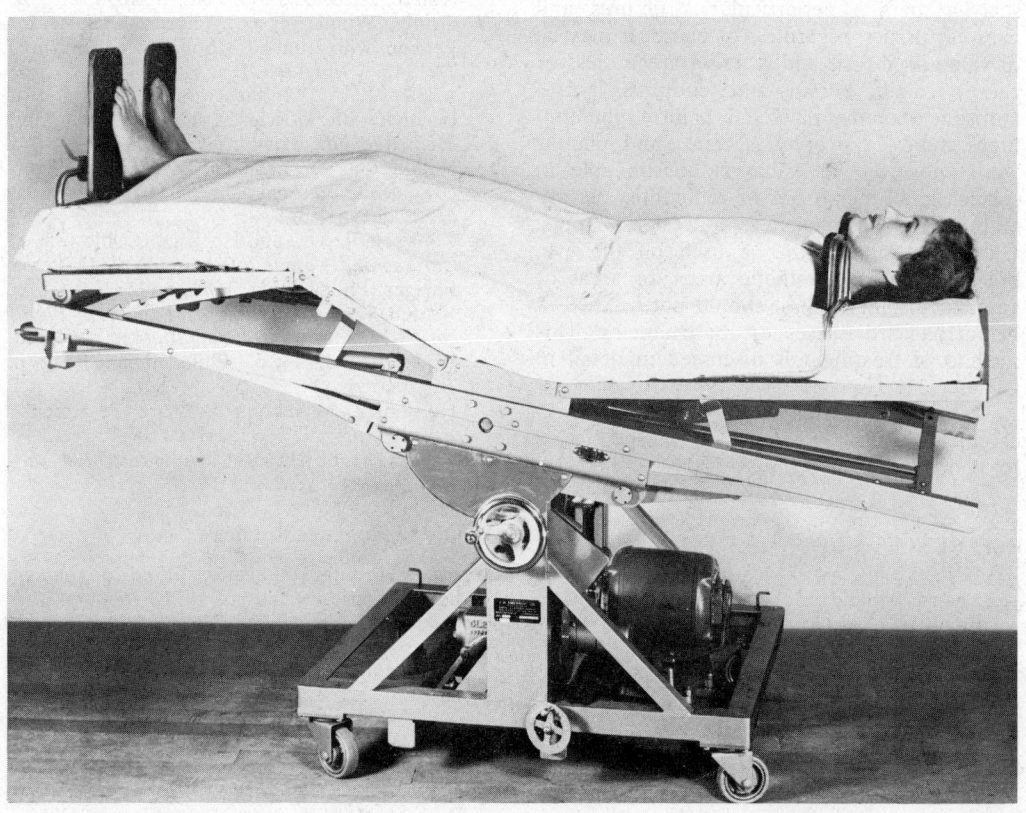

Figure 30-11. An oscillating bed. Note supports for shoulders and feet. (Courtesy of Emerson Co., Cambridge, Mass.)

some time in a respirator; it is, therefore, a valuable adjunct in the transition period when a patient is learning that he or she can breathe without such mechanical assistance. The oscillating bed was originally called the rocking bed because of its motion. The latter term may be used in some areas today.

4. ULTRASOUND

An ultrasound generator bears some resemblance to a short-wave diathermy generator. The ultrasound head is applied to the body or to the surface of a pan of water in which the hand or foot rests; it is a form of energy, and when waves are applied to the skin, changes have been noted by numerous scientists. The effects of ultrasound are thought to be caused by heat it generates; the degree of heat may be regulated through the amount of ultrasound used and the techniques employed.

Following an analysis of biologic and physiologic research conducted by many scientists, Frank H. Krusen and associates [20] concluded that treatment by ultrasound is effective in joint contractures resulting from tightness and scarring of the periarticular structures and capsular tissues, regardless of cause. It may be of value in fibrosis and scarring (regardless of cause), calcific bursitis and tendinitis, hydrocortisone therapy, pain and painful phantom limbs, reflex dystrophy, sprains, and plantar warts; however, its value is questionable in sciatica and other forms of radiculitis, peripheral arterial insufficiency, and nerve roots. Ultrasound should *not* be used on the eye, pregnant uterus, anesthetic areas, or areas of vascular insufficiency; it should not be used in hemorrhagic diatheses or malignancies. This method of treatment is discussed in detail in Chapter 31.

Treatment by ultrasound is given in a physical therapy department by specialists in this form of therapy.

REFERENCES

1. Knapp, Miland E.: "Massage," in Krusen, Frank H., et al.: *Handbook of Physical Medicine and Rehabilitation,* 2nd ed. W. B. Saunders Co., Philadelphia, 1971, p. 381.
2. Beard, Gertrude, and Wood, Elizabeth C.: *Massage: Principles and Techniques.* W. B. Saunders Co., Philadelphia, 1964, p. 46.
3. Covalt, Nila Kirkpatrick: *Bed Exercises for Convalescent Patients.* Charles C Thomas, Publisher, Springfield, Ill., 1968, p. 31.
4. Knapp, Miland E.: *op. cit.,* p. 384.
5. Covalt, Nila Kirkpatrick: *op. cit.*

5a. Goldthwait, Joel E., et al.: *Essentials of Body Mechanics—In Health and Disease,* 5th ed. J. B. Lippincott Co., Philadelphia, 1952.
6. Kottke, Frederic J.: "Therapeutic Exercise," in Krusen, Frank H., et al.: *Handbook of Physical Medicine and Rehabilitation,* 2nd ed. W. B. Saunders Co., Philadelphia, 1971, p. 385.
6a. Surdyk, F., et al.: "Strengthening Exercises for the Knee (Home Program)," *Am. Correct. Ther. J.,* **29:**143, (July–Aug.) 1975.
6b. Drummond, Rees A.: "Stabilizing Neck Exercises," *Physiotherapy,* **60:**244, (Aug.) 1974.
7. Gardiner, M. Dena: *The Principles of Exercise Therapy,* 3rd ed. Macmillan Publishing Co., Inc., New York, 1963, p. 26.
8. Kelly, Mary M.: "Exercises for Bedfast Patients," *Am. J. Nurs.,* **66:**2209, (Oct.) 1966.
9. Schultz, Lucie C. M.: "The Nursing Care of the Patient with a Stroke," *Ala. J. Med. Sci.,* **5:**27, (Jan.) 1968.
10. ———: "Nursing Care of the Patient with a Stroke," in Tantorski, Edward P., and Morphis, Maxine R.: *Principles in the Treatment of Stroke.* The Connecticut Stroke Program, Gaylord Hospital, Wallingford, Conn., 1972, Section IV, p. 1.
11. Brower, Phyllis, and Hicks, Dorothy: "Maintaining Muscle Function in Patients on Bed Rest," *Am. J. Nurs.,* **72:**1250, (July) 1972.
12. Kottke, Frederic J.: *op. cit.,* p. 389.
13. Griffin, Winnie, et al.: "Group Exercise for Patients with Limited Motion," *Am. J. Nurs.,* **71:**1742, (Sept.) 1971.
14. Muller, E. A.: "Influence of Training and of Inactivity on Muscle Strength," *Arch. Phys. Med. Rehabil.,* **51:**449, (Aug.) 1970.
15. Huddleston, O. Leonard: *Therapeutic Exercises, Kinesiotherapy.* F. A. Davis Co., Philadelphia, 1961, p. 23.
16. Conn, Hadley L., and Horwitz, Orville (eds.): *Cardiac and Vascular Diseases,* Vol. II. Lea & Febiger, Philadelphia, 1971, p. 153.
17. Krusen, Frank H., et al.: *Handbook of Physical Medicine and Rehabilitation,* 2nd ed. W. B. Saunders Co., Philadelphia, 1971, p. 707.
18. Hobson, L.: "Suction Pressure Treatment," *Am. J. Nurs.,* **37:**1091, (Oct.) 1937.
19. Krusen, Frank H., et al.: *op. cit.,* p. 704.
20. *Ibid.,* p. 316.

Additional Suggested Reading

American Hospital Association: *Winds of Change.* The Association, Chicago, 1971.
Boyer, John L., and Kasch, Fred W.: "Exercise Therapy in Hypertensive Men," *J.A.M.A.,* **211:**1668, (Mar. 9) 1970.
Brunnstrom, Signe: *Clinical Kinesiology,* 3rd ed. F. A. Davis Co., Philadelphia, 1972.
Colson, John: *Progressive Exercise Therapy in Rehabilitation and Physical Education,* 2nd ed. John Wright & Sons, Ltd., Bristol, Eng., 1969.
Duffield, M. H. (ed.): *Exercise in Water.* Bailliere, Tindall & Cassel, Ltd., London, 1969.
Hicks, Dorothy J., et al.: "Increasing Upper Ex-

tremity Function," *Am. J. Nurs.,* **64:**69, (Aug.) 1964.

Jackson, Bettie Springer: "Chronic Peripheral Arterial Disease," *Am. J. Nurs.,* **72:**928, (May) 1972.

Kendall, Henry O., et al.: *Muscles, Testing and Function,* 2nd ed. Williams & Wilkins Co., Baltimore, 1971.

Kraus, Hans: *Clinical Treatment of Back and Neck Pain.* McGraw-Hill Book Co., New York, 1970.

———: *Therapeutic Exercises,* 2nd ed. Charles C Thomas, Publisher, Springfield, Ill., 1963.

Lee, J. M., et al.: "Ice, Relaxation and Exercise in Reduction of Muscle Spasticity," *Physiotherapy,* **60:**296, (Oct.) 1974.

Licht, Sidney (ed.): *Therapeutic Exercise,* 2nd ed. Elizabeth Licht, Publisher, New Haven, Conn., 1965.

MacDonald, E. M. (ed.): *Occupational Therapy in Rehabilitation,* 3rd ed. Bailliere, Tindall & Cassel, Ltd., London, 1970.

Maitland, G. D.: *Peripheral Manipulation.* Appleton-Century-Crofts, New York, 1970.

Merton, P. A.: "How We Control the Contraction of Our Muscles," *Sci. Am.,* **226:**30, (May) 1972.

Morehouse, Laurence E., and Miller, August T.: *Physiology of Exercise,* 5th ed. C. V. Mosby Co., St. Louis, 1967.

Mundale, M. O.: "The Relationship of Intermittent Isometric Exercise to Fatigue of Hand Grip," *Arch. Phys. Med. Rehabil.,* **51:**532, (Sept.) 1970.

Murakami, I., et al.: "Proceedings: Reflex Vasodilation of the Central Nervous System in Response to Heat," *J. Physiol. Soc. Jap.,* **36:**392, (Sept. 1) 1974.

Nilsson, S., et al.: "Physical Work Capacity and the Effect of Training on Subjects with Long-Standing Paraplegia," *Scand. J. Rehabil. Med.,* **7:**51, (No. 2) 1975.

Pollock, D.: "Progressive Resistive Exercise Device for Quadriplegic," *Phys. Ther.,* **55:**992, (Sept.) 1975.

Powell, Mary: *Orthopaedic Nursing.* Churchill Livingstone, London, 1976.

Rusk, Howard A.: *Rehabilitation Medicine.* C. V. Mosby Co., St. Louis, 1971.

Smith, Genevieve W.: *Care of the Patient with a Stroke.* Springer Publishing Co., New York, 1967.

Thompson, Clem W.: *Kranz-Manual of Kinesiology,* 5th ed. C. V. Mosby Co., St. Louis, 1965.

Gladys Nite
Virginia Henderson

CHAPTER 31

Radiation Energies and Therapeutic Applications

1. BASIC CONCEPTS AND DEFINITIONS

Energy in its electronic form, according to Albert Szent-Györgyi, is a basic unit of life. He says "A molecule is, essentially, a cloud of electrons, held together by nuclei, and so its energy can be no other than electronic energy." *

The study of electronic energy forms and their harnessing for common utilization, medical data gathering, patient monitoring, and for therapeutic use is a twentieth-century endeavor. In the 1890s, Roentgen first produced x-rays by forcing a beam of electrons to hit a target in a vacuum tube, and a short while later, Becquerel first observed the emission of energy from the atomic nucleus. These events opened up a new era in therapeutics, and x-ray became a popular tool for attempting cures of all kinds of illnesses, some simple and some complex, until the dangers of its overadministration came to be recognized. After the work of Madame Curie, atomic radiation was tapped for therapy in the forms of radium and radon but it was not until after 1933, when Frederick and Irene Joliot-Curie first demonstrated the technique for creating artificial radioactive isotopes, that the emanations from other isotopes could be utilized.

Recognition of the importance of these therapeutic forms as a medical specialty was slow but today there is a new discipline known as Nuclear Medicine. M. J. Chamberlain says

"Nuclear Medicine, the application of radioactive materials to the diagnosis and treatment of patients and the study of human disease, has recently been declared a viable if not lusty infant, almost 40 years after its birth." * According to him, "Clinical Nuclear Medicine had its beginning in 1937 in San Francisco when Dr. John Lawrence gave radioactive phosphorus to a patient in an attempt to treat a form of cancer from which she suffered." *

The energy forms to be described in this chapter come from three main sources: (1) the nucleus of the atom (nuclear radiation); (2) light waves (the electromagnetic spectrum, including laser); and (3) sound waves (vibrations of particles in a material medium, also known as mechanical radiation). Also discussed will be the new field of biologic radiation.

Nuclear Radiation. Although today it is known that the atomic nucleus contains and emits many diverse particles or energies, only four emanations are of importance for therapeutics. They are the alpha ray or particle, the beta ray or particle, the gamma ray or photon, and the neutron.

The *alpha ray or particle* has been described by Paul N. Goodwin and his associates. They say that "Two protons and two neutrons form a stable combination called an alpha particle. Alpha rays from radioactive substances are streams of such particles." They go on to say, "all elements with atomic weight greater than

* Szent-Györgyi, Albert: *The Living State, wtih Observations on Cancer.* Academic Press, New York, 1972, p. 44.

* Chamberlain, M. J.: "Nuclear Medicine: What Is it?" *Alumni Gazette Univ. Western Ont.,* **52**:6, (Fall) 1975.

309 or atomic number greater than 83 have unstable nuclei; they are said to be radioactive." * In disequilibrium an unstable atom (radioactive) occasionally emits an alpha particle from the nucleus. These elements include actinium, polonium, uranium, radium, and many others. While it is possible for an artificially produced radioactive isotope to emit an alpha particle, it very rarely happens. The great majority of the artificial radioactive isotopes do not emit alpha particles.

In the early days of nuclear medicine an alpha emitter, such as radium, was mixed with a salve or placed in a small box or plaque. These were applied externally to the body and directly on the spot to be radiated. However, this type of application was proven ineffective and went rapidly into disuse. On the other hand, alpha particles, when ingested, are highly dangerous. In the body they act like calcium and go to bones. This is believed to be the prime reason for the development of osteosarcoma in so many of the radium dial painters. They ingested small amounts of radium daily as they moistened paint brushes with the tongue. In atomic nuclear disaster such ingestion can be prevented by using only bottled or canned foods and fluids.

Since the alpha particle consists of two protons and two neutrons, it can also be defined as "the nucleus of the helium atom." It has no orbital electrons and this makes it unstable. If it had two orbital electrons, it would be a helium atom. Consequently, it travels only a very short distance in air before it picks up two electrons and becomes an atom of the inert gas, helium. Therefore, we know it as a heavy particle (it has a weight of 4) having a short range. Alpha particles move at about 5 to 7 per cent of the velocity of light. Alpha particles are stopped by a few centimeters of air, a thin sheet of aluminum, or even by an ordinary sheet of paper. Radiation precautions (time, distance, and shielding) are not considered necessary for alpha emission.

The *beta ray or particle* is a fast-moving electron. It is extremely light and has considerable energy. Therefore, it can correctly be called a particle because of its weight, or a ray because of its energy. Goodwin and associates state, "The nucleus is made up of protons and neutrons: the electron is not one of its components. The expelled negative electron must then result from the separation of a neutron into a proton and an electron." † It is impor-

tant for nurses to realize that emission of an electron from the nucleus of the atom is *beta radiation*. Displacement of an atomic orbital electron, on the other hand, is *ionization*. The air path of a beta particle is usually several meters, and its penetrating power is greater than that of an alpha particle having the same energy. Even so, its penetrating power is only about 2½ cm or less. Therefore, Charles F. Behrens and associates [1] state that beta radiation's usefulness is limited to beta emitters that may be taken internally.

Today certain beta emitters retain their popularity and therapeutic usefulness. They are phosphorus 32, (P-32) which is useful for treatment of blood dyscrasias, and iodine 131 (I-131), which is useful for direct radiation of iodine-absorbing tissue of the thyroid. Both phosphorus 32 and iodine 131 are taken by mouth. Gold 198 (Au-198) is also an excellent beta emitter and is useful for direct radiation within cavities and in soft tissue tumors. There are usually no radiation precautions necessary for beta radiation since its penetration power is so limited. However, if the beta emitter is also a gamma emitter, then radiation precautions are indicated to protect against the gamma radiation. In nuclear disaster, no food or beverage contaminated with "fallout" should be ingested since beta radiation is harmful.

Gamma rays are *photons* which are quanta (bits) of high-frequency radiation. In the atomic nucleus, when an alpha or beta particle is emitted, such emission is accompanied by a burst of energy known as *gamma radiation*. Goodwin and associates state, "They represent excess nuclear energy remaining after the expulsion of some component, and the rearrangement of the others." * Atomic gamma radiation is identical with gamma radiation of the electromagnetic spectrum and *is by nature a high velocity x-ray*. Gamma radiation is the most penetrating of the three types of radioactive emission. Complete shielding requires thick layers of lead. When an isotope taken internally is a gamma emitter, such as Au-198 or I-131, radiation precautions should be taken for all patient "contacts." Isotopes emitting gamma rays are more frequently used in teletherapy (external radiation from a machine like an x-ray machine). The most commonly used isotopes for teletherapy are cobalt 60 (Co-60) and cesium 137 (Cs-137). In nuclear disaster, strict precautions should be taken against the ingestion of any gamma emitters in nuclear fallout. All gamma emitters are dangerous when taken internally.

The *neutron* can be used therapeutically, al-

---

* Goodwin, Paul N., et al.: *Physical Foundations of Radiology,* 4th ed. Harper & Row, New York, 1970, p. 221.
† *Ibid.,* p. 222.

* *Ibid.,* p. 222.

though such instances are very rare. John G. Taylor says, "Rutherford had already conjectured in 1920 that the electron-proton pairs that were in the nucleus might combine to make a neutral massive particle, which he called the neutron." * Its reality was confirmed in 1932 by James Chadwick.

Neutrons are available *only* at an atomic pile. Any therapeutic use of them would take place at medical research facilities located nearby. Direct neutron therapy is not satisfactory because skin ulceration is a frequent sequel. William H. Blahd [2] describes "neutron capture therapy." The customary procedure is to give the patient a stable isotope, which is absorbent to neutrons. Boron has been used in such a way in the past. Then the patient is subjected to bombardment by a stream of fast neutrons which renders the stable isotope radioactive. From this point on, the therapy continues from the newly made artificial radioisotope now in the patient's body, not from the neutrons themselves. However, many problems have arisen in the past with this technique, two of which are the chemical toxicity of the boron, and the difficulty in measuring the radiation dose. So this type of therapy quickly fell into disuse, although research along these lines continues.

Neutrons are hazardous only where there is an atomic pile; they constitute an occupational hazard to atomic pile workers. An atomic pile is composed of many rods containing isotopes emitting neutrons. These rods are usually shielded by water and further protection is afforded by careful technical handling.

The Electromagnetic Spectrum. The concept of the electromagnetic spectrum is fundamental to an understanding of radiation, either as a natural phenomenon or as a source of therapeutic energy. All observant people develop early in life a beginning conceptualization of this spectrum because they have seen and admired the natural beauty of a rainbow. A rainbow is a minute portion of the spectrum; it is the visible light wavelength which has been further differentiated into its component wavelengths by the refractive effect of light passing through water (raindrops). When looking at one edge of the rainbow a band of red color is seen which is the infrared wavelength of visible light. On the opposite edge a violet color is seen, which is the ultraviolet wavelength of visible light. But this is not the entire story. O. S. Heavens says "Electromagnetic waves [are] a whole range of waves of which light forms a minute part." † For a broader compre-

hension of some of the components in the electromagnetic spectrum, see Figure 31-1.

Electromagnetic radiation travels through space in all directions from its source, at the speed of light, which is 186,000 miles per second. This is the maximum speed at which energy can be transferred. Electromagnetic radiation is generated when an electric charge is accelerated. It always involves energy loss from the source of the radiation. The quantity of energy lost is related to the frequency of the radiation and so to the wavelength—the higher the energy value given off, the shorter the wavelength. The longer wavelength just beyond visible light is infrared. Still longer wavelengths are microwaves and radiowaves, also known as Hertzian waves. These have very long wavelengths and very low energy values. On the other side of visible light waves, where wavelengths become shorter and energy values higher, are, first, ultraviolet, then x-rays, gamma rays, and cosmic rays.

In order to fully understand this spectrum the behavior of light waves should be understood. *Radiation* is the means by which energy is transferred through space, which is accomplished by wave motions. The most common type of wave found in nature is the sine or sinusoidal wave (see Fig. 31-2).

There are various terms relating to specific characteristics of wave motions that are useful to know. A *cycle* is defined as the motion from one point on a wave to the exact point on the next wave (b). The *length* of a wave is the straight-line distance from peak to peak. The wavelength between points P_1 and P_2 is indicated by the line (a). The number of times

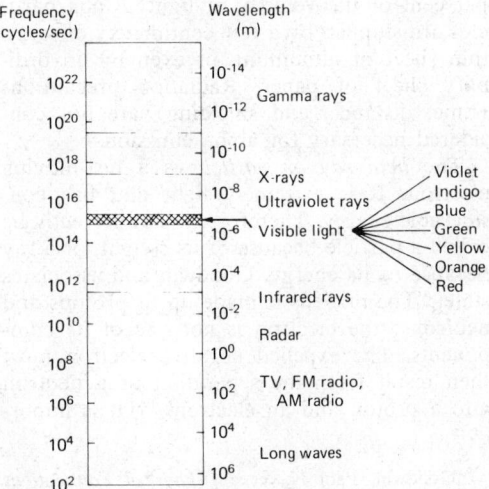

Figure 31-1. The electromagnetic spectrum. The portion that is visible to the human eye is only a small part of the total spectrum.

* Taylor, John G.: *The New Physics.* Basic Books, Inc., New York, 1972, p. 58.

† Heavens, O. S.: *Lasers.* Charles Scribner's Sons, New York, 1971, p. 10.

Figure 31-2. The sine (or sinusoidal) wave shown diagrammatically. The wave length (*a*) is the distance from P_1 to P_2; a cycle (*b*) is one complete wave; the frequency is the number of cycles that occur in 1 second (*c*) (in this case the frequency is 1¾ cycles per second); and the amplitude (*d*) is the height of the wave. As can be seen from Figure 31-1, visible light waves have a frequency of approximately 10,000,000,000,000,000 cycles per second and a wavelength of approximately 0.000,000,1 meters.

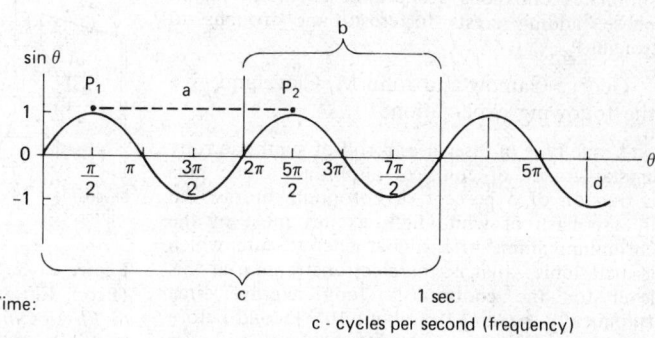

per second that a given wave repeats its cycle is called *frequency,* commonly abbreviated as cps (cycles per second) (c). The *amplitude* of a wave is the distance of the peak from the midline about which the wave oscillates (d). *Velocity* or speed is the time taken for the wave to travel in space.

Electromagnetic radiation exhibits wavelike properties under some experimental conditions and behaves like a stream of particles under other conditions. The particle-like behavior of light is most pronounced at the high frequencies of gamma radiation. Such a particle of radiation energy is known as a photon.

Atoms of all matter are in continual vibration (thermal motion) and they are continually radiating electromagnetic waves. Every gas, liquid, or solid object at temperatures above absolute zero degrees gives off radiant energy. Thermal radiation has a broad range of frequency corresponding to the continuum of frequencies of oscillating atoms or molecules. The higher the temperature of the material, the more violent the atomic vibrations, and although at lower temperatures the effects of these vibrations are not visible, at about 500 degrees, bodies become "red hot," emitting red light. The sun, which is the earth's natural source of radiant energy, emits radiations continuously over a very wide range of the spectrum. However, in the passage of sunlight through the atmosphere to the earth, many of the sun's rays are absorbed and scattered. The ozone absorbs the ultraviolet; water vapor absorbs some of the infrared lengths; and smoke, dust particles, and water vapor scatter the rays, especially the shorter ones. Solid objects emit almost continuous spectra.

Today, scientists have learned how to harness the energies of the electromagnetic spectrum for man's use. Our homes contain many objects utilizing these energies. A few illustrations are radio, television, electric lights, sun lamps, heating pads, and microwave ovens. Medical science has harnessed for therapeutic use microwaves (diathermy), infrared, ultraviolet, and x-rays. The specific use of each of these will be developed later in this chapter.

Paradoxically, while the energies of the electromagnetic spectrum benefit mankind, they also present hazards, some of them lethal. Care must be taken to prevent electric shock. Today there is concern over hazardous radiation emissions from some microwave ovens and some color television sets. However, safety standards are constantly being reviewed for all home appliances and this means continual improvement from the standpoint of safety. Most national governments set and maintain safety standards for all therapeutic equipment to minimize the hazards of using this kind of equipment. (See also Chapter 15.)

Laser is a newcomer to the therapeutic utilization of the visible light wavelength of the electromagnetic spectrum. It is defined by Heavens [3] as "_l_ight _a_mplification by the _s_timulated _e_mission of _r_adiation." Its name is formed from the first letters of the words in its definition as underlined above.

Man's ability to amplify light was first demonstrated in 1960 and the exploration of this field has developed rapidly since. Heavens describes the laser as "a device which produces an intense, highly directional beam of light of a very pure color" and goes on to say "The laser beam also possesses the property of coherence, which indicates a certain regularity of the waves in the beam." *

Arthur W. Wiggins describes more fully how the laser is developed by saying:

Atoms are pumped to a higher energy level by shining radiation of just the right wavelength on them; when they jump back to their original

---

* *Ibid.,* p. 2.

energy level, the radiation each atom gives off stimulates emissions from another atom, all in phase, adding crests to crests and troughs to troughs.*

George Gamow and John M. Cleveland give the following explanation:

. . . one type of laser uses a rod of synthetic ruby crystal—made of colorless aluminum oxide plus a fraction of a percent of chromium atoms. An intense flash of white light excites most of the chromium atoms to a higher energy state which is metastable—that is, the electrons remain at this level for the enormously long average time (atomically speaking) of about 10^{-3} second before spontaneously dropping back to a level of lower energy.†

Hessel Howard Flitter [4] stresses that the dropping back to a lower level releases the energy which is the laser beam itself.

Gamow and Cleveland continue to describe the laser apparatus:

. . . the synthetic ruby is made in the shape of a cylinder, with its ends exactly flat and exactly parallel. These ends are now silvered—one completely, to reflect as perfectly as possible; and the other only partially, so that a fraction of the incident photons may escape. An early spontaneous photon, that is of just the right wavelength and is exactly perpendicular to the silvered ends, will be reflected back and forth between them to set up a standing wave. This stimulates the emission of other photons, which follow it exactly in both phase and direction, and these stimulate others, and so on until this standing wave grows to enormous intensity. Photons from this standing wave that leak through the partially silvered end constitute the actual laser beam. This is a beam of coherent light. All the photons are in phase with each other, and all are traveling in the same direction. Such a coherent beam will spread very little. It can be focused by lenses or mirrors to a tiny point of concentrated energy, able to burn through steel, to make microscopic welds, or to sear living tissues in bloodless surgery.‡

For a schematic diagram of the ruby laser, see Figure 31-3.

Laser beams as a therapeutic tool have already been used successfully in some types of ophthalmologic work and are being used experimentally in the so-called "bloodless surgery" field. Also, the destruction of malignant tissues is being attempted by their use. Laser is

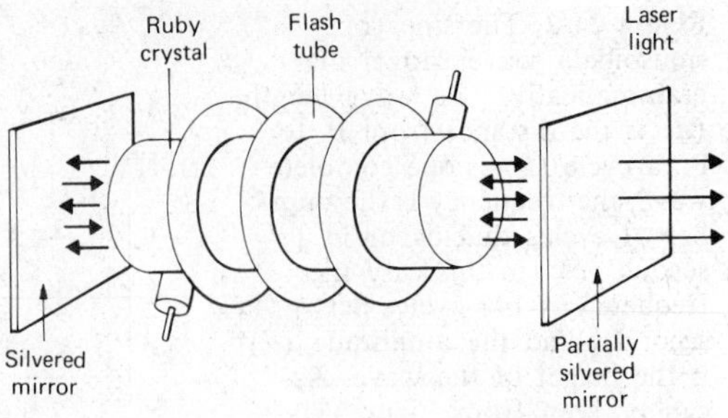

* Wiggins, Arthur W.: *Physical Science with Environmental Applications.* Houghton Mifflin Co., Boston, 1974, p. 264.

† Gamow, George, and Cleveland, John M.: *Physics, Foundations and Frontiers,* 2nd ed. Prentice Hall, Inc., Englewood Cliffs, N.J., 1969, p. 429.

‡ *Ibid.,* p. 429.

Figure 31-3. Schematic diagram of the ruby laser. (From Flitter, Hessel Howard: *An Introduction to Physics in Nursing,* 6th ed. C. V. Mosby Co., St. Louis, 1972, p. 249.)

a tool of extraordinary power and man needs time to develop its full potential.

Mechanical Radiation. This refers to a wave motion passing *through a medium,* such as the mechanical wave motions of water, and sound waves in air, water, or other substances. These are relatively slow waves. Sound waves in air travel at 1100 ft per second in all directions from their source. Sound waves and shock waves (air movement) originate when part of a medium adjacent to a moving object is displaced from its state of equilibrium. Since every small part of the medium is elastically connected with its neighboring part, the disturbance is transmitted throughout the medium. The object causing the original disturbance expends energy in doing so, and this energy is propagated through the medium by the waves.

Biologic Radiation. While radiations from nonliving substances have been studied by physicists and other natural scientists, it is only recently that the full range of the radiations from biologic material and living organisms, their electrical and magnetic fields, have been given much serious attention. A fuller understanding of bioelectricity may hold great promise in the study of man in his environment and his health. Harold Saxton Burr, whose work is discussed elsewhere in this book, pioneered in this field while at Yale University over 40 years ago. Leonard Ravitz, a psychiatrist who studied with Burr, continued his work, and Russian scientists have done much in this field.[5] An example of the evidence of the electric field produced by and surrounding the body is shown in photographs of fingertips (see Fig. 31-4) produced through a special electrophotographic process developed by a Russian husband and wife team.[6] These photographs were taken by the second author in studies she is conducting with the technique.

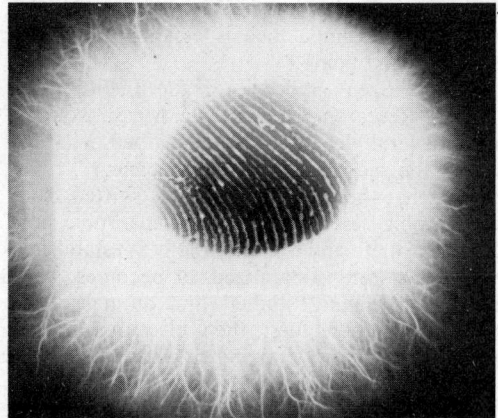

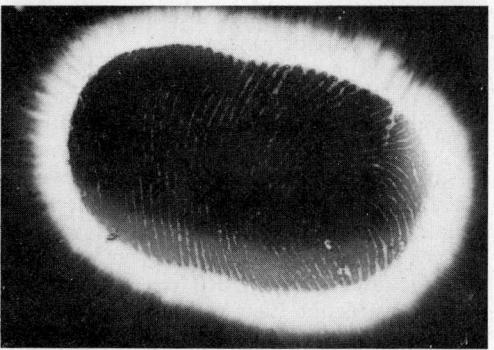

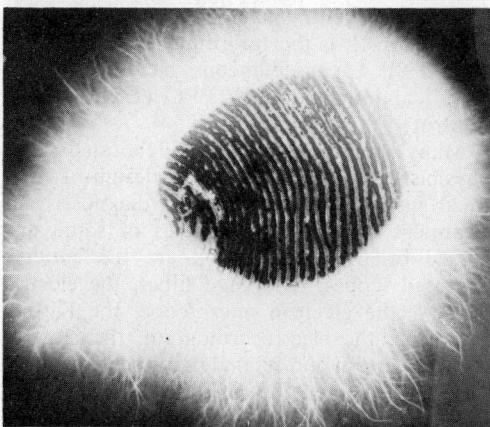

Figure 31-4. Kirlian photographs of fingertips showing the electric field produced by and surrounding the body. (Photograph courtesy of Dorothy Harrison.)

The technique is presently being studied by scientists all over the world in an effort to determine its full significance and use.

As more and more of the body's electric properties are investigated by scientists, advances can be made in the care of the ill. Ap-

plications in the form of biomedical electronic instruments will help the nurse in the care and monitoring of the ill. It should be pointed out that the following pertains not so much to "radiation" as to use of the body's electric properties in general.

The oldest and most widely known and used electronic monitoring device is the electrocardiograph (ECG) for the study of the electric properties, and hence functioning, of the heart. Perhaps a close second would be the electroencephalograph (EEG) for the monitoring of the brain waves. One of the most recent uses of this principle is a device left at the bedside of an unconscious patient which monitors brain wave output and so alerts the nurse to their cessation, or to death.* Bedside patient monitoring systems are now standard equipment in intensive care and coronary care units. The basic components in this setting are the electrocardiograph attached to an amplifying system, an alarm device, and a rate meter. More complex units are also used in the operating room with a complete surgical monitoring system.

Muscular activity and its nerve stimulation is also monitored with electromyographs (EMG). These can monitor electric waves from a single cell to a group of fibers or a complete muscle.

Techniques available now to monitor functions by telemetery are called biotelemetry. This is the measurement of biologic or physiologic events from a distance. Typical applications are the radiofrequency transmissions for the monitoring of astronauts in space. More closely related to nursing care is the use of telephone links to the transmission of electrocardiograms, and the monitoring of patients in an ambulance or other locations away from the hospital.

New devices are appearing on the market daily so that it is well nigh impossible to give a complete listing of the many available. The nurse would be well advised to keep up with the literature in this field. *Biomedical Instrumentation and Measurements* [7] by Leslie Cromwell and associates is a useful source with which to begin.

Bioelectric Medicine. There are perhaps no branches of the health sciences more exciting right now than biophysics, medical electronics, and medical engineering. Attention was called in Chapters 5 and 19 to the work of Harold Saxton Burr who, with his associates, demonstrated the following—as he expressed it:

* The Life Watch, Humetrics Corp., Los Angeles, Calif.

". . . the organism possesses a [electro-dynamic] field as a whole which embraces subsidiary or local fields, representing the organism's component parts." * With Eugen Kahn, Leonard J. Ravitz, Jr., and others, Burr showed that body states in health and markedly abnormal behavior paralleled deviations in electrometric examination. Both the normal process of ovulation and the abnormality of malignant growths, for example, were reflected in measurable variations in the flow of energy in the body. Burr spoke of "the field as a signpost." [7a] The following is the Foreword of his summary volume *The Electric Fields of Life.*

The Universe in which we find ourselves and from which we cannot be separated is a place of Law and Order. It is not an accident, nor chaos. It is organized and maintained by an Electro-dynamic Field capable of determining the position and movement of all charged particles.

For nearly half a century the logical consequences of this theory have been subjected to rigorously controlled experimental conditions and met with no contradictions.†

Burr's work clearly demonstrated the electrodynamic basis of life and that a balance between the positively and negatively charged elements are essential to life. It is of interest to note that this concept is akin to the ancient Chinese concept that a balance between the Yin-Yang, or male and female elements in the body, is necessary to health and life. The effectiveness of acupuncture, an ancient medical art, can be explained as an electrodynamic phenomenon.

The work of Galvani and Faraday in the nineteenth century led to the demonstration that electric currents affect the nervous system and this is said to have "opened the door to the development of neurophysiology." ‡ However, Greek and Roman physicians seem to have understood that electricity had a pain-killing effect. Scribonius Largus in A.D. 46 is reported to have used the electric ray, or torpedo fish, to treat headache and gout.[7b]

In recent decades there has been general recognition of the necessity of maintaining a balance between the negatively and positively charged ions in body fluids. Whole curricula have been built around the concept of homeostasis, or the maintenance of "steady states" in the organism. This is partly dependent on the electrolytes in the circulating fluids, or substances capable of conducting an electric current. Actually homeostasis is theoretical since tension from imbalance is essential to a dynamic, living being.*

Albert Szent-Györgyi, of the Institute for Muscle Research, Woods Hole, Mass., working over several decades, has developed what he calls "the electronic theory of cancer." † He thinks that the cell of cancer has shifted from the aerobic resting state to the anaerobic proliferative state and that pathology is established when this state is stabilized, or becomes "constitutive." Having studied first animals, then cells, then molecules, then electrons, Szent-Györgyi is now studying movement within cells and what substances may inhibit movement, or cell division.[7c] He believes the hope for cancer control lies in reversing the proliferative state rather than in using agents that destroy the cells of cancer.

Electric pain control may be as old as acupuncture and the sting of the torpedo fish, but in modern Western medicine it is relatively new. An editor of *Emergency Medicine,* discussing "a new approach to pain," notes that in the late nineteenth century "crude electrical devices sprang up in quantity." There were so many false claims made for them that the manufacturers were forced out of business. The claims for the Electreat, patented in 1918 by a "naturopath," were modified so it weathered the storm of disapproval and demonstrated the potential value of electric cutaneous stimulation. It is the forerunner of the Neuromod TNS (Transcutaneous Neural Stimulator ‡), and the Stimtech EPC (Electric Pain Control).§

Many physicians have collaborated with physicists and engineers in the design of electrical instruments used in the diagnosis and treatment of disease. Examples of some discussed briefly in this book are the battery-operated scopes, or lighted tubes, the electric cautery, the electron microscope, the Kirlian "camera," the electrocardiogram, the electroencephalogram and related monitoring devices, the brain scanner, the cardiac pacemaker, the

---

* Viktor E. Frankl questions this striving for equilibrium on philosophical grounds. He makes the following observation:

I consider it a dangerous misconception of mental hygiene to assume that what man needs in the first place is equilibrium or, as it is called in biology, "homeostasis," i.e., a tensionless state. What man actually needs is not a tensionless state but rather the striving and struggling for some goal worthy of him. (Frankl, Viktor E.: *Man's Search for Meaning.* Pocket Books, New York, 1975, p. 166.)

† Szent-Györgyi is best known for his discovery of ascorbic acid (vitamin C).

‡ Made by Medtronic, Inc., of Minneapolis, Minn.

§ Made by Stimulation Technology, Minneapolis, Minn.

---

* Burr, Harold Saxton: *The Electric Fields of Life.* Ballantine Books, New York, 1972, p. 85.

† Burr, Harold Saxton: *op. cit.,* p. 1.

‡ "A New Approach to Pain," *Emergency Med.,* (Mar.) 1974.

artificial kidney, and the respirator. Many nurses learn to use such instruments and may find themselves involved in their design. The School of Nursing of the Health Sciences Center, State University of New York at Stony Brook presented a one-day program in 1975 entitled "The Nature and Nurture of Life." A physicist, an engineer, biologists, a respiratory technologist, a geocosmic researcher, statisticians, psychologists, psychiatrists, philosophers, oncologists, other physicians, and nurses met to discuss such subjects as the use of the electric field theory in medicine, states of awareness, biofeedback, mother-child biorhythms, rates of aging, and "a 20th Century Look at the Ancient Arts." Nurses who have studied and worked with those in many branches of science and the healing arts are more able than those who have not had this opportunity to see the possibilities in bioelectric medicine and what may be a "scientific explanation" of why an empirical practice is effective. Some nurses are involved in research along these lines. All nurses use some of the instruments mentioned above and, with special instruction, a few nurses may be involved in the use, and possibly the design, of many of them. As shown in Chapter 49 nurses in one pain rehabilitation center manage electric skin stimulation with the physician as a consultant.[7d] Nurses are conducting many tests that depend upon electronic equipment; they interpret the recording of monitors and they operate respirators and other therapeutic machinery. The procedures involved are so dependent on the design of the equipment, and those designs are so often changed, or improved, that operators must depend largely on the instructions issued with the instruments or machines. It seems impractical to suggest methods in this chapter. The intent here is to point out the importance of bioelectric medicine and the extent to which it invades the province of diagnosis and that of treatment. Even children of today, looking at a television program such as *The Incredible Machine,* have seen red blood cells passing in single file through a capillary and the scavenger activity of a white blood cell; they have seen differences in skin temperature showing up as vividly contrasting colors. Programs on genetics are making terms like chromosomes and DNA common. Average citizens will know that bioelectric techniques have diagnostic value. Patients in, and visitors to, intensive care units see monitors in constant use. Knowledge of respirators and pacemakers is common and, if electric skin stimulation for pain fulfills its promise, these instruments will be as well known. It seems likely that in the near future there will be more systematic preparation of nurses in the bioelectric aspects of health care.

2. HELIOTHERAPY

Definition. Heliotherapy is the exposure of the body to the rays of the sun, *helios* being the Greek word for sun.

Therapeutic Uses. The stimulating effect of the sun's rays on the growth of plants is well known. Plants show their need by turning toward the sun and by their sickly appearance if deprived of sunlight. Radiations of different lengths are given off by the sun and include the ultraviolet rays (shorter waves), the luminous rays of the visible spectrum, and the near infrared rays (longest rays). Therefore, sunlight has both the chemical effect of light and ultraviolet rays and the heat effect of infrared radiation. An overdose of sunlight produces the same toxic symptoms that result from excessive exposure to ultraviolet and infrared rays, although what we call sunburn (overexposure in humans) is produced by the ultraviolet irradiation. Arthur L. Watkins [8] says that ultraviolet rays stimulate the production of a histamine-like substance that dilates the skin capillaries and produces erythema. He also says that irradiation has an effect on some amino acids, one of which is tyrosine. Tyrosine produces pigment which is deposited in the horny layers of the epidermis and results in tanning. Ultimately, the superficial layer of the skin thickens.

From ancient times both the healing and destructive effects of the sun's rays have been recognized. Exposure to intense heat and light from the sun withers plants and burns and prostrates animals and human beings. To avoid this, the toleration of the organism must be carefully developed. The minimal erythemal dose (M.E.D.) for the sun is variable with the time of day, time of year, latitude, and the condition of the atmosphere. The amount of pigmentation in the skin of the patient will also influence the length of exposure. Exposure should be gradual. F. Daniels and associates [9] recommend starting with a period of about 15 minutes when the treatment is instituted, and gradually increasing the length of exposure over a period of weeks. The rate of increase varies with each patient, depending on the skin reaction. In the past, heliotherapy was used for erysipelas, furunculosis, and extrapulmonary tuberculosis; however, such conditions are now treated with other types of therapy such as chemicals and antibiotics. Exposure to the sun is still considered useful, especially in early childhood, for the prevention of rickets, and in convalescence for its general beneficial effect.

Ultraviolet rays are believed to be completely absorbed by the skin, and any harmful effect is thought to be due to chemical changes effected there. Likewise, injuries to the eye from sunlight are the result of its effect on the conjunctiva and cornea. Extreme exposure may ulcerate the cornea, causing permanent impairment of vision.[10] Medical scientists admit the generally wholesome effect of sunlight and the dependence upon it of most living organisms; however, today it is not looked upon as a specific in the treatment of disease.[11]

One of the more common types of skin cancer is the basal cell carcinoma, occurring mainly on the face, and in some patients it seems to be associated with too prolonged exposure to the sun since its highest incidence is in outdoor workers such as farmers and seamen. The action of sunlight and its effect on health is discussed in more detail in Chapter 14.

Regulation of Dosage. Just as much care must be taken to prevent overexposure to sunlight as to other types of radiation. The physician prescribes the desired length of exposure, usually short at first, increasing the period from a few minutes daily to an hour or more if tolerance is developed and if the treatment seems beneficial. Reddening of the skin is an indication of the patient's tolerance. Nature's protective device is the production of the dark pigment, melanin.[12] Some persons, for example, redheads, often lack this capacity and never get a "suntan" but continue to redden and blister. The eyes may be protected with dark glasses, or the head shaded, if the sunlight is intense or exposure prolonged. A method of zoning is ordinarily used; that is, the area of exposure is increased from day to day until the whole body is exposed. A covering is provided for the genitalia.

Symptoms of overexposure, other than erythema, are headache, elevation of body temperature, nausea, and vomiting, and in severe cases, collapse. Heliotherapy is rarely ordered if the patient is febrile or has a gastrointestinal disorder.

The skin should be protected against the rays of the sun when conditions necessitate prolonged exposure and especially when the skin lacks protective pigments. Ointments and suntan preparations are temporarily effective because they prevent or reduce the passage of the ultraviolet rays to the skin area on which the suntan preparation has been applied. However, if the preparation is to provide effective protection against sunburn, it is advisable to reapply the preparation after each exposure as well as every 2 or 3 hours of exposure thereafter. Daniels and associates[13] say that protection against sunburn by special preparations is only partial.

Suggested Procedure. Help patients as necessary to undress and put on very brief garments for modesty. Short trunks for men and bikinis for women might be useful. Protect them adequately while going to a porch, roof, or yard—wherever the treatment is to be given. Their condition and the facilities available determine whether they should walk or be conveyed by chair, stretcher, or bed. Shield the patient from drafts, shade the head, and if necessary protect the eyes with dark glasses. If there is any indication of overexposure, terminate the treatment and report the symptoms to the physician. Daily exposure is usually prescribed and it should fall between the hours of 10 A.M. and 2 P.M. When the radiation (the difference between the temperature in the shade and the sun) is over $-6.67°C$ $(20°F)$, the time of exposure is usually cut to two-thirds the prescribed period. In very cold climates exposure to the sun in front of a window made of special glass (fused quartz), which does not screen out all the ultraviolet rays, is of some value but is not as effective as outdoor exposure. Specific directions should be given to patients for the use of ultraviolet energy from the sun if heliotherapy is to be carried out in the home.

Recording the Treatment. Note the patient's condition, especially any symptoms that indicate an unfavorable reaction to the treatment; indicate the time, duration, intensity, radiation, and body zones exposed. In some hospitals a special form is used for recording such treatments.

3. ELECTRIC LIGHT BATHS (HEATED AIR BATHS)

Definition. An electric light bath is the exposure of the body to light from incandescent lamps (ordinary electric light bulbs) inserted in a cabinet that has a reflecting metal lining. This may be constructed so that the patient can lie or sit. From 20 to 50 lights are provided; a few or all of them may be used in the treatment. A partial electric light bath is administered by exposing any portion of the body to ordinary artificial light. Bulbs are inserted in the roof and sides of a cradle or box (see Fig. 31-5) and are as a rule 60-watt bulbs.[14] There are many such devices. Bulbs suspended from an ordinary cradle make an effective substitute for the commercial type illustrated. The bulbs should be 30 cm (11½ inches) or more from the skin area.

Therapeutic Uses. The action of an artificial light bath, using ordinary incandescent bulbs, and a natural sun bath is the same except that the sun's ultraviolet radiation effect is lacking. An ultraviolet unit can, of course, be added to

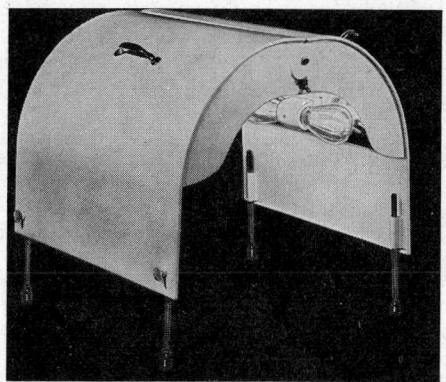

Figure 31-5. Electric-light cradle used for a partial light bath. (Courtesy of Burdick Corp., Milton, Wisc.)

any cabinet or baker, but such a device should be considered under the heading of ultraviolet therapy. As compared to ultraviolet lamps, the action of these ordinary light bulbs is mild. However, if sufficiently powerful bulbs are used and placed close to the skin, burns can result. Actually, this treatment is an application of infrared radiation. The effect is like that of a hot pack, the result of surrounding the body with a blanket of still hot air. Sweating is profuse, and the blood vessels of the skin are dilated.

There is a difference of opinion on the value of hot air baths, particularly systemic baths. The water loss from excessive sweating is admittedly dangerous unless the subject makes up for fluid loss by drinking. Some of the values of hot air baths are said to be that they lower blood pressure, increase blood alkalinity, relax muscles, and put the patient in a condition to benefit from massage and passive exercise. General hot air baths have been most frequently prescribed in nervous and mental disorders. They are so rarely used now that the method is not described in this text. Local hot air baths are used in arthritis, rheumatism, gout, lumbago, and neuritis; to promote healing of wounds, burns, excoriation, and skin eruptions; to stimulate circulation in the extremities; and postoperatively in the treatment of fractures after a cast has been bivalved or while the patient is in traction. In such cases a moderate temperature, not higher than 80°C (176°F) is used.

Suggested Procedure for a Partial Electric Light Bath. Give patients a suitable explanation of the treatment. Adjust the posture so that it is a comfortable one because they may be obliged to stay in this position for some time. Support a painful extremity on pillows or pads; place a blanket directly under the part. Protect the part to be treated from contact with metal. (If the head is to be treated, patients must wear dark glasses.) Place the baker in position over the part to be treated. Draw the blanket that is under the part over the box or cradle, and snugly around the opening, to prevent admission of air. An additional blanket over the top of the cradle may be needed according to the size and nature of the apparatus.

Maintain the prescribed temperature of the air inside the cradle for a designated period. For this purpose all bakers and heated cradles must be provided with a thermometer. Watkins[15] states that research has shown that heat within a cradle or baker comes from three sources simultaneously. First, the electric light bulbs give off measurable heat; second, the glass and the metal of the bulbs get hot and after a time give off their own heat; and third, if the baker has metallic sides these get increasingly hot and reach their maximum reflective power in about an hour. Consequently, as time passes, the amount of heat the patient receives steadily increases. During the treatment the nurse should visit the patient frequently to check the thermometer and to observe the patient's condition. If the skin gets very reddened or if the patient complains of being uncomfortably warm, one or more bulbs can be turned off until the patient is comfortable, but the temperature should not be reduced too much.

The duration of the treatment varies. It may be resorted to daily or several times a week, and each treatment may last from a few minutes to several hours (usually 1 hour), depending upon the temperature used, the sensations of the patient, and the nature of the case under treatment. In the treatment of wounds and burns, it may be necessary to maintain a temperature slightly above that of the body for periods of days or weeks.

If a high temperature has been maintained inside the baker, subsequent chilling should be prevented. After removing the baker, keep the part wrapped in blankets until the circulation has returned to normal and sweating has ceased.

Some cradles are equipped with a heating unit that is thermostatically controlled. Such a device may be used over long periods since the air inside the cradle never goes below the prescribed temperature. Such a gentle heat is believed to be particularly valuable in the treatment of peripheral vascular disease.

Recording the Treatment. Note the time the treatment was given, the area exposed, the duration, the temperature used, and the patient's reaction.

4. INFRARED RADIATION

Definition. Infrared radiation is the exposure of the body to an electrically heated unit capable of emitting therapeutic doses of infrared rays. Pauline M. Scott[16] describes these heated units as of two types—the nonluminous and the luminous. The nonluminous type gives off less heat than the luminous and may be simply a wire wound around some insulating material. This type is most commonly seen in the ordinary household heater. Or, the wire may be embedded in or placed behind a disc of fireclay or porcelain. This disc is usually colored black but when heated gives off a dull red glow. A third type is a metal cylinder or rod that encases the heating unit. All these devices when heated give off infrared rays. The luminous type, as its name suggests, is always a light bulb and is known as an infrared lamp. The wattage may be from 100 watts to 1500 watts or even higher. Any infrared bulb over 300 watts is considered potentially explosive, and when in a reflector, the open side of the reflector should be covered with a fine wire mesh to catch glass fragments should there be an explosion.

Therapeutic Uses. The application of infrared radiation has the effect produced by any form of heat; it is therefore used in the same conditions as those for which conductive types of heat are prescribed (see Chapter 28). Infrared radiation dilates blood vessels, and relaxes connective tissue and muscles. In some conditions it relieves pain. Its advantages over hot applications that transmit heat by conduction are that dosage can be regulated easily, the application has no weight, and the patient can be made more comfortable throughout the treatment. This is the type of home treatment prescribed for some skin diseases, and patients can easily be taught to use it safely. As more specific methods of treatment are developed, use of infrared radiation therapy decreases.

Regulation of Dosage. In order to prevent burning the skin with infrared radiation, the intensity of the heat at the source, the distance of the heating unit from the skin, the sensitivity of the patient, and the duration of the treatment must be considered.

Infrared lamps are usually placed from 30 to 60 cm (1 to 2 ft) above the skin area, depending on the size and intensity of the heating unit. A sensation of pleasant warmth should be produced, and with the responsible patient the subjective reaction is a guide; with infants and irrational adults, the operator cannot rely on this. The color of the skin must be closely watched; burns may result through a failure to do so. It is dangerous to allow the skin to get too red. It is helpful to place the bulb of a bath thermometer within the heated area at the same distance from the heating unit as the skin. A temperature of 46°C (114.8°F) is a safe one and will not burn the patient. The treatment ordinarily ranges in duration from 20 to 40 minutes and may be given once or twice daily, or, if mild enough, may be extended to several hours. Excessive reddening of the skin, pain, or discomfort are indications for discontinuing the treatment or reducing the dosage.[17]

Suggested Procedure. Place patients in a position they can maintain comfortably for the duration of the treatment. Expose the area to be irradiated and protect the rest of the body with suitable covering. Adjust the heating unit at a distance from the skin area that gives the patient a pleasant sensation of warmth. (If the distance is correctly estimated, it is not necessary to keep the heating unit in motion to avoid burning; but if lamps are used that throw their rays on a small area, it may be necessary to move the lamp several times during the treatment in order to cover the prescribed area.) Increase the distance between the heating unit and the skin if there is marked flushing, or if the patient complains. Some patients think if a little is good, more is better. In their desire to get relief they may ask for more intense heat; therefore, the operator must not rely entirely on the patient's reaction at first. Ultimately, the patients and their families must be taught to use an infrared lamp when they are ambulatory and the treatment drawn out. After the heating unit is removed, cover the area with warm clothing or bedding, and protect the part treated from exposure to cold air until normal circulation is reestablished.

Recording the Treatment. Note the area treated, the hour and duration, the distance of the unit from the skin, and the patient's reaction.

5. ULTRAVIOLET RADIATION

Definition. Ultraviolet radiation is understood to mean exposure of the body to an electrically heated unit that gives off ultraviolet rays in therapeutic doses. Less powerful but nevertheless therapeutically effective ultraviolet radiation may be accomplished by exposure to the sun.

Therapeutic Uses. Ultraviolet rays have little power of penetration and therefore affect the superficial, rather than the deeper, tissues. However, ultraviolet rays are absorbed by protoplasm and physical and chemical changes take place which are only manifested hours later. Its therapeutic value and its uses have been pointed out in the discussion of heliotherapy (page 1387).

Regulation of Dosage. Serious injury may be done patients if the dosage of ultraviolet rays is not carefully regulated. In many hospitals radiation therapy (with the exception of heliotherapy) is entirely in the hands of special therapists; in other institutions nurses are expected to give this treatment, and therefore they should understand the underlying principles and the techniques involved. Watkins [18] says that the use of ultraviolet lamps in the home should be discouraged.

Ultraviolet radiation produces an erythema that does not appear until several hours after the treatment. The reaction may be so intense as to burn and blister the skin. This effect is seldom desired except in a skin disease, such as erysipelas, when the physician may actually want to kill bacteria and destroy infected tissue. The degree of erythema produced by artificial means depends upon the source, the distance between the lamp and the patient's skin, the duration of exposure, the area of the body treated, and the sensitivity of the individual. The lamps vary greatly; each one should indicate the M.E.D. (minimal erythemal dose) or seconds of exposure. The physician prescribes so many M.E.D.'s, using a specific piece of equipment. The size of the dose may be increased from 1 to 10 or more minutes daily, according to the lamp. Physicians must decide whether ultraviolet radiation is to be used, what source is best, what area is to be treated, what dose should be used initially, how often they wish the treatment given, and how to increase the exposure.

The following is a method of testing the patient's sensitivity: Cut a series of holes 2 cm in diameter in a large piece of white paper. Place this paper over the medial surface of the forearm or thigh. (The area must be untanned.) Cover all but the lowest opening and expose the underlying skin to the action of the lamp for a period of 15 seconds; at the end of this time uncover the next opening and expose the underlying skin to 15 seconds of exposure; uncover the next and the last openings in the same manner so that the first area radiated will have been exposed for one minute. At the end of 18 to 24 hours, note the erythema produced on these four spots, and in giving the treatment use the length of exposure that produces the desired skin reaction; or increase the exposure if one minute is not long enough. Generally speaking, men tolerate larger doses than women, brunettes are less sensitive than blonds, and a tanned skin tolerates far larger doses than an untanned skin. (Blondness as used here refers to a fair skin, not to the color of the hair.) As the skin becomes pigmented, the dosage is increased. *Both the patient and the operator must wear dark glasses* (see Fig. 31-6) to avoid irritation of the conjunctiva and cornea.

Suggested Procedure. Except for the protection of the eyes with goggles, the preparation of patients is the same as for infrared radiation. However, because there is no sensation of heat as

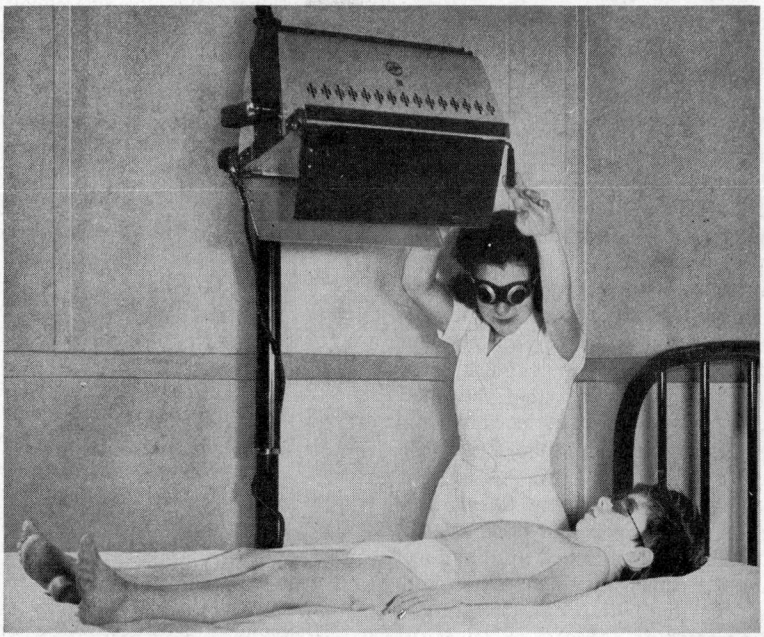

Figure 31-6. Ultraviolet treatment in the hospital. Note that both the patient and physical therapist are wearing protective goggles. (Courtesy of National Society for Crippled Children & Adults, Inc., Chicago, Ill.)

there is with infrared radiation, patients' reactions do not protect them, and ultraviolet radiation must therefore be even more carefully applied than infrared radiation. Neither is there immediate reddening of the skin to guide the operator; the erythema appears several hours later. If the test for sensitivity has been properly carried out and the results considered in administering the treatment, there need be no fear of burning the patient.

If it seems advisable to prescribe treatment with an ultraviolet lamp at home, patients must be thoroughly taught how to use it. They should be warned of the danger of excessive use and the danger of being burned if they fall asleep while under the lamp.

6. X-RAY (ROENTGEN RAY) THERAPY

Definition. X-rays, also known as roentgen rays, are *generated* rays. They are produced (created) by the passage of a high-voltage electric current through a glass-walled tube under vacuum conditions. When the electrons in the electric current strike a target in the tube, x-rays are produced. Soft radiation is low-voltage radiation of about 50 kilovolts (kV). W. J. Meredith and J. B. Massey [19] state that 50 kV therapy is considered superficial radiation and is useful for superficial tumors, such as skin tumors. These authors go on to say that a middle range of radiation is at the 250 kV or 300 kV level. This strength of energy penetrates to the location of tumors of average depth, such as breast tumors, and some head and neck tumors. Deep therapy, or hard radiation, may be 1 million electron volts (MeV) and up. Rays of this velocity and strength penetrate into deep abdominal tissues and into parts of the body where tumors are deeply embedded. All the above kilovolt or million electron volt radiation sources require different machines for their generation.

In the present-day x-ray therapy department, one finds two other therapy machines. One is the linear accelerator and the other is the betatron. The linear accelerator machine operates on the same principle as the ordinary x-ray therapy machine except that the x-ray tube is much longer. When the electrons from the electric current enter the tube, because it is so long, they can be speeded up, or accelerated, in a straight line, or linearly, through the use of magnets, microwaves and other devices placed in the tube that will speed up the movements of these electrons within it. Meredith and Massey [20] say that with linear acceleration, therapeutic energies of 4 MeVs to 10 MeVs can be generated and can be manipulated for tumor destruction with great precision and effectiveness. The betatron is known as a

"cycle" machine. Instead of a straight passageway for the speeded-up electrons, as in the linear accelerator, the passageway is circular and the electrons can be forced to go around and around until they have accelerated to extremely high energies. The betatron produces therapeutic energies from 20 to 35 MeVs, according to Meredith and Massey.[21]

Therapeutic Uses.* The therapeutic value of radiation is due to its destructive effect on living cells. Goodwin and his associates describe this process by saying:

Generally the effects observed are swelling of the cell, increased acidity of protoplasm, clumping of chromosomes, and retarding of cell division. These changes may be temporary, and followed by apparent recovery, or they may be precursors of more drastic organic deterioration.†

Therefore, in x-ray therapy, since it is desirable to kill as many malignant cells as possible, it is customary to give many small doses over a long period rather than a large dose at any one time. This process is known as fractionated dosage or therapy, and is designed to affect as many cells as possible.

There is always the question in radiation therapy about the degree to which normal cells are affected if they receive any radiation meant for malignant cells. Goodwin and his associates state that

. . . after each irradiation, all the cells recover to some extent, but the normal ones more than the diseased ones. Thus, the differential between their conditions constantly increases, until finally a state is reached in which the normal tissues can recover, and the tumor cannot.‡

Some cancer cells are known to be radioresistant, and consequently, x-radiation as a therapy is seldom used for their destruction. The higher the degree of radiosensitivity of cellular tissue, the greater the effectiveness of the therapy.

Radiation Precautions. The amount of radiation received from any source is affected by three conditions: (1) the distance of the person from the radiation source; (2) the time the person remains in the presence of the radiation source; and (3) the amount of shielding existing between the radiation source and the person receiving the radiation. Today much is known about the hazards of radiation and about protective devices that minimize danger to personnel working in these departments. Furthermore, good personnel health practices

---

* Diagnostic x-ray is discussed in Chapter **7.**
† Goodwin, Paul N., et al.: *Physical Foundations of Radiology*, 4th ed. Harper & Row, New York, 1970, p. 287.
‡ *Ibid.*, p. 289.

RADIATION THERAPY RECORD

(If out-patient get correct and complete address and telephone number)

Family Name | First Name | Middle Name | Occupation | Room No. | Hosp. No.

Address | City | Zone | State | Home Phone | Age | Date | X-ray No.

Date	Target skin distance [in cm.]	Added filters [in mm.]	Kv. P.	Half value layer [in mm. of cu.]	Effective wave length	Ma.	r per minute	Time [in min.]	r to field	Total r to the field	Size of field [in cm.]	Location of field	Operator

FORM F-602 | PHYSICIANS' RECORD CO., BERWYN, ILLINOIS - PRINTED IN U.S.A. | RADIATION THERAPY RECORD

Figure 31-7. A radiation therapy record form. (Courtesy of Physicians' Record Co., Berwyn, Ill.)

are recommended by Earnest F. Gloyna and Joe O. Ledbetter,[22] such as requiring the use of radiation monitoring devices (film badges worn by all employees exposed to unusual amounts of radiation in their work) which help to show when any person has received up to his or her quota of "safe radiation." When this happens, a job shift for health safety is indicated. Also, the requirement of routine health examinations provides opportunity for the detection of symptoms of radiation overdose. And, the use of lead-lined protective devices, such as gloves and aprons in fluoroscopy rooms, dentists' offices, and other places where workers are exposed to high radiation, tend to protect patient and practitioner alike from the dangers of overdosage.

Suggested Procedure. Physicians determine the dosage of radiation therapy desired for their patients. They send their requests to the x-ray department where the roentgenologist assumes responsibility from this point on. A plan of therapy is developed specifying the kind and number of treatments. The patient is given an appointment schedule and the area to be radiated is marked with an indelible body marking pencil or a small tattoo (see Fig. 31-8). Patients and nurses must be very careful never to remove these marks since they outline the portal of entry ("port") into the body of the x-ray beam. If necessary, patients are measured or fitted for some kind of body protective shields and these are made up for them, identified with their name and kept in the x-ray department until their course of therapy is completed. Then they are destroyed. Thin strips of flexible pure lead have been used for many years for this

purpose and are still in use today. However, the use of the protective body mold, as mentioned above, is becoming more common since it is considered more effective for this purpose.

At the time of the treatment the x-ray technician greets patients and takes them to the machine prepared for their therapy dosage. Patients are then placed in position on the table and the protective devices previously made for them are applied. The machine is carefully placed over or near patients according to the prescription for the therapeutic dose, and the roentgenologist is notified. The roentgenologist checks the following conditions of the therapy before therapy is administered: the position of the patient, the position of the machine, the provisions for shielding, and the exposure of the "ports." When the roentgenologist is satisfied that the procedure is correct, he or she approves its administration. Then the technician closes the door * and returns to the control room where the machine is activated by remote control and the patient observed on a television monitor. Treatments vary from a few seconds to a few minutes, but by and large none of them are of long duration. Goodwin and his associates [23] signify this time as "rate per minute" (R/min). Therefore, the patient can be comforted by being told of the shortness of the treatment.

The size of the machine and the idea of being left in the room alone are likely to make patients apprehensive or even frighten them very much. Knowing that there is an intercommunication system over which they may talk with the technician or that the technician is always able to see them helps to allay their fears.

After the treatment is completed, the technician returns to the patient, pushes the machine away, removes the protective devices, and stores them in readiness for the next visit. Technicians then help patients on to the stretcher or into a wheelchair for return to the hospital bed or to a conveyance if they are to go home.

Goodwin and his associates [24] say that with large doses of radiation, there may be a *skin reaction*. The appearance and intensity of the symptoms usually depend on the site and volume of irradiated tissue, rate of administration, and the patient's skin sensitivity. If patients express anxiety, the nurse may reassure them by reaffirming what the doctor has already told them, which is usually that the dose of radiation needed to treat the illness often cannot be delivered without affecting the skin in some degree and that the reaction will fade in time. Such an area should be referred to as a skin reaction or erythema, *not* as a burn.

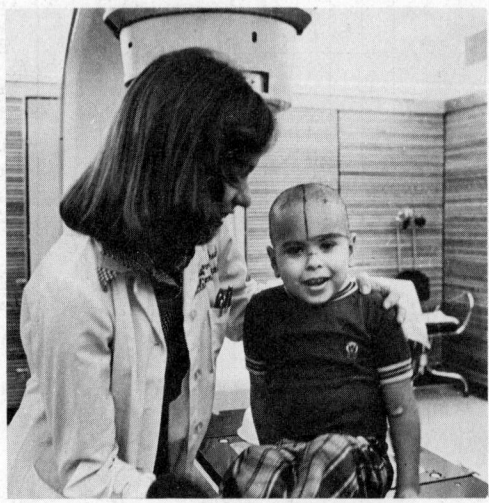

Figure 31-8. Young patient, with lines on the head to indicate area for supervoltage radiation therapy of deep tumor, is helped on the table by technician. (From *The Healing Arts. A Report from Stanford University Medical Center,* **5:**11, [Winter] 1975.)

* The closing of the door activates a red warning light, which turns on near the door, and a safety latch, which permits the machine to be operated by remote control. If by accident a person enters the room while the therapy is being administered, the inactivation of the safety latch by the door opening automatically turns off the x-ray machine inside.

Several factors influence the degree of skin reaction. Since people vary in their sensitivity to radiation, as in the case of ultraviolet rays producing sunburn, the fair-skinned persons may be expected to have a skin reaction more quickly and more marked than the dark-skinned. Different parts of the body, such as the face, are more sensitive to radiation than other areas.

The patient should be told at the start of the treatment that there will probably be a skin reaction during or soon after the course of treatment and that all forms of irritation (mechanical, thermal, or chemical) which will increase the severity of the reaction are to be avoided. The patient should be cautioned not to wash the part under treatment. The radiated part should be covered with soft clothing and any excessive exposure to sunlight, such as sunbathing, avoided. When the jaw area of a man's face is being treated, he should be told not to shave until the reaction has disappeared.

In *first- and second-degree skin reactions* the chief complaint is usually itching. Early application of a simple starch powder * relieves the itching and helps control the reaction since the patient will not be inclined to touch and further irritate the part under treatment. In *third- and fourth-degree skin reactions,* dressings may be needed to prevent infection. If blistering (vesication) should occur, the area may be treated with bland ointments such as boric acid ointment or vitamin A and D ointment; this will facilitate the removal of any dressings which are apt to adhere to the skin when there is serous oozing. Too thick an application of an ointment is to be discouraged since it hinders the natural discharges and so might promote infection. Discharges may be removed gently with mineral oil and cotton applicators. Even though the area is not sterile it is advisable to use sterile equipment, if available, to prevent secondary infection. Fourth-degree reactions are treated in the same manner as third-degree reactions, but they respond more slowly to treatment.

When the course of radiation therapy is completed and the skin reaction subsides, the treated skin is more sensitive and therefore more liable to damage. Patients should be cautioned against further irritation from sunburn, hot-water bottles, strong winds, excessive cold, or other special irritants. Exposed parts, such as the hands, or parts subject to friction, such as the feet, need special protection.

Gloyna and Ledbetter [25] describe a second kind of reaction, a systemic reaction, which is most often seen when large doses of radiation are administered or when there is prolonged therapy. This is known as *radiation sickness* and may take many forms from a simple nausea to severe and prolonged vomiting and diarrhea. When such a reaction develops after the treatment, the degree of reaction and time of appearance vary greatly because of individual patient tolerance. When the area of irradiation is small, milder symptoms such as headache, some mental depression, and general lassitude may develop. The symptoms generally clear up in a matter of days after the treatment is terminated. Neither the physician nor the nurse should suggest or imply that such symptoms are to be expected, but inpatients and outpatients should be led to report at each visit on loss of appetite or any discomfort.

If there is a systemic reaction, medications such as pyridoxine and dimenhydrinate (Dramamine), prescribed for "motion sickness," may help prevent nausea and loss of appetite. Anxiety states may be managed by the use of tranquilizers. Today no particular drug can be depended upon to control the symptoms of radiation sickness. It has been found that sedative drugs can be useful and that several of the vitamins, especially B and C, can be of value. Fluids lost by vomiting should be replaced by intravenous fluids, otherwise the dehydration may prolong nausea and vomiting.

When patients are followed in the outpatient department the tiny tattoo mark or colored lines ordinarily used for showing the center of the skin ports must not be removed. Most doctors ask that no water or aqueous solution come in contact with the skin ports until the treatment is terminated. Nurses explain this to patients and help them understand that their cooperation is essential. Patients should be encouraged to drink more liquids than usual— 1 to 2 quarts more than usual. Fluid can be taken in the form of fruit drinks, soda water, milk, tea, coffee, or water. Loss of appetite may be a temporary symptom. A nourishing diet, with frequent small meals, is more likely to be tolerated than three large meals. In any event, the daily diet should be a complete one, including fresh fruits and vegetables, and meat, fish, eggs, or cheese.

7. RADIUM AND RADON THERAPY

Definition. Radium is one of the most important of the earth's radioactive elements. Radioactivity results from the emission of penetrating rays during the slow disintegration

---

* Ordinary dusting powders should not be used since many of them contain the metal zinc and the presence of zinc in the powder will give rise to secondary radiation which will only irritate the skin further.

of a radioactive element, in this case, radium. For therapeutic purposes, radiation is obtained from the element itself (radium) and from a gas (radon) which results from the continuous disintegration of radium. Blahd [26] states that radium is commonly applied in needles, applicators, and plaques. Radon, which is a gas, is trapped in the lumen of gold wires about the size of a No. 18 needle. The wires are cut into small pieces and these pieces are then known as gold seeds. Gold seeds are usually implanted directly into tumor tissue under surgical conditions. Blahd [27] describes this as interstitial radiation and says that customarily they are never removed.

Therapeutic Uses. Radium was extremely popular as therapy in the first half of the twentieth century, but with the development of artificial radioisotopes its popularity has waned. The chief reason for its falling into disfavor is that it has a half-life * of 1620 years. Its long half-life and the fact that it emanates gamma rays (as powerful as high-voltage x-rays) demand special storage and shielding facilities. Then, since radium is a very rare element and exists in such small quantities, its monetary value is very high. The most common use of radium currently is in gynecology.

Radon, in contrast with radium, has a half-life of 4 days, so long-term storage problems do not exist as they do with radium. But, since radon is a gas and is only available as a product of radium decay, its availability and use are limited. Today, radon is used mainly as implants for mouth and tongue tumors and for bladder tumors.

Suggested Procedure. In radium therapy, nurses usually carry more responsibility than in x-ray therapy, since they often help with the insertion and removal of the radium appliance and they care for the patient while it is in place. The dose and time required to give the necessary amount of exposure are calculated by the doctor, and specific information on the location of the radium and exact time at which it is to be removed by the doctor must be noted in the chart when the nurse assumes responsibility for the care of the patient. Any shifting of the position of the radium applicator, whether suspected or seen, should be reported immediately to the doctor for it may decrease the dosage to the affected area and irradiate normal tissues. In treatments of, or near, pelvic organs the applicator containing the radium

is usually inserted in the selected body cavity under surgical conditions in the operating room, or in a special room prepared for this kind of therapy. According to newer techniques in the process of development, patients are prepared in the operating room for the therapy by having inserted the empty applicator or other devices suitable for holding radium for therapy. Then patients are returned to their unit or a specially prepared radiation-safe room for afterloading of the radium. This technique is designed to reduce the radiation hazard to all personnel. Gold seeds may be implanted in the operating room or in a treatment room if patients are not hospitalized.

Besides assisting with the insertion and removal of radium applicators and giving nursing care to patients while the radium is in place, the nurse's responsibility includes preventing loss of the radium itself. Radium is a very rare element and is extremely costly. Also, it constantly emanates gamma rays which are of the nature of x-rays, only more powerful, and therefore are extremely hazardous to any persons unknowingly exposed to them. "Lost" radium constitutes an emergency and should be guarded against rigorously. Radium applicators and radon seeds should be kept in thick lead-lined containers until they are prepared for use. These items are then transferred to portable lead carriers; radon seeds are later transferred to a small lead chamber in which they can be sterilized in preparation for insertion. Whenever nurses handle a radium applicator they hold it at arm's length by means of a long-handled forceps and place it promptly in the portable lead carrier. When working with radon seeds, nurses should always handle them with long forceps, preferably working behind a lead shield.

When a radium applicator is removed from the patient's body, nurses should provide at the bedside a lead-lined container in which the applicator is stored after removal, a small bowl of warm soapy water, a long-handled forcep, and a long-handled brush. When the applicator is removed by the physician the long-handled forcep is used. Then, using the long-handled brush and the soapy water, either the physician or the nurse washes off any blood or mucus adhering to the applicator before placing it in the lead-lined container. The radium should *never,* under any circumstances, be removed from the applicator. To help prevent loss, all sinks in areas where radium appliances and radon seeds are used should be equipped with special traps; this will prevent the introduction of radioactive material into the sewer system.

Patients receiving radium treatment should not be allowed bathroom privileges because of the increased danger of loss of radium. Some of the following practices may be indicated; their use is determined by the length of time the radium applicators remain in place and their location in the body.

1. Use a hamper frame with a laundry bag so that linen used during the treatment may be discarded into it.
2. Provide a waste can lined with a heavy paper

---

* Half-life is the decay rate of any given radioisotope. Each radioisotope has its own decay rate; this means "the time taken by any amount of a radioactive substance to undergo the decay of half of its atoms." (Graham, E. C. [ed.]: *The Basic Dictionary of Science.* Macmillan Publishing Co., Inc., New York, 1965, p. 174.)

bag and operated by a foot pedal for discarded dressings and other similar waste.

3. Use a large bottle so that urine may be discarded into it through a funnel placed in the neck of the bottle.

4. Provide a galvanized pail with a tight-fitting cover for the disposal of feces and a second pail for the disposal of vomitus if the radium or radon has been inserted into the mouth area.

The items listed above are placed in a bathroom which adjoins the patient's room where they are convenient and yet inconspicuous to the patients and their visitors. All soiled linen, dressings, waste, and excreta should be kept until the radium has been removed from the patient and accounted for. If the waste containers are to be emptied before the radium is removed and there is any doubt about the location of the radium, the nurse notifies the physicist who will see that the contents are monitored for possible loss of radium and who will supervise the disposal of the material.

A radiation symbol (see Fig. 31-9) should be placed on patients' doors or, if they are in an open ward, the symbol should be put where it can easily be seen. Nurses assigned to provide care to these patients should be aware of all precautionary measures in practice. Nursing care plans should include the additional precaution of checking on the radium location in the patient's body at all tour-of-duty or shift changes.

The exposure of medical personnel to radium and radon (applicators, needles, and seeds) can be reduced and controlled by in-telligent application of principles and by using suitable equipment and accessories. Containers for the transportation of applicators, etc., are designed to protect personnel during transit time only and should not be considered adequate for permanent storage. All workers who are exposed to radiation should be monitored or tested for the presence of accidental, accumulative radioactive contamination by means of personnel-monitoring instruments. Blahd [28] says that these instruments are the pocket chamber or dosimeter, which resembles a fountain pen and can be carried in the pocket, and the film badge, which is attached to the outer clothing. Both of these devices measure the amount of radiation the wearer receives within a given time period. They should be kept in the administrative unit of the patient care location and should be identified with the wearer's name. (This unit is in different places in different hospitals, often at the head nurse's station or near the entrance of the patient care location.) Wearers should attach their monitoring device to their clothing before giving care to patients receiving radiation. At the completion of the patient contact, the monitoring device should be returned to the administrative unit where radiation safety personnel collect it and take it to a laboratory for determining the extent of that day's exposure. It is then replaced by an unused instrument. If nurses have a number of patients to care for who are receiving radiation they usually turn in their monitoring instrument at the end of their tour of duty for that day.

Differential and total white-cell counts are often required for personnel having close contact with sources of radiation. These counts are made at regular intervals such as once a month, or more often at the discretion of the personnel health department.

Possible dangers of unwarranted radiation to bed patients and hospital personnel should be checked routinely by radiation department personnel. A Geiger-Müller counter is used whenever there is a question of contamination, and especially after the discharge of a patient before personnel clean the room and dispose of linen, dressings, and excreta.[29]

Nurses who regularly care for patients being treated should perform their duties keeping in mind the radiation precautions of "time" and "distance." Limitation of time for the nurse near the radiation product may be affected by carefully preplanning the work to be done. Equipment can be assembled and necessary materials for nursing care conveniently placed. Then, nurses should perform work as expeditiously as possible but should avoid the appearance of undue haste. General conversa-

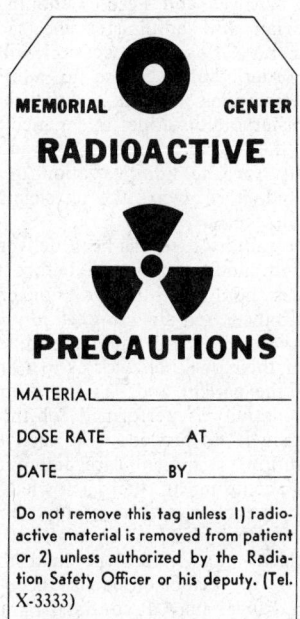

Figure 31-9. The distinctive radioactivity symbol.

tions with patients can be conducted 5 or 6 ft away from them. Visitors are usually restricted to immediate family members or close personal friends and they are cautioned to stay at least 6 ft from the patient.

It must be remembered that patients with a radium implant do not present a dangerous exterior. The danger comes from the radiation emanations from the implant within them. They should, of course, be provided with entertainment such as radio, television, books, or newspapers. During the time they are on "radiation precautions," patients may feel isolated. Nurses should be aware of this and make a special effort to keep up their morale.

8. ARTIFICIAL RADIOISOTOPE THERAPY

Definition. A radioisotope or radioactive isotope is an isotope exhibiting the property of spontaneous decomposition or disintegration by the emission of a particle or ray from its nucleus. All elements have a number of isotopes. An isotope is characterized by having the same atomic number as its element but a different atomic weight. The difference in weight is governed by the number of neutrons in the nucleus. All elements with an atomic number larger than 83 are naturally radioactive. Radon and radium fall into this class. However, when authorities speak of a radioactive isotope in medical therapy they are usually referring to isotopes of stable elements (lead with the atomic number of 82 and below) which have been rendered radioactive by artificial means. Today, the most common way of making a stable element radioactive is to subject it to bombardment by fast neutrons in an atomic pile. In this way almost any element can be made to yield one or more artificially produced radioactive isotopes and these isotopes can be shipped anywhere in the world for therapeutic or research purposes. (Diagnostic tests involving radioactive isotopes are discussed in Chapter 7.)

Therapeutic Uses. Curiously enough, the number of artificial radioisotopes used therapeutically, according to Blahd,[30] is quite small. Those commonly taken orally by the patient are iodine (I-131), used in the treatment of thyroid disorders, and phosphorus (P-32), commonly used in the blood dyscrasias. Gold (Au-198), a colloidal liquid, is very useful for instillation into the thoracic or abdominal cavity for direct radiation to cancerous tissue therein and for controlling the production of cavity fluid. Gold (Au-198) is also, on occasion, injected into soft tissue tumors. Iridium (Ir-192) is usually applied exteriorly. The iso-

tope is placed in a polyethylene or nylon tube and sutured into place over the cancer tissue to be radiated. At the end of the treatment the tube is removed. Cobalt (Co-60) and cesium (Cs-137) usually do not come into contact with the patient at all. They are used in teletherapy. Their emanations are like high-voltage x-rays, so a measured amount of the radioisotope is placed in a machine in the x-ray department. Then, patients are treated in the same fashion as though they were receiving an x-ray treatment. However, when the electricity is turned on for the therapy, instead of x-rays being generated, shutters open and powerful gamma radiation is emitted into the exposed "port" area. This ceases when the shutters are closed.

Suggested Procedure. Most hospitals today have a health physics department where trained physicists or technicians handle and store all radioactive products. In such cases, medicine or nursing is not responsible for either. However, for a complete understanding of how radioisotopes are stored and handled "behind the scenes" in any agency, nurses should visit the department and learn about these practices.

When desiring radioisotopes to be used therapeutically, physicians send prescriptions to the health physics department (except for Co-60 and Cs-137, which are in the x-ray department). The health physicist or technician prepares the requested doses and delivers them to the patients' units at the requested times. They arrive suitably protected in lead-lined containers. Nurses should have ready disposable equipment for administration. For doses to be swallowed, paper cups may be used. For those to be instilled into a cavity, disposable syringes and needles should be used. The physician will administer the radioisotope himself or herself, or on occasion will leave a "doctor's order" for a nurse to administer it. In other situations trained technicians prepare and administer radioisotopes under medical supervision. If the therapy requires entrance into a body cavity for the administration of a radioactive colloid, it is always the physician who administers the therapy.

After the radioisotope has been delivered to the patient's unit, and immediately before the treatment, nurses should institute radiation precautions of time, distance, and shielding. *A physician's order is unnecessary* for such precautions since nurses alter their own behavior as to (1) the *time* spent with the patient and (2) the *distance* from which any activity is performed for the patient's benefit. There is no procedure as such for radiation precautions in patient care and nurses practice them according to their knowledge of the physiologic behavior of the isotope in the patient's body, the kind of emanations, and the isotope's decay rate. After the final therapeutic treatment of the radioisotope has been given to the patient, nurses may discontinue radiation precautions on their own authority *providing* the radioisotope has decayed to a safe level of emanations and all environmental safety conditions have been met.

If a patient dies and the body is known to contain a radioisotope, the body should have attached to it, in a prominent place, a radiation sign. A note should also be attached to the body with the following information for all subsequent handlers of the body: (1) the name of the radioisotope administered to the patient; (2) its date of administration; (3) its method of administration; and (4) its half-life. In the case of gold (Au-198), if a dressing is adhering to the body at the site of injection, it should be inspected for cleanliness. A dressing contaminated with radioactive gold (cherry-red color) should be removed and the skin bathed by a nurse wearing rubber gloves. A clean dressing should be applied over the wound and information should be attached to the body stating that this was done and warning against contaminated dressings on which there may be seepage.

Specific Isotopes Commonly Used in Therapy and Some Suggestions for Nursing Care. *
Iodine (I-131) according to Henry H. Wagner [31] is a beta and a gamma emitter and has a half-life of 8 days. It is ingested and is usually mixed with drinking water for this purpose. Paper cups should be used and then destroyed under radiation precautions. Immediately after ingestion, patients are considered "hot" and nurses and all other personnel attending them should practice radiation precautions. Iodine is excreted from the body in the urine and in perspiration. [32] All urine must be collected in bottles marked with a radiation symbol and kept in the patient's unit, preferably behind some kind of shielding. These should *never* be kept in a utility room or on an open ward. A hamper should be kept in the patient's room for linen soiled with the droplets of urine or for an incontinent or perspiring patient. Linen may be removed from a patient's room by dropping it into a clean bag held by a nurse as in medical asepsis. However, linen contaminated with an isotope should be marked with a radiation sign and processed for laundering according to procedures arrived at by the administrators of the nursing department, the laundry, and the health physics department. After discharge, the patient's room should be carefully cleaned according to procedures arrived at by the administrators of the nursing department, the housekeeping de-

partment, and the health physics department. Special attention should be paid to all places that could have inadvertently been contaminated by droplets of urine such as the floor, bedpans, urinals, or a toilet seat. Finally, when the cleaning is completed the room should be carefully monitored for safety by personnel from the health physics department using Geiger counters or other such monitoring devices. [33]

Phosphorus (P-32), according to Blahd, [34] is a beta emitter and has a half-life of 14.3 days. It is ingested, is usually mixed with ordinary drinking water, and is given in paper cups that are immediately destroyed under radiation precautions. Since P-32 is a beta emitter only, there are usually no further radiation precautions. However, any material vomited immediately after swallowing should be considered contaminated and handled accordingly. It is not unusual to give P-32 on an outpatient basis.

Gold (Au-198), according to Blahd, [35] is a beta and a gamma emitter. He also describes it as being a colloidal liquid of a cherry-red color with a half-life of 2.7 days. Au-198 is very useful for treating tiny tumor implants in the thoracic and abdominal cavities, especially when such implants are causing pleural effusion or abdominal ascites. In its administration the cavity is first drained by thoracentesis or paracentesis. Immediately following drainage of the cavity the Au-198 is instilled into the cavity through the thoracentesis or paracentesis needle which has been left in place for this purpose. A disposable syringe should be used and destroyed thereafter under radiation precautions. It is important medically that the entire interior of the cavity be coated with the colloidal fluid. Such coating enhances the possibility that tiny tumor implants existing within the cavity are subjected to direct beta radiation with a good chance that they will be destroyed. Also, excess fluid production in the cavity is greatly lessened by this therapy. Therefore, patients should be told to turn the body from side to side at frequent intervals after the treatment and the reasons for doing so should be explained. Every 10 or 15 minutes for an hour or two should be sufficient. If patients are unable to turn themselves the nurses should turn them.

After the Au-198 has been instilled into a cavity or injected into any soft tissue tumors, there is a possibility of seepage. The nurse should check the dressings for the appearance of any cherry-red color. If there is seepage, the nurse, wearing rubber gloves, applies another dressing *over* the contaminated dressing and repeats the procedure if necessary. The

* The number of radioisotopes used therapeutically is constantly increasing. Only the more commonly used ones are covered here. If nurses in their practice encounter one unknown to them, they should refer to an authoritative text. They should especially acquaint themselves with the method of administration, the emanations, and the half-life of the radioisotope so that they can plan safe nursing care for patients and themselves.

physician should be notified immediately, since the therapeutic dose is now being changed by seepage loss. If nurses are asked to remove the dressing, they should wear rubber gloves and handle the dressing with long-handled forceps. The dressing should be placed in a disposable container and marked with a radiation sign. Customarily, the health physics department of the hospital collects and disposes of these contaminated materials. If not, the nurse should follow any routines set up by the hospital for personnel safety. Since Au-198 is a gamma emitter, all nursing care should be administered under radiation precautions of time, distance, and shielding until the isotope has decayed to a safe level of emanation and all environmental safety conditions have been met.

Tracers are minute quantities of a large number of radioisotopes that are used for diagnostic and research work. When nurses are told that the isotope is a "tracer," they should know that it is being used in such infinitesimal quantities that no possible danger can exist. Therefore, it is a general rule that for all "tracer" work, no radiation precautions are necessary.

9. ELECTROTHERAPY

Definition. The passage of any electric current through living tissue for chemical, physical, or heat effects falls under the general classification of *electrotherapy*. If an electrical current is used to cauterize or destroy tissue cells, the process is referred to as *electrosurgery*. The usual classifications of electrotherapy include:

I. High-frequency currents (heat action)
  A. Surgical
    1. Electrocoagulation
    2. Desiccation
    3. Fulguration
    4. Radiocutting knife
  B. Medical
    1. Conventional (long-wave) diathermy
    2. Short waves (90 to 30 meters)
    3. Ultrashort waves (6 meters and below)
II. Low-frequency currents (mechanical or chemical action)
    1. Galvanic current
    2. Faradic current
    3. Sinusoidal current
    4. Static current

Infrared and ultraviolet radiation from artificial sources also belong in a classification of electrotherapy, but they have been discussed at length and are not referred to in this section (see p. 1389). The forms of electrotherapy may be used alone or in combination.

At the present time, nurses, unless they are also physical therapy technicians, are rarely responsible for the operation of electrotherapy apparatus, other than that used for infrared radiation. They often prepare patients for treatment and take care of them during the treatment and afterward. Nurses should, therefore, have some knowledge of the principles and methods involved.

Diathermy. If alternating high-frequency currents are passed from one electrode to another through living tissue, the process is called *medical diathermy*. The resistance offered by the tissues to the passage of the current produces heat. With an alternating current of high frequency, the ions in the body fluids move to and from the electrodes so rapidly that there is no appreciable chemical change in the tissues. The only therapeutic result is believed to be the heat effect. This may be mild and produce a moderate hyperemia or may be so intense as to coagulate or "cook" the tissues. In medical diathermy the strength of the current is regulated in such a way that the temperature changes within the tissues fall within a therapeutically effective range. Its advantage over other forms of heat is that it affects all the tissues of the body lying between the electrodes. Internal organs can therefore be treated as easily as superficial tissues. Because different types of tissue offer varying amounts of resistance to electric currents, the effect is not uniform throughout the body, and some tissues respond more favorably to treatment with diathermy than others.

Diathermy may be used for any condition in which heat is indicated. Many physicians claim to have seen excellent results in a number of inflammatory conditions, for example, bronchitis, bronchial asthma, pleurisy, arthritis, and neuritis. It is also useful for joint injuries and nerve injuries.

Diathermy is used in fever therapy, often in combination with infrared radiation. The operation of the apparatus is always in the hands of a physician or special technician. Nursing care of the patient is the same, regardless of the medium employed to produce artificial fever therapy. Because it is so seldom used, the procedure is not described here.

When diathermy is prescribed by physicians to treat a "frozen" shoulder or other joint with limited motion, they may prescribe exercises for the patient. Nurses help the patient with such exercises; if there are untoward effects, such as increased severe pain, the reaction should be reported to the physician.

Electrosurgery might be termed *surgical diathermy,* for high-frequency alternating currents also are used for this purpose. The chief difference between this and medical diathermy is the strength of the current. It is used to desiccate, coagulate, or cut tissue, and to limit the area of injury the electrodes used must be of appropriate shapes and sizes, and there must be a nice adjustment of the strength of the current.

Surgical diathermy is used for the destruction or removal of warts, moles, and papillomas. It is rarely used in removing large growths or for major surgery.

Low-Voltage Currents. Alternating (sine wave), galvanic, and pulsating direct currents are low-voltage currents used in electrotherapy. Their effects may be mechanical or chemical or a combination of the two. Sine wave, or sinusoidal, currents stimulate involuntary muscle movements and in this way produce the mechanical action of passive exercise or massage. The galvanic current produces chemical changes or ionization within the tissues as it passes from one electrode to the other; an astringent effect is produced at the positive pole (anode) and a relaxing effect at the negative pole (cathode). The astringent effect is antihemorrhagic. Ionization of metallic salts in human tissue is another effect aimed at in electrotherapy.

Electric currents are commonly used to test the function of muscles and nerves when those structures have been injured or an injury is suspected.

Nurses, unless trained as technicians in physical therapy, are not expected to operate apparatus used in electrotherapy. (More detailed discussions of this subject are found in texts on therapeutics and monographs on this aspect of physical therapy.)

10. SONAR (ULTRASOUND) THERAPY

Definition. Scott [36] describes sound waves as longitudinal waves in matter that consist of a to-and-fro movement of particles in the direction in which the waves are traveling. In this they differ from electromagnetic or light waves which consist of an up-and-down movement of the ether. Sound waves require some material medium through which to travel, whereas light waves move freely through space. Ultrasound is a mechanical vibration identical with that of sound except it is of a much higher frequency and therefore cannot be heard by the human ear. It is produced in a machine called an ultrasonic generator. In this machine, high-frequency electric current (light waves) are directed against quartz, causing it to oscillate. This in turn causes a metal diaphragm to vibrate and emit sound waves.

Therapeutic Uses. Ultrasound is a form of diathermy and its main therapeutic purpose is deep heating. Since misuse can result in tissue damage it should be administered only by trained personnel. Its use in diagnosis is discussed in Chapter 7.

Regulation of Dosage. Most ultrasound generators need a warming-up period before use. By the use of dials and timers the prescribed treatment can be regulated. The applicator, which is usually known as the sound head, can be placed directly on the part of the body to be treated. If so, there must be some medium through which the sound waves are transmitted. This is known as "coupling," and mineral oil is a good conductor. Also, it is well known that water conducts sound waves. For body prominences or small body parts such as fingers, therapy can be instituted through underwater coupling, with the part to be treated immersed in water and the sound head placed in the water and directed at the part to be treated. Watkins [37] describes an improvement in technique which has led to the development of a diasonic applicator. This applicator is "fixed" on an adjustable arm attached to the ultrasound generator. It can be attached to a prescribed position on the neck, back, shoulder, etc., and through the use of mineral oil for coupling can be left in place until the treatment time is terminated.

Suggested Procedure. Explain to the patient that ultrasound therapy and diathermy are very similar and that the desired effect of the treatment is the production of heat. Place patients in a comfortable position that can be maintained for the length of treatment. Expose the body part to be treated and protect the other body parts against exposure with suitable covering. If oil coupling is to be used it is important to protect the patient's clothing from the oil. Fairly bulky and absorbent turkish towels may be needed for this purpose. After the treatment is completed gently remove the oil remaining on the skin with soap and water and take care that none is left to soil the patient's undergarments. If the underwater coupling method is used, provide towels to dry the patient's body parts immersed in the water bath.

REFERENCES

1. Behrens, Charles F., et al.: *Atomic Medicine,* 5th ed. Williams & Wilkins Co., Baltimore, 1969, p. 95.
2. Blahd, William H.: *Nuclear Medicine,* 2nd ed. McGraw-Hill Book Co., New York, 1971, p. 662.

3. Heavens, O. S.: *Lasers.* Charles Scribner's Sons, New York, 1971, p. 1.

4. Flitter, Hessel Howard: *An Introduction to Physics in Nursing,* 6th ed. C. V. Mosby Co., St. Louis, 1972, p. 249.

5. Pressman, A. S.: *Electromagnetic Fields and Life.* Plenum Press, New York, 1970.

6. Kirlian, S. D., and Kirlian, V. K.: *Photography and Visual Observation by Means of High-Frequency Currents.* Zhurnal Nauchnoy i Prikladnoy Fotografii i Kinematografii, Vol. 6, No. 6, 1961, pp. 397–403. (Translation Services Branch, Foreign Technology Division, WP-AFB, Ohio.)

7. Cromwell, Leslie, et al.: *Biomedical Instrumentation and Measurements.* Prentice Hall, Inc., Englewood Cliffs, N.J., 1973.

7a. Burr, Harold Saxton: *The Electric Fields of Life.* Ballantine Books, New York, 1972, pp. 85, 93.

7b. "A New Approach to Pain," *Emergency Med.,* (Mar.) 1974.

7c. Szent-Györgyi, Albert: *The Living State, with Observations on Cancer.* Academic Press, New York, 1972, p. 100.

7d. Indeck, Walter, and Printy, Andrea: "Skin Application of Electrical Impulses for Relief of Pain in Chronic Orthopaedic Conditions," *Minn. Med.,* **58:**305, (Apr.) 1975.

8. Watkins, Arthur L.: *A Manual of Electrotherapy,* 3rd ed. Lea & Febiger, Philadelphia, 1968, p. 40.

9. Daniels, F., et al.: "Sunburn," *Sci. Am.,* **219:**38, (July) 1968.

10. Watkins, Arthur L.: *op. cit.,* p. 60.

11. *Ibid.,* p. 38.

12. Daniels, F., et al.: *op. cit.*

13. *Ibid.*

14. Watkins, Arthur L.: *op. cit.,* p. 21.

15. *Ibid.,* p. 22.

16. Scott, Pauline M.: *Clayton's Electrotherapy and 'Actinotherapy,* 7th ed. Bailliere, Tindall & Cassell, London, 1975, p. 259.

17. Licht, Sidney (ed.): *Therapeutic Heat and Cold,* 2nd ed. Elizabeth Licht, Publisher, New Haven, Conn., 1965, p. 236.

18. Watkins, Arthur L.: *op. cit.,* p. 61.

19. Meredith, W. J., and Massey, J. B.: *Fundamental Physics of Radiology,* 2nd ed. Williams & Wilkins Co., Baltimore, 1972, p. 365.

20. *Ibid.,* p. 498.

21. *Ibid.,* p. 501.

22. Gloyna, Earnest F., and Ledbetter, Joe O.: *Principles of Radiological Health.* Marcel Dekker, Inc., New York, 1969, p. 285.

23. Goodwin, Paul N., et al.: *Physical Foundations of Radiology,* 4th ed. Harper & Row, New York, 1970, p. 288.

24. *Ibid.,* p. 296.

25. Gloyna, Earnest F., and Ledbetter, Joe O.: *op. cit.,* p. 201.

26. Blahd, William H.: *op. cit.,* p. 788.

27. *Ibid.,* p. 792.

28. *Ibid.,* p. 164.

29. *Ibid.,* p. 166.

30. *Ibid.,* p. 664.

31. Wagner, Henry N.: *Principles of Nuclear Medicine.* W. B. Saunders Co., Philadelphia, 1968, p. 275.

32. *Ibid.,* p. 361.

33. Blahd, William H.: *op. cit.,* p. 166.

34. *Ibid.,* p. 760.

35. *Ibid.,* p. 775.

36. Scott, Pauline M.: *op. cit.,* p. 342.

37. Watkins, Arthur L.: *op. cit.,* p. 241.

Additional Suggested Reading

Barckley, V.: "Cancer Consultant to Nursing Homes," *Am. J. Nurs.,* **70:**804, (Apr.) 1970.

————: "A Visiting Nurse Specializes in Cancer Nursing," *Am. J. Nurs.,* **70:**1683, (Aug.) 1970.

Barnes, Priscilla, and Rees, David: *A Concise Textbook of Radiotherapy.* J. B. Lippincott Co., Philadelphia, 1972.

Barnett, Mark: "The Nature of Radiation and Its Effect on Man," *Nurs. Clin. North Am.,* **2:**11, (Mar.) 1967.

Boeker, Elisabeth H.: "The Nurse in Radiation Protection," *Nurs. Clin. North Am.,* **2:**23, (Mar.) 1967.

————: "Radiation Safety," *Am. J. Nurs.,* **65:**111, (Apr.) 1965.

Braestrup, Carl Bjorn, and Vikterlöf, K. J.: *Manual on Radiation Protection in Hospitals and General Practice.* World Health Organization, Geneva, 1974.

Burns, Patricia, and Parker, Helen: "Precautions Are Necessary When Radioactive Iodine or Gold Is Used," *Am. J. Nurs.,* **56:**1404, (Nov.) 1956.

Chadwick, D. R.: "Radiation in Perspective," *Nurs. Clin. North Am.,* **2:**3, (Mar.) 1967.

Craytor, Josephine K., and Fass, Margot O.: *The Nurse and the Cancer Patient.* J. B. Lippincott Co., Philadelphia, 1970.

Day, John E., and Lightfoot, David A.: "OR Radiation Hazards," *AORN J.,* **20:**249, (Aug.) 1974.

Deeley, Thomas: *Modern Trends in Radiotherapy—2.* Appleton-Century-Crofts, New York, 1972.

Donovan, Marilee, and Pierce, Sandra: *Cancer Care Nursing.* Appleton-Century-Crofts, New York, 1976.

Eicherly, Elizabeth E.: "Nursing in Thermonuclear Disaster," *Nurs. Clin. North Am.,* **2:**324, (June) 1967.

Fenner, Matthew L.: *Elementary Clinical Radiotherapy.* Appleton-Century-Crofts, New York, 1968.

Garde, Sister Mariana: "Cancer of the Thyroid," *Am. J. Nurs.,* **65:**98, (Nov.) 1965.

Ginsberg, Frances: "Where Nurses Err While Handling Radium," *Mod. Hosp.,* **99:**138, (Sept.) 1962.

Gohr, Frank A.: "Safety Is Everybody's Business," Part IV, *Hosp. Manage.,* **100:**50, (Nov.) 1965.

Gribbons, Carol A., and Aliapoulios, M. A.: "Treatment for Advanced Breast Carcinoma," *Am. J. Nurs.,* **72:**678, (Apr.) 1972.

Hilkemeyer, Renilda: "Nursing Care in Radium

Therapy," *Nurs. Clin. North Am.,* **2:**83, (Mar.) 1967.

Johnson, Philip C.: "Benefits and Risks in Nuclear Medicine," *Am. J. Public Health,* **62:**1568, (Dec.) 1972.

Kautz, Harold, et al.: "Radioactive Drugs," *Am. J. Nurs.,* **64:**124, (Jan.) 1964.

Kendall, Elizabeth: "Care of Patients Treated with Sealed Sources of Radioisotopes," *Nurs. Clin. North Am.,* **2:**97, (Mar.) 1967.

Korsos, Ruth: "Nursing Care of the Patient with Radiation Sickness," *J. Pract. Nurs.,* **14:**24, (Oct.) 1964.

Licht, Sidney (ed.): *Therapeutic Electricity and Ultraviolet Radiation.* Physical Medicine Library Vol. 4. Elizabeth Licht, New Haven, Conn., 1967.

Love, Robert A.: "Care of the Patient Exposed to Radiation," *J. Pract. Nurs.,* **14:**22, (Oct.) 1964.

Maynard, C. Douglas: *Clinical Nuclear Medicine.* Lea & Febiger, Philadelphia, 1971.

Mould, R. F.: "Physics and Radiotherapy. 4. Radiation Protection," *Nurs. Times,* **70:**468, (Jan. 12) 1974.

Norwood, William D.: "Radiation Casualties— Emergency Plans and Medical Care," *Arch. Envir. Health,* **23:**129, (Aug.) 1971.

Nowak, Patricia Ann: "Inservice Education in Radiation Health," *Nurs. Clin. North Am.,* **2:**107, (Mar.) 1967.

Quimby, Edith H.: "What Nurses Should Know About Radiation Hazards," *Int. Nurs. Rev.,* **11:**19, (July–Aug.) 1964.

Ring, Sister M. Alanna: "Cobalt-60 Teletherapy," *Hosp. Prog.,* **47:**111, (Aug.) 1966.

Rummerfield, Philip S., and Rummerfield, Marilyn J.: "What You Should Know About Radiation Hazards," *Am. J. Nurs.,* **70:**780, (Apr.) 1970.

Sameer, Rafla, and Rotman, Marvin: *Introduction to Radiotherapy.* C. V. Mosby Co., St. Louis, 1974.

Sellars, Jacqueline H.: "Clinical Applications of Unsealed Radioisotopes," *Nurs. Clin. North Am.,* **2:**61, (Mar.) 1967.

Selman, Joseph: *The Fundamentals of X-Ray and Radium Physics,* 5th ed. Charles C Thomas, Publisher, Springfield, Ill., 1972.

Szent-Györgyi, Albert: *The Living State, With Observations on Cancer.* Academic Press, New York, 1972.

Thomas, Dolores A.: "The Nurse's Contribution in a Radiation Therapy Outpatient Department," *Nurs. Clin. North Am.,* **2:**49, (Mar.) 1967.

Underhill, R. A.: "Ultrasound in Obstetrics," *Nurs. Times,* **69:**1278, (Oct. 4) 1973.

Vahey, Sister Mary Hope: "Clinical Applications of Unsealed Radioisotopes," II, *Nurs. Clin. North Am.,* **2:**73, (Mar.) 1967.

Walker, Elizabeth: "Responsibilities of the Hospital Nurse in the Clinical Use of Radiation," *Nurs. Clin. North Am.,* **2:**35, (Mar.) 1967.

Watson, John C.: *Patient Care and Special Procedures in Radiologic Technology,* 4th ed. C. V. Mosby Co., St. Louis, 1974.

Welch, Marion S.: "Comfort Measures During Radiation Therapy," *Am. J. Nurs.,* **67:**1880, (Sept.) 1967.

Zaino, Costantino: "Eliminating the Hazards from Radiation," *Am. J. Nurs.,* **62:**60, (Apr.) 1962.

Katherine Nelson
Dorothy Harrison
Virginia Henderson

CHAPTER 32

Processing Sterile Supplies and Equipment Used in Patient Care and Treatment

1. PROCESSING SUPPLIES AND EQUIPMENT IN ANY TREATMENT SETTING

In Chapters 15 and 44 the principles of disease control are discussed. It is pointed out that extreme youth and old age, lowered body resistance, "intrusive therapy," and communal living are among the conditions that predispose the human being to infection. Because all of these conditions are found in hospitals, this chapter describes the way in which supplies and equipment are processed there. While less meticulous methods which may not be as effective are often used in other treatment settings, the procedures recommended for hospitals can be used, and are standards to which all clinic, school, corrective institution, industrial, home care, and other health services should aspire.

In technologically developed and affluent societies commercially processed (sterilized and packaged) disposable supplies are used in all types of health services. In countries where commercial products are not available or are too costly, adaptations of the methods described in the following pages for processing supplies must be used. Suggestions for processing supplies in the home are included at the end of this chapter.

The authors have relied heavily on the findings and opinions of John J. Perkins, a physician and bacteriologist, who has devoted years to the investigation of aseptic practice.

2. THE CENTRAL SERVICE DEPARTMENT OF A HOSPITAL

Development of Central Services in Institutions. For many years, processing of sterile supplies was carried out in the department or area where they were to be used. Hospitals had separate sterilizers on every clinical unit, or supplies, packaged on the units, were sent to the operating room for autoclaving. Much of this work was done by nursing personnel.

Under such conditions it was hard to standardize supplies and techniques throughout the hospital. *Standardization* is necessary because danger and confusion result when the same kind of dressing is called a "compress" on one package and a "sponge" on another, when needles fit one syringe but not another, or when solutions in identical containers are both suitable and unsuitable for intravenous use. In the United States the American Hospital Association, the US Bureau of Standards, the American College of Surgeons, and the US Public Health Service have collaborated in promoting standardization of products and processes.

The Central Service Department, as we know it today, is an outgrowth of an attempt to standardize surgical dressings and centralize the preparation of all surgical supplies in one unit * and also to separate nonnursing from nursing functions. This department is variously known as Central Medical and Surgical Supply Service, Central Supply Room, Central Sterile Supply Department, Central Dispatch, or Central Distribution. Perkins [1] suggests the name Central Service Department because it more accurately describes the work performed. Its function is highly complex and important in the total task of providing quality patient care. The department not only promotes standardization and uniform *quality of supplies and equipment,* but by making possible more effective use of personnel and materials it helps *reduce costs.* In addition, by providing centralized decontamination, cleaning, and resterilization of used equipment it *reduces the hazard of cross-infection.*

Functions of the Central Service Department. Specific functions of the Central Service Department vary from hospital to hospital, but in general it *receives, collects, sorts, processes, stores, issues,* and *distributes all supplies and equipment* used in the care and treatment of the patient. Nadean E. Wright [2] says that the over-all objective of central supply is to have the right item, at the right place, at the right time, in the right condition. Among the supplies and equipment handled by the Central Service Department are plastic, rubber, and shellacked goods, sterile dressings, sterile solutions for external and parenteral use, intravenous administration sets, surgical instruments, utensils such as bath basins and bedpans, sterile linen supplies, large portable equipment such as cardiac arrest carts, and,

in some hospitals, orthopedic and inhalation therapy equipment.[3,4] The pharmacy may be in some cases under the same director and adjacent to the Central Service Department.

Another function of the Central Service Department in some hospitals is testing and evaluating new products to determine the advisability of their purchase by the hospital. This is usually done in cooperation with the hospital's Standardization Committee.[5] Product testing and evaluation is an important function; a product's usefulness and acceptability to patients and staff should be evaluated by those who use it before it is purchased in quantity.

In some hospitals, Central Service Departments are taking on new responsibilities involving direct patient contact. In these instances, nursing and other personnel work as teams to provide intravenous therapy, inhalation therapy, surgical preparation of the patient, and patient transport under the administration of the Central Service Department.[6]

Some hospitals employ nurses as directors of Central Service Departments. Other hospitals consider nursing skills to be wasted in that capacity unless, as noted above, the department gives direct patient care. Stocking, storing, and preparing supplies involve technical processes almost entirely. Except for the management of the personnel, operating a central supply service consists of manipulating inanimate objects. The person in charge of the central supply service has need of managerial ability and enough knowledge of economics, physics, chemistry, bacteriology, and hospital management to enable him or her to use consultants in these fields wisely.

Regardless of the background of the person in charge, supervision and training of personnel is an important component of central service management. A break in technique by someone working in the Central Service Department could cost the life of a susceptible patient even if that employee never comes in contact with the patient. Central Service Department employees are "at risk," as well, every time they handle materials contaminated with pathogenic organisms. Employees must be able to tell the difference between safe and dangerously contaminated equipment, especially when the equipment doesn't look contaminated. In order to protect themselves and others, they must have fairly extensive knowledge about communicable disease, its cause, the way it is spread, and methods of control. Everyone who processes supplies must acquire a way of thinking about microorganisms and their relationship to personnel, patients, supplies, and equipment.[7]

Central Service Department personnel (and

---

* Some hospitals of very recent construction are building each floor or clinical division as an autonomous unit. In such cases there is a service department on each division. The service department and the pharmacy for the division may be under the same director, a pharmacist. This is a modification of the Friesen design briefly described in Chapter 15.

all hospital employees) should be free from transmissible infection manifested by fever, colds, boils or other skin eruptions, and diarrhea while on duty, and should be grounded in the elements of personal hygiene. Some may have to be taught the importance of handwashing or the necessity of covering the nose and mouth when sneezing. Even if nurses are not in charge of the Central Service Departments they may be called on to function as teachers.

3. COLLECTION AND DISTRIBUTION OF SUPPLIES AND EQUIPMENT

Supplies are transported to and from the Central Service Department by carts, vertical conveyors, dumbwaiters, elevators, pneumatic tubes, and by messenger, used singly or in combination. Care must be taken, whichever method is used, to protect personnel performing this function and to avoid spreading infectious disease. The principle of separating "clean" and "dirty," or used, equipment, should apply to all conveyors. The person collecting used equipment should not deliver clean equipment at the same time. The practice of exchanging "clean for used" should therefore be discouraged. There should be separate areas on the patient unit for clean and used supplies. (See discussion of separation of clean and soiled items under the Friesen Concept in Chapter 15.)

Some hospitals transport supplies throughout the hospital in automated battery powered carts (AMSCAR) that move unaided through tunnels on guideline tracks buried in the floor. The carts are programmed and electronically guided anywhere in the hospital at the turn of a dial and push of a button. They are capable of delivering 90 per cent of all supplies, including food and laundry. They can return soiled items and refuse to Central Service, and finally propel themselves through an automatic wash, emerging clean and ready for another round of distribution.

Because all equipment coming in contact with patients is potentially contaminated with pathogenic organisms, cleaning or rinsing gross soil from equipment on the patient unit should be avoided (with the possible exception of rinsing blood or other body fluid out of a reusable syringe) because of the possibility of contaminating sinks, other equipment, and personnel. Soiled reusable equipment on the unit should be placed in containers with disposable liners. Needles and sharp instruments, if to be reprocessed, should be transported in closed containers that cannot be perforated. Equipment from patients with infectious disease should be double-bagged, labeled CONTAMINATED, and bear a label identifying the contents. (See page 898, Chapter 15, for a description of double-bagging.)

In hospitals where patients' bedside utensils such as bath basins and bedpans are not processed in the Central Service Department, they are usually washed and sanitized for reissue by being soaked in a disinfectant solution on the patient care unit by nursing or housekeeping personnel, or they may be washed by housekeeping personnel, assembled in paper bags, and delivered to the Central Service Department for sterilization.

Efficient collection and distribution of supplies and equipment not only helps control infection, but also ensures that equipment is immediately available when needed. Its rapid delivery may be a matter of life or death for a patient whose recovery depends on it. Suggestions for a system of equipment control can be found in *The Central Service Technician,* published by the International Association of Hospital Central Service Management.[8]

4. CENTRAL DECONTAMINATION AND CLEANING OF SUPPLIES AND EQUIPMENT

Defined Areas. The Central Service Department should have separate processing areas for the following activities: receiving, assembling and packaging, sterilizing, storing, and dispensing. Since all used equipment is potentially contaminated with infectious organisms, there should be a central decontamination area as well—a space in or adjacent to the central service. In the decontamination area, soiled articles are received, sorted, and rendered safe for further handling. Ideally, this area should be separated by a physical barrier from other sections of the department.

Methods of Decontaminating and Cleaning. Equipment should be decontaminated before handling. Items are selected according to type and, if not damaged by water and heat, are placed in a *washer-sterilizer* which preferably has two doors, one that opens into the decontamination area and the other into the clean work area on the other side of the barrier. In some hospitals, unopened bags of contaminated equipment are run through the autoclave before handling. Articles that are sensitive to heat are decontaminated by chemical disinfection and cleaned manually before being transferred to the clean work area through a pass-through window. Equipment that cannot be sterilized by steam or liquids, such as electrical equipment, is bagged separately for gas sterilization. Large contaminated items of portable equipment, such as suction machines, are wiped off with a phenol, or other, disinfecting solution and covered with a plastic bag before being returned to the Central Service Department for processing.

Modern mechanical equipment has simplified cleaning procedures considerably. Devices such as ultrasonic cleaners and washer-sterilizers have greatly improved the efficiency of processing sterile supplies and equipment. Some hospitals have mechanical washers to clean and disinfect transportation carts before returning them to storage or dispatch areas.

The washer-sterilizer is designed to clean and decontaminate a variety of articles: instruments, scrub brushes, trays, bowls, soap dishes, basins, bedpans, ice bags, hot-water bags, and assorted glassware. In this machine, equipment is washed in a detergent solution while being sterilized with saturated steam. The process takes about 15 minutes. Being enclosed, the washer-sterilizer prevents dissemination of aerosols commonly created by manual scrubbing and cleaning.[9]

Another commonly used cleaning device is the *ultrasonic cleaner* which cleans but does not sterilize. For this reason, equipment from infectious patients should not be put into the ultrasonic machine until after the equipment is decontaminated either by autoclaving or by chemical disinfection.* The ultrasonic cleaner is used primarily for surgical instruments and syringes. In this machine, instruments are immersed in a detergent solution and subjected to energy created by high-frequency sound waves. This process is followed by a rinse-and-dry cycle. Ultrasonics initiates cavitation, which is the formation of minute bubbles that expand,

---

* Some manufacturers claim that certain chemical solutions will *sterilize* equipment when used in an ultrasonic cleaner. Claims should be substantiated before such solutions are relied on for sterilization.

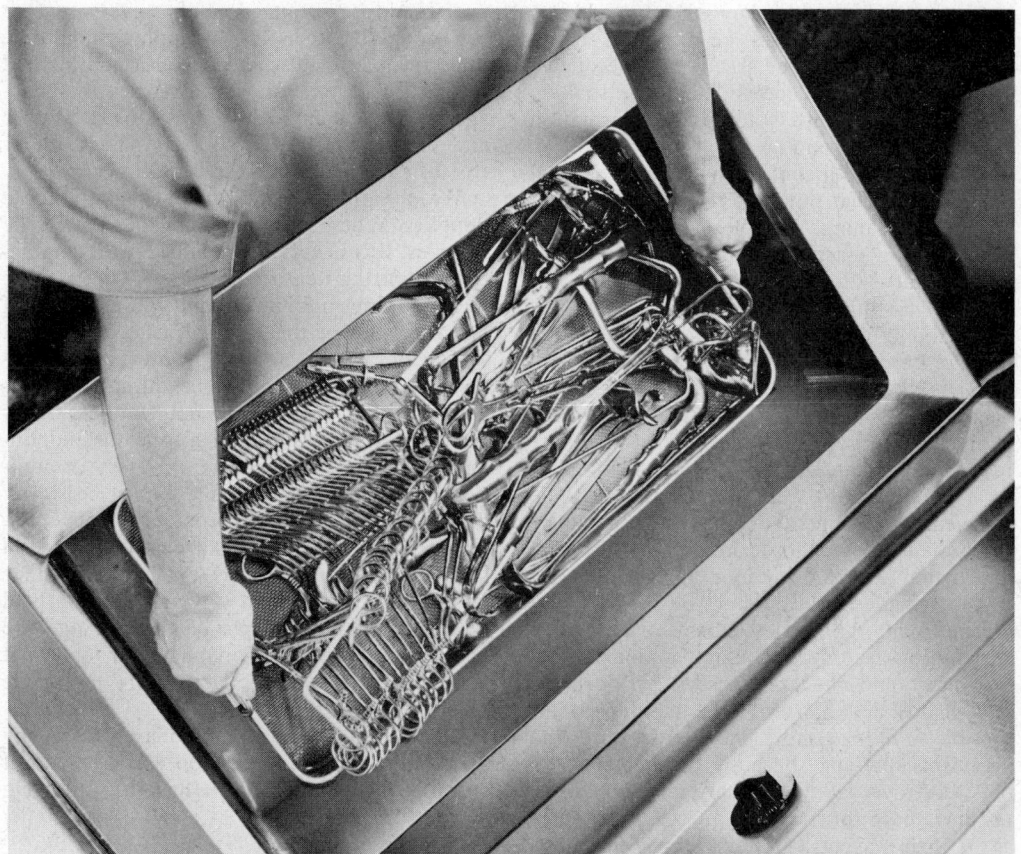

Figure 32-1. Tray of instruments assembled for effective processing in sonic cleaner. (From American Sterilizer Company: "Processing of Surgical Instruments," *J. Hosp. Res.,* **2:**9, [Aug.] 1970. Courtesy of American Sterilizer Company, Erie, Pa.)

become unstable, and collapse. The resulting implosion (opposite of explosion) produces localized vacuum areas that are responsible for dislodging soil from surfaces (see Fig. 32-1). The minute cavitation bubbles rush in between surfaces so small they are not easily apparent. Ultrasonic cleaning is superior to hand brushing since cavitation penetrates areas that the bristles of a brush are too coarse to penetrate. Like all mechanical equipment, the ultrasonic cleaner must be used correctly and must be maintained properly.[10-12]

Cleaning the Equipment. Thorough cleaning is essential for effective sterilization of equipment. Equipment must be free from soil, particularly oil and organic substances such as pus, blood, or other secretions. Disinfectants will not penetrate organic materials, and heat sterilization tends to coagulate protein, "baking" the soil firmly onto surfaces. No one detergent is suitable for all cleaning purposes. The choice of detergent and cleaning technique depends on the nature of the soil, the kind of equipment, water hardness, and other factors. When cleaning is done by hand rather than by machine, soaking may be helpful to loosen soil. Cool water should be used on blood stains, or an alkaline detergent capable of dissolving blood should be added to the soaking solution. (See page 877 for more information about cleaning agents.)

One major difficulty in cleaning medical equipment is that much of it cannot be taken apart for cleaning. Complex machinery such as heart-lung machines, kidney dialysis units, and inhalation therapy equipment often contains valves, tubing, and inaccessible crevices. Surgical instruments have serrations and hinges that are hard to clean.[13]

Chemical agents used to destroy harmful bacteria are commonly called disinfectants, germicides, and bactericides. When they are used on inanimate objects, they are referred to as *disinfectants* because the contact can be sufficiently prolonged and the surfaces can be smooth enough to allow penetration and make destruction of most microorganisms possible; when used (properly diluted) on the skin and mucous membranes, chemical agents are called *antiseptics* because the contact cannot be very prolonged and the skin has many openings into glands and hair follicles, making it impossible to destroy more than a fraction of the organisms present. Because disinfectants do not destroy all harmful microorganisms (mainly spore forms), they are not referred to as sterilizing agents. Glutaraldehyde is an exception; when correctly used, glutaraldehyde will kill all microorganisms, including spores, fungi, and viruses. Glutaraldehyde is used on cutting-edge instruments, or instruments with delicate lenses, and on anesthesia and inhalation-therapy equipment. It does not affect the sharpness of blades, or interfere with the electric conductivity of nonconductive rubber. An automated machine that cleans and sterilizes respiratory equipment using activated (buffered) glutaraldehyde (Cidex) as the sterilizing agent is available.*

5. METHODS OF WRAPPING, PACKAGING, MARKING, AND STORING SUPPLIES

To prepare materials for sterilization, equipment which has been properly cleaned is assembled in compact units, wrapped, secured, and labeled before being put into an autoclave or gas sterilizer. During the sterilizing process, Perkins says there must be direct steam or gas contact with all surfaces, as well as "every strand, fiber, or particle of the substance undergoing sterilization." † The wrapping material must, therefore, be permeable to the sterilizing agent, and the contents of the package should be arranged so that every surface can be permeated. The wrapping should be impermeable to dust and bacteria and applied so that it will maintain sterility when the package is opened and while it is stored. Before and during packaging, supplies should be as free of microorganisms as possible.[14]

Wrapping Materials for Packaging Sterile Supplies. When selecting a wrapper for sterile supplies, it is necessary to consider the characteristics of the item to be wrapped. In general, the wrapping must not inhibit the entrance of steam or gas, or the elimination of air, and it should not be affected by the sterilizing process. The wrapping should be durable, preferably reusable, and should not tear, crack, or puncture easily. It should also withstand humidity during storage. The wrapper, in addition to serving as a dust filter, must be sturdy enough to protect the contents from contamination when the package is handled and to protect it from insects or vermin.[15] Since the wrapper must often serve as a sterile field from which the contents of the package are handled, it should be soft and tend to lie flat rather than to spring back over the sterile object.

Canvas should not be used as a wrapping for sterile supplies as it is too dense to permit entrance of steam. *Muslin* has the following

---

* The cidematic sterilizing machine made by Arbrook, Inc., Arlington, Tex.

† Perkins, John J.: *Principles and Methods of Sterilization in Health Sciences,* 2nd ed. Charles C Thomas, Publisher, Springfield, Ill., 1969, p. 111.

advantages: it permits steam penetration; it can be laundered many times; when opened on a flat surface, a muslin wrapper may serve as a sterile field; it does not tear easily; and it protects contents from damage in handling or in accidental falls. When used, muslin should be of double thickness, with layers stitched together. *Plastic* has the advantage of being impermeable to dust and of allowing contents to be visible. *Paper* makes a good wrapper because it is convenient, inexpensive, and may be discarded after use. The main drawback of paper is its lack of pliability. Kraft paper (brown wrapping paper) is not recommended because it is brittle, which leads to defects that allow contamination. Dennison wrap is a crepe paper that is strong and permeable to steam, but it is hard to make a flat surface with this product. Patapar is a paper product that is satisfactory at first but decreases in usefulness as the drying period is prolonged. Glassine covers are soggy during the sterilization process and brittle afterward. They are easily punctured, but are widely used for disposable articles sterilized in ethylene oxide. Waxed paper is not acceptable. Aluminum foil is good only in dry heat sterilization; it is often the most convenient for home use, particularly for sterilization of syringes. The use of *plastic film* has increased, especially in gas sterilization of new products. Polyethylene is the film of choice for ethylene oxide gas sterilization because it allows rapid penetration and dissipation of the gas; it is not suitable for steam sterilization. Nylon film is acceptable for steam sterilization when an extended drying period is used, but is not satisfactory for gas. Saran wrap is minimally acceptable for gas sterilization because the pores are extremely fine. (Permeability is decreased as pore size decreases.) Cellophane has been used to wrap packages for gas sterilization, but it cracks easily in handling and storage. If cracks in cellophane develop, the article should be rewrapped and resterilized.[16]

Packaging of Materials to Be Sterilized. Permeation of the interior of the bundle depends on the size of the bundle and the density of the pack. *Bundles* should not exceed 12 by 12 by 20 inches in size and 12 lb in weight. Packages of this size can have uniform steam penetration when sterilized at 121°C (250°F) for 30 to 60 minutes. Basins should not be packaged with fabrics as they may interfere with air elimination, cause excess condensation, and prevent effective drying following sterilization. The contents of the pack should be arranged in an orderly manner in order of use. Gauze sponges, if included, should be located near the center to break up close contact between the other more closely woven fabrics. Gauze, being light and porous, readily admits steam through the center of the pack. Each succeeding layer of linen is placed crosswise on the one below to promote free circulation of steam. When the materials are assembled, the covers should not be drawn up too tightly, only enough to hold the contents together for a reasonable amount of handling. Articles must be completely covered, with the corners of the wrapper turned in. A small cuff on the under fold (the first fold to be turned over the contents) provides a safe area to grasp when the package is opened, to avoid contaminating the contents. The inner cover of a pack is used as a sterile field when the package is opened. An outer cover or wrapper is secured with cord or tape.

When it is necessary to reduce the size and density of a *pack*, sheets and table covers ("drapes") should be the first to be eliminated; because of their density when folded, they are the most difficult items to sterilize. Such articles should be wrapped separately in packs containing no more than two "drapes" or two sheets. Towels and gowns do not present a problem, as towels, being coarse, offer little resistance to steam, and gowns, because of the loose arrangement of the fabric, are not particularly dense, even when folded.[17]

Dressing-drums, jars, canisters, or cans, should *not* be used for packaging sterile supplies. Compact arrangement of the material prevents free access of steam and expulsion of air when sterilized in a steam autoclave, and gas will not penetrate the container. Moreover, after "sterilization," while the container is in use, each time the container is opened to remove materials, contaminating microorganisms are inevitably admitted. Gauze sponges, and all other supplies, should be packaged for individual, one-time use, rather than in bulk.

Rubber sheets and other impervious materials should not be folded for sterilization, as steam cannot penetrate them. The rubber sheet should be covered with a piece of fabric the same size and, together, loosely rolled before wrapping.

Weck sterilizing tubing, a tube of transparent material, is widely used for packaging catheters, drains, and other items. It is economical, easy to use, and by permitting visibility of contents, eliminates the need for labeling. A variation with nylon front and paper back which can be sealed with a heat-sealer, or tape, has printing that turns green when steam autoclaved. While steam and gas readily penetrate the tubing during sterilization, it is impervious to contamination during storage.[18]

Securing the wrapper and labeling is done in several ways. Wrapped packages may be secured with twine, heavy cord, or pressure-sensitive tape. Some kinds of plastic can be sealed with a heat-sealer. Tape can be written on to identify contents. Sterilizer-indicating tape that changes color during autoclaving has the added advantage of identifying packages that have been through the sterilizing process. This does not ensure sterility of contents, however. (See page 1411 for description of such safeguards.)

Pins should *not* be used to secure wrappings, as they permit contamination to enter, shorten the life of the covering fabric, increase the tendency to tear, and encourage tight wrapping. All packs and items should be clearly labeled, using waterproof marking material, with the date, name of tray or item, and initials of the person preparing the package.

Packaging Treatment Trays or Sets. Equipment for every kind of surgical procedure and medical treatment is prepared and packaged on individual trays for sterilization. Space does not permit detailed instructions for tray preparation here, but this information can be found in many source books.[19-21]

Numerous prepackaged, disposable, sterile treatment trays are available commercially. They are widely used and have many advantages: they remain sterile indefinitely unless the package is damaged, and they do not have to be resterilized every 30 days if not used; they are of uniform size convenient for stacking; the name of the tray and itemized contents are printed on the outside; they minimize cross-contamination due to improper cleaning or inadequate sterilization, and in situations where labor costs are high, can be less expensive than reusable trays. Generally speaking, commercial sterilization methods are reliable and therefore reduce the risk of infection, but the second great advantage of disposable trays is the saving of time and labor in preparation. Like all disposable items, they have the following disadvantages: they pose a serious disposal problem and they require more storage space than reusable trays which can be torn down or reprocessed after each use.[22]

Storing Sterilized Supplies and Equipment. Sterile packages should be stored on clean, enclosed shelves, protected from moisture. The length of time packages remain sterile depends on the porosity of the wrapping and protection from outside contamination. Numerous studies have been made in an attempt to establish *"shelf life"* (the length of time equipment remains sterile if not opened or damaged) of sterile articles. Paul Standard and his associates[23] found that single-wrap muslin (two layers stitched together) allows bacteria to enter the package as early as 3 days when stored on open shelves, while double-wrap muslin (four layers stitched together) and two-way crepe paper (single layer) remain growth-free for up to 28 days. They also found that handling of the articles decreases shelf life. G. A. Nichols[24] reported that materials sealed in plastic showed no bacterial growth after 18 months.

E. Reilly and F. Ginsberg[25] suggest that, in general, muslin- and paper-wrapped packages may be stored 30 days. Plastic sacks or wraps around muslin or paper packages increase the shelf life to 3 months, while heat-sealed packages may be stored from 6 months to a year. Peelback polyethylene film-covered packages may be stored indefinitely.

Articles in damaged or torn covers, or packages exposed to moisture, should be considered contaminated and should be opened and reprocessed if reusable, or thrown away if they are disposable. Commercially packaged disposable equipment should not be resterilized with ethylene oxide gas because a highly toxic compound may be formed (see page 1413).

6. STERILIZING SUPPLIES AND EQUIPMENT—METHODS

Current Methods. A more complete discussion of sterilization is presented in Chapter 15. This section deals mainly with techniques of loading and operating sterilizers.

There are several effective methods of sterilization; in each instance, the method selected should be appropriate for the material to be sterilized. The common methods used in hospitals are *steam under pressure* (autoclaving), *ethylene oxide gas,* and *dry heat.*

Sterilizing by Steam Under Pressure (Autoclaving). Heat destroys bacteria by coagulating cell protein. Coagulation is hastened by the addition of moisture, but steam or boiling water alone are inadequate for sterilization; pressure to increase the temperature of the steam is necessary to make it effective. Autoclaving, a process using steam under controlled pressure, is suitable for articles such as fabrics or paper that would be damaged by dry heat at high temperatures. In the autoclave, all air must be replaced by steam, and equipment must be packaged and loaded so that steam reaches all surfaces of the materials being sterilized.[26,27,28]

Loading the autoclave is a critical step. All packs and other items should be put on edge and arranged in the chamber so that steam passes through the whole load. Rubber goods should not be sterilized in the same load with items requiring a longer sterilization time. Packages containing gloves should rest on edge with thumbs uppermost. All jars, tubes, and other containers must be placed horizontally to permit displacement of air and allow steam to flow inside. Utensils and packaged treatment trays should be put on edge to facilitate drying. Instruments should be placed in trays with perforated bottoms. Utensils should not be nested, and hard goods, when sterilized in a load with fabrics, should be put on the lowest shelves with linen packs above. Small items, such as syringes, should be sterilized in wire mesh baskets. Solutions should be sterilized separately from other supplies. To avoid overcrowding the sterilizer, there should be free space on all sides and at least 3 inches at the top (see Fig. 32-2). Each type of article has its own physical and chemical properties, and its own requirements for sterilization. All personnel using the autoclave

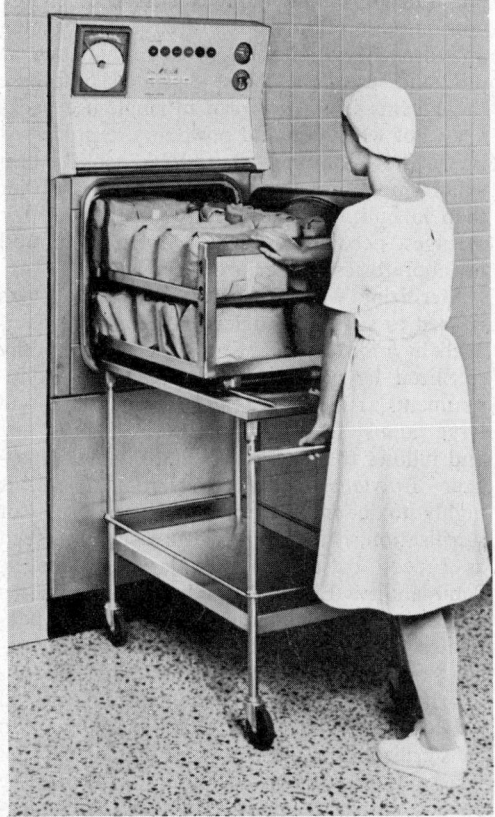

Figure 32-2. An example of good loading practice for large surgical supply sterilizer. All packs are resting on edge with some space between them for free circulation of steam. (Courtesy of American Sterilizer Company, Erie, Pa.)

must be familiar with these requirements and with the operation of the autoclave. The manufacturer's instructions should be closely followed.

Moist packages require a drying period before removal from the autoclave. Even when packages are well dried out in the sterilizer, sudden cooling may result in condensation of residual vapor inside the package. Freshly sterilized packages should not be put on a cold surface such as a metal table top, as "sweating" may occur, causing the package to become damp and subject to contamination. It is good practice to leave supplies on the carriage for 15 or 20 minutes following removal from the chamber. If no loading carriage is used, packages should be laid out on edge, on a wire mesh or slotted wood surface which is covered with several layers of muslin to absorb moisture.[29] Enclosing freshly sterilized packages in plastic after they are thoroughly dry will increase their shelf life.

Finally, it is important to note that *temperature is the important factor* in sterilizing by autoclave, not pressure. Although increased temperature and pressure go hand in hand, moist heat is the sterilizing agent. Pressure is significant because it raises the temperature of the steam. The sterilizing period must be measured from the moment the thermometer in the discharge line indicates a minimum temperature of 121°C (250°F); it should *not* begin when the pressure gauge indicates 15 or 20 lb pressure. Table 32-1 indicates minimum exposure periods for sterilization of supplies.

Sterilization controls must be used in autoclaving. Because of the possibility of sterilization failure, a system of controlling the process to confirm the sterility of a particular article, or to evaluate the effectiveness of a sterilizer, is essential. There are three types of controls: (1) mechanical devices, such as recording and indicating thermometers (see Fig. 32-3) to identify and prevent operational malfunction; (2) biologic controls, such as spore strips (live spores on paper strips); and (3) chemical controls which detect cool air pockets at the center of the load. A biologic control consists of placing live spores in the densest part of a pack during sterilization, then sending them to the laboratory for incubation to see whether they are alive or dead. One kind of chemical control consists of putting a small glass tube containing pellets which melt when conditions of time and temperature are favorable in the center of bundles in different parts of the autoclave. Another chemical control is to place a dye-impregnated card which changes color when steam of a given temperature is in contact with it for a given length of time. A third

Table 32-1.   Minimum Exposure Periods for Sterilization of Supplies *†

Article	250–254° F (121°– 123° C) minutes	270°F (132° C) minutes
Brushes in dispensers, and/or individually wrapped cans	30	10
Dressings, wrapped in paper or muslin	30	10
Dressings, in canisters (on sides)	30	10
Flasked solutions		
75 ml–250 ml	20	—
500 ml–1000 ml	30	—
1500 ml–2000 ml	45	—
Glassware empty, inverted	15	3
Instruments, metal only, any number	15	3
Instruments, metal combined with other materials	15	7
Instruments, metal only, in covered and/or padded tray	15	7
Instruments, metal combined with other materials, in covered and/or padded tray	20	10
Instruments, wrapped in double-thickness muslin	20	10
Linen, packs, 12 by 12 by 20 inches or less	30	—
Needles, individually packaged in glass tubes or paper (lumen moist)	30	10
Rubber gloves, wrapped in muslin or paper	20	—
Rubber catheters, drains, tubing, etc., individually packaged in muslin or paper (lumen must be moist)	20	—
Rubber catheters, drains, etc., unwrapped	20	10
Treatment trays, wrapped in muslin or paper	30	10
Utensils, unwrapped	15	3
Utensils, wrapped in muslin or paper	20	10
Syringes, unassembled, individually packaged in muslin or paper	30	10
Sutures, silk, cotton, or nylon, wrapped in paper or muslin	30	10

* American Sterilizer Company: *Technique Manual.* The Company, Erie, Pa., 1965.

† Using steam under pressure in standard type hospital sterilizers.

type of chemical control is to use a sterilizer-indicating tape which, by developing dark stripe marks, shows that a pack or article has been through the sterilizing process. While mechanical and chemical controls are useful to ensure that the sterilizing process has been successfully completed, they are not a guarantee of sterility. Only biologic controls can indicate sterility.[30]

Sterilizing with Boiling Water. Boiling water is inadequate as a sterilizing medium because it does not kill spores. When necessary to use it in the home (where better methods are unavailable) it can be made more effective by adding sodium carbonate (sal soda) to make a 2 per cent solution. This reduces the hydrogen ion concentration. Rubber goods and glassware must not be boiled in sodium carbonate, however, as it is destructive to both. Articles to be boiled must be clean and free from grease. They must be placed in the container of water so that no air is trapped inside. Sharp instruments should not be boiled because the edges will be dulled in the process.[31] (See page 1427 for more information about home disinfection.)

Sterilizing with Dry Heat. In sterilization with dry heat, hot air at 160°C (320°F) is applied for 1 hour or longer, depending on the type of item being sterilized. This is not the method of choice for most items because the prolonged time and high temperatures required are destructive to some materials, and are time-consuming and expensive in energy consumption. Dry heat is used for sterilizing anhydrous (without water) materials such as oils and powders. Most hospitals purchase these items in sterile form in single-use packages, but when oils and powders are processed in the hospital, they should be packaged in small amounts in individual containers rather than in bulk. Dry heat is frequently used for syringes, needles, and sharp instruments, and in laboratories to sterilize glassware.[32]

Sterilizing with Gas (Ethylene Oxide). Gas is used to sterilize articles that would be damaged by moisture or heat. Articles commonly sterilized by gas include delicate surgical instruments, rubber or plastic equipment, and large items such as bassinettes, incubators, and pillows that will not fit into a steam sterilizer. Ethylene oxide, a bactericidal gas, is highly toxic and flammable. When used for sterilization, it is mixed with an inert gas such as Freeon or carbon dioxide to reduce its flammability. Ethylene oxide kills all known microorganisms, including spore forms; it penetrates porous substances such as fabrics, paper, and polyethylene. Nylon, however, is poorly penetrated by ethylene oxide and should not be used as wrapping material for items to be sterilized by gas. Ethylene oxide will not penetrate glass, but can be used to sterilize the outside of glass vials or ampoules of medication. Such ampoules must be examined for minute cracks, as ethylene oxide, if permitted to enter and mix with the solution inside the ampoule, may cause a change in chemical composition.[33]

Because of the toxicity of ethylene oxide,

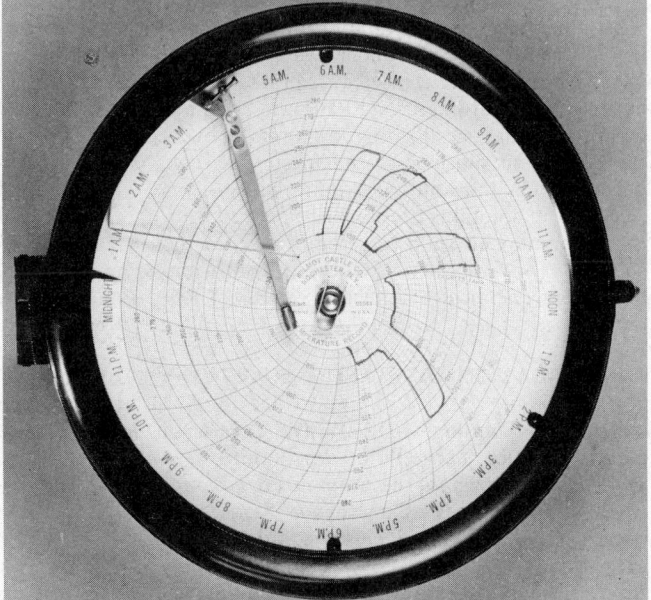

Figure 32-3. Temperature recording chart, a mechanical control to show that steam autoclave is operating effectively. Temperature inside the sterilizing chamber is recorded automatically on paper disk. Record shows repeated and regular sterilizing periods. (Courtesy of Wilmot Castle Co., Rochester, N.Y.)

equipment must be aerated following exposure, particularly porous materials such as rubber or plastic. Air admitted to the sterilizer at the end of the cycle partially aerates the load, but an additional aeration period is necessary until the gas dissipates. Ethylene oxide is a vesicant (causes blisters) if it comes in contact with the skin; if inhaled, it causes eye and nose irritation. Long exposure may result in nausea, vomiting, and dizziness. The gas is soluble in water, and must be completely eliminated from tubing such as intravenous catheters before use. Manufacturers of sterilizing equipment recommend the length of aeration periods for various kinds of materials.[34] An ethylene oxide aerator which removes residual gas following sterilization will decrease the aeration period.

Ethylene oxide sterilization is more expensive than steam sterilization and it requires a longer exposure period. Items that are to be gas-sterilized should be tagged "for gas," to avoid their inadvertently being steam-sterilized. Donald Vesley and V. W. Greene[35] say ethylene oxide should never be used to resterilize disposable items that have been commercially sterilized by gamma radiation, as a highly toxic compound, *ethylene chlorhydrin,* may be formed.

Only skilled personnel should be assigned to the ethylene oxide sterilizer as it requires exact knowledge of proper blending of gases with the humidity, temperature, and the time of exposure. All of these factors—temperature, humidity, and time of exposure—are important in successful sterilization. It is imperative that the manufacturer's instructions be fol-

lowed, and it is also necessary to study the literature of the manufacturers of delicate instruments for information about sterilization of each.

Irradiation Sterilization. Irradiation by radiant energy (electron beam or cobalt) is one of the newer methods of sterilization of medical supplies. At the present time it is mainly used commercially as it is too costly for hospital use.[36]

Ultraviolet rays are not considered a sterilizing agent. Effectiveness of the rays depends on the distance of the source of light and the nature of the item being exposed. Ultraviolet rays have little penetrating power, although if properly placed, they may kill some airborne organisms.[37,38]

Chemical Disinfection. Disinfectant solutions are sometimes used to sterilize products which are injured by heat and cannot be penetrated by steam or gas, but this is to be discouraged in most instances. Most chemical disinfectants are just that—they disinfect, but do not sterilize; that is, they kill vegetative forms of bacteria, but do not kill resistant spores or capsule-forming organisms such as tubercle bacilli. Some disinfectant solutions will harbor and permit the growth of some organisms. Fatal outbreaks of infection have been traced to improper sterilization of instruments in benzalkonium chloride (Zephiran), a disinfectant which is ineffective against gram-negative bacteria and which becomes inactivated in the presence of organic matter such as feces, pus, mucus, blood, cotton, gauze, soap, and some plastics.

As noted earlier in this chapter, activated glutaraldehyde is one liquid disinfectant that actually sterilizes. Sold under the trade name Cidex, it is commonly used to sterilize lenses, cutting-edge instruments, and anesthesia equipment. Following sterilization in glutaraldehyde, the equipment must be rinsed in sterile water before use, as the solution is toxic. Since items sterilized in solutions are not wrapped, sterility is not maintained following removal from the solution. (See Chapter 15 for more information about chemical disinfection.)

7. PREPARATION OF STERILE SOLUTIONS

Types of Solutions—Descriptive Terms. In clinical practice, sterile fluids or solutions have many uses. They may be administered parenterally * into veins, subcutaneous tissue, and bone marrow. In some cases, solutions used externally should be sterile. *Parenteral solutions* are administered to replace normal body fluid and to supply nutrients. *External solutions,* also referred to as irrigation solutions, topical solutions, or surgical solutions, are used for application to the skin and for irrigation of wounds and body cavities, as well as for moistening sponges, compresses, and dressings.

Sterile solutions are fluids in which distilled water (usually) is a solvent for one or more solutes. Sterile solutions for external use must be prepared with the same meticulous technique as parenteral solutions because any solution used to irrigate a wound or body cavity, or to bathe tissues where there is a break in their integrity, can carry microorganisms into the bloodstream. Solutions used externally like those used parenterally must be free of impurities and be *isotonic* with body fluids and with blood. A *hypotonic* fluid such as distilled water, on entering the bloodstream, will cause the red cells to swell and burst. A *hypertonic* solution, on the other hand, may cause crenation (shrinkage with notching of the edges) of red cells. An isotonic solution, or one compatible with blood and body fluids, is easily absorbed by the blood and lymph and should not destroy blood cells. The *United States Pharmacopoeia* refers to an isotonic solution as one containing not less than 0.85 per cent and not more than 0.95 per cent of sodium chloride in water. Commonly called normal, or physiologic, saline, it is the most generally used solution for replacing fluids in the body, as well as for external use.[39] (Blood and plas-

mas are, of course, given parenterally instead of saline in certain conditions.)

Preparing Parenteral Solutions. Although in most hospitals of the United States, commercially prepared intravenous solutions are used, some of which are packaged in plastic bags rather than flasks (see Fig. 32-4), some hospital staffs prefer to prepare their own. Commercial preparation, although by and large more reliable than hospital preparation, is not an absolute guarantee of sterility. Several outbreaks of fatal infection have been traced to commercially prepared solutions.

There are several *dangers* or *causes* of error. Improperly prepared solutions, if introduced into the blood stream, may cause mild or severe febrile reactions. Death can result from unsterile and chemically toxic solutions. Errors that may occur in the preparation of solutions are inadequate distillation of water, the introduction of a toxic substance during distillation or sterilization, the inaccurate measurement of substances that make up the solution, in-

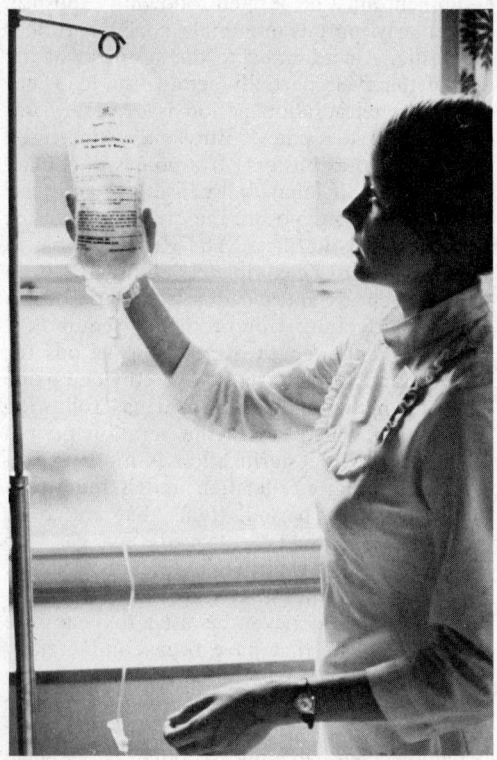

Figure 32-4. Intravenous solutions packaged in plastic bags offer several advantages over glass bottles. The bag is unbreakable, lightweight, easier to set up, has a built-in hanger, and provides a closed system as no venting is necessary. (Courtesy of Travenol Laboratories, Inc., Morton Grove, Ill.)

---

* Parenteral is derived from the Greek (*para* = beside, *enteron* = intestine) and means other than by way of the alimentary tract.

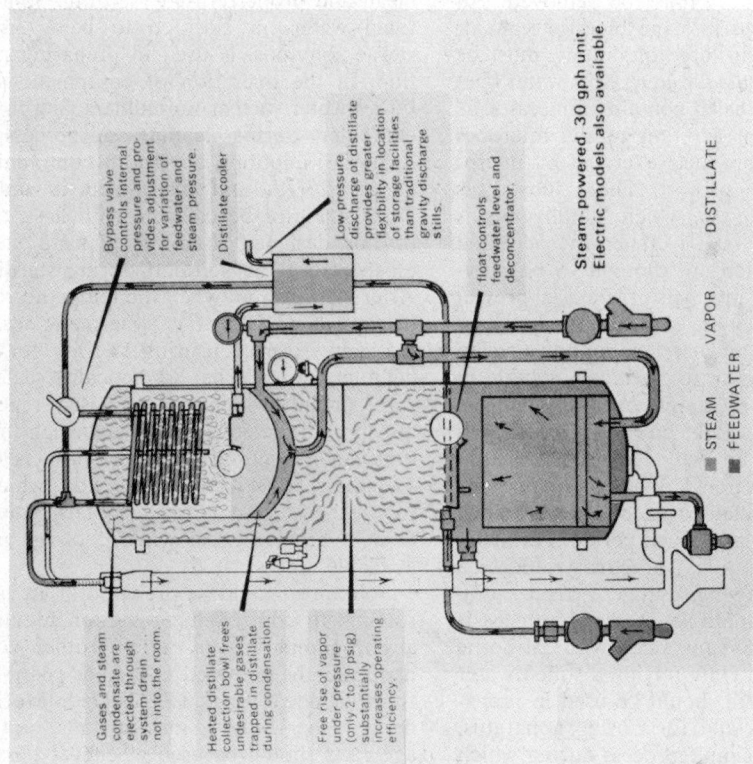

B

Bypass valve controls internal pressure and provides adjustment for variation of feedwater and steam pressure.

Distillate cooler

Low pressure discharge of distillate provides greater flexibility in location of storage facilities than traditional gravity discharge stills.

float controls feedwater level and deconcentrator.

Steam-powered, 30 gph unit. Electric models also available.

Gases and steam condensate are ejected through system drain—not into the room.

Heated distillate collection bowl frees undesirable gases trapped in distillate during condensation.

Free rise of vapor under pressure (only 2 to 10 psig) substantially increases operating efficiency.

■ STEAM ■ VAPOR ░ DISTILLATE
▨ FEEDWATER

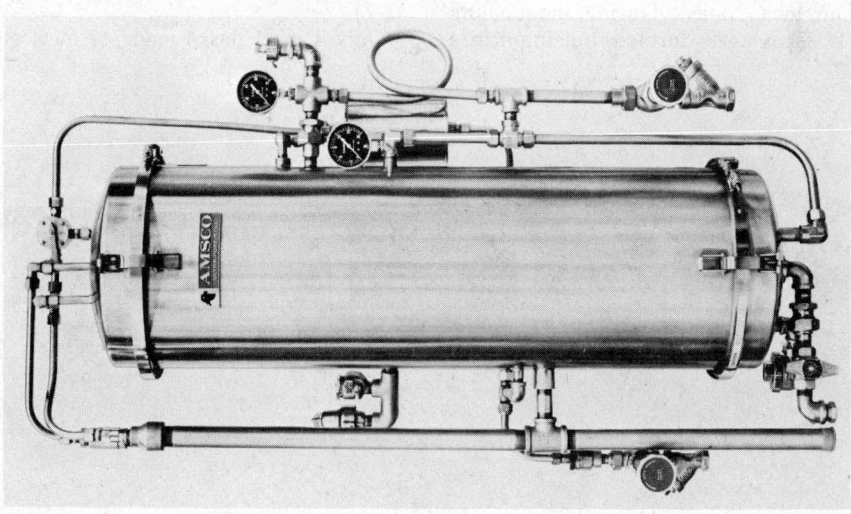

A

Figure 32-5. *A.* All-stainless steel water still. (Courtesy of American Sterilizer Company, Erie, Pa.) *B.* Sectional view of water still. (From Perkins, John J.: *Principles and Methods of Sterilization in Health Sciences,* 2nd ed. Charles C Thomas, Publisher, Springfield, Ill., 1969, pp. 420, 421.)

complete sterilization, contamination of the solution after sterilization, and mistakes in marking flasks. Reactions may result also from careless preparation of the apparatus through which the solution runs. Whatever method is used, *toxic* substances must be removed. All solutions introduced into the blood stream or under the skin, if in large quantities, must be prepared with *distilled water*. Any water that filters through the earth contains mineral salts and is unsterile. In addition to the microbes themselves, toxic products excreted by microorganisms may be present. These substances are known as *pyrogens,* which literally means "fever-producing." It is generally accepted that pyrogens, which are thought to be polysaccharides, are by-products of bacterial growth or metabolism. They are closely related to bacterial O antigen and are commonly called endotoxins. Pyrogens are extremely soluble in water. They cannot be removed by passage through a Berkfeld filter, but may be removed by adsorption on an activated asbestos filter, or on activated charcoal. Pyrogens cannot be destroyed by autoclaving except at very high temperatures for a prolonged period. Perkins [40] says sterilization is of no practical value as a safeguard in removing pyrogens from solutions. One of the main sources of pyrogens is distilled water contaminated with airborne pyrogenic bacteria. Only freshly distilled water from an efficient still should be used in preparation of solutions and for rinsing apparatus.

Distillation is a simple process during which water in a still is heated by boiling until it turns into steam, then cooled. During the cooling process, water is again formed, but impurities are left behind. Stills are available for hospital use in sizes ranging from 5- to 150-gal capacities. A conductivity meter checks the water for purity as the still is used. In order to give safe, adequate service, water stills must be kept clean and properly used (see Fig. 32-5). Distilled water, in addition to being used for sterile solutions, is used in preparing medication, in the operation of equipment that requires water such as humidifiers, and in rinsing equipment during cleaning and processing.

Sterile solutions are most commonly prepared, stored, and distributed in individual *flasks* made of borosilicate with flask closures or lids designed to allow air and vapor to escape from the solution during sterilization. After sterilization, when the temperature drops below 100°C (212°F), a hermetic seal automatically forms, ensuring sterility for an indefinite period. The hermetically sealed closure, or lid, which can be used repeatedly, also provides a sterile lip over which the solution can be poured when the flask is opened (see Fig. 32-6). Disposable lids, which also free exhaust vapors during sterilization and form a hermetic seal when cooling, are also available.

Solutions should be prepared in an enclosed room with controlled circulation to minimize airborne microorganisms and other contaminants, and be prepared as soon as possible after fresh distilled water is collected. Mechanical flask washers, fillers, mixing units, and drainage carts should be used whenever possible to lessen the possibility of human error (see Fig. 32-7).

Only Type I flasks made of hard glass that

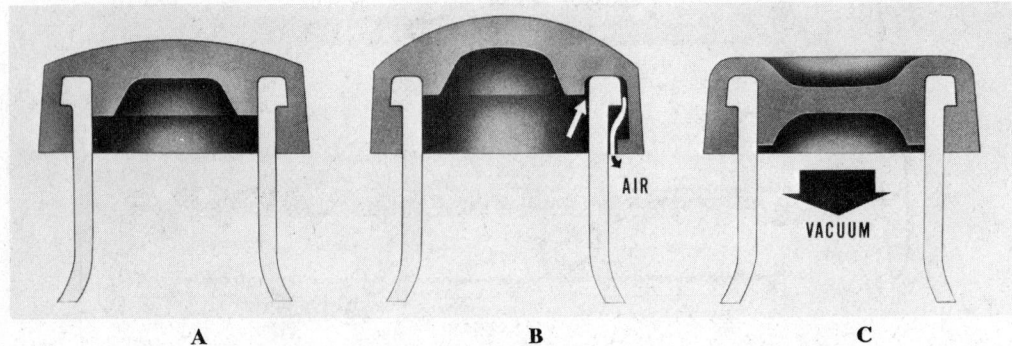

Figure 32-6. *A*. Automatic sealing and venting closure. This shows position of cap on collar before sterilization. *B*. Position of cap on collar showing pathway for escape of air from flask when 1½ lb. pressure has developed in flask during sterilization. *C*. Position of cap automatically sealed on collar by vacuum after solution has been sterilized. (From American Sterilizer Company: "Preparation of External Solutions in Hospitals," *J. Hosp. Res.,* **1**:15, [Jan.] 1963.)

A

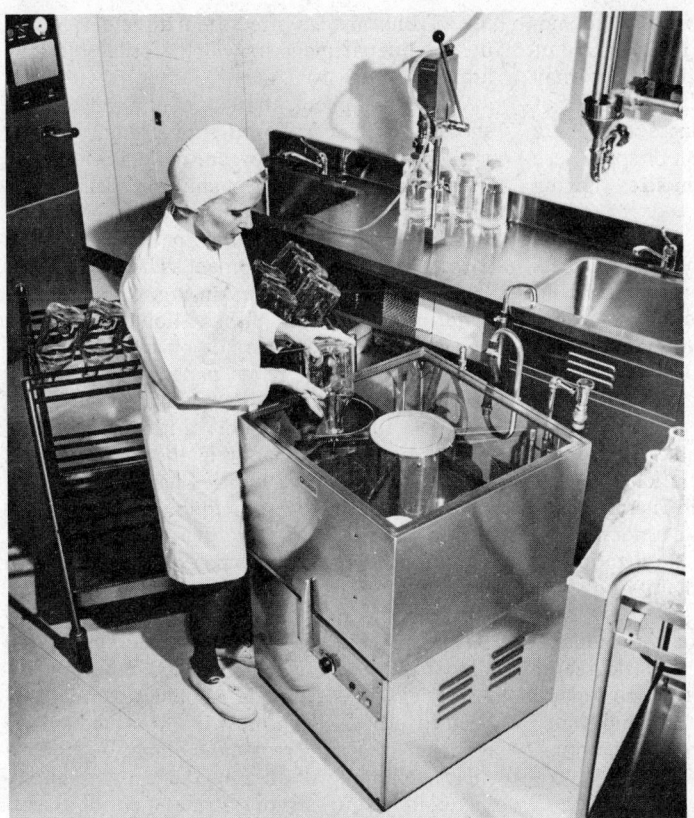

B

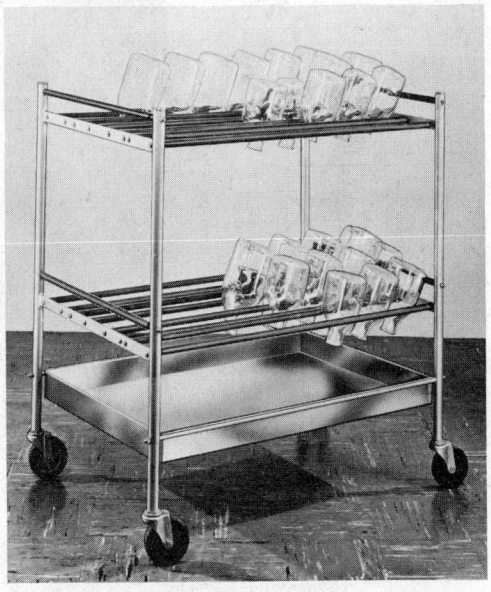

Figure 32-7. *A*. Automatic flask washer. *B*. Flask drain cart. (From American Sterilizer Company: "Preparation of External Solutions in Hospitals." *J. Hosp. Res.,* **1:**15, [Jan.] 1963; revised Apr. 1967.)

is alkaline free and resistant to heat and mechanical shock should be used. Flasks made of soft glass having a high alkali content may change the pH of solutions and start a series of chemical reactions. Solution flasks of square design provide the best utilization of space (see Fig. 32-8). They are available in sizes ranging from 75 ml to 2000 ml.

Reclaimed flasks or bottles, such as commercial intravenous solution bottles or glass containers used for food and beverages, should never be used for the preparation of sterile solutions. They are made of soft glass which chips and breaks easily; and the glass itself breaks down after repeated exposure to intense heat and chemicals.

Identification labels are available for distilled water and for all isotonic solutions. Flasks should be dated, even though hermetically sealed solutions remain sterile indefinitely. Dates should be stamped after sterilization to provide a fast, easy means of identifying sterilized flasks.

Chemical ingredients used for the preparation of solutions should be of a high degree of purity and be free of pyrogenic substances. The solute to be added to the distilled water should be measured and prepared in the pharmacy. Pharmacists are often directors of the hospital department in which sterile solutions are prepared.

New equipment, flasks, caps, and collars should be given a thorough preliminary cleaning to eliminate microorganisms that may have been introduced during manufacture and shipping. An ideal cleaning agent for glassware should clean with ease and speed and be safe for both user and equipment. The final cleaning step is a thorough rinsing with distilled water. After rinsing, flasks should be placed inverted on a drain cart or on a surface covered with lint-free Kraft paper. There should be no cloth towels or other lint-producing materials in the solution room during processing, as any particulate matter in the air may be a source of contamination. Flasks should be closed immediately after filling, and sterilized within an hour. No more than 10 or 20 flasks should be filled and exposed to air at one time.[41,42]

Flasks of solutions are *sterilized* in the autoclave for varying periods depending on the size of the flasks. Different sizes, requiring different exposure periods, should not be sterilized together. Steam must be exhausted slowly to avoid the danger of caps popping off. Premature opening of the autoclave door, allowing cold air to rapidly strike the hot flasks, could make them explode. After the steam is exhausted, the loading cart should be removed from the sterilizer and held until cold in an area free from drafts. Solutions are usually stored at room temperature, but those requiring higher temperatures can be kept in reserve in thermostatically heated cabinets.[43]

8. CARE AND STERILIZATION OF INSTRUMENTS, NEEDLES, AND SUTURES

Instruments. Surgical instruments are expensive, but high quality instruments will last for many years if handled properly. When subjected to rough handling and injurious cleaning techniques, their life expectancy is sharply reduced. Instruments should be used only for the purpose for which they were intended. They should be *cleaned* as soon as possible after use to avoid rusting or pitting, and to remove soil before it can harden in the serrations and crevices. Instruments should be opened or taken apart for cleaning, which should preferably be done in an instrument washer or ultrasonic washer. Ordinary soap and abrasives should be avoided; soap leaves an insoluble alkali film, and abrasives roughen the surface. In general, moderately alkaline,

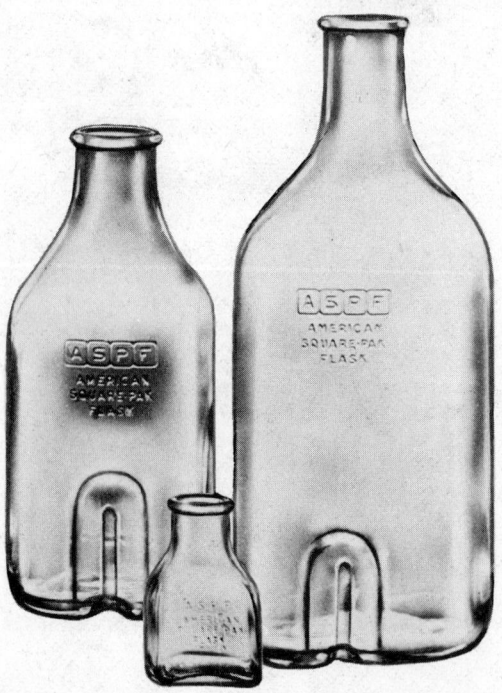

Figure 32-8. Solution flasks of square design. For use in preparation of external or parenteral solutions. (From American Sterilizer Company: "Preparation of External Solutions in Hospitals," *J. Hosp. Res.,* **1**:15, [Jan.] 1963.)

low-sudsing detergents such as Edisonite, Reliance Solvent, or Haemosol are satisfactory detergents. Ultrasonic cleaner manufacturers usually recommend a specific detergent to be used with the machine. A special detergent made with a coconut oil base has been developed for use in the washer-sterilizer.*

Oiling instruments is not recommended because oil prevents steam and disinfectant solutions from penetrating to the surface. Stiff instrument joints may be loosened by applying a drop or two of pHisohex and working it in or by applying commercial silicone oil compounds such as Surgeo-Sil.†

Autoclaving is the method of choice for sterilization of instruments. The destruction of spores requires that instruments be subjected to saturated steam under pressure at a temperature of 121°C (250°F) for a minimum of 12 minutes, or 132°C (270°F) for 2 minutes, with direct steam in contact with all surfaces. Before being put into the autoclave, all jointed instruments must be open or unlocked and placed in an instrument tray with a wire-mesh bottom to allow steam to reach all surfaces.

If sterilized instruments are to be held in temporary storage, the entire tray should be wrapped with double-thickness muslin and additional time should be added to the sterilization procedure to allow for penetration of steam through the wrapper.

For *emergency sterilization* of instruments when rapid sterilization is necessary, Perkins [44] recommends a high-speed pressure instrument sterilizer, adjusted for operation at 132°C (270°F) and 27 to 28 lb pressure for 3 minutes.

Proctoscopes, cystoscopes, bronchoscopes, and all *telescopic instruments containing lenses* must be sterilized in such a way that the lens and the substance used to hold it in place are not affected. Some of the newer "scopes" have been designed to withstand steam sterilization, but unless this is known to be the case, such instruments should be sterilized with ethylene oxide gas, Cidex, or Bard-Parker solution which consists of alcohol and formaldehyde. When instruments are sterilized in solutions, the chemical must be removed with sterile water before the instrument is used.

Needles. Commercially sterilized disposable needles are a boon to patients and health workers but they are relatively expensive. Many individuals and institutions elect to process and reuse needles. Reusable needles used for aspiration or injection of fluids are available in a wide range of sizes. They are scaled according to their length and diameter. Figure 32-9 shows the actual size of commonly used needles of this type. Points (or bevels) should be short or long, according to the purposes for which the needle is used. Needles are made of platinum, iridium, gold, nickel, steel with chromium plate, and stainless steel. Platinum and gold needles are too costly for ordinary use; some metals are so soft that it is difficult to make and preserve a sharp point. Stainless steel is relatively noncorrosive, takes a good point, is strong and moderately flexible, and probably makes the most desirable needle.

When needles are to be processed for reuse they require meticulous attention. The bore is so fine that it gets hopelessly clogged unless cleaned each time it is used; the points of needles are so delicate that the slightest contact with a hard surface may bend them backward, or produce a "burr."

Needles should be *cleaned* as soon as possible after use, paying special attention to the inside of the hub. When cleaned manually, they must be *decontaminated* before handling. This is essential for protection of personnel.

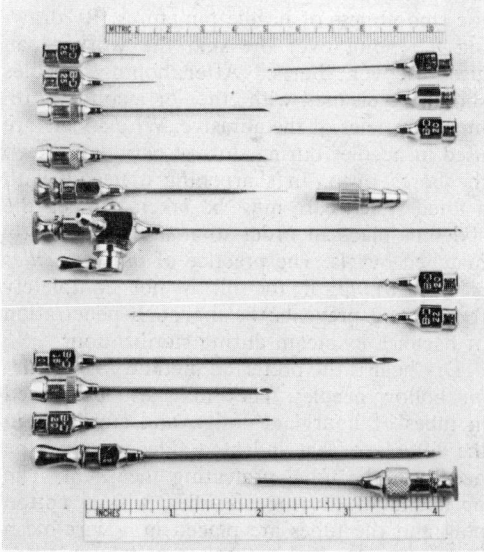

Figure 32-9. Various needles of different gauges and lengths, and several adapters. *Left, top to bottom:* Intradermal and hypodermic needles; two intravenous needles; Lindemann needle; needle and stopcock, used in venous pressure; three aspirating needles; trocar and cannula. *Right, top to bottom:* Three intramuscular needles; adapter; two needles used in infiltration anesthesia; biopsy needle. (Courtesy of Becton-Dickinson & Co., Rutherford, N.J., and Clay-Adams Co., New York, N.Y.)

---

* A product of American Sterilizer Company, Erie, Pa.
    † V. Mueller and Company, Chicago, Ill.

To decontaminate, they are placed in a deep tray containing 2 per cent trisodium phosphate solution and the tray is put in the autoclave for 30 minutes at 121°C (250°F). After decontamination, if needles are processed by hand, they are rinsed under running water and a stylet is inserted through the hub, not from the point. The needle is then washed inside and outside with an alkaline detergent, flushed well, and the hub is cleaned with a tightly wound cotton applicator before it is rinsed with distilled water and inspected for cleanliness and sharpness. Manual cleaning of needles is difficult and time consuming; a mechanical needle cleaner saves time and cleans more effectively. The machine cleans out the hub with a power-driven swab and forces three separate cleaning liquids through the cannula.[45]

Needles must often be *sharpened* before reusing. The temper is tested by flexing the shaft. If brittle, a break usually occurs at the junction of the shaft and hub. The point is examined with a magnifying glass, and if it is dull it should be honed on an oiled Arkansas stone, or in a sharpening device, with care to preserve the bevel. A cake of fine abrasive, such as Bon Ami, is a fairly satisfactory substitute for an Arkansas stone. A piece of chamois stretched over hoops is useful to test the smoothness of needle punctures. By drawing the point over the skin the worker can also discover "burrs." After honing, needles should be cleaned with éther or alcohol to remove particles of the abrasive. Wire stylets are used in needles during storage periods to keep the bores open. In sharpening a needle with a fitted stylet, care must be taken to keep the stylet in place in order to maintain perfectly matched bevels. The practice of *oiling needles is undesirable;* if the oil is not completely removed, it prevents the thorough penetration of bacteria by steam during sterilization.

Dry heat is the preferred method for *sterilizing* hollow needles. They may also be placed in tubes of hourglass design and sterilized in the autoclave. The indented sides suspend the needle in the tube, protecting the point. The open end of the tube is filled with a cotton plug and the tubes are placed in a wire-mesh basket for loading into the sterilizer. When needles are autoclaved, they should be flushed with distilled water before being put into the autoclave, and should be placed in a horizontal position to allow for air escape and free circulation of steam inside and out.[46]

Suture needles used in the repair of tissues are made in many shapes and sizes. In order to prevent undue trauma, they must have sharp points; the shafts may be rounded or more or less triangular, with cutting edges. The needle selected depends upon the tissue to be repaired, the size and position of the wound, and the kind of suture with which the needle is to be threaded. Suture needles are treated as described for other sharp instruments.

Sutures. Sutures are used for the following important functions: hemostasis, wound approximation, bowel and vascular anastomosis, retention, identification of specimens, securing drains, and application of pressure dressings.[47] There are basically two kinds of suture, *absorbable* and *nonabsorbable*. An absorbable suture is digested and absorbed by enzymes during the process of wound healing and is made of surgical gut; a nonabsorbable suture which is not digested and absorbed by the body becomes encapsulated with fibrous tissue and remains in the body. Unabsorbable sutures are made of silk, cotton, nylon, polyethylene, silver, stainless steel, and synthetics such as dacron and polyester.

Absorbable sutures are packaged by the manufacturer in sealed glass tubes or in plastic envelopes. If labeled "boilable gut," the tube or the envelope may be *autoclaved;* if labeled "non-boilable gut," the exterior of the tube must be sterilized by *chemical "sterilization."* When silk, cotton, and nylon suture materials are purchased nonsterile, they must be wrapped in muslin and sterilized in an autoclave at 121°C (250°F) for 30 minutes or 132°C (270°F) for 15 minutes.

If sutures are subjected to superheating, the tensile strength is affected. To avoid superheating, it is necessary to hydrate the suture material by moistening with distilled water before sterilizing. Sutures should not be resterilized more than three times. Monofilament stainless steel suture can be effectively sterilized by saturated steam. It should be sterilized in pre-cut lengths, or wrapped around a reel to prevent kinking.[48]

9. CARE AND STERILIZATION OF RUBBER, SHELLACKED, AND PLASTIC ARTICLES

General Principles. Rubber deteriorates with age and exposure to light, heat, and chemicals. As a rule, rubber goods do not wear out; they are destroyed. Substances harmful to rubber, latex, and certain plastic materials are: alcohol, ether, oil (vegetable or mineral *), phenols, cresols, lubricating agents such as pe-

---

* Rubber is a hydrocarbon, as is mineral oil, kerosene, gasoline, and benzine. Hydrocarbons are soluble in each other. Rubber cement (or glue) is a solution of rubber in one of these liquid hydrocarbons. When rubber equipment is lubricated with mineral oil, a comparable process is started.

troleum jelly, cleaning agents such as green soap, cleaning fluids, oxidizing agents, copper and manganese, and ozone which is generated by electric motors, diathermy machines, and fluorescent lights.

Gloves. Single-use, disposable gloves are widely used, but some institutions continue to reprocess reusable gloves. For this group, Perkins[49] recommends the following procedures: New gloves should be washed before packaging and sterilizing to remove any powder or residue. Soaking in a 5 per cent solution of sodium carbonate for 15 minutes will remove irritants occasionally present. Immediately following use, gloves should be rinsed in cold running water before removal from the hands. This should be done with caution to avoid splashing and the release of aerosols. If a brush is used, the action should take place with the hands and brush both submerged under water. Following removal, the gloves should be placed in a plastic container for delivery to the Central Service Department or the laundry for machine washing. Soaking for long periods is not recommended.

Washing, turning, and drying gloves by hand is an outmoded technique. Automatic washers, glove conditioners, dryers, and testers are efficient and economical. If possible, gloves should be processed in a glove processing room as part of the Central Service Department. Rubber gloves should be *washed,* preferably in a commercial rotary washer, in water at a temperature of 32° to 41°C (90° to 105°F) with a mild, low-sudsing detergent and *dried* in a mechanical dryer. The drying temperature should not exceed 38°C (100°F) or the gloves will become sticky ("tacky"). After washing, rinsing, and drying, gloves should be allowed to "rest" for 8 hours to regain tensile strength. Latex rubber is weakest when wet; testing before adequate drying and rest may produce defects. Gloves are inspected for defects and *tested* by inflating them by hand or by using a machine to distend them with nitrogen gas. Glove *powder* is a harmful substance and should be used with caution. Talcum powder, being nonabsorbable in a wound, may cause adhesions and granulation of tissue. Also, powder contaminates the air. Liquid and cream *lubricants* have been developed as a substitute for glove powder. Gloves should be *packaged* in such a way that no two surfaces are in close contact. Where the wrist section is folded back to form a cuff, a band of gauze should be inserted under the fold, and a pad of gauze or muslin inserted in the palm to hold apposing surfaces apart and to promote escape of air and penetration of steam. Surgical gloves are wrapped in an inner wrap, then in steam-permeable paper, or double-thickness muslin

cover. Packaged gloves are *sterilized* in saturated steam at 121°C (250°F) for 20 minutes, or in ethylene oxide gas followed by an aeration period of 96 hours. If sterilized in a prevacuum, high-temperature sterilizer, the manufacturer's instructions should be followed. Gloves should be held in *temporary storage* after sterilization for a minimum of 24 hours, preferably 48 hours, before distribution, to permit restoration of tensile strength. They should always be stored where they will be protected from excessive light or heat.

Catheters, Tubing, and Drains. These items are very difficult to process. If it is economically feasible it is recommended that they be used only once and disposed of. If this is not possible, they should be *decontaminated,* then soaked for 2 hours in warm water with a low-sudsing type of detergent such as trisodium phosphate or Oakite, then attached to a multiple spout and flushed thoroughly with water, or they should be *washed* in a commercial or glove washer and rinsed through three cycles.[50] The manufacturer's directions for processing special catheters should be followed. Before assembling the decontaminated, cleaned items, they should be flushed with distilled water if they are to be steam *sterilized,* as catheters and tubes, like hollow needles, require interior moisture which can be converted to steam. Soft, flat drains should not be folded when packaged, as steam must circulate through the lumen; they should be *packaged* in paper, muslin, or plastic wrappers, or placed in individual gusset-type paper catheter bags. When they are packaged in paper or cellophane tubing, one end of the tubing is left open to provide access for steam and to prevent bursting of the tube. Catheters and rectal tubes should be marked for size. Figure 32-10 shows sizes in the French scale, approximate sizes in the English scale, and actual diameters in millimeters.

Woven Catheters, Bougies, and Filiforms. Woven catheters are coated with a synthetic resinous material (shellac) which absorbs water, especially in the presence of heat. Before sterilization, they should be *cleaned* in a solution free from alkali or organic solvents. Water containing a mild soap is recommended. Green soap containing glycerin or phenol, or solutions of trisodium phosphate, should *not* be used as they cause deterioration of woven catheters. The cleaning agent should be flushed through the lumen using a syringe or siphon. Copious rinsing should be avoided to prevent forcing too much moisture into the catheter surface. Catheters should be *packaged* without bending or coiling and *sterilized* with steam under pressure at 121°C (250°F) for 20 minutes.[51]

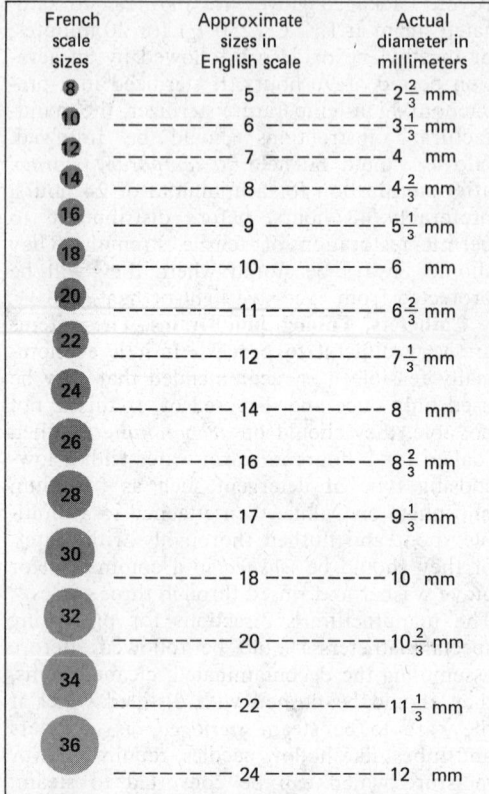

French scale sizes	Approximate sizes in English scale	Actual diameter in millimeters
8	5	$2\frac{2}{3}$ mm
10	6	$3\frac{1}{3}$ mm
12	7	4 mm
14	8	$4\frac{2}{3}$ mm
16	9	$5\frac{1}{3}$ mm
18	10	6 mm
20	11	$6\frac{2}{3}$ mm
22	12	$7\frac{1}{3}$ mm
24	14	8 mm
26	16	$8\frac{2}{3}$ mm
28	17	$9\frac{1}{3}$ mm
30	18	10 mm
32	20	$10\frac{2}{3}$ mm
34	22	$11\frac{1}{3}$ mm
36	24	12 mm

Figure 32-10. Scale for rubber catheters; sizes in the French scale, approximate sizes in English scale, and actual diameter in millimeters are given. (Courtesy of Meinecke and Co., New York.)

10. CARE AND STERILIZATION OF GLASSWARE, ENAMELED WARE, AND STAINLESS STEEL UTENSILS

General Principles. The necessity of sterilizing glass articles used in medical care and all public services makes it important to select a hard glass that is resistant to heat and mechanical shock. Pyrex, a borosilicate glass, is an example. Glass used for solutions should be alkaline free; soft glass may change the pH of liquids in contact with it and start a series of chemical changes. To reduce reactions between glass and other materials, and to facilitate cleaning, glass should have a hard smooth surface, or be properly annealed. Such a surface is relatively impervious to the action of water or steam and may be sterilized in the autoclave; ground glass as used in syringes is very susceptible to erosion by water or steam and should be sterilized with dry heat. Soaps and detergents erode the smooth surface of glass

and attack ground-glass surfaces readily. Abrasives of all sorts are to be avoided in cleaning glass. After use, *immediate rinsing under cold running water to remove organic soil* from glass articles is essential in prolonging their usefulness. If blood or body discharges dry on glass they are dislodged with difficulty. Rinsing with force, as in a mechanical washer, is the preferred method of cleaning glass. A non-etching, low sudsing detergent, buffered to maintain neutral pH, is best suited for cleaning glassware, particularly syringes. Contact with detergent should be limited to the time essential for cleanliness. Glassware used for parenteral therapy and for solutions used to irrigate a wound or body cavity, or to bathe tissues, should be rinsed in freshly distilled water and inverted on racks to drain. If a flask or a beaker is clean, distilled water leaves an unbroken film on the surface; if there is a greasy soil, the film will be broken and droplets will form.

Heat-resistant glass will withstand steam under pressure, and dry heat around 160°C (320°F). Flaming is tolerated, and water may be boiled in Pyrex flasks, but exposure to sudden wide variation in temperatures is likely to crack even a high grade of glass. Soft glass breaks readily in extremes of temperature, or with rapid changes.

Syringes. Even though disposable syringes and needles are among the most commonly used disposable items, many hospitals continue to supplement their use with reusable syringes. Many syringes used for special purposes are too costly to be replaced after each use. Diabetics and others who use syringes in self-care find the purchase of disposable syringes beyond their means.

Metal, glass, plastic, and rubber are all used alone, or combined, in reusable syringes. There are standard designs with standard names illustrated in Figure 32-11.

When sterilizing *Asepto syringes,* remove the rubber bulb from the glass barrel. This facilitates penetration of the sterilizing agent and keeps the rubber from sticking to the glass, as it is likely to do when very hot. The bulb and the glass portion should be wrapped in the same package to avoid difficulty later in fitting them together, which is accomplished more easily if the neck of the rubber bulb is moistened. The woven plunger of the *Triumph syringe* also is difficult to fit into the glass barrel unless it is wet. In sterilizing this type of syringe, the two parts should be separated but wrapped in the same cover.

Luer syringes are costly and perishable because of their shape, the ground-glass surfaces, and the handling and high temperatures to

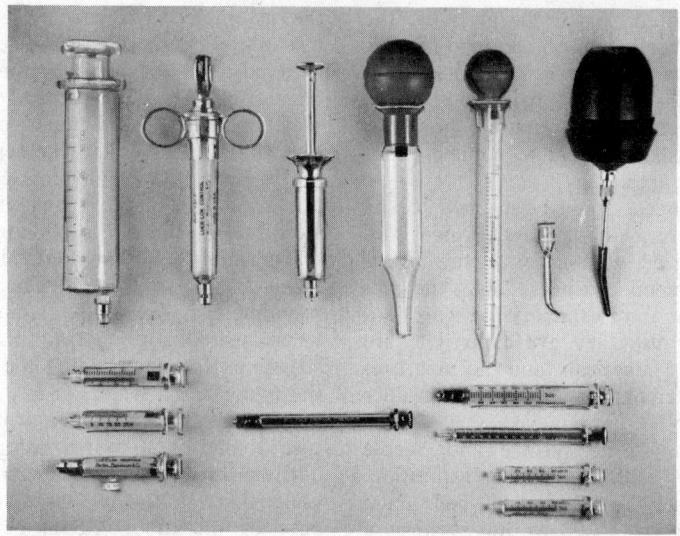

Figure 32-11. Various types of reusable syringes. *Top, left to right:* 50-ml (cc) eccentric tip, graduated glass syringe; Luer-Lok glass syringe with metal tip and metal finger rings; all-metal irrigating syringe with flanged finger holder; Asepto glass syringe with detachable rubber bulb, 1 oz mark indicated; graduated irrigating glass syringe with detachable rubber bulb; curved irrigating needle; injection syringe with hypodermic needle and hard-rubber tip. *Bottom, left:* Hypodermic syringe with center glass tip, 20 ml hypodermic syringe with center glass tip, 25 ml; Luer-Lok hypodermic syringe. *Bottom, center:* Insulin, long tuberculin type, blue plunger syringe with metal tip. *Bottom, right:* Insulin, 125-unit glass syringe (3 ml); insulin, long tuberculin type, blue plunger syringe with glass tip; insulin, short type, glass syringe with glass tip (80 units); insulin, short type, glass syringe with glass tip (40 units). (Courtesy of Becton-Dickinson & Co., Rutherford, N.J., and Clay-Adams Co., New York, N.Y.)

which they are exposed. They must be made of alkaline-free and heat-resistant glass.

Tips of all syringes should be of a standard size in order that they may be used with standard needles. Tips that are not centered in the end of the barrel are called eccentric. Syringes with eccentric tips are sometimes preferred for injecting veins. *Luer-Lok syringes* are distinguished by a metal tip made in such a way as to lock the needle on the syringe. Reputable firms have been careful to make tips and needles of standard patterns, so that all needles fit either the slip type of tip or the locking tip. A *Kaufman syringe* is one that has a second outlet on the side to which rubber tubing may be attached either for draining the syringe or for the injection of a solution. The *Tubex* closed-injection hypodermic syringe (see Figs. 22-3 and 22-4, Chapter 22) is a reusable stainless steel implement into which a sterile cartridge-needle unit containing the solution to be injected is inserted each time it is used. With this system, only the empty vial and the used disposable needle need be discarded.

Rinsing a reusable syringe immediately after

use is a big factor in lengthening the life of a syringe. If this is not done, cleaning is difficult, and the barrel is likely to stick to the plunger. Stuck syringes may be forced apart with a B-D syringe opener, an all-metal syringe which will loosen any frozen Luer-Slip or Luer-Lok syringe. If such an instrument is not available, boiling the syringes for 10 minutes in a 25 per cent aqueous solution of glycerin is effective, if the parts are separated while they are hot. Soaking in a weak solution of nitric acid may be used also. If the needle is stuck to the hub of the syringe, immersing it in boiling water will make the metal expand, facilitating removal from the glass tip. Boiling in the glycerin solution is likewise effective.

Blood and organic matter may be removed with "Haemosol." Soaps and detergents are erosive to ground glass and should be avoided if possible.

In sterilizing syringes, barrels and plungers that are paired should be kept together to avoid wasting time later in matching parts. Some authorities say that the plunger and barrel should always be separated (but kept in the same package) during the sterilizing period; others maintain that if the glass has the same expansion coefficient, the syringe may be sterilized with the plunger in place in a hot-air sterilizer. Separation of parts is essential when steam or chemicals are used, however, to allow the sterilizing agent to come in contact with all surfaces.

All metal syringes should be cleaned by the same process described for glass syringes and should be sterilized with other metal instruments. While metal syringes have the advantage of being unbreakable, they are not widely used because they are expensive, are more difficult to keep clean, and the metal reacts with a greater number of drugs than does glass.

Since a fresh, sterile syringe and needle must be used for each injection or aspiration, it is estimated that the average 200-bed, acute hospital may use from 200 to 300 syringes a day.[52] For the busy hospital using reusable syringes, a centralized syringe and needle service is essential, as is a *mechanical ultrasonic syringe cleaner,* an ideal, rapid, efficient means of cleaning syringes.

When *manual cleaning of syringes* is necessary, the barrel and plunger should be separated immediately after use and rinsed in cold water if the syringe has been used for aspiration of blood or body fluids. Both parts should then be gently washed in warm detergent solution which must be forced through the tip.* Syringes should be rinsed in three changes of water to make sure that all traces of detergent are removed. The final rinse should be distilled water.

Dry heat is considered the most satisfactory agent for *sterilizing* syringes. Autoclaving is also recommended, but boiling in water or soaking in alcohol between patients in health care institutions is condemned. This, however, may be the only method available to people who give themselves insulin or other preparations subcutaneously. It should be recognized that in this case the risk of infection is reduced because only one person is using the syringe.

The syringe should be separated for *packaging* and both parts wrapped in one muslin cover. A needle can be embedded in gauze and wrapped in the same package. With this method of preparation, the exposure time should not be less than 1 hour, preferably 2 hours at 160°C (320°F). Another method of preparation for dry-heat sterilization is to put the assembled syringe into a slightly larger test tube. Perkins describes a technique recommended by Carl Walter using a disposable plastic shield placed over the syringe tip.* The plastic shield seals off the tip of the syringe so that the plunger cannot be removed until the seal is broken. Specially fabricated paper bags are also available for packaging syringes for sterilization, and are in wide use today.[53]

Thermometers. The principle of thermometry is based on the well-established physical principle that gases, liquids, and solids expand when heated and contract when cooled. Instruments for determining the temperature of the living body, water, drugs, foods, materials of all sorts, and for measuring the temperature of the air in rooms, oxygen tents, ovens, and sterilizing chambers usually consist of a scaled glass tube that has a liquid inside the bore of the tube. (Metal coils that expand when heated also are used, but the care of these is rarely one of the nurse's problems.)

Mercury, a liquid metal, is ordinarily used because it is very heavy and has a low coefficient of expansion, so that a short scale measures a wide range of temperatures. Lighter liquids are used in thermometers made to show temperatures of room air.

Self-registering thermometers have a constriction in the bore above the reservoir that supports the column of liquid as it rises in the bore of the tube and keeps it from falling back into the reservoir as the instrument cools; vigorous shaking or jarring is required to make the liquid fall to the bulb or reservoir. This type of instrument is used for measuring body temperatures; chemical, dairy, and room thermometers are not self-registering and must be read while they are surrounded by the medium whose temperature they are measuring.

In *using, cleaning,* and *sterilizing* thermometers, the worker should remember that the instrument must not be exposed to temperatures above those that the thermometer is designed to measure because if the liquid expands beyond the capacity of the inner bore it may break the glass. Thermometers used to measure body temperatures have a short scale from 33.3° to 43.3°C (92° to 110°F), and therefore must not be washed in hot water or sterilized by heat. Some chemical thermometers register temperatures as high as 100° to 150°C (212° to 302°F). Such instruments may be sterilized by boiling, or in the case of a thermometer registering 150°C, it may be sterilized by steam under pressure.

Ordinary thermometers that cannot tolerate

* Gloves should be worn when handling blood or blood-contaminated equipment to protect against infectious agents, particularly the virus causing hepatitis.

* Plastic tips are available from Macbick Company, Wilmington, Mass.

high temperatures must be sterilized by ethylene oxide gas or by chemical agents that are effective against disease-producing microorganisms transmittable through the respiratory and gastrointestinal tracts. This rules out most agents except glutaraldehyde (Cidex), the iodophors, and ethyl alcohol 70 to 80 per cent combined with iodine.[54] Regardless of the type of disinfectant, thermometers must be thoroughly cleaned with a cleaning agent such as green soap, using friction, and rinsed in cool water before immersing in the disinfectant solution. Only water-soluble lubricants should be used for rectal thermometers because removal of an oily lubricant is difficult and the oily film protects the thermometer from the action of the disinfectant.

An electronic thermometer with disposable, one-time-use probes is available, as is a reusable, battery-operated electronic thermometer probe to be used with plastic sheaths that fit over the probe. The soiled sheath is discarded, and a clean sheath applied each time the electronic probe is used.

Enameled Ware. Many qualities of enameled ware are on the market. The better grades are less affected by heat and mechanical blows than the poorer ones. The finish on all enameled ware is eroded by heat, mercuric salts, acids, alkalis, and many other chemicals. Even the best qualities are subject to chipping. Generally speaking, enameled ware is an unsatisfactory material for surgical procedures, because it is soon destroyed by the repeated exposure to high temperatures. Sterile forceps used for handling enameled ware should have the gripping ends protected by rubber; otherwise there is danger of chipping the enamel.

Stainless Steel Utensils. Better grades of stainless steel are moderately heavy and are not easily dented; they are not visibly affected by high temperatures and are resistant to corrosion. Because it is easily cleaned, heat resistant, and unbreakable, stainless steel is the material of choice for cups, bowls, and trays used in surgery, and for patients' bedside utensils.

Basins and other containers to be used in surgery should be wrapped in muslin and *sterilized* in the autoclave, after thorough decontamination and cleaning, preferably in a washer-sterilizer. Patient bedside utensils— bath basins, emesis basins, bedpans, and urinals should be washed and *decontaminated* in a washer-sterilizer and packaged in paper bags if the cost and waste disposal problems do not prohibit this practice. If a washer-sterilizer is not available, they should be soaked in a disinfectant solution and washed in a mild detergent solution before *packaging* and *steri-*

lizing. Disposable plastic bedside utensils are used in some hospitals.

11. STERILIZATION OF SURGICAL DRESSINGS, CLOTHING, AND DRAPING FABRICS

Processing Linen Supplies. The term "linen" is used here to designate a plain, closely woven cotton fabric, usually bleached or unbleached muslin. Effective *sterilization* of linen (as for all sterile supplies) depends upon correct methods of *cleaning* and *packaging*, proper loading of the sterilizer, and its conscientious operation.

The processing of sterile linen begins in the laundry. Before packaging, linen must be carefully inspected, preferably over an illuminated glass top table. Pinholes and other defects are encircled with a pencil and sent to the sewing room to be repaired with thermo-type patching equipment. Linen should be inspected and folded in an area separated from the Central Service Department because handling linen releases lint and dust particles into the air. When it is necessary to carry out these functions in the Central Service Department, a separate, enclosed area with effective air conditioning should be provided.

Uniform folding of the same kinds of linen articles the same way helps to standardize linen supplies. A simplified method of producing towels of uniform size, for example, is to fold each in half, then right over left, and left over right. Gowns are folded inside-out in three or four folds, taking care to contain all tapes within the folds. The gowns are then rolled or folded from each end to the center. When the gown is opened, whatever end is grasped the gown will only unroll halfway and not touch the floor. Folded linen is sorted and stocked on shelves according to the way it will be used in the assembling and wrapping process. The term "packs" refers to linen assembled in bundles for use in specific operations. In addition to standard packs such as "abdominal" or "delivery" packs, items such as gowns, towels, or sheets are wrapped separately.

Processing Dressings. The term "dressing" refers to various materials applied for the protection of wounds (see also Chapter 33). It includes coverings of various styles, sizes, textures, or weaves. The material may be either gauze, cotton, cellulose, cloth, wool, paper, plastic, or sponge. The terms "flats" or "sponges" refer to folded gauze in sizes ranging from 2 by 2 inches to a large laparotomy pad 18 by 18 inches.[55] Sponges (folded squares of gauze) used in body cavities should be all gauze and x-ray detectable. Sponges should be *packaged* individually or bought prepackaged. Large bulk quantities are a potential source of contamination. (See page 1409, packaging of materials to be sterilized.)

12. STERILIZATION OF ANHYDROUS MATERIALS: OINTMENTS, OILS, GAUZE IN PETROLEUM JELLY, AND POWDERS

General Principles of Sterilizing Oils and Nonaqueous Supplies. Shallow *containers* such as petri dishes are suitable for sterilizing petroleum jelly and ointments that are not normally liquid at room temperature, but shallow containers are not suitable for oils because the shallow depth increases the possibility of spilling. Small cylindrical containers are suitable for oil.

Petroleum Gauze. The preparation and sterilization of petroleum gauze is a troublesome, difficult procedure. The purchase of sterile, single-use packets from a medical supply house is a more satisfactory way to obtain it. If processed in the hospital, twenty strips of gauze bandage, each 6 to 8 inches long and 2 inches wide, are put in a steel catheter tray 2½ inches wide, 8 inches long, and 1¼ inches deep. Each strip of bandage is folded over at one end so that the corners can be easily grasped with sterile forceps in removing the preparation from the container. The gauze is then covered with 4 oz of petroleum, previously liquefied by heating; this should form a layer ½ inch deep with a thin layer of petroleum over the top strip. The container is *sterilized* in a hot air sterilizer at 160°C (320°F) for 2½ hours.[56] Because of the possibility of contaminating the contents while being used, this type of bulk packaging is not recommended.

Powders. Due to the slow rate of heat transfer through containers of powder, it should not be sterilized in amounts of more than 1 oz. The quantity should be restricted to a ¼-inch layer in a petri dish or similar type of container. Ideally, powder is sterilized in single-use paper envelopes. Test tubes with cotton plugs, individually wrapped, are also suitable containers. Sulfonamide powders may be heated to a temperature of 155°C (311°F) for 1½ hours. This is close to the melting point of sulfonamide; however, Perkins[57] recommends 140° to 150°C (285° to 300°F) for 3 hours. Zinc peroxide should be sterilized at 140°C (285°F) for 4 hours. Other chemicals such as kaolin, zinc oxide, mercurous chloride, and bismuth subnitrate can be dry-heat sterilized at 170°C (340°F) for 1 hour or 160°C (320°F) for 2 hours.

13. PROCESSING LARGE PORTABLE EQUIPMENT

An average Central Service Department is said to handle 50 to 75 types of portable equipment, ranging from an intravenous stand to a circular electric bed. It is imperative that all equipment be available and in working condition and safe to use when needed. Mechanical and electric equipment that has not had proper maintenance may be more of a hazard than a help. (See Chapter 15 for more about electric equipment hazards.)

Cleaning Portable Equipment. All large, movable equipment should be *cleaned* with a suitable detergent followed by a topical application of a *chemical disinfectant*. All reusable parts such as drainage bottles, connectors, and tubing should be washed and sterilized. If part of the equipment is heat sensitive, gas sterilization or, if this is unavailable, chemical disinfection, is used. Attached tubes that have been inserted in the body should be discarded. After cleaning and disinfecting, all equipment should be *inspected* and *checked* to be sure it is in working condition, electrical cords and plugs especially. Equipment and accessories are then *reassembled;* ends of connecting tubing and connectors are sealed with plastic or a paper bag, and the entire unit *covered* with a plastic bag before its return to storage.[58]

Special Precautions in Processing Anesthesia and Respiratory Therapy Equipment. Control and prevention of infection associated with anesthesia and respiratory equipment is dependent on its proper cleaning and processing, and this particular kind of equipment is among the most difficult to decontaminate. Inhalation therapy equipment using reservoir nebulizers is capable of generating aerosols containing large numbers of microorganisms. The source of contamination may be the jet of the nebulizer, improper cleaning and sterilization of the reservoir, or contaminated solutions or medications used in the nebulizer. Proper care requires that all contaminated components be removed, thoroughly *cleaned, dried,* and *sterilized* by steam under pressure or ethylene oxide gas every 8 to 12 hours, and *always* between patients. Detachable equipment that cannot be autoclaved or sterilized with gas should be thoroughly cleaned with hot water and a detergent and soaked in an *effective germicide,* then rinsed and dried. Activated glutaraldehyde (Cidex) is the recommended agent of choice. If that is not available, 70 to 90 per cent isopropyl alcohol, or phenolic or iodophor germicides may be used. Disinfecting solutions must be changed frequently, at least every other week for activated glutaraldehyde, and as often as every day for some products. After soaking, the equipment should be rinsed in sterile water, *dried thoroughly,* and *wrapped* and *stored,* using sterile technique.* Disposable anesthesia equipment is available and recommended if budget permits.

14. PROCESSING STERILE SUPPLIES IN THE HOME

When supplies are sterilized in the home, procedures and techniques must be adapted to fit the available materials and equipment, and adapted to what the family is able to do. Ruth B. Freeman [59] says that a procedure carried out in the home by a nurse is a teaching activity because family members often watch and copy what they see. Procedures should, therefore, be as simple as possible, safe, low in cost of equipment and supplies, and high in teaching potential. Most of the methods of sterilization described earlier in this chapter may be simplified and adapted for home use.

Moist Heat Sterilization in the Home. While *boiling water* is probably the most common method of disinfecting supplies in the home, it is not as effective as other methods. The maximum temperature that can be reached by boiling water is 100°C (212°F) or less, depending on the altitude. For this reason, boiling water is considered a method of *disinfection* rather than *sterilization*. It is suitable for the destruction of vegetative bacteria, but cannot be relied on to kill resistant spore forms or viruses which withstand this temperature, even with lengthy exposure. Boiling water may be used to decontaminate bedside utensils and contaminated dishes used by a patient with an infectious disease, but it is not the preferred method for the preparation of instruments used to penetrate the skin or otherwise come in contact with wounds.

Several factors influence the effectiveness of boiling water as a disinfecting agent. At altitudes higher than sea level, the boiling point is decreased, thereby decreasing the effectiveness of the boiling process. The hydrogen ion concentration of the water also affects its bactericidal efficiency. Addition of an alkali such as sodium carbonate (sal soda) to make a 2 per cent solution, or sodium hydroxide (caustic soda) to make $\frac{1}{10}$ per cent solution, increases the hydrogen ion concentration and the disinfecting power of the water as it boils.

Boiling time also affects the efficiency of the process. The safe minimum period for disinfection in boiling water at sea level without the addition of alkali is 30 minutes. At higher altitudes the exposure period must be increased.[60]

All articles to be disinfected must be completely submerged during boiling so that every surface is exposed. The objects to be disinfected and the container in which they are boiled must be clean and free from soil, especially grease that would prevent the moist heat from reaching bacteria. Equipment should be removed from the water as soon as the boiling period is completed; if allowed to remain, the article will be contaminated as steam condenses. Deposits of inorganic salts on the equipment may be reduced by the addition of a water softener such as Calgonite, by wrapping the articles in gauze or other fabric, or by boiling the water before placing the objects in the container.

Steam under pressure as a sterilizing process is available in the home by using a pressure cooker as a substitute for a steam autoclave. A pressure cooker may be used for sterilizing all types of supplies including surgical instruments and dressings. Materials that hold water can be dried in the oven after removal from the pressure cooker.

Dry Heat Sterilization in the Home. A household oven can be used for dry heat sterilization of syringes and needles, instruments, and other heat-resistant supplies. Equipment may be wrapped in aluminum foil and processed in the oven alone, or while the oven is being used to prepare food.

Flaming, by holding a sharp instrument or steel needle in an open flame for 20 seconds, is an emergency method of sterilizing an instrument to be used to penetrate the skin. This method has little value, however, if it damages or dulls the edge of the instrument.

Chemical Disinfection in the Home. When heat is not available, clean equipment may be soaked in 70 to 90 per cent alcohol, or an iodophor solution such as Betadine. (For more information about chemical disinfection see page 882.)

Processing Sterile Dressings in the Home. If a sterile dressing is needed in an emergency, gauze (or other fabric) may be boiled and used wet, or wrung as dry as possible using sterile forceps or gloved hands. If a dry sterile dressing is necessary, a fabric may be ironed with a very hot iron.

* Recommendation of the Center for Disease Control, US Public Health Service, Atlanta, Ga.

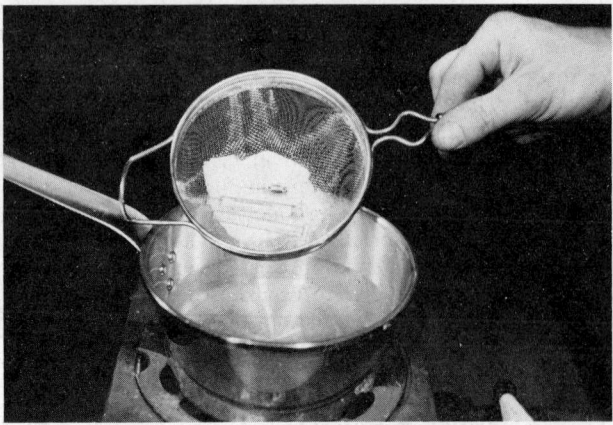

Figure 32-12. Sterilization of syringe and needle in the home. The syringe is taken apart and placed with the needle in a strainer lined with a gauze square. The strainer is then put into a pan of water. Water is added to cover syringe and needle. This is heated and then boiled for 10 minutes. After boiling, the strainer is lifted out, the water poured from the pan, and the strainer returned to the pan until the syringe and needle have cooled. (Courtesy of Dr. Henry Dolger and New York Diabetic Association, New York, N.Y., and Clay-Adams Co., New York, N.Y.)

Processing Syringes and Needles in the Home. Even though boiling water is not an effective method of sterilization, a syringe and needle used by only one person may be safely and easily disinfected using the following procedure: After a thorough washing and rinsing, the dismantled syringe and needle are placed in a wire strainer lined with a gauze square. The strainer is then put into a pan with enough water to cover the needle and syringe, and heated, then boiled for 10 minutes. After boiling, the strainer is lifted out, the water is poured from the pan, and the strainer is returned to the pan until the equipment is cool enough to handle. This method is shown in Figure 32-12.

Cindy Kurey [61] suggests the following procedure for sterilizing a syringe and needle set by the dry heat method in an oven: A clean, dry, assembled syringe and needle are placed in the center of two thicknesses of 8- by 10-inch aluminum foil. The barrel of the syringe is protected with a cotton ball, and the needle inserted into a second cotton ball (see Fig.

32-13). After the foil is securely but loosely wrapped around the syringe with the edges of the foil double-folded, the package is placed in a 177°C (350°F) oven for 30 minutes on a disposable aluminum foil pan with holes punched in the bottom to allow penetration and circulation of heat. After "baking" and cooling, the package should be marked to indicate that it has been sterilized. When needed, the package is unwrapped (with washed hands) and alcohol is poured over the cotton balls, one of which is used to clean the vial and the other to clean the injection site. This method has the advantage of permitting sterilization at the most convenient time, rather than immediately before use, and because the syringe and needle are assembled before sterilization, there is no need to assemble the set later, using sterile technique.

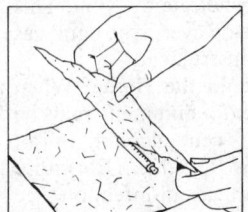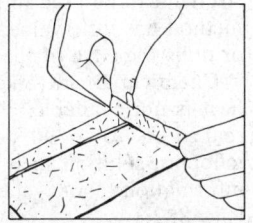

Figure 32-13. Double-thickness aluminum foil encloses assembled syringe and needle before sterilization in home oven. Ends and sides are sealed by a double fold to prevent contamination. (From Kurey, Cindy: "Baked Insulin Syringes. Ideas that Work," *Am. J. Nurs.,* **70:**1310, [June] 1970.)

REFERENCES

1. Perkins, John J.: *Principles and Methods of Sterilization in Health Sciences,* 2nd ed. Charles C Thomas, Publisher, Springfield, Ill., 1969, p. 363.
2. Wright, Nadean E.: *Central Supply Procedure Manual.* Catholic Hospital Association, St. Louis, 1972, p. 1.
3. McGibony, John, et al.: *A Study of Hospital Central Medical and Surgical Supply Services.* US Government Printing Office, Washington, D.C., 1965, p. 14 (PHS Pub. No. 930-C-10).
4. US Public Health Service, Division of Hospital and Medical Facilities: *A Manual for Hospital Central Medical and Surgical Supply Services.* US Government Printing Office, Washington, D.C., 1966, p. 7 (PHS Pub. No. 930-C-13).
5. Kelly, Nan K.: "Product Testing and Evaluation," in US Public Health Service, Division of Hospital and Medical Facilities: *Adminis-*

trative Aspects of Hospital Central Medical and Surgical Supply Services. US Government Printing Office, Washington, D.C., 1966, p. 18 (PHS Pub. No. 930-C-12).

6. Perkins, John J.: *op. cit.*

7. International Association of Hospital Central Service Management: *The Central Service Technician.* Clissold Books, Chicago, 1969, p. 43.

8. International Association of Hospital Central Service Management: *op. cit.,* p. 54.

9. Perkins, John J.: *op. cit.,* p. 239.

10. Vesley, Donald, and Greene, V. W.: "Sterilization, Disinfection, and Cleaning Techniques," in Bond, Richard, et al. (eds.): *Environmental Health and Safety in Health-Care Facilities.* Macmillan Publishing Co., Inc., New York, 1973, p. 62.

11. American Sterilizer Company: "Processing of Surgical Instruments," *J. Hosp. Res.,* **2:**8, (July) 1964 (revised Aug. 1970).

12. Perkins, John J.: *op. cit.,* p. 245.

13. Vesley, Donald, and Greene, V. W.: *op. cit.,* p. 61.

14. Rubbo, S. D., and Gardner, J. F.: *A Review of Sterilization and Disinfection: As Applied to Medical, Industrial, and Laboratory Practice.* Lloyd-Luke, Ltd., London, 1965, p. 26.

15. Perkins, John J.: *op. cit.,* p. 200.

16. Reilly, E., and Ginsberg, F.: "Modern Central Service: How New Packaging Materials Work," *Mod. Hosp.,* **116:**100, (Jan.) 1971.

17. Perkins, John J.: *op. cit.,* p. 205.

18. Berry, Edna, and Kohen, M. L.: *Introduction to Operating Room Technique,* 4th ed. McGraw-Hill Book Co., New York, 1972, p. 28.

19. International Association of Hospital Central Service Management: *op. cit.,* pp. 82, 124.

20. Wright, Nadean E.: *op. cit.,* pp. 27, 111.

21. US Public Health Service, Division of Hospital and Medical Facilities: *op. cit.,* p. 26.

22. Wright, Nadean E.: *op. cit.,* p. 111.

23. Standard, Paul, et al.: "Microbial Penetration of Muslin and Paper-Wrapped Sterile Packs Stored on Open Shelves and in Closed Cabinets," *Appl. Microbiol.,* **22:**432, (Sept.) 1971.

24. Nichols, G. A. "Sterile Shelf Life Prolonged by Use of Plastic Outer-Wrap," *Hosp. Top.,* **46:**123, (Feb.) 1968.

25. Reilly, E., and Ginsberg, F.: "Modern Central Service: Here Are Guidelines for Package Shelf Life," *Mod. Hosp.,* **116:**112, (Feb.) 1971.

26. Berry, Edna, and Kohen, M. L.: *op. cit.,* p. 29.

27. Perkins, John J.: *op. cit.,* p. 95.

28. Lawrence, Carl A., and Block, Seymour: *Disinfection, Sterilization, and Preservation.* Lea & Febiger, Philadelphia, 1968, p. 714.

29. Perkins, John J.: *op. cit.,* p. 211.

30. US Public Health Service, Division of Hospital and Medical Facilities: *op. cit.,* p. 82.

31. Berry, Edna, and Kohen, M. L.: *op. cit.,* p. 30.

32. Perkins, John J.: *op. cit.,* p. 286.

33. International Association of Hospital Central Service Management: *op. cit.,* p. 52.

34. Berry, Edna, and Kohen, M. L.: *op. cit.,* p. 34.

35. Vesley, Donald, and Greene, V. W.: *op. cit.,* p. 52.

36. International Association of Hospital Central Service Management: *op. cit.,* p. 53.

37. *Ibid.*

38. Lawrence, Carl A., and Block, Seymour: *op. cit.,* p. 761.

39. American Sterilizer Company: "Preparation of External Solutions in Hospitals," *J. Hosp. Res.,* **1:**8, (Jan.) 1963 (revised Apr. 1967).

40. Perkins, John J.: *op. cit.,* p. 431.

41. *Ibid.,* p. 437.

42. American Sterilizer Company: "Preparation of External Solutions in Hospitals," *J. Hosp. Res.,* **1:**8, (Jan.) 1963 (revised Apr. 1967).

43. *Ibid.*

44. Perkins, John J.: *op. cit.,* p. 259.

45. *Ibid.,* p. 307.

46. *Ibid.,* p. 308.

47. Sindik, M.: "Surgical Sutures," *AORN J.,* **14:**57, (Sept.) 1971.

48. Perkins, John J.: *op. cit.,* p. 261.

49. *Ibid.,* p. 220.

50. US Public Health Service, Division of Hospital and Medical Facilities: *op. cit.,* p. 16.

51. Perkins, John J.: *op. cit.,* p. 228.

52. *Ibid.,* p. 304.

53. *Ibid.,* p. 302.

54. Taylor, Joyce W., et al.: "For Effective Thermometer Disinfection," *Nurs. Outlook,* **14:**56, (Feb.) 1966.

55. Perkins, John J.: *op. cit.,* p. 193.

56. *Ibid.,* p. 299.

57. *Ibid.,* p. 297.

58. US Public Health Service, Division of Hospital and Medical Facilities: *op. cit.,* p. 23.

59. Freeman, Ruth B.: *Public Health Nursing Practice,* 3rd ed. W. B. Saunders Co., Philadelphia, 1966, p. 175.

60. California State Department of Health: *Cleaning, Disinfection, and Sterilization; A Guide for Hospitals and Related Facilities.* The Department, Sacramento, 1965, p. 14.

61. Kurey, Cindy: "Baked Insulin Syringe," *Am. J. Nurs.,* **70:**1310, (June) 1970.

Additional Suggested Reading

American Sterilizer Company: "Prevacuum High Temperature Steam Sterilization," *J. Hosp. Res.,* July, 1963.

———: "Chemical Disinfection and Antisepsis in the Hospital," *J. Hosp. Res.,* Feb., 1972.

———: "The Hospital Environment and Infection," *J. Hosp. Res.,* July, 1968.

———: "Ethylene Oxide Sterilization," *J. Hosp. Res.,* Nov., 1971.

———: *Tips for Improving Your Sterilizing Techniques—Steam Sterilizers.* The Company, Erie, Pa., 1968 (Brochure).

———: *Sterilizing Aids.* The Company, Erie, Pa., 1968 (Brochure).

————: *Wrapping Materials for Sterilizing and Storing Supplies.* The Company, Erie, Pa., 1968 (Brochure).

Atkinson, L. J.: "O. R. Fact and Principle," *AORN J.,* **6:**83, (Nov.) 1967.

Central Nursing Supply Service. Central Nursing Supply Headquarters, US Air Force, Washington, D.C. (USAF Manual No. 160-9).

Central Supply Service Procedural and Instructional Manual. Hospital Logistics Management, Rantoul, Ill.

Centralized Material Service. US Government Printing Office, Washington, D.C., 1974 (US Army Manual St. 8-275).

Driscoll, J.: "Many Variables Influence Packaging and Pre-Sterilization," *South. Hospitals,* **34:** 40, (Jan.) 1966.

Dyer, E. D., et al.: "Bacteriologic Study of Muslin and Parchment Wrapped Sterile Supplies," *Nurs. Res.,* **15:**79, (Winter) 1966.

Ginsberg, Frances, et al.: *A Manual of Operating Room Technology.* J. B. Lippincott Co., Philadelphia, 1966.

Grief, E. E., et al.: "Quality Control Procedures for Packaging Sterile Supplies," *Hosp. Pharmacy,* **4:**4, (Jan.) 1969.

Huckins, D. D.: "New Concepts in Economy of Supplies and Equipment," *Hosp. Pharmacy,* **4:**9, (Jan.) 1969.

Samuels, T. M., et al.: "Study Shows Hospital Applicability of Industrial Sealing Techniques," Part I, *Hosp. Top.,* **46:**75, (Sept.) 1968; Part II, **46:**101, (Oct.) 1968.

Scully, K. J.: "Hospital Adaptation of Industrial Packaging Equipment and Devices," *Hosp. Manage.,* **106:**87, (July) 1968.

Shooter, R. A.: "Packaging and Its Problems," *Br. Hosp. J. Soc. Serv. Rev.,* (June 30) 1967, p. 1207.

Julina P. Rhymes
Virginia Henderson

The authors wish to thank Marie M. Lech, Hospital Nurse Consultant, US Public Health Service, Rockville, Md., for supplying valuable references for this chapter.

CHAPTER 33

Application of Surgical Dressings

1. PURPOSE OF DRESSINGS

Protecting the Wound, Preventing Infection, and Promoting Healing. Surgeons and other physicians prescribe dressings to protect wounds against mechanical injury and as barriers against contamination by pathogenic organisms in the environment. If wound healing is to take place as rapidly and as completely as possible, protection of wounds is essential, although some authorities think dressings are not necessarily an essential aspect of this protection (see page 1433). Application of a dressing to the wound supports the surrounding tissue and holds wound edges immobile. Most surgeons think a dressing is protection against infection which retards the healing process. A wound infection may also develop into septicemia and cause death. Dressings on a draining wound absorb the drainage and remove a media which supports the growth of pathogens. However, to be effective, dressings to a draining wound must be changed frequently. A dressing saturated with drainage establishes a wet-path (strike-through) from the outer surface of the dressing. Chances of secondary contamination are enhanced by the wet-path. E. J. L. Lowbury and A. M. Hood [1] demonstrated that organisms such as *Pseudomonas pyocyanea* and *Bacillus proteus* passed very quickly through thick absorbent material in which a wet-path had been created.

Adequate circulation in the affected area promotes wound healing. It is important for nurses to make sure that dressings, either those applied by themselves or others, are not so tight, or restricting, that they interfere with the circulation. But at times dressings are applied with pressure to prevent swelling and accumulation of blood in the incised area. Particularly in plastic surgery, where grafting has been done, serum collection and hematomas can hinder healing and accentuate suture marks.[2]

Pressure and *position* are frequently used to regulate and promote venous circulation. In treating ulcers of the leg, for instance, the part is usually elevated and a tight bandage applied to prevent congestion in a dependent part and to promote the return of venous blood.

2. THE NURSE'S RESPONSIBILITIES IN APPLYING DRESSINGS

Applying the Initial Dressing. While this chapter is concerned primarily with dressings applied following surgery in hospital, clinic, or doctor's office, the same principles apply to dressing accidental wounds or skin lesions where the protection of a dressing is indicated. Those who nurse in homes, industries, schools, corrective institutions, ships, and other settings where physicians may be available only periodically or as consultants, have the responsibility for selecting and applying the initial dressing; those who nurse in hospitals, clinics, and doctor's offices are usually responsible for changing dressings that were applied by physicians or surgeons. Many surgeons, however, prefer to dress the wounds of their patients until satisfactory healing is assured and the nurse's responsibility is minimal. Nurses in remote areas, nurses on islands, for example, where there are no physicians, may perform minor surgery. They may incise a boil or remove a foreign body embedded in the skin and underlying tissue. In daily living and in emergencies, anyone may be called on to apply dressings. The general principles of wound protection should be common knowledge, as is stressed in Chapter 43. It should be studied in conjunction with this chapter.

Frequency of Change. The surgical dressings applied by the surgeon in the hospital operating room, the clinic, or the office may be changed by the surgeon or other physicians associated with him or her or by nurses. If no discharge is expected a dry sterile gauze dressing is applied and secured with elastic adhesive. Generally there is no need to disturb the initial dressing until the sutures are removed. Healing of the wound usually occurs by "first intention" or without suppuration and granulation. In many instances sutures are removed on the fifth or seventh day after surgery.

Most surgeons change the dressing the first time after surgery. Thereafter, dressing the wound is often the responsibility of the nurse rather than the surgeon or other physician. Wounds with drainage or other conditions that delay healing are usually dressed by the surgeon the first day after operation and daily thereafter. Nurses would change the outer dressings of a draining wound as soon as they notice a soiled dressing. This decreases the chance of secondary contamination as mentioned above.

When helping physicians with dressings, nurses prepare the materials to be used, and if they are dressing the wounds of more than one patient, nurses plan the dressing sequence and procedure that will provide for asepsis, for the comfort of patients, and for such assistance as ensures that wounds may be dressed by surgeons with the greatest ease and efficiency. Whether dressing the wound or helping surgeons, nurses should know the nature and results of the operation involved: the kind of wound (whether clean or with drainage); the type of dressing; and any special equipment required; when the first dressing after operation is likely to be done; and the time scheduled for dressings.

Observations. When caring for the patient with a surgical wound, dressed or undressed, the nurse is responsible for observing it and for noting anything unusual in the healing process. An *assessment* of the initial condition of the wound or dressing will help establish a *baseline* for comparison with later observations. For example, if a blood stain is apparent on a dressing, a line should be drawn around it when first observed. Any increase in the size of the stain, which might be indicative of continued or renewed bleeding, can then be readily detected.

During a dressing change the wound is observed for the approximation of its edges. Also

noted, if present, are local symptoms of infection (redness, tenderness, heat, swelling). An elevated temperature and increased pulse are systemic symptoms of infection. Dressings removed from the wound are examined for the presence of discharge. It is not unusual for a wound to exude some serous drainage immediately after surgery. The amount of discharge that is considered normal varies according to size and type of wound. Yellow or green drainage, often thick and having an unpleasant odor, of course, indicates infection.

3. PRINCIPLES OF ASEPSIS IN SURGICAL DRESSINGS

Sterilization and Aseptic Preparation of Equipment and Supplies. Dressing a wound is a surgical procedure which should be carried out with the precision and care of an operation. All materials used should be sterile. The method chosen to sterilize an article depends on its properties. A detailed discussion of the preparation of sterile supplies is found in Chapter 32. If economically feasible, commercially prepared, prepackaged, disposable sterile items, which are used for one patient only and then discarded, are believed most effective in reducing cross contamination. When such supplies are unavailable, everything that comes in direct contact with a wound should be sterilized by one of the following methods: steam under pressure (autoclaving), ethylene oxide gas, or dry heat. See Chapter 32 for a discussion of these methods.

There are many places in the world where none of the above three sterilization methods are available to the person who is dressing a wound. Boiling materials in water for an extended period will destroy most bacteria, but it will not kill their spores. If there is any reason to suspect the presence of pathogenic spores, particularly those causing the dreaded wound infections of gas gangrene and tetanus, boiling water is not a satisfactory method of preparing equipment for wound care. Some spore-forming microorganisms, such as the *Clostridium welchii*, are prevalent and harmless on the intact tissue but dangerous after its integrity has been destroyed.

It is important to note that sterilization procedures can be modified more safely in the home because the patient usually has developed immunities to organisms existing in his or her environment. (See also Chapter 32.)

In addition to the aforementioned sterilizing agents, high-energy electron beam and gamma radiation are possible agents in sterilizing equipment, but they are expensive and available in few settings.

Handling Equipment and Supplies Used in Surgical Dressings. Before handling equipment and supplies used in surgical dressings, nurses should wash their hands thoroughly. It must be remembered, however, that hands can never be made sterile. In order to maintain the sterility of objects that come in contact with wounds it is necessary to handle them with sterile forceps or sterile gloves. Manipulation with instruments is by far the most efficient way to handle sterile surgical materials. However, instruments used for one dressing cannot be used for another with safety until they have been resterilized.

There is always danger of contamination of articles exposed to the air, especially air exhaled by human beings. For this reason masks are often worn by surgeons, nurses, and other attendants,[3] dressings are not changed for at least 15 minutes after the room has been swept or cleaned, and the practice of storing dressings in large jars or drums, opened and closed frequently during the day, has been discontinued. Individually wrapped sterile dressings and equipment provide the greatest safety for the patient.

Sterile draping around the wound is not essential, if unsterile bedding does not come in contact with the wound or in close proximity to it. Clean draping that protects the bedding and clothing is desirable. The bed may be protected from cleaning and irrigating solutions by the proper use of basins, plastic sheeting, or impervious paper with a layer of absorbent cellucotton over it. Such materials should be discarded after each dressing. Basins used should be resterilized. During the procedure, the nurse works carefully and avoids contaminating the patient's skin, clothing, and bedclothing with soiled instruments or dressings.

Unsterile articles, such as binders and pins used to hold dressings in place, bandages, scissors, and basins for the collection of waste should be handled with clean hands. To prevent infection of the wound, it is necessary to keep unsterile objects from coming in contact with it. To prevent the spread of disease generally, it is important that clean and contaminated equipment be kept separate and that all medical attendants wash their hands after every service to the patient that requires handling the body discharges, clothing, or bedding.

The practice of keeping transfer forceps in containers of disinfectant solution has been discontinued in most health agencies. Instead, individually wrapped sterile forceps are used to transfer sterile items to a sterile field at each time the dressing is changed. If transfer forceps in disinfectant solution are used in a health agency the nurse should observe the following practices: (1) if the forceps touch an unsterile item, resterilize them before returning them to the container; (2) if the forceps are held tips up so that the disinfectant solution touches the unsterile handle and then flows back down to the sterile part, resterilize them; and (3) sterilize the forceps and container and use fresh solution at least once daily.

4. TYPES OF DRESSINGS USED IN CARE OF WOUNDS

The type of a dressing applied to a wound varies according to the surgical procedure, the size of the wound, the presence of drainage, and the signs of infection. The type of dressing applied should coincide with the purpose of the dressing. For example, simple protection of a clean wound might be best accomplished by using a Band-Aid * or a single thickness of gauze with adhesive tape. Tape alone may serve to draw two sides of a wound together without the use of sutures; a butterfly dressing (a piece of tape or gauze bandage which is narrow in the middle and wide at either end, see Fig. 33-1) would accomplish this purpose. If a wound is expected to drain profusely, a Penrose, or cigarette drain (gauze encircled by rubber or plastic tubing), is inserted at the time of surgery. Such a wound requires multilayered absorbent compresses and frequent dressing changes. Sometimes a Hemovac closed suction apparatus is attached to a drainage catheter in the wound. This apparatus allows the removal of exudate from the wound by application of gentle suction, and permits the application of fewer dressings on the wound.

Classification of Dressings. There are two main classifications of dressings—*nonantiseptic* and *antiseptic*. Nonantiseptic dressings are sterile, unmedicated dressings applied to a fresh wound to protect it from infection. Antiseptic dressings are impregnated with such medications as iodine (Iodoform) and boric acid. They are applied to wounds already infected to limit the septic processes. They were introduced and commonly used in the last century when less was known about preventing infection with asepsis than is known today. Dressings may also be classified as wet, dry, occlusive, adhesive, fixed, porous, etc. Some dressings are classified according to their inventors' names, as, for example, a Jones dressing or a Carrel-Dakin dressing.[4] (See page 1435

* Johnson & Johnson, New Brunswick, N.J.

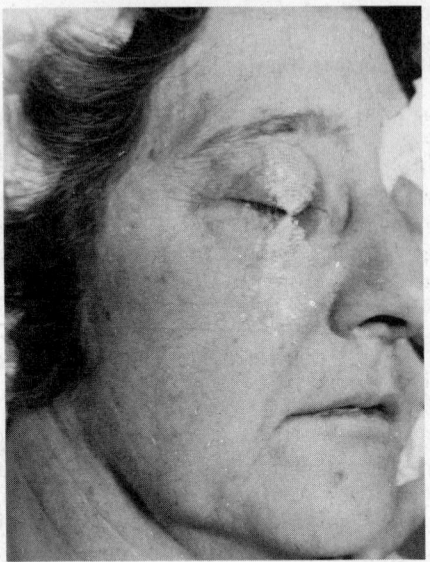

Figure 33-1. A butterfly dressing made with a small piece of bandage and collodion. This keeps the eye shut and protects it when the corneal reflex is absent. (Courtesy of Neurological Institute of the Columbia-Presbyterian Medical Center, New York, N.Y., and Clay-Adams Co., New York, N.Y.)

for a description of the latter.) The Jones dressing was devised in 1919 by Sir Robert Jones for the purpose of immobilizing joints after orthopedic surgery. The updated and modified version of this dressing consists of layers of gauze, rolled cotton, a conforming gauze, and an Ace bandage.[5]

Undressed Wounds. Although it is not a new idea, some surgeons have recently been leaving wounds completely undressed. I. F. Mac-Laren[6] suggests that exposed wounds heal satisfactorily and show no higher incidence of wound complications than dressed wounds. It is now common practice in the United States to omit the dressing once consistently applied to the severed umbilical cord of the newborn infant. Other advantages of not dressing wounds are that the patient is less uncomfortable, the wound is easily inspected, and the cost of dressings is saved. An ad hoc committee of the Committee on Trauma, American College of Surgeons,[7] issued the statement in 1964 that the site of the undressed wound is an influencing variable in the occurrence or non-occurrence of sepsis. To illustrate this point, P. B. Wood[8] found that undressed sutured wounds of the hand became infected twice as often as those with dressings, whereas Mac-Laren's study demonstrated that the undressed wounds of 137 persons with femoral and inguinal herniorrhaphies and 146 persons with ab-

dominal surgery for peptic ulcer showed no difference in incidence of wound complications from those of persons with dressed wounds who had similar surgery.

Sealed Dressings. Sometimes wounds are sealed with collodion or a clear plastic spray material so that the need for any other dressing is eliminated.

Dry Dressings. So-called *clean wounds* are dressed with two to eight layers of gauze, folded into a suitable shape and size. This dressing is held in place by strips of adhesive, a bandage, or a binder. If adhesive is used it should be porous to prevent the underlying skin from becoming moist. If nonporous adhesive is used a small hole should be cut in the center of the adhesive so the wound can "breathe." Before applying adhesive the nurse should ask whether the patient is allergic to adhesive. Nonallergic tape * or scotch tape can often be used if a patient is allergic to adhesive.

To avoid infection, the dressing and wound should be kept dry. It should not be swabbed with any type of solution. Many surgeons believe that if a wound shows signs of healing satisfactorily, the less that is done to it the better.

Pressure Dressings. When there is danger of bleeding or when there may be seepage from a wound, the surgeon is likely to use a pressure dressing. This is a thick sterile pad made of gauze or gauze and cellulose applied with a firm bandage (Elastoplast †) or binder. While the many-tailed abdominal (scultetus) binder is still used, some surgeons believe it restricts the movement of the diaphragm, which results in shallow breathing, and they consequently disapprove of its use.

Wet Dressings. If wounds are infected, wet dressings are often used to soften the discharge and promote drainage. The viscous exudate of an infected wound tends to coagulate on the surface of the wound and interferes with drainage. The moisture of a wet dressing prevents this. A wet dressing is also used to conduct heat to tissue. Wet heat is more penetrating than dry heat. It can be beneficial in localizing the infection into an area that can be incised and drained. Erle Peacock[9] discusses the value and effects of wet dressings in a chapter on wound healing in the *Manual of Preoperative and Postoperative Care* prepared by a committee of the American College of Surgeons.

When dressed, infected wounds are thoroughly cleaned with sponges saturated in saline solution or in a mild antiseptic; they may be

---

* 3 M Company, St. Paul, Minn., under the brand name of MICROSPORE.

† Duke Laboratories, Inc., South Norwalk, Conn.

irrigated with a syringe, and the surgeon may want to probe the wound with an instrument or to insert a wick or packing. Wet dressings or compresses are made of many layers of gauze or a pad of cellucotton covered with gauze. An impervious material, such as plastic sheeting, should be used to hold the dressing in place. Obviously, the protector must itself be sterile. The skin around the wound area is sometimes protected with strips of gauze impregnated with petroleum jelly or zinc oxide ointment which prevents maceration of the skin by the wet dressing. Aqua-flo,* a fine-mesh gauze impregnated with "wettable" petroleum which prevents maceration of the skin, is a commercial product that can be used for the application of wet dressings. Current techniques employed to keep wet dressings warm consist of either the application of a hot water bottle, or a chemical pad (Lightingpak †), or a circulating pad (Aquamatic-K Pad ‡) as the source of external heat. In some instances, rubber sheeting, aluminum foil, or plastic is also used for insulation.[10]

Carrel-Dakin Dressings. During World War I a technique for treating deep infected wounds was developed by Alexis Carrel, a physician, and H. D. Dakin, a chemist. This technique is still used occasionally. The object of the dressing is to provide either frequent or constant flushing of the wound. A tube, closed at the end and having fine holes along the sides for a short or longer distance according to the size of the wound, is inserted in the wound; the irrigating solution is then introduced through this tube, which is held in the wound by gauze packed lightly around it. Soft, thick compresses are laid over the wound to absorb the drainage. The compresses are soon saturated and must be changed frequently to avoid soiling the clothing and bedding. Usually, the skin area around the wound is protected with strips of gauze saturated with petroleum jelly.

Various types of solutions are used for irrigating the wound. Today, many contain antibiotics. The solution used by Carrel was a preparation of sodium hypochlorite developed by Dakin. Any fluid used for irrigation may be introduced periodically with a syringe inserted into the end of the tube, which lies outside the dressing (see Fig. 33-2), or continuously by attaching the end of the tube to a reservoir, such as an intravenous bottle.

When this type of dressing is used, the tubes and packing are replaced daily, since the purulent material from the wound tends to saturate the packing and clog the holes of the

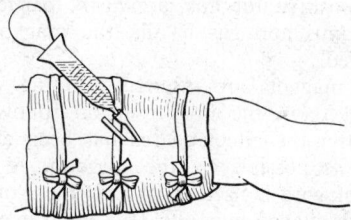

Figure 33-2. Diagram showing one method of irrigating infected wounds, using the Carrel-Dakin technique. (After Mason, R. L.: *Preoperative and Postoperative Treatment.* W. B. Saunders Co., Philadelphia, 1937.)

drainage tubes. As the compresses get soggy, they are replaced from time to time throughout the day, as often as necessary for the comfort of the patient.

Occlusive Dressings. This type of dressing is used over burns when exposure of the burn is not thought desirable or practicable. A single layer of gauze impregnated with petrolatum, with wax and carbon (carbogauze), or with antibacterial ointment is used, or a dry, fine-meshed gauze is placed next to the burn wound. A bulky layer of washed fluffy gauze is applied next and this is followed by large abdominal pads, all held in place with an elastic or crepe bandage. The dressings are applied evenly and with compression to eliminate dead space, give vascular support, and produce a splinting effect.

Biologic Dressings. Recently biologic dressings have been used as temporary wound coverings for extensive burns and denuded areas. The sources of biologic materials are fresh homografts, pig (porcine) skin, bovine embryo skin, and preserved canine heterografts.[11,12] Zeno-Derm * is an example of a porcine epidermal dressing. For a discussion of the treatment of burns, see Chapter 42.

The Therapeutic Use of Maggots in Wounds. Maggots (grown from eggs of the bluebottle fly) have been applied to sloughing, suppurative wounds in osteomyelitis, because they are supposed to digest dead necrotic material, and they are able to differentiate the dead from the living tissues more minutely than can the human eye. The flies are kept in cages in the laboratory and fed entirely on sterile food. Their eggs are placed in a sterile culture medium and allowed to hatch in an incubator kept at 38°C (100.4°F). Maggots thus produced are kept for 24 to 48 hours, during which time cultures are taken from the medium in which they are living. If cultures prove

* Chesebrough-Pond, Greenwich, Conn.
† Elbert Co., Newton, Mass.
‡ Gorman-Rupp Industries, Belleville, Ohio.

* Hancock Laboratories, Orange, Calif., distributed by Chesebrough-Pond, Greenwich, Conn.

to be positive for any organism, particularly the tetanus and gas bacilli, the maggots are discarded.

The maggots are inserted into the wound every 4 days, the first insertion following 8 days after the infected area has been cleaned as far as possible by the surgeon. A shield made of wire is used to protect the wound; a cradle is placed over the area and an electric light bulb suspended from the roof of the cradle. Since maggots turn from the light, this is used to keep them from working out of the incision, or to regulate their position in relation to the wound. A severe constitutional reaction follows, generally about 24 hours after the application. For this and other reasons, many surgeons do not use this method of treatment. Psychologically, it is hard for the patient and the family to accept.

The nurse's responsibilities consist in constant supervision of the patient, in the aspiration or withdrawal of the large amounts of secretion in the wound that follows the use of maggots, in the provision for drainage of the wound, and in the adjustment of the bedding, screen, cradle, and light. This treatment is now extremely rare.

5. EQUIPMENT FOR SURGICAL DRESSINGS

Hospital Practice. Materials used in hospitals for surgical dressings are stored in the same area on a unit so that they can be gathered up and brought to the bedside with the least possible effort. The dressing carriage of old is no longer brought to the bedside for dressing changes as this technique was found to promote cross-infections. Where carriages still exist they serve only as storage tables for surgical dressing supplies. Supplies that are necessary for surgical dressings, which should be stored together in a convenient area, are: sterile towels; gauze-and-cotton sponges; dressings of various sizes; gauze packing of different widths; drains made of tubing; rubber tubes and syringes for irrigating wounds; bottles of solutions; cups and bowls of different sizes; instruments such as forceps, scissors, scalpels, and probes; ointments; strips of gauze impregnated with petroleum jelly; and other items such as wooden spatulas, applicators, bandages, binders, adhesive, pins, and paper bags for the reception of waste. If the nurse is sufficiently familiar with the needs of the patient and the preferences of the surgeon, she or he should be able to assemble what is required without difficulty.

The specific equipment needed for a dressing change depends upon the kind of wound.

The safest aseptic technique is that carried out by using individually packaged sterile items which can be opened at the bedside or in the ward dressing room. If a bottled solution is required for a dressing, it should not be taken from one patient to another. In many hospitals in the United States, non-nursing personnel place the dressings to be used daily for each patient in a cabinet that opens both into a corridor and into the patient area or room (a "nurserver") (see Fig. 15-6), nurses specifying what they need. In like manner, non-nursing personnel collect daily or oftener, from a similar but different cabinet the used dressings which have been put in a waterproof bag.

For changing wound dressings it is necessary to have a receptacle for the old dressing. A waxed paper bag or plastic bag serves this purpose well. Any receptable holding soiled dressings should not be left in the patient's room but should be discarded in special containers in the work room unless the "nurserver" system is used.

Home Nursing. Prepackaged sterile dressing equipment is available for use in the home just as it is in hospitals, industries, schools, offices, and all other settings where wounds are dressed. In the United States such equipment can be purchased at most local drugstores. For parts of the world where a similar situation does not exist and a dry sterile dressing is not available, a substitute can be made by ironing pieces of soft and absorbent fabric of suitable sizes, not allowing anything that has not also been subjected to some sterilizing process to touch the dressing between the time it is ironed and applied to the wound. Since moist heat is more effective than dry heat in sterilizing, it is desirable to wet the cloth before ironing it. A moist cloth laid over a hot iron and allowed to dry is perhaps the cleanest dry dressing that can be produced in the home. Gauze sponges for cleaning may be made nearly sterile in a pressure cooker or by boiling in a pan in the kitchen; they may be used directly from the container in which they are sterilized. The pan in which instruments are boiled serves as a sterile tray after the water is poured out. In this procedure the essentials of asepsis are observed, although it is very simple and the protection not so complete as that afforded when all sterile articles used in the dressing have been autoclaved.

6. PROCEDURE FOR DRESSING WOUNDS

Ward Dressing Rooms. Robert A. Roaf and Leonard J. Hodkinson [13] recommend that there be a room on patient units reserved for dressings and related sterile procedures since there is always an element of risk when a person's wound is dressed in a room with other patients. The ventilation and heating of the room can be designed so that dust and droplets are driven away from rather than toward sterile areas. The walls and floors in this type of room can be cleaned more easily and frequently than those in a patient's room. Storage in the room should be minimal and it is desirable to have excellent natural and artificial light.

Preparing a Patient and the Environment for a Dressing. Before dressings are begun, the patient's unit or room should be in order, with no unnecessary articles in the way, but dressings should not be changed for at least 15 minutes after the room has been cleaned or floors swept to allow time for airborne particles to settle. Windows and doors should be closed to eliminate drafts. Curtains should be drawn around the patient to provide privacy, and the bedside table or overbed table should be cleared so there is sufficient space to set up a sterile field and to place needed supplies and equipment.

Patients are told that the dressing is to be changed, who will change it, and what will be expected of them during the procedure. Light anesthetics are given for some very painful dressings, for example, dressings of extensive burns. The position of the patient depends on the area to be dressed, but unless contraindicated, is dorsal recumbent. Patients should be made as comfortable as possible and free from all strains. For instance, they should not be obliged to raise the head or an extremity for the application of a dressing or bandage without support. At the same time, positions should be convenient ones for those applying the dressings. The bed should be at a comfortable height so that the physician or nurse has to neither stoop nor reach. The patient's hands should be out of the way and in no danger of contaminating or interfering with the dressing. It is wise to suggest to those patients who have indicated a fear of looking at their wound to turn their head away during the dressing procedure. During the procedure, the nurse, a friend, or a relative placing a hand on the patient's arm or shoulder and making a comment that acknowledges the presence of pain, often helps patients tolerate it better. Allowing an infant to be held by a parent or nurse may be a comforting measure for both parent and child. If it is anticipated that a dressing procedure will produce great pain for the patient, an appropriate analgesic should be administered at least 15 minutes prior to the procedure. In case a wound is to be irrigated,

the patient should be drawn to the side of the bed. When extra pillows, a back rest, or Gatch frame interferes with the dressing, the pillows should be removed or the back rest lowered.

The arrangement of the clothing depends upon the area to be dressed, but in all cases the following principles should be observed: With the exception of the top sheet, the upper clothing should be turned back neatly and smoothly so as to allow a free area around the wound for the dressing, with no bulky folds to interfere with it; the upper sheet should then be turned back, forming one thin flat fold at the margin of the area. Unnecessary exposure and chilling of the patient should be avoided. If the dressing is on an abdominal wound, the spread and blanket should be turned back neatly and smoothly to the thighs. If the weather is cool, or if there is any danger of chilling, a chest protector, or folded bath blanket, should first be placed across the chest. The sheet should be folded down to expose the area to be dressed, the patient's gown tucked back out of the way. If drainage from the wound is free, or if the wound is to be irrigated, plastic or rubber sheeting should be used to protect the bed and bedding, and suitable basins provided to collect the discharge.

After preparing for the dressing, as above, the bandage or binder confining the dressing is removed; cast or splints and other appliances are removed when necessary. The adhesive strapping is loosened on one side or both. If a daily dressing change is necessary, it is more comfortable for the patient if tape strapping— adhesive to which tape is fastened and tied over the dressing (Montgomery straps)—is used (see Fig. 33-3). When removing adhesive, pull it on each side toward the wound to prevent strain on the sutures or wound. Satu-

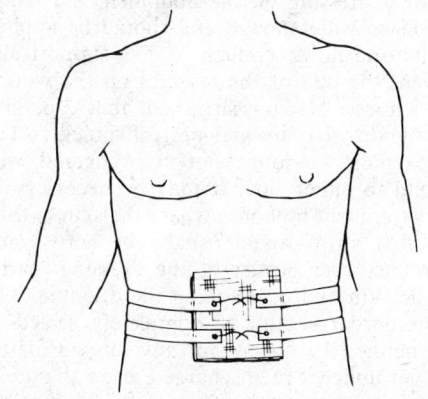

Figure 33-3. Montgomery straps: adhesive straps are used to secure dressings that must be changed frequently.

rating the adhesive with a hydrocarbon, such as benzine, acetone, or ether, makes its removal more comfortable. Removing adhesive quickly is much less painful than removing it slowly, but this should be explained to the patient as it gives the impression of a ruthless act. Removal of adhesive is most painful if hairs were not shaved from the skin before its application. Many persons have very sensitive, delicate skin and the removal of the adhesive may leave a raw or inflamed area. Only extreme care and the use of nonallergic adhesive can prevent great discomfort.

Dressings may be removed from noninfected wounds by touching the outer layer of gauze only. If the wound is infected the dressing is removed with sterile gloves or forceps. If the dressing adheres to the wound, moistening it with physiologic saline or hydrogen peroxide will loosen it for removal. Adherence of a dressing to the wound can be prevented through the use of a special dressing, Telfa,* which has a nonadherent inner surface. A new sterile dressing is applied over the wound, preferably with sterile gloves or forceps.

Completing the Dressing and Making the Patient Comfortable. Dressings are held in place by the application of scotch tape, adhesive strapping, binders, or bandages.

In order to apply scotch tape or adhesive strapping over the dressing, first remove any adherent particles of adhesive with benzine or alcohol—these particles are unsightly and irritating. If the skin is abraded, hot water may be used.

As previously noted, adhesive strapping is applied to hold dressings in place, to draw the edges of the wound together and relieve strain on sutures, and to give support to the muscles of the abdomen, especially if the muscle wall is thick and pendulous.

For a dressing on the abdomen, the straps should be wide enough and should be applied tightly and firmly enough to give support and prevent the pull of the muscles on the wound and sutures. Narrow strips cut the skin, give no support, dry up, and peel off quickly. The straps must be long enough to extend well around to either side. It may be necessary to pad prominent hipbones where the skin is thin. The first strip should usually be across and over the lower border of the dressing, partly on the skin and overlapping the dressing. The lower border should be completely sealed so that neither the fingers nor any foreign matter can get under it or discharge escape to spread infection. The other strips are applied in the

same way from below toward the waist. To apply the strap, first fasten securely on the opposite side, then draw it toward the operator over the dressing with one hand and with the other gently but firmly press the abdominal wall toward the wound (away from the operator), and quickly and securely fasten the adhesive in place. This draws the edges together, relieves strain, and gives support. The patient is more comfortable, does not feel as though he or she were falling apart, and is not afraid to move. Adhesive must never be applied over an abraded skin. When a daily dressing is necessary, to prevent irritation of the skin and pain and discomfort to the patient caused by the daily removal of adhesive, tape strappings (Montgomery straps) are fastened on either side and tied over the dressing. If used the tapes should be removed as soon as they are soiled, the edges are curled, or adhesion is lost.

Binders and bandages are frequently used to secure dressings in place and for support. They are discussed and different types illustrated in the next section of this chapter.

A liquid adhesive is available that is convenient for certain dressings. It is said to be less irritating than adhesive tape. As soon as the dressing has been fixed in position, the dressing rubber or plastic protector and towels are removed, the bedding straightened, pillows adjusted, and bedside table replaced, if moved. Soiled linen is placed in the appropriate container. Soiled instruments are collected in a basin; used dressings are placed in a paper bag and immediately disposed of in a waste container in the work room or in the "nur-server."

If patients are expected to change their own dressings eventually, they should know this from the outset, be encouraged to watch the procedure, and to ask questions during it. A time schedule should be agreed upon, so that both patient and nurse are working toward the same goal. Allowing patients more and more responsibility for the dressing change will ensure the build-up of confidence in their own abilities. Gradually the nurse should become the observer and the patient the operator.

7. PRINCIPLES UNDERLYING THE SELECTION AND APPLICATION OF BANDAGES AND BINDERS

Purposes for Which Bandages Are Used. Bandages are used in first-aid treatment, and in orthopedic and general surgery. They are applied for the following purposes: (1) to hold surgical dressings, medicinal applications,

* Curity product available from Kendall Co., Edison, N.J.

or splints in place; (2) to apply pressure on various parts in order to control bleeding, to support weak-walled blood vessels, to relieve congestion, to promote the absorption of fluid or exudates, and to prevent or reduce edema or swelling; and (3) to immobilize a part, to afford support and protection to injured limbs and joints, and to correct deformity.

Materials of Which Bandages Are Made. Various materials are used, the most common being gauze, muslin, elastic webbing, woven cotton, felt, flannel, and crinoline impregnated with plaster of Paris or other substances. The material selected must be suitable for the purpose for which the bandage is applied.

Crinoline impregnated with starch, plaster of Paris, or plastics is used to immobilize a broken limb or joint. It is also used as a means of support in diseases of bones or joints, such as osteomyelitis of the leg or a tuberculous ankle. Space is left to allow for dressings. (For further discussion of casts, see Chapter 34.)

Elasticized bandages (webbing) are used for even pressure over varicose veins, and for limitation of motion at joints. Polyurethane plastic synthetic fiber is incorporated into the weaving of the bandage. These bandages are commonly referred to as Ace bandages. The PEG (pressure elastic grip) Ace bandage adheres to itself so that no hooks or clips are needed * (see Fig. 33-4).

Elastoplast is a woven bandage with an adhesive side. It is useful when pressure should be maintained for a relatively long period.

Felt is used under splints and plaster-of-Paris bandages to protect the skin.

Flannel is soft and elastic, and may be applied smoothly and with even pressure using simple spiral turns; it is warm and absorbent. Flannel is applied to painful joints and extremities in rheumatism and gout for comfort. Outing (Canton) or cotton flannel is used for abdominal and many-tailed bandages or scultetus binders. These binders are also made of cotton twill.

Gauze is thin, light, soft, porous, and cool. It can be readily adjusted with an even pressure and is suitable for holding dressings and splints in place. It is always used to retain wet dressings in place, and is usually preferred to muslin in applying bandages to children. Gauze is more pliable and stays on better, but it should be remembered that the soft tissues of children can tolerate little pressure and any bandage should be applied with special care.

Kling * is a gauze which has been woven so that it will stretch and conform to body contours. It has a crepelike texture and since it tends to stick to itself it retains its position on highly movable parts of the body such as the extremities.

Unbleached muslin is heavier and firmer and may be used to apply pressure, to give support, to limit motion, and to hold splints in place. Sometimes sheet wadding is first wrapped around the extremity when muslin bandages are applied for pressure and support.

Types of Bandages and Their Uses

1. The *triangular bandage* is used as a sling to support the hand and arm, and may be

* Becton-Dickinson, Rutherford, N.J.

* Johnson & Johnson, New Brunswick, N.J.

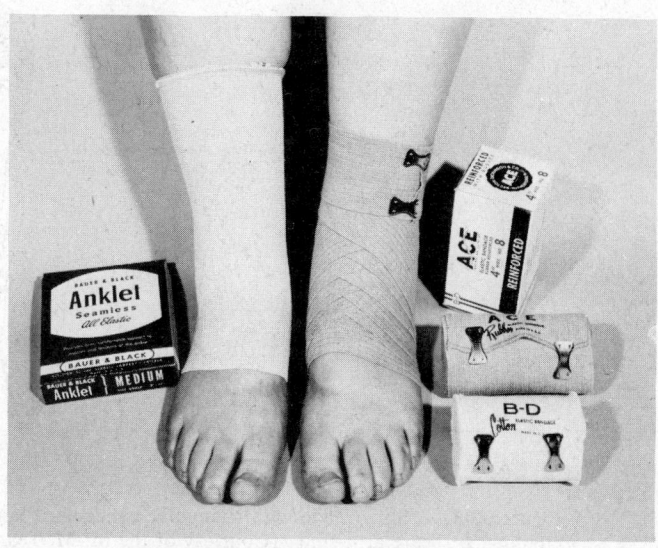

Figure 33-4. Cotton elastic bandage applied to an ankle and elastic anklet, both used for support of a sprained ankle. (Courtesy of Bauer & Black, Chicago, Ill.)

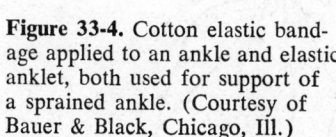

used to hold dressings in place on the shoulder, hand, foot, hip, breast, or buttocks.

2. The *cravat bandage* is a triangular bandage with the apex first folded to the base and the material then rolled or loosely folded to the base, making a bandage of the desired width. It is used as a sling to support the hand and in first-aid treatment to hold dressings in place on such parts as the axilla, groin, or back of the neck.

A *sling* is a swinging bandage most commonly used to support the hand, forearm, and elbow. It may be made of a roller bandage, a cravat, or a triangular bandage. The *triangular bandage* is the sling generally used. It may be made of any firm, pliable material, but is usually made by folding a piece of muslin a yard square into a triangle. Slings for ambulatory patients should be made of inconspicuous (usually dark) materials.

Before applying the sling, the injured arm is extended horizontally across the body, in the semiprone position—that is, with the thumb up. The triangle is placed under the injured arm so that the hand rests on the base and the apex extends beyond the elbow. The corner of the base of the triangle that rests against the body is carried up over the shoulder of the injured side while the other portion is carried up over the opposite shoulder. The two ends are then tied around the neck. The apex at the elbow is then folded neatly and pinned securely to the body of the bandage. Some surgeons prefer to pin it to the posterior portion while others pin it to the anterior portion. See Figure 33-5 for a commercially available sling that can be adjusted so that there is minimal pressure on the back of the neck.

The cravat sling is used when it is necessary to support the wrist and hand only.

3. The *handkerchief bandage* is made of thin, pliable material cut in squares of different sizes, folded in the shape of a triangle or cravat, and readily adjusted to different parts of the body. The ends can be securely tied or pinned. The handkerchief bandage has been used for centuries. It is especially useful to hold temporary dressings on the head, hand, foot, knee, or elbow in first-aid and emergency work and for applications that require frequent attention.

4. *Tailed bandages* consist of a body and one or many tails. The most commonly used are the *single-T,* or the *double-T* bandage (see Fig. 33-7), and the *many-tailed* bandages. They are used to hold dressings on various parts of the body. They are particularly useful if the patient is confined to bed, if a dressing requires frequent attention and changing, or if it is applied to a part that must be disturbed as little as possible, as in the treatment of a wound in a fractured arm or leg. The body of the bandage is used to cover the dressing, and the tails are used for fastening.

The *single-T bandage* or *binder* consists of a single upright strip that extends at right angles from the middle of a horizontal strip, thus forming the shape of a letter *T*. It is sometimes made of outing (Canton) or cotton flannel, but is usually made of double unbleached muslin stitched around the edges. It is used to hold dressings in position over the rectum and external genitals, and occasionally for pressure.

A single-T binder is used for female patients. A double-T binder may be used for

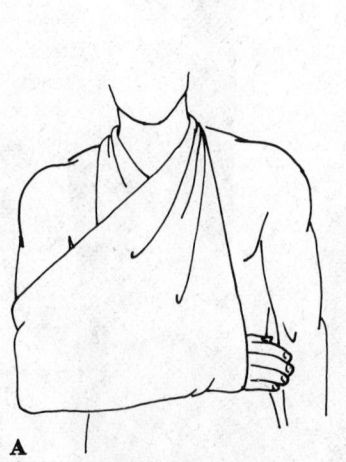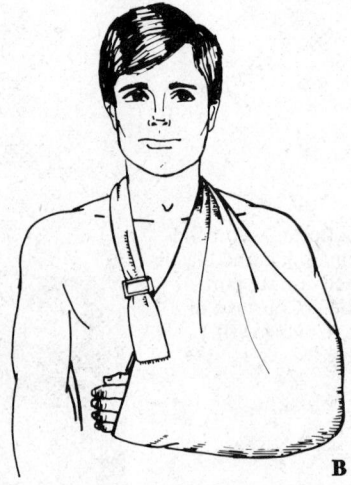

A   **B**

Figure 33-5. *A*. Sling made with triangular bandage; it is usually applied over the clothing. *B*. Teare arm sling. (Courtesy of the M. M. Teare Co., Buffalo, N.Y.)

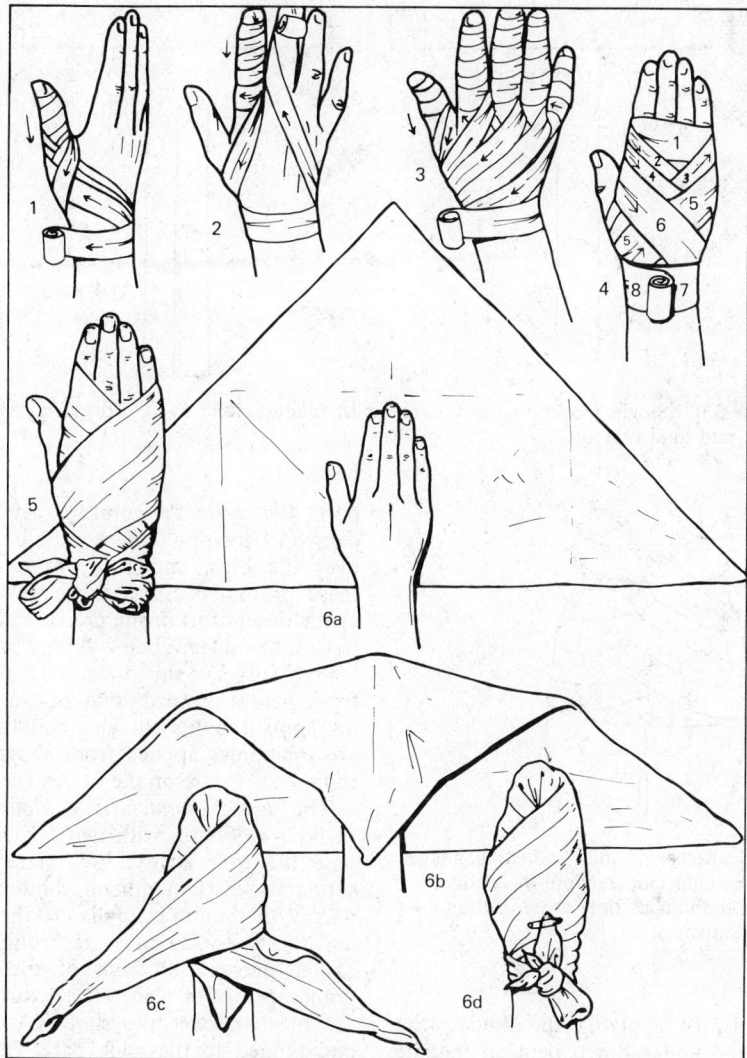

Figure 33-6. Hand and finger bandages.

dressings over the male genitalia or rectum. The belt or horizontal strip that fastens around the waist should be wide enough for comfort. The upright strip or strips that pass between the thighs over the external genitals must be wide enough to cover the dressing and hold it securely in place in such a way that the dressing or wound will not become infected from external sources. This strip should be fastened securely to the belt with safety pins. In male patients, a double-T binder may be arranged to leave the penis uncovered if there is no dressing over it.

These binders must be changed immediately when soiled or dampened from perspiration or discharge from the wound.

The *scultetus,* or *many-tailed, binder* is used

on the abdomen to hold dressings and to give added support following abdominal operations. It is used particularly after extensive operations if the muscle walls are thick or flabby or if the abdomen is pendulous, and the patient inclined to be restless. It prevents tension on the sutures and wound. If properly applied, it adds greatly to the comfort of the patient. If not properly applied, it is loose, hot, and untidy, and a source of discomfort.

The binder is made by putting together five strips of Canton, or cotton, flannel, three inches wide and about a yard and a half (1.4 meters) long so that each strip overlaps a half of the one below. The strips are then sewn together for about a quarter of a yard. This forms the body of the bandage, the balance

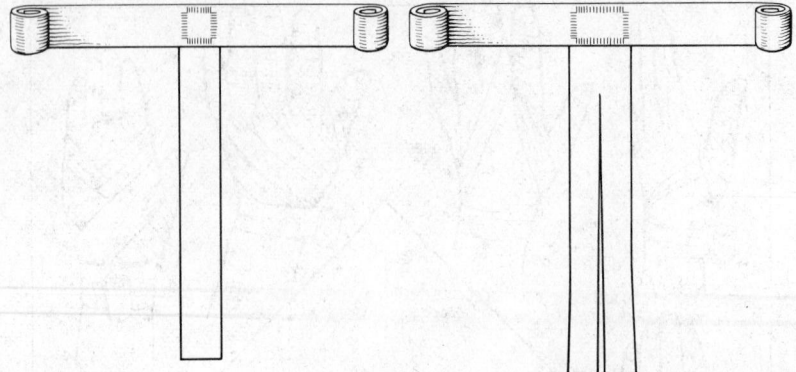

Figure 33-7. Single-T and double-T bandage or binders, used to hold dressings over pubic and anal regions.

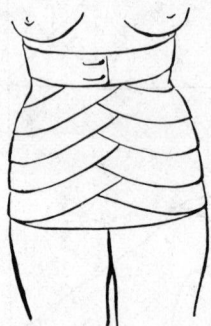

Figure 33-8. Scultetus, or many-tailed, bandage used as an abdominal binder. Note the oblique direction given the tails as they cross in the midline of the abdomen.

being the tails. In applying the binder, the center is placed under the patient so that its lower border comes well down over the hips but does not interfere with the use of a bedpan. The strips are then brought one by one from either side obliquely over the abdomen, crossing each other in the midline. Considerable traction is used in order to give firm support, the patient's comfort determining the degree of traction. There must be no wrinkles over the hips, and strips must not end on these prominences, as the ends are likely to cause discomfort from pressure if the patient lies on the side. When a binder is applied following surgery, the pressure is usually made from below upward; that is, the lowest tails are applied first. Following childbirth, the tails are sometimes applied from above downward, to make pressure on the uterus (see Fig. 33-8).

The *breast binder* is a *double-T binder* (8-inch-wide strip with two 2-inch strips sewn onto the wide strip). It is generally used to support breasts of nursing mothers. The wide part of the binder is applied to the upper back, and the two wide ends are brought under the axillae across the front of the breasts and pinned firmly in place. The two narrow strips are brought over the shoulders to the front and pinned to the wide part. Darts must be pinned under the breast to make the binder fit (see Fig. 33-9).

5. The *roller bandage* is the one most commonly used. It is made by cutting or tearing any of the above mentioned materials into long narrow strips and rolling them into a compact

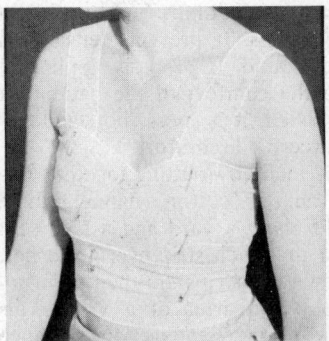

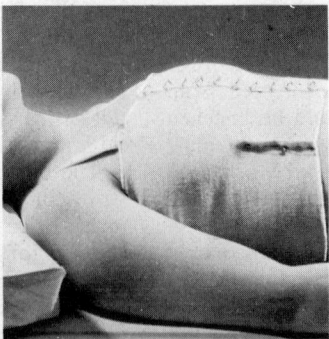

Figure 33-9. Ace bandage used as breast binder. (Courtesy of Johnson & Johnson, New Brunswick, N.J.)

cylinder. The width and length of the bandage depends upon the part of the body to which it is to be applied.

Variations in Width and Length of the Roller Bandage. The width and length will usually vary as follows:

	Width (Inches)	Length (Yards)
Finger	¾ to 1	1 to 5
Hand	1 to 2	3
Arm	2 to 2½	7 to 9
Head	2 to 2½	6
Eye	2	3
Foot	1½ to 3	3
Leg	2½ to 3	9
Body	3 to 6	9 to 10

To make a roller bandage by hand, fold one end of a bandage upon itself again and again until a small stiff roll is formed, firm enough to grasp between the thumb and finger without bending. If this roll, or core, is not tight, it will be impossible to make a well-rolled bandage. This roll is then grasped between the thumb and index finger of the left hand, and the free end is held tightly and firmly between the thumb and index finger of the right hand. The cylinder is revolved by the left hand, the right hand holding the free end firmly and acting as a guide to keep the bandage even. Some may find it easier to reverse this order, holding the roll in the right hand and the free end between the thumb and index finger of the left hand.

6. *Stockinet* is a bandage dispensed as a tube so that a body part may be inserted into it. It is useful in holding dressings on the head. *Surgitube,* a product made like stockinet, is effective for finger bandages (see Fig. 33-10). *Surgifix* is not used as a dressing, but it is used to hold dressings in place after amputations of extremities, mastectomies, and other operations. It can be used to hold wet dressings in place and may be used for slings.

7. *Elastic stockings* are capable of applying even pressure to the leg from the foot to mid-thigh. Commonly used over varicose veins, they have an advantage over Ace bandages in that they are more easily applied and removed. Elastic wristlets and anklets are also available and are useful to support injured wrists and ankles.

Principles to Observe in the Application of Bandages. Bandaging requires practice to acquire the necessary skill and dexterity. In applying the bandage, comfort and durability should have first attention. A bandage should never be uncomfortable. In addition, the aim should be to acquire ease in applying, economy

in time and materials, and a neat, finished appearance. Only clean bandages should be used.

Comfort, durability, and neatness can be attained only by observing the following rules:

Place the patient in a comfortable position which is convenient for the operator who, in most cases, must stand *directly in front of the patient* in applying the bandage. Support the parts that are also elevated while being bandaged—foot, leg, pelvis, or head. Sandbags, pillows, or special rests may be used for the heel, ankle, elbow, or pelvis.

Place the part in a functional position and apply the bandage. For instance, in applying a bandage to the elbow, flex the arm at the elbow, not extended.

Before applying a bandage see that the part is clean and dry. Dust it lightly with powder. Two skin surfaces must never be allowed to come in contact. Absorbent cotton should be used, for example, under the breasts, between the toes or fingers, between the arms and body, and behind the ear. Joints, bony prominences, and angles, such as in the axilla, groin, bend of the elbow or of the knee, where the bandage is likely to press or cut, should always be padded. Hollows should also be padded.

In applying a bandage, hold the roll uppermost. The outer surface of the initial extremity of the bandage is placed on the part to be bandaged and is held in place by the fingers of the left hand and the body of the bandage is held by the right hand. Never unwind more bandage than is absolutely necessary (unwind gradually as required), and bandage from right to left if right-handed. Always anchor a bandage securely by making two circular turns around the part. The second turn fixes, or anchors, the first.

In bandaging an arm or a leg, begin at the extremity and work toward the trunk. This is in order to avoid congestion, swelling, and possible gangrene of the part below. Fingers and toes are usually left exposed so that they may be observed from time to time as a guide to the condition of the circulation. If they become pale, cold, blue, tingling, or numb, the bandage is applied too tightly and must be removed to prevent gangrene.

Each turn of a bandage should be applied with even pressure or tension. The comfort of the patient and durability of the bandage depend to a large extent on the tension used. Good judgment is required in each case to know just how much pressure to make, and considerable practice in bandaging is necessary before good judgment is acquired. The patient's comfort is one of the best guides. The operator should always question the patient

A

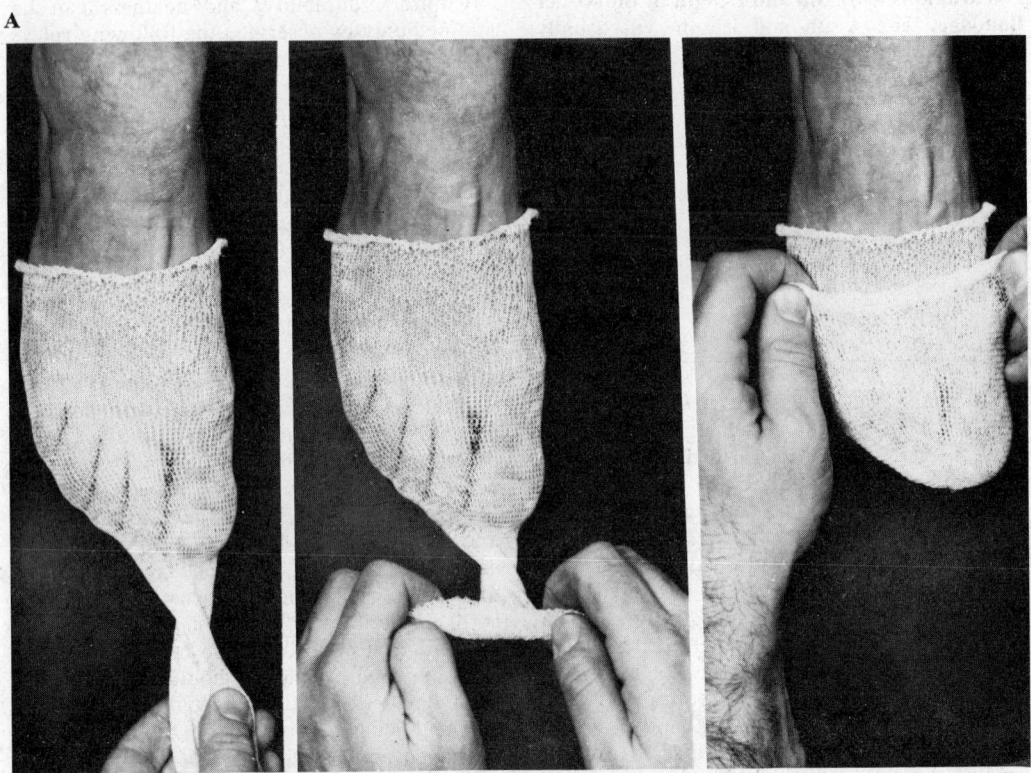

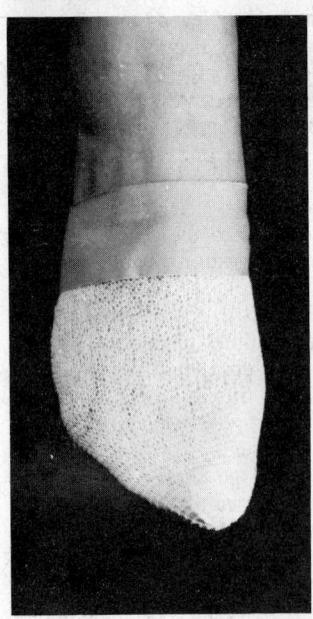

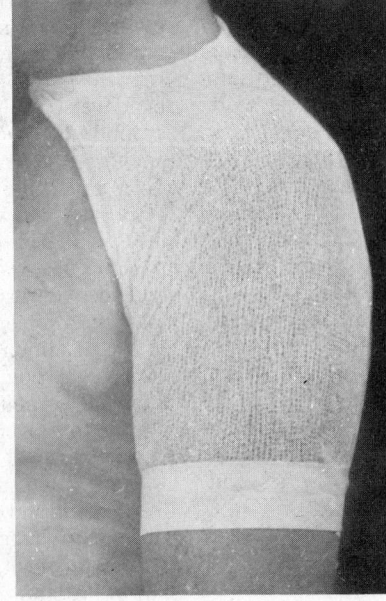

Figure 33-10. *A, B.* Application of Surgitube to foot. Surgitube may be used as a clean dressing when ointments are applied or it may be used over a sterile dressing instead of a roller bandage to hold it in place. *C.* Completed dressing of the same material, applied to the shoulder. (Courtesy of Surgitube Products Corp., New York, N.Y.)

B

C

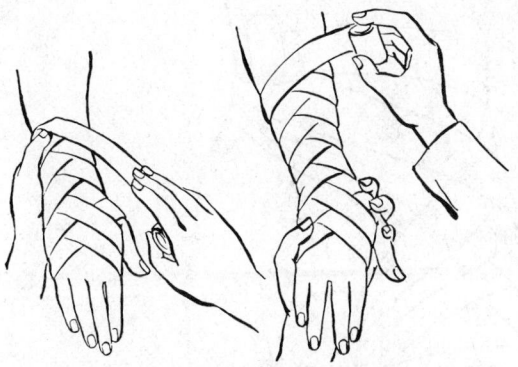

Figure 33-11. *Left:* Spiral-reverse bandage of the forearm, showing effective position of the hands in reversing the bandage. *Right:* Figure-of-eight bandage of the forearm, showing the oblique direction the bandage should take.

on comfort, both during the procedure and after its completion.

Pressure should not be used over inflamed, painful tissues, and especial care should be taken in applying bandages to infants and young children. Care should be taken also in bandaging wet dressings in place, for this bandage when dry will shrink and be unbearably tight. The bandage should be tight enough to ensure permanency but not tight enough to interfere with the circulation.

In bandaging, avoid useless turns. This makes the part uncomfortably hot, wastes the bandage, and makes the pressure uneven— each turn over the same region nearly doubles the pressure. Use a second bandage if necessary to complete a bandage, but do not make extra turns just to use all the bandage. Each turn should overlap exactly the same area of the preceding turn; the area covered is usually one half or two thirds. Reverses and crosses should always be even or in a straight line. Portions of skin (gaps between the turns) should never be left uncovered.

If the preceding rules are observed, the desired pattern and a finished appearance follows.

Fundamental Bandages. These are the circular, spiral, spiral-reverse, figure of eight, spica, and recurrent. These, together with combinations or modifications of these turns, are the basis for the greater number of bandages used. The form chosen will depend on the part of the body to be bandaged and the purpose of the bandage.

The *circular bandage* consists of several circular turns of a roller bandage around a part, each turn exactly covering the preceding one. It is used to hold dressings on such parts as the neck, wrist, or forehead, and one or two circular turns are always made to anchor the initial end of a bandage. Each turn holds the preceding one firmly in place.

The *spiral bandage* is applied to parts of uniform circumference, such as the upper arm, fingers, or trunk. It consists of simple oblique turns around the part, each turn ascending (or sometimes descending) higher than the preceding one and overlapping it one half or two thirds.

The *spiral-reverse bandage* consists of the spiral bandage in which reverses are made (see Fig. 33-11). By means of these the bandage may be made to fit parts that are tapering or of uneven circumference, such as the forearm or leg. When it is necessary to make a reverse in order to have the bandage fit, place the thumb of the left hand on the bandage where the reverse is to be made; with the right hand holding the roll, unwind the latter about 6 inches. Then pronate the hand so that the bandage is directed downward instead of upward (reversed). Then carry the bandage around the limb with firm traction. Continue the turns, making sure that the reverses are uniform and in line and that each turn covers the same area as the preceding one; otherwise the bandage will be uncomfortable and will not fit or stay on, and the pressure will not be even. Reverses should not be made over bony prominences or joints, as they increase the pressure.

The bandage is used to retain dressings or splints in place and to apply pressure and afford support. It is used chiefly on the arms and legs.

The *figure-of-eight bandage* consists of oblique turns that alternately ascend and descend after encircling the part (see Fig. 33-12). Each turn crosses the preceding one in front, making a figure of eight, and overlaps it one half or two thirds. This bandage is used to hold dressings in place, to apply pressure and afford support, and is particularly useful in immobilizing joints, such as the elbow, ankle, knee, wrist, thumb, hip, neck, and axilla, or the head and neck. In affording support to a limb, it is often combined with the spiral-reverse.

The *spica bandage* derives its name from the fact that the turns are supposed to resemble the arrangement of the husks of an ear of corn (see Fig. 33-13). It is applied to the thumb, shoulder, groin, and foot. Each turn follows the preceding turn, covering two thirds of it and either going higher or lower, according to whether the bandage is an ascending or descending spica. The turns cross each other, forming an angle or spica.

The *recurrent bandage* is used chiefly to

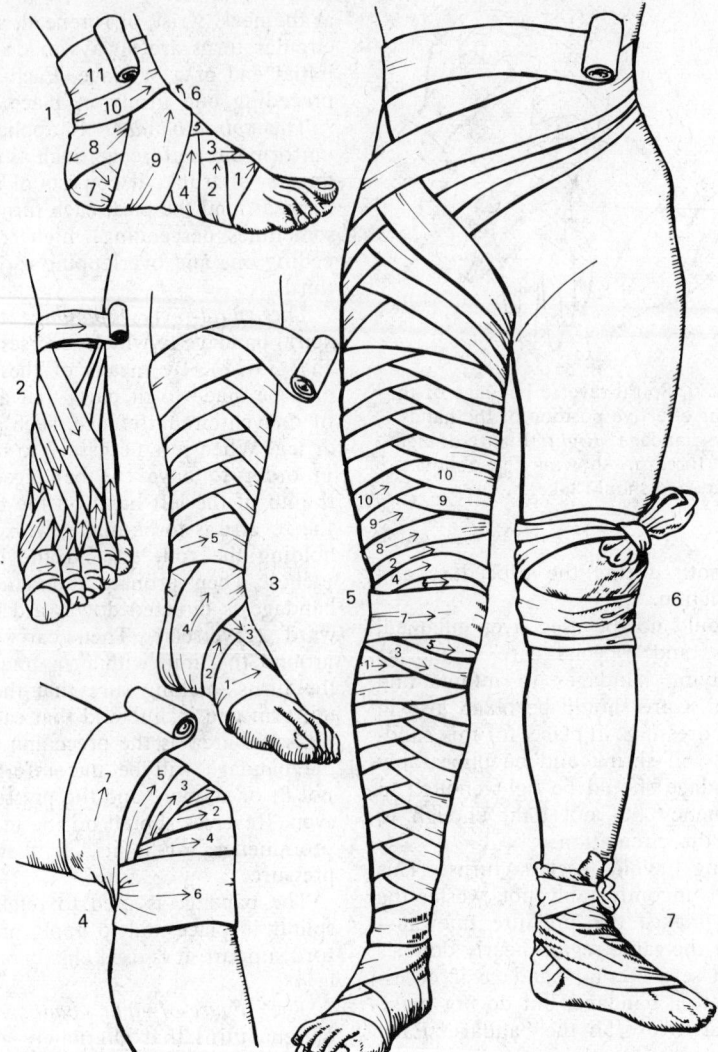

Figure 33-12. Feet, toes, ankle, leg, and knee bandages.

retain dressings on the ends of the fingers, the head, or the stump of an amputated extremity. It consists of a series of turns, the first turn usually being in the middle and the following turns passing back and forth over the part, first on one side, then on the other, each time returning (or recurring) to the starting point, until the whole area is covered. Each turn covers one half to two thirds the preceding one. The ends are bound down firmly with several circular turns.

Method of Securing a Bandage. A bandage may be secured by pinning, sewing, tying, or by adhesive strapping. It should never be pinned or tied in the following places: (1) over an injured part or inflamed surface; (2) over a bony prominence, or on the inner surface of a limb; (3) over a part that the patient may lie on; (4) over a part where there is likely to be friction or where it may cause discomfort in any way. Body bandages should be pinned in front, and head bandages over the temple.

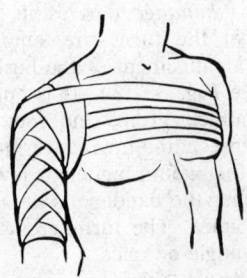

Figure 33-13. Spica of the shoulder.

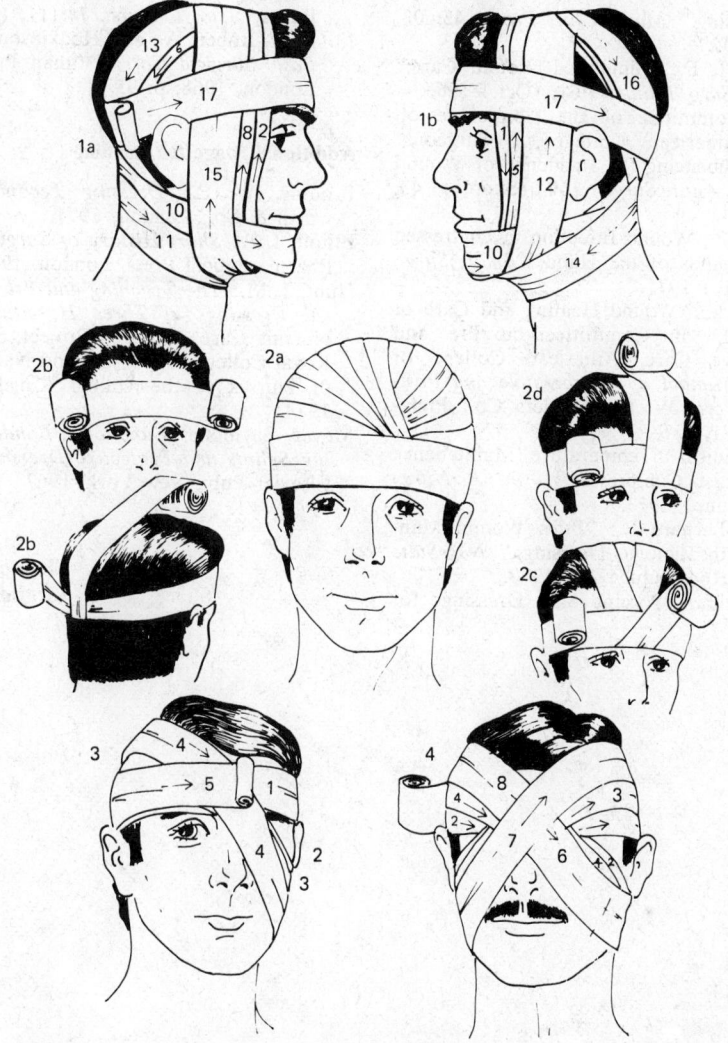

Figure 33-14. Head, forehead, lateral eye, and bilateral eye bandages.

Small safety pins are preferable to large ones. Pins should be inserted in the long axis of the bandage so that friction or straining will not remove but rather make it more secure. To tie a bandage: tear the terminal end the required distance, which depends upon the circumference of the part, twist or tie the ends to prevent further tearing, and pass them around the part in opposite directions and tie at the starting point.

Method of Removing a Roller Bandage. The bandage may be cut (with bandage scissors) if necessary to avoid pain or fatigue, to save time in an emergency, or when the bandage is soiled. In all cases where the bandage is to be used again, unfasten the terminal end and unwind, gathering the loose turns as unwound and passing them from hand to hand; otherwise, the bandage will become entangled about the extremity. This method also saves time and prevents the bandage from soiling.

REFERENCES

1. Lowbury, E. J. L., and Hood, A. M.: "A Disinfectant Barrier in Dressings Applied to Burns," *Lancet,* **2:**899, (May 3) 1952.
2. Sharpe, Charles: "Surgical Dressing Technique: Two Examples," *Aust. NZ J. Med.,* **38:**360, (May) 1969.
3. Nash, D. F. E.: *The Principles and Practice of Surgery for Nurses and Allied Professions.* Edward Arnold, Ltd., London, 1969, p. 428.
4. Bishop, William J.: *A History of Surgical Dressings.* Robinson & Sons, Ltd., Chesterfield, Eng., 1959.
5. Schlein, A. P., et al.: "The Modified Robert

Jones Dressing," *Mayo Clin. Proc.,* **45**:602, (Aug.) 1970.

6. MacLaren, I. F.: "Simplified Wound Care," *J. R. Coll. Surg. Edinb.,* **9**:61, (Oct.) 1963.

7. Ad Hoc Committee of the Committee on Trauma, American College of Surgeons: "Factors Influencing the Incidence of Wound Infection," *Ann. Surg.,* **160** (Suppl): 43, (Aug.) 1964.

8. Wood, P. B.: "Wound Infection in Undressed Sutured Wounds of the Hand," *Br. J. Surg.,* **58**:543, (July) 1971.

9. Peacock, Erle: "Wound Healing and Care of the Wound," in Committee on Pre and Postoperative Care, American College of Surgeons: *Manual of Preoperative and Postoperative Care.* W. B. Saunders Co., Philadelphia, 1971, p. 9.

10. Petrello, Judith: "Temperature Maintenance of Hot Moist Compresses," *Am. J. Nurs.,* **73**:1050, (June) 1973.

11. Bromberg, Bernard E.: "Burn Wound Management with Biologic Dressings," *NY State J. Med.,* **70**:1645, (June 15) 1970.

12. Stinson, Velda: "Porcine Skin Dressings for Burns," *Am. J. Nurs.,* **74**:111, (Jan.) 1974.

13. Roaf, Robert A., and Hodkinson, Leonard J.: *Basic Surgical Care.* Pittman Publishing Co., London, 1968, p. 95.

Additional Suggested Reading

Broome, W. E.: *Dressing Techniques.* Butterworth & Co., London, 1971.

Elliott, I.: *A Short History of Surgical Dressings.* Pharmaceutical Press, London, 1964.

Hunt, J. M.: *The Teaching and Practice of Surgical Dressings in Three Hospitals.* (Study of Nursing Care, Research Project, Ser. 1 No. 6.) Royal College of Nursing and National Council of Nurses of the United Kingdom, London, 1974.

Meyer, Seymour: *Functional Bandaging, Including Splints and Protective Dressings.* American Elsevier Pub., New York, 1967.

Eleanor Taggart
Virginia Henderson

CHAPTER 34

Application of Restraints, Splints, Casts, and Traction for Protection and Support

1. INTRODUCTION

Restraints, splints, and casts are all used to immobilize a person, or a segment of his or her body. The limitation of movement needed may range from the use of a single wristlet restraint during an intravenous infusion, to almost total immobilization as with a plaster of Paris hip spica cast. The purpose of these devices is preventive in the first case, therapeutic in the second. Restraints are applied to prevent persons' injuring themselves or others; splints and casts are applied to immobilize a part of the body. They are therapeutic agents in nerve, muscle, or bone pathology.

While bone growth is fostered more by "stress" than immobilization, the latter serves to maintain a position that is the best anatomically so that injured parts will be most functional when they are healed. And by immobilizing a part during the healing process, injury to newly formed tissue may be prevented.

All forms of restraint or immobilization are psychologically distasteful to living organisms. Hypomobility is physiologically harmful as well. Its effects are discussed at some length in Chapters 12 and 38. Health workers should promote hypomobility only when necessary and then should make every effort to counteract the adverse responses of those subjected to it.

2. RESTRAINTS

Purposes. Since the purpose of restraints is protection of the person rather than rigid maintenance of a position for healing, they are made of flexible materials and are not applied for long periods of time.

Conditions That May Require Limitation of Movement. *Irrational states* from any cause may make persons' movements dangerous to themselves or others. High temperatures with delirium, anesthesia, injury, operations on nerves, and functional mental diseases are some conditions in which it may be necessary to restrain movement.

Paralysis, and temporary conditions like anesthesia, result in *limitation of motor power or muscular coordination.* Conscious or semiconscious, the partially paralyzed or anesthetized person may fall out of bed while trying to get something from a table or while trying to change position. They may require the protection of restraining sheets, safety belts, safety vests, or side rails on the bed when continuous nursing care is unavailable.

When an intravenous fluid or blood is administered to children or semiconscious adults, arm or leg movements must be restrained so that the needle does not come out of or move and injure the vein. The wrists or hands of irrational or semiconscious persons with nasogastric tubes, catheters, or chest tubes may also have to be restrained so that these tubes are not withdrawn by the patient.

People, particularly children, who have itching skin must often have their hands restrained to keep them from scratching, removing crusts, and exposing the skin to injury and infection from the many organisms on the hands and under the nails. Even cooperative patients will scratch the skin when half asleep. In some *surgical conditions where disturbance of the dressing* would be disastrous, as, for example, in the operation for cataract or harelip, devices

1449

may be used that keep the patient from touching it.

Devices Used to Limit Movement. When it is necessary to limit motion of the entire body, as, for example, in irrational states, canvas, wooden, or metal side boards may be attached to the bed.* If the person is very active, these are not adequate. Occasionally a patient needs total immobilization for a brief period of time. In such situations, restraining sheets may be used, or a special restraining net with belts attached may be used to hold the arms and legs.

Wide belts, vests, or jackets are among the devices that may be chosen to limit movement. Safety *belts* made of electrically nonconductive materials are frequently used on stretchers and operating room tables. Safety *vests* made of cotton, nylon, or dacron mesh that do not cover the arms are suitable for supporting the trunk of partially paralyzed patients in a wheelchair. They are also appropriate for restraint of the upper part of the body of the patient in bed. Some of the safety vests have openings arranged so that they may be crisscrossed in front, giving maximum safety to the patient, or crisscrossed at the back to give maximum freedom. *Jacket* restraints usually enclose the upper body, and both arms and hands. They are infrequently used these days and require a physician's written prescription.

Ankle and wrist restraints may be padded leather straps, nylon webbing, tightly woven twill, orthopedic felt, cotton flannel, or gauze bandaging. Since these last three types of "limb-holders" do not withstand strong pull, they are generally used when patients simply need reminding that they are not to move a particular part of the body. When the condition of patients is such that the leather restraints are necessary for their safety or that of others, a written statement by the physician is required in most institutions and agencies before the restraints can be applied.

A common restraint for a young child is a cuff which is tied on the arm so that he or she cannot bend the elbow. It is made of cotton or flannel material with small pockets at regular intervals in which tongue blades can be inserted. Safety vests with straps at the shoulders

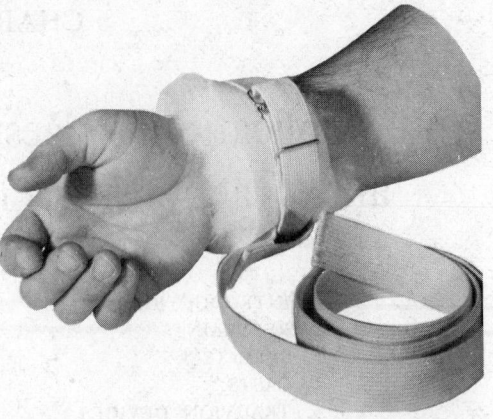

Figure 34-1. One type of commercially made limb-holder. Padding under the wristlet prevents pressure sores and skin abrasions. (Courtesy of Posey Co., Pasadena, Calif.)

and waist that can be attached to the head and side of the bed, and crib nets that cover the top of the crib are other devices used to protect children when an adult cannot be with them continuously.

Nursing Care. While many sick persons tend to be quiet and even need encouragement to move as much as is good for them, in some circumstances movements are irrational and injurious. In such instances protective devices must be employed, and whether patients are rational or irrational, the physician or the nurse should tell them why their movements are restricted.

Devices limiting movement cannot be used legally in many states without a physician's prescription. In some mental hospitals the physician is required to fill in a form, stating why a restraining sheet, a safety jacket, or solitary confinement is necessary. In general hospitals as well as psychiatric institutions, physicians and nurses try to gain the patient's cooperation, thus making restraint unnecessary.

Almost always, restraint of motor activity is distasteful. Many sick persons limit their movements voluntarily for comfort, but limitation of movement enforced by another person nearly always meets with mental if not physical resistance. The restrained individual feels frustrated mentally and physically, and if kept in one position very long, begins to suffer from physical fatigue. The natural reaction to restraint is so violent and in some cases so injurious that, as we have noted, laws have been passed in many states to protect the patient from its injudicious use. The word

---

* Unwisely used, side rails can be dangerous or futile. A very elderly, confused patient was found not long ago padding barefooted and in his nightshirt down a hospital corridor with his side rails in his hands. Meeting the night nurse, he said, "Miss, couldn't you find some place to store these things? People keep putting them on my bed and they get in my way." It was fortunate that he was neither hurt by climbing over them nor exhausted by the effort of bringing them to the nurse.

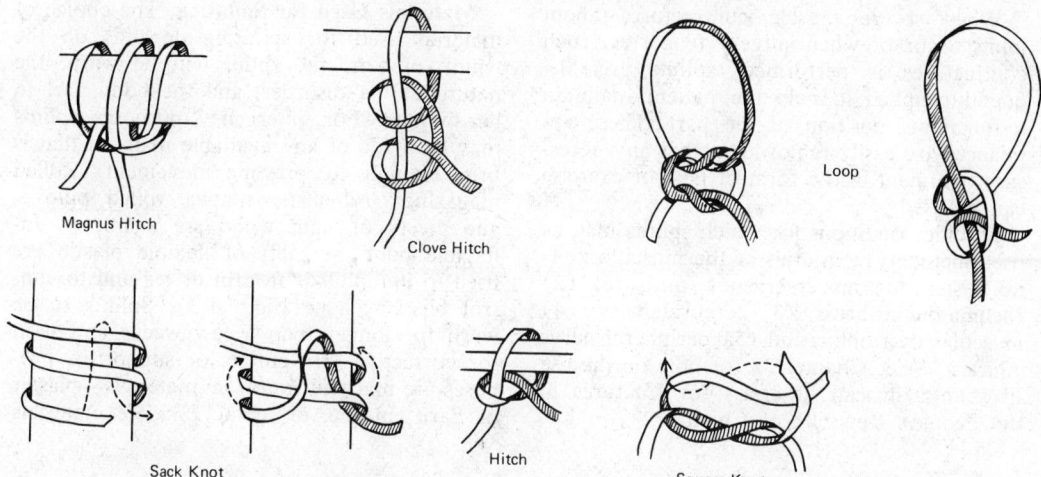

Figure 34-2. These are effective knots for use when securing safety straps and are easy to learn. (Courtesy of Posey Co., Pasadena, Calif.)

restraint is seldom heard because of its distasteful connotation, and a sincere effort is being made to limit motion only when this is necessary for the *protection of the patient*.

Protective devices should be as unnoticeable to patients as possible and should allow as much motion as can be permitted without injury to them. Since patients often struggle against a device that limits motion, care must be taken to prevent skin abrasions. Metals and rough materials should not be used in the construction of such equipment, and any surfaces likely to cause friction or pressure should be padded with absorbent cotton, lamb's wool, or some other soft material. Any type of restraint that causes pressure on underlying tissues should be removed at intervals and normal circulation re-established before it is again applied. If the patient has more than one arm or leg restrained and is irrational, the nurse can loosen one restraint at a time in order to permit bathing and exercise, and to allow increased circulation to the part before reapplying the restraint.

When soft-tie restraints are used the nurse should take care that these are not tied with knots that will tighten and reduce circulation to the part if the patient pulls against the restraint. The square knot and clove hitch knot are shown in Figure 34-2 and are two knots that do not tighten or loosen with the movement of the patient. They are somewhat difficult to untie, and in the event of an emergency the ties may be cut in order to remove the device. Figure 34-2 also describes pictorially other types of knots that can be used to fasten the ties of safety belts and vests to bed rods or wheel chair supports.

3. SPLINTS

Purposes. Splints are appliances used to partially and, in most cases, temporarily support an injured body part. They are made so that they maintain immobilization, but at the same time permit easy inspection or treatment of the part. The purpose of some types of splints is emergency immobilization. Other types are used to correct muscle contractures, to support weak muscles, to prevent stretching of temporarily paralyzed muscles, or to protect bone and other tissues during healing. Splints such as the Thomas splint, the Bohler-Braun splint, the Murray-Jones splint, and the Keller-Blake splint are used with traction to maintain the reduction of long bone fractures.

Therapeutic Uses. Splints are often necessary following an accident when there is an injury or suspected injury to the musculoskeletal system. These splints are temporary and serve to prevent further movement of the injured part while the person is taken to a hospital.

Splints may be used to relieve pain and muscle spasm when there is damage to soft tissues surrounding a bone or joint, as in sprains, strains, and dislocations. They are used instead of a complete cast when there is a fracture with little if any displacement of bone. There are occasions when a fracture has healed to the point of clinical union but the fracture site needs continued protection while bone consolidation takes place. At such times a cast may be removed or traction discontinued and a splint applied. This allows patients to have greater mobility and is usually more comfortable for them.[1]

When severe muscle contractures about joints occur or when surgery to correct such contractures is performed, splints are frequently applied to help the patient maintain a functional position of the part. These appliances are easily removed so that any necessary treatment in the form of heat or exercise can be used.

Specific conditions for which splints may be used include (1) injuries of the musculoskeletal system as an emergency measure; (2) rheumatoid arthritis; (3) cerebral palsy; (4) muscular dystrophy; and (5) peripheral nerve injuries.[1a] (See Chapter 38 for note on the use of splints [instead of casts] for fractures in the People's Republic of China.)

Materials Used for Splinting. The choice of material used for splinting depends on the length of time the splint will be worn, the nature of the disorder, and the body part to be splinted. For emergency purposes splints may be made of any available material that is firm enough to prevent movement. Rolled magazines, rolled newspaper, rolled pillows, and pieces of light wood are examples. Inflatable boots or cuffs of flexible plastic are used to immobilize an arm or leg and to control bleeding (see Fig. 34-3). Splints to be worn for longer than a few weeks and used for corrective, preventive, or supportive purposes are made of *inflexible* materials—plaster of Paris, plastic, or metal. *Flexible* materials

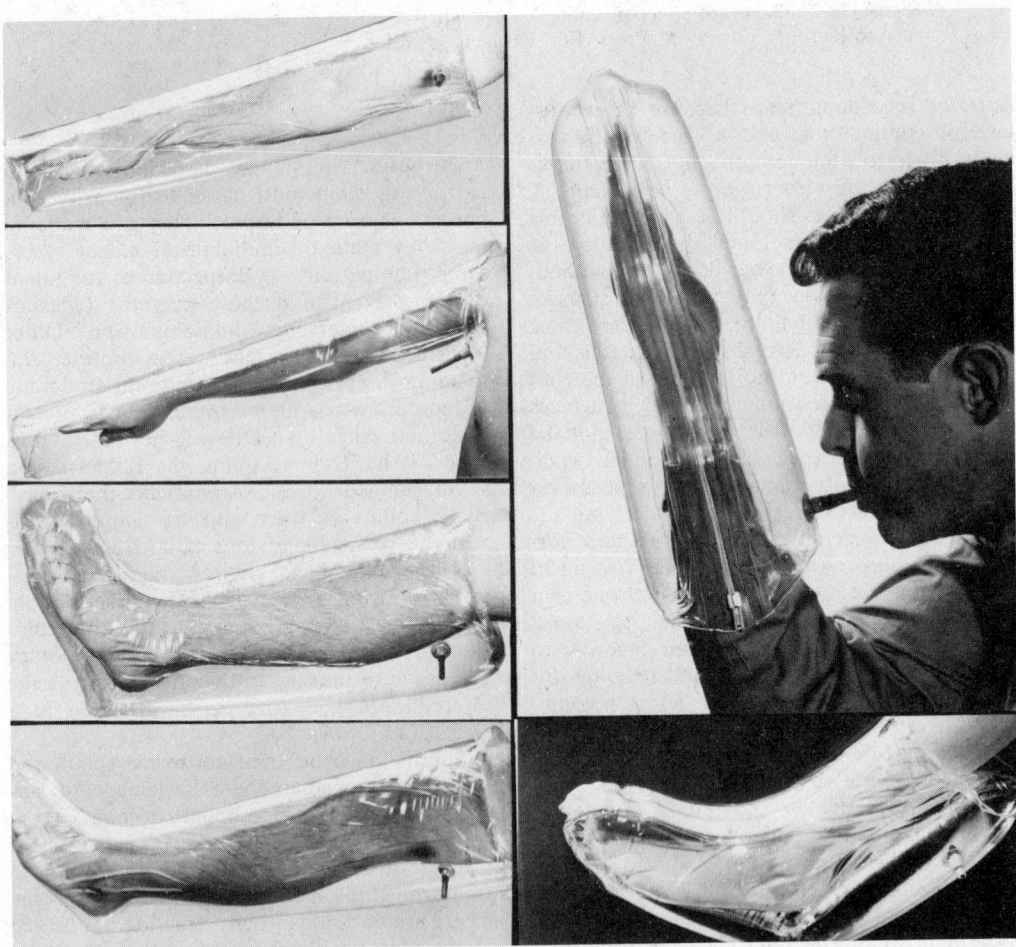

Figure 34-3. Plastic, inflatable splint slipped over the injured part, zippered closed, and inflated. Such a splint provides firm support, controls bleeding, and has the advantage of permitting x-rays to be taken through the material. These splints come in six sizes. (Courtesy of the Mine Safety Appliance Company, Pittsburgh, Pa. From: Mahoney, Robert F.: *Emergency and Disaster Nursing,* 2nd ed. Macmillan Publishing Co., Inc., New York, 1969, p. 127.)

—adhesive strapping, woven elastic bandaging, stockinet, or a heavy canvas bandage—are used in conditions that do not demand prolonged immobilization and where protection is the major requirement, for example, the support of an arm when there is an incomplete fracture in the shoulder girdle.

Plaster of Paris is the least expensive of those materials used to form a rigid, contoured splint, and can be accurately molded to provide the best support. However, splints made of plaster are heavy, easily cracked or broken, and hard to keep clean. The reader will find methods of protecting plaster cast (or splint) edges and methods for cleaning such casts on page 1458 of this chapter.

Many of the plastic materials now being used for splinting have the advantage of being light in weight, do not crack or break easily, and can be cleaned with warm soapy water. The disadvantage of these materials is that they are malleable only at high temperatures and, therefore, cannot be placed directly on the patient but must be formed over a mold of the part of the subject's body. This increases the cost of the splint to the patient.[1b]

A laminated plaster-plastic bandage splint seems to combine the advantages of plaster splints and plastic splints. Its construction involves sandwiching a plaster of Paris shell, formed to the contour of the extremity, between two layers of plastic bandage. Straps of elastic with Velcro * at the ends are attached to the outer layer of the splint so it can be held securely on the arm or leg. The plastic bandage is a combination of woven fiberglass strands impregnated with cellulose acetate.[2] The setting process of the bandage is initiated by dipping it into a solution that has an acetone base. Since the solution is inflammable and irritating to the mucous membrane and the skin, precautions must be taken during its use to assure adequate ventilation in the room and the absence of an open flame or electric fire. If the plastic bandage (sold under the brand name Aire-Cast in the United States) is used alone and contoured about the extremity rather than the plaster shell, the patient's skin should be protected with a sheet of transparent plastic food wrap. The transparent wrap is removed later from the splint surface. This plastic bandaging when used without the plaster "filling" has the advantage of being

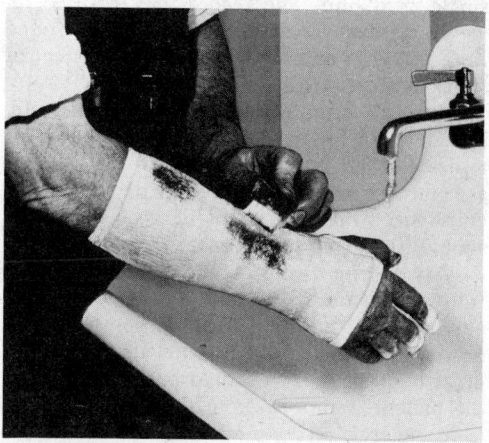

Figure 34-4. A cast made of Aire-Cast is light in weight and not damaged by water; therefore, it has some advantages over plaster of Paris for convalescent casts or splints. (Courtesy of Tower Co., Seattle, Wash.)

water repellent, transparent to x-ray, and porous enough to be comfortable in warm weather [3] (see Fig. 34-4).

Nursing Care. Since injuries requiring emergency splints rarely occur in hospitals, and since the immediate treatment of the accident victim is of utmost importance, there should be common knowledge of splints and splinting. Splinting as a part of first aid is taught to Scout troops or their equivalents, to policemen, to firemen, and to the military in most countries. The Red Cross here and abroad sponsors courses for the public that include this subject, and nurses often teach such courses. The nurse in industry, in schools, on ships, in penal institutions, working in a shelter because of a natural disaster, or present at the time of any accident should have fundamental knowledge about first aid and methods of splinting various kinds of injuries. Although nurses in the United States seldom work in emergency ambulance services, in some countries they are members of mobile health units that respond to calls in all sorts of emergencies.

The first concern for victims of an accident must be for their life. The person giving first aid examines them to see whether they are having difficulty breathing, are hemorrhaging, or are in shock. The extent of these problems must be estimated and if threatening they must be treated before skeletal injuries are identified.[4] If, however, patients are in such a position that the nature of respirations and bleeding cannot be determined, they should be presumed to have a spinal injury and moved or turned so that their body is maintained as a

---

* Velcro is the brand name for a nylon tape used as a fastening material. It consists of two pieces of tape, one containing nylon hooks and the other nylon loops. When the two surfaces are pressed together a strong fastening is made. The tape may be cleaned with soap and water without losing its adhering property.

single rigid unit. The reader may wish to review emergency resuscitation measures found in Chapter 35 and the emergency treatment of shock and hemorrhage in Chapter 45.

Once the initial examination has been completed and life-saving treatment instituted as indicated, the nature and extent of possible skeletal injuries can be identified. It must be emphasized that all victims of major accidents should be given emergency treatment as if they had spinal injuries and should be carefully placed on a solid surface, which acts as a splint, before they are transported to a hospital. If splints of any kind are needed on other body parts they should be applied before the patient is moved from the area.

In general, an extremity should be temporarily splinted in a position of comfort for the patient. The joint above and the joint below the injury should be included in the supporting device because the motion of either may cause pain and movement of the bone fragments. The position of comfort in the case of an injured arm is usually one of flexion and support across the body of the patient; however, if the bone of the upper arm (humerus) is injured the position of extension may be the most comfortable. A simple sling will frequently suffice as a splint when there is an arm injury. Any splint applied to the arm should support the hand but leave the fingertips visible so that a watch can be kept on the circulation of the hand[5] and indirectly the arm.

When splinting an injured lower extremity, the splint should not put extreme pressure on the lateral popliteal areas, since blood vessels and nerves pass through this region and are near enough the surface to be damaged by prolonged pressure. For more detailed information about the use of specific splints in emergencies the reader is referred to *Emergency Care: Surgical and Medical* by Warren H. Cole and Charles B. Puestow,[6] and to the section on first aid in Avice Kerr's *Orthopedic Nursing Procedures.*[7]

Since many patients who require the use of a splint over a prolonged period are not hospitalized or confined to bed, it is often a clinic, a school, or industrial or district nurse who is responsible for follow-up care. With any patient wearing a splint, nurses in all settings should look for signs of developing pressure areas or circulatory impairment. This is a potential problem if there is much swelling or if a splint is too tightly applied. The nurse must know whether the physician has directed that the splint be worn intermittently or constantly and whether patients are responsible for the application and reapplication of their own splint. It is the nurse's responsibility to make

certain that either he or she, the physical therapist, or the occupational therapist has taught the patient how to do this. The proper application of a splint for supporting the wrist and hand is particularly important because repeatedly misplaced straps may completely immobilize the fingers and result in stiffness of the phalangeal and metacarpal joints. Straps repeatedly fastened too tightly cause circulatory restriction, swelling, pain, neuropathy, and, eventually, lessened touch discrimination of the fingers.[8] The most effective way for the nurse to determine the patient's ability to apply the splint is to arrange for him or her to demonstrate the procedure.

If adhesive strapping is to be used for splinting the part, the patient's skin should be cleaned and dried before the adhesive tape is applied. Ether used after the soap and water cleaning helps remove any natural oils left on the skin and dries the part thoroughly so the tape adheres well. Although shaving the part to be strapped makes the removal of the tape more comfortable for the patient, many physicians request that body hair be clipped, when there is a large amount, rather than shaved. Clipping the hair is thought to minimize trauma to the skin and prevent infection of the hair follicles (folliculitis). If the part is shaved in preparation for strapping, care must be taken to avoid the small lacerations that frequently accompany the use of a razor. Before the tape is applied, tincture of benzoin is often painted on the skin because it is mildly antiseptic, checks minor capillary bleeding that sometimes occurs after shaving, and leaves a resinous film that protects the skin and improves tape adherence. Some physicians prefer to use a commercial aerosol adhesive that protects the skin and makes the splinting or skin traction tape stickier.[9]

When a Velpeau bandage is used to immobilize the bones of the arm, forearm, hand, and shoulder girdle, the nurse must be certain there is a protective pad inserted between the arm and the chest, that is, where there is skin-to-skin contact. If stockinet is used for this type splint the protective pad is unnecessary.[10]

The Arm Immobilizer is a substitute for the Velpeau bandage and sling. It is especially appropriate when intermittent mobilization is indicated, or when the physician wants the patient to exercise the hand and arm to some extent at intervals. It is the type of splint most easily applied by the patient.

Braces. Braces are appliances that are freely or partially movable at a joint as contrasted with splints which are defined by Maxwell H. Bloomberg[11] as appliances that do not provide for motion of at least one joint.

Braces are frequently used to enable patients to walk when they might otherwise be chair-bound because of their condition as, for example, cerebral palsy or poliomyelitis with partial paralysis. Braces may also be used to prevent or correct mild deformities or the tendency to deformity and in the treatment of orthopedic conditions of long duration. At best, they are uncomfortable, and unless made to fit and properly adjusted, they may do more harm than good.

Braces should never be used unless prescribed by the physician who is giving follow-up care of the patient. Muscles that are supported, and hence have no work to do, lose their tone. This may be prevented in most cases by removing the braces at regular intervals for massage and exercise. Such treatment must also be prescribed by the physician.

Braces are usually combinations of metal supports and canvas or leather cuffs that are strapped and buckled in place. Most braces have delicate mechanisms at the joints which require proper oiling. Because their construction requires skilled labor, braces are expensive. Nurses should, therefore, treat them with respect and teach the patient how to care for the joints, the cuffs, the metal supports, and the straps. Nothing should rest on the brace when not in use, since it can be bent out of shape. The regular use of a soap made for cleaning leather keeps such parts malleable and free from odors, while the canvas parts can be scrubbed with ordinary soap and water.

The nurse who is working with a person using a brace should routinely check for irritation of the skin; excessive motion of the brace joint due to wear; noisy joints due to inadequate oiling or poor alignment; worn or missing parts; worn heels and soles on shoes used with leg braces; brittle, soiled, or stiff leather pieces.[12]

4. CASTS

Purposes. Casts are devices that encase the injured part and permit a high degree of immobilization. They maintain the reduction of a fracture (alignment of broken ends) until clinical union of the bone has occurred.*

Orthopedists in the United States use casts when they believe that immobilization should be uninterrupted for weeks or, in some cases, months. If there is swelling underneath the cast or in the hand or foot protruding from the

cast, or unexplained pain, the physician may remove the cast and correct any defects in reapplying the cast. "Bone setters" in some countries use a bivalved type of cast that is removed at frequent intervals for skin care and massage, which is thought to reduce discomfort and hasten rehabilitation. Bivalved casts are often used in the United States when the correction of a deformity requires use of the cast for months—perhaps at night only.

Therapeutic Uses. Casts are applied when there is bone pathology that requires rigid immobilization to permit healing or to correct a bone deformity, such as scoliosis. Fractures are frequently held in the proper position by casts after realigning the fractured bone ends without surgery (a closed reduction).*

Immobilization of a fracture by a cast or any other means relieves the pain associated with it because muscle spasm is relieved and the movement of bone fragments through soft tissues, the periosteum, and endosteum are prevented. Continuity of the fractured bone is reestablished by an "explosion" of the specialized osteoblast cells, the formation of a calcified matrix or callus, and finally the consolidation of this matrix into fully mineralized bone containing osteoblasts, osteocytes, and osteoclasts. As soon as the callus is so firm that there is no movement of the fracture fragments and the fracture line is barely discernible by x-ray, the fracture is said to be "clinically united" and the cast is usually removed. A return to the original strength of the bone, however, will take additional time.[13] The rapidity with which clinical union occurs depends on the age of the patient, the location of the fracture, the amount of initial displacement of the fracture, and the blood supply to the fragments.[14]

Materials Used for Casts. Casts are made of materials such as plaster of Paris or plastics of various kinds. These materials are soft and malleable when moistened with water or a chemical solution, but are hard and durable when dry.

Application of a Cast. Whether the cast is applied for treating a fracture or a spinal deformity, the materials used and the application of the cast are essentially the same. The required articles are (1) sheet wadding—a starch-covered layer of unabsorbent cotton webbing; (2) tubular stockinet which comes in sizes from 2 inches to 18 inches; (3) felt

---

* In modern practice an x-ray is used to verify the physician's judgment that the broken ends are united by new growth of bone (callus).

* Some fractures, because of their location or extent of injury to the bone or surrounding soft parts, must be realigned by a surgical procedure (open reduction). In such cases metal pins and/or plates to immobilize and strengthen the fracture site may be used.

or sponge rubber for protection of bony prominences; (4) reinforcing materials such as yucca board, wire mesh, or aluminum strips; (5) plaster bandages *; (6) a deep basin or pail lined with newspapers or old pieces of cloth and filled with tepid water between 35° and 40.5°C (95° and 105°F); and (7) gloves and gown for the physician.

The bandages are *applied* by the surgeon. The nurse's responsibility is usually limited to preparing the patient and articles required and to helping with the application. In some orthopedic clinics nurses are playing a larger role in the application of casts. First, the part to be bandaged is washed, dried thoroughly, and powdered. The bed or table and floor should be protected. A rest should be provided to elevate and support the part, which must be kept in the proper position—that is, the position in which it is to remain after the application is completed. (Frequently casts are applied in the operating room and special tables used that support the body but leave the affected parts accessible to the surgeon.)

Stockinet of the proper size is used next to the skin. It protects the skin and lines the cast. A long strip of gauze bandage may be slipped under the stockinet at this time. After the cast is completed the ends of the gauze can be tied on top of the cast and the bandage slid back and forth to function as a "scratcher." Sheet wadding may also be used next to the skin, but is more often applied over the stockinet as a light-weight padding. When the plaster bandages are applied, a portion of the stockinet and sheet wadding is left uncovered. Later this material can be turned back to form a cuff over the rough edges of the cast which prevents irritation of the skin and crumbling of the edge of the cast (see Fig. 34-5).

Plaster bandages are applied when wet. They are removed from the vessel of water in which they have been immersed as soon as bubbles

cease to rise. They should not be squeezed as this removes the plaster. Paper-wrapped bandages may be thoroughly wetted by placing them on edge in the basin of tepid water. The nonwrapped bandages should be immersed in a horizontal position with the hands of the nurse cupped over the ends of the roll.* Only a few bandages should be placed in the basin at any one time since the crystallization of the plaster begins as soon as the bandage is saturated and has stopped bubbling. Before the bandage is handed to the physician the end is unrolled for a few inches.

After the cast has been applied, the pail of water used to saturate the bandages should be allowed to stand for a short time so that the plaster may settle to the bottom. The water may then be safely discarded into a hopper which has a trap in the waste pipe. The trap collects whatever plaster may not have settled to the bottom of the basin and protects the plumbing. The paper or cloth lining of the basin may then be discarded with the largest portion of the excess plaster in it.

Nursing Care. It is possible for the nurse caring for a patient in a large cast to classify the problems as those *currently* present for the patient because of bone pathology and maintaining normal functions of living; those problems *potentially* present because of the cast, because of the immobility of the patient, or because of the age of the patient; and, finally, those problems that may *possibly* develop because of the individuality of the patient.[15]

Current Problems. Since a *current* problem of a patient in a cast is that of bone pathology, the care of the new cast is immediately important for the desired outcome of a well knit, functional bone. In order that the cast may be effective and comfortable as possible for the patient, his or her normal body curves must be maintained, and the cast must be well supported until it is dry. Boards placed lengthwise or a full-size bed board under the mattress are necessary for the patient who has a body cast or hip spica cast. However, until the cast is completely set, pillows to support the curved areas of the cast are also essential. A series of boards the width of the bed, instead of the length of the bed, may be placed under the mattress for a patient in a long leg cast. Short boards are easier to handle and store than large boards and they permit the upper part of the bed to be raised slightly when the patient uses the bedpan.

---

* Before these bandages were made commercially, the nurse frequently prepared them in the following way: the crinoline was first cut into strips of the desired width and length and rolled into roller bandages. The table and floor were protected. The required amount of plaster was placed on the table. The crinoline bandage was placed on the table opposite the operator, with the body uppermost and the initial end drawn toward the operator. The plaster was spread over the crinoline freely and rubbed smoothly and evenly into all its meshes with a spatula or with the heel of the hand. The strip was loosely rolled as each portion was finished. Each bandage was wrapped separately and securely in waxed paper as soon as it was prepared. Then the bandages were stored in an airtight box or container and not handled individually until used. The wrapper helped prevent deterioration of the plaster from exposure to the moisture of the air and prevented the sifting out of plaster.

---

* Some physicians prefer that the nonwrapped bandage be held at an approximately 45-degree angle since this appears to allow more thorough wetting and prevent the trapping of air bubbles in the bandage layers.

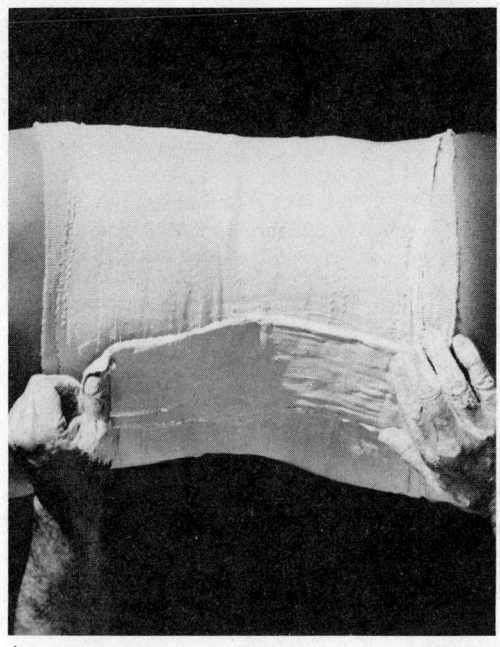

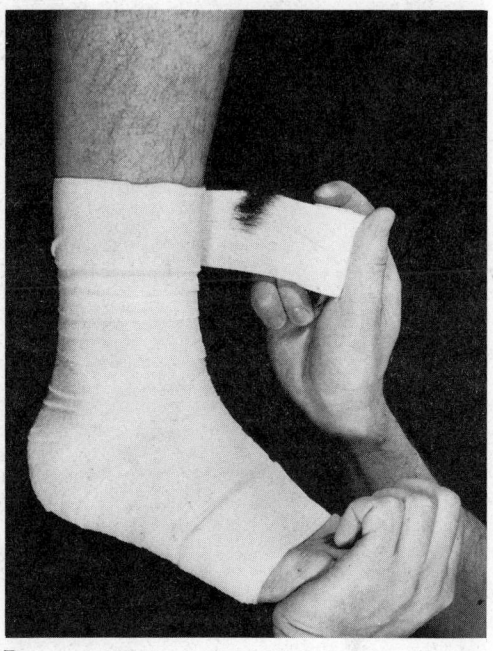

A   B

Figure 34-5. *A.* A body plaster-of-Paris cast being applied. Note the stockinet between the body and the cast to protect the skin. The stockinet will be turned over the edges of the cast to protect the patient from the rough edges. *B.* Sheet wadding being used to cover an extremity and to protect the skin prior to the application of a cast. Stockinet and sheet wadding are sometimes used in combination when applying a cast. (Courtesy of Bauer & Black, Chicago, Ill.)

Commercial fracture beds have canvas straps stretched across the metal framework to support the patient. A firm mattress and wire springs are placed directly under such canvas straps. Each canvas strap can be tightened with a special device at the side, or loosened and removed. A middle section of the mattress can be lowered without affecting the upper and lower sections. These features make it possible to remove the straps under the buttocks, lower the mattress, and introduce the bedpan without necessitating a change in the patient's position and without removing the support from the rest of the body.

The bed should also have a Balkan frame attached (see Fig. 34-6). From this a trapeze (a metal or wooden bar suspended on ropes) can be hung to enable patients to lift and move themselves when they become accustomed to the cast. The Balkan frame is also a necessary part of the bed for a patient in traction.

Plastic or rubber-covered pliable pillows are used to support the curves of the cast in order that these curves will not flatten or crack. It is particularly necessary that the cast be supported in such a way that it does not flatten over the sacrum or back of the heel, and through pressure damage the soft tissues of these parts. The supporting pillows should be arranged so there is no sharp break in their alignment that might make the cast sag at certain points. The pillow for the patient's head should be pulled down beneath the shoulders so that good alignment of the cervical spine is maintained, and so that the thorax and upper abdomen do not press against the edge of the cast. After the cast has dried, pillows are no longer needed to support it, but may be used for the comfort of the patient and to relieve pressure points.

While the cast is drying the patient should be covered or kept warm; however, the cast itself should not be covered since this will prevent air circulation and the evaporation of moisture from the plaster. A thorough drying of the cast may take from 24 hours to 3 days, depending on the size of the cast, the weather, and/or the equipment used to hasten drying. The nurse should explain to the patient that as the crystallizing process of the plaster takes place heat will be generated but will stop once the plaster has set. Drying the cast with a small watt bulb suspended from a bed cradle or with a commercial dryer to blow warm air over the cast should not be started until the plaster has set. If a cradle with a light bulb

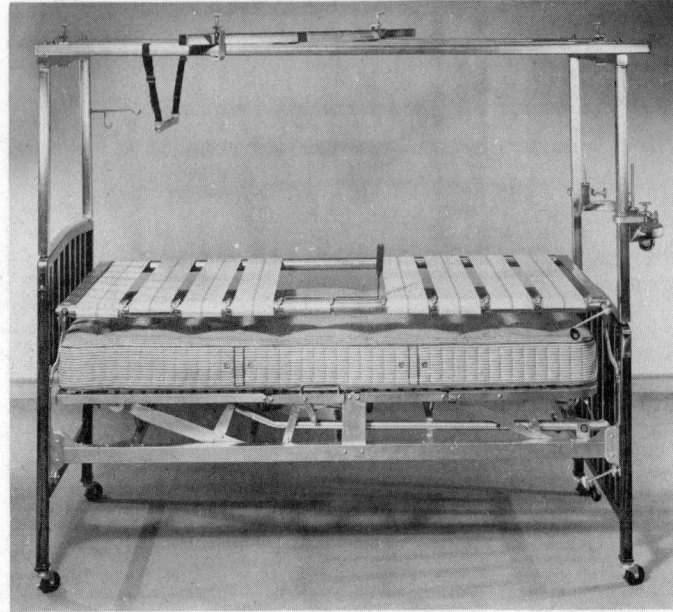

Figure 34-6. A Balkan frame with a trapeze bar. A fracture bed frame is placed over the mattress to facilitate caring for the patient in a cast. (Courtesy of Simmons Co., New York, N.Y.)

attached is used it should be completely uncovered, or if that is not possible, the ends should be uncovered to allow for air circulation. If the temperature of the drying equipment is too high the outside layer of the cast may dry too quickly and leave the underlying layers damp. This predisposes to a weakening of the cast and the growth of a fungus, or mildew.

All the edges of the cast should be protected so they do not break off in small pieces and cause discomfort. If stockinet has been used for the cast lining, it should be turned over the edges of the cast and taped in place. This method of making a smooth edge for the cast is not possible, however, if sheet wadding has been used for the lining. Instead, petals of adhesive tape may be cut and attached over the cast edge. On the underside of the cast the tape will adhere to the sheet wadding, and may be fastened securely on the outside by a moistened strip of plaster of Paris bandage placed over the tape ends. If the single layer of plaster of Paris bandage is not used to hold the stockinet or adhesive tape strips in place, the cast must be completely dry and the tape ends pressed tightly to the cast so they will not roll and adhere to the bedclothes.

Body casts and hip spica casts should have plastic or adhesive tape petals about the perineal area to protect them from soiling. Strips of thin plastic waterproofing material may be placed around the cast opening so that their edges overlap. They may then be fastened on the outside of the cast with adhesive tape or a plaster of Paris strip, and the free end tucked

well inside the cast opening. For young children this is a good method for preventing soiling of the cast since these strips are not only waterproof but can be pulled out, cleaned, dried, and reinserted.

In order to help keep the cast as clean as possible, the entire cast is sometimes waterproofed by painting it with shellac, varnish, or lacquer. These materials must not be used until at least 48 hours after the cast is completely dry. Casts without this kind of waterproofing should be cleaned very carefully with an almost dry cloth and a mildly abrasive cleanser. If a large area of the cast is soiled, Carroll B. Larson and Marjorie Gould recommend the following procedure:

From a plaster bandage of suitable width a double thickness is cut to fit exactly over the soiled area. This pattern is swiftly immersed in water so that it is barely moistened through when it is lifted from the pan. The pattern is applied directly over the soiled area and is carefully rubbed into the cast. It must be well incorporated by rubbing, or it will peel off later like an onion skin. Some orthopedists advise that the cast be roughened slightly with a nail file or scissors before the pattern is applied. A generous sprinkling of baby powder rubbed into the moistened plaster will remove the odor that may accompany soilage.*

They also suggest that if the inside of the cast is soiled and stockinet has been used for a

* Larson, Carroll B., and Gould, Marjorie: *Orthopedic Nursing,* 8th ed. C. V. Mosby Co., St. Louis, 1974, p. 60.

lining it may be carefully detached from the cast, pulled down, and the soiled part trimmed away. It should, of course, be retaped so that the edge of the cast is covered with the clean stockinet that is stretched to cover it.

Another *current* problem for the patient in a cast is that of using the bedpan. Because urinating and defecating are considered, in our culture, a private and personal affair the patient who is hospitalized for the first time may have considerable apprehension about performing these necessary acts when they are complicated by the rigidity of the cast. If the person is sufficiently apprehensive he or she may suppress the need to defecate or urinate until supremely uncomfortable. If, on the other hand, nurses anticipate this possibility, they can explain before the need arises how elimination is managed and verbally empathize with the person about the lack of privacy and the awkward position necessary for use of the bedpan. When the bedpan is placed under the patient who is in a cast, but not on a commercial fracture bed or Bradford frame, the buttocks must not be higher than the head. Elevating the head of the bed very slightly and placing another pillow under the back will help to keep the urine from flowing back under the cast (see Fig. 34-7). Another precaution that may be taken is placing an absorbent pad on that part of the bedpan placed under the sacral area. The use of the fracture bedpan with its more compatible shape is helpful to many patients. Pillows can be arranged under both legs so that the patient is comfortably balanced on the bedpan. To avoid the possibility of breaking the cast the nurse must take care that sharp angulation at the groin does not occur.

Children who have acquired little or no bladder control can be given upper trunk support with plastic-covered pillows, and a perineal pad made of a folded diaper held in place with a regular diaper used instead of a bedpan. Of course, the diaper must be checked frequently and changed as soon as possible after it is wet so that the cast does not get damp, soft, and odorous.

Potential Problems. Patients in casts often develop a number of problems that are preventable and so can be viewed by the nurse as *potential*, rather than current, patient problems. Individuals who are immobilized for any reason or by any means are potentially candidates for the many pathologic effects of hypoactivity. These effects and the nursing care to prevent them are discussed later in this chapter and in Chapters 12 and 38. Two other potential problems of a patient in a cast are pressure on a superficial nerve and/or con-

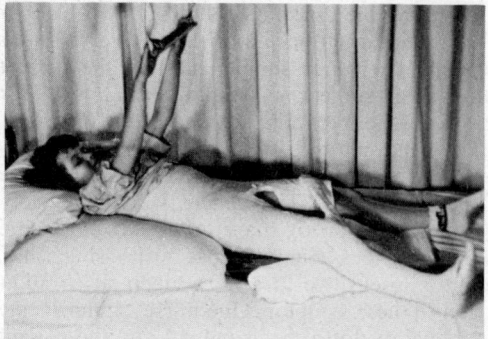

Figure 34-7. Patient with a plaster cast on the bedpan. Note the adequate support by the use of pillows. (Courtesy of Frederick J. Knocke and Lazelle S. Knocke, and Clay-Adams Co., New York, N.Y.)

stricted blood vessels. These problems are particularly important because they develop rapidly and, if not corrected soon enough, can result in permanent paralysis or amputation of an extremity.[16] Still other potential problems are pressure sores that may occur on areas covered by the cast, at cast edges, or on the elbows and heels of patients in a body cast when they use them to change their position. Finally, the problems of itching under the cast and skin irritation at cast edges, if they occur, are intensely annoying and uncomfortable for the patient.

Adults with arm casts or lower leg casts and young children are often hospitalized only until the plaster is completely dry and the effects of any anesthesia are gone. In these instances nurses should be sure that when the patient or family leaves the hospital they understand the symptoms that indicate blood vessels are being constricted or nerves are being compressed, and that they understand how to prevent the other potential problems named above.

Even though a patient's arm or leg cast is carefully applied, the binding force of the bandaging material reinforced by the drying plaster may cause pressure on a superficial nerve or constrict blood vessels. If the cast is applied within the first 24 hours following injury, or if it is applied over a seeping surgical wound, pressure and constriction may be the result of tissues swelling against the unyielding cast or against the combination of cast and blood-soaked dressing. In order to prevent problems of nerve and circulatory pressure, some orthopedists apply only a posterior splint or plaster half cast. While this lessens the risks of constriction and pressure on the extremity, it also reduces the adequacy of the immobilization.

During the 24 hours following a cast application and then once or twice in every 8-hour period, the nurse should question the patient to get at subjective symptoms and look for signs of poor circulation and nerve pressure. The hand or foot below the cast should be inspected for warmth, color, swelling, or the blanching sign.* The patient who is developing constriction of the arteries has pale, cool fingers or toes, a nailbed that flushes sluggishly, and is insensitive to a light touch. If in addition to these symptoms the nurse cannot locate a radial or dorsal pedis pulse † and the patient has little or no movement of the fingers or toes, circulatory constriction should be relieved *immediately* by cutting the plaster bandage and all layers of the underlying padding along the length of one or both sides of the cast.[17,18] This is called "bivalving" the cast. Lessened sensation to touch and an inability to move the fingers or toes are indications that the patient's arm or leg has had prolonged (more than 4 hours) inadequate circulation. When these symptoms are present but there are no other indications of circulatory obstruction the problem is nerve injury due to pressure from the cast. In this case the cast must be windowed at the point it compresses the nerve, or, if this is not possible, it must be bivalved.

Pressure sores or decubiti are a potential problem for any patient who is unable to move freely in bed, and may develop whenever bony prominences are thinly protected by overlying soft tissues. Decubiti are especially troublesome if they occur under a cast or at the cast edges. Pressure from the cast compresses skin and subcutaneous tissue against the bone and causes a localized site of circulatory impairment. If the patient complains of pain in any area likely to be a pressure point such as the sacrum, buttocks, shoulder blades, heels, or elbows, and later does not complain, the nurse should suspect the development of a pressure sore. Tissues that develop localized circulatory impairment are painless after the

---

* The blanching sign indicates the rapidity with which capillaries refill at the tested site. The nailbed of the thumb or great toe (depending on the extremity involved) is compressed and the return flow observed. The nailbed should change from white to pink *immediately* after the pressure has been removed. (Larson, Carroll B., and Gould, Marjorie: *op. cit.,* p. 51.)

† Some physicians cut a square or circular opening in the cast (a window) when it is applied to allow for pulse taking. If the cast has a window and doctors have requested frequent pulse rate reports, they are particularly interested in the condition of the affected arm or leg. They, therefore, expect the pulse rate to be taken at the window and not on the unaffected extremity.

first stage of tissue destruction. The nurse can prevent the potential problem of a pressure sore from becoming a current problem by turning the patient once every hour after the cast has dried, and by massaging with alcohol-moistened finger tips as far inside the cast as she or he can reach.

The initial turning of the patient in a new cast from the supine to the prone position should be done at least by the evening of the day the cast is applied—it may be done earlier if so prescribed by the physician. This initial turning is necessary for the patient's comfort as well as for drying the posterior of the cast. The shoulders of a patient in a body cast can be rubbed at this time, and the areas under and at the edges of the cast can be stimulated with massage for better circulation.

When patients have become accustomed to the cast and learned how to use the trapeze to lift themselves in bed, one nurse can help them turn; however, the first time or two the patient is turned it is necessary to have at least three people help them. This not only permits the patient and cast to be turned as a single unit, but reassures the patient who will almost certainly be afraid of falling out of the bed. The patient is gently pulled to the side of the bed corresponding to the leg in plaster. (A turning or lifting sheet as described and illustrated in Chapter 12 facilitates this.) One or more assistants move to the opposite side of the bed and arrange the pillows to receive the cast. The patient is told exactly what is to be done. He or she is asked to place the arms at the side or over the head; one person supports the hip and shoulder; another supports the thigh and the foot of the leg in the cast; and the third person gently pulls the underlying shoulder through and helps lower the patient onto his or her face. While turning patients nurses should use the palms of their hands rather than their fingertips to prevent molding the cast, and should *never use the crossbar of the spica cast as a handle for turning.* After the patient is in the prone position the nurse should check to see that he or she is in good alignment; that the pillows supporting the cast and the patient's head do not cause the cast edges to press into either the abdomen or the back; and that there is no pressure on the toes or dorsum of the foot.

Frequently body areas not covered by the cast develop pressure sores. The most common of these areas are (1) the heel of the unaffected leg which patients may use to push themselves toward the head of the bed, and (2) the elbows because patients use them to prop themselves so that they can see what is going on around them. To prevent ulcerations from developing at these vulnerable sites patients should be taught to grasp the trapeze bar with both hands, to place their unaffected foot flat on the bed, and then to move themselves in the bed. (See Chapter 12 for a full discussion of decubiti and their prevention.)

When itching occurs under the cast, the "scratcher" provided when the cast was applied can be untied and the bandage moved about to create friction. These strips may be replaced at any time by tying a clean piece of bandage to one end of the used piece and drawing it under the cast into position. Gauze dampened with alcohol and drawn under the cast in this fashion further alleviates itching. There is some doubt as to whether scratchers should be used for children, because it suggests to them putting all sorts of things under the cast.

Irritation of the skin about the cast edges can be prevented by covering the rough edges in ways described earlier in this chapter, and by keeping the skin immediately above and below the cast edges clean and dry. A small hand vacuum cleaner used with caution is helpful in removing minute pieces of irritating material that get under the cast.

In addition to observing the condition of the patient's skin, using the sense of touch to detect moisture, wrinkling, or pieces of irritating materials, the nurse should learn to use the sense of smell to detect abnormal odors that may indicate a sloughing area under the cast. Larson and Gould [19] say that the nurse who is checking the patient's cast for unusual odor should get her or his nose within an inch of it instead of standing upright and sniffing.

Studies made of the reaction of adults to body casts have shown the following to be among the common complaints: a feeling of being restricted; a sense of helplessness and dependence on others; a fear of falling out of bed on turning; depression at the thought of the time required by the treatment; fear that the injured part is not healing properly; a physical sensation of pressure in some areas; itching underneath the cast; excoriation of the skin around the groin; a sense of uncleanliness; and fatigue that is caused by the restricted position.

With skillful care most of these difficulties can be partially or even fully overcome. A way of turning the patient comfortably and safely has already been discussed, as have the nursing measures to achieve cleanliness and to relieve itching and irritation of the skin and pressure from the cast.

Restricting the movement of the patient with a skeletal or spinal cord injury is a necessary part of therapy, but it is also potentially hazardous physiologically and psychologically. The *potential* problem due to hypomobility is as important to combat in the orthopedic patient, who may be immobilized from 6 weeks to 12 months, as it is in the patient suffering from a myocardial infarction or a stroke. The plan of care should be designed to help patients find a balance between rest and activity so that they have maximum physical and psychologic energy available for recovery. Too frequently nurses caring for orthopedic patients focus their activities on the current (and not inconsiderable) problems of cast care or traction maintenance with little regard for the potential physiologic and psychologic difficulties the patients are facing, and the kinesthetic deprivation they are experiencing.

In the last 15 years the dangers of prolonged hypomobility have been explored and are well documented. (For a full discussion of this, see Chapters 12 and 38.) Some of the disabilities resulting from limitation of motion for an extended time period are disturbances of circulation, respiration, and elimination (urinary and fecal); stiffness and pain in joints and muscle; atrophy of muscle; demineralization of bone; and breakdown of skin.[20]

The elderly patient is in more danger physiologically from immobilization than are younger patients. Aging persons have already undergone some degenerative changes in the systems most vitally affected by prolonged hypomobility, and although they may tolerate stress better initially than a younger person, this tolerance lasts for a very limited period of time. Skin care for the elderly immobilized patient is considered by Jesse T. Nicholson [21] to be second in importance only to the necessity for an adequate fluid intake. Muscle contractures and increased osteoporosis develop quickly in the immobilized elderly. Good bed posture with daily range-of-motion exercises are essentials.

Physicians, physical therapists, and nurse specialists stress the value of exercise as a preventive measure in the immobilized patient. They advocate for bedfast patients a planned exercise program and say that such programs can markedly reduce the frequency and severity of the complications listed above.[22,23] The nurse can encourage the patient who is in a large cast, whatever his or her age, to use isometric * exercises for muscles enclosed by the cast, and range-of-motion and isotonic ex-

---

* Isometric exercises are sometimes spoken of as "setting exercises." They require the alternate tightening and relaxing of muscles without joint motion. Isotonic exercises require the active use of muscles to move a joint. These exercises are most effective when the muscle works against a resistive force.

ercises for unaffected body parts. Peter J. Karpovich [24] reports that clinicians have observed a "cross-education" effect when isotonic exercises were used, that is, the training of a muscle in one limb through isotonic exercise increased the strength of a similar muscle on the other side of the body. An exercise program for a patient in a cast should not only focus on preventing the complications of immobilization, but should also be directed toward preparing the patient for ambulation with crutches or a walker. The uses of exercise for the bedfast patient are discussed in more detail in Chapter 30.

Observant nurses have frequently seen intense psychologic reactions from patients who are undergoing enforced limitation of movement; however, we have found experimental studies of this phenomenon only within the last two decades. In these studies immobilized animals showed deficient visual-spatial performance, learning ability (maze running), and motor coordination. Immobilized human subjects showed a definite loss of manual dexterity, kinesthetic sensitivity,* intellectual activity, and color discrimination. These effects appeared even though the subjects, unlike patients in body casts or traction, were released from the immobilizing apparatus at mealtimes, throughout the night, and for toileting (once a day) during the week of the experiment.[25]

C. Wesley Jackson and associates,[26] who applied the findings of deprivation studies to the clinical situation, reported the responses of two patients, one a man 34 years old and one a woman 60 years old, immobilized as a result of skeletal injuries. The patients' normal active days were changed abruptly to days of inactivity, sedation, and relative social isolation. Both patients exhibited psychotic-like hallucinations and delusions during this period of reduced sensory stimulation. Analgesics given to relieve the patients' pain and tranquilizers given to calm their manifest anxiety also dulled their perceptions and awareness of stimuli. In addition, their medication-lowered agitation required less bedside attention from the nursing and medical staffs. When tranquilizers and analgesics were discontinued, when the patients were moved to rooms where there was opportunity for more companionship than in the semiprivate rooms, when more frequent visits from relatives were encouraged, when occupational therapy was instituted, and when nurses gave more attention to the pa-

tients than had previously been thought necessary, the psychotic-like behavior of the patients diminished and then disappeared. It seems obvious that as the nursing staff became more aware of and actively involved in helping these immobilized patients carry out activities they would have normally performed unaided the patients' health improved.

Immobilization has different psychologic meanings for, and elicits different responses from, various age groups. Elderly hospitalized patients have frequently exhibited psychotic-like behavior which was not directly related to their illnesses. Carter R. Rowe [27] cites the instance of an 84-year-old woman who was disoriented and unmanageable following orthopedic surgery. She was discharged from the hospital to be nursed at home. Several days later, when seen by the physician, she was completely reoriented, cooperative, and apparently quite happy.

Whether such behavioral responses of the elderly patient result from immobilization, too high or too low a level of visual and auditory stimulation from the hospital environment, or from a loss of the known stimulation of the home environment, is not known.*

School-age children and early teen-agers react to limitation of movement more frequently with anger and aggression than they do with the hallucinatory, disoriented behavior of the older person. Florence Erickson suggests that for the school-age child the "inability to move is a threat to self-preservation, and this is anxiety- and aggression-producing. It reactivates the dependence-independence struggle, the activity-passivity struggle." † For the child in this age group the achievement and socially acceptable use of motor skills are essential for the development of a healthy body-image, and, perhaps more importantly, the development of a healthy self-image.[28,29] When one of their most important ways of coping with the normal developmental crises is severely limited through immobilization, and the anxiety and fears of illness and hospitalization are added, they react with the kind of behavior often labeled "bad," or with apathy, hopelessness, and submission.

While nursing care for immobilized children must still be directed toward a therapeutic

---

* Kinesthetic sensitivity was tested by asking subjects to bend their elbows to either a 20° or 60° angle and to discriminate between several small cubes slightly different in weight.

* An investigation by Sylvia Carlson indicates that lack of sensory stimulation rather than immobilization was the basis for the apathetic behavior of a small group of elderly women hospitalized with hip fractures. (Carlson, Sylvia: "Selected Sensory Input and Life Satisfactions of Immobilized Geriatric Female Patients," in *ANA Clinical Sessions, 1967.* Appleton-Century-Crofts, New York, 1968, p. 117.)

† Erickson, Florence: "When 6- to 12-Year-Olds Are Ill," *Nurs. Outlook,* 13:48, (July) 1965.

balance of rest and activity, more of the latter is indicated for children than for adults. In addition to activity which is more vigorous than using the ubiquitous coloring book, children should be with other children of their age group, and should have the opportunity to talk about their feelings and fears with an adult they trust. Since parents are the most important adults in any child's life, the nurse should talk with them about his or her health problems as well as the current developmental problem, and to encourage them to talk with their child about his or her fears and fantasies. Working together, they will be better able to give the child the help he or she needs.

Immobilization for the preschool child has many of the same meanings as for the older child. However, because preschoolers have a very limited ability to cope with the anxiety of separation from their mother and the unknown and frightening environment, they are in greater danger of losing ground in their over-all developmental progress than is the older child.[30] The nurse should provide for the continued presence of the mother or another adult whose presence the child can count on. The nurse should give the mother the help she needs and wants in caring for her child in the hospital setting and especially providing for the child appropriate large muscle activities some part of each day.

The effect of immobilization on the newborn child or infant has been little studied. However, the need for appropriate sensory stimulation of all kinds in adequate amounts beginning in the first months of life has been well documented. A recent study by Luz S. Porter[31] has shown that 20 minutes per day for 2 months of passive cycling-motion exercises of all extremities resulted in a significant increase in the growth and development of normal, well children who were 1 month through 9 months of age. One can speculate, then, that when the natural movements of the infant are curtailed through immobilization the rate of growth and development is markedly slowed. On the basis of this evidence the nurse should pay particular attention to exercising the upper extremities of the young child who may be in a cast for the correction of club foot or a congenital hip anomaly.

5. TRACTION DEVICES

Purposes. Patients with bone pathology may be immobilized for therapeutic reasons through the use of traction rather than a cast. The purpose of traction is to apply a pull-force and a counter-force to the bone so that

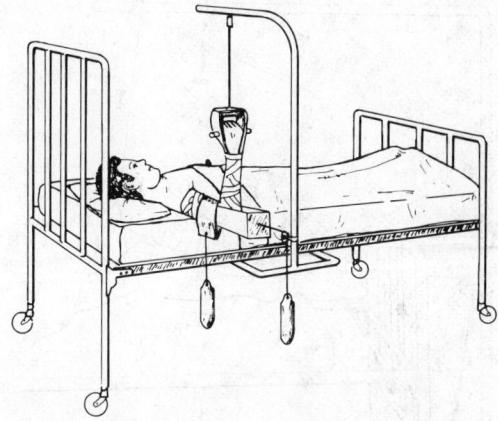

Figure 34-8. A side-traction apparatus that is useful for fractures of the clavicle, the head and neck of the humerus, shaft of the humerus, or the supracondylar process. Note that in order to maintain traction in the anatomic line of the shoulder and arm the patient must be without a pillow. (Adapted from Larson, Carroll B., and Gould, Marjorie: *Orthopedic Nursing,* 7th ed. C. V. Mosby Co., St. Louis, 1970, p. 231.)

the direction and amount of tissue stretching remains constant. This may be accomplished *indirectly* by applying traction to the skin or *directly* by applying traction to the bone. The latter requires surgically inserted pins or tongs. Pull may also be exerted by a halter on the chin, a sling or belt about the pelvis, or an anklet around the ankle. To be effective, the pull exerted by weights attached to the various traction devices must maintain the anatomic line of the part being treated (see Fig. 34-8).

Methods Used to Apply Traction. Traction tapes or pins are applied to that section of the fracture farthest from the trunk (the distal fragment) because this fragment is more easily aligned than the less movable fragment nearer the trunk (the proximal fragment).[32] Traction pull may be in a straight or running line, as with Bryant traction or Buck's extension. Straight, or running, traction exerts pull without a hammock or splint supporting the affected part.

Another type of traction applies a pull-force, either through skin tapes or skeletal pins, in combination with the elevation of the arm or leg in a hammock or splint (balanced suspension). Examples are the Russell traction and the Thomas splint with Pearson attachment (see Fig. 34-9).

Whatever kind of traction is used, pulleys with their hanging weights, attached to the end of the bed or a bed frame, should extend far enough for the weights to hang free, but

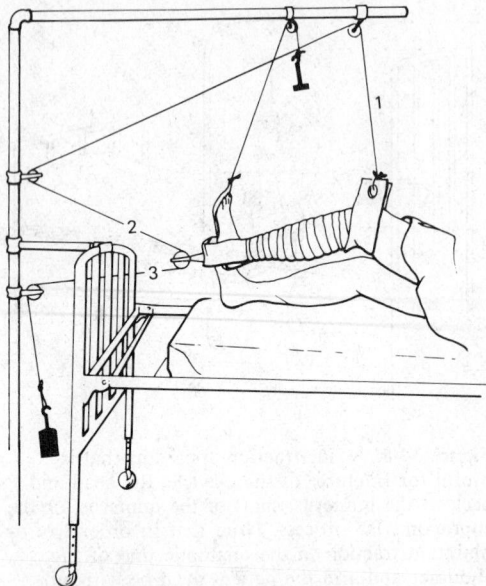

Figure 34-9. An adaptation of the Russell splint. The foot end of the bed is raised to provide countertraction and the weight hangs free so the pull is not reduced. (Adapted from Flitter, Hessel Howard: *An Introduction to Physics in Nursing,* 6th ed. C. V. Mosby Co., St. Louis, 1972, p. 19.)

not so far they are in the way of passers-by. Weights may be metal discs of different sizes, measured and prefilled sandbags, or plastic water bags marked to indicate the amount of water needed to produce the required pull-force.

Countertraction is provided by tilting the bed on blocks and sliding the patient away from the traction. Nurses should periodically examine patients to make sure there is enough tilt to their bed to keep them away from the traction. If the patient slides so the weights come to rest on the bed or floor traction is, of course, eliminated.

Skin Traction. Skin traction is applied indirectly to bones of the arm or leg by placing synthetic sponge, moleskin, or adhesive tape on the skin, attaching these tape strips to either side of a spreader block, and attaching ropes and weights to a hook on the bottom of the block. Since the development of synthetic sponge strips for use as traction tape, problems of skin irritation and infection from moleskin or adhesive tape have been reduced. Some of the newer tapes have an adhesive coating on the attaching side, while others rely on the friction of the sponge surface for adherence to the skin. These tapes are hypoallergenic, allow perspiration to evaporate under the tape, and can be removed and replaced if necessary.

Preparation of the skin for skin traction is the same as for application of a bandage splint of adhesive tape described on page 1454.

Skin traction tape withstands 10 pounds of pull for about 4 weeks before it starts slipping down the arm or leg.[33] Buck's extension, straight line skin traction with horizontal pull, is used with adults since they have enough body weight to provide effective countertraction. However, because more than 4 weeks is usually necessary for healing adult bone, the skin tapes may have to be replaced one or more times. Children less than 6 years old, on the other hand, do not have enough body weight to provide countertraction to the horizontal pull of Buck's extension. Therefore, the ropes, pulleys, and weights are arranged so the traction force is applied vertically with Bryant traction, and the child's hips are at a right angle to the trunk (see Fig. 34-10). In addition, the bones of the young heal quickly and traction is usually discontinued before the tapes begin to slip.

Skeletal Traction. Skeletal traction is that applied directly to the skeletal system by attaching the traction apparatus to pins or wires inserted through the bone of an extremity, or to tongs anchored in the parietal bones of the skull. The most commonly used materials for skeletal traction are the Steinmann rustless steel pin, the Kirschner piano wire or chromic steel, and Crutchfield or Vinke tongs. The pins,

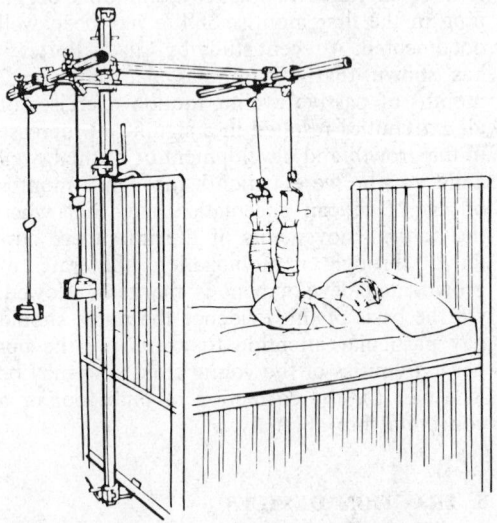

Figure 34-10. Bryant's traction. Note that the buttocks are slightly elevated from the mattress and all weights are out of the child's reach. (Adapted from Leifer, Gloria: *Principles and Techniques in Pediatric Nursing,* 2nd ed. W. B. Saunders Co., Philadelphia, 1972, p. 171.)

wires, or tongs are inserted, using surgically aseptic technique, in the operating room. The skin is ordinarily prepared under aseptic conditions and a dressing applied in advance of the procedure. After the pins have been inserted the physician decides whether or not to use dressings over the insertion site. The tips of the pins or wires, however, should be covered with cork or adhesive to protect the patient and nurse from accidental injury.

Traction with Splints. Splints of various kinds are also used when treating a fracture with traction. Some of the most common types are the Thomas and Murray-Jones splints, their modifications, aeroplane splints, and the Bahler frame. These splints are light in weight, having a slender metal framework and a ring that is padded and covered with leather. Because this ring is held against the groin or the axilla, it should be protected from soiling by a waterproof fabric covered with soft absorbent cotton material and particular attention given to skin care in this area. The leg or arm is supported on a hammock made by

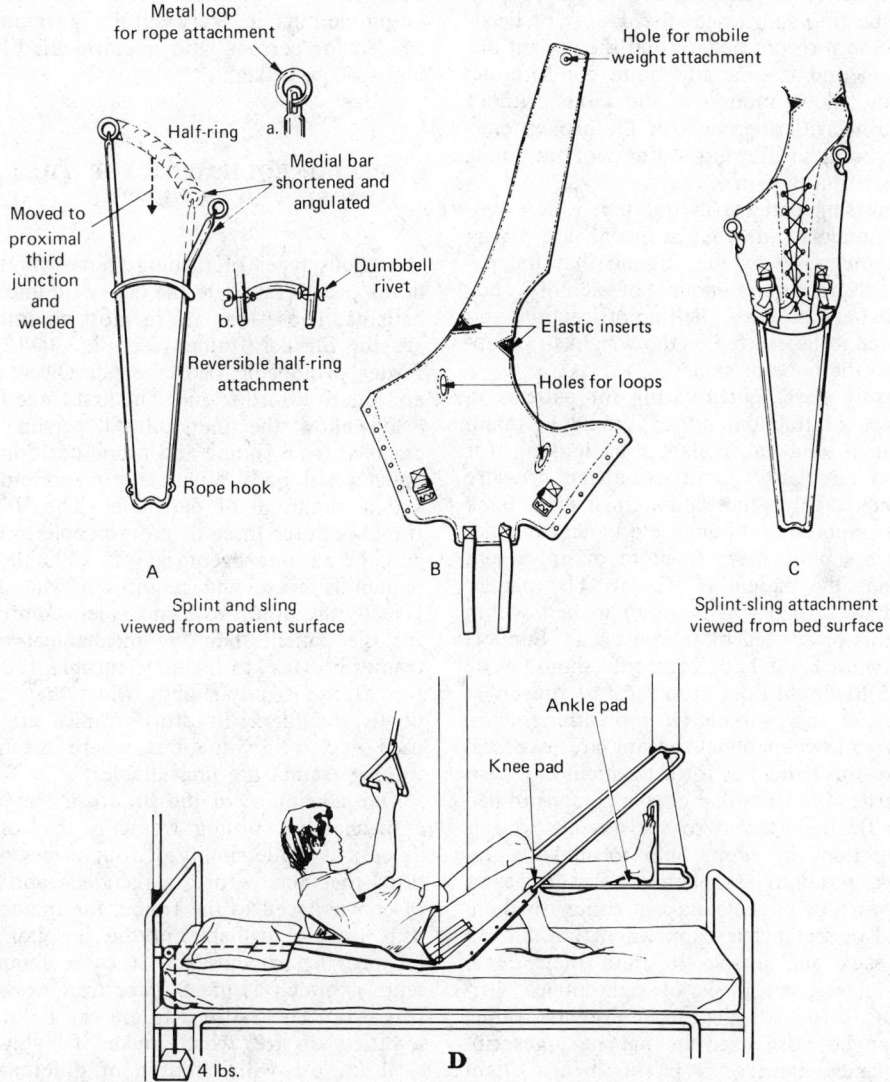

Figure 34-11. *A, B, C.* Ringless splints replace the usual metal ring with a canvas sling and offer more comfort to the patient. The sling can also be washed or replaced when it becomes soiled. *D.* The canvas sling goes under both the patient and his pillow. (Adapted from Bailey, Joseph A.: "Tractions, Suspensions and a Ringless Splint," *Am. J. Nurs.,* **70**:1724, [Aug.] 1970.)

weaving a Canton flannel bandage or cravat bandages over the metal framework.

A splint has been developed that replaces the ring with a canvas sling contoured to prevent soiling at the perineal area. A portion of the canvas extends under the patient to the head of the bed where weights can be attached for countertraction.[34] This kind of traction splint is relatively comfortable for the patient and prevents many of the discomforts of the ring in the groin (see Fig. 34-11).

There are several advantages of the open traction method of treatment over the use of plaster casts. Having the arm or leg exposed ensures better circulation, and therefore promotes healing and lessens the danger of decubiti. Some surgeons believe that the patient has less pain and is generally more comfortable. Traction allows motion in the joints without interfering with alignment of the broken ends of bone and so prevents stiffness of the joints and loss of function.

In nursing patients in traction, it is essential to understand what surgeons are trying to do, the positions they intend that the patients assume, the amount of activity they want patients to have, the line of traction, and the force to be exerted or the weight to be applied to the bone or skin.

Nursing Care. When caring for patients in any type of traction, nurses should maintain the same kind of vigilance in looking for signs of circulatory constriction and pressure that they use for the patient in a cast. Back care is important, although the patient in traction has slightly more freedom of movement than has the patient in a cast. The patient should be turned and elevated in bed within the limits prescribed by the physician. Support and alignment of body segments should have special attention. Foot drop must be prevented by exercise and position. Deep breathing, exercising, and occupational therapy are as necessary for this patient as for the patient in a cast.

Overhead mirrors that enable persons in bed to see themselves and to see anyone who is coming into the room help to make a restrictive position less onerous. Prism glasses when worn by patients make it easier for them to read or watch television when they are on their back and unable to raise their head. Prism glasses are made of right-angled (triangular) prisms attached to an eyeglass frame, and can be worn over the patient's prescription glasses. Because a prism "bends" light rays by internal reflection, persons wearing such glasses can apparently be looking at the ceiling but seeing objects at right angles to them. Overbed tables with reading desks also make patients more independent; pockets for

writing materials, toilet articles, and other objects hung on the bed within reach add greatly to the patient's comfort. Wisely selected occupational therapy does more than any other one thing to make time pass quickly. Patients with crippling orthopedic conditions often learn a useful trade from the occupational therapist. During the convalescent period, special forms of occupation and recreation may be prescribed for their value in muscle training. Music is a great resource and reading can be both educational and recreational. For its effect on the mental outlook of the patient, some form of occupational therapy is desirable for all patients whose physical condition permits it. Very special programs are needed for persons with impairments of hearing, speech, or sight.

6. SPECIAL EQUIPMENT FOR THE IMMOBILIZED PATIENT

Various types of turning frames have been developed to facilitate the care of immobilized patients. Those that are in most common use are the Stryker frame (see Fig. 34-12), the Foster orthopedic bed, the CircOlectric bed, and the Bradford frame. The first three frames listed allow the immobilized person to be changed from supine and prone positions with undisturbed body alignment, maximum ease, and a minimum of personnel. The Bradford frame requires three or more people to turn it and the turning becomes very difficult if the patient is obese and requires a wide frame. Usually the Bradford frame is less comfortable for the patient than the mechanical turning frames because, to facilitate turning, the Bradford frame is only slightly wider than the patient's shoulders. Bradford frames are never used except in situations where mechanical turning frames are unavailable.

One advantage of the Bradford frame over a mechanical turning frame is that of cost. Since it is made simply of four pieces of pipe fitted together to form a rectangle and pieces of canvas laced to the frame, the material for it is usually available in the hospital maintenance department, and it costs about one-tenth as much as the Stryker frame or Foster bed. Also the Bradford frame can be made in a variety of sizes which makes it highly practical for use with children of different ages.

The CircOlectric bed (see Fig. 38-8, Chapter 38) differs from the other frames in that the patient can be turned vertically rather than laterally. Since electric power is used to turn the bed, the patient can adjust his or her own position, although this is not always desirable. The patient can be changed from a supine position, to a standing position, to a prone position, or any degree in between. In addition, the bed is made so that the occupant can be in the sitting or Trendelenburg positions.[35] Although electric beds are not generally considered hazardous to patients, any electric equipment can become dangerous if some of its component parts are defective or if the hospital wiring system does not have proper electric grounding. The most common defect of electric beds, as well as other generally used equipment such as lamps, radios, or television sets, is a frayed or broken power cord or plug. Nurses caring for patients in a CircOlectric bed should inspect the cable frequently to see that it has no worn or broken areas, that it is coiled rather than sharply flexed, and that the cable is arranged so heavy objects do not pass over it. The three-pronged plug should be checked to see that the ground prong (slightly longer than the two power-conducting prongs) is not broken off, and fits snugly into the wall outlet. The cable should be unplugged immediately if any tingling sensations are felt by the nurse when touching the bed. If other electric devices are to be used on or by the patient in the CircOlectric bed they should be plugged into the same group of wall outlets so there is a common ground for all equipment. Water pitchers and basins should be kept away from the hand control that operates the bed, and the patient should be kept dry.[36]

Therapeutic Uses. The therapeutic reasons for the use of a frame are the same for all types. Since mechanical frames are easy to turn, patients who require prolonged immobilization, as in Pott's disease, angulation fractures of the spine, or spinal cord injuries, benefit from their use because they can be turned more frequently and much more easily than when on a bed. Patients in traction, particularly cervical traction, patients with pelvic fractures, and patients with spinal fractures who require hyperextension can be given effective nursing with fewer persons and less time and effort if a frame is used. The frames can be adapted for patients with severe burns, extensive decubitus ulcers, or wounds with excessive drainage because specific areas of pressure are relieved without loss of support.

Equipment Used. All of the turning frames have both an anterior and posterior frame, canvas coverings and sheets with varying kinds of fasteners, and safety straps. Additional accessories such as footboards, arm supports, a utility tray for serving meals or holding diversional material, and traction attachments are available from the manufacturers of these frames.

Nursing Care. When patients are turned, they are sandwiched between the two frames. The frame on which they lie prone is called the anterior frame, that on which they lie supine the posterior frame. Both are fitted with sectioned canvas covers laced on tightly. Both frames have middle sections that can be removed for the use of the bedpan. (The middle section for the anterior frame can be merely fenestrated for the male patient.) The upper section of the canvas on the anterior frame extends from the shoulder girdle to the symphysis pubis, allowing the face and head freedom. The lower section of the canvas extends 4 inches below the symphysis pubis to the internal malleolus, leaving the feet free. The forehead is supported by a padded canvas strip, a folded towel pinned tightly to the frame, or a head piece made by the manufacturer.

Patients should have a thorough explanation of the frame before they are placed on it. A demonstration with a member of the staff as subject is desirable. When patients are turned they should be secured between the frames with the canvas strips provided for this purpose and should be told to grasp the rod underneath the frame. They should know when the quick turn will be made and in which direction. Until they feel very secure it is wise to have two persons in whom they have confidence adjust the frames and operate the swivel.

The nurse working with a patient on a frame who is in traction must be sure that the weights do not rest on the floor after the patient has been turned. In addition, she or he must be certain that countertraction is maintained throughout the procedure.

7. INSTRUCTION FOR PATIENTS IN A CAST OR IN TRACTION

During hospitalization of patients in a cast the nurse should be continually explaining to them what is happening. They should participate in making their plan of care if they are rational and wish to do so. They should know the purpose of the cast and/or traction, the ways in which the nurse will help them maintain as many normal functions as is possible under the circumstances, and the ways in which they can promote a rapid recovery.

For many patients, one explanation is not sufficient because their fears and other intense feelings may interfere with their listening ability. They, therefore, need "review" sessions when their understanding can be evaluated,

A

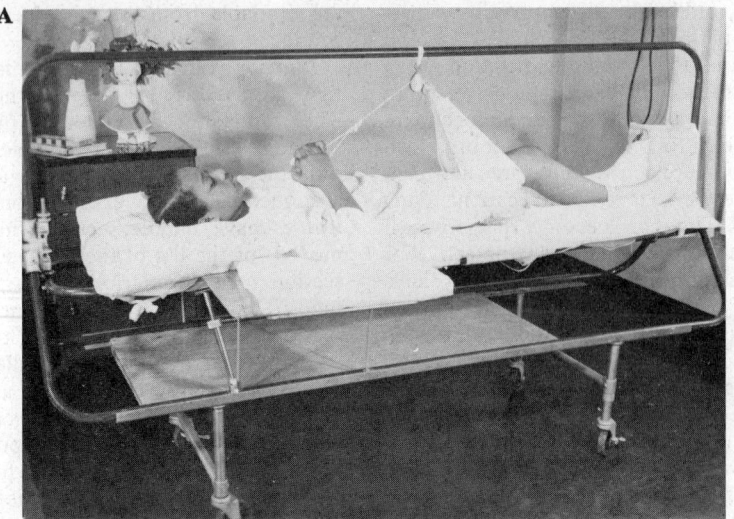

B

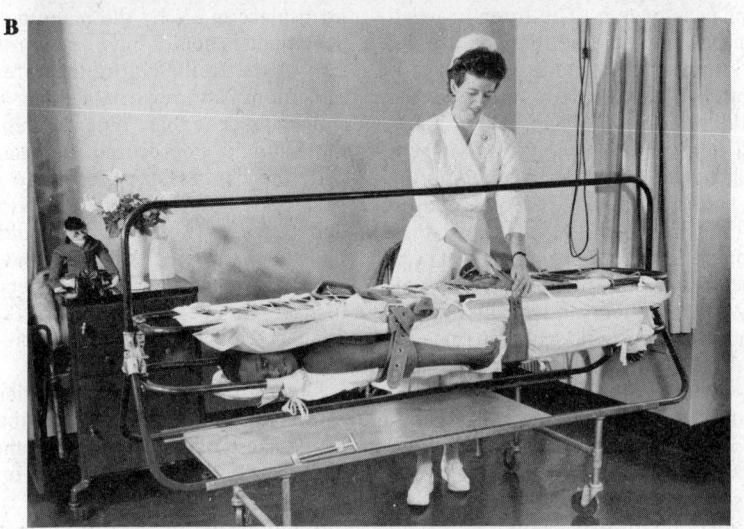

C

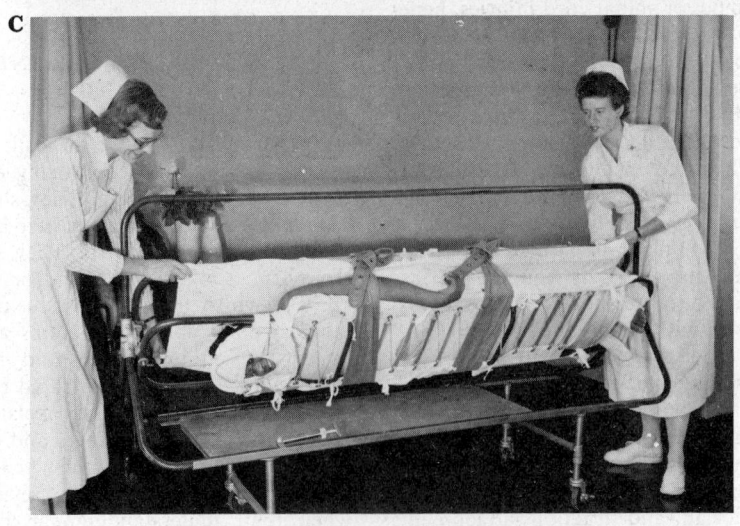

D

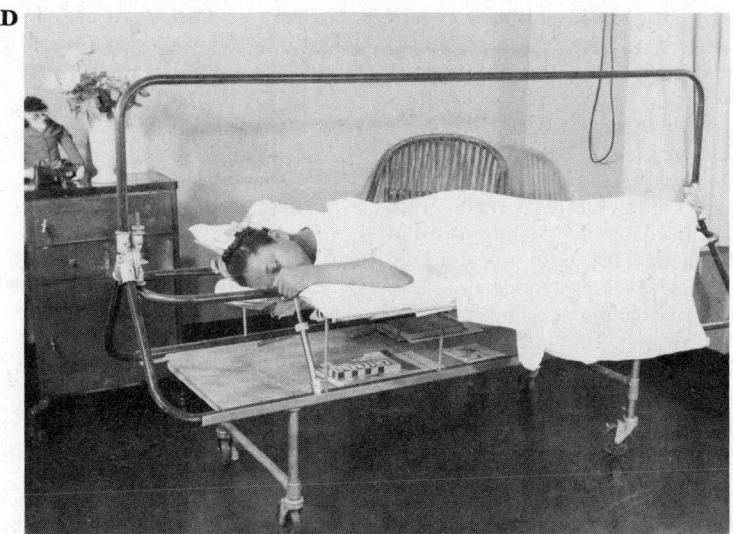

E

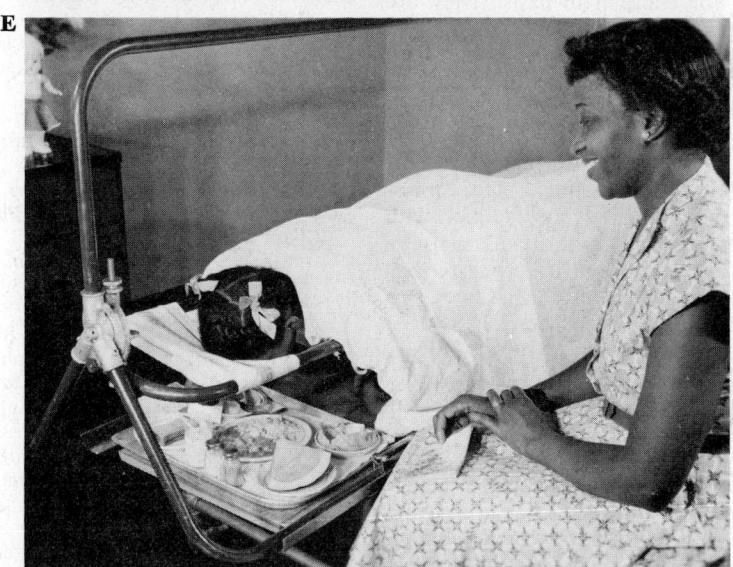

Figure 34-12. *A*. The Stryker frame. The patient is in the supine position with the arms supported on rests and the feet maintained in a position to prevent foot drop. (The sling around the thigh is used to enable the patient to exercise an injured leg; it is not part of the Stryker frame.) *B*. The nurse is preparing to change the patient from the prone to the supine position. She is sandwiching the patient between the upper and lower frames. *C*. Although one nurse can turn the patient, it gives the patient more confidence to have a second nurse at the head of the frame the first few times the patient is turned. *D*. The patient is in the prone position for sleeping, with the arm rests adjusted. The head is supported on a covered ring, suspended between the bars of the frame. *E*. In the prone position with the arm rests removed, the patient is able to feed herself, to read, or to play such games as checkers. Note the use of a towel pinned over the frame as a head support. Many persons prefer this to the rubber ring. (Courtesy of Columbia-Presbyterian Medical Center, New York, N.Y., and Clay-Adams Co., New York, N.Y.)

and they can be given an opportunity to ask about those things that puzzle them. The old adage "what he doesn't know, won't hurt him," applies to few persons who are ill or disabled; it is particularly inapplicable to the patient with a skeletal injury.

In addition to verbal explanations, patients in casts and/or traction derive benefit from demonstrations of what is happening or what will happen to them. One head nurse of an orthopedic unit has developed models of dolls in various kinds of traction to show patients, their families, and new employees what the traction system is like, and the why and how of procedures carried out for the patient in traction.[37]

Teaching a patient about his or her care is not something delayed until the day of discharge, but should begin when the nurse first meets the patient and the family. This is particularly true for children in casts. They are often sent home for a large part of their treatment period and parents should understand the "whys" and "wherefores" of the child's care since they will give most of it. Nurses who can imaginatively put themselves in the mother's place can make suggestions for home care that are compatible with the treatment plan, care of the cast, and the mother's home situation with its many demands on her time and energies. Many adults are sent home in leg casts they can walk on or with an arm in a sling or a splint. Canvas shoes may be worn over the foot if the patient has a leg cast (or when surgery of the foot has been done), and arm slings support the hand and wrist without putting pressure on the back of the neck. They should be given specific (written) directions or plans. Home visits from the hospital nursing staff or from community or district nurses are desirable. Nurses in industries, schools, and penal institutions may have to collaborate with nurses in hospitals on plans for follow-up care. Rehabilitation methods discussed in Chapter 8 are particularly applicable to patients with bone, muscle, and nerve injuries treated with immobilizing devices.

REFERENCES

1. Sarmiento, Augusto, and Sinclair, William F.: "Fracture Orthosis," in American Academy of Orthopedic Surgeons: *Atlas of Orthotics. Biomechanical Principles and Application.* C. V. Mosby Co., St. Louis, 1975, p. 245.

1a. Kennedy, Joan M.: *Orthopedic Splints and Appliances.* Williams & Wilkins Co., Baltimore, 1974, p. 4.

1b. Rotstein, Jerome: *Simple Splinting.* W. B. Saunders Co., Philadelphia, 1965, p. 103.

2. Granger, Carl V., et al.: "Laminated Plaster-Plastic Bandage Splints," *Arch. Phys. Med. Rehabil.,* **46:**585, (Aug.) 1965.

3. Rotstein, Jerome: *op. cit.,* p. 49.

4. Currie, D. J.: "Early Management of the Critically Injured," *Can. Med. Assoc. J.,* **95:**862, (Oct. 22) 1966.

5. Kerr, Avice: *Orthopedic Nursing Procedures,* 2nd ed. Springer Publishing Co., New York, 1969, p. 70.

6. Cole, Warren H., and Puestow, Charles B.: *Emergency Care: Surgical and Medical,* 7th ed. Appleton-Century-Crofts, New York, 1972.

7. Kerr, Avice: *op. cit.,* p. 65.

8. Adams, John C.: *Outline of Orthopaedics.* Churchill-Livingstone, London, 1971, p. 264.

9. Cozen, Lewis Nathan: *Office Orthopedics,* 4th ed. Charles C Thomas, Publisher, Springfield, Ill., 1974, p. 30.

10. Gilchrist, Don K.: "A Stockinette-Velpeau for Immobilization of the Shoulder Girdle," *J. Bone Joint Surg.* [*Am*], **49-A:**750, (June) 1967.

11. Bloomberg, Maxwell H.: *Orthopedic Braces.* J. B. Lippincott Co., Philadelphia, 1964, p. 12.

12. Stewart, John D. M.: *Traction and Orthopedic Appliances.* Churchill Livingstone, New York, 1975, p. 129.

13. Robinson, Robert A.: "Bone Physiology in Relation to Structure," in Blakemore, William S., and Fitts, William T. (eds.): *Management of the Injured Patient.* Harper & Row, New York, 1969, p. 63.

14. DePalma, Anthony F.: *The Management of Fractures and Dislocations,* Vol I, 2nd ed. W. B. Saunders Co., Philadelphia, 1970, p. 10.

15. Mayers, Marlene G.: *A Systematic Approach to the Nursing Care Plan.* Appleton-Century-Crofts, New York, 1972, p. 30.

16. Salter, Robert B.: *Textbook of Disorders and Injuries of the Musculoskeletal System.* Williams & Wilkins Co., Baltimore, 1970, p. 378.

17. Apley, A. Graham: *A System of Orthopaedics and Fractures,* 4th ed. Butterworth & Co., London, 1973, p. 373.

18. DePalma, Anthony F.: *op. cit.,* p. 123.

19. Larson, Carroll B., and Gould, Marjorie: *Orthopedic Nursing,* 7th ed. C. V. Mosby Co., St. Louis, 1970, p. 47.

20. Kottke, Frederic J.: "The Effects of Limitation of Activity upon the Human Body," *J.A.M.A.,* **196:**117, (June 6) 1966.

21. Nicholson, Jesse T.: "Symposium: Surgical Care of the Elderly Patient Is Different," *J. Bone Joint Surg.* [*Am*], **47-A:**1036, (July) 1965.

22. Karpovich, Peter J.: "Exercise in Medicine: A Review," *Arch. Phys. Med. Rehabil.,* **49:**66, (Jan.) 1968.

23. Kelly, Mary M.: "Exercises for Bedfast Patients," *Am. J. Nurs.,* **66:**2209, (Oct.) 1966.

24. Karpovich, Peter J.: *op. cit.*

25. Zubek, John P. (ed.): *Sensory Deprivation: Fifteen Years of Research.* Appleton-Century-Crofts, New York, 1969, p. 248.

26. Jackson, C. Wesley, et al.: "The Application of Findings from Experimental Sensory Deprivation to Cases of Clinical Sensory Deprivation," *Am. J. Med. Sci.*, **243**:558, (May) 1962.

27. Rowe, Carter R.: "Symposium: The Management of Fractures in Elderly Patients Is Different," *J. Bone Joint Surg.* [*Am*], **47-A**:1043, (July) 1965.

28. Nash, John: *Developmental Psychology—A Psychological Approach.* Prentice-Hall, Englewood Cliffs, N.J., 1970, p. 460.

29. Blake, Florence: "Immobilized Youth," *Am. J. Nurs.*, **69**:2364, (Nov.) 1969.

30. Wolfe, Barbara S.: "The Language Development of a 3-Year-Old Immobilized Child," in *ANA Clinical Sessions, 1966.* Appleton-Century-Crofts, New York, 1967, p. 109.

31. Porter, Luz S.: "The Impact of Physical-Physiological Activity on Infants' Growth and Development," *Nurs. Res.*, **21**:210, (May–June) 1972.

32. DePalma, Anthony F.: *op. cit.*, p. 125.

33. Schmeisser, Gerhard: *A Clinical Manual of Orthopedic Traction Techniques.* W. B. Saunders Co., Philadelphia, 1963, p. 3.

34. Bailey, Joseph A.: "Tractions, Suspensions, and a Ringless Splint," *Am. J. Nurs.*, **70**:1724, (Aug.) 1970.

35. Brobsky, Arthur: "The Patient on a Circ-Olectric Bed," *Am. J. Nurs.*, **71**:2352, (Dec.) 1971.

36. Sovie, Margaret D., and Fruehan, C. Thomas: "Protecting the Patient from Electrical Hazards," *Nurs. Clin. North Am.*, **7**:469, (Sept.) 1972.

37. Anderson, Faye A.: "Traction Explanations Made Easy," *Am. J. Nurs.*, **70**:2377, (Nov.) 1970.

Additional Suggested Reading

Abramson, Arthur S., and Delagi, Edward F.: "Influence of Weight-Bearing and Muscle Contraction on Disuse Osteoporosis," *Arch. Phys. Med. Rehabil.*, **42**:147, (Feb.) 1961.

American College of Surgeons, Committee on Trauma: *The Management of Fractures and Soft Tissue Injuries,* 2nd ed. W. B. Saunders Co., Philadelphia, 1965.

————: *Early Care of the Injured Patient.* W. B. Saunders Co., Philadelphia, 1972.

Anderson, Helen C.: *Newton's Geriatric Nursing,* 5th ed. C. V. Mosby Co., Philadelphia, 1971.

Bame, Kathleen B.: "Halo Traction," *Am. J. Nurs.*, **69**:1933, (Sept.) 1969.

Brower, Phyllis, and Hicks, Dorothy: "Maintaining Muscle Function in Patients on Bed Rest," *Am. J. Nurs.*, **72**:1250, (July) 1972.

Chodil, Judith, and Williams, Barbara: "The Concept of Sensory Deprivation," *Nurs. Clin. North Am.*, **5**:453, (Sept.) 1970.

Eyre, Mary K.: "Total Hip Replacement," *Am. J. Nurs.*, **71**:1384, (July) 1971.

Gartland, John J.: *Fundamentals of Orthopedics,* 2nd ed. W. B. Saunders Co., Philadelphia, 1974.

Griffin, Winnie, et al.: "Group Exercises for Patients with Limited Motion," *Am. J. Nurs.*, **71**:1743, (Sept.) 1971.

Hilt, Nancy E., and Schmitt, E. William, Jr.: *Pediatric Orthopedic Nursing.* C. V. Mosby Co., St. Louis, 1975.

Howe, Jeanne: "Children's Ideas About Injury," in *ANA Regional Clinical Conferences, 1967.* Appleton-Century-Crofts, New York, 1968.

Johnson & Johnson: *Professional Uses of Adhesive Tape.* The Company, New Brunswick, N.J., 1972.

Lane, Phyllis A.: "A Mother's Confession—Home Care of a Toddler in a Spica Cast: What It's Really Like," *Am. J. Nurs.*, **71**:2141, (Nov.) 1971.

Leifer, Gloria: *Principles and Techniques in Pediatric Nursing,* 2nd ed. W. B. Saunders Co., Philadelphia, 1972.

Linton, Patrick H.: "Sensory Deprivation in Hospitalized Patients," *Ala. J. Med. Sci.*, **2**:256, (July) 1965.

O'Donoghue, Don H.: *Treatment of Injuries to Athletes.* W. B. Saunders Co., Philadelphia, 1976.

Orthopedic Nurses Association: *Standards of Orthopedic Nursing Practice.* The Association, New York, 1975.

Powell, Mary: *Orthopaedic Nursing.* Churchill Livingstone, London, 1976.

Reid, Robert L., and Gamon, Robert S.: "The Cast Syndrome," *Clin. Orthop.*, **79**:85, (Sept.) 1971.

Senf, Harriet R.: "Caring for the Patient in the CircOlectric Bed," *Am. J. Nurs.*, **60**:227, (Feb.) 1960.

Stryker, Ruth P.: *Rehabilitative Aspects of Acute and Chronic Nursing Care.* W. B. Saunders Co., Philadelphia, 1972.

Catherine Temple
Virginia Henderson

PART V

Common Problems—
Symptomatic Nursing

CHAPTER 35

Marked Disturbance of Intake and Output of Gases Demanding Medical Intervention or First Aid

1. INTRODUCTION

Respiration, in the broadest sense of the word, refers to all the processes involved in the intake and utilization of oxygen and the production and elimination of carbon dioxide. Oxygen is utilized and carbon dioxide is produced at the cellular level by a myriad of chemical reactions collectively termed metabolism. Normal respiration and the help most people need with maintaining it are discussed in Chapter 9. Its contents should be studied in conjunction with this chapter that deals with pathologic respiration.

Many of the signs and symptoms associated with impaired pulmonary function, and common to a variety of respiratory disorders, are related to the harmful cellular effects of oxygen deprivation and abnormal carbon dioxide tensions with the associated acid–base imbalances. The body responds to alterations of these important gases by massive recruitment of compensatory mechanisms directed toward reestablishing a normal internal milieu or intercellular fluid. An important responsibility of the nurse caring for patients with a marked disturbance in respiratory gas exchange is properly assessing the patient's needs, then instituting nursing actions that reinforce the body's innate ability to restore normal respiration.

Between the external environment and the cells of the body are the ventilatory and gas transport apparatus. Provision of adequate oxygen and efficient removal of carbon dioxide depend on alternating pressure gradients between the alveoli and external environment, a patent, unobstructed airway to the alveolar level, absence of a barrier to diffusion of gases from alveoli to blood and from blood to alveoli, and a gas transport system that can acquire sufficient oxygen and discharge excess carbon dioxide during the less than 1 second spent by erythrocytes in the pulmonary capillaries. Disease or injury of any part of the ventilatory or transport systems or mechanisms can disturb the intake and output of gases and impair the function or endanger the life of the patient.

Regardless of the medical diagnosis, patients with marked disturbance in the intake and output of gases will have specific problems requiring critical nursing assessment, careful nursing action, and continuous evaluation of the effectiveness of the nursing care. Patients with respiratory impairment may experience dyspnea (difficult breathing), hypoxia (deficient oxygen), hypocapnia (deficient carbon dioxide), hypercapnia (excessive carbon dioxide), or asphyxia (suffocation), singly or in various combinations. Respiratory impairment may be acute and fulminating, as in pulmonary infarction, but more often it is chronic and insidious, as in chronic obstructive emphysema. In order to successfully care for patients with respiratory conditions and accurately assess their response to that care, the nurse must understand both the physiology of respiration and the pathology involved in the condition, recognize signs that indicate improvement or deterioration in the patient's status, and, especially if the disease is a chronic one, appreciate the economic, social, and psychologic impact on the patient and his or her family.

2. DYSPNEA

Few patients present the distress and apprehension equal to that seen in dyspneic patients. Air hunger and the inability "to catch the breath" frighten them and aggravate their dyspnea. Nursing care of these patients includes not only the administration of medically prescribed treatments such as oxygen administration, drugs, or ventilatory support, but also kindness, understanding, and the psychologic support of the nurse's presence. Although dyspnea is frequently associated with cardiac and pulmonary diseases and trauma, all the factors contributing to it are not fully understood, and it has a definite subjective component. Julius H. Comroe has said of dyspnea:

Let me start with my concept of what dyspnoea *is* and *is not*. It is *not* tachypnoea, which is rapid breathing; it is *not* hyperpnoea, which is increased ventilation in proportion to increased metabolism; it is *not* hyperventilation, which is ventilation in excess of metabolic requirements. Instead, dyspnoea *is* difficult, laboured, uncomfortable breathing; it is an unpleasant type of breathing, though it is not painful in the usual sense of the word. It is subjective and, like pain, it involves both perception of the sensation by the patient and his reaction to the sensation.*

It has not been possible to attribute dyspnea to any single cause or physiologic alteration. Although dyspnea is not unexpected in patients with airway obstruction or decreased amounts of functioning lung tissue (for example, pulmonary fibrosis), the degree of discomfort experienced by the patient is not necessarily proportional to the extent of his or her respiratory embarrassment. Dyspnea seems to be more closely related to the patient's awareness of difficulty in moving air into and out of the lungs than to altered blood gases. In the report of an interesting experiment in which he was voluntarily paralyzed by *d*-tubocurarine, M. Scott Smith commented, after recovery, "I felt that I would give anything to be able to take one deep breath." † He had a feeling of shortness of breath despite the fact that pulmonary ventilation and oxygenation were adequate.

Attempts have been made to correlate the patient's dyspneic distress with some measurement such as maximum breathing capacity (MBC), or maximum voluntary ventilation (MVV), and these attempts have led to the concept of a dyspnea index.[1,2] Andre Cournand and Dickinson W. Richards [3] have suggested that dyspnea occurs when the actual ventilation (in liters per minute) reaches a certain fraction of the maximum breathing capacity. Thus, an athletic young man with a maximum breathing capacity of 200 liters per minute may be dyspneic when his ventilation reaches 60 liters per minute after exercise, whereas a severely emphysemic patient with a maximum breathing capacity of only 20 liters per minute will be dyspneic when ventilating only 6 liters per minute. This latter value of ventilation is characteristic of quiet breathing in normal adults and indicates that what a healthy individual is relatively unaware of becomes a conscious, total effort for the dyspneic patient. It seems that expiratory flow measurements such as the maximum midexpiratory flow (MMF) may provide better correlation with the dyspnea experienced by a patient than maximum breathing capacity.[4] That is, the sensation of dyspnea may be more closely related to how rapidly patients can expel air from their lungs than to how much air they can move into and out of their lungs.

The respiratory act itself requires muscular energy that is normally a very small part of the total metabolic expenditure.[5] For patients with pulmonary dysfunction, however, the work of breathing is increased, and more of the oxygen inhaled is consumed by the respiratory muscles themselves. Furthermore, this oxygen consumption increases disproportionately with ventilation.[6] So, the more strenuously the patient ventilates in an attempt to supply the body's oxygen needs, the greater is the amount of oxygen consumed by the respiratory muscles. A vicious circle develops as the increased work of breathing leads to muscle fatigue and increasing dyspnea.

As fatigue and dyspnea increase, breathing may become rapid and shallow. A portion of the air moved during each respiratory cycle is confined to the anatomic dead space, that part of the tracheobronchial tree across which no gas exchange with the blood occurs. Dead space averages about 150 cc in the normal adult, and this volume must be subtracted from the tidal volume (TV), the amount of air moved into and out of the respiratory passages during each respiratory cycle, to determine the alveolar ventilation (AV), the volume of air actually reaching the alveoli each minute and exchanging oxygen and carbon dioxide with the blood. The simple example shown in Table 35-1 illustrates how different values of alveolar ventilation can occur with the same minute respiratory volume (MRV), and how rapid, shallow breathing can reduce the amount of respiratory gas exchange while increasing muscular fatigue and dyspnea.

* Comroe, Julius H., Jr.: "Some Theories of the Mechanism of Dyspnoea," in Howell, J. B. L., and Campbell, E. J. M. (eds.): *Breathlessness.* Blackwell Scientific Publications, Oxford, 1966, p. 1.

† Smith, Scott M., et al.: "The Lack of Cerebral Effects of *d*-Tubocurarine," *Anesthesiology,* **8**:1, (Jan.) 1947.

Table 35-1. Alveolar Ventilation (AV) with the Same Minute Respiratory Volume (MRV) Produced by Different Respiratory Rates and Tidal Volumes (TV)

Rate	TV	MRV	(TV − Dead Space) × Rate = AV
10/min	600 cc	6 L/min	(600 − 150) × 10 = 4.5 L/min
12/min	500 cc	6 L/min	(500 − 150) × 12 = 4.2 L/min
20/min	300 cc	6 L/min	(300 − 150) × 20 = 3.0 L/min
40/min	150 cc	6 L/min	(150 − 150) × 40 = 0.0 L/min

Some Conditions Associated with Dyspnea. A variety of conditions, some of which are listed below, can interfere with the free, easy movement of gases into and out of the lungs, increase the work of respiration, bring the act of breathing from the subconscious to the conscious level, and predispose to dyspnea.

Chronic obstructive emphysema is one of the major health problems in the United States today.[7] It is believed to begin with chronic inflammatory processes of the air passages.[8,9] The condition seems to be aggravated by environmental air pollution and cigarette smoking and is, therefore, largely preventable. Destruction of alveolar septa, hypersecretion of a thick, tenacious mucus, and edema of tissues lining the respiratory passages combine to impede the normal flow of air. Expiration is usually more difficult than inspiration because the elasticity of the lung tissue, which normally facilitates expiration, is decreased, and increased intrathoracic pressure during expiration further diminishes the diameter of the narrowed airways.[10] Patients will often purse their lips during expiration in an attempt to maintain an intrapulmonary pressure adequate to postpone the expiratory collapse of the air passages. Air trapped within the lungs beyond the points of obstruction leads to increasing alveolar distention and disruption and results in the development of a "barrel chest." Figure 35-1A shows the damage produced in the lungs by emphysema and Figure 35-1B illustrates both the method and the effect of pursed lip breathing.

Cor pulmonale is dilation, hypertrophy, and even failure of the right ventricle of the heart secondary to destructive changes in the pulmonary capillary bed and lung parenchyma. It can occur in patients with chronic obstructive emphysema. This serious complication is often accompanied by increased dyspnea.[11]

Bronchial asthma can affect persons of all ages. Acute attacks are usually due to an allergic reaction between antibodies in the sensitized bronchial mucosa and an antigen.[12] Since the onset of acute attacks is usually sudden, nurses in schools, industries, and clinics often have to care for patients suffering an acute asthmatic attack. The immunologic response results in constriction of bronchiolar smooth muscle, increased secretion of a thick mucus, and mucosal edema. Dyspnea is often pronounced, and the accessory respiratory muscles may be recruited to increase ventilation. Since expiration further narrows obstructed air passages, this phase of respiration is usually more difficult for the patient than inspiration. The acute attack subsides when the offending antigen is removed, the bronchiolar constriction relieved, and the thick mucus expectorated. If bronchial asthma becomes chronic, the structural changes in the lungs and the symptoms presented by the patient may be similar to those of chronic obstructive emphysema. Chronic bronchial asthma has been implicated by some as an etiologic factor in the development of emphysema.[13]

Pulmonary fibrosis is not a single entity, but results from a variety of conditions in which normal lung tissue has been replaced by fibrous connective tissue. The lungs become more rigid and difficult to ventilate. Pulmonary fibrosis may be secondary to pneumonia, tuberculosis, collagen diseases, long-term inhalation of industrial dusts, and numerous other conditions. Fibrosis results in restricted respiratory movements and decreased pulmonary compliance, which increase the work of breathing and can lead to dyspnea.

Pulmonary edema is caused by a number of cardiac and pulmonary conditions and can literally drown patients in their own secretions.[14] Alveolar spaces can be filled with blood, serum, or excess mucus following a chest wound or the inhalation of irritating gases and substances to which the patient is allergic. Pulmonary infections, uremia, heroin poisoning, and smoke inhalation are noncardiac factors which can produce pulmonary edema.[15] The direct cause of the outpouring of fluid from the capillaries is an increased permeability of their walls. What makes this often sudden change in the capacity of the capillaries to contain their contents is not thoroughly understood. As fluid leaks from the capillaries into

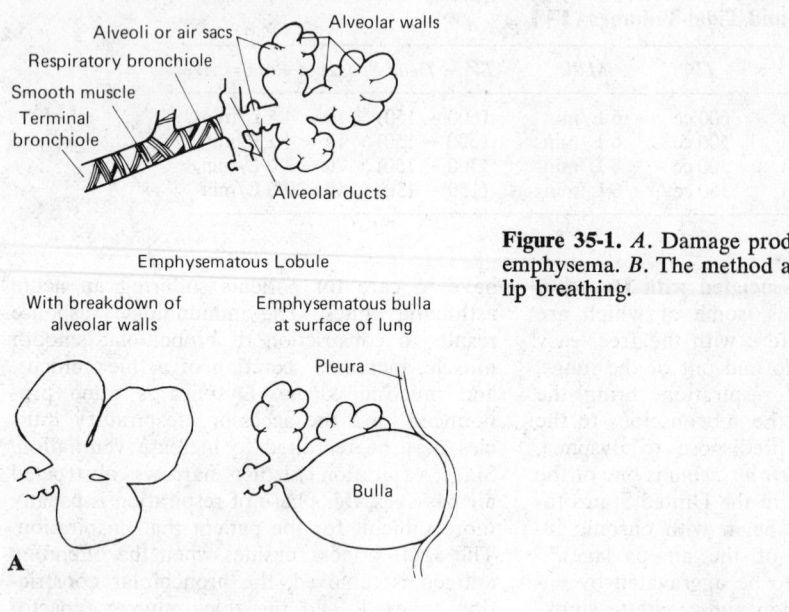

Normal Primary Lobule
(after Miller)

Alveoli or air sacs
Respiratory bronchiole
Smooth muscle
Terminal bronchiole
Alveolar walls
Alveolar ducts

Emphysematous Lobule

With breakdown of alveolar walls
Emphysematous bulla at surface of lung
Pleura
Bulla

A

Other alveoli
Pursed lips
Bronchiole

Compression of bronchiole on forced expiration
B
Bronchiole kept open by positive pressure during expiration

Figure 35-1. *A.* Damage produced in the lungs by emphysema. *B.* The method and the effect of pursed lip breathing.

the interstitial spaces and the alveoli themselves, two factors contribute to the patient's dyspnea. The tissue pressure of the lungs increases, thereby increasing the difficulty with which the lungs expand and deflate, and accumulation of fluid within the alveoli and interstitial spaces retards gas exchange.

The onset of pulmonary edema is usually sudden and is said to be, in some cases, unheralded by warning signs. The feeling of oppression in the chest may, however, develop gradually, with mounting anxiety, whereas with a sudden onset and outpouring of fluid into the tissues the pain may be so great that the patient cries out in stark fear. A conspicuous symptom is an incessant cough producing a frothy, sometimes blood-tinged, sputum. The sputum gets increasingly copious until, if the condition is not controlled, the fluid gushes from the nose and mouth. Rales can be felt and heard all over the chest, and the breathing

is increasingly moist, or crackly, as in the "death rattle." Breathlessness and cyanosis progress until the patient is gasping for air. The face is covered with cold sweat, the pulse gets steadily weaker, and the blood pressure falls. Attacks are said to be more common at night or in the early morning, and may be confused with asthma. It has been said that pulmonary edema may be fatal in a few hours or that symptoms may persist for 12 to 24 hours and then disappear. When fatal, pulmonary edema usually develops slowly and is accompanied by coma; the prognosis is always grave. It is one of the most dreaded emergency states.

Airway obstruction due to foreign bodies lodged in the airway is a common source of acute dyspnea. A great variety of objects have been removed from the airways of small children and adults. The immediate seriousness of foreign bodies in the respiratory tract depends

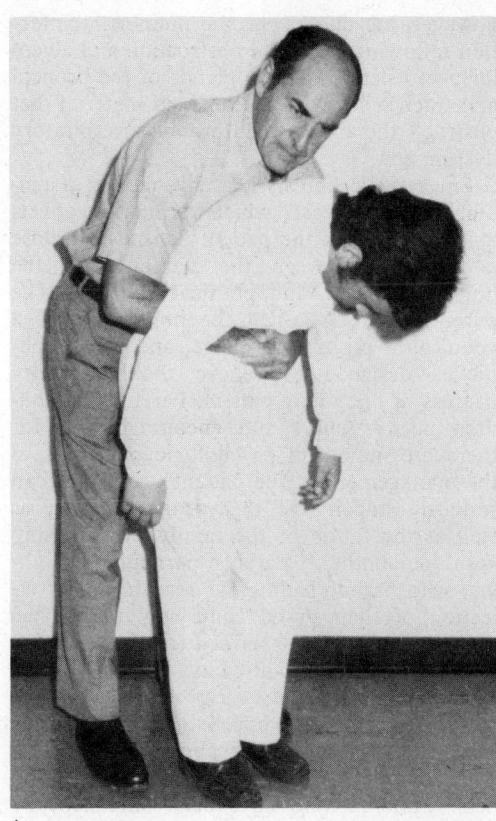

A

B

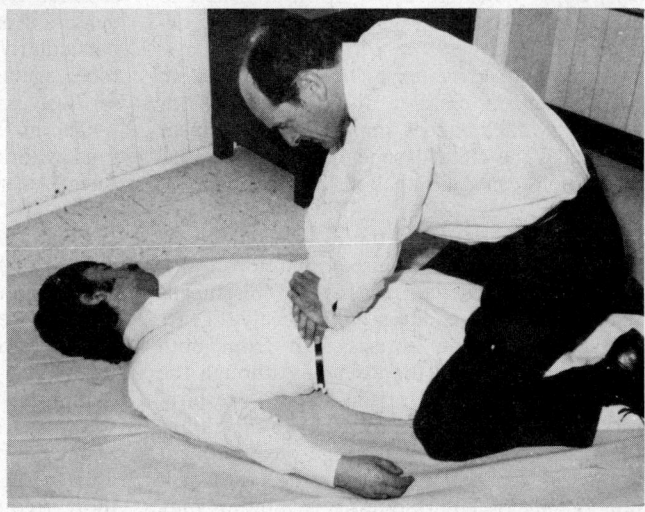

Figure 35-2. Applying the Heimlich maneuver with the victim in (*A*) the standing position; (*B*) the supine position. (Courtesy of Dr. Henry J. Heimlich, The Jewish Hospital, Cincinnati, Ohio.)

upon where the obstruction occurs. For example, an occluded trachea is more of an emergency than an occluded bronchus because the latter allows ventilation of at least one lung. However, an occluded bronchus is by no means harmless.

An emergency measure called the *Heimlich maneuver* has been described for removing aspirated food from the airway.[15a,15b] This maneuver may be effective in saving the victim's life when the obstructing material is lodged too deeply in the air passages to be removed manually. The underlying principle of the Heimlich maneuver is compression of the air behind the foreign body, and its expulsion, by forcible upward movement of the diaphragm.

The Heimlich maneuver may be performed on the victim in a standing, sitting, or supine position. When the victim is in the standing position, the rescuer places his arms around the victim's waist from behind and grasps his one fist with his other hand (see Fig. 35-2*A*). The upper part of the victim's body is allowed to hang forward. The rescuer positions his grasped fist over the abdomen slightly above the umbilicus and exerts a quick upward thrust on the diaphragm. If the first attempt to clear the airway is unsuccessful, the maneuver should be repeated. The same technique is used when the victim is seated in a chair.

The Heimlich maneuver may also be applied to a victim in the supine position. With the victim lying on his back, the rescuer positions himself astride the victim as shown in Figure 35-2*B*. The heel of one hand is placed on the victim's abdomen slightly above the umbilicus, and the other hand is placed on top of the first. A quick upward thrust is applied to the abdomen and repeated as necessary to dislodge the obstruction.

Unconsciousness and death will occur within a few minutes of airway obstruction. Therefore, there must be no delay in applying the Heimlich maneuver to a choking victim. If a person aspirates a large food particle and no help is available, he or she should immediately apply quick, forceful, upward thrusts to his or her own diaphragm to dislodge the obstruction.

Acute obstructive laryngitis (*croup*) is seen more often in children than in adults. Inflamed, swollen tissues impede air movement and make the child dyspneic. In severe cases, ventilation can be impaired to the point of asphyxia.

Cystic fibrosis (sometimes referred to as CF) is a genetically acquired condition, transmitted as a mendelian recessive.[16] This means that only those children who receive genes carrying the cystic fibrosis trait from both parents will develop the disease. Although the disease affects many organ systems, respiratory symptoms often appear early in the child's life, and early diagnosis and vigorous treatment are necessary to prevent severe, permanent lung damage.[17] The respiratory symptoms may be mild or severe, with dyspnea, paroxysmal cough, and intercostal and suprasternal retraction. The mother may report to the nurse that she is able to pull thick, stringy mucus from the child's throat.[18]

In addition to the involvement of the lungs, the pancreas is frequently involved, and there are attendant nutritional disturbances. In fact, the disease was first identified as one of the pancreas.[19] Most deaths from cystic fibrosis,

however, are due to chronic pulmonary infection following bronchial obstruction and alveolar overdistention.[20] The glands of the bronchi and trachea secrete a thick viscid material that obstructs the airways and produces respiratory dysfunction.[21]

Since cystic fibrosis is a chronic and potentially fatal disease which primarily affects children, care of the patient depends on close cooperation between the parents and the nurse, physician, and physical therapist. The parents must be taught the proper use of a nebulizer,* postural drainage, and other techniques designed to relieve the respiratory distress of the young patient. Parents and children need support and encouragement, for there are important psychologic overtones to the management of the patient's care that can seriously impair the therapeutic regimen as well as the fabric of the family's relationship with one another.[22] Parents, particularly mothers, who harbor feelings of resentment or rejection of their cystic child may permit the child to resist the prescribed treatment or fail to keep clinic appointments. Overprotectiveness or denial of the severity of the illness by parents may impair effective communication between them and their child and interfere with educating the child about his or her illness. Children who have been unrealistically shielded from the facts of their illness may develop a sense of shame about their illness and, particularly as they reach adolescence, may rebel against their treatments to the point of seriously endangering themselves.

The air surfaces of normal alveoli are covered with a film of surfactant, a material produced by some of the epithelial cells (type II cells) of the alveoli themselves.[23] Surfactant facilitates alveolar inflation, and when surfactant is *absent or insufficient* alveolar ventilation decreases and the work of breathing increases. Respiratory distress syndrome of the newborn, or hyaline membrane disease, seems to involve insufficient or abnormal surfactant. Symptoms include tachypnea, cyanosis, inspiratory retraction, and expiratory grunting. Such symptoms appear within a few hours after birth.[24] Premature infants are affected more frequently than those delivered at term, and the mortality rate is high. Alveolar hypoventilation contributes to decreased oxygen and increased carbon dioxide in the blood, but with a proper regimen of assisted mechanical ventilation, many more of the affected infants

---

* Some physicians may prescribe mist tents, but their value has recently been questioned, one writer claiming that there is only one center left in the United States that uses them (see Chap. 20).

may survive.[25] George A. Gregory and associates [26] used continuous positive airway pressure in the treatment of 20 infants seriously ill with idiopathic respiratory distress syndrome. They reported that 16 of these infants, including seven with birth weights of less than 1500 gm, survived. (See Chapter 20 for a discussion of mechanically assisted ventilation.)

Cellular immaturity seems to be an important cause of decreased surfactant production, but other factors can also reduce the amount of this important product of alveolar cells. Abnormal surface tension of lung tissue from adults suggests decreased surfactant production, especially as a result of decreased pulmonary blood flow such as can occur with pulmonary embolism or cardiopulmonary bypass. Surfactant is thought to play some role in keeping the lungs free of excessive fluid accumulation, and pulmonary edema has been noted in conjunction with increased surface tension, but whether the pulmonary edema resulted from decreased surfactant synthesis or vice versa has not been totally resolved.[27]

Increased intrapleural pressure is another cause of dyspnea. Inspiratory air flow results from a decreased intrapleural pressure expanding the lungs and creating a pressure gradient from the atmosphere to the alveoli. Even at end-expiration, intrapleural pressure is less than atmospheric pressure, and this negative pressure keeps the lungs slightly expanded and opposes their natural tendency to collapse. Whenever air gains access to the pleural space either through a traumatic or surgical wound in the thoracic wall or through a ruptured bulla, intrapleural pressure increases and the lung on the affected side may collapse. Air in the pleural cavity is called a pneumothorax. Impaired ventilation due to a pneumothorax can produce dyspnea, because the more deeply the patient inspires, the more air he or she draws into the pleural space to further compress the affected lung.

Fluid (hydrothorax) or blood (hemothorax) in the pleural space also increases the intrapleural pressure, restricts lung expansion, and decreases ventilation. Pulmonary blood flow is usually shunted from the collapsed to the unaffected lung, and, in patients with no other pulmonary involvement, adequate gas exchange and blood oxygenation is usually maintained. However, in the presence of additional pulmonary complications, decreased ventilation secondary to increased intrapleural pressure may produce severe dyspnea.

Weakness of the respiratory muscles or skeletal deformities of the thorax can limit respiratory excursions and reduce ventilation. Neuromuscular diseases such as amyotrophic lateral sclerosis, Guillain-Barré syndrome, and myasthenia gravis are not accompanied by a dulled sensorium; therefore, the patient is conscious of the increased respiratory difficulty and this awareness, coupled with a decreased ability to ventilate, sets the stage for dyspnea. It is particularly important for the nurse to give close attention to these patients and provide ventilary assistance when necessary, for they would breathe if they could, but they truly cannot.

Anxiety, stress, or depression can cause dyspnea. The sighs of a depressed person are attempts to get a deep breath. In Chapter 20 reference is made to the euphoria seen in patients with respiratory distress when they are put in a room with a high oxygen content.

Nursing Assessment and Measures in Caring for the Dyspneic Patient. Careful, astute observation of the patient will enable the nurse to more accurately identify particular needs of the individual and institute nursing actions designed to reduce or alleviate them. Because dyspnea occurs in so many conditions, nurses in all types of settings—the home, hospitals, clinics, schools, industrial plants, penal health services, and other institutions—will encounter patients with this problem. Discussions with the patient and the family provide information valuable to the nurse in assessing the patient's needs. The nurse should carefully observe the degree to which the patient uses the accessory respiratory muscles of the shoulder girdle and neck to help in breathing. Extensive use of these muscles suggests difficulty in ventilating adequately. Flared nares, pursed lips, and an apprehensive or pained facial expression also indicate marked ventilatory effort.

Respiratory difficulty can be greatly exaggerated by any posture that reduces the size of the rib cage or puts pressure from the abdominal organs on the lungs. In helping persons with ventilatory difficulties—and their families—nurses should always include assessment of posture and exercise. If patients are confined to bed and under the care of nurses, this assessment is continuous.

Dyspneic patients will naturally assume the posture that allows them to breathe with minimum difficulty and discomfort and with maximum efficiency. It is important that nurses recognize this and allow the persons to assume positions most comfortable for them, regardless of how uncomfortable or unnatural they may appear. Upright or sitting positions are usually favored over the supine position. The upright or sitting position helps to prevent the abdominal organs from pressing upward on the diaphragm and lungs and allows for easier expansion of the lungs. The nurse should determine the most comfortable position and provide adequate support for the upper part of the patient's body. A pillow placed on an overbed table provides support for the arms of a patient sitting upright; however, the level of the table should be high enough to allow full expansion of the thorax. Leaning on a table that is positioned too low restricts thoracic expansion and increases the work of an already overtaxed ventilatory mechanism.

Observations of nurses and the information they get from the patient and family will help identify activities or situations that provide or aggravate dyspneic episodes. Measures can then be instituted to minimize these factors. If, for example, meals are often associated with increased dyspnea, it may benefit the patient to have smaller amounts of food at more frequent intervals, to have a rest period free from all activity and visitors before each meal, and to be served foods that are easy to chew and swallow. Certain "visitors" or companions may, however, help rather than harm the patient so that generalizations about them are questionable.

In acute conditions nurses may decide to feed patients to conserve their energy—or need for oxygen—or they may help a member of the family or an intimate friend to do this. Seeing that the head is elevated and that patients are in comfortable positions in bed or in a chair is very important. It is also important for them to eat slowly. For patients subject to coughing, eating can be dangerous, for if they cough with food in their mouths the food may be insufflated and, if not coughed up, the material can cause a lung infection. The importance of feeding a patient slowly cannot be overemphasized.

The difficulty some victims of long-term respiratory disease have in eating may discourage them from going out to restaurants or even joining the family for meals. Nurses can help in suggesting that they eat small meals often, eat slowly, take small mouthfuls, and avoid talk while food is in the mouth to reduce coughing during a meal or other dangers of eating. Withdrawing from family meals is especially undesirable from the standpoint of morale.

Persons with respiratory difficulty of psychogenic origin may suspect that their feeling of breathlessness is a form of indigestion. They may be tempted to put themselves on a restricted diet that is ultimately lacking in the necessary nutrients. In such cases the nurse can help them seek diagnostic tests and help them understand and accept the findings. Those who have insight into the cause of psychogenic dyspnea are more likely to eat a normal diet and avoid overeating and distention of the stomach.

It goes without saying that persons with pathology of the respiratory system are more likely to effect a cure if they eat a well-balanced diet. Overweight exaggerates respiratory difficulties by overtaxing the heart muscles and by making all body movement demand a high oxygen expenditure.

In the assessment of the person who is acutely dyspneic as the result of a foreign body in the airway, the nurse should learn, if possible, the nature of the offending material, the length of time since aspiration, and the severity of the symptoms indicating the degree of alteration in the intake and output of oxygen and carbon dioxide. (See page 1490 for a description of the stages of asphyxia.) The presence or absence of breath sounds, as well as their character, over various parts of the lungs can indicate the extent of pulmonary ventilation.

The age, mental alertness, and general appearance, as well as the state of nutrition and hydration of every patient with respiratory distress, should be determined and recorded by the nurse. The duration and increasing or decreasing severity of the signs and symptoms presented by the patient provide important information and should be included in the record.

As mentioned previously, dyspnea occurs in a variety of diseases and conditions; therefore, knowledge of the specific cause is a prime requisite for the provision of effective nursing care. Much of the anxiety and apprehension of the dyspneic patients can be allayed by understanding nurses who have a calm but concerned supportive attitude toward them as they give nursing care. Nursing care for dyspneic patients should include the assurance that their calls for assistance will be promptly answered. Fear on the part of patients that they will be unable to continue breathing and that no one will come when needed can increase their anxiety and decrease the effectiveness of their respiratory efforts.

Measures to reduce airway obstruction should be instituted by the nurse in order to decrease the work of breathing and increase the amount of air reaching the alveoli. Patients with pulmonary disorders often accumulate large amounts of thick mucus in the respiratory passages that impede airflow. Nurses can help patients get rid of this mucus by teaching them to take several deep breaths before coughing and to use the abdominal muscles and diaphragm to increase the pressure against the lung bases. This procedure increases the effectiveness of the cough and helps move secretions into the larger airways from which they can be more easily expectorated or suctioned. An opaque container with a tight-fitting lid should be provided for collecting the sputum so the nurse may see its amount and character. The color of the sputum should be noted—whether it is pink or brownish in color, indicating fresh or old blood; whether it is frothy, suggesting pulmonary edema; and whether it is purulent or foul-smelling, which would suggest the presence of an infection such as a lung abscess.[28] The sputum container should be removed from the bedside at frequent intervals to reduce the unpleasant odors that would tend to take away the patient's appetite or be a source of embarrassment. With many respiratory difficulties, there is a cough which may be paroxysmal, violent, and frightening or almost constant. A cough can be dry and hacking and sound like a mere habit, or moist and productive, suggesting an infection of the respiratory tract.

All coughing is, in a sense, antisocial. Those who love the victims suffer with them; those who don't tend to be annoyed or apprehensive and to avoid their company.* Victims of sinusitis, emphysema, or other conditions inducing a productive cough are naturally interested in the nature of the discharge and they sometimes form the habit of spitting on a handkerchief and looking at the excrement. In their concern over the possibility that they may, for instance, be bleeding, they forget that that practice is unesthetic or even repulsive to others. A productive cough may suggest tuberculosis or some other communicable disease to the person who has it and to those who are present. Anxiety, or fear, accompanies coughing.

Helping those affected with a cough or a discharge from the nose is often difficult. People can, however, learn to suppress a cough, to seek privacy when coughing purposely to clear the airway, or when clearing nasal passages. Patients with severe respiratory difficulties who are confined to bed should, if possible, be in private rooms. If they must share rooms with others, unesthetic or (to some) repellent treatments, such as postural drainage, should not be scheduled near meal hours; screening patients helps to protect oth-

ers and to suggest to those going through the process that privacy is desirable.

Meticulous and frequent mouth care reduces odors and the unpleasant taste which may result from mouth-breathing and frequent expectoration. A clean mouth, free of offensive taste and odors, refreshes the patient, stimulates the appetite, and removes a possible source of embarrassment, and therefore, social withdrawal. Patients should be encouraged to brush their teeth at regular intervals, and a mouthwash of the patient's choice should be readily available for use as desired, especially after expectoration of foul-smelling or foul-tasting sputum and before meals. Dentures should be cared for as carefully as the patient's natural teeth. (See Chapter 14 for a more detailed discussion of mouth care.)

Several nursing measures can help patients clear the respiratory passages and facilitate the movement of air to and from the lungs. One of these is to keep patients well hydrated. Adequate intake of fluids helps keep the mucus thin, watery, and easier to expectorate; it also replaces the fluids lost by mouth-breathing and producing large amounts of sputum. Many patients quickly tire of water so the nurse should offer fruit juices, carbonated drinks, bouillon, or whatever patients want and that their diet, if they are on a special one, permits.

To ensure optimal airflow the airway must be kept free of obstructing secretions by judicious nasotracheal suctioning applied as often as the signs and symptoms presented by the patient indicate the need. Before introducing the suction catheter, the patient should be allowed to rinse the mouth, gargle, and blow the nose. To reduce the possibility of introducing infectious material into the patient's airway, a sterile catheter should be used and sterile gloves should be worn by the nurse. The catheter should be gently passed through the nares into the trachea, advancing the catheter into the trachea during inspiration.[29] Entry of the catheter into the trachea will be signalled by vigorous coughing. Negative suctioning pressure should be applied only as the catheter is being withdrawn to avoid sucking the lining of the trachea against the opening of the suction catheter and damaging these fragile tissues as the catheter is introduced. The negative pressure should be no more than is necessary to remove the secretions, and the suctioning periods should be short, allowing the patient the opportunity to breath air or oxygen between suctioning periods, because suctioning removes not only accumulated secretions, but also oxygen, from the airway.

Patients may have an artificial airway such as an endotracheal or tracheostomy tube. (See

---

* A man the second author knew was so irritated by what he considered the bad manners of persons clearing out their respiratory tracts that he would say to a stranger making this racket, "The bathroom is the place to do that!" And a woman she knows goes to the bathroom to use a handkerchief and, when questioned about it, said she thought emptying the nose in company nearly as unpleasant as emptying the bladder in public.

Chapter 20 for detailed tracheostomy procedure.) Effective suctioning of these patients requires that the suction catheter be passed into the airway beyond the end of the tube. Secretions that accumulate within the tube may dry and obstruct it, thereby eliminating any benefit of the tube. By keeping the patient adequately hydrated, instilling a small amount of sterile saline solution prior to suctioning, and carefully removing secretions from the inner lumen of the tube, the nurse can help keep the artificial airway patent and functional. Patients with an artificial airway are unable to speak since the larynx is bypassed. The nurse should carefully explain the suctioning treatment, and all other treatments, to patients to allay their apprehension and answer the questions they are unable to ask verbally. A pad and pencil on which they can write questions or observations is useful for those who are able to write. (See Chapter 48.)

Those with severe respiratory difficulties tend to be silent because talking is a tremendous effort. They seem withdrawn to their families and friends because all their energy is focused on their fight for life. Nurses can explain this to their associates, if it seems necessary, and they can suggest to members of the family and intimate friends who are with those sick persons that they try on their visits to do the talking, or perhaps read aloud when patients are able to enjoy it, or simply sit with them quietly as a comforting presence, listen to music, or, perhaps, watch a television program that interests the patient.

Bronchodilating drugs, nebulized detergents, and mucolytic agents increase the lumen of the airway and help liquefy secretions that can then be more easily expectorated. A variety of agents is administered to patients to increase airway patency, and the nurse should be knowledgeable about the actions of each of these. Normal saline administered through a nebulizer moistens the tissues lining the respiratory passages and loosens accumulated secretions, while nebulized distilled water is a mild irritant that stimulates coughing. Detergents such as Alevaire liquefy secretions.[30] Bronchodilators such as isoproterenol (Isuprel) and epinephrine act by relaxing bronchiolar muscle spasms. Proteolytic agents may be administered as aerosols, but they are effective only when the secretions are purulent or proteinaceous, which mucus itself is not.[31]

Nurses cannot know too much about the action of drugs. However, their study should be directed toward classes of drugs, or those with similar effects. There are so many preparations now that the pharmacist has been added to the clinical team in some hospitals. In Chapter 50 on death and dying the value of collaboration between nurse, pharmacist, and physician is discussed. The process of dying involves respiratory failure. In a long-drawn-out death, dyspnea is one of the most distressing and frightening conditions. Bronchodilators or drugs that liquefy, reduce, or drain fluid from the respiratory tract can bring immediate relief to dying persons and to those who watch someone they love struggling to breathe.

Postural drainage utilizes gravity to help remove accumulated secretions from air passages. The patient may be placed in a variety of positions (see Fig. 35-3) to direct secretions from different lobes and regions of the lungs into the trachea from which they can be expectorated. The nurse must see that the patient is in a safe and comfortable position for postural drainage. Adults for whom this treatment is prescribed at home should be taught to manage it independently; parents should be taught to help the child with it.

The psychologic implications cannot be neglected in the care of the patient whose dyspnea is associated with a chronic disease such as emphysema. Since this condition affects males more frequently than females, there may be marked changes in the family structure. When the patient is incapacitated to the point where he is no longer able to work as before, his position as "head of the family" may be threatened. Financial burdens associated with a decreased income and increased expense may force a wife who has never worked during the marriage to seek employment; savings may be consumed and plans for a college education for the children or a comfortable retirement may never be realized. Faced with these changes and the chronicity of the disease, the patient may become irritable, stubborn, and even suicidal.[32] Helping the patient and family cope with their psychologic and financial burdens, as well as providing the patient with the continuing medical and nursing care needed, should be shared by the nurse, social worker, physician, and the family's spiritual adviser. The impact on the family of a chronically ill mother can be severe. Children are deprived of the physical care and attention of their mother that they have come to depend upon. Young children may be unable to comprehend the mother's inability to function as before, and they may become frightened and confused. Older children may have to help care for their ill mother and assume many of the household responsibilities formerly carried by her. The time available for school work and study and associating with friends may be drastically reduced, and the children may resent the demands on their time necessitated by the moth-

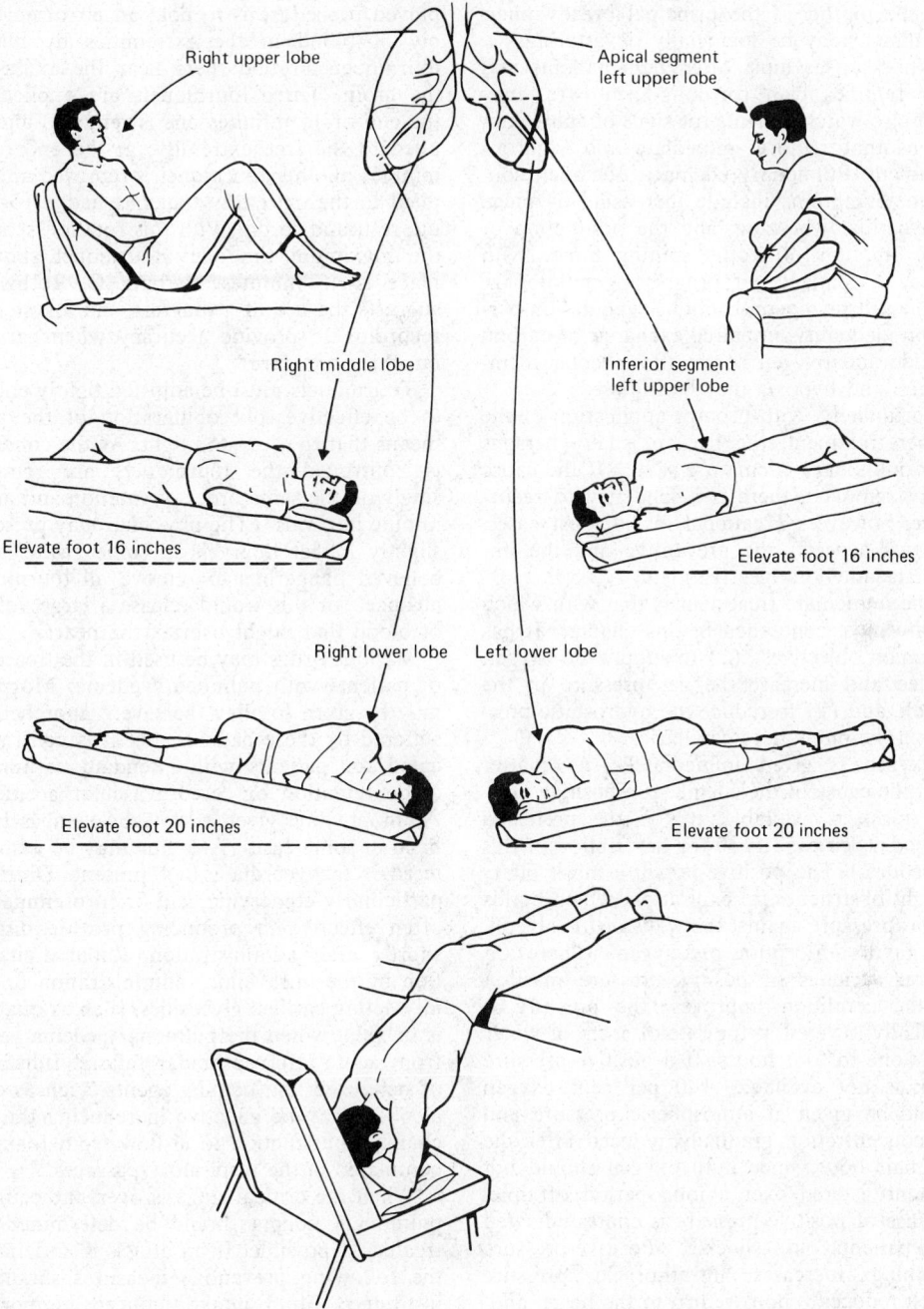

Right upper lobe

Apical segment
left upper lobe

Right middle lobe

Inferior segment
left upper lobe

Elevate foot 16 inches

Elevate foot 16 inches

Right lower lobe Left lower lobe

Elevate foot 20 inches

Elevate foot 20 inches

Figure 35-3. Postural drainage.

er's illness. The husband will find that his wife is no longer able to assume her former share of the family responsibilities. Loss of the assistance of his wife in the management of the home and family and the change in his wife's role from one of active participation and responsibility to one of dependence can place a great burden upon the husband.

Financial difficulties resulting from the mother's illness should be recognized, especially since many women today work outside the home and contribute to the family's income. Absence of a second income, as well as the additional expense of medical care and salaried household help, will often change the family's standard of living. If, as in many families, the mother is the principal breadwinner, her illness may be financially devastating.

While nurses must often help patients and their families plan for long-term care, they must also watch patients for signs of acute conditions that require immediate and vigorous treatment. Pulmonary edema is one such condition. Symptoms include increasing dyspnea, tachycardia, wheezing, and the production of large amounts of frothy sputum tinged with blood. A sequence of progressing pulmonary edema, bronchoconstriction, ventilation-perfusion inequality, impaired exchange of carbon dioxide and oxygen across the alveolar membranes, and hypoxia may be initiated.[33]

Fortunately, with prompt application of the proper treatment, the lives of many persons with pulmonary edema are saved. If the cause is not removed, there is a tendency to recurrence, however. Treatment, as in most cases, has two aspects: the preventive and the immediate ameliorative treatment.

The immediate treatment is that with which we are most concerned in this chapter. It has two main objectives: (1) to supply the oxygen needed and increase the gas pressure in the alveoli, and (2) to reduce the hydrostatic pressure in the pulmonary capillaries.

Oxygen is given immediately, no matter what the cause of the edema. If a positive pressure mask is available, this is the preferred method. (See page 1110 for description of this procedure.) The positive-pressure mask offers a slight obstruction to expiration, which builds up gas pressure against the walls of the alveoli. This favors absorption of oxygen. (There are several varieties of positive-pressure masks.) As the condition improves, the pressure is gradually lowered at the rate of 1 cm of water every one to four hours. If a positive-pressure mask is not available, 100 per cent oxygen should be given at atmospheric pressure and the concentration gradually reduced after the first half hour, since pure oxygen should not be administered over a long period of time. The use of positive pressure is contraindicated for patients in shock.[34] Positive-pressure breathing increases intrathoracic pressure which reduces venous return to the heart, and, therefore, the amount of blood available to be pumped to the body by the left ventricle. Blood pressure should be monitored and positive pressure breathing discontinued if the blood pressure falls markedly.[35] Administration of oxygen is discussed in detail in Chapter 20.

As soon as oxygen therapy is instituted, steps should be taken to reduce hydrostatic pressure in the lungs by decreasing the blood volume. Venesection (phlebotomy), with the removal of 500 to 700 ml of blood, is advocated for hypertensive patients. A more universally employed procedure is to hold an abnormal supply of blood in the extremities by placing tourniquets around them near the axilla and the groin. Three tourniquets are applied. At the end of 15 minutes one is removed and applied to the free extremity; at the end of 30 minutes another tourniquet is removed and applied to the extremity that has had a 15-minute rest, and so on. With this rotation scheme, the maximum time any tourniquet stays in place is 45 minutes. Barbara C. Rothwell[36] suggests the use of a diagram and a system of recording to provide accuracy when carrying out this procedure.

Tourniquets must be adjusted tightly enough to be effective, but obliteration of the pulse means that they are too tight. As the condition is controlled the tourniquets are removed singly, in the same order of rotation and at 15-minute intervals. (The physician may prescribe slightly longer intervals in some cases.) It is believed dangerous to remove all tourniquets at once, for this would release a large volume of blood that might overtax the heart.

Various drugs may be used in the treatment of patients with pulmonary edema. Morphine may be given to allay the severe apprehension suffered by these patients, but it is contraindicated for patients with attendant carbon dioxide retention or cerebrovascular accident.* Aminophylline given slowly, by vein, is beneficial in some cases. Atropine may be administered if tachycardia is not present. Diuretics, particularly ethacrynic acid or furosemide, are often effective in producing profuse diuresis shortly after administration. Rapid digitalization by the intravenous administration of rapidly acting cardiac glycosides, such as ouabain, is of value when the pulmonary edema results from acute left ventricular failure. Inhalation of nebulized antifoaming agents, such as ethyl alcohol, may be effective in reducing the mechanical obstruction to airflow from foam accumulated in the respiratory passages.[37]

When the critical stage is over, the cause of pulmonary edema should be determined and treated, if possible. If an attack is anticipated, the following preventive measures should be instituted: Fluid intake reduced temporarily and 100 per cent oxygen administered for 30 minutes at 30-minute intervals. Bed rest and warmth are also advocated.

3. HYPOXIA

The blood has unique capabilities for transporting oxygen from the lungs to all the body

---

* Many persons have adverse reactions to morphine, and the elderly are especially susceptible.

cells in amounts adequate for their metabolic activities and returning the carbon dioxide produced by the cells to the lungs for excretion. A variety of factors that alters the ventilatory movement of air in and out of the lungs can cause the following: (1) decreased diffusion of gases across the alveolar and pulmonary capillary membranes (alveolar-capillary block); (2) changes in the gas transport capabilities of the blood; (3) shunting of blood to poorly ventilated regions of the lung or of air to poorly perfused regions (ventilation-perfusion abnormalities); and (4) marked alterations in blood gases. Under normal conditions the oxygen tension (pO_2) of arterial blood is about 95 mm Hg and about 40 mm Hg in mixed venous blood.[38] The hemoglobin in blood leaving the left ventricle is usually only slightly less than 100 per cent saturated with oxygen. Under certain conditions and in a number of disease states, a change in blood gases can lead to changes in all the organs of the body and produce signs and symptoms that reflect functional modifications at the cellular level.

Hypoxia implies an availability of oxygen that is less than the cells need. The term anoxia is often used interchangeably with hypoxia, but anoxia really means an absence of oxygen. Profound physiologic alterations occur in hypoxic states, long before true anoxia is reached, and most symptoms presented by patients with an inadequate oxygen supply are due to hypoxia, not anoxia.

Most of the oxygen carried in the blood is transported in combination with hemoglobin, not in simple solution in the plasma. The percentage of hemoglobin saturated with oxygen depends on the oxygen tension (pO_2) in the nonlinear fashion represented by hemoglobin saturation curves. The amount or volume of oxygen in each 100 ml of blood (volumes %) depends on both the hemoglobin concentration of the blood and the per cent saturation of the hemoglobin. The hypoxia associated with respiratory conditions is usually due to decreased hemoglobin saturation rather than decreased amounts of hemoglobin. In fact, patients with chronic hypoxia often have compensatory increases in the number of red blood cells and hemoglobin concentration.

All the disease entities described earlier as giving rise to dyspnea can produce hypoxia if there is an attendant reduction in the amount of oxygen inspired or diffusing across the alveolar and capillary membranes. Hypoxia can also occur when the oxygen-carrying capabilities of the blood are reduced by anemia (decreased hemoglobin) or carbon monoxide inhalation which displaces oxygen from hemoglobin. Depression of the respiratory center in the medulla by drugs or infections predisposes

to hypoxia as do neuromuscular defects and thoracic injuries in which pain or structural damage prevent normal ventilatory movements and reduce the amount of oxygen reaching the alveoli. Head injuries that result in increased intracranial pressure or actual trauma to the medullary respiratory neurons can depress respiration and cause hypoxia.[39]

Nursing Assessment and Measures in Caring for the Hypoxic Patient. Every one of the body's billions of cells use and require oxygen. Hypoxia, therefore, adversely affects the entire body and can produce other than strictly respiratory symptoms. Assessment of the patient, so vital to effective nursing, is based on the nurse's own observations and information given by the family. The rate, depth, and character of respiratory movements are important to note and report accurately. Audible respirations such as stridor (harsh, whistling sounds associated with air being forced past an obstruction) or rales (gurgling sounds heard over the lungs as air flows over fluids) are clues to the cause of the hypoxia and indicate what should be done. Tachypnea (rapid respiration) may be seen in acute hypoxia, but severe hypoxia of long duration is indicated by severely altered, periodic breathing patterns such as *Cheyne-Stokes* respiration and *Biot's* breathing. *Cheyne-Stokes* respiration is characterized by alternating periods of apnea (cessation of breathing) and respirations in which there is an increase in tidal volume followed by a decrease in tidal volume.[40] *Biot's* breathing is similar to *Cheyne-Stokes* in that it is alternating periods of apnea and respiration, but each breath is of about the same size, not a waxing and waning of the tidal volume during the respiratory periods. Both these respiratory patterns usually indicate involvement of the medullary respiratory neurons.

Hypoxia is often accompanied by altered blood pH and carbon dioxide tension. These changes in blood chemistry affect the cells of the brain, and the patient's altered mental state may often provide the earliest indication for nursing intervention. Drowsiness, decreased mental alertness, or coma may be seen in the hypoxic patient; however, restlessness and agitation can also result from other changes in blood gases. Prolonged hypoxia affects organs other than the brain and can produce anorexia, headache, tachycardia, and increased temperature, systolic blood pressure, and renal output.[41] Since the patient's behavior and expression provide one of the earliest signs of decreased oxygen availability, the nurse must carefully record changes in the patient's mental state (such as drowsiness and confusion) and share this information with all members of the health care team.

Hypoxia stimulates cardiovascular changes that attempt to increase the oxygen supply to the hypoxic cells.[42] An increased heart rate occurs in hypoxia, so a rapid pulse may suggest to the nurse the need for suctioning or getting the patient to cough to remove secretions interfering with normal gas exchange or oxygen administration.

Accumulated tracheobronchial secretions are a common cause of hypoxia. They obstruct air passages and decrease the amount of oxygen reaching the alveoli and oxygenating the venous blood. It is the nurse's responsibility to show patients how to cough up the secretions and to encourage them to do this at regular intervals. Although coughing and deep breathing may be prescribed by the physician every 2 hours, the nurse must be alert to signs that indicate a need for these measures at more frequent intervals. The use of intermittent positive pressure breathing (IPPB) with the administration of nebulized saline, bronchodilators, or mucolytic agents, and postural drainage may help patients remove accumulated secretions.

Tracheal suctioning periods should be short (less than 10 seconds) and the suction (negative pressure) should be no more than is necessary because it removes not only mucus but oxygen from the airway. Hypoxia increases the irritability of the myocardium and serious alterations in cardiac electrical activity may result from overvigorous suctioning.[43]

Oxygen may be administered by mask, catheter, or tent to increase the low oxygen tension of the patient's blood. However, an airway free of excessive secretions is still necessary for the oxygen to reach the respiratory surfaces of the alveoli, and the nurse must not neglect attention to this aspect of care simply because the patient is receiving increased concentrations of oxygen. The percentage of oxygen and the rate at which it is given depend upon the method of administration and on the reason for administering it. Oxygen should be administered with care to hypoxic patients, especially those with elevated arterial carbon dioxide tensions.[44] Carbon dioxide is normally the stimulus for the respiratory center in the brain, but when the carbon dioxide has been elevated for a period of time the respiratory center loses its sensitivity to it. In patients with respiratory insufficiency, that is, those with an arterial oxygen tension of less than 50 mm Hg and a carbon dioxide tension of more than 50 mm Hg, the stimulus for cyclic respiratory activity is low oxygen tension, rather than high carbon dioxide tension.[45] Therefore, injudicious administration of oxygen that increases arterial oxygen tension without a concomitant decrease in carbon dioxide level of the blood may re-

move the patient's only respiratory stimulus and lead to cessation of respiration (this is referred to as removing the hypoxic drive). Hypoxic patients with elevated carbon dioxide tensions who are receiving oxygen require critical nursing observation and evaluation, for although it is important that the patient be adequately oxygenated respiratory depression must be avoided and early signs of this detected.

Active persons consume oxygen at a higher rate than inactive ones. Rest, therefore, reduces the oxygen demands of the body. A balanced program of rest and activity based upon the patient's respiratory capabilities eliminates excessive demands on his or her ventilatory system. Some activity is necessary to prevent physiologic and psychologic complications caused by inactivity. Victims of chronic respiratory pathology, such as emphysema, find themselves breathless when they exercise, so they tend to be less and less active until this very inactivity initiates a series of pathologic consequences. If patients are helped to understand the physiologic—and psychologic—consequences of inactivity, they may plan the expenditure of their energy more wisely. Solitude and inactivity with its sensory deprivation will eventually produce the mute persons seen in so many nursing homes. Talking is, in a sense, a respiratory stimulant. If persons are not encouraged to talk, they come to think themselves unable to talk, and finally those around them begin to treat them as mutes.

Exercises of the arms, legs, head, and trunk while lying in bed or on the floor can keep most persons in fair condition. Such exercise is tolerated by many who could not tolerate exercise in a standing position and who cannot walk any distance without discomfort. Mental agitation increases oxygen consumption; the nurse should try to identify sources of irritation and reduce these to a minimum.

4. HYPOCAPNIA AND HYPERCAPNIA

The normal carbon dioxide tension (pCO_2) in arterial blood is about 40 mm Hg and about 46 mm Hg in mixed venous blood. Hypocapnia and hypercapnia mean decreased and increased levels of carbon dioxide in the blood and may be used interchangeably with the terms respiratory alkalosis and respiratory acidosis.

When a patient hyperventilates, carbon dioxide is removed from the body at a rate in excess of its production. The carbon dioxide tension of the blood decreases, the patient becomes hypocapnic, and a respiratory alkalosis is produced. Infectious processes, thyrotoxicosis, overdosage of salicylates, hysteria, and anxiety can produce hyperventilation and hypocapnia. The improper use of mechanical respirators may also result in the removal of excess amounts of carbon dioxide from the body.

Carbon dioxide is hydrated, under the influence of the enzyme carbonic anhydrase, to form carbonic acid (H_2CO_3). Carbonic acid dissociates into hydrogen ions (H^+) and bicarbonate ions (HCO_3^-). The carbonic acid-bicarbonate system is one of the most important buffering systems in the body. In hypocapnia, renal compensation for decreased carbon dioxide provides for excreting additional bicarbonate ions and thereby reducing the alkalinity of the blood. Renal compensation is not a rapid process and hypocapnia, especially that associated with hysteria, is more easily and rapidly corrected by calming patients and having them rebreathe their expired air (and carbon dioxide) from a bag placed over the nose and mouth.

Hypercapnia can be caused by anything that sufficiently decreases ventilation and promotes carbon dioxide retention. Trauma to the chest, obstruction of the airway, drugs that depress respiration, injury of the head, loss of functional lung tissue, and abnormalities of the neuro- and skeletomuscular systems affecting the thoracic cage are some of the causes of carbon dioxide retention and, consequently, hypercapnia. Hypoventilation and the concomitant accumulation of carbon dioxide in the body fluids upsets the normal ratio of bicarbonate to carbonic acid and increases the acidity of the body fluids. This condition is called respiratory acidosis.[46]

An important compensatory mechanism in respiratory acidosis is increased renal production of bicarbonate ions and excretion of hydrogen ions; however, this requires time and may not always provide adequate compensation. Measurement of hydrogen ion concentration (pH) and carbon dioxide tension of arterial blood are important in assessing the patient's compensatory mechanisms and evaluating the effectiveness of therapy. Other laboratory examinations that determine total carbon dioxide content, carbon dioxide combining power, standard bicarbonate, buffer base, and serum electrolytes also provide valuable information on the patient's status, the degree of compensation, and the presence or absence of an acid–base disturbance of metabolic origin superimposed on that of respiratory origin.[47]

Nursing Assessment and Measures in Caring for Patients with Hypo- and Hypercapnia. Even though all the organs and tissues of the body are adversely affected by acid–base disequilibrium, the nervous system is the most

sensitive, and the earliest signs of altered blood gases may be a change in the patient's expression or behavior. Acid–base abnormalities can be due to pulmonary or metabolic causes or both. Laboratory examination of blood for pH, oxygen and carbon dioxide tensions, and bicarbonate levels is necessary to determine whether the patient is suffering from respiratory acidosis (excessive retention of carbon dioxide) or respiratory alkalosis (excessive removal of carbon dioxide) compensated for or complicated by renal factors involved in the defense of body pH, but nurses can identify symptoms in the patient's physiologic state that indicate the need for immediate treatment. Such symptoms include tachycardia, weakness, drowsiness, slurred speech, and coma.

Hypercapnia can occur in obstructive conditions such as emphysema. Persons with this condition expire against resistance and this favors retention of excess carbon dioxide. Within limits, carbon dioxide in the blood provides an important and potent stimulatory drive to the respiratory center in the medulla, as has been noted several times; however, when hypercapnia is severe or of long duration, the medullary respiratory neurons may no longer recognize it as a stimulus. Nurses can themselves report, and help the family to recognize and report, changes in the rate and depth of the person's respirations and his or her mental alertness (usually a decrease), both of which suggest developing respiratory acidosis.

Medical treatments and nursing actions for the hypercapnic patient are directed toward removing excess carbon dioxide from the body. Ventilation may be improved by intermittent positive pressure breathing devices; mucolytic, detergent, and bronchodilating agents decrease airway resistance, while suction, tracheostomy, and mechanically assisted ventilation can facilitate removal of accumulated carbon dioxide.[48] The hypoventilatory state that contributes to carbon dioxide retention may also cause hypoxia. We repeat for emphasis that oxygen must be given to hypercapnic patients with care, since in severely hypercapnic patients, hypoxemia provides the primary stimulus to respiration. If the hypoxemia is corrected without an associated decrease in carbon dioxide tension, the patient will lack the respiratory stimulus it provides and may become apneic. Oxygen therapy is, nevertheless, important in the treatment of patients with increased levels of carbon dioxide, and high carbon dioxide levels can be tolerated for prolonged periods if the patient is adequately oxygenated.[49] Oxygen should be administered to these patients in low concentrations—about 25 to 30 per cent, and at low flow rates.[50,51] The nurse must watch the hypercapnic patient receiving oxygen closely for signs of impaired or reduced ventilation.

Narcotics, most hypnotics, and some other drugs depress the respiratory center. Such drugs must be given with caution to patients with respiratory impairment.

Respiratory alkalosis, or hypocapnia caused by hyperventilation, is seen less frequently than respiratory acidosis. Strong emotion can produce psychogenic dyspnea in those with no abnormality of their ventilatory apparatus and can markedly reduce the blood carbon dioxide tension. As the level of carbon dioxide in the blood decreases, so does the physiologic drive upon the respiratory center, and a compensatory reduction in respiration results that allows the level of carbon dioxide to return to normal. This compensatory reduction in ventilation may be interpreted by extremely sensitive and nervous persons as some respiratory impairment and so make them panic and consciously overbreathe, thus perpetuating and worsening the hypocapnia.[52] In such cases, blood becomes more alkaline, and the pH rises, as excessive amounts of carbon dioxide are "blown off." These changes in the acid–base components of the blood can cause restlessness, blurred vision, and neuromuscular irritability which may result in painful, powerful spasms that begin in the muscles of the face, fingers, and toes.[53] These spasms, if severe, can make the arms or legs assume grotesque positions. This will, of course, be uncomfortable and alarming and further aggravate the hyperventilation. Nurses in schools, clinics, and hospitals may see people with acute respiratory alkalosis from hyperventilation. Their presence with the patient during these episodes and the institution of relief measures can reduce the duration and severity of hyperventilation and the resulting respiratory alkalosis. A critical part of the nursing assessment is recognizing the emotionally labile individual. Nurses can help all concerned to identify and prevent situations that are likely to initiate or exacerbate hyperventilation episodes. An understanding, kind, yet firm, behavior on the part of nurses or others who are with them can often break the vicious circle of hyperventilation-hypocapnia-alkalosis-panic-hyperventilation. Assuring such excited persons that their condition can be relieved quickly, dispelling their panic, and having them rebreathe expired carbon dioxide from an ordinary paper bag held over the nose are effective in reducing the alkalosis resulting from psychogenic hyperventilation.

Not every case of respiratory alkalosis results from psychogenic hyperventilation, however; the acute lowering of carbon dioxide tension in the blood by use of a respirator may produce alkalosis. A person using a respirator should be carefully assessed both for adequate ventilation and signs of respiratory alkalosis such as muscle twitching, hyperactivity, convulsions, and acute cardiac arrhythmias.[54] The kidneys and lungs work together to maintain a normal pH of body fluids. For example, hyperventilation can compensate for an acidosis resulting from abnormal metabolism or kidney function (metabolic acidosis), while hypoventilation can help reduce the pH in metabolic alkalosis.[55] In some instances, therefore, changes in a patient's pattern of ventilation are not detrimental, but compensatory and beneficial. It is the responsibility of nurses to know patients' diagnoses and problems so that they can institute nursing measures consistent with prescribed therapy and with the over-all plan to help patients and their families with the identified problems.

5. ASPHYXIA

Asphyxia comes from the Greek prefix, *a,* absence of, and *sphyxis,* pulse. It is a condition of unconsciousness, due to suffocation or interference of any kind with the oxygenation of the blood. Asphyxia may result from any of the following conditions that produce severe hypoxia: mechanical interference with the entrance of air into the lungs caused by inflammation and swelling of the throat and larynx or the formation of a membrane, as in diphtheria; edema of the glottis in diphtheria, tuberculous laryngitis, cardiac and renal diseases; foreign bodies in the respiratory tract; pressure on the trachea or bronchi from goiter, tumor, or aneurysm; water and mucus in the respiratory tract, as in drowning. The inhalation of smoke, or poisonous gases, such as coal gas, ammonia, nitric acid, and carbon monoxide, which traumatize the respiratory passages or displace oxygen from hemoglobin, as well as diseases of the heart and lungs that decrease the amount of air and oxygen reaching the alveoli or the amount of blood flowing through the lungs, can reduce the availability of oxygen to the body's cells to the point of asphyxia. Other causes of asphyxia are weakness of the respiratory muscles from disease, trauma of the respiratory center in the medulla, fatigue from convulsive spasms or the protracted coughing of croup or whooping cough, and failure of the lungs to expand in the newborn.

The symptoms of asphyxia develop in three stages. In the *first stage* altered oxygen and carbon dioxide tensions of the blood stimulate the respiratory center, making the breathing more rapid (hyperpnea), labored (dyspnea), and distinctly audible. Respiratory muscles not used in quiet breathing are forced into action. The appearance of the patient is alarming—the lips are blue, the face is congested, the eyes are prominent and bloodshot, and the expression is anxious. These alterations may also stimulate peripheral vasoconstriction and raise the blood pressure. This stage lasts about one minute.

In the *second stage,* convulsions occur as a result of further stimulation of the centers in the medulla, and are soon followed by coma.

The *third stage* is characterized by exhaustion. The patient's muscles are flaccid and the pupils widely dilated; blood pressure falls and as the heart fails, the pulse is almost imperceptible. The inspirations are prolonged and sighing, and the intervals between increase until breathing finally ceases. Death results from gradual exhaustion and paralysis of the centers in the medulla. Death from asphyxia may follow in 5 to 10 minutes after the onset of these grave symptoms.

Asphyxia is an emergency situation and there is no time for elaborate assessment. Treatment must be begun immediately. This consists in removing anything that might interfere with breathing, in establishing natural respiration with the least possible delay, and in treating the patient for shock. The first step is to remove any obstruction to the free passage of air, if possible. Foreign bodies, such as false teeth or a partial plate, should be removed from the mouth or throat. Mucus should be wiped out or removed with suction. The patient's position must be such as to keep the air passages wide open and to allow for free expansion of the lungs.

When fluid obstructs the lungs and bronchi, as in drowning, clothing should be loosened about the neck, chest, and waist and the patient then turned on his or her face, and the body raised at the waistline with a folded blanket or clothing. Pressure should then be applied, with both hands outspread over the lower ribs. Fluid from the stomach and lungs will run out by gravity from the esophagus and the trachea through the mouth and nose. Mucus should be removed from the nose, mouth, and throat.

In asphyxia caused by closure of the larynx it may be necessary to introduce an airway. A rubber, plastic, or metal tube can be inserted to keep the respiratory channel sufficiently open to allow the patient to breathe until the obstruction can be removed. Tracheal intubation is indicated whenever an obstruction to breathing is causing, or is in danger of causing,

marked dyspnea, cyanosis, or exhaustion of the patient.*

Articles required for intubation are a mouth gag, an intubator or introducer, an extubator for the removal of the tube, and a set of hard-rubber tubes graded to correspond to the size of the larynx of patients at various ages. Each tube is threaded with silk thread and attached to an obturator.

Successful treatment depends largely on having the patient in a position that will facilitate insertion of the tube. An adult is placed horizontally on the bed or table, with the head perfectly straight and firmly held. A small child is wrapped and confined closely in a sheet, and is held upright by the nurse, with the back of the child's head resting on the nurse's shoulder and the feet securely held between the nurse's knees. Another person should hold the child's head up and backward as far as possible with the chin in a straight line with the trachea. This person also holds the mouth gag in place. The operator (a doctor if he or she is available) sits directly opposite the patient.

A good light is essential. The doctor may wear a head mirror from which the light is reflected into the child's throat; otherwise, the child is held so that the artificial light or light from a window will shine directly into the throat.

Inserting the tube stimulates the secretion of mucus or it may have already collected. The head should be held to one side to allow this to escape or the mouth and throat suctioned. If the tube is properly inserted in the larynx, one or two coughs will be followed soon by quiet breathing and improved color. The subject, worn out with struggling, usually falls asleep. If the tube is passed into the esophagus by mistake coughing will not occur, the color and breathing will not improve, and the string (attached to the tube and left hanging from the mouth) will gradually recede as the peristaltic action carries it down the esophagus. The string or silk thread should be left hanging from the mouth and watched for about 10 minutes; it is then either removed or passed around the ear and fastened to the cheek with Scotch tape. One objection to leaving the silk attached is that it is possible for a child, if not carefully guarded, to reach it and pull the tube out. Removal of the silk thread does not increase the danger from the tube passing into the trachea, because the whole tendency is to cough the tube up and out; however, the silk thread may

* Tracheotomies by courageous laymen have been reported when they found it impossible to dislodge the obstructing object in the throat.

be useful in removing the tube should it go into the esophagus.

The insertion of the tube should take only about two or three seconds. It should not last more than 15 seconds, because the breathing is obstructed during the introduction of the tube. Speedy and successful insertion depends to a great extent upon the assistance, judgment, and presence of mind of those present—physicians, nurses, or others.

In some cases of asphyxia a tracheotomy is performed. This is described on page 1115.

The *aftercare* in asphyxia is very important, and is the particular responsibility of the nurse. The intubation tube is usually left in 2 to 7 days, according to the cause of the asphyxia and the patient's condition. During this time he or she should be constantly watched and given the best nursing care, with particular attention to nutrition. The usual method of feeding is by nasal gavage. Special precautions must be taken to see that the catheter is in the esophagus, and also to prevent any liquid from accidentally entering the tube in the trachea. When nasal feeding is not used, the patient's head is sometimes held much lower than the body, and liquids are given by mouth with a spoon. If there is difficulty in feeding without having liquid enter the tracheal tube, intravenous feeding must be used.

In removing the tube from the respiratory passage, the position of the patient is the same as for its introduction. After its removal, the patient must be closely and continuously watched for any swelling of the throat, or for renewed difficulty in breathing. In hospitals the physician may wait, or be within call, for at least 1 hour.

The administration of oxygen may be indicated in the treatment of asphyxia. Opiates are contraindicated as are all drugs that depress the respiratory center.

In cases of asphyxia in which the larynx and trachea are open and there is no interference with the passage of air to and from the lungs, *artificial respiration* is indicated. If used, it should be started immediately. There are several methods of giving artificial respiration—that is, reestablishing respiration when it has ceased.

The technique of *mouth-to-mouth* resuscitation is not new, but there has been a resurgence in its use, and it is now considered a highly satisfactory method of artificial respiration.[56] Advantages of mouth-to-mouth resuscitation include the facts that it can be rapidly instituted if even one person is present, it delivers a greater tidal volume than most manual methods, and it permits the resuscitator to observe the patient's chest movements and determine if air is moving into and out of his or her lungs. Surprising as it may seem, the operator's expired air contains sufficient oxygen to supply the patient's basal needs.

A patent upper airway, free of any obstruction or secretions, should be assured before beginning mouth-to-mouth resuscitation. The patient's head should be extended and the lower jaw should be lifted upward and backward. This straightens the airway and helps prevent the tongue from falling backward and occluding the airway. A pillow may be placed under the patient's back and shoulders for support and to maintain the extended position of the neck.

The operator inspires deeply, tightly pinches the patient's nostrils shut, places his or her widely opened mouth tightly over the patient's open mouth, and forcibly exhales. The patient's chest will noticeably rise if an adequate tidal volume has been delivered. The operator then removes his or her mouth from the patient's and allows the patient to passively exhale (see Fig. 35-4). The procedure should be repeated 12 to 20 times each minute. During mouth-to-mouth resuscitation, pressure should be applied to the epigastrium to prevent gastric distention by air that the operator may force down the esophagus.[57]

If, for some reason, the operator is unable to form a tight seal over the patient's mouth, mouth-to-nose resuscitation may be employed [58] (see Fig. 35-4). When resuscitating small children, care must be exercised to avoid excessive pressure during inflation, for it could rupture alveoli.

During the application of mouth-to-mouth resuscitation, the operator hyperventilates, and, as a result, may have symptoms of hypocapnia, such as vertigo. Ideally, there should be a relief operator, but if none is available, decreasing the force of exhalation can reduce the loss of carbon dioxide and allow the operator to continue efforts to save the victim of asphyxia.

Mouth-to-mouth (or mouth-to-nose) resuscitation is universally favored now and has supplanted the Schäfer, Sylvester, Holger-Nielsen, and Schäfer-Emerson-Ivy methods, all of which depended on encouraging drainage and alternately expanding and compressing the chest by manipulation of the body. Anyone interested in descriptions of these methods may consult the fifth edition of this text.

Mechanical ventilators (available on beaches where there are lifeguards, in police and fire stations, and in other institutions) provide the most efficient means of artificial respiration, but there should be no delay in instituting other methods of artificial respiration. If pa-

Mouth-to-Mouth Resuscitation

Inspiration   Expiration

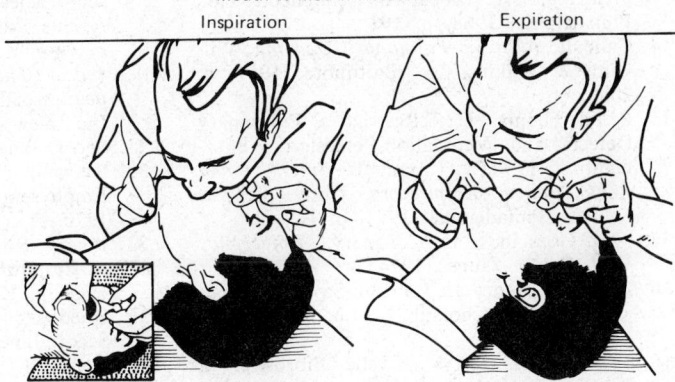

Figure 35-4. Techniques for mouth-to-mouth and mouth-to-nose resuscitation. (Adapted from Secor, Jane: *Patient Care in Respiratory Problems.* W. B. Saunders Co., Philadelphia, 1969.)

Mouth-to-Nose Resuscitation

Inspiration   Expiration

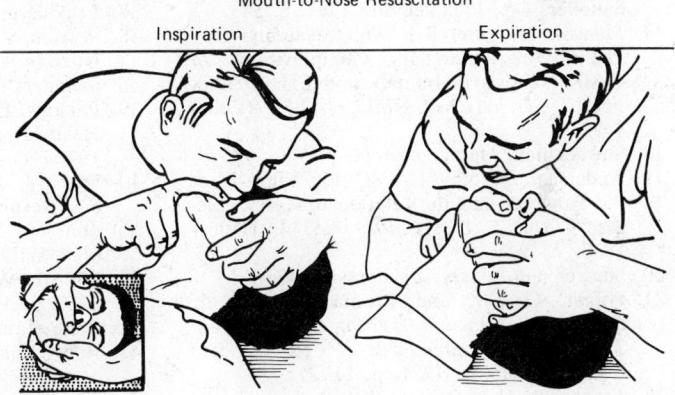

tients are to survive asphyxia or apnea with all their mental faculties intact, they must be oxygenated during the time required to get a respirator or until they can resume spontaneous respiration. Speed in action and perseverance are essential.

REFERENCES

1. Snider, Gordon L.: "Physiologic Causes of Dyspnea," in Banyai, Andrew L., and Gordon, Burgess L. (eds.): *Advances in Cardiopulmonary Diseases,* Vol. IV. Year Book Medical Publishers, Chicago, 1969, p. 156.
2. Hyatt, Robert E.: "Dynamic Lung Volumes," in Fenn, Wallace O., and Rahn, Hermann (eds.): *Handbook of Physiology,* Section 3, *Respiration,* Vol. II. American Physiological Society, Washington, D.C., 1965, p. 1395.
3. Cournand, Andre, and Richards, Dickinson W., Jr.: "Pulmonary Insufficiency. I. Discussion of a Physiological Classification and Presentation of Clinical Tests," *Am. Rev. Tuberc.,* **44:**26, (July) 1941.
4. Leuallen, Edmund C., and Fowler, Ward S.: "Maximal Midexpiratory Flow," *Am. Rev. Tuberc.,* **72:**783, (Dec.) 1955.

5. Otis, A. B.: "The Work of Breathing," in Fenn, Wallace O., and Rahn, Hermann (eds.): *Handbook of Physiology,* Section 3, *Respiration,* Vol. I. American Physiological Society, Washington, D.C., 1965, p. 463.
6. Lukas, Daniel S.: "Dyspnea," in MacBryde, Cyril Mitchell, and Blacklow, Robert Stanley (eds.): *Signs and Symptoms; Applied Pathologic Physiology and Clinical Interpretation.* 5th ed. J. B. Lippincott Co., Philadelphia, 1970, p. 343.
7. Nett, Louise M., and Petty, Thomas L.: "Why Emphysema Patients Are the Way They Are," *Am. J. Nurs.,* **70:**1251, (June) 1970.
8. Guyton, Arthur C.: *Textbook of Medical Physiology,* 5th ed. W. B. Saunders Co., Philadelphia, 1976, p. 576.
9. Secor, Jane: *Patient Care in Respiratory Problems.* W. B. Saunders Co., Philadelphia, 1969, p. 10.
10. Cherniack, Reuben M., et al.: *Respiration in Health and Disease,* 2nd ed. W. B. Saunders Co., Philadelphia, 1972, p. 323.
11. Friedberg, Charles K.: *Diseases of the Heart,* 3rd ed. W. B. Saunders Co., Philadelphia, 1966, p. 1565.
12. Lukas, Daniel S.: *op. cit.,* p. 350.
13. Houston, J. C., et al.: *A Short Textbook of*

Medicine, 3rd ed. J. B. Lippincott Co., Philadelphia, 1968, p. 191.

14. Callcutt, John S.: *Pulmonary Oedema.* Williams & Wilkins Co., Baltimore, 1969, p. 208.
15. Petty, Thomas L.: "Restrictive Pulmonary Defects and Ventilation-Perfusion Abnormalities," in Petty, Thomas L.: *Intensive and Rehabilitative Respiratory Care.* Lea & Febiger, Philadelphia, 1971, p. 129.
15a. "Pop Goes the Cafe Coronary," *Emergency Med.,* **6:**154, (June) 1974.
15b. Heimlich, Henry J.: "A Life-Saving Maneuver to Prevent Choking," *J.A.M.A.,* **234:**398, (Oct. 27) 1975.
16. Shwachman, Harry: "Cystic Fibrosis," in Kendig, Edwin L., Jr. (ed.): *Disorders of the Respiratory Tract in Children.* W. B. Saunders Co., Philadelphia, 1967, p. 543.
17. Mearns, Margaret B.: "Treatment and Prevention of Pulmonary Complications of Cystic Fibrosis in Infancy and Early Childhood," *Arch. Dis. Child.,* **47:**5, (Feb.) 1972.
18. Shwachman, Harry: *op. cit.,* p. 550.
19. Andersen, Dorothy H.: "Cystic Fibrosis of the Pancreas and Its Relation to Celiac Disease," *Am. J. Dis. Child.,* **56:**344, (Aug.) 1938.
20. Shwachman, Harry: *op. cit.,* p. 547.
21. Polgar, George, and Promadhat, Varuni: *Pulmonary Function Testing in Children: Techniques and Standards.* W. B. Saunders Co., Philadelphia, 1971, p. 219.
22. Tropauer, Alan, et al.: "Psychological Aspects of the Care of Children with Cystic Fibrosis," *Am. J. Dis. Child.,* **119:**424, (May) 1970.
23. Scarpelli, Emile M.: *The Surfactant System of the Lung.* Lea & Febiger, Philadelphia, 1968, p. 1.
24. *Ibid.,* p. 177.
25. Reynolds, E. O. R.: "Effect of Alterations in Mechanical Ventilator Settings on Pulmonary Gas Exchange in Hyaline Membrane Disease," *Arch. Dis. Child.,* **46:**152, (Apr.) 1971.
26. Gregory, George A., et al.: "Treatment of the Idiopathic Respiratory-Distress Syndrome with Continuous Positive Airway Pressure," *N. Engl. J. Med.,* **284:**1333, (June 17) 1971.
27. Said, Sami I.: "Metabolic Events in the Lung," in Frohlich, Edward D. (ed.): *Pathophysiology.* J. B. Lippincott Co., Philadelphia, 1972, p. 173.
28. Secor, Jane: *op. cit.,* p. 41.
29. Tyler, Martha L., et al.: "Intensive Nursing, Inhalation Therapy, and Physical Therapy," in Petty, Thomas L.: *Intensive and Rehabilitative Respiratory Care,* 2nd ed. Lea & Febiger, Philadelphia, 1974, p. 81.
30. Swinyard, Ewart A.: "Demulcents, Emollients, Protectives and Adsorbents, Antiperspirants and Deodorants, Absorbable Hemostatics, Astringents, Irritants, Sclerosing Agents, Caustics, Keratolytics, Anti-

seborrheics, Melanizing and Demelanizing Agents, Mucolytics, and Certain Enzymes," in Goodman, Louis S., and Gilman, Alfred (eds.): *The Pharmacological Basis of Therapeutics,* 5th ed. Macmillan Publishing Co., Inc., New York, 1975, p. 997.
31. Secor, Jane: *op. cit.,* p. 42.
32. Schwaid, Madeline C.: "The Impact of Emphysema," *Am. J. Nurs.,* **70:**1247, (June) 1970.
33. Peters, Richard M.: *The Mechanical Basis of Respiration.* Little, Brown & Co., Boston, 1969, p. 124.
34. Friedberg, Charles K.: *op. cit.,* p. 427.
35. Secor, Jane: *op. cit.,* p. 59.
36. Rothwell, Barbara C.: "Nursing Care in Pulmonary Edema," *Am. J. Nurs.,* **48:**700, (Nov.) 1948.
37. Friedberg, Charles K.: *op. cit.,* p. 426.
38. Watson, Jeannette E.: *Medical-Surgical Nursing and Related Physiology.* W. B. Saunders Co., Philadelphia, 1972, p. 264.
39. Parsons, L. Claire: "Respiratory Changes in Head Injury," *Am. J. Nurs.,* **71:**2187, (Nov.) 1971.
40. Seabury, John H.: "Pulmonary Ventilation and Respiration; Tests of Respiratory Function," in Sodeman, William A., and Sodeman, William A., Jr.: *Pathologic Physiology,* 4th ed. W. B. Saunders Co., Philadelphia, 1967, p. 527.
41. Secor, Jane: *op. cit.,* p. 46.
42. Riley, Robert L.: "Gas Exchange and Transportation," in Ruch, Theodore C., and Patton, Harry D. (eds.): *Physiology and Biophysics,* 19th ed. W. B. Saunders Co., Philadelphia, 1965, p. 785.
43. Jacquette, Germaine: "To Reduce Hazards of Tracheal Suctioning," *Am. J. Nurs.,* **71:**2362, (Dec.) 1971.
44. Arnold, Winslow H., Jr., and Grant, Joseph L.: "Oxygen-Induced Hypoventilation," *Am. Rev. Resp. Dis.,* **95:**255, (Feb.) 1967.
45. Traver, Gayle A.: *Nursing the Patient with Respiratory Insufficiency,* League Exchange No. 96. National League for Nursing, New York, 1972.
46. Bigelow, D. Boyd: "Acid-Base and Electrolyte Abnormalities in Respiratory Failure," in Petty, Thomas L.: *Intensive and Rehabilitative Respiratory Care,* 2nd ed. Lea & Febiger, Philadelphia, 1974, p. 69.
47. Beerel, F. R., and Vance, J. W.: "A Simplified Method for Presenting Acid-Base Balance Situations," *Chest,* **5:**480, (May) 1970.
48. Secor, Jane: *op. cit.,* p. 51.
49. Bigelow, D. Boyd: *op. cit.,* p. 76.
50. Traver, Gayle A.: *op. cit.,* p. 3.
51. Secor, Jane: *op. cit.,* p. 49.
52. Lukas, Daniel S.: *op. cit.,* p. 347.
53. Weiner, Michael W., and Epstein, Franklin H.: "Signs and Symptoms of Electrolyte Disorders," in Maxwell, Morton H., and Kleeman, Charles R. (eds.): *Clinical Disorders of Fluid and Electrolyte Metabolism,*

2nd ed. McGraw-Hill Book Co., New York, 1972, p. 653.

54. Peters, Richard M.: *op. cit.*, p. 301.
55. Makoff, Dwight L.: "Acid-Base Metabolism," in Maxwell, Morton H., and Kleeman, Charles R. (eds.): *Clinical Disorders of Fluid and Electrolyte Metabolism*, 2nd ed. McGraw-Hill Book Co., New York, 1972, pp. 328, 333.
56. Stephenson, Hugh E., Jr.: *Cardiac Arrest and Resuscitation*, 4th ed. C. V. Mosby Co., St. Louis, 1974, p. 257.
57. Secor, Jane: *op. cit.*, p. 161.
58. Stephenson, Hugh E., Jr.: *op. cit.*, p. 261.

Additional Suggested Reading

Asmundsson, Tryggi, and Kilburn, Kaye H.: "Survival of Acute Respiratory Failure," *Ann. Intern, Med.*, **70**:471, (Mar.) 1969.

Bader, Mortimer E., and Bader, Richard A.: "Intermittent Positive Pressure Breathing," in Banyai, Andrew L., and Gordon, Burgess L. (eds.) *Advances in Cardiopulmonary Diseases*, Vol. IV. Year Book Medical Publishers, Chicago, 1969.

Belinkoff, Stanton: *Emphysema and Chronic Bronchitis*. Little, Brown & Co., Boston, 1971.

Bhagwanani, S. G., et al.: "Prediction of Neonatal Respiratory Distress by Estimation of Amniotic-Fluid Lecithin," *Lancet*, **1**:159, (Jan. 22) 1972.

Byers, Virginia B.: *Nursing Observation*. Wm. C. Brown Co., Dubuque, Iowa, 1968.

Chang, Nora, and Levison, Henry: "The Effect of a Nebulized Bronchodilator Administered with or Without Intermittent Positive Pressure Breathing on Ventilatory Function in Children with Cystic Fibrosis and Asthma," *Am. Rev. Resp. Dis.*, **106**:867, (Dec.) 1972.

Cherniack, Reuben M.: "Ventilation, Perfusion and Gas Exchange," in Frohlich, Edward D. (ed.): *Pathophysiology*. J. B. Lippincott Co., Philadelphia, 1972.

Cournand, Andre, et al.: "The Oxygen Cost of Breathing," *Trans. Assoc. Am. Physicians*, **67**:162, 1954.

Davenport, Horace W.: *The ABC of Acid-Base Chemistry*, 5th ed. University of Chicago Press, Chicago, 1969.

Early, Mary: "The Gaseous Exchange Process: Nursing Implications," in Kintzel, Kay Corman (ed.): *Advanced Concepts in Clinical Nursing*. J. B. Lippincott Co., Philadelphia, 1971.

Featherby, Elizabeth A.: "Use of Pulmonary Function Tests in Asthma and Cystic Fibrosis," *Proc. R. Soc. Med.*, **64**:582, (May) 1971.

Feldman, Stanley A., and Crawley, Brian E.: *Tracheostomy and Artificial Ventilation*, 2nd ed. Williams & Wilkins Co., Baltimore, 1972.

Foley, Mary F.: "Pulmonary Function Testing," *Am. J. Nurs.*, **71**:1134, (June) 1971.

Foley, Robert E.: "The Management of Acute Pulmonary Edema," *Med. Clin. North Am.*, **53**:327, (Mar.) 1969.

Gross, Paul, and Detreville, Robert T. P.: "The Lung as an Embattled Domain Against Inanimate Pollutants," *Am. Rev. Resp. Dis.*, **106**:684, (Nov.) 1972.

Hsieh, Yuan-Ching, et al.: "The Effect of Cold Air Inhalation on Respiratory Gas Exchange During Exercise in Patients with Chronic Obstructive Pulmonary Disease," *Chest*, **57**:18, (Jan.) 1970.

Johnson, Paul C.: "Nervous and Chemical Control of Respiration," in Selkurt, Ewald E. (ed.): *Physiology*, 3rd ed. Little, Brown & Co., Boston, 1971.

Karpatkin, Margaret, et al.: "Respiratory-Distress Syndrome and Disseminated Intravascular Coagulation in Two Siblings," *Lancet*, **1**:102, (Jan. 8) 1972.

Knowles, John H.: *Respiratory Physiology and Its Clinical Application*. Harvard University Press, Cambridge, Mass., 1959.

Lloyd, Thomas C., Jr.: "Respiratory Gas Exchange and Transport," in Selkurt, Ewald E. (ed.): *Physiology*, 3rd ed. Little, Brown & Co., Boston, 1971.

Lowry, Thomas P. (ed.): *Hyperventilation and Hysteria*. Charles C Thomas, Publisher, Springfield, Ill., 1967.

McFadden, E. R., Jr., and Linden, David A.: "A Reduction in Maximum Mid-Expiratory Flow Rate," *Am. J. Med.*, **52**:725, (June) 1972.

McGregor, Maurice, and Becklake, Margaret R.: "The Relationship of Oxygen Cost of Breathing to Respiratory Mechanical Work and Respiratory Force," *J. Clin. Invest.*, **40**:971, (June) 1961.

Mitchell, Robert A.: "Control of Respiration," in Frohlich, Edward D. (ed.): *Pathophysiology*. J. B. Lippincott Co., Philadelphia, 1972.

Moore, Francis D., et al.: *Post-Traumatic Pulmonary Insufficiency*. W. B. Saunders Co., Philadelphia, 1969.

Morgan, Thomas E.: "Pulmonary Surfactant," *N. Engl. J. Med.*, **284**:1185, (May 27) 1971.

Nelson, Nicholas M.: "Of HMD, ICU'S, CPAP and Jenner," *N. Eng. J. Med.*, **284**:1376, (June 17) 1971.

Pace, William R., Jr.: *Pulmonary Physiology in Clinical Practice*, 2nd ed. F. A. Davis Co., Philadelphia, 1970.

Paget, V.: "Bronchial Lavage and ıermittent Positive-Pressure Ventilation," *Nurs. Times*, **65**:1200, (Sept. 18) 1969.

Porter, Ruth (ed.) *Breathing: Hering-Breur Centenary Symposium*, a Ciba Foundation Symposium. J. & A. Churchill, London, 1970.

Rodman, Theodore, and Sterling, Francis H.: *Pulmonary Emphysema and Related Lung Diseases*. C. V. Mosby Co., St. Louis, 1969.

Rosenblatt, Milton B.: "Emphysema: Historical Perspective," *Bull. N.Y. Acad. Med.*, **48**:823, (July) 1972.

Sedlock, Stephanie Ann: "Detection of Chronic Pulmonary Disease," *Am. J. Nurs.*, **72**:1407, (Aug.) 1972.

Selkurt, Ewald E., and Johnson, Paul C.: "Respiratory and Renal Regulation of Acid-Base Balance," in Selkurt, Ewald E. (ed.): *Physiology*, 3rd ed. Little, Brown & Co., Boston, 1971.

Sheffer, Albert L., and Valentine, Martin D.:

"The Treatment of Bronchial Asthma," *Med. Clin. North Am.,* **53:**239, (Mar.) 1969.

Sinha, R., and Bergofsky, E. H.: "Prolonged Alteration of Lung Mechanics in Kyphoscoliosis by Positive Pressure Hyperinflation," *Am. Rev. Resp. Dis.,* **106:**47, (July) 1972.

Slonim, N. Balfour, and Hamilton, Lyle H.: *Respiratory Physiology,* 3rd ed. C. V. Mosby Co., St. Louis, 1976.

Tuttle, W. W., and Schottelius, Byron A.: *Textbook of Physiology,* 17th ed. C. V. Mosby Co., St. Louis, 1973.

Waligora, Sister Barbara Marie: "The Effect of Nasal and Oral Breathing upon Nasopharyngeal Oxygen Concentration," *Nurs. Res.,* **19:**75, (Jan.–Feb.) 1970.

West, John B.: "Causes of Carbon Dioxide Retention in Lung Disease," *N. Engl. J. Med.,* **284:**1232, (June 3) 1971.

LaNelle E. Geddes
Virginia Henderson

CHAPTER 36

Marked Disturbance of Nutrition, Fluid and Electrolyte Balance— Starvation-Undernutrition, Obesity, Vomiting and Diarrhea

1. STARVATION-UNDERNUTRITION
2. OBESITY
3. VOMITING
4. DIARRHEA

1. STARVATION-UNDERNUTRITION

Starvation may be general or specific. General starvation of the body implies being without food for long periods and is most often seen in poverty, famine, droughts, wars, and some chronic diseases, including advanced neoplasms and anorexia nervosa. Specific starvation refers to a severe deficiency of a specific nutrient (if any), for instance, protein, resulting in kwashiorkor, which is widespread in the Far East, Africa, and Latin America.

Undernutrition, which borders on starvation in more situations than most people would like to admit, may be defined as any deviation below good nutrition whenever it can be demonstrated that a nutrient is responsible for subnormal response to any of the following: (1) normal growth; (2) normal development, maintenance, and function of all body organs and tissues; (3) reproduction; (4) optimal work efficiency; (5) necessary calories for energy requirements; (6) ability to repair injury; and (7) maximal resistance to infection.[1] The term malnutrition may be used to imply undernutrition or overnutrition—obesity, for example.

Undernutrition, semistarvation, or starvation are physical conditions that result from a negative nutritive balance; they occur when metabolic utilization and excretion of one or more essential nutrients exceeds intake.

Fortunately, the human body has a remarkable capacity for surviving on limited intake and even without food for long periods. The fasting period of 40 days and 40 nights by Jesus as recorded in the Bible has been shown repeatedly to be within the capability of a healthy adult. For example, Terence Mac-Swiney, the Irish revolutionist and mayor of Cork, in his hunger strike in a British prison in 1920 survived for 74 days before dying of starvation.[2]

Ancel Keys, in his book *The Biology of Human Starvation*[3] (1950), gives us the most comprehensive review of world literature including reports of his own important experiments. Descriptions of severe undernutrition in concentration camps and prisons of World War II as well as famines in so many parts of the world have been provided by others. Most of these publications were available to members of various health groups—not to the general public—and the American scientists who were concerned with clinical aspects of nutrition usually focused their attention on the underdeveloped countries where the problems are acute. Such research is supported by a number of American and international agencies—it is said to be less disturbing than domestic research that raises social issues on a local, state, and national level.

However, the picture changed radically during the 1960s when the disgraceful state of hunger and poverty in the United States was exposed to all the people by the Southern Christian Leadership Conference, a group dedicated to improving the life of poor blacks, led by Martin Luther King. Jean Mayer, chairman of the White House Conference on Food, Nutrition and Health of December 1969, describing the contribution of Dr. King and his group says:

That the national conscience was awakened slowly is attributable in part to the failure of professionals in the health field to recognize the extent -of this nation's nutrition problems. Indeed, it was not the experts but rather a small, heterogeneous group of concerned citizens who took the first steps toward eliminating hunger among the black agricultural workers in the deep South.*

Gradually, a growing number of concerned Americans became aware of the fact that many were hungry, malnourished, or actually starved. To identify "hunger counties" where malnutrition was a way of life, a board of inquiry titled National Council on Hunger and Malnutrition in the United States was established under the leadership of the Field Foundation and it included other concerned organizations. Some members of Congress, including Joseph Clark and George McGovern and the late Robert Kennedy, took up the cause, and a number of dedicated individuals like Dorothy Height, Robert Choate, John Kramer, Leslie Dunbar, and the late Walter Reuther spoke on the problem before many groups all over the country. Finally, newspapers and television and radio networks publicized it. Journalists published pioneering articles and books. A notable example is *Let Them Eat Promises* by Nathan Kotz.[4] This was followed by a CBS television documentary titled "Hunger in America"—a vivid description of the findings of the National Council and other investigative bodies. Recognition of poverty, so real to so many people, became public. Too much emphasis on the rising average income and the ever-increasing gross national product had lulled people into thinking that there was no poverty in the United States.

It is impossible to describe in a work such as this the poverty and associated problems of malnutrition and starvation that continue to exist in the United States and other countries. We suggest, therefore, that references at the end of this chapter be consulted and that all persons, particularly members of all health groups, read *Poverty, Ethnic Identity, and Health Care* by Bonnie Bullough and Vern L. Bullough[5] and *U.S. Nutrition Policies in the Seventies,* edited by Jean Mayer.[6]

Incidence. According to Sohan L. Manocha,[7] undernutrition and malnutrition among adults and children on all continents has been so acute during the past few decades that the eugenic effects cannot be ignored. Approximately half of the present population has managed to survive a period of severe nutritional deprivation during childhood; and of all the children of the world, more than half are said

to be "at risk" from the serious effects of malnutrition.[8] Manocha estimates that "more than 350 million children, or seven out of ten children under the age of six in the entire world, are affected by some degree of malnutrition which leads to impaired learning potential and hence deterioration of the genetic quality of the human species." * He notes that protein and protein-calorie malnutrition is now the most widespread nutritional disease, causing an alarming number of deaths especially in the developing countries. Clinical diseases characterized by protein deficiency, notably kwashiorkor and marasmus, have been reported among American Indians and migrant farm workers in Florida.[9,10] (See Fig. 36-1 for a listing of the signs and symptoms of these two diseases.)

In the United States about one person in eight (or 26 millon persons of the present population of 210 million) is inadequately nourished, and the majority of these are children. Authorities consistently note that poverty is the most common cause of malnutrition in the United States (as well as many other countries). This is a great tragedy, since the United States has available the technology and resources to produce and distribute all necessary nutrients for all its people, plus much more for export to other less fortunate peoples.[11]

Hunger is a problem in all age groups and affects all races. As we have said, infants and children—the helpless—are affected most often. Studies have shown that a family of one aged person or an elderly couple were more likely to experience hunger than other families because their incomes fall below the poverty line.[12] One of the most troubled regions in the United States is the southern Appalachians, encompassing approximately 80,000 square miles and including parts of Alabama, Georgia, Kentucky, North Carolina, Virginia, and West Virginia. Maryland and South Carolina are on the fringe of the area. Migrant farm workers, composed of ethnic minority groups, consist of three major streams, according to Bullough and Bullough, who say:

One group spends the winter in Florida and Georgia, harvesting winter crops and moving northward through the Atlantic states in the summer and returning late in the fall; a second group moves northward from Texas and spreads out through the central states, while a third stream is centered in California and the Pacific states.†

* Mayer, Jean (ed.): *U.S. Nutrition Policies in the Seventies.* W. H. Freeman & Co., San Francisco, 1973, p. 2.

* Manocha, Sohan L.: *Malnutrition and Retarded Human Development.* Charles C Thomas, Publisher, Springfield, Ill., 1972, p. 5.
† Bullough, Bonnie, and Bullough, Vern L.: *Poverty, Ethnic Identity, and Health Care.* Appleton-Century-Crofts, New York, 1972, p. 115.

Figure 36-1. Schematic representation of the interrelationship of kwashiorkor and marasmus. At the left of the pyramidal base, the intensity of the stippling suggests the frequency with which the signs and symptoms listed appear in marasmus. At the right, the occurrence of the same signs and symptoms in "classic" kwashiorkor are portrayed. In between are all combinations between these two extremes. The severity of the signs and symptoms is indicated by the distance from the apex. (From Manocha, Sohan L.: *Malnutrition and Retarded Human Development*. Charles C Thomas, Publisher, Springfield, Ill., 1972, p. 19.)

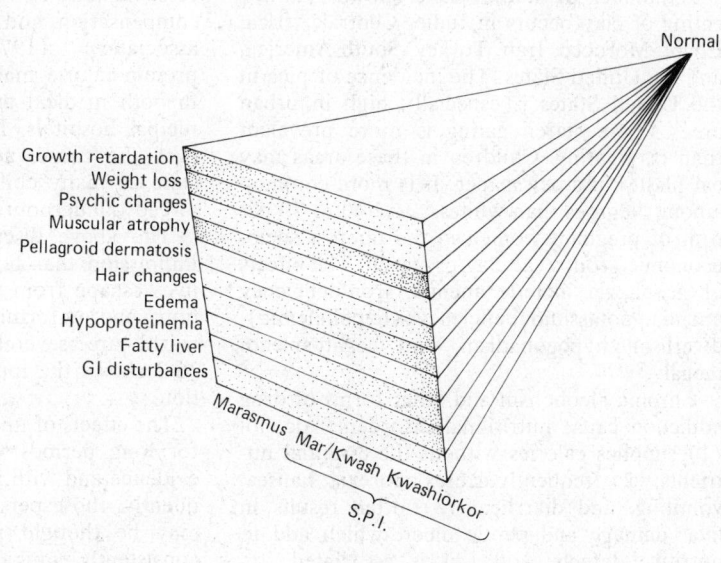

Not only do many of these persons suffer from hunger but also from poor sanitation, housing, medical care, and education. The plight of the American Indian has been told repeatedly in the press and on radio and television networks as has that of those (both blacks and whites) in the slums of large cities. Many people have periods of going without a meal and most eat only one meal a day.

Causes and Effects. The primary cause of undernutrition, semistarvation, or starvation is an insufficient intake of nutrients or interference with absorption or storage of these to meet the metabolic needs of the body, resulting in a negative caloric balance.

Poverty and *ignorance* are consistently listed as the two most common factors contributing to undernutrition of the world's population, including affluent societies. Unfortunately, the poor and uneducated in many countries constitute the large majority of the population. These people often do not have the money to purchase an optimal diet, the best foods are not always available to them because of distribution problems, and frequently, when proper foods are available, both economically and physically, they are not chosen because of lack of information, misinformation, inconvenience, habit, or local, religious, or ethnic customs that prohibit the choice. Cyril M. MacBryde, criticizing the literature on nutrition, says:

In the United States one might mistakenly think from reading nutrition manuals that we are all Anglo-Saxon in our eating habits. The truth is instead that our people are heterogeneous in racial and social backgrounds and customs; food choices differ widely in various groups and localities. Foods considered pleasing to the palate are often widely different between Spanish-Americans, Chinese-Americans, Italo-Americans, Afro-Americans, Anglo-Saxon Americans, Jewish-Americans. . . .*

The diets of the poor consist primarily of carbohydrates, such as corn, wheat, rice, and potatoes; they are lacking in foods supplying fats and "protective" nutrients (proteins, vitamins, and minerals) found in meat, eggs, milk, vegetables, and fruits, which are more costly because they are hard to produce and distribute.

Food faddism of all types, including vegetarianism, is not uncommon and may cause many different types of deficiencies. Another form of undernutrition results from ingestion of abnormal substances because of an individual idiosyncrasy, custom, or severe hunger. The term *pica* means eating any foreign substance, including earth, dirt, clay, dried paint and putty, and starch. *Geophagia* means the eating of grass, leaves, dirt, and other substances. This occurs throughout the world, especially among the poor and malnourished who do it to allay hunger pains.

* MacBryde, Cyril M.: "Weight Loss and Undernutrition," in MacBryde, Cyril M., and Blacklow, Robert Stanley (eds.): *Signs and Symptoms; Applied Pathologic Physiology and Clinical Interpretation*, 5th ed. J. B. Lippincott Co., Philadelphia, 1970, p. 873.

A number of studies have shown that the eating of clay occurs in India, Central Africa, Egypt, Morocco, Iran, Turkey, South America, and the United States. The incidence of pica in the United States is especially high in urban areas where starch eating is more prevalent than clay eating. Children in these areas may eat plaster and newspaper. It is more common among Negroes than whites,* and 40 to 70 per cent of pregnant women in the poorest socioeconomic groups eat clay or starch. The effects of geophagia include anemia, iron-deficiency anemia, potassium deficiency (hypokalemia), dwarfism, hypogonadism, and hepatosplenomegaly.[13-15]

Chronic alcoholism and other forms of drug addiction cause nutritional disorders. Alcohol (1) supplies calories without the essential nutrients; (2) frequently causes anorexia, nausea, vomiting, and diarrhea; (3) often results in liver damage and peptic ulcer, which add to nutritive defects; and (4) is associated frequently with neglected diets. All alcoholics suffer from malnutrition to some degree. They lose interest in food and eventually find it repugnant. Addictive drugs of all kinds tend to reduce activity and alter judgment about diet selection.

Organic diseases of many types may cause undernutrition (mild or severe). Diseases of the mouth, the tongue, and the pharynx may restrict diets to liquids over a long period. Diseases of the gastrointestinal tract, including inflammatory, ulcerative, neoplastic, and obstructive diseases, or surgery on the tract, usually interfere with normal food intake. Anorexia, nausea, or vomiting associated with these conditions frequently add to undernutrition (specific or general).

In the *malabsorption syndrome,* a term used to designate a group of diseases that include tropical sprue, nontropical sprue, idiopathic steatorrhea, and celiac disease, there is severe chronic diarrhea with loss of important nutrients.

Any *psychic disorder* can affect the function of the alimentary canal as well as interest in food. In anorexia nervosa, the person actually shuns food and will only pick at once favored dishes. Intravenous and gastrointestinal feedings are not uncommon to sustain life.

In certain physical disorders the total body metabolism may be increased so that a much greater supply of nutrients than normal is required. Examples of such conditions are fevers, neoplasms, hyperthyroidism, cardiac decompensation, and trauma. B. R. Bristrian and associates[15a] (1976) report that significant protein-calorie malnutrition occurs commonly in both medical and surgical patients in municipal hospitals. Low-grade infections, whatever the cause, add to the poor nutritional state of many children in the world who are already undernourished.

The above discussion leaves one with the impression that few persons throughout their lives escape from some degree of undernutrition; and unfortunately many people in the world are severely undernourished. Figure 36-2 shows the multiple etiology of malnutrition.

The effects of undernutrition may be obscure for long periods with little, if any, physical evidence and with ill-defined symptoms; consequently, those persons who seek health advice may be thought psychoneurotic. Authorities consistently emphasize the importance of early detection of undernutrition before marked signs appear.

MacBryde[16] describes five distinguishable stages of nutritional failure. Stage I is called negative balance. The demand for one or more nutrients is so great that supply cannot keep pace or it is deficient.

Stage II is called tissue depletion. Stored nutrients are used up and supplies in the cells, tissues, and fluids are drawn on. The tissue depletion stage may proceed for considerable periods before other effects are evident and symptoms appear, because as a rule, the body carries certain protective reserves.

Stage III is recognized as a biochemical disturbance. It occurs when abnormalities in the fluids and tissues reach a point where chemical changes in the blood and tissues may be measured. In protein deficiency, for example, total serum protein falls, especially the albumin fraction, with a smaller decrease in serum globulin. A disturbance in electrolytes may occur with a decrease in chloride, sodium, potassium, and magnesium; sodium bicarbonate is reduced in the presence of ketosis. Notable changes in vitamins may occur, such as low levels of ascorbic acid in deficiencies of vitamin C and a lengthened prothrombin time with the lack of vitamin K. Calcium or phosphorus levels may be low in rickets, while the phosphate level may be elevated. These are the findings of some of the chemical tests that are helpful in detecting early stages of undernutrition before functional or anatomic evidence is present.

In stage IV, where there are functional changes, victims are finally aware of disturbance of function, although at first neither they

---

* Such comparisons are questionable since the two groups are not equally affluent. It is possible that this habit is associated with poverty rather than any racial characteristic.

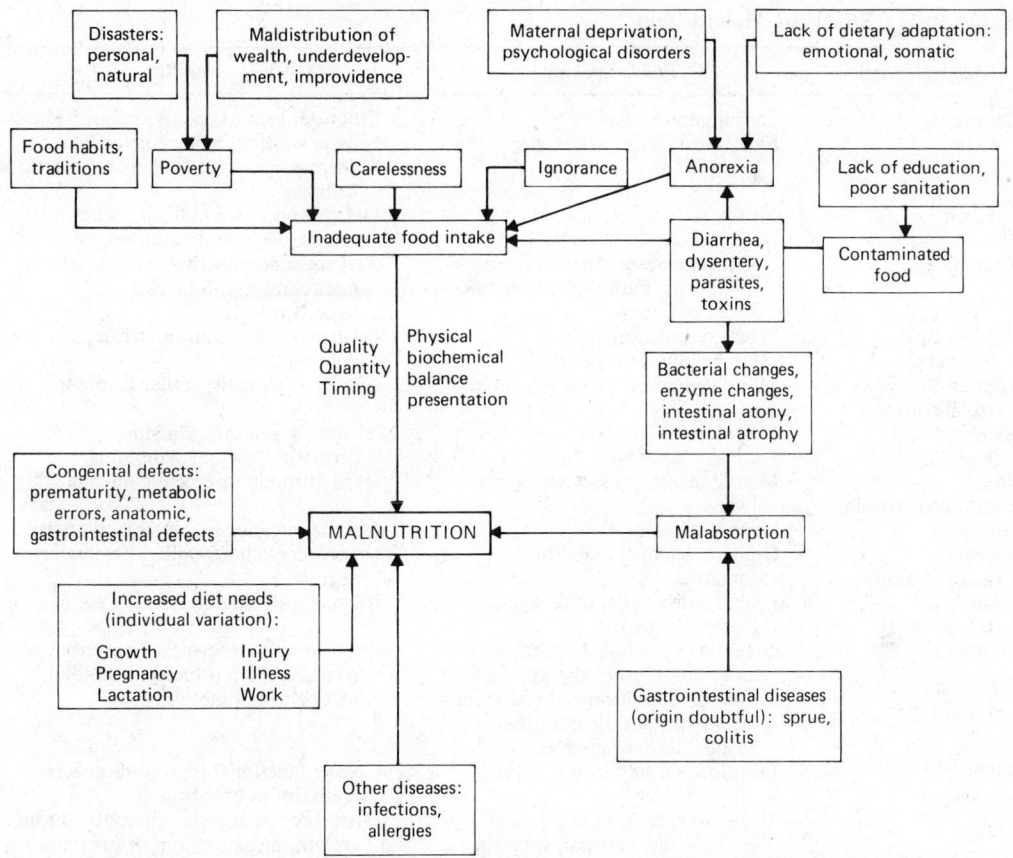

Figure 36-2. The multiple etiology of malnutrition. (From Manocha, Sohan L.: *Malnutrition and Retarded Human Development.* Charles C Thomas, Publisher, Springfield, Ill., 1972, p. 18.)

nor their therapist may recognize the disturbed function as a stage of tissue depletion and biochemical disturbance, for they are present over long periods. Some of the first symptoms may be characteristic. Aching legs in children (called growing pains) is, for example, a sign of rickets; sore gums is characteristic of scurvy; paresthesiae (or leg pains), of thiamine deficiency; or a disturbed mental state, of pellagra. In more advanced starvation, symptoms indicating functional changes include lack of energy, fatigue, dizziness, faintness, a tendency to collapse on prolonged standing, leg ache, backache, chilliness, and numbness. Vital signs are affected. For example, the pulse rate may be as low as 40 beats per minute, systolic blood pressure reduced to 80 mm of mercury, and body temperature lowered to 35°C (95°F).

Stage V, characterized by anatomic lesions, is difficult to separate from stage IV (functional changes), since they are part of the same process and functional disturbances may

be present for long periods before physical manifestations appear. Weight loss is the most common physical sign; at first it may be slight and slow but if uncorrected it will progress to emaciation. There is muscle waste after fat padding is lost. Pallor is usually present and there may be hemorrhages into the skin, dermatitis, edema of the legs, and collapse of vertebrae. The effects of severe undernutrition in various deficiency states are given in Table 36-1 of this chapter and Table 10-1, Chapter 10. Extreme undernutrition may be fatal. In advanced nutritional failure, there is extreme emaciation, loss of practically all body fat, muscle atrophy, and extreme weakness. The skin loses its elasticity, is dry, rough, and wrinkled; the hair is dry, brittle, and gray and breaks and falls out; the gums may bleed and atrophy; and the teeth may be carious, loose, and even fall out.

The effects of undernutrition are devastating to the very young. If it occurs during the critical stages of rapid growth, changes in the

Table 36-1.　Effects of Malnutrition *

Factor Lacking	Foods Lacking	Results
Calories	Carbohydrates, fats	Thinness, lack of energy, failure to grow
Protein	Eggs, meat, milk, wheat, corn, rice, peas, beans	Muscle wasting, hypoproteinemia, anemia, edema, osteoporosis, fractures of bone
Calcium	Milk	Defective bones and teeth, rickets; osteomalacia and tetany in pregnancy
Vitamin A	Green vegetables, carrots, tomatoes, milk, eggs, butter, fish-liver oils, sweet potatoes	Xerosis of conjunctiva and cornea, nightblindness, follicular hyperkeratosis
Vitamin B_1 (thiamine)	Whole cereals, milk, meat (especially liver and pork)	Beriberi, polyneuritis, anorexia, constipation
Vitamin B_2 (riboflavin)	Milk, eggs, liver, green vegetables	Cheilosis, glossitis, ocular disorders
Nicotinic acid (niacin)	Milk, lean meat, liver	Pellagra, stomatitis, glossitis, dermatitis, mental symptoms
Vitamin B_{12} (cyanocobalamin)	Muscle meats, eggs, wheat germ, liver	Hyperchromic macrocytic anemia
Folic acid	Leafy vegetables, liver	Macrocytic anemia, glossitis, diarrhea
Vitamin C (ascorbic acid)	Oranges, lemons, grapefruit, tomatoes	Scurvy, capillary fragility, hemorrhages, anemia
Vitamin D (calciferol)	Fish, fish-liver oils, milk, eggs, liver (sunlight)	Rickets, osteomalacia
Vitamin K	Green leaves: spinach, cabbage, kale, cauliflower; also egg yolk, liver; *plus* exclusion of bile from intestinal tract, or intestinal lesions, or liver disease	Prothrombin deficiency; hemorrhages resulting from prolonged bleeding and clotting time
Iodine	Fish, iodized salt	Goiter; functional thyroid disorders; cretinism in offspring
Iron	Meat, liver, eggs, beans, prunes, peas, wheat, oatmeal, spinach	Hypochromic anemia, especially during growth, menstruation, or pregnancy; blood loss

* MacBryde, Cyril M.: "Weight Loss and Undernutrition," in MacBryde, Cyril M., and Blacklow, Robert Stanley (eds.): *Signs and Symptoms; Applied Pathologic Physiology and Clinical Interpretation,* 5th ed. J. B. Lippincott Co., Philadelphia, 1970, p. 899.

central nervous system may result in loss of brain weight, decreased size, and a cell deficit. Anatomic and biochemical changes in the neurons and neuroglial cells as well as interruption in the process of myelination may occur. An adult suffering from the same degree of undernutrition, however, may experience only minimal effects on the brain.[17,18] Manocha says:

If the period of malnutrition happens to be a few weeks prior to birth (due to severe maternal nutritional deprivation) and is continued to a few weeks or months of postnatal life (due to lactation failure or nonavailability of good quality uncontaminated milk), the brain is left with a permanent deficit in cell number, incomplete organization, and serious and most probably permanent impairment of its functional ability.*

Not only do undernourished infants and children gain weight slowly, but they remain short in stature and the skeletal structures develop

slowly. They have poor resistance to infection and, according to most authorities consulted, they may be mentally retarded. Studies show that intellectual development and learning ability is impaired.[19]

Prevention and Clinical Management. An adequate intake of calories, protein, and all other essential nutrients is the only effective means of preventing and treating undernutrition (mild or severe). Obviously, as the above discussion shows, this is easier said than done because of the complexity of the problem. Manocha says:

The future of man's fight against prevalent malnutrition depends on our determination to fight with all the resources at our command and consists mostly of (1) removing ignorance; (2) augmenting food supplies of both energy-yielding and high-quality proteinaceous foods, with special emphasis on the latter; and (3) controlling the exploding human population.*

* Manocha, Sohan L.: *op. cit.,* p. 88.

* *Ibid.,* p. 300.

In an effort to combat ignorance, authorities consistently emphasize that new and intensive educational programs must begin with very small children before they enter school and continue throughout their lifetime so that they may keep abreast of new knowledge of food technology and nutrition since these will affect their choice of food. A variety of educational sources is available. They include television, newspapers, advertisements, family, friends, and teachers. Advanced educational preparation in nutrition is stressed for all health workers but particularly nutritionists, dietitians, dentists, nurses, physicians, and teachers of home economics, health education, physical education, and recreation, as well as agricultural extension workers.[20]

The very best educational program will not serve its intended purpose unless people have the money to buy needed food. The US Department of Agriculture estimated that a family of four in the United States should spend about $1570 a year for a modest but varied nutritious diet. However, at the poverty level a family of four is limited to about $600 yearly for food.[21] Several governmental programs to combat hunger at the local, state, and federal levels include school breakfasts and lunches, camps, and day care. Health workers and other interested persons should do everything they can to see that these programs benefit the poor and that they are established in all locations where children go hungry. In the spring of 1971, at least 600,000 of 6.6 million needy children were not getting free or reduced-price lunches even though monies had been appropriated by the Congress. Of the nation's 100,000 public schools, 23,000 still provided no school lunches.

Family feeding programs consist of two major activities: direct distribution of commodities, and food stamps. It is estimated that the commodities program operates in approximately 1000 of the nation's 3100 counties, feeding some 3.8 million people. As the foods available in this program are the country's excess food items, it is doubtful that the recipients are eating a nutritious diet. The food stamp program, started in 1961 by the late President John F. Kennedy, enables the poor to purchase food stamps for less than face value for use at retail food markets (see Table 36-2).

These programs should be improved if they are to serve the purpose for which they are intended. For example, approximately 300 very poor counties do not have any program because local authorities will not ask the US Department of Agriculture for assistance, and some existing programs are discontinued at harvest time to ensure abundant labor at sub-

Table 36-2. The 1972 Schedule of Food Stamp Benefits per Month (Abbreviated) *

Monthly Net Income (After Deductions)	Purchase Requirement	
	Four Persons in Household (Coupon Allotment: $112.00)	Eight Persons in Household (Coupon Allotment: $192.00)
$ 0 to 19.99	$ 0.00	$ 0.00
20 to 29.99	0.00	0.00
30 to 39.99	4.00	5.00
40 to 49.99	7.00	9.00
50 to 59.99	10.00	12.00
60 to 69.99	13.00	16.00
—	—	—
150 to 169.99	45.00	45.00
170 to 179.99	47.00	51.00
—	—	—
360 to 389.99	88.00	108.00
390 to 419.99	can't buy	117.00
630 to 659.99	can't buy	152.00
—	—	—
over 659.99	can't buy	can't buy

* Mayer, Jean (ed.): *U.S. Nutrition Policies in the Seventies.* W. H. Freeman & Co., San Francisco, 1973, p. 227.

sistence wages.[22] A guaranteed adequate family income to ensure a nutritious diet for all people (and hence the prevention of undernutrition) has been proposed by many congressmen, civic leaders, and health workers. Many people view this as a necessary long-term goal. Some authorities are convinced that malnutrition (mild and severe) in the world will not be eradicated until the ever-increasing human population is controlled. Nurses, other health workers, and interested laymen should be actively involved on the local, state, and federal levels in eradicating hunger.

In states of severe undernutrition, such as calorie-protein deficiency, treatment consists of correcting fluid and electrolyte imbalances, giving an appropriate diet, and treating infections. Oral and parenteral solutions containing glucose and electrolytes may be given, especially if diarrhea is present, and antibiotics if infections are present. Initially, frequent small feedings should be given as neither the gastrointestinal tract nor the cardiovascular system is able to cope with the effects of large feedings. Fortunately, undernourished persons have an appetite that is easily satisfied. Dietary intake may be increased as small quantities are tolerated.

Current knowledge of the physiology of starvation, according to Vernon R. Young and Nevin S. Scrimshaw, shows that the brain switches from glucose to ketone bodies as its main energy source for preservation of the body's integrity. They say:

All that can be suggested is that in a food-shortage emergency it may be best to spread out the consumption of the limited supply of protein and/or carbohydrate over the day, taking nibbles at frequent intervals, so that the periods of fasting and consequent breakdown of body protein for glucose synthesis will be shortened.*

For nurses and others to be successful in helping the undernourished, they must recognize that changing food habits is a slow process, eating is more social and psychologic than intellectual, knowledge of good nutrition is only one factor in change, and criticism arouses resistance. Of course, health workers must know what is eaten and why as a basis for any help they offer since the causes of malnutrition are so numerous and varied.

2. OBESITY

The term *obesity* derives from the Latin word *obesus,* meaning to devour. It is commonly defined as an accumulation of excess body fat stored in adipose tissue. A man is usually termed obese when his body weight

* Young, Vernon R., and Scrimshaw, Nevin S.: "The Physiology of Starvation," *Sci. Am.,* **225**:14, (Oct.) 1971.

exceeds 20 per cent of the standard weight listed in height-weight-age tables, while a woman is said to be obese when her body weight exceeds 25 per cent of the listed standard. See Table 36-3 for desirable weights for men and women age 25 and over. Most authorities recognize that the recommended body weight of these tables does not provide an accurate assessment of body fat because of the wide range of body build in the general population. As body weight is composed of bone, muscle, fat, other tissues, and fluid, this measure may provide only a rough index of obesity in some persons who are mildly overweight. However, the severely overweight person is recognizable and the condition presents a serious health problem.[23] (See Tables 36-4 and 36-5.) Most authorities say the best way to determine actual body fatness is by measuring skinfold thickness with calipers (see Fig. 36-3). Norms for this measurement have not been established, however.

For the past 25 years, emphasis has been placed on weight reduction in the United States; yet, according to Albert J. Stunkard, "we have no evidence of any decrease in the incidence of severity of obesity." * He believes

* Stunkard, Albert J.: "The Obese: Background and Programs," in Mayer, Jean (ed.): *U.S. Nutrition Policies in the Seventies.* W. B. Freeman & Co., San Francisco, 1973, p. 29.

Table 36-3.   Desirable Weights in Pounds for People 25 or Over *†

	Men				Women		
Height ‡ Ft. In.	Small Frame	Medium Frame	Large Frame	Height ‡ Ft. In.	Small Frame	Medium Frame	Large Frame
5 2	112–120	118–129	126–141	4 10	92– 98	96–107	104–119
5 3	115–123	121–133	129–144	4 11	94–101	98–110	106–122
5 4	118–126	124–136	132–148	5 0	96–104	101–113	109–125
5 5	121–129	127–139	135–152	5 1	99–107	104–116	112–128
5 6	124–133	130–143	138–156	5 2	102–110	107–119	115–131
5 7	128–137	134–147	142–161	5 3	105–113	110–122	118–134
5 8	132–141	138–152	147–166	5 4	108–116	113–126	121–138
5 9	136–145	142–156	151–170	5 5	111–119	116–130	125–142
5 10	140–150	146–160	155–174	5 6	114–123	120–135	129–146
5 11	144–154	150–165	159–179	5 7	118–127	124–139	133–150
6 0	148–158	154–170	164–184	5 8	122–131	128–143	137–154
6 1	152–162	158–175	168–189	5 9	126–135	132–147	141–158
6 2	156–167	162–180	173–194	5 10	130–140	136–151	145–163
6 3	160–171	167–185	178–199	5 11	134–144	140–155	149–168
6 4	164–175	172–190	182–204	6 0	138–148	144–159	153–173

* Kogan, Benjamin A.: *Health: Man in a Changing Environment.* Harcourt, Brace & World, New York, 1972, p. 292.
† These figures are based on the person's wearing indoor clothing. For nude weight, women should subtract 2 to 4 lb; men 5 to 7 lb. Girls between the ages of 18 and 25 should subtract 1 lb for each year under 25.
‡ Height is measured with shoes on: 1-inch heels for men, 2-inch heels for women.
Source: Metropolitan Life Insurance Company. Derived primarily from data of the Build and Blood Pressure Study, Society of Actuaries, 1959.

that instead of directing attention to the prevalence of severe obesity among the poor, whose condition presents a real health hazard, large numbers of mildly overweight persons in the United States have been worried by the emphasis on reducing diets. While throughout history, obesity has been restricted to the "privileged classes," in the United States it is now associated with lack of wealth and status.

According to E. R. Buskirk,[24] almost one-half the population of the United States is obese, a condition associated with the following health problems:

1. Changes in the regulation of various body functions.
2. An increase in incidence of particular diseases such as arteriosclerosis, hypertension, coronary artery disease, and diabetes mellitus.
3. An increase in complications of severity of a disease.
4. Development of psychologic disorders that may alter physiologic function as well as impair mental health.
5. Limitation of mobility because more energy is required to move one's excessively fat body.

These and other problems associated with obesity are discussed later in this chapter.

Incidence. Obesity is said to be a major public health problem in North America today and the incidence of overweight is increasing, affecting all age groups. At least 15 to 20 per cent (10 million) teenagers are overweight.[25] The proportion of obesity is highest in adults because it includes those whose patterns of obesity continue as well as an additional group of persons who become overweight after the age of 25. After 40 years of age, 30 per cent of all men and 40 per cent of all women are more

Table 36-4. Overweight and Excess Mortality *†

Overweight (Per Cent)	Excess Mortality (Per Cent)	
	Men	Women
10	13	9
20	25	21
30	42	30

* Kogan, Benjamin A.: *Health: Man in a Changing Environment.* Harcourt, Brace & World, New York, 1972, p. 292.
† Compared with mortality of standard risks (mortality ratio of standard risks equals 100 per cent).
Source: Metropolitan Life Insurance Company. Derived from data of the Build and Blood Pressure Study, Society of Actuaries, 1959.

Table 36-5. Overweight and Excess Mortality from Some Major Diseases *†

Disease	Excess Mortality (Per Cent)	
	Men	Women
Heart disease	43	51
Cerebral hemorrhage	53	29
Malignant cancers	16	13
Diabetes	133	83
Digestive system diseases (gallstones, cirrhosis, etc.)	68	39

* Kogan, Benjamin A.: *Health: Man in a Changing Environment.* Harcourt, Brace & World, New York, 1972, p. 292.
† Compared with mortality of standard risks (mortality ratio of standard risks equals 100 per cent). These data apply to people about 20 per cent or more overweight.
Source: Metropolitan Life Insurance Company. Derived from data of the Build and Blood Pressure Study, Society of Actuaries, 1959.

than 20 per cent overweight. Part of their weight gain can be attributed to a fairly constant food intake over a long period while actual needs are steadily decreasing. Nancy L. Wilson and associates say "A 10-calorie-per-day surplus becomes 3650 calories in 1 year or an increase of about 1 pound of body weight; in 10 years this increase becomes the 10-pound general trend in body weight increase for the population." *

To explore attitudes toward weight and diet, according to Johanna T. Dwyer and Jean Mayer,[26] surveys of the population of the United States were conducted in 1950, 1956, and 1966. Findings show that concern with weight has been widespread within the population during this 20-year period. Women were more concerned with weight and more likely to do something about excess weight than men. Concern was more prevalent in "both sexes among better as opposed to less well educated persons, and in higher as opposed to lower class men." Approximately 14 per cent of the women and 7 per cent of the men reported they were dieting at the time of the surveys.

Within the recent past, a series of studies has shown, to a remarkable degree, that the prevalence of obesity in the general population is related to social class, particularly in women. Three studies of urban populations in the United States and Great Britain are frequently

* Wilson, Nancy L., et al.: "The Development and Perpetuation of Obesity: An Overview," in Wilson, Nancy L. (ed.): *Obesity.* F. A. Davis Co., Philadelphia, 1969, p. 5.

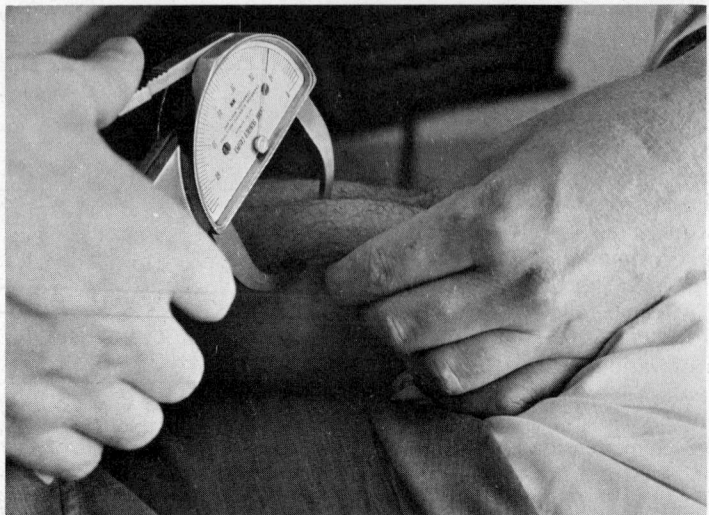

Figure 36-3. A skinfold measurement is made by means of a caliper. This determines the amount of subcutaneous fat of an individual and is an indicator of total body fat. (Courtesy of *Roche Medical Image,* Hoffmann LaRoche, Inc.)

cited. The Midtown Manhattan study consisted of 1660 adults (out of a group of 110,000 individuals) between 20 and 59 years of age who were rated, "low," "medium," and "high" according to their socioeconomic status. Findings show that the prevalence of obesity among the women of lower socioeconomic status was 30 per cent, decreasing to 16 per cent among those of middle status, and to only 5 per cent in the upper status group. This means that obesity in the lower class women was six times that found in the upper class. The differences among men were less marked; 32 per cent in the lower status group and 16 per cent in the upper status group.[27,28]

A recent study conducted in London paralleled the findings of the Manhattan study showing an inverse relationship between social class and obesity.[29] Finally, L. E. Hinkle,[30] in a sample of executives of the Bell Telephone System, found that socioeconomic status and upward social mobility were inversely related to coronary heart disease (the opposite of the stereotype of coronary disease) as the result of the drive for achievement and the stress of responsibility. In addition, obesity was inversely correlated with social status, which explains in part the distribution of heart disease.

Causes and Effects. Because of the complexities of the problem and the complexities of personality, there is no single or simple answer to cause or treatment of obesity. Authorities generally agree that obesity, a disturbance of the whole person, is best viewed as having multiple causes, which means that prevention and treatment should be individualized.

Although obesity *genes* have been identified in several animals, including the mouse, rat, dog, and chicken, they have not been identified in man. However, obesity, especially in its extreme form, tends to be familial. It is much more common in children when both parents are obese than when neither parent is obese. The interaction of genetic factors and environmental factors such as cooking, eating, and habitual activity of the family makes it difficult to determine the contribution of each. It is thought that those children who are obese at birth probably have an "obesity gene." Heavy children usually become heavy adults, and they are of shorter stature, have greater breadth of trunk, and smaller hands and feet than lean persons. An example of genetically determined localized adiposity is the massive adipose tissue over the buttocks of some Bushmen, called "Hottentot bustle." This example suggests that genetically a given number of adipose cells may be allotted to each person and that the number and location of these cells determines to some degree the magnitude and the character of the obesity.[31]

In support of the concept of "obesity genes" in man, Buskirk says "Adopted children who are thin may not become obese even though their foster parents are obese, and twins separated from their parents or from each other when young often retain obesity trait even though raised in an environment favorable to weight reduction." * Prenatal nutrition, the earliest contributing factor, may stimulate

* Buskirk, E. R.: "Obesity," in Downey, John A., and Darling, Robert C.: *Physiological Basis of Rehabilitation.* W. B. Saunders Co., Philadelphia, 1971, p. 231.

a genetic tendency toward overweight. There is a 50 per cent chance that a child will be obese when one parent is overweight and the probability increases to 80 per cent when both parents are overweight; this tendency, however, is not seen in children adopted at an early age, according to Wilson and associates.[32]

Although *metabolic* and *endocrine* factors leading to the development of obesity have not been well defined, some authorities suspect there are abnormalities in the rate fat is deposited in or mobilized from adipose tissue. Other suggested abnormalities include the rate of absorption of foodstuffs from the gastrointestinal tract, the rate of synthetization of metabolic products into adipose tissue, and the rate of metabolism of nutrients in the peripheral tissues. The question of whether the many reported endocrine and metabolic abnormalities in obese persons are cause or effect is not known, according to Margaret J. Albrink.[32a]

While it is known that insulin promotes the synthesis of fat, large increases in postcibal insulin concentration (hyperinsulinism) are characteristic of the obese, resulting in an insensitivity of the tissues to insulin. The pancreas in response to insulin insensitivity increases concentration of the hormone which is ineffective in restoring substrate (such as certain amino acids, glucose, and probably others) levels to normal. Although the explanation for insulin insensitivity of the obese is unknown, it is related to increased cell size. When body weight is reduced the cell size returns to normal and insulin sensitivity is restored. The increased insulin production, over a period of years in the obese, places a burden on the pancreas and may result in pancreatic exhaustion and diabetes, which accounts for the association between obesity and diabetes.

Pathologic concentrations of various adrenal hormones are reported in some obese persons; however, the overactivity of the adrenal cortex is not believed to cause simple obesity. The thyroid gland functions normally in the obese and there is no evidence that thyroid deficiency plays a role in the etiology of simple obesity. Even though thyroid hormone is prescribed for some obese persons, weight loss occurs only with toxic doses.

Sex hormones are thought to affect the amount and distribution of fat, especially female sex hormones. For instance, there is a greater amount of subcutaneous fat in women than men. As parity increases so does obesity, and frequent gain of weight occurs during the menopause. The absence of male sex hormones in eunuchs is thought to be the cause of obesity in these persons. Hypogonad obesity occurs during childhood but disappears at puberty when fat begins to be distributed in the adult pattern of men and women.

The role of the central nervous system in regulating food intake is gaining attention because most authorities believe that metabolic abnormalities of the obese are the result rather than the cause of obesity. Overfeeding of young rats may "set" the regulatory centers in the hypothalamus, resulting in an irreversible number of fat cells that persist throughout life. The extent to which variations in balance between the satiety center, located in the central medial hypothalamus, and a neighboring feeding center contribute to ordinary obesity is unknown.[33]

The role of *cultural, behavioral,* and *psychologic* factors in the development of obesity is well established. As in previous centuries, the most obvious cause of caloric imbalance, leading to increased obesity in all age groups, is decreased physical activity. Unfortunately, North Americans rely on electrical appliances and machines to accomplish tasks that were done with muscle power in the past. Work-saving devices are far too common in the average home—vacuum cleaners, carpet sweepers, dishwashers, electric blenders and beaters, ice crushers, and even toothbrushes. The automobile is in common use by all members of the family, even for going to neighborhood shops within walking distance for the average person. It is rare for children to walk to school; they ride with a parent, relative, or neighbor, or in a school bus. Sunday hikes are no longer fashionable and the people of the United States have become spectators rather than participants of recreational activities. There is less and less difference between life in the country and in cities. Complex machinery is used in cultivating the land and harvesting its yield; cattle, on some ranches, are herded from one area to another by helicopter rather than by the man on horseback.

Many women, especially housewives with young children, are more active than men. They shop, carry groceries and other purchases, care for the children, and do housework, all of which keep them on their feet and moving most of the day. The activity of many men, on the other hand, is limited because many of them ride to and from work, spend the day in a sedentary occupation, and watch television in the evening.

Authorities agree that exercise is the only factor that leads to a major increase in expenditure of energy and that food intake does not necessarily increase with increased exercise. Regular participation in exercise programs has been shown to reduce body weight in fat persons.[34-36] Unfortunately, people tend to maintain ancestral eating habits and regular exercise has never been popular with most obese persons, so a positive balance of calories results. D. Jacobs and associates [37] and B. A. Bullen and associates,[38] in studies of children and adolescents, found that although the obese ate less than the nonobese they also were less active. A study at the University of Edinburgh showed that the calorie intake was not increased sufficiently to account for the increase in weight gain of adults but it was thought that a reduction of physical activity was the major causal factor in the obese persons studied.[39] It can be assumed that as excessive weight increases, physical activity tends to decrease. It is known that the basal metabolism rate of fairly inactive persons is about 10 per cent lower than the normal rate of the active person.

Family and cultural eating habits are established at an early age. In families in which great emphasis is placed on food, most members tend to overeat. Success is equated with obesity in some cultures; consequently, the ambitious person strives to gain a comfortable corpulence. The dietary habits of some families such as those who like predominantly calorie-rich foods, snacks between meals, and the major meal in the evening, all contribute to the development and maintenance of adiposity.

An increasing number of clinicians believe that emotional factors are often the primary cause of obesity in a large number of individuals. The psychologic responses to stress, unfortunately, lead to increased intake of food and drink and decrease in physical and social activity, both changes leading to an increase in weight gain. In a recent book, *The Psychology of Obesity; Dynamics and Treatment,*[40] the works of psychoanalysts, psychiatrists, psychologists, sociologists, anthropologists, demographers, internists, and nutritionists are delineated in an attempt to solve the puzzle of obesity. Norman Kiell, in the introduction to this publication, says:

. . . there is now general agreement that persistence in overeating has its basis in unresolved emotional problems and that the overeating serves as a substitute for other satisfactions. This finding is comparatively recent. One of the roadblocks to the understanding of obesity has been the failure to acknowledge the psychological aspects involved. The mind-body dichotomy that permeated so much of pre-Freudian medical thinking, and is still clung to by doctors more comfortable with the palpable soma than the spooky psyche is much in evidence when it comes to obesity. The traditional medical view blames the failure of the obese to diet simply on the inability to control food intake, a view that is as helpful as stating that alcoholics cannot control their liquor consumption. But a more enlightened outlook perceives the adipose person as the victim of social and unconscious forces which compel him to persist in a repetitive, self-destructive pattern.*

Noting that there is no single or simple answer to obesity, he believes that at this time the problem of obesity should be viewed as having multiple causes: metabolic, neurologic, psychologic, and socioeconomic.

The effects (or as some authorities say "hazards") of obesity are great and include the following: (1) the life expectancy of the obese is lower than that of the nonobese and is directly proportional to the degree of obesity; (2) the mortality rate of obese persons with any medical illness is higher than in nonobese persons; (3) the obese are more likely to suffer from a variety of medical diseases than the nonobese, for example, hypertension and gallbladder disease are twice as common, diabetes is three times as common, arthritis, lung diseases, angina, and sudden death are all much more common; and coronary heart disease is more common among the obese, increasing in severity with increased obesity.[41-43] Although these and other diseases place obesity near the top of the list of public health problems in the United States, obesity is different because there is uncertainty that obesity in itself has serious ill effects. Stunkard says "It is the way one becomes obese in America—by diminished physical activity and by the consumption of a high-calorie, high-fat diet—that has been implicated in coronary heart disease and other degenerative illnesses." †

In contrast to so many other forms of pathology, almost, if not all, of the adverse effects of obesity can be reversed. For instance, diabetes and high blood pressure disappear completely in many persons when they lose excess fat. In those persons who successfully lose weight and maintain the weight loss, life expectancy is increased to what it would have been had they never been obese, according to life insurance studies.[44]

A distinctive type of disturbance in body image that affects only some obese persons seems to persist for long periods, is unaffected by weight reduction, and is relieved only by psychotherapy, although this may not be effective. In a study of 74 randomly selected obese persons, Stunkard and V. Burt [45] report the following findings: (1) many patients were repelled by the sight of their bodies,

* Kiell, Norman (ed.): *The Psychology of Obesity; Dynamics and Treatment.* Charles C Thomas, Publisher, Springfield, Ill., 1973, p. x.
† Stunkard, Albert J.: *op. cit.,* p. 31.

almost unable to look in a mirror; (2) they were intensely self-conscious in general and even held misconceptions of how they were viewed by others, relating all occurrences, real and imaginary, to their weight; and (3) they were self-conscious with the opposite sex, avoiding contact and in some instances hatefully devaluating them. In addition, the disturbances of body image occurred almost exclusively in those who were obese in childhood. Disturbances were found in half of those with onset of obesity during childhood or adolescence (frequently called the "juvenile obese"), while none of the 40 persons with obesity starting in adulthood showed a severe body image disturbance.

Studies show that the impressionable years of adolescence are a critical period for the development of these disturbances. The importance of preventing obesity during childhood and treating it promptly should be stressed. In a study of nearly 2000 children who were followed for 30 years, "the odds against an obese child becoming a normal weight adult were 4 to 1; for those who did not reduce during adolescence they were more than 28 to 1!" *

The stigma of obesity, closely associated with body image disturbances, is prevalent among many groups and interferes with effective treatment. In a study of 650 boys and girls (age 10 and 11), N. S. Richardson and associates [46] report that the normal child was the most preferred while the obese child was least preferred among those with physical disabilities. Other disabled children with whom the obese child was compared were a child sitting in a wheelchair with both legs covered, or wearing a brace, using crutches, having a missing hand, or a disfigurement on one side of the face. G. L. Maddox and associates,[47] in a study of selected adults, who are thought to be indifferent to societal preference for leanness (those with low incomes, Negro men, and the elderly), also selected the picture of the obese child as least desirable and likable.

Negative attitudes toward obesity have been found in physicians who often describe these persons as being "awkward," "ugly," and "weak-willed." And attitudes toward obesity have been shown to influence admission to colleges. Those who were obese were less likely to be accepted even though there was no difference in academic achievement, motivation, and social class.[48,49] It is important for all

health workers to understand the nature and characteristics of obesity if they are to be successful in the prevention and treatment of this major health problem.

Because of the consequences of juvenile-onset obesity, it deserves special mention. There is sufficient evidence to suggest that fat tissue of those who become obese during childhood differs from those with adult-onset obesity in that it is composed of connective tissue embedded with specialized cells for fat storage. Authorities generally agree that the number of fat cells are determined early in life and that overeating during childhood influences the development of fat tissue containing a large number of fat cells. With increasing age, fat tissue progressively loses its ability to grow by increasing the number of cells; consequently, increase in body size is attained by an increase in the size of each individual cell. Weight reduction, therefore, is the result of a decrease in the size of cells rather than a decrease in their number.

When persons with juvenile-onset obesity attempt weight reduction, they are confronted with a double burden, that is, more and larger fat cells. This may explain why they find it more difficult to lose weight and maintain a normal weight than do other obese persons. Another reason for giving special attention to juvenile-onset obesity is that the associated emotional problems are more numerous and harder to solve than are those of persons with adult-onset obesity. As discussed above, disturbances in body image are common and the young obese view their bodies as loathsome, believing that others view them with contempt. Finally, the compulsive, even bizarre, eating patterns that are seen in some obese persons are almost always found in those whose obesity began in childhood.

Prevention and Clinical Management. Because the results of medical treatment are consistently poor, emphasis is placed on preventive measures by most authorities. The majority of obese persons will not enter treatment programs; those who do will not lose a significant amount of weight; and of those who lose weight, most regain it. Albrink [50] says "within 5 years almost certainly" weight is regained—obesity seems to be self-perpetuating. The results of membership in self-help groups are more encouraging and are discussed later.

It is obvious that prevention, especially if begun during childhood, is easier than treatment. The reduction of food intake and the increase of energy expenditure are the only preventive measures available until the cause of obesity in each person is determined.

The selection of a diet for weight control

---

* Penick, Sidnor B., and Stunkard, Albert J.: "Newer Concepts of Obesity," in Kiell, Norman (ed.): *The Psychology of Obesity; Dynamics and Treatment.* Charles C Thomas, Publisher, Springfield, Ill., 1973, p. 11.

must be nutritionally sound (see Chapter 10). The likes, dislikes, and eating practices of the individual and family must be considered. Some persons consistently overeat at night. This practice should be discouraged, but it may be better to suggest controlled food intake at the habitual time than to try to change a well-established pattern. Breakfast should not be skipped by the dieter as it prevents symptoms of hypoglycemia and hyperketonemia during the day. Some persons do well on frequent small feedings, especially those who cannot tolerate any restriction on food intake; while those who cannot stop eating once they start, do poorly. Individual differences in hunger and satiety patterns should be considered in the size and frequency of meals.

If prevention of obesity is to be effective, education of all the people in our already diet-conscious civilization about nutritive and caloric values of foods is absolutely essential. Education should start with prenatal classes, for mothers are responsible for establishing life-long dietary patterns in their children. Teaching of children can begin in public and private schools. Federal school lunch and breakfast programs afford an excellent opportunity to demonstrate proper nutritional practices. Institutions, such as the various branches of the armed services, responsible for feeding large segments of the population, are in a good position to establish new eating habits as well as prevent weight gain in men and women during their service. Public and private agencies should intensify their efforts in educating the public and all health workers. Educational programs should include the most recent and most reliable information on obesity; they should identify and counteract the widespread misinformation and faddism now so prevalent. Stunkard says:

Where misinformation extends to questionable practices and outright fraud, the Food and Drug Administration and other federal agencies must intervene more forcefully than has been their custom. We need to expand programs designed to control inappropriate diets, drugs, and "reducing machines," and to combat the practices of unscrupulous entrepreneurs.*

Probably the least achievable but most important aspect of preventing and controlling obesity is discontinuing the promotion by the various food industries of high-caloric foodstuffs having low nutritional value. Rich pastries and other delicacies, composed of purified fats and carbohydrates, are the worst offenders. Finally, an adequate income for purchasing necessary foods must be available

* Stunkard, Albert J.: *op. cit.*, p. 36.

to all persons. It is most difficult, if not impossible, to prepare nutritious diets from foods now available to the poor in the United States, and in consequence, to prevent obesity and associated illness.

Physical activity can go a long way in preventing overweight, especially in those persons who have difficulty in controlling food intake. Regular activity such as walking, jogging, swimming, bicycling, and skating reduces weight. Emphasis should be placed on the importance of exercise and physical work in maintaining optimum health and preventing obesity during the early years of life. The young should be encouraged to learn skills that involve the use of their bodies, such as hiking, cross-country skiing and bicycling, skating, swimming, and gardening. The goal for weight control and prevention of obesity is to establish and maintain a regular exercise program of reasonable intensity within one's physical capabilities.[51-53]

Successful treatment of obesity requires considerable change in life style, including dietary and physical activity patterns. This change is achieved only by highly motivated persons. All health workers, if they are successful in helping others, must realize that it is most difficult for individuals to change their pattern of living. Also, it is of equal importance for the obese person to recognize these facts, and to understand that weight reduction is achieved by decreasing food intake, increasing physical activity, or both, in many situations. The obese must reduce intake of calories below that expended in body metabolism and activity.

A careful history of weight gain and dietary practices of the client is essential. If poor dietary habits are established, the familial, economic, and psychologic background for these habits should be explored. Patterns of appetite and satiety, as well as physical activity, must be identified so that the energy balance of the person may be made. In a few persons, obesity is caused by endocrine disorders. Examples are hypothyroidism, hypogonadism, and hyperadrenocorticism. Obesity is also caused by fluid retention as in renal dysfunction and congestive heart failure. The underlying cause must, of course, be treated also. Characteristics of those without a demonstrable disease who are most likely to benefit from a weight reduction program include the following: slightly or moderately overweight, adult-onset obesity, first serious attempt to lose weight, highly motivated, and sufficiently well adjusted to pursue this goal which is *his* or *her* goal.[54]

A balanced, low-calorie diet, consisting of foods usually available and that can be continued following weight reduction, is the simplest way to reduce food intake, yet it is the most difficult kind of diet to follow during weight reduction. Diets that provide about 1000 kcal per day for women and 1500 kcal per day for men are usually successful for most of these persons and lead to a weight reduction of 0.45 kg (or 1 lb) per week with a yearly loss of 23.2 kg (or 52 lb). Diets that provide less than the amounts listed above are poorly tolerated over a long period; however, some have been successful in controlled situations, such as hospital wards and clinics. The initial weight loss, regardless of type of diet, is primarily water, but as time passes more fat is metabolized and cell substance, including protein matrix, is lost also.

It is important for dieters to know the caloric values of foods included in their diets, what is a usual serving or portion of food, and the value of restricting all alcoholic beverages because of their high caloric content. If the restricted diet is well balanced, the food is fresh and of good quality, vitamin supplements are not necessary, according to authorities consulted on obesity. There are, however, physicians such as Linus Pauling who believe every one living in Western cultures benefits from vitamin supplements. (See Chapter 10.)

Restriction of sodium chloride is often associated with reducing diets and may be indicated, especially if hypertension or water retention and edema are present. While artificial sweeteners were used in the immediate past, they are no longer available since the restriction of cyclamates (see Chapter 10). Probably their greatest advantage was psychologic. Although saccharin continues to be used, its safety is under investigation and consumers are cautioned to limit their intake to one gm a day. The use of liquid reducing diets, once popular, is declining because dieters have found them impractical on a long-term basis.

Many obese persons find total starvation relatively easy to tolerate for the following reasons: hunger ceases after the seventh day, weight loss is rapid, compulsive eating is more easily controlled, and fasting seems simpler than dieting, according to E. J. Drenick.[55] Medical supervision is necessary for those who are fasting because of the many physiologic and metabolic effects, including postural hypotension due to potassium, sodium, and water excretion, and continued potassium excretion with possible depletion. Additional effects include reduced gastric secretory activity and bowel function, ketoacidemia and metabolic acidosis (including lactacidemia and citric acidosis), magnesium loss with possible muscle irritability and cramping, depletion of protein stores, contraction of red blood cell mass,

plasma, and blood volumes, hyperuricemia, and acute gout.[56-58] Emotional disturbances associated with fasting are common. As noted, weight loss is rapid in total starvation, but almost invariably the weight is regained.

Andrew Malleson, a general practitioner turned psychiatrist, has very little faith in the physician's ability to help the obese, and a great deal of faith in the self-help movement, which is in essence group therapy.* In his chapter on "healthy doctoring," he has this and much more to say about self-help:

For years doctors have been struggling to make their fat patients thin. Seldom do they succeed, though they often manage to get them hooked on slimming-pills in the process. The obese are prima donnas in the art of diet cheating, and doctors are far too naive to catch them out. In 1961, a fat Long Island housewife discovered that fat people are much more effective in helping fat people lose weight than are doctors—other munchers know at once when someone is bluffing on their calories. Jean Nidetch made this discovery when her obesity clinic issued her with an ultimatum: "Stick to your diet or leave the clinic." Ever since she was 10, Jean Nidetch had been trying to lose weight and had been excusing her failures with words like "glandular" and "metabolic." Threatened with expulsion from her clinic, Mrs. Nidetch collected some fat friends with whom she could follow the clinic's diet. They met weekly to see how well they were all doing. So started "Weight Watchers." Now it has 1,500,000 slimmed-down fatties as its members in countries throughout the world. [Nidetch, Jean: *The Story of Weight Watchers.* World Publishing Co., New York, 1970.] The overweight are now giving each other tons of encouragement and between them they are losing tons of surplus fat.†

Almost everybody who has had any experience with them believes that self-help groups such as Weight Watchers and TOPS (Take Off Pounds Sensibly) are making a significant contribution to the control of obesity. Such groups offer an opportunity for the obese to relate to others with the same problem, which is a source of moral support. Sandra Shumway and Marjorie Powers[59] describe a group-centered approach to the problem of obesity used with ten selected patients attending a hypertension outpatient clinic. The approach included involving group members in as many decisions as possible, discussing cultural, social, and environmental factors related to problems of overweight among them, and encouraging the use of emotional support. Associated

---

* See the Appendix for names and addresses of these organizations or agencies.
† Malleson, Andrew: *Need Your Doctor Be So Useless?* George Allen & Unwin, London, 1973, p. 212.

articles describing the problems and behavior of one patient should be helpful to all nurses.[60,61] To avoid stigmatizing the obese, Beatrice J. Kalisch[62] suggests group sessions for staffs in hospitals and other health agencies to explore their feelings so that they will be more helpful to their patients and clients. Similar sessions have been used successfully with nursing personnel.[62a]

The largest single factor for expenditure of energy is exercise or physical work; metabolic rate can be increased up to 20 times the resting level during peak work loads. Buskirk, noting that regulation of food intake seems to be closely related to energy expenditure in non-obese persons, says:

This relationship may not hold, however, for obese men and women, for it has been repeatedly shown that if obese subjects exercise the equivalent of 300 Kcal per day or more, a slow reduction in body fat stores occurs, even though the subjects have free choice of meals.*

Ability to work hard physically is reduced in the obese because their ability to deliver oxygen to working muscles (aerobic capacity) is low; consequently, they keep their activities at a low level. Understandably, they find difficulty in establishing good habits of physical activity. Obese men show a lower negative caloric balance than expected when a combination of exercise and diet restriction is employed because they usually eat more when exercising. The obese subjects, however, lose more weight when they exercise than when they do not.[63,64] George V. Mann, in his article titled "Obesity, the Nutritional Spook," emphasizes exercise in the control of obesity rather than drugs, and notes that the "arithmetic of reducing is quite simple" (see Table 36-6). The need for regular, vigorous exercise is obvious. It results in a loss of weight, increased physical fitness, and the chance to produce some useful work.

* Buskirk, E. R.: *op. cit.*, p. 238.

Table 36-6.   The Arithmetic of Reducing *

1 lb body fat   3250 kcal
1 lb wgt loss/week is safe max.
$$\frac{3250}{7} = 464 \text{ kcal loss/day}$$
1 hr walking on level costs 350 kcal
1 hr workout may cost 800 kcal
4 workouts/week = 3200 kcal—*no diet*

* Mann, George V.: "Obesity, the Nutritional Spook," *Am. J Public Health,* **61**:1497, (Aug.) 1971.

In answer to the question "What is the proper management of obesity?" he says:

. . . obesity has two sides, underactivity and overeating. Overeating in an abundant culture requires neither courage, skill, learning, nor guile. Gluttony demands less energy than lust, less effort than avarice. We have no proper anorectant. We rarely see obesity in cultures where physical work is necessary. Our only effective treatment, whether preventive or curative, is physical activity. The role of the professional is to explain these realities to concerned people . . . . There is no gain in driving fat people to faddists, or to drink or to eternal anguish. There is no more sense to an ileal bypass for the treatment of obesity than in treating a cigarette-smoker by cutting off his hands.*

There is no justification for the use of appetite-suppressant drugs, or the amphetamine group, in the treatment of obesity. These drugs are effective for a few weeks, but dependency on their stimulating effects makes withdrawal a serious problem. The use of these drugs began in 1937 when M. H. Nathanson[65] synthesized amphetamine and showed that it was a central stimulant. In 1938, M. F. Lesses and A. Myerson[66] reported that it impaired appetite. The drug houses quickly began to promote its use in the treatment of obesity; and, because it effectively elevated the client's mood, the volume of amphetamine sold was out of proportion to the prevalence of obese people. Eight billion doses were produced in the United States only 20 years later.[67] Addiction and a "bootleg market" for these drugs are well established in various countries, deriving from so-called obesity treatment.[68,69] The uses, effects, and abuses of these drugs are discussed in more detail in Chapters 21 and 41.

Some drugs are used in obesity for the purpose of correcting accompanying pathology. Diuretics may be prescribed for those who retain excess water and sodium because of a cardiovascular or renal dysfunction, and thyroid hormones may be prescribed for those with an established thyroid deficiency.

Plastic surgery, or removal of excess adipose tissue, has been employed cosmetically for the obese. Surgical bypass (removal of a portion of the small intestines) to reduce the absorption of foodstuffs has been used in the treatment of severe obesity with some success, resulting in a weight loss of 8 to 12 pounds every month for the first year or so, at which time a satisfactory plateau is reached by most. Complications include vitamin and mineral

* Mann, George V.: "Obesity, the Nutritional Spook," *Am. J. Public Health,* **61**:149, (Aug.) 1971.

deficiencies (especially deficiencies in potassium and calcium), disturbances in liver function, poor absorption of medicines, and alcohol intolerance.[70-73]

In summary, the solution to the problem of obesity is a nutritionally sound diet and regular physical activity so that the energy balance is maintained. Treatment must be individualized as the role of *cultural, behavioral,* and *psychologic* factors in the development of obesity is well established. The importance of education, began in early childhood, in prevention and treatment is recognized by most authorities.

3. VOMITING

Loss of appetite (anorexia), nausea, and vomiting are three closely related protective mechanisms. Anorexia and nausea reduce ingested material or stop eating altogether, and vomiting removes food from the gastrointestinal tract after it has been swallowed.

Anorexia is usually described as a loss of the desire to eat even when the person is obviously in need of food. It is commonly seen in persons with diseases of the gastrointestinal tract and liver, in severe extraintestinal diseases, such as congestive heart failure, uremia, and pulmonary failure, and in psychogenic disturbances, such as depression and anxiety. Anorexia nervosa, a disease that may be life-threatening, is attributed to psychogenic factors and is characterized by a voluntary and marked reduction in the intake of food, ultimately leading to undernutrition. It is a classic example of anorexia in the severest form.

Nausea is a disagreeable sensation characterized by a revulsion to food and may be defined as a psychic experience; it gives rise to the feeling of wanting to vomit, usually a sensation in the epigastrium or the throat. Nausea, which often precedes or accompanies vomiting, is usually associated with decreased functional activity of the stomach and changes in the motility of the small intestines, especially the duodenum. Symptoms of altered autonomic, especially parasympathetic, activity are evidenced by increased perspiration and salivation, pallor, and tachycardia. When the vagus nerve is stimulated, hypotension and bradycardia may be present.[74,75] Nausea can be more unbearable than pain. It is often accompanied by dizziness. The victim of seasickness often says "Let me die." They declare that they had no fear of dying, only a longing for relief from the overwhelming misery of seasickness.

Vomiting is a forceful expulsion of the contents of the stomach, duodenum, and proximal jejunum through the mouth. *Retching,* which frequently precedes emesis, is characterized by labored rhythmic respiratory activity. *Projectile* vomiting, a special type of vomiting, is extremely forceful, occurring without warning; it is especially significant as it indicates increased intracranial pressure.

The *vomiting center,* located in the dorsal portion of the lateral reticular formation in the medulla oblongata, is stimulated by impulses initiated by sensory receptors and transmitted by the vagus and sympathetic afferent nerves. Sensory receptors are located within as well as outside the alimentary canal. Those within the alimentary canal are located in the fauces, pharynx, stomach, and intestines; those outside the alimentary canal are located in the uterus, kidneys, heart, and semicircular canals. These receptors may be stimulated by excessively irritating substances or by overdistention or even overexcitability of an organ supplied with sensory receptors. Impulses from the cerebral cortex that stimulate certain areas of the hypothalamus also cause vomiting, although the exact neuronal connections for these effects are unknown. Various psychic stimuli, such as disagreeable odors, sounds, and sights, can cause vomiting. Finally, the chemoreceptor trigger zone, located bilaterally on the floor of the fourth ventricle, outside the vomiting center, may be stimulated by humoral agents including certain toxins, resulting in vomiting. Certain drugs, including apomorphine, morphine, copper sulfate, and toxic dosages of digitalis, can initiate vomiting by direct stimulation of the chemoreceptors.[76,76a]

The Act of Vomiting. When the vomiting center is sufficiently stimulated, motor impulses are transmitted through the 5th, 7th, 9th, 10th, and 12th cranial nerves to the upper gastrointestinal tract and through the spinal nerves to the diaphragm and abdominal muscles. Immediately preceding and during the act of vomiting there are usually extreme vasomotor and autonomic disturbances; these include sudden and excessive salivation, increased perspiration, pallor, faintness, weakness, and dizziness, and on occasion hypotension with slow pulse (bradycardia). James E. McGuigan describes the sequence of events during the act of vomiting as follows:

. . . the upper half of the stomach and the region of the gastroesophageal sphincter relax. Peristaltic contractions from the midportion of the stomach proceed to the angulus of the stomach, where a violent contraction occurs. The diaphragm undergoes violent descent, with simultaneous contractions of the abdominal muscles expelling gastric contents up into and through the esophagus. Descent of the diaphragm and acute contraction

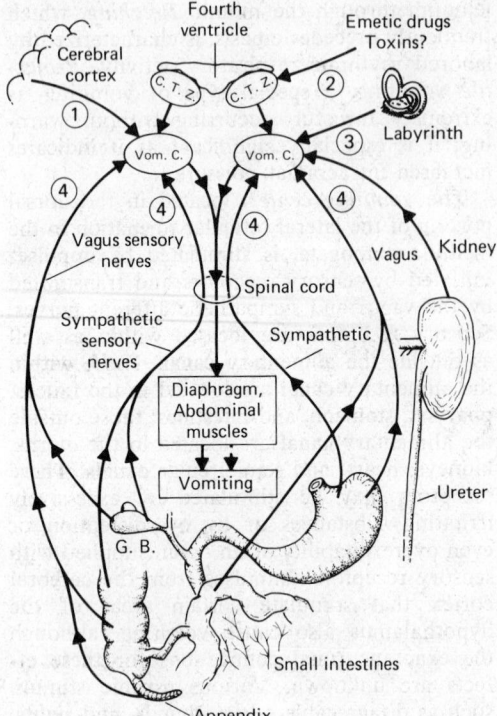

Figure 36-4. Mechanisms in the initiation of vomiting. C.T.Z., chemoreceptor trigger zone; Vom. C., vomiting center; G. B., gallbladder; *1,* cerebral stimulation of vomiting center; *2,* drug stimulation of chemoreceptor trigger zone; *3,* labyrinthine (motion, etc.) stimulation of vomiting center; *4,* visceral afferent stimulation of vomiting center. (Adapted with permission from Beland, I., and Passos, J.: *Clinical Nursing,* 3rd ed., Macmillan Publishing Co., Inc., New York, 1975.)

of the abdominal muscles operate in concert to elevate acutely the intra-abdominal pressure. During the forceful expulsion of food up and out through the esophagus the glottis is closed, respirations cease, and the soft palate is thrust upwards against the nasopharynx.*

During states of unconsciousness, regardless of cause, the glottis does not close during vomiting. The unconscious person should therefore be put in a position that favors drainage through the mouth from the tracheobronchial tree, otherwise the vomitus is drawn back into the lungs (insufflated). This can cause suffocation or, in some cases, a fatal infection.

* McGuigan, James E.: "Anorexia, Nausea, and Vomiting," in MacBryde, Cyril M., and Blacklow, Robert Stanley (eds.): *Signs and Symptoms; Applied Pathologic Physiology and Clinical Interpretation,* 5th ed. J. B. Lippincott Co., Philadelphia, 1970, p. 373.

Causes and Possible Effects of Vomiting. As indicated above, the variety of sites containing sensory receptors that if stimulated cause vomiting and the types of conditions likely to stimulate them suggest that vomiting occurs in many diseases. Vomiting may be associated with practically all organic diseases of the alimentary tract and its appendages, as well as organic diseases of almost every organ in the body, derangements of the autonomic nervous system, and functional as well as psychologic disturbances. Some diseases or conditions in which vomiting is a common symptom are appendicitis, cholecystitis, intestinal obstruction, peritoneal irritation, Addison's disease, uremia, congestive heart failure, brain tumor, Ménière's disease, and in pregnancy.[77] Vomiting is common in a variety of febrile infectious diseases. Experimental administration of microgram quantities of staphylococcal enterotoxin and enterobacteriaceal endotoxin in cats induces vomiting. In the rhesus monkey the staphylococcal endotoxin induces vomiting and it appears that it affects receptors in the abdominal viscera.[78,79]

Although nausea and vomiting in the postoperative state are discussed in Chapter 48, it seems appropriate to note here also certain factors that are thought to be related to postoperative vomiting. In a survey of 1713 patients, Ian E. Purkis [80] reports the highest incidence of vomiting occurred in the age groups from 0 to 19 and 40 to 59 years; there was an increased incidence of vomiting in the adult female as compared with the male; and short, thick-set patients were more prone to vomit than tall, thin types. Patients who had experienced motion sickness or nausea and vomiting with previous surgery showed a higher incidence of vomiting than those who had had no such experience. The disease state also had some influence on postoperative vomiting. Any physiologic disturbance causing nausea or vomiting before anesthesia, unless relieved by the operation or treatment, tended to produce symptoms of nausea and vomiting postoperatively, as for example, uremia, ketosis, or electrolyte imbalance. Also there was a higher incidence of vomiting in accident or emergency cases than in patients having elective surgery. Certain sedatives and anesthetic agents such as morphine, ether, and cyclopropane seemed to produce vomiting.

As noted earlier in this chapter, anorexia nervosa, an emotional disturbance, may be associated with anorexia and also with vomiting. Vomiting may be transitory or may persist with a psychic disturbance. Oscar Hill,[81] in a study of 42 patients, reports that vomiting was related to a variety of psychologic factors.

Those most common were marital sexual problems, the health and habits, such as alcoholism, of a close relative, loss of parental affection, and problems with a difficult aging relative. In over 50 per cent of the subjects, there was an inescapable, hostile relationship between the patient and the family. For these patients, vomiting symbolically represented a way of ridding themselves of their problem. In a later publication, Hill notes that contact between close family members is often inescapable at mealtime and if hostility exists, vomiting is a likely symptom. Allowing these individuals to bring their feelings out in the open with a trusted person is often the best method of treatment.[82] Infants and children subjected to stress during meals often respond by vomiting what they eat.

Nausea that results in vomiting is often caused by movement of fluid in the semicircular canals as in seasickness. Nausea may be caused by odors. Those who stay in the fresh air while on a rolling boat or ship are not nearly as subject to nausea as those who stay below deck. A skunk's ejection can produce violent nausea and vomiting.

Severe and persistent vomiting (as a result of physiologic or psychologic causes) may result in a number of metabolic disturbances. To understand these metabolic consequences, it is essential to know the properties of gastric juice. Under normal conditions, the daily volume of gastric juice secreted by the resting stomach is from 1 to 1½ liters, but it may increase to approximately 2½ liters under the stimulation of food intake and ordinary activity. Gastric juice is a complex and variable mixture of water, inorganic ions, hydrochloric acid, bicarbonate ions (when hydrochloric acid is absent), several enzymes, mucus, and the intrinsic factor. Cations found in the gastric juice include sodium, magnesium, calcium, and potassium. All except potassium are present in concentrations at or below their respective levels in other body fluids. Potassium, however, is usually present in a concentration 2 to 4 times that of the blood plasma. Loss of gastric juice, therefore, is a common cause of potassium depletion. Anions present include predominantly chloride with some phosphate and sulfate.[83-85]

Because of the nature of gastric juice, vomiting results in the loss of many electrolytes as well as fluid. Vomiting of the stomach contents alone leads to a loss of hydrogen and chlorides and ultimately to metabolic alkalosis. On the other hand, because the duodenal contents are predominantly alkaline, vomiting of contents from the intestinal tract causes a loss of alkali and this results in a metabolic acidosis. At the same time, vomiting of any origin results in a decreased carbohydrate intake, glycogen depletion, and ultimately ketosis, which also leads to metabolic acidosis.[86,87]

Vomiting confined to the gastric contents results not only in metabolic alkalosis but in a number of other disturbances, namely, a decrease in the chlorides in the blood (hypochloremia) a decrease in potassium in the blood (hypokalemia), and ultimately, excessive amounts of nitrogenous bodies in the blood (hyperazotemia), as a result of the following events. First, because of the loss of hydrochloric acid, there is a rise in bicarbonate in the extracellular fluid which causes a rise in body pH (alkalosis). In an attempt to offset the alkalosis, the kidney excretes bicarbonate; however, it also excretes sodium and potassium which are in combination with the bicarbonate. Because of this further loss of sodium, water also is lost, resulting in an increase in dehydration. In response to the alkalosis, potassium leaves the intracellular space, establishing a vicious circle in which the loss of potassium enhances the alkalosis, which, in turn, depletes the potassium. Although the kidney is capable of ridding the plasma of excessive potassium, it is not efficient in conserving this ion; consequently, as long as the kidney is capable of increasing the output of urine (diuresis), potassium may be lost in the urine despite a progressive depletion in the cells and serum. Finally, renal function is impaired by the dehydration which results in a decreased blood volume and a diminishing glomerular filtrate. There is consequently a retention of urea nitrogen which is reflected in the hyperazotemia. Although the renal loss of potassium is reduced with impaired kidney function, the net result is disadvantageous because the failing kidney can no longer excrete bicarbonate to combat the alkalosis. In this phase, there is marked oliguria, as well as a marked ketosis due to a lack of intake of carbohydrates and metabolism of fats.[88,89]

In addition to affecting the acid-base balance of the body, loss of potassium inhibits nerve impulses which ultimately results in muscular weakness and paralysis. In addition to a low serum potassium level in the blood, the electrocardiogram may be useful in detecting a low potassium level, as there is a depression and broadening of the T wave and a prolonged QT interval.[90,91]

Vomiting of gastric contents alone, which results in disturbances of metabolism discussed above, may occur in any condition in which the pyloric sphincter is obstructed, as, for example, an inflamed peptic ulcer, carcinoma of the stomach, congenital pyloric obstruction, pylorospasm, and adhesions of the duodenum to a chronically inflamed gallbladder.

In any condition where vomiting occurs, the amount of emesis should be measured, and the presence of food, gastric juice, mucus, bile, blood, and foreign bodies should be noted as well as its odor. Emesis, or vomitus, should have the penetrating odor of hydrochloric acid. If no odor is present, the absence of hydrochloric acid should be suspected. On the other hand, vomitus may have an odor of feces. This suggests intestinal obstruction, gastrocolic fistula, or peritonitis. If food particles are found 8 to 10 hours after eating, an obstruction at the pyloric sphincter may be present. A large amount of food residue containing bile suggests obstruction below the opening of the common bile duct (ampulla of Vater). If vomitus consists entirely of large amounts of pure gastric juice, which has the appearance of clear fluid, an active duodenal ulcer with hypersecretion and pylorospasm may be suspected. Excessive mucus with gastric juice might indicate chronic gastritis or rhinopharyngitis. The presence of blood is of great significance since it suggests a bleeding ulcer, ruptured esophageal varices, or carcinoma, all of which present a threat to life and may indicate the need for surgery.[92]

Treatment and Nursing Care. Treatment of the patient is based on the cause and effects of vomiting. For example, if vomiting is associated with ingestion of contaminated food, then the obvious treatment is removal of the stomach contents by irrigation. On the basis of the above discussion of causes, treatment is directed toward relieving vomiting in the following ways: (1) removal of all irritating substances from the stomach; (2) relief or prevention of distention of the stomach; (3) discontinuance of all drugs that stimulate the chemoreceptor trigger zone; (4) correction of all fluid and electrolyte imbalances; (5) correction of all metabolic disorders in which circulating "toxins" activate the chemoreceptor trigger zone; and (6) diminishing the sensitivity of the chemoreceptor trigger zone.

Irritating materials may be removed from the stomach and small intestines by gastric lavage or nasogastric suction, and from the large intestine by enemas.[93] (See Chapter 23 for a discussion of these procedures.) Nasogastric suction is usually used when the stomach is distended, as it prevents severe and prolonged vomiting that may result in disturbances in fluid and electrolytes.

There are several antiemetic drugs, including chlorpromazine, dimenhydrinate (Dramamine), trimethobenzamide (Tigan), and the barbiturates, that raise the threshold of the chemoreceptor trigger zone to stimulation. These drugs may be given in the treatment of vomiting and in the prevention of motion sickness.[94] According to John Adriani and associates,[95] antiemetics should be withheld until the need is established. In a study of 1625 postoperative patients, they found that 26 per cent vomited once, while only 15 per cent had persistent vomiting. If antiemetics are given prophylactically or routinely after the first vomiting, many patients receive a drug unnecessarily.

A number of physical and chemical agents may induce vomiting. Treatment with x-ray or radioactive isotopes frequently causes nausea and vomiting. However, treatment with radioactive substances is usually continued even when vomiting persists. Drugs are frequent offenders in nausea and vomiting. Narcotics such as morphine and meperidine (Demerol) may induce vomiting, especially in susceptible persons.* Toxic dosages of digitalis also cause vomiting. Drugs should be discontinued when it is evident that they are responsible for vomiting or when there is a likelihood of it.

Regardless of the cause of nausea and vomiting, nurses can help the victim by keeping the surroundings quiet. Visitors should be prohibited except for intimates who will refrain from talking. Nauseated persons are usually more comfortable lying flat with a pillow under the knees to relax the abdomen. Sometimes they want to lie on the abdomen for warmth and pressure. They dread movement and especially sudden movement. A hot-water bottle at the feet, sometimes on the abdomen, is comforting. A cold cloth on the forehead or an ice cap is often welcome.

For some patients it may be necessary to direct treatment toward restoring fluid and electrolyte balance. If vomiting persists and the patient is unable to take fluids, dehydration may be severe. Initially, isotonic intravenous solutions such as normal saline may be given to restore the fluid volume and improve kidney function. Of course, if there is hypernatremia (too much salt) the patient should be given a hypotonic solution; if there is hyponatremia (too little salt), the patient should be given a hypertonic solution. The amount of fluid given is based on the history, physical examination, laboratory reports, and the responses to therapy. When kidney function has been restored to a satisfactory urine output (approxi-

---

* Some persons are so sensitive to these drugs that they should carry with them a statement to this effect. Accidents can result in unconscious states in which the patient is unable to pass on this information.

mately 50 to 60 ml per hour), potassium chloride may be given intravenously. The daily dose of potassium chloride should be about 100 mEq, but larger doses may be necessary if depletion is severe. The metabolic alkalosis will ultimately be corrected by the administration of potassium chloride because the increase in body chlorides will reduce the amount of bicarbonate necessary to maintain balance in body fluids.[96,97]

Diet therapy may also be used to restore and maintain fluid and electrolyte balance. Initially, fluids should be given in the form of a clear liquid diet consisting of bouillon, clear broth, consommé, gelatin, sugar, weak tea, and water. However, it should be emphasized that this diet is inadequate in every respect and should not be used for more than 48 hours. The patient may then be given cereal, gruel, toast, crackers, skimmed milk, and ginger ale, and later a regular diet. Orange juice should not be taken initially as it increases peristalsis. If necessary, foods that are high in potassium may be included. Some of these are flavored meat extract, all coffee, especially instant Nescafé, dry whole milk, tea, cheese, and bananas. As the patient is progressively able to tolerate a diet orally, the intravenous fluid replacement can be decreased.[98,99]

Because fats are a common offender in vomiting, foods with high fat content should be restricted in the early stage of nausea and vomiting. Fluids taken at meals may also precipitate vomiting. Small meals consisting of foods such as thickly cooked cereals, melba toast with jelly, saltine crackers, and baked potato at 2-hour intervals may be well tolerated. Fluids should not be given during the meal but may be given 1 hour before and after eating. Skimmed milk should be taken rather than whole milk. Lean meats, fish, chicken, hardcooked eggs, and desserts such as arrowroot cookies, sponge cake, and pound cake may be added.

If vomiting continues over a long period, there may be dental erosion. The teeth become very white, worn, sensitive, and eroded.[100] Dental erosion is probably caused by the acid pH of the vomitus, according to A. C. McLundie and associates.[101] Frequent cleaning will prevent erosion and remove the taste of the vomitus. Rinsing the mouth with a carbonated drink such as ginger ale is refreshing to some patients. Chapter 14 discusses effective mouth care in detail.

The patient's environment should be as odorless as possible. It is very important that it be free of strong and offensive odors such as those from dressings, emesis, cleaning materials, and perfumes. The room should be well ventilated. As soon as the patient vomits, the emesis basin should be emptied, washed, and placed within reach but out of sight (if possible) because the sight of it may elicit vomiting. After vomiting, the patient should rinse the mouth. If the bed linens are soiled, they should be changed in such a way that the patient's position is moved slowly, as sudden movement may precipitate an attack of nausea and vomiting. On occasion, the vomiting reflex may be suppressed by deep breathing, swallowing, and cold applications to the throat.

As stated earlier, emotional care is important in the prevention and treatment of vomiting. Rhetaugh Dumas and Robert Leonard[102] have shown that emotional care is helpful in preventing vomiting in the postoperative period. In a study of 51 patients, nursing care was directed toward helping the patient attain a calm acceptance of surgery. They attempted to find out whether patients were in a state of psychologic stress, then explored the causes and what was needed to relieve the distress. The patients were seen at least 1 hour before surgery and the nurse researcher went with them to the operating room and stayed until patients were put on the operating table. Results showed that only 16 per cent of the patients receiving this treatment vomited, while 84 per cent of the control group vomited during the postoperative period. This suggests that helping the patient relieve fears and apprehensions before surgery results in a less stressful postoperative period physically as well as psychologically.

It is obvious that a number of measures may be necessary to control vomiting. At all times, the patient should be encouraged in the belief that vomiting can and will be controlled.

4. DIARRHEA

As the physiology underlying gastrointestinal function and elimination is discussed in Chapter 11, and a general discussion of causes, effects, prevention, and management of diarrhea is presented in Chapter 37, the discussion here is limited to severe diarrhea, resulting in disturbances in fluids and electrolyte balance, with emphasis on bacterial diarrhea.

The devastating effects of severe diarrhea in the past have been shown to change the course of history. For instance, during the Greek and Persian wars of the fifth century B.C., Xerxes' army was reduced 50 per cent by dysentery. In 1227, the crusade of Frederick II of Germany failed because he and his son were stricken with severe dysentery. In 1270, while en route to the Crusades, both Louis II of France and his son died of the same disease in Tunis, and Henry V of England and 75 per cent of his army lost their lives. During World War II, the victory of the British Army at El Alamein is attributed more to dysentery in the German and Italian military forces than to any other factor.[103,104]

Prior to and after the isolation of the organisms for cholera, salmonellosis, and shigellosis at the end of the nineteenth century by Robert Koch, Theobald Smith, and Shiga, a variety of therapies have been tried with varying degrees of success. Gerald Keusch makes the following observation: "It was only with the discovery of potent antimicrobials that specific therapy could be offered; and antimicrobials created additional new problems." *

Authorities consistently emphasize the importance of determining the specific causative agent. If the cause is unknown, the condition is described as "acute diarrheal disease" or "acute undifferentiated diarrhea." Organisms such as *Vibrio cholerae, Shigella, Staphylococcus, Salmonella, Escherichia coli,* and *Vibrio parachemolyticus* may cause a cholera-type diarrhea—profuse, painless, rice-water stools —and dysentery with scanty, mucoid, bloody stools with severe abdominal cramps. The only way to determine the specific etiology is by laboratory demonstration of the infecting agent or rising titer of specific antibodies.

Although it is hard to distinguish diarrhea from dysentery in many situations, such an attempt should be made, as an etiologic diagnosis is useful in treatment. Diarrhea is usually defined as an increase in the frequency of the stools over the customary habits of the individual, or a difference in their consistency. Diarrhea may vary from the elimination of several liters of feces to one loose stool in 24 hours. Dysentery is usually characterized by diarrhea with mucus-bloody feces, tenesmus, fever, abdominal tenderness, and colic—all of these symptoms are more severe than in diarrhea. While dysentery is associated with marked involvement of the colon, diarrhea involves the small intestine.[105,106]

Some Causes and Effects. It is difficult to say that a particular type of diarrhea (bacterial or nonbacterial) always causes an excessive loss of fluid. For instance, C. Benyajati[107] reports that when two volunteers were fed bacteria-free cholera toxin, one lost nearly 15 liters of liquid feces in 48 hours, while the other passed a single loose stool.

David W. Watson[108] believes volume overload of the colon, resulting in diarrhea, is the

most common of gastrointestinal afflictions. In cholera (which is, however, not an example of a common condition), the massive flux of sodium and fluid into the bowel lumen exceeds the reabsorptive capacity of the small intestines and the colon; consequently the colon fills to capacity and watery diarrhea follows. While patients with severe cholera ordinarily produce watery stools at the rate of 500 ml per hour, ordinarily the colon can be filled with a barium suspension to 1500 ml when examined by x-ray. The colon is capable of absorbing up to 300 ml of fluid daily—about 125 ml per hour, or a little more than 2 ml a minute. Obviously, a volume load can exceed these limits in a short period. As the volume of the watery feces increases, so does the loss of some electrolytes—sodium, potassium, chloride, and bicarbonate.

Some of the more common types of volume overload of the colon include diarrhea of travelers, viral gastroenteritis, enteropathogenic *E. coli* infection, *Clostridium* and staphylococcal toxin-contaminated foods, and the use of cathartics. Other infectious diarrheas that may result in fluid and electrolyte imbalance include salmonella enteritis and shigellosis. The bacteria causing these diseases are widely distributed in nature and may be found in contaminated foods, for instance in meats, poultry, dried eggs, and milk, and also water. Poor sanitation, low standards of personal hygiene, and crowded living conditions favor the spread of these infections.[109-112a]

Additional causes of diarrhea are not included in this chapter as they are discussed in Chapter 37. It should be remembered that the effects of diarrhea, regardless of cause, can result in dehydration accompanied by loss of sodium, potassium, chloride, and bicarbonate.[113]

Diarrhea frequently results in dehydration, and excessive loss of potassium (hypokalemia) and metabolic acidosis. Symptoms of dehydration include dry skin and mucous membranes, with furrows of the tongue; weight loss, which may be in excess of 10 per cent in the infant or in excess of 5 per cent in the child or adult; oliguria or anuria; drop in body temperature; and lassitude. There is an increase in the red blood cell count, packed cell volume, and hematocrit because the plasmal volume is decreased owing to the decrease in extracellular fluid volume. Severe diarrhea is one of the most frequent causes of metabolic acidosis, according to Arthur C. Guyton, because of excessive loss of gastrointestinal secretions which normally contain large amounts of sodium bicarbonate. The bicarbonate buffer system shifts toward the acid side, resulting in

---

* Keusch, Gerald: "Bacterial Diarrheas," *Am. J. Nurs.,* **73:**1028, (June) 1973.

metabolic acidosis. He makes the following statement: "In fact, acidosis resulting from severe diarrhea can be so serious that it is one of the most common causes of death in young children." * The major effect of acidosis is *depression of the central nervous system*. As the serum pH falls below 7.0, the nervous system is so depressed that the patient is weak and lethargic; he or she may then progress to disorientation, and finally from stupor to coma. The respirations are deep and rapid. With excessive loss of potassium (hypokalemia), the following symptoms occur: abdominal distention from collection of gas in the intestine; soft, flabby muscles; weakness, tremors; flaccid paralysis; paresthesia of the extremities; disorientation; and later, heart block and cardiac arrest. Of course, the severity of symptoms depends on the degree of potassium loss.

Prevention and Management of Diarrhea.
The immediate treatment of severe diarrhea is replacement of fluid and electrolytes. If the patient does not have renal failure, the urine output is an important index of hydration; however, the degree of hydration is best measured by the hemoconcentration, according to Leighton E. Cluff. Discussing treatment of cholera, he makes the following observation: "Plasma protein concentration, and particularly plasma specific gravity, can usually serve as a reliable index for administration of fluids and electrolyte." † Other laboratory examinations, including serum potassium, sodium, chloride, bicarbonate, glucose, pH, and hematocrit are usually considered necessary. When the patient is first seen, large volumes of physiologic saline and 5 per cent glucose may be given to correct hydration while the various examinations are made.

Isotonic alkalinizing solutions are used to correct metabolic acidosis. These include sodium lactate ⅙ M, Butler's solution, and lactated Ringer's solution. For some patients, the physician may elect to add specific amounts of various electrolytes to the solution.

In a study of 53 children with severe cholera and noncholera diarrhea, Dilip Mahalanabis and associates [114] report two methods of treatment that were equally effective. To one group, only lactated Ringer's solution was given intravenously, while additional water, glucose, and potassium were being given by mouth; to the other group, three different intravenous solutions (with various amounts of electrolytes) were given to meet all fluid and electrolyte requirements. About 15 per cent of the children treated in the first group were subject to prolonged stupor and vomiting and were unable to take a sufficient quantity of glucose by mouth; consequently, a hypotonic glucose-saline solution as an intravenous supplement was necessary. These investigators are convinced that lactated Ringer's solution is suitable as the sole intravenous solution for children with acute diarrhea (cholera or noncholera) if oral supplements as described are tolerated.

Accurate measurement of all fluid losses is mandatory in the acute phase—watery feces, urine, and vomitus (if any). Daily weight is important and should be taken if bed scales are available for those who are bedfast. Discussing the importance of the relationship of fluid output to treatment in cholera, Charles C. J. Carpenter has the following to say:

The same fluids should subsequently be infused in quantities equal to the gastrointestinal losses. If losses cannot be measured accurately, intravenous fluids should be given at a rate sufficient to maintain a normal radial pulse and normal skin turgor. Overhydration can be avoided by careful observation of neck venous filling and auscultation of the lungs. Close observation is mandatory during the acute phase of the illness, because the cholera patient can lose as much as 1 liter of isotonic fluid per hr during the first 24 hr of the disease. Inadequate or delayed restoration of fecal fluid losses may result in a very high incidence of acute renal failure.*

The same statements apply to patients with other forms of severe diarrhea, although the amount of fecal fluid loss is not usually as high as in cholera. (See Chapter 11, page 714, for an example of Intake and Output Records.)

During the acute stage of diarrhea, the gastrointestinal tract is usually put to rest by giving glucose, electrolytes, and fluids parenterally; however, oral therapy is instituted as quickly as possible. Oral electrolyte solutions are useful because glucose in the lumen of the small bowel facilitates absorption of water and salts, counterbalancing that lost in the stools.[115] Frequent, high-caloric feedings with large amounts of fluids should be encouraged. Foods that are high in calories and proteins, such as custards, puddings, and milk, are well tolerated by most persons. Additional foods are added until the patient is able to eat a normal diet. The reader should consult Chapter 37 for

---

* Guyton, Arthur C.: *Textbook of Medical Physiology*, 5th ed. W. B. Saunders Co., Philadelphia, 1976, p. 497.

† Cluff, Leighton E.: "Cholera," in Beeson, Paul B., and McDermott, Walsh (eds.): *Textbook of Medicine*, 14th ed., Vol. I, W. B. Saunders Co., Philadelphia, 1975, p. 375.

* Carpenter, Charles C. J.: "Cholera," in Wintrobe, Maxwell M., et al. (eds.): *Harrison's Principles of Internal Medicine*, 7th ed., Vol. I. McGraw-Hill Book Co., New York, 1974, p. 856.

a more detailed discussion of dietary management of diarrhea.

Currently, a number of antimicrobial agents may be used in the treatment of bacterial diarrheas. Noting that the choice of drugs differs with the physician, Louis Weinstein, writing in Louis S. Goodman and Alfred Gilman's text, makes the following observation:

. . . the current availability of a number of drugs that are approximately equally effective makes an order of choice very difficult, if not impossible. To complicate matters, sensitivity patterns of a number of microorganisms often vary with the hospital or clinic in which they are isolated; in some instances, this reflects a varying degree of exposure to specific agents.*

Neomycin, tetracycline, or ampicillin are usually given when the diarrhea is caused by the organism *E. coli;* in shigellosis (caused by one of the species of *Shigella* bacilli), ampicillin, chloramphenicol, or tetracycline may be used. Tetracycline is the drug of choice in the treatment of cholera (caused by *Vibrio cholerae*) when prompt replacement of the large loss of water and electrolytes does not stop the diarrhea. The dosage varies with the age and condition of the patient and the severity of the disease.[116] Currently there is no evidence that antibiotic therapy is effective in diarrhea caused by the microorganism *Salmonella,* according to Edward W. Hook.[117]

Medication to control diarrhea and dysentery or inhibit bowel movements may be necessary. Most authorities consulted say that opium or its derivatives such as paregoric, morphine, codeine, or diphenoxylate hydrochloride may reduce abdominal discomfort and tenesmus but should be used cautiously. The use of antibiotics that destroy organisms causing frequent or copious bowel movements has almost replaced the use of drugs that inhibit the elimination of the offending bowel content. See Chapter 37 for additional information.

Until preventive measures, including public education and protective legislation, are given as much attention as medical treatment for the major worldwide health problems discussed in this chapter, it is doubtful whether health personnel can be very effective in their efforts to build a healthy, productive world citizenry. T. D. Luckey and B. R. Maier, in their article "A Holistic Approach to the Interruption of the Diarrhea-Malabsorption-Malnutrition Cycle," note that with increased dietary supplements, food packaging, and relatively good rainfall in the past few years, the condition of children in underdeveloped countries has probably improved in the last decade; however, no real impact has been made on the incidence of malnutrition in 1 billion people. They list the following conditions that must be considered:

The holistic view of infantile and childhood diarrhea must consider vectors of a) environmental management including cleanliness and a reduction of counter-productive bacterial inocula from the environment; b) nutrition with or without supplements; c) therapeutic drugs to break the cycle of diarrhea-malabsorption-malnutrition; d) a positive microbic input; and e) education toward changing habits, albeit with a minimum of perturbation of present activities. Success of a program would be read in reduced mortality and would present the political problem of a 5% increase in population growth.*

Luckey and Maier stress the importance of improving sanitation and cleanliness. The reasons for and against the use of antibiotics are discussed in considerable detail. It has been known for a long time that when people are malnourished they are subject to all types of infections. A healthy state is dependent on being well nourished and knowing what a good diet is; on having essential foods available; and on having the will to use both knowledge and food to maintain the health of children and adults, the weak, and the elderly. What has been said about the problems of people in underdeveloped nations applies equally to many poverty-stricken areas in the most advanced nations of the world.

REFERENCES

1. MacBryde, Cyril M.: "Weight Loss and Undernutrition," in MacBryde, Cyril M., and Blacklow, Robert Stanley (eds.): *Signs and Symptoms; Applied Pathologic Physiology and Clinical Interpretation,* 5th ed. J. B. Lippincott Co., Philadelphia, 1970, p. 872.
2. Young, Vernon R., and Scrimshaw, Nevin S.: "The Physiology of Starvation," *Sci. Am.,* **225:**14, (Oct.) 1971.
3. Keys, Ancel: *The Biology of Human Starvation.* University of Minnesota Press, Minneapolis, 1950.
4. Kotz, Nathan: *Let Them Eat Promises.* Doubleday & Co., Garden City, N.Y., 1971.
5. Bullough, Bonnie, and Bullough, Vern L.:

* Weinstein, Louis: "Antimicrobial Agents. General Considerations," in Goodman, Louis S., and Gilman, Alfred (eds.): *The Pharmacological Basis of Therapeutics,* 5th ed. Macmillan Publishing Co., Inc., New York, 1975, p. 1096.

* Luckey, T. D., and Maier, B. R.: "A Holistic Approach to the Interruption of the Diarrhea-Malabsorption-Malnutrition Cycle," *Am. J. Clin. Nutr.,* **25:**612, (June) 1972.

Poverty, Ethnic Identity, and Health Care. Appleton-Century-Crofts, New York, 1972.

6. Mayer, Jean (ed.): *U.S. Nutrition Policies in the Seventies.* W. H. Freeman & Co., San Francisco, 1973.

7. Manocha, Sohan L.: *Malnutrition and Retarded Human Development.* Charles C Thomas, Publisher Springfield, Ill., 1972, p. 3.

8. Winich, M.: "Nutrition and Mental Development," *Med. Clin. North Am.,* **54:** 1413, (Nov.) 1970.

9. *Hunger, U.S.A.: A Report by the Citizen's Board of Inquiry into Hunger and Malnutrition in the United States.* Beacon Press, Boston, 1968, p. 20.

10. Delgado, Graciela, et al.: "Eating Patterns Among Migrant Families," *Public Health Rep.,* **76:**349, (Apr.) 1961.

11. MacBryde, Cyril M.: *op. cit.,* p. 873.

12. Orshansky, Mollie: "The Poverty Roster," in Ralston, Richard M. (ed.): *Sources: A Blue Cross Report on the Health Problems of the Poor.* Blue Cross, Chicago, 1968, p. 10.

13. Halsted, J. A.: "Geophagia in Man: Its Nature and Nutritional Effects," *Am. J. Clin. Nutr.,* **21:**1384, (Dec.) 1968.

14. Minnich, V., et al.: "Pica in Turkey. Effect of Clay upon Iron Absorption," *Am. J. Clin. Nutr.,* **21:**78, (Jan.) 1968.

15. Ronaghy, H., et al.: "Controlled Zinc Supplementation for Malnourished Schoolboys: A Pilot Experiment," *Am. J. Clin. Nutr.,* **22:**1279, (Oct.) 1969.

15a. Bristrian, B. R., et al.: "Prevalence of Malnutrition in General Medical Patients," *J.A.M.A.,* **235:**1567, (Apr. 12) 1976.

16. MacBryde, Cyril M.: *op. cit.,* p. 897.

17. Chase, P. H., et al.: "The Effect of Malnutrition on the Synthesis of a Myelin Lipid," *Pediatrics,* **40:**551, (Oct.) 1967.

18. Davison, A. N., and Dobbing, J.: "Myelination as a Vulnerable Period in Brain Development," *Br. Med. Bull.,* **22:**40, (No. 1) 1966.

19. Latham, Michael C., and Cobos, Francisco: "The Effects of Malnutrition on Intellectual Development and Learning," *Am. J. Public Health,* **61:**1307, (July) 1971.

20. Goldsmith, Grace A.: "Professional and Para-Professionals," in Mayer, Jean (ed.): *U.S. Nutrition Policies in the Seventies.* W. H. Freeman & Co., San Francisco, 1973, p. 193.

21. Choate, Robert: "Special Problems of the Poor," in Mayer, Jean (ed.): *U.S. Nutrition Policies in the Seventies.* W. H. Freeman & Co., San Francisco, 1973, p. 188.

22. Manocha, Sohan L.: *op. cit.,* p. 297.

23. Buskirk, E. R.: "Obesity," in Downey, John A., and Darling, Robert C.: *Physiological Basis of Rehabilitation.* W. B. Saunders Co., Philadelphia, 1971, p. 229.

24. *Ibid.*

25. Maddox, G.: *Slim Down, Shape Up Diets*

for Teen-Agers. Avon Books, New York, 1963.

26. Dwyer, Johanna T., and Mayer, Jean: "Attitudes Toward Body Weight and Dieting Behavior; Potential Dieters: Who Are They?" *J. Am. Diet. Assoc.,* **56:**510, (June) 1970.

27. Moore, Mary E., et al.: "Obesity, Social Class, and Mental Illness," *J.A.M.A.,* **181:** 962, (Sept. 15) 1962.

28. Goldblatt, P. B., et al.: "Social Factors in Obesity," *J.A.M.A.,* **192:**1039, (June 21) 1965.

29. Silverton, J. T., et al.: "Social Factors in Obesity in London," *Practitioner,* **202:**682, (May) 1969.

30. Hinkle, L. E., Jr.: "Occupation, Education and Coronary Heart Disease," *Science,* **161:**238, (July) 1968.

31. Albrink, Margaret J.: "Obesity," in Beeson, Paul B., and McDermott, Walsh (eds.): *Textbook of Medicine,* 14th ed., Vol. I. W. B. Saunders Co., Philadelphia, 1975, p. 1376.

32. Wilson, Nancy L., et al.: "The Development and Perpetuation of Obesity: An Overview," in Wilson, Nancy L., et al. (eds.): *Obesity.* F. A. Davis Co., Philadelphia, 1969, p. 3.

32a. Albrink, Margaret J.: *op. cit.*

33. Knittle, J. L., and Hirsch, J.: "Effect of Early Nutrition on the Development of Rat Epididymal Fat Pads: Cellularity and Metabolism," *J. Clin. Invest.,* **47:**2091, (Oct.) 1968.

34. Buskirk, E. R.: "Increasing Energy Expenditure: The Role of Exercise," in Wilson, Nancy L., et al. (eds.): *Obesity.* F. A. Davis Co., Philadelphia, 1969, p. 163.

35. ———, et al.: "Energy Balance of Obese Patients During Weight Reduction: Influence of Diet Restriction and Exercise," *Ann. N.Y. Acad. Sci.,* **110:**918, 1963.

36. Moody, D. L., et al.: "The Effect of a Moderate Exercise Program on Body Weight and Skinfold Thickness in Overweight College Women," *Med. Sci. Sports,* **1:**75, (Jan.) 1969.

37. Jacobs, D., et al.: "Obesity. Prevention," *J.A.M.A.,* **186:**28, (Jan. 10) 1963.

38. Bullen, B. A., et al.: "Physical Activity of Obese and Nonobese Adolescent Girls Appraised by Motion Picture Sampling," *Am. J. Clin. Nutr.,* **14:**211, (Apr.) 1964.

39. Wilson, Nancy L., et al.: *op. cit.,* p. 6.

40. Kiell, Norman (ed.): *The Psychology of Obesity; Dynamics and Treatment.* Charles C Thomas, Publisher, Springfield, Ill., 1973.

41. Stunkard, Albert J.: "The Obese: Background and Programs," in Mayer, Jean (ed.): *U.S. Nutrition Policies in the Seventies.* W. B. Freeman & Co., San Francisco, 1973, p. 29.

42. Best, Charles H., and Taylor, Norman B.: *The Physiological Basis of Medical Prac-*

tice, 8th ed. Williams & Wilkins Co., Baltimore, 1966, p. 1410.

43. "Overweight and Hypertension," *Nutr. Rev.,* **27**:168, (June) 1969.

44. Stunkard, Albert J.: *op. cit.,* p. 31.

45. Stunkard, A. J., and Burt, V.: "Obesity and the Body Image. II. Age at Onset of Disturbances in the Body Image," *Am. J. Psychiatry,* **123**:1443, (May) 1967.

46. Richardson, N. S., et al.: "Cultural Uniformity and Reaction to Physical Disability," *Am. Sociol. Rev.,* **26**:241, (Apr.) 1961.

47. Maddox, G. L., et al.: "Overweight as Social Deviance and Disability," *J. Health Soc. Behav.,* **9**:287, (Dec.) 1968.

48. Maddox, G. L., and Liederman, V.: "Overweight as a Social Disability with Medical Implications," *J. Med. Educ.,* **44**:214, (Mar.) 1969.

49. Canning, M., and Mayer, J.: "Obesity— Its Possible Effect on College Acceptance," *N. Engl. J. Med.,* **275**:1172, (Nov. 24) 1966.

50. Albrink, Margaret J.: *op. cit.,* p. 1457.

51. Mayer, J., and Thomas, D. W.: "Regulation of Food Intake and Obesity," *Science,* **156**:328, (Apr.) 1967.

52. Moody, D. L., et al.: *op. cit.*

53. Van Itallie, T. B.: "Management of Obesity," in Southward, H., and Hofman, F. G. (eds.): *Columbia-Presbyterian Therapeutic Talks,* Vol. I. Macmillan Publishing Co., Inc., New York, 1963, p. 163.

54. Buskirk, E. R.: "Obesity," in Downey, John A., and Darling, Robert C.: *Physiological Basis of Rehabilitation.* W. B. Saunders Co., Philadelphia, 1971, p. 235.

55. Drenick, E. J.: "Starvation in the Management of Obesity," in Wilson, Nancy L., et al. (eds.): *Obesity.* F. A. Davis Co., Philadelphia, 1969, p. 191.

56. Gilder, H., et al.: "Components of Weight Loss in Obese Patients Subjected to Prolonged Starvation," *J. Appl. Physiol.,* **23**:304, (Sept.) 1967.

57. US Public Health Service, Division of Chronic Diseases: *Obesity and Health: A Source Book of Current Information for Professional Health Personnel.* US Government Printing Office, Washington, D.C., 1966.

58. Kjellberg, Jan, and Reizenstein, Peter: "Effect of Starvation on Body Composition in Obesity," *Acta. Med. Scand.,* **188**:171, (Sept.) 1970.

59. Shumway, Sandra, and Powers, Marjorie: "The Group Way to Weight Loss," *Am. J. Nurs.,* **73**:269, (Feb.) 1973.

60. Ryan, Geraldine C.: "Ms. S.," *Am. J. Nurs.,* **73**:273, (Feb.) 1973.

61. Willacker, Jean: "Follow-up of Ms. S.," *Am. J. Nurs.,* **73**:275, (Feb.) 1973.

62. Kalisch, Beatrice J.: "The Stigma of Obesity," *Am. J. Nurs.,* **72**:1124, (June) 1972.

62a. Loxsom, Rosalind: "Changing Obesity Patterns," *Nurs. Outlook,* **23**:711, (Nov.) 1975.

63. Buskirk, E. R.: "Increasing Energy Expenditure: The Role of Exercise," in Wilson, Nancy L., et al.: (eds.): *Obesity.* F. A. Davis Co., Philadelphia, 1969, p. 163.

64. ———, et al.: "Energy Balance of Obese Patients During Weight Reduction: Influence of Diet Restriction and Exercise," *Ann. N.Y. Acad. Sci.,* **110**:918, 1963.

65. Nathanson, M. H.: "The Central Action of B-aminopropylbenzene (Benzedrine)," *J.A.M.A.,* **108**:528, (Feb. 13) 1937.

66. Lesses, M. F., and Myerson, A.: "Human Autonomic Pharmacology: Benzedrine Sulfate as an Aid in the Treatment of Obesity," *N. Engl. J. Med.,* **218**:119, (Jan. 20) 1938.

67. Luria, D. B.: *The Drug Scene.* McGraw-Hill Book Co., New York, 1968.

68. Perman, E. S.: "Speed in Sweden," *N. Engl. J. Med.,* **283**:760, (Oct. 1) 1970.

69. "And Pep in America" (editorial), *N. Engl. J. Med.,* **283**:761, (Oct. 1) 1970.

70. Payne J. H., and DeWend, L. T.: "Surgical Treatment of Obesity," *Am. J. Surg.,* **118**:141, (Aug.) 1969.

71. Heydman, Abby Hitchcock: "Intestinal Bypass for Obesity," *Am. J. Nurs.,* **74**:1102, (June) 1974.

72. Scott, H. W., Jr., et al.: "Experience with a New Technique of Intestinal Bypass in the Treatment of Morbid Obesity," *Ann. Surg.,* **174**:560, (Oct.) 1971.

73. "Is the Intestinal Bypass Operation an Accepted Method of Treatment for Obesity," *J.A.M.A.,* **223**:1281, (Mar. 12) 1973.

74. Isselbacher, Kurt J., and Shumaker, Jay B.: "Anorexia, Nausea, and Vomiting," in Wintrobe, Maxwell M., et al., (eds.): *Harrison's Principles of Internal Medicine,* 7th ed., Vol. I. McGraw-Hill Book Co., New York, 1974, p. 210.

75. Faigenblum, M. J.: "Retching, Its Causes and Management in Prosthetic Practice," *Br. Dent. J.,* **125**:485, (Dec. 3) 1968.

76. Guyton, Arthur C.: *Textbook of Medical Physiology,* 5th ed. W. B. Saunders Co., Philadelphia, 1976, p. 899.

76a. Kirsner, Joseph B.: "The Stomach," in Sodeman, William A., Jr., and Sodeman, William A.: *Pathologic Physiology, Mechanisms of Disease,* 5th ed. W. B. Saunders Co., 1974, p. 711.

77. McGuigan, James E.: "Anorexia, Nausea, and Vomiting," in MacBryde, Cyril M., and Blacklow, Robert Stanley (eds.): *Signs and Symptoms; Applied Pathologic Physiology and Clinical Interpretations,* 5th ed. J. B. Lippincott Co., Philadelphia, 1970, p. 369.

78. Martin, W. J., and Marcus, S.: "Relation of Pyrogenic and Emetic Properties of Enterobacteriaceal Endotoxin and of Staphylococcal Enterotoxin," *J. Bacteriol.,* **87**:1019, (May) 1964.

79. Sugiyama, H., and Hayama, T.: "Abdominal Viscera as Site of Emetic Action for Staphylococcal Enterotoxin in the Monkey," *J. Infect. Dis.*, **115**:330, (Oct.) 1965.

80. Purkis, Ian E.: "Factors That Influence Post-Operative Vomiting," *Can. Anaesth. Soc. J.*, **11**:335, (Apr.) 1964.

81. Hill, Oscar: "Psychogenic Vomiting and Hypokalemia," *Gut*, **8**:98, (Apr.) 1967.

82. ———: "Psychogenic Vomiting," *Gut*, **9**:348, (June) 1968.

83. Best, Charles H., and Taylor, Norman B.: *op. cit.*, p. 1086.

84. Howe, C. T., and LeQuesne, L. P.: "Pyloric Stenosis: The Metabolic Effects," *Br. J. Surg.*, **51**:923, (Dec.) 1964.

85. Ellis, Harold: "Stenosis Due to Duodenal Ulceration," *Postgrad. Med. J.*, **42**:778, (Dec.) 1966.

86. Guyton, Arthur C.: *op. cit.*, p. 497.

87. Bland, John: *Clinical Metabolism of Body Water and Electrolytes.* W. B. Saunders Co., Philadelphia, 1963, p. 188.

88. Welt, Louis G.: "Acidosis and Alkalosis," in Wintrobe, Maxwell M., et al. (eds.): *Harrison's Principles of Internal Medicine,* 7th ed., Vol. II. McGraw-Hill Book Co., New York, 1974, p. 1365.

89. Nathan, Galloway, et al.: "Hypokalemic Neuropathy of Vomiting," *South. Med. J.*, **57**:1303, (Nov.) 1964.

90. Cantor, Meyer: "Ileus," *Am. J. Gastroenterol.*, **47**:461, (June) 1967.

91. Brusilow, Saul, and Cooke, Robert: "Fluid Therapy of Diarrhea and Vomiting," *Pediatr. Clin. North Am.*, **11**:889, (No. 4) 1964.

92. Bockus, Henry L.: *Gastroenterology,* Vol. I. W. B. Saunders Co., Philadelphia, 1963, p. 45.

93. Rapoport, Morton I.: "Food Poisoning," in Conn, Howard F. (ed.): *Current Therapy, 1973.* W. B. Saunders Co., Philadelphia, 1973, p. 19.

94. Jarvik, Murray E.: "Drugs Used in the Treatment of Psychiatric Disorders," in Goodman, Louis S., and Gilman, Alfred: *The Pharmacological Basis of Therapeutics,* 5th ed. Macmillan Publishing Co., Inc., New York, 1975, p. 169.

95. Adriani, John, et al.: "Postanesthetic Vomiting," *Am. J. Surg.*, **103**:2, (Jan.) 1962.

96. Howe, C. T., and LeQuesne, L. P.: *op. cit.*

97. Welt, Louis G.: *op. cit.*

98. Turell, Robert: *Diseases of the Colon and Anorectum.* W. B. Saunders Co., Philadelphia, 1969, p. 168.

99. Wohl, Michael, and Goodhart, Robert: *Modern Nutrition in Health and Disease.* Lea & Febiger, Philadelphia, 1968, p. 836.

100. Allen, Douglas: "Dental Erosion from Vomiting," *Br. Dent. J.*, **136**:311, (Apr. 1) 1969.

101. McLundie, A. C., et al.: "Studies of the Effects of Various Ions on Enamel Solubility," *Arch. Oral Biol.*, **13**:1321, (Nov.) 1968.

102. Dumas, Rhetaugh, and Leonard, Robert: "The Effect of Nursing on the Incidence of Post-Operative Vomiting," *Nurs. Res.*, **12**:12, (Winter) 1963.

103. Felsen, Joseph: *Bacillary Dysentery, Colitis and Enteritis.* W. B. Saunders Co., Philadelphia, 1945, p. 1.

104. Gear, H. S.: "Hygiene Aspects of the El Alamein Victory, 1942," *Br. Med. J.*, **1**:383, (Mar. 18) 1944.

105. Gorbach, S. L., et al.: "Intestinal Microflora in Asiatic Cholera: Part 2. The Small Bowel," *J. Infect. Dis.*, **121**:38, (Jan.) 1970.

106. Beaty, Henry N., and Patersdorf, Robert G.: "Shigellosis (Bacillary Dysentery)," in Wintrobe, Maxwell M., et al. (eds.): *Harrison's Principles of Internal Medicine,* 7th ed. McGraw-Hill Book Co., New York, 1974, p. 811.

107. Benyajati, C.: "Experimental Cholera in Humans," *Br. Med. J.*, **1**:140, (Jan. 15) 1966.

108. Watson, David W.: "The Small Intestine," in Sodeman, William A., Jr., and Sodeman, William A. (eds.): *Pathologic Physiology, Mechanisms of Disease,* 5th ed. W. B. Saunders Co., Philadelphia, 1974, p. 759.

109. Schroeder, A. S., et al.: "Epidemic Salmonellosis in Hospitals and Institutions. A 5 Year Review," *N. Engl. J. Med.*, **279**:674, (Sept. 26) 1968.

110. Mallory, A., and Gangarosa, E. J.: "Salmonella Surveillance 1968," *J. Infect. Dis.*, **121**:87, (Jan.) 1970.

111. Giannella, Ralph A., et al.: "Salmonella Enteritis. II. Fulminant Diarrhea in and Effects on the Small Intestine," *Digestive Dis.*, **16**:1007, (Nov.) 1971.

112. Cluff, Leighton E.: "Shigellosis," in Beeson, Paul B., and McDermott, Walsh (eds.): *Textbook of Medicine,* 14th ed., Vol. I. W. B. Saunders Co., Philadelphia, 1975, p. 371.

112a. Sack, R. Bradley: "Human Diarrheal Disease Caused by Enterotoxigenic *Escherichia coli*," *Annu. Rev. Microbiol.*, **29**:333, (Mar.) 1975.

113. Gamble, John R., and Wilbur, Dwight L.: *Chemistry of Digestive Diseases.* Charles C Thomas, Publisher, Springfield, Ill., 1961, p. 85.

114. Mahalanabis, Dilip, et al.: "The Use of Ringer's Lactate in the Treatment of Children with Cholera and Acute Non-Cholera Diarrhoea," *Bull. WHO,* **46**:311, (No. 3) 1972.

115. Hirschiorn, N., et al.: "Decrease in Net Stool Output in Cholera During Intestinal Perfusion with Glucose-Containing Solutions," *N. Engl. J. Med.*, **279**:176, (July 25) 1968.

116. Weinstein, Louis: "General Considerations," in Goodman, Louis S., and Gilman,

Alfred (eds.): *The Pharmacological Basis of Therapeutics,* 5th ed. Macmillan Publishing Co., Inc., New York, 1975, p. 1090.

117. Hook, Edward W.: "Salmonella Infections Other Than Typhoid Fever," in Beeson, Paul B., and McDermott, Walsh (eds.): *Textbook of Medicine,* 14th ed., Vol. I. W. B. Saunders Co., Philadelphia, 1975, p. 366.

Additional Suggested Reading

Barnes, H. V., et al.: "An Approach to the Obese Adolescent," *Med. Clin. North Am.,* **59:**1507, (Nov.) 1975.

Bray, George A.: "The Myth of Diet in the Management of Obesity," *Am. J. Clin. Nutr.,* **23:**1141, (Sept.) 1970.

Bruns, Thomas W.: "Nutritional Factors in Disease," in Sodeman, William A., Jr., and Sodeman, William A.: *Pathologic Physiology, Mechanisms of Disease,* 5th ed. W. B. Saunders Co., Philadelphia, 1974.

Christakis, George: "Obesity and Nutrition Education," *Minn. Med.,* **52:**1279, (Aug.) 1969.

Curtis, Diane E., and Bradfield, Robert B.: "Long-term Energy Intake and Expenditure of Obese Housewives," *Am. J. Clin. Nutr.,* **24:**1410, (Dec.) 1971.

Fisher, A., et al.: "Obesity: Its Relation to Anesthesia," *Anaesthesia,* **30:**633, (Sept.) 1975.

Hollifield, Guy, and Parson, William: "Metabolic Adaptations to a 'Stuff and Starve' Feeding Program. I. Studies of Adipose Tissue and Liver Glycogen in Rats Limited to a Short Daily Feeding Period," *J. Clin. Invest.,* **41:**245, (Feb.) 1962.

James, J. Walter: "Longitudinal Study of the Morbidity of Diarrheal and Respiratory Infections in Malnourished Children," *Am. J. Clin. Nutr.,* **25:**690, (July) 1972.

Kopacz, M. S., et al.: "Through a Glass Darkly," *Am. J. Nurs.,* **75:**2159, (Dec.) 1975.

Levitan, Ruven: "Colonic Absorption of Electrolytes and Water," *Am. J. Clin. Nutr.,* **22:**315, (Mar.) 1969.

Low-Beer, T. S., and Read, A. E.: "Progress Report, Diarrhoea: Mechanisms and Treatment," *Gut,* **12:**1021, (Dec.) 1971.

Melton, Janet Hornell: "A Boy with Anorexia Nervosa," *Am. J. Nurs.,* **74:**1649, (Sept.) 1974.

Mendeloff, Albert I.: "Constipation, Diarrhea, and Disturbances of Anorectal Function," in Wintrobe, Maxwell M., et al. (eds.): *Harrison's Principles of Internal Medicine,* 6th ed. McGraw-Hill Book Co., New York, 1970.

Murrell, T. G. C., et al.: "Pig-Bel: Enteritis Mecroticans, A Study in Diagnosis and Management," *Lancet,* **1:**7431, (Jan. 29) 1966.

"Nutrition," *Public Health Rep.,* **84:**211, (Mar.) 1969.

Robson, J. R. K.: "Zen Macrobiotic Dietary Problems in Infancy," *Pediatrics,* **53:**326, (Mar.) 1974.

Schmidt, Mary P. W., and Duncan, Beverly A. B.: "Modifying Eating Behavior in Anorexia Nervosa," *Am. J. Nurs.,* **74:**1646, (Sept.) 1974.

Scrimshaw, Nevin S.: "Undernutrition, Starvation, and Hunger Edema," in Beeson, Paul B., and McDermott, Walsh (eds.): *Cecil-Loeb Textbook of Medicine,* 13th ed. W. B. Saunders Co., Philadelphia, 1971, p. 1437.

Seltzer, Carl C., et al.: "Reliability of Relative Body Weight as a Criterion of Obesity," *Am. J. Epidemiol.,* **92:**339, (June) 1970.

Stare, Fredrick J.: "Overnutrition," *Am. J. Public Health,* **53:**1795, (Nov.) 1963.

Truelove, S. C., and Reynell, P. C.: *Diseases of the Digestive System,* 2nd ed. Blackwell Scientific Publications, Oxford, London, 1972.

Gladys Nite
Virginia Henderson

CHAPTER 37

Marked Disturbance of Elimination— Constipation, Diarrhea, Retention or Suppression of Urine, Incontinence of Urine or Feces

1. CONSTIPATION
2. DIARRHEA
3. RETENTION OF URINE
4. SUPPRESSION OF URINE
5. INCONTINENCE OF URINE OR FECES

1. CONSTIPATION

To understand the problem of constipation, its causes, prevention, and correction, one must understand the underlying physiology. As the subject has been discussed in Chapter 11, only a brief description is given here. This chapter should be studied in conjunction with Chapter 11.

When food enters the stomach (as when eating an ordinary meal), it begins to pass into the duodenum within a few minutes. The process takes 3 or 4 hours and leaves the stomach empty. The rate of gastric emptying depends on a number of factors, the chief ones being the amount and type of food eaten, the time intervals between eating, and the person's nutritional and emotional state. Chyme moves rapidly in the duodenum and jejunum, more slowly in the ileum, taking 6 to 9 hours to reach the large intestine. The consistency of chyme in the small intestine is semiliquid; a great deal of water is absorbed but is also replaced, to some extent, by the secretions of the intestinal mucosa (succus entericus), pancreatic juice, and bile. Formation of the stool, eventually discharged from the rectum, is accomplished in the colon, especially the cecum and transverse colon where maximum water absorption takes place.[1] Motility of the small intestine and colon is influenced by the autonomic nervous system; motility may be increased by parasympathetic action or decreased by the sympathetics. The following types of movement or contraction propel the food residue through the gastrointestinal tract: segmenting, pendular, kneading, peristaltic, and mass. Control of the segmenting and pendular movements is inherent in the muscles.

N. C. Hightower, Jr., and Henry D. Janowitz describe the composition of feces as follows:

. . . adult on an average diet excrete from 75 to 170 grams of feces daily, about 25 to 30% of which is made up of solids; the remainder is water. If the diet is rich in vegetables the quantity is greater, especially if the vegetables are eaten raw. Bacteria comprise about one-third of the dry weight of the feces under average conditions. The pH is 7.0 to 7.5. . . . The organic material is principally cellulose, protein and fats. About half the protein nitrogen of the feces is of bacterial origin; the remainder represents unabsorbed intestinal secretions and digestive fluids, mucus, and desquamated epithelial cells from the mucosa. Only a small amount is actual food residue. Enzymes are also present but in very small quantities. . . . Fats comprise from 5 to 25% of the feces under normal circumstances. . . .*

The feces normally is a brown, soft, plastic mass. It is colored by stercobilin and urobilin, derivatives of bilirubin. The characteristic odor is derived from products of bacterial action, which varies according to the type of food eaten and the person's colonic bacterial flora. Indole, skatole, mercaptans, and hydrogen sulfide are the odoriferous products.[2]

Definition. Henry L. Bockus defines constipation as "an abnormal retention of fecal mat-

* Hightower, N. C., Jr., and Janowitz, Henry D.: "Movements of the Alimentary Canal," in Brobeck, John R., et al. (eds.): *Best and Taylor's Physiological Basis of Medical Practice,* 9th ed. Williams & Wilkins Co., Baltimore, 1973, pp. 2–120.

ter in the intestinal canal or an undue delay in the discharge of excreta from the rectum." * There is wide variation in defecating patterns. Some persons defecate once daily, others 2 or 3 times, while there are those who normally defecate once every 2 to 3 days. When the stool is dry and hard and defecation is uncomfortable, the person is said to be constipated. If the proximal end of the feces is as hard as the distal end, obviously, the person is constipated.

Causes and Effects of Constipation. Authorities give many causes of constipation, or delayed defecation. Malcolm L. Peterson[3] classifies them under three headings as follows, but notes some overlapping: (1) *Neurogenic constipation* is induced by direct stimulation or inhibition of the autonomic nervous system, with the impulses arising in the brain, the hypothalamus, the medulla, the cord, or the peripheral nerve endings. Examples are lack of regularity or failure of the individual to respond to the reflex impulse, excessive tone (spastic colon), psychogenic disturbances, such as grief, anger, or fear, acute infectious disease, traumatic lesions and organic disease of the nervous system, and drugs such as morphine, codeine, and atropine. (2) *Muscular constipation* is caused by problems or diseases that interfere with the motility of the bowel. Examples are lack of sufficient bulky foods to stimulate reflex activity, excessive use of laxatives that overstimulate the bowel, thus "wearing out" the reflex, inflammation of the abdominal and pelvic viscera, intrinsic lesions of the ileum and colon, and extra-alimentary tumors, resulting in narrowing of the bowel lumen by compression. (3) *Mechanical constipation* is caused by problems or diseases that interfere with the ability of the bowel to move the chyme or fecal matter distally at its usual rate. Some of these are weakness of the bowel muscles, weakness of the voluntary muscles of defecation, an abnormal consistency of the bowel content as in severe dehydration, mechanical obstruction of the bowel lumen, and megacolon.

Bockus[4] stresses the adverse effects of civilization on defecation. He believes that modern living has fostered constipation for the following reasons: (1) most persons eat a diet lacking in roughage; (2) few persons train the child at an early age to establish the habit of defecating at a regular time, while both young and old neglect the defecation urge; (3) few assume the squatting position for defecation that increases intra-abdominal pressure which, in turn, helps expel the fecal mass; (4) few provide sufficient toilet facilities to maintain good sanitation in public places, institutions, schools, and business offices, which interferes with immediate response to the defecation urge, thereby blunting or eliminating it; and (5) many persons abuse laxatives and enemas. Unfortunately this practice is begun in childhood in many families. It results in constipation for a day or two, followed by more purging or enemas, until there are bowel movements.

Most authorities consulted recognize the importance of the following four muscular structures: the diaphragm, abdominal wall, pelvic floor, and intestinal musculature. They say that weakness or lack of tone in any one of these can be a cause of constipation. However, they think the loss of rectal defecation reflex caused by failure to heed the defecation urge or by repeated use of strong laxatives is probably the most frequent cause of simple constipation. They also emphasize medicinal agents, such as antacids (calcium carbonate, aluminum hydroxide), opiates, alcohol, and sedatives as causes of constipation. The role that these drugs play in inducing constipation should be stressed, as so many persons in our society today have access to at least some of these—if not directly by way of the corner drugstore and liquor store, indirectly by appeal to the physician. Antacids may be bought at any drugstore and many people purchase these, using them indiscriminately for "nervous stomach" and functional and organic disorders. Unfortunately, more and more people rely on sedatives and tranquilizers as a substitute for solving their personal problems. To get most of these medications, a medical prescription is necessary. Even so, it is not uncommon in a social setting to hear individuals comparing the type and effectiveness of sedative or tranquilizer they are using. The escape through alcoholism is commonplace. Those of us who are familiar with current hospital practices know the frequency with which sedatives and tranquilizers are used so that the "patient gets a good night's sleep," "rests better," "isn't so nervous," "isn't so depressed."

Early in this chapter we noted that emotions can cause constipation. Frederic R. Stearns reports that "many individuals who have chronic constipation are known to have a tendency to angry responses." * Moses Paulson[5] thinks *life stress* and *emotional conflict*

---

* Bockus, Henry L. (ed.): *Gastroenterology*, Vol. II, 3rd ed. W. B. Saunders Co., Philadelphia, 1976, p. 936.

* Stearns, Frederic R.: *Anger, Psychology Physiology Pathology*. Charles C Thomas, Publisher, Springfield, Ill., 1972, p. 11.

are often associated with the development of the irritable colon. He says this phenomenon has been observed by clinicians and supported by scientific investigations. The incidence of colitis is high in the United States, and it is possible that the same stresses in our culture that have led to an increase in frank psychoses are producing such somatic conditions as ulcers of the stomach, the irritable, hyperactive, ulcerative colon, and even the atonic hypoactive colon with its associated constipation.*

Fecal impaction occurs when overdry feces is tightly wedged into the colon or rectum. The mass is most commonly found in the rectum, but may extend into the distal colon. The size of the mass is variable, and may be as large as 5 to 6 cm (about 2 inches). The mass can be palpated through the abdominal wall and is hard, movable, and nonpainful.[6] A fecal impaction develops because there is an incomplete evacuation of feces from the rectum. The fecal matter continues to accumulate in the colon and rectum, and as long as the mass remains in contact with the bowel mucosa, it loses fluid through absorption. The result is a firm, large mass of stool that cannot be mechanically expelled through the anal sphincter. Occasionally, a patient has frequent, small, watery stools, although the rectum is still partially obstructed.

Conditions that induce severe or prolonged constipation may result in a fecal impaction; the more common predisposing conditions are (1) bed rest, especially in the elderly person who has been constipated previously and in some surgical patients who are not ambulated early; (2) debilitation, especially in the aged and others because of muscular atony and lack of physical exercise, as in the orthopedic patient; (3) mental illness, when the psychotic person fails to heed the defecation urge; (4) use of drugs, those that influence the character of the stools, hardening them (aluminum and bismuth used as antacids and barium used in x-ray examinations, and hydrophilic colloids and bran, in some instances), and those that slow bowel motility (anticholinergic group used for peptic ulcer); and (5) organic causes

that block the passage of solid feces such as congenital megacolon, strictures, and anal disease, including spasm.[7] Impaction is common among alcoholics for they have frequent periods of near coma when they fail to respond to any stimuli.

Although fecal impactions may occur more frequently than we would like to believe possible in general and special hospitals, including mental institutions, nursing homes which are growing in number almost daily, and in private homes where we find many elderly persons whose activity is limited, the complications that result, according to Edward C. Raffensperger, are rare. He says:

> The most serious [complication] is perforation. Bizarre manifestations of perforation have been reported, such as fecaloma in a fallopian tube and in a dermoid. Dystocia caused by fecal impaction has been reported. Rarely complete obstruction by fecal impaction may require operation. Under these circumstances operation may have been performed because of an erroneous diagnosis of tumor. Goodall reported a jejunal obstruction from a calcium soap fecalith in a patient who had multiple duodenal and jejunal diverticula. Fecal impaction in the elderly male with prostatism may give rise to difficulty in urination and at times urinary retention. These symptoms are relieved by the breaking up and evacuation of the impaction.*

Because persons with a fecal impaction usually strain excessively when trying to expel the feces, pathologic conditions such as cerebrovascular accidents, heart block, hemorrhoids, fissures, ulcers, and rectal prolapse may occur at or near the time of defecating.[8]

It seems safe to say that the incidence of constipation, a symptom of so many disorders of the body and mind, probably affects all persons, male and female, of all ages, in health and in sickness. I. Phillips Frohman [9] believes that more men are affected than women because they are more subject to stress; women who have had children are also prone to develop constipation (possibly from muscle impairment); and tense children anywhere are also likely candidates.

Most authorities consulted mention the high incidence of constipation in the aged. Theodore Chohen and Leo Gitman,[10] in a study of 102 elderly patients who had clinical evaluation of the gastrointestinal tract, report the most common complaint was constipation—43.1 per cent. Contributing factors were decreased intestinal secretions, decreased peristalsis, loss of

---

* J. Clark Maloney compares the 400 mentally ill per 100,000 population in the United States in 1949 with the 80 mentally ill per 100,000 in 1880. He also compares figures for the United States with the 49 mentally ill per 100,000 in Japan in 1940. The suggestion is that the rigid infant toilet training in the United States may be a contributory factor. (Report of the Sakuraga-Oka, Hoyoin or Cherry Hill Asylum, Tokyo.) (Senn, Milton J. [ed.]: *Problems of Infancy and Childhood; Transactions of the Fourth Conference, New York, March, 1950.* Josiah Macy, Jr. Foundation, New York, 1951.)

* Raffensperger, Edward C.: "Fecal Impaction of the Colon and Rectum," in Bockus, Henry L. (ed.): *Gastroenterology,* Vol. II, 2nd ed. W. B. Saunders Co., Philadelphia, 1964, p. 1075.

abdominal wall tone, and decreased nervous sensibility.

In the care of infants and small children, the mother or her substitute usually attaches great importance to any sign of constipation; in fact, it is overstressed. Lack of bulky food may cause constipation at any age but according to Waldo E. Nelson and associates,[11] constipation in breast-fed infants who receive an adequate amount of milk is practically unknown and is rare in those who are fed artificially. Additional causes that he mentions in the child are (1) spasticity of the intestine resulting from irritation by cathartics or too much residue, and fissures or hemorrhoids causing spasm of the rectal sphincter; (2) lack of muscular tone of the intestinal and abdominal muscles which may occur in malnutrition, rickets, anemia, any protracted illness, lack of exercise, and following long, continued use of laxatives, enemas, and suppositories; (3) anatomic abnormalities such as various forms of incomplete intestinal obstruction, enteroptosis, anal stenosis, megacolon, and an unduly long or tortuous sigmoid; and (4) a faulty habit pattern of defecation, including irregular habits of evacuation and injudicious use of suppositories, enemas, and laxatives.

Common signs and symptoms associated with constipation are multiple and vary in individuals. The most important are the type and quality of the feces. The typical stool of the constipated is hard and dry, including the distal end, and there is more or less difficulty in defecating. Frequently, there is straining with excessive use of the voluntary muscles. Bockus says:

In simple constipation (dyschezia) symptoms are rare until one of the following has occurred:

1. A fecal mass in the rectum or sigmoid has achieved great size producing local or reflex symptoms.
2. A lesion has developed in the anal canal owing to pressure of the fecal mass, or to frequent movements following the ingestion of laxatives, or to irritation from an enema tube, or to trauma from the passage of hard stools.
3. Abdominal symptoms have appeared because of irritation of the intestines due to the use of laxatives and enemas.*

Local symptoms in rectal constipation (dyschezia) include a sensation of fullness or pressure in the rectum, tenesmus (spasmodic contraction of anal sphincter) accompanied by a frequent desire to move the bowels, and unsuccessful attempts at defecation. When these symptoms occur, the fecal mass is so large that even with straining it is difficult to eject

through the anal canal. In chronic constipation, complications such as hemorrhoids, fissures, ulcers, inflamed anal papilla, and a diffuse anusitis are common. Abdominal symptoms usually occur after the person has become habituated to the use of laxatives or enemas. They include epigastric fullness and discomfort, belching, regurgitation, and nausea. Those addicted to laxatives have abdominal distention, excessive flatus, and migratory abdominal pains.

Reflex symptoms are now thought to be caused by distention of the rectum and pressure of the feces on the anterior divisions of the third, fourth, and fifth sacral nerve roots rather than by intestinal toxemia. Common reflex manifestations are pain in the region of the sacrum, buttocks, back of the thighs, and the hip joint as well as headache and vertigo. With prolonged constipation, Bockus notes that there are systemic manifestations and he suggests that a state of low-grade toxemia may exist; however, it is difficult to prove that toxins absorbed from the intestinal tract produce systemic effects. Symptoms most often cited include anorexia, nausea, bad taste, coated tongue, malaise, chronic fatigue, dull headache, vertigo, pains in the muscles and joints, slight anemia, low-grade nutritional deficiencies, and occasionally a sallow, brownish complexion of the skin. Most persons presenting these symptoms are addicted to laxatives and, in fact, may have gone for many years without having a well-formed stool.

It is of interest to note the amount of money spent on laxatives. Writing on the subject in 1955, Frohman says:

Last year the American public spent $85,000,000 for proprietary laxatives. An additional $20,000,000 was probably spent on laxatives prescribed by physicians, since it is fairly safe to assume that 1 out of every 10 patients has some bowel dysfunction which requires such a prescription. American people, then, spend $105,000,000 yearly to move their bowels! *

Ten years later (1965), Keith W. Sehnert[12] reports that retail drugstores and hospital pharmacies bought $34.8 million (wholesale) worth of bowel evacuants and laxatives in 1 year. When one considers the physiologic and psychologic damage that results from continued use of artificial help in defecating, one wonders why, in this enlightened age, people continue to buy these laxatives and evacuants (spending an exorbitant amount of money) and why they are prescribed and given so routinely and freely to patients in hospitals of

* Bockus, Henry L. (ed.): *op. cit.,* p. 941.

* Frohman, I. Phillips: "Constipation," *Am. J. Nurs.,* **55:**65, (Jan.) 1955.

all types, nursing homes, clinics, and private homes. It seems as though the American people, health workers included, are far too concerned about the bowel and far too inclined to use artificial rather than natural means of stimulating its movements.

Prevention and Management of Constipation. It is obvious from the above discussion that prevention is important; all efforts should be directed toward helping people, sick or well, to avoid the *routine* use of laxatives, enemas, and suppositories. Once the habit is established, it is difficult to break. Constipation must be recognized as a symptom and if treatment is to be successful, the cause must be identified and removed. Bockus says:

The most important principles of management include: (1) an attempt to eradicate the underlying cause, (2) the education of the patient in the physiology of defecation, (3) stopping the use of strong laxatives and enemas, and (4) the institution of a regimen to re-establish normal hygiene.*

A superficial glance at these principles may lead one to conclude that implementation of them is easy and that results will be immediate, but this is not true. Most authorities say that to reestablish normal defecation habits in a person takes a long time (2 to 4 weeks for some) and a great deal of patience.

Any person suffering from constipation must understand the physiology of defecation. One explanation is not sufficient. In fact, repeated instruction may be needed. Visual aids, including diagrams, may be helpful. The patient is the most important member of the health team and it is doubtful if any therapeutic program is effective for a long period unless the person (or, in the case of an infant or small child, the parent) is willing to cooperate fully in all aspects. And, the more the patient or the parent knows, the better equipped he or she is to deal with the problem.

The diet plays a major role in preventing and managing constipation. Patients should understand that if they omit or eat too little breakfast, bowel peristalsis may not be stimulated. A well-balanced diet including sufficient fibrous and laxative foods is desirable. Foods that have a high fibrous content are kale, cabbage, celery, raw vegetable salads, raw and cooked fruits, and whole-grain cereals and breads.[13] Prunes are thought by some to have a more laxative effect than any other food, probably because they have an active principle like di-hydroxyl-phenyl isatin. Bedfast coronary patients who drank prune juice, 150 to 200 ml, before breakfast reestablished their normal defecation patterns more quickly than did a similar group who did not drink prune juice.[14]

Neil Stamford Painter [15,16] recommends a high-residue diet including bran to prevent constipation in persons with diverticular disease because it is "known that a low-residue diet produces the disease." For those persons with an "irritable colon" who are forced to eat a "bland" diet, bananas are an excellent food because they have a high fibrous content but are nonirritating to the mucosa of the colon. The addition of milk sugar (lactose) is another means of increasing the laxative quality of the diet. Foods that should be avoided are those that are highly refined and concentrated, and excessive amounts of rough bran and seasoning. Thomas P. Almy [17] believes that the quantity and quality of food taken at breakfast is more important than the bulk of the over-all residue of the daily diet or the total amount of daily fluid intake since one purpose of breakfast is to produce a peristaltic rush, culminating in a vigorous gastrocolic reflex. He suggests that everyone eat a large breakfast, as for example, fruit juice, stewed prunes or other cooked fruit, cereal with milk and sugar, toast, jam, and coffee. The importance of such a diet is certainly understandable when one knows the physiology of stool formation and defecation.

Conditioning of the defecation reflex should be established. Shortly after eating a large breakfast the person should sit on the toilet for at least 10 minutes, his or her condition permitting. The environment should be relaxing if possible. It may be necessary for an adult to get up earlier than usual and rearrange the early morning's activities. If there are activities that ordinarily promote relaxation, such as reading or browsing through a favorite magazine, these should be encouraged. It will probably be helpful for the nurse to review with the patients their early morning activities. Then, together, a realistic regimen may be planned and opportunity provided for clarifying any misunderstanding and asking any questions. As mentioned earlier, some physicians say that it may take as long as 4 weeks to reestablish normal defecation patterns. Patients must be involved in setting the therapeutic goal and accept the length of time it may take to reach it.

For a detailed discussion of toilet training of infants and small children, the reader is referred to Chapter 11. Probably all that needs to be said here is that tension in the child, mother, or attendant interferes with conditioning of the defecation reflex. As with the

---

* Bockus, Henry L. (ed.): *op. cit.,* p. 944.

adult, the child needs an environment that is conducive to relaxation. Most authors, discussing constipation, speak of the "tense person" as having a "tense intestine." *When the defecation urge occurs, regardless of time, the person should heed it,* lest the reflex is weakened.

Posture and exercise are important factors in defecation. The sitting position should be used with the feet flat on the floor. If the feet are supported on a stool or block of wood to produce a squatting position, this is even more effective since intra-abdominal pressure, necessary for expelling feces, is increased. (However, straining at stool distends blood vessels and can cause hemorrhage or dislodge clots or plaques on the vessel walls in those suffering from cardiovascular disease.) The height of toilets should be given more attention. The infirm find it difficult to get on and off very low seats, and the high seat is disadvantageous to the "bearing down" act. An adjustable footstool may be the best solution of the problem until an adjustable toilet seat is developed. Exercise and its importance in elimination is frequently overlooked. Any activity that improves muscle tone should be encouraged. Walking and swimming are helpful, but it is especially important to strengthen the abdominal and perineal muscles with exercises designed to accomplish this.

Most authors refer to the abuse of laxatives and enemas or the laxative habit and enema habit. It is worth repeating that far too many laxatives and enemas are used in the home and hospital. Unfortunately, their dangers aren't stressed. Certainly all health workers should question their continued use and every effort should be made to substitute harmless practices. This is not to say that some persons, under certain circumstances, should not be given laxatives or enemas. But the routine laxative given before bedtime is highly questionable. The use of mineral oil over a period of time is believed by some authors to cause lipoid pneumonia and loss of vitamins, minerals, and ingested calories.[18] Nurses should do all they can to help patients break the laxative or enema habit and should certainly not contribute to the formation of either.

If laxatives are necessary, the bulk-forming laxatives are recommended by most authorities. Hydrophilic colloids or gummy agents that tend to swell when combined with fluid and to form an emollient gel or viscous solution keep the feces softened and hydrated. It is thought that peristalsis is stimulated reflexly by this indigestible residue. Although the full effect of these agents may not occur until the second or third day, it is usually evident within 12 to 24 hours. Copious amounts of water (at least 8 glasses in 24 hours) should be taken with all bulk-forming laxatives.[19] Some of the popular brand names are Metamucil, Siblin, Mucidose, Plancillo, Calogel, and Konsyl.

Manigel, a powder containing mannitol, pectin, and dehydrated citrus fruit juices, was found to be an effective laxative in a study of 39 patients, ranging in age from 15 to 70 years. The average daily dose was 3 to 4 heaping tsp of powder stirred into a glass of water, fruit juice, lemonade, or milk. A cup of hot tea or coffee or a glass of plain water immediately after taking the powder improved results.[20]

Stool softeners are helpful for those persons who may be susceptible to fecal impactions, especially the elderly and bedridden and those with active anal disease or anal and rectal strictures. In such persons the fecal mass is likely to be large, well formed, or hard, necessitating considerable straining at stool which may precipitate a cardiovascular crisis. Dioctyl sodium sulfosuccinate is reportedly successful in such patients because it softens the fecal material without irritating the bowel.[21]

Other laxatives or cathartics that may be given to those with a long history of constipation—those who have used enemas and strong laxatives repeatedly—include the following: (1) irritants—cascara, senna, rhubarb, bisacodyl, phenolphthalein, castor oil; (2) saline cathartics—magnesium hydroxide (milk of magnesia), magnesium sulfate, magnesium citrate solution, sodium phosphate; and (3) emollients—mineral oil, light or heavy. None of these drugs should be used over long periods; each is credited with some harmful side effects. Uncomfortable griping may occur with the irritants; saline cathartics cause excessive loss of water and electrolytes; and the emollients (oil in the form of a laxative) interfere with the absorption of vitamins A and B and may cause lipoid pneumonia.[22,22a]

Although suppositories and enemas may be used for some persons, authorities are in agreement that their continued use must be discouraged. Eric Hudson[23] (in 1961) says he is convinced the "old methods" will eventually die; that is, enemas and laxatives will not be used to treat constipation. Marcelle F. Dunning and Fred Plum[24] report the development of severe potassium depletion in a patient with poliomyelitis following repeated prolonged enemata. Potassium loss seemed to be greatest when contact between infused fluid and the dilated atonic bowel was prolonged. The reader should consult Chapter 23 for a detailed discussion of the methods and therapeutic uses of enemas and suppositories.

Education of the individual, sick or well, is probably the most important contribution of all health workers, including the nurse, in the prevention and management of constipation. Everybody should understand the physiology of defecation and the conditions that promote normal bowel habits as well as those that contribute to the development of constipation. The routine use of laxatives should be discouraged in hospitals, and other measures, discussed in the preceding pages, used to facilitate normal bowel movements. Observation of the frequency, type, amount, and consistency of stool should be noted. An assessment of the patient's "normal" defecation pattern should always be made, otherwise treatment may be instituted for some persons who really have no defecation problem.

2. DIARRHEA

Definition. Diarrhea, the opposite of constipation, is an abnormal precipitant passage of fecal material in the intestinal canal resulting in loose stools. The frequency of bowel movements is ordinarily increased, and the person may have abdominal cramping, or tenesmus.

Some Causes and Effects of Diarrhea. Diarrhea, like constipation, is a symptom of many ills, physical and emotional. Various classifications of diarrhea are used, based on etiology, site of involvement, and on its acute or chronic nature. Peterson[25] gives the following four causes of diarrhea under pathophysiologic mechanisms, noting some limitations with this arrangement: (1) *Malabsorption* of water, fats, proteins, or carbohydrates or various combinations of these may be caused by a defect or temporary inflammatory changes of the mucosa of the small intestine, lack of certain enzymes, and derangement of bile salt activity, resulting in diarrhea. Examples are pancreatitis, regional enteritis, lactase deficiency, metallic poisons, and cholera. (2) *Neurogenic basis of diarrhea,* the results of dysfunction of the sympathetic system, the parasympathetic system, or muscular tissue, may be caused by atony or increased motility of the intestines. Because motility is under neural and endocrine control, a variety of conditions and medications can cause diarrhea, for instance, postvagotomy, diabetic enteropathy, irritable colon, narcotic withdrawal, and excessive doses of some drugs (colchicine, quinidine). (3) *Mechanical diarrhea,* associated with incomplete obstruction of the bowel, may be caused by stenosis, adhesions, tumors, and fecal impaction (especially in the elderly,

bedridden, and postoperative patient). (4) *Inflammatory diarrhea* is caused by mucosal damage from organisms or their toxins. Examples are salmonellosis, turista, ulcerative colitis, amebiasis, and tropical sprue.

E. Clinton Texter[26] reports that 50 per cent of all patients with gastrointestinal problems who consult physicians have functional motor disturbances of the bowel and these are second only to the common cold as a cause of disability. He says disturbances of any of the primary functions of the small intestines (motility, secretion, digestion, and absorption) or of the large intestine (motility, absorption, storage, and excretion) may result in diarrhea. Following an extensive review of the literature (226 references), T. S. Low-Beer[27] reports more than 4 million working days were lost in England and Wales in the year 1966–1967 (with similar rates in the United States) owing to acute diarrhea. While acute diarrhea is usually mild and self-limiting in adults, it may be dangerous in infants. Organisms identified in a minority of cases include *E. coli* (in serious infantile epidemics), *Salmonellae,* and some viruses. In tropical countries, however, acute diarrhea can be very serious, as for example, cholera may kill up to 60 per cent of those infected, sometimes within 4 hours of the onset of symptoms. The staphylococcus organism, associated with acute gastroenteritis, is seen in two forms of infection. Staphylococcal food poisoning, a virulent illness, is the most common bacterial food poisoning in the United States. Foods such as custards, processed meat, potato salad, and chicken salad have been most often reported as responsible for the infection. Within 1 to 6 hours after eating the contaminated food, the subject has severe cramping abdominal pain, vomiting, and profuse diarrhea. Headaches, fever, and dehydration are not uncommon; however, recovery is usually rapid for most young or middle-aged adults (in about 24 hours). The elderly, those suffering from other serious disease, or debilitated persons may die, according to Harold P. Lambert.[28] The other form of infection caused by an overgrowth of *Staphylococcus aureus* (not usually pathogenic in the gastrointestinal tract) in patients who have received antibiotic therapy may result in acute diarrhea. Nurses should be aware of this possibility.

Discussing the extent of the problem of acute diarrhea, Mervin Silverberg and Murray Davidson write:

Epidemics of acute diarrhea are still common, are usually associated with excessive waves of endemic diarrheal disease, natural disasters and sewage pollution and occur in vulnerable groups, such as newborns, mental retardates and newly aggregated and migrant populations. Among infants, even in well developed societies, acute diarrhea still ranks among the five most common causes of death. In older children and adults, in whom it is usually milder, it is exceeded only by upper respiratory infections as the most frequent cause of disease. One of every six illnesses of adults in the United States is a digestive disorder, and episodes of diarrhea are among the most common gastrointestinal complaints.*

Functional diarrhea (or nonorganic diarrhea) is usually thought to have a psychosomatic basis but authorities disagree on whether the emotional or the somatic influences are most important. The generic term "irritable colon" is frequently used for conditions such as "mucous colitis, mucous diarrhea, spastic colon, spastic diarrhea, nervous diarrhea and colonic neurosis," according to Silverberg and Davidson.[29] Arthur C. Guyton [30] says psychogenic or emotional diarrhea is precipitated by nervous tension, as for instance, when a student is taking an examination or when soldiers go into battle. In such situations, there is excessive stimulation of the parasympathetic nervous system, resulting in increased motility and secretion of mucus in the colon. In fact, in tense states, large quantities of water and electrolytes may be lost when the chyme in the small intestine is flushed into the large intestine and on through the anus. In ulcerative colitis the motility of the colon is often so great that mass movements occur most of the time (rather than the usual 10 to 20 minutes each day) and the secretions are also increased. Ulcerative colitis is like neurogenic diarrhea in this respect as well as being associated with different states of nervous tension. In both conditions the person has repeated diarrheal bowel movements.

Nervous or emotional diarrhea, according to Bockus,[31] occurs most often in persons who are nervous, sensitive, and emotionally unstable. Bouts of diarrhea may continue for days and even weeks in some cases, usually follow emotional stress (fear or grief), tension, anxiety, and nervous shock. Stools, in the morning after breakfast and after other meals, are liquid in consistency. The person may be a semi-invalid if the diarrhea persists over a long period of time. Bockus thinks that persons suffering from mucous colitis exhibit characteristics that are not necessarily evident in those with a spastic colon. Emotional tension is severe; anxiety, resentment, and guilt are common; and the patient may exhibit depressive, neurasthenic, and hypochondriac features.

The cause of ulcerative colitis remains unknown but a number of theories, yet to be validated by experimental research, include infection (bacteria, viruses, fungi), destructive enzymes (mucinase, proteolytic), lack of "protective" substance in the colon, allergy and hypersensitivity (food allergy as with milk, bacterial endotoxin), and psychovisceral (colonic motor disturbances, vascular disturbances, autonomic nervous imbalance). The onset of the condition may occur at any age, infancy to old age, but seems to be more common between the ages of 20 and 40 years.[32,32a] Diarrhea, cramping abdominal pain, and rectal bleeding are a consequence of the inflamed and ulcerated colon. Large amounts of plasma proteins and electrolytes (especially potassium) are lost by way of the raw colon surface. James L. A. Roth says, "These losses in the exudate of ulcerative colitis may create profound deficits, manifest clinically and in the laboratory." * The first symptom is diarrhea, and the stools contain bloody mucus; constipation may follow. The severity of diarrhea may vary from three to four stools in one day or as often as every 1 to 2 hours during the 24-hour period. As the condition persists the character of the stool may change to a "soft formed, mushy, or a loose, brick-red slush and mixture of blood" and defecation is associated with urgency and incontinence in some circumstances. The rectal area may be excoriated, causing considerable discomfort. Abdominal pain, colicky or crampy, usually occurs in the left lower abdominal quadrant. Anorexia, fullness, nausea, epigastric discomfort, and vomiting (probably reflexly initiated) may occur and to such a degree that it is difficult to maintain normal nutrition. It is not surprising that persons with severe ulcerative colitis lose weight and strength. The temperature may or may not be elevated, but when it is, dehydration may be a contributing factor.

Following an extensive survey of the literature, Roth concludes that if one accepts the concept that ulcerative colitis is a manifestation of constitutional disturbances, anything that affects the body as a whole can cause a recurrence. Causes discussed by authorities cited include the following: (1) emotional or psychic disturbances, with some believing that 50 per cent of recurrences are on this basis; (2) upper respiratory and intercurrent infec-

---

* Silverberg, Mervin, and Davidson, Murray: "Functional and Organic Causes of Diarrhea," in Turell, Robert (ed.): *Diseases of the Colon and Anorectum,* Vol. II, 2nd ed. W. B. Saunders Co., Philadelphia, 1969, p. 847.

* Roth, James L. A.: "Ulcerative Colitis," in Bockus, Henry L. (ed.): *Gastroenterology,* Vol. II, 3rd ed. W. B. Saunders Co., Philadelphia, 1976, p. 654.

tions, including gastrointestinal infections such as "food poisoning," dysentery and "virus," tonsillitis, tooth infection, and occasionally systemic infections, have been attributed to a relapse or reoccurrence; (3) dietary indiscretion, especially food or drink to which the person is unaccustomed; also food sensitivity (such as seafood, milk, chocolate, eggs) and the use of bowel irritants, strong laxatives, or other irritating drugs (colchicine, antibiotic-mycins); (4) pregnancy, especially if the child is unwanted; and finally (5) less common causes are thought to be stress due to exertion, physical fatigue, surgical procedures, or endocrine and allergic factors. In summary, the importance of emotion in recurrence of this condition is obvious.

Some of the colonic complications include pseudopolyposis, stricture, perianal abscess or fistula, massive hemorrhage, carcinoma, toxic megacolon, and perforation; systemic complications are arthritis, skin lesions, and liver disease. Obviously, the effects of ulcerative colitis may be many, varied, and of a serious nature. Effective management and prevention of recurrence is the major concern of all health workers if the serious consequences of this condition are to be avoided.

The importance of the role of defective carbohydrate digestion and absorption in the production of diarrhea in infants, children, and adults is emphasized by authorities. Lactose (a reducing disaccharide found principally in the milk of all mammals and constituting practically all the carbohydrates in the mother's milk) intolerance is a condition in which the body is unable to utilize ingested lactose. This results in nutritional failure and chronic diarrhea. The stools are watery, have an acid reaction, smell sour, and appear frothy.[33-35]

It is well known that a considerable portion of the world's population does not get enough to eat; many go to bed at night in a state of hunger. The United States also has its share of poverty. Salvador Zubiran (1962) notes that malnutrition may be caused by gastrointestinal diseases and disturbances. His studies of the Mexican population show that the majority have a deficient diet. In a special study on 92 adults with primary malnutrition, he found that 86 per cent had diarrhea. He says:

Diarrhea was the outstanding clinical finding in the majority of cases. The clinical syndrome is similar to the malnutrition diarrhea or "hunger diarrhea" observed in famines and in concentration camps. The number of bowel movements per day varied.

Stools contained mucus and blood in 41 per cent of the patients, suggesting the possibility of a primary intestinal disease. However, results of stool studies for intestinal parasites and pathogenic bacteria were negative.

In 28 per cent of the patients, gross fat and undigested food particles were present in the stools. These findings have often been described in the literature and the pathogenesis has been widely discussed. This diarrhea should probably be attributed to deficient intestinal absorption brought about by malnutrition and probably involves no constant morphologic alterations.*

Diarrhea is said to be a troublesome complication following treatment of duodenal ulcer by vagotomy. Some studies suggest that diarrhea is related to the type of surgical procedure, while others suggest it is related to gastric stasis.[36,37]

As noted throughout this discussion, the effects of diarrhea can be serious. According to John R. Gamble and Dwight L. Wilbur,[38] diarrhea, regardless of cause, can result in dehydration "accompanied by loss of sodium, potassium, chloride and bicarbonate." Acidosis may occur, especially in children; however, alkalosis does also occur, but less often. In chronic diarrhea the potassium loss may be greater than expected because of loss by the urine as well as feces. The severity of dehydration and hypokalemia may be increased by an inadequate intake, so common among persons with diarrhea. The subject of fluid and electrolyte disturbances is discussed in greater detail in Chapter 36.

Prevention and Management of Diarrhea. It is frequently necessary, according to Almy,[39] to relieve the diarrhea or its consequences before the causes can be identified and treated. Diarrhea helps rid the body, at least in part, of the offending agent in most acute infectious diarrheas. Replacement of fluid and electrolyte loss by infusion of physiologic saline and 5 per cent glucose is usual. The amounts and proportions are "guided by measurements of urinary output and plasma volume." Replacement of potassium and other adjustments of acid-base balance is dependent on the serial determinations of serum sodium, potassium, chloride, and bicarbonates.

If the person can tolerate oral fluids, warm weak tea, broth, and ultimately thin cooked cereals should be given in sufficient quantity to maintain a urinary output in excess of 1500 ml per day. Cold liquids and concentrated sweets should *not* be taken as they are poorly tolerated. Following this dietary regimen, a low-residue diet is given. Foods that leave

* Zubiran, Salvador: "Nutritional Aspects of Gastrointestinal Disease," in McHardy, Gordon: *Current Gastroenterology.* Harper & Row, New York, 1962, p. 197.

little, if any, residue in the intestinal tract include tender beef, veal, chicken, hard-cooked eggs, boiled or steamed rice, strained fruit juices, and broth.[40]

The opium alkaloids, according to Louis S. Goodman and Alfred Gilman,[41] are the most effective agents in treating dysenteries and exhaustive diarrhea. It is important to recognize that dependency on the drug may occur when used over a long period. Almy [42] believes that bismuth, pectins, and kaolin (binding agents) are not too effective. Those that are effective include aluminum hydroxide gel (20 to 40 ml four times a day), codeine sulfate 0.03 to 0.06 gm or morphine sulfate 0.008 to 0.015 gm every 3 to 4 hours during acute diarrhea, diphenoxylate hydrochloride (a synthetic opiate) 5 to 10 mg three times daily before meals and at bedtime, or camphorated tincture of opium (paregoric) 4 ml after each bowel movement until diarrhea is controlled. Opium and its derivatives are nauseating to many persons, however, and are therefore useless. Pectin is helpful in controlling some diarrhea; it may be administered in the form of ground raw apple. The successful treatment with yogurt of 15 patients with antibiotic-induced diarrhea has been reported.[43] If the diarrhea is caused by food or drug poisoning, of course, the toxic agent should be evacuated, usually by laxatives, but in some cases of drug poisoning by gastric lavage.

As we have said, authorities agree that emotions affect motility of the gastrointestinal tract and this is especially true in persons suffering from "nervous or emotional diarrhea," "mucous colitis," "irritable colon," and ulcerative colitis. In addition to the treatment discussed above, these persons need a great deal of help in identifying those personal problems that may be a factor in the cause of diarrhea as well as some assistance in dealing with them. Psychotherapy may be necessary for some, especially for those with ulcerative colitis. Surgical intervention (ileostomy) may also be necessary. Such patients are often found on psychosomatic services.

The character and quantity of the feces are two of several indices used by the nurse, physician, and patient in determining the cause of diarrhea. The feces should be observed for color, odor, consistency (formed, mushy, liquid, frothy), and presence of foreign matter such as mucus, blood, pus, and worms. Patients may have a great urge to defecate, one that they cannot control, resulting in partial expulsion of fecal matter before they can get to the toilet. This sense of urgency may be accompanied by cramping, pain, or tenesmus on defecation. Following defecation, there may be a feeling of not having completely emptied the rectum. There may be complaints of weakness during the defecating act. The terms "large stool" and "small stool" diarrheas are frequently used in discussing the cause of the condition. Richard W. Sherbaniuk writes:

Large stool diarrhea is caused by disease of the small intestine or proximal colon and is probably due to irritating intestinal contents or those of large volume stimulating a functionally normal distal colon. The stimulus is thus similar to a dose of salts. Stools are likely to be pale, foul, watery, frothy or greasy, and free of gross blood. If pain is present as an accompanying symptom, it is likely to be perumbilical or right lower quadrant in location (small bowel or cecal reference).

In small stool diarrhea, the patient may have the urge to defecate frequently but passes abnormally small quantities of feces. Disease or disorder is present in the left colon or rectum, with diminished storage function and increased irritability, so that much smaller quantities of stool than normal trigger a defecation reflex. Stools tend to be mushy, dark, rarely foul, and may be mixed with mucus or blood. Often urgency and tenesmus are present.*

An analysis of this description suggests that a great deal can be done for the person with diarrhea, such as replacement of fluids and electrolytes, administration of medications to control diarrhea, giving food that is nonirritating to the intestine, helping to relieve emotions that aggravate the condition, and noting accurately the character of the feces which may help to identify the cause. Of course, the patient should be made as comfortable as is possible under the circumstances. An environment conducive to rest is important and all disturbing conditions should be eliminated if possible. An effort should be made to control odors, especially those from the feces. Following defecation, the anal area should be washed and if the skin is irritated, an ointment may be applied, as for example, A and D ointment. The patient should be encouraged to lie flat in bed. A hot water bottle or heating pad on the abdomen is helpful; however, heat should not be used on those who, for some reason, are unable to detect heat.

The importance of preventing diarrhea cannot be overemphasized. Once the cause has been identified, the patient should be helped to understand the importance of avoiding any condition that may contribute to a recurrence. As patients acquire understanding they are

* Sherbaniuk, Richard W.: "Symposium on Inflammatory Disease of the Intestine: The Physiology of Diarrhea," *Can. Med. Assoc. J.*, **91**:1, (July 4) 1964.

able to cope more effectively with all their health problems.

3. RETENTION OF URINE

Definition. Retention of urine may be defined as an inability to expel urine from a full bladder or to completely empty the bladder. In the latter situation, the urine remaining in the bladder is called *residual* urine. Less than 15 to 20 ml is not too significant, according to John G. Keuhnelian and Virginia E. Sanders,[44] but if the amount is 60 ml or over, the bladder is decompensating. The number of times a person voids during the 24-hour period varies, but since the average adult man excretes about 1500 ml in amounts of approximately 300 ml, he usually voids about five times daily. The woman usually voids less often in the 24-hour period as her bladder is somewhat larger than that of a man.

Some Causes and Effects of Retention. Urinary retention is a complication experienced at the following times or for the following reasons by many individuals: (1) operative procedures, especially those performed in the lower part of the abdominal cavity; (2) obstructive lesions of the lower urinary tract caused by anatomic factors (strictures and hypertrophy of the prostate) or functional factors (for example, spasm of the urethral sphincters and atony of the detrusor muscle); (3) neurogenic vesicle dysfunction caused by disorders within the brain (trauma or tumor for instance) and the spinal cord (trauma, infections, neoplasms, degenerative lesions, and congenital anomalies); and (4) serious emotional illness.[45,45a] This list shows a variety of conditions that may cause retention of urine in the bladder, although the list is probably incomplete.

Charles Creevy,[46] writing in Campbell and Harrison's *Urology*, attributes postoperative urinary retention to a combination of factors, such as inability to void in the unnatural recumbent position; pain around the incision when attempting to urinate postoperatively; decreased tone of the detrusor urinae muscle caused by spinal anesthesia or antispasmodic drugs; increased tone of the internal sphincter caused by use of opiates, such as morphine, codeine, and Demerol; and "latent obstruction at the vesical neck." With further elaboration, he says:

An initial retention due to these factors is often prolonged unreasonably by the thoughtlessness, neglect, or fear of the catheter exhibited by the surgeon who writes "Do not catheterize unless absolutely necessary," or who, having ordered two liters of fluid intravenously, then writes "Catheterize every 8 hours if necessary," forgetting that by the end of 8 hours the bladder will be enormously distended.*

It is equally important to recognize that persons who have practiced voluntary retention (failure to respond to the signal to micturate) for one reason or another fail to empty the bladder completely after surgery. All the conditions noted above must be taken into account by nurses as they give postoperative care.

Because of the difficulties of voiding after intestinal operations, Edward N. Cook and associates [47] undertook a study of more than 4000 patients who had bowel surgery at the Mayo Clinic during 1951 through 1955. An analysis of data on 869 patients (443 men and 426 women) showed that 167 had a residual volume of urine of 100 ml or more, which is evidence of disturbed vesical function; the incidence of retention was higher in men than in women, regardless of the type of operation; the level of operation was highly significant, regardless of sex, since retention of urine occurred more frequently in both men and women following perineal resection and less frequently in those operations done on the bowel at a higher level. Retention was more common in the older groups (60 years and above for those with perineal resection and 55 years and above with anterior resection of the bowel), regardless of sex. Further examination of the data by the investigators showed that the presence or absence of the uterus in the woman or before prostatectomy in the man did not influence urinary retention. Discussing their findings, they say:

Any attempt at etiologic explanation requires consideration of the primary problem: an imbalance between the forces tending to expel urine and those tending to retain it. . . . Unquestionably there is a neurogenic disturbance, and we believe that this is manifested more as abnormal sensation than as motor inability to contract the vesical wall. Many of these patients experience no urge to urinate. They should be firmly instructed to try to void every 2 hours when their catheter is removed. As Campbell suggested, a degree of edema and fixation in the form of pericystitis undoubtedly occurs, and we believe that this is proven by the fact that the passage of time after operation is conducive to the regaining of ability to void. Mechanical blockage due to an obstructed vesical neck may be positive or, at times, relative. This latter type accounts, we believe, for the appreciable number of men who had little or no obstructive

---

* Creevy, Charles: "Urinary Retention," in Campbell, Meredith F., and Harrison, J. Hartwell: *Urology*, Vol. III, 3rd ed. W. B. Saunders Co., Philadelphia, 1970, p. 2283.

disease preoperatively and only minimal prostatic enlargement but who, because of inability of the vesical wall to contract satisfactorily, experienced postoperative urinary difficulty.*

Other authors note, as does Cook, that urinary retention occurs more frequently in men than in women after surgery; however, following gynecologic operations, inability to void for several days does occur.

Acute urinary retention is seen in some gynecologic disorders, such as pelvic abscess, uterine myomas, cystocele, and hematocolopos (accumulation of blood in the vagina in girls with an inperforate hymen). Postpartum retention is less common today than in the past, probably because of early ambulation.

Any disorder of the vesical neck that involves the internal urinary meatus and sphincter, the prostate gland and prostatic urethra, or the urogenital diaphragm, will hinder emptying the bladder and may ultimately produce an obstructive uropathy above it. The first symptom of obstruction at the vesical neck is interrupted urination at first morning voiding, followed by nocturia, a small stream, hesitancy, and increased diurnal frequency. Consequently, acute retention may occur or the residual urine may become so great that overflow incontinence and renal insufficiency result. If the residual urine is in excess of 700 ml, atony of the bladder may also be suspected. The problem may become complex when there are spasms of the sphincters so that it is impossible to insert a catheter without the use of a local, regional, or general anesthetic. Of course, strictures are also a complicating factor.[48] When the patient cannot void at all or, at best, can manage to express (with effort) only a few drops of urine at frequent intervals, the condition (retention) must be differentiated from that of *anuria* (cessation of urine production).[49] Disease of the prostate gland is a common cause of acute and chronic retention.

Reed M. Nesbit says urinary obstruction in children is a common occurrence in both sexes, especially with contracture of the bladder neck, but that its early symptoms are frequently overlooked by physicians and parents alike. It is finally recognized following recurrent urinary infection and enuresis. Contrasting the difference between normal and abnormal urination of male infants, he writes:

. . . [he] urinates a forceful high trajectory stream which is at once the object of curious pride to his mother as well as the envy of his father; and he empties his bladder with a continuous stream. Any male infant who does not emulate the boy made famous in the statue in Brussels and who urinates with an interrupted stream must be regarded with grave suspicion.*

Urinary retention associated with emotional disturbances in women, according to James W. Larson and associates [50] (1963), has been recognized for some time. In a study of 37 women complaining of urinary retention who had no objective evidence of organic disease, the onset of retention was shown to be related to medical or psychologic trauma and the subjects usually had multiple somatic complaints and had undergone many surgical procedures. Psychologic tests showed that these women were severely ill emotionally, the most frequent diagnosis being conversion hysteria and schizophrenia. As one might suspect, vesical neck resection did not relieve retention. Psychogenic urinary retention in women usually follows some psychologic or social trauma, for instance divorce, incest, self-punishment toward a resented parent or relative, or surgery. Hydronephrosis has occurred in severe cases.[50a,50b]

G. F. J. Goddard [51] describes "urinary retention lasting 27 days after 15 days' treatment with amitriptyline hydrochloride (Tryptizol)" in a woman suffering from depression. He emphasizes the necessity for daily examination for urinary retention of patients who are taking amitriptyline hydrochloride and especially for those who are unable to make observations of retention and report them.

Neurogenic vesical dysfunction, which may be caused by any disorder, disease, infection, trauma, or congenital defect of the brain, spinal cord, or peripheral nerves, can result in urinary retention. In a mechanized society, injuries of the spinal cord are the most frequent cause of the neurogenic bladder. The term "cord" bladder indicates that the bladder lacks tone or is atonic; there is retention of urine or inability to void even when there are sensations of a full bladder.[51a]

The person who has retention is usually very anxious—concerned about his or her inability to urinate—and has intense suprapubic pain. A hard mass is usually palpable above the symphysis pubis. Urinary infection is frequently associated with retention and it probably results from injury to the mucosa from stretching the bladder and the constant presence of urine, which is an excellent media for bacterial growth. Hemorrhage if it is present devitalizes the tissues. Some electrolytes may be absorbed from the bladder in prolonged re-

---

* Cook, Edward N., et al.: "Urinary Retention Following Operations on the Bowel," *J. Urol.*, **89**: 259, (Feb.) 1963.

* Nesbit, Reed M.: "Urinary Obstructions in Children," *Surg. Gynecol. Obstet.*, **102**:748, (June) 1956.

tention. In a study of ten patients with acute urinary retention, D. E. M. Taylor [51b] reports a rise in blood pressure with isometric bladder contraction in all the patients and a fall in blood pressure in eight during passive bladder decompression by catheterization.

Prevention and Management of Urinary Retention. All workers who are directly concerned with health teaching or the care of the sick should understand the physiology of micturition, be able to recognize early symptoms of urinary retention, help the person micturate if this is possible, and teach others (sick and well, including parents of children) to recognize these symptoms and seek medical help when needed.

When urinary retention is suspected, the following should be noted: the amount of urine excreted in 24 hours, the amount at each voiding, the force of the urinary stream, changes in the size of the stream, and difficulty in urination such as straining, hesitancy, or intermittent stopping of the stream. Nocturia, posturinary dribbling, and incontinence are also important observations. One or several of these may indicate the presence of retention. The patient may be catheterized to determine the volume of residual urine but catheterization is associated with infection so often that it is avoided if possible. Other methods used include intravenous urography, Diodrast labeled with I [131], and phenolsulfonphthalein test.[52]

There are a number of measures that may help prevent urinary retention postoperatively. The position that one ordinarily assumes when voiding is best, but when this is not possible the head of the bed should be raised to a 45-degree angle if the patient's condition permits. The man patient may be permitted to stand by the side of the bed, with assistance, and attempt to void in the urinal. Sedatives and narcotics should be given only in limited amounts as they tend to interfere with micturition; of course, the person must have taken a sufficient amount of fluids. Stroking, pinching, or scratching the trigger areas (genitalia, perineum, or anterior thighs) may cause expulsion of part or all of the urine. Placing the patient's hands in water, letting the patient listen to running water, or applying heat over the bladder area also may be helpful. Of course early ambulation is desirable. Stimulation of the bladder may be accomplished by the use of choline drugs by mouth and instilling irritating solutions such as gentian violet or Mercurochrome into the bladder.

Urinary retention, acute and chronic, may necessitate other relief measures such as intermittent catheterization or an indwelling catheter that provides drainage and irrigation. The closed system should be used because fewer urinary infections are associated with its use as compared to the open drainage. Suprapubic puncture and transurethral resection may be thought necessary. Suprapubic puncture is used when it is impossible to insert the catheter because of strictures or severe spasms of the sphincters. Transurethral resection is performed when treatment by indwelling catheter of patients with bowel surgery has been unsuccessful in resolving the problem of retention. Most authors consulted stress the importance of using conservative measures. Any "intrusive therapy" of the bladder is risky. Insertion of an indwelling catheter, followed by intermittent catheterization, control of infection with drugs, use of vesical stimulants such as bethanechol (Urecholine) or carbachol (Doryl) administered orally or intramuscularly, and lavage of the bladder with gentian violet, mercurochrome, or silver nitrate are all used in combating retention before there is a resort to surgery.

A detailed discussion of the possibility of developing a urinary infection with the use of the catheter, methods of prevention, and treatment may be found in Chapter 24.

4. SUPPRESSION OF URINE

Definition. Urinary suppression refers to a reduction in the formation of urine by the kidneys out of proportion to the intake of fluids. Two terms are commonly used to describe the extent of the suppression: *oliguria* is a deficient secretion of urine resulting in a total volume of 400 ml or less of urine in 24 hours; *anuria* is a complete failure to secrete urine.

Some Causes and Effects of Urinary Suppression. When the kidneys fail to secrete urine (anuria) or the formation of urine is markedly suppressed, nitrogenous and other waste products, normally excreted by the kidneys, are retained in the blood and there is a profound disturbance of fluid and electrolyte balance. All this produces a state of toxicity. Any condition or factor that diminishes the glomerular filtration rate in the kidneys or interferes with the reabsorption of fluid in the tubules, as well as the exchange of metabolites, can result in urinary suppression, usually called acute renal failure. According to John P. Merrill [53] and William Boyd,[54] the causes of acute renal failure may be summarized into the following categories: *prerenal, renal,* and *postrenal.* Such a classification emphasizes the fact that prerenal and postrenal factors may be corrected immediately by specific means, whereas in renal failure the acute lesions of the renal parenchyma must heal spontaneously. *Prerenal* failure, due to an inadequate blood volume and pressure, results in severe functional changes without damage to the kidneys' essential tissues (parenchyma). The decreased glomerular filtration rate and subsequent decreased excretion of solutes are the result of acute circulatory insufficiency. Shock, hemorrhage, burns, and dehydration (as, for example, in excessive diarrhea, vomiting, and sweating) are conditions associated with this type of urinary suppression. Postoperative gastric suction over a period of time without adequate replacement of fluid and electrolytes may also cause prerenal failure. Regardless of cause, it is reversible if recognized and treated early.

Postrenal failure is due to mechanical obstruction to the escape of urine. This obstruction may be the result of calculi, blood clots, tumors, or strictures at any point between the renal pelvis and the ureteral orifices. In such conditions, complete anuria is present, usually preceded by renal colic, although this may not always be the case. If the cause is identified and treated, the state of anuria may be corrected.

Renal failure results in severe functional changes with acute structural damage of the kidney parenchyma. The causes are numerous; however, most authorities say nephrotoxic drugs or chemicals and systemic injury or illness can cause acute tubular necrosis. Drugs often mentioned include the sulfonamides and other commonly used antimicrobial drugs such as kanamycin, bacitracin, neomycin, and cephaloridine. Nephrotoxic chemicals include organic solvents (such as carbon tetrachloride) and inorganic mercurials and other heavy metals (such as bismuth and lead). Systemic injury or illness, resulting in acute tubular necrosis, include severe trauma (as for example crushing injuries and major operations), severe febrile illnesses, complicated pregnancies, and incompatible blood transfusions.[55] Most authorities say there is an overlapping of causes in two categories (prerenal and renal) as noted above and believe as does Merrill that "different patients, or even the same patient at a different time, may respond differently to the same insult." *

The onset of acute renal failure varies from hours to as long as 2 days after the inciting event. The oliguric phase, which may last from a few hours to 3 or more weeks is followed by the diuretic phase (lasting from a few days to a week or more) and finally by the recovery phase if renal function is restored.

If the urinary suppression (regardless of cause) is allowed to progress or is irreversible, the patient is seriously ill and presents a variety of symptoms such as headache, weakness, pallor, restlessness or drowsiness, muscular twitching, anorexia, nausea, vomiting, pruritus, skin eruptions, dehydration or edema, hypertension or hypotension, pericarditis, confusion, and finally coma and death. Laboratory findings usually include an elevation in the blood nonprotein nitrogen, urea, creatinine, and potassium.

Prevention and Management of Urinary Suppression. On examining the causes or conditions that may impair renal function—resulting in oliguria or anuria—the importance of

* Merrill, John P.: *The Treatment of Renal Failure,* 2nd ed. Grune & Stratton, New York, 1965, p. 127.

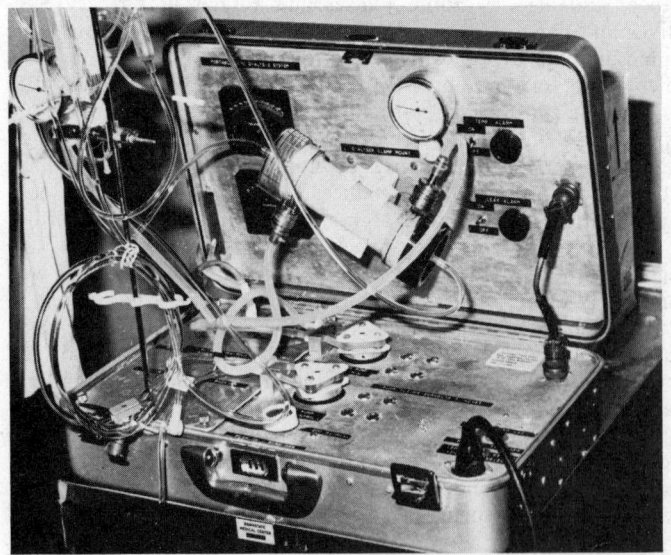

Figure 37-1. "Suitcase Kidney," weighing about 20 lb. (Briefel, G. R., et al.: "Compact Travel Hemodialysis System," *Proc. Clin. Dial. Transplant Forum,* 5:61, [Nov.] 1975. From: Dr. Eli A. Friedman, State University of New York, Downstate Medical Center.)

prevention is obvious. Preventive steps include the following: (1) all poisons and drugs should be stored so they are not accessible to children who for one reason or another may ingest them; (2) any person taking sulfanilamide or other nephrotoxic drugs should be told their dangers and the toxic signs and how to prevent them, especially measuring fluid intake and output; (3) health workers should make careful observation on blood volume and pressure on all surgical patients (before, during, and after surgery) so that the condition may be detected and corrected immediately; (4) any person under health supervision who is likely to sweat excessively or have diarrhea or vomiting should be told the dangers involved and the need for seeking medical attention as quickly as possible; and (5) the nurse or attendant who has under his or her care a patient, regardless of diagnosis, who excretes 500 ml or less of urine in 24 hours, should report this information to the physician immediately.

Although the kidneys have the ability to recover from insult, the final outcome depends on the severity of the underlying cause, its early detection, and immediate treatment. Most authorities emphasize the importance of establishing the *cause* lest treatment be superficial. Treatment is directed toward removing the cause and maintaining (insofar as possible) normal fluid and electrolyte balance, adequate nutrition (low in protein, high in carbohydrates), and suppression of nitrogenous breakdown so that the kidneys are given a chance to recover their normal function.

During the oliguric phase, the fluid intake is limited to 400 ml daily plus an amount equal to the urine excreted in the preceding 24 hours. If the patient has vomited or perspired excessively, these amounts must be calculated as accurately as possible so that the fluid intake is increased accordingly. An accurate daily record of all fluid intake, output, and body weight is essential. An indwelling catheter may be used in some patients so that the hourly production of urine can be determined (see Fig. 37-2*A–C*). Authorities repeatedly state that forcing fluids cannot make a diseased kid-

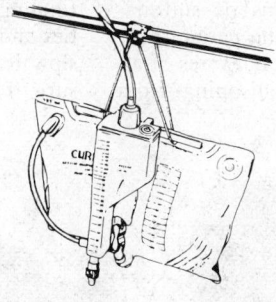

A.
To properly position unit, attach collection bag to bed by threading cord hanger around frame and fastening to clasp on cord loop *or* use metal hook provided.

Drainage tubing may be anchored to bed clothing by the quick-fastener device attached.

Figure 37-2. Urine collection device with Urine-Meter. (Courtesy of Kendall Co., Hospital Products Div., Chicago, Ill.)

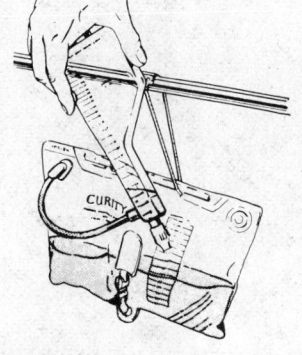

B.
To transfer contents of Urine-Meter to collection bag, lift and tilt Meter. *Note:* Urine in connecting tube is included in calibration.

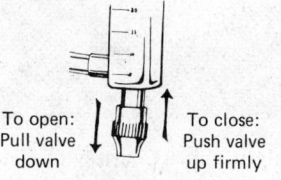

To open:
Pull valve down

To close:
Push valve up firmly

C.
To collect urine sample or to drain meter, *pull valve down—to close, push valve up firmly.*

ney function normally. The patient should be given an explanation of the reasons for fluid restriction and should be encouraged to help distribute the amounts over the 24 hours. The type of parenteral fluids given depends on the serum electrolyte concentrations. In most cases potassium is restricted. Sodium chloride may be required for those patients with vomiting or diarrhea but limited for others.

Most authorities recommend a diet low in protein (20 gm or less) and high in carbohydrates (minimum of 100 to 200 gm), with vitamin supplements to supply adequate nutrients and reduce the amount of tissue protein and fat broken down for energy (catabolism). If the patient is unable to eat because of poor appetite or because of nausea and vomiting, glucose and vitamins may be given parenterally. The importance of *rest* cannot be overemphasized. Activity is restricted so that the production of metabolic wastes is minimized.

Treatment of pathologic conditions due to a sudden reduction in blood volume such as diarrhea, vomiting, sweating, burns, and hemorrhage includes parenteral administration of blood plasma and/or electrolyte or glucose solutions. In hemolytic reactions or sulfonamide and uric acid poisoning, the patient may be given sodium bicarbonate for purposes of alkalinization. In heavy metal poisoning from

mercury, bismuth, or uranium, dimercaprol (BAL) may be used. If the patient is anuric, dialysis may be necessary to rid the body of these "bound" substances. If the poison remains in the stomach, gastric lavage can be used effectively.

When conservative measures fail, other means for extracting retained waste products from the blood include cation exchange resin (oral or rectal administration), gastric and intestinal lavage, and dialysis (hemodialysis and peritoneal dialysis) (see Fig. 37-3). Hemodialysis and peritoneal dialysis are discussed in Chapter 24.

Some authorities believe that cation exchange resin enemas are more effective in removing excess potassium from the blood stream than glucose and insulin. Oral resins may also be given if the patient is not vomiting. Continuous gastric or intestinal lavage or suction may be used. Drainage of the small intestine is most effective as the potassium content of the secretions of the small intestine is greater than that of the gastric juice. Potassium intoxication, a common complication in renal failure, is characterized by muscular weakness, tingling sensation or numbness in the extremities and around the mouth, shallow respiration, slow irregular pulse, and a fall in blood pressure. The nurse should report such symptoms

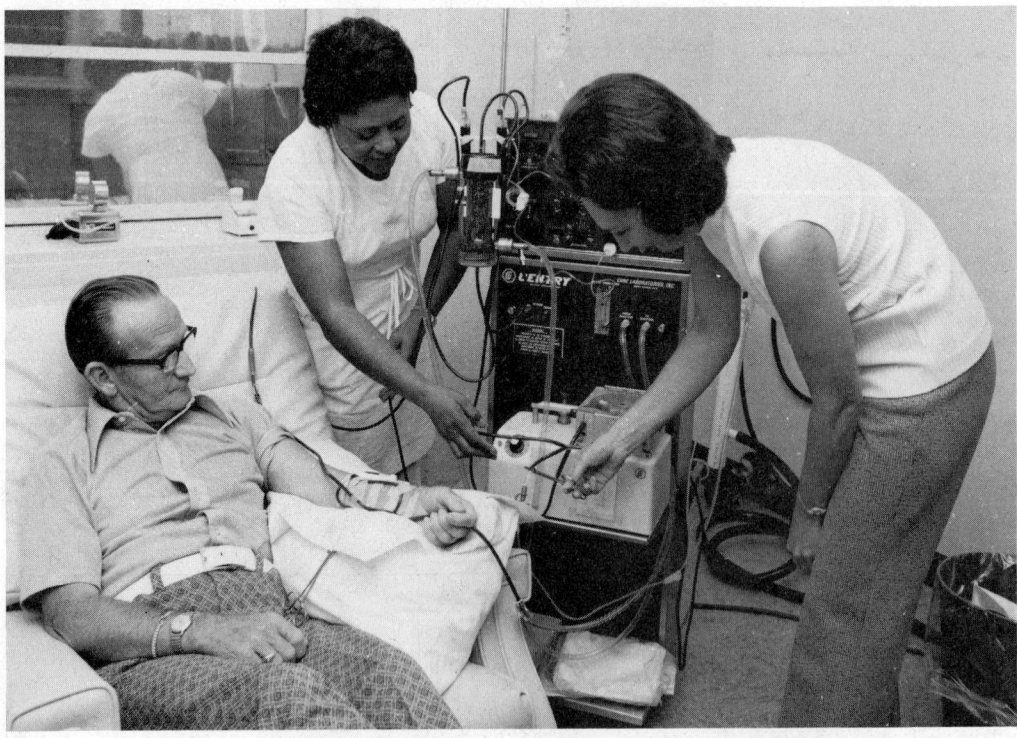

Figure 37-3. Hemodialysis unit. (Courtesy of Veterans Administration Hospital, Houston, Tex.)

so that treatment may be instituted immediately.

Uremic patients are prone to pulmonary complications and infections. Of the two, pulmonary complications are probably the more common and the effects are serious. The fact that uremic patients are also prone to infections adds to its dangers. Because the pulmonary secretions are viscous and tenacious, the cough reflex depressed, and the diaphragm elevated and restricted, measures should be instituted to prevent obstruction of the airway, atelectasis, and pneumonia. Patients should be encouraged to cough deeply, spitting out all mucus; their position should be changed frequently and the head tilted forward so that mucus is not aspirated. If nasopharyngeal and tracheal suction is used, the utmost care must be exercised to avoid traumatizing the tissues and predisposing them to infection. For the same reasons, good oral hygiene is of the utmost importance. An unclean mouth in the uremic patient, who frequently has sore, bleeding oral mucous membranes, is an excellent medium for bacteria growth. A mouth infection may lead to a bacterial pneumonia. Oral hygiene is discussed in detail in Chapter 14. Since the problem of infection is so great in the uremic patient, everything possible should be done to protect the patient from all organisms. It may be necessary to put the patient in semi-isolation and restrict all persons (hospital personnel and visitors) from the room who have any type of infection, including the common cold. All treatments should be carried out under aseptic conditions.

Before patients leave the hospital, nurses fulfill an important function in teaching them and their families all aspects of care that they need to know to ensure recovery.[55a,55b] They must understand the importance of diet and what they should and should not eat. In addition, all restrictions on fluid intake should be carefully explained as well as any need for increasing fluid intake. The importance of an accurate daily intake and output should also be stressed. Finally, patients should understand the importance of gradually increasing their activities, getting plenty of rest, and avoiding infections. Arrangements should be made for the next visit to the physician or clinic, and in some instances a referral to the Visiting Nurse Association for care in the home is indicated.

5. INCONTINENCE OF URINE OR FECES

Causes of Partial and Complete Loss of Bladder and Bowel Control—Enuresis and Incontinence. The lack of bowel and bladder control of the newborn baby or infant concerns no one. However, when a child continues to lack control after the age when most children have completed these tasks, parents, schoolteachers, nurses, and physicians are concerned. The age at which children are expected to be continent is cultural, but in the Western world more or less adult behavior in controlling micturition and defecation is expected by the age of 2 to 4 years.

Bowel training can be started when the child is able to stand upright and starts walking, which shows that enough neurologic development has taken place so that learning to "hold on" and "let go" at the proper time and place can begin. Consistent bowel control is usually accomplished by boys at 22 months, and by girls at 20 months.

Bladder training can only begin when the child's bladder has grown enough to hold 85 ml of urine (in an infant, the bladder holds only 15 ml) and bladder sensation has developed. This usually occurs between the ages of 1½ and 2½ years. Between the ages of 2½ and 4½ years the child's bladder grows enough to hold 250 ml, and he or she learns to control the reflex activity that relaxes some muscles and contracts others so that detrusor muscles are stimulated and voiding takes place under his or her control.[56]

Making these reflex acts voluntary ones is easier for children when they are awake than when they are asleep; therefore, reflex night voiding, or bed wetting, persists in childhood beyond the age when they wet their clothing by day. *Enuresis,* which means literally "incontinence of urine," when coupled with the word *nocturnal,* is the medical term for bed wetting after the age at which the child usually acquires complete control over the bladder. In our own culture, bed wetting often persists throughout childhood and occasionally into adult life. Nelson and his associates[57] note that many children do not develop nocturnal bladder control until the ages of 5, 6, or 7 years. In fact, 10 to 20 per cent may occasionally wet the bed as late as 9 or 10 years.

Leon Eisenberg[58] says that despite the many studies done on nocturnal enuresis, the cause and psychophysiology remain obscure. Harold P. McDonald,[59] reporting his experience with more than 2000 children in 25 years, says 75 per cent with urinary symptoms or enuresis showed a narrow urethral meatus. Eisenberg[59a] points out that in some cases of nocturnal enuresis parents have simply not made consistent efforts at training because of their own developmental backgrounds. He goes on to say that for each of a number of suggested causes of nocturnal enuresis, there are exceptions. For instance, it has been suggested that a very deep level of sleep is the cause, but many children respond favorably to sedation; that defects of the genitourinary system have been indicted, but these are rarely found; that nocturnal enuresis is the result of a psychologic disturbance, but the enuresis may be the child's only symptom; or that there is a failure to develop an adequate bladder capacity, but the child does not wet the bed when visiting overnight.

Enuresis is classified as primary and secondary by Robert E. Cooke.[59b] He defines primary enuresis as a delay in the development of bladder control that is due to the interaction of genetic background and environmental and physical factors. The importance of the genetic factor was shown by studies of twins. From a group of 30 pairs of identical twins, both children in 21 pairs were enuretic; however, there was only a random incidence of enuresis among the children of 10 pairs of fraternal twins. The effect of environmental factors became apparent in a population study of children 7¾ years old when 14 per cent of the children in the lower socioeconomic group were found to be enuretic while only 7 per cent of those in the higher socioeconomic group were. Among a group of 218 enuretic children 5 years of age, 54 per cent had bladder ages from 0 to 2 years, and 43 per cent had bladder ages from 2 to 3 years.

Treatment of primary enuresis is directed toward hastening maturation of functional control of the bladder. The goal is to gradually increase the capacity of the bladder so that larger and larger amounts of urine can be retained. Fluids should be encouraged consistently, and weekly measurements made of the amount voided. When a capacity of 300 to 400 ml is reached there is less chance of bedwetting. The child should be encouraged to practice starting and stopping the urine stream in order to make control a more conscious effort.

Secondary enuresis, according to Cooke, seems to be highly psychologic. It frequently occurs after a number of years of nighttime control, and often is associated with the birth of a sibling. If no evidence of a physical disorder is found with a urologic examination, the parents of the child should be encouraged to help him or her see his or her importance to the family and refrain from any punishment.

While *incontinence* is synonymous with enuresis in the dictionary, it is used in medical parlance for the inability to retain urine or feces because of a cerebral or spinal lesion, or the loss of control over the sphincters guarding either the bladder, the rectum, or both during the day and night. The term is not applied to infants since sphincter control is actually immature in babies.

After infancy, control of elimination by bowel and bladder depends upon a normal neuromuscular mechanism. Congenital malformations, injuries, growths, spontaneous hemorrhages, and poisoning by chemicals or bacterial toxins may temporarily or permanently destroy the nerve pathways producing incontinence. The following types of urinary incontinence are described by Bernard Lytton and Franklin H. Epstein[60]: congenital, acquired, and paradoxic incontinence. The first occurs when there is some congenital abnormality such as bladder exstrophy, epispadias, or defects in the spinal cord associated with spina bifida and meningomyelocele. The second, acquired incontinence, may develop when the nerve supply to the bladder or rectum is interrupted or destroyed by disease in the central nervous system (brain and spinal cord) or in the nerves leaving and entering the cord to and from the bladder and rectum; it may be due to irradiation injuries that produce openings (fistulas) between the bladder and vagina or the ureters and vagina; it may be due to loss of urethral resistance following the birth of a baby if the structures of the pelvic floor and perineum are overstretched or torn; it may be due to injury of the sphincter mechanism after a pelvic fracture or prostatic surgery in the elderly; or it may occur as stress incontinence. The third type, paradoxic incontinence, accompanies bladder distention with urinary retention. The distention is caused by some kind of obstruction or neurologic impairment that allows small frequent "overflow" voidings, but does not allow emptying of the bladder.

In rare cases, congenital defects or growths make storage and discharge of urine by the bladder impossible. The surgeon will then make a permanent or temporary opening from the bladder to the skin; he or she will attach the ureters to the rectum, or attach their outlets to the skin surface of the trunk. Under the latter circumstances the person is saddled for the rest of his or her life with a type of incontinence difficult to manage, since there is not even an incompetent sphincter to guard the outlet.

Many otherwise healthy and normal persons are incontinent or "spill urine" in emotional states. "Stress incontinence" is fairly common, particularly in women.[61] According to Jack Lapides,[62] it is caused by the abnormally short urethra. Other factors such as intravesicular pressure, status of the urethral epithelium, and tonicity of the muscle and elastic tissues in the wall of the urethra may be implicated. He says the urethra is a mobile structure whose length varies with activity. Many women "spill urine" when coughing, laughing, or straining while lifting a heavy object.

In John C. Brocklehurst's study of bladder incontinence in about 3000 old people in hospitals, he says: "The incidence has proved to be twice as common among females as among males." He suggests the following as possible explanations: (1) women live longer than men, and senile changes are therefore more often seen; (2) mental confusion was twice as common in the women as in the men, possibly for the same reason as in item one; (3) men can keep some sort of urinal in position, which may relieve the anxiety about wetting; and (4) the difference in anatomic structure. He cites the conclusion of William T. Kennedy, based on surgery and dissection, that the female urethra opens as the result of muscle contraction rather than relaxation, as was generally believed. As Brocklehurst says:

The short female urethra does make the woman more liable to stress incontinence, . . . the external sphincter may take the form of a Muscle of Micturition [Kennedy's] in the female, and any increase in the tone of the muscle . . . would tend to open up the urethra, instead of closing it more tightly as a true external sphincter would do.*

There is a close relationship between sexual arousal and bladder function. "Honeymoon cystitis" is a condition characterized by urgency, frequency, and sometimes by incontinence.

Treatment of Bladder Incontinence. Treatment of incontinence of the urinary bladder depends upon its cause and the supposed duration. Sometimes the abnormal condition, therefore the incontinence, is curable; sometimes it is permanent.

Marguerite E. Pennefather and Elizabeth R. Tanner report that the reeducation of pelvic floor muscles has been helpful to many women who have stress incontinence. They suggest that women who are already familiar with postnatal exercises should again practice them daily. In addition,

1. The patient is encouraged to try to stop the flow of urine while she is sitting on the lavatory by tightening the muscles of the perineum, and also those on the lower part of the abdomen.
2. The patient should choose some firm surface in her home, for example, the edge of the kitchen sink, a firm table or back of a chair, and, placing the palms of her hands on it, try to "push it through the floor." The patient should stand close to the object she is pushing down and be careful not to bend forward at her hips. Ideally,

the surface should be at a level somewhere between the top of the pelvis and the hip joint.*

When incontinent patients are nonambulatory, caring for them becomes a major nursing problem. Any accident, growth, or disease severe enough to interfere with the function of the pelvic organs is likely to interfere with the blood supply, hence nutrition, of the skin, and often to limit motor activity. Pressure sores or bedsores (discussed more fully in Chapter 12) are the inevitable result of lying in one position too long. Their formation is hastened by poor nutrition and by maceration and irritation of the skin by moisture and chemicals in the urine and stool. It is imperative that the patient be kept clean and dry. Pressure sores can be cured only by correcting the conditions that provoke them; it is therefore wise to institute these measures early enough to prevent the breakdown of the skin.

Treatment goals for incontinent patients are to (1) prevent urine from contact with the skin and so prevent skin excoriation; (2) help the patient maintain a socially acceptable level of personal hygiene; and (3) prevent back pressure of urine into the ureters and kidneys (vesico-ureteral reflux) when the incontinence is of the "overflow" type.

To prevent contact between the urine and skin, a catheter is inserted and held in the bladder, the ureter, or even the pelvis of the kidney. This is called an "indwelling catheter," and the procedure is described in Chapter 24. Another means of diverting urine from the skin in the male patient is to attach a bag to the penis. A variety of bags are used (see Fig. 37-4). They can be purchased from commercial firms or can be made by the patient or a family member from small plastic sandwich bags or shower caps.[63-65] Although many devices have been developed and tried for women, most have been unsatisfactory. However, a recent report by Derek Schofield [66] (in England) says that pads containing water-soluble cellulose colloids and shaped like an ordinary sanitary pad have been successful for an 8-hour period in 50 per cent of a group of 27 incontinent women, and effective for overnight use in 80 per cent of them.

Indwelling catheters, accompanied by several types of irrigation to stimulate bladder function and combat infection, are extensively used until the degree of bladder disability is determined, and for patients whose condition limits life. In such cases the low-grade bladder infection accompanying so-called catheter life may be more tolerable than the struggle with

---

* Brocklehurst, John C.: *Incontinence in Old People*. E. & S. Livingstone, Ltd., Edinburgh, 1951, p. 102.

* Pennefather, Marguerite E., and Tanner, Elizabeth R.: "Spending a 'New Penny,'" *Nurs. Times*, **67**:640, (May 27) 1971.

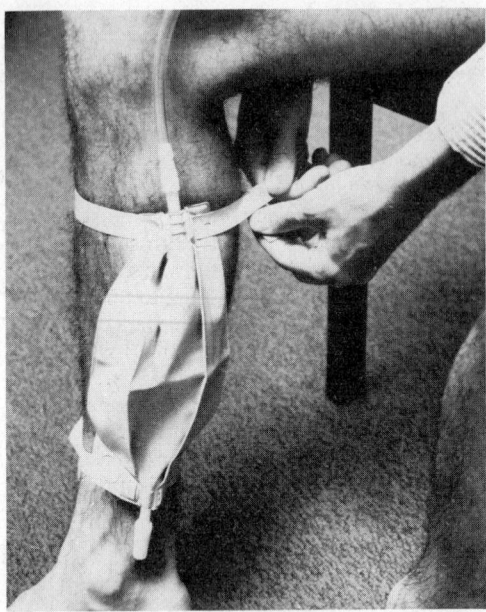

Figure 37-4. Urinary leg bag that may be worn on the thigh or on the calf of the leg. The bag holds up to 740 ml (cc), has a one-way valve to prevent back flow, and is easily emptied by removal of the bottom drain cap. (Courtesy of Chesebrough-Pond's, Inc., Hospital Products Division, Greenwich, Conn.)

wet and foul clothing and bedding. However, it is increasingly common to see experts in the care of patients with a stroke urging that catheters *not* be used. All those with temporary incontinence are fortunate if they escape catheterization, which so often leads to infection. Methods to reduce the intensity or incidence of bladder infections due to an indwelling catheter are discussed in Chapter 24.

Intermittent catheterization, that is, catheterizing the patient on a regular schedule throughout the day and night and employing a strict sterile technique, is being used with success in a number of rehabilitation centers. Comparing this method to a bladder training program, A. Estin Comarr says:

. . . it is the method of choice for treatment of the traumatic cord bladder * since (1) more patients are discharged with sterile urine specimens, (2) the incidence of penoscrotal pathology is negligible, (3) those patients who respond to this management become catheter-free more quickly, (4) patients with incomplete lesions become cathe-

ter-free more quickly and (5) more quadriplegics become catheter-free.*

He also says that the intermittent catheterization program is limited to 90 days, because studies show the majority of patients, regardless of the type of their lesion, will recover bladder function within this time. Ascorbic acid, Mandelamine, and bethanechol chloride are usually given, and the patient's fluid intake is adjusted according to his or her renal output in order to prevent an overdistention of the bladder. If 300 to 400 ml of urine is taken from the bladder at the time of the scheduled catheterization, the patient's intake and output are thought to be adequately balanced.[67] This balance requires a restricted intake of fluids so that hourly catheterization is not needed. Before each catheterization the patient is encouraged to void and when residual urine is acceptably low (50 to 100 ml), catheterization is discontinued.[68] Chapter 24 has a more detailed discussion of the use of intermittent catheterization.

If intermittent catheterization is unsuccessful after a period of 90 days, an indwelling catheter is inserted and bladder training is attempted. Obviously, this habit training is easiest with young, otherwise healthy persons.

Alice B. Morrissey points out patients' psychologic handicap; they are naturally embarrassed that they cannot control elimination, and after a few "accidents" they may "take refuge in withdrawal behavior and refuse to cooperate with further attempts toward rehabilitation."

Therefore, the first step . . . is on the psychological level. . . . The nurse must approach the problem with realism, tact, patience and knowledge. She must gain the patient's co-operation and confidence. . . . Sometimes, simply extending the hope that it is possible to overcome these difficulties is sufficient. . . . In urinary and bowel rehabilitation, as in other rehabilitation procedures, the disabled person must learn to do most of the work himself. When success is finally achieved, the rewards and satisfactions are great.[†]

Embarrassment is reduced if the nurse and patient are of the same sex, but the fact that they are not should never keep the nurse from giving the patient the help he or she needs.

Most patients with central nervous system lesions above the sacral segment of the spinal cord develop an *automatic* bladder after the initial period of spinal shock (diaschisis) has

---

* The terms "cord bladder" or "neurogenic bladder" are used to describe bladder impairment that results from brain or spinal cord lesions.

* Comarr, A. Estin: "Intermittent Catheterization for the Traumatic Cord Bladder Patient," *J. Urol.,* **108:**79, (July) 1972.
† Morrissey, Alice B.: *Rehabilitation Nursing.* G. P. Putnam's Sons, New York, 1951, p. 104.

subsided. Then the typical micturition reflex returns and when the bladder becomes sufficiently distended, the reflex is stimulated, the bladder contracts, and voiding takes place. No voluntary control can occur, however, because nerve pathways to the brain have been interrupted. Bladder training in this situation requires the removal of the catheter, an intake of 800 to 1000 ml over a 2-hour period, and stimulation of the bladder using the trigger areas (genitalia, perineum, or anterior thighs). If the patient voids, the residual urine is checked, and if it is under 100 ml, the procedure continues. The patient continues to drink large amounts of fluid, 200 ml each hour, and is stimulated to void every 2 to 3 hours. Although the patient no longer has a conscious urge to urinate he or she learns to interpret other signals of a full bladder such as sweating, restlessness, chills, flushing, or a vague feeling of fullness.

The patient who has an injury or lesion to the sacral segment of the spinal cord develops the *autonomous* bladder. The micturition reflex is lost and bladder training consists of teaching the patient to take a deep breath to tighten the abdominal muscles, to strain down, and use manual pressure suprapubically (as with Crede's method) to help empty the bladder. The amount of fluid taken by the patient during waking hours is about 2000 ml. This is in contrast to the patient with an automatic bladder who may need as much as 3000 to 4000 ml.[69-72] Accurate records of the patient's intake and output must be kept by the patient and nurse. Mildred J. Allgire [73] summarizes the major points in the management of urinary habit training which includes an intake and output report that can be used for patients in hospitals, nursing homes and private homes (See Fig. 37-5*A*). This combined instruction sheet and record can be useful to health workers, the patient, and the family.

Patients who are undergoing bladder training decrease their fluid intake early in the evening, but are helped to void once or twice before bedtime. Some are eventually able to remain dry throughout the night; others may wear some external drainage appliance described earlier.

Thomas S. Wilson [74] succeeded in helping those with *senile urinary incontinence* to control the desire to void. His method was to fill the bladder very slowly with an antiseptic solution. The very excitable bladder responds with waves of contraction, which the patient interprets as a desire to micturate. It may be urgent enough to seem painful to the subject. The physician asks the patient to bear this discomfort or hold the urine. If the patient can control the impulse to void, the contractions will cease and the patient will be relieved. Wilson believed that if the patient could be convinced that relief follows inhibiting the impulse, as well as giving in to it, he or she could reduce the excitability of the bladder or train it to hold more urine. This same sort of retraining applies to any patient who has habituated the bladder to holding only small amounts.

Brocklehurst, comparing incontinence among comparable populations of old people in different institutions, concluded that morale had a direct bearing on the incidence. He says: "There is no doubt that the status of the nurses in charge of these old people, and the nursing methods they use have a direct bearing on the incidence of incontinence." * It was highest in a hospital staffed with untrained personnel; it was lowest in that giving what he believed to be the best nursing care. Old people who are occupied and encouraged to "keep on their feet" are not nearly so likely to be incontinent as the bedfast. Ability to go to the bathroom is a great stimulus to keep dry, and this privilege should be maintained as long as possible. Brocklehurst found little difference between the incidence of incontinence in the age groups 60 to 69, 70 to 79, and 80 years and over. He did not find that organic disease of the nerves played a part, although he noted a high incidence of blood pressure elevation and spastic muscular contraction. The incidence was high in the mentally confused if they were inactive and confined to bed. A great injustice is done many persons who are incontinent when they are not gotten into wheelchairs or encouraged to lead as normal a life as possible.

Any bladder training is a long and tedious process, and during this time there may be leakage or spilling between voidings. If the patient is out of bed, urosheaths for men and protective pants and pads for women are necessary. If the patient is bedfast, the mattress is protected with a full-length waterproof cover. The usual bottom sheet is then adjusted. On top of this another waterproof rectangle covered with a cotton sheet is placed so that it extends from the neck to the knees and is tucked in at the sides. On this and directly under the buttocks is a waterproof rectangle, covered with a heavy absorbent material like cellucotton. Smaller absorbent pads should be placed between the legs and over the rectum. If the cellucotton pads are changed often enough, the larger sheets are never soiled, but there must be several layers of protectors for the mattress.

Frequent washing and, particularly, drying

* Brocklehurst, John C.: *op. cit.,* p. 100.

HABIT TRAINING FOR URINARY BLADDER CONTROL
(Do only with medical approval)

Management of Urinary Habit Training

1. Patient should attempt to urinate at regular intervals, starting with a rigid one- or two-hour schedule. If dry at the end of one or two hours, increase to a three-hour schedule; then later to a four-hour schedule.

2. A sitting or standing position helps in emptying the bladder.

3. Some paralyzed patients have warning when the bladder is ready to empty: some sense a fullness of the bladder; others may perspire, have "goose pimples," or other warnings.

4. Some patients have a "trigger point"; if this area is stroked, it stimulates urination. It may be the perineum, the foot, or the abdomen. Hearing water run may also stimulate urination. Voluntary sighing or breathing through the mouth helps others.

5. Urinary habit training may require several months. A record of progress for the entire period required to train the bladder should be kept.

6. Urinal or padding is worn when away from home to prevent possible soiling.

Procedure for Establishing Urinary Bladder Habit

1. Patient takes one or two 8-ounce glasses of fluid one hour before attempting to urinate. (Adult paraplegics need 2 quarts of fluid on cool days and 3 or more on hot days.)

2. No fluids should be taken between 6 P.M. and 6 A.M. if no urinating at night is desired.

3. Alcoholic drinks are contraindicated.

4. Coffee, tea, and soft drinks should be avoided.

5. All fluid taken by mouth (including soup, gelatin, ice cream, etc.) should be measured and the amounts recorded.

6. All urine voided should be measured and the amounts recorded.

SAMPLE RECORD OF URINARY BLADDER TRAINING FOR ONE WEEK

DATE	Sunday		Monday		Tuesday		Wednesday		Thursday		Friday		Saturday	
TIME	In-take	Out-put	In-take	Out-put	In-take	Out-put	In-take	Out-put	In-take	Out-put	In-take	Out-put	In-take	Out-put
6 A.M.	8													
7 A.M.		12												
8 A.M.	16													
9 A.M.		10												
10 A.M.	16													
11 A.M.		11												
12 Noon	16	A												
1 P.M.		4												
2 P.M.	16													
3 P.M.		10												
4 P.M.	8													
5 P.M.		7												
6 P.M.	8													
7 P.M.		6												
8 P.M.														
9 P.M.–6 A.M.														
Total ounces in 24 hours	88	60												

Under "Intake" record (in ounces) all fluids taken by mouth.
Under "Output" record (in ounces) all urine passed. Record "A" for accidental urinating.

A

Figure 37-5. *A*. Major aspects and procedure for urinary bladder training with a sample record for one week. This chart may be used by children and adults in hospitals, nursing homes, and private homes. *B*. Management of bowel habit training, including procedure and a sample record for one week. The chart may be used by adults as well as children in hospitals, nursing homes, and private homes. (From Allgire, Mildred J.: *Nurses Can Give and Teach Rehabilitation,* 2nd ed. Springer Publishing Co., New York, 1968, pp. 48, 49, 50, 51.)

HABIT TRAINING FOR BOWEL CONTROL
(Do only with medical approval)

Management of Bowel Habit Training

1. Patient should adhere to strict schedule of diet and elimination.

2. An accurate record, as indicated on chart below, should be kept.

3. Bowel movement is not necessary every day for all patients; however, a regular habit of every day or every other day should be established.

4. Leaning forward in a sitting position on side of bed or on commode for evacuation is helpful; patient may rest arms on back of a chair.

5. Patient may stimulate evacuation by inserting a gloved finger into the rectum.

6. Enemas are to be avoided; they delay habit training. If ordered, they should be given at the hour scheduled for evacuation.

7. Many patients establish the habit of emptying the bowels in the evening. If habit trained for morning evacuation, it may make the person late for work or school.

8. Allow time; for some patients habit training requires only a few days, for other many weeks are needed.

Procedure for Establishing Bowel Habit

8 A.M. — Patient takes 4 ounces of prune juice; also medication may be given but only if ordered by the doctor.

6 P.M. — Insert glycerine suppository into the rectum well plast the sphincter muscle (some patients need two suppositories). Teach patient to insert the suppository as soon as he can do it.

7 P.M. — Have patient attempt evacuation; allow adequate time.

SAMPLE RECORD OF BOWEL TRAINING FOR ONE WEEK

Month	Sunday	Monday	Tuesday	Wednesday	Thursday	Friday	Saturday
DATE							
Time of Prune Juice	8 AM	8 AM	8 AM	8 AM	8 AM	8 AM	8 AM
Time of Medication				8 AM			
Time of Suppository	6 PM	6 PM	6 PM	6 PM	6 PM	6 PM	6 PM
Time X, A, or E Results	7 PM X	7 PM X		7 PM X	7 PM X	8 PM X	7 PM X

Record X for evacuation. Record A for accident. Record E for enema.

B

of the skin is, of course, necessary. A number of commercial products are available that act as protective agents, and cornstarch is sometimes successfully used. Any powder that is used must not be allowed to cake in skin folds. A lanolin-based cream or A and D ointment may be used to coat the clean skin and delay the softening, or macerating, effect of later contact with urine.

The control of odor from the incontinent patient is a difficult problem. Andrea E. Dory reports that the use of a high-potency chlorophyllin medication (Derifil) has eliminated the odor associated with incontinence in a large nursing home. She says:

Derifil tablets have now been used by these and other incontinent patients for a period of two years. There has been no diminution in the effectiveness of the odor control. Nor has any patient experienced undesirable side effects. Some patients chew rather than swallow the tablets as instructed, but the temporary green staining of the mouth is of no consequence.*

* Dory, Andrea E.: "The Control of Odor in Urinary Incontinence," *Nurs. Homes*, **20**:28, (Oct.) 1971.

Treatment of Bowel Incontinence. The same therapeutic principles discussed above underlie the treatment of bowel incontinence (see Fig. 37-5B). If the rectum and anus are intact, rehabilitation can usually be effected. Two types of damage to the sphincter muscle can occur following a spinal cord lesion—atonic, a loss of tone of the sphincter muscle, or hypertonic, a spastic (tight) sphincter muscle. Incontinence occurs in the former as the rectum is dilated and there also is a loss of propulsive action. The internal anal sphincter, controlled by the autonomic nervous system, can be trained to take over the work of the external sphincter whose function is temporarily or permanently lost along with that of other voluntary muscles.

For the paralyzed patient all conditions that regulate bowel movements under ordinary circumstances are even more important; namely, (1) freedom from stress, (2) a regular time for defecation, (3) a diet that results in a soft, formed stool, (4) exercise to strengthen abdominal muscles used in defecation, and (5) a semisquatting position if condition permits. Patients should be taught exercises they can carry out in bed and encouraged to get up and move about as soon as possible.

Medications should be used only when more natural means of encouraging evacuations are ineffective. The gums such as tragacanth or senna leaves that produce bulk are probably the most desirable. Cascara, mineral oil, milk of magnesia, and other preparations will, however, be prescribed. Impactions are not uncommon. In such case the injection of oil followed in several hours by an enema or an irrigation may remove the impaction; often it must be removed with the gloved hand.

Unless patients can be helped to train the bowel function, their independence and usefulness are sadly curtailed. If they cannot accomplish regular and more or less normal bowel habits with diet, exercise, position, and manual pressure over the lower abdomen as they bear down in defecation, they may find that glycerin suppositories will stimulate an evacuation. Patients should be taught to insert from one to three suppositories about one-half to three hours before the usual time for defecation, depending upon the sensitivity of the colon. Glycerin is mildly irritating and stimulates contraction of the colon by drawing fluid into the rectum, increasing and at the same time softening the bulk of the stool. Dulcax suppositories are also used. The physician may prescribe small, evacuating enemas until regularity is established.

Brocklehurst found that 70 per cent of the old people who had bladder incontinence also suffered from incontinence of the rectum. He believed rectal incontinence in the aged had a physiologic basis, but, like bladder incontinence, the chief causes were (1) paralysis, (2) bedfastness, and (3) confusion.

The writers' summary presents Brocklehurst's opinion on senile incontinents:

Incontinence is commonly described by neurologists as "loss of sphincter control." It would appear, however, that the function of the sphincter is a subsidiary one, certainly less important than the tone and movements of the bladder and large bowel. Between intervals of defecation the presence of a constantly filled rectum suggests at once senile incontinence as well as colonic overactivity; but the uninhibited contractions of the rectum cause the evacuation of only a part of the intra-rectal mass. Although the rectum is hyperexcitable in this condition and empties itself at a smaller volume of contents than normal, residual feces are almost always found within the rectum because defecation in senile incontinents is precipitate and can usually be neither facilitated nor retarded by the patient's use of his accessory muscles (recti, abdominis, diaphragm, etc.).

In terminal illness where bowel training is not possible, regular bowel movements can still be encouraged with the same means as those just described. In such cases the nurse may have to assume the entire responsibility for the program prescribed by the physician. See Chapter 50 for a discussion of bowel function in the last stage of terminal illness.

REFERENCES

1. Peterson, Malcolm L.: "Constipation and Diarrhea," in MacBryde, Cyril M., and Blacklow, Robert S. (eds.): *Signs and Symptoms; Applied Pathologic Physiology and Clinical Interpretation,* 5th ed. J. B. Lippincott Co., Philadelphia, 1970, p. 381.
2. Guyton, Arthur C.: *Textbook of Medical Physiology,* 5th ed. W. B. Saunders Co., Philadelphia, 1976, p. 892.
3. Peterson, Malcolm L.: *op. cit.,* p. 383.
4. Bockus, Henry L. (ed.): *Gastroenterology,* Vol. II, 3rd ed. W. B. Saunders Co., Philadelphia, 1976, p. 937.
5. Paulson, Moses: *Gastroenterologic Medicine.* Lea & Febiger, Philadelphia, 1969, p. 1189.
6. Raffensperger, Edward C.: "Fecal Impaction of the Colon and Rectum," in Bockus, Henry L. (ed.): *Gastroenterology,* Vol. II, 2nd ed. W. B. Saunders Co., Philadelphia, 1964, p. 1071.
7. *Ibid.,* p. 1074.
8. McCarthy, Joyce A.: "Effects on Gastrointestinal Function," *Am. J. Nurs.,* **67:**785, (Apr.) 1967.
9. Frohman, I. Phillips: "Constipation," *Am. J. Nurs.,* **55:**65, (Jan.) 1955.

10. Chohen, Theodore, and Gitman, Leo: "Clinical Evaluation of the Gastrointestinal Tract in the Aged," *Am. J. Gastroenterol.,* **33:**422, (Apr.) 1960.

11. Nelson, Waldo E., et al. (eds.): *Textbook of Pediatrics,* 9th ed. W. B. Saunders Co., Philadelphia, 1969, pp. 144, 697.

12. Sehnert, Keith W.: "Review of Pharmacology of Bowel Evacuants and Laxatives," *Nebr. State Med. J.,* **50:**54, (Feb.) 1965.

13. Robinson, Corinne H.: *Proudfit-Robinson's Normal and Therapeutic Nutrition,* 14th ed. Macmillan Publishing Co., Inc., New York, 1972, pp. 341, 461.

14. Nite, Gladys, and Willis, Frank N.: *The Coronary Patient, Hospital Care and Rehabilitation.* Macmillan Publishing Co., Inc., New York, 1964. p. 155.

15. Painter, Neil Stamford: "Diverticular Disease of the Colon and Constipation and Their Relationship to Our Diet I," *Nurs. Times,* **68:**536, (May 4) 1972.

16. ————: "Diverticular Disease of the Colon and Constipation and Their Relationship to Our Diet II," *Nurs. Times,* **68:**564, (May 11) 1972.

17. Almy, Thomas P.: "Management of Chronic Constipation," in Turell, Robert (ed.): *Diseases of the Colon and Anorectum,* Vol. II, 2nd ed. W. B. Saunders Co., Philadelphia, 1969, p. 859.

18. Magnuson, Charles: "The Geriatric and Bedridden Patient and the Large Bowel," *Nebr. State Med. J.,* **50:**73, (Feb.) 1965.

19. Fingl, Edward: "Cathartics and Laxatives," in Goodman, Louis S., and Gilman, Alfred (eds.): *The Pharmacological Basis of Therapeutics,* 5th ed. Macmillan Publishing Co., Inc., New York, 1975, p. 978.

20. Seneca, H.: "A Mannitol-Pectin-Fruit Juice Preparation (Manigel) with Mild Laxative Action," *J. Am. Geriatr. Soc.,* **12:**95, (Jan.) 1964.

21. Bockus, Henry L. (ed.): *op. cit.,* p. 947.

22. Sehnert, Keith W.: *op. cit.*

22a. Corman, Narvin L., et al.: "Cathartics," *Am. J. Nurs.,* **75:**273, (Feb.) 1975.

23. Hudson, Eric: "Bowel Management: Modern Methods," *Nurs. Times,* **57:**1597, (Dec. 8) 1961.

24. Dunning, Marcelle F., and Plum, Fred: "Potassium Depletion by Enemas," *Am. J. Med.,* **20:**789, (May) 1956.

25. Peterson, Malcolm L.: *op. cit.,* p. 387.

26. Texter, E. Clinton, Jr.: "Pathophysiologic Basis for Diarrhea," *Am. J. Gastroenterol.,* **40:**284, (Sept.) 1963.

27. Low-Beer, T. S.: "Progress Report—Diarrhoea: Mechanisms and Treatment," *Gut,* **12:**1021, (Dec.) 1971.

28. Lambert, Harold P.: "Food Poisoning," in Beeson, Paul B., and McDermott, Walsh (eds.): *Textbook of Medicine,* Vol. I, 14th ed. W. B. Saunders Co., Philadelphia, 1975, p. 47.

29. Silverberg, Mervin, and Davidson, Murray: "Functional and Organic Causes of Diarrhea," in Turell, Robert (ed.): *Diseases of the Colon and Anorectum,* Vol. II, 2nd ed. W. B. Saunders Co., Philadelphia, 1969, p. 854.

30. Guyton, Arthur C.: *op. cit.,* p. 898.

31. Bockus, Henry L. (ed.): *op. cit.,* p. 899.

32. Roth, James L. A.: "Ulcerative Colitis," in Bockus, Henry L. (ed.): *Gastroenterology,* Vol. II, 2nd ed. W. B. Saunders Co., Philadelphia, 1964, p. 818.

32a. Jackson, Bettie: "Ulcerative Colitis from an Etiological Perspective," *Am. J. Nurs.,* **73:**258, (Feb.) 1973.

33. Durand, P.: *Disorders Due to Intestinal Defective Carbohydrate Digestion and Absorption.* Grune & Stratton, New York, 1964, p. 107.

34. Littman, A., and Hammond, J. B.: "Diarrhea in Adults Caused by Deficiency in Intestinal Disaccharidases," *Gastroenterology,* **48:**239, (Feb.) 1965.

35. Lifshitz, Fima, et al.: "Carbohydrate Intolerance in Infants with Diarrhea," *J. Pediatr.,* **79:**760, (Nov.) 1971.

36. Cox, Alan G., and Bond, Michael R.: "Bowel Habit After Vagotomy and Gastrojejunostomy," *Br. Med. J.,* **1:**460, (Feb. 27) 1964.

37. Burge, H. W., et al.: "Selective Vagotomy in the Prevention of Post-Vagotomy Diarrhea," *Lancet,* **2:**897, (Oct. 21) 1961.

38. Gamble, John R., and Wilbur, Dwight L.: *Chemistry of Digestive Diseases.* Charles C Thomas, Publisher, Springfield, Ill., 1961, p. 85.

39. Almy, Thomas P.: "Disorders of Motility," in Beeson, Paul B., and McDermott, Walsh (eds.): *Textbook of Medicine,* Vol. II, 14th ed. W. B. Saunders Co., Philadelphia, 1975, p. 1188.

40. Robinson, Corinne H.: *op. cit.,* p. 508.

41. Goodman, Louis S., and Gilman, Alfred: *The Pharmacological Basis of Therapeutics,* 5th ed. Macmillan Publishing Co., Inc., New York, 1975, p. 263.

42. Almy, Thomas P.: *op. cit.,* p. 1188.

43. Shapiro, Shepard: "Control of Antibiotic-Induced Gastrointestinal Symptoms with Yogurt," *Clin. Med.,* **7:**297, (Feb.) 1960.

44. Keuhnelian, John G., and Sanders, Virginia E.: *Urologic Nursing.* Macmillan Publishing Co., Inc., New York, 1970, p. 17.

45. Creevy, Charles: *Outline of Urology.* McGraw-Hill Book Co., New York, 1964, pp. 113, 194, 341.

45a. Raz, Shlomo, and Smith, Robert B.: "External Sphincter Spasticity Syndrome in Female Patients," *J. Urol.,* **115:**443, (Apr.) 1976.

46. Creevy, Charles: "The Care of the Urological Patient Before and After Operation," in Campbell, Meredith F., and Harrison, J. Hartwell: *Urology,* Vol. III, 3rd ed. W. B. Saunders Co., Philadelphia, 1970, p. 2106.

47. Cook, Edward N., et al.: "Urinary Retention Following Operations on the Bowel," *J. Urol.,* **89:**255, (Feb.) 1963.

48. Creevy, Charles: *op. cit.,* p. 123.
49. Keuhnelian, John G., and Sanders, Virginia E.: *op. cit.*
50. Larson, James W., et al.: "Psychogenic Urinary Retention in Women," *J.A.M.A.,* **184:** 697, (June 1) 1963.
50a. Knox, S. J.: "Psychogenic Urinary Retention After Parturition Resulting in Hydronephrosis," *Br. Med. J.,* **2:**1422, (Nov.) 1960.
50b. Margolis, G. J.: "A Review of Literature of Psychogenic Urinary Retention," *J. Urol.,* **94:**257, (Mar.) 1965.
51. Goddard, G. F. J.: "Prolonged Retention of Urine Due to an Antidepressant Drug," *Am. J. Psychiatry,* **119:**476, (Nov.) 1962.
51a. Pearman, John W.: *The Urological Management of the Patient Following Spinal Cord Injury.* Charles C Thomas, Publisher, Springfield, Ill., 1973, p. 27.
51b. Taylor, D. E. M.: "Cardiovascular Disturbances in Acute Retention of Urine," *Lancet,* **2:**1033, (Nov. 16) 1963.
52. Lindbjerg, I. F., and Brandt, N. J.: "Indirect Determination of the Volume of Residual Urine with 131-I-labelled Hippuran," *Acta. Chir. Scand.,* **127:**675, 1964.
53. Merrill, John P.: *The Treatment of Renal Failure,* 2nd ed. Grune & Stratton, New York, 1965, p. 118.
54. Boyd, William: *A Textbook of Pathology, Structure and Function in Disease,* 8th ed. Lea & Febiger, Philadelphia, 1970, p. 671.
55. Bricker, Neal S.: "Acute Renal Failure," in Beeson, Paul B., and McDermott, Walsh (eds.): *Textbook of Medicine,* Vol. II. 14th ed. W. B. Saunders Co., Philadelphia, 1975, p. 1107.
55a. Hekelman, Francine P., and Ostendarp, Carol A.: "Nursing Approaches to Conservative Management of Renal Disease," *Nurs. Clin. North Am.,* **10:**431, (Sept.) 1975.
55b. Bazzato, Giorgio, and Onesti, Gaddo: *Hemodialysis in the Home; Techniques and Clinical Results.* Charles C Thomas, Publisher, Springfield, Ill., 1975.
56. Cooke, Robert E.: "The Bladder," in Cooke, Robert E. (ed.): *The Biologic Basis of Pediatric Practice.* McGraw-Hill Book Co., New York, 1968, p. 1056.
57. Nelson, Waldo E., et al. (eds.): *op. cit.,* p. 1109.
58. Eisenberg, Leon: "The Preschool and School Age Child—Psychological Considerations," in Cooke, Robert E. (ed.): *The Biologic Basis of Pediatric Practice.* McGraw-Hill Book Co., New York, 1968, p. 1579.
59. McDonald, Harold P.: "Enuresis," in Conn, Howard F. (ed.): *Current Therapy.* W. B. Saunders Co., Philadelphia, 1964, p. 338.
59a. Eisenberg, Leon: *op. cit.*
59b. Cooke, Robert E.: *op. cit.*
60. Lytton, Bernard, and Epstein, Franklin H.: "Dysuria, Incontinence, and Enuresis," in Wintrobe, Maxwell M., et al. (eds.): *Harrison's Principles of Internal Medicine,* 6th ed. McGraw-Hill Book Co., New York, 1970, p. 271.

61. Lapides, Jack: "Neuromuscular Vesical and Ureteral Dysfunction," in Campbell, Meredith F., and Harrison, J. Hartwell (eds.): *Urology,* Vol. III, 3rd ed. W. B. Saunders Co., Philadelphia, 1970, p. 1373.
62. ———: "Stress Incontinence," *J. Urol.,* **85:** 291, (Mar.) 1961.
63. Hurwitz, Sidney P., et al.: "Preparation of an Incontinence Bag," *J. Urol.,* **73:**1103, (June) 1955.
64. Ream, W. Dale, and Feldman, Daniel J.: "A Modified Urinary Drainage Apparatus for the Neurogenic Male Bladder," *Arch. Phys. Med. Rehabil.,* **45:**428, (May) 1964.
65. Brunkow, Clarence W.: "Male Incontinence: Plastic Bag Receptacle for Mild Cases," *Northwest Med.,* **71:**616, (Aug.) 1972.
66. Schofield, Derek: "Management of Urinary Incontinence," *Nurs. Mirror,* **131:**39, (Aug. 21) 1970.
67. Bors, Ernest, and Comarr, A. Estine: *Neurological Urology.* University Park Press, Baltimore, 1971, p. 293.
68. Abramson, Arthur S.: "Advances in the Management of the Neurogenic Bladder," *Arch. Phys. Med. Rehabil.,* **52:**143, (Apr.) 1971.
69. Pratt, Rosalie: "Management of the Bladder," *Nurs. Times,* **67:**604, (May 20) 1971.
70. Delehanty, Lorraine, and Stravino, Vincent: "Achieving Bladder Control," *Am. J. Nurs.,* **70:**312, (Feb.) 1970.
71. Bergstrom, Doris A.: *Care of Patients with Bowel and Bladder Problems; A Nursing Guide.* American Rehabilitation Foundation, Minneapolis, 1968, p. 20.
72. Stryker, Ruth P.: *Rehabilitative Aspects of Acute and Chronic Nursing Care.* W. B. Saunders Co., Philadelphia, 1972, p. 74.
73. Allgire, Mildred J.: *Nurses Can Give and Teach Rehabilitation,* 2nd ed. Springer Publishing Co., New York, 1968, p. 48.
74. Wilson, Thomas S.: "Incontinence of Urine in the Aged," *Lancet,* **2:**374, (Sept.) 1948.

Additional Suggested Reading

Boone, Elizabeth T.: "Nursing Care of the Paraplegic Using an Experimental Electronic Spinal Neuroprosthesis to Activate Voiding," *J. Neurosurg. Nurs.,* **4:**61, (July) 1972.
Broad, John N.: "Urinary Incontinence—A New Method of Control," *Nurs. Times,* **68:**1212, (Sept. 28) 1972.
Calapinto, V., and McCallum, R. W.: "Urinary Continence After Repair of Membranous Urethral Stricture in Prostatectomized Patients," *J. Urol.,* **115:**392, (Apr.) 1976.
Caldwell, K. P. "Sphincter Stimulators to Prevent Incontinence," *Nurs. Times,* **69:**1524, (Nov. 15) 1973.
Comarr, A. Estin, and Gunderson, Bernice B.: "Sexual Function in Traumatic Paraplegia and Quadriplegia," *Am. J. Nurs.,* **75:**250, (Feb.) 1975.
Cornell, Sudie A., et al.: "Comparison of Three Bowel Management Programs During Rehabili-

tation of Spinal Cord Injured Patients," *Nurs. Res.,* **22**:321, (July–Aug.) 1973.

Culp, Patricia: "Nursing Care of the Patient with Spinal Cord Injury, *Nurs. Clin. North Am.,* **2**: 447, (Sept.) 1967.

Degroot, Jane, and Kunin, Calvin M.: "Indwelling Catheters," *Am. J. Nurs.,* **75**:448, (Mar.) 1975.

Dische, Sylvia: "Bedwetting and Its Treatment," *Nurs. Mirror,* **134**:46, (Feb. 25) 1972.

Dodge, Warren F., et al.: "Nocturnal Enuresis in 6–10 Year Old Children," *Am. J. Dis. Child.,* **120**:32, (July) 1970.

Drew, L. R. H.: "Drug Control of Incontinence in Adult Mental Defectives," *Med. J. Aust.,* **2**:206, (July 29) 1967.

Feustel, Delycia: "Autonomic Hyperreflexia," *Am. J. Nurs.,* **76**:228, (Feb.) 1976.

Grosicki, Jeannette P.: "Effect of Operant Conditioning on Modification of Incontinence in Neuropsychiatric Geriatric Patients," *Nurs. Res.,* **17**:304, (July–Aug.) 1968.

Gross, James B., and Kokkro, Julia P.: "The Influence of Increased Tubular Hydrostatic Pressure of Renal Function," *J. Urol.,* **115**:427, (Apr.) 1976.

Harrington, Joan D., and Brener, Etta Rae: *Patient Care in Renal Failure.* W. B. Saunders Co., Philadelphia, 1973.

Johnson, H. Katheryn, et al.: "Nursing Care of the Patient with Acute Renal Failure," *Nurs. Clin. North Am.,* **10**:421, (Sept.) 1975.

Keegan, Lynn: "Fecal Incontinence Bag," *Nurs. Homes,* **20**:40, (Mar.) 1971.

Leonard, Martha: "Health Issues and Primary Nursing in Nephrology Care," *Nurs. Clin. North Am.,* **10**:413, (Sept.) 1975.

Lindan, Rosemary, and Bellamy, Virginia: "The Use of Intermittent Catheterization in a Bladder Training Program. Preliminary Report," *J. Chronic Dis.,* **24**:727, (Nov.) 1971.

Mihalov, Thelma R.: "Bowel and Bladder Management of Children with Myelomeningocele," *Nurs. Clin. North Am.,* **3**:459, (Sept.) 1966.

Murphy, John J.: "Urologic Management of the Patient with Spinal Cord Injury," in Austin, George (ed.): *The Spinal Cord,* 2nd ed. Charles C Thomas, Publisher, Springfield, Ill., 1972.

Reif, Laura: "Managing a Life with Chronic Disease," *Am. J. Nurs.,* **73**:261, (Feb.) 1973.

Smith, Jim, and Bullough, Bonnie: "Sexuality and the Severely Disabled Person," *Am. J. Nurs.,* **75**:2194, (Dec.) 1975.

Tudo, Lea L.: "Bladder and Bowel Retraining," *Am. J. Nurs.,* **70**:2391, (Nov.) 1970.

US Public Health Service: *Renal Disease and Hypertension.* Proceedings of 14th Annual Conference, Apr. 1975, San Francisco, Calif. US Government Printing Office, Washington D.C., 1975 (DHEW Pub. No. [HSA] 6–2001).

Whitehead, Elizabeth: "Coping with Female Incontinence," *Nurs. Mirror,* **131**:38, (Aug.) 1970.

Woodward, Sister M. Hilary: "Urinary Incontinence in the Physically Handicapped Child," *Nurs. Times,* **66**:1098, (Aug. 27) 1970.

Gladys Nite
Virginia Henderson

CHAPTER 38

Motor Disturbances—Hypoactivity, Immobilization

1. INTRODUCTION

Hypoactivity and *immobilization* are terms that define themselves. The hypoactive person is less active than is normal for him or her, while the immobile person is unable to move. Both hypoactivity and immobilization may be of psychic origin just as either may result from organic disease. Anything that depresses people, that turns their thoughts inward, tends to reduce their involvement in life and make them hypoactive; strong emotion, as, for example, intense fear, can immobilize its victims. In catatonia, a severe condition associated with schizophrenia, there is such muscular rigidity that patients will hold any position in which they are placed for hours (catalepsy). Conversion reactions can produce paralyses of the whole or parts of the body.

Hypoactivity and immobilization result from so many forms of organic illness that it is impractical to try to list specific causes. However, examples are febrile, debilitating diseases that prostrate patients and make them inactive unless forced by necessity to move, and circulatory and respiratory conditions that reduce the oxygen supply to the cells, making inactivity a means of conserving the amount of available oxygen. Disease of the muscles or nerves supplying them can cause hypoactivity or inability to move the whole or a part of the body. For example, pressure on motor areas in the brain or spinal cord as a result of hemorrhage can bring about hypoactivity or immobilization from complete paralysis; injuries to any part of the body may lessen or completely destroy motor power by severing the nerves supplying the muscles. Chemicals, or drugs, are one of the commonest causes of hypoactivity and their use and misuse are discussed later in this chapter and also in Chapters 21, 22, 49, and 50.

Actually, it is hard to think of any disease that isn't accompanied by hyperactivity or hypoactivity, more often the latter. For this reason, and because rest may be prescribed as treatment, the management of hypoactivity and immobility is a critical aspect of nursing. Whether hypoactivity or immobility is self-imposed or prescribed, it affects the body and spirit. Doris Carnevali and Susan Brueckner [1] in "reassessing" the concept of immobilization as "prescribed or unavoidable restriction of movement in any area of a patient's life" emphasize, as do many others, the sensory deprivation it entails. The effects of hypoactivity can be predicted and, particularly if the cause is identified, can be mitigated to a considerable extent by imaginative and skillful nursing. As in all symptomatic nursing, excellent care is individualized care.

Hypoactivity and its extension *immobility* are discussed in one chapter because they are so closely related, but actually the care needed by a 75-year-old woman who has developed mutism and progressive hypoactivity in a nursing home has little in common with that required by an otherwise healthy 10-year-old boy in a body cast who is being treated for fractures by immobilization.

Frederick Leboyer, a physician who is well known for his method of delivering infants designed to minimize the trauma of birth, is the author of an illustrated book on infant massage which is used to counteract the effects of immobility in the newborn. The title of the book is *Loving Hands—The Traditional Indian Art of Infant Massage* (Alfred A. Knopf, Inc., New York, 1976). Until the infant can turn, or during the first six months of life, women of India spend about one-half hour daily massaging their infants and flexing the arms and legs. Photographs of the infant taken throughout this procedure show it to be a satisfying experience for him (see Fig. 38-1*A* and *B*) and suggest the intuitive wisdom of Indian mothering. From infancy to old age the baleful effects of hypoactivity must be combatted by those who value health.

There is no doubt that the effect of the massage is emotionally satisfying as well as physically beneficial. The harmful effect of depriving infants of touching, or caressing, has been thoroughly investigated. Lytt I. Gardner reports some studies on this subject. He also

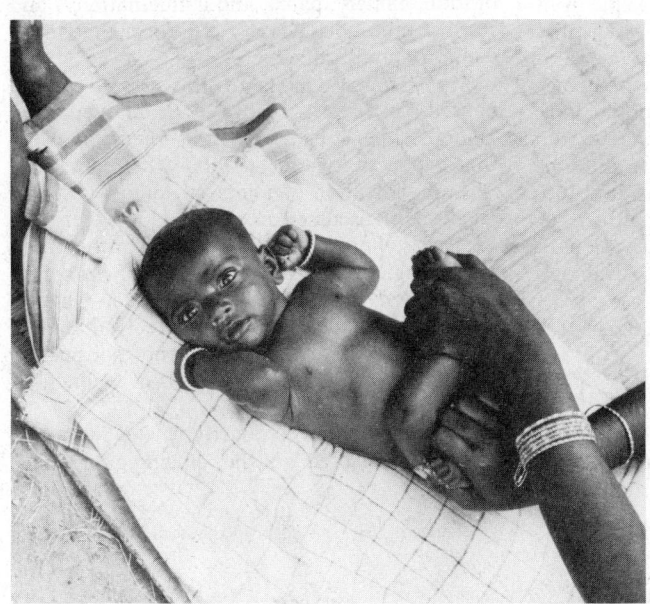

A

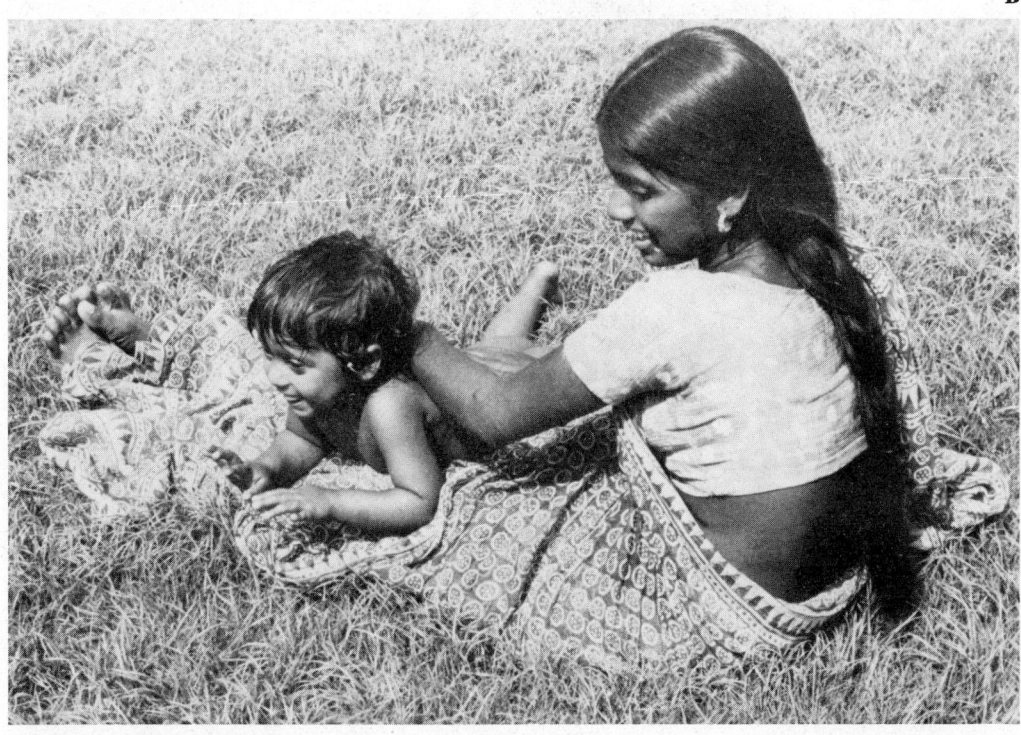

B

Figure 38-1. *A*. Mother flexing legs of infant following massage. *B*. Shows mother massaging infant's older sister who has been watching (perhaps enviously) the massage of the infant. (From Leboyer, Frederick: *Loving Hands —The Traditional Indian Art of Infant Massage.* Alfred A. Knopf, New York, 1976, p. 84.)

reports his investigation, with Robert Gray Patton, of six patients from "disordered family environments." They concluded that children raised in an emotionally deprived environment (which involved hypoactivity and little mental stimulation) can have their growth stunted by it.* Research on inactivity in man is paralleled by studies of inactivity in animals. Mark R. Rosenzweig and his associates, for example, give evidence that rats kept in a lively environment for 30 days show "distinct changes in brain anatomy and chemistry compared with animals in a dull environment." These authors believe researchers should look "more penetratingly" for such changes in the human brain as a result of living in a dull environment.† Leo Goldberger, writing in 1966, said "The experimental study of the effects of perceptual isolation or sensory deprivation in human beings is of relatively recent origin." ‡

* Gardner, Lytt I.: "Deprivation Dwarfism," *Sci. Am.,* **227**:76, (July) 1972.
† Rosenzweig, Mark R., et al.: "Brain Changes in Response to Experience," *Sci. Am.,* **226**:22, (Feb.) 1972.
‡ Goldberger, Leo: "Experimental Isolation: An Overview," *Am. J. Psychiatry,* **122**:774, (Jan.) 1966.

His review of the literature up to 1966 should be useful for interested readers. Articles by nurses on sensory deprivation appear more and more frequently in nursing journals. A good example is Judith Chodil's and Barbara Williams' discussion in *Nursing Clinics of North America* (**5**:435, [Sept.] 1970). They list types of patient behavior (boredom, inactivity, slowness of thought, daydreaming, thought deterioration, anxiety, panic, and hallucinations) and suggest nurse behavior or the form that intervention should take.

Many nursing texts of this era stress the hazards of bedrest. Figure 38-2, adapted from Nancy Roper's text, diagrams them, showing that hypoactivity affects all body systems.

Immobilization of joints by splints, casts, or traction is discussed in Chapter 34 where the emphasis, however, is on method rather than psychologic or physiologic effects of immobilization. Body mechanics is discussed in Chapter 12 and the point is made repeatedly that free, enjoyable body movement and normal posture are essential to the highest levels of wellness of mind and body.

This chapter on hypoactivity and immobilization is devoted to the effects of reduced

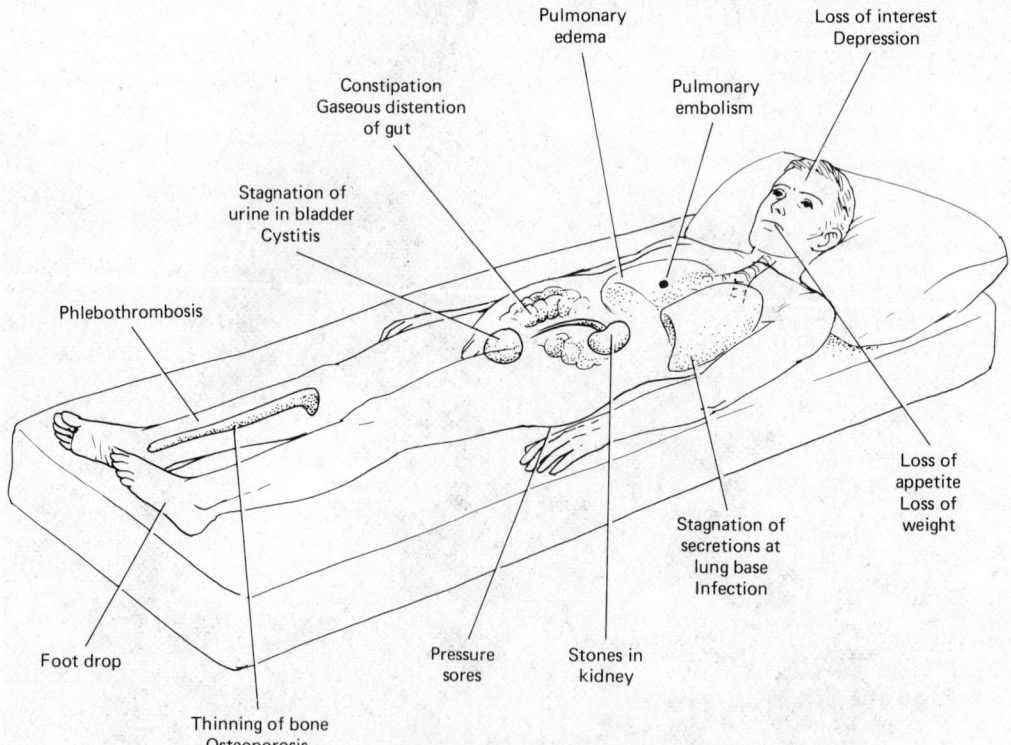

Figure 38-2. Diagram showing the hazards of prolonged bedrest on various body systems. (Adapted from Roper, Nancy: *Principles of Nursing,* E. & S. Livingston, Ltd., Edinburgh and London, 1967, p. 182.)

activity from any cause. It discusses some of the problems immobilization poses for patients, the special help they need in dealing with these problems and, most particularly, the help nurses can give hypoactive or immobilized patients and their families.

Nurses' concepts of hypoactivity and immobilization affect the way they deal with the inactive patient. If they believe that motor activity has only physical effects, they will treat hypoactivity as a purely physical handicap; if they think of all paralysis as caused by hemorrhages in the central nervous system, they may associate helplessness with the chronically ill and older patient. If, on the other hand, nurses have had experience in their family with hysterical paralysis or with young persons whose war injuries, for example, have reduced them to a wheelchair existence, or if they have had an alcoholic father who spent his evenings in bed or on a sofa, they will of necessity bring a broader understanding of the subject under discussion here. Nurses' concepts of bedrest as altogether beneficial or potentially harmful will also affect the ways in which they manage hypoactivity and immobilization.

If the goal of health care is helping people to realize their full potential, hypoactivity must be regarded as a serious symptom. Nurses have always been family health counselors, and in this capacity they can be alert to hypoactive behavior, whether it be a sign of organic pathology, unhealthy human relations, or an unhealthy environment.

It is helpful to trace how inactivity has been associated with illness and helplessness in the minds of both the givers and receivers of care. "Bedrest" has been the treatment for many illnesses without scientific evidence that it is helpful. A physician writing on bedrest calls attention to the jargon of illness that emphasizes the bed—"bedrest," "bedside manner," and hospital size as measured by the number of beds.[2] When persons are sick, they are often put to bed. To some, this is a welcome prescription, but for a young child or an active adult, it can be a difficult one to accept. In the last three decades the hazards of immobility have been increasingly emphasized. Numerous studies have shown that in diseases such as tuberculosis, hepatitis, and myocardial infarction, total bedrest has been ineffective in altering the course of the disease.[3-5] It has been demonstrated that early ambulation decreases complications of surgery, but it is hard to alter the commonly held belief that bedrest will make the sick better.[6] Changing this concept is especially difficult in a hospital where beds are the most obvious piece of furniture and where traditions are entrenched.

It is easier for some nurses to care for patients in bed or up in a chair for part of the day than for patients who must be helped to dress and who will then need help in finding suitable occupation and companionship.

2. GENERAL CAUSES OF HYPOACTIVITY AND IMMOBILIZATION

Hypoactivity and immobilization result from disease, trauma, and disability. Both are prescribed as treatment and both may result from maltreatment. Medical and nursing education has focused on hypoactivity and immobility as prescribed treatment. One of the first procedures a nurse learns is to bathe patients and make their beds, disturbing them as little as possible. The rehabilitation of the disabled with all or part of their bodies immobilized began to get attention in World War I, and since World War II it has had major attention. Physical rehabilitation in the United States had its genesis in military hospitals. Immobilization as a result of psychic trauma is familiar to all who have seen the depressed inactive patients in mental health institutions. Hypoactivity is visible in large cities where "nodding" drug addicts (including alcoholics) hardly move or respond.

Hypoactivity and immobilization are prescribed as therapy to promote healing, provide protection, or reduce pain. Physicians may advise patients to decrease motion in a part of the body—to rest an infected hand in a sling or to rest a fractured patella by making the knee immobile with a cast. Physicians may advise hypoactivity of the body as a whole, as in the treatment of myocardial infarction, acute rheumatoid disease, or prostrating infections such as lobar pneumonia or meningitis. Some people are confined to beds or rooms not so much because their condition demands it, but because they have a communicable disease, and limiting the activity of the infected persons makes it easier to prevent the transmission of their infections to others.

Hypoactivity and Immobility as Prescribed Treatment. The history of rest and immobilization as prescribed treatment shows the dramatic effects of clinical research (including pharmacologic studies) on patient care. Physicians of the nineteenth century and early part of the twentieth century tended to treat many, if not most, illnesses with bedrest. R. A. J. Asher[7] wrote in 1947 on the "dangers of going to bed." Before the development of antibiotics, the prostration resulting from most infections kept those with infectious disease in bed. Before disease-specific chemotherapy, such as penicillin for pneumococcal pneumonia and isoniazid (INH) or streptomycin for tuberculosis, many infections were fatal. A person with tuberculosis might be kept in bed for months, even years; a child with rheumatic fever and a serious heart impairment might spend much of his or her short life in bed.

Before the development and general use of antibiotics and sulfonamides, surgery was frequently complicated by infection. Postoperatively, patients were treated with bedrest because it was the common belief that immobility reduced morbidity and mortality. William Dock * was one of the first surgeons to stress early ambulation postoperatively. In 1945, he wrote that long-term bedrest might cause hypo-

* Dr. William Dock, a nephew of the noted American nurse Lavinia Dock, used to shock nursing audiences by saying that "good" nurses had killed more patients than many dread diseases. While he exaggerated to make a point, his contention was that nurses were taught to anticipate patients' needs and to do everything they could *for* them rather than encourage activity and independence. He also said that the medical students he taught were so impressed with the dangers of rest that they were "afraid to go to bed." (Personal communication with the second author.)

static pneumonia, acute pulmonary collapse, pulmonary edema, general edema, constipation, and inability to void.[8] As chemotherapy improved and as studies showed that early ambulation prevented many complications of surgery and hastened the healing process, the length of time the person having surgery was allowed to stay in bed became shorter and shorter. Now it is common practice to get every surgical patient out of bed within the first 24 hours, even those having extensive surgery.

Until recently, patients who had a myocardial infarction were kept in bed for varying but long periods. There is still a wide diversity of medical opinion on the length of prescribed bedrest following an acute myocardial infarction, but the length of time is considerably shorter than the traditional 4- to 6-week period prescribed in the past.[9] In a controlled trial of early mobilization and discharge from the hospital in uncomplicated myocardial infarction, Jane E. Harper and associates[10] found that patients who were up out of bed after 7 days fared no worse than those kept in bed for 20 days. There was no difference between the two groups in mortality, complication rates, or oc-

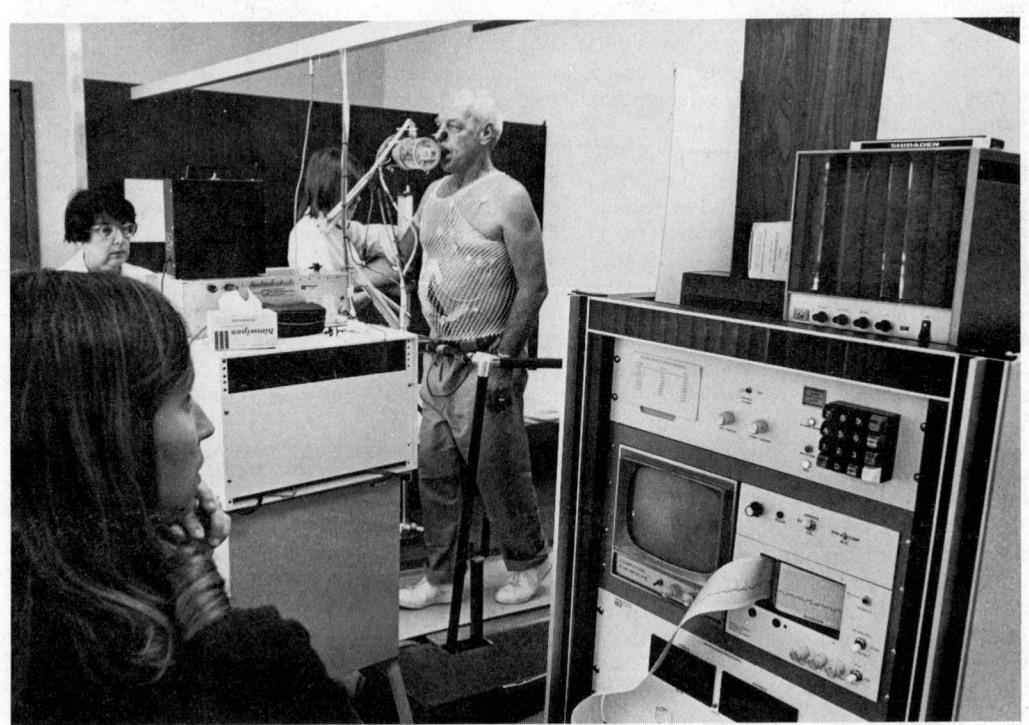

Figure 38-3. Participant of Stanford cardiac rehabilitation program's sponsored pilot heart disease prevention seminar taking an exercise tolerance test on treadmill. (From *The Healing Arts. A Report from Stanford University Medical Center,* **5**:11, [Winter] 1975.)

currence of ventricular aneurysms. Similarly, D. C. Boyle and associates [11] found that patients classified as "not at risk" tolerated discharge from the hospital within 10 days. These patients had less deep vein thrombosis, postural hypotension, and "cardiac neurosis" than those kept in bed for longer periods. Also, early discharge from the hospital meant a better utilization of hospital beds as long as the safety of patients was ensured. Rehabilitation of cardiac patients involves testing their tolerance of exercise (see Fig. 38-3) and some believe nothing is more important than exercise in preventing heart disease (see Fig. 38-4).

Hepatitis was another disease usually treated with lengthy periods of bedrest and inactivity. The prevailing practice of prescribing extended rest for patients with hepatitis is slowly changing. Once patients feel better and have less malaise, physicians advise them to gauge their own activity. Total bedrest has been shown ineffective in altering the course of the disease, and exercise for the patient with hepatitis has had no untoward effects.[12,13]

Immobilization is prescribed for skeletal injuries in the form of casts or splints for broken bones or torn cartilages. Such immobility provides the necessary rest and support for the injury to heal and decreases pain and makes patients feel more comfortable.*

Hypoactivity and Immobility as a Result of Disability or Trauma. Hypoactive infants, children, or adults may be mentally retarded, malnourished, or emotionally starved.† Lytt I. Gardner [14] discussed "deprivation dwarfism"

* The second writer has been told by visitors to China and Japan that often in the treatment of fractures immobilization is reduced to a minimum. Frederick F. Kao, a physician who has recently visited the People's Republic of China, says: "The treatment of fractures is being radically transformed. Instead of using casts to immobilize the limbs in plaster, the ancient Chinese method of treating fractures includes the employment of small splints for some immobilization of the limbs, thus avoiding bed sores and stiffening of the joints. The fracture reduction is simultaneously coupled with movement of the limbs." (Kao, Frederick F.: "Chinese Medicine and the Chinese Medical System," *Am. J. Chinese Med.,* **1:**1, [Jan.] 1973.)

† Hypoactive children may be the "battered children" so often mentioned in the news media. People are even urged if they see a child abused to call a special number (911) in those communities where all emergency services respond to this number.

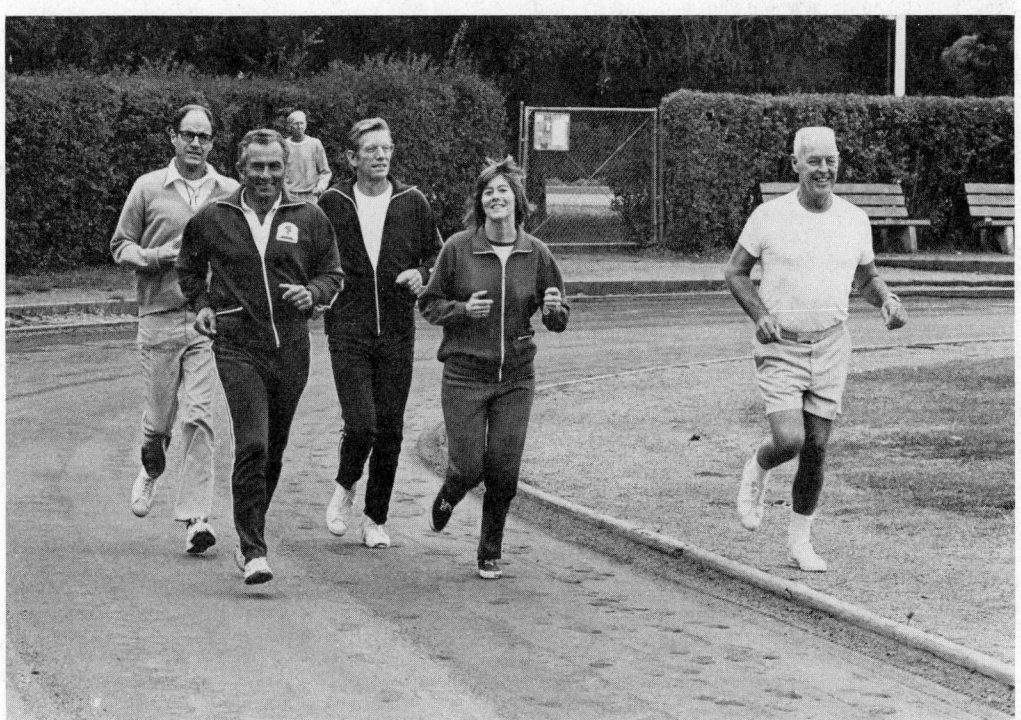

Figure 38-4. Stanford cardiac rehabilitation program sponsored a pilot heart disease prevention seminar for members of the community in 1975. Physician Robert DeBusk (third from right), program director, and nurse Nancy Houston participate. (From *The Healing Arts. A Report from Stanford University Medical Center,* **5:**11, [Winter] 1975.)

in *Scientific American* in 1972. Hypoactive children or adults may have a brain tumor, an infection, or an endocrine imbalance. Hypoactivity or immobility as a result of disease is probably associated in the minds of most persons with victims of stroke (cerebral hemorrhage) or injuries of the spinal cord. Tumors may produce the same symptoms as hemorrhages. Both may produce temporary or permanent paralysis depending on their locations in the central nervous system, on their size, and ultimately on whether the hemorrhage is absorbed, whether it has destroyed areas of the brain, or whether tumors can be removed or irradiated (see Chapter 44). Surgery to prevent or arrest hemorrhage is increasingly common, and with improved techniques, is more and more effective.* Brain pathology may be accompanied by disturbances of consciousness and orientation. These are discussed in Chapter 40. The nursing care of an unconscious or disoriented person poses different problems from those in nursing the inactive or immobile, although one person may present both types of problems. Loss of consciousness or marked disorientation makes activity impossible in one

* The much-discussed return to the stage of Patricia Neal, a well-known actress, who had surgery and skilled care following a stroke has given some needed publicity to the possibility of rehabilitating stroke victims. V. H.

case and hazardous in another, so such patients are of necessity cared for in bed or in a confined space. Such patients include anesthetized persons.

Until the development of the polio vaccine in 1954, poliomyelitis left many who contracted it either partially or totally paralyzed.[15] Other viral and bacterial infections of the brain and its covering may cause temporary paralysis.[15a] In the United States, a major cause of paralysis is neuromotor injuries, and accidents are a major cause of disability.[15b] Also, as a result of about 18 years of war in the twentieth century, many young men have become paraplegics and quadriplegics. Even outside hospitals it is not uncommon to see these people on crutches and in wheelchairs. A tremendous effort has been made to keep the paralyzed and partially paralyzed military victims in the stream of life through such provisions as motorized wheelchairs and specially constructed cars.

There are innumerable devices for reducing the isolation of immobilized or hypoactive people and for encouraging independence. Engineers and others at the American Telephone and Telegraph Company have worked with personnel of the Institute of Rehabilitation Medicine, New York University Medical Center, to construct instruments and equipment that further independence of the handi-

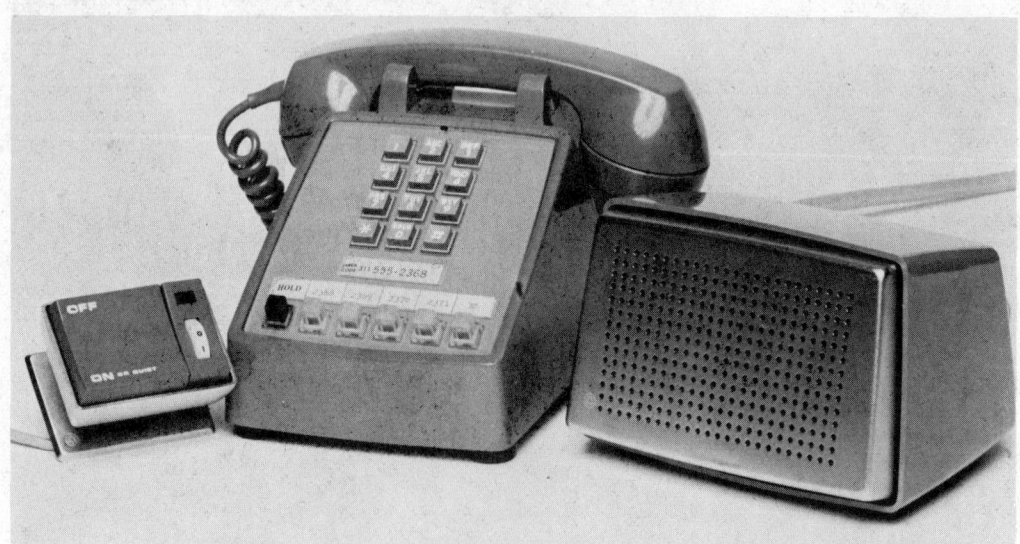

Figure 38-5. Speakerphone for persons with motor disability enables them to converse by pushing a button and without removing handset from cradle. (Photograph from American Telephone and Telegraph Company: *Telephone Services for the Motion Handicapped.* [Prepared with the cooperation of the Institute of Rehabilitation Medicine, New York University Medical Center.] The Company, New York, 1968, p. 128.)

capped. Figure 38-5 shows a Speakerphone that enables a person to converse by pushing a button without removing the handset from the cradle. Figure 38-6*A* and *B* shows persons with motor handicaps using a telephone where the handset is held with several types of "jacks."

Figure 38-7 shows a young man who, after suffering a broken neck in a driving accident, had paralyzed arms and legs. He is in a work area where, by shrugging his shoulder and using hand prostheses, he can operate the control stick of the motor-driven armchair. This enables him to use the Speakerphone, operate a tape recorder, and use a tape recorder.

Psychic trauma is another cause of hypoactivity or even paralysis, and effective treatment

A

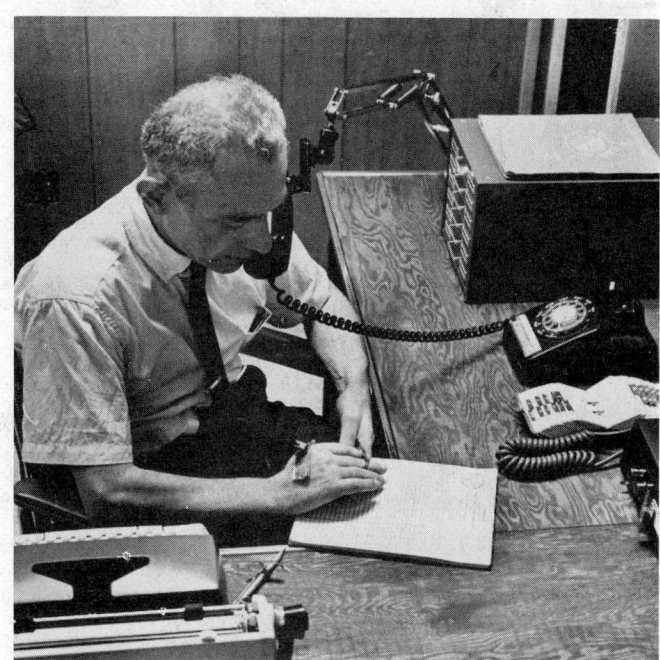

Figure 38-6. Persons with partial function in the hands. *A*. Man using a writing device and an extension arm that holds a standard handset. *B*. Woman with a "Wear-It-Or-Hold-It" handset. (Photographs from American Telephone and Telegraph Company: *Telephone Services for the Motion Handicapped*. [Prepared with the cooperation of the Institute of Rehabilitation Medicine, New York University Medical Center.] The Company, New York, 1968, pp. 18, 5.)

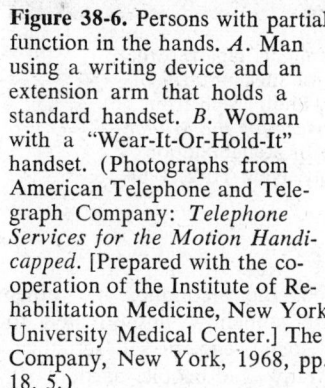

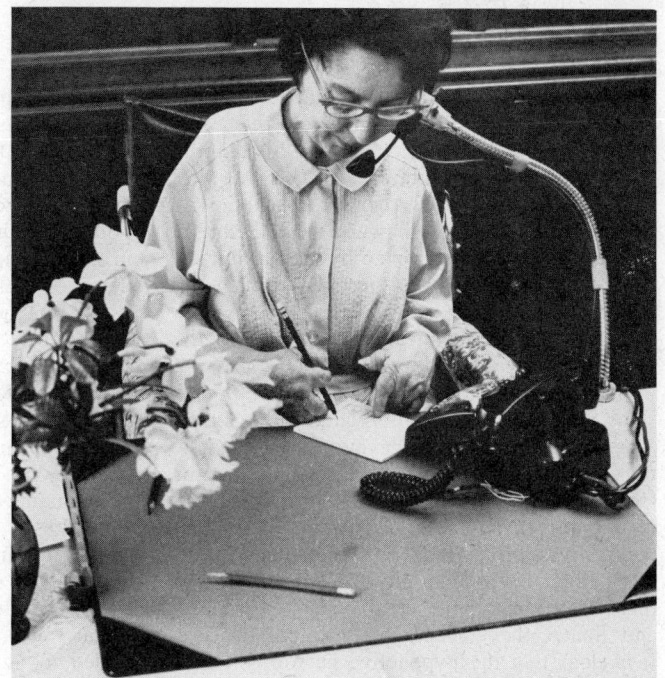

B

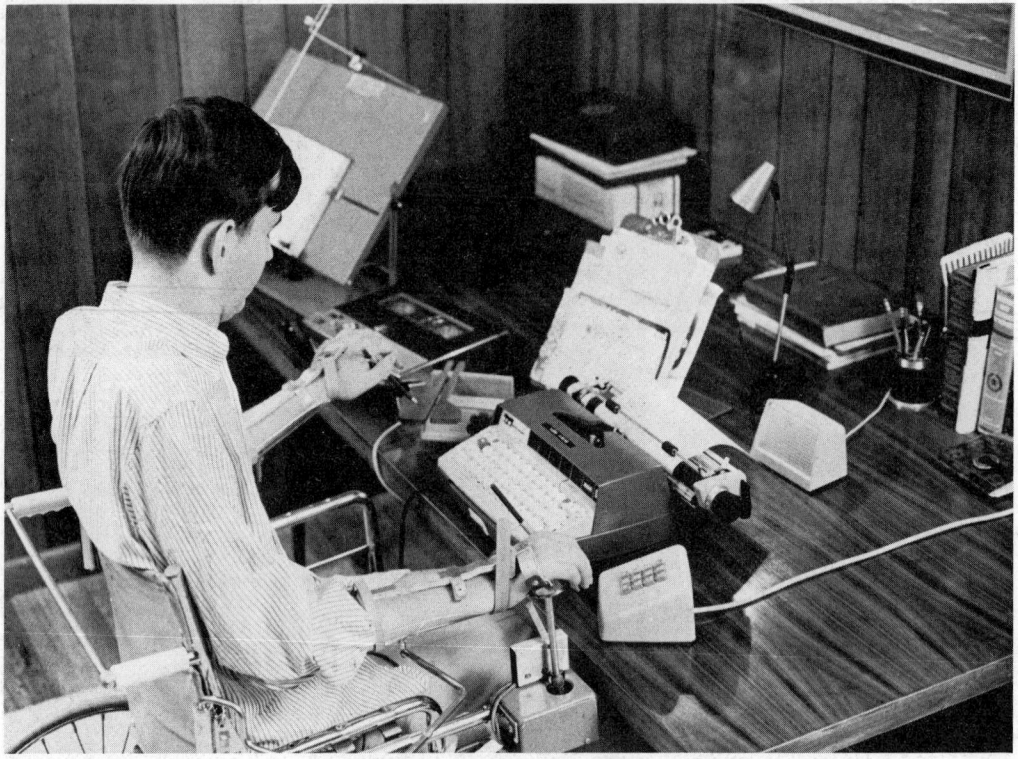

Figure 38-7. Working area with wheelchair, typewriter, speakerphone, tape recorder, and electric page turner, all operated by quadriplegic by control stick on arm of chair which he can move with shrugging motions of shoulder. (Photograph from American Telephone and Telegraph Company: *Telephone Services for the Motion Handicapped.* [Prepared with the cooperation of the Institute of Rehabilitation Medicine, New York University Medical Center.] The Company, New York, 1968, p. 15.)

usually depends on skillful psychiatric and supportive care. It is interesting to note that early in the 1900s S. Weir Mitchell,[16] a Philadelphia physician, was well known for his hospital where the victims of a "nervous breakdown" or "nervous prostration" were treated chiefly with bedrest, their care given by special nurses. This costly practice was accepted but never generally adopted, if for no other reason than because it was economically impossible for the average family.

Inactivity is often a person's choice; he or she is not stimulated or motivated to be active. Abraham Maslow[17] has developed a theory of motivation based on the premise that it stems from the urge to meet a successive hierarchy of human needs. Only when persons have met their physiologic needs can they proceed to meet their needs for physical safety. From there they meet their social needs, ego needs, and finally their needs for self-actualization. It is clear that the hypoactive person—including the depressed, the alcoholic, and other drug addicts—are somehow unmotivated to have either their social, ego, or self-actualization needs met. Many aged people, particularly in Western cultures, do not realize their full potential. The tendency to segregate the aged in retirement communities and nursing homes deprives them of their opportunity to remain useful, to love and be loved by their families and friends. Personnel who can and do show affection for patients go a long way toward making up for the loss of living with a family.

Through the use of alcohol and other drugs, numerous members of society in most countries try to make their lives pleasanter and more manageable. In the United States, with what Leslie Farber[18] calls an "addicted society," it is imperative that drugs be used more responsibly since irresponsible and excessive use has produced incalculable human suffering, social waste, apathy, and inactivity. Once addicted to any drug, including alcohol, people expend most of their energy in satisfying their physiologic craving for the drug; proceeding toward self-actualization is out of the question.*

Drugs, including alcohol, are used, generally, to alter consciousness—to relax and slow down, to get "high." The excessive use of drugs has been associated with rapidly changing and urbanized society, particularly in the United States. David Musto [19] writes about drug addiction as "The American Disease." Numerous social experiments on how to deal with the drug problem have been made and are in progress: prohibition, religious revivalism, and the provisions of treatment centers, to name a few. The answer, some believe, lies between motivation and meaningful activity, through programs such as those provided within Alcoholics Anonymous or Synanon, or vocational training and social revolution.

Malleson,[19a] a Canadian psychiatrist who was once a general practitioner in England, believes that physicians overuse drug therapy, but he thinks the public is also to blame because they expect, and have undue faith in, the prescribed drug. One chapter in his book *Need Your Doctor Be So Useless?* is on "Doctors for the Mind." He believes psychiatrists are especially prone to prescribe tranquilizers, opiates, hallucinogens, and antianxiety, antidepressant and stimulating drugs. He thinks they should instead help people accept and deal with anxiety, fear, and depression and feelings of dominance and inferiority as common, biologically useful, facts of life. He reviews the historical use of opiates and alcohol in the treatment of the "insane," their condemnation, the subsequent use of chloral and paraldehyde, the recent use of barbiturates and their current replacement by "the more expensive C.N.S. [central nervous system] depressant drugs. . . . Meprobamate (Miltown) was the first of these new drugs" † and this has been followed by a long list of addictive drugs. Malleson names 13 "trendy pharmaceutics," that most literate persons would recognize. He says:

Anxiety is unpleasant. Nobody likes it. The more effective a drug is at relieving it, the more it will be a drug of addiction. There can only be one safe drug for the treatment of anxiety: that is a drug that does not work. A brain chronically intoxicated with depressant drugs does not function well. By giving these drugs to patients who are already having difficulties in managing their lives doctors just add to their patients' problems. They are not being useful.*

People under the influence of depressant drugs are now found everywhere: in homes, at work, in schools, in nursing homes, in general hospitals, in specialized hospitals, and, of course, in psychiatric hospitals. Physical restraint and sedation with hydrotherapy have been replaced by chemical restraint, and hypoactivity is a symptom from which almost all these drug-users suffer. (See also Chapter 21 for a discussion of drug abuse.)

Malleson, building a case for the development of self-reliance in patients and the effectiveness of self-help, cites many studies that show the increase in mental illness and the dubious value of current psychiatric treatment. Malleson thinks that the old "insane asylum" surrounded by a farm may have at least offered inmates useful occupation and "nursing" personnel that were at least interested in and helpful in teaching patients a variety of indoor and outdoor skills. Through work—or activity—patients might have more easily achieved responsible behavior than under the present conditions of chemically induced hypoactivity. Currently, those who provide milieu therapy, or try to provide a therapeutic environment, recognize its importance and view work and other activity as instrumental in altering maladaptive behavior and strengthening ego functions.[19b]

Whether or not the reader is convinced by Malleson's carefully documented argument, few will deny that inactivity and dependence are initiated and fostered by many forms of treatment as well as by disease. Nurses have more opportunity than any other health workers to promote optimum activity and help patients achieve optimum rehabilitation. They should be particularly knowledgeable about the causes of hypoactivity and how they may be eliminated, especially the treatment-centered causes.

3. PHYSIOLOGIC AND PATHOLOGIC EFFECTS OF HYPOACTIVITY AND IMMOBILIZATION

In order to appreciate the various effects of immobility, one must realize that "use" of any organ is essential to its function, as Frederick J. Kottke [20] points out in discussing "deterioration of the bedfast patient." Because "disuse" of any organ decreases its efficiency,

---

* Andrew Malleson says " 'Psychiatric drugs can cause a lot of trouble." He shows a photograph of a gallon jar full of tablets and capsules that are "mostly hypnotics" which he says were collected within 10 days by a coroner investigating sudden deaths in North London. (*Need Your Doctor Be So Useless?* George Allen & Unwin, London, 1973, p. 136.)

† Malleson, Andrew: *op. cit.*, pp. 61, 62.

* *Ibid.*, p. 62.

it is important to evaluate the effects of immobilization on each part of the body. Kottke describes eight major types of deterioration in an immobile person: deterioration of motor ability, muscle strength, circulation, metabolic balance, skin condition, urinary tract function, respiration, and intellectual and emotional response.[21] Consequently, if a person were immobilized following a stroke or heart attack, much more than the paralyzed limb or the heart muscle would be put at "rest," and changes in all immobile organs would be expected. The issue in prescribing hypoactivity and immobilization as treatment for any illness or condition is one of balancing benefit and risk.

The last part of this chapter deals with care of the hypoactive or immobilized person. Some of the major physiologic and pathologic effects of immobility are pointed out, especially as they relate to nursing. These may include hypostatic pneumonia, thromboembolism, decubitus ulcers, contractures, osteoporosis, urinary retention and renal calculi, constipation, and numerous emotional difficulties. Asher [22] and Edith V. Olson and her associates [23] discuss these effects.

In medicine, there has probably been more research on the relation of activity to heart disease than to any other entity. The fact that people with some heart ailments were more comfortable sitting than lying led to early controversy over the relative merits of these postures. In 1928, Thomas Lewis,[24] a British physician, described a bedstead for use in treating cardiac patients suffering from congestive heart failure which was so designed that it could be converted into a chair. Thereafter, many physicians reported on the harmful effects of recumbency and the lowered mortality rate when cardiac patients were allowed some activity.[25,26] In 1959, Bessie L. Lendrum and her associates [27] reported that early return to activity had no ill effects on 360 children with rheumatic fever who had been followed for 2 years. Concurrently studies showed fewer complications for cardiac patients when specified periods of activity were allowed. Research on physiologic changes attributable to hypoactivity showed that all cardiac functions increase in supine subjects, well and sick, and that the recumbent position permits greater venous return and requires 74 per cent greater cardiac output than the sitting position.[28]

Since 1835, bedrest and immobilization of inflamed joints have been the major treatment for rheumatoid arthritis.[29] In 1971, J. A. Mills and associates [30] reported no significant differences in improvement of acute rheumatoid arthritis for patients randomly assigned to a group treated with 10 weeks of extensive bedrest and a group that encouraged ambulation as the patients desired. This study clearly illustrated the importance of questioning and testing the prescription of immobilization for many diseases in which bedrest has been the accepted "nonspecific" treatment.

Health workers are getting better acquainted with the dangers of bedrest, immobilization, and the maintenance of any position for an extended period. Articles and books now stress the positive value of group and individual exercise and of adult exercise programs for prone patients and for patients with limited motion.[31-33]

However, in stressing the harm that may result from inactivity, there is danger in seeming to condemn repose and other valuable states of mind and body associated with it. The importance of sleep and rest are discussed in Chapter 13 and the Eastern philosophies that teach relaxation and mind control are referred to in various chapters.

The physiologic effects of meditation add an important dimension to knowledge of relaxation, even immobility. Robert Wallace and Herbert Benson [34] discuss Transcendental Meditation as an efficient, easily learned way to control physiologic reactions to psychologic events. It is particularly promising as a method of preventing and treating such common problems as hypertension, central nervous system disorders, and anxiety. In a study of 36 volunteer subjects in the United States with an average of 2 to 3 years' experience in meditation, it is reported that there was reduced metabolic rate during meditation.[35] It was observed that the significant fall in blood-lactate level during meditation could have a beneficial psychologic effect since anxiety has been associated with high blood-lactate levels. Reduced oxygen consumption, carbon dioxide elimination, and rate and volume of respiration, along with the increase of alpha and theta waves during meditation, produce this "wakeful, hypometabolic" state. D. Bright and associates [36] say that Transcendental Meditation, based on introspection and nurturing individual identity, may be useful in counteracting the anxiety that prevails in technologic society.

4. PSYCHOLOGIC EFFECTS OF HYPOACTIVITY AND IMMOBILIZATION —SENSORY DEPRIVATION

In a general text it is impossible to examine closely the profound psychologic effects that inactivity and confinement of movement can have on a person of any age. For most, the idea of punishment is inextricably associated with restriction of movement. A child who has "misbehaved" is often separated from playmates and sent to his or her room or to bed. Youths and adults who break the law may be sent to corrective institutions (jails, prisons, or reformatories). In prison, solitary confinement (now euphemistically called "maximum protection") is the most severe punishment except death itself.[37] It does not seem farfetched, therefore, to say that many persons put to bed in the daytime, in some cases deprived of outdoor clothing, may wonder what they have done to deserve this fate; they almost certainly feel sorry for themselves and as if they had been plunged suddenly into a world that separates them from those dressed in street clothes, up and about, and free to do as they choose. The chasm between health and illness is almost proportionate to the degree of restriction the illness or disability puts on people's movements—on their freedom to do what they wish with whomever they choose.

A child in a spica cast, a burned or paralyzed person on a Stryker frame, or an inmate in solitary confinement experiences intense psychologic changes that should be understood by health workers and others who are trying to help them. A significant portion of people's response to any major change is affected by their experience and state of mind, but immobilization or confinement invariably produces feelings of isolation, dependency, and low self-esteem. Disabled or inactive persons are victims of countless fears of rejection and loss. Immobilization is a threat to their independence and authority. People who care for inactive persons recognize that depression and pessimism are natural reactions to loss of self-esteem. Quadriplegics, paraplegics, and others with major incapacitating illnesses frequently go through a period of denial and then anger before accepting their limitations. Carnevali and Brueckner[38] say that immobilized persons commonly respond with protest, despair, and detachment before they are able to participate in their rehabilitation. The process of adjustment varies for the individual, depending on his or her personality, social support, and the understanding and therapeutic skills of those giving care.

The psychologic response to confinement, whether in prison or on a Stryker frame, may be passive resignation and apathy, or it may be protest, agitation, increased anxiety, claustrophobia, or more severe neuroses. The more social isolation imposed by the hypoactivity and immobility, the more sensory deprivation experienced and the more profound its effects.

Hospitals necessarily impose some sensory deprivation. Patients in intensive care units may be overloaded with new sensations and actually kept from rest or sleep by the continuous activity and noise of machinery; they are, at the same time, deprived of the comfort of a familiar presence. Most hospitals, clinics, and nursing homes provide stark and unchanging environments. There is an increasing awareness of the psychic needs of immobile patients, particularly those who are monitored, their bodies invaded by tubes, subjected to confusing sensations, and deprived of adequate sleep. Attempts should be made to help patients understand their experiences and to constantly evaluate the meaning of the illness to them.[39] Linda R. Thompson, a nurse, gives the following description of her reactions as a patient on an intensive care unit where she experienced hallucinations, delusions, emotional lability, and frightening dreams in the course of her acute illness:

My first impression was of a huge ward, with me on a mattress of logs in a pit in one corner, away from everyone else. Actually, I was in a four-bed unit. The walls on my left and behind me were decorated with many cards and get-well wishes. To my right was a patient. The curtain between us was usually closed so that my view of the window was blocked. At the foot of my bed, the Kiil dialyzer and tank, a monstrous machine, obstructed my view of the rest of the room.*

Eugene Ziskind and his associates [40] studied the hypnagogic (drowsiness preceding sleep) symptoms of 88 patients who had bilateral eye-patching postoperatively. They described the components of these patients' sensory deprivation as visual and proprioceptive deprivation and social isolation. "Mental" symptoms were reported in 100 per cent of patients operated on for detached retina (whose eyes were patched longer) and 30 per cent of those operated on for cataracts. These symptoms included removing the patches from their eyes against advice, restlessness, perceptual distortion, mood changes, and thinking disturbances. There was a higher incidence of hemorrhage in those who had such mental symptoms. An important finding of the study was that disturbances were more common in persons who did not speak English, had a hearing deficit, a history of alcoholism, or antecedent organic brain damage.

Outside the hospital, particularly in convalescent, nursing, and rest homes, where the average patient is elderly, there is great sensory

* Thompson, Linda R.: "Sensory Deprivation: A Personal Experience," *Am. J. Nurs.,* **73:**266, (Feb.) 1973.

deprivation. Just as immobilization and less than optimal care produce the contractures, decubitus ulcers, and pneumonia that bring the elderly into the general hospital, the immobilization and sensory deprivation of the aged ill are often responsible for their disorientation and deterioration. When people who have been independently managing their own homes and daily activities are put into a nursing home or hospital, their self-image is drastically changed.[41] Dependency and loss of their usual social stimuli result in loneliness and hopelessness. Unable to identify these feelings, or perhaps unwilling to acknowledge them, patients may express loneliness and hopelessness by being demanding or irritable. Eventually, they become apathetic as mental and physical deterioration proceed, often at a rapid pace.

The US Department of Health, Education, and Welfare estimates that three-fourths of the noninstitutionalized population over 65 have one or more chronic conditions.[42] Almost half of these are hypoactive as a result. If any of these people are put to bed or go to a nursing home, certain consequences are almost inevitable. The elderly person with minimal problems of circulation or ambulation, if kept in bed for any ailment, becomes totally dependent and suffers the harmful effects of inactivity described in the preceding pages of this chapter. Besides loss of muscle strength and electrolytic imbalance, the elderly person in such institutions is often overtranquilized or sedated. They may be given an effusive, infantilizing type of sympathy that may anger them—or worse, lower their self-esteem. Malleson[42a] says "help can be lethal" and he refers to the "baby help" that fosters dependence and degrades the adult.

All people in nursing homes feel the effects of hypoactivity and sensory deprivation. There is little to stimulate them to be active. Dorothea Jaeger and Leo W. Simmons[42b] report a series of patient studies suggesting that nursing homes offer little opportunity for living normal lives and that their staffs have limited understanding of the elderly person's initial anger and frustration at being in a strange, lonesome environment. In attempting to satisfy their basic emotional needs, patients may "act out" their feelings to show that their needs are not being met.[43] Emotional, spirited expression, no matter how negative it seems, is an important ingredient of active involvement in the new situation. Without such involvement, the elderly in nursing homes tend to pass to a phase of resignation and apathy to protect themselves from forces they cannot control. This apathy further exaggerates the sensory

deprivation they feel and should be the most dreaded reaction to institutional life.

It is essential that the staff and family members and friends who visit those in nursing homes recognize the importance of activity and the maintenance of personal relationships in retaining the quality of life for the elderly. All nursing homes should offer work and recreational programs. Families and friends should be encouraged to visit patients and to take them away from the institution for outings overnight or for weekend visits, if feasible. One reason there is so much fear of the nursing home is that it is looked upon as a point of no return. Patients who believe they can resume a more normal life when they can take care of themselves have a different attitude toward a rehabilitative program from that of persons who expect to be institutionalized for life.

Alexander Leaf[43a] studied healthy, elderly people over the age of 100 in regions of Ecuador, Russia, and Kashmir. These centenarians said they believed that remaining active and having a feeling of continuity with their families who came after them were responsible for their longevity.

Many types of health workers, including nurses, have studied the causes and symptoms of sensory deprivation in the immobilized and hypoactive. Judith Chodil and Barbara Williams,[44] two nurses, are among those who believe that many of the psychologic problems associated with hypoactivity can be prevented and managed with skillful, enlightened, and attentive care.

5. CARE OF HYPOACTIVE OR IMMOBILIZED PATIENTS

Assessing the Patient's Needs. As has been said, hypoactivity may be prescribed as an aspect of the treatment of the disease or condition from which the patient is suffering, as, for example, myocardial infarction or rheumatoid arthritis; or one or more parts of the body may be immobilized to promote healing after an injury. The underlying reason for the patient's inactivity or immobility is important for patients, their families, and all health personnel caring for them to understand. Such understanding is essential in helping patients with rehabilitation or gaining optimum independence. Specific knowledge of their problems helps patients cooperate effectively with the health worker or family members caring for them. When patients know their strength and limitations, whether prescribed or a result of motor dysfunction, they are more likely to develop the necessary motivation to help plan and to actively participate in constructive programs. The time and effort required of the nurse to discuss patients' problems, help them identify and cope with their overriding anxieties, and elicit their active cooperation are well worthwhile. Listening, discussing, and explaining help to prevent further disability and to develop the feeling of self-worth that comes with a return to independence.

Since nurses are with patients for more hours than other health workers, they are usually able to find out why a person has slowed down, lost interest in normal activities, or even prefers to sit in a chair or stay in bed. For the same reason nurses are likely to know whether patients accept prescribed hypoactivity or immobilization; whether they understand the need for it; and whether they are making an adequate adjustment to the treatment. Effective care depends upon an accurate assessment of the cause of self-imposed hypoactivity and the person's response to prescribed hypoactivity and immobilization.

It is obviously impossible in a general work such as this to discuss the individual modifications in nursing care according to types of conditions or particular types of patients. In the following pages an effort is made to point out the more general problems of hypoactive and immobilized patients and to suggest some of the measures that have been found effective in helping people cope with reduced activity and immobilization. As in all aspects of nursing, the care of the patient is adapted to sex, chronologic and intellectual age, to his or her culture, life experience, habits and, of course, to the particular pathology from which the patient suffers.

Respiration. The immobile person can easily acquire a respiratory problem. Persons who do not move themselves, inhale deeply, or cough are not likely to expand their lungs adequately or remove the secretions from the respiratory passages. Efficient exchange of oxygen and carbon dioxide and full aeration of the lungs are essential in preventing bronchitis or hypostatic pneumonia. Hypoactive and immobile patients have decreased respiratory movements and decreased elimination of mucus from the respiratory tract. The stagnant mucus thickens, clogs the respiratory passages, and further decreases respiratory efficiency. Lower lobe pneumonia is a common hospital-acquired condition. It is often the result of injudicious use of sedation and restraint of patients; both reduce respiratory movements. If a bedridden patient seems uncomfortable or looks agitated he or she may be suffering from oxygen want. In any event, there is an underlying reason for

his or her discomfort. Taking the time to determine the reason and satisfy the patient's need prevents unnecessary sedation or restraint and subsequent respiratory difficulties.

To promote normal breathing, frequent changes in body position are important, whether the patient is sitting or lying flat. Patients should be taught deep breathing with prolonged expiration, and coughing to expel accumulated secretions. The nurse should note any sign of labored respiration and cyanosis and institute necessary treatment immediately. Not only teaching patients how to breathe deeply but seeing that they do is often necessary; also helping them to move into a different position at least hourly is essential. Hypoactive and immobile patients should be encouraged to undertake whatever self-care they can, for this is an excellent way to ensure lung expansion, ease of breathing, and the use of other muscles. Revolving beds and frames for the totally immobile are helpful (see Fig. 38-8); the patient's position can be changed with ease, and chest expansion is encouraged. Suctioning may be necessary if patients have an obstructed airway that they cannot clear by coughing. Some immobilized patients require oxygen administration. Serious respiratory disorders are discussed in Chapter 35 and inhalation therapy in Chapter 20.

Nutrition. Hypoactivity decreases the desire for food, and eating and drinking are difficult for the patient whose hands or arms are immobile. Persons who cannot manage to feed themselves feel dependent and inadequate; their self-esteem suffers. If patients are totally helpless, it is the nurse's or family's responsibility to feed them what they need and want in a manner that is unhurried and natural.[45] Those feeding immobile patients should be sure that food is hot, palatable, and cut into manageable portions. Taking extra care in the preparation and serving of food can minimize patients' anxiety about their disability and can help them get the necessary caloric and fluid intake. Feeding the sick, including the helpless, is also discussed in Chapter 10.

With paralyzed patients, it is important to check the swallowing reflex by giving them a teaspoon of water. If patients do not choke and they swallow the water without difficulty, they may be given fluids and solids as indicated by their nutritional needs. The position for eating or drinking is a sitting or semi-sitting one. If this is not possible and the patient must remain flat on the back, the neck should not be bent with a plump pillow. It is possible to drink in a side-lying position but obviously food tends to fall out of a spoon or off a fork with the patient in this position.

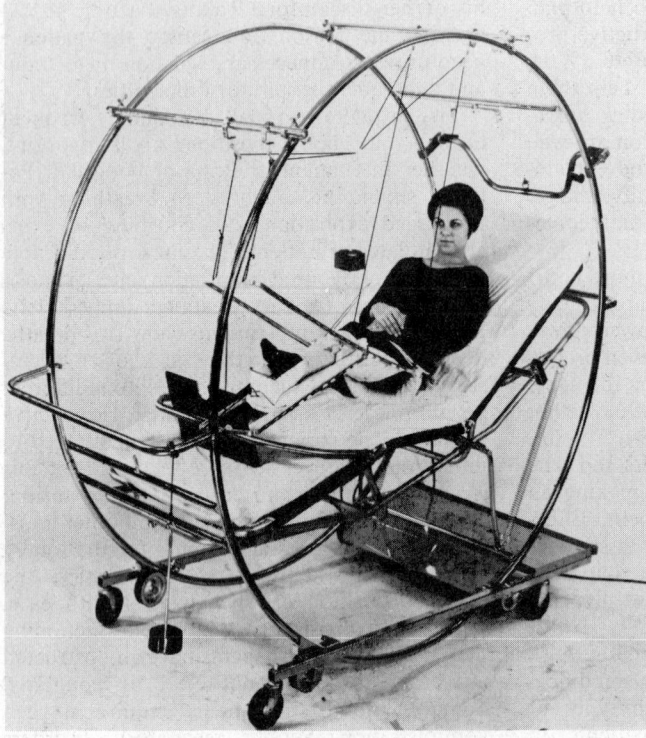

Figure 38-8. Revolving bed in upright sitting position. (CircOlectric bed, courtesy of Stryker Corp., Kalamazoo, Mich.)

Irene Beland[46] says, however, that the side-lying position is safer. She thinks choking more likely in the supine position and that it is hard to help people quickly enough if they aspirate food while lying on their backs. Patients who have use of their hands and arms can sit up in bed and eat their meals after the food is prepared so that it is easy to manage. Hemiplegic patients may have defective vision in a part of their visual field (hemianopsia).[47] When eating, they may take only a small portion of that served because they cannot see the remaining food on the plate. Simply rotating the plate so that the food is in their visual field will demonstrate whether or not the food is left uneaten intentionally. Any inactive patients may suffer from loss of appetite (anorexia) because of a negative nitrogen balance produced by accelerated catabolic activity.[48,49] It is important to explain the cause of the anorexia to the patient in understandable terms; it may help him or her to take more frequent and smaller meals. Favorite foods are most readily eaten but appetites of the hypoactive are capricious.

A high-protein diet is frequently prescribed for the immobile patient, especially one who is paralyzed and prone to pressure sores.[50] Donald Griffith,[51] writing in *Aerospace Medicine*, says that there is some evidence that a 1-gm sodium diet in combination with a diuretic decreases immobilization hypercalciuria. Also,

since immobilization results in a decrease in bone tissue (osteoporosis), it is important that the patient receive adequate amounts of vitamin C, since deficiency of vitamin C hinders bone formation.

In any institution, the immobile and inactive should be helped and encouraged to eat in communal dining areas. With appropriate teaching about dietary needs of the patient, families can be encouraged to bring in especially liked foods, even prepare them in designated cooking areas. In some countries a member of a family stays in the hospital and prepares the patient's food. Elizabeth Barnes, reporting a study of "people in hospital," says:

. . . in communities where family life is powerful and closely-knit, hospitals find they cannot keep relatives away however much they may wish to. The relatives insist on coming into hospital with the patient and would never dream of leaving him alone. They provide all his food, attend to his bodily needs and, in some cases, one of them sleeps under his bed at night.*

Chapters 22 and 23 discuss parenteral and tube feedings. Hypoactive and immobile patients may require such measures, but if the

* Barnes, Elizabeth: *People in Hospital.* (A study in nine countries conducted under the sponsorship of the International Council of Nurses, the International Hospital Federation, and the World Federation of Mental Health.) Macmillan & Co., Ltd., London, 1961, p. 123.

swallowing reflex is present, they should not be necessary. It may take considerable ingenuity to motivate and help a depressed, paralyzed, or hysterically frightened person to eat, but this is an important function of the nurse. Serving small, manageable portions of food is desirable so that the patients aren't frustrated by the amount and the waste that results if they don't eat. Whether or not patients are helpless, it is often a good thing to stay with them to encourage their eating and to reinforce the progress they make in feeding themselves. Members of the family or good friends who come at mealtimes may make them pleasanter occasions.

Elimination. Inactivity is a major cause of faulty elimination. The auxiliary muscles of defecation lose tone or atrophy with immobility. The greater the restriction of movement, the more difficult it is for patients to respond to the defecation reflex in their accustomed manner. For patients who cannot assume a sitting posture, defecation is especially difficult. Emptying the bladder while lying down is hard for many persons and emptying the rectum even more difficult. Eating fruits and vegetables and using fecal-softening agents are helpful. Routine exercises should include those that strengthen abdominal muscles. The usual time of defecation in health offers a clue to the schedule that should be followed when the person is immobile. However, if daily bowel movements do not occur the patient should be helped to understand that less frequent bowel movements are usual with inactivity and reduced food intake. It is increasingly thought that patients should use the commode or the toilet rather than the bedpan if either is possible.[52,53] There is less straining, energy expenditure, and anxiety when the patient uses a commode or the toilet. If a patient is on an electric Stryker frame, a bedpan is fitted in place without lifting him or her.

Immobilized patients should be catheterized only if it is essential. Many patients, especially after a stroke, lose bladder control only temporarily, so catheterization should never be a routine measure for incontinence alone. Helen Large and her associates,[54] describing care in "the first stroke intensive care unit," say that catheterization, with the almost inevitable consequence of chronic cystitis, is avoided. The use of an indwelling catheter also necessitates bladder retraining, as noted by Paul B. Beeson[55] writing on "The Case Against the Catheter." For further discussion of the dangers of catheterization, see Chapter 24.

Few patients cannot move themselves or help nursing personnel who are turning or lifting them. An overhead trapeze (see Fig. 38-9) which the patient can grasp enables

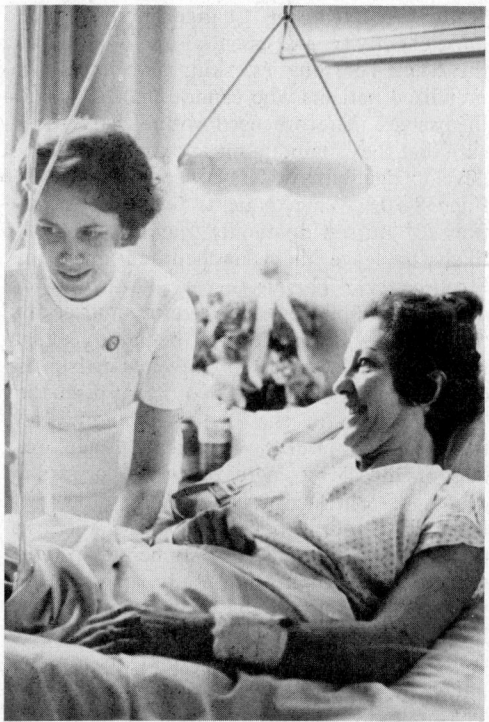

Figure 38-9. Overhead bar is an asset for patients who can use one or both arms in turning, pulling themselves up in bed or into a sitting posture. (Courtesy of Loyola University Medical Center, Maywood, Ill. Bev Montgomery, Photographer.)

many patients who could not otherwise do so to sit up in bed, to move toward the head of the bed, or to change their position in a variety of ways.

Genrose Alfano, nurse director of Loeb Center for Nursing and Rehabilitation, writes "There are no routine patients. Adaptation to the aging process results in diminished capacity; for some it results in chronic illness. But it need not result in helplessness." * She describes the "independence with support" supplied by the highly individualized program of care in the Center.

For patients whose hypoactivity makes them subject to bedsores, a water mattress may be provided to equalize pressure. The "Aquapedic" mattresses and chair pads are good examples. An inside balloon holds the water; a heavy vinyl outer covering resists pin punctures. The head of the mattress is solid foam rubber which keeps the occupant from feeling a floating sensation.†

* Alfano, Genrose J.: "There Are No Routine Patients" *Am. J. Nurs.*, **75:**1804, (Oct.) 1975.
† Available from Scientific Management Association, Summit, N.J.

Moving, Exercising. Changes in position and muscle activity are essential for maintaining the health of muscles, skin, and joints. Immobilized patients who cannot change position themselves therefore need special care to ensure that they maintain muscle tone and do not develop decubitus ulcers or contractures (see Fig. 38-10). When patients feel sick and depressed, nurses or family members are too likely to leave them undisturbed until they "feel better." This is a very hazardous decision. Immobile patients require muscle and joint activity from the very beginning of immobilization in order to prevent further discomfort and disability. Kottke,[56] discussing "Deterioration of the Bedfast Patient," says that when a muscle is kept at complete rest, loss of muscle strength occurs at a rate of 10 to 15 per cent per week of inactivity. Immobility fosters bone destruction and osteoporosis. Patients may not cooperate in doing range-of-motion exercises daily at prescribed periods, especially if they are trying to deny incapacitation. In such cases, the nurse's careful explanation and allowing patients to ventilate their anger or frustration are important.

To avoid pressure sores, patients in bed and unable to turn themselves should be turned hourly, although some nurses writing on the subject may say that such frequent turning is unnecessary.[57,58] During the morning bath and thereafter when the nurse comes to turn the patient or give him or her other kinds of care, the extremities should be put through the range-of-motion exercises. The gentle insistence of the nurse may be necessary. If there is pain, a mild analgesic given before muscle and joint movement may be helpful. Hemiplegic patients can be taught to exercise their affected side using the unaffected arm. If given this responsibility and encouragement, they will probably take pride in exercising diligently and efficiently. The benefits of continued passive and active exercise cannot be overestimated in preventing more severe disability, and the activity should be increased as rapidly as the patient's condition allows.

Turning sheets and lifting devices can be used with completely immobilized persons. "Sheet burns" and continuous pressure on bony prominences causing inflamed or ulcerated areas of the skin must be avoided. If patients are transferred to a wheelchair or stretcher, they can go or be taken to another room. The benefits of movement, exercise, and changing position are then augmented by the pleasure of being in a different environment. Figure 38-10 shows a lifting device that also transports a patient. It can be converted from a stretcher into a chair and a commode.

Exercise for the bedfast patient helps prevent venous stasis, thrombosis, and emboli.[59] Exercise serves the same purpose for the weightless astronaut in space. When hypoactivity is self-imposed, the relationship of mood to activity is clear, and it is necessary to deal with the emotional basis of the inactivity whether it is depression, addiction, or the social isolation of the aged. Newly institutionalized patients may refuse to move because they do not understand the new environment and they may feel insecure. For the chronic inactive patient, behavior modification has been used successfully to reinforce and encourage participation of once-helpless people in their activities of daily living. (For further discussion of exercise, see Chapters 8 and 14.) As mentioned in Chapter 14, it is desirable to provide all patients with a movable chair, one in which by push buttons or levers they can change their position from an erect to a reclining position with support for the legs. Figure 38-10A, B, C shows a stretcher that can be converted into a wheelchair. Use of the "Stretchair" would simplify transporting a helpless patient or taking them into another room or outdoors for a refreshing change of scene. Figure 38-11 shows a bed that can be converted into a chair and a commode that can replace a mattress section for bedfast patients who cannot get to the bathroom. The company making this bed-chair offers commodes and armchairs equipped with a motorized device that pushes the person who has trouble getting up and down into a standing position. Other moving and lifting devices are shown in Chapters 12 and 14.

Rest and Sleep. Hypoactive and immobilized patients lie on the back or side according to habit, but patients in casts may suffer acutely from being forced to lie in positions not habitual to them. They may sleep during the day because they are bored, depressed, or anxious. Sleep is a retreat from a reality they'd like to forget. Nights can be restless, empty hours. Changing the patients' positions and helping or encouraging them to sit up in bed or a chair if at all possible provide exercise and give patients a change that relieves boredom. While sitting, patients can play a game, read, or do some handwork. Since patients have been involved in making plans of care, they can look forward to the periods when they will be turned, helped to sit up, get out of bed, or participate in some activity. If their day is spent in activities interspersed with needed rest periods, patients sleep better at night. Companionship and recreation help decrease the tension and anxiety so frequently seen in people who are either hypoactive or immobile. The difficulty of sleeping in a prescribed posi-

A

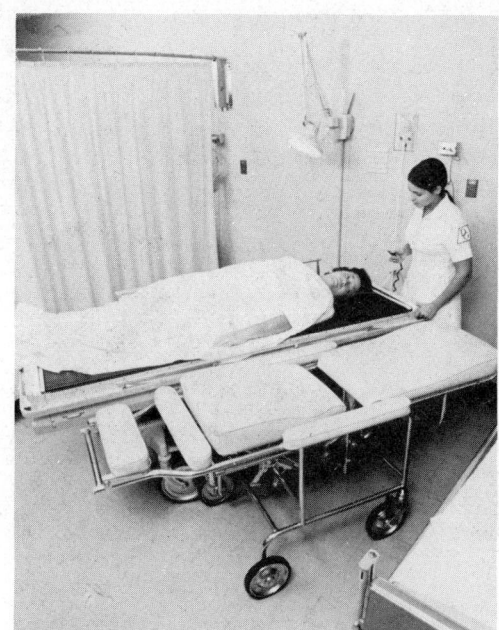

B

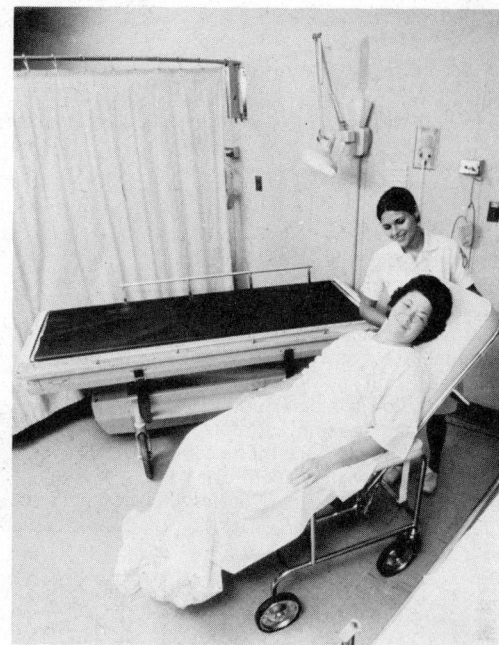

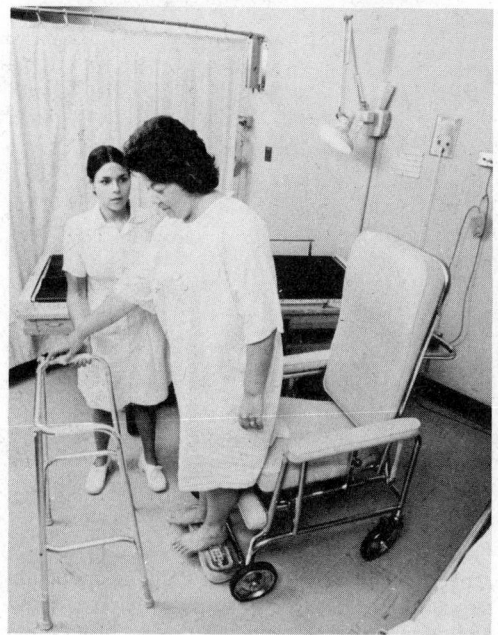

C

Figure 38-10. "Stretchair"—chair that can be converted into a stretcher, and vice versa, is helpful in transporting patients but also simplifies changing the position of a hypoactive person. (Courtesy of Mobilizer Medical Products, Inc., Summit, N.J.)

tion when in traction or a cast is described in Chapter 31.

Hypoactivity is closely associated with depression. Ernest L. Hartmann, discussing research on sleep and his conclusions on the function of sleep, says:

Depression is more complicated [than mania]. The textbook picture of a severely depressed patient involves disturbed and reduced sleep. Indeed, sleep laboratory studies of hospitalized depressed patients have generally found low total sleep, especially low SWS [synchronized-sleeping, waking, sleeping], and many awakenings—in other words, very poor sleep. Results on D-time [desynchronized or dreaming sleep or Rapid Eye Movement, or REM] have been mixed. I have found hypersomnia in most neurotic or mild de-

A

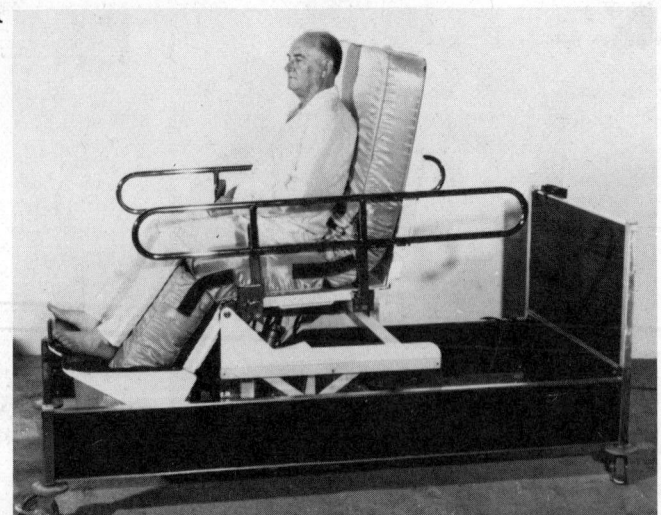

Figure 38-11. A bed that simplifies the care of a helpless patient in a hospital or at home. By pushing a button the patient can be put into a sitting (*A*) or standing (*B*) position. With the occupant in a lying position a section of the mattress can be removed, replaced with a commode, and the bed adjusted so that the patient can sit on the commode (*C*). (Courtesy of Burke, Inc., Mission, Kans.)

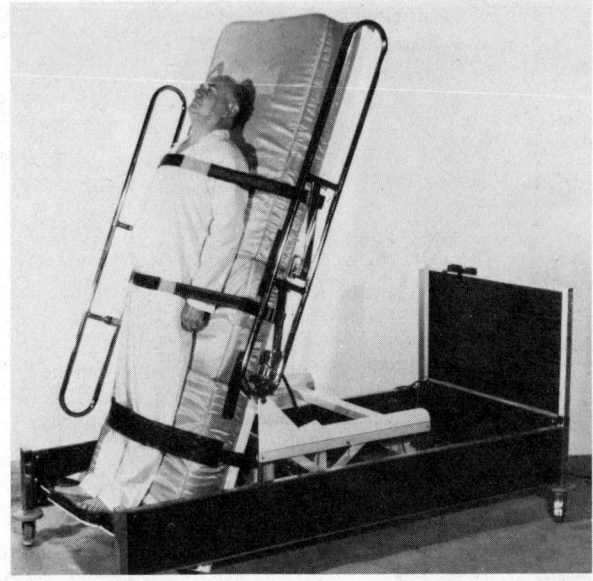

B

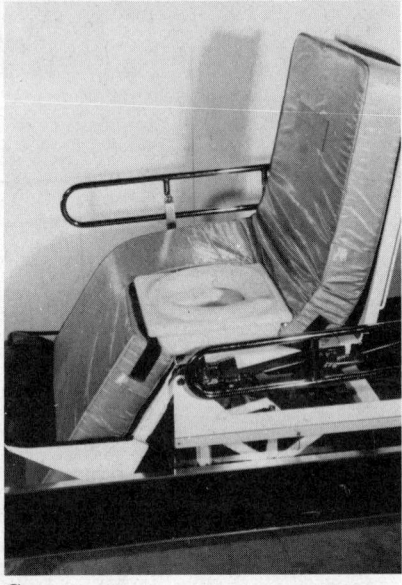

C

pressions. . . . My conclusion is that depression is usually characterized by a tendency toward requirement for more sleep and more D-time. . . .*

According to Hartmann and other authorities, a normal night's sleep includes both S and D sleep. Exercise, with attendant physical fatigue, induces S sleep. Without exercise, it is hard to achieve balance, and drugs may still further disturb the normal sleep pattern. There are few

* Hartmann, Ernest L.: *The Functions of Sleep.* Yale University Press, New Haven, Conn., 1973, p. 91.

aspects of nursing care that demand more understanding and creativity than helping hypoactive and immobilized persons to order their lives in such a way as to promote healthy rest and sleep.

Keeping Clean and Well Groomed. Dressing and Undressing. Protecting the Skin. Many hypoactive patients lose interest in appearance, grooming, and cleanliness; immobilized patients have difficulty both in keeping clean and in dressing. Since a goal of nursing care stressed throughout this book is to help individuals care for themselves, there should be little need to discuss bathing or dressing here.

It might be assumed that patients will be helped to maintain or acquire optimum independence. However, the immobile patient, whether paralyzed or in a cast, needs encouragement and teaching and at first may need considerable help. It is very easy for nurses to forget the goal of self-care and do the bathing and dressing for patients, especially if patients are frustrated or angry over their disabilities. But even when patients are very weak they can wash their own faces if nurses or family members wring out the washcloth for them. However small or time consuming the effort, it helps patients to feel some degree of ability and independence if they perform any part of their daily care.

Special attention should be paid to cleaning the mouth of helpless people to help prevent deterioration of gums and subsequent loss of teeth. An electric toothbrush may be useful. All too frequently, elderly people in the hospital or in a nursing home are given inadequate mouth care, particularly if they are thought of as "difficult." Actually, the elderly need especially good mouth care since they are likely to have dentures and often have low resistance to infection. It is imperative that those giving care to the inactive patient realize the rapidity of tooth and gum destruction if the mouth is not cleaned and rinsed regularly. Proud persons are reluctant to ask nurses, family members, or friends to brush their teeth or clean their dentures, so it is up to the skillful, attentive nurse or family member to assume this responsibility when patients are not able to perform these tasks themselves.

There are devices to help paralyzed people dress themselves. Chapter 12 includes a discussion of various rehabilitation procedures and shows that the hemiplegic can learn to dress and undress. The partially paralyzed person learns to use the unaffected arm to dress the affected side first. Clothing should be easy to put on and remove, and it is important to have the person in a secure position so that falling can be avoided and frustration reduced to a minimum.

Immobilizing devices may make modification in clothing necessary. For example, a leg with a cast on it needs a special sock to keep the exposed foot warm; a protective boot is useful for a walking cast. Patients on a Stryker frame should have gowns that open in the back to facilitate frequent back care and use of the bedpan. (See also Chapter 34 for a discussion of such questions.)

The prevention of pressure sores is discussed in Chapter 30. Some authorities maintain that with sufficient care, pressure sores can be prevented; others say that immobilized patients may develop decubitus ulcers when every known means is used to prevent them. Rosalie Pratt [60] says these measures include a high protein diet, adequate vitamin intake, good skin care, frequent turning, and rapid attention to and relief of pressure from any reddened area that does not fade in one hour.

Families should be encouraged to help hypoactive and immobilized persons dress in daytime clothing to keep them living as normal a life as possible. The act of dressing gives muscles needed exercise. An unkempt and careless appearance may be a result of depression. In these cases it takes considerable nursing skill to keep the patients looking well while helping them deal with their underlying hopelessness and despair.

Protection from Danger. Immobile patients require special protection from hazards in the environment since they are physically unable to remove themselves from danger. It is of major importance that they know they will not be harmed or deserted. They feel defenseless and they must trust those responsible for their care. Anxious patients may constantly call for a nurse or family member just to assure themselves that they are cared for—both physically and emotionally. It is especially important to realize that hemiplegia may be characterized by irresponsible behavior. Joan Birchenall and her associates [61] say that confusion and disorientation are particularly frequent when the left side is affected. The usual precautions are necessary. Bed rails give patients a secure bar to hold so that they can move from side to side when they wish if they have the strength. Rails undoubtedly prevent some falls but the disoriented can climb over them and have a more serious fall. Some patients detest bed rails. They may offer security and independence to one person but represent infantile restriction to another. Bed rails should be used on the bed of hypoactive and immobilized persons after careful assessment of personal preference and safety factors.

Work, Occupation, Recreation. Reeducation is a fundamental need of hypoactive or immobile persons if they are to be rehabilitated (see Chapter 8). In self-imposed hypoactivity, people lack purpose; in prescribed hypoactivity, they lack alternatives to their usual work and recreation. Immobilized people may have to learn many new skills before they acquire any measure of independence. The nurse can work with other members of the health team to help patients with reeducation. In hospitals, visiting nurse agencies, and rehabilitation facilities, specialists in physical therapy, occupational therapy, vocational counseling, and other specialties are available to evaluate people's strengths and weaknesses, or assets and liabilities, and help patients find appropriate work and recreation.

Activities that involve friends and family should be encouraged. A family can prepare a favorite meal to be eaten with the patient. Entertainment and outings can be planned. In the home the family plays the major role in seeing that the quality of life of the immobile or inactive family member is good or constructive. Calendars help a person keep track of the passing of time; events and accomplishments can be noted on them. Clocks, newspapers, and judicious use of radios and television all help to orient hypoactive and immobilized persons and fill their time with purposeful and pleasurable activity.

It is difficult for the handicapped to find employment, particularly when there are high unemployment rates. Certain industries make an effort to recruit workers who have certain disabilities. War veterans with motor handicaps have received special attention because of the difficulty they find getting employment. Vocational training is essential and should be offered by all rehabilitation agencies.

Communication, Human Relations. There are many types of communication difficulties that hypoactive or immobile persons must overcome. Those with self-imposed hypoactivity are usually depressed, anxious, or fearful, and burdened by lowered self-esteem. They may be withdrawn and even resort to mutism. Nurses and other health workers skilled in communication can give them a sense of reality. The importance of listening cannot be overstressed. Also, the acceptance of silence without anxiety or inappropriate interruption is important.

Inactive or incapacitated people are often treated in an infantile, patronizing manner. Earlier reference was made to what Malleson calls "baby help," which he thinks fosters regression and irresponsibility. Nurses frequently call older patients by their first names with the justification that it is what the patient prefers. In many instances, the patient's preference has not been elicited, and he or she is talked to and treated as a child. While humor and warmth are important in communication, they should not be used at the expense of respect for the patient.

It should always be assumed that a motionless, unresponsive person can hear, since the ability to hear is said to be retained longer than any other sense. Speaking to those who can't or don't want to respond is a skill that requires special patience and understanding. Nurses and family members should be helped and encouraged to develop this skill. Aphasic persons present a somewhat similar problem in that they are unable to respond verbally or answer questions correctly. In some cases communication must take place on a nonverbal level, and gestures become very meaningful. Madeline J. Fox [62] discusses talking with patients who can't answer. She suggests a number of exercises that can help aphasic patients as they slowly regain their ability to talk. It is important to speak in simple and direct sentences to the patient, always looking for signs of understanding or confusion. A useful exercise is to have patients complete sentences or find the missing word for common phrases. Hemiplegic patients may have perceptual as well as speech deficits.[63] Difficulty in seeing things as others see them can be very frustrating. Here, as in all relearning, efforts should be made to involve patients in rehabilitation from the beginning of the illness so that they can see their progress. D. A. Foster [64] describes handwriting exercises for those with motor disturbances that help improve communication and physical rehabilitation. Therapists can prescribe special programs which visiting nurses and family members can help patients to follow. Essential manual skills such as dialing the telephone or turning the television on and off have to be relearned. Patients need encouragement to master those tasks that allow them to communicate with others.

Physical, occupational, and speech therapists and vocational guidance counselors are available in large rehabilitation centers, but nurses in many situations must give patients help that specialists would give were they available.

Worship. It is important to make it possible for people to maintain their customary religious interests and practices. Inactive or immobilized persons will require special help either in getting transportation to a religious service or in arranging for the religious rites to be brought to them. In many communities there are agencies such as the Red Cross or FISH, that provide transportation. Many health institutions have on their staff full-time or part-time religious advisers. When they do not, nurses can take the initiative in finding out whether patients would like to see their ministers, priests, rabbis, or other religious representative. Nurses may talk with such representatives or communicate through families or social workers. Hospitals, nursing homes, and other institutions may have religious services or take patients to services in the community. Radio and television programs and books can, in many cases, supply religious and spiritual needs.

REFERENCES

1. Carnevali, Doris, and Brueckner, Susan: "Immobilization—Reassessment of a Concept," *Am. J. Nurs.*, **70**:1502, (July) 1970.
2. Asher, R. A. J.: "The Dangers of Going to Bed," *Br. Med. J.*, **2**:967, (Dec. 13) 1947.
3. Chalmers, Thomas C.: "Rest and Exercise in Hepatitis," *N. Engl. J. Med.*, **281**:1421, (Dec. 18) 1969.
4. Repsher, L. H., et al.: "Effects of Early and Vigorous Exercise in Recovery from Infectious Hepatitis," *N. Engl. J. Med.*, **281**: 1393, (Dec. 18) 1969.
5. Browse, Norman L.: *The Physiology and Pathology of Bed Rest.* Charles C Thomas, Publisher, Springfield, Ill., 1965.
6. Asher, R. A. J.: *op. cit.*
7. *Ibid.*
8. Dock, William: "The Undesirable Effects of Bedrest," *Surg. Clin. North Am.*, **25**:437, (Apr.) 1945.
9. Duke, Martin: "Bedrest in Acute MI. A Study of Physician Practices," *Am. Heart J.*, **82**:486, (Oct.) 1971.
10. Harper, Jane E., et al.: "Controlled Trial of Early Mobilization and Discharge from Hospital in Uncomplicated Myocardial Infarction," *Lancet*, **2**:1331, (Dec. 18) 1971.
11. Boyle, D. C., et al.: "Early Mobilization and Discharge of Patients with Acute Myocardial Infarction," *Lancet*, **2**:57, (July 8) 1972.
12. Chalmers, Thomas C.: *op. cit.*
13. Repsher, L. H., et al.: *op. cit.*
14. Gardner, Lytt I.: "Deprivation Dwarfism," *Sci. Am.* **227**:76, (July) 1972.
15. Sabin, A. D.: "Commentary on Report on Oral Poliomyelitis Vaccines," *J.A.M.A.*, **190**: 52, (Oct. 5) 1964.
15a. Shafer, Kathleen N., et al.: *Medical-Surgical Nursing*, 6th ed. C. V. Mosby Co., St. Louis, 1975, p. 899.
15b. "Impairments Due to Injury, U.S., 1971," in *Vital and Health Statistics. Data from the National Health Survey.* US Department of Health, Education, and Welfare, Washington, D.C., 1971, p. 20 (Series 10, no. 87).
16. Mitchell, S. Weir: *Fat and Blood: An Essay on the Treatment of Certain Forms of Neurasthenia and Hysteria.* J. B. Lippincott Co., Philadelphia, 1911, p. 57.
17. Maslow, Abraham: *Motivation and Personality.* Harper & Row, New York, 1970.
18. Farber, Leslie: "Ours Is the Addicted Society," in Matheson, Douglas, and Dairson, Meridin (eds.): *The Behavioral Effects of Drugs.* Holt, Rinehart & Winston, New York, 1970, p. 18.
19. Musto, David: *The American Disease.* Yale University Press, New Haven, Conn., 1973.
19a. Malleson, Andrew: *Need Your Doctor Be So Useless?* George Allen & Unwin, Ltd., London, 1973.
19b. Robinson, Lisa: *Psychiatric Nursing as a Human Experience.* W. B. Saunders Co., Philadelphia, 1972, p. 236.

20. Kottke, Frederick J.: "Deterioration of the Bedfast Patient," *Public Health Rep.*, **80**: 437, (May) 1965.
21. *Ibid.*
22. Asher, R. A. J.: *op. cit.*
23. Olson, Edith V., et al.: "The Hazards of Immobility," *Am. J. Nurs.*, **67**:779, (Apr.) 1967.
24. Lewis, Thomas: "Bedstead for Use in Treating Cardiac Patients Suffering from Congestive Failure," *Br. Med. J.*, **2**:977, (Dec. 1) 1928.
25. Levine, Samuel A.: "Some Harmful Effects of Recumbency in the Treatment of Heart Disease," *J.A.M.A.*, **126**:80, (Sept. 9) 1944.
26. Beckworth, Julian, et al.: "The Management of Myocardial Infarction with Particular Reference to the Chair Treatment," *Ann. Intern. Med.*, **41**:1189, (Dec.) 1954.
27. Lendrum, Bessie L., et al.: "Relation of Bedrest in Acute Rheumatic Fever to Heart Disease Present Two to Fourteen Years Later," *Pediatrics*, **24**:389, (Sept.) 1959.
28. Rosenbaum, F. F., and Belknap, E. L.: *Work and the Heart.* Paul B. Hoeber, Inc., New York, 1959.
29. "Immobilization and Bedrest in Rheumatoid Arthritis" (editorial), *Lancet*, **1**:1281, (June 19) 1971.
30. Mills, J. A., et al.: "Value of Bed Rest in Patients with Rheumatoid Arthritis," *N. Engl. J. Med.*, **284**:453, (Mar. 4) 1971.
31. Cureton, Thomas K.: *The Physiological Effects of Exercise Programs on Adults.* Charles C Thomas, Publisher, Springfield, Ill., 1969.
32. Etter, Mildred F.: *Exercise for the Prone Patient.* Wayne State University Press, Detroit, 1968.
33. Griffin, Winnie, et al.: "Group Exercise for Patients with Limited Motion," *Am. J. Nurs.*, **71**:1742, (Sept.) 1971.
34. Wallace, Robert, and Benson, Herbert: "The Physiology of Meditation," *Sci. Am.*, **226**:85, (Feb.) 1972.
35. *Ibid.*
36. Bright, D., et al.: "What School Physicians, Nurses, and Health Educators Should Know About Transcendental Meditation," *J. Sch. Health*, **43**:192, (Mar.) 1973.
37. Mitford, Jessica: *Kind and Usual Punishment.* Alfred A. Knopf, New York, 1973.
38. Carnevali, Doris, and Brueckner, Susan: *op. cit.*
39. Worrell, Judith D.: "Nursing Implications in the Care of the Patient Experiencing Sensory Deprivation," in Kintzel, Kay C. (ed.): *Advanced Concepts in Clinical Nursing.* J. B. Lippincott Co., Philadelphia, 1971, p. 137.
40. Ziskind, Eugene, et al.: "Observations on Mental Symptoms in Eye Patched Patients: Hypnagogic Symptoms in Sensory Deprivation," *Am. J. Psychiatry*, **116**:893, (Apr.) 1960.
41. Carnevali, Doris, and Brueckner, Susan: *op. cit.*

42. *Working with Older People: A Guide to Practice.* US Public Health Service, Rockville, Md., 1971, p. 1.

42a. Malleson, Andrew: *op. cit.,* p. 115.

42b. Jaeger, Dorothea, and Simmons, Leo W.: *The Aged Ill. Coping with Problems in Geriatric Care.* Appleton-Century-Crofts, New York, 1970.

43. Hulicka, Irene M.: "Fostering Self-Respect in Aged Patients," *Am. J. Nurs.,* **64:**83, (Mar.) 1964.

43a. Leaf, Alexander: "Search for the Oldest People," *Nat. Geographic Mag.,* **143:**98, (Jan.) 1973.

44. Chodil, Judith, and Williams, Barbara: "The Concept of Sensory Deprivation," *Nurs. Clin. North Am.,* **5:**453, (Sept.) 1970.

45. Cornelison, Sophia: "Guidelines to Feeding the Helpless Patient," *J. Psychiatr. Nurs.,* **2:** 184, (Mar.–Apr.) 1964.

46. Beland, Irene, and Passos, Joyce: *Clinical Nursing: Pathophysiological and Psychosocial Approaches,* 3rd ed. Macmillan Publishing Co., Inc., New York, 1975.

47. Birchenall, Joan, and Streight, Mary E.: *Care of the Older Adult.* J. B. Lippincott Co., Philadelphia, 1973, p. 162.

48. Olson, Edith, and McCarthy, Joyce A.: "Immobility—Effects on Gastrointestinal Function," *Am. J. Nurs.,* **67:**785, (Apr.) 1967.

49. Browse, Norman L.: *op. cit.*

50. Pratt, Rosalie: "Caring for the Paralyzed," *District Nurs.,* **13:**49, (June) 1970.

51. Griffith, Donald: "Immobilization Hypercalciuria: Treatment and a Possible Pathophysiologic Mechanism," *Aerosp. Med.,* **42:** 1322, (Dec.) 1971.

52. Harper, Jane E., et al.: *op. cit.*

53. Lavin, Mary Ann: "Bed Exercises for Acute Cardiac Patients," *Am. J. Nurs.,* **73:**1227, (July) 1973.

54. Large, Helen, et al.: "In the First Stroke Intensive Care Unit," *Am. J. Nurs.,* **69:**76, (Jan.) 1969.

55. Beeson, Paul B.: "The Case Against the Catheter" (editorial), *Am. J. Med.,* **24:**1, (Jan.) 1958.

56. Kottke, Frederick J.: *op. cit.*

57. Pratt, Rosalie: *op. cit.*

58. Large, Helen, et al.: *op. cit.*

59. Lavin, Mary Ann: *op. cit.*

60. Pratt, Rosalie: *op. cit.*

61. Birchenall, Joan, and Streight, Mary E.: *op. cit.*

62. Fox, Madeline J.: "Talking with Patients Who Can't Answer," *Am. J. Nurs.,* **71:**46, (June) 1971.

63. Burt, Margaret M.: "Perceptual Deficits in Hemiplegia," *Am. J. Nurs.,* **70:**1026, (May) 1970.

64. Foster, D. A.: "Handwriting Rehabilitation for a Spastic Paraplegic," *Nurs. Mirror,* **130:** 28, (May 1) 1970.

Additional Suggested Reading

Browder, Phyllis, and Hicks, Dorothy: "Maintaining Muscle Function in Patients on Bed Rest," *Am. J. Nurs.,* **72:**1250, (July) 1972.

Cockburn, Kathleen: "Sensory Stimulation in the Nursing Care of Chronic Schizophrenic Patients," in *ANA Regional Clinical Conferences, 1967.* Appleton-Century-Crofts, New York, 1968.

Evans, Beryl: "Multiple Sclerosis and Melancholia," *District Nurs.,* **13:**217, (Feb.) 1971.

Gage, Frances B.: "Suicide in the Aged," *Am. J. Nurs.,* **71:**2153, (Nov.) 1971.

Guerrieri, Belga O.: "Survey of the Knowledge of the Nurse in Direct Care Services Concerning Proper Bed Positioning of the Patient with Hemiplegia," *Nurs. Res.,* **17:**157, (Mar.–Apr.) 1968.

Kelly, Mary M.: "Exercises for Bedfast Patients," *Am. J. Nurs.,* **66:**2209, (Oct.) 1966.

Kupfer, D. J.: "Sleep and Depressive Syndromes," *N. Engl. J. Med.,* **285:**1490, (Dec. 23) 1971.

Ogg, Elizabeth: *Milestones in Muscle Disease Research.* Muscular Dystrophy Association of America, New York, 1971.

Powell, Mary: *Orthopaedic Nursing.* Churchill Livingstone, London, 1976.

Slater, Marianne C.: "Nursing Intervention for the Patient with CNS Dysfunction," in Kintzel, Kay Corman (ed.): *Advanced Concepts in Clinical Nursing.* J. B. Lippincott Co., Philadelphia, 1971.

Catherine Forrest
Virginia Henderson

CHAPTER 39

Motor Disturbances—Hyperactivity

1. TYPES OF HYPERACTIVITY

In Chapter 12, which deals with posture and movement, the point was made that these states of being express thought, mood, or emotion. Throughout most of the preceding chapters the impossibility of separating thought and feeling from action has been stressed. People move in response to a desire to take another position or to go from where they are to where they want to be. Even when a person is still, parts of the body, such as the heart, are in constant motion, and individual cells, if adequately magnified, can be seen to move. Striated muscles are called voluntary (also skeletal) because they are attached to bones and their lengthening and shortening enable people to move according to their wishes (*voluntary* meaning will); unstriated muscle is called involuntary (also visceral) because it was believed that the will could not control such functions as the heart beat or the action of the intestines. While visceral muscles respond mainly to chemical changes in the fluid surrounding the muscle cells, it has been demonstrated that visceral activity is very much affected not only by strong emotions but also by the human will in response to various rewards or punishments. For examples, a child who learns that he or she can avoid going to school by self-induced vomiting or diarrhea can utilize these symptoms to frighten and control his or her mother; it has been suggested that there are even some individuals who can will their death, or the cessation of the heart beat.* Laboratory experimentation has demonstrated that animals will control visceral activity for some reward or punishment. The foregoing observations suggest the interrelationship of thoughts, emotions, and actions, and suggest that skeletal and visceral muscles are both under the influence of the "mind" or "spirit."

This chapter deals with hyperactivity, or disturbance of skeletal and visceral muscle function, from a symptom-oriented rather than a disease-oriented point of view. The following types of hyperactivity are included in this general work because nurses see them in all ambulatory and institutional settings and because the victims of such disturbances and their families often need help from nurses. By accurate observation and description, nurses also can play an important role in determining the cause of the motor disturbance. In many situations nurses must act immediately on the basis of their assessment. Disease entities with which persistent and severe hyperactivity are associated are discussed fully in texts on neuromuscular and psychiatric disorders. Some of these texts are listed at the end of this chapter and should be consulted by the reader who wants to know more about the symptoms discussed in the following pages.

There are a number of ways to classify those motor disturbances reflected in agitated, overactive, or excessively energetic behavior, either as the total or partial body response to stimuli. The sudden contraction of a group of muscles is called a *spasm*. Spasms that are habitual are called *tics* and may affect an eye, the mouth, the side of the face, an arm, or a leg. If the muscle of the diaphragm is involved, the spasm is called *hiccups*. Trembling is a normal body response to cold or strong emotion but persistent *tremors* of any part of the body are pathologic. While tremors are often confined to the hands, they may include the head or pervade the whole body. They may even affect

---

* Discussed by Neal Miller, a psychologist at Rockefeller University, during a talk he gave in New Haven in 1966. Willing death is a subject treated by many anthropologists. See especially Chapters 38 and 50 for psychic control of visceral function, although the interrelation of mind and body is stressed throughout this work.

speech. Hyperactivity that affects the whole body commonly is seen in personalities who are *habitually hyperactive* or those who have *cyclic hyperactivity* alternating with periods of hypoactivity. Cyclic overactivity is associated with mild or severe euphoria (called mania if very marked) and alternately mild or severe depression. *Delirium,* with its alternating states of consciousness and attention, is marked by emotional instability, restlessness, and agitation in response to an acute organic condition. A transitory but severe, generalized, and involuntary hyperactivity with aimless motion is called a *convulsion* (from *convellere,* to shake) and is always a condition to be taken seriously, although the underlying pathology, especially in the young, may not be serious.

2. SPASMS, TICS, AND HICCUPS

Spasms. According to Cyril Mitchell Mac-Bryde, a spasm is "a marked, if not violent, contraction of a muscle or group of muscles which is often but not always painful." * Ordinary "muscle cramps" are the usual example, but spasm also occurs in such conditions as tetany, Bell's palsy, viral infection, poisoning, or degenerative neuromuscular diseases. An ordinary cramp can be relieved by massaging or passively extending the affected arm or leg, or by actively exercising the extremity. However, one must be cautious about using massage if it is known or suspected that the person has a vascular disease because there is danger of dislodging a blood clot.

Treatment of spasm related to a particular disease is determined by the underlying cause of the disease. For example, specific antidotes are used to treat poisoning, and calcium is used to treat tetany. Helping people understand the importance of diet in preventing tetany is a nursing function. Milk is the most obvious source of calcium, but cheese and eggs are also excellent sources; many fruits and vegetables have a high calcium content. However, regulating calcium intake is not the whole story. Many people must also learn, for example, that vitamin D is a necessary activating substance for calcium metabolism and that sunshine, fish, egg yolks, and butter are important sources of vitamin D.

Where the cause of spasm is unknown, it is often impossible to relieve the symptom. Though spasms may be uncomfortable and a nuisance, they rarely interfere with the usual activities of daily living or body function.

---

* MacBryde, Cyril Mitchell (ed.): *Signs and Symptoms,* 4th ed. J. B. Lippincott Co., Philadelphia, 1964, p. 654.

Tics. Any brief and repetitious, involuntary movement that involves a small part of the body is known as a *tic* or a *habit spasm.* Such movements can be associated with organic problems, but more frequently the cause is emotional. The most common tics are facial grimacings, blinkings, shoulder shrugging, or small spasms of the head and neck. From a psychologic point of view, tics are thought to be little protective ceremonies to ward off unconscious impulses that are stereotyped by repetition.

Tics often make their first appearance during childhood. They should be taken seriously. Not only the child but also the parents may need help to understand and change the attitudes, behaviors, and values that contribute to this symptom. Intensive, investigative psychotherapy frequently is helpful, but successful outcomes are dependent on motivation and on the severity of the underlying problem, and for some people it is prohibitively expensive. The popularity of parent-education programs and the strong interest that nurses and other health-care practitioners have in working with and understanding disturbed family relations suggest acceptance of responsibility for improving the environment in which such people live. The nurse who is alert to problems in family relations and who knows the community resources for help can be an invaluable consultant and teacher. Early detection is essential to the prevention of chronicity and irreversible patterns of maladaptive behavior. It is important for the nurse to determine the extent to which the tic interferes with ordinary relationships and activities, the problems of communication, and how much capacity the patient has for insight into the problem. If the circumstances that tend to make the tic worse can be determined, it is possible to reduce the seriousness of the symptom by avoiding those situations. A psychologically related kind of problem is known as "occupational" spasm, one example of which is writer's cramp. This spasm causes progressive disability since it involves muscles essential to the person's occupational skills. Again, psychotherapy often is helpful. Sometimes merely making a favorable change in one's life situation may be effective.

Hiccups. Hiccups (singultus) is a peculiar phenomenon with an etiology and physiologic mechanism that are poorly understood. According to an editorial in the *British Medical Journal:*

It appears to serve no useful purpose as vomiting does, for instance. Most people have experienced it. Few have seriously considered its mechanism, for the symptom is usually transient, the cause is usually obvious (at least to the mind of the hiccupper), and the treatment is merely to wait for it to stop or to try and arrest it by bizarre manoeuvres most of which have in common a temporary cessation of respiration. However, . . . persistent hiccup can be serious, intractable, and exhausting, and its cause often obscure.*

Though many observers suggest the possibility of a psychogenic basis, intractable hiccuping most often is associated with such toxic states as renal disease, certain cardiac conditions, brain-stem injury or lesion, encephalitis, and lesions near the diaphragm.

The specific mechanism is assumed to be involuntary and probably is related to the "combined action of the respiratory and phrenic centres, together with the hypothalamic sympathetic centre, and may actually perform the work of a specific centre." † Hiccup is an involuntary clonic spasm of some portion of the diaphragm and related inspiratory muscles, followed by an abrupt closure of the glottis.

Ordinary hiccups can occur in anyone, especially after eating or drinking. They usually are short-lived and there are many well-known remedies. Each person seems to have his or her favorite maneuver, the most common of which include holding the breath while swallowing cold water, chewing ice, breathing deeply, rebreathing from a paper bag, applying finger pressure on the eyeballs through closed lids for several minutes, drinking hot liquids, taking mild digestive stimulants, and preparing household concoctions too numerous to cite. One group of observers corresponding with the *New England Journal of Medicine* reports that: "One teaspoonful of ordinary white granulated sugar, swallowed 'dry,' resulted in immediate cessation of hiccups in 19 of 20 patients. Twelve of these patients were otherwise in good health and had suffered from their hiccups for less than 6 hours. . . . The remaining eight patients had suffered from persistent hiccups for 24 hours to 6 weeks." ‡ The mechanism of action for this symptomatic relief is unknown.

For those more serious, persistent cases of hiccup, the treatment is as varied as the underlying cause. When the etiology is obscure and the physiology is so poorly understood as is the case with persistent hiccups, any treatment method has only limited success and is bound to have debatable merits. Drugs [1] such as ami-

triptyline, haloperidol, edrophonium, methylphenidate, and chlorpromazine have been reported successful in the relief of some persistent cases. These drugs are known primarily for their effects on the central nervous system and frequently are used in the treatment of psychoses and depressions. Additionally, however, they act on the autonomic nervous system to effect neuromuscular, adrenergic, or vagal blockage. The mechanism of action is not very well understood, but these drugs do sometimes relieve hiccups. Benzedrine, which relaxes smooth muscle, and quinidine, which has properties of vagal blockage and muscle relaxation, are sometimes tried, but are generally regarded as ineffective. Barbiturates and inhalations of carbon dioxide/oxygen can be particularly useful in early treatment, though the mechanism of action is unclear. Applications of a galvanic sinusoidal current have been useful for slowing the rate, but are relatively ineffective in later stages of an attack. Ethyl chloride sprays to the neck and deep anesthesia have been tried, but generally are not recommended. Hypnosis may be helpful in the prevention of hiccups in a susceptible person in whom psychogenic influences play a major part; however, it is not useful during an acute phase. Local anesthesia, such as Xylocaine, used as a phrenic nerve block, particularly on the left side, has been known to interrupt a severe case of hiccups. When everything else fails, dissection of either the phrenic circle, the sympathetic, or the lower thoracic or upper lumbar nerve may be indicated.

3. TREMORS

Tremors are rhythmic and relatively continuous quivering or shaking movements due to individual muscle contractions. The many causes of tremulousness include shivering from cold, senility, anxiety, chronic alcoholism, Parkinson's disease (paralysis agitans), degenerative neuromuscular diseases, liver disease, hyperthyroidism, and midbrain tumors and lesions. Tremors may involve any body part—arms, legs, hands, feet, head, throat and neck, facial muscles. Obviously, the treatment varies with the underlying etiology.

Severe tremors, such as those observed in Parkinsonism, affect many body functions and can interfere seriously with activities of daily living. Drinking from a glass or cup can be so difficult that it is necessary to provide a straw or tube to prevent spilling. Similar difficulties exist with ordinary eating utensils. If nurses anticipate some of these problems, they can prepare appropriate finger foods, cut meat and

---

* "Hiccup," *Br. Med. J.,* **2**:234, (May 1) 1971.

† Samuels, Lester: "Hiccup: A Ten Year Review of Anatomy, Etiology and Treatment," *Can. Med. Assoc. J.,* **67**:315, (Oct.) 1952.

‡ Engleman, Edgar G., et al.: "Granulated Sugar as Treatment for Hiccups in Conscious Patients" (correspondence), *N. Engl. J. Med.,* **285**:1489, (Dec. 23) 1971.

vegetables into manageable pieces, and arrange meals so that they can be taken with minimal distress or embarrassment to the incapacitated person. It is equally important, however, to allow and encourage as much independent function as possible. It is a delicate thing to know when and how to assist someone who cannot adequately dress or undress, wash or feed himself or herself, or safely move from one place to another. Severe tremors can interfere with all of these activities, and individuals vary markedly in their needs and wishes for help. It is not easy for most persons to express their emotions, concerns, or needs, and the nurse should be alert to ways of encouraging and fostering adequate communication patterns. Sleep and rest can be problematic because tremors sometimes are present when the person is inactive. Supporting arms and legs in good body alignment fosters relaxation. Too much attention or concentration on a particular activity as well as emotional stress can exaggerate a tremor. Persons afflicted with tremors must learn to recognize these situations and avoid them, as must their associates. Normal exercise and recreation should be encouraged, not only because of their effect on motor performance but also because activities tend to improve mood and outlook.

Some drugs provide symptomatic relief of the tremors associated with Parkinson's disease. However, there is only 20 to 30 per cent effectiveness in about 60 to 80 per cent of all cases, and the best results occur with combinations of drugs.[2] Three drugs in particular are useful in the treatment of Parkinsonian tremors—trihexyphenidyl, benztropine, and ethopropazine. Trihexyphenidyl is often the initial drug of choice because of its low toxic threshold. Benztropine eases the pain associated with muscle spasm and cramping; it also is long acting and has mildly sedative properties. Ethopropazine is especially good for tremors. There is no optimum dose of these drugs for a particular person, and drug changes frequently are needed both in kind and amount. Additionally, all drugs mentioned have adverse effects on mood, but appropriate stimulants, sedatives, or tranquilizers can be given to counteract the emotional side effects. In a small number of carefully selected cases, neurosurgery has been known to effect symptomatic relief, but surgery is still regarded essentially as a last resort.

4. HYPERACTIVE BEHAVIOR

Definition. Hyperactivity is a word that has emotional connotations and lacks specificity. It is a "symptom" that is hard to define, though in general it refers to both kind and amount of activity, with associated social and psychologic characteristics. In some ways it is undefinable because so much of its meaning is relative. For example, people physically active, outgoing, cheerful, always "on the go," engaged in many undertakings, and demonstrating a keen mind and acute awareness are said to have hyperkinetic personalities. Most people would consider such traits within the range of healthy or normal behavior. Some might advise such a person to slow down. Exaggerate hyperkinetic traits to the point where that person is unable to sleep, is irritable and even tremulous, is almost always in motion, overreacts to every stimulus, and keeps shifting focus or attention, and it is probable that he or she is in serious enough difficulty to require some special care and attention. Furthermore, the person and the family should be helped to identify the cause of the hyperactivity so that proper care and treatment can be made available. If it is due to some toxic disease, a different treatment is indicated from that provided for hyperactivity with a nontoxic cause. However, once such therapeutic judgments are made, nursing care frequently becomes a critical factor in determining the outcome. Hyperactive behavior may be associated with any number of disease processes as, for example, endocrine disorder, renal failure, chorea, manic-depressive illness, senility, alcoholism, drug reaction, or acute schizophrenia. Some common signs of hyperactivity are increased motor and verbal activity, with pressured speech, increased social involvement, intrusiveness, increased expression of anger, provocativeness, marked sleeplessness, euphoria, and delusions of grandeur.

Nursing Care. Because hyperactive states are characterized by lack of control, one overriding principle of care is to provide external controls within the environment. This is no easy task, since many of these patients resist control and restriction of activity even in its most subtle form. Often the patient tends to antagonize others, and to deal with that tendency requires enormous tact and patience. The nurse's ingenuity and endurance are inordinately challenged when he or she assumes responsibility for the care of such a person.

In many societies those who are seriously lacking in control, or those considered asocial in their behavior, are cared for behind barred windows and locked doors. Since felons and criminals are also incarcerated, this extreme form of restraining a person's activity naturally elicits resentment and hostility. Those who are confined suffer, and health workers

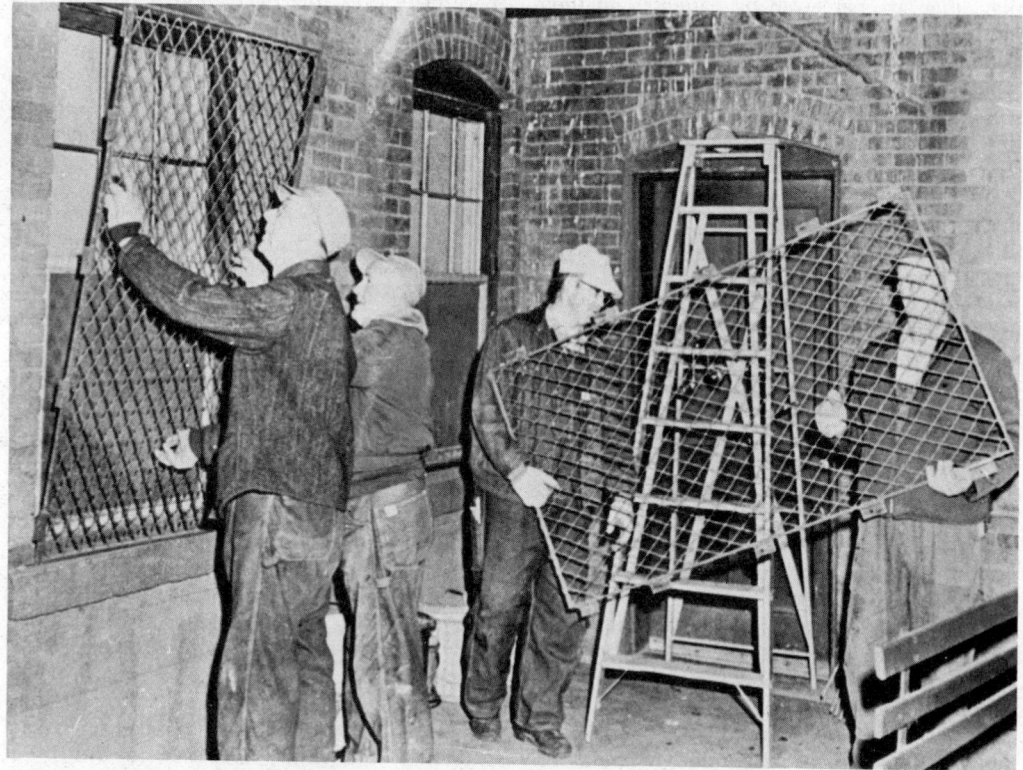

Figure 39-1. Workers in 1960 removing heavy iron grilles from windows of the Connecticut Valley Hospital. (From Carini, Esta, et al.: *The Mentally Ill in Connecticut: Changing Patterns of Care and the Evolution of Psychiatric Nursing, 1936–1972.* Connecticut Department of Mental Health, Hartford, 1974, p. 78.)

also suffer, for they must enter and leave the clinical area through a locked door, which gives them the unhappy sense of being jailors rather than therapists. More and more psychiatric hospitals are abolishing restraints. Esta Carini and associates, discussing the "increasingly liberal attitude toward the hospitalized mentally ill" in Connecticut, say: ". . . the 'open door policy' was very gradually put into effect during the sixth decade of the twentieth century." * Figure 39-1 shows workers in the 1960s removing heavy iron window grilles from a large state hospital. The grilles were replaced with detention screens which were "less formidable" and "less prison-like." Some psychiatric hospitals have no restraining characteristics that physically differentiate them from general hospitals.

It is sometimes necessary to protect hyper-

active persons from environmental stimulation both inside and outside the hospital; occasionally they also may have to be secluded and their activities restricted. Adequate ventilation and lighting, quiet, restriction of visitors, reduction of stimulation and excitement in any form are all important considerations in selecting and controlling the environment. Some agitated people cannot tolerate solitude for even limited periods. For such people, it may be crucial that some nonstimulating person who can set firm limits be in constant attendance. Often these general measures may produce a sedative effect immediately. However, they are rarely sufficient for prolonged relief.

With people who are very angry and suspicious during an extreme hyperactive state, it may be necessary to physically restrain them to prevent injury to self or others. If it is necessary to restrain them in bed, the side rails should be padded to ensure protection. Most hyperactive persons will climb over side rails, so restraining sheets or garments may be used. Such measures are a last resort, since

* Carini, Esta, et al.: *The Mentally Ill in Connecticut: Changing Patterns of Care and the Evolution of Psychiatric Nursing, 1936–1972.* Connecticut Department of Mental Health, Hartford, 1974, p. 73.

they often are perceived by patients and their family as punitive. They tend to increase the patient's agitation.

Nursing measures that would tend to have a soothing or sedative effect are very important, particularly in the acute phase of a hyperactive state. For example, a warm bath followed by a hot drink before going to bed in a quiet, darkened room may induce sleep. Individual idiosyncrasies must be considered—idiosyncrasies about the amount and kinds of light, noise, and sensate qualities that are soothing to a particular person. (See also Chapter 13 where sleep induction is discussed.)

For an individual who is extremely agitated and hyperactive, a prolonged bath may have a calming effect. Water should be regulated to a continuous flow that will keep the temperature at 35.5° to 36.6°C (96° to 98°F). If such bathing is used repeatedly, the skin should be oiled to prevent undue softening or drying. An air pillow under the head or behind the neck contributes to the patient's comfort. Sometimes the contrasting temperature of an ice cap to the forehead or scalp plus cool water and liquid foods to drink enhances the desired effect. Pulse rate and skin color must be checked frequently to determine body response to the water and temperature. Whenever the person is too hot or too cold, immediate removal from the bath is indicated. The person should be wrapped in warm, dry towels and then covered with a blanket. Any conversation during this bath should be restricted to easy, peaceful topics and kept to a minimum.

Children. Hyperactive behavior in childhood represents a very complicated problem of diagnosis and treatment. There is little agreement on definition. J. S. Werry defines hyperactivity in childhood as "a chronic, sustained, excessive level of motor activity which is the cause of significant and continued complaint both at home and at school." * Though this operational definition fits with most clinical observations, Barbara K. Keogh tells us that "there is only limited evidence to document quantitative differences in activity levels of hyperactive and normal children. . . . [It] is not just the amount of motor activity, but also the character of the activity which defines . . . [the problem]." † The situational or social appropriateness of the behavior seems to

be a critical factor. Even though high activity levels increase the probability of inappropriate behavior, they also are characteristic of some people of high achievement.[3] Though definition is imprecise, most parents and professionals do seem to recognize the problem when they see it.

Etiology is unknown, but childhood hyperactivity commonly is associated with abnormal function of the central nervous system and with developmental defects or unfavorable environmental influences. One recent hypothesis suggests that the cerebral dysfunction may be the result of faulty metabolism of norepinephrine.[4] Other postulates about origin include direct injury to the central nervous system, anoxia, infections, or hemorrhage associated with accidents of the birth process or accidents in early childhood.[5] The most widely accepted premise is that hyperactivity results from the interaction of multiple biologic and environmental factors.

Normal children very often become restless, overactive, or distractible when they are tired. Only when those behaviors are excessive or persistent are they regarded as signs of developmental immaturity. Even when hyperactivity is severe enough to require special attention, the child's response to drugs, remedial education, or sociopsychiatric treatment depends on his or her age and the severity of the mental disorder.

Problems of care and management abound, and long-term assistance to both parents and children is essential. Camilla M. Anderson and H. B. Plymate [6] have suggested that one of the most important aspects of management is the prevention of complications that arise through inadequate early care, particularly care during adolescence. The very nature of the problem makes for difficult parent-child relations from the beginning, and adequate care and treatment must reflect concern and attention to the family as a unit.

So far as medical needs are concerned, the findings of a complete neurologic examination and electroencephalogram frequently fail to demonstrate any abnormality, though an underlying neurologic impairment generally is assumed to exist as the basis for a number of maladaptive symptoms. Treatment of hyperactivity with drugs is common and stimulants are reported to be helpful in from half to two-thirds of all cases. However, when medication is given as the *only* treatment, with the expectation of easy relief, there is inevitable disappointment. Furthermore, many children resent the idea of having to take medication in order to "get along" in school and tend to omit doses or arbitrarily discontinue the medi-

* Werry, J. S.: "Diagnosis, Etiology, and Treatment of Hyperactivity in Children," in Hellmuth, J. (ed.): *Learning Disorders,* Vol. 3. Special Child Publications, Seattle, Wash., 1968, p. 171.

† Keogh, Barbara K.: "Hyperactivity and Learning Disorders: Review and Speculation," *Except. Child.,* **71:**101, (Oct.) 1971.

cine as they grow older. Nevertheless, various energizers and stimulants have been demonstrated as useful adjuncts to educational and psychologic management. The amphetamines are widely used and generally regarded as valuable; methylphenidate (Ritalin), dextroamphetamine (Dexedrine), and diphenhydramine (Benadryl) are the most commonly used drugs. With judicious use, improved behavior has been demonstrated and, in some instances, improved cognitive functioning. A decrease in restlessness and impulsivity has important value for social acceptance and approval, which undoubtedly enhances self-esteem. Such success may even influence motivation for learning. In addition, if impulsivity and restlessness interfere with accurate intake of information and lead to rapid decision-making, the results are likely to be many errors and poor problem-solving. Thus medication may influence learning by that process as well. Since toxicity does occur over a wide range of dosages, it is very important to know and recognize signs of overdose. These include constant twisting and turning, purposeless movement, mumbling, hyperirritability, tremulousness, confusion, delirium, hallucination, and panic. Since there is no antidote, treatment of overdose is symptomatic.

Though many hyperactive children have a high incidence of learning problems, more than half of them never receive any remedial education to supplement their regular schooling. This state of affairs obviously reflects a lack of public understanding and a dearth of planning and programming rather than a lack of need for special facilities. An additional problem is that very few teachers have had the kind of training necessary to meet the needs of these children. Taxpayers and citizens should look at the whole pattern of public education and be resourceful and imaginative in changing the system so that social and emotional damage to handicapped children will be prevented. Educational authorities should be encouraged to play a more effective role in the development of special services and programs. Hyperactive children need small classes in a supportive environment with interested, caring, patient teachers who will help them to learn at their own pace.

So far as social and psychologic problems are concerned the greatest emphasis belongs on prevention. Often it is the public health nurse in the school or the home who can detect potential problems and who can counsel teachers and parents accordingly. Chapter 5 on diagnosis and the physical examination discusses the nurse's role in routine examination. Assessing this condition very early in life is crucial so that parents and professionals can be alerted to potential behavior problems. Parental mismanagement is rarely, if ever, the primary cause of hyperactive behavior, though many bewildered parents feel guilty and resent their misfortune in having a hyperactive child. The nurse can be helpful by providing the encouragement and clarification such parents need in order to provide the healthiest possible home climate. Parents should be helped to learn what kinds of difficulties to expect and how best to deal with them. Through discussion and well-selected readings they can be persuaded that they are not to be blamed for their child's problems so that they can feel less angry and less helpless about dealing with him or her on a day-to-day basis. They can realize that being firm and setting limits is every bit as important as being warm and loving if the child is going to learn how to cope with impulsiveness and overactivity. They must learn that useful habits and routines will provide an external structure to counteract the lack of internal control. They must also

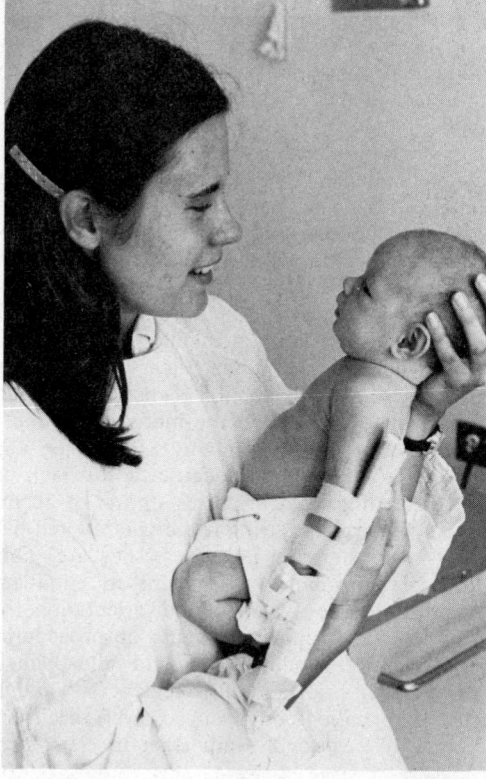

Figure 39-2. When an infant must be restrained, the harmful effects can be minimized by special attention from relatives and health personnel. (Courtesy of Children's Memorial Hospital, Chicago, Ill.)

learn how to be patient about repeatedly showing and demonstrating rather than telling the child how to accomplish a given task—how to keep things simple, concrete, and within the child's grasp. This kind of patience is particularly difficult for those parents who themselves are bright and quick in their grasp of abstract ideas.

Children themselves should be prepared to see themselves as somewhat different from other children so that they can learn to accept the rejection and criticism that inevitably come from others and to recognize their own limitations in order to avoid constant frustration and unhappiness. Simultaneously, hyperactive children must be helped to develop compensatory behavior patterns, a task that requires inordinate sensitivity and ingenuity on the part of everyone concerned. It is especially important to provide and encourage true peer associations so that these children are not always perceived as "out-group" persons. This contact should not be too difficult to arrange because hyperactivity in childhood is not a rare condition. In spite of the best possible efforts, there are some hyperkinetic children whose growth and development may be so stunted or retarded that they may never be able to live without special supports and a protective environment, either within the family or an institution. Whenever indicated, such special placements should be very carefully and thoughtfully arranged.

5. DELIRIUM

Delirium is an acute reaction to some organic state. Alternative states of consciousness, emotional instability, extreme restlessness, and agitation are among its most prominent features. Its most common causes include infection, trauma, misuse of drugs including alcohol, lack of vitamins, disturbances of metabolism, and just about any organic brain disorder.

With delirium, a general discomfort, restlessness, sleeplessness, and mental irritability may last for only a few hours or for a few days, after which increased restlessness, marked tremulousness, hallucinations, and delusions can develop very rapidly. There are three characteristic motor abnormalities that Jerome B. Posner describes as the most important physical signs for distinguishing organic brain disease from either structural brain lesion or psychiatric illness. These signs are: (1) a coarse, irregular *tremor* that usually is absent at complete rest; (2) an abnormal, involuntary jerking in the hands, known as *asterixis,* and elicited by dorsiflexion of the wrist and extension of the fingers; and (3) sudden nonrhythmic, nonpatterned, gross muscle contractions that occur during rest, primarily in the face and shoulders, known as *multifocal myoclonus.*[7]

While organic brain disease is fairly common and easy to diagnose, often delays and mistakes are made because some of its behavioral manifestations evoke resentment and anxiety. Posner identifies this problem in the following vivid description of delirium:

. . . the fearful, uncooperative, combative person who thrashes about in bed and either cries for help or shouts loud, obscene, or plaintive imprecations, meanwhile resisting or actually striking out at all who try to help him (invites diagnostic errors and delays). It takes a remarkably clear clinical head to resist meeting such obstreperousness immediately with sedation and incarceration and to consider that grave metabolic disease may be the cause, not just "schizophrenia," "hysteria," or plain "cussedness." Parenthetically, such unfortunate patients, often inadvertently, abet the misdiagnosis by expressing fears of "going crazy," a frequent delusion of metabolic brain disease. . . .*

Treatment of delirium involves correcting the underlying or causal systemic disorder. Nursing care is as variable as the vast array of additional signs and symptoms that may be present and the personal, or individual, needs of the patient.

Since noise and activity further stimulate agitated and restless patients, they should be in as quiet a place as possible. Because darkness often accentuates confusion and disorientation if constant, and can keep the knowledge of night and day from patients, rooms should be lit by the sun during the day and dimly lit with a lamp at night.

The confusion and fearfulness of delirious patients make it difficult, if not impossible, for them to understand the motives of others. Even if they are not combative, they often will reject the care offered because of this lack of understanding. When nurses approach them, it can be very reassuring if they merely tell patients who they are and where they are. This kind of information also helps to eliminate some of the confusion and disorientation. In addition, if specific treatments or procedures are to be performed, they should be explained carefully, in brief and clear sentences. Though such explanations ought to be given to all patients, it is especially important to clarify, as

---

* Posner, Jerome B.: "Delirium and Exogenous Metabolic Brain Disease," in Beeson, Paul B., and McDermott, Walsh (eds.): *Cecil-Loeb Textbook of Medicine,* 13th ed. W. B. Saunders Co., Philadelphia, 1971, p. 93.

much as possible, understanding of what is to be done during delirium.

If patients are extremely restless and fearful, they may need someone constantly with them. Arrangements should be made to have special nurses or members of the family in attendance. Those intimately acquainted with patients often can calm them where others fail, and out of a stream of talk an intimate often can make sense when a stranger cannot. If they are confused or overactive to the point of harming themselves, and if it is impossible to have constant attendance, then it may be necessary to use physical restraints. (Restraints are discussed also in Chapter 34.) However, such belts, cuffs, and harnesses should be used judiciously and as a very last resort. They should be applied as loosely as possible, with padding to prevent excoriation of the skin around the wrists and ankles. If it is necessary to restrain patients over a period of several hours, the devices should be removed frequently for skin care and the area over which they are applied inspected for signs of interference with circulation. Physical restraints have long been among the most abused aids to patient care. These writers cannot overemphasize the importance of using them cautiously. Kenneth Dewhurst describes the most common physical restraints as follows:

Bodyband restraint is like a slimming device designed for an obese Egyptian belly dancer. A wide belt of reinforced webbing is applied tightly over the abdomen, while a similar strap firmly secures the patient to the bed.

The Posey belt, made of 6 inch (15 cm.) wide reinforced webbing, is also used to strap the patient to the bed. It may also serve to strangle him should he try too hard to wriggle out.

Wrist and ankle restraints are now made of webbing rather than iron, but they serve the same function as in Pinel's day. In extremely restless patients there is always the danger of injuring the secured limb.

The safety vest is another name for a strait jacket. This device enables the victim to be firmly secured in either an upright chair or a wheelchair. With cynical abandon, it is recommended to enable the nursing staff to "proceed with other duties confident of the patient's well-being, comfort and safety."

The V-type restraining harness passes around the patient's neck and secures him to the bed. Death by misadventure has been recorded when such a harness, used to quieten a restless child, got entangled causing death by asphyxiation.*

A warm bath might be indicated for its soothing, sedative effect. Because sedative

* Dewhurst, Kenneth: "The New Methods of Restraint," *Nurs. Times*, **66:**751, (June 11) 1970.

drugs can depress circulation, cause constipation, and accentuate delirium, their use is to be discouraged. However, small doses of paraldehyde or chlordiazepoxide may be prescribed to quiet patients.

Because their behavior can be so trying, it often is difficult for nurses and families to be patient, calm, and reassuring with a delirious person. Nevertheless, the attitude of nurses and their desire to be comforting, in spite of rejection, obnoxious and provocative behavior, are crucial to reducing the fear and confusion that so much determine the degree of agitation and hyperactivity.*

Feeding delirious persons can be very problematic. During lucid moments they can feed themselves with minimal assistance. However, when the delirious phase is acute, it frequently is impossible to feed them anything by mouth. Tube or intravenous feeding then are used. (Tube feeding is discussed in Chapter 23 and intravenous feeding in Chapter 22.) With tube feedings, nurses must be especially alert to the problem of aspiration. People who are very restless or combative may easily end up with the tube leading into their lungs rather than their stomachs. With intravenous feeding, nurses must watch carefully for signs of infiltration and must prevent patients from pulling the needles out of veins.

6. CONVULSIONS

While the modern-day public image is slowly changing, people who have convulsive disorders still are shunned all too often as strange or mentally unsound. This reaction results in a restricted personal life for the victims. They feel uncertain and fear disapproval. An increasing body of knowledge is developing to explain many types of convulsive disorders on specific etiologic grounds such as low calcium blood levels, tumors, head injuries, hypoglycemia, childhood fever, drug or alcohol withdrawal, or encephalitis. In fact, just about any disease or structural abnormality of the brain may be associated with convulsions. When etiology is unknown, however, which is true more than half the time, the term "idiopathic epilepsy" may be used and the cause assumed to be genetic. To further

* When delirium is caused by alcohol or other drug abuse, nurses and families sometimes make moral judgments that color attitudes and behavior toward the delirious patient. Management of alcoholic "delirium tremens" with medication has so reduced the noisy and unreasoning behavior of patients in most situations that the condition is not so difficult a problem as it once was.

confuse the classification picture, there are nonconvulsive seizures, in which the altered state of consciousness, or awareness, is minimal.

Convulsions have been reported in an estimated 2 to 5 per cent of all children under 5 years of age. One-third of all childhood convulsive disorders are associated with fever caused by common viral and bacterial infections, and are most common in white, male children.[8]

Physiologic and environmental triggering factors in recurrent convulsive disorders frequently are unique and reproducible in a particular patient. The triggering specificity probably reflects the anatomy and physiology of the seizure focus in that person. According to Gilbert H. Glaser, it is likely that several factors combine to produce a given attack:

. . . a genetically determined predisposition, an increased cerebral excitability related to a general metabolic disturbance, the presence of a focal brain lesion or a tendency to vascular insufficiency, and a triggering disturbance such as an emotional crisis or an excessively flickering light. Each patient, therefore, must be evaluated from many different aspects in order to establish causation on different levels and to develop appropriate total therapy.*

Broadly speaking, recurrent convulsive disorders can be classified into three types, each with its own characteristics, as follows: (1) grand mal or generalized, major seizures; (2) petit mal or minor seizures; and (3) focal or partial seizures. Nursing care and medical management vary with the type of convulsive disorder.

Grand mal seizures have a wide range of causes and occur in all age groups. It is this disorder that is associated in most minds with the term convulsion. The attack usually has a pattern or sequence that includes a prodromal phase, a convulsion, and the phase following the convulsion. The prodromal phase may last for a few seconds or even a few hours, with subtle changes in emotional response during that time. The *aura,* a brief and unusual sensation of sight, sound, odor, or fear, immediately precedes a state of unconsciousness and generalized tonicity. Sometimes there is a simultaneous cry or loud vocal sound just as the convulsion begins. Though this tonic episode lasts for only a few seconds, it can be very frightening to an observer who witnesses a rigid body, clenched teeth, distorted features, dilated pupils, and respiratory distress. Very

quickly this tonic behavior shifts to a clonic episode that may last for several minutes. It is characterized by heavy, difficult breathing, rhythmic jerking of the arms, legs, and trunk, facial spasms, intense cyanosis, frothing at the mouth, biting the tongue (often severely enough to cause bleeding), and frequently bowel and bladder incontinence. Gradually the convulsive movements get less severe and frequent, the color clears, breathing is more normal, and there are signs of returning consciousness. During the last phase, the patient is confused and groggy, and may sleep for a while. Headache and irritability sometimes persist for a few hours. Though he or she may remember the prodromal phase or aura, the patient usually is amnesic during the second, or convulsive, phase. Whether or not a person is unconscious during a convulsion is debatable. In any event, it is a mistake for those with the patient to assume that he or she is unconscious and to say things they would not otherwise say.

Nursing care during a convulsion is geared toward the prevention of injury and careful, detailed observation. Even though many hospitalized patients may be in bed at the start of an attack, most often persons (especially epileptics who are leading active lives) fall into immediate unconsciousness wherever they happen to be. Hard objects and furniture should be pushed aside, and a coat or pillow put under the head. If neither is available, it may be helpful to cushion the head against one's own thighs. If there is a warning, it is useful to put either a handkerchief or a padded tongue blade between the person's teeth to prevent him or her from biting the tongue. However, since jaws clench immediately at the start of an attack, there is no way to prevent injury to the tongue if it was between the patient's teeth. Furthermore, to force a mouth gag at that moment can do nothing but harm in the form of bruised gums or broken teeth, though it may be helpful to hold the jaws open (by pulling down on the lower jaw and chin) if that is possible. Because breathing is impaired, it is important to ensure an open airway. Tight clothing, such as a collar or belt, should be loosened and the head turned to the side so that the tongue can fall forward and saliva run out. Suffocation or aspiration can be checked by watching for food, vomitus, dentures, or bed covers around the face and mouth. By this time the clonic phase of the seizure is well under way, and one can only protect the patient's head, arms, and legs from pounding against hard surfaces. Restraint is not advisable because bones may be fractured by strong muscular contractions.

* Glaser, Gilbert H.: "The Epilepsies," in Beeson, Paul B., and McDermott, Walsh (eds.): *Cecil-Loeb Textbook of Medicine,* 13th ed. W. B. Saunders Co., Philadelphia, 1971, p. 263.

No attempt should be made to move the patient until after the attack is over. If there has been any fecal or urinary incontinence or excessive sweating, a bath should be provided in such a way that embarrassment for the patient is minimized. If the body temperature is elevated, it can be reduced with a sponge bath and with aspirin. Afterward, the person should be helped to a comfortable, quiet place where he or she can sleep or rest until able to resume normal activities.

Nurses, or anyone present, should report and record exactly what they have observed. Such details as number of seizures and time of day, nature of onset, general body position, location and type of movements and how they spread, arousal level, color, pulse, pupils, and breathing are all significant cues to identifying the etiology and deciding on subsequent medical management. Very often the keen eye of the nurse, mother, or other observer is crucial to such determination and to the patient's future welfare.

Petit mal seizures consist of a sudden, very brief lapse of consciousness, with no convulsive movements and representing no more than a momentary blank stare, slight purposeless and rhythmic movement of the face or hands, a slight lapse of focus, or a fading voice. None of these lasts for more than a few seconds. It is a disease of childhood with no specific etiology and a declining incidence after puberty. Medical therapy is the most important consideration for this condition, and will be discussed later under treatment and prevention.

Focal or partial seizures are typical of an acquired convulsive disorder caused by pathology of a specific brain area. The attack usually involves only a certain part of the body. Sometimes a focal (or partial) seizure may develop into a more generalized convulsion. Typically, there is some loss of memory, but not total unconsciousness or amnesia. "Jacksonian march," for example, is the classic designation for this kind of seizure. It usually starts with the fingers, toes, or the corner of the mouth, as a twitching movement, and gradually spreads to the trunk of the body. Though this kind of seizure usually remains partial, it may become more general. Patients subject to these attacks often have time to lie down or put a gag in the mouth before they lose consciousness.

A very thorough diagnostic evaluation is necessary to determine both etiology and precipitating circumstances of any seizure disorder, convulsive or otherwise, with particular effort to identify a causative illness or lesion. Laboratory tests, electroencephalogram, x-rays,

a health history, and a physical examination are essential to an accurate diagnosis. Frequently the nurse has invaluable information about and observations of the patient to contribute. Once a specific cause has been determined, it can be treated directly. For example, a tumor can be surgically removed or a metabolic disturbance can be treated with appropriate diet and drugs. However, since etiology is unknown in the majority of cases, anticonvulsant drugs are most often used in the control and prevention of attacks. The amount and kind of medication vary with the individual and with the character, frequency, and severity of the seizure disorder that he or she has. Glaser [9] makes the following recommendations about drug treatment: Petit mal seizures respond best to succinimides or oxazolidinediones (methadiones). Grand mal and some focal seizures respond to the hydantoins and phenobarbital, with most effective control produced by combining the two medications. Acetazolamide can be used as an adjuvant with any type of seizure, but should be used intermittently because tolerance develops. Though careful attention to individual details results in satisfactory or complete control of most seizures, there are a number of people who suffer from side effects of drugs or from increasing social and psychologic difficulties.

Dietary restrictions or specific dietary preparations are not particularly valuable to most people with a convulsive disorder. However, a ketogenic diet, one high in fats and low in proteins and carbohydrates, is sometimes helpful as an adjunct to drugs in the management of intractable petit mal seizures.[10] This dietary regime is based on the theory that an artificially produced acidosis (ketosis) tends to decrease seizures. When more fats than carbohydrates are used during the metabolic process, ketone bodies are produced. In order to determine the amount of ketosis and dietary effectiveness, frequent urinalysis for acetone and dietetic acid is indicated. Food must be weighed and kept in the following balance: 8 per cent carbohydrates, 8 per cent protein, and 84 per cent fat. Unfortunately, this diet is monotonous and unappetizing, making it difficult to maintain. It requires ingenuity to make a ketogenic diet variable and attractive. In addition to a restricted diet, people prone to convulsive disorders are advised to stay away from alcohol, avoid fatigue, get sufficient sleep, and eat regular meals.

Occasionally, after careful evaluation of those cases that do not respond to medical management, surgical intervention may be indicated. Small tumors, vascular lesions, or scars can be removed if they are not too large and not located in a brain site that would leave the patient with some additional neurologic impairment after surgical removal of the growth.

While nursing care of a person during convulsion can be protective and the nurse can make observations that can help the physician identify the cause, it is perhaps in the social and psychologic area of management that the nurse can play the most significant role. Because there is still so much social stigma attached to convulsions, many of their victims have problems in life adjustment and other serious psychologic problems. It is well known that emotional disturbances or stress is likely to precipitate a given attack. Patients and their close associates must be taught what to do during a seizure, how to avoid stressful or disturbing situations, and how to overcome a number of unnecessary fears and misconceptions. They must learn to understand the importance of medication in the control of seizure activity. Psychologic needs vary with age and social circumstances, but it is extremely important for nurses to be attuned to individual variations and to counsel patients accordingly, so that they can overcome their anxiety, fear, shame or self-consciousness, and sense of futility if seizures, or the threat of them, are interfering with a productive, satisfying life.

Most people with convulsive disorders are able to go to regular schools and develop productive careers and live in much the same fashion as ordinary persons. Very few require a special, protective environment with intensive medical, psychologic, educational, and vocational training programs. So far as occupational choice is concerned, only those that involve potentially dangerous activities are contraindicated, as for example jobs that involve the use of strong chemicals or electrical equipment or ones that require hazardous climbing. Though many people with convulsive disorders have difficulty finding and keeping a job, in fact, very few of them have seizures frequent or severe enough to interfere with any activity.

REFERENCES

1. Goodman, Louis E., and Gilman, Alfred: *The Pharmacological Basis of Therapeutics,* 5th ed. Macmillan Publishing Co., Inc., New York, 1975.
2. *Ibid.,* p. 241.
3. Keogh, Barbara K.: "Hyperactivity and Learning Disorders: Review and Speculation," *Except. Child.,* **71:**101, (Oct.) 1971.
4. Silver, L. B.: "A Proposed View of the Etiology of the Neurological Learning Disability Syndrome," *J. Learning Disabilities,* **4:**123, 1971.
5. Laufer, Maurice W.: "Cerebral Dysfunction and Behavior Disorders in Adolescents," *Am. J. Orthopsychiatry,* **32:**501, (Apr.) 1962.
6. Anderson, Camilla M., and Plymate, H. B.: "Management of the Brain-Damaged Adolescent," *Am. J. Orthopsychiatry,* **32:**496, (Apr.) 1962.
7. Posner, Jerome B.: "Delirium and Exogenous Metabolic Brain Disease," in Beeson, Paul B., and McDermott, Walsh (eds.): *Cecil-Loeb Textbook of Medicine,* 13th ed. W. B. Saunders Co., Philadelphia, 1971, p. 91.
8. Millichap, J. G.: *Febrile Convulsions.* Macmillan Publishing Co., Inc., New York, 1968, p. 34.
9. Glaser, Gilbert H.: "The Epilepsies," in Beeson, Paul B., and McDermott, Walsh (eds.): *Cecil-Loeb Textbook of Medicine,* 13th ed. W. B. Saunders Co., Philadelphia, 1971, p. 269.
10. *Ibid.,* p. 271.

Additional Suggested Reading

Beland, Irene L., and Passos, Joyce Y.: *Clinical Nursing: Pathophysiological and Psychosocial Approaches,* 3rd ed. Macmillan Publishing Co., Inc., New York, 1975.
Carozza, Virginia J.: "Understanding the Patient with Epilepsy," *Nurs. Clin. North Am.,* **5:**13, (Mar.) 1970.
Craig, Eleanor: *P. S. You're Not Listening.* New American Library, New York, 1973.
Cruickshank, William, et al.: *A Teaching Method for Brain-Injured and Hyperactive Children,* University of Syracuse Press, Syracuse, N.Y., 1961.
Fish, Barbara: "Treating Hyperactive Children" (editorial), *J.A.M.A.,* **218:**1427, (Nov. 29) 1971.
Howell, J. B. L.: "The Diaphragm," in Beeson, Paul B., and McDermott, Walsh (eds.): *Cecil-Loeb Textbook of Medicine,* 13th ed. W. B. Saunders Co., Philadelphia, 1971.
Kenny, Thomas J., et al.: "Characteristics of Children Referred Because of Hyperactivity," *J. Pediatr.,* **79:**618, (Oct.) 1971.
Korczyn, A. D.: "Hiccup," *Br. Med. J.,* **2:**590, (June 5) 1971.
Strauss, Alfred, and Lehtinen, Laura: *Psychopathology and Education of the Brain-Injured Child.* Grune & Stratton, New York, 1951.
Strauss, Hans: "Epileptic Disorders," in Arieti, Silvano (ed.): *American Handbook of Psychiatry,* Vol. 2. Basic Books, Inc., New York, 1959.
Weiss, Gabrielle, et al.: "Studies on the Hyperactive Child: Five-year Follow-up," *Arch. Gen. Psychiatry,* **24:**409, (May) 1971.
Werry, John: "Studies on the Hyperactive Child. VII. Neurological Status Compared with Neurotic and Normal Children," *Am. J. Orthopsychiatry,* **42:**441, (Apr.) 1972.

Roberta Spurgeon
Virginia Henderson

CHAPTER 40

Disturbances of Consciousness and Orientation

1. CONSCIOUSNESS

Consciousness has been described as awareness of one's self and one's environment. The conscious person is not only fully awake but also able to use all his or her mental faculties and perceptions to interpret what is happening and to draw on stored memories.[1,2]

Consciousness has two major components. One is wakefulness or awareness, and the other is a composite of thoughts, memories, feelings, and language called the *content* of consciousness.[3] Wakefulness and arousal are in large part controlled by the reticular activating system in the brain stem, while the processes of thought, memory, language, and the analysis of sensory perceptions are mainly under the control of the cerebral cortex. However, because of the constant reciprocal interaction of these systems, both must be intact for a fully functioning consciousness.[4]

Since the publication of William James' *Principles of Psychology* (Holt, Rinehart & Winston, New York, 1890), student of personality have distinguished between conscious and unconscious thought and the influence of both. James conceived of all experience as stored in "the mind" as persons might store the possessions they acquired through life in a huge dark building. Those possessions the individual might see if he or she carried a candle through the building would be a minute fraction of the whole and might represent the focus of the conscious mind; those that exist unseen but can be brought to light at any time represent the potential focus of the unconscious mind and are just as real as those on which the light of the candle (or consciousness) is focused at the moment. Gordon W. Allport, a contemporary student of personality, in *Pattern and Growth in Personality* has more references to James than to any other writer except Sigmund Freud. Both writers should be read by those who wish to know more about states of consciousness than can be discussed here.

Allport shows diagrammatically the proportions of conscious, preconscious, and unconscious thought in "purposive planning and reality testing," "normal creativity and imagination," "creativity in the neurotic," and "distortion of reality in the insane." About this diagram he makes the following observation:

A diagram adapted from Kubic [see Figure 40-1] represents the wide difference that exists between lives ordered largely by conscious plans, purposes, and intentions (autonomous ego) and lives driven primarily by unconscious compulsions and neurotic formations.

The diagram calls attention to the presence of the preconscious in all lives. It suggests that this region of available memories is especially important in creativity. The creativeness of the normal person depends more on the cooperation of the preconscious and the conscious than is the case with neurotics, where the unconscious enters more compulsively and in larger proportions.

The diagram also recognizes a continuous series of personalities from those almost completely dominated by their conscious purposes and in continuous contact with reality, through personalities with less insight and less integration and somewhat more dominated by both preconscious and unconscious functions, to the clearly abnormal cases whose lives are more and more controlled by dissociated and unconscious systems.*

Present-day methods of locating brain lesions with brain scans, of stimulating the exposed brain during surgery, of studying the effect of drugs on the brain are leading to greater understanding of human behavior, especially speech, the most characteristic attri-

---

* Allport, Gordon W.: *Pattern and Growth in Personality.* Holt, Rinehart & Winston, New York, 1961, p. 153.

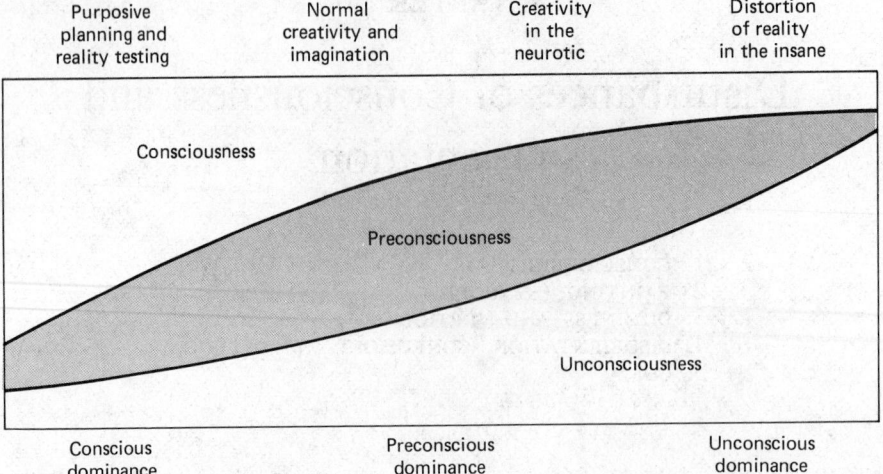

Figure 40-1. Varying proportions of conscious and unconscious dominance in personalities. (Allport, Gordon W.: *Pattern and Growth in Personality*. Holt, Rinehart & Winston, New York, 1965, p. 153; adapted by Allport from Kubie, L. S., "The Neurotic Process as the Focus of Physiological and Psychoanalytical Research," *J. Ment. Sci.*, 1958, p. 104.)

bute of humans.[4a] Some psychologists have referred to this as "the age of the unconscious."

A healthy individual's level of consciousness normally varies throughout the 24-hour day. Sleep, occurring under predictable and regular circumstances, is the most obvious of these variations. Insofar as sleeping persons give no evidence of being aware of themselves or their surroundings, they are unconscious. However, this unconsciousness is easily reversible and a return to complete awareness is the normal response to stimulation. (See Chapter 13 for a more detailed discussion of sleep.) Throughout the wakeful part of the day, an individual's state of consciousness may range from alert responses to a variety of external and internal stimuli to deep concentration or daydreaming when he or she is responding to internal (thought and memory) stimulation.

Fluctuations in an individual's state of consciousness are detectable to some extent by changes in the electrical impulses of the brain recorded on the electroencephalogram (EEG). Much of the time, according to Arthur C. Guyton,[5] brain waves are irregular and without a particular pattern; however, at other times, both in health and illness, distinct patterns occur. In normal persons there are four classifications of brain wave patterns, and there is a general relationship between these patterns and cerebral activity. For instance, delta waves appear during sleep, surgical anesthesia, stupor, and in infants; theta waves occur in infants and in heightened psychomotor condi-

tions of adults; alpha waves are present in quiet, relaxed states; and beta waves appear during intense mental activity.*

Interestingly, the alpha and beta wave patterns most associated with mental activity make their appearance only gradually during childhood. They reach adult frequencies when a person is between the ages of 14 and 16, when the cerebral cortex is thought to be mature.[6] The wakefulness of infants, then, is a rather special case of consciousness. They respond to internal physiologic stimuli and most external stimuli, but have not yet developed any of the content—thoughts, memories, and language—of consciousness. A somewhat similar situation is that of adults who have aphasia (an inability either to comprehend language or to express themselves in language), amnesia (inability to remember), or a severe emotional disorder. They are generally considered conscious because they are fully awake; however, they are unable to make use of portions of the consciousness content that had been available to them in the past.

Level of Consciousness. Of most concern to nurses in the hospital setting is the patients'

---

* Gerald Jonas reports that studies of hypnotized persons and those in Zen meditation show altered EEGs. During transcendental meditation (which the subjects can induce and terminate), there is a "wakeful hypometabolic state" that explains how a person may survive burial for hours or days. It may be a factor in the long life of some semicomatose patients. (Jonas, Gerald: *Visceral Learning; Toward a Source of Self Control*. Viking Press, New York, 1973, p. 107.)

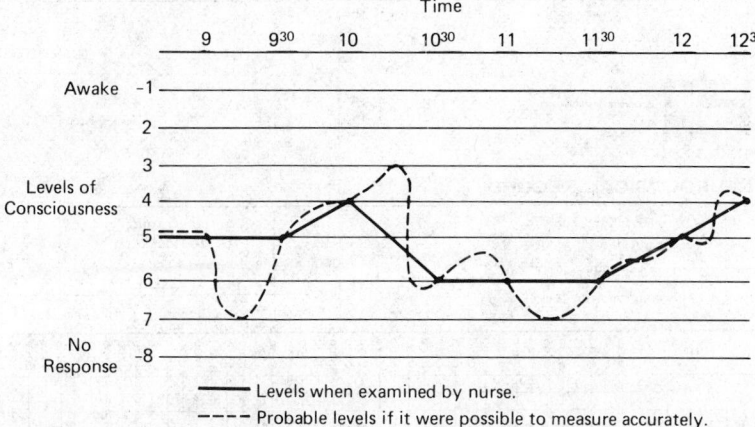

Figure 40-2. Possible variations in level of consciousness in a semiconscious patient. (From Quesenbury, Jeanne H., and Lembright, Pamela: "Observations and Care for Patients with Head Injuries," *Nurs. Clin. North Am.*, 4:239, [June] 1969.)

level of consciousness, or the completeness with which they can respond to various stimuli. It is possible for patients to be aware of themselves and their environment but be unable to respond. On the other hand, they may be able to respond to tactile sensations through reflex action but be deeply unconscious.

In order to have as objective a description of a patient's level of consciousness as possible, the following definitions of eight stages of response are often used:

1. Alert, awake. The patient is alert and initiating appropriate conversation.
2. Oriented to time, place, and person. When questioned as to time, place and person, the patient responds with orientation in all spheres. The progression of disorientation occurs first in time, then place and then person . . . if the patient is becoming more alert . . . he will need reorientation as to time and place.
3. Restless. The patient shows restlessness or agitation by thrashing about or picking at himself, attached equipment, or bedclothes. He is uncooperative when stimulated.
4. Sleeplike state. The patient becomes less responsive to questioning and acts drowsy or lethargic. This is not comparable to a normal sleep from which a patient can be aroused and be expected to respond appropriately in a short period of time. During this level, incontinence may occur in a patient who has been continent up to this time.
5. Responds to verbal command. When the examiner commands the patient to perform some activity (usually a one-level command, i.e., "lift your right arm off the bed"), the patient carries it out correctly.
6. Responds to painful stimuli in a purposeful manner.
7. Responds to painful stimuli in a nonpurposeful manner. The patient may grimace or move an extremity but will not push away the noxious stimulus in a purposeful manner. Decerebrate posturing may also be the response to painful stimulus.
8. No response, no gag or cough reflex.*

Because the level of a patient's consciousness fluctuates during even short periods of time, he or she should have repeated evaluations. Jeanne Quesenbury and Pamela Lembright[7] say that the pattern of change in level of consciousness is more significant than an observation at any one time. If the rating of the level of consciousness is placed on a graph (see Fig. 40-2), it helps to determine at a glance whether the patient is progressively more conscious or unconscious. Figure 40-3 is an example of a neurologic record for recording neurologic signs.

2. FAINTING (SYNCOPE)

The most common type of unconsciousness is *fainting* or *syncope*. It is a transient condition that may last from a few seconds to several minutes. Although fainting has been reported as occurring in 25 to 30 per cent of young men, it is considered to be more frequent among adolescents and women.[8]

Causes and Treatment. Following a study of 510 patients with syncope, H. H. Wayne[9] concludes that its general causes are (1) diminished blood supply to the brain; (2) changes in

---

* Quesenbury, Jeanne H., and Lembright, Pamela: "Observations and Care for Patients with Head Injuries," *Nurs. Clin. North Am.*, **4:**239, (June) 1969.

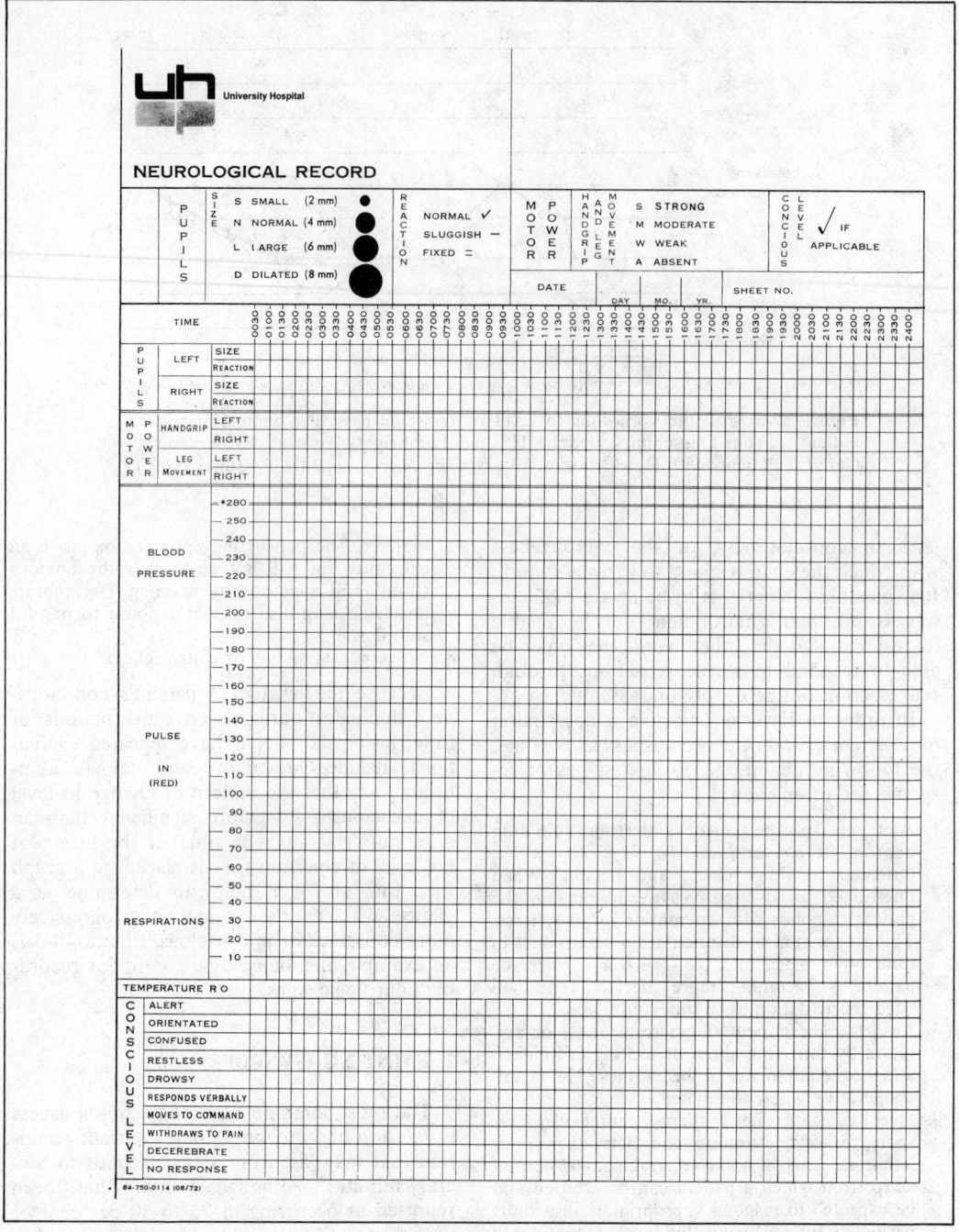

Figure 40-3. A neurological record used when monitoring neurological signs. (Courtesy of University Hospital, University of Western Ontario, London, Ont.)

the chemical composition of the blood in cerebral vessels; and (3) effects of multiple stimuli on the pattern of central nervous activity. In each category there are specific conditions that bring about syncope. Some of these are benign in that they are only temporary imbalances

in the body system, while others may indicate a serious and perhaps progressive imbalance.[9a]

Among the benign or temporary conditions that cause fainting, vasodepression is the most common.[10] This is the result of a widespread loss of normal resistance in peripheral arteries and veins with a pooling of blood in these dilated vessels. Less blood is returned to the heart, and consequently there is a diminished supply to the brain. Vasodepressor syncope may occur after a person has been standing for a long time as happens when watching a parade, or it may occur when a patient gets out of bed for the first time or two following an illness.

A premonition usually precedes fainting. There is a feeling of weakness and dizziness, often nausea, before the person falls to the ground. The face and lips blanch; the skin gets cold and clammy; there is complete relaxation with closure of the eyelids, although the pupils will react to light if the eye is opened. The pulse rate is increased, the respirations are shallow, and the blood pressure falls. All of these symptoms are of brief duration in typical syncope.

The treatment of this condition is simply placing the person in the horizontal position. If he or she is vomiting, the patient should be placed face down with the head turned to one side and resting on the back of one hand. The collar or clothing should be loosened about the neck and the subject should have free access to fresh air. Bathing the person's face with cold water and administering spirits of ammonia or other olfactory stimulants may be helpful. It might be said that the individual has initiated treatment himself or herself, since falling to the ground immediately changes the pull of gravity on the circulatory system. If the person gives warning that he or she feels faint, an attack may be prevented by having the person sit down and bend the head toward the knees, or kneel on one knee and bend forward as if tying a shoelace.[11]

Benign causes of syncope in which a change in the chemical composition of blood is involved are reduced oxygen intake because of a high altitude, or hyperventilation due to excitement or anxiety, or a mild hypoglycemia because of a long period without food. This last condition usually brings about faintness and dizziness but not loss of consciousness unless there is some underlying metabolic pathology. Known diabetics who are taking insulin may develop hyperinsulinism (hypoglycemia) and faint if they do not get their meals at regular times, or if they get very excited, or exercise strenuously. Faintness from hyperventilation can be relieved by having the individual breathe into a paper bag or hold the breath for a short time. Faintness from high altitude oxygen deficiency can be relieved by less activity until the body's compensating mechanisms have made the necessary accommodation.[12,13]

Other common and essentially nonpathologic causes of syncope are changes in central nervous system activity. It is not unusual for persons to faint at the sight of a bleeding wound or from fear during vaccination. The emotion that induces fainting, however, may be one of relief or joy on hearing that a beloved person is alive who was reported dead. The mechanism of this type of syncope is thought to be an "inhibition of the normal activity of the vasoconstrictor center of the brain by reflex stimuli from the cerebral cortex." * The symptoms and treatment of vasodepressor syncope apply to this type of fainting also.

Nurses caring for patients who may require the removal of large amounts of fluid from the pleural cavity, peritoneal cavity, or bladder should be aware that fainting may occur during these procedures. Although the mechanism involved is not known, it is thought that there is a pooling of blood in the venous system as pressure is abruptly decreased by removal of the fluid or urine.

Hysterical fainting (the mid-Victorian "drawing-room swoon") is most frequently seen in young women. The individual loses consciousness and slumps gracefully to the floor, usually in the presence of others. There is no change in heart rate, respiratory rate, arterial pressure, or the electroencephalogram in the individual, and nausea, pallor, and sweating are not present.

More serious causes of fainting are hemorrhage, heart disease, pathology of the carotid arteries or carotid sinuses, orthostatic hypotension in disease of the autonomic nervous system, obstructive emphysema, hypoglycemia in adrenocortical insufficiency or liver disease, and epilepsy. Syncope in these conditions, except orthostatic hypotension, does not respond to the simple treatment discussed earlier. A physician should see the patient as soon as possible so the underlying cause can be treated.[14,15]

3. DIZZINESS AND VERTIGO

Dizziness and vertigo are terms used to describe symptoms of a mildly altered consciousness because of impaired balance or equilibrium. These terms should not be used interchangeably, for they have different meanings. A clear definition and understanding of each is important, since the treatment of the two conditions differs.

* Cole, Warren H., and Puestow, Charles B.: *Emergency Care—Surgical and Medical*, 7th ed. Appleton-Century-Crofts, New York, 1972, p. 359.

Dizziness is an inclusive term sometimes used by patients to describe sensations of whirling, but more frequently they mean giddiness, faintness, weakness, confusion, lightheadedness, or a swimming sensation in the head. *Vertigo,* on the other hand, is a specific term that describes the sensation of motion when there is no movement. The sensation may be one of turning or spinning, either of one's self or one's environment, or it may be a sensation of side-to-side movement, front-to-back movement, up-and-down movement, or a sensation of falling; any hallucination of motion is defined as vertigo.[16]

To help patients describe more accurately the sensations they are having, a number of techniques can be used. Patients can be asked to describe in as much detail as possible what they mean by "dizziness," or if this is too difficult for them, they can be asked to describe the specific circumstances under which they feel "dizzy." Another method of getting an accurate description consists of three simple tests that cause either giddiness (dizziness) or vertigo, and asking patients to compare their sensations after each test with those they have had at other times. In one test, patients are asked to breathe deeply for 3 minutes (hyperventilation), after which giddiness is felt; in another test they are asked to stoop over for one minute and then straighten up which results, again, in giddiness; and, finally, they are asked to turn rapidly in one direction ten times after which the sensation they feel is vertigo.[17]

Dizziness. Although the commonly experienced sensation of dizziness or giddiness often has no clinical significance, frequently experienced episodes should be investigated, the cause determined, and treatment instituted. Physiologic changes that cause fainting may also cause dizziness. Dizziness frequently follows head injury. It is thought to be both a physical effect of and a psychologic response to injury.

Dizziness associated with hypertension may be attributed to the nervousness, fear, or anxiety associated with the diagnosis; it may be caused by transient changes in the cranial vessels; or it may be attributed to both sources. Dizziness in anemia is probably due to a mild brain hypoxia. This is caused by a decrease in the red blood cells and a reduction in hemoglobin.

Postural dizziness is a common complaint, especially among the elderly, those in poor physical health, and those confined to bed over a period of time. Such persons feel giddy or sway after stooping over, or when sitting on the side of the bed after being in the recumbent position. They may also have blurred vision or spots before the eyes. The condition is thought to be caused by a temporary failure of reflex vasoconstriction of the peripheral vessels which allows temporary pooling of blood in the extremities. This pooling reduces the amount of blood available for nourishment of the brain. As a result of decreased cerebral blood flow, dizziness and visual symptoms can occur. A more common type of postural dizziness occurs in some healthy individuals after standing for some time or after rising suddenly from a sitting or recumbent position. A healthy person may also be dizzy after a hot bath. During pregnancy, women often complain of "dizzy spells" on getting out of bed quickly.

Dizziness is common in psychoneurotic states and particularly in introspective persons who have an overawareness of various parts of the body. It is a frequent complaint of anxious persons; however, it may be that the anxiety is produced because the victims don't know why they have the repeated dizzy spells, or because they fear they cannot carry out their usual activities safely or adequately.[18] W. R. Brain[19] emphasizes that physiologic factors must be investigated and eliminated before the cause of patients' symptoms of dizziness can be considered psychogenic.

Vertigo. Any hallucination of motion is called vertigo and results from some disorder of the complex mechanisms for maintaining balance (equilibrium). Healthy individuals adjust equilibrium continually on the reflex level and are ordinarily unaware of doing so. The membranous labyrinths of the inner ear, particularly the semicircular canals and utricles, play an important part in helping to maintain balance. Hair tufts projecting from hair cells in the utricles and semicircular canals provide signals, by bending, for detecting the position and movement of the head. Information necessary for keeping the head in position with the rest of the body also comes from the proprioceptive * joint receptors of the neck. Additional information on position in space comes through what is seen. All this information is integrated and sorted through the vestibular nuclei and vestibular pathways located, for the most part, in the brain stem. When there is a disorder of the membranous labyrinth of the ear, the proprioceptors of the neck, vision, the vestibular nuclei, or the vestibular pathways, vertigo is likely to occur. The brain stem contains complex neural circuits and specialized motor and sensory nuclei that control eye movements; support the body against gravity; and that flex, extend, turn, and rotate the body.

---

* Information arising from stimuli that originate in the body rather than outside the body.

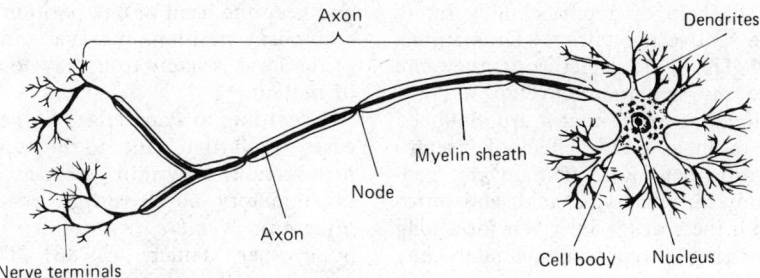

Figure 40-4. A neuron.

The brain stem contains nerves that affect respiratory, cardiovascular, and gastrointestinal function. The anatomic proximity of all these cells and neural circuits in the brain stem allows abnormal stimuli from the apparatus of equilibrium to influence many functions. Figure 40-4 shows a neuron (nerve cell) and Figure 40-5 shows a synapse where a nervous impulse is transmitted from one neuron to another. Symptoms associated with vertigo include nystagmus,* staggering, and nausea.[20]

Michael M. Paparella [21] says that 85 per cent of the patients with vertigo have a disorder of the inner ear. In healthy individuals, each movement of the head stimulates the labyrinth of one ear and suppresses the other. When the signals from both ears combine, the individual has necessary information about his or her position in space. Sudden and severe change

* "When a person rotates his head, his eyes must rotate in the opposite direction if they are to remain 'fixed' on any one object long enough to gain a clear image. After they have rotated far to one side, they jump suddenly in the direction of rotation of the head to 'fix' on a new object and then rotate slowly backward again. This sudden jumping motion forward and then slow backward motion is known as nystagmus. The jumping motion is called the *fast component* of the nystagmus, and the slow movement is called the *slow component*." (Guyton, Arthur C.: *Textbook of Medical Physiology*, 4th ed. W. B. Saunders Co., Philadelphia, 1971, p. 667.)

in the ability of either labyrinthine mechanism to respond to stimuli with excitation or suppression causes vertigo. If the function of one labyrinth is totally lost, the person learns to interpret the unopposed signal from the remaining labyrinth. After this accommodation takes place, symptoms formerly present at time of motion subside. There may be temporary vertigo, however, whenever the person is quiet.[22] Many persons with complete destruction of both labyrinths have almost normal equilibrium as long as they can see what position they are in.[23]

There are numerous *causes* of vertigo. A common cause of a mild and fairly transient vertigo is "motion sickness." It is an individual response of an oversensitive labyrinth to constant or violent agitation of the fluid in the semicircular canals. Some persons are much more susceptible than others. Those affected by the motion of a boat do not necessarily get carsick, and some people may be inexplicably free from motion sickness under conditions that usually cause marked distress. It is thought that the emotional state, therefore, may help to induce the characteristic vertigo and nausea. When vomiting is added to these symptoms, the subject may be very ill unless the resulting dehydration is corrected. The cause and the generally benign nature of motion sickness are so well recognized by the

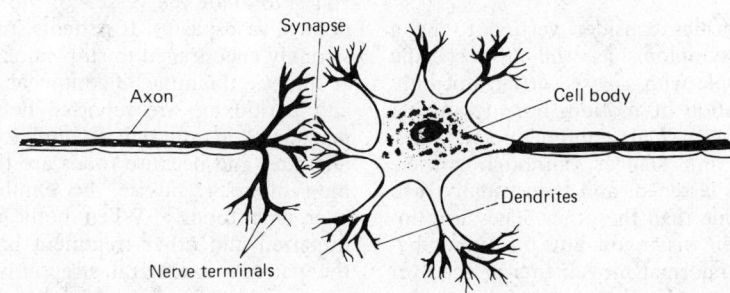

Figure 40-5. The synapse or junction between two or more neurons. It is believed that a nerve impulse is carried across the synaptic space by chemical transmitters.

public that the help of a physician is rarely sought. The antivertigo drugs Dramamine, Bonine, and Tigan are effective if they are taken before any symptoms develop.[24]

Nurses should be aware that a drug-induced vertigo can result as a side effect of streptomycin, dihydrostreptomycin, kanamycin, gentamicin, viomycin, ethacrynic acid, and nitrogen mustard if these drugs are given for a long time. Nurses should report immediately any indication of vertigo in patients who are receiving these medications so that they can be discontinued.[25]

Fractures of the temporal or occipital bones, tumors of the vestibular apparatus, and arteriosclerosis of the blood vessels associated with the labyrinth may be causes of labyrinthine vertigo.[26] Some disorders not of the membranous labyrinth such as epilepsy, multiple sclerosis, whiplash injuries, and acute vascular accidents in the brain stem account for 15 per cent of those who suffer from vertigo. Vertigo may result from the necessity of adapting to an unusual visual environment, as in looking down from a height or adjusting to bifocal lenses in eyeglasses. Vertigo can be a symptom in the early stages of an ocular muscular paralysis.[27]

When patients seek the help of a physician because of vertigo, the caloric test is commonly used to determine the adequacy of the membranous labyrinth. Either cold air or ice water (2 to 5 ml) is introduced into one auditory canal when the patient's head is tilted 30 degrees backward. The cold water increases the density of the endolymph in the semicircular canal, and the endolymph sinks downward. This results in slight movement of the fluid in the canal, causing nystagmus and a sensation of rotating. If the labyrinth being tested is normal, it becomes the more active one, and the individual feels as if he or she were rotating in the direction of the side being tested. More accurate and sophisticated methods of testing vestibular function are carried out with the use of electronystagmographic recordings of eye movements.[28]

Some authorities consider vertigo to be a syndrome of symptoms as well as a specific symptom. People with severe vertigo not only have hallucination of motion, but are unable to stay balanced when standing erect. They tend to reel and stagger, although muscle strength is not lessened, and they usually turn more to one side than the other. They are unable to fix their vision on any one point because of the abnormal movements of the eyeball, and frequently there are nausea and vomiting. The severity of the vertigo lessens if the person can lie down with the eyes closed and keep the head in one position. Even in the recumbent position, however, any movement of the head is likely to aggravate the sensation of motion.[29]

According to Paparella,[30] 75 per cent of the cases of vertigo, due to impairment of the membranous labyrinth, are classified as noninflammatory aural vertigo called *Ménière's disease* or *Ménière's syndrome*, first described by Prosper Ménière in 1861. The syndrome consists of three essential symptoms—vertigo, fluctuating hearing loss, and tinnitus (ringing, buzzing, and roaring in the ear). Ménière's disease affects both men and women and usually begins in middle life. Its cause is unknown. Etiologic theories include an overproduction or a diminished reabsorption of the endolymph circulating in the labyrinth; a vasomotor disturbance of the inner ear; an endocrine disturbance; an emotional disturbance; and various allergies. Most authorities agree that the symptoms are initiated by a sudden rise of endolymphatic pressure in the membranous labyrinth.[31,32]

Spontaneous attacks of Ménière's disease occur at intervals, and patients may have remissions that last for a few hours or several years. During an acute attack persons are often prostrated. They are pale, sweating, and have nystagmus. Nausea and vomiting, varying in degree, often accompany episodic attacks. The disturbed hearing associated with the vertigo in Ménière's disease has some specific characteristics—sounds of low intensity are not heard, sounds that are heard are distorted, music is dysharmonic, speech is jumbled, and loud sounds appear too loud. After repeated attacks, there is some permanent hearing loss.

Since the specific cause of Ménière's disease has not been determined, many forms of *treatment* are used. A low-sodium diet is often prescribed in an attempt to increase absorption of the endolymph and, for the same reason, diuretics are sometimes used. Nicotinic acid 50 to 100 mg four times daily is prescribed during acute attacks, as well as in later chronic stages to dilate the vessels of the inner ear and control vasospasms. If patients smoke, they are strongly encouraged to stop smoking. Vitamins A and C, thiamine, nicotinic acid, riboflavin, and pyridoxine are reported helpful to older persons. Some physicians emphasize testing for allergies, and because foods are the most common offender, advise the elimination of all allergenic foods.[33] When both labyrinths are impaired and other treatment has not helped the patient, parenteral streptomycin is sometimes used. This drug selectively concentrates in the labyrinth and, if given over a period of several weeks, destroys the vestibular function.

Surgical treatments that have been moderately successful are drainage of the endolymphatic sac and the surgical removal of the entire affected membranous labyrinth.[34]

When patients are having an acute attack of vertigo, they need help in finding a comfortable recumbent position, preferably in a darkened, quiet room. Noise and sudden jarring of the bed or patient should be avoided. Such patients need help with many of their activities of daily living. Some persons are almost completely helpless. Getting out of bed unaided may result in a fall with a serious injury. Following an acute attack, daily activities should be resumed gradually, as well as congenial social and recreational activities. Since the hearing difficulties and loss of equilibrium are not always apparent to the patient's family and friends, they should have some explanation of what the patient is experiencing, so that they can modify their conversation with the patient accordingly.[34a]

Vertigo caused by a labyrinthitis from viral or bacterial invasions of the inner ear is less common than the noninflammatory type. Vertigo from an infection of the labyrinth is severe but is usually self-limiting and recovery is complete. In such cases the person may wake in the morning with vertigo, a vague sensation of fullness in one ear, nausea, and, in some instances, vomiting. There is usually no hearing loss, but if the vestibular nerves associated with hearing are affected, permanent damage is likely.[35]

4. DISORIENTATION, CONFUSION, AND DELIRIUM

Patients admitted to hospitals have many gradations of consciousness, and it may range from complete alertness (with fully functioning perceptions, memory, thought, and appropriate emotional responses) to deep coma where only the vegetative functions are in operation. Disorientation, confusion,* and delirium are terms frequently used to describe a level of consciousness when there is less than full alertness, but not total unresponsiveness. The terms are, however, ambiguous and often difficult to interpret. Nurses should, therefore, report the details of their observations when assessing consciousness rather than their belief that the patient is disoriented, confused, or delirious. In full recognition of the nonspecific nature of these terms the discussion in this

section is, nevertheless, based on common usage, because it is convenient to organize current knowledge about diminished consciousness around them.

Disorientation. When a person is unable to recognize the temporal, spatial, and interpersonal relationships (time, place, and person) of the physical and social environment, he or she is said to be *disoriented*. Louis Linn [36] says that, in general, the capacity to maintain *orientation* to one's surroundings depends on (1) the availability of sensory information, (2) the availability of recent memory information, and (3) a commitment to the demands of reality, which is a part of the mature adult's emotional equipment.

Brief periods of disorientation to time and place are not uncommon in a healthy person, may even seem to be planned as part of one's recreational activity, and often occur as a part of the preschool period of development. Disorientation in healthy individuals can be present for a very short time after waking from a deep sleep in strange surroundings, or after a real and vivid dream. The person who becomes completely engrossed in a stage play, movie, or television program often requires a brief period of reorientation to his or her surroundings when the drama has ended; and the imaginary friend of the young child is a common form of childhood disorientation partially due to an immature ability to entirely differentiate reality from fantasy. The sometimes indiscriminate use of drugs, including alcohol, is another way in which individuals "encourage . . . flights from reality and facilitate rapprochement with the world of make believe." *

Disorientation among the seriously ill is usually a symptom of organic brain disorder but may also be a functional or psychologic disorder. Stephen M. Ayres and Stanley Giannelli [37] believe that a decrease in oxygenation of brain cells, either through diminished cerebral blood flow or diminished oxygen content of the circulating blood, results in disorientation as well as other symptoms. Psychologic bases for disorientation include a subconscious wish to return to a less troubled time and place; a denial of illness or the seriousness of an illness; or escape from a developmental crisis the patient is facing—adolescence, for example —at the onset of illness. Deprivation of sleep and sensory stimulation may cause disorientation.[38]

Although many hospitalized persons don't

---

* Some authorities use the terms *confusion* and *delirium* interchangeably, others consider delirium a stage of consciousness between confusion and coma, while still others think delirium a separate entity.

* Linn, Louis: "Clinical Manifestations of Psychiatric Disorders," in Freedman, Alfred M., *et al.* (eds.): *Comprehensive Textbook of Psychiatry,* Vol. I, 2nd ed. Williams & Wilkins Co., Baltimore, 1975, p. 801.

know what day or week it is, this is a transient condition and readily corrected. Even this temporary state might be eliminated if each patient had a calendar and a clock within sight.* If, however, the patient makes an error about the time of day for a particular meal, that is, mistakes lunch or dinner for breakfast, organic brain damage may be suspected. And, if the patient consistently makes the same error in naming the year, emotional factors may be playing an important part in his or her disorientation.

Disorientation of place may take the form of calling the hospital a hotel, or restaurant, or one's home. Some patients correctly identify the hospital, but make a serious error in the distance between hospital and home.[39]

According to Alfred M. Freedman and his associates,[40] orientation for one's self generally remains, even though time and place orientation are disturbed. However, if a person with an organic brain disorder does not know who he or she is, it is a serious symptom suggesting progressive deterioration.

To *assess* the extent of disorientation when some is obvious, health workers should question patients about time, place, and person because many patients do not ask the kind of questions that would alert the nurse to their difficulty. Raymond D. Adams and Maurice Victor suggest the following to determine a patient's orientation:

Orientation: What is your name? What is your occupation? Where do you live? Are you married?

Place: What is the name of the place where you are now? How did you get here? What floor is it on? Where is the bathroom? What are you doing now?

Time: What is the date today? What time of day is it? What meals have you had? When was the last holiday? †

Confusion. According to Adams and Victor,[41] the term *confusion* has two meanings for neurologists. The first is a state in which there are drowsiness and *sensorial clouding,* that is, a general reduction in alertness—an inattention to environmental stimuli, and an inability to "take in" during a short space of time all the elements of a situation. Common features of

confusion used in this (commonest) sense are impaired reasoning, memory loss, and a short attention span. Frequently the stimuli responded to by the patient are misinterpreted (illusions), and some patients see, hear, or feel external objects when there are no such real objects (hallucinations). The second meaning of the term confusion refers to *slowness and inefficiency in thinking with an impairment of memory for recent events.*

The *causes* of confusion are multiple. Confusion in the sense of the first meaning, sometimes called primary mental confusion, may occur in acute illnesses or trauma, and often precedes or follows recovery from coma. Usually primary mental confusion is a reversible condition, although it can progress to irreversible coma. Some causes are circulatory or metabolic disturbance; toxemia in systemic infection, drugs, especially alcohol, or poisons; brain trauma; or brain tumors. In some disease processes, confusion is caused by interference with the metabolic activities of the cerebral cortex cells, a reduction of cerebral oxygen, excessive electric discharges from the cells of the brain, and sometimes destruction of brain cells.[42]

The mechanisms within the nervous system leading to disturbed consciousness are not fully known, although findings of biochemical research on the brain are shedding considerable light on behavior. For instance, because cerebral hypoxia is so important in disturbed consciousness, a method to determine the rate of cerebral blood flow and cerebral metabolism has been developed. Values for the cerebral metabolic rate and the rate of cerebral blood flow in humans have now been determined for healthy persons and for some with specific disease processes.[43] *

Indications of confusion are both quantitative and qualitative. Mildly confused patients may seem to be quite normal except that they fail to recall events of the past few hours or days, and may appear "upset." As confusion progresses their reactions get slow and indecisive. They spend their time in idleness because of lowered initiative and a short attention span. It is difficult for them to keep a conversation moving, and their responses are often abrupt, brief, and mechanical, or slow and incoherent. Because their alertness and perceptions are decreased, they are usually disoriented to time and place. Confused, bewildered persons ask the same question or make the same remark over and over. In ad-

---

* It has been suggested that daily announcements over a communication system of the date and the outside temperature might be helpful in some institutions.

† Adams, Raymond D., and Victor, Maurice: "Derangements of Intellect and Behavior Due to Diffuse and Focal Cerebral Disease," in Wintrobe, Maxwell M., et al. (eds.): *Harrison's Principles of Internal Medicine,* 7th ed. McGraw-Hill Book Co., New York, 1974, p. 164.

* Guy Owens maintains that strokes might be prevented and a more exact location of cerebral bleeding detected with improved techniques for such measurements. (Personal communication, V.H.)

dition, they often misinterpret voices, the action of others, and various objects.

Those in a deeper state of confusion are extremely drowsy and notice little that happens; however, when they respond, it is with irritation or suspicion and with single words or phrases. The degree of confusion may vary throughout the day, and much that happens leaves no trace in the patient's memory.

In the discussion of communication and age (see Chapter 16), it was noted that many old people remain oriented as long as they are in familiar surroundings, but get disoriented in nursing homes and other institutions. This is thought to be the result of the monotony of the life (lack of sensory stimulation) and a loss of interest in life. The old person is denying life and is making as little effort to live as possible. If taken back into family life, they may recover their sense of identity, their awareness of time and place. Many of the tranquilizing drugs, used so freely for the elderly, are responsible for their confusion.[43a]

Sensory deprivation, high fever with an inadequate fluid intake, immobility, inadequate lung ventilation, sleeplessness, and anxiety all tend to influence a hospitalized patient's response to an acute illness and may be major factors that lead to a state of confusion. Relief of each of these factors is largely under the control of the nurse, and, if adequately planned for, may prevent the confusion.[44]

Patients who have hearing or seeing difficulty, although not totally deaf or blind, need more planning for perceptual stimulation than do those who hear or see well (although all hospitalized patients require such stimulation). Encouraging patients to drink, to cough and turn, to go through range-of-motion exercises (with which they will need help) are all common nursing measures that should be carried out for all patients, but especially for the confused and the acutely ill elderly patient. The sleepless patient and the anxious patient may need appropriate medication, but they may also need an opportunity to talk about their concerns, or to have explanations they can understand. No drug affecting behavior has yet been discovered that has no undesirable effects if used over long enough periods. Effective nursing can often prevent the necessity for such drugs.

To preserve the link between themselves and their world, patients who become confused because of an acute disorder or because of accompanying environmental and psychologic factors should be cared for by the same personnel and have repeated orientation to time and place. The behavior of many confused patients is understandable to those who know them best but is incomprehensible to others. If nurses keep in mind that patients may be reacting to internal stimuli and that all behavior has meaning, they may be able to find ways to alter the apparently senseless behavior. Although most patients who have an acute episode of confusion have little memory of events that occurred during the confusion, this is not true of all patients or all events. The following report by Alma C. Ware and Mary N. Chelgren of a patient's account of her experience during a period of confusion illustrates these points:

I thought I was in a sardine factory. The employees weren't packing sardines in little tins, but rather were packing people like sardines into kidney-shaped cans. The packing was going on in the basement and people would be sent down this narrow slide into the cans. The door to the slide was just outside my room. I decided that if I hung onto the rails on my bed very tightly, it would jam the slide and they couldn't push me down. So, I hung on. I can tell you the name of the nurse who helped me come out of this. It was Miss _____ and I remember after she said, "Mrs. Blane, let go of the side rails, and hold on to my arm, I'll not let anything happen to you," I knew I had a friend and someone I could trust. Before that I thought the doctors, nurses, even my sister and son were all against me, and trying to get rid of me by getting me to let go of those rails. Also I couldn't see very well for a while. Everything looked blurred and I couldn't tell who anyone was and many times didn't know when someone was in the room. They'd bring me food on a tray and I couldn't see what was there so I wouldn't eat. I guess I was really sick, and you must think I'm a terrible person for the way I acted.*

Confusion, defined as inefficiency in thinking, with memory impairment, is often caused by progressive, degenerative brain disorders, and may develop during middle age. Examples of such conditions are Alzheimer's disease, Pick's disease, Huntington's chorea, cerebral arteriosclerosis, prolonged toxic conditions (alcoholism), inflammatory disease (encephalitis), trauma, and tumors.[45]

Confused behavior that is similar to the confusion of brain disorders may be seen in some elderly persons. However, the causes of their behavior may not be degenerating central nervous system disease or change, but sociocultural and psychologic factors related to aging and the aged. Dorothy V. Moses says, "senility is not an inevitable biologic state in the life cycle, but is, rather, a cultural artifact. Senility is the inevitable culmination of the

---

* Ware, Alma C., and Chelgren, Mary N.: "When 'Holding on' Brought Change," *Nurs. Clin. North Am.,* **6:**125, (Mar.) 1971.

combined social rejection of the aged person and the senescent person's self-rejection." *

The earliest indications of confusion that result from a progressive brain disease or the aging process are often difficult to differentiate from fatigue or boredom. These persons lose some of their mental quickness, spontaneity, and initiative. They seem slow and lacking in energy. As the condition causing confusion progresses, there is the loss of memory for recent events without loss of memory for events long past. Such persons forget appointments or conversations, become lost in familiar surroundings, find it difficult to think through a new task, cannot understand complex directions, have difficulty making decisions, and often misinterpret the actions of others. They may be able for a time to seem normal by using their customary social manners and habitual way of speaking. However, their language begins to lack precision and pertinence, and they fail to follow the gist of a conversation.

As patients become aware of their inability to perform many mental tasks that were once simple for them, they begin to be afraid they are losing their mind. Some of their behavior then becomes a reaction to that catastrophic possibility. They try to hide their difficulty by withdrawing from people, and so they appear asocial and apathetic. They may insist on excessive orderliness and develop rituals for daily living activities in an effort to make up for their failing memory, and they may become apprehensive, gloomy, or irritable because of their dissatisfaction with their restricted life.

In later stages, patients lose their memory of the distant past, fail to care for themselves or appreciate their surroundings, and do not recognize even their nearest relatives. They often become bedridden, incoherent, irrational, and incontinent.[46] Drug users, including alcoholics, have many of the characteristics just listed. In the treatment of confusion, the first step may be the immediate or gradual withdrawal of all drugs.

Adams and Victor say that if patients are asked the following questions, a reasonable evaluation of their thinking and memory impairment can be made:

Memory:
Remote: Tell me the names of your children and their birth dates. When were you married? What was your mother's maiden name? What was the name of your first school teacher? What job have you held?
Recent Past: Tell me about your recent illness (compare with previous statements). What did you have for breakfast today? What is my name or the nurse's name? When did you see me for the first time? . . . What were the headlines in the newspaper today? . . .
Immediate Recall: Repeat these numbers after me (give series of 3, 4, 5, 6, 7, 8 digits at speed of 1 per second). Now when I give a series of numbers, repeat them in reverse order.
Visual Span: Show the patient a picture of several objects and then ask him to name what he has seen and to note any inaccuracies.
General Information: Ask about names of presidents, well known historic dates, the names of large rivers, or large cities, etc.
Capacity for sustained mental activity:
Calculation: Test ability to add, subtract, multiply, and divide. Subtraction of serial 7s from 100 is a good test of calculation as well as of concentration.
Abstract Thinking: See if the patient can detect similarities and differences between classes of objects, or explain a proverb or a fable.*

Nursing care can help to relieve confusion. When a patient's confusion is of the impaired thinking and memory type, a number of general points should be kept in mind by the nurse planning and giving care. Although some of these patients are of middle age, many more are elderly. Authorities on aging have pointed out that while older persons have more memories and a longer history than does a younger one, they should be helped to live in the present. Although older persons have less physical ability to influence their world, they still have the human desire and capacity for control. In spite of the fact older persons may have lost those they loved because of death or distance, they need to love and be loved; and though older persons may have no friends left, they still have a capacity for friendship. Finally, while older persons' actions may be childlike, they need continuing respect for their past accomplishments as well as their current abilities.

To lighten the burden of failing memory and slowness in thinking for confused patients, a consistent approach and plan should be used by each health worker caring for them. The environment should be kept as set and familiar as possible. Patients should have the same room, bed, furniture placement, and the same persons giving them care. When changes have to be made, as, for instance, a new nurse assigned to them, patients should meet them first and have sufficient time to "take in" the coming change.[47]

As a means of fostering patients' orientation, they should be gently corrected when they

---

* Moses, Dorothy V.: "The Older Patient in the General Hospital," *Nurs. Clin. North Am.,* **2:**705, (Dec.) 1966.

* Adams, Raymond D., and Victor, Maurice: *op. cit.*

make errors about time, place, or persons. Lilyan T. Weymouth [48] says patients are often testing their own sense of reality and subtly asking for confirmation or correction of their ideas. They may need to have some events of their past recalled, and family members should be encouraged to help them in this respect. In fact, relatives and intimate friends can reduce confusion and help patients, nurses, and others, for they can often interpret what may seem incomprehensible remarks or behavior of patients.

It is often helpful to establish and make known to confused patients expectations of some consistent behavior from them, as well as some limitations on their behavior. Whenever possible, these should be cooperative decisions made with patients rather than those arbitrarily imposed on them. The development of a "pattern of living" for confused patients should take into account their social history and living habits as well as their present problems. Any pattern of living developed with patients should help them maintain regular habits of dressing, toileting, eating, resting, and participating in recreational activities.[49,49a]

Directions should be given simply, clearly, and slowly so that patients can hear them easily and have sufficient time to organize their thinking. It is often necessary to repeat what has been said for unobtrusive reinforcement. Written directions may be necessary. Diagrams and color codes have been used to make it easier for confused persons to follow directions for taking drugs at home, for example.

Delirium. Some authorities characterize delirium as a state of confusion with overactivity, excitement, sleeplessness, tremulousness, illusions, and hallucinations. Other authorities believe that the early symptoms of delirium are like those of primary mental confusion—drowsiness, loss of recent memory, bewilderment, short attention span—and that the very excitable stage, commonly identified as delirium, develops later. Still other authorities believe there are two types of delirium. One type is characterized mainly by drowsiness and reduced awareness (hypokinetic delirium), while the other has excitement, tremulousness, and hallucinations (hyperkinetic delirium) as its main characteristics.

There are numerous *causes* of delirium. John A. Aita [50] says that delirium is "everyman's psychosis," because so many different conditions can result in delirium. He lists as causative agents 21 pathologic classifications having 82 subcategories, with many of the subcategories divided still further. He says delirium is compounded of the following abnormal conditions:

1. Biochemical defects at the highest cortical neuronal levels.
2. Predisposing deficits (as, for example, drug dependency, prior cerebral damage, or circulatory insufficiency, emphysema).
3. Personality and emotional makeup of the individual.
4. Current emotional stresses and problems.
5. Experience of illness, dependency, hospitalization, diagnostic and therapeutic procedures, sensory deprivation, sleep deprivation, immobilization, exhaustion.*

It has been estimated that 10 per cent of all patients who are hospitalized will develop delirium or a period of acute confusion. The same organic disturbances that cause disorientation and confusion can lead to delirium. There are, however, some conditions that seem to be more frequently associated with hyperkinetic delirium than are others, for instance, drug abuse or withdrawal (particularly alcohol), barbiturates, and tranquilizers; infections and high fevers; the early postoperative period; and the intensive care unit.

The classical picture of delirium is the one presented by alcoholic patients. According to Adams and Victor,[51] patients talk incessantly and incoherently and appear to have vague notions that they are pursued by someone or something that intends harm. It is evident that they misinterpret ordinary objects and have vivid, often unpleasant, hallucinations of vision, hearing, and touch. They usually have tremors and restless movements that may be violent. The end of the attack of delirium is indicated by the occurrence of sound sleep and increasingly lengthy periods of lucidity. Recovery is usually complete.

Postoperative delirium was studied by Robert M. Morse and Edward M. Litin.[52] They found there were significant differences between a group of 60 delirious patients and a group of 57 nondelirious patients who had been matched on the basis of age, sex, and type of surgery. As might be expected, the incidence of organic disorder following surgery (metabolic and electrolyte disturbances, cardiac failure, cardiovascular disease, infection, senile brain syndrome, alcohol or drug intoxication) was significantly higher in the delirious patients. The length of the surgery (over 4 hours), whether it was an emergency procedure, whether more than five drugs of any kind were being taken during the recovery period, and whether the patient required more than 2 units of transfused blood during the surgery were factors more frequently found

* Aita, John A.: "Everyman's Psychosis—The Delirium, Part II," *Nebr. State Med. J.*, **53**:425, (Sept.) 1968.

among the group of delirious patients. Morse and Litin found, in addition, that the delirious patients were significantly different psychosocially from the control group. For example, those who developed delirium consciously feared death; had hearing or sight deficiencies; had a verified history of alcoholism (not necessarily a current drinking problem); they were depressed; had preoperative insomnia; or had retirement problems. An interesting finding was that patients who denied they were afraid before surgery were found more often in the nondelirious group. Morse came to the conclusion that "delirium may be a function of psychosocial factors if organic disorder exists. Vulnerability to delirium may then depend on the residual capacity of the subject to tolerate stress of any kind at that time." *

Studies of patients in intensive care units or coronary care units show that after a lucid period of from 3 to 5 days, many patients begin to have symptoms of delirium. According to Donald S. Kornfeld and his associates,[53] this change in mental status may be the first indication that a pathologic shift in a basic physiologic process has occurred.† They also say that the unique environment of these special units may be the cause of, or at least add to, the patient's state of delirium:

The concern for psychologic factors is not a mere nicety. These patients are critically ill. The physiological manifestations of emotional disturbance can tip the balance in their medical course, e.g., an increase in cardiac irritability secondary to anxiety; a withdrawal and lack of cooperation; secondary depression; a psychotic agitation: all these can have serious and perhaps fatal consequences. It is, therefore, necessary that we be alert to the possible impact of these rooms on their occupants.‡

It is obvious that nursing care is most important to lessen the impact of the intensive care unit environment. Kornfeld and associates say the monotonous and rhythmic sounds of oxygen tents, air conditioners, and monitoring equipment should be reduced as much as they can be; for example, monitoring equipment may be maintained outside the patient's room.

To give the patient as much mobility as feasible, one should remove all unnecessary wires and tubes. Each patient should have access to a window on an outside wall, a clock, a calendar, and patient-controlled radio or television.

Prior to surgery, nurses should see the patients for the purpose of learning about their individual needs, as well as telling them what to expect in the intensive care unit. Children are shown unfamiliar hospital furnishings and equipment in a preoperative visit. Many adult patients might profit from the same sort of orientation but this decision should be an individual one. Once patients have entered the unit the plan of care should allow for a maximum number of uninterrupted sleep periods that maintain the day-night cycle as nearly as possible. In addition, frequent explanations of treatments and procedures together with time and place orienting cues should be given.

Nevin M. Katz and his coworkers [54] found that from a group of 35 patients with an average stay of only 2 days in the intensive care unit, 11 patients became delirious and 9 of these had delirium caused by organic abnormalities, whereas the other 2 patients suffered severe sensory monotony. Some delirium from physiologic causes can be prevented by appropriate medical treatment which can be instituted in early stages if nurses report the first sign of confusion. Katz and associates developed a short "mental status" test with a total of 12 points (see Table 40-1) that they believe gives early indication of impending delirium. They found that nondelirious patients scored, on the average, between 8.8 and 9.2 points. Delirious patients, on the other hand, scored between 1.4 and 3.4 during periods of hallucination or confusion, and between 7.8 and 9.3 points during lucid intervals. They also found that questions asked to determine the patient's orientation to place, although not included in the score, differentiated between patients whose delirium related to sensory and sleep deprivation and those whose delirium was organically based. The sensory and sleep-deprived patients scored high on the recall and mental manipulations part of the test, but were disoriented about where they were (place or spatial orientation).

When a patient is delirious, most authorities emphasize the need for sufficient light in the room to eliminate shadows because they increase the incidence of hallucinations, illusions, and fear. Because patients in delirium are in such poor contact with their environment, H. H. Garner believes verbal communication with them should be direct and forceful, for instance, "I have a glass of orange juice for you! Sit up and drink it!" He says that giving the

* Morse, Robert M.: "Postoperative Delirium: A Syndrome of Multiple Causation," *Psychosomatics,* **11**:168, (May–June) 1970.

† At the University of Kansas Medical Center, cardiac care units have been decentralized, and the same team of doctors and nurses cares for the patient throughout the illness. This system is believed to improve patient care as well as the education of medical and nursing students.[53a]

‡ Kornfeld, Donald S., et al.: "Psychological Hazards of the Intensive Care Unit," *Nurs. Clin. North Am.,* **3**:41, (Mar.) 1968.

Table 40-1.   A Short Mental Status Test That Can Be Used to Determine Quickly the Patient's Level of Confusion: A Score of 8–12 Points Is Normal.*†

Mental Status Test—Scoring Form	
I Year	
Correct = 1 point	
II Month	
Correct = 1 point	
III Counting backward from 20 to 10	
20,19,18,17,16,15,14,13,12,11,10	
No errors with ease	= 3 points
No errors with difficulty	= 2 points
One error with ease	= 2 points
One error with difficulty	= 1 point
Two errors with ease	= 1 point
Two or more errors	= 0 point
IV Repeating digits in reverse order	

Digits	Span Length	Digits	Span Length
3 7		25973	
	2		5
4 9		83469	
635		518723	
	3		6
283		694152	
9352		2597183	
	4		7
5846		6429315	

* Katz, Nevin M., et al.: "Delirium in Surgical Patients Under Intensive Care," *Arch. Surg.,* **104:**310, (Mar.) 1972.
† Score = highest span length repeated backward correctly.

patient "reality based data in a forceful, succinct verbalization is the psychotherapeutic element in treatment." * Additional aspects of the nursing care of delirious patients are discussed in Chapter 39.

5. COMA

Definition. A seriously ill person may move from a stage of mild disorientation, confusion, and perhaps delirium into a semicomatose or

* Garner, H. H.: "Confrontation Technique—Applied to Delirium and Confusional States," *Ill. Med. J.,* **137:**72, (Jan.) 1970.

comatose state. *Coma* comes from the Greek *kōma,* deep sleep. It is defined as unconsciousness from which the patient cannot be aroused; *coma vigil* is a condition in which the patient lies with the eyes open but is unconscious.

Characteristics of Coma. Patients in a *semicoma* appear deeply asleep and unresponsive to their surroundings, but they still have corneal, pupillary, pharyngeal, tendon, and plantar reflexes. They may be aroused enough to stir or moan if they are shaken vigorously or called in a loud voice, or if they get uncomfortable from a distended bladder, or if the area around the lips is massaged vigorously, or if the anterior axillary fold is pinched, or the sternum is compressed by the examiner's knuckle. Any movements or sounds they make, as well as the specific stimuli to which they respond, should be completely described and recorded by the nurse.

Patients in a *coma* have lost the reflexes mentioned above and cannot respond to either external or internal stimuli. Their sense of self-preservation is so damaged that it is the nurse who must supply the consciousness, the physical energy, and the will that the patient lacks in providing for daily physical needs. Coma may be of short duration and of a critical nature; on the other hand, it may last for weeks, months, or years. In such cases those who nurse the comatose may feel that the patient's life is more theirs than his or hers. They are as dependent upon a nurse as the newborn is upon his or her mother.

The same long list of disease conditions that may lead to confusion or delirium is associated with coma. Many of these diseases are so severe that, in the past, death inevitably followed coma. With the current advances in medical science and therapy, support for failing respiratory and circulatory systems can be given and patients maintained for long times in a state of deep coma. Questions are now posed about the religious, ethical, and legal rightness of maintaining a patient for whom there is believed to be no hope of recovery (*irreversible coma*). In an effort to establish criteria that all can use as the basis for continuing or discontinuing heroic medical treatment, the Ad Hoc Committee of the Harvard Medical School [55] reported that when the brain is permanently nonfunctioning, it can be considered dead, and the criteria for irreversible coma must define the characteristics of such a nonfunctioning central nervous system. They concluded that irreversible coma is present when (1) there is complete unresponsiveness, and a total unawareness of both externally applied stimuli and inner needs; (2) during observations of at least 1 hour, there are no spontaneous muscular movements, or spontaneous respirations, or responses to stimuli such as pain, touch, sound, or light; (3) there are no reflexes such as pupillary reaction, blinking, swallowing, yawning, or vocalization; and (4) there is a flat electroencephalogram. (See Chapter 50 for complete report of the Ad Hoc Committee.)

Many physicians believe that the patient's family should make the final decision about whether medical measures should be continued or discontinued. Increasingly, individuals are making such decisions themselves long before the need arises, and informing their families of their wishes by means of the "Living Will" (see page 1937 in Chapter 50).

Treatment and Nursing Care of the Person Who Is Unconscious. Not all persons who develop coma are in a hospital, and a problem sometimes faces the responsive person who comes across a comatose person sitting in a car or lying in the street. The problem is one of distinguishing between alcoholic stupor or stupor from any drug and other forms of coma. This is not easy. A few clues are that (1) the alcoholic can usually be aroused, (2) there is no irregularity in the pupils, and they will respond to light, and (3) paralysis of one side of the body, with a distortion of the face, is not present as it is likely to be in "a stroke," "apoplexy," *brain hemorrhage,* or "cerebral accident" as the condition is variously termed. Regardless of the cause, all comatose persons should be observed medically; needless deaths have occurred because passersby have assumed the unconscious or confused person to be "drunk." The odor of alcohol on the breath, or its absence, is a relatively unimportant sign since the person with a cerebral hemorrhage may very well have had a drink just before the accident occurred; nor is it always possible to recognize the odor of alcohol (for example, vodka) on the breath of the inebriated. The comatose person should be taken to a hospital or to his or her home where medical attention is available.

Coma is always a symptom of some disease process, and Adams[56] says the physician must approach an unconscious patient who is not known to him or her in a methodical way so that all the common and treatable causes are investigated. He says that therapeutic emergency measures take precedence over any diagnostic measures; however, if the patient does not seem to be suffering from asphyxia, hemorrhage, or shock he or she is transported to a place where adequate medical and nursing care can be given. If there is any reason to suspect injury to the cervical vertebrae, the person should be moved in the supine position with the head extended; otherwise, the prone position is advised to facilitate mouth drainage. Good alignment of body segments is important. The patient should be rolled "log-fashion," not lifted, onto the stretcher. Figure 40-6 shows a stretcher designed to reduce handling to a minimum.

When making a diagnosis, the physician does a very thorough physical examination that includes neurologic and reflex tests. There may be many contributory factors in coma; therefore, the physician is likely to x-ray the skull and to test the spinal fluid, blood, and urine. Liver function tests and estimates of the basal metabolic rate will be ordered. If there is fever or any sign of infection, suitable cultures will be made. An electrocardiogram and an electroencephalogram may be ordered. If there is reason to suspect poisoning, the stomach may be suctioned and washed out by lavage.

In the examinations and tests, nurses play an important role, as described in Chapters 5 and 6; in providing for the patient's hourly and daily physical needs they play the star role, and few persons survive prolonged coma without good nursing. Table 40-2 shows a comprehensive description of the patient's neurologic problems with nursing actions.

Whether a comatose patient has been newly admitted to the hospital or coma has developed during hospitalization, the same kinds of observations and examinations are necessary to help determine changes in his or her condition. Skilled nursing care is based on the nurse's knowledge of the diagnosis, his or her assessment of the patient's changing condition, the patient's physiologic needs, and the psychosocial needs of both the patient and the family.

For any comatose or semicomatose patient, the maintenance of adequate *respiration* is of

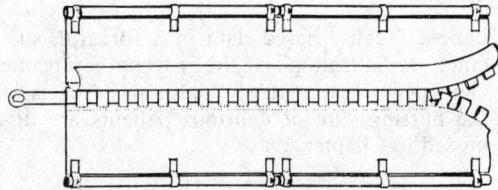

Figure 40-6. Separating stretcher to reduce movement of seriously injured patients to a minimum is of strong canvas construction, 28 by 74 inches. Halves interlock easily and are held together by a long metal strip. Used for ambulance patients and for operative eye, ear, and nose as well as other types of general cases, since the stretcher halves can be slid easily from under the patient. There are four rigid wood poles. (Courtesy of Melrose Hospital Uniform Co., Inc., Brooklyn, N.Y.)

utmost importance. Frequently, the respiratory center and the cough reflex are depressed; therefore, the rate, depth, and character of respirations, as well as the kind and amount of respiratory secretions, should be observed and reported. Placing the patient on the side and slightly over on the chest (semiprone position) is a most effective way to allow for drainage of mucus. Unconscious patients should not be left on their backs, because the relaxed tongue may fall over the glottis, and mucus cannot drain from the mouth while they are in this position. As they recover they are turned on the back for certain periods, if they prefer this position.

Should the patient require suctioning, the nurse must be able to suction the mouth skillfully and be aware of the dangers of the procedure, especially for the patient with a head injury. Suctioning of the nasopharynx can cause gagging or vomiting, and these activities can, in turn, increase intracranial pressure. If the patient has a tracheostomy, special care must be taken to keep the tube clean and to make certain the air is moist enough to prevent drying bronchotracheal secretions, for this increases the difficulty of removing them.

Blood pressure, pulse rate and character, pulse pressure, skin color, temperature, and general appearance all can indicate the condition of the patient's *circulatory* system. The patient whose blood pressure is increasing and whose pulse rate is decreasing may have rising intracranial pressure. However, if the reverse is true—that is, a decreasing blood pressure and increasing pulse rate—the patient is likely hemorrhaging. The condition of the patient's skin may not only indicate the adequacy of the patient's peripheral circulation, but may also show areas of excessive pressure that can develop into decubiti.

Maintaining a normal state of *nutrition* is perhaps the most difficult problem. Unless the swallowing reflex is present and patients in, at least partial, contact with reality, it is impossible to feed them by mouth. They may not suck on a drinking tube and food put in the mouth will stay there or, worse, be drawn into the respiratory passage. There are three choices used for feeding comatose patients: intravenous feeding, nasogastric intubation, or an incision into the stomach (gastrostomy) that makes it possible to put food directly in the stomach. Fluids given by nasal tube can be prepared so that they provide a complete diet. They can be bought ready for use or made in the hospital or home. Intravenous feeding will ultimately traumatize the veins, just as the passage of the nasal tube will traumatize the nose, pharynx, and esophagus. Intubation must

be skillfully managed to avoid insufflation of food and mucus when the tube is withdrawn. Authorities recommend oral feeding in small amounts as soon as the swallowing reflex is re-established. The quantity fed by mouth is increased as rapidly as the patient tolerates it until tube feeding can be dispensed with. (Nasal gavage is described in detail in Chapter 23.)

Gastrostomy feeding is indicated when the patient cannot take food orally for a long time. The gastrostomy tube is placed in the stomach through a surgical incision in the upper abdomen, and sutured in place. It is essential that the area of skin around the tube be kept clean and dry. Foods given through the gastrostomy tube are the same as those given by nasogastric tube, and the same amounts given at the same intervals (see Chapter 23).

There are many commercial preparations available for tube feedings. A regular diet made to a fine puree with a blender is often the best since it is most likely to produce normal stools. Protein and vitamins are essential for tissue repair and wound healing; therefore a complete diet is especially important when these are involved. Esta Carini and Guy Owens [57] recommend a high-vitamin, high-protein feeding of 2500 to 3000 calories in 2500 to 3000 ml of fluid in each 24 hours for an adult, unless the physician prescribes otherwise. Regurgitations of tube feedings with the possibility of respiratory aspiration can be lessened by giving small, frequent feedings. Nurses should realize that any other method than oral feeding is a poor substitute for normal eating. As soon as it is safe to do so they should start feeding the patient; first liquids and then solids, gradually increasing the amounts until intubation or intravenous feeding can be discontinued.

The maintenance of *fluid and electrolyte balance* depends upon the nature of the feeding, the amount taken, and the functioning of the organs of elimination. Excessive sweating, vomiting, and diarrhea can seriously upset the balance. Nurses must be aware of these dangers and assume their share of the responsibility for seeing that fluid and electrolyte balance is maintained either by intubation, intravenous infusions, or oral feeding.

The body's normal mechanisms for maintaining fluid and electrolyte balance are discussed in detail in Chapter 10, and methods and medications or nutrients used to manage disturbances of this balance are discussed in Chapters 22 and 23. A patient's loss of fluid through the urinary tract, mucous membranes, or skin, or through vomitus or feces should be measured or estimated as accurately as possible

[*Text continues on page 1610.*]

Table 40-2. Standard Care Routine—Neurological Record *

Problem	Outcome	Deadline	Nursing Actions
Deterioration in level of consciousness due to 1. Wide and direct depression of the function of *both* cerebral hemispheres (i.e., metabolic disorder—drugs ↓ sugar ↑ O₂ ↑ or ↓ sugar ↑ CO₂ or mass effect) (by pressure from above). 2. Depression or destruction of the brainstem-activating systems (reticular activity system).†	Early detection and reporting of change (this is usually first sign noticed by the nurse). Patient is alert and oriented.	Check with NSR	Evaluate present testing in terms of previous testing referring to the following categories and S.O.A.P. any changes on progress notes. *Eye Opening* 1. *Spontaneous opening.* When the patient is first approached he may have his eyes open. This finding implies that the arousal mechanisms in the reticular activating system of the brainstem are functioning. Of course, at times, such a patient will sleep and have his eyes closed. In some brain-damaged patients the natural diurnal rhythm may be reversed, the patient being alert during the night and asleep during the day. 2. *Opening to speech.* When the patient's eyes are not open at the start of the examination the nurse should first speak and then if necessary shout to him. Usually the patient's name is called and he is requested to open his eyes, but if this occurs the important point is that it is in response to stimulation by sound rather than to any specific command. 3. *Opening to pain.* If verbal stimulation is unsuccessful in achieving eye opening, physical stimulation is applied. The most useful method is to exert pressure on the patient's fingernail bed by means of a pen or pencil. It is seldom of practical value to attempt more subtle distinctions such as whether only a light shaking or various grades of pressure or pain are required. 4. *No eye opening.* Absence of opening of even one eye in response to painful stimulation implies a marked degree of depression of the arousal system. *Best Verbal Response* 1. *Oriented.* After arousing the patient the nurse asks him who he is and also where he is and what the year and month are. If accurate answers are obtained, the patient is recorded as being oriented. It is unreasonable to expect the patient to give the exact date of the month, as even nurses and doctors sometimes forget this. 2. *Confused conversation.* This is recorded when the patient is capable of producing language, for instance, phrases, sentences, and even conversational exchanges, but is unable to give the correct answers to questions about orientation.

1604

3. *Inappropriate words*. The patient speaks or exclaims only a word or two (often swear words). Such a response is usually obtained only by physical stimulation rather than a verbal approach, although occasionally a patient will shout obscenities or call relatives' names for no apparent reason.

4. *Incomprehensible sounds*. The patient's verbal responses consist of groans, moans, or indistinct mumbling and do not contain any intelligible words.

5. *No verbal response*. Prolonged and, if necessary, repeated stimulation does not produce any phonation. The patient's verbal response may be impaired as a result of a single focal lesion of the speech area in the dominant hemisphere, that is, "aphasia." The assessment of such a patient's language ability can include written instructions and written replies. The level of verbal response achieved should still be indicated, but an appropriate note may be made that the impairment is considered to be due to dysphasia (D = dysphasia).

Best Motor Response

1. *Obeys commands*. This requires an ability to appreciate instructions, usually given in the form of verbal commands but sometimes by gestures, or even in writing. The patient is required to perform the specific movements requested. After the patient has been maximally aroused, a variety of commands may be tried: "open your eyes," "put out your tongue," "hold up your arms."

   A commonly used test is to ask the patient to squeeze the examiner's fingers, but this suffers from a number of disadvantages. A nonspecific sound stimulus may induce a reflex contraction of the patient's fingers or, alternatively, such a reflex response can result from the physical presence of the examiner's fingers against the palm of the patient. Before it is accepted that the patient is truly obeying commands, it is wise to test that the patient will also release and squeeze again to repeated commands.

2. *Response to pain*. If the patient does not obey commands, physical stimuli are applied. First, the fingertips are stimulated in the same manner as when testing for eye opening to painful stimulation. Subsequently it may be appropriate to test for "localizing" by stimulating the patient's head by pressure over the supraorbital notch, or pinching the opposite shoulder.

Table 40-2. Standard Care Routine—Neurological Record (Continued)

Problem	Outcome	Deadline	Nursing Actions
			3. *Localizes pain.* This is recorded when the patient moves a limb in such a way as to locate the painful stimulus on head or trunk, in an attempt to remove it.
			4. *Flexion response.* After painful stimulation at the fingertip the arm bends at the elbow but does not achieve a localizing response when stimulated at other sites.
			5. *Extension response.* In response to stimulation, the elbows straighten. In some instances the extension of the elbow is accompanied by inward rotation at the shoulder and in the forearm with the wrist being flexed and the fingers straightened. The limbs may even adopt this posture without stimulation. This response corresponds to what is often termed "decerebrate rigidity," but using this term without a clear definition can give rise to confusion. Also decerebrate carries the implication of a lesion of the midbrain, which in many cases is erroneous.
			6. *No response to pain.* This is scored when repeated and varied stimulation elicits no detectable movement or change in tone of the limbs. The scale of responses to pain is applicable to the movements of the arms. Record the better of the two sides of the body if there is a difference between them.
Any change in pupil size and/or reaction of one or both pupils due to impairment of: 1. Optic nerve (extremely rare) 2. Third nerve and its brainstem connections 3. Sympathetic fibers to eye (Horner's syndrome) 4. Drugs—i.e., narcotics, pilocarpine, atropine, etc.	Early detection and reporting of changes.	Check with NSR	*On Testing Pupils* Make certain that there is an even distribution of light in the room. Ask the patient to open his eyes and look at the nurse, or open them if he cannot. By observation note whether the pupils are equal in size or whether one side is larger than the other. Examine both eyes at same time for equality of size (look at both eyes without flashlight). Using a flashlight and shining it into the patient's eyes (one at a time) from the side, check to see that the pupil constricts (becomes smaller) with the added light. 1. *Size:* the size is measured by comparing it with the series of circulamillimeter measures on the chart. 2. *Reaction:* when assessing pupil reaction use a bright light and have dim surroundings—if the light is not bright enough and the surroundings too bright, an absent response may be mistakenly obtained—record only the presence or absence of reaction.

Impaired limb movement due to lesion of the opposite cerebral cortex and/or its connections (usually weakness appears on the opposite side of the body to where the lesion is).

Early detection and reporting of change.

Check with NSR and PRN

Consider whether the patient is right- or lefthanded.

Check for "drift" in both arms, i.e., have patient close his eyes and extend both arms perpendicular to his chest for 15–20 seconds to see whether either arm falls even slightly.

Test hand grips by crossing your own arms so that your left hand is in contact with patient's left hand and your right hand with the patient's right. This helps you to remember which side, if any, is weak.

Present your first two fingers for the patient to grip.

Ask the patient to squeeze your fingers.

Check to see that the patient is able to release the grip on command.

Test strength of legs by patient's ability to lift them off the bed and wriggle his toes.

1. *Normal power* is recorded when the examiner considers that the limb movements are appropriate to the normal muscle strength for that patient.

2. *Weakness of movement* covers a wide range between normal and no response. It is difficult to make absolute distinctions between various degrees of weakness. These are, in practice, less important than making comparisons between the limbs on either side or detecting a change in an individual limb between successive examinations. Sufficient information for this purpose is conveyed by recording either (a) mild or (b) severe weakness. If one limb appears to show normal power but its opposite is less strong, mild weakness is recorded; if the difference is very marked, severe weakness is recorded. If the strength on both sides is reduced but to different degrees, mild and severe weakness would indicate the stronger and weaker side respectively.

The preceding terms can be applied both to movement to command and after painful stimulation.

3. *Spastic flexion* describes a movement of the arm which is slow and accompanied by stiffness. The limb tends to take up a "hemiplegic" position with the forearm and hand held against the body. This is obviously different from both normal withdrawal response and severe weakness. In the withdrawal response, although the elbow flexes, the movement is rapid, the arm is drawn away from the trunk, and stiffness of the muscles is not found. In severe weakness the limb is generally limp.

Table 40-2. Standard Care Routine—Neurological Record (*Continued*)

Problem	Outcome	Deadline	Nursing Actions
			4. *Extension*—the limb is straightened at the elbow or knee joint, and in the upper limb there is marked inward rotation of the hand.
			5. *No response* is recorded if the limb is limp and does not respond in any way to stimulation.
			The arms and legs are divided into different sections: spastic flexion is recorded only for the arms. When the two sides are the same, recordings are made in the normal manner, but when differences exist, right and left can be recorded independently with the letters **R** and **L**, respectively.
Increase or decrease of 30 mm in blood pressure due to pressure on vasodilator and vasoconstrictor centers in the medulla or increase in pulse pressure (difference between systolic and diastolic).	Early detection and reporting of significant change. Blood pressure is within normal limits for the individual patient.	Check with NSR	Position patient flat in bed with head down (unless contraindicated). Recheck blood pressure to make certain you are accurate. (Systolic is the first beat heard; diastolic is the last beat heard.) Give antihypertensive drugs as ordered and chart when they are given on the NSR sheet in red.
Decrease or increase in pulse rate due to change of pressure within the arteries (pulse becomes full and bounding) or as pressure is exerted upon them.	Early detection and reporting of significant changes outside the normal range for the individual patient (60–100 beats per minute in an adult is considered to be normal).	Check with NSR and/or blood pressure	Rouse patient before taking pulse (pulse is decreased when sleeping). Note strength and rhythm of pulse as well as rate. Feel for apical, femoral, carotid, or pedal pulse if unable to get a radial pulse. Take pulse for 60 seconds.
Change in rate, type, and character of respirations due to effects on various areas of brain.	Early detection and reporting of changes in respirations. Respirations are maintained within the accepted limits for the individual patient.	Check with NSR and PRN	Observe and record rate, depth, and character of respirations for a full minute—changes in respiration, in coma (i.e., Cheyne-Stokes, stridor). Note patient's color, i.e., cyanotic, etc. Maintain patent airway by suctioning and/or changing position (both head and body) on the patient's side or semi-prone. Insert airway if indicated. Check to see if change is related to medications and/or treatment.

1608

Increase in temperature due to pressure on the temperature-regulating center in the hypothalamus.

Temperature within normal range, 36–37.5 °C.

Check with NSR or q4h

Temperature is taken **BID** routinely, orally or rectally. The manner and frequency are determined by the patient's condition or frequency at neurologic testing.

Use rectal thermometers for seizure patients, children, restless patients, patients with lowered conscious level, tracheostomy patients, and postoperative patients.

Remove any extra clothing and linen if temperature is elevated. Tylenol or A.S.A. as ordered (rectally depending on the patient). Sponge with alcohol, alcojel, untinted savlon 1:100, cooling blanket if available. Push fluids if not contraindicated.

Chart temperature in red on **NSR** record (because at times systolic pressure and temperature may run into each other).

---

* (Courtesy of University Hospital, University of Western Ontario, London, Canada.)
† Network of gray matter and interlacing fibers of white matter found in medulla, midbrain, and pons.

so that fluid intake and output can be kept in balance.

Elimination is a serious problem during comatose states. Sphincter control of the urinary bladder and rectum is often lost. The care of the incontinent patient is described in Chapter 37. Little can be added here to that discussion. An indwelling catheter will protect the skin from repeated contacts with urine which predisposes the patient to pressure sores; it will reduce the amount of linen and the quantity of Cellucotton, etc., needed; on the other hand, a catheter is a foreign body in the bladder and its presence almost inevitably results in the development of a stubborn low-grade cystitis which makes rehabilitation very difficult. More and more authorities on the care of the unconscious are advising against the use of catheters. Cranberry juice may be given to the patient to increase urine acidity and lessen the possibility of bacterial growth in the urinary system. Again, it is a question of a choice of two imperfect practices. Some physicians and nurses prefer to use a catheter of the Foley type, with tidal drainage that provides automatic filling and emptying of the bladder so bladder muscle tone is maintained and the hazard of pressure sores from constantly wet skin is reduced. Normal elimination should be reestablished as soon as possible.

Daily bowel elimination should be encouraged by including laxative foods in the tube feeding. Prune juice, for example, is very effective. If indicated, mild laxatives may be added to the feedings, and, if necessary, a colonic lavage given daily until the bowel resumes its tone and normal functionings. The bowel movement should be induced at the patient's regular hour for defecation, if this is known, and observed for amount, consistency, and color. Feces can easily accumulate in the rectum until they are impacted if the nurse does not make sure that there is adequate daily elimination. If the rectum is impacted, Carini and Owens [58] recommend hydrogen peroxide retention enemas.

When the patient is deeply unconscious and motionless, the nurse must move the patient every hour. *Body movement* is essential for normal maintenance of many functions, but the nurse's most immediate concern is the prevention of hypostatic pneumonia and pressure sores which can develop very rapidly. Change of position, adequate nutrition, and cleanliness are the chief means of reducing the latter hazard.

Contractures must be prevented during unconscious states by change of posture, placing the patient in physiologic positions, rather than contracted ones, and occasionally by splinting joints when there is a tendency to flexion. The patient is kept in side-lying positions chiefly (see Chapter 12). Turning sheets reduce the effort involved and help to keep the body segments in good alignment. In some cases the surgeon gives specific directions about the position of the patient and how he or she should be turned. Figure 40-7 *A–D* shows the use of a lifting sheet in turning the patient with a spinal injury.

Range-of-motion exercises to all extremities, hips, and shoulders should be carried out daily unless contraindicated by the nature of the illness or injury. Massage, however, is not recommended because of the possibility that venous stasis with thrombus formation exists and fatal emboli could be dislodged.

With returning consciousness, patients should be encouraged to participate in, and finally take responsibility for, exercising unless they are completely paralyzed. Patients should not remain bedfast any longer than is necessary. Even if they must be lifted, it is desirable to get them into a chair or move them by stretcher. They need both the activity and the change of scene as their condition improves.

Except for convulsive movements, the deeply unconscious patient is motionless, but many comatose patients are also restless. They may vary from hour to hour or day to day in their awareness or depth of unconsciousness, and for this reason it is rarely safe to assume that the stuporous, irrational, and disoriented may not be in danger of falling from bed or otherwise subjecting themselves to injury if left alone. *Protection of the unconscious* from injury is an essential part of the nursing program. Bedsides, or homemade substitutes for them, should be used when it is necessary to leave the patient unattended. Restraints should always be used with caution since they often cause severe restlessness in patients who are unconscious or in a decreasing state of consciousness. Straining against restraints can also cause increased intracranial pressure in a patient who has cerebral injury.

Intuitive nurses who can discover the cause of the restlessness and relieve it often reduce the need for restraint to a minimum. They should explain to the patient what is going to happen and what is happening and hope that he or she understands enough to relieve some of the anxiety. Nurses should, of course, remove causes of physical discomfort that lead to restlessness, if this is possible.

A firm bed is desirable. Sponge-rubber mattresses reduce the difficulty of preventing pressure sores, and sponge-rubber pads can be used in a variety of ways for support. There are also alternating pressure mattresses available and in wide use for preventing continuous pressure and possible decubiti on any body part. Waterbeds (hydrobeds) are also used.

Because patients cannot say that they are hot or cold, they are dependent upon the nurse for this aspect of their physical comfort or protection. The body temperature is measured by rectum during coma, as one might suppose. This is some guide in clothing and covering the patient adequately and in regulation of the room temperature. Feeling the feet, as one would a baby's, tells the nurse whether the patient is overheated, comfortable, or cold. External heat should be applied with particular caution since patients cannot protect themselves from burns.

Cleanliness for unconscious patients is not easily achieved. As in infancy, they are dependent upon the nurse. A daily bath is important for the stimulation of the circulation and to prevent skin lesions. Soap should be avoided and neutral cleansing agents substituted. Skin lubricants, such as the commercial preparation "Alpha Keri" lotion, vegetable oils, or lanolin should be applied. Alcohol is drying, and therefore contraindicated in most cases. Incontinence should be managed, if possible, so that the bed is not soiled repeatedly, but if this occurs the patient should be sponged, dried, and the bed linen changed at once. Many of the infant care products are good for the protection of the skin and cornstarch is an inexpensive and highly effective product to apply to the buttocks and other areas where moisture may collect.

It is important to clean the mouth of the unconscious even more carefully than that of most patients. (Removable dentures should not be worn until consciousness returns.) During the process patients should lie on the side with the head tilted so that water put into the mouth runs out into a basin, rather than down the throat. If this occurs, there is little danger in rinsing the mouth with fluid introduced with a syringe. Motorized mouth suction is so helpful in caring for the unconscious that the apparatus should be rented when it is not otherwise available. Figures 14-11 *A–C* in Chapter 14 shows the nurse using a toothbrush to clean the mouth of a comatose woman. A soft rubber catheter, size #20 or #22 French, is used in suctioning. The teeth should be brushed two or three times daily, and the mouth rinsed every few hours with water or a mouthwash. The lips should be lubricated with cold cream to prevent drying and cracking.

Since the patient cannot blow his or her nose, the passages may be occluded by encrusted mucus. Unless there is bleeding from the nose, or a head injury that contraindicates the procedure, the nurse should clean the nostrils as described in Chapter 14. Following a head injury, spinal fluid may drain from the nose. Any sign of this should be reported at once.

With deep unconsciousness the winking reflex may be absent; this takes away the patient's involuntary means of protecting the cornea and conjunctiva from injury. In such cases the eye can be protected by closing the lids with a dressing such as that shown in Figure 33-1, Chapter 33. The dressing should be removed and the eye examined every few days. Untreated irritation may lead to permanent injury. The physician will order medication and possibly irrigation, if conjunctivitis develops.

Ears should be examined for bleeding if there has been a brain injury. Sterile cotton may be kept in them. Any cleaning done should be very gentle and aseptic precautions taken. The surgeon should approve the method used. Evidence of bleeding or meningeal fluid draining from the ears should be reported at once.

For the family's sake, if not for the patient's, the hair should be brushed and combed becomingly. In cases of brain surgery it may be necessary to cut the hair or even shave the head. A head covering can be devised that is quite attractive. Shampoos cause minimum disturbance if given skillfully by several workers who, in helping each other, can shorten the time required for the procedure. There are several commercial dry shampoos that may be substituted for wet shampoos.

It is not unusual to find unconscious patients in a gloomy environment, others assuming that they are unable to enjoy their surroundings. The writers believe this an unwise position to take. In the first place, there is no exact measure of the patient's awareness, and,

Figure 40-7. Turning a patient with a cervical cord injury to his left side with the aid of a draw sheet. This is done in four steps: *A.* Draw sheet is pulled tight beneath the patient. *B.* Patient is rolled toward his left. *C.* Patient is turned on his left side at the edge of the bed. *D.* Patient is moved to the center of the bed. Note the attendant turning the patient's head throughout the procedure. (From Munro, Donald: *The Treatment of Injuries to the Nervous System.* W. B. Saunders Co., Philadelphia, 1952.)

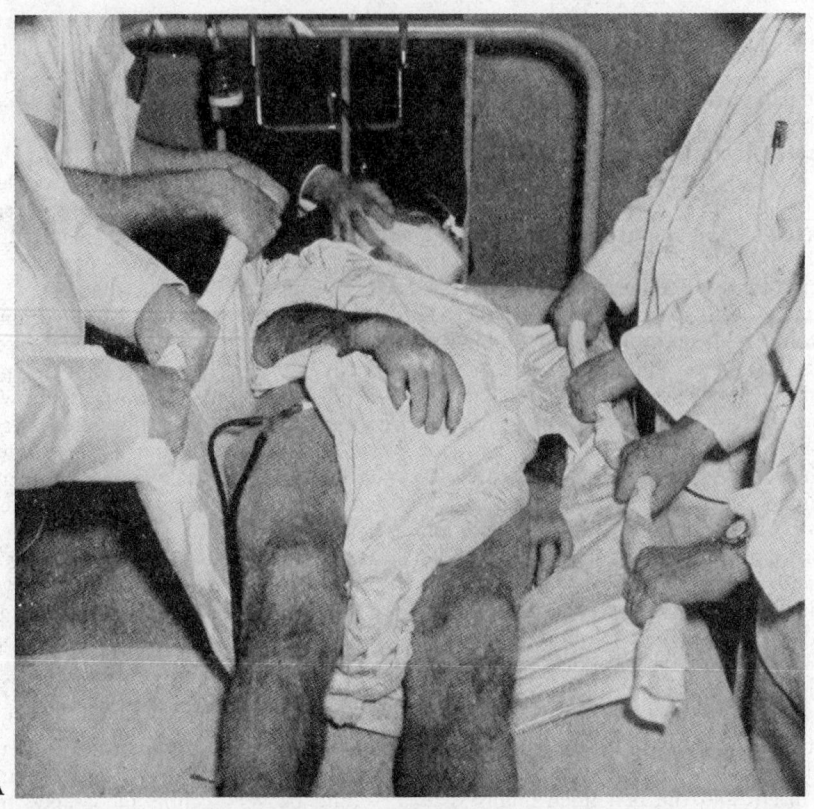

A

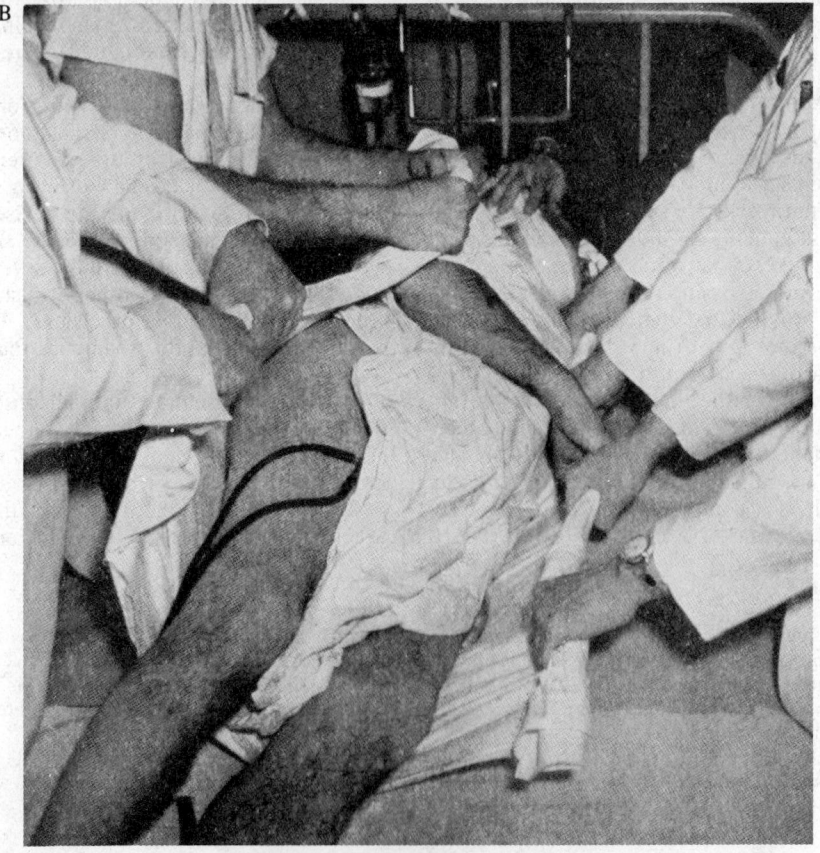

B

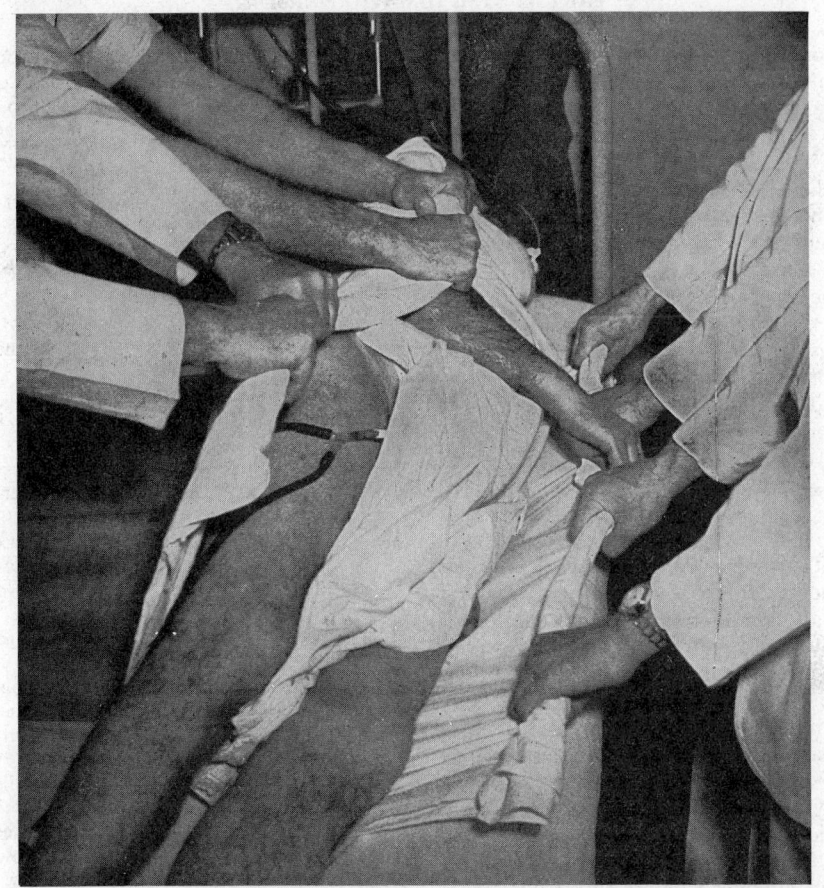

C

D

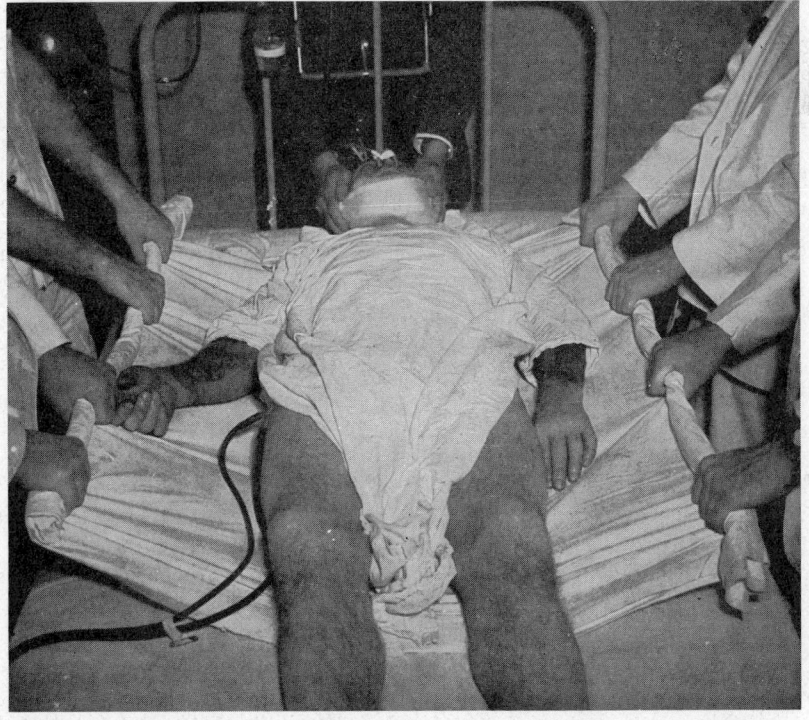

in the second place, the environment reacts on the patient's family and friends and on those in attendance upon him or her. The room should be kept at a comfortable temperature. It should not only be free from unpleasant odors and sights, but made attractive to the senses. The more normal and cheerful the environment, the less confusing it is to the person as consciousness returns, and the more normal the outlook of those who care for him or her. Positive factors such as change of furnishings, music, and perfumes might be studied for their effect on the comatose, particularly if the state is believed to have a psychogenic origin and is prolonged.

The *psychologic aspects* of nursing the unconscious are more often neglected than the physical aspects. Medical workers, friends, and families make the *serious* mistake of talking in the patient's presence as if he or she could not hear.* They often speak discouragingly about the patient's condition or perhaps complainingly of the care required. Even if they do not commit one of these gross blunders, they increase the confusion in the patient's mind by saying things he or she cannot understand. It is wise to assume at all times that patients may be able to hear and, therefore, to refrain from saying anything in their presence that should not be said to them. As patients seem to recover, but still cannot speak, a conversation between their intimates who are sitting with them may be encouraging, interesting, or entertaining, if they try to make it so.

A program of rehabilitation should be planned and initiated at once if there is a chance that the patient will survive the condition underlying the unconscious state. This optimism will communicate itself to the patient, and he or she will be encouraged to fight for a return to health, if others seem to expect it.

REFERENCES

1. Adams, Raymond D.: "Coma and Related Disturbances of Consciousness," in Wintrobe,

---

* Various methods of communication with aphasic patients have been devised. In one method the alphabet has been divided into quarters, and then the individual letters identified by numbers. The patient is asked, "First, second, third, or fourth." Then, when the correct portion of the alphabet has been identified by the patient's nodding the head, he or she is asked, "First, second, etc., letter." This method is laborious, but in short-term illnesses has proved useful. Another method is based on the sign language; however, instead of using signs for individual letters, the various gestures represent phases such as "I am thirsty."

Maxwell M., et al. (eds.): *Harrison's Principles of Internal Medicine,* 7th ed. McGraw-Hill Book Co., New York, 1974, p. 716.
2. Freedman, Alfred M., et al.: *Modern Synopsis of Psychiatry.* Williams & Wilkins Co., Baltimore, 1972, p. 190.
3. Plum, Fred: "Consciousness and Its Disturbances," in Beeson, Paul B., and McDermott, Walsh (eds.): *Textbook of Medicine,* Vol. I, 14th ed. W. B. Saunders Co., Philadelphia, 1975, p. 540.
4. Guyton, Arthur C.: *Textbook of Medical Physiology,* 5th ed. W. B. Saunders Co., Philadelphia, 1976, p. 729.
4a. Geschwind, Norman: "Language and the Brain," *Sci. Am.,* 226:76, (Apr.) 1972.
5. *Ibid.,* p. 734.
6. Nash, John: *Developmental Psychology: A Psychobiological Approach.* Prentice-Hall, Inc., Englewood Cliffs, N.J., 1970, p. 100.
7. Quesenbury, Jeanne H., and Lembright, Pamela: "Observations and Care for Patients with Head Injuries," *Nurs. Clin. North Am.,* 4:239, (June) 1969.
8. Elbert, R. V.: "Syncope," *Circulation,* 27: 1148 (June) 1963.
9. Wayne, H. H.: "Syncope. Physiological Consideration and an Analysis of the Clinical Characteristics in 510 Patients," *Am. J. Med.,* 30:418, (Mar.) 1961.
9a. Patten, John P.: "Faints and Falls," *Nurs. Times,* 68:967, (Aug. 3) 1972.
10. Stead, Eugene A.: "Fainting (Syncope)," in MacBryde, Cyril M., and Blacklow, Robert S. (eds.): *Signs and Symptoms; Applied Pathologic Physiology and Clinical Interpretation,* 5th ed. J. B. Lippincott Co., Philadelphia, 1970, p. 712.
11. Cole, Warren H., and Puestow, Charles B.: *Emergency Care—Surgical and Medical,* 7th ed. Appleton-Century-Crofts, New York, 1972, p. 358.
12. Heyman, Albert: "Hyperventilation," in Beeson, Paul B., and McDermott, Walsh (eds.): *Textbook of Medicine,* Vol. I, 14th ed. W. B. Saunders Co., Philadelphia, 1975, p. 629.
13. Adams, Raymond D., and Braunwald, Eugene: "Faintness, Syncope, Episodic Weakness," in Wintrobe, Maxwell M., et al. (eds.): *Harrison's Principles of Internal Medicine,* 7th ed. McGraw-Hill Book Co., New York, 1974, p. 72.
14. Heyman, Albert: "Syncope," in Beeson, Paul B., and McDermott, Walsh (eds.): *Textbook of Medicine,* Vol. I, 14th ed. W. B. Saunders Co., Philadelphia, 1975, p. 626.
15. Adams, Raymond D., and Braunwald, Eugene: *op. cit.*
16. Simonton, Kinsey M.: "Dizziness, Vertigo and Imbalance," *Okla. State Med. Assoc. J.,* 64:63, (Feb.) 1971.
17. Victor, Maurice, and Adams, Raymond D.: "Dizziness, Vertigo and Disorders of Gait," in Wintrobe, Maxwell M., et al. (eds.): *Harrison's Principles of Internal Medicine,* 7th

ed. McGraw-Hill Book Co., New York, 1974, p. 94.

18. Hyland, H. H.: "Vertigo and Dizziness," in MacBryde, Cyril M., and Blacklow, Robert S. (eds.): *Signs and Symptoms; Applied Pathologic Physiology and Clinical Interpretation,* 5th ed. J. B. Lippincott Co., Philadelphia, 1970, p. 741.
19. Brain, W. R.: "Vertigo of Central Origin," *Proc. R. Soc. Med.,* **55:**361, 1962.
20. Guyton, Arthur C.: *op. cit.,* p. 700.
21. Paparella, Michael M.: "The Dizzy Patient," *Postgrad. Med.,* **52:**97, (Aug.) 1972.
22. Simonton, Kinsey M.: *op. cit.*
23. Guyton, Arthur C.: *op. cit.*
24. Musser, Ruth D., and O'Neil, John J.: *Pharmacology and Therapeutics,* 4th ed. Macmillan Publishing Co., Inc., New York, 1969, p. 486.
25. Paparella, Michael M.: *op. cit.*
26. Barber, H. O.: "Dizziness and Head Injury," *Can. Med. Assoc. J.,* **92:**974, (May 1) 1965.
27. Victor, Maurice, and Adams, Raymond D.: *op. cit.*
28. Maddox, H. Edward: "Advances in the Evaluation of the Dizzy Patient," *Tex. Med.,* **67:**66, (Aug.) 1972.
29. Simonton, Kinsey M.: *op. cit.*
30. Paparella, Michael M.: *op. cit.*
31. Lindsay, J. R.: "Pathology of Vestibular Disorders, *Ann. Otol.,* **76:**193, 1968.
32. Hallpike, C. S., and Crains, H.: "Observations on the Pathology of Meniere's Syndrome," *J. Laryngol. Otol.,* **53:**625, (Oct.) 1938.
33. Simonton, Kinsey M.: *op. cit.*
34. Paparella, Michael M.: *op. cit.*
34a. Blancher, Gertrude C.: "My Trip Through the Semicircular Canals," *Am. J. Nurs.,* **74:**1842, (Oct.) 1974.
35. Drachman, David A.: "Dizziness and Vertigo," in Beeson, Paul B., and McDermott, Walsh (eds.): *Textbook of Medicine,* 14th ed. W. B. Saunders Co., Philadelphia, 1975, p. 623.
36. Linn, Louis: "Clinical Manifestation of Psychiatric Disorders," in Freedman, Alfred M., et al. (eds.): *Comprehensive Textbook of Psychiatry,* Vol. I, 2nd ed. Williams & Wilkins Co., Baltimore, 1975, p. 801.
37. Ayres, Stephen M., and Giannelli, Stanley: *Care of the Critically Ill.* Appleton-Century-Crofts, New York, 1967, p. 90.
38. Linn, Louis: *op. cit.*
39. *Ibid.*
40. Freedman, Alfred M., et al: *op. cit.,* p. 191.
41. Adams, Raymond D., and Victor, Maurice: "Derangements of Intellect and Behavior Due to Diffuse and Focal Cerebral Disease," in Wintrobe, Maxwell M., et al. (eds.): *Harrison's Principles of Internal Medicine,* 7th ed. McGraw-Hill Book Co., New York, 1974 p. 156.
42. *Ibid.,* p. 156.
43. *Ibid.*
43a Jaeger, Dorothea, and Simmons, Leo W.: *The*

Aged Ill. Appleton-Century-Crofts, New York, 1970.
44. Gerdes, Lenore: "The Confused or Delirious Patient," *Am. J. Nurs.,* **68:**1228, (June) 1968.
45. McHugh, Paul R.: "Dementia," in Beeson, Paul B., and McDermott, Walsh (eds.): *Textbook of Medicine,* Vol. I, 14th ed. W. B. Saunders Co., Philadelphia, 1975, p. 558.
46. Adams, Raymond D., and Victor, Maurice: *op. cit.,* p. 156.
47. Moses, Dorothy V.: "The Older Patient in the General Hospital," *Nurs. Clin. North Am.,* **2:**705, (Dec.) 1967.
48. Weymouth, Lilyan T.: "The Nursing Care of the So-Called Confused Patient," *Nurs. Clin. North Am.,* **3:**709, (Dec.) 1968.
49. Smith, Barbara G.: "Patterned Program Nursing for the Confused," in *ANA Clinical Sessions, 1970.* Appleton-Century-Crofts, New York, 1971, p. 93.
49a. Fowler, Roy S., and Fordyce, Wilbert: "Adapting Care for the Brain-Damaged Patient," *Am. J. Nurs.,* **72:**2056, (Nov.) 1972.
50. Aita, John A.: "Everyman's Psychosis—The Delirium, Part I," *Nebr. State Med. J.,* **53:** 389, (Aug.) 1968.
51. Adams, Raymond D., and Victor, Maurice: *op. cit.,* p. 164.
52. Morse, Robert M., and Litin, Edward M.: "Postoperative Delirium: A Study of Etiologic Factors," *Am. J. Psychiatry,* **126:**136, (Sept.) 1969.
53. Kornfeld, Donald S., et al.: "Psychological Hazards of the Intensive Care Unit," *Nurs. Clin. North Am.,* **3:**41, (Mar.) 1968.
53a. Burk, Mary Louise: "Critical-Care Nursing in the Docent Team Concept," *Heart Lung,* **1:**490, (July–Aug.) 1972.
54. Katz, Nevin M., et al.: "Delirium in Surgical Patients Under Intensive Care," *Arch. Surg.,* **104:**310, (Mar.) 1972.
55. Ad Hoc Committee of Harvard Medical School: "A Definition of Irreversible Coma," *J.A.M.A.,* **205:**85, (Aug. 5) 1968.
56. Adams, Raymond D.: *op. cit.,* p. 116.
57. Carini, Esta, and Owens, Guy: *Neurological and Neurosurgical Nursing,* 6th ed. C. V. Mosby Co., St. Louis, 1974, p. 144.
58. *Ibid.,* p. 111.

Additional Suggested Reading

Alter, Milton: "Examination of the Comatose Patient," *Minn. Med.,* **51:**1175, (Sept.) 1968.
Brooks, Helen L.: "The Golden Rule for the Unconscious Patient," *Nurs. Forum,* **4:**12, (No. 3) 1965.
Bruya, Margaret Auld, and Bolin, Rose Homan: "Epilepsy: A Controllable Disease. Part I. Classification and Diagnosis of Seizures," *Am. J. Nurs.,* **76:**388, (Mar.) 1976.
———: "Epilepsy: A Controllable Disease. Part II. Drug Therapy and Nursing Care," *Am. J. Nurs.,* **76:**393, (Mar.) 1976.
Chambers, Carolyn: "Senility or Deprivation?" in *ANA Clinical Sessions, 1966.* Appleton-Century-Crofts, New York, 1967.

Clipper, Margaret: "Nursing Care of Patients in a Neurologic Intensive Care Unit," *Nurs. Clin. North Am.,* **4:**211, (June) 1969.

Field, William E., and Ruelke, Wylma: "Hallucinations and How to Deal with Them," *Am. J. Nurs.,* **73:**638, (Apr.) 1973.

Gardner, M. Arlene Martin: "Responsiveness as a Measure of Consciousness," *Am. J. Nurs.,* **68:**1035, (May) 1968.

Gelperin, Abraham, and Gelperin, Eve A.: "The Inebriate in the Emergency Room," *Am. J. Nurs.,* **70:**1494, (July) 1970.

Hayter, Jean: "Patients Who Have Alzheimer's Disease," *Am. J. Nurs.,* **74:**1460, (Aug.) 1974.

Hedburg, Allan G., and Schlong, Audrey: "Eliminating Fainting by School Children During Mass Inoculation Clinics," *Nurs. Res.,* **22:**352, (July–Aug.) 1973.

Hoskins, Lois M.: "Vascular and Tension Headaches," *Am. J. Nurs.,* **74:**846, (May) 1974.

Lindsay, John R.: "Postural Vertigo," *Minn. Med.,* **50:**1013, (June) 1967.

Mays, E. Truman, et al.: "Metabolic Changes in Surgical Delirium Tremens," *Surgery,* **67:**780, (May) 1970.

McNally, W. J.: "The Assessment of Vertigo," *Minn. Med.,* **50:**1003, (June) 1967.

Meinhart, Noreen T., and Aspinall, Mary Jo: "Nursing Interventions in Hypovigilance," *Am. J. Nurs.,* **69:**994, (May) 1969.

Miller, Jean: "Cognitive Dissonance in Modifying Families' Perceptions," *Am. J. Nurs.,* **74:**1468, (Aug.) 1974.

Moraczewski, Albert: "The Hopelessly Unconscious Patient," *Postgrad. Med.,* **44:**126, (Dec.) 1968.

Morris, Magdelena, and Rhodes, Martha: "Guidelines for the Care of Confused Patients," *Am. J. Nurs.,* **72:**1630, (Sept.) 1972.

Rubinstein, David, and Thomas, John K.: "Psychiatric Findings in Cardiotomy Patients," *Am. J. Psychiatry,* **126:**360, (Sept.) 1969.

Skelly, Madge: "Re-Thinking Stroke, Aphasic Patients Talk Back," *Am. J. Nurs.,* **75:**1140, (July) 1975.

Slater, Marianne Costopoulos: "Nursing Intervention for the Patient with Central Nervous System Dysfunction," in Kintzel, Kay Corman (ed.): *Advanced Concepts in Clinical Nursing.* J. B. Lippincott Co., Philadelphia, 1971.

Wallace, James F.: "Infectious Delirium," *Southwest. Med.,* **50:**181, (Oct.) 1969.

Williams, Henry J.: "The Episodic Vertigoes," *Minn. Med.,* **50:**1008, (June) 1967.

Gladys Nite
Catherine Temple
Virginia Henderson

CHAPTER 41

Anxiety, Depression, Insomnia

1. ANXIETY
2. DEPRESSION
3. INSOMNIA

1. ANXIETY

Anxiety is commonly defined as a diffuse, unpleasant, vague feeling of apprehension, nervousness, or dread expressed both somatically and psychically. Many investigators think that, like fear, it is a reaction to a threat; however, unlike fear—a response to a known, definite, external, and immediate danger—anxiety is felt as a threat from something unknown, vague, internal, and in the future.

Anxiety is considered by some authorities to be entirely disruptive, handicapping, and destructive because it severely limits the efforts of individuals to manage their lives in constructive ways. Most psychiatrists believe that anxiety plays a major role in the psychologic origin (psychogenesis) of emotional illness and is, in fact, its central problem. On the other hand, anxiety is thought to be extremely important in the normal development of individual character and personality and, therefore, has played a positive role in the history of man. From this standpoint anxiety is seen as normal and helpful since it can heighten the use of persons' capacities and sharpen perceptions so that behavior can be constructively modified. Between these two extremes of pathology and normality is an in-between state or level of anxiety, where individuals have limited ability to focus on what is really happening around them, and their efforts to manage their anxiety result in inappropriate but not necessarily destructive behavior. For example, they may withdraw from others or be unable to participate in some common everyday experiences; they may create angry, tense situations or complain or argue; or they may have numerous bodily symptoms for which no causative agent can be found.

It is estimated that some 5000 articles and books have been written about anxiety in the last two decades. The reader should, therefore, be aware that authors have often included different components and aspects of anxiety in their definitions of the phenomena under study, and the terminology and results of the reports may not be completely comparable. For instance, Isidore Portnoy,[1] in 1959, used the term "anxiety state" to describe a pattern of symptoms characterized by chronic apprehensiveness with repeating episodes of acute anxiety. He differentiated these states from transitory periods of anxiety that occur in relatively healthy individuals during times of stress. Currently, however, researchers are using the term "anxiety state" in the opposite way to define a transitory level of anxiety that may either improve one's response to a situation or interfere with it. They are using the term "anxiety trait" to characterize a relatively stable personality trait that predisposes one to react to a wide variety of nondangerous situations as if they are highly dangerous.[2]

Prevalence of Anxiety. Frieda Fromm-Reichmann has said: "The most unpleasant and at the same time the most universal experience, except loneliness, is anxiety." * And, according to Rollo May,[3] the recognition of anxiety as a powerful force in the day-to-day living of the twentieth century is apparent not only in the emphasis given to it as the central problem of emotional disturbances, but also as a central theme in literature, social, political, and economic thought, education, religion, and philosophy. He cites as examples the novels of Thomas Wolfe, Franz Kafka, and Herman Hesse; the poetry of W. H. Auden; the writings of theologian-philosophers Paul Tillich and Reinhold Niebuhr; and the comments of journalist-editor Norman Cousins. To this list might be added the publications of psycho-analyst-philosopher Erich Fromm and the symphony composed by Leonard Bernstein, *Age of Anxiety*. Ivan H. Scheier [4] says that this is not only an age of anxiety, but is an age of anxiety about anxiety.

Estimates of the incidence of anxiety vary

* Fromm-Reichmann, Frieda: "Psychiatric Aspects of Anxiety," in Stein, M., et al. (eds.): *Identity and Anxiety*. Free Press, Glencoe, Ill., 1960, p. 129.

because of the different criteria used to define it. However, Raymond B. Cattell and Ivan H. Scheier have developed and verified a questionnaire-based battery of tests that is used extensively to measure anxiety in groups and individuals, according to Oscar K. Buros.[4a] From studies using these questionnaires, Cattell [5] reports that people working as newspaper editors, artists, and air cadets in training have high anxiety levels, whereas policemen, clerical workers, and engineers have lower anxiety levels. Although nursing was not one of the occupations studied, the presence of high anxiety levels particularly among the specialized groups of nurses working in Intensive or Coronary Care Units has been described in a number of articles written by nurses and others.[6-8] Cattell further reports "Anxiety fluctuates in early childhood, rises most consistently in adolescence, and declines considerably through adulthood until it rises again after 60 or 65." * Surprisingly, when questionnaire scores of persons in India, Italy, Japan, the United Kingdom, and the United States were compared, Americans showed the lowest level of anxiety. Cattell believes this finding suggests Americans may have more "effort stress" (his term) than anxiety.

Physicians and nurses generally believe there is a high level of anxiety in many of the patients they see. A survey of 291 Iowa physicians in private practice showed that 18.5 per cent of the patients they treated were thought to have high emotional components in their illnesses, and that anxiety-tension was the most frequent symptom.[9]

Origins of Anxiety. The origins of anxiety are generally thought to lie in the psychology of the individual, and treatment has consisted of some form of psychotherapy. However, because of the effective use of tranquilizing drugs in the treatment of anxious patients, many investigators have studied the possible neurochemical causes, and in the last several years other researchers have theorized that cognitive appraisal (use of thought processes) is responsible for the arousal of anxiety. Lydia C. Rapoport [10] says that any stress situation perceived as being a threat to one's fundamental needs or sense of wholeness is met with anxiety.

Many explanations of the origins of anxiety are psychoanalytical and based on the work of Sigmund Freud. Freud pioneered in exploring man's inner life and demonstrated the existence of an unconscious mind and the mechanism of repression. He is usually credited with being the first to demonstrate and apply the principle that human behavior has its cause in the past experience of the individual whether this cause is consciously known or remembered.

A portion of psychoanalytic theory deals with a three-part structure of the mind—the id, ego, and superego. Freud postulated that the psyche of a newborn infant has only an id, that is, instinctual drives that seek gratification. The infant cannot delay, control, or satisfy these drives and is dependent on others both physically and psychically for survival. Freud further postulated that the id is modified by pressures from the external world to form the ego which, in turn, influences the id to accept the substitution of the "reality principle" for the "pleasure principle." He described the chief functions of the ego as maintaining a sense of reality, reality testing, and adapting to reality. The superego develops as the child identifies with and internalizes his or her parents' values and goals, thereby acquiring a conscience.[11]

Discussing the origin of anxiety, Freud theorized that the "ego is the sole seat of anxiety." In each age of development, the ego, through maintaining a relationship with the external world, is faced with "danger." Freud thought that when the biologic and emotional needs of infants are not gratified, they feel frustrated, angry, and anxious; and when early preschool children are separated from their mothers or mother substitutes, whom they recognize as the source of support and gratification of their needs, they feel anxious. Freud further postulated that boys in the late preschool period feel anxiety because they fear castration, and that girls of this age feel anxiety because they fear the loss of love. Finally, he thought school-age children are anxious because they fear the guilt aroused by the superego or conscience. He said:

In the course of development the old determinants of anxiety should be dropped, since the situations of danger corresponding to them have lost their importance owing to the strengthening of the ego. But this only occurs most incompletely. Many people are unable to surmount the fear of loss of love; they never become sufficiently independent of other people's love and in this respect carry on their behaviour as infants. Fear of the super-ego should normally never cease, since, in the form of moral anxiety, it is indispensable in social relations, and only in the rarest cases can an individual become independent of human society.*

---

* Cattell, Raymond B.: "The Nature and Measurement of Anxiety," *Sci. Am.*, **208:**96, (Mar.) 1963.

* Freud, Sigmund: *The Complete Introductory Lectures on Psychoanalysis.* (Translated and edited by James Starchey.) W. W. Norton & Co., New York, 1966, p. 552.

Freud was certain that the persons he described as "neurotic" had not overcome childhood anxiety-producing experiences, but had repressed and changed them so that any thoughts, feelings, wishes, or drives that were considered unacceptable called forth an expectation of loss of love and approval or an expectation of punishment.

Other theorists and clinicians in the field of psychoanalysis such as Harry S. Sullivan, Karen Horney, and Rollo May have discussed anxiety from the standpoint of cultural and interpersonal influences on the person. They are essentially in agreement that anxiety is connected with fear of punishment and disapproval, withdrawal of love, disruption of interpersonal relationships, and isolation or separation.[12]

Abraham H. Maslow,[13] describing the safety needs of neurotically anxious adults, says they act as if they were afraid of being spanked or abandoned. In other words, they appear to have been unaffected by learning and growing-up and are always ready to react as children do in the same kind of threatening or "dangerous" situations.

Study of the biophysiologic basis of emotional disorders was given great impetus with the use of tranquilizers in the successful treatment of hospitalized mental patients starting in 1955. However, the interest in the relationships between neurophysiology, neurochemistry, and emotion began much earlier with the study of comparative neuroanatomy and brain-damaged patients. Alfred M. Freedman and his associates [14] believe that while various drugs, intracerebral electrodes, and refined techniques of stereotactic surgery * are currently used to some extent in the investigation and modification of emotions, future psychiatric research will focus even more on electrical, chemical and possibly surgical alterations in subcortical sections of the brain in order to understand and treat emotional problems.

Available neurophysiologic evidence indicates that physiologic reactions and symptoms associated with fear, a part of the emotional pattern of anxiety, are dominated by the sympathetic nervous system. The sympathetic system, as well as other body systems, requires both nervous and hormonal chemical messengers for the integration of experience and behavior, and the principal chemical transmitter of the sympathetic system is norepinephrine. This hormone comes mainly from the medulla of the adrenal gland, but the end-knobs of some sympathetic neurons also secrete norepinephrine.

Other brain structures and neural systems under investigation as affecting emotion or components of the emotional states are the limbic system and the reticular activating system. Current knowledge of these structures and systems does not expressly link them to anxiety, but to emotional states in general.

The limbic system is composed of structures located on the medial and ventral portions of the cerebral hemispheres, and of subcortical structures such as the hypothalamus. As more evidence about various portions of this system accumulate, it appears that different areas of the system perform specific functions. The hypothalamus, for instance, secretes a number of substances that affect the anterior pituitary gland and the autonomic nervous system. Recently, it has been learned that many hypothalamic and related structures are centers for pain and pleasure sensations.

The reticular activating system beginning in the lower brain stem controls the over-all degree of central nervous activity. It has an excitatory portion that alerts the brain to complete wakefulness. This portion has the ability to select those stimuli to which it is essential that the organism react. For example, a mother hears her baby cry, but does not hear the telephone ring. The reticular system also has an inhibitory portion that, when stimulated, produces sleep and, when destroyed, produces insomnia.[15-17]

Biochemical knowledge on the etiology of emotions or their biochemical components is scant and contradictory at the present time. According to some authorities, research is proceeding along two general lines. One is the influence of electrolytes (sodium, potassium, calcium, magnesium, and lithium) on nervous activity, and the other is the metabolism of neurohormones in the central nervous system (norepinephrine, acetylcholine, dopamine, and serotonin) as transmitters of impulses across nerve synapses.[18,19]

A third point of view about the origins of anxiety is being explored by "cognitive theorists." * Richard S. Lazarus and his associates say that any emotional state is presumed to have behavior-organizing properties, but they believe "It is the cognitive processes leading to emotion that organize behavior and not the

---

* A modification of psychosurgery consisting of making small lesions in selected portions of the brain.

* Cognition is the process of knowing. The cognitive theorist is a person studying the process of thought, or reasoning, and its effect. (Here is another question of the chicken and the egg. Which comes first, the thought or the emotion?)

emotions themselves." * Lazarus assumes people are evaluating organisms, judging each stimulus in their environment for its relevance and significance in fulfilling needs or desires. He defines the thought process (cognitive process) intervening between the environmental situation and the emotional reaction as appraisal, and differentiates the following kinds: primary appraisal, secondary appraisal, and reappraisal. He says, "Primary appraisal refers to the judgment that a situation is relevant or irrelevant, or that it will have either a beneficial or harmful outcome. Secondary appraisal is a judgment about the forms of coping available for mastering anticipated harm, or for facilitating potential benefits. Reappraisal involves changed evaluations based on new cues, feedback from one's re-

sponse or the effects of the response, or further reflection about the evidence on which the original appraisals were based." *

Lazarus theorizes that anxiety results when a stimulus is appraised as a threat to ideas, concepts, or values to which the person is committed; or when stimuli are appraised as being without structure or meaning and so become threatening; or when appraisal results in uncertainty about the nature of the threat and, consequently, about what might be done about it.

Within each of the three broad points of view about the origins of emotion and anxiety that are described above, there are many fine distinctions. The reader who wishes to pursue this subject may consult the references listed at the end of the chapter.

Manifestations of Anxiety. The manifestations of anxiety as reported in psychologic, psychiatric, medical, and nursing literature are many and varied. Some of them are objective in the sense that nurses and others can see them; some are subjective or must be reported by the affected person (see Fig. 41-1). Some manifestations of anxiety are so hidden from

---

* Lazarus, Richard S.: "Cognitive and Personality Factors Underlying Threat and Coping," in Appley, Mortimer H., and Trumbull, Richard: *Psychological Stress.* Appleton-Century-Crofts, New York, 1967, p. 152. Carroll E. Izard criticizes this point of view and says, "This view appears to violate observations from both ontogenetic and phylogenetic development. In ontogeny emotional processes appear to precede cognitive processes such as appraisal and reappraisal. From an evolutionary point of view, the cognitive position would require that the animal be able to think or appraise before being able to have emotion. The reverse seems much more plausible." (Izard: Carroll E: *Patterns of Emotions.* Academic Press, New York, 1972, p. 80.)

* Lazarus, Richard S., and Averill, James R.: "Emotion and Cognition: With Special Reference to Anxiety," in Spielberger, Charles D. (ed.): *Anxiety: Current Trends in Theory and Research,* Vol. II. Academic Press, New York, 1972, p. 242.

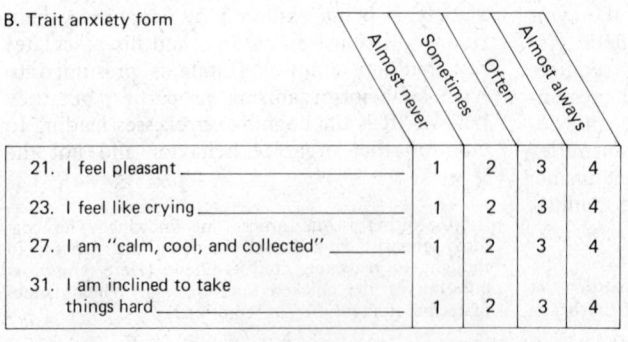

A. State anxiety form

	Not at all	Somewhat	Moderately so	Very much
1. I feel calm	1	2	3	4
3. I am tense	1	2	3	4
9. I feel anxious	1	2	3	4
20. I feel pleasant	1	2	3	4

B. Trait anxiety form

	Almost never	Sometimes	Often	Almost always
21. I feel pleasant	1	2	3	4
23. I feel like crying	1	2	3	4
27. I am "calm, cool, and collected"	1	2	3	4
31. I am inclined to take things hard	1	2	3	4

Figure 41-1. Statements from Spielberger's "Self-Analysis Questionnaire" illustrating the state, *A,* and trait, *B,* forms of the instrument. (Reproduced by special permission from Spielberger, C. D.: *The State–Trait Anxiety.* Consulting Psychologists Press Inc., New York, 1969.)

both the observer and the anxious person that they must be inferred from answers given to various kinds of questions.

If, as some authorities speculate, emotions have as one component a specific innate neural foundation, stimulation of the sympathetic portion of the autonomic nervous system appears to produce many manifestations of what is generally called "anxiety." For instance, increased heart rate and blood pressure, increased sweating (particularly palms of the hands), pallor or flushing of the face, loss of appetite, nausea, vomiting, muscle tension, blinking of the eyes, and dilation of the pupils —usually considered indications of anxiety— are also direct or indirect effects of sympathetic stimulation. At the same time, stimulation of the parasympathetic system seems to be involved also because diarrhea and frequent urination are often associated with anxiety.

Although not specifically related to activity of the autonomic nervous system, alterations in speech patterns and voice quality are commonly reported as signs of anxiety; for example, rapid, staccato speech with frequent interruption of another speaker; hesitating and slow speech; shifts in the tempo of speech; shifts in the tone of voice; loud or high-pitched voice; increased hoarseness; or an unsteady quavering voice. Other frequently listed signs of anxiety are irritability, or general impatience; restlessness, inappropriate alertness; nail- or lip-biting; tremors of the hands; twitching of various parts of the body; stiffness of posture; and strained facial expression. Subjective symptoms reported by some patients, voluntarily or with questioning, are that they feel tense and cannot relax. They feel something is going to happen. They cannot think or concentrate on the activity of the moment. They have a "lump" in their throat, or "butterflies" in their stomach. Some persons say "I feel as if I could jump out of my skin." Anxious persons usually sleep poorly and have nightmares.

Everyone has experienced some level of anxiety at some time. Nurses tend to "diagnose" this condition in a patient subjectively on the basis of their own experience, rather than on a more objective analysis. However, since no one has all or even most of the anxiety manifestations listed above, it is difficult to determine which behaviors are truly expressive or typical of anxiety. In studies of medical-surgical patients that attempted to correlate nurses' perceptions of who were the anxious patients with physicians' perceptions and psychometric scales, little agreement was found about who was anxious. In one study in which nurses were asked to describe the basis of their

conclusions about medical-surgical patients' anxiety, it was apparent that nurses relied heavily on the seriousness of the patient's diagnosis, his or her knowledge of the diagnosis, the prognosis, and the necessary therapy.[20,21]

Cattell and his associates,[22] over a period of 12 years, described many of the objective and subjective manifestations commonly associated with anxiety and then intercorrelated these manifestations. They found that among persons who experienced anxiety as a fluctuating state rather than as a personality trait there was a raised cholinesterase (a neural enzyme) level, high respiratory rate, high heart rate, increased systolic pulse pressure, high steroid hormone level, high willingness to admit common faults, and high irritability.

In a study of 70 surgical patients, Lois E. Graham and Elizabeth M. Conley [23] reported the patients' verbal expressions of anxiety plus elevated systolic pulse pressure were the most significant indicators of preoperative anxiety. With the large number of possible manifestations of anxiety and the general uncertainty about which of these have consistent diagnostic value, the conclusions reached in this study may be the best basis (at the present time) on which nurses can judge the presence or absence of a patient's anxiety.

Precipitating Factors of Anxiety. Psychologic stress is said to be the precipitating factor of an anxiety attack. Samuel Silverman writes, "Psychological stress derives particularly from interaction with other human beings and from reaction to the social, economic, and cultural settings which man has created. If stresses from these sources are sufficiently intense and sustained, it may be assumed that any individual will react strongly. Most stresses, however, are those which are associated with the unpredictable vicissitudes of everyday life and are minor conflicts." * He goes on to name situations that are stressful and that occur in the lives of many, such as illness and hospitalization; the death of a close relative or friend; or anniversaries of one kind or another. In addition, he discusses everyday happenings, such as differences or arguments with colleagues, friends, or relatives; anticipation of new and unknown experiences; and, for students, the common experience of writing or "taking" examinations.

It is generally conceded that hospital medical workers are constantly under stress and at the same time it is almost axiomatic to say

* Silverman, Samuel: *Psychological Aspects of Physical Illness.* Meredith Corp., New York, 1968, p. 23.

that their psychologic state, no less than their technical expertise, influences the effectiveness of the care they provide. Nurses are confronted with the impact of illness, death, and disability—as few people are—and the related tasks are often distasteful or frightening.[24-25a]

In addition to their own reaction to stress, nurses must work with the reactions of patients and their families, and of professional colleagues. Many patients and relatives are appreciative of and grateful for the care the ill person is receiving, but some are critical of that care and unreasonably demanding. Some want to take over the patient's care, while others symbolically abandon the patient by withdrawing their physical presence and support, and leave complete responsibility for him or her to the physician, the nurse, and other members of the health team. These are some conditions in the work situation that may arouse very strong and mixed feelings in the nurse. Isabel E. P. Menzies describes the conflicting feelings of "pity, compassion, and love; guilt and anxiety; hatred and resentment of the patients who arouse these strong feelings; envy of the care given the patient." * It would seem that the nature of nursing puts its practitioners at considerable risk of being flooded by intense and unmanageable anxiety.

According to Menzies,[26] the traditions of nursing service, though subconsciously designed to relieve the nurse's anxiety, in reality increase it. Because it is traditional for nurses to evade recognition of their feelings, they can do little to change or lessen them. Some of the ineffective practices that have developed over a period of time in nursing service are (1) keeping the nurse-patient relationship on a superficial level through the use of task assignments or frequent changes in assignment; (2) depersonalizing, categorizing, and denying the significance of the individual through such devices as talking about a patient by bed number or diagnosis; (3) detaching and denying feelings through the use of brisk, directing behavior such as saying to a nurse colleague "Don't become too involved" or "Pull yourself together" (sometimes said to a patient as well as to another nurse); (4) attempting to eliminate decisions by ritual task performance or standing orders, rules, and regulations; and (5) reducing the weight of responsibility in decision-making by checks and counterchecks. These long-standing methods of evading anxiety should be condemned. They have resulted in lessening the ability of the nurse to confront

situations that produce anxiety, and to work through them constructively. This has had an unfortunate effect on nursing care.

Illness and hospitalization make most persons anxious. This kind of anxiety concerns nurses and physicians because it is believed that anxiety requires the use of somatic and psychic energy that cannot then be used in the process of recovery. In recent studies it has been concluded that 20 to 25 per cent of the hospitalized medical patients suffer anxiety from illness or hospitalization.[27]

Minna Field, in her frequently quoted book *Patients Are People,* describes the circumstances in which the average patient finds himself:

The patient is subjected to examinations and tests, the purpose of which he does not understand and the results of which are not explained. A nurse comes in and sticks him with a needle, another puts a thermometer in his mouth; a strange looking machine is wheeled to his bedside and connected with his arms and legs; he is put on a stretcher and wheeled through long corridors and passageways. Some of the tests to which he is subjected are unfamiliar, some are painful, many are frightening, but nobody tells him what they mean. And nobody tells him whether the results are favorable or unfavorable. The patient is afraid to ask questions because everyone seems so busy, so intent on what he is doing, or perhaps the patient is afraid to ask because he is afraid to know the answer. Whatever the reasons, the unasked questions remain unanswered, and uncertainty and fear prey on his mind. *

In addition, patients are usually subjected to unfamiliar sounds and peculiar medical language (or maybe a foreign tongue); required to meet a schedule of daily living (not of their own making) different from the one to which they are accustomed; allowed to see their families only when the hospital permits it; and surrounded by a "team" of strangers. It is little wonder that of every five hospitalized patients one is moderately or severely anxious. Many of these sources of stress can be modified by nurses, reducing the level of anxiety experienced by hospitalized patients.[27a] Nurses may not, however, be in a position to influence sources of stress for patients who enter the hospital because they are overwhelmed by anxiety.

Alleviating Anxiety. Psychotherapy of one kind or another has often been used to help people with distress that results from illness or the effects of social or emotional crises. Many

* Menzies, Isabel E. P.: "A Case-Study in the Functioning of Social Systems as a Defence Against Anxiety," *Hum. Rel.,* **13**:95, (May) 1960.

* Field, Minna: *Patients Are People,* 3rd ed. Columbia University Press, New York, 1967, p. 58.

of these therapies have been derived from Freud's psychoanalytic methods and theories, and they use, as major components of the therapeutic process, verbal interactions and the client-therapist relationship. Izard[28] reports there is clinical evidence to suggest that anxiety with its fear-related base responds more readily to relationship or predominantly verbal-cognitive psychotherapy and conditioning-learning techniques than does depression. He believes the positive response to the treatment occurs because the anatomic location of the sympathetic system ganglia, which are so influential in fear-related emotions, places the neurons under the relatively direct and immediate influence of the brain and central nervous system.

It would seem that nurses are in a particularly advantageous position to use verbal-cognitive therapeutic relationships to help alleviate the mild to moderate levels of anxiety experienced by patients; in other words, to help patients understand the origin of their anxiety. While skill in developing and maintaining such relationships is important, at least one therapist, Carl R. Rogers,[29] believes the skill of the professional person is secondary to the attitude of warmth and "realness" felt toward, and conveyed to, the patient.

In a rather general way, psychotherapies may be divided into four broad classifications. These classifications are overlapping in some characteristics but are a framework for discussing ways in which anxiety can be alleviated. One group of "insight therapies" has as its main goal the reconstruction of emotional reactions and personality structure. An example of this classification is psychoanalysis. A second group of insight therapies has as its main goal reeducation in new and better ways to deal with stress that are based on awareness of one's motive and psychologic make-up. Client-centered therapy is an example of this classification. Supportive therapies that have as the main goal restoring or strengthening psychologic defenses or integrative abilities that were disrupted by a temporary crisis are a third type of therapy. Crisis intervention, brief psychotherapy, and the cognitive approach for dealing with disruptive emotions are examples of supportive therapy. A final group of therapies are the behavioral therapies based mainly on B. F. Skinner's[29a] point of view that behavior is shaped and maintained by its consequences—behavior is repeated if its consequences are satisfying and vice versa. These therapies have as their main goals the modification of current behaviors without reference to the underlying causes. Desensitization with relaxation and positive reinforce-

ment therapies are examples of the approach advocated by Skinner.

Psychoanalytic therapists who use the first type of insight therapy focus on one of three central therapeutic goals in working with anxious patients. One therapeutic goal is to guide people in understanding, accepting, and learning to live with as well as to utilize mild degrees of anxiety. In the case of more intense states of anxiety, the psychotherapeutic goal is to help patients uncover, resolve, and integrate the causes of these anxieties in order to prevent the development of mental symptoms used as defenses against the awareness of these anxiety states. For example, some patients may develop obsessive behavior patterns, such as counting marks on the wall or some similar repetitive acts, which tend to modify the experience of anxiety. When anxiety is so severe that patients develop mental symptoms or mental illness, the therapeutic goal should be to help them develop insight into the emotional roots of their anxiety and of their symptomatology, and to face, work through, and eventually vanquish their excess anxiety using psychoanalytically-oriented dynamic psychotherapy. Fromm-Reichmann warns that caution is indicated regarding the timing and dosage of therapeutic intervention and enlightenment, lest patients be made to face more dynamic insight into their anxiety than they can accept at a given time.

The arduous nature of the practice of psychoanalysis that uses the patient's anxiety as a cue or avenue to the patient's neurosis is described by Donald M. Kaplan.[30] He says that in psychoanalysis the analyst listens to the patient but he also listens for the influence that his listening has on what the patient is saying. The analogy Kaplan uses to describe the patient-therapist relationship is that of creating and maintaining an electrical circuit. He says it is like picking up an invisible wire attached to the patient to complete the circuit, and holding on to the "wire" without relenting. To drop it would mean the end of the analytic dialogue and the beginning of ordinary conversation. This relationship is not easy to maintain. It depends on the analyst's own emotional and intellectual suitability for psychoanalysis. The relationship can traumatize the patient.

Client-centered psychotherapy as insight therapy with the major goal that of reeducation was developed by Carl R. Rogers.[31] It is based in part on his belief that each individual has growth tendencies toward self-actualization that are increased by the therapeutic climate. Rogers views the client-centered therapeutic relationship as a special instance of all interpersonal relationships, and the growth and change occurring in therapy as a special instance of growth and development that can and does occur in all people. It is, perhaps, for these reasons that the client-centered approach has been used by diverse groups of professional persons in a variety of settings. Nurses find the principles of this therapy applicable to the care of most patients, and the suggestions that follow for developing a therapeutic nurse-patient relationship in any nursing situation are based on what is often referred to as the Rogerian method.

Nurses should attempt to provide three conditions in their relationship with patients that basically come from their belief in the worth and dignity of the individual. These three conditions are genuineness; unconditional positive regard for, or acceptance of, patients; and the emotional appreciation of patients' feelings (empathy). Genuineness in this context means the nurses are their actual selves and their words, feelings, and actions or nonverbal communications do not subtly contradict one another. They (nurses) do not say one thing and mean or imply another. They do not operate behind a front or play a role. Patients feel they can trust them. Unconditional positive regard implies that nurses care for patients and that what happens to them concerns the nurse. This caring does not involve judgment of the patient as a person, his or her personality or status, but simply a warm acceptance of them as they are at the moment. This condition allows patients freedom to have their own feelings, whether positive or negative. Empathy means that nurses are able to sense the patient's feelings of fear, anger, rage, or whatever he or she is feeling and to convey this understanding to the patient. Nurses enter into the meaning of the emotion without entering into the emotion itself—the nurse is neither fearful nor angry.[32] This is a very sensitive endeavor and demands that nurses be comfortable with their own feelings, and that they not impute their feelings to patients or treat them as objects. These three attitudinal conditions are basic for a therapeutic nurse-patient relationship.

Crisis intervention is an example of a supportive therapy, developed within the past few decades, for persons who are overwhelmed by anxiety or depression from problems of daily living. Its premises come from the work of many human behavior theorists—Sigmund Freud, Heinz Hartman, Sandor Rado, Erik Erikson, Erich Lindeman, and Gerald Caplan, to name a few. The techniques of crisis intervention are based on the concept that a crisis occurs when individuals are faced with a "hazardous" situation perceived as a threat, a loss, or a challenge that is entirely new to them and for which their usual problem-solving activities are not adequate. The tension and discomfort that develop are felt as anxiety, fear, guilt, shame, and helplessness. It is believed that when a person's relative psychologic equilibrium is upset, he or she is susceptible to even a small amount of influence from others and that it can help him or her master the situation or move toward failure.[33]

Since a major change in personality structure is not the purpose of crisis intervention, it is short-term therapy that rarely lasts longer than 6 weeks and often for much less time. The therapeutic goal is to help individuals resolve their immediate problems so that as a minimal result they are able to function at the same level at which they functioned before the crisis. The maximal therapeutic goal of crisis intervention is to help people improve their ability to function above the precrisis level.

Studies of responses to stressful situations have shown that in many of the common human crises there are well-defined, characteristic patterns of behavior. The "generic" approach to crisis intervention focuses on a particular kind of crisis and its characteristic course rather than the intrapsychic processing —the individual approach *—of the person in crisis. The emphasis in this kind of supportive therapy is on problem-solving. Therefore, the first step is to help clients gain an intellectual understanding of the relationship between their discomfort and the event or series of events that preceded it. The second step is to help them bring into the open their present feelings and to be aware of them. The third step is to help them examine past solutions to problems that might be helpful in this crisis and to look for new ways to cope with it. The use of other persons, agencies, or institutions as resources for help with the tasks and feelings involved may be developed. The fourth, and last, step is to summarize the progress the individual has made in order to help him or her reexperience and reconfirm it; help him or her, if necessary, make realistic plans for the future; and discuss ways in which the present experience might help in future crises.[34,34a]

Nurses are in a strategic position to make use of the steps involved in crisis intervention and to positively influence mental health. They

---

* The use of the individual approach in crisis intervention requires that the therapist have a "solid background in psychodynamics, and [can make] a professional assessment of the unique intrapsychic and interpersonal processes" that have been activated. (Morley, Wilbur E., et al.: "Crisis: Paradigms of Intervention," *J Psychiatr. Nurs.,* 5:531, [Nov.–Dec.] 1967.)

are usually present or available in critical times, for instance, when a husband and wife are entering parenthood, when parents and children are experiencing common growth crises,* when people are ill and hospitalized, and when families and individuals face death and bereavement. Because a crisis constitutes a transitional period, during which even a small amount of appropriate help leads to personality growth, the nurse has an incomparable opportunity to practice preventive mental health.

To help reduce the severe anxiety of a patient who has been hospitalized because of it, Hildegarde Peplau[35] has suggested four steps that can be used in the nurse-patient relationship. These steps are similar to those of crisis intervention but have as the goal preparing the patient for further intensive psychotherapy. The steps suggested in this technique are (1) encourage patients to identify the anxiety or to recognize when they are experiencing it; (2) encourage patients to identify their relief-giving patterns and to connect these to their awareness of anxiety; (3) encourage patients to identify situations and interactions that occur before the increase in anxiety is experienced and verbalize these to the nurse; and (4) encourage patients to formulate the probable or immediate and situational causes for the increased anxiety.

Another kind of supportive therapy for patients (not classified as psychiatric) who are apprehensively anticipating some aspect of their hospitalization or treatment has been termed "the cognitive approach." Anxiety is often precipitated in patients because they lack knowledge and understanding of their illness or hospitalization. Explaining hospital routines to them, pointing out the location of specific patient facilities, describing the use of equipment provided, and describing a treatment before it is given have long been advocated as a part of effective nursing care. However, since patients have apparently been too little affected by this rather minimal information, other more complex explanatory approaches to relieve the apprehensive anticipation of patients are being investigated.

Mary E. Meyers[36] reports that it is the content of nurse-patient communication that is important in the reduction of tension and anxiety. She says that distracting, irrelevant conversation is not helpful to patients, whereas specific information upon which they can struc-

ture impending stressful events is. In a study conducted by Arlene M. Putt,[37] 36 hospitalized patients with peptic ulcers were given instruction on an individual basis and with the help of a booklet "What You Should Know About Healing Your Ulcer." * Such instructed patients had significantly fewer hours of discomfort and shorter hospitalizations than did a group who had no such instruction. The effectiveness of still another level of specificity of information was demonstrated in a study conducted among 99 patients by Jean E. Johnson.[38] She found that when patients were given descriptions of the *sensations* that they were likely to have with a gastrointestinal endoscopy examination, they needed less medication for sedation during the procedure. In addition, those patients who heard the description of sensations were far more relaxed than the group who had heard only about the procedure.

Nurses, in addition to increasing their skill in the use of therapeutic relationships, must recognize the influence of environment on reducing or increasing anxiety. One goal of the nursing team in a hospital, according to Gladys Nite and Frank N. Willis,[39] is to provide a setting that is as much like a home environment as possible. This involves such things as encouraging the patient's family to bring some of the patient's personal belongings to the hospital; making the furnishing of rooms attractive; supplying conversation and social stimulation that would ordinarily be part of the patient's day if he or she were not hospitalized; making the patient's meal a social occasion; and introducing a pattern of recreation appropriate to the patient's tastes and phase of recovery. Also, more attention is given to organizing the unit so that patients can make use of their anxiety to promote growth and avoid unhealthy psychologic solutions. There is increasing emphasis on making conditions flexible and giving patients more to say about them. For example, consumers are members of policy-making bodies—or boards of directors—and there is patient government in many health services. Elizabeth Barnes[39a] describes the "patient community organization" of the Cassel Hospital, London, England, that seems to have been very fruitful. Such organizations are especially desirable in extended care facilities, such as nursing homes, and in health services of corrective agencies where rehabilitation is the ultimate purpose.

The preceding discussion about ways to reduce anxiety has focused on therapeutic behaviors of the nurse toward and with the anxious patient. However, as noted earlier,

---

* Examples of growth crises are the beginning independence of the 2-year-old ("the terrible twos"), the 6-year-old entering school, or the critical attitude of adolescents toward parents.

* Wyeth Laboratories, Philadelphia, 1955.

nurses, themselves, are highly vulnerable to anxiety and may not know how to reduce or modify it. Conscious recognition by nurses of their anxiety and their feeling of helplessness in many patient care situations is, of course, the first step. Beyond that step, Pamela A. Holsclaw says the nurse should develop understanding of herself and develop constructive defenses against the emotional risks of nursing —"She cannot do this alone; as the initial risk to self involves at least two persons, so must the measures for safeguarding the self." *

It has been suggested by nurses and others that arrangements be made for a psychiatric consultant to work with nursing personnel so they can talk about their feelings and learn to understand the dynamics of interpersonal aspects of their nursing care. Such conferences provide nurses with an opportunity to realize that fears, doubts, guilt, uncertainty, and anger arising from their work are shared, acceptable feelings; to work through feelings that cannot be expressed immediately because such expression would be inappropriate then; to share approaches others have found helpful in dealing with human relations; to develop constructive solutions for other problems associated with the work setting; and to make suggestions to the hospital administration when necessary. It should be recognized that a periodic withdrawal of nurses, particularly from patient units that involve high emotional risks, is necessary for them to regroup their emotional forces. This withdrawal might take the form of leaves of absence, temporary transfer to another patient unit, or the care of patients who present problems with lower emotional risk. Nurses and hospital administrators are just beginning to make use of these kinds of activities that when utilized benefit both patients and nurses.[40,41]

The biochemical approach to the relief of anxiety has resulted in an unprecedented increase in the use of tranquilizers in the past 20 years. These are potent drugs that reduce anxiety temporarily. Their effects are *palliative, not curative*. Because physicians have misunderstood these drugs or have been unable to control anxiety in any other way, or because patients are convinced that there are "pills" to cure any discomfort, tranquilizers have often been prescribed indiscriminately.[42] Even though the use of these drugs has sometimes been abused, most persons recognize their value in the treatment of emotional disorders. Frank J. Ayd[43] says that 1 year after tranquilizers were first used on a large scale to treat hospitalized

psychiatric patients, the population in hospitals decreased for the first time in 175 years.

The major tranquilizer groups such as rauwolfia derivatives, the phenothiazines, and the thioxanthenes are most useful in the treatment of *psychoses* in which severe anxiety, tension, agitation, hallucinations, delusions, and psychomotor excitement are prominent.[44,45] The minor tranquilizers are especially useful in the management of acute anxiety and tension in helping prevent chronic neuroses and in restoring psychologic equilibrium in patients under stress. The most frequently used minor tranquilizers are diazepam, chlordiazepoxide, oxazepam, meprobamate, tybamate, and doxepin.*[46,47]

Tranquilizers have, as do many potent drugs, a number of undesirable side effects. These reactions vary with the chemical structure of the drug and with its potency. Space does not allow a complete description of these medications and their action, but readers are urged to study the literature so they may learn to use these drugs safely and correctly. Perhaps it should be stressed again that such drugs should be used as a temporary measure. They are a poor substitute for treatment that enables persons to understand the reason why they are anxious and to modify their lives so that the cause of the anxiety is removed or they learn to live comfortably with the provocation.

2. DEPRESSION

Although the phenomenon of depression has been recognized and discussed in medical literature since the time of Hippocrates it is hard to find a definition with which all authorities agree. Some believe that depression is a well-defined illness with a characteristic and specific set of symptoms to identify it. Others, including Aaron T. Beck[48] (who offers a Depression Inventory), think that severe depression is an exaggeration, in particularly susceptible persons, of the "blue moods" experienced by nearly everyone. Nurses and nonpsychiatric physicians frequently see "depression" as a symptom among other symptoms of a debilitating, life-threatening, or life-terminating illness. Henry P. Laughlin[49] says it is the intensity, duration, and depth of depression that affect the way in which it is categorized, that is, as an illness, an exaggeration of mood, or a symptom. Sometimes it is simply the reaction of a person who gives up, who hasn't learned

---

* Holsclaw, Pamela A.: "Nursing in High Emotional Risk Areas," *Nurs. Forum*, 4:36, (No. 4) 1965.

* Valium; Librium; Serax; Miltown and Equanil; Solacen and Tybatran; and Sinequan are the trade names of the drugs listed above. The trade names are in the same order as the drugs named.

to fight back. Recent studies indicate that it may be possible to define depression on the basis of excreted metabolic products of neurohormones or other biochemical substances.

Depression and grief are thought to be similar in many ways; however, there are some differences. For instance, the loss of self-esteem that almost invariably occurs in depression is not present with normal grief. Also, the low spirits prevalent in depression are generally thought to originate internally rather than externally as does the consciously recognized loss associated with grief. And finally, the despondency of depression seems to the outside observer to be out of proportion to the situation while that of grief seems to be appropriate and proportional to the loss.[49a]

Prevalence of Depression. Of the authorities consulted, most agree that depression is a problem of considerable magnitude, but the number of depressed persons in the community has not been determined with any accuracy.* William G. and Gerald C. Crary[50] estimate that depression afflicts millions of Americans annually; however, of this number only 30,000 have the condition recognized and treated. Nathan S. Klein[51] says that recent information indicates 15 per cent of the American population between the ages of 18 and 74 have significant depressive symptoms, but that only 5 per cent of this number are, in fact, diagnosed and treated. The figure for the number of depressions treated reflects the point of view that depression is a disease entity. The larger figure probably includes depressions that are of low intensity and duration, or that are "masked" by physical symptoms or deviant behavior.

Although most of the evidence about the frequency with which depression occurs in specific groups of people is contradictory and inconclusive, some points can be made: (1) depression seems to be more common among women than men, and this is so whether the depression is evaluated as a feeling, as neurotic depression, or as depressive psychosis; (2) seasonal peaks of the onset of depression have been noted in March and September, with the lowest occurrence in the summer months; (3) the syndrome of depression rarely occurs in infancy and childhood, but does appear in adolescence, increases in frequency in young adulthood, reaches its greatest occurrence in the middle years, and declines somewhat in the later years.[52] However, suicide rates in the United States are highest in the over-sixty age group.[52a]

While the adult syndrome of depression is not seen in infants or children, René A. Spitz[53] has described what he called "anaclitic depression" * among infants less than a year old. Harry Bakwin[54] and John Bowlby[55] have described similar depressive behavior in institutionalized infants or those who for some reason were deprived of mothering. Child psychiatrists now believe that many behavior problems, including delinquency, failure to achieve in school, school phobia, and childhood psychosomatic illnesses, are indications of depressive feelings in children, but are not recognized as depression.[56,57]

Manifestations of Depression. Many persons who have a "one-day depression" or "blue mood" complain of coldness of their hands and feet, of fatigue, a lack of energy, a "let down" feeling, or a temporary loss of interest in life. Some individuals show depression through more physiologic routes that Laughlin[58] calls "depressive-equivalents" and other authorities call "masked depression," such as excessive sleeping, loss of appetite, shifting body complaints, or even the common cold.

Depression in its more intense or profound states is expressed by the *whole person*. There is a lowering or reduction of all body processes—feeling, activity, thought, and function. Depressed persons feel sad, helpless, hopeless, worthless, and lose interest in people, the environment, and their usual activities. Sandor Rado[59] says their sustained gloomy mood is complicated by feelings of guilty fear, anger, and blame. Unfortunately, these feelings make the person less lovable. Relatives and friends tend to withdraw from the person who is silent, unappreciative, unresponsive, and sometimes tearful. This establishes a vicious circle with the depressed and their associates having less and less opportunity for intellectual or emotional satisfaction, which only deepens the depression.

Depressed persons may express (verbally or nonverbally) the wish to die, since the present and future hold little for them. They show obvious difficulty in concentrating, making decisions, or carrying on conversations. In fact, the extent of what they say may well be limited to hesitant answers to questions. Their dress also reflects their feelings. Clothes they wear tend to be uninteresting, dull, dark, and often unclean. The most conspicuous sign of depression may be the person's loss of his or her normal appearance.

---

* Two journalists reviewing the literature title their article "Depression: The Common Cold of Mental Ailments" (*The New York Times Magazine*, Nov. **25,** 1973, p. 38).

* Derived from the Greek *anaklisis,* a lying back. In psychiatry, state of emotional dependence.

Many depressed persons complain of fatigue and pain. Any body organ or system may be the focal point, but the gastrointestinal system is most often affected. There is a general slowing of body functions; for instance, the motility of the gastrointestinal tract slows down. This results in poor appetite, a feeling of fullness in the stomach, and constipation. The respiratory rate is slowed and it may be difficult to get a deep breath. Depressed persons are often seen to "heave great sighs." Muscle tension decreases throughout the body and this affects posture and gait. Depressed persons get progressively less active until they finally sit or lie down most of the time. This lack of exercise affects every other function of the body, but it badly disrupts the normal pattern of sleep. Many authorities believe that so-called dawn insomnia is a characteristic sleep disturbance of depression. Some psychiatrists ask nurses to make graphic charts of sleep in badly depressed patients because change indicates worsening or improvement in the patient's condition. (Insomnia and depression are also discussed in a following section.)

Precipitating Factors of Depression. Depression may follow internal conflicts or specific events that represent significant loss. Persons during their middle years often suffer from depression (and/or anxiety) following some type of crisis.[59a,b] It has been seen to accompany almost all types of illness whether their origin is infectious, metabolic, endocrine, toxic, malignant, degenerative, or traumatic. Influenza, infectious hepatitis, and infectious mononucleosis have all been described as being complicated by feelings of depression. Potassium deficiency due to an inadequate diet or prolonged maintenance on potassium-free intravenous fluids has frequently led to depression. The endocrine disorders that have depression associated with them are Cushing's syndrome, Addison's disease, and hypopituitarism. Drug-induced depression has been reported with the use of reserpine and the phenothiazines.[60,61]

Depression in persons who have cancer, degenerative disease, mutilating operations such as an amputation, or spinal cord injury is widely recognized. Laughlin[62] says that, broadly speaking, depression may be regarded as reaction to loss. The loss may be sudden or anticipated, actual or symbolic, specific or obscure. A relationship between loss, depression, and the life-threatening or life-terminating conditions mentioned above is almost self-evident.

Some recent studies show that rather nebulous, but still detectable, precipitating causes of depression are the number of "life-changes" in the person's recent past. Such changes may not seem especially depressive but just ordinary happenings, such as a son or daughter leaving home, trouble with in-laws, a change in financial status, kind of work, residence or school, or a vacation, or retirement, and curiously, an outstanding personal achievement. Early investigations showed that if an individual faced a series of events each of which required new, adaptive, or coping behavior, and the events were clustered within a 2-year period, then, illness developed. While such events were not considered as direct causes of illness, their accumulation was thought to produce enough stress to bring about illness.[63,64] From this information the investigators developed a scale based on the importance of each event. Later studies using such life-change scales and comparing groups of depressed persons to those not depressed found that life-change scores were significantly higher among the depressed than the nondepressed.[65,66]

Origins of Depression. The specific cause of depression has not yet been determined. Theories about its cause come from psychiatry, studies of biogenetics, neurophysiology, biochemistry, and sociology.* Although the theories of psychoanalysis are possibly the best known and have been the basis for much of the treatment of depression, neurochemical theories are currently receiving a great deal of attention. Studies of the neurochemistry of the brain have been stimulated by (1) the idea that with changes in feeling (mood) there are likely to be changes in the central nervous system, autonomic nervous system, and endocrine system; and (2) by a desire to understand how or why psychotropic drugs work. A number of hypotheses to explain the neurophysiology and biochemistry of depression (as well as other emotional disorders) are being proposed. The catecholamines † hypothesis, first stated by Joseph H. Schildkraut, is perhaps the best known. This hypothesis is that "Some, if not all, depressions are associated with an absolute or relative deficiency of catecholamines, particularly norepinephrine, at functionally important receptor sites in the

---

* Since the incidence of depression (and suicide) varies from country to country and age to age, the culture or state of society, must influence it. This century has produced rootless societies and alienation, as described by Alvin Toffler in *Future Shock* and by Vance Packard in *A Nation of Strangers.* The sociologic approach to the study of depression is the most comprehensive. (Toffler, Alvin: *Future Shock,* Bantam Books, Inc., New York, 1970; Packard, Vance: *A Nation of Strangers,* David McKay Co., Inc., New York, 1972.)

† The three catecholamines usually considered of physiologic importance are norepinephrine, dopamine, and epinephrine.

brain. Elation, conversely, may be associated with an excess of such amines." *

The evidence that supports this assumption comes from many behavioral-pharmacologic experiments with animals, and studies of human reactions to a variety of drugs. Some of these drugs (reserpine, chlorpromazine) are known to interfere with the metabolism of norepinephrine so that depression results, while others (monoamine exidase inhibitors, amphetamine, tricyclic drugs, and cocaine) are known to activate it and depression is lessened. Electroconvulsive shock treatment of animals has also been shown to increase brain norepinephrine.[67]

Although most of the evidence about catecholamines is indirect, James W. Maas and his associates [68] have found more direct evidence to support the hypothesis by showing that a specific metabolic product of brain norepinephrine (3-methoxy-4-hydroxy-phenolglycol, MHPG) appears in smaller amounts in the urine in some depressed patients than in nondepressed persons. They also report that when these depressed patients were given dextroamphetamine or imipramine (a tricyclic drug), their depression lessened and the level of urinary MHPG rose. Depressed patients whose MHPG levels were normal or higher than normal showed little or no change in behavior or MHPG levels.[69] Schildkraut and his co-workers [70] found that this latter group seemed to improve with the use of a different tricyclic drug, amitriptyline. Researchers point out that since patients in both groups had similar psychiatric diagnoses of depression, the determination of the level of urinary MHPG may be a more specific way to classify, diagnose, and treat this condition than has been available before. In addition, it shows the relationship between norepinephrine and depression.[71]

There is other biochemical research on the relationship between adrenocortical steroid hormones, electrolytes, and indoleamines (principally serotonin) and depression. According to Joseph Mendels and James L. Stinnett "a meaningful biological hypothesis of affective disorders should explain the interrelationships between biogenic amines, the endocrine system, electrolytes, and adenyl cyclase activity." †

Psychoanalytic theory explains the origin of depression as a breakdown in self-esteem and self-image. One's self-image is thought to come initially through adequate and appropriate oral gratification. In the first years of life, or development, response to frustration of oral needs is rage. If rage is met with insufficient parental acceptance and love, infants unconsciously fear retaliation, but they also subconsciously recognize that the object of their anger is also the object of their love on whom they are totally dependent. Should the infant continue to experience excessive and premature frustrations, and consistent parental devaluation, with the constant possibility of parental retaliation through withdrawal of love, the foundation for a pattern of response to disappointment or frustration is developed. Because infants are unable to clearly differentiate their sense of "self" and their sense of "others," the anger and aggression felt toward others are subconsciously turned inward. Rado [72] says the behavior of the depressed person is a cry for love that is brought about by a real or imagined loss that threatens emotional security.

A specific sociologic theory about the cause of depression has not yet been proposed; however, attempts have been made to find relationships between depression and social class, urban versus rural residence, ethnic membership, and family background. Although little consistency has been found between these circumstances and depression, some authorities report that ethnic membership or family background does influence its occurrence.[73] Izard [74] points out that these factors may be confused with hereditary factors. On the other hand, abnormal home environments have been implicated in the alteration or suppression of pituitary growth hormone in children, resulting in marked retardation of growth and emotional development, and hypopituitarism has been cited as a "cause" of depression.[75]

Samuel H. Kraines,[76] as well as other researchers, believe the origins of depression are in the genes, that is, that a physiologic predisposition toward depression is inherited. In an attempt to identify heredity as a cause of depression, many researchers have investigated its incidence among the family members of depressed patients who were hospitalized, and among sets of identical and fraternal twins. Although there is evidence that inherited factors contribute to the etiology of depression as a disease entity, the evidence is not adequate enough to fit into any known genetic model. It is possible that in the future specific links between heredity and the neurochemistry of depression will be found.

---

* Schildkraut, Joseph H.: "The Catecholamine Hypothesis of Affective Disorders: A Review of Supporting Evidence," *Am. J. Psychiatry*, **122**:509, (Nov.) 1965.

† Mendels, Joseph, and Stinnett, James L.: "Biogenic Amine Metabolism, Depression, and Mania," in Mendels, Joseph (ed.): *Biological Psychiatry*. John Wiley & Sons, New York, 1973, p. 81.

The influence of women's endocrine-physiologic processes on depression has been widely studied, and psychologic changes associated with the menstrual cycle described. Mild depression, restlessness, or tension a few days before the menstrual period are common feelings for many women. Findings of some studies suggest, however, that this endocrine activity may influence *when* severe emotional reactions occur in women rather than explain *why* they occur.[77]

A common cause of depression is drug addiction. Addictive drugs, including alcohol, are depressants. By depressing inhibitions, they produce a "high" period during which fear, pain, embarrassment, and self-consciousness are relieved so they are often referred to as "stimulants." They may allow repressed eroticism to assert itself and so produce sexual excitement. Some drug users feel "transported" and many writers have attempted to describe mystic experiences under the influence of drugs. Whatever the immediate effect, the ultimate result is a deep depression, with all its emotional consequences that ultimately result in death.

Since there are an estimated 9 to 10 million alcoholics in the United States and probably as many or more persons misusing other addictive drugs, the possibility of some sort of drug addiction as the cause of depression should always be considered. The man, woman, or child who is progressively dependent on drugs to put them to sleep will ultimately suffer from some degree of depression just as surely as will the person who misuses alcohol, cocaine, heroin, or other "hard line" drugs.

The depression associated with the use of an addictive drug fluctuates according to whether the person under its influence is forcibly taken off the drug or is voluntarily "withdrawing." In a culture that frowns on drug dependence, the addict is always affected by social disapproval. However, depression is a logical outcome with a physiologic explanation, for addictive drugs are, as a class, cerebral depressants. Most articles on alcoholism, while discussing the effect of alcohol on the liver, on sleep, memory, anxiety, or human relations, refer to depression as if it was an accepted accompaniment of the disease of addiction. For example, Laverne C. Johnson,[77a] studying sleep patterns in chronic alcoholics (patterns that, incidentally, resemble those of depressed persons), says that at the end of a 10-day withdrawal period, patients reported feeling "less depressed." Milton M. Gross and associates, also studying sleep disturbances in 100 alcoholics, noted in a check list, or "factor

analysis of daily clinical course, that 48 subjects suffer from depression." * David Davis,[77b] studying mood changes in alcoholic subjects with programmed and free-choice experimental drinking, reports they include depression and show a high incidence, as Peter E. Nathan and his associates also reported.[77c] The latter investigators note that alcoholics say they use alcohol to decrease their anxiety and depression but they note that it does not actually do this. Peter Steinglass and Sheldon Weiner say:

Such generally accepted notions as that of the alcoholic's drinking in order to relieve anxiety and depression have not borne up under direct clinical scrutiny. Instead, repeated observations of alcoholics during prolonged drinking bouts have demonstrated increasing levels of tension and anxiety, the emergence of suicidal ideation, and clinical and verbal evidence of profound depression.†

Alfonso Paredes and his associates, who filmed subjects who had drunk 120 ml of 80-proof vodka, say, "The effects more commonly expressed were depression, anxiety and anger." ‡ To summarize, depression accompanies addiction for physiologic and psychologic reasons. Addicts eventually reduce their activity. With hypoactivity, sensory stimulation is diminished. Finally, addicts sit or lie in one place, often cut off from family and old friends. Their associates tend to be other addicts and their activity is limited to that required to get the drug they crave. All addicts suffer, consciously or subconsciously, from social disapproval, lowered self-esteem, and guilt. Depression is an inevitable accompaniment of addiction in most, if not all, cultures.

Treatment of Depression. Authorities agree that the tendency of the depressed person, except for the most seriously psychotic and the persistent drug addict, is toward gradual and spontaneous recovery. (Whether this is recovery or simply a remission is a matter of

---

* Gross, Milton M., et al.: "Sleep Disturbances in Alcoholic Intoxication and Withdrawal," in Mello, Nancy K., and Mendelson, Jack H. (eds.): *Recent Advances in Studies of Alcoholism.* (National Institute on Alcohol Abuse and Alcoholism.) US Government Printing Office, Washington, D.C., 1971. (Pub. No. [HSM] 71–9045.)

† Steinglass, Peter, and Weiner, Sheldon: "Familial Interactions and Determinants of Drinking Behavior," in Mello, Nancy K., and Mendelson, Jack H. (eds.): *Recent Advances in Studies of Alcoholism.* (National Institute on Alcohol Abuse and Alcoholism.) US Government Printing Office, Washington, D.C., 1971. (Pub. No. [HSM] 71–9045.)

‡ Paredes, Alfonso, et al.: "Filmed Representations of Behavior and Responses to Self-Observation in Alcoholics," in Mello, Nancy K., and Mendelson, Jack H. (eds.): *Recent Advances in Studies of Alcoholism.* (National Institute on Alcohol Abuse and Alcoholism.) US Government Printing Office, Washington, D.C., 1971. (Pub. No. [HSM] 71–9045.)

some debate.) However, therapeutic measures are usually instituted when depression is diagnosed because the depressed are unbearably uncomfortable (mentally and physically) and, untreated, the danger of suicide is high. Leonard Cammer [77d] says the depressed person can be saved. Kline [77e] believes the problem is that society doesn't provide the effective treatment that is now available.

Pharmaceuticals are playing an increasingly important part in the therapy of all psychiatric disorders. Depression is no exception. In fact, some persons look upon the use of the following two groups of drugs as the major "breakthrough" in the treatment of depression. One is the tricyclic group of which imipramine (the first psychotropic drug used to treat depression) is a member. The exact biochemical mechanism through which these drugs are effective is not completely known, but it is thought they increase or activate brain norepinephrine. In general they have a more rapid action than do drugs in the second major group —the monoamine oxidase inhibitors. Both groups of drugs, however, have a period of from 1 to 4 weeks during which their effects are not noticeable. Some psychiatrists begin treatment with dextroamphetamines or electroconvulsive shock therapy, and later change to the tricyclic drugs. These medications as a group are short-acting and noncumulative, although there are some differences between specific drugs in this group.

The monoamine oxidase inhibitor (MAOI) group of drugs are generally used when the patient is treated in a hospital rather than on an outpatient basis because there is danger of hypertensive crisis and cerebral hemorrhage. These drugs are thought to prevent the oxidation of norepinephrine and serotonin (as well as other normal chemical compounds that have one amino group in their structure) in the brain. Drugs in this group should be used cautiously because they intensify the effects of a number of other commonly used drugs such as the antihistamines found in cold remedies. They also cause severe hypertensive reactions if certain foods are eaten during the time the drug is taken or for 1 to 2 weeks after the drug is discontinued. Foods to be avoided until monoamine oxidase is again synthesized by the patient's body are cheese, wine (especially Chianti), yeast products, yogurt, broad beans, chicken liver, and pickled herring. These foods contain large amounts of tyramine that raises the blood pressure, and that is normally destroyed in the body by monoamine oxidase.[78,79]

Drugs in both the tricyclic group and MAOI group can cause death if taken in large enough amounts. For this reason nurses should make certain that patients have access to a limited supply at any one time and that the drug is taken by the patient rather than "saved." The psychotropic drugs are considered so useful and are being used so frequently that anyone concerned with depression is encouraged to read extensively about their administration and effects.

Psychotherapeutic measures are considered by many psychiatrists to be the best approach to treatment. The basic ideas of some psychotherapies are discussed in the earlier section about anxiety. When intensive psychotherapy is started, its goals are to provide support for self-esteem through recognition, approval, and appropriate use of environmental conditions; to help patients readjust their levels of aspiration toward alternate goals in keeping with their abilities; to soften the dictates of their harsh consciences; and to help them reach a gradual recognition, acceptance, and examination of the hostility and anger that is a part of their depression.[80,80a] Psychiatric nurses with advanced preparation often act as primary therapists with depressed patients in psychiatric units either with individuals or groups. However, many patients on medical-surgical nursing units are depressed and need help from nurses. Beck [81] believes that much can be accomplished by supportive therapy with an empathetic, accepting person. He suggests that the emphasis should be placed on honestly reassuring patients that they will in time feel better. He also suggests that patients be encouraged to talk about the situations and relationships that are bothering them, and to cry if this is a natural result of their talking about their difficulties. A third suggestion is to plan activity for patients on a scheduled hourly basis in order to provide them with a tangible, daily structure, and to prevent their staying in one place and brooding.

A well-planned program of occupational and recreational activity for any person must be based on an understanding of that person. Age, sex, tastes, interests, experience, cultural prejudices, and his or her physical condition should be taken into account. Work at something that is productive is especially helpful as it results in a feeling of achievement and self-worth.* Books, movies, and television pro-

---

* Work that engages the whole man or woman is, of course, most therapeutic. Actually, such an occupation is play as well as work since the person enjoys it. Many of the crafts offered patients in occupational therapy departments are seen as yielding almost worthless products and so the patient scorns them. Marshall McLuhan [82] makes the point that work
(Continued)

grams help the person forget his or her worries for a time. They can be valuable aspects of therapy, but rarely take the place of a consuming task. Since depressed persons feel they are "failures," it is important that the work they undertake be something at which they can succeed.

Although electroconvulsive therapy (ECT) is used infrequently now, at one time it was the only effective treatment for depression. Some psychiatrists continue to use this method if the individual is severely depressed, or if rapid symptomatic improvement is the treatment goal. They also say some patients respond better to psychotherapy after several electroconvulsive treatments. Since electroconvulsive shocks increase the levels of norepinephrine and serotonin in the brain, they may have an effect like that of psychotropic drugs. Other biochemical changes with ECT are reported by Gunnar Holmberg.[83] There is hyperglycemia (lasting from 1 to several hours after the treatment), increased blood nitrogen compounds, potassium, calcium, phosphorous, and steroids, but there is no change in the activity of the brain monoamine oxidizing enzymes.

ECT consists of passing an electric current to the brain through small electrodes placed on the temporal areas of the head. The electric stimulation produces a convulsive seizure that is controlled through the use of pretreatment muscle relaxant medications. According to Holmberg,[84] the use of muscle relaxants and oxygen increases the therapeutic effect of the treatment.

During the treatment a brief anoxia occurs, the heart rate is frequently rapid and irregular, and there may be extreme fluctuations in blood pressure. Salivary and bronchial secretions are increased, and there is psychomotor restlessness. Following ECT, there is a varying amount of memory loss. This may range from mild forgetting to severe confusion, and if treatments are too close together, there may be increasing confusion.

When patients are to have ECT, the nurse is responsible for preparing them physically and mentally, for being with the patient during the treatment, and for safeguarding and reassuring him or her afterward. In most circumstances, people are better able to tolerate stressful events if they know what to expect

and what is expected of them. Therefore, patients should be told when the treatment will be given; what premedications will be given and by whom; * the general pattern of the treatment; and who will be with them during the treatment. Patients' questions should be answered as honestly as possible, and an opportunity provided for them to see the treatment room and have the equipment explained, if they want an explanation.

Food and fluids are restricted before ECT, and patients are asked to empty the bladder, and to remove glasses, contact lenses, and dentures. During the treatment the chin is supported and the arms held close to the chest to prevent movement and possible injury. Immediately following the electroshock convulsion, the patient's head should be turned to the side to prevent aspiration of saliva. After the treatment, when the patients have returned to their rooms, they should be safeguarded so that in their confusion and possible hyperactivity they do not hurt themselves. They should also be reassured that their memory loss is not permanent, reintroduced to those things they may have forgotten, and helped to participate in the current unit activities.[85]

Depression and Suicide. Because the depressed person feels discouraged, despondent, worthless, and hopeless, the possibility that suicide will be attempted or achieved is very high. Jacques Choron [86] says that approximately half of the estimated annual 30,000 suicides in the United States are committed by individuals who have had or are having a recognized depression. No one can be *sure* that the other half were not depressed when they took their lives. The very fact of wanting to die indicates depression. But this is not saying that all or even most of the persons with depression commit suicide, only that the rate of suicide among the depressed is 500 times the national rate.† Unfortunately, it is hard to determine whether or not a patient is depressed and suicidal. Not all depressed patients show the classic symptoms of depression; some conceal their feelings and low spirits, and mask the depression with shifting physi-

---

doesn't exist in a nonliterate world. He thinks primitive hunters or fishermen didn't know whether they were working or playing, and he says the painter or poet of today makes no distinction. His point is that there is no work if the whole man is involved. This should be the goal in finding occupation for the depressed.

* Anesthesiologists administer the intravenous sedation, muscle relaxants, and a cholinergic blocking agent such as atropine. They also administer oxygen if it is needed or at the end of the treatment for a rapid resuscitation.

† While there are official statistics for the number of suicides committed each year, most experts believe the figures are too low. The reasons given for this underreporting are religious or social, that is, the protection of the person from blame. In some circumstances, it is hard to know whether a death is accidental or suicidal.

Table 41-1. Outline of Types of Suicide and Suggested Preventive Treatments *

Logical Type	Personal Characteristics	Psychologic Label	Suggested Mode of Treatment
Logical. The process of reasoning is acceptable according to Aristotelian standards.	Individuals who are typically older, widowed, and who are in physical pain.	*Surcease suicide.* Person desires surcease from pain and reasons that his death will give him this.	Treatment is in terms of giving freedom from pain through use of analgesics and sedatives, and providing companionship by means of active milieu therapy such as clubs, activities, home placement.
Paleologic. Makes logical identifications in terms of attributes of the predicates rather than of the subjects.	Individuals who are delusional and/or hallucinatory.	*Psychotic suicide.* Not all suicides are psychotic, but psychotics can be unpredictably suicidal.	Treatment has to do primarily with the psychosis and only subsequently with suicidal tendencies (if remaining). Treatment should include protecting the individual from his own impulses.
Thanatologic. The logical or semantic error is in the overemphasis on the self as experienced by others.	Individuals whose beliefs permit them to view suicide as a transition to another life or as a means of saving reputation.	*Cultural suicide.* The belief concerning the concept of death in relation to the self plays a primary role in the suicide.	Treatment has to do with deeply entrenched religious and cultural beliefs and would have to deal with and clarify the semantic implications of the concept of death.
Catalogic. The logic is destructive. It confuses the self as experienced by the self with the self as experienced by others.	Individuals who feel lonely, helpless, fearful, and pessimistic about making meaningful personal relationships.	*Referred suicide.* The confusion in logic and in the psychologic identification is "referred" (like referred pain from other root problems).	Treatment would consist of psychotherapy wherein the goal would be to have the patient establish a meaningful, rewarding relationship so that his search for identification would not be barren.

* Shneidman, Edwin S., and Farberow, Norman L.: "Suicide and Death," in Feifel, Herman (ed.): *The Meaning of Death.* McGraw-Hill Book Co., New York, 1965, p. 299.

1633

cal symptoms. Laughlin says, "the outward evidence of, or degree of, the depression is by no means necessarily indicative of the degree of probability, or even the possibility, of the occurrence of suicide." * Longitudinal and follow-up studies of mental disorders indicate that it is frequently the person recovering from a diagnosed "depression" who commits suicide. Robert J. Bahra [86a] discusses four mechanisms that underlie suicide attempts: (1) ego destruction, (2) ego withdrawal, (3) displaced hostility, and (4) response to delusions. He notes that erosion of self-esteem to the point that a person considers self-destruction can occur under a variety of influences.

Authorities studying suicide agree that depressed persons often talk about suicide with others close to them, but if they do not they should be asked forthrightly if they have such thoughts, impulses, or plans. Nurses should know there is a four-level hierarchy of increasing suicidal danger: suicide thoughts, suicide plans, suicide preparations, and finally suicide attempts.[87]

Suicide studies conducted since 1960 at the Veterans Administration Hospital in Los Angeles indicate that, except for patients with neuropsychiatric disorders, the greatest number of suicides occurred in patients with diagnoses of long-term illness. Table 41-1 shows the types of suicide and suggested preventive treatments. From a study of 90 patients (45 suicides and 45 matched nonsuicides) with

* Laughlin, Henry P.: *Neuroses.* Appleton-Century-Crofts, New York, 1967, p. 195.

cardiorespiratory illnesses, a profile for the patient who was potentially suicidal was developed. In general, the patient most likely to commit suicide was more emotionally disturbed than his or her matched counterpart, had poorer relationships with the hospital staff and family, and was seen as both highly dependent and highly dissatisfied. While in the hospital this patient was described as hostile, agitated, apprehensive, depressed, complaining, and constantly demanding special attention from the hospital personnel.[88] Suicide notes are not uncommon. Table 41-2 shows the number and percentage of 619 suicide notes classified according to Menninger's hypothesis.

Table 41-3 shows the rate of suicide per 100,000 population in the United States of various age groups of white and nonwhite men and women for the years 1956–1957 and 1966–1967. The highest rate is among white men over age 64, while the greatest increase is among young men and women between the ages of 15 and 24 years, and women 25 to 44 years of age.[89] A study conducted at the Royal Infirmary of Edinburgh in Scotland found that the rates for *attempted* suicide were highest in the late teens and early 20s. This study also found that suicide rates reached a peak in the spring and autumn much like the incidence rates of depression, and reported that in the United States the use of drugs as the means for suicide had increased dramatically.[90] Figure 41-2 shows the total number of suicides in England and Wales for 1945–1970 and the most common methods used.

It appears that the most potent forces for

Table 41-2. Numbers and Percentages of 619 Suicide Notes Classified According to Menninger's Hypothesis *

Ages	Sex	To Kill		To Be Killed		To Die		Unclassifiable	
		Number	Per Cent	Number	Per Cent	Number	Per Cent	Number	Per Cent
20–39	Male	31	31	27	27	23	23	18	18
	Female	12	32	8	21	8	21	10	26
40–59	Male	50	23	35	16	75	35	55	26
	Female	15	29	9	17	15	29	13	25
60+	Male	20	11	18	10	99	57	38	22
	Female	6	15	2	5	30	75	2	5
	Total male	101	21	80	16	197	40	111	23
	Total female	33	25	19	15	53	41	25	19
	Totals	134	22	99	16	250	40	136	22

* Shneidman, Edwin S., and Farberow, Norman L.: "Suicide and Death," in Feifel, Herman (ed.): *The Meaning of Death.* McGraw-Hill Book Co., New York, 1965, p. 295.

Table 41-3. Rates of Suicide per 100,000 Population in U.S.A. by Age, White and Nonwhite, Male and Female, for Years 1956–1957 and 1966–1967 *

Age		15–24 yrs			25–44 yrs			45–64 yrs			65+ yrs	
		1956-57	1966-67	+ or –	1956-66	1966-67	+ or –	1956-57	1966-67	+ or –	1956-57	1966-67	+ or –
Male	White	6.4	10.4	+ 60%	16.0	20.0	+25%	34.2	32.9	–3%	50.0	40.3	–19%
	Nonwhite	5.5	8.4	+ 50%	11.5	15.6	+35%	11.3	13.3	+17%	15.6	13.5	–13%
Female	White	1.9	3.3	+74%	5.8	9.5	+64%	9.6	12.5	+30%	8.4	9.0	+5%
	Nonwhite	1.3	3.5	+115%	2.6	5.0	+92%	2.7	3.5	+30%	†	†	†

* Abstracted from the Metropolitan Life Insurance Company *Statistical Bulletin,* August 1972.
† No figures given.

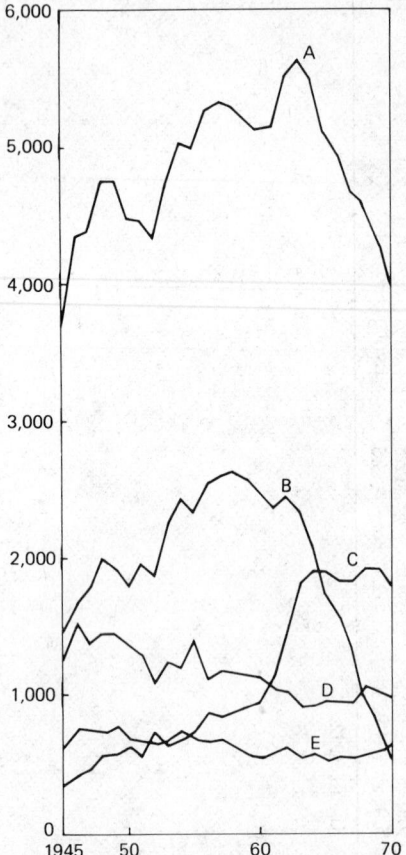

Figure 41-2. Total number of suicides in England and Wales for the years 1945–70 and the number of deaths for the most common methods used. *A.* Total number of suicides each year. *B.* Suicides by domestic gas poisoning. *C.* Suicides by drowning, firearms, jumping from high places, cutting, and other unspecified methods. *E.* Suicides by hanging and strangulation. (From Malleson, Andrew: *Need Your Doctor Be So Useless?* George Allen & Unwin, Ltd., London, 1973, p. 72.)

preventing suicide are (1) persuading the distressed persons that other people care what happens to them, and (2) helping them believe there is realistic hope that their disturbed feelings can be modified through treatment. Various suicide prevention centers and *Hot Line telephone services* * developed since the

early 1960s are based on these principles. Such centers operate on the basic assumptions that help should be available to persons in crisis, and the helper should be able to respond with competency and resourcefulness.[91]

Some persons who call crisis centers are unwilling or unable to meet with a therapist or other helping persons even after they have asked for help. For these individuals and their families, home visits by nurses are used increasingly to help the potentially suicidal person.[92]

Hospitalized patients identified as potentially suicidal benefit from nurses who like people, respect patients' individual personalities, and show concern for their individual welfare. According to reports from Norman L. Farberow and his associates,[93] the incidence of suicide was low on units staffed with such nurses, while the potentiality for suicide increased on units where the attitude of the nursing personnel was impersonal, distant, or uninterested. Sidney M. Jourard believes, as do others, "That some self-destructive mechanisms are always present in our bodies, and that there are agents in the environment that can release these mechanisms . . . anything that diminishes a person's experience of hope, meaning, and value in his continued existence simply releases the activity of the self-destructive mechanisms to a far greater degree than might be expected from ordinary wear and tear." *

3. INSOMNIA

Insomnia is ordinarily defined as the inability to sleep, and more particularly defined as a lessening of the duration or depth of sleep. It is the frequent companion of a disease and is nearly always present when a person is anxious or depressed. Researchers speculate that particular patterns of insomnia are associated with particular illnesses as the "dawn insomnia" mentioned earlier is thought to accompany severe depressions. Recent investigations indicate that it may not be the

---

* In Chapter 2, Emergency Medical Services Communication Systems (EMS) were discussed. It was pointed out that between January, 1968, and June, 1972, approximately 230 communities in the United States adopted the medical emergency telephone number 911. Communities not organized this way may have special numbers that suicidal or alcoholic persons may call or to which persons seeing a child "abused" may report the incident. Telephone opera-

tors are given these numbers and trained to help the public. Alcoholics Anonymous, Al-Anon (for families of alcoholics), and Alateen (for teenagers who have alcoholic parents) usually have listed numbers in large communities in most countries. In the United States, these organizations have national headquarters in New York City which can supply telephone numbers for local chapters if they are not listed in telephone directories (A.A., P.O. Box 459, Grand Central Station; Al-Anon and Alateen, P.O. Box 182, Madison Square Station). Local mental health centers and psychiatric hospitals provide such information as well as emergency treatment for the suicidal.

* Jourard, Sidney M.: "Suicide—An Invitation to Die," *Am. J. Nurs.*, **70:**269, (Feb.) 1970.

total amount of time spent sleeping that is the critical factor of insomnia, but that the duration of the various stages of sleep may be what is important for restful sleep. Authorities on sleep such as Nathaniel Kleitman[94] in the United States and Ian Oswald[95] in England agree there is a need for many well-conducted investigations of insomnia focused on the relationships between different types of insomnia and different types of illness. We believe that nurses are in an excellent position to study insomnia, as well as other disorders of sleep, since they are the health workers responsible for and available to patients during customary times of sleeping.

Prevalence of Insomnia. The number of individuals who have difficulty in sleeping is not known, but it is estimated that more than $100 million per year is spent in the United States for sleep medication.[96] One can assume from this that insomnia is a problem affecting large numbers of persons. Since many sleep-inducing drugs can be bought without prescription, they provide an uncontrollable health hazard.

The determination of whether an individual is suffering from insomnia is frequently a subjective judgment. If people believe that 8 hours of sleep are necessary but they are getting only 6 or 7, they may consider themselves as much insomniacs as those who are getting 3 or 4 hours of sleep. There are instances reported of healthy individuals who slept only 3 hours in each 24, or who had only "cat naps" between two full-time jobs at a factory.[97,98]

It appears that sleep disturbances occur in all age groups. While infants under 3 months of age ordinarily sleep from 14 to 16 hours each day, less sleep than this is associated with errors in handling them, rigid feeding schedules, as well as premature discontinuance of nighttime feedings. Nursing mothers can produce insomnia in their infants by drinking coffee, tea, Coca Cola, or eating foods that contain stimulants. With nursing or bottle-fed infants over 3 months, poor daily routines, colic, or infections may lessen sleep. Causative factors in children 9 months to 3 years of age include too much excitement and activity, and in older children, fear of the dark, irregular sleep routines, and overtiredness. At the opposite end of the age scale, older persons with little to do, perhaps receiving minimal stimulation from their environment or others, and sitting in a chair dozing a large part of the time, are prone to insomnia.

Causes of Insomnia. The causes of insomnia are frequently classified as being exogenous, or primarily outside the individual, and endogenous, or primarily internal to the in-

dividual. Exogenous factors are environmental; for instance, a change in accustomed night sounds (traffic versus no traffic), or the hardness or softness of the bed, or more or less light, or more or less heat than usual. Another exogenous factor is thought to be the occupation; for instance, the sleep pattern is broken when there are frequent changes in required work hours and accompanying changes in available sleep hours. The individual's circadian rhythm (see Chapter 6) is involved in adjusting to a changing work schedule. Given sufficient time, this rhythm changes to meet the new requirements. However, if the schedule for work and available sleep time is changed too often, insomnia is likely to persist, since body rhythms are in a state of almost constant flux. (Nurses assigned to short periods of "night duty" often have great difficulty in sleeping during the times available for sleep.) Other exogenous causes of insomnia, according to Kleitman,[99] are faulty habits of hygiene, climatic conditions, and meteorologic conditions.

Endogenous factors that may cause insomnia are physiologic, psychologic, a combination of the two, or idiopathic (unknown). Many disease conditions and their associated symptoms have been found to interfere with sleep, for instance, pain associated with duodenal ulcers; cough, bronchospasm or dyspnea associated with respiratory disease; and frequent urination associated with prostatic disease. In addition, fever, a central nervous system lesion (particularly in the reticular activating system), cardiovascular pathology, or hepatic insufficiency * usually produces insomnia.[100]

Another physiologic cause of insomnia under investigation is body temperature as it affects the quality of sleep. Gay G. Luce reported that the temperatures of good sleepers began to fall at bedtime and continued to fall to a low point in the early morning. "About an hour or two before they awakened in the morning, their temperatures began to climb, and were normal by the time they got up. By contrast, the temperatures of the poor sleepers declined less and were still declining when they arose in the morning." † Luce suggests that poor sleepers may have a body rhythm that is longer than a normal 24-hour rhythm so that they are continually out of synchrony with a 24-hour day.

---

* All patients with hepatitis whom the writers have known suffered fairly persistent insomnia and depression.

† Luce, Gay G.: *Body Time—Physiological Rhythms and Social Stress.* Pantheon Books, New York, 1971, p. 81.

Psychologic symptoms and their relationship to insomnia are also being studied. Depression and its apparently typical pattern of falling asleep easily but awaking very early is being investigated in conjunction with each stage of sleep. (Chapter 13 discusses normal stages of sleep.) The studies have shown that while depressed persons might have either very large or very small amounts of REM sleep, they characteristically had an erratic pattern quite different from the predictable REM rhythm of normal persons. In addition, instead of having deep stage IV sleep early in the night, the depressed person did not fall into stage IV sleep until early morning. The total amount of time in stage IV sleep was, therefore, less than normal.[101,102] H. W. Agnew and his associates[103] say that studies carried out to determine and compare the effects of stage IV and REM sleep deprivation suggest that individuals who were deprived of stage IV sleep developed depression and a reduction in their ability to function. Those persons deprived of REM sleep became more irritable and unstable in their reactions.* Gerald W. Vogel[103a] (in 1975) presents a comprehensive review of the literature on REM sleep deprivation.

Manifestations of Insomnia. Most persons have had a night of limited sleep and know the "torture" of sleeplessness, but for the insomniac these feelings are intensified. As insomnia persists, affected individuals, in spite of all they can do, are unable to interrupt this self-energizing mechanism. As night approaches and bedtime draws nearer, fear of being unable to sleep increases. The writers have seen some insomniacs who were in despair as night approached. Their thoughts were bent on being unable to sleep although they were droopy-eyed and yawning continually. In general, the behavior of the insomniac is like that of persons undergoing experimental sleep deprivation. This is described in more detail in Chapter 13.

There are at least the three following patterns of insomnia: (1) "initial," "predormitional," or difficulty in falling to sleep after going to bed; (2) intermittent, waking throughout the night; and (3) early morning waking. In the first or initial insomnia, which is the most common type, the onset of sleep is delayed for long periods of time. Patients complain that they are unable to get to sleep when others are sleeping and everything is quiet.

Oswald notes that this type of insomnia is understandable in persons with anxiety or, for that matter, in persons with an overactive mind. He says they are experiencing an "excitatory corticofugal bombardment of the reticular formation." * The second type of insomnia, intermittent (lacunary) insomnia, waking one or more times during the night, is attributed to poor sleep habits, but it can be associated with nightmares or unpleasant dreams. Some people have been able to break this habit once they recognized the nature of the problem. The third type of insomnia, terminal (postdormitional) insomnia, is characterized by early waking and the inability to get back to sleep.

Relief of Insomnia. In general, authorities agree that the underlying causes of insomnia must be identified if treatment or care is to be effective. Nurses can play a major role in discovering the cause of insomnia. By talking with patients, they can get a past and current description of their sleep patterns, and can find out whether they have or have had any of the conditions thought to be associated with insomnia. Nurses can help patients identify fears and worries, and finally, they can learn what drugs, if any, have been taken. After the causes or possible causes of insomnia are identified, a plan of care made by the patient, physician, and nurse can then be instituted. The plan may include the use of techniques to induce relaxation, reduce stimuli to all the senses, and reduce or eliminate factors producing fears and worries.† Perhaps the most important aspect of any program is exercise. Exciting exercise, as in games, should not be scheduled near bedtime, but rhythmic monotonous exercises can be highly soporific (see Chapter 13).

Hydrotherapy and massage can induce sleep, and general physical and hygienic measures that increase a person's comfort and sense of well-being are important.

Hypnotics, tranquilizers, and tricyclic antidepressant drugs may be used when other measures fail. Many techniques to help patients sleep are discussed in detail in Chapter 13. The difficulty of inducing restful sleep with drugs and the dangers of habitually using medication to induce sleep are also discussed in that chapter.

The insomniac requires health workers, family, and associates who understand him or her and who recognize that the difficulty may

---

* Some investigators think the relationship between the amount of sleep a depressed patient gets and his or her catecholamine metabolism will determine the best treatment for the individual. (Kupfer, David J.: "Sleep and Depressive Syndromes," *N. Engl. J. Med.,* **285:**1490, [Dec. 23] 1971.)

* Oswald, Ian: *Sleeping and Waking.* Elsevier Publishing Co., New York, 1962, p. 193.

† Many programs for alcoholics (who suffer greatly from insomnia) regularly include group classes in techniques to induce relaxation.

not be readily resolved in spite of their best efforts. It may be helpful for all those concerned with relieving insomnia to know that some experts claim there is little evidence that chronic insomnia results in any physiologic pathology,[104] no matter how distressing it is subjectively. Some highly productive persons have used many hours when most people are sleeping to do their best work. Thomas Edison is known to have slept for only about 4 of the 24-hour cycle, and the writers have known persons with comparable sleeping patterns. They advocate reading, taking exercises, or otherwise occupying wakeful hours rather than lying in bed and worrying that sleep doesn't come. Undoubtedly, most persons have much to learn about mental hygiene or control of the mind. All religions and many philosophies, especially those from the East, teach serenity. Sleep has a mysterious and mystical aspect about which volumes have been written. No function of the body is more complex or harder to understand.

REFERENCES

1. Portnoy, Isidore: "The Anxiety States," in Arieti, Silvano (ed.): *American Handbook of Psychiatry,* Vol. I. Basic Books, Inc., New York, 1959, p. 308.
2. Spielberger, Charles D. (ed.): *Anxiety: Current Trends in Theory and Research,* Vol. II. Academic Press, New York, 1972, p. 482.
3. May, Rollo: "Centrality of the Problem of Anxiety in Our Day," in Stein, M., et al. (eds.): *Identity and Anxiety.* Free Press, Glencoe, Ill., 1960, p. 120.
4. Scheier, Ivan H.: "Experimental Results to Date from the Standpoint of the Clinician," *Ann. N.Y. Acad. Sci.,* **93:**840, (Oct. 10) 1962.
4a. Buros, Oscar K. (ed.): *Personality Tests and Reviews.* Gryphon Press, Highland Park, N.J., 1970, p. 1061.
5. Cattell, Raymond B.: "The Nature and Measurement of Anxiety," *Sci. Am.,* **208:**96, (Mar.) 1963.
6. Michaels, Davida R.: "Too Much in Need of Support to Give Any?" *Am. J. Nurs.,* **71:**1932, (Oct.) 1971.
7. Kornfeld, Donald S., et al.: "Psychological Hazards of the Intensive Care Unit," *Nurs. Clin. North Am.,* **3:**41, (Mar.) 1968.
8. Vreeland, Ruth, and Ellis, Geraldine L.: "Stresses on the Nurse in an Intensive-Care Unit," *J.A.M.A.,* **208:**332, (Apr. 14) 1969.
9. Finn, Richard, and Huston, Paul E.: "Emotional and Mental Symptoms in Private Medical Practice," *J. Iowa Med. Soc.,* **56:** 138, (Feb.) 1966.
10. Rapoport, Lydia C.: "The State of Crisis: Some Theoretical Considerations," in Parad,

Howard J. (ed.): *Crisis Intervention: Selected Readings.* Family Service Association of America, New York, 1965, p. 25.
11. Freedman, Alfred M., et al.: *Modern Synopsis of Psychiatry.* Williams & Wilkins Co., Baltimore, 1972, p. 108.
12. *Ibid.,* p. 139.
13. Maslow, Abraham H.: *Motivation and Personality,* 2nd ed. Harper & Row, New York, 1970, p. 40.
14. Freedman, Alfred M., et al.: *op. cit.,* p. 36.
15. Gellhorn, E.: "The Neurophysiological Basis of Anxiety: A Hypothesis," *Perspect. Biol. Med.,* **8:**488, (Summer) 1965.
16. Guyton, Arthur C.: *Textbook of Medical Physiology,* 5th ed. W. B. Saunders Co., Philadelphia, 1976, p. 758.
17. Izard, Carroll E.: *Patterns of Emotions.* Academic Press, New York, 1972, p. 10.
18. Crammer, J. L.: "A Biochemical Approach to Affective Illness," in Mandelbrote, B. M., and Gelder, M. G. (eds.): *Psychiatric Aspects of Medical Practice.* Staples Press, London, 1972, p. 14.
19. Frazer, Alan, and Stinnett, James L.: "Distribution and Metabolism of Norepinephrine and Serotonin in the Central Nervous System" in Mendels, Joseph (ed.): *Biological Psychiatry.* John Wiley & Sons, New York, 1973, p. 35.
20. Schwap, John J., et al.: "The Differential Perception of Anxiety in Medical Patients: Sociodemographic Aspects," *Psychiatr. Med.,* **1:**151, (Apr.) 1970.
21. Lagina, Suzanne M.: "A Computer Program to Diagnose Anxiety Levels," *Nurs. Res.,* **20:**484, (Nov.–Dec.) 1971.
22. Cattell, Raymond B.: *op. cit.*
23. Graham, Lois E., and Conley, Elizabeth M.: "Evaluation of Anxiety and Fear in Adult Surgical Patients," *Nurs. Res.,* **20:**113, (Mar.–Apr.) 1971.
24. Menzies, Isabel E. P.: "A Case-Study in the Functioning of Social Systems as a Defence Against Anxiety," *Hum. Rel.,* **13:**95, (May) 1960.
25. Barton, David, and Kelso, Margaret T.: "The Nurse as a Psychiatric Consultation Team Member," *Psychiatr. Med.,* **2:**108, (Apr.) 1971.
25a. Grace, Mary J.: "The Psychiatric Nurse Specialist and Medical-Surgical Patients," *Am. J. Nurs.,* **74:**481, (Mar.) 1974.
26. Menzies, Isabel E. P.: *op. cit.*
27. Schwap, John J., et al.: *op. cit.*
27a. Burkhardt, Marti: "Response to Anxiety," *Am. J. Nurs.,* **69:**2153, (Oct.) 1969.
28. Izard, Carroll E.: *op. cit.,* p. 10.
29. Rogers, Carl R.: "Client-Centered Therapy," in Arieti, Silvano (ed.): *American Handbook of Psychiatry,* Vol. III. Basic Books, Inc., New York, 1966, p. 184.
29a. Skinner, B. F.: *Beyond Freedom and Dignity.* Alfred A. Knopf, New York, 1971.
30. Kaplan, Donald M.: "The Decline of a Golden Craft," *Harper's Magazine,* **234:**41, (Feb.) 1967.

31. Rogers, Carl R.: *op. cit.*, p. 193.

32. *Ibid.*, p. 183.

33. Rapoport, Lydia C.: *op. cit.*

34. Aguilera, Donna, et al.: *Crisis Interventions: Theory and Methodology.* C. V. Mosby Co., St. Louis, 1970, p. 47.

34a. Hitchcock, Janice Marland: "Crisis Intervention, The Pebble in the Pool," *Am. J. Nurs.,* **73:**1388, (Aug.) 1973.

35. Peplau, Hildegarde: "Interpersonal Techniques: The Crux of Psychiatric Nursing," *Am. J. Nurs.,* **62:**53, (June) 1962.

36. Meyers, Mary E.: "The Effect of Types of Communication on Patients' Reactions to Stress," *Nurs. Res.,* **13:**126, (Spring) 1964.

37. Putt, Arlene M.: "One Experiment in Nursing Adults with Peptic Ulcers," *Nurs. Res.,* **19:**484, (Nov.–Dec.) 1970.

38. Johnson, Jean E.: "Effects of Structuring Patients' Expectations on Their Reactions to Threatening Events," *Nurs. Res.,* **21:**499, (Nov.–Dec.) 1972.

39. Nite, Gladys, and Willis, Frank N.: *The Coronary Patient; Hospital Care and Rehabilitation.* Macmillan Publishing Co., Inc., New York, 1964, p. 173.

39a. Barnes, Elizabeth (ed.): *Psychosocial Nursing. Studies from the Cassel Hospital.* Tavistock Publications, London, 1968.

40. Holsclaw, Pamela A.: "Nursing in High Emotional Risk Areas," *Nurs. Forum,* **4:**36, (No. 4) 1965.

41. Hay, Donald, and Oken, Donald: "The Psychological Stresses of Intensive Care Unit Nursing," *Psychosom. Med.,* **34:**109, (Mar.–Apr.) 1972.

42. Kaufman, Arthur, et al.: "Tranquilizer Control," *J.A.M.A.,* **221:**1504, (Sept. 25) 1972.

43. Ayd, Frank J., Jr.: "The Chemical Assault on Mental Illness—The Major Tranquilizers," *Am. J. Nurs.,* **65:**70, (Apr.) 1965.

44. *Ibid.*

45. Kline, Nathan S., and Davis, John M.: "Psychotropic Drugs," *Am. J. Nurs.,* **73:**54, (Jan.) 1973.

46. *Ibid.*

47. Morgan, Arthur J.: "Minor Tranquilizers, Hypnotics, and Sedatives," *Am. J. Nurs.,* **73:**1220, (July) 1973.

48. Beck, Aaron T.: *Depression.* Harper & Row, New York, 1967, p. 9.

49. Laughlin, Henry P.: *Neuroses.* Appleton-Century-Crofts, New York, 1967, p. 137.

49a. Jackson, Pat Ludder: "Chronic Grief," *Am. J. Nurs.,* **74:**1288, (July) 1974.

50. Crary, William G., and Crary, Gerald C.: "Depression," *Am. J. Nurs.,* **73:**472, (Mar.) 1973.

51. "Many Reported Sufferers of Depression," *Houston Post,* June 18, 1973.

52. Silverman, Charlotte: *The Epidemiology of Depression.* Johns Hopkins Press, Baltimore, 1968, p. 73.

52a. Chinn, Austin B. (ed.): "Working With Older People," in *Clinical Aspects of Aging,* Vol. IV. US Government Printing Office, Washington, D.C., 1971. (PHS Pub. No. 1459).

53. Spitz, René A.: "Anaclitic Depression—An Inquiry into the Genesis of Psychiatric Conditions in Early Childhood, II," in Freud, Anna, et al. (eds.): *The Psychoanalytic Study of the Child,* Vol. II. International Universities Press, New York, 1949, p. 313.

54. Bakwin, Harry: "Emotional Deprivation in Infants," *J. Pediatr.,* **35:**512, (Oct.) 1949.

55. Bowlby, John: *Maternal Care and Mental Health.* World Health Organization, Geneva, 1951. (Monograph Series No. 2.)

56. Glaser, Kurt: "Masked Depression in Children and Adolescents," in Chess, Stella, and Thomas, Alexander (eds.): *Annual Progress in Child Psychiatry and Child Development, 1968.* Brunner/Mazel Publishers, New York, 1968, p. 345.

57. Malmquist, Carl P.: "Depressions in Childhood and Adolescence," in Chess, Stella, and Thomas, Alexander (eds.): *Annual Progress in Child Psychiatry and Child Development, 1972.* Brunner/Mazel Publishers, New York, 1972, p. 502.

58. Laughlin, Henry P.: *op. cit.,* p. 154.

59. Rado, Sandor: "Psychodynamics of Depression from the Etiologic Point of View," in Gaylin, Willard (ed.): *The Meaning of Despair.* Science House, New York, 1968, p. 96.

59a. Peplau, Hildegard E.: "Mid-Life Crises," *Am. J. Nurs.,* **75:**1761, (Oct.) 1975.

59b. Hargreaves, Anne G.: "Making the Most of the Middle Years," *Am. J. Nurs.,* **75:**1772, (Oct.) 1975.

60. Silverman, Charlotte: *op. cit.,* p. 112.

61. Kety, Seymour: "Brain Catecholamines, Affective States and Memory," in McGaugh, James L. (ed.): *The Chemistry of Mood, Motivation and Memory.* Plenum Press, New York, 1972, p. 76.

62. Laughlin, Henry P.: *op. cit.,* p. 184.

63. Wyler, Allen R., et al.: "Magnitude of Life Events and Seriousness of Illness," *Psychosom. Med.,* **33:**115, (Mar.–Apr.) 1971.

64. Rahe, Richard H.: "Life-change Measurement as a Predictor of Illness," *Proc. R. Soc. Med.,* **61:**1124, (Nov.) 1968.

65. Thomson, Kay C., and Hendric, Hugh C.: "Environmental Stress in Primary Depressive Illness," *Arch. Gen. Psychiatry,* **26:**130, (Feb.) 1972.

66. Paykel, Eugene S., et al.: "Life Events and Depression," *Arch. Gen. Psychiatry,* **21:**753, (Dec.) 1969.

67. Kety, Seymour: *op. cit.*

68. Maas, James W., et al.: "Catecholamine Metabolism, Depressive Illness, and Drug Response," *Arch. Gen. Psychiatry,* **26:**252, (Mar.) 1972.

69. Fawcett, Jan, et al.: "Depression and MHPG Excretion," *Arch. Gen. Psychiatry,* **26:**246, (Mar.) 1972.

70. Schildkraut, Joseph H., et al.: "Effects of Tricyclic Antidepressants on Norepinephrine Metabolism: Basic and Clinical Stud-

ies," in Ho, Beng T., and McIsack, William W. (eds.): *Brain Chemistry and Mental Disease*. Plenum Press, New York, 1971, p. 217.

71. Mendels, Joseph, and Stinnett, James L.: "Biogenic Amine Metabolism, Depression, and Mania," in Mendels, Joseph (ed.): *Biological Psychiatry*. John Wiley & Sons, New York, 1973, p. 68.

72. Rado, Sandor: *op. cit.*

73. Silverman, Charlotte: *op. cit.*, p. 73.

74. Izard, Carroll E.: *op. cit.*, p. 220.

75. Gardner, Lytt I.: "Deprivation Dwarfism," *Sci. Am.*, **227:**76, (July) 1972.

76. Kraines, Samuel H.: *Mental Depressions and Their Treatment*. Macmillan Publishing Co., Inc., New York, 1957.

77. Silverman, Charlotte: *op. cit.*

77a. Johnson, Laverne C.: "Sleep Patterns in Chronic Alcoholics," in Mello, Nancy K., and Mendelson, Jack H. (eds.): *Recent Advances in Studies of Alcoholism*. (National Institute on Alcohol Abuse and Alcoholism.) US Government Printing Office, Washington, D.C., 1971. (Pub. No. (HSM) 71–9045.)

77b. Davis, David: "Mood Changes in Alcoholic Subjects with Programmed and Free-Choice Experimental Drinking," in Mello, Nancy K., and Mendelson, Jack H. (eds.): *Recent Advances in Studies of Alcoholism*. (National Institute on Alcohol Abuse and Alcoholism.) US Government Printing Office, Washington, D.C., 1971. (Pub. No. (HSM) 71–9045.)

77c. Nathan, Peter E., et al.: "Comparative Studies of the Interpersonal and Affective Behavior of Alcoholics and Nonalcoholics During Prolonged Experimental Drinking," in Mello, Nancy K., and Mendelson, Jack H. (eds.): *Recent Advances in Studies of Alcoholism*. (National Institute on Alcohol Abuse and Alcoholism.) US Government Printing Office, Washington, D.C., 1971. (Pub. No. (HSM) 71–9045.)

77d. Cammer, Leonard: *Up From Depression*. Simon & Schuster, New York, 1969.

77e. Kline, Nathan S.: *Depression: Its Diagnosis and Treatment; Lithium: the History of Its Use in Psychiatry*. S. Karger, White Plains, N.Y., 1969.

78. Kline, Nathan S., and Davis, John M.: *op. cit.*

79. Morgan, Arthur J.: *op. cit.*

80. Laughlin, Henry P.: *op. cit.*, p. 210.

80a. Penalver, Meg: "Helping the Child Handle His Aggression," *Am. J. Nurs.*, **73:**1555, (Sept.) 1973.

81. Beck, Aaron T.: *op. cit.*, p. 315.

82. McLuhan, Marshall: *Understanding Media —The Extension of Man*. McGraw-Hill Book Co., New York, 1964.

83. Holmberg, Gunnar: "Biological Aspects of Electro-convulsive Therapy," *Int. Rev. Neurobiol.*, **5:**389, 1963.

84. *Ibid.*

85. Cohen, Roberta: "EST + Group Therapy =

Improved Care," *Am. J. Nurs.*, **71:**1195, (June) 1971.

86. Choron, Jacques: *Suicide*. Charles Scribner's Sons, New York, 1972, p. 76.

86a. Bahra, Robert J.: "The Potential for Suicide," *Am. J. Nurs.*, **75:**1782, (Oct.) 1975.

87. Mintz, Ronald S.: "Basic Considerations in the Psychotherapy of the Depressed Suicidal Patient," *Am. J. Psychother.*, **25:**56, (Jan.) 1971.

88. Farberow, Norman L., et al.: "Suicide Among Patients with Cardiorespiratory Illness," *J.A.M.A.*, **195:**128, (Feb. 7) 1966.

89. Grove, W. R.: "Suicide—International Comparisons," *Stat. Bull. Metropol. Life Ins. Co.*, **53:**3, (Aug.) 1972.

90. McCulloch, J. Wallace, and Philip, Alistair E.: *Suicidal Behavior*. Pergamon Press, Oxford, 1972.

91. Haughton, Anson B.: "Suicide Prevention Programs—The Current Scene," *Am. J. Psychiatry*, **124:**114, (June) 1968.

92. Kloes, Karen B.: "The Suicidal Patient in the Community: A Challenge for Nurses," in *ANA Clinical Sessions, 1968*. Appleton-Century-Crofts, New York, 1968, p. 36.

93. Farberow, Norman L., et al.: *op. cit.*

94. Kleitman, Nathaniel: *Sleep and Wakefulness*, rev. ed. University of Chicago Press, Chicago, 1963, p. 274.

95. Oswald, Ian: *Sleeping and Waking*. Elsevier Publishing Co., New York, 1962, p. 193.

96. Pilling, Loran F.: "Clinical Disturbances of Sleep," *Postgrad. Med.*, **41:**178, (Feb.) 1967.

97. Jones, Henry S., and Oswald, Ian: "Two Cases of Healthy Insomnia," *Electroencephalogr. Clin. Neurophysiol.*, **24:**378, (Apr.) 1968.

98. Wheatley, David: "Sleep," *Proc. R. Soc. Med.*, **62:**149, (Feb.) 1969.

99. Kleitman, Nathaniel: *op. cit.*, p. 275.

100. Williams, Donald H.: "Sleep and Disease," *Am. J. Nurs.*, **71:**2321, (Dec.) 1971.

101. Hauri, Peter, and Hawkins, David R.: "Phasic REM, Depression, and the Relationship Between Sleeping and Waking," *Arch. Gen. Psychiatry*, **25:**56, (July) 1971.

102. Mendels, Joseph, and Hawkins, David R.: "Sleep and Depression," *Arch. Gen. Psychiatry*, **16:**344, (Mar.) 1967.

103. Agnew, H. W., Jr., et al.: "Comparison of Stage Four and 1-REM Sleep Deprivation," *Percept. Mot. Skills*, **24:**855, 1967.

103a. Vogel, Gerald W.: "A Review of REM Sleep Deprivation," *Arch. Gen. Psychiatry*, **37:**749, (June) 1975.

104. Plum, Fred: "Sleep and Its Disorders," in Beeson, Paul B., and McDermott, Walsh (eds.): *Textbook of Medicine*, Vol. I, 14th ed. W. B. Saunders Co., Philadelphia, 1975, p. 522.

Additional Suggested Reading

Allekian, Constance I.: "Intrusion of Territory and Personal Space: An Anxiety-Inducing Factor for Hospitalized Persons—an Exploratory Study," *Nurs. Res.,* **22:**236, (May–June) 1973.

Barnes, Corinne M., et al.: "Measurement in Management of Anxiety in Children for Open Heart Surgery," *Pediatrics,* **49:**250, (Feb.) 1972.

Beck, A. T., et al. (eds.): *The Prediction of Suicide.* Charles Press Publishers, Bowie, Md., 1974.

Drye, Robert C., et al.: "No-Suicide Decisions: Patient Monitoring of Suicidal Risk," *Am. J. Psychiatry,* **130:**171, (Feb.) 1973.

Dyrud, Jarl: "Treatment of Anxiety States," *Arch. Gen. Psychiatry,* **25:**298, (Oct.) 1971.

Farberow, Norman, et al.: *Techniques in Crisis Intervention—A Training Manual.* Suicide Prevention Center, Inc., Los Angeles, 1968.

Fisher, S. A.: *Suicide and Crisis Intervention; Survey and Guide to Services.* Springer Publishing Co., New York, 1973.

Francis, Gloria M., and Munjas, Barbara: *Promoting Psychological Comfort.* Wm. C. Brown Co., Dubuque, Iowa, 1968.

Gage, Frances Boland: "Suicide in the Aged," *Am. J. Nurs.,* **71:**2153, (Nov.) 1971.

Gorman, M. Leah: "Conscious Repatterning of Human Behavior," *Am. J. Nurs.,* **75:**1752, (Oct.) 1975.

Jung, Carl G., et al.: *The Meaning of Death.* McGraw-Hill Book Co., New York, 1959.

Karakan, Ismet (ed.): "Proceedings of Sleep Symposium Held at 19th Annual Academy Meeting," *Psychosomatics,* **14:**14–124, (Mar.–Apr.) 1975.

Kogan, Benjamin A.: *Health; Man in a Changing Environment.* Harcourt, Brace & World, New York, 1970.

Kolb, David A., and Boyatzis, Richard E.: "On the Dynamics of the Helping Relationship," *J. Appl. Behav. Sci.,* **6:**267, (July–Aug.–Sept.) 1970.

Kora, Takehisa, and Ohara, Kenshiro: "Morita Therapy," *Psychology Today,* **6:**63, Mar.) 1973.

Maas, J. W., et al.: "A Kinetic Study of the Disposition of Circulating Norepinephrine in Normal and Depressed Subjects," *J. Psychosom. Med.,* **31:**451, 1969.

Mark, F. R.: "A New Project for Nursing Homes to Combat Loneliness, Anxiety, Boredom," *Nurs. Homes,* **22:**32, (Apr.) 1973.

Melton, Arthur W., and Martin, Edwin (eds.): *Coding Processes in Human Memory.* John Wiley & Sons, New York, 1972.

Mendelson, Mary Adelaide: *Tender Loving Greed.* Alfred A. Knopf, New York, 1974.

Millon, Theodore: *Theories of Psychopathology and Personality.* W. B. Saunders Co., Philadelphia, 1973.

Pai, Mangalore Narasimha: *Searchlight on Sleep Disorders.* Literary Services and Production, Ltd., London, 1969.

Peitchinis, Jacquelyn A.: "Therapeutic Effectiveness of Counseling by Nursing Personnel: Review of the Literature," *Nurs. Res.,* **21:**138, (Mar.–Apr.) 1972.

Penfold, Kathleen McNally: "Supporting Mother Love," *Am. J. Nurs.,* **74:**464, (Mar.) 1974.

Pierce, C. M., et al.: "Enuresis and Dreaming," *Arch. Gen. Psychiatry,* **4:**166, (Feb.) 1961.

Powers, Mary Ann E., and Storlie, Frances: "The Apprehensive Patient," *Am. J. Nurs.,* **67:**58, (Jan.) 1967.

Pride, L. Frances: "An Adrenal Stress Index as a Criterion Measure for Nursing," *Nurs. Res.,* **17:**292, (July–Aug.) 1968.

Redmond, D. E., Jr., et al.: "Changes in Primate Social Behavior Following Treatment with Alpha Methyl Tyrosine," *J. Psychosom. Med.,* **32:**551, 1970.

————: "Changes in Primate Social Behavior After Treatment with Alpha Methyl Para Tyrosine and Para Chloraphenylalamine," *Fed. Proc.,* **30:**711, 1971.

Renshaw, Domeena C.: "Psychiatric First Aid in an Emergency, *Am. J. Nurs.,* **72:**497, (Mar.) 1972.

Robishon, Paulette: "The Challenge of Crisis Theory for Nursing," *Nurs. Outlook,* **15:**28, (July) 1967.

Saper, Beatrice: "Patients as Partners in a Team Approach," *Am. J. Nurs.,* **74:**1844, (Oct.) 1974.

Schoen, Eugenia A.: "Clinical Problem: The Demanding, Complaining Patient," *Nurs. Clin. North Am.,* **2:**715, (Dec.) 1967.

Sims, Mary, et al.: "Drug Overdoses in a Canadian City," *Am. J. Public Health,* **63:**215, (Mar.) 1973.

Stephens, Kathleen Schmidt: "A Toddler's Separation Anxiety," *Am. J. Nurs.,* **73:**1553, (Sept.) 1973.

Vallen, Karen Helm, and Watson, Charles G.: "Suicide in Relation to Time of Day and Day of Week," *Am. J. Nurs.,* **75:**263, (Feb.) 1975.

Wacker, Margaret S.: "Analogy: Weapon Against Denial," *Am. J. Nurs.,* **74:**71, (Jan.) 1974.

Westercamp, Twilla M.: "Suicide," *Am. J. Nurs.,* **75:**260, (Feb.) 1975.

Whitney, William, et al.: "Depressive Symptoms and Academic Performance in College Students," *Am. J. Psychiatry,* **128:**122, (Dec.) 1971.

Williams, James G., et al.: "Behavioral Measurement of Severe Depression," *Arch. Gen. Psychiatry,* **27:**330, (Sept.) 1972.

Gladys Nite
Catherine Temple
Virginia Henderson

The authors acknowledge the assistance of Laurie M. Gunter, R.N., Ph.D., Professor, School of Nursing, Pennsylvania State University, in the preparation of the section on anxiety.

CHAPTER 42

Hyperthermia or Hypothermia as a Result of Exposure to Extreme Environmental Temperatures or as Prescribed Treatment

1. ENVIRONMENTAL EFFECTS OF CLIMATIC TEMPERATURES ON MAN
2. EFFECTS OF EXTREMES OF CLIMATIC HEAT ON MAN
3. BURNS
4. EFFECTS OF EXTREMES OF CLIMATIC COLD ON MAN
5. HYPOTHERMIA AS PRESCRIBED TREATMENT

1. ENVIRONMENTAL EFFECTS OF CLIMATIC TEMPERATURES ON MAN

Man, as well as other mammals and birds, is a homeotherm, which means that they all have mechanisms for the maintenance and regulation of a constant body temperature even when environmental temperatures are at extreme variance with that of the body. Constancy of body temperature is necessary to normal metabolism. Homeotherms are free to pursue their activities rather than have their activities determined for them by their environments.[1]

Effects of Climate on Health. Climate with its variations in temperature affects man's living habits and health. Differences exist among men living in tropical climates, temperate climates, and arctic climates. These climates profoundly affect man's adaptation and his way of life.

Clarence A. Mills[2] in *Climate Makes the Man* develops the thesis that since even the food in cold and tropical climates differs chemically, man, played on by this and other climatic influences, has a set of characteristics typical of the cold, temperate, and tropical zones. One characteristic of the northerner, who, according to Mills, has better food, is his abundant energy or drive. Arteriosclerosis and other degenerative diseases are thought by Mills to be associated with this temperament. He believes the peoples of cold climates wear themselves out. The less well-fed but easygoing southerner Mills thinks less susceptible to degenerative disease but an easy

prey for the bacteria and protozoa surrounding him in such profusion. Marston Bates, in a study of the tropics, *Where Winter Never Comes*, questions most of our preconceived notions about hot countries. He points out that the "profusion of nature" in the tropics is reflected in the variety of indigenous diseases, mostly infectious. He also points out that "modern medicine" is a product of Western civilization and that it has consequently been most successful in nontropical areas. He adds:

In other words, disease conditions in the tropics are in part dependent on the cultural environment rather than the climatic environment. Diseases that we now think of as primarily tropical were once much more widely spread. Malaria, for instance, was common a hundred years ago in places like Denmark, Sweden, England, Connecticut, and Michigan. Bubonic plague was one of the diseases that swept across medieval Europe with disastrous effect. Yellow fever . . . was [once] the cause of a great epidemic in Philadelphia.*

He goes on to say that "with the methods presently available, there is no technical reason why the tropics should not be just as healthy as any other part of the earth's surface." Bates thinks that many of the ills suffered by the nonnative in tropical climates result from bringing into a hot climate habits of living unsuited to it. There is, on the other hand, a general acceptance of the theory that the white man is more susceptible than his dark-skinned brother to the excessive ultraviolet

* Bates, Marston: *Where Winter Never Comes.* Charles Scribner's Sons, New York, 1952, pp. 136, 153.

irradiation near the equator. Harold F. Blum [3] concludes that the higher incidence of cancer of the skin and lips in the southern part of the United States than is found in the northern part can be attributed to the difference in ultraviolet irradiation in these regions. Certainly, white races living in tropical countries develop more skin pigment, which is evidently nature's protection.

The studies of George E. Burch and Nicholas P. DePasquale [4] show that a hot, humid environment increases the stroke volume, cardiac output, mechanical and physical work of the heart, and the tension on the ventricles. The degree of thermal stress on the individual by the environment is analogous to that produced by physical exercise. In a patient with a decreased cardiac reserve due to heart disease, heat stress may produce acute left ventricular failure. The incidence of myocardial infarction seems to be associated with climatic stress. In northern climates of the United States the stress of the climate is at its peak during the winter months and the number of myocardial infarctions is increased, while in the South climatic stress is greater during the summer months and the number of myocardial infarctions increases at this time.

The ideal climate as described by Burch and DePasquale [5] exists when the environmental wet bulb * temperature is between 10°C (50°F) and 15.5°C (60°F), but becomes uncomfortable when the wet bulb temperature is above 21.1°C (70°F). The amount of clothing worn by the person and the activity he or she performs also must be taken into consideration, and habits and traditions affect the preferred temperature. In the United States, the preferred room temperature is higher than that of England and lower than that of Singapore. [6]

Effects of Heat. Man can lose or conserve heat, within limits, by physiologic changes. When these limits are exceeded, hot or cold environments can be fatal. Heat is lost by

* Wet bulb temperature is calculated from the temperature, humidity, and wind velocity.

man through the excreta and expired air but chiefly from the surface of the body by radiation, conduction-convection, and evaporation of perspiration (see Fig. 42-1). In a hot environment the heart beats more rapidly, and the blood vessels dilate to bring more blood to the surface of the body where it can be cooled; sweating is increased so that heat can be lost from the body through its vaporization. Heat loss is further induced by voluntarily seeking a cooler environment, by removing clothing that surrounds the body with insulating jackets of still air, and by cutting down muscular activity or the metabolic rate. Man can increase and conserve body heat by increasing the metabolic rate with shivering, by reducing the circulating fluids in the skin by contracting the blood vessels and slowing the heartbeat, and by decreasing the activity of sweat glands. Exposed to a cold environment, man seeks warmth, hunches himself to reduce the body surface, puts on more clothing, and increases metabolism with voluntary muscular exercise.

Radiation provides for heat transfer from one body to another regardless of intervening media. Heat is transmitted from the sun in the form of ultraviolet and infrared energy. Man, too, can lose heat in the form of radiation, or receive it from his surroundings. [7] All mass in the universe that is not at absolute zero temperature radiates heat energy. As long as body temperature remains above the temperature of the surroundings, heat will be radiated from the body, but when the surroundings become hotter than the human body, heat will be radiated to the body. [8]

Heat is lost or gained by man, also, through conduction-convection. Heat is conducted from one source to another by direct contact between the objects. When a person touches a cooler object, heat is transferred to the cooler object and the opposite occurs when a warm object is touched. Convection is the flow of heat as a result of contact with the physical movement of gas or liquid. Rapidly moving air currents, or wind, is a good example of a source of heat transfer by convection. For ex-

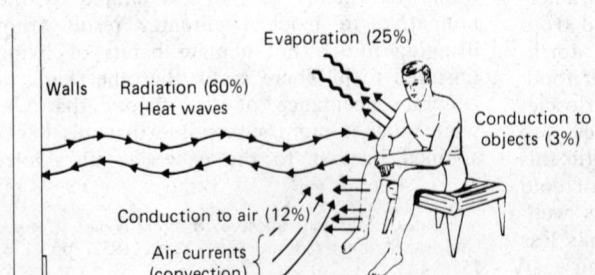

Evaporation (25%)

Walls   Radiation (60%)
         Heat waves
                                    Conduction to
                                    objects (3%)

Conduction to air (12%)

Air currents
(convection)

Figure 42-1. Mechanisms of heat loss from the body. (From Guyton, Arthur C.: *Textbook of Medical Physiology*, 4th ed. W. B. Saunders Co., Philadelphia, 1971, p. 832.)

ample, skin coming in contact with cool wind currents is cooled because as the air in contact with the skin is warmed it is constantly being replaced by more cool air.[9] Conduction and convection are often considered together because they both require direct contact for transfer of heat.

The third method of heat exchange by man is through evaporation of water from the surface of the skin. This channel of heat exchange is thought to result only in the loss of heat by the body, while the other two methods of exchange could produce heat gain or loss. Total evaporative heat loss is accounted for by evaporation from the respiratory tract, diffusion of water vapor through the skin, and perspiration, which is sensible wetness of the skin.[10] Perspiration supplements insensible water vapor loss from the skin, in reaction to increases in environmental temperature, and plays a particularly important role in the body's response to excessive environmental heat.

During resting conditions, approximately two-thirds of heat loss is accomplished by radiation and conduction-convection. Evaporation of water that diffuses insensibly through the skin makes up the remaining avenue of heat loss. Increased heat loss necessitated by exposure to hot environmental temperatures or increased amounts of work is accomplished only through an increase in the production of sweat, the evaporation of which can provide heat losses at the rate of 600 calories per liter. Increases in heat losses through conduction-convection and radiation brought about by circulatory vasodilation are inconsequential.[11]

Man has learned to adapt to extremely cold conditions through the use of such cultural adaptations as fire, clothing, and shelter. Consequently, there has been little need for him to become physically acclimatized to cold. However, man has not been as successful in his cultural adaptation to heat. Man can tolerate far less extremes of heat than cold. The process of heat acclimatization, therefore, assumes greater importance than acclimatization to cold.

Jerome W. Conn defines acclimatization as "that process of adaptation which occurs when man is exposed to an environment hotter than that to which he is accustomed and which, when completed, results in a remarkable increase in his capacity to live and work in heat without distressing symptoms." * Artificial acclimatization to heat may be achieved by exposing an individual to higher environmental

temperatures for 2-hour periods daily for as little as 14 days.[12]

When individuals are asked to work hard in an industrial environment or exercise under hot-wet conditions, their tolerance is low. Their skin rapidly becomes flushed, respirations increase to the point of hyperventilation, temperature rises, and they soon experience hypotensive collapse. On the first exposure they may be unable to work, but with subsequent exposures they find work easier and, if exposed daily over the next 2 to 3 weeks, they become fully acclimatized. The physiologic changes that bring about the increased adaptation involve the circulation, sweat production, respiration, and the less obvious changes in sweat composition and kidney and endocrine function. The fact that changes do occur has been known for many years but the reasons why they occur remain unclear. The first time persons are exposed to extremes of environmental heat they become flushed, the heart rate increases, and they experience hypotension and may faint. This reaction is caused by the sudden peripheral vasodilation and increased vascular bed in response to heat without adequate compensation by the body. After a few days, however, the pulse of such persons slows, their postural hypotension passes, and they are able to work harder and longer. Peripheral vasoconstriction, increased sweat production, and other compensatory mechanisms combine to provide an increased tolerance by the body to heat stress.[13]

The first responses of the circulatory system to acclimatization to heat are peripheral vasoconstriction and increased cardiac output; however, the most important adaptive response of the body is the increased effectiveness of the sweat mechanism. On first exposure to heat the maximum amount of sweat produced by a healthy adult man is approximately 1.5 liters per hour, but this amount gradually doubles after 10 days, and increases to about 2½ times as much in 6 weeks. This is due to an increased output of the sweat glands. The concentration of sodium chloride in the sweat decreases as the body attempts to conserve salt, which is attributed primarily to the increased production of aldosterone.[14] Conn[15] states that the results of acclimatization to heat can be explained almost entirely by increased production and activity of aldosterone.

The production of sweat is not an immediate response to heat. Sweating may not occur until the body temperature reaches 38°C (101°F) and does not begin all over the body at the same time. There is a dermatomal recruitment of sweat glands beginning at the extremities and progressing to the trunk and

* Conn, Jerome W.: "Some Clinical and Climatological Aspects of Aldosteronism in Man," *Trans. Am. Clin. Climatol. Assoc.,* **74:**61, 1962.

face. The sweat production increases with the rising body temperature until it reaches a maximum level. With progressive exposure to heat over a period of days, sweating begins at a lower body temperature and the maximum rate increases; however, at no degree of acclimatization are maximum sweat rates maintained. After about an hour of continuous production the sweat rate falls off.[16] This phenomenon has been termed *hidromeiosis* and occurs under conditions of humid heat. While the exact mechanism by which hidromeiosis occurs is unknown, it is thought to be related to the soaking of the skin. Hidromeiosis is described by Harwood S. Belding [17] as a homeostatic mechanism because it enables the body to conserve fluid when high rates of sweat production would be of no avail.

Activation of the sweat glands at lower body temperatures is thought to be the key in the process of acclimatization. Initiation of sweating enables the body to release heat prior to significant circulatory strain and rises in core body temperature.* [18,19]

Human tolerance and responses to heat have been studied mainly in young, physically fit men; there is less known about the responses of others. A few studies on women suggest they can acclimatize but that they tolerate work in heat less readily than men; however, it is also stated that women may tolerate heat during rest more readily than men. The ability of 100 elderly persons (men and women) to tolerate a combined stress of work and heat was studied by Austin Henschel and associates,[20] who report that "these elderly people were capable of developing heat acclimatization and physical conditioning and were, in fact, very responsive to moderate changes in their thermal environment and level of physical activity . . . for moderate levels of physical and environmental stress, age, *per se*, does not severely restrict adaptive capacity." † Since the incidence of acute and chronic illness is higher with increasing age, the incidence of heat intolerance among the aged would naturally be higher. An increased mortality rate among aged individuals has been reported during a sudden heat wave.[21]

Extremes of environmental heat can be ex-

pected to affect man's ability to work. The effects of heat stress on performance have been studied extensively because of the practical implications for those industries where heat stress exists. It is well known that performance deteriorates above a certain level of air temperature, wind velocity, and humidity. However, a useful index by which the level of heat stress could be predicted in a variety of such working conditions is yet to be developed. As Cyril H. Wyndham states:

. . . there is at present no index of heat stress which can be used to predict, reliably, the physiologic reactions of men engaged in physical work, at different rates, in various conditions of heat stress. It is also true that the physiologic criteria used for judging when men either have reached the limits of their tolerance to heat stress or are in danger of heat stroke are still a matter of contention among physiologists.*

Wyndham,[22] working with the Human Sciences Laboratory in Johannesburg, South Africa, has reported a number of studies involving the process of acclimatization of thousands of Bantu laborers in the gold mines of South Africa. From these studies, he has developed a scale for use with this particular population that shows the incidence of heatstroke and the changes in work productivity as the effective temperature † increases. He states that similar curves could be developed for other hot industries. If heatstroke is not a problem, then the relationship of other heat-induced illnesses, such as heat cramps or heat exhaustion, to effective temperature could be demonstrated, which could prove useful to those whose job it is to regulate the environment in hot industries.

Based on the existing knowledge of man's ability to respond and adapt to heat, certain measures can be identified to improve the tolerance to heat. Sweating, for example, can be highly detrimental if fluid is not replaced. Through sweating an individual may lose as much as 2 liters or more per hour. This must be replaced to prevent dehydration. Every liter lost represents 1½ per cent body weight, and death may occur when 18 to 20 per cent of the body weight is lost in this manner.[23] When the person makes a conscious effort to replace the fluids and salts lost, sweating is less dangerous. Working in high temperatures where 5000 to 8000 ml (5 to 8 qt) of sweat is lost per day, a person should take at least 15 gm

---

* The temperature of the internal body organs, the heart, lungs, abdominal organs, and brain. At rest the skin temperature is ideally 4°C (7.2°F) lower than the core temperature; however, the difference may reach as much as 20°C (35.7°F). (Astrand, Per-Olof, and Rodahl, Kaare: *Textbook of Work Physiology.* McGraw-Hill Book Co., New York, 1970, p. 492.)

† Henschel, Austin, et al.: "Heat Tolerance of Elderly Persons Living in a Subtropical Climate," *J. Gerontol.,* **23:**17, (Jan.) 1968.

* Wyndham, Cyril H.: "Adaptation to Heat and Cold," *Environ. Res.,* **2:**442, (Oct.) 1969.

† The temperature of air saturated with water vapor that produces the same sensation as the environment being studied. It is used as a measure of discomfort.

(225 gr) of sodium chloride. A day's diet supplies two-thirds of this amount; in addition, 5 gm (75 gr) should be supplied by drinking 5000 ml (5 qt) of 0.1 per cent sodium chloride solution or by taking the 5 gm (75 gr) of sodium chloride in tablets spaced throughout the day.[24] However, heavier salting of food is currently recommended to replace salt lost during periods of extra heavy sweating. An awareness of the need for increased salt by military and industrial leaders is believed to have led to the decreased evidence of heat cramps.[25] Suggested supplements of salt are presented in Table 42-1.

Effects of Cold. Heat is lost from the body, as discussed previously, by radiation, conduction-convection, and evaporation. Man can protect himself physiologically from losing heat to the environment through peripheral vasoconstriction and shivering. By vasoconstriction of the skin's blood vessels, blood flow is diverted to the deeper blood vessels, therefore, much of the warm blood is not exposed to the cooler surface. Through this effort a sixfold increase in the insulating capacity of the skin is achieved. Peripheral vasoconstriction is most pronounced in the toes and fingers; these peripheral tissues may approach the temperature of the environment, and are consequently prone to damage by the cold.[26] A second means of conserving body heat is to increase the body metabolic rate through shivering. Shivering is brought about by reflex contraction of virtually all muscle groups. Heat is produced at a relatively high rate and the metabolic rate may be increased 2 to 4 times. Active work may further increase heat production.[27]

Man has been able to successfully adapt to cold through the use of shelter, fire, and clothing. But it appears that the adaptive mechanisms for physiologic response to cold are not as developed as they are for heat. Even the Eskimo living in arctic conditions has developed clothing and shelter to enable him to maintain a body temperature similar to that of man in temperate regions. As O. G. Edholm and H. E. Lewis [28] state, to develop adaptation to cold one must be exposed to cold temperatures for certain lengths of time. Men stationed on the bases of Antarctica are out of doors for less than 10 per cent of the time, and their clothing is efficient enough to maintain body heat, except in the extremities, for this time. Findings of man's ability to adapt to cold are inconclusive at present. However, this "should not be interpreted to mean that man cannot adapt to cold, only that man in polar areas in present circumstances may have an inadequate stimulus to develop a degree of cold adaptation sufficient for measurement." *

A certain measure of local acclimatization to cold has been demonstrated. When the hands are exposed to cold repeatedly for periods of 30 minutes daily over a few weeks, the blood supply increases so that they remain comparatively warm. While this means that a greater amount of heat will be lost from the hands, it will enable them to do work of a more precise nature.[29]

Because man has developed effective shelter and clothing, he is able to tolerate the polar environment; without this protection he would

* Edholm, O. G., and Lewis, H. E.: "Terrestrial Animals in Cold: Man in Polar Regions," in Dill, D. B., et al. (eds.): *Handbook of Physiology: Adaptation to the Environment*. American Physiological Society, Washington, D.C., 1964, p. 445.

Table 42-1. Recommended Daily Salt Addition to Normal Diet *

Conditions	Acclimatization	Work	Addition, gm
Warm humid	Acclimatized	Moderate to heavy	0
Warm humid	Unacclimatized	Moderate to heavy	7
Hot dry	Acclimatized	Sedentary	0
Hot dry	Acclimatized	Moderate to heavy	7
Hot dry	Unacclimatized	Moderate	7
Hot dry	Unacclimatized	Heavy	14
Very hot †	Acclimatized	Moderate to heavy	14
Very hot †	Unacclimatized	Moderate to heavy	21

* Lee, Douglas H. K.: "Terrestrial Animals in Dry Heat: Man in the Desert," in Dill, D. B., et al. (eds.): *Handbook of Physiology: Adaptation to the Environment*. American Physiological Society, Washington, D.C., 1964, p. 565.

† High air temperatures or radiant heat as occurs in some industries, combined with hot dry conditions away from work.

not survive. The Eskimo shelter built of slabs of ice provides effective insulation because the ice traps air, an excellent insulator. Clothing, as a measure to improve tolerance to extremes of cold, must allow for the escape of water vapor, provide small "pockets" for trapped air as insulation, and provide an outer windproof layer. Warmth of a garment depends on how much air is trapped in the fibers. The addition of filling, such as down, cotton, or fur, allows for trapping air. Several layers of lighter clothing offer more protection than one heavy garment. When an individual must work actively in the cold he will sweat, and this sweat must be allowed to evaporate. If the water vapor cannot pass through the clothing, it will condense inside; it may freeze, and this will greatly decrease the protective value of the clothing, because ice conducts body heat much more readily than air. The outer garment will have to be unbuttoned or unzipped periodically during work to allow for water vapor to escape and refastened before too much cooling takes place. The inhabitants of cold environments must continually guard against getting their clothing wet. Water in the air spaces of cloth increases the conductivity of heat twenty times and the protective value of the clothing is lost.[30,30a]

When it is not possible to provide patients with comfortably warm surroundings, they should be given several layers of clothing or bedding that holds air in its fibers and they should be encouraged to exercise. Warm socks and mittens are particularly helpful because skin temperature is always lowest in the extremities. Tight clothing should be avoided because it interferes with circulation. An outer windproof layer of clothing should be used when there is strong air movement.

Patients with heart disease are particularly vulnerable to extremes of cold or heat and should be cautioned about this. The greatest degree of stress occurs during the first few days of very warm or very cold weather. During periods of hot, humid weather, individuals should remain in an air-conditioned environment, or at least have their bedrooms air-conditioned, if possible. When hospitalized, they should be placed in a comfortable environment. If the hospital is not air-conditioned they could be placed in a cooled oxygen tent for greatest comfort. During extremely cold weather, the heart disease patient should be

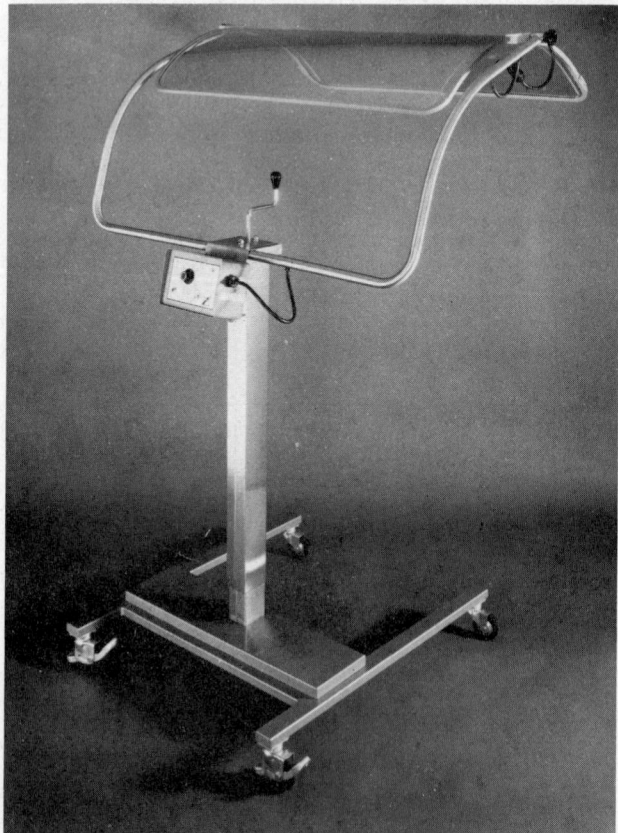

Figure 42-2. Patient warmer. An electrically heated canopy, made of transparent plastic, provides a neutral environment for burn, postoperative, and neonatal patients. By counterbalancing convective, radiant, and evaporative heat loss, the canopy eliminates need for blankets, undesirable clothing, frames, or restraints. The neutral environment promotes minimum oxygen consumption and enables the patient to conserve energy and avoid shivering thermogenesis. The canopy can be applied to any resuscitation or intensive care station to provide controlled warmth. Position adjustments provide access to patient for x-rays, exchange transfusions, or treatment without loss of temperature control. (Courtesy of Cavitron/KDC Medical Sales, New York, N.Y.)

cautioned against strenuous physical work, for example, shoveling snow. Clothing should be light and warm. Because changes in weather can be predicted in advance in most situations, patients with heart disease should be taught to pay attention to weather forecasts and to modify their activities accordingly.[31]

2. EFFECTS OF EXTREMES OF CLIMATIC HEAT ON MAN

Heat Syncope. Heat syncope is a self-limiting condition caused by heat exposure. The causative factor is an unfavorable distribution of blood. Circulating blood pools in the peripheral vessels. If the person is standing for a prolonged period blood pools in the lower extremities. In such cases the blood pressure falls and there is an inadequate supply of oxygen to the brain.[32] The person so affected should be removed from the heat and placed in a recumbent position with the legs elevated. Consciousness and equilibrium are quickly regained.

Heat Exhaustion. A more serious circulatory condition resulting from heat exposure is heat exhaustion. It is described as circulatory collapse resulting from the failure of the body to compensate for the peripheral vasodilation and dehydration that occur in high temperatures not necessarily associated with exposure to the sun's rays. The symptoms of heat exhaustion range from very mild ones, such as dizziness, fatigue, and headache, to complete collapse and unconsciousness. Body temperature varies from subnormal to a slight fever. The blood pressure is low at the time of collapse. The skin is pale and sweating is profuse.

The ingestion of sodium chloride and ample fluids will usually prevent this condition, and it is relieved by saline and glucose solutions. If the subject is conscious, fluids may be given orally; if not, they are administered intravenously. Drugs, such as cardiac stimulants, may be indicated in severe collapse, but re-establishment of blood volume is usually adequate treatment.

Heat Cramps. Painful muscle cramps in the voluntary muscles of the extremities can occur following heavy work at high temperatures. Heat cramps result from salt depletion due to profuse sweating with the intake of large quantities of water. As a result the body fluids become dilute, although the total volume is maintained. The painful cramps are relieved with the ingestion of salt. For relief in severe cases intravenous saline solutions may be required. Heat cramps can be prevented with extra intake of salt (about 3 gm—¾ dram—

extra per day) added to food at mealtimes or taken separately in tablets or saline solution.[33]

Heatstroke or Sunstroke. Heatstroke, heat pyrexia, or sunstroke occurs as a result of a failure in the body's heat-regulating mechanism. Exposure to high environmental temperature and humidity are the usual precipitating factors; however, cases have occurred under temperate conditions. During periods of exercise the body may produce large amounts of heat that it is incapable of dissipating. According to Ezra Sohar and associates:

Body temperature rises when the total heat load of the body exceeds its capacity to dissipate heat, whether this heat load is caused by external heat, by physical work, or by a combination of both. The term "heat" in heatstroke is best divorced from *external heat* and should denote excessive *body heat* (body temperature) per se.*

The primary cause of the failure of the heat-regulating mechanism remains unclear. The sweat glands are usually affected because sweat production ceases. However, heatstroke may occur in the presence of continued sweating, as reported by Sohar.[34] As the temperature rises, cardiac output increases and then drops at temperatures above 42°C (107.6°F). Oxygen consumption increases over 40 per cent, but also falls above 42°C (107.6°F). With prolonged exposure, cell death is evident[35] (see Fig. 42-3).

The patient's temperature is markedly elevated to a height of 41.1°C (106°F) or higher. The blood pressure may be low and pulse rate rapid and weak. The skin usually feels hot and dry. In fatal cases reported, a disturbance in sensorium is present, which is characterized by coma and convulsions with or without delirium. The liver is easily damaged by heat and consequently the level of serum enzymes is elevated. This is accompanied by a prolonged prothrombin time and hypofibrinogenemia. The serum potassium is low initially, but rises if renal failure develops. Acidosis is present owing to the buildup of lactate and pyruvate. In severe cases spontaneous hemorrhage into body tissues develops.[36]

Robert G. Petersdorf states that heatstroke "requires heroic emergency measures." † Since fatal tissue changes in heatstroke appear to result from excessive body temperature, the aim of therapy is to reduce fever. Immersion of the

---

* Sohar, Ezra, et al.: "Heatstroke Caused by Dehydration and Physical Effort," *Arch. Intern. Med.*, **122:**159, (Aug.) 1968.
† Petersdorf, Robert G.: "Disturbances of Heat Regulation," in Thorn, George W., et al. (eds.): *Harrison's Principles of Internal Medicine*, 8th ed. McGraw-Hill Book Co., New York, 1977, p. 56.

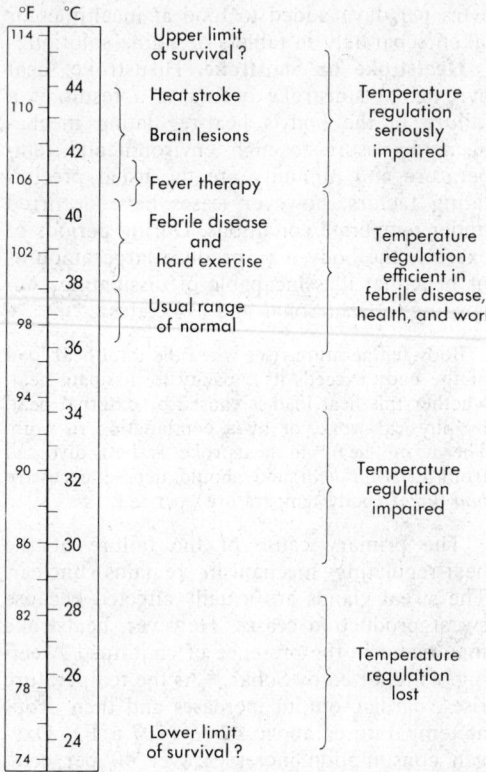

Figure 42-3. Extremes of human body temperature with an attempt to define the zones of temperature regulation. (From Dubois, Eugene F.: *Fever and the Regulation of Body Temperature.* Charles C Thomas, Publisher, Springfield, Ill., 1948.)

body in ice water, or cold water as available, is the most effective method. After the removal of the patient from the bath, the body should be kept moist and fans played on it to produce evaporation. Rubbing, or vigorous massage, increases the cooling effect, for the peripheral circulation is often stagnant. Ice caps applied to the head, axilla, and groin are helpful. Rectal temperature should be taken at frequent intervals and the cooling measures discontinued when it falls to 38.9°C (102°F). (If cold colonic irrigations are used, as is sometimes the case, the mouth temperature may be a more reliable index. The delirium that accompanies hyperpyrexia prohibits the taking of mouth temperature in most cases.) A drop in temperature does not mean that the temperature may not soar again, calling for a repetition of the measures just described. Oxygen is helpful in reducing tissue anoxia and acidosis. Intubating and suctioning the airway to remove secretions at frequent intervals may be necessary. Shivering must be controlled since

it increases the metabolic rate. Repeated doses of chlorpromazine or diazepam (Valium) are helpful in reducing muscle tension. Valium will also control seizures, if they are a problem. Fluid administration must be carefully monitored to prevent overloading the circulation. Complications that may develop include renal failure, central nervous system damage, and liver necrosis.

Prognosis is said to depend on the promptness and effectiveness of relief measures. Untreated cases of heatstroke result in death. Joseph M. Quashnock [37] states that one-third of treated uncomplicated cases may result in death as well. A correlation seems to exist between the outcome and how high the temperature is for how long.

Malignant Hyperthermia. A condition described with increasing frequency is termed malignant hyperthermia, which occurs under general anesthesia. The temperature of the affected individual rises at an alarming rate, apparently triggered by the anesthetic agent. The condition is similar to heatstroke in that the heat production by the body outstrips its ability to dissipate heat, and the body temperature rises rapidly. Treatment, as in heatstroke, is aimed at decreasing the temperature.

The etiology of the two conditions is different, however. Malignant hyperthermia appears to result from unknown and perhaps multiple causes.[38] One explanation frequently mentioned is that the anesthetic agent triggers an abnormal reaction in the muscle tissues, releasing large amounts of heat. M. B. Barlow and H. Isaacs [39] report that more than 40 per cent of the cases are familial, that is, due to an inherited muscle defect. Mortality is as high as 70 to 80 per cent.

Certain physical findings are typical, but may not be seen in every case. Often the patient is young, healthy, and undergoing elective surgery. Increased muscle tone and rigidity are many times present in spite of the administration of succinylcholine, a muscle relaxant. The skin becomes hot and dry. The sweating mechanism is usually ineffective because belladonna preparations have been given preoperatively. The body attempts to compensate by increased cardiac output and vasodilation. As the metabolic rate rises, oxygen consumption becomes greater than oxygen intake and the tissues get hypoxic. Hypoxia and acidosis lead to vascular collapse and finally heart failure.

The rapid increase in temperature to a fatal height (the temperature may increase −0.56°C [1°F] every 15 minutes or oftener) makes early detection and vigorous treatment mandatory. Therapy is directed at lowering the temperature, supplying oxygen sufficient to meet the demand, and correcting acidosis and other electrolyte imbalances. As soon as the condition is diagnosed, the anesthetic agent must be stopped and the surgical procedure rapidly terminated. Cooling is most effectively accomplished by immersion in iced water. Chlorpromazine is administered to counteract shivering and promote vasodilation. The patient must be hyperventilated with 100 per cent oxygen to combat tissue hypoxia. Buffer solutions are administered intravenously. When the esophageal temperature measures 38.3° to 37.7°C (101° to 100°F) the patient should be removed from the water bath to allow for downward drift of the temperature, which accompanies hypothermic measures. The patient will require intensive nursing care until temperature and metabolic equilibrium are regained.

Because of the rapid progression and high mortality rate with malignant hyperthermia, preventive measures are imperative. Abby M. Heydman and Mary Ruth Stegman,[10] who are nurses and one of whom survived malignant hyperthermia, suggest that the nurse can learn preoperatively if any of the patient's family have developed fever or died while under anesthesia. A history of therapy with tranquilizers is important, as they may accentuate hyperthermia. Continuous monitoring during surgery to show temperature increases is recommended.

Hyperthermia as Prescribed Treatment. Before the introduction of antibiotics, fever therapy was a dramatic method used to combat certain infections. Fever was induced artificially in a patient (by introducing pyrogens into the body) with the hope that the high temperature produced would destroy the original infection. Donald L. Rose[41] states that fever therapy was abandoned with the introduction of antibiotics. Other reasons were the change from disease-oriented to concept-oriented treatment methods and the inherent dangers of this type of therapy.

Fever therapy, perhaps better termed hyperthermia, has not been given up completely, however. There are reports in the current literature of its use in cancer therapy. Tumor cells are known to be destroyed by heat more easily than normal cells; the reason is not completely understood. It is thought that tumor cells under hyperthermia cannot maintain growth because their metabolism is increased beyond their nutritional supply.[42] Use of hyperthermia in the treatment of cancer has been hindered by inadequate methods of application. It is hard to raise the internal temperature (by application of heat to the outside) without burning the surface of the body. M. A. Henderson and R. T. Pettigrew[43] describe a technique developed to apply hyperthermia in the palliative treatment of malignancies. Heat is transmitted to the body through ventilation with a warmed combination of oxygen and helium. The alveolar surface, which is 20 times that of the skin, is utilized for heat transfer. At the same time heat loss is prevented by almost total covering of the body with liquid paraffin at 45°C (113°F) which solidifies and effectively insulates the body. The body temperature rises 5 to 6°C (9° to 10.7°F) in 20 to 40 minutes. Hyperthermia has been used in the treatment of 19 patients with terminal cancer, most of these being treated with the above method. When the temperature rise was successful, all the patients reported improvement in a feeling of well-being as well as reduction or elimination of pain. The authors state that this method is safe when the patient is carefully monitored, when oxygen is given at a high level, and when fluid and salts are adequately replaced.

Holger Ehlers[44] reports the use of hyperthermia in the treatment of aestival conjunctivitis, a disease of young men. In 19 episodes of this condition, hyperthermia has produced complete reversal of inflammatory symptoms, although the nature of the reversed process is unknown. Body temperature was elevated in these cases by injecting a coli vaccine.

3. BURNS

Burns are caused by the exposure of the body to a very high temperature of either dry or moist heat, electricity, x-ray, radium, or corrosive poisons. The extent and depth of the burn wound and the presence of epithelial tissue are the criteria used for classification of burns. The terms commonly used now are "partial-thickness," "deep-dermal," and "full-thickness," which describe the depth of the injury (see Fig. 42-4). (They have also been called first-, second-, and third-degree burns.) "Partial-thickness" burns are those involving the epidermis and/or the upper dermal tissue, as, for example, sunburn. The epithelializing elements remain. The hair follicles and sweat and sebaceous glands remain intact, and healing occurs spontaneously with no need for grafting. "Deep-dermal" burns are partial-thickness burns penetrating the lower levels of dermal tissue. Some dermal appendages (hair follicles and sweat glands) penetrate this level into subcutaneous fat and may regenerate epithelial tissue. In the past, infection of the wound destroyed any epithelial tissue re-

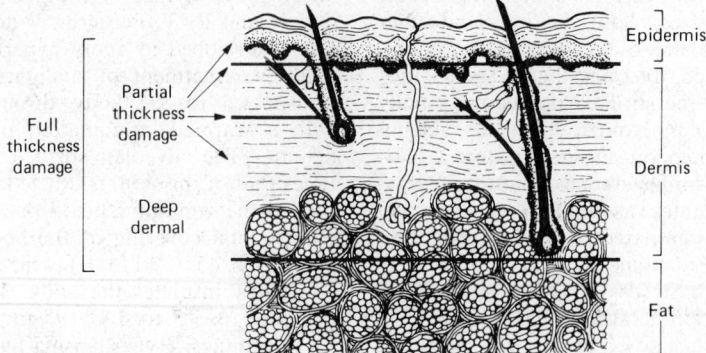

Figure 42-4. Diagram of skin, showing depth of burn. (From Jacoby, Florence Greenhouse: *Nursing Care of the Patient with Burns.* C. V. Mosby Co., St. Louis, 1972, p. 10.)

maining and converted this burn to a full-thickness wound, whereas, with present topical treatment, sufficient dermal tissue may remain to resurface the wound. In "full-thickness" burns, all epithelial tissue is destroyed and the subcutaneous fat tissue is involved. These wounds cannot heal spontaneously and must have skin grafts applied for optimum return of function.[45] Douglas MacG. Jackson [46] recommends that the initial depth of damage be assessed by the patient's sensitivity to pinprick. He states that this method "provides the easiest and most reliable measure of the depth of necrosis in a new burn." * Feeling of the pinprick as sharp indicates that the burn will heal in 3 weeks without grafting. Analgesia, or inability to feel the pinprick as sharp, indicates that the area either may spontaneously heal in 3 weeks or more or involves all layers of skin, and skin grafting will be necessary.

Burns are also classified according to the extent of the body surface injured. The Rule of Nines is a common method used for determining the extent of the burned surface. The body surface is divided into multiples of nine and rapid calculation of the per cent of surface involved can be made. The Lund and Browder chart and table (see Fig. 42-5) make a more accurate estimate of burned surface possible because body size is taken into consideration.[47]

The extent of the body surface burned and the depth of the burns are determining factors in categorizing the burn as minor, moderate, or major. A minor burn is a partial-thickness burn of less than 15 per cent or a full-thick-

ness burn of less than 2 per cent of body surface, excluding the critical areas of feet, face, hands, and genitalia. A moderate burn is a partial-thickness burn of 15 to 30 per cent or a full-thickness burn of less than 10 per cent of body surface. A major burn is a partial-thickness burn over 30 per cent of body sur-

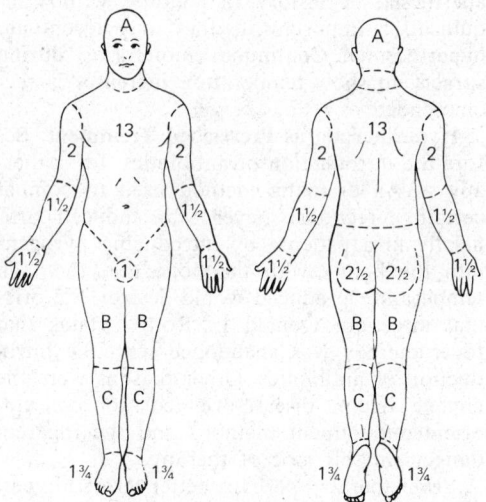

Relative Percentage of Areas Affected by Growth

| | Age in Years | | | | | |
	0	1	5	10	15	Adult
A ½ of head	9½	8½	6½	5½	4½	3½
B ½ of one thigh	2¾	3¼	4	4¼	4½	4¾
C ½ of one leg	2½	2½	2¾	3	3¼	3½

Figure 42-5. Lund and Browder Chart. (From Artz, Curtis P.: "The Burned Patient: Newer Concepts of Medical and Nursing Management," in Kintzel, Kay Corman [ed.]: *Advanced Concepts in Clinical Nursing.* J. B. Lippincott Co., Philadelphia, 1971, p. 323.)

* Jackson, Douglas MacG.: "In Search of an Acceptable Burn Classification," *Br. J. Plast. Surg.,* **23:** 219, (July) 1970.

face. It may also be a full-thickness burn of 10 per cent or more in a child or 15 per cent or more in an adult. Full-thickness burns of the face, hands, feet, or genitalia are considered major. Complicating factors such as respiratory injury, fractures, or internal injuries, or predisposing illnesses such as heart disease, metabolic disorders, or renal disease make the burn injury a major one. Any burn in a victim under 18 months or over 65 years can be a serious injury.[48]

An immediate first-aid treatment of a burn is the application of cold. Dressings soaked in cold water or ice may be applied. Greasy ointments should be avoided initially until the burn can be evaluated by a physician because they tend to cover the wound and are difficult to remove. Harvey Kravitz[49] recommends that the general public should be made aware of ice-cold water as a first-aid treatment for burns, through first-aid courses and the mass media. Nurses should be particularly aware of this first-aid measure and incorporate it in any first-aid classes or individual teaching of parents and other clients.

Any burns except the smallest accidental injuries should be treated in an emergency room or other treatment facility if possible. Minor burns may be treated on an outpatient basis. Cold is usually applied initially to lessen pain and edema; the wound is then cleaned and a bulky, occlusive dressing is applied and changed every 2 to 5 days.[50] Because these wounds frequently become infected, Francis C. Nance and associates[51] recommend frequent dressing changes, using a light, lubricated dressing with or without an antiseptic topical agent. In the 106 patients studied, clinical infection of the burn wound was virtually absent and patients were easily taught to change their dressings twice daily. The use of light, lubricated dressings which are changed frequently appears to lower the rate of infection of minor burns. Nurses working in outpatient or emergency care facilities can teach patients how to change the burn dressing and keep the wound clean.

With a moderate or major burn, immediate therapy is directed toward respiratory care, maintenance of fluid balance, and local care of the wound. The patient must be closely observed for signs of respiratory distress which include restlessness, hoarseness, coughing, rapid respirations, or crowing noises.[52] A tracheostomy may even be performed to insure an adequate airway. The nurse must be alert for signs of respiratory distress and report significant changes to the physician immediately.

Heat injury causes the capillaries to be damaged in such a way that the permeability of the membrane no longer is selective, and fluid flows into the tissues with resulting edema. The fluid changes can produce hypovolemic shock. Consequently, fluid therapy is always begun in a patient with a major burn. Lynn D. Ketchum and associates[53] report that the development of successful fluid resuscitation formulas has resulted in decreasing the mortality rate of acute burns from 75 per cent in the 1950s to less than 25 per cent in 1971.

Electrolytes, colloids, and water are lost by seepage into the burned tissue. These components must be replaced in order to prevent hypovolemic shock. To facilitate this, an intravenous catheter is inserted into a vein. Controversy exists over the optimum amount of each fluid component to be given; however, most authorities say a sufficient quantity of fluid is mandatory. The Evans formula and the Brooke formula are in wide usage; each recommends 2 ml (½ dram) of fluid per kilogram body weight for each per cent of burned body surface. The Brooke formula recommends a 1:3 ratio of colloid to electrolyte. The Evans formula recommends a 1:1 ratio. Both formulas allow for 2000 ml (2 qt) of water for adults.[54] The formulas are calculated for the first 24 hours. One-half of the total fluid is infused during the first 8 hours, one-fourth during the second 8 hours, and one-fourth during the third 8 hours. Fluids are infused rapidly at first; the hourly urine output provides the best guide to fluid balance.[55] Nurses caring for a severely burned patient must keep accurate records of fluid intake and output. Each bottle of fluid given should be numbered. Whole blood is infrequently used during the resuscitative period. Urinary output should be measured hourly and maintained at 30 to 50 ml (1 to 1⅔ oz) per hour. Central venous pressure monitoring provides a measure of fluid balance. A rising central venous pressure indicates pulmonary edema, a complication of fluid overload. (See Chapter 35 for a discussion of pulmonary edema.)

Patients with major burns should be given nothing by mouth for the first 24 to 48 hours, because of the incidence of vomiting and gastric dilation. After about 2 days they are given clear liquids as tolerated and solid foods are added until they are taking a high-protein, high-caloric diet. Metabolic rates of burned patients increase significantly as the body attempts to repair itself. Evaporation of water through the unprotected burn eschar produces heat loss at the rate of over 0.5 kilocalorie per milliliter of water evaporated.[56] To meet the energy requirements for evaporation of water, fat stores are utilized and eventually muscle tissue. In order to maintain a positive nitrogen balance. an intake of 5000 to 6000 calories per day is necessary. Because patients often have no appetite (are anorexic) nurses should devote great effort and imagination in helping them eat prescribed diets (see Chapter 10). Parenteral hyperalimentation has been recommended as a method of providing sufficient calories and protein for the victim of burns so that additional tissue will not be broken down.[57,58]

After fluid therapy is begun and the patient is breathing adequately, attention may be given to the care of the burn. The burn wound is not sterile and organisms can gain entry and multiply in the wound itself. Tetanus prophylaxis is routine with all seriously burned patients. Because the wound made by a burn is avascular, systemic antibiotics have little effect in preventing infection of the wound. Attention has been focused in the past few years on developing and utilizing topical agents to control infection. A variety of methods of local wound care are described, such as occlusive dressings, exposure treatment, silver nitrate dressings, and the application of sulfamylon acetate cream. In many cases more than one type of local treatment may be used with the same patient. The choice of treatment depends in part on the extent and depth of the burn, other associated injuries, the part of the body burned, and the facilities and personnel available.[59] Although the dressings and agents used, physical facilities, and timing of procedures vary greatly, Florence Greenhouse Jacoby says the results are similar if the following principles are applied:

1. Keep the patient's general condition as stable as possible by meeting his physical and emotional needs.
2. Keep infection to a minimum.
3. Pursue an aggressive course of definitive care, with close attention to the details of a particular treatment.*

Initially, all burns must be cleaned and dead tissue and dirt removed. A mild soap solution can be applied with gauze pads and rinsed off with water. Tar and oily substances can be removed with benzene. Gentle cleaning is essential to avoid damaging existing epithelium.

Occlusive dressings are usually recommended for the outpatient with a burn of less than 10 to 15 per cent. The danger of burn wound sepsis is great with burns over a larger surface and therefore other measures are preferable. Occlusive dressings may be used

for hospitalized patients as well. A gauze impregnated with a water-soluble ointment or Furacin is placed over the burn and covered with a bulky layer of gauze. A semielastic covering such as stockinet or Ace bandage is then applied over the whole dressing. It should provide even compression over the entire wound. The extremity should be elevated to increase the reabsorption of fluid. The patient should be cautioned against getting the dressing wet, as moisture provides an entry for bacteria. The dressing should be changed about every 5 days or immediately should the surface be wet. Disadvantages of the occlusive dressing technique are that dressing changes are very painful, as there is usually an offensive odor and there is less control over infection than with other types mentioned.[60]

Burns may be treated by the exposure method with or without the use of topical antibacterial agents. Many second-degree or partial-thickness burns do well with exposure alone, especially burns of the face, neck, and perineum. Because of the great danger of infection, deep-dermal and full-thickness burns are best treated by exposure and a topical antibacterial agent.[61]

Following initial cleaning the patient is placed in bed on clean sheets in a comfortable position. A crust forms on the surface of partial-thickness burns formed by the drying exudate. If uninfected, the crust falls off in 14 to 21 days, leaving a healed surface. The thickened dead skin of a full-thickness burn is called an eschar. Burns of the face do well when exposed because of the good blood supply to the area. Circumferential burns are best exposed with the use of a turning frame. Stryker frames or CircOlectric beds offer the patient greater comfort in turning, during elimination, and when bed linen is changed. Burns can be exposed adequately if the patient is turned every 2 to 4 hours. A further advantage of a turning frame is that the patient may be moved on the frame to recreation areas or even out-of-doors, as his or her condition permits.

Burns treated by exposure have a tendency to adhere to the sheets and make turning painful. Curtis P. Artz and John A. Moncrief[62] recommend the use of a plastic, nonadherent dressing called Microdon (see Fig. 42-6). It may be placed next to the patient and pulled away easily from burned surfaces after turning. A small amount of water or saline is helpful in releasing sheets or dressings that adhere to the wound. Some type of tent or cradle should be put over the exposed area to protect the skin from drafts. Heat may be added by a heat lamp or a hair dryer circulating warm air.

* Jacoby, Florence Greenhouse: *Nursing Care of the Patient with Burns.* C. V. Mosby Co., St. Louis, 1972, p. 25.

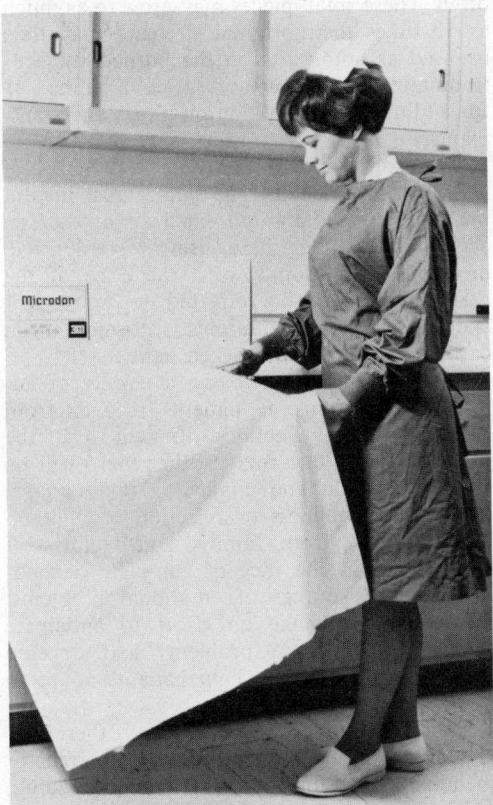

Figure 42-6. Nonstick sheeting made by 3M Company. Whenever burns are exposed and an antibacterial ointment is used, certain portions of the body frequently stick to the bed. As shown in the photograph, this sheeting comes in a large roll and can be placed over the patient's bed and changed each day. (Courtesy of 3M Company, New York. Also see Artz, Curtis P.: "The Burned Patient: Newer Concepts of Medical and Nursing Management," in Kintzel, Kay Corman [ed.]: *Advanced Concepts in Clinical Nursing.* J. B. Lippincott Co., Philadelphia, 1971, p. 329.)

The crust of the partial-thickness burn should be inspected for cracks and signs of infection daily. Loose crust should be removed and the area protected with fine gauze.[63]

The exposure method in conjunction with topical antibacterial agents is the recommended treatment of large burns. Infection is the major cause of death in patients with extensive burns. Bacterial invasion of the burn that spreads to surrounding healthy tissue is termed "burn wound sepsis."[64] Two agents commonly used to treat burns are silver nitrate solution and sulfamylon cream. Others will undoubtedly be discovered or developed.*

* Pigskin is being used as a dressing over wounds and the Chinese report good results with dressings of

Silver nitrate is used in a 0.5 per cent aqueous solution. Gauze dressings are applied to the burn and are saturated with the solution. Stockinet may be used to hold the dressings in place. The patient is then covered with a cotton sheet and cotton blanket to prevent chilling. The dressings should be resoaked with warmed 0.5 per cent silver nitrate solution every 2 hours as necessary. Continuous wet dressings are necessary to maintain the action of the silver nitrate so that it does not become caustic. Dressings may be changed once a day until the eschar begins to separate, after which they are changed more often. The nurse should help the patient move his or her arms and legs during dressing changes to maintain joint action. Dressing changes can be tedious and painful. The nurse can attempt to distract the patient through conversation, and by working gently and slowly to cause as little discomfort as possible.

The serum electrolytes of patients receiving silver nitrate should be monitored routinely as sodium, potassium, and calcium deficits can occur.[65] Silver nitrate stains everything it comes in contact with when exposed to light an ugly brown. It is our opinion that the staining, though unpleasant, should not be an insurmountable problem. The floors, walls, and furniture of the patient's room should be protected with plastic covering or other protective material. Linen should be kept separate from other laundry. Nurses caring for the patient should wear protective gowns and foot coverings. Plastic gloves should be worn when changing dressings. William W. Monafo[66] recommends the following solution for removing silver nitrate stains from clothing and skin:

Ammonium chloride crystals	60 gm (2 oz)
Bichloride of mercury crystals	150 gm (5 oz)
Water	1000 ml (1 gal)

Mattresses, beds, and furniture, if permanently stained, may still be used for the care of patients with burns.

Sulfamylon cream is an effective topical agent recently developed for the treatment of extensive burns. A 10 per cent concentration of sulfamylon acetate in a water-soluble base has been found to be effective against a wide variety of pathogens. The nurse can apply the cream directly to the burned surface with a sterile glove. The cream should be removed each day, preferably by placing the patient in

leaves. It is not possible in this chapter to discuss the great variety of methods used in the treatment of burns.

a Hubbard tank or other large tub. This allows the patient to move and improves his or her sense of well-being. The cream itself may cause some immediate pain on application, therefore, it may be necessary to give an analgesic.[67] No dressings should be applied over the cream. The water bath allows for debridement as the eschar softens. Sulfamylon cream has been found to be highly effective in preventing sepsis, particularly from the organism *Pseudomonas*.[68] * Many burns that were thought to be subdermal heal spontaneously from dermal appendages when infection is prevented using the topical application of sulfamylon cream or silver nitrate solution.

Contracture formation is a major problem in the treatment of patients with burns. Development of contractures can be lessened by keeping patients in positions that prevent them, by the use of splints and traction, and by exercise. The burned patient tends to assume the position of greatest comfort, which usually means that the neck, elbows, and knees and hands are flexed. Any extremity can be contracted or fixed in a flexed position. The patient is especially vulnerable during sleep. Splints are often used on the neck, arms, legs, and hands and should be in place at all times, except for periods of exercise. Pillows should not be used under the patient's head because they cause neck flexion and contraction formation. Following skin grafting the traction may be applied to the extremity to allow for exposure and immobilization.[69]

Skin grafting is begun after all dead tissue is removed and the area underneath begins to heal. Three types of grafts may be used: heterografts, grafting of skin taken from another species; homografts, grafting of skin taken from a cadaver of the same species; and autografts, grafting of healthy skin taken from the burned individual. Homografts and heterografts are often used to provide temporary coverage to the burned area to lessen the chance of infection and prevent insensible water loss. After the patient's general condition improves autografts may be applied surgically to the burn wound.[69a] Burns of the hands and face are grafted first so that individuals may participate in their care; after these heal, burns over joint areas are grafted. Aaron Freeman and associates [69b,69c] suggest a new method of skin grafting in which small pieces of skin are removed from the burned subject and cultured. These small pieces may grow to as much as 50 times their original size and may then be used as autografts on the burned subject's traumatized skin surface. (See Chapter 43 for additional information on grafts and transplants.)

Skin grafts and donor sites alike heal best when exposed to air. The nurse must inspect the graft areas daily and expel air or exudate accumulated under these, using a sterile swab in a rolling motion toward the edge of the graft. The reader is referred to more specialized texts for additional information on care of skin grafts in burned patients.[69d,69e]

Nurses may expect to see a variety of adjustment problems as patients recover from extensive burns. Feelings of guilt over the cause of the injury, anxiety that there will be loss of function and change in body image, feelings of loneliness or rejection brought on by separation from family, and feelings of helplessness in the face of complete dependency are all sources of emotional problems. Nurses should make an effort to anticipate and recognize these problems and develop positive approaches to help patients adapt to injury.

Isolation should be avoided and, therefore, grouping burned patients has been recommended. Diversions, as for example reading, music, and television, should be started early. Nurses can help patients by focusing on future plans and on their individual strengths.[70] Patients with facial burns causing swollen, closed eyelids and impaired hearing, taste, and smell experience sensory deprivation. Every effort must be made to foster contact with reality since without sensory stimulation they can easily become disoriented. Nurses can provide stimulation by speaking clearly and directly to patients and by touching unburned areas. Patients may be terrified that their vision is lost and need reassurance that this is not likely, that edema is making it impossible to open their eyes.

N. J. C. Andreasen and A. S. Norris,[71] in a study of the long-term adjustment mechanisms of severely burned patients, offer useful suggestions to help them recover their emotional equilibrium. They studied 20 male and female adults (from 1 to 5 years following the injury) who had an average total body surface burn of 37 per cent. They describe the reaction of a severely burned person as an identity crisis because he or she must face a new and possibly overwhelming change in life style in addition to a radical change in body image. They say: "His basic adjustment problem is learning how to rally new coping and defense mechanisms that will help him resolve this

---

* *Pseudomonas*, one of the gram-negative organisms, can produce what is called "gram-negative shock"—an infection so virulent and rapid in its development that a severely burned child can die from it within 24 hours.

crisis within his sense of identity and maintain his sense of continuity and sameness." * They state that the patient's reestablishment of his or her role in the family is the strongest factor in recovering a sense of continuity. Therefore, the nurse should be aware of the importance of family contacts and the emotional support given by close family members. The spouse and other family members should be helped to be aware of the importance of their visits and the positive encouragement they provide the patient. If possible, children should be allowed to visit their parents.

Patients should not be discouraged from talking about their injuries and the pain and suffering they feel. Physicians and nurses tend to expect patients to be stoic. However, this attitude denies patients the safety valve of expression and may foster repression of painful feelings. Patients in the sample studied were able to adapt to their injury successfully for the most part by focusing on their positive internal, nonphysical qualities. In another study by Shizuko Fagerhaugh of 21 burned patients on an intensive burn care unit, the subjects reported that being informed about what to expect during different phases in their recovery helped reduce the pain by reducing the accompanying anxiety. The patients also stated that other patients were their greatest source of support.[71a]

Because pain is an unavoidable accompaniment of extensive burns, there is a tendency to overdo the use of narcotics, and so drug addiction may be added to the patient's troubles. The emotionally depressing effect of painkilling drugs should be more generally recognized and their use carefully guarded.

The preceding discussion of the treatment and nursing care of burns should be augmented by the study of specialized texts and articles. The following suggestions on the treatment of special types of burns may be helpful.

In *burns caused by corrosive poisons*, the chemical substances may be *acids* or *alkalies*. Burns caused by acids should be irrigated freely with alkaline solutions to neutralize the acid. Limewater, weak ammonia, or a solution of bicarbonate of soda may be used. Carbolic acid or creosote should be neutralized by alcohol (or whisky), after which a dressing of alcohol or a soothing ointment may be applied. Oil should not be used, as it hastens the absorption of carbolic acid. Burns caused by alkalies (caustic soda, caustic potash, or am-

monia, etc.) should be treated with boric acid, vinegar and water, or diluted lemon juice. The amount of the solvent is more important than the neutralizing agent in it. If the appropriate solvent is not immediately available, the area should be flooded with copious amounts of water.

Burns of the hands occur frequently because the hands are involved in combating a fire, or exposed to other sources of heat. The main objective in treatment is to maintain optimum function of the hand. Exposure is advocated for this reason; if it is used, the patient should be encouraged to move the hands in helping with his or her care. Motion can be encouraged by bathing the hands in a whirlpool bath. When not being exercised the hands should be elevated to reduce edema. If dressings are applied the hand should be placed in the position of function.[71b] Nurses should anticipate the needs of patients having both hands bandaged. Some sort of signal should be devised that patients can manipulate with head or foot. Even without the use of their hands patients should be encouraged to do as much for themselves as possible.

Burns of the eye are especially dangerous. Thermal burns of the lids are treated by irrigating with saline solution, then drying and applying a bland substance, such as castor oil —unless the patient can be taken to the doctor at once. When pain is severe, a wet dressing lessens the pain.

Burns of the conjuntiva and cornea are sometimes caused by boiling water, steam, lime, mortar, acids, powder, or molten metal. They occur most frequently among industrial workers. Treatment consists in the complete removal of the irritating substance as soon as possible. The conjunctival sac is irrigated with a solution that neutralizes the substance or renders it insoluble. A very weak tannic acid solution is used to remove lime, mortar, and other caustic alkalies. A weak solution of bicarbonate of soda may be used to remove acids. Robert A. Ralph and Harvey H. Slansky state that immediate and copious irrigation of the chemically burned eye is the most important factor for a favorable prognosis. The actual solution used is of less significance than the fact of removing the caustic material and diluting the irritating chemical.[71c] Solids are removed, as are foreign bodies, after which the sac is irrigated and precautions are taken to prevent infection. Cold compresses are usually ordered to relieve inflammation and prevent swelling and pain. Atropine is used as a sedative, and also to dilute the pupil and prevent adhesions. A bandage is occasionally applied in order to protect the eyes.

---

* Andreasen, N. J. C., and Norris, A. S.: "Long-Term Adjustment and Adaptation Mechanisms in Severely Burned Adults," *J. Nerv. Ment. Dis.*, **154:** 352, (May) 1972.

About 7.5 persons per 1000 are burned annually by hot objects or open flames. Three-fourths of the deaths are attributed to fires in the home.[72] These statistics do not show the tremendous human suffering and the loss of wage-earning power caused by burns. The fact that many of these accidents are *preventable* makes them all the more tragic. Nurses can play a major role in helping the public learn to prevent burns in the home. People can learn safety measures in schools, hospitals, public health centers, and industrial centers. Space heaters and other household heaters should be properly protected as these constitute a major hazard. Many types of clothing, particularly children's nightwear, are highly flammable. The use of flame-resistant clothing should be encouraged. Nurses can work to support legislation providing for safer heating appliances and for flameproofing children's clothing. Ways of eliminating fire hazards can be included in health teaching efforts by nurses for children, parents, and other clients.*

4. EFFECTS OF EXTREMES OF CLIMATIC COLD ON MAN

Accidental Hypothermia. Accidental hypothermia may be defined as a condition in which the rectal temperature unintentionally falls below 35°C (95°F) as opposed to hypothermia induced for medical or surgical treatment. It is life-threatening when the temperature reaches 32.2°C (90°F).[73]

Body temperature falls if heat loss exceeds heat production. Hypothermia may result from an increase in heat loss, a decrease in heat production, or both.[74] Heat loss is brought about by overexposure to cold environmental temperature or exposure to wind, rain, or snow. Heat production can be decreased by a variety of factors; G. M. Wilson[75] identifies the following: starvation and malnutrition; failure of the shivering mechanism; endocrine disorders, such as hypothyroidism and hypopituitarism; immobility in conditions such as coma, paralysis, parkinsonism, and arthritis; and severe circulatory failure. All age groups may be affected, but the very young and the very old seem to be more susceptible to extremes of cold.

* Burns are a major cause of injury and death— the leading cause of death for children aged 1 to 11. A September 12, 1973, issue of *HEW News* reports that under a 3-year contract with the University of Texas Southwestern Medical School at Dallas and the Texas Woman's University a program (master's or doctoral) is being developed to prepare nurse practitioners and researchers who will be specialists in "the burn field."

The physiologic effects of hypothermia include reduced oxygen consumption, respiratory depression, metabolic acidosis, and a profound cardiovascular disturbance. The electrocardiographic changes are characteristic and diagnostic of the condition. Other clinical features include cyanosis and vasoconstriction which give the patient a gray, dusky, appearance. Reflexes are sluggish and response to questioning is slow.[76-78] Warren C. Hunter[79] reports that the lethal effects of cold are due to the changes it brings about—hemoconcentration, edema, pulmonary congestion, and, most important, electrocardiographic changes in the form of ventricular or atrial fibrillation. These lead to cardiac arrest.

James Freeman and Griffith Pugh[80] identify symptoms of hypothermia occurring as a result of prolonged exposure. The affected person becomes fatigued and may experience mental changes, such as apathy or uncooperative behavior. Muscular weakness and collapse develop and are followed by stupor and rigidity. Death may ensue in 1 to 2 hours. When stress from cold is combined with fatigue and other discomfort, the point of exhaustion is reached earlier than when these operate in isolation. Fatigue and mental impairment may prevent a search for shelter and other safety measures; so a series of events leads to fatal accidents and death from hypothermia.[81]

Accidental hypothermia is not, however, a condition confined to the presence of extremes of environmental temperature. Keith G. Tolman and Arthur Cohen[82] report a study of 11 patients with accidental hypothermia in Houston, Texas, where the climate is subtropical. They point out that hypothermia should be suspected in the comatose, hypotensive patient. The condition may often be missed because clinical thermometers used have 35°C (95°F) as the lowest reading. If the condition is suspected, the temperature should be measured rectally with thermocouple rectal probe or pediatric incubator thermometer. A thermometer designed to measure lower body temperatures is, therefore, an important part of the equipment used in emergency treatment facilities. Because hypothermia may mimic other clinical states, its presence may be overlooked entirely unless the physician or nurse working in such facilities remembers to take the patient's temperature rectally.[83] The electrocardiogram is another important diagnostic measure, because it may demonstrate the presence of typical changes, particularly the "J" waves, occurring in profound hypothermia.[84] Prompt recognition of accidental hypothermia through these measures is vital to successful treatment.

Warming the hypothermic patient is a critical process and little agreement has been found on how it is best accomplished. In hypothermia there is a large difference between the temperature of the surface of the body, where marked vasoconstriction exists, and the temperature of the viscera, or the body core. With the application of external heat, as with rapid rewarming, vasodilation of the skin's blood supply is brought about and the cool blood trapped in the body surface returns to the body core cooling internal organs, such as the heart, even more.[85] The danger of fibrillation and cardiac arrest may be increased. The profound vasodilation caused by the application of heat also produces the risk of what is called "rewarming shock." Hunter [86] suggests that rapid rewarming be used only in acute hypothermia of rapid onset and less than 12 hours in duration; while in chronic hypothermia, slower in onset and over 12 hours in duration, he recommends gradual rewarming primarily by the patient's own body heat. Siv Anderson and associates [87] agree that the longer the patient has been exposed to hypothermia, the slower should be the rewarming process. Hunter,[88] however, suggests that if the body temperature is in the range of 20° to 25°C (68° to 77°F) some form of artificial rewarming be instituted until the body temperature reaches 30° to 31.6°C (86° to 89°F), at which time the spontaneous rewarming by the patient be allowed to proceed.

D. M. Davies and associates [89] report successful treatment of an 82-year-old woman who was comatose owing to hypothermia by use of extracorporeal circulation, which means that the blood was drawn from the body, warmed, and returned to the body. This method obviates the danger of external rewarming, but the necessary equipment and supplies may not be available in most settings.

Management of persons with accidental hypothermia requires prompt action and usually intensive medical and nursing care. Victims of hypothermia may also develop a metabolic acidosis from tissue hypoxia and depletion of glycogen reserve. Pulmonary functioning is also impaired, with slow and shallow respirations. Respiratory depression may be corrected by assisted ventilation with the addition of oxygen. Parenteral fluid administration will help to correct the hypotension and oliguria. Acidosis should be treated by the administration of bicarbonate or other buffer solutions as well as by the use of a respirator to help the body rid itself of excess carbon dioxide. Low-molecular-weight dextran has been used to help expand the plasma volume. It is believed to be helpful in preventing intravascular thrombosis, a common complication.[90] Continuous monitoring of the patient's vital signs and taking an electrocardiograph are important during the rewarming phase to detect fatal arrhythmias and the presence of shock. Infections and metabolic imbalances often follow hypothermia.

The treatment of accidental hypothermia has been generally unsatisfactory. Favorable prognosis seems to depend more on the degree of hypothermia, the age of the patient, and the presence of underlying disorders than on any one method of treatment.[91] The mortality rate is around 50 per cent for those with severe hypothermia—when the body temperature falls to 32.2°C (90°F) or below.

Because of its high mortality rate and the difficulty of treating accidental hypothermia, prevention is of utmost importance. Those especially susceptible—such as the elderly, the very young, the infirm, and those living alone—should be recognized.[92] The use of thermometers that register low temperatures by those caring for the elderly in their homes and treatment centers would identify hypothermia in its early stages. Contributing factors such as poorly heated quarters, insufficient nutrition, improper clothing, and relative isolation can be identified by nurses working with the elderly in homes, clinics, and hospitals. When these factors are combined with chronic illness and the use of alcohol or other depressants the risk of hypothermia is increased.[93] Regular visiting of the aged individuals who live alone may help prevent injury from cold. The nutritional status of these people should be noted and their diets supplemented if necessary.

In working with infants and their families in all situations, the nurse should also be watchful for hypothermia. Again, the low-registering thermometer should be used. Hypothermia in infants can occur when the delivery is in a cold room. Those helping the mother in a home delivery should see that the room is heated to at least 18.3°C (65°F).[94] The ritual of daily bathing for the infant in a cold environment must be discouraged, and the very young infant should not be left out-of-doors in a buggy or pram for any length of time during cold weather.

Mark C. Rogers and associates [95] report three cases of neonatal cold injury following the infants' discharges from a hospital. Within 10 days at home the infants became lethargic and failed to eat adequately. On readmission the rectal temperature was less than 32.2°C (90°F). Treatment included gradual rewarming and intravenous and oral feedings. Infants appear to be susceptible to cold stress during the early stage of development and when this is combined with malnutrition they are in a precarious state. Infants in this report were exposed to cold, inadequately heated rooms, or rooms inappropriately air-conditioned. The nurse can help parents understand the dangers of cold during the neonatal period. The practice of swaddling can further prevent heat production because warmth produced by shivering is decreased.

Because accidental hypothermia can occur even in young and healthy individuals, adequate precautions against development of the problem must be taken. For example, those organizing outdoor excursions during the winter months should make adequate preparations. Accidental hypothermia under conditions of exposure can be prevented by keeping dry, taking shelter, and resting. If hypothermia occurs on an excursion, Freeman and Pugh [96] recommend treatment of the individual on the spot rather than risking sudden death during the journey to a treatment center. The exhausted individual should find shelter out of the wind and try to stay dry and conserve energy rather than continue exposure to cold. Waterproof outer garments of bright color should be worn and a change of clothing carried in a plastic bag.[97] Adequate head covering should also be worn to protect against heat loss from the head.

Frostbite. Frostbite is caused by prolonged exposure to extreme cold. The parts of the body that are most commonly affected are the extremities because they are most distant from the blood-warming viscera and the ears, nose, and cheeks because they are unprotected by hair and clothing.

The pathologic changes in frostbite remain inconclusive. Two schools of thought are reported on the primary mechanism of tissue damage. One states that the tissue damage is a direct result of cold injury to the cells; the other states that damage to tissue is secondary to injury to the blood vessels.[98] Frostbite causes ice crystals to form in the extracellular spaces and the crystals create a hypertonicity of the interstitial fluid. Water, therefore, leaves the cells in an attempt to maintain isotonicity; but the isotonic fluid freezes and the cycle continues. The cellular membrane, as a result, can no longer function with selective permeability. Upon thawing, the cells are damaged and massive interstitial edema results. The circulatory system responds to the cold by vasoconstriction, which slows and cools the blood and produces venous stasis. The stasis and "sludging" of the blood lead to tissue anoxia and resultant biochemical changes.[99]

The symptoms of frostbite are the following:

the part tingles, aches, and feels cold at first but is soon numb and painless. The subject is often unaware of the danger, for when all sensation is lost the tissues have been seriously injured. Because vasodilation is the initial response to cold the area looks red at first, but vasoconstriction follows rapidly and then the area looks dead white. At this point it is "frostbitten."

The US Army has developed a classification system describing four degrees of frostbite. Practically, it is difficult to discriminate between the degrees of injury, and a more restrictive classification using the terms "superficial" and "deep" has been suggested.[100] Superficial frostbite involves only the skin and subcutaneous tissues. Following rewarming, blisters form in 24 to 36 hours. Deep frostbite involves muscles, nerves, and sometimes the bone; blisters form in from 3 to 7 days and the extremity may remain swollen for weeks. With superficial injury the blister fluid is reabsorbed and an eschar is formed. The tissue sloughs in 2 to 3 weeks, leaving a reddened, partially healed surface. In deep frostbite, the tissue turns blue or gray, is swollen, and gangrene may develop.

The treatment of frostbite seems to be controversial. The objective of first-aid treatment is to prevent any further injury. In the past it has been recommended that the part be rubbed with snow or cold water applied. These practices are now discouraged because they will produce further injury to already damaged tissue. The part should be rested, not massaged or exercised. The person should be transported to a warm environment and additional treatment begun as soon as possible.[101]

Donald G. Sessions and associates [102] recommend the rapid method of rewarming the frozen part, as opposed to slow rewarming. They and others say that this method is gaining acceptance. Sessions further states: "Experimental and clinical evidence indicates that the time-honored concepts of frostbite treatment should be discarded in favor of a more physiological approach." * Rapid rewarming through the use of a warmed water bath produces less tissue damage and reduces the amount of tissue loss as compared with slow rewarming of the part.[103,104] It is recommended that the extremity be placed in a water bath at 41.6° to 43.3°C (107° to 110°F) for 15 to 20 minutes and that an analgesic be given to lessen pain. Sessions and associates [105] recommend thawing the frostbitten ear by surrounding it with cotton pledgets maintained at 37.7° to 42.2°C (100° to 108°F). Following rewarming the part should

---

* Sessions, Donald G., et al.: "Frostbite of the Ear," *Laryngoscope,* **81**:1223, (Aug.) 1971.

be elevated and immobilized to help control edema. Excess fluid in the affected area will be reabsorbed if the tissue is not severely damaged and if the blebs that form remain intact. If the blebs are broken the chances of infection are greater. Whirlpool baths are recommended as a means of mechanical debridement and facilitating motion of the injured part.[106] Following this treatment the extremity is wrapped in sterile dressings to decrease the chance of infection. The success of therapy depends on prevention of further damage to the tissues; therefore, gentle handling throughout the treatment procedure is imperative. Amputation should be delayed until the true line of demarcation appears. Many times only the surface tissues are damaged, and the extent of damage is difficult to evaluate initially. Jacques LeBlanc reports that the infusion of low-molecular-weight dextran has been shown even more beneficial than rapid rewarming in conserving frozen tissue. To be effective, the infusion must be started immediately upon thawing.[106a]

Sympathectomy, which may seem like a radical measure, has been found in some cases to reduce tissue loss and pain in the affected site. For maximum benefit it should be done within the first 2 to 3 days. Anticoagulants, vasodilators, and cortisone have proven to be of little value in the treatment of frostbite. Tobacco in any form should be discouraged because of its vasoconstricting effects. Wide-spectrum antibiotics are recommended in the event of infection.

Health teaching of the public by nurses and others is particularly important if injury from frostbite is to be prevented. How to dress in cold weather is one aspect of the educational program. For example, people can learn that clothing should be nonrestricting and should allow for the evaporation of perspiration. Foot gear should be impermeable to water. Gloves should be loose, and mittens offer better protection for the fingers than gloves. During cold weather the diet should contain extra carbohydrate and fat to increase the body's production of heat.[107] The consumption of alcohol and other depressant drugs in combination with exposure to cold should be avoided because alcohol leads to vasodilation, ataxia, impaired psychomotor functioning, and faulty judgment by reducing self-control.[108]

5. HYPOTHERMIA AS PRESCRIBED TREATMENT

Induced Hypothermia. Induced hypothermia is the reduction of body temperature, in a controlled manner, as an adjunct to medical or surgical treatment. The purpose is to reduce metabolic rate of various organs in the body and thereby decrease their need for oxygen. Oxygen consumption by the tissues decreases at a rate of 6.7 per cent per degree (centigrade) of drop in temperature. At a body temperature of 28°C (82.4°F) oxygen consumption has therefore decreased from that of normal body temperature—37°C (98°F)—by approximately 50 per cent. As the temperature decreases the cardiac rate and output also decrease. The walls of the ventricles cool at different rates, because of the differing muscle masses, and this predisposes to arrhythmias at 28°C (82.4°F) or below. The hematocrit level of the blood increases as the viscosity of the blood increases. The urine output of patients treated by hypothermia increases. This is thought to be the result of a decrease in the insensible water loss by the body.[109]

Hypothermia has been effectively used as an adjunct to open heart and neurologic surgery, because it decreases the circulation and reduces the oxygen requirements of the cells. Hypothermia is also used nonsurgically in the treatment of neurologic injury because it decreases cerebral oxygen consumption and blood flow. In addition, it decreases cerebrospinal fluid pressure and cerebral edema, and it prevents hyperthermia which is a frequent complication of brain injury.[110] It has further been used in the control of hyperpyrexia, in the treatment of burns, and in conjunction with surgery for the treatment of cancer. The three methods of inducing hypothermia described most frequently are external skin cooling, extracorporeal cooling, and localized cooling of selected organs. Each of these will be described in greater detail.

As stated earlier, heat is lost from the body by radiation, conduction-convection, and evaporation. The first two processes are important in the production of hypothermia. The body radiates heat to the surrounding environment when the environmental temperature is lower than that of the body. Heat is conducted from the body when it comes in contact with a cold object. Usually, the loss of heat is minimal as the object warms to approximate body temperature. With the application of external hypothermia, however, conduction is a main avenue of heat loss as the body is in direct contact with a continually cold surface. In order to facilitate heat loss by radiation and conduction in inducing hypothermia externally, the heat-conserving mechanisms of peripheral vasoconstriction and shivering are blocked. This is accomplished through the intramuscular or intravenous administration of a combination of drugs, such as chlorpromazine (Thorazine), promethazine hydrochloride (Phenergan), and meperidine hydrochloride (Demerol). This particular combination of drugs is referred to as the "lytic cocktail" and as a single means of hypothermia may reduce the body temperature by 2.24°C (4°F). Chlorpromazine has a direct effect on the hypothalamus and its thermoregulating mechanisms. It acts as vasodilator and reduces muscle tone; the latter inhibits shivering. Promethazine is given for its sedative action, reducing the amount of narcotics needed. Meperidine also produces sedation and helps control shivering. These drugs may be given in equal or varying amounts, either by diluted intravenous drip or intramuscularly.[111]

The first report found of induced hypothermia in this era is by Lawrence W. Smith and Temple Fay.[112] They discuss the successful utilization of total body hypothermia in the treatment of malignancies for the relief of pain. Early use of hypothermia in cardiac surgery utilized cooling of body surface to 28° to 30°C (82.4° to 86°F). This allowed the interruption of circulation safely for 6 to 8 minutes. This method was replaced by the use of bloodstream cooling through extracorporeal circulation. The blood is cooled directly and the core temperature drops rapidly. Through this means hypothermia may be induced efficiently and shivering is much less of a problem than it was with the first method. Although deep levels of hypothermia may be achieved —to 10°C (50°F)—if necessary, the moderate level of 28° to 30°C (82.4° to 86°F) is most often used because of the lessened incidence of complications. Blood from the patient passes through a "heat exchanger" unit which is placed in the circuit of the pump oxygenator. The blood may also be rewarmed as it passes through the heat exchanger back to the patient.[113] Deep surface-induced hypothermia— to 25°C (77°F)—in conjunction with extracorporeal bypass has been recommended for the surgical correction of congenital cardiac defects in infants. This method is thought to be particularly important because of the high mortality rate in infants associated with extracorporeal bypass.[114]

Induced hypothermia has been found to have important applications in the field of neurosurgery. Body temperature was lowered previously by surface cooling of the entire body with cooling blankets, and ice-water baths. However, ventricular fibrillation was a serious complication with these measures. Nerve tissue can tolerate temperature as low as 5°C (41°F) while cardiac complications may occur at 32°C (89.6°F). A lower degree of hypothermia is more desirable in neurosurgical procedures.[115]

Therefore, attempts have been made to develop a method of local application of cold to the brain while the temperature of the rest of the body remains normal. A series of studies has been reported by Juan Negrin[116] demonstrating the effective use of extravascular perfusion of cold solutions to the brain and spinal cord. In this way local hypothermia of the nerve tissue can be effected without lowering the general body temperature. The instrument that has been developed for this purpose is called the hypothermostat. A catheter directs the cooled fluid around the brain or spinal cord exposed by craniotomy or laminectomy. Fluids used include normal saline, glycerol solutions, cerebrospinal fluid, or Ringer's solution. The temperature of the circulating bath can be maintained from "room temperature" to 5°C (41°F). Local hypothermia has been used effectively in the removal of neoplasms invading the third and fourth ventricles of the brain, in the management of vascular aneurysms and other lesions, and in the treatment of trauma. An unexpected and favorable side effect has been the suppression of intractable seizures in epileptic patients following local cerebral hypothermia.

The use of local hypothermia for spinal cord injuries was a logical consequence of its use in cerebral cooling. During a laminectomy the cord may be bathed by cold fluid through specially placed catheters in the epidural and/or subarachnoid spaces. Using this technique, Negrin[117] has reported remissions in spasticity, paraplegia, and pain following acute or chronic spinal cord injuries. In another study, he reports the relief of spasticity and intractable pain in patients with multiple sclerosis.[118] This technique may be used postoperatively at the bedside through the specially placed catheters or needles. It does not require the facilities offered in operating rooms. The exact mechanism in relieving spasticity and intractable pain requires further study.[119]

Total body hypothermia during surgery has been used in conjunction with intra-arterial perfusion of alkylating agents in the treatment of cancer involving the head and neck. Alkylating agents are toxic to the bone marrow and therefore the dosage must be limited when the patient's temperature is normal. Induced hypothermia is thought to decrease the blood supply and metabolism of the bone marrow, thereby protecting it from damage by larger doses of alkylating agents.[120] H. A. Condon[121] reports a study of 31 patients in which total body hypothermia was used along with the intra-arterial perfusion of an alkylating agent. In addition to the protection to the bone marrow, and the increased effectiveness of the drug on tumor activity, he found that pain was relieved in 88 per cent of the patients having pain.

Externally Induced Hypothermia. External hypothermia may be applied using ice bags, blankets wrung from cold water, and the commercially available hypothermia blanket. This blanket is a large piece of synthetic material through which cooling fluid circulates. The temperature of the cooling agent may be controlled only with the hypothermia blanket and therefore its use is more generally accepted than ice bags and wet blankets.[122] Figure 42-7 illustrates a type of hypothermia machine with blankets or pads coiled and not in use.

Prior to the induction of external hypothermia, the patient must be prepared both physically and mentally. The procedure and its indications and technique must be explained to the patient and the family. This will help to lessen alarm and anxiety on the part of both and encourage the patient to cooperate in his or her care. Physical preparation involves cleaning the patient's skin thoroughly. Partial baths during hypothermia may be all that is needed. The skin may further be prepared by the application of lanolin, mineral oil, or lotion. This provides a thin layer of lubricant that protects the skin and fosters conduction of cold from the blanket. A Foley catheter may be inserted to empty the patient's bladder. Monitoring of the patient's output and the specific gravity of the urine is helpful in detecting renal damage. Intravenous fluids should be started to provide for fluid intake but also as a means of administering drugs, if needed. The vital signs (temperature, pulse, respirations, and blood pressure) are taken at least twice before initiating hypothermia to establish a baseline for later comparison. Other observations of the patient's status include presence of edema, level of consciousness, condition of the skin, and regularity of the heart rate. The blanket is placed under the patient. A cotton blanket or sheet is placed next to the patient's skin to protect it from contact with the synthetic blanket. Another cooling blanket may be placed over the patient with a sheet next to the patient's skin. Kerlix or cotton padding may be used between the toes to prevent frostbite. The machine is turned on and the control is set for the desired temperature as prescribed by the physician. Temperature is monitored by a thermometer device placed in the esophagus or rectum.

June Abbey and others report a method of controlling shivering without the use of drugs. Seventeen incidences of the use of the hypothermic blanket on 15 patients were studied.

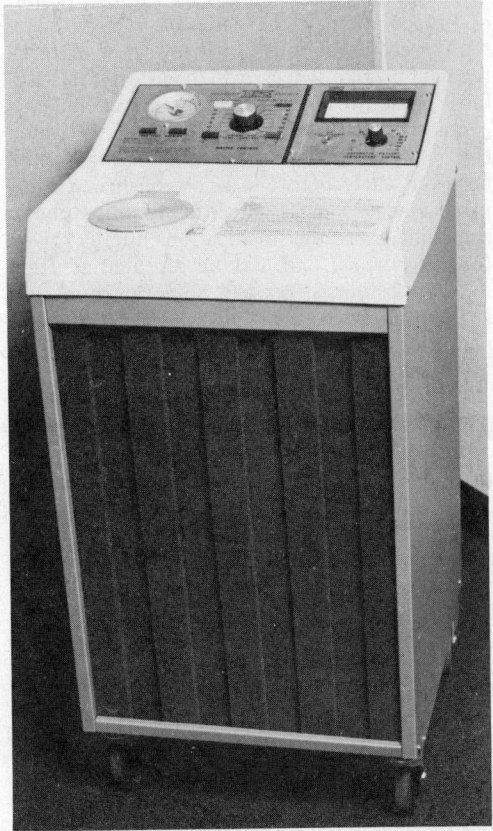

Figure 42-7. Externally induced hypothermia may be obtained through use of a hypothermia machine. Illustrated is the Gorman-Rupp RK-300 hypo-hyperthermia unit. (Courtesy of Gorman-Rupp Industries, Belleville, Ohio.)

Both upper and lower extremities were wrapped from the elbows to the fingertips and from the knees to the tips of the toes with three thicknesses of terry cloth toweling clamped with wooden clothespins. The toweling was changed whenever it became damp. Wrapping the extremities decreased the incidence of shivering from the usual incidence of 75–100 per cent to 24 per cent without the use of shiver-suppressive drugs.[122a]

Care during hypothermia includes provisions for the patient's comfort and maintaining the effectiveness of the hypothermia. The shivering response to cold must be controlled during the induction phase. Shivering causes an increase in the metabolic rate to such an extent that hypothermia is difficult to effect and it also produces increased intracranial pressure and increased oxygen consumption. The nurse may see the earliest signs of shivering by watching the patient's chest for muscle tremor, or fasciculation. If the patient's ECG is being monitored continuously, it may show fine, irregular, bizarre waves, which distort the baseline. These are due to muscle tremor and this is another early sign of shivering to watch for.[123] Medication to control shivering should be given early before it is established. Chlorpromazine (25 mg), which is an antipsychotic tranquilizer, is the medication usually given for this purpose and may be repeated as often as every 2 hours if needed. Shivering stops and is followed by general muscle rigidity at temperatures of 30° to 33°C (86° to 91.4°F).[124]

The blood pressure and pulse rate may show a temporary rise due to vasoconstriction during the induction of hypothermia. As the temperature falls, however, blood pressure and pulse rate also drop. When the temperature reaches 30°C (86°F) or below, the danger of ventricular fibrillation markedly increases. Cardiac resuscitation equipment, a tracheostomy tray, a respirator, and emergency drugs should be close at hand. The temperature, pulse, respiration, and blood pressure should be taken and recorded every 5 minutes depending on the patient's condition. A decrease in blood pressure and pulse can be expected during hypothermia. In addition, the nurse should be aware of the patient's disease process and how it affects his or her temperature, blood pressure, and pulse rate.[125] The respiration rate decreases during hypothermia and assisted ventilation may be required. Suction equipment should be available. Nasopharyngeal suction is applied if the patient cannot control secretions from the nose and mouth. Pupillary reaction, level of consciousness, and movement of extremities should be observed and recorded. Seizures may occur and be difficult to control.[126] Maurice Bloch,[127] in a study of 71 episodes of prolonged hypothermia in 25 patients who had minimal impairment of function from brain tumor, found that consciousness progressively decreases as temperature falls.* At temperatures of 30° to 32°C (86° to 89.6°F) most patients remained alert, and others lapsed into light sleep but were easily aroused. He noted that the principal mental difficulties were the inability to concentrate and the inability to retain freshly acquired information. At 26.6°C (80°F) the patient loses control of voluntary movement and is unable to respond to verbal stimuli. The corneal reflexes are usually affected. Care of the eyes should be provided by use of eyedrops or an irrigating solution, such as normal saline. Eye patches may add further protection. The

nurse should take particular care to maintain a quiet environment—to reduce all stimuli to a minimum. Patients are reassured when nurses work confidently and when they show respect for them as individuals. Care should be explained before it is carried out. In this way communication is maintained even though the patient may be unable to respond verbally. The patient may have many fears about hypothermia and its possible results and the nurse's presence alone, as someone known and trusted, is reassuring.[128] It is comforting to think that decisions will be made by competent individuals and that one is in "safe hands."

Fluid and electrolyte balance is maintained through either intravenous fluids or tube feedings. The latter must be given slowly because peristalsis is diminished in hypothermia. Fluid requirements are decreased because of the decrease in body metabolism. The average adult requirements at temperatures of 30° to 32°C (86° to 89.6°F) are provided for by 1000 ml (1 qt) of 5 per cent dextrose in water and 1000 ml (1 qt) of 5 per cent dextrose in 0.2 per cent saline solution for 24 hours.[129] Cleaning and rinsing the patient's mouth are important because he or she is unable to control secretions and is taking no food or liquid by mouth. The mucous membranes of the mouth should be swabbed or wetted periodically with water or water and mouthwash. The lips should be lubricated with a thin coat of cold cream or petroleum jelly, especially if the patient is breathing through the mouth. Teeth should be brushed for the patient periodically and excess water and secretions removed by suctioning if the patient cannot spit.

The effects of hypothermia on the action of many drugs is unknown. Hypothermia tends to modify drug action by decreasing absorption and excretion, and increasing potency. Massaging the injection site facilitates absorption. Nurses must be aware of the action of the drugs they are administering and watch for cumulative side effects.

The patient's position should be changed every hour if not more frequently, and the skin over the bony prominences massaged, to prevent skin breakdown. Passive range-of-motion exercises may be carried out to prevent circulatory stasis. If conscious, the patient should be encouraged to breathe deeply and cough frequently. The signs of respiratory infection and other complications may be masked by hypothermia.

The cooling device is usually turned off at about 1.11° or 1.67°C (2° or 3°F) above the desired temperature. This is because the body temperature will continue to go down at least this amount after the cooling device is turned

---

* Death by freezing is said to be an easy one for this reason.

off. This phenomenon is termed "downward drift" and is explained by the fact that the skin and periphery of the body are cooler than the body core. Blood coming from the viscera to the skin is cooled by the cold periphery, even after external cooling has stopped, and when the blood returns to the center of the body, the internal organs are cooled even more.[130] Some factors that affect the amount of "downward drift" of the temperature are the patient's age and size, muscle tone, degree of peripheral vasodilation, thermoregulatory response, and core temperature.[131] Some cooling devices will cut off automatically when a set temperature is reached and turn on as the body temperature drifts upward.

Certain complications can occur with hypothermia. Some individuals are hypersensitive to the treatment. As with an allergic reaction the person develops urticaria, increased pulse rate, decreased blood pressure, and dyspnea.

Frostbite is another complication of hypothermia. Frostbite occurs when the skin and subcutaneous tissue actually freeze or when ice crystals form on them. Following rewarming, the skin appears reddish blue and edematous. The nurse caring for the patient during hypothermia should pay particular attention to the color of the skin, watching for a white, red, or blue discoloration, particularly on the coccygeal area, that indicates beginning tissue damage. Another sign of frostbite is a complaint by the patient of numbness or tingling in the area.[132]

The patient may develop fat necrosis while under surface hypothermia. Subcutaneous fat solidifies, feeling hard and immobile. Fat necrosis is most likely when cold is applied to the tissues for long periods. Massaging susceptible areas and turning the patient frequently helps prevent this complication.

The simplest and safest way to rewarm the patient is to discontinue the hypothermia and allow the patient to warm spontaneously. The hypothermia blanket may also be used to gradually rewarm the patient in which case it is turned off when the body temperature reaches 34.4° to 35°C (94° to 95°F).[133] This allows for the tendency of the temperature to drift upward before it stabilizes within normal limits. It may be desirable to rewarm the person by immersion in warm water, covering with warm blankets, or using a heat cradle. With these measures the patient's skin must be observed closely for damage as cold skin is especially susceptible to burns. The patient's temperature, pulse, respiration, and blood pressure should be monitored at least every 30 minutes until they stabilize. With rapid rewarming shock may develop from peripheral vasodilation and a decrease in peripheral resistance.[134]

Gastric Hypothermia. The application of hypothermia locally to control massive gastrointestinal bleeding has been reported as a useful adjunct to surgery, or as a method of controlling bleeding when surgery is contraindicated. Surgical intervention is the treatment of choice in most cases of gastric hemorrhage. However, if the patient is elderly, has an unassociated systemic disease, or is in shock from blood loss, the risk of surgery is greatly increased. In these patients gastric hypothermia has certain advantages: it allows for diagnostic tests, it allows for stabilization of the patient's condition in preparation for elective surgery, and on occasion it controls the hemorrhage so that the need for surgery is obviated.[135]

Continuous gastric lavage using iced saline is one means of achieving gastric hypothermia.[136] (Gastric lavage is described in Chapter 23.) Discomfort can be prevented by keeping the patient warm and by administering sedatives. The nasogastric tube may require continuous irrigation to keep it free from clots. Monitoring the temperature, pulse, respirations, and blood pressure is particularly important during gastric lavage as shock is often present. Because the cooling fluid passes near the heart, arrhythmia may develop. The rectal temperature shows whether or not normal body temperature is being maintained.

In some patients more extreme measures of hypothermia are necessary to control bleeding. The use of gastric balloon hypothermia as developed by O. H. Wangensteen is frequently reported as a useful measure. In 1958, the technique was first described and has since been modified. R. F. Edlich and associates[137] describe hypothermia along with tamponade with a balloon which conforms to the contours of the human stomach. The balloon provides contact with the walls of the stomach and hemostasis is achieved partially through compression of the blood vessels in the gastric mucosa. The tube leading to the balloon has four lumens: two to provide circulation of cold water within the balloon, one to provide aspiration of drainage from the duodenum, and the fourth to aspirate the regurgitated blood and gastric juice from the esophagus. The iced water cooling fluid flows by gravity into the system.

To introduce the balloon the posterior pharynx is sprayed with a topical anesthetic and a nasogastric tube is inserted. Any blood clots present in the stomach are removed through lavage with iced saline. Blood clots in the stomach would prevent adequate contact of the cooling device with the stomach lining. The balloon is wrapped around the four-lumen tube and is well lubricated. It is passed under fluoroscopy until the tip can be seen to reach the antrum of the stomach. The balloon is then slowly inflated with cooled water. Continuous suction is applied to the gastroduodenal and esophageal outlets.

The patient's systemic temperature is maintained at 35°C (95°F) with an electric blanket. Blood pressure, pulse, and respirations are checked frequently, again observing for arrhythmia. Hemoglobin determinations should be made every 4 hours. With the continuous aspiration of the esophagus the serious complication of aspiration pneumonia is prevented. The hypothermia is continued for 24 hours following cessation of bleeding. After balloon removal the patient receives a continuous drip of antacid to control acid and pepsin. Utilizing this technique, Edlich and associates report cessation of bleeding in eighteen out of twenty patients. Further, because of improvement over previous techniques, many of the complications of balloon gastric hypothermia have been eliminated.

Cryotherapy. The therapeutic use of extremes of cold is a new and rapidly expanding field. The use of freezing temperatures has been widely applied to a variety of surgical procedures where tissue excision and cautery have been used in the past. Anna E. Marks says: "Cryosurgery is the technique wherein cellular structure is altered reversibly or irreversibly by the rapid, profound application of intense cold down to −190°C (−310°F) for varying periods of time. It is the calculated destruction of unwanted cells and tissues." * Cryotherapy has been successfully used in clinical services or neurosurgery, in the treatment of parkinsonism and brain tumors; otolaryngology, in the treatment of angiofibroma, epistaxis, and for tonsillectomy; ophthalmology, for retinal detachment and eye tumors; urology, for prostate and bladder surgery; gynecology, in the treatment of intractable menorrhagia and cervicitis; and dermatology, for the removal of cutaneous tumors. One widely used and adaptable instrument makes use of the freezing properties of liquid nitrogen at a temperature of −196°C (−320.8°F). The liquid nitrogen flows from the reservoir through an insulated cannula and probe. The probe is insulated except for the very tip. Freezing takes place when this tip comes in contact with the tissue. The temperature at the tip of the probe is constantly monitored. The technique allows for complete control by the operator of the degree of cold being applied.[138] The procedure is relatively simple and has marked benefits for the patient. In the areas listed above in which it has been utilized, cryotherapy produces adequate control of hemorrhage, lessens the analgesia required, and lessens or eliminates the need for anesthesia. Operating room nurses can become skilled in the operation of cryotherapeutic devices and their clinical uses.

An example of the use and benefits of cryotherapy follows: Julius Hicks[139] describes the use of the technique in the treatment of epistaxis. A balloon containing cooled circulating alcohol was applied to the nasopharynx for less than 30 minutes with the patient in modified Fowler's position (see Fig. 42-8). In comparing 26 patients with epistaxis treated with cryotherapy to 16 patients treated with nasal packing, he found that 20 per cent of the patients receiving cryotherapy required narcotics as opposed to 44 per cent of those treated with nasal packing. The duration of hospitalization for those having cryotherapy averaged 4.27 days as compared with 7.06 days for those having nasal packing. The five patients treated with both methods stated that the pain associated with cryotherapy was infinitely less than that with nasal packing.

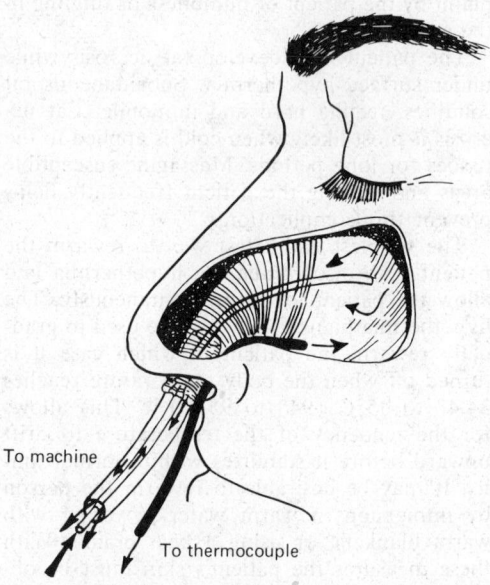

To machine

To thermocouple

Figure 42-8. Placement of thermocouple and rubber balloon in patient's nose. The thermocouple monitors the temperature of the circulating coolant. (From Hicks, Julius N.: "Cryotherapy for Severe Posterior Nasal Epistaxis," *Laryngoscope,* **81:**188, [Dec.] 1971.)

* Marks, Anna E.: "Cryogenics: The Indications and Implications for Nursing," *Am. Assoc. Ind. Nurses J.,* **15:**7, (Oct.) 1967.

Refrigeration Anesthesia. Cold in the form of ice as an anesthetic agent has been previously utilized in patients needing amputations for whom general anesthesia was believed very risky. Refrigeration anesthesia has fallen into disuse perhaps because of its difficulties and the improvements made in other anesthetic techniques.[110] The use of dry ice refrigeration as adjunct to regional or general anesthesia for amputation of an ischemic lower extremity is described currently in the literature. J. F. Gorman and J. C. Rosenberg[111] report a series of 72 patients requiring above-knee amputation for ischemic gangrene. In approximately half of these, dry ice refrigeration was used preoperatively for its bacteriostatic effects and because time was gained to prepare the patient physically.

The technique is described as follows: Clothing is removed from the affected limb and stockinet is applied to the leg and secured with tape 3 to 4 inches above the extent of gangrene. A double layer of rubber sheeting is placed under the leg and 10 to 15 pounds of chipped dry ice or solid carbon dioxide at $-45°C$ ($-49°F$) is placed around the leg. The rubber sheet is wrapped around the leg, secured with safety pins, and covered with a wool blanket (see Fig. 47-3 in Chapter 47). The uninvolved extremity is wrapped in a sheet and a board is placed between the legs. The dry ice is kept in place for a minimum of 24 hours. Dry ice is not as cumbersome as wet ice and is more economical and available than hypothermic units. The mortality rate for patients with infected limbs not treated with dry ice was 46 per cent, as compared with 6 per cent in the treated group whose legs were infected. The causes of death in both groups were pulmonary embolism, congestive heart failure, and pneumonia. German and Rosenberg recommend that dry ice refrigeration prior to surgery be employed for those patients in whom gangrene is complicated by sepsis. For further discussion of this subject, see Chapter 47.

REFERENCES

1. Belding, Harwood: "Resistance to Heat in Man and Other Homeothermic Animals," in Rose, Anthony H. (ed.): *Thermobiology*. Academic Press, New York, 1967, p. 479.
2. Mills, Clarence A.: *Climate Makes the Man*. Harper & Row, New York, 1942, p. 9.
3. Blum, Harold F.: "The Physiological Effect of Sunlight on Man," *Physiol. Rev.*, **25**:483, (July) 1945.
4. Burch, George E., and DePasquale, Nicholas P.: *Hot Climates, Man and His Heart*. Charles C Thomas, Publisher, Springfield, Ill., 1962, p. 153.
5. Burch, George E., and DePasquale, Nicholas P.: *op. cit.*, p. 7.
6. Astrand, Per-Olof, and Rodahl, Kaare: *Textbook of Work Physiology*. McGraw-Hill Book Co., New York, 1970, p. 515.
7. Newman, Russell W.: "Why Man Is Such a Sweaty and Thirsty Naked Animal: A Speculative Review," *Hum. Biol.*, **42**:12, (Feb.) 1970.
8. Guyton, Arthur C.: *Textbook of Medical Physiology*, 5th ed. W. B. Saunders Co., Philadelphia, 1976, p. 956.
9. Newman, Russell W.: *op. cit.*
10. *Ibid.*
11. Clothier, J. Guthrie: "Work in Hostile Climates," *Ann. Occup. Hyg.*, **14**:197, (June) 1971.
12. *Ibid.*
13. Ladell, William S. S.: "Terrestrial Animals in Humid Heat: Man," in Dill, D. B., et al. (eds.): *Handbook of Physiology, Adaptation to the Environment*. American Physiological Society, Washington, D.C., 1964, p. 625.
14. Guyton, Arthur C.: *op. cit.*, p. 835.
15. Conn, Jerome W.: "Some Clinical and Climatological Aspects of Aldosteronism in Man," *Trans. Am. Clin. Climatol. Assoc.*, **74**:61, 1962.
16. Ladell, William S. S.: *op. cit.*, p. 628.
17. Belding, Harwood S.: "Research on Problems of Work in Heat," *Arch. Environ. Health*, **15**:660, (Nov.) 1967.
18. *Ibid.*
19. ———: "Resistance to Heat in Man and Other Homeothermic Animals," in Rose, Anthony H. (ed.): *Thermobiology*. Academic Press, New York, 1967, p. 498.
20. Henschel, Austin, et al.: "Heat Tolerance of Elderly Persons Living in a Subtropical Climate," *J. Gerontol.*, **23**:17, (Jan.) 1968.
21. *Ibid.*
22. Wyndham, Cyril H.: "Adaptation to Heat and Cold," *Environ. Res.*, **2**:442, (Oct.) 1969.
23. Newman, Russell W.: *op. cit.*
24. Maxcy, Kenneth F. (ed.): *Rosenau's Preventive Medicine and Hygiene*, 7th ed. Appleton-Century-Crofts, New York, 1951, p. 175.
25. Belding, Harwood: *op. cit.*
26. Astrand, Per-Olof, and Rodahl, Kaare: *op. cit.*, p. 496.
27. *Ibid.*, p. 498.
28. Edholm, O. G., and Lewis, H. E.: "Terrestrial Animals in Cold: Man in Polar Regions," in Dill, D. B., et al. (eds.): *Handbook of Physiology, Adaptation to the Environment*. American Physiological Society, Washington, D.C., 1964, p. 435.
29. Astrand, Per-Olof, and Rodahl, Kaare: *op. cit.*
30. Edholm, O. G., and Lewis, H. E.: *op. cit.*, p. 437.
30a. LeBlanc, Jacques: *Man in the Cold*. Charles C Thomas, Publisher, Springfield, Ill., 1975, p. 9.

31. Burch, George E., and DePasquale, Nicholas P.: *op. cit.,* p. 155.

32. Astrand, Per-Olof, and Rodahl, Kaare: *op. cit.,* p. 515.

33. Quashnock, Joseph M.: "Heat and Cold," in Beeson, Paul B., and McDermott, Walsh (eds.): *Cecil-Loeb Textbook of Medicine,* 13th ed. W. B. Saunders Co., Philadelphia, 1971, p. 30.

34. Sohar, Ezra, et al.: "Heatstroke Caused by Dehydration and Physical Effort," *Arch. Intern. Med.,* **122:**159, (Aug.) 1968.

35. Eichler, Allen C., et al.: "Heat Stroke," *Am. J. Surg.,* **118:**855, (Dec.) 1969.

36. *Ibid.*

37. Quashnock, Joseph M.: *op. cit.*

38. Hogg, Charles E.: "Malignant Hyperpyrexia," *Int. Anesthesiol. Clin.,* **10:**111, (Spring) 1972.

39. Barlow, M. B., and Isaacs, H.: "Malignant Hyperpyrexial Deaths in a Family," *Br. J. Anaesth.,* **42:**1072, (Dec.) 1970.

40. Heydman, Abby M., and Stegman, Mary Ruth: "One in Ten Thousand," *Am. J. Nurs.,* **71:**1944, (Oct.) 1971.

41. Rose, Donald L.: "Change Is Not Necessarily Progress" (editorial), *Arch. Phys. Med. Rehabil.,* **50:**595, (Oct.) 1969.

42. Beeks, John W.: "Hyperthermia as an Adjunct to the Treatment of Neoplasms," *J. Kans. Med. Soc.,* **67:**521, (Oct.) 1966.

43. Henderson, M. A., and Pettigrew, R. T.: "Induction of Controlled Hyperthermia in Treatment of Cancer," *Lancet,* **1:**1275, (June 19) 1971.

44. Ehlers, Holger: "Fever Therapy in Aestival Conjunctivitis," *Acta Ophthalmol.,* **46:**284, 1968.

45. Jacoby, Florence: "Current Nursing Care of the Burned Patient," *Nurs. Clin. North Am.,* **5:**563, (Dec.) 1970.

46. Jackson, Douglas MacG.: "In Search of an Acceptable Burn Classification," *Br. J. Plast. Surg.,* **23:**219, (July) 1970.

47. Artz, Curtis P.: "The Burned Patient: Newer Concepts of Medical and Nursing Management," in Kintzel, Kay Corman (ed.): *Advanced Concepts in Clinical Nursing.* J. B. Lippincott Co., Philadelphia, 1971, p. 321.

48. Jacoby, Florence: *op. cit.*

49. Kravitz, Harvey: "First-Aid Therapy for Burns—Cool It!" *Clin. Pediatr.,* **9:**695, (Dec.) 1970.

50. Artz, Curtis P.: *op. cit.,* p. 325.

51. Nance, Francis C., et al.: "Aggressive Outpatient Care of Burns," *J. Trauma,* **12:**144, (Feb.) 1972.

52. Larson, Duane, and Gaston, Rita: "Current Trends in the Care of Burned Patients," *Am. J. Nurs.,* **67:**319, (Feb.) 1967.

53. Ketchum, Lynn D., et al.: "Burn Treatment Advances," *J. Kans. Med. Soc.,* **72:**133, (Mar.) 1971.

54. Jacoby, Florence: *op. cit.*

55. Artz, Curtis P.: "The Brooke Formula," in Polk, Hiram C., Jr., and Stone, H. Harlan (eds.): *Contemporary Burn Management.* Little, Brown & Co., Boston, 1972, p. 43.

56. Ketchum, Lynn D., et al.: *op. cit.*

57. *Ibid.*

58. Liljedahl, S. O., and Birke, G.: "The Nutrition of Patients with Extensive Burns," *Nutr. Metab.,* **14:**110, (Suppl.) 1972.

59. Artz, Curtis P., and Moncrief, John A.: *The Treatment of Burns,* 2nd ed. W. B. Saunders Co., Philadelphia, 1969, p. 142.

60. *Ibid.,* p. 151.

61. *Ibid.,* p. 102.

62. *Ibid.,* p. 159.

63. *Ibid.,* p. 160.

64. *Ibid.,* p. 162.

65. Monafo, William W.: *The Treatment of Burns.* Warren H. Green, Inc., St. Louis, 1971, p. 120.

66. *Ibid.,* p. 262.

67. Artz, Curtis P.: "The Burned Patient: Newer Concepts of Medical and Nursing Management," in Kintzel, Kay Corman (ed.): *Advanced Concepts in Clinical Nursing.* J. B. Lippincott Co., Philadelphia, 1971, p. 329.

68. Artz, Curtis P., and Moncrief, John A.: *op. cit.,* p. 165.

69. Larson, Duane L., et al.: "Splints and Traction," in Polk, Hiram C., Jr., and Stone, H. Harlan (eds.): *Contemporary Burn Management.* Little, Brown & Co., Boston, 1972, p. 419.

69a. Artz, Curtis P.: *op. cit.,* p. 335.

69b. Freeman, Aaron, et al.: "A New Method for Covering Large Surface Area Wounds with Autografts," *Arch. Surg.,* **108:**721, (May) 1974.

69c. Igel, Howard J., et al.: "A New Method for Covering Large Surface Area Wounds with Autografts II," *Arch. Surg.,* **108:**725, (May) 1974.

69d. Lackmann, Joan, and Sorensen, Karen Creason: *Medical-Surgical Nursing: A Psychophysiologic Approach.* W. B. Saunders Co., Philadelphia, 1974, p. 1277.

69e. Jacoby, Florence Greenhouse: *Nursing Care of the Patient with Burns.* C. V. Mosby Co., St. Louis, 1972.

70. Artz, Curtis P., and Moncrief, John A.: *op. cit.,* p. 282.

71. Andreasen, N. J. C., and Norris, A. S.: "Long-Term Adjustment and Adaptation Mechanisms in Severely Burned Adults," *J. Nerv. Ment. Dis.,* **154:**352, (May) 1972.

71a. Fagerhaugh, Shizuko: "Pain Expression and Control on a Burn Care Unit," *Nurs. Outlook,* **22:**645, (Oct.) 1974.

71b. Artz, Curtis P., and Moncrief, John A.: *op. cit.,* p. 249.

71c. Ralph, Robert A., and Slansky, Harvey H.: "Therapy of Chemical Burns," *Int. Ophthalmol. Clin.,* **14:**171, (Winter) 1974.

72. Artz, Curtis P.: "The Burned Patient: Newer Concepts of Medical and Nursing Management," in Kintzel, Kay Corman (ed.): *Advanced Concepts in Clinical Nurs-*

ing. J. B. Lippincott Co., Philadelphia, 1971, p. 322.

73. Hutchinson, James H.: "Hypothermia in Infancy," *Med. Sci. Law,* **9:**224, (Oct.) 1969.

74. Wilson, G. M.: "Hypothermia in Clinical Medicine," *Med. Sci. Law,* **9:**231, (Oct.) 1969.

75. *Ibid.*

76. Trevino, Alfonso, et al.: "The Characteristic Electrocardiogram of Accidental Hypothermia," *Arch. Intern. Med.,* **127:**470, (Mar.) 1971.

77. Clements, Stephen D., Jr., and Hurst, J. Willis: "Diagnostic Value of Electrocardiographic Abnormalities Observed in Subjects Accidentally Exposed to Cold," *Am. J. Cardiol.,* **29:**729, (May) 1972.

78. Wilson, G. M.: *op. cit.*

79. Hunter, Warren C.: "Accidental Hypothermia, Part III," *Northwest Med.,* **67:**837, (Sept.) 1968.

80. Freeman, James, and Pugh, L. Griffith C. E.: "Hypothermia in Mountain Accidents," *Int. Anesthesiol. Clin.,* **7:**997, (Winter) 1969.

81. Hunter, Warren C.: *op. cit.*

82. Tolman, Keith G., and Cohen, Arthur: "Accidental Hypothermia," *Can. Med. Assoc. J.,* **103:**1357, (Dec. 19) 1970.

83. Hunter, Warren C.: *op. cit.*

84. Schamroth, Leo, and Perlman, Moses M.: "The Electrocardiographic Manifestations of Hypothermia," *Heart & Lung,* **1:**233, (Mar.–Apr.) 1972.

85. Hunter, Warren C.: *op. cit.*

86. *Ibid.*

87. Anderson, Siv, et al.: "Accidental Profound Hypothermia," *Br. J. Anaesth.,* **42:**653, (July) 1970.

88. Hunter, Warren C.: *op. cit.*

89. Davies, D. M., et al.: "Accidental Hypothermia Treated by Extracorporeal Blood-Warming," *Lancet,* **1:**1036, (May 13) 1967.

90. Tolman, Keith G., and Cohen, Arthur: *op. cit.*

91. Phillipson, Eliot A., and Herbert, F. A.: "Accidental Exposure to Freezing: Clinical and Laboratory Observations During Convalescence from Near-Fatal Hypothermia," *Can. Med. Assoc. J.,* **97:**786, (Sept. 23) 1967.

92. Wilson, G. M.: *op. cit.*

93. Hunter, Warren C.: "Accidental Hypothermia, Part I," *Northwest Med.,* **67:**569, (June) 1968.

94. Hutchinson, James H.: *op. cit.*

95. Rogers, Mark C., et al.: "Cold Injury of the Newborn," *N. Engl. J. Med.,* **285:**332, (Aug. 5) 1971.

96. Freeman, James, and Pugh, L. Griffith C. E.: *op. cit.*

97. Hunter, Warren C.: "Accidental Hypothermia, Part III," *Northwest Med.,* **67:**837, (Sept.) 1968.

98. Sessions, Donald G., et al.: "Frostbite of

the Ear," *Laryngoscope,* **81:**1223, (Aug.) 1971.

99. Carter, Joey M., and Bevin, A. Griswold: "Frostbite of the Extremities," *N.C. Med. J.,* **31:**447, (Dec.) 1970.

100. Sessions, Donald G., et al.: *op. cit.*

101. Beal, John M.: "Frostbite," *Ill. Med. J.,* **136:**592, (Nov.) 1969.

102. Sessions, Donald G., et al.: *op. cit.*

103. Beal, John M.: *op. cit.*

104. Carter, Joey M., and Bevin, A. Griswold: *op. cit.*

105. Sessions, Donald G., et al.: *op. cit.*

106. Carter, Joey M., and Bevin, A. Griswold: *op. cit.*

106a. LeBlanc, Jacques: *op. cit.,* p. 40.

107. Cavanaugh, Daniel G.: "The Pathogenesis and Treatment of Frostbite," *J. Kans. Med. Soc.,* **71:**11, (Jan.) 1970.

108. Meyers, Frederick H., et al.: *Review of Medical Pharmacology,* 3rd ed. Lange Medical Publications, Los Altos, Calif., 1972, p. 229.

109. Nealon, Thomas F., Jr., and Gosin, Stephen: "Hypothermia: Physiologic Effects and Clinical Application," *Med. Clin. North Am.,* **49:**1181, (Sept.) 1965.

110. Hickey, Mary Catherine: "Hypothermia," *Am. J. Nurs.,* **65:**116, (Jan.) 1965.

111. *Ibid.*

112. Smith, Lawrence W., and Fay, Temple: "Observation of Human Beings with Cancer, Maintained at Reduced Temperatures of 75°–90° Fahrenheit," *Am. J. Clin. Pathol.,* **10:**1, (No. 1) 1940.

113. Nealon, Thomas F., Jr., and Gosin, Stephen: *op. cit.*

114. Gray, T. Cecil, and Graham, G. R.: "Hypothermia," in Gray, T. Cecil, and Nunn, J. F.: *General Anaesthesia,* 3rd ed. Appleton-Century-Crofts, New York, 1971, p. 406.

115. Negrin, Juan, Jr.: "Hypothermia of the Central Nervous System," *Trans. N.Y. Acad. Sci.,* **33:**557, (June) 1971.

116. *Ibid.*

117. *Ibid.*

118. Negrin, Juan, Jr.: "Spinal Cord Hypothermia to Relieve Muscle Spasticity in Multiple Sclerosis: Preliminary Observations," *J. Nerv. Ment. Dis.,* **144:**430, (No. 5) 1967.

119. ——: "Hypothermia of the Central Nervous System" *Trans. N.Y. Acad. Sci.,* **33:**557, (June) 1971.

120. Harrison, D. F. N.: "The Use of Hypothermia in Intra-Arterial Chemotherapy for Head and Neck Cancer," *J. Laryngol. Otol.,* **81:**173, (Feb.) 1967.

121. Condon, H. A.: "Hypothermia and Cancer Chemotherapy," *Anesth. Analg.,* **48:**92, (Jan.–Feb.) 1969.

122. Hickey, Mary Catherine: *op. cit.*

122a. Abbey, June, et al.: "A Pilot Study: The Control of Shivering During Hypothermia by a Clinical Nursing Measure," *J. Neurosurg. Nurs.,* **5:**78, (Dec.) 1973.

123. Schamroth, Leo, and Perlman, Moses M.: *op. cit.*

124. Hickey, Mary Catherine: *op. cit.*

125. *Ibid.*

126. Rosomoff, Hubert, and Safar, Peter: "Management of the Comatose Patient," in Safar, Peter (ed.): *Respiratory Therapy.* F. A. Davis Co., Philadelphia, 1965, p. 255.

127. Bloch, Maurice: "Cerebral Effects of Rewarming Following Prolonged Hypothermia: Significance for the Management of Severe Cranio-Cerebral Injury and Acute Pyrexia," *Brain,* **90:**769, (Dec.) 1967.

128. Gregg, Dorothy: "Reassurance," in Skipper, James K., and Leonard, Robert C. (eds.): *Social Interaction and Patient Care.* J. B. Lippincott Co., Philadelphia, 1965, p. 127.

129. Rosomoff, Hubert, and Safar, Peter: *op. cit.,* p. 255.

130. Hickey, Mary Catherine: *op. cit.*

131. Stevens, Virginia C.: "Clinical Hypothermia: Some Nursing Concepts," *J. Neurosurg. Nurs.,* **4:**33, (July) 1972.

132. Hickey, Mary Catherine: *op. cit.*

133. Carini, Esta, and Owens, Guy: *Neurological and Neurosurgical Nursing,* 5th ed. C. V. Mosby Co., St. Louis, 1970, p. 96.

134. Hickey, Mary Catherine: *op. cit.*

135. Edlich, R. F., et al.: "Gastric Tamponade as an Adjunct to Cooling for Massive Upper Gastrointestinal Tract Hemorrhage: A Preliminary Report of a New Technique," *Surgery,* **66:**669, (Oct.) 1969.

136. Given, Barbara A., and Simmons, Sandra J.: *Nursing Care of the Patient with Gastrointestinal Disorders.* C. V. Mosby Co., St. Louis, 1971, p. 122.

137. Edlich, R. F., et al.: *op. cit.*

138. Marks, Anna E.: "Cryogenics: The Indications and Implications for Nursing," *Am. Assoc. Ind. Nurses J.,* **15:**7, (Oct.) 1967.

139. Hicks, Julius N.: "Cryotherapy for Severe Posterior Nasal Epistaxis," *Laryngoscope,* **12:**188, (Dec.) 1971.

140. Hussain, S. Amjad, et al.: "Preoperative Freezing for Sepsis Complicating Gangrene," *Int. Surg.,* **48:**515, (Dec.) 1967.

141. Gorman, J. F., and Rosenberg, J. C.: "Dry Ice Refrigeration for Above-Knee Amputations," *Am. J. Surg.,* **113:**241, (Feb.) 1967.

Additional Suggested Reading

Britt, B. A., et al.: "Hereditary Aspects of Malignant Hyperthermia," *Can. Anaesth. Soc. J.,* **16:**89, (Mar.) 1969.

Clowes, George H. A., and O'Donnell, Thomas F.: "Heatstroke," *N. Engl. J. Med.,* **291:**564, (Sept. 12) 1974.

Davidson, Shirlee Proctor: "Nursing Management of Emotional Reactions of Severely Burned Patients," *Heart & Lung,* **2:**370, (May–June) 1973.

Feller, Irving, et al.: "The Team Approach to Total Rehabilitation of the Severely Burned Patient," *Heart & Lung,* **2:**701, (Sept.–Oct.) 1973.

Friedman, Steven Arthur, and Hirsch, Stuart E.: "Extreme Hyperthermia After LSD Ingestion," *J.A.M.A.,* **217:**1549, (Sept. 13) 1971.

Hummel, Robert P., and McConnell, Conn M.: "Jailhouse Burns," *J. Trauma,* **16:**232, (Mar.) 1976.

Ingram, D. L., and Mount, L. E.: *Man and Animals in Hot Environments.* Springer-Verlag, Inc., New York, 1975.

Koepke, George H.: "The Role of Physical Medicine in the Treatment of Burns," *Surg. Clin. North Am.,* **50:**1385, (Dec.) 1970.

Moncrief, John A.: "Topical Therapy," *Surg. Clin. North Am.,* **50:**1301, (Dec.) 1970.

Morgan, Alfred P., and Kundsin, Ruth: "Absolute Isolation in Burn Care," *Surg. Clin. North Am.,* **50:**1267, (Dec.) 1970.

Popovic, Vojin, and Popovic, Pava: *Hypothermia in Biology and Medicine.* Grune & Stratton, New York, 1974.

Pugh, L. G. C. E.: "Accidental Hypothermia in Walkers, Climbers, and Campers: Report to the Medical Commission on Accident Prevention," *Br. Med. J.,* **1:**123, (Jan. 15) 1966.

Schaman, Stanley H.: "Patterns of Urban Heat-Wave Deaths and Implications for Prevention: Data from New York and St. Louis During July, 1966," *Environ. Res.,* **5:**59, (Sept.) 1971.

Shibolet, S., et al.: "Heatstroke: Its Clinical Picture and Mechanism in 36 Cases," *Q. J. Med.,* **36:**525, (Oct.) 1967.

Ward, M.: "Frostbite," *Br. Med. J.,* **1:**67, (Jan. 12) 1974.

Whitner, Willamay, and Thompson, Margaret C.: "The Influence of Bathing on the Newborn Infant's Body Temperature," *Nurs. Res.,* **19:**30, (Jan.–Feb.) 1970.

Willis, Barbara A., et al.: "Positioning and Splinting the Burned Patient," *Heart & Lung,* **2:**696, (Sept.–Oct.) 1973.

Zinn, Willard J.: "Hypothermia on the Critical Care Unit," *Heart & Lung,* **2:**58, (Jan.–Feb.) 1973.

Shirley M. Morrison
Virginia Henderson

CHAPTER 43

Local Injury or Wound with Infection

1. TYPES OF WOUNDS
2. REACTION OF THE BODY TO TRAUMA, NATURE OF INFLAMMATION, WOUND INFECTION
3. IMMEDIATE CARE, OR FIRST AID TO THE WOUNDED
4. HEMORRHAGE AND GENERAL TREATMENT
5. LATER CARE OF THE WOUNDED
6. TRANSPLANTS OF TISSUES AND ORGANS—BANKS AND PROGRAMS FOR PRESERVING AND DISTRIBUTING TRANSPLANTS

1. TYPES OF WOUNDS

Definition. A wound is defined as "a disruption in continuity of an external or internal surface of the body." Physical trauma, defined as a "wound or injury," occurs when a physical agent acting on the body causes tissue damage. W. D. Snively and Donna R. Beshear report that trauma is "the leading cause of death in persons between the ages of 1 and 37 years, and in all age groups it ranks fourth as the cause of death and first as the cause of disability." [*]

Trauma is an all-inclusive term that may be applied to any type of injury such as thermal, electric, mechanical, emotional, sound, pressure, and radiation injuries. This chapter is concerned mainly with trauma resulting from mechanical forces. Burns are discussed in Chapter 42.

Classification. Wounds are classified according to the part wounded, their cause, and their size and shape. They are also classified as clean or infected and poisoned wounds, but this perpetuates the misconception that a wound can be completely protected from bacteria. It is safe to say that all wounds are infected to some extent. Infection that threatens the general health and delays wound healing is rightly considered a special problem; in this sense the classification of clean and infected wounds is helpful. Breaks in tissue continuity made by animals and insects are sometimes put in the special category of poisoned wounds. Surgery produces a wound that must be treated in the same way as an accidental wound except

that it is less exposed to infection. This suggests the classification, surgical and accidental wounds.

For purposes of treatment the wounded in any catastrophe might be divided into two groups—those who are seriously wounded, showing signs of shock, and those who are not. They might be further divided into those with wounds of the head, the chest, abdomen, or extremity; into those with obvious fractures or those with injuries of soft tissues. Injuries from burns might be still another classification. They may be caused by heat, electricity, x-rays, radioactive substances, and caustic chemicals. Since burns are included in the definition "a disruption in continuity . . ." wounds are sometimes classified as mechanical, electric, irradiated, or chemical injuries.

Terms Used in Describing Accidental Wounds. Accidental wounds may be abrased, contused, incised, lacerated, stab, punctured, fractured, or poisoned wounds (see Fig. 43-1).

An *abrased wound* is one in which the epidermal cells are torn away by friction. While any break in "external continuity" can admit infectious agents, these injuries are usually of little consequence and heal quickly without scarring. There is minimal bleeding.

A *contused wound* is made by a blunt instrument. The skin is ruptured, crushed, or split, and the surrounding tissues are bruised. Blood is released inside the tissue but usually there is no surface bleeding. The age of the injury is easily identified by color. A fresh contusion is red. The color changes to purple and finally to blue as the red cells break down. The color disappears as white cells clean up the hemorrhage. In very large bruises, a yellow hue may result from decomposition of some blood cells.[1]

An *incised wound* is caused by a sharp, cut-

[*] Snively, W. D., Jr., and Beshear, Donna R.: *Textbook of Pathophysiology.* J. B. Lippincott Co., Philadelphia, 1972, p. 75.

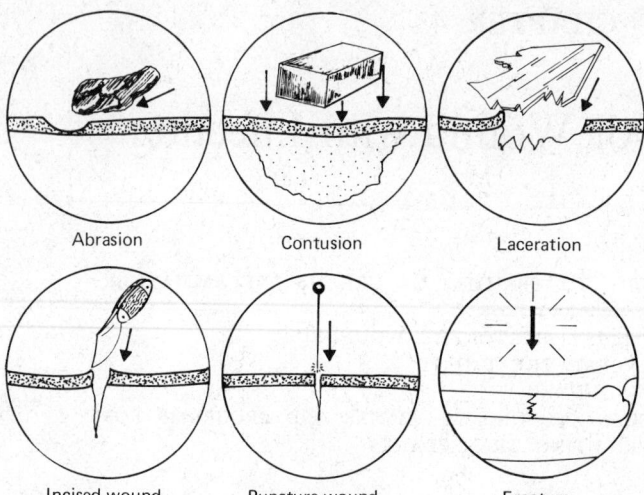

Figure 43-1. Types of tissue injury. (From Snively, W. B., Jr., and Beshear, Donna R.: *Textbook of Pathophysiology.* J. B. Lippincott Co., Philadelphia, 1972, p. 76.)

ting instrument, such as a razor, which severs the tissues and vessels so that they gape open. Damage is usually confined to the severed tissues and vessels and does not involve adjacent structures. Wound margins are smooth.

A *lacerated wound* is one in which the tissues are torn apart—the edges are roughened and jagged, and there is more or less contusion around it. Examples are the wound caused by the bite of an animal, the torn knuckles of a fighter caused by striking the mouth and teeth, the injury of a fisherman when a hook is drawn through the tissues, and industrial wounds caused by machinery. There may be laceration of internal structures without skin or subcutaneous tissue damage. Structures frequently lacerated are muscles, ligaments, and blood vessels. The damage is usually caused by excessive stretching.

A *stab wound* is caused by a sharp, cutting, pointed instrument, such as a dagger or knife. Along with puncture wounds, this category is highly susceptible to dangerous infections, especially tetanus. Access of air to a wound discourages growth of microorganisms and exclusion of air encourages it. For this reason, stab and puncture wounds are particularly dangerous.

A *puncture wound* is made by a sharp, narrow, pointed instrument, such as a needle, splinter of wood, or a nail. A rusty nail is more dangerous because, being rough, it injures the tissues more and also holds more dirt and bacteria. A *gunshot wound* is a special type of puncture. Tate M. Minckler says:

Bullet wounds have special characteristics by virtue of the added influence of rotary motion imparted to the missile by a rifle barrel. . . . Because of this rotational energy, bullet wounds produce a cylinder of injury along the path of the

bullet. This tract might extend several inches in all directions and can fracture bones not in the direct path of the bullet. A frequent complication of bullet wounds is the production of secondary missiles from splinters of fractured bone.*

A *fracture* is a disruption in the continuity of bone caused by mechanical force exceeding the strength of the bone. A simple fracture occurs when there is no accompanying break in the skin; a compound fracture involves penetration of the skin by the broken bone ends; an incomplete fracture occurs when the fracture line does not produce two separate pieces; a complete fracture occurs when there are two separate pieces of bone; a comminuted fracture causes a shattering of bone resulting in more than two separate pieces; and a compound comminuted fracture is one occurring when there are at least three distinct pieces of bone and an open wound at the site of injury.

Poisoned wounds may be caused by the bites of poisonous snakes or spiders, a rabid dog, and insect bites and stings. If the bite is that of a poisonous snake, pain, swelling, and discoloration appear within a few minutes; septicemia, prostration, and collapse may follow very quickly. The victim must have first-aid treatment at once and antivenin as soon as possible. The purpose of the treatment is to prevent the poison's entrance into the general circulation and to relieve shock. Several tourniquets are applied at different levels above the fang marks, and the wound is freely incised lengthwise of the arm or leg; sometimes suction is applied to the incision, and bleeding is encouraged. The wound may be swabbed with pure

* Minckler, Tate M.: "Physical Agents in Disease," in Minckler, Jeff, et al.: *Pathobiology, An Introduction.* C. V. Mosby Co., St. Louis, 1971, p. 295.

carbolic acid or cauterized. Potassium permanganate has been used with some success. As the snake venom is not dangerous unless it enters the bloodstream, the practice of sucking the wound has been advocated when other means of suction are not at hand. There is slight danger to the person who sucks the wound if there is an abrasion on the lips or mouth. Complete rest, external heat, and stimulants are necessary to counteract shock. The tourniquets are removed one at a time (the one nearest the body first) if no symptoms of general poisoning appear.

Persons exposed to the danger of snakebite are advised to provide themselves with a protective serum or antivenin for the species they are likely to encounter. Unfortunately, this protective serum is not available for all types of poisonous snakes, nor is it easily procured in every community in every country. There is, however, a single antivenin (Nearctic-Crotalidae) which can be used for the bite of any and every North American poisonous snake, except the Gulf region coral snake (there is a special treatment for a coral snake bite).

Bites from poisonous spiders are treated in the same manner as snakebite. Bees, wasps, and other insects inject formic acid with their stings, and they are therefore treated with neutralizing alkaline solutions, such as ammonia water, bicarbonate of soda, soap and water, or a paste of baking soda. The sting, if visible in the tissue as a fine bristle, should be removed. This can be done by pressing firmly on the tissues around the wound with a round, hollow object, such as a key. Compresses moistened with an alkaline solution should be applied— hot applications are frequently more soothing. Shock is often marked when there are multiple stings. Bromides and morphine are given to relieve nervousness and pain. If the bites result in severe itching, a weak solution of carbolic acid, which is a mild local anesthetic, relieves it.

2. REACTION OF THE BODY TO TRAUMA, NATURE OF INFLAMMATION, WOUND INFECTION

The reaction of the body to trauma is the same wherever it occurs although it varies so much in degree that the condition of the mildly and seriously injured may pose very different problems. Henry K. Beecher, in 1951, urging that what has been learned about the military wounded be applied to civil life, said:

The consequences to the human body are the same whether an artery is severed by a shell fragment or a broken windshield. . . . There is

a universality in these cause and effect relationships, a universality, too, in the principles of treatment that makes them apply to thousands of victims of atomic violence as well as to a child whose tonsillectomy wound [continues to] bleed.

. . . It will be tragic if medical historians can look back on the World War II period and write of it as a time when so much was learned and so little remembered.*

Bleeding. The immediate and visible response to injuries is bleeding. If capillaries only are injured, in very superficial wounds blood will edge away from the surface; if larger vessels or veins are severed, blood will stream from the wound, while it will spurt from an artery. Bleeding results in formation of a clot, unless there is an uncontrolled and, therefore, fatal hemorrhage. In any event, the circulating blood volume is reduced which, of course, decreases the oxygen-carrying capacity of the blood. This volume reduction of blood is the chief activator of the metabolic response to trauma.[2] Bleeding and control methods are discussed later in this chapter and in Chapter 45.

Metabolic Response to Trauma. Metabolic response to trauma varies greatly in duration and extent depending on the nature and extent of the injury, general health of the victim, pain, fear, time lapse between injury and treatment, and other conditions.[2a]

During recent decades, the metabolic response of the body to injury has been studied extensively. Morton H. Maxwell and Charles R. Kleeman, recognizing the importance of making a "gross assessment" of the magnitude of the injury, suggest that the system proposed by Francis D. Moore should be used. This system divides stimuli into three groups on a scale of ascending magnitude:

Group I, called "threshold stimuli," is made up of stimuli that initiate minor and/or transient endocrine and metabolic changes, and includes minor tissue injury (e.g., elective repair of a small inguinal hernia), anesthesia and drugs, immobilization, starvation, fear, pain, cold and fatigue. Group II, called "threatening challenges," consists of stimuli that produce a near maximal metabolic response and require treatment. Included in Group II are extensive tissue injury (e.g., gastrectomy, colectomy, pneumonectomy), replaced or transient blood or plasma loss, fluid accumulation, traumatic edema, desalting water loss, anoxia, and hypercapnia. Group III, called "tissue-killing injury," consists of stimuli which add the products of tissue degeneration to the trauma, greatly speed the rate of bodily wasting, produce a maximal metabolic response, and demand intensive treatment.

---

* Beecher, Henry K.: *Early Care of the Seriously Wounded Man.* Charles C Thomas, Publisher, Springfield, Ill., p. 1; also *J.A.M.A.,* **145:**196, (Jan.) 1951

Group III includes very extensive tissue injury, invasive sepsis, necrosis of tissue, and shock with prolonged deficiency of blood flow.*

Maxwell and Kleeman[3] also describe four phases of metabolic response to injury. In *phase I,* called "adrenergic-corticoid phase" or "phase of injury," there is a significant release of adrenergic and adrenocortical hormones. The duration of this phase, following major trauma, is from 2 to 4 days. *Phase II,* called the "corticoid-withdrawal phase" or the "turning point," appears between the third and seventh days, lasting about 2 days. If there is a lot of tissue necrosis this phase may not be identifiable, but it can be recognized clinically because the patient looks and feels better. *Phase III,* the "phase of muscular strength," is characterized by muscle rebuilding and a return of strength and energy, lasting 2 to 5 weeks. Finally, *phase IV,* "phase of fat gain," is characterized by replenishment of fat lost previously and lasts for several months.

There is clear evidence of endocrine hyperactivity during phase I, including stimulation of the adrenal medulla, anterior pituitary, and sympathetic nervous system. Transient increases of growth hormone secretion immediately following injury have been reported. Although the growth hormone's exact role in the response to injury is unknown, it is thought to influence protein synthesis and mobilization of carbohydrate and fat. Hypersecretion of adrenocorticotropic hormone (ACTH) invariably occurs. Prolonged hypersecretion of ACTH accompanies extensive tissue injuries, septic wounds, and shock. The hypersecretion of antidiuretic hormone (ADH) results in abnormal urinary retention. During the second phase, however, ADH secretion is brought under control and diuresis often occurs. Aldosterone, the chief electrolyte-regulating hormone, is secreted almost immediately after a major injury. There seems to be no change in the secretion of thyroid hormone or the sex hormones (the estrogenic and androgenic hormones). Changes in gonadal function following severe trauma have been noted, however, as for example, loss of sex drive, amenorrhea, and irregular menses. Finally, there are increases in the consumption of oxygen, production of carbon dioxide, and conversion of energy.[4]

Local Inflammatory Reaction to Injury. Inflammation may be defined as "a vascular and cellular response designed to defend the body against alien substances and to dispose of dead and dying tissue preparatory to the repair process." * The features of inflammation have been recognized since earliest times. Celsus, a nonmedical Roman (first century A.D.), recorded the four cardinal signs of inflammation —redness, swelling, heat, and pain—to which Galen, a Greek physician (A.D. 130–200) added a fifth—loss of function. Inflammation was considered a disease until John Hunter (1728–1793) convinced the medical world that it was a nonspecific defense reaction. Julius Cohnheim (1839–1884) pointed out the important role played by the small blood vessels, emphasizing that the venules rather than the capillaries were responsible. Elie Metchnikoff (1891) maintained that phagocytosis (the engulfing destruction of bacteria by white blood cells) was the essential part of the inflammatory process in contrast to the prevailing view that protection of the organism came primarily from escape of plasma. In our century, Valy Menkin (1901–1960) carried on extensive research, despite opposition, into the cellular nature of inflammation. A. G. Macleod credits him with the modern concept of inflammation, stating:

He brought together the vascular reactions emphasized by Cohnheim, the phagocytic activities discovered by Metchnikoff, and the importance of the biochemical mediators and immune phenomena that are the principle subjects of research today. . . . While the biochemical mediators Menkin described and named are no longer adequate to explain the accumulated experimental data they pointed the direction which modern research is following.†

Most authorities now recognize that the *acute* inflammatory process includes two phases. In the first phase there is an immediate but brief increase in vascular permeability, whereas the second phase is prolonged and, according to Macleod,[5] consists of the following body responses: increased vascular permeability; lining up or margination of the white blood cells along the vessel wall and the resultant "sticking" to the wall; emigration or diapedesis (passage of blood cells through an intact vessel wall) of the leukocytes and engulfing of foreign particles, including bacteria, by these cells (phagocytosis); linkage of fibrinogen and platelets from the vessels with fibrin deposited in the injured area; intravascular clotting and destruction of some vessels; disposal of most of the necrotic debris by mac-

---

* Maxwell, Morton H., and Kleeman, Charles R.: *Clinical Disorders of Fluid and Electrolyte Metabolism,* 2nd ed. McGraw-Hill Book Co., New York, 1972, p. 1068.

* Peacock, Erle E., Jr., and Van Winkle, Walton, Jr.: *Surgery and Biology of Wound Repair.* W. B. Saunders Co., Philadelphia, 1970, p. 1.
† Macleod, A. G.: *Aspects of Acute Inflammation.* Upjohn Co., Kalamazoo, Mich., 1969, p. 5.

rophages; and finally migration of fibroblasts, and the development of normal cells (proliferation) to fill in, or bridge, the break in the continuity of tissue.

Increased vascular permeability is the key to all subsequent events of the inflammatory process. Current research findings indicate that histamine action is largely responsible for the increased vascular permeability of the initial and transient first phase of the inflammatory response, whereas kinins have been identified as belonging to that group of substances activating the second phase. Kinins are polypeptides (leukotaxin—the first chemical mediator identified by Menkin was a polypeptide) with strong pharmacologic actions. According to Macleod, they "strongly affect the contraction of smooth muscle, produce hypotension, cause increased vascular permeability in small blood vessels, and induce severe pain when injected." * Among other substances involved in the second phase are lysolecithin, ribonucleic acid (RNA), and a material extracted from lymph node cells called lymph node permeability factor (LNPF).

If the process of inflammation is seen microscopically, it will be noted that, although the vessels remain dilated, more resistance seems to be made to the flow of blood and the stream slows down. (The nature of this resistance is not understood, but is thought to be some change in the endothelial lining of the blood vessels.) With the slowing of the stream, white cells are carried by their own weight to the sides of the vessels; in the venules they are seen rolling along close to the walls, then adhering to them, and finally passing through by active ameboid movements into the tissue spaces. It is thought that an endogenous material is produced at the time of injury which induces the migration of leukocytes and possibly "attracts" them to the site of injury. This movement, influenced by a specific chemical stimulus, is called chemotaxis.[6] The predominant type of white blood cell initially found at the injury site is the polymorphonuclear leukocyte. It is generally thought that mononuclear cells and polymorphonuclear cells begin emigration at the same time. However, mononuclear cells are slower-moving, which accounts for the predominance of polymorphonuclear cells. In older inflammatory reactions, monocytes may predominate, since polymorphonuclear cells are very short-lived (perhaps less than 24 hours). Another cell found at the injury site fairly early is the lymphocyte.[7] Current studies indicate that substances that induce emigration of the leukocyte are not responsible for inducing emigration of the lymphocyte—an entirely different chemical seems to be involved.[8]

Red cells in varying numbers also are found outside the vessels. How they get out is unknown. It is thought that they have no power of motion, but they are compressible and may passively follow the leukocytes, a process called diapedesis. The red cells are soon destroyed if they escape from the blood vessels. The breakdown of red blood cells is indicated by the discoloration of the part. Outside the blood stream these cells swell or shrink, clutter up the zone, and are picked up and carried away by the white blood cells.

At the same time, and probably before the passage of cells, fluid oozes out into the tissues; the lymphatics and lymph spaces, before invisible, are seen to be engorged with fluid (edema) distending the tissues, crowding the cells, and pressing on the sensitive nerve endings. So the third physical symptom—*swelling*—and the fourth symptom—*pain*—are explained. The swelling of the injured part, pain, and, more important, nature's effort to avoid increasing irritation and pain by movement together cause the fifth symptom—*loss of function*. This loss of function, although a matter of inconvenience, may not be very serious if it merely involves a finger or even the temporary loss of the use of a hand; but it is a matter of great seriousness if it involves a vital organ, such as the heart or lungs.

Not all bacteria and foreign particles are engulfed (phagocytosis) with equal ease. Because of the protective capsules of virulent organisms, they are more slowly disposed of than the less virulent. Fortunately, a group of antibodies, opsonins, instead of reacting with antigens, become attached to the surface of the bacteria, making it easier for the leukocytes to attack them.[9]

Inflammation has long been regarded as a protective process. The more that is known about it, the more certain this seems. It represents the struggle of the body to overcome an injurious agent. Brought to a successful termination it results in healing, but healing may never occur and the systemic effects of unresolved inflammation may be fatal.

Inflammation becomes *chronic* when its duration is prolonged by the persistence of the causative agent. The tubercle bacillus, for instance, can be walled off and contained, but not destroyed. The walling off protects the organism as a whole, but the local inflammatory process goes on. There is a marked difference in the vascular picture of the chronic condition as compared with the acute inflammatory condition. The main cells in chronic inflamma-

* Macleod, A. G.: *op. cit.*, p. 14.

tion include lymphocytes, monocytes, plasma cells, and eosinophils.

Infection. Wound infection is presently a serious problem. W. A. Altemeier [10] (1971) reports that an average of $7000 was spent per patient developing wound sepsis. Included in this figure were additional hospitalization costs and treatment, temporary and permanent disability, and insurance settlements. Wound infection occurs only when a living organism finds its way into a traumatized tissue. Pathogenic organisms frequently found in wounds are staphylococci, gram-negative enteric bacilli, and occasionally group A hemolytic streptococci. In accidental wounds clostridia may be found.[11]

Microorganisms may enter through the skin or mucous membrane, or they may be brought to the area by the circulating fluids from other parts of the body.[11a,11b] If there is a high degree of resistance in the tissues there may be no visible signs of infection—that is, the body defenses may immediately destroy the invading organisms; if, on the other hand, the resistance is low or the invaders strong and numerous, symptoms of inflammation will soon appear.

There are many factors that influence wound contamination and growth of bacteria. *The nature and location of the wound* is important. For example, wounds of the pulmonary and urogenital systems and alimentary tract are predisposed to infection because of their endogenous bacteria. Extensive wounds are associated with large amounts of tissue damage which make ideal culture mediums for bacteria. Stab and puncture wounds are especially susceptible to infection caused by the aerobic bacilli. *Impaired blood supply* to the wound area regardless of cause contributes to development of infection. W. Bruce Conolly and J. Englebert Dunphy say that wound susceptibility to infection "is probably due to decreased nutritive blood flow, secondary to changes in blood volume, blood viscosity, or both. . . ." * A number of factors associated with *faulty surgical technique* are related to the incidence of wound infection; these include inadequate debridement and control of hemorrhage, rough handling of tissue, and leaving a dead space which permits formation of a hematoma. According to Seymour I. Schwartz and associates,[12] adequate debridement is the most important factor in the care of contaminated wounds because dead tissue has a poor blood supply and is heavily contaminated. *Inadequate resistance of the host* is also known

to influence the development of infection. The very young and very old are more susceptible to wound infection than individuals in other age groups; malnutrition, obesity, metabolic conditions (such as leukemia, anemia, and diabetes) lower a person's resistance to infection as does some drug therapy (steroids, cancer chemotherapy).

Friction and pressure from the outside or presence of an insoluble foreign body inside the tissues destroys and irritates cell bodies, thereby lowering their resistance to infection. Nature may in some cases wall off a foreign body with fibrous tissue in such a way as to protect the surrounding structures (chronic inflammation); more often the object is forced to the surface of the body or to the wall of a cavity, breaks through it, and is ejected from the body. If this happens, it is often accompanied by infection even before the skin or mucous membrane is ruptured. The predisposing cause of infection is irritation, and the direct cause is the bacteria that may have been present on the foreign body or that later enter the wound from the skin or mucous surface.

Termination of Inflammation and the Healing Process. If the injury has been slight, the inflammatory reaction will be mild. Fluid that oozes out from injured vessels will quickly cause the sides of the wound to grow together; leukocytes will carry away dead cells; and digestive enzymes will liquefy the dead tissue which will then be absorbed. When the area is cleared of debris in this manner, inflammation is said to end by *resolution,* and the tissues are said to be resolving.

Injury to the tissues may be so severe, or the wounded area so extensive, that the damaged tissues can be neither revitalized nor carried away fast enough by the process of resolution. The same tissue will then die and form a slough that will separate by degrees from the living tissues, leaving an ulcer that must be filled in by the formation of new tissue.

If the irritated or injured area is invaded by bacteria there are living cells opposed to each other and struggling for existence. If the tissue cells are weak, or if the bacteria are very virulent, or attack in great numbers, they destroy large numbers of living cells. Serum and fibrin permeate the devitilized tissue; ferments from dead leukocytes and cells gradually liquefy it, forming a zone of thick, yellowish fluid (pus). Finally, the whole mass is liquefied into a circumscribed collection of pus, or an abscess. When this occurs the inflammatory process is said to progress to *suppuration.*

Suppuration terminates in various ways according to the extent of the process, the virulence of the organisms, and other conditions. Some of the exudate and toxins are ab-

---

* Conolly, W. Bruce, and Dunphy, J. Englebert: "Influence of Distant Trauma on Local Wound Infection," *Surg. Gynecol. Obstet.,* **128:**713, (Apr.) 1969.

sorbed into the lymph stream by resolution; or the abscess, if superficial, may rupture on the body surface and drain; a boil may rupture the skin; if the suppuration is in the lung, some of the pus will be coughed up. If the abscess is deep it may form a sinus or tract to the surface; or it may have to be incised and the fluid withdrawn by drainage or aspiration. The pressure may help to form an outlet of discharge for the pus, or may force it into the tissues, pushing it along the lines of least resistance. An extension of the inflammatory process into a large surrounding area is known as cellulitis.

All inflammatory exudates caused by bacteria are not purulent, however. Microorganisms that cause pus formation are called pyogenic microorganisms. Because of their significance, from a diagnostic and prognostic standpoint, physicians have given names to exudates that indicate their chief characteristics. The adjectives commonly used are serous, mucoid, fibrous, and purulent; all of them except the last, which has been defined, are self-explanatory.

The *healing process* depends on the nature, extent, and location of the injury and the types of cells injured. It also depends upon the age and vitality of the host. The term *regeneration* is used when healing is accomplished primarily by proliferation of the parenchymal (essential

as distinguished from supporting) elements of the tissue and the organ or area is completely restored to its original condition. When healing is accomplished chiefly by the nonspecialized elements of connective tissue, fibrosis or scarring results and the term *repair* is used. Healing of this kind may take place either by primary or secondary union (intention).[13] (See Fig. 43-2.)

The wound made in a surgical operation, if infection does not already exist, is a clean, incised wound. It is made by a sterile, sharp, cutting instrument, and the tissues are cleanly divided without tearing or laceration. When the edges of such a wound are brought together, it should heal by direct primary union, or "first intention." This means that the cut edges grow together or heal, with the slightest possible inflammatory reaction and with minimum new tissue.

When, for any reason, the edges of a wound cannot be brought together, and a gap remains between them that must be filled in, repair is said to take place by indirect union, or "secondary intention." The new tissue is called granulation tissue.

Granulation tissue consists of abundant blood vessels and young connective tissue cells spread apart by fluid and fibrin. When healthy it is soft, gray or grayish red, gelatinous, and translucent, with an irregular, velvety surface,

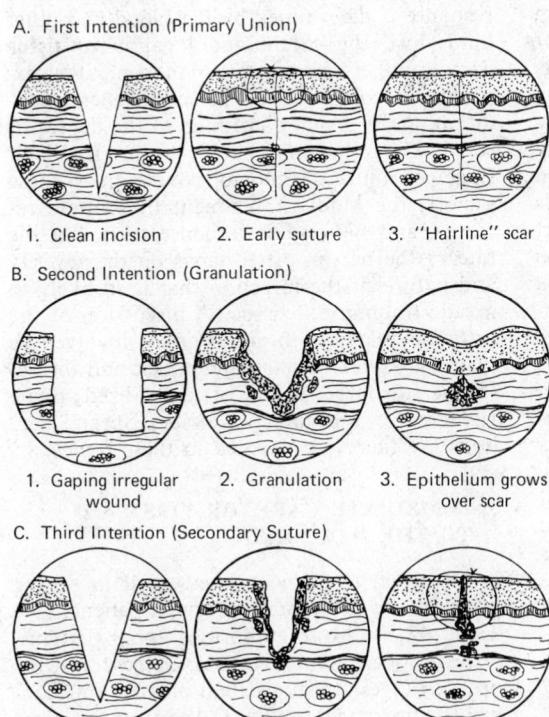

A. First Intention (Primary Union)

1. Clean incision   2. Early suture   3. "Hairline" scar

B. Second Intention (Granulation)

1. Gaping irregular wound   2. Granulation   3. Epithelium grows over scar

C. Third Intention (Secondary Suture)

1. Wound   2. Granulation   3. Closure with wide scar

Figure 43-2. Chronologic course of wound healing by first, second, and third intention. In the final stage of second-intention healing the underside of the epithelium is smooth and not serrated as normally. In the healing by second intention, the important role of contraction, which occurs in the patient in three dimensions, as seen in *B, 2* and *B, 3* in two, is shown. Contraction also plays a role in third-intention healing (*C, 2* and *C, 3*). The skin islands shown under the epithelium in *B, 2* and *C, 2* are typical of this phase of early healing. In *C, 3* an early phase is shown. Later the granulation tissue will be incorporated as a wide, fibrous scar. (From Allen, K. G.; et al.: *Surgery Principles and Practices.* J. B. Lippincott Co., Philadelphia, 1961, p. 8.)

bleeding readily, but quite insensitive to pain because it contains no nerves. Although the surface of a healthy granulating wound offers great resistance to bacterial invasion, this resistance may be broken down by very slight injuries, such as probing, or the removal of a dressing, particularly a dry dressing that sticks to the surface. Skin edges also tend to turn inward and may act as a wick, carrying infection into the wound. Some surgeons now use so-called closed dressings on even badly infected wounds because they want to avoid injury to the granulating tissue. Others insist on excision of that portion of a scab where purulent material is found. Erle E. Peacock says, ". . . scabs are used primarily as biological dressings for wounds which require only epithelization to heal." *

Sometimes healing is delayed or "indolent." When this occurs the tissue is pale, dry, shrunken, flabby, and unhealthy looking. Sometimes it grows too fast, and is soft and bleeds easily. It is then said to be "redundant." Granulation should form from the bottom and sides of the wound, until even with the surface, but sometimes it grows above the surface and must be removed; or sometimes there is a tendency to close in at the top leaving an open channel, or sinus, underneath. A wick or drain in the wound prevents healing from the top because it keeps the wound open.

When the gap in a surface wound is nearly filled, a thin, grayish-blue film of epithelium may be seen spreading from the edges to cover the surface. The epithelial cells behind divide, multiply, and push the others forward until the surface is finally covered. At first the tissue looks bluish or purplish under the pearly epithelium because of the abundant blood vessels; later many of the new blood vessels are pressed shut and disappear, and the part becomes hard and very white because of the lack of specialized pigment cells. At this stage it is called a cicatrix or scar. Specialized structures, such as secreting glands, hair, and pigment cells, are not formed. When a wound is extensive, or the formation of new epithelium is slow, a graft of living tissue is usually applied.

Repair by indirect union may be a mere patchwork; it may be quite unsightly and fail to restore the function of the part because several kinds of tissue are injured, and tissues vary greatly in their power to regenerate themselves. Connective and epithelial tissue form the bulk of new material for repair. The con-

nective tissue produced by the body in the healing process is fibrous tissue that is strong but not elastic and poorly supplied with blood vessels. Because the tissue is inelastic it contracts the part. Extensive scar tissue causes deformity, or a partial loss of function unless that is prevented.

To summarize, wounds may heal cleanly and neatly by first intention when there is a minimum of infection present; seriously infected areas heal with one or more of the following results or complications: (1) An ulcer—a raw surface caused by necrosis of skin or mucous membrane resulting from such conditions as poor circulation, poor nutrition, and from interference with the nerve supply; (2) an abscess with sinus formation—a channel extending from an abscess to the skin, mucous membrane, or wound; (3) scar formation, with deformity and loss of function; and (4) keloid—an actual tumor formed in the surface of a scar owing to overactivity of the connective tissues. All treatment of wounds is designed to promote complete healing without appreciable derangement of function or disfigurement.

Systemic Reaction. The effect of trauma on the total organism can scarcely be discussed without dividing it into the immediate and later reactions, and without considering separately the effect of slight trauma and the profound effect of severe injury. The immediate response is determined by the blood and other fluids lost, the extent and location of tissue damage, the emotional component, the exposure to cold, and the person's general condition, all of which contribute to the degree of shock. The systemic effect during the later stages of injury depends of course on all these factors, the kind of treatment the patient receives, and his or her response to it, but the fate of the person often hangs on the severity and nature of the infection that is so likely to invade traumatized tissue. A discussion of the systemic reaction to injury may involve the reaction to hemorrhage and shock and the response to large areas of devitalized tissue (gangrene) and infected tissue. Special sections are therefore devoted to these topics.

3. IMMEDIATE CARE, OR FIRST AID TO THE WOUNDED

An initial assessment is essential in setting priorities for the care of wounded patients (see Table 43-1). Most authorities agree that priorities of care should be set in the following order: (1) establish a patent airway, (2) control hemorrhage, and (3) prevent or treat shock. Other aspects of emergency care include treatment of the wound, relief of pain

---

* Peacock, Erle E., Jr.: "Wound Healing and Care of the Wound," in American College of Surgeons, Committee on Pre and Postoperative Care: *Manual of Preoperative and Postoperative Care,* 2nd ed. W. B. Saunders Co., Philadelphia, 1971, p. 8.

Table 43-1. Critical Injury Index * †

System	Abnormal	Severely Abnormal
1. Airway	Obstructed, partially by foreign object	Obstructed completely by injury
2. Breathing	Shallow or uneven	Labored or undetectable
3. Respirations	24–36 per minute	Below 16, above 40 per minute
4. Bleeding	Minor, controllable by external pressure	Massive, uncontrollable by simple pressure
5. Pulse	90–120 per minute	Irregular or none, below 60 or above 120 per minute
6. Wounds	Superficial multiple lacerations, or abrasions	Major, deep, or with loss of body parts
7. Fractures	Deformed extremity, stable, closed	Bone exposed, unstable, open
8. Extremity sensation	Any change in feeling, tingling, burning	Loss of feeling (anesthetic)
9. Extremity movement	Any limitation of voluntary motion or weakness	Loss of functions (paralyzed)
10. Mental state	Excited, intoxicated	Depressed, unconscious (coma)

* Romano, Teresa, and Boyd, David R.: "Illinois Trauma Program," *Am. J. Nurs.*, **73**:1004, (June) 1973.
† *The first attendant reaching accident victims identifies their most severe injuries, using the Critical Index, reports by two-way radio to a trauma center professional, and receives orders for the victim's care.*

and mental stress, and provision of appropriate transportation to a medical treatment center.[13a] Figure 43-3 shows a patient identification tag that is attached to the patient.

Deprived of oxygen, the subject will, of course, suffocate in a very short time. Insertion of an oropharyngeal tube which keeps the tongue away from the pharynx may be necessary. Turning the patient into the prone position may allow the relaxed tongue to fall forward or it may drain obstructive fluid from the mouth; or turning the head to one side may be sufficient. The mouth may need to be inspected for foreign bodies, and if found, removed before adequate oxygenation occurs.

Hemorrhage should be controlled by pressure dressings directly over the wound, by manual pressure over the bleeding points, by elevating the bleeding area, and by tourniquets (see Fig. 43-4). (See page 1685.) Hand pressure on a dry sterile dressing directly over the wound while elevating the injured part usually provides satisfactory control. Sterile dressings are preferred in controlling hemorrhage; however, if they are not available, clean substitutes, such as handkerchiefs or towels, may be used. If these items are not immediately available the next best choice is the patient's own blood-stained clothing. "Sucking" chest wounds must be closed with the best dressing material available.* Some authorities advocate direct finger pressure in the case of a massive hemorrhage that cannot be controlled by any other means. The risk of continuous bleeding outweighs the danger from contamination or risk of wound infection from using unsterile and unclean

means of control.[14-15b] Dressings should never be removed en route to the hospital since this might dislodge any clots already formed and increase bleeding. As dressings are saturated with blood they should always be reinforced rather than removed.

The body of an accident victim should be thoroughly examined for all kinds of bleeding. Many persons die because covert bleeding is unnoticed. Since hemorrhage is a specific problem in the immediate care of the wounded it is treated in some detail in a following section.

Shock is a complex of symptoms that results from injury and other causes. It must be included in any complete discussion of wounds because the patient's life depends on a reversal of the physiologic changes in the shock syndrome. However, because the circulatory collapse typical of traumatic shock is believed to be so similar to the circulatory collapse that occurs in many diseases, and because the treatment and nursing care of the patient in shock are highly specialized, Chapter 45 is devoted to this subject.

The threat of shock may be lessened by elevating the lower extremities above the trunk of the body, and by giving electrolyte solutions intravenously until plasma and whole blood are available. The Committee on Trauma of the American College of Surgeons states that "there is sufficient clinical evidence that plasma expanders and electrolyte solutions can expand blood volume adequately until type-specific, cross matched blood is available." * To prevent hypovolemic shock, G. Tom Shires and Ronald C. Jones [16] suggest that intravenous in-

* Negative pressure during inspiration sucks material from the wound into the pleural cavity or the lung itself if it has been pierced.

* American College of Surgeons, Committee on Trauma: *Early Care of the Injured Patient.* W. B. Saunders Co., Philadelphia, 1972, p. 28.

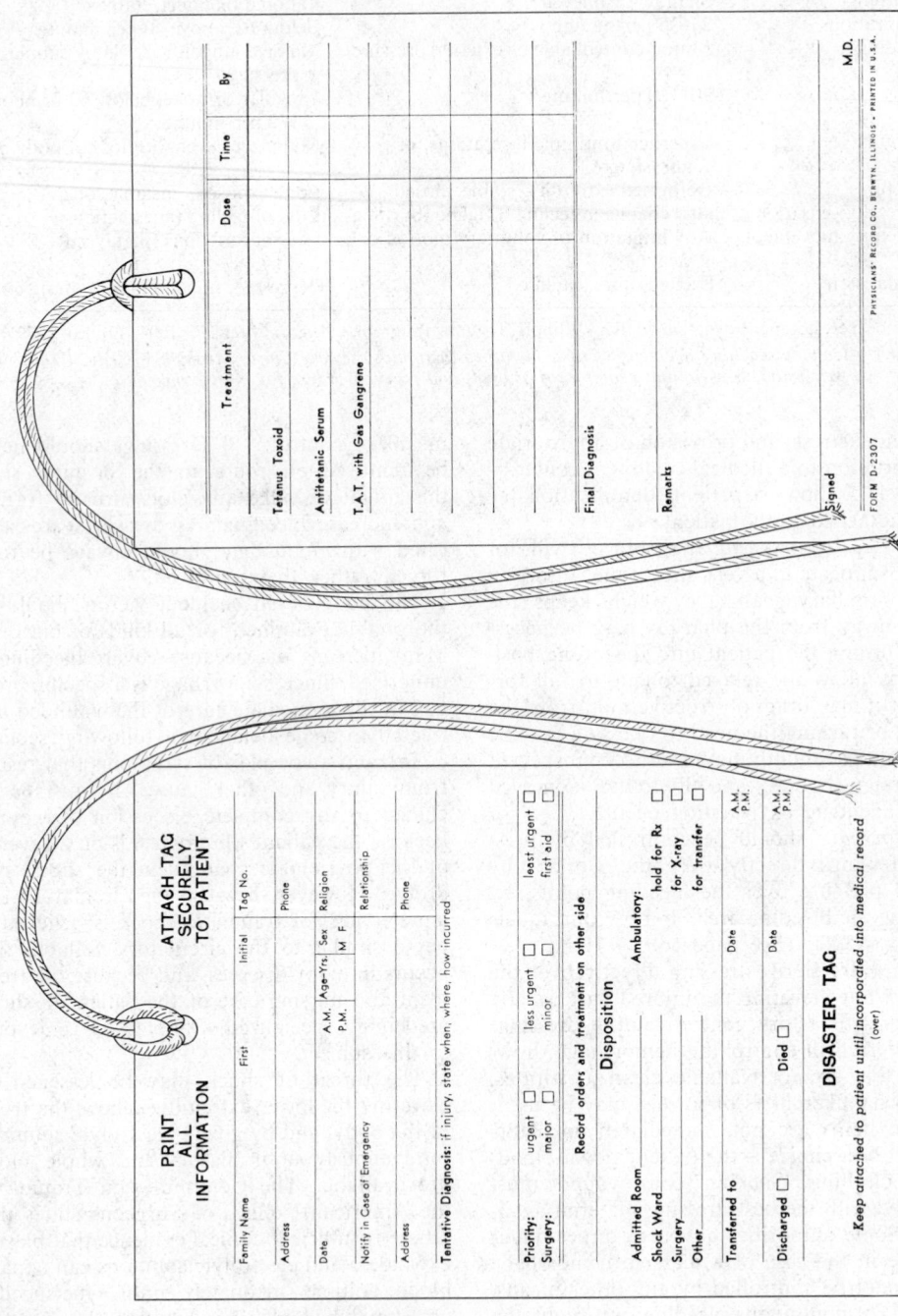

Figure 43-3. Patient identification used in disaster nursing. (Courtesy of Physicians' Record Co., Berwyn, Ill.)

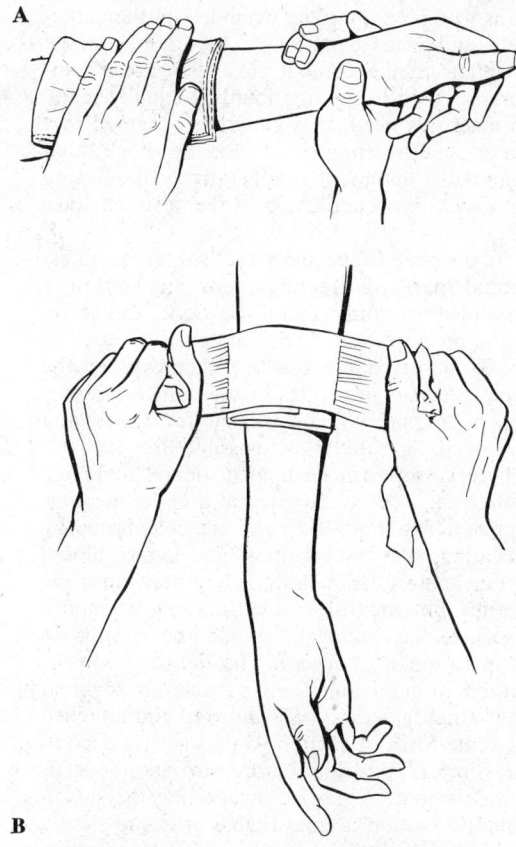

Figure 43-4. Control of hemorrhage. *A*. The nurse applies pressure to the wound with bandage over a dressing on the wound. *B*. Preparation for securing the bandage with pressure. (From Aaron, J. E.; Bridges, A. F.; and Ritzel, D. O.: *First Aid and Emergency Care*. Macmillan Publishing Co., Inc., New York, © 1972.)

fusions should be administered in two extremities simultaneously to the severely injured patient. In "crushing" injuries the application of elastic or pressure bandages immediately after release of the injured part may help to prevent shock (crushing syndrome) or will, at least, lessen its effect.[17]

After an airway is established, bleeding is controlled, and shock is being treated, attention can be given to care of the wound. Dry, sterile dressings should be applied to all wounds to prevent further contamination. Loose foreign bodies may be removed from wounds, but no attempt should be made to remove foreign bodies unless they are easily dislodged as doing so may only cause further injury. Instead, the wound should be filled in with dressings and built up and then a pressure bandage applied so as not to cause extreme pressure against the foreign body. This is especially true in the case of head injuries. Unless dressings are heavily padded, bone fragments left in the wound may be pushed farther into brain tissue, causing irreversible damage.

In the case of amputated extremities or other body parts (such as an ear), a pressure bandage should be applied over the stump, and the amputated part should be covered with sterile dressings or placed in a clean pillowcase and sent along with the patient to the hospital. It is also helpful to surround the dressed part with plastic bags of ice or an air splint.[18] Through the efforts of expert surgical teams, reimplantation or reattachment of upper extremities have been successful in a number of instances. According to the Committee on Trauma, American College of Surgeons, "excellent emergency care before the patient and the severed extremity reach the hospital will favor a successful reimplantation." *

Transportation of the injured is very important. In an effort to give effective treatment to injured persons as soon as possible after an injury, a number of cities are developing radio and radio-telephone communication links between city hospitals, area hospitals, and various public safety groups such as ambulance services and police and fire departments. In many of these communities ambulances are equipped to provide a full range of emergency services with medical supervision provided through biomedical telemetry. Where state laws allow it, emergency medical technicians administer intravenous fluids, perform defibrillation of the heart, and give skillful first aid. By means of a two-way communication system between the ambulance and hospital the emergency medical technician can request advice that will help stabilize the condition of the injured person before transporting him or her to the hospital. In addition, the ambulance crew can report the patient's condition en route to the hospital, any special requirements he or she might have, and other pertinent information.[18a,b]

Movement should be limited until the nature of the injury is known. If there are fractures, some splinting is desirable before any gross body movement and always before transportation. Splinting helps to prevent shock by keeping the part still which reduces irritation and the likelihood of dislodging an already formed clot. Air splints are now used frequently for fractures of the extremities, especially the ankle, wrist, and forearm. They not only prevent movement of a joint but provide pressure and therefore help control bleeding from open wounds. Thomas splints have traditionally been used for upper leg fractures and their use continues. Spine boards should be used for

* *Ibid.*, p. 401.

those patients suspected of having a back injury. Short and long spine boards are essential equipment for ambulances and should be kept in hospital emergency departments to be exchanged with arriving ambulances so that patients need not be transferred from the spine board on which they arrive. When such boards are unavailable, a table top or a door may be substituted.

Any patient with wounds of the face, head, shoulder, or any unconscious patient could have a cervical spine injury and should be handled accordingly. Sandbags should be applied to each side of the head.

Morphine is available in some ambulances and to soldiers in some battle areas in case of severe pain following injury, and the attendants (including soldiers) are taught to give it to others and themselves (soldiers). Beecher in 1952 and others more recently say that morphine should be used with great care and in the smallest effective doses. If given intramuscularly it may be very slowly absorbed, and if repeated can produce delayed poisoning with the characteristic depression of respiration. Infants and the elderly often react atypically to morphine. Their response should be tested before normal doses are given. Barbiturates are recommended as treatment of the anxiety and hysteria sometimes seen in the wounded. When pain is severe, morphine is indicated, and may be given intravenously for rapid and sure absorption. Most authorities consulted recommend a dosage of morphine sulfate 10 mg (⅙ gr) and never more than 15 mg (¼ gr). They think "stimulants," the vasoconstrictors, of little use and contraindicated in large dosage. Pain can often be relieved if clothing is loosened or cut over swollen areas. When Thomas splints are adjusted over shoes, the latter should be unlaced and split.

Beecher found in his study of the military wounded that, to his great surprise, only 23.7 per cent of a total of 215 seriously wounded men had "bad pain." Only 27.0 per cent wanted relief therapy; 32.1 per cent said they had no pain. Beecher concluded that morphine is often unnecessary and should never be given except for severe pain since its effect as a respiratory depressant and its tendency to nauseate make the anesthetic more hazardous. Morphine should not be given to the patient in shock. Sometimes the respiratory system is in such a precarious condition that no pain medication can be given at all, but the suffering of the wounded is not confined to pain, and relief should be aimed at its source. What is said to give reassurance is of great importance for anxiety over the outcome of the wound is often extreme. For this reason chaplains who go among the wounded on the battlefield and who see them as they come to the hospitals in the combat zone give great comfort. Civilian hospitals should be equally ready to meet this need. It is generally accepted that there is a psychogenic factor in shock; that fear and excitement preoperatively predispose to shock postoperatively. (See also Chapter 45.)

It is stressed repeatedly that surgery is an essential part of treatment for the seriously wounded. Nothing should be done, therefore, while giving first aid or treatment for shock to make surgery dangerous or difficult. When the wounded person arrives at the clinic or hospital, he or she will be treated for shock and prepared as rapidly as possible for surgery, where vessels will be ligated, debris removed, bones set, wounds closed, and aseptic dressings applied. The wounded, who are dehydrated by sweating, possibly vomiting, and loss of blood, suffer acutely from thirst. They may rinse the mouth, but should be given nothing by mouth because the stomach should be empty in preparation for surgery. The danger of insufflation of fluid and food particles is so great that a nasogastric tube is inserted and attached to some form of suction so that gastric decompression is possible before an anesthetic is administered. A gastric lavage may be substituted if suction is unavailable or is too slow a means of emptying the stomach before emergency surgery. Rapid intravenous infusion of either saline or lactated Ringer's solution should be started with every patient with actual or impending shock. As much as 1 to 2 liters may be given in 15 minutes. However, Theodore Drapanas and Martin S. Litwin recognize that the "best primary therapy for hemorrhagic shock" is adequate replacement of crossmatched, type-specific whole blood, but low-titer, Rh-negative, type O blood can be administered until type-specific blood is available. Summarizing the priorities in the initial management of a person with multiple injuries, they say:

. . . first, the airway should be maintained; second, hemorrhage should be controlled; third, open or sucking chest wounds should be sealed; fourth, adequate treatment for shock should be instituted; fifth, fractures should be splinted; sixth, a more complete examination of all the body viscera should be performed; and finally, seventh, the patient should be under continuous observation for as long as is necessary to be absolutely certain that he has no other injuries.*

* Drapanas, Theodore, and Litwin, Martin S.: "Trauma: Management of the Acutely Injured Patient," in Sabistan, David C., Jr. (ed.): *Davis-Christopher Textbook of Surgery; The Biological*

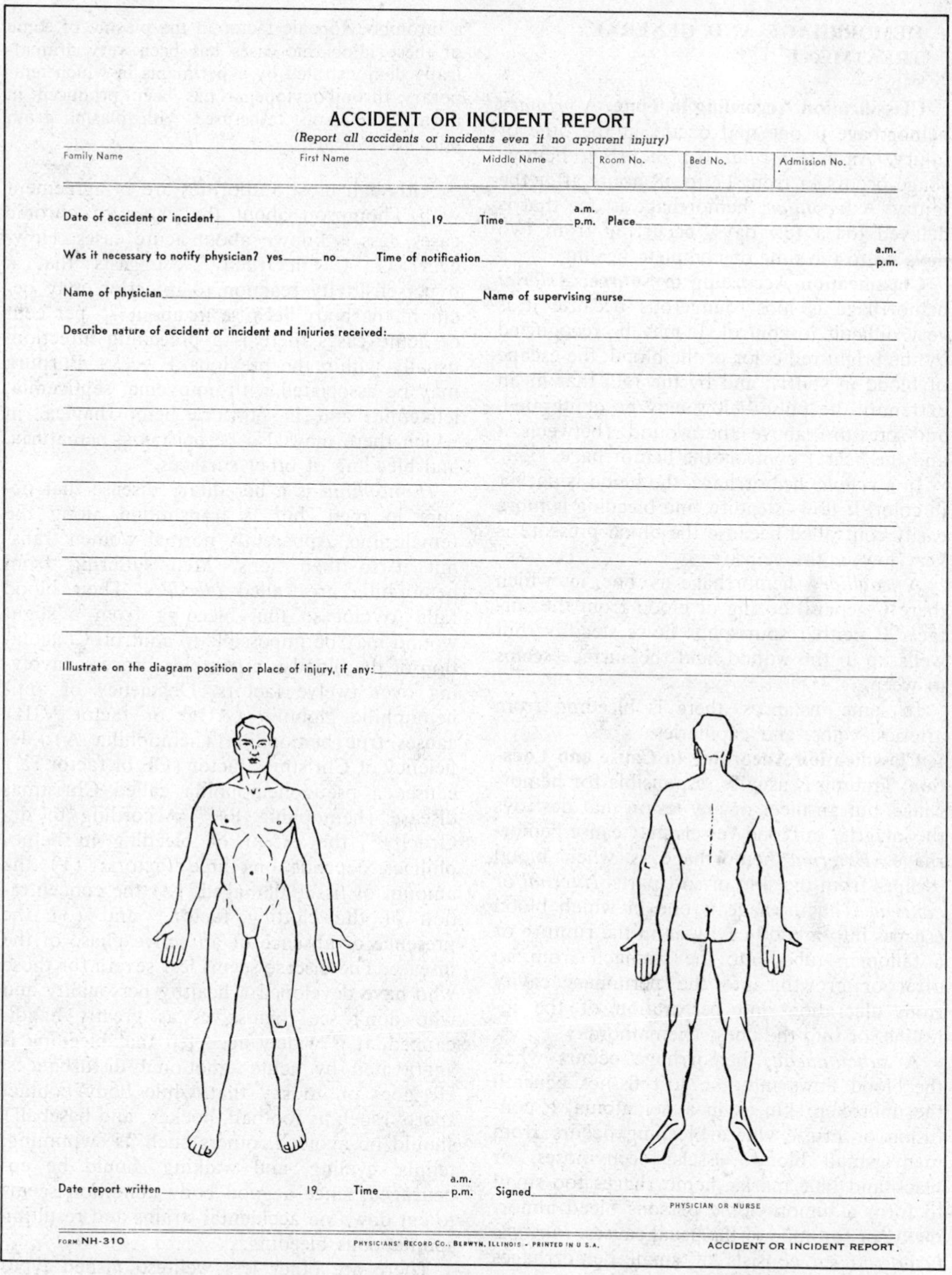

ACCIDENT OR INCIDENT REPORT
(Report all accidents or incidents even if no apparent injury)

Family Name	First Name	Middle Name	Room No.	Bed No.	Admission No.

Date of accident or incident_____ 19____ Time_____ a.m. p.m. Place_____

Was it necessary to notify physician? yes____ no____ Time of notification_____ a.m. p.m.

Name of physician_____ Name of supervising nurse_____

Describe nature of accident or incident and injuries received:_____

_____

_____

_____

_____

_____

_____

_____

Illustrate on the diagram position or place of injury, if any:_____

Date report written_____ 19____ Time_____ a.m. p.m. Signed_____

PHYSICIAN OR NURSE

FORM NH-310   PHYSICIANS' RECORD CO., BERWYN, ILLINOIS · PRINTED IN U.S.A.   ACCIDENT OR INCIDENT REPORT

Figure 43-5. A form that is used by a physician or nurse when reporting an accident or incident even if there is no apparent injury to the victim. (Courtesy of Physicians' Record Co., Berwyn, Ill.)

Since hemorrhage and shock are specific problems in the immediate care of the wounded, hemorrhage is treated in some detail in the following section and shock is discussed in Chapter 45.

The nurse or physician should prepare a written report of all accidents or incidents even though there is no apparent injury to the victim (see Fig. 43-5).

Basis of Modern Surgical Practice, 10th ed. W. B. Saunders Co., Philadelphia, 1972, p. 355.

4. HEMORRHAGE AND GENERAL TREATMENT

Classification According to Time. A *primary* hemorrhage is one that occurs at the time of injury. An *intermediate* or *recurrent* hemorrhage occurs in from 12 to 48 hours after the injury. A *secondary* hemorrhage is one that is delayed for a few days, occurring from two days up to the time of complete healing.

Classification According to Source. *Arterial* hemorrhage is most dangerous because it is very difficult to control. It may be recognized by the bright red color of the blood; the escape of blood in spurts; and by the fact that in an extremity the pulse below may be obliterated, and pressure above the wound (between it and the heart) controls the hemorrhage.

In a *venous* hemorrhage, the blood is darker in color. It flows steadily, and bleeding is more easily controlled because the blood pressure is very low in the veins.

A *capillary* hemorrhage is one in which there is general oozing of blood from the surface. It neither spurts nor flows steadily, but wells up in the wound, and the surface seems to weep.

In some instances, there is bleeding from arteries, veins, and capillaries.

Classification According to Cause and Location. Trauma is usually responsible for hemorrhage, but an ulcer or any lesion that destroys the integrity of blood vessels may cause hemorrhage. *External* hemorrhage is when blood escapes from the skin or soft parts. *Internal* or *concealed* hemorrhage is one in which blood escapes into a body cavity as in the rupture of a fallopian tube, into the stomach from an ulcer or growth, into the peritoneal cavity from ulceration and perforation of the intestine, or into the chest (hemathorax).

A *subcutaneous* hemorrhage occurs when the blood flows into the soft tissues beneath the unbroken skin as in a hematoma, a contusion or bruise where bleeding occurs from many small blood vessels; ecchymoses, or black and blue marks, hemorrhages too small to form a tumor. Some persons bleed abnormally, or for none of the usual causes. *Purpura hemorrhagica* consists of small hemorrhages under the skin. Pinpoint bleeding points are called petechiae. The spots are at first bright red but get darker as the hemoglobin disintegrates. They usually occur in groups, especially on the upper chest, neck, arms, and legs. The most pronounced feature of this condition is a reduction in the circulating blood platelets (thrombocytopenia). R. B. Thompson writes:

. . . the thrombocytopenia is often due to the development of platelet agglutinins. The presence of a thrombocytopenic factor in the plasma of some of these idiopathic cases has been very dramatically demonstrated by experiments in which temporary thrombocytopenia has been produced in normal recipients transfused with plasma from purpuric patients.[*]

Although most authorities are in agreement with Thompson about the cause of chronic cases, less is known about acute cases. However, G. C. deGruchy[19] suggests that a hypersensitivity reaction to infection may occur in the body because in about 75 per cent of acute cases there is a preceding infection, usually within the previous 3 weeks. Purpura may be associated with empyema, septicemia, leukemia, and in purpura hemorrhagica, in which there may also be epistaxis, hematuria, and bleeding of other surfaces.

Hemophilia is a hereditary disease that occurs in men, but is transmitted along the female line. Apparently normal women transmit it to their sons. Men suffering from hemophilia are called *bleeders*. Their blood fails to clot so that bleeding from a slight wound may be impossible to control. Coagulation of the blood is a complex process, involving over twelve factors. Deficiency of antihemophilic globulin (AHG or factor VIII) causes true hemophilia (hemophilia A); deficiency of Christmas factor (CF or factor IX) causes a pseudohemophilia called Christmas disease (hemophilia B).[20] According to deGruchy[21] the extent of bleeding in hemophiliacs depends on three factors: (1) the amount of tissue damaged, (2) the concentration of the clotting factor,[†] and (3) the presence or absence of an active phase of the disease. The disease seems less severe for those who have developed a healthy personality and who don't see themselves as greatly handicapped. It is widely accepted that bleeding is aggravated by acute emotional disturbances. He goes on to say that while body contact sports (such as football, hockey, and baseball) should be avoided, others such as swimming, tennis, cycling, and walking should be encouraged, since a good body condition seems to cut down on accidental strains and resulting spontaneous bleeding.

There are other less well-established types of abnormal bleeding whose etiology is also obscure. A deficiency of any of the factors in

---

[*] Thompson, R. B.: *A Short Textbook of Haematology*, 3rd ed. J. B. Lippincott Co., Toronto, 1969, p. 338.
[†] When the concentration of the clotting factor is at least 3 per cent of the normal value, bleeding is usually mild, but when it is under 1 per cent, bleeding is severe.

the physiologic chain action of clotting can delay or prevent it. Deficiencies are found in prothrombin, fibrinogen, bile, and vitamin K. Overdoses of heparin, an anticoagulant, large amounts of intravenous stored blood, and liver disease may cause bleeding. Because these examples are limited, the reader should consult hematology texts for a more detailed discussion of the subject.

Classification According to Severity and Danger. Hemorrhage may be *slight, severe,* or *profuse,* according to the extent of the injury, the size and number of vessels cut, and the amount of blood and rapidity with which it is lost. A severe hemorrhage from a large artery or vein is always accompanied by shock. The degree of shock is usually in direct proportion to the blood lost. A sudden loss is much more dangerous than a gradual loss, because the body has insufficient time for the necessary adjustment; however, gradual loss, as from hemorrhoids, may cause a very severe anemia.

Nature's Way of Reacting to Loss of Blood. When a small vessel is cut, its walls contract, making its lumen smaller, and at the same time it shrinks within its outer elastic sheath, which then partially or completely closes over the opening. The blood, meeting this resistance and coming in contact with air, soon begins to coagulate, forming clots around the opening and extending into the lumen so that bleeding is checked before a serious loss occurs. If this natural response did not take place, the merest untreated scratch would be fatal.

Clotting occurs very quickly in small vessels, especially the veins, because their walls collapse more readily than those of the arteries and thus prevent a serious loss of blood. When large vessels are injured, clots cannot form at first because of the force of the blood current. As blood continues to escape, however, the volume is so depleted that the blood pressure is lowered. As the force of the current is reduced, the blood is usually able to clot and plug the opening before death occurs.

Later the blood-forming organs manufacture and deliver to the blood an increased number of cells to make up for those lost, but nature's reaction alone is not in many cases sufficient to check a hemorrhage or to repair rapidly the damage caused by a serious loss of blood. To prevent loss of life, the following steps must be taken.

Local Treatment of Hemorrhage. Hemorrhage may be controlled by pressure, position, extreme heat or cold, astringents or styptics, ligation, torsion, sutures, and cautery.

Pressure may be made with the fingers (digital pressure), a tourniquet, compresses or packing, and a tight bandage. A tourniquet may be used as a last resort when all other methods to control hemorrhage have failed. The bleeding must be controlled by whatever means are at hand. Pressure with the fingers along the course of the bleeding vessel will control a hemorrhage temporarily, even from a large vessel. Lay persons as well as health workers are being taught to know exactly where and how pressure may be made on large vessels, such as the facial, carotid, subclavian, axillary, brachial, and femoral arteries. They may learn this by feeling their own bodies to discover where each artery approaches the surface and where it lies against a bone—that is, where its pulse may be most easily felt and compressed.

So-called pressure points for the control of hemorrhage, or for counting pulsations of the artery, include: (1) temporal artery, for wounds in region of the temple; (2) facial artery, for wounds of the face below the temple; (3) carotid artery, for wounds in upper part of the neck; (4) subclavian artery, for wounds of the shoulder and upper part of the arm; (5) brachial artery, for wounds in the arm below this point; and (6) femoral artery, for wounds in the leg (see Fig. 43-6).

Bleeding from the forearm can be checked only by pressure on the vessels in front of the elbow or on the brachial artery, because the radial and ulnar arteries are too deeply embedded in the tissues to be easily compressible. Their branches also anastomose freely. The same is true of bleeding from the vessels of the lower leg.

In bleeding from an artery, pressure must be made above the wound—that is, between it and the heart. In bleeding from a vein, digital pressure must be made below the bleeding point—that is, between it and the periphery. Also, all tight constricting bands (tight clothing, elastic garters, etc.) between the bleeding point and the heart must be removed to allow the blood to return to the heart by the deep veins.

The *tourniquet* is one of the most successful means of controlling bleeding from a large artery in an extremity, but because it is dangerous, it is a last resort. It is applied above the bleeding point, but as low as possible on the extremity. Especially constructed tourniquets are made either of rubber or of heavily braided material. Improvised tourniquets may be used —rubber tubing, a folded handkerchief, a necktie, or a leather strap (a belt) serves the purpose. In all cases the tourniquet must be of sufficient width not to cut the skin, and pressure must never be made on nerve trunks. A hard, firm compress is placed over the line of the artery (where digital pressure is made).

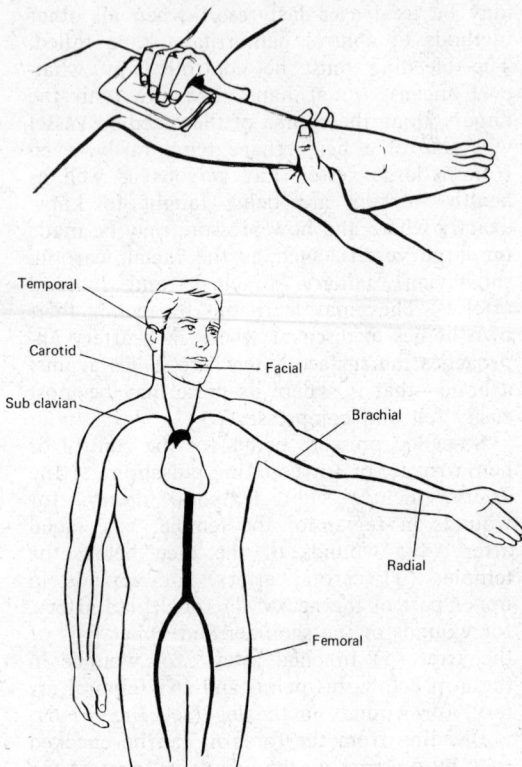

Figure 43-6. Use of pressure points to control bleeding. (From Aaron, J. E.; Bridges, A. F.; and Ritzel, D. O.: *First Aid and Emergency Care.* The Macmillan Publishing Co., Inc., New York, © 1972.)

The compress should be wrapped with several layers of cloth about 3 inches wide before applying the tourniquet to help prevent bruising the skin and muscles and causing irreversible nerve damage because it widens the pressure area. A tourniquet must be tight enough to control the hemorrhage, if necessary tight enough to obliterate the pulse. It is never left on longer than necessary. Some authorities suggest loosening the tourniquet every 30 minutes for 5 minutes. If bleeding increases, then both the tourniquet and release time intervals should be shortened. If there is minimal oozing or no bleeding after a 5-minute release interval, the tourniquet should be removed. Prolonged pressure causes severe pain and results in severe injury. Since the region below the tourniquet is deprived of all circulation, gangrene may set in. According to the Committee on Trauma, American College of Surgeons, "the prolonged application of a tourniquet gravely jeopardizes the success of reconstructive surgery, and it makes amputation almost

inevitable." * If tourniquets are applied at the site of an accident, they may be left on too long because they are forgotten. Therefore, a part of the tourniquet should always be exposed under the blankets covering the victim. Another suggestion is to write the letters *TK* across the patient's forehead or tag the victim in some other way to alert the ambulance drivers and emergency room personnel. It should also be noted that a tourniquet too loosely applied actually increases the bleeding. There are some reports of crush syndrome after release of tourniquets. It is thought also that in some instances the tourniquet itself causes severe muscle damage and that at the time of tourniquet release myoglobin (muscle pigment) is released into the circulation.[22] A tourniquet is used only when a pressure dressing and other methods of control have failed; therefore, it usually must remain on the extremity until the bleeding vessels can be ligated on the operating table, even though gangrene results.

Systemic Treatment of Hemorrhage. Major methods of treating hemorrhage systemically include *transfusions* and *drugs.* The patient should be kept as quiet as possible and in the recumbent position with the head lowered and the trunk and extremities elevated to increase the blood supply to the brain. Direct transfusions should be started as soon as possible. (When a populace is threatened, everyone should have his blood typed so that in a catastrophe blood transfusions can be started with the least possible delay.) In capillary hemorrhage, continuous transfusions are sometimes given to make up for the constant loss of blood.

Transfusion is indicated as treatment for bleeding from known causes but it is also used to maintain blood volume after severe blood loss in hemophiliacs. However, to correct the patient's deficit temporarily, normal plasma or fractions of plasma rich in antihemophilic factor is the treatment of choice, according to Oscar D. Ratnoff.[23] In obstructive jaundice or biliary fistula where a prothrombin deficiency delays clotting, vitamin K administered parenterally will usually check bleeding and consequently transfusions are usually not necessary. However, in diffuse hepatic disease where fibrinogen may also be depleted, vitamin K has little if any corrective effect whereas transfusions of fresh blood or fresh-frozen plasma will provide temporary correction of the coagulation defect.[24] When bleeding is caused by overdoses of heparin (anticoagulant), prota-

* American College of Surgeons, Committee on Trauma: *op. cit.,* p. 385.

mine sulfate is recommended by deGruchy. He says that protamine inactivates heparin in ratios of 1:1. Accordingly, he suggests:

When reversal of the effect of heparin is required within minutes of its intravenous injection, a full neutralizing dose of protamine (1 mg of protamine to 100 units [1 mg] of heparin) should be given. If neutralization is required 30 minutes after heparin injection, 50 per cent of the full neutralizing protamine dose should be given, and if required after one hour, 25–30 per cent is given. . . . The administration of protamine sulphate may have to be repeated because the drug is cleared from the blood stream more rapidly than heparin.*

In coagulation disorders, an accurate diagnosis is most important because the drugs used to correct the abnormalities are usually specific and can only be successfully used when matched with the appropriate disorder. In addition to those mentioned above, other drugs include calcium gluconate, epsilon aminocaproic acid, and trasylol.[25]

Bleeding from Special Areas and Methods of Control. Epistaxis, or bleeding from the nose, is a capillary hemorrhage from a deeply congested mucous membrane.

The great vascularity of the nose accounts for the frequency of nasal bleeding and for occasional difficulty in controlling it.

The *causes of epistaxis* are *local*—traumatism, ulceration, foreign bodies, new growths, and picking and scratching with the fingers; or *constitutional*—hemophilia, the onset of certain infectious diseases, venous congestion in cardiac or pulmonary or cerebral diseases. Nasal bleeding is seen in puberty in some children, especially those with a rheumatic tendency. There may be a hereditary tendency to epistaxis.

Epistaxis may occur during sleep, the blood swallowed being vomited later and thus confused with hematemesis; or the blood may be coughed up and so confused with hemoptysis.

In the *treatment* of epistaxis the patient's head should be kept erect or elevated, or the head of the bed elevated, in order to aid the venous return. He or she should not bend over a basin. The clothing, especially the collar, should be loosened. Raising the arms above the head will lessen the blood supply to the nose.

The blood tends to clot and thus spontaneously check the bleeding. The patient should be warned not to blow his or her nose or in any way loosen the clot until control of bleed-

ing is established. Pressing the outer aspect of the nares against the septum for 5 or 10 minutes usually arrests bleeding. Ice or ice compresses may be applied to the forehead, the bridge of the nose, and the back of the neck. Ice may be pressed against the nose.

Compression may be made on the facial artery by pressure on the superior maxilla near the nose on the bleeding side. The anterior nares may be packed with sterile gauze or cotton, but this should be lubricated with petroleum jelly so that it will not disturb the clot when it is removed. It is obvious that the blood must not be allowed to run down into the throat. This is one reason why patients with face injuries are transported in the prone position which allows fluids to drain from the mouth.

When first-aid measures fail to control nasal bleeding the physician may apply Adrenalin or silver nitrate (a cauterizing agent) solution or stick to the bleeding point. When the site of bleeding cannot be found the nose may be sprayed with cocaine and Adrenalin solutions and postnasal packing inserted. The packing is removed 24 hours later.

Hemorrhages of the stomach and *of the lung* are considered together because they are often confused. The term *hematemesis* refers to the vomiting of blood; *hemoptysis* means the spitting of blood from the larynx, trachea, or lungs (see Table 43-2).

The *causes of gastric hemorrhage* may be *local* or *constitutional*. Local causes include (1) cancer, ulcer, diseases of blood vessels (miliary aneurysms and varicose veins), acute congestion, and operations on the stomach; (2) passive congestion, caused by obstruction of the portal system as in cirrhosis of the liver, thrombus in the portal vein, and enlarged spleen, or pressure on the portal veins from without by tumors; and (3) traumatism from wounds and corrosive poisons. Hemophilia and severe anemia are constitutional causes of gastric hemorrhage.

The *causes of lung hemorrhage* are (1) diseases of the lungs—pulmonary tuberculosis, pneumonia, cancer, abscess, gangrene, and ulceration of the bronchi, trachea, or larynx; (2) certain diseases of the heart, particularly mitral lesions that dam blood in the left atrium, then into the pulmonary vessels and cause marked pulmonary congestion; (3) erosion of an aneurysm of a large blood vessel; and (4) trauma to the lungs, such as puncture of the lung caused by a fractured rib.

It is often difficult to differentiate the symptoms of gastric hemorrhage from those of pulmonary hemorrhage. The vomiting of blood is not always a sign of bleeding from the

---

* deGruchy, G. C.: *Clinical Haematology in Medical Practice*, 3rd ed. Blackwell Scientific Publications, Oxford, 1970, p. 699.

Table 43-2.   Differentiation Between Hematemesis and Hemoptysis (Osler)

Hematemesis	Hemoptysis
1. Previous history points to gastric, hepatic, or splenic disease.	1. Cough or signs of some pulmonary or cardiac disease precedes, in many cases, the hemorrhage.
2. The blood is brought up by vomiting, prior to which the patient may experience a feeling of giddiness or faintness.	2. The blood is coughed up, and is usually preceded by a sensation of tickling in the throat. If vomiting occurs, it follows the coughing.
3. The blood is usually clotted, mixed with particles of food, and has an acid reaction. It may be dark, grumous, and fluid.	3. The blood is frothy, bright red in color, alkaline in reaction. If clotted, rarely in such large coagula, and mucopus may be mixed with it.
4. Subsequent to the attack the patient passes tarry stools, and signs of disease of the abdominal viscera may be detected.	4. The cough persists, physical signs of local disease in the chest may usually be detected, and the sputa may be bloodstained for many days.

stomach, because blood from the nose, throat, or lungs may be swallowed and later vomited.

When red blood cells stay in the stomach for a short time, they are disintegrated by the action of gastric juice, setting free the hemoglobin. Hemoglobin is in turn disintegrated forming hematin, a brown pigment. The same thing happens in the intestines. This accounts for the clotted, dark-brown or "coffee-ground" vomitus and also for the tarry stool some time after hemorrhage in the alimentary tract. Blood from the stomach will have an acid reaction.

In the *treatment for gastric hemorrhage*, the patient should lie quietly. Morphine is often prescribed, but a barbiturate that does not predispose to nausea and other undesirable effects is preferable. Usually a nasogastric tube is inserted into the stomach and continually irrigated with an iced saline solution until bleeding stops and all clots are removed. In the case of a stress ulcer, when bleeding stops, R. N. McClelland says that "the patient may be placed on a constant intragastric drip of cold half-and-half milk and cream containing about 10 oz liquid antacid preparation per quart of milk and cream mixture. This is given at the rate of 4 oz per hour." * The advantage of this method over the traditional oral Sippy regime is that rebleeding can be recognized almost immediately by frequent aspiration of the nasogastric tube. In addition, the tube is already in place should the administration of iced saline be indicated. Surgery may be necessary for some of these patients. Anticholinergic drugs are usually prescribed and coagulant drugs may be given hypodermically. No stimulants are given because of the danger of in-

creasing the hemorrhage. Blood transfusions are indicated if there is appreciable blood loss.

In *treatment of pulmonary or lung hemorrhage* nurses should recognize that the patient is usually frightened. Those with the patient should reassure and encourage him or her. Continuous bleeding of the lung is rare because of low pressure normally found in the pulmonary artery.

Patients should be turned on the affected side, if this can be determined, as the blood is then less likely to enter the unaffected lung. If they want to sit up, however, and can breathe more easily and are less anxious or alarmed when in that position, it is better to allow them to do so. To lessen the nervous excitement one of the barbiturates is usually prescribed. Some physicians allow the patient to suck pieces of ice, but when immediate surgery is possible, oral intake is contraindicated.

Immediate treatment is the aspiration of blood from the pleural cavity which may be accomplished by a thoracentesis. If bleeding continues, however, closed tube drainage is recommended. Tubes should remain in place at least 24 hours past cessation of any drainage. When the blood clots within the pleural cavity cannot be aspirated, enzymes (for example, Varidase) can be used to dissolve the clots. Robert R. Shaw and Watts R. Webb [26] recommend that the tubes be clamped 4 to 6 hours after administration of enzymes. Blood drainage will come forth after a release of the clamps. High febrile states usually accompany the use of Varidase so antipyretic drug therapy is recommended, also. Massive uncontrolled bleeding is an immediate indication for thoracotomy (surgical incision of the chest wall).

An extensive or prolonged hemorrhage of any sort is always treated with whole blood if available.

---

* McClelland, R. N.: "Stress Ulcers," in Shires, G. Tom (ed.): *Care of the Trauma Patient.* McGraw-Hill Book Co., New York, 1966, p. 663.

Menorrhagia is a profuse or prolonged menstrual flow; *metrorrhagia* is loss of blood in the intervals between menstruation; a *post-partum hemorrhage* is one occurring after childbirth or a miscarriage. Lesions, tumors, foreign bodies, displacements, and systemic disorders and visceral diseases, such as diseases of the heart, may cause vaginal bleeding.

Any irregular bleeding from the uterus or unusually profuse menstrual flow, particularly after the age of 35, should be reported to a surgeon *without delay*. It may result from cancer in which the only hope of control is an early diagnosis and surgical interference. If such a condition is brought to the attention of the nurse, she should urge an immediate medical examination. People are usually alarmed at the sight of blood or a hemorrhage from the nose, lungs, stomach, or any other organ, but women are likely to be confused as to the cause of bleeding from the uterus and so ignore the early symptoms of disease. Nurses share with doctors and other health workers the responsibility for teaching the lifesaving effect of early treatment.

The *immediate treatment* of vaginal bleeding depends on the cause. In all cases of marked bleeding the patient should be put to bed and kept quiet. The buttocks should be elevated and an ice bag applied to the lower abdomen. Ergot or oxytocic substance (Pitocin) may be prescribed to contract the uterus. Vaginal tampons or uterine tampons are frequently inserted to check bleeding by pressure. In the giving of douches or in the packing of the vagina or uterus, everything must be sterile. Packing the uterus is never attempted by a nurse, except as a last resort after all other measures have failed and only when it is impossible to get the services of a doctor.

Surgical treatment consists in removal or correction of the causes, such as tumors, foreign bodies, or displacements, by operative procedure and/or radium therapy. Systemic treatment is the same as in all severe hemorrhage.

Injury to the female reproductive system occurs sometimes following "blunt trauma," such as one might expect in a car accident. Rupture of the uterus is more likely to occur if the woman is pregnant. A ruptured uterus constitutes a severe medical emergency. There is abrupt and massive hemorrhage into the peritoneal cavity and immediate shock. Treatment for shock and exploratory laparotomy are begun simultaneously. Even though there is great surgical risk when the patient is in severe shock, surgery must be attempted since it is necessary to stop bleeding.

Cerebral hemorrhage is discussed in the section devoted to head injuries (see page 1687).

Primary bleeding generally occurs at the time of trauma or operation. It may be a steady oozing from capillaries which involve a large operative area, or it may occur from the small blood vessels which were not tied off in surgery.

Intermediate or *recurrent* bleeding happens normally within a few hours after trauma or operation, when the circulation and blood pressure have returned to normal. At the time of operation, owing to the depressing effect of the anesthetic upon the circulation, bleeding from the capillaries may be very slight and easily controlled by the normal clotting of blood; bleeding from small blood vessels may be so slight as to be overlooked by the surgeon and not be tied off; or a ligature around a large vessel may be tied too near the cut edge, or not tied securely. As the depressing effect of the anesthetic wears off, the heartbeat becomes stronger and the blood pressure is increased, so that blood clots are easily displaced and bleeding begins from the capillaries and small blood vessels. The increased blood pressure may cause a ligature to slip, so that bleeding may occur from a large vessel. Restless movements of the patient increase the rate and force of the heartbeat, and raise the blood pressure, thus increasing the danger of hemorrhage.

Secondary bleeding may happen any time after the first 24 hours up to the time of complete healing of the wound. A secondary hemorrhage is likely to be severe, as it usually occurs from a large vessel, the smaller vessels being occluded after the first 24 to 48 hours. In surgery it may result from the slipping of an insecurely tied ligature, and should be watched for, particularly in infected wounds, where there is sloughing of the tissues, sloughing or slipping of ligatures, or erosion of the walls of blood vessels.

Local or external hemorrhage happens at the site of a visible wound. Direct pressure or tying the offending blood vessel with a ligature is usually sufficient to control it. In internal bleeding, as, for example, when a wound is closed or tightly packed, with no means of drainage, the blood will flow into the tissues or into a body cavity with little or no local evidence but it will cause systemic symptoms and eventual shock. It is comparatively easy to see and report a patient's visible blood loss, but it requires keener observation on the part of the nurse to detect the signs indicative of early internal bleeding.

In general, both the local wound area and the patient's systemic condition should be taken into account when watching a patient for signs of hemorrhage. Nurses should be familiar with the character and amount of drainage expected with various types of surgery, so that they can differentiate between normal postoperative bleeding and hemorrhage. In some cases external evidence of bleeding is minimal or absent. The hematocrit reading is not a dependable means of measuring a patient's current blood status since a patient hemorrhaging loses plasma and red blood cells in equal amounts. The hematocrit ratio, therefore, could remain normal and yet there could be massive internal bleeding. Not until 10 or 12 hours later would the hematocrit indicate that there is a problem. Other manifestations of hemorrhage must then be relied on. These are restlessness, apprehension, rapid pulse, respiratory distress, pallor, weakness, and thirst. If prolonged or severe, hemorrhage produces shock, with a fall in blood pressure, weak rapid pulse, cold clammy perspiration, and apathy. If bleeding is severe, death follows rapidly. It has been said that death follows the loss of one half the volume of blood; but a hemorrhage of a smaller amount, accompanied by other complications, may also be fatal.

Summary. Since hemorrhage is the cause of shock and loss of life in accidental trauma and surgery, it is essential for nurses to understand its physiology and be able to recognize early the signs and symptoms.

It is estimated that a healthy man weighing 75 kg (165 lb) may lose blood amounting to 3 per cent of the body weight and still recover. Blood loss can usually be treated successfully, and the patient's life saved, provided the hemorrhage is noticed in time.

Since blood transfusions are so commonly used, it is the practice of most hospitals to type the blood of the surgical patient before the operation is performed, so that a transfusion may be given in as short a time as possible, should the need arise. Since the advent of the blood bank, it is possible for friends and relatives of prospective surgical patients to donate blood for future use.

Control of hemorrhage is the immediate concern of all present. The patient should be kept quiet, and a sedative administered. Local treatment may include inspection of the wound and ligation of a blood vessel, applying a pressure dressing, elevating the bleeding extremity, packing the wound, or using styptics or vasoconstrictors. The head of the bed is usually lowered to prevent shock; and blood loss is estimated and replenished by blood transfusions. When a blood transfusion is not immediately possible, intravenous solutions of Ringer's lactate, plasma, saline, or glucose may be used as substitutes. If the site of the hemorrhage is deep-seated or if bleeding is difficult to control, it may be necessary to reopen a surgical wound and ligate the blood vessels in the operating room. In slow bleeding, preparations which encourage the clotting of blood, such as calcium and vitamin K, and drugs for specific conditions are given. Cold applications are also used to control capillary bleeding. Bleeding areas are in a few cases cauterized. Prevention and control of shock are discussed fully in Chapter 45.

5. LATER CARE OF THE WOUNDED

First aid of the wounded has been discussed. It is assumed that, if indicated, all clothing has been removed, the extent of the injury assessed, and asphyxia, hemorrhage, or shock resulting from the wound controlled or treatment instituted. Now the health team turns its attention to repair of the wounded area, preventing infection, and building up the individual's general health, if the wound is a threat to it. The local treatment of a deep or extensive injury may require major surgery. In such cases the patient must be prepared as for any emergency operation; slight injuries often require additional treatment besides the first-aid treatment that has been described. Some wounds may appear to be insignificant and yet demand special caution. The particular dangers of even slight head injuries are discussed on page 1682. Injuries that destroy nerves may cause paralysis, and signs of nerve injury must be watched for; stabs and punctures are particularly dangerous because microorganisms are driven into the deeper tissues.

Anaerobic bacilli of gas gangrene and tetanus multiply rapidly in tissues without access to air as "anaerobic" indicates. The patient must be specially treated to reduce this hazard. A pinprick can be lethal if it carries into the tissues a sufficient number of deadly organisms. Tetanus is a disease caused by the anaerobic organism *Clostridium tetani* and its toxins, characterized by local convulsive spasms of the voluntary muscles. The incidence of tetanus could be eliminated by universal immunization. The use of tetanus toxoid is now stressed for all penetrating traumatic wounds, serious burns, and also for animal and human bites. The physician determines for each patient individually what protection against tetanus is necessary. The Committee on Trauma, American College of Surgeons, has recommendations for prophylactic treatment of tetanus according to the severity of the wound and the patient's past immunization record (see Table 43-3). Passive immunization is recommended for

Table 43-3. Prophylactic Treatment of Tetanus * †

Type of Wound	Patient Not Immunized or Partially Immunized	Patient Completely Immunized Time Since Last Booster Dose		
		1‡ to 5 years	5 to 10 years	10 years +
Clean minor	Begin or complete immunization per schedule; tetanus toxoid, 0.5 ml	None	Tetanus toxoid 0.5 ml	Tetanus toxoid 0.5 ml
Clean major or tetanus prone	In one arm: Human tetanus-immune globulin § 250 mg In other arm: Tetanus toxoid 0.5 ml, complete immunization per schedule §	Tetanus toxoid 0.5 ml	Tetanus toxoid 0.5 ml	In one arm: Tetanus toxoid § 0.5 ml In other arm: Human tetanus-immune globulin § 250 mg
Tetanus prone, delayed or incomplete debridement	In one arm: Human tetanus-immune globulin § 500 mg In other arm: Tetanus toxoid § 0.5 ml complete immunization per schedule thereafter Antibiotic therapy	Tetanus toxoid 0.5 ml	Tetanus toxoid 0.5 m. Antibiotic therapy	In one arm: Tetanus toxoid § 0.5 ml In other arm: Human tetanus-immune globulin § 500 mg Antibiotic therapy

* American College of Surgeons, Committee on Trauma: *Early Care of the Injured Patient.* W. B. Saunders Co., Philadelphia, 1972, p. 39.

† Note: With different preparations of toxoid, the volume of a single booster dose should be modified as stated on the package label.

‡ No prophylactic immunization is required if patient has had a booster within the previous year.

§ Use different syringes, needles, and sites.

those persons *without* previous active (tetanus toxoid) immunization. In the past, either equine or bovine antitoxin was used; however, because problems frequently arose (serious allergic reactions, rapid elimination from the body, and delayed serum sickness syndrome), their use is now totally discouraged. Currently, human tetanus-immune globulin (Hypertet), a safer preparation than equine or bovine antitoxin, is recommended and should be administered intramuscularly—*never intravenously.* Hypertet protects the person for approximately 30 days. If human globulin is not available, however, either the horse or bovine preparations may be used. Before the dose of antitoxin is given, a few drops should be injected intradermally. If the patient is sensitive to the serum, there will be a reddened area around the wheal. Persons sensitive to horse serum may tolerate the bovine preparation.

X-ray films are made to determine the extent of injury. This is particularly important in severe injuries such as gunshot wounds, stab wounds, and those caused by nonpenetrating blunt objects. X-ray films should be attempted only if the patient's condition is stable. They are used to locate pieces of for-

eign matter thought to be lodged within the body such as bullets, needles, and fishhooks. (Sometimes when a fishhook is embedded in the tissues it can only be removed by further trauma.) X-ray films can sometimes help diagnose the presence of gas gangrene when taken at intervals of from 2 to 4 hours. When an early diagnosis is made, treatment can begin at once and amputation avoided.[27]

Contused and lacerated wounds may require excision of hopelessly injured tissue that, potentially necrotic, will act as a foreign body in the wound. Living tissue tends to protect itself from alien material by walling it off in a fibrous capsule or by forming pus around it. When the abscess drains, the foreign body is extruded from the wound. Nature's remedy is obviously a long-drawn-out process during which the patient may die. Thorough cleaning and surgical debridement are an essential part of the treatment of many wounds. Poisoned wounds require special care as described earlier in this chapter.

As we have indicated, treatment by a surgeon should be sought at once, especially for dangerous or disfiguring wounds. When this is impossible for hours or days, steps must be taken to clean the wound after bleeding has been controlled. The operator should scrub his hands in the usual way for a sterile procedure if no sterile instruments are available for handling articles that come in contact with the hand. The wound should be covered with sterile gauze, and the area around it should be shaved if necessary and cleaned with a detergent. Under no circumstances should an antiseptic solution containing detergent be used on the wound itself since it is very harmful to tissue and actually increases the wound's susceptibility to infection. Following a study of the effectiveness of pHisoHex and Betadine surgical scrub solutions, Joseph Custer and associates say:

The deleterious effects of these scrub solutions appear to be the result of their detergent content. The antiseptic agents contained in these scrub solutions exerted a favorable influence on the contaminated wound but their beneficial effects did not eliminate the harmful influences of the detergent.*

Betadine and pHisoHex may still be used on the skin preoperatively and surrounding a wound as a cleansing solution. Two per cent iodine in alcohol is as effective as any other agent used to prepare the skin for wound care, according to the Committee on Pre and Postoperative Care, American College of Surgeons. After the skin is cleaned, the wound itself should then be gently irrigated with a sterile saline solution or a very mild antiseptic. Some surgeons recommend peroxide of hydrogen 1:3 because with its bubbling effect and its penetrating quality it brings dirt to the surface; however, in cases of hemorrhage it should not be used because of its dissolving effect on clots. In a hospital or clinic where equipment is available and surgical debridement of the contaminated wound must be delayed for several hours, the Committee on Pre and Postoperative Care, American College of Surgeons, recommends the use of hydrodynamic flushing. Adequate volume and force are key factors in achieving debridement. They report that by forcibly injecting a large volume of isotonic solution onto the surface or into the cavity of a wound, a large number of bacteria and other contaminants can be flushed away. Others say that bacterial contamination is not greatly lessened by this technique but major necrotic debris is flushed away. Forceful irrigation is recommended only when no serious hemorrhage has occurred, or hemorrhage has been

stopped by hemostats or temporary ligation. Disinfecting solutions strong enough to destroy bacteria are likely also to destroy the tissue cells; however, dressings impregnated with the sulfonamides and antibiotics are well tolerated and have markedly increased the speed with which some wounds heal. Dry and wet sterile dressings are also used, depending on the objectives of treatment. Peacock says:

Artificial dressings should be selected specifically to promote drainage, prepare a granulating surface for grafting, or protect a wound surface during natural closure. Selection of the proper dressing material requires unerring diagnostic accuracy in assessing what is occurring in the wound as well as a clear-cut idea of what the objectives of wound healing are.*

General Therapeutic Measures and Nursing Care. With the development of the sulfa drugs and antibiotics the practice of giving them routinely to prevent or control threatened infection has grown up. Some surgeons give penicillin in all major surgery as a protective measure and for the same reason would employ it in treating accidental wounds. Some authorities believe that this trend is regrettable for the following reasons: (1) the surgical team may be lulled into a false sense of security and therefore relax its efforts to make the surgical procedure really aseptic; (2) bacteria that are now sensitive to antibiotics may develop strains resistant to drugs too commonly encountered; and (3) therapeutic agents should be prescribed on a specific rather than a general basis. The question of prophylactic use of antibiotics continues to be a moot question; however, there seems to be a trend away from their indiscriminate prophylactic use, because bacterial resistances have developed. Stephen E. Smith[28] says the bacterial resistance may be the result of using too small a dosage and for too short a time. It is important, therefore, that persons take the full course of a prescribed drug—not only to prevent infection from flaring up again but to prevent development of bacterial resistance. This is extremely important because the person may need the drug again. William R. Sandusky recommends that drug prophylaxis be limited to situations in which risk is great, such as

1. Wounds resulting from trauma which are heavily contaminated or for which thorough debridement and mechanical cleansing are not possible or are delayed.
2. Burns.
3. Operative sites associated with heavy contamination or established infection.

* Custer, Joseph, et al.: "Studies in the Management of the Contaminated Wound, V. An Assessment of the Effectiveness of pHisoHex and Betadine Surgical Scrub Solutions," *Am. J. Surg.,* **121**:572, (May) 1971.

* Peacock, Erle E., Jr.: *op. cit.,* p. 11.

4. Preparation of the large intestine for operation.
5. Operations requiring the insertion of permanent prostheses.
6. Surgical procedures on patients prone to infection because of factors such as impoverished local blood supply, the carrier state, undernutrition, pre-existing infection remote from the operation site, or therapy which may alter host defense mechanisms.*

Most authorities agree that if prophylaxis is chosen, the drug (in order to be optimally effective) must be started before the incision is made—otherwise, it is not considered prophylactic treatment.

How resistance occurs remains unknown except in one particular case. Some strains of staphylococci have developed an enzyme identified as penicillinase which destroys penicillin. Smith reports "Twenty years ago benzylpenicillian (penicillin G) was useful in all staphylococcal infections; today in hospital practice it works in hardly any of them." † Resistance of bacteria can be overcome by treating infections with combinations of antibiotics and by using certain drugs *only* for infections by organisms that are known to be resistant to drugs in common use. Altemeier says that accumulated data of studies suggest that large doses of broad-spectrum antibiotics may "impair host resistance by decreasing phagocytosis, intracellular killing of bacteria, and antibody synthesis." ‡

Medical literature abounds in reports on the relative merits of the known sulfa compounds and antibiotics. Almost any opinion cited is, however, out-of-date before it can be published. New agents are developed so rapidly that it is impossible to keep abreast of knowledge in this field. Statements that any one preparation is *the* most therapeutic agent should be considered tentative.

Sandusky[29] discusses the following five principles that are implicit in the selection and continued use of drugs to combat infection: (1) the organism causing the infection must be identified and its sensitivity to the drug selected determined; (2) the drug used must come in contact with the organism; that is, if applied locally it must reach every part of the lesion and if given systemically the blood supply must be sufficient to transport an effective concentration of the drug to the site of infection; (3) the drug should be as free as possible from unfavorable side effects and those who care for the individual must be able to recognize and treat the adverse effects of the treatment; (4) no body substance should be present at the site of infection that will inhibit action of the drug; for instance, sulfonamides are ineffective if suppuration and necrosis are present; and (5) the natural defenses of the body of the host against infection must be active.

Ideally, cultures are made and drugs prescribed on the basis of the laboratory findings. This is essential in the selection of antisera. In some cases the facilities for making cultures are not available, and often the physician or surgeon believes that he or she can judge the probable nature of the threat of infection from the location of the wound. It is common practice, therefore, to give one of the antibiotics to the wounded in protective doses, especially in severe trauma wounds. Cultures of the wound should be taken as soon as possible so that in the event the antibiotic chosen is not successful in combating the developing infection a satisfactory alternative can be chosen. It is also recommended that cultures of wounds be taken throughout the healing process, especially when healing is prolonged. The possibility exists of developing secondary infections as well as resistance to the antibiotics in use. When an elevation of body temperature and other symptoms indicate that a wound is seriously infected, most surgeons think it is gross neglect to fail to discover, if possible, the chief invading organisms.

Because there are literally hundreds of chemotherapeutic and antibiotic agents on the market, it is not possible to include many important details on administration of these drugs. It is important, however, to say that nurses as well as physicians should be familiar with the various ways that antimicrobial agents work in combating bacteria. Smith[30] describes three ways these drugs work. First, drugs such as penicillin G, ampicillin, cephalexin, and polymyxin disrupt the cell wall, causing the cell to break up. These drugs are called bactericidal. Second, drugs by interfering with DNA in the cell nucleus of the bacteria prevent cell division. Most of these drugs are bacteriostatic and include tetracycline, chloramphenicol (Chloromycetin), Erythrocin, and streptomycin. Finally, drugs may interfere with cell metabolism, for example the sulphonamides which have a bacteriostatic effect.

In Chapter 44, there appears a table on the current use of major antibiotics and sulfon-

* Sandusky, William R.: "Infection and Antimicrobial Agents," in American College of Surgeons, Committee on Pre and Postoperative Care: *Manual of Preoperative and Postoperative Care,* 2nd ed. W. B. Saunders Co., Philadelphia, 1971, p. 117.

† Smith, Stephen E.: "Antibacterial Drugs," *Nurs. Times,* **67:**177, (Feb. 6) 1971.

‡ Altemeier, W. A.: "Current Infection Problems in Surgery," in *Proceedings of the International Conference on Nosocomial Infections,* Center for Disease Control, August 3–6, 1970. American Hospital Association, Chicago, 1971, p. 86.

amides in systemic infections (see page 1726).

Enzymes are currently used in some cases to quickly reduce hematomas and edema. They are given either intramuscularly or sublingually because they are protein substances and are destroyed in the digestive tract. When they are given intramuscularly, the nurse should expect some reaction since they are of plant or animal origin. Although much is still not known about the exact mechanisms involved, it is thought that the enzymes dissolve fibrin clots, thereby preventing the occlusion of capillaries and lymph vessels responsible for the edema. One disadvantage should be especially noted. Since these enzymes dissolve fibrin they should not be used when hemorrhage must be controlled.

Promoting Drainage and Closure of Infected Wounds. The sulfonamides and antibiotics have worked miracles in the control of infections associated with wounds. Conditions that would have taken months to control heal in a few days or weeks with the "wonder drugs." Sometimes, however, even they fail, and a life is lost or the wound continues to drain. In such cases hot wet dressings, irrigations, or suction of the wound may be prescribed; surgeons may incise walled-off pockets of pus, or they may remove the abnormal tissue around the wound and attempt a fresh closure or a plastic repair.

Specific Aspects of Treatment and Nursing Care. Processes of repair are greatly influenced by diet, as has been repeatedly emphasized in this book. A high-caloric, high-protein, high-vitamin diet with increased mineral content is stressed. If, for any reason, the patient's oral intake is inadequate it must be supplemented by nutritious parenteral fluids. There is no greater service the nurse can give patients than accurately observing and reporting what they eat. It is often necessary to feed severely wounded persons. This need is obvious if their hands are injured, or if their position makes eating difficult; it is not so obvious when they fail to eat because the effort of getting the food to their mouths is so great that they decide "it isn't worth it." The nurse is the person who should take the initiative; few patients will ask to be fed.

A high fluid intake is important. If they are diluted, chemicals produced in the healing process are less irritating to all tissues, and particularly to the kidneys that excrete them. While serious infections are usually prevented with modern treatment, few patients run a completely afebrile course. A high fluid intake replaces the fluid lost in sweating associated with fever and the dehydrating effect of drainage from the wound, when this is appreciable. The care of a person who is running a high temperature is described in more detail in

Chapter 44. Exercise should be specifically prescribed for the seriously wounded. The dangers of immobility were discussed in Chapters 12 and 30. The wounded have special need of therapeutic exercises to combat contractures or deformity. Such measures are described in Chapter 30. They are initiated by the physical therapist, if one is available. Usually the exercises must be continued by the nurse and, of course, the patient. In some cases the nurse must assume the function of the physical therapist.

Rest and sleep, induced by a good hygienic regime rather than drugs, are, of course, important. Without variety, occupation, and some satisfaction of emotional needs from congenial companionship, relaxation is difficult to achieve. Each patient's program should provide an opportunity for diverting, and productive or creative, activities and for association with friends, family, and other patients, according to his or her tastes and needs.

Rehabilitation of the wounded may involve very little or a complicated program requiring the cooperation of almost every type of medical worker. Patients with wounds that leave functional handicaps or ones whose mutilating effects are visible demand particular care. The plastic surgeon, the maker of prostheses, the vocational expert, and often the psychiatrist and psychologist must be added to the regular members of the health team. The rehabilitation program should be started, ideally, on the patients' admission to the hospital; otherwise they may have much to unlearn and many an unnecessary physical handicap to overcome.[31,32]

Occupational health (industrial) nurses work with adults who are in many cases subjected to risks of injury. Texts on emergency health care and articles in nursing and medical journals on treatment of injuries are often addressed to occupational health personnel. While the principles of treating trauma are the same everywhere, the available personnel and facilities affect the methods used, as do state compensation laws. Occupational health nurses should be familiar with the literature, examples of which are included in the references of this chapter. (For further discussion of occupational health nursing see Chapter 3.)

6. TRANSPLANTS OF TISSUES AND ORGANS—BANKS AND PROGAMS FOR PRESERVING AND DISTRIBUTING TRANSPLANTS

Introduction.[33-36] An understanding of terms used in various classifications of tissue and organ transplants is necessary for effective nursing practice with patients and their families. The terms *transplant* and *transplantation* are used to describe the partial detachment or removal of a part of the body and its implantation onto or into the body of a different or the same person. Usually, *host* and *recipient* are synonymous, as are *graft* and *transplant*. Transplantation does not include the use of prostheses (made of synthetic materials) that may be attached within or onto the body.

There are four classes of transplants between donor and recipient that are determined by their genetic relationship:

1. *Autograft,* or *autogenous transplant ("auto"* pertaining to self), is a graft or transplantation of tissue taken from another site in or on the body of the organism receiving it. This type of graft or transplant, made of the person's own tissues, is usually successful. A common autograft is a split-skin graft consisting of half the skin thickness.
2. *Isograft, syngenetic graft,* or *isotransplant* is the exchange of tissue between genetically identical individuals of the same species, as between monozygotic twins or between animals of a highly inbred strain. Isografts are more likely to be successful than allografts.
3. *Allograft, homograft,* or *homotransplant* is a graft or transplantation of tissue or organ removed from the body of another animal of the same species but with a genotype differing from that of the recipient, as transplantation of bone or blood vessel from two unrelated persons. While these are usually successful, a heart transplant from unrelated persons is usually unsuccessful unless potent immunosuppressive measures are used. There are great differences in the extent and type of allograft rejection following transplants.
4. *Zenograft (heterograft)* is defined as transplantation or graft of tissue between species, as from a monkey to a man. These tissues are quickly rejected because vascular anastomoses are rarely established.

Transplants may also be classified according to site of implantation: *orthotopic* or *heterotopic*. Orthotopic transplants are those that are located in the same part of the body or surrounded by the same kind of tissue after transplantation as before, for instance, corneal transplant. Other transplants are heterotopic, for example, a graft of a kidney or liver to the lower pelvic region or the lower abdomen. Grafts may be *viable* or *nonviable* at time of implantation. Nonviable grafts of blood vessels, bone, and cartilage are therapeutically

functional even though their nonviability has been caused by preservative processes. There are many other less common ways of classifying transplants that are not included here.

The concept and reality of organ and tissue transplantation, widely publicized by the press during the 1960s following transplantation of a human heart in Cape Town, South Africa, in December, 1967, are not new. The accomplishments during the past decade rest on the works of many scientists throughout the world over several centuries. John Marquis Converse and Phillip R. Casson, in a review of the historical background of transplantation, write:

> The replacement of diseased, worn out, or injured tissues and organs with sound parts has stimulated the imagination of man for many centuries. Mention is made in Greek mythology of transplants from animals to man, and early Christian legends and folk tales of the Middle Ages tell of successful transplants of noses and even of whole limbs from one individual to another. During the Renaissance, Gaspare Tagliacozzi, a Bolognese anatomist and surgeon, considered the possibility of using flesh from another person to reconstruct the nose but discarded the idea. . . .*

Tagliacozzi, an internationally known surgeon, described in his treatise *De Curtorum Chirurgia per Institionem,* published in 1596, a technique he used to restore a person's nose to near normality by using a flap from the upper arm; this technique, known as the Tagliacotian flap, is used today.

Baronio, who is credited with the first scientific approach to the subject of transplantation in 1804, reported successful autogenous skin grafts in sheep as well as allegedly successful grafting experiments between animals of the same and different species; other workers were unable to achieve his success, however. A successful skin transplant by Bunger, who in 1823 used a free graft from the thigh to reconstruct part of a woman's nose, was the first published clinical report in modern medical literature; however, it is alleged that similar transplants were employed hundreds of years earlier in India.

Paul Bert, an early worker in transplantation research and student of Claude Bernard, published over 200 scientific papers and books; Converse and Casson write:

> He [Bert] recognized the differences between the behavior of autografts, allografts, and xenografts, but did not exclude the possibility of a successful outcome in allografts and also cautioned against

* Converse, John Marquis, and Casson, Phillip R.: "The Historical Background of Transplantation," in Rapaport, Felix T., and Dausset, Jean (eds.): *Human Transplantation.* Grune & Stratton, New York, 1968, p. 3.

applying the results of such animal experiments to man.*

The idea that homograft rejection is mediated by a process of active immunity is attributed to Jensen (1903) by Sir Peter Medawar in London. Medawar's classic experiments and their results form the basis for modern transplantation research (1945, 1946, and 1947). Considerable advances have been made since that time in transplantation immunology and consequently successful transplantation of tissues and organs in humans. Many scientists throughout the world, especially in Europe and the United States, have contributed to our present knowledge of this subject but it is not practicable to include a description of their work in this book. Interested readers can consult references at the end of this chapter.

All health professionals caring for families and individuals who are considering donating or receiving an organ or tissue are responsible for giving them current information. Nurses who work directly with patients and their families must be prepared to help them deal with many of the medical, moral, and legal issues that are openly discussed in today's society. A great deal of information is now available on donating an organ or body, storing tissues or organs for later use, and distributing donor tissues or organs to recipients.

Procurement of Organs and Tissues. Skin grafts, blood transfusions, bone grafts, and corneal transplants have been done for many years and are acceptable forms of treatment to most persons; getting these tissues to meet transplant needs does not generally present a problem. However, getting and distributing whole organ transplants, such as the kidney, heart, and liver, have raised moral, ethical, and legal questions for the public, theologians, lawyers, and health professionals. Jean Hamburger and Jean Crosnier, in 1968, write:

Does the physician have the moral right to accept from a healthy individual who desires to amputate a vital portion of his body, such a gift, so as to prevent the death of one of his fellow men? Does the surgeon have the right to remove a liver, a heart, or a kidney from a cadaver in order to practice what [J. R.] Elkinton [37] (1964) has termed "cannibalizing," in reminiscence of the wartime art of recreating new cars with spare parts obtained from two useless vehicles?†

Although these questions have been discussed and the problems analyzed for years by physicians, moralists, and jurists and a Symposium of the Ciba Foundation was devoted to the subject in 1966, there continue to be worldwide differences of opinion. Hamburger and Crosnier [38] think these differences should be expected because of the "wide divergence between judicial or administrative customs" in different countries as well as within a particular country.

There are two sources of organs and tissue: (1) *living donors* (related and unrelated) and (2) *cadaver donors*. Authorities consistently emphasize that it is inconceivable that any vital organ other than the kidney might be removed from a healthy *living donor* for transplantation into the body of another person.

Major concern must always be shown for donors. Above all, they should be volunteers who clearly understand the nature of the procedure and its possible consequences.

The situation of living donors raises questions that are different from that of persons who become donors on dying. One question in particular about living donors is the nontherapeutic removal of an organ—"Is it justifiable to possibly endanger a person's life through the removal of a healthy organ?" Medical science is unable to predict with absolute certainty in every case the results of surgical intervention. Physicians, however, must consider all possible outcomes and share these with donors so that they may give what is called "informed consent." Informed consent is not limited to an explanation. The idea of informed consent also is dependent on the ability of the donor to understand what has been said about the risks involved and to be emotionally capable of enduring the postoperative period. [39]

According to Folkert O. Belzer and associates [40] (1975), approximately 5000 individuals have donated one kidney during the last decade. Within a few months after removal of a kidney in young donors, the remaining kidney hypertrophies, providing 75 to 80 per cent of the original renal function. Anesthesia and the operation itself are the main risks to the donor. Mortality rate is estimated to be 0.1 to 0.5 per cent. Postoperative complications in living kidney donors have been pneumothorax, hypotension, and urinary tract and wound infection. [41] Belzer and associates note that "renal failure occurred postoperatively in one of our donors, but cleared spontaneously." *

A large percentage of donations from living

---

* *Ibid.,* p. 4.

† Hamburger, Jean, and Crosnier, Jean: "Moral and Ethical Problems in Transplantation," in Rapaport, Felix T., and Dausset, Jean (eds.): *Human Transplantation.* Grune & Stratton, New York, 1968, p. 37.

* Belzer, Folkert O., et al.: "Organ Transplantation," in Dunphy, J. Englebert, and Way, Lawrence W.: *Current Surgical Diagnosis and Treatment,* 2nd ed. Lange Medical Publications, Los Altos, Calif., 1975, p. 1070.

donors are made to family members; consequently, it is most important that all health workers understand that at times undue pressure is placed on donor candidates. Frequently, the emotional reaction to the possibility of losing a beloved relative may lead members of a family to value the donor candidate less than the dying member who is in need of the transplant. Consent given under such duress is not "free informed consent." Because pressure is sometimes brought to bear on potential donors, institutions that perform organ transplantation require assessment of the entire family situation by a clinical psychologist or psychiatrist before getting written consent from the living donor.

The kidney donor is admitted to the hospital for special studies *only* after he or she has been judged to be a true volunteer and the complications and risks have been explained and understood by the donor. Following a comprehensive history and physical examination, the following routine work-up is done: chest x-ray, electrocardiogram, urinalysis, serum bilirubin, creatine clearances, blood urea nitrogen, and fasting blood sugar. If these tests are normal, an intravenous urogram is performed and, if normal, then a renal arteriogram is made. The person is judged an acceptable donor if the renal arteriogram is normal.[42]

The importance of tissue typing in transplantation is emphasized by most authorities. The degree of histoincompatibility determines the success of tissue grafts between individuals of the same species. Clinical guidelines that have proved successful in the selection of donors, based on tissue typing, are as follows, according to Belzer and associates:

1. Verification of ABO compatibility and a negative leucocyte cross-match to avoid hyperactive rejections during surgery must be the first step. If a more sensitive technic were available, it might be possible to prevent some losses that occur in the first 3 weeks after operation.
2. If the donor is a sibling, the best choice is an identical genotype based on a family study. Lacking a family study, the second choice is an identical phenotype.
3. In parent-child combinations, matching (other than ABO) is not mandatory, but the information derived from matching may be useful in determining which antigens (if any) are most active in rejection.
4. The value of HL-A typing in unrelated donors is still controversial.*

There is some disagreement among authorities on the necessity of a psychiatric evaluation

of all donors. Some believe that all that is needed is an adequate evaluation by the donor's own physicians while others believe that the donor should undergo a thorough psychiatric evaluation—a common practice in the early days of transplantation.

A person who becomes a donor in death is known as a *cadaver donor*. (See also Chapter 50.) This may be accomplished in two ways: (1) a person may, prior to death, sign a consent willingly expressing a desire to donate his or her body, or certain organs needed for transplantation, or (2) upon the death of an individual the next of kin may sign for consent of the body or certain organs, providing the donor made no directive otherwise while alive.

Prior to the enactment of the Uniform Anatomical Gift Act of 1968, individuals in the United States did not have the authority to give their body for medical purposes, because their next of kin were legally entitled to the possession of the body at the time of death. The Uniform Anatomical Gift Act, enacted by the National Conference of Commissioners on Uniform State Laws on July 30, 1968, places the issue of organ donation solely in the hands of the individual. Any person of sound mind and 18 years of age or older may donate all or part of his or her body to medical science. The gift takes effect after the individual's death. The consent of the individual is usually given in the form of a will. However, the Act has recently been interpreted as providing that donation by an individual can be made by any written document which "may be a card designed to be carried on the person." (See Figure 43-7). The card must be signed by the donor and witnessed by two persons. The card is an advantage in emergencies when time is limited, when the prospective donor is unconscious, and when the existence of a will is unknown.[43] At present, laws based on the Uniform Anatomical Gift Act have been adopted in all 50 states and the District of Columbia. National organizations such as the National Kidney Foundation, the Eye Bank Association of America, and the American Medical Association will provide information immediately on how an individual can go about signing up as a tissue or organ donor.

The cadaver donor has certain rights which should be known and respected by all health workers. Discussing these rights, George W. Miller writes:

The Reverend Raymond F. Collins, professor of moral theology, Pope John XXIII National Seminary has numbered five rights which he feels are due the donor. They are (1) a right to life, (2) a right to die, (3) a right to freedom and personal

* *Ibid.,* p. 1068.

UNIFORM DONOR CARD

OF _____
                    Print or type name of donor

In the hope that I may help others, I hereby make this anatomical gift,
if medically acceptable, to take effect upon my death. The words and
marks below indicate my desires.

I give: (a) ____ any needed organs or parts
         (b) ____ only the following organs or parts

                    Specify the organ(s) or part(s)
for the purposes of transplantation, therapy, medical research
or education;
         (c) ____ my body for anatomical study if needed.

Limitations or
special wishes, if any: _____

Signed by the donor and the following two witnesses in the presence
of each other:

_____   _____
    Signature of Donor   Date of Birth of Donor

_____   _____
    Date Signed   City & State

_____   _____
    Witness   Witness

This is a legal document under the Uniform Anatomical Gift Act or
similar laws.

Figure 43-7. This card was developed
through the work of an Ad Hoc
Committee on Medical-Legal Problems of the National Academy of
Sciences–National Research Council
Committee on Tissue Transplantation,
with the assistance of other related
groups. The card is valid under the
Uniform Anatomical Gift Act, is
simple to use, covers all medical needs
for tissues and organs, and is usable
by all relevant groups.

autonomy, (4) the right to privacy, (5) the right
to bodily respect.*

Sanctity of life and dignity of death are
rights due every human being. As has been
said so frequently and by so many—"There is
a time to live and a time to die." Potential donors must in no way be neglected by the medical profession; they must be provided with all
the benefits of medical science if there is a
possibility that such measures may lead to
their survival. Furthermore, donors must be
protected against a premature pronouncement
of death. All who are interested in the issues
raised by organ transplantation recognize that
a conflict of interest could arise if the same
physicians care for both the donors and the recipients. Consequently, health institutions
(universally) accept the fact that potential
donors and recipients must be cared for by
different physicians. To protect donors against
a premature pronouncement of death, it is
agreed that the determination of death be entrusted to a team of doctors that is not the
surgical transplant team.

The necessity of providing a fresh organ for
transplantation and assuring that no organ is

removed until the donor is dead has resulted
in an attempt by medicine to redefine death.
Previously, death was defined as the cessation
of the circulation of blood (the heart) and
other vital signs. Now, the definition of death
is an involved process, especially when transplantation of a vital human organ is planned.
Death is a gradual process at the cellular level
with tissues varying in their ability to withstand
deprivation of oxygen. Physicians are not so
interested in preservation of isolated cells and
the point of death of individual organs as the
certainty that the process of death has become
irreversible by available techniques of resuscitation. Consequently, no single criterion is
entirely satisfactory in determining that death
exists. In determining the legal time of death,
however, the final criterion when an organ
transplant is contemplated is death of the
brain. Definition of brain death has been studied by a variety of ad hoc medical and legal
committees: Harvard Medical School, Institute of Forensic Science of Duquesne University School of Law, and American Electroencephalographic Society. The criteria of brain
death accepted by these groups include (1) unreceptivity and unresponsitivity, (2) no breathing movements, (3) no reflexes, and (4) a flat
EEG (electroencephalogram).[44]

Medicine's attempt to redefine death is being

---

* Miller, George W.: *Moral and Ethical Implications of Human Organ Transplants.* Charles C
Thomas, Publisher, Springfield, Ill., 1971, p. 42.

studied by moral philosophers. They contend that to redefine death so that a physician will know with a higher degree of certainty that death has occurred (and it is therefore permissible to remove a fresh, or viable, organ) is one thing but to redefine death for the purpose of obtaining more organs for transplantation is another matter. (See also Chapter 50 for a discussion of defining death.)

The right to personal autonomy has been provided the donor by the enactment of the Uniform Anatomical Gift Act, as discussed above. The Act gives the individual the legal authority to decide what medical science can and cannot do with his or her body and its parts at death.

The right of the donor for privacy is a moral and ethical issue. It is unfortunate that so much publicity in national and local television programs, newspapers, and popular magazines accompanied each transplantation of a vital organ, especially the heart, during the 1960s. The question has been raised as to what real value there is in publishing the name of the donor. Many times this undue publicity serves only as an infringement of the privacy of the donor and an added burden for the grieving family.

The right to respectful treatment of the body after death has always been emphasized in nursing. It is mentioned here to remind readers that although the deceased voluntarily donated his or her body or parts of it for medical purposes, donors do not relinquish the inherent right to the proper treatment of their bodies.

Preservation of Tissues and Organs. Successful attempts at tissue and whole organ transplants have created the need for reliable means of preserving and storing tissues and organs of various sizes and types for later use. Methods such as simple freezing or freeze-drying permit long-term preservation of connective and structural tissues, such as bone, dura, heart valves, and fascia. These and other tissues, such as skin, tendons, and cornea, are stored in special laboratories known as *tissue banks.* The primary function of tissue banks are to collect, process, store, and dispense, for grafting, various types of tissues noted above. In most instances, graftings are not life-saving measures as are organ transplantations, but they are helpful in salvaging many members of society who otherwise would live disfigured and disabled.

Before the establishment of multitissue banks, monobanks that stored only one type of tissue existed, and in most instances these were for tissues of the eye. They were called *eye banks,* although the whole eyes were not used, only tissues from them. The first eye bank was established in 1944 at the Manhattan Eye, Ear, and Throat Hospital in New York City. Today, eye banks are located in 67 major cities in the United States and Canada, and 55 are located in 51 foreign countries.[45]

The United States Navy tissue bank in Bethesda, Md., was the first multitissue bank established in the United States (in 1949). Originally it stored bone, skin, fascia, and tendons; today, it stores these in addition to other tissues. The Navy now has a bank in San Diego, Calif., as well as in Bethesda. Since the establishment of the Bethesda bank, over 6600 patients have received tissues from it (see Table 43-4) and each year over 240 new patients are recipients of stored tissues. Tissues are dispensed to the whole of the United States as well as foreign countries. For example, United States Navy Tissue Banks supplied 3000 square inches of human skin to fire victims in Brazil.[46,47]

The second tissue bank was established in 1952 at the regional Institute of National Health, Hrádec Králove, Czechoslovakia. In 1971, R. Klen[48] reported that this bank, over an 18-year period, supplied 19 different kinds of preserved tissues for transplant to 163 hospitals in Czechoslovakia and 23 hospitals in different parts of the world. For the most part, shipments outside of Czechoslovakia were made to developing countries where Czechoslovakian surgeons were working. Recently, this service has been extended, through the assistance of the World Health Organization,

Table 43-4. Tissue Collected and Dispensed from May 1950 to May 1970, Navy Tissue Bank, Bethesda, Md.*

	Tissue Processed	Tissue Dispensed
Skin	7,062	4,635
Cartilage	528	302
Eyes	95	81
Fascia	1,021	755
Dura	515	404
Tendon	31	1
Nerve	157	38
Bone	14,585	10,360
Artery		176
Heart valve	117	80
Totals	24,111	16,832
	Total sterile tissue procurement	
Total recipients 6669	procedures	903

* Sell, Kenneth W.: "Long-Term Tissue and Organ Preservation," *Transplant. Proc.,* **3:**274, (Mar.) 1971.

Table 43-5. Problems Encountered in Attempts to Freeze Whole Organs *

1. Condition of the organ at the start of the procedure
   Need proper preparation of donor
   Optimal when donor has an intact cardiovascular system
2. Quality of perfusion
   Simple flushing techniques inadequate
   Need the very best perfusion methods and media
3. Toxicity of the cryoprotective agents
4. Control of freezing and thawing rates
5. Removal of cryoprotective agents
6. Vascular endothelial cell damage
7. Specific requirements of different cell types

* Sell, Kenneth W.: "Long-Term Tissue and Organ Preservation," *Transplant. Proc.,* **3:**276, (Mar.) 1971.

Table 43-6. Reasons for Discarding 56 Machine-Perfused Human Cadaveric Kidneys Without Transplantation *

Good reasons		29
Poor or borderline perfusion	23	
Accidental injury to or contamination of kidney	4	
Donor disease discovered at autopsy	2	
Borderline reasons		6
Harvesting damage to kidney	6	
Questionable reasons		21
Unfounded concern with perfusion flows and pressures	10	
No local recipients	5	
Multiple vessels or ureters	4	
Donor creatinine level elevated	2	

* Moore, Thomas C., et al.: "Factors Involved in Discarding Cadaveric Kidneys Preserved by Machine Perfusion," *Surg. Gynecol. Obstet.,* **138:**545, (Apr.) 1974.

to a number of leprosaria in Brazil, Burma, India, Mexico, and Tanzania.

In 1953, a bank of human tissue for clinical use was established at the Harrison Department of Surgical Research at the University of Pennsylvania. Blood vessels, fascia, and skin tissues were freeze-dried and supplied by this bank until 1958 when emphasis shifted to the development of a viable organ bank for long-term or semipermanent preservation.[49]

Although the principles for preservation of organs are the same as those for tissues, techniques to preserve whole organs have not met with great success (see Table 43-5). The major reason that large organs cannot be successfully frozen is the inability to control the rate of freezing and subsequent warming of tissue mass. If tissue cells are frozen too rapidly, intracellular water crystallizes and ice crystals produce damage. The addition of cryoprotective agents such as glycerol and DMSO (dimethylsulfoxide) reduces crystallization.[50] Many people are trying to solve the problem of long-term organ preservation in 42 organ transplant and preservation laboratories in the United States.[51] Noting that storage of organs, a young science, is confronted with an unusual number of challenges, M. D. Turner says:

True hibernating mammals accomplish whole body self-preservation at refrigerator temperatures for periods of weeks, and even months, a feat yet to be duplicated by the human body or other warm-blooded nonhibernators. Perhaps we shall learn from the hibernators how to store a complex part, or even the whole, of any mammalian body above freezing for long periods. By far the most successful means of kidney storage is actually the culture of that organ at hypothermic temperatures. However, during hibernation the differentiated tissues of hibernating mammals are still under a complex interplay of hormonal influences, and the fate of isolated organs in the prolonged absence of these factors is not yet known.*

A short-term storage system has been developed for the kidney. The Belzer Preservation Unit, a $21,000 machine that keeps kidneys viable and functioning for up to 36 hours, was developed by Dr. Fred Belzer in San Francisco in the late 1960s. The machine "works by drawing on a reserve of frozen human plasma which is thawed and filtered by the machine and then pumped through the organ." † Utilizing the Belzer Unit, short-term kidney storage programs have been initiated in San Francisco, Calif., the Cleveland (Ohio) Clinic, and the Cornell University Medical School in New York City, according to David Rovik (1971).[52]

Thomas C. Moore and associates[53] report that 56 of 334 human cadaveric kidneys preserved on a Belzer machine were discarded during a 27-month period (March 1971–July 1973). Table 43-6 lists the reasons for discarding these kidneys. The authors emphasize the importance of getting these organs under circumstances that ensure a maximum number of good quality. A regional organ preservation laboratory (Organ Preservation Laboratory, Interhospital Organ Bank at Boston, Mass.) for 13 transplant centers in the New England area has been established. During the period July 1972 to May 1973, 107 kidneys were preserved. Of these, 14 kidneys were dis-

* Turner, M. D.: "Organ Storage," in Hardy, James (ed.): *Human Organ Support and Replacement.* Charles C Thomas, Publisher, Springfield, Ill., 1971, p. 35.
† Rovik, David: *As Man Becomes Machine.* Doubleday & Co., Inc., Garden City, N.Y., 1971, p. 64.

carded while 93 kidneys were transplanted; 53 per cent functioned immediately, 44 per cent developed tubular necrosis, and 3 per cent never functioned and were removed. Preservation of cadaver kidney (up to 50 hours) has been achieved, according to Sang In Cho and associates.[54]

The survival rate of the graft and recipient continues to increase. C. M. Balch and associates, in 1975, reported 94 per cent survival at 3 years in 18 patients with end stage congenital renal disease requiring kidney transplantation. After analyzing survival data from 9900 patients in the Organ Transplant Registry (Chicago), they say:

> The overall five year *patient survival* was 69.3 percent for those receiving the kidney from a living related donor and 50.1 percent for those receiving a cadaveric kidney. . . .
> The overall five year *allograph survival* was 53.3 percent for kidneys from living related donors and 30.9 percent for cadaveric kidneys.*

The Organ Transplant Registry, which was under the American College of Surgeons and the National Institutes of Health, was dissolved in 1976.

Distribution of Tissues and Organs. Distributing tissues does not seem to present the problems of organs for transplantation. Because connective and structural tissues such as bone, dura, heart valves, fascia, tendons, and cornea can be stored by freezing or freeze-drying methods, they can be taken in quantity from cadaver donors. Furthermore, tissue rejection is not usually seen with grafts of structural or connective tissue. Storage by freeze-drying reduces histoincompatibility and antigenicity, so tissue-typing, or matching of donors and recipients, is not necessary.[55] The Tissue Graft Registry (Bethesda, Maryland) helps individual tissue banks in the United States by providing a systematic follow-up of patients who receive tissue transplants; records are kept for further evaluation and follow-up studies.

Severe shortage of vital organs for transplantation has created two major problems in distributing organs for transplantation. The first problem, among recipients, is who will receive a transplant and who will not. The second problem is providing an effective and equably distributed communication system throughout a country or the world so that all

potential recipients have an equal chance at access to available organs.

The problem of recipient selection is both a medical and a moral problem. Physicians and moral philosophers generally agree that before any patient (recipient) can be considered as a candidate for an organ transplant, the person must meet certain medical qualifications. That the recipient has no reasonable hope for survival without the operation must be determined, yet he or she should not be so critically ill that survival of the transplant is questionable. Consideration is also given to associated conditions of the recipient, especially a chronic disease of any other organ system that could gravely complicate recovery.

Physicians generally take the position that the most important consideration in the selection of a recipient is biomedical. Experience has shown that if success is to be anticipated in organ transplantation, tissue-typing and tissue-matching are prime factors in the selection of a recipient. However, when more than one patient is waiting for a transplant attempt, the decision as to who receives the organ must be made. In such a situation, selection of the recipient is based on social as well as biomedical criteria. Some authorities have suggested that committees be set up to help select recipients on the basis of their worth to society. Many medical centers have established psychiatric screening for potential recipients to assess their mental health as well as their ability to withstand lifelong treatment.

To ensure tissue-matching for organ transplants a surgeon must look for a recipient identical in tissue type to that of the donor. If an identical match cannot be found, a donor-recipient combination as nearly identical or compatible as possible is sought. As organ transplants have grown in volume, authorities have realized that the search for recipients and donors for matching could be greatly facilitated by pooling such information. Such a pooling of information occurs in the Eurotransplant Program.[56] Recipients in this program are typed before donor organs are available. Information from this typing, along with other facts about the recipient such as age, sex, blood type, and state of disease, is fed into a computer. Recipient lists are updated and distributed monthly to tissue-typing centers in the program. More than 28 medical centers in Belgium, Germany, the Netherlands, England, Italy, the Scandinavian countries, and Switzerland participate in the Eurotransplant Program. The Computing Center of the Eurotransplant Foundation is located at the University of Leiden in the Netherlands.

A program like the Eurotransplant Program

---

* Balch, C. M., et al.: "Kidney Transplantation in Patients with End Stage Congenital Renal Disease. Report of Eighteen Cases and Review of the Organ Transplant Registry," *Am. J. Surg.*, **130**:304, (Sept.) 1975.

was established in the United States at the University of California at Los Angeles in 1970. This program, the National Transplant Communications Network, maintains a computerized file of all waiting recipients in the United States and Canada. The file includes complete information on the physical condition and histocompatibility of the waiting recipient. File information is updated daily. Another communications network that pools information on tissue-typing of potential recipients is the National Cadaver Recipient Pool. More than 60 hospitals in the United States and Canada that perform transplantation surgery belong to this program.[57]

In addition to the above communications systems, there are registries that collect biologic information in the new science of organ transplantation for the purpose of evaluating the diverse efforts in the field. The earliest of such registries established in the United States was the Human Kidney Transplant Registry operated in Boston, Mass. In mid-1970, this registry merged with the newly organized American College of Surgeons/National Institutes of Health Organ Transplant Registry. The ACS/NIH Organ Transplant Registry is located in the Chicago headquarters of the American College of Surgeons. The registry maintains an accurate census for each type of organ transplant. Data related to transplantations of kidneys, hearts, livers, lungs, and pancreata are collected from all over the world and analyzed. The registry distributes reports on this medical data to contributors and other interested persons in the health professions.[58]

REFERENCES

1. Minckler, Tate M.: "Physical Agents in Disease," in Minckler, Jeff, et al.: *Pathobiology, An Introduction.* C. V. Mosby Co., St. Louis, 1971, p. 294.
2. Moore, Francis D.: "Convalescence: The Metabolic Sequence After Injury," in American College of Surgeons, Committee on Pre and Postoperative Care: *Manual of Preoperative and Postoperative Care,* 2nd ed. W. B. Saunders Co., Philadelphia, 1971, p. 28.
2a. Lal, S. K., et al.: "Variation of Some Plasma Components After Closed Fractures," *J. Trauma,* **16:**206, (Mar.) 1976.
3. Maxwell, Morton H., and Kleeman, Charles R.: *Clinical Disorders of Fluid and Electrolyte Metabolism,* 2nd ed. McGraw-Hill Book Co., New York, 1972, p. 1068.
4. *Ibid.,* p. 1069.
5. Macleod, A. G.: *Aspects of Acute Inflammation.* Upjohn Co., Kalamazoo, Mich., 1969, p. 5.
6. Curran, R. C., and Codling, B. W.: "Acute Inflammation," in Curran, R. C., and Harnden, D. G. (eds.): *The Pathological Basis of Medicine.* W. B. Saunders Co., Philadelphia, 1972, p. 35.
7. Cappell, D. F., and Anderson, J. R.: *Muir's Textbook of Pathology,* 9th ed. Edward Arnold, Ltd., London, 1971, p. 41.
8. Macleod, A. G.: *op. cit.,* p. 20.
9. *Ibid.,* p. 21.
10. Altemeier, W. A.: "Current Infection Problems in Surgery," in *Proceedings of the International Conference on Nosocomial Infections,* Center for Disease Control, August 3–6, 1970. American Hospital Association, Chicago, 1971, p. 86.
11. Sandusky, William R.: "Infection and Antimicrobial Agents," in American College of Surgeons, Committee on Pre and Postoperative Care: *Manual of Preoperative and Postoperative Care,* 2nd ed. W. B. Saunders Co., Philadelphia, 1971, p. 118.
11a. Dineen, P., and Drusin, L.: "Epidemics of Post-operative Wound Infections Associated with Hair Carriers," *Lancet,* **2:**7157, (Nov. 24) 1973.
11b. Walter, Carl W., et al.: "The Airborne Component of Wound Contamination and Infection," *Arch. Surg.,* **107:**588, (Oct.) 1973.
12. Schwartz, Seymour I., et al. (eds.): *Principles of Surgery,* Vol. I. McGraw-Hill Book Co., New York, 1969, p. 162.
13. Anderson, W. A. D., and Scotti, Thomas M.: *Synopsis of Pathology,* 7th ed. C. V. Mosby Co., St. Louis, 1968, p. 55.
13a. Compton, Carol Yank: "War Injury: Identity Crisis for Young Men," *Nurs. Clin. North Am.,* **8:**53, (Mar.) 1973.
14. Cole, Warren H., and Puestow, Charles B.: *Emergency Care: Surgical and Medical,* 7th ed. Appleton-Century-Crofts, New York, 1972, p. 117.
15. Gardner, A. Ward, and Roylance, Peter J.: *New Essential First Aid.* Little, Brown & Co., Boston, 1971, p. 55.
15a. O'Boyle, Catherine M.: "Sports Injuries in Adolescents: Emergency Care," *Am. J. Nurs.,* **74:**1732, (Oct.) 1975.
15b. Ostaszewski, Teresa M., and Marshall, John L.: "Prevention and Treatment of Sports Injuries," *Am. J. Nurs.,* **75:**1737, (Oct.) 1975.
16. Shires, G. Tom, and Jones, Ronald C.: "Initial Management of the Severely Injured Patient," *J.A.M.A.,* **213:**1872, (Sept. 14) 1970.
17. Paradies, Louis H.: "Injuries to the Hand," in Shires, G. Tom (ed.): *Care of the Trauma Patient.* McGraw-Hill Book Co., New York, 1966, p. 466.
18. American College of Surgeons, Committee on Trauma: *Early Care of the Injured Patient.* W. B. Saunders Co., Philadelphia, 1972, p. 401.
18a. US Health Services and Mental Health Administration, Division of Emergency Health Services: *Emergency Medical Services Communications Systems.* US Government Print-

ing Office, Washington, D.C., 1972 (DHEW No. [HSM] 73–2003).

18b. LaZae, Jean E.: "Community Health Services Emergency Planning," in International Council of Nurses: *Focus on the Future.* Proceedings of the 14th Quadrennial Congress of the Council. Montreal, Canada, June 22–28, 1969. S. Karger, New York, 1970.

19. deGruchy, G. C.: *Clinical Haematology in Medical Practice,* 3rd ed. Blackwell Scientific Publications, Oxford, 1970, p. 623.

20. Thompson, R. B.: *A Short Textbook of Haematology,* 3rd ed. J. B. Lippincott Co., Toronto, 1969, p. 348.

21. deGruchy, G. C.: *op. cit.,* p. 674.

22. Baxter, Charles R.: "Myoglobinuria," in Shires, G. Tom (ed.): *Care of the Trauma Patient.* McGraw-Hill Book Co., New York, 1966, p. 669.

23. Ratnoff, Oscar D.: "Classic Hemophilia," in Beeson, Paul B., and McDermott, Walsh (eds.): *Textbook of Medicine,* Vol. II, 14th ed. W. B. Saunders Co., Philadelphia, 1975, p. 1567.

24. ———: "Acquired Disorders of Blood Coagulation," in Beeson, Paul B., and McDermott, Walsh (eds.): *Textbook of Medicine,* Vol. II, 14th ed. W. B. Saunders Co., Philadelphia, 1975, p. 1570.

25. deGruchy, G. C.: *op. cit.,* p. 667.

26. Shaw, Robert R., and Webb, Watts R.: "Trauma to the Chest," in Shires, G. Tom (ed.): *Care of the Trauma Patient.* McGraw-Hill Book Co., New York, 1966, p. 322.

27. American College of Surgeons, Committee on Trauma: *op. cit.,* p. 46.

28. Smith, Stephen E.: "Antibacterial Drugs," *Nurs. Times,* **67:**177, (Feb. 6) 1971.

29. Sandusky, William R.: *op. cit.,* p. 121.

30. Smith, Stephen E.: *op. cit.*

31. Rose, Mary Ann: "Home Care After Peripheral Vascular Surgery," *Am. J. Nurs.,* **74:**260, (Feb.) 1974.

32. Norsworthy, Edith: "Nursing Rehabilitation After Severe Head Trauma," *Am. J. Nurs.,* **74:**1246, (July) 1974.

33. Stickel, Delford L., and Seigler, H. F.: "Transplantation. Historical Aspects," in Sabiston, David C. (ed.): *Davis-Christopher Textbook of Surgery,* 10th ed. W. B. Saunders Co., Philadelphia, 1972, p. 425.

34. Rapaport, Felix T., and Dausset, Jean (eds.): *Human Transplantation.* Grune & Stratton, New York, 1968.

35. Calne, R. Y.: *Renal Transplantation.* Edward Arnold, Ltd., London, 1967.

36. Woodruff, M. F. A.: *The Transplantation of Tissues and Organs.* Charles C Thomas, Publisher, Springfield, Ill., 1960.

37. Elkinton, J. R.: "Moral Problems in the Use of Borrowed Organs, Artificial and Transplanted," *Ann. Intern. Med.,* **60:**309, (Mar.) 1964.

38. Hamburger, Jean, and Crosnier, Jean: "Moral and Ethical Problems in Transplantation," in Rapaport, Felix T., and Dausset, Jean (eds.): *Human Transplantation.* Grune & Stratton, New York, 1968, p. 37.

39. Lyons, Catherine: *Organ Transplants. The Moral Issues.* Westminster Press, Philadelphia, 1970, p. 85.

40. Belzer, Folkert O., et al.: "Organ Transplantation," in Dunphy, J. Englebert, and Way, Lawrence W.: *Current Surgical Diagnosis and Treatment,* 2nd ed. Lange Medical Publications, Los Altos, Calif., 1975, p. 1068.

41. Bergan, John: "Current Risks to Kidney Transplant Donor," *Transplant. Proc.,* **5:** 1131, (June) 1973.

42. Belzer, Folkert O., et al.: *op. cit.,* p. 1070.

43. Sadler, Alfred M., Jr., and Sadler, Blair L.: "Recent Developments in the Legal Aspects of Transplantation in the United States," *Transplant. Proc.,* **3:**293, (Mar.) 1971.

44. Miller, George W.: *Moral and Ethical Implications of Human Organ Transplants.* Charles C Thomas, Publisher, Springfield, Ill., 1971, p. 26.

45. Hamilton, Mary Jo: "What the Nurse Should Know About Eye Banks," *Nurs. Clin. North Am.,* **5:**483, (Sept.) 1970.

46. Sell, Kenneth W.: "Long-Term Tissue and Organ Preservation," *Transplant. Proc.* **3:** 274, (Mar.) 1971.

47. Isler, Charlotte: "The World of Transplants —Part 1," *RN,* **35:**36, (Nov.) 1972.

48. Klen, R.: "Research Report 1952–1970 of the Tissue Bank," *Folia Biologica,* **17:**348, (Oct.) 1971.

49. Lehr, Herndon, et al.: "A Viable Organ Bank," *Pa. Med.,* **73:**57, (Oct.) 1970.

50. Turner, M. D.: "Organ Storage," in Hardy, James (ed.): *Human Organ Support and Replacement.* Charles C Thomas, Publisher, Springfield, Ill., 1971.

51. Isler, Charlotte: "The World of Transplants —Part 2," *RN,* **35:**40, (Dec.) 1972.

52. Rovik, David: *As Man Becomes Machine.* Doubleday & Co., Garden City, N.Y., 1971, p. 63.

53. Moore, Thomas C., et al.: "Factors Involved in Discarding Cadaveric Kidneys Preserved by Machine Perfusion," *Surg. Gynecol. Obstet.,* **138:**545, (Apr.) 1974.

54. Cho, Sang In, et al.: "Regional Organ Preservation Program in the New England Area," *Surgery,* **75:**528, (Apr.) 1974.

55. Sell, Kenneth W.: *op. cit.*

56. Van Rood, J. J., et al.: "Eurotransplant," *Transplant. Proc.,* **3:**933, (Mar.) 1971.

57. Isler, Charlotte: *op. cit.*

58. Bergan, John: "Structure and Function of the Organ Transplant Registry of the American College of Surgeons," *Transplant. Proc.,* **3:**298, (Mar.) 1971.

Additional Suggested Reading

Ahern, M. S.: "Reflections of an Occupational Health Nurse as 'Safety Engineer'," *Occup. Health Nurs. (NY),* **17:**22, (Oct.) 1969.

Baxter, C. R.: "The Current Status of Burn Research," *J. Trauma,* **14:**1, (Jan.) 1974.

Bellack, Janis Peacock: "Helping a Child Cope with the Stress of Injury," *Am. J. Nurs.,* **74:** 1491, (Aug.) 1974.

Bock, James E.: "Trauma—Skiing and Nursing," in Anderson, Edith H., et al. (eds.): *Current Concepts in Clinical Nursing,* Vol. 4. C. V. Mosby Co., St. Louis, 1973.

Bouzarth, W. F.: "Management of Head Injury by Industrial Nurses," *Ind. Med. Surg.,* **39:**21, (Jan.) 1970.

Boyd, David M., et al.: *The Critically Injured Patient. Concept and the Illinois Statewide Plan for Trauma Centers.* Illinois Department of Public Health, Springfield, 1972.

Bruckner, Walter L., and Longmire, William P.: "Wound Healing: A Local Reaction on a Systemic Process," *J. Surg. Res.,* **9:**279, (May) 1969.

Brunius, Ulf: "Wound Healing Impairment from Sutures," *Acta Chir. Scand. Suppl.,* **396:**4, (June 16) 1969.

Cannavo, J. J.: "The Industrial Nurse's Role in Occupational Health Safety," *Occup. Health Nurs. (NY),* **22:**7, (Feb.) 1974.

Cobey, James C., and Cobey, Janet H.: "Chronic Leg Ulcers," *Am. J. Nurs.,* **74:**258, (Feb.) 1974.

Detroit Industrial First Aid Advisory Committee: *First Aid Guide for the Small Establishment.* Wayne State University Press, Detroit, 1967.

Edlich, Richard F., et al.: "Studies in Management of the Contaminated Wound. III. Assessment of the Effectiveness of Irrigation with Antiseptic Agents," *Am. J. Surg.,* **118:**21, (July) 1969.

Frobisher, Martin, and Fuerst, Robert: *Microbiology in Health and Disease,* 13th ed. W. B. Saunders Co., Philadelphia, 1973.

Fu, W.: *Angiography of Trauma.* Charles C Thomas, Publisher, Springfield, Ill., 1971.

Gallaher, Hazel L., et al.: "The Occupational Health Nurse and the Patient with Trauma," *Nurs. Clin. North Am.,* **5:**609, (Dec.) 1970; *Occup. Health (London),* **23:**197, (June) 1971.

Hafey, Lucile W., and Keane, Barbara A.: "Patient with Acute Insult to the Central Nervous System," *Nurs. Clin. North Am.,* **8:**743, (Dec.) 1973.

Hannah, B., et al.: "Infection Control: Viewpoints of the Nurse, Physician, and Administration," *Can. Hosp.,* **48:**38, (Sept.) 1971.

Hekmatpanah, Javad: "The Management of Head Trauma," *Surg. Clin. North Am.,* **53:**47, (Feb.) 1973.

Hruza, A.: *Resistance to Trauma.* Charles C Thomas, Publisher, Springfield, Ill., 1971.

Jensen, Ole B., et al.: "Factors Influencing the Frequency of Post-Operative Wound Sepsis," *Acta Chir. Scand. Suppl.,* **396:**84, (Jan. 5) 1969.

————: "Post-Operative Wound Sepsis in General Surgery, III. An Evaluation of the Post-Opera-

tive Administration of Antibiotics," *Acta Chir. Scand. Suppl.,* **396:**94, (Jan. 5) 1969.

Myers, M. Bert: "Sutures and Wound Healing," *Am. J. Nurs.,* **71:**1725, (Sept.) 1971.

Piskozub, Z. T.: "The Efficiency of Wound Dressing Materials as a Barrier to Secondary Bacterial Contamination," *Br. J. Plast. Surg.,* **21:** 387, (Sept.) 1968.

Quesenbury, Jeanne N., and Hammes, Sara: "Immediate Nursing Care Following Cervical Cord Injury," in Anderson, Edith H., et al. (eds.): *Current Concepts in Clinical Nursing,* Vol. 4. C. V. Mosby Co., St. Louis, 1973.

Read, Donald A., and Greene, Walter H.: *Health and Modern Man.* Macmillan Publishing Co., Inc., New York, 1973.

Rieser, Mary, et al.: "Intensive Care Nursing," in Kintzel, Kay Corman (ed.): *Advanced Concepts in Clinical Nursing.* J. B. Lippincott Co., Philadelphia, 1971.

Romano, T.: "Trauma Nurse Specialist," *Am. J. Nurs.,* **73:**1008, (Jan.) 1973.

Ross, Russell: "Wound Healing," *Sci. Am.,* **220:** 40, (June) 1969.

Royce, Judith A.: "Shock—Emergency Nursing Implications," *Nurs. Clin. North Am.,* **8:**377, (Sept.) 1973.

Shreve, A. J.: "Care of the Open Injury," *Am. Assoc. Ind. Nurses J.,* **16:**15, (Oct.) 1968.

Sproul, Carmen Warner, et al. (eds.): *Emergency Care.* C. V. Mosby, St. Louis, 1974.

Stinson, Velda: "Porcine Skin Dressings for Burns," *Am. J. Nurs.,* **74:**111, (Jan.) 1974.

Taylor, Lord: *First Aid in the Factory,* 4th ed. Churchill Livingstone, London, 1973.

Trafford, H. S.: "Infections of the Hand," *Practitioner,* **201:**723, (Nov.) 1968.

US Department of Labor, Bureau of Labor Standards: *Elements of a Safety Program.* US Government Printing Office, Washington, D.C., 1967.

————: *The Fundamentals of Accident Prevention.* US Government Printing Office, Washington, D.C., 1969.

Waterman, Norton G.: "Tissue Temperatures in Localized Pyogenic Infections," *Am. J. Surg.,* **118:**31, (July) 1969.

Weed, Robert I., et al. (eds.): *Hematology for Internists.* Little, Brown & Co., Boston, 1971.

Gladys Nite
Virginia Henderson

The authors acknowledge the assistance of Eleanor Taggart, Assistant Professor of Medical-Surgical Nursing, Yale University School of Nursing, New Haven, Conn., in preparing the section on Transplants of Tissues and Organs—Banks and Programs for Preserving and Distributing Transplants.

CHAPTER 44

Systemic Infection — A Communicable Condition Transmitted by Various Channels, With or Without Febrile States

1. DEVELOPMENT OF CONCEPTS

Historical Perspective. In the history of medicine there are no more exciting chapters than those that tell of the conquest of infectious disease. This is often considered modern medicine's greatest accomplishment, and programs aimed at elimination of communicable disease are its cornerstone. Many effective methods of controlling infectious disease were known in ancient times. The Law of Moses contains certain regulations that recognized the communicability of diseases such as leprosy and the "discharge from his body" that we think was gonorrhea.* We believe that the methods suggested before the microscopic origin of disease was understood were based on trial and error rather than on knowledge of the underlying principles. Early scientists were aiming in the dark, sometimes hitting their mark, while scientists of the last few centuries have thrown so much light on the study of communicable disease that it is no longer necessary to shoot blindly. Today's scientist considers it essential, in order to understand thoroughly the prevention and control of a transmissible disease, to complete the following steps: isolate the organism causing the disease (so as to learn as much as possible about the characteristics of that organism), determine its mode of transmission (how it attacks the host), and find out where and how long it survives in the environment.

New Insight. Some present-day practices have been known for centuries (for example, isolation of an infected person), and yet the scientific control of communicable disease is,

in some respects, still in an early stage. Modern life has presented us with new problems. For example, jet travel has complicated disease control by making it possible for people to go halfway around the world during the incubation period of many infectious diseases. Because the development of vaccines and potent antibiotics has given medical science the tools with which to prevent and treat the major infections of man, many epidemic diseases have disappeared from the Western world in the past half century, but modern travel may bring them back to a population unprotected by natural immunity.

The Chinese have made remarkable changes in the health of 600 million people by eliminating many communicable diseases in their country. According to Victor W. Sidel and Ruth Sidel,[1] venereal disease has been eliminated, and cholera, plague, smallpox, and most nutritional diseases have disappeared. Opium addiction has been eliminated through community efforts. Through mobilization of the people against pests such as flies, mosquitoes, rats, sparrows, and bedbugs, other communicable diseases have disappeared. (See Chapter 2, p. 126).

Not only is there a specific understanding of control measures for diseases of known origin, but there are hypotheses for research where an organism is unknown. It is possible, therefore, to proceed more systematically in dealing with any communicable disease. (The spectrum of disease is shown in Fig. 44-1.)

But communicable disease can *never* be conquered once and for all. Many writers warn against complacency. Evaluation of the results of treatment with antimicrobial agents and the greatly increased use of these drugs

---

* See Leviticus 13 and 14, 15:1–13.

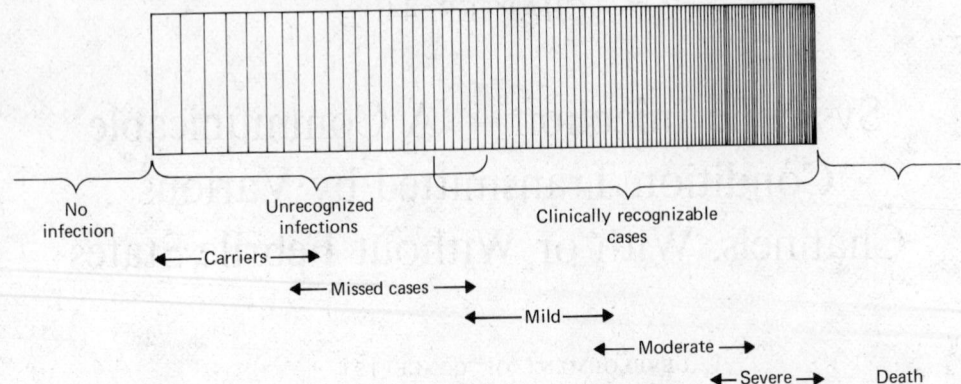

Figure 44-1. Spectrum of disease. (From Anderson, Gaylord W., et al.: *Communicable Disease Control,* 4th ed. Macmillan Publishing Co., Inc., New York, 1962.)

have shown that microorganisms will adapt themselves to an environment and resist antibiotics, or allow other organisms to replace them, making the challenge of controlling infectious disease an ever-present reality. A. McGehee Harvey says: "The apparent retreat of epidemic disease from the West may in part represent a phase of the natural biologic cycle rather than the result of 'modern' methods of disease control." *

Notwithstanding all the advances that have been made, however, there were about

* Harvey, A. McGehee, et al.: *The Principles and Practice of Medicine,* 18th ed. Appleton-Century-Crofts, New York, 1972, p. 1001.

1,143,000 cases of reportable diseases (excluding streptococcal sore throat and scarlet fever) in the United States in 1973, of which approximately 932,000 were venereal diseases.[2] And in 1974 the Center for Disease Control in Atlanta, Georgia, reported over 30,000 new active cases of tuberculosis.[2a] (See Figs. 44-2, 44-3, and 44-4.) Data from the World Health Organization indicate that there were nearly 17,000 cases of diphtheria, an entirely preventable disease, among the world's population in 1970.[3] The high incidence of communicable disease is due partly to our unapplied scientific findings and partly to the limitations of scientific discovery. That there are outbreaks of diphtheria, smallpox, cholera, and typhoid fe-

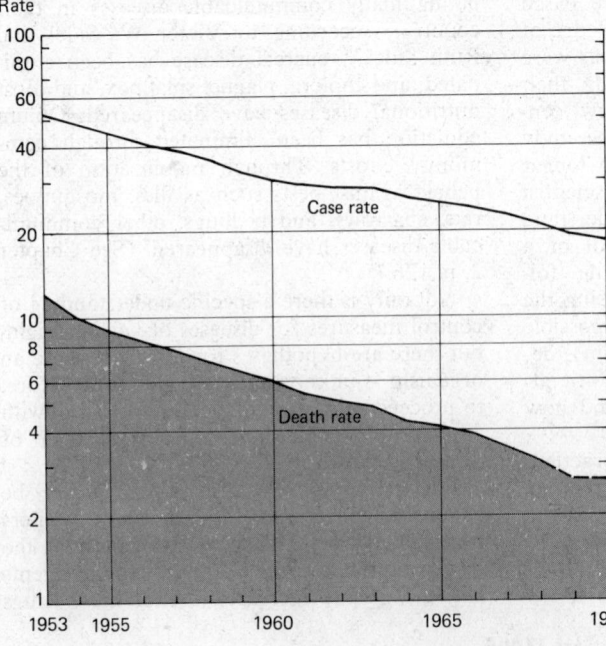

Figure 44-2. Tuberculosis case rate and death rate, United States, 1953 to 1970. (*Reported Tuberculosis Data 1970.* DHEW Pub. No. [HSM] 72–80961. US Department of Health, Education, and Welfare, Public Health Service, Health Services and Mental Health Administration, Center for Disease Control, Atlanta, Ga.)

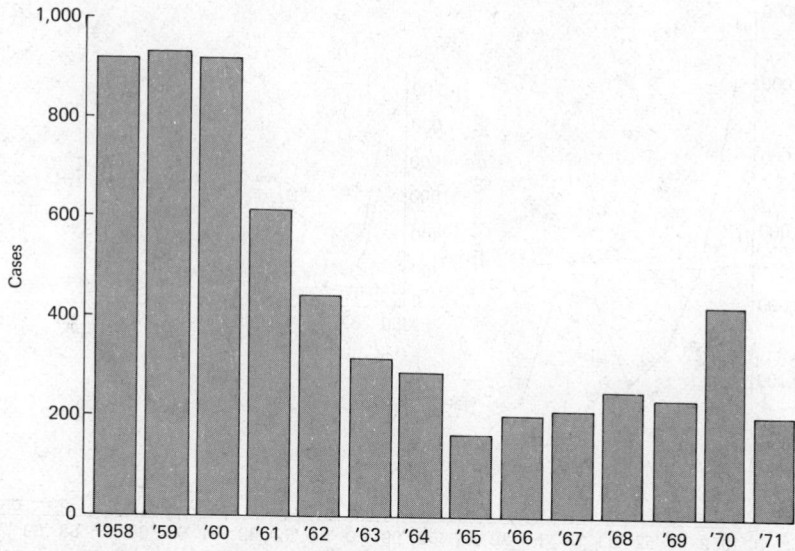

Figure 44-3. Pertussis—reported cases, United States, 1950–1971, showing the dramatic effect of control measures. (*Morbidity and Mortality Weekly Report*, Annual Supplement, Summary 1971. US Department of Health, Education, and Welfare, Health Services and Mental Health Administration, Center for Disease Control, Atlanta, Ga.)

ver in the world today is wholly the result of failure to use available preventive measures; but the high incidence of viral diseases, such as influenza and the common cold, can be attributed to limited knowledge of prevention and control. Although Linus Pauling, a Nobel prize winner in chemistry, has suggested the use of vitamin C in the prevention of the common cold, his findings are challenged by other authorities.[4-6]

Michael B. Gregg,[7] at the time chief of the Epidemic Intelligence Service, US Public Health Service, classified communicable diseases as follows:

The Disappearing Diseases
 Bacterial: diphtheria, pertussis, tetanus, tuberculosis
 Viral: poliomyelitis, measles, smallpox
The Elusive Diseases
 Influenza, hepatitis
The Emerging Diseases
 Viral infection, nosocomial infection *

This classification illustrates trends in communicable disease control and suggests the

* Nosocomial infection refers to one that develops in a patient during hospitalization and is not believed to be present or incubating at the time of hospital admission. Occasionally, the infection may not present symptoms until after the patient is discharged from the hospital. (Definition from the *Outline for Surveillance and Control of Nosocomial Infections*, USPHS, Center for Disease Control, Hospital Infections Section, Atlanta, Ga., revised September 1970.)

importance of recognizing the ever-changing character of infectious disease. As Gregg says, the interaction of the varying host population, the endlessly adapting agent (parasitic organism), and the constant pressure from a man-made environment each shape the other, but no one of these is strong enough to control the other two. This endless push and pull of forces poses a profound challenge to all health workers trying to prevent and control infection.

In spite of the existence of a safe and effective means for preventing measles, for example, reports indicate a rise in the prevalence of this disease simply because children are not immunized properly.[8,9] Doctors, nurses, and other health workers should bear in mind that there is a lag between scientific discovery and its application, and that our practices should be held up to scrutiny at frequent intervals to see whether they are consistent with newer knowledge. Health workers, and also the general public, should be informed about programs aimed at eradicating disease.

For many years scientists have been studying viruses as a possible cause of cancer in humans. Certain viruses have been found to be associated with Hodgkin's disease and carcinoma of the cervix. These organisms have also been suggested as causative agents of human leukemia, breast cancer, and sarcomas. If it is determined that viruses are the source of all forms of cancer, it may not be long before

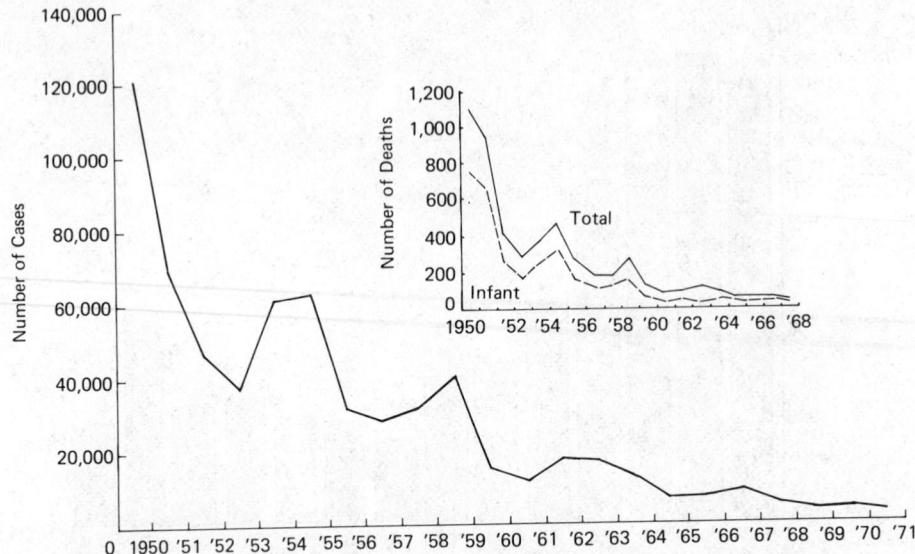

Figure 44-4. Diphtheria—reported cases, United States, 1958–1971, showing the varying effect of control measures. (*Morbidity and Mortality Weekly Report,* Annual Supplement, Summary 1971. US Department of Health, Education, and Welfare, Health Services and Mental Health Administration, Center for Disease Control, Atlanta, Ga.)

human virus vaccines are developed to prevent this disease.[10]

Currently immunologists are conducting research into the linkage between the body's natural ability to fight infections and its ability to fight cancer through its own defense mechanisms. Immunotherapy provides new treatment methods for the control of cancer. One method uses vaccines prepared from tumors to stimulate the body to reproduce its own antibodies. Another method uses the bacillus of Calmette and Guerin (BCG) to stimulate the body's immune system as a whole.[11] The prospect of this way of controlling neoplasms makes immunology an exciting field for research.

Lewis Thomas, in 1976 president of the Memorial Sloan-Kettering Cancer Center, predicted at a 1958 symposium that the body's ability to reject transplants and its ability to fight off cancer are related to the immune system. He made the following observation:

Perhaps the phenomenon of homograft rejection will turn out to represent a primary mechanism for natural defense against neoplasia. . . . If this were the case, one might expect that a defect in the mechanism of delayed-type hypersensitivity would result in special susceptibility to cancer.*

* Lawrence, H. Sherwood (ed.): *Cellular and Humoral Aspects of the Hypersensitive States.* A Symposium held at the New York Academy of Medicine. Paul B. Hoeber, New York, 1959, p. 530.

There is today an increasing body of evidence that supports the validity of Thomas's prediction.

Albert Szent-Györgyi's theory about the cause and control of cancer, which is different from that of most researchers, is discussed briefly in Chapter 31 (see page 1386). He is searching for an agent that will inhibit the proliferation of cells, on the assumption that a cancer cell with its pathogenic tendency to multiply could be restored to a normal resting state.[12]

It is entirely conceivable that many systemic infections and cancer (if it is proved to belong in this category of disease) might be eradicated by an extension and application of what is known about vaccines and serums that produce immunity, drugs that cure early cases, diets that help to develop a resistance to disease, environmental factors, and methods and materials used to destroy pathogenic organisms.

Changing Emphases. It is an old story that, when bacteria were first found to cause disease, physicians and sanitarians thought the secret of control lay chiefly in the use of strong chemicals. Disinfection of the air was attempted. The public began to associate the smell of coal-tar products, such as carbolic acid and cresol, with safety from disease-producing bacteria, and hospitals were likely to reek of such drugs. A great variety of chemicals was manufactured, each one of which was believed to be effective in destroying all microorganisms. Fumigation with poisonous gases was used routinely in disinfecting rooms vacated by patients with communicable disease. Chemical disinfection was widely applied, and great confidence was placed in its efficacy.

Besides the emphasis on chemical disinfection, there was a general belief that bacteria thrived in dirty places, so that, in the attempt to control an epidemic of any kind, a great effort was made to clean up cities, towns, and individual houses. Edward Jenner demonstrated the effectiveness of vaccination with cowpox as a protection against smallpox in 1796, but the scientific principles of vaccination against any disease were laid down by Louis Pasteur and his associates during the 1870s and 1880s in what might be called the beginning of the modern program of communicable disease control. Shortly afterward came the knowledge that insects transfer infectious material from the sick to the well, and strenuous campaigns were launched against flies and mosquitoes.

Although none of these theories or practices has been discredited, some of them have been modified so that control measures are becoming more specific as more is learned about the nature of the organisms causing disease, their portals of entry to the body, the ways in which they are transmitted from person to person, and their resistance to physical and chemical agents.

Presently, emphasis is placed on the following preventive measures: (1) developing immunity to disease by general hygienic living, paying particular attention to an adequate diet; (2) using vaccines, particularly during periods of especial susceptibility; (3) isolating the sick individual, using a technique adapted to the type of disease from which the patient is suffering; (4) disinfecting (with a physical agent such as heat or light) or destroying contaminated dishes, toilet articles, linens, and other objects used by persons in common; (5) disposing of paper handkerchiefs in incinerators or general sewage system; (6) reducing bacterial content of air by natural ventilation and treating room air with ultraviolet light; (7) cleaning floors with a disinfectant solution, a chemically treated dust mop, or a filtered wet vacuum pick-up machine [13]; and (8) destroying the breeding places of insects and rodents that spread disease. These practices may vary from place to place and, of course, according to the disease in question. Physicians studying the control of tuberculosis, for example, think that much effort is wasted trying to disinfect objects used by a patient with this disease.[14] Currently, very few precautionary measures are suggested for hospitalized tuberculosis patients on drugs who learn how to cover their nose and mouth when coughing and sneezing.[15]

The value of light (particularly sunlight) in disinfecting room air has been accepted for many years; the use of ultraviolet rays, reverse isolation procedures, and Laminar Air Flow Rooms are some of the newer ways to protect patients from infections.

A Laminar Air Flow Room is a room within a room containing approximately 8½ by 10 ft of protective living space. The inner room has transparent walls, glove ports for patient access, and a bank of air filters. Normal room air passes through a prefilter, then through a bank of high efficiency particulate air filters before entering the inner room. The air then passes out through an open doorway and returns to the prefilter. Automatic controls permit the patient to operate a curtain that gives privacy, window curtains, and a television set, all of which are located outside the inner room.[16]

The results of numerous studies show these practices all have merit but they also have limitations. (See Chapter 15 for a discussion of making the environment relatively free from pathogenic microorganisms.)

2. CONTROL OF COMMUNICABLE DISEASE

Principles. The first step in communicable disease control (after initial identification) is to report it to the local health authority. Administrative practice as to which diseases are reported and how varies so much from one region to another that an American Public Health Association Committee has prepared a manual (now in its 12th edition) for health workers and others concerned with controlling infectious disease.[17]

Because uniformity in reporting permits comparison of data within a country and between nations, it is important to recognize that a system of reporting operates at four levels:

1. Collecting basic data in the local community where the disease occurs.
2. Assembling data at district, county, state, or provincial level.
3. Collecting total data nationally.
4. Reporting certain diseases by nations to the World Health Organization.[18]

The aforementioned manual distributes communicable diseases among five classes according to what practical benefit is to be derived from the reporting process. The classes and disease examples are as follows:

Class 1: Case Report Universally Required by International Health Regulations
Examples: cholera, plague, smallpox, yellow fever, typhus fever, relapsing fever, paralytic poliomyelitis, malaria

Class 2: Case Report Regularly Required Wherever the Disease Occurs (A. Report by telephone, telegraph; B. Report by most practical means)
Examples: typhoid fever, diphtheria, brucellosis, leprosy

Class 3: Selectively Reportable in Recognized Endemic Areas (A. Report by telephone, telegraph; B. Report by most practical means; C. Report by mail)
Examples: tularemia, scrub typhus, coccidioidomycosis, sandfly fever

Class 4: Obligatory Report of Epidemics—No Case Report Required
Examples: food poisoning, infectious keratoconjunctivitis, influenza

Class 5: Official Report Not Ordinarily Justifiable
Examples: common cold [19]

If any attack on communicable diseases is to be successful, it must be global; for in this way, worldwide assaults can be mounted that aim at eradicating disease. Coordination is now the responsibility of the World Health Organization in Geneva, Switzerland. This organization has established a worldwide network of institutions that can provide their national counterparts with such services as consultation, collection and analysis of information, assistance in the establishment of standards, production and distribution of standard or reference material, exchange of information, training, and organization of collaborative research.[20]

Gaylord W. Anderson and associates suggest that it is important for health workers to recognize the following six factors essential to the development of an infectious disease:

1. A causative or etiological agent
2. A reservoir or source of the causative agent
3. A mode of escape from the reservoir
4. A mode of transmission from the reservoir to the potential new host
5. A mode of entry into the new host
6. A susceptible host *

They say these represent a logical sequence of conditions that are essential to the development of infectious disease. If any one of these links is missing, disease will not ensue even though the other conditions may be present. Further discussion of the process by which diseases are transmitted can be found in this reference and under Additional Suggested Reading at the end of this chapter.

* Anderson, Gaylord W., et al.: *Communicable Disease Control.* Macmillan Publishing Co., Inc., New York, 1962, p. 19.

Factors Modifying Methods of Control. There are several factors affecting the ways in which nurses approach control of systemic infection. Among these are variations in methods used in different institutions, the seriousness of the disease under consideration, susceptibility of individuals or groups to be protected, and mode of transmission of the invading organism. Another factor modifying control—the susceptibility of different microorganisms to disinfecting agents—is discussed in Chapter 15.

It is often puzzling to see one set of precautions taken in handling a patient with one type of disease and an entirely different set followed in caring for a person with another communicable condition. And certain measures may be used to prevent infections among infants that are not used for adults. All health workers should be fortified with a knowledge of the underlying principles of microbiology so that they themselves can judge the reliability of procedures and build up their own method based on reason rather than cut-and-dried rules taught them by someone else.

Rules can be inadequate guides because methods must be adapted to the conditions as they exist; it is impossible to make a sufficient number of rules to fit all the situations nurses are likely to encounter. It is true that many of the differences in methods of communicable disease control are unjustifiable and represent confusion in the work and writings of those who should speak with authority, but certain differences in method indicate a thoughtful adaptation of practice to the demands of a particular set of circumstances.

When certain *serious diseases* are hard to detect and treat early, as, for example, leprosy, or when the disease rapidly assumes epidemic proportions in barracks, camps, ships, or schools, as, for example, meningococcal meningitis, more drastic efforts are made to isolate the person having the disease than when the condition tends to be a mild one, such as ringworm (dermatophytosis) or the common cold.

Leprosy is not highly infectious, and yet in some parts of the world lepers are segregated because the disease requires persistent treatment, is disfiguring, and evokes horror from the public. State laws to control leprosy differ. In New York, for example, persons with leprosy are not isolated; in others, as for example, Florida, isolation is "required." In Montana, admission to a national leprosarium is "advised" in most cases, although Montana's 1965 Regulation No. 40 specifies that treatment in the home community may be authorized with the approval of the health officer.[21-23] Since leprosy is endemic in warm rather than cold climates and seems to progress more rapidly in hot countries, there is a possibility that climate should be taken into account in the treatment of the disease.

Meningococcal meningitis is transmitted only on direct contact with the infected individual, and more often with carriers than with active cases; however, in many hospitals, the patient with this disease is completely isolated initially, even though invasion rarely causes systemic disease.

Ringworm, although unpleasant and hard to eradicate, is not considered a serious infection nor is it especially repellent in many of its forms. Therefore persons infected with ringworm are allowed to mix freely in society, although with severe cases of ringworm of the scalp (tinea capitis), the hair is covered with a cap after treatment, and children with ringworm of the body (tinea coporis) are excluded from gymnasiums and swimming pools.

The common cold, on the other hand, is highly contagious, but since this condition is often a mild one, many persons disregard methods of control. These examples illustrate the point that, whether it is sound reasoning or not, in practice, we usually stress measures of control and follow stricter regimens for persons having dangerous conditions than for those having highly communicable but milder diseases.

There are many circumstances that make *individuals susceptible* to infections. Newborns are particularly vulnerable, so that workers in hospital nurseries pay scrupulous attention to handwashing, often wear gowns, and isolate infants with infections; workers use extra precautions when caring for premature infants. It goes without saying that any worker who contracts an infection should stay away from newborn infants and others until the infection is over. The process of labor and delivery often predisposes a mother to infection. Special techniques are used in caring for the mother to prevent transmission of disease.

There are other conditions that make individuals susceptible to communicable disease in general or to some type of infection. Among them are: certain diseases such as diabetes mellitus, cancer, or blood disease; burns; treatment with certain drugs or radiation therapy that cause suppression of the immunologic process; organ-transplant surgery; open-heart surgery; and hemodialysis. Malnutrition lowers the resistance to almost any disease invasion, and this is also true of conditions that interfere with normal circulation. Children with certain anomalies are more prone to infections than others. Smoke from fires and irritating gases—such as ether—predispose the lungs to pneumonia, and anything that destroys the integrity of the skin invites infection. Old age, chronic debilitating disease, shock, coma, and trauma (accidental or surgical) also influence susceptibility. Nurses should be familiar with all well-established theories of infection proneness and should be alert to the necessity for special protection of vulnerable individuals or groups.

The *modes of transmission,* or routes by which pathogenic organisms leave the body of the sick and enter the body of the well person, are important factors to consider in setting up measures of prevention and control. Beland and Passos [24] suggest that health workers ask and try to answer the following questions each time they are faced with the question of disease transmission: Who should be protected from whom? From what and for how long is protection necessary? The answers can then become the basis for intelligent action.

Communicable diseases and appropriate measures of prevention may be grouped according to the manner in which the causative organisms are transmitted from the infected person to another individual. In *wound infections,* disease organisms leave the sick through discharges from the wound and enter the body of the second person through a break in the skin or mucous membrane. It is obvious that measures of control consist in keeping infected wounds covered; handling used dressings with forceps and gloves and immediately destroying them by disposing of them in a tightly closed, impervious plastic bag and then burning; disinfecting all instruments that come in contact with the wound; careful handwashing before and after patient contact; use of two sets of gloves—changing gloves and washing hands between removal of the old dressing and application of the new one; and taking every precaution to prevent breaks in the skin, particularly those of the hands. When wounds are dressed it is possible for microorganisms to pass from dressings and linen into the air and for the contaminated air to infect wounds. It is important, therefore, to use dust-suppressive measures and for workers to wear gowns when changing dressings (masks may be necessary also). Linen is disposed of through use of the double-bagging technique * and every effort is made to avoid vigorous movements when changing linen so as to minimize the dissemination of living microorganisms into the air.

---

* Double-bagging refers to a method for removing contaminated items from a contaminated to a clean area by placing those items in a securely closed bag which is then placed in a clean bag held by a "clean" individual just outside the patient's room. (See Chapter 15.)

In *infectious skin disease* everything the patient's skin touches—bedding, clothing, personal articles, and dishes—is handled as it would be if the patient had a contaminated wound or skin infection, using secretion and discharge precautions. (See Summary Table of Data, page 1752.) Workers who are obliged to handle contaminated objects are protected by wearing gloves or, if they are unavailable, by thorough hand-scrubbing with soap and water. Gowns, and sometimes masks, are worn to protect the worker caring for the patient with infectious skin disease, depending upon the amount of drainage and kind of organism present. In 1976, the Communicable Disease Center of the USPHS recommended strict isolation for wounds contaminated by *Staphylococcus aureus* and group A streptococcus microorganisms.[25]

Infections of the alimentary canal—diseases transmitted by discharges from the intestinal tract—comprise a third group. These are controlled by disinfecting dishes and toilet articles, or using disposable items; by double-bagging linens before removal for laundering; by disposal of urine, feces, liquids, and semisolid food waste into the general sewerage system for treatment, or disinfecting waste with an antimicrobial agent when a safe disposal system is unavailable. Patients' attendants wear gowns and often gloves when in direct contact with contaminated secretions, excreta, or equipment, and are careful to wash their hands after caring for the patient.

A similar category, or group, is *communicable diseases of the genital tract,* in which the danger lies in the discharges from this tract coming in contact with the mucous membranes of the well person. The *conjunctiva covering the eye* is susceptible to infection from the same bacteria that invade the genital tract— for example, the gonococcus and the staphylococcus. Attendants often wear eyeglasses when giving treatments such as irrigations, where splattering of infectious material is likely to occur. Articles containing discharges from either the genitalia or the eyes are disposed of in tightly closed plastic bags and then are incinerated. As in skin and intestinal diseases, any clothing, bedding, dishes, or other articles that may be soiled with discharges from the genitalia or eyes are handled with particular care. The attendants wear gowns and gloves while in actual contact with patients and wash their hands thoroughly after leaving them.

The last group includes *communicable diseases of the respiratory tract.* These diseases are spread by discharges from almost any portion of the respiratory mucosa. The organisms may be discharged through the mouth, nose, and the ears if the latter become infected and the drums are ruptured. Obviously, diseases of this class may be contracted by the well person if the causative organisms are deposited in the mouth or nose. Control consists of putting up a barrier, in the shape of a mask, between the noses and mouths of the sick and the well. Either the sick or the well person may wear the mask, however, occasionally it is more practical to mask the patient. Infected persons are taught to cover the nose and mouth with a paper handkerchief when coughing or sneezing, later to destroy it. The use of paper handkerchiefs, which can be burned or placed in toilets and hoppers, is now happily almost a routine habit among the sick and well. In addition to these precautions, special care is taken to dispose of in an impervious plastic bag, or to incinerate all articles containing secretions from the nose, throat, eyes, and ears; all dishes and toilet articles, unless disposable, are disinfected; linen is double-bagged and mattresses and pillows are covered with an impervious plastic material which can either be laundered or cleaned with a germicidal solution. Attendants are careful to wash their hands before and after leaving the patient with a communicable respiratory disease. Dust control by disinfecting floors and bedding and the reduction of air bacteria by sunlight, ultraviolet light, and air filters may also be part of the program. Some hospitals have built special "life-island" units to completely isolate a patient with an infection, or with susceptibility to an infection, such as a faulty immunologic system, by enclosing him or her in four walls of plastic with their own filtered, sterilized air supply. A child in a Texas hospital has lived in such an isolated environment from birth to school age without serious psychological impairment. The previously described Laminar Air Flow Room (see page 1709) is an example of a method of protecting the patient from contracting an infection. There are advantages and disadvantages to the attendants and the patient under these circumstances.

It is important, however, if the mode of transmission of an organism is undetermined, to observe strict precautions. It was the practice in some institutions to get cultures from the nose, throat, and stool of all new employees, and sometimes routinely thereafter, so as to discover persons who are carriers of infectious organisms. It is thought now, however, that routine culturing of employees is unnecessary unless an outbreak of infection occurs.

A summary of information from a manual developed by the USPHS Center for Disease Control, Atlanta, Ga., is presented in Table 44-1. It is noticeable that one safeguard is

Table 44-1. Isolation Techniques for Use in Hospitals *

Classification	Examples of Diseases	Private Room	Gowns	Masks	Hand Washing	Gloves	Special Handling of Articles
Isolation							
1. Strict	Burns, extensive infected Staphylococcal pneumonia Diphtheria	X	X	X	X	X	X
2. Respiratory	Tuberculosis, pulmonary (positive sputum) Mumps Rubella	X		X	X		X
3. Protective	Agranulocytosis Patients receiving immunosuppressants Severe dermatitis	X	X	X	X	X	X†
Precautions							
4. Enteric	Cholera *E. coli* gastroenteritis Hepatitis, viral (infectious or serum)	X‡	X		X	X	X
5. Wound and Skin	Impetigo Wound infections Burns, extensive, uninfected	X§	X	X‖	X	X	X
6. Discharges							
A. Secretion— lesion	Gonorrhea				X		X
B. Secretion— oral	Streptococcal pharyngitis				X		X
C. Excretion	Poliomyelitis				X		

* Summarized from US Public Health Service: *Isolation Techniques for Use in Hospitals.* (Prepared by Center for Disease Control, Hospital Infections Section, Bacterial Diseases Branch, Epidemiology Program, Atlanta, Ga.) US Government Printing Office, Washington, D.C.,1970 (PHS Pub. No. 2054).
† Possibly some exceptions to disinfecting articles brought into the patient's room.
‡ Private room for children only.
§ Private room desirable.
‖ Masks worn during dressing changes.

common to all groups, namely, that the attendants *always wash their hands* before and after caring for a patient "on isolation" or "on precautions." As a matter of fact, it is generally agreed that for sanitary reasons all health workers should wash their hands before and after giving care to any patient or handling any objects that they have touched, whether they are believed to have communicable diseases or not. Undoubtedly *handwashing* is the single most important preventive measure to employ when caring for any patient with any infection.[26]

Further description of current methods of control may be found in a later section of this chapter.

Although the mode of transmission deter-mines very largely *what* shall be disinfected, it is the type of organism to be killed that influences the selection of the disinfecting agent. Dishes and linens should be so handled in communal living, or in public places, that they are decontaminated after each use. Again, the reader is referred to Chapter 15 for a discussion of the susceptibility of different microorganisms to various disinfecting agents.

3. PREVENTION

Epidemiology. The contributions of epidemiology to preventive medicine have been universally recognized and accepted. Hugh R. Leavell and E. Gurney Clark [27] call epidemiology an orderly means of describing what is known about the natural history of a disease and also suggest that it is a scientific method for filling in gaps in knowledge about factors in the natural history. Epidemiologic methods of studying infectious diseases have been developed that, if universally practiced, would control, if not eradicate, diseases caused by living organisms. So dramatic are the results of these methods that they have come to be the basis for controlling other conditions, as, for example, nutritional deficiencies, cardiovascular disease, cancer, mental disorders, and accidents. As the approach developed in this field has been adapted to others, however, it has also been modified so that there is equal emphasis on conditions within and without the human organism.

The modern concept of epidemiology derives from *epidēmios*, which, literally translated from the Greek, means "upon the population." Philip E. Sartwell[28] defines it as the study of the distribution and dynamics of diseases in human populations. John R. Paul says epidemiology is

. . . concerned with measurements of the circumstances under which diseases occur, where diseases tend to flourish, and where they do not. Such circumstances may be microbiological or toxicological; they may be based on genetic, social, or environmental factors; even religious or political factors may come under scrutiny, provided they are found to have some bearing upon disease prevalence.*

Leavell and Clark also say it is "a field of science which is concerned with the various factors and conditions that determine the occurrence and distribution of health, disease, defect, disability, and death among groups of individuals."† No matter which definition is applied, the differences are seen to be ones of degree only. Whether the focus is on the disease or if disease is included in a broader spectrum of human concern, the definitions indicate a multiplicity of influencing factors.

Ecology, the study of mutual relations among organisms and between them and their environment, also recognizes the multiform causation of disease. This science acknowledges poor environment, for example, or deficient genetic endowment as underlying contributors to disease, but implies an interaction of people with their environments that is not yet fully understood.[29] In contrast, the emphasis in epidemiology is on the interaction between the host, the agent, and the environment, and its description relies upon the characteristics of time (when) and place (where) and the persons themselves affected (who).[30]

One of the early epidemiologic studies was John Snow's classic description of a cholera epidemic in London in 1854. He pointed to the Broad Street pump, which was supplying water to his dying patients, as the culprit, even though the organism causing cholera had not yet been identified.[31] Florence Nightingale herself could be considered an epidemiologist. At about the time of Snow's investigation she was nursing soldiers in the Crimea, and, knowing nothing of "the germ theory," was able to reduce the death rate among the men simply by keeping the environment clean with soap and water, using clean linens, feeding patients clean food and drink, and in general providing humane treatment.

Present-day epidemiologic research includes studying the incidence of the defect or disease in a totally defined population group, encompassing both its sick and well members. An example of modern-day epidemiologic research was the attempt in 1976 to determine the cause of "Legionnaire's Disease," a mysterious illness causing sickness and death among a population of conventioneers in Philadelphia, Pa.[31a] It also includes analyses of the distribution of disease according to climate, season, weather, geographic units such as city, state, or nation, and age, sex, race, occupational, socioeconomic, marital, and often educational status. Some studies have involved detailed physical measurements that might serve as a basis for typing the individuals or temperaments susceptible to carcinoma of the cervix, tuberculosis, hypertension, or schizophrenia, for example.

Modern epidemiology not only tells us what diseases are found where and in what numbers, but it goes further in suggesting diagnostic procedures and treatment. Just as these studies led to the recognition of the mosquito as the carrier of malaria or viral encephalitis, the epidemiologic studies of lung cancer suggested its relationship to smoking and the respiratory irritants in urban life. Research in schizophrenia offered some clues to the social conditions that may have produced it, and studies of accidents pointed to internal states that made the individual "accident prone."

Prevention of disease follows the same pattern regardless of the cause, although modern man has been most successful in preventing the infectious diseases, because his knowledge of their causes is most specific. After the identification of the agent of disease, and the conditions within the environment and the host that

---

* Paul, John R.: *Clinical Epidemiology*, rev. ed. University of Chicago Press, Chicago, 1966, p. 4.

† Leavell, Hugh R., and Clark, E. Gurney: *Preventive Medicine for the Doctor in His Community*, 3rd ed. McGraw-Hill Book Co., New York, 1965, p. 40.

make it possible for the agent successfully to invade and attack the host, a preventive program can be launched that (1) removes or destroys the agent or (2) renders the host immune to its attack. Most programs are a combination of these measures. One disease after another has been brought under control in this way. In the United States, diphtheria, smallpox, and typhoid fever are no longer feared, chiefly because the host has been immunized against the agent of the disease through the use of vaccines; dysenteric disease, hookworm, and malaria are examples that, on the other hand, are less feared because the conditions in the environment that enabled the agent to invade the host have been modified by improved sanitation.

In Chapter 2 it was pointed out that in 1900 pneumonia, tuberculosis, diarrhea and enteritis, and diphtheria were included among the ten leading causes of death, whereas in 1973 only the acute and chronic respiratory infections—influenza and pneumonia, and bronchitis, emphysema, and asthma—remain on the list. In order of rank this group now is preceded by major cardiovascular diseases, malignancies, and accidents.[32] Even with so great accomplishment to the credit of bacteriologists, sanitarians, health legislators, and health workers, however, there are still many thousands of preventable deaths caused by infectious diseases or their sequelae. As mentioned earlier, we need not only an extension of knowledge but also a more thorough application of measures whose values have been demonstrated. USDHEW's Center for Disease Control (Atlanta, Ga.) periodically publishes recommendations, for example, for syphilis treatment, which an Advisory Committee establishes after consultation with therapy experts.[32a]

Science can never rest on its laurels. There is evidence that flies and other insect vectors have acquired an immunity to DDT, and that DDT itself has a devastating effect on the environment. All of this means that the struggle against disease is an unending one and that it is probably a mistake to think of any disease as conquered once and for all. Prevention, therefore, depends upon epidemiologic and clinical research, the implementation of these findings, and most particularly *public education*. In our judgment more depends on what the average citizen knows and does than what the expert knows and does. Observers in mainland China often comment on the attitudes and behavior of children that help account for the reduced incidence of disease.[33-35]

Nurses have taken an increasingly active part in all aspects of preventive programs. For example, they have played a major role in mass immunization campaigns to protect the public against polio, measles, and rubella. They have participated in blood donor activities designed to help prevent serious complications following trauma or surgery. The success of public health nurses in finding persons infected with communicable disease is admittedly second to none, and their daily contacts with individuals everywhere has done more to teach the average citizen the means of controlling infection than any other form of education. A large part of the successful care of infectious patients is the protection of others. In the United States nurses, more than any others, enforce rigid aseptic techniques to prevent the spread of disease.

Nurses must continually extend their knowledge as the causes of disease are discovered and as methods of prevention and treatment are developed. This is such a rapidly developing field that health agencies often prepare nurses to act as communicable disease specialists and to direct the periodic revision of control practices within the agency. The nurse-epidemiologist in the hospital is one example of such a specialist. In a 1967 Conference on the Legal Aspects of Infection Control, it was recommended that an active Infection Control Committee become a part of every modern hospital system. The Committee's charge was to support a nurse-epidemiologist whose function would be to prevent epidemics of infections in hospitals.[36] Today most large hospitals have carried out this recommendation.

Public health nursing agencies have now come to rely less on nurse specialists in communicable disease control, but they incorporate the principles of disease control in all of their nursing practice. There should be continuing education programs on disease control available to health workers and interested citizens in every community.

Aspects of Prevention. Prevention can be thought of as consisting of three levels where preventive measures are applied, as shown in Figure 44-5. The first level—primary prevention—consists of health promotion and specific prevention, some examples of which are health education, counseling, and immunization. Secondary prevention, at level two, consists of early diagnosis and prompt treatment, and disability limitation. At this level an effort is made to find and treat disease and to prevent complications. Rehabilitation, at level three, is tertiary prevention where the potential of each individual is maximized through retraining and work therapy programs.[37]

Among the measures used in the control of infectious disease, the following factors should be stressed. They demand the establishment of

THE NATURAL HISTORY OF ANY DISEASE OF MAN

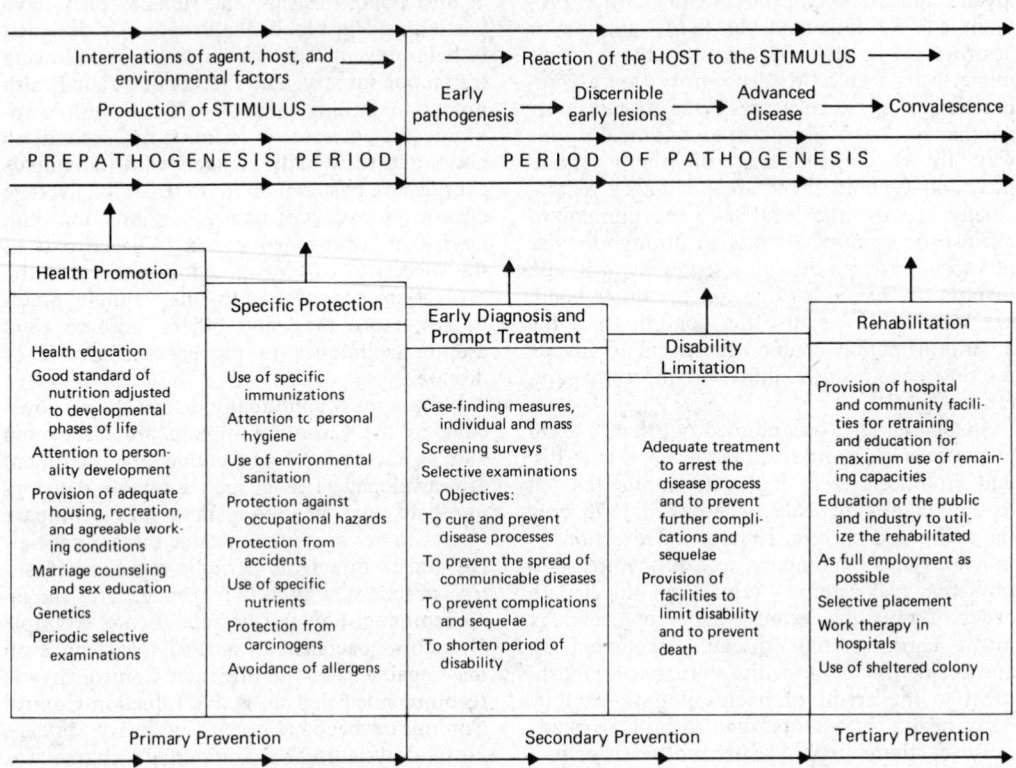

Figure 44-5. Levels of application of preventive measures in the natural history of disease. (Leavell, Hugh R., and Clark, E. Gurney: *Preventive Medicine for the Doctor in His Community,* 3rd ed. McGraw-Hill Book Co., New York, 1965, p. 21.)

laws and public health regulations to enforce many of them.

1. Providing a sanitary environment including clean food, milk, and water, safe disposal of sewage and waste, and satisfactory vector control.
2. Reporting infectious disease, the use of isolation and quarantine, selective immunization by administration of protective vaccines and sera, and the use of effective control techniques.
3. Health education in homes, industry, schools, and health agencies.
4. A system of records and statistics, and epidemiologic research.
5. A program of detection or case finding through multiphasic screening, with emphasis on recognition of early symptoms, predisposition, or susceptibility to disease.
6. Health promotion through adequate nutrition, healthful living, satisfactory housing,

recreation, and working conditions, and protection from excessive fatigue and emotional stress.

Current Methods. The provision of a sanitary environment has been discussed in Chapter 15, and might be reviewed in conjunction with this chapter. Reporting infectious disease is the responsibility of the physician or nurse who makes the diagnosis, or their associates. Nurses (in fact, any citizen) are negligent if they do not report to the physician, or to a public health official, a client who they have reason to believe is suffering from an untreated communicable disease.

The American Public Health Association defines *isolation* as

. . . the separation, for the period of communicability, of infected persons or animals from others, in such places and under such conditions as will prevent the direct or indirect conveyance of the infectious agent from those infected to those who are susceptible or who may spread the agent to others.*

After isolation, there may be required immunization of persons known to have been in contact with the infected individual, as in smallpox, for example, or an investigation of those persons in contact with someone having been diagnosed as having pulmonary tuberculosis, for example. Ordinarily, however, there are few requirements for isolation or quarantine of "contacts" or associates of an infected person.

As described in Table 44-1, isolation, when practiced in the hospital, can be classified into three groups: strict isolation, respiratory isolation, and protective isolation. Precautions, also, can be subdivided into three groups: enteric precautions, wound and skin precautions, and secretion and discharge precautions (including lesion and oral secretions and excretions).

Strict isolation requires (1) that the patient be in a private room protected from vectors of disease and provided with both handwashing and toilet (including bathing) facilities; (2) that there be restriction of visitors to the immediate family, only two at a time, and that they understand and use strict gown, mask, and glove techniques; (3) that attendants and visitors wear a fresh gown and mask on entering the room and that hands be washed before entering and after leaving (and as otherwise indicated during patient care), and that gloves be used routinely by all personnel before entering and until leaving the room; (4) that personnel caring for the patient maintain up-to-date immunization status; (5) that provision be made for disposition in impervious plastic bags of all dressings and tissues soiled with discharges from the patient, and that they be subsequently incinerated; (6) that there be special handling of linens and patient's clothing after use through double-bagging technique and sterilization; (7) that there be disinfection of objects contaminated by the patient prior to their removal from the contaminated areas; (8) that disposable needles and syringes be used, and, if possible, disposable thermometer, dishes, water carafe and drinking glass, or subsequent disinfection or sterilization of these articles; (9) that there be disposal of the patient's urine and feces into the regular sewerage system, or, if a portable utensil is used, thorough cleaning of it before replacing it at the bedside; (10) that there be double-bagging of

* Benenson, Abram S. (ed.): *Control of Communicable Diseases in Man,* 12th ed. American Public Health Association, Washington, D.C., 1975, p. 382.

laboratory specimens labeled *Contaminated* to warn laboratory personnel of potential danger; and (11) that there be concurrent cleaning and terminal disinfection of the patient's room by using disposable wiping cloths and cleansing solution, and disinfection of the cleaning equipment. Some diseases for which strict isolation is required are inhalation anthrax; extensive, staphylococcal, or streptococcal (group A) infected burns; diphtheria; generalized and progressive vaccinia; disseminated herpes zoster; varicella (chickenpox); Lassa fever; Marburg virus disease; rabies; congenital rubella syndrome; variola (smallpox); major *Staphylococcus aureus* and streptococcus (group A) wound infections; staphylococcal pneumonia; streptococcal pneumonia.[38]

As can be seen in Table 44-1 on page 1713, respiratory isolation omits the use of a gown and gloves but requires a mask and disinfection of articles contaminated with secretions. Protective isolation omits special handling of excreta and secretions and of some articles brought into the patient's room but requires that a gown and mask be worn by all persons entering the room, and gloves by those having direct patient contact. Precautions for enteric diseases, and wound, skin, and secretion discharges require the use of different methods for each.

Currently there is a trend away from caring for patients with infectious diseases in specialized communicable disease hospitals or tuberculosis sanatoria and more emphasis on caring for them in the general hospital or at home. In public health practice, isolation follows most of the above requirements. Modified isolation, however, is often indicated and, in such instances, the local health officer prescribes the isolation technique to be followed, depending upon the disease. In New York State, for example, authorities urge families to keep at home those with the most highly communicable diseases (examples are measles, chickenpox, streptococcal sore throat) if they are uncomplicated by conditions that demand hospitalization.[39]

Quarantine is a term derived from the practice of keeping offshore for forty days a ship suspected of carrying infection. Now it is used to mean limiting the freedom of a person who has been exposed to a communicable disease until the incubation period has passed. Some state laws require quarantine for more diseases than others. California, for example, confined its list in 1971 for *complete quarantine* to persons exposed to cholera, plague, and smallpox, and to infants exposed to enteropathogenic diarrhea and diarrhea of the newborn; for *modified quarantine* to diphtheria until nose and throat cultures are negative, and "contacts" handling food or working with children; to measles in sparsely settled, nonendemic areas; to whooping cough for nonimmune children; to salmonellosis, shigellosis, and typhoid fever for contacts acting as food handlers; for *personal surveillance* to meningococcal meningitis; to louse-borne typhus fever and relapsing fever until after application of insecticide with residual effect; for *segregation* in those instances when it is important to remove susceptible children to homes of immune persons, or establishment of a sanitary boundary to protect uninfected from infected members of a population.[40]*

Incubation period is generally defined as the time interval between the exposure of an individual to an infectious agent and the appearance of the first sign or symptom of the disease. Learning the supposed incubation periods of the communicable diseases is difficult. It is often helpful to consult a manual such as the one published by the American Public Health Association † or manuals supplied by many local or state health departments. The Summary Table of Data on page 1742 also lists incubation periods, which are approximations, of course. The length of the incubation period depends upon the nature of the parasite, the strength of the invading agent, and the response of the host. Sartwell says:

Each disease has its characteristic incubation period, which seems to depend largely on the rate of proliferation of the particular agent. It also depends, with some exceptions, on whether the agent multiplies exclusively at or near the portal of entry, in which case it is usually brief (e.g., staphylococcal skin infections, gonorrhea, diphtheria) or at remote sites (typhus fever, infectious hepatitis) when it tends to be longer. The speed with which host defenses are mobilized also can play a role not only in the incubation period but in the type of response; thus the previously sensitized host reacts faster and in different fashion at the site of infection with tubercle bacilli or vaccinia virus than the one experiencing such infection for the first time.

. . .

Dosage of the infectious agent is a factor which demonstrably affects the length of the incubation period, but experimental work indicates that this is not the only factor, for variation persists when the infective dose is kept as constant as possible.‡

* Definitions for these terms can be found in Benenson, Abram S. (ed.): *Control of Communicable Diseases in Man,* 12th ed., American Public Health Association, Washington, D.C., 1975, p. 384.
  † Benenson, Abram S. (ed.): *op. cit.,* p. 382.
  ‡ Sartwell, Philip E. (ed.): *Maxcy-Rosenau Preventive Medicine and Public Health,* 10th ed. Appleton-Century-Crofts, New York, 1973, p. 42.

Immunization to communicable disease is so generally practiced these days that most adults have some knowledge of the procedure even though they may not understand the biologic process involved. Each of the infectious diseases is a *specific disease;* that is, each has a specific cause and the organism causing it has its own characteristics, its definite mode of attack, its mode of living, and its means of transmission. Protection of the individual from each disease, whether by natural immunity or immunity acquired by artificial means, is also specific. A newborn baby is born with immunity, or antibodies derived from its mother's body fluids that temporarily protect it from some diseases. Examples of these are measles and mumps. The infant is highly susceptible to the pathogen *Escherichia coli,* the viruses of herpes simplex, and the protozoan of toxoplasmosis.[41] A Classification of Immunity is presented in Table 44-2 and the reader may refer to this summary. If readers wish more detailed information than is provided in Table 44-2, they should consult one of the texts listed at the end of this chapter.

In giving vaccines and serums, one must decide whether active or passive immunity is indicated. Being vaccinated or having had actual attacks of the disease excites the body to form agents (antigens) that stimulate the production of antibodies that protect it against the bacteria or virus. This is what is meant by active immunity. Immune serums or serums containing the specific antibodies that were produced in other persons or in animals when introduced into another body confer immunity. This process is known as passive immunity. It is not dependent upon the reaction of the body to the organism.

Nurses work with physicians, and, in some cases, independently, in giving tests and vaccines, noting reactions to the various materials, helping to dissipate ignorance of and apathy toward immunization, and promoting a desire on the part of individuals and families for prophylactic measures. Immunization practice is continuously changing, and nurses must be able to understand and interpret the changes. Mothers will often disregard immunization of young infants and may ignore medical advice unless they can be helped to understand the reasons for these preventive measures.

In 1975 the Committee on Infectious Diseases of the American Academy of Pediatrics recommended the immunization schedule shown in Table 44-3.

Perhaps all persons should have an immunization record as part of the health history that remains in their possession. This might include data kept by schools and employing agencies.

Table 44-2.   Classification of Immunity *

Natural Immunity			Acquired Immunity		
Naturally Acquired	Inherited	Naturally Acquired	Artificially Acquired		
Passive	Species	Active	Active		Passive
Example: newborns with transplacental antibodies from mother	Racial Individual Example: resistance of Jewish race to tuberculosis	Example: an attack of measles, mumps, or chickenpox	Vaccines Toxoids a. Nonreplicating antigens (killed bacteria, rickettsiae, or viruses) Examples: typhoid, typhus, pertussis, or rabies vaccine b. Inanimate antigens (toxoids and polysaccharides) Examples: diphtheria or tetanus toxoid; pneumococci polysaccharide c. Replicating antigens (living bacteria and viruses) Examples: bacillus Calmette-Guerin (BCG) for tuberculosis; yellow fever, smallpox, measles, mumps, polio (Sabin), or rubella vaccine		Antitoxins Antiserums Immune serums: a. Antibacterial Example: pneumonia b. Antitoxic Examples: diphtheria, tetanus, or gas gangrene c. Gamma globulin Examples: measles, rubella, or hepatitis d. Hyperimmune gamma globulin Example: pertussis

* Summarized from Johnson, Dorothy F.: *Essentials of Communicable Disease with Nursing Principles.* C. V. Mosby Company, St. Louis, 1968, pp. 41–45; and Leavell, Hugh R., and Clark, E. Gurney; *Preventive Medicine for the Doctor in His Community,* 3rd ed. McGraw-Hill Book Company, New York, 1965, p. 140.

Figure 44-6 shows the form used by the Mobil Oil Corporation on which the immunization records of its employees are kept.

For persons who are traveling from one country to another and who wish to know what protection they should seek, a periodical is prepared yearly by the US Public Health Service titled *Health Information for International Travel* (DHEW Pub. No. [CDC] 76–8280, Supplement to *Morbidity and Mortality Weekly Report,* Vol. 24, Dec. 1975, Center for Disease Control, Atlanta, Ga.). It provides information on required and recommended immunizations for international travel in over 160 countries as agreed upon in that committee of the World Health Organization concerned with communicable disease control. Because some countries change requirements from time to time as the incidence of disease warrants,* it is wise to get the current edition of the booklet or ask local or state health departments or the Bureau of Epidemiology of the Center for Disease Control (Atlanta, Ga. 30333) for specific directions. A summary of US Public Health Service recommendations is presented in the Appendix.

The nurse is usually responsible for giving immunizing agents. Pediatric and family nurse practitioners and often community health nurses are now determining when tests and vaccines are indicated, and are providing these

* In 1971, the US Public Health Service, for example, lifted the requirement for smallpox vaccination for all travelers reentering the United States, except those coming from a foreign country where smallpox had not been eradicated. Only Ethiopia has reported any smallpox in 1976.

Table 44-3. Schedule for Active Immunization and Tuberculin Testing of Normal Infants and Children in the United States Recommended by the American Academy of Pediatrics *

Age	Vaccines and Toxoide
2 months	Diphtheria and tetanus toxoids combined with pertussis vaccine (DTP) (injectable) Trivalent oral poliomyelitis virus vaccine (TOPV) (Suitable for breast-fed as well as bottle-fed infants)
4 months	Repeated as above
6 months	Repeated as above
1 year	Tuberculin test. Frequency of test depends on risk of exposure and prevalence of tuberculosis in the population. Measles vaccine or combined vaccines: measles-rubella or measles-mumps-rubella
1–12 years	Rubella vaccine or combined as above Mumps vaccine or combined as above
1½ years	Diphtheria and tetanus toxoids combined with pertussis vaccine (DTP) (injectable) Trivalent oral poliomyelitis virus vaccine (TOPV) (Repeated at this age as supplementary doses to increase immunity, called "boosters")
4–6 years	Repeated as above
14–16 years	Combined tetanus and diphtheria toxoids (adult type) (Td) (Repeated every 10 years)

* Adapted from "Revised Schedule for Active Immunization and Tuberculin Testing of Normal Infants and Children in the United States." A 1975 addendum to the *Report of the Committee on Infectious Diseases,* 16th rev. ed. American Academy of Pediatrics, Evanston, Ill., 1970, p. 5.

immunizations as part of well-child care. In all instances nurses are responsible for examining the patient before administration and after giving these agents to evaluate the local and systemic response. Explicit directions for their administration accompany most biologic preparations. It is important that the preparation be fresh, and used before the expiration date specified on the container. Biologic agents should be stored at the temperature recommended by the manufacturer and, once opened, discarded within the designated time limit. Unused yellow fever vaccine, for example, is discarded within 1 hour of its reconstitution as it loses its effectiveness if held open longer.[42] Agents should be given at room temperature because they are less irritating than when they are injected cold.

Education of the public in the control of disease has progressed to such a point in this country that even school children are aware of the dangers of using drinking vessels in common, or of failing to protect a wound. Teachers, biologists, sanitarians, health legislators, doctors, nurses, and nearly all categories of health workers have contributed toward the public awareness, but probably none of them is called upon more consistently than the nurse for specific information and particularly for

personal instruction and demonstration of control measures. Federal, state, and local public health agencies have a wealth of teaching materials, as do voluntary health agencies devoted to the control of particular diseases such as tuberculosis. A number of life insurance companies spend large sums on educational materials. The nurse is most effective when she has command of an extensive body of information that enables her to answer accurately the questions that patients and their families ask. Since, however, she cannot hope to have all the data they need at the tip of her tongue, nor has she time to impart it, she should be able to use and suggest to others the printed and audiovisual sources of information that are available. Medical libraries, designed primarily to serve physicians, are giving way to health science libraries designed to serve all those concerned with health promotion, disease prevention, and treatment. Some health science libraries are now open to the public. As knowledge of health becomes more general the interests of health workers and the public merge, and it is increasingly difficult to separate books, articles, and audiovisual materials for "professional" and "lay" consumption.

There is a division, or department, of research or disease investigation in every health

IMMUNIZATION RECORD

CO-1949A (6-64)

EMPLOYEE

DATE	REMARKS	INITIALS	DATE	REMARKS	INITIALS
	SMALL POX				
	TYPHOID-PARATYPHOID				
	TETANUS & DIPHTHERIA TOXOIDS				
	POLIO				
	CHOLERA				
	TYPHUS				
	YELLOW FEVER				

Figure 44-6. Employee immunization record form. (Courtesy of the Mobil Oil Corporation, New York, N.Y.)

agency concerned with communicable disease control, although the programs range from very limited to very extensive ones. All nurses employed in these agencies contribute to these programs through the records they keep; some nurses are employed full time on investigation. There is a great need for nurses trained to take an active part in this kind of research.

Case finding or detection is an integral part of all communicable disease programs. In this,

EMPLOYEE

DATE	REMARKS	INITIALS	DATE	REMARKS	INITIALS
ALLERGIES					
OTHER					

Figure 44-6. (Continued).

interviewing is a skill that is particularly important to nurses who are trying to find persons who have been exposed to infectious disease, especially tuberculosis, syphilis, and gonorrhea. Actually, skillful interviewing is a tool that every nurse should possess.[43]

Finally, communicable disease, as is the case with all disease, must be controlled by improving the individual health status. It is the theory of the "organic gardener" that the production of healthy plants, rather than insect control, is the key to good crops. While it is debatable whether healthy plants and animals can always resist invasion of parasitic organisms, the resistance of the host is a major factor in all infections. The known susceptibility of certain pathogenic microorganisms to the slightest change in the pH of laboratory culture media suggests the basis on which overindulgence in sweets, for example, may predispose a person to infection. The known relationship between disease and dietary deficiencies has been discussed in Chapter 10 and elsewhere. The provision of an adequate diet is the cornerstone on which every health program rests. Another body state that affects susceptibility to all diseases, including those produced by microorganisms, is fatigue, whether it is caused by lack of sleep, overexertion, or nervous tension. The effects of these conditions have been discussed in Chapter 13 and elsewhere in this text and will not be elaborated upon here. Every student of physiology is probably ready to accept the existence of a relationship between physical and emotional fatigue and almost every classification of disease.

4. TREATMENT AND NURSING CARE

General Principles. Therapy in communicable disease has many common elements because the diseases have a common causation —a living organism. Therapy is aimed at killing or destroying the potency of such organisms. When the causative organism has been isolated and/or when a therapeutic agent has been discovered, the plan of therapy is relatively simple; when the organism is unknown and when there is no effective therapeutic agent, treatment can only be symptomatic. Organisms producing disease in man vary so greatly in their character and in the tissues they affect that the symptoms, or the pathologic changes, have a wide range. They can, however, be categorized into (1) local tissue changes and (2) the systemic manifestations produced by the toxic products of the causative organisms. These toxins are carried throughout the body in the circulating fluids. "Symptoms" of infection are interrelated and are most realistically seen as syndromes. Of these groups of related symptoms, *fever* is the most common. Unchecked infections of certain organisms may produce bacteremia or septicemia.

When an effective therapeutic agent is known and available, therapy is usually simple and recovery rapid. Nursing care in such cases is relatively less complex and less important than when recovery depends on supporting nature in her defensive mechanisms. In the past few years, the number of infections that fail to respond to drugs and antimicrobial agents has rapidly diminished, yet new organisms and new drugs to combat them have appeared. A fictional description of modern medicine's fight to battle an obscure infection against overwhelming odds is contained in a chapter of Michael Crichton's book *Five Patients—The Hospital Explained.*[44] This experience shows why nursing care in systemic infections poses a constant challenge.

The development of chemicals and antibiotics that have a specific effect upon pathogenic organisms has not only shortened the duration of illness but has cut down the period of communicability of the disease so that many isolation and quarantine regulations have been abandoned. Few state or local health departments have applied all the new developments in clinical microbiology, and there continues to be wide variation in public health regulations. While this lag in the application of knowledge may be inevitable, it can be reduced by constructive criticism and suggestion. Informed nurses in administration are helping to change the regimen of patients in hospitals and homes by presenting new methods based upon research in nursing and medicine.

Regardless of the nature of the infection, the following principles apply to treatment and nursing care:

1. Identifying the invading organism, if possible.
2. Administering a therapeutic agent that kills, destroys, or decreases the pathogenicity of the organism, if the organism is identified and a specific agent is available. (The therapeutic agent may be applied locally or given by mouth and/or parenterally.)
3. Identifying and relieving symptoms, particularly those of fever.
4. Giving supportive care essential in any illness when the patient is unable to provide for his needs.
5. Preventing the transmission of the patient's infection to other persons.

The responsibility for carrying out the foregoing is shared by the members of the health team, the patient, and his family, as discussed in Chapter 8. Diagnostic methods were discussed in Chapter 7, and to some extent in Chapter 5. Details about particular diseases can be found in texts listed at the end of this chapter.

Because it plays such a prominent role in the program of communicable disease control, and because it is always changing, the use of chemotherapeutic agents and antimicrobial agents is summarized in the following pages.*

Chemotherapy of Microbial Diseases. Louis S. Goodman and Alfred Gilman *define* antibiotics as "chemical substances produced by various aspects of microorganisms (bacteria, fungi, actinomyces) that suppress the growth of other microorganisms and may eventually destroy them." Although the total number of antibiotics now extends into the hundreds, over 40 have been developed to the stage where they are of value in the therapy of infectious diseases.

A note of caution about these agents has been introduced by John M. Adams, who warns that widespread indiscriminate use of drugs, particularly antibiotics, for most respiratory infections is *not* indicated. He says that when secondary or complicating signs are evident or suspected, wise choice of an antibiotic can usually be made.[45]

Some of the major antimicrobial agents in use today are found in Table 44-4. Goodman and Gilman stress that choice of specific agents for the treatment of various infections is always subject to some disagreement among physicians. They also say that it is important to recognize that as more information accumulates, as newer drugs are used over a longer period of time, and as newer agents are discovered, some modifications will inevitably be made in these choices.

1. *Sulfonamides and Trimethoprim-Sulfamethoxazole.* The sulfonamides were the first effective chemotherapeutic agents to be employed for the prevention and cure of bacterial infections in man. Today they continue to occupy an important yet relatively small place in the therapeutic regimen but, in some instances, are more effective than other antimicrobial agents. They include a number of derivatives of para-amino-benzene-sulfonamide (sulfanilamide). More than 5400 congeneric substances were synthesized and studied in the 10-year period following the discovery of sulfanilamide, which was first prepared in 1908. However, less than a score of the sulfanilamides have attained any therapeutic importance. Now sulfonamide-resistant organisms have reduced the effectiveness of these drugs but they are useful agents in the management of uncomplicated infections of the urinary tract and certain other infections such as nocardiosis and chan-

croid, and as an alternative drug in other instances. The introduction of trimethoprim in combination with sulfamethoxazole is an important advance, demonstrating that these drugs together produce a supra-additive effect and broader therapeutic usefulness.

2. *Penicillins and Cephalosporins.* Penicillin, discovered by Fleming in 1928, is one of the most important antibiotics and probably the one most widely used in the treatment of infections. The first clinical trial of penicillin in the United States was given at New Haven Hospital (Yale University) in 1942 for a patient with septic abortion. Several of the early natural penicillins (designated by Roman numerals in England and by capital letters in the United States) proved to be inferior to the penicillin discovered and given the letter G. Penicillin G became the master standard for unit dosage in 1944 and all major classes of penicillin preparations contain mainly, or only, penicillin G for parenteral administration. Penicillin V is preferred for oral treatment of infections. Penicillin is one of the most potent of all the antimicrobial agents and is very effective in the treatment of streptococcal and staphylococcal infections, and diseases caused by gram-positive and certain gram-negative bacilli. Among diseases in which it is the drug of choice are meningococcal meningitis, pneumococcal pneumonia, anthrax, tetanus, gas gangrene, erysipelas, diphtheria, Weil's disease, gonorrhea, actinomycosis, syphilis, and yaws. It is used as a prophylaxis in patients who have had rheumatic fever and those with rheumatic or congenital heart disease who are undergoing certain surgical procedures. It is the drug of choice in *Salmonella typhi* carriers. Some of the penicillins are penicillin V, phenethicillin, methicillin, oxacillin, cloxacillin, dicloxacillin, floxacillin, nafcillin, ampicillin, amoxicillin, carbenicillin, and carbenicillin indanyl. The cephalosporins (designated P, N, and C) were discovered in 1948 and act against certain gram-positive and gram-negative bacteria. Cephalothin is a semisynthetic derivative of cephalosporin C and is a powerful antimicrobial agent. Other drugs in this group are cefazolin, cephapirin, cephaloridine, cephalexin, cephradine, and cephaloglycin.

3. *Streptomycin, Gentamicin, and Other Aminoglycosides.* Streptomycin was discovered in 1944 by Schatz, Bugie, and Waksman following a well-planned, scientific search for antibacterial substances effective against gram-negative microorganisms. This drug inhibits the growth of the tubercle bacillus (but is no longer the drug of first choice in this disease) and certain other kinds of multiplying bacteria. In addition to its use as an alternative drug in

* The summary is based on Chapters 55–61 in Goodman, Louis S., and Gilman, Alfred (eds.): *The Pharmacological Basis of Therapeutics*, 5th ed. Macmillan Publishing Co., Inc., New York, 1975; *The Medical Letter on Drugs and Therapeutics*, Medical Letter, Inc., New Rochelle, N.Y., Vol. 18, No. 3, Jan. 30, 1976 (Issue 445); and *Handbook of Antimicrobial Therapy*, rev. ed., Medical Letter, Inc., New Rochelle, N.Y., 1976.

tuberculosis, it is effective in the treatment of bubonic plague, tularemia, and glanders. A major disadvantage of streptomycin is the development of bacterial resistance. Gentamicin is a broad-spectrum antibiotic studied by Weinstein in 1963 and Rosselot in 1964. It is used successfully against gram-negative organisms of *Pseudomonas aeruginosa, Escherichia coli, Klebsiella,* and *Enterobacter (Aerobacter).* Tobramycin, kanamycin, neomycin, and paromomycin are other aminoglycoside antibiotics in this group.

4. *Tetracyclines and Chloramphenicol.* The tetracyclines are effective in rickettsial diseases such as Rocky Mountain spotted fever, typhus fever, murine fever, Brill's disease, Q fever, and rickettsialpox, and in other bacterial infections such as chancroid, brucellosis, cholera, granuloma inguinale, psittacosis, relapsing fever, and inclusion conjunctivitis. The first antibiotic in this group, chlortetracycline, was discovered in 1948 (then called Aureomycin) and two years later oxytetracycline became available (earlier called Terramycin). The third member of this group, tetracycline, followed in 1952, and in 1959 demeclocycline became available for general use. The next drug to appear was rolitetracycline, then methacycline in 1961, doxycycline in 1966, and minocycline in 1972, all semisynthetic derivatives. The tetracyclines are of proven value as an alternative antimicrobial in many infections. They are used as prophylaxis in chronic bronchitis and in bowel surgery. Chloramphenicol, first isolated in 1947, is used mainly in severe typhoid fever, in certain intestinal and nervous system infections, and initially in *Haemophilus influenzae* meningitis and epiglottitis in children. It has been in limited use since 1950 because it can cause fatal blood dyscrasias.

5. *Drugs Used in the Chemotherapy of Leprosy and Tuberculosis.* The treatment of infections caused by acid-fast bacteria is still an important and challenging problem in chemotherapy because of (1) the inadequacy of defense mechanisms in man, (2) the metabolic characteristics of mycobacteria, (3) the development of drug-resistant strains, (4) the lack of bactericidal activity of some of the available drugs, and (5) the untoward effects produced by the therapeutic agents.

All forms of leprosy are most effectively managed through the use of the *sulfones,* which were first tried clinically in 1941. Derivatives of *dapsone,* the sulfones are moderately toxic but may be given safely for many years if proper precautions are taken. Treatment is usually begun with small doses orally and then gradually increased. Patients on therapy (often for years) must be constantly

supervised because reactions to the sulfones can be very severe. The *thiosemicarbazones* (chiefly amithiozone) have been used for leprosy since 1946. They are important because their discovery led to the development of isonicotinic acid hydrazide (isoniazid), presently one of the most effective agents for treatment of tuberculosis. *Clofazimine* is now considered to be the chief drug for use in sulfone-resistant patients.

Streptomycin, discussed earlier on page 1724, was the first clinically effective drug used to treat tuberculosis. Far from ideal, this drug was found to suppress, not eradicate, the tubercle bacillus and to give rise to resistant strains of it. For best effect, streptomycin is given in combination with other tuberculostatic drugs, and, because of its toxicity, is commonly administered in small doses intramuscularly once or twice weekly.

Aminosalicylic acid (PAS, para aminosalicylic acid), discovered by Lehmann in 1946, is highly specific for *M. tuberculosis.* Its effectiveness is increased by the addition of either streptomycin or isoniazid. Because it is a gastric irritant and produces hypersensitivity reactions, the drug is used now only as a second-choice antimicrobial.

The fortuitous discovery of *isoniazid* (INH) in 1945 provided a drug more effective than any known synthetic or antibiotic agent against tuberculosis. INH is valuable not only in the treatment of tuberculosis but alone as a prophylactic agent. Peripheral neuritis is a common reaction to INH and, because of this, pyridoxine is often administered concurrently. Adverse effects are relatively infrequent even with 1 or 2 years of treatment, but liver damage occasionally occurs and requires monitoring of liver function tests during administration.

Ethambutol, discovered by Thomas and co-workers in 1961, produces very few untoward reactions except optic neuritis, and has been used with considerable success in treating tuberculosis; it is now preferred to PAS. *Rifampin,* first isolated in 1959, is an oral agent of great effectiveness and infrequent toxic effects, approaching isoniazid in its usefulness. It is used only in combination with other antituberculosis drugs.

There are a number of tuberculostatic drugs called "second-line" drugs because they are usually administered when drug-resistant strains of the *M. tuberculosis* organism develop. After treatment with the primary drugs described above, these agents are given with caution because of their high toxicity: *cycloserine, viomycin, pyrazinamide, ethionamide, kanamycin,* and *capreomycin.* All drugs
[*Text continued on page 1736.*]

Table 44-4. Current Use of Antimicrobial Agents in the Therapy of Infections

I. Gram-Positive Cocci	Diseases	Drug Order of Choice		
		1st [1]	2nd [1]	3rd [1]
Staphylococcus aureus *	Penicillin G sensitive: Abscesses, Bacteremia, Endocarditis, Pneumonia, Meningitis, Osteomyelitis	Penicillin G	A cephalosporin [2]	Clindamycin [2], Erythromycin, Gentamicin, Lincomycin, Vancomycin [4]
	Penicillin G resistant	A penicillinase-resistant penicillin		
	Methicillin resistant	Vancomycin	A cephalosporin ± kanamycin [3]	A tetracycline [5]
Streptococcus pyogenes (groups A, B, C)	Pharyngitis, Scarlet fever, Otitis media, sinusitis, Cellulitis, Erysipelas, Pneumonia, Bacteremia, Other systemic infections	Penicillin G, Penicillin V	A cephalosporin [2], Clindamycin [2], Erythromycin, Lincomycin	A tetracycline [5]
Streptococcus (viridans group) *	Dental infections, Subacute endocarditis, Urinary tract infection, Meningitis	Penicillin G ± streptomycin	A cephalosporin [2], Erythromycin	Vancomycin
Streptococcus faecalis * (enterococcus)	Urinary tract infection, Bacteremia, Meningitis, Brain abscess	Ampicillin, Penicillin G + an aminoglycoside	Vancomycin	Erythromycin ± an aminoglycoside
Streptococcus bovis	Endocarditis, Urinary tract infection, Bacteremia, Meningitis, Brain abscess	Penicillin G	Erythromycin	Vancomycin
Streptococcus (anaerobic species) *	Bacteremia, Endocarditis, Brain and other abscesses	Penicillin G [6]	Chloramphenicol, Clindamycin, Erythromycin, A tetracycline	—

I. Gram-Positive Cocci

Diseases	Drug Order of Choice		
	1st	2nd [1]	3rd [1]
Streptococcus (Diplococcus) *pneumoniae* (pneumococcus) — Pneumonia, Meningitis, Endocarditis, Arthritis	Penicillin G	A cephalosporin [2] Chloramphenicol Clindamycin [2] Erythromycin Lincomycin	A tetracycline [7]

II. Gram-Negative Cocci

Diseases	Drug Order of Choice		
	1st	2nd [1]	3rd [1]
Neisseria gonorrhoeae (gonococcus) — Genital infections, Arthritis, Meningitis, Endocarditis	Penicillin G	Ampicillin Spectinomycin [8]	A cephalosporin [2] Erythromycin A tetracycline
Neisseria meningitidis (meningococcus) — Meningitis, Bacteremia	Penicillin G	Chloramphenicol	Erythromycin A sulfonamide [9]
Carrier state	Rifampin A sulfonamide [9]	—	—

III. Gram-Positive Bacilli

Diseases	Drug Order of Choice		
	1st	2nd [1]	3rd [1]
Bacillus anthracis * — "Malignant pustule", Pneumonia, Meningitis	Penicillin G	Erythromycin A tetracycline	A cephalosporin [2] Chloramphenicol Lincomycin
Corynebacterium diphtheriae [10] (Klebs-Loeffler bacillus) — Pharyngitis, Laryngotracheitis, Pneumonia, Other local lesions, Carrier state	Penicillin G	Erythromycin	A cephalosporin Lincomycin Rifampin
Corynebacterium species, aerobic and anaerobic * (diphtheroids) — Endocarditis, Hepatic disease, Wound infections	Penicillin G	Erythromycin	—

Table 44-4. Current Use of Antimicrobial Agents in the Therapy of Infections (Continued)

III. Gram-Positive Bacilli

Diseases	Drug Order of Choice		
	1st	2nd [1]	3rd [1]
Listeria monocytogenes — Meningitis, Bacteremia, Endocarditis, Recurrent abortion	Ampicillin ± streptomycin; Penicillin G ± streptomycin	Erythromycin; A tetracycline	Chloramphenicol
Erysipelothrix rhusiopathiae — Erysipeloid	Penicillin G	Erythromycin; A tetracycline	Chloramphenicol
Clostridium perfringens and other species — Gas gangrene	Penicillin G [11]	Erythromycin; A tetracycline	A cephalosporin; Chloramphenicol
Clostridium tetani — Tetanus	Penicillin G [12]	A tetracycline	Erythromycin

IV. Gram-Negative Bacilli

Diseases	Drug Order of Choice		
	1st	2nd [1]	3rd [1]
Escherichia coli * — Urinary tract infection [13]	Ampicillin; Nitrofurantoin; A sulfonamide; Trimethoprim-sulfamethoxazole	Carbenicillin indanyl; A cephalosporin; Methenamine mandelate; Nalidixic acid; A tetracycline	Chloramphenicol
Escherichia coli * — Other infections	Ampicillin; Gentamicin	A cephalosporin [2]; Chloramphenicol; A tetracycline	Colistimethate; Kanamycin; Polymyxin B
Diarrhea due to enteropathogenic strains [14]	Ampicillin; Gentamicin; Polymyxin B	A cephalosporin; Kanamycin; Neomycin	——
Enterobacter (Aerobacter) aerogenes * — Urinary tract and other infections	Gentamicin	Carbenicillin; Chloramphenicol; Kanamycin; A tetracycline	Colistimethate; Polymyxin B
Alcaligenes faecalis * — Urinary tract and other infections	Chloramphenicol; A tetracycline	Colistimethate; Polymyxin B	Gentamicin; Kanamycin

IV. Gram-Negative Bacilli

	Diseases	Drug Order of Choice		
		1st	2nd [1]	3rd [1]
Proteus mirabilis	Urinary tract and other infections	Ampicillin Nitrofurantoin [15] A sulfonamide [15]	A cephalosporin [2] Gentamicin Kanamycin	Chloramphenicol A tetracycline
Proteus, other species *	Urinary tract and other infections [16]	Carbenicillin Kanamycin	Gentamicin	Chloramphenicol Streptomycin A tetracycline
Pseudomonas aeruginosa *	Urinary tract and other infections	Carbenicillin [17] Gentamicin ± carbenicillin [17]	Colistimethate Polymyxin B	—
Klebsiella pneumoniae * (Friedlander's bacillus)	Pneumonia Urinary tract infection Biliary tract infection Osteomyelitis	A cephalosporin [18] Kanamycin or gentamicin ± a cephalosporin	Chloramphenicol A tetracycline	Colistimethate Polymyxin B
Salmonella *	Typhoid fever Paratyphoid fever Bacteremia Acute gastroenteritis	Ampicillin [19] Chloramphenicol [19]	Trimethoprim-sulfamethoxazole	—
Shigella *	Acute gastroenteritis [20]	Ampicillin Chloramphenicol	Kanamycin [21] Polymyxin B [21] A tetracycline	A sulfonamide [22] Trimethoprim-sulfamethoxazole
Serratia *	Variety of opportunistic infections, primarily in patients receiving immunosuppressive therapy	Gentamicin	Chloramphenicol Kanamycin	Carbenicillin Colistimethate Nalidixic acid Polymyxin B Trimethoprim-sulfamethoxazole
Haemophilus influenzae *	Pharyngitis Otitis media Epiglottitis Laryngotracheobronchitis Pneumonia Meningitis	Ampicillin [23] Chloramphenicol [23]	Streptomycin A sulfonamide A tetracycline [24]	—

1729

Table 44-4. Current Use of Antimicrobial Agents in the Therapy of Infections (Continued)

IV. Gram-Negative Bacilli	Diseases	Drug Order of Choice		
		1st	2nd[1]	3rd[1]
Haemophilus ducreyi	Chancroid	A tetracycline	A sulfonamide	Erythromycin Streptomycin
Acinetobacter * (*Mima-Herellea* group)	Urethritis Bacteremia Endocarditis Meningitis	Gentamicin Kanamycin	Carbenicillin Colistimethate Polymyxin B	—
Brucella	Brucellosis	A tetracycline ± streptomycin[25]	Chloramphenicol ± streptomycin[25]	—
Yersinia (Pasteurella) pestis	Bubonic plague	Streptomycin ± a tetracycline	A tetracycline	Chloramphenicol A sulfonamide
Francisella (Pasteurella) tularensis	Tularemia	Streptomycin	A tetracycline	Chloramphenicol
Pasteurella multocida	Abscesses Bacteremia Meningitis	Penicillin G	A tetracycline	—
Vibrio cholerae (comma)	Cholera[26]	A tetracycline	Chloramphenicol Furazolidone	Erythromycin Trimethoprim- sulfamethoxazole
Flavobacterium meningosepticum	Meningitis	Erythromycin	Rifampin	—
Pseudomonas (Actinobacillus) mallei	Glanders	Streptomycin + a tetracycline	Streptomycin + chloramphenicol	—
Pseudomonas (Actinobacillus) pseudomallei	Melioidosis	A tetracycline ± chloramphenicol	Chloramphenicol	Trimethoprim- sulfamethoxazole
Bacteroides[27] (intestinal)	Brain abscess Other abscesses Empyema Bacteremia	Chloramphenicol Clindamycin[2]	Lincomycin A tetracycline	Ampicillin Penicillin G[28]

IV. Gram-Negative Bacilli

Diseases		Drug Order of Choice	
	1st	2nd [1]	3rd [1]
Fusobacterium nucleatum (*fusiforme*) Ulcerative pharyngitis Lung abscess, empyema Genital infections Gingivitis	Penicillin G	Chloramphenicol	Clindamycin Erythromycin Lincomycin A tetracycline
Calymmatobacterium (*Donovania*) *granulomatis* Granuloma inguinale	A tetracycline	Streptomycin	Ampicillin
Streptobacillus (*Haverhillia*) *moniliformis* Bacteremia Arthritis Endocarditis Abscesses	Penicillin G	Erythromycin A tetracycline	A cephalosporin

V. Acid-Fast Bacilli

Diseases		Drug Order of Choice	
	1st	2nd [1]	3rd [1]
Mycobacterium tuberculosis (human type) Pulmonary, miliary, renal, meningeal, and other tuberculosis infections	Isoniazid + ethambutol [29] Isoniazid + ethambutol + streptomycin [30]	Rifampin [31]	Aminosalicylic acid [31] Cycloserine [31] Ethionamide [31] Pyrazinamide [31]
Atypical mycobacteria [32] Lymphadenitis Pulmonary and other lesions	Isoniazid + ethambutol Isoniazid + ethambutol + streptomycin	Erythromycin Rifampin	Aminosalicylic acid Cycloserine Ethionamide Pyrazinamide
Mycobacterium leprae (Hansen's bacillus) Leprosy	A sulfone	Amithiozone	———

VI. Spirochetes

Diseases		Drug Order of Choice	
	1st	2nd [1]	3rd [1]
Treponema pallidum Syphilis	Penicillin G	A tetracycline	Erythromycin
Treponema pertenue Yaws	Penicillin G	A tetracycline	Erythromycin

Table 44-4. Current Use of Antimicrobial Agents in the Therapy of Infections (Continued)

Diseases	Drug Order of Choice		
	1st	2nd[1]	3rd[1]
VI. Spirochetes			
Borrelia recurrentis — Relapsing fever	A tetracycline	Penicillin G	Chloramphenicol
Leptospira — Weil's disease, Meningitis	Penicillin G	A tetracycline[33]	——
VII. Actinomycetes	1st	2nd[1]	3rd[1]
Actinomyces israeli — Cervicofacial, abdominal, thoracic, and other lesions	Penicillin G[34]	Erythromycin, A tetracycline	A cephalosporin, Chloramphenicol, Lincomycin
Nocardia * — Pulmonary lesions, Brain abscess, Lesions of other organs	A sulfonamide + streptomycin	A sulfonamide + ampicillin	A tetracycline + cycloserine, Trimethoprim-sulfamethoxazole
VIII. Miscellaneous Agents	1st	2nd[1]	3rd[1]
Mycoplasma pneumoniae (Eaton agent) — "Atypical viral pneumonia"	Erythromycin, A tetracycline	——	——
Mycoplasma hominis — Nonspecific urethritis, Pelvic abscess, Septicemia	Clindamycin[35], A tetracycline	Chloramphenicol, Erythromycin[36], Gentamicin, Streptomycin	Kanamycin
Rickettsia — Typhus fever, Murine typhus, Brill's disease, Rocky Mountain spotted fever, Q fever, Rickettsialpox	A tetracycline	Chloramphenicol	——
Chlamydia psittaci — Psittacosis (ornithosis)	A tetracycline	Chloramphenicol	——

Drug Order of Choice

VIII. Miscellaneous Agents

Diseases	1st	2nd [1]	3rd [1]
Lymphogranuloma venereum	A sulfonamide + a tetracycline	A tetracycline	Chloramphenicol
Chlamydia trachomatis Trachoma	A sulfonamide + a tetracycline [37]	Erythromycin A tetracycline [37]	Chloramphenicol
Inclusion conjunctivitis (blennorrhea)	A tetracycline [38]	Chloramphenicol [39]	——

Drug Order of Choice

Diseases	1st	2nd [1]	3rd [1]
IX. Fungi			
Candida albicans Skin and superficial mucous membrane lesions	Amphotericin B [40] Nystatin [40]	——	——
Candida albicans **Cryptococcus neoformans** **Aspergillus** Pneumonia Meningitis Skin lesions Isolated lung lesions	Amphotericin B ± flucytosine [41]	Flucytosine	
Coccidioides immitis **Histoplasma capsulatum** **Mucor** Bone lesions Disseminated disease	Amphotericin B	——	
Blastomyces dermatidis Blastomycosis (North American) [42]	Amphotericin B	Hydroxystilbamidine	
Microsporum **Trichophyton** **Epidermophyton** Skin, hair, and nail infections (tinea)	Griseofulvin	——	
Sporothrix (Sporotrichum) schenckii Sporotrichosis	Iodides	Amphotericin B Griseofulvin	

X. Viruses	Diseases	Drug Order of Choice		
		1st	2nd[1]	3rd[1]
Herpes simplex virus	Keratoconjunctivitis Encephalitis	Idoxuridine[43]	—	—
Influenza virus	Influenza	Amantadine[44]	—	—

(Based on Table 55-1 from Goodman, Louis S., and Gilman, Alfred: *The Pharmacological Basis of Therapeutics*, 5th ed. Macmillan Publishing Co., Inc., New York, 1975, pp. 1097–1103.)

Presentation of choices of specific agents for the treatment of various infections is always provocative of discussion and disagreement because such choices often represent the distillate of personal experiences that may not duplicate those of others. In addition, the current availability of a number of drugs that are approximately equally effective makes an order of choice very difficult, if not impossible. To complicate matters, sensitivity patterns of a number of microorganisms often vary with the hospital or clinic in which they are isolated; in some instances, this reflects a varying degree of exposure to specific agents. The material presented in this table represents not only the practice of the author, based on his experience with the management of these infections, but also that of other experts in the United States. It is important to stress that, as more information accumulates, as recently introduced drugs are used for longer periods, and as entirely new agents are developed, some of the recommendations will require modification not only in the order of choice but even in the specific drugs that are suggested.

Taxonomy is not a static field, and nomenclature of microorganisms changes as further insight into their relationships is obtained. The system used in this table and textbook is that of the eighth edition of *Bergey's Manual of Determinative Bacteriology* (Buchanan and Gibbons, 1974). Older generic and specific names are indicated parenthetically in italic type.

* All strains must be examined *in vitro* for sensitivity to various antimicrobial agents.

[1] Drugs included for second and third choices are (a) indicated in patients hypersensitive to equally or more effective agents, (b) potentially more dangerous than equally active drugs, (c) less likely to produce the desired therapeutic response, or (d) in need, in some cases, of further study in order to allow a valid evaluation of their efficacy.

Lists of drugs within each box are given alphabetically since they are approximately equally effective.

[2] Therapeutic concentrations of this drug are not achieved in the cerebrospinal fluid, and alternative agents should be used to treat infections of the central nervous system.

[3] Not all strains are sensitive to this combination.

[4] As indicated, vancomycin is the drug of first choice for methicillin-resistant staphylococci, since these microorganisms are usually also resistant to all other less toxic antimicrobials.

[5] About 10 to 30% of strains of group-A *Strep. pyogenes* are insensitive to tetracyclines.

[6] Large doses of penicillin G may be required.

[7] Some strains of pneumococci are resistant to tetracyclines.

[8] Spectinomycin is useful for genital infections only.

[9] Although many strains are resistant, sulfonamides are effective for sensitive microorganisms.

[10] Antibiotics alone do not alter the clinical course of diphtheria, but drugs can eradicate the carrier state.

[11] Adequate debridement is absolutely essential. Antitoxin therapy is advisable, but newer evidence suggests that this may not play an important role in cure. At least 30 million units of penicillin G should be administered daily.

[12] Ten to 20 million units of penicillin G daily, with debridement and adsorbed tetanus toxoid. Human tetanus immune globulin administration may be advisable.

[13] Sulfonamides, trimethoprim-sulfamethoxazole, and urinary tract antiseptics are particularly useful for acute urinary tract infections, especially cystitis, in the patient without obstructive uropathy or in whom the disease has not become chronic. These agents also prove useful for chronic suppressive therapy in patients with recurrent urinary tract infection. Some clinicians prefer to reserve the antibiotics for cases in which there are systemic manifestations—particularly in acute pyelonephritis.

[14] For toxigenic noninvasive strains of *E. coli*, poorly absorbed antibiotics (polymyxins, aminoglycosides) are administered orally by some physicians. There is, however, no convincing

evidence of the efficacy of antibiotic therapy. For invasive strains, there is debate as to the relative efficacy of systemic antibiotic therapy versus treatment with agents confined to the gastrointestinal tract.

15 Acute lower urinary tract infection can often be controlled by the use of sulfonamide or nitrofurantoin.

16 Some strains are sensitive to chloramphenicol, tetracyclines, or streptomycin. In serious infections, it is best to begin treatment with carbenicillin while the microorganisms are being examined for sensitivity to other drugs. If they prove to be susceptible to other agents, one of these should constitute the therapy of choice.

17 For all serious infections with *Pseudomonas*, many clinicians prefer gentamicin in combination with carbenicillin, but not in the same solution.

18 An increasing number of strains are becoming resistant to the cephalosporins.

19 Chloramphenicol is the drug of choice for the treatment of typhoid fever. Ampicillin may be used as initial treatment for other types of salmonella infection. However, many strains of this microorganism are presently resistant to a wide variety of drugs; sensitivity testing is mandatory.

20 Many strains of *Shigella* are now resistant to ampicillin, and some are also resistant to chloramphenicol and tetracyclines.

21 Administered orally; poorly absorbed.

22 May be used if responsible strain is sensitive to sulfonamide.

23 Ampicillin-resistant strains have been reported in many parts of the United States. This requires the concurrent use of penicillin G and chloramphenicol in the *initial* treatment of children with bacterial meningitis. Chloramphenicol can be discontinued if cultures demonstrate *Strep. pneumoniae or N. meningitidis*. If *H. influenzae* is causative, sensitivity tests are necessary to determine if ampicillin may be substituted for chloramphenicol.

24 This agent may be effective when given alone in infections of the pharynx, larynx, trachea, and lungs. In meningitis, it does not produce as good results as when it is combined with streptomycin or as does ampicillin or chloramphenicol.

25 Such combined therapy is useful in severe infections.

26 The primary treatment of cholera is prompt replacement of the large loss of water and electrolytes; although this is all that is required, antimicrobial agents will usually shorten the course of the disease. Furazolidone, listed as a second-choice drug for cholera, is no longer generally available in the United States; its pharmacology is discussed in the *fourth edition* of this textbook.

27 Surgical drainage of abscesses is necessary when they are present.

28 Many strains of *Bacteroides fragilis* are resistant to conventional doses of penicillin G. Other species of *Bacteroides (e.g., B. melaninogenicus)* are sensitive to penicillin G.

29 For pulmonary tuberculosis. For advanced disease, some experts favor isoniazid plus rifampin.

30 Recommended by many clinicians for more severe forms of tuberculosis, such as meningitis and the disseminated (miliary) disease. Other physicians use only two of these agents, combining isoniazid with streptomycin, or isoniazid with one of the second- or third-choice drugs.

31 Always combined with another effective tuberculostatic agent. Capreomycin, viomycin, and kanamycin are additional alternatives.

32 Atypical mycobacteria are variably sensitive to tuberculostatic drugs. While a number of strains are sensitive to isoniazid and streptomycin, most are resistant to aminosalicylic acid. Scotochromogens may be sensitive to erythromycin. Cycloserine, ethionamide, or pyrazinamide may need to be used and should be given with another drug. All strains must be tested for sensitivity. About 85% of *M. scrofulaceum* and nearly all *M. kansasii* are sensitive to 0.5 to 2 μg/ml of erythromycin. Strains of *M. intracellulare* vary in sensitivity.

33 Some physicians favor a tetracycline over penicillin G as the drug of first choice.

34 If abscesses are present, they should be drained, regardless of the antibiotic administered.

35 Active against all strains, including T strains.

36 Most active against T strains.

37 A tetracycline may be given orally alone, or it may be applied locally in the conjunctival sac while a sulfonamide is being administered orally.

38 Topical or oral administration.

39 Topical application.

40 Applied locally.

41 Many clinicians give this combination regularly for severe infections due to these microorganisms. There is some evidence that, when a microorganism is resistant to flucytosine, the drug may suppress the activity of amphotericin B.

42 For South American blastomycosis (*Blastomyces brasiliensis*), amphotericin B is the drug of first choice, while a sulfonamide is an alternative.

43 Idoxuridine is of proven value in the therapy of keratoconjunctivitis when applied locally. It is of questionable effectiveness when used in other types of infection due to herpes simplex, including herpetic encephalitis.

44 No evidence of an important therapeutic effect, but apparently effective as prophylaxis for Asian A_2 influenza virus.

mentioned here for the treatment of tuberculosis are usually given in combination for greatest effectiveness.

6. *Miscellaneous Antibacterial Agents, Antifungal, and Antiviral Agents*

A. *Antibacterial*

Erythromycin, discovered by McGuire in 1952, is an orally effective antibiotic possessing few adverse effects. It is used in mycoplasma pneumonia and as an alternative drug to penicillin in a variety of gram-positive infections.

Lincomycin, developed in 1962 from soil collected near Lincoln, Nebraska, appears to be highly effective in chronic osteomyelitis but can cause diarrhea in as many as 20 per cent of patients. A derivative, *clindamycin,* may cause not only diarrhea but the more serious complication of colitis. Its usefulness is limited to those infections where it is clearly the superior agent (*Bacteroides* and *Mycoplasma hominis*).

Spectinomycin has been in limited use for acute genital and rectal gonorrhea, especially in penicillin-sensitive patients.

Polymixin B is one of several antibiotics discovered in 1947 (polymixins A, B, C, D, E) and is useful in gram-negative infections, especially those caused by *Pseudomonas* affecting the kidney. Its toxicity is high, and it is replaced now by gentamicin and carbenicillin. Topical polymixin can be used in combination with other agents for infected wounds or otitis externa.

Colistin (polymixin E) is usually used parenterally and for infections caused by *Pseudomonas aeruginosa.*

Vancomycin (1956) is primarily active against gram-positive bacteria but produces serious untoward effects, especially ototoxicity and nephrotoxicity. Its use is limited to severe disease produced by methicillin-resistant staphylococci.

Bacitracin, produced from the Tracy-I strain of *Bacillus subtilis,* was isolated in 1943 from a septic compound fracture in a young girl named Tracy; it is in current use only as a topical ophthalmic or dermatologic ointment.

Tyrothricin is used only as an ointment or local solution to treat infected surface ulcers and wounds, pyodermas, and infections of the eye, nose, and throat.

B. *Antifungal*

Nystatin inhibits the growth of a variety of yeasts and fungi and does not affect bacteria, protozoa, or viruses. It is employed primarily to treat *Candida* infections of the skin, mucous membrane, and intestinal tract.

Amphotericin B, available as an injection only, possesses a large number of untoward effects. Over 80 per cent of persons given this drug develop decreased renal function. It is effective, however, in a variety of fungal infections that prior to its availability were invariably fatal. Its usefulness extends to patients with blastomycosis, coccidioidomycosis, and histoplasmosis.

Flucytosine, converted in fungal cells to fluorouracil, is an oral agent that is less toxic than amphotericin B but not as effective against yeasts and fungi.

Griseofulvin was first isolated in 1939 but was not given attention until 1946 as an antifungal agent. It is especially effective against fungal disease of the skin, hair, and nails and has a greater affinity for diseased tissue than normal; as diseased tissue is shed, the new growth is entirely free of infection. Given orally, treatment requires long periods of time but is associated with infrequent serious reactions.

C. *Antiviral*

Although the search for antiviral agents has been long and intensive, very few have been discovered that are clinically useful. *Idoxuridine* is used for herpes simplex keratitis; *amantadine* can be employed as a prophylactic agent against the Asian (A_2) influenza virus; *methisazone* is a synthetic that may be useful against two complications of smallpox, vaccinia gangrenosa and eczema vaccinatum; and *cytarabine* is useful to treat herpes virus (type 2) infections.

The dramatic effect of antimicrobial drugs should not be emphasized to the exclusion of old and new drugs in other categories. The general effectiveness of vitamins in helping prevent infections and hastening recovery from avitaminoses was stressed in Chapter 10. Earlier in the present chapter reference was made to a recent controversial report of the use of vitamin C in preventing the common cold. There is reason to hope that there will continue to be improvements in pharmaceutical agents that will increase their toxicity to the invading organism and decrease the danger to man. Few nurses can keep abreast of the research in therapeutics, but they can grasp every opportunity to participate in it and to learn about it, particularly as it relates to the care of their patients. All nurses can be familiar with reliable handbooks such as those listed in Chapter 21. It is becoming more and more important for practicing nurses, particularly nurse specialists, to have thorough knowledge of each therapeutic agent. While physicians prescribe most medications, nurses usually are responsible for administering the therapeutic agent, or teaching the patient about it, and this cannot be done intelligently without knowledge of the nature and effect of each drug.

Symptomatic and Supportive Care of the Patient with a Fever. The treatment and nursing care of persons with local infections, both inflammatory and suppurative processes, were dealt with in Chapter 43. One or both of these are present in many acute systemic infectious diseases. Examples are the inflamed pharyngeal tissues of tonsillitis and pharyngitis, the skin lesions of chicken pox and impetigo, and the lesions of syphilis that are present on either the exterior or interior of the body, sometimes both. In a few of the acute generalized infections, the local manifestation is the only troublesome symptom as, for example, the pustules of chicken pox; in others it is a rash of very limited duration that demands no local treatment except, perhaps, a soothing bath, lotion, or ointment. Such rashes are seen in scarlet fever, rubella, and roseola infantum (exanthem subitum).

Infections may be typified by capillary hemorrhage produced either by their dilation or by a fragility of the wall that is a result of the infection. When capillaries are affected by infectious disease, the resulting petechiae may predominate on the trunk and extremities as in meningococcemia.[46] Local treatment of petechial lesions is rare except to allay itching if present. Very smooth bedding and clothing are helpful in reducing irritation.

The lesions of impetigo are treated as infected wounds. It is common practice to remove the crusts from impetigo pustules because they protect the organisms from the action of the prescribed antiseptic ointment or lotion.

Inflammation of the mucous membranes of the eyes, ears, nose, and throat is common in many acute systemic infections. When the eyes are inflamed, as in measles and some upper respiratory conditions, they should be kept at rest and protected from bright lights with an eyeshade or dark eyeglasses.

Symptomatic and supportive care in most infections is directed toward *combating the harmful effects of fever.* While it is now realized that fever is one of the body's means of making itself uninhabitable to the invading microorganisms, it is generally believed that if this reaction is prolonged or very severe, the body tissues as well as the invading organisms may suffer. Artificially produced fever (fever therapy) was used in the 1930s and 1940s in the treatment of gonorrhea and other infections, but is rarely used now. In 1948, Eugene F. DuBois in his classic monograph on fever said:

A temperature of 41°C (105.8°F) may be harmful and temperatures over 42°C (107.6°F) dangerous if prolonged a few hours. It is doubtful if a temperature of 40°C (104°F) even over a period of days can be considered harmful in itself, though of course it is usually an indication of severe infection accompanied by many other deleterious factors. Fever is only a symptom and we are not sure that it is an enemy. Perhaps it is a friend.*

Most of us have experienced fever or have watched someone else with it. Knowledge of its effect on body functions suggests the nursing needs. The following is a classical picture of a typical febrile patient.

The respiratory rate is increased, as is the pulse rate; there is a vague or marked feeling that something is wrong; there may be headache and nausea, so the victim instinctively seeks rest and seclusion; he feels groggy and seems to sleep a great deal; he may have dreams, and when the fever is highest he has a sense of unreality; the dreams may merge into waking fantasies so that it is said that the patient is "delirious." (A delirium usually occurs more often in elderly patients and when the fever is over 40°C [104°F].) [47] The patient's skin feels hot and dry, and he looks flushed when the fever is at its height. With fevers that fluctuate and just before the onset of a sudden fever, there is a sensation of chilliness or a shaking chill that is not relieved by external warmth. Profuse sweating precedes a drop in the body temperature; the clothing and even the sheets may be soaking wet. The appetite is usually poor in a patient with fever, but thirst is a prominent feature and fluids should be encouraged.

Since fever weakens the patient and dulls the judgment, he or she may get severely dehydrated, and, if neglected, lose weight rapidly. The lips are parched or cracked, and crusts form on them and in the nose. The nasal air passages are often occluded, and the patient breathes through the mouth; the tongue is coated, often swollen, and if the fever persists and its effects are not successfully combated, the gums swell and bleed easily and the margins may be discolored. Febrile patients are usually uncomfortable, restless, and irritable; they lose interest in those around them. In a "delirium" they may pose questions that no one can answer satisfactorily, and this adds to their confusion. If the fever is not too intense or prolonged, the brain dysfunction is only temporary, but a prolonged fever can produce irreversible brain damage. Unless the patient is hydrated, urine output is scanty because there is excessive water loss through sweating. Constipation or diarrhea may be present according

* DuBois, Eugene F.: *Fever and the Regulation of Body Temperature.* Charles C Thomas, Publisher, Springfield, Ill., 1948, p. 57.

to the patient's intake and the effect of the infection on the alimentary canal.

Many of these symptoms can be identified as signs of a neglected febrile patient; they can be forestalled and the picture greatly modified by effective care, especially adequate treatment. DuBois, discussing "the management of fever patients," says, "In the first place a good nurse is required." *

If the foregoing is an accurate description of the febrile state, the following symptomatic nursing care is suggested:

Bed rest is indicated when there is sufficient rise in temperature to affect appreciably the respiratory and pulse rates. It is usually prescribed when the adult's oral temperature exceeds 38°C (100.4°F), although a persistent temperature of even less than this suggests the need for more than the average amount of rest and sleep.

Quiet surroundings are indicated by the tendency to headache, nausea, and irritability and by the need for extra sleep. If there is photophobia, dark glasses, an eyeshade, or a silk scarf tied over the eyes is welcome. This is to be preferred to darkening the room, although the latter may be desirable in some cases. A dark, gloomy room is depressing, particularly so to the confused or the delirious person. It is also more difficult for nurses to give effective care if they cannot see the patient's response to treatment or see clearly the equipment with which they are working.

Sleep should be encouraged by removing the sources of discomfort, if possible. Sedatives may induce sleep, but they increase the patient's mental confusion and depression and, as in all cases, tend to develop a dependence on drugs. A skillfully given sponge bath, a back rub, a cool, smooth bed, relief of thirst, and cleaning the mouth and removing crusts that obstruct the nose or mouth will induce a more natural, restful sleep than medications.

Reassurance should be given anxious and delirious patients. The presence of anyone they trust is reassuring, but if the nurse can anticipate their needs and discover the sources of their worries and in what way they are disoriented, their anxiety can be reduced appreciably. Patients may, for example, fail to distinguish between reality and optical illusions, or even hallucinate. This situation requires a nurse who understands the fears that often accompany fever. Restraint of the febrile patient may be necessary but is never desirable. Disoriented persons struggle against restraint and increase their energy consumption. Reducing patients' physical discomfort usually reduces

* *Ibid.,* p. 55.

restlessness. For example, nurses should be sure that bedclothes are not too warm or restricting, or that patients are not thirsty or feeling the urge to urinate or defecate. Rooms of febrile patients should be cool but free from drafts. Patients who are isolated feel deprived of human contact unless nurses make an extra effort to provide companionship and encourage visits from families. Radio and television programs, and, as patients recover, books, games, and handcrafts, can relieve the tedium of convalescence.

Reducing extremes of body temperature is a responsibility shared by physicians and nurses. While physicians ordinarily prescribe many of the measures to be used, they expect them to be adapted to patients' needs by nurses. Antipyretic drugs were commonly employed in the first part of the century but are given less often now for antipyresis than for some other therapeutic effect. Aspirin (acetylsalicylic acid), for example, reduces the temperature but is often used for its mildly sedative rather than its antipyretic action. Sponge baths are still used routinely in many areas for protracted fevers of 39°C (102.2°F) and over. While temperatures of less than 40.6°C (105°F) are not likely to cause permanent injury to nerve tissue, they are likely to produce intense discomfort and signs of delirium. Alcohol or tepid sponge baths and other forms of cooling therapy, such as ice packs or refrigerated blankets, are prescribed for patients with high temperatures. These procedures are described in Chapter 42. They are discontinued, of course, if the patients respond unfavorably. If patients have a low-grade fever and are not on bed rest, ordinary clothing is appropriate. It is often wise, however, and more practical, to dress sick children so that they do not have to stay under bedclothes for warmth.

The profuse sweating that accompanies fever demands frequent cleansing baths and changes of clothing. Alcohol applied to the skin has a cooling effect, and the odor is refreshing to most persons. During a chill, extra covers and external heat are welcomed by patients, but they may have no effect on the paroxysm. Absorbent cotton clothing is likely to feel less clammy than synthetic fibers, but personal preferences should be considered.

Combating water loss and electrolyte imbalance and other forms of malnutrition is the nurse's major task in caring for the patient with fever. The febrile patient usually eats reluctantly and, if nauseated, cannot even tolerate fluids, while, as was pointed out in Chapter 42, fever speeds up metabolism and the body requires more nourishment. Elisha Atkins [48] suggests there is roughly a 7 per cent metabolic increase for each degree Fahrenheit (above 98.6°F); for example, at a temperature of 105°F (40.6°C), the basal metabolism is about 50 per cent above normal. It is important for the nurse to see that the febrile patient is provided with ample fluids, protein, and calories to maintain a level of resting metabolism during any prolonged temperature elevation.

During brief periods of fever, there is little probability of dangerously increasing the dehydration with a lowered fluid intake. Infants and young children are, however, very susceptible to dehydration, and even with adults, it is unwise to allow the urinary output to fall below 1000 ml (1 qt) per day. Since a diet complete in all food elements except fat can be given parenterally, there are few cases in which patients in modern hospitals need be exposed to the dangers of inadequate diet and fluid intake. Where patients must depend on mouth feeding, the nurse's skill may be taxed to the utmost, and if vomiting is persistent, parenteral feeding is essential. This is a particular problem in any disease accompanied by coughing, since coughing may induce vomiting. It is helpful in this instance to feed the patient after a paroxysm, to avoid overloading the stomach, and to reduce tension during feeding periods as much as possible. Insufflation of food in the mouth during a coughing spell is a serious danger. This is a particular hazard for the elderly, the infant, and the disoriented. Oral feeding of such persons requires considerable nursing judgment.

No effort should be spared in providing the nutritional requirements during the febrile period. It is well known that starvation in itself can produce fever and that a poor appetite is one of the signs of a vitamin deficiency. The cracked lips, the swollen gums, and furry tongue (sordes), so common in protracted febrile states in years past, were unquestionably signs of a vitamin lack, since it was customary to "starve a fever." Malnutrition starts a vicious circle which, once established, is hard to interrupt.

Elimination by the skin, bowels, and bladder should be observed by nurses and their observations reported. Excessive sweating, as has been noted, often reduces elimination by the kidneys to a dangerous point. Nurses keep an accurate record of intake and output so that physicians can prescribe parenteral fluids if there is an inadequate intake by mouth. Nurses themselves should, however, realize that for an adult a daily output of less than 1000 ml is a danger signal, as is dark, concentrated urine. Bowel elimination is regulated by diet, if possible. Cathartics may increase the tendency to

nausea and they hurry food through the intestines before optimum absorption has occurred. Suppositories, stool softeners, or low enemas may be prescribed for constipation when diet is ineffective and cathartics contraindicated. With the well-recognized dangers of bed rest in mind, physicians are more likely to permit patients bathroom privileges even though they have a fever. However, the use of the bedpan is necessary in most cases unless a private bathroom is available, so as to prevent the patient from transmitting disease, if infectious, to others.

Skin care, or bodily cleanliness, is a special problem, because excessive sweating may keep any person feeling "unclean." Frequent baths are often desirable for their refreshing as well as their antipyretic effect. Starch baths are soothing in eruptive diseases, such as measles and hives, but unless there is a private bathroom available to the patient it is difficult to provide a comforting starch bath without subjecting others to inconvenience.* When immersion baths are contraindicated by the existence of skin lesions that physicians think will be adversely affected by water, nurses should bathe those portions of the body where lesions are not present, particularly the face and hands, the axillae, pubic area, and feet. If such body parts are bathed well, patients feel very much as they might if the whole body had been bathed. Often, turning patients frequently, exposing the skin to air, and applying an antipruritic lotion are helpful nursing measures. Frequently, open, wet dressings are ordered to soothe irritating and pruritic skin lesions.

Care of the eyes, nose, mouth, and ears is a simple or difficult problem according to the patient's age, the duration of the fever, and the effect of the specific infection on the mucous membrane. If the microorganism causing fever does not also produce lesions of the mucous membrane, care of the eyes, nose, and mouth may not differ from that given in health, although cleaning processes may be required at more frequent intervals. "Fever blisters" may occur in certain febrile diseases but are caused by a separate organism—the virus of herpes simplex—which may be activated by the rise in body temperature.[49] Because sordes (crusts on lips and gums) accompanied fever more or less regularly in the past, mouth lesions were looked upon as inevitable, and it was customary to replace the toothbrush with cotton applicators that were believed to clean more gently. With adequate feeding and with per-

* Aveeno is a patented preparation of starch available in a convenient form for this purpose.

sistent and effective use of the toothbrush, sordes can be prevented. The authors doubt whether the teeth are ever thoroughly cleaned unless a brush is used. A refreshing mouthwash is helpful, and the lips should be lubricated with cold cream or its equivalent. Gargles and warm throat irrigations may be prescribed when there is an infection of the mouth or pharynx.

Crusts should be removed from the nose with a cotton-tipped applicator that has been slightly moistened with an emollient, such as vegetable oil. The eyes may need cleaning frequently if there is a discharge. If this is tenacious and has a tendency to dry and hold the lids closed, sterile cotton and water may loosen the crusts, and a small amount of sterile petroleum jelly on the lid margins may keep them separated. Photophobia may be relieved by protecting the patient from bright lights (see page 1792).

The ears require no special care unless the infection invades them. The nurse should be alert to the early symptoms of an ear involvement since this complication occurs frequently in many of the acute systemic infections unless patients respond to treatment in the early stages.

Providing companionship, diversion, and occupation is a major problem in fever and communicable disease nursing. During the acute phase when there is prostration, physical discomfort, and anxiety, patients need someone with them almost constantly in order to supply them with water, nourishment, and other bodily wants, as well as to provide reassurance. As patients recover and are able to do more and more for themselves, the seclusion forced on them by the communicability of the disease may be depressing and, to the small child, frightening and frustrating. The companionship of other patients with the same disease is usually helpful but not always available. In any event, nurses should consider the provision of diversion and occupation a part of the responsibility they share with the family and other members of the health team. The *rehabilitation* of the person with infectious disease should begin during the early stages; however, the special problems involved cannot be discussed adequately in this text.

Role of the Nurse in Different Settings. It is important to recognize the significance of the nurse who works outside and inside the hospital in the conquest of infectious disease. It was pointed out in Chapter 3 that the nurse works in homes, hospitals, clinics, nursing homes, doctors' offices, schools, colleges and universities, industries, camps, ships, trains, planes and spacecraft, homes for the mentally

retarded, and prisons or houses of correction. In all of these settings, the nurse can help prevent and control communicable disease and give care to its victims.

Community or district nurses and "health visitors" have a vital role to play. It is often they who may recognize a communicable disease in its early stages. They are in a position to minimize the effects of the infection by teaching families how to prevent its spread. In doctors' offices, in hospitals and clinics, nurses can enlist the help of physicians in screening for tuberculosis and venereal diseases and immunizing against preventable diseases. Many opportunities are available to nurses working in schools, colleges, universities, camps, and industrial plants to lessen the incidence and prevalence of communicable disease. Nurses in all these settings should (1) familiarize themselves with the local and state regulations controlling communicable disease, (2) determine the immunization level present in the population and recommend ways of improving it, and (3) determine the state of knowledge of the population and of those responsible for these groups and institute educational and preventive programs if indicated.

Nurses working in nursing homes, homes for the mentally retarded, houses of correction, and other domiciliary institutions have an especially vulnerable group of clients under their care. By such simple and obvious methods as seeing that adequate handwashing and other sanitary facilities are available, by teaching habits of covering mouth and nose when coughing and sneezing, and by arranging for and participating in preventive services such as vaccination for influenza, nurses can help reduce the rates of infectious disease.

While nurses have an important role, they and physicians can take too much credit for reducing disease rates and increasing the life span of man. Elsewhere we have noted that:

The average life span in the United States . . . has risen from about 50 years in 1900 to about 71 years in 1969, chiefly because infant mortality has dropped dramatically and because children die far less often from infectious diseases in this century than in the last. This drop in infant and child mortality is not so much because doctors and nurses have given good medical and nursing care to infants and children, but because the water they drink and the food they eat is cleaner, and because protective sera, antibiotics, and specific drugs have been developed to protect the young against the pathogenic organisms that in the last century could and sometimes did, wipe out even large families.

Those who have so greatly increased the life span therefore include not only doctors and nurses, but bacteriologists, chemists, sanitarians, and legislators—all who have identified dangers in the environment, developed controlling agents, and devised protective legislation. Credit is also due biological scientists and educators who have raised the general level of nutrition.*

In summary, it might be said that nursing patients with systemic infections rarely presents new problems. It demands an understanding of concepts, control, prevention, and epidemiology of communicable diseases. It also requires knowledge of the effects of fever and requires nurses to practice (and teach others to practice) a more rigid aseptic technique than is necessary elsewhere. The distressing symptoms of infection are seen everywhere and they are relieved by measures nurses use quite commonly. Effective care in communicable disease depends on identifying the causative organism, if possible, accurate diagnosis and appropriate treatment, anticipation of patients' needs, and an understanding of how to control the spread of infection as well as prevent disease. Complications of infectious disease such as glomerulonephritis, otitis media, and pneumonia are rarely seen now, but avoidance of these complications is not the ultimate goal. As with all categories of disease, the health team should not feel satisfied until a patient has been rehabilitated and has assumed an effective place in the life of the community. Patients' illnesses can often be made valuable learning experiences for them and their families.

The Summary Table of Data which follows will, it is hoped, give the reader the specific information needed in providing controls for the more common communicable diseases. It should be clear from these data that the recommended measures depend upon the avenues through which the infection enters and leaves the human body, the incubation period of the organism, the period of communicability, and the immunity conferred after recovery.

For more details, the reader should refer to books and articles listed at the end of this chapter.

* Henderson, Virginia: "Health Is Everybody's Business," *Can. Nurse,* **67**:31, (Mar.) 1971.

5. SUMMARY TABLE OF DATA

Presenting in Simplified Form the Important Aspects of Control in Selected Communicable Diseases *

Disease	Causative Organism	Classification of Reportable Diseases †	Portal of Entry and Mode of Transmission	Incubation Period	Period of Communicability	Immunity after Recovery	Immunization	Isolation	Control Measures
A. Caused by Bacilli									
Diseases Spread Mainly Through Discharges from the Mouth and Nose									
1. Diphtheria	*Corynebacterium diphtheriae* (Klebs-Loeffler bacillus)	Class 2A	Tonsils, pharynx, larynx, nose, or other mucous membranes or skin (may affect wounds). Contact with a patient or carrier or with articles soiled with discharges from mucous membranes of nose and nasopharynx, and from skin and other lesions of infected persons. Raw milk can be a vehicle	Usually 2–5 days, occasionally longer	Variable, until virulent bacilli have disappeared from secretions and lesions; usually 2 weeks or less, seldom more than 4 weeks. Carriers may shed organisms for 6 months or more	Usually, but clinical attack not always followed by persisting immunity	Active immunization of all children with diphtheria toxoid (usually combined with tetanus toxoid and pertussis vaccine: DTP); beginning at 2 months of age, three intramuscular injections are given at 6–8 week intervals, a booster dose is given 1 year after third injection and again at school entrance; after 6 years of age, booster doses of tetanus and diphtheria toxoids (Td) are given every 10 years	For period of communicability and until 2 cultures each from throat and nose fail to show diphtheria bacilli; cultures to be taken not less than 24 hours apart and after cessation of antimicrobial therapy	Concurrent disinfection, of all articles in contact with patient and all articles soiled by discharges of patient; terminal cleaning; strict isolation under hospital conditions; all intimate contacts are placed under modified quarantine until nose and throat cultures are negative; all contacts are immunized and carriers and atypical cases searched for; educational measures and efforts to immunize on a population basis, with emphasis on infants, preschool children, and high-risk adults.

* Data compiled from Benenson, Abram S.: *Control of Communicable Diseases in Man*, 12th ed. American Public Health Association, Washington, D.C., 1975.
† See scheme of reporting diseases, classes 1–5, page 1710.

Disease	Causative Organism	Classification of Reportable Diseases †	Portal of Entry and Mode of Transmission	Incubation Period	Period of Communicability	Immunity after Recovery	Immunization	Isolation	Control Measures
A. Caused by Bacilli			*Diseases Spread Mainly Through Discharges from the Mouth and Nose*						
2. Tuberculosis (pulmonary)	*Mycobacterium tuberculosis* (human tubercle bacillus	Class 2B	Nose, mouth. Contact with bacilli in pulmonary secretions or sputum of infected persons; spread predominantly by airborne route; of no importance is indirect contact with contaminated articles or dust	From infection to demonstrable primary lesion, about 4–6 weeks; to progressive pulmonary or extra pulmonary tuberculosis may be years: first 6–12 months after infection is most hazardous period	As long as infectious tubercle bacilli are being discharged; extra pulmonary or extra pulmonary tuberculosis is not generally communicable	Disease is arrested; relapses may occur and disease can become reactivated at any time during life	BCG vaccination of tuberculin-negative household contacts under special circumstances	Prompt antimicrobial therapy reduces infectiousness rapidly; treatment in hospital or home with sputum precautions	Handwashing and good housekeeping practices; no special precautions necessary for handling fomites; disinfection of air by ultraviolet light and ventilation; preventive treatment of high-risk contacts with isoniazid; periodic tuberculin-testing of high-risk groups; health education and intensive follow-up of cases, contacts.
3. Whooping cough (pertussis)	*Bordetella pertussis*	Class 2B	Nose, mouth. Direct contact with discharges from laryngeal and bronchial mucous membranes of infected persons by droplet spread; indirectly by con-	7–21 days; almost uniformly within 10 days	Highly communicable in catarrhal stage from 7 days after exposure until 3 weeks after onset of typical paroxysmal whoop; when treated with	Immune after one attack although exposed adults occasionally have second attacks	Active immunization of all children with pertussis vaccine (usually combined with diphtheria and tetanus toxoids: DTP, as described under diphtheria);	Separation of patient from susceptible children and exclusion from school and public places for 14 days after exposure; booster immunization to	Concurrent disinfection as in diphtheria; active immunization in infancy is most effective control measure

5. SUMMARY TABLE OF DATA (Continued)

Disease	Causative Organism	Classification of Reportable Diseases †	Portal of Entry and Mode of Transmission	Incubation Period	Period of Communicability	Immunity after Recovery	Immunization	Isolation	Control Measures
A. Caused by Bacilli			Diseases Spread Mainly Through Discharges from the Mouth and Nose						
			tact with articles freshly soiled with discharges		erythromycin or ampicillin, infectious only 5–7 days after onset of therapy		pertussis vaccine is not given after 6 years of age	children under 3; erythromycin or ampicillin to nonimmunized children	
B. Caused by Cocci and Other Organisms									
1. Meningitis meningococcal	Neisseria meningitidis (N. intracellularis) groups A, B, and C, groups X, Y, and Z	Class 2A	Nose, mouth. Direct contact, including droplet spread, with discharges from nose and throat of infected persons, more often with carriers than cases; commonly occurs among persons living under crowded conditions in barracks and in institutions; indirect contact is of questionable significance	2–10 days, commonly 3–4 days	Until organism disappears from discharges of nose and mouth	Type-specific immunity of unknown duration probably follows even a subclinical infection	None; experimental vaccines are under investigation	Until 24 hours after start of chemotherapy	Concurrent disinfection as in diphtheria; health education in personal hygiene, prevention of overcrowded living and working spaces (especially in barracks, camps, ships, and schools); careful surveillance of cases and contacts when an outbreak of disease occurs; selective use of prophylactic agents in epidemics

B. Caused by Cocci and Other Organisms

Diseases Spread Mainly Through Discharges from the Mouth and Nose

Disease	Causative Organism	Classification of Reportable Diseases †	Portal of Entry and Mode of Transmission	Incubation Period	Period of Communicability	Immunity after Recovery	Immunization	Isolation	Control Measures
2. The pneumonias a. Pneumococcal	*Streptococcus pneumoniae* (pneumococci), types I to XXXII	Class 4	Nose, mouth. Droplet spread by direct contact with patients or carriers, or indirectly through articles soiled with discharges	Not well determined; believed to be 1–3 days	Unknown, presumably until discharges of mouth and nose no longer contain virulent form of agent; penicillin eliminates organism in 3 days	Immunity usually follows an attack and may last months or years	Immunization with bacterial polysaccharides is under investigation	Of limited value; institute secretion precautions for duration of illness	Concurrent disinfection as in diphtheria; chemoprophylaxis for outbreaks in institutions; whenever practicable, avoid overcrowded living and sleeping quarters, particularly in institutions and on shipboard
b. Bacterial	*Streptococcus pyogenes* (group A hemolytic) *Staphylococcus aureus, Klebsiella pneumoniae Haemophilus influenzae Pseudomonas aeruginosa Escherichia coli*	Class 4	As above	1–3 days	As above; antibiotic therapy greatly decreases period of communicability	Varies with infectious agent	Against influenza in adults and against measles in children may be useful	Strict for staphylococcal and streptococcal pneumonias; secretion precautions for others	As above; chemoprophylaxis for streptococcal infections

5. SUMMARY TABLE OF DATA (Continued)

Disease	Causative Organism	Classification of Reportable Diseases †	Portal of Entry and Mode of Transmission	Incubation Period	Period of Communicability	Immunity after Recovery	Immunization	Isolation	Control Measures
B. Caused by Cocci and Other Organisms			Diseases Spread Mainly Through Discharges from the Mouth and Nose						
c. Mycoplasmal (pleuro-pneumonia-like group of organisms: PPLO)	*Mycoplasma pneumoniae* (Eaton agent)	Class 4	As above	14–21 days	Probably less than 10 days	Indefinite	None	None	As above
3. Streptococcal disease, beta hemolytic (scarlet fever, streptococcal sore throat, and other related infections)	*Streptococcus pyogenes*, group A of at least 60 types	Class 4	Nose, mouth. By direct or intimate contact with patient or carrier, rarely by indirect contact with contaminated objects; nasal carriers are especially important in disease transmission; outbreaks of streptococcal sore throat may follow ingestion of contaminated milk or other food	1–3 days	10–21 days in untreated uncomplicated cases; untreated with purulent discharges lasts weeks or months; with adequate penicillin therapy, transmission is eliminated in 24 hours	Immunity develops only for the specific M-type of group A streptococcus and lasts for years; second attacks of scarlet fever rarely occur; repeated attacks of streptococcal sore throat by different types of organisms frequently occur	Not practicable	May terminate 24 hours after initiation of antibiotic therapy if continued for 10 days	Concurrent disinfection of purulent discharges and all articles soiled therewith; terminal cleaning; pasteurization of milk; exclusion of infected persons from handling food and milk; public education in methods of control; penicillin chemoprophylaxis; strict asepsis in obstetric procedures; provision of adequate laboratory facilities

C. Caused by Filtrable Viruses

Diseases Spread Mainly Through Discharges from the Mouth and Nose

Disease	Causative Organism	Classification of Reportable Diseases †	Portal of Entry and Mode of Transmission	Incubation Period	Period of Communicability	Immunity after Recovery	Immunization	Isolation	Control Measures
1. Respiratory disease, acute viral									
a. Acute febrile respiratory disease	Parainfluenza virus, types 1, 2, 3, and 4; respiratory syncytial virus; adenovirus, types 1, 2, 3, 4, 5, 7, 14, and 21; rhinoviruses; certain coronaviruses; certain types of coxsackievirus, groups A and B, echoviruses, groups A and B, and *M. pneumoniae*	Class 4	Mouth, nose. Direct oral contact or by droplet spread; indirectly by articles freshly soiled by discharges of nose and throat of infected person (some viruses are discharged in feces and may be involved in transmission)	From a few days to 1 week or more	For duration of active disease	Infection induces specific antibodies; reinfection commonly occurs with syncytial and parainfluenza viruses but illness is milder or absent	Non	Of no established value; infected persons should avoid exposure to others; bed rest in acute stage accomplishes modified isolation; isolation may be helpful in institutions	Concurrent disinfection of eating and drinking utensils; sanitary disposal of mouth and nose discharges; education of public in personal hygiene; avoid overcrowding
b. Common cold	89 or more rhinovirus serotypes, several coronaviruses, and some other known respiratory viruses	Class 5	As above	12–72 hours, usually 24 hours	From 24 hours before onset to 5 days after onset	Not immune	Not available	As above	As above
2. Rubella (German measles)	Virus of rubella	Class 3B	Nose, mouth. By droplet spread or direct contact with patients or by indirect contact with freshly	14–21 days, usually 18 days	1 week before and at least 4 days after onset of rash	One attack usually confers permanent immunity	A single dose of live attenuated rubella virus vaccine to all prepubertal children over 1 year of age;	Impractical, unless contacts include nonimmune pregnant women	Rubella immune globulin (human) containing high titers of specific antibody is under

5. SUMMARY TABLE OF DATA (Continued)

Disease	Causative Organism	Classification of Reportable Diseases †	Portal of Entry and Mode of Transmission	Incubation Period	Period of Communicability	Immunity after Recovery	Immunization	Isolation	Control Measures
C. Caused by Filtrable Viruses			Diseases Spread Mainly Through Discharges from the Mouth and Nose						
			soiled articles; possible transmission through blood, urine, or feces; infants with congenital rubella syndrome transmit virus through excretions				immunization of pregnant women is strictly contraindicated		clinical trial; in case of natural infection in pregnancy or vaccine given to a susceptible pregnant woman, abortion is considered because of risk of damage to fetus
3. Influenza	Influenza virus, types A, B, and C	Class 1 under WHO surveillance; class 4 in other areas	Direct contact through droplet infection or by articles freshly soiled with discharges from mouth and nose; probably airborne transmission	24–72 hours	Limited to 3 days from clinical onset	Immunity to specific type of infecting virus	Immunization with vaccine of prevailing strain of virus; limited to certain groups of individuals in years when epidemics are anticipated	None recommended, may isolate highly susceptible individuals from acutely ill patients	Concurrent disinfection of discharges from nose and throat; education of public in personal hygiene; health planning to avoid disruptive effects of influenza epidemic; community surveillance for outbreaks of disease; prompt reporting and identification of causative virus

C. Caused by Filtrable Viruses

Diseases Spread Mainly Through Discharges from the Mouth and Nose

Disease	Causative Organism	Classification of Reportable Diseases †	Portal of Entry and Mode of Transmission	Incubation Period	Period of Communicability	Immunity after Recovery	Immunization	Isolation	Control Measures
4. Measles (rubeola)	Virus of measles	Class 2B	Nose, mouth. Transmission as in influenza	About 10 days, varying from 8 to 13 days; rash usually appears on 14th day	From beginning of prodromal period to 4 days after rash appears	Immune	A single dose of live attenuated vaccine is given at 1 year of age	Impracticable in community; in institutions isolate to protect other children	Vaccinate contacts on day of exposure; if contraindicated give measles immune serum globulin; health education of public in importance of vaccination
5. Mumps (infectious parotitis)	Virus of mumps, a myxovirus	Class 3C	As above	12–26 days, commonly 18 days	About 48 hours before parotid gland enlargement	Immune	A single dose of live attenuated vaccine is given to children over 1 year of age and to selected susceptible adolescents and adults; available also as a combination measles-mumps-rubella vaccine	For 9 days after onset of swelling, less if swelling has subsided	Concurrent disinfection of articles soiled with nose and throat discharges; presently unknown if mumps immunization prevents disease; mumps hyperimmune globulin of questionable effectiveness
6. Poliomyelitis (infantile paralysis)	Poliovirus, types 1, 2, and 3	Class 1	Direct contact with pharyngeal secretions or feces of infected persons through close association	Commonly 7–12 days, with a range of 3–21 days	Cases are most infectious from 7 to 10 days before and after onset of symptoms; virus persists in throat 1 week and in feces	Type-specific immunity	Oral poliovirus vaccine containing all 3 types is given to all susceptible persons; infants are immunized with first dose usu-	For not more than 7 days (in hospital management); of little value at home	Concurrent disinfection of throat discharges and feces, and of articles soiled therewith; health education of public

5. SUMMARY TABLE OF DATA (Continued)

Disease	Causative Organism	Classification of Reportable Diseases †	Portal of Entry and Mode of Transmission	Incubation Period	Period of Communicability	Immunity after Recovery	Immunization	Isolation	Control Measures
C. Caused by Filtrable Viruses			Diseases Spread Mainly Through Discharges from the Mouth and Nose						
					for 3–6 weeks or longer		ally at 6–8 weeks, second dose at 4 months, third dose at 6 months, and with boosters 1 year after third dose and at school entrance		toward early immunization; community vaccination programs at earliest indication of an outbreak
7. Smallpox (Variola)	Variola virus	Class 1	Nose, mouth, and lesions of skin and mucous membranes. Transmission also occurs through recently contaminated articles, through bedding and other linens	7–17 days, commonly 10–12 days to illness onset and 2–4 days more to onset of rash	From development of earliest lesions to disappearance of all scabs, about 3 weeks	Immune; after vaccination immunity gradually wanes	In endemic countries a single vaccination with potent smallpox vaccine using techniques of multiple pressure, multiple puncture, or jet injection; recent WHO directive removes requirement for primary vaccination, revaccination, or vaccination for travel, in smallpox-free coun-	Until all scabs have disappeared; strict isolation under hospital conditions	Strict isolation; concurrent disinfection as in diphtheria; terminal cleaning of room with disinfecting agents known to kill poxviruses; quarantine of all close contacts for 17 days; prompt vaccination of all contacts; search for source of infection; immediate public education

Disease	Causative Organism	Classification of Reportable Diseases †	Portal of Entry and Mode of Transmission	Incubation Period	Period of Communicability	Immunity after Recovery	Immunization	Isolation	Control Measures
							tries; where disease is endemic, primary vaccination is advised for infants soon after birth, at 1 year of age, and then every 5 years		

Diseases Spread Mainly Through Discharges from the Mouth and Nose

Disease	Causative Organism	Classification of Reportable Diseases †	Portal of Entry and Mode of Transmission	Incubation Period	Period of Communicability	Immunity after Recovery	Immunization	Isolation	Control Measures
8. Chickenpox-herpes zoster (varicella-shingles)	Varicella-zoster virus (V-Z virus)	Class 3B	Nose, mouth, skin lesions. Direct contact, droplet, or airborne spread of secretions from respiratory tract of infected persons; indirectly through freshly soiled articles by discharges from vesicles. Scabs are noninfective. Susceptibles may contract disease from patients with herpes zoster	2–3 weeks, commonly 13–17 days	5 days before skin eruption to 6 days after first crop of vesicles appears	Long immunity conferred; second attacks rare; infection may recur years later as herpes zoster; disease more severe in adults than in children	None	None; school exclusion for 1 week after first eruption occurs	Concurrent disinfection of articles soiled with discharges of nose, throat, and skin lesions; Zoster Immune Globulin (ZIG) may prevent or modify disease in high-risk contacts

5. SUMMARY TABLE OF DATA (Continued)

Disease	Causative Organism	Classification of Reportable Diseases †	Portal of Entry and Mode of Transmission	Incubation Period	Period of Communicability	Immunity after Recovery	Immunization	Isolation	Control Measures
			Diseases Spread Mainly Through Discharges from Skin and Mucous Membranes						
1. Chancroid	*Hemophilus ducreyi*	Class 2B	Genitourinary tract. Direct sexual contact with discharges from open lesions; indirect transmission is rare; accidental inoculation of children is known; evidence of asymptomatic infections in women	From 3–5 days, up to 14 days	As long as infectious agent persists in original lesion or discharging lymph nodes	None	None	None; avoid sexual contact until all lesions are healed	Personal cleanliness; investigation of contacts 2 weeks before and after onset of disease; general health promotional measures; control of prostitution and indiscriminate sexual promiscuity; provision of early detection and treatment facilities
2. Dermatophytosis a. Ringworm of the scalp (tinea capitis)	Various species of *Microsporum* and *Trichophyton* (fungi)	Class 4	Skin. Direct or indirect contact, especially with backs of seats used by the public, barber instruments, toilet articles, or clothing contaminated with hair from infected animals or man	10–14 days	As long as lesions remain and spores persist on contaminated materials	Not immune	None	Impractical	In epidemics, examination of heads of school children with ultraviolet light (Wood's filter); in severe cases, wash and cover scalp with cap; discard or boil cap after use; education of children, par-

Diseases Spread Mainly Through Discharges from Skin and Mucous Membranes

Disease	Causative Organism	Classification of Reportable Diseases †	Portal of Entry and Mode of Transmission	Incubation Period	Period of Communicability	Immunity after Recovery	Immunization	Isolation	Control Measures
									ents, and school personnel; study household contacts and pets for source of infection
b. Ringworm of the body (tinea corporis)	Various species of *Microsporum* and *Trichophyton;* also *Epidermophyton floccosum*	Class 4	Direct or indirect contact with skin and scalp lesions of infected persons, lesions of animals, contaminated floors, shower stalls, beaches, etc.	10–14 days	As above	Not immune	None	Infected children are excluded from gymnasiums and swimming pools	Frequent laundering of clothing; sterilization of towels used in gymnasiums; general cleanliness of showers; disinfection of floors and benches with a fungicidal agent; public health education
c. Ringworm of the foot (tinea pedis)	*Trichophyton rubrum, T. mentagrophytes, Microsporum* species	Class 5	Direct or indirect contact with skin lesions of infected persons or contaminated floors, shower stalls	Unknown	As above	Not immune; second attacks are frequent	None	None	As above. Special care in drying between toes after bathing; regular use of a fungicide powder; boil socks of severely infected person; expose feet to air by wearing sandals

5. SUMMARY TABLE OF DATA (Continued)

Disease	Causative Organism	Classification of Reportable Diseases †	Portal of Entry and Mode of Transmission	Incubation Period	Period of Communicability	Immunity after Recovery	Immunization	Isolation	Control Measures
Diseases Spread Mainly Through Discharges from Skin and Mucous Membranes									
d. Ringworm of the nails (tinea unguium)	Various species of *Trichophyton*; also *Epidermophyton floccosum* and *Candida albicans*	Class 5	As above, but usually no transmission even to close family associates	Unknown	As above, possibly	Not immune; reinfection frequent	None	None	As for tinea corporis
3. Gonococcal disease a. Gonorrhea	*Neisseria gonorrhoeae*	Class 2B	Genitourinary tract by sexual contact with exudates from mucous membranes of infected persons	Usually 2–5 days, sometimes 9 days or longer	For months or years unless treated, especially in females	Not immune	None	None; avoid sexual contact with untreated previous sexual partners	As in chancroid, care in disposal of discharges from lesions and articles soiled therewith; rigorous investigation for and treatment of contacts of infectious patient; public education
b. Gonococcal vulvovaginitis of children	As above	As above	Intimate direct contact with exudates from infected adults; direct sexual contact and occasionally contact with contaminated articles, instru-	3–9 days	While discharges persist, usually 3–6 months	Not immune	None	Until 24 hours after initiation of antibiotic	As above. Prompt search for source of infection within the institution or group affected; rigid enforcement of hygienic principles and early

Disease	Causative Organism	Classification of Reportable Diseases†	Portal of Entry and Mode of Transmission	Incubation Period	Period of Communicability	Immunity after Recovery	Immunization	Isolation	Control Measures
			ments, foreign bodies, or rectal thermometers						sex education; education of those caring for children
Diseases Spread Mainly Through Discharges from Skin and Mucous Membranes									
c. Gonococcal ophthalmia neonatorum	As above	As above	Contact with infected birth canal during delivery	36–48 hours	For 24 hours following treatment or until eye discharges cease	Not immune	None	Until 24 hours after initiation of antibiotic	Use of chemoprophylactic agent in eyes of newborn; routine cervical and rectal gonococcal culture during third trimester of pregnancy; care in disposal of conjunctival discharges and articles soiled therewith
4. Staphylococcal disease a. In the community (boils, abscesses, generalized infections)	Various coagulase-positive strains of *Staphylococcus aureus*	Class 4	Anterior nares; autoinfection and shedding of organism through nasal secretions of asymptomatic carrier; contact with purulent lesion; role of contaminated objects is overstressed; airborne spread is rare	Commonly 10–14 days	As long as purulent lesions continue to drain or carrier state persists	Not well understood	None	Not practical in communities; avoid contact with infants and debilitated individuals	Education in personal hygiene, especially handwashing; burn or dispose of dressings from open lesions; prompt treatment of infected persons; search for nasal carriers

5. SUMMARY TABLE OF DATA (Continued)

Disease	Causative Organism	Classification of Reportable Diseases †	Portal of Entry and Mode of Transmission	Incubation Period	Period of Communicability	Immunity after Recovery	Immunization	Isolation	Control Measures
Diseases Spread Mainly Through Discharges from Skin and Mucous Membranes									
b. In hospital nurseries (impetigo of the newborn)	As above	As above	As above; spread by hands of hospital attendants	As above	As above	Not immune	None	Immediate isolation in hospital nursery	Strict asepsis in hospital techniques; thorough handwashing; use of a rotational system in nursery; surveillance and supervision by an active Hospital Infections Control committee; examination of and exclusion of carriers from work until cultures are negative; prompt investigation of nursery outbreaks
c. In hospital medical and surgical wards (wound infections, generalized sepsis)	As above	As above	As above	As above	As above	Not immune	None	Strict isolation under hospital conditions for generalized sepsis; wound and skin precautions for duration of illness	As above Collect and burn dressings; autoclave linens before laundering; terminal cleaning of room; search for additional cases among patients

Diseases Spread Mainly Through Discharges from Skin and Mucous Membranes

Disease	Causative Organism	Classification of Reportable Diseases †	Portal of Entry and Mode of Transmission	Incubation Period	Period of Communicability	Immunity after Recovery	Immunization	Isolation	Control Measures
5. Syphilis a. Venereal	Treponema pallidum	Class 2A	Genitourinary tract, mucous membrane of mouth and skin. Direct contact in heterosexual or homosexual activity with exudates from moist lesions, body fluids, and secretions of infected persons; indirect contact with contaminated articles is possible but rare; can be transmitted after fourth month of pregnancy through placenta; occasionally by transfusion	10 days–10 weeks, usually 3 weeks	Variable and indefinite; during primary and secondary stages intermittently for 2–4 years	No natural immunity; infection leads to gradual resistance to certain strains of Treponema	None	None. To avoid reinfection, partners should refrain from sexual contact with previous partners not under treatment	Same as for chancroid and gonorrhea. Serologic test for syphilis (STS) premaritally, in pregnancy, and as part of a general physical examination. For contact investigation, stage of disease determines criteria: 1. *Primary*— all sexual contacts of preceding 3 months 2. *Secondary*— those contacts of preceding 6 months 3. *Early latent* —those contacts of preceding year 4. *Late and late latent*—sexual partners and children of infected mothers

Diseases Spread Mainly Through Discharges from Skin and Mucous Membranes

Disease	Causative Organism	Classification of Reportable Diseases †	Portal of Entry and Mode of Transmission	Incubation Period	Period of Communicability	Immunity after Recovery	Immunization	Isolation	Control Measures
									5. *Congenital*—all immediate family members
b. Nonvenereal (Bejel)	As above	3B	Direct or indirect contact with infectious early lesions of skin and mucous membranes; common use of eating and drinking utensils	2 weeks–3 months	During moist eruptions of skin; several weeks or months	As above	None	None; avoid intimate contact	General health promotional measures; intensive control activities; provision of facilities for early detection and treatment; treatment of family contacts
6. Herpes simplex	Herpes simplex virus, types 1 and 2	Class 5	Mouth. Direct contact with virus in saliva of carrier; transmission of type 2 by sexual contact	Up to 2 weeks	Secretion of virus in saliva as long as 7 weeks after recovery; can also be isolated from saliva in asymptomatic adults	Not immune	None	Persons with herpetic lesions isolated from newborns, children with eczema or burns, and immunosuppressed patients	Personal hygiene and health education toward minimizing transfer of infectious material; care to avoid contaminating skin of eczematous patients with infectious material

Diseases Spread Mainly Through Discharges from the Gastrointestinal Tract

Disease	Causative Organism	Classification of Reportable Diseases †	Portal of Entry and Mode of Transmission	Incubation Period	Period of Communicability	Immunity after Recovery	Immunization	Isolation	Control Measures
1. Amebiasis (amebic dysentery)	*Entamoeba histolytica*	Class 3C	Mouth. Spread through contaminated water containing cysts from feces of infected persons; hand to mouth transfer of fresh feces; by contaminated raw vegetables, flies, and soiled hands of food handlers, and perhaps water	Variable, from a few days to several months or years, commonly 2–4 weeks	During intestinal infection which may continue for years	Immunity not clearly demonstrated	None	None; exclusion of known cyst passers from food handling until completion of treatment	Sanitary disposal of feces; protection of public water supply; health education of public; control of flies; regular supervision of public eating places
2. Shigellosis (bacillary dysentery)	30 serotypes of *Shigella*, groups A, B, and C, and *Sh. sonnei*, group D	Class 2B	Mouth. Transmission by fecal-oral route from infected patient or carrier; indirectly by objects soiled with feces; by contaminated food, milk, or water; by flies	1–7 days, usually less than 4 days	During acute infection and until infectious agent is no longer present in feces; rarely carrier state may persist for 1 year or longer	Unknown	Evidence of protection with type-specific live vaccines	During acute illness; rigid enteric precautions by attendants; nonemployment as food handlers until rectal cultures are negative 2 days after cessation of therapy	As for amebiasis. Public education in personal hygiene, scrupulous cleanliness in food preparation; pasteurization or boiling of milk supply
3. Paratyphoid fever	*Salmonella paratyphi*, types A, B, and C	Class 2A	Mouth. Direct or indirect contact with feces or urine of patient or carrier; vehicles of transfer indi-	1–3 weeks for enteric fever; 1–10 days for gastroenteritis	As long as infectious agent persists in excreta, commonly 1–2 weeks, but may be permanent	Partial species-specific immunity	Not proved to be effective	Exclusion of infected persons as food handlers and from caring for young children and elderly un-	As for typhoid fever (see column below)

Diseases Spread Mainly Through Discharges from the Gastrointestinal Tract

Disease	Causative Organism	Classification of Reportable Diseases †	Portal of Entry and Mode of Transmission	Incubation Period	Period of Communicability	Immunity after Recovery	Immunization	Isolation	Control Measures
			rectly are food, milk, milk products, shellfish, water, contaminated hands, and flies					til stool cultures are negative on 3 successive days	
4. Typhoid fever	*Salmonella typhi*, about 50 types	Class 2A	Mouth. As in paratyphoid fever especially unsafe raw fruits and vegetables, milk, and milk products; contaminated imported canned meat	Dependent on size of infecting dose, usual range 1–3 weeks	As long as typhoid bacilli appear in excreta, usually from first week throughout convalescence; thereafter, variable; 10% of infected persons discharge bacilli for 3 months, 2–5% become permanent carriers	Resistance usually follows recovery	Typhoid vaccine is given in a primary series of 2 injections spaced by several weeks; preference is given to those subject to exposure through occupation or travel, those living in endemic areas, and those in institutions where maintenance of good sanitation is difficult; periodic single reinforcing injection is desirable every 3 years in such instances	Hospitalization in fly-proof room with enteric precautions; patient remains under supervision of health authority until three negative stool and urine cultures are obtained at least 24 hours apart and not earlier than 1 month after onset of illness	Concurrent disinfection of feces and urine and articles soiled therewith; use of vaccine in outbreaks not recommended; exclusion of suspected food; intensive search for case or carrier; protection of public water supply; fly control; sanitary disposal of excreta; boiling or pasteurization of milk and dairy products; control of shellfish supply; supervision of public eating places;

Diseases Spread Mainly Through Discharges from the Gastrointestinal Tract

Disease	Causative Organism	Classification of Reportable Diseases †	Portal of Entry and Mode of Transmission	Incubation Period	Period of Communicability	Immunity after Recovery	Immunization	Isolation	Control Measures
									identification of chronic carriers; public health education, particularly of food handlers
5. Hepatitides, viral									
a. Infectious, (hepatitis A)	Filtrable agent, with characteristics of an enterovirus or parvovirus	Class 2A	Mouth. Person-to-person contact by fecal-oral route; outbreaks related to contaminated water, food; can be spread by ingestion or by parenteral inoculation of infected blood or blood products	Dose related; from 15–50 days, average 28–30 days	During latter half of incubation period through few days, after onset of jaundice	Unknown, but presumed to be long-lasting	None. Immune serum globulin may be given prophylactically to travelers to highly endemic areas, to household contacts, and to staff and newly admitted patients to mental institutions	Enteric precautions during first 2 weeks of illness and at least 1 week after onset of jaundice	Sanitary disposal of feces and urine; public health education toward good sanitation and personal hygiene; proper sterilization of syringes, needles, or use disposable units; epidemiologic investigation of outbreak
b. Serum, (Hepatitis B)	A virus of probable DNA nucleic acid content	As above	Skin. Transmitted by parenteral innoculation of human blood, plasma, serum, and other blood products of an infected person; by contami-	45–160 days, usually 60–90 days	Possibly many weeks before symptom onset through clinical course of disease; chronic carrier state may persist for years	Not yet defined	None	Enteric precautions for hospital patients	As above Avoid indiscriminate use of transfusions; strict supervision of blood donors and blood banks; surveillance of all cases of

Disease	Causative Organism	Classification of Reportable Diseases †	Portal of Entry and Mode of Transmission	Incubation Period	Period of Communicability	Immunity after Recovery	Immunization	Isolation	Control Measures
		Diseases Spread Mainly Through Discharges from the Gastrointestinal Tract							
			nated needles and syringes; may be spread through contamination of wounds or lacerations or by ingestion of infective blood						post-transfusion hepatitis; disinfection of all equipment contaminated with blood
6. Cholera	*Vibrio cholerae*	Class 1	Mouth. Spread through ingestion of water contaminated with feces or vomitus of patients; or of feces of carriers, food contaminated by water, soiled hands, or flies	From a few hours to 5 days, usually 2–3 days	Unknown, but presumably for duration of stool-positive carrier state lasting only a few days after recovery; carrier state may persist for several months	Infection results in significant antibodies, immunity acquired by most persons in endemic areas by early adulthood	Cholera vaccine available and provides partial active immunity (50% protection); vaccine lasts only few months and does not prevent asymptomatic infection	Desirable under hospital management during presence of acute symptoms; strict isolation not necessary	As in typhoid fever; active immunization of little value as control measure

Disease	Causative Organism	Classification of Reportable Diseases †	Portal of Entry and Mode of Transmission	Incubation Period	Period of Communicability	Immunity after Recovery	Immunization	Isolation	Control Measures
			Diseases Transmitted to Wounds by Organisms from Various Sources						
1. Tetanus (lockjaw)	Clostridium tetani	Class 2A	Wounds, skin; spores introduced into body during injury, usually puncture wound contaminated with soil, street dust, or animal feces; through burns and trivial wounds; and infection of umbilicus	4 days to 3 weeks, average 10 days	Not directly transmitted from person to person	Not immune; second attacks occur	Active immunity with tetanus toxoid in infancy (as described under diphtheria); recommended booster dose on day of injury if more than 3–5 years has elapsed since last dose; persons never immunized are given 2 doses of toxoid 4 weeks apart, a booster dose 8–12 months later, then every 10 years; immunization is recommended for international travelers, for workers in contact with soil or domestic animals, members of military forces and policemen, and for pregnant women in tetanus-prevalent areas;	None	Health education of public in importance of immunization; licensing and supervision of attendants at childbirth to ensure strict asepsis; thorough cleansing of wounds

5. SUMMARY TABLE OF DATA (Continued)

Disease	Causative Organism	Classification of Reportable Diseases †	Portal of Entry and Mode of Transmission	Incubation Period	Period of Communicability	Immunity after Recovery	Immunization	Isolation	Control Measures
							passive immunization with tetanus-immune globulin (human) or tetanus antitoxin (equine or bovine) is given in special instances		
Diseases Transmitted to Wounds by Organisms from Various Sources									
Diseases Spread Mainly by Infected Animals									
1. Anthrax (malignant pustule)	*Bacillus anthracis*	Class 2A	*Skin:* direct contact with tissues of animals dying of this disease; contaminated hides, hair, soil, biting flies, and vultures; *Respiratory tract:* inhalation of spores that float in air *Gastrointestinal tract:* ingestion of contaminated uncooked meat	Within 7 days, usually 2–5 days	Never reported as transmitted from man to man; articles and soil contaminated with spores may remain infective for years	Uncertain; no well-documented second attack reported	A cell-free vaccine is available in special instances to prevent anthrax in high-risk persons such as veterinarians and industrial workers	For inhalation anthrax, strict isolation procedures; for cutaneous anthrax, wound isolation until lesions are free of bacillus	Concurrent disinfection of discharges from lesions and articles soiled therewith; spores require steam sterilization or burning; education of workers who handle potentially contaminated articles; dust control, ventilation, medical care, handwashing and adequate eating facilities for employees; disinfection of hair, wool,

Disease	Causative Organism	Classification of Reportable Diseases†	Portal of Entry and Mode of Transmission	Incubation Period	Period of Communicability	Immunity after Recovery	Immunization	Isolation	Control Measures
									hides, and bone meal before processing; control of industrial wastes; disposal by burning infected carcasses; treatment and vaccination of animals

Diseases Spread Mainly by Infected Animals

Disease	Causative Organism	Classification of Reportable Diseases†	Portal of Entry and Mode of Transmission	Incubation Period	Period of Communicability	Immunity after Recovery	Immunization	Isolation	Control Measures
2. Brucellosis (undulant or Malta fever)	Various biotypes of *Brucella abortus, Brucella canis, Brucella melitensis,* and *Brucella suis*	Class 2B	Mouth, abrasions in skin or mucous membranes; contact with tissues, blood, urine, vaginal discharges, aborted fetuses of infected animals (especially placentas); by ingestion of milk or dairy products (cheese) from infected animals; airborne infections may occur; also laboratory transmission	Highly variable and difficult to ascertain, usually 5–21 days, occasionally several months	No evidence of communicability from person to person	Of uncertain duration	None	None	Concurrent disinfection of purulent discharges; health education of workers in slaughterhouses, packing plants, and butcher shops; control of infection among livestock; meat inspection; milk pasteurization or boiling; infection tracing to determine source

5. SUMMARY TABLE OF DATA (Continued)

Disease	Causative Organism	Classification of Reportable Diseases †	Portal of Entry and Mode of Transmission	Incubation Period	Period of Communicability	Immunity after Recovery	Immunization	Isolation	Control Measures
			Diseases Spread Mainly by Infected Animals						
3. Rabies	Virus of rabies, a rhabdovirus	Class 2A	Bite of rabid animal and (rarely) skin scratches; virus-laden saliva of rabid animal, including dog, fox, coyote, wolf, jackal, cat, skunk, racoon, mongoose, and bat; airborne spread in bat caves is rare	Usually 2–8 weeks, depending on extent of laceration, site of wound in relation to richness of nerve supply and distance from brain, amount of virus introduced, clothing and other factors	In dogs and other biting animals, 3–5 days before clinical onset and during course of disease; bats may shed virus for weeks without illness	Unknown; invariably a fatal disease	Administration of antirabies serum and/or vaccine upon injury, following published USPHS recommendations	Strict isolation for duration of illness	Concurrent disinfection of saliva and articles soiled therewith; immediate and thorough cleansing with soap and water of all animal bites, public education in necessity of restriction, vaccination, and registration of dogs, reporting of bites, and procurement of medical attention; detention and observation of biting animals for 7–10 days; establishment of rabies control measures with wildlife conservation and animal health authorities

REFERENCES

1. Sidel, Victor W., and Sidel, Ruth: *Serve the People, Observations on Medicine in the People's Republic of China.* Beacon Press, Boston, 1973, pp. 23, 107.

2. US Department of Commerce, Bureau of the Census: *The U.S. 1976 Fact Book, American Almanac, Statistical Abstract of the U.S.,* 96th ed. Grosset & Dunlap, New York, 1976, p. 87.

2a. US Department of Health, Education, and Welfare, Public Health Service, Center for Disease Control, Tuberculosis Control Division: *1974 Tuberculosis Statistics: States and Cities.* Atlanta, Ga., July 1975, p. 3.

3. *World Health Statistics Report* **25:**8, World Health Organization, Geneva, 1972.

4. Pauling, Linus: *Vitamin C and the Common Cold.* W. H. Freeman & Co., San Francisco, 1970.

5. ———: "Ascorbic Acid and the Common Cold," *Am. J. Clin. Nutr.,* **24:**1294, (Nov.) 1971.

6. Goldsmith, Grace A.: "Common Cold: Prevention and Treatment with Ascorbic Acid Not Effective," *J.A.M.A.,* **216:**337, (Apr. 12) 1971.

7. Gregg, Michael B.: "Communicable Disease Trends in the United States," *Am. J. Nurs.,* **68:**88, (Jan.) 1968.

8. Conrad, J. L., et al.: "The Epidemiologic Rationale for the Failure to Eradicate Measles in the United States," *Am. J. Public Health,* **61:**2304, (Nov.) 1971.

9. Hinman, Alan R.: "Resurgence of Measles in New York," *Am. J. Public Health,* **62:**498, (Apr.) 1972.

10. Allen, David W., and Cole, Philip: "Viruses and Human Cancer," *N. Engl. J. Med.,* **286:**70, (Jan. 13) 1973.

11. Silberstein, Melvin J., and Morton, Donald L.: "Cancer Immunotherapy," *Am. J. Nurs.,* **73:**1178, (July) 1973.

12. Szent-Györgyi, Albert: *The Living State, With Observations on Cancer.* Academic Press, New York, 1972.

13. Litsky, Bertha Y.: "Scientific Housekeeping and the Professional Nurse," *Nurs. Clin. North Am.,* **5:**99, (Mar.) 1970.

14. McLean, Ross L.: "How Contagious Is Tuberculosis?" *Natl. Tub. Assoc. Bull.* **49:**10, (Dec.) 1963.

15. "Guidelines for the General Hospital in the Admission and Care of Tuberculosis Patients," *Am. Rev. Resp. Dis.,* **99:** [Apr.] 1969. A statement prepared by Ad Hoc Committee of USPHS and National Tuberculosis and Respiratory Disease Association.

16. *Nursing Care of Patients in the Laminar Air Flow Room.* A Nursing Clinical Conference presented by the Nursing Department of the Clinical Center, National Institutes of Health. US Department of Health, Education, and Welfare, Washington, D.C., 1971 (DHEW Pub. No. [NIH] 72–93).

17. Benenson, Abram S. (ed.): *Control of Communicable Diseases in Man,* 12th ed. American Public Health Association, Washington, D.C., 1975.

18. *Ibid.,* p. xxii.

19. *Ibid.,* p. xxiv.

20. *Ibid.,* p. xviii.

21. *New York State Sanitary Code.* Chapter 1, Title 10, Section 2.28, Albany, N.Y., 1963.

22. Florida State Board of Health: *Rules of State Board of Health,* [St. Petersburg, 1972], Chapter 170 B-1, p. 14.

23. Montana State Board of Health: *Communicable and Other Reportable Diseases.* The Board, Helena, 1965, p. 19.

24. Beland, Irene L., and Passos, Joyce Y.: *Clinical Nursing: Pathophysiological and Psychosocial Approaches.* Macmillan Publishing Co., Inc., New York, 1975, p. 174.

25. *Isolation Techniques for Use in Hospitals,* USPHS Communicable Disease Center, Atlanta, Ga., 1975, p. 7.

26. Steere, A. C., and Mallison, G.: "Handwashing Practices for the Prevention of Nosocomial Infections," *Ann. Intern. Med.,* **83:**683, (Nov.) 1975.

27. Leavell, Hugh R., and Clark, E. Gurney: *Preventive Medicine for the Doctor in His Community,* 3rd ed. McGraw-Hill Book Co., New York, 1965, p. 39.

28. Sartwell, Philip E. (ed.): *Maxcy-Rosenau Preventive Medicine and Public Health,* 10th ed. Appleton-Century-Crofts, New York 1973, p. 1.

29. Kilbourne, Edwin D., and Smillie, Wilson G. (eds.): *Human Ecology and Public Health,* 4th ed. The Macmillan Company, Collier-Macmillan, Limited, London, 1969, p. 1.

30. Goerke, Lenor S., and Stebbins, Ernest L.: *Mustard's Introduction to Public Health,* 5th ed. Macmillan Publishing Co., Inc., New York, 1968, p. 116.

31. Rosen, George: *A History of Public Health.* MD Publications, Inc., New York, 1958, p. 286.

31a. US Department of Health, Education, and Welfare, Public Health Service, Center for Disease Control: *Morbidity and Mortality Weekly Report,* **25:**270, (Sept. 3) 1976.

32. US Department of Commerce, Bureau of the Census: *op. cit.,* p. 64.

32a. US Department of Health, Education, and Welfare, Public Health Service, Center for Disease Control: *Morbidity and Mortality Weekly Report,* **25:**101, (Apr. 9) 1976.

33. Sidel, Victor W., and Sidel, Ruth: *op. cit.*

34. Wegman, Myron E. et al. (eds.): *Public Health in the People's Republic of China.* Josiah Macy, Jr. Foundation, New York, 1973.

35. Kessen, William: *Childhood in China.* Yale University Press, New Haven, Conn., 1975.

36. Horsh, Donald: "Legal Aspects of Infection Control." Paper presented at Conference on Infection Control in Hospitals and Institutions, October, 1967. US Public Health Service, Center for Disease Control, Atlanta, Ga., March 1971.

37. Leavell, Hugh R., and Clark, E. Gurney: *op. cit.,* p. 20.

38. US Department of Health, Education, and Welfare, Public Health Service: *Isolation Techniques for Use in Hospitals,* 2nd ed. US Government Printing Office, Washington, D.C., 1975.

39. New York State Department of Health, Bureau of Epidemiology: *Requirements for Communicable Diseases* (Form CD-205). Chart prepared for the New York State Department of Education, Albany, 1970.

40. California State Department of Public Health: *A Manual for the Control of Communicable Diseases in California.* The Department, Sacramento, 1971, p. 496.

41. Schaffer, Alexander J., and Avery, M. E.: *Diseases of the Newborn,* 3rd ed. W. B. Saunders Co., Philadelphia, 1971, p. 632.

42. US Department of Health, Education, and Welfare: *Morbidity and Mortality Weekly Report.* Vol. 18, No. 21. The Department, Center for Disease Control, Atlanta, Ga., (Oct.) 1969.

43. Wolff, Ilse S.: "Interviewing in Public Health Nursing: An Examination of Attitudes," Part I. *Nurs. Outlook,* 6:267, (May) 1958; "An Examination of Skills and Methods," Part II. *Nurs. Outlook,* 6:320, (June) 1958.

44. Crichton, Michael: *Five Patients—The Hospital Explained.* Alfred A. Knopf, New York, 1970, p. 35.

45. Adams, John M.: *Viruses and Colds, the Modern Plague.* American Elsevier Publishing Co., New York, 1967, p. 13.

46. DeGowin, Elmer L., and DeGowin, Richard L.: *Bedside Diagnostic Examination,* 3rd ed. Macmillan Publishing Co., Inc., New York, 1975, p. 447.

47. Atkins, Elisha: "Fever," in MacBryde, Cyril Mitchell and Blacklow, Robert Stanley: *Signs and Symptoms,* 5th ed. J. B. Lippincott Co., Philadelphia, 1970, p. 461.

48. *Ibid.,* p. 459.

49. *Ibid.*

Additional Suggested Reading

Ahern, Cheryl: "I Think I Have VD," *Nurs. Clin. North Am.,* 8:77, (Mar.) 1973.

American Social Health Association: *Today's VD Control Problem, 1974.* Symposium sponsored by American Public Health Association, American Social Health Association, American Venereal Disease Association, and Association of State and Territorial Health Officers, 1974.

Atkinson, M. C., et al.: *Patient Care in Tuberculosis.* National League for Nursing, New York, 1973.

Brown, H. W.: *Basic Clinical Parasitology.* Appleton-Century-Crofts, New York, 1975.

Corrigan, Marjorie J., and Corcoran, Lucille E. (eds.): *Epidemiology in Nursing.* Catholic University of America Press, Washington, D.C., 1961.

Council for International Organizations of Medical Sciences: *Communicable Diseases: Provisional International Nomenclature. A List of Names of Diseases Recommended for International Use as a Complement to the WHO International Classification of Diseases.* (Simen Btesh, ed.) CIOMS, % WHO, Geneva, 1973.

DeWeese, David, and Saunders, W. H.: *Textbook of Otolaryngology.* C. V. Mosby Co., St. Louis, 1973.

Dubos, René J., and Hirsch, James G. (ed.): *Bacterial and Mycotic Infections of Man,* 4th ed. J. B. Lippincott Co., Philadelphia, 1965.

Edson, Lee: "A Secret Weapon Called Immunology," *New York Times Magazine,* (Feb. 17), 1974, p. 10.

Eisen, Abraham H.: "The Role of Infection in Allergic Disease," *Pediatr. Clin. North Am.,* 16:67, (Feb.) 1969.

Garner, Julia S., and Kaiser, Allen B.: "How Often Is Isolation Needed?" *Am. J. Nurs.,* 72:733, (Apr.) 1972.

Grissom, D. K.: *Communicable Diseases.* Little, Brown & Co., Boston, Mass., 1971.

Hilleboe, Herman E.: "Modern Concepts of Prevention in Community Health," *Am. J. Public Health,* 61:1000, (May) 1971.

Horsfall, Frank L., and Tamm, Igor (eds.): *Viral and Rickettsial Infections of Man,* 4th ed. J. B. Lippincott Co., Philadelphia, 1965.

Jekel, James F.: "Communicable Disease Control and Public Policy in the 1970s—Hot War, Cold War, or Peaceful Coexistence?" *Am. J. Public Health,* 62:1578 (Dec.) 1972.

Krugman, Saul, and Ward, Robert: *Infectious Diseases of Children and Adults,* 5th ed. C. V. Mosby Co., St. Louis, 1973.

Lerner, Phillip I., et al. (eds.): "Symposium on Infectious Diseases," *Med. Clin. North Am.,* 58, (May) 1974.

Lester, Mary: "Every Nurse an Epidemiologist," *Am. J. Nurs.,* 57:1434, (Nov.) 1957.

McGrath, P., et al.: "Level of Basic Venereal Disease Knowledge Among Junior and Senior High School Nurses in Massachusetts: A Survey," *Nurs. Res.,* 23:31, (Jan.–Feb. 1974.)

McInnes, M. E.: *Essentials of Communicable Disease,* 2nd ed. C. V. Mosby Co., St. Louis, 1975.

Merson, M. H.: "Turista," *N. Engl. J. Med.,* 292:969, (May 1) 1975.

Monif, Gilles (ed.): *Infectious Diseases in Obstetrics and Gynecology.* Harper & Row, Medical Department, Hagerstown, Md., 1974.

Morrison, Shirley T., and Arnold, Carolyn R.: *Landon and Sider's Communicable Diseases,* 9th ed., F. A. Davis Co., Philadelphia, 1969.

Mudd, Stuart, (ed.): *Infectious Agents and Host Reactions.* W. B. Saunders Co., Philadelphia, 1970.

National League for Nursing: *Infection Control.* Papers presented at a workshop conducted by CHRINS in cooperation with the ALA Nursing Department at NLN, Mar. 1975. The League, Council of Hospital and Related Institutional Nursing Services, New York, 1975.

Payne, A. M. M.: "Approaches to Communicable Disease Control," *WHO Chron.,* 22:3, (Jan.) 1968.

Pinneo, Lily, and Pinneo, Rose: "Mystery Virus

from Lassa," *Am. J. Nurs.,* **71:**1352, (July) 1971.

Proceedings of the International Conference on Nosocomial Infections, 1970. American Hospital Association, Chicago, 1970.

Roberts, Doris E.: "Strengthening Nursing Practice Through Epidemiology," in *ANA Regional Clinical Conferences, 1967.* Appleton-Century-Crofts, New York, 1968.

Scrimshaw, N. S., et al.: "Interactions of Nutrition and Infection," *WHO Monogr. Ser.* No. 57. World Health Organization, Geneva, 1968.

"Symposium on Infection and the Nurse," *Nurs. Clin. North Am.,* **5:**85, (Mar.) 1970.

Top, Franklin H., Sr., and Wehrle, Paul F.: *Communicable and Infectious Diseases: Diagnosis, Prevention, Treatment,* 8th ed. C. V. Mosby Co., St. Louis, 1976.

Top, Franklin H. (ed.): *Control of Infectious Diseases in General Hospitals.* American Public Health Association, Washington, D.C., 1968.

Winslow, C.-E. A.: *The Conquest of Epidemic Disease—A Chapter in the History of Ideas.* Princeton University Press, Princeton, N.J., 1943.

Youmans, G. P., et al.: *The Biologic and Clinical Basis of Infectious Diseases.* W. B. Saunders Co., Philadelphia, 1975.

Patience Wilson
Virginia Henderson

CHAPTER 45

Shock or Collapse, With or Without Hemorrhage

1. INTRODUCTION

Some Historical Aspects. The word *shock* has been in use for more than two centuries in all clinical disciplines to describe a progressive collapse of vital organ functions after injury or surgery; it was first used medically by the unnamed translator of Henry François Le Dran's *A Treatise of Reflections Drawn from Experiences with Gunshot Wounds*. By the end of the 1800s, surgeons recognized shock when they saw it.[1]

Much of our present-day understanding of traumatic and hypovolemic * shock is based on the first extensive experimental studies by George W. Crile (in 1899), who concluded that the characteristics of hypovolemic shock were failure of venous return, low central venous pressure, and favorable response of venous pressure to infusions of warm saline, with resulting increase in cardiac output. His work and that of others (physiologists, biochemists, and pathologists) who focused on animal experimentation dominated the field for the next half century. All of these investigators adopted the term *shock* to describe the subject of their studies. The major accomplishments of this era are described by C. J. Wiggers[2] in *Physiology of Shock* (1950).

In 1910, Yandell Henderson in the following statement clearly stated the relationship between venous return, cardiac output, and arterial pressure:

Because of the diminished venous supply the heart is not adequately distended and filled during diastole. Hence the picture of a "failing heart" revealed by the pulse. For the same reason arterial pressure ultimately sinks in spite of an intense activity (not because of failure) in the vasomotor nervous system, and in spite of an extreme con-

striction (not because of relaxation) of the arterioles.*

Noting that these observations on hemodynamic mechanisms were important contributions to the understanding of shock, Max Harry Weil,[3] writing in 1967, saw no clearer statement of the basic events responsible for the decline of arterial pressure could be made then.

During World War I, W. B. Cannon and W. M. Bayliss initiated the team approach for investigating and treating patients in shock. They were assisted by American and British physiologists and clinicians in collecting clinical descriptions and measuring physiologic and biochemical phenomena in patients who were in shock. Comparable studies made concurrently on animals tended to reinforce their findings. Although some of the conclusions of these studies were misleading, others were not. For instance, the relationship of shock and its severity to deficits in circulating blood volume was established and came to be generally recognized.

Interest in shock declined after World War I, but during World War II several special units to study battle casualties were established. Lloyd D. MacLean writes: "Notable among these was a board headed by [Henry K.] Beecher, which concluded that the major cause of shock was *hemorrhage and fluid loss*, which in turn led to metabolic acidosis when the condition was severe and protracted." †

Through the efforts of the Minnesota group,

---

* Henderson, Yandell: "Acapnia and Shock—III. Failure of the Circulation," *Am. J. Physiol.*, 25:152, (Jan. 1) 1910.

† MacLean, Lloyd D.: "Shock: Causes and Management of Circulatory Collapse," in Sabiston, David C., Jr. (ed.): *Davis-Christopher Textbook of Surgery; The Biological Basis of Modern Surgical Practice*, 10th ed. W. B. Saunders Co., Philadelphia, 1972, p. 67.

---

* Blood volume less than normal.

Table 45-1. Some Historic Landmarks in Shock *

1743 *Henri François Le Dran*—Shock is progressive deterioration following injury.

1831 *Thomas Latta*—First use of intravenous saline for hypovolemic shock.

1895 *John Collins Warren*—Shock is an adaptive response to life-threatening injury.

1899 *George W. Crile*—First extensive experimental studies of shock; defined dangers of hemorrhage, hypothermia, anesthesia, and fluid loss in surgical shock; noted value of measurement of central venous pressure in hypovolemic shock.

1908 *Yandell Henderson*—"Venous pressure is . . . the fulcrum of the circulation. Shock as surgeons use the word is failure of the fulcrum."

1917 *Edward Archibald and W. S. McLean*—"While a low blood pressure is one of the most constant signs of shock, it is not the essential thing, let alone the cause of it . . . we have focused our attention far too much on blood pressure, so much so as unconsciously to have come to regard it as almost causal."

1917 *W. B. Cannon*—Noted correlation between hypotension and reduction in alkali reserve. Postulated accumulation of fixed acids (lactic acid) due to impaired oxygen transport.

1919 *N. M. Keith*—The severity of shock is correlated with the magnitude of decrease in blood volume.

1923 *W. B. Cannon and W. M. Bayliss*—Organizers and leaders of first shock team. Best clinical descriptions and first battlefield measurements of physiologic and biochemical phenomena in patients in shock.

1930 *A. Blalock and D. B. Phemister*—Demonstrated conclusively that traumatic shock is due to hypovolemia. There was no suggestion of a toxic factor such as histamine as a causal factor in their well planned studies.

1943 *A. Cournand and D. W. Richards*—First measurements of cardiac output in patients in shock.

* MacLean, Lloyd, "Shock: Causes and Management of Circulatory Collapse," in Sabiston, David C., Jr. (ed.): *Davis–Christopher Textbook of Surgery*, 10th ed. W. B. Saunders Co., Philadelphia, 1972, p. 66.

led by Wesley Spink, bacterial (or septic) shock was recognized as a discrete clinical entity after 1955. This group concluded that endotoxin was the cause of bacterial shock. Some of the historical landmarks in present-day understanding of shock are summarized in Table 45-1. For additional information, the reader should consult references at the end of this chapter.

Recent Definitions. There has been a tendency in the past to designate a related group of symptoms following injury as "shock" and to describe a similar bodily state as "collapse" when it is not associated with accidents or surgery. Currently, the term *shock* is applied to the syndrome characterized by acute prostration and circulatory collapse from almost any cause. In 1968, Robert M. Hardway [4] compiled a list of more than 100 types of shock discussed in the literature, which include allergic, cardiogenic, endotoxic, hematogenic, paralytic, traumatic, dehydration, electric, and psychic. He questioned their having anything in common.

At this writing, there seems to be no universally accepted definition of shock. The term, however, is commonly used to refer to a group of signs and symptoms that usually include pale, cold, and clammy skin, weakness, mental stupor, a rapid and thready pulse, low blood pressure, oliguria, and prostration.

Recognizing that many physiologists think there is no single definition for circulatory shock, because it has so many causes, Arthur C. Guyton and associates say one common denominator is always present; that is, the "cardiac output is insufficient to supply the tissues of the body with their normal nutritive needs." * MacLean believes an appropriate definition is simply "inadequate blood flow to vital organs or failure of the cells of vital organs to utilize oxygen." † Although most authorities consulted emphasize the role of impaired tissue perfusion in shock, others believe that shock is related to or caused by inadequate cellular metabolism that may or may not be caused by inadequate tissue perfusion but by other factors such as the direct cellular effects of endotoxin.

Eugene D. Jacobson defines shock as follows:

. . . acute circulatory insufficiency characterized by cardiac output inadequate to provide normal perfusion for the major organs. Whether shock is associated with generalized increased resistance to blood flow, widespread pooling or loss of blood, marked hypotension or inability of the heart to force enough blood peripherally is immaterial.‡

Jacobson emphasized that the end result is the same—an insufficient circulating blood volume to ensure adequate tissue perfusion.

Many degrees of shock have been observed clinically. Henry K. Beecher and associates (in 1947) described the signs and symptoms

* Guyton, Arthur C., et al.: *Circulatory Physiology. Cardiac Output and Its Regulation*. W. B. Saunders Co., Philadelphia, 1973, p. 372.

† MacLean, Lloyd D.: "The Patient in Shock," in American College of Surgeons, Committee on Pre and Postoperative Care: *Manual of Preoperative and Postoperative Care*, 2nd ed. W. B. Saunders Co., Philadelphia, 1971, p. 211.

‡ Jacobson, Eugene D.: "A Physiologic Approach to Shock," *N. Engl. J. Med.*, **278**:834, (Apr. 11) 1968.

Table 45-2.   Grading of Shock *

| Degree of Shock | Blood Pressure (Approx.) | Pulse Quality | Skin | | | Thirst | Mental State |
			Temperature	Color	Circulation (Response to Pressure Blanching)		
None	Normal	Normal	Normal	Normal	Normal	Normal	Clear and distressed
Slight	To 20% increase	Normal	Cool	Pale	Definite slowing	Normal	Clear and distressed
Moderate	Decreased 20–40%	Definite decrease in volume	Cool	Pale	Definite slowing	Definite	Clear and some apathy unless stimulated
Severe	Decreased 40% to non-recordable	Weak to imperceptible	Cold	Ashen to cyanotic (mottling)	Very sluggish	Severe	Apathetic to comatose, little distress except thirst

* Beecher, H. K., et al.: "The Internal State of the Severely Wounded Man on Entry to the Most Forward Hospital," *Surgery,* **22:**672, 1947.

of shock according to severity—slight, moderate, and severe, as shown in Table 45-2. Shock also has been termed *irreversible* when all known treatment fails to reverse the cell pathology.[5]

"Electric shock" and "insulin shock" are common medical and lay terms. Nobody would hesitate to say that a friend was so "shocked" by bad news that he or she fainted. In none of these cases is the cause physical trauma in the ordinary sense. In the first case it is an electric charge, in the second a chemical, and in the third a psychic stimulus. It might be helpful in summary to point out that *shock* is the more general term used to describe a depressed bodily state of varying severity and duration; symptoms may vary from sensations of weakness, dizziness, and nausea, typical of fainting, to the disturbance of consciousness and the profound prostration of all vital functions seen in a person who has been hemorrhaging, in one who has been thrown from a moving vehicle, or in the diabetic whose early signs of insulin shock have been unrecognized and untreated. In each case, a "shock syndrome" is present as the vital organs are deprived of circulating fluids of physiologic quantity or quality.

Classification of Shock. Because there are so many unrecognized clinical abnormalities that cause shock, the need for a working clinical classification has been recognized for years. Various classifications have been proposed and continue to be used by physicians in the diagnosis and treatment of shock. The etiologic

classification developed by Alfred Blalock in 1934 is still considered useful and functional by most authorities. This classification as given by F. A. Simeone in 1966 consists of the following categories: (1) hematogenic shock, secondary to blood loss; (2) neurogenic shock, secondary to vasodilation and reflex inhibition of the heart; (3) cardiogenic shock, secondary to cardiac failure; and (4) vasogenic shock, caused by dilation of blood vessels secondary to humoral (for example, vasoactive substances) rather than nervous factors.[6]

On the basis of current knowledge, it is now clear that shock results from abnormalities in one or more of four basic components of the circulatory system: the heart, the blood vessels, the blood volume, and the blood viscosity.[7] Guyton says that, since shock results ultimately from inadequate cardiac output, any factor that may reduce cardiac output may also cause clinical shock. The many conditions that reduce cardiac output he groups into the following categories:

1. Those that decrease the ability of the heart to pump blood.
2. Those that tend to decrease the venous return.*

The first category includes any condition (myocardial infarction, for example) that damages the heart so severely that it cannot pump adequate quantities of blood to perfuse the vital organs. The second category includes all those

* Guyton, Arthur C.: *Textbook of Medical Physiology,* 5th ed. W. B. Saunders Co., Philadelphia, 1976, p. 357.

conditions that reduce venous return, including reduced blood volume, decreased vasomotor tone, and increased resistance to blood flow.

2. CAUSES AND EFFECTS

The most common cause of shock is diminished blood volume (*hypovolemia*). Loss of blood (hemorrhage) is said to be the most common cause of *hypovolemic shock*. Loss of whole blood may result from external or internal injuries or from nontraumatic internal hemorrhage. Two examples are bleeding peptic ulcer and ruptured varices. Other causes of hypovolemic shock include loss of plasma and blood in crushing injuries and fractures, loss of plasma and hemolysis of red cells in extensive burns, and loss of plasma into body cavities, as seen in peritonitis. Most authorities note that dehydration, loss of fluid from all body compartments, may cause hypovolemic shock. Guyton makes the following observation:

. . . [dehydration] can reduce the blood volume and cause hypovolemic shock very similar to that resulting from hemorrhage. Some of the causes of this type of shock are: (a) excessive sweating; (b) fluid loss in severe diarrhea or vomiting; (c) excess loss of fluid by nephrotic kidneys; (d) inadequate intake of fluid and electrolytes; (e) destruction of the adrenal cortices, with consequent failure of the kidneys to reabsorb sodium, chloride, and water; and (f) loss of the secretion of antidiuretic hormones by the supraoptico-hypophyseal system.*

The diminished circulating blood volume, regardless of cause, *decreases the mean systemic pressure* and consequently decreases the venous return to the heart. The cardiac output, therefore, begins to fall and shock develops. According to Louis L. Smith and Max Harry Weil,[8] the hemodynamic and biochemical effects of hemorrhage are determined by the rate, quantity, and duration of blood loss. If less than 100 ml of blood per day is lost gradually over a period of days, circulatory failure is prevented by expansion of the plasma volume through compensatory mechanisms, and by the maintenance of normal red cell mass, as long as the iron stores are adequate. On the other hand, rapid loss of 50 per cent of the blood volume in a healthy young person results in profound shock and usually death unless immediate and vigorous treatment is instituted.

The second most common type of shock is caused by impaired cardiac pumping, termed

cardiogenic shock. MacLean defines it as "inadequate blood flow to vital organs due to inadequate cardiac output despite a normal cardiac filling pressure." * The body tries to compensate for this state of decreased blood pressure by increased heart rate (tachycardia), peripheral vasoconstriction, anaerobic production of adenosinetriphosphate (ATP), and release of a large number of erythrocytes into the circulation. Cardiogenic shock may be seen in a wide variety of surgical and medical patients, and according to MacLean, may be due to any one of the following conditions:

(1) Myocardial infarction, (2) arrhythmias, (3) cardiac tamponade, (4) delayed and inadequate volume replacement in hypovolemia, (5) inappropriate volume replacement in hypovolemia with the creation of a high hematocrit, (6) epidural anesthesia with resultant cardiac sympathectomy, and (7) adrenal insufficiency.†

After hemorrhage and myocardial infarction, sepsis is the next most frequent cause of shock and is usually termed *septic* or *bacterial shock*. Although the mechanism of this type of shock is incompletely understood, Jack A. Barnett and Jay P. Sanford have the following to say about its pathogenesis:

. . . endotoxin, a complex lipopolysaccharide common to the cell wall of all gram-negative bacteria, plays a major role in initiating the hemodynamic events. Most experimental evidence supports the view that endotoxin effects a redistribution of blood within the vascular bed in a manner precluding the maintenance of an adequate circulating blood volume. Consequences of this pooling include poor oxygenation of tissues resulting in anaerobic metabolism with lactic acidemia and, ultimately, loss of cellular integrity within vital structures. The nature of the unfavorable redistribution of blood within the vascular bed varies with the animal species. The patterns of hemodynamic responses in septic shock in man are much less stereotyped than in animals. In some patients there is marked reduction in cardiac output and prolongation of circulation time, with total peripheral resistance (TPR) normal or increased. In other patients with hypotension of comparable degree, however, there is relatively normal or high cardiac output and normal or shortened circulation time, with TPR reduced.‡

Gram-negative bacteria, *Escherichia coli* followed by *Aerobacter aerogenes*, *Proteus*, and *Pseudomonas aeruginosa*, are the most

---

Ibid., p. 365.

* MacLean, Lloyd D.: "The Patient in Shock," in American College of Surgeons, Committee on Pre- and Postoperative Care: *Manual of Preoperative and Postoperative Care*, 2nd ed. W. B. Saunders Co., Philadelphia, 1971, p. 220.

† *Ibid.*, p. 222.

‡ Barnett, Jack A., and Sanford, Jay P.: "Bacterial Shock," *J.A.M.A.*, **209**:1514, (Sept. 8) 1969.

common offending organisms; however, other organisms such as fungi, rickettsiae, viruses, and gram-positive bacteria may cause the shock syndrome. G. Tom Shires and associates [9] say that the most frequent source of gram-negative infections is the genitourinary system. Almost half of these patients have had an associated operation or instrumentation of the urinary tract. (The dangers of urinary infections and methods of prevention are discussed in detail in Chapter 24.) The respiratory system is the second most frequent site of origin. Many of these patients have an associated tracheostomy. The third most frequent site is the alimentary system, especially in the presence of diseases such as peritonitis, intra-abdominal abscesses, and biliary tract infections. Instrumentation is always a source of infection. An increasingly important source of contamination is the indwelling venous catheter used for monitoring and hyperalimentation, especially when its use is prolonged. In a study of 398 patients (during a 12-year and 2-month period) with gram-negative sepsis, W. A. Altemeier and associates [10] report that an increase in incidence was noted during the last 2 years of the study. This was thought to be related to the rapid expansion of new and complex surgical procedures to elderly and other poor-risk patients, whose resistance was lowered by extensive trauma, associated chronic diseases, and treatment with steroids, immunosuppressive agents, and anticancer drugs. In Chapter 15, reference was made to the death of infants and children with gram-negative sepsis who may not survive 24 hours after the condition is recognized. It has been estimated that about 75 per cent of these infections are hospital acquired. Shock developing during the course of sepsis may result from any one or any combination of the following: (1) cardiac failure, (2) hypovolemia, or (3) failure of the capillary circulation.[11]

Anaphylactic shock develops immediately after an antigen to which the person has been previously sensitized enters the circulatory system. According to K. Frank Austen,[12] the chemical mediators of anaphylaxis that are specifically formed and released by the antigen-antibody interaction include amines, such as histamine and serotonin, small peptides, such as bradykinin, and an acidic lipid which is called a "slow-reacting substance of anaphylaxis," or simply "SRS-A." Each of these mediators is capable of performing two specific functions—causing contraction in a particular group of smooth muscles and increasing vascular permeability. Austen explains that histamine and serotonin are released from the tissues in which they exist in their biologic form; bradykinins and SRS-A, however, are

formed and released as a result of the antigen-antibody reaction. Patients are known to exhibit at least three distinct patterns of reaction within the anaphylactic syndrome: respiratory distress due to edema of the nasopharynx and larynx or as a result of severe bronchospasm, with hypotension occurring secondary to the hypoxia, or primary vascular collapse without prior respiratory distress. There has been some speculation that the pattern of laryngeal edema is mediated by the release of histamine, that the intractable bronchospasm is mediated by the SRS-A, and that the primary vascular collapse is mediated by bradykinin.

Martin D. Valentine and Albert L. Sheffer say, "substances which incur the risk of anaphylaxis are heterologous proteins, large polysaccharides, or simple chemicals which when associated with a host protein molecule act as immugenic haptens." * (Hapten: a partial antigen that is incapable of stimulating antibody production when injected into an animal and that reacts with an antibody only within an artificial environment.) Some of the common proteins include antiserums (horse), such as tetanus and diphtheria antitoxins, and hormones, such as insulin and ACTH. The polysaccharides include dextran and iron-dextran substances. Diagnostic agents, such as the iodinated organic contrast agents, and antibiotics, particularly penicillin, tetracycline, and streptomycin, are included in the hapten class.

Neurogenic shock, as defined by Shires and associates, "is that form of shock which follows serious interference with the balance of vasodilator and vasoconstrictor influences to both arterioles and venules." † This is the type of shock that is seen with "syncope" (fainting) and may occur when a person is exposed to unpleasant events, such as seeing blood, hearing sad news, or experiencing sudden pain. It may also occur in patients after a high spinal anesthesia because of paralysis of vasomotor influences and in patients after acute gastric dilation because of interruption of reflex nerve impulses.

Neurogenic shock differs from hypovolemic shock in that the low blood pressure is usually accompanied by a pulse rate that is slower than normal and the skin is usually warm, dry, and flushed; whereas in hypovolemic shock the pulse rate is rapid and the skin is cold, clammy, and pale. The cardiac output is reduced; however, there is a decrease in the resistance of the arteriolar vessels and a de-

* Valentine, Martin D., and Sheffer, Albert L.: "The Anaphylactic Syndromes," *Med. Clin. North Am.,* **53:**249, (Mar.) 1969.

† Shires, G. Tom, et al.: *Shock.* W. B. Saunders Co., Philadelphia, 1973, p. 149.

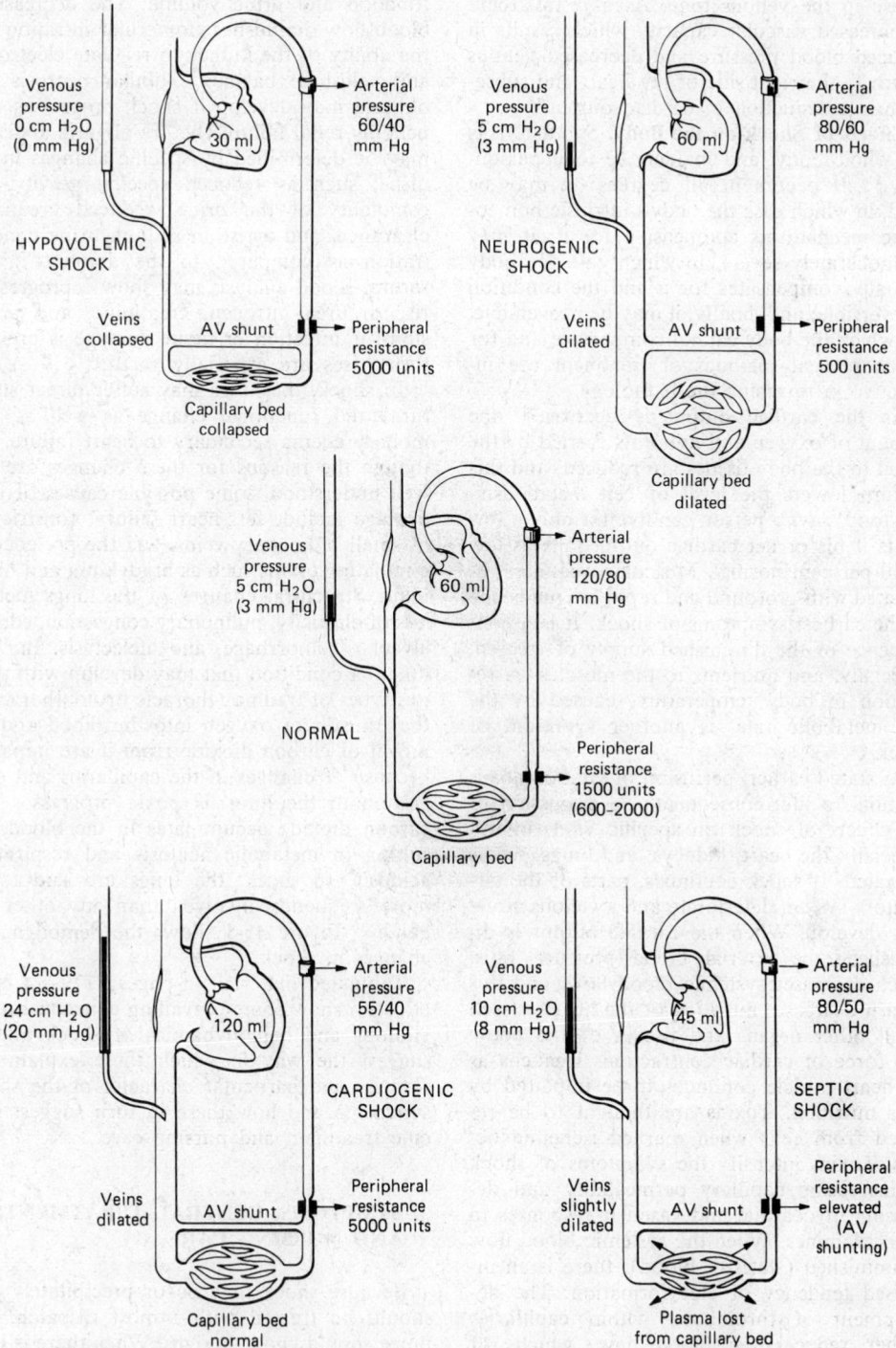

Figure 45-1. Hemodynamic changes in shock. (Blaisdell, F. William: "Shock," in Dunphy, J. Englebert, and Way, Lawrence W. [eds.]: *Current Surgical Diagnosis and Treatment*. Lange Medical Publications, Los Altos, Calif., 1973, p. 213.)

crease in the venous tone. As a result, there is increased vascular capacity which results in reduced blood pressure and decreased venous return to the right side of the heart and subsequently a reduction in cardiac output.[13]

Effects of Shock on the Body. Shock affects the whole body, and in fact the total personality.[13a] It occurs in all degrees: it may be mild, in which case the body's intrinsic homeostatic mechanisms compensate for it; it may be moderately severe, in which case the body partially compensates for it and the condition is reversible; and, finally, it may be irreversible, for which the body cannot compensate and for which present methods of treatment are ineffective in reversing the pathology.

As the cardiac output is decreased, the amount of oxygen and nutrients carried by the blood to the body tissues are reduced, and this in turn lowers the level of cell metabolism. Guyton[14] says a person can live for only a few hours if his or her cardiac output falls as low as 40 per cent normal. Muscular weakness associated with profound and rapid fatigue is one of the earliest symptoms of shock. It is a consequence of the diminished supply of oxygen, especially, and nutrients to the muscles. A reduction in body temperature, caused by the low metabolic rate, is another symptom of shock.

As stated earlier, perfusion of vital organs is essential to life; consequently, a discussion of the effects of shock on specific vital organs, especially the heart, kidneys, and lungs, seems indicated. If shock continues, parts of the circulatory system deteriorate and a vicious circle may develop. When the cardiac output is diminished, the arterial blood pressure falls, which decreases systemic blood flow, and this in turn decreases nutrition of the heart as well as all other organs and tissues of the body. The force of cardiac contractions weakens as the heart muscle continues to be impaired by poor nutrition. Toxins are thought to be released from cells when marked ischemia occurs. Toxins intensify the symptoms of shock by increasing capillary permeability and depressing myocardial and vascular responses to catecholamines. When the systemic blood flow is diminished (stasis of blood), there is an increased tendency of clot formation. The development of thrombosis within capillaries further reduces the blood flow, which, of course, contributes to the progression of shock. A vicious circle may be initiated, each factor intensifying the severity of the preceding one.[15]

Renal perfusion is decreased in shock because the afferent and efferent arterioles of the kidney are constricted, shunting the blood away from the glomeruli which reduces renal function and urine volume. The decrease in blood flow diminishes glomerular filtration and the ability of the kidney to regulate electrolyte and acid-base balance. Tubular necrosis and oliguria may develop if shock progresses. Impending renal failure (before oliguria appears) may be determined by specific changes in the urine, such as reduced specific gravity and osmolality of the urine, reduced creatinine clearance, and a rise in sodium urine concentration as compared to the amount in the serum. Blood analysis may show a progressive rise in urea nitrogen, creatinine, and potassium; if infection or tissue damage is present, these rises are especially rapid.[16]

In shock, the lungs may suffer direct structural and functional change as well as pulmonary edema secondary to heart failure. Although the reasons for these changes are not well understood, some possible causes of lung damage include left heart failure, constriction of small pulmonary veins, and the presence of circulating toxins such as bradykinin and histamine. Structural changes of the lungs include loss of elasticity, pulmonary congestion, edema, alveolar hemorrhage, and atelectasis. In "wet lung," a condition that may develop with various types of trauma (thoracic or nonthoracic), the transfer of oxygen into the blood and removal of carbon dioxide from it are impaired because of changes in the capillaries and congestion in the lung. Hypoxia progresses and carbon dioxide accumulates in the blood, resulting in metabolic acidosis and respiratory acidosis. In shock, the lungs are said to be more frequently involved than any other organ.[17-19] Figure 45-1 shows the hemodynamic changes in shock.

Tabulated material on pages 1779–84 is an effort to show some prevailing concepts on the etiology and hemodynamics of shock and to suggest the way in which these explain the severity and particular character of the shock syndrome and how these in turn suggest specific treatment and nursing care.

3. SYMPTOMS, GENERAL TREATMENT, AND NURSING CARE

Because shock may occur precipitately and should be treated with utmost dispatch, the nurse should know its signs. When there is likelihood of shock, the patient should be under constant observation—as, for example, after major surgery, traumatic injury, myocardial infarction, pancreatitis, or other serious illness. With the rising incidence of gram-negative sepsis with its attendant shock, nurses must be alert to its signs and symptoms. Even with early and heroic treatment, the condition may be fatal. A lowered blood pressure and a weak rapid pulse are probably the most important signs of shock. The systolic and diastolic blood pressures are indicative of the degree of shock from which the patient is suffering. A systolic pressure below 90 mm Hg should be considered dangerous. The vital centers are considerably damaged if the systolic pressure remains below 50 mm Hg for long. Such a condition is usually terminated by death. When the systolic pressure is as low as 80 mm, it is often impossible to determine the diastolic pressure, but the lower the diastolic reading, the more profound the state of shock. Other signs of shock are apathy, pallor, and cold, moist skin. Generally, the patient is quiet and listless, but may be anxious and apprehensive. This is particularly true if he or she knows life is threatened by hemorrhage. The temperature is frequently subnormal, and the respirations may be rapid and shallow, or deep. Patients, especially those in hypovolemic shock, are very thirsty. The mouth feels parched because fluids are drawn into the vascular compartment from the interstitial spaces. There may be decreased urinary output. Amounts lower than 25 ml per hour are considered serious. Cyanosis may follow marked loss of blood cells. The patient does not usually lose consciousness unless the shock is severe or prolonged. Table 45-3 shows the hemodynamic and metabolic differences in various types of shock.

Treatment of the condition, once it develops, depends on the underlying cause. Since reduction of blood volume, by one means or another, is by far the most common cause of shock, it is essential that the volume of blood be restored as quickly as possible. Intravenous infusions of whole blood, plasma, or a plasma volume expander (such as dextran) are given

as quickly as possible. Blood is usually the preferred solution, especially when bleeding is not, or cannot be, arrested. Plasma, dextran (high and low molecular weight), or electrolyte solutions (such as Ringer's lactate) are used in disorders such as burns, peritonitis, and pancreatitis. Frequent laboratory studies of relative volumes and concentrations of blood cells, hemoglobin, plasma protein, and electrolytes are made so that treatment may be determined and administered on the basis of the physiologic needs. Central venous pressure (see Chapter 6 for an explanation of the procedure) is measured continuously in most patients in shock because it is the best gauge for estimating the adequacy of fluid replacement.

While in the recent past the Trendelenburg (head-down) position was used as an adjunct in the treatment of hypovolemic shock, recent studies have demonstrated that this position does not improve cardiac output. James Taylor and Max Harry Weil report that in "patients in a state of shock, decrease rather than an increase was noted in the intra-arterial blood pressure, and more often a decrease in the cardiac index when the patients were placed in a head-down posture." * Because patients with multiple trauma frequently sustain injuries of the abdomen and chest, the head-down position may interfere with respiratory exchange far more than the supine position, according to Shires and associates.[20] Simeone[21] recommends that patients lie supine with their legs elevated to a 45° angle, knees straight and the pelvis slightly higher than the thorax. The head should be placed in a comfortable

* Taylor, James, and Weil, Max Harry: "Failure of the Trendelenburg Position to Improve Circulation During Clinical Shock," *Surg. Gynecol. Obstet.*, 122: 1009, (May) 1967.

Table 45-3.　Hemodynamic and Metabolic Differences in Various Types of Shock *†

	Blood Pressure	Pulse Rate	CVP	Cardiac Index	Urine Flow	Response to Volume Load	Arterial pO₂	Arteriovenous O₂ Difference	Arterial Blood Lactate
Hypovolemic shock	↓	↑	↓	↓	↓	↑	↓	↑	↑
Cardiogenic shock	↓	↑ or ↓	↑	↓	↓	↓	↓	↑	↑
Peripheral pooling	↓	↑	↓	↓	↓	↓	↓	↑	↑
Septic shock (hyperdynamic)	↓	↑	↑	↑	↓	↓	↓	↓	↑

* MacLean, Lloyd D.: "Shock: Causes and Management of Circulatory Collapse," in Sabiston, David C., Jr. (ed.): *Davis-Christopher Textbook of Surgery; The Biological Basis of Modern Surgical Practice*, 10th ed. W. B. Saunders Co., Philadelphia, 1972, p. 72.

† ↑ Increased; ↓ decreased.

position on a pillow. Some forms of shock, particularly neurogenic shock, will respond to the head-down position; the effect of posture on cerebral circulation has not been clearly defined in hypovolemic shock.[22] Since the circulation is very unstable in shock, patients should not be turned or moved and the head should not be raised during the time the blood pressure is very low or fluctuating within a low range.

Vasopressor drugs are given less frequently now than in the past; however, they continue to be administered when the physician believes that vasoconstriction is insufficient to maintain blood flow, particularly to the heart and brain. Metaraminol (Aramine) and norepinephrine (Levophed) are perhaps the most frequently used of a number of vasopressor agents. These drugs are usually given intravenously, but the latter may be given intramuscularly also. The dosage and rate of intravenous flow are regulated according to the blood pressure, which must be taken at least every 15 minutes and, at times, more frequently.[23,23a]

Vasodilators are used in selected cases. Phenoxybenzamine (Dibenzyline), phentolamine (Regitine), and chlorpromazine are reportedly effective in treatment of shock in man and animal. When these drugs are used, patients must be observed closely for evidence of circulatory improvement or failure. Central venous pressure must be monitored and blood volume increased as needed. One or more liters of additional fluid may be required to fill the additional vascular capacity created by the vasodilator drug.[24,25]

The importance of deficient ventilation and oxygenation in the development of shock is stressed by most authorities consulted. An adequate supply of oxygen and removal of carbon dioxide are essential to life. The airway must be kept open and functioning at all times. Patients in severe respiratory failure may need ventilatory support from a respirator; an endotracheal tube may be inserted or, after a tracheostomy is performed, a cuffed tracheostomy tube inserted. Oxygen is given at the lowest concentration that will maintain an oxygen tension (pO_2) of 60 mm Hg because high concentrations of oxygen are known to damage the lungs.[26]

Since pain may aggravate shock, it must be controlled. In the early stages of shock, morphine given intravenously (about one-half the usual dose) is advocated by most authorities for the relief of pain, but it markedly depresses the vital centers and predisposes to nausea, vomiting, and later to constipation and other undesirable reactions. When shock is caused by cerebral injury, analgesics and sedatives are *not* used. Since many persons have an idiosyncratic response to morphine, it must be used with care. Patients in shock are rarely alert enough to warn doctors, nurses, and others against the use of drugs to which they respond unusually.

The patient should be kept comfortably cool with the aim of reducing body metabolism. Light blankets may be used to prevent loss of body heat, but sweating must be avoided, since it results in a loss of valuable body fluids.

There is no better test of nurses' ability to act effectively under pressure than the first aid they give patients during incipient shock and the care they give them later. The importance of the control of the environment for the benefit of the patient must be emphasized here as it is throughout this book. An attitude of "caring" that is evident to the patient and family is important. Far too many former patients and family members get the impression that nurses and physicians are more concerned with "life-saving equipment" including monitoring devices than with patients during their stay in intensive care units and other treatment settings.

Shock is a threatening state; more or less so according to its severity. Those in a state of shock *feel* threatened, or afraid. If taken into an intensive care unit, they are surrounded by strangers and, to some persons, by very frightening sights and sounds. When it does not interfere with life-saving measures, a near relative or close friend should be allowed to stay with the patient.

"Heroic" life-saving measures often involve risk, and the patient, if in a condition to make decisions, has the right to refuse them. If patients cannot give "informed consent," it should be given by the family or friends who bring them to the treatment setting. There have been many cases in which persons who haven't considered themselves very ill have through "intrusive therapy" left the hospital with a stubborn infection or some other even more serious iatrogenic condition.

In this chapter, shock is discussed as a mild, serious, or fatal condition. It must be treated in any setting where the person happens to be, since delay in treatment may be disastrous. Everyone should know the principles of treatment and they are taught in all first aid courses. Lives have been saved by informed lay persons as well as by health personnel.

In areas supplied with mobile health units, milder forms of shock may be successfully treated without institutionalizing the patient. Treatment for severe shock may be started in mobile units or ambulances, especially those that have telephonic or even video connections with medical centers. In such cases, specialists can advise ambulance and mobile unit crews.

Nurses in industry, in schools, in hospitals, and in remote areas where there are no resident physicians have to use whatever knowledge and resources are available to help persons in shock. The methods outlined in the following pages are not available to all those persons who suffer from shock. And since such treatment is very costly, it should be reserved for those in severe shock. In fact, unduly expensive and elaborate treatment cannot be justified even if it is available.

When a person's life is threatened and he or she realizes it, every effort should be made to see that, according to their wishes and those of the family, a religious adviser or clergyman of their choice is available. On the battlefields of World War II, Beecher and his associates concluded that the presence of chaplains contributed to the recovery of men in shock from battle wounds. There seems no reason to think that the state of mind of the person who faces the possibility or likelihood of death differs materially in war and peace.

Research on the shock states continues and discoveries are made almost daily. Because of the efforts of researchers and clinicians, more patients with shock survive than a few years ago. Fortunately, an increasing number of specialized units are staffed by knowledgeable physicians and nurses who work as a team in giving expert medical and nursing care.

4. TABULATION OF SPECIFIC TREATMENT BASED ON SPECIFIC CAUSE [27-34]

Causes	Hemodynamics	Signs and Symptoms	Treatment and Nursing Care
1. *Inadequate circulating blood volume* with decreased venous return to right atrium due to a. Hemorrhage, internal or external, following accidents, surgery, and disease that ruptures blood vessels—"Hypovolemic Shock" or "Hematogenic Shock" (most common form of shock)	Inadequate circulating blood volume ↓ Decrease venous return to right atrium ↓ Decreased cardiac output ↓ Reduced tissue perfusion and cellular hypoxia ↓ Increased peripheral venous constriction ↓ Tendency of blood cells to clump in minute vessels (sludging) ↓ Further decrease in venous return ↓ Further decrease in cardiac output. ↓ Increased sludging and metabolic acidosis (increase in lactate accumulation) ↓ Decreasing venous return ↓ Impaired myocardial efficiency ↓	Early indications: Complaints of chest pain or inability to breathe Apprehensiveness and restlessness Complaints of feeling cold Weakness and fatigue Faintness in upright position Dizziness Dimness of vision Nausea and vomiting Thirst Later indications: Restlessness changing to confusion and apathy with insensitivity to stimuli Intense thirst Continued nausea and vomiting Rapid, thready pulse (over 100) Systolic pressure (under 90 mm Hg) falls more than diastolic, resulting in reduced pulse pressure Central venous pressure low (under 2 cm of water) Cool, clammy, pale or mottled skin Nail beds fill slowly when emptied by	Control hemorrhage or remove underlying cause at the same time treatment for shock is given Place in supine position with legs elevated 10–20° to promote perfusion of brain and heart Move or turn patient slowly and gently to prevent sudden blood volume shifts, for which depressed circulatory reflexes cannot compensate Provide quiet environment to promote rest Work quietly and confidently to avoid excitement. Do not leave patient unattended. Let relative or close friend stay with patient (especially if an infant or child) unless they interfere with life-saving measures Cover the patient with blankets to conserve body heat, but do not apply extra warmth that will cause sweating and dilation of the peripheral vessels. (Sweating further depletes the low blood volume and peripheral vasodilation deprives vital organs of their share of an already lowered blood supply.) Give oxygen when early symptoms of shock appear in patients with traumatic injuries or other conditions likely to lead to shock. (Lack of oxygen to vital tissues is thought to lead to progressive shock by contributing to deterioration of the heart, other parts of the circulatory system, and respiratory inadequacy.) Observe for signs of respiratory distress. Endotracheal intubation or tracheostomy with positive pressure ventilation may be necessary. Use positive pressure respirators with great care because of the risk of impeding venous return to the heart

Causes	Hemodynamics	Signs and Symptoms	Treatment and Nursing Care
	Additional decrease in cardiac output ↓ Additional decrease in tissue perfusion	pressure Urinary output falls below 25 ml per hour Laboratory findings: Moderately elevated blood lactate (20–30 mg per 100 ml of blood) Decreased hematocrit	Give whole blood in large amounts in a shorter time than usual. If typed and cross-matched blood is not immediately available, give Ringer's lactate solution, isotonic saline, or plasma expanders such as dextran or human albumin until blood is available

Provide for monitoring circulatory effectiveness and make available equipment for introduction of a catheter into the right atrium to determine CVP: a catheter placed in an artery for serial determination of blood pressure and to collect blood samples for PaO_2, $PaCO_2$, and pH levels. Have available a retention catheter to put in the bladder to monitor urine output. (Although a patient in shock may present an emergency situation, all catheters must be inserted using strict aseptic technique.)

With a CVP above 10–15 cm of water, it is likely blood volume is too high and the heart is being overtaxed. In such cases measure urine output and record at hourly intervals

Some authorities recommend sedatives rather than opiates intravenously to relieve restlessness and apprehension. If opiates are given for pain, give small doses and repeat them if necessary. Ask patient how he or she responds to morphine before giving it. Do not give a normal dose of morphine to a patient who is semiconscious or unconscious without testing his or her response with a very small dose

Allow patient to rinse the mouth, but give nothing by mouth unless prescribed by the physician. To guard against aspiration of vomitus turn the patient's head to the side and have suction equipment available

Although arterial blood pressure is no longer considered the best indicator of the shock patient's circulatory condition, a series of readings is helpful in determining circulatory improvement if hypotension was present before transfusions or fluid therapy was started. Apply a blood pressure cuff to the patient's arm and record the pressure at 5-minute intervals unless the patient is obviously improving

The patient is improving when alert and responsive to stimuli; the skin warm and pink; the pulse rate slowed and of good quality; urine output increased to 50 ml per hour; and arterial blood pressure returned to normal

| b. Plasma lost from circulating fluids as in burns | | A patient in shock caused by seepage of plasma from a burned area (sec- | Since plasma loss is in direct relation to the area burned, and it progresses at an established rate, secondary shock in burns may be prevented by the paren- |

Causes	Hemodynamics	Signs and Symptoms	Treatment and Nursing Care
		ondary shock of burns) presents the picture just described, but the blood findings differ from shock caused by loss of whole blood Here the hematocrit is raised; or the cell count and hemoglobin are high in relation to the blood plasma, although there is loss of cells. The total volume of circulating fluid is reduced to as dangerous a point as in massive hemorrhage	teral administration of water, electrolyte solutions (particularly Ringer's lactate solution), plasma, and other appropriate solutions. The aim of the physician is to give the type and amount of fluid necessary to restore specific deficits

c. Dehydration or loss of water and electrolytes as in
  Excessive sweating
  Diarrhea
  Vomiting
  Nephrotic kidneys
  Inadequate fluid and electrolyte intake
  Addisonian Crisis
  Heat exhaustion
		Here the volume of circulating fluid is low owing to loss of water and electrolytes; blood analysis shows a high hematocrit. The nature of the electrolyte loss depends on the cause of the dehydration	Shock caused by dehydration without the conflicting factor of endocrine deficiency is treated chiefly by plasma intravenously and water and electrolytes by mouth or vein until blood findings approach normal values. Control of this type of shock is relatively simple

2. *Decreased cardiac output due to myocardial dysfunction:*
  Myocardial infarction
  Acute arrhythmias, especially severe tachycardia
  Unrecognized or untreated valvular disease
  General anesthesia
  Epidural anesthesia resulting in cardiac sympathetic block—"Cardiogenic Shock," second most common type of shock
	Decreased cardiac output
	↓
	Increased left or right atrial pressure
	↓
	Increased venous pressure
	↓
	Increased peripheral resistance
	↓
	Continuing low cardiac output
	↓
	Continuing decrease of tissue perfusion
		Early symptoms include restlessness, agitation, and then progression to listlessness, apathy, and extreme weakness
		Later symptoms include low blood pressure, rapid, thready pulse, decreased pulse pressure, peripheral cyanosis, mental confusion, high or low central venous pressure, oliguria, normal hematocrit
			Make careful use of cardiac glucosides (digitalis), isoproterenol, and norepinephrine to improve the strength of myocardial contraction
			Administer intravenous fluids judiciously with continuous monitoring of CVP
			Monitor ECG continuously to detect heart block and arrhythmias
			Insert indwelling catheter in bladder and monitor hourly urine excreted
			Cyclic intra-aortic balloon pump may be inserted. (A polyurethane three-chambered balloon [which is inserted by a femoral arteriotomy and positioned in the descending aorta] may be inflated to 20 to 40 ml of gas. The inflated balloon increases the amount of blood flowing into the coronary arteries.)
			Arrhythmias may be treated with isoproterenol, lidocaine, Pronestyl, and occasionally, external or internal pacemakers
			Ventilation and external cardiac compression should be started as soon as arrest occurs

Causes	Hemodynamics	Signs and Symptoms	Treatment and Nursing Care
3. *Diminished perfusion of arterial blood in microcirculation,* termed "Septic Shock" and most often due to Gram-negative bacterial endotoxins from the following organisms: *E. coli* *Pseudomonas* *Klebsiella-enterobacter* *Proteus* *Mima-Herella* bacteria Conditions predisposing to gram-negative infections: Diabetes Cirrhosis Leukemia Arteriosclerotic vascular disease Burns Recent manipulation and/or infection of the genitourinary tract Childbirth Respiratory infection Skin infections Male over 60 Newborn infants Hospitalization ("Septic Shock" is the third most common type of shock and is increasing rapidly.)	Endotoxin production by gram-negative bacteria ↓ Inhibited cellular use of oxygen ↓ Intense arteriolar and venous spasm ↓ Immobilization of blood in capillaries of lungs, spleen, and kidneys ↓ Stagnant anoxia in tissues of these organs ↓ Development of localized acidosis in tissues of these organs ↓ Relaxation of arteriolar sphincter while venule remains constricted ↓ Blood pools in capillaries ↓ Plasma leaks into interstitial fluid ↓ Decrease in venous return to the heart ↓ Decrease in cardiac output ↓ Systemic arterial hypotension ↓ Further vasoconstriction ↓ Reduction of blood flow to kidneys, lungs, and skin ↓ Sludging of blood and intravascular coagulation possibly caused by red cell agglutination due to bacterial endotoxins	Early indications: Sudden onset of chills and fever Skin warm, dry, and red Consciousness varies from normal to lethargy and confusion Rapid respirations —hyperventilation Mild respiratory alkalosis Pulse increased but regular, full, and bounding Blood pressure begins to fall 6–18 hours after onset Urine flow adequate but concentrated Later indications (hours to days): Skin cool, pale, and moist Respirations rapid and shallow Pulse rapid, weak, and thready Hypotension Urine flow decreased Hyperthermia replaced by hypothermia Less obvious early symptoms: Unexplained rapid respirations, lethargy, confusion, nausea, vomiting, diarrhea, or abdominal distention Laboratory findings: Hematocrit normal in early stages—increased in later stage Blood lactate increased Blood glucose increased	In early stages when circulatory collapse has not occurred, therapy consists o taking cultures from likely foci to determine the specific bacteria involved Until bacteriologic reports are available, a broad-spectrum, bactericidal antibiotic such as cephalosporin with a poymyxin may be used Give Ringer's lactate solution or normal saline to restore adequate blood volume. If central venous pressure and arterial pressure increase, no other treatment is needed Give vasodilator drugs (phenoxybenzamine, phentolamine, and chlorpromazine) or isoproterenol if the CVP rises, peripheral resistance remains high (vasoconstriction), and cardiac output is low Isoproterenol is not given if the pulse rate exceeds 120 because it stimulates myocardial contractility. No vasodilators are given until blood volume has been restored to normal and the CVP is in the high normal range. When vasodilators are used, additional fluids must be given to offset the increased peripheral venous capacity If there is evidence of venous pooling of blood, give small doses of alpha-adrenergic drugs (metaraminal and norepinephrine) that lead to increased cardiac output (positive inotropic effect) and slight increase in peripheral resistance Although sludging of blood and intravascular coagulation occur in other forms of shock, they are frequently found in septic shock. Dextran and heparin is often given to prevent or modify many of the effects of intravascular coagulation Massive doses of corticosteroids have been advocated, but their usage is still controversial

Causes	Hemodynamics	Signs and Symptoms	Treatment and Nursing Care
4. *Decreased vaso-motor tone or in-creased vascular capacity* called "Neurogenic Shock" and due to Decreased vaso-motor tone: Deep general anesthesia Spinal anes-thesia Brain damage Fainting Occasionally —pain Increased vas-cular capacity: Rapid re-moval of ascites fluid Removal of large ab-dominal tumor	"Pooling" of blood in peripheral ves-sels ↓ Decreased venous return to the heart ↓ Decreased cardiac output	Pale, warm, dry skin Lowered blood pres-sure Rapid, weak pulse Rapid, shallow res-pirations Restlessness and ap-prehension	Give oxygen until medical help arrives Elevate patient's lower extremities (but not entire body) to promote venous re-turn Administer intravenous fluids to correct the relative blood volume reduction, and monitor by observing central ve-nous pressure Give vasoconstrictor drugs to restore vas-cular tone Monitor blood pressure, pulse, and respi-ration every 15 minutes Neurogenic shock caused by the common faint is usually benign and self-limiting unless an injury is sustained
5. *Decreased cardiac output and arterial pressure with ve-nous dilation* called "Anaphylactic Shock" and due to: Antigen-anti-body reaction that takes place imme-diately after an antigen to which the person is sen-sitive has en-tered the cir-culation	Antigen-antibody re-action may dam-age the vascular walls or cardiac muscle ↓ Histamine or hista-mine-like sub-stance released by reaction damaged tissues ↓ Venous and arteriole dilatation ↓ Increased vascular capacity ↓ Decreased arterial pressure ↓ Decreased venous return to the heart ↓ Damaged cardiac muscle and de-creased output	Signs and symptoms as described above in various types of shock showing acute respiratory insufficiency and cardiovascular collapse	Immediate discontinuation of the aller-gens Give Ringer's lactate solution or normal saline infusion Give intravenous antihistamines If response is slow, give epinephrine, aminophylline, and corticosteroids Relieve intense bronchospasm by addi-tional epinephrine or isoproterenol by nebulizer Use intermittent positive pressure breath-ing if helpful
6. *Blocking of venous return to heart,* termed "Obstruc-tive Shock," due to Sudden occlu-sion of the vena cava Severe valvular stenosis	Mechanical blocking of venous return to the heart or me-chanical interfer-ence with atrial or ventricular flow ↓ Inadequate cardiac output ↓	Same as those for "Neurogenic Shock"	Relieve mechanical obstruction by sur-gery if indicated Use closed chest drainage or pericardial paracentesis if indicated Restore adequate blood flow by appropri-ate fluids as determined by the physi-cian

Causes	Hemodynamics	Signs and Symptoms	Treatment and Nursing Care
Ball-valve atrial thrombi Intracardiac tumors Pulmonary emboli Sudden shifts of the mediastinum due to tension pneumothorax or hemothorax Rapid accumulation of fluid in the pericardial sac (pericardial tamponade)	Decreased tissue perfusion ↓ Decreased venous return		

REFERENCES

1. MacLean, Lloyd D.: "Shock: Causes and Management of Circulatory Collapse," in Sabiston, David C., Jr. (ed.): *Davis-Christopher Textbook of Surgery; The Biological Basis of Modern Surgical Practice,* 10th ed. W. B. Saunders Co., Philadelphia, 1972, p. 65.
2. Wiggers, C. J.: *Physiology of Shock.* Commonwealth Fund, New York, 1950.
3. Weil, Max Harry: "General Concepts and Definitions," in Weil, Max Harry, and Shubin, Herbert (eds.): *Diagnosis and Treatment of Shock.* Williams & Wilkins Co., Baltimore, 1967, p. 5.
4. Hardway, Robert M., III: *Clinical Management of Shock, Surgical and Medical.* Charles C Thomas, Publisher, Springfield, Ill., 1968, p. 5.
5. Ebert, Paul A.: "Shock and Hemorrhage," in Cole, Warren H., and Zollinger, Robert M. (eds.): *Textbook of Surgery,* 9th ed. Appleton-Century-Crofts, New York, 1970, p. 237.
6. Simeone, F. A.: "The Nature of Shock," *Am. J. Nurs.,* **66:**1287, (June) 1966.
7. Dietzman, Ronald H., et al.: "Shock: Mechanisms and Therapy," *Can. Anaesth. Soc. J.,* **14:**276, (July) 1967.
8. Smith, Louis L., and Weil, Max Harry: "Shock Due to Blood Loss," in Weil, Max Harry, and Shubin, Herbert (eds.): *Diagnosis and Treatment of Shock.* Williams & Wilkins Co., Baltimore, 1967, p. 113.
9. Shires, G. Tom, et al.: *Shock.* W. B. Saunders Co., Philadelphia, 1973, p. 152.
10. Altemeier, W. A., et al.: "Gram-Negative Septicemia: A Growing Threat," *Ann. Surg.,* **166:**530, (Oct.) 1967.
11. Nardi, George L.: "Shock," in Nardi, George L., and Zuidema, George D. (eds.): *Surgery; A Concise Guide to Clinical Practice,* 3rd ed. Little, Brown & Co., Boston, 1972, p. 208.
12. Austen, K. Frank: "Introduction to Clinical Immunology," in Wintrobe, Maxwell M., et al. (eds.): *Harrison's Principles of Internal Medicine,* Vol. I, 7th ed. McGraw-Hill Book Co., New York, 1974, p. 347.
13. Shires, G. Tom, et al.: *op. cit.,* p. 149.
13a. Compton, Carol Yank: "War Injury: Identity Crisis for Young Men," *Nurs. Clin. North Am.,* **8:**53, (Mar.) 1973.
14. Guyton, Arthur C.: *Textbook of Medical Physiology,* 5th ed. W. B. Saunders Co., Philadelphia, 1976, p. 367.
15. Lillehei, Richard C., et al.: "The Pharmacologic Approach to the Treatment of Shock," *Geriatrics,* **27:**73, (July) 1972.
16. Fishman, Alfred P.: "Shock," in Beeson, Paul B., and McDermott, Walsh (eds.): *Textbook of Medicine,* Vol. II, 14th ed. W. B. Saunders Co., Philadelphia, 1975, p. 902.
17. Olcott, C., et al.: "Diagnosis and Treatment of Respiratory Failure After Civilian Trauma," *Am. J. Surg.,* **122:**260, (Aug.) 1971.
18. Bredenberg, C. E., et al.: "Respiratory Failure in Shock," *Ann. Surg.,* **169:**392, (Mar.) 1969.
19. Martin, Arthur M.: "Pathologic Anatomy of the Lungs Following Shock and Trauma," *J. Trauma,* **8:**687, (Sept.) 1968.
20. Shires, G. Tom, et al.: *op. cit.,* p. 127.
21. Simeone, F. A.: *op. cit.*
22. Shires, G. Tom, et al.: *op. cit.,* p. 126.
23. Goodman, Louis S., and Gilman, Alfred (eds.): *The Pharmacological Basis of Therapeutics,* 5th ed. Macmillan Publishing Co., Inc., New York, 1975, p. 507.
23a. Moyer, John H., and Mills, Lewis C.:

"Vasopressor Agents in Shock," *Am. J. Nurs.,* **75:**620, (Apr.) 1975.

24. Wilson, R. F., et al.: "The Usage of Dibenzyline in Clinical Shock," *Surgery,* **56:**172, (July) 1964.

25. Hakstian, R. W., et al.: "Pharmacological Agents in Experimental Hemorrhagic Shock," *Arch. Surg.,* **83:**335, (Sept.) 1961.

26. Wilson, John N.: "The Management of Acute Circulatory Failure," *Surg. Clin. North Am.,* **43:**469, (Apr.) 1963.

27. Blaisdell, F. William: "Shock," in Dunphy, J. Englebert, and Way, Lawrence W. (eds.): *Current Surgical Diagnosis and Treatment.* Lange Medical Publications, Los Altos, Calif., 1973, p. 212.

28. Conn, Julius: "Shock," in Beal, John M., and Eckenhoff, James E. (eds.): *Intensive and Recovery Room Care.* Macmillan Publishing Co., Inc., New York, 1969, p. 111.

29. Fishman, Alfred P.: *op. cit.,* p. 968.

30. Gius, John Armes: *Fundamentals of Surgery.* Year Book Medical Publishers, Chicago, 1972, p. 81.

31. Guyton, Arthur C.: *op. cit.,* p. 357.

32. Hayes, Morton F., et al.: "Diagnosis and Treatment of Hemorrhagic and Septic Shock," *Int. Surg.,* **58:**299, (May) 1973.

33. Petersdorf, Robert G.: "Septic Shock," in Wintrobe, Maxwell M., et al. (eds.): *Harrison's Principles of Internal Medicine,* 6th ed. McGraw-Hill Book Co., New York, 1970, p. 736.

34. Frazee, Sharry, and Nail, Lillian: "New Challenges in Cardiac Nursing: The Intra-aortic Balloon," *Heart Lung,* **2:**526, (July–Aug.) 1973.

Additional Suggested Reading

Amsterdam, Ezra A., et al.: "Evaluation and Management of Cardiogenic Shock. Part III. The Roles of Cardiac Surgery and Mechanical Assist," *Heart Lung,* **2:**122, (Jan.–Feb.) 1973.

Bechamps, Gerald J., and Van Heerden, Jonathan A.: "Shock, a Brief Review with Emphasis on Septic Shock," *Va. Med. Mon.,* **99:**1287, (Dec.) 1972.

Beland, Irene L., and Passos, Joyce Y.: *Clinical Nursing: Pathophysiological and Psychosocial Approaches,* 3rd ed. Macmillan Publishing Co., Inc., New York, 1975, p. 799.

Clark, N. F.: "Pump Failure," *Nurs. Clin. North Am.,* **7:**539, (Sept.) 1972.

Cohn, Jay N.: "Monitoring Techniques in Shock," *Am. J. Cardiol.,* **26:**565, (Dec.) 1970.

Conference on the Dynamics of Septic Shock in Man, Albert Einstein College of Medicine: *Septic Shock in Man.* Little, Brown & Co., Boston, 1968.

Conference on Shock, Glasgow, 1970: *Proceedings.* C. V. Mosby Co., St. Louis, 1972.

Foster, Sue B.: "Pump Failure," *Am. J. Nurs.,* **74:**1830, (Oct.) 1974.

Goldberg, Leon I., and Talley, Robert C.: "Current Therapy of Shock," *Adv. Int. Med.,* **17:** 363, 1971.

Hartford, Charles E.: "The Early Treatment of Burns," *Nurs. Clin. North Am.,* **8:**447, (Sept.) 1973.

Johns, Lois A.: "An Experimental Approach to Vigilance in Nursing-Patient Monitoring," in Downs, Florence S., and Newman, Margaret A.: (eds.): *A Source Book of Nursing Research.* F. A. Davis Co., Philadelphia, 1973.

Kahn, Herman, and Bruce-Briggs, B.: *Things to Come. Thinking About the Seventies and Eighties.* Macmillan Publishing Co., Inc., New York, 1972.

Kornfield, Donald: "Psychiatric View of the ICU," *Brit. Med. J.,* **1:**108, (Jan. 11) 1969.

Koumans, A. R. J.: "Psychiatric Consultation in an Intensive Care Unit," *J.A.M.A.,* **194:**633, (Nov. 8) 1965.

Lang, Tzu-Wang, et al.: "New Concepts in Temporary Circulatory Assist for Treatment of Cardiogenic Shock," *Geriatrics,* **26:**90, (Sept.) 1971.

MacLean, Lloyd D., et al.: "Patterns of Septic Shock in Man—A Detailed Study of 56 Patients," *Ann. Surg.,* **166:**543, (Oct.) 1967.

Mitty, William F., et al.: "Treating Shock in the Emergency Room," *Am. Fam. Physician,* **5:**76, (June) 1972.

Mueller, Hiltrud S., et al.: "The Evaluation and Treatment of Cardiogenic Shock," *Med. Times,* **98:**137, (July) 1970.

Rieser, Mary, et al.: "Intensive Care Nursing," in Kintzel, Kay Corman (ed.): *Advanced Concepts in Clinical Nursing.* J. B. Lippincott Co., Philadelphia, 1971.

Royce, Judith A.: "Shock, Emergency Nursing Implications," *Nurs. Clin. North Am.,* **8:**377, (Sept.) 1973.

Shinn, Arthur F., et al.: "Drug Interactions of Common CCU Medications," *Am. J. Nurs.,* **74:**1442, (Aug.) 1974.

Silva, J. F.: *Management of Neglected Trauma.* Charles C Thomas, Publisher, Springfield, Ill., 1972.

Studi, Carol: "Cardiogenic Shock," *Am. J. Nurs.,* **74:**1636, (Sept.) 1974.

Symposium on Fundamental Mechanisms of Shock, Oklahoma City, Oct. 1971: *Proceedings.* Plenum Press, New York, 1972.

Toffler, Alvin: *Future Shock.* Bantam Books, New York, 1970.

Weber, Karl T., et al.: "Left Ventricular Dysfunction Following Acute Myocardial Infarction," *Am. J. Med.,* **54:**697, (June) 1973.

Weil, Max Harry, and Shubin, Herbert: "Changes in Venous Capacitance During Cardiogenic Shock—A Search for the Third Dimension," *Am. J. Cardiol.,* **26:**613, (Dec.) 1970.

Gladys Nite
Virginia Henderson

The authors acknowledge the assistance of Marie Anderson, R.N., M.S., in review of literature of selected topics in this chapter.

CHAPTER 46

Disorders of Communication Attributable to Impairments of Sight, Hearing, and Speech

1. INTRODUCTION
2. IMPAIRMENTS OF SIGHT
3. IMPAIRMENTS OF HEARING
4. IMPAIRMENTS OF SPEECH

1. INTRODUCTION

Abilities to see, hear, and speak are taken for granted until there are impairments in these functions. The loss of external input has many implications, dependent on (1) whether it is the sense of sight, hearing, or speech that is impaired; (2) whether one or more of the senses are impaired; (3) the degree to which they are impaired; and (4) the age at which the impairment occurs. The effects of sensory impairments also vary according to the following conditions: (1) the affected person's ability to relate to the external environment of other people and objects; (2) the affected person's ability to master the developmental stages of life; and (3) the ability of those associated with the affected person to relate to those with the sensory impairment.

In order really to help people with sensory deficits, those who relate to them must understand the enormously painful process they go through in dealing with themselves and their environment. Having these deficits is stressful enough, but the stress of illness, treatment, and hospitalization can reach panic proportions. Institutionalized persons with sensory impairment must adapt to routine and to strange people on whom they are dependent.

Consequently, the main focus of this chapter is on the meaning of the impairments to those so impaired. It is hoped that this will help nurses and others who care for such persons to understand them better. Unless caretaking persons understand the basic problems of sensory deficits, they cannot even begin to understand the reactions to illness of persons so handicapped. Explicit suggestions are made on how to relate or respond to the handicapped. This chapter also briefly discusses some causes and treatments of such sensory impairments and some aids or devices useful to those so impaired. For further information on the physical aspects of sensory impairments, the reader is referred to comprehensive medical texts such as *Harrison's Principles of Internal Medicine,* edited by M. M. Wintrobe and his associates.[1] This chapter should be read in conjunction with Chapter 16 that deals with communication and human relations.

2. IMPAIRMENTS OF SIGHT

Legal Blindness. Normal vision, 20/20 vision, refers to the ability the majority of people have in reading letters of a standardized size on an eye chart when they are 20 ft from the chart. A *definition of legal blindness* is the inability to see the largest letter on the eye chart at 20 ft.[2] The National Association for the Prevention of Blindness defines blindness as a central visual acuity of 20/200 or less in the better eye with correcting glasses, or a field defect in which the peripheral field has contracted so that the widest diameter of the visual field subtends an angular distance no greater than 20 degrees.[3] This latter type of blindness is tunnel vision, or the inability to see objects at the periphery.[4]

It is a common misconception that those registered as blind have no remaining sight. This is largely true for the war blind, but not for civilians.[5] Visual disability means that daily activities are severely interfered with.[6] According to the above definition, many blind persons see light, and some read newspaper headlines and can identify distant objects. Such people can use light in corridors, windows, doorways, and the like to guide them.[7] In other words, there are many types of "blindness."

In spite of the efforts that have been made to prevent blindness, its *incidence* is still high. As of mid-1973, about 10 million people in the United States had some visual disability. Of these, about 1.5 to 2 million were so disabled that they could not hold a regular job. Of these, about 500,000 were considered legally blind and eligible for benefits.[8]

According to L. Riley,[9] discussing the *causes* of sight impairment, most total blindness in the United States is caused by glaucoma. John G. Bellows [10] says about 2 million people over age 35 in the United States are threatened with this disease. Glaucoma is characterized by elevation of intraocular pressure leading eventually to optic nerve damage and irreversible field loss unless it is prevented or controlled. The increase in intraocular pressure is related to an imbalance between the production of aqueous humor (a fluid formed constantly by filtration from the capillaries) and its escape through the normal exit channels. Obstruction to the outflow of intraocular fluid appears to be mainly responsible for this imbalance.[11-13]

Causes of primary glaucoma are unknown. Vasomotor and emotional instability, hyperopia, and heredity are among the predisposing factors. Glaucoma should be suspected in persons over 35 years of age who have the following symptoms: need for frequent change of lenses, mild headaches, vague visual disturbances, seeing halos around electric lights, or impaired dark adaptation. Routine eye examinations in persons over 35 should include examination with a tonometer to check the intraocular pressure.[14]

Defective vision is also caused by cataracts (a major reason for impaired vision in adults over age 65),[15] degeneration of the retina, other retinal affections, optic nerve atrophy, uveitis, myopia, affections of the cornea or sclera, keratitis, and retrolental fibroplasia. Causes of less than normal vision also include senile degeneration, congenital defects, diabetes, vascular disease, injuries and poisonings, infectious disease, and neoplasms.[16] Overillumination may also injure the retina. Ophthalmologists have begun to question the belief that most light is the best light. Maternal viral infections such as rubella, rubeola, and cytomegalic inclusion diseases can be transmitted to the fetus during pregnancy and cause various degrees of blindness in the unborn child.[17] Pregnant women, especially in the first trimester, should try to avoid exposure to infectious disease. H. Robert Blank [18] says the most frequent cause of newborn blindness during the 1940s through the middle 1950s was excessive use of oxygen resulting in retrolental fibroplasia associated with premature births.

Occasionally, total or partial blindness is a conversion reaction. The disturbance is then an expression of an unconscious conflict. The affected person blinds himself or herself to whatever threatens to reactivate a conflict that arouses intolerable anxiety. Norman Cameron [19] says that if the blindness is total, it is usually confined to one eye. A conversion reaction may mimic true visual loss but usually can be detected either by lack of proper history for sudden visual loss, by inconsistencies with known anatomic lesions, or by what Darrell D. Franks [20] calls "La Belle indifference."

Congenitally Blind Children. Because the problems of congenitally blind children intensify *developmental difficulties* that are sometimes evident to lesser degrees in children without this deficit, and because the problems of the congenitally blind also are like the difficulties that partially blind persons or those who become blinded later in life face to varying degrees, the difficulties of the congenitally blind child are discussed here in some detail.

George S. Klein [21] says there are critical periods in the life of a child during which certain forms of stimulation with accompanying learning must take place or it is likely that intractable consequences for adulthood will result. Congenitally blind children have difficulty in reality testing and in mastering themselves and their environment. They have problems in gross motor development, in adaptive hand behavior, in verbalization, in developing interpersonal relations, and in developing body image and self-image concepts. They have difficulty in achieving an adequate sense of reality, in dealing with language and abstract functions, and in controlling and expressing emotions.[22-24]

Blind and sighted children follow a roughly parallel developmental course for about 12 to 16 weeks. Then, in moving from the passive oral phase to a more active phase (see page 570 for developmental table), the blind child's ego development pursues a course resulting in passive self-centeredness and lack of striving toward mastery at later ages.[25] Selma Fraiberg and David A. Freedman,[26] who studied the ego development of the congenitally blind child, say that for blind persons the mouth functions as a discriminatory sensory organ throughout life.

Since the blind infant depends on cutaneous and other senses as substitutions for vision, it is critical to develop to the greatest degree all the infant's sensory resources from birth. But since it is easier and safer to see and hear than to smell, taste, and touch forbidden things, it is difficult for adults to help young infants use these latter senses to the fullest extent. The sense of smell suffers most from repression and atrophy because of its close association with anality and genitality. For the same reason, there is some repression of touch.[27]

The usual *parental reaction* to discovering that their baby is blind (usually within the first few weeks after birth) is depression, and the mother often seems to suffer more acutely than the father. Unfortunately, this can lead to emotional withdrawal from the child, which has far-reaching consequences.[28] The fact that blind babies listen intently and become quiet often makes the mother feel that she is not needed by her child. When she feels unneeded, she is less involved. Yet it is essential for her to take part in developing the infant's hearing if she is to continue to stimulate his or her interest. Dorothy Burlingham[29] emphasizes the importance of hearing in the maturation of blind children.

Fraiberg[30] found that birth of blind babies was a disaster for their families. Old wounds in the femininity and masculinity of the young mothers and fathers were opened. Some of the fathers became impotent. The unconscious revulsion of the parents to the defective infant took the form of avoidance so that they touched the baby only when it was absolutely necessary. Fraiberg and her group, studying the problem, concluded that it was essential that they help establish communication between blind babies and their parents, and help the parents with their feelings, if the child's development was to proceed along healthy lines.

As blind babies develop into active children, their blindness overtaxes their parents' resources, evokes their latent conflicts, and frequently precipitates anxiety, hostility, and guilt against which they mobilize defense mechanisms and compensatory reactions. The most common of these are overprotectiveness and a marked displacement of anxiety toward blindness as the cause of their difficulties. Under such circumstances the relationships of the parents and children are greatly distorted. Health workers learn that a parental request for help must first be examined as an indication of the parent's need, an indication of his or her emotional problem, as well as an indication of the child's problem.[31]

As a direct consequence of the difficulties in mastery that blind children encounter, they tend to concentrate their attention on their own body experiences rather than on sources of external stimulation. There is evidence that all children blind from birth show a degree of fixation to the earliest phase of development in which the passive experience of bodily gratification is dominant.[32]

The blind infant's first toy, the first learning tool, is himself or herself. Carroll B. Parten[33] says it is important to develop body awareness in order to build a self-concept. Without vision, the blind babies are not attracted by toys and other inanimate objects. They revert to interest in their own bodies and that of their mothers and other people, and animals surrounding them. This *heightened attachment to bodily interests* including body movement and contact with animate and inanimate objects continues to provide a much needed respite for blind children in their task of coping with the world. The maternal care blind infants receive determines the degree of their progress toward mastery of the external environment, but Doris M. Wills,[34] Anne-Marie Sandler,[35] and others say that the basic tendency toward self-centeredness and the modes of gratification characteristic of the first phase of life will always be present.

The blind baby must find adaptive substitutes for vision in order to achieve a coherent sensorimotor organization. When *hands must substitute for vision*, they are the bridge between the body ego and the objective world. Without this bridge the personality may remain frozen on the level of body centeredness and nondifferentiation of self and not self. Fraiberg's[36] group found that it was important to educate the blind baby's hands. They built into the child's day rich tactile experience and tactile differentiation, using toys and other interesting objects. They encouraged the parents of these children to play games that would help the children bring their hands together at the midline. They sought toys that united tactile and sound qualities. They encouraged the mothers to place their baby's hands on the bottle during feeding. They suggested patty-cake games and hand-clapping games with songs. And when the baby was lying down they encouraged the use of cradle gyms and dangling toys. This process was started as early as 5 or 6 months and continued throughout the baby's early development. Only when babies could coordinate sound and grasping were they on their way to the next developmental stage. Fraiberg thinks that if one can reach blind children even as late as the second year—if their hands can be brought into a coherent sensorimotor organization—then they will continue to develop as they should. But if the hands of blind children do not engage at the midline of their bodies, a complex sequence leading to hand reciprocity and coordinate use of the hands may not evolve.

Fraiberg found that for congenitally blind

children *creeping and walking was delayed* by several months or even several years, for it is vision that initiates the creeping pattern. Seeing arouses curiosity and movement toward the objects seen. Sound from objects not seen does not by itself arouse curiosity expressed by reaching out to touch the objects. No babies in Fraiberg's sample learned to creep before they could reach an object on sound cue alone. This is a different conceptual experience than that of using sight. The baby must actually acquire a concept of an object in which the form connotes the thing. Sighted babies can usually grasp an object on sight between 5 and 6 months. No blind baby in Fraiberg's group could demonstrate responding to sound cues as the sighted child responded to sight cues. The average age for reaching on sound cue alone was 10 months.

Fraiberg[37] found that once the blind baby had the maturational readiness for creeping and could also demonstrate reaching on sound cue, then he or she could usually find the creeping pattern or could be taught how to creep with various lures. The difficulty in learning to creep for the congenitally blind child should not be underestimated. The majority of the blind babies studied could not creep or walk with support until they were about 15 months of age.

There is another delay between the first steps and walking freely, because walking freely for blind children is walking into a void. The average age for free walking in the children studied by Fraiberg[38] was 17 months. However, once the child achieved mobility by walking, there was a great push toward discovering things and toward discovering the organization of space. A healthy blind child in his or her second year will be into everything.[39] However, the blind child will, of course, be handicapped. One can reasonably expect some delay in his or her development, since in the second year of life vision serves more efficiently than the other senses for differentiation of one's self from others, of external objects from one another, for classifying and conceptualizing, and for mastering the problems of mobility.[40]

Blind children have more *fear of the environment* than sighted children because they do not have the visual warning that prevents them from getting into accidents. Such children need a mother who teaches them to use hearing and touching as protection.[41] Inability to test reality by means of sight increases and intensifies the fear of being observed, of the toilet, of the dark, of stillness, and great fear of being left alone. Night is especially frightening for blind children. These children are continually at the mercy of those who take

care of them. They have to trust others implicitly, for they themselves are unable to detect danger or to keep out of harm's way. When caretakers go to bed, blind children feel forsaken and left to meet real and fantasied dangers alone. They may fall into a state of helplessness and despair, sometimes terror or panic.[42]

Blind children *have great need for assistance from others,* for the use of others' eyes. Because they fear not getting the help they need, they fear displeasing others and so tend to repress those characteristics and traits that would be likely to alienate those whom they need most. They tend to repress aggression and awareness of aggression in others.[43] Wills[44] and her staff, studying blind children's understanding of their world, were struck by the compliance, passivity, and inhibition of aggression of the children. Since blind children have special difficulty with anger and aggression, it is important that adults help such children express aggression and tensions in socially acceptable ways. Elders should not cramp such children's expressions of anger and aggression in order to have "good children."

Blind children are in a state of permanent alertness to external dangers that must be mastered. Distress, danger, or extreme anxiety may immobilize them. A new environment may have the same effect. They stay still in order to orient themselves, collecting as much information as possible through various sense organs, especially the ear. As with blind babies, blind children sometimes seem very passive when actually they may be extremely active listening and attending to what is going on in the external environment. Unfortunately, this passivity may be interpreted by adults as withdrawn, inattentive behavior. A sad consequence is that these children may even be scolded for their behavior.[45]

There is no question that in their dealings with the external world blind children are constantly exposed to and must tolerate excessive frustrations because of their helplessness.[46] When they are anxious and trying to cope, there is a great pull exerted by *regressive tendencies,* a need to cling to old forms of need satisfaction. And when blind children are anxious they tend to seek close body contact with those on whom they are dependent, which is not surprising when we know that their tendency to understand the world is in bodily terms.[47] At such times they should be cuddled and helped to talk about what they are experiencing. Fraiberg[48] noted that the condition of helplessness produces transient pathologic states in the young blind child that are relatively independent of the quality of mothering. Regression remains the chief defense of the young blind child. It is not blindness alone that imperils the child's development, but the absence of vision as an organizer of experience.

One of the most striking impressions one gets when observing blind nursery school children is the ease with which they stop playing and withdraw into simple primitive activities unless an adult constantly stimulates and supports their interest. Yet play is an activity very necessary for the mastery of the blind child's inner and outer world. The blind child's mother remains the mediator far longer than does the mother of the sighted child. She is crucially important to the blind child in ways not so necessary for the sighted child. The blind child has intense feelings invested in people rather than in objects for two main reasons: (1) they produce a relatively understandable sensory impression; and (2) they are necessary for these children as auxiliary egos to provide for their physical needs and to help them cope with and understand their world.[49]

Blind children love bodily games and rhythmic games. They need simple repetitive *play* to help them master situations. Left to their own devices, they play safe and repeat the familiar, such as opening and shutting doors, turning light switches off and on, and playing with water faucets or filling and emptying containers. They do not progress without individual help in a one-to-one relationship. These children need ways to discharge their instinctual feelings and should be given the opportunity to play with safe objects that have meaning such as those previously stated. Much experience common to the child with sight is strange to blind children. They have great difficulty in mastering common experiences and the excitement they arouse. The adult can help the children in coping with their impulses by helping them verbalize what they are experiencing as they relate to new objects and events.[50]

Since it is easier for blind children to respond to inner sensations and inner reality, they prefer *fantasy*.[51] It is therefore hard to find toys for blind children that have meaning. Whatever they choose that enable them to play more directly with adults or with themselves should be used. Such toys allow for displacement and externalization of aggressive and sexual fantasies. The perpetual human task of keeping inner and outer reality separate yet interrelated is one in which play has a major role for all children, but especially for blind children. By age 6, blind children should be able to differentiate between pretending and actual fact—for example, that animals do not really talk. This ability appears earlier in children with sight.[52]

A Blind Child in the Hospital or Other Health Institution. Much has been written about the traumatic effects of hospitalization on children. One of the major factors is the *separation of small children from those upon whom they depend,* especially their mothers. However, if they can be with their mothers in the institution, the experience has a completely different effect upon their psychic development. Blind children may think that their handicap is what made their mothers abandon them, especially if mothers spend little time visiting them. They feel no longer loved as they did at home. If children are newly blinded, their mothers will likely have profound and often prolonged periods of depression. The mother's ability to perceive and respond to the child's needs will be markedly impaired. The newly blinded and institutionalized children will therefore suffer not only from their blindness, but also from the loss of their mother when they most need her.[53-55] Sigmund Freud[56] noted that if mothers are absent or have withdrawn their love from their children, the children are no longer sure of the satisfaction of their needs. They are then exposed to the most distressing feelings of tension.

As has been previously emphasized, it is crucial that adults help blind children understand, conceptualize, and verbalize their inner overwhelming experiences and affects so they can acquire appropriate means of expressing their feelings. Before blind children are hospitalized, they should be *prepared for hospitalization*—helped to understand the reason for going to the hospital and anticipate the experience; otherwise they have great difficulty in accepting hospitalization and may see it as punishment.

Alice B. Colonna[57] suggests that before going to the hospital it can be helpful to make a book about hospital life that contains actual objects the blind child can feel and discuss. Visiting the hospital and meeting the staff can also be helpful as long as the experience is kept within the child's toleration limits. The following comments on *hospitalization* relate especially to blind children. More specific suggestions for all blind persons are in the section titled "Helping Those with Impairment of Sight." When in the hospital, blind children need careful orientation to time, their room, the bathroom, and where needed objects are that can be reached and used. If they are unable to be up and about, children should know where toys are. They long for their own playthings, so they should be allowed to have their own clothes, toys, and any other important familiar possessions. They need a schedule that enables them to anticipate events. This helps them stay in the real world at this traumatic time instead of turning to what can be a fearful fantasy world. But a schedule given to blind children obligates adults to adhere to it. Parents and friends should visit at prearranged times. Meals and routine nursing procedures should be done as regularly as possible. Colonna also suggests that during visits it is helpful for families and friends to walk with the blind children around their rooms and units to help them get oriented. This adds to their reassurance as long as the orientation is adjusted to the child's mastering abilities.

Cyril E. Williams,[58] describing a children's unit in a British hospital, says that play is the chief need of hospitalized children since play is the child's major way of mastering strange new experiences. Even in an acute medical or surgical ward, there are a fair number of children who are ambulatory. In the extended care facility, Williams thinks that the provision for play should take precedence over almost any other. But even when confined to bed, children can be helped to play with appropriate toys.

If the child is hospitalized for an operation to make him or her see, Aliza Segal and Frederick H. Stone,[59] describing the emotional sequelae of an operation for bilateral congenital cataracts, say the problem should be diagnosed early and the operation should be done as soon as is surgically possible after birth since it is very traumatic for children to begin to see for the first time. They are flooded with new stimuli that can be overwhelming when added to the internal chaotic feelings they are already experiencing from hospitalization. Segal and Stone suggest that if these children or those prematurely blind have special difficulty with hospitalization, a therapist who is familiar with problems of blind children should work with the staff and the parents.

Reactions to Sudden Blindness. Blank[60] thinks that the reaction to sudden blindness can be divided into two stages: (1) immediate shock, and (2) subsequent recovery (the definitive stage). The initial shock consists of depersonalization followed by depression. Depersonalization usually lasts from 2 to 7 days. At first, patients are almost immobile, their expressions are blank, and, if they speak at all, they speak slowly and softly. If they talk about their feelings they say they have none, or they feel that they or the world is unreal. Depersonalization seems to be an emergency defense against the threat of dissolution of the ego by the eruption of overwhelmingly painful affects.

Roy G. Fitzgerald,[61] in his study of adults with recent loss of sight (partial or full), noticed that many of them reported initial absolute disbelief that they were losing their sight or in fact had lost it. Various behaviors demonstrated that a partial denial or protest of their condition was initially present or even persisted with a longing for the sighted state. The initial defense mechanism of denial should not be tampered with. George L. Adams and Jerome T. Pearlman[62] say it is necessary and adaptive.

The affects thereafter tend to emerge slowly in order for the ego to handle them a little at a time. The depression that follows the depersonalization may blend with it. The depression is a state of mourning for the loss of sight. The mourning must take place for these persons to recover and be rehabilitated. They must be helped to mourn the loss. It is inappropriate to insist upon high morale at this stage. Actually, if such patients totally deny or seem only slightly disturbed by their new state of blindness, they may have a latent psychosis or a severe neurotic need for punishment.[63]

Fitzgerald[64] found that, with patients he studied, disbelief and protest slowly gave way and were gradually, suddenly, intermittently, or concomitantly replaced with depression and other forms of intrapsychic distress. These varied in intensity from a moderate upset to frequent and severe incapacitating states in which depression with suicidal ideation, anxiety, weight loss, sleep disturbance, and even paranoid thinking occurred.

When this *early psychologic reaction* spontaneously ends, patients enter a stage of *adjusting to an unseen environment* which is comparable to the experience of children learning about their environment. The recently blinded begin the process of becoming different persons with different adaptive possibilities. This process is crucial to adequate adjustment. Dependent needs of newly blinded persons must be met, and responsibilities and demands must be gradually and judiciously placed upon them as with children. They must begin to learn how to adjust to their environment as blind persons. Training in how to adapt without sight should now be initiated.[65]

Almost one-third of the persons studied by Fitzgerald[66] who showed loss of sight could have anticipated their blindness, but became as depressed and anxious as did those who were not able to anticipate it. The turning point in improvement of 62 per cent was associated with increased self-esteem from attempting and mastering self-sufficient acts and with establishing positive interpersonal relationships with those caring for them and with other blind persons. Using the white cane was also regarded as a good indicator of adjustment even though only one-half of the subjects studied by Fitzgerald were willing to use it for travel and identification.

Fitzgerald [67] reports that one-fourth of the blind persons he studied had special and continuous visual experiences ("visual phenomena") seemingly outside their control. These included sensations such as changing, flashing, or kaleidoscopic effects. One man, otherwise well adjusted, commented that the display of flickering lights was often so absorbing that they kept him awake at night. Visual hallucinations during the early weeks after sudden loss of sight were thought by Fitzgerald to be associated with maladaptive coping. Hallucinations have often been reported in the recently blinded. It is the first author's experience that such hallucinations are not necessarily evidence of an incipient psychosis and should not be so considered.

Many of the persons studied by Fitzgerald [68] commented on the changes in their *dreams* after their loss of sight. Three-fourths of the dreamers said their dreams were more vivid, colors were more intense, or that there was a change in content; dreams often contained visual experiences from the remote past; and one-fifth of the subjects dreamed about loss of sight, about blindness, darkness, or others going blind. Visual preoccupations and *daydreaming* as a pastime were common; two-thirds of the group had eyestrain, tearing, and headaches; half of the group were aware of straining to see things they knew they could not see—tending to do this rather than concentrate on nonvisual cues. Felix Deutsch [69] implies that the majority of blind persons do not accept their loss, are not reconciled to it, and are always ready to flee from reality to fantasy.

Especially important in adjusting to blindness is the ability to handle the inherent dependency. Franks [70] says it may be that the person's adjustment to an overtly dependent role is not so much accepting it as recognizing the existence of dependency to which he or she had not previously admitted. Preexisting personality traits play an important role in determining social adjustment after the onset of blindness. Blindness in itself does not seem to cause psychotic or neurotic personality disorders, but the *blindness may be a precipitating factor in decompensation from preexisting personality disorders*.

Blank [71] notes that *permanent reactions* to blindness include nearly every kind of psychopathology. The following are the most common: prolonging the depressive phase of the shock into a chronic state of masochistic depression, with self-recrimination and bitterness toward the world and God (these people remain dependent and resentful of those on whom they depend); character disorders that are often an aggravation of preexisting traits (the most common is chronic dependency); and many who seem successfully adjusted and productive identify themselves with other blind persons in a defensive self-protective minority against what they consider to be the hostile inconsiderate world of those who can see. If blind persons show a really undiscriminating prejudice toward those who see, then Blank suggests that they are unconsciously sharing the hostile attitudes toward themselves that they attribute to those who are not blind.

Persons whose vision changes slowly over time must continually adjust. They anxiously face an uncertain future. Helen M. Mehr and associates [72] say there seems to be a greater incidence of adjustment difficulties in the *partially blind* than in those who are totally blind. The partially blind tend to feel that they are in limbo—neither blind nor sighted. They talk of people criticizing them with exasperation for not using their partial vision more effectively.

The ambiguity of the partially blind makes it difficult for them to acquire a realistic self-concept. They tend to cling tenaciously to the identity of a seeing person. Mehr and associates [73] say their patterns of adjustment include the following: denial of having a marked visual handicap; an overly independent reaction where the handicap is recognized privately, but is minimized publicly, with attempts at normal behavior; a defensive reaction such as rationalization and projection; a pseudoparanoid tendency; a lack of trust in others with devastating effects on family relationships; withdrawals from frustrating situations; and behavioral reactions that foster a continual inability to deal with everyday living problems.

Use of a cane and Braille are so strongly symbolic of the totally blind that many partially blind people will not use them despite their intrinsic value. Franks [74] noted that those partially blinded from World War II showed a higher rate of emotional maladjustment than those totally blinded. Those with slight vision or light perception in one eye were unwilling to accept the certainty of this disability. They continued to express hope for recovery of their lost vision, or anxiety over the possibility of losing their remaining vision. They had false hopes that medicine or religion would miraculously restore their sight. P. M. Duke-Elder and E. Wittkower [75] report another study of soldiers blinded in one eye who had great fear of total blindness, which seemed to be responsible for eyestrain, eye ache, and photophobia.

All the partially blind persons studied by Mehr and associates [76] seemed to tire sooner than the normally sighted people because they continually tried to interpret their environment with defective visual equipment. All of them had problems with illumination and changes in illumination. It seems obvious that the partially blind need extra rest.

Mehr and associates found that *group discussion* was helpful to all who attended. The group included partially blind patients, their families, and close friends. Leaders were from various professions. The best size for the group was thought to be eight to ten people. Meetings were held fortnightly. Emphasis was on the present and on expressing feelings. Through discussion of mutual problems, fears, and doubts, misperceptions and embarrassments were lessened. Members were comforted to find they were not alone and welcomed the opportunity for exchanging ideas on feelings, social experiences, visual aids, and other problems. The discussions especially helped the partially sighted deal with depression, anxiety, guilt, loneliness, and their role in life.

Effects of Bilateral Eye Patching. A number of studies have shown that the behavior of patients who have bilateral eye patching is significantly different from that of those not patched.[77-79] Louis Linn and associates [80] noted that the most common change in behavior was increased psychomotor activity. There was restlessness, tearing off the mask, and attempts to climb over side rails. Nearly one-third of their patients (patched following cataract extractions) had paranoid delusions. About one-fifth had somatic complaints or showed elation or both. A little over one-third showed some degree of spatial disorientation. About one-fifth showed temporal disorientation. A small number had hallucinations. Almost all showed more than one of the previously mentioned *behavior reactions,* but those who showed a severe reaction tended to manifest more than one type. Frequently these reactions occurred simultaneously, in some cases increasing in severity on successive nights. There seemed to be a relationship between the presence and degree of organic brain disease and the development of disturbed behavior. Also, older patients were more apt to show disturbances. However, Linn and associates say that the premorbid personality seemed unrelated to the incidence of the altered behavior, even though it determined to some extent the particular type of pattern exhibited. They noted that removing the mask resulted in prompt improvement in about one-third of their patients and gradual improvement in others, yet some continued to show disturbances after the mask was removed.

Glenn O. Dayton and associates [81] found that a proportionately higher frequency of behavioral disturbances occurred during the evening than during any other time in both bilaterally patched and unpatched patients. The bilaterally unpatched patients on medications showed a lower frequency of symptoms than when not on medications; the reverse was true for the bilaterally patched patients. Possibly, this is because with medication the bilaterally patched patient feels less in control and less able to relate to reality. Patients on medication received sleeping pills every night, tranquilizers every day, and Demerol for pain, or both, longer than 1 day postoperatively.

Eugene Ziskind and his associates [82] found that bilaterally patched patients frequently failed to obey the physician's two major instructions: to lie on their backs, and to leave the patches in place. Failure by patients to follow instructions has often been attributed to lack of cooperation, but eye patched patients are highly motivated to cooperate because their vision is at stake. Despite pain or discomfort, they do not usually remove the patches or change their position when they are fully conscious. The noncompliance would seem to occur primarily when these patients are sleeping or beginning to awake—that is, in periods of reduced awareness. Other possible causes of the *noncompliance* were not as significant as the *state of reduced awareness.* With reduced awareness, there were concomitant hypnagogic hallucinations which also occurred during the daytime when patients were in periods of light sleep. Awareness is more easily reduced in the bilaterally patched patient than in those whose eyes aren't covered. The data suggest eye-patched patients are in a clouded state, not in a conscious noncooperative state.

Symptoms of eye-patched patients include all, or most of those, that have been reported for persons in sensory deprivation experiments. Consequently, the effects of bilateral patching and of not allowing visitors (which also seemed to contribute to the sensory deprivation and resultant symptoms) should be carefully weighed, since the negative effects seem inevitable and the opposite of what the patching is intended to do, which is to keep the patient still.[83]

Helping Those with Impairment of Sight. In countries where educational and health care systems are well developed, a network of services is available for those with impaired vision. There are special schools for the blind or special classes in regular schools. In schools and classes for the blind a wide variety of special equipment is available to encourage normal activity. (See Figure 46-5 for example.)

Many books are printed in Braille or in large type. Figure 46-1 shows two children with impaired vision reading an enlarged edition of a book. Volunteer workers all over the United States and other countries are helping to convert the printed word into records or tapes to which the blind may listen. Totally blind students using "talking books" are graduating from professional schools as teachers, lawyers, and even doctors. Health workers should know about the resources available within their communities, and within the nation, that are available to those with impaired vision.

Patients in hospitals or other health institutions who are partially sighted or blind require special care. Although all patients deserve this consideration it is especially important that those with vision impairments be told who will be taking care of them and what will be done. It is particularly hard on such patients when

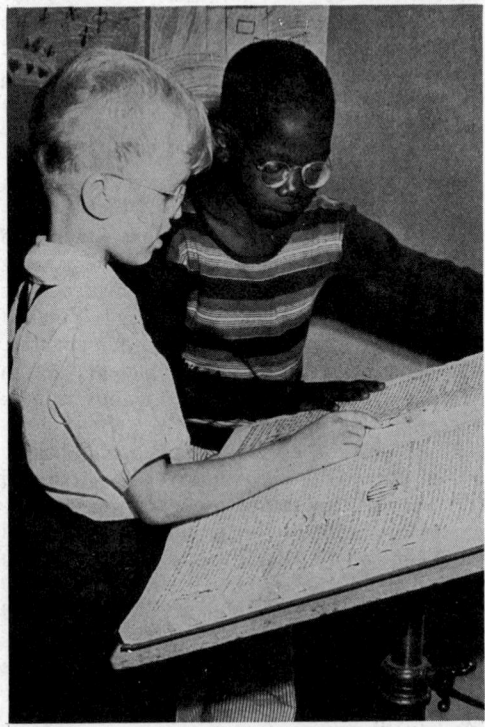

Figure 46-1. Children with impaired vision enjoy reading an enlarged edition of a book. (Courtesy of Michigan State Normal College, Kalamazoo, Mich.)

doctors and nurses fail to discuss their illnesses and treatments with them. Unanswered questions allow the worst fears to be magnified. Unhurried discussion of the patients' concerns, which may be the source of great mental suffering, can help them deal with reality more effectively. However, it is well known that sighted persons who are forced to be in contact with the blind are often shy, embarrassed, and even sometimes feel dislike and repulsion. Burlingham[84] has noted that blind children confronted with such reactions soon realize that they are avoided and pitied, that people without their handicap are sometimes revolted by and fear them. So it is important to have staff members who are comfortable in the presence of the visually handicapped work with these patients. It can be helpful to talk with persons, such as educators for the blind, who are familiar with these problems and to have staff conferences on the special help needed by the blind. The remainder of this section is devoted to some suggested practices. They must be tailored to how ill patients are and their limitations.

Always identify yourself when you approach patients.[85] If they are blind or severely limited in vision, touch an arm or grasp a hand.[86] Since they cannot see you, it is helpful if they can both hear and touch you. Describe yourself and others since patients generally feel more at ease knowing how people look. However, if patients' worries are paramount, they take priority over orientation to the external environment and should be addressed as soon as they are identified. Shouting is unnecessary unless patients have hearing as well as sight problems. Allow people to ask for help; don't rush toward them with exaggerated helpfulness and never leave without telling them.[87]

If patients are partially blind, it is important to find out how much they can see. If totally blind, persons shuffle slowly and hesitatingly with head bent forward, veering from side to side with arms extended to find objects for guidance; they may have had little rehabilitation and will need more assistance than those who have had the benefit of a good program. To escort the blind, allow them to take your arm lightly above your elbow with the thumb on the outside. This places them about half a step behind you and protects them. They can feel slight movements and anticipate directional changes. As you reach stairs, inclines, or other major changes, describe them so that the blind person can make the necessary adjustments. Include the blind in conversations held in their presence. Most blind persons will ask questions so they can orient themselves and behave as independently as possible.[88]

G. D. Jackson,[89] a psychologist blinded since age 5, thinks that one should not hesitate to offer help to a blind person who is walking. The assistance offered is almost always appreciated since it minimizes the extra time and nervous tension of the blind person in traveling alone. When helping blind persons cross the street, do not leave until they are safely on the other side. If helping them into a car or mounting the stairs of a bus, help them by putting their hands on the rail or other appropriate guide, and help them until they actually reach a seat and sit down.

Inactivity is as bad for the blind as for anyone else. (See Chapter 12 on body mechanics and Chapter 38 on the motor disturbances of hypomobility and immobility.) It is, however, harder to provide opportunity for the blind to get the exercise they need. When the nursing staff cannot find the time to walk with the blind or otherwise help them exercise, volunteer workers can usually be found to do this.

If blind persons are hospitalized, help them become familiar with their rooms by letting them move about, touching the furniture and equipment.* They should be encouraged to arrange and organize their rooms, closets, and drawers to suit their convenience. The furniture should be sturdy and solid so it won't slip. Once organized, the objects in the room and the patient's belongings should be kept in the same location.[90] If patients have partial vision, all activities should be from the side of the best eye; the bedside table and chair should also be on that side.[91] I. L. Fraser,[92] writing on understanding blindness, suggests that the blind person be given a roommate who can give verbal assistance.

It is important to help them stay oriented to time. Fraser thinks that a Braille watch is essential. A radio can be helpful in telling the time as well as keeping patients in touch with current events. Having people read newspapers or magazines aloud can also help the blind maintain interest in the world surrounding them.[93] The still of the night is often the most lonely and frightening time, as was observed earlier in this chapter. It is important to keep the blind persons' doors open so that

---

* It is ideal to make preadmission visits to the hospital with a planned orientation program.

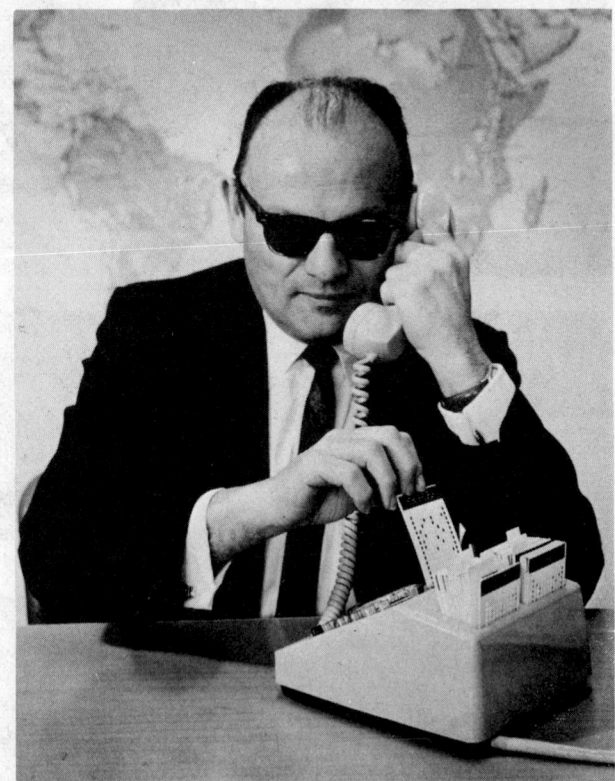

Figure 46-2. Card dialer for those who have motor difficulty in dialing. Each telephone number the person uses often is prepunched on an individual card. When the card is inserted into the telephone and the start bar is pressed, the number is dialed automatically. For the blind, the number can be put on the card in Braille; for the aphasic who cannot remember numbers, a photograph of the person being dialed can be put on the card. (American Telephone and Telegraph Company: *Telephone Services for the Motion Handicapped.* [Prepared with the cooperation of the Institute of Rehabilitation Medicine, New York University Medical Center.] The Company, New York, 1968, p. 149.)

they can hear the routine noises of the unit which they have, hopefully, learned to recognize through talking with others.[94] Sudden, loud, unexpected noises can be especially frightening and should be explained.[95]

Allow patients to care for themselves as much as possible. It is important to find out what they can do and only offer help as needed. But if a patient hesitates and clearly needs help, then do not hesitate to offer it. A matter-of-fact attitude is helpful. Patients should be allowed to dress themselves. If they dress inappropriately, tell them; they will ap-

preciate it. Jackson[96] suggests that the words "see" or "blind" need not be avoided. Those with poor vision or no vision are used to them.

Food should be arranged in clockwise fashion such as meat at 6 o'clock and potatoes at 3. But always check with patients to see whether they already have a system. It can be helpful to comment about the food on the plate and what it looks like; unidentified food can be unappetizing. Blind persons will not be able to butter rolls easily or cut meat, and would usually rather have it done for them than make

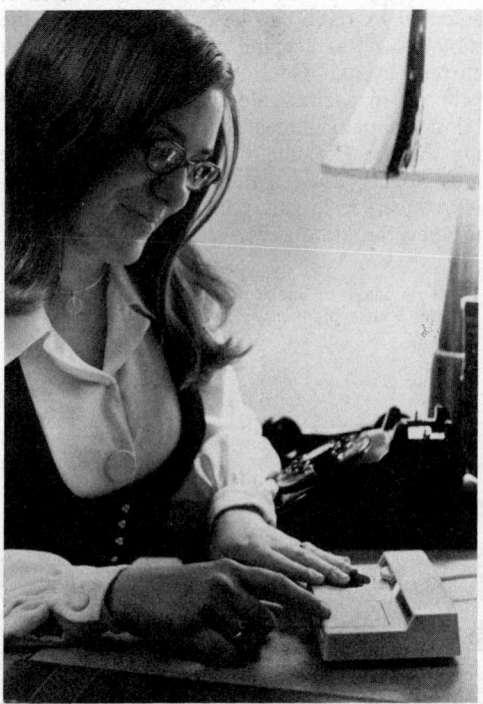
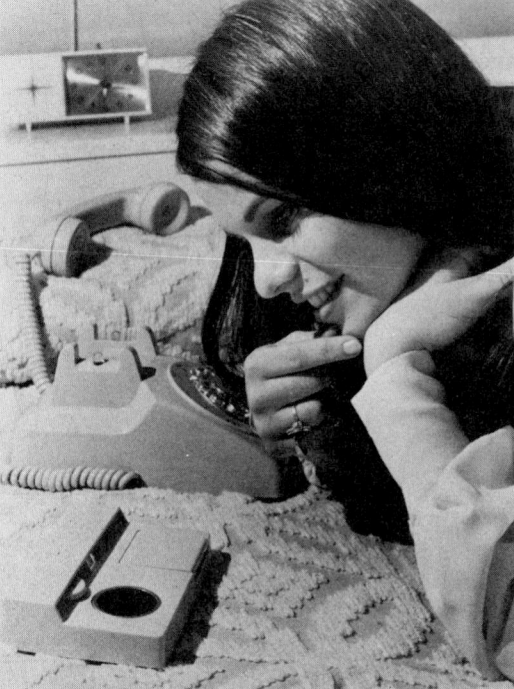

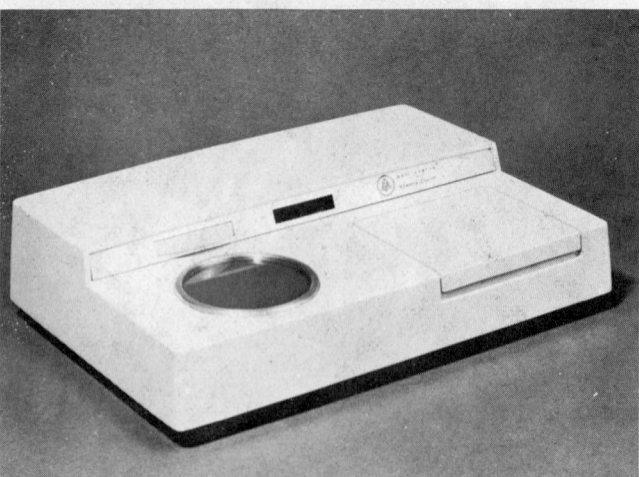

Figure 46-3. Deaf and deaf blind communicating with the use of the Code-Com set. The instrument converts sound into sight signals by a flashing light and into touch signals by vibrations on a half-dollar-size disc. If signals are coded in a prearranged way, such as dots and dashes, the deaf person can read them by watching the flashing light or feeling the disc. The person who is blind and deaf depends upon touch alone. (Photographs courtesy of American Telephone and Telegraph Co., New York, N.Y.)

a mess of it.[97] Emma D. Condl [98] suggests that a cup, glass, or bowl should never be served completely full; nor should hot liquids be poured without telling the patient. Place the person's hand on the container of liquid to show where it is. Condl suggests that using the back of the hand can be helpful in finding hot liquids. Knowing where liquids are prevents spills and wet fingers. For one who has little or no vision, all food should be ready to eat—milk cartons opened, meat cut, and salt and pepper added as the patient desires. Most persons, except small children, prefer eating with a fork. If they must be fed, then ask them what they would like to eat first. Give them foods they can pick up in their fingers for this helps them feel more in control of the situation.

When the patient with severely limited vision or no vision is in the hospital and is clearly not rehabilitated, a rehabilitation program, which involves the services of a variety of professional workers, should be instituted. Most organized communities have special services for the blind, and talking books are delivered on request for the legally blind by the postal service. The Bell System has developed a telephone for the use of the blind that makes dialing unnecessary for numbers the blind person uses often. A punch card with the number in Braille at the top is inserted in the telephone and with a start bar the number is dialed automatically (see Fig. 46-2). If professional health workers cannot devote the necessary time for helping the blind with learning what they need to know and occupying their time with suitable work or recreation, they should seek out other professionals who can or volunteer workers who may, though untrained, be quite effective. Anyone who has seen the articles made in workshops for the blind knows that they can learn to make a wide range of useful and beautiful objects. Hospitalization, or treatment in health care institutions, need not interfere with anyone's purposeful activity that gives life its fullest meaning. Also developed by the Bell System is a method of telephone communication for the deaf and the deaf blind. A Morse Code type of signals is used instead of speech (see Fig. 46-3).

Carter C. Collins and Paul Bach-y-Rita in 1973 described a "portable electronic projection seeing-aid system" (see Fig. 46-4) that might, if found practicable, affect the future management of blindness.

Blind patients, when able, should be taken to religious services of their choice. The clergy or representatives of their faith should be notified when they are admitted to a health institution and visits from them encouraged when it

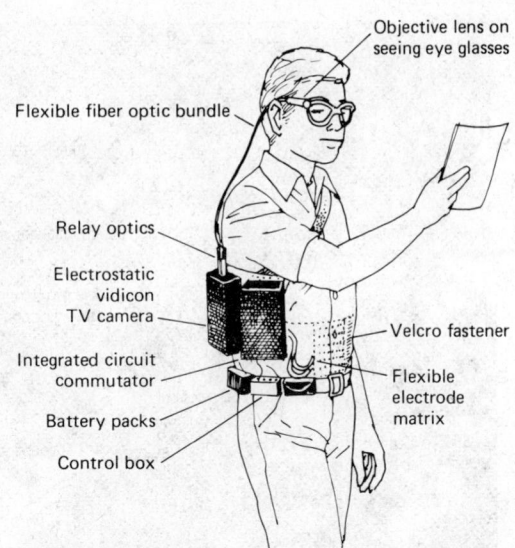

Figure 46-4. Sketch of a prototype portable electronic image projection seeing-aid system. The flexible fiberoptic bundle mounted on a pair of glasses permits the object at which the subject points his head to be imaged on the lightweight television camera. This image is converted into a pattern of electronic pulses applied to the skin by an array of small concentric electrodes in a flexible conducting plastic sheet in contact with the skin. (From Collins, Carter C., and Bach-y-Rita, Paul: "Transmission of Pictorial Information Through the Skin," *Adv. Biol. Med. Phys.,* **14:**285, 1973.)

is apparent that patients take comfort in them. Attendance at schools for those with sensory handicaps should be encouraged. Special equipment of all sorts is used to develop interests and skills. Figure 46-5 shows, for example, blind children playing with a "beeping" ball that enables those who can't see the ball to follow it by the beep.

3. IMPAIRMENTS OF HEARING

Deafness—Definition, Incidence, Causes, and Types. Leonard Diller [99] says deafness is *defined* as an impairment of hearing that results in impaired communication with others. People whose hearing is defective but functional, with or without a hearing aid, are considered partially deaf.

David M. Luterman and Judith Chasin [100] estimate that one infant per 1000 is born with impaired hearing. Diller [101] says it has been estimated that in the United States there are 3,000,000 children with some type of auditory

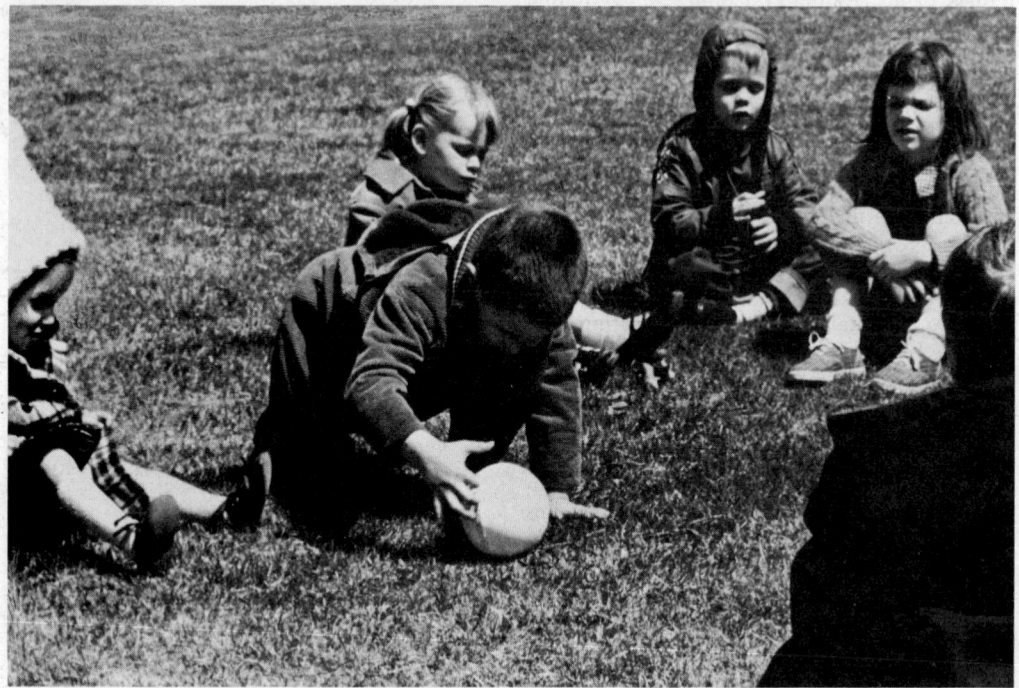

Figure 46-5. Blind children at the Colorado School for the Deaf and Blind playing catch with the Audio Ball, developed and produced by the Telephone Pioneers. A sound chamber buried in the center of the ball gives off a constant "beep," enabling the blind child to hear where it goes. (Courtesy of Morris F. Tyler Chapter #9, Telephone Pioneers of America, New Haven, Conn.)

defect. An estimate for England is approximately 100,000 people who are totally deaf and 15,000 who are deaf and mute. Some form of deafness is believed to handicap 2,000,000 persons.[102] The actual *incidence* of impaired hearing in any country is unknown, since it is taken for granted in the elderly and is rarely reported.

Approximately 60 per cent of hearing difficulties are from congenital causes; 40 per cent are acquired.[103] Congenital deafness occurs because of hereditary defects or injury to the fetus during pregnancy.[104] The major causes of deafness (meningitis, prenatal rubella, complications of the RH factor, premature births, and genetic factors) also cause such conditions as cerebral palsy, aphasia, organically caused behavioral disorders, mental retardation, and visual problems. Deaf people often have multiple handicaps.[105] Meningitis is one of the commonest causes of acquired deafness. The hearing impairments associated with meningitis are especially severe.[106] John C. Denmark[107] says that many diseases that cause deafness also cause brain damage with intellectual impairment.

C. J. Roberts[108] notes recent studies that suggest a higher degree of relationship between congenital deafness and visual defects than was previously recognized. Congenital cataracts are the most common primary medical problem of impaired vision. Laszlo K. Stein and Mary Briggs Green[109] suggest that a large number of deaf-blind children between ages 1 and 7 are victims of maternal rubella. They may also have cardiac problems, mental retardation, and psychotic or autistic behavior. Primary cardiac defects, as well as primary visual defects, are usually identified soon after birth and can be treated during the first 2 years of life.

Norman Cameron[110] notes that people can use selective, partial, or complete deafness to express forbidden impulses, as a defense against impulses, and as self-punishment. This selective deafness is used to screen out what has been forbidden or is unacceptable. Under such circumstances, complete deafness is rare. H. I. Harris,[111] writing on the range of psychosomatic disorders in adolescence, says up to 45 per cent of hearing loss can be expected from the effects of rock bands, especially when there are concomitant psychologic problems.

There are two general categories or *types* of hearing loss: conductive and sensorineural.

Conductive hearing loss is caused by conditions in the external and middle ear. Most of them can be corrected by surgical techniques or by wearing a hearing aid. According to Craig Linnell and associates,[112] the hearing problem in conductive hearing loss is lack of loudness.

Otitis media is a common cause of temporary conductive hearing loss in young children. The episodes are usually infrequent and of short duration. But in some children the episodes begin during the first few months and often recur. Many of these children continue to have recurrent and chronic otitis media, accompanied by fluctuating hearing acuity throughout the years critical for language development. In such cases, language development can be severely affected. These children will understand what is being said only under the most favorable circumstances—with people facing them and speaking loudly at close range.[113]

The sensorineural type of hearing loss involves the inner ear. This type cannot be corrected by surgery and poses a special diagnostic and rehabilitative problem. In addition to lack of loudness, this type of hearing loss has a built-in distortion factor due to defects of the sense organ (cochlea) or to the neural pathway to the temporal lobe of the brain, or to both. A hearing aid will overcome the loudness problem for those with a conductive hearing loss, but for those with a sensorineural type of hearing loss, the distortions of sound will also be apparent through the hearing aid, so special training is also required.[114]

Importance of Hearing for Language Development. Language development is critical for the congenitally deaf, as it is for everyone, since language is not only necessary for communication but for total personality development.[115] Kathleen A. Wilson and M. Carlisle,[116] discussing specialized psychiatric services for the deaf, point out some of the problems associated with these relationships. After birth, a baby who can hear is bombarded with auditory input so necessary for the development of language. Without hearing, language and speech develop only to a limited degree or not at all.

Figure 46-6 shows areas of the human brain associated with language. Norman Geschwind reviews the research that has led to identification of these areas, which are named after those who identified them. Writing in 1972 he said:

Effective and safe methods for studying cerebral dominance and localization of language function in the intact, normal human brain have begun to appear. Doreen Kimura of the University of Western Ontario has adapted the technique of dichotic listening to investigate the auditory asym-

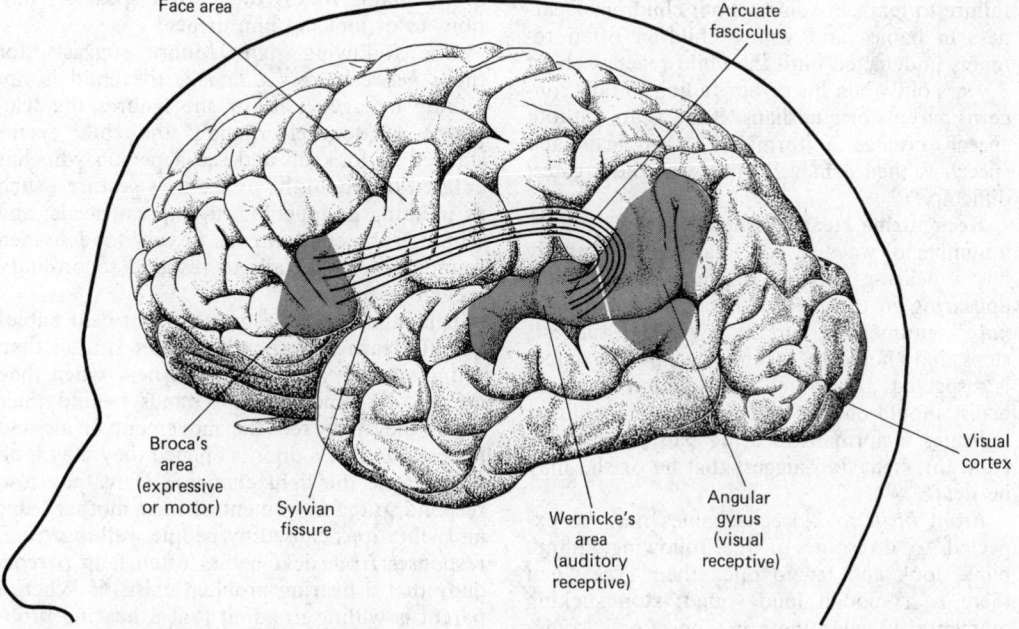

Figure 46-6. Primary language areas of the human brain. These areas are thought to be located in the left hemisphere because only rarely does damage to the right hemisphere cause language disorders. (Adapted from Geschwind, N.: "Language and the Brain," *Sci. Am.,* **226:**76, 1972.)

metries of the brain. More recently several investigators have found increased electrical activity over the speech areas of the left hemisphere during the production or perception of speech. Refinement of these techniques could lead to a better understanding of how the normal human brain is organized for language. A deeper understanding of the neural mechanisms of speech should lead in turn to more precise methods of dealing with disorders of man's most characteristic attribute, language.*

There seems to be good evidence of the asymmetry of the human brain and the dominance of one hemisphere over the other. A good deal has been learned about special training for children who are born with neural defects but who have the capacity for developing compensatory mechanisms; adults with aphasia may also be helped to improve their speech.

Birth to 16 months is the best age period for beginning language development. Linnell and associates [117] point out that unfortunately many hearing deficits are not recognized until later. The peak time of language acquisition is between 2 and 4 years. M. S. Kent [118] says that after this highly receptive period the capacity for language acquisition diminishes sharply. Lack of speech is usually equated with mental retardation. Denmark [119] notes that the congenitally deaf, especially if also mute, are often mistakenly diagnosed as mentally retarded.

Undetected deafness as well as undiagnosed visual impairment is known to be a cause of disturbed behavior in young children and of failure to learn in some school children. Deafness in babies and young children often remains undetected until the child reaches about 3 years old when his or her failing to talk concerns parents or guardians. But 3 years without speech creates a formidable handicap and speech is then achieved only with the greatest difficulty.[120]

Recognizing Hearing Impairment. There are a number of ways an adult can tell that a baby has a hearing defect. An anonymous article appearing in the *New Zealand Nursing Journal* [121] enumerates certain signs and suggests steps that should be taken. If a hearing defect is suspected, a thorough investigation by a specialist should be made. The following behavior indicates a normally hearing baby; deviations from this behavior suggest that he or she may be deaf.

From birth to 2 weeks babies may be expected to do some of the following: jump, blink, look and try to open their eyes when there is a sudden loud sound; stop sucking momentarily when there is a noise or if someone begins to talk; stir in their sleep when there is a noise nearby; jump or blink when there is a sudden soft click (such as from a light switch when the room is quiet); stop crying when a person begins to talk; and appear to seem aware of someone speaking.

From 2 to 10 weeks babies may be expected sometimes to do some of the following: stop crying when someone talks to them; stop their movements when someone enters the room; seem aware of a person's voice; and cry, blink, or jerk at sudden loud noises.

From 2½ to 6 months babies may be expected to react in some of the following ways: coo with pleasure when a person begins to talk; turn their eyes toward the speaker; know when their fathers come home and wriggle in welcome; seem to enjoy a soft musical toy; cry when exposed to sudden, loud, unexpected noise; stop moving when a new sound is introduced; try to turn in the direction of a new sound or a person who starts to talk; make many different babbling sounds when alone; and respond to sounds that indicate that food or the bottle is being prepared.

Mary Virginia Moore,[122] discussing the diagnosis of deafness, offers the following signs of hearing loss that can be noticed *before age 1:* it is difficult to awaken the baby without touching or shaking him or her; he or she responds to comforting only when held; the sound of speech fails to get a response; little interest is shown in musical toys or noisemakers unless held by the baby; and the baby ignores his or her name unless the person speaking motions to or looks at him or her.

The following signs Moore suggests for those *between ages 1 and 2:* the child is not talking by age 2; he or she ignores the telephone or doorbell ringing; the child seems startled to look up and see a person who has entered the room; he or she uses gestures, such as pointing or touching, to express needs; and although the child attends to very loud sudden sounds he or she fails to respond to ordinary speech or to music.

It is important to remember that deaf babies quickly learn to respond to other stimuli than sound, so they may appear to hear when they do not. If someone claps hands behind their heads they may feel the movement of air and look around. If a door is opened they may look up because the light changes. They may also respond to the movement of their mothers' lips and vibrations caused by people walking. Such responses from deaf babies often help parents deny that a hearing problem exists.[123] When a parent is willing to admit that a hearing problem may exist and is concerned enough to tell medical personnel, it is usually certain that such a problem in fact does exist. The concern should not be taken lightly.[124]

* Geschwind, Norman: "Language and the Brain," *Sci. Am.,* **226:**76, (Apr.) 1972.

Early testing of babies will greatly reduce the number of children whose deafness discovered too late becomes a major handicap to the development of speech and social adjustment.[125] M. P. Downes,[126] describing a newborn infant screening program, says that nurses working in newborn nurseries can detect hearing loss with a remarkable degree of accuracy. Babies said to be "at risk" are those with a family history of deafness, those whose mothers contracted rubella during the first 16 weeks of pregnancy, and those born prematurely. In the anonymous article cited earlier,[127] A. C. Miller states that one child in 20 suffers from some degree of deafness, but, by discovering this early, 90 per cent can be cured or helped by simple means. Total deafness is rare. Even a 3-month-old baby can use a hearing aid. Since it is better for a baby to hear specific sounds, such as talking, laughing, crying, doors opening and closing (even if they are fuzzy), than not to hear at all, a hearing aid is necessary.

Signs of deficient hearing in children of *2 years or more* are usually manifested by lack of development or by gradual or sudden changes in their behavior. Slowness or absence of normal speech development is evident. Sounds may be produced poorly or unintelligibly. Deaf children may gesture to express themselves. Behavior disturbances such as hyperactivity, shyness, nervousness, silence, inattentiveness, temper tantrums, or nightmares may occur.[128] Deaf children may overreact when tapped on the shoulder or if approached from behind.[129] School-age children are often slow learners and, unfortunately, often considered stupid, queer, preoccupied, self-centered, or frightened.[130]

Failure to react to sound is not, however, necessarily an indication of deafness. It may reflect the child's lack of attention, or it may indicate a more serious disorder such as mental retardation, brain damage, or severe emotional disturbance. Like babies with hearing defects, children who seem to hear a loud noise may actually be responding to a vibration or to air pressure changes rather than to sound. They may appear to react to sound when they are actually responding to visual cues such as movement by others who are responding to sound.[131]

Behavioral changes may also be evident in *adults* with deficient hearing and are usually more apparent than the behavioral changes in the child. Speech may be inappropriately softer or louder depending on that person's perception of his or her voice. There may be defective enunciation. In an attempt to communicate effectively, deaf persons may be especially alert to gestures and reactions of others. They are often emotional and apprehensive in their attempts to understand and be understood. E. Levine,[132] discussing the psychology of deafness, says that increased tension in interpersonal relationships may produce various somatic complaints such as headaches or back or neck pains. The greater the degree of hearing loss, the more likely it is that people will feel isolated from or rejected by their families and friends. They may express such a feeling by irritability, hostility, or hypersensitivity.[133]

While deafness in infants and children has been stressed, the fact should also be emphasized that deafness can occur at any age. Infections or hemorrhages precipitate deafness. In both cases the condition may clear up or persist. It is, of course, a frightening experience for anyone to find that, often very suddenly, he or she cannot hear. While patients and families shouldn't be given false hopes, it is rarely possible to say with certainty that hearing will not return. A period of hope—even if it diminishes—gives the subject time to accept the idea of rehabilitative measures.

Characteristics of the Deaf. Deaf babies have a loss of the auditory stimuli that help them perceive nurturing qualities they so sorely need during the early phase of development. The guilt, sorrow, mourning, and anger which mothers of deaf babies often feel tend to keep them from relating warmly to them. Deaf children from 18 months to 3 years often show feeding and toilet training problems. Parents are afraid to let them be independent despite the advice of professional health workers to do so. Hilde S. Schlesinger and Kathryn P. Meadow [134] say this is less true if the parents are themselves deaf, for they appear more comfortable with their children and describe fewer problems at this stage.

In the period from 3 to 6 years, parents should provide answers to their children's endless questions, yet the deaf child is often inhibited because he or she has a paucity of symbols and so asks fewer questions. However, as Anny Katan [135] says, children deprived of the ability or opportunity to express powerful feelings in words usually erupt in actions. Expression through motor behavior is potentially increased for deaf children, but even this is often inhibited by the innumerable safety limits adults place on them during the very period that their bodies crave motor activity. Such forced inactivity places on many of these children an added stress that may inhibit learning.[136]

Because deaf children are greatly handicapped by a lack of the verbal symbols by which to express what they think, feel, and need, they also show a relative inability to receive the necessary feedback from others about their behavior and its effects on others.[137] This results in a lack of empathy which in turn creates a seeming bluntness in their social relationships.[138]

It has also been noticed that deaf children have a high threshold of response to pain. They appear impassive to injuries. Yet these children will howl if their desires are not immediately understood and gratified. This impassivity is closely related to their proneness to hyperactivity, which, however, reverses rapidly with the acquisition of language or other modes of communication. These early characteristics of hyperactivity, relatively passive response to pain, and blank faces sometimes result in their being mistakenly diagnosed as autistic, retarded, or brain damaged.[139] Behavioral characteristics discussed here should suggest hearing problems and careful evaluations should be made.

The following are various psychologic characteristics in the deaf. They seem to exhibit a high degree of emotional immaturity. E. S. Levine,[140] in *Youth in a Soundless World: A Search for Personality,* thinks this is expressed as egocentricity, irritability, impulsiveness, and suggestibility. H. R. Myklebust[141] found that the deaf were immature in caring for others. Kenneth Z. Altshuler[142] characterized the deaf as egocentric, lacking in empathy, grossly coercive-dependent, impulsive, and lacking in thoughtful introspection. When children are deaf at an early age, their impulsivity is said to be relatively free of anxiety or guilt.[143] This tendency toward impulsivity suggests that their rage lies close to the surface and is not internalized.[144]

The most common psychopathologic response to hearing loss is suspicion of others, which can progress to paranoia. Deaf persons see people talking and smiling, but since they cannot hear them, they tend to suspect that they are being talked about and laughed at. Harris[145] says that adolescents who lose their hearing have more difficulty than other age groups with this because all adolescents are normally preoccupied with themselves. Loss of hearing (whether gradual or sudden) creates an acute sensory deficit because sound input is normally continuous.

A common characteristic of the deaf is the admixture of doubt and uncertainty that coexists with rigidity and obstinacy. This characteristic is like that seen in people with an obsessive compulsive personality disorder. However, the major underlying dynamics of the obsessive compulsive are related to unconscious conflicts with aggression and sex. The obstinacy of the obsessive is related to a battle with authority. Their doubts stem from

rapid swings between rage and fear, their ambivalences from fluctuations between love and hate. But doubt in the deaf, with its accompanying rigidity and obstinacy, stems from insecurity about what they perceive and what others perceive about them. It extends to a doubt about what they think others feel about them.[146] With their handicap, their rigidity and obstinacy allow them some degree of security and individuation.[147]

It has also been noted that the deaf frequently lack insight about their interpersonal difficulties and frequently blame others for such problems. McCay Vernon[148] says that because they tend to blame others for their difficulties rather than holding themselves responsible, their motivation for treatment is, unfortunately, sometimes very limited.

The effects of deafness on character depend, of course, on whether persons are born deaf or whether deafness comes on during childhood, youth, adulthood, middle or old age; and then whether it comes on gradually or suddenly. The effects can be modified in all cases by the willingness and ability of the deaf and their families to accept treatment, to use hearing aids, or to learn new ways of communicating.

Parent-Child Relations and the Importance of Manual Communication. The immaturity of the person who is born deaf or who acquires deafness in childhood is a necessary consequence of auditory deprivation. Schlesinger and Meadow[149] say there is a complex interplay of school and family environmental factors in the characteristically immature personality patterns of many deaf persons. Early marked deafness frequently leads to disturbed parent-child relations. Denmark[150] thinks much of the guidance given parents is overoptimistic, leading them to believe erroneously that their child will completely overcome his or her handicap. The child's failure to attain the parents' goals often makes them feel guilty and too protective, or the parents think the child has failed and they reject him or her.[151]

Prelingual "profound" deafness presents such a handicap to total development that every channel of communication must be fully utilized, especially in the early years. Profoundly deaf children require special education.[152] B. Fisher[153] has shown that a school child with even a very slight loss of hearing may suffer educationally and wrongly be thought inattentive, preoccupied, and dull.

The educational achievement of the deaf is appallingly low as compared with their intelligence. Inadequate rehabilitative and educational programs and opportunities are seen as the primary reason for this discrepancy. Low achievement begins early in the family life of young deaf children where communication is inadequate. Many effects of early deprivation are irreversible, so the early diagnosis of deafness and the institution of an immediate and effective program of training in communication are crucial.[154]

Vernon[155] believes strongly that the communication needs of the deaf must be met by total manual and oral techniques from infancy through adulthood if achievement levels of the deaf are to rise. Research has shown that using oral methods to the exclusion of manual (sign) methods is a dismal failure. Combining oral and manual techniques can greatly increase the present low academic achievement levels.

Studies have demonstrated that children with early manual communication are more advanced when they enter school, and they maintain this edge throughout the early school years.[156] Despite the fact that deaf persons need to communicate through signs, through manual communication, they are often discouraged from it. The reason often given is that the deaf must learn to communicate in a hearing, verbal society. Arthur I. Alterman[157] says that there is a mistaken idea that manual communication prevents the development of oral communication. It is striking that in spite of all discouragement, manual communication has subversively persisted in classrooms, playgrounds, and dormitories.[158] If profoundly deaf children are to have any chance of adequately communicating in a world where communication is so essential, they must not only be allowed to develop sign language, but helped to do so.[159]

Unfortunately, many teachers are totally unaware that manual communication is important for blind children's perceptions and interpretations of their environments.[160] Adults' attitudes are crucial. A. Beasley and associates,[161] writing for parents, say that they should not try to make a deaf child an imitation of a hearing child. Despite the findings of studies showing that these children must be allowed to develop manual communication if they are to have any hope of developing along appropriate developmental lines, parents have been and still are advised by many professionals not to teach manual communication.[162] It is not surprising, therefore, that parents are confused and often feel that health personnel lack understanding of deafness as it affects children and parents. Group discussion with professionals who are familiar with the latest findings in the field should be available to parents and to others who work with deaf children.[163]

Disturbed Relationships in Later Life When There Is Deafness. Gradual loss of hearing is a common affliction of the elderly. Sudden and complete deafness is infrequent but, unfortunately, not a rare occurrence. Most with hearing defects fall into one of the following categories: (1) those who can hear only low notes; (2) those who can hear only high notes; and (3) those who cannot hear particular frequencies. E. C. Naylor-Strong[164] says most are in the first category. The rest of this discussion on hearing in old age is based on his observations.

The high notes are lost first. A person may notice that he or she does not hear a telephone, whistling kettle, or squeaking door, but does hear a buzzer, distant thunder, or rumbles and vibrations of traffic. This difficulty tends to increase with age. High notes are more audible if the person cups the ear with the hand.

The masking or interference of one sound with another leads to difficulty in localizing the source and direction of sound. In senile deafness, the high frequency sound will be misunderstood more often than will the low frequency sound. Simply raising volume is not helpful because, beyond a certain point, it has the opposite effect of that intended. It is helpful in talking to the elderly to speak slowly, finish every word, and enunciate clearly.

Another common difficulty for the elderly is an inability to locate the source of sound and to tell its direction. Two ears are needed to do this, but often one ear is more defective than the other; for certain sound levels only one ear functions. Consequently, certain sounds cannot be localized. This problem exists whether or not the person is wearing a hearing aid.

Understanding speech depends upon hearing consonants, not on hearing the low frequency sounds in the vowels. When the elderly miss the high tones, they often fail to hear the consonants, which results in many misinterpretations and misunderstandings. The deaf person often wrongly guesses the whole trend of a conversation. Those who communicate with them should be aware of this common difficulty and alert to such misunderstandings.

Another condition, which is not restricted to senile deafness, is tinnitus aurium (noises in the head). The noises are often so persistent that many deaf persons say the noises have made them deaf. This is questionable. However, it is known that patients with this condition often show a high tone deafness when tested, though they have not been aware of this. Sometimes the noise is a persistent drone. Persons with this condition will often seek noisy places or switch on the radio to drown out the inner noise. In a few cases a hearing aid, in partly restoring the hearing, will overcome tinnitus.

Relating to the Deaf. Most deaf children can be taught to talk. H. Bakwin and R. M. Bakwin [165] and other authorities who have dealt with the deaf encourage all who come into contact with deaf babies and children to respond to the babbling and cooing of infants and to talk to them a great deal throughout infancy and childhood. Babies should be talked to when they are held in one's arms and while looking into one's face. They learn from seeing changes of expression and often respond. It is also important to talk about what they can see and feel. For example, touch the baby's nose with his or her fingers and say, "Here is your nose"; then touch your own nose with their fingers and comment.[166]

Deaf children should be encouraged to participate in conversations to help them with lipreading and social contacts. Talking is helpful if it is close to their ears. Also point to or let them touch and see what you are talking about, or do both. It is important for parents or nurses to keep the head still so as not to distract the baby or child from the difficult task of watching the lips. The face should be kept at a level with that of the infant or child. Whole sentences and good pronunciation are important. The deaf learn to fill in what they miss.[167]

It is helpful to the deaf if other persons observe the following [168]: always face them when talking; make certain that they are in adequate light without shadows or glares so that they can see the face of the respondent distinctly; speak naturally, simply, and enunciate clearly; speak in a lower rather than a higher pitch (deaf people can understand a man better than a woman because a man's voice has a lower pitch) [169]; and if the deaf person does not understand (but can read), use paper and pencil. Avoid speaking too slowly, shouting, grimacing, and speaking without actually using the voice. Smoking, eating, chewing gum, moving the head or face out of the deaf person's visual field, or obstructing the face with something can add to his or her difficulty in understanding what is said.

It is important to continually assess whether the person understands. Look for puzzled expressions or inappropriate or irrelevant responses. Also note frequent requests for clarification or turning one side toward the speaker or leaning forward. Misunderstandings must be immediately corrected, especially if the speaker is giving directions that are important to the patient's care. If the deaf person does not understand, rephrase what was said, using simple language. Try not to communicate too much at a time.[170] Gerald R. Popelka and Kenneth W. Berger [171] stress using appropriate gestures and encouraging the deaf to watch and use gestures if they do not already do this.

Let's Talk

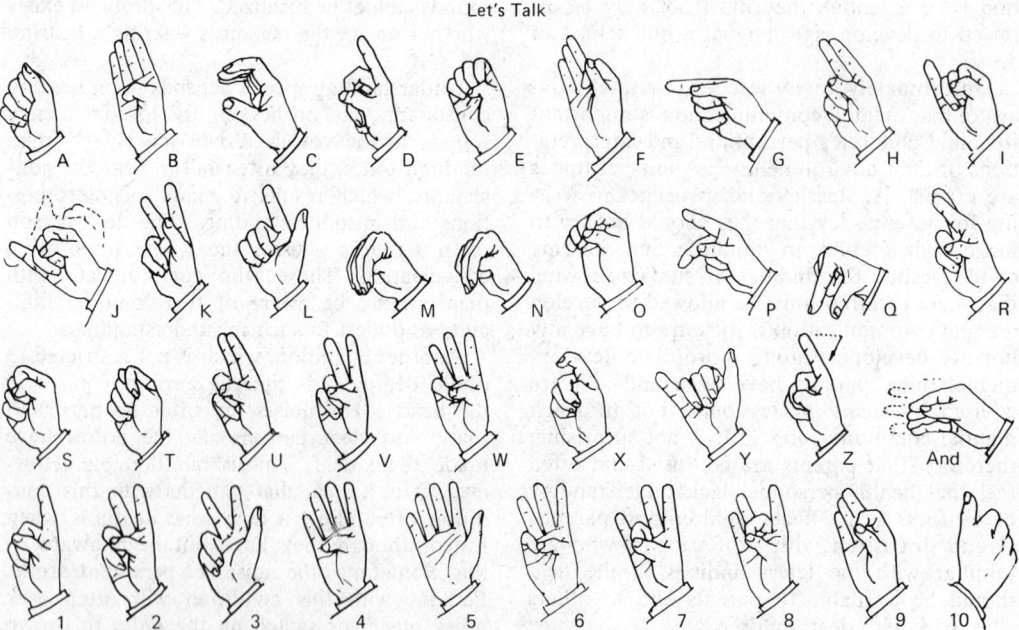

Figure 46-7. The American manual alphabet. (From Doctor, Powrie Vaux [ed.]: *Communication with the Deaf. A Guide for Parents of Deaf Children.* American Annals of the Deaf, Washington, D.C., 1969, p. 35.)

The sensitivity of the deaf person to non-verbal behavior can be an asset to nurses who use it effectively, but nurses should be acutely aware of their behavior to avoid misinterpretation. For example, try not to talk to someone else in front of the deaf and exclude them. If there is a conversation in their presence, explain what the conversation was about.[172]

Learning New Ways of Communicating. While most deaf infants and children can be taught to talk, learning to talk is not the major problem for adults who gradually or suddenly face deafness. Those who become deaf gradually may find it hard to admit their handicap to themselves and to others. At first they bluff a good deal and, having heard only a few words, keep up a conversation in which the responses are often inappropriate, sometimes ludicrous. Finally, when any sort of conversation is difficult or impossible, they tend to withdraw from their friends and family, and this withdrawal may be mutual since shouting and being misunderstood are hard on those who try to converse with them.

Persons who suddenly become deaf suffer a severe shock. They, too, may withdraw from society or, if literate, may take so much satisfaction in written responses from family and friends that they enjoy being in company, but since communication is a two-way process, the companions of the deaf as well as the deaf themselves must be willing to make the necessary effort to converse.

There are schools for the deaf in most communities. In these, students and teachers learn to talk with each other fluently, and family

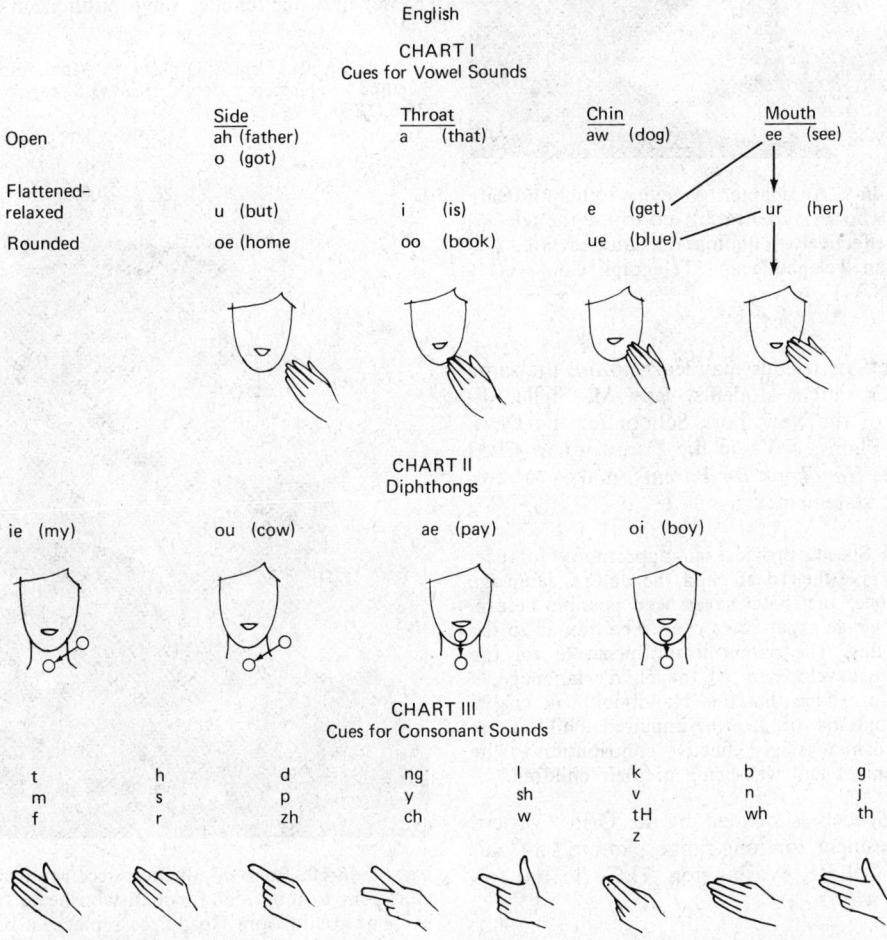

Figure 46-8. Charts used at Gallaudet College, Washington, D.C., to teach parents (and others) to communicate with the deaf. (From Doctor, Powrie Vaux [ed.]: *Communication with the Deaf. A Guide for Parents of Deaf Children.* American Annals of the Deaf, Washington, D.C., 1969, p. 67.)

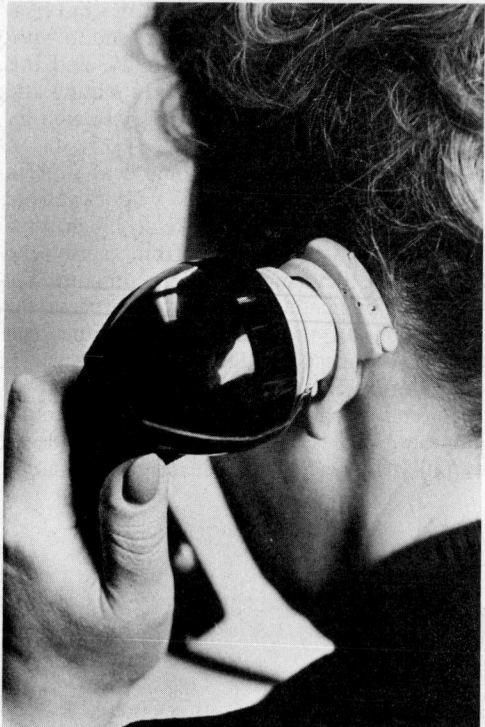

Figure 46-9. An adapter. A device to help a deaf person who wears a hearing aid to use the telephone effectively. (Photograph courtesy of American Telephone and Telegraph Co., New York, N.Y.)

The result of my attempts to find a new and better method is Cued Speech, a method of communication in the visual equivalent of spoken English, through the combination of speech (with or without sound) with "cues." These cues are not signs in the usual sense, since they have no meaning without simultaneous observation of the movement of the lips. They cannot be used for "manual" communication.*

Cued Speech has assumed so much importance in rehabilitating the deaf that the Cued Speech Program of Gallaudet College has published *Cued Speech News* three times a year since 1967. Gallaudet College is said to be the only college for the deaf in the United States.

Figure 46-7 shows the American Manual Alphabet and Figure 46-8, Cued Speech. Families and friends concerned about the rehabilitation of the deaf may be motivated to learn enough about this system to use it.

The dramatic accomplishments of Helen Keller and her teacher have publicized widely

* Cornett, R. Orin: "Oralism vs Manualism—The Method Explained . . . ," *Hearing Speech News,* 35:6, (Sept.) 1967.

members or friends may learn to use the same methods taught students. Roy M. Stelle, director of the New York School for the Deaf, White Plains, N.Y., in the Foreword to *Cued Speech: Handbook for Parents,* makes the following statement:

Cued Speech provides an opportunity for parents to give their deaf child the natural language experiences that have never been possible before. The language experiences cannot be limited to the school day. The parent is indispensable for the complete development of the child's language.

It is my hope that this Handbook will enable many parents of hearing-impaired children to make an increasingly effective contribution to the development and well-being of their children.*

Cued Speech is defined by R. Orin Cornett, vice-president for long-range planning at Gallaudet College, Washington, D.C., in the following way:

* Stelle, Roy M.: "Foreword," in *Cued Speech: Handbook for Parents.* Gallaudet College, Cued Speech Program, Washington, D.C., 1971.

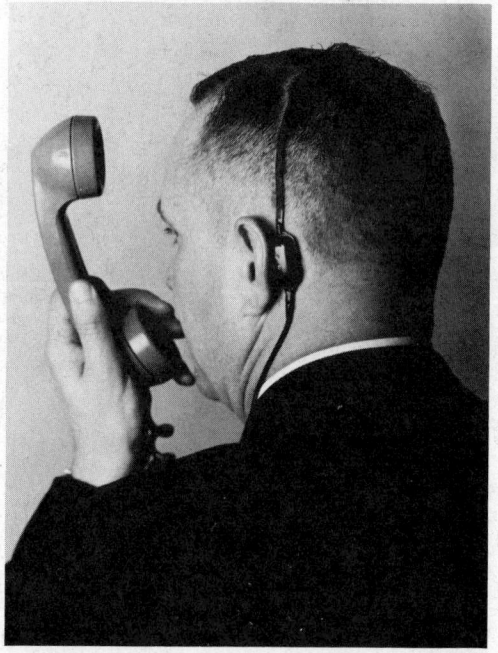

Figure 46-10. Bone conduction receiver transmits vibrations to inner ear for man who hears better by bone conduction. Headpiece replaces a bone conduction hearing aid worn habitually, during a telephone conversation. (Photograph courtesy of American Telephone and Telegraph Co., New York, N.Y.)

the possibility of teaching the most seriously handicapped persons to communicate with others. Attention has been called to the program in Gallaudet College where a deaf student can earn a master's degree. Health workers, but most particularly school nurses, should be informed about the learning resources for the partially or totally deaf.

Types and Use of Hearing Aids. Nurses should be aware of resources available for people who require hearing aids and for instruction in their use and care. Two basic types of aids are *the body type* and *the postauricular type*. The former is about the size of a small compact and is usually carried in a pocket, clipped to a tie, or pinned to a brassiere. The postauricular (shrimp) type may be worn behind the ear or it may be incorporated in the earpiece of eyeglasses, either for one ear or for binaural use.[173] All aids have a basic construction—a microphone to pick up the sound, an amplifier to make it louder, and an earpiece to reproduce it.[174] R. W. Bailie [175] says that some elderly patients get more help from an ear trumpet than from other types of hearing aids.

Body types of hearing aids are cheaper to buy and maintain. They have the disadvantage of a cord which may produce a background noise from friction of the cord against the clothing, but this noise can be minimal. The body types are usually more powerful than the postauricular and they often have a greater frequency range. The smaller postauricular type of hearing aid worn behind the ear is less noticeable to others than the body type, is usually more convenient for the user, and is free from the cord-produced background noise. But it is more likely to be dropped or damaged when dislodged through accidents. The postauricular aid is also more expensive to buy and maintain.[176]

Learning how to use hearing aids effectively may take many months. The function of a hearing aid is to amplify sound, but the lack of intensity of sound is often not the only problem. Many deaf persons have other problems too, such as problems in discriminating between words. Hearing aids tend to distort sound, which adds to the difficulty in learning to use them.[177]

Persons who are deaf in only one ear find hearing aids of questionable value. They are confused by the difference in sound between the two ears. Naylor-Strong [178] says it is sometimes more helpful to put the hearing aid on the better side with the volume low than on the deafer side with the volume high. The reason for this is that there is increased clarity and less distortion.

The following are important points in using a hearing aid: do not turn the volume too high (the deaf have lived in a quiet world for some time and it may take months to get used to a noisy world); do not leave the switch on when the aid is not being used, as it may whistle from "feedback" in the instrument (deaf persons may not hear it, normally hearing persons usually can) [179]; turn it off before removing the ear mold, or the receiver, from the ear; see that the ear mold, or receiver, fits correctly (squealing can be caused by a loose-fitting ear mold, incorrect volume, or a defective transmitter); wash the ear mold in warm soapy water (wax in the ear mold canal can be removed by gently running a pipe cleaner through the opening); avoid exposing the hearing aid to radiation or x-ray; remove batteries when it is not in use for periods of time; store batteries in a cold, dry location and do not put them on a metal surface; and clean the case with a slightly damp cloth rather than alcohol, acetone, or cleaning fluid.[180]

Those dependent on hearing aids may have difficulty using the telephone. The Bell System has developed a device called an "adapter" which, inserted into the telephone, enables

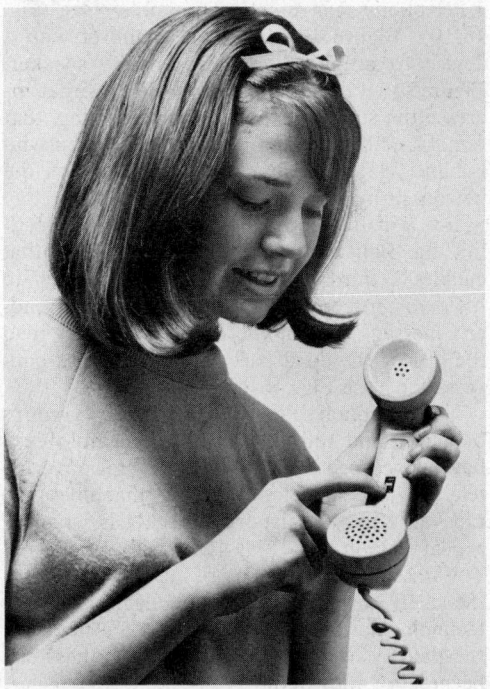

Figure 46-11. Hard-of-hearing handset provides amplification of the voice of the speaker at the other end of the telephone so that the handicapped person can hear him. (Photograph courtesy of American Telephone and Telegraph Co., New York, N.Y.)

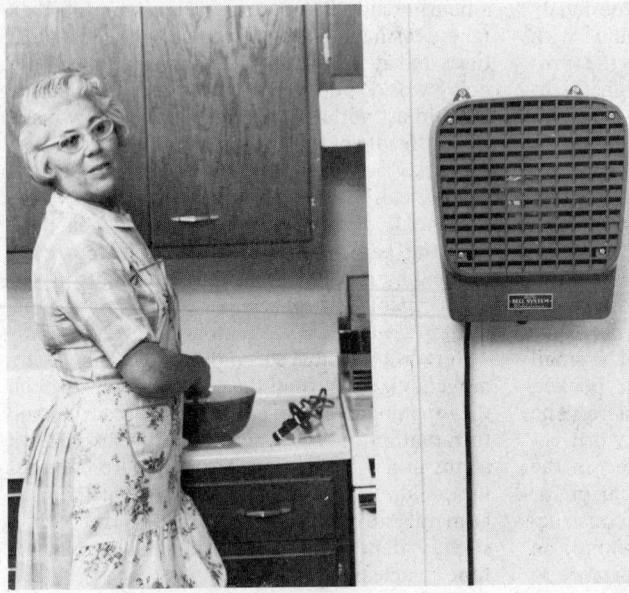

Figure 46-12. Loud 8-in. gong telephone signal useful to the deaf. All telephones are equipped with a device that enables the customer to make the bell louder, but the gong pictured above is a more arresting noise than the regulation bell. (Photograph courtesy of American Telephone and Telegraph Co., New York, N.Y.)

those with some types of disability to hear with the aid in place (see Fig. 46-9). For those who hear best by bone conduction, a headpiece that replaces the hearing aid worn habitually makes a telephone conversation possible (see Fig. 46-10). Figure 46-11 shows a handset with a device to amplify the voice of the speaker. Figures 46-12 and 46-13 show devices that increase the sound of the telephone ringing, that signal a call with a light or, for the person who is blind, a fan blowing a current of air on the person sitting near the telephone.

For a deaf executive dependent on lip reading, the Bell System designed a receiver that enables a third party, such as a secretary, to listen to the conversation and repeat the sender's message so that the deaf person can read the lips of the third party and carry on a conversation (see Fig. 46-14).

The Telephone Pioneers of America (groups of active and retired Bell System employees) have developed a method of using converted teletypewriters (often obsolete machines) to type messages received over the telephone of a deaf person (see Fig. 46-15).

With the development of more schools for the deaf, with theater for the deaf, and with technological advances such as those made by the Bell System, the handicap of deafness can be greatly mitigated.

4. IMPAIRMENTS OF SPEECH

Definitions. Early Language Development. W. Johnson[181] defines speech disorders as deficiencies, distortions, or disturbances of speech that make a significant difference to the speaker, to the listener, or to both in their attempts to communicate with each other.

Imitation and association are important in the development of speech. When young children imitate adults they choose the important words and omit the redundant ones. They add words by degrees. Language maturity is related to vocabulary size and length of utterance, but the best single index of language development is the latter. Children select from all the sounds to which they are exposed those that most closely represent things having importance to them.[182]

Comprehended vocabulary is much larger than used vocabulary in both children and adults. The most important single factor in speech comprehension is the age at which training in sound discrimination begins. If children are older than 2 before attempts are made to introduce speech sounds, they are never able to discriminate adequately. This suggests that speech discrimination is learned and depends on exposure at an optimal period.[183]

D. R. Davis[184] says there is a good deal of evidence to show that the *security of the child is important to early language development*. Children's mothers are their primary love object and their language model. Disruption of the mother-child relationship results in severe trauma to the child, whether the disruption is the result of physical separation or psychologic withdrawal of the mother from the child. Actually, any early and severe anxiety or conflict when language is not firmly established tends to disrupt speech. Like all biologically new functions, it is highly vulnerable.[185] Disruptions in communication during infancy and early childhood can have lasting effects on personality development and intellectual achievement.[186]

Children vary greatly in their ability to withstand stress. Some handle it more easily than others. Stress varies in intensity with the situation. Stress may be so severe that even the psychologically healthy cannot integrate it.[187]

The first word is expected at about 1 year of age. C. Van Riper and J. V. Irwin,[188] in a monograph, *Voice and Articulation,* say that any child who is not using at least a few understandable two-word phrases or sentences by age 2½ should be immediately referred to a physician or speech therapist. C. Worster-Drought[189] states that most normal children use short sentences by age 2, though there are some exceptions where otherwise normal children do not acquire average linguistic ability until the end of their third year. Sometimes this is a family characteristic. Worster-Drought says that if children do not speak by age 3, some defect in their speech mechanism is usually present. In general, therefore, it is expected that the child will use at least two simple related words by 2½ to 3 years of age. Between ages 2 and 3, most children have a

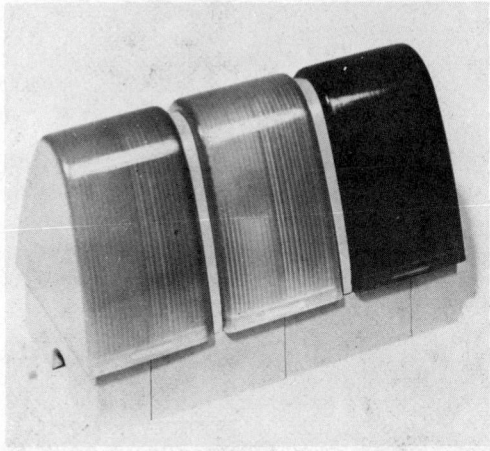

Figure 46-13. For those who cannot hear the telephone ring a lighting device attached to the telephone can signal a call. A "Signalman" can be attached to a lamp that will make it go on every time the telephone rings if the lamp is off and go off each time it rings if the lamp is on. For a person who is blind and deaf, a small electric fan plugged into the Signalman unit will announce that the telephone is ringing with a current of air. (Photograph courtesy of American Telephone and Telegraph Co., New York, N.Y.)

vocabulary of several hundred words. By ages 4 or 5, nearly all normal youngsters can usually express themselves quite well.[190]

Development of Speech in Handicapped Children. Myklebust[191] says the *development of speech in deaf and hard-of-hearing children* consistently lags behind that of normal children of the same age, though the basic pattern of acquisition is similar. In both groups, for instance, girls mature more quickly than boys. Deaf children tend to reach a plateau at a level equivalent to the normal 11- to 13-year-old, and continue thereafter to use shorter sentences with a greater proportion of nouns. They tend to be less flexible in their sentence structures and to repeat "carrier phrases," as, for example, "I see dog, I see boy." This characteristic is seldom seen in those with normal hearing. But what the deaf lose in speech they tend to gain in writing, making fewer mistakes and being superior to those with normal hearing in their use of punctuation.[192]

Mentally subnormal persons tend to show the following abnormalities of speech: poor articulation, small vocabulary, and lack of association between words or speech (crossmodal association) and other aspects of behavior such as movement. Compared to those with normal intelligence, they use a higher proportion of nouns and a higher proportion of vowel sounds. C. E. Renfrew[193] says identifying and comprehending consonants may be faulty, especially word endings. For example, they may identify *tray, sea,* and *you* (with vowels at the end of the word), but not be able to distinguish *cart* from *calf* or *sheet* from *sheep* (with consonants at the end of the word). They also have difficulty in grasping concepts represented by prepositions, for example, *down, under,* and *after.*[194]

*Autistic * and psychotic children show a lack of desire to communicate* or form emotional relationships with others. They appear unaware of their own identities. They seem preoccupied with particular objects or parts of objects without regard to their accepted functions, and they tend to show lack of or excessive responsiveness to sensory stimuli.[195] B. Furneaux,[196] in an article on the autistic child, says they examine objects by touch, smell, and taste rather than by vision. Sounds often evoke no response, and it seems as if these children cannot localize and register sounds in the usual way.[197] Some who exhibit many classical autistic signs are still able to communicate verbally. There is some evidence that such children acquire some understanding of words

* Autism means a morbid tendency to concentrate on oneself.

when mute, as the first words uttered by mute children are often fairly mature in form.[198] However, it is rare for these children to acquire normal adult speech.[199] The most common residual defects are referring to themselves in the third person as, for example, "John" or "He wants to . . ."; reversal of pronouns; repeating words meaninglessly (echolalia); and talking in a pedantic elaborate way called by Furneaux "officialese." [200]

Basic Types of Speech Disorders. There are two main types of speech disorders: *aphasia and dysphasia,* which have to do with comprehension, or brain function, and *dysarthria,* which has to do with articulation which is dependent upon the integrity of the nerve and muscular structures of speech. Pathology in areas of the brain concerned with language or their connections results in aphasia (loss or impairment of the capacity to use words as symbols of ideas), or in lesser degrees dysphasia (difficulty in speaking or in understanding language). When the speech defect is due to faulty articulation caused by nerve defects,

dysarthria is the term used.[201] Disorders of articulation involve omission of sounds, as, for example, *pay* for *play,* substitution of one sound for another, for instance, *wan* for *ran,* or distortion of sound as a whistled *s* sound. The rate of speech may be too rapid, too slow, or uneven. Speech may vary in fluency, such as in hesitancy and repetitiveness, both of which are involved in stuttering. A third type of speech disorder, in which only the voice is affected, is *dysphonia,* manifested by hoarseness, breathiness, harshness, and excessive nasality, or *aphonia,* where the voice is completely lost.[202] Dysphonia is often associated with dysarthria.[203] There can also be problems with loudness, or pitch, or both. Speech may be too high, too low, or monotonous.[204]

Disorders of articulation are the most frequent and potentially handicapping of all speech disorders. Disorder patterns can be divided into articulatory immaturity patterns (those reflecting late, slow, or incomplete development), and articulatory dysmaturity patterns (those reflecting disturbed development).

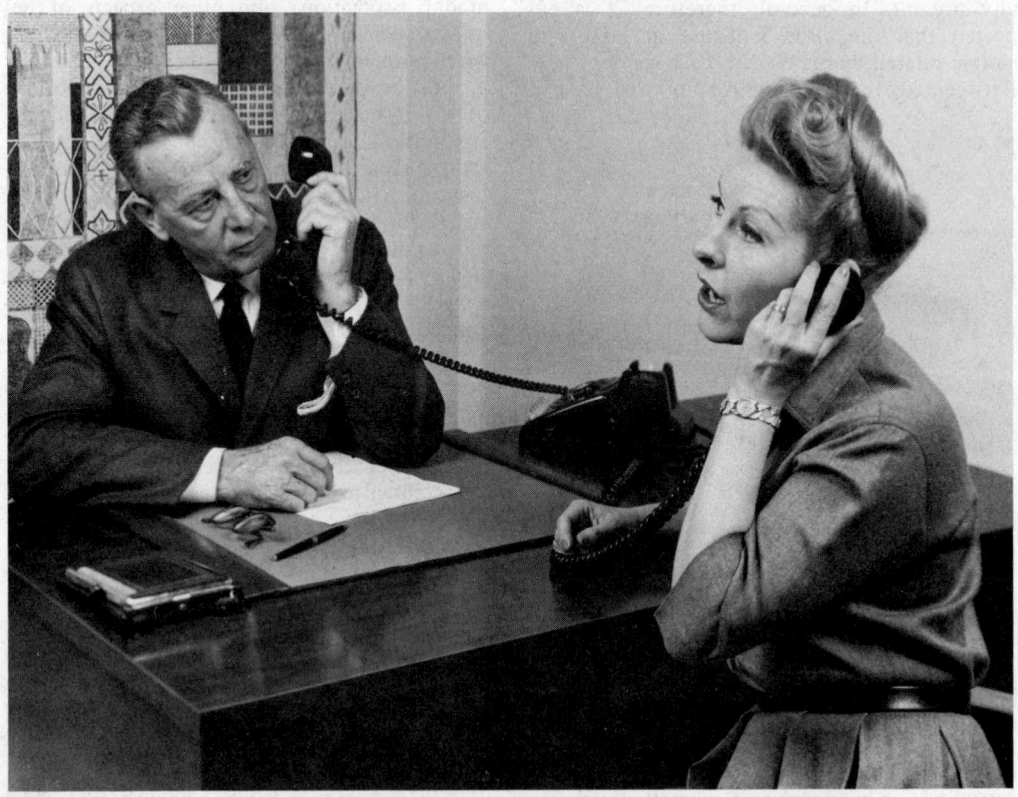

Figure 46-14. Deaf executive carrying on a conversation with the help of a third party, who, using a watch case receiver, can hear and is repeating the incoming message so that the deaf person can read her lips and participate in the conversation. (Photograph courtesy of American Telephone and Telegraph Co., New York, N.Y.)

Articulatory immaturity patterns are those in which speech sound patterns typical of a younger child persist into youth and adulthood, and where they continue to persist unless there is therapeutic intervention. The problem can range from mildly immature to completely unintelligible speech.[205]

M. H. Powers [206] identifies two principal forms of *speech immaturity:* infantile "perseveration" and delayed speech. The former is an inability to hear or produce speech sounds accurately; the latter is delayed speech with various oral deficiencies.

Edward D. Mysak,[207] in *Manual of Child Psychopathology,* says articulatory dysmaturity involves interference with normal maturational processes by such factors as hearing loss, problems in auditory discrimination, or anatomic anomalies in the speech apparatus.

Vocal immaturity refers to conditions that may retard the maturation and function of the laryngeal structures, and vocal dysmaturity refers to conditions that may directly interfere with the development and function of the laryngeal structures. One reason for vocal immaturity in a postpubertal adolescent would be dysfunction of the sex glands that inhibit laryngeal growth and development. There are also known cases of prepubertal or pubertal hoarse-husky voices that appear related to the onset of maturity. Mysak [208] notes that children aged 10 to 12 are often referred to school speech therapists because they have hoarse or husky voices. Actually, these characteristics often disappear after puberty.

There are many conditions that may affect speech through the pubertal period. A. B. Schwartz [209] noted the infantile voice of congenital laryngeal stridor, the possible causes of which are immaturity of the larynx, abnormally shaped larynx, and excessive rehearsal of the laryngeal closing reflex during aquatic fetal life. Mysak [210] gives other causes of childhood voice problems as complete or partial loss of the larynx in childhood from cancer or trauma (rare), allergies, asthmatic conditions, and physical weakness.

Van Riper and Irwin [211] discuss various laryngeal pathologies that may affect the voice. They say vocal nodules are the result of abuse of the voice. F. S. Brodnitz [212] and D. K. Wilson [213] say it is not uncommon to find "screamer's nodes" and hoarseness in childhood. Margaret C. L. Greene [214] observes that children who shout and yell excessively between ages 5 and 10 are often chronically hoarse. Hoarseness from inflammation of the vocal cords during colds is also common in children.[215] Uncommon in children are contact ulcers (attributed to misuse and abuse of the cords),[216] laryngeal webs (often congenital but possibly sometimes caused by diphtheria),[217] and neurogenic involvement of the larynx (except in cerebral palsy cases).[218]

Hypernasality is a common voice disorder in children, one cause of which is congenital cleft

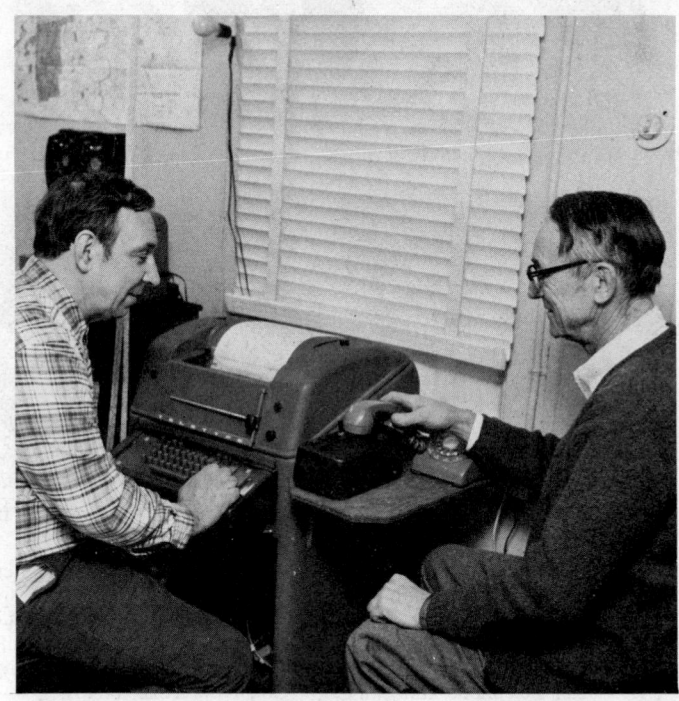

Figure 46-15. The teletypewriter in use by a deaf person in his home is typing a message being sent via teletype signals passing over telephone lines. (Courtesy of Morris F. Tyler Chapter #9, Telephone Pioneers of America, New Haven, Conn.)

palate.[219] Transient hypernasality (lasting 4 to 6 weeks) may follow an adenotonsillectomy.[220] It may be due to an anatomic or physiologic problem, or it may follow bulbar poliomyelitis or diphtheria.[221]

Mutism, Stammering, and Stuttering. *Mutism* is most frequently caused by lack of sound perception. Deaf-mutism is one of the most common forms; congenitally, it occurs 15 per cent more in boys than in girls. Other forms of mutism are found in the following categories of people: the severely retarded (without deafness), children with psychoses, infantile autism, the hysterical, and those who are voluntarily silent. *Elective mutism* is rare. Children who elect mutism are usually sensitive, shy, and susceptible to teasing and ridicule. Milton S. Adams,[222] discussing "a case of elective mutism," says there is always a risk that mute children will be classified as mentally defective in the absence of a full investigation of their condition.

Several authors have been impressed with the fact that several etiologies interact in elective mutism.[223-225] Most commonly implicated are combinations of conditions such as a constitutional hypersensitivity to instinctual drives which may be manifested by social reticence; traumatically experienced events during critical periods of language development, such as being belittled when first learning to speak; insecure environment, such as from overprotective or abusive parents; a psychologic fixation, such as utilizing mutism as the principal fear reduction mechanism; and a neurotic symptom compromise arising out of familial conflicts involving talking, openness, and dependency, such as concern with family secrets.[226]

Werner I. Halpern and associates [227] review elective mutism in children and suggest readings for those who wish to study the subject further. They indicate through their review that the following treatment methods have sometimes been successful: suggestion alone or in combination with other forms of therapy; changing the home environment where parental behavior is believed to be a major cause of the child's mutism; milieu therapy in residential schools; and individual or collateral

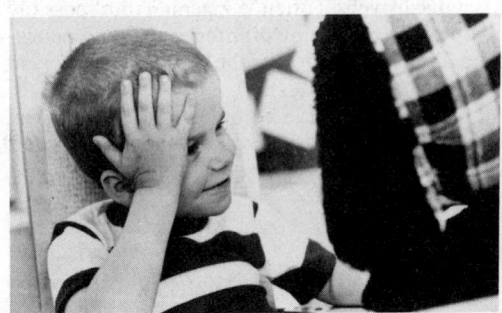

"You want me to pinch your nose?"

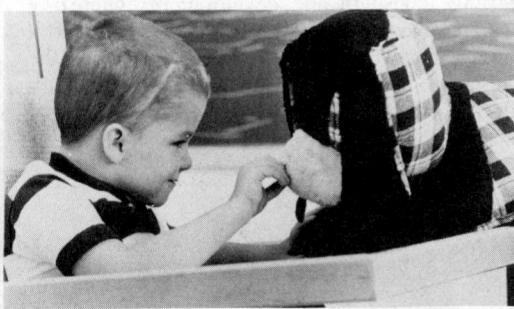

"All right, if you want me to."

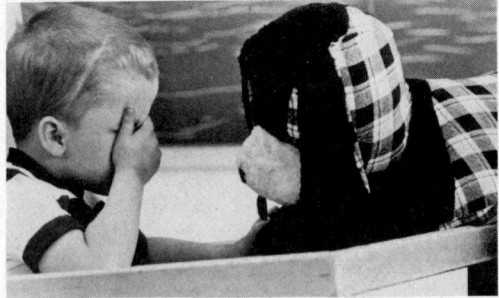

"I didn't mean to to hurt you."

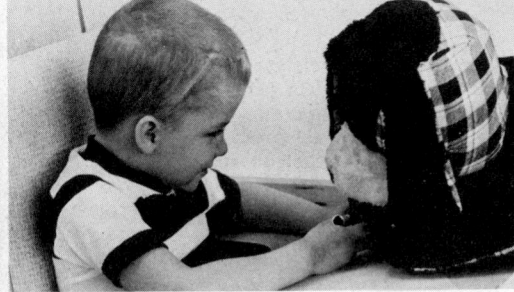

"Are we still friends?"

Figure 46-16. A toy dog equipped with a "walkie-talkie," enabling teachers to communicate better with retarded children or those who have speech difficulties. A normal child is illustrating the use of this device. At the Special Education Center, Reading, Pa., it has been demonstrated that even when children realize it is the teacher talking, they still respond to "Mike" the dog. (Photograph courtesy of American Telephone and Telegraph Co., New York, N.Y.)

family therapy. For the children to give up mutism, they must eventually take the chance of becoming vulnerable through speech. They must learn that speech reduces rather than produces anxiety. The Bell System has developed for the Special Education Center, Reading, Pa., a mechanical dog through which the teacher talks to the child who is having difficulty learning to talk (see Fig. 46-16). A child who will not respond to a person may respond to the "talking" animal. Other anxiety-reducing techniques may have the same effect.

It is not necessarily abnormal to lose the voice when under stress. This phenomenon can occur in situations such as having to speak to an audience for the first time. In such cases, loss of speech is usually temporary and does not bring relief from anxiety. But sudden more *intractable mutism* is a dramatic conversion symptom which helps the person deal with a forbidden impulse to speak of something that would cause great anxiety and guilt if he or she could speak. Mutism is therefore welcomed. Norman Cameron [228] says psychiatric treatment is indicated for those who behave in this way. Cameron also indicates that *stammering, stuttering,* and the *inability to speak above a whisper* when there is no demonstrable organic cause have similar symbolic meanings to elective mutism. Milton J. E. Senn and Albert J. Solnit [229] say it is not uncommon for stammering to occur in children who are in a hurry to express themselves—or those whose thoughts come faster than their words. This type of stammering usually disappears as the child gains control and better coordination of his or her thought and speech. They suggest that parents and teachers ignore this type of stammering or tell the child to slow down. *Lisping* and other infantile mannerisms may be learned and may persist if parents reinforce the behavior by showing amusement. Stammering may also be a form of withholding emotions.

Children may become mute as a way of demonstrating opposition or negativism, though muteness in children is more often associated with deafness or other physical defects. Infants may be slow to speak because they are not stimulated by hearing others. A preschool child may regress or become mute after a traumatic event, such as hospitalization, the birth of a sibling, or the death of a parent. Mutism may be a means of asserting power over adults, and silent children will often speak again when they no longer feel threatened by a lack of power. Senn and Solnit [230] suggest that giving the child more individual attention can be helpful, especially if the attention comes from those upon whom he or she depends.

It is important to note that lisping, stammering, and other articulatory deficiencies are not true impairments but characteristics of normal children under ages 5 or 6. Such speech "defects" are best handled by treating children who have them as if they were normal, being patient, and giving them time to speak and learn. [231]

Stuttering is usually first noticed between ages 2 and 4 when children begin to struggle with complex grammatical forms. At that age their neurophysiologic maturation may lag behind their emotional and intellectual needs for expressing relatively complex thought. Concomitantly, children of this age have to renounce early instinctual gratifications, aggressive impulses are discouraged, and a new sibling often threatens their place in the family; their ties to the mother are loosening. *Primary stuttering* (with its easy effortless repetition of syllables, sounds, and words) usually disappears as the child's neurophysiologic maturation enables him or her to cope with a heavy linguistic load. [232]

Stuttering is not inherited, but a tendency to a *labile language organization* may be. More boys than girls stutter. Katrina de Hirsch [233] suggests that it may be because physiologic maturity comes later for boys. In older children, stuttering with its severe blocking, tension, and avoidance rituals becomes part of the ego's defensive system. It is rarely amenable to treatment by speech therapy alone. A. M. Freedman and associates [234] say it must be regarded as a psychiatric disorder to be treated by psychotherapy. De Hirsch [235] says that intervention with psychiatric consultation is essential because the symptom itself arouses so much anxiety in both parents and child that it tends to be self-perpetuating.

Cluttering, Dyslalia, Cleft Palate. Greene [236] says *cluttering* is a constitutionally determined, severe linguistic disturbance with a familial origin which often persists into adulthood. De Hirsch [237] says cluttered speech is characterized by excessive rate, fluctuations in rhythm, monotony, frequent repetitions of syllables and sounds, articulatory instability, and a tendency to reverse the order of sounds and words.

Cluttering is apparent when children begin to form sentences. They are unaware of their hesitation in speech, they are very talkative and lively, and they constantly repeat words or the first syllable of words. [238] In contrast to those who stutter, clutterers have little awareness of their difficulty. They do not seem anxious about the symptom.

Cluttering is basically a disassociation between thinking and speaking. Cluttering children or adults, as described by D. Weiss,[239] are driven to talk but get lost in the middle of their sentences. They seem unable to plan ahead, to anticipate what the sentence will say; the tempo of their speech is speeded up by racing thoughts, sequencing is faulty, and articulation is undifferentiated. Those with cluttered speech show immaturity in other ways. They have short auditory memory and diffuse auditory discrimination, many are tone deaf and lack rhythm, and feedback mechanisms seem faulty. Such persons have poor motor coordination, their motility patterns are primitive, and they have reading and spelling difficulties.[240] Children may outgrow cluttering if the parents do not correct them, but speak slowly to them and encourage them to take time to speak while also helping them to improve their language abilities.[241]

Dyslalia * is another constitutionally determined linguistic disturbance. Between ages 4 and 7, dyslalic children have difficulty in making themselves understood because they cannot articulate normally. They omit words, substitute words, telescope words, and distort sounds, all of which obscures more subtle receptive language deficits which include short auditory memory span, diffuse auditory discrimination, and problems with the sequential ordering of incoming information. Dyslalic children usually understand others, but they may be unable to interpret the small, grammatical words that represent spatial, causal, and temporal relationships. As such children mature, their speech usually improves, but subtle residual problems with formulation and organization of language usually remain.[242]

M. Pannbacker[243] reviews studies on the language skills of children with *cleft palates* and finds that they are, to some degree, deficient in them. In numerous studies it has been found that the incidence of hearing loss is substantially greater among individuals with cleft palates than among those with normal palates, but because there is some question as to the possibility of biased samples the above generalization is only tentative. Conditions that may adversely influence the language development of children with cleft palates include the following: inadequate language stimulation and reinforcement; frequent long periods of hospitalization and convalescence or both; and self-consciousness about speech or appearance or both. Several investigators have indicated that children with cleft palates are not usually maladjusted or emotionally disturbed, though they

may have some difficulty with social acceptance. This suggests the importance of stimulating the child's speech and helping parents to do so. It may be necessary for parents to work through some of their feelings about their handicapped children before they can be adequate role models for these children. Nurses have more opportunities than any other health workers to help these children through helping the parents. It is often visiting nurses, or district nurses, who help parents realize the need for surgical repair of the cleft palate. They know the resources of the community and are able to tell the parents where such surgery is performed.

Aphasia and Associated Problems. *Childhood aphasia* refers to the speech of children which is abnormally delayed or impoverished in the absence of any other defects, such as hearing defects. Many authors object to this term on the grounds that aphasia rightly applies to the loss of an established skill rather than the inability to acquire it. However, Moyra Williams[244] says the term is so widely used this way that health workers should be aware that it is.

There is some evidence that aphasic children are lacking in the ability to receive and decode speech so they cannot make the necessary integration for normal speech development.[245] Children with aphasia have difficulty in focusing on and discriminating single sounds,[246] suggesting failure in the mechanism that filters out extraneous stimuli.[247] Aphasic children's auditory retention is poor and they have difficulty associating sounds with action[248]; they can distinguish between single vowels in words only when there are consonants on either side. For example, *a* and *e* are often distinguishable but *bat* and *bet* are not. Aphasic children do, however, tend to have good visual retention[249]; they can understand written material better than spoken material, but they usually have difficulty with comprehension and generalization, and they articulate poorly.[250] Childhood aphasia is often misdiagnosed as mental retardation or deafness even though it usually involves no intellectual impairment.[251]

The basic processes leading to writing or speech may be divided into the three following functions: (1) The sensory or receptive function, which requires using the ears and auditory nerves to convey sounds to the brain, and using part of the temporal lobes to interpret sounds as sounds. (2) The central or integrating function, which is carried on in the cerebral hemispheres and involves an appreciation of the symbols intended by the various sounds (the ability to make sense of what is heard, to

---

* According to Gould's medical dictionary, "Impairment of the power of speaking due to a defect in the organs of speech."

decide what should be said in reply, and to mentally produce the words that are to be spoken). This requires an ability to think constructively, to arrange thoughts in some order, to select words representing appropriate ideas, and to initiate the complex processes needed to convert the mental images of words into a series of coordinated responses. (3) The motor or expressive function, which involves sending impulses from the cerebral hemispheres through the peripheral nerves to muscles of the face, mouth, throat, and respiratory system involved in speech. Essential to this is the coordination of the movements of these muscles. When they function properly, words can be spoken.[252]

Aphasia is the loss of the ability to transmit ideas of language in any of its forms (reading, writing, speaking) or failure to understand the written, printed, or spoken word.[253] The following are common causes of aphasia in the adult: hemorrhage of the blood vessels of the brain, blocking of the blood vessels of the brain, hardening of the arteries, outside injury to the brain, or involvement of some degenerative disease.[254]

All aphasic patients are not alike in the loss of language they suffer. Elizabeth W. Reeves [255] says that a speech pathologist's diagnosis will usually classify a patient as having one of the following: *expressive aphasia, receptive aphasia,* or *expressive-receptive aphasia.* Impairments known as receptive aphasia are generally subclassified as *auditory aphasia* (difficulty in hearing) and *alexia* (difficulty in reading). Subclassifications of expressive aphasia are *motor aphasia* (difficulty in speaking) and *agraphia* (difficulty in writing). There are other subclassifications, but these are ones the nurse is most likely to encounter.

In aphasia, the areas of the brain concerned with the comprehension of spoken language, or those controlling speech, are undeveloped or disordered by disease. The higher intellectual processes continue to function, though in some cases imperfectly. Aphasia, therefore, can be a disorder in comprehension and formulation of speech, or only a defect in the latter—comprehension remaining normal, or adequate. In both comprehending speech and talking, memory is essential. Aphasic patients, unless their mental faculties are also impaired, can usually communicate quite well by means of signs and gestures.[256]

There are two types of receptive aphasia: (1) Auditory aphasia, in adults, is an inability to understand spoken language owing to loss of a developed ability, or in children, a difficulty and lateness in learning to do so, though hearing is intact. This condition is known as word-deafness. (2) Visual aphasia is an inability to interpret, or a difficulty in learning to appreciate, written or printed language when sight and general intelligence are normal. This disorder is also termed word-blindness, *alexia* or *dyslexia.* It is one of the varieties of reading difficulties.[257]

Temporary aphasia is known to occur in association with idiopathic epilepsy, especially in temporal lobe epilepsy, usually following a seizure or series of seizures. Usually such aphasia disappears after an interval of variable length but may recur following further epileptic seizure. In some cases, a hearing defect and impairment of comprehension (receptive aphasia) has occurred before the epileptic seizure. The aphasia may then be persistent. Even the milder cases are slow to improve despite intensive speech therapy. Worster-Drought [258] says that aphasia in association with idiopathic epilepsy in children is a rare disorder.

Two other types of aphasia that are often seen in the general hospital are *motor aphasia* and *dysarthria.* With motor aphasia the patients are unable to combine speech sounds into words and syllables, even though they still have the ability to recall words. Dysarthria is the inability to pronounce or articulate accurately owing to a loss of muscle control. Barbara E. Miller [259] notes that patients with dysarthria frequently have difficulty chewing and swallowing for the same reason.

It is typical of dysarthria that speech is mildly unintelligible and gets worse when the person uses polysyllables and long sentences; when short sentences are used, the person's speech is usually understandable. People with dysarthria tend to draw out their words. W. E. Jones and D. R. Mittlestedt [260] say there is a definite muscular difficulty that makes speech halting and slurred. With persons who have this problem the listener should respond to the content of communication and not the quality. When word-finding difficulties are apparent, nurses must to some extent sense the patient's need, and in meeting it, tell him or her the interpretation that has been made and the intent of the response.[261]

Lesions in the dominant cerebral hemisphere may be followed by language disorders (dysphasia), but Williams [262] says that loss of language is seldom total. The ability to communicate is severely disrupted because the person has difficulty in finding appropriate words at the right moment, or in stringing these together in accepted syntactical sequence. These disorders of expression may or may not be accompanied by loss of comprehension.

D. H. Howes and N. Geschwind [263] noted

that expressive dysphasics (those with severe reduction of output but little disturbance of comprehension) are more common than jargon dysphasics (those with a tendency to talk jargon in whom disorders of comprehension are also evident). When the term *dysphasics* is used, it usually refers to expressive dysphasics, which is how the term is used here. Speech of dysphasics follows normal statistical laws, but there is a severe restriction of vocabulary. R. C. Oldfield and A. Wingfield [264] say that common words and words in common contexts are more easily accessible than rare words or words in rare contexts. H. Schuell [265] says that if expression is grossly abnormal then comprehension is almost always impaired to some degree.

G. Rochford and M. Williams [266] note that a word that cannot spontaneously be found in response to a request to name an object will often surface if the person is given a cue, as, for example, "We bite with our . . ." or if the word itself is produced in a different context, as "In a comb these are teeth too."

Dysphasic adults don't seem to have lost the basic word or its organization, but only parts of it. When they fail to find a correct word they tend to describe the subject by its use or to give a word associated with it. Children who have aphasia caused by brain pathology, such as a temporal lobe lesion, tend to remain more mute than children with aphasia from other causes, as described earlier. Yet adults with similar lesions nearly always make some attempt to verbalize even if it is inappropriate. Compared with adults, children have no well-rehearsed words to fall back on. [267]

Because of focal lesions, the *language disorders seen in patients with senile dementia* are different from those seen in dysphasics. In the early stages of senility, speech usually remains fluent, grammatical, and appropriate, though there is a lack of precision and some difficulty in naming objects. In the next stage, speech is reduced to simple phrases in which sounds and prepositional forms remain intact, but there is little meaning. Speech tends to go on endlessly and to be repetitive. Such patients can comprehend the general trend of a conversation but they miss the details. In the final stage, speech is limited to one or two sensible utterances in a stream of inarticulate jargon. [268]

Compared to dysphasic patients, senile patients are often better at naming pictures than in selecting a named picture from alternatives, and better at reading lists of words aloud than at matching written words to pictures. On matching tasks, it seems that they fail to grasp what they are supposed to do rather than that they are unable to do it. Completely erroneous responses are often accompanied by a loose verbal confabulation, [269] and errors made by senile patients, when they fail to correctly name objects, show perceptual as well as linguistic defects. For example, dice are called boxes with seeds in them. Naming things that can be identified with less difficulty (such as body parts) shows less error. [270]

In senile dementia, language breakdown doesn't parallel normal language function or the development of language in normal children. It is not accessibility to words that seems to be the problem, but inability to select the correct word, both in expression and comprehension. It has been suggested that maybe the wrong semantic field is alerted, possibly through faulty perception. [271]

Diseases or Injury of the Larynx. It is beyond the scope of this chapter to discuss the types of infections of or types of mechanical or chemical injuries to the larynx or the tumors that might affect it. Any of these that change the structure or function of the vocal cords affect speech. The effect may be temporary or permanent. Those who cannot temporarily communicate by speaking, or for whom silence is prescribed as part of medical treatment, may resort to writing or sign language; those whose speech is permanently affected should have a planned program of rehabilitation. They may join a self-help organization (see the Appendix) and get support from others with a similar handicap. The Bell System has developed a battery-powered electronic larynx that substitutes electronic vibrations for the natural vibrations of the voice (see Fig. 46-17). This device can be used for those who have a temporary or permanent disability.

Attitudes of Families to Those with Aphasia. There seems to be a relationship between family attitudes and the recovery made by persons with aphasia. Relatives tend to experience any of the following: guilt, unrealistic expectations, rejection, overprotection, and social withdrawal. In a study reported by R. L. Malone and associates, [272] conferring with speech pathologists and medical personnel (physicians, nurses, and physical therapists) did not seem to have a demonstrable effect on such feelings in spouses of aphasics. Most of these spouses had also talked with social workers and occupational therapists. It is noteworthy that all these spouses felt that the information given them was inadequate in content or presentation. It seemed that these feelings might be partly the result of inaccurate information or understanding of the disorder and its impact on the family. This study suggests that families of aphasics need at least the following help: (1) accurate information about aphasia effectively presented; (2) effective counseling to achieve a realistic understanding of the aphasic person and his or her impact on the family; and (3) a program of counseling that focuses on helping relatives (and friends) with their feelings in order that they may respond more realistically to the person with aphasia.

Helping Persons with Speech Problems. F. A. Griffith,[273] writing in the journal *Rehabilitation Record,* says any training program should be based on an assessment of the patient's knowledge, assets, and limitations. What is important is early identification of speech, hearing, and language problems (or any combination of them), followed by as intensive a regimen of treatment as the patient can tolerate and as is justified by the potential recovery or improvement. It is not reasonable, for example, to try to help patients develop writing or reading skills they never had prior to the illness that is believed to be the source of their writing or reading difficulties.[274]

Evaluation of a patient's aphasia is first needed. The following are several ways to evaluate comprehension. Give a simple direction, as for example, "Point to your nose." If the patient points to something else, then the evaluator knows he or she can point, but cannot understand the latter part of the command. If the person can understand a simple command, next try one that requires two responses, as, for example, "Raise your right hand and place it on your head." To evaluate visual recognition, have a few items on a table or tray, for instance, a comb, pencil, key, and coin, and ask the person to point to the object named. In showing the object, also show the printed word which the person may recognize by sight. The evaluator can test the subject's ability to read and comprehend written instructions by writing simple instructions and seeing if he or she can follow them. Miller[275] says apparent lack of understanding of the spoken or written words, or inability to recognize objects, usually indicates that the person has a receptive aphasia.

Whether or not patients seem to understand

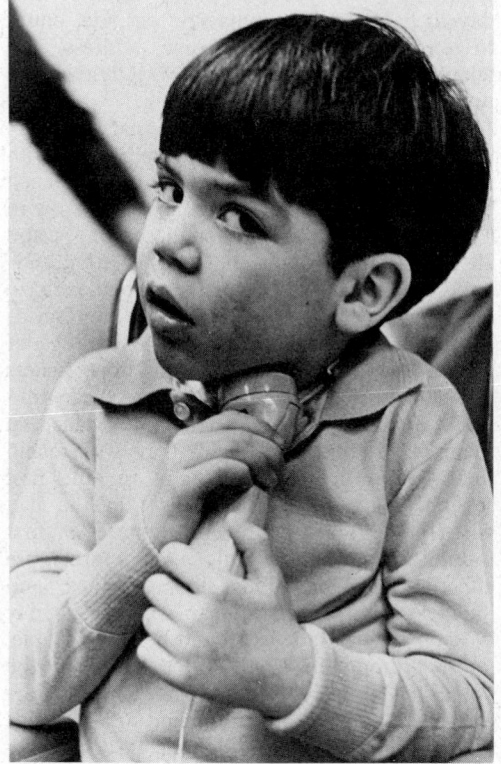

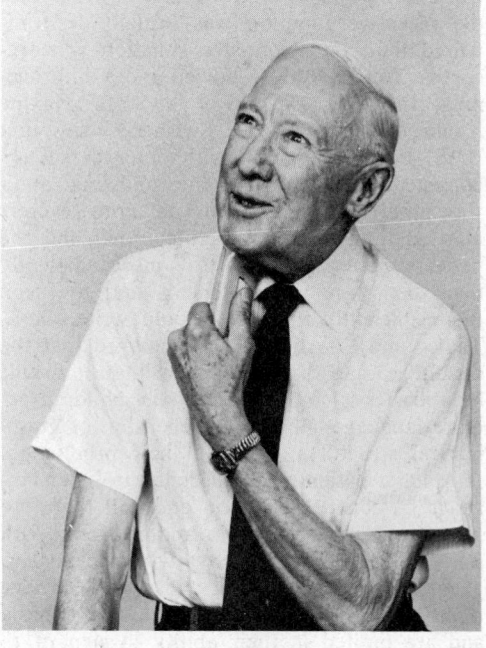

A   B

Figure 46-17. Battery-powered electronic larynx for those who have temporarily or permanently lost the use of the larynx. It substitutes electronic vibrations for the natural vibrations of the voice. *A.* Child recovering from an injury to the vocal cords using an electronic larynx modified for him. *B.* Adult using electronic larynx. (Photographs courtesy of American Telephone and Telegraph Co., New York, N.Y.)

and respond to written, spoken, or visual stimuli, the health worker (or family) can continue to evaluate them in the following ways: ask them to count from 1 through 10, to name days of the week, or the months of the year. If patients can count forward but not backward, it suggests that the response is automatic rather than the result of thinking. Another way to test this is to ask the patient to count by 2 or by 5. Other manifestations of automatic speech are the spontaneous and often repetitive use of such speech forms as profanity, interjections, or exclamations. Spontaneous responses may sound logical on the surface but the evaluator should not be deluded into believing that the patient no longer has aphasia. Test patients by asking them to tell time using a clock or watch or using a large cardboard clock; have them count money and make change; and find out whether they can write and spell.

If patients have difficulty writing, spelling, telling time, or counting, it may indicate that they have expressive aphasia. If they seem to have equal difficulty in speaking, understanding, and writing, they may have a combination expressive-receptive aphasia. Miller says almost all aphasic patients have a combination of defects.

In his study of aphasic patients with and without treatment, L. A. Vignolo [276] found that the receptive function was initially less impaired than the expressive function. The receptive function also showed more improvement than the expressive function. Maxine Kenin and Linda Peck Swisher [277] say that B. E. Porch's research with aphasic patients consistently demonstrated the following: auditory input was more often and more severely affected than visual or tactile input, and the patients were able to gesture more efficiently than they were able to speak, and to speak more efficiently than they could write. O. L. Taylor and C. Anderson [278] observed that the dissolution and reacquisition of linguistic skills by aphasics is similar to the way children acquire language—that comprehension of grammatical structures precedes their production.

Aphasic patients have a deficit in inner language or conceptualization and will therefore have the same difficulty in finding words with sign language that they have with spoken language. A large majority of aphasic adults have right hemiplegia associated with the aphasia and are limited in their ability to sign or to spell with the finger. If a person's linguistic ability is poor, his or her right (dominant) hand will not be very useful. [279]

Some aphasics can express themselves reasonably well with written language in combination with speech. If such patients are capable of spelling words with their fingers, they are capable of writing words. Many aphasics become skillful pantomimists. A hungry or thirsty patient can learn to express the need for food and drink very easily through pantomime accompanied by isolated words or sounds of varying pitch and loudness. Silence is not helpful for these patients even though they have difficulty talking. Health workers, family, and friends should talk with them. Using the basic words to express basic needs is a helpful form of communication [280] and helps keep life as normal as possible for them. When one talks to people with speech problems, it is important to stand directly in front of them or at the better functioning side if there is a difference.

It is helpful to aphasic patients if words used relate to what the worker, family member, or friend is doing, as, for example, "Here is some water," or "Here is the bell cord." It is especially important to incorporate early in their rehabilitation words they must use to meet their immediate needs—words such as *doctor, nurse, drink,* or *bedpan.* Reeves thinks that if their attendants take a few minutes each day to help these patients say the date, count to ten, and repeat their name, address, and telephone number, such daily activities can promote progressive improvement.

Nurses can explain to patients that they wish to have short daily sessions to help them with words and reading. Patients may stare back blankly or burst into tears. Many persons with aphasia have marked personality changes and alterations in self-concept. They tire quickly, are often irritable, and have a tendency to laugh or cry. Patients' tears at the mention of speech retraining may be due to feelings of gratitude and appreciation or of hopelessness and resignation. Since it will not be clear until later, if then, what the behavior means, let them cry it out. Eventually they will regain their composure and be ready for the first session. Have the sessions early in the day when patients are fresh. Five minutes at first is long enough; short daily sessions are more effective than occasional long sessions, and having the session at the same time each day is also helpful. Patients should be comfortable, lighting should be good, and there should be no distractions. [281] It is difficult enough for aphasic patients to directly attend to a stimulus without listening to or looking at distracting stimuli. [282]

Receptive aphasics need work concentrated on recognition of the spoken or written word. An initial goal in working with expressive aphasics is to elicit some form of verbal sound from them.

Miller [283] suggests the following as methods of retraining: Buy or make cards, each of which has printed on it the name of a common object, as for example an orange, a comb, a pencil. Also have these same objects or pictures of the objects. Group the words and corresponding items or pictures together in separate units of related items, as for instance food, clothing, toilet articles. Use one group of words at a time and ask the patient to match the items with the words or reverse the procedure (matching the words with the items).

Another procedure suggested by Miller is to show patients an item or a picture of the item and ask them to print its name. It may be helpful for patients to first trace over the printed letters. As people progress in matching items and words, ask them to repeat the words as the nurse says them, and do not be concerned if the pronunciation is imperfect. Encourage patients judiciously and keep the training plan within their tolerance limits, which may differ on consecutive days owing to fatigue, discouragement, and other conditions. More complex retraining can include having learners respond to short instructions, as, for example, "Pick up the pen." Writing, spelling, and arithmetic can be encouraged later if patients had these skills before they were ill. Some who did not may still be taught rudimentary practices.

To help patients with speech, first give them a few tongue and lip exercises, as, for example, ask them to move the tongue from side to side and up and down, and purse the lips as in whistling and blowing. If the person can make sounds at all, these exercises may give encouragement. Then work on one vowel or consonant at a time. Show the patient how to use the lips and tongue by letting him or her watch you. A large mirror can help patients see what they are doing. Sound drills can be given next. Move from simple to complex words, simple to complex phrases, and sentences. Miller reminds the worker that with all retraining it is important to finish a lesson with exercises the patient can do well.

Aphasic people may have trouble getting into telephonic communication when left alone. The Bell System has developed an instrument which will dial the number automatically if a punch card is inserted in it and the starter pressed (see Fig. 46-2). A picture of the person to whom the aphasic person wants to speak is attached to the card since the aphasic may not recognize, or be able to dial, numbers.

It is uncomfortable for many persons to work with those who have the handicaps described in this chapter. It should be remembered that for everyone, health workers as well

as patients, it is important that they have someone with whom they can discuss their feelings. Seminars and conferences where experts are brought in as consultants may be helpful to students and staff in the health professions and to families. Patients themselves are often discouraged and tend to withdraw. They should be given an opportunity to openly acknowledge their feelings and helped to talk about what they might do to gain the skills they so sorely need to function adequately or keep "in the stream of life." As patients gain skills, they will be motivated to reach their potential achievement, while health workers, families, and friends will be motivated to help them reach this goal. The rewards for all concerned are immeasurable.

REFERENCES

1. Wintrobe, M. M., et al. (eds.): *Harrison's Principles of Internal Medicine,* 7th ed. McGraw-Hill Book Co., New York, 1974.
2. "All About Your Eyes—And How to Save Them" (Interview with Dr. Carl Kupfer, National Eye Institute), *U.S. News & World Report,* (June 11) 1973, p. 67.
3. Diller, Leonard: "Psychological Aspects of Physically Handicapped Children," in Wolman, Benjamin B. (ed.): *Manual of Child Psychopathology.* McGraw-Hill Book Co., New York, 1972, p. 599.
4. Condl, Emma D.: "Ophthalmic Nursing: The Gentle Touch," *Nurs. Clin. North Am.,* **5:**467, (Sept.) 1970.
5. Fitzgerald, Roy G.: "Reactions to Blindness: An Exploratory Study of Adults with Recent Loss of Sight," *Arch. Gen. Psychiatry,* **22:**370, (Apr.) 1970.
6. "All About Your Eyes—And How to Save Them," *op. cit.*
7. Condl, Emma D.: *op. cit.*
8. "All About Your Eyes—And How to Save Them," *op. cit.*
9. Riley, L.: "The Epidemiology of Partial Sight," *Am. J. Optom.,* **47:**587, (Aug.) 1970.
10. Bellows, John G.: "Contemporary Practices in Ophthalmology," *Ill. Med. J.,* **138:**47, (July) 1970.
11. Seaman, Florence W.: "Nursing Care of Glaucoma Patients," *Nurs. Clin. North Am.,* **5:**489, (Sept.) 1970.
12. Greisheimer, Esther M.: *Physiology and Anatomy,* 7th ed. J. B. Lippincott Co., Philadelphia, 1955, p. 357.
13. Lyght, Charles E. (ed.): *The Merck Manual of Diagnosis and Therapy.* Merck Sharp & Dohme Research Laboratories, Rahway, N.J., 1961, p. 495.
14. *Ibid.*
15. Bellows, John G.: *op. cit.*
16. Riley, L.: *op. cit.*
17. Bellows, John G.: *op. cit.*

18. Blank, H. Robert: "Psychoanalysis and Blindness," *Psychoanal. Q.*, **26**:1, 1957.

19. Cameron, Norman: *Personality Development and Psychopathology.* Houghton Mifflin Co., Boston, 1963, p. 316.

20. Franks, Darrell D.: "Adjustment to Acquired Blindness," *J. Kans. Med. So.*, **72**:238, (May) 1971.

21. Klein, George S.: "Blindness and Isolation," *Psychoanal. Study Child*, **17**:82, 1962.

22. Burlingham, Dorothy: "Some Notes on the Development of the Blind," *Psychoanal. Study Child*, **16**:121, 1961.

23. Fraiberg, Selma: "Intervention in Infancy: A Program for Blind Infants," *J. Am. Acad. Child Psychiatry*, **10**:381, (July) 1971.

24. Wills, Doris M.: "Vulnerable Periods in the Early Development of Blind Children," *Psychoanal. Study Child*, **25**:461, 1970.

25. Sandler, Anne-Marie: "Aspects of Passivity and Ego Development in the Blind Infant," *Psychoanal. Study Child*, **18**:343, 1963.

26. Fraiberg, Selma, and Freedman, David A.: "Studies in the Ego Development of the Congenitally Blind Child," *Psychoanal. Study Child*, **19**:113, 1964.

27. Blank, H. Robert: *op. cit.*

28. Sandler, Anne-Marie: *op. cit.*

29. Burlingham, Dorothy: "Hearing and Its Role in the Development of the Blind," *Psychoanal. Study Child*, **19**:95, 1964.

30. Fraiberg, Selma: *op. cit.*

31. Blank, H. Robert: *op. cit.*

32. Sandler, Anne-Marie: *op. cit.*

33. Parten, Carroll B.: "Encouragement of Sensory Motor Development in the Preschool Blind," *Except. Child*, **37**:739, (Summer) 1971.

34. Willis, Doris M.: "Problems of Play and Mastery in the Blind Child," *Br. J. Med. Psychol.*, **41**:213, (Part 3) 1968.

35. Sandler, Anne-Marie: *op. cit.*

36. Fraiberg, Selma: *op. cit.*

37. Fraiberg, Selma: "Parallel and Divergent Patterns in Blind and Sighted Infants," *Psychoanal. Study Child*, **23**:264, 1968.

38. ———: "Intervention in Infancy: A Program for Blind Infants," *J. Am. Acad. Child Psychiatry*, **10**:381, (July) 1971.

39. ———: "Parallel and Divergent Patterns in Blind and Sighted Infants," *Psychoanal. Study Child*, **23**:264, 1968.

40. Blank, H. Robert: *op. cit.*

41. Omwake, Eveline, and Solnit, Albert J.: "It Isn't Fair: The Treatment of a Blind Child," *Psychoanal. Study Child*, **16**:352, 1961.

42. Burlingham, Dorothy: "Psychic Problems of the Blind," *Am. Imago*, **2**:43, 1941.

43. *Ibid.*

44. Wills, Doris M.: "Vulnerable Periods in the Early Development of Blind Children," *Psychoanal. Study Child*, **25**:461, 1970.

45. Burlingham, Dorothy: "Hearing and Its Role in the Development of the Blind," *Psychoanal. Study Child*, **19**:95, 1964.

46. Nagera, Humberto, and Colonna, Alice B.: "Aspects of the Contribution of Sight to Ego and Drive Development," *Psychoanal. Study Child*, **20**:267, 1965.

47. Wills, Doris M.: "Some Observations on Blind Nursery School Children's Understanding of Their World," *Psychoanal. Study Child*, **20**:344, 1965.

48. Fraiberg, Selma: "Parallel and Divergent Patterns in Blind and Sighted Infants," *Psychoanal. Study Child*, **23**:264, 1968.

49. Wills, Doris M.: "Problems of Play and Mastery in the Blind Child," *Br. J. Med. Psychol.*, **41**:213, (Part 3) 1968.

50. *Ibid.*

51. Burlingham, Dorothy: "Psychic Problems of the Blind," *Am. Imago*, **2**:43, 1941.

52. Willis, Doris M.: *op. cit.*

53. Spitz, Rene A.: "Hospitalism," *Psychoanal. Study Child*, **1**:53, 1945.

54. ———: "Hospitalism," *Psychoanal. Study Child*, **2**:113, 1946.

55. Colonna, Alice B.: "A Blind Child Goes to the Hospital," *Psychoanal. Study Child*, **23**:391, 1968.

56. Freud, Sigmund: *New Introductory Lectures on Psychoanalysis.* W. W. Norton & Co., New York, 1933, p. 121.

57. Colonna, Alice B.: *op. cit.*

58. Williams, Cyril E.: "The Mary Sheridan Unit," *Nurs. Mirror*, **131**:57, (Oct.) 1970.

59. Segal, Aliza, and Stone, Frederick H.: "The Six-Year Old Who Began to See: Emotional Sequelae of Operation for Congenital Bilateral Cataract," *Psychoanal. Study Child*, **16**:481, 1961.

60. Blank, H. Robert: *op. cit.*

61. Fitzgerald, Roy G.: *op. cit.*

62. Adams, George L., and Pearlman, Jerome T.: "Emotional Response and Management of Visually Handicapped Patients," *Psychiatry Med.*, **1**:233, (July) 1970.

63. Blank, H. Robert: *op. cit.*

64. Fitzgerald, Roy G.: *op. cit.*

65. Cholden, L. S.: *A Psychiatrist Works with Blindness.* American Foundation for the Blind, New York, 1958, p. 52.

66. Fitzgerald, Roy G.: *op. cit.*

67. Fitzgerald, Roy G.: "Visual Phenomenology in Recently Blind Adults," *Am. J. Psychiatry*, **127**:1533, (May) 1971.

68. *Ibid.*

69. Deutsch, Felix: "The Sense of Reality in Persons Born Blind," *J. Psychol.*, **10**:121, (July) 1940.

70. Franks, Darrell D.: *op. cit.*

71. Blank, H. Robert: *op. cit.*

72. Mehr, Helen M., et al.: "Psychological Aspects of Low Vision Rehabilitation," *Am. J. Optom.*, **47**:605, (Aug.) 1970.

73. *Ibid.*

74. Franks, Darrell D.: *op. cit.*

75. Duke-Elder, P. M., and Wittkower, E.: "Psychological Reactions in Soldiers to Loss of Vision in One Eye and Their Treatment," *Br. Med. J.*, **1**:155, (Feb. 2) 1946.

76. Mehr, Helen M., et al.: *op. cit.*

77. Dayton, Glenn O., Jr., et al.: "Overt Behavior Manifested in Bilaterally Patched

Patients," *Am. J. Ophthalmol.*, **59**:864, (May) 1965.

78. Linn, Louis, et al.: "Patterns of Behavior Disturbance Following Cataract Extraction," *Am. J. Psychiatry*, **110**:281, (Oct.) 1953.

79. Ziskind, Eugene, et al.: "Observations on Mental Symptoms in Eye Patched Patients: Hypnagogic Symptoms in Sensory Deprivation," *Am. J. Psychiatry*, **116**:893, (Apr.) 1966.

80. Linn, Louis, et al.: *op. cit.*

81. Dayton, Glenn O., Jr., et al.: *op. cit.*

82. Ziskind, Eugene, et al.: *op. cit.*

83. *Ibid.*

84. Burlingham, Dorothy: *op. cit.*

85. Kramer, C. H., and Dunlop, H. E.: "Insight for the Sighted," *Geriatr. Nurs.*, (Feb.) 1968, p. 17.

86. Condl, Emma D.: *op. cit.*

87. Kramer, C. H., and Dunlop, H. E.: *op. cit.*

88. Condl, Emma D.: *op. cit.*

89. Jackson, G. D.: "The Needs of the Visually Handicapped," *Nurs. Outlook*, **13**:34, (Sept.) 1965.

90. Kramer, C. H., and Dunlop, H. E.: *op. cit.*

91. Condl, Emma D.: *op. cit.*

92. Fraser, I. L.: "Understanding Blindness," *Nurs. Mirror*, **130**:44, (Dec.) 1969.

93. Kramer, C. H., and Dunlop, H. E.: *op. cit.*

94. Fraser, I. L.: *op. cit.*

95. Kramer, C. H., and Dunlop, H. E.: *op. cit.*

96. Jackson, G. D.: *op. cit.*

97. Kramer, C. H., and Dunlop, H. E.: *op. cit.*

98. Condl, Emma D.: *op. cit.*

99. Diller, Leonard: *op. cit.*, p. 600.

100. Luterman, David M., and Chasin, Judith: "The Deaf Child," *Am. Fam. Physician*, **3**:88, (Mar.) 1971.

101. Diller, Leonard: *op. cit.*, p. 601.

102. Anonymous: "The Five Senses. Hearing. These Are the Deaf," *Dist. Nurs.*, **14**:93, (Aug.) 1971.

103. Diller, Leonard: *op. cit.*

104. Bailie, R. W.: "Deafness—A Problem of Communication," *Nurs. Times*, **68**:923, (July) 1972.

105. Vernon, McCay: "Potential, Achievement, and Rehabilitation in Deaf Population," *Rehabil. Lit.*, **31**:258, (Sept.) 1970.

106. Diller, Leonard: *op. cit.*

107. Denmark, John C.: "Developmental Disorders of Communication with Special Reference to Deaf Children with Additional Handicaps," *Br. J. Disord. Commun.* **6**:113, (Oct.) 1971.

108. Roberts, C. J.: "Visual Handicaps in Congenitally Deaf Children," *Dev. Med. Child Neurol.*, **12**:32, (Feb.) 1970.

109. Stein, Laszlo K., and Green, Mary Briggs: "Problems in Managing the Young Deaf-Blind Child," *Except. Child*, **38**:481, (Feb.) 1972.

110. Cameron, Norman: *op. cit.*

111. Harris, H. I.: "The Range of Psychosomatic Disorders in Adolescence," in Howells, J. G. (ed.): *Modern Perspectives in Adolescent*

Psychiatry. Brunner/Mazel Publishers, New York, 1971, p. 240.

112. Linnell, Craig, et al.: "The Hearing-Impaired Infant. Diagnosis and Rehabilitation," *Nurs. Clin. North Am.*, **5**:507, (Sept.) 1970.

113. Holm, Vanja A., and Kunze, LuVern H.: "Effects of Chronic Otitis Media on Language and Speech Development," *Pediatrics*, **43**:833, (May) 1969.

114. Linnell, Craig, et al.: *op. cit.*

115. Wilson, Kathleen A., and Carlisle, M.: "Specialized Psychiatric Services for the Deaf," *Nurs. Mirror*, **133**:28, (Sept.) 1971.

116. *Ibid.*

117. Linnell, Craig, et al.: *op. cit.*

118. Kent, M. S.: "Are Signs Legitimate?" *Am. Ann. Deaf*, **115**:497, (Sept.) 1970.

119. Denmark, John C.: "Psychiatry and the Deaf," *Curr. Psychiatr. Ther.*, **11**:68, 1971.

120. Anonymous: "Deaf Babies," *N.Z. Nurs. J.*, **63**:18, (Mar.) 1970.

121. *Ibid.*

122. Moore, Mary Virginia: "Diagnosis: Deafness," *Am. J. Nurs.*, **69**:297, (Feb.) 1969.

123. Anonymous: *op. cit.*

124. Luterman, David M., and Chasin, Judith: *op. cit.*

125. Anonymous: *op. cit.*

126. Downes, M. P.: "Organization and Procedures of a Newborn Infant Screening Program," *Hearing & Speech News*, **35**:26, (Mar.) 1967.

127. Anonymous: *op. cit.*

128. Conover, Mary, and Cober, Joyce: "Understanding and Caring for the Hearing-Impaired," *Nurs. Clin. North Am.*, **5**:497, (Sept.) 1970.

129. Luterman, David M., and Chasin, Judith: *op. cit.*

130. Conover, Mary, and Cober, Joyce: *op. cit.*

131. Luterman, David M., and Chasin, Judith: *op. cit.*

132. Levin, E.: *The Psychology of Deafness*. Columbia University Press, New York, 1960.

133. Conover, Mary, and Cober, Joyce: *op. cit.*

134. Schlesinger, Hilde S., and Meadow, Kathryn P.: "Development of Maturity in Deaf Children," *Except. Child*, **38**:461, (Feb.) 1972.

135. Katan, Anny: "Some Thoughts About the Role of Verbalization in Early Childhood," *Psychoanal. Study Child*, **16**:184, 1961.

136. Schlesinger, Hilde S., and Meadow, Kathryn P.: *op. cit.*

137. Goldfarb, W.: *Childhood Schizophrenia*. Harvard University Press, Cambridge, Mass., 1961.

138. Lesser, Stanley R., and Easser, B. Ruth: "Personality Differences in the Perceptually Handicapped," *J. Am. Acad. Child Psychiatry*, **11**:458, (July) 1972.

139. *Ibid.*

140. Levine, E. S.: *Youth in a Soundless World: A Search for Personality*. New York University Press, New York, 1956.

141. Myklebust, H. R.: *The Psychology of Deafness, Sensory Deprivation, Learning and Ad-*

justment. Grune & Stratton, New York, 1960.

142. Altshuler, Kenneth Z.: "Personality Traits and Depressive Symptoms in the Deaf, in Wortis, J. (ed.): *Recent Advances in Biological Psychiatry 6.* Plenum Press, New York, 1964, p. 63.

143. Rainer, John D., and Altshuler, Kenneth Z. (eds.): *Psychiatry and the Deaf.* US Government Printing Office, Washington, D.C., 1967.

144. Altshuler, Kenneth Z.: op. cit.

145. Harris, H. I.: *op. cit.,* p. 241.

146. Lipton, E. L.: "A Study of the Psychological Effects of Strabismus," *Psychoanal. Study Child,* **25**:146, 1970.

147. Lesser, Stanley R., and Easser, B. Ruth: *op. cit.*

148. Vernon, McCay: "Sociological and Psychological Factors Associated with Hearing Loss," *J. Speech Hear. Res.,* **12**:541, (Sept.) 1969.

149. Schlesinger, Hilde S., and Meadow, Kathryn P.: *op. cit.*

150. Denmark, John C.: "Psychiatry and the Deaf," *Curr. Psychiatr. Ther.,* **11**:68, 1971.

151. Denmark, John C., and Eldridge, Raymond W.: "Psychiatric Services for the Deaf," *Lancet,* **2**:259, (Aug.) 1969.

152. *Ibid.*

153. Fisher, B.: M. Ed. Thesis, Manchester, Eng. 1965.

154. Vernon, McCay: "Potential, Achievement, and Rehabilitation in Deaf Population," *Rehabil. Lit.,* **31**:258, (Sept.) 1970.

155. *Ibid.*

156. Howse, Jean M. DeSalle, and Fitch, James L.: "Effects of Parent Orientation in Sign Language on Communication Skills of Preschool Children," *Am. Ann. Deaf,* **117**:459, (Aug.) 1972.

157. Alterman, Arthur I.: "Language and the Education of Children with Early Profound Deafness," *Am. Ann. Deaf,* **115**:514, (Sept.) 1970.

158. Kent, M. S.: op. cit.

159. Alterman, Arthur I.: op. cit.

160. Cicourel, Aaron V., and Boese, Robert J.: "Sign Language Acquisition and the Teaching of Deaf Children," *Am. Ann. Deaf,* **117**:27, (Feb.) 1972.

161. Beasley, A., et al.: "Suggested Readings for Parents of Preschool Deaf Children," *Am. Ann. Deaf,* **117**:431, (Aug.) 1972.

162. Vernon, McCay: "Sociological and Psychological Factors Associated with Hearing Loss," *J. Speech Hear. Res.,* **12**:541, (Sept.) 1969.

163. Beasley, A., et al.: op. cit.

164. Naylor-Strong, E. C.: "Deafness in the Elderly," *Nurs. Mirror,* **129**:50, (July) 1969.

165. Bakwin, H., and Bakwin, R. M.: *Clinical Management of Behavior Disorders in Children.* W. B. Saunders Co., Philadelphia, 1963.

166. Anonymous: op. cit.

167. Diller, Leonard: op. cit.

168. Conover, Mary, and Cober, Joyce: op. cit.

169. Bessinger, Mary J.: "My Personal Experiences with Mr. H.," *Bedside Nurse,* **2**:36, (Nov.–Dec.) 1969.

170. Conover, Mary, and Cober, Joyce: op. cit.

171. Popelka, Gerald R., and Berger, Kenneth W.: "Gestures and Visual Speech Reception," *Am. Ann. Deaf,* **116**:434, (Aug.) 1971.

172. Conover, Mary, and Cober, Joyce: op. cit.

173. *Ibid.*

174. Naylor-Strong, E. C.: op. cit.

175. Bailie, R. W.: op. cit.

176. Naylor-Strong, E. C.: op. cit.

177. Conover, Mary, and Cober, Joyce: op. cit.

178. Naylor-Strong, E. C.: op. cit.

179. *Ibid.*

180. Conover, Mary, and Cober, Joyce: op. cit.

181. Johnson, W.: "Speech Disorders," in Deutsch, A., and Fishman, H. (eds.): *The Encyclopedia of Mental Health,* Vol. 6. Franklin Watts, Inc., New York, 1963, p. 1952.

182. Williams, Moyra: "Development and Breakdown of Speech," in Howells, J. G. (ed.): *Modern Perspectives in International Child Psychiatry, No. 3.* Brunner/Mazel Publishers, New York, 1971, p. 550.

183. *Ibid.,* p. 553.

184. Davis, D. R.: "Interact and Communicate," The Fifth Jansson Memorial Lecture of the College of Speech Therapists, *Br. J. Disord. Commun.* **6**:3, (Apr.) 1971.

185. de Hirsch, Katrina: "Stuttering and Cluttering. Developmental Aspects of Dysrhythmic Speech," *Folia Phoniatr.,* **22**:311, 1970.

186. Davis, D. R.: op. cit.

187. de Hirsch, Katrina: op. cit.

188. Van Riper, C., and Irwin, J. V.: *Voice and Articulation.* Prentice-Hall, Inc., Englewood Cliffs, N.J., 1958, p. 108.

189. Worster-Drought, C.: "Speech Disorders in Children," *Dev. Med. Child Neurol.,* **10**:427, (Aug.) 1968.

190. Adams, Milton S.: "A Case of Elective Mutism," *J. Natl. Med. Assoc.,* **62**:213, (May) 1970.

191. Myklebust, H. R.: op. cit.

192. Williams, Moyra: *op. cit.,* p. 555.

193. Renfrew, C. E.: "Development of Speech in Mentally Retarded Children," in White, F. A. (ed.): *Children with Communication Problems.* Pitman Medical Publishing Co., London, 1965.

194. Williams, Moyra: *op. cit.,* p. 556.

195. *Ibid.,* p. 558.

196. Furneaux, B.: "The Autistic Child," *Br. J. Disord. Commun.* **1**:85, (Apr.) 1966.

197. Taylor, I. G.: "The Deaf and the Non-Communicating Child," in White, F. A. (ed): *Children with Communication Problems.* Pitman Medical Publishing Co., London, 1965.

198. Furneaux, B.: op. cit.

199. Williams, Moyra: *op. cit.,* p. 558.

200. Furneaux, B.: op. cit.

201. Worster-Drought, C.: op. cit.

202. Johnson, W.: *op. cit.*
203. Worster-Drought, C.: *op. cit.*
204. Johnson, W.: *op. cit.*
205. Mysak, Edward D.: "Child Speech Pathology," in Wolman, B. B. (ed): *Manual of Child Psychopathology.* McGraw-Hill Book Co., New York, 1972, p. 625.
206. Powers, M. H.: "Functional Disorders of Articulation—Symptomatology and Etiology," in Travis, L. E. (ed.): *Handbook of Speech Pathology.* Appleton-Century-Crofts, New York, 1957, p. 718.
207. Mysak, Edward D.: *op. cit.*, p. 627.
208. *Ibid.*, p. 630.
209. Schwartz, A. B.: "Congenital Laryngeal Stridor—Speculations Regarding Its Origin," *Pediatrics,* **27:**477, (Mar.) 1961.
210. Mysak, Edward D.: *op. cit.*, p. 630.
211. Van Riper, C., and Irwin, J. V.: *op. cit.*, p. 185.
212. Brodnitz, F. S.: *Vocal Rehabilitation.* Whiting Press, Rochester, Minn., 1959, p. 61.
213. Wilson, D. K.: "Children with Vocal Nodules," *J. Speech Hear. Disord.* **26:**19, (Feb.) 1961.
214. Greene, Margaret C. L.: *The Voice and Its Disorders.* Pitman Medical Publishing Co., London, 1957, p. 69.
215. Mysak, Edward D.: *op. cit.*, p. 630.
216. Van Riper, C., and Irwin, J. V.: *op. cit.*, p. 193.
217. Mysak, Edward D.: *op. cit.*, p. 630.
218. Worster-Drought, C.: *op. cit.*
219. Mysak, Edward D.: *op. cit.*, p. 630.
220. Greene, Margaret C. L.: "Speech of Children Before and After Removal of Tonsils and Adenoids," *J. Speech Hear. Disord.,* **22:** 361, (Sept.) 1957.
221. Worster-Drought, C.: *op. cit.*
222. Adams, Milton S.: *op. cit.*
223. Morris, J. V.: "Cases of Elective Mutism," *Am. J. Ment. Defic.* **56:**661, (Apr.) 1953.
224. Reed, G. F.: "Elective Mutism in Children: A Reappraisal," *J. Child Psychol. Psychiatry,* **4:**99, 1963.
225. Salfield, D. J.: "Observations on Elective Mutism in Children," *J. Ment. Sci.,* **96:**1024, (June) 1950.
226. Halpern, Werner I., et al.: "A Therapeutic Approach to Speech Phobia: Elective Mutism Re-examined," *J. Am. Acad. Child Psychiatry,* **10:**94 (Jan.) 1971.
227. *Ibid.*
228. Cameron, Norman: *op. cit.*, p. 309.
229. Senn, Milton J. E., and Solnit, Albert J.: *Problems in Child Behavior and Development.* Lea & Febiger, Philadelphia, 1968, p. 47.
230. *Ibid.*
231. *Ibid.*
232. Freedman, A. M., et al.: *Modern Synopsis of Comprehensive Textbook of Psychiatry.* Williams & Wilkins Co., Baltimore, 1972, p. 608.
233. de Hirsch, Katrina: *op. cit.*
234. Freedman, A. M., et al.: *op. cit.*, p. 609.
235. de Hirsch, Katrina: *op. cit.*

236. Greene, Margaret C. L.: "Early Detection of Speech Difficulty: (2) Danger Signals," *Nurs. Times,* **65:**1170, (Sept.) 1969.
237. de Hirsch, Katrina: *op. cit.*
238. Greene, Margaret C. L.: *op. cit.*
239. Weiss, D.: "Cluttering," *Folia Phoniatr.,* **19:** 233, 1967.
240. de Hirsch, Katrina: *op. cit.*
241. Greene, Margaret C. L.: *op. cit.*
242. Freedman, A. M., et al., *op. cit.*, p. 608.
243. Pannbacker, M.: "Language Skills of Cleft Palate Children: A Review," *Br. J. Disord. Commun.,* **6:**37, (Apr.) 1971.
244. Williams, Moyra: *op. cit.*, p. 559.
245. Anonymous: "Research into Childhood Aphasia," *Nurs. Mirror,* **132:**40, (Apr.) 1971.
246. Lea, J.: "Children Suffering from Receptive Aphasia," *Speech Pathology Ther.,* **8:**58, 1965.
247. Treisman, A.: "Verbal Responses and Contextural Constraints," *J. Verbal Learning Verbal Behavior,* **4:**118, (Apr.) 1965.
248. Williams, Moyra: *op. cit.*
249. Eisenson, J.: "Perceptual Disorders in Children," *Br. J. Disord. Commun.,* **1:**21, (Apr.) 1966.
250. Williams, Moyra: *op. cit.*
251. Anonymous: *op. cit.*
252. Brocklehurst, J. C.: "Guidelines for Rehabilitating Stroke Patients. Number 1. Dysphasia and the Nurse," *Nurs. Mirror,* **133:**17, (Oct.) 1971.
253. Freedman, A. M., et al.: *op. cit.*, p. 607.
254. Reeves, Elizabeth W.: "The Aphasic Patient," *Nurs. Outlook,* **11:**522, (Nov.) 1963.
255. *Ibid.*
256. Worster-Drought, C.: *op. cit.*
257. *Ibid.*
258. Worster-Drought, C.: "An Unusual Form of Acquired Aphasia in Children," *Dev. Med. Child Neurol.,* **13:**563, (Oct.) 1971.
259. Miller, Barbara E.: "Assisting Aphasic Patients with Speech Rehabilitation," *Am. J. Nurs.,* **69:**983, (May) 1969.
260. Jones, W. E., and Mittlestedt, D. R.: "Surveying Speech and Hearing Problems, (Part 2)," *Geriatric Nurs.,* (Jan.) 1968, p. 16.
261. Goda, S.: "Letters to the Editor: Manual Communication for Aphasics," *Arch. Phys. Med. Rehab.,* **53:**344, (July) 1972.
262. Williams, Moyra: *op. cit.*, p. 560.
263. Howes, D. H., and Geschwind, N.: "Statistical Properties of Aphasic Language," *Excerpta Medica Int. Congress,* Series #38, VIIth International Congress of Neurology, Rome, 1961.
264. Oldfield, R. C., and Wingfield, A.: "Response Latencies in Naming Objects," *Q. J. Exp. Psychol.,* **17:**273, (Part 4) 1965.
265. Schuell, H.: "Aphasia in Adults in Relation to Language Disturbances in Children," *Br. J. Disord. Commun.,* **1:**33, (Apr.) 1966.
266. Rochford, G., and Williams, M.: "The Development and Breakdown of the Use of Names," *J. Neurol. Neurosurg. Psychiatry,*

25:222, (Aug.) 1962; **26:**377, (Aug.) 1963; **28:**407, (Oct.) 1965.

267. Williams, Moyra: *op. cit.,* p. 559.
268. Mayer-Gross, W., et al.: *Clinical Psychiatry.* Cassell Publishing Co., London, 1960.
269. Rochford, G., and Williams, M.: "The Measurement of Language Disorders," *Speech Pathology Ther.,* **7:**1, (Oct.) 1964.
270. Rochford, G.: "Organic Speech Disorders," Ph. D. Thesis, Oxon, Eng. 1966.
271. Williams, Moyra: *op. cit.,* p. 564.
272. Malone, R. L., et al.: "Attitudes Expressed by Families of Aphasics," *Br. J Disord. Commun.,* **5:**174, (Oct.) 1970.
273. Griffith, F. A.: "Communication as a Prime Handicap," *Rehabil. Rec.,* **12:**36, (Jan.–Feb.) 1971.
274. Reeves, Elizabeth W.: *op. cit.*
275. Miller, Barbara E.: *op. cit.*
276. Vignolo, L. A. "Evolution of Aphasia and Language Rehabilitation: A Retrospective Exploratory Study," *Cortex,* **1:**344, (Dec.) 1964.
277. Kenin, Maxine, and Swisher, Linda Peck: "A Study of Pattern Recovery in Aphasia," *Cortex,* **8:**56, (Mar.) 1972.
278. Taylor, O. L., and Anderson, C.: "Neuropsycholinguistics and Language Learning," Communications at the Conference of Language Training for Aphasics, Ohio State University, Columbus, 1968.
279. Goda, S.: *op. cit.*
280. Reeves, Elizabeth W.: *op. cit.*
281. Miller, Barbara E.: *op. cit.*
282. Reeves, Elizabeth W.: *op. cit.*
283. Miller, Barbara E.: *op. cit.*

Additional Suggested Reading

Altshuler, Kenneth Z., and Rainer, John D. (eds.): *Mental Health and the Deaf: Approaches and Prospects.* US Government Printing Office, Washington, D.C., 1969.
Buck, McKenzie: *Dysphasia: Professional Guidance for Family and Patient.* Prentice-Hall, Inc., Englewood Cliffs, N.J., 1968.
Carroll, Thomas J.: *Blindness: What It Is, What It Does, and How to Live with It.* Little, Brown & Co., Boston, 1961.
Cholden, Louis S.: *A Psychiatrist Works with Blindness.* American Foundation for the Blind, New York, 1958.
Clark, F. Le Gros: *Blinded in War.* Priory Press, Ltd., Royston, Hertfordshire, Eng., 1969.
Cullen, Irene C.: Techniques for Teaching Patients with Sensory Defects," *Nurs. Clin. North Am.,* **5:**537, (Sept.) 1970.

Dorward, Barbara: *Teaching Aids and Toys for Handicapped Children.* Council for Exceptional Children, Washington, D.C., 1960.
Griffith, Jerry (ed.): *Persons with Hearing Loss.* Charles C Thomas, Publisher, Springfield, Ill., 1969.
Herth, Kaye: "Beyond the Curtain of Silence," *Am. J. Nurs.,* **74:**1060, (June) 1974.
Horwitz, Betty: "An Open Letter to the Family of an Adult Patient with Aphasia," *Rehab. Lit.,* **23:**141, (May) 1962.
Irwin, John V., and Marge, Michael (eds.): *Principles of Childhood Language Disabilities.* Appleton-Century-Crofts, Education Division, Meredith Corp., New York, 1972.
Keller, Helen: *The Story of My Life.* Doubleday, Page & Co., New York, 1903.
Lehman, Jean Utley: *Do's and Dont's for Parents of Pre-School Deaf and Hard of Hearing Children.* National Easter Seal Society for Crippled Children and Adults, Chicago, 1967.
Levine, Edna Simon: *The Psychology of Deafness.* Columbia University Press, New York, 1960.
Myklebust, Helmer R.: *The Psychology of Deafness: Sensory Deprivation, Learning and Adjustment,* 2nd ed. Grune & Stratton, New York, 1964.
———: *Your Deaf Child: A Guide for Parents.* Charles C Thomas, Publisher, Springfield, Ill., 1950.
Sataloff, Joseph: *Hearing Loss.* J. B. Lippincott Co., Philadelphia, 1966.
Smith, Genevieve W.: *Care of the Patient with a Stroke.* Springer Publishing Co., New York, 1959.
Taylor, Martha L.: "Speech Problems of Hemiplegic Patients," a paper presented at 1962 Annual Convention of National Easter Seal Society for Crippled Children and Adults.
US National Center for Health Statistics: *Hearing Status and Ear Examination: Findings Among Adults, United States, 1960–62.* US Government Printing Office, Washington, D.C., 1972 (Vital and Health Statistics Series 11, No. 32).
Ventry, Ira M., et al. (eds.): *Hearing Measurement. A Book of Readings.* Appleton-Century-Crofts, New York, 1971.
Westlake, Harold, and Rutherford, David: *Speech Therapy for the Cerebral Palsied.* National Easter Seal Society for Crippled Children and Adults, Chicago, 1961.

Mimi Dye
Virginia Henderson

CHAPTER 47

The Preoperative State

1. INTRODUCTION

It is estimated that between 12 and 15 million people a year undergo a surgical operation in the United States.[1] While there are still risks associated with this form of treatment, surgery and supportive care can be undertaken with greater assurance of an uneventful recovery than has ever been possible before. The problems that beset surgery from ancient to modern times may be difficult for young nurses to grasp because there have been such significant advances in this century. Unless they have studied the history of medicine they have no idea of the hazard of surgery in earlier centuries.

In his book, *Surgery: Old and New Frontiers,* Robert G. Richardson,[2] himself a surgeon, describes some problems of the past. He says that until the modern era the critical concern was whether the patient lived or died, regardless of the possibility of mutilation. The inability to recognize the relationship between cleanliness and the development of infection led to the prevailing thought that pus was an inevitable part of the healing process. Therefore, "laudable pus" was an expression that pervaded the seventeenth-century literature, and the concept that pus was even "laudable" or beneficial retarded progress in the efforts to control infection. Styptic powders, red hot cauteries, and boiling pitch slapped on stumps of amputated legs and arms were among the remedies used to control bleeding. Such treatment, combined with ineffective methods of producing anesthesia, made severe and prolonged pain and its devastating effect an accompaniment of surgery. Fortunately, these practices and their associated problems have been largely overcome.

Inactive nurses often say that they would be "afraid" to nurse surgical patients because their care has changed so greatly in the last decades. This fear is justified to a large extent, and to get an overview of these changes it might be helpful to mention the developments that have made modern surgery one of the marvels of the century. Sir Cecil Wakeley,[3] discussing "the changing face of surgery," in 1950 expressed the opinion that scientific surgery was based on the knowledge of the human body acquired by dissection. This opportunity has been available to the surgeon for a relatively short time historically. Asepsis was developed in the nineteenth century along with anesthesia, both cornerstones of effective surgery. All of us are familiar with these developments. Few health workers, however, can keep up with the change in physiologic concepts on which are based the present practices in maintaining electrolyte and acid-base balance or in maintaining normal nutrition through parenteral therapy and improved oral and gastric feeding. The expanded use of x-rays, radium, other radioactive elements, and light amplification (laser) in diagnosis and therapy necessitates the use of new pre- and postoperative techniques. Microscopic photography and photography of internal organs have made diagnoses possible that never were before. The expanding list of chemotherapeutic agents, specifically the antibiotics used to treat infections, make it almost impossible for anyone outside the field of pharmacy to know the latest arrival in the antibiotic family, even though methods of administering them have been greatly simplified. People unfamiliar with hospital care during the last 10 years are amazed to see a progressively shorter time interval between the operation and ambulation (getting out of bed). Rehabilitation and the phrase "early ambulation" come easily; both have had wide publicity. However, older nurses often find it difficult to believe that patients who have had their stomach removed are expected to flex and extend their legs a few hours after recovery from anesthesia, turn themselves, and be prepared to get to their feet and perhaps walk, either the day of or the day after operation, even though they may have a tube in the nose and a cannula in an arm vein ready for the next bottle of fluid. Emphasis on the use of whole blood and blood products (packed red cells, fibrinogen, plasma), antibiotics, and pressure dressings has hastened the process of tissue repair and, in many cases, revolutionized treatment of trauma and wounds. Management of burns is now an area for specialized practice. There is increasing success in controlling infection and using plastic surgery to reduce scarring, distortion, and loss of function in burned areas. (See Chapter 42 for full discussion of the treatment of burns.) Identification and use of steroids and new developments in the field of immunology have enabled people to undergo operations that would have been fatal in the past. Today's surgeons have at their disposal a wide array of techniques and equipment that permit operations on parts of the body that were previously thought inaccessible to surgery, as, for example, the heart and the blood vessels entering and leaving it, and certain areas of the brain.

With few exceptions, anatomic barriers have disappeared. Not very long ago, patients with mitral stenosis would grow progressively short of breath and very often death would be a welcome relief. Now it is not only possible to repair diseased hearts but also possible to replace them. Tissue and organ transplants and replants (reattachment of limbs to the owner's body) led to the successful completion of the first heart transplant in 1967 by Dr. Christian Barnard in Capetown, South Africa. These procedures are not yet routine because of problems associated with the production of antibodies that lead to the rejection of foreign tissue and to the problems of getting healthy organs for transplantation.* There are signs, however, that a solution to tissue rejection may soon be forthcoming. One example of pertinent research is that of Ralph A. Reisfeld and Barry D. Kahan.[4] These investigators have identified in the cells of each individual unique protein "markers" that distinguish the "self"

from the "not self" and that prompt the body to reject cells that are not labeled with the appropriate markers. Identification of these "markers of biological individuality" may lead to solution of the major problems associated with tissue rejection and therefore help in the management of human organ transplants.

Brain surgery has also progressed rapidly in recent years. Today it is possible to destroy brain tumors by a "knifeless, bloodless" method that utilizes a powerful magnetic field to fix microscopic iron pellets in capillaries that feed a brain tumor. This method, described by Robert W. Rand, a neurosurgeon, and James A. Mosso,[5] his associate, may provide significant relief for patients who have surgically inaccessible angiomas, and may reduce the blood loss in surgery on more accessible hypervascular tumors. Important advances in the use of microscopy in surgery now help the surgeon work on some of the tiniest structures imaginable. A case of lifesaving corrective surgery performed on the minuscule biliary ducts of a young infant by Keijiro Suruga, a Japanese surgeon, was reported in *Time Magazine* in 1973.[6] This case of "microsurgery" was performed on biliary ducts that averaged 1/500 of an inch in diameter with the aid of a surgical microscope at 20- to 40-power magnification. Continued advances in microsurgery are enabling surgeons to transplant tissue by microvascular anastomosis. This has been particularly beneficial in surgery to replant traumatically amputated digits and limbs in animals and humans.[7,8] In addition to the improvements in treatment, newer methods for diagnosing conditions that require surgery are being developed that will not only speed up the diagnostic process but reduce the cost as well. For example, it is now possible for physicians to use computers to help them reach a diagnosis and also to determine whether the treatment should be medical or surgical.[9]

With these advances come new and more complex responsibilities for all who participate in the care of people who are about to undergo operations. It is well to remember that the best technical efforts of the most able surgeon may be severely undermined by poor or inadequate preoperative care. While modern surgery is often referred to as one of the miracles of this era, it is not without dangers and disadvantages. Some critics of medical care say that because surgical risks have been so greatly reduced, today's surgeons undertake it too readily. Newspapers and popular journals have carried excerpts from surveys showing that in certain centers the rate of elective operations, for example, hysterectomies, is higher

---

* The ethical aspects of organ transplantation are widely discussed in professional and popular books and journals, as well as its economics. Such surgery is very costly and some persons believe that the money spent on (possibly) prolonging the life of persons in seriously impaired health might be better spent on preventing disease or treating disease in which there is less risk.

among affluent than among impoverished patients. There is evidence in some of the recent professional literature of the serious concern over the number of operations that are performed unnecessarily.[10-12] This suggests that some surgeons may be motivated by their earnings rather than the patient's need for surgery. Popular as well as professional literature has stressed the increased danger of "nosocomial infections" as more and more difficult surgery is performed that demands what is called "intrusive therapy." Chapter 15 particularly, but also Chapters 20, 22, 23, 24, 26, 33, 37, 43, 44, and 48 discuss the dangers of such procedures as intravenous injections, blood transfusions, tissue transplants, catheterizations, and inhalation therapy, to mention just a few of the risky treatments.

Nurses must realize that in this era informed people come to the hospital well aware of some of the dangers of therapy, and it is useless to dismiss their fears as unfounded. While the patient's tumor may be successfully removed or the normal body contour restored by plastic surgery, he or she may leave the hospital with a stubborn bladder, respiratory, or bone infection. Many older persons facing radical surgery may look with skepticism on the extension of their life which will, nevertheless, be a useless or painful one. (See Chapter 50 for further discussion of this subject.)

Nurses, more than any other health workers, have opportunities to hear patients and their families discuss their fears and reservations about the recommended surgery and to provide assistance as appropriate. This information is important to others who share responsibility for the patient's care and should, therefore, be reported—especially to the physician and surgeon. No patient should feel that he or she has been coerced into surgery. The advantages and risks should be discussed honestly with the patient and the family. The choice or decision is always, at least legally, theirs. If delay may be fatal, as in certain emergencies, some person must be responsible for deciding what to do immediately, and this may involve surgery.

2. GENERAL PRINCIPLES OF PREOPERATIVE CARE

Illness, hospitalization, and surgery are disruptive life experiences that are perceived by most people as threats to survival and well-being. The significance of the preoperative period lies in the assumption that people can be prepared for potentially stressful life events in ways that may enable them to develop effective resistance for withstanding stress—in this case, the stress associated with surgery—and that this preparation will improve their chances for survival and optimum recovery. As we have already said, no matter how "modern" the methods, there are risks involved in operation and anesthesia. While these cannot be eliminated, they can be greatly reduced by appropriate attention to the details of preoperative care. Ideally, this care begins the moment the decision is made to operate and continues up to the time of the surgical incision. The time boundaries vary. Surgical emergencies often dictate a short preparatory period; elective procedures allow more flexibility. In either case, the major objective is to help the person prepare the mind to cope effectively with the potentially stressful psychologic stimuli and help the body make the physiologic adjustments necessary to meet the special metabolic demands and altered functions incident to the surgical experience. This is a period for assessing the general condition of the patient—the psychologic and social adjustment as well as the general physiologic state. It is a period for identifying and treating special problems, and, in general, planning and providing the technical and supportive care that will help the patient be as ready for surgery as possible. There is a growing body of evidence in the literature to support the proposition that competent and creative care in this period will set the stage for an easier anesthetic induction, a smoother operation, and a more rapid recovery.

Social and Psychologic Aspects. Hospitalization and surgery pose a number of problems for patients, their families, and close friends, such as *separation* from family and friends and adjustment to an *unfamiliar environment and regimen. Fears of pain, body mutilation,* or *death* are predominant sources of anxiety, and in addition, adults often worry about the *cost of surgery, loss of time from work,* or the possibility that *they can't return to previous occupation and care for dependents.* Many persons may worry over providing for *convalescence* and *rehabilitation. Children's fears* may seem less well defined but even more pervasive and overwhelming since they have less knowledge with which to combat them. The important implications of the psychosocial aspects of preoperative care have been stressed in the literature through the years.[13-16] During the past 10 years, studies by nurses and their associates have focused on the psychologic or social care of surgical inpatients. In 1963, Rhetaugh G. Dumas and Robert Leonard[17] emphasized the need for psychologic preparation of surgical patients and reported improvement in postoperative recovery in a group of patients who received special preparation as part of preoperative nursing care. Since that time there has been a stream of studies by nurses on preoperative care and related problems.[18-28] Although they differ in their focus and findings, the general conclusions reached in most of these studies support the statements that (1) social and psychologic reactions have important implications for the welfare of surgical patients; (2) the nurse is capable of identifying these reactions and helping patients with them; and (3) preoperative nursing that deals with the psychosocial aspects of care can provide comfort for the patient, help prevent postoperative complications, and reduce the length of postoperative hospitalization.

The importance of first impressions on admission to an institution was discussed in Chapter 8. The behavior of those with whom the patient has initial contact influences his or her sense of security and general reaction to the illness, the hospital or clinic environment, and course of treatment. The following are some psychosocial goals that nurses might set up as part of preoperative care: fostering human relations that will enable patients to express their desires, hopes, fears, and other concerns and emotions; regulating the environment and adapting routines in such a way as to reduce tension as much as possible and help the patient cope with anxiety, discomfort, and disability; promoting patient understanding of the help available from religious counselors, social workers, psychiatric personnel, family, and friends, as the need for such help arises.

In certain types of surgery, the psychosocial problems far outweigh the physical ones. All mutilating surgery is a threat to the patient's personality, and acceptance is very difficult. Surgery designed to transform a person who has lived as a woman into one who will live as a man, or vice versa, demands a highly specialized type of preoperative care. Such surgery is preceded by months or years of psychotherapy and hormonal treatment (the use of estrogens and progestins). Changing from a man to a woman, and vice versa, affects all human relations and even the legal status of the subject.* Programs to help in-

dividuals establish their true sexual identity are so established that a national organization in the United States (the Erickson Foundation) has been set up for further understanding of the subject. Not only do such specialized journals as *Sexology, Erickson Foundation Newsletter,* and *Medical Aspects of Human Sexuality* carry articles on the subject, but so do the official journals of medical and nursing organizations as well as popular journals.[29-33] While types of surgery cannot be discussed in this chapter, references listed at the end of it provide sources for readers with special interests. Suggested surgical nursing texts go far more thoroughly into the specifics of preoperative care than is possible here.

Preoperative instruction and counseling should be available and easily accessible to patients who are anticipating anesthesia and surgery as soon after the decision to operate as is possible. Few surgeons have, or take, the time for detailed explanations of preoperative and postoperative procedure. Within surgical departments, committees composed of surgeons, anesthetists, nurses, social workers, physical therapists, nutritionists, chaplains, and others should develop a preoperative teaching program that would eliminate unnecessary fear of surgery and prepare the patient to participate more effectively in the postoperative program.

In some hospitals, preoperative orientation and instruction of inpatients begin prior to hospital admission; in others, this part of the patient's preparation begins shortly after admission. In any case, preoperative instruction and counseling comprise the first stage of the rehabilitation program. Figure 47-1 shows a nurse teaching a preoperative patient how she will manage bowel movements through the abdominal wall rather than through the anus. The patient is to have an operation in which the lower part of the colon is removed and the end of the colon attached to the abdomen (a colostomy). All preoperative instruction and counseling must be individualized for maximum effectiveness. However, group discussion is often a valuable aspect of the program.

In Chapters 8 and 15, references are made to prehospitalization visits for children. If children are to have surgery they are shown the operating and recovery rooms and, if possible, they meet the members of the staff who will care for them. Instruments such as stethoscopes, thermometers, and syringes are shown them and they may be allowed to handle them or even play with them. Nancy Lockwood [34] reported that doll-play reduced the anxiety levels postoperatively with children of only certain ages. Differences among children of age, culture, sex, and other factors de-

---

* Christine Jorgensen was a soldier named George Jorgensen. Her successful treatment in Europe in the 1950s was given wide publicity, and she has since lectured in many universities in this country.[28a] It is estimated that about 1500 of the 10,000 transsexuals (not to be confused with homosexuals or transvestites) have changed their gender. Surgery involves amputation of the penis and scrotum with creation of a vagina, or, for a woman who wants to be a man, removal of the breasts and the creation of a rudimentary penis from the clitoris.

mand that approaches be individualized. Separation from parents and the strangeness of the hospital environment are sources of psychic trauma in children. Rooming-in for parents and efforts toward prehospitalization orientation often reduce the trauma. The trend toward *"outpatient" surgery* is especially helpful for children.[35] Many hospitals have been moving in this direction over the last 10 years and it is now estimated that the number of operations for adults and children done on an outpatient basis greatly outnumber those requiring inpatient hospitalization. The facilities where outpatient surgery is performed have been variously labeled: *"come and go surgical facilities," "ambulatory surgery units," "surgicenters,"* and *"outpatient surgical units."* Some are parts of traditional hospital outpatient departments; others may be located in separate buildings designed specifically for this type of surgery. This relatively new concept minimizes the trauma, reduces the disruption in the patient's family, cuts down on the possibility of cross-infections, and reduces the costs of surgical service. In addition, it makes more hospital beds available for those people who really need them.[36-38]

The preoperative care of *surgical outpatients* should begin before the time the patient comes to the surgical unit. The physical examination and general "workup" are done most often in the physician's office and the laboratory work is done in a certified laboratory. Detailed descriptions of the preoperative workup, admission procedure, and the anticipated course of recovery are given patients before they come for surgery. Some programs give patients written instructions that are supplemented and explained by the surgeon. The patient shares a

great deal of responsibility for the preparation for this type of surgery and it is of utmost importance that clear instructions are given and that the patient is able to follow them. The nurse in these units must be prepared to make necessary home visits to counsel and help patients with the preliminary preparation. In describing their program for adults, Burton S. Epstein and associates say that

Most preadmission instructions for patients receiving general or regional anesthesia include at least the following directions: before surgery, the patient must take no food or liquid after midnight, and he must notify the surgeon of any change in his physical condition; the patient is advised that, after surgery he must arrange for a responsible adult to accompany him. He also is instructed to avoid ingestion of alcoholic beverages for 24 hours, to refrain from driving a car for 24 hours, and to delay important decision-making until he makes a full recovery.*

Some programs for adults are quite comprehensive and cover a wide range of topics, issues, and procedures through formal and informal individual or group presentations and discussions. Others may provide a simple explanation of hospital procedures and the patient's course of treatment. Certain hospitals distribute leaflets offering explanations and directions. Patients with recent surgical experience can often contribute helpful suggestions for what should be included in preoperative information and instruction. For example, the second writer heard a man who had seemed calm the day after operation tell

* Epstein, Burton S., et al.: "Outpatient Surgery, Guidelines for Organization of Unit and for Selection of Patient and Surgical Procedure," *Hospitals,* **47**:80, (Sept. 1) 1973.

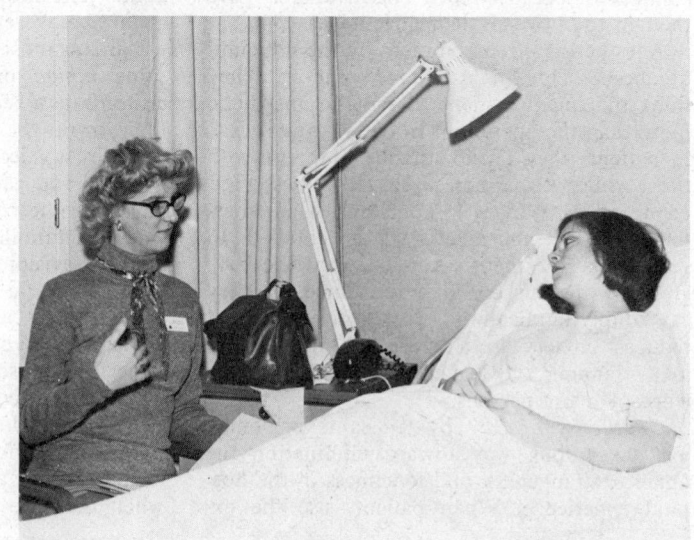

Figure 47-1. A nurse explaining a colostomy irrigation to a patient who knows she is to have a colostomy. (Courtesy of Columbia–Presbyterian Medical Center, New York, N.Y., and Clay-Adams Co., New York, N.Y.)

the participants in a nursing clinic much later that he had on that day thought he was dying because he had found himself in a room rather than in his accustomed place on the clinical division when he woke to consciousness after the operation. He said that had someone thought to tell him before the operation that he would be put there to be near the night nurse he would have been spared this mental anguish. Actually, patients are often the best teachers for those undergoing operations such as the removal of part of the colon necessitating a colostomy, or a laryngectomy necessitating a tracheotomy.

It should be explained to patients and their families that blood transfusions, intubations, or other procedures that may be fearsome to them are used routinely and that such treatments do not necessarily mean that the patient is in a critical condition. If procedures such as using the bedpan or doing postoperative exercises are explained and taught preoperatively, there is far less resistance to them and more effective results from them postoperatively. If patients are shown side rails and told that they will probably be put on the bed the first night, they may not be frightened by looking through bars in one of their first conscious moments. Likewise, if patients are to be put in a recovery room, its nature and advantages sh6uld be explained because they may be badly frightened by the sight of other postoperative patients; indeed, if they are awake in the recovery room, there may be no way to keep them from being frightened by what they see. In Chapter 48 there is a discussion of the advantages and disadvantages of recovery rooms and attention is called to the program at one university medical center where they, and intensive care units, have been eliminated because their disadvantages are thought to outweigh their advantages.

Anesthetists often comment on the difficulty of anesthetizing the frightened patient. They think that many patients dread the anesthetic more than the operation. In one or more visits to patients they try to establish rapport with them while, at the same time, they assess their condition as a basis for deciding what anesthesia to give, and what risks are entailed. In such visits anesthetists can enhance the help given by the surgeon and the nurse, or they can simply duplicate it. Preoperative care that reduces anxiety to a minimum necessitates joint planning and a nice coordination of the work of many persons.

Continuity of care by the same personnel will go a long way toward eliminating the anxiety, strangeness, and loneliness in the hospital experience. When patients use the expression "my doctor" or "my nurse" and show trust in them, it is a sure sign that their loads are lightened. As one surgeon [39] puts it, confidence is the "sheet anchor" for patients, and once this is established they "cease to worry." They cannot establish this relationship with a "battalion of workers." It is very desirable, therefore, to have the same nurses assigned to patients for the preoperative and postoperative periods, and highly desirable to have them go with patients to the operating room. (Postoperative care is simplified for nurses if they can watch the operation, but there is seldom enough personnel to make this possible except in private nursing practice.) In medical practice this principle of *continuity* of medical care is so thoroughly established that it needs no comment here.

Attention paid the family and explanation of rules and routines that may seem unpleasant or unreasonable react favorably on patients who may be as unhappy on the family's account as on their own. From the beginning, an effort should be made to prevent misunderstanding about the visiting hours or the number of visitors likely to benefit the patient. The family also should feel that their convenience is taken into account. Time may be as precious to them as to hospital personnel. When a long treatment is to be done or a lengthy examination made, it is thoughtful to tell visitors who are waiting; this enables them to go out for a meal or make some other use of their time, and it relieves impatience. The smaller the nursing circle, the easier it is for them to form friendly and helpful relationships with the family. Relatives are always happier when they are assured that at least a few of the patient's attendants know him or her and are interested in "the person" as well as "the patient." The importance of individualized care cannot be overemphasized.

Nurses must understand that patients of some *ethnic* or *racial* groups have *values, customs,* and *behavioral norms* that differ from their own. An understanding of cultural differences is necessary to provide the best care possible for each patient.[40,40a] For example, plans for the care of patients from close-knit extended families, such as gypsies, should include provision for many visitors. Assigning the patient to a room near an outside wall will provide easy access and minimize potential disturbance to others on the unit.[41] A Mexican-American nurse has pointed out that patients who are members of this subculture are likely to perceive admission to a hospital as a sign that they are in a serious condition. For them hospitals are places where people go only when they are very ill or dying.[42] Clarifying information and giving support and reassurance are especially important for these patients. Similarly, people from groups that have been systematically excluded from full participation in the society-at-large, such as the American Blacks, Spanish-speaking Americans, Asian-Americans, and American Indians, are likely to be suspicious of hospital personnel and afraid to entrust them with any aspect of their care. Patients themselves and often members of the family will try to prevent neglect by maintaining a constant vigil. In some cases, it is important to let family or friends stay with the preoperative patient until they are convinced by what they see and hear that it is safe to leave the patient in the care of the unit staff. *Religious practices* of some subcultures may require special rites for the ill. It may be important, therefore, to help the patient and family or friends arrange for the rites before the patient goes to the operating room.[43] In his book, *Psychological Aspects of Nursing Care,* Morton A. Seidenfeld[44] stresses "therapeutic answers" to patients' questions. He thinks that what nurses say as well as what they do is important. He also believes that such questions as "How am I getting along?" or "Do you think I'll pull through, Doc?" may represent "a wealth of emotional disturbance" and that fear will not be dissipated by a guarded or superficial reply. He thinks people want specific information, even statistics sometimes on their "chances." Nurses, who are with the patient so much more than the surgeon, are in a particularly favorable position to recognize signs of fear and their sources. Ordinarily, the nurse doesn't answer questions about diagnosis or prognosis, but he or she can bring these questions to the attention of the surgeon in written or oral reports, and there are many queries nurses can answer fully and helpfully. Listening and showing interest in what the patient says are themselves therapeutic.

Nurses, who are chiefly young, healthy men and women, need considerable imagination in working with the individual who is about to have mutilating surgery. Virginia Dericks,* Irving L. Janis,[44a] and others have wisely remarked that people must be permitted a period of grief. It is a mistake to try to jog them out of it with a superficial cheerfulness.

A brief discussion, such as this, of the social and psychologic preoperative problems is obliged to be superficial. We hope that it is not misleading. Nurses are face to face with the fear of death, disfigurement, disability, separation from family and friends, the dread of unconsciousness, of pain, of temporary loss of freedom, and all the unknown and, to many, frightening experiences of hospitalization. Mature and dominating executives may suddenly realize that temporarily at least they will be helpless and their very lives will depend on the judgment of nurses and doctors who may seem to them both young and inexperienced. Even the best medical team, with the greatest goodwill, cannot dispel all preoperative anxiety; they can, however, minimize it and in so doing set the stage for an easier anesthesia, a better operation, and a more rapid recovery.[44b]

Physiologic Aspects. It is not uncommon for preoperative patients to have diseases or disorders that are unrelated to the condition that is to be treated by surgery. These conditions may affect the risk of surgery and must be identified and evaluated before the operation. It is, therefore, very important that the surgeon see the patient as soon as possible after admission to the hospital, not only to reassure and encourage him or her, but also to thoroughly evaluate the patient's condition and weigh carefully the risks of the operation against its expected benefits. No matter how thorough the initial diagnostic examination, this does not take the place of the immediate preoperative evaluation. In some cases, the operation must be done despite other complicating conditions; in others, the risk may be too great and the operation must be postponed until corrective treatment reduces the risk. The operation may be canceled if corrective treatment is not feasible. Patients with conditions such as pulmonary or cardiac disease, metabolic, endocrine, or blood disorders, or marked dehydration or malnutrition may have an extended preoperative period to allow for complete "workup" and corrective treatment.

Nurses often arrange for the physical examination. It is important that they exercise good judgment in determining whether the patient wants to talk privately to the surgeon before or after the examination. Interns or resident physicians often assume responsibility for the medical examination. Nurses may assist throughout, or physicians may do most of the examination without assistance. When nurses do participate, it gives them a chance to assess the amount and kind of nursing the patients need, and it can make certain aspects of the examination easier for patients and physicians. In hospitals where there are no interns or resident physicians, nurses or clerks may record the general data for the medical record (also referred to in some places as the "data base"). The doctor in charge of the case then performs all other medical duties.

---

* Personal communication with second author.

The physical examination is discussed in Chapter 5 and, as it relates to surgery, there is more discussion of it in this chapter. However, assessment of the patient's physiologic status is not limited to the medical examination. Nurses make an assessment from their observations, interviews, and informal conversations with patients and their family and friends. This is a very significant aspect of the total assessment of the patient. For example, it may be the nurse (especially in emergency admissions) who finds that a patient is a *heavy smoker, chronic alcoholic,* or a *drug addict* or *drug abuser.* All these problems may have important implications for the care and management of the patient. Because of the lung involvement, patients who smoke heavily are advised to discontinue smoking a few days before surgery. Acute alcoholic intoxication may not present a serious problem, but chronic alcoholism always does. Chronic alcoholic patients usually have a high tolerance for anesthesia and certain other drugs, such as paraldehyde or the barbiturates; for this reason, they are potential candidates for overdose of anesthesia. In addition, they are likely to have liver impairment and reduced myocardial contractile force, Jonathan E. Rhoads and his associates [45] say. These surgeons recommend that "cured" drug addicts not be given narcotics preoperatively or postoperatively. Instead, for pain, they should be given nonaddicting analgesics, such as methotrimeprazine or pentazocine. Patients who are currently addicted must be maintained on the abused drug to suppress withdrawal symptoms. According to Rhoads and associates, narcotic addicts are easy to maintain, often on half of their usual dosage. Barbiturate-dependent patients pose additional problems. It is hard to establish their usual dosage and so "maintenance" is difficult. If the drug is withheld, the patient will most likely go into withdrawal syndrome characterized by tremors, agitation, nausea, vomiting, weakness, and hyperreflexia. The patient may also hallucinate. Patients who are under the influence of LSD may be calmed with small doses of pentobarbital given intramuscularly.[46,46a] To our knowledge, very little has been reported on the consequences of the use of LSD or marijuana in surgical patients.

Ethical and Legal Issues. Nurses share with others on the surgical team the responsibility of seeing that every patient receives the best care that is available, under the safest conditions possible, and at the lowest cost. Care should include comprehensive services that cover the total welfare insofar as this is possible. The welfare of health workers must also be considered, for there is growing concern with the protection of the rights of all human beings. Legislation in the field of health care is increasing in quantity and importance every year. Helen Creighton,[47] a nurse who is also a lawyer, urges nurses to study the legal framework of their practice in order that they can assess the consequences of their options and make wise and prudent choices in the practice of their profession. Accidents occurring in the course of medical care are the principal concern of nurses and doctors, say Irene A. Murchison, a nurse, and Thomas S. Nichols,[48] a lawyer. "A patient injured on the operating table through an improper or negligent act of a surgeon or nurse is, of course, equally the victim of accident as is the person injured in an automobile collision. In neither case is injury intended, but in both cases it is brought about by a failure to act responsibly." * The victims suffer losses as a consequence and society has methods to provide them with recompense for their losses by shifting the loss to whoever is finally determined to be responsible for the loss. The branch of law that deals with allocation of accident losses is called *tort law.* "The overriding objective of the tort law," according to Murchison and Nichols, "is to provide a means for compensating those injured by the wrongful conduct of another." † The wrong conduct may be unintentional, or it may be intentional. *Intentional,* according to law, does not merely refer to conduct that had as its purpose to harm or produce a specific result. An injury that could have been foreseen by a wise and prudent person or "a reasonable man" as likely to occur is, according to the law, intentional.[49,50] Tort law then is of particular significance in surgical care because of the high risks and potential liabilities. Surgical treatment ranks highest among the areas for malpractice claims or suits. Anesthesiologists and surgeons are subject to malpractice claims more frequently than physicians in other specialties.[51,52] Nurses who assume positions as independent contractors are also subject to malpractice claims. Creighton says: "The nation [US] has experienced a growth in the number of malpractice claims against doctors, hospitals, nurses, and other health providers in recent years. . . . increases of 100 to 200 per cent in a single year are not unknown." ‡

---

* Murchison, Irene A., and Nichols, Thomas S.: *Legal Foundations of Nursing Practice.* Macmillan Publishing Co., Inc., New York, 1970, p. 74.

† *Ibid.,* p. 72.

‡ Creighton, Helen: "The Medical Malpractice Commission. In Accountability of the Nurse. Are There Legal Barriers to Assuming Professional Responsibility?" (Speeches presented at the 48th Convention, American Nurses' Association.) The Association, Kansas City, Mo., 1973, p. 9.

The nature of the contract between patients and their physicians, their nurses, and others who participate in their care should be clear and mutually acceptable to all parties involved. The patient should understand the nature of the treatment that is planned, and be informed about the risks involved and the probable consequence of failing to carry out the treatment as planned. Given these conditions, the patient's written consent should be gotten. In other words, no surgical procedure should be done without the informed consent of patient or guardian. Every hospital or clinic has a form for such *written consent* (see Fig.

University Hospital

CONSENT TO OPERATION - PATIENT

I, _____
(Name in full)

of _____
(Address and municipality)

hereby consent to undergo the operation or procedure of _____

to be performed by Dr. _____ and his surgical team, the nature and

effect of which have been explained to me by Dr. _____ and are understood by me.

I also consent to such further or alternative operative procedures as in the opinion of Dr. _____
are immediately necessary, and to the administration of any general or other anaesthetic for any of these purposes.

I also agree that University Hospital or any of its medical staff may retain for the purpose of study, diagnosis, education or research any tissues, parts or organs removed from me and/or may dispose of any of the same in accordance with the Hospital's customary practice.

TIME: _____

DATE: _____   _____
                                                  (Signature of patient)

Read over and explained to _____ the patient, who acknowledges that
                            (Name of patient)
he/she understood the contents and signed his/her name in my presence.

_____
(Signature of witness)

EMERGENCY OPERATION

I hereby certify that I believe that the delay that would be caused by obtaining the consent in writing to the

performance of the surgical operation specified hereunder on _____
would endanger the patient's life.

Operation or Procedure _____

TIME: _____   _____
                                                  Witness

DATE: _____   _____
                                                  Signature of Operating Surgeon

84-750-0073 (03/73)

Figure 47-2. Patient consent form for surgical procedures. (Courtesy of University Hospital, University of Western Ontario, London, Ont.)

AUTHORIZATION FOR MEDICAL AND/OR SURGICAL TREATMENT

I, the undersigned, a patient in————————————————————— Hospital, hereby authorize

Dr.————————————————(and whomever he may designate as his assistants) to administer such treatment as is

necessary, and to perform the following operation————————————————,

NAME OF OPERATION

and such additional operations or procedures as are considered therapeutically necessary on the basis of findings during the course of said operation.

I also consent to the administration of such anesthetics as are necessary, with the exception of————————,

NONE, SPINAL ANESTHESIA, OR OTHER

Any tissues or parts surgically removed may be disposed of by the hospital in accordance with accustomed practice.

I hereby certify that I have read and fully understand the above **Authorization for Medical and/or Surgical Treatment**, the reasons why the above named

surgery is considered necessary, its advantages and possible complications, if any, as well as possible alternative modes of treatment, which were ex-

plained to me by Dr.————————————. I also certify that no guarantee or assurance has been made as to the

results that may be obtained.

Date————————   Signed————————————————

                                    PATIENT

Witness————————————   Or————————————————

                                    NEAREST RELATIVE

Relationship to Patient————————————

> **Both authorizations must be signed by the patient, or by the nearest relative in the case of a minor or when patient is physically or mentally incompetent.**

AUTHORIZATION FOR RELEASE OF INFORMATION

Authorization is hereby granted to release to the————————————————

                          NAME OF INSURANCE COMPANY OR COMPANIES
such information as may be necessary for the completion of my hospitalization claims.

Date————————   Signed————————————————

                                    PATIENT

Or————————————————

                                    NEAREST RELATIVE

Relationship to Patient————————————

Figure 47-2. (continued).

47-2). Some of these forms provide a space for listing the specific operation to be performed; others make only general reference to "an operation" or "surgery." Only in extreme emergencies in which it is impossible to get written consent are patients taken to surgery without it. In these cases, consent is "implied." Emanuel Hayt [53] points out that this written operative permit or "release" does not necessarily protect the surgeon from charges of malpractice, but he thinks that in case the operation leads to litigation there is less room for controversy. The main purpose of consent is to protect the physician against claims of unauthorized operations and to protect the patient against unsanctioned surgery. Authorization may be the physician's best legal defense.

Consent does not imply that the surgeon may perform unnecessary surgery. No matter how broad or general the authorization may be, the burden is upon the physician to be reasonably certain the operation was pathologically indicated.

All members of the surgical staff should be aware of potential dangers to the *physical safety of patients,* and take the necessary precautions to prevent accidents. Explosions in the operating room rarely happen but are a dreaded hazard. The possibility of this happening must not be ignored. Most of the agents used in general anesthesia are volatile—divinyl ether, diethyl ether, ethyl chloride, ethylene, and cyclopropane will explode in the presence of gases that support combustion (oxygen, nitrous oxide) and a source of ignition. In Chapter 15 attention is called to a report of an intestinal rupture when gas in the colon was ignited by cauterization of the bladder. To prevent explosions, it is important to avoid using combustible substances in situations where x-ray, cautery, or other equipment that might throw sparks is used. Explosive substances should be properly stored away from sources of heat and in well-ventilated places. Hydrocarbons should be stored away from oxygen and nitrous oxide. Explosive gases should be mixed with the minimum dilution of oxygen or nitrous oxide, in such ratio that will make them nonexplosive, and administered through "closed systems" that do not permit the gas to escape. Static sparks should be prevented. The humidity of the operating room is important in preventing sparks. The drier the operating room, the more conducive to static sparks. It is important to ground all persons and objects in the room. This means that operating room personnel must wear special shoes or pull nonconductive covers over regular shoes. They are also required to wear cotton rather than rayon or nylon clothing because the synthetics conduct static electricity. Nurses who go with patients to and from the operating room must also observe this regulation.

As new machines and equipment are introduced into the hospital, it is important that nurses learn their potential dangers in and outside operating rooms. *Electrical shocks and fires* are among these dangers. Inspection of the equipment, plugs, and outlets is important and any sign of impairment should be recorded and the objects repaired immediately.

(See Chapter 15 for detailed discussion of electrical hazards.)

In the case of an accident, patients should receive prompt and appropriate care. A complete report of the details of the accident should be made in writing by the unit administrator to the director of the institution or agency. The importance of *records* cannot be overemphasized. Patients' charts and records are used as a source of evidence in cases of accidents and injury claims.

There are legal implications in many injuries requiring surgical treatment. These might, for example, involve the patient's insurance company or workmen's compensation benefits; or, in the case of violence, such as gunshot, stabbing, or automobile accidents, the police and the courts. Making and keeping accurate records of examination and treatment are mandatory. The kinds of records depend somewhat on the setting, but those in hospitals, schools, and industrial health services have common characteristics. Those used in penal institutions may be designed with special consideration for the protection of the staff against charges of negligence.

There are obviously a number of other considerations of ethical and legal significance that are not covered in this discussion. The advent of organ transplants, legal abortions, the use of lobotomy and other surgical techniques to control behavior, and transsexual surgical procedures are a few examples. The performance of unnecessary elective surgery has always existed, but many writers imply that it happens more and more often.

3. PREOPERATIVE EXAMINATION

Hospital Inpatients. As soon as the patient is admitted to the hospital for surgery, the surgeon and the intern on the service are notified. In cases where there are no interns, the patient's regular physician is notified. The patient is helped to get ready for the physical examination. (See Chapter 5.) The intern takes a complete history and makes a thorough examination of the patient, although nurses may play a major role in getting the history. Types of histories are discussed in Chapter 5. Although surgeons may differ in what laboratory studies they request, and there are variations among hospitals as to what is considered "routine," they usually include the following: complete blood counts (i.e., hemoglobin, hematacrit, counts of red and white blood cells, cell differential); test for syphilis; clotting time; blood type and cross-match; serum chemistries (i.e., calcium, potassium, sodium, carbon dioxide, blood urea nitrogen); blood sugar (particularly when diabetes mellitus is known or suspected).[54,55] Urinalysis is made for all patients and it is often the nurse's responsibility to collect a specimen when the patient arrives on the unit. Chest x-rays are usually taken routinely unless the patient's condition prohibits this. Some hospitals include an electrocardiogram among the routine tests for newly admitted patients. Special attention is given to specific aspects of the physical examination depending on the history, age of patient, and type of operation to be performed. All patients are observed for signs of cardiac or pulmonary problems, such as dyspnea, edema, rapid heart rates, lung rales, cyanosis, clubbing of fingers, and poor tolerance of exercise. Children are examined for signs of dehydration, malnutrition, infection, and fever. Fever is a contraindication for surgery in both children and adults. Surgeons generally insist that it be reduced before undertaking surgery. W. Gerald Austen says that "there are very few areas where an infection has greater catastrophic implications than in cardiac surgery." * Patients who are scheduled for cardiac surgery are screened very carefully for signs of infection. Some surgeons are so strict about this that they will have teeth with cavities filled or capped before operation. Few surgeons will operate on any patient—with perhaps the exception of the surgical emergency —until a thorough study has been made.

In surgical emergencies, the physical examination and other aspects of the preoperative evaluation must be carried out with the greatest dispatch. If the patient is hemorrhaging or if there is severe intercranial pressure, it may be necessary to omit parts of the examination and many of the usual tests may not be feasible. Physicians may measure the patient's temperature, pulse, and blood pressure during the medical examination or they may ask that nurses make these measurements. Since nurses will be making these measurements frequently during the postoperative period, it is desirable for them to know their preoperative characteristics as a basis for comparison.

Outpatients. As soon as the surgeon and patient agree to the operation, the date and time are scheduled. The history may be taken and the physical examination made in the clinic or the physician's office. Laboratory studies may be made in a private facility or clinic laboratory. Occasionally, the laboratory work is performed on admission to the surgical facility a few hours before the surgery is to be performed. This arrangement might at first glance seem to be more convenient for patients; however, it does not permit the surgeon to identify abnormal results before admission of the patient. In cases where the results contraindicate surgery on that day, patients are greatly inconvenienced because they are discharged to return again after the problem is cleared up. Nurses working in an outpatient surgical facility may or may not see patients before they arrive for surgery. Whenever they do, however, it is important that the nurse check to be sure that patients have had a physical examination and that the results of the examination and laboratory work are available to the surgeon before the operation is performed—preferably before the patient is admitted for surgery. Nurses working in physicians' offices often play important roles in taking the history, collecting specimens for laboratory studies, and in assisting with or performing the physical examination. Ideally, there should be communication between nurses in physicians' offices and those in the facility where the surgery is to be performed to assure that all preliminary preparation is complete and that the nurses in the "surgicenter" are appropriately prepared to receive patients.

Many surgeons perform minor surgery in their offices. They, and the nurses associated with them, have highly individualized admission and treatment regimens. This is also true of some industrial health clinics. Chapter 3 deals briefly with major settings in which nurses function and the nature of nursing practice in those settings. References listed at the end of Chapter 3 include texts on these specialized types of nursing. They include something on the nurse's role in surgery that is performed outside of hospitals.

General efforts during physical examination to assure that patients are in the best condition for surgery and to reduce the possibility of preoperative and postoperative complications may often entail a much more extensive list of diagnostic tests and longer preoperative treatment regimen in hospitals or outside hospitals than is suggested in this chapter. Surgical texts should be used in conjunction with the material given here.

4. ANESTHESIA

Much of the progress in modern surgery has been possible by improved anesthesia. Not only have new agents been found, but also the number of physicians with special training in

---

* Austen, W. Gerald: "Cardiac Surgery," in American College of Surgeons: *Manual of Preoperative and Postoperative Care.* W. B. Saunders Co., Philadelphia, 1971, p. 310.

anesthesia is increasing. Their cooperation with surgeons and the discovery of new drugs have made many operations possible that were formerly impossible, and have improved pre- and postoperative care. Except in cases of emergency, administration of an anesthetic lies outside traditional nursing; however, it seems desirable for all nurses to have a practical knowledge of anesthetic agents and their relative merits. In most states there are laws prohibiting the administration of an anesthetic by anyone other than a person specially trained in anesthesia, except in extreme emergencies. There have been, and still are, many nurse anesthetists who have special preparation. There is in the United States an Association of Nurse Anesthetists that has an official journal. It is becoming more common, however, for physician anesthetists to take charge of this work. The physician anesthetist can be of great help to the surgeon by assuming part of the medical responsibility for the patient's condition during the operation and also by prescribing the immediate postoperative care. The importance of the anesthetist's preoperative evaluation as a basis for selecting the anesthetic and minimizing its risks is emphasized in everything one sees in current books and articles on anesthesia and surgical care. While anesthetists study the patient's record and use the opinions and findings of other medical personnel, they make certain tests and measurements themselves and assess the patient's emotional makeup and attitude toward the operation and the anesthetic. When anesthetists are prepared to assume the major responsibility for the patient's general condition during the operation, the surgeon is able to give his or her complete attention to the intricacies of the operation itself.

Patients who can recall having general anesthesia 25 years ago, on having it today, are amazed at the ease with which they "go under." Now they often have no recollection of the anesthetic. Premedication makes them drowsy, and in this state they are taken, sometimes in their beds, to an anteroom off the operating suite where an anesthetist induces anesthesia by a scarcely felt intravenous injection. In their next conscious moment they realize that the operation is over and that many hours have elapsed. In some cases, anesthetists bring drugs used for induction of anesthesia to the patient's room, and in these cases the patient cannot even remember going to the operating room. From the patient's point of view, this represents one of the most outstanding advances in anesthesia.

Giving different drugs by different routes has greatly reduced the risks of anesthesia.

One drug may be a respiratory depressant, another may be toxic to the kidneys. When they are combined, less is needed of each one and the danger of each is reduced. Patients who have had anesthetics in years past often notice that the effects are now briefer and milder than they were.

Inhalation Anesthesia. *Ethyl ether* used by William Morton in 1846 was the first successful anesthetic. John A. Paulson and John S. Lundy [56] in 1950, Henry K. Beecher [57] in 1952, and Robert D. Dripps and associates [58] in 1972 say that it is still the safest agent for most patients in the hands of most anesthetists. Ether may be inhaled from a cone or mask on which the liquid is dripped or from a vaporizing machine. Often its vapor, mixed with oxygen, is insufflated from a tube passed into the pharynx or trachea, although these mixtures may also be breathed in through masks over the nose.* The average patient, in thinking about anesthesia, rejects ether because of its unpleasant effects as used years ago. The induction was stormy and anesthesia was deep. Postoperatively, there were unpleasant thoughts, laryngospasms, vomiting, headache, and dehydration. Today, ether, well managed, need not have these effects. [59]

Vinyl ether (Vinethene), which has the combined properties of *ethyl ether* and *ethylene*, and *cyclopropane* are substitutes for ethyl ether. Vinyl ether is recommended for short surgical procedures where a quick pleasant induction and a rapid recovery are needed.

Nitrous oxide gas produces an anesthesia quickly and easily and has been called "laughing gas." Like *ethyl chloride* and *ethylene*, it is used for short surgical procedures where complete relaxation is unnecessary. Cyclopropane has had ardent advocates and is still used. The period of induction is shorter and pleasanter than that of ether, and there is no suffocation or falling sensation. It is not a circulatory depressant and the respirations are not labored, making it especially desirable for upper abdominal and chest surgery. Recovery from cyclopropane anesthesia is rapid and usually uncomplicated. It has a major disadvantage in that, since so much oxygen is given, the patient's color remains good regardless of his or her condition. Other common symptoms, such

---

* Intratracheal anesthesia is desirable when the surgeon must work around the patient's head and neck, making it almost impossible for an anesthetist to hold a mask in place. Nurses often notice that following brain surgery tracheotomies are necessary. One reason is that the pharynx and trachea have been irritated by the tube as well as by the anesthetic, and the resulting swelling and accumulation of mucus block the airway.

as changes-in-the-eye reactions, are obscured, and for these reasons only a highly experienced person should administer cyclopropane.

Chemists have continued to find more effective drugs for anesthesia. Their progress has led to the synthesis of *fluorine, halothane,* and *methoxyflurane.* These are called the halogenated inhalation anesthetics and have been widely used in the past 10 years. They provide for more rapid induction than ether (perhaps slower than nitrous oxide and cyclopropane) and ventricular arrhythmias are rare. Elimination of these drugs is delayed. In general, neuromuscular blockers must be used because most of these drugs provide poor muscular relaxation.[60]

Intravenous Anesthesia. *Hexobarbital (Evipal), thiopental (Pentothal), thiamylal (Surital),* and *methohexital (Brevital)* are some of the drugs given intravenously to produce general anesthesia. Thiopental (Pentothal) is the most commonly used of these drugs and is administered alone or in combination with other anesthetics. The terms *neuroleptic anesthesia* and *dissociative anesthesia* are used to describe *newer trends* in intravenous anesthesia. The administration of one of the butyrophenone series (similar to the phenothiazine group) and a powerful opioid produces a state of reduced motor activity, reduced anxiety, and indifference in which the patient can respond appropriately to command. This drug combination is adrenolytic, antiemetic, and anticonvulsant. The fixed combination that is being used currently is called Innovar.[61,61a]

Dissociative anesthesia is described as acting at specific sites in the central nervous system and having far-reaching effects on the brain. Ketamine is a drug used for this purpose. Patients having this anesthetic look awake but are not aware of what is happening and won't remember it. The drug is related to hallucinogenic drugs like LSD. Patients may have unpleasant dreams under its influence and the effects may extend into the postoperative period.

Current research includes investigation of steroids for producing general anesthesia. In laboratory animals, steroids have been used to produce anesthesia characterized by rapid induction, brief duration, and smooth recovery. These drugs have yet to be tested for similar effects in man.[62] Problems of solubility, side effects, and potency have continued to plague investigators.[62a]

Intravenous and inhalation anesthetics are frequently used together. In addition, drugs such as *diazepam (Valium)* and *meperidine (Demerol)* have been administered intravenously to supplement nitrous oxide when used in outpatient surgery.[63]

Regional Anesthesia. Almost any area of the body can be made insensitive to pain by applying anesthetics to the skin or mucous membrane or by injecting anesthetics in variout parts of the body. The location and size of the area that is made insensitive are governed by the site of the injection or application. Regional anesthesia is classified anatomically by James E. Eckenhoff and Edward A. Brunner[64] as *topical, local infiltration, field block, peripheral nerve block, epidural, spinal,* and *intravenous regional.* In describing each type, the authors say topical and local anesthesia involve sensory perceptors. All other types except intravenous involve nerve conduction and are frequently called *conduction anesthesia. Topical anesthetics* are applied with a dropper, an atomizer, or a cotton swab directly to a small area of the body. This type of anesthesia, when using aqueous solutions, is effective only if the skin is inflamed or diseased, because healthy intact skin prevents the penetration of the solution through the epidermis. Ointments containing anesthetic agents are effective on healthy skin. Aqueous solutions containing salts of cocaine, lidocaine, or tetracaine are effective for mucous membranes. These are often used for anesthesia of the conjunctiva and cornea of the eye, the nose, mouth, throat, and the urethra and anus. Topical anesthetics applied to mucous membranes are rapidly absorbed. Therefore, the amount of anesthetic used is much less than that for infiltration.

Local infiltration also affects the sensory nerve endings. This type of regional anesthesia permits the injection of anesthetics directly into the operative site to render insensitive those nerve endings that may be stimulated by the operation. Local infiltration is frequently used for simple dental surgery, for incision and drainage of an abscess, and similar procedures. In the *field block,* the objective is to circumscribe the operative field with anesthetics in order that the nerve fibers supplying the operative site be blocked and the field desensitized. The field block covers a larger area of the body than do the topical or local infiltration methods. The *peripheral nerve block* is made possible by injecting the anesthetic in proximity to major nerve trunks. This method may be combined with local infiltration. It permits larger areas of the body to be anesthetized than any of the previous methods discussed. For example, by the blocking of the brachial plexus, the arm and hand can be anesthetized. Similarly, the entire lower extremity can be made insensitive by blocking the femoral, sciatic, and obturator nerves. A combination of other nerve blocks can be used to provide anesthesia for abdominal surgery.

In *epidural anesthesia,* the anesthetic agent is deposited in the extradural space of the vertebral canal. The epidural space may be penetrated at any level. When the anesthetic is introduced at the sacrococcygeal hiatus, it is termed caudal anesthesia. This technique is used to relieve pain in labor and delivery and for rectal operations. The lumbar region is most frequently used because it is an easy point of entry and there is less danger that the spinal cord will be injured. The cervical and thoracic areas are not used so often because there is more danger of injuring the spinal cord. The major advantage of using epidural anesthesia rather than spinal anesthesia is that the former produces extensive anesthesia and minimizes the hazards of spinal cord injury and the contamination of the cerebrospinal fluid. *Spinal anesthesia* is the injection of anesthetics into the cerebrospinal fluid so that the drug bathes all of the peripheral nerve roots. Because spinal anesthesia is used frequently and many patients have questions about it (some are very afraid of it), the subject is discussed here in more detail than other forms of regional anesthesia.

Recent advances in spinal anesthesia have kept pace with inhalation anesthesia. According to P. C. Lund,[65] spinal anesthesia has had a stormy course in its relatively short history. There are contraindications for spinal anesthesia, and complications attributed to it include serious nerve injuries. Lund says that practically all of these complications are preventable. Many of the neurologic complications attributed to spinal anesthesia in the past are said by some authorities to have other causes. Spinal anesthesia is indicated for geriatric patients and for other patients who have concomitant pathology that precludes inhalation anesthesia or makes it risky.[66] The list of drugs used for spinal anesthesia increases. Today, many on the list are rarely used. Some of the older ones are losing popularity because they are cytotoxic, give too brief an anesthesia, or are inactivated by glucose; some of the newer ones are infrequently used because their use has been inadequately studied. *Tetracaine (Pontocaine), lidocaine (Xylocaine),* and *mepivacaine (Carbocaine)* are used extensively.[67] The equipment and procedure used for spinal anesthesia are like those described for lumbar puncture followed by a medication (see Chapter 22). The duration of spinal anesthesia is hard to control. Vasopressin (Pitressin), epinephrine, and other vasoconstrictors may be given with the anesthetic to prolong the effect, or spinal anesthesia may be supplemented by intravenous anesthetics or analgesics.

Regional anesthesia has the advantage of enabling the patient to be conscious and to follow directions during surgery. It also prevents the disagreeable or potentially dangerous physiologic consequences of inhalation anesthesia. The patient is able to move about and take nourishment sooner and this reduces the incidence of complications attributed to immobility. Occasionally, a patient is given a general and regional anesthetic. This may reduce the amount of general anesthetic needed for the surgery involved. Some types of regional anesthesia have been useful in controlling intractable pain. Local anesthetics have developed so rapidly in recent years that it is impractical to try to list all these drugs. A few examples are *tetracaine (Pontocaine), lidocaine (Xylocaine), mepivacaine (Carbocaine), dibucaine (Nupercaine), procaine (Novocain),* and *cocaine.* Cocaine was first used in 1884, but because of its toxicity and habit-forming properties it is not used frequently in therapy now. It is one of the drugs currently used by addicts.

Actually, all anesthetics are toxic and idiosyncratic reactions to them are not uncommon. The second author of this chapter has seen a patient die from an injection of novocaine almost before the surgical team realized what was happening. A small fraction of the therapeutic dose should be given first to test the individual's response to the drug. A few minutes should elapse between the injection of the local anesthetic and surgery to allow time for the drug to act. The time to be allowed depends on the agent, the method of administration, and the patient. Because nurses often help surgeons in using local anesthetics and may prepare them, they should have references available that enable them to check dosage. In fact, anyone involved in giving an anesthetic should be familiar with the dosage. When new drugs are used, physicians prescribing them should assume responsibility for making reports available on their nature, action, and dangers.

Rectal or Colonic Anesthesia. Dripps and his associates [68] say that intravenous anesthesia has probably reduced the use of rectal or colonic methods, primarily because in the giving of anesthesia by rectum, control of absorption of the drug is both uncertain and unpredictable. With inhalation and intravenous anesthesia, absorption is more or less controllable. David D. Cohen and John B. Dillon [69] say this method is still used primarily in outpatient surgery and for pediatric surgery. They give thiopental or thiamylal, 25 to 35 mg/kg in 10 per cent solution, as the usual dosage. Tribromoethanol (Avertin) is perhaps more familiar to nurses who have been out of practice for a while. It was one of the popular agents for rectal anesthesia in pediatric surgery and for the hyperthyroid patient when it was necessary to "steal the goiter." When rectal or colonic anesthesia is used, nurses prepare the colon by giving enemas or colonic irrigations to clear it of feces. This must be done a few hours before the administration of the anesthetic; otherwise, the drug will be expelled by contractions stimulated by the enema or irrigation.

Refrigeration Anesthesia (*Hypothermia*). It has long been known that lowering the temperatures of tissues makes them insensitive. F. M. Allen [69a] says it is an anesthesia of protoplasm instead of a mere anesthesia. In recent years some surgeons have advocated ice anesthesia. When, for any reason, general anesthesia is contraindicated and local anesthetic or nerve block impracticable, they refrigerate the tissue and operate with no other means of controlling pain except an analgesic, such as morphine. This method has been advocated for amputation when there is threatened gangrene, especially when the subject is an elderly person who will tolerate anesthetics poorly.

Ludwig H. Segerberg [70] in 1943 reported a lowered mortality with this refrigeration anesthesia in arterioslerotic and diabetic gangrene. Bertram Cook [71] in 1950 wrote that he used it in severe accidents with a view to "stalling" until he could get the patient ready for radical surgical treatment. Then ice anesthesia procedure was seen so rarely that one must conclude that it was either not generally accepted as the best method or that it was thought impractical. Cynthia Van Blarcom, discussing the nursing care in 1943, said, "the postoperative course of these patients is astounding . . . postoperative nursing care is simplified one-hundred fold."* Segerberg reported that such operations did not produce shock because the loss of blood was minimal and the limb had been gradually separated, metabolically, from the body. Little pain was suffered after the operation; the patient could eat a meal immediately on return to the clinical unit. Wounds were said to heal normally in spite of tissue refrigeration.

Prior to the writings of any of the above authors, we are told that local refrigeration was used to permit painless amputation during the Napoleonic wars. And, since 1950, hypothermia has been used not only for amputation, but also in the treatment of congenital heart defects, congenital aneurysms of cerebral vessels, and occasionally for cerebral vascular tumors.[72,73] R. G. Nugent [74] says this method

of anesthesia reduces metabolic activity slowly and methodically and allows a severely impaired organ to survive because its blood requirements are lessened under the newly created conditions. There are certain dangers involved in the use of deep hypothermia. Cardiac arrest is the most severe of these. Others include the following: shivering, which may lead to exhaustion of liver and muscle glycogen from hyperventilation and increased metabolic activity of the brain; burns, which may result from using hot water bottles when the temperature goes below the desired level during hypothermia treatment, or when getting body temperatures back to normal after the treatment is terminated. Edema, fat necrosis, seizures, and drug reactions may occur from slowed metabolism and the resultant failure of the body to detoxify and excrete drugs properly. In an article discussing the nursing care of patients in hypothermia, Nancy Graves [75] emphasizes the importance of skin care, checking intake and output hourly, giving bladder irrigations to prevent infection and loss of bladder tone, and checking vital signs every 15 minutes. Graves reports patients staying in hypothermia from 3 to 7 days at a body temperature as low as 30° to 33°C (86° to 89°F). She warns against the use of hot water bottles, saying that even tepid water may burn. She, in fact, advises that they not be used at all. When hypothermia is temporarily or finally terminated, the patient should be allowed to warm at his or her own rate, under blankets that have *not* been warmed. The blankets are removed as the patient's temperature rises. Good oral hygiene, eye care (especially important because of decreased corneal reflexes), putting the patient in good anatomic positions to prevent deformities, and turning every 2 hours are among the other essentials of nursing care of patients in deep hypothermia.

Techniques for use of this anesthesia for *arm or leg amputation* are briefly these: After the usual systemic preparation of the patient, including an analgesic and the local skin cleaning and shaving, elevate the head of the bed and protect the mattress with a full-length waterproof sheet. It may be helpful to put a cotton blanket over this sheet and under the patient. Put a layer of chipped ice 2 inches deep (or solid carbon dioxide at −45° to −49°C) in the bottom of a galvanized tank or rubber trough, large enough to hold the arm or leg, first having removed the sharp edges from the chipped ice (if ice is used) by passing it through water. Gently lift the limb onto the ice (J. F. Gorman and J. C. Rosenberg [75a] recommend first covering the extremity with stockinet and they also recommend solid car-

---

* Van Blarcom, Cynthia: "Nursing Care in Ice Anesthesia," *Am. J. Nurs.*, 43:799, (Sept.) 1943.

bon dioxide rather than ice). (See Fig. 47-3.) Surround the limb up to the groin or armpit with ice. Use a sponge-rubber cuff at the proximal end of the limb. (The amount of ice required for anesthetizing the leg is about 150 lb.) Elevate the head of the bed so that the water from the ice, as it melts, will drain away from the body. (An electric refrigeration unit reduces the expenditure of time and energy and results in more complete anesthesia of the upper third of the thigh, when this is important.) If the leg is under treatment, protect the genitalia and the unaffected leg with bath towels and a board placed between the legs.* About 2 hours before the operation, the surgeon applies a tourniquet, protecting the skin under it with a folded towel. Ice bags may be applied over the area exposed in this process. Transport the patient to the operating room in his or her bed. Gorman and Rosenberg

---

* Some authorities recommend the use of hot water bottles applied to untreated areas for comfort, but, as noted earlier, Graves says even tepid water may burn.

advocate the application of dry ice (carbon dioxide) for 24 hours; Graves reports much shorter periods (4½ hours) used with "wet ice."

A dramatic illustration of the use of deep hypothermia by a team of surgeons at the University of Chicago's Wyker Children's Hospital was recently reported in *Time Magazine*.[76] The patient was 1 year old. To prepare him for surgical correction of a congenital heart defect, his body was packed in ice bags and suspended over a tank of cold water until his temperature was reduced to 18.3°C (65°F). His heart was injected with potassium solution that stopped the beat, leaving his body in a state that resembled death. As shown in a film of the operation,[77] this condition enabled the surgeon, Robert Replogle, to operate without the risk of heavy bleeding and without the impediment of a beating heart. The surgical part of the 5-hour procedure took only 31 minutes, following which a heart-lung machine pumped warm blood through the patient's body, washed out the potassium, and restored his heart beat to normal within 30 minutes.

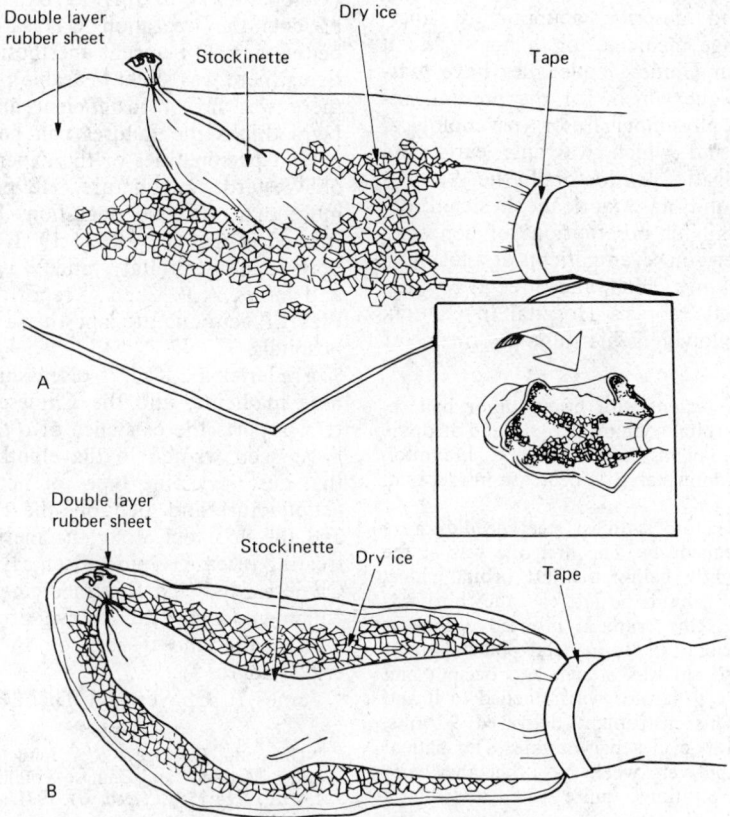

Figure 47-3. One method of refrigeration anesthesia.

The operation was uncomplicated and, at the time of the published report, the child was described as doing "quite well." Deep hypothermia is being used in surgery more and more frequently around the world.[78-82] (See Chapter 42 for further discussion of hypothermia.)

Acupuncture. Acupuncture is a form of Chinese therapy that dates back to ancient Chinese theories about the anatomy and physiology of the human body. It utilizes techniques that involve pricking designated parts of the body with tiny needles. This form of treatment and its use in rendering parts of the body insensitive to pain are controversial in some countries. Physicians have traveled from other countries to various parts of the Occident and the Orient to try to learn more about this technique. Their accounts appearing in the professional literature in the United States confirm the effectiveness of acupuncture in the cases that they observed, and leave unexplained the physiologic or psychologic basis for high rates of success that are reported. In summarizing his opinion of acupuncture based on observations in several hospitals in China, P. E. Brown, a general practitioner from Gravesend, Kent, England, states: "It would be very wrong, . . . to describe acupuncture anesthesia as 'fringe medicine' or 'a hoax' . . . it seems that our Chinese colleagues have mastered a technique which, for the present, defies normal physiological or psychological explanation; and which warrants early and careful investigation by doctors in the West." * E. Grey Dimond, an American physician, describes in detail his observations of acupuncture and surgery on seven patients at a teaching hospital in Peking, China, and three at Kwangtung Provincial People's Hospital in Canton, China. The following is his summary of one of the cases:

Case 1. The patient with brain tumor had received phenobarbital sodium, 0.1 gm, and atropine at bedtime the night before surgery. Mannitol, 20% ml, was administered to decrease intracranial pressure.

Three acupuncture stainless steel needles were inserted subcutaneously. The first one was at the inner side, slightly below the left orbital ridge; the second was behind the left ear; the third was at the vertex of the cranium inserted obliquely, right and anterior. Finally a metal plate approximately 4 × 4 sq cm was attached to occiput and a biphasic pulse generator was attached to it and the needles. This instrument delivered 9 volts, from 120 to 180 cycles per minute. The patient was conscious but very weak. No other anesthesia was used. Respirations, pulse rate, and blood pressure were carefully monitored and recorded. Holes, made with burrs, craniotomies, and lobectomies were carried out uneventfully.*

Acupuncture is preferred by those Chinese physicians who use it because it provides greater comfort for the patient; it is reported to be absolutely safe; there is no alteration in patients' hydration; fluids and food need not be withheld from patients; there are no unpleasant aftereffects (common with some other types of anesthesia) such as vomiting and nausea; and acupuncture does not lower the blood pressure. And postanesthesia respiratory tract complications, seen with respiratory anesthetics, are not a problem in acupuncture anesthesia. On the basis of his personal observations in the People's Republic of China, Dimond said that "acupuncture anesthesia has found an acceptable place in medical practice in China" † and he predicted that intensive ongoing research in this form of treatment and method of anesthesia might bring useful surprises to the rest of the world. Since this statement, considerable investigation has gone forward along these lines.

Nguyen Van Nghi,[82a] reporting on the first 50 cases of acupuncture anesthesia in France (October 1971 to July 1972), said that in 32 patients the operation was satisfactory with better than 90 per cent anesthesia; with 11 patients there was slight bearable pain; in 7 cases there was no or insufficient anesthesia. Van Nghi thinks the failures can be attributed to patient personalities or the experimental phase of Western acupuncture. He points out that more than 400,000 operations had been performed in China by June 1971. Van Nghi reports a study in Italy, and Wayne Y. H. Ho and James Y. P. Chen [82b] report two successful uses of acupuncture anesthesia in California hospitals.

Frederick F. Kao,[82c] discussing China, Chinese medicine, and the Chinese medical system, reports the existence of a text thought to have been written in the eighth century B.C. that describes nine types of needles used for acupuncture and mentions the 12 "meridians" and the 365 loci along the meridians used in treating disease. Guido Fisch says "Traditional Chinese Medicine is a medicine of energetics which endeavors to resolve problems of human health and disease on the basis of energy (Chi)." ‡

James F. Chaves and Theodore X. Barber,

---

* Dimond, E. Grey: "Acupuncture Anesthesia, Western Medicine and Chinese Traditional Medicine," *J.A.M.A.,* **218:**1558, (Dec. 6) 1971.
  † *Ibid.*
  ‡ Fisch, Guido: "The Triple-Burner and Its Significance in Energy Pathogenics," *Am. J. Chinese Med.,* **1:**99, (Jan.) 1973.

* Brown, P. E.: "Use of Acupuncture in Major Surgery," *Lancet,* **1:**1328, (June 17) 1972.

two psychologists, have examined ". . . the mystery of acupuncture and Chinese meridians." They say "Although this ancient theory of acupuncture still appears to have many advocates in China, it certainly is acceptable to few if any Western-trained scientists. It isn't even accepted by all Chinese surgeons." * They go on to summarize a number of reports by Western and Chinese surgeons. They discuss the possibility that the relief of pain by acupuncture works on the basis of "the gate theory" (see Chapter 49) but point out that the gate theory is still speculative. Chaves and Barber say that when acupuncture is used as an anesthetic the needles are twirled or attached to a weak electric current which produces a counterirritation, which is accepted, East and West, as giving relief from pain. They suggest that the following may explain the successful use of acupuncture: (1) the subjects believe it will prevent pain and their anxiety is relieved; (2) the special preparation accompanying the use of acupuncture by surgeons (it is never used in emergency operations) relieves anxiety and tends to establish trust in the surgeon; (3) the suggestion begun before operation is reinforced by the acupuncturist during surgery; (4) the needles are a distraction, or counterirritation; (5) narcotic analgesics, local anesthetics, and sedatives are often used with acupuncture; and (6) surgery may not be as painful as it has been thought to be.

Harold S. Burr and his associates have in this century plotted the electromagnetic fields of the body and have measured with a voltmeter the changes in the negative and positive charges in body areas during ovulation and in mood swings, to mention a few physiologic states. There is considerable medical research in China, not only on Western methods but on traditional Chinese medicine; the latter in an attempt to explain its merits scientifically. It is interesting to speculate on the relationship (suggested by Burr and F. S. C. Northrup, a philosopher, in their joint works [52d,82e]) between China's ancient art of healing and the electromagnetic field theory of this era.

The literature on acupuncture in Western countries is growing rapidly. Manako Yoshio and Ian A. Urquhart have published *The Layman's Guide to Acupuncture* (Weatherill, New York, 1972); Mary Austin has published *Acupuncture Therapy* (Asi Publishers, New York, 1972); and Margaret E. Armstrong has written an article "Acupuncture," (*Am. J. Nurs.,* **72:**1584, [Sept.] 1972) especially for nurses.

* Chaves, James F., and Barber, Theodore X.: "Needles and Knives—Behind the Mystery of Acupuncture and Chinese Meridians," *Hum. Behavior,* **2:**19, (Sept.) 1973.

The *American Journal of Nursing* takes note of changes in the law affecting acupuncture, as for example, the statement "Licensure for Acupuncture Authorized in Nevada" (**73:**1157, [July] 1973). Readers who wish to pursue this subject will find no dearth of sources.

5. PHYSICAL PREPARATION OF THE PATIENT FOR SURGERY

Medical Directions or "Preoperative Orders." The surgeon's directions for preoperative management, traditionally called "orders," represent what he or she sees as significant in getting the patient in the best condition possible to promote smooth and uneventful anesthesia and surgery, rapid uninterrupted wound healing, and a complete and uncomplicated recovery if this is possible. The physical preparation of the patient should vary according to the patient's individual needs, the preferences of the surgeon and anesthetist, and the resources and regulations of the hospital, other institution, office, or agency where surgery is performed. However, in all cases the following are guidelines: (1) supply nutrients, fluids, and other essential blood elements as needed; (2) eliminate sources of infection; (3) correct or control, if possible, preexisting pathology that might complicate the surgical procedure; and (4) minimize physical and mental tension.

The surgeon's and anesthetist's "orders" relate to feeding, or its omission; evacuation of the contents of the stomach, bowel, and bladder; the administration of parenteral fluids; and the use of hypnotics, analgesics, and other preoperative medication. Laboratory tests and the preparation of the operative site are usually included. In some institutions the skin is shaved and cleaned and made as free from microorganisms as is possible after the patient gets to the operative suite. In many hospitals there is a routine procedure or regimen for the preparation of patients undergoing certain operations, and if no deviation from this program is indicated in the surgeon's "orders," the staff is expected to follow the routine. Grave emergencies may reduce the immediate preoperative care. The patient may be taken immediately to the operating room. In the following discussion it is assumed that time is available for optimum preparation which may take place over a period of hours, days, or weeks. It may begin before the patient is admitted for the surgery, especially in the case of outpatient surgery.

Administration of Food and Water Orally and Parenterally. Patients who have been eating well and have no significant nutritional or fluid and electrolyte imbalances are given no special food, drinks, or intravenous feeding. They are usually given the regular or routine diet of the home or hospital and are encouraged to drink water freely. Adults are encouraged to drink fluids at the rate of 1000 ml every 24 hours up to the time that oral intake is prohibited. Malnutrition and severe imbalance in fluids and electrolytes increase surgical risks and are reasons for postponing the operation until a balance is restored, except in emergencies where postponement of surgery might be fatal. Obese patients are "surgical risks" since they have a tendency to develop pulmonary or cardiovascular complications. The caloric intake of these patients is often restricted preoperatively. Whenever possible, the nutritional requirements should be met through oral intake. Since this is not always possible up to and immediately after surgery, *parenteral therapy* is believed necessary by surgeons especially as the stomach should be empty when the patient is taken to the operating room. When inhalant anesthetics are used, they stimulate coughing, choking, and vomiting, and the patient is always in danger of aspirating the stomach contents.

Surgeons allow patients who are having general anesthesia to take foods and fluids by mouth from 4 to 6 hours before the operation. Anesthetists are, by and large, inclined to be more cautious. Beecher, in 1953, made the following comments and recommendations:

The commonest preventable fatal accident to occur in any operating room is probably the aspiration of vomitus under anesthesia. It ought not to happen. It would not happen if stomachs were properly emptied. In most cases this can be accomplished only by carefully withholding all food or fluids for 12 to 18 hours preoperatively. In emergency cases it can be accomplished only by taking active steps to empty the stomach by inducing vomiting. Aspiration through the largest tube which can be inserted into the stomach should not be neglected, but the size of chunks of food individuals ordinarily swallow can often not be aspirated through the largest tubes employed for the purpose.*

If all food and fluid is withheld for 18 hours prior to operation, the patient will obviously be dehydrated unless water and nutrients are given parenterally. Surgeons differ considerably in their methods of supplying food and fluid preoperatively. It is the nurse's responsibility to see that the doctor's wishes are carried out. Nurses should, however, understand the physiology of water and electrolyte balance and be prepared to discuss the patient's needs with the

doctor if they think they are not being met.

Electrolyte and water balance with maintenance of adequate nutrition by parenteral injection has been discussed in Chapters 10 and 22. Nurses might be reminded, however, that anything inhibiting the normal body urges or the patient's ability to satisfy them upsets this balance. With food and drink prohibited, and with a period of anxiety, inactivity, and usually unconsciousness forced on patients, they will inevitably suffer from imbalance unless the health team prevents it. Articles or texts by Ralph E. Homann,[83] Irving M. Ariel and Arnold J. Kreman,[84] Henry T. Randall et al,[85] John H. Bland,[86] Henry K. Beecher,[87] and many others [88-90] discuss in detail parenteral methods of supplying nutritional needs. Water and electrolytes are nearly always given; protein hydrolysates and glucose are often added. The value of whole blood or packed red blood cells and, in fact, the demand for it preoperatively when the oxygen-carrying elements of the blood are low are stressed throughout the literature. A total of 2000 to 4000 ml or more (2 to 4 qt) of parenteral fluids in the 24 hours preceding operation is said to be needed by some (adult) patients.

Bland, discussing parenteral fluids for surgical patients in 1952, emphasized that in preoperative care, nutritional deficits must be met and shock prevented with fluids and electrolytes. He said:

Fluid and electrolytes by mouth is the most physiologic of all methods and should be used as much preoperatively as is practicable and as soon postoperatively as possible. There remains enough unknown about fluid and electrolyte balance by parenteral means to make it necessary to provide insofar as is possible calories, water and electrolyte in the most physiologic manner we know, and a return to full and normal diet should be stressed. . . . The caloric and protein requirements particularly should be calculated. . . . If oral feedings are not sufficient to make up necessary caloric and protein requirements, parenteral protein hydrolysate may be used to make up the difference. If the caloric and protein requirements must be met entirely by the parenteral route, this may be accomplished by using protein hydrolysate, whole blood, glucose solutions and human serum albumin; alcohol has recently been added. . . . The vitamins, particularly ascorbic acid, thiamine hydrochloride, nicotinic acid, riboflavin and vitamin K, should be provided. . . . Parenteral therapy is always second best and is to be used either when the oral route is contraindicated or as an emergency measure.*

He thought most preoperative patients grossly "undertreated," although in some cases they

---

* Personal communication. Henry K. Beecher, Department of Anesthesia, Massachusetts General Hospital, Boston, March, 1953.

* Bland, John H.: *The Clinical Use of Fluid and Electrolyte.* W. B. Saunders Co., Philadelphia, 1952, p. 145.

might be given more water than they needed. He thought potassium depletion particularly common and believed it accounted for a great deal of the postoperative lassitude. These concerns are still important today.

No aspect of preoperative care is more important than supplying water, nutrients, and oxygen-carrying blood elements as needed. There may be considerable loss of blood during the operation, and in many cases, water loss may occur through sweating and vomiting. Nutritional balance helps prevent shock, nausea, thirst, and many other dangers and discomforts of surgery.

Elimination. Under general anesthesia and some types of regional anesthesia, the patient loses control of sphincter muscles, and contents of the rectum and the bladder may be expelled on the operating table. To prevent this possibility of contamination of the operative field, the bladder and bowels should be emptied before the operation. Also, full organs are more easily punctured than empty ones, which is another important reason to see that the stomach, intestines, and bladder are not distended.

A *cathartic* is sometimes ordered the day before the operation, but this practice has been discontinued by many surgeons for the following reasons: free catharsis depletes the patient's strength, robs the tissues of water, relaxes and lowers the tone of the intestinal muscles, and is believed to predispose the patient to postoperative distention. Castor oil or mineral oil is sometimes given, especially when patients have had barium or similar substances. A surgeon may order a mild laxative, alone or to be followed by an enema. So much depends upon the nature of the surgery that is to be performed. For example, the most extensive preparation of the intestinal tract is required in gastrointestinal surgery. Intestinal antiseptics may be given by mouth for several days before the operation. Usually, a *cleansing enema* is given the night before the operation. In addition to cleaning the colon, an enema prevents fecal impaction or straining with bowel movements postoperatively. If the result of the preoperative enema is not satisfactory, it may be necessary to repeat it; sometimes, particularly for operations on the vagina, colon, or perineum, enemas are given until the return is clear, showing a thorough cleansing. The enema is usually given 6 hours before an operation to allow peristalsis to subside. In an emergency operation, the enema is often omitted. Patients should use the toilet in expelling the enema rather than the bedpan, unless their conditions contraindicate this.

The most important principle common to all surgery of the alimentary tract is to see that it is empty for the surgery and kept empty during the immediate postoperative period. The stomach is emptied by nasogastric tube and low suction. Richard L. Varco [91] suggests that inserting a 9-holed gastric tube and applying continuous, gentle suction on the evening before the operation permits the surgeon to work with a collapsed bowel. He proposes that this approach might be used for major intra-abdominal operations, repair of a pendulous ventral hernia, and for abnormally apprehensive individuals who are prone to swallow excessive amounts of air.

Elimination from the bladder usually takes care of itself, but if there is any possibility of urinary retention the patient is *catheterized,* in spite of the inherent danger of infection from catheterization. Some surgeons suggest that the patient be sent to the operating room with a clamped-off indwelling catheter, or an ordinary catheter held in position with adhesive. The bladder can then be emptied immediately before the operation and the catheter removed after the operation. As preparation for bladder operations, cleansing and antiseptic irrigations are often prescribed. See Chapter 24 for a description of methods and steps that can be taken to minimize the risks of catheterization.

Mouth Care. A clean mouth will obviously reduce the risks of postoperative infections, particularly those of the lungs and salivary glands. A prophylactic treatment by the dentist or oral hygienist is desirable if time is available; if not, the nurse can supplement the patient's efforts as indicated by his or her particular needs. The principles and technique of mouth cleansing are discussed in Chapter 14.

Bathing and Care of the Hair. For esthetic reasons it is desirable that the patient have a bath either the night before or the morning of the operation. Encrusted dirt should be removed, and skin irritations or lesions of any sort cleared up before the operation. This is particularly important if afterward the patient must be inactive. The nails should be cleaned and nail polish removed so that the anesthetist and surgeon can see color changes in the nail bed. Fastidious persons usually have a shampoo before admission for an operation. To those not so careful the nurse may suggest one. Since washing the hair may be uncomfortable for some time postoperatively, this seems a reasonable procedure. Baths and shampoos are of course contraindicated when patients are in shock or when they are being prepared for an emergency operation.

Preparation of the Site of the Operation. The objectives in preparing the operative site are to remove hair and pathogenic organisms. Hair carries keratin and bacteria into the wound, as does the skin. While it is impossible to destroy the bacteria on the skin completely, they can be greatly reduced in number (see Chapters 15, 33, 43, and 44). Attention should be called to the disadvantages of shaving the skin as well as its advantages. Because it is thought that shaving irritates the skin, removes some of the superficial cells, and opens up hair follicles that contain bacteria, some surgeons believe shaving increases the risk of infection. Even when an episiotomy is anticipated or found necessary, some obstetricians and midwives leave the pudenda unshaven, as do some

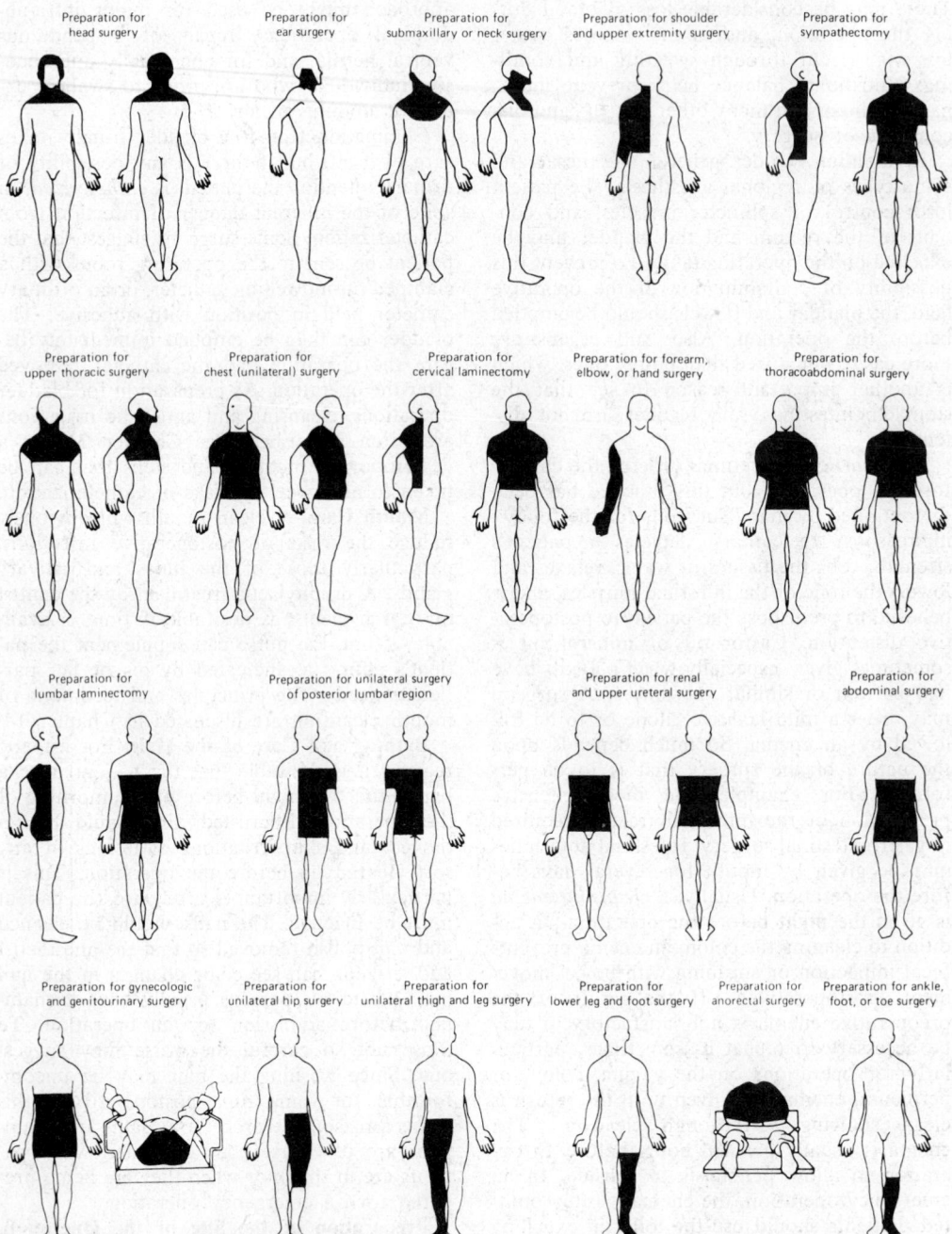

Figure 47–4. The skin areas to be prepared for surgery as determined by the type of operation. (Courtesy of the Purdue Frederick Co., Yonkers, N.Y.)

gynecologists operating on the vulva and perineum.[92-95b] Some obstetricians and midwives want the perineum shaved but not the vulva, calling this a "mini-prep."

Skin preparation is begun on the surgical unit and completed in the operating room immediately before the surgical incision is made. The location and extent of the area to be prepared depend upon the impending operation and the preferences of the surgeon. Figure 47-4 shows typical skin areas prepared for some specific operations. If the operation is new or nurses are unfamiliar with their preferences, surgeons may use a diagram of the body part and shade the area they want prepared.

There are different opinions on what constitutes effective skin preparation. However, most surgeons direct that the area be shaved and the skin cleaned with soap and water on the evening before the day of the operation. A topical bactericidal agent is applied in the operating room just before the incision is made. Erle E. Peacock,[96] writing in the American College of Surgeons' *Manual of Preoperative and Postoperative Care,* recommends a 2 per cent solution of iodine and alcohol as a most effective bactericidal agent. (For other discussions of skin disinfection, see Chapters 14, 33, and 43.)

Care should be taken to protect the patient's privacy, and certain esthetic considerations are also important. For example, it is considerate to postpone shaving the head (if this is necessary) until the patient gets to the operating room and preferably until the patient is anesthetized. Peacock says, "Loss of hair is associated with loss of dignity, and the few extra minutes required to prepare the scalp after the patient is asleep is a thoughtful gesture that most surgeons can afford to make in the interest of preventing embarrassment." * Peacock advocates shaving rather than clipping the hair but says that care should be exercised to avoid abrasions. If the skin is nicked or cut, the lesion should be treated with an antiseptic to reduce the possibility of infection. Inspection of the general condition of the skin for evidence of abrasions and unclean areas are points to be emphasized. In rare cases, body lice and pubic lice are present and must, of course, be eliminated before a person is sent to the operating room. It may sometimes be difficult to thoroughly clean the skin of patients who have not bathed for a long time, but irritating substances and stiff brushes must be avoided. Special preparation extending over

* Peacock, Erle E., Jr.: "Wound Healing and Care of the Wound," in American College of Surgeons: *Manual of Preoperative and Postoperative Care.* W. B. Saunders Co., Philadelphia, 1971, p. 5.

several days may be prescribed by the surgeon for some operations such as skin grafts and orthopedic procedures.

In surgery of the eye, nose, throat, and genitourinary and alimentary tracts, where mucous membrane predominates, the problem of preparing the site of operation is one of trying to make the operative field clean rather than sterile. The surgeon writes specific directions for the preparation of these areas, or a routine is set up on these special services for particular operations.

Promoting Sleep and Rest. Preoperative medication is a much discussed subject. It is generally agreed that a good night's rest before the day of operation is important. Sometimes pain may interfere with sleep, but in most cases the control of anxiety is all that is necessary. Many surgeons recommend one of the barbiturates the night before the operation. Morphine, if used at all, is reserved for preanesthetic medication. Because of the harmful effects of morphine, some surgeons urge the substitution of other drugs unless control of pain is the first and foremost consideration. Many persons have an idiosyncratic response to morphine, as, for example, nausea and vomiting. Patients should be asked whether they have ever had morphine and if so how it affects them. The second author saw an elderly patient die from what was thought to be the effect of a single average dose of morphine sulfate. Nurses should use every art at their disposal to promote sleep and rest preoperatively. Chapter 13 discusses these arts; a repetition here seems unnecessary.

Preparation for Postoperative Exercises. Respiratory and circulatory complications following surgery continue to be of concern for surgeons, anesthetists, and nurses.[97-99] It is generally believed that the incidence of such complications might be reduced by postoperative exercises that will help patients in clearing the trachea and bronchi of mucus secretions that promote pulmonary ventilation, and ones that discourage sluggish circulation leading to excess blood, or venous stasis, in the lower extremities. It is important that nurses help patients understand the importance of postoperative exercises and learn how to do them before the operation. If people learn the exercises in the preoperative period, they will be better able to attend to directions in the postoperative period when they are likely to be "groggy" from the anesthesia and also distracted by various discomforts.

Deep breathing, coughing, turning, and leg and foot movements make up the basic exercises. Equipment used (such as respirators for positive pressure breathing), procedures for the exercises, and teaching methods vary. It is important that nurses who provide preoperative care be familiar with the purposes and methods for the exercises and see that the patient is able to do them whether or not they will be with the patient during the postoperative period. Figure 47-5 shows a nurse teaching leg and foot movements preoperatively that are shown in an illustrated pamphlet given the patient. Ideally, patients should be taught by those nurses or other personnel (i.e., inhalation therapists) who will be responsible for this aspect of their care during the postoperative period. The merits of the postoperative exercises are discussed in the professional literature [100-103] and studies testing various approaches for their relative effectiveness are being undertaken by nurses.[104,105] See Chapter 48 for a more detailed discussion of the postoperative exercises.

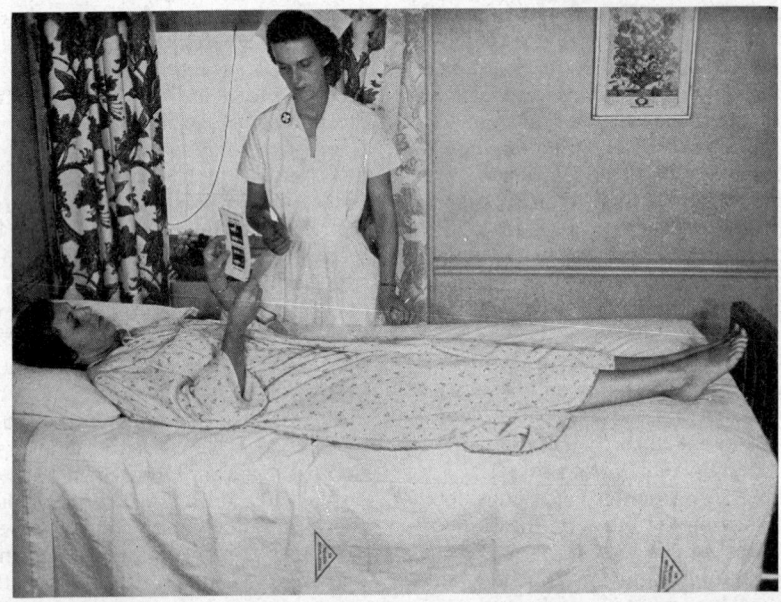

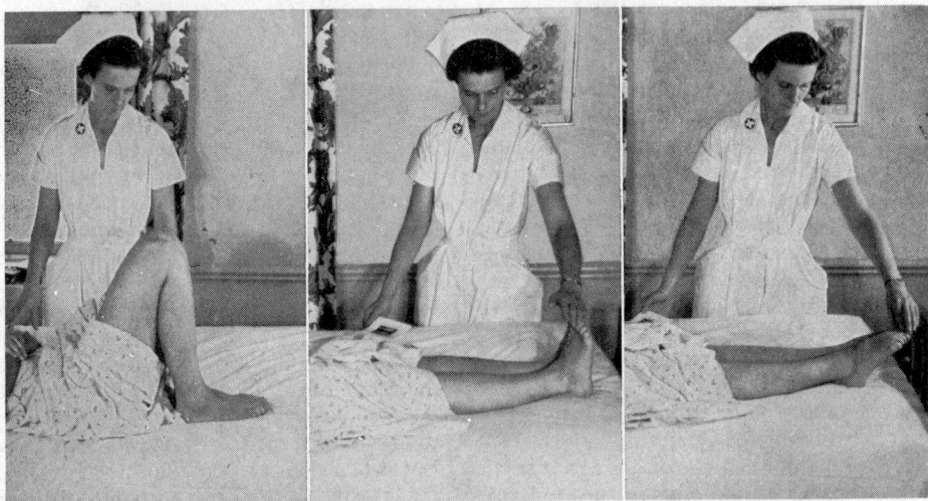

Figure 47-5. (*Top*) A patient looking at illustrations of the exercises she will be asked to do postoperatively. (*Bottom*) The nurse supervises: the first exercise is flexion of the knees, the second is flexion of the ankles and toes, and the third is extension of the ankles and toes. (Courtesy of Columbia–Presbyterian Medical Center, New York, N.Y., and Clay-Adams Co., New York, N.Y.)

6. STEPS TO BE TAKEN JUST BEFORE SURGERY

Final Observations of Patient's Condition. On the morning of the operation, the body temperature, pulse, and respiratory rates are assessed and recorded as usual. If the body temperature is elevated, it is reported to the doctor. When "taking" the temperature, nurses look for any sign of a cold, sore throat, or obstruction of breathing. Some surgeons postpone surgery, even at the last hour, if there are symptoms of an upper respiratory infection.

It is expected that most patients will be somewhat nervous or anxious just before surgery. However, any unusual nervousness or emotional distress should be reported. The operating room nursing staff should report immediately any change in the hour set for the operation so that patients may stay in their rooms or wards as long as possible. Nothing makes a person so nervous and fearful as waiting in the anterooms or corridors of the operating suite for an undue length of time.

Nurses in charge of the preoperative patient know that their patient is scheduled for surgery at a particular time; they should plan their work accordingly. Early morning hours are considered desirable for operations, but it is not possible to give everyone this advantage. Patients should not be made ready too far in advance of a midmorning or afternoon operation. Judgment and experience are required for accurate timing of nursing procedures, and consideration of the patient should have precedence over hospital routines.

Grooming and Dressing. Ordinarily patients have *preoperative baths* the day before, but additional bathing, which does not interfere with the prepared area or unduly tire the patient, is often relaxing. *The hair* should be combed and arranged in a comfortable style. Hair is most easily controlled and tangles are prevented by braiding. Hair that is long enough can be arranged in two braids, one on each side of the head. Shorter hair, if braided, requires more braids using smaller portions of hair. Close-cropped hair styles may be too short for braids and should be combed and brushed thoroughly. All pins, combs, and clips must be removed because of the danger of their sticking into the patient while he or she is unconscious.

While the hair is being combed, even though an inspection for head lice has previously been made, further examination is indicated in some cases. This can be done tactfully and without the knowledge of the patient. It is not safe to depend on the social position of a person as a criterion for the necessity of this inspection. Even well-groomed persons may accidentally be infested.

Wigs or hairpieces should be removed before the patient leaves the unit and stored according to the hospital's policy for the care of valuables. Most hospitals provide turbans or towels for patients to wear to the operating room. These serve the double purpose of preventing the straying of loose hair in the operating room and of keeping the patient's hair clean and in place during the operation. If the hair is not covered before the patient leaves the clinical unit, the anesthetist will wrap the hair in a towel.

Clothing worn to the operating room varies, but a clean hospital gown is generally worn. If the legs must be put in stirrups (as in operations on the pelvis) leggings are used. Actually, there is room for improvement in the way patients are dressed for surgery from the standpoint of esthetics, ease in changing garments, and in protecting the body from exposure and chilling.

Because the color of the face, lips, and nailbeds is watched carefully by the anesthetist for cyanosis and signs of oxygen want during surgery, patients are asked to remove facial makeup and nail polish.

Protection of Valuable Belongings. Although it is the policy in most hospital divisions to ask patients to send valuable articles home or to put them in the hospital safe, they may elect to keep such things as small amounts of money, a watch, a clock, or a ring. These must be protected. Since most patients who wear a wedding ring wish to keep it on, the common practice is to secure it with a strip of adhesive tape.

All other valuable articles should be put in an envelope on which is written the patient's name, room number or unit, and the date. In some cases the envelope is left with the nurse administrator, who places it in a locked drawer or cabinet in his or her office. In other instances it is put in the hospital safe until the patient can again assume responsibility for his or her possessions.

Valuable articles are lost in hospitals from time to time; their loss and replacement cause embarrassment and expense to the personnel and hospital authorities. Every precaution should be taken to prevent such losses.

Before a patient is anesthetized, false teeth, detachable bridges, and chewing gum must be removed. This should be done when the mouth is cleaned shortly before the patient is transferred. Some anesthetists now prefer that plates be left in the mouth because, when the cheeks are filled, the mask used in administering the anesthetic fits more snugly, and the anesthetic is given more easily. An occasional patient will have artificial teeth that look removable but actually are not. Plates and bridges should be recorded on the chart and called to the attention of the anesthetist, since a valuable denture may be broken if the anesthetist tries to remove it when the patient is too drowsy to explain or protest. The presence of loose teeth also should be noted on the chart.

Good care should be taken of dentures, contact lenses, artificial eyes, and other protheses which must be removed before an operation. These articles are costly. They should be wrapped and labeled in the event that the patient is to be transferred to another unit postoperatively. If the patient is to return to his or her original unit, these articles should be left in suitable places. Dentures are stored in covered containers.* Most institutions supply special disposable denture cups. An artificial eye may also be taken care of in this way, provided that gauze or cotton is used to line the container to prevent scratching, chipping, or breaking. All articles in the room or unit that might be damaged or lost or that might injure patients while they are unconscious are removed. A satisfactory explanation should be given patients so that they will understand why valuables, for example, a wristwatch, are taken away temporarily. Since little things of this kind seem to make a great difference, every effort should be made to consider patients' wishes.

Removal of Urine from the Bladder. The bladder should be emptied 5 to 15 minutes before patients leave the unit, to prevent both the possibility of their voiding on the operating table and an accidental puncture of a distended bladder if there is an abdominal operation.

Sometimes patients may be unable to void before they are transferred to the operating room. Catheterization in some cases is necessary but should be avoided if possible. To prevent delay in getting the patient to the operating room, one should determine the necessity for catheterization in advance of the appointed time for transfer. Some surgeons prefer to have the catheterization done in the operating room so that they may be assured that the bladder is empty. The use and serious dangers of catheterization, especially those from indwelling catheters, were discussed in Chapter 24.

Preliminary Medication. Preanesthetic medication is used to allay anxiety, to inhibit certain undesirable reflexes during anesthesia (such as gagging, coughing, and swallowing), to dry up secretions, and, in general, to promote a state of relaxation in preparation for the anesthesia. The drugs chosen depend a great deal on the age and condition of the patient and the type of anesthetic to be used. For example, narcotics are frequently given when Pentothal or nitrous oxide is used. However, narcotics are avoided for the very young and the elderly patient. Kathleen Shafer and associates [106] point out that older patients are often given chloral hydrate, ethinamate (Valmid), or glutethimide (Doriden); atropine alone is the drug usually ordered for infants. Occasionally, antibiotics are given for their prophylactic effect.

For their sedative effects, the barbiturates are often used. Pentobarbital (Nembutal) or secobarbital (Seconal Sodium) are frequently prescribed. Tranquilizers such as diazepam or hydroxyzine may be given intramuscularly. Narcotics—morphine or meperidine (Demerol)—are used primarily to reduce metabolism and make for easier anesthetic induction. One of the belladonna derivatives may be used to reduce secretions in the mouth and respiratory tract and to limit reflexes. Atropine is the most commonly used drug in this category. Some of the new anesthetics do not stimulate secretions and atropine is not always given. When used, atropine is administered with one of the barbiturates, an opiate, or a tranquilizer, not less than 30 minutes before the operation. Beecher, who studied the care of wounded men in World War II, proposed that morphine be reserved for the person in severe pain. He said:

> Morphine is not to be used to treat the restlessness arising from fear, apprehension, a confused mental state, anoxia, anemia, low blood volume, low blood pressure, hemorrhage or shock.
> . . . The outstanding effect of overdose with morphine is respiratory depression with anoxia. This is followed by circulatory damage. Less severe poisoning than the above, even therapeutic doses, often complicates treatment of the patient. Morphine by causing anorexia, nausea and vomiting limits the intake of food and fluids by mouth and increases fluid loss in vomitus and sweat. (Its needless use in shock is to be condemned.) Severe constipation is produced.*

Beecher went on to say that if the circulation is sluggish, absorption of morphine given intramuscularly or subcutaneously may be delayed and its action may be most marked during surgical operations when depression of the

---

* It is desirable to store dentures submerged in water (or a dilute mouthwash), since the composition of the material in which teeth are set may get brittle or warp if subjected to dry atmospheres. (See Chapter 14.)

* Beecher, Henry K.: *Early Care of the Seriously Wounded Man: The Management of Traumatic Shock.* Charles C Thomas, Publisher, Springfield, Ill., 1949, p. 23.

respiration is decidedly dangerous. He advocated the intravenous administration of morphine when pain demands it and suggested that not more than 15 mg (¼ gr) be given. He thought its maximum analgesic effect is produced by 10 mg (⅙ gr). Another objection to morphine is the well-known idiosyncrasy that the very young and elderly have to this drug. Today nurses will find surgeons substituting for morphine preoperatively such drugs as pentobarbital (Nembutal), amobarbital (Amytal), secobarbital (Seconal), or meperidine (Demerol). There is general agreement that some drug that makes patients less aware of what is happening should be used. In this detached state, the anesthetic can be given much more easily; also, their memory of events preceding the operation will not be so vivid.

After patients are given sedatives, they should be quiet. If a member of the family or a close friend is present, the importance of allowing the drug to act should be explained in order to discourage conversation.

Emotional Support for Patient's Family. As the time for the operation grows close, the anxiety level of patients and their families usually rises. Things that might seem trivial at other times take on greater significance to patients who are awaiting operations. They are very likely to misinterpret what they see and hear and very often take strange bodily sensations like dryness of the mouth and dizziness to mean that something is seriously wrong with them. A grimace or frown on the face of the nurse while taking their blood pressure might make patients think that their blood pressure is abnormal. It is very important, therefore, that nurses be aware of these possibilities and that they provide patients and their families with the needed support and reassurance. A simple explanation that the preoperative medication causes dryness and why this is necessary might be very reassuring to the worried patient. In many cases there are unavoidable periods of waiting either on the unit or in the operative suite—a waiting period between the time patients have the last-minute preparation on the clinical unit and the time that they are taken to the operative suite, or between the time that they arrive in the operating suite and the time that the operation is begun. Waiting may be almost unbearable to patients and to relatives who have come to be with them. Every minute seems like an hour; often they cannot gauge time or find any but tragic explanations for the delay. One of the kindest things nurses can do is to learn why there is the delay so that they can inform and encourage patients and their relatives. Sometimes an operation takes longer than was ex-

pected or for some other reason the patient stays in the operating room longer than was anticipated. If nurses can learn how things are progressing, they can explain and encourage waiting relatives. It does not matter so much whether the nurse administrator, staff nurse, special nurse, or student does this so long as it is done effectively. Hospital regulations and duties may determine who will do it. Tact, good judgment, and real sympathy are needed. Some hospitals have gone so far as to allow a member of the family or a close friend to go to the operating suite with the patient. They also provide sitting rooms where the family can wait during the operation, and members of the operating room staff see that reports are relayed from time to time on the progress of the operation and the patient's condition. Whatever the approach, emotional support for patient and family is a very vital part of the preoperative and operative regimen.

Transporting Patients to Operative Site. Modern hospital construction and equipment allow patients to be transferred to the operating room in their beds—a very comfortable, expedient method. In such cases the bed can be warmed and protected while the operation is proceeding, and at its completion, the patient need be moved only once. Many hospitals, however, still use stretchers. Nurses should remember that the preoperative medication may make patients lightheaded or dizzy and therefore uncertain of themselves on a narrow stretcher. Medicated patients have most disagreeable sensations when they are wheeled down a corridor, when the stretcher is pushed into an elevator, or when it accidentally bumps into something. There is no remedy for the sensations, but it helps to have stretchers that can be easily steered, handled by attendants strong enough to manage them and move them at an even pace. Sudden stops should be avoided. The elevator should be precisely at floor level, and neither started nor stopped with a jerk. Whenever the stretcher must be pushed up or down an incline, patients should be warned, if they are awake. In any event, the stretcher should be steadied. It is a regulation in most hospitals to strap patients to the stretcher in going to or returning from the operating room.

Fear and premedication (especially narcotics) may cause nausea; therefore, the nurse who accompanies the patient to the operating room should provide squares of soft paper and a basin. Paper handkerchiefs are useful for patients who perspire excessively, as is often the case when morphine is administered. A paper bag for waste should be at hand.

It may be inappropriate for nurses to discuss

the operation with patients while transferring them or to talk to patients who obviously want to be undisturbed; nurses should, however, explain to patients what will happen during the transfer, step by step. Unexpected motion is disagreeable enough when one is fully conscious, and may be highly disturbing to the confused mind of the drugged patient. In most hospitals, orderlies transport patients to the operating room, but it is desirable to have a nurse or an anesthetist known to the patient in constant attendance.

Hospital facilities should include, when possible, waiting or anesthesia rooms that can be quiet and comfortable. Even if such provision has not been made, thoughtful nurses can do a great deal to bring about these conditions wherever patients must wait.

Whenever possible, nurses should watch the operation performed on their patients in order that they may be better prepared to care for them. Complications may be encountered; emergencies may occur; or, the diagnosis leading to surgery may be changed after the surgeon's exploration; operative findings will be known which may mean that nurses can take more intelligent postoperative care of the patient.

7. RECORDS OF PREOPERATIVE CARE AND SURGERY

Recording Preoperative Care. All significant procedures entering into the preparation of patients for operations are recorded on their charts: for example, nurses note a cleansing enema, *if given;* the time and amount of last voiding; the way in which the area of operation was treated; the administration of prescribed medication; and the time at which patients were taken to the operating room. They also note the presence of dentures in the mouth and they record any symptoms or reactions of patients that might influence the administration of the anesthesia or the operative procedure. The patient's record is sent to the operating room with him or her.

Recording the Operation. All reputable hospitals require anesthetists to make a full written report of the administration of the anesthetic and all surgeons to make an equally detailed report of the operative procedure. Throughout the operation, data are recorded by appointed members of the departmental staff, and immediately after the operation, the anesthetist and the surgeon incorporate them into a formal written report. Sample forms of operative reports are shown in Chapter 48. The surgeon's postoperative orders and the

patient's chart are sent to the clinical division with him or her; the operative report is added to the patient's record within a few hours. The medical and nursing staff assigned to the care of the patient should be familiar with the contents of these reports if they expect to give the most effective care. The legal implications of record-keeping were discussed in Chapter 4. Surgical records are among the most critical, or among those most likely to be used in lawsuits.

REFERENCES

1. Williams, Lawrence B.: *How to Avoid Unnecessary Surgery.* Nash Publishing Co., Los Angeles, 1971.
2. Richardson, Robert G.: *Surgery: Old and New Frontiers.* Charles Scribner's Sons, New York, 1968.
3. Wakeley, Sir Cecil: "The Changing Face of Surgery," *Lancet,* **249:**6641, (Dec.) 1950.
4. Reisfeld, Ralph A., and Kahan, Barry D.: "Markers of Biological Individuality," *Sci. Am.,* **226:**28, (June) 1972.
5. Rand, Robert W., and Mosso, James A.: "Ferromagnetic Silicone Vascular Occlusion in a Superconducting Magnetic Field: Preliminary Report," *Bull. Los Angeles Neurol. Soc.,* **37:**67, (Apr.) 1972.
6. "Microsurgery in Japan," *Time Magazine,* (Feb. 19) 1973, p. 68.
7. Furnas, D. W.: "Growth and Development in Replanted Forelimbs," *Plast. Reconstr. Surg.,* **46:**445, (Nov.) 1970.
8. Horn, J. S.: "The Reattachment of Severed Extremities," in Apley, A. Graham (ed.): *Recent Advances in Orthopedics.* Williams & Wilkins Co., Baltimore, 1969, p. 49.
9. Knill-Jones, R. P., et al.: "Use of Sequential Bayesian Model in Diagnosis of Jaundice by Computer," *Br. Med. J.,* **1:**530, (Mar. 3) 1973.
10. Williams, Lawrence B.: *op. cit.*
11. Gerber, Alex: "Surgical Pros and Cons," *Surg. Gynecol. Obstet.,* **135:**431, (Sept.) 1972.
12. Knowles, John H.: "Surgical Pros and Cons," *Surg. Gynecol. Obstet.,* **135:**432, (Sept.) 1972.
13. Ilgenfritz, Hugh C.: *Preoperative and Postoperative Care of Surgical Patients.* C. V. Mosby Co., St. Louis, 1948, pp. 103, 108.
14. Eckenhoff, J. E.: "Some Preoperative Warnings of Potential Operating-room Deaths," *N. Engl. J. Med.,* **255:**1075, (Dec. 6) 1956.
15. Janis, Irving L.: *Psychological Stress.* John Wiley & Sons, New York, 1958.
16. Egbert, L., et al.: "Reduction of Postoperative Pain by Encouragement and Instruction of Patients," *N. Engl. J. Med.,* **270:**825, (Apr. 16) 1964.
17. Dumas, Rhetaugh G., and Leonard, Robert: "The Effect of Nursing on the Incidence of

Postoperative Vomiting," *Nurs. Res.,* **12:**12, (Winter) 1963.

18. Downs, H.: "The Control of Vomiting," *Am. J. Nurs.,* **66:**76, (Jan.) 1966.

19. Carnevali, Doris: "Preoperative Anxiety," *Am. J. Nurs.,* **66:**1536, (July) 1966.

19a. Felton, G., et al.: "Preoperative Nursing Intervention with the Patient for Surgery, Outcomes of Three Alternative Approaches," *Int. J. Nurs. Stud.,* **13:**83, 1976.

20. Healy, Kathryn: "Does Preoperative Instruction Make a Difference?" *Am. J. Nurs.,* **68:**62, (Jan.) 1968.

21. Johnson, Barbara, et al.: "Research in Nursing Practice: The Problem of Uncontrolled Situational Variables," *Nurs. Res.,* **19:**337, (July–Aug.) 1970.

22. Johnson, Jean, et al.: "Psychosocial Factors in the Welfare of Surgical Patients," *Nurs. Res.,* **19:**18, (Jan.–Feb.) 1970.

23. ————: "Contribution of Emotional and Instrumental Response Processes in Adaptation to Surgery," *J. Pers. Soc. Psychol.,* **20:**55, (Oct.) 1971.

24. Lindeman, Carol: "Nursing Intervention with the Presurgical Patient: The Effectiveness and Efficiency of Group and Individual Preoperative Teaching," Monograph, Luther Hospital, Eau Claire, Wis., 1971 (*Nurs. Res.,* **21:**196, [May–June] 1972).

25. ————, and Van Aernam, Betty: "Nursing Intervention with the Presurgical Patient: The Effects of Structured and Unstructured Preoperative Teaching," *Nurs. Res.,* **20:**319, (July–Aug.) 1971.

26. Dumas, Rhetaugh G., and Johnson, Barbara A.: "Research in Nursing Practice: A Review of Five Clinical Experiments," *Int. J. Nurs. Stud.,* **9:**137, (Aug.) 1972.

27. Shetler, Mary: "Operating Room Nurses Go Visiting," *Am. J. Nurs.,* **72:**1266, (July) 1972.

28. Wolfer, John A., and Davis, Carol E.: "Assessment of Surgical Patients' Preoperative Emotional Condition and Postoperative Welfare," *Nurs. Res.,* **15:**402, (Sept.–Oct.) 1970.

28a. "The Sexes. Prisoners of Sex," *Time Magazine,* (Jan. 21) 1974, p. 63.

29. Pauly, I. B.: "Current Status of the Change of Sex Operation," *J. Nerv. Ment. Dis.,* **147:**460, (Nov.) 1968.

30. Erickson Educational Foundation: *Legal Aspects of Transsexualism and Information on Administrative Procedures,* rev. ed. The Foundation, Baton Rouge, La., 1972.

31. Anonymous: "My Daughter Changed Sex," *Good Housekeeping,* (May) 1973.

32. Stinson, B.: "A Study of Twelve Applicants for Transsexual Surgery," *Ohio State Med. J.,* **68:**245, (Mar.) 1972.

33. Benjamin, Harry, and Ihlenfeld, Charles L.: "Transsexualism," *Am. J. Nurs.,* **73:**457, (Mar.) 1973.

34. Lockwood, Nancy: "The Effect of Situational Doll Play upon Preoperative Stress Reactions of Hospitalized Children," in *ANA Clinical Sessions, 1970.* Appleton-Century-Crofts, New York, 1971.

35. Condon, Sherrilyn R.: "Day-Time Hospital for Children," *Am. J. Nurs.,* **72:**1431, (Aug.) 1972.

36. Epstein, Burton S., et al.: "Outpatient Surgery, Guidelines for Organization of Unit and for Selection of Patient and Surgical Procedure," *Hospitals,* **47:**80, (Sept. 1) 1973.

37. Edelson, Edward: "The New 'Come-and-Go' Surgery," *Fam. Health,* (Sept.) 1973, p. 41.

38. "One-Day Surgery—An Economical, Fast, Less Worrisome Approach to Hospital Stays," *Health Care Today,* (July–Aug.) 1973, p. 1.

39. Wakeley, Sir Cecil: *op. cit.*

40. Leininger, Madeleine: "Becoming Aware of Types of Health Practitioners and Cultural Imposition," in *Becoming Aware of Cultural Differences in Nursing.* American Nurses' Association, Kansas City, Mo., 1972, p. 9.

40a. Jefferson, Roland: "The Psychiatric Assessment of Candidates for Cosmetic Surgery," *J. Nat. Med. Assoc.,* **68:**411, (Sept.) 1976.

41. Anderson, Gwen, and Tighe, Bridget: "Gypsy Culture and Health Care," *Am. J. Nurs.,* **73:**282, (Feb.) 1973.

42. Gonzalez, Hector Hugo: "Health Beliefs of Some Mexican-Americans," in *Becoming Aware of Cultural Differences in Nursing.* American Nurses' Association, Kansas City, Mo., 1972, p. 1.

43. Mosley, Doris: "The Experience of Some Blacks with the Health Care System," in *Becoming Aware of Cultural Differences in Nursing.* American Nurses' Association, Kansas City, Mo., 1972, p. 7.

44. Seidenfeld, Morton A.: *Psychological Aspects of Nursing Care.* Charles C Thomas, Publisher, Springfield, Ill., 1946, p. 123.

44a. Janis, Irving L.: *op. cit.*

44b. Henderson, Arthur R.: "Psychology of Hospitalized Patients," *J. Nat. Med. Assoc.,* **68:** 378, (Sept.) 1976.

45. Rhoads, Jonathan E., et al.: *Surgery: Principles and Practice,* 4th ed. J. B. Lippincott Co., Philadelphia, 1970, p. 246.

46. *Ibid.*

46a. Haller, D. M., et al.: "Anesthetizing the Drug Abuser," *J. Am. Assoc. Nurse Anesth.,* **40:**227, (Aug.) 1972.

47. Creighton, Helen: *Law Every Nurse Should Know,* 3rd ed. W. B. Saunders Co., Philadelphia, 1975.

48. Murchison, Irene A., and Nichols, Thomas S.: *Legal Foundations of Nursing Practice.* Macmillan Publishing Co., Inc., New York, 1970.

49. Creighton, Helen: *op. cit.*

50. Murchison, Irene A., and Nichols, Thomas S.: *op. cit.*

51. *Medical Malpractice.* Report of the Secretary's Commission on Medical Malpractice, US Department of Health, Education, and Welfare. US Government Printing Office, Washington, D.C., Jan. 1973, p. 8.

52. Lewis, Howard R., and Lewis, Martha: ". . . And Surgeons Go Astray," in *The Medical Offenders*. Simon & Schuster, New York, 1970, p. 207.

53. Hayt, Emanuel: "A Signed Permit for Surgery Is Safest," *Hospitals,* **24**:56, (June) 1950.

54. Varco, Richard L.: "Principles of Preoperative and Postoperative Care," in Davis, Loyal (ed.): *Christopher's Textbook of Surgery,* 9th ed. W. B. Saunders Co., Philadelphia, 1968, p. 173.

55. Gilchrist, R. K.: Surgery of the Colon and Rectum," in American College of Surgeons: *Manual of Preoperative and Postoperative Care.* W. B. Saunders Co., Philadelphia, 1967, p. 346.

56. Paulson, John A., and Lundy, John S.: "Anesthesia," *Annu. Rev. Med.,* **1**:303, 1950.

57. Beecher, Henry K.: *Early Care of the Seriously Wounded Man.* Charles C Thomas, Publisher, Springfield, Ill., 1952, p. 26.

58. Dripps, Robert D., et al.: *Introduction to Anesthesia: The Principles of Safe Practice,* 4th ed. W. B. Saunders Co., Philadelphia, 1972, p. 130.

59. *Ibid.,* p. 130.

60. *Ibid.,* p. 137.

61. *Ibid.,* p. 165.

61a. Conahan, Thomas J.: "New Intravenous Anesthetics," in Wollman, Harry, and Greenhow, D. Eric (eds.): *Surgical Clinics of North America; Recent Developments in Anesthesia.* W. B. Saunders Co., Philadelphia, 1975, p. 851.

62. *Ibid.,* p. 160.

62a. Conahan, Thomas J.: *op. cit.*

63. Cohen, David D., and Dillon, John B.: *Anesthesia for Out-Patient Surgery.* Charles C Thomas, Publisher, Springfield, Ill., 1970, p. 34.

64. Eckenhoff, James E., and Brunner, Edward A.: "Anesthesia," in Sabiston, David C. (ed.): *Davis-Christopher Textbook of Surgery,* 10th ed. W. B. Saunders Co., Philadelphia, 1972.

65. Lund, P. C.: *Principles and Practice of Spinal Anesthesia.* Charles C Thomas, Publisher, Springfield, Ill., 1971, p. xi.

66. *Ibid.,* p. xii.

67. *Ibid.,* p. 198.

68. Dripps, Robert D., et al.: *op. cit.,* p. 114.

69. Cohen, David D., and Dillon, John B.: *op. cit.,* p. 33.

69a. Allen, F. M.: "Reduced Temperature in Surgery; Surgery of Limbs," *Am. J. Surg.,* **52**:225, (May) 1941.

70. Segerberg, Ludwig H.: "Ice Anesthesia," *Am. J. Nurs.,* **43**:897, (Sept.) 1943.

71. Cook, Bertram: "Experience with Refrigeration Anesthesia in General Practice," *Med. J. Aust.,* **1**:467, (Apr.) 1950.

72. Brickman, R. D., et al.: "Circulatory Arrest During Profound Hypothermia for Treatment of Complicated Disease of Major Vessels," *Arch. Surg.,* **103**:259, (Aug.) 1971.

73. Matsuki, A., et al.: "Operation under Hypothermia in a Pregnant Woman with an Intracranial Arteriovenous Malformation," *Can. Anaesth. Soc. J.,* **19**:184, (Mar.) 1972.

74. Nugent, R. G.: "Prolonged Hypothermia," *Am. J. Nurs.,* **60**:967, (July) 1960.

75. Graves, Nancy: "Nursing During Prolonged Hypothermia," *Am. J. Nurs.,* **60**:969, (July) 1960.

75a. Gorman, J. F., and Rosenberg, J. C.: "Dry Ice Refrigeration for Above-Knee Amputations," *Am. J. Surg.,* **113**:241, (Feb.) 1967.

76. "Frozen Heart," *Time Magazine,* (Jan. 29) 1973, p. 44.

77. Replogle, Robert: "A Treatment of Complex Cardiac Anomaly in Infancy Using Profound Hypothermia and Cardiac Arrest," Film, University of Chicago's Wyker Children's Hospital, 950 E. 59 St., Chicago, Ill. 60637.

78. Puig, Flores J. A.: "Hypothermia and Extracorporeal Circulation in Intra-cranial Vascular Surgery," *Rev. Esp. Anestesiol. Reanim.,* **20**:74, (Jan.) 1973.

79. Banders, L. A., et al.: "Surgical Treatment of Congenital Heart in Infants with Superficial Hypothermia, Short Extra-corporeal Circulation and Circulatory Arrest," *G. Ital. Cardiol.,* **3**:165, 1973.

80. Tsybaneva, N. G., et al.: "Changes in the Electrocardiogram During Correction of Congenital Heart Defects Under Conditions of Deep Hypothermia by the Method of Surface Cooling 24–23 Degrees," *Kardiologiia,* **11**:96, (July) 1971. (English abst.)

81. Mori, A., et al.: "Deep Hypothermia Combined with Cardiopulmonary By-Pass for Cardiac Surgery in Neonates and Infants," *J. Thorac. Cardiovasc. Surg.,* **64**:45, (July) 1972.

82. Tsuiki, T., et al.: "Removal of Tracheal Adenoid Cystic Carcinoma Under Hypothermia," *Otolaryngology,* **43**:1013, (Dec.) 1971.

82a. Van Nghi, Nguyen: "Acupuncture Anesthesia," *Am. J. Chinese Med.,* **1**:135, (Jan.) 1973.

82b. Ho, Wayne Y. H., and Chen, James Y. P.: "Acupuncture Anesthesia. A Report of Two Cases," *Am. J. Chinese Med.,* **1**:151, (Jan.) 1973.

82c. Kao, Frederick F.: "China, Chinese Medicine and the Chinese Medical System," *Am. J. Chinese Med.,* **1**:1, (Jan.) 1973.

82d. Burr, H. S., and Northrop, F. S. C.: "The Electro-dynamic Theory of Life," *Q. Rev. Biol.,* **10**:322, 1935.

82e. Northrop, F. S. C., and Burr, H. S.: "Experimental Findings Concerning the Electro-dynamic Theory of Life and an Analysis of Their Physical Meaning," *Growth,* **1**:78, 1937.

83. Homann, Ralph E.: "Fluid and Electrolyte Therapy in Surgical Patients," *Am. J. Surg.,* **81**:10, (Jan.) 1951.

84. Ariel, Irving M., and Kreman, Arnold J.: "Compartmental Distribution of Sodium Chloride in Surgical Patients Pre- and Post-

operatively," *Ann. Surg.,* **132:**1009, (Dec.) 1950.

85. Randall, Henry T., et al.: "Sodium Deficiency in Surgical Patients and Failure of Urine Chloride as a Guide to Parenteral Therapy," *Surgery,* **28:**182, (Aug.) 1950.
86. Bland, John H.: *The Clinical Use of Fluid and Electrolyte.* W. B. Saunders Co., Philadelphia, 1952, p. 147.
87. Beecher, Henry K.: *Resuscitation and Anesthesia for Wounded Men: The Management of Traumatic Shock.* Charles C Thomas, Publisher, Springfield, Ill., 1949, p. 56.
88. Dudrick, S. J., et al.: "Renal Failure in Surgical Patients. Treatment with Intravenous Essential Amino Acids and Hypertonic Glucose," *Surgery,* **68:**180, (July) 1970.
89. Geyer, R. P.: "Parenteral Nutrition," *Physiol. Rev.,* **40:**150, (Jan.) 1960.
90. Meng, H. C., and Law, D. H.: *Parenteral Nutrition.* Charles C Thomas, Publisher, Springfield, Ill., 1970.
91. Varco, Richard L.: *op. cit.,* p. 183.
92. Seropian, R., and Reynolds, B. M.: "Wound Infections After Preoperative Depilatory Versus Razor Preparation," *Am. J. Surg.,* **121:**25, (Mar.) 1971.
93. Beland, Irene L., and Passos, Joyce Y.: *Clinical Nursing: Pathophysiological and Psychosocial Approaches,* 3rd ed. Macmillan Publishing Co., Inc., New York, 1975, p. 927.
94. Brunner, Lillian Sholtis, et al.: *Medical-Surgical Nursing.* J. B. Lippincott Co., Philadelphia, 1975, p. 160.
95. Dison, Norma Greenler: *An Atlas of Nursing Techniques,* 2nd ed. C. V. Mosby Co., St. Louis, 1971, p. 33.
95a. Bryant, Richard, and Overland, Anna E.: *Obstetric Management and Nursing.* F. A. Davis Co., Philadelphia, 1964, p. 222.
95b. Reeder, Sharon R., et al.: *Maternity Nursing.* J. B. Lippincott Co., Philadelphia, 1976, p. 310.
96. Peacock, Erle E., Jr.: "Wound Healing and Care of the Wound," in American College of Surgeons: *Manual of Preoperative and Postoperative Care.* W. B. Saunders Co., Philadelphia, 1971, p. 4.
97. Bendixen, H. H., et al.: *Respiratory Care.* C. V. Mosby Co., St. Louis, 1965, p. 85.
98. Varco, Richard L.: *op. cit.,* p. 191.
99. Mezzanotte, Elizabeth: "Group Instruction in Preparation for Surgery," *Am. J. Nurs.,* **70:**89, (Jan.) 1970.
100. Dripps, Robert D., and Deming, Margery: "Postoperative Atelectasis and Pneumonia," *Ann. Surg.,* **124:**94, (July) 1946.
101. Dripps, Robert D., and Walters, R. M.: "Nursing Care of Surgical Patients. 1. The Stir-up," *Am. J. Nurs.,* **41:**530, (May) 1941.
102. Healy, Kathryn: *op. cit.*
103. Lindeman, Carol, and Van Aernam, Betty: *op. cit.*
104. Healy, Kathryn: *op. cit.*
105. Lindeman, Carol, and Van Aernam, Betty: *op. cit.*
106. Shafer, Kathleen N., et al.: *Medical Surgical Nursing,* 6th ed. C. V. Mosby Co., St. Louis, 1975, p. 202.

Additional Suggested Reading

Aiken, L. H.: "Systematic Relaxation to Reduce Preoperative Stress," *Can. Nurse,* **68:**38, (June) 1972.

Berry, Edna Cornelia, and Kohn, Mary Louise: *Introduction to Operating Room Technique,* 4th ed. McGraw-Hill Book Co., New York, 1972.

Buck, Barbara, and Lee, Allen: "Amputation: Two Views," *Nurs. Clin. North Am.,* **11:**641, (Dec.) 1976.

Campbell, W. Norris: *A Nurse's Guide to Anaesthetics, Resuscitation and Intensive Care,* 6th ed. Churchill Livingstone, New York, 1975.

Cole, Warren, and Puestow, Charles (eds.): *Emergency Care: Surgical and Medical,* 7th ed. Appleton-Century-Crofts, New York, 1972.

Condon, Robert E.: *Manual of Surgical Therapeutics,* 2nd ed. Little, Brown & Co., Boston, 1972.

Devney, Ann Marie, and Kingsburgh, Barbara: "Hypothermia in Fact and Fantasy," *Am. J. Nurs.,* **72:**1424, (Aug.) 1972.

Dlin, B. M.: "Sex After Ileostomy or Colostomy," *Med. Aspects Human Sexuality,* **6:**32, (July) 1972.

Dormandy, K. M.: "Preoperative Investigation and Management During Surgery of Patients with Bleeding Disorders," *Ann. R. Coll. Surg. Engl.,* **48:**26, (Jan.) 1971.

Dundee, J. W., et al.: "Studies of Drugs Given Before Anaesthesia. XIX. The Opiates," *Br. J. Anaesth.,* **42:**54, (Jan.) 1970.

Egbert, L. E.: "Psychological Support for Surgical Patients," in Abram, H. S.: *Psychological Aspects of Surgery.* Little, Brown & Co., Boston, 1967.

Fogel, L. N.: "Outpatient Presurgical Care Conserves Inpatient Days," *Hospitals,* **43:**51, (Jan.) 1969.

Fream, W. C.: *Notes on Surgical Nursing.* E. & S. Livingstone, Edinburgh, 1971.

Friedman, R. C., et al.: "Reassessment of Homosexuality and Transsexualism," *Annu. Rev. Med.,* **27:**57, 1976.

Gabrieli, E. R.: "Computer-oriented Documentation of Surgical Patients," *Gynecol. Obstet.,* **28:**539, (Mar.) 1969.

Goulding, Erna I., and Koop, C. Everett: "The Newborn, His Response to Surgery," *Am. J. Nurs.,* **65:**84, (Oct.) 1965.

Hicks, Dorothy J.: "An Incidence Study of Pressure Sores Following Surgery," in *ANA Clinical Sessions, 1969.* Appleton-Century-Crofts, New York, 1970.

Irving, M. H., and Rishman, G. B.: "Parenteral Nutrition for the Surgical Patient. A Review of Indications and Current Practice," *Anaesthesia,* **26:**450, (Oct.) 1971.

Kapsar, P. P.: "The Preoperative Visit—O.R. Nurses and Patients Interact," *Hospitals,* **50:**87, (Apr. 16) 1976.

Kornfeld, D. S.: "Psychiatric Aspects of Patient Care in the Operating Suite and Special Areas," *Anesthesiology,* **31:**166, (Aug.) 1969.

Kowalyshyn, T. J., et al.: "A Review of the Present Status of Preoperative Hemoglobin Requirements," *Anesth. Analg. (Cleve.)* **51:**75, (Jan.–Feb.) 1972.

Lemaitre, George D., and Finnegan, Janet A.: *The Patient in Surgery. A Guide for Nurses.* W. B. Saunders Co., Philadelphia, 1970.

Levine, D. C., and Fiedler, J. P.: "Fears, Facts, and Fantasies about Pre- and Postoperative Care," *Nurs. Outlook,* **18:**26, (Feb.) 1970.

Lisboa, J. M.: "Role of the Special Care Unit Nurse in a Preoperative Teaching Program," *Nurs. Clin. North Am.,* **7:**389, (June) 1972.

Midgley, Jan, and Osterhage, Sister Ruth Ann: "Effects of Nursing Instruction and Length of Hospitalization on Postoperative Complication in Cholecystectomy Patients," *Nurs. Res.,* **22:**69, (Jan.–Feb.) 1973.

Modell, J. H., et al.: "Acupuncture Anesthesia— A Clinical Study," *Anesth. Analg. (Cleve.),* **55:**508, (July–Aug.) 1976.

Morbidelli, R., et al.: "The Behavior of the Hospitalized Child Awaiting a Surgical Operation," *Minerva Pediatr.,* **27:**79, (Jan. 28) 1975. (Eng. abstr.)

Morris, Jan: *Conundrum.* [Autobiographical Account of Changing from a Man to a Woman.] Harcourt Brace Jovanovich, New York, 1974.

Morrison, J. D.: "Studies of Drugs Given Before Anaesthesia. XXII. Phenoperidine and Fentanyl, Alone and in Combination with Droperidol," *Br. J. Anaesth.,* **42:**1119, (Dec.) 1970.

Morrison, J. D., et al.: "Studies of Drugs Given Before Anaesthesia. XXI. Droperidol," *Br. J. Anaesth.,* **42:**730, (Aug.) 1970.

Nichols, R. L., and Condon, R. E.: "Antibiotic Preparation of the Colon: Failure of Commonly Used Regimens," *Surg. Clin. North Am.,* **51:**223, (Feb.) 1971.

Pauser, G., et al.: "Clinical and Experimental Results with Acupuncture Analgesia," *Anaesthetist,* **25:**215, (May) 1976. (Eng. abstr.)

Pockley, E. V.: "The Pros and Cons of Microsurgery," *Trans. Ophthalmol. Soc. NZ,* **28:**101, 1976.

Polycratis, G. S., et al.: "Preoperative Preparation of the Patient in Different Fields of Surgery. A Greek Panel Reports," *Int. Surg.,* **51:**277, (Apr.) 1969.

"Preoperative and Postoperative Physiotherapy," *Lancet,* **2:**646, (Sept. 26) 1970.

Rose, R. A.: "Effective One-day Colon Preparation for Colonoscopy and Polypectomy," *Hawaii Med. J.,* **35:**199, (July) 1976.

Roseman, D. L.: "Improving the Survival of the Critically Ill Surgical Patient," *Surg. Clin. North Am.,* **50:**517, (Apr.) 1970.

Ryan, D. W.: "A Questionnaire Survey of Preoperative Fears," *Br. J. Clin. Pract.,* **29:**3, (Jan.) 1975.

Scahill, M.: "Preparing Children for Procedures and Operations," *Nurs. Outlook,* **17:**36, (June) 1969.

Schmitt, Florence E., and Wooldridge, Powhatan J.: "Psychological Preparation of Surgical Patients," *Nurs. Res.,* **22:**108, (Mar.–Apr.) 1973.

Shaw, J.: "Volunteers Prepare Children for Surgery Through Puppet Therapy," *Mod. Hosp.,* **114:**126, (June) 1970.

Shetler, M. G.: "Operating Room Nurses Go Visiting," *Am. J. Nurs.,* **72:**1266, (July) 1972.

Shine, K. I.: "Preoperative Cardiac Evaluation," *Urol. Clin. North Am.,* **3:**217, (June) 1976.

Shojania, A. M.: "Preoperative Bleeding and Clotting Time," *Can. Med. Assoc. J.,* **100:**1061, (June 14) 1969.

Smith, Dorothy W., et al.: *Care of the Adult Patient—Medical Surgical Nursing,* 3rd ed. J. B. Lippincott Co., Philadelphia, 1971.

Smith, Stephanie Hamilton: *Nil by Mouth? A Descriptive Study of Nursing Care in Relation to Preoperative Fasting.* Royal College of Nursing and National Council of Nurses of the United Kingdom, London, 1973.

Sovie, Margaret D., and Fruehan, C. Thomas: "Protecting the Patient from Electrical Hazards," *Nurs. Clin. North Am.,* **7:**469, (Sept.) 1972.

"Symposium on Current Surgical Nursing," *Nurs. Clin. North Am.,* **8:**107, (Mar.) 1973. (Series of eight papers on special operative procedures.)

Watson, Jeannette E.: *Medical Surgical Nursing and Related Physiology.* W. B. Saunders Co., Philadelphia, 1972.

Wilson, W. E.: "Preoperative Anxiety and Anesthesia: Their Relation," *Anesth. Analg. (Cleve.),* **48:**605, (July–Aug.) 1969.

Young, D. D., et al.: "Preparing a Patient for Surgery: Consent, Information, and Emotional Support," *Clin. Obstet. Gynecol.,* **19:**431, (June) 1976.

Rhetaugh G. Dumas
Virginia Henderson

CHAPTER 48

The Postoperative State

1. INTRODUCTION

Phases of the Postoperative State. The postoperative period is often thought of as the time immediately following the end of the operation. It does begin then, but continues through recovery from surgical trauma and until the patient is rehabilitated to as wide a range of normal activities as possible. The *immediate postoperative* or *postanesthetic* phase is a critical period, with possible complications of asphyxia and respiratory or circulatory collapse. All patients, therefore, who have had a general anesthetic should have close and continuous observation. Patients who have had spinal or epidural anesthesia also should have constant observation until the effects of the sympathetic block have worn off, complete sensation has returned, and the danger of circulatory collapse is past (approximately 2 to 4 hours). In addition, many anesthetists recommend placing under constant postanesthetic observation patients who have topical or local anesthetics for respiratory tract examinations or cardiac catheterizations.

Recovery from general anesthesia may take anywhere from 30 minutes to 5 hours. It has been called the "twilight zone" because patients are neither fully anesthetized nor fully awake. During this time their protective reflexes are only partially present. For example, normal vasoconstrictor responses to movement and pain are lessened. Respiration may be inhibited by the aftereffects of neuromuscular blocking drugs, or by obstruction or aspiration because of inactive gag reflexes.[1]

One type of anesthetic reported to have little or no adverse effect on the protective reflexes is acupuncture. Acupuncture, which is not widely used in the Western world, is actually hypoalgesia because the patient's pain threshold is raised while consciousness and other sensations are not altered.[2] (Acupuncture is discussed in Chapter 47 as well as other methods of producing anesthesia.) According to E. Grey Dimond,[3] some mild postoperative reactions to acupuncture have been seen. A Chinese anesthetist at Peking Medical College who used acupuncture anesthesia for approximately 4900 patients has reported slight soreness and moderate bruising (ecchymosis) at the needle sites with some patients. The same anesthetist also noted an increase in white cells and an increase in pulse rate, without a rise in temperature, following acupuncture with many patients.

Recovery from surgical trauma occurs in what may be called the second postoperative phase. During this time, the wound heals and body systems return to normal function. The length of time required to complete this phase varies with patients' ages, their past and present physical conditions, the type and extent of surgery performed, and the type and quality of medical and nursing care. The majority of surgical patients have "uneventful" recoveries or do not require heroic life-saving measures. Later sections of this chapter discuss nursing care that promotes optimal functioning of body systems so recovery from the surgery proceeds as smoothly and quickly as possible.

Although *rehabilitation* of an ill or injured

person is often thought of as a third stage of recovery, the authors have continually emphasized throughout these pages that rehabilitation should begin as soon as care is started. Rehabilitation of postsurgical, or any other, patients involves preventing unnecessary damage to operative, injured, or diseased tissues, preventing deterioration of apparently uninvolved tissues and organs, and helping patients to modify or return to as normal a life as possible. (See Chapters 8 and 17.) Many times nurses caring for surgical patients in the postanesthetic period are unaware of ways they might help patients with rehabilitation. "Stir-up" * regimens, usually a routine part of postanesthetic care, are early rehabilitative measures since they promote better functioning of respiratory and cardiovascular systems—preventing pneumonia and thrombi. During the time patients are recovering from the surgery they can start many activities they perform without help at home. For instance, a person who has had a colostomy must learn how to care for the stoma (artificial anus); a person having transsexual surgery must learn to act like persons of the other sex. Men or women who have lost a leg must be helped to work through their grief over the mutilation of their body and to develop muscular strength for and skill in using crutches.

Recovery Rooms and Intensive Care Units. The *purpose* of a recovery room is to provide an area where postanesthetic patients can be continuously observed and given the skilled care that prevents immediate postoperative complications. The advantages of concentrating patients, nursing care, and special equipment for this critical period were demonstrated during World War II in frontline hospitals. Intensive care units (ICUs) as an extension of recovery rooms were developed when it became apparent that some postoperative patients benefited from the same constant observation and care after recovering from anesthesia. Surgical intensive care units were duplicated, in turn, by those for nonsurgical patients who were critically ill or injured. Some hospitals now have separate units for surgical patients, patients with burns, patients with coronary disease, and so forth. Other hospitals combine recovery rooms and intensive care units, and still others have neither recovery rooms nor intensive care units.

According to John M. Beal and James E.

Eckenhoff, the basic difference between a recovery room and a general intensive care unit is that the former admits all patients who have had a general or regional anesthetic and some patients with a local anesthetic; the intensive care unit, on the other hand, admits only seriously ill medical or surgical patients and especially those with severe circulatory, respiratory, or intracranial pathology. They also say:

A special care unit is not simply a convenient area in which to accumulate patients so that fewer nurses can observe them more easily. These units are parts of the hospital in which the optimum in medical care for unconscious or critically ill patients can be provided by bringing together the resources of physicians, nurses, and other personnel who have the necessary special skills and experience, as well as the appropriate equipment with which to work.*

Whether recovery rooms or intensive care units are new and specifically planned for their purposes or are areas that have been converted to this use, each patient-space has its own oxygen supply as well as its own suction outlets. Individual blood pressure equipment is available so no time is spent moving it from patient to patient. It may be wall-mounted or attached to a wall rail behind each bed. Overhead tracks with movable hooks may be provided for hanging infusion bottles and other equipment, or intravenous standards may be inserted in devices fixed to the frame of the bed.

The *floor plans* of these postoperative units allow for continuous observation of each patient from the nursing station. Because both men and women are admitted to the same unit there is also provision for privacy when that is needed. In addition, some single rooms are provided for patients who must be isolated for their own protection or the protection of others. Utility rooms and areas for storing equipment and supplies are a part of the unit so personnel do not have to leave to find anything necessary for giving skillful nursing care. In some hospitals emergency supplies of drugs, disposable syringes, and tracheotomy tubes are hung on wall pegboards where they are easily accessible. Many of these special units have a small laboratory located nearby so that blood gases and other critical blood tests can be made quickly and patients' care modified accordingly.

Various kinds of patient *monitoring devices* are a part of the special unit equipment. Stanton Belinkoff [4] says that at the minimum the recovery room should have a cardioscope, a

---

* "Stir-up" regimens consist of deep breathing exercises, coughing, turning from side to back to side, and either passive (done by nurse) or active (done by the patient) exercises of the arms and legs. As noted in Chapter 47, patients should be taught this regimen preoperatively if there is time and they are rational.

* Beal, John M., and Eckenhoff, James E. (eds.): *Intensive and Recovery Room Care.* Macmillan Publishing Co., Inc., New York, 1969, p. vi.

pacemaker, and a defibrillator. Intensive care units, as well as some recovery rooms, have additional equipment such as blood pressure and pulse monitors, central venous pressure monitors, and electroencephalogram machines. Other emergency equipment includes tracheotomy and phlebotomy sets, mechanical and hand-controlled resuscitators, positive pressure breathing machines, and electronic equipment to control the patient's temperature (hypothermia blankets).

Nurses who are assigned to recovery rooms or intensive care units have *special preparation* that is often provided by the hospital.* Such preparation includes all or most of the following: intensive reviews of the respiratory, cardiovascular, and neuromuscular systems; practice in emergency resuscitative measures such as artificial respiration and external cardiac massage; additional knowledge and skill in interpreting the information obtained from various electronic monitors; review of laboratory data such as enzyme levels, electrolyte balance, and reports of blood gases; use of special equipment such as respirators, central venous pressure and arterial pressure monitors, and electrocardiographs; and information about emergency and other drugs commonly used in the special unit. In many in-service programs, emphasis is placed on helping patients understand their condition, the sights and sounds of the unit, and the various activities that make up their care plan.[5-9]

The *advantages* of special care units include a lower mortality rate for patients who are critically ill or injured, a more economical use by the hospital of specially prepared personnel and expensive, complex equipment, and an increased opportunity, particularly for physicians, for research.

Critical care units also have a number of *disadvantages* for both patients and personnel. For instance, the financial cost to patients who are in these units for several days is extremely high; some patients have adverse psychologic reactions to the sights and sounds of the unit or to the change in circadian rhythms; some patients who become reliant on the monitors and constant presence of nurses develop great fear and anxiety when they are transferred to a medical or surgical floor with a smaller staff of nurses; and because patients rarely see the intensive care unit nurses after they leave the

unit, the opportunity for developing a continuous nurse-patient relationship is absent. Perhaps the greatest psychologic disadvantage of the surgical recovery room is the fact that patients come out of anesthesia with no familiar faces around them.

Nurses assigned to special care areas are under great and almost constant stress because of the critical, often emergency, nature of patients' conditions, and if a staff member resigns it is frequently difficult to find a replacement who has the specialized skills required. Another disadvantage of the concentration of seriously ill patients with specially prepared nurses is that nurses on the general care units often become deficient in the knowledge and skill required to carry on the care of patients coming from the intensive care units who still need intensive nursing.[10-13]

Currently, there is debate about the advantages of the coronary care unit. At least one medical center has discontinued such units and has reorganized the entire staff of health workers into teams headed by a "physician-scholar." All patients admitted to the hospital are assigned to a "docent team" for as long as they require medical attention and the coronary patients are cared for within the medical ward.[14] This continuity of care by physicians, nurses, and others is thought by this center to promote patient welfare and staff satisfaction.

Recovery in Private or Multiple Occupancy Rooms and Open Wards. Some hospitals have neither a recovery room nor an intensive care unit, and patients are returned to their own wards or rooms from the operating room. *Close observation during the postanesthetic phase is very necessary no matter where the patient is located.*

Postanesthetic patients who are in rooms with convalescing patients need some privacy, and convalescing patients, in turn, should be shielded from the sights and sounds of the postanesthetic period. While patients in private rooms are not faced with this problem, there is a danger on a busy surgical unit that constant attendance on the patient may not be possible for as long a period as is desirable.

Recovery in Day Care Surgical Units and Homes. An increasing number of surgical patients are being admitted to day care units for operations such as tonsillectomies, herniorraphies, diagnostic dilation and curettage (D & C), dental repair, myringotomies, and rectal surgery that require some anesthesia but are believed not to demand professional medical and nursing attention after the day of operation. Patients enter the unit early in the morning and leave by 6:00 P.M. the same day. (Chapter 47 describes the preoperative prepa-

---

* Many physician administrators of special units believe the nursing skills required are so exacting that undergraduate nurses do not profit from a brief experience in the unit. Nurses who are assigned to these units usually have an orientation and a continuing in-service program especially designed to develop the necessary skills.

ration of day care surgical patients.) Burton S. Epstein and his associates say the advantages of these units are "reduction of medical care costs, increase in the availability of hospital beds for those who need them, and the opportunity to offer patients the same quality care administered to inpatients without such associated inconveniences and potential hazards as the disruption of the family unit and cross infection." * In addition, these patients, with generally minor surgical procedures, are not inadvertently "lost" among those requiring more intensive, complex care. Nurses have sufficient time so they can help identify and relieve patients' fears and concerns. This, in turn, helps patients feel more confident and secure.

The postanesthetic recovery period of a surgical day care patient is 3 to 5 hours. Patients are discharged when judged by the anesthetist to be able to walk without assistance. A responsible adult must escort them home. At the time of discharge, patients are given a prescription for pain medication, if the surgeon so indicates; they are advised to take only liquids (except alcoholic beverages) the first 6 hours after they are home, to rest or reduce their activities for at least a day, and to postpone important decisions until they have fully recovered.

During the postanesthetic period, patients in the "surgicenters" are watched as carefully as if they were in the usual hospital units. However, because they have little or no presurgical medication and either a light inhalant or local anesthetic, immediate postoperative complications are infrequent. Should a complication such as vomiting and aspiration, bleeding, or severe headache occur, patients are admitted to a general inpatient division of the hospital.

As part of the patient care plan, nurses who work in these surgical day care units often visit or telephone patients the day following surgery. In this way they get a report about the patient's recovery, are able to answer questions and resolve minor problems, and can reassure patients about their progress.[15-17]

2. POSTANESTHETIC CARE

Transporting the Patient from the Operating Room. When surgery is completed, patients are returned to their own rooms or to a recovery room. The patient's own bed or a stretcher may

* Epstein, Burton S., et al.: "Outpatient Surgery—Guidelines for Organization of Unit and for Selection of Patient and Surgical Procedure," *Hospitals,* **47**:80, (Sept.) 1973.

be used as a conveyance. Using the patient's bed minimizes the amount of lifting and moving of an unconscious patient; it enables the operating team to put the patient in a desirable position immediately after surgery; it also increases the element of safety during transportation. Many hospitals use a bed especially designed for recovery rooms. It is narrower than the regular hospital bed and has attached side rails, large wheels, a low head board, and a device making it possible to put patients in Trendelenburg and other positions.

If the *patient's own bed or a recovery room bed* is used for transportation, the coverings differ very little from the ordinary bed. The foundation is the same except for an additional strip of rubber or plastic sheeting covered by a cotton drawsheet that is placed across the upper part of the mattress to protect it from any vomitus, mucus, or blood which may drain from the mouth. Usually the upper bedding is not tucked in, but is folded to the edge of the mattress on one side so the patient may be easily transferred (see Fig. 48-1). In cold weather, hot-water bottles may be added to the bed to insure warmth, but if the hospital hall or room temperatures are 23.9°C (75°F) or higher this is undesirable. Placing patients between warm blankets and/or in a room at/or above 23.9°C induces sweating, with loss of fluid and electrolytes, and makes the patient uncomfortable. It may be necessary, however, to provide a warmed postoperative bed for some patients. Infants, debilitated patients, and aged persons tend to develop temperatures below 36°C (97°F) following surgery (postoperative hypothermia). Air-conditioned operating rooms with temperatures below 21°C (70°F), the length of time a body cavity is opened and exposed to cool air, the amount of unwarmed blood given during surgery, and certain methods of administering anesthesia also lower body temperatures of both children and adults. When the depth of hypothermia is planned and controlled, as it is with patients undergoing some kinds of cardiac surgery or neurosurgery, the accompanying decrease in metabolism is beneficial to the patient. (See Chapter 42.) Less anesthesia is needed, less oxygen is used by body tissues, and respirations are decreased. Other effects of hypothermia that include increased clotting time, lower blood pressure, decreased potassium excretion, and the development of metabolic acidosis can be corrected and controlled with appropriate treatment. When, however, unintentional hypothermia develops, the decrease in metabolism prevents the patient from overcoming the effects of the anesthetic and neuromuscular blocking agents, frequent shiv-

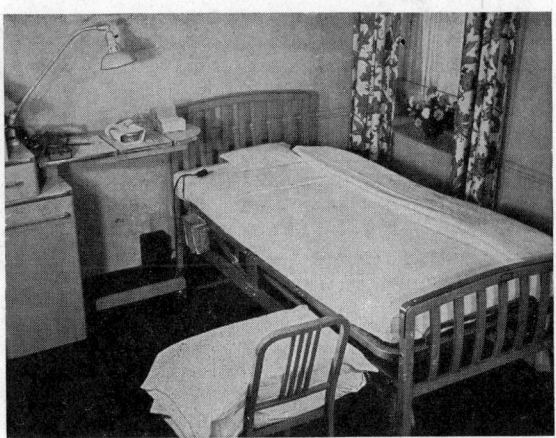

Figure 48-1. Clinical unit prepared for the postoperative patient. Note the protection of the bedding, the fanned bedclothes, and the pillows to be used to keep the patient in a desirable position. A blood pressure apparatus, a record for vital signs, emesis basins, water and drinking tubes, and paper handkerchiefs are on the bedside stand. Nearby are several plastic airways. (Courtesy of Columbia-Presbyterian Medical Center, New York, N.Y., and Clay-Adams Co., New York, N.Y.)

ering increases heart work and oxygen consumption that, in turn, can cause hypoxia, and metabolic acidosis may go unsuspected.[18-22]

When *stretchers* are used to move patients from the operating room, the pads are usually covered with a disposable or cotton sheet and patients are covered with a cotton blanket. Requirements of warmth for patients are the same whether they are transported on a stretcher or their own beds.

Transfer of the patient to bed or stretcher should be accomplished with as little jarring and strain as possible to avoid overtaxing the circulatory system and prevent undue strain on the operative area. Because anesthetics and many drugs used preoperatively are cardiovascular depressants, the patient's peripheral vascular system has a lessened ability to compensate for sudden changes in position. Rough handling may, therefore, bring about a sudden lowering of blood pressure.[23]

While patients are moved, their bodies should be kept straight, with the extremities, head, and trunk well-supported so an arm or leg is not caught between the operating table and the stretcher and so that any needles that have been inserted in veins are not dislodged. At the same time there should be no undue strain on those who are moving patients. Lifting patients is easily and quickly accomplished when several persons support the patient's weight with a lifting sheet that extends the full length of the body or by using an electrical lifting device. (Additional details about lifting and transporting patients are found in Chapter 12.)

Immediately after a patient has been transferred to the bed or stretcher, blood pressure and pulse should be checked to see that they are within normal limits. While patients are transported, the neck and chin should be extended to prevent the tongue from falling into the pharynx, and the head turned so any vomitus or secretions can drain out and not obstruct the airway. Because patients may develop hypoventilation from the effects of muscle relaxants used during surgery, or hypoxia with the change from a high concentration of oxygen to room air, it is desirable for the anesthetists to accompany patients to recovery units in order to observe their conditions during the transfer and before relinquishing their care to the nurse[24]; when this is not possible, nurses should accompany patients from the operating room. If an infusion is running, a special standard designed so that the base may be tucked under the mattress is useful for supporting the bottle during transportation.

Stretchers are so much narrower than beds that guard rails should always be up while transporting a patient, and safety belts should be fastened securely across the patient's legs. Care should be taken that patients' arms or elbows are at their sides so they are not accidentally injured when the stretcher is moved through doorways. Any drainage tubes patients may have, such as those in the chest or bladder, are ordinarily clamped shut while the patient is being transferred from the operating room.

Patients who are taken to the recovery area by stretcher should be moved to the bed in the same way they were moved from the operating table to the stretcher. Their blood pressure and pulse should be rechecked and they should be put in a comfortable position and one that prevents respiratory obstruction (see Fig. 48-2).

Administering Postanesthetic Care. It is the nurse's responsibility to see that all *equipment needed* for postoperative care is assembled and ready for use before the patient returns from the operating room. In addition to

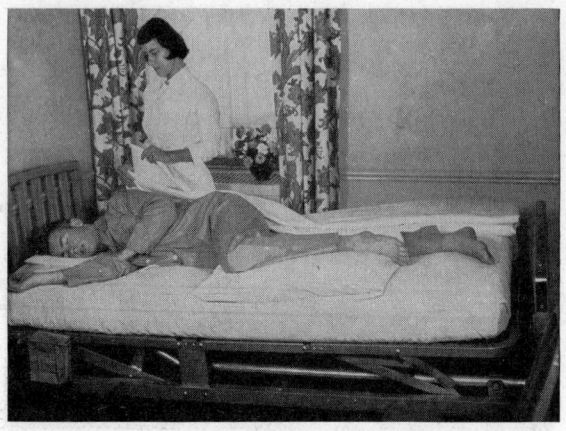

Figure 48-2. Postoperative position that favors drainage from the mouth as well as abdominal relaxation. A pillow can be placed against the abdomen to support the patient's left arm and to expand the chest. A pillow at the patient's back tends to keep him from rolling over but is contraindicated in operations on the spine. (Courtesy of Columbia–Presbyterian Medical Center, New York, N.Y., and Clay-Adams Co., New York, N.Y.)

equipment permanently in place such as oxygen and suction outlets, there should be a sphygmomanometer, mouth gag, tongue forceps, artificial airway, emesis basin, paper handkerchiefs, and a pad and pencil for keeping notes.

As soon as the patient is brought to the recovery unit, the nurse should *check the patient's condition* with the anesthetist or nurse who transferred him or her. This should include the patient's color and body warmth, as well as blood pressure, pulse, and respirations. Nurses should get from the anesthetist or operating room nurse a short verbal report about the operative procedure, the kind of anesthetic and medication used, any problems that occurred during surgery, and the general condition of the patient. An extremely important part of the postoperative nursing care is observation of the patient. Since this care is a continuation of that received at the time of operation, the nurse should know what operative procedure was performed as well as how the patient withstood the procedure. It may not be possible for recovery nurses to be present at the operation, but they should familiarize themselves with the records kept by the anesthetist and surgeon. This information will enable them to give postoperative care more specifically adapted to the needs of the patient. Figure 48-3*A–D* shows samples of an operating room record, an anesthetist's record, a surgeon's operative record, and an anesthetist's postoperative visit record.

In the immediate postoperative period the patient's face is usually flushed and the skin moist and warm, because most anesthetics dilate the superficial capillaries. The *blood pressure, pulse,* and *respirations* are taken immediately, and at short intervals thereafter (usually every 15 to 20 minutes) until the patient has fully reacted, and then every hour or less often as his or her condition improves and if the blood pressure stays fairly constant. (For normal figures, see page 465.) Any marked variation from the average blood pressure is reported to the anesthetist or surgeon, for it may indicate a complication, such as shock or hemorrhage. In order to determine whether or not the blood pressure is abnormally low or high, the nurse should know what the patient's blood pressure was prior to surgery. This may be determined from the notes on the chart. Usually a drop in blood pressure can be expected postoperatively owing to the loss of blood and to the effect of the anesthetic and preoperative medications. Many anesthetists believe that a change of less than 20 mm Hg from preoperative blood pressure values is not harmful, but danger exists if the blood pressure continues to either fall or rise.[25,26] Edward A. Brunner and James E. Eckenhoff[27] say that systolic blood pressures below 90 mm Hg and above 180 mm Hg in patients who previously had normal blood pressure are "to be viewed with concern." Nurses should be aware that when patients are lying on their sides both the systolic and diastolic blood pressure recorded from the uppermost arm will be lower than when patients are on their backs.[28] Evaluation of the blood pressure changes should always be made on an individual basis and depend on the patient's general condition and preexisting pressure.

The pulse and respiratory rates are also indicators of the patient's condition that may be determined easily and quickly. They are generally taken at the same interval with the blood pressure, but in some cases more frequently. After surgery the pulse is usually more rapid and sometimes weaker, with a regular volume and rhythm. Pulse rates above 110 may be due to hemorrhage, inadequate oxygenation, shock, apprehension, or pain.

University Hospital

OPERATING ROOM RECORD

COMPLETE BY O.R. AFTER OPERATION	REGISTER NO.		
EMERGENCY ☐	TEACH ☐	O.R. NURSE CHECKING CHART	

DATE			O.R.	ANAESTHETIST	ANAESTHETIST ASSISTANT
DAY	MO.	YR.			

			TIME STARTED	TIME FINISHED

ANAESTHETIC: ☐ GENERAL ☐ LOCAL ☐ OTHER

OPERATION PERFORMED

	TIME STARTED	TIME FINISHED

PRE-OP DIAGNOSIS

POST-OP DIAGNOSIS

SURGEON	FIRST ASSISTANT	OTHERS

CHARGE NURSE	SCRUB NURSE

CIRCULATING ASST.

NARCOTICS	MEDICINES (OTHER THAN THOSE GIVEN BY THE ANAESTHETIST)

I.V. SOLUTIONS

BLOOD		RIGHT TIME ON	TOURNIQUETS TIME OFF	TIME ON	LEFT TIME OFF
SPONGE COUNT	X-RAY 4X4	STRINGS	YOUNGS	FOWLERS	INTESTINALS
	X-RAY 8X4	PATTIES	TAPES	PINS	PLUGS	REELS

NEEDLE COUNT	FREE	ATRAUMATIC	BLADES

COUNT CORRECT YES ☐ NO ☐	SIGNATURE OF CHARGE NURSE	SIGNATURE OF SCRUB NURSE

IF NOT CORRECT SURGEON NOTIFIED BEFORE END OF CASE YES ☐ NO ☐	IF INCORRECT X-RAY TAKEN YES ☐ NO ☐	COMMENTS

SPECIMEN SENT TO	CYTOLOGY YES ☐ NO ☐	PATHOLOGY YES ☐ NO ☐	BACTERIOLOGY YES ☐ NO ☐	OTHER

CATHETERS	PACKING

DRAINS

WOUND CLASSIFICATION	CLEAN ☐	CLEAN CONTAMINATED ☐	CONTAMINATED ☐	SEPTIC ☐	NONE ☐

REMARKS

SIGNATURE OF NURSE IN CHARGE OF CASE

84-750-0156 (01/75)

Figure 48-3. *A*. An example of the record kept by nurses in the operating room. It has information on the anesthetic, operation, and medications, as well as the placement of drains, catheters, and packing. (Courtesy of University Hospital, University of Western Ontario, London, Ont.)

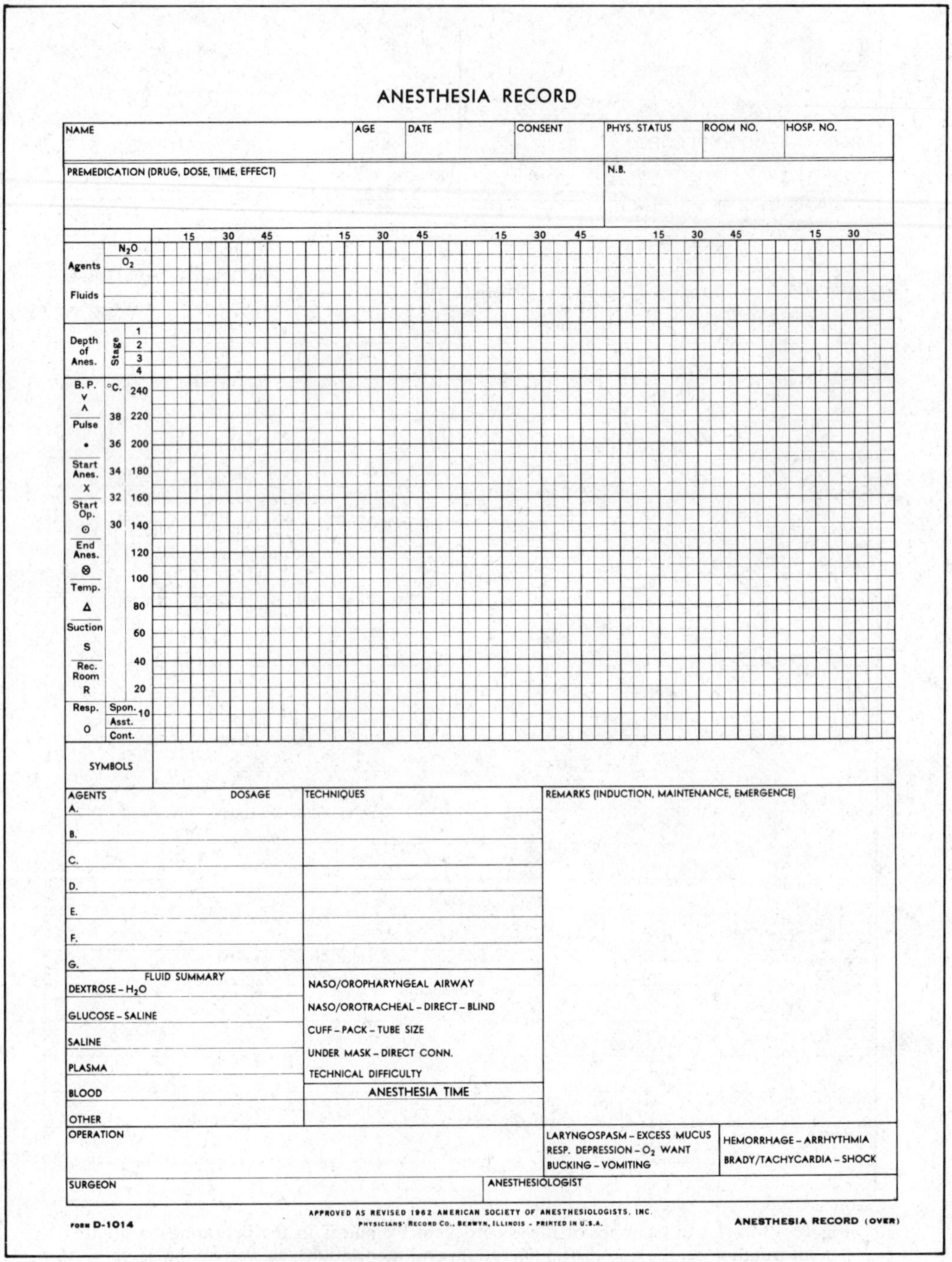

ANESTHESIA RECORD

NAME	AGE	DATE	CONSENT	PHYS. STATUS	ROOM NO.	HOSP. NO.

PREMEDICATION (DRUG, DOSE, TIME, EFFECT)

N.B.

15 30 45   15 30 45   15 30 45   15 30 45   15 30

Agents — N_2O / O_2

Fluids

Depth of Anes. — Stage 1 2 3 4

B.P. ∨ ∧ — °C. — 240
Pulse • — 38 — 220
— 36 — 200
Start Anes. X — 34 — 180
Start Op. ⊙ — 32 — 160
— 30 — 140
End Anes. ⊗ — 120
Temp. △ — 100
Suction S — 80
— 60
Rec. Room R — 40
— 20
Resp. Spon. O Asst. Cont. — 10

SYMBOLS

AGENTS	DOSAGE	TECHNIQUES	REMARKS (INDUCTION, MAINTENANCE, EMERGENCE)
A.			
B.			
C.			
D.			
E.			
F.			
G.			

FLUID SUMMARY
DEXTROSE – H_2O
GLUCOSE – SALINE
SALINE
PLASMA
BLOOD
OTHER

NASO/OROPHARYNGEAL AIRWAY
NASO/OROTRACHEAL – DIRECT – BLIND
CUFF – PACK – TUBE SIZE
UNDER MASK – DIRECT CONN.
TECHNICAL DIFFICULTY
ANESTHESIA TIME

OPERATION

LARYNGOSPASM – EXCESS MUCUS
RESP. DEPRESSION – O_2 WANT
BUCKING – VOMITING

HEMORRHAGE – ARRHYTHMIA
BRADY/TACHYCARDIA – SHOCK

SURGEON

ANESTHESIOLOGIST

APPROVED AS REVISED 1962 AMERICAN SOCIETY OF ANESTHESIOLOGISTS, INC.
PHYSICIANS' RECORD CO., BERWYN, ILLINOIS - PRINTED IN U.S.A.

FORM D-1014

ANESTHESIA RECORD (OVER)

Figure 48-3. *B.* A sample of the record used by the anesthetist during surgery. (Courtesy of Physicians' Record Co., Berwyn, Ill.)

NAME					HOSP. NO.		WARD OR ROOM NO.	
DIAGNOSIS							O. R.	
OPERATION PROPOSED							TIME	
AGE		M F	HT.	WT.		B. P.		
TEMP.		PULSE		RESP.		HB.	W.B.C.	
URINE								
BLOOD CHEM.							B.M.R.	
RESPIRATORY FUNCTION						ASTHMA SPUTUM		
CARDIAC FUNCTION								
NECK				TEETH		DRUG ALLERGY		
MENTAL STATUS						ATARACTIC		
PREVIOUS ANESTHETICS						CORTICOIDS		

PREOPERATIVE COMPLICATIONS

OPERATIVE COMPLICATIONS

POSTOPERATIVE COMPLICATIONS

(D-1014 BACK)

Figure 48-3. *B*. (Continued)

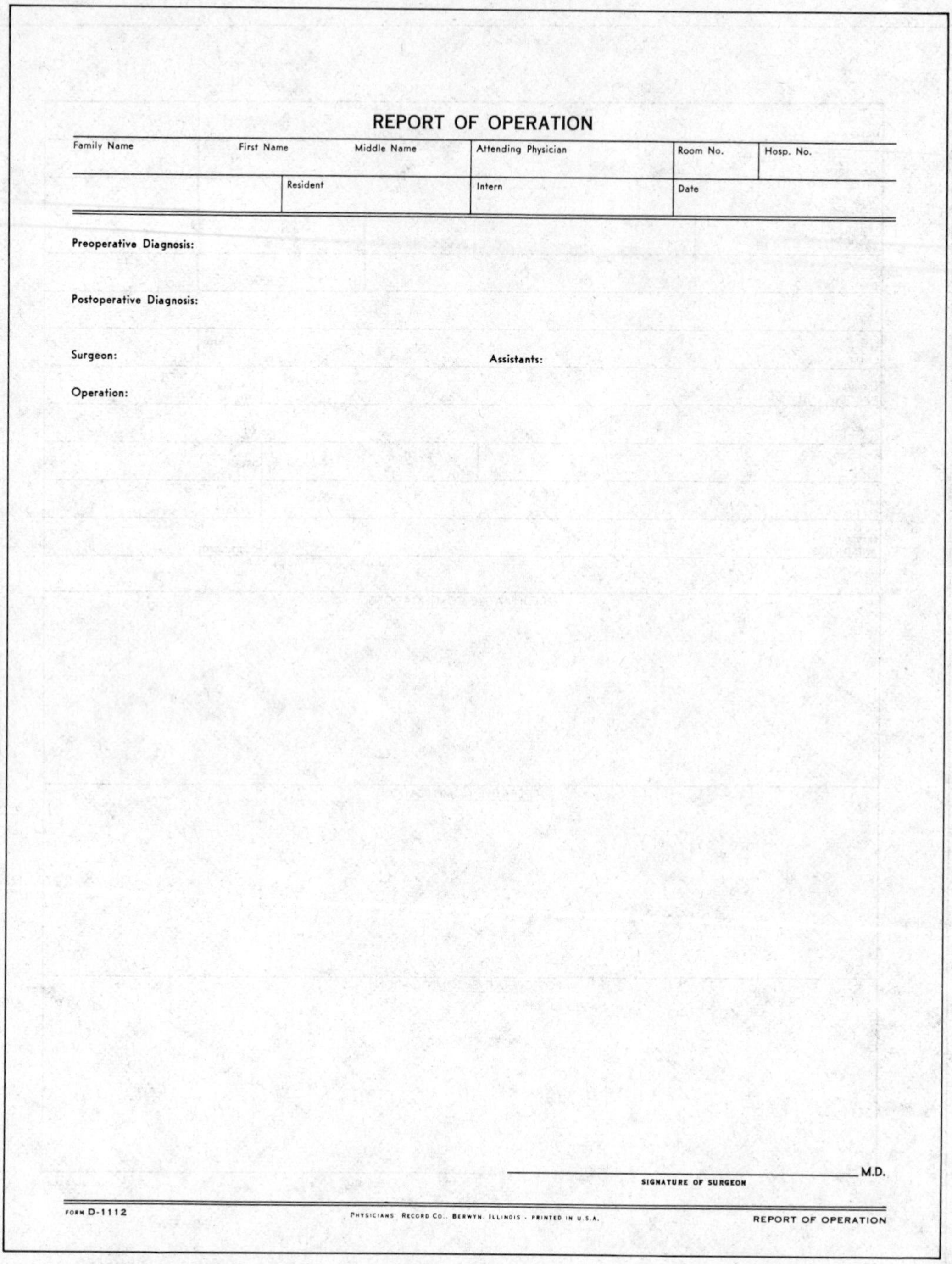

REPORT OF OPERATION

Family Name	First Name	Middle Name	Attending Physician	Room No.	Hosp. No.
		Resident	Intern	Date	

Preoperative Diagnosis:

Postoperative Diagnosis:

Surgeon: **Assistants:**

Operation:

_____ M.D.
SIGNATURE OF SURGEON

FORM D-1112   PHYSICIANS RECORD CO., BERWYN, ILLINOIS · PRINTED IN U.S.A.   REPORT OF OPERATION

Figure 48-3. *C*. A sample of the record used by the surgeon to describe the operative procedure. It may or may not accompany the patient to the recovery room. (Courtesy of Physicians' Record Co., Berwyn, Ill.)

uh University Hospital

POST–OPERATIVE VISIT BY THE ANAESTHETIST

Pre-Anaesthetic Condition and Complications: ____________________

Post-Anaesthetic Condition: ____________________

Post-Operative Visit:

Date: ____________ Anaesthetist ____________ M.D.

Remarks: ____________________

SPEEDISET MOORE BUSINESS FORMS LTD

84-750-0141 (09/72)

CHART

Figure 48-3. *D.* A sample of an anesthetist's postoperative visit record. (Courtesy of University Hospital, University of Western Ontario, London, Ont.)

Pulse rates below 60 are sometimes caused by the continuing action of drugs used during anesthesia.[29]

Respirations are often noisy until the patient is conscious. Any change should be noted, such as excessively shallow, rapid, or difficult breathing. If the difficulty is due to an obstructed air passage, immediate measures, such as those to be discussed later, should be instituted. If the character, rate, or rhythm of the respirations continues to be inadequate, the surgeon or anesthetist should be notified. It may be that the lungs are poorly ventilated and oxygen is needed.*

Unless the surgeon fears a disturbance in the body's heat mechanism, *the temperature* is ordinarily not measured as often in the immediate postoperative period as is the blood pressure, pulse, and respiratory rate. In most cases, it is taken every 4 hours for the first 24 hours, and then less frequently if it is not elevated to an unusual degree. A slight elevation in body temperature usually exists for about the first 3 days after an operation. While the cause has not been definitely determined, endogenous pyrogenic material released from white blood cells trapped in the surgically traumatized tissues may be responsible.[30,31] Some authorities believe a "low-grade fever," where there is no infection, may be due to a slight increase in basal metabolic heat production together with a slight decrease in heat loss due to vasoconstriction.[32]

During the postanesthetic period, the very young and the elderly may have higher-than-normal temperature if they are in overheated rooms or have excessive bed coverings. Malignant hyperthermia (body temperature over 41°C [105.6°F]) is a rare febrile reaction that may occur during anesthesia and surgery. (The critical care required for patients with this condition is described in Chapter 42.) Elevated temperatures in the later postoperative period may be due to wound infections, pulmonary or urinary infections, drug idiosyncrasies, or thrombi and emboli.

Lower-than-normal body temperatures (hypothermia) due to air-conditioned operating rooms have already been mentioned. They usually occur during the immediate postanesthetic period rather than in the later postoperative period. In Chapters 42 and 47 the nursing care of patients who are placed in a hypothermic state for the purpose of cardiac or neurologic surgery is discussed.

Since hemorrhage is a constant danger during the first 24 hours, *the dressings* should be checked at frequent intervals during this period. Nurses should be familiar with the character and amount of drainage expected with various types of surgery, so that they can differentiate between normal drainage and hemorrhage. Blood will, of course, flow by gravity to the lowest point, so that the upper dressing may not be stained although the bed beneath the patient may be. Should a dressing be stained with blood, the size of the stain should be checked frequently to determine whether or not it increases. This can be seen easily if the stained area is measured or outlined with a pencil and any increase in size noted. If this does occur, the doctor should be immediately notified. A small amount of bleeding from the superficial capillaries is of no significance; on the other hand, a severe hemorrhage at the operative site is very serious. The dressings are only reinforced by the nurse if there is an appreciable amount of drainage, because surgeons usually prefer to have the original dressing kept in place until their arrival.

The length of time required for patients to *regain consciousness* and the way they react from the anesthetic are also important observations. During the unconscious phase, patients do not respond to questioning or painful stimuli. As they pass into the semiconscious phase, they often respond to painful stimuli by restlessness and moaning or loud talking. With the return of the gag and swallowing reflexes, there may be vomiting and expectoration of mucus. In order to know when patients have fully reacted, it is necessary to be sure that they are oriented to their surroundings. They should be able to answer questions related to their identity, time, and familiar happenings. It should be remembered, however, that in determining reaction from anesthesia one must compare the expected mental and physical response postoperatively with the patient's response in the preoperative period. It is desirable to allow the patient to return to consciousness naturally rather than jog him or her or talk loudly in an effort to hasten return to consciousness. Speaking distinctly, close to the ear, and at the same time pressing on patients' arm or hand usually suffice to elicit a satisfactory response if they are reacting.

Some anesthetists recommend a method of evaluating the postanesthetic patient that is based on a 10-point score. This method is similar to the one developed by Virginia Apgar

---

* For this reason, anesthetist Robert D. Dripps and his associates recommend that oxygen be given routinely to patients in the postanesthetic period unless the attending anesthetist states otherwise. (Dripps, Robert D., et al.: *Introduction to Anesthesia; The Principles of Safe Practice.* W. B. Saunders Co., Philadelphia, 1972, p. 395.)

to evaluate newborn infants.[33] A patient's *activity, respiration, circulation, consciousness,* and *skin color* are given ratings of 0, 1, or 2 according to the character of each as listed in Figure 48-4. Postanesthetic patients with scores of 10 are in the best possible condition. Most patients with scores of 8 to 10 are considered to have recovered from the anesthetic and, if in a recovery room, are discharged to their own rooms. Patients with total scores of 7 or less should continue to have close observation. Some anesthetists and surgeons believe postanesthetic patients should be evaluated every 5 minutes, while others think that when patients are closely observed scoring evaluation can be done every 15 to 30 minutes depending on the patients' condition, type of surgery, and anesthetic.[34-36] Because most hospitals have recovery rooms, postoperative patients recovering from anesthesia have continuous observation. It is unsafe to leave such patients alone. In unusual situations, where medical workers are not available for constant attendance, a member of the family or a friend may be allowed to stay with the patient until he or she is conscious.

Although mechanical, routine nursing care of any patient is to be deplored, nurses who consistently use a well-thought-out "routine" to evaluate a postanesthetic patient assure both the patient and themselves that nothing is being overlooked during this critical period. The nurse should make sure that (1) the patient's airway is open and respirations are adequate; (2) the patient is in such a position that vomitus, blood, or mucus will not be aspirated; (3) blood pressure and pulse are taken, recorded, and, if they indicate pathology, reported immediately; (4) any intravenous fluids or blood transfusions are observed for the prescribed rate of flow and type of fluid, and whether there is any infiltration; (5) the presence and location of any drainage tubes are determined and they are connected to the correct suction outlets or drainage bottles; (6) the operative site is checked for bleeding; (7) the patient's skin is observed for color, temperature, and moisture; and (8) the patient's level of consciousness is evaluated.

While most patients in the immediate postoperative period appear dull and confused, Charles Winkelstein and his co-workers [37] found that they were able to give intelligible and intelligent answers to interview questions a very short time after having general anesthesia. They found, also, that 24 hours later

	At arrival	1 hour	2 hours	3 hours
Able to move 4 extremities voluntarily or on command = 2 " " " 2 " " " " " = 1 Activity " " " 0 " " " " " = 0				
Able to deep breathe & cough freely = 2 Dyspnea or limited breathing = 1 Respiration Apneic = 0				
BP ± 20% of preanesthetic level = 2 BP ± 20–50% of preanesthetic level = 1 Circulation BP ± 50% of preanesthetic level = 0				
Fully awake = 2 Arousable on calling = 1 Consciousness Not responding = 0				
Pink = 2 Pale, dusky, blotchy, jaundiced, other = 1 Color Cyanotic = 0				
Totals				

Study # _____
Name _____ Age ____ Sex ____ Hospital number _____
Date _____ Preanesthetic risk _____ Arrival time to RR _____
Type of surgery _____
Anesthetic agents _____
Muscle relaxants other than for intubation _____
Anesthesia time _____ Anesthesiologist _____

Figure 48-4. Postanesthetic recovery score data sheet. (From Aldrete, J. Antonio, and Kroulik, Diane: "A Postanesthetic Recovery Score," *Anesth. Analg.,* **49:**924, [Nov.–Dec.] 1970.)

90 per cent of the patients recalled with accuracy the postanesthetic interview. Nurses should be aware, as has been emphasized before in these pages, that even when patients are not fully alert they absorb and remember much of what is going on about them. Explanations about procedures should, therefore, be given even though the patient may not appear to be awake, and personal, animated conversations should be held in areas well away from patients.

The nurse's *postoperative notes* should include a concise record of the observations discussed, in order to give a progressive picture of the patient's recovery. Concurrent notes should be kept on the vital signs, color, body warmth, condition of the dressing, presence of nausea and vomiting, reaction from the anesthetic, and evidences of pain or discomfort. A written record of the treatments administered should also be made. Fluids administered, medications, irrigations, and similar treatments should all be included in the postoperative record. Actually, the record for the postoperative patient is like that for any other patient except that notes are made more frequently in accordance with the patient's condition.

3. PROMOTING NORMAL RESPIRATIONS AND PREVENTING RESPIRATORY COMPLICATIONS

Promoting Normal Respirations. In the immediate postoperative period, it is obviously of great importance to protect and reinforce the patient's own tendencies toward adequate respiration. Providing an airway free from mechanical obstruction is of first concern; however, restrictions or a partial paralysis of the respiratory muscles, or depression of the respiratory center due to medication, should not be overlooked as likely obstacles to normal pulmonary function.

Mechanical obstructions of the upper respiratory tract due to accumulated secretions or a relaxed tongue are the most frequent hindrances to breathing in unconscious or semiconscious patients.

Unless contraindicated, patients should be placed on their side as shown in Figure 48-2, until the swallowing and gag reflexes return. For additional support, a pillow may be placed along the back, against the abdomen, or between the knees, making fuller relaxation possible. Leaving a patient on the back while unconscious is quite hazardous because with diminished swallowing and gag reflexes, mucus or vomitus may be aspirated into the bronchi, or the breathing may be obstructed if the re-

laxed tongue falls back into the throat ("swallowing the tongue"). With the patient in the lateral position, the tongue drops to the side of the mouth, air passes above it, and the respirations are improved. If, for some reason, it is advisable for an unconscious patient to remain on the back, the danger of aspiration can be lessened by turning the head to one side when vomiting occurs, suctioning the secretions or vomitus from the throat as required, and observing for respiratory obstruction so that the proper measures may be employed promptly.

Obstruction of the airway should be suspected if there are exaggerated movements of the chest and abdomen with very little air flow felt against a hand held over the nose or mouth, or if breathing is noisy or snoring. An old medical axiom says *noisy breathing is always obstructed breathing, but not all obstructed breathing is noisy.*[38]

The tongue falling back into the pharynx is frequently the cause of obstruction. This can be relieved by pressing on the angle of the lower jaw, and pushing it forward, at the same time keeping the teeth separated. If an unobstructed air passage cannot be maintained in this way, it may be necessary to insert an artificial airway. On certain occasions, grasping the tongue and pulling it forward will allow for a free passage of air (a gauze square covers the nurse's fingers and enables her to hold the tongue firmly). (See Fig. 48-5.) Use of a mouth wedge whenever it is necessary to take hold of the patient's tongue or force the teeth apart will safeguard the nurse's fingers against injury. Most wedges are made of wood, soft enough to lessen the possibility of the patient's breaking a tooth if the jaws should

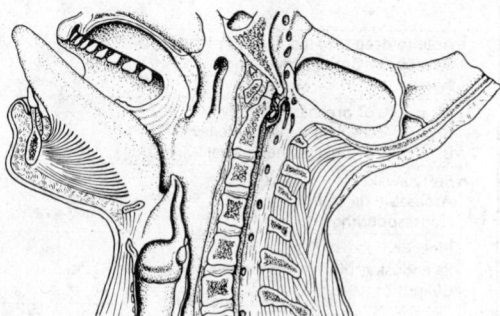

Figure 48-5. Median section of portion of head and neck showing that upward traction on the tip of the tongue draws the epiglottis away from the glottis opening and permits free ingress of air. (Redrawn from Hare, H. A.: *Practical Therapeutics.* Lea & Febiger, Philadelphia, 1927.)

tighten. A satisfactory mouth wedge may be made by wrapping several tongue blades together, and padding them with gauze and adhesive tape.

Because there is a constant danger of the patient's aspirating secretions, blood, or vomitus into the lungs when he or she cannot spit, it is desirable to suction this material from the throat at frequent intervals as it accumulates. This may be accomplished by means of a whistle-tip catheter connected to an electric or wall suction or other suitable type of negative pressure. The catheter should be inserted into the pharynx through the mouth, but occasionally if the patient's mouth cannot be opened, it may be inserted through the nostril. If the nostril is used, care should be taken to pinch off the catheter during insertion and removal so that the nasal mucosa will not be damaged by suction. The catheter should be left in place only long enough to suction the secretions, and then removed. Nurses are reminded that some oxygen is taken from the respiratory tract along with the accumulated secretions whenever the airway is suctioned.

Often, as an added precaution, the patient will have an artificial airway inserted before or after going to the recovery unit. The purpose is to hold the tongue forward by means of a hollow tube and thus ensure unobstructed breathing. Endotracheal tubes are also used to ensure an open airway, although they do not hold the tongue forward. (Types of airways are illustrated in Fig. 48-6.) Suctioning can be carried out by inserting the catheter directly through the airway. When the patient begins to gag or push the airway out with the tongue, it can usually be removed, as this indicates a return of the swallowing and gag reflexes. William M. Stahl[39] warns, however, that many patients who spontaneously remove their endotracheal tubes can still develop hypoxia and cardiac arrest because they may be unable to breathe deeply enough to inflate all alveoli and allow an adequate exchange of oxygen and carbon dioxide.

Tracheotomy (once a last-resort, emergency, life-saving measure) is more often used by today's surgeons to give easier access to the patient's tracheobronchial tree, and to allow more complete suctioning of secretions that interfere with respiration. The surgeon may perform a tracheotomy at the close of the operation if the patient's presurgical history has indicated there are likely to be postoperative respiratory complications, as, for example, in the case of a heavy smoker. When patients enter the recovery unit without a tracheotomy, the nurse's careful observation and early reporting of any respiratory difficulty allow the physician to perform a planned, controlled procedure if other aspirating or ventilating methods prove ineffective. Chapter 20 describes the care of patients with tracheotomies and the details are not repeated here.

Some postanesthetic patients continue to have *inadequate respirations* even though they have an open airway. One cause is partial paralysis of the respiratory muscles when neuromuscular blocking drugs are used during the operation. Many of today's surgical procedures are carried out with the assistance of muscle-relaxing drugs (in addition to the anesthetics) that block nerve impulses at the point the nerve ending and muscle cell meet. This point is called the motor end-plate, synapse, or neuromuscular junction. The use of these drugs results in greater relaxation of abdominal muscles than can be effected with anesthesia alone, and patients need not be as deeply anesthetized as they were in the past. Neuromuscular blocking agents such as *d*-tubocurarine, gallamine, pancuronium, or succinylcholine produce paralysis first in muscles innervated by the cranial nerves, next in muscles of the trunk, arms and legs, and lastly in muscles of respiration. Recovery occurs in the reverse order. Although the paralyzing effects of these agents are relatively short, that is, 20 to 45 minutes following the injection, some patients cannot excrete or metabolize all the drug in that length of time, or they may

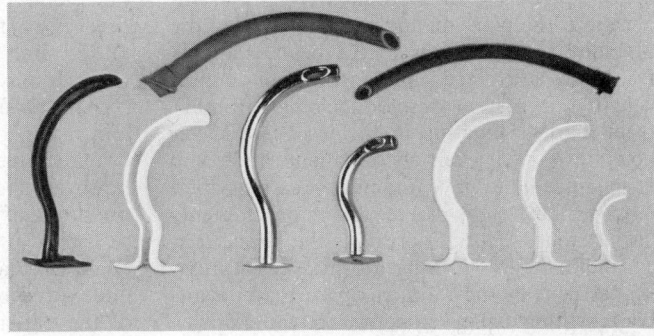

Figure 48-6. Plastic, hard-rubber, soft-rubber, and metal airways in a variety of sizes. (Courtesy of Clay-Adams Co., New York, N.Y.)

have been given additional injections throughout the surgery and almost to the end of the operation. The action of curariform blocking agents and gallamine can be shortened or reversed by giving injections of neostigmine, but polarizing agents like succinylcholine have no known antagonists so patients may react with a prolonged respiratory block.[40] For patients who have a residual effect from these drugs, mechanical respirators or ventilators (see Chapter 20) are necessary to ensure adequate pulmonary function and to keep arterial oxygen and carbon dioxide ratios normal until competent, spontaneous respirations are regained. When patients can raise their heads and maintain a firm hand grip, the effects of the drugs are diminishing. However, use of a respirometer is a better guide to adequate ventilation, and determination of blood-gas ratios is the most certain. Patients who have a partial respiratory paralysis from neuromuscular blocking drugs need repeated reassurance that their feeling of wanting to, but being unable to, take a deep breath is temporary, as is the use of the ventilator or resuscitator.

Inadequate respiration may also occur if constrictions of the chest wall or abdomen interfere with normal movements of the respiratory muscles. Postoperative pain, especially with abdominal or thoracic surgery, may limit movement of the chest wall and produce rapid, shallow respirations with the chest kept in the expiratory position. Obese patients, those who have had upper abdominal surgery, or those with tight surgical dressings of the abdomen have increased abdominal pressure that limits the downward motion of the diaphragm during inspiration. Unless contraindicated, tight abdominal dressings can be loosened, and obese patients or those with upper abdominal surgery may have respiratory help with the use of hand-operated positive pressure equipment. (See Chapter 20.)

Postanesthetic patients often have the foot of their beds tilted up 24 to 45 cm (10 to 18 inches). The head-lower-than-hips position (Trendelenburg) makes use of gravity to encourage drainage of secretions from the trachea into the pharynx and to increase the flow of blood from the legs to the heart. Patients frequently are placed in this position to prevent the formation of blood clots (thrombi) from blood stagnating in the leg vessels (venous stasis); however, obese patients and some of medium build have difficulty breathing then because the weight of the abdominal contents against the diaphragm prevents the chest from expanding fully. During normal respiration, 75 per cent of the thoracic space made available for lung expansion comes from the downward movement of the diaphragm and abdomen, while only 25 per cent comes from outward movement of the rib cage. When patients are in a head-down position, the diaphragm cannot move as freely as it should and the thoracic muscles must work harder to expand the chest. This increases the amount of energy used in respiration (oxygen cost of the work of breathing) and puts an extra burden on the circulation. In addition, there is a danger, particularly in obese persons, that the lung may partially collapse from mechanical interference with breathing. To promote good circulation in the legs but prevent respiratory inadequacy, one should elevate only the legs, rather than the whole bed, of obese patients until consciousness returns.[41]

Anesthetics and preoperative medications may be the cause of inadequate respiration since they usually slow the respiratory rate and depress the respiratory center in the medulla. For this reason nurses must be cautious about giving additional narcotics for pain in the postanesthetic period. One-third to one-half the usual amount of medication should be given the first time pain medication is administered. Overuse of a narcotic may lead not only to further respiratory depression, but to constant volume respiration with no deep, sighing breaths. This, in turn, may result in many small areas of unexpanded alveoli in the lungs (miliary atelectasis) and hypoxia.[42-44]

Patients with a drug-induced inadequate ventilatory drive have a depressed respiratory center that cannot respond enough to overcome an abnormal increase in arterial carbon dioxide (hypercapnia), and hypoxia results. The increase of arterial carbon dioxide often develops when anesthesia with a high concentration of oxygen is discontinued and the patient is required to breathe the lower concentration of oxygen in room air.

Patients with unobstructed airways but inadequate ventilation may have fast and shallow, or abnormally slow, respirations. In the early stages of respiratory inadequacy, the pulse is usually full, bounding, and rapid, and the blood pressure raised. If the inadequacy progresses, the blood pressure falls while the pulse rate continues to increase. Conscious patients may get more and more restless, confused, and drowsy. The skin may be red, hot, and moist, or the fingernails and lips may be cyanotic due to inadequate oxygen. Cyanosis, however, should not be relied on as a primary symptom of poor oxygenation. Cyanosis may be owing to a decreased hemoglobin or inadequate circulation. Cyanosis may be present but undetected because of the color and thickness of the patient's skin.[45]

Whatever the reason for the inadequate respirations, the nurse's first step, after making sure the airway is open, is to help the patient to breathe. As a temporary measure or until the cause of the difficulty is determined, self-inflating bags, such as the Ambu bag or the Ohio self-inflating bag,* can be used. These devices may be attached to an oxygen supply and oxygen administered by compressing the bag at the end of each inspiration.

Oxygen, like most substances used to treat disease conditions, can be harmful if used carelessly or unwisely. For example, if oxygen is given patients with severe hypercapnia without regard for oxygen concentration or rate of flow, the patient's only respiratory stimulus, the hypoxic drive, may be removed and respiration arrested. Furthermore, prolonged exposure (over 24 hours) to 100 per cent oxygen can lead to pulmonary irritation, edema, and fibrotic lung changes. Patients developing an adverse reaction to oxygen may complain of a feeling of tightness in the chest and have a dry, nonproductive cough and increasing dyspnea; however, the most reliable evidence that oxygen toxicity is developing is a decreasing arterial oxygen tension in spite of increasing oxygen consumption.[46-49] Chapters 6, 9, 20, and 35 have additional details about normal and abnormal respirations as well as the promotion of and treatments leading to adequate respiration.

Preventing Postoperative Respiratory Complications. Atelectasis, pneumonia, and pneumothorax are common postoperative respiratory complications. *Atelectasis* means an incomplete expansion or the collapse of some part of the lung. Currently it is thought that nearly 80 per cent of postoperative patients have some atelectasis because they neither sigh at normal intervals nor take periodic deep breaths. Under these circumstances, small groups of alveoli scattered throughout the lung fail to expand (miliary atelectasis). A large atelectic area may result from a mucous plug that entirely closes a bronchi. In this case, the air that is in the alveoli beyond the plug absorbs and the alveoli collapse. If these small or large areas are allowed to stay collapsed, ventilation is reduced, secretions remain in the nonfunctioning areas, infection develops, and pneumonia results. Atelectasis may also develop if air, blood, or fluid enters the intrapleural space and compresses the lung. Possible causes of this type of atelectasis are ruptured alveoli, tracheotomy, surgery immediately under the diaphragm, carelessly connected chest drainage tubes, or accidentally

disconnected drainage tubes. (See Chapter 35 for a further discussion of pneumothorax.)

Nursing measures essential to the prevention of atelectasis, from lack of sighing or the accumulation of secretions, are encouraging patients to take deep breaths, to cough up secretions, and to turn from side to back to side at hourly intervals—unless the patient is getting much-needed sleep. Because both deep breathing exercises and coughing are likely to be uncomfortable or even painful after surgery, it is desirable to give first small amounts of an analgesic. This lessens the pain and decreases the amount of natural thoracic "splinting" that is the result of pain. Furthermore, patients should be sitting in as upright a position as possible in order to promote optimum chest expansion during deep breathing and coughing. Other measures that prevent atelectasis are reminding patients of their preoperative instructions for deep breathing and coughing exercises, helping them with the procedures, and continually persuading them that these uncomfortable activities will hasten their recovery.

A number of procedures can be used to encourage the *deep breathing* so essential to patients' postoperative welfare. The simplest is to ask patients to take a series of deep breaths. Marie E. Collart and Janice K. Brenneman,[50] who studied the subject, report that five consecutive, deep breaths are the maximum most patients can tolerate without a brief rest. Intermittent positive pressure machines (see Chapter 20), rebreathing implements, and blow bottles are devices that are also used to help patients periodically hyperinflate their lungs.[51-53]

Rebreathing devices are intended to increase the dead air space of respiration by approximately 1 liter, and so increase arterial carbon dioxide tension and the depth and rate of respiration. They may be 30- to 40-inch lengths of wide-bore tubing with a mouthpiece or mask at one end (the Dale-Schwartz rebreather) or a series of compartments in a compact, closed cuplike device (the Adler rebreather). Oxygen may be added to either aid if the patient is hypoxic.

Blow bottles may be of two types. One type requires patients to blow against water pressure to create bubbles. Water pressure against which the patient blows is established by the insertion of a piece of bent glass tubing (in a two-hole rubber stopper) to a depth of 37½ cm (15 inches) in a large bottle filled with water. The other type requires patients to blow a prescribed amount of water from one bottle to another in as few breaths as possible. There is no current evidence to indicate that

* Ohio Medical Products, Madison, Wisc.

one method more than another increases ventilation in all patients.* However, because patients are individuals differing in age, alertness, general condition, and other attributes, nurses may find that one method is more effective with one person than another. A cooperative decision between the patient, nurse, and physician about the method to be used may, therefore, be very important.

Coughing naturally follows the patient's deep breathing exercises in most cases. If it does not, the cough reflex may be stimulated to help bring tracheobronchial secretions up into the pharynx. For instance, a cough can be externally stimulated by putting a finger firmly on the trachea just above the bony prominences of the clavicle (the manubrial notch) and rubbing up and down. This gentle, but firm, friction creates an irritating sensation that initiates the cough reflex. A cough can be produced by internal stimulation by teaching patients to slowly but forcefully exhale all the air their lungs hold. The prolonged expiration dries the tracheal mucosa, builds up some carbon dioxide tension, and produces coughing. As a third measure, nurses can teach patients to exhale all the air possible, to inhale as deeply as possible, and then cough. † It goes without saying that these techniques should always be explained to patients and their families before they are used. When family members know the importance of coughing and how to help bring it about, they can encourage, remind, and help patients with the procedure.[54,55]

Patients' fear of injuring an abdominal or chest incision sometimes inhibits deep, productive coughing. This fear can be relieved and the discomfort associated with coughing reduced if a hand or arm (the nurse's or patient's) is placed over the incision and light pressure applied. A cough belt as shown in Figure 48-7 is helpful to patients when used in the same way. The flat surface is placed between the patient's back and the bed and the loops are crossed in front. With a loop in each hand the nurse or patient pulls in an outward direction when the patient coughs.[56]

Keeping patients well hydrated with oral fluids and keeping the surrounding air well humidified help dilute tenacious secretions.

This, in turn, makes the secretions easier to dislodge by coughing.

Pneumothorax with an accompanying atelectasis may be an inevitable part of the patient's operation, as, for instance, with cardiac surgery, or it may develop slowly during the postoperative period from ruptured alveoli or from surgery about but not in the chest. Tension pneumothorax, the name given to the latter type, is infrequent but more serious because of its insidiousness, the gradual decrease in functioning lung tissue, and the impairment of venous blood return to the heart if there is a shift of the mediastinal contents to the side opposite the pneumothorax.

After most thoracic operations the surgeon makes provision for removal of air or fluid from the chest with a drain or drains connected to a water-seal drainage apparatus, a Pleur-evac * thoroseal apparatus, or a thoracic pump. With a tension pneumothorax, however, there is no exit for air accumulating in the pleural space. The physician, therefore, must provide a way to remove the air. The first measure used may be the insertion of a thoracentesis needle into the pleural space (see Chapter 26 for a discussion of thoracentesis and the risks of "intrusive therapy"), followed by the insertion of a chest tube to be attached to a water-seal drainage system. The purpose of the water-seal system, also called *closed chest drainage,* is to allow air or fluid to escape from the pleural space with each exhalation and to prevent air from entering through the chest drain with each inhalation. (The mechanics of respirations and negative thoracic pressure are discussed in Chapter 9.)

Whether the chest drain is inserted in the operating room or at the patient's bedside, the same equipment used for a thoracentesis (see Chapter 26) should be ready with the addition of a sterile thoracotomy tray, sterile chest drains of different sizes, adhesive tape, and the water-seal drainage system. A one-bottle system consists of a 1-gal bottle with approximately 1000 ml sterile saline or water, a tightly fitting two-hole stopper, a glass tube long enough to go no more than 2 cm (1 inch) below the level of the water, and a short glass tube to act as an air vent from the bottle. The level of the water should be marked so that any fluid coming from the pleural space can be measured.

The long glass tube is connected to the chest drain tubing. Air or fluid enters the bottle when the patient exhales, but is prevented from returning to the pleural space by the water acting as a seal. Air coming from the patient

---

* Most physicians consider blow bottles to be dangerous for patients with a pneumonectomy because too much pressure may be put on the bronchial stump. In some patients, intermittent positive pressure machines can create too high an intrathoracic pressure with a serious decrease of venous blood return to the heart.

† Preoperative preparation includes this instruction, as was stressed in Chapter 47.

* Deknatel Company, Queensville, N.Y.

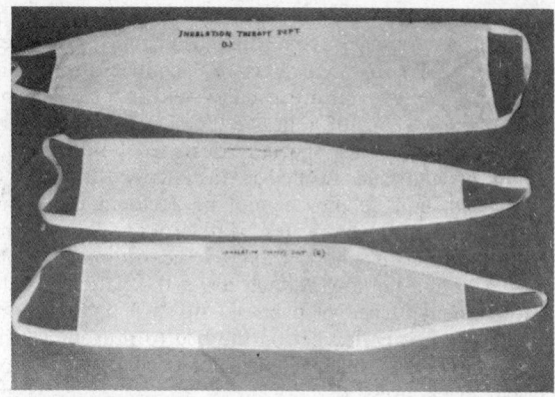

A

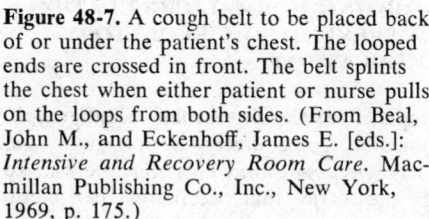

Figure 48-7. A cough belt to be placed back of or under the patient's chest. The looped ends are crossed in front. The belt splints the chest when either patient or nurse pulls on the loops from both sides. (From Beal, John M., and Eckenhoff, James E. [eds.]: *Intensive and Recovery Room Care.* Macmillan Publishing Co., Inc., New York, 1969, p. 175.)

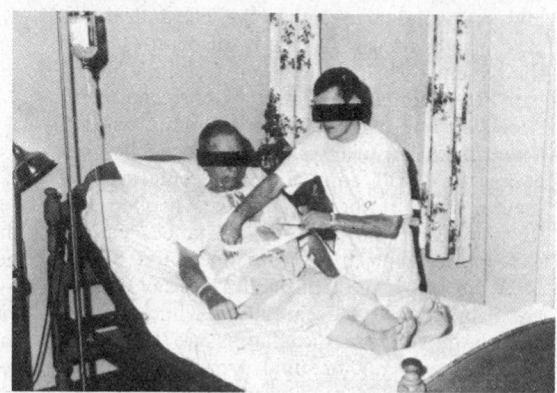

B

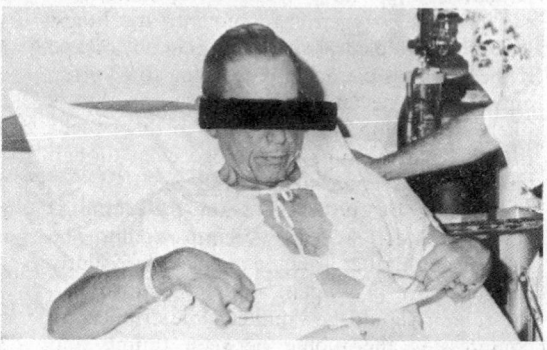

C

is kept from building up pressure in the bottle by the short air-vent tube. Some physicians prescribe the attachment of an Emerson * suction machine, set at 15 to 20 cm water, negative pressure, to the air-vent tube. When the system is operating properly, a small amount of water is drawn into the long tube when the

* J. H. Emerson Company, Cambridge, Mass.

patient inhales and air bubbles or drainage fluid is seen in the water when the patient exhales.[57,58]

Closed-chest drainage systems consisting of two or three bottles are often used with continuous suction. Both arrangements have one bottle that is the water seal and another bottle filled with water to varying levels that provides a break in the continuous suction action. The third bottle in the three-bottle system is used to collect drainage from the chest tube. In any of these arrangements all connections must be airtight and are usually held in place with narrow strips of adhesive tape. All bottles should be fixed in a specially designed holder hung on the bed frame or fastened to the floor with tape so they cannot be accidentally overturned and the water seal broken. The tubing from the chest drain to the drainage bottle should be long enough to let the patient move about in bed or even get up in a chair, and should be coiled flat on the bed to prevent a hanging loop that can obstruct drainage or create back pressure.

A usual practice when patients have closed chest drainage is to have one or two hemostats always available to clamp the chest drain in case the drainage system is disconnected or the patient is turned; however, Calvin V. Morgan and Thomas W. Orcutt [59] say this is unnecessary and even dangerous for the patient. They maintain clamps are unnecessary because the small amount of air entering the pleural space if the water seal is broken (by knocking over the bottle, for instance) can be expelled by the patient with one good breath after the seal is reestablished. They say clamps are dangerous if they are used while the patient is moved and the clamps are forgotten. This prevents air or fluid from leaving the pleural space and tension pneumothorax develops or redevelops. Clamps are most dangerous if they are used for any reason while the patient is on positive pressure ventilation. In this instance, oxygen is forced into the lungs, leaks into the pleural space, and cannot escape if the tubing is clamped. According to Morgan and Orcutt, the tension pneumothorax that is likely to develop is more lethal to the patient than leaving the tube unclamped even though temporarily disconnected.

Clogging of the chest drain or tubing is common and it acts as a clamp would. The tubing should, therefore, be checked frequently to make sure it is open, and, if not draining, the tubing should be "milked" or stripped by compressing the tubing between thumb and fingers and using alternate hands to "milk" the tube toward the bottle.

Chest drains are removed when air and fluid are no longer coming from the pleural space. The tube is removed quickly at the end of a full inspiration or during expiration to prevent air from being sucked into the pleural space while the tube is withdrawn. Usually a dressing of petrolatum gauze covered with a dry gauze square is taped firmly in place.

Patients with respiratory inadequacy are generally apprehensive, and the addition of chest drainage equipment only adds to their fears. Nurses' careful explanation of the purpose and nature of the treatment, their honesty in answering patients' and families' questions, and their concern and manner of caring for patients will do much to relieve anxiety.

Older patients with a fractured femur or pelvis, which necessitates a long stay in bed, may develop *hypostatic penumonia*. Early physical signs include a slight temperature elevation, increased pulse and respiratory rates, and occasionally a slight cough. It is important for the nurse to help or encourage the patient to change position at least hourly. It is also important that the posture allow for full chest expansion (see Chapter 12). In most cases the person breathes more easily if the head and shoulders are elevated.

4. PROMOTING NORMAL CIRCULATION AND PREVENTING CIRCULATORY COMPLICATIONS

Postoperative Cardiovascular Changes. In the immediate postoperative period, many patients have *hypotension*. This may be caused by an anesthetic that decreases peripheral vascular resistance or the contractility of heart muscle, or to spinal or epidural anesthetic that results in temporary sympathectomy. A subnormal blood pressure may also be due to blood lost during surgery, or to postoperative bleeding or hemorrhage. A number of physicians believe that if patients have warm, dry skin, and pink mucous membranes with a normal urine output, the hypotension is not dangerous. However, patients should be kept in a horizontal position or have their legs elevated, and should be moved or turned slowly and gently while regaining consciousness to prevent a sudden pooling of blood in the *relaxed peripheral blood vessels*. Rough handling can cause a sudden shift of blood volume away from the heart, a relative decrease of blood volume, and unexpected cardiovascular collapse.[60-62]

An actual postoperative *decrease in circulating blood volume* can occur because the blood loss during surgery was estimated inaccurately and, consequently, replaced inadequately. Although many patients are given a single postoperative transfusion on the assumption that this replaces blood lost during surgery, there is current debate on the wisdom of giving only one transfusion to any patient. According to J. Garrott Allen,[63] patients who are thought to require only one transfusion will probably have their blood volume needs met satisfactorily by the administration of plasma volume expanders, and will also avoid the possible risks of a transfusion. However, he also says that while the dangers and possible errors of multiple transfusions increase at an arithmetical rate, when a large amount of blood is needed, it should be given. In these instances every precaution for blood collection, storage, and administration must be followed so there is minimal risk to the patient.[64]

Intravenous fluids other than blood are often given throughout surgery and postoperatively to maintain normal fluid and electrolyte balance, as well as blood volume. Although nurses are not responsible for determining the kinds and amounts of intravenous fluids necessary for postoperative patients, they are responsible for understanding the mechanisms involved and for noting and reporting signs indicating the need for intravenous fluids. They should keep in mind that during the first 48 postoperative hours the body responses to trauma tend to conserve both sodium and water. Therefore, unless there is an unusual loss (over 500 ml) of fluids and electrolytes, as for instance through a nasogastric tube or excessive vomiting, 2000 to 3000 ml of dextrose and water is ordinarily given to replace urinary and insensible fluid losses. If excessive water is given during this early postoperative period, the patient may develop a subnormal concentration of sodium in the blood (hyponatremia). A reduced attention span, apathy, lack of appetite, nausea, vomiting, and backache are its only symptoms, even with a very low blood sodium concentration. Excessive water administration may also lead to overdilution of plasma protein (hypoproteinemia) resulting in edema of the brain, lungs, and peripheral tissues, with patients usually becoming more and more apprehensive, irritable, and restless.[65,66]

About the third postoperative day the diuretic phase of the body response begins and water and electrolytes are excreted by the kidneys. At this time it may be necessary to add sodium, a small amount of potassium, and vitamins B and C to the intravenous fluids.[67] For the above reasons, surgeons are vitally interested in the patient's intake and output. Through a study of these relationships and by tests on the blood and urine, they are able to prescribe the parenteral feedings needed. In general, patients are supported by intravenous feedings until they are able to take a full-liquid diet by mouth. As they gradually increase their oral intake, they are given less by vein. Nurses give an invaluable service when they keep an accurate record of patients' oral and parenteral intake, as well as their urinary output and the fluid loss through vomitus, feces, and drainage from any body area.

Because of the need for fluid postoperatively, and because it cannot always be administered simultaneously with the body's natural urge to drink, patients are usually thirsty, which is the body's physiologic response to the need for fluids. If there is an inadequate amount present, water is drawn from the tissues to compensate, leaving the mouth dry and coated. Nurses should realize, however, that thirst can be quenched with the administration of fluids by the parenteral route as well as the oral. It is, of course, more desirable to give as much of the fluid as possible orally, for it is the natural, and likewise the most pleasant and comfortable, way of receiving it. Frequent attention to mouth care helps relieve a dry mouth, as will be discussed later.

Simple explanations and instructions on the necessity of measuring fluids and excreta contribute toward a wholesome and relaxed attitude on the part of the patient. In addition, provision should be made for rest and change of position while infusions are running. A padded arm board should be used whenever the needle is inserted at a site where the joint should not be moved, such as the elbow or wrist. Even when these sites are used, there is no reason why the arm should be completely immobilized. With caution, patients may be helped to tighten and relax the arm muscles and to flex the uninvolved joints at periodic intervals. They should also be encouraged to change position from side to side, and if their condition permits, the nurse can help them to walk by protecting the involved arm as they get out of bed, and by supporting the solution bottle as they walk together.

Postoperative patients who were in fairly good health before surgery make up fluid and electrolyte deficits rapidly when they begin to eat, drink, and move. Chapter 22 has further discussion of fluid and electrolyte balance.

Postoperative bleeding or hemorrhage can be prevented to some extent by careful consideration of the patient's preoperative history and the laboratory reports of blood analysis. It may be necessary for nurses to call to the surgeons' attention the patient's account of bruising easily or having had difficulty in stopping blood flow from a minor cut. Nurses should make certain the surgeon sees all the patient's laboratory reports, particularly those for blood typing and coagulation factors, and knows about any drugs the patient has been taking (such as Dicumarol) that might interfere with clotting mechanisms. Surgeons have the major responsibility for preventing postoperative bleeding or hemorrhage through the appropriate use during the operation of ligatures, sutures, packs, topical thrombin, locally applied vasoconstrictors, and other hemostatics such as Gelfoam and Oxycel.

Nurses are responsible for the *detection of postoperative bleeding* and should check surgical dressings frequently (as described earlier in this chapter) in order to determine the presence and character of visible bleeding. Patients prone to bleed freely should be watched with special care. The detection of invisible, internal hemorrhage is often difficult and takes keen observation of patients' total behavior and appearance.

It is obvious that a loss of blood from what is normally a closed circulatory system reduces the amount of fluid the heart can pump and, consequently, reduces the arterial blood pressure. There are, however, several *physiologic mechanisms,* taking a few seconds to an hour to be completely mobilized, that help the body compensate for this condition. Sympathetic reflexes prompted by the decreased arterial pressure cause the constriction of arterioles, veins, and venous reservoirs so that arterial pressure is raised again, and venous blood return to the heart is maintained. In addition, the heart pumps faster in an effort to deliver sufficient blood to vital tissues, and respirations quicken to increase the availability of oxygen.[68] The symptoms patients exhibit with this chain of events are hypotension, pallor, increasing pulse rate, increasing respiratory rate, and if oxygen is not given, increasing apprehension and restlessness as vital brain cells receive less oxygen. As the blood reserves of the systemic venous system are mobilized, particularly the splenic and pulmonary reserves, "patients inspire sharply as though surprised. Fine tremors develop and gross movements weaken. Perspiration spreads from forehead and palms. Shivering starts in the masseter jaw muscles." *

Should bleeding continue without treatment, other adjustments for returning blood volume to normal begin to operate. These include the absorption of large amounts of fluid from the intestinal tract and interstitial spaces, and additional conservation of renal water and salt. The patient then becomes very thirsty and has a reduced urine output.

A cause of decreased cardiac output other than lowered peripheral vascular resistance and loss of blood is a *loss of plasma* due to intestinal obstruction, severe burns, and dehydration. Postoperative dehydration, in turn, may result from excessive sweating, severe vomiting, inadequate intake of fluids and electrolytes, and renal insufficiency.[69] If, during a 24-hour period, the circulating fluid loss exceeds 60 per cent of the total blood volume, and if blood, plasma expanders, or fluids are not given promptly in adequate amounts, the patient's condition progresses to irreversible shock and death. (Shock is discussed in Chapter 45 and additional information about hemorrhage can be found in Chapter 43.)

Infants, young children, and the elderly are readily dehydrated and have a limited capacity to adapt to blood volume changes. The compensatory mechanisms of the very young have not fully developed, and those of the aged mobilize sluggishly. Furthermore, the elderly are often hypertensive, and unless comparisons between their postoperative and preoperative blood pressure levels are made, the postoperative measurements may be unreliable indicators of their actual condition. Both groups should have especially close observation in the early postoperative period.

To *control* severe postoperative *external or internal hemorrhage,* patients are usually returned to the operating room so the surgeon can find the exact point of bleeding and take appropriate steps. Whole blood and other fluids must then be given to increase the volume of the cardiac output.

The intravenous administration of whole blood, as well as blood substitutes and other intravenous fluids, is discussed at length in Chapter 22; however, some of the precautions for giving *transfusions* cannot be emphasized too frequently and are, therefore, repeated here. The nurse should make certain there is a record of the patient's blood type and that a cross match has been made with the donor's blood. Before blood is given, it should be inspected for gas bubbles indicating bacterial growth, and for any abnormal color or cloudiness indicating hemolysis or clotting. In most hospitals two persons must check the container of donor blood for the correct patient's name with identifying hospital number * and the attending physician's name against the requisition slip and patient's chart. In addition, the blood type, Rh factor, expiration date, and blood unit number of the donor blood should be checked by the same two persons. Blood bank procedures are sufficiently refined so that mismatching does not often occur from laboratory errors; however, mistakes continue to happen with blood intended for one patient

---

* Abbey, June C.: "Nursing Observations of Fluid Imbalance," *Nurs. Clin. North Am.,* **3:**77, (Mar.) 1968.

* Allen says, "The author has been both surprised and terrified by the frequency with which the full name of the recipient and, indeed his diagnosis, will correspond exactly to that of another patient hospitalized at the same time." (Allen, J. Garrott: "Blood Transfusions and Related Problems," in Rhoads, Jonathan E., et al. [eds.]: *Surgery; Principles and Practice,* 4th ed. J. B. Lippincott Co., Philadelphia, 1970, p. 164.)

administered to another because identifying information was not adequately given or checked.[70]

Hemolytic reactions take place in about 0.53 per cent of the transfusion recipients. Immediate reactions are the most serious and begin after only 25 to 50 ml of blood have been infused. The patient has a sensation of stinging or burning along the vein; there are flushing of the face, chills and fever, acute dyspnea or a feeling of pressure in the chest, headache, pain in the lumbar region, rapid pulse, and perhaps shock. Nurses should remain with patients for at least the first 15 minutes of a transfusion or until 50 ml have been infused to guard against this precipitous reaction.

If a patient has a hemolytic reaction, the transfusion should be discontinued immediately without removing the needle. Because peripheral vascular collapse is often a part of the transfusion reaction, valuable time may be lost in trying to reintroduce a needle into a collapsed vein in order to give an infusion of glucose and water. Oxygen should be started if the patient is not already receiving it, and the physician, if absent, notified in order to get instructions for additional procedures thought necessary.

Allergic and pyrogenic reactions sometimes occur near the completion of a transfusion if the recipient reacts to certain proteins in the donor's blood, or if the blood given is more than 10 to 12 days old * and has bacterial growth. Redness at the site of the needle insertion, itching, hives, wheezing, or a fever of 39.4°C (103°F) or above should all be watched for and, if any of these are present, the transfusion should be discontinued. Any blood unused because of a patient's adverse response to it should be returned to the blood bank immediately so it can be analyzed to determine the reason for the reaction.[71,72]

Cardiac arrhythmias (see Chapter 6), indicating a change in the heart pacing and conductive systems, occur with relative frequency during anesthesia and in the postoperative period. Joseph Kuner and his associates [73] report that in a group of 154 consecutively anesthetized patients, 95 had some form of arrhythmia during anesthesia. Arrhythmias were particularly common with a general anesthetic and most frequent with neurosurgical or

thoracic operations, when the trachea was intubated, or when the patient was hyperventilated. Physical condition, age, sex, and preexisting heart disease were not significantly related to the arrhythmia. Postoperatively, hypoxia, hypoventilation, and hyperventilation appear to be instrumental in bringing about an arrythmia.

Stahl says that of the several arrhythmias a slow heart beat (bradycardia) can be best tolerated by patients unless the rate falls below 40 beats per minute, at which point external pacing must be started. A fast beat (tachycardia) can be tolerated up to 140 to 150 beats per minute if the patient has normal heart muscle reserve. He also says:

. . . atrial tachycardia, atrial flutter, and atrial fibrillation rarely are emergency problems if ventricular rates are maintained within the normal range. . . . Such atrial arrhythmias may be serious, however, in the patient with recent myocardial infarction. . . . Ventricular tachycardia and fibrillation are serious arrhythmias and can cause sudden death.*

Although every cardiac irregularity should be reported to the anesthetist or surgeon, more and more nurses are being prepared to act immediately if the patient should need defibrillation or cardiac resuscitation. Drugs, pacemakers, and precordial shock are used to treat patients with arrhythmias, and the reader is referred to other texts for more detailed information.

Preventing Cardiovascular Complications. *Phlebitis* (inflammation of a vein) that is related to intravenous infusion or indwelling venous catheters is becoming a frequent cardiovascular complication for postoperative as well as other patients who are given intravenous fluids. When fluids are given through a needle inserted into the vein, the site of the insertion and the upper part of the vein often become red, warm, and painful. Physiologic solutions presently used have an acid pH which is thought to contribute to the development of the phlebitis. However, Eric W. Fonkalsrud and his associates [73a] say that commercially prepared glucose fluids (in most countries universally used) cannot be manufactured at physiologic acid-base level for practical as well as technical reasons. Nurses and physicians at University of California at Los Angeles Medical Center found that when 20 ml of a 1 per cent sodium bicarbonate solution was added to either hospital-prepared or commercially prepared intravenous solution given to 160 post-

---

* Allen says that "Another hazard of aged blood is that certain of the gram-negative bacterial contaminants, when present, may reach fairly luxuriant growth by the 21st day of refrigerated storage. Whereas, by the 10th day their growth and endotoxic products are minimal and may be tolerated, the same blood may cause a fatality if allowed to incubate at 2° to 6°C. for 18 to 21 days." (Allen, J. Garrott: *op. cit.,* p. 171.)

* Stahl, William M.: *Supportive Care of the Surgical Patient.* Grune & Stratton, New York, 1972, p. 139.

operative patients just before the fluid was to be administered, the incidence of infusion phlebitis was reduced by 30 to 50 per cent. If this procedure is used, both physicians and nurses should be reminded that some drugs are inactivated when added to a neutral solution.[74] Chapter 22 discusses other causes of infections from intravenous infusions.

Recent studies indicate that *thrombi* (abnormal clots in blood vessels) develop in approximately 30 per cent of the patients having major surgery. Whether this is due to venous stasis, to changes in the coagulation mech-

anisms of the blood, or changes in the vein wall is not definitely known. It seems likely that with different persons any one or a combination of these changes may be the cause. It is thought that many thrombi are formed and absorbed within the first two postoperative weeks without any signs or ill effects. The major danger of thrombi formation comes from the possibility that sections of the clot may break away (emboli) and be carried to the lungs and plug the pulmonary arteries (pulmonary embolism) or other small vessels elsewhere in a vital organ such as the heart or

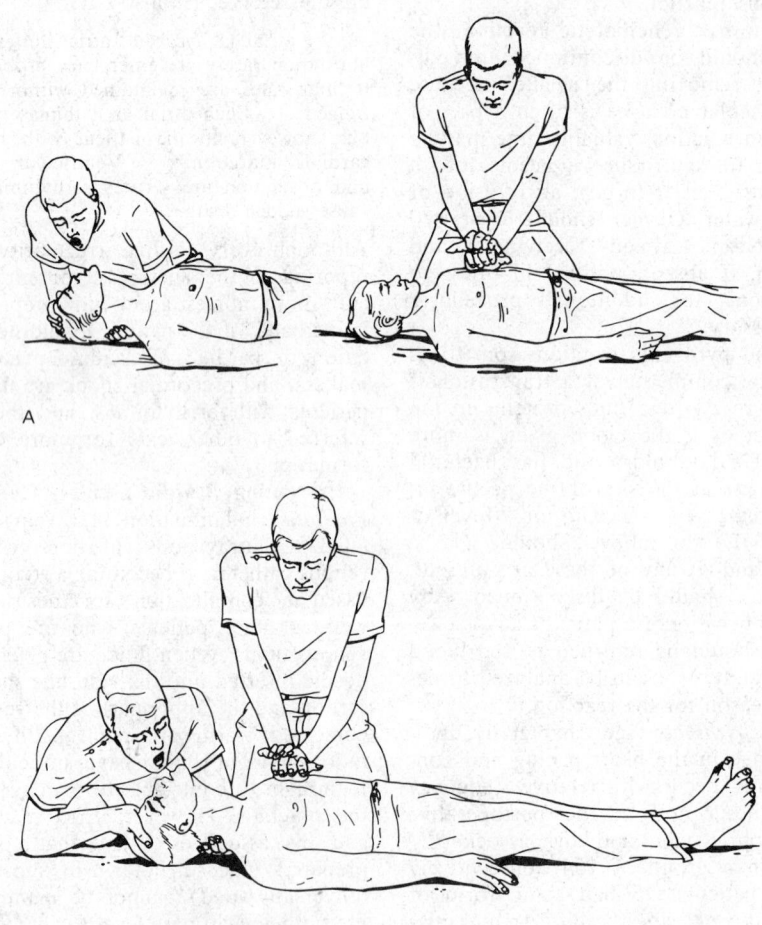

Figure 48-8. *A*. Cardiopulmonary resuscitation by one rescuer using 15:2 ratio of compression to ventilation. *B*. Cardiopulmonary resuscitation by two rescuers using 5:1 ratio of compression to ventilation. Ventilation is by mouth-to-mouth method. *C*. Cardiopulmonary resuscitation by two rescuers using 5:1 ratio of compression to ventilation. Ventilation is by mouth-to-nose method. *D*. Cardiopulmonary resuscitation by two rescuers using 5:1 ratio of compression to ventilation. Ventilation is by bag-valve-mask device. *E*. Child in lateral position for external cardiac compression by index and middle fingers of rescuer. Head is extended to provide open air passage.

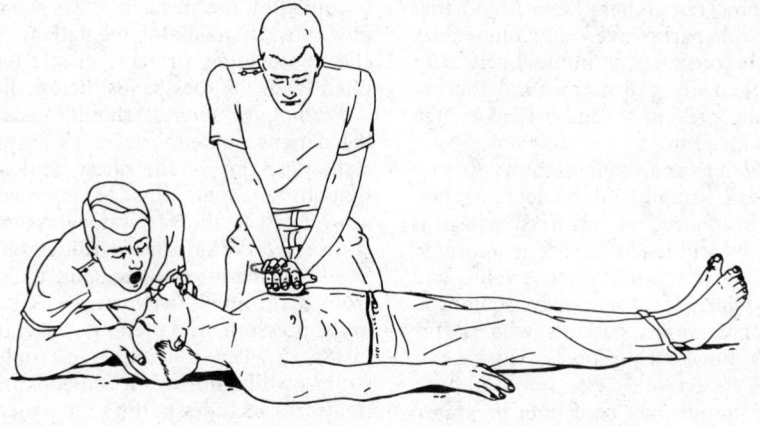

C

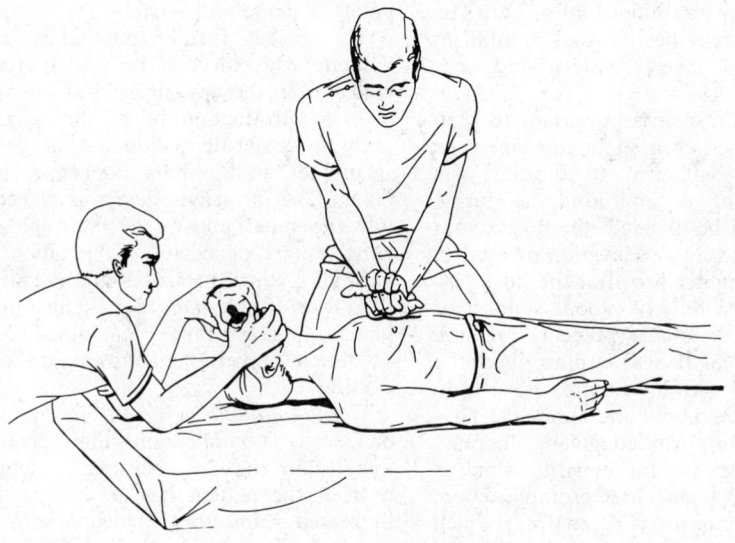

D

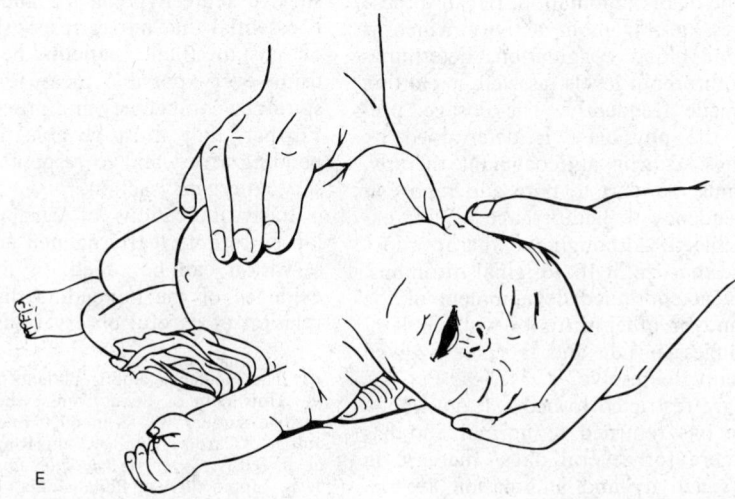

E

the brain.[75] Some researchers have found that small doses of heparin given subcutaneously 8 to 12 hours before surgery, immediately after surgery, and then every 6 hours until the patient is walking, prevent thrombosis in a high percentage of patients.[76]

Thrombophlebitis is an inflammatory disease of the vein wall, usually in the legs, accompanied by thrombosis. A primary cause is venous stasis which tends to occur more in the elderly, in persons with varicose veins, and among those who are prone to muscular inactivity as, for example, patients who sit for a long time in Fowler's position or in a chair with the knees flexed.

The first symptom may be a pain or cramp in the calf which the patient reports to the nurse during morning care. When this happens, the nurse should see that the patient stays in bed until the doctor examines him or her. The initial discomfort may be followed by mild to moderate swelling, fever, redness, and continuing pain.

In thrombophlebitis, it is important to keep the leg at rest, since even slight movement or exertion may be sufficient to dislodge the thrombus. Straining of any kind, as during defecation, should be avoided. On no account is the leg to be massaged. Elevation of the leg, on soft pillows, slightly flexed at the knee, encourages the return flow of blood. Support of the bedclothes by a cradle prevents pressure on the affected area. If heat is prescribed, the cradle is equipped with light bulbs.

In addition to the above measures, the physician may institute anticoagulant therapy. Anticoagulant drugs include heparin, which is given intravenously and has prompt action, and bishydroxycoumarin (Dicumarol), which may be given orally and has a delayed (24 hours) but prolonged action. The drugs may be used alone or in combination. Because these drugs depress prothrombin activity which is necessary for blood coagulation, determinations of prothrombin levels, as well as clotting time, are made frequently. The dosage, prescribed by the physician, is determined by these findings. During anticoagulant therapy, the nurse must be alert to note and report at once any tendency to hemorrhage as, for example, nosebleed. Although the therapy does not decrease the size of the original thrombus, it does prevent continued development of the thrombus and/or other thrombi while inflammatory changes subside and the clot is given an opportunity to resolve.

Patients are restricted to bed rest until body temperature has returned to normal and has remained there for several days. Increase in the patient's activity and ambulation are determined by the physician. To promote venous flow, physicians may have patients wear cotton elastic stockings or have elastic bandages applied from the toes to just below the knee.

Pulmonary emboli should be suspected if the patient suddenly develops dyspnea, cough, stabbing pains in the chest, and anxiety. Although the symptoms of pulmonary emboli are related to the respiratory system, its cause is usually within the cardiovascular system. Small segments are thought to break away from a thrombus when there is increased venous pressure and venous distention as, for instance, when a patient gets out of bed or strains while sitting on a bedpan. Immediate treatment includes putting the patient in a comfortable upright position and giving oxygen. The physician may prescribe a small amount of morphine or a tranquilizer to reduce the patient's panic and anxiety.

To prevent further pulmonary emboli in patients who survive the initial attack, anticoagulation therapy, ligation of the vena cava, or the introduction of an intracaval device such as a silastic balloon, a dacron-covered spring, or an umbrella filter may be undertaken. The intracaval device is placed just below the renal portion of the vena cava and either filters or occludes the blood flow. As with all medical measures that are strange and therefore frightening to patients, nurses' explanation, reassurance, and quiet competency do much to help patients endure these procedures.[77]

Cardiopulmonary arrest is an extremely dangerous complication that occurs infrequently in the postoperative patient; * however, if the patient has an unrecognized and untreated respiratory inadequacy or a period of persistent hypotension, cardiac arrest may result. Because human brain cells can only survive acute hypoxia for about 3 minutes, it is essential that nurses responsible for the care of postanesthetic patients be zealous about using every possible measure to improve respiratory competency and prevent hypotension. Further, they must be able to recognize impending arrest and to respond with the necessary emergency action.[78]

Early indications of cardiopulmonary collapse are not clearly defined and no single observation can be relied on to give sufficient evidence of the impending disaster. The correlation of careful observations, frequently re-

* The incidence among patients at the Hospital of the University of Pennsylvania who were not having cardiac surgery was 1 in 6000 operations. (Johnson, Julian: "Cardiac Surgery," in Rhoads, Jonathan E., et al. [eds.]: *Surgery; Principles and Practice*, 4th ed. J. B. Lippincott Co, Philadelphia, 1970, p. 1295.)

corded, is therefore necessary to determine when treatment is needed. Indications that cardiopulmonary collapse is threatening are (1) a rapid deterioration of skin color, pallor, or cyanosis; (2) absent or weak carotid pulse; (3) venous distention; (4) dyspnea; (5) sudden laryngeal stridor; (6) gurgling respirations; (7) delirium or disorientation; (8) restlessness; (9) garrulousness; (10) rapidly dilating pupils; and (11) loss of consciousness.

The resuscitation phase of cardiopulmonary arrest involves three steps: (1) establishing a patent airway; (2) giving mouth-to-mouth resuscitation (described in Chapter 35) or using a hand-controlled ventilator; and (3) starting external cardiac massage.* If, after 3 to 5 effective lung inflations, the patient is not breathing spontaneously and there is no carotid pulse, external cardiac compression should be started. For cardiac massage, the patient must be on a hard surface, that is, on a board between patient and mattress, or on the floor. Pressure is applied with the heel of one hand placed on the lower half or third of the sternum and the other hand pressed over the first with all fingers off the chest wall. The heart is compressed in a "head-ward" direction because the attachment of the pericardium prevents sideward compression. The sternum must move 3½ to 5 cm (1½ to 2 inches) toward the spine about 60 times per minute. The downward movement should be quick, held for approximately half a second, and then released immediately to allow the chest to recoil. While 80 to 100 lb of pressure is needed for the adult male, any greater pressure may cause additional injury to the heart or surrounding tissues.

For children the heel of only one hand is used, for babies the tips of middle and index fingers, and for tiny infants the chest is circled with the hands and both thumbs are used to apply pressure. The compression rate in these instances should be 100 per minute.

External cardiac massage is useless if ventilation is not continued simultaneously with heart compression. A ratio of 4 to 5 sternal compressions to 1 ventilation of the lungs is recommended in order to adequately circulate oxygenated blood. Figure 48-8*A–D* shows various methods of providing ventilation for a patient in cardiac arrest, and Figure 48-8*E* shows how external cardiac compression is used for infants. When the resuscitation effort is effective the patient's color improves immediately, the carotid pulse can be felt with

each sternal compression, and the pupils of the eyes begin to constrict. After ventilation and circulation have been reestablished, various drugs are given to increase peripheral vascular constriction, to stimulate the heart muscle, and to correct the metabolic acidosis.

Postresuscitation measures are aimed at diagnosing and correcting the cause of the arrest. Whatever the cause, the pulmonary, cardiovascular, renal, and central nervous systems are continuously monitored and observed. Usually minute-to-minute treatment is required.[79,80]

Patients who survive this major biologic insult are often confused and disoriented when they regain consciousness. Nurses must continually reorient them to time, place, and self, and describe or explain the numerous tubes, bottles, and machines. When nurses calmly carry out nursing measures with dexterity and confidence they communicate a sense of safety and reassurance to patients which, in turn, lessens their anxiety and apprehension. Families of patients who have undergone cardiopulmonary arrest also are relieved when they see nurses functioning competently and are given the same kind of explanations given patients.

5. PROMOTING ADEQUATE NUTRITION

The importance of good nutritive food for tissue repair after an operation or an accidental injury is well established. Loss of body protein and increased nitrogen excretion result from either moderate or severe tissue damage; consequently, more than the normal requirement of protein must be supplied in the postoperative diet. Furthermore, studies show that the healing wound needs additional glucose for the first 3 or 4 days after injury, and that vitamin C (ascorbic acid), essential to healing, leaves the plasma and is concentrated at the operative site. Most patients can, however, tolerate 24 to 48 hours without food if their fluid and electrolyte balance is maintained with appropriate intravenous solutions.[81-84]

For Patients Who Have Not Had Surgery of the Alimentary Tract. *Following a general anesthetic,* water may be given as soon as nausea and vomiting cease or when peristaltic sounds are heard in the abdomen. The first or second day after the operation clear liquids such as tea, bouillon, and ginger ale, or fruit-flavored or bouillon gelatin are given to patients as often as they want them. Drinks high in fermentable carbohydrates or amino acids, such as orange juice or milk, are ordinarily

---

* These steps are sometimes called the ABC's of cardiopulmonary resuscitation, that is, Airway, Breathing, Circulation.

not given until the third or fourth day. These foods tend to produce gas and abdominal distention because the sluggish intestine allows a longer time for bacterial fermentation to take place.[85] The fluids administered should be cool, not iced or tepid. It is believed that very cold fluids cause distention by lessening peristalsis, and that ice chips increase the patient's thirst unless they are made from physiologic salt solution. Tepid water may act as an emetic, increasing nausea and vomiting.

By the third or fourth postoperative day, most patients tolerate a liquid diet that includes milk and fruit juices. Usually from this time on the diet plan progresses rapidly through a soft or light diet (simply prepared foods low in residue) to a "general," "regular," "full," or "house" diet that has almost all the foods ordinarily eaten by healthy persons, but is higher in protein. In contrast to patients with abdominal surgery, those with chest, renal, or neurosurgery may progress through the above sequence in a shorter period. By the second or third postoperative day they may be eating a regular diet with some modification of the amount of salt or other electrolytes.

Following a local or regional anesthetic, perhaps used for a bronchoscopy or herniotomy, patients are usually able to eat as they wish as soon as the effects of the anesthetic disappear.

Following acupuncture, patients are able to eat a full meal immediately after the operation. In fact, nurses and physicians who have been observers in Chinese hospitals report that patients are frequently given fruit to eat while still undergoing surgery.[86,87]

Although parenteral solutions for supplying necessary nutrition to critically ill patients are continually being improved, Jonathan E. Rhoads says, "It must be emphasized again and again that the alimentary canal, if normal or only moderately impaired, is the best route for alimentation." * Robert Elman[88] has said that intravenous feedings compete only with starvation and cannot compete with oral feedings. The *advantages eating and drinking have over parenteral feedings* include (1) a larger variety of nutrients are made available to the patient for healing and recovery, as well as the better absorption and assimilation of these nutrients through the physiologic mechanism "designed" for that purpose; (2) the dangers involved with repeated "intrusive" intravenous therapy are avoided and patients are spared the ordeal of combating infections

they may acquire through these procedures; and (3) food and drink are made available in the normal way, and this means for most patients that improvement is taking place and they are on the road to recovery.

Flexibility in the diet through the use of a daily selective menu takes into consideration patients' preferences, and in that way helps increase their comfort and promote recovery. Patient preferences alone, however, may not suffice to give patients the necessary nutrients. Because they often cannot eat or do not relish all the foods served on a hospital diet, the foods consumed by the average postoperative patient tend to be deficient in protein and vitamins, so necessary for tissue healing. Nurses, then, should consider the dietary intake of patients as conscientiously as they consider the administration of an important medication. When patients make poor food choices or do not eat the protein- and vitamin-rich foods served to them, nurses can encourage better food habits by explaining the value of these nutrients and their importance for recovery.

Nurses should realize that a number of drugs commonly given in the postoperative period are likely to decrease the patient's appetite. Morphine, meperidine (Demerol), and codeine tend to cause nausea and consequently make the patient uninterested in eating; they also delay gastric emptying time for 12 hours or more; sedatives given indiscriminately make the patient too sleepy to be interested in food; and aspirin and antibiotics may cause a loss of appetite for some patients. All of these are constipating and may be a factor in loss of appetite. Nurses should question patients who do not eat zestfully to find out if medications are responsible. They should then consult with the physician about discontinuing the drug, reducing the dosage or frequency, or prescribing a different drug.

Every effort should be made to serve foods appetizingly and to arrange the surroundings attractively. Convalescing patients need particular attention if they have a room partner who is retching or vomiting. A pleasant eating area can often be arranged in a solarium, or a plan for a patients' dining room instituted.

Postoperative nausea and vomiting with general anesthesia are thought to occur less frequently now than in the past. Various reports place the incidence from 3.6 per cent to 60 per cent of the patients studied.[89,90] Nausea is the desire to vomit, but it may or may not result in this explosive movement which often relieves nausea. It is often accompanied by increased salivation, sweating, a faster pulse rate, and variations in the rate, depth, and regularity of respirations. Retching occurs when

---

* Rhoads, Jonathan E.: "Nutrition," in Rhoads, Jonathan E., et al. (eds.): *Surgery; Principles and Practice,* 4th ed. J. B. Lippincott Co., Philadelphia, 1970, p. 108.

the stomach is empty or nearly so, while vomiting occurs when there are gastric contents. Both consist of a series of movements, initiated in the vomiting center of the medulla, that squeeze the relaxed stomach between the descending diaphragm and the contracting abdominal muscles, open the sphincters between the stomach and the mouth, and close the glottis to protect the trachea.[91]

Postoperative nausea with or without vomiting often (but not necessarily) occurs when the gag reflex returns. It may last from 1 to several hours, and has various causes. The most common is the anesthetic or the drugs given preoperatively or during the operation. Patients anesthetized through a mask rather than an endotracheal tube are particularly prone to postoperative nausea and vomiting because the mask technique requires deeper anesthesia, and the stomach is easily distended with the anesthetic. Obese patients not only vomit more frequently than do lean persons, but often for a longer time because the anesthetic is retained in fat deposits. Patients with abdominal surgery which included manipulation of the intestines, women patients, and patients between the ages of 26 and 56 are more likely to have nausea and vomiting than are men, children, or the elderly. And, finally, vomiting occurs frequently with nervous persons who vomit easily, those who have a history of motion sickness, or who have had a past experience of vomiting after an anesthetic.[92,93] Vomiting does not usually persist beyond the first day, but if it does, more serious complications, such as peritonitis or intestinal obstruction, should be suspected.

Nausea and vomiting cause considerable discomfort, to say the least. Retching and vomiting may also be hazardous if they place undue strain on the suture line, or if the vomiting becomes excessive with an accompanying loss of fluids and electrolytes. Dehydration and electrolyte loss cause further nausea and vomiting and hinder the body's reparative processes. In some cases, the surgeon anticipates these events and introduces a gastrointestinal tube preoperatively or immediately following the surgery. At other times, the intubation is done when the patient's vomiting cannot be controlled by other means. Fluids and electrolytes must then be replaced through intravenous solutions. If excessive vomiting occurs, nurses' observations and records of the type, amount, and frequency of vomitus as well as the amount of fluid taken by mouth are important for planning the patient's continuing treatment.

Various measures may be used to prevent or relieve postoperative nausea and vomiting, although no one method is effective with every patient. Nurses should turn patients carefully and slowly, because movement of the head, even in patients not prone to motion sickness, tends to increase nausea in the postanesthetic patient. Patients taught to take a series of deep breaths often find this helpful. Sometimes the administration of a sedative, such as phenobarbital, decreases nausea by inducing rest; however, morphine or meperidine may increase the nausea. A number of drugs that contain antihistamines, phenothiazines, or butyrophenones have been developed for the control of nausea and vomiting within recent years. Those most commonly used are chlorpromazine (Thorazine), promethazine (Phenergan), and perphenazine (Trilafon). These drugs vary with individuals in their effectiveness. In addition, their side effects may be more harmful than the vomiting itself because they include hypotension, extrapyramidal reactions, and respiratory depression if the drugs are given with a narcotic. Dimenhydrinate (Dramamine) is also given to relieve nausea and seems to be most effective with patients prone to motion sickness or those who have had surgery on or near the vestibular labyrinth.[94,95]

Because the presence of nausea and vomiting may depend on the person's general reaction to stressful situations rather than specific physiologic causes, Elman's comment in 1951 is still valid. He said:

In a few patients solid foods will be tolerated better than liquids. Anything very much desired by the patient is not apt to produce nausea. A patient who is allowed up and about early is not as likely to suffer nausea and vomiting as much as one who must remain in the horizontal position.*

Rhetaugh G. Dumas and Robert C. Leonard [96] report that the incidence of postoperative vomiting is considerably reduced when nurses, during the preoperative period, identify and relieve any overt or covert distress the patient may be having. (See Chapter 47 for further discussion of this subject.)

The head of the patient who is vomiting should be turned to one side and an emesis basin conveniently placed. By supporting the patient's head firmly, the nurse can prevent excessive movement and relieve some of the strain involved. It is undesirable to keep an emesis basin within sight of the patient, because the power of suggestion may in itself induce vomiting. The basin should, however, be easily reached. A cool damp cloth to clean

* Elman, Robert: *Surgical Care: A Practical Physiological Guide.* Appleton-Century-Crofts, New York, 1951, p. 308.

the patient's face, a pleasant-tasting mouth rinse, a well-ventilated room free from odor, and the reassuring presence and concern of the nurse all help to make the nauseated or vomiting patient more comfortable.

Thoughtful nursing can contribute greatly to alleviation of the symptom. Although it is not always possible to differentiate the psychogenic causes from the physical ones, it should nevertheless be realized that emotional response to factors such as a disagreeable odor, foul-tasting mouth, fear, or resentment can certainly aggravate or perpetuate an "upset stomach" no matter what the original cause. It is therefore wise for the nurse to use a combination of physical and psychologic measures in caring for patients with this disturbing symptom.

For Patients Who Have Had Surgery of the Alimentary Tract. Providing adequate nutrition for patients who have had *surgery on the mouth or throat* can be a temporary, rather simple task or a long-term complicated one. Patients who have had a large number of teeth extracted, who are waiting for dentures, or who are becoming accustomed to dentures often need help with planning a nutritious liquid or soft diet. Since their digestion of foods is not impaired, any foods can be taken in a fluid form, or ground so they require little chewing. Electric blenders are very useful in such cases. Most of the commercially prepared baby foods are good temporary substitutes until chewing can be resumed comfortably.

After a tonsillectomy, the temperature and consistency of foods given the first few days are most important. Very cold and mild-flavored liquids offer the most comfort to the patient and prevent bleeding from the tonsillar fossa. Ice cream and popsicles are favorite choices of children. Warm, soft foods, such as a poached egg, milk toast, or strained vegetables may be added the second or third day, and hot foods cautiously added after 4 or 5 days. Within a week to 10 days the patient will have returned to a normal diet.[97]

Postoperatively, patients who have extensive surgery of the mouth, neck, or esophagus not only require that food be of a special consistency, but also frequently require a completely different way of ingesting food, that is, intravenously or by way of a tube. If the patient will be unable to chew or swallow after the operation, a cervical esophagostomy tube is often inserted at the time of surgery. After patients with this kind of feeding tube come from the operating room, the tube is attached to intermittent suction for 24 to 48 hours in order to prevent gastric distention and vomiting, and then tube feeding diets are started. The tube should be marked in some way so it is not confused with other drainage tubes in this area of the neck.

Once these patients are no longer nauseated or vomiting, they are given foods in the same sequence as general surgical patients who are not fed through a tube: water and clear liquids are given through the tube first, then more nutritious fluids, and finally liquified ("blenderized") regular diets. Cervical esophagostomy tubes are usually removed after 2 or 3 weeks.

Some patients with extensive head and neck surgery are able to swallow but not chew postoperatively; consequently, they may first take fluids using a straw, and then be gradually introduced to a liquified or soft diet as chewing and swallowing improve. Tables 48-1,

Table 48-1.   Standard Pureed Gavage (basically a normal diet in pureed form, with 1 cal/ml; adequate in all nutrients if enough calories are taken)*

Ingredients	Approximate Household Measure	Amount	Calories	Carbohydrate (gm)	Protein (gm)	Fat (gm)
Baby veal	5⅓ oz	160 gm	146		24.8	4.3
Baby peas	4½ oz	130 gm	70	11.1	5.5	0.3
Baby peaches	4½ oz	130 gm	105	26.3	0.8	0.3
Skim milk powder	9 tbsp	70 gm	254	36.6	25.1	0.7
Oil (corn, etc.)	2 tbsp	30 gm	265	0.0	0.0	30.0
Dextrose (dark label Karo)	2 tbsp	30 gm	110	30.0	0.0	0.0
Poly-Vi-Sol (Mead Johnson)		0.6 ml				
Add water to make 1 qt (unused portions must be refrigerated)		1000 ml	950	104.0	56.2	35.6

* Diets adapted from *A Handbook for Writing Modified Diets.* Department of Pediatrics, Indiana University Medical Center, Bloomington, 1969.

Table 48-2. Standard Milk-Base Gavage (a maintenance or supplemental milk-base diet; should not be used for a long time since it is not as nutritionally complete as standard pureed gavage)*

Ingredients	Approximate Household Measure	Amount	Calories	Carbohydrate (gm)	Protein (gm)	Fat (gm)
Homogenized milk	3¾ cup	900 ml	585	44.1	31.5	31.5
Skim milk powder	7 tbsp	50 gm	182	26.2	18.0	0.4
Dextrose (dark label Karo)	4 tbsp	60 gm	220	59.7	0.0	0.0
Poly-Vi-Sol (Mead Johnson)		0.6 ml				
Fer-In-Sol (Mead Johnson)		0.6 ml				
Water to make: (unused portions must be refrigerated)	1 qt	1000 ml	987	130.0	49.5	31.9

48-2, and 48-3 show diets that can be made for hospitalized patients or those cared for at home who have had operations of the head and neck.[98-100]

Nutrition for patients who have *surgery of the stomach or intestines* is also provided by intravenous or tube feedings. A nasogastric tube, gastrostomy tube, or duodenal tube may be inserted. Chapter 23 discusses the basic procedures that are used when patients are intubated for feeding. It also describes the methods of instilling formulas in the tube; consequently, those procedures are not repeated here.

If a feeding tube is inserted into the jejunum, the patient's physiology may require a longer time to become accustomed to this method of receiving nutrients than if the tube is higher in the alimentary tract. During the immediate postoperative period, the tube is connected to low suction or allowed to drain by gravity. Usually, after 24 hours a normal saline solution is introduced into the tube by continuous drip. Following this, a solution of equal parts of boiled skimmed milk and lime water (U.S.P.) may be given, and if this is well tolerated, a high-protein, high-carbohydrate, low-fat, low-residue liquid diet is begun. Skimmed or evaporated milk is used in these formulas because fresh, whole milk tends to cause gas and distention.[101]

Any diet formula given through a jejunostomy tube must be introduced slowly, or cramps, diarrhea, or the "dumping syndrome" are likely to develop. The dumping syndrome with nausea, cramps, vomiting, pallor, sweating, and faintness occurs when a larger than usual amount of undiluted food enters the jejunum, whether from the stomach or an ostomy feeding. While the causes of this syndrome are not well understood, it is partially due to the mechanical distention of the jejunum and the shifting of body fluids into the intestine to make the contents isotonic. Should

Table 48-3. High-Protein Nourishment (high calorie–high protein feeding; one 8-oz glass provides 425 calories) *

Ingredient	Approximate Household Measure	Amount	Calories	Carbohydrate (gm)	Protein (gm)	Fat (gm)
Half and Half cream	3 oz	100 ml	134	4.6	3.2	11.7
Milk	2 cups	480 ml	317	23.5	16.8	17.8
Eggs	4	180 ml	293	1.6	23.2	20.7
Skim milk powder	2½ cups	180 gm	653	94.1	64.6	1.4
Dextrose (dark label Karo)	6 tbsp	90 gm	330	89.6	0.0	0.0
Vanilla extract	1 tbsp	1 tbsp				
Total (unused portions must be refrigerated)	1 qt	1000 ml	1727	213.4	107.8	51.6

* Diets adapted from *A Handbook for Writing Modified Diets.* Department of Pediatrics, Indiana University Medical Center, Bloomington, 1969.

this condition occur, the formula is discontinued, dextrose in water is given intravenously, and the use of the skimmed milk and lime water solution is resumed.[102]

Most patients who are fed postoperatively through a tube are able to dispense with that method of "eating" before they are discharged from the hospital. However, during the time a feeding tube is in place nurses should take precautions so that a treatment designed to help patients regain a measure of health does not instead cause additional injury. For instance, if nurses are responsible for inserting the nasogastric tube, they must know the anatomy of the alimentary tract, must be certain the tube is in the stomach, and, should the tube be left in place for some days, must make sure the tube is taped to the side of the patient's face so there is no pull and no pressure on the nostril. The freshness, temperature, and rate of administration of the formula must all be carefully regulated, and the tube kept from clogging with a rinse of isotonic saline solution after each feeding. The ingenuity of nurses is taxed to the utmost to provide the emotional satisfactions of eating and mealtime for patients who are fed through a tube for a long time. Since these patients can no longer enjoy food for its flavor, consistency, or pleasing aroma, other aspects of mealtime such as attractive serving containers, attractive tray covers, and pleasant companionship can be provided.

If a patient with a nasogastric tube is nauseated and vomiting, care must be taken, particularly with an unconscious patient, that none of the vomitus is aspirated. The same *measures to control nausea and vomiting* that were described earlier are applicable to intubated patients. If antiemetic medications are given, they are easily instilled through the feeding tube in liquid form.

Some patients are so critically ill or so debilitated from the preoperative disease that neither oral nor tube feedings provide enough protein, calories, vitamins, and minerals for recovery. In these situations, a concentrated solution of nutrients may be given intravenously (*parenteral hyperalimentation*). Stanley J. Dudrick and Jonathan E. Rhoads say:

The primary aim of total parenteral nutrition is to provide suitable carbohydrates, protein moieties, and other essential nutrients exclusively by vein for prolonged periods of time in quantities substantially greater than the basal requirements for caloric and nitrogen equilibrium. . . . The solution must not contain pyrogens or cause fever for any other reasons. It must exert at least sufficient total osmotic pressure to avoid injury to the cellular elements of the blood. The foodstuff must be in forms that normally travel in the circulatory system, such as glucose, fructose, amino acids, or peptides of very short chain length. It must preserve or permit the body to maintain normal concentrations of the various biologic ions such as sodium, potassium, chloride, calcium, phosphorus, and bicarbonate, with a resultant pH in the normal range. The method must avoid the production of thrombosis and embolism and should not necessarily confine the patient to bed or other forms of inactivity. The technique of infusion must include stringent precautions against infection and must be sufficiently safe and stable that administration apparatus can be left in place and kept functioning for several days or weeks when required.*

In order to achieve these goals, a small catheter is introduced under sterile conditions into a subclavian vein and then into the superior vena cava. The first responsibility of nurses in this procedure is to explain it to patients. The explanation includes (1) what is going to be done; (2) that a slight head-down position with the face turned to one side and absolute stillness are necessary; (3) that a small pinprick will be felt at the collar bone when the local anesthetic is given; and (4) that sterile towels, or cloths, will be placed over the area and partially cover the face for a short time. After the physician inserts the catheter, the nurse explains that the dressing covering the catheter insertion should not be removed and should be kept dry. In addition, patients are encouraged to move freely in bed and to walk as much as possible using a rolling intravenous stand to hold the feeding solution. Further nursing responsibilities with patients having parenteral hyperalimentation are to maintain the sterility of the infusing fluid, to redress periodically (approximately every other day) the insertion site and change all of the intravenous tubing except the catheter, using a sterile technique, and to make certain the rate of flow is constant over each 24-hour period. Extreme care is needed to maintain conditions of sterility so that infections do not occur either locally at the site of the catheter insertion or systemically from the solution. A constant rate of flow is essential to an optimum utilization of the glucose in the solution. A strictly accurate intake and output record and a daily weight record are necessary to help the physician determine the patient's fluid balance.[103,104]

* Dudrick, Stanley J., and Rhoads, Jonathan E.: "Metabolism in Surgical Patients: Protein, Carbohydrate, and Fat Utilization by Oral and Parenteral Routes," in Sabiston, David C., Jr. (ed.): *Davis-Christopher Textbook of Surgery*, 10th ed. W. B. Saunders Co., Philadelphia, 1972, p. 159.

Some patients require surgical removal of nearly all or some portion of the stomach. In the immediate and early postoperative periods, nutrients are usually provided by parenteral hyperalimentation until the patient is able to take sufficient food by mouth. Long-term dietary problems with partial gastrectomy result from the loss of gastric storage capacity, inadequate mixing of food with digestive enzymes, loss of intrinsic factor (important in the prevention of pernicious anemia), and interference with iron absorption. There is much debate about whether excessive weight loss following gastrectomy is due to inadequate caloric intake or inadequate digestion and/or absorption. Some diets, consequently, are high in protein, fat, and carbohydrates, while others are high in protein and fat, but low in carbohydrates. In any case, frequent small meals are recommended and vitamins and inorganic iron salts are usually prescribed.[105] Nurses, with the physician, dietitian, and patient, should discuss the diet, keeping in mind the goal of providing simple, easily digested, mild-flavored foods to give the alimentary tract a chance to perform its normal functions.

Adequate nutrition is provided for patients who have had an ileostomy in essentially the same way as for general surgical patients during the immediate and early postoperative periods. Once these patients have progressed past the liquid diet stage, they are usually given, for a limited time, a diet that is easily digested and has little residue. After a period of 3 to 12 weeks, the discharge from the ileostomy stoma becomes pastelike rather than liquid, and patients may add other foods to the diet. Individuals who have had an ileostomy for some time are able to eat entirely normal meals. A few foods such as fish, onions, and eggs may be omitted because they produce odors; cooked cabbage, prune juice, and baked beans may be omitted because they are likely to increase the amount of ileostomy drainage; and corn, popcorn, and berries with large seeds should be omitted because they tend to block the ileostomy stoma. Patients with ileostomies should be encouraged to eat any foods that appeal to them, but be reminded that all foods must be thoroughly chewed. In addition, well-salted food and extra amounts of water at meals and between meals must be taken to offset water and sodium loss through the ileostomy.[106]

Patients who have a colostomy opening on the abdomen follow essentially the same sequence in dietary progression as do other surgical patients. Some will need assistance in planning diets to eliminate individualized reactions, such as diarrhea, to specific foods.

6. PROMOTING ADEQUATE ALIMENTARY ELIMINATION

For Patients Who Have Not Had Surgery of the Alimentary Tract. Most surgical patients have a decrease in bowel function for the first 2 or 3 postoperative days. This is largely due to the anesthetic agent, the cumulative effect of the surgical trauma, and the lack of bulk in the intestine. Because the lack of alimentary tract motility allows the accumulation of gas in the intestines, many surgeons routinely insert a postoperative nasogastric tube which is connected to continuous suction for 48 to 72 hours. Other surgeons insert such a tube if the patient vomits excessively or develops a distended abdomen in the postoperative period. Frequently, the discomfort of abdominal distention is more distressing than the operation itself.

Distention with gas may be due to a variety of causes: extensive exposure and handling of the intestine during surgery, morphine, codeine, atropine, or anticholinergic drugs, postoperative inactivity, inflammatory processes, and too early an introduction of food, especially gas-producing foods such as orange juice and milk. Although cutting and burning the intestine produce no painful sensation, stretching it, as occurs with gas distention, is extremely painful.

It is estimated that about 70 per cent of all gas reaching the gastrointestinal tract comes from swallowed air.[107] Under normal conditions, 5 to 15 per cent of this air is absorbed in the small intestine, and the remainder is transported to the large intestine. The average healthy, active person has 7 to 10 liters of gas entering or forming in the large intestine every day, but expels only 0.5 liters.[108] The remainder is absorbed through the intestinal mucosa. Postoperatively, when peristalsis is decreased and patients' activity limited, the gas is neither absorbed nor expelled, and the accumulation may stretch the intestine to an enormous size. Also, segments of the bowel often undergo spastic contractions, causing the pain to be intermittent and cramplike in character.

Gas pains can usually be minimized, and in many cases prevented or relieved, by conscientious nursing. Eliminating gas-forming foods from the diet and teaching the patient how to swallow less air, especially while drinking, are helpful measures. Frequent changes in position and ambulation will help prevent the accumulation of gas, and will also help in its expulsion. Inserting a tube in the rectum is often sufficient to start the expulsion of gas. Application of heat to the abdomen may give relief, and can be used alone or in conjunction with a rectal tube. Occasionally, the surgeon will prescribe drugs to stimulate the contraction of the intestinal muscles, such as vasopressin (Pitressin), surgical vasopressin (surgical Pituitrin), and bethanechol (Urecholine), given usually in combination with the insertion of a rectal tube.

The surgical patient's ability to expel gas and have a bowel movement spontaneously indicates that normal function has returned to the gastrointestinal tract. Although gas may be expelled earlier, a spontaneous bowel movement does not usually occur until about the fourth or fifth postoperative day. Some surgeons prescribe an enema or cathartic on the second or third postoperative day. Others prefer to wait for a natural movement, provided the delay is not prolonged. The management of postoperative defecation espoused by Elman [108a] more than two decades ago is generally accepted practice today. He said that it is unwise to hasten defecation by artificial means, such as enemas, cathartics, or peristaltic stimulants. This is because postoperative cessation of peristalsis serves as a physiologic protective mechanism to keep the gastrointestinal tract at rest, just as immobilization of an injured arm is a voluntary protective mechanism to keep the arm at rest. He considers that a delay in defecation of 4 or 5 days following surgery produces no harmful effects, and that methods of routine postoperative purging may not only produce harm, but also are "just as illogical as whipping a tired horse," besides causing needless pain and distress to the patient. If proper attention is paid to postoperative exercise, ambulation, nutrition, and to the patient's physical and psychogenic needs, such as privacy, normal position, and timing with the urge to defecate, there is generally no problem.

In cases where the feces remain in the rectum longer than usual, as can be determined on rectal examination, or the patient feels the urge to defecate without being able to expel adequate amounts, some assistance is usually required. This occurs more frequently with elderly patients and children. The simplest methods of promoting a bowel movement may be tried first, such as mild cathartics, the introduction of a thin glycerin suppository, or a small oil retention enema followed by a small cleansing enema. If the feces are impacted, more drastic measures may be needed, such as digital removal or instrumental removal through an anoscope. Very small bowel movements or diarrhea should be noted and reported to the surgeon, for either may indicate the presence of fecal impaction.

For Patients Who Have Had Surgery of the Alimentary Tract. Patients with operations of the esophagus or stomach usually have little difficulty with fecal elimination once they can have semisolid or solid foods. Some surgery of the intestinal tract, however, requires a diversion of feces from the diseased or injured colon, rectum, and anus through the creation of a colostomy or an ileostomy. This is done by bringing a part of the intestine through an abdominal opening (stoma).

A *temporary colostomy* (an abdominal anus fashioned from a section of the colon) is usually made when the surgeon's goal is to decompress the bowel in preparation for later resection and reconstruction of the distal colon, or when the goal is to divert intestinal contents from a perforated section of the colon, or a rectovaginal fistula. Once healing of the distal colon occurs, the colostomy ends are sutured and replaced in the abdomen. Defecation can then take place in the usual way. A *permanent colostomy* is made if the entire rectum and anus must be excised because of a malignant growth. Helping patients cope with the emotional shock of this change in body function, whether temporary or permanent, is discussed in Chapter 23. Other aspects of the preoperative, postoperative, and rehabilitative care of patients with colostomies are also discussed in that chapter and are not repeated here. Articles written by nurses that will be helpful to the especially interested reader are listed at the end of this chapter.[109-115]

An ileostomy (an abdominal anus made from a section of the ileum) is nearly always a permanent anatomical change because it is only occasionally possible to leave part of the colon and rectum for later reconstruction. Ileostomies are generally the last recourse for treatment of patients with ulcerative colitis or familial polyposis.* Marshall Sparberg describes the differences between an ileostomy and a colostomy as follows:

Ileostomy	Colostomy
1. For ulcerative colitis or multiple polyposis	1. For rectal carcinoma or diverticular disease
2. Stoma protrudes [from abdomen]	2. Stoma [is] flush [with abdomen]
3. Right sided	3. Left sided
4. Effluent [is] liquid	4. Effluent [is] solid
5. Effluent [is] corrosive	5. Effluent [is] inert
6. Appliance required	6. Appliance optional
7. Irrigation unnecessary	7. Irrigation required *

* Sparberg, Marshall: *Ileostomy Care.* Charles C Thomas, Publisher, Springfield, Ill., 1971, p. vi.

* Polyposis is a rare disease characterized by the presence of polyps of varying sizes in the colon and frequently occurs in several family members because it has a genetic origin.

The intestinal contents expelled through an ileostomy are liquid for the first 3 to 4 months after surgery, and although always loose become semisolid as the ileum adapts and absorbs some of the water once absorbed by the colon. Because this discharge cannot be regulated as can the discharge from a colostomy, and it is rich in enzymes capable of digesting skin, an ileostomy appliance must be worn at all times.

The ileostomy prosthesis consists of two parts. Although there are variations in design, it consists of a pouch or bag to hold the effluent and a face plate to attach the appliance over the stoma. The main differences between temporary appliances and permanent appliances are the materials used for the pouch and face plate, and the presence or absence of attachments for a belt. Temporary appliances are made of plastic or some other transparent disposable material and have adhesive already on the face plate. This adhesive, while effective for many hours, finally softens and allows leaking and soiling around the stoma. The permanent appliance is made of heavy opaque rubber or plastic and the face plate is attached over the stoma with a special cement used each time the prosthesis is changed. A belt to give additional support to the appliance is attached to hooks on either side of the face plate. The bottom of the bag has an opening that is rolled and closed with a rubber band or clip after the bag has been emptied. (Some temporary appliances also are constructed in this way.) Figure 23-16 shows the removal and reapplication of a permanent ileostomy appliance.

A temporary appliance is placed over the stoma before the patient leaves the operating room so the condition of the stoma can be observed without removing the bag and so none of the effluent touches the skin. The seal between the skin and appliance plate or adhesive material must be absolutely leak-proof, and whenever the appliance is changed a new leak-proof seal must be provided. It is far easier to prevent excoriated skin than to cure it.

Temporary bags are less desirable for posthospitalization use than permanent bags because they sometimes develop leaks, the thinner bag material breaks if the wearer is very active, and the cost eventually becomes very high. Some patients prefer them, however, because of the ease of their use.

The importance of preventing skin irritation for the ileostomy patient must be constantly emphasized, because ulcerated or irritated skin around the stoma prevents patients from wearing any kind of appliance that, in turn, is essential to a life of activity and productiveness.

Karaya gum powder or Karaya washers next to the patient's skin are considered the most useful of any materials used for skin protection.* Karaya gum powder is made from the resin of the *Sterculia urens* tree in India. It is healing, absorbs moisture, is not greasy, and is resistant to pancreatic enzymes. In addition, it has an adherent quality that makes its use in the first few weeks of care important because cements do not have to be used. Karaya washers consist of Karaya powder and glycerin baked into rings of various sizes with varying sized openings. When the patient is active again, a thin layer of cement may be painted over the washer or moistened powder to give additional assurance that the appliance is firmly attached.[116]

Immediate postoperative care of the patient with an ileostomy differs from that of other surgical patients only in the scrupulous care given the peristomal skin, careful measurement and recording of fluids lost through the ileostomy, and attention to the perineal wound. The perineal wound is usually painful the first several postoperative days and may have packs or catheters in the area formerly occupied by the rectum. To promote healing from the inside out, meticulous perineal hygiene with frequent soap and water washing and frequent sitz baths are usually prescribed. (Sitz baths are discussed in Chapter 29.)

Since space does not permit discussion here of many important details of late postoperative ileostomy care, readers are referred to Marshall Sparberg's book, *Ileostomy Care,*[116a] written for health personnel, and the *Manual for Ileostomy Patients*[116b] published for individuals with ileostomies by the Ostomy Association of Boston, Inc.

7. PROMOTING ADEQUATE URINARY ELIMINATION

For Patients Who Have Not Had Surgery of the Urinary System. A competently functioning renal system is extremely important to any patient's well-being, and this is especially true for the postoperative patient. The generally accepted level of *adequate postoperative renal function* is the production each hour of 30 to 50 ml of urine with a normal specific gravity. This measurement is not only an effective measure of kidney functioning but also of an adequate circulating blood volume and

---

* Sprays of plastic film that create a thin layer of material between the skin and cement or any leaking ileal discharge have been developed in recent years; however, their effectiveness in preventing skin irritation has not yet been tested among enough individuals to know whether they are as useful as Karaya powder.

adequately functioning cardiopulmonary systems. If the surgeon suspects that a patient's kidney function may be in more danger than usual in the postoperative period, a retention catheter is inserted in the bladder before the patient leaves the operating room. This makes hourly monitoring of urine output more precise. Catheters inserted for this reason are generally removed in a few days. They must be inserted under strict aseptic conditions and connected with sterile closed-drainage collection equipment (see Chapter 24). Recent research shows that with careful adherence to aseptic procedures when emptying or changing any part of the closed-drainage equipment, the incidence of bacteriuria in patients with retention catheters for less than a week is considerably reduced from the 95 per cent incidence found with patients having the open-drainage system of several years ago. Vincent T. Andriole [117] and Robert E. Desautels [118] say that from 80 to 90 per cent of patients having catheters less than 7 to 10 days do not develop bacteriuria when (1) the connection between the catheter and drainage tubing is not broken after it is established under aseptic conditions; (2) the collecting bag is emptied every 8 hours and the outlet tube cleaned with aqueous Zephiran solution; (3) the bag is not inverted so that urine touches or goes into the drainage tubing; and (4) perineal care with soap and water or aqueous Zephiran solution is given at least twice daily to women and once a day to men. Dennis G. Maki and his associates [119] say that in addition there should be mandatory handwashing by nurses and physicians between contacts with all patients and especially catheterized persons. Their research indicates that patients with indwelling catheters should not be in the same rooms or their beds close to one another in a ward because bacteriuria organisms are so easily transferred from one patient to another.

The combined effects of surgical trauma, blood loss, and anesthetic in the early postoperative period activate a body fluid conservation system that decreases the amount of urine, saliva, sweat, and gastrointestinal juice, as well as the sodium level of these body fluids. It is generally thought that this reduction of urine formation lasts about 48 hours, and patients with minor surgery and little blood loss need no special treatment.[120] Most patients who have had major operations, however, are given appropriate fluids. Thomas V. Berne and Benjamin H. Barbour [121] believe that the vigorous treatment of low blood volume with fluids and diuretic therapy has prevented renal failure in many patients having general surgery.

The ability to empty the bladder after surgery is of more immediate concern to patients than is kidney function. The details of muscle and nerve interaction leading to *normal voiding* are discussed in Chapter 11. Postoperatively, the bladder tends to hold the urine which has accumulated in it for longer periods than under ordinary conditions. Besides causing the patient considerable discomfort and restlessness, *retention of urine* also predisposes to the development of cystitis. Several reasons are given why urinary retention tends to occur postoperatively. Most authorities agree that diminished sensitivity after general anesthesia permits the bladder to fill more completely than under ordinary circumstances, and also that psychic phenomena play a definite role. Besides this, Vernon S. Dick suggests that overdistention of the bladder may occur more quickly than is realized following surgery because of the rapid administration of fluids. This in turn causes a decrease in muscle tone of the bladder, with later difficulty in urination.

Adding to these circumstances is the fact that the voluntary abdominal and perineal muscles play a much greater part in the act of micturition than many people realize, and if the operative site is so located that pain is produced by effort to contract these muscles, further interference of vesical emptying is produced.*

Many patients are unable to void, even though the bladder feels full, because of the unnatural position the use of a bedpan or urinal requires. In addition, the presence of other patients and nurses may trigger long forgotten childhood admonitions and restrictions about proper times and places to urinate. However, if given appropriate privacy and helped to be as comfortable as possible most patients are able to void. Chapter 11 describes nursing measures that can be used to stimulate voiding.

Frequently, patients will suffer from retention as long as they remain in bed, and be relieved immediately when allowed to get up and assume the normal position for voiding. In a study of postoperative urinary retention, Charles W. McLaughlin and John R. Brown [122] studied 1964 young men undergoing surgery. In one group, the patient was not permitted to stand to void but received doses of neostigmine (Prostigmin). The incidence of urinary retention under these conditions was 3 per cent. When injections of saline were substituted for neostigmine, the incidence remained essentially the same. In the second group, the patient was permitted up to void and received the same doses of neostigmine as the first

* Dick, Vernon S.: "Management of Postoperative Urinary Retention," *Lahey Clin. Bull.,* **7:**57, (Oct.) 1950.

group. Under those conditions, the incidence of urinary retention was only 0.76 per cent, and did not significantly change when saline was substituted for the neostigmine.

With early ambulation, then, and with conditions simulating a normal atmosphere for the function of elimination, urinary retention is not as common a problem as it was when patients were kept in bed for longer periods. However, it is still an important function of the nurse to safeguard the patient against this untoward development, for it is through intelligent and sympathetic nursing that the incidence of urinary retention and its complications can be reduced.

Most surgeons will make provision, in case a patient is unable to void, for catheterizing him or her within 8 to 10 hours after the operation. Some allow a shorter period, and others a longer interval; but the aim is always to catheterize the patient before the bladder becomes distended, provided other measures are unsuccessful. (See Chapter 24 for basic catheterization procedures and the risks of bladder infection.) Many authorities believe that when the bladder is allowed to become overdistended, and is then decompressed, there is congestion and edema of the mucous membrane, and the tendency to develop cystitis increases. The residual urine then serves as a culture medium for the growth of bacteria upon introduction of a catheter. Also, stretching of the vesical wall may induce atony and interfere with later resumption of normal tone and voiding.

Heonir Rocha says:

It seems that the condition of the bladder at the time of catheterization greatly influences the subsequent incidence of bacteriuria. The normal bladder, because of highly effective defense mechanisms, delays the onset of bacteriuria and is more capable of cleansing itself of infection. Single catheterization in healthy ambulatory persons results in very few cases of bacteriuria.*

Should the patient continue to have difficulty with urination, the surgeon may prescribe a drug to stimulate the parasympathetic nervous system. Two drugs that are used for this purpose are carbachol (Doryl) and bethanechol (Urecholine).

For Patients Who Have Had Surgery of the Urinary System. The most common surgical procedure of the urinary system is the transurethral prostatectomy, and the least common is the kidney transplantation. Although the specialized equipment and procedures of urology

---

* Rocha, Heonir: "Epidemiology of Urinary Tract Infection in Adults," in Kaye, Donald (ed.): *Urinary Tract Infection and Its Management.* C. V. Mosby Co., St. Louis, 1972, p. 147.

and urologic nursing are not detailed here, some general comments about maintaining the urinary elimination of patients who have surgery of the renal tract can be made.

In almost any surgical procedure involving the kidneys, ureters, bladder, or urethra, the urinary output is directed away from the operated part by catheters and drains into sterile containers. In the case of a nephrostomy, the tube comes from the operative site through the skin of the flank; with a reimplantation of ureters in the bladder, ureteral catheters and a suprapubic cystotomy catheter drain urine to the outside; with surgery of the bladder, a cystotomy tube comes from the bladder through the abdominal wall; and with transurethral surgery, a retention catheter in the urethra drains the bladder of urine. In all of these conditions, the amount of urine in the drainage container or on saturated dressings must be carefully measured or estimated and matched with the patient's intake.

All catheters placed after urologic surgery must be kept open and free of blood clots. Only very small amounts of irrigating fluid should be used (0.5 ml for the renal pelvis and 30 ml for the bladder) to determine if the catheter is unobstructed. *The procedure should be carried out using the best aseptic technique.* The end of the catheter should be cleaned with an antiseptic solution before gently injecting sterile intravenous solution with a sterile syringe. If the drainage tubing becomes contaminated when disconnected from the catheter, the tubing and container must be changed. If the irrigating fluid does not return, the physician must be notified immediately.

Some patients require an operation that permanently drains urine from the bladder (the bladder may or may not be removed). The most common of these surgical procedures is the ileal conduit in which a small portion of the ileum is used to make a tube to hold the ureters. A permanent opening is then made on the abdomen and urine constantly flows through this stoma. In addition to making certain that adequate amounts of urine are coming through the stoma, skin care is of utmost importance, and requires the same careful, conscientious treatment as in the case of an ileostomy.[122a,122b] Readers needing information on the care of patients having these operations should consult specialized texts.

8. PROMOTING REST AND SLEEP

Relieving Fear and Anxiety. Rest and sleep at regular intervals and for specific but individualized lengths of time are the first rules of health learned by children. Throughout a person's life, restful sleep relieves fatigue, restores health, and preserves sanity. Although freedom from fear and worry is most conducive to rest and sleep, this ideal state can only occasionally be reached by the postoperative patient. In spite of this, nurses and other health workers can do much to relieve patients' anxieties by their *constant, concerned attendance* during the early postoperative periods. Many seriously ill patients, particularly children and those with tracheostomies, should be told that when nurses must leave the bedside, they will return in a specific length of time. If the nurse's absence will be longer than a few minutes, patients should be introduced to the person who will be substituting.

Perhaps one of the most reassuring measures nurses can take is simply to sit beside the patient and hold a hand. Dosia Carlson, who has written feelingly about one of several experiences as a patient in an intensive care unit, says:

Understanding, concern, empathy—these essential qualities could never be communicated by impersonal machines, no matter how streamlined their construction. . . . In contrast to the cold steel of my respirator or transparent glass of my suction jar, I wanted the touch of a warm, human hand.*

Whether patients are in the recovery room, their own rooms, or an intensive care unit, careful *explanations* of medical and nursing measures, as well as honest and accurate answers to patient questions, also help relieve fear and worry by bringing the "unknown" into the "known." Patients' families should have frequent reports and explanations, with the opportunity to ask questions and have answers. Too often the busy ICU nurse forgets that families' anxieties may be communicated to patients even though their visits last only 5 minutes.

Many patients are far from home when hospitalized in a medical center. Nurses can suggest the hospital chaplain, local priest, minister, rabbi, or other religious adviser if the patient or the patient's family indicate this would be of help.

For more than 20 years it has been known that hospitalization is psychologically less harmful to children under 5 years of age if their mothers are with them. For this reason many children's hospitals now allow mothers to stay with children immediately before and after an operation. At least one study indicates that adults, too, respond with relief when

health personnel who were with them before surgery are with them after surgery [123] and some hospitals allow family members to stay near patients when this seems best for the patient.

Controlling Noise, Activity, and Light. A dark, cool, quiet room with a comfortable bed and sleeping clothes are ordinary arrangements that healthy persons make when going to bed at night. Hospitals, however, are busy places with noise, activity, and lights, even at night, and patients frequently find it difficult to sleep there. Personnel of recovery rooms and intensive care units have learned that as the level of noise increases, more patients require pain medication.[124] Monitors should, therefore, be placed so their various clicks, ticks, or beeps are less audible to patients, exuberant conversation and laughter should be relegated to areas away from patients, and various pieces of equipment should have well-oiled wheels and tight parts to prevent rattling. For at least part of the night, lights should be dimmed. If there are many critically ill patients in the unit at one time and lights and noise are inevitable, it may be possible to supply eyeshades and earplugs for the other patients. (See Chapter 15 for other environmental factors that influence patients' recovery while in the hospital.)

Conversations in the unit should be carried on quietly, and movement about the unit reduced as much as possible. Patient care measures that are essential during the night should be carried out at the same time, as much as possible, so patients have longer periods of rest without interruptions. At least two nursing studies indicate that patients in postcardiac surgical units rarely have enough time free from intrusions to complete a normal number of sleep cycles.[125,126] (Chapter 13 has a more detailed discussion of rest and sleep.)

Promoting Relaxation. During the postanesthetic and early postoperative period, patients are turned every hour or two. Each time they should be placed in positions (such as those illustrated in Figs. 12-5, 12-6, 12-7 in Chapter 12) that favor relaxation. If the patient's surgery requires a special position, even slight modification can have a relaxing effect. When a patient cannot be moved a great deal, gentle massage of the neck, back, sacrum, and buttocks often relieves soreness and tension. Of course, patients who have freedom of movement profit from relaxing massage also.

Most patients in the early postoperative period appreciate having their face and hands washed, teeth cleaned, hair brushed, gown or pajamas changed, and bed tightened and freshened during the evening hours or about

---

* Carlson, Dosia: *The Unbroken Vigil: Reflections on Intensive Care.* John Knox Press, Richmond, Va., 1968, p. 81.

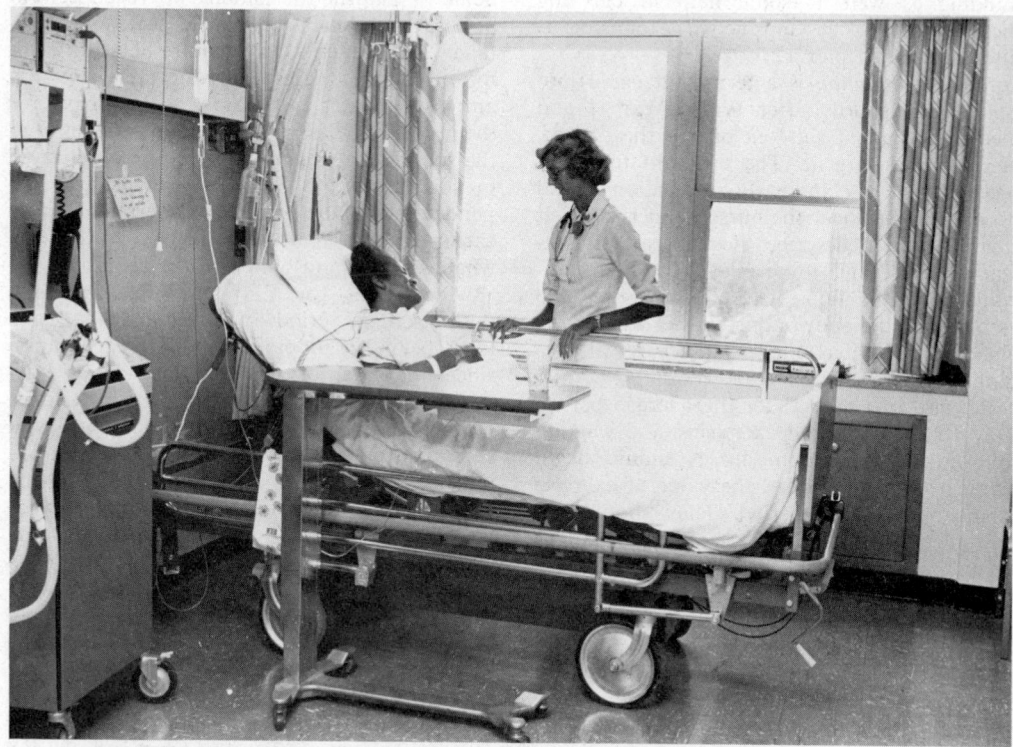

Figure 48-9. Intensive care unit of Rush University Hospital, Chicago, Ill., shown here because patients have view from windows that orients them to time of day and place. Some ICU's and surgical recovery rooms are windowless, which contributes to disorientation. (Courtesy of the hospital.)

the time they ordinarily go to bed. Frequently, at this time they can be encouraged to try systematic relaxation. One method to help patients with this is to tell the patient to take a deep breath, curl the toes, and tighten the muscles of one leg, then to release the breath slowly and at the same time relax the whole leg and foot. An important point is to encourage patients to compare consciously the feelings of tension and relaxation. The second leg, each hand and arm, and the face are tightened and relaxed in turn.* Some patients need a great deal of practice to learn to relax the whole body, while others learn it very quickly. One nursing study of a small group of patients (4) scheduled for cardiac surgery found that preoperative teaching of systematic relaxation and its use postoperatively resulted in fewer postoperative psychiatric complications.[127]

* A number of years ago, the first author observed a group of expectant mothers learning to relax in this way in preparation for "natural childbirth." After approximately 10 minutes, half the group was asleep.

Exercise and Walking (Ambulation). Healthy individuals know that after a day of sufficient exercise, sleep comes easily and is deep and restful, and there is a general sense of well-being. Postoperative patients also need and benefit from a program of *exercise,* although the initial purpose may be to improve circulation and respirations rather than promote sleep.

During the time the patient is reacting from the anesthetic, passive exercises are commonly used as a part of the "stir-up" regimen. The exercises are carried out by the nurse who moves the patient's arms and legs through a series of normal movements. These passive exercises are carried out at frequent intervals until the patient is awake. When postoperative patients are critically ill for several days, passive exercises should be continued until the patients can exercise actively or get out of bed. Active exercises are of greater value to patients than passive exercises because muscles actually work to move the part and circulation is more markedly improved. Patients who have been taught bed exercises and their value during the preoperative period often need reminding as well as some help in carrying them out. (Passive and active exercising is discussed in Chapter 12.)

Early ambulation is a term that came into general use shortly after World War II and means the patient gets out of bed the day of, or after, the surgery. The program for postoperative exercise and early ambulation should be carried out under the nurse's supervision. It is important to describe the program in sufficient detail, and to give each patient individual consideration. Through exercise and ambulation, the body is quickly restored to the physical state interrupted by the surgical procedure.

Because it is natural for the average person to feel reluctant about exercising and walking following an operation, nurses should begin helping the patient to see the value of exercise in the preoperative period. They should not wait, as did one nurse who said to her patient postoperatively: "I will help you get up now." The patient replied: "Certainly not. Don't you know I've had an operation?"

For the first day or two after an operation, many surgeons advise against sitting in a chair except for very short periods, such as required for making the bed. They think that sitting compresses the popliteal and femoral veins and a dependent position of the extremities may cause venous stasis and thrombosis. In general, it is more desirable for patients to be either walking or in bed. After a few days, they are usually able to get about freely by themselves and should be encouraged to do so.

With many types of surgery, the patient will have one or more tubes attached to the body for urinary or other types of drainage, or for the infusion of parenteral fluid. In walking with these patients, the nurse must use caution to prevent dislodging the tube or allowing the drainage to soil the patient's clothing. When there is a catheter or open drainage tube in place, it may be attached to a small bottle or plastic bag or other appropriate receptacle for walking. When an infusion is running, the nurse can support the bottle in one hand as he or she walks along with the patient.

It should be remembered that, although postoperative patients are up and about and can bathe themselves, their wounds and general physical condition will not always permit a full range of activities. If they have a sterile dressing on the body, they cannot take a shower or a tub bath (unless some means is provided for keeping the dressing dry) (see Fig. 14-2, Chapter 14), so they are often dependent on the bed bath or sponge bath at the hand basin. With many types of surgery it is difficult or painful for patients to reach certain body areas such as the back, feet, and genitalia. Also, patients may require help in reaching or lifting articles from the table. For example, the water carafe may be too heavy for them to lift. Plastic tubing that reaches into the supply of drinking water may be indicated in some cases. A wise nurse will take dependency factors into consideration while caring for ambulatory patients, and provide whatever help and guidance are required.

Medications for Rest and Sleep. In the postanesthetic period, sedatives and analgesics must be given to patients with great caution since they depress further the already depressed vascular and respiratory systems. However, if patients thrash about with wild shouting (emergence delirium), narcotics are indicated. The doses should be small, and the patient closely observed for developing hypotension or respiratory depression.

We are currently said to be living in a "drug culture" that provides, and even advocates, drugs for every conceivable ill, real or imagined. Nurses, unfortunately, must share some of the blame for encouraging widespread use of drugs to induce sleep. Too often a sedative is offered to sleepless patients before any attempt is made to discover what is bothering them, or before using other measures (discussed in Chapters 13 and 49) to promote relaxation.

A somewhat different aspect of the problem is described by a former patient. When a nurse was asked if the "sleeping pill" that was offered contained a barbiturate, the reply was "I don't know." This patient was particularly concerned, because at one time in the past the danger of being addicted to ("hooked on") barbiturates had been very real. Caring nurses can only agree with the statement "A patient always has the right to protect himself from drugs that may harm him." * Readers are encouraged to read pages 765–66 in Chapter 13 and pages 1128–38 in Chapter 21 that discuss in greater detail the overuse of sedatives and drug abuse.

9. RELIEVING PAIN

The Nature of Pain. Many nurses and physicians have come to the conclusion that "Pain is what the patient says hurts." † When nurses caring for postoperative patients accept this as

---

* Long, Edna S.: "How to Survive Hospitalization," *Am. J. Nurs.,* **74**:486, (Mar.) 1974.

† Parkhouse, James, and Holmes, C. M.: "Assessing Postoperative Pain Relief," *Proc. R. Soc. Med.,* **56**: 579, (July) 1963.

a basic premise, they can focus on determining, with the patient, the probable causes of the pain and find ways to relieve it as much as possible instead of trying to determine *if* the patient has pain. Patients who are able to describe their pain often use such terms as sticking, flashing, shooting, or stabbing to indicate brief sensations of different intensity (sticking seems to be less severe than stabbing but of approximately the same duration). Longer-lasting or recurring pain sensations are often said to be burning, throbbing, cramping, twisting, or crushing, and pain provoked by touch, motion, or pressure is frequently described as soreness or tenderness. The use of such descriptive terms implies there is more to pain than abnormal stimulation of various pain end organs. Chapter 49 explores the "pain experience," various theories of pain physiology, and the many influences that effect pain sensations and reactions.

Postoperative Pain and Its Causes. A number of researchers report that approximately 20 to 30 per cent of surgical patients have little or no pain postoperatively, 30 to 60 per cent have fairly acute pain, and 20 to 30 per cent have severe pain. Patients having upper abdominal or thoracic surgery are more likely to have moderate to severe pain than are those with lower abdominal or superficial surgery. Children and the elderly seem to be generally tolerant of postoperative pain and are kept most comfortable with loving, concerned care rather than analgesics.[128,129]

Although the exact *physiologic mechanisms* that cause pain after tissue is traumatized are not known, it is believed that bradykinin and histamine, released as part of the body response to cell damage, are partially responsible. Other causes are thought to be muscle spasm and tissue ischemia (a localized anemia from loss of blood supply). Muscle spasm produces a diminished blood supply and, consequently, a relative ischemia in the body part. Ischemia, in turn, is believed to produce large amounts of pain-arousing lactic acid or bradykinin and histamine.[130]

Psychologic influences, such as the patient's expectations, fears, motivations, perceptions, anticipation, suggestibility, and past experiences, contribute to the total pain sensation and are impossible to separate from it. Henry K. Beecher's [131] often-cited study of wounded men in World War II shows this relationship. He found that pain caused by severe battle wounds was less in soldiers than in civilians with the same injuries. He concluded that for the soldier, the wound represented release from the battlefield, while for the civilian, it represented loss of income and additional ex-

penses. Lawrence D. Egbert and his associates [132] found that patients who had preoperative instruction about the likelihood of pain postoperatively, its probable character and duration, its causes, and ways in which the patients themselves could relieve the pain through relaxation had less medication the first 5 postoperative days and were discharged almost 3 days sooner than patients who did not have such instruction. An important part of this "treatment" was the reinforcement and encouragement of the patient each day until pain medication was no longer needed. When Laura Archer Copp [133] asked 148 patients in intensive care units to characterize their pain, they used such emotion-laden words as treacherous, sneaky, degrading, strong, and tempting. The comments of the same patients when asked what doctors and nurses can do to relieve pain gave many suggestions that nurses will find helpful, and these are listed in Chapter 49.

Postoperative Pain Reduction. As the effects of the anesthetic wear off, the patient is increasingly aware of pain, discomfort, and outside stimuli. James E. Gildea [134] says the greatest need for *narcotic analgesia* to reduce pain is between 12 and 36 hours postoperatively, and that after 48 hours the presence of pain usually indicates complications. As the patient is waking from the anesthesia, there may be an inclination to talk and express some of the fears, confusion, or pain that the patient naturally experiences. Reassurance and explanations given repeatedly will relieve his or her anxiety and reduce the response to pain. Patients should be asked about the methods they have used in the past to manage either oncoming or present pain. Many of these methods can be used in the hospital setting and should be encouraged if they are not injurious.

The writers have had experience in a number of cases where no analgesic or narcotic was required or desired after major surgery. In these instances patients were given careful instruction as to what their role would be in the postoperative recovery period, and emphasis was placed on turning and having patients exercise the extremities and breathe deeply every 1 or 2 hours during the first 24-hour period, both day and night. Aside from inducing early mobilization, this regimen prevents the severe pain that results from the motion of muscles that have been abnormally splinted in an unchanged position for hours at a time.

Pain should always be regarded as an individual matter, however, and depends largely on the patient's tolerance, the type and extent of surgery performed, and the complications encountered. Good nursing care can do much to minimize pain. Frequent changes of position, the use of pillows, correct anchorage of drainage tubes, and similar nursing measures all contribute greatly to the patient's general comfort. Chapter 49 describes other effective nursing measures that take into account patients as feeling, thinking, acting persons who are capable of taking part in relieving their pain.

The practice of keeping the patient asleep or in a dozing (i.e., depressed) condition for the first 48 hours after operation, common 25 years ago, is now thought undesirable. The objective should be to eliminate pain and discomfort, preferably by physical or psychologic means, helped if necessary by mild sedatives and analgesics. It follows then that narcotics, when used, should not be administered routinely, but only as required for pain that cannot otherwise be prevented or relieved. This will enable the body to function as normally as possible without the influence of depressing drugs. Most surgeons will make provision for administering a narcotic such as morphine or meperidine hydrochloride, every 4 hours as required for pain for the first day or two following surgery. The frequency with which it is given is usually left to the discretion of nurses and they are once again reminded of the necessity of giving smaller-than-usual doses during the early postoperative period. Untoward effects of narcotics should be carefully observed, especially respiratory depression, hypotension, continued nausea and vomiting, and an abnormal dependence on drugs.

Acupuncture analgesia is being explored by a number of physicians and others as an antidote to pain. Up to this time, however, Kenneth L. Casey[135] says no neurophysiologic search has been done that establishes a cause-and-effect relationship between acupuncture and current Western theories of pain physiology. Nevertheless, the use of acupuncture is apparently increasing, and one study has reported that four patients who had acupuncture as anesthesia for herniorrhaphies had no complaints of pain for at least 4 hours after surgery.[136]

Postoperative Pain and Complications. In Chapter 31, "Radiation Energies and Therapeutic Applications," bioelectric medicine is discussed and acupuncture is assumed to be an electrodynamic process. Uses of the latter in anesthesia are discussed in Chapter 47, "The Preoperative State." In Chapter 49, which deals with "Pain—Its Meaning, Prevention, and Relief," transcutaneous neural stimulation, or electric pain control, is described and some of the devices used are shown. Attention is

drawn in all these chapters and in Chapter 50, "Death and Dying," to the work of physicians in various centers in the United States and one center in England using electric pain control. In several Minneapolis, Minn., hospitals, the work of Alan C. Hymes and his associates (including A. L. Printy, a nurse) in controlling postoperative pain and preventing atelectasis and paralytic ileus is of special interest. In 1974 they reported a series of 213 patients having abdominal and thoracic surgery who were treated with electric surface stimulation. When these patients were compared with controls who did not have this treatment, the results were striking. Hymes et al. summarize this experience, which extends over several years:

Reduction of postoperative pain allows deep breathing and coughing, resulting in the reduction of postoperative atelectasis. The restoration of the appropriate parastalsis may be a direct effect on the autonomic nervous system or on the gastrointestinal tract itself, resulting in a new noninvasive modality for the prevention and treatment of ileus.*

A 1973 report shows that in 20 patients who already had abdominal distention with no audible bowel tones, 5 minutes after the application of electric stimulation gastrointestinal tract activity increased. The postoperative ileus of 15 of these patients was relieved the same day electrical stimulation was started.[136a] In 1975, Avram M. Cooperman and his associates (including Barbara Hall, a nurse) report a series of 50 patients in whom the suggestive effect of electric stimulation in control of postoperative pain was tested. They used stimulators with and without current and report "good to excellent results in 77% of the patients when stimulators with current were used; a good result with only 34% of the cases when stimulators without a current were used." However, they said that "Pain relief was significantly better ($p < .008$) when stimulators with current were used.† Unlike Hymes et al., they found no significant difference in the incidence of postoperative atelectasis or paralytic ileus using either type of stimulator.

While the results of the reported studies are in conflict, there seems to be sufficient success in both cases to warrant further use of electric stimulation for the prevention or relief of postoperative pain, especially as it has none of the disadvantages of drugs or the dangers of "intrusive therapy" (severance of nerves, destruc-

* Hymes, Alan C., et al.: "Electrical Surface Stimulation for Treatment and Prevention of Ileus and Atelectasis," *Surg. Forum,* **25**:222, 1974.

† Cooperman, Avram M., et al.: "Use of Transcutaneous Electrical Stimulation in Control of Postoperative Pain," *Surg. Forum,* **26**:77, 1975.

tion of nerve roots, or injection of nerves). Those who are interested might study the growing body of literature on this subject. No claim is made here to an exhaustive review of the data.

10. PROVIDING FOR CLEANLINESS AND GROOMING

Care of the Mouth. After *general anesthesia,* mouth care is an important hygienic need of the patient. A dry mouth and lips cause great discomfort to postoperative patients, and if the lingering aftertaste of vomitus is added, the discomfort is compounded. Dryness of the oral mucosa is the result of a number of generalized as well as specific influences. Preoperative medications such as atropine and scopolamine decrease secretions of the mouth and respiratory tract; the normal physiologic reaction to trauma results in conservation of extracellular fluid and a decrease in saliva as well as other body fluids for approximately 48 hours; frequent suctioning of the mouth and pharynx mechanically removes secretions; and continuous administration of oxygen, particularly through a nasal catheter, and open-mouth breathing dry the mucous membranes by rapid evaporation of moisture.

One nurse who subjected herself to a 5-hour test of nasal catheter oxygen, open-mouth breathing, continuous suction, and no liquids, reported at the end of 4 hours:

My entire mouth feels coated. The roof of my mouth feels very numb. . . . My tongue feels very thick and burning continues at the tip. . . . The corners of my lips feel cracked. My lips are dry and they burn. . . . It feels like there is debris all over my teeth. . . . It is very difficult to talk now.*

During the fifth hour of testing, tooth brushing with glycerin and lemon was used twice at 30-minute intervals while the oxygen, suctioning, and mouth breathing continued. At the end of the test the nurse subject was able to say, "There seems to be a lot more saliva and the burning at the tip of my tongue is gone. My mouth feels pretty normal except for the cracks in my lips." † However, 48 hours were needed to recapture the normal ability of discriminating flavors other than tartness.

When tooth brushing and mouth rinses as described in Chapter 14 are started in the re-

covery period, the postoperative discomfort described above is avoided. Furthermore, halitosis and surgical parotitis are prevented. One cause of halitosis has been reported to be the presence of stagnant saliva that allows the growth of gram-negative organisms with the production of malodorous breath. Because even a small amount of glucose inhibits the growth of these gram-negative organisms, chewing gum may be helpful for the conscious patient. The chewing also increases the flow of saliva and prevents its stagnation.[137] Parotitis is not as common as it once was, but if there is no stimulation of parotid secretions from chewing, the inactive glands may be exposed by way of the parotid duct to a massive invasion of microorganisms from the mouth.

Patients who have surgery of the head and neck or those with oral surgery may be able to have only warm salt rinses, with the solution removed by suction and a soft catheter. If the teeth are wired together, a very soft nylon brush with even bristles may be used. The cheek on one side and then the other should be gently pulled back with a tongue blade and the brush used with short, vertical, vibrating strokes to clean between the wires and elastics. Each application of the brush should end with a sweeping motion toward the crowns of the teeth, followed by a final rinse and suctioning. "Water-pics" that direct tiny, high-pressure jets of water against the teeth and gums are often useful for patients who cannot use a toothbrush, or who need frequent rinses of the mouth.[138,139] Patients who have had *local or regional anesthesia* are usually able to take fluids and to keep their mouths hydrated and clean with minimal help.

Care of the Skin. Postoperative sweating may be profuse and patients made uncomfortable from damp clothing and bed sheets. Since dry, clean skin tends to prevent infection as well as add to patient comfort, partial baths with back rubs and changes of clothing may be given during the postanesthetic period. Full bed baths are not usually given until the patient has completely reacted to the anesthetic because hypotension and vomiting may result from excessive turning.

Occasionally, eruptions appear around the operative site and the area itches. This is likely due to the antiseptic solution used in the operating room, and is relieved by washing the area with alcohol, then soap and water, and drying the skin thoroughly.

Decubitus ulcers are not generally associated with the early postoperative period; however, a survey of the postoperative records of 100 patients showed that when patients were on hard-surfaced operating tables over 4 hours,

---

* DeWalt, Evelyn M., and Haines, Sister Ann Kathleen: "The Effects of Specified Stressors on Healthy Oral Mucosa," *Nurs. Res.,* **18**:22, (Jan.–Feb.) 1969.

† *Ibid.*

the likelihood they would develop pressure sores was high.[140] Nurses caring for postanesthetic patients should, therefore, make sure the areas of pressure are well massaged, are kept dry, and that the patient is turned away from those sites as much as possible. In Chapter 12 there is a detailed discussion of decubitus ulcers.

Care of the Hair. Patients with long hair are usually prepared for surgery by braiding the hair so it is confined but comfortable. After surgery, it is wise to braid it because if vomiting occurs, the vomitus will not be caught in the hair.

When patients sweat profusely, brushing the hair and using a dry cloth around the hairline may make them more comfortable. Since pillows often hold unpleasant odors, folded bath towels in their place may be more satisfying and restful for patients. Some patients find that a covered hot-water bottle filled with about two cups of cool water makes a pleasant "water-pillow."

Postoperative Clothing. In the immediate postoperative period, patients are usually clad in the clothing provided by the hospital. Because these garments are often stained and damp following surgery, they should be changed as soon as possible. Of course, any time they are soiled with vomitus or wet from excessive sweating they should be changed.

Ordinarily, gowns are short and open in the back, with wide long sleeves. Many hospitals are using pastel colors to make them somewhat more attractive, while other hospitals provide long-legged pants to go with the tops. When patients have been transferred to their own rooms, they generally feel better when they can use their own clothing. Nurses should take care that the patient's clothing is not sent to the hospital laundry since the methods of washing often are harsh and the clothing may be lost. A few hospitals are using disposable paper clothing that is attractive in color and looks and feels like cloth.

11. PROTECTING THE PATIENT AGAINST ENVIRONMENTAL HAZARDS

Preventing Injuries and Falls. Many patients reacting from a general anesthetic undergo a period of *restlessness* and mental confusion before consciousness is regained, and injuries can occur at this time. This restlessness seems to be related to age, physical status, preoperative medications, anesthetic, and the operative procedure. Young persons, those who are relatively muscular, and those who expect intense pain or mutilation from their surgery are most likely to be excited postoperatively. However, respiratory inadequacy or hypoxia should not be forgotten as possible causes of restlessness, and adequate oxygenation should be assured the patient before other measures are tried.[141]

As patients become more conscious, this behavior subsides, but if they are receiving an infusion, there is the possibility that they may injure themselves by uncontrolled movements; and during this time some form of *minor restraint* may be indicated until they are sufficiently conscious to benefit by explanations and reassurance. A padded arm board may be used to prevent flexion of the elbow or wrist. Care should be taken to pad the extremity before tying it, and to release the restraint at frequent intervals to provide for a change in position.

To safeguard the patient from falling out of bed, *side boards* should be used. These are usually left in place through the first postoperative night in case the patient is still under the effects of the anesthetic or is confused by narcotics.

Usually, with attentive care and repeated explanations, the above methods will afford the patient adequate protection. If restlessness is very severe, it may be necessary to use a more limiting type of restraint, for it seems more sensible to provide this than to expect nurses of ordinary strength to prevent large and vigorous patients from falling out of bed or otherwise injuring themselves. However, it is natural even when semiconscious to struggle against restraint, and so it must be avoided if possible and only used judiciously.

It is always necessary for the nurse to be with patients who are *getting out of bed* for the first time or are taking their first steps after surgery. Should patients feel dizzy or faint after a few minutes of sitting on the edge of the bed, further attempts to get up should be delayed and the patient helped to lie down again.

Hospital beds that can be lowered allow patients getting up to reach the floor with ease and safety. If the beds cannot be lowered, sturdy, nonskid footstools of the proper height must be provided, and the wheels of the bed braked to prevent rolling.

Patients beginning to walk after surgery often need physical support from the nurse. The nurse's arm linked through the patient's arm in such a way that the nurse bears some of the patient's weight seems to give more confidence to the patient than an arm about the waist. In order to prevent falls from a too-loose slipper, it is usually wise for patients to wear their own slippers or shoes when walking at any time and especially after surgery. Chapter

12 discusses other ways to safeguard patients when they are ambulatory or being transported from place to place.

Infections. The incidence of hospital-acquired (nosocomial) disease continues to increase in spite of an ever-growing list of anti-infectious drugs, and the use of sophisticated and complicated mini-environments. The surgical patient is particularly vulnerable since many of the body's natural defenses are temporarily impaired by the operation or depleted by the condition requiring the operation. Prevention of these nosocomial conditions is complex because their incidence and dispersion throughout the ward or hospital depend in part on the virulence of the organisms, the method of their spread, and the susceptibility of the potential hosts.

The most frequent kinds of postsurgical infections that threaten patients are urinary tract infections following catheterization, phlebitis from indwelling venous catheters, respiratory infections, and wound infections.[142] Since many organisms may be carried on objects inserted into the body, nurses' constant and scrupulous attention to the use of sterile techniques with catheterizations and bladder drainage equipment and with infusion equipment can go a long way toward reducing additional burdens of infection for the already susceptible postoperative patient. *Urinary tract infections* of hospitalized patients have been associated with contamination of the hands of health workers, fluids used for bladder irrigation, lubricating material used for catheter insertion, bedpans, rectal thermometers, and the dust and air of the hospital environment.[143] (See Chapters 15 and 24.) The major method of the transmission of urinary infections is considered to be the hands of nursing personnel. Maki and associates,[144] in random surveys in the Miami (Fla.) Veterans Administration Hospital, found that a particular organism cultured from patients with urinary tract infections was also cultured from the hands of nursing personnel 50 per cent of the time. It cannot be emphasized too strongly that *hands must be washed before attending to each patient.* This important measure of aseptic technique applies not only to patients with infections, but to all care given to all patients.

The occurrence and treatment of nosocomial infections *following parenteral therapy* have been related to the length of time the catheter was left in the vein, the size of the vein used, the size of the catheter, the rate of infusion, the pH of the solution, and the use of antibiotics at the site of the needle insertion. Chapter 22 discusses these matters more fully.

Most of the postoperative *respiratory infec-tions* are thought to be transferred by ventilators and resuscitators so often needed by surgical patients. Many large hospitals have inhalation therapy departments that are responsible for maintaining this equipment and making certain pathogenic organisms do not reach the patient through this means. However, when such specialized personnel are not available, nurses are usually responsible for preventing pulmonary infection from breathing or oxygenation equipment. Providing fresh filters and autoclaved parts prior to each treatment with an IPPB (intermittent positive pressure breathing) machine or changing these parts every 8 hours if the treatment is long-term is essential to prevent upper respiratory tract infection.[145] Chapter 20 describes in more detail the prevention of ventilator-carried respiratory infections, and Chapter 15 discusses institutional ventilation systems that reduce the incidence of these nosocomial illnesses.

The frequency of postoperative *wound infection* continues to rise and to increase the patient's length of stay in the hospital with its additional costs. In an effort to prevent nosocomial wound infection, a 5-year survey of 23,649 surgical wounds was done at a Canadian hospital.[146] Some of the recommendations made by the researchers after the survey were (1) the patient's preoperative stay should be as short as possible, since the longer the hospitalization prior to surgery, the greater the incidence of wound infection; (2) a hexa-chlorophene detergent shower should be given before surgery; (3) shaving and even clipping hair on the body surface should be kept to a minimum, with an electric razor or depilatory used for hirsute patients; (4) contamination of any kind should be scrupulously prevented during the surgery; and (5) particular care should be taken in the treatment of the elderly, the obese, the malnourished, and the diabetic. Chapter 43 discusses many of the drugs used to combat infected wounds and Chapter 15 discusses hospital environmental conditions that relate to this problem.

Equipment Hazards. Patients in recovery rooms and intensive care units are in an "electric environment" and often are near or in contact with electrical devices. This is particularly hazardous for those with cardiac problems or pacemakers, and great caution must be taken to prevent electrical leakage from flowing through the patient rather than into the ground. Elizabeth A. Trought says:

Unsubstantiated claims have been made that 1200 patients a year are accidentally electrocuted in hospitals. Most qualified authorities think this number is an exaggeration. Since there is rarely any specific evidence of electrical death at au-

topsy, no certain figures can be expected. Nevertheless, prevention of electric shock to both patients and staff is an attainable goal which every health care facility should actively strive for.*
(See Chapter 15 for electrical safety measures.)

All kinds of equipment as well as its improper use may present risks to the hospitalized patient. In general, hazardous equipment falls into two categories: (1) devices that cause direct injury or death, such as improperly grounded electrical equipment, and (2) devices that perform inadequately, such as suction pump with insufficient suction, or poorly calibrated devices for regulating infusion rates.

A testing laboratory at the Emergency Care Research Institute † (ECRI),[147] established in 1968, comparatively evaluates medical equipment and shares with hospitals its findings about hazards, limitations, deficiencies, and cost-effectiveness. Over the past 5 years the testing laboratory has discovered such deficiencies as defibrillator paddles that shock both patient and staff, respirators in which the ventilatory rate varies with electrical power variations, and alternating air pressure mattresses that only alternate air pressure when there is no patient on them.

Fire Hazards. The prevalence of oxygen therapy, potential spark-producing equipment, and an environment conducive to static electricity formation combine to make hospital fires a dreaded possibility. In order to keep the danger at a minimum, many hospitals hold regular inspections to detect fire hazards and have periodic fire drills and regular examinations of emergency fire-fighting equipment. The section on hospital fire hazards in Chapter 15 should be reviewed carefully by all nurses and students of nursing.

12. REHABILITATION AND CONTINUING CARE

For Patients with Uncomplicated Surgery. Most surgical patients are discharged from the hospital before they are fully convalescent, and many need explanations concerning the extent

---

* Trought, Elizabeth A.: "Equipment Hazards," *Am. J. Nurs.,* 73:858, (May) 1973.

† The Institute is a nonprofit organization that does not accept advertising or support from any manufacturers. A membership fee provides for a monthly report, *Health Devices,* as well as such services as telephone consultation regarding the selection of equipment, and periodic workshops on equipment safety, operation, selection, inspection, and maintenance. The Institute also provides consultation and personnel training programs to hospitals that request them.

of their activities once they are home. Physicians often discuss with patients the limitations they will have, but if the physician does not, nurses should make sure patients have this information. When giving such information or advice, nurses should take into account the patient's usual health habits, living arrangements, or family relationships. If nurses query patients and their families about ways in which they expect to handle any necessary limitations, encouragement can be given or substitutions suggested and a plan the patient is likely to follow can be developed. Because arrangements to accommodate the patient's restrictions, even though short-term, may have to be made before the patient leaves the hospital, discussions about plans should be started well in advance of the discharge date, and not an hour or two before the patient leaves. Ordinarily, the patient who has had uncomplicated surgery will be given an appointment for 4 to 6 weeks later to see the physician in an office or clinic for a follow-up examination. A telephone number for the use of patients if unexpected events occur between hospitalization and follow-up examination adds to the patients' security and sense of continuing care.

For Patients Discharged with Indwelling Tubes. Some patients are discharged after surgery with indwelling catheters or feeding tubes. Nurses are responsible for teaching patients and families how to use these devices. They are also responsible, with the physician's approval, for referring patients to the liaison nurse if there is one, or to visiting or district nurses where they are available. In a few areas throughout the United States, groups of nurses are arranging independent nursing practices and are helpful to patients with problems such as those described above.

For Patients with Permanently Changed Body Functions. Space does not permit an extensive discussion of the many rehabilitative measures available for patients who have had amputations, permanent tracheotomies, or ostomies for feeding or elimination purposes. There are, however, three main categories of nurse activities that are necessary to help patients during convalescence and rehabilitation: (1) helping patients to become as independent as possible by teaching them how to care for and manage their changed physical functions; (2) helping patients to have hope for the future by introducing former patients with a like disability, and using social service workers to help resolve economic and emotional problems; and (3) acquainting patients with various organizations that were created by persons with a similar problem to exchange information, answer questions, and provide emotional support for rehabilitation and productive living. (See the Appendix for a partial list of these organizations.)

Surgery and Human Sexuality. Although it is often said that Western cultures are more open now in their sexual relationships than in the past, nurses and physicians seldom give attention to the effect illness has on patients' sexual responses or activities.[148] Linbania Jacobson says:

When it comes to human sexuality, nursing is still in the Dark Ages—ignorant and prudish about this important aspect of patient care. Little or no attention has been given by nursing to how a patient's sexuality may be altered, affected, or denied during the acute or chronic phases of illness. Drugs, procedures, and conditions that can modify the physical or the emotional aspects of sexuality are seldom if ever discussed with patients, their spouses, or families.*

She points out that in order to counsel patients with sensitivity, the nurse must have (1) knowledge of the ways surgery or the disease process may affect sexual performance; (2) familiarity with all forms (coital and noncoital) of the expression of physical love; (3) a nonjudgmental attitude with empathy and warmth for others; and (4) a sense of self as a sexually expressive person.

Patients with transsexual surgery must learn to understand the sexuality of their new status. Before surgery, they should have learned what forms of physical sexuality will be possible for them; the ways they can acquire the characteristics of the opposite sex, and the extent to which this is possible. Nurses should read books and articles written by persons such as Jan Morris,[149] Dawn L. Simmons,[150] and Christine Jorgenson[151] to get a firsthand knowledge of how they might help these patients. Nurses should also be in a position to suggest books and articles to families on whose understanding and support patients are dependent. Concern about new sex role behavior when changed from man to woman may be expressed in such questions as

How does one want to behave when she goes out with a boy. I've never gone out with a boy as a girl before. Are most girls "easy"—is that OK? My hair is such a mess. Could you help me with curlers and stuff? How does it feel to urinate this way? Do I just sit, or what? †

Women changing to men have similar questions. With sensitive and warm nurses and physicians acting as role models, the rehabilitation of these patients can proceed smoothly.

* Jacobson, Linbania: "Illness and Human Sexuality," *Nurs. Outlook,* **22**:50, (Jan.) 1974.
† Strait, Joyce: "The Transsexual Patient After Surgery," *Am. J. Nurs.,* **73**:462, (Mar.) 1973.

REFERENCES

1. Holley, H. Steele: "Immediate Postoperative Management," in Beal, John M., and Eckenhoff, James E. (eds.): *Intensive and Recovery Room Care.* Macmillan Publishing Co., Inc., New York, 1969, p. 53.
2. Kao, F. F., et al.: "Acupuncture Anesthesia in Herniorrhaphy," *Am. J. Chinese Med.,* **1**:327, (No. 2) 1973.
3. Dimond, E. Grey: "Acupuncture Anesthesia," *J.A.M.A.,* **218**:1563, (Dec. 6) 1971.
4. Belinkoff, Stanton: *Manual for the Recovery Room.* Little, Brown & Co., Boston, 1967, p. 33.
5. Miller, Joan E.: "Staff Development in the Intensive Care Unit," *Nurs. Clin. North Am.,* **7**:323, (June) 1972.
6. Schmitt, Yvonne: "A Program for Inservice Education in an Intensive Coronary Care Unit," *Nurs. Clin. North Am.,* **3**:87, (Mar.) 1968.
7. Fochtman, Dianne: "Nursing Care in the Pediatric Intensive Care Unit," in Beal, John M., and Eckenhoff, James E. (eds.): *Intensive and Recovery Room Care,* Macmillan Publishing Co., Inc., New York, 1969, p. 41.
8. Committee on Guidelines of the Society of Critical Care Medicine: "Guidelines for Organization of Critical Care Units," *J.A.M.A.,* **222**:1532, (Dec. 18) 1972.
9. Tanser, A. R., and Wetten, B. G.: "Multipurpose Intensive Care Unit in a District General Hospital," *Br. Med. J.,* **3**:227, (July 28) 1973.
10. Kornfeld, Donald S.: "Psychiatric Aspects of Patient Care in Operating Suite and Special Areas," *Anesthesiology,* **31**:166, (Aug.) 1969.
11. Klein, Robert F., et al.: "Transfer from a Coronary Care Unit," *Arch. Intern. Med.,* **122**:104, (Aug.) 1968.
12. Strauss, Anselm: "The Intensive Care Unit: Its Characteristics and Social Relationships," *Nurs. Clin. North Am.,* **3**:7, (Mar.) 1968.
13. Hay, Donald, and Oken, Donald: "The Psychological Stresses of Intensive Care Unit Nursing," *Psychosom. Med.,* **34**:109, (Mar.–Apr.) 1972.
14. Wiley, Loy (ed.): "Innovations in Nursing: Decentralizing the Coronary Care Unit," *Nursing '72,* **2**:6, (Oct.) 1972.
15. Chandrakant, R. Shan, et al.: "Day Care Surgery for Children: A Controlled Study of Medical Complications and Parental Attitudes," *Med. Care,* **10**:437, (Sept.–Oct.) 1972.
16. Taylor, Dorothy H.: "Medical-Surgical Day Care Unit," *Am. J. Nurs.,* **73**:2109, (Dec.) 1973.
17. Efurd, Nancy J., and Hartman, Harold W.: "In-Hospital Care in the Outpatient Center," *Am. J. Nurs.,* **73**:678, (Apr.) 1973.
18. Klingensmith, William: "Inadvertent Hypo-

thermia During Surgery," *Tex. Med.*, **67**:52, (May) 1971.

19. Morris, Roger H., and Wilkey, Brian R.: "The Effects of Ambient Temperature on Patient Temperature During Surgery Not Involving Body Cavities," *Anesthesiology*, **32**:102, (Feb.) 1970.

20. Goldberg, Michael J., et al.: "Temperature Changes During Anesthesia and Operations," *Arch. Surg.*, **93**:365, (Aug.) 1966.

21. Harrison, G. G., et al.: "Temperature Changes in Children During General Anaesthesia," *Br. J. Anaesth.*, **32**:60, (Jan.) 1960.

22. Roe, C. Francis, et al.: "Heat Loss in Infants During General Anesthesia and Operations," *J. Pediatr. Surg.*, **1**:266, (June) 1966.

23. Stark, David C. C. (ed.): *Practical Points in Anesthesiology*. Medical Examination Publishing Co., New York, 1973, p. 61.

24. Dripps, Robert D., et al.: *Introduction to Anesthesia; The Principles of Safe Practice*, 4th ed. W. B. Saunders Co., Philadelphia, 1972, p. 395.

25. Norris, Walter, and Campbell, Donald: *Anaesthetics, Resuscitation, and Intensive Care*, 4th ed. Churchill-Livingstone, London, 1974, p. 149.

26. Danner, Charles A., et al.: "Recovery Scoring Revisited," *South. Med. J.*, **66**:865, (Aug.) 1973.

27. Brunner, Edward A., and Eckenhoff, James E.: "Anesthesia," in Sabiston, David C., Jr. (ed.): *Davis-Christopher Textbook of Surgery*, 10th ed. W. B. Saunders Co., Philadelphia, 1972, p. 211.

28. Foley, Mary K.: "Variations in Blood Pressure in the Lateral Recumbent Position," *Nurs. Res.*, **20**:64, (Jan.–Feb.) 1971.

29. Brunner, Edward A., and Eckenhoff, James E.: *op. cit.*

30. Hardy, James D. (ed.): *Critical Surgical Illness*. W. B. Saunders Co., Philadelphia, 1971, p. 77.

31. Curran, R. C., and Harnden, D. G.: *The Pathological Basis of Medicine*. W. B. Saunders Co., Philadelphia, 1972, p. 386.

32. Stahl, William M.: *Supportive Care of the Surgical Patient*. Grune & Stratton, New York, 1972, p. 42.

33. Apgar, Virginia: "Evaluation of the Newborn Infant—Second Report," *J.A.M.A.*, **168**:1985, (Dec. 13) 1958.

34. Aldrete, J. Antonio, and Kroulik, Diane: "A Postanesthetic Recovery Score," *Anesth. Analg.*, **49**:924, (Nov.–Dec.) 1970.

35. Danner, Charles A., et al.: *op. cit.*

36. Holzgrafe, Robert E.: "A Postanesthesia Recovery Score," *Wis. Med. J.*, **71**:239, (Nov.) 1972.

37. Winkelstein, Charles, et al.: "Psychiatric Observations on Surgical Patients in Recovery Room—Pilot Study," *N.Y. J. Med.*, **65**:865, (Apr. 1) 1965.

38. Norris, Walter, and Campbell, Donald: *op. cit.*, p. 146.

39. Stahl, William M.: *op. cit.*, p. 22.

40. Goodman, Louis S., and Gilman, Alfred: *The Pharmacological Basis of Therapeutics*, 5th ed. Macmillan Publishing Co., Inc., New York, 1975, p. 580.

41. Marshall, Robert: "The Nursing Position After Operation and the Work of Breathing," *Thorax*, **24**:330, 1969.

42. Holley, H. Steele: *op. cit.*

43. Stahl, William M.: *op. cit.*, p. 21.

44. Dripps, Robert D., et al.: *op. cit.*

45. Guyton, Arthur C.: *Textbook of Medical Physiology*, 5th ed. W. B. Saunders Co., Philadelphia, 1976, p. 580.

46. Kinney, John M.: "Ventilation and Ventilatory Failure," in American College of Surgeons, Committee on Pre and Postoperative Care: *Manual of Preoperative and Postoperative Care*, 2nd ed. W. B. Saunders Co., Philadelphia, 1971, p. 187.

47. Nett, Louise, and Petty, Thomas L.: "Oxygen Toxicity," *Am. J. Nurs.*, **73**:1557, (Sept.) 1973.

48. Brannin, Patricia Kay: "Oxygen Therapy and Measures of Bronchial Hygiene," *Nurs. Clin. North Am.*, **9**:111, (Mar.) 1974.

49. Winter, Peter M., and Smith, Graham: "The Toxicity of Oxygen," *Anesthesiology*, **37**:210, (Aug.) 1972.

50. Collart, Marie E., and Brenneman, Janice K.: "Preventing Postoperative Atelectasis," *Am. J. Nurs.*, **71**:1982, (Oct.) 1971.

51. Adler, Richard N., and Brodie, Stella L.: "Postoperative Rebreathing Aid," *Am. J. Nurs.*, **68**:1287, (June) 1968.

52. Collart, Marie, and Brenneman, Janice K.: *op. cit.*

53. Colgan, Frank J., et al.: "Resistance Breathing (Blow Bottles) and Sustained Hyperinflations in the Treatment of Atelectasis," *Anesthesiology*, **32**:543, (June) 1970.

54. Ungvarski, Peter: "Mechanical Stimulation of Coughing," *Am. J. Nurs.*, **71**:2358, (Dec.) 1971.

55. Brannin, Patricia Kay: *op. cit.*

56. Barsch, John, and Kamen, Jack: "Special Problems in Respiratory Therapy," in Beal, John M., and Eckenhoff, James E. (eds.): *Intensive and Recovery Room Care*. Macmillan Publishing Co., Inc., New York, 1969, p. 164.

57. Morgan, Calvin V., Jr., and Orcutt, Thomas W.: "The Care and Feeding of Chest Tubes," *Am. J. Nurs.*, **72**:305, (Feb.) 1972.

58. Kersten, Laura: "Chest-tube Drainage System—Indications and Principles of Operation," *Heart and Lung*, **3**:97, (Jan.–Feb.) 1974.

59. Morgan, Calvin V., Jr., and Orcutt, Thomas W.: *op. cit.*

60. Holley, H. Steele: *op. cit.*, p. 63.

61. Harvey, James D.: "Operative Surgical

Care," in Rhoads, Jonathan E., et al. (eds.): *Surgery; Principles and Practice,* 4th ed. J. B. Lippincott Co., Philadelphia, 1970, p. 291.

62. Smith, R. Brian, et al.: "In a Recovery Room," *Am. J. Nurs.,* **73**:70, (Jan.) 1973.

63. Allen, J. Garrott: "Blood Transfusions and Related Problems," in Rhoads, Jonathan E., et al. (eds.): *Surgery; Principles and Practice,* 4th ed. J. B. Lippincott Co., Philadelphia, 1970, p. 175.

64. *Ibid.,* p. 176.

65. "Hazards of Postoperative Fluid Therapy," *Drug Ther. Bull.,* **10**:47, (June 9) 1972.

66. Stillman, John D.: "Fluid, Electrolytes, Acid-Base Abnormalities," in Bushnell, Sharon S. (ed.): *Respiratory Intensive Care Nursing.* Little, Brown & Co., Boston, 1973, p. 168.

67. Dillard, David H.: "Preoperative and Postoperative Care," in Harkins, Henry N., and Nyhus, Lloyd M. (eds.): *Surgery of the Stomach and Duodenum,* 2nd ed. Little, Brown & Co., Boston, 1969, p. 487.

68. Guyton, Arthur C.: *op. cit.,* p. 358.

69. *Ibid.,* p. 365.

70. Child, Judy, et al.: "Blood Transfusions," *Am. J. Nurs.,* **72**:1602, (Sept.) 1972.

71. Walter, Carl W.: "Blood Donors, Blood and Transfusions," in American College of Surgeons, Committee on Pre and Postoperative Care: *Manual of Preoperative and Postoperative Care.* W. B. Saunders Co., Philadelphia, 1971, p. 146.

72. Allen, J. Garrott: *op. cit.,* p. 168.

73. Kuner, Joseph, et al.: "Cardiac Arrhythmias During Anesthesia," *Dis. Chest,* **52**:580, (Nov.) 1967.

73a. Fonkalsrud, Eric W., et al.: "Reduction of Infusion Thrombophlebitis with Buffered Glucose Solutions," *Surgery,* **63**:280, (Feb.) 1968.

74. Pederson, Betty M.: "A Solution for Post-Infusion Thrombophlebitis," *Am. J. Nurs.,* **70**:325, (Feb.) 1970.

75. Becker, Jorgen: "Post-operative Venous Thrombosis," *Acta. Chir. Scand. (Suppl.)* **431**:1, 1972.

76. Neuschatz, Joel, and Crosby, William H.: "The Prevention of Postoperative Thrombosis—A Simple, Safe Approach," *Arch. Intern. Med.,* **130**:966, (Dec.) 1972.

77. Daly, Catherine R., and Kelly, Elizabeth A.: "Prevention of Pulmonary Embolism: Intracaval Devices," *Am. J. Nurs.,* **72**:2004, (Nov.) 1972.

78. Norris, Walter, and Campbell, Donald: *op. cit.,* p. 205.

79. Collard, George M., and Jude, James R.: "Cardiopulmonary Resuscitation in the Cardiac Care Unit," *Nurs. Clin. North Am.,* **7**:573, (Sept.) 1972.

80. Gildea, James E.: "Cardiovascular Resuscitation," in Beal, John M., and Eckenhoff, James E. (eds.): *Intensive and Recovery Room Care.* Macmillan Publishing Co., Inc., New York, 1969, p. 127.

81. Randall, H. T.: "Diet and Nutrition in the Care of the Surgical Patient," in Goodhart, Robert S., and Shils, Maurice E. (eds.): *Modern Nutrition in Health and Disease: Dietotherapy,* 5th ed. Lea & Febiger, Philadelphia, 1973, p. 950.

82. Stahl, William M.: *op. cit.,* p. 41.

83. MacBryde, Cyril M.: "Weight Loss and Undernutrition," in MacBryde, Cyril M., and Blacklow, Robert Stanley (eds.): *Signs and Symptoms; Applied Pathologic Physiology and Clinical Interpretation,* 5th ed. J. B. Lippincott Co., Philadelphia, 1970, p. 897.

84. Moore, Francis D.: "The Endocrine and Metabolic Basis of Surgical Care," in Rhoads, Jonathan E., et al. (eds.): *Surgery; Principles and Practice,* 4th ed. J. B. Lippincott Co., Philadelphia, 1970, p. 349.

85. "Postoperative Distention and Fruit Juices," *J.A.M.A.,* **194**:476, (Oct. 25) 1965.

86. Dimond, E. Grey: *op. cit.*

87. Chang, Margaret K.: "A Visit to the Peking Children's Hospital," *Am. J. Nurs.,* **72**:2219, (Dec.) 1972.

88. Elman, Robert: "Protein Needs in Surgical Patients," *J. Am. Diet. Assoc.,* **32**:524, (June) 1956.

89. Janhunen, L,, and Tammisto, T.: "Postoperative Vomiting and Different Modes of General Anesthesia," *Ann. Chir. Gynaecol. Fenn.,* **61**:152, 1972.

90. Lutz, H., and Immick, H.: "Antiemetic Effect of Benzaquinamide in Postoperative Vomiting," *Curr. Ther. Res.,* **14**:178, (Apr.) 1972.

91. Guyton, Arthur C.: *op. cit.,* p. 899.

92. Holley, H. Steele: *op. cit.,* p. 68.

93. Wylie, W. D., and Churchill-Davidson, H. C.: *A Practice of Anaesthesia,* 3rd ed. Year Book Medical Publishers, Chicago, 1972, p. 1314.

94. *Ibid.,* p. 1315.

95. Lutz, H., and Immick, H.: *op. cit.*

96. Dumas, Rhetaugh G., and Leonard, Robert C.: "The Effect of Nursing on the Incidence of Postoperative Vomiting," *Nurs. Res.,* **12**:12, (Winter) 1963.

97. Robinson, Corrine H.: *Normal and Therapeutic Nutrition,* 14th ed. Macmillan Publishing Co., Inc., New York, 1972, p. 500.

98. Hennon, David K., et al.: "Nutritional Considerations for Maxillofacial Patients," in Chalian, Varoujan A., et al. (eds.): *Maxillofacial Prosthetics.* Williams & Wilkins Co., Baltimore, 1971, p. 257.

99. Hartwell, Shattuck W., Jr., and Cole, Owen R.: "The Feeding Oesophagostomy in the Management of Head and Neck Cancer," *Aust. N.Z. J. Surg.,* **39**:241, (Feb.) 1970.

100. Welty, Mary Jane, et al.: "The Patient with Maxillofacial Cancer," *Nurs. Clin. North Am.,* **8**:137, (Mar.) 1973.

101. Sawyer, Robert B.: "Jejunostomy for Feeding or Decompression," *Surg. Clin. North Am.,* **49:**1311, (Dec.) 1969.

102. Thompson, James C.: "The Stomach and Duodenum," in Sabiston, David C., Jr. (ed.): *Davis-Christopher Textbook of Surgery,* 10th ed. W. B. Saunders Co., Philadelphia, 1972, p. 849.

103. Grant, Jo Ann N.: "Patient Care in Parenteral Hyperalimentation," *Nurs. Clin. North Am.,* **8:**165, (Mar.) 1973.

104. Irving, M. H., and Rushman, G. B.: "Parenteral Nutrition for the Surgical Patient," *Anaesthesia,* **26:**450, (Oct.) 1971.

105. Thompson, James C.: *op. cit.*

106. Sparberg, Marshall: *Ileostomy Care.* Charles C Thomas, Publisher, Springfield, Ill., 1971.

107. Varco, Richard L.: "Principles of Preoperative and Postoperative Care," in Davis, Loyal (ed.): *Christopher's Textbook of Surgery,* 9th ed. W. B. Saunders Co., Philadelphia, 1968, p. 202.

108. Guyton, Arthur C.: *op. cit.,* p. 901.

108a. Elman, Robert: *Surgical Care: A Practical Physiological Guide.* Appleton-Century-Crofts, New York, 1951.

109. Dericks, Virginia C.: "Rehabilitation of Patients with Ileostomy," *Am. J. Nurs.,* **61:**48, (May) 1961.

110. Gallagher, Ann M.: "Body Image Changes in the Patient with a Colostomy," *Nurs. Clin. North Am.,* **7:**669, (Dec.) 1972.

111. Gibbs, Gertrude E., and White, Marilyn: "Stomal Care," *Am. J. Nurs.,* **72:**268, (Feb.) 1972.

112. Gutowski, Frances: "Ostomy Procedure: Nursing Care Before and After," *Am. J. Nurs.,* **72:**262, (Feb.) 1972.

113. Katona, Elizabeth A.: "A Patient-Centered, Living-Oriented Approach to the Patient with an Artificial Anus or Bladder," *Nurs. Clin. North Am.,* **2:**623, (Dec.) 1967.

114. Lenneberg, Edith, and Mendelssohn, Alan N.: "Colostomies: A Guide for the Patient," *Dis. Colon Rectum,* **12:**201, (May–June) 1969.

115. Murray, Barbara S., et al.: "The Patient Has an Ileal Conduit," *Am. J. Nurs.,* **75:**1560, (Aug.) 1971.

116. Ostomy Association of Boston, Inc.: *Manual for Ileostomy Patients,* 7th ed. The Association, Boston, 1972.

116a. Sparberg, Marshall: *op. cit.*

116b. Ostomy Association of Boston, Inc.: *op. cit.*

117. Andriole, Vincent T.: "Care of the Indwelling Catheter," in Kaye, Donald (ed.): *Urinary Tract Infection and Its Management.* C. V. Mosby Co., St. Louis, 1972, p. 263.

118. Desautels, Robert E.: "The Causes of Catheter-Induced Urinary Infections and Their Prevention," *J. Urol.,* **101:**757, (May) 1969.

119. Maki, Dennis G., et al.: "Prevention of Catheter-Associated Urinary Tract Infection," *J.A.M.A.,* **221:**1270, (Sept. 11) 1972.

120. Moore, Frances D.: "Homeostasis: Bodily Changes in Trauma and Surgery," in Sabiston, David C., Jr. (ed.): *Davis-Christopher Textbook of Surgery,* 10th ed. W. B. Saunders Co., Philadelphia, 1972, p. 37.

121. Berne, Thomas V., and Barbour, Benjamin H.: "Acute Renal Failure in General Surgical Patients," *Arch. Surg.,* **102:**594, (June) 1971.

122. McLaughlin, Charles W., Jr., and Brown, John R.: "Postoperative Urinary Retention," *US Naval Med. Bull.,* **42:**1025, (May) 1944.

122a. Keuhnelian, John G., and Sanders, Virginia E.: *Urologic Nursing.* Macmillan Publishing Co., Inc., New York, 1970, p. 168.

122b. Grayhack, John T., and Dahl, Douglas S.: "The Urologic Patient," in Beal, John M., and Eckenhoff, James E. (eds.): *Intensive and Recovery Room Care.* Macmillan Publishing Co., Inc., New York, 1969, p. 204.

123. Winkelstein, Charles, et al.: *op. cit.*

124. Minckley, Barbara Blake: "A Study of Noise and Its Relationship to Patient Discomfort in the Recovery Room," *Nurs. Res.,* **17:**247, (May–June) 1968.

125. Walker, Betty Boyd: "The Postsurgery Heart Patient: Amount of Uninterrupted Time for Sleep and Rest During the First, Second, and Third Postoperative Days in a Teaching Hospital," *Nurs. Res.,* **21:**164, (Mar.–Apr.) 1972.

126. Woods, Nancy Fugate: "Patterns of Sleep in Postcardiotomy Patients," *Nurs. Res.,* **21:**347, (July–Aug.) 1972.

127. Aiken, Linda H., and Henrichs, Theodore F.: "Systematic Relaxation as a Nursing Intervention Technique with Open Heart Surgery Patients," *Nurs. Res.,* **20:**212, (May–June) 1971.

128. Gildea, James E.: "The Relief of Postoperative Pain," *Med. Clin. North Am.,* **52:**81, (Jan.) 1968.

129. Copp, Laura Archer: "The Spectrum of Suffering," *Am. J. Nurs.,* **74:**491, (Mar.) 1974.

130. Guyton, Arthur C.: *op. cit.,* p. 664.

131. Beecher, Henry K.: "Relationship of Significance of Wound Pain Experienced," *J.A.M.A.,* **161:**1613, (Aug. 25) 1956.

132. Egbert, Lawrence D., et al.: "Reduction of Postoperative Pain by Encouragement and Instruction of Patients," *N. Engl. J. Med.,* **270:**825, (Apr. 16) 1964.

133. Copp, Laura Archer: *op. cit.*

134. Gildea, James E.: "The Relief of Postoperative Pain," *Med. Clin. North Am.,* **52:**81, (Jan.) 1968.

135. Casey, Kenneth L.: "The Neurophysiologic Basis of Pain," *Postgrad. Med.,* **53:**63, (May) 1973.

136. Kao, F. F., et al.: *op. cit.*

136a. Hymes, Alan C., et al.: "Electrical Surface Stimulation for Control of Acute Postoperative Pain and Prevention of Ileus," *Surg. Forum,* **24:**447, 1973.

137. McNamara, Thomas F., et al.: "The Role

of Microorganisms in the Production of Oral Malodor," *Oral Surg.,* **34:**41, (July) 1972.

138. Tarsitano, John J., et al.: "Nursing Care After Oral Surgery," *Am. J. Nurs.,* **69:**1493, (July) 1969.

139. Newcombe, Barbara: "Care of the Patient with Head and Neck Cancer," *Nurs. Clin. North Am.,* **2:**599, (Dec.) 1967.

140. Hicks, Dorothy J.: "An Incidence Study of Pressure Sores Following Surgery," in *ANA Clinical Sessions, 1970.* Appleton-Century-Crofts, New York, 1971, p. 49.

141. Eckenhoff, James E., et al.: "The Incidence and Etiology of Postanesthetic Excitement," *Anesthesiology,* **22:**667, (Sept.–Oct.) 1962.

142. Feingold, David S.: "Hospital Acquired Infections," *N. Engl. J. Med.,* **283:**1384, (Dec. 17) 1970).

143. Rocha, Heonir: "Epidemiology of Urinary Tract Infection in Adults," in Kaye, Donald (ed.): *Urinary Tract Infection and Its Management.* C. V. Mosby Co., St. Louis, 1972, p. 142.

144. Maki, Dennis G., et al.: *op. cit.*

145. Dyer, Elaine D., and Peterson, Daryl E.: "Safe Care of IPPB Machines," *Am. J. Nurs.,* **71:**2163, (Nov.) 1971.

146. Cruse, Peter J. E., and Foord, Rosemary: "A Five-Year Prospective Study of 23,649 Surgical Wounds," *Arch. Surg.,* **107:**206, (Aug.) 1973.

147. "ECRI—What It Is and What It Does," *Am. J. Nurs.,* **73:**860, (May) 1973.

148. Dlin, Barney M., and Perlman, Abraham: Sex After Ileostomy or Colostomy," *Med. Aspects Hum. Sexuality,* **6:**32, (July) 1972.

149. Morris, Jan. *Conundrum.* Harcourt, Brace, Jovanovich, New York, 1974.

150. Simmons, Dawn L.: *Man into Woman.* Manor Books, New York, 1971.

151. Jorgenson, Christine: *Christine Jorgenson: A Personal Autobiography.* Bantam Books, New York, 1968.

Additional Suggested Reading

Betson, Carol, and Ude, Linda: "Central Venous Pressure," *Am. J. Nurs.,* **69:**1466, (July) 1969.

Bryant, Lester R., et al.: "Reappraisal of Tracheal Injury from Cuffed Tracheostomy Tubes," *J.A.M.A.,* **215:**625, (Jan. 25) 1971.

Chapman, Jacqueline S.: "Effects of Different Nursing Approaches upon Selected Postoperative Responses of Male Herniorrhaphy Patients," in Downs, Florence S., and Newman, Margaret A.: *A Source Book of Nursing Research.* F. A. Davis Co., Philadelphia, 1973.

Conner, George H., et al.: "Tracheostomy," *Am. J. Nurs.,* **72:**68, (Jan.) 1972.

Danilowicz, Delores A., and Gabriel, P. H.: "Postoperative Reactions in Children: 'Normal' and Abnormal Responses after Cardiac Surgery," *Am. J. Psychiatry,* **128:**185, (Aug.) 1971.

Drury, John H., Jr.: "Handbook of Range-of-Motion Exercises," *Nursing '72,* **2:**19, (Apr.) 1972.

Durr, Carol A.: "Hands That Help . . . But How?" *Nurs. Forum,* **10:**392, (No. 4) 1971.

Elms, Roslyn R.: "Recovery Room Behavior and Postoperative Convalescence," *Nurs. Res.,* **21:**390, (Sept.–Oct.) 1972.

Elsberry, Nancy L.: "Psychological Responses to Open Heart Surgery: A Review," *Nurs. Res.,* **21:**20, (May–June) 1972.

Fuchs, Peter C.: "Indwelling Intravenous Polyethylene Catheters; Factors Influencing the Risk of Microbial Colonization and Sepsis," *J.A.M.A.,* **216:**1447, (May 31) 1971.

Gernet, Carolyn F., and Schwartz, Stephanie: "Pulmonary Artery Catheterization," *Am. J. Nurs.,* **73:**1182, (July) 1973.

Jarvis, Dorothy: "Open Heart Surgery: Patients' Perception of Care," *Am. J. Nurs.,* **70:**2591, (Dec.) 1970.

Layne, Otis, and Yudofsky, Stuart: "Postoperative Psychosis in Cardiotomy Patients," *N. Engl. J. Med.,* **284:**518, (Mar. 11) 1971.

Liao, Sung J.: "Acupuncture—An Appraisal," *Conn. Med.,* **37:**506, (Oct.) 1973.

Melzack, Ronald, and Chapman, C. Richard: "Psychologic Aspects of Pain," *Postgrad. Med.,* **53:**69, (May) 1973.

Peters, Gustavus A., and Marcoux, J Paul: "Some Adverse Drug Reactions Common in the Postoperative Period," *Surg. Clin. North Am.,* **49:**1123, (Oct.) 1969.

Powell, Mary: "An Environment for Wound Healing," *Am. J. Nurs.,* **72:**1862, (Oct.) 1972.

Reitz, Marie, and Pope, Wilma: "Mouth Care," *Am. J. Nurs.,* **73:**1728, (Oct.) 1973.

Ross, S. Ann: "Infusion Phlebitis," *Nurs. Res.,* **21:**313, (July–Aug.) 1972.

Schauerhamer, Robert A., et al.: "Studies in the Management of the Contaminated Wound," *Am. J. Surg.,* **122:**74, (July) 1971.

Schultz, Nancy V.: "How Children Perceive Pain," *Nurs. Outlook,* **19:**670, (Oct.) 1971.

Tinker, John H., and Wehner, Robert: "The Nurse and the Ventilator," *Am. J. Nurs.,* **74:**1276, (July) 1974.

Wallace, Gladys, and Hayter, Jean: "Karaya for Chronic Skin Ulcers," *Am. J. Nurs.,* **74:**1094, (June) 1974.

Wiley, Loy (ed.): "Innovations in Nursing: Patterns of Pain—Do They Affect Medications?" *Nursing '72,* **2:**11, (Aug.) 1972.

Wolfer, John A.: "Definition and Assessment of Surgical Patients' Welfare and Recovery; Selected Review of the Literature," *Nurs. Res.,* **22:**394, (Sept.–Oct.) 1973.

Woodrow, Kenneth M., et al.: "Pain Tolerance: Differences According to Age, Sex, and Race," *Psychosom. Med.,* **34:**548, (Nov.–Dec.) 1972.

Catherine Temple
Virginia Henderson

CHAPTER 49

Pain—Its Meaning, Prevention, and Relief

1. THE PAIN EXPERIENCE: A DEFINITION
2. FACTORS INFLUENCING PAIN SENSATION AND REACTION
3. NURSING CARE AND TREATMENT
4. PREVENTION

1. THE PAIN EXPERIENCE: A DEFINITION

In 1857, Robley Dunglison devised what is probably the most indefinite definition in existence when he termed pain "a disagreeable sensation which scarcely admits of definition" [1]; yet he put his finger on the elusive quality of this concept. Though pain is something anyone can describe, scientists have failed to propose a comprehensive and satisfying definition of it. *Pain* remains a catchall term for a wide range of experience. But pain is recognized as *the* primary signal that something is wrong with the body. In the form of a midnight earache or a mother's spanking, pain may also be the first thing a child learns to fear. Pain can be an unwelcome reminder of mortality, but it can also be of tremendous diagnostic value in pinpointing pathology. Pain can make people feel vulnerable and alone, or they may feel pain when they are alone and vulnerable. For some, pain is a code name for any totally unpleasant experience, "Pain, it was all pain!" Others use body language to describe feelings and relationships—"She's a pain in the neck"; "All he wants to do is hurt me." A survey of the literature substantiates W. K. Livingston's statement that "the chief difficulty encountered in a search for a satisfactory definition for pain, is the fact that it can be encountered from either a physiologic or a psychologic approach." † Pain as a manifestation of disease is intertwined with the ethical interpretation of suffering. As a result, pain is related to such polarities as good-bad, reward-punishment,* love-hate, triumph-defeat, innocence-guilt.[2]

* Livingston, W. K.: *Pain Mechanisms.* Macmillan Publishing Co., Inc., New York, 1943, p. 62.
† The word *pain* is derived from the Latin, Greek, and French words for punishment—*poena, poinē, peine.* Whether pain is a sequel to bodily damage or emotional loss, patients normally wonder, "What did I do to deserve this?"

Primary Conceptualizations of Pain. In 1952, J. D. Hardy and associates [3] listed the following primary conceptualizations of pain in the nineteenth and twentieth centuries: (1) a feeling state that is the opposite of pleasure; (2) the result of strong stimulation of any sensory mechanism; (3) a sensation having its own specialized neural mechanisms; and (4) a complex phenomenon involving both a feeling state and a sensation with its own properties. Today, most theorists (whether they approach pain from an anatomist's or a psychiatrist's point of view) would agree that *pain is always a psychosomatic event* because pain refers both to perceived unpleasant sensations *and* the meaning the patient attaches to this real, threatened, or phantasized injury.

Thomas Szasz's [4] (1957) analysis of pain at three distinct symbolic levels was one of the first attempts to bridge the gap between pain as a strictly physiologic phenomenon and pain as an expression of psychic distress. He distinguished among (1) the person registering the fact that there is damage to his or her body, (2) the communication of this pain in asking someone else for relief, and (3) pain as a nonspecific request for help or a complaint about being unfairly treated. If one accepts his distinctions, it is clear that nurses are *never* asked to deal with "purely" physical pain; they respond to the statements made by patients about their pain. People invariably react to pain as an insult to their functional integrity, and they also have feelings about having to ask for help, and these feelings become part of anything they say about their symptoms. Possible differences in the meaning of the threat to the body as understood by patients and by nurses necessitate ongoing validation of the complete significance of the complaint of pain.

Physiologic Theories. Physiologic theories of pain have also varied in how much they assumed a direct-line communication of pain from the skin to the brain, and the influence

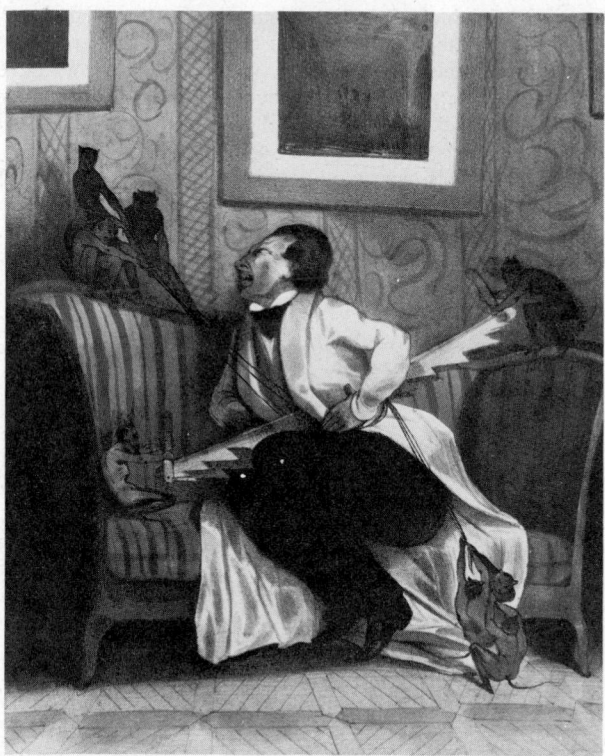

Figure 49-1. A nineteenth-century artist's conception of pain.

of psychologic factors on the triggering of pain perception. The specificity theory (which maintains that pain is a unique modality with specific pain receptors in body tissues that send messages to a pain center in the thalamus) and the pattern theory (which holds that pain is produced by intense stimulation of nonspecific receptors) were challenged in 1965 by the "gate control" theory. This last theory assumes a regulatory process that screens sensory input before it evokes pain perception and response [5] (see Fig. 49-2). Ronald Melzack and Patrick D. Wall's "gate control" theory has the merit

of showing how emotions, memories, attitudes, and expectations have an effect on the actual transmission of pain signals. According to them, the substantia gelatinosa (SG) in the dorsal horn of the spinal cord acts as a "gating" mechanism controlled by the balance of input from large peripheral fibers (L) which inhibit and small peripheral fibers (S) which conduct. If the impulses reaching the "gating" mechanism achieve a critical point, they are conducted to the central transmission (T) cells, where they trigger the pain action system. Pain is prevented by stimulation of large af-

Figure 49-2. Diagram of the gate-control theory of pain. *L:* Fibers of large diameter. *S:* Fibers of small diameter. These project to substantia gelatinosa (*SG*) and the main secondary afferent neuron or first central transmission cell (*T*). (From Melzack, Ronald, and Wall, Patrick D.: "Pain Mechanisms: A New Theory," *Science,* **150:**971, [Nov.] 1965.)

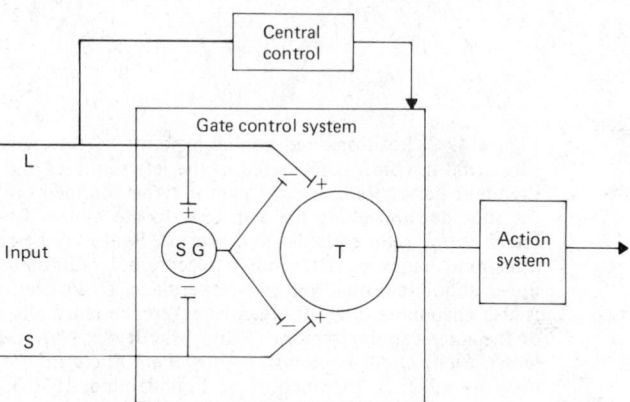

ferent fibers which normally inhibit the smaller pain-carrying fibers in the spinal cord; the system can also be modified by conditions that affect the descending efferent fibers.

Since the Melzack-Wall model suggests that pain response is triggered after the cutaneous sensory input has been modulated by both sensory feedback mechanisms and the influences of the central nervous system, many regard it as the best theory to date for explaining the following gamut of events that result from unexpected damage to the skin: (1) a startle response; (2) a flexion reflex; (3) postural readjustment; (4) vocalization; (5) orientation of the head and eyes to examine the damaged area; (6) autonomic responses; (7) evocation of past experience in similar situations and prediction of the consequences of the injury; and (8) other behaviors that diminish the sensory and affective components of the whole experience as, for example, biting the lips.[6] Whether the "gate control" theory remains forevermore the prevailing explanation or not, it has already produced a renaissance in thinking about pain because it has led to the development of innovative, physiologically nondestructive ways of blocking pain (for example, electrical stimulation).

A Working Definition. Nurses should be familiar with the many conceptualizations of pain because they all have some effect on treatment of the person in pain. However, the recurring emphasis in the professional literature on pain as a private, subjective experience makes Margo McCaffery's definition seem most relevant to nursing care. She says, "Pain is whatever the experiencing person says it is and exists whenever he says it does." * But "to understand it as the patient 'feels' it" (as one patient described such an attitude) † anyone trying to help should be familiar with the many conditions that modify physical sensation and emotional reaction.

2. FACTORS INFLUENCING PAIN SENSATION AND REACTION

Innumerable factors influence how a specific pain feels, and make different people even react differently to the same kind of pain. Pain can be described according to location, radiation, duration, intensity, frequency, precipitating and aggravating factors, associated symptoms, and the reactions generated by each of these descriptors in the affected person. Variations in age, sex, religion, intellectual ability, ethnic heritage, family size, and threat to life style have been correlated with different behavior patterns. Certain psychologic traits also influence pain tolerance and the response to painful stimuli.

* McCaffery, Margo: *Nursing Management of the Patient with Pain.* J. B. Lippincott Co., Philadelphia, 1972, p. 8.
† Cashatt, Barbara: "Pain: A Patient's View," *Am. J. Nurs.,* **72:**281, (Feb.) 1972.

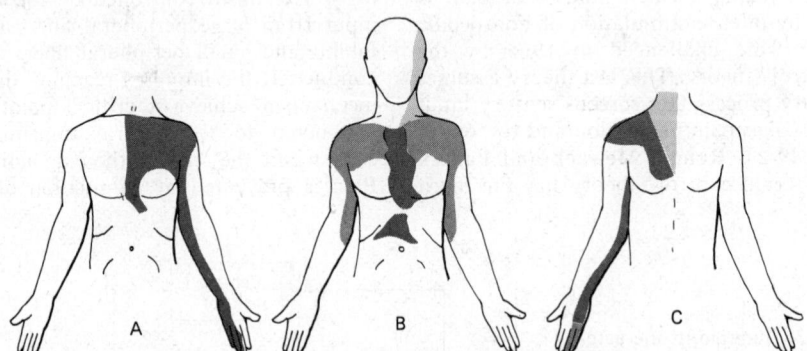

Figure 49-3. Positions and common points of reference of cardiac pain. *A.* Area of substernal discomfort projected to the left shoulder and arm over the distribution of the ulnar nerve. Reference of pain may be confined only to the left shoulder, or to the shoulder and along the arm only to the elbow. Less frequently pain may be referred to the right shoulder and arm. *B.* Pain may be referred to both shoulders, arms, and hands simultaneously. Occasional radiation to the epigastrium and right upper abdominal quadrant may take place. *C.* Projection of anginal pain to the back is also encountered less frequently; reference is usually to the area of the left scapula or the interscapular region. (From MacBryde, Cyril M., and Blacklow, Robert S. [eds.]: *Signs and Symptoms. Applied Pathologic Physiology and Clinical Interpretation,* 5th ed. J. B. Lippincott Co., Philadelphia, 1970.)

Location, Radiation. Superficial somatic structures are richly innervated and so skin pain, for example, can be precisely located. Deeper somatic structures and viscera are more sparsely innervated and so such pain is likely to be diffuse, poorly localized, and referred (or felt in another area) according to the distribution of its innervation. For example, cardiac pain is not felt precisely where the heart is located, but may be felt over the distribution of the ulnar nerve [7] (see Fig. 49-3). Injury that can be seen and monitored may be less disturbing than injury that cannot be seen. Localized pain may be dismissed as minor, but radiating pain may be exaggerated because it seems to be "all over." Pain with a discernible cause is less disturbing than pain of unknown etiology; broken bones can be fixed, but with nonspecific pain "it could be *anything.*" Cutaneous pain, which is bright and pricking in quality, tends to elicit "fight or flight" responses on both the physiologic and behavioral levels, while visceral pain, which usually has a dull, gripping quality, seems to have a depressing effect. It is as if there is no running away from the enemy within.[8]

Postural and Environmental Influences. Understanding the relationship between body activities and physiologic processes is helpful in identifying the nature of the pathologic process responsible for the pain. The subcutaneous tissues are sensitive to stretching and to chemical irritants; muscles react to the accumulation of waste normally removed by the circulating blood. Bones, joints, bursae, and tendons give rise to pain on movement, and there is relief when the parts are at rest; nerve pain is intensified by any posture that makes a bone impinge on the involved nerve or root. Pain from pleura and trachea correlates with the extent of respiratory movements; gastrointestinal pain tends to increase with peristaltic activity. Encapsulated organs (e.g., liver, kidneys, spleen, pancreas) are usually painful when even slightly swollen because pressure is felt as soon as they are compressed. Environmental conditions can also modify pain. Drafts may cause severe pain to burned patients because exposed nerve endings are stimulated. Slight cold can trigger paroxysms of pain in those suffering from trigeminal neuralgia. Sulfur gas in the atmosphere can irritate sensitive mucous membranes and be very painful to the patient with chronic lung disease. Strenuous exercise in hot weather, leading to excessive sodium chloride depletion through perspiration, can produce sudden muscle cramp.

Intensity. Trauma to several areas does not result in an arithmetically compounded perception of pain. There is a maximum amount of pain that can be felt, and beyond that point an increase in stimulus will not cause greater pain, though extensive injuries may increase the patient's anxiety and doubts about whether recovery is possible. In fact, a number of different pain impulses can close the hypothetical "gate" in the spinal cord because it is the "balance" of inhibiting and conducting nervous fibers that triggers the pain action system rather than the total number of injuries sustained. Resisting the insult of the dentist's drill with fingernails jabbed into the hands is an everyday example of pain countering pain.

Meaning of Affected Body Part. Certain parts of the body have special meaning for the patient. After a hysterectomy, a woman may "feel" the pain of physical trauma and the loss of her fertility. If a man's parents died from cardiac failure, chest pain of any sort can be taken as a sign that he will suffer the same fate. Gashes on the face and head, sites central to body image, will generate more of a reaction than will comparable wounds on the feet. Hemorrhoids are painful, but the embarrassment of calling attention to a part of the body that is commonly labeled unclean may increase the patient's discomfort.

Precipitating and Aggravating Factors. Back pain may be described by the patient as "moderate," and minutes later as "severe" if blood is seen in the urine. Once pain is described as burning or gnawing, the "being consumed" image conjured up by these words can be distressing in its own right. Everyone knows that pain at 2 A.M., when there is little to distract a person's attention from it or to divert him or her from the imagination run wild, seems much more sinister than the same pain in broad daylight. Responses to pain also vary with the level of consciousness: head injury, cerebral oxygen depletion, and central nervous system infections are organic states that diminish awareness of noxious stimuli, while some drugs chemically alter perceptions. The interval between attacks and the duration of discomfort —minutes, hours, days, years—further affect how the person handles the experience.

Threat to Life. Patients with chronic pain do not become accustomed to it. Short-term pain is tolerable because there is an end in sight. Protracted pain, since it is so often associated with general weakness, malnutrition, interrupted family life, fatigue, sleep deprivation, curtailed activities, and anxiety, is physically and psychologically debilitating. Anticipation of unlimited pain can paralyze all sense of coping—"I can take it now, but can I take *more* (or take it *forever*)?" A young nurse who was treated for cancer described these feelings very eloquently:

Severe or continued moderate pain was very depressing to me, especially when I could see no end to it in the near future—or possibly ever. Even though I gained a two- or three-hour relatively pain-free period from some analgesics, I knew the pain would be there again when the medication wore off. I began to wonder if I would ever again be free of pain. My mind became obsessed with my pain. I could think of very little else, and when I could concentrate on something else, it was only for a short time. My patience and my tolerance ran short. Little things seemed big—sometimes too big to handle. After continued coping with pain, even the smallest amount of added discomfort seemed too much to tolerate.

.   .   .

The pain affected my emotions in ways other than depression. When the nurse was delayed in bringing me something for pain I began to think she just did not care or that she thought I really had no pain . . . I began to wonder if my pain was real or if I really was imagining it. I began to take out my feelings of frustration on the staff or on some member of my family.*

If pain means possible or certain death, or is perceived as "the worst ever" and interferes with the pleasures of daily living, it frequently monopolizes the patient's complete attention and takes on an all-pervasive quality.† Such pain is hard to influence because care must be geared to meet the patient's needs at various levels. The anxiety, depression, frustration, anger, and paranoia that *normally* color the patient's responses must be treated just as much as the obvious physical problems.

Powerlessness and Self-determination as They Affect Pain. Control over the termination of the painful stimulus has repeatedly been shown to have considerable influence on the amount of discomfort experienced. In laboratory experiments, discomfort ratings were lower in studies where the subjects could push a button and turn off the pain stimulus; the pain threshold (minimal point at which pain is aroused) was significantly lower when the subject was deprived of control over the stimulus.[9] Pain in a terminal illness may be seen as excruciating because it represents the ultimate "no escape" condition. Cardiac pain is unbearable because it becomes intense so quickly that the individual is unable to achieve any control over it. However, nurses should remember that with adequate preparation a person can be taught to handle slowly rising pain.[10] Feelings of powerlessness, whether first prompted by a poor prognosis or by health personnel who encourage passivity as the cor-

rect patient attitude, will have a less insidious, debilitating effect if patients are subsequently shown that they can relieve some of the pain themselves.

Knowing that the pain "makes sense" and that one can do something to control it has a profound effect on the individual's progress through an experience of pain. A good example is the pain of labor. The "natural childbirth" movement is based on the notion that mothers should understand that labor hurts because the uterus is contracting to expel the baby and that they can help themselves by using specific relaxation techniques to avoid fighting the contractions. This concept was also borne out in a study of patients with abdominal surgery who were shown the possibilities for self-help. They needed half as much postoperative narcotic and were discharged $2\frac{7}{10}$ days sooner than patients with the same sort of surgery who did not get this instruction. The "special-care" group was told where they would feel pain, how severe it would be, and how long it would last, and they were reassured that having pain was normal after abdominal surgery. It was explained that pain is caused by spasm of the muscles under the incision and that *they could relieve most of the pain themselves* by relaxing these muscles. They were taught deep-breathing and what positions allow the abdominal wall to relax, and they were reminded that if they could not achieve a reasonable level of comfort, they should ask for medication.[11] Instead of being encouraged to regard medication as the *principal* source of pain relief, as so often happens, these patients were urged to play an active role in their convalescence—with dramatic results. The emphasis on self-determination and on doing what would promote healing of the wound is a sharp contrast to swallowing a pill and passively waiting for it to "take effect." Since individuals may use their own behavior in response to an aversive stimulus as a basis for deciding whether the stimulus was painful, patients who find they *can* relax themselves may then rate the total experience as much less unpleasant than they expected it to be.[12]

Past Associations. The analgesic potential of different types of instruction has also been demonstrated in the very use of the word *pain* for unpleasant sensations. Once ambiguous experiences are described as pain, instead of referring to them by a more neutral term, patients may have lower pain thresholds than if a less loaded word is used.[13] A patient may assume that a nurse's mention of the word *pain* is proof that there is or will be pain. Readers might consider their own reactions to being asked about a "head pain" or a "headache"—

* *Ibid.*
† There are many medical cartoons showing the rest of the body as a mere appendage to an area that hurts; a toe with gout may be drawn ten times its normal size.

the former conjures up images of serious pathology, but the latter sounds as if it refers to an everyday experience. Uterine pain and menstrual cramps may be used to describe the same discomfort, but the two phrases evoke different responses from a woman. The reason for this phenomenon is that past painful experiences condition everyone's reactions to the concept "pain." Just thinking about pain can make a person feel vulnerable and more sensitive. Memories and fears can be triggered in the absence of physiologic stimulation, just as remembered relief can be activated by the attention of a sympathetic nurse if the patient has previously been helped by a nurse. The nurse's ministrations may also recall previous satisfying parental concern—"Mother makes the hurt go away."

Patients with Increased Tolerance for Pain. "Pain tolerance" (the amount of pain a person is able to endure beyond the point where it began to hurt) and "pain expression" (style of responding to a painful stimulus) are phrases that are sometimes linked, yet the factors that influence one do not necessarily affect the other. Richard A. Sternbach described persons with the greatest tolerance for pain as

. . . those whose perceptual judgments of other stimuli err on the small side (perceptual reduction), whose unconscious body images have definite boundaries, who are extraverted, not neurotic, and have relatively low anxiety. Pain tolerance decreases with lowered sensory input and an exposure to frequent pain experiences. Pain tolerance increases with motivation associated with group membership, voluntarily submitting to pain (cognitive dissonance), attention to another task, and with anxiety reduction.*

This summarization was based on laboratory and clinical studies, as, for example, the following: A. Petrie proposed that individuals could be ranked along a continuum from "reducers," who minimize stimulus input, to "augmenters," who exaggerate sensory input. Subjects who appeared to tolerate pain least manifested greater apprehension of pain.[14] Extraverts have higher thresholds to sensory stimuli than introverts. Extraversion is, however, associated with "exaggerated" expression of pain. The garrulous may find it beneficial to talk their way through the discomfort instead of bottling up their feelings inside of them. Making use of the Eysenck Personality Inventory, Cornell Medical Index, and Whiteley Index of Hypochondriasis, M. R. Bond[15] found that patients respond to symptoms of

disease according to their basic personality structure; denial is strong in all patients, and the spectrum of hypochondriacal attitudes increases in the presence of pain and other symptoms. A. H. Buss and N. W. Portnoy[16] found that strong group identification increased tolerance for pain; American subjects who were goaded to think that Russians had a greater tolerance for pain than Americans endured pain well beyond their established thresholds, apparently out of some sense of competition. B. B. Wolff and A. A. Harland[17] tested the effect of suggestion on endurance; individuals who already indicated that they could stand no more pain were able to increase their tolerance for pain after imagining that they would receive $1000 if they endured the shock a little longer.

Cultural Factors. Sternbach described those most likely to complain of pain as "older, neurotic, intropunitive, had more pain experiences, more siblings and come from laboring class families." * This profile calls to mind Szasz's third conceptualization of pain, which we considered earlier in this chapter. Complaint behavior does seem more likely if it is a nonspecific request for help—as it might very well be with the old, the anxious, the self-punishing, and the chronically ill. Large and taciturn families are known to communicate at times through physical symptoms. T. A. Gonda[18] pointed out that pain is a signal of distress in large families. Pain can be a way of eliciting sympathy, preventing loneliness, forestalling criticism, controlling the actions of others, and getting attention.

Ethnic affiliation is another important factor in accounting for pain reaction differences. In his classic 1952 study of four ethnic groups, Mark Zborowski[19] came to the following conclusions: (1) the Old American (Yankee) has a phlegmatic, "the doctor will help me" viewpoint; (2) Jews are expressive, concerned about the implications of pain, future-oriented, think the patient knows best, and see the doctor as only a consultant; (3) Italians view pain as a disease in itself, want immediate pain relief, and enjoy conversation and activity as means to forestall depression; (4) Irish perceive suffering as something to be hidden—you do not share your trouble with others just as you would not expect them to share theirs with you—and needing a doctor is regarded as a final capitulation to the pain. R. A. Sternbach and B. Tursky[20] replicated Zborowski's study with a group of housewives and got similar results: Italians were least able to take pain; Yankees were matter-of-fact; Yankees and

---

* Sternbach, Richard A.: *Pain—A Psychophysiological Analysis.* Academic Press, New York, 1968, p. 151.

* *Ibid.,* p. 77.

Irish were both undemonstrative but from different attitudes; Italians and Jews were demonstrative but for different reasons.

Other Variables. One could go on at length citing conditions that influence pain sensation and reaction. H. Merskey and F. G. Spear [21] report racial differences as significant when considering sensitivity to pain—Negroes have lower pain thresholds than Caucasians—yet Gracia S. McCabe [22] found that Southern Negroes hesitate to ask for pain relief. Children are commonly allowed more leeway in the expression of pain than adults; women are permitted to be more demonstrative than men, though members of each sex are conceded more freedom as they grow older. A person's religion may influence his or her behavior. Pain viewed as a punishment will affect the patient differently from pain seen as purifying character; pain perceived as a meaningless inconvenience will have still another effect. Finally, the individual's knowledge and understanding make a difference. Young children, with little language ability, find even the prick of an injection very distressing because they do not understand either the purpose of the procedure or the reason why loving parents submit them to such hostile treatment. Similarly, if a person does not understand the concept of time, even short-term pain can seem unending.

Ever-Changing Influences. This litany of factors influencing pain sensation and reaction can be overwhelming to nurses if they feel compelled to make use of all this information in each encounter with a patient. That would be impossible. Facts that help the nurse evaluate an individual's unique experience are important, but many differences are not important in themselves, though they do underscore the many things that affect any outcome. These factors have been listed to sensitize nurses to the many needs a person in pain may have and to the necessity of conceptualizing treatment so that as many as possible of the emotional, intellectual, social, and physiologic needs of the patient are met. However, nurses must guard against falling into the trap of automatically categorizing people according to current knowledge, just as they must sort out whether some facts seem to contradict others.* For example, older patients show

pain more easily and the elderly experience less pain than younger patients with similar disorders. Analysis will show in this instance that the first fact is speaking to pain expression while the second one deals with pain tolerance.[23,24]

When authors speak of women having lower pain thresholds, it is not always clear whether they are referring to increased sensitivity to pain or greater social freedom in expressing such feelings. One wonders whether this is another example of women "acting out" the accepted role of female weakness (an attitude that may change with the advent of role liberation for both sexes) or whether there actually are differences in sensitivity between the sexes. Black persons are also said to have low pain thresholds. Maybe a low pain threshold is in part a minority group phenomenon; after all, pain is a common conversion symptom.[25] Perhaps through sensitivity to pain the disadvantaged communicate a message of social importance. Consider the following questions: As individuals identify less and less with a specific religion or ethnic group, what differences will this make to pain expression or repression? As families become smaller and more sophisticated about interpersonal relations, will pain cease to be a way of getting attention and controlling the actions of others? These questions are meant to be provocative; they suggest that nurses should always be open to new information as they assess what nursing care is indicated in a specific situation.

3. NURSING CARE AND TREATMENT

Since pain is essentially a subjective experience and since, we believe, the patient's subjective experience is the primary focus of nursing, nurses are as a group more concerned with day-to-day care of the patient in pain than is any other profession. The physician focuses first and foremost on diagnosis and cure, and spends comparatively little time with patients; it is the nurse who helps the patient deal with bouts of pain—including the anxiety and depression that surface when arriving at a diagnosis becomes a long-drawn-out process and the pain seems increasingly ominous.* Perhaps it is this sustained contact with pain that accounts for the high percentage of studies on the nursing care of patients in pain in the research of the last decade. Efforts include de-

---

* Since many findings are based on small sample sizes and the attitudes of only a few ethnic groups have ever been examined, categorizing can easily become ludicrous. A married woman may have an Irish surname, but be a second-generation Swede. Her religion may be listed as Roman Catholic, but she may not be a regular churchgoer. When a person is in pain, it is hard to evaluate whether he or she is an extravert, an introvert, or a neurotic. Frequently, such labels make nurses judgmental of patients without being of any benefit whatsoever.

* A middle-aged bank president was heard to exclaim to a strange woman, sitting beside him when both were waiting, dressed in hospital nightshirts, for abdominal x-rays, "How in the world can you read Boswell's *Life of Johnson* when your life is hanging in the balance?!"

scribing ministering to patients in pain; surveys of the literature; programmed instruction for students on how to care for the patient in pain; and designs for clinical experiments that test the effectiveness of specific nursing approaches.[26-29]

A Brief Review of Nursing Studies. M. A. Bochnak and associates,[30] in their study, suggested that medication is not always necessary for the alleviation of pain. They found that if nurses determined the meaning of the pain to the patient, only 31 per cent of the patients sampled needed medication. Doctors' expectations of nurse action in the use of PRN medication orders were surveyed by M. Dorsch and associates.[31] Eighty-four per cent of the doctors interviewed expected nurses to utilize nursing measures such as talking to patients and changing their positions to relieve or minimize pain prior to, or in conjunction with, prescribed PRN medication orders. Yet A. Buckeridge and associates [32] studied nurse action when Darvon and Darvon compound were prescribed for PRN administration, and found relatively few incidents in which the nurse offered verbal support or comfort measures. Apparently, many nurses see the drug as an adequate solution to the patient's needs without further intervention on their part. There is some evidence that patients share this stereotyped view of relief.[33,34] However, in a study by the first writer involving 36 surgical patients, fully one-third attached importance to the relationship between their pain and its psychologic implications. One patient said, "Pain makes you crabby and say things you don't mean." [35]

Fay T. Moss and Burton Meyer [36] reported a clinical experiment in which the nurse succeeded in altering patients' perceptions of the stimuli associated with pain by changing their attitudes toward the stimuli. Meyer, this time in conjunction with B. Caleen Walike,[37] considered the relation among self-strength, dependency, and level of anxiety, and responses to placebo therapy.* They suggested that nurses themselves may produce a placebo effect in their activity and interaction with patients. Wilda G. Chambers and Geraldine G. Price [38] tested the effect of suggestion and distraction on pain relief, but their findings were inconclusive. Karen S. Billars,[39] on the other hand,

found that the suggestion of pain relief when associated with a nursing intervention was a major variable in reducing the pain of the 30 patients she studied. Three interrelated inquiries, involving a total of 96 patients, found that nursing approaches that take into account the "whole" patient, as a feeling, thinking, doing person, are more likely to produce pain relief than approaches that systematically eliminate one or more dimensions. The results can be seen after brief interactions (15 minutes or so), and if medication is given, its effect with nursing is greater than the effect of medication *alone*.[40] All of these clinical experiments point to the nurse as an important therapeutic agent in the alleviation of pain. In the words of one article, the nurse *is* the additive to the analgesic.[41]

There is also considerable agreement on what good nursing care actually includes. In 1962, Dorothy Crowley and associates [42] first spelled out for the nurse three phases in the effective management of pain: (1) assessment of the situation, (2) active intervention, and (3) evaluation of the intervention. Ten years later, Margo McCaffery [43] elaborated on these stages of nursing care in book form and urged nurses to meet the patient's needs through all three time periods—anticipation, the actual experience of pain, and the aftermath.

Assessment. Over the years, assessment has come to mean two things: assessment of what is troubling the patient and evaluation of nurse bias in the assessment of the patient. What is troubling the patient can be determined by asking the patient to describe his or her pain according to (1) location and radiation (cutaneous, visceral, localized); (2) onset (time of day, under unique circumstances, gradual or sudden); (3) severity ("worst ever," interference with sleeping, concentration, eating); (4) duration (seconds, minutes, hours); (5) frequency (interval between attacks); (6) character (burning, gnawing, dull, colicky, knifelike, constant); (7) precipitating factors (certain kinds of food, emotion, unusual exercise, accident); (8) associated symptoms (nausea, fever, syncope); (9) ameliorating or aggravating factors (meals, position, weather); and (10) response to initial treatment efforts (cold, warmth, repositioning, immobilization, distraction). The words patients use to describe their experiences can be of great diagnostic value. For example, causalgic pain is frequently described as burning; the stabbing or cramping quality of visceral pain can provide the key to diagnosis; hemorrhoids are well known to have smarting, itching qualities.[44] Every effort should be made to find out what the person thinks is wrong and what he or she thinks will help. If the patient is a child

---

* *Placebo* refers to a drug that is pharmacologically inert, and is given simply to please the patient. "Placebo effect" is a phrase that has come to mean the psychologic benefit of any medication or procedure given with therapeutic intent, but which is independent of, or minimally related to, the pharmacologic effect of the medication or the specific effect of the procedure. The placebo effect, however, is notoriously short-lived. The beneficial results infrequently last even one week, much less over a month.

or infant, it is important to get an accurate description from the parents of the child's or infant's behavior and what the parents believe is wrong. With unconscious, mentally defective, deaf, or mute persons, assessment of pain is particularly difficult and requires a special study of their behavior.

The Ohio State University study of nurse action in the relief of pain suggested the following as the primary indicants of pain: (1) attention—degree of preoccupation, patient's awareness of environment; (2) anxiety—amount of tension, irritability, and worry seen in daily activities; (3) verbal expression of pain; (4) skeletal muscle response—increase in motor activity and restlessness; (5) respirations—regular or irregular; and (6) perspiration—marked, some, or normal.[45] Pain inhibits gastrointestinal motility; there can be increased oxygen consumption and respiration rate. Muscle tension increases in the area of pain stimulation, accompanied by accelerated blood flow to the muscles of that area. There frequently is marked elevation of both systolic and diastolic pressures, pulse rate, and stroke volume, and increased peripheral vasoconstriction.[46] According to Zborowski,[47] pain responses can be arranged as follows: (1) motor responses (wiggling, twisting); (2) vocal responses (moaning, crying); (3) verbal responses (cursing, complaining); (4) social responses (withdrawal, changes in manners); and (5) the absence of manifest behavior (hiding discomfort, suppressing external signs of pain). Once the nurse perceives what is bothering the patient (for example, he got a "splitting" headache after being told that surgery will have to be postponed), how profoundly it is affecting the person (for instance, he is restless, irritable, sweating all over), and what changes the pain experience itself has produced (elevated blood pressure, added muscle tension), a nursing diagnosis can be made and treatment can be conceptualized.

Nurse Bias. Before nurses actually decide what intervention is indicated, it is always wise to consider whether any bias has limited their ability to assess the patient's needs correctly. There is considerable evidence that a nurse's own age influences how he or she assesses the pain tolerance of patients in various age groups; young nurses rate the pain of the young as more severe, just as older nurses are inclined to believe that patients of their age are more sensitive to pain. Nurses who believe that people should stand some pain before taking a drug tend also to believe that patients tolerate pain well.[48] It is reported that nurses infer greater physical pain when patients are verbal about their discomfort and that there may be a corresponding tendency to give less attention to nonvocal patients. However, nurses are said to infer greater psychologic distress when the patient gives nonverbal clues.[49] Health professionals are inclined to rate the onset stage of the patient's illness as the most painful and psychologically distressing.[50] There is some evidence that inferences of suffering differ according to the cultural background of the nurse, and the patient's socioeconomic background and diagnosis. Puerto Rican nurses, for example, tend to describe the same patient as in much greater distress than American Negro nurses do. Upper class patients are perceived as suffering significantly less than middle or lower class patients. Leukemia patients are automatically assumed to have more pain than diabetic patients.[51] Some judgments are, of course, made on the basis of valid knowledge and clinical experience, but many nurse judgments are conditioned responses that have no basis in fact. Pain is such a serious patient problem that nurses should do everything to avoid being moralistic when they should be open.

Intervention. Pain sufferers seek help in different quarters. Partly because physicians in many countries are in short supply or poorly distributed and partly because medical care in some countries, such as the United States, is very costly, many get advice from persons other than physicians. Some avoid a doctor because they fear an accurate diagnosis that threatens life or freedom or they dread the loss of control over their lives that comes too often with an admission to a hospital. The corner druggist and the chiropractor may be consulted. The first may suggest drugs, the second manipulative therapy. In Eastern countries, and more and more often in the Western world, *acupuncture* operators offer relief through the implantation of fine needles.[52] Though the 1958 discovery that acupuncture could be used to induce sufficient analgesia for major surgery astonished the Western medical world, acupuncture has been used in the treatment of pain for thousands of years in Eastern countries and, while not recognized by organized medicine in the West, has been recognized by some individuals as effective. For instance, Sir William Osler in 1892 said, "For lumbago acupuncture is, in acute cases, the most efficient treatment," and discussing various ways of treating sciatica he says, "acupuncture may also be tried. . . ." * He is specific in stating

* Spoerel, W. E., and Leung, C. Y.: "Acupuncture in a Pain Clinic," *Can. Anaesth. Soc. J.*, **21**:221, (Mar.) 1974; Osler, William: *The Principles and Practice of Medicine.* D. Appleton & Co., New York, 1892, pp. 282, 820.

the area in which the "needles" should be inserted and the length of time they should stay in position. Skepticism about acupuncture persists, and the reader might review an article by James F. Chaves and Theodore X. Barber [52a] reported on in some detail in Chapter 47, "The Preoperative State."

Physical therapy in various forms may be tried; for example, the use of radium or cobalt, and diathermy, massage, exercise, and applications of heat and cold. These modalities have been and still are used by the public to combat pain. In most Western countries, schools of physical therapy and radiology are conducted under the auspices of medical schools, but some practitioners operate independently. Chapters 28, 29, 30, 31, and 42 describe physical therapeutic procedures and discuss the physiologic basis for their use, as, for example, the virtue of cold applications when swelling of an area causes pain and interferes with function. Cold, by decreasing the caliber of blood vessels, reduces pressure causing pain and loss of function; heat, by decreasing muscular contraction that causes pain, can sometimes bring immediate relief. The use of heat and cold for pain is well known to most cultures, and animals instinctively use cold water or the hot sun as therapy. A domestic animal will use a hot stove indoors for the same purpose.

Not infrequently, people consult a nurse they happen to know, or a district or visiting nurse, or a family health practitioner. The role of the nurse in health assessment and diagnosis of disease is discussed in Chapter 5. The point was made there and earlier in this chapter that pain is *a serious symptom.* Acute abdominal pain may be caused by the violent contraction of the intestine in response to excessive gas formation, or it may indicate an obstructed area that will rupture without surgical intervention; head pain may be caused by a temporary dilation of cranial vessels or the presence of a tumor that must be excised. As the role of nurses "expands," they must assume increasing responsibility for giving advice on pain and for using therapeutic measures. Nurses in schools, in industries, in homes, and in many health services without resident physicians operate under so-called standing orders of medical consultants or physicians employed by the services. These include the administration of mild analgesics for pain. Effective use of such blanket prescription has always carried with it a grave responsibility. The difficulty and importance of developing clinical judgment and making an accurate assessment of the patient's problems and need for help are discussed in Chapters 5 and 8, but it might be re-peated here with reference to pain. Acute, and particularly persistent, pain must never be taken lightly.

Certain methods of relieving or controlling pain are strictly within the physician's domain. Some examples are surgical removal of a growth, surgical interruption of a specific nerve pathway, numbing nervous tissue with an alcohol block, or the implantation of electronic devices to "short-circuit" pain.[53,54] If the patient accepts the physician's advice (or the parents accept the advice for their child), the nurse's responsibility is confined to explaining the rationale behind the procedure to the patient and, after the treatment, evaluating whether the transmission of pain signals has actually been interrupted. In many situations, however, methods of pain control, even in hospitals where physicians are in attendance, are used at the nurse's discretion (e.g., PRN analgesics, PRN warm compresses, PRN ice bags) or perhaps not used unless the nurse initiates them. Nurses have traditionally underestimated the repertoire of treatment possibilities that they have under their command, but they are considerable. To begin with, the nurse should give serious thought to Thomas Aquinas's advice that pain can be "assuaged by pleasure, tears, sympathy of friends, contemplating the truth, sleep and baths." *

When Aquinas mentioned *pleasure,* he was reflecting the thinking of his period in which pain was seen simply as the opposite of pleasure. While complex physiologic and psychologic theories have made us wary of talking about "giving" a patient pleasure, it still makes sense to *fight one sensation with another one.* In fact, many interventions are based on this principle. Since pain tolerance increases with attention to another task, providing other sensory input is one method of pain control.† Auditory stimulation, together with strong suggestion that it abolishes pain, provides an effective stratagem for achieving "control" over pain if the pain does not rise suddenly and sharply.[55] Concentration on the competing sensory stimulation provided by loud stereophonic music has enabled countless dental patients to handle drilling better. Burned patients have profited by listening to "white noise" which has the scratching sound of amplified static, through headphones during dressing changes; irritating the ears with un-

---

* Merskey, H., and Spear, F. G.: *Pain—Psychological and Psychiatric Aspects.* Bailliere, Tindall & Cassell, London, 1967, p. 5.

† It is a commonplace in theatrical circles that actors can be in great pain before and after a performance but unconscious of it while they are on the stage.

pleasant sounds diverts the person from what is hurting his skin. Reading murder mysteries, watching television, crocheting, or concentrating on crossword puzzles can be of some assistance in helping patients cope more effectively with slowly fluctuating postsurgical pain. Screaming, humming, biting the lips, pinching the ear lobes, squeezing the hand hard—all help. The more a patient's other senses are involved—vision, hearing, touch—the more effective relief may be.

Distraction is not a stratagem that should be discounted as too trivial to be of consequence. Everyone has had some firsthand experience with feeling miserable in the morning and not noticing the discomfort nearly as much once at work. This does not mean that the original pain was "in the head." It means that one cannot give complete attention to pain and think about something else at the same time. The woman in labor who focuses her attention on a "concentration point" cannot by definition give her "whole" attention to the pain. The boy who wiggles his toes during an ear examination is distracted from the discomfort of metal touching his ear. The woman who is encouraged to describe in detail what she did on her last vacation cannot feel the pain of suture removal as much as she would if she had nothing else to do but look at the wound as the stitches come out.

Breathing exercises developed in the Lamaze method of preparation for childbirth—slow chest breathing, panting, and blowing—can be applied to a number of other clinical situations. Not only do these exercises distract the patient, but also they are ways of counteracting pain with relaxation. Asking patients to describe wall hangings, their children, or past happy times can help them through unpleasant situations even if they get angry with the nurse for asking them a question that seems trivial at such a moment. It is important to remember that even anger is a way of handling pain. Once the pain has passed, nurses who use this technique can explain their intent and encourage patients to help themselves by using the same device. In fact, the "pleasure" of being able to help oneself may be the greatest of all!

Two other treatment concepts are related to distraction. *Waking-imagined analgesia* is the name given to trying deliberately to imagine something pleasant in the place of something unpleasant. Patients have reported tolerating the first stage of labor or myelograms by imagining sexual intercourse. Pretending that a blinding headache was due to someone they loved pressing his or her fingers on the scalp has helped other patients.[56] Patients have experienced less discomfort when encouraged to substitute one sensation for another one in their minds; imagining numbness, coolness, or pressure is preferable to thinking of pain. *Desensitization,* using the principles of behavior therapy, can also help. If potentially frightening equipment is shown to the patient when relaxed, a future painful procedure employing that equipment may prove to be less uncomfortable than it might have otherwise been. Prepared childbirth classes teach the husband to simulate a contraction by squeezing the wife's arm or leg in increasing then decreasing intensity as a preparation for the actual experience. Discomfort that people are trained to handle is clearly easier to deal with than that which catches them off guard.

Distraction, waking-imagined analgesia, and desensitization are nursing techniques that can be invaluable adjuncts to therapy, but they will not work if the nurse does not have confidence in them. Patients rely on the nurse for new ideas about how to handle problems. Just giving the patient new ideas is as much of a treatment as the notion itself may be. Nurses need not feel like charlatans when they offer suggestion instead of a sedative; these techniques are based on solid behavioral concepts. It is important to remember that the most potent drugs are in part placebos because their effectiveness also is enhanced by the expectation of relief.

On the surface, *encouraging tears and giving sympathy* do not seem like especially rigorous nursing interventions. Yet a nurse-patient who was hospitalized for months echoed similar needs when she listed the things that helped her most.

1. The people who showed me they cared.
2. The people who took the time to listen.
3. A very good, interested, and caring physician.
4. Being able to have family and friends near when I felt I needed them.[57]

Access to family support, concerned friends, and caring professionals—these are essential to patients and of paramount importance in the care of the chronically ill, since anxiety and depression are a feature of all pain experiences.

When people hurt, they feel hurt. Patients who can communicate their feelings to an understanding nurse will experience relief on a number of levels. The release of tension is considerable that crying, cursing, or just describing how they feel produces. Patients may understand their own feelings better once they are said out loud, and voicing concerns may lead to solving the inherent problems. For example, talking about financial worries may lead to new information about how to deal with them; saying that they are scared that the pain will drive them crazy may make people appreciate how self-possessed they really are.

Nurses act more effectively if they are sensitive to the factors contributing to anxiety and depression in patients with pain. Some of these are fear of the unknown, a sense of estrangement from family and friends, loneliness, fear of losing control over their behavior, being reminded that death is inevitable, fear of becoming so quarrelsome that they cease to be lovable, fear of losing their cherished independence, and ambivalence toward physical dependence. One way in which these issues can be worked out is by sharing an observation on "how this might make you feel" and then asking the patient for validation of the perception. For example, "I would imagine getting used to a colostomy bag is sometimes harder on you than the pain you had following the operation itself. Is it?" or "Do you sometimes find that just lying in bed is more painful than the pain itself?" or "Do you feel that your worries about the pain are actually worse than the pain itself?" or "It must be awfully hard on you having all those tubes in you; there's the pain around the stitches but the tubes themselves must be a pain. Ever feel that way?" Comments like these often lead patients to elaborate on how they are feeling and can have a therapeutic effect in their own right because they reaffirm the important fact that there are times when it is reasonable to be troubled by negative feelings.[58]

The therapeutic aspects of the nurse-patient relationship can be enhanced if the nurse conveys the notion that "I know this is hard on you, but you're handling it well." Such an attitude helps patients feel that they are coping individuals. Taking into account the patient's expectations is also important to the nurse-patient relationship. If a nurse senses that a patient is more concerned about the future implications of pain rather than about his or her present experience, their conversation will differ from that of the patient who wants *immediate* relief and cares about nothing else. Patients may think that if nothing is being done for the pain, then nothing can be done. How patients report their experience can be revealing. The choice of language may indicate how disassociated the patient has become from the pain, as, for example, *"the* stomach hurts." Not all patients can communicate their distress verbally (children may use dolls to act out their feelings), and not all patients feel appreciably better after letting emotions show, but offering to be of help can help. The very process of asking patients to describe their problems, sharing your own observations, and finding out what the patient thinks will help is usually comforting.

Contemplating the truth may not literally "set you free," but knowing what kind of pain to expect and how discomfort can be relieved can free patients to the point where anxiety is minimal and they are better able to tolerate the pain. Kathryn M. Healy's [59] preoperative-instruction study of 321 patients is evidence that teaching patients about pain can result in their needing fewer narcotics in general and fewer parenteral narcotics in particular. In this study, pain was referred to as discomfort or ache so the suggestion of an intolerable sensation would be avoided. Patients were taught exercises to avoid "gas pains" and aching legs; they were shown how to move so as to avoid sudden pain. However, Healy assumed the desirability of analgesia in the immediate postoperative period on the grounds that patients require the euphoria of medication to facilitate ease of movement. Being able to move without undue discomfort has the added benefit of proving to patients that they are improving—a perception that has its own curative value. In the Healy study, analgesia was given late in the evening whenever possible so patients could avoid a long restless night and could greet the morning refreshed.

Though the nurse should be sensitive to the fact that information can be anxiety producing when too much is given for the patient to absorb or when it is given so far ahead of time that it makes the period of anticipation seem interminable, it is important to consider asking each patient, "Do you think that you would feel better if you knew more about what is causing the pain?" In answering this question, a truck driver who was labeled "difficult" because he kept complaining of pain showed that he was confused about the nature of his scheduled surgery. He said his surgeon always seemed to be in a hurry when the patient thought of asking for an explanation, and the patient was embarrassed to confront the doctor with his questions because he did not know the "right words." With help from the nurse, three questions were formulated, written, and taped to the patient's i.v. pole. The following day, the patient read these three questions to the doctor, got his answers, and felt considerably more relaxed.[60]

Knowing that fluorides ease bone pain because fluoride binds with calcium and thickens bone structure can make a patient more willing, and even eager, to take prescribed fluoride preparations.[61] Once therapy is understood, patients may actually notice less pain with each dose because they have the satisfaction of actually doing something to hasten recovery. Some of the information a patient needs may be so obvious that it goes unnoticed. Much of the pain around a surgical incision is due to spasm of muscles that have been cut, yet patients are frequently unprepared to understand, and therefore tolerate, this common problem. If nurses deliberately remind patients that pain is a part of the "normal" healing process, they may have a completely different attitude from the one they have if left alone to ponder the horrors that lurk behind a bulky, oozing dressing. And if nurses assure patients that these traumatized muscles can be relaxed by applying moist heat (by use of the Hydrocollator Steam Pack, for example), they enhance their comfort considerably.[62] General discussion of pain is often most effective in small groups where common concerns can be shared in such a way as to underline how normal are both the anxious feelings and the physical experiences.

Though the importance of *sleep and relaxation* is discussed at length in Chapters 13 and 17, their relations to pain should be emphasized here. Interference with both is probably the highest toll exacted by pain, for a lack of sleep increases muscular tension and makes pain less tolerable. All comfort measures, especially those that involve touch, can be effective in countering pain or inducing relaxation and finally sleep.[63] Since pain increases muscle tension, there are sound physiologic reasons why nurses respond to pain with the offer of a back rub. Even if the patient cannot be turned over, the back of the neck and temples can be massaged and this can be effective because muscle tension is so often felt there. With increasing evidence that pain can be controlled by the stimulation of large afferent fibers, hydrotherapy and massage take on a renewed therapeutic importance. The "cures" attributed to the hydrotherapeutic measures of Roman baths and Victorian spas can be explained on a physiologic as well as a psychologic basis.

A number of nursing interventions result from the principle of decreasing noxious stimuli. Some examples are splinting an incised area to avoid strain; lying flat to correct cerebrospinal fluid imbalance and headache from this cause; drinking milk to soothe a stomach ulcer; repositioning to take pressure off a sensitive area; applying an ice compress to minimize edema following trauma; massaging to increase blood flow and improve muscle tone; applying heat to induce vasodilation, remove waste products, and improve nutrition; filtering the air to relieve the labored breathing of an asthmatic patient.

Thomas Aquinas's list of treatments may have omitted mention of *drugs,* but few modern nurses can ignore their widespread use. As everyone knows, physicians prescribe drugs to control pain, and nonprescription drugs are used by many persons at their own discretion for this purpose. There is something very appealing (even magical) about taking a pill or getting an injection and having all of one's miseries disappear for a few hours, but it takes considerable skill to make sure patients receive the right medication, in the correct amounts, at proper intervals, for no longer than they need it. In Chapter 21 the illegal use of prescription drugs is discussed and the whole question of drug dependency treated briefly. It is impossible to say how many persons habitually misusing drugs can trace the formation of their habit to an illness when dependence on hypnotics, analgesics, and narcotics was sanctioned, but physicians, nurses, and students of the drug problem are aware that this can happen.

Drug dependency is one of the major concerns of this age in many countries. National, state (or provincial), and local commissions have been set up to study the problem and it is so complex that a general text of this sort can only deal with it superficially. However, to discuss pain without reference to drug abuse and drug addiction suggests that they are unrelated. Few would question a relationship.

Analgesics, hypnotics, and narcotics are used to escape from pain, fear, anxiety, stress, tension, sleeplessness, or simply dissatisfaction with things-as-they-are (reality).* It is also believed that healthy and relatively contented persons who take drugs because their associates are doing it can become habitués after a few experiences if they find the removal of inhibitions or the sensations they have after taking the drug are exciting or pleasant. It is also easy for health workers to create the impression that a drug is the first line of defense against pain, anxiety, sleeplessness, and even just reality.

In some hospitals, almost any patient can get a hypnotic or an analgesic by asking for it and there are few health services in schools and industries that deny a request for aspirin or a comparable "non-habit-forming" drug. Most hospitals, regardless of those they serve, have nurses on active duty at night. In Chapter 13, "Rest and Sleep," attention is called to studies made at the Cassel Hospital (for neurotics) in London which convinced its staff that the Hospital's climate was creating unnecessary

* Helen H. Nowlis, director of the National Association of Student Personnel Administrators' Drug Education Project, under contract with the US Food and Drug Administration, in 1968 observed that "Man has used drugs throughout the ages to escape from discomfort and misery but it is interesting to note that in our society [which she calls a "pill society"] misery is a condition familiar not only to the socially and economically depressed but also to those in the very midst of 'success.' " She says, "the real problem is not drugs but people who use drugs." She thinks the principal task in stopping drug abuse is education. (Nowlis, Helen H.: "Why Students Use Drugs," *Am. J. Nurs.,* **68:**1680, [Aug.] 1968.)

dependence on drugs. The conclusion was reached that the night nurse on the clinical unit was unnecessary if one could sleep on the service and be "on call" (an "orderly" is on duty at night). After this change, lights were put out at bedtime and patients tended to sleep all night as most families do. The use of drugs was greatly reduced when a study showed that analgesics and hypnotics were often given because nurses—rather than the patients themselves—could no longer tolerate the patient's anxiety or agitation.[64] There is little doubt that physicians prescribe and nurses give drugs for pain or sleeplessness when they cannot think of any other way to help patients, or when, for one reason or another, they are unable or unwilling to make the effort to take a more individualized approach.

Any discussion of the use of drugs must avoid overemphasizing their efficacy because addiction to pain medications (in the form of either a physical need or just a distorted confidence in what they can do) is such a serious problem, but also must avoid being excessively moralistic about how abstemious drug usage should be because withholding needed medication can further increase patients' anxieties. What is necessary is an over-all care plan, worked out between the physician and nurse, which meets the patient's present needs and simultaneously avoids long-term complications. The specifics of such a plan will be determined by many factors, especially by whether the cause of the pain can be eliminated by treatment.

The use made of drugs for the relief of pain can be one thing for the person whose condition can be relieved by treatment; it can be another for patients with cancer, for example, in its terminal stages. In Chapter 50 the conclusions reached by Cicely Saunders (nurse, social worker, and physician) on control of pain by drugs in terminal illness are discussed. She has made a long study of the subject and is able to relieve patients of the *fear of pain* by giving enough narcotic at regular time intervals to control pain, by changing the drugs used if a tolerance is developed, and by adjusting dosage to the demands of each person.* Saunders questions the wisdom of PRN prescriptions when dealing with chronic pain. She thinks that if patients have to convince the persons caring for them—and controlling the drugs—that their pain is severe enough to warrant "a shot" they are likely to develop a craving for drugs. When analgesics are given routinely to prevent pain from occurring (rather than to control it when it is already present), patients become much less dependent on the staff and on drugs, and may even forget about the pain. Pain should be kept constantly in remission because pain itself is the strongest antagonist to successful analgesia.

Overmedication is what is to be avoided at all costs. Rational patients or guardians of those who are not should know the nature of the drugs, their therapeutic action, and their harmful as well as their helpful effects. Drugs may elevate the pain threshold, interrupt the transmission of pain impulses, modify the central perception of pain, or alter the reaction to the sensation, but even the most potent medication should not be viewed as *the* treatment for the relief of pain. Some drugs are very effective with specific kinds of pain (e.g., ergotamine for migraine headaches, colchicine for the pain of gout, Pyridium for urinary tract discomfort). Some drugs relieve a variety of types of pain, for example codeine, morphine, aspirin. (Table 49-1 shows types of drugs for the control of pain and their actions.) Pain cannot automatically be assumed to be due to the patient's primary disease process, so an accurate diagnosis should precede selection of a drug. For example, pain due to constipation may call for an enema, just as the pain accompanying dyspnea may call for bronchodilators and steroids, rather than narcotics. Tranquilizers often prove more effective in the treatment of chronic pain than opiates because depression may need treating even more than the physical sensation does.* (However, different persons respond in different ways to tranquilizers.) While chemotherapy is an essential element in modern nursing care, the nurse has to guard against succumbing to the stereotyped thinking that television commercials perpetuate. Few, if any, drugs can offer the patient "complete" relief, if for no other reason than that it is impossible to maintain a "steady" amount of medication in the patient's system unless the drug is given intravenously. Since the patient will be making "optimal" use of the drug for about 1 hour out of every 4 hours (when medication is given

---

* A film, "Paula," made in St. Christopher's Hospice in London, shows a physician interviewing a 38-year-old woman who died 6 weeks later. Although cancer has invaded many organs of her body and both fractured legs are in traction, Paula is alert, talks freely about her experience, and shows that she is able to enjoy her life in the Hospice. She says that here for the first time in several years her pain is controlled with drugs that don't make her "feel dopey." Paula feels that the important thing is that she is given her drugs regularly every 4 hours without having actually to request relief.

* A heavy reliance on alcoholic beverages may also develop with the chronically ill. Alcohol may be used to try to forget a poor prognosis (real or imagined), and nurses should be alert to the possibility that a drinking problem may have started as a defense against real physical pain.

Table 49-1.   A Comparison of Narcotic Analgesics with Respect to Dosage and Duration of Action *†

Nonproprietary Name	Trade Name	Dose (mg)	Duration of Action (hr)
Morphine		10	4 to 5
Heroin (diacetylmorphine)		3 (2 to 8)	3 to 4
Hydromorphone (dihydromorphinone)	Dilaudid, etc.	1.5	4 to 5
Oxymorphone (dihydrohydroxymor-phine)	Numorphan	1.0 to 1.5	4 to 5
Metopon (methydihydromorphinone)	Metopon	3.5	4 to 5
Codeine		120 (8 to 20)	(4 to 6)
Hydrocodone (dihydrocodeinone)	Hycodan, etc.	(5 to 10)	(4 to 8)
Dihydrocodeine	Paracodin	60	4 to 5
Oxycodone (dihydrohydroxycodeinone)	Percodan	10 to 15	4 to 5
		(3 to 5)	(4 to 5)
Pholcodine (β-morpholinylethyl-morphine)		(10 to 15)	(4 to 5)
Levorphanol	Levo-Dromoran	2 to 3	4 to 5
Phenazocine ‡	Prinadol	3	4 to 5
Methadone ‡	Dolophine, etc.	7.5 to 10	3 to 5
Dextromoramide ‡	Palfium	5 to 7.5	4 to 5
Dipipanone ‡§	Pipadone	20 to 25	4 to 5
Phenadoxone §	Heptalgin, etc.	10 to 20	1 to 3
Meperidine	Demerol, etc.	80 to 100	2 to 4
Alphaprodine	Nisentil	40 to 60	1 to 2
Anileridine	Leritine	30 to 40	2 to 3
Piminodine	Alvodine	7.5 to 10	2 to 4

* Based on table from *The Pharmacological Basis of Therapeutics,* 5th ed., by Louis S. Goodman and Alfred Gilman, Macmillan Publishing Co., Inc., New York, 1975, p. 256.
† Dose shown is the amount given *subcutaneously* that produces approximately the same analgesic effects as 10 mg of morphine administered subcutaneously. The figures in *parentheses* are the *doses* and the *duration* of action for oral, antitussive doses; they are not necessarily equieffective doses. *Duration of action* shown is for *subcutaneous* administration; after *intravenous* administration, peak effects are somewhat more pronounced but overall effects are of shorter duration.
‡ May exhibit cumulative effects on repeated dosage.
§ Marked irritation at injection sites.

every 4 hours), the nurse must learn not to develop an excessive reliance on chemotherapy. Nurses have to be familiar with the properties of specific drugs so they can know what relief can *reasonably* be anticipated.

It is important to bear in mind that the analgesic given at 10 A.M. can bring some immediate relief because the patient is getting attention. Confidence in the eventual effectiveness of the drug can prompt the patient to take a shower and put on fresh makeup. Feeling refreshed, the patient may decide to write some letters which provide her with a sense of accomplishment, just as walking to the shower unassisted did an hour before. This same patient may decide to take a nap after lunch because she feels relaxed and may awaken at 3 P.M. still feeling better than she did at 10 A.M. Was it the medication that kept her comfortable, or the cumulative effect of chemotherapy, expectation, distraction, warm water, and sleep?

Finally, Thomas Aquinas's list of treatments made no mention of *electric pain control,* but that is a form of intervention fast gaining popularity, though the method is still in the experimental stage. In Chapter 31 there is a section on bioelectric medicine in which the use of electricity for the control of pain is mentioned as one of the oldest therapeutic agents, while in modern "Western medicine" it is one of the newest therapeutic agents.

Acupuncture, an ancient art of Oriental medicine used to relieve or prevent pain, is now practiced on every continent. While we have not found a completely satisfactory explanation of its action, it is generally conceded that the needles, inserted at key points along the body's electric field, jam the pain signals traveling along the nerve pathways before they reach the brain. Neurologists and neurosurgeons have come to recognize it as one form of electric pain control.*

* Albert W. Cook and Stanley P. Weinstein have reported ". . . significant modification of abnormal neurological signs and dysfunction in patients with

The following statement is taken from a 1974 editorial on electric pain control:

For centuries medicine has searched for an innocuous, nondestructive way of relieving pain that's both efficient and practical—and all it's come up with are drugs, with their inevitable side effects, and neurosurgical destruction, with its associated morbidity and mortality. The ability to knock out pain at will without knocking out its victim would be one of the greatest boons ever accorded mankind.

Electrical neural stimulation may give us that ability, say three neurosurgeons: Dr. C. Norman Shealy, director of the Pain Rehabilitation Center at St. Francis Hospital in LaCrosse, Wis., who has devoted the past seven years to investigating the association of electrical stimulation and the control of pain and who was responsible for the original development of an electronic device to test that association; and Drs. Charles V. Burton, associate professor of neurosurgery at Philadelphia's Temple University Health Sciences Center, and Donlin M. Long, professor and chairman of neurosurgery at Johns Hopkins Hospital, both of whom have worked extensively with the device since it first became generally available two years ago. All three agree that the process involved may very well turn out to be a major medical milestone.*

Shealy and his associates have numerous reports of their work, a few of which are included in the references for this chapter.[65-68] Discussing the "pain patient," Shealy makes the following summary statement:

Destructive procedures, cordotomy, posterior root section and cingulumotomy are primarily useful in cancer pain. In the disk syndrome, rhizotomy of the articular nerve of the spinal facets relieves pain in most patients. Electrical stimulation, either transcutaneous or of the dorsal columns, is the procedure of choice in benign pain and in unilateral cancer pain for which no other procedure is satisfactory. When no surgical procedure seems practical, operant conditioning will allow the patient to reach his maximum potential.†

Shealy discusses the erosive effects of pain, the excessive amounts of money spent by patients seeking relief,‡ the hostility of some physicians who, he says, "look upon the pain patient as they do the alcoholic." Shealy says,

"The average pain patient *can* be rehabilitated without mind-shattering drugs and crippling or destructive surgery." * Mentioning, or discussing briefly, the uses of rest, corrective exercises, x-ray therapy, metabolic poisons, narcotics, cold and hot applications, massage, nerve blocks, severance of nerves, destruction of nerve roots with a radiofrequency needle, and bone surgery to relieve pressure on a nerve, Shealy describes dorsal column stimulation in some detail. He shows a silicone-rubber electrode that was inserted and sutured between the dura and the arachnoid in the spinal column and the external transmitter and antenna for the dorsal column stimulator.†

For some conditions, Shealy says transcutaneous electric stimulation (TNS) is the most useful technique. This consists of applying two electrodes to the appropriate skin area and teaching the patient how to operate a battery-powered stimulator to which the electrodes are attached.

Walter Indeck, a physician and Andrea Printy, a nurse, report the results of using transcutaneous electric stimulation for the relief of pain in chronic orthopedic conditions. Forty persons were admitted to "a pain ward"; 50 were treated in an outpatient setting. Electrodes were placed on either side of the vertebral column and the stimulator attached to the top of the trousers for an ambulatory patient. Skin irritation from the electrodes is said by Indeck and Printy to be reduced by using a carbonized rubber electrode applied with a tincture of benzoin interface.[69]

D. M. Long in 1973 reported the results of using electric stimulation to treat ten patients for pain caused by nerve injury. He concluded that "While the technique appears to be quite promising, at the present time it should be reserved for patients not satisfactorily treated by other means. Prolonged or continued patient evaluations over many years will be required before widespread clinical use can be recommended." ‡

In 1974, P. W. Nathan and P. D. Wall reported treating postherpetic neuralgia in 30 patients with the following results:

The results of treating patients with severe post-herpetic neuralgia with prolonged self-administered electric stimulation from a portable apparatus were good in 11 out of 30 patients. None of these patients had had as good relief of pain

MS," [multiple sclerosis] following "chronic dorsal column stimulation with a neuropacemaker." They say this is also effective for relief of pain. ("Chronic Dorsal Column Stimulation in Multiple Sclerosis," *NY State J. Med.*, **73**:2868, (Dec. 15) 1973, and personal communication.)

* "A New Approach to Pain," *Emergency Med.*, (Mar.) 1974.

† Shealy, C. Norman: "The Pain Patient," *Am. Fam. Physician*, **9**:131, (Mar.) 1974.

‡ He cites one patient who reported that the cost to his insurance carrier was $450,000.

* Shealy, C. Norman: *op. cit.*

† Instruments used for electric pain control are being improved so rapidly that it seems inappropriate to show a photograph of this device.

‡ Long, D. M.: "Electrical Stimulation for Relief of Pain from Chronic Nerve Injury," *J. Neurosurg.*, **39**:718, (Dec.) 1973.

with other forms of treatment. In 10 patients some effects from stimulation continued after stimulation stopped. In eight there was an improvement in the course of the neuralgia, and in two there was a cure.*

Since "all forms of therapy" were said to have failed for these patients, the effect of electric stimulation in this instance is striking.

In Chapter 48, the control of pain after surgery is discussed and attention drawn to the reports by Alan C. Hymes and his associates in 1973 and 1974 on the use of transcutaneous electric stimulation for the control of pain and the treatment and prevention of ileus (a non-functioning bowel) and atelectasis (imperfect expansion of the lungs). Compared with controls, the results with 213 patients were impressive. Hymes et al. observed in the study reported in 1973 that

. . . the incidence of atelectasis and ileus were strikingly reduced . . . the length of stay in the ICU was significantly reduced . . . the majority [of patients] reported a subjective reduction [in pain] of 60% to 80%.†

The studies cited and others listed in the references for this chapter indicate a growing confidence in the control of pain with electricity.[70-76] In 1974, Long noted its relative effectiveness in a variety of conditions and the fact that its only serious disadvantage is the skin irritation which remains a problem. He makes the following comment on the nurse's major role in the use of the stimulator:

The use of the device is primarily managed by a nurse well trained in dealing with pain patients and skilled in the use and theory of the instrument. A clinic has been established where these patients can come both for initial evaluation and instruction in the use of external electrical stimulation and for continued help with the resolution of their long term management. It is not necessary for a physician to be involved in this phase of the patient's care except on a consultative basis and the majority of the difficulties can be solved by a combination of expert nursing care and the availability of technical assistance with the stimulator.‡

Hypnosis for pain is gradually being accepted by Western physicians. Harold B. Crasilneck, a clinical psychologist, and James A.

Hall, a psychiatrist, review the history, the theories, and techniques of hypnosis in a 1975 publication. They discuss its use in surgery, in the treatment of psychosomatic illness, and in almost every clinical setting. In the chapter on hypnosis for the control of pain, studies over the past thirty years are cited. They conclude with the summary statement:

Management of pain problems remains one of the first and most enduring uses of hypnosis. It should be used with care by persons aware of the diagnostic and treatment problems of organic illness. In proper perspective hypnosis can alleviate much otherwise unapproachable pain and can help maintain the functional ability and dignity of many patients otherwise dependent on large quantities of medication.*

Laurel Archer Copp gives the following summary of patients' responses when asked what nurses and doctors could do about pain:

"Slow down, don't hurry so, you can't hurry pain."
"What is more important than talking to patients about pain?"
"Be prompt. Try to understand. Make more of an effort."
"Stop telling people they don't have pain when they actually do. Don't try to feel for people when you can't know if they hurt or not."
"Don't make judgments when you don't know and haven't hurt."
"Don't ignore patients in pain and give them the brushoff—we aren't a bunch of neurotics."
"Have confidence you can help the pain—if you had more confidence we would, too."
"Be realistic about pain. Don't be too casual or flip."
"Don't assume the shot or pill helps."
"If you had hurt just once, you wouldn't hand out this 'it won't hurt a bit' routine."
"I'd like one doctor and one nurse each shift. There isn't enough energy to describe the pain over and over again."
"See patients as individuals and not textbook pictures."
"Don't be callous. You treat patients like a garage repairman but we aren't automobiles."
"Prescribe fewer pain pills and shots and get down to the cause." †

Evaluation of Effectiveness. Once the patient's needs have been assessed, the intervention has been determined with the patient's involvement, and the treatment has been carried out, its effectiveness should be evaluated. The physiologic manifestations, what the patient says, and the behavior which originally made the nurse believe that the patient was in pain should have changed by the conclusion of the nursing treatment. If the patient looks

---

* Nathan, P. W., and Wall, P. D.: "Treatment of Post-Herpetic Neuralgia by Prolonged Electric Stimulation," *Br. Med. J.,* **3:**645, (Sept. 14) 1974.

† Hymes, Alan C., et al.: "Electrical Surface Stimulation for Control of Acute Postoperative Pain and Prevention of Ileus," *Surg. Forum,* Vol. 24, Fifty-ninth Annual Clinical Congress, 1973, p. 447.

‡ Long, D. M.: "External Electrical Stimulation as a Treatment of Chronic Pain," *Minn. Med.,* **57:**195, (Mar.) 1974.

* Crasilneck, Harold B., and Hall, James A.: *Clinical Hypnosis: Principles and Applications.* Grune & Stratton, New York, 1975, p. 78.

† Copp, Laurel Archer: "The Spectrum of Suffering," *Am. J. Nurs.,* **74:**491, (Mar.) 1974.

more comfortable * and verbally corroborates this, nursing care has been successful. If the patient's pain is unchanged or if the patient is in less distress but clearly would like something else to be done, the nurse should reassess the patient's needs and try other interventions. The patient might be asked, "Can you think of anything else that we might try to make you even more comfortable?"

In evaluating effectiveness, the nurse should consider whether the goal for the individual is comfort, relief from pain, or both. Patients can feel more comfortable without experiencing total relief from pain; patients can feel less pain and still not feel comfortable. There is some evidence that pain relief with no increase in comfort is less acceptable to the patient than comfort without relief from pain.[77] Patients sometimes describe themselves as "feeling so much better; even though the pain is still there, it doesn't bother me so much." This distinction should not surprise nurses if they remember that pain is part physical sensation and part emotional reaction. Often a person can handle noxious stimuli once his or her anxiety is under control.

Degree of effectiveness is, of course, related to the severity of pain prior to intervention. Mild or moderate pain can be relieved more absolutely than severe or chronic pain, because the latter is inevitably colored by strong reactions to the experience. Curative treatment is one thing; palliative treatment is another. Chest pain due to infection can be eradicated by antibiotics. The pain caused by cancer will not go away completely so long as the malignant growth remains the same size or increases in size. Effectiveness is also tempered by the importance pain has assumed in the individual's way of living; some patients cannot give up their pain because it has come to have a certain positive value in their lives, even though such ambivalent feelings are usually unconscious. Finally, effectiveness is contingent on the state of the science and art of therapy; some pain cannot be alleviated until more is known about what causes it.

4. PREVENTION

One element of nursing care that deserves special attention is prevention. Implicit in all the references to teaching the patient about pain, changing the patient's response to unpleasant stimuli from passive acceptance of care given by others to active involvement in treatment, and extending the patient's repertoire of pain-relief methods is the important notion that some pain can be avoided. Those who have angina can limit tightness in the chest by learning to use nitroglycerin and avoiding overexertion; women prone to cystitis can be shown how to avoid infection from germ-carrying tampon strings; persons subject to gas pains may prevent some by lying on their stomachs; those who suffer from gallbladder attacks can be shown how to restrict their intake of fatty foods, just as those with gastric ulcers can learn to shun spicy dishes and those with diverticulitis to give up nuts and corn if they want to avoid attacks of pain. After one bout with pain, a patient may be ready to learn how to handle the next experience better; a woman may be very receptive to the idea of learning breathing exercises and relaxation techniques during her second pregnancy because she knows what to expect from the pain of labor.

Assessing Attitudes about Pain. Nurses should consider assessing a patient's attitudes toward pain and using such information in helping the patient prepare for pain. Ada Jacox, a nurse at the University of Iowa who is studying pain, suggests that if patients were asked to state whether they agreed or disagreed with statements such as the following, the nurse would have a definite impression of the patient's expectations on which to base care:

1. If you ignore most pains they will soon go away.
2. It helps to discuss your pain with others.
3. If something painful is going to happen to me, I would like to know ahead of time.
4. Patients should be permitted to take an active part in deciding how to care for their own pain.
5. Most nurses expect patients to stand too much pain.
6. When a patient in the hospital, I would prefer to call for the nurse myself if I need something for pain, rather than wait to be asked.
7. It is a sign of weakness for a person to admit to having pain.
8. I like to have someone with me when I am in pain.
9. We are punished for our wrongdoing by being made to suffer pain.
10. Most nurses don't like it if patients complain of pain too often.
11. When I am in pain, I prefer to be alone.
12. It doesn't help to talk with others about your pain.
13. When I am in pain, it helps to keep busy.

---

* There is some danger in equating the sleeping patient with the comfortable patient. Some patients feign sleep so nurses will leave them alone. All too often a narcotic may induce drowsiness yet not provide the REM sleep (so called because rapid eye movements accompany these periods of dreaming) that is considered to be most refreshing.

14. People should stand some pain before they take pain medicine.
15. When I am in pain, I don't want to know why it hurts, I just want the pain to go away as soon as possible.*

While these statements might not be the ones every nurse practitioner would want to use with patients, some knowledge of the patient's personal beliefs is necessary for planning long-range care.

Pain is not usually an isolated happening; it is a problem most persons face from time to time throughout their lives. Developing a profile of each patient's expectations and past experiences is a logical step toward developing strategies for meeting therapeutic needs. If nurses assess feelings about pain before pain becomes a reality for the patient beginning therapy, it has the added benefit of showing nurse concern right from the start. Such information could also be used in helping the patient deal with the aftermath of pain. When nurses are aware of patients' attitudes toward pain as a life experience, they can help resolve misgivings that surface when patients feel that they did not handle the experience well. Handling the experience of pain well is important to most people because it is an inevitable part of living and one that is considered by many a test of character.

REFERENCES

1. Behan, Richard: *Pain.* Appleton-Century-Crofts, New York, 1920, p. 19.
2. Engel, George L.: "Pain," in MacBryde, C. M., and Blacklow, R. S. (eds.): *Signs and Symptoms,* 5th ed. J. B. Lippincott Co., Philadelphia, 1970, p. 50.
3. Hardy, J. D., et al.: *Pain Sensations and Reactions.* Williams & Wilkins Co., Baltimore, 1952, p. 24.
4. Szasz, Thomas: *Pain and Pleasure.* Tavistock Publications, Ltd., London, 1957, p. 103.
5. Melzack, Ronald, and Wall, Patrick D.: "Pain Mechanisms: A New Theory," *Science,* **150:**971, (Nov.) 1965.
6. *Ibid.*
7. Engel, George L.: *op. cit.,* p. 52.
8. McCaffery, Margo: *Nursing Management of the Patient with Pain.* J. B. Lippincott Co., Philadelphia, 1972, p. 40.
9. Murray, John B.: "Psychology of the Pain Experience," *J. Psychol.,* **78:**193, (July) 1971.
10. Melzack, Ronald, and Wall, Patrick D.: *op. cit.*
11. Egbert, Lawrence D., et al.: "Reduction of Postoperative Pain by Encouragement and Instruction of Patients," *N. Engl. J. Med.,* **270:**825, (Apr. 16) 1964.
12. Bandler, R. J., Jr., et al.: "Self-Observation as a Source of Pain Perception," *J. Pers. Soc. Psychol.,* **9:**205, (No. 3) 1968.
13. Blitz, B., and Dinnerstein, A. J.: "Effects of Different Types of Instructions on Pain Parameters," *J. Abnorm. Psychol.,* **73:**276, (No. 3, Pt. I) 1968.
14. Petrie, A.: *Individuality in Pain and Suffering.* University of Chicago Press, Chicago, 1967.
15. Bond, M. R.: "The Relation of Pain to the Eysenck Personality Inventory, Cornell Medical Index and Whiteley Index of Hypochondriasis," *Br. J. Psychiatry,* **119:**671, (Dec.) 1971.
16. Buss, A. H., and Portnoy, N. W.: "Pain Tolerance and Group Identification," *J. Pers. Soc. Psychol.,* **6:**106, (No. 1) 1967.
17. Wolff, B. B., and Harland, A. A.: "Effect of Suggestion upon Experimental Pain," *J. Abnorm. Psychol.,* **72:**402, (No. 5, Pt. I) 1967.
18. Gonda, T. A.: "The Relation Between Complaints of Persistent Pain and Family Size," *J. Neurol. Neurosurg. Psychiatry,* **25:**277, (Aug.) 1962.
19. Zborowski, Mark: *People in Pain.* Jossey-Bass, Inc., San Francisco, 1969.
20. Sternbach, R. A., and Tursky, B.: "Ethnic Differences Among Housewives in Psychophysical and Skin Potential Responses to Electric Shock," *Psychophysiology,* **1:**241, (Jan.) 1965.
21. Merskey, H., and Spear, F. G.: *Pain—Psychological and Psychiatric Aspects.* Bailliere, Tindall & Cassell, London, 1967, p. 147.
22. McCabe, Gracia S.: "Cultural Influences on Patient Behavior," *Am. J. Nurs.,* **60:**1101, (Aug.) 1960.
23. Sternbach, Richard A.: *Pain—A Psychophysiological Analysis.* Academic Press, New York, 1968, p. 77.
24. Bond, M. R.: *op. cit.*
25. Merskey, H., and Spear, F. G.: *op. cit.,* p. 43.
26. Kaufmann, M., and Brown, D.: "Pain Wears Many Faces," *Am. J. Nurs.,* **61:**48, (Jan.) (1961).
27. Smith, Mary Margo: "Nursing Knowledge and Activity in Relation to the Period of Anticipation of Pain in the Adult," in *Solving "Difficult" Problems in Nursing Care,* A.N.A. Monograph #20, New York, 1962, p. 25.
28. "Pain—Part I of Programmed Instruction: Basic Concepts and Assessment," *Am. J. Nurs.,* **66:**1085, (May) 1966.
29. "Pain—Part II of Programmed Instruction: Rationale for Intervention," *Am. J. Nurs.,* **66:**1345, (June) 1966.
30. Bochnak, M. A., et al.: "Comparison of Two Types of Nursing Activity on the Relief of Pain," in *Innovations in Nurse-Patient Relationships: Automatic or Reasoned Nurse*

---

* These (selected) statements are based on the "Orientation to Pain" Inventory being developed by Ada Jacox at the University of Iowa (US Public Health Service Grant No. 00387–02.)

Actions, A.N.A. Monograph #6, New York, 1962, p. 5.

31. Dorsch, M., et al.: "Doctors' Expectations of Nurse Action and Judgment in the Use of PRN Medication Orders," in *Evaluation of Nursing Intervention,* A.N.A. Monograph #3, New York, 1964, p. 26.

32. Buckeridge, A., et al.: "A Study of Overt Nurse Action when Darvon and Darvon Compound Are Prescribed for PRN Administration," in *Evaluation of Nursing Intervention,* A.N.A. Monograph #3, New York, 1964, p. 44.

33. Whiting, J. F.: "Patients' Needs, Nurses' Needs and the Healing Process," *Am. J. Nurs.,* **59:**664, (May) 1959.

34. McBride, Mary Angela B.: " 'Pain' and Effective Nursing Practice," in *ANA Clinical Sessions, 1966.* Appleton-Century-Crofts, New York, 1967, p. 75.

35. ———: "The Additive to the Analgesic," *Am. J. Nurs.,* **69:**974, (May) 1969.

36. Moss, Fay T., and Meyer, Burton: "The Effects of Nursing Interaction upon Pain Relief in Patients," *Nurs. Res.,* **15:**303, (Fall) 1966.

37. Walike, B. Caleen, and Meyer, Burton: "Relation Between Placebo Reactivity and Selected Personality Factors," *Nurs. Res.* **15:**119, (Spring) 1966.

38. Chambers, Wilda G., and Price, Geraldine G.: "Influence of Nurse upon Effects of Analgesics Administered," *Nurs. Res.,* **16:**228, (Summer) 1967.

39. Billars, Karen S.: "You Have Pain? I Think This Will Help," *Am. J. Nurs.,* **70:**2143, (Oct.) 1970.

40. Diers, Donna, et al.: "The Effect of Nursing Interaction on Patients in Pain," *Nurs. Res.,* **21:**419, (Sept.–Oct.) 1972.

41. McBride, Mary Angela B.: *op. cit.*

42. Crowley, Dorothy, et al.: *Pain and Its Alleviation.* University of California School of Nursing, Los Angeles, 1962.

43. McCaffery, Margo: *op. cit.*

44. Melzack, R., and Torgerson, W. S.: "On the Language of Pain," *Anesthesiology,* **34:**50, (Jan.) 1971.

45. Newton, M., et al.: *A Study of Nurse Action in Relief of Pain.* U.S. Public Health Service Grant #NU–00004–02. Ohio State University, Columbus, 1964.

46. Sternbach, Richard A.: *op. cit.,* p. 151.

47. Zborowski, Mark: *op. cit.,* p. 18.

48. Jacox, Ada: "Analysis of Factors Influencing Nurses' Assessment of Pain," presented at the A.N.A. Convention, Detroit, 1972.

49. Baer, Eva, et al.: "Inferences of Physical Pain and Psychological Distress: I. In Relation to Verbal and Nonverbal Patient Communication," *Nurs. Res.,* **19:**388, (Sept.–Oct.) 1970.

50. Lenburg, Carrie B., et al.: "Inferences of Physical Pain and Psychological Distress: II. In Relation to the Stage of the Patient's Illness and Occupation of the Perceiver," *Nurs. Res.,* **19:**392, (Sept.–Oct.) 1970.

51. Davitz, Lois Jean, et al.: "Nurses' Inferences of Suffering," *Nurs. Res.,* **18:**100, (Mar.–Apr.) 1969.

52. "Pins Against Pain," *Time,* (June 12) 1972, p. 44.

52a. Chaves, James F., and Barber, Theodore X.: "Needles and Knives—Behind the Mystery of Acupuncture and Chinese Meridians," *Hum. Behavior,* **2:**19, (Sept.) 1973.

53. White, James C., and Sweet, William H.: *Pain and the Neurosurgeon.* Charles C Thomas, Publisher, Springfield, Ill., 1969.

54. "Easing Wallace's Pain," *Newsweek,* (Jan. 15) 1973, p. 49.

55. Melzack, R., et al.: "Stratagems for Controlling Pain: Contributions of Auditory Stimulation and Suggestion," *Exp. Neurol.,* **8:**239, 1963.

56. McCaffery, Margo: *op. cit.,* p. 171.

57. Cashatt, Barbara: "Pain: A Patient's View," *Am. J. Nurs.,* **72:**281, (Feb.) 1972.

58. McBride, Mary Angela B.: "Nursing Approach, Pain, and Relief: An Exploratory Experiment," *Nurs. Res.,* **16:**337, (Fall) 1967.

59. Healy, Kathryn M.: "Does Preoperative Instruction Make a Difference?" *Am. J. Nurs.,* **68:**62, (Jan.) 1968.

60. McBride, Mary Angela B.: "The Additive to the Analgesic," *Am. J. Nurs.,* **69:**974, (May) 1969.

61. "Fluorides Ease Bone Pain," *Am. J. Nurs.,* **69:**1178, (June) 1969.

62. Halsell, Marilyn: "Moist Heat for Relief of Postoperative Pain," *Am. J. Nurs.,* **67:**767, (Apr.) 1967.

63. McCaffery, Margo, and Moss, Fay: "Nursing Intervention for Bodily Pain," *Am. J. Nurs.,* **67:**1224, (June) 1967.

64. Barnes, Elizabeth (ed.): *Psychosocial Nursing.* Tavistock Publications, Ltd., London, 1968.

65. Shealy, C. Norman, et al.: "Six Years' Experience with Electrical Stimulation for Control of Pain," *Adv. Neurol.,* Vol. 4, 1974.

66. Shealy, C. Norman, and Mortimer, J. T.: "Dorsal Column Electroanalgesia," in Rejnolds, D. N., and Sjoberg, A. E. (eds.): *Neuroelectric Research. Electroneuroprosthesis, Electroanesthesia and Non-Convulsive Electrotherapy.* Charles C Thomas, Publisher, Springfield, Ill., 1971.

67. Shealy, C. Norman: "Transcutaneous Nerve Stimulation for the Control of Pain," *Surg. Neurol.,* **2:**45, (Jan.) 1974.

68. ———: "Transcutaneous Electroanalysis," *Surg. Forum,* **23:**419, 1973.

69. Indeck, Walter, and Printy, Andrea: "Skin Application of Electrical Impulses for Relief of Pain," *Minn. Med.,* **58:**305, (Apr.) 1975.

70. Sternscheim, B. A., et al.: "Causalgia," *Arch. Phys. Med. Rehabil.,* **56:**58, (Feb.) 1975.

71. Winter, A., et al.: "Pain Relief—Transcutaneous Nerve Stimulation," *J. Med. Soc. N.J.,* **71:**365, (May) 1974.

72. Campbell, J. N., and Taub, A.: "Local Analgesia from Percutaneous Electrical Stimula-

tion; A Peripheral Mechanism," *Arch. Neurol.,* **28:**347, 1973.

73. Loeser, J. D., et al.: "Relief of Pain by Transcutaneous Stimulation," *J. Neurosurg.,* **42:**308, (Mar.) 1975.

74. Long, D. M.: "Cutaneous Afferent Stimulation for the Relief of Pain." Congress of Neurosurgery, Honolulu, Vol. 21, Chap. 22. Williams & Wilkins Co., Baltimore, [1974].

75. Sweet, W. H. "Stimulation of Peripheral Pain Suppressor Mechanisms," presented at International Symposium on Pain, Seattle, Wash., 1973.

76. Taub, A., and Campbell, J. N.: "Percutaneous-Local Electrical Analgesia: Peripheral Mechanisms," presented at International Symposium on Pain, Seattle, Wash., 1973.

77. McCaffery, Margo: *op. cit.,* p. 218.

Additional Suggested Reading

"Acupuncture," *Am. J. Nurs.,* **74:**503, (Mar.) 1974.

Brena, S.: *Pain and Religion; A Psychophysiological Study.* Charles C Thomas, Publisher, Springfield, Ill., 1972.

Breugel, Mary A.: "Relationship of Preoperative Anxiety to Perception of Postoperative Pain," *Nurs. Res.,* **20:**26, (Jan.–Feb.) 1971.

Copple, Dionna: "What Can a Nurse Do to Relieve Pain Without Resort to Drugs?" *Nurs. Times,* **68:**584, (May 11) 1972.

Drakontides, Anna B.: "Drugs to Treat Pain," *Am. J. Nurs.,* **74:**508, (Mar.) 1974.

Evans, Frederick J.: "The Power of a Sugar Pill," *Psychology Today,* **7:**54, (Apr.) 1974.

Gaumer, William R.: "Electrical Stimulation in Chronic Pain," *Am. J. Nurs.,* **74:**504, (Mar.) 1974.

Glazer, Henry: "Pain," *J. Emotional Educ.,* **11:** 277, (Fall) 1971.

Goloskov, Joan, and LeRoy, Pierre: "Use of the Dorsal Column Stimulator," *Am. J. Nurs.,* **74:** 506, (Mar.) 1974.

Hilgard, Ernest R., and Hilgard, Josephine R.: *Hypnosis in the Relief of Pain.* W. Kaufman, 1975.

International Symposium on Pain, Rottach-Egein, Ger., 1969: *Pain.* Williams & Wilkins Co., Baltimore, 1972.

Jacox, Ada, and Stewart, Mary: *Psychosocial Contingencies of the Pain Experience* (Monograph). University of Iowa, Iowa City, 1973.

Keele, Kenneth O.: "Pain: How It Varies from Person to Person," *Nurs. Times,* **68:**890, (July) 1972.

McLachlan, Eileen: "Recognizing Pain," *Am. J. Nurs.,* **74:**496, (Mar.) 1974.

Markham, M. M.: "The Relief of Pain," *Nurs. Times,* **66:**1579, (Dec. 10) 1970.

Marks, Richard M., and Sachar, Edward J.: "Undertreatment of Medical Inpatients with Narcotic Analgesics," *Ann. Intern. Med.,* **78:**173, (Feb.) 1973.

Mastrovito, René C.: "Psychogenic Pain," *Am. J. Nurs.,* **74:**514, (Mar.) 1974.

Melzack, Ronald: *The Puzzle of Pain.* Basic Books, New York, 1973.

———, and Perry, Campbell: "Self-regulation of Pain: The Use of Alpha-feedback and Hypnotic Training for the Control of Chronic Pain," *Exp. Neurol.,* **46:**452, (Mar.) 1975.

Merskey, H.: "Pain," *Nurs. Times,* **67:**988, (Aug. 12) 1971.

Morgan, Arthur James: "Minor Tranquilizers, Hypnotics, and Sedatives," *Am. J. Nurs.,* **73:** 1220, (July) 1973.

"Nurse, It Hurts," *Nurs. Times,* **67:**975, (Aug. 12) 1971.

Rogers, A.: "Pain and the Cancer Patient," *Nurs. Clin. North Am.,* **2:**671, (Dec.) 1967.

Sarbin, Theodore R.: *Hypnosis. A Social Psychological Analysis of Influence Communication.* Holt, Rinehart & Winston, New York, 1972.

Saunders, Cicely: "The Management of Terminal Illness; Physical Distress in the Dying Patient," *Hosp. Med.,* **1:**317, (Jan.) 1967.

———: "The Symptomatic Treatment of Incurable Malignant Disease," *Prescribers' J.,* **4:**68, (Oct.) 1964.

Schultz, N. V.: "How Children Perceive Pain," *Nurs. Outlook,* **19:**670, (Oct.) 1971.

Siegele, Dorothy S.: "The Gate Control Theory," *Am. J. Nurs.,* **74:**498, (Mar.) 1974.

Sobel, David: "Love and Pain," *Am. J. Nurs.,* **72:**910, (May) 1972.

Storlie, Frances: "Pain: Describing It More Accurately," *Nursing '72,* **2:**15, (June) 1972.

Strassberg, D. S., and Klinger, B. I.: "The Effect on Pain Tolerance of Social Pressure Within the Laboratory Setting," *J. Soc. Psychol.,* **88:** 123, (Oct.) 1972.

Strauss, Anselm: *Anguish.* San Francisco Sociology Press, San Francisco, 1970.

Swafford, L. I., and Allan, D.: "Pain Relief in the Pediatric Patient," *Med. Clin. North Am.,* **52:** 135, (Jan.) 1968.

Turnbull, F.: "Pain and Suffering in Cancer," *Can. Nurse.,* **67:**28, (Aug.) 1971.

Woodforde, J. H., and Merskey, H.: "Personality Traits of Patients with Chronic Pain," *J. Psychosom. Res.,* **16:**167, (June) 1972.

Angela Barron McBride
Virginia Henderson

CHAPTER 50

Death and Dying

1. BELIEFS, ATTITUDES, CUSTOMS, AND CONDITIONS AFFECTING DEATH AND DYING

Death as a Part of Life. Death is often referred to as the final act in the drama of life. It is an inescapable reality which many refuse to face until their lives, or the lives of those they love, are threatened. Lewis Thomas, a physician and philosopher who calls himself a "biology watcher," writing about the death of all living things, marvels at the invisibility of death. He makes the observation that billions of insects die unnoticeably; he calls attention to the instinct animals have for "performing death alone, hidden." He says:

It is a natural marvel. All of the life of the earth dies, all of the time, in the same volume as the new life that dazzles us each morning, each spring. All we see of this is the odd stump, the fly struggling on the porch floor of the summer house in October, the fragment on the highway. I have lived all my life with an embarrassment of squirrels in my backyard . . . and I have never seen, anywhere, a dead squirrel.

I suppose it is just as well. If the earth were otherwise, and all the dying were done in the open, with the dead there to be looked at, we would never have it out of our minds. We can forget about it much of the time, or think of it as an accident to be avoided, somehow. But it does make the process of dying seem more exceptional than it really is, and harder to engage in at the times when we must ourselves engage.

Having commented on the way in which we humans conform, "as best we can," to the rest of nature in having most of the 50 million deaths a year take place in relative secrecy, he says:

Less than a half century from now, our replacements will have more than doubled the numbers. It is hard to see how we can continue to keep the secret, with such multitudes doing the dying. We will have to give up the notion that death is catastrophe, or detestable, or avoidable, or even strange. We will need to learn more about the cycling of life in the rest of the system, and about our connection to the process. Everything that comes alive seems to be in trade for something that dies, cell for cell. There might be some comfort in the recognition of synchrony, in the information that we all go down together, in the best of company.*

In *Medical Nemesis, The Expropriation of Health* Ivan Illich includes a chapter entitled "Death Against Death." He traces the changing attitudes toward death from the fourth to the present century. He says, "In every society the dominant image of death determines the prevalent concept of health. . . . A society's image of death reveals the level of independence of its people, their personal relatedness, self-reliance and aliveness." † Illich thinks that the image of a "natural death," a death that ought to come under medical care and find us in good health and old age is a recent idea and he traces the five stages in its development from the fourteenth century "dance of death" through death under intensive hospital care. Illich notes that in primitive societies death is the outcome of someone's evil intentions and from the fourth century onward the Christian church struggled against "the pagan tradition of crowds dancing in cemeteries; naked,

---

* Thomas, Lewis: *The Lives of a Cell. Notes of a Biology Watcher.* Viking Press, New York, 1974, pp. 98–99.
† Illich, Ivan: *Medical Nemesis. The Expropriation of Health.* Pantheon Books. New York, 1976, p. 122.

frenzied and brandishing swords. . . . The dance with the dead over their tombs was an occasion for affirming the joy of being alive and a source of many erotic songs and poems." With the acceptance of "the church triumphant in heaven man faced death differently and his aim was to die well." Illich refers to *Ars Moriendi* as "one of the first printed do-it-yourself manuals," which he said was a "best seller for 200 years."

A sermon by John Donne was published in 1632 under the title *Death Duell or A Consolation to the Soule Against the Dying Life and Living Death of the Body.** Another book, written by W. C. London, published by William Stansky in 1931, was entitled *La Danse Machabre or Deaths Duell.* The title page shows the living overcoming death by dance and Father Time determining the close of life for every human, regardless of the station of life and the promise of life after death in heaven. (See Fig. 50–1.)

Michel de Montaigne, a seventeenth-century philosopher with a flair for lighthearted observations on profound subjects, said we should not make death a stranger but should think of it daily without fear, directing our thoughts toward the prolongation of our work rather than life itself.

The end of our cariere is death, it is the necessarie object of our aim; if it affright us, how is it possible we should step one foot farther without an ague? The remedie of the vulgar sort is not to thinke on it. . . . Let us learne to stand, and combat her with a resolute minde. . . . Let us remove her strangeness from her, let us converse frequent, and acquaint ourselves with her, let us have nothing so much in minde as death. . . . He who hath learned to die hath learned to serve. There is no evill in life for him who hath well conceived, how the privation of life is no evill. To know how to die doth free us all from subjection and constraint. . . . I would have a man to be doing and to prolong his lives offices as much as lieth in him, and let death seize upon me, whilst I am setting my cabiges, careless of her dart, but more of my unperfect garden.

For the aged and for the hopelessly ill, death is, indeed, as he says, "no evill"; for the religious who believe in life hereafter, there is no fear or dread. Doctors, nurses, and ministers of wide experience tell of many who are happy and exalted in death. Death can be made beautiful by the courage with which the person and those around him or her face it. Montaigne, quoting Epaminondas, implied that dying well is the ultimate test of a man. He

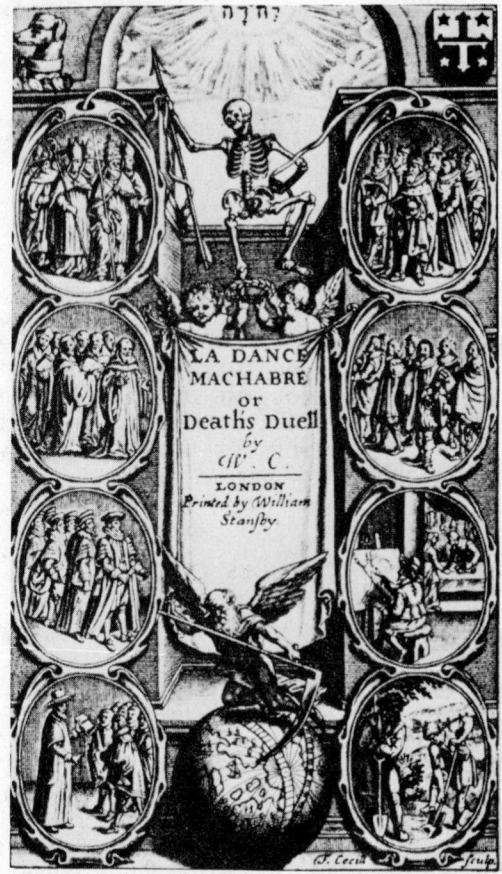

Figure 50-1. Cecill's engraving of La Danse Machabre depicts three chronologic sequences—first, the living overcome death by dance; second, Father Time determines the close of life of every human regardless of the station of life; and third, the promise of life after death in heaven. (Donne, John: *Deaths Duell. A Sermon.* Edited with a postscript by Geoffrey Keynes. David R. Godine, Boston, 1973.)

said: "Epaminondas being demanded which of the three he esteemed most, either Chabrias, or Iphicrates, or himselfe; 'It is necessary,' said he, 'that we be seene to die, before your question may be well resolved. Verily we should steale much from him, if he should be weighed without the honour and greatness of his end.' " *

The writers (believing that death is part of life and, as Montaigne said, not to be feared) emphasize in this chapter helping people to live as fully as possible up to the moment of death, helping them and those who love them to accept death and to make it as easy as

---

* Donne, John: *Death Duell. A Sermon.* Edited with a postscript by Geoffrey Keynes. David R. Godine, Boston, 1973, p. 47.

* Montaigne, Michel E. de: *Essayes.* Modern Library, Random House, New York, 1928, pp. 47–56.

most students of dying think it should be. Lois Jaffe, who has acute leukemia and is a social worker by profession, speaking at a Right to Life Conference, in 1974, observed that

The one thing that has impressed me most about all of these dialogues is that over this two year period, there has been a subtle shift in our conversations from a focus on death and dying to what it means to live a full, rich life, in whatever time we have left. I believe this shift in focus, along with the recent plethora of books, public discussions, articles, and television programs, reflects a beginning recognition that while a person may be dying, he also is very much living, and that death need not be thought of as pathology and disease, but rather as a vital part of life. This shift obviously reflects, too, my own change of perspective from a concern about quantity of life to quality.*

Studies on Death and Dying. Historians, philosophers, theologians, anthropologists, psychologists, biologists, sociologists, social workers, lawyers, doctors, pharmacists, dentists, nurses, novelists, journalists, poets, dying persons, and their families have all studied and written about death and dying; about the attitudes toward death in different cultures and eras; about the effect of religion—especially the belief in an afterlife; about the relationship between the status and care of the aged and of the dying in a society; and about the effect of war and catastrophes, such as decimating plagues, floods, and famines. Current literature includes reports of efforts to assess the effect on humans of realizing that atomic warfare makes possible the immediate destruction of this civilization, and reports of efforts to assess the effect of interplanetary travel—the possibility of encountering life on other planets which can challenge some religious convictions.

Thanatos is an ancient Greek personification of death; *thanatology* has been adopted as a term to encompass the study of death. Several important bibliographies on the subject exist, many of them recently published. Robert Kastenbaum, Professor of Psychology, University of Massachusetts, Harbor Campus, in Boston, has compiled a retrospective bibliography which, at this writing, is ready to be published. Other important bibliographic collections have been prepared by Richard Kalish of the Graduate Theological Union; Robert Fulton of the University of Minnesota; Michael Simpson, formerly at McMasters Medical School in Hamilton, Ont., but now at The Royal Free Hospital, London, Eng.; Austin

and Lillian Kutscher of the Foundation of Thanatology at the College of Physicians and Surgeons, Columbia University, New York City; Richard Torpie of Philadelphia; LeRoy Walters (*Bibliography of Bioethics*), Kennedy Institute, Georgetown University, Washington, D.C.; and finally the *Bibliography of Society, Ethics and the Life Sciences* prepared by the Hastings Center, Hastings-on-Hudson, N.Y.

Important writings are so widely published in professional journals of theology, ethics, medicine, nursing, sociology, and anthropology, as well as in magazines, newspapers, and books read by the general public, that members of the International Work Group on Death and Dying are presently doing a feasibility study to determine whether one central bibliography is needed to cite all the literature in one periodical.

The most superficial study of the literature on death and dying shows readers the "multifarious faces" of death and makes them leery of generalizations. While there are biologic commonalities in the process of dying, each life is different and each death, as part of that life, is unique.

People who have had a brush with death have described their experiences; others have left minute records of their terminal illnesses. Parents, spouses, and children have written equally vivid descriptions of the last months, weeks, days, and hours with those they loved. Some are reports of carefully structured research and a number of such reports are cited in appropriate sections of this chapter.

The wish to die while living and the wish to live after death are the same throughout the centuries. Poets in every age put these timeless thoughts into memorable words. Ted Rosenthal, who was born in 1938 and died of leukemia in 1972, left a poignant record of his experience as "a man who knows death." He says, "I speak only truth to those who will listen." He says he feels "so all alone abandoned" but he urges his readers to "never yield a minute to despair," to love life, to love people—"It's love. It's your only path." He ends a long poem with these lines:

We cross the stream and walk up the slope
See, the hawk is diving
The plain stretches out ahead, then the hills, the
    valleys and the meadows
Keep moving people. How could I not be among
    you? *

Irving E. Alexander and Arthur M. Adlerstein, psychologists writing in 1965, say that this is an "era of greater awareness of death"

---

* Jaffe, Lois: *Making Time Count.* [Keynote address, Right to Life Conference.] Mercy Hospital, Pittsburgh, Pa., November 20, 1974, processed.

* Rosenthal, Ted: *How Could I Not Be Among You.* George Brazilier, New York, 1973.

and that in consequence "there is an increased trend toward religion." *

Throughout the centuries and in many cultures, mankind has also demonstrated fear of death. Even when life seems to hold little chance of happiness, death may not be welcomed.† Hamlet's soliloquy includes the following which strikes a familiar chord for most readers:

But that the dread of something after death,
The undiscover'd country from whose bourn
No traveller returns, puzzles the will,
And makes us rather bear those ills we have
Than fly to others that we know not of? ‡

Societal Viewpoints. Humans have always treasured a belief in immortality. Robert J. Lifton and Eric Olson, social scientists, think a "sense of immortality is expressed in five modes or categories: biological, creative, theological, natural, and experiential." § *Biological* means that people live on in their progeny; *creative* means that they live on through their works; *theological* means that people accept a religious concept of eternal life; *natural* means that they have faith in the endurance of nature, of which man is part; and *experiential transcendence* means that they accept "moments of ecstasy as being beyond . . . life and beyond death." Perhaps what Wordsworth meant by "intimations of immortality."

In some cultures even today, death as a cessation of being is denied. The ancient practice of putting food, clothing, jewels, household utensils, even wives and slaves in the tombs of the pharaohs is an example of the unwillingness to accept death in ancient times by providing the body in burial with commodities and companions for life to come. It has also been noted that in Greek mythology the gods are described as going from heaven (Olympus) to the earth and back again and to hell (Hades) and back to earth. Certain American Indian tribes, even in this century, mourn the dead but also fear them, believing that they still exist in some form that enables them to take vengeance on those who have wronged them.[1]

Elisabeth Kübler-Ross, a physician, has come to support the belief that there is life after death. A philosopher and medical student, Raymond Moody,[1a] gives his evidence— a large number of persons who have told of their experiences when they were given up for dead and subsequently revived. The explanation for these vivid and ecstatic impressions of persons who returned to life after, apparently, dying is also being examined by psychologists and psychiatrists. Russell Noyes and Roy Kletti [1b] suggest that the individual shields himself from the threat of death by depersonalization.

Spiritualists all over the world claim to be in communication with those who have died, and students of bioelectric phenomena, such as Harold Saxton Burr, maintain that the bioelectric field of every living organism is indestructible. In a scientific sense, this parallels the mystic's concept of a "soul" that has life everlasting and the Eastern (Hindu) concept of transmigration with the ultimate merging of the perfected life with an eternal, all-inclusive Being or Reality.[2] While the dominant beliefs of major religions are discussed in more detail in Chapter 18, it seems obvious to most people that they affect attitudes of the faithful toward dying and death. Some studies do not support the statement that the religious person is less anxious about death than the nonreligious. For example, in a study of healthy young men, Jews and Christians, by Alexander and Adlerstein,[3] there was little difference between the religious and the nonreligious. John Hinton [3a] differentiated between those who were firmly convinced either in religious faith or no faith and those who waver or are unsure. Those convinced were less anxious.

Religious beliefs and ethical values certainly affect the way people treat death and dying, and custom, or what is thought seemly, affects both. In cultures where families of three and four generations live together in one house, or in a compound, dying and death cannot be hidden, and concern for the dying is usually shared by a dozen or more persons. In tribal life or in religious communities, the concern may be shared by hundreds. In some primitive societies and undeveloped countries, where little is known about the cure of disease and the relief of its symptoms, death from disease may involve undue suffering from those symptoms; on the other hand, in modern societies, undue suffering may be caused by the heroic life-saving measures.

In primitive society, the family or members of the community are more likely to stay with

---

* Alexander, Irving E., and Adlerstein, Arthur M.: "Death and Religion," in Feifel, Herman (ed.): *The Meaning of Death*. McGraw-Hill Book Co., New York, 1965, p. 282.

† Persons who believe in a life hereafter and expect to rejoin those they love in heaven accept death most easily. Many persons express a wondering faith in the essential goodness and continuity of life. Annie W. Goodrich, when she was about 80, expressed regret that she had survived a serious operation. She said, "I was ready and now I'll have to go through that all over again. Anyway, I can't wait to see what's on the other side!"

‡ Shakespeare, William: *The Tragedy of Hamlet, Prince of Denmark*, Act III, Scene i.

§ Lifton, Robert J., and Olson, Eric: *Living and Dying*. Praeger Publishers, New York, 1974, p. 76.

the dying and mitigate the almost inevitable feeling of loneliness. The term *family* as used here always means those who are closest to or live with the patient; they are not necessarily blood kin since some patients will have outlived their relatives or lived apart from their relatives for years, but may have friends who play an essential role in the patient's life, as the patient does in theirs. The term *significant key others* (SKO) is used frequently to identify these persons.

Reference is often made to the chasm that separates the sick and the well. While all persons know that they face death ultimately, some who believe that they have only a few years, months, weeks, or days to live seem, in most cases, to be "doomed." People facing death may seem "different." When friends and family know that a person's death is imminent, they are often unnatural in their presence. In the novel *The Years,* Virginia Woolf [3b] describes the awkwardness of the children and husband of a woman who is dying in the prime of her life.

In some sophisticated cultures there are those who stay with or near the dying as a friendly duty—or privilege. Madame de Sévigné, in *Letters to Her Daughter,* written in the seventeenth and eighteenth centuries, described many death scenes. A citizen of Paris and a welcome visitor at Versailles, she was often there to help one of her friends in this Royal Commune through a terminal illness.

In many European, Asian, South American, and Central American countries the elderly live and die in their own homes or in the homes of their children. The word pictures drawn by Madame de Sévigné might even today seem familiar to rural families in China, Brazil, Greece, India, or Russia, but strange indeed to North Americans, particularly urban dwellers.* In today's United States, the family is typically composed of parents and children of school age living in a small apartment or a small house. Grown children establish independent homes, and grandparents tend to move into small apartments, communities for the retired, or institutions for the elderly. Disease is treated in hospitals so that as sick people imperceptibly become dying people they are even more likely to disappear from family life.

Religious beliefs, ethical values, and customs in any culture affect dying and death. Economics is also a powerful influence. Anthropologists point out that among nomadic people the sick and dying, the weak and elderly, threaten the survival of the tribe if its movements are hampered by them. In rural cultures, on the other hand, where a family's welfare depends on the number of healthy children who can work the land, every effort is made to prevent the death of children and youths, especially the deaths of sons. In most cultures, young adults, especially young parents, have the highest social worth, and their deaths are accounted the greatest social loss.[4]

Where and How Death Occurs. Some Morbidity and Mortality Statistics Showing Where, When, and How People Die. It is not practicable in a book such as this to attempt to give a worldwide picture of when, how, and where deaths occur. Enough may have been said to suggest that attitudes toward death, and customs in helping those who are dying, vary with the culture—its religious beliefs and ethical values, the size and character of the family or communal unit, how people live, and the resources available to them.

The following data on "When, Why, and Where People Die" apply to the United States and may not represent worldwide trends.

The Russell Sage Foundation published *The Dying Patients,* a report edited by Orville G. Brim and associates, in 1970.[5] In this volume, Monroe Lerner showed (see Table 50–1) that between 1900 and 1966 the mortality rates per 1000 of the population fell from 17.2 to 9.5, that the drop was lower for females than males, and that the most striking change was the drop under 1 year of age from 162.4 (both sexes) to 23.1 (both sexes). In other words, the death of babies in 1966 was far more unusual than in 1900, while the death rate for those 85 years and over was not so different in 1966 from that in 1900. The implications are that now and in the foreseeable future persons will be dying in later life and after a prolonged period of sickness and debilitation.

Lerner gives data on selected causes of death in institutions in 1949 and 1958 in the United States and some comparative figures by geographic area.* He shows that while in 1949

---

* Geri Berg, in a letter to F. W., January 23, 1976, with reference to teaching through art, makes the following observation: "Material from the history of art is used to sharpen observational and critical inquiry skills and to provide an avenue for learning about cultural attitudes towards children, the self, body image, aging and death and dying. Edvard Munch's *Death in the Sickroom,* 1893, depicts the pervasive melancholy and incommunicability that characterizes one family's reactions to death. This work provides a good example of the kind of visual and biographical material that can be used by students to examine the personal and cultural attitudes towards death which confront practitioners and patients."

* See Chapter 2, page 140, for table showing principal causes of death in different decades of this century.

Table 50-1. Mortality Rates per 1000 Population by Age and Sex, United States, 1900 and 1966 *

Age (years)	1900			1966		
	Both Sexes	Males	Females	Both Sexes	Males	Females
All ages	17.2	17.9	16.5	9.5	11.0	8.1
Under 1	162.4	179.1	145.4	23.1	25.7	20.4
1–4	19.8	20.5	19.1	1.0	1.0	0.9
5–14	3.9	3.8	3.9	0.4	0.5	0.4
15–24	5.9	5.9	5.8	1.2	1.7	0.6
25–34	8.2	8.2	8.2	1.5	2.0	1.0
35–44	10.2	10.7	9.8	3.1	3.9	2.3
45–54	15.0	15.7	14.2	7.3	9.7	5.1
55–64	27.2	28.7	25.8	17.2	23.6	11.2
65–74	56.4	59.3	53.6	38.8	52.0	28.1
75–84	123.3	128.3	118.8	81.6	98.5	69.5
85 and over	260.9	268.8	255.2	202.0	213.6	194.9

* Lerner, Monroe: "When, Why and Where People Die," in Brim, Orville G., Jr., et al. (eds.): *The Dying Patient*. Russell Sage Foundation, New York, 1970, p. 11.

deaths occurred as frequently outside as inside institutions (50.5 to 49.5 per cent), in 1958 they occurred much less frequently outside than inside institutions (39.1 to 60.9 per cent). Lerner gives more recent figures from the Maryland State Health Department: institutional deaths, 64.4 per cent in 1957, 71.8 per cent in 1966.[6] Of the institutional deaths in the United States in 1958, most occurred in *general hospitals* (47.6 per cent of all deaths), with deaths in convalescent and nursing homes the next most usual institutional setting (6 per cent of all deaths). *Nervous and mental hospitals, chronic disease, convalescent and other special hospitals, tuberculosis, and maternity hospitals* are other sites, in this order of frequency (see Table 50-2). Current figures would probably show a greater proportion of deaths in *nursing homes* today than in 1958, since nursing home beds have increased at a spectacular rate. However, patients in these beds are frequently transferred to hospitals at the end, because of the difficulty in care, so that while the dying process is in the nursing home, the death statistic is recorded in the hospital.

Patients who die in the general hospital are likely to be in the *emergency room* or in the *intensive care unit*. In contrast to these divisions of the acute hospital are the small specialized units where extended, personalized care helps patients and their families come to terms with illnesses which no longer respond to curative treatment. Palliative treatment for symptoms and spiritual support for patients and families help them to cope with the reality of death. These units can be part of a hospital or a separate facility. As noted in Chapter 3, there are in England between 20 and 30 facilities of this sort; some are called *hospices;* this kind of care is spreading in the United States and Canada.

Death may occur in any of these contrasting institutional settings, in any part of a medical center, in any sort of hospital, in a nursing home, in a private home, in a school, in an occupational setting, in the street, or, in fact, anywhere. The effect of the setting on the care that it is possible to give is discussed later in this chapter.

In any setting, the family and friends of the dying patient require help. They can play an important role. Most persons are comforted by the presence of those they particularly love, so, for the patient's benefit, family and friends should be part of the dying scene. Nurses and physicians may have to focus on the patient, but they should not forget that relatives and friends of the dying are suffering and, as they face being left behind, need physical and psychologic help. In fact, they are likely to need such help both before and after the patient's death; it is for this reason that almost as much space is devoted in this chapter to a discussion of helping relatives and friends as to helping the dying patient. A 1976 film *Dying*, made by WGBH in Boston for the Public Broadcasting System, shows four persons who are terminally ill and the response of their families. In Figure 50-2 a single picture and a cited statement

Table 50-2. Number and Per Cent of Deaths Occurring in Institutions by Type of Service of Institution, United States, 1949 and 1958 *

Type of Service of Institution	1958		1949	
	Number	Per Cent	Number	Per Cent
Total deaths	1,647,886	100.0	1,443,607	100.0
Not in institution	644,548	39.1	728,797	50.5
In institution	1,003,338	60.9	714,810	49.5
Type of Service of Institution				
General hospital	784,360	47.6	569,867	39.5
Maternity hospital	1,862	0.1	2,249	0.2
Tuberculosis hospital	9,097	0.6	13,627	0.9
Chronic disease, convalescent, and other special hospitals	24,180	1.5	12,402	0.9
Nervous and mental hospitals	57,675	3.5	45,637	3.2
Convalescent and nursing homes, homes for the aged, etc.	98,444	6.0	22,783	1.6
Hospital department of institutions, and other domiciliary institutions	3,646	0.2	41,841	2.9
Type of service not specified	24,074	1.5	6,404	0.4

* Lerner, Monroe: "When, Why and Where People Die," in Brim, Orville G., Jr., et al. (eds.): *The Dying Patient*, Russell Sage Foundation, New York, 1970, p. 11.

from each of the vignettes suggest striking differences in the way that the dying person and the families respond to approaching death.

The *cost of institutional terminal care* is a factor that influences where death occurs, particularly death following prolonged efforts to extend life. Robert J. Glaser,[7] then dean of the medical school, Stanford (Calif.) University, reported in 1970 that the costs of "heroic operations," such as heart and kidney transplants are, in the United States, usually paid for out of research funds. The National Heart Institute in the US Public Health Service estimated the minimum cost of a heart transplant as $20,000 for the period of hospitalization plus several hundred dollars a day thereafter for an indefinite period of recovery. If and when the investigative period of such surgery ends and research funds are no longer available, a heart transplant might spell financial ruin for the average family whose health insurance does not cover such contingencies. Glaser emphasizes the "enormous economic and emotional cost of prolonging life in the presence of irreversible disease."[8]

As the movement to build hospices in the United States is getting under way, analysis of costs for 3 months of a coordinated interdisciplinary service for patients and their families, that includes an average of 21 home care visits and 18 inpatient days, would cost about

$2600 in an urban New England community.* Comparatively, the cost is greater than nursing home care but less than hospital care in the same region. Cost estimates at St. Christopher's Hospice in England parallel these figures.

Prolongation of Life. Suicide, Euthanasia, and Homicide. Hospice care and palliative treatment are alternatives to be distinguished from *prolonging life* that has lost its meaning and from *euthanasia* which solves the dilemma by shortening life. The distinction between hospice care and euthanasia is of utmost importance. The purpose of a hospice is to make life livable again and so provide the patient and family with time for growth and achievement. Medical, psychosocial, pharmacologic, and nursing assessment of the person's symptoms and relief through palliative treatment is the essential first step.

Many critics of medical management that appears to deny death—keeping the patient alive when life is purposeless and often uncomfortable or painful—use the expression *prolonged dying*. Many people who dread weeks, months, or maybe years in an institution where

* These estimates are based on per diem costs calculated for New Haven by a hospice planning staff in collaboration with the Connecticut Hospital Association.

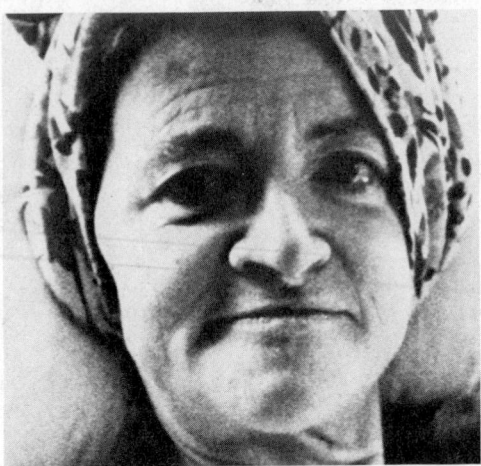

A. The story of Sally. "Before I was sick, I was a big, healthy redhead climbing mountains all over and having a wonderful time and mowing lawns and just having a nice time. And then, down, down, down. . . ."

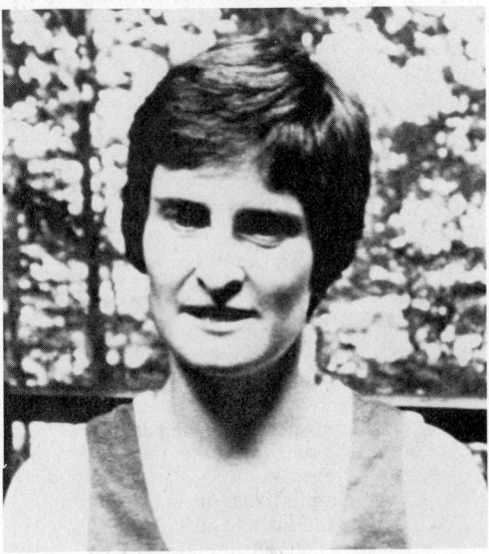

C. The story of Sandy and Mark. "In a strange way it was a good day. We were able to share things. I read to Mark. I gave him his last bath. Then in the early evening he kissed me and said, 'Let's call it quits, Pooh.' And he died about a half-hour later."

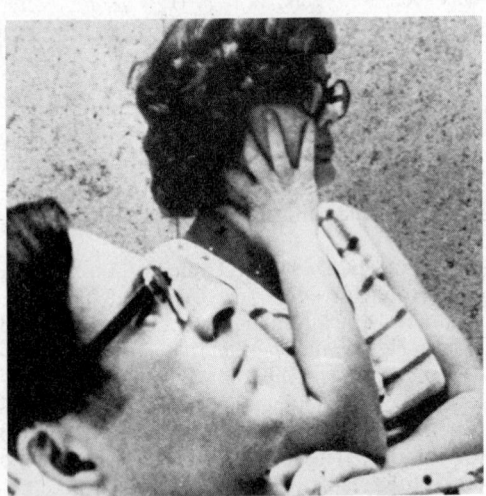

B. The story of Harriet and Bill. "And he even said, 'What happened to the sweet girl I married?' And I said, 'The sweet girl you married is being tortured by this cancer.'"

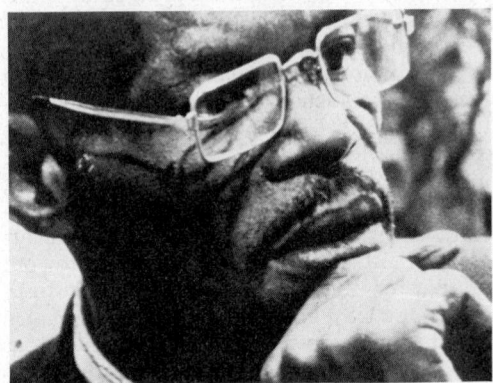

D. The story of the Reverend Bryant. "I can say right now that I'm living some of the greatest moments in life. If I should use a name—I don't think that Rockefeller could be as happy a man as I am. I am the most happiest man in the world. Even though the doctor has told me that I didn't have long to live, the time that I have on the topside of this earth, I'm going to live out the happiest and best that I know how."

Figure 50-2. Four approaches to death as told by the subjects and their families. (From the film *Dying*, a production of WGBH of Boston for Public Broadcasting System. Courtesy WGBH and PBS. Film Director, Michael Roemer. 1976.)

they are kept alive with infusions, drugs, and oxygen, are signing the statement called *A Living Will.* Marya Mannes,[9] in *Last Rights,* reports that in 1972 more than 50,000 persons wrote to the Euthanasia Educational Fund in New York City for free copies of this will and that the number of requests is rising steadily. The "Will" is a statement addressed to the subject's family, physician, and clergyman (see Fig. 50-3). At the time of this writing the Living Will is not legally binding, but it is not apt to be ignored by those to whom it is addressed, and attempts are being made in courts of law to make it legal. During the writing and publication of this book too many cases and state decisions were reported to keep information current and complete.

Many major works on death and dying discuss the social, ethical, moral, religious, and legal aspects of allowing a person to die, of withholding life-prolonging treatment, and even of terminating life when it seems purposeless and painful, but it is impossible here to review the various points of view. J. H. Hall and D. D. Swenson [10] say that Alexis Carrel and C. C. Guthrie, in 1905, demonstrated in animals the feasibility of transplanting veins and organs. The achievements in human surgery since then are well known.

Lifton and Olson [11] think "the most absolute effort to stave off final extinction" is *freezing bodies* immediately after death on the assumption that they can be brought back to life and cured when effective treatment for the disease causing death is discovered.

*Cryptobiosi*s is the term applied to the death-

TO MY FAMILY, MY PHYSICIAN, MY LAWYER, MY CLERGYMAN
TO ANY MEDICAL FACILITY IN WHOSE CARE I HAPPEN TO BE
TO ANY INDIVIDUAL WHO MAY BECOME RESPONSIBLE FOR MY HEALTH, WELFARE OR
AFFAIRS

Death is as much a reality as birth, growth, maturity and old age—it is the one certainty of life. If the time comes when I, _____ can no longer take part in decisions for my own future, let this statement stand as an expression of my wishes, while I am still of sound mind.

If the situation should arise in which there is no reasonable expectation of my recovery from physical or mental disability, I request that I be allowed to die and not be kept alive by artificial means or "heroic measures". I do not fear death itself as much as the indignities of deterioration, dependence and hopeless pain. I, therefore, ask that medication be mercifully administered to me to alleviate suffering even though this may hasten the moment of death.

This request is made after careful consideration. I hope you who care for me will feel morally bound to follow its mandate. I recognize that this appears to place a heavy responsibility upon you, but it is with the intention of relieving you of such responsibility and of placing it upon myself in accordance with my strong convictions, that this statement is made.

Signed _____

Date _____

Witness _____

Witness _____

Copies of this request have been given to _____

_____

_____

_____

Figure 50-3. Called a "Living Will," this is a formal request to the signer's family or others concerned with the signer's wish to avoid "heroic" measures to prolong life in the face of irreversible illness. (Reprinted with permission of the Euthanasia Educational Council, 250 W. 57th St., New York, N.Y. 10019.)

like state of certain animals that have been almost completely dehydrated. Even after decades, when such animals are moistened they survive. John H. Crowe and Alan F. Cooper [12] say that some nematodes have been revived after 39 years in a dried condition. They note that Anton van Leeuwenhoek was aware in 1702 of suspended animation due to water loss and the revival of the organism when moistened. This phenomenon suggests that suspension of metabolism can't be used as a criterion of death in certain forms of life. Crowe and Cooper suggest that for such organisms the loss of structural integrity must be the criterion of death. Freezing and cryptobiosis are not, so far as we know, seriously considered for human beings, but discussion of them has given rise to fiction and drama based on their possibilities. *

Nurses, like anyone else, may wonder whether prolonging life is merciful, or ethically defensible, especially when patients seem to be hopelessly ill and when the nurses believe that the patients and their families are ready to accept death. While nurses may themselves suffer in such situations, they must realize that physicians, who bear a heavy load in reaching crucial therapeutic decisions, are equally troubled. No aspect of medical practice is more difficult than decisions on prolonging life in the face of weakness, disease, or the wishes of patients to terminate life. The training of a physician is focused on prolongation of life, and it is often remarked that for a physician death spells defeat. It is usually said that the Hippocratic Oath taken by many graduating classes of medical students commits them to the principle of prolonging life, but only in the following paragraph is this even suggested:

I will follow that system of regimen which, according to my ability and judgment, I consider for the benefit of my patients, and abstain from whatever is deleterious and mischievous. I will give no deadly medicine to anyone if asked, nor suggest any such counsel; and in like manner I will not give to a woman a pessary to produce abortion. With purity and with holiness I will pass my life and practise my Art.†

Some medical schools have substituted in commencement exercises the Maimonides Physician's Prayer [12a] which includes many of the ethical principles in the Hippocratic Oath but is not as binding in respect to prolonging life as the Hippocratic Oath is considered to be. David Israel Macht, in his 1905 memorial address, gives the following version of this "invocation" which Maimonides was "said to have repeated daily."

And now, I turn unto my calling;
Oh, stand by me, my God, in this truly important task!
Grant me success! For—
Without Thy loving counsel and support,
Man can avail but naught.
Inspire me with true love for this my art
And for Thy cre-a-tures,
Oh, grant—
That neither greed for gain, nor thirst for fame, nor vain ambition,
May interfere with my activity.
For these, I know, are enemies of Truth and Love of men,
And might beguile one in profession
From furthering the welfare of Thy creatures.
Oh, strengthen me!
Grant energy unto both body and the soul,
That I may e'er unhindered ready be
To mitigate the woes,
Sustain and help,
The rich and poor, the good and bad, the enemy and friend,
Oh, let me e'er behold in the afflicted and the suffering,
Only the human being! *

Morris Wessel, in an article describing newly developing medical approaches to the terminally ill, used the words of Edward Trudeau, eminent tuberculosis expert, "To cure sometimes, to relieve often, to comfort always" in the title of his article published in the *Yale Alumnae Magazine* (June, 1972, p. 19).

Bayless Manning, dean of the law school at Stanford (Calif.) University, who discusses "Legal and Policy Issues in the Allocation of Death," notes that today's life-saving technology forces doctors to make decisions on the following: drugs, surgical techniques, implements and therapies in attacking the patient's problem. He says doctors must decide "which of these to draw upon, to what extent, and for how long, where." He adds:

The effect of the treatment will be to prolong the circulatory and respiratory life of the patient, but will leave him permanently comatose.

The effect of the treatment will be to preserve his "life" in the sense that the patient will be conscious and able to communicate, but will also permanently strip him of all physical mobility, forcing him to complete dependence upon full-time attendants for all his bodily wants.

---

* Woody Allen's American film *Sleeper* is a comedy based on the possibility of making viable after decades a human body held in suspended animation by lowered temperature.

† Jones, Harold Wellington, et al. (eds.): *Blakiston's—The New Gould Medical Dictionary*, 1st ed. Blakiston Co., Philadelphia, Pa., 1949, p. 465.

* Macht, David Israel: "Moses Maimonides (In Memoriam 1205–1905 C.E.)," *Johns Hopkins Hosp. Bull.*, **17**:1, (No. 187) (Oct.) 1906.

The effect of the treatment will be to restore his bodily activity and his mental competence to communicate, but will completely destroy the existing personality structure.

The effect of the treatment will be the economic obliteration of the patient and his entire family.

The effect of the treatment will be to divert to the permanent monopoly use of this patient scarce equipment or resources, thus producing the certain death of other patients.

The effect of the treatment will be to restore the patient to a state of life and health which he has already found intolerable and which he, and all members of his family, implore the doctor not to restore.*

Manning points out that termination of treatment at patients' requests can be interpreted as helping them commit suicide and in so doing physicians risk "civil liability." He adds: "Consent by the next of kin to the termination of medical care is not likely to stand the doctor in any better stead in the event of indictment" under the Wrongful Death Statute. While Manning thinks physicians' decisions are "not easy," now he also believes that they may be yet more difficult when the public fully realizes the power residing in medical technology to improve the quality and increase the length of life. He thinks society will eventually realize that "the widespread application of that technology [including genetics] would produce a wholly different society. No aspect of economic or social life would stay as it is today."

Manning thinks the length of life today depends largely on economic status, certainly in relation to developed countries.† He says, "it has always been true that the well-to-do have been able to command better medical attention than other men, and that their chances of health and long life are better." He thinks that "so long as medical services are privately financed by the patient, rapid advances of medical technology will make it glaringly apparent that the rich can live longer but the poor must die." ‡

Manning is asking for recognition of the complexity of the problem, for centers where such problems would be identified and studied,

and for a democratic system that would give mankind equal treatment when it comes to decisions on the quality and length of life. Any health worker inclined to question the judgment of physicians should realize that physicians are subject to charges of neglect and to civil and criminal liability. To quote Manning:

The doctor and his co-workers are as subject to the laws of homicide as other citizens, and the doctor's patient is as entitled to the protection of the homicide laws as any other victim. In fact, however, very few indictments have ever been brought against doctors for murdering patients, or even for manslaughter. Where such situations have arisen the circumstances have differed entirely from the topic at hand; the homicide charge might have arisen, for example, out of a love triangle, and the manslaughter charge out of the doctor's allegedly inept performance of his medical responsibilities. Occasionally one hears reports of doctors involved in "mercy killing," but so far at least criminal prosecutions on that theory have not found their way into the recorded cases.

What does the future hold in store on this point? One suspects that the heightened public perception of the physician's effective power to allocate death will tend to reduce the traditional unquestioning confidence in the physician's position, and may in time, lead some . . . prosecutor to file a homicide indictment against the physician.*

In January 1977, Joseph M. Healy, a lawyer on the faculty of the University of Connecticut, reported at a Colloquia on the Humanities and Death that there are already eight published volumes on legal decisions in the Karen Quinlan case.

Quakers are known throughout the world for their respect for life, their pacifism, and their simultaneous acceptance by both armies of warring countries just as Red Cross workers are accepted as neutral agents. In 1970 a committee composed of six physicians, a medical social worker, and a Protestant minister wrote a report for the American Friends Service Committee titled *Who Shall Live? Man's Control Over Birth and Death*. Among the committee's "answers for today" is the following statement:

We approve withholding therapy or withdrawing the supportive therapy that is keeping an unconscious person alive if, by evidence of brain death or such other evidence as the medical profession deems valid, it is the best judgment of the medical profession that the patient's brain is irreparably damaged and he will never recover consciousness.†

* Manning, Bayless: "Legal and Policy Issues in the Allocation of Death," in Brim, Orville G., Jr., et al. (eds.): *The Dying Patient*. Russell Sage Foundation, New York, 1970, p. 257.

† Victor R. Fuchs would question this. He says: "A second profound change is the disappearance of the traditional relationship between life expectancy and per capita income. As with medical care a certain minimum level of income is important, but beyond that there is little correlation between mortality and income across and within industrialized countries." (Fuchs, Victor R.: *Who Shall Live? Health, Economics, and Social Choice*. Basic Books, New York, 1974, p. 31.)

‡ Manning, Bayless: *op. cit.*, pp. 271, 273.

* *Ibid.*, p. 257.

† American Friends Service Committee: *Who Shall Live? Man's Control Over Birth and Death*. Hill & Wang, New York, 1970, p. 70.

Joseph F. Fletcher, a professor of Christian ethics, believes that the decision to prolong or shorten the dying process should not be made by the physician alone. He makes the following statement:

I would myself agree with Pope Pius XII, and with at least two Archbishops of Canterbury (Lang and Fisher) . . . that the doctor's technical knowledge, his "educated guesses" and experience, should be the basis for deciding the question as to whether there is any "reasonable hope." . . . But, having determined that a condition is hopeless, I cannot agree that it is either prudent or fair to physicians as a fraternity to saddle them with the onus of alone deciding whether to let the patient go. Here is a point at which, if the patient is beyond competent consent, the family and friends must accept their share of the responsibility of loving relationship, just as they would for a child or a psychotic or a patient in coma.*

This plea for shared responsibility in decisions on prolonging life (or prolonging the process of dying) would probably be echoed by many physicians. While under the present laws they may be held most responsible, relatives, friends, and nurses who are with patients most constantly may have more intimate knowledge of the patients' suffering and of their readiness to die than has the doctor.

Bills to legalize *euthanasia* in England in 1936 and 1969 were defeated in the House of Lords, according to Hinton. Hinton, a physician who has devoted much of his life to studying the care of the terminally ill, opposes it, and says, "It seems a terrible indictment that the main argument for euthanasia is that many suffer unduly because there is a lack of preparation and provision for the total care of the dying" † Fred Rosner [12b] surveys the varying national attitudes toward, and laws on, euthanasia. According to him, Switzerland had the most lenient legislation at the time he was writing.

Earlier in this chapter, reference was made to the fact that helping a person to die can be interpreted as helping him to commit *suicide*, which is punishable by law.‡ It is an antisocial act in most cultures and most eras, and it is sometimes noted that animals, in contrast to humans, never take their own lives. This is debatable, however. Sick dogs often disappear from a household where every effort is being made to help them. It is commonly thought, as Thomas [13] has suggested, that they instinctively hasten death and seek the hidden way of dying.

Suicide, chiefly as an escape from depression, is discussed in Chapter 41. Sidney M. Jourard [14] thinks suicide is the answer to "an invitation to die" from relatives, friends, or society in general. The guilt felt by others when a person commits suicide helps explain society's condemnation of the act. It was pointed out in Chapter 41, however, that in some cultures and certain eras, suicide has been commendable under some circumstances. Socrates chose the self-administered cup of hemlock and, according to the record of his followers, who spent hours before his death in philosophic discourse, died a heroic death.[15] Prominent Romans, in disfavor with their rulers, were thought nobler if they died by their own hands than if they accepted death by Caesar's edict; and their wives often chose to die with them. The Japanese, even in recent times, have elected suicide rather than dishonor their country or their family by dying at the hands of their enemy.

Melba W. Shepard,[16] a nurse of this era, suggests that the elderly in contemporary society have every reason to prefer suicide to an aimless existence and lingering death in a hospital or nursing home. Another contemporary viewpoint on suicide is Lael T. Wertenbaker's [17] account of the illness leading up to her husband's suicide and her role in helping him end his life.* Both of these publications were answered by a representative of the Roman Catholic faith. Sister Bernadette Armiger says in "Reprise and Dialogue":

Christian ethics teaches that it is not necessary to use extraordinary means, such as a heart transplant, to *preserve* life. But to take positive means to terminate life by injection, or pill, with or without the consent of the patient, is contrary to both divine and human law.

. . .

As nurses who are deeply committed to societal needs, let us bend our professional strength to help right the wrongs in the geriatric wards of city hospitals and nursing homes. These are not impossible dreams, but if they may seem to be, we may strive to "exhaust the field of the possible" in order to assist the aging to live out their last years in tranquility and prepare peacefully for unending life.†

---

* Fletcher, Joseph F.: "Anti-dysthanasia: The Problem of Prolonging Death," in Reeves, Robert B., Jr., et al. (comps. and eds.): *Pastoral Care of the Dying and Bereaved: Selected Readings.* Health Sciences Publishing Corp., New York, 1973, p. 157.

† Hinton, John: *Dying,* 2nd ed. Penguin Books, Harmondsworth, Eng., 1972, p. 148.

‡ The literature on suicide is extensive. C. Killick Millard, in 1931, reviewed the literature, in poetry and prose, on suicide with special attention to "The Legislation of Voluntary Euthanasia" (*Public Health* [*London*], **45**:39, [Nov.] 1931.)

* This book was dramatized into a successful play starring Henry Fonda.

† Armiger, Sister Bernadette: "Reprise and Dialogue," *Nurs. Outlook,* **16**:26, (Oct.) 1968.

Arnold A. Hutschnecker, discussing personality factors in dying patients, quotes Bernard Shaw, an avowed agnostic, as saying when he was 94: "The will to live is wholly inexplicable. Rationally I ought to blow my brains out, but I don't and I won't." * This will to live is believed by most persons to be "normal," whatever that is, and death by suicide abnormal, unusual, or wrong. Health workers are committed to saving the lives of those they find attempting suicide, and should be prepared to offer special help to surviving relatives and friends in both abortive and successful suicide attempts because they are so traumatic.

Dictionaries equate *euthanasia* (*eu* = well, good, or pleasant, *thanatos* = death) with *"mercy killing"*—the act of putting to death painlessly a person suffering from an incurable and painful disease. Like suicide, contraception, and abortion, it has been opposed on religious grounds as being contrary to the natural, or divine, order.

According to Mannes,[18] the Euthanasia Society of London (Eng.) was formed in 1935 (Rosner says by a doctor [19]), the American Euthanasia Society incorporating the Euthanasia Educational Fund in 1938, and the Euthanasia Society of the Netherlands in 1973. Mannes, spokesman for euthanasia and for allowing all citizens to choose the manner in which they die, in *Last Rights* speaks eloquently against the prolongation of life past its useful or satisfying stage—most particularly delaying the death of the person in irreversible coma. Quoting several poets, she says that "the open dialogue of death is [now] far more pragmatic than poetic because machines control the timing—*and* definition—of death." † She cites the observation of Henry Beecher, a physician, who said recently that we are entering an era "where to do nothing is far more radical than to do something." He cites the case of a 21-year-old woman in Montreal who was kept alive for 12 years in an unconscious state, keeping 312 patients out of the hospital bed she occupied.[20] This is an age in which violent death by warfare is still condoned, but physicians may be prosecuted if they terminate oxygen administration or intravenous feedings for the hopelessly ill. Shirley J. Braverman,[21] a young nurse, gives a poignant description of her own suffering as she watched "the death

of a monster." While she realized that this pitifully deformed, scarcely viable infant could never live in the true sense of the word, she felt guilty in not trying to prolong his life.*

While Mannes [22] thinks there is a "rising chorus" in support of euthanasia, she admits that "religious scruples" are not the only barriers to euthanasia. She thinks moral and ethical codes prohibit it for many, and few have the courage to carry out their convictions. She sees in the hospice movement, as described on page 176, an "alternative" for euthanasia and credits certain chronic disease hospitals, such as Calvary in New York City and Youville in Cambridge, Mass., as offering patients hope of what might be called a good death.

Margaret Mead, an anthropologist who is fully aware of the ways in which various cultures have limited their populations for the sake of survival, discusses the "right to die" in this society. While she thinks medical workers should respect the patient's right to refuse treatment and questions keeping people alive when their "brains" have ceased to function and thinks that the threat of this "hangs over all Americans," she seems in the following statement to question mercy killing:

Yet it is an essential part of our present medical progress that physicians and nurses are pledged to preserve life, in every person, regardless of age or sex, race or status, as long as the last breath of life flickers within him. Without this pledge, we would not have modern medical care. But with it we face this new problem of the stricken or the elderly who are preserved far beyond what they or those who love them would choose for them.

We cannot ask either physician or nurse for relief. They must remain absolutely pledged to life. But there is another recourse. If an individual is conscious, he may refuse an operation, or a blood transfusion, or any other medical remedy that is recommended. And just as it is possible to make a will, stating that one is of sound mind, many years before one's death, so it is possible to make a legal statement—while one is of sound mind—forbidding medical intervention which may result in states, which, while called life, nevertheless mean a life without meaning, when one is only a burden to others. Just as a physician honors a patient's refusal of surgery, so such a duly executed statement can be honored. Once made, it means that the old can live out their lives without the haunting fear of witless dependency.†

* "Off-duty" at last and freed from the dying infant's wails, she describes her return to the room where he was, the way the infant grasped her hair and uniform as she took him in her arms, and how he, in that moment, died—quietly. She was comforted by having offered a compassionate response to his suffering and having evoked a response, even though she knew it was only a reflex movement.

† Mead, Margaret: "The Right to Die," *Nurs. Outlook,* **16:**22, (Oct.) 1968.

---

* Hutschnecker, Arnold A.: "Personality Factors in Dying Patients," in Feifel, Herman (ed.): *The Meaning of Death.* McGraw-Hill Book Co., New York, 1959, p. 247.

† Mannes, Marya: *Last Rights. A Case for the Good Death.* William Morrow & Co., New York, 1974, pp. 57, 58.

Many persons think it a risky business to legalize euthanasia. Manning [23] says that while most animals display an inhibition against killing their own kind, "Man has little such reluctance." While he is certainly not suggesting that patients are in danger of being killed by medical personnel, he does imply that both patients and the physician are protected by the latter's scrupulous adherence to the principle of prolonging life.

Homicide, or *death by violence,* has been made commonplace in this age through world wars and the proliferation of communication networks, but it does not seem to have brought an acceptance of death. Lifton and Olson are among the social scientists who think this an era that stresses youth, rejects the aged, and denies death. They say, "Death has now become unacceptable because it is associated with images of absurd holocaust and annihilation and because our lives have become rootless and disconnected." * Philippe Ariès [24] makes the point that the role played by the elderly differs from age to age and within each age according to the culture to which dying persons belong. In the Middle Ages the dying played the central role in a supernatural drama, whereas he says modern man has been "robbed" of the experience; we die in the isolation of hospital, alone, except for medical technicians who are strangers. We are often drugged into unconsciousness. While contemporary man may die in isolation and many persons may grow to adulthood without seeing the dying process, television has made death by violence a common sight.† Ours is often referred to as a violent age but it may be forgotten that it has never before been possible to see violence and its aftermath on a worldwide scale. This constant exposure to the sight of violence is thought by some persons to make people indifferent to suffering and death; it is also thought to make people more aware and fearful of death. Since this immediate exposure to worldwide death is a relatively new phenomenon, it is obviously hard to assess its effects accurately. Meanwhile, educational and experimental television programs are also beginning to deal with death. CBS has devoted several panel discussions to it, with professionals caring for dying persons expressing varied points of view, and NET has prepared documentaries showing the relationships possible when a whole family works to make it possible for a grandparent to live and die at home.

Personnel in emergency rooms of large urban hospitals have what amounts to, in some cities, an overwhelming exposure to homicide and the nearly lethal effects of violence. Jan de Hartog's [25] description in *The Hospital* of an emergency room in a Texas hospital includes a report of staff illness and turnover, clearly indicating the strain of trying to save the mangled bodies and tortured minds. While people may develop a technique that lessens the drain on their feelings and makes them seem callous, it is doubtful whether health personnel can be unaffected by the sights and sounds of suffering. At conferences for persons who are professionally involved in caring for the dying, a recurring theme is care for the caregivers. In lecturing Elisabeth Kübler-Ross has proposed that a "screaming room" be made available for staff members where they can release their feelings.* The architect, Lo-Yi Chan,[25a] includes a staff screaming room in his design of the Hospice in Branford, Connecticut. It is a completely carpeted space at the top of the building with a view of the sky through a dome—no other windows and no furnishings except pillows and beanbags.

Michael Crichton, in *Five Patients. The Hospital Explained,* says that the modern (general) hospital in recognizable form is less than 50 years old. He thinks it is changing rapidly and that more and more it will be devoted to the care of the acutely ill and to research. Crichton describes a series of emergency room admissions at the Massachusetts General Hospital during one night. He quotes an undergraduate college student, working on a computer project, as saying: "I don't know how anybody can stand to work here." Crichton says:

The ER is the place where the haste, the crowding, and impersonality [of the hospital] are seen

---

* Lifton, Robert Jay, and Olson, Eric: *op. cit.,* p. 29.

† According to Fuchs, "Accidents, suicide, homicide—deaths from violence in one form or another account for *three out of every four* male deaths in this age group [15 to 24 years]. Twenty years ago, the overall death rate among this age group was 15 percent lower, and the rate for violent deaths was 40 percent lower! The increase since then can hardly be attributed to a deterioration in medical care. On the contrary, the treatment of trauma is an area of medicine that has seen particularly significant advances, and there are undoubtedly many victims of violence being saved today who would have died two decades ago. Numerous theories have been advanced to explain the increase in violent deaths among the young—affluence, the Vietnam war, the decline in religious belief, overly permissive parents, and so on—but the only thing we can be certain of is the increase itself. The suspicion also exists that the self-destructiveness of the young is a symptom of more widespread problems in society at large." (Fuchs, Victor R.: *op. cit.,* p. 42.)

* Discussed at the International Work Group in Death, Dying and Bereavement, Columbia, Md., Nov. 1974.

in their most exaggerated form. . . . Its growth in recent years has been phenomenal. Its patient load is increasing steadily at the rate of 10 per cent per year. . . . It now treats more than 65,000 patients a year.*

In the past decade palliative treatment for patients with terminal illness, particularly with cancer, has been developed as an alternative method of care when aggressive curative treatment does not change the course of the disease and does further reduce the patient's quality of life to a miserable existence. Cicely Saunders, Medical Director of St. Christopher's Hospice, has been the prime force in this movement which links expert medical management with spiritual support for patient and family. Because this treatment improves the quality of life, the need to turn to euthanasia or suicide is diminished.

Any consideration of the care of the dying and attitudes toward death must take into account the great variety of settings in which death occurs and the difficulty that is encountered in giving life-saving care, and at the same time attending to the psychosocial needs of those involved—patients, their relatives, and friends. Nevertheless, it is important that health workers try to develop conditions in emergency rooms, in industrial health services, in military field stations, in prisons and everywhere death occurs that make it possible to work through some of the stress suffered by those involved. The work of Mother Teresa and her Missionaries of Charity in taking care of the destitute and dying in Calcutta may be the ultimate example. Malcolm Muggeridge's acount in an illustrated paperback, *Something Beautiful for God*,[25b] describes her work.

Preparing Health Workers to Help the Terminally Ill. It is hard to say when special preparation for giving terminal care began. The example set by saintly individuals and religious groups in serving the hopelessly ill and dying throughout history has been a potent influence on society. Most present-day hospices include spiritul care for patients and, even though the search for the meaning of life varies among patients, those involved must have time and support in that search. Persons far from home or without wealth often went to such hospices to die or, if they had the means, sought the help of workers trained in them. But the present-day emphasis on palliative treatment in terminal care is of recent origin. William Osler [26] and Alfred Worcester [27] are physicians now dead whose teaching and writing have influenced medical workers through-

out this century. Richard C. Cabot, a physician, and Russell L. Dicks, a clergyman, collaborated on a text, *The Art of Ministering to the Sick*,[28] that stressed the psychosocial and religious needs of the dying. Saunders, a nurse, social worker, and physican, has been writing for the last two decades on care of the dying with special attention to palliative treatment and spiritual care, and being available and able to answer questions patients ask about their condition.[29-33] Most large hospitals have chapels and visiting or resident clergy available to the critically ill. Internships and residencies for hospital chaplains are not new, but they are increasingly common, and a body of literature is developing around the function of spiritual ministry for the sick.

In 1959, under the editorship of Herman Feifel, *The Meaning of Death* was published, which he implies is the first "multifaceted" approach. Contributions from "anthropology, art, literature, medicine, philosophy, physiology, psychoanalysis, psychiatry, psychology, and religion" were included in this "common area," * and suggest the need for preparing everyone to face death and dying, but particularly those who are cast in helping roles. Gardner Murphy, discussing or summarizing the contents of this volume, comes to the following conclusions:

I would think that we face a great big job, and I think Dr. Feifel in organizing this has started us on our way. I would think, however, that perhaps the next few jobs to be done would all involve, in various ways, the study of the . . . complexity of this attitude syndrome, the . . . undefined factors—psychological, biological, cultural . . . in the . . . system of ideas, including the limitations of each one of us, depending upon his own special bias to the subject.†

During and since the publication of this volume, the proliferation of books and articles about death, dying, and bereavement continues to document interdisciplinary efforts; some are reports of carefully structured investigations that focus on preparing health workers to recognize and help meet the needs of the dying patient. The *Archives of the Foundation of Thanatology* has been published since 1968, and *Omega, the Journal on Death and Dying* was started in 1969. Both publications stress the inclusion of this subject in health curricula and in health science libraries.

In 1967, Jeanne C. Quint, a nurse and sociologist, published *The Nurse and the Dying*

---

* Crichton, Michael. *Five Patients. The Hospital Explained.* Alfred A. Knopf, New York, 1970, p. 20.

* Feifel, Herman (ed.): *The Meaning of Death.* McGraw-Hill Book Co., New York, 1959, p. vii.
† Murphy, Gardner: "Discussion," in Feifel, Herman (ed.): *The Meaning of Death.* McGraw-Hill Book Co., New York, 1959, p. 339.

Patient,[34] which was part of a 5-year investigation of death and dying in the San Francisco area under the direction of Anselm L. Strauss, a sociologist. With Barney G. Glaser, his co-author, Strauss published *Awareness of Dying*[35] in 1965 and *Time for Dying*[36] in 1968. Read in conjunction, these volumes and related articles give a discouraging picture of the care of dying patients in general hospitals. Glaser, Strauss, and Quint found that health workers withdrew from the dying patient and changed the subject or cut off conversations in which patients hinted at or talked openly about death and dying. One student nurse questioned by Quint writes:

Two days later I found another patient dead, which was really something. I found the staff very helpful. When the one nurse told me to go ahead into the utility room, they didn't seem to look down on me because I was having a little problem with this—expecting it, getting used to it. They seemed to take it matter-of-factly, which at the time I wasn't. Nothing was ever said afterward about my not taking my responsibilities after this person died, since he was my patient.*

While it may have been a most unusual circumstance, the fact that one student, within 2 days, found two patients who had died alone bears out the investigator's impression that medical workers did, indeed, withdraw from dying patients in this institution. Quint's emphasis is more on the nurse than the patient, and her "implications for change" focus on the education of nurses and interdisciplinary education; reassessment of "cultural values" and nursing practices; the importance of the nurse assuming responsibility for her acts; the development of better communication between nurses, physicians, and others; greater recognition of the psychosocial needs of patients; planned instructions on care of the dying person by prepared faculty who can act as role models when students have assigned experience in situations where it is possible to supply the kind of care that dying patients need. Quint [37] noted that nurse-teachers stressed the individual nurse's responsibility for what happens to dying patients, but that in practice it was almost impossible for the young nurse to accept the responsibility and act upon it. Curricula of nursing and medical schools offered little on the moral, ethical, and legal aspects of care in terminal illness, especially the patient's right to know when his or her own life is at stake (one of the recently listed rights in the American Hospital Association's *A Patient's Bill of Rights*).[38] In addition to scoring

curricula for little attention to the care of the dying, Quint noted that poor communication between physician and nurse, and an absence of professionals to serve as role models, made it nearly impossible for the nurse to accept responsibility and accountability for the care of the dying patient. Many changes since then are helping physicians, nurses, and other health workers to meet the needs of dying patients and their families, but Balfour M. Mount's [39] study of attitudes toward death and dying made in 1974 in a teaching hospital (the Royal Victoria Hospital, Montreal, Canada) shows that conditions still leave much to be desired. Noting that the majority of nurses and doctors did not respond to the questionnaire he circulated, Mount interprets this as a form of denial, and he reported that those who did answer the questionnaire showed, in many cases, that they avoid discussion of death.

In the Western world there are numerous seminars, workshops, and other kinds of learning sessions on death and dying. The Foundation of Thanatology in New York, the Society for Health and Human Values and the Ars Moriendi in Philadelphia, and the Equinox Group in Boston are some of the interdisciplinary bodies with regular forums for the exchange of ideas. Saunders has spoken on many continents. Kübler-Ross, whose work with the dying in Chicago hospitals has been widely publicized, has given lectures, seminars, and workshops throughout North America, bringing new insights to thousands of caregivers. St. Christopher's Hospice in England with its fifty-six inpatient service and a home care program for an even greater number of patients, serves as a teaching center for nurses, physicians, clergymen, social workers, and interested laymen. Work experience there, as well as discussions and guided tours, is helping society to see where dying fits into life and how health professionals, and society in general, can respond to such questions as "Shall we never stop trying?" and "How can we help those who face death?"

As other hospices have developed throughout Great Britain and in the United States, several now share the responsibility for teaching and evaluation. The founders of the Hospice in New Haven, Conn., of the Palliative Treatment Unit in the Royal Victoria Hospital in Montreal, Canada, and of the Hospice Center, St. Luke's Hospital in New York City all spent many months at St. Christopher's studying its approach.

Medical and nursing schools have introduced courses of varying lengths into their curricula. Bernard Schoenberg and Arthur C. Carr report in 1972 surveys conducted by the

---

* Quint, Jeanne C.: *The Nurse and the Dying Patient.* Macmillan Publishing Co., Inc., New York, 1967, p. 137.

Foundation of Thanatology of 168 medical schools and 97 nursing schools in the United States to see whether professionals are educated in the psychosocial care of the terminally ill. Responses indicate that their preparation is far from adequate in any respect. For instance, 48.1 per cent of the respondents reported that the requirements for the diagnosis of death were not "included formally" in the medical school curriculum and over one third of the respondents said that the physician's responsibility for the care of the bereaved was not included in the curriculum. While data from the nursing schools indicate that neither faculty nor students are satisfied, Schoenberg and Carr make the following comparison:

Results of a similar survey of the deans of ninety-seven nursing schools support the impression that nursing schools probably are much more concerned, both theoretically and in a practical way, with training students to handle and console dying patients and the bereaved than are medical schools.*

Austin H. Kutscher, a dental educator at the Columbia University School of Dental and Oral Surgery, New York City, reports that a survey has been made of dental schools to see what is being taught and what should be taught about dental care for dying patients, with special emphasis on the needs of patients with cancer. He thinks "The training of such

a corps of dental practitioners and dental hygienists will require efforts similar to those which should be employed for physicians and nurses." *

In 1974, at the University of Washington School of Nursing, Seattle, Jeanne Quint Benoliel taught a two-term course for graduate nurses titled Death Influence in Clinical Practice.[40] Melvin Krant, medical director of the Cancer Unit while at Lemuel Shattuck Hospital, Boston, Mass., described an interdisciplinary program designed to increase the competence of various clinicians "in the context of dying"—"to develop new approaches for a teaching institution." [41] He and Sandra Bertman have developed a library of vignettes in the form of video tapes showing patients with advanced cancer in interaction with professionals so that they can evoke discussion about the humanistic dimensions of medical care.

At Yale University, New Haven, Conn., David Duncombe,[41a] chaplain of the Medical School, instituted an interdisciplinary seminar on death and dying in 1968. Faculty and students from the nursing, medical, law, and divinity schools and other parts of the university have participated. Patients and families who have chronic illness and face death are the teachers for the students, helping them "gain a good grasp of the sick person's world." The issues and their impact are discussed in weekly supervisory conferences with the students'

---

* Schoenberg, Bernard, and Carr, Arthur C.: "Educating the Health Professional in the Psychosocial Care of the Terminally Ill," in Schoenberg, Bernard, et al. (eds.): *Psychosocial Aspects of Terminal Care.* Columbia University Press, New York, 1972, p. 7.

* Kutscher, Austin H.: "The Psychosocial Aspects of the Oral Care of the Dying Patient," in Schoenberg, Bernard, et al. (eds.): *Psychosocial Aspects of Terminal Care.* Columbia University Press, New York, 1972, p. 130.

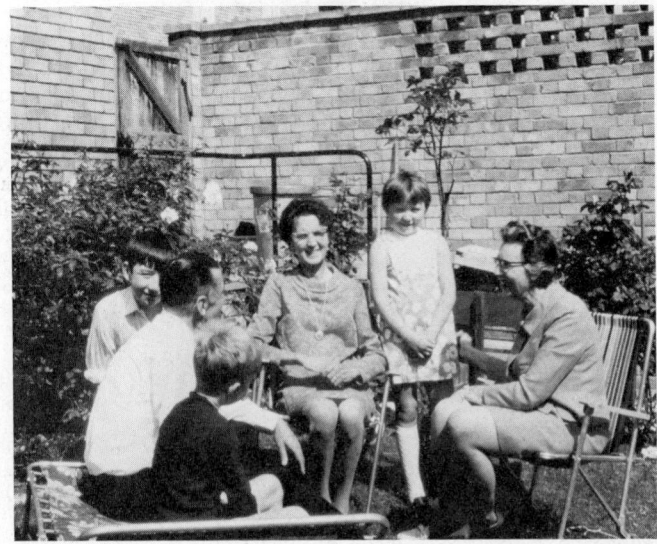

Figure 50-4. A patient referred for admission to a British hospice. After control of the physical symptoms and the establishment of confidence, she went home and is shown here taking part in family life. (Courtesy of St. Christopher's Hospice, London, England.)

peers and the course leaders. There is at Yale, to some persons, a surprising interest in studying death and dying. In the spring of 1975, James P. Carse, Visiting Lecturer in Religious Studies, offered a course, "The Meanings of Death." [42] There were 275 applicants for the 20 openings in this course. Carse taught a course on death in television's "Sunrise Semester" in 1974.

Dying is a separation. Some will face death unexpectedly, others with little notice, a few will have a long period of dying, either alert to the end or comatose. Hinton, discussing physical distress in terminal illness, gives a good deal of data on its length. While it is somewhat conflicting and confusing, he concludes by saying:

It is hard to draw any firm, simple conclusion from these diverse data, collected from different sources in various ways and with the terminal phase of an illness often difficult to define. I hope it will not be too vague or misleading a summary

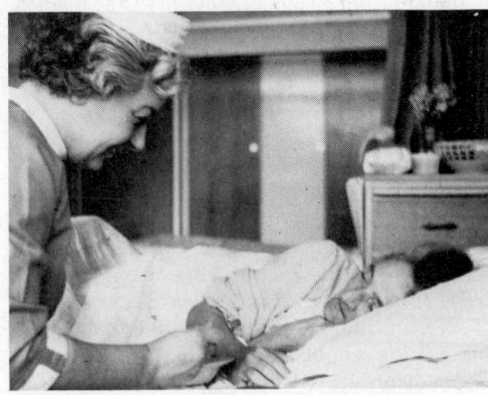

Figure 50-6. Nurse of the staff of St. Christopher's Hospice helping a patient to eat. (Courtesy of St. Christopher's Hospice, London, England.)

to say that although a small proportion are struck down suddenly and a small proportion have months of being seriously ill before they die, the majority will have a terminal period requiring special care lasting a few days or weeks and not usually exceeding three months.*

The essential ways of coping with the separation of the living and the dead are to know the physical and psychologic forces in play, to acquire the skills that mitigate pain and discomfort, to develop the ability to express and accept feelings of sadness and loss. Patients and families live through these crises each in accord with the way they cope, helping one another and using help from the outside (see Figs. 50-4, 50-5, and 50-6). Colin Murray Parkes says, "the pain of grief is just as much a part of life as the joy of love; it is, perhaps, the price we pay for love, the cost of commitment." †

The following statement by Krant may express the hope of all those who are trying to learn how to see and accept dying and death as part of life:

Our struggle is to place the human endeavor in proper perspective. From sunrise to sunset and through the dark hours, we participate in the living of a day and night. The beauty of the day culminates in the splendor of a sunset and the peace of the night. And so too with living and dying—our challenge is to bring dignity and peace to the twilight hours and into the night that follows.‡

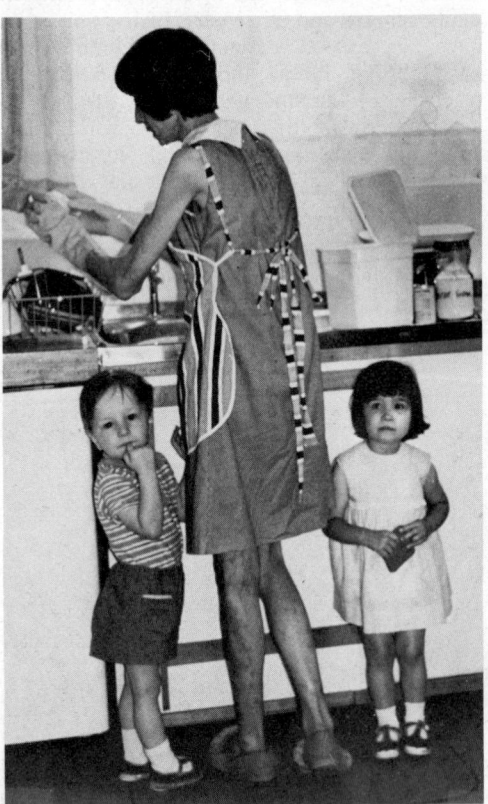

Figure 50-5. A mother and her children in their home. A picture taken three weeks before the mother's death following a two-day hospitalization at St. Christopher's Hospice. (Courtesy of St. Christopher's Hospice, London, England.)

* Hinton, John: *op. cit.*, p. 69.
† Parkes, Colin Murray: *Bereavement: Studies of Grief in Adult Life.* International Universities Press, New York, 1972, p. 5.
‡ Krant, Melvin: "In the Context of Dying," in Schoenberg, Bernard, et al. (eds.): *Psychosocial Aspects of Terminal Care.* Columbia University Press, New York, 1972, p. 209.

2. SIGNS OF APPROACHING DEATH

The Multifarious Ways of Death. There are many kinds of death, and many variations in the way its approach is manifested. George Draper, a physician who was a student of the personality, said: "And finally at the end, because his passage on earth is determined according to the patterns of his individual constitution, each man dies in a notably personal way." * Someone has said that death may come as quietly and easily as snuffing out a candle. Death may come suddenly, a few moments after the individual seemed in good health; in other cases, a person may be on the borderline between life and death for weeks. In sudden death there is no time for the failing circulation to bring about those changes in the appearance and behavior seen when death comes at the end of an illness. Worcester [43] has given a striking description of the process of death when it comes slowly and the care that should be given the dying. He does not believe that it is possible to say in any case just when the process of dying begins. He comments on the "multifarious" ways in which "death triumphs," and cautions the young doctor against expecting every patient to follow the textbook description.

A number of people have tried to find out what it is like to die suddenly. Noyes and Kletti reviewed the literature on dying from falls and translated a study reported by Albert von St. Gallen Heim, a geologist, "Remarks on Fatal Falls," published in 1892. Heim witnessed fatal falls in mountain climbing and had a near-fatal fall himself. He interviewed persons in a variety of occupations, each of whom had a brush with death. He came to the following conclusion:

In nearly 95 percent of the victims there occurred, independent of the degree of their education, thoroughly similar phenomena, experienced with only slight differences. In practically all individuals who faced death through accidental falls, a similar mental state developed. It represented quite a different state than that experienced in the face of less suddenly occurring mortal dangers. It may be briefly characterized in the following way: no grief was felt, nor was there paralyzing fright of the sort that can happen in instances of lesser danger (e.g., outbreak of fire). There was no anxiety, no trace of despair, no pain; but rather calm seriousness, profound acceptance, and a dominant mental quickness and sense of surety. Mental activity became enormous, rising to a hundred-fold velocity or intensity. The relationships of events and their probable outcomes were overviewed with objective clarity. No confusion entered at all. Time became greatly expanded. The individual acted with lightning-quickness in accord with accurate judgment of his situation. In many cases there followed a sudden review of the individual's entire past; and finally the person falling often heard beautiful music, and fell in a superbly blue heaven containing roseate cloudlets. Then consciousness was painlessly extinguished, usually at the moment of impact, and the impact was, at the most, heard but never painfully felt. Apparently hearing is the last of the senses to be extinguished.*

Heim maintained that sudden death was far more painful for the onlooker than the subject. Thomas in an essay on death reaches the same conclusions, which he puts in the following terms:

In a recent study of the reaction to dying in patients with obstructive disease of the lungs, it was concluded that the process was considerably more shattering for the professional observers than the observed. Most of the patients appeared to be preparing themselves with equanimity for death, as though intuitively familiar with the business. One elderly woman reported that the only painful and distressing part of the process was in being interrupted; on several occasions she was provided with conventional therapeutic measures to maintain oxygenation or restore fluids and electrolytes, and each time she found the experience of coming back harrowing; she deeply resented the interference with her dying.

I find myself surprised by the thought that dying is an all-right thing to do, but perhaps it should not surprise. It is, after all, the most ancient and fundamental of biologic functions, with its mechanisms worked out with the same attention to detail, the same provision for the advantage of the organism, the same abundance of genetic information for guidance through the stages, that we have long since become accustomed to finding in all the crucial acts of living.†

While sudden death and lingering death may be different, there is reason to believe that at the end they may have much in common.

Most people seem to realize that they are going to die even before signs of death are apparent to their medical attendants, although in a few instances patients appear to be unaware of their condition up to the last. This foreboding of death, when it is present, produces as profound changes in the mental outlook of the person as in the physical functions of the body. Tolstoy's story, *The Death of Ivan Ilych*,[44] is often cited as an accurate picture of the dying man's state of mind. The

---

* Draper, George, et al.: *Human Constitution in Clinical Medicine.* Paul B. Hoeber, Inc., New York, 1944, p. 74.

* Heim, Albert von St. Gallen: "Remarks on Fatal Falls," quoted in Noyes, Russell, Jr., and Kletti, Roy: "The Experience of Dying from Falls," *Omega*, 3:45, 1972.

† Thomas, Lewis: *op. cit.*, p. 51.

description of Ivan's physical suffering is less typical of this age when more is known about relieving physical symptoms.

Realization that they are dying is most likely to occur to patients while they and those caring for them—family, friends, and health workers—are under severe stress. This stress makes communication, both listening and talking, difficult. Few patients ask the direct question, "Am I dying?"; they are likely to say, "I feel I am slipping" or they may ask, "What's coming next?," "As my hand grows cold, will you hold it in your warm hand?," or "Will it be long?" These oblique messages require sensitivity to interpret and courage to answer. Oblique messages are probably a form of the symbolic language used by anyone anxious and fearful. Such direct or oblique requests that someone stay at the bedside must be seriously considered as a sign that the patient feels death is not far off. If the family is not ready to let go, its members may have great difficulty in hearing these words, and even greater difficulty in answering them. Nurses can help those involved by answering questions that others cannot, and by seeing that the person or persons whom patients want most can be with them. Nurses can support patients, family, and friends during this period of intense feeling associated with the pain of separation and the necessity of facing death in many ways.

Acceptance of Death by the Patient, the Family and Friends, and Medical Workers. The Question of Whether and When to Tell the Truth. * Many clinicians have written about the experience of dying patients in the last decade. In the United States, the writings and workshops of Kübler-Ross have greatly influenced the concepts of what it is like to die and how the dying can be helped. Kübler-Ross, a psychiatrist, has talked with thousands of terminally ill patients. At the Billings Hospital, University of Chicago, half of the 400 patients she talked with had never been told they had a serious illness, but all of them knew that they were dying. She and her colleagues believe that dying patients go through the following stages:

The stages don't always follow one another; they overlap sometimes and sometimes they go back and forth. Most patients react with shock and denial, the second most important and common response is anger, then there is the stage of bargaining, after a while the patients become silent and grieve. When the patient says, "I have now

finished all of my unfinished business. I have said all the words that have to be said. I am ready to go," the patient has reached the stage of acceptance.*

The impression she sometimes gives, that the stages occur in a regular sequence, is questioned by other physicians, as, for example, Avery D. Weisman and Cicely Saunders, and by some nurses, as, for instance, the first author of this chapter. These clinicians speculate that while dying patients show the behaviors Kübler-Ross calls "stages," the stages have no regular sequence. Expecting sequential steps can hamper more than help the physician, nurse, or family member who uses these stages as a guide. If the patient's anger is accepted as a stage or a phase that will pass, then the patient's immediate frustration over an unmet need may not be recognized, as, for example, relief from pain, getting a hot cup of coffee, or opportunity to talk frankly and openly with the physician. Another problem with the concept of stages is that if acceptance is seen as the final and ultimate goal, family, friends, physicians, and nurses may believe they have failed when patients do not accept death. Weisman uses the term "readiness to relinquish," describing it in the following terms:

. . . a conflict-less decision to relinquish life *after* primary pain and secondary suffering have been relieved. This aspect of the terminal phase is not the same as desperately wishing to die as a way out of unremitting anguish. Readiness to relinquish means that the patient is prepared to hand over decision to the counter-control of people in whom he has confidence.†

Weisman's psychiatric study of terminality, *On Dying and Denying,* is instructive for all doctors and nurses anywhere. He, in association with others, including William Worden, Robert Kastenbaum, and Thomas Hackett, has studied denial of death in patients at the Massachusetts General Hospital for years. Weisman discussed what he believed to be common misconceptions about death and denial and common fallacies about dying patients. He thought that while man recognizes the universality of death, he cannot imagine his own death. Weisman differentiates between fear of dying and the fear of death; between "annihilation anxiety" and "alienation anxiety." He thinks that fear of dying and fear of death "seldom afflict people who are face-to-face

---

* Telling the patient the truth is also discussed under the heading "Getting the House in Order" (see page 1956) and under the roles of the doctor, the nurse, and others discussed on pages 1956–67.

* Adapted from Kübler-Ross, Elisabeth: "What Is It Like to Be Dying?" *Am. J. Nurs.,* **71:**54, (Jan.) 1971.
† Weisman, Avery D.: *On Dying and Denying; A Psychiatric Study of Terminality.* Behavioral Publications, Inc., New York, 1972, p. 134.

with literal death" and he says that "To tell or not to tell is seldom an urgent question." He believes that, "contrary to popular expectations, to be informed about a diagnosis, especially a serious diagnosis, is to be fortified, not undermined." Weisman thinks that hope means that a person has confidence in the desirability of survival; but it does not depend on survival, while hopelessness is associated with diminished self-respect. He sees no conflict between hope and acceptance of death. In fact, he says, "Hope and acceptance of death are natural accompaniments of each other." [45]

Sister Madeleine Clemence Vaillot calls hope "the restoration of being"—"a plenitude of being that is always possible in spite of biologic limitations against which medicine is helpless." *

Kübler-Ross [46] makes the point that people who face death do not necessarily lose hope, but that their hopes are modified by their condition—"he . . . will alter his hopes to something which will be realistic in the face of his imminent death." Dying persons may hope to live until after Christmas or some other holiday when the family gathers; they may hope to live until a grandchild is born or until a relative comes back from overseas; the very sick and suffering may even hope that death is not far away. Certainly the sick and well think of death differently. Stewart Alsop, writing about his experience with leukemia in *Stay of Execution,* makes the following comparison:

In short, for people who are sick, to be a bit sicker—sick unto death itself—holds far fewer terrors than for people who feel well. Both Cy Sulzberger and Bill Attwood wrote me letters in which they referred to death as the Greek god, Thanatos. It was at this point that I began to think of death as Uncle Thanatos. When I felt sick enough, I even felt a certain affection for Thanatos, and much less fear of him than I had before.

I was never "half in love with easeful Death," and I suspect John Keats wasn't either. Only a psychotic really wants to die. But at least the thought of death was more easeful, and far less terrible, than it had been. Afterward, when I felt well again and believed I was cured, the thought again became very terrible.†

Some patients cared for by the first author of this chapter have found the pain, anxiety, or other symptoms of their disease so all-consuming that they have said they wished life would end. However, when palliative treatment was successful in reducing the discomfort, these same patients would sometimes retract that statement. The effects and methods of palliative treatment are discussed in a later part of this chapter.

Hinton, a British physician of wide experience with the terminally ill, has surveyed the literature on dying and death and presents a summary of his findings and those of others on "awareness and denial: struggle and acceptance." Hinton quotes Saunders as saying in *Care of the Dying:*

In my own experience I find that the truth dawns gradually on many, even most, of the dying even when they do not ask and are not told. They accept it quietly and often gratefully but some may not wish to discuss it and we must respect their reticence.*

Hinton's observations of patients in general hospitals have led him to the same conclusion. He believed acceptance of death brought peace of mind but progress toward it may be "uneven and wayward." With acceptance, an alert patient "may be quite content . . . [with] the little events of the day. . . . Many dying . . . become . . . more noble in spirit. . . . They can often accept more completely than those around them that they are about to die." †

Many who have studied terminal care recognize fear or dread of death and dying, its denial, and acceptance as part of the dying process for most persons. These states of mind are experienced by patients, their relatives and friends, and by health workers.

Studies by Glaser, Strauss, and Quint showed how difficult it is for health workers to develop an acceptance of death. They also showed that the hope of making all of life worth living for the dying enables caregivers to face death with patients and those close to them. The withdrawal of families and health workers from patients and the latter's consequent loneliness, is believed to be one of the psychosocial symptoms of death and dying. This withdrawal appears to result from a sense of helplessness and a sense that nothing more can be done. The extent to which this loneliness can be mitigated by a family member is described by Jocelyn Evans,[47] a wife who had the strength and the desire to avoid withdrawing and who nursed her husband while he was dying at home. Cicely Saunders,[47a] Thelma Ingles,[47b] Florence S. Wald and Joan Craven,[47c] and Barbara McNulty [47d] have described the care given in hospices and in the patient's

---

* Vaillot, Sister Madeleine Clemence: "Hope: The Restoration of Being," *Am. J. Nurs.,* **70:**268, (Feb.) 1970.

† Alsop, Stewart: *Stay of Execution.* J. B. Lippincott Co., Philadelphia, 1973, pp. 134, 135.

* Hinton, John: *op. cit.,* p. 95.

† *Ibid.,* 93–107.

home. In such settings, staff and family face death with the patient; first physical symptoms, including pain, are relieved. This means that life can indeed be lived until the end and the emphasis can be on living rather than on dying.

Physical Changes Signaling Death. In addition to the symptoms caused by specific diseases, with associated organic pathology, there are signs or conditions indicating the approach of death. First, there is a general slowing of the circulation shown by the fact that the feet, especially, and later the hands, ears, and nose are cold to the touch. Shakespeare noted this in *Henry V* as Mistress Quickly described the death of Falstaff—"So a' bade me lay more clothes on his feet: I put my hand into the bed and felt them, and they were as cold as any stone; then I felt to his knees, and they were as cold as any stone, and so upward, and upward, and all was as cold as any stone." * While it is true that the skin of dying persons is usually cold to the touch, they may feel hot, for they often pull at the bedclothes as if they wanted to get rid of them. Often there is excessive sweating, the reason for which has not yet been explained.

Respiration may be rapid, shallow, irregular, or abnormally slow. Periods of rapid breathing separated by pauses (called Cheyne-Stokes respiration) are common. Difficult respiration (dyspnea) may have many causes—excessive pulmonary secretions with or without a persistent cough, pulmonary or cardiac failure, or both, pleural effusion, pulmonary infection, bronchospasm, spread of a malignancy through the lymphatics, or any combination of these conditions. Mental distress (apprehension, fear, or worry of any sort) can cause dyspnea and exaggerate the effect of any other predisposing physical condition.†

As the muscles lose their tone, the body falls into the supine position, the jaw may sag as the patient breathes through the mouth with flaccid lips and cheeks. The lips are dry, swallowing becomes difficult, and mucus collects in the throat. All of this may account for the noisy breathing spoken of as the "death rattle."

Loss of muscle tone makes speech difficult. Inability to speak creates the impression that dying persons are unconscious, especially as they may also close their eyes. But hearing, as discussed later on page 1981, may be intact and *it should never be assumed that the dying cannot hear*.* The rapidity with which vision fails during the dying process is not known. Some dying persons may keep their eyes closed for days, as if they wanted to close out the living world; others keep their eyes open and seem to want to be aware until the end.

With loss of muscle tone, there may be urinary and rectal incontinence. There may also be retention and impaction of feces, especially if the patient is receiving regular doses of tranquilizers, hypnotics, and narcotics, many of which decrease motility of the digestive tract.

During the dying process, there is usually little if any interest in eating and drinking. Taste and smell are frequently altered. Preferences for particular foods change. Many patients develop an aversion for meat, but favor sweet dishes. The pace of eating is slow. Swallowing is difficult, and with mouth breathing it is easy to strangle on food put in the mouth. There may be nausea and vomiting, and with vomiting there is always the danger of insufflation of vomitus. Dryness of the mouth, often due to side effects of drugs, is a frequent symptom which interferes with eating and talking.

In long debilitating diseases, such as advanced cancer, there is a period of weakness and a sense of helplessness. Many fight sleep, hoping to stay conscious—they even say "I want to be alive when I die"; others hope to die in their sleep.

The writers believe that people differ in their wish to have family and friends nearby —there is no one answer. "It's so hard on my family," is a recurrent theme, deeply felt by the patient, so that often death occurs just after the family members have gone out for a much-needed break, as if the patient wanted to spare them the pain of the last moment. Other patients drift off with a son or daughter, husband or wife—the one or two persons closest to them—at their side. They are often quiet, communicating with one another with a lift of the eyebrow, pressure of the hand, or a carefully chosen word.

In old age, especially, the very sick may seem to die more than once. The preceding signs herald death, and the family may as-

---

* Shakespeare, William: *The Life of King Henry V*, Act II, Scene iii.

† It is not uncommon for people to fear suffocation as the immediate cause of death. In Chapter 41 attention was called to the fact that fear, or an attempt to bring respiration under voluntary control, results in embarrassed breathing.

* People who have almost died in shock or in cardiac or respiratory failure, and have been resuscitated, tell about hearing what those around them were saying while they were unable to respond. Patients coming out of anesthesia or other periods of unconsciousness have the same experience. Those who care for the sick seem to forget quite often that a person's hearing and comprehension may be intact when the response is lacking or inappropriate.

semble to say farewell and support each other. Suddenly, for no apparent reason, the patient rallies and may live for weeks or months.* Many persons, young and old, may live for years following recovery from accidents and episodes of acute illness.

Medical and nursing care of the dying may involve heroic life-saving measures, discussed elsewhere in this book, intended to reverse the dying process, but when this is not thought possible or desirable, care is directed toward assessment and relief of the components of suffering—loneliness, apprehension, anxiety, dyspnea, pain, weakness, dehydration, nausea, inability to move and to speak.

The first author of this chapter has within recent years given or participated in the care of approximately 100 terminally ill patients in their homes, in nursing homes, and in general hospitals in the United States.† She has also been a participant observer in the care of the terminally ill at St. Christopher's Hospice in London, Eng. The discussion in the following section of symptomatic care of the dying patient has taken these experiences into account as well as the work of others in this field.

3. CARE OF THE DYING PERSON—THE SETTING

The Effect of the Setting on the Kind of Care That Is Possible. If most people want to die at home, care anywhere else may be less than ideal.‡ In the United States, more people die in hospitals than anywhere else, and the number that die in nursing homes is increasing.

As has been noted, patients who die in the general hospital are likely to be in the emergency room or in the intensive care unit, both

organized and equipped for heroic life-saving measures. Some patients are brought to the emergency room for the physician to confirm or "pronounce" their death; others arrive mortally sick or injured, and for these persons measures designed to arrive at an immediate diagnosis and vigorous resuscitation are mobilized. When a patient is managed as an acute emergency, physicians and nurses don't have time to note that these may be the last moments of the patient's life, that family and friends who are there should be instantly summoned, and that they should be given professional support. Many hospitals have an individual, such as an ombudsman, or staff member in a department of religious ministry available who can help the emergency personnel meet the needs of the patient and the family. Some hospitals have social workers or psychiatrists especially prepared to help families and friends of patients.

While many clients of the emergency room will have been well up until the moment of a heart attack or an accident that brought them to the hospital, other patients will arrive just as ill, yet quite aware and prepared for death. A patient may have been at home or in another institution, such as a nursing home, and have to come to the emergency room either because help was needed for symptoms, such as air hunger, weakness, or hemorrhage, or because the family or those caring for needed physical or psychologic support through the very last phases of life. Thus the emergency room staff is confronted with patients who are dead or dying, but whose ways of coming to terms with death are completely unknown to the staff. Emergency room workers must decide quickly, with little information, whether to resuscitate the patient or to give supportive care only.

In sharp contrast with the emergency room of the acute hospital are the small specialized units where extended, personalized care helps patients and their families come to terms with an illness that no longer responds to curative treatment. From the moment the patient is greeted at the door by the nurse who will be giving care, the approach is human being to human being. As noted in Chapter 3, there are in England between 20 and 30 facilities of this sort; some are called hospices. One of the most widely known is St. Christopher's Hospice in London. There the treatment of choice is palliative, that is, skillful management of the symptoms of disease. By minimizing such symptoms as pain, weakness, anxiety, and nausea, patients facing death are kept comfortable, alert, and able to sustain activity and social relationships. In a setting such as this, nurses can at-

---

* One of the writers saw an elderly man who had been this close to death live in an ambulatory state for 3 months. During this time, he sent for an old friend because he wanted to tell him "how easy it was to die."

† *A Nurse's Study of Care for Dying Patients.* U.S.P.H.S. Nursing Resources Grant NU 00352–01, 02, Sept. 1, 1969–Aug. 30, 1971 (report in preparation).

‡ Reed Nelson, formerly research coordinator at Hospice, Inc., New Haven, Conn., interviewed 100 close relatives of persons who died of cancer in New Haven between 1968 and 1971. Of these, 42 died in the hospital but only 21 had wanted to go there. Another 20 died in a nursing home while only 7 had wanted to go there. Only 38 died at home, although 65 had said they would like to stay at home with their families. Of the 100 persons interviewed, 72 were unable to keep the sick family member at home although 61 of them said they would have liked to do so had adequate support been available. (*Hospice* [Newsletter], Oct. 1974. p. 3.)

tend to the particular needs of the dying with little conflict and confusion, and the patient and the family can be helped to live fully until the end. The majority of these institutions offer home care as well as an inpatient service and so provide both alternatives.

Death may occur in either of these contrasting institutional settings. Wherever it occurs, the family and friends of the dying patient, if they are present, require help. As will be discussed later, involvement of family is important. Most persons are comforted by the presence of those they love, so, for the patients' benefit as well as for their sake, family and friends should be part of the dying scene. Nurses and physicians may have to focus on the patient but they should not forget that relatives and friends of the dying are suffering and when left behind will need physical and psychologic help. In fact, such help should be available before as well as after the patient's death. Bereavement is discussed later in this chapter but it is emphasized that preparation for bereavement starts early. The principles of care being developed by persons working in hospices state that the patient-family is their client.

Even if patients come to terms with death and are ready to relinquish life, those around them may not reach that point at the same time. Family members or the patient's helpers (nurses, physicians, and others) may be ready to "let go" before or after the patient is ready. If nurses understand this, they can sense, mitigate, or relieve the tension emanating from a conflict created by differing expectations between themselves and others. Clues to such conflicts are varied. For example, a child said her mother would not have died "If only she had put up a better fight!" Another 6-year-old referred to his father with childish disappointment in saying, "Mean Daddy, he died on me." Both of these children expressed natural feelings of disappointment and loss of a very significant person in their lives.

The feeling of being left behind or abandoned is often a cause of suffering and a reason for the relative's or friend's need to cling to the patient. Equally understandable is the family's desire to see the end of a life that has come to be meaningless. For example, a 40-year-old husband whose wife had been comatose for a month following cardiac arrest on the operating table and who realized hope for her recovery was not realistic, did not want her death delayed. To him and to his teenage daughters, the wife and mother was already dead, but to the staff of the nursing home where every other patient was over 65 this young and beautiful woman was very much alive. The staff's well-meant efforts to prolong the patient's life with tube feedings were painful for the family to watch or to accept as useful, but the nursing home staff thought she deserved their concentrated attention, more perhaps than the old persons there, even though the young woman was unresponsive and their older patients were responsive.

Differences in the expectations and attitudes of those concerned with the dying person create tensions that charge the atmosphere with emotion. Decisions are difficult and differences between right and wrong are not obvious. Whether in the hospital or at home, nurses must be capable of providing suggestions about who should be called, what help professionals, friends, and family can give, and what help all involved need, including the staff. Nurses and doctors often overlook the impact of the loss of a patient on themselves, or feel that, as professionals, they should not show their emotions. In studies by Glaser and Strauss and by Quint and others, this observation was made repeatedly, partially accounting for what is interpreted as the withdrawal of the staff from the patient and the family. In homes or in homelike institutional settings such as hospices, it is possible for everyone to behave more naturally, more individually, more personally than in large hospitals. Saunders, talking about a setting in which a person (in this case, a child) can feel secure says: "Gossiping is very important and I suppose playing and reading with a child are its equivalents. I am sure I do not have to emphasize the importance of delight, of beauty and fantasy, and of parties." *

T. S. West, deputy medical director of St. Christopher's Hospice, makes the following observation on individualizing care:

Death has become a fashionable subject to talk about and to write about. It is clothed with such words as "dignity" and many who approach the subject hope that "the specialists in death" will have some formula that can be handed round to make the "dignity" a reality.

There is no such formula.

Members of an institution whose main concern is to care for people whose terminal disease is causing them suffering know only too well that no formula can be applied to more than one patient. At St. Christopher's we have begun to learn that just as each patient will approach death in his own particular way, so each member of staff must find his own and special way to approach each patient. We know that patients and staff have to

---

* Saunders, Cicely: "The Management of Fatal Illness in Childhood," *Proc. R. Soc. Med.*, **62:**550, (June) 1969.

learn to deal not only with each other, but also with themselves.*

Wherever care is given the dying patient, the *environment* is important. In private homes it may be desirable for the patient to be in a room on the ground floor so that he or she can walk or be wheeled outdoors and eat meals with the family as long as possible. Nearby bathroom facilities are important, and the cheerfulness and comfort of the furnishings of the patient's room. Familiar and beloved objects in the room to which they are accustomed, may, however, make persons prefer not to move to another seemingly more suitable room.

In general hospitals or nursing homes, every effort should be made to provide privacy when it is desirable for patients and their families. If death is imminent, a private room is often preferred. However, if patients are expected to live for weeks or possibly months, they may be happier in a multiple-bed unit where they will not feel isolated between visits from family or friends. Multiple-bed units are especially desirable for solitary persons who have no visitors.

Henry Wald, who has studied the architectural designs of hospices and special units for the terminally ill, thinks that the preference in acute care hospital design for private rooms for most, if not all, patients does not apply to hospices. In his 1971 master's thesis for the Columbia University School of Architecture, he supports the following US Department of Health, Education, and Welfare recommendation for four-bed units:

The terminal phase of life is an area that has just begun to be investigated in an objective way, and the results raise some surprising psychological issues. Reactions to imminent death vary as much as reactions to familiar life circumstances. But research has shown that during the last few months of life the individual has an increased feeling that his body is inadequate. The dying person experiences a growing feeling of helplessness because of loss of influence over his environment but he has an increased interest in other people. A study comparing interviews (1) with persons who died within a year and (2) with those who survived, showed that the individuals closest to the time of their death, showed a much greater interest in their immediate environment. Information such as this suggests that perhaps the greatest disservice that can be done to the dying person is to isolate him.

To deny the dying person access to others and to the information of his normal environment, therefore, would seem to reduce the likelihood that he will resolve his own departure with dignity. Isolation of the dying is, perhaps, a reflection of the attitudes of younger professionals who are disquieted by their own unresolved conflicts. The social and psychological, as well as the physiological, concomitants of dying should be considered carefully in design services for the terminally ill persons.*

The architect's model and the floor plan for ten four-bed units now being designed for the hospice in Branford, Conn., are shown in Chapter 3. Craven and Wald, describing the design of the hospice, say that

The four single rooms will be used as alternatives for those who are not helped by the multi-bed arrangement—a teenager who may need lots of loud companions, a writer trying to get work done, a couple who face the end of life simultaneously.†

They point out that the scale of the hospice "is human" and designed to help patients continue "life as usual"; to feel a part of on-going life. Patients have easy access to the outdoors, as well as to other parts of the hospice, including the chapel. They see children going to and from the nursery school within the hospice for children of personnel, and volunteers of all ages going about their various activities—gardening, folding linen, serving tea and coffee, etc.

In general hospitals it is common practice to hide the sight and sound of death. Saunders, in discussing the program at St. Christopher's Hospice, London, Eng., describes the acceptance of death on the ward as one of its advantages. One or more members of the staff, as well as family members, are present, and a prayer is usually said at the end. Other patients, who may never have witnessed death, see that it comes easily and that they will not be alone when they die. Patients can sometimes help each other and frequently want to do so. Just the presence of someone else is support for the dying, and in turn, those who see this as a more distant but inevitable event are reassured to know that dying patients are appropriately treated.

In the last days of life, though the pace is slower, patients' appreciation of peace, quiet, and beauty are frequently heightened. A flower or a beloved object put at close range, where it is seen by the dying, gives pleasure. Ample and comfortable seating should be available to make the patient's visitors feel they are wanted and seats arranged so that the patient

---

* West, T. S.: "Symposium on Care of the Dying. Approach to Death," *Nurs. Mirror,* **139**:56, (Oct. 10) 1974.

* US Department of Health, Education, and Welfare: *Working With Older People,* Vol. II. US Government Printing Office, Washington, D.C., Apr. 1970 (PHS Pub. No. 1459), p. 7.

† Craven, Joan, and Wald, Florence: "Hospice Care for Dying Patients," *Am. J. Nurs.,* **75**:1816, (Oct.) 1975.

can easily see and hear them. In any setting, every effort should be made to prevent disagreeable odors in the room. (See Chapter 15 for full discussion of this subject.) If anything is used to mask unavoidable odors, it should probably have an aromatic smell, like that of ammonia or camphor, rather than either an acrid or sweet smell. For the sake of patients and their families, whatever makes for beauty in the environment should be kept until the end. It is possible that music might help many who are dying. They should be surrounded with what they most like at the last.

4. CARE OF THE DYING PERSON— PRINCIPLES AND GOALS

Principles and Goals of Terminal Care in Any Setting. The principles and goals of terminal care are emerging from those who are providing and evaluating care in hospices, hospitals, at home, and in nursing homes. They are applicable to any setting.

An interdisciplinary group called the International Work Group on Death, Dying and Bereavement has prepared a working document on standards of care and will develop outcome measures, using these standards as working hypotheses.*

The standards in this working document touch upon the need for palliative treatment of highest quality; the need for spiritual support, care and respect for the family; open communication, shared decision-making and support for the patient's family who are searching for meaning. The document also emphasizes need for an interdisciplinary team and an atmosphere of concern and support.

Saunders, writing about the management of fatal illness in childhood, and the unusual strain it put on the staff, says: "We are all concerned . . . in trying to come to terms . . . with our own feelings of guilt and fear in the presence of death. It is easier when we know we are not alone. We . . . need frequent, informal meetings. *I would give for the first principle of terminal care co-operation or, perhaps better, community.*" [Italics ours] †

Edward Henderson, a physician, discussing the approach to patients with incurable diseases, makes the following points:

In summary, those caring for the patient with an incurable illness should (a) provide him with knowledge as to the reasonable expectations and limitations imposed by his disease; (b) help him thoroughly and thoughtfully to obtain the greatest possible rewards from his truncated existence; (c) maintain as much as possible an emotional and social environment consistent with his pre-diagnosis status; and (d) preserve his self-esteem and self-recognition for as long as his illness permits, both by allowing and requiring of him a role and voice in the decisions of his life.*

In the following pages an effort is made to describe some ways in which these goals can be met.

Influence of Age on the Care of the Dying Person. It is easy to say that it is the quality rather than the length of a life that is important but almost everyone sees the death of a much wanted *infant* or the death of a beloved *child* as particularly sad. Some students of medicine and nursing who planned to specialize in child care have given up the idea because they couldn't cope with their own suffering and feeling of helplessness when faced with the fatally ill and dying child. Health workers share with parents the fear that more might have been done, a cure found, or the life prolonged until a cure was discovered. It is hard to help parents to accept the inevitability of death and to know when and how to face it with the child. Ida Martinson † has been giving nursing care and psychologic support to dying children and their parents. Most of her patients have had leukemia. Many of them with her help, have been able to stay at home longer and even die at home. Many children might die more happily at home if parents weren't clinging to the hope that a medical miracle would save them. But hospital life for sick children is becoming more bearable as institutions encourage parents to participate in the child's care, even making provision for parents to stay overnight.

There seems to be general agreement that children after the age of 5 know what death means. Before this, they may not think of death as a permanent separation. Children, like adults, sense the imminence of death and ask questions which, if not answered adequately and truthfully, isolate them with their fears of death. Wessel says, "The basic need for a grieving child is to have open and honest relationships with trusted adults." ‡ Their fears

* Working Document, International Work Group on Death, Dying and Bereavement, Yale University, 1976 Conference. Not available for publication in 1976.

† Saunders, Cicely: "The Management of Fatal Illness in Childhood," *Proc. R. Soc. Med.,* **62:**550, (June) 1969.

* Henderson, Edward: "The Approach to the Patient with an Incurable Disease," in Schoenberg, Bernard, et al. (eds.): *Psychosocial Aspects of Terminal Care.* Columbia University Press, New York, 1972, p. 61.

† Martinson, Ida Marie (ed.): *Home Care for the Dying Child, Professional and Family Perspectives.* Appleton-Century-Crofts, New York, 1976.

‡ Wessel, Morris A.: "A Death in the Family. The Impact on Children," *J.A.M.A.,* **234:**865 (Nov. 24) 1975.

may be so much worse than the reality of death that protecting children from the sight of dying and death may be a great disservice. Saunders reports the following conversation between a nurse and a dying child:

A boy with sarcomatosis died with us not very long ago. Towards the end of his four months' stay with us Sister suddenly knew that the time had come to speak directly while she was doing something practical for him. She just said quietly: "Are you afraid about dying, David?" "Yes," he said. "You've seen other people here. . . . You know we won't let you down. It will be all right." He said: "Yes, it *is* all right" and never needed to say anything else.*

This conversation suggests the importance of allowing the child to see others die—easily and supported by those they love. Maria H. Nagy,[48] Delphie J. Fredlund,[49] and Erna Furman,[50] among others, have studied the meaning of death to children.† Readers will find their reports helpful. Special chapters in texts on child care describe the care of the dying child and helping parents in more detail than can be included here.

While the death of those who haven't had a chance to live fully is particularly sad, the death of *young adults,* and especially young parents, is also hard to accept. They weigh heavily in the scale of social worth emphasized by Glaser and Strauss. Like fatally ill children, they are likely to get the best physical care available in a general hospital. Heroic life-saving measures may be used long after the staff realizes these measures are useless.

The difficulty of facing death with the parent and with the children may result in complete avoidance of the subject. This isolates the fatally ill patients with their instinctive knowledge that death is imminent. W. E. Wynant,[51] a clergyman, describes the help he was able to give a husband in facing death with his dying wife and the support he gave her in seeing her children who had withdrawn from their mother, feeling themselves unloved and forsaken by her.

Death in *middle* and *old age* rarely has the poignancy that death in youth has. However, age is not a matter of years alone. In some cultures, men and women are old at 45 or 50; in others, they retain their zest for living far beyond the Biblical threescore years and ten. In every culture, there are individuals whose death at 80, or even older, is a social loss. For example, there are statesmen and scientists whose life work is nearing fruition, artists who are producing masterpieces in their maturity, and men and women who are, for one reason or another, holding families together. In 1945, Leo W. Simmons published a study of the aged in primitive society [52] and in 1970, with Dorothea Jaeger, he reported a study of the care of the aged in the United States.[53] Such works should be consulted for data on this subject, but the generalization may be justifiable that isolation and withdrawal in the care of the dying apply particularly to the elderly. On the other hand, the aged may not be subjected to prolonged dying through the use of respiratory aids and artificial feeding. Kastenbaum, under the title "While the Old Man Dies: Our Conflicting Attitudes Toward the Elderly," describes the thoughts of the son who has witnessed the death of a father when they could not communicate with each other:

The core problem is the one to concentrate upon: many of us have misgivings about the prospects of our own aging and death, and we have mixed feelings about people in our own lives who are aged. We are quick to project our own attitudes and expectations upon elderly men and women. This projection can exert powerful influence over the lives and deaths of the elderly as we are generally in a position of greater socioeconomic leverage. If we are convinced it is right or necessary for an old person to die, then we may be making it extraordinarily difficult for him to live. We may fail to bolster his chances of remaining in good health, we may fail to recognize when, in fact, his preterminal process has begun, and we may remain so closeted in our own assumptions that we do not bother to find out what it is that he really needs in his last hours.
And then, one of these days, there is somebody over us with all the ignorant benevolence we have taught him . . .*

Such experiences represent not only an unsatisfactory end to a life but a lasting source of unhappiness to the witness.

If the staff can give the kind of care to the elderly that relieves them of pain and discom-

---

* Saunders, Cicely: "The Management of Fatal Illness in Childhood," *Proc. R. Soc. Med.,* **63**:550 (June) 1969.

† David Maddison and Beverley Raphael say that "Before the age of five years, death is equated with sleep and is not considered final. Through the years from five to nine, death is often personified and may be thought of as an event contingent upon the aggressive fantasies or actions of others. It is only after the age of nine that death is seen as a process dependent upon natural laws and characterized by the permanent cessation of vital bodily functions. Fear of death in children is variously seen as a fear of the aggressive retaliation of others, together with a fear of emotional deprivation possibly related to separation anxiety. (Maddison, David, and Raphael, Beverley: "The Family of the Dying Patient," in Schoenberg, Bernard, et al. [eds.]: *Psychosocial Aspects of Terminal Care.* Columbia University Press, New York, 1972, p. 187.)

* Kastenbaum, Robert: "While the Old Man Dies: Our Conflicting Attitudes Toward the Elderly. Concluding Note," in Schoenberg, Bernard, et al. (eds.): *Psychosocial Aspects of Terminal Care.* Columbia University Press, New York, 1972, p. 124.

fort and that makes them feel wanted, and if the institution encourages the presence of relatives (adults and children, and, Saunders says, "even the dog"), it is unlikely that the death of an elderly parent will leave this traumatic memory. In the same way, families caring for the elderly at home can be helped by the clergy, by doctors, and by nurses on a home care staff to give the elderly a chance to die in peace and dignity. The family that observes its older members face death with equanimity can see the ultimate achievement and so experience strength and pride, and the person who has so died may be an inspiration to those who go on.

5. CARE OF THE DYING PERSON— ROLES OF CAREGIVERS

Helping the Patient with "Getting the House in Order." * A peaceful death is difficult as long as the persons who are dying are struggling to complete unfinished tasks; as long as they feel there are persons they have injured to whom they have never made amends; as long as relatives or friends who have depended on them are not provided for. Giving the dying person an opportunity to complete the tasks of life, as nearly as this is possible, is one of the principal arguments for giving them the best professional assessment of the time they have left. Saunders titles an article on the care of the dying person "The Moment of Truth" and she gives the following explanation:

The title . . . includes far more than the question "Who should tell—or should you tell—a patient that his death is near?" I think that the title includes many more of the realities and challenges of the situation. It is a situation that concerns all of us, whether we are doctors, nurses, psychiatrists, psychologists, social workers, or theologians. (I have deliberately made the list alphabetical, because all are of equal importance.) Perhaps most of all the situation concerns us when a member of our family or a friend is dying. This is or should be, a "moment of truth.". . . it is the patient who is, or who should be, in the center. The question is *his* because it is his situation and he is the person who matters.†

One of the practical aspects of "getting the house in order" is making or changing a will, as the patient often wants to do. State laws require wills to be signed in the presence of two

or three witnesses. The nurse may be asked to witness a signature on a will and to get one or more persons to act in this capacity. It is unwise for medical personnel to witness signatures unless there is no alternative. There may be subsequent litigation that will require their presence in court and that will interrupt the work for which they are best fitted. In addition to the patient's attorney, the hospital nurse can turn to its ombudsman, the hospital's attorney, social worker, or administrator; outside the hospital, nurses can guide the patient or family to the Legal Aid Society or its equivalent if they don't have their own attorney.

Putting the house in order, arriving at the point where death can be faced calmly—and even gratefully for some—may require the help of family, friends, and professionals. The roles of the various workers who may be involved in the care of the dying are discussed briefly in the following paragraphs. Their roles are overlapping and they may have to substitute for each other according to who is available when help is needed. The importance of working together, of coordinating the various competences represented in a community and reaching decisions in harmony, cannot be overstressed. Coordination is most likely when, as Saunders says, everyone sees the dying as "the person that matters."

Role of the Family and Friends. There is no substitute for the presence of the family at the bedside of dying persons when they want them there. Those closest to patients can communicate with them effortlessly; a word, a question, a glance can speak volumes. Expressions of family love and loyalty can make persons who are not particularly proud of their accomplishments realize that their life has not been wasted and that they will live on in the memory of their kin. The presence of intimate friends can be equally important. Those who are experienced in the care of dying patients say that the patient and family should be treated as a unit. Craven and Wald make the following observations:

A family group can be compared to a mobile made up of infinite numbers and kinds of members suspended from a single strand. Each member can move and change independently to some degree, but every shift cannot help but precipitate movement of every other member and the whole. Terminal illness has immediate and long-range effects on this equilibrium.*

When a person dies at home, the family may give some part, even most, of the physical care.

---

* This is a term which patients in my study frequently used. [F. W.]

† Saunders, Cicely: "The Moment of Truth: Care of the Dying Person," in Pearson, Leonard (ed.): *Death and Dying: Current Issues in the Treatment of the Dying Person.* Press of Case-Western Reserve University, Cleveland, 1969, p. 49.

* Craven, Joan, and Wald, Florence S.: "Hospice Care for Dying Patients," *Am. J. Nurs.,* **75:**1816 (Oct.) 1975.

The role of professional health workers is to share their skills with the family and help them learn how to relieve pain and discomfort; also to identify the tension and conflicts that illness creates and to help the family solve or cope with their problems. When people die in hospitals, nursing homes, and hospices, the staff can encourage the family and friends to participate in the care of the patient. Every effort should be made to sense when they would like to be left alone with each other and when the presence of another person enables them to do or say something that they want to have done or said.

Patients and families have taken the initiative themselves in forming mutual aid and support. In the United States Orville Kelly and his family have built a nationwide network of patients and their families who are facing death. In addition to providing mutual support, its members (particularly Orville Kelly and his wife Wanda) have lectured to community groups and health workers. This organization is called "Make Today Count."

The founders of The Foundation of Thanatology, Austin and Lillian Kutscher, developed that institution because of the experiences both had in the loss of a spouse.

One of the characteristics of present-day hospices that help account for the contentment expressed by patients is the welcome they offer the family and friends; the opportunity to share the life of the dying patient. Rooms are available where family members can stay overnight. As Saunders put it, a family "moved in" to the room of a youth who was dying, bringing games and pets—anything that would make his last days as normal and content as possible.

Later in this chapter bereavement is discussed, but the treatment of the bereaved begins while the patient is living, for bereavement is least traumatic for those who can believe that they have done everything that was possible for the one who has died.

Books such as John Gunther's *Death Be Not Proud*,[54] Jocelyn Evans' *Living with A Man Who Is Dying*,[55] and C. S. Lewis' *A Grief Observed*[56] describe the satisfaction there is in sharing the pain of separation but living each day as fully as possible until the end.

Role of the Clergy. The role of the clergy is important. Death strikes at the roots of people's lives; it sometimes shakes but also strengthens their faith, and, if they have time to think, impending death makes them question their ethical values. A religion may or may not include belief in an afterlife. In a sample of 30,000 Americans, E. S. Shneidman[57] reported in 1971 that 43 per cent were convinced there was life after death or tended

to believe in it. Only 11 per cent preferred not to believe in an afterlife. Ninian Smart,[58] writing in *Man's Concern with Death,* edited by Arnold Toynbee and his associates, estimated that about half the people in Great Britain believed in life after death. Alan L. Berman,[59] reviewing other studies and his own data, concluded that "religiously active Catholics and Protestants" are more likely to believe in an afterlife than inactive members of these faiths. Fewer Jews, whether they are active or inactive, believe in an afterlife. Lifton and Olson contrast the teachings of Freud and Jung in the following excerpt from their chapter on symbolic immortality:

Jung described the psychic vitality of "primitive" peoples who live in tune with archetypal truth. And he observed the positive effects of belief in myths for persons nearing death. He said that when man's conscious thinking is in harmony with the deep truths of the unconscious revealed in mythology, then fear of death is no longer overwhelming. Life can then be lived to the fullest until the end. Therefore, Jung, in contrast to Freud, encouraged belief in religious teachings because he thought such belief was, in his words, "hygienic—necessary for healthy living." He wrote: "When I live in a house that I know will fall about my head within the next two weeks, all my vital functions will be impaired by this thought, but if, on the contrary, I feel myself to be safe, I can dwell there in a normal comfortable way." *

There are certain observances and religious practices that help persons of each faith. Ministers of all denominations are expected to give the services of their church to the dying, and will administer them at the patient's request whether they are at home or in an institution. Some religions have no sacraments; others have sacraments of vital significance. This is, however, not the only, or chief, reason why sick people may want to see their ministers. When a relationship exists between the sick and their religious representative, a patient's faith can be strengthened. The clergyman can be a friend and confidant who will discuss with the dying their hopes and fears, their plans for their families, the fact that they are dying, and the consequences of their death. (See Fig. 50-7.) The ability of the clergy to help patients and families in crisis varies widely and is affected by religious and social issues. Many members of a congregation may be at odds with their clergyman over changes in forms of worship or the church's involvement with current events. An example of the first case is the modernization of Roman Catholic or Protes-

* Lifton, Robert Jay, and Olson, Eric: *op. cit.,* p. 73.

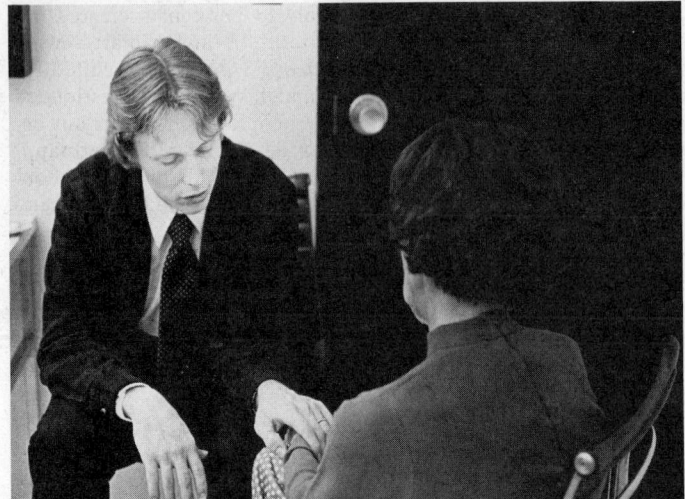

Figure 50-7. Chaplain of a tumor program treatment team at the Yale–New Haven Hospital talking with a patient. (From "Caring for the Cancer Patient—A New Approach," *Focus,* Summer 1976. Office of Public Relations. Photograph by Don Kleinberg.)

tant liturgies; an example of the second, the church's position on women's rights or on wars such as those in Israel, Vietnam, Ireland, Lebanon, or Angola. Some clergymen have had so little experience with seriously ill and dying persons that they have not learned how to give adequate help. It is easier for the priest, minister, rabbi, swami, or other religious representative to help patients if they have been seeing them throughout their illness. If there are resident chaplains in the hospitals, their visits are made routinely; if not, the family, the doctor, or the nurse should help find an appropriate person, whether clergy or lay person, who will give the patient spiritual comfort.

Patients should know that a minister is coming to see them. If nurses have any reason to believe that patients do not realize the seriousness of their condition and might assume that a visit from a clergyman means they are thought to be dying, nurses may assure them that patients are often visited by clergymen on a hospital service. In Chapter 18, where working with the clergy was discussed at some length, it was pointed out that the Catholic Church adopted the term "sacraments of the sick" in 1968 to replace the "sacraments of the Viaticum" (last rites) in order to avoid the finality of "last rites."

Communities where ministries reach out to help people in need regardless of religious creed provide patient, family, and health workers with support that spans all creeds and acknowledge the patient's need to be cared for with or without ritual. It is worth repeating that the clergy, the patient, the family, and other health workers should have as long a time to know one another as possible.

On the clergyman's first visit to the patient,

nurses can help by telling them what they think will be helpful about the patient's physical condition, problems, and needs, and, in turn, ask the clergyman what relevant information he has. The minister, priest, rabbi, swami, or other religious representative may prefer to go to the patient unaccompanied, but nurses should offer to take them to patients and make the introduction. It is desirable for this visit to be so timed that the patients are as alert and rational as possible. Among Christians, the Catholics—Roman, Western Non-Roman, and Eastern Orthodox—attach the greatest importance to the sacraments. The Episcopalian, Lutheran, and Moravian are spoken of as "bridge faiths" between Catholicism and Protestantism and have some sacraments and rituals in common. If patients belong to any of these groups, it is desirable to have ready a few simple things the clergyman will need for the administration of the sacraments—usually a table covered with a white cloth and on it a glass, a small bowl of water, a spoon, and a linen napkin or a towel. A glass, a tube, and fresh drinking water should be on the bedside table. Most ministers bring what is needed; if not, they may ask the nurse for certain articles. In denominational hospitals, sacred objects, such as holy oil and crucifixes, are kept in a special place ready for use. If nurses of the same faith are available, they may be of special help to the patient, the family, and the clergyman.

Those involved should be asked whether they prefer privacy or sharing the ritual with others. It can be a rewarding and moving experience for the staff and other patients to see or participate in the ritual, even though they are not of the same faith. The religious observance can be a bridge for others on the periphery to share the suffering of patient and family and the offered help. When privacy is preferred, this should be provided with screens or curtains in an open space, or by putting signs on doors of private rooms.

The sacraments have been described in Chapter 18, but it might be repeated here that the Roman Catholics especially believe that the sacraments are essential to a "state of grace" and admission to heaven. The sacraments administered to the dying are Baptism (if the person has not been baptized), Penance (Confession), Holy Eucharist (Communion), formerly called Viaticum when received by a dying person, and Extreme Unction. If the dying person is a Roman Catholic and has not been baptized (as in the case of an infant), nurses should make every effort to get a priest to baptize the person. If this is not possible, a Roman Catholic member of the staff should be asked to administer the sacrament. In the last resort, a non-Catholic can do so.

It is not possible to describe the ministrations of the spiritual adviser to the various Protestant, Catholic, Jewish, Hindu, Mohammedan, and other faiths, but nurses should know something about all the great religions. Their understanding, as stressed in Chapter 18, would be broadened by reading sources listed at the end of that chapter and some at the end of this chapter. In this decade (1970–1980) many people have a belief in faith healing and laying on of hands. Nurses serve dying patients best by seeing that the proper representatives of their churches are present and then by providing the clergymen as nearly as they can with the conditions they indicate are essential

to, or helpful to, their ministry. Visits of clergymen should be recorded. The name of the person administering the sacraments, and the time at which they were received, should be included in the record.

Dicks [60] long ago warned those who attend dying persons against trying to make them conform to their theological beliefs, and contemporary writers are emphatic on this score.[61-63]

Role of Doctors. The role of doctors has been touched on throughout this chapter. Traditionally they bear the professional responsibility for deciding when it is inappropriate to continue using so-called heroic measures to prolong life. Many opinions have been cited on this subject and the reader is referred to Hinton's volume *Dying* [64] that includes a review of the literature up to 1972. The volume, *The Dying Patient,* [65] edited by Orville Brim, Jr., and his associates includes discussions of the physician's role by Osler Peterson and by Anselm Strauss and Barney G. Glaser. Avery D. Weisman, a physician who has devoted years to the study of the psychosocial aspects of dying, makes the following observation:

What the Doctor can do about death has two sides, professional and personal. As a professional, he tries to diagnose and treat. If he cannot, then he relieves anguish. But if this, too, fails, he continues to give of himself. Then, when death approaches, he stands by, guiding, assisting, ameliorating. [See Fig. 50–8.] This is his "professional" responsibility, which can be assigned to others, but cannot be routinely relegated. Like most ethical ideals, it can rarely be fulfilled. Lacking time as well as training, he may perform the essentials of his skill, and allow competent paraprofessionals to take over. However, the Doctor

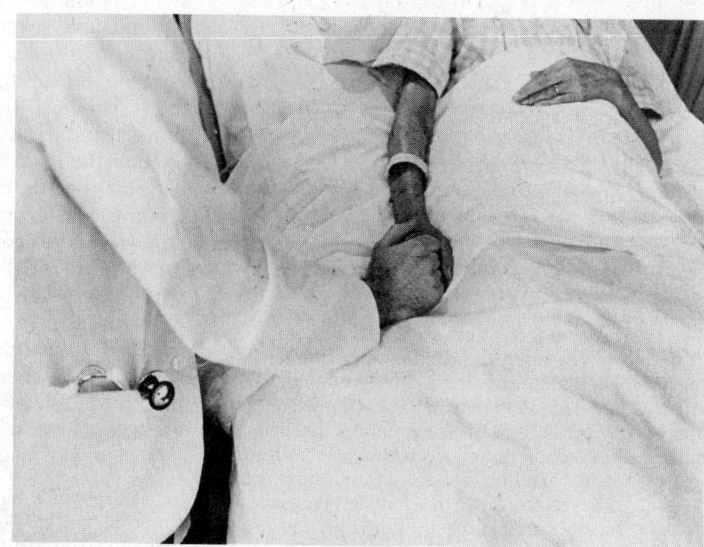

Figure 50-8. Physician and patient. (From "To Comfort Always," *Yale Alumni Magazine,* June, 1972, p. 19. Photograph by Jerry L. Thompson, New Haven, Conn.)

may not realize that he cannot fulfill his own ethical expectations. His traditional role at the pinnacle of the professional pyramid may create an illusion that everything is under his control, because he has not assigned his job to anyone else. What has happened is that having other obligations prevents the Doctor from following his obligations to the dying. He does not delegate; he has already forfeited.*

Edmund Pellegrino, who has spoken and written widely on the importance of a humane and authentic relationship between patients and health workers, especially physicians, includes the following in a 1975 lecture:

For most of its history, the relationship of physician and patient has been dominated by the physician's point of view. Ethical codes have been established more on the basis of the obligation physicians feel than those patients may impose. The image of physicians which dominates the profession and society is still based in the Hippocratic ideal. . . . Hippocratic physicians assume responsibility as set forth in the Oath—not to harm patients, not to induce abortion, not to practice euthanasia, to preserve confidentiality, and to take a paternal interest in their students as the future members of a select group. . . . *The Law, Decorum, The Physician,* and *Precepts.* . . . enjoin physicians to attend carefully to their comportment, to be dignified, and reserved, to use common sense, to be moderate, and to reveal nothing of their secrets to those outside of the brotherhood, or even to their patients.

. . .

We no longer have consensus as a nation about what we expect from physicians and from medicine. Our attitudes about the authority, privileges and superiority of professional groups have changed drastically. In a democratic society, we expect everyone to participate in decisions which will affect them.

In a democratic society . . . the crucial issues [are] how to enable people to participate as free individuals in the choices which affect them.

. . .

There are particular features of illness which diminish and obstruct patients' capacity to live a specifically human existence to its fullest. These features create a relationship of inherent inequality between two human beings—one a physician, the other a patient.

By virtue of the event of illness, these patients lose their freedom to act; they lack the knowledge upon which to make rational choices or to regain their freedom to act; they must place themselves in the power of another human, as petitioners, to regain their humanity, their integrity—i.e., self-image. . . . The sick person lacks knowledge of almost all the essential information needed to make rational choices and decisions of the utmost importance to his life. He does not know what is wrong; he is not sure of how he became ill, or why; he does not know how serious his prob-

lem may be, whether he can recover, what treatments are available, whether they are effective, and with what risk, cost, pain or loss of dignity.

[And so,] in making his competence available to the patient, the physician must also attend to the other deficiencies created by illness. His technical decisions must be congruent with the patient's needs to participate in the choices as freely and rationally as education, time and the circumstances permit. Disclosure of the facts of the illness, the degree of its gravity, the alternatives open, their relative effectiveness, costs and dangers, the physician's own experience and skill in comparison with others, and the likelihood of success or failure must all be explicated. Only with the closing of the information gap can patients approach truly valid consent, one which permits participation as a human and enables the patient to incorporate the decision into his own value system.*

Krant, a medical educator, in the following statement makes a plea for the preparation of physicians who can and will share the responsibility for decision-making with others:

Care of the dying patient and of his family obviously involves extensive professional performance, and frequently the best caregivers may be nurses, aides, psychologists, social workers, and others who come to know the patient and family. Yet it is the physician who is the ultimate power in any unit, and he can effectively block an open program of care. The physician may view himself as the lonely, solitary figure in decision-making and care-giving. In a way, the educational process he is put through fosters such an exclusiveness.†

While it is part of the physician's traditional role to discuss the imminence of death with the patient's family and to notify the family when death occurs, systems in which the physician bears sole responsibility for telling the patient have severe critics. Hinton [66] called attention to studies showing that the majority of doctors (80 to 90 per cent) say they rarely tell their patients the illness is terminal even though studies have also shown that 80 per cent of the patients interviewed want to be told.

Some health care practitioners argue that patients will crumble if the truth is disclosed. Other practitioners express opposing views and present practical difficulties that result from withholding the truth; for instance, patients die without getting their affairs in order. There are also ethical and moral issues and the legal right of the patient to be informed and participate in decisions affecting him or her is transgressed. Those who can continue to talk to the end can add an important dimension to their

---

* Weisman, Avery D.: *op. cit.,* p. 201.

* Pellegrino, Edmund D.: *The Humanistic Base of Professional Ethics in Medicine.* Jubilee Lecture, Memorial University of Newfoundland, Canada, May 13, 1975.

† Krant, Melvin: *op. cit.,* p. 203.

lives and help those around them to understand what it is like to be dying.

Saunders puts the principle in practical and clear terms: "Every patient needs an explanation of his illness that will be understandable and convincing to him if he is to cooperate in his treatment or be relieved of the burden of unknown fears. This is true whether it is a question of giving a diagnosis in a hopeful situation or of confirming a poor prognosis." *

Physicians are changing their views on informing patients. For example, Oliver Cope,[67] professor emeritus of surgery at Harvard University, has recommended that when cancer of the breast is suspected, patients should be included in decisions, beginning with diagnostic procedures. He recommends that the diagnostic process have sequential steps, which begin with telling the patient that no therapy will be prescribed until a biopsy is made and until the pathology report can be reviewed by a team of physician-surgeon, oncologist, radiologist, and pathologist. The nature and extent of the pathology will be discussed by the team and the following questions answered: Is there blood vessel invasion? What is the chance of the disease spreading by way of the lymphatics? What are the relative merits of available types of treatment (modalities)? After consideration of these issues, the conferring physicians and pathologists agree on what treatment is best and why. At this point, the primary physician discusses the findings with the patient and they reach a decision, and so the patient can give an "informed consent" to treatment.

Alfred S. Ketchan, writing on a surgeon's approach to advanced cancer, expressed the following opinion:

The doctor who takes it upon himself to be less than honest with the mentally alert cancer-bearing patient, who has family or financial responsibilities, is treading deeply in the realm of the Supreme Being. Although there is nothing sweeter to the ears of the physician than the words, "Thank you Doctor, for curing me," or "Here I am Doc, it's been five years since you told my wife I was going to die," it can be almost as satisfying and heart-warming to hear the sincere and heartfelt expression of the patient, "Thank you, Doctor, for being honest and frank with me in telling me what I need to know, if I am to properly prepare for what lies ahead of me." †

These changing views are amply supported in *A Patient's Bill of Rights*,[68] published by the American Hospital Association, which include the patient's right to know about treatment, the risks involved, and the right to refuse the treatment recommended. (See also Chapter 3.)

Richard Lamerton, a physician of the Home Care Service of St. Joseph's Hospice, Hackney, Eng., puts the responsibility for deciding when to "abandon cure" (but not *care*) on the doctor, who "must decide who is dying." He says the next question is "who shall be told, and when." Lamerton says that patients tend to ask first-year nurses and medical students rather than the medical consultant and he makes the following observation:

If the doctors will not be realistic . . . the nurses can find themselves required to deceive patients who are not fooled, and having to ask nurses from the previous shift which lie they are supposed to be supporting.

Ward sisters should have a completely free hand to confirm or reassure as they see fit, and junior nurses should have had the opportunity to discuss in advance what their response should be. Patients . . . sooner or later . . . will lose faith in any one who deceives them.

This kind of approach demands good communication between the nurses and doctors, and also with any other member of the caring team whom the patient may choose as his confidante.

Lamerton thinks that the caring team, including the chaplain and the social worker, should have access to all the information there is on diagnosis and prognosis and that regular conferences are essential. He says:

Only in this way can we really function as a team, learning to trust one another, and to serve the patient properly.*

In addition to making a diagnosis and a prognosis on the length of life and telling the patient and the family, it is traditional for the doctor to prescribe the medical management of symptoms and to pronounce death. While the physicians prescribe drugs for pain, nausea, dyspnea, and other symptoms, it is the nurses who give them and have the best opportunity to see their effects. As in the psychosocial aspects of care there is much to be gained by pooling judgment, by conferring frequently, and by inviting the opinion of the most experienced caregivers regardless of their appointed roles.

Pronouncement of death is discussed later, but it is by law the function of the physician.

---

* Saunders, Cicely: "Telling Patients," *Dist. Nurs.*, **8**:149, (Sept.) 1965.

† Ketchan, Alfred S.: "A Surgeon's Approach to the Patient with Advanced Cancer. Who Should Know," in Schoenberg, Bernard, et al. (eds.): *Psychosocial Aspects of Terminal Care*. Columbia University Press, New York, 1972, p. 97.

* Lamerton, Richard: "Symposium on Care of the Dying. Ethical Questions in the Care of the Dying," *Nurs. Mirror*, **139**:61, (Oct. 10) 1974.

Robert H. Moser, discussing the doctor's role, notes what he calls "the new ethics." He makes the following observation on defining the border between life and death and contemporary problems:

But there is now a new dimension. Our engineers and technologists have provided us with machines that have prodded and crowded Death onto a strange, unfamiliar terrain. The delicate yet definable border between life and death that existed in the past now has new, ill-defined interfaces with philosophy and ethics. We are denied a simple physiological endpoint for death. What morality applies in choosing live donors for organ transplantation? When is the donor of an unpaired organ dead? Must we designate some arbitrary waiting period before removing critical organs that are becoming ischemic? Is it a violation of Hippocratic ethic to dialyze or infuse mannitol into the patient dying from a head injury just to preserve his kidneys for graft purposes? Dare we remove vital organs from a patient who is not judged, by all criteria, to be totally and irrevocably dead? Who will make the decision? Just what is our obligation to potential donors and potential recipients, for example, the mother of three who just happens to be the most compatible donor for a fourth child with end-stage kidney disease?

In this same article Moser says:

The shifting, perhaps slightly tattered image of the physician in the public eye continues to evoke much thought and comment. When the tumult subsides, one thing will not have changed since the first aboriginal mother took her dying child to the village shaman: the status of the physician as life and death decisionmaker. Of his many roles, this role has always been the most difficult for the physician.*

Saunders, also discussing the inescapable distress for physicians in the care of the dying, says it is more difficult than the nurse's role because the latter can do something for the patient with their hands. This giving by touching is mutually comforting, it makes nurses feel useful to patients, while the doctors, with all their authority, feel frustrated and helpless. Perhaps the answer lies in shared decisions, always remembering that "informed patients" and their families should have the last word.

Among physicians, no specialists seem to have shown more interest in research on death than *psychiatrists*. They may be on the staff of institutions and home care services for the purpose of studying the meaning of death, the psychosocial needs of the dying, the reaction of others to the dying person, or the effect of bereavement. Psychiatrists may also have staff appointments so that they can be accessible to patients and their families or as consultants to the other physicians, to nurses, or to anyone involved in patient care. Psychiatrists in psychiatric hospitals are, of course, responsible for the total medical care of terminally ill patients. The staff also needs support so psychiatrists indirectly help the patient when they help the caregiver.

Role of Pharmacists. Pharmacists have a special role in institutions and agencies providing terminal care since the medical management of symptoms is in many cases dependent on knowledge of drugs, their actions and interactions.[68a] This is particularly true in the case of cancer. This era is characterized by proliferation of drugs. It is hard for physicians to keep up with the development of pharmacology. Doctors and nurses are more than ever inclined to consult pharmacists and use their special competence in the preparation of drugs and in assessing their interaction. In other eras nurses may have been expected to operate the pharmacy in the afternoon and at night after the pharmacist left for the day; in this age the danger of having any but experts prepare and dispense drugs (which was always present) is so generally recognized that pharmacists are available on a full-time basis. They may often participate in patient conferences. Many medical centers have a research pharmacist who can gather relevant data quickly and, using a computer, can make comprehensive up-to-date information available. The pharmacist increasingly helps the physician and nurse relieve the symptoms so that patients can lead a more active and comfortable life.

Role of the Nurse. The nurse's role in the care of dying patients depends upon whether the patients are at home or in an institution and on the amount of care family or friends want and are able to give. How nurses function depends also on how others expect or permit them to function, the environment created by administrative officers of an institution, the limiting, or inhibiting, rules and regulations, and time available to nurses for meeting the needs of dying patients.

Either directly or by teaching others, it is the function of the nurse to give patients the help they need with the activities of daily living (see Chapter 8), to help them maintain their independence as long as possible, and to make it possible for patients to have what they consider a good death.* It is also the function

---

* Moser, Robert H.: "The New Ethics," in Schoenberg, Bernard, et al. (eds.): *Psychosocial Aspects of Terminal Care*. Columbia University Press, New York, 1972, p. 43.

* It is interesting that Jocelyn Evans, a wife who took care of her dying husband, says that this role of the nurse, which she read in the *ICN Basic Principles of Nursing Care*, "reflects my attitude abso-

of the nurse to minimize any pain or discomfort associated with the dying process by helping patients and families use effectively the measures prescribed by physicians. In situations where physicians are unavailable, as in most emergencies, nurses may have to assume responsibility for using a relief measure that has not been prescribed. Physicians' directions ("orders") may stipulate a discretionary role of the nurse in relation to certain treatments.

In institutions and in some home care services, nurses are with the patient more than other trained health workers so it is they who have the best opportunity to sense patients' needs and wishes, their symptoms and responses to treatment, their fears and anxieties, their hopes and the way they want to die (see Fig. 50-9). Saunders repeatedly refers to the

lutely. 'The unique function of the nurse,' it says, 'is to assist the individual, sick or well, in the performance of those activities contributing to health or its recovery (or to peaceful death) that he would perform unaided if he had the necessary strength, will or knowledge.' The nurse assists her patient, it explains, by contributing to 'what is—to *him*—a good death.'" (Evans, Jocelyn: *Living with a Man Who Is Dying.* Taplinger Publishing Co., New York, 1971, p. 109.)

tendency of patients to "confide in the nurse." Ronald Gibson,[69] a British physician, says few nurses appreciate what they mean to patients and their families. Nurses are accessible and the physical care they give patients evokes a confidential relationship.

So many articles on nursing care of the dying have appeared recently in the *American Journal of Nursing* that Mary H. Browning and Edith P. Lewis compiled them in a volume—*The Dying Patient: A Nursing Perspective.*[70] Reports given at ANA Clinical Conferences have focused on care of the dying.[71,72] Reference has been made to Jeanne C. Quint's (Benoliel) study [73] and to the course she is teaching at the University of Washington School of Nursing, to a program at the University of Florida School of Nursing, described by Ramona Powell Davidson,[74] and to the experience of the first author of this chapter in an investigation of terminal nursing care.[75] Counterparts of the American articles appear in nursing journals around the world.[76-82] Saunders' writings, dating from the 1950s, stress the importance of the nurse's (the "Sister's") role and she pays special tribute to the nurses in the Irish Order of the Sisters of

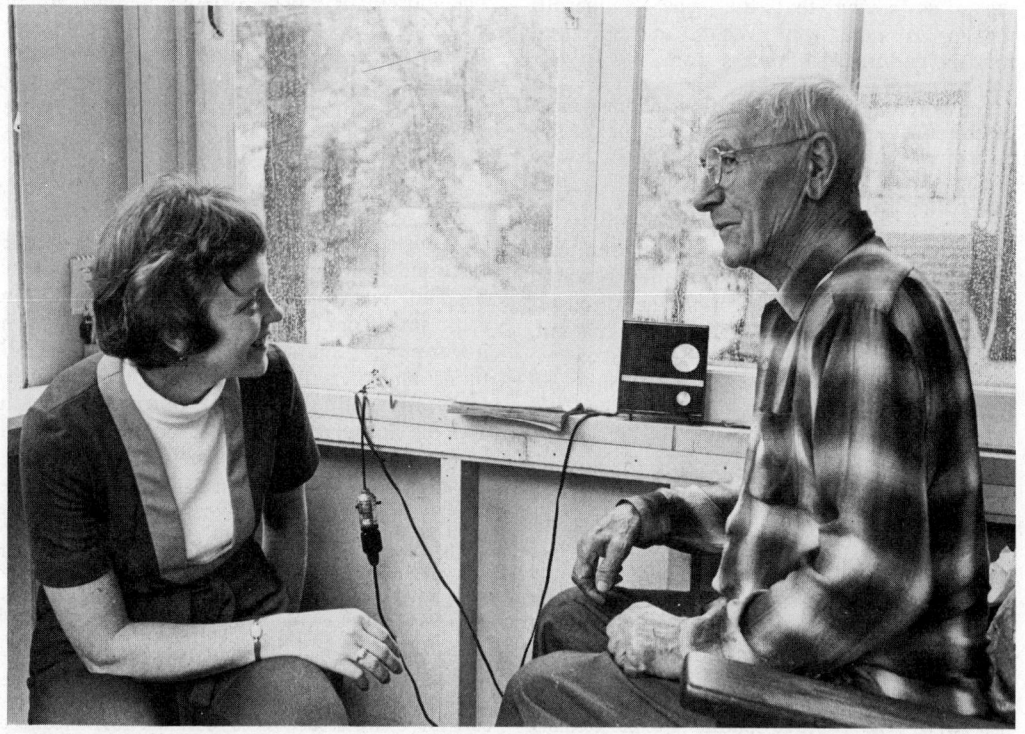

Figure 50-9. Nurse member of the Hospice Home Care Team talking with a patient during a home visit. (Courtesy of Hospice, Inc., New Haven, Conn. Photograph by George B. Gibbons, Jr., New Haven, Conn.)

Charity, who, at St. Joseph's Hospice in London, demonstrated their skilled and sensitive care of the dying—care on which she, as its founder, has based the program at St. Christopher's Hospice in London.

Barbara J. McNulty, nursing officer of the Domiciliary Service at St. Christopher's, hopes it will be part of every nurse's skill to give [effective] terminal care. She stresses the importance of nurses realizing that they are members of "a team" which means that the nurse may be the most important person to some patients, but "the back-up" for other workers in other cases. McNulty thinks it essential that nurses understand their attitudes toward death; that they individualize their care of patients and help to relatives; and that they learn to "feel without being overwhelmed, to care without being overcome, to participate without being identified." * Earlier, for an American audience, McNulty described St. Christopher's and its home care program.[83] And there is an illustrated description of Christmas there which shows how nurses join with other members of the staff in creating a "joyous" atmosphere.[83a]

D. H. Summers, another member of St. Christopher's nursing staff, discussing the role of the nurse in 1974, quotes Florence Nightingale as saying that the most dangerous maxim for a nurse is "What can't be cured must be endured." Summers says:

Let us refute this statement [that nothing more can be done] and accept the challenge that at this point everything can and must be done, not to prolong life, but to improve the quality of [life in] the time that remains.†

Summers thinks nurses can be effective in their role if they become involved, if they function as one of a concerned group. She discusses the way the nurse "shares" with the patient, the family, other nurses, doctors, the clergy, social workers, nutritionists, occupational and physical therapists—the various health workers serving the patient.

No rules can be laid down for the nurse's behavior with the dying and their families or what they do for them since no two situations are alike. And so much depends on the age of the patient; whether the death comes suddenly or after a long illness; on the setting in which the death occurs; and on the availability of other health workers. Even though nurses have

had no previous experience with death, they need not fear self-consciousness or embarrassment if they turn their entire attention to their helping task. A great deal depends upon their sensitiveness to people, their judgment, and taste; or, in other words, the nurse's personality. People cannot give something they do not themselves possess. Nursing skills can be learned that relieve or lessen the patient's physical discomfort and therefore the family's distress, but everyone concerned is supported by the nurse's willingness to go with them through an experience with death. This willingness is an attitude which is expressed in thoughtful actions even more than words. If present, it helps the patient and family make use of the nurse's professional sustaining competence. Carol Ren Kneisl, a nurse, discussing thoughtful care for the dying, stresses the importance of simply being with the patient. She thinks that dying people suffer most from a sense of isolation and abandonment. She notes that "the ancient Greeks believed the most fearful event was not dying but dying alone." * Ilse S. Wolfe, a psychiatric nurse, years ago, illustrated with clinical incidents this willingness to walk beside the patient. She called this "The Magnificence of Understanding." [84] Listening is, of course, essential to understanding. The most experienced persons in the care of the dying keep saying that directly or obliquely most patients will let caregivers know their needs if they will sit quietly and listen.

When death is imminent, nothing is more reassuring to patients and their families than the promise that someone will be there when the patient needs a comforting presence. And, it goes without saying that such promises must be realistic so that they can be kept. Reference was made on page 1944 to reports of solitary hospital deaths and the literature abounds in criticism of doctors who are not present, even in hospitals.† Nurses have the greatest opportunity and therefore should have the responsibility for noting signs of approaching death and the authority to call the physician, and in

---

* McNulty, Barbara J.: "Symposium on Care of the Dying. The Nurse's Contribution in Terminal Care," *Nurs. Mirror*, **139**:59, (Oct. 10) 1974.

† Summers, D. H.: "The Role of the Nurse," presented at Thanatology Nursing Symposium, New York City, Nov. 1–2, 1974.

---

* Kneisl, Carol Ren: "Thoughtful Care for the Dying," *Am. J. Nurs.*, **68**:550, (Mar.) 1968.

† Dorothy P. Geis, a nurse who interviewed 26 mothers who had lost a child, found that the doctor was present in 13 instances, the nurse in 8, the father and mother in 5, the mother alone in 4, the father in 1, others in 6 cases, and in 4 cases the mother did not know. The mothers thought physicians most helpful (11), the clergy next, and the nurse third. In 5 cases, no one was "most helpful." The sample is too small to have much significance but data of this sort are badly needed as a substitute for unfounded inferences on the needs of patients and families and who can and will meet them. (Geis, Dorothy P.: "Mothers' Perceptions of Care Given Their Dying Children," *Am. J. Nurs.*, **65**:105, [Feb.] 1965.)

his absence, or with his approval, the family and the clergy or a spiritual adviser of the patient's choice. While nurses cannot legally pronounce death, in the physician's absence and in the normal course of open communication with the family they should share their opinion that life is over. Nurses prepare the body to go to the undertaking establishment; this is discussed in a later section, as is their role in helping the bereaved.

Role of Social Workers. Social workers, Ruth D. Abrams says, are the most available counselors in many medical settings. They collaborate with chaplains, doctors, nurses, and others in helping patients and their relatives with a variety of problems. In some countries and in certain eras, the preparation and work of the public health nurse and the social worker are combined; in the United States, visiting nurse associations often have social workers on their staffs.

Abrams thinks there are common misconceptions about the role of the social worker whose function she sees as follows:

Many people think of the social worker as a person who gives advice on how to manage the financial aspect of the illness. If they do not need such help, their first reaction is to reject the suggestion that such a person can be useful. I believe that changing the term "social worker" to "family counselor" would be a giant step toward ensuring acceptance by health workers and by the family. Her help should include practical matters, to be sure, but it goes well beyond that.*

Abrams,[85,86] through excerpts from case studies, shows the problems and describes the kinds of help social workers at the Massachusetts General Hospital give patients with cancer and the families of these patients. Social workers may help them cope with financial problems or with the changes in the way the family lives when either parent dies. Knowing the resources in the community, social workers may be the best prepared persons to help patients and families make use of them. As, through regular visits and participation in patient conferences, they come to know the patients, their relatives, and friends, they may be in an admirable position to help patients' families to live as normally as possible during a terminal illness and to return to normal community life after the period of acute grief.

Role of Nutritionists. Since the maintenance of good nutrition can minimize the severity of almost any pathology, the nutritionist or dietician can play a very important role in relieving symptoms that may accompany the dying process. In the last analysis, poor nutrition may precipitate death when symptoms of the disease include loss of appetite (anorexia), nausea, and vomiting. In some cases patients may be able to enjoy eating and drinking to the end. Meals and "snacks" may be among the remaining pleasures left. Eating alone is not, for most people, conducive to the enjoyment of meals. Nutritionists in administrative positions can help plan facilities that foster communal meals and that make it possible for patients and their families to share favorite dishes and even prepare them.

Patients' appetites have unexpected shifts. While they may eat little for days at a time, they may also have a sudden urge to eat a hearty meal. Fortunately, hospital kitchens can now be designed to make and freeze meals so that it is possible to respond to an unexpected request. At Calvary Hospital in the Bronx, New York City, a kitchen staff with well-prepared nutritionists has menu plans that allow for such changes.

It is one of the functions of nutritionists in home care services and in institutions to visit patients and to discuss their nutritional needs, their dietary habits, and their eating and drinking problems. Participation by nutritionists or dietitians in patient care conferences is often crucial in making the adjustments in hospital or nursing home practices essential to the welfare of the dying patient. One of the aspects of hospice's programs that excites admiring comment is the excellent, homelike, and individualized meals, the availability night and day of certain nutrients patients may need, and the "snack bars" where patients and family may purchase things to eat and drink as they sit outdoors together or in common rooms. One note of caution discussed further is that urging a patient to eat when he or she doesn't feel like it can create tension between patients and others.

In almost every culture, food and drink are essential elements of almost any celebration. For dying patients, their birthday, Christmas, New Year's, Chanukah, Easter, a christening, bar mitzvah, wedding or other high day may be of great importance. Nutritionists, working with nurses, occupational therapists, volunteers, and others can help to make high days happy occasions for everyone and healing memories for bereaved families.

Role of Occupational and Recreational Therapists. While the occupational and recreational therapists are in the best position to suggest how specific ideas for occupation and recreation can be carried out, nurses, social workers, volunteers, and families may help in this aspect of care.

---

* Abrams, Ruth D.: *Not Alone With Cancer.* Charles C Thomas, Publisher, Springfield, Ill., 1974, p. 14.

Terminally ill patients are faced with their own mortality, and for this reason the search for meaning in life absorbs much of their time. Each individual approaches this question in a different way. Individual interests, capabilities, beliefs about life after death, and ties to relatives and friends must be understood so that the patient has a sense of fulfillment. Just whiling away the hours is not enough.

Weakness, flagging strength, increasing helplessness, and the realization that families, friends, and caregivers are sore pressed by the patient's illness put a heavy burden on the patient. Most patients have a strong desire to give to others and do for others in return for help given them. Patients want to be active participants in life, despite the fact that their energies come in spurts. Therefore, whatever they choose to do should be appropriate to the surge and lapse of strength and to the time they have left.

As Lifton points out, one way that people come to terms with their own mortality is to know that their works and contributions will live after them, and another way is to realize that they are a significant link in the human chain; that they live in the memories of family and friends and in their progeny.

Some patients may take comfort in helping other patients; especially when family or staff don't understand the patient's point of view. If it is hard for a patient to sit up or to do physical work, it is still possible to reminisce with members of the family and hand down the family lore. A mother or grandmother may pass on recipes; any patient might enjoy arranging snapshots in the family album, and identifying the subjects.

Many patients have taken the role of teacher by writing about their experiences as patients (Jaffe, Alsop, Rosenthal) and by speaking to caregivers and students about what has helped and what has hindered them. Others have contributed in the making of films that tell viewers what it is like to die.* The ideas and recommendations of patients and their families provide a different and essential perspective on the environment. (See Fig. 50-10.)

A professional person, writer, artist, musician, whose work has been interrupted by illness may need time, space and the freedom to finish that work if and when it is possible.

Heightened appreciation may accompany terminal illness, so flower arranging and flower care, listening to music, and playing an instrument are all important.

* Mike Rohmer's film "Dying"; "Paula," a patient at St. Christophers, and "I Have Lived a Life," at St. Christopher's Hospice, Inc.; Children's Hospital, Philadelphia, also has films on dying.

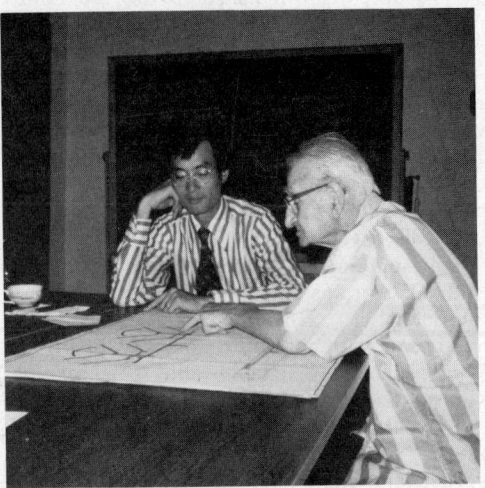

Figure 50-10. A patient, plumber by occupation, reviews the plans for the inpatient facility of the hospice to be built in Branford, Conn., with the architect Lo-Yi Chan. (Courtesy of Hospice, Inc., New Haven, Conn. Photograph by Shirley Dobihal, L.P.N.)

Occupational and recreational therapists are specialists who are prepared to provide the conditions, tools, and materials that enable persons to engage in purposeful activity, or work, and in recreational activities. Patients receiving palliative treatment may suddenly find themselves comfortable and able to maneuver once again, so that in a hospice, such as St. Christopher's, patients may be able to do something in which they are interested up to a few days or hours of their death. A work laboratory, or occupational therapy department, facilitates a work program at least by providing space for storing materials so that they are easily available.

It is the role of these therapists to know patients, to discuss their interests and capabilities, and to make it possible for them to follow those interests and make optimum use of their capabilities as long as possible. Too often the public thinks of the occupational therapist as a person who teaches crafts, the products of which have doubtful artistic or practical merit, and the recreational therapist as a person who works with children in playgrounds. But some dying patients enjoy learning how to make an object they can give to a beloved relative or friend whether or not it has much practical or artistic merit. Some patients may want conditions provided that enable them to continue the tasks or activities with which they have been occupied in health—reading, writing, listening to, making, or composing music, painting, organizing a collection, designing and making clothing or decorative objects, and playing games.

By talking with patients, studying their records, and taking part in patient care conferences, occupational and recreational therapists in institutions are often in the best position to help. Because patients' interests and competence are so varied and no one worker can encompass all these areas of interest and competence, these special therapists can expand the scope of the program by enlisting help of volunteers who can work with patients in many areas. Strength that suddenly waxes and wanes is to be expected, so that work which is proposed should be realistic.

Role of Physical Therapists. Terminal illness may force inactivity and weakness on many persons and predispose them to contractures, fractures, and nerve atrophy or injury. Physical therapists specialize in the prevention and treatment of such conditions. It is most desirable for a hospital, nursing home, or a hospice to have a department or laboratory in which specialized equipment facilitates the work of the physical therapist. As with occupational and recreational therapy, this is not essential, for there is much that physical therapists can do in patients' rooms and ward units.

Physical therapists must work closely with doctors who, after consultation with the therapist, prescribe appropriate treatment. Physical therapists should also work closely with nurses, or, in home care programs, with nurses and families, who must continue or maintain the treatment initiated by the therapist. A physiotherapy regimen must take into account what the patient can *realistically* achieve in light of irreversible tissue degeneration and/or in the case of advanced care, the knowledge that pathologic fractures may give way under certain prescribed movements.

Participation in patient care conferences is, in some cases, as important for the physical therapist as it is for the nutritionist or any other specialized worker.

Role of Volunteers. In hospices, in many hospitals, and possibly in some nursing homes, volunteers play important roles. There is usually a department for volunteer service with an administrative head. There are so many things that volunteers do, or could do, that it is hard to describe their roles. They can visit and talk and write letters for patients, they can transport patients and relatives or take them on recreational excursions, they can act as interpreters, they can distribute mail, arrange flowers and water plants, cultivate gardens, provide library services and clerical services, run shops, or give assistance in almost any department including the department of nursing. Many volunteers have found work in health services so rewarding that they have made it a full-time occupation; many recruits into professional health schools were originally volunteers. Many lay persons have, through their own experiences in losing a husband, wife, or child, an enriching experience that makes them of particular help. In the United States the Widow to Widow programs, and the Make Today Count program have chapters in many communities. Such organizations are discussed more fully under the heading of bereavement. Hospices, hospitals, and nursing homes are settings in which community members can learn what it is like to be dying, and how others can help the person who is dying.

Role of Administrators. In institutions and home care services, administrators facilitate the roles of all types of workers—those whose roles have been discussed and the many other categories of personnel that are employed in institutions and agencies giving terminal care. In Chapter 3 it is stated that the importance of the administrator's philosophy can't be overemphasized. Before terminal care can be materially improved in this or any other country, administrators of health care services must understand the needs of the dying and their families and the needs of those who serve them. They, and interested citizens on governing boards, must decide whether existing institutions and agencies or departments in them can be modified to this end or whether new ones must be created.

Patricia A. Downie, a British physical therapist, says that in Great Britain:

. . . the dying and the progressively ill are cared for either in the essentially religious foundation staffed by religious personnel with secular assistance, in the newer type of hospice which is essentially lay but with a strong emphasis on spiritual help, or in homes run by specific charities representing specific disease, which are endeavoring to plug a gap in the hospital services.*

Downie, returning from a visit to Canada and the United States, notes the numbers of groups in both countries who are now meeting to discuss ways and means of changing the care of the dying and who are studying British institutions. She quotes Ivan Illich's saying "Only the very rich in the United States can now afford what all people in poor countries have—personal attention round the death bed." But she describes some programs, most notably

* Downie, Patricia A.: "Symposium on Care of the Dying. A Personal Commentary on the Care of the Dying on the North American Continent," *Nurs. Mirror,* **139:**68, (Oct. 10) 1974.

that of Calvary Hospital in "one of the seamier parts" of New York City where the kind of care is given that is seen in twenty or more British institutions. She makes the following observation:

The concept of care is clearly seen: it is a normal approach to a natural event. Frankness is the keynote to this approach. With five full-time doctors each patient is assured of very personal care and, once a good rapport is established, openness and honesty can be practised.

As I walked round it was apparent that each patient was very much an individual who was assessed and treated in the way he preferred. For the first time in their lives, some of these patients were experiencing love in its fullest sense.*

Here and in the other places mentioned on page 1953 those who cannot visit the European hospices can see the various givers of care filling the roles discussed in this section. Mannes,[87] comparing Youville (Cambridge, Mass.) and Calvary Hospitals with St. Christopher's Hospice, says they are "primarily hospitals" while St. Christopher's is different—it is a home for the end of life, a family, a community where drugs are used to anticipate rather than relieve pain. Saunders [88] describes it as "a therapeutic community." The mutual respect shown patients, families, and all types of paid and volunteer workers makes it therapeutic for everyone. Muggeridge, in his tribute to Mother Teresa of Calcutta, describes a therapeutic community she and other Sisters of the Missionaries of Charity created for lepers and other "poorest of the poor." Speaking of the Home for the Dying, as shown in the film he made of Mother Teresa's work, he says:

One thing everyone who has seen the film seems to be agreed about is that the light in the Home for the Dying is quite exceptionally lovely. This is, from every point of view, highly appropriate. Dying derelicts from the streets might normally be supposed to be somewhat repellent, giving off stenches, emitting strange groans. Actually, if the Home for the Dying were piled high with flowers and resounding with musical chants —as it may well have been in its Kali days—it could not be more restful and serene. So, the light conveys perfectly what the place is really like; an outward and visible luminosity manifesting God's inward and invisible omnipresent love. This is precisely what miracles are for—to reveal the inner reality of God's outward creation. I am personally persuaded that Ken recorded the first authentic photographic miracle.†

There may be places in other continents where the needs of the dying are as fully met. No claim is made here to a worldwide survey of institutions or practices and, as elsewhere in this book, the writers take the position that people can learn from all cultures and that none has a corner on the instinctive or acquired ability to provide conditions under which a person can die well.

6. CARE OF THE DYING PERSON— SYMPTOMATIC MANAGEMENT

Helping Patients Cope with Disturbed Functions. Descriptions of the management of the dying patient may be as old as any written medical works but a study of the literature, comprehensive or superficial, gives the impression that because, by the nature of their training, doctors feel defeated by death, few have written about the care of the dying. Until recently, few nurses have written about it. Sir William Osler, studying "the art and act of dying" in 500 patients, reported that only 18 per cent had pain and only 2 per cent apprehension. He speaks of "how rarely agony" is seen and he says "The hard process of nature's law is for most of us mercifully effected . . ." * Previously cited are the opinions along these lines of Worcester, a contemporary of Osler and a student of the dying process, and the experience of Lewis Thomas, who said that he had seen agony only once "in a patient with rabies." †

Saunders, founder of St. Christopher's Hospice, emphasizes the way in which physical symptoms can be controlled so that repose is possible and she often speaks of the ease with which the end comes. Noyes, writing on "the care and management of the dying," after reviewing the meaning of death to Greek philosophers, people of the Middle Ages, the Renaissance, and the present day, makes the following observations:

Dying persons do not regularly agonize over their departure. The misconception that they do results, perhaps, from the wish among those of us living vigorously that the dying should suffer, lest in not doing so they should seem to show a disdain for the life which we cherish, or should seem happy to leave us behind.‡

Eric Wilkes, British medical educator, as well as medical director and founder of St. Luke's Nursing Home in Sheffield, Eng., discussing

---

* *Ibid.*
† Muggeridge, Malcolm: *Something Beautiful for God. Mother Teresa of Calcutta.* Collins-Fontana Books, London, 1973, page 44.

* Osler, William: "Thoughts on Dying," *Can. Med. Surg.,* **16:**511, 1888.
† Thomas, Lewis: *op. cit.,* p. 50.
‡ Noyes, Russell, Jr.: "The Care and Management of the Dying," *Arch. Intern. Med.,* **128:**299, (Aug.) 1971.

Table 50-3. Terminal Care: The Ten Major Symptoms After Admission (296 Cases) * †

Pain	58%	Bedsores	15%
Incontinence	38%	Vomiting	13%
Confusion	21%	Open wounds	13%
Dyspnea	17%	Cough	5%
Nausea	16%	Dysphagia	3%

* Wilkes, Eric: "Symposium on Care of the Dying. Relatives, Professional Care, and the Dying Patient," *Nurs. Mirror,* 139:54, (Oct. 10) 1974.
† Note: Symptoms such as insomnia, anorexia, depression, and anxiety are excluded since, although often diagnosed, they were rarely complained of even when present, nor did they often impress the observer as a major symptom.

"Relatives, Professional Care, and the Dying Patient," reports a study of 296 patients who died of cancer, giving the incidence of the "10 major symptoms" that were "complained of" after admission to the hospital (see Table 50-3).

In a series of articles on care of the dying published in *Nursing Times* and afterward in a reprinted booklet,[89] Saunders discusses control of pain in terminal cancer as primarily the physician's problem because it involves prescription of drugs. "Mental distress" and "mental pain" are presented as a challenge to all who attend the dying patient. Under "the nursing of patients dying of cancer" the following symptoms and their treatment are discussed, in this order: intractable vomiting, dysphagia, fungating growths, (sore or painful) mouth, pathologic fractures, fits, urinary complications, bowel (complications), (disordered) sleep, bedsores, hiccoughs, persistent coughs, and asphyxia and dyspnea. Craven and Wald[90] list pain, depression, anorexia, weakness, lethargy, breathlessness, and gastrointestinal disturbances as "common symptoms" associated with cancer. Emotional support and control of physical symptoms are the essential elements in palliative treatment of terminal care, so that the patient can be unburdened and live as naturally as possible.

Throughout this book, the position is taken that mind and body are inseparable or that thought has a physical response. It may therefore be artificial and misleading to separate mental and physical symptoms or even to speak of symptom control *and* emotional support as if they weren't to some extent interdependent. The effect of emotional support on minimizing pain is stressed in Chapter 49 and the fact mentioned that pain is pushed out of conscious thought by powerful emotions or an overwhelming sense of purpose in accomplishing a task.

The extent to which symptoms, mental and physical, are interrelated is debatable; but few would claim that any symptom is a separate entity. By discussing symptoms as aberrations of normal body function, an effort is made in the following pages to show relationships. McNulty[91] urges that *all* symptoms be taken seriously, maintaining that it is hard to know which one, or which ones, are really disturbing the patient. Robert G. Twycross urges physicians and nurses to practice according to the "Ten Commandments":

1. Thou shalt not assume that the patient's pain is due to the malignant process.
2. Thou shalt try simple analgesics in the first instance.
3. Thou shalt not be afraid of narcotic drugs.
4. Thou shalt not prescribe inadequate amounts of any analgesic.
5. Thou shalt not use the abbreviation p.r.n.
6. Thou shalt take into account the patient's feelings.
7. Thou shalt provide support for the whole family.
8. Thou shalt not limit thy approach simply to the use of drugs.
9. Thou shalt not be afraid to ask colleagues' advice.
10. Thou shalt have an air of quiet confidence and cautious optimism.*

Problems Associated with Breathing. People who talk about their fear of the dying process sometimes say that they are afraid of suffocation. Difficulty in breathing (*dyspnea*) was found by Wilkes in 17 per cent of 296 patients (see Table 50-3). *Breathlessness* or a feeling of *suffocation* in malignancies may be due to pleural effusion which can be aspirated. The patient's anxiety, which always accompanies dyspnea, is relieved by sedatives, and, according to Saunders, sedatives (amylobarbitone) (Amobarbital, Amytal) 30 gm or chlordiazepoxide hydrochloride (Librium) 5 to 10 gm, given two or three times daily, should be combined with any other treatment of breathlessness. Wilkes[92] suggests Librium and diazepam (Valium) and diamorphine (heroin). Noyes[93] recommends both and thinks they are free of the "troublesome side effects" of the phenothiazines (Prolixin) and tricyclic antidepressants (Elavil).

Saunders says antibiotics should be given if there is *purulent sputum* with or without a *persistent cough*. While they are not likely to prolong life at this stage, they make the last weeks or days more comfortable. Chloramphenicol is said to be "most effective." She says

* Twycross, Robert G.: "Principles and Practice of the Relief of Pain in Terminal Cancer," *Update, From the Postgraduate Centers,* July 1972, p. 82.

patients "like" cough mixtures, which alone justifies their use. She thinks linctus, especially if diluted with boiling water, effective, and "nothing replaces" linctus diamorphine (heroin).

Bronchospasm may be treated with ephedrine and oxtriphylline (choline theophyllinate) (Choledyl) [or theophylline itself which is just as effective and less expensive;] and they sometimes help when there is no clinical evidence of bronchospasm. Saunders says that when dyspnea cannot be relieved, an effort should be made to lift its oppression. Even when there is bronchospasm "nothing but the opiates will relieve the intolerable feelings of suffocation. . . . Small doses should be given initially, combined with sedation."

Dryness of the respiratory passages and *excessive secretions* may be causes of dyspnea and stridor. Humidity control helps to relieve dryness in some cases. Cold cream, petroleum jelly, or petroleum jelly with vitamins A and D, applied to the nose and lips, are comforting. Physicians may prescribe an antihistamine, such as Benadryl, to decrease secretions; if excessive secretion is the cause of dyspnea, Benadryl may relieve the attendant anxiety. Mucus that collects in the mouth may be removed with sponges held in a forceps, but more efficiently with a catheter attached to a motorized suction apparatus.

Administration of oxygen may or may not be indicated. No techniques are free from disadvantages. Oxygen rooms and tents isolate the patient and may deepen their anxiety; masks over the face and tubes in the nose are uncomfortable, and motor-driven equipment is noisy and interferes with the communication of patients with family, friends, and staff. With collaboration between patients, doctors, pharmacists, and nurses, a drug, or a combination of drugs and other treatment modalities, for example appropriate use of oxygen, can usually be found that controls respiratory difficulties. If the patient is isolated and lacks the reassurance of a comforting presence, no drugs may be effective.

In prolonged illness, there is a possibility that an old tubercular lesion may become active. For this reason, routine diagnostic chest x-rays should be a part of medical assessment in managing symptoms, as well as protecting other patients, families, and staff.

Persistent hiccoughs, caused by spasms of the diaphragm, are among the most distressing symptoms. They are nerve-racking, for they interfere with rest and sleep. If present while patients are eating or drinking, they may make them insufflate solids or liquids. Various relief measures are discussed in Chapter 39. Saunders suggests the administration of carbon dioxide or having the patient breathe in and out of a paper bag, adding that injections of chlorpromazine are sometimes effective. A simple but effective agent is 1 tsp of dry granulated sugar. The small crystals flowing over the esophagus are believed to effect a change.[93a]

Asphyxia, the end result of dyspnea, when the supply of oxygen is so reduced that it will not support life is, in a sense, always present at the end of life. In some accidents, as, for instance, carbon monoxide poisoning or drowning, the principal life-saving measure is immediate relief, since irreparable brain damage and death result from inadequate oxygen for even short periods. Heroic resuscitation (such as that described in Chapter 35) is seriously questioned in the treatment of the person who is dying of an illness that is believed to be irreversible.

Problems Associated with Eating and Drinking. A *loss of appetite* (*anorexia*) is common in terminal illness. Pain, fear and anxiety, insomnia, inactivity, and separation from many of life's normal activities, including work, tend to diminish appetite. Solitary meals or anything that detracts from the pleasure of eating, decreases appetite. Saunders says that more than one third of those admitted to St. Christopher's suffer from anorexia, but it frequently disappears with pain relief and a change of diet. Persistent loss of appetite is treated with an antiemetic, with alcoholic drinks before or with meals, and with small doses of steroids (prednisolone or prednisone, 5 mg three times daily).

Diminished food intake over any length of time for any reason tends to decrease the appetite. A high-caloric, high-vitamin diet may increase the appetite but the diet should be in a form that appeals to the patient and preferably is easily digested. Many patients prefer ethnic foods—pizza, spaghetti and meatballs, tacos, stuffed grape leaves. Even if the patient has difficulty in swallowing the blender can be used so that the wanted flavor can be had in a blended food. The dietary department at Calvary Hospital has been particularly successful in serving meals which terminally ill patients enjoy and can eat. The company of close relatives and friends and communal meals may improve the appetite unless patients have eating problems that make them self-conscious or that are anxiety-provoking.

When patients require help in eating, it is of the utmost importance for their helpers to be skillful in giving the needed help but also to be unhurried. It goes without saying that the quality of the food and the appropriateness of the service directly affect appetite. Small, frequent feedings rather than full meals may be indicated, and every effort should be made to cater to the patient's likes and dislikes. However, family and caregivers should anticipate the sudden appearance of a craving for a specific meal or large intake. Patients, families, friends, nurses, and nutritionists should collaborate with the physician in combating loss of appetite. Good nutrition minimizes most pathology and poor nutrition has the opposite effect.

According to Saunders, one third of the admissions to St. Christopher's (most of whom are terminally ill cancer victims) suffer from *nausea* and *vomiting,* and even more from loss of appetite.* These figures are said to "illustrate one of the reasons for our use of diamorphine." Nauseated and vomiting patients should have constant attendance and the environment should be as free as possible from noise and unpleasant sights and odors. Aromatic odors such as camphor or ammonia may be tolerated, or even welcomed. Coolness, sometimes an ice cap or cold cloth on the head, is refreshing. Cool drinks or chips of ice help, and carbonated drinks, such as ginger ale, vichy, or soda water may be retained when nothing else by mouth is tolerated. Sherbets are more likely to be acceptable than ice cream, and milk added to ginger ale, to give it more food value, may also be acceptable. These helpful tasks may prove a good way for family to participate in care.

Persistent nausea and vomiting make the patient miserable as well as those who, helplessly, watch their suffering. Every effort should be made to remove the cause when this is possible. Pressure from malignant growths or bleeding may, in some cases, be relieved by surgery, irradiation, or chemotherapy, but the uses of such treatment have usually been exhausted in the terminal phase of the illness. Hinton [94] says that vomiting can be a sign that the kidneys or liver are ceasing to function adequately. In a group of patients he studied who suffered from these symptoms, one third could not be relieved. He believes these symptoms and impaired swallowing are less easily controlled than pain and summarizes the treatment as adjustment of the diet, antiemetic drugs, and surgical relief of obstruction. However, in the past few years the use of antiemetic drugs (Compazine, Dramamine) before radiation or chemotherapy has proved successful.

In discussing the use of opiates when there is intractable vomiting, Saunders says that they do not cause vomiting as often when the patient is in bed and in pain as they do with normal people, but that their use is undoubtedly responsible for some of the nausea and vomiting seen in terminal illness. She thinks diamorphine is the least likely to cause nausea but suggests that different drugs in the opium group be tried until the most satisfactory one is found. Arthur Lipman [94a] points out "that narcotic analgesics induce nausea through both medullary and middle ear mechanisms." Accordingly, if the patient is more active and is moving about, the nausea is exacerbated. Reducing activity may relieve the nausea, or an even better solution is to use a phenothiazine antiemetic and an antihistamine antiemetic such as cyclazine. In that way, the patient is able to be active without discomfort. Of course other reasons for nausea must also be considered such as involvement of the gastrointestinal tract by the malignancy or involvement of the central nervous system. When vomiting continues, drugs by mouth are stopped and analgesics given hypodermically. Analgesic suppositories are used occasionally. Several antiemetics should also be tried to see which works best. Saunders says that some patients have an amazing response to reassurance—"They have probably been vomiting because of pain and misery." If vomiting persists, the stomach contents may be removed by suction through a nasal tube. This prevents the constant retching. Saunders suggests replacing the fluid with a rectal infusion but this is often ineffective. (See Chapter 23.)

Dysphagia, or *difficulty in swallowing,* may be caused by obstructive growths, by weakness of the muscles of deglutition, or by an emotional disorder. The second author saw a man suffering from a paralysis of these muscles who lived for several years with a drain in the mouth when up or suction when he was in bed because he could not swallow the saliva. He was able to swallow semisolid foods and was kept alive on puréed (baby) foods. When swallowing is painful, Saunders says that a local anesthetic jelly before a meal may help and that in dysphagia, iced water is "the most welcome drink." * Many persons with such difficulties have been sustained with tube feeding. Carbonated drinks may help to keep tubes clear. Cold carbonated drinks used as a mouth wash are welcome in some cases. They can be alternated with the patient's favorite antiseptic rinse. Mouth cleanliness, discussed later, is of

---

* Families or staff, in an effort to express concern and wanting to help, may press a patient to eat when they cannot, and the end result is tension between patient and others, or disappointment. Steroids, for example prednisone, used to control symptoms of cancer, also stimulate the appetite. F. W.

* Treatments attributed to Saunders on this and preceding pages are from Saunders, Cicely: *Care of the Dying. Nursing Times Reprint.* Macmillan Journals, Ltd., London, [1970]; and Saunders, Cicely: "The Symptomatic Treatment of Incurable Malignant Disease," *Prescribers J.,* **4:**68, (Oct.) 1964.

special importance to such patients. Dryness of the mouth can also be caused by side effects of anticholinergic components in drugs such as phenothiazines and tricyclic antidepressants. Reducing the dosage, or offering small sips of fluid or making hard candy available will enable the patient to relieve dryness of the mouth.

Patiently and consistently giving liquids will usually prevent dehydration and is likely to be appreciated by most people. In hospitals often an intravenous feeding is almost routine on admission. This practice is highly questionable when there is no hope of recovery unless there is no family member or enough staff to prevent dehydration. Noyes makes the following statement which would apply here:

Decisions regarding life-prolonging procedures should, whenever possible, be placed in the hands of patients themselves and, when this is not reasonable, in the hands of the family.*

Problems Associated with Elimination. Elimination by bowel, bladder, or skin may be affected in the dying patient. A daily *bowel movement* is habitual for many persons and interruption of this habit may make them anxious.† Saunders makes the following statement: "Patients regard a regular action as their birthright and will wear themselves out over it but some can be persuaded that once or twice weekly may be quite in order for them."‡

Methods of preventing, controlling, and managing constipation, diarrhea, and fecal incontinence discussed in Chapters 11 and 37 apply here. Regulation by fluid and food intake is increasingly difficult as appetite wanes, particularly if nausea and vomiting drastically curtail intake of fluids and food. Consideration of the medications being used that affect mobility of the bowels is essential. Bisacodyl (Ducilax) often prevents constipation. It must always be kept in mind that a physical blockage somewhere along the digestive tract may be the reason there is no bowel movement. Prune juice, when tolerated, is useful and a high liquid intake is desirable except at night when emptying the bladder frequently inter-

feres with sleep. Marked *constipation* may result in *impaction of feces* that requires manual removal (see Chapter 37). Heavy mineral oil (liquid paraffin) by mouth (to be distinguished from light mineral oil, which is less effective and causes uncomfortable leaking from the rectum), vegetable oil rectal injections, and paraffin suppositories are all useful. Another useful approach is to increase and soften the fecal bulk with a medication such as Colace. It goes without saying that keeping active just as long as possible is of great importance in preventing constipation. Finding sedatives and analgesics that are least likely to cause constipation is desirable, but almost any drug that reduces pain reduces activity and appetite, and in turn causes constipation.

Diarrhea is an accompaniment of some malignancies of the intestinal tract. Its management is discussed in Chapter 36 and the same principles apply here except that in terminal illness it may be impossible to eliminate the cause. Antibiotics may be used effectively for diarrhea caused by microorganisms; a bland diet may control diarrhea caused by irritating foods. Drugs by mouth may be terminated one by one to see which one is the irritant.

Diarrhea is not only dehydrating and exhausting, but can be accompanied by pain because it results in a very sore anus. A soothing ointment, such as Vaseline with vitamins A and D added, may be healing to the anus and surrounding skin.

Frequent bowel movements can be of psychic origin. In such cases, it is essential that the patient have ready access to a toilet, a commode, or a bedpan. The fear of soiling clothing, bedding, or furniture is a source of anxiety to most people but can be an obsession for the fastidious. Increasing weakness, helplessness, and loss of control of the dying patient can be overwhelming. Patients may ask for and use a bedpan within an hour or two of death and ask the nurse for help that will prevent soiling. Reassurance that they will not be left alone may in itself relieve diarrhea of psychic origin. Relief of pain may also relieve the mental stress that has upset the intestinal function.

Urinary elimination is affected by most pathology that causes a protracted terminal illness. Methods of preventing, controlling, and managing *urgency, frequency, retention, incontinence, anuria, bladder spasm,* and *renal colic* discussed in Chapters 11 and 37 may apply here. Like the problems of bowel elimination, they may be caused by growths that cause pressure, by infections, by bleeding, by irritating foods or drugs, or by fear and anxiety that affects function. Treatment should be

---

* Noyes, Russell, Jr.: *op. cit.*

† One elderly lady in her 90s who had failed for several days to have her usual daily bowel movement said to the nurse with an alarmed finality, "I'm sealed up." A colonic irrigation was used to show her that the bowel contents could be removed even when her strength was not sufficient to propel feces through the anus.

‡ Saunders, Cicely: *Care of the Dying. Nursing Times Reprint.* Macmillan Journals, Ltd., London, [1970], p. 25.

directed toward the elimination of the cause if this is possible. By the terminal stage of illness, surgical measures are rarely appropriate. Antibiotics and sulfonamides may be used for infections. As with intestinal problems of psychic origin, the reassurance of an understanding presence may be enough to relieve urinary symptoms caused by fear, anxiety, and embarrassment over dependence on others in using toilets, commodes, bedpans, or urinals.

In addition it should be noted that drugs such as phenothiazines, tricyclic antidepressants, antihistamines, and anticholinergic agents will cause urinary retention. Bethanechol (urecholine) can be prescribed to ease this condition.[94b]

As the muscles lose their tone, the bladder and rectum may leak their contents. To avoid embarrassing patients, the bedpan—the urinal in the case of a man or a boy—should be put in position periodically. Even though patients have too little strength to ask for them they may be able to use them.* The bed should be protected by soft pads of cellucotton that have a waterproof paper base. These can be changed frequently without much inconvenience to patients. In some cases the bladder is distended by a failure to void. A retention catheter relieves the sensation of pressure and avoids the necessity of moving on and off a bedpan, which is so difficult for the weak patient, but patients may find the presence of the catheter unpleasant and it makes the patient more vulnerable to infection. The problems associated with elimination are lessened if the patient is ambulatory. Every effort should be made to keep the dying from being bedfast, as is stressed throughout this chapter.

Problems Associated with Body Movement. Neuromuscular pathology includes inactivity, weakness, fractures, contractures, tremors and seizures, and pressure sores. The discussion of body mechanics in Chapter 12 and of hypo- and hyperactivity in Chapters 38 and 39 apply here. The symptoms listed may be of organic, functional, or psychic origin. With the relief of pain, improved nutrition, and effective management of elimination, patients who had been confined to bed often stay relatively active until the last few days or hours of life.

Putting institutionalized patients to bed in night clothes tends to encourage isolation and *inactivity*. It also encourages *contractures* that make movement difficult and finally impossible. Inactivity also produces *pressure sores*

(*bedsores* or *decubiti*).* It follows, therefore, that with a few exceptions every effort should be made to prevent bedfastness and isolation even though a growing weakness and depression may tempt the patient to accept both. Moving from room to room and going outdoors, even going for a drive, is possible for some patients until the last days or hours of life. When staying in bed is, or seems, inevitable, frequent change of position is essential to prevent contractures and bedsores.

Weakness and helplessness are as much causes of the dying patient's discomfort as pain or nausea, and for several reasons they may be more difficult to deal with. There are many medications that prevent pain and, in some cases, prevent or control nausea, both of which wax and wane, but there is no medication to directly affect weakness and its relentless progression.

Patients who can pace themselves, and be content with doing less and resting more, have an advantage over those who continue to live beyond their strength. The young dying mother who sees her children doing for themselves and her husband overworked finds it harder to slow down when it is so obvious that her active involvement is needed. An unanticipated observation by the first author in the conduct of her study was that mothers and fathers, husbands and wives feel a sense of guilt that they are leaving loved ones "flat." It is often hard to decide when patients should stay in bed. Helping them to the bathroom can be time consuming and risky because a fall may result in a sprain, dislocation, or fracture. On the other hand, the feeling of independence that using the bathroom gives patients may make that risk worth taking. A back rub, tub bath, shower, or shampoo can sap limited energy but also be comforting, refreshing, and revitalizing. The nurse should carefully consider the appropriate pace and look for ways to avoid procedural steps that don't benefit the patient. Nurses should try in this respect as in all others to see the situation from the patient's and family's perspective. At the last, if soiled sheets, an unattended pressure sore, or a wound causes the patient or the family dis-

---

* The practice of leaving exposed bedpans and urinals on bedside stands is to be decried. If kept near the patient, they should be covered for esthetic reasons.

* The prevention and treatment of pressure sores are discussed in detail in Chapter 12. While their prevention is more difficult in the terminally ill, it is possible and should be the goal of all caretakers. Nurses should be flexible and able to assess whether the patient is aware of the bedsore, and whether it is the patient's need or the nurse's need to continue vigorous routines that requires frequent turning of the patient when it is painful and/or debilitating. One way to solve the dilemma is to provide analgesics prior to the turning of the patient so he or she suffers minimally because of the procedure.

comfort, the nurses should attend to it, but if it is only nurses who suffer because they are not demonstrating ostensibly "good nursing care," then the sheets, the sore, or the wound should be disregarded.

Terminally ill patients have unexpected spurts of energy. It is just as important for the staff to know when to step aside and help the patients enjoy these moments as it is to know when to step in. On Friday a patient may be limp as a rag, but on Saturday he or she may feel vigorous, especially if there is to be a celebration, a family reunion, or a significant event. Advice on rest and activity must be flexible, to say the least.

It is hard to make rules about the treatment of *fractures* of the terminally ill. If the patient is near death and if the fracture does not cause pain or interfere with activity in which the patient finds satisfaction, those concerned may decide not to use traction or apply a cast. Some form of immobilization is, however, nearly always necessary to prevent pain.

Nonspecific "fidgets," *tremors, spasms,* and *convulsions,* their causes and medical management, are discussed in Chapter 39. They would be treated the same way in the dying, should they occur, except that less effort might be made to determine the cause and, if anything, more effort made to help patients and families cope with the conditions. Weakness which may be accompanied by tremors is common in the terminal phase of illness and may make it necessary for patients to accept help with their toilet, with dressing and undressing, with their meals, and with most of the activities of daily living. It is the responsibility of nurses to give this help, or to help family members, friends, or volunteer workers do so.

Convulsions are especially painful for families and friends to watch. Since it is very difficult to know when the person loses and regains consciousness, it should be an unbroken rule that nothing is said by those present that the patient would be distressed to hear. The patient should always be addressed as if conscious. (For further discussion of the care of patients with convulsions, see Chapter 39.)

Dying patients are often seen lying on the back, which is probably the *least* comfortable position for them. In this posture the relaxed tongue falls against the pharynx, mucus collects in the mouth, and the effect of both is to close off the respiratory passage. If patients are turned on the side, the tongue falls forward and the mouth drains more satisfactorily. When there is little muscular control left, the body must be well supported by pillows. Patients often prefer to have the head elevated, feeling that they can breathe more easily in this position. Several writers of long experience in medical practice say that the dying wish to be turned toward the light and that the room should never be darkened because of the patient's dimming vision and the natural desire to see their surroundings until the end of life. The room should be airy as well as light, for patients breathe more easily if the air is in movement.

Problems Associated with Rest and Sleep. *Bad dreams, insomnia, restlessness,* and *night confusion* are common problems for the terminally ill as their life habits are interrupted and as their peace of mind is dispelled by worry over unfinished tasks, dependents inadequately provided for, dread of separation from all they love, and, often, fear of the process of dying —or death itself. People even in good health who, for one reason or another, are inactive or are attempting to solve a difficult problem find it hard to sleep at night. Inactive patients tend to nap during the day and they may not realize how much sleep they get this way that decreases the need for sleep at night.

Help in solving problems and providing companionship and activity until the last encourages normal sleep. Many of the ways of inducing sleep, described in Chapter 13, apply here—use of the toilet or bedpan, cleanliness, including mouth care, a back rub, a smooth bed, warmth (a hot-water bottle if necessary), quiet and darkness, or shaded lights, induce sleep. A hot drink may help, and Saunders thinks that "alcohol works splendidly with some patients." Low doses of hypnotics earlier in the evening will add immensely to the effect of a last sedative such as diazepam (Valium), or flurazepam (Dalmane).* The knowledge that someone will be there if help is needed also helps. For this reason, round-the-clock services, 7 days a week, with immediate telephone response to questions, is considered a requisite in services at home or in hospice institutions.

Natural sleep is always more refreshing than drug-induced sleep, but sedatives are not withheld from the terminally ill if they need and want them. Patients who are experienced in transcendental meditation may use it to refresh themselves. Barbiturates may, according to Saunders, give hangovers and make the elderly, particularly, restless. At St. Christopher's Hospice, a syrup of chlorpromazine is used and unlike most general hospitals and

---

* Saunders, Cicely: *Care of the Dying. Nursing Times Reprint.* Macmillan Journals, Ltd., London, 1970, p. 26. (Saunders thinks alcohol as a sedative is especially effective for men. This may be because many men have a habit of drinking at bedtime.)

nursing homes, the patient is rarely confined by bed sides, although bed sides may be left attached to help the patient change position without calling someone. Tranquilizers are used to prevent restlessness, and sleepless nights are a rarity unless the patient is troubled. The importance of the night nurse, available to talk with the patient about his concerns, cannot be stressed too much.

Problems of Cleanliness and Grooming. Cleanliness and appearance are important until the end. Even though some patients may seem to be uninterested in their appearance, most are affected, as are their relatives, friends, and caregivers. The other important question nurses must ask themselves about the patient's grooming is, "Am I doing this for the patient and/or family or for myself?"

Cleanliness of the skin helps prevent lesions, including pressure sores. As long as they have the strength, patients should be helped to take their own baths or showers. It is, however, most important when they lose this independence that those who help them make them feel that they take satisfaction in doing so. Some persons are fortunate in having been self-sufficient since their youth and men, especially, are embarrassed and humiliated by dependence on others in performing their toilet. It is particularly difficult for the aged and the weak to keep their fingernails and toenails trimmed and cleaned; long and jagged toenails can cause scratches that get infected and heal slowly. In some cases the services of a podiatrist may be indicated, but nurses can usually trim even the heaviest toenails if the feet are first soaked. Many patients with cancer are aware of bad, disagreeable odors, even though others may seem not to notice them. Air fresheners in the room, rinsing the mouth, and cleaning areas where there is discharge and using Chloromycetin gauze on sloughing wounds help overcome odors.

Clean hair, becomingly cut or arranged, goes a long way toward making most people feel that they look their best. If the disease or treatment makes patients lose their hair, "hair pieces" or wigs may raise their morale. Scarves can be arranged as turbans or in other becoming styles. Barber shop and beauty parlor equipment and services should be made available to institutionalized patients, but skilled nurses can give a shampoo to a bed patient and shave men patients when it is necessary. (See Chapter 14.)

Cleanliness of the mouth is, physically and psychologically, important. Kutscher, a dentist and president of the Foundation of Thanatology, calls attention to the fact that the mouth is the first area of gratification and is likely to be the last. He makes the following observation that as strength fails

. . . the mouth becomes the sole remaining modality by which a dying patient can anger or please, demand, request, beg, entreat, command, or even, in the larger sense, still affect for good or ill the lives of others whom he loves or hates— through expressions ranging from heartfelt words . . . to a whim . . . or making changes in a will.[*]

Dentists are needed for the replacement of teeth and the adjustment of plates. As consultants, they can help nurses devise modifications of usual techniques (see Chapter 14) when there are growths in or on the mouth or other conditions that make mouth care difficult. Patients should be encouraged to use a toothbrush as long as they have the strength to do so. Nurses, at the last, may have to manipulate the brush. Applicators provide so little friction that they do not make the teeth feel as clean as does a brush, but in some cases they must be used as a last resort. Antiseptic mouth washes of the patient's choice should be available. Motorized suction, available in institutions, should be gently used; a rubber-tipped syringe can be substituted in home care. The excessive dryness caused by mouth breathing can be relieved by coating the mucous membrane with a thin layer of oil applied with a cotton applicator or with an atomizer after gentle cleansing. Water, or some refreshing liquid, should be given in small amounts at short intervals to keep the mouth moist. By putting the finger over one end of a drinking straw after it is in a glass of water, suction is created and water is held in the straw. Small amounts can be given the patient from this straw. It is believed that the dying suffer from dehydration as discussed earlier. It has been shown that they can drink enough to control it and avoid the infusions so routinely used in hospitals.

The care of the mouth may be complicated by oral cancer. E. V. Zegarelli and associates [95] have described the care of patients with mouth cancer. Specialized articles and texts should be consulted by those caring for patients with diseases of the mouth or for those who have had mouth surgery.

Wearing apparel is as important at the end as at any other period of life. If the terminally ill wear *daytime clothing* it is easier for them to remain a part of family life and to live normally. The second author remembers with

---

[*] Kutscher, Austin H.: "The Psychosocial Aspects of the Oral Care of the Dying Patient," in Schoenberg, Bernard, et al. (eds.): *Psychosocial Aspects of Terminal Care.* Columbia University Press, New York, 1972, p. 127.

admiration and wonder a physician, a stranger to her, who died of cancer 10 days after taking a fish bone out of her throat with consummate skill and in a manner that gave no hint of his condition. Another man in his place might have been lying around a hospital in pajamas waiting for death to overtake him. It is, of course, not possible for everyone to "die with their boots on," but those who want to should be helped, rather than hindered. There is no question that purposeful activity holds in abeyance much of the mental and even physical distress of dying and that clothing affects the ability to stay in the stream of life.

Death usually comes to those with a debilitating disease when they are in bed. Covering should be light but warm enough for comfort. Attention has been called to the changes that occur as the circulatory mechanism fails. It is customary to try to warm the cooling extremities by the application of blankets and hot-water bottles. This should be done with great care. Worcester [96] attributes much of the restlessness and pulling at the bedclothes seen in the dying to the fact that they themselves feel hot even though the skin may feel cold to the touch. If patients can respond, they should be asked whether they would like additional warmth. A gown wet with perspiration should be changed. Rubbing the skin gently with alcohol may have a refreshing effect, but a quiet, comforting presence may be all that is wanted at the last and should be tried first.

Controlling Pain. The management of pain, and especially pain in the last stages of cancer, has been studied for years. Chapter 49 is devoted to a review of theories on the nature of pain and measures of control. The emphasis in that chapter is on the psychosomatic nature of pain, the definition by Margo McCaffery that "pain is whatever the experiencing person says it is and exists whenever he says it," and the three phases in dealing with pain: first assessment, then intervention, followed by evaluation; all this is as true for the dying patient as it is for every patient. If the reader has not read that chapter recently it might be helpful to do so now. Most of the symposia on death cited in this chapter include a discussion of pain, its management, and the difficulty of assessing its intensity when patients are at the same time suffering from the "mental pain" of fear, anxiety, depression, and the uncertainty engendered by false hopes or a lack of candor from those on whom they depend for help.

Hinton believes pain is the symptom associated with death that is most commonly feared. While admitting that it is an inherent part of some incurable diseases, he thinks it is by no means an inevitable accompaniment of the dying process, and that few "in this culture are allowed to follow the 'natural' course of a distressing mortal disease." * Hinton reviews studies on pain in terminal illness beginning with Osler's record of 500 deaths in which only 18 per cent suffered bodily pain or distress. He notes Beecher's work with the wounded and dying in World War II where only 25 per cent of the wounded wanted analgesics and where pain seemed influenced by the hopefulness of the outcome of the battle. On the other hand, Hinton reports his own experience with a group of terminally ill patients visited in a general hospital where 66 per cent were liable to pain that required treatment and he notes a review of 7000 cancer patients nursed at home by district nurses in England where more than two thirds had moderate or severe suffering.[97]

Noyes, in his discussion of the care and management of the dying, says:

> The experience of pain is profoundly influenced by a patient's interpretation of its meaning and by anxiety. In addition to recognizing the source of anxiety and providing appropriate reassurance, it may be controlled by the use of the minor tranquilizing medications such as chlordiazepoxide hydrochloride (Librium) or diazepam (Valium). These agents are also effective in reducing the symptoms of grief and are free of many of the troublesome side effects of the phenothiazines and tricyclic antidepressants.†

Saunders, who, as nurse, social worker, and physician, has studied care of the dying for years, has described explicitly the methods used at St. Joseph's and St. Christopher's to control the pain which patients with advanced cancer suffer. Saunders illustrates her points with patients' histories. Describing the care of a woman who was in "continuous, severe pain" on admission and who was given drugs regularly from the start, she makes the following observation:

> It is my opinion that this is the cardinal rule in the treatment of pain in this type of patient. Pain should never be allowed to take control and regular doses of analgesic should be given as soon as a patient is at all worried by it. It is not safe to rely on patients to ask, for either they will wait too long (and once pain has become really severe it is a potent antagonist to any drug) or else they will ask too soon and addiction may become a problem. If a patient receives prompt relief from the beginning and knows that he can rely on the next dose appearing on time he does not increase his own pain by fear and tension. There must, of course, be some latitude and no

* Hinton, John: *op. cit.,* p. 69.
† Noyes, Russell, Jr.: *op. cit.*

Table 50-4. Narcotic Analgesics Used in Terminally Ill Patients *†

Drug	Route	Dose (mg)	Average Duration of Action (hr)
Alphaprodine	s.c.	20–60	2–3
(Nisentil)	i.v.	10–30	1–2
Hydromorphone	p.o.	2–4	3–4
(Dilaudid)	p.r.	3–6	3–4
	i.m., s.c.	3–4	3–4
	i.v.	2–3	3–4
Levorphanol	p.o.	2–3	6–8
(LevoDromoran)	s.c.	2	6–8
	i.v.	2	4–6
Meperidine	p.o.	100–150	3
	i.m., s.c.	75–100	3
Methadone	p.o.	5–15	6–8
(Dolophine)	i.m., s.c.	5–15	4–6
Morphine sulfate	p.o.	10–20	3–4
	i.m., s.c.	5–15	4–6
	i.v.	5–8	3–4
Oxymorphone	p.r.	2–5	4
(Numorphan)	i.m.	1–1.5	4

* Lipman, Arthur G.: "Drug Therapy in Terminally Ill Patients," *Am. J. Hosp. Pharm.*, **32**:270, (Mar.) 1975.
† Approximate equianalgesic doses.

one should be kept in pain until the "right time." (Sometimes a milder analgesic by mouth in between injections is enough.)

We should begin with drugs by mouth when possible and mild and moderate pain is often surprisingly well controlled by aspirin or tablets of codein compound. A most effective mixture is made by dissolving these with 15–30 minims of Nepenthe.*

Other drugs including some mentioned by Saunders are pethidine; meperidine (Demerol), which she says is disappointing by mouth (and is short-acting, 3 hours); methadone; dihydrocodeine bitartrate (30 to 60 mg); dipipanone hydrochloride (10 to 20 mg); and phenazocine hydrobromide (4 mg) (the last three drugs are not available in the United States). She says, as noted earlier, "nothing can replace the opiates." She prescribes them in small doses (2.5 to 5 mg of diamorphine, for instance) in earlier stages of the illness than the stages at which such drugs are used in a general hospital. She maintained in 1964 that of 1100 patients only 2 per cent had acquired an "emotional dependence" (addic-

* Saunders, Cicely: *op. cit.*, p. 13.

tion) or a demand for an increased dose or more frequent injections without any evidence of increased pain. "Addiction, the continual craving for injections, hardly ever occurs" Saunders reported and "we are finding that the rare patient who develops it responds almost immediately when amiphenazole is added to morning and afternoon doses of the opiate." Saunders also believes that the practice of rapidly increasing the dose of the opiate immobilizes patients, making them unable to respond and unable to interact with family and friends. She thinks that rapidly increasing the dose of an opiate is hard on patient, family, and friends and does "a very great disservice." [98,99]

Tolerance for drugs is said by Saunders to develop rarely during a terminal illness, morphine in doses of 1 gm being very unusual, and in some cases the size of the dose is reduced. The patient's confidence in the doctor's ability to control the pain relieves the anxiety so effectively that less drug is needed. Twycross,[99a] while a physician in charge of the Department of Clinical Studies at St. Christopher's, studied the fluctuations in dosages of diamorphine (heroin) in 115 patients with advanced cancer. The data support the hypothesis that increases in dose are necessitated by increased pain rather than tolerance. As mentioned earlier, they should not be used as sedatives or hypnotics and all of these drugs should be prescribed and administered so that patients do not feel "doped," but can remain aware and as active as their conditions permit. Adjuvant use of antidepressants and other drugs used to relieve other symptoms help to keep doses to a minimum.

While pain is usually controlled with drugs when a person is dying, some physicians believe that other methods that do not have the disadvantages of drugs should be considered. C. Norman Shealy, of the Pain Rehabilitation Center, LaCrosse, Wis., says "The average pain patient *can* be rehabilitated without mind-shattering drugs and crippling or destructive surgery." * He says "Destructive procedures, cordotomy, posterior root section and cingulumotomy are primarily useful in cancer pain." † He thinks surgery may be indicated for treatment of disk [vertebral] syndrome, but he says "Electrical stimulation, either transcutaneous or of the dorsal columns, is the procedure of choice in benign pain and in unilateral cancer pain for which no other procedure is satisfactory." He adds "When no surgical procedure seems practical, operant

* Shealy, C. Norman: "The Pain Patient," *Am. Fam. Physician*, **9**:131, (Mar.) 1974.
† *Ibid.*

conditioning will allow the patient to reach his maximum potential." *

Discussing cancer pain in more detail, Shealy says that it is usually caused by "nerve plexus or bony involvement." Noting that "x-ray therapy, metabolic poisons and narcotics are used extensively," he observes that some patients "still may suffer needlessly." He suggests spinal nerve blocks with iced saline irrigations in pelvic cancer and thinks phenol in glycerine may occasionally be of value, but with the latter there is a risk of bowel and bladder paralysis. He thinks that at least 80 per cent of cancer patients with unilateral pain can be relieved by cordotomy, but he acknowledges the risk of paralysis of leg, arm, or bladder and thinks "painful cordotomy paresthesias may be worse than the original pain."

In Chapters 31, 48, and 49, the use of electric control of pain is discussed. Studies reported by Alan C. Hymes and his associates, D. M. Long and P. W. Nathan, and P. D. Wall are cited. In a 1974 Symposium, "The Spectrum of Suffering," reported in the *American Journal of Nursing*,[99b] electric control of pain was included in the discussion. Orderly assessments of the effectiveness of electric cutaneous stimulation in the control of pain are relatively new, but one device for applying an electric current to the skin, the Electreat, was patented in 1918 and is still in use. The ancient art of acupuncture, an intrusive form of treatment as compared with cutaneous stimulation, is accepted as an effective anesthetic in some surgery and as a form of electric therapy in the treatment of pain, which thousands of persons claim is effective.

While the majority of health workers in Western medicine may know more about pain control with drugs than with any other agent, everybody interested in helping the dying patient should welcome the opportunity to study any method that is meeting with success. No attempt can be made here to present exhaustive data on any method.

Problems of Communication and Human Relations. The relief of pain and physical discomfort goes a long way toward enabling patients to cope with the mental and emotional distress of dying. Helping patients and their families with problems of communication and human relations is perhaps the most difficult of the caretakers' tasks. It requires understanding and a willingness to be involved, to be honest, to work with and through others, to collaborate and cooperate.

Nurses, many of whom have been taught to refer all questions on diagnosis, prognosis, and

therapy to the physician, may find it hard to answer patients' questions, and yet it is repeatedly observed by those studying the dying process that patients tend to question nurses rather than doctors. It may be because nurses are with them for so many more hours than are doctors and it also may be that the nurse's answer isn't the final verdict they fear from the physician.

In discussions on care of the dying, nurses frequently raise the question "How should we answer the patient who asks 'Am I dying?'" It may be reassuring to the nurse who fears being put in this position to know that patients rarely say this directly but instead they ask why they are having pain, why the weakness doesn't go away, or how long will it last. In one form or another, they say, "What will happen next?" They don't know what to expect next. These questions are not difficult to answer; in fact, they open the way for a patient to develop confidence in the nurse, when the nurse has experience and may know more than the patient; for both the question may help to plan ways of meeting difficulties encountered during the relationship.

Saunders says that all patients need an explanation of their illness that will be understandable and convincing to them if they are to cooperate in their treatment or be relieved of the burden of unknown fears.[99c] She also makes the point that others, including nurses, share with the doctor the responsibility for answering questions honestly so that patients feel that they can trust those around them. If those who care for the dying accept this postulate, then each question patients ask can help those who care for them to understand what they are experiencing, what symptoms demand relief, what fantasies patients have about the outcome of their illness, and whether these fantasies are justified. If nurses and other health workers are to answer patients' questions constructively, they must know the diagnosis, the cause of symptoms, and how to relieve symptoms; they must also have a capacity for understanding that patients handle the experience of dying in different ways and that they have the right to choose the one that is bearable and significant to them—that contributes to their peace of mind.

Because they are trained in assessment and are with patients in private homes, nursing homes, hospitals, and hospices more constantly than any other professional health workers, nurses are in a position to advise the family, the friends, the clergyman, and the physician about what is happening to patients and when patients want to see them. Nurses are responsible for reporting changes that indicate ap-

* *Ibid.*

proaching death. Hospitals and hospices are staffed so that a doctor can always be available, but in private homes and nursing homes, physicians are likely to be absent at the very end, leaving dying patients and families in the hands of nurses. Physicians can usually be reached by telephone even though visits are a rarity. Worcester, writing in 1935, made the following statement about the physician's helping role at births and deaths:

During the last half century, as we all know, there has been vast improvement in midwifery. But instead of any progress in the art of caring for the dying, medical practice seems to have deteriorated. In fact many doctors nowadays, when the death of their patients becomes imminent, seem to believe that it is quite proper to leave the dying in care of the nurses and sorrowing relatives. This shifting of responsibility is unpardonable. And one of its bad results is that as less professional interest is taken in such service, less and less is known about it.*

Nurses can help physicians maintain a relationship with patients and their families throughout the dying process despite the fact that physicians vary in the time they will give to patients whose conditions do not respond to treatment. For example, a physician may answer the nurse's call that the patient is "getting worse," "sinking," or "critical" by asking "What can *I* do?" The tone of the question may sound harsh or irritated. Nurses should realize that some physicians are, perhaps unconsciously, irritated when they believe they have nothing more to offer patients and families. Therefore, nurses are in an excellent position to suggest ways physicians can help and so change the pattern of withdrawal by the physician. For instance, the nurse, who has seen the patient light up when the doctor comes in the room, can tell the doctor how much it means to the patient to just see him or her—and to the family. The nurse's report of specific symptoms may suggest that a change in therapy is needed. For example, incipient respiratory distress and restlessness may signal the need for an agent that will dry secretions. The physician and nurse who collaborate in choosing a mild sedative, such as the antihistamine or benedryl which relieves the respiratory distress and restlessness, are more likely to maintain their respective helping relationships with the patient until the end. Selecting medications for dying patients is usually necessary if they are to get optimum help in being comfortable and alert until death

comes. Nurses as well as physicians should know about new pharmacologic agents, their actions, and side effects. They should be able to discuss and choose the most appropriate agent considering the patient's ability to circulate, metabolize, and excrete drugs, and understand the effects of other agents given simultaneously. Prescriptions may be written by physicians in such a way as to enable nurses to use their judgment in administering them. Pharmacists who work closely with doctors and nurses in using drugs can contribute significantly and this requires the pooling of knowledge and judgment.[99d]

In some settings, interprofessional relationships are sustained between the clergy, physicians, nurses, and social workers from the time of referral through the bereavement of the family after the patient's death. St. Christopher's Hospice in London, Eng., and St. Luke's Nursing Home in Sheffield, Eng., have, for example, such interdisciplinary teams. Craven and Wald review the hospice movement in an article titled "Hospice Care for Dying Patients." [100] They describe several centers in the United States whose professional staffs provide care and maintain contact with patient and family through the dying process and with the family during bereavement. Calvary Hospital in New York City, Youville Hospital in Cambridge, Mass., Hospice, Inc., in the greater New Haven area in South Central Connecticut, and the Nursing Homes of the Order of Rose Hawthorn are examples of such centers providing some or all of these services. Patients cared for by professionals who work together in this way can ask any member of that team questions about their condition. Any member of the team who has the needed information and is also able to give the patient the emotional support to hear the answer may respond to the patient's question.

The diagnosis of physical and psychologic pain or discomfort and knowing how the patient wants and is able to cope with that suffering is one part of the picture; assessment of the suffering of family members and friends, and the capacity of the whole group to deal with the suffering of each of its members is equally important. As long as "the team" supports the policy of open communication, then the social worker, the clergy, the physician, the lawyer, the nurse, or any member of "the team" may assume the responsibility for including family members and friends in patient care, for sharing information, and for helping relatives and friends communicate openly with the patient. However, patterns of communication, especially "telling" the patient about his or her illness and prognosis, are

* Worcester, Alfred: *The Care of the Aged, the Dying and the Dead.* Charles C Thomas, Publisher, Springfield, Ill., 1935, p. 33.

likely to have started at the time the first symptom was noted and the therapy prescribed. Glaser and Strauss [101] say that the usual pattern is for the physician to be more open with the family than with the patient, which in turn establishes a pattern of communication that is closed or partially closed. A health team caring for the patient weeks, months, or years after that initial diagnosis confronts an established pattern of communication that is difficult to reshape. There is great variation, therefore, in when and how much the patient who is terminally ill and the family can be open with everyone involved.

If the nurse is to succeed in being responsible and accountable to both patient and family, he or she must know where each of the family members, and the patient, "is at." In fact, each involved person should keep in communication with the others in talking about the impending separation and how hard "letting go" will be. An excellent way to help the family members is to encourage them to take an active role in the nursing care. This is easy when the patient is at home and the family has adequate support from health professionals. In hospitals or nursing homes, problems of limited visiting hours and institutional rules prohibiting visitors from cooking, staying overnight, and attending staff conferences discourage family involvement. The nurse in such settings may be able to find ways to amend these rules or regulations, or to promote the establishment of new settings that encourage family involvement. Many settings still adhere to the traditional practice of allowing only the physician to tell the family that the patient's condition is critical. Even in the physician's absence, the nurse is not permitted to exercise this responsibility. Patients may ask nurses about their condition. Nurses can begin by asking the patients what the doctors have told them. The more truthful the nurse, the better, because then the patient-nurse relationship can be more open.

In Chapter 16, Communication, Human Relations, Learning, Health Goals and Guidance, it was observed that one of the commonest, and perhaps the greatest, trial imposed by illness, as it is experienced today, is separation of the sick human being from those they love. For institutionalized patients, sexual activities are interrupted. Unless privacy is provided for patients and their visitors, any physical manifestations of love are so embarrassing to most persons that they are completely unable to show affection or tenderness. Many young people assume that the need for the physical expression of love of one's mate does not exist in middle and old age. Studies cited in Chapter 16 refute this concept. Readers will find it helpful to refer to page 937 and to consult references in this chapter.[101a-102]

As pointed out in Chapter 16, nurses are in a position to promote home care, visits of institutionalized patients to their homes, and the provision of privacy in hospitals and nursing homes. Patients and their wives or husbands may need sexual counselling, and nurses are in a position to suggest this on occasions when it seems appropriate.

The couple facing an end to a loving relationship may need sex more than ever as a release of tension, as a way of giving mutual support, and as an affirmation of love. However, the weakness of the patient and the general anxiety both have about the illness and its sequela may prevent or disturb the sexual component of the relationship. Disfigurement from the disease, or fear that the disease may be catching, also interferes. Jaffe, a social worker at the University of Pittsburgh, has lived three years with the knowledge that she has acute leukemia. She continues to lecture, teach health care professionals and lay persons and is preparing papers for publication. Three of her major papers are to be published soon. She recognizes that health professionals know too little about the function and dysfunction of sexual relationships and urges better education and development of the initiative in helping patients and their families.

"Getting the house in order" has been discussed, but it might be stressed here again because this involves the patient in talking with family and friends, the clergy, possibly social workers, and often a lawyer. There may be persons important for the dying person to see and messages to be given. As the patient's strength wanes, nurses should help friends and relatives visit him or her at the best time, and as often as is good for the patient. This can vary greatly from individual to individual, and from day to day. Though a patient seems to be dying, there may suddenly come a day or an hour when the presence of a roomful of visitors can be a great joy to all involved. The more flexible and open everyone is, the better. While there is much poignancy and grief at the end of life, there is also opportunity for laughter and warmth. Sometimes this may seem to deny or mask the prevailing sadness; at other times these two opposite moods coexist. Patients have made remarks to the first author such as "I'm going to lick this cancer, if it kills me," and then burst out laughing with tears flowing freely. Frances Storlie reports the last conversation with Gloria, a dying friend (a nurse), who sees humor in life until the end. Gloria tries to tell Frances what it is like to be dying: "Frances, once in a while I feel like two people, one who is dying and the other—an identical twin, watching the whole business. Now THAT'S being beside yourself." * Frances, sitting in the chapel at Gloria's funeral, remembers that she "laughed genuinely" after this remark, and thinks to herself, "you could almost say this woman died laughing." It helps dying patients to be with those who can laugh and cry with them. In any event, there are ups and downs for the dying and their families and friends. C. S. Lewis describes how those "ups" can provide joy even at the very end: "It is incredible how much happiness, even how much gaiety, we sometimes had together after all hope was gone. How long, how tranquilly, how nourishingly, we talked together that last night!" †

There are advantages in having relatives or close friends help in the physical care of patients. In addition to keeping them involved with one another, patients or family members may find that if a third person is present, they feel "safe" in giving important, yet emotionally charged, directions, as, for example, who is to inherit a piece of jewelry or what clothes the patients wish put on them after death. Those close to patients can help nurses understand instructions that seem cryptic. They can explain the "private language" of patients, for example, translating a foreign language, or words that have particular meanings to intimates. Some families have the strength and sufficient understanding of physical and psychologic needs, either by intuition or by professional education, to require little help. It is sufficient if caregivers offer reassurance, are available when decisions are hard to reach, or when another pair of hands is needed.

In contemporary society many people are learning to deal with death, dying, and bereavement as a fact of life, albeit a difficult time. Alfred Leslie's painting, "The Death of My Mother, 1957," illustrates innate family strength. (See Fig. 50-11.)

Patients may be moved to leave a possession with the nurse, and this can create difficulties. When patients express such an intention, nurses should express their thanks but they can say that they realize how important it is for grieving family members or friends to receive concrete assurances of the patients' affection and in this way discourage the bequest to the nurse. Judgment and tact may be

needed to prevent embarrassment over the disposition of material mementos. In the early stages of bereavement, it is often difficult for survivors to accept death and to believe that separation is final. During this time, things the patient has valued have special significance. In addition to tears and grief, one must be equally prepared for *love* and *humor*. Nurses must be capable of receiving as well as giving. Families, as well as patients, find relief in expressing their appreciation of all that is done for them. If nurses can accept patients' ideas, their words, and their thanks as gifts, it will help patients see that their relationship with the nurse is what is important and that material expressions of appreciation are unnecessary.

In addition to leaving the customary will which indicates guardianship of children and distribution of worldly goods, many persons make their wishes known about events preceding death if the time comes when they can no longer speak and events after death when they are no longer present to participate in making decisions. The "Living Will" (see page 1937) prepared by the Euthanasia Educational Council and signed by the patient may be discussed with family, physician, clergyman, or lawyer before death. Patients may ask nurses to witness their signatures to a document that leaves parts of the body, or the whole body, to an institution. Patients may consult nurses on such decisions so it is desirable that they know about such processes. It is important that people have an opportunity to tell their next of kin, physicians, and nurses about such intentions, since appropriate forms must be signed, and in the case of donated body tissues, procedures for preserving them set in motion, especially if they have not done so before. Finally, most patients want to discuss funeral arrangements with family and friends. Nurses can provide emotional support to those involved in such discussions by a quiet presence or by helping relatives and friends express their wishes freely, to hear one another despite the emotions evoked, and to reach a mutually acceptable decision.

Resuscitated patients have told about hearing remarks made by persons who, because the patient could not talk, thought they could not hear. Hearing is certainly possible after the power to speak is gone. Because hearing probably gets less acute, people should stand near the dying person and speak quietly but distinctly. *Nothing should be said in the room that the patient should not hear, for no one knows how much seemingly unconscious persons can hear. Whispering, especially, should be avoided. Patients may see the lips move*

---

* Storlie, Frances: "Gloria," *Am. J. Nurs.*, **75**:1188, (July) 1975.

† Lewis, C. S.: *A Grief Observed*. Seabury Press, New York, 1961, p. 14.

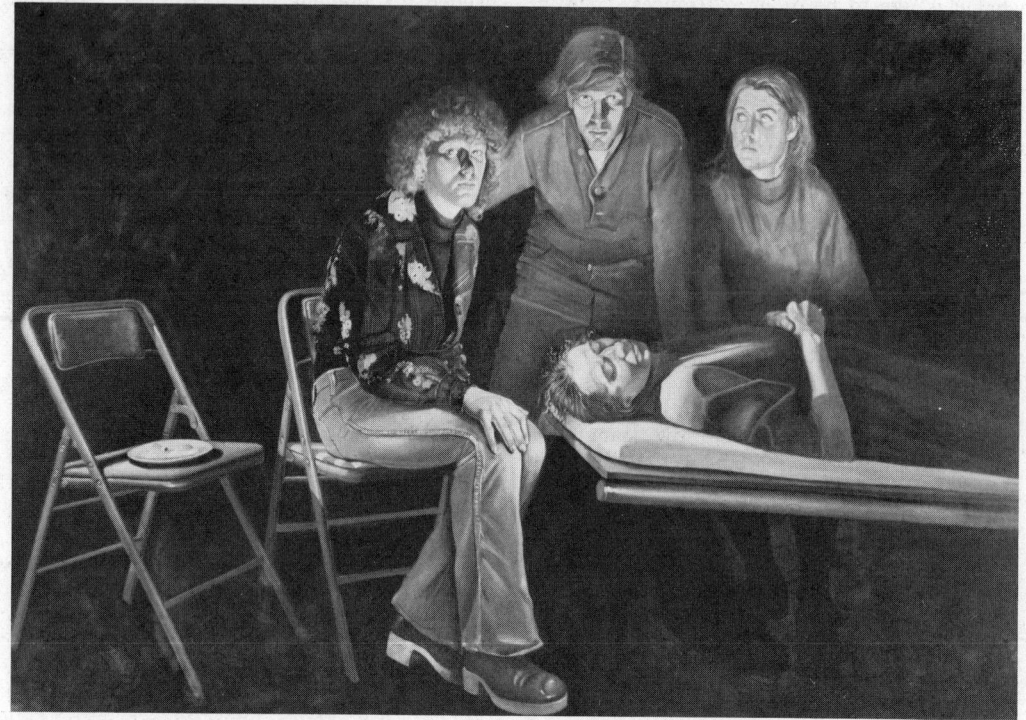

Figure 50-11. Alfred Leslie's "The Death of My Mother, 1957" was painted in 1976 and like most of his works presents a life situation. Robert Rosenbaum comments that his paintings "compel us to stare hard and close up at the most rock bottom visual experiences." (Museum of Fine Arts, Boston. Hirshhorn Museum and Sculpture Garden, Smithsonian Institution, Washington, D.C., Alfred Leslie Exhibition Catalogue, 1976.) (Courtesy of Allan Frumkin Galleries and Alfred Leslie.)

and be distressed that they cannot hear what is being said. The following story has been told of the clergyman who was dying and thought by two nurses to be incapable of hearing. One nurse whispered to the other, "Feel his feet, the feet of dying people grow cold first." The patient opened one eye and said distinctly, "Joan of Arc's feet didn't." Many persons can talk, think, keep a sense of humor, be with those they love, and participate in various aspects of life until the end.

Nurses stay with patients as long as they show signs of life except for short periods when they may want to be left with a friend, a member of the family, the physician, or the religious representative. During this time, the nurse will be needed to help the family, as well as the patient. Relatives and friends need support, answers to questions, and assistance in "letting go."

Cessation of breathing is generally considered the ultimate sign of death, and the exact time when this occurs should be reported and recorded on the patient's chart. The heart may beat after respiration has ceased, but the physician, who is the one to pronounce death, usually bases his or her decision on the latter sign. In cases of asphyxia or drowning, every effort is made to reestablish the respiration as long as the heart functions; however, this is not desirable when the patient is hopelessly ill and it is only a question of prolonging life for a few hours or days.

When breathing ceases, if the physician is not present, the nurse reports this fact immediately and asks the physician to come. After the physician certifies the death of the patient and the family is ready to leave the body in their hands, nurses prepare the body for the undertaker, who is notified as soon as possible. Family and even the health care professional need time to absorb the shock that the patient has died. In busy hospitals it may be difficult to allow an hour or more to let the family alone in a quiet spot to answer questions and collect belongings; yet it is so important. There also must be time for staff and other patients to express their feelings.

Certain conditions surrounding death may complicate its pronouncement. In the following pages an effort is made to explain recent developments in medical practice and reevaluation of historical data that have complicated the definition of death and the procedure in pronouncing and reporting death.

7. DEFINING, PRONOUNCING, AND REPORTING DEATH

Defining and Pronouncing Death. In 1972 the Task Force on Death and Dying of the Institute of Society, Ethics, and the Life Sciences made a report [103] in which it was noted that new technological powers of sustaining the signs of life in the severely ill and injured make the determination of death difficult. The heartbeat can be stimulated electrically and a mechanical pump can keep the lungs expanding and contracting. Obviously these facts pose philosophical, ethical, and moral questions. The Task Force proposed eight criteria by which to measure "good criteria of death" and applied them to the criteria of the Ad Hoc Committee of the Harvard Medical School to Examine the Definition of Brain Death published in 1968. The Task Force questioned using any one criterion, and specifically "brain death," as an adequate basis for determining the boundary between life and death.

The Ad Hoc Committee stated its "primary purpose is to define irreversible coma as a new criterion for death." Its definition follows:

1. *Unreceptivity and Unresponsitivity:* There is a total unawareness to externally applied stimuli and inner need and complete unresponsiveness. . . . Even the most intensely painful stimuli evoke no vocal or other response, not even a groan, withdrawal of a limb, or quickening of respiration.
2. *No Movements or Breathing:* Observation covering a period of at least one hour by physicians is adequate to satisfy the criteria of no spontaneous muscular movements or spontaneous respiration or response to stimuli such as pain, touch, sound, or light. After the patient is on a mechanical respirator, the total absence of spontaneous breathing may be established by turning off the respirator for three minutes and observing whether there is any effort on the part of the subject to breathe spontaneously. (The respirator may be turned off for this time provided that at the start of the trial period the patient's carbon dioxide tension is within the normal range, and provided also that the patient had been breathing room air for at least 10 minutes prior to the trial.)
3. *No Reflexes:* Irreversible coma with abolition of central nervous system activity is evidenced in part by the absence of elicitable reflexes. The pupil will be fixed and dilated and will not respond to a direct source of bright light. . . . Ocular movement (to head turning and to irrigation of the ears with ice water) and blinking are absent. There is no evidence of postural activity (decerebrate or other). Swallowing, yawning, vocalization are in abeyance. Corneal and pharyngeal reflexes are absent.

. . .

4. *Flat Electroencephalogram:* Of great confirmatory value is the flat or isoelectric EEG. We must assume that the electrodes have been properly applied, that the apparatus is functioning normally, and that the personnel in charge is competent. . . .

All of the above tests shall be repeated at least 24 hours later with no change.*

In a report prepared for the American Friends Service Committee in 1970, the following definition of death (which emphasizes circulatory failure) is quoted from *Black's Law Dictionary:* "The cessation of life; the ceasing to exist; defined by physicians as a total stoppage of the circulation of the blood and a cessation of the animal and vital functions consequent thereupon, such as respiration, pulse, etc." †

Kastenbaum says that with R. B. Aisenberg he has studied "psychological death" and in this connection they made a partial survey of the literature on interrupted or completed premature burial. They concluded "although many of these reports are to be doubted, it is probable that a substantial percentage of them were accurate." ‡

The possibility that anybody can be buried alive makes a valid determination of death, in any place, in any age, most important; it is no wonder that society puts on the doctor—the most highly educated class of health workers— the responsibility for pronouncing death. Cessation of breathing, stoppage of the circulation, and brain death would seem to be adequate

---

* Harvard Medical School, Ad Hoc Committee to Examine the Definition of Brain Death: "A Definition of Irreversible Coma. Report of the Ad Hoc Committee . . ." *J.A.M.A.,* **205:**337, (Aug. 5) 1968. (This is a slightly shorter version of the published statement with only some explanatory details omitted.)

† *Who Shall Live? Man's Control Over Birth and Death.* A Report Prepared for the American Friends Service Committee. Hill and Wang, New York, 1970, p. 110. (The definition quoted is said to be from *Black's Law Dictionary,* 4th ed., 1951, West Publishing Co., St. Paul, Minn. The definition did not seem to be in later editions.) This definition also appears in the Harvard Medical School Ad Hoc Committee's report cited above.

‡ Kastenbaum, Robert: "Psychological Death," in Pearson, Leonard (ed.): *Death and Dying. Current Issues in the Treatment of the Dying Person.* Press of Case–Western Reserve University, Cleveland, 1969, p. 6.

RESPONSIBLE PERSON OR AGENCY	BIRTH CERTIFICATE	DEATH CERTIFICATE	FETAL DEATH CERTIFICATE (Stillbirth)
Physician, Other Professional Attendant, or Hospital Authority	1. Completes entire certificate in consultation with parent(s). Physician's signature required. 2. Files certificate with local office of district in which birth occurred.	1. Completes medical certification and signs certificate. 2. Returns certificate to funeral director.	1. Completes or reviews medical items on certificate. 2. Certifies to the cause of fetal death and signs certificate. 3. Returns certificate to funeral director. 4. In absence of funeral director, files certificate.
Funeral Director		1. Obtains personal facts about deceased. 2. Takes certificate to physician for medical certification. 3. Delivers completed certificate to local office of district where death occurred and obtains burial permit.	1. Obtains the facts about fetal death. 2. Takes certificate to physician for entry of causes of fetal death. 3. Delivers completed certificate to local office of district where delivery occurred and obtains burial permit.
Local Office (may be Local Registrar or City or County Health Department)	1. Verifies completeness and accuracy of certificate. 2. Makes copy, ledger entry, or index for local use. 3. Sends certificates to State Registrar.	1. Verifies completeness and accuracy of certificate. 2. Makes copy, ledger entry, or index for local use. 3. Issues burial permit to funeral director and verifies return of permit from cemetery attendant. 4. Sends certificates to State Registrar.	

City and county health departments use certificates in allocating medical and nursing services, followups on infectious diseases, planning programs, measuring effectiveness of services, and conducting research studies.

State Registrar, Bureau of Vital Statistics	1. Queries incomplete or inconsistent information. 2. Maintains files for permanent reference and as the source of certified copies. 3. Develops vital statistics for use in planning, evaluating, and administering State and local health activities and for research studies. 4. Compiles health related statistics for State and civil divisions of State for use of the health department and other agencies and groups interested in the fields of medical science, public health, demography, and social welfare. 5. Prepares copies of birth, death, and fetal death certificates or records for transmission to the National Center for Health Statistics.
Public Health Service National Center for Health Statistics	1. Prepares and publishes national statistics of births, deaths, and fetal deaths; and constructs the official U.S. life tables and related actuarial tables. 2. Conducts health and social–research studies based on vital records and on sampling surveys linked to records. 3. Conducts research and methodological studies in vital statistics methods including the technical, administrative, and legal aspects of vital records registration and administration. 4. Maintains a continuing technical assistance program to improve the quality and usefulness of vital statistics.

Figure 50-12. Chart showing the various persons and agencies responsible for reporting vital statistics and the uses made of these statistics.

criteria if it weren't for the question as to whether one or all of these functions can be revived. If tissues or organs of the dying patient are to be donated, the determination of death is still further complicated.

In Chapter 43, the laws governing donation of tissues and organs were discussed. Attention was called to the [U.S.] Uniform Anatomical Gift Act (July 1968) which was endorsed by the American Bar Association and the American Medical Association. The law attempts to reconcile conflicting interests; it states that accredited hospitals, medical schools, organ and tissue banks, surgeons, physicians, or any individual specified by donors (who must have been 18 years of age and of sound mind when they wrote the bequest) can receive the anatomic gift. The Act specifies that the time of death must be determined by the physician attending the donor at the time of death and that he or she shall not participate in the transplantation.

The World Health Organization in 1969 reviewed laws in a number of countries governing questions related to transplants, showing that they differ widely.[104] Health workers should have access to such publications and be aware of the legal complications that are involved. Moser, a physician, discussing "the new ethics" in relation to death, says:

. . . the issue [definition of death] is far from settled. There have been columns of prose, often elegant, but mostly tedious, in both medical and lay literature debating the role of clergyman, lawmaker, judge, and family members in the life-death decision, but as indicated earlier, the weight cannot be lifted from the sagging, often reluctant shoulders of the physician.*

* Moser, Robert H.: *op. cit.,* p. 44.

Perhaps the only way to define death is to say that it is a subjective judgment of a physician, or if he or she is not available, the judgment of others that the signs of life, such as breathing and the heart beating, are absent. When a physician is not with the dying patient, nurses must make this judgment. They usually assume that the patient is dead when respirations cease. When the patient's illness is accepted by all concerned as irreversible, nurses do not try to resuscitate the patient but get a doctor as quickly as possible to pronounce death. Resuscitation of patients whose illness may be reversible is discussed on page 1492 and nurses in many situations are performing this function.

Edmund V. Cowdry, writing on the aging process, says that when the heart continues to beat after respiration ceases the physician bases his decision on the latter. However, he notes that a human being is not "wholly dead" because some cells continue to live for varying periods. He says: "Death is always piecemeal for humans. . . . Death is disorganization of living matter which makes permanently impossible any and all vital phenomena. . . ." *

Embalming, discussed later as one aspect of the care of the body after death, prevents the burial of a living body, one of the unhappy outcomes still possible in countries where embalming is not practiced.

Reporting Death. It is the physician's function to pronounce death and to report it in writing to the local health department (see Fig. 50-12). Reports of births and deaths furnish data on which all vital statistics in developed countries are based and some of the

* Cowdry, Edmund V. (ed.): *Problems of Aging: Biological and Medical Aspects,* 2nd ed. Williams & Wilkins Co., Baltimore, 1942, p. 364.

Figure 50-13. International form of medical certificate of cause of death. (From World Health Organization: *Medical Certification of Cause of Death,* 3rd ed. The Organization, Geneva, 1968, p. 7.)

INTERNATIONAL FORM OF MEDICAL CERTIFICATE OF CAUSE OF DEATH

CAUSE OF DEATH		Approximate interval between onset and death
I *Disease or condition directly leading to death* *	(a) .... due to (or as a consequence) of	....
Antecedent causes Morbid conditions, if any, giving rise to the above cause, stating the underlying condition last	(b) .... due to (or as a consequence) of (c)	....
II *Other significant conditions* contributing to the death, but not related to the disease or condition causing it	....	....

* This does not mean the mode of dying, e.g., heart failure, asthenia, etc. It means the disease, injury, or complication which caused death.

Name .... Unit No. ....

Address ....

Birth Date .... Accommodation ....

POST-MORTEM EXAMINATION PERMISSION AND CONSULTATION REQUEST*

SECTION "A"

PERMISSION FOR POST-MORTEM EXAMINATION

Date: _____ , 19____   Time: ____   A.M. / P.M.

I hereby grant permission for a post-mortem examination on the remains of:

_____
Name of Patient

I also authorize the Hospital to remove and retain such tissues or parts as may be deemed necessary for this examination. Such removed tissues or parts may be preserved for scientific or teaching purposes or otherwise be disposed of.

Signed: _____ Relationship to Deceased: _____

Address: _____

Witness: _____
Doctor obtaining permission

Remarks: _____

SECTION "B"

TELEPHONE PERMISSION FOR POST-MORTEM EXAMINATION

Date: _____ , 19____   Time: ____   A.M. / P.M.

I have spoken by telephone with _____
Name

the _____ of _____ and I have obtained
Relationship   Name of Patient

permission to perform a post-mortem examination. The following statement was read to and agreed to by the above named person:

"I authorize _____ to conduct a post-mortem examination on the remains of _____ for whom I assume responsibility
Name of Patient

for burial. I also authorize the Hospital to remove and retain such tissues or parts as may be deemed necessary for this examination. Such removed tissues or parts may be preserved for scientific or teaching purposes or otherwise be disposed of."

Signature: _____
House Officer or Responsible Physician obtaining permission

Witness' Signature: _____
Person who monitors telephone conversation

(*Consultation Request on the back of this page to be completed by the physician.)

Figure 50-14. Form authorizing permission for post-mortem examination.

SECTION "C"

AUTHORIZATION BY PUBLIC OFFICIAL

Date: _____, 19_____ Time: _____ A.M.
P.M.

The undersigned, _____, _____,
_____ Name _____ Title

authorizes that a post-mortem examination be performed on the remains of:

_____.
_____ Name of Patient

Signature: _____ Title: _____

State's Attorney, Ass't State's Attorney, Coroner,
Chief Medical Examiner, authorized Ass't Medical
Examiner.

SECTION "D"

CONSULTATION REQUEST FOR POST-MORTEM EXAMINATION

Service _____ Date of Admission _____ Date and Time of Death _____

Primary Diagnosis: _____

_____

_____

Other Diagnoses: _____

_____

_____

Major Surgical Operations: _____

_____

Major Complications: _____

_____

Brief clinical summary indicating special problems and areas of interest: _____

_____

_____

_____

_____

_____

Terminal Event: _____

_____

Name of Attending physician(s) _____

_____

_____

Requested by signed: _____ M.D.

Figure 50-14. (continued).

data for morbidity, longevity, and other studies. They are part of the legal record of every citizen.

The World Health Organization publishes a *Manual of the International Statistical Classification of Diseases, Injuries, and Causes of Death* (Vol. 1, 1967, Vol. 2, 1969). This work, based on recommendations of the Eighth Revision Conference in 1965, was adopted at the 19th World Health Assembly. This and the pamphlet *Medical Certification of Cause of Death* (3rd ed 1968) are guides for health agencies around the world (see Fig. 50-13).

The death certificate is made out by the physician, the undertaker, and the pathologist if an autopsy is performed. Families are often asked by physicians to allow an autopsy, or postmortem examination, and to sign a release slip (see Fig. 50-14). Such decisions are influenced by many things, but perhaps the known wishes of the person who has died carry greatest weight. Laws and public health regulations on autopsies vary from state to state, and health workers should be familiar with them.

8. CARE OF THE BODY AFTER DEATH

Immediate Care. The nurse or nurses who have been with patients at the moment of death usually prepare the body for removal to an undertaking establishment.

Margaret Aasterud [105] thinks the primitive taboo of death is continued in modern society in postmortem care. She notes that two nurses usually work together and refer to "the body" in hushed tones. She thinks people demonstrate their aversion to and fear of death in hiding the sight of the dead body and by saying only good things about the dead. Quint, [106] with excerpts from reports by student nurses, showed that 10 years ago students showed fear in touching the body and were unhappy when they saw the body callously handled by experienced hospital workers.

In hospitals where a physician is present or can be gotten immediately to pronounce death, the nurse takes no steps toward caring for the body until this has been done. This may in part account for the previously noted observation of dead patients being "found" by other members of staff. In home nursing, hours may elapse before the physician's visit. Patients are not legally dead until the physician has certified death, and nothing should be done that would interfere with life, as there is always a possibility of life remaining in the body. The undertaker, for example, cannot legally accept the body or prepare it for burial before this official pronouncement has been made.

Transplants were discussed as a problem related to defining and pronouncing death. They also affect the immediate care of the body since surgical removal of an organ or tissue for transplantation should be made as soon after the pronouncement of death as possible.* L. K. Christopherson and D. T. Lunde, [107] discussing "the selection of cardiac transplant recipients and their subsequent psychosocial adjustment," think anonymity is important. The donor family should not meet the recipient family. They think donor families have special needs that the institution must be prepared to meet. Removal of organs or tissues for donation should not leave the body mutilated in appearance. [108] Figure 50-15 shows a form issued by the State of Connecticut incorporated in a driver's license that facilitates donation of organs.

Hibernation in animals has demonstrated that lowering the body temperature reduces metabolism to the minimum consistent with the maintenance of life. It is also known that drying can give a living organism the appearance of death over decades. [109] These principles are used in organ and tissue transplants and in the maintenance of *tissue banks*.

Nurses preparing the body after death should know whether there is to be an autopsy or an inquest; whether there is to be a donation of the body for research, or a donation of organs. They should know state laws governing these matters and the particular regulations of the institution or agency in which they are employed.

Custom varies in relation to the care of the body after death, but certain principles should be kept in mind. Bodies are usually embalmed, or chemically preserved, and made to look as natural as possible. Congestion and clotting within the blood vessels before or after death can interfere with the embalming process if there is a long delay between the patient's death and the embalming. Distortion, discoloration, or scarring of the body is distressing to the family and friends and should therefore be prevented. The body itself should be

---

* David D. Sanders asks, "what claims to cadavers by what persons should be recognized and protected by society?" in an article titled "Medical Advance and Legal Lag: Hemodialysis and Kidney Transplantation," (*UCLA Law Review,* 15:357, 1968). Andie L. Knutson reviews practices with relation to autopsies in many cultures, noting that there are eras in which they are allowed, others in which they are banned. Mohammedans, Hindus, and Hebrews may oppose them on religious grounds. A coroner may, however, have a legal right to perform an autopsy to determine cause of death in some cases. Bodies of criminals may, in some societies, be given to hospitals or medical schools for dissection. (Knutson, Andie L.: "Cultural Beliefs on Life and Death," in Brim, Orville G., Jr., et al. [eds.]: *The Dying Patient.* Russell Sage Foundation, New York, 1970.)

PRINT NAME (Donor)

DATE OF BIRTH | OPERATOR LICENSE NO.

I hereby make the following anatomical gift(s), shown below and/or on the reverse of this stub if medically acceptable, to take effect upon my death.

Signed by donor in the presence of (2) two witnesses set forth below:

SIGNATURE OF DONOR
X
SIGN BY WITNESS
X
SIGN BY WITNESS
X

This is a legal document for your wallet, under the Anatomical Gift(s) Act.

ORGAN DONOR PROGRAM

Connecticut law provides an opportunity for any person, 18 years of age or over, to designate on the driver's license that upon death he or she wishes to donate body organs.

IF YOU DO NOT WISH TO BECOME A DONOR, destroy this card. Complete your application for driver's license and return to the Motor Vehicle Department with the appropriate license fee.

IF YOU WISH TO BECOME AN ORGAN DONOR:

1. Complete the stub of this form and sign it in the presence of two witnesses.

2. Have the two witnesses sign it in the appropriate spaces, in your presence.

3. Sign your license renewal application, check the box on the application, and print ORGAN DONOR on the license stub.

4. Return the signed renewal and the appropriate license fee to the Motor Vehicle Department.

5. Retain the stub of this flyer on your person, as notice of donation.

The donor's stub constitutes, upon your death, sufficient legal authority for the removal of body organs, if medically acceptable. The designation may be removed from your operator's license stub at any time upon 30 days written notice to the Motor Vehicle Department.

B-142 ANATOMICAL DONATION FLYER NEW 8-75   IBM Z25321

Figure 50-15. Form providing for the donation of body organs, to be filled in and attached to driver's license. Form is designated a legal document under the Anatomical Gift(s) Act. (Courtesy of State of Connecticut.)

clean and wrapped in clean covering when sent to the undertaking establishment, and should be plainly marked to avoid mistakes in identity.

In order to keep the normal position of the features and form, the eyes if not already closed are closed immediately, as in sleep, and the body is straightened with the arms laid at the sides; the mouth is closed and any dentures that have been removed for the patient's comfort are replaced; the head is elevated on one pillow, and a folded towel is used to prop the chin in position for a short time until the process of death stiffens the features.* (Bandages have been used to hold the jaw firm, but at the present time undertakers prefer to have this omitted because the bandage may indent or discolor the skin.) An important possession to find is the patient's hairpiece or wig, and to make sure a responsible family member, friend, or undertaker will see that this is available when preparing the patient's body for funeral services. (Chemotherapy, radiation therapy, and the sequelae of disease often cause the falling out of hair.) All of this may be done before the physician's certification of death, if it is impossible for him to see the patient for several hours or more after the nurse believes that death has occurred.

Before proceeding with any necessary bathing of the body, all rings (including wedding rings), earrings, bracelets, beads, or other articles worn should be removed and placed in a separate package with other articles of value, such as money, jewelry, receipts, eyeglasses, letters, keys, and any emblem of sacred or religious meaning. If the death has occurred in the hospital, an itemized list of such valuables should be made, and later, together with the package, taken to the administrative office if the family is not present. When the family is there, they should take the items and review and sign the receipt. Nothing is too small to be listed. What may seem of trivial value to the nurse may be, on account of its association, of untold value to a family. When earrings or rings cannot be removed, a note to this effect should be made on the list of valuables. When it is requested by members of the family that a wedding ring or like article remain on the body, it should be securely tied on with a bandage. In institutions, it is wise to have requests of this kind in writing, and such written requests should be left in the main office.

Soiled dressings should be replaced with fresh dressings (adhesive marks should be removed with benzine). In hospitals, a pad of cellucotton, lined on one side with waterproof paper, and a diaper of old muslin are applied to prevent the escape of urine and feces from the relaxed meatus and anus. In some hospitals, a mortuary gown is put on the body; in others it is omitted. A tag containing the patient's name, the clinical division, and the date is attached to one wrist. When the toilet is complete, the body is wrapped in a shroud that is usually made of a very large square of muslin or paper. This square is arranged diagonally.

---

* Stiffness (or *rigor mortis*) passes, and after hours (differing in number according to the age of the person) the body is malleable. Some undertakers say that the position of the body when they receive it is immaterial.

A tag is attached to the outside bearing the same information as that attached to the wrist. A stretcher is prepared, and the body should be placed on it and covered in such a way that it cannot easily be distinguished from that of a living person, but must be securely fastened to the stretcher. In the hospital the removal of the body from the clinical division to the morgue is usually conducted inconspicuously and with respect and dignity. The nurse may be confronted with joking or heartless words and behavior. The first author in the course of her study (previously noted) sometimes found herself in this position. It was at first difficult to accept such dehumanized behavior involving the patient with whom she had been talking less than an hour before. However, she was usually able to minimize the coarseness by telling the person responsible for transporting the body to the morgue something about the patient. The coarse behavior seems to result from embarrassment—not knowing how to act. As far as possible, all the details of death, aftercare, and removal of the body are spared other patients in hospitals.

In hospices, a death is treated differently. Since patients know each other and are involved with others in their clinical units, secretiveness and avoidance are inappropriate.

There is disagreement as to whether bodies of the dead should be camouflaged or hidden from veiw as they are taken to the morgue or to a room from which they are removed by undertakers. Some families have the body, after it is treated by the undertaker, brought home and laid on the bed, as if in sleep, until the funeral or interment. Some hospices are trying to develop flexible practices designed to give the bereaved the greatest possible comfort. Family and friends may want to stay with the body until the undertaker removes it. It is often desirable for nurses to bathe the body, comb the hair, and arrange the clothing and bedding before the family and friends part with the body so that in their mind's eye they see the person looking as normal as possible in death. Some family members may want to do this themselves. The nurse or the undertaker or both should give the family any help they may need in doing so. Many funeral directors and clergy throughout the country are adapting their procedures to include family in preparing the body, in taking an active part in the ritual and service, and even in the interment.

All clothing and other personal property of the patient should be listed, wrapped neatly in a bundle, properly tagged, and taken to the office or given to the family according to the regulations of the institution.

In homes, the body is left dressed in some soft gown until the undertaker comes. A large sheet should be available for wrapping the body if it is to be removed from the dwelling to be prepared for burial.

Later Care and Disposal of Bodies. There are great cultural differences in the way bodies are prepared for their ultimate disposition. In most societies, the procedure is in the hands of specialists—people trained in the arts of embalming, or in the ways of preserving the body in a lifelike state for days, weeks, months, or years. In some cultures, bodies are regularly burned or cremated, as is the practice of Hindus in India; or bodies may be exposed to the elements and carrion birds, as is the practice of Zoroastrians in Iran (known as Parsees in India). Today, as in past centuries, people are buried in tombs, vaults, and mausoleums above ground. Some of the most beautiful and interesting structures in the world are tombs of rulers, often built during their lifetime. Not only was the body buried in the tomb but also, in the case of powerful rulers, wives and servants might be buried with them to serve them in a life after death. More often, the servers took the form of life-size figures or small figurines of wood, stone, or pottery.

Russian excavations of the burial mounds of the nomadic Scythians confirm descriptions by Herodotus of their funeral customs. Rudolph Chelminski, describing some of the treasures taken from these mounds, makes the following observation:

The harsh conditions of nomadic life on the steppe seem to have created a most exacting loyalty to chieftain and king, one which demanded that many of his subjects join him in his grave. A Scythian of great importance was embalmed at his death (an herbal mixture of chopped cypress, frankincense, parsley seed and anise seed was stuffed in the abdominal cavity, after which the body was encased in wax) and taken around his territory for 40 days. The cart bearing his body was followed by ostentatiously grieving subjects, who engaged in all manner of self-mutilation and choruses of wailing, shouting and jingling bells. The burial chamber was dug deep below ground level, buttressed by wooden beams and topped off with an immense earthen mound. Inside the tomb the chieftain was dressed in his finest gold-sewn clothes, surrounded by his gold treasure and left with his weapons to defend it.

But he did not go to the afterlife alone. Far from it. It was common practice for the ruler's favorite concubine and closest servants to be sent with him, persuaded by the gentle art of strangulation and themselves adorned in their best gold. Accompanying them all on their voyage were his horses, put to ritual death—as many as 360 have been found in a single grave—and lain around them in procession, themselves bedecked in leather and gold and felt. One final practice completes the macabre picture: One year after a king's death, up to 50 of his young bodyguards would be volunteered for strangulation, along with a similar number of horses. They were then impaled with wooden lances atop their mounts and propped up in a circle around the grave— ghostly riders of a ghostly honor guard.*

Burial customs of ancient Egyptians paralleled those of the Scythians in some respects. Both indicate a belief in a life after death for which provision was made according to a person's means.

John B. Noss,[110] in his study *Man's Religions,* reviews burial customs from primitive to modern times, showing clearly the relationship between the religious or philosophic beliefs of peoples and the disposition of the body. People of this age tend to look upon practices in earlier ages as "primitive," "barbaric," or "superstitious," but a worldwide survey of present-day practices shows that they vary widely. Even today, the burial practice one culture thinks comforting, important, or even necessary to the welfare of the body, the spirit, or the memory of the departed, may be thought "primitive," "barbaric," or "superstitious" by another culture. Those who cannot accept the reality of death may fear the return of the dead; some fear their ghosts; some believe that the spirit of the dead survives, having either malevolent or benign powers, or both. In some cultures, the body must be buried immediately, or before sundown of the day of death; in other cultures, this would be considered unseemly haste.

Evelyn Waugh [111] in *The Loved One* satirizes the "Hollywood" attitude of the people of the United States toward death. It can be called a form of denial because undertakers, with cosmetics, transform the appearance of the dead, a euphemistic language is adopted, and the costly, ostentatious funerals and mausoleums suggest accomplishments by the dead and human relations that did not exist. Jessica Mitford [112] in *The American Way of Death* takes somewhat the same position and justifiably questions the high cost of funerals and the pretense involved. It is possible, however, that the wish to be remembered, the fear of being buried in "a pauper's grave" (in Potter's Field), and the desire to honor the dead are to some extent universal.†

When patients have families and friends, they assume responsibility for making funeral arrangements; institutions may have to assume this responsibility when a patient dies who is not known to have either. State or municipal sanitary codes usually describe the procedure to be followed. Funeral directors or manufacturers of vaults and caskets publish booklets that contain helpful information on subjects such as funeral customs, planning a funeral, making a will, and Social Security and veterans' benefits. The National Selected Morticians (identified as an International Society of Independent Funeral Directors) published a *Code of Good Funeral Practice* in which, among other things, they pledge themselves to "respect all faiths, creeds and customs . . ." and "to be responsive to the needs of the poor, serving them within their means." They also provide a form "Suggestions to Those Who Plan My Funeral" which, if filled out, helps survivors by giving them such information as persons to notify; biographic data; membership in organizations that pay benefits; social security number; where a will and valuables are found; and wishes about the place of burial and the funeral ceremonies.* Health care personnel who have known the patient through home care, hospice care, or nursing home care may become that patient's family when no friends or family are there.

While there are great differences in the disposition people wish to have made of their bodies, and equal differences in the wishes of the survivors, many students of bereavement think that the religious rites and customary ceremonies have healing powers for relatives and friends. The wishes of the deceased should not be completely disregarded, but the funeral should be planned so that it attests to the worth of the individual who has died and gives those in the family and community who have known and loved them the greatest possible comfort and satisfaction.[112a] It is becoming more common for the family to take an active role in the funeral rites and work to be done. For example, three sons who survived their father, a college professor, made the coffin for him, a beautiful work to see.

Public Health Regulations on the Disposition of the Body After Death. While there are differences dictated by religion, custom, and personal preference in the disposition of the body after death, there are also health laws and regulations. In some countries these are

---

* Chelminski, Rudolph: "USSR Lends Its Dazzling Scythian Gold for American Exhibitions," *Smithsonian,* **6**:29, (Apr.) 1975.

† A visitor to Naples, Italy, who asks a native for a list of the city's most important sights may be surprised at the emphasis put on seeing the cemetery. It is a collection of monuments ranging from simple ones to a replica, in miniature, of the beautiful cathedral in Milan. Perhaps the most memorable monument is a life-size statue of "the nut woman," a detailed Victorian work in white marble showing this little woman who spent her life selling strings of

nuts on the streets of Naples. She commissioned and paid for the statue during her lifetime (just as Hadrian built his tomb, in Rome) to insure a lasting memorial to her brief tenure on this earth.

* National Selected Morticians, 1616 Central St., Evanston, Ill. 60201

national laws and regulations; in others they are provincial or state laws. However, there is a growing tendency to adopt federal standards and even international standards developed by the World Health Organization. To facilitate compilation of international statistics, the World Health Assembly in 1948 recommended the specific medical information requested on the certificate of death. These recommendations have been accepted by all states in the United States.[113,114] In hospitals, some of these data are gotten for physicians by other personnel; in homes, the physicians usually assume responsibility for all items in the report except those for which the undertaker and pathologist are responsible.

State laws regulate the disposition of both unidentified and identified bodies. In getting permission for autopsies when an unidentified person dies in a hospital, the local health department is notified, and this agency assumes responsibility for trying to determine the identity of the body and for making arrangements for burial. Some states rule that bodies may be available for study and research by a recognized medical group, if they are not identified within a stated period, usually 48 hours, after death. When a person has a family or is in the custody of friends, most state laws require that the permission of the nearest of kin or the custodial friend be obtained before an autopsy is performed. If there is a question of poisoning, however, or any other circumstance in connection with the death that necessitates a coroner's inquest, the state is permitted to conduct an autopsy without the consent of the relatives of the deceased.[115]

The local health departments set up special regulations governing the treatment of bodies of persons who die of certain communicable diseases. The Sanitary Code of New York City[116] stipulates that undertakers must not expose or hold the bodies of persons who die of cholera, bubonic plague, diphtheria, poliomyelitis, scarlet fever, or smallpox. Such bodies must be placed in the coffin, which is sealed immediately.

9. GRIEF—BEREAVEMENT

Universality of Grief in Bereavement. Descriptions of grief and bereavement in animals and humans appear through the ages in poetry and prose. Separation from those they love, or from those on whom life's patterns depend, is a crisis to which everyone must learn to adjust. Some *birds* and *animals* demonstrate grief over the loss of mates or their young. The goose, for example, is monogamous and will stay with its sick and dying mate while the flock migrates without them. Dogs grieve over the loss of their masters or mistresses. Charles Darwin's study, *The Expression of Emotions in Man and Animals*,[117] was published in 1872 and included the study of grief. Infants and small children grieve over the absence of their parents, especially their mothers, which they may fear is a final separation. Sigmund Freud[118] observed that a child does not distinguish between temporary absence and permanent loss.

There are numerous studies of the child's reaction to death. Humberto Nagera,[119] a child psychiatrist, reviews these, beginning with the reports of Sigmund, and later Anna, Freud. Nagera notes that John Bowlby thought the reaction of infants separated from an important object was identical with adult mourning, but that Anna Freud questioned it, and that both Anna Freud and Helene Deutsch thought "the process of mourning" differs in adults and children. There is great disagreement on the age at which children are capable of mourning. Bowlby said that infants from 6 months onward could mourn, in the adult sense, while M. Wolfenstein said that this is not possible until adolescence has been resolved. Nagera more or less concurs in this. He and others see death of a close relative as a traumatic event that interferes with the child's or the youth's development. He uses patient histories to illustrate the effect of the death of a child's love-object at different ages.[120-130]

A sensitive pediatrician, Morris Wessel, writes of children's needs, from those of toddlers to those of adolescents. The child's ability to master a task in growth, to gain confidence and trust in others in the early stages, to gain self-reliance and independence in the teens will be affected by the mourning process when a loved one (a parent) dies. The child's problem is compounded when other important adults are lost in grief. A pediatrician, nurse, family friend, social worker, or the clergy can be helpful in filling the void. They can help the children in a grief-stricken family.[130a-130c]

Maria H. Nagy,[131,132] also taking a developmental approach, studied the child's view of death. She asked children ages 3 to 10 living in Budapest to write down everything that came to their minds about death. She studied these compositions and concluded that in the first stages (3 to 5 years) children deny death as a regular and final process; in the second stage (5 to 9 years) death is personified, that is, they know and admit that a person has died but they try to "keep it distant from themselves"; and in the third stage (9 to 10 years) death is recognized as something that happens to all of us and that ends in the dissolution of the body.

Nagy's study was made on children in one city in the middle of this century. Children in other cultures in other eras might respond differently. Jill Miller's [133] review of the psychoanalytic literature on the death of a parent gives a range of views. Nothing is more certain than individuality, from infancy onward, and it has been stressed throughout this book. Infants, children, and adolescents deserve the health workers' earnest efforts to understand their particular reaction to death and dying and the particular needs of each child or youth.

It is generally conceded that children who have seen pets die, who have seen relatives in final illnesses and who have gone to their funerals, and children who have seen a normal process of grieving are less likely to have a neurotic response to the loss of a beloved object or person than those who have been protected from the sight of illness and death. Nagy, in her study, makes this concluding observation:

A final thought based on clinical experience is that it is really not possible to conceal death from the child nor should concealment be permitted. Natural behavior in the child's presence can greatly diminish the impact of his acquaintance with death.*

Margaret Mead,[134] an anthropologist who has studied many cultures, decries the protection of children and youths growing up in America from the sight of the dying and the dead because it leaves them, as adults, less prepared than they might be to cope with these inescapable aspects of life.

While the loss of one or both parents is not uncommon in childhood and youth, and is usually the most traumatic experience people of this age have with death, the loss of an infant or child by an adult—the experience in reverse—is also crippling. A great deal depends on the age of the parents, whether the infant or child is the first child, whether it is an only child, and whether, in the case of a newborn, the pregnancy was welcome or unwelcome. In cultures where there is insufficient food and where families consider sons who can work the land an asset but daughters a liability, infanticide has been widely practiced. In cultures where late marriages and small families are customary, the loss of an infant or a child is more likely to be a tragedy for parents who may spend the rest of their lives childless.

Myra Estrin Levine,[135] a nurse, describes what it means to lose a much-wanted newborn soon after its birth and how she worked through the stages of her bereavement. Rothlyn Zahourek and Joseph S. Jensen,[136] nurse and physician, interviewed 25 mothers who had lost an infant just before, during, or immediately after birth, trying to differentiate between normal and pathologic mourning. Susan A. Yates,[137] a nurse, reports on mothers' reactions to stillbirth and what health workers can do to mitigate the inescapable suffering. Joan Marie Johnson,[138] also a nurse, describes her own response to a stillbirth.

Because doctors and nurses may actually feel guilty when an infant is lost, or at least feel that they have failed the parents, they may unconsciously withdraw from the saddened mother and father. The bereft mother may fear that the infant died through some fault of hers and she may also suffer from guilt. If the mother cannot bring herself to look at the dead infant, she may fear that it was abnormal and this may make her afraid to have other children.*

Joan Kron[139] describes her experience in the loss of an older child and the healing effect of working in a seminar on death and dying in a Philadelphia hospital—a kind of organization springing up in many areas to help parents and other bereaved persons. Sylvia A. Mann,[140] a psychiatric nurse, studied the parents' dilemma in coping with a child's fatal illness, noting that they have to work through acknowledging the inevitability of death, their anger, bitterness, blame, and guilt, while, at the same time, trying to help make as happy as possible the months, weeks, or days left to the child. Mann warns nurses that if they are to give parents optimum help through understanding they must be prepared to share the parents' suffering to some extent. Sister Marie Bernadette Maxwell,[141] a nurse, describes the terminal illness of an adolescent and how the nursing staff helped the parents and each other cope with bereavement before death and during the first 8 months of loss through visits and telephone calls.

The adolescent whose parent is dying is in an unusually difficult situation. At the time of life when he or she is working to develop a life style and to loosen the ties to parents, the

---

* Nagy, Maria H.: "The Child's View of Death," in Feifel, Herman (ed.): *The Meaning of Death.* McGraw-Hill Book Co., New York, 1959, p. 98.

* A mother who had a stillbirth told the second author that her reaction was one of anger which was directed at the infant and the doctor. Because she would not look at the child and could not for some time believe the doctor or her husband, the fear that "something was wrong with it" made her reluctant to have another child. Eight years later she did have a normal birth and healthy baby.

illness, weakness, anxiety, and depression of the patient compound the situation. The adolescent is caught in a tug-of-war between a longing for independence and a dread of final separation from parent. The writings of Wessel discuss this issue in greater detail.[141a]

There have been many studies of grief and bereavement in adult life. Thomas B. Elliot,[142] in 1932, wrote on bereavement as a crisis for individuals and families; Peter Marris[143] studied widows and their families in London; Helena Z. Lopata[114] studied the life of 300 older widows in Chicago; John Bowlby's[145] psychoanalytic study of attachment and loss, the first volume of which was published in 1969, is still in progress and has influenced a great deal of the work on bereavement. In most subsequent studies on bereavement, reference is made to Erich Lindemann's 1944 report, "Symptomatology and Management of Acute Grief."[146] *

It is not possible to mention all the research on bereavement but much of it has been conducted under the auspices of the Tavistock Institute of Human Relations, in England, the US National Institute of Mental Health, numerous hospitals in the United Kingdom, the United States, Canada, and other countries. Most studies corroborate Lindemann's concept of bereavement as a typical life crisis; however, Gerald Caplan, director of the Laboratory of Community Psychiatry, Harvard Medical School, thinks this an "oversimplification." He thinks the work of Ira O. Glick, Robert S. Weiss, and C. Murray Parkes at Harvard shows that adjustment to widowhood may involve a series of crises but is more appropriately conceived of as a period of transition. Early work suggested that if a widow "managed her grief work adequately" she might "recover" in about 6 weeks; he makes the following statement:

We now realize that most widows continue the psychological work of mourning for their dead husbands for the rest of their lives. During the turmoil and struggles of the first one to three years most widows gradually learn how to circumscribe and segregate this mourning within their mental economy and how to continue living despite its burden. After this time they are no longer actively mourning, but their loss remains a part of them and now and again they are caught up in a resurgence of feelings of grief. This happens with decreasing frequency as time goes on, but never ceases entirely.*

This study by Glick and his associates of 58 widows and 27 widowers does not contradict and may later validate earlier studies claiming that widowhood increases the risk of mental illness. David Maddison and Wendy L. Walker[147] found that among widows in the United States and Australia 20 to 30 per cent were suffering physical or psychologic ill health as compared with 7 per cent of a matched sample of married women. If most studies of adult bereavement seem to stress widowhood, it may be because widows are, according to Hinton,[148] less likely to remarry than widowers, which suggests a stronger monogamous bond in women. Widows have a tendency to commune with their dead husbands. American and English widows often report a "sense of presence," and in a study of Japanese widows it was reported that 90 per cent of the widows had this experience.

In general, the studies of grief, separation, and bereavement suggest that the human response is universal, although Glick and his associates[149] say that religious beliefs encouraging people to maintain a relationship with the dead, as do Shintoism and Buddhism, can result in different expressions of grief.

Widows and widowers have themselves written about their experiences and feelings. For example, C. S. Lewis,[150] a theologian who lost his wife, titles his subjective study *A Grief Observed*. Lynn Caine[151] writes about the practical problems encountered by widows as well as the emotional aspects of losing a husband. Phyllis R. Silverman[152] has developed a self-help organization called the Widow-to-Widow Program which has its counterpart in many communities. The death of a spouse has been stressed as the most significant loss for adults. The death of an unmarried mate can be as significant a loss in some cases and so can the death of a beloved friend. Adults who continue to live with parents and whose lives are intertwined with theirs may find the loss of a mother or father devastating. Patient histories reported by psychiatrists make it very clear that the degree of dependence determines the emotional reaction; nevertheless, studies of widowhood seem to be far more numerous and systematic than studies of any other bereaved state.

The publications mentioned in the preceding pages are only examples of the numerous research reports, literature surveys, autobio-

---

* Lindemann's study (with Stanley Cobb) included many of those bereaved in the famous Cocoanut Grove fire in Boston, Mass. (Cobb, S., and Lindemann, E.: "Neuropsychiatric Observations After the Cocoanut Grove Fire," *Ann. Surg.,* **117**:819, (June) 1943.)

* Caplan, Gerald: Foreword in Glick, Ira O., et al.: *The First Year of Bereavement*. John Wiley & Sons, New York, 1974, p. viii.

graphical books, and articles now appearing on the subject of bereavement. Every conference on dying and death includes one or more persons who have made a study of it so the conference proceedings usually include the report of a session devoted to this topic. The romantic terminology of "swooning with grief" and "dying of a broken heart" has given way to descriptions of physical changes observed in the survivors of those who die suddenly, to descriptions of "anticipatory grief," to "immediate and delayed responses to loss," and to "resolved and unresolved grief." There is a growing acceptance of a relationship between unresolved grief and mental illness and a realization that the family should indeed be "the patient" for the caretakers of the dying.

Symptoms of Grief. It is not easy to list the physical symptoms and typical behavior of persons experiencing grief. Survivors of those who die suddenly may go into shock, as discussed in Chapter 45; relatives and friends of those who die after a long illness may, through anticipatory grief, reach the stage of acceptance before death occurs. In such cases, the acute and even the later stages of grief come with the diagnosis of a fatal condition and in adjusting to the subsequent stages of the illness. If the patient has been unconscious for weeks, months, or perhaps years, the survivors may feel guilty when relief is the dominant emotion they feel. This is also true when the patient's pain or discomfort have been unrelieved or the personality has been distorted. Family and friends often find that seeing either of these conditions is almost unbearable. But deaths in which the dominant response is relief may also bring an overpowering sense of guilt which can be as devastating in its way as sorrow, a point made later in discussing "anticipatory grief."

The grieving response is affected most by the emotional involvement and by the age of the patient, or the extent to which he or she seemed to have arrived at fulfillment. The death of a young person is, in most cases, harder to accept than the death of the elderly. Obviously, the loss is greater for the survivors if the death of a relative or friend means that their way of life must change drastically. A woman with children who loses a husband whose earnings were the family's sole means of support faces a crisis that is quite different from that faced by a wealthy childless widow; an old man who knows that he will be put into a nursing home at the death of his wife is in a different position from that of an old man whose children have already provided a protective home environment for him.

Taking into consideration these and many

other conditions influencing the reaction to death and emphasizing the possible fallacy of any "typical reaction," the following are some symptoms as reported by those who have studied bereavement.

Parkes,[153] in *Bereavement—Studies of Grief in Adult Life,* looks upon intense grief over the death of others as a form of mental illness, even though it is a normal response to this stress which, while occurring rarely in each life, is common to all lives. Like Lindemann, Parkes speaks of the "stages of grieving" with their differing characteristics, but he stresses that the stages may have varying lengths and manifestations according to the individual and the circumstances surrounding death. The fact that widows and widowers (as well as unmarried men and women) have a higher death rate than married men and women supports the theory that unresolved grief has the physical consequences of prolonged stress, or at least the effect of aggravating latent disease.

Lewis, writing subjectively in *A Grief Observed,* begins by saying:

No one ever told me that grief felt so like fear. I am not afraid, but the sensation is like being afraid. The same fluttering in the stomach, the same restlessness, the yawning. I keep on swallowing.

At other times it feels like being mildly drunk, or concussed. There is a sort of invisible blanket between the world and me. I find it hard to take in what anyone says. Or perhaps, hard to want to take it in. It is so uninteresting. Yet I want the others to be about me. I dread the moments when the house is empty. If only they would talk to one another and not to me.*

Parkes concurs, and says that in acute grief people respond to grief with the following symptoms that Walter B. Cannon (in *Bodily Changes in Pain, Hunger, Fear and Rage,* 2nd ed., Appleton-Century-Crofts, London and New York, 1929) attributed to alarm, or the fight or flee syndrome:

This response includes changes in body function under the control of the sympathetic part of the autonomic nervous system, which improve muscular performance (increase heart and respiratory rate, transfer blood to the muscles from other organs, increase muscular tension), improve vision (by dilation of the pupil and retraction of the eyelids), assist heat loss (increase sweating), cause the bristling of hair characteristic of "threatening" (by contraction of erector pili muscles), and mobilize reserves of energy (convert glycogen in the liver to glucose). It also results in inhibition of activities of the parasympathetic system which controls digestion and other non-priority functions (by stopping the flow of saliva, relaxing the bowel

* Lewis, C. S.: *op. cit.,* p. 7.

and bladder, reducing the flow of secretion in the bowel, and increasing the tone of the sphincter muscles). . . . Clearly, sympathetic stimulation and parasympathetic inhibition have the useful function of putting the animal into a state of readiness for instant action.

Little has been added to Cannon's original description, which still serves to summarize the effects of stress. Typically these changes occur whenever the animal is alarmed, but the more sensitive elements, such as sweating and heart rate, have been shown to alter as the result of minimal stimuli, for example, when an animal passes from a state of inattention to a state of focused attention. It is these sensitive changes that have been closely studied in recent years.*

Parkes gives as stages of grief: alarm; searching (for the lost person); mitigation, or finding sources of comfort; anger and guilt; and gaining a new identity, or adjustment to loss. He also describes atypical or unresolved grief where there is so inadequate an adjustment that the person may be hospitalized.

Following a sudden death, the period of alarm may be preceded by a period of shock, complete inability to act, or even to comprehend what has happened. Just as in shock from any other cause (see Chapter 45), the person is in a critical state which can end fatally or precipitate death if the person's health is already precarious. Partly for this reason health workers should break the news of death as gently as possible and preferably in the presence of a group of supportive relatives or friends.

The term *anticipatory grief* is attributed to Lindemann by Robert Fulton and Julie Fulton,[154] who discuss this topic in a compendium, *Psychosocial Aspects of Terminal Care.* Relatives and friends of patients who have extended terminal illnesses may do what Freud called "the work of mourning" before the person dies.† The adjustment to separation is completed and all that is seen at death is what Glick and associates call a "low-key" grief. While Parkes[155] thinks anticipatory grieving can never be complete, the family and friends may feel guilty that their sorrow is not acute —that they cannot act as society expects them

to act on the death of a close relative or intimate friend.

Regardless of the nature or stage of grief or the behavior of the survivors, they deserve the support of health workers. Nurses, social workers, doctors, and others who have the broadest knowledge of social custom may find it easiest to understand the outward behavior of relatives and friends. Studies by present-day anthropologists, such as those of Margaret Mead, Leo W. Simmons, and E. H. Volhart, are helpful sources. However, historians, as, for example, Herodotus, and essayists, such as Montaigne, have much to say that seems applicable to modern man. Many experts in this field quote Shakespeare's wise observations.

In some cultures it may be so important to demonstrate sorrow that neighbors or professional mourners are invited by the family or even employed to wail or to "keen." Relatives may spend hours or days in this expression of grief. Geoffrey Gorer[156] cites the Shivah, the Orthodox Jew's 7 days of mourning, as a supportive ritual; others question its value. In the case of public figures, whole communities may participate in this demonstration.* George R. Krup and Bernard Kligfeld[157] think funerals are designed to maintain the integrity of a community and to force the bereft to work through their grief. There are cultures in which a stoical control of emotion is admired and even the nearest and dearest relatives and friends manage to stifle every sign of it.

Some persons consider grief such a private affair that they avoid any public ceremony; in fact, some men and women leave requests that they be cremated and that the ashes be disposed of so that no markers are left to show that they have lived on this earth. In the United States, undertakers provide booklets in which those who want to help relatives and friends plan their funeral, or its substitute, can express their wishes as well as provide survivors with biographic data and other helpful information. Allusion has been made to public figures who have built their tombs and planned the ceremonies surrounding their death down to the last detail. No fact may be better known about Sarah Bernhardt, the great French actress, than that she bought her coffin before death and kept it in her home. Preplanning of a funeral by the principal, according to the way it is done, can either help or make things more difficult for the family and friends.

---

* Parkes, Colin Murray: *op. cit.,* p. 30.

† Glick and his associates make this interesting comment about anticipatory grief: "Some writers on the topic have suggested that the anticipation of a death enables grief to start in advance of the event and that one aim of preparation should be the expression of this grief. We are unconvinced of this. Although it may be possible for a person to grieve in advance of a death, we suspect that this can only be done by the person so far withdrawing from the dying patient that the patient is treated as effectively dead. To do this to a living person might well later give rise to corresponding feelings of guilt in the mourner." (Glick, Ira O., et al.: *op. cit.,* p. 294.)

---

* Whole communities may feel that their spiritual or material welfare depends on a leader. Only this can explain the outpouring of sorrow in this century when, for example, Mahatma Gandhi, Franklin D. Roosevelt, and John F. Kennedy died.

In summary it should be stressed that while the emotional response to the death of a beloved relative or friend—or even a public figure—is to some extent the same all over the world, the strength of the attachment, the dependency of the bereaved on the deceased, the age of those who die, and the circumstances of their illness and death affect the emotional response. The way in which the bereaved demonstrate emotion or behave under its influence depends very largely on custom, on practices prescribed by the religion they profess, or by the social class to which they belong. Occasionally, of course, highly independent individualists may disregard religious practice and social convention but, generally speaking, both comfort the bereaved and have evolved for this purpose.

Helping the Bereaved. Krup and Kligfeld [158] define the following "problems" with which people in any culture need help: an explanation of death; dealing with the fear of death; fear of dead bodies, of ghosts; hostilities engendered by death; attempts to recover the lost persons—to continue interaction with them through dreams or other means; the quest for immortality; the effect of death on the community; and how to deal with the loss.

The symptoms of "normal" grief with which the bereaved must cope, as defined by Lindemann, Weisman, Glick, Parkes, Bowlby, and others have been listed in the previous section. Pathognomonic grief, as defined by Lindemann, [159] is an exaggeration or persistence of the following symptoms of normal grief: somatic distress; preoccupation with the image of the deceased; guilt; hostile reactions; and loss of patterns of contact.

Efforts to help the bereaved should *encourage* the expression of normal grief—the resolution of grief—and should *discourage* the development of pathological, abnormal, or persistent grief. Programs to mitigate grief belong to a community rather than to health workers alone but the latter play an important role. The family, friends, the clergy, funeral directors, members of concerned organizations, and neighbors all contribute.

Parkes, in *Bereavement—Studies of Grief in Adult Life* (1972) says:

If bereavement can have detrimental effects upon physical and mental health, what can be done to prevent these effects from occurring? Most doctors and clergy would regard it as one of their roles to give help and advice to the dying and the bereaved but they have, in the past, received little formal training in this area of service and it is only in recent years that bereavement counselling has become recognized as worthy of special attention. Not that there is as yet much clear evidence

concerning the effectiveness of bereavement counselling. At the time of writing no research aimed at evaluating counselling programmes has been published and such programmes are still at an early state of development.*

Since the publication of this work, with its chapter "Helping the Bereaved," Parkes has collaborated with Glick and Weiss in a study, *The First Year of [Conjugal] Bereavement* (1974). [160] Excerpts from recorded interviews with 49 widows and 19 widowers corroborate many of the inferences in earlier studies about the effects of bereavement and ways in which the pain of grief can be mitigated and practical help provided.

So much has been written about conjugal bereavement that many communities in the United States and abroad have organized agencies to help the bereaved and their children. The Widow's Aide Program of Boston, Mass. (organized by the social worker Phyllis Silverman) has been mentioned already; Parents Without Partners; THEO, Inc. (Pennsylvania); Post-Cana (Washington, D.C.); and the Big Brother and Big Sister organizations represent some of the American efforts. In the United Kingdom, Cruse is one of the most important. This agency provides professional counseling of mothers and children by social workers, doctors, and the clergy, and organizes groups of widows for self-help during the transitional period. Cruse is not intended as a final refuge for those who would like to withdraw from normal life. The director of Cruse (Mrs. Alfred Torrie) is author of the book *Begin Again*, [161] which gives information on death grants, pensions, insurance, and other subjects. Also in England there is an experimental program, reported by Parkes, [162] in the London Borough of Camden through a cooperative effort of the Camden Council of Social Service and the Tavistock Institute of Human Relations. Here an offer is made, by mail, of emotional support and practical advice to all bereaved persons in that area. This seems to be the most comprehensive of the helping programs and if successful and practicable may be replicated all over England and be a model for any country. Other British organizations include the Society of Compassionate Friends, founded by Simon Stephens, a minister, and The Samaritans, also founded by a Protestant minister. The Samaritans help despairing persons, especially those contemplating suicide.

While these organizations have as their sole purpose helping the bereaved and depressed, many institutions, organizations, and

---

* Parkes, Colin Murray: *op. cit.*, p. 149.

agencies to which the persons who have died or their survivors belong have formal or informal programs that help the bereaved. In the United States, those who qualify for Social Security get "benefits" that help meet funeral costs; qualified veterans, through the Veterans Administration, have a specified "benefit" that helps meet the cost of the funeral; the VA provides a flag for the casket, space in a national cemetery, and grave markers; the Odd Fellows, the Elks, the Masons, and other fraternal orders offer financial assistance and other kinds of support in some cases. Religious congregations and orders supply spiritual counseling, friendly support, and often material assistance.[163] These are only a few examples of the sources of help within the community. Those who live in big cities, especially newcomers, may have little help of this sort in the early or later stages of bereavement but established members of friendly neighborhoods may be astounded at the expressions of concern and offers of assistance of all kinds—especially in the first stages, or immediately after the death occurs. Parkes makes the comment that health workers should enlist the help of relatives, friends, and neighbors rather than trying to supplant them for these are more permanent relationships for the survivors and it is important that friends and neighbors feel needed and wanted and that the bereaved feel that they can rely on their help.

There is some question as to when health workers should begin to help mitigate the suffering of bereavement. It is suggested that it should begin in childhood. As stressed earlier, if children have learned to respect life but to accept, as a part of it, the death of plants, animals, and humans, they are most likely to be prepared as adults to accept the death of someone they love. If they have seen normal grief expressed and seen its resolution, this is what they are most likely to expect of themselves. The Equinox Group in Boston, under the leadership of Krant, is teaching children in secondary schools and in agencies dealing with children.

Parkes, Glick, Weiss, and other students of bereavement think there is reason to believe that persons whose questions have been answered honestly by the physician and other health workers, who have known what to expect, who have faced the imminence of death with the relative or friend throughout the terminal illness, and who have had time to think about what life will be like without the sick person, are best able to bear the suffering of final separation and best able to resolve their grief. The work of the first author leads

to the assumption that family and friends who have participated in the care of the patient and in decision-making are less prone to blame and guilt and more certain that everything was done that could be done. There is also some reason to believe that widows who have helped take care of their sick husbands are least traumatized by their death and this may be true for everyone who loses someone they love. In any event, health workers—and nurses have the greatest opportunity to make this possible —should encourage the participation of relatives and friends in terminal care. For those who are with the patient in death, it comes as no shock. For those who are not present, it is most important that they learn it in the presence of other members of the family and that the news be broken gently. It is generally agreed that the public still expects or wants the doctor to be present at death and to accept the responsibility of talking with the next of kin. Since physicians must sign death certificates, they legally pronounce death. In many cases they are not present when death occurs, and in some cases there is no professional health worker to assume the responsibility for telling the family and friends. Abrupt, harsh, or insensitive treatment at this time is especially traumatic and gives rise to a long-lasting anger which, under the best conditions, may be one of the crippling symptoms of bereavement.

When the patient's life is over, the family and friends should be the focus of the health worker's attention. A relative may want to help the nurse prepare the body for the undertaker. Members of the family may want to stay with the body or they may want to be in a room where they can talk with and comfort each other—where they can cry without attracting attention. It should be possible for intimate friends and the clergy to be with the bereaved if they need them.

When there has been sufficient warning of death, plans for the funeral or disposition of the body are usually made before it occurs; if not, the near relatives, who may be in a state of shock, will need a good deal of help in arranging for the disposal of the body. Mention has been made of booklets given to families by undertakers that help them collect the information that will be needed and to make necessary plans.

In sudden deaths, young families especially may not have a burial plot or may not, in fact, have decided on cremation or burial, on public or private funeral, on the choice of an undertaker, or a clergyman to conduct a service. Parkes [164] mentions his "favorite" cemetery in Boston, Mass., where people can buy their graves in advance and where a public relations officer (a widow) is available to offer support and advice to bereaved women. The public relations officer actually has annual conferences on a variety of topics relevant to widowhood. This is a Jewish cemetery and the point is made that preplanning is most important for persons who, as in the case of Jews, believe that the body should be buried within the first 24 hours after death.

Close relatives or friends may be dazed and find it hard to make any decisions, so that others may be obliged to act for them in notifying the undertaker, other relatives, and friends, in preparing notices for the paper, and in making decisions about the ceremonies, or "rites of passage." Decisions should not, however, be taken out of the hands of the nearest kin unless they want to relinquish them.

Previous experience and custom determine, to a large extent, the effect on the bereaved of seeing the person in death prepared for cremation or burial. While, as noted earlier, there has been widespread criticism of elaborate funerals and excessive use of cosmetics to make the person look healthy and to hide the signs of age, a beautiful ceremony may be healing for the family and friends, and if in a violent death the face has been mutilated it may be comforting to relatives if the face is repaired. Parkes [165] reports that in several studies of conjugal bereavement wives and husbands were about equally divided on whether seeing the corpse of their spouse was traumatic or helpful.*

Funerals, rituals, and *ceremonies* that sur-

round the bereaved with assurance that the dead person was valued, admired, or beloved offer comfort. Mead [166] notes that in many of the developing countries rituals are "protecting, purifying and healing." In the Western world, the family and friends may be especially pleased if doctors, nurses, and others who have taken care of the dead are present at funeral or memorial services. Private nurses may stay on with the family until after the funeral in some cases, acknowledging the need of the bereft for continued help. More and more health professionals are attending services for patients who have been under their care, not only for the sake of the family, but also for their own sake, to allow themselves to grieve for the human being who came to them as a patient.

Because somatic symptoms and sleeplessness may accompany acute grief, physicians often prescribe analgesics, hypnotics, or tranquilizers for the bereaved. Those who haven't experienced acute grief may be alarmed by its intensity and may be afraid they are "going crazy." Parkes, who is a psychiatrist, thinks that the danger of suicide is real in some cases, and that if persons can talk about their fears it may minimize them. He says:

It is common enough for a bereaved person to say "I wouldn't care if I died tomorrow," and such remarks need not cause alarm, but a person who has thought seriously of killing himself or herself should always see a psychiatrist. . . . People are often afraid to mention suicide as if, by doing so, they could bring it about. But a simple question, "Has it been so bad that you have thought of killing yourself?" is more likely to save a life than to take one.*

A distressing symptom that appears in the first month or two is the bereaved hearing the voice of the person who has died; or the bereaved may automatically set the table to include the person who has died. These fantasies subside but can be frightening and lead those who have them to think themselves mentally ill.

Drugs may bring immediate relief and drug-induced sleep. However, since people must work through and resolve their grief, drugs may only slow this process, or postpone resolution. Parkes [167] comments that tobacco and alcohol are the drugs most commonly used to assuage grief. In the Harvard study of widows and widowers, 40 per cent of the young widows and 37 per cent of the young widowers were smoking more in the first year of bereavement, and corresponding figures were 38 and 31 per cent for alcohol consumption. Parkes

* The Judaic position on "viewing the remains" and the cosmetology of undertaking is expressed in the following terms by Maurice Lamm and Naftali Eskreis: "It is a perversion of the true religious import of the funeral to disguise the reality of death. The display of the dead in the most lifelike appearance, the semblance of life through the use of cosmetics, the clothing in gowns or tuxedos, the propping of the head and use of pillows, the facsimile of a happy person asleep is contrary to the spirit that religion seeks to engender. Man does not, as the happy phrase has it, merely 'go to sleep with his forefathers.' Man dies and decays and his physical existence is no more. His good works live on after him, but his body returns to the earth as it was. His personality, his goodness go on to a greater dimension of existence; the chemical elements decompose and return to their original state.

From the standpoint of psychotherapy, the idea of viewing the corpse as standard funeral procedure because of the therapeutic value inherent in the practice has not been proved clinically and, in fact, appears to contradict the very basic thrust of its method." (Lamm, Maurice, and Eskreis, Naftali: "Viewing the Remains: a New American Custom," in Reeves, Robert B., Jr., et al. [eds.]: *Pastoral Care of the Dying and Bereaved: Selected Readings.* Health Sciences Publishing Corp., New York, 1973.)

* Parkes, Colin Murray: *op. cit.,* p. 165.

thinks addiction to alcohol is a real danger. He makes the following observation:

The GP who can recognize grief as the painful process through which a family must pass in becoming another kind of family is aware that the symptoms to which it gives rise must be seen in perspective. By showing his willingness to accept their need to mourn, he may help them more positively than he would by taking the easier course of prescribing anti-depressives and tranquillizers.*

Clergymen often play an important role in bereavement and are most helpful if they have seen the family from time to time during the terminal illness of the dying relative or friend. If present at the death of the patient, they may say a prayer; later they officiate at the burial services and, according to their relationship with the bereaved, they may give counsel and support during the grieving process. If a man or woman has lost his or her spouse and if children have lost a parent, especially if young children have lost a mother, there is a radical change in the family's pattern of living, and everyone involved may need help in adjusting to it. Visiting nurses and social workers may find homemakers for the family or in other ways help those whose lives are disrupted to meet their needs.

The programs in British hospices and in the newly established units for terminal care in the United States provide individual services to the bereaved just as they provide individual care of the dying patient. This service begins with the admission of the patient and is continued in some form as long as the family needs, or seems to want, help from the hospice staff. Much of the support of hospices is given by relatives and friends who have had this help and some return to take part in the program as paid or volunteer workers.

Summary. The proliferation of information on death in print and nonprint materials is noted, as are the difficulty of adequately describing the changing attitudes toward death and the care of the dying and the ways in which society faces and copes with death. Delaying death with technology is discussed and the desire of both the public and health workers to prevent the unnatural extension of a meaningless existence. Attention is called to the importance of health services that enable families, when they wish it, to keep the dying person at home. Hospices are described —places where caregivers and the environment encourage the dying, their families, and friends to make the end of life a period of growth and achievement—a period when the dying enjoy friends and relatives, when "the house is put in order," and when the patient and the family are helped with the process of "letting go" of life.

Palliative symptomatic management is presented in detail. While it is recognized that this is most highly developed for the person with cancer, the suggested methods have general application. The point is made that when pain and discomfort are controlled by skillful medical and nursing management, patients and those who love them are able to make the end of life constructive and rewarding. The importance of continuous collaboration is stressed —of taking cues from the patient and the family, allowing people to express their fears, needs, and wishes and to have a "good death" as they see it.

The possible roles of physicians, special therapists and pharmacists, nurses, social workers, the clergy, and others (including volunteers) are outlined. The emotional strain for caretakers of working with patients, their families, and friends during terminal illness is recognized and ways of reducing this strain suggested. Helping families and friends when death occurs and immediately thereafter is discussed and a special section devoted to bereavement. Emphasis is placed on preparing relatives and friends for loss, giving them an opportunity to participate in the care of the dying, which seems to mitigate the shock of death. Attention is called to the organizations for the bereaved where members help each other in the resolution of their problems. Readers with special interest in terminal care and bereavement are directed to bibliographic projects that facilitate continuing study of this subject.

---

* *Ibid.*, p. 174.

REFERENCES

1. Opler, Morris E.: "An Interpretation of Ambivalence of Two American Indian Tribes," *J. Soc. Psychol.,* 7:82, (Feb.) 1936.
1a. Moody, Raymond: *Life After Life.* Mockingbird Books, Covington, Ga., 1976.
1b. Noyes, Russell, and Kletti, Roy: "Depersonalization in the Face of Life-Threatening Danger. An Interpretation," *Omega,* 7:103, (No. 2) 1976.
2. Noss, John B.: *Man's Religions,* 4th ed. Macmillan Publishing Co., Inc., New York, 1969, p. 102.
3. Alexander, Irving E., and Adlerstein, Arthur M.: "Death and Religion," in Feifel, Herman (ed.): *The Meaning of Death.* McGraw-Hill Book Co., New York, 1965.
3a. Hinton, John: *Dying,* 2nd ed. Penguin Books, Harmondsworth, Eng., 1972.

3b. Woolf, Virginia. *The Years.* Harcourt, Brace & World, New York, 1937, p. 21.

4. Glaser, Barney G., and Strauss, Anselm L.: *Time for Dying.* Aldine Press, Chicago, 1968.

5. Brim, Orville G., Jr., et al. (eds.): *The Dying Patient.* Russell Sage Foundation, New York, 1970.

6. Lerner, Monroe: "When, Why and Where People Die," in Brim, Orville G., Jr., et al. (eds.): *The Dying Patient.* Russell Sage Foundation, New York, 1970, p. 22.

7. Glaser, Robert J.: "Innovations and Heroic Acts in Prolonging Life," in Brim, Orville G., Jr., et al. (eds.): *The Dying Patient.* Russell Sage Foundation, New York, 1970, p. 119.

8. *Ibid.,* p. 125.

9. Mannes, Marya: *Last Rights. A Case for the Good Death.* William Morrow & Co., New York, 1974, p. 127.

10. Hall, J. H., and Swenson, D. D.: *Psychological and Social Aspects of Tissue Transplantation.* US Department of Health, Education, and Welfare, Chevy Chase, Md., 1968 (Supplement No. 1, 1969).

11. Lifton, Robert Jay, and Olson, Eric: *Living and Dying.* Praeger Publishers, New York, 1974, p. 35.

12. Crowe, John H., and Cooper, Alan F., Jr.: "Cryptobiosis," *Sci. Am.,* **225**:30, (Dec.) 1971.

12a. Bratton, Fred Gladstone: *Maimonides— Medieval Modernist.* Beacon Press, Boston, 1967, p. 81.

12b. Rosner, Fred: "Euthanasia," in Schoenberg, Bernard, et al. (eds.): *Psychosocial Aspects of Terminal Care.* Columbia University Press, New York, 1972, p. 315.

13. Thomas, Lewis: *The Lives of a Cell. Notes of a Biology Watcher.* Viking Press, New York, 1974.

14. Jourard, Sidney M.: "Suicide: An Invitation to Die," *Am. J. Nurs.,* **70**:269, (Feb.) 1970.

15. Livingstone, R. W.: *Portrait of Socrates; Being the Apology, Crito and Phaedo of Plato in an English Translation with Introduction and Notes.* Oxford University Press, London, 1938.

16. Shepard, Melba W.: "This I Believe . . . About Questioning the Right to Die," *Am. J. Nurs.,* **68**:22, (Oct.) 1968.

17. Wertenbaker, Lael T.: *Death of a Man.* Random House, New York, 1957.

18. Mannes, Marya: *op. cit.*

19. Rosner, Fred: "Euthanasia," in Schoenberg, Bernard, et al. (eds.): *Psychosocial Aspects of Terminal Care.* Columbia University Press, New York, 1972, p. 312.

20. Mannes, Marya: *op. cit.,* p. 58.

21. Braverman, Shirley J.: "Death of a Monster," *Am. J. Nurs.,* **69**:1682, (Aug.) 1969.

22. Mannes, Marya: *op. cit.*

23. Manning, Bayless: "Legal and Policy Issues in the Allocation of Death," in Brim, Orville G., Jr., et al. (eds.): *The Dying Pa-*

tient. Russell Sage Foundation, New York, 1970, p. 253.

24. Ariès, Philippe: *Western Attitudes Toward Death: From the Middle Ages to the Present.* (Translated by Patricia M. Ranum.) Johns Hopkins Press, Baltimore, 1974.

25. de Hartog, Jan: *The Hospital,* Atheneum Publishers, New York, 1964.

25a. Chan, Lo-Yi: "Hospice. A New Building to Comfort the Dying," *Am. Inst. Arch. J.,* (Dec.) 1976, p. 42.

25b. Muggeridge, Malcolm: *Something Beautiful for God. Mother Teresa of Calcutta.* Collins-Fontana Books, London, 1973.

26. Osler, William: *Science and Immortality.* Constable & Co., Ltd., London, 1906.

27. Worcester, Alfred: *The Care of the Aged, the Dying and the Dead.* Charles C Thomas, Publishers, Springfield, Ill., 1935.

28. Cabot, Richard C., and Dicks, Russell L.: *The Art of Ministering to the Sick.* Macmillan Publishing Co., Inc., New York, 1936.

29. Saunders, Cicely: "Mental Distress in the Dying," *Nurs. Times,* **55**:1067, (Oct. 30) 1959.

30. ———: "Control of Pain in Terminal Cases," *Nurs. Times,* **55**:1031, (Oct. 23) 1959.

31. ———: "Should a Patient Know," *Nurs. Times,* **55**:954, (Oct. 16) 1959.

32. ———: "The Treatment of Intractable Pain in Terminal Cancer," in *Proceedings of the Royal Society of Medicine.* The Society, London, 1963.

33. ———: "The Symptomatic Treatment of Incurable Malignant Disease," *Prescribers J.,* **4**:68, (Oct.) 1964.

34. Quint, Jeanne C.: *The Nurse and the Dying Patient.* Macmillan Publishing Co., Inc., New York, 1967.

35. Glaser, Barney G., and Strauss, Anselm L.: *Awareness of Dying.* Aldine Press, Chicage, 1965.

36. ———: *Time for Dying.* Aldine Press, Chicago, 1968.

37. Quint, Jeanne C.: *op. cit.,* p. 230.

38. American Hospital Association: *A Patient's Bill of Rights.* The Association, Chicago, 1972.

39. Mount, Balfour M., et al.: "Death and Dying; Attitudes in a Teaching Hospital," *Urology,* **4**:741, (Dec.) 1974.

40. Benoliel, Jeanne Quint: *Death Influence in Clinical Practice.* [Course Outline] University of Washington School of Nursing, Seattle, 1974, processed.

41. Krant, Melvin: "In the Context of Dying," in Schoenberg, Bernard, et al. (eds.): *Psychosocial Aspects of Terminal Care.* Columbia University Press, New York, 1972, p. 207.

41a. Duncombe, David C.: "Five Years at Yale: 'The Seminar on the Chronically Ill,' " *J. Pastoral Care,* **28**:152, (Sept.) 1974.

42. "The Meanings of Death," *Yale Alumni Mag.,* **38**:12, (Apr.) 1975.

43. Worcester, Alfred: *op. cit.*

44. Tolstoy, Leo: *The Death of Ivan Ilych and Other Stories.* New American Library, New York, 1960.

45. Weisman, Avery D.: *On Dying and Denying; A Psychiatric Study of Terminality.* Behavioral Publications, New York, 1972, pp. 13, 14, 17, 22.

46. Ross, Elisabeth K. [Kübler-Ross]: "Hope and the Dying Patient," in Schoenberg, Bernard, et al. (eds.): *Psychosocial Aspects of Terminal Care.* Columbia University Press, New York, 1972.

47. Evans, Jocelyn: *Living with a Man Who Is Dying.* Taplinger Publishing Co., New York, 1971.

47a. Saunders, Cicely: "The Moment of Truth: Care of the Dying Person," in Pearson, Leonard (ed.): *Death and Dying.* Press of Case Western Reserve University, Cleveland, 1969, p. 49.

47b. Ingles, Thelma: "St. Christopher's Hospice," *Nurs. Outlook,* **22:**759, (Dec.) 1974.

47c. Craven, Joan, and Wald, Florence S.: "Hospice Care for Dying Patients," *Am. J. Nurs.,* **75:**1816, (Oct.) 1975.

47d. McNulty, Barbara: "St. Christopher's Outpatients," *Am. J. Nurs.,* **71:**2328, (Dec.) 1971.

48. Nagy, Maria H.: "The Child's View of Death," in Feifel, Herman (ed.): *The Meaning of Death.* McGraw-Hill Book Co., New York, 1959.

49. Fredlund, Delphie J.: "A Nurse Looks at Children's Questions About Death," in *ANA Clinical Conferences, 1970.* Appleton-Century-Crofts, New York, 1970.

50. Furman, Erna: *A Child's Parent Dies. Studies in Childhood Bereavement.* Yale University Press, New Haven, 1974.

51. Wynant, W. E.: "Dying But Not Alone," *Am. J. Nurs.,* **67:**574, (Mar.) 1967.

52. Simmons, Leo W.: *The Role of the Aged in Primitive Society.* Yale University Press, New Haven, Conn., 1945.

53. Jaeger, Dorothea, and Simmons, Leo W.: *The Aged Ill; Coping with Problems in Geriatric Care.* Appleton-Century-Crofts, New York, 1970.

54. Gunther, John: *Death Be Not Proud.* Harper & Brothers, New York, 1949, pp. 250, 251.

55. Evans, Jocelyn: *op. cit.*

56. Lewis, C. S.: *A Grief Observed.* Seabury Press, New York, 1961.

57. Shneidman, E. S.: "You and Death," *Psychology Today,* **5:**43, (June) 1971.

58. Smart, Ninian: "Death and the Decline of Religion in Western Society," in Toynbee, Arnold, et al. (eds.): *Man's Concern With Death.* McGraw-Hill Book Co., New York, 1968.

59. Berman, Alan L.: "Belief in Afterlife, Religion, Religiosity, and Life-Threatening Experiences," *Omega,* **5:**127, (Summer) 1974.

60. Dicks, Russell L.: *Who Is My Patient?* Macmillan Publishing Co., Inc., New York, 1941.

61. Feifel, Herman (ed.): *The Meaning of Death.* McGraw-Hill Book Co., New York, 1959.

62. Hinton, John: *Dying,* 2nd ed. Penguin Books, Harmondsworth, Eng., 1972.

63. Schoenberg, Bernard, et al. (eds.): *Psychosocial Aspects of Terminal Care.* Columbia University Press, New York, 1972.

64. Hinton, John: *op. cit.*

65. Brim, Orville G., Jr., et al. (eds.): *op. cit.*

66. Hinton, John: *op. cit.*

67. Cope, Oliver: "Has the Time Come for a Less Mutilating Treatment?" *Radcliffe Q. Rev.,* June 1970.

68. American Hospital Association: *op. cit.*

68a. Lipman, Arthur C.: "Drug Therapy in the Care of Terminally Ill Patients," *Am. J. Hosp. Pharm.,* **32:**270, (Mar.) 1975.

69. Gibson, Ronald: "Symposium on Care of the Dying. Caring for the Bereaved," *Nurs. Mirror,* **139:**65, (Oct. 10) 1974.

70. Browning, Mary H., and Lewis, Edith P. (comps.): *The Dying Patient: A Nursing Perspective.* American Journal of Nursing Co., New York, 1972 (Contemporary Nursing Series).

71. Aguilera, Donna Conant: "Crisis: Death and Dying," in *ANA Clinical Sessions, 1968.* Appleton-Century-Crofts, New York, 1968.

72. Wald, Florence S.: "Development of an Interdisciplinary Team to Care for Dying Patients and Their Families," in *ANA Clinical Conferences, 1969.* Appleton-Century-Crofts, New York, 1970.

73. Quint, Jeanne C.: *op. cit.*

74. Davidson, Ramona Powell: "To Give Care in Terminal Illness," *Am. J. Nurs.,* **66:**74, (Jan.) 1966.

75. Wald, Florence S.: *A Nurse's Study of Care for Dying Patients,* U.S.P.H.S. Nursing Resources Grant NU 00352–01, 02, Sept. 1, 1969–Aug. 30, 1971 (report in preparation).

76. Henderson, I., and Henderson, J. E.: "Psychological Care of Patients with Catastrophic Illness," *Can. Nurse,* **61:**899, (Nov.) 1965.

77. Craig, Y.: "The Care of a Dying Child. The Needs of the Nurses, the Patient, and Parents," *Nurs. Mirror,* **137:**14, (Sept. 28) 1973.

78. Cramond, W. A.: "The Psychological Care of Patients with Terminal Illness," *N.Z. Nurs. J.,* **66:**27, (Sept.) 1973.

79. Bennett, M. B.: "Care of the Dying," *S. Afr. Med. J.,* **47:**1558, (Sept. 1) 1973.

80. Goldfogel, L.: "Working with the Parents of a Dying Child," *Nurs. J. India,* **62:**8, (Jan.) 1971.

81. Kono, H.: ["Death and Nursing"], *Jap. J. Nurs.,* **37:**98, (Jan.); 1046, (Aug.) 1973.

82. Cramond, W. A.: "The Psychological Care of Patients with Terminal Illness," *N.Z. Nurs. J.,* **66:**23, (Oct.) 1973.

83. McNulty, Barbara J.: "St. Christopher's Outpatients," *Am. J. Nurs.,* **71:**2328, (Dec.) 1971.

83a. ———: "Christmas at St. Christopher's," *Am. J. Nurs.,* **71:**2325, (Dec.) 1971.

84. Wolfe, Ilse S.: "The Magnificence of Understanding," in Standard, Samuel, and Nathan, Helmut (eds.): *Should the Patient Know the Truth.* Springer Publishing Co., New York, 1955.

85. Abrams, Ruth D.: "The Responsibility of Social Work in Terminal Cancer," in Schoenberg, Bernard, et al. (eds.): *Psychosocial Aspects of Terminal Care.* Columbia University Press, New York, 1972.

86. ———: *Not Alone with Cancer.* Charles C Thomas, Publisher, Springfield, Ill., 1974.

87. Mannes, Marya: *op. cit.,* p. 118.

88. Saunders, Cicely: "A Therapeutic Community: St. Christopher's Hospice," in Schoenberg, Bernard, et al. (eds.): *Psychosocial Aspects of Terminal Care.* Columbia University Press, New York, 1972.

83a. McNeil, D.: "A Death at Home," *Can. Nurse,* **70:**17, (Mar.) 1974.

89. Saunders, Cicely: *Care of the Dying. Nursing Times Reprint.* Macmillan Publishing Journals, Ltd., London, [1970].

90. Craven, Joan, and Wald, Florence: "Hospice Care for Dying Patients," *Am. J. Nurs.,* **75:**1816, (Oct.) 1975.

91. McNulty, Barbara J.: "Symposium on Care of the Dying. The Nurse's Contribution in Terminal Care," *Nurs. Mirror,* **139:**59, (Oct. 10) 1974.

92. Wilkes, Eric: "Symposium on Care of the Dying. Relatives, Professional Care, and the Dying Patient," *Nurs. Mirror,* **139:**54, (Oct. 10) 1974.

93. Noyes, Russell, Jr.: "The Care and Management of the Dying," *Arch. Intern. Med.,* **128:**299, (Aug.) 1971.

93a. Engleman, Edgar C.: "Management of Persistent Hiccup," *Drug Therapy,* July 1972.

94. Hinton, John: "The Physical and Mental Distress of the Dying," *Q. J. Med.,* **32:**1, (Jan.) 1963.

94a. Lipman, Arthur C.: *op. cit.*

94b. *Ibid.*

95. Zegarelli, E. V., et al.: "Maintaining the Oral and General Health of the Oral Cancer Patient," Parts 1 and 2, in *Oral Care for Oral Cancer Patients.* US Government Printing Office, Washington, D.C., June 1968.

96. Worcester, Alfred: *op. cit.*

97. Hinton, John: *Dying,* 2nd ed. Penguin Books, Harmondsworth, Eng., 1972, pp. 71, 72, 73.

98. Saunders, Cicely: "The Symptomatic Treatment of Incurable Malignant Disease," *Prescribers J.,* **4:**68, (Oct.) 1964.

99. ———: *Care of the Dying, Nursing Times Reprint.* Macmillan Journals, Ltd., London, [1970], p. 26.

99a. Twycross, Robert G., and Wald, Shari: "The Long Time Use of Diamorphine in Advanced Cancer," Proceedings of 1975 International Association of Pain.

99b. "The Spectrum of Suffering," (Symposium), *Am. J. Nurs.,* **74:**491, (Mar.) 1974.

99c. Saunders, Cicely: "Telling Patients," *Dist. Nurs.,* **8:**145, (Sept.) 1965.

99d. Lipman, Arthur C.: *op. cit.*

100. Craven, Joan, and Wald, Florence: *op. cit.*

101. Glaser, Barney G., and Strauss, Anselm L.: *Time for Dying.* Aldine Press, Chicago, 1968.

101a. Fontaine, Karen Lee: "Human Sexuality: Faculty Knowledge and Attitudes," *Nurs. Outlook,* **24:**174, (Mar.) 1976.

101b. Elder, M. S.: "Unmet Challenge—Nurse Counseling on Sexuality," *Nurs. Outlook,* **18:**38, (Nov.) 1970.

102. Jacobson, Linbania: "Illness and Human Sexuality," *Nurs. Outlook,* **22:**50, (Jan.) 1974.

103. Institute of Society, Ethics, and the Life Sciences, Task Force on Death and Dying: "Refinements in Criteria for the Determination of Death: An Appraisal," *J.A.M.A.,* **221:**48, (July 3) 1972.

104. World Health Organization: *Use of Human Tissues and Organs for Therapeutic Purposes: A Survey of Existing Legislature.* The Organization, Geneva, 1969.

105. Aasterud, Margaret: "Defenses Against Anxiety in the Nurse-Patient Relationship," *Nurs. Forum,* **1:**48, (Summer) 1962.

106. Quint, Jeanne C.: "Nursing Services and the Care of Dying Patients, Some Speculations," *Nurs. Sci.,* **2:**432, (Dec.) 1964.

107. Christopherson, L. K., and Lunde, D. T.: "The Selection of Cardiac Transplant Recipients and Their Subsequent Psychosocial Adjustment," *Semin. Psychiatry,* **3:**(1) 1971.

108. Buda, Joseph A.: "Organ Transplantation Workshop," in Schoenberg, Bernard, et al. (eds.): *Psychosocial Aspects of Terminal Care.* Columbia University Press, New York, 1972.

109. Crowe, John H., and Cooper, Alan F., Jr.: *op. cit.*

110. Noss, John B.: *Man's Religions,* 4th ed. Macmillan Publishing Co., Inc., New York, 1969.

111. Waugh, Evelyn: *The Loved One.* Chapman & Hall, London, 1948.

112. Mitford, Jessica: *The American Way of Death.* Hutchinson & Co., Ltd., London, 1963.

112a. Nichols, Roy, and Nichols, Jane: "Funerals: A Time for Grief and Growth," in Kübler-Ross, Elisabeth (ed.): *Death the Final Stage of Growth.* Prentice-Hall, Inc., Englewood Cliffs, N.J., 1975.

113. *Physicians' Handbook on Medical Certification: Death, Fetal Death, Birth.* US Government Printing Office, Washington, D.C., 1973 (DHEW Pub. No. [HRA] 75–1108).

114. Sartwell, Philip E. (ed.): *Maxcy-Rosenau's Preventive Medicine and Hygiene,* 10th ed. Appleton-Century-Crofts, New York, 1973.

115. Hayt, Emanuel, and Hayt, Lillian R.: *Law*

of Hospital, Physician, and Patient, 3rd ed. Physicians' Record Co., Berwyn, Ill., 1972.

116. New York City. Board of Health: *New York City Health Code.* The Board, New York, 1959.

117. Darwin, Charles: *The Expressions of Emotions in Man and Animals.* John Murray, London, 1872.

118. Freud, Sigmund: *Inhibitions, Symptoms and Anxiety.* Hogarth Press, London, 1959.

119. Nagera, Humberto: "Children's Reactions to the Death of Important Objects," *Psychoanal. Study Child,* **25**:360, 1970.

120. Deutsch, Helen: "Absence of Grief," *Psychoanal. Q.,* **6**:77, 1937.

121. Bowlby, John: "Childhood Mourning and Its Implications for Psychiatry," *Am. J. Psychiatry,* **118**:481, (Dec.) 1961.

122. ———: "Pathological Mourning and Childhood Mourning," *J. Am. Psychoanal. Assoc.,* **11**:500, 1963.

123. ———: "Grief and Mourning in Infancy and Early Childhood," *Psychoanal. Study Child,* **15**:9, 1960.

124. Freud, Anna, and Burlingham, D.: *Infants Without Families.* International Universities Press, New York, 1944.

125. ———: *War and Children.* International Universities Press, New York, 1943.

126. Nagera, Humberto: *Early Childhood Disturbances, the Infantile Neurosis, and the Adulthood Disturbances.* International Universities Press, New York, 1966.

127. Wolfenstein, M.: "Death of a Parent and Death of a President," in Wolfenstein, M., and Kliman, G. (eds.): *Children and the Death of a President.* Doubleday & Co., New York, 1965.

128. Robertson, J.: *Young Children in Hospital.* Tavistock Publications, London, 1958.

129. Shambaugh, B.: "A Study of Loss Reactions in a Seven-Year-Old," *Psychoanal. Study Child,* **16**:510, 1961.

130. Wolf, A. W. M.: *Helping Your Child to Understand Death.* Child Study Association, New York, 1958.

130a. Furman, Edna: *A Child's Parent Dies.* Yale University Press, New Haven, 1974.

130b. Wessel, Morris: "The Bereaved Child," *Family Health,* August 1975.

130c. ———: "Adolescents and the Death of a Parent," in Roswell, Ballagher J., et al.: *Medical Care of the Adolescent,* 3rd ed. Appleton-Century-Crofts, New York, 1976.

131. Nagy, Maria H.: "The Child's Theory Concerning Death," *J. Genet. Psychol.,* **72**:26, (Mar.) 1948.

132. ———: "The Child's View of Death," in Feifel, Herman (ed.): *The Meaning of Death.* McGraw-Hill Book Co., New York, 1959.

133. Miller, Jill: "Children's Reactions to the Death of a Parent: A Review of the Psychoanalytic Literature," *J. Am. Psychoanal. Assoc.,* **19**:697, (Oct.) 1971.

134. Mead, Margaret: *op. cit.*

135. Levine, Myra Estrin: "Benoni," *Am. J. Nurs.,* **72**:466, (Mar.) 1972.

136. Zahourek, Rothlyn, and Jensen, Joseph S.: "Grieving and the Loss of the Newborn," *Am. J. Nurs.,* **73**:836, (May) 1973.

137. Yates, Susan A.: "Stillbirth—What a Staff Can Do," *Am. J. Nurs.,* **72**:1592, (Sept.) 1972.

138. Johnson, Joan Marie: "Stillbirth—A Personal Experience," *Am. J. Nurs.,* **72**:1595, (Sept.) 1972.

139. Kron, Joan: "Learning to Live With Death," *Omega,* **5**:5, (Spring) 1974 (Reprinted from *Philadelphia Mag.,* Apr. 1973).

140. Mann, Sylvia A.: "Coping With a Child's Fatal Illness," *Nurs. Clin. North Am.,* **9**:81, (Mar.) 1974.

141. Maxwell, Sister Marie Bernadette: "A Terminally Ill Adolescent and Her Family," *Am. J. Nurs.,* **72**:925, (May) 1972.

141a. Wessel, Morris A.: *op. cit.*

142. Elliot, Thomas B.: "The Bereaved Family," *Ann. Am. Acad. Political Soc. Sci.,* **160**:184, 1932.

143. Marris, Peter: *Widows and Their Families.* Routledge and Kegan Paul, London, 1958.

144. Lapata, Helena Z.: *Widowhood in an American City.* Schenkman, Cambridge, Mass., 1973.

145. Bowlby, John: *Attachment and Loss.* Basic Books, New York, 1969, 3 vol.

146. Lindemann, Erich: "Symptomatology and Management of Acute Grief," *Am. J. Psychiatry,* **101**:141, (Sept.) 1944.

147. Maddison, David, and Walker, Wendy L.: "Factors Affecting the Outcome of Conjugal Bereavement," *Br. J. Psychiatry,* **113**:1057, 1967.

148. Hinton, John: *Dying,* 2nd ed. Penguin Books, Harmondsworth, Eng., 1972.

149. Glick, Ira O., et al.: *The First Year of Bereavement.* John Wiley & Sons, New York, 1974, p. 11.

150. Lewis, C. S.: *op. cit.*

151. Caine, Lynn: *Widow.* William Morrow & Co., Inc., New York, 1974.

152. Silverman, Phyllis R., et al.: *Helping Each Other in Widowhood.* Health Sciences Publishing Corp., New York, 1973.

153. Parkes, Colin Murray: *Bereavement; Studies of Grief in Adult Life.* International Universities Press, New York, 1972, pp. 5, 7, 16.

154. Fulton, Robert, and Fulton, Julie: "Anticipatory Grief: A Psychosocial Aspect of Terminal Care," in Schoenberg, Bernard, et al. (eds.): *Psychosocial Aspects of Terminal Care.* Columbia University Press, New York, 1972.

155. Parkes, Colin Murray: *op. cit.,* p. 152.

156. Gorer, Geoffrey: *Death, Grief and Mourning.* Doubleday & Co., Garden City, N.Y., 1965; Cresset Press, London, 1965.

157. Krup, George R., and Kligfeld, Bernard: "The Bereavement Reaction—A Cross-Cultural Evaluation," in Reeves, Robert B.,

Jr., et al. (comps. and eds.): *Pastoral Care of the Dying and Bereaved; Selected Readings.* Health Sciences Publishing Corp., New York, 1973.

158. Krup, George R., and Kligfeld, Bernard: op. cit., p. 3.
159. Lindemann, Erich: "Symptomatology and Management of Acute Grief," in Reeves, Robert B., Jr., et al. (comps. and eds.): *Pastoral Care of the Dying and Bereaved; Selected Readings.* Health Sciences Publishing Corp., New York, 1973.
160. Glick, Ira O., et al.: *op. cit.*
161. Torrie, M. (Mrs. Alfred): *Begin Again: A Book for Woman Alone.* J. M. Dent & Sons, Ltd., London, 1970.
162. Parkes, Colin Murray: *op. cit.,* p. 167.
163. *Facts Every Family Should Know.* Wilbert, Inc., Forest Park, Ill. (undated).
164. Parkes, Colin Murray: *op. cit.,* p. 153.
165. ———: *op. cit.,* p. 157.
166. Mead, Margaret: *Culture, Health, and Disease. Social and Cultural Influences on Health Programmes in Developing Countries.* J. B. Lippincott Co., Philadelphia, 1966.
167. Parkes, Colin Murray: *op. cit.,* p. 171.

Additional Suggested Reading

Abrams, Ruth: "Denial and Depression in the Terminal Cancer Patient," *Psychiatr. Q.,* **45:** 394, (No. 3) 1971.

Agee, James: *A Death in the Family.* Avon Books, New York, 1956.

American Medical Association, Task Force on Death: "Task Force on Death and Dying of the Institute of Society, Ethics, and the Life Sciences," *J.A.M.A.,* **221:**48, (July) 1972.

Arnold, J. D., et al.: "Public Attitudes and the Diagnosis of Death," *J.A.M.A.* **206:**1949, (Nov. 25) 1968.

Ayd, F. J.: "What Is Death?" *Med. Counter Point,* **1:**7, (Mar.) 1969.

Barton, D., et al.: "Death and Dying: A Course for Medical Students," *J. Med. Educ.,* **47:**945, (Dec.) 1972.

Beck, Frances: *The Diary of a Widow. Rebuilding a Family After the Funeral.* Beacon Press, Boston, 1966.

Benoliel, J. Q.: "Talking to Patients About Death," *Nurs. Forum,* **9:**254, 1970.

Bermann, Eric: *Scapegoat; The Impact of Death-Fear on an American Family.* University of Michigan Press, Ann Arbor, 1973.

Blewett, L. J.: "To Die at Home," *Am. J. Nurs.,* **70:**2063, (Dec.) 1970.

Boase, T. S. R.: *Death in the Middle Ages. Mortality, Judgment and Remembrance.* McGraw-Hill Book Co., New York, 1972.

Breuer, Paul H.: "Should the Patient Be Told the Truth?" in Skipper, James J., Jr., and Leonard, Robert C.: *Social Interaction and Patient Care.* J. B. Lippincott Co., Philadelphia, 1965.

Burnside, Irene Mortenson: "You Will Cope, of Course . . ." *Am. J. Nurs.,* **71:**2354, (Dec.) 1971.

Burton, Lindy: *Care of the Child Facing Death.* Routledge & Kegan, London, 1974.

Cancer Care, Inc.: *Catastrophic Illness in the Seventies. Proceedings of the Fourth National Symposium.* National Cancer Foundation, New York, 1971.

Carson, J.: "Learning from a Dying Patient," *Am. J. Nurs.,* **71:**333, (Feb.) 1971.

Choron, Jacques: *Death and Western Thought.* Crowell Collier & Macmillan, New York, 1963.

———: *Modern Man and Mortality.* Macmillan Publishing Co., Inc., New York, 1964.

Christopherson, L. K., and Lunde, D. T.: "Experiences with Heart Transplant Donors and Their Families," *Semin. Psychiatry,* **3:**(1), 1971.

Collins, V. J.: "The Right to Die; Limits of Medical Responsibility in Prolonging Life," *J. Am. Assoc. Nurse Anesth.,* **41:**27, (Feb.) 1973.

Cook, Sarah Sheets, et al.: *Children and Dying: An Exploration and a Selective Bibliography.* Health Sciences Publishing Corp., New York, 1973.

Crane, Diana: "Dying and Its Dilemmas as a Field of Research," in Brim, Orville G., Jr., et al. (eds.): *The Dying Patient.* Russell Sage Foundation, New York, 1970.

———: *The Sanctity of Social Life: Physicians' Treatment of Critically Ill Patients.* Russell Sage Foundation, New York, 1975.

Craytor, Josephine K., and Fass, Margot O.: *The Nurse and the Cancer Patient.* J. B. Lippincott Co., Philadelphia, 1970.

Dempsey, David: "Learning How To Die," *New York Times Mag.,* Nov. 14, 1971.

Dobihal, Edward F.: "Talk or Terminal Care?" *Conn. Med.,* **38:**364, (July) 1974.

Drummond, Eleanor E.: "Communication and Comfort for the Dying Patient," *Nurs. Clin. North Am.,* **5:**55, (Mar.) 1970.

Duff, Raymond S., and Hollingshead, August B.: *Sickness and Society.* Harper & Row, New York, 1968.

Dunlop, Hope E.: "Family and the Dying Patient," *Geriatric Nurs.,* **3:**15, (June) 1967.

Engel, George L.: "Grief and Grieving," in Browning, Mary H., and Lewis, Edith P.: *The Dying Patient: A Nursing Perspective.* American Journal of Nursing Co., New York, 1972.

Epstein, Charlotte: *Nursing the Dying Patient; Learning Processes for Interaction.* Reston Publishing Co., Reston, Va., 1975.

Folta, Jeannette R.: "Perception of Death," *Nurs. Res.,* **14:**234, (Summer) 1965.

Fox, S.: "The Death of a Child," *Nurs. Times,* **68:**1322, (Oct. 19) 1972.

Futterman, Edward H., et al.: "Parental Anticipatory Mourning," in Schoenberg, Bernard, et al. (eds.): *Psychosocial Aspects of Terminal Care.* Columbia University Press, New York, 1972.

George, Maureen McGrath: "Long-Term Care of the Patient with Cancer," *Nurs. Clin. North Am.,* **8:**623, (Dec.) 1973.

Gibson, Ronald: "Caring for the Bereaved," *Nurs. Mirror,* **139:**65, (Oct.) 1974.

Glaser, Barney G., and Strauss, Anselm: The Social Loss of Dying Patients," *Am. J. Nurs.,* **64:**
141, (June) 1964.

Golbally, B. P.: "Resuscitation and Euthanasia,"
Aust. Nurses J., **2:**26, (June) 1973.

Gordon, David Cole: *Overcoming the Fear of
Death.* Macmillan Publishing Co., Inc., New
York, 1970.

Gray, V. Ruth: "Dealing with Dying," *Nursing
'73,* **3:**26, (June) 1973.

Griffin, Jerry J.: "Family Decision," *Am. J. Nurs.,*
75:794, (May) 1975.

Grollman, Earl A.: *Concerning Death: A Practical Guide for the Living.* Beacon Press, Boston, 1974.

Group for the Advancement of Psychiatry: *The
Right to Die. Decision and Decision Makers.
Proceedings of a Symposium.* The Group, New
York, 1973.

Guimond, J.: "We Knew our Child Was Dying,"
Am. J. Nurs., **74:**248, (Feb.) 1974.

Gyulay, J. E.: "The Forgotten Grievers," *Am. J.
Nurs.,* **75:**1476, (Sept.) 1975.

Hammond, H. M.: "Psychotherapy with a Dying
Patient," *Voices: The Art & Science of Psychotherapy,* **8:**4, (Summer) 1972.

Henry, C.: "A Time to Live and a Time to Die,"
Nurs. Times, **67:**1016, (Aug. 19) 1971.

Hershey, Nathan: "On the Question of Prolonging Life," *Am. J. Nurs.,* **71:**521, (Mar.) 1971.

Hertzberg, Leonard J.: "Cancer and the Dying
Patient," *Am. J. Psychiatry,* **128:**806, (Jan.)
1972.

Hetzler, Florence: *Death and Creativity.* Health
Sciences Publishing Corp., New York, 1976.

Hoffman, Esther: "Don't Give Up on Me!" in
Browning, Mary H., and Lewis, Edith P.: *The
Dying Patient: A Nursing Perspective.* Ameri-
can Journal of Nursing Co., New York, 1972.

Hunt, Gladys: *The Christian Way of Death.* Zon-
dervan Publishing House, Grand Rapids, Mich.,
1971.

Jackson, Edgar N.: *Understanding Grief.* Ashley
Books, Port Washington, N.Y., 1957.

Johnson, A. G.: "The Right to Live or the Right
to Die?" *Nurs. Times,* **67:**573, (May 13) 1971.

Jung, Carl G., et al.: *The Meaning of Death.* Mc-
Graw-Hill Book Co., New York, 1959.

Kalish, R. A.: "Life and Death: Dividing the Indivisible," *Soc. Sci. Med.,* **2:**249, 1968.

Kastenbaum, Robert, and Aisenberg, Ruth: *The
Psychology of Death.* Springer Publishing Co.,
New York, 1972.

Kavanaugh, Robert E.: *Facing Death.* Nash Publishing Co., Los Angeles, 1972.

Kelly, Orville E., and Becker, W. R.: *Make Today
Count.* Delacorte Press, New York, 1975.

Kierkegaard, S.: *Fear and Trembling; The Sickness Unto Death.* Doubleday & Co., Garden
City, N.Y., 1954.

Kluge, Eike-Henner: *The Practice of Death.* Yale
University Press, New Haven, Conn., 1976.

Knight, Aldrich C.: "The Dying Patient's Grief,"
J.A.M.A., **184:**329, (May 4) 1963.

Knudson, Alfred G., et al.: "Participation of
Parents in the Hospital Care of Fatally Ill
Children," *Pediatrics,* **26:**482, (Sept.) 1960.

Kobrzycki, Paula: "Dying with Dignity at
Home," *Am. J. Nurs.,* **75:**1312, (Aug.) 1975.

Kron, Joan: "Learning to Live with Death,"
Omega, **5:**5, (Spring) 1974 (reported from
Philadelphia Magazine).

Kübler-Ross, Elizabeth: "Anger Before Death,"
Nursing '71, **1:**12, (Dec.) 1971.

————: *Death the Final Stage of Growth.* Prentice-Hall, Inc., Englewood Cliffs, N.J., 1975
(Human Development Series).

————: *On Death and Dying.* Macmillan Publishing Co., Inc., New York, 1969.

————: "The Right to Die with Dignity," *Bull.
Menninger Clin.,* **36:**302, (May) 1972.

Kutscher, Austin H.: *Caring for the Dying Patient and His Family.* Health Sciences Publishing Corp., New York, 1972.

————, et al. (eds.): *Psychopharmacologic Agents
in the Care of the Terminally Ill and the Bereaved.* Columbia University Press, New York.

————: *Religion and Bereavement; Council for
the Physician—Advice for the Bereaved;
Thoughts for the Clergyman.* Health Sciences
Publishing Corp., New York, 1972.

Kutscher, Austin H., Jr., and Kutscher, Austin H.:
*A Bibliography of Books on Death, Bereave-
ment, Loss, and Grief.* Health Sciences Publishing Corp., New York, 1969.

Labby, Daniel H. (ed.): *Life or Death; Ethics
and Options.* University of Washington Press,
Seattle, 1968.

Lamerton, Richard: *Care of the Dying.* Priory
Press, London, 1973.

————: "Ethical Questions in the Care of the
Dying," *Nurs. Mirror,* **139:**61, (Oct. 1) 1974.

Lamont, Corliss: *Humanist Funeral Service.*
American Humanist Association, San Francisco, Calif. (n.d.).

Lederer, Henry: "Notes on a Dying Professor,"
Nurs. Outlook, **20:**502, (Aug.) 1972.

LeShan, L., and LeShan, E.: "Psychotherapy in
the Patient with a Limited Life Span," *Psychiatry,* **24:**4, (Nov.) 1961.

Levinston, P.: "On Sudden Death," *Psychiatry,*
35:160, (May) 1972.

Lifton, Robert J.: *Death in Life. Survivors of
Hiroshima.* Simon & Schuster, New York, 1967.

Lloyd, J. W.: "The Role of Pain in Terminal
Care," *Nurs. Mirror,* **137:**36, (Aug. 24) 1973.

McNulty, B.: "The Problem of Pain in the
Dying Patient," *Queens Nurs. J.,* **16:**152, (Oct.)
1973.

McNulty, B. J.: "Domiciliary Care of the Dying
—Some Problems Encountered," *Nurs. Mirror,*
136:29, (May 18) 1973.

Maxwell, Sister Bernadette: "A Terminally Ill
Adolescent and Her Family. How Staff Mem-
bers Helped Them and Each Other," *Am. J.
Nurs.,* **72:**925, (May) 1972.

Mead, Margaret: "The Right to Die," *Nurs. Outlook,* **16:**22, (Oct.) 1968.

Mervyn, Frances: "The Plight of Dying Patients
in Hospitals," *Am. J. Nurs.,* **71:**1988, (Oct.)
1971.

Meyer, J. E.: *Death and Neurosis.* (Translated
by Margarete Nunberg.) International Universities Press, New York, 1975.

Miller, M. B.: "Decision-Making in the Death Process of the Ill Aged," *Geriatrics,* **26:**105, (May) 1971.

Mills, G. C., et al.: *Discussing Death: A Guide to Death Education.* Available from E. T. C. Publications, Homewood, Ill. (n.d.).

Montagu, Ashley: *Touching.* Harper & Row, New York, 1971.

Moody, Raymond A., Jr.: *Life After Death.* (With an introduction by Elisabeth Kübler-Ross.) Mockingbird Books, Atlanta, Ga., 1975.

Moustakas, Clark E.: *Loneliness.* Prentice-Hall, Inc., Englewood Cliffs, N.J., 1972.

Neale, Robert E.: *The Art of Dying.* Harper & Row, New York, 1975.

Noyes, Russell, Jr.: "The Experience of Dying," *Psychiatry,* **35:**183, (May) 1972.

Parkes, Colin Murray, and Brown, R. J.: "Health After Bereavement," *Psychosom. Med.,* **34:**449, (Sept.–Oct.) 1972.

Patterson, Robert D., et al.: "Psychiatric Aspects of Adaptation, Survival, and Death," in Granick, Samuel, and Patterson, Robert D. (eds.): *Human Aging II. An Eleven-Year Follow-up Biomedical and Behavioral Study.* US Government Printing Office, Washington, D.C., 1971 (DHEW Pub. No. [HMSO] 71–9037).

Piepgras, Ruth: "The Other Dimension: Spiritual Help," *Am. J. Nurs.,* **68:**2610, (Dec.) 1968.

Pine, Vanderlyn R.: *Caretaker of the Dead.* Halstead Press, New York, 1975.

Porter, J. V.: "A Therapeutic Community for Dying," *AORN J.,* **21:**838 (Apr.) 1975.

Rees, W. D., and Lutkins, S. G.: "Mortality of Bereavement," *Br. Med. J.,* **4:**13, (Oct. 7) 1967.

Saunders, Cicely: "The Last Stages of Life," *Am. J. Nurs.,* **65:**70, (Mar.) 1965.

———: "Watch with Me," *Nurs. Times,* Nov. 26, 1965, p. 1615.

Scientific Publications Section, Office of Public Information, National Institute of Child Health and Human Development: *Sudden Infant Death Syndrome; Selected Annotated Bibliography 1960–1971.* US Government Printing Office, Washington, D.C., 1972 (DHEW Pub. No. [NIH] 72–237).

Scott, Frances G., and Brewer, Ruth M. (eds., comps.): *Confrontation of Death; A Book of Readings and Suggested Method of Instruction.*

Continuing Education Publications, Corvallis, Ore., 1971.

Shillinglow, B.: "Caring for the Terminal Patient in Her Home," *Aust. Nurses J.,* **2:**24, (June) 1973.

Shneidman, Edwin: *Death: Current Perspectives.* Mayfield Publishing Co., 1975.

Shusterman, L. R.: "Death and Dying—A Critical Review of the Literature," *Nurs. Outlook,* **21:**465, (July) 1973.

Silverman, Phyllis R., et al.: *Helping Each Other in Widowhood.* Health Sciences Publishing Corp., New York, 1974.

Smith, JoAnn Kelley: *Free Fall.* Judson Press, Valley Forge, Pa., 1975.

Solnit, A. J., and Green, M.: "The Pediatric Management of the Dying Child, Part III: The Child's Reaction to the Fear of Dying," in Solnit, A. J., and Provence, S. A. (eds.): *Modern Perspectives in Child Development.* International Universities Press, New York, 1963.

Solzhenitsyn, Alexander: *Cancer Ward.* (Translated by Nicholas Bethell and David Burg.) Bantam Books, New York, 1968.

Spitzer, Stephan P., and Folta, Jeannette R.: "Death in the Hospital: A Problem for Study," *Nurs. Forum,* **3:**85, (No. 4) 1964.

Strauss, Anselm: *Anguish.* San Francisco Sociology Press, San Francisco, 1970.

Waechter, Eugenia H.: "Children's Awareness of Fatal Illness," *Am. J. Nurs.,* **71:**1168, (June) 1971.

Weber, L. J.: "Ethics and Euthanasia: Another View," *Am. J. Nurs.,* **73:**1228, (July) 1973.

Weissman, Avery D.: *The Psychological Autopsy.* Human Sciences Press, New York, 1972.

———: "On the Value of Denying Death," *Pastoral Psychology,* **23:**24, (June) 1972.

Weller, M. F.: "Bereavement," *Aust. Nurses J.,* **4:**5, (Aug.) 1975.

Wilson, J. B.: *Death by Decision.* Westminster Press, Philadelphia, 1975.

Yelverton, T.: "A Study in Terminal Care," *Nurs. Times,* **67:**293, (Mar. 11) 1971.

Zeligs, Rose: *Children's Experience with Death.* Charles C Thomas, Publisher, Springfield, Ill., 1974.

Florence S. Wald
Virginia Henderson

Appendixes

Appendixes

Special Enemas

Anthelmintic Enema. This is an injection of a solution containing a drug capable of destroying or expelling worms from the intestines. Pin, thread, or seat worms may be destroyed and expelled by repeated injections of an infusion of quassia, using 15 gm (½ oz) of chips to 600 ml (20 oz) of water. About 250 ml (½ pt) is the amount usually used, and the treatment is given daily until the worms are destroyed. Before the treatment is given, the bowel should be cleaned by a soap solution, so that the drug may come in direct contact with the worms and the lining of the intestines. Quassia is an astringent. It contracts the tissues and blood vessels, checks bleeding and inflammation, lessens the amount of mucus in which the worms may lodge, shrivels and destroys the worms. The patient should be encouraged to retain the solution for 15 to 30 minutes.

Astringent Enema. Usually alum, 60 gm (2 oz) dissolved in 1000 ml (2 pt) of hot water. The enema is not to be retained.

Other *astringents*, such as tannic acid 2 gm in 500 ml of water (30 gr in 1 pt), are sometimes used to destroy worms, or microorganisms in dysentery or cholera, and to relieve inflammation. They are usually given in the form of rectal or colonic irrigations. The solution is allowed to run in very slowly and gently and to return immediately in order to avoid distention, pain, and irritation of the inflamed wall.

Carminative Enemas. Given to prevent or relieve distention, a carminative enema is an injection into the rectum of a solution containing drugs that have a carminative action. Such drugs by their antiseptic action prevent the formation of gases and by their irritant action on nerve endings in the lining of the intestines cause the contraction of their muscular walls (reflex action) and expulsion of the gas causing the distention. Turpentine, asafetida, and alum are the drugs commonly used as in the following: (1) *Turpentine.* From 8 to 16 gm (2 to 4 drams) of turpentine may be added to 1000 ml (2 pt) of soap solution. The turpentine must be thoroughly mixed and dissolved. This enema is not to be retained. *Milk and Molasses.* To prepare the enema, according to the amount ordered, heat from 96 to 256 ml (3 to 8 oz) of milk. To this add slowly an equal amount of molasses, stirring it in well and heating to 71.1°C (160°F) to mix thoroughly. The temperature of the solution when given should be from 38° to 40°C (100.4° to 104°F). The carminative action is due to the fact that the sugar in molasses is irritating to the lining of the intestines and the sugar and milk together produce gas that distends the intestines and causes pressure, peristalsis, and defecation.

Rectal injections for a carminative effect are usually given as hot as the patient can stand (43°C or 109.4°F), the heat being a powerful stimulus to peristalsis and expulsion of gas. The injections should be given slowly, and when small amounts are used, the patient should be encouraged to retain the enema for 10 to 30 minutes, or as long as possible. As the treatment is given for the relief of distention, note and record the amount of flatus expelled— little, moderate, or large.

Emollient Enema. This is an injection of some bland solution for the purpose of checking diarrhea or soothing and relieving irritation of an inflamed mucous membrane. Starch is commonly used. To prepare the solution, dissolve 4 gm (1 dram) of starch in a little cold water making a smooth paste. Then add slowly 192 ml (6 oz) of boiling water, stirring constantly. Allow the solution to cool to 40°C (104°F) and give with a catheter. The enema is to be retained. Laudanum (tincture of opium) is sometimes added to a starch enema to check secretions and peristalsis and to relieve pain and local irritation in diarrhea. When ordered, laudanum should be added just before the enema is given. Be sure that the full amount ordered is given. To ensure this, sometimes the drug is added to a small portion of the starch solution. After this is injected, the remaining solution is given.

Oil Enema. Before a soapsuds enema is given, an injection of oil is sometimes necessary to soften hard feces. Oil enemas are also frequently given before the first bowel movement after operations on the rectum or perineum, such as a hemorrhoidectomy or a perineorrhaphy, to avoid straining and injury to the wound. The enema may consist of 192 ml (6 oz) of olive oil, or to this may be added 64 ml (2 oz) each of castor oil and glycerin, to increase the softening effect. The oil is prepared by warming it to a temperature of 38°C (100.4°F). An oil enema should be retained. It may be followed in 1 hour by a soapsuds enema or it may be retained from 2 to 6 hours before the cleansing enema is given.

Purgative Enemas. In obstinate constipation rectal injections of cathartics may be necessary to hasten evacuation. The cathartics commonly used are glycerin, *fel bovis*, or ox gall, Rochelle and Epsom salts (magnesium sulfate). Glycerin and ox gall both act as softening agents on fecal masses and by their irritating effect on the mucous lining stimulate peristalsis and evacuation. The amount ordered, usually from 8 to 16 ml (2 to 4 drams) of glycerin or ox gall, may be added to a soapsuds enema or may be given in a small amount of warm water or normal saline solution and followed in 1 hour by a soapsuds enema. A small enema consisting of 96 ml (3 oz) each of glycerin and soapsuds thoroughly mixed is sometimes used; this is to be expelled. *Compound Medicated.* Turpentine 16 ml (4 drams), asafetida 8 gm (2 drams), ox gall 16 gm (4 drams), glycerin 128 ml (4 oz) with 1000 ml (2 pt) of soapsuds. To prepare the enema, first mix the ox gall, if in crystals, with the turpentine, otherwise it will not dissolve. Also see that the utensils used are dry. Add the other ingredients and thoroughly mix with the soapsuds. The temperature of the solution when given should be 43°C (109.4°F).

Saline Enemas. Rochelle and Epsom salts may be given in a dilute or concentrated form. From 120 to 180 gm (4 to 6 oz) of Rochelle salts or from 15 to 120 gm (½ to 4 oz) of magnesium sulfate are the usual amounts prescribed for rectal injections. To prepare the solution, the amount ordered is added to sufficient hot water to dissolve the salts thoroughly. An enema (commonly called a 1.2.3 enema), consisting of magnesium sulfate 30 gm (1 oz), glycerin 64 ml (2 oz), and hot water 96 ml (3 oz), is frequently used. When given in this form, the concentration of salts in the intestines is greater than that in the blood and tissues. Fluid is therefore drawn from the blood and tissues by osmosis. The resulting accumulation of fluid in the intestines induces peristalsis and evacuation.

The saline cathartics are sometimes given in dilute form by adding the amount ordered, first thoroughly dissolved in hot water, to a tap-water enema. When given in this dilute form, the concentration of salts in the intestines is less than that in the blood and tissues; the salts are not absorbed but they prevent the absorption of the water. The intestines are therefore distended with fluid, inducing peristalsis, and evacuation.

Rectal injections of the saline cathartics are thought by some of value in nephritis and cardiac conditions when there is an accumulation of fluid in the tissues (edema).

APPENDIX II

Weights and Measures

Tables of Equivalents

Dry Measure

Metric		Apothecaries'		Household
16.0	grams	4 drams		1 tablespoonful
8.0	grams	2 drams		1 dessertspoonful
4.0	grams	1 dram		1 teaspoonful
2.0	grams	½ dram		½ teaspoonful
1.0	gram	15	grains	
0.6	gram	10	grains	
0.3	gram	5	grains	
0.2	gram	3	grains	
0.1	gram	1½	grains	
0.06	gram	1	grain	
0.03	gram	1/2	grain	
0.015	gram	1/4	grain	
0.008	gram	1/8	grain	
0.004	gram	1/16	grain	
0.0032	gram	1/20	grain	
0.0027	gram	1/25	grain	
0.0022	gram	1/30	grain	
0.0016	gram	1/40	grain	
0.0013	gram	1/50	grain	
0.0011	gram	1/60	grain	
0.001	gram	1/64	grain	
0.0006	gram	1/100	grain	
0.0005	gram	1/120	grain	
0.0004	gram	1/150	grain	
0.0003	gram	1/200	grain	

Fluid Measure

Metric	Apothecaries'	Household
1.0 ml (cc)	15 minims	¼ teaspoonful
4.0 ml (cc)	1 fluid dram	1 teaspoonful
32 ml (cc)	1 fluid ounce	2 tablespoonfuls
500 ml (cc)	1 pint	2 8-oz glassfuls
1000 ml (cc)	1 quart	

Units of Length *

English System	Metric System
	10 millimeters = 1 centimeter
12 inches = 1 foot	10 centimeters = 1 decimeter
3 feet = 1 yard	10 decimeters = 1 meter
5½ yards = 1 rod	10 meters = 1 decameter
1,760 yards = 1 mile	10 decameters = 1 hectometer
5,280 feet = 1 mile	10 hectometers = 1 kilometer
	10 kilometers = 1 myriameter

Tables of Equivalents (continued)

Units of Mass *

English System		Metric System	
Troy Units		10 milligrams	= 1 centigram
24 grains	= 1 pennyweight	10 centigrams	= 1 decigram
20 pennyweights	= 1 ounce	10 decigrams	= 1 gram
12 ounces	= 1 pound	10 grams	= 1 decagram
Avoirdupois Units		10 decagrams	= 1 hectogram
27.34 grains	= 1 dram	10 hectograms	= 1 kilogram
16 drams	= 1 ounce	1,000 kilograms	= 1 metric ton
16 ounces	= 1 pound		
25 pounds	= 1 quarter		
4 quarters	= 1 hundredweight		
20 hundredweight	= 1 short ton		
2,240 pounds	= 1 long ton		
Apothecaries' Units			
20 grains	= 1 scruple		
3 scruples	= 1 dram		
8 drams	= 1 ounce		
12 ounces	= 1 pound		

Approximate Equivalents Used in Converting Dosage *

1 grain	= 60 to 64 milligrams
15 grains	= 1 gram
1 minim	= 0.06 milliliter
15 or 16 minims	= 1 milliliter
1 dram	= 4 grams
1 fluid dram	= 4 milliliters
1 ounce	= 30 grams
1 fluid ounce	= 30 milliliters

Useful Equivalents *

Length
Centimeter 0.032808 foot = 0.3937 inch = 0.01 meter
Foot 12 inches = 0.3048 meter
Inch $\frac{1}{12}$ foot = $\frac{1}{36}$ yard = 25.40005 millimeters
Meter 39.37 inches = 1.093611 yards = 3.290833 feet
Micron 39.37 millionths of an inch
Millimeter 0.03937 inch = 0.001 meter
Yard 3 feet = 36 inches = 0.91440183 meter

Weight
Kilogram 2.2046223 pounds = 1,000 grams
Milligram 0.0000352739 ounce = 0.001 gram
Pound 16 ounces = 453.5924 grams

Volume
Gallon 4 quarts = 8 pints = 3.7853 liters
Liter 1.056710 quarts = 0.035316 cubic foot = 1,000 milliliters
Milliliter 0.001 liter = 1 milliliter
Pint (liquid) $\frac{1}{2}$ quart = 16 fluid ounces = 0.473167 liter
Quart (liquid) 2 pints = 32 fluid ounces = 0.946333 liter

* From Flitter, Hessel Howard: *An Introduction to Physics in Nursing*, 6th ed. C. V. Mosby Co., St. Louis, 1972, pp. 8, 11.

Table for Solutions

Prescribed Strength	Amount of Crude Drug	Fluid to Be Added
1:1000	1 teaspoonful	to 1 gallon
1:1000	15 drops	to 1 quart
1/10 of 1%	15 drops	to 1 quart
1:500	2 teaspoonfuls	to 1 gallon
1:500 ⎫	30 drops	to 1 quart
1/5 of 1% ⎭	30 drops	to 1 quart
1:200	5 teaspoonfuls	to 1 gallon
1:200 ⎫	1¼ teaspoonfuls	to 1 quart
½ of 1% ⎭	1¼ teaspoonfuls	to 1 quart
1:100 (1%)	2½ teaspoonfuls	to 1 quart
1:50 (2%)	5 teaspoonfuls	to 1 quart
1:25 (4%)	2½ tablespoonfuls	to 1 quart
1:20 (5%)	3 tablespoonfuls	to 1 quart

Alphabetized List of Measurements and How to Convert Them *

Multiply Number of	By	To Get
British thermal units	0.2520	Kilograms-calories
British thermal units	777.5	Foot-lb
Centigrams	0.01	Grams
Centiliters	0.01	Liters
Centimeters	0.3937	Inches
Centimeters	0.01	Meters
Centimeters	10.00	Millimeters
Centimeters of mercury	0.01316	Atmospheres
Centimeters of mercury	27.85	Lb./sq. ft.
Centimeters of mercury	0.1934	Lb./sq. inch
Cubic centimeters	3.531×10^{-5}	Cubic feet
Cubic centimeters	6.102×10^{-2}	Cubic inches
Cubic centimeters	10^{-6}	Cubic meters
Cubic centimeters	2.642×10^{-4}	Gallons
Cubic centimeters	10^{-3}	Liters
Cubic centimeters	2.113×10^{-3}	Pints (liq.)
Cubic centimeters	1.057×10^{-3}	Quarts (liq.)
Cubic feet	2.832×10^{4}	Cubic cm.
Cubic feet	1728	Cubic inches
Cubic feet	0.02832	Cubic meters
Cubic feet	0.03704	Cubic yards
Cubic feet	7.48052	Gallons
Cubic feet	28.32	Liters
Cubic feet	59.84	Pints (liq.)
Cubic feet	29.92	Quarts (liq.)
Cubic inches	2.143×10^{-5}	Cubic yards
Cubic inches	4.329×10^{-3}	Gallons
Cubic inches	1.639×10^{-2}	Liters
Cubic inches	0.03463	Pints (liq.)
Cubic inches	0.01732	Quarts (liq.)
Cubic meters	10^{6}	Cubic centimeters
Cubic meters	35.31	Cubic feet
Decigrams	0.1	Grams
Deciliters	0.1	Liters
Decimeters	0.1	Meters
Dekagrams	10	Grams
Dekaliters	10	Liters
Drams	27.34375	Grains
Drams	0.0625	Ounces
Drams	1.771845	Grams
Feet	30.48	Centimeters
Feet	12	Inches
Feet	0.3048	Meters

Alphabetized List of Measurements and How to Convert Them *

Multiply Number of	By	To Get
Feet	1/3	Yards
Gallons	3785	Cubic centimeters
Gallons	0.1337	Cubic feet
Gallons	231	Cubic inches
Gallons	3.785×10^{-3}	Cubic meters
Gallons	3.785	Liters
Gallons	8	Pints (liq.)
Gallons	4	Quarts (liq.)
Grains (troy)	0.06480	Grams
Grains (troy)	2.0833×10^{-3}	Ounces (troy)
Grams	15.43	Grains
Grams	10^{-3}	Kilograms
Grams	10^{3}	Milligrams
Grams	0.03527	Ounces
Grams	0.03215	Ounces (troy)
Grams	2.205×10^{-3}	Pounds
Hectograms	100	Grams
Hectoliters	100	Liters
Hectometers	100	Meters
Hectowatts	100	Watts
Inches	2.540	Centimeters
Inches of mercury	0.03342	Atmospheres
Inches of mercury	1.133	Feet of water
Inches of mercury	70.73	Lb./sq. ft.
Inches of mercury	0.4912	Lb./sq. inch
Inches of water	0.002458	Atmospheres
Inches of water	0.07355	Inches of mercury
Inches of water	25.40	Kg./sq. meter
Inches of water	0.5781	Ounces/sq. inch
Inches of water	5.202	Lb./sq. ft.
Inches of water	0.03613	Lb./sq. inch
Kilograms	2.205	Pounds
Kilograms	10^{3}	Grams
Kiloliters	10^{3}	Liters
Kilometers	10^{5}	Centimeters
Kilometers	3281	Feet
Kilometers	10^{3}	Meters
Kilometers	0.6214	Miles
Kilometers	1094	Yards
Kilowatts	56.92	B.T.U./min.
Kilowatts	1.341	Horsepower
Kilowatts	10^{3}	Watts
Kilowatts-hours	3415	B.T.U.
Liters	10^{3}	Cubic centimeters
Liters	0.03531	Cubic feet
Meters	100	Centimeters
Meters	3.281	Feet
Meters	39.37	Inches
Meters	10^{-3}	Kilometers
Microns	10^{-6}	Meters
Miles	1.609	Kilometers
Milligrams	10^{-3}	Grams
Milliliters	10^{-3}	Liters
Millimeters	0.1	Centimeters
Millimeters	0.03937	Inches
Ounces	16	Drams
Ounces	437.5	Grains
Ounces	0.0625	Pounds
Ounces	28.349527	Grams
Ounces	0.9115	Ounces (troy)
Ounces	2.790×10^{-5}	Tons (long)
Ounces	2.835×10^{-5}	Tons (metric)

Alphabetized List of Measurements and How to Convert Them *

Multiply Number of	By	To Get
Ounces (troy)	480	Grains
Ounces (troy)	20	Pennyweights (troy)
Ounces (troy)	0.08333	Pounds (troy)
Ounces (troy)	31.103481	Grams
Ounces (troy)	1.09714	Ounces (avoir.)
Ounces (fluid)	1.805	Cubic inches
Ounces (fluid)	0.02957	Liters
Pennyweights (troy)	24	Grains
Pennyweights (troy)	1.55517	Grams
Pennyweights (troy)	0.05	Ounces (troy)
Pennyweights (troy)	4.1667×10^{-3}	Pounds (troy)
Pounds	16	Ounces
Pounds	256	Drams
Pounds	7000	Grains
Pounds	453.5924	Grams
Pounds	1.21528	Pounds (troy)
Pounds	14.5833	Ounces (troy)
Pounds (troy)	5760	Grains
Pounds (troy)	12	Ounces (troy)
Pounds (troy)	373.24177	Grams
Pounds (troy)	0.822857	Pounds (avoir.)
Pounds (troy)	13.1657	Ounces (avoir.)
Quarts (dry)	67.20	Cubic inches
Quarts (liq.)	57.75	Cubic inches
Square centimeters	0.1550	Square inches
Square centimeters	10^{-4}	Square meters
Square centimeters	100	Square millimeters
Square feet	929.0	Square centimeters
Square feet	144	Square inches
Square inches	6.452	Square centimeters
Square inches	6.944×10^{-3}	Square feet
Square inches	645.2	Square millimeters
Square millimeters	0.01	Square centimeters
Square millimeters	1.550×10^{-3}	Square inches
Temperature (°C) + 273	1	Abs. temp. (°C)
Temperature (°C) + 17.78	1.8	Temp. (°F)
Temperature (°F) + 460	1	Abs. temp. (°F)
Temperature (°F) − 32	5/9	Temp. (°C)
Watts	0.05692	B.T.U./min.
Yards	91.44	Centimeters
Yards	3	Feet
Yards	36	Inches
Yards	0.9144	Meters

* Adapted from *Carr Lane Handy Multipliers and Trigonometry Tables for Engineers.* Carr Lane Manufacturing Co., St. Louis, Mo., 1971.

Note: For comprehensive information on conversion of measurements see Hodgman, Charles D. (ed.): *Handbook of Chemistry and Physics,* 34th ed. Chemical Rubber Publishing Co., Cleveland, Ohio, 1952.

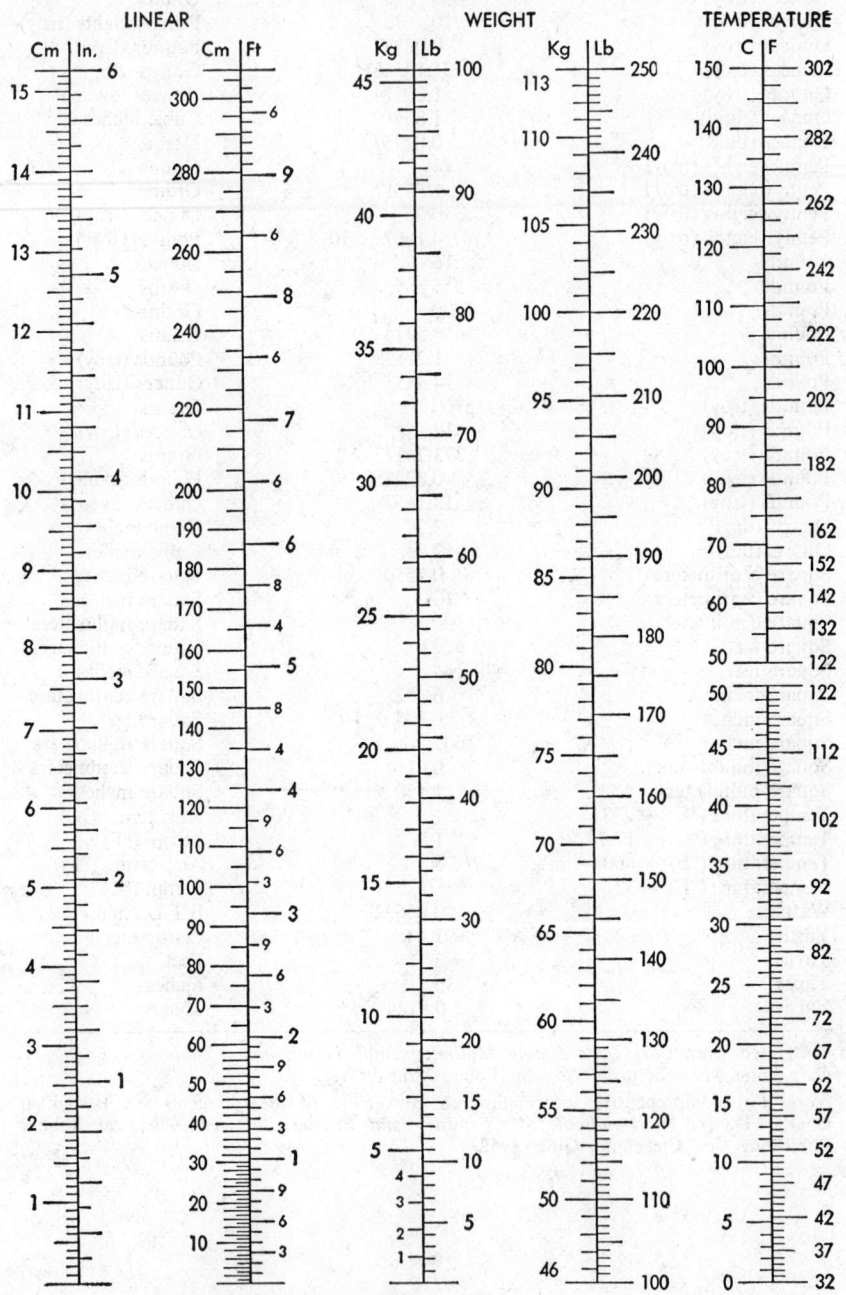

Comparative scales of measures, weights, and temperatures.
2.5 cm = 1 in.   2.2 kg = 1 lb

To convert centigrade to Fahrenheit,
multiply by 9/5 and add 32

To convert Fahrenheit to centigrade
subtract 32 and multiply by 5/9

APPENDIX III

Abbreviations and Symbols

Abbreviation	Derivation	Meaning
Preparations of Drugs		
Aq.	aqua	water
aq. dest.	aqua destillata	distilled water
Comp.	compositum	compound
Conf.	confectio	confection
D.	detur	give
Dil.	dilutus	dilute
Empl.	emplastrum	plaster
et	et	and
Fl.	fluidum	fluid
Inf.	infusum	infusion
Lin.	linimentum	liniment
Liq.	liquor	liquid
Lot.	lotio	lotion
Mist.	mistura	mixture
N.N.R.		new and nonofficial remedy
Ol.	oleum	oil
Pil.	pilula	pill
Pulv.	pulvis	a powder
S. fr.	spiritus frumenti	whisky
Sp.	spiritus	spirit
S. v. r.	spiritus vini rectificatus	alcohol
S. v. g.	spiritus vini gallici	brandy
Syr.	syrupus	syrup
Tinct.	tinctura	tincture
Troch.	trochiscum	lozenge
Ung.	unguentum	ointment
Vin.	vinum	wine

Prefixes and Symbols Approved for Use with SI Units * by the General Council on Weights and Measures for Metric Units †

Prefix	Symbol	Power	Value
Tera	T	10^{12}	1,000,000,000,000
Giga	G	10^{9}	1,000,000,000
Mega	M	10^{6}	1,000,000
Kilo	k	10^{3}	1,000
Hecto	h	10^{2}	100
Deca	da	10^{1}	10
Deci	d	10^{-1}	.1
Centi	c	10^{-2}	.01
Milli	m	10^{-3}	.001
Micro	μ	10^{-6}	.000001
Nano	n	10^{-9}	.000000001
Pico	p	10^{-12}	.000000000001
Femto	f	10^{-15}	.000000000000001
Atto	a	10^{-18}	.000000000000000001

* International System of Units, abbreviated to SI Units.
† From Flitter, Hessel Howard: *An Introduction to Physics in Nursing,* 6th ed. C. V. Mosby Co., St. Louis, 1972, p. 9.

Time of Administration

Abbreviation	Derivation	Meaning
A.c.	ante cibum	before meals
Alt. die.	alternis diebus	alternate days
Alt. hor.	alternis horis	alternate hours
Alt. noct.	alternis noctes	alternate nights
A.M.	ante meridiem	morning
B.i.d.	bis in die	twice a day
H.	hora	hour
H.d.	hora decubitus	at bedtime
H.s.	hora somni	at sleeping time
M. et N.	mane et nocte	morning and night
O.d.	omni die	daily
O.m.	omni mane	each morning
O.n.	omni nocte	each night
P.c.	post cibum	after meals
P.M.	post meridiem	afternoon
P.r.n.	pro re nata	when required
Q.h.	quaque hora	every hour
Q.2 h., Q.3 h. Q.4 h.		every two, three, or four hours
Q.i.d. or 4 i.d.	quater in die	four times a day
Stat.	statim	at once
T.i.d.	ter in die	three times a day

Hours of Administration

4 i.d.	8 A.M., 12 N., 4 P.M., 8 P.M.
Q.2 h.	6, 8, 10, 12, etc.
Q.3 h.	9, 12, 3, 6, etc.
Q.4 h.	8, 12, 4, etc.
Q.6 h.	6, 12, etc.
B.i.d.	10 A.M., 4 P.M.
T.i.d.	10 A.M., 3 P.M., and 6 P.M.
A.c.	½ hour before meals—6:30 A.M., 12:30 P.M., 4:30 P.M.
P.c.	8 A.M., 2 P.M., 6 P.M.
O.d.	10 A.M.
O.m.	6 A.M.
O.n.	8 P.M.

Dosage and Application

Abbreviation	Derivation	Meaning
āā	ana	of each
Add.	adde	add to
Add. part. dol.	adde partem dolente	to the painful part
ad. lib.	ad libitum	as much as desired
C.	congius	gallon
C	Celsius	Celsius, or centigrade
c̄	cum	with
cc	cubic centimeter	cubic centimeter
Cap.	capiat	let him take
cm	centimeter	one hundredth of a meter
Contin.	continuatur	let it be continued
Dim.	dimidius	one half
D. in p. aeq.	dividatur in partes aequales	divide in equal parts
Div.	dividatus	divide
Dur. dolor.	durante dolore	while the pain lasts
F	Fahrenheit	Fahrenheit
Ft.	fiat	let it or them be made
ft	foot	foot, feet
gal	gallon	gallon, gallons
gm	gram	gram, grams
gr	granum, grana	grain, grains
gtt	gutta	drop, drops
Garg.	gargarisma	gargle
Kcal	kilocalorie,	a thousand calories
kg	kilogram	thousand grams
L.	liter	liter
lb	libra	pound
M.	misce	mix
m.	minimus	minim
mcg	microgram	one millionth of a gram
mg	milligram	one thousandth of a gram
ml	milliliter	one thousandth of a liter
mm	millimeter	one thousandth of a meter
N.b.	nota bene	note well
No.	numero	number
O	octarius	pint
oz	uncia	ounce
Part. vic.	partibus vicibus	in divided doses
pt	pint	pint, pints
Q.s.	quantum sufficit	as much as is sufficient
qt	quart	quart, quarts
℞	recipe	take
s̄	sine	without
S. or Sig.	signa	give the following directions
S.o.s.	si opus sit	if necessary
Ss	semi	one half
tsp	teaspoon	teaspoonful
tbsp	tablespoon	tablespoonful
ʒ	drachma	dram
℥	uncia	ounce
℈	scrupulum	scruple

Tables of Normal Values*

Many of the normal values in this table, according to Davidsohn and Henry, are based on the experience in the Department of Pathology, Mount Sinai Hospital, Chicago, Illinois, and the Division of Clinical Pathology, State University Hospital, State University of New York, Syracuse, New York. Actual values may vary with different techniques or in different laboratories. Appropriate chapters in Davidsohn and Henry should be reviewed for further details on age and other variables that may yield different values.

Abbreviations Used in Tables

<	= less than	mI.U.	= milliInternational Unit
>	= greater than	mOsm.	= milliosmole
dl.	= 100 ml.	mμ	= millimicron
gm.	= gram	ng.	= nanogram
I.U.	= International Unit	pg.	= picogram
kg.	= kilogram	μEq.	= microequivalent
mEq.	= milliequivalent	μg.	= microgram
mg.	= milligram	μI.U.	= microInternational Unit
ml.	= milliliter	μl.	= microliter
mM.	= millimole	μU.	= microunit
mm. Hg	= millimeters of mercury		

Whole Blood, Serum, and Plasma (Chemistry)

Test	Material	Normal Value	Special Instructions
Acetoacetic acid, qualitative	Serum	Negative	
quantitative	Serum	0.2–1.0 mg./dl.	
Acetone, qualitative	Serum	Negative	
quantitative	Serum	0.3–2.0 mg./dl.	
Albumin, quantitative	Serum	3.2–4.5 gm./dl. (salt fractionation) 3.2–5.6 gm./dl. by electrophoresis 3.8–5.0 gm./dl. by dye binding	
Alcohol	Serum or whole blood	Negative	
Aldolase	Serum	Adults: 3–8 Sibley-Lehninger U/dl. at 37°C. Children: Approximately 2 times adult levels Newborn: Approximately 4 times adult levels	
Alpha-amino acid nitrogen	Serum	3–6 mg./dl.	
δ-Aminolevulinic acid	Serum	0.01–0.03 mg./dl.	
Ammonia	Plasma	20–150 μg./dl. (diffusion) 40–80 μg./dl. (enzymatic method) 12–48 μg./dl. (resin method)	Collect with sodium heparinate; specimen must be analyzed immediately
Amylase	Serum	60–160 Somogyi units/dl.	
Argininosuccinic lyase	Serum	0–4 U./dl.	

* From Davidsohn, Israel, and Henry, John H. (eds.): *Todd-Sanford Clinical Diagnosis by Laboratory Methods*, 15th ed. W. B. Saunders Co., Philadelphia, 1974, pp. 1376–92.

Whole Blood, Serum, and Plasma (Chemistry) (continued)

Test	Material	Normal Value	Special Instructions
Arsenic	Whole blood	<3 µg./dl.	
Ascorbic acid (vitamin C)	Plasma Whole blood	0.6–1.6 mg./dl. 0.7–2.0 mg./dl.	Analyze immediately
Barbiturates	Serum, plasma, or whole blood	Negative	
Base excess	Whole blood	Male: −3.3 to +1.2 Female: −2.4 to +2.3	
Base, total	Serum	145–160 mEq./L.	
Bicarbonate	Plasma	21–28 mM./L.	
Bile acids	Serum	0.3–3.0 mg./dl.	
Bilirubin	Serum	Up to 0.3 mg./dl. (direct or conjugated) 0.1–1.0 mg./dl. (indirect or unconjugated) Total: 0.1–1.2 mg./dl. Newborns total: 1–12 mg./dl.	
Blood gases pH pCO_2 pO_2		7.38–7.44 arterial 7.36–7.41 venous 35–40 mm. Hg arterial 40–45 mm. Hg venous 95–100 mm. Hg arterial	
Bromide	Serum	0–5 mg./dl.	
BSP (bromsulfonphthalein) (5 mg./kg.)	Serum	$<6\%$ retention after 45 min.	
Calcium	Serum	Ionized: 4.2–5.2 mg./dl 2.1–2.6 mEq./L. or 50–58% of total Total: 9.0–10.6 mg./dl. 4.5–5.3 mEq./L. Infants: 11–13 mg./dl.	
Carbon dioxide (CO_2 content)	Whole blood, arterial	19–24 mM./L.	
	Plasma or serum, arterial	21–28 mM./L.	
	Whole blood, venous	22–26 mM./L.	
	Plasma or serum, venous	24–30 mM./L.	
CO_2 combining power	Plasma or serum, venous	24–30 m.M./L.	
CO_2 partial pressure (pCO_2)	Whole blood, arterial	35–40 mm. Hg	
	Whole blood, venous	40–45 mm. Hg	
Carbonic acid	Whole blood, arterial	1.05–1.45 mM./L.	
	Whole blood, venous	1.15–1.50 mM./L.	
	Plasma, venous	1.02–1.38 mM./L.	
Carboxyhemoglobin (carbon monoxide hemoglobin)	Whole blood	Suburban nonsmokers: $<1.5\%$ saturation of hemoglobin Smokers: 1.5–5.0% saturation Heavy smokers: 5.0–9.0% saturation	

Whole Blood, Serum, and Plasma (Chemistry) (continued)

Test	Material	Normal Value	Special Instructions
Carotene, beta	Serum	40–200 μg./dl.	
Cephalin cholesterol flocculation	Serum	Negative to 1+ after 24 hours 2+ or less after 48 hours	
Ceruloplasmin	Serum	23–50 mg./dl.	
Chloride	Serum	95–103 mEq./L.	
Cholesterol, total	Serum	150–250 mg./dl. (varies with diet and age)	
Cholesterol, esters	Serum	65–75% of total cholesterol	
Cholinesterase Pseudocholinesterase	Erythrocytes Plasma	0.65–1.00 pH units 0.5–1.3 pH units 8–18 I.U./L. at 37°C.	
Citric acid	Serum or plasma	1.7–3.0 mg./dl.	
Congo red test	Serum or plasma	>60% after 1 hour	Severe reactions may occur if dye is injected twice; check patient's record
Copper	Serum or plasma	Male: 70–140 μg./dl. Female: 85–155 μg./dl.	
Cortisol	Plasma	8 A.M.–10 A.M.: 5–25 μg./dl. 4 P.M.–6 P.M.: 2–18 μg./dl.	
Creatine	Serum or plasma	Males: 0.2–0.6 mg./dl. Females: 0.6–1.0 mg./dl.	
Creatine phosphokinase (CPK)	Serum	Males: 55–170 U./L. at 37°C. Females: 30–135 U./L. at 37°C.	
Creatinine	Serum or plasma	0.6–1.2 mg./dl.	
Creatinine clearance (endogenous)	Serum or plasma and urine	Male: 123 ± 16 ml./min. Female: 97 ± 10 ml./min.	
Cryoglobulins	Serum	Negative	Keep specimen at 37°C.
Electrophoresis, protein	Serum	<table><tr><td></td><td>per cent</td><td>gm./dl.</td></tr><tr><td>Albumin</td><td>52–65</td><td>3.2–5.6</td></tr><tr><td>Alpha-1</td><td>2.5–5.0</td><td>0.1–0.4</td></tr><tr><td>Alpha-2</td><td>7.0–13.0</td><td>0.4–1.2</td></tr><tr><td>Beta</td><td>8.0–14.0</td><td>0.5–1.1</td></tr><tr><td>Gamma</td><td>12.0–22.0</td><td>0.5–1.6</td></tr></table>	
Fats, neutral	Serum or plasma	0–200 mg./dl.	
Fatty acids, total free	Serum Plasma	9–15 mM./L. 300–480 μEq./L.	
Fibrinogen	Plasma	200–400 mg./dl.	
Fluoride	Whole blood	<0.05 mg./dl.	
Folate	Serum Erythrocytes	5–25 ng./ml. (bioassay) 166–640 ng./ml. (bioassay)	
Galactose	Whole blood	Adults: none Children: < 20 mg./dl.	
Gamma globulin	Serum	0.5–1.6 gm./dl.	

Whole Blood, Serum, and Plasma (Chemistry) (continued)

Test	Material	Normal Value	Special Instructions
Globulins, total	Serum	2.3–3.5 gm./dl.	
Glucose, fasting	Serum or plasma Whole blood	70–110 mg./dl. 60–100 mg./dl.	Collect with heparin-fluoride mixture
Glucose tolerance, oral	Serum or plasma	Fasting: 70–110 mg./dl. 30 min.: 30–60 mg./dl. above fasting 60 min.: 20–50 mg./dl. above fasting 120 min.: 5–15 mg./dl. above fasting 180 min.: fasting level or below	Collect with heparin-fluoride mixture
Glucose tolerance, IV	Serum or plasma	Fasting: 70–110 mg./dl. 5 min:. Maximum of 250 mg./dl. 60 min.: Significant decrease 120 min.: Below 120 mg./dl. 180 min.: Fasting level	Collect with heparin-fluoride mixture
Glucose-6-phosphate dehydrogenase (G-6-PD)	Erythrocytes	250–500 units/10^9 cells 1200–2000 mI.U./ml. of packed erythrocytes	
γ-Glutamyl transpeptidase	Serum	2–39 U./L.	
Glutathione	Whole blood	24–37 mg./dl.	
Growth hormone	Serum	<10 ng./ml.	
Guanase	Serum	<3nM./ml./min.	
Haptoglobin	Serum	100–200 mg./dl. as hemoglobin binding capacity	
Hemoglobin	Serum or plasma	Qualitative: Negative Quantitative: 0.5–5.0 mg./dl.	
Hemoglobin	Whole blood	Female: 12.0–16.0 gm./dl. Male: 13.5–18.0 gm./dl.	
Hemoglobin A₂	Whole blood	1.5–3.5% of total hemoglobin	
α-Hydroxybutyric dehydrogenase	Serum	140–350 U./ml.	
17-Hydroxycorticosteroids	Plasma	Male: 7–19 μg./dl. Female: 9–21 μg./dl. After 25 USP units of ACTH I.M.: 35–55 μg./dl.	Perform test immediately or freeze plasma
Immunoglobulins IgG IgA IgM IgD IgE	Serum	 800–1600 mg./dl. 50–250 mg./dl. 40–120 mg./dl. 0.5–3.0 mg./dl. 0.01–0.04 mg./dl.	
Insulin	Plasma	11–240 μI.U./ml. (bioassay) 4–24 μU./ml. (radioimmunoassay)	
Insulin tolerance	Serum	Fasting: Glucose of 70–110 mg./dl. 30 min.: Fall to 50% of fasting level 90 min.: Fasting level	Collect with heparin-fluoride mixture
Iodine, butanol extraction (BEI)	Serum	3.5–6.5 μg./dl.	Test not reliable if iodine-containing drugs or radiographic contrast media were given prior to test
protein bound (PBI) (BEI)	Serum	4.0–8.0 μg./dl.	

Whole Blood, Serum, and Plasma (Chemistry) (continued)

Test	Material	Normal Value	Special Instructions
Iron, total	Serum	50–150 μg./dl.	Hemolysis must be avoided
Iron-binding capacity	Serum	250–450 μg./dl.	
Iron saturation, per cent	Serum	20–55%	
Isocitric dehydrogenase	Serum	50–250 U./ml.	
Ketone bodies	Serum	Negative	
17-Ketosteroids	Plasma	25–125 μg./dl.	
Lactic acid	Whole blood (venous)	5–20 mg./dl.	Draw without stasis
	Whole blood (arterial)	3–7 mg./dl.	
Lactate dehydrogenase (LDH)	Serum	80–120 Wacker units 150–450 Wroblewski units 71–207 I.U./L.	
Lactate dehydrogenase isoenzymes	Serum	Anode: LDH_1 17–27% LDH_2 27–37% LDH_3 18–25% LDH_4 3–8% Cathode: LDH_5 0–5%	
Lactate dehydrogenase (heat stable)	Serum	30–60% of total	
Lactose tolerance	Serum	Serum glucose changes are similar to those seen in a glucose tolerance test	
Lead	Whole blood	0–50 μg./dl.	
Leucine aminopeptidase (LAP)	Serum	Male: 80–200 Goldbarg-Rutenburg units/ml. Female: 75–185 Goldbarg-Rutenburg units/ml.	
Lipase	Serum	0–1.5 Cherry-Crandall U./ml. 14–280 mI.U./ml.	
Lipids, total	Serum	400–800 mg./dl.	
cholesterol		150–250 mg./dl.	
triglycerides		10–190 mg./dl.	
phospholipids		150–380 mg./dl.	
fatty acids		9.0–15.0 mM./L.	
neutral fat		0–200 mg./dl.	
phospholipid phosphorus		8.0–11.0 mg./dl.	
Lithium	Serum	Negative Therapeutic level: 0.5–1.5 mEq./L.	
Long-acting thyroid-stimulating hormone (LATS)	Serum	None	
Luteinizing hormone (LH)	Plasma	Male: <11 mI.U./ml. Female: Midcycle peak >3 times baseline value Premenopausal: <25 mI.U./ml. Postmenopausal: >25 mI.U./ml.	
Macroglobulins, total	Serum	70–430 mg./dl.	
Magnesium	Serum	1.5–2.5 mEq./L. 1.8–3.0 mg./dl.	
Methemoglobin	Whole blood	0–0.24 gm./dl. 0.4–1.5% of total hemoglobin	
Mucoprotein	Serum	80–200 mg./dl.	

Whole Blood, Serum, and Plasma (Chemistry) (continued)

Test	Material	Normal Value	Special Instructions
Nonprotein nitrogen (NPN)	Serum or plasma Whole blood	20–35 mg./dl. 25–50 mg./dl.	
5′Nucleotidase	Serum	0–1.6 units	
Ornithine carbamyl transferase (OCT)	Serum	8–20 mI.U./ml.	
Osmolality	Serum	280–295 mOsm./L.	
Oxygen Pressure (pO$_2$)	Whole blood, arterial	95–100 mm. Hg	
Content	Whole blood, arterial	15–23 volumes %	
Saturation	Whole blood, arterial	94–100%	
pH	Whole blood, arterial	7.38–7.44	
	Whole blood, venous	7.36–7.41	
	Serum or plasma, venous	7.35–7.45	
Phenylalanine	Serum	Adults: <3.0 mg./dl. Newborns (term): 1.2–3.5 mg./dl.	
Phosphatase, acid, total	Serum	0–1.1 U/ml. (Bodansky) 1–4 U/ml. (King-Armstrong) 0.13–0.63 U/ml. (Bessey-Lowry) 1.4–5.5 U/ml. (Gutman-Gutman) 0–0.56 U/ml. (Roy) 0–6.0 U/ml. (Shinowara-Jones-Reinhart)	Hemolysis must be avoided; perform test without delay or freeze specimen
Phosphatase, alkaline, total	Serum	Adults: 1.5–4.5 U/dl. (Bodansky) 4–13 U/dl. (King-Armstrong) 0.8–2.3 U/ml. (Bessey-Lowry) 15–35 U/ml. (Shinowara-Jones-Reinhart) Children: 5.0–14.0 U/dl. (Bodansky) 3.4– 9.0 U/ml. (Bessey-Lowry) 15–30 U/dl. (King-Armstrong)	
Phospholipid phosphorus	Serum	8–11 mg./dl.	
Phospholipids	Serum	150–380 mg./dl.	
Phosphorus, inorganic	Serum	Adults: 1.8–2.6 mEq./L. 3.0–4.5 mg./dl. Children: 2.3–4.1 mEq./L. 4.0–7.0 mg./dl.	Separate cells from serum promptly
Potassium	Plasma	3.8–5.0 mEq./L.	

Proteins, total
  albumin
  globulin
	Serum	6.0–7.8 gm./dl.
		3.2–4.5 gm./dl.
		2.3–3.5 gm./dl.	

Protein fractionation	Serum		See Electrophoresis
Protoporphyrin	Erythrocytes	15–50 μg./dl.	
Pyruvate	Whole blood	0.3–0.9 mg./dl.	
Salicylates	Serum	Negative Therapeutic level: 20–25 mg./dl.	

Whole Blood, Serum, and Plasma (Chemistry) (continued)

Test	Material	Normal Value	Special Instructions
Sodium	Plasma	136–142 mEq./L.	
Sulfate, inorganic	Serum	0.2–1.3 mEq./L. 0.9–6.0 mg./dl. as SO_4	Hemolysis must be avoided
Sulfhemoglobin	Whole blood	Negative	
Sulfonamides	Serum or whole blood	Negative	
Testosterone	Serum or plasma	Male: 400–1200 ng./dl. Female: 30–120 ng./dl.	
Thiocyanate	Serum	Negative	
Thymol flocculation	Serum	0–5 units	
Thyroid hormone tests	Serum		

		Expressed as Thyroxine	Expressed as Iodine
T_4 (by column)		5.0–11.0 µg./dl.	3.2–7.2 µg./dl.
T_4 (by competitive binding —Murphy-Pattee)		6.0–11.8 µg./dl.	3.9–7.7 µg./dl.
Free T_4		0.9– 2.3 ng./dl.	0.6–1.5 ng./dl.
T_3 (resin uptake)		25–38 relative % uptake	
Thyroxine-binding globulin (TBG)		10–26 µg./dl. (expressed as T_4 uptake)	

Test	Material	Normal Value	Special Instructions
Transaminases: GOT	Serum	8–33 U/ml.	
GPT	Serum	1–36 U/ml.	
Triglycerides	Serum	10–190 mg./dl.	
Urea nitrogen	Serum	8–18 mg./dl.	
Urea clearance	Serum and urine	Maximum clearance: 64–99 ml./min. Standard clearance: 41–65 ml./min. or more than 75% of normal clearance	
Uric acid	Serum	Male: 2.1–7.8 mg./dl. Female: 2.0–6.4 mg./dl.	
Vitamin A	Serum	15–60 µg./dl.	
Vitamin A tolerance	Serum	Fasting: 15–60 µg./dl. 3 hr. or 6 hr. after 5000 units vitamin A/kg.: 200–600 µg./dl. 24 hr.: fasting values or slightly above	Administer 5000 units vitamin A in oil per kg. body weight
Vitamin B_{12}	Serum	Male: 200–800 pg./ml. Female: 100–650 pg./ml.	
Unsaturated vitamin B_{12} binding capacity	Serum	1000–2000 pg./ml.	
Vitamin C	Plasma	0.6–1.6 mg./dl.	Collect with oxalate and analyze within 20 minutes
Xylose absorption	Serum	25–40 mg./dl. between 1 and 2 hr.; in malabsorption, maximum approximately 10 mg./dl. Dose: Adult: 25 gm. D-xylose Children: 0.5 gm./kg. D-xylose	For children, administer 10 ml. of a 5% solution of D-xylose per kg. of body weight
Zinc	Serum	50–150 µg./dl.	
Zinc sulfate turbidity	Serum	<12 units	

Urine

Test	Type of Specimen	Normal Value	Special Instructions
Acetoacetic acid	Random	Negative	
Acetone	Random	Negative	
Addis count	12-hr. collection	WBC and epithelial cells: 1,800,000/12 hr. RBC: 500,000/12 hr. Hyaline casts: 0–5,000/12 hr.	Rinse bottle with some neutral formalin; discard excess
Albumin, qualitative quantitative	Random 24 hr.	Negative 10–100 mg./24 hr.	
Aldosterone	24 hr.	2–26 μg./24 hr.	Keep refrigerated
Alkapton bodies	Random	Negative	
Alpha-amino acid nitrogen	24 hr.	100–290 mg./24 hr.	
δ-Aminolevulinic acid	Random 24 hr.	Adult: 0.1–0.6 mg./dl. Children: <0.5 mg./dl. 1.5–7.5 mg./24 hr.	
Ammonia nitrogen	24 hr.	20–70 mEq./24 hr. 500–1200 mg./24 hr.	Keep refrigerated
Amylase	2 hr.	35–260 Somogyi units per hour	
Arsenic	24 hr.	<50 μg./L.	
Ascorbic acid	Random 24 hr.	1–7 mg./dl. >50 mg./24 hr.	
Bence Jones protein	Random	Negative	
Beryllium	24 hr.	<0.05 μg./24 hr.	
Bilirubin, qualitative	Random	Negative	
Blood, occult	Random	Negative	
Borate	24 hr.	<2 mg./L.	
Calcium, qualitative (Sulkowitch) quantitative	Random 24 hr.	1 + turbidity Average diet: 100–250 mg./24 hr. Low calcium diet: <150 mg./24 hr. High calcium diet: 250–300 mg./24 hr.	Compare with standard
Catecholamines	Random 24 hr.	0–14 μg./dl. <100 μg./24 hr. (varies with activity)	
Chloride	24 hr.	110–250 mEq./24 hr.	
Concentration test (Fishberg)	Random after fluid restriction	Specific gravity: >1.025 Osmolality: >850 mOsm./L.	
Copper	24 hr.	0–30 μg./24 hr.	
Coproporphyrin	Random 24 hr.	Adult: 3–20 μg./dl. 50–160 μg./24 hr. Children: 0–80 μg./24 hr.	Use fresh specimen and do not expose to direct light; preserve 24-hr. urine with 5 gm. Na_2Co_3
Creatine	24 hr.	Male: 0–40 mg./24 hr. Female: 0–100 mg./24 hr. Higher in children and during pregnancy	

Urine (continued)

Test	Type of Specimen	Normal Value	Special Instructions
Creatinine	24 hr.	Male: 20–26 mg./kg./24 hr. 1.0–2.0 gm./24 hr. Female: 14–22 mg./kg./24 hr. 0.8–1.8 gm./24 hr.	
Cystine, qualitative	Random	Negative	
Cystine and cysteine	24 hr.	10–100 mg./24 hr.	
Diacetic acid	Random	Negative	
Epinephrine	24 hr.	0–20 µg./24 hr.	
Estrogens, total	24 hr.	Male: 5–18 µg./24 hr. Female: Ovulation: 28–100 µg./24 hr. Luteal peak 22–105 µg./24 hr. At menses: 4–25 µg./24 hr. Pregnancy: Up to 45,000 µg./24 hr. Postmenopausal: 14–20 µg./24 hr.	Keep refrigerated
Estrogens, fractionated Estrone (E1) Estradiol (E2) Estriol (E3)	24 hr.	Nonpregnant, midcycle 2–25 µg./24 hr. 0–10 µg./24 hr. 2–30 µg./24 hr.	
Fat, qualitative	Random	Negative	
FIGLU (N-formiminoglutamic acid)	24 hr.	<3 mg./24 hr. After 15 gm. of L-histidine: 4 mg./8 hr.	
Fluoride	24 hr.	<1 mg./24 hr.	
Follicle-stimulating hormone (FSH)	24 hr.	Adult: 6–50 mouse uterine units/24 hr. Prepubertal: <10 MUU/24 hr. Postmenopausal: >50 MUU/24 hr.	
Fructose	24 hr.	30–65 mg./24 hr.	
Glucose, qualitative	Random	Negative	
quantitative: copper-reducing substances total sugars glucose	24 hr.	0.5–1.5 gm./24 hr. Average: 250 mg./24 hr. Average: 130 mg./24 hr.	
Gonadotropins, pituitary (FSH and LH)	24 hr.	10–50 MUU/24 hr.	
Hemoglobin	Random	Negative	
Homogentisic acid	Random	Negative	
Homovanillic acid (HVA)	24 hr.	<15 mg./24 hr.	
17-Hydroxycorticosteroids	24 hr.	Male: 5.5–14.5 mg./24 hr. Female: 4.9–12.9 mg./24 hr. Lower in children After 25 USP units ACTH, I.M.: a 2- to 4-fold increase	Keep refrigerated
5-Hydroxyindoleacetic acid (5-HIAA), qualitative	Random	Negative	Some muscle relaxants and tranquilizers interfere with test
5-HIAA, quantitative	24 hr.	<9 mg./24 hr.	

Urine (continued)

Test	Type of Specimen	Normal Value	Special Instructions
Indican	24 hr.	10–20 mg./24 hr.	
Ketone bodies	Random	Negative	Fresh, keep cool
17-Ketosteroids	24 hr.	Male: 8–15 mg./24 hr. Female: 6–11.5 mg./24 hr. Children: 12–15 yr., 5–12 mg./24 hr. <12 yr., <5 mg./24 hr. After 25 USP units ACTH, I.M.: 50–100% increase	Keep refrigerated; tranquilizers interfere with test
Androsterone		Male: 2.0–5.0 mg./24 hr. Female: 0.8–3.0 mg./24 hr.	
Etiocholanolone		Male: 1.4–5.0 mg./24 hr. Female: 0.8–4.0 mg./24 hr.	
Dehydroepiandrosterone		Male: 0.2–2.0 mg./24 hr. Female: 0.2–1.8 mg./24 hr.	
11-Ketoandrosterone		Male: 0.2–1.0 mg./24 hr. Female: 0.2–0.8 mg./24 hr.	
11-Ketoetiocholanolone		Male: 0.2–1.0 mg./24 hr. Female: 0.2–0.8 mg./24 hr.	
11-Hydroxyandrosterone		Male: 0.1–0.8 mg./24 hr. Female: 0.0–0.5 mg./24 hr.	
11-Hydroxyetiocholanolone		Male: 0.2–0.6 mg./24 hr. Female: 0.1–1.1 mg./24 hr.	
Lactose	24 hr.	12–40 mg./24 hr.	
Lead	24 hr.	<100 μg./24 hr.	
Magnesium	24 hr.	6.0–8.5 mEq./24 hr.	
Melanin, qualitative	Random	Negative	
3-Methoxy-4-hydroxyman-delic acid (VMA)	24 hr.	1.5–7.5 mg./24 hr. (adults) 83 μg./kg./24 hr. (infants)	No coffee or fruit 2 days prior to test
Mucin	24 hr.	100–150 mg./24 hr.	
Myoglobin, qualitative quantitative	Random 24 hr.	Negative <1.5 mg. L.	
Osmolality	Random	500–800 mOsm./L.	May be lower or higher, depending on state of hydration
Pentoses	24 hr.	2–5 mg./kg./24 hr.	
pH	Random	4.6–8.0	

Phenolsulfonphthalein (PSP)	Urine, timed after 6 mg. PSP I.V.
	  15 min.
	  30 min.
	  60 min.
	  120 min.
		
		20–50% dye excreted
		16–24% dye excreted
		9–17% dye excreted
		3–10% dye excreted	

Phenylpyruvic acid, qualitative	Random	Negative	
Phosphorus	Random	0.9–1.3 gm./24 hr.	Varies with intake

Urine (continued)

Test	Type of Specimen	Normal Value	Special Instructions
Porphobilinogen, qualitative quantitative	Random 24 hr.	Negative 0–2.0 mg./24 hr.	
Potassium	24 hr.	40–80 mEq./24 hr.	Varies with diet
Pregnancy tests	Concentrated morning speci- men	Positive in normal pregnancies or with tumors producing chorionic gonadotropin	
Pregnanediol	24 hr.	Male: 0–1 mg./24 hr. Female: 1–8 mg./24 hr. Peak: 1 week after ovulation Pregnancy: 60–100 mg./24 hr. Children: Negative	Keep refrigerated
Pregnanetriol	24 hr.	Male: 1.0–2.0 mg./24 hr. Female: 0.5–2.0 mg./24 hr. Children: <0.5 mg./24 hr.	Keep refrigerated
Protein, qualitative quantitative	Random 24 hr.	Negative 10–100 mg./24 hr.	
Reducing substances, total	24 hr.	0.5–1.5 mg./24 hr.	
Sodium	24 hr.	80–180 mEq./24 hr.	Varies with die- tary ingestion of salt
Solids, total	24 hr.	55–70 gm./24 hr. Decreases with age to 30 gm./24 hr.	
Specific gravity	Random	1.016–1.022 (normal fluid intake) 1.001–1.035 (range)	
Sugars (excluding glucose)	Random	Negative	
Titratable acidity	24 hr.	20–50 mEq./24 hr.	Collect with toluene
Urea nitrogen	24 hr.	6–17 gm./24 hr.	
Uric acid	24 hr.	250–750 mg./24 hr.	Varies with diet
Urobilinogen	2 hr. 24 hr.	0.3–1.0 Ehrlich units 0.05–2.5 mg./24 hr. or 0.5–4.0 Ehrlich units/24 hr.	
Uropepsin	Random 24 hr.	15–45 units/hr. 1500–5000 units/24 hr.	
Uroporphyrins, qualitative quantitative	Random 24 hr.	Negative 10–30 μg./24 hr.	
Vanillylmandelic acid (VMA)	24 hr.	1.5–7.5 mg./24 hr.	
Volume, total	24 hr.	600–1600 ml./24 hr.	
Zinc	24 hr.	0.15–1.2 mg./24 hr.	

Synovial Fluid

Test	Normal Value
Blood-synovial fluid glucose difference	<10 mg./dl.
Differential cell count	Granulocytes <25% of nucleated cells
Fibrin clot	Absent
Mucin clot	Abundant
Nucleated cell count	<200 cells/μl.
Viscosity	High
Volume	<3.5 ml.

Seminal Fluid

Test	Normal Value
Liquefaction	Within 20 min.
Morphology	>70% normal, mature spermatozoa
Motility	>60%
pH	>7.0 (average 7.7)
Sperm count	60–150 million/ml.
Volume	1.5–5.0 ml.

Gastric Fluid

Test	Normal Value
Fasting residual volume	20–100 ml.
pH	<2.0
Basal acid output (BAO)	0–6 mEq./hr.
Maximal acid output (MAO) after histamine stimulation	5–40 mEq./hr.
BAO/MAO ratio	<0.4

Hematology

Test	Normal Value		
Hemoglobin A$_2$	1.5–3.5%		
Hemoglobin F	<2%		
Osmotic fragility			% Lysis (after 24-hr. incubation at 37° C.)
	% Na Cl	% Lysis (fresh)	
	0.20		95–100
	0.30	97–100	85–100
	0.35	90–99	75–100
	0.40	50–95	65–100
	0.45	5–45	55–95
	0.50	0–6	40–85
	0.55	0	15–70
	0.60		0–40
	0.65		0–10
	0.70		0–5
	0.75		0
Platelet count	150,000–400,000/μl.		
Reticulocyte count	0.5–1.5%		
	25,000–75,000 cells/μl.		
Sedimentation rate (ESR) (Westergren)	Men under 50 yr.: <15 mm./hr.		
	Men over 50 yr.: <20 mm./hr.		
	Women under 50 yr.: <20 mm./hr.		
	Women over 50 yr.: <30 mm./hr.		
Viscosity	1.4–1.8 times water		
Complete blood count (CBC)			
Hematocrit	Male: 40–54%		
	Female: 38–47%		

Hematology (continued)

Test	Normal Value	
Hemoglobin	Male: 13.5–18.0 gm./dl.	
	Female: 12.0–16.0 gm./dl.	
Red cell count	Male: 4.6–6.2 × 10⁶/µl.	
	Female: 4.2–5.4 × 10⁶/µl.	
White cell count	4,500–11,000/µl.	
Erythrocyte indices		
Mean corpuscular volume (MCV)	82–98 cu. microns (fl)	
Mean corpuscular hemoglobin (MCH)	27–31 pg.	
Mean corpuscular hemoglobin concentration (MCHC)	32–36%	

White blood cell differential (adult)	*Mean Per Cent*	*Range of Absolute Counts*
Segmented neutrophils	56%	(1800–7000/µl.)
Bands	3%	(0–700/µl.)
Eosinophils	2.7%	(0–450/µl.)
Basophils	0.3%	(0–200/µl.)
Lymphocytes	34%	(1000–4800/µl.)
Monocytes	4%	(0–800/µl.)

Test	Normal Value
Blood volume	Male: 69 ml./kg.
	Female: 65 ml./kg.
Plasma volume	Male: 39 ml./kg.
	Female: 40 ml./kg.
Coagulation tests	
Bleeding time (Ivy)	1–6 minutes
Bleeding time (Duke)	1–3 minutes
Clot retraction	½ the original mass in 2 hr.
Dilute blood clot lysis time	Clot lyses between 6 and 10 hr. at 37°C.
Euglobin clot lysis time	Clot lyses between 2 and 6 hr. at 37°C.
Partial thromboplastin time (PTT)	60–70 seconds
Kaolin activated	35–50 seconds
Prothrombin time	12–14 seconds
Venous clotting time	
3 tubes	5–15 minutes
2 tubes	5–8 minutes
Whole blood clot lysis time	None in 24 hr.

Amniotic Fluid

Test	Normal Value	
	Early Gestation (Before 28 Weeks)	*Term*
Appearance	Clear	Clear or slightly opalescent
Absorbance difference at 450 nm.	<0.05	<0.02
Albumin	0.04 (no S.D. given)	0.05 (no S.D. given)
Bilirubin	<0.075 mg./dl.	<0.025 mg./dl.
Chloride	Approx. equal to serum chloride	Generally 1–3 mEq./L.; lower than serum chloride
Creatinine	0.8–1.1 mg./dl.	1.8–4.0 mg./dl. (generally greater than 2.0 mg./dl.)
Estriol	Below 10 µg./dl.	>60 µg./dl.
Osmolality	Approx. equal to serum osmolality	<250 mOsm./L.
pCO₂	33–55 mm. Hg	42–55 mm. Hg (increases toward term)
pH	7.12–7.38	6.91–7.43 (decreases toward term)
Protein, total	0.60 ± 0.24 gm./dl.	0.26 ± 0.19 gm./dl.
Sodium	Approx. equal to serum sodium	Generally 7–10 mEq./L. lower than serum sodium
Staining, cytologic		
Oil red O	<10%	>50%
Nile blue sulfate	0	>20%
Urea	18.0 ± 5.9 mg./dl.	30.3 ± 11.4 mg./dl.
Uric acid	3.72 ± 0.96 mg./dl.	9.9 ± 2.23 mg./dl.
Volume	450–1200 ml.	500–1400 ml. (increases toward term)

Miscellaneous

Test	Specimen	Normal Value
Bile, qualitative	Random stool	Negative in adults; positive in children
Chloride	Sweat	4–60 mEq./L.
Clearances	Serum and timed urine	
Creatinine, endogenous		115 ± 20 ml./min.
Diodrast		600–720 ml./min.
Inulin		100–150 ml./min.
PAH		600–750 ml./min.
Diagnex blue (tubeless gastric analysis)	Urine	Free acid present
Fat	Stool, 72 hr.	Total fat: <5 gm./24 hr. and 10–25% of dry matter Neutral fat: 1–5% of dry matter Free fatty acids: 5–13% of dry matter Combined fatty acids: 5–15% of dry matter
Nitrogen, total	Stool, 24 hr.	10% of intake or 1–2 gm./24 hr.
Sodium	Sweat	10–80 mEq./L.
Trypsin activity	Random, fresh stool	Positive (2+ to 4+)
Thyroid ^{131}I uptake		7.5–25% in 6 hr.
Urobilinogen, qualitative	Random stool	Positive
quantitative	Stool, 24 hr.	40–200 mg./24 hr. 30–280 Ehrlich units/24 hr.

Serology

Test	Normal Value
Antibovine milk antibodies	Negative
Antidesoxyribonuclease (ADNAase)	<1:20
Antinuclear antibodies (ANA)	<1:10
Antistreptococcal hyaluronidase (ASH)	<1:256
Antistreptolysin O (ASLO)	<160 Todd units
Australia antigen	See hepatitis-associated antigen
Brucella agglutinins	<1:80
Coccidioidomycosis antibodies	Negative
Cold agglutinins	<1:32
Complement, C′3	100–170 mg./dl.
C-Reactive protein (CRP)	0
Fluorescent treponemal antibodies (FTA)	Nonreactive
Hepatitis-associated antigen (HAA or HBAg)	Negative
Heterophile antibodies	<1:56
Histoplasma agglutinins	<1:8
Latex fixation	Negative
Leptospira agglutinins	Negative
Ox cell hemolysin	<1:480
Rheumatoid factor	
sensitized sheep cell	<1:160
latex fixation	<1:80
bentonite particles	<1:32
Streptococcal MG agglutinins	<1:20
Thyroid antibodies	
antithyroglobulin	<1:32
antithyroid microsomal	<1:56
Toxoplasma antibodies	<1:4
Trichina agglutinins	0
Tularemia agglutinins	<1:80
Typhoid agglutinins	
O	<1:80
H	<1:80
VDRL	Nonreactive
Weil-Felix (Proteus OX-2, OX-K, and OX-19 agglutinins)	Fourfold rise in titer between acute and convalescent sera

Cerebrospinal Fluid

Test or Constituent	Normal Value	Special Instructions
Albumin	10–30 mg./dl.	
Albumin/globulin ratio	1.6–2.2	
Calcium	2.1–2.9 mEq./L.	
Cell count	0–8 cells/μl.	
Chloride	Adult:　　118–132 mEq./L. Children: 120–128 mEq./L.	These values are invalidated by admixture of blood
Colloidal gold curve	0001111000	
Globulins, qualitative (Pandy)	Negative	
quantitative	6–16 mg./dl.	
Glucose	45–75 mg./dl.	
Lactate dehydrogenase (LDH)	Approximately $\frac{1}{10}$ of serum level	
Protein, total CSF	15–45 mg./dl.	
ventricular fluid	8–15 mg./dl.	
Protein electrophoresis		
Pre-albumin	$4.1 \pm 1.2\%$	
Albumin	$62.4 \pm 5.6\%$	
Alpha-1 globulin	$5.3 \pm 1.2\%$	
Alpha-2 globulin	$8.2 \pm 2.0\%$	
Beta globulin	$12.8 \pm 2.0\%$	
Gamma globulin	$7.2 \pm 1.1\%$	
Xanthochromia	Negative	

Emergency First-Aid Items for a Family of Four Persons or Less *†

First-Aid Item	Quantity	Substitute	Use
1. *Antiseptic solution:* Benzalkonium chloride solution. 1 to 1000 parts of water.	3 to 6 oz. bottle	Organic mercurial compounds in water. Drug stores have them under several trade names.	*For open wounds,* scratches and cuts. Not for burns.
2. *Aromatic spirits of ammonia*	1 to 2 oz. bottle	None	*For faintness,* adult dose ½ teaspoonful in cup of water; children 5 to 10 drops in ½ glass of water. As smelling salts hold bottle under nose.
3. *Table salt*	1 box	Sodium chloride tablet, 10 grains.	*For shock*—dissolve 1 teaspoonful salt and ½ teaspoonful baking soda in 1 qt. water. Have patient drink as much as he will. Don't give to unconscious person or semiconscious person. If using substitutes dissolve six 10-gr. sodium chloride tablets and six 5-gr. sodium bicarbonate (or sodium citrate) tablets in 1 qt. water.
4. *Baking soda*	8 to 10 oz. box	Sodium bicarbonate or sodium citrate tablets, 5 grains	*For some slight protection against nerve gas*—dissolve 4 teaspoonfuls of baking soda in 1 qt. water. Wash parts of body exposed to nerve gas with it or saturate cloth and place over face as gas mask.
5. *Triangular bandage* compressed, 37 × 37 × 52 in., folded, with 2 safety pins.	4 bandages	Muslin or other strong material. Fold to exact dimentions. Wrap each bandage and 2 safety pins separately in paper.	*For a sling; as a covering; for a dressing.*
6. *Large bath towels*	2	None	*For bandages or dressings:* Old soft towels and sheets are best. Use as bandages or dressings. Cut in sizes necessary to cover wounds. Towels are burn dressings. Place over burns and fasten with triangular bandage or strips of sheet. Towels and sheets should be laundered, ironed, and packaged in heavy paper. Relaunder every 3 months.
7. *Small bath towels*	2	None	
8. *Bed sheet*	1	None	

* Federal Civil Defense Administration: *Emergency Action to Save Lives,* Publication PA-5. U.S. Government Printing Office, Washington, D.C., 1951.
† These emergency first-aid items are assembled and then wrapped in a moistureproof covering that is placed in an easily carried box. A copy of the chart should be pasted inside the box cover; the box is then placed in the shelter area prepared.

Item	Number	Alternative	Use
9. Medium first-aid dressing 8 in. by 7½ in., folded, sterile with gauze enclosed cotton pads. Packaged with muslin bandage and 4 safety pins.	2	Must be bought	For open wounds or for dry dressings for burns. These are packaged sterile. Don't try to make your own.
10. Small first-aid dressing 4 in. by 7 in., folded, sterile with gauze enclosed cotton pads and gauze bandage.	2	Must be bought	
11. Paper drinking cups	25 to 50	Envelope or cardboard type	For administering stimulants and liquids.
12. Eye drops, castor oil	½ to 1 oz. bottle with dropper	Bland eye drops sold by druggists under various trade names	For eyes irritated by dust, smoke or fumes. Use 2 drops in each eye. Apply cold compresses every 20 minutes if possible.
13. Flashlight	1	Must be bought	Electric lights may go out. Wrap batteries in moisture proof covering. Don't keep in flashlight.
14. Safety pins, 1½ in. long	15	None	For holding bandages in place.
15. Razor blades, single edge	3	Sharp knife or scissors	For cutting bandages and dressings, or for removing clothing from injured part.
16. Toilet soap	1 bar	Any mild soap	For cleansing skin.
17. Splints, plastic, wooden, ⅛ to ¼ in. thick, 3½ in. wide by 12 to 15 in. long.	12	A 40-page newspaper folded to dimensions, pieces of orange crate sidings, or shingles cut to size.	For splinting broken arms or legs.
18. Tongue blades, wooden	12	Shingles, pieces of orange crate, or other light wood cut to approximately 1½ in. × 6 in.	For splinting broken fingers or other small bones and for stirring solutions.
19. Water purification tablets	Bottle of 100	Iodine tablets: chlorine tablets; chlorine capsules sold under various trade names	For purifying water when it can't be boiled, but tap water officially declared radioactive must not be used for any purpose.
20. Measuring spoons	1 set	Cheap plastic or metal	For measuring or stirring solutions.

APPENDIX VI

Questions of Concern to Nurses on Communicable Disease Control

Formulated from materials received from state health departments in response to our request for communicable disease information (1972). Survey was made to show comparison among the states and not to reflect current practices.

	Al*	Ak	Az	Ar	Ca	Co	Ct	De*	DC	Fl	Ga	Hi	Id	Il	In	Ia	Ks	Ky
1. Does the state regulate																		
a. Communicable disease control?	x	x	x	x	x	x			x	x	x	x	x	x	x	x	x	x
b. Water/milk supply?					x		x					x				x		
c. Sewage/refuse disposal?							x					x					x	x
d. Food handling?					x	x	x					x					x	x
e. Sanitation of camps, hospitals, other institutions?							x		x				x	x				
2. Does the state protect the public against radiation dangers?							x							x				
3. Does the state regulate maternal and child health through																		
a. Protection of the eyes of the newborn?	x			x		x					x			x	x	x		
b. Control over midwifery services?							x										x	
c. Lead poisoning reporting?																		
4. Are certain immunizations recommended?	x	x	x	x	x	x	x	x	x	x	x		x	x	x	x	x	x
5. Are certain immunizations required by law for school entrance?		x																
Diphtheria?										x	x					x	x	
Pertussis?										x	x					x	x	
Tetanus?										x	x					x	x	
Smallpox?											x					x	x	
Polio?						x				x	x					x	x	
Measles?						x				x	x					x	x	
Rubella?								x		x	x					x		
6. Is there special provision for																		
a. Tuberculosis control?				x	x	x			x	x				x	x	x	x	
b. Venereal disease control?				x	x	x			x	x				x	x	x	x	
c. Cancer reporting?										x							x	x
7. Are there regulations governing care of bodies after death?				x	x	x			x	x				x			x	x

	La	Me	Md*	Ma	Mi	Mn*	Ms	Mo	Mt	Nb	Nv*	NH	NJ	NM*	NY	NC	ND
1. Does the state regulate																	
a. Communicable disease control?	x	x		x	x		x	x	x	x		x	x		x	x	x
b. Water/milk supply?		x		x			x					x	x		x	x	
c. Sewage/refuse disposal?							x					x	x		x	x	
d. Food handling?		x		x			x					x	x		x	x	
e. Sanitation of camps, hospitals, other institutions?		x		x			x					x	x		x		
2. Does the state protect the public against radiation dangers?		x															
3. Does the state regulate maternal and child health through																	
a. Protection of the eyes of the newborn?	x	x			x								x		x		
b. Control over midwifery services?																	
c. Lead poisoning reporting?																	
4. Are certain immunizations recommended?	x	x		x	x		x	x	x	x	x	x	x	x	x	x	x
5. Are certain immunizations required by law for school entrance?																	
Diphtheria?							x	x			x		x		x		
Pertussis?							x				x		x		x		
Tetanus?							x				x		x		x		
Smallpox?							x	x							x		
Polio?							x	x			x		x		x		
Measles?							x	x					x		x		
Rubella?							x	x			x			x			
6. Is there special provision for																	
a. Tuberculosis control?		x		x	x			x	x			x	x		x	x	
b. Venereal disease control?		x		x	x			x	x			x	x		x	x	
c. Cancer reporting?				x													
7. Are there regulations governing care of bodies after death?		x		x								x	x		x	x	

	Oh	Ok	Or	Pa	RI	SC*	SD*	Tn	Tx	Ut	Vt*	Va	Wa	WV	Wi	Wy*
1. Does the state regulate																
a. Communicable disease control?	x	x	x	x	x			x	x	x		x	x	x	x	
b. Water/milk supply?		x	x				x							x		
c. Sewage/refuse disposal?		x	x			x	x							x		
d. Food handling?		x	x			x	x							x	x	
e. Sanitation of camps, hospitals, other institutions?		x	x			x	x							x		
2. Does the state protect the public against radiation dangers?		x					x							x		
3. Does the state regulate maternal and child health through																
a. Protection of the eyes of the newborn?	x	x	x	x	x				x			x	x	x		
b. Control over midwifery services?														x		
c. Lead poisoning reporting?				x												
4. Are certain immunizations recommended?	x	x	x	x	x		x	x	x	x	x	x	x	x	x	
5. Are certain immunizations required by law for school entrance?																
Diphtheria?		x					x	x				x		x		
Pertussis?		x						x				x		x		
Tetanus?		x					x	x				x		x		
Smallpox?							x							x		
Polio?		x					x	x				x		x		
Measles?		x					x	x				x		x		
Rubella?		x						x				x				
6. Is there special provision for																
a. Tuberculosis control?	x	x	x	x	x			x	x		x	x	x	x		
b. Venereal disease control?	x	x	x	x	x			x				x	x	x		
c. Cancer reporting?														x		
7. Are there regulations governing care of bodies after death?							x	x						x	x	

* Information not received or incomplete at time of the 1972 request.

APPENDIX VII

Recommended Schedule for Active Immunization of Normal Infants and Children *

2 mo	DTP [1]	TOPV [2]
4 mo	DTP	TOPV
6 mo	DTP	TOPV
1 yr	Measles [3]	Tuberculin Test [4]
	Rubella [3]	Mumps [3]
1½ yr	DTP	TOPV
4–6 yr	DTP	TOPV
14–16 yr	Td [5]	and thereafter every 10 years

* Source: American Academy of Pediatrics, Evanston, Ill., July 1975.

[1] DTP—diphtheria and tetanus toxoids combined with pertussis vaccine.

[2] TOPV—trivalent oral poliovirus vaccine. This recommendation is suitable for breast-fed as well as bottle-fed infants.

[3] May be given at 1 year as measles-rubella or measles-mumps-rubella combined vaccines.

[4] Frequency of repeated tuberculin tests depends on risk of exposure of the child and on the prevalence of tuberculosis in the population group. The initial test should be at the time of, or preceding, the measles immunization.

[5] Td—combined tetanus and diphtheria toxoids (adult type) for those more than 6 years of age in contrast to diphtheria and tetanus (DT) which contains a larger amount of diphtheria antigen. *Tetanus toxoid at time of injury:* For clean, minor wounds, no booster dose is needed by a fully immunized child unless more than 10 years have elapsed since the last dose. For contaminated wounds, a booster dose should be given if more than 5 years have elapsed since the last dose.

Storage of Vaccines

Because vaccines vary in stability, the manufacturers' recommendations for optimal storage conditions (e.g., temperature, light) should be carefully followed. Failure to observe these precautions may significantly reduce the potency and effectiveness of the vaccines.

APPENDIX VIII

Vaccination Requirements and Recommendations for Cholera, Yellow Fever, and Smallpox, by Country *

I means vaccination certificate required of travelers arriving from *all countries*, except as indicated in notes for individual countries.

II means vaccination certificate required of travelers arriving from *infected areas*, except as indicated in notes for individual countries. (Readers are advised to consult booklet *Health Information for International Travel 1976* for additional information.)

Ages shown indicate vaccination certificate required only of travelers of that age or older.

Country	Cholera	Yellow Fever	Smallpox
Afars and the Issas, French Territory of the	None	II 1 yr	I 3 mo
Afghanistan	II	None	I
Albania	II 6 mo	II 1 yr	I 6 mo
Algeria	None	II 1 yr	I
Angola	II	II 1 yr	I 3 mo
Antigua	None	II 1 yr	I
Argentina	None	None	I
Australia	None	II	II 1 yr
Austria	None	None	I 1 yr

Country	Cholera	Yellow Fever	Smallpox
Azores	None	II 1 yr	II 6 mo
Bahamas	None	II 1 yr	II
Bahrain	None	II 1 yr	I
Bangladesh	None	II	I
Barbados	None	II 1 yr	I 1 yr
Belgium	None	None	II
Belize (formerly British Honduras)	None	II	I
Benin, People's Republic of (formerly Dahomey)	None	I 1 yr	I 1 yr
Bermuda	None	None	I
Bolivia	None	None	I
Botswana	None	II	I 1 yr
Brazil	None	II	I 3 mo
British Solomon Islands	None	II by air	I
Brunei	II 6 mo	II 1 yr	I
Bulgaria	None	None	I 6 mo
Burma	Only to countries that require a certificate	II	I
Burundi	None	II 1 yr	I 1 yr
Cambodia (formerly Khmer Republic)	None	II	I
Cameroon, United Republic of	None	I 1 yr	I
Canada	None	None	II 1 yr
Canal Zone	None	None	I
Canary Islands	None	None	II
Cape Verde Islands	II	II 1 yr	I 3 mo
Cayman Islands	None	None	I
Central African Republic	None	I 1 yr	I

* Adapted from the booklet, *Health Information for International Travel 1976*. Published as a Supplement to the *Morbidity and Mortality Weekly Report,* US Department of Health, Education, and Welfare, Public Health Service, Center for Disease Control, Atlanta, Ga., 1976 (DHEW Pub. No. [CDC] 76–8280). This booklet tabulates data on risk of contracting malaria by country, by area in country, by altitudes and months of the year, and contains various health hints on travel.

Sources used in preparation of the booklet: *International Health Regulations 1969, Second Annotated Edition.* World Health Organization, Geneva, 1974; *Vaccination Certification Requirements for International Travel*—situation as of January 1976. World Health Organization, Geneva 1976; *Weekly Epidemiological Record.* World Health Organization, Geneva, 1976; *Collected Recommendations of the Public Health Service Advisory Committee on Immunization Practices* (AICP), *Supplement to the Morbidity and Mortality Weekly Report,* Vol. 21, No. 25, June 1972.

Country	Cholera	Yellow Fever	Smallpox
Chad	None	II 1 yr	I 1 yr
Chile	None	None	I
China, People's Republic of	No official information received		
China, Republic of (Taiwan)	No official information received		
Christmas Island (Indian Ocean)	II 1 yr	II	I 1 yr
Colombia	None	None	I 3 mo
Comoro Archipelago	None	None	I
Congo	None	I 1 yr	I 6 mo
Cook Islands	None	None	I by air 3 mo
Costa Rica	None	None	II
Cuba	None	II	II
Cyprus	None	II	I 1 yr
Czechoslovakia	None	None	I
Denmark	None	None	I
Dominica	None	II 1 yr	I
Dominican Republic	None	None	II
Ecuador	None	II	I
Egypt	II 1 yr	II 1 yr	I 3 mo
El Salvador	None	II 6 mo	I 1 yr
Equatorial Guinea	None	II	I
Ethiopia	None	I	I
Falkland (Malvinas) Islands	None	None	I
Faroe Islands	None	None	I
Fiji	II	II by air 1 yr	I by air
Finland	None	None	II
France	None	None	I
French Guiana	None	I 1 yr	I
French Polynesia (Tahiti)	None	II 1 yr	I
Gabon	None	I 1 yr	I 6 mo
Gambia	None	II 1 yr	I 1 yr
German Democratic Republic (East)	None	None	I
Germany, Federal Republic of (West)	None	None	I
Ghana	None	I 1 yr	I 1 yr
Gibraltar	None	None	II 3 mo
Gilbert and Ellice Islands	None	II 1 yr	I
Greece	None	II 6 mo	I
Greenland	None	None	I
Grenada	None	None	I
Guadeloupe	None	II 1 yr	I
Guam	None	None	II
Guatemala	None	None	I
Guernsey, Alderney and Sark	None	None	II
Guinea	None	II 1 yr	I 1 yr
Guinea-Bissau	II	I 1 yr	I 3 mo
Guyana	None	II	I 3 mo
Haiti	None	II	I
Honduras	None	II	I 1 yr
Hong Kong	None	None	I
Hungary	None	None	I
Iceland	None	None	I
India	Only to countries that require a certificate	II	Only to countries that require a certificate
Indonesia	None	II	I 1 yr
Iran	II 6 mo	II 1 yr	I
Iraq	None	II	I 1 yr
Ireland	None	None	I 1 yr
Isle of Man	None	None	II
Israel	None	None	II
Italy	II 1 yr	None	II
Ivory Coast	None	I 1 yr	I
Jamaica	None	II 1 yr	I 1 yr
Japan	None	None	II
Jersey	None	None	II
Jordan	None	None	I
Kenya	None	II 1 yr	I
Korea, Republic of (South)	None	None	I 1 yr
Kuwait	II 1 yr	II	I 3 mo
Laos	II	II	I
Lebanon	None	II by air	I
Lesotho	None	II	I 13 mo
Liberia	None	I	I
Libyan Arab Republic	II 1 yr	II 1 yr	I 1 yr
Liechtenstein	None	None	II
Luxembourg	None	None	II

Country	Cholera	Yellow Fever	Smallpox
Macao	None	II / 1 yr	I / 3 mo
Madagascar	II / 6 mo	II / 1 yr	I / 3 mo
Madeira	None	II / 1 yr	II / 6 mo
Malawi	I	II	I
Malaysia	None	II / 1 yr	I / 6 mo
Maldives	I	II	I
Mali	II	I	I
Malta	None	II / 6 mo	I
Martinique	None	II / 1 yr	I
Mauritania	None	I / 1 yr	I
Mauritius	None	II / 1 yr	I
Mexico	None	II / 6 mo	I
Monaco	None	None	None
Mongolian People's Republic	None	None	I
Montserrat	None	II	I / 1 yr
Morocco	None	None	I
Mozambique	None	II / 1 yr	I / 3 mo
Namibia	None	II / 1 yr	I
Nauru	II / 1 yr	II / 1 yr	I / 6 mo
Nepal	None	II	I
Netherlands	None	None	II
Netherlands Antilles	None	II / 6 mo	I / 3 mo
New Caledonia and Dependencies	None	II	I
New Hebrides	None	II / 1 yr	II / 1 yr
New Zealand	None	None	II / 3 mo
Nicaragua	None	None	I
Niger	None	I / 1 yr	I / 6 mo
Nigeria	Only to countries that require a certificate	I / 1 yr	I / 3 mo
Norway	None	None	I / 1 yr
Oman	II / 1 yr	II	I
Pacific Islands, Trust Territory of the USA	None	None	I
Pakistan	II	II	I
Panama	None	None	I
Papua New Guinea	I / 1 yr	II	I / 1 yr
Paraguay	None	II	I / 6 mo
Peru	None	II / 6 mo	I / 6 mo
Philippines	None	II / 1 yr	I
Pitcairn Island	II	II / by air / 1 yr	I / by air
Poland	None	None	I
Portugal	None	II / 1 yr	II / 6 mo
Portuguese Timor	None	I / 1 yr	I / 3 mo
Puerto Rico	None	None	II
Qatar	II	II	I
Reunion	None	II / 1 yr	I
Rhodesia	None	II	I
Romania	None	None	I
Rwanda	None	II / 1 yr	I / 6 mo
Ryukyu Islands	II	II	I
Saint Helena	II / 1 yr	None	I / 1 yr
Saint Kitts-Nevis-Anguilla	None	II / 1 yr	I / 3 mo
Saint Lucia	None	II / 1 yr	I
Saint Pierre and Miquelon	None	None	I
Saint Vincent	None	None	I / 3 mo
Samoa, American	None	None	II
Samoa, Western	None	II / 1 yr	I
Sao Tome and Principe	None	I / 1 yr	I / 3 mo
Saudi Arabia	I	II	I
Senegal	None	I / 1 yr	I / 6 mo
Seychelles	I	II / 1 yr	I
Sierra Leone	None	I / 1 yr	I
Singapore	None	II	I / 1 yr
Somali	None	II	I
South Africa	None	II	I
Spain	None	None	II
Spanish Sahara	None	None	II
Sri Lanka (formerly Ceylon)	None	II / 1 yr	I
Sudan	None	I / 1 yr	I
Surinam	None	II	I
Swaziland	II	II	I
Sweden	None	None	II
Switzerland	None	None	II
Syrian Arab Republic	None	II	I / 6 mo

Country	Cholera	Yellow Fever	Smallpox	Country	Cholera	Yellow Fever	Smallpox
Tanzania, United Republic of	None	II 1 yr	I	Upper Volta	None	I 1 yr	I
Thailand	None	II 1 yr	I	Uruguay	None	None	I 1 yr
Togo	None	I 1 yr	I 1 yr	Venezuela	None	None	I 6 mo
Tonga	None	II 1 yr	I	Viet-Nam, South, Republic of	None	II by air 1 yr	I 6 mo
Trinidad and Tobago	None	II 1 yr	II	Tunisia	None	II 1 yr	II 1 yr
Virgin Islands (USA)	None	None	II
Turkey	None	None	I	Wake Island	None	None	II
Uganda	None	I 1 yr	I	Yemen	None	II 1 yr	I
Union of Soviet Socialist Republics	None	None	I	Yemen, Democratic	None	II 1 yr	I
United Arab Emirates (formerly Trucial Sheikhdoms)	None	II	I 3 mo	Yugoslavia	None	None	II 1 yr
Zaire	None	II 1 yr	I 3 mo
United Kingdom	None	None	II	Zambia	II 1 yr	II 1 yr	I 6 mo
United States of America	None	None	II

Selected List of Self-Help Groups and Addresses of National Headquarters

The following are established self-help groups, listed alphabetically. Local groups are listed in local telephone directories.

Al-Anon Family Groups (for families of alcoholics)
P.O. Box 182, Madison Square Station
(115 East 23rd St.), New York, N.Y. 10010

Alateen (for teenage family members of alcoholics)
P.O. Box 182, Madison Square Station
(115 East 23rd St.), New York, N.Y. 10010

Alcoholics Anonymous
Box 459, Grand Central Station
New York, N.Y. 10017

Association for Children with Learning Disabilities
2200 Brownsville Road
Pittsburgh, Pa. 15210

Child Abuse Listening Mediation, Inc. (C.A.L.M.)
P.O. Box 718
Santa Barbara, Calif. 93102

Cruse, The Organization for Widows and Their Children
The Charter House
6 Lion Gate Gardens
Richmond, Surrey, Eng.

Diet Workshop
28 Merrick Ave.
Merrick, N.Y. 11566

Five-Day Plan (to stop smoking)
Box 4390
Washington, D.C. 20012

Gam-Anon (for spouses of gamblers)
P.O. Box 4549
Downey, Calif. 90241

Gamblers Anonymous
P.O. Box 17173
Los Angeles, Calif. 90017

International Association of Laryngectomees
219 East 42 St.
New York, N.Y. 10017

Mongoloid Development Council
P.O. Box 1089
Kansas City, Kans. 66117

Nar-Anon Family Group Headquarters, Inc.
(for families of drug abusers)
P.O. Box 2562
Palos Verdes Peninsula, Calif. 90274

Narcotics Anonymous
P.O. Box 622
Sun Valley, Calif. 91352

National Foundation for Sudden Infant Death, Inc. (S.I.D.)
1501 Broadway
New York, N.Y. 10036

Parents Anonymous
2009 Farrell Ave.
Redondo Beach, Calif. 90278

Neurotics Anonymous
1341 G. St., N.W.
Washington, D.C. 20005

Overeaters Anonymous
3265 Westwood Blvd.
Westwood, Calif.

Parents Without Partners (for bereaved persons)
80 Fifth Ave.
New York, N.Y. 10011

Post-Cana, Family Life Movement (for bereaved persons)
1721 Rhode Island Ave., N.W.
Washington, D.C. 20006

Reach for Recovery (a subsidiary of the American Cancer Society)
777 Third Ave.
New York, N.Y. 10017

Recovery, Inc. (for people who are "nervous" and need help)
116 S. Michigan Ave.
Chicago, Ill. 60603

The Samaritans (for bereaved persons)
Church of St. Stephen's Walbrook
London EC4, Eng.

SmokeEnders, Inc.
3435 Camino Del Rio South
San Diego, Calif. 92108

Smoke Watchers International, Inc.
605 Third Ave.
New York, N.Y. 10016

The Society of Compassionate Friends (for bereaved persons)
℅ Rev. Simon Stephens
27a St. Columba's Close
Coventry, Warwickshire, Eng.

Synanon
2240 24th Street
San Francisco, Calif.

Therapeutic Communities of America
624 South Michigan Ave.
Chicago, Ill. 60605
(A national association of self-help programs, including *Abraxas Foundation*, Marionville, Pa.; *Aliviane*, El Paso, Tex.; *Cedu Foundation*, Running Springs, Calif.; *Daytop Village*, New York, N.Y.; *Eagleville Hospital & Rehabilitation Center*, Eagleville, Pa.; *The Family House*, Seattle, Wash.; *Gateway Houses Foundation*, Chicago, Ill.; *Gaudenzia*, Philadelphia, Pa.; *Habilitat*, Kaneohe, Hawaii; *Integrity*, Newark, N.J.; *Logos Center*, Bronx, N.Y.; *Marathon House*, Providence, R.I.; *New Arizona Family*, Phoenix, Ariz.; *Odyssey House*, New York, N.Y.; *Phoenix House Foundation*, New York, N.Y.; *The Portage Program*, Montreal, Que.; *Project R.E.T.U.R.N. Foundation*, New York, N.Y.; *The Renaissance Project*, New Rochelle, N.Y.; *Samaritan Halfway Society*, Jamaica, N.Y.; *Second Genesis*, Bethesda, Md.; *Spectrum House*, North Grafton, Mass.; *The Village South*, Miami, Fla.)

TOPS Club, Inc. (Take Off Pounds Sensibly)
4575 S. Fifth St.
Milwaukee, Wis., 53207

United Ostomy Association, Inc.
1111 Wilshire Blvd.
Los Angeles, Calif. 90017

Weight Watchers International, Inc.
175 East Shore Rd.
Great Neck, N.Y. 11023

Some Diets in Current Use*

Diets for Healthy Persons and Some Whose Disease States Are Under Control. A *regular,* or *unrestricted, diet* is the most commonly prescribed diet. For those who are overweight the caloric content may be reduced and the protein content increased proportionately. A *prudent diet* is a term used by some persons to describe a regular diet in which foods high in cholesterol, saturated fats, and concentrated sweets are generally avoided.

Diets Regulated for Consistency. A *liquid diet* can be restricted to *clear liquids* or may include a *full range of liquids* and foods that liquefy at body temperature. For persons who cannot chew but can digest a regular diet the diet can be liquefied by putting it through a blender. This is called a *nonchew diet.* When patients must be fed through a nasal or gastric tube over long periods the *liquid tube feeding* must furnish a complete or regular diet. It is possible to make a regular diet of a consistency that will go through a nasal tube, but there are many commercial firms that make products which alone or in combination can provide complete diets. Examples are *Casec* (Mead Johnson Laboratories), *Citrotein* (Doyle Pharmaceuticals), *Hycal* (Beecham-Massengill Pharmaceuticals), *Isocal, Lonalac, MCT Oil* (Mead Johnson Laboratories), *Meritene* (Doyle Pharmaceuticals), *Portagen* (Mead Johnson Laboratories), *Precision LR, Precision High Nitrogen* (Doyle Pharmaceuticals), *Sustacal* (Mead Johnson Laboratories), *Vivonex* and *Vivonex High Nitrogen* (Eaton Laboratories). For convenience many institutions use such feedings rather than preparing a diet and putting it through a blender.

Diets Used in the Treatment of Persons with Cardiovascular Disease. *Sodium-restricted diets* are prescribed with daily allowances of sodium specified—2000 to 3000 mg (30 to 45 gr), a mild restriction, and less than 1000 mg (15 gr), a severe restriction. Dietary fat-restricted diets used to lower the triglyceride, cholesterol, and carbohydrate concentration in the plasma are called *hyperlipoproteinemia diets* and classified types I to V.

Diets Used in the Treatment of Persons with Diabetes Mellitus (Disorders of Carbohydrate Metabolism). These include the "prudent," or modified regular, diet and those with calories and amounts of carbohydrate, protein, and fats prescribed.

Diets Used in the Treatment of Persons with Gastrointestinal Disorders. These include a *bland diet* or a *peptic-ulcer-regimen* that restricts irritants; a *low-fiber diet* to decrease fecal bulk in preoperative and postoperative states and in acute phases of diverticulitis and ulcerative colitis; a *high-fiber diet* to increase fecal bulk in some chronic intestinal disorders, especially constipation; and diets that *restrict* the content of *gluten, lactose,* or *fats.*

Diets in the Treatment of Persons with Renal Disease. These include diets with caloric, protein, sodium, potassium, phosphorus, and volume of liquid restrictions.

Diets in the Treatment of Persons with Burns. It is usual to stress high-calorie and high-protein diets. Diets are estimated on the basis of area of body surface burned and amount of seepage.

Diets Used for Persons Having Diagnostic Tests. Tests for *glucose tolerance,* for *motility of the intestinal tract,* for *absorption of fats,* and tests involving *barium meals or barium enemata* are some tests for which there are dietary prescriptions.

Commonly Prescribed Diets. Regular, prudent, light, soft, clear liquid and full liquid, high-fiber and low-fiber diets are commonly prescribed. These are outlined briefly in this Appendix. For more complete descriptions of these and all diets prescribed in health and disease see the following texts and manuals (the sources used in preparing this Appendix):

Bowes, A., and Church, C. F.: *Food Values of Portions Commonly Used,* 11th ed. J. B. Lippincott Co., Philadelphia, 1970.

Church, C. F., and Church, H. N.: *Food Values of Portions Commonly Used,* 12th ed. J. B. Lippincott Co., Philadelphia, 1975.

Dietetic Service Staff, J. Hillis Miller Health Center, W. A. Shands Teaching Hospital and

---

* Adapted from *Manual of Diets* used by Departments of Dietetics, Hospital of St. Raphael, Veterans' Administration Hospital, Yale–New Haven Hospital, Yale–New Haven Medical Center, New Haven, Conn., 1972, p. 42.

Clinics: *Guide to Normal Nutrition and Diet Modification Manual.* University of Florida, Gainesville, 1973.

Food and Nutrition Board, National Research Council: *Recommended Dietary Allowances,* 8th ed. rev. National Academy of Sciences, Washington, D.C., 1974.

Goodhart, R. S., and Shils, M.: *Modern Nutrition in Health and Disease.* Lea & Febiger, Philadelphia, 1973.

Mitchell, Helen S., et al.: *Nutrition in Health and Disease,* 16th ed. J. B. Lippincott Co., Philadelphia, 1976.

National Heart and Lung Institute: *Dietary Management of Hyperlipoproteinemia. A Handbook for Physicians and Dietitians.* The Institute, Bethesda, Md., 1974.

Nutrition Department, The Johns Hopkins Hospital: *Manual of Applied Nutrition,* 6th ed. Johns Hopkins University Press, Baltimore, 1973.

Robinson, Corinne H., and Lawler, Marilyn: *Normal and Therapeutic Nutrition,* 15th ed. Macmillan Publishing Co., Inc., New York, 1977.

Weinsier, R. L., et al.: "High and Low Carbohydrate Diets in Diabetes Mellitus," *Ann. Intern. Med.,* **80:**332, (Mar.) 1974.

White, P. L., and Nagy, M. E.: *Total Parenteral Nutrition.* Publishing Sciences Group, Inc., Acton, Mass., 1974.

REGULAR OR NORMAL DIET (ADULT)

Characteristics and Principles. No foods are restricted. The number of calories are based on body size, build, and activity (2000 to 2200 is average). Foods are chosen to include Basic Four Food Groups according to Recommended Dietary Allowances of the Food and Nutrition Board of the National Research Council. A minimum of 75 gm (2.5 oz) of protein should be included. During pregnancy and lactation the caloric requirement and protein content should be increased and vitamins D, B12 and folic acid may be prescribed.

Type of Food	Foods Allowed	Foods Restricted
Beverages	All	None
Breads	All Four servings of bread (or cereal) recommended	None
Cereals and cereal products	All Interchangeable with bread—whole grain, enriched, recommended	None
Dairy products	All Milk, 500 ml (1 pt or 2 cups) recommended Butter, 16 gm (½ oz or 1 tbs) recommended	None, but a "prudent diet" restricts or limits whole milk, cream, and butter, and cheeses made of whole milk
Desserts	All Fruit desserts recommended	None, but a "prudent diet" restricts or limits concentrated sweets and pastries
Eggs	One daily recommended	None
Fats	All Recommended allowance of fortified margarine same as butter or substituted for butter	None, but a "prudent diet" restricts fatty meats and cheeses made from whole milk and substitutes margarine for butter
Fruits	All Two servings recommended	None
Meats, fish, and poultry	All Two servings, 150 gm (5 oz) recommended	None, but a "prudent diet" restricts heavily marbled meats, bacon and other fatty meats
Seasonings	All	None, but a "prudent diet" restricts or limits salt and highly spiced foods
Soups and broths	All	None, but a "prudent diet" restricts or limits use of creamed soup
Sweets, candy, honey, jelly, and syrup	All Natural sweets, such as honey and molasses rather than refined sugars recommended	None, but a "prudent diet" restricts or limits use of sweets
Vegetables	All, including potatoes Three servings recommended	None

Note. A regular diet is the basis for a *high-caloric diet.* No foods are restricted but eating low-caloric, filling foods is discouraged and the size of the servings of high-caloric foods is increased. A regular diet is also the basis for a *high-protein* diet. The size of the servings of high-protein foods is increased and those of foods with high carbohydrate and high fat content are proportionately decreased. High-protein diets are often used for weight reduction.

REGULAR OR NORMAL DIET (INFANTS—CHILDREN)

Characteristics and Principles. After the age of 3 years children can eat the adult diet but fried and highly spiced foods should be avoided. Infants and children have high nutritional requirements per unit of body weight. Only strained foods should be given infants until they have teeth; after this, foods should be chopped until there is full chewing ability. Infants require frequent feedings which are gradually reduced in number until, as children of about 3 years, they share meals with the family.

Type of Food	Foods Allowed	Foods Restricted
Beverages	All fruit juices (and milk)	Tea, coffee, and bottled drinks containing a drug of any sort
Breads	Toasted enriched bread recommended, three to four servings, interchangeable with cereals	Freshly baked bread
Cereals and cereal products	Whole grain, enriched cereals and breads are recommended	None
Dairy products	Milk, 750 ml to 1000 ml ($\frac{3}{4}$–1 qt) Butter (or fortified margarine), 8 gm ($\frac{1}{4}$ oz or 2 tsp), creamed or cottage cheese Cream in small amounts	Strong or spiced cheese
Desserts	Custards, jellies, and fruit desserts Ice cream	Concentrated sweets, pastries, rich desserts
Eggs	One daily recommended	Fried egg not recommended
Fats	Fortified margarine (or butter), 8 gm ($\frac{1}{4}$ oz or 2 tsp)	Fatty meats or fowl, fried foods
Fruits	Two servings (1 citrus), strained or chopped, cooked or raw, daily	None
Meats, fish, and poultry	Ground or chopped meat, fowl, or fish One serving daily, 60 gm (2 oz)	Marbleized meats and other fatty meats and fowl
Seasonings	Salt in moderation	Spices and strong seasonings
Soups and broths	All strained soups with meat or cream bases	Highly seasoned soups
Sweets, candy, honey, jelly, and syrup	Natural sweets—honey, molasses in small amounts	Rich candies Refined sugars should be avoided
Vegetables	Potato, rice, or pasta, one serving Other vegetables, strained or chopped, one to two servings	None
Miscellaneous	Smooth peanut butter	

Note. The preceding diet can be given babies up to 18 months. Solid foods are gradually added to the milk diet of the first weeks or months. (Experts hold different views as to how soon to start this process.) Dietary requirements for children up to 3 years are about the same but the size of servings is increased and the number of feedings, or meals, decreased until children eat their meals with adults.

CLEAR LIQUID DIET

Characteristics and Principles. This diet is composed of water-based liquids used to relieve thirst and provide some nourishment with minimal stimulation of the gastrointestinal tract. It does not provide a complete diet and should not be used for more than three or four days unless diet supplements are added. Fluids are given at frequent intervals (about six feedings daily) or as requested.

Type of Food	Foods Allowed	Foods Restricted
Beverages	Coffee or substitutes, tea, and carbonated drinks, such as ginger ale	All, other than those shown under beverages allowed
Breads	None	All
Cereals and cereal products	None	All
Dairy products	None	All
Desserts	Flavored clear gelatin	All (other than clear gelatin)
Eggs	None	All
Fats	None	All
Fruits	Strained fruit juices	All, other than strained fruit juices
Meats, fish, and poultry	None	All
Seasonings	Salt in broths	All spices
Soups and broths	Clear broths	All milk-based soups
Sweets, candy, honey, jelly, and syrup	Sugar in tea or coffee, honey and hard (clear) candy	All, other than those shown
Vegetables	None	All

Note: 576 ml (18 oz) of the supplement *Citrotein* added to a clear liquid diet provides about 380 calories, one-half the protein, some of the mineral, and most of the vitamin requirements of the Recommended Dietary Allowances of the Food and Nutrition Board of the National Research Council. (Other available supplements are *Hycal, Precision LR,* and *Vivonex*.) For those who must use a liquid diet over a period of weeks, months, or years, a liquid feeding should be used that meets all dietary requirements and that is tolerated by the gastrointestinal tract.

FULL LIQUID DIET

Characteristics and Principles. Besides water-based liquids, this diet includes milk-based liquids and solid foods that liquefy at body temperatures. It can provide a complete diet and is prescribed for persons who cannot or will not chew. Those who cannot or will not swallow are fed a similar diet through a tube introduced into the gastrointestinal tract through the nose, the mouth, or an abdominal incision.

Type of Food	Foods Allowed	Foods Restricted
Beverages	Any, according to taste	None
Breads	None	None
Cereals and cereal products	All cooked and strained	Dry cereals
Dairy products	All that can be liquefied—milk, cream, yogurt (plain or without fruit with pulp and seeds)	None
Desserts	Jello, ice cream, sherbet, custard, junket, tapioca, puddings	All that will not liquefy at body temperature
Eggs	Poached, soft boiled, eggnog	Fried or hard-cooked eggs
Fats	Cream, butter, or fortified margarine on cereals	Any that will not liquefy at body temperature
Fruits	Strained juices	All in solid form
Meat, fish, and poultry	Meat, fish, or poultry broths	All except in the form of broths
Seasonings	Any according to taste in moderate amounts	None
Soups and broths	Any strained meat, fish, poultry, or vegetable soups, clear or creamed	All containing solid foods None in strained form
Sweets, candy, honey, jelly, and syrup	Any according to taste (in moderation)	Concentrated sweets should be used in moderation and rich sweets avoided
Vegetables	Tomato and other strained vegetable juices	None in strained form

Note. If carefully planned and prepared, a full liquid diet can provide the Recommended Dietary Allowances of the Food and Nutrition Board of the National Research Council. If prescribed because the person cannot chew a complete and varied diet it can be put through a blender. Food supplements mentioned on page 2050 can be added to a full liquid diet to increase its nutritional value in a variety of ways.

TUBE-FED DIET (LIQUID NUTRITION)

Characteristics and Principles. When people, for any of a variety of reasons, cannot take food by mouth a liquid diet can be given through a nasal tube that meets all the Recommended Dietary Allowances of the Food and Nutrition Board of the National Research Council. Foods are prepared in a blender or, if a blender is not available, put through a sieve. It is convenient to have them prepared so that 1 ml (16 m) provides 1 calorie. To save labor, commercially prepared liquid feedings may be used in hospitals and homes. The Barnes Hospital *Handbook of Nutrition Care* lists a number of commercial supplements and gives their composition. Commercially prepared tube feedings that are said to be nutritionally complete are *Isocal, Meritene,* and *Precision LR.*

Tube Feeding to Be Prepared in Blender

Ingredient	Metric	Apothecary	Household
Bread (whole wheat)	60 gm	2 oz	2½ slices
Egg	50 gm	1⅘ oz	1 egg
Farina (enriched, cooked)	100 gm	3⅓ oz	½ cup
Liver, strained	100 gm	3⅓ oz	½ cup
Milk, skim	375 ml	12 oz	1½ cup
Milk, nonfat, dry	15 gm	½ oz	2 tbs
Orange juice concentrate (frozen)	70 ml	2⁴⁄₁₀ oz	⅓ cup
Peaches, strained	100 gm	3⅓ oz	½ cup
Vegetable oil	20 gm	⅔ oz	4 tsp
Water to make	1000 ml	1 quart	4 cups

SOFT DIET

Characteristics and Principles. This diet provides a complete diet and a wider range of foods than the liquid diet. It is prescribed for those who have trouble, for various reasons, in chewing and swallowing. Soft diets may be differentiated into *nonchew diet* and *mechanical soft diet*. Foods must be selected in each case according to the patient's taste and tolerance. See note below for *light diet*.

Type of Food	Foods Allowed	Foods Restricted
Beverages	Any	None
Breads	Any including pancakes, waffles, and French toast	None
Cereals and cereal products	Any	"Crunchy" cereals may not be tolerated
Dairy products	Any	None
Desserts	Any that are tolerated	All that contain nuts or "crunchy" foods
Eggs	Any	None
Fats	Any	None
Fruits	Any fresh, canned, or frozen fruits or fruit juices as tolerated	Some raw fruits may not be tolerated
Meat, fish, and poultry	Tender meat, fish, or poultry—whole, chopped, ground, or pureed as tolerated	None, if tolerated. Smooth peanut butter and beans, peas, and lentils can be used as meat extenders
Seasonings	All, as tolerated	None, if tolerated
Soups and broths	All	None
Sweets, candy, honey, jelly, and syrup	Any, according to taste, used in moderation	None
Vegetables	All, fresh, canned, or frozen vegetables as tolerated	None, if tolerated

Note. All foods included in the *soft diet* are allowed in the *light diet* which is sometimes called *convalescent diet*. It is a modification of the *regular diet* in which foods are prepared so that they are easily digested. Fried foods and pastries are eliminated, as well as nuts and fatty foods such as avocados and fatty salad dressings. Bran, raw vegetables and fruits, and gas-forming vegetables, such as beans and the cabbage family, are avoided.

RESTRICTED SODIUM DIET

Characteristics and Principles. Foods high in sodium are restricted or limited and salt is not added as foods are cooked and served. This diet reduces water retention (edema). The diet prescription specifies 250, 500, 700, and 2000– 4500 mg of sodium. (A person in health may eat 6–12 gm or even 20 gm of salt daily.) Tables showing the sodium content of foods must be used in planning diets according to prescription. The diet should be complete and may be made more palatable for some persons by the use of a salt substitute.

Type of Food	Foods Allowed	Foods Restricted
Beverages	Coffee, tea, Postum, and most carbonated drinks	Whole milk may be restricted and sodium-free milk prescribed
Breads	Salt-free breads	All breads made with salt
Cereals and cereal products	Most cereals can be used freely if not prepared with salt	No cooked cereals if prepared with salt. A few dry cereals are restricted that have an appreciable sodium content
Dairy products	500 ml milk daily. Unsalted butter or margarine	Low-sodium milk may be prescribed and foods made with milk limited or restricted
Desserts	Most desserts if prepared without salt. Fruits recommended	Commercial desserts made with salt
Eggs	One daily	
Fats	Unsalted butter or fortified margarine. Mayonnaise (unsalted)	Commercial salad dressing prepared with salt
Fruits	All—amounts served are determined by sodium content	None
Meats, fish, and poultry	None, if prepared with salt	Canned meats put up with salt and all dried and salted meats and fish
Seasonings	Salt substitutes may be prescribed. Herbs may be used to flavor foods so that salt-free dishes are more palatable	Salt (sodium chloride)
Soups and broths	All if made at home or commercially without salt	Most canned broths and soups restricted unless low sodium is specified
Sweets, candy, honey, jelly, and syrup	All in discreet amounts, if made at home or commercially without salt	Commercial candies containing salt
Vegetables	All that have low-sodium content and that are cooked without salt. Amount served depends on sodium content	Frozen or canned if processed with salt —vegetables high in sodium (see lists giving sodium content)

Note. Light salting of foods may be allowed for diets prescribing more than 2000 mg of sodium.

RESTRICTED FAT DIETS
(HYPERLIPOPROTEINEMIA DIETS)

Characteristics and Principles. Restricted fat diets are of five types with slightly different characteristics and used for different purposes as follows: *Type I*—To decrease the dietary fat available and so lower the triglyceride concentration of the blood plasma. *Type IIa*—To decrease the dietary fat so that the level of triglyceride is lowered in the blood plasma. *Type IIb*—To decrease the dietary cholesterol and carbohydrate, to control the cholesterol and triglyceride concentration in the blood plasma. *Type III*—To decrease the amount of dietary cholesterol and carbohydrate, to control the concentration of cholesterol and triglyceride in the blood plasma. *Type IV*—To control weight, to restrict the amount of carbohydrate and cholesterol in the diet and so reduce the level of prebetalipoproteins of the blood plasma. *Type V*—To restrict calories, fat, and cholesterol to reduce chylomicron and prebetalipoprotein in the blood plasma.

For detailed directions the reader should refer to booklet prepared by the National Heart and Lung Institute. See page 2051 for references listed at the beginning of this section on diets.

	Type I	Type IIa	Type IIb and Type III	Type IV	Type V
Diet Prescription	Low fat—25–30 gm (¾ to 1 oz)	Low cholesterol—polyunsaturated fat increased	Low cholesterol—about 20% protein, 40% fat, 40% carbohydrate	Controlled carbohydrate—45% of calories—moderately restricted cholesterol	Low fat—30% of calories, carbohydrate 50%—moderately restricted cholesterol
Calories	Unrestricted	Unrestricted	Sufficient to maintain or reach "ideal" weight		
Protein	Unrestricted	Unrestricted	Increased protein	Limited to amount that maintains or achieves "ideal" weight	Increased protein
Fat	Kind unrestricted Amount restricted to 25–30 gm (¾ to 1 oz)	Limited amount of saturated fat allowed; polyunsaturated fat increased	Controlled so that 40% of calories come from polyunsaturated fats	Limited to amount that maintains or achieves "ideal" weight (polyunsaturated fats recommended)	Limited so that 30% of calories come from (polyunsaturated) fats
Cholesterol	Unrestricted	Limited; only that in meat allowed	Limited to less than 300 mg from meat in diet	Limited to 300–500 mg (5–8 gr)	
Carbohydrate	Unrestricted	Unrestricted	Restricted—concentrated sweets not allowed		
Alcohol	Restricted	Discreet amount allowed	2 drinks allowed if substituted for carbohydrates		Restricted

BLAND DIET

Characteristics and Principles. This diet is a regular diet from which foods are omitted that mechanically or chemically irritate the gastrointestinal tract. Some institutions have dropped the designation "bland," but all provide a nonirritating dietary regimen which may start with frequent small feedings of milk, dishes made with milk, cereals, starches, and jello. Other foods are added, as tolerated, until the diet meets the Recommended Dietary Allowances of the Food and Nutrition Board of the National Research Council. Some institutions list bland diets I through IV.

Type of Food	Foods Allowed	Foods Restricted
Beverages	Milk, whole or skim, and drinks made with milk	Coffee, tea, carbonated beverages, and seasoned broths, chocolate drinks
Breads	Toasted bread and crackers made of refined flour, rusk, and zweiback	Whole-grain breads and crackers. Freshly baked bread
Cereals and cereal products	Cereal gruel, strained	Whole-grain cereals unless strained
Dairy products	Whole or skim milk, yogurt, butter, junket, cheese—cottage, cream, Cheddar	Rich cheeses
Desserts	Custards, jello, ice cream, sherbet	Any desserts made with nuts or fruit with skins or seeds. Rich pastries
Eggs	One or two daily, soft boiled, poached, or in eggnog	Fried egg
Fats	Butter, fortified margarine	All fried foods and fatty meats
Fruits	Strained fruit juices. Fresh or cooked peeled fruits without seeds as tolerated	Unpeeled fruits and fruits with seeds and fibers like pineapple; some raw fruits may not be tolerated
Meat, fish, and poultry	All omitted at first but tender nonfatty meats, fish, and poultry are added as tolerated	Tough, fried, spiced, or fatty meats, fish, or poultry
Seasonings	Salt to taste	Spices and condiments generally
Soups and broths	None allowed at first but gradually added if made without irritating foods	Commercial soups containing spices, or any restricted seasonings
Sweets, candy, honey, jelly, and syrup	Clear candies, honey, jelly, and syrup in small amounts	Chocolate candies, coconut candies, and excessive use of concentrated sweets
Vegetables	Rice, potato (without skin) added first with gradual addition of carrots, peas, spinach, asparagus, and other non-irritating vegetables	Gas-forming vegetables such as the cabbage family, beans, corn, cucumber, peppers, onions
Miscellaneous		Nuts, pickles

LOW- OR MINIMAL-FIBER DIET

Characteristics and Principles. A diet designed to reduce residue or fecal bulk in the intestines and to reduce mechanical irritation of the intestinal wall. It may be prescribed before and after surgery on the gastrointestinal tract and during inflammation of the intestines where distention causes pain or in ulcerative conditions where perforation is feared. (In constipation, chronic diverticulitis, and some other bowel disorders a high-fiber diet is believed by many to be indicated (see Note). A minimal-fiber diet may be deficient in thiamine and vitamin B6. Both of them may be prescribed.

Type of Food	Foods Allowed	Foods Restricted
Beverages	Any	None
Breads	Any breads, pancakes, or waffles made with refined flour or meal	Bran breads made with coarsely ground flour or meal
Cereals and cereal products	Cooked and raw cereals made with finely ground grains	Cereals made with bran or any coarsely ground grain
Dairy products	Any	None
Desserts	Any without skin and seed of fruit, nuts, or coarsely ground grain	Any with skin or seeds of fruit, nuts, or coarsely ground grain
Eggs	Any	None
Fats	Any	None
Fruits	Strained fruit juices	All whole fruits
Meat, fish, and poultry	Any	None
Seasonings	Any	Pickles, relishes, olives
Soups and broths	Any clear or strained soup	Soups made with vegetables or any restricted food
Sweets, candy, honey, jelly, and syrup	Any without nuts, seeds, or skins of fruit	Any with nuts, seeds, or skins of fruits
Vegetables	None	All vegetables

Note. A *high-fiber diet* is one in which the restricted foods on the *low-fiber* diet (fruits, vegetables, and whole-grain breads and cereals) are not only allowed but stressed.

Names and Addresses of Selected Nursing and Other Health Organizations*

INTERNATIONAL NURSING ORGANIZATIONS

International Council of Nurses (with which is associated the Florence Nightingale International Foundation)
37 rue de Vermont
1202 Geneva, Switzerland
(mail address: P.O. Box 42, Ch-1211
Geneva 20, Switzerland)
International Committee of Catholic Nurses
Square Vergote 43
B 1040, Brussels, Belgium
World Federation of Neurosurgical Nurses
% Judith Wills, Sec.
Sparshott House, Royal Infirmary
Oxford Road
Manchester M139W2, England

OFFICIAL NATIONAL NURSING ORGANIZATIONS OF THE WORLD

Members of the International Council of Nurses arranged alphabetically by country. (Personal communication with the Council May 1977.)
Federación Argentine de Enfermeria
Casilla de Correo No. 59
Sucursal 53
Buenos Aires, Argentina
Royal Australian Nursing Federation
132–136 Albert Road
South Melbourne
Victoria 3205, Australia
Osterreichischer Krankenpflegeverband
A-1180, Mollgasse 3a
Vienna, Austria
The Nurses Association of the Bahamas
P.O. Box 1691
Nassau, Bahamas

* Names and addresses in this listing are taken from the following sources: Annual directories published in the American Journal of Nursing, Nursing Outlook, *and Union of International Organizations:* Yearbook of International Organizations, *15th ed. (Published by the Union, 1 rue aux Laines, Brussels 1000, Belgium, 1974.) For fuller information on private and public health organizations, agencies, and institutions, see these sources. Many countries, cities, and smaller communities have directories of social agencies or social welfare yearbooks that include directories.*

Barbados Registered Nurses Association
"Gibson House," Spry Street
Bridgetown 5, Barbados
Fédération Nationale des Infirmier(ière)s Belges
18, rue de lâ Source
B-1060, Brussels, Belgium
Bermuda Registered Nurses Association
P.O. Box 1466
Hamilton 5, Bermuda
Asociación Nacional de Enfermeras Profesionales de Bolivia
Casilla No. M-17
La Paz, Bolivia
The Nurses Association of Botswana
P.O. Box 126
Gaborone, Botswana
Associação Brasileira de Enfermagem
Av. L-2 Norte, Modulo B
Quadra 603
CEP 70,000 Brasilia, Brazil
Burma Nurses Association
% The Lady Health Visitors Training School
11, East Bazaar Road
Rangoon, Burma
Canadian Nurses Association
50, The Driveway
Ottawa, Ontario, Canada
Colegio de Enfermeras de Chile
Correo Central
Casilla No. 9752
Santiago, Chile
Asociación Nacional de Enfermeras de Colombia
Carrera 17 No. 58-B-17
Bogota D.E., Colombia
Colegio de Enfermeras de Costa Rica
Apartado 5085
San José, Costa Rica
The Danish Nurses' Organization
Vimmelskaftet 38
DK 1161
Copenhagen K, Denmark
Asociación Ecuatoriana de Enfermeras
Apartado 3523
Quito, Ecuador
Egyptian Nursing Association
5 Sarai Street
Manial
Cairo, Egypt

Ethiopian Nurses Association
  P.O. Box 467
  Addis Ababa, Ethiopia
Fiji Registered Nurses Association
  C/-GPO Box 1364
  Suva, Fiji
The Finnish Federation of Nurses
  Töölöntullinkatu 8
  00250 Helsinki 25, Finland
*Association Nationale Française des Infirm-
  ières et Infirmiers Diplômés et Elèves*
  24, Avenue de la Republique
  F-75011, Paris, France
The Gambian Nurses Association
  P.O. Box 347
  Banjul, Gambia
Deutscher Berufsverband für Krankenpflege
  Heinrich-Hoffmann Str. 3
  D-6000, Frankfurt 71
  Federal Republic of Germany
Ghana Registered Nurses Association
  P.O. Box 2994
  Accra, Ghana
*Hellenic National Graduate Nurses Associ-
  ation*
  Athens Tower (C. Building)
  11 Athens 610, Greece
Guyana Nurses Association
  178, Alexander & Charlotte Streets
  Lacytown, Georgetown, Guyana
*Association Nationale des Infirmières Licen-
  ciées d'Haiti*
  Boite Postale 410
  Port-au-Prince, Haiti
Hong Kong Nurses Association
  P.O. Box 3868
  Sheung Wan, Hong Kong
Icelandic Nurses Association
  Thingoltsstr. 30
  Reykjavik, Iceland
Trained Nurses Association of India
  L-16 Green Park
  New Delhi 110016, India
Iranian Nurses Association
  P.O. Box 33/405
  Shemran, Tehran, Iran
National Council of Nurses of Ireland
  20, Lower Leeson Street
  Dublin 2, Ireland
National Association of Nurses in Israel
  The Histadrut
  93 Arlosoroff Street
  Tel-Aviv, Israel
*Consociazione Nazionale delle Associazioni
  Infermiere-Infermieri ad altri Operatori
  Sanitario-Sociali*
  Via Arno 62
  I-00198, Rome, Italy
The Nurses Association of Jamaica
  Mary Seacole House

  72, Arnold Road
  Kingston 5, Jamaica
Japanese Nursing Association
  8–2, 5-Chome
  Jingumae, Shibuya-ky
  Tokyo, Japan
Jordan Nurses & Midwives Council
  P.O. Box 10076
  Amman, Jordan
National Nurses Association of Kenya
  P.O. Box 49422
  Nairobi, Kenya
Korean Nurses Association
  88–7 Sang Lim Dong
  Choong Ku
  Seoul, Korea
L'Ordre des Infirmières du Liban
  % American University of Beirut
  Beirut, Lebanon
Liberian Nurses Association
  P.O. Box 1608
  Monrovia, Liberia
*Association Nationale des Assistantes d'Hy-
  giene Sociale, Assistantes Sociales et In-
  firmières Hospitalières Graduées*
  10, avenue Guillaume
  Luxembourg
Malaysian Trained Nurses' Association
  % School of Nursing
  General Hospital
  Kuala Lumpur, Malaysia
Nursing Association of Mauritius
  159 Royal Road
  Beau Bassin, Mauritius
Colegio Nacional de Enfermeras, A.C.
  Czda. Obrero Mundial 229
  Apartado Postal 12–986
  Mexico 12 D.F., Mexico
*Association Nationale Marocaine des Infirmiers
  et Infirmerières Diplômés d'Etat*
  B.P. 33 RP
  Rabat, Morocco
Trained Nurses Association of Nepal
  Mahabaudha Campus for Nurses
  Kanti Path
  Kathmandu, Nepal
*National Organization of Professional Health
  Workers*
  P.O. Box 2087
  Haarlem, The Netherlands
New Zealand Nurses' Association
  C.P.O. Box 2128
  Wellington, New Zealand
Colegio de Enfermeras Nicaragüenses
  Apartado No. 3289
  Managua, Nicaragua
*The Professional Association of Trained Nurses
  of Nigeria*
  P.O. Box 5194
  Lago, Nigeria

Norwegian Nurses Association
Postboks 3649
Gamlebyen-Oslo 1, Norway

Pakistan Nurses Federation
% College of Nursing
Jinnah Postgraduate Medical Centre
Karachi 35, Pakistan

Asociación Nacional de Enfermeras de Panamá
Apartado 52 72
Panama 5, Panama

Asociación Paraguaya de Enfermeras
Dte. de Enfermeria y Obstetricia
Ministerio de Salud Publica y B.S.
Brasil y Petirossi
Asunción, Paraguay

Federación Peruana de Profesionales de Enfermería
Jirón Washington No. 1651—Oficini No. 201
Apartado No. 5866
Lima, Peru

Philippine Nurses Association
1663, Kansas Avenue
Malate
Manila D-2801, Philippines

Polskie Towarzystwo Pielegniarskie
Koszykowa 8
00–564 Warsaw, Poland

Associaçäo das Enfermerias e dos Enfermeiros Portugueses
Rua Dúque de Palmela No. 27–4° D
Lisbon, Portugal

Colegio de Profesionales de la Enfermería de Puerto Rico
Calle Arrigoitia Esq. Salaman Rossevelt
Hato Rey
Puerto Rico 00918

Rhodesia Nurses' Association
P.O. Box 1202
Bulawayo, Rhodesia

St. Lucia Nurses Association
P.O. Box 819
Castries, St. Lucia

Asociación Nacional de Enfermeras Salvadoreñas
Casa de la Enfermera
Reparto "Los Heroes"
Gabriel Rosales y Matias Alvarado No. 157
San Salvador, El Salvador

Association Nationale des Infirmiers et Infirmières d'Etat du Senegal
Hôpital A. Le Dantec, B.P. 353
Dakar R.P., Senegal

Sierra Leone Nurses Association
P.O. Box 971
Freetown, Sierra Leone

Singapore Trained Nurses' Association
Professional Centre
Block 23, Outram Park
Singapore 3

Asociación Profesional de Enfermeras Espanolas
Consejo Nacional de Auxiliares Sanitarios y ATS
Buen Suceso, 6–2°
Madrid 8, Spain

Sri Lanka Nurses Association
Post-Basic School of Nursing
E.W. Perera Mawatha
Colombo 10, Sri Lanka (Ceylon)

Sudan Professional Nurses Association
P.O. Box 1063
Karthoum, Democratic Republic of Sudan

Swaziland Nursing Association
% King Sobhuza II Health Centre
P.O. Box 53
Manzini, Swaziland

Swedish Nurses Association
P.O. Box 5277
S-102 46
Stockholm 5, Sweden

Association Suisse des Infirmières et Infirmiers Diplômés
Choisystrasse 1
CH-3008 Berne, Switzerland

The Nurses Association of the Republic of China
89, Nei Chiang Street
Taipai, Taiwan (Republic of China)

Tanzania Registered Nurses' Association
P.O. Box 4357
Dar es Salaam, Tanzania

The Nurses Association of Thailand
21/12 Soi Rang Nam, Rajchaprarob Road
Bangkok, Thailand

Trinidad & Tobago Registered Nurses Association
8, Mon Chagrin Street
San Fernando, Trinidad, W.I.

Turkish Nurses Association
Türk Hemsireler Dernegi Genel Merkezi
Saglik Sokak No. 36/4
Ankara, Turkey

Uganda National Association of Registered Nurses and Midwives
P.O. Box 5456
Kampala, Uganda

The Royal College of Nursing of the United Kingdom
1, Henrietta Place
Cavendish Square
London WIM OAB, England

American Nurses' Association
2420 Pershing Road
Kansas City, Missouri 64108 (U.S.A.)

Asociación de Nurses del Uruguay
Colonia 1342
2° Piso, Esc. 5
Montevideo, Uruguay

Colegio de Profesionales de Enfermería de
    Venezuela
    Av. Luiz Roche 8a y 9a
    Transversal Altamira
    Caracas, Venezuela
Western Samoa Registered Nurses Association
    Public Hospital
    P.O. Box 192
    Apia, Western Samoa
Nurses Association of Yugoslavia
    Lole Ribara 8
    42000 Varázdin, Yugoslavia
Association des Infirmiers du Zäire
    B.P. 12.156
    Kinshasa I, Republic of Zaire
Zambia Nurses Association
    P.O. Box 2104
    Kitwe, Zambia

NATIONAL NURSING ORGANIZATIONS OF THE UNITED STATES

American Association of Colleges of Nursing
    Eleven Dupont Circle, Suite 430
    Washington, D.C. 20036
American Association of Critical Care Nurses
    2192 Martin, Suite 200
    Irvine, Calif. 92664
American Association of Nephrology Nurses
    and Technicians
    2 Talcott Road, Suite 8
    Park Ridge, Ill. 60068
American Association of Neurosurgical Nurses
    5813 Westhaven Drive
    Indianapolis, Ind.
American Association of Nurse Anesthetists
    111 E. Wacker Drive, Suite 929
    Chicago, Ill. 60601
American Association of Occupational Health
    Nurses
    79 Madison Avenue
    New York, N.Y. 10016
American College of Nurse Midwives
    1000 Vermont Avenue, N.W., Suite 500
    Washington, D.C. 20005
American Indian Nurses Association
    2241 W. Lindsey, Suite 502
    Norman, Okla. 73069
American Nurses' Association
    2420 Pershing Road
    Kansas City, Mo. 64108
American Nurses' Foundation
    2420 Pershing Road
    Kansas City, Mo. 64108
Association of Operating Room Nurses
    10170 E. Mississippi Avenue
    Denver, Colo. 80231

Association of Pediatric Oncology Nurses
    % Lorraine Bivalec
    Children's Hospital of Stanford
    520 Willow Road
    Palo Alto, Calif. 94304
Association of Rehabilitation Nurses
    1132 Waukegan Road
    Glenview, Ill. 60025
Emergency Department Nurses Association
    P.O. Box 1566
    East Lansing, Mich.
National Association of Pediatric Nurse As-
    sociates/Practitioners
    Box 1034
    Evanston, Ill. 60204
National Association for Practical Nurse Edu-
    cation and Service
    122 East 42 Street
    New York, N.Y. 10019
National Black Nurses Association
    P.O. Box 8295
    Canton, Ohio 44711
National Federation of Licensed Practical
    Nurses
    250 West 57 Street, Suite 323–25
    New York, N.Y. 10019
National League for Nursing
    10 Columbus Circle
    New York, N.Y. 10019
National Nurses for Life
    1998 Menold
    Allison Park, Pa. 15101
National Student Nurses' Association
    10 Columbus Circle
    New York, N.Y. 10019
Nurses Association of the American College of
    Obstetricians and Gynecologists
    One East Wacker Drive, Suite 2700
    Chicago, Ill. 60601
Nurses Coalition for Action in Politics
    1030 15th Street, N.W.
    Washington, D.C. 20005
Nurses Educational Funds
    10 Columbus Circle
    New York, N.Y. 10019
Oncology Nursing Society
    155 East 91 Street, Apt. 3-B
    New York, N.Y. 10028
Orthopedic Nurses Association
    1938 Peachtree Street, Suite 501
    Atlanta, Ga. 30309

STATE NURSING ORGANIZATIONS OF THE UNITED STATES

Appear in annual directories in American Journal of Nursing.

HEALTH ORGANIZATIONS OF WHICH NURSING IS AN INTEGRAL PART OR IN WHICH THERE ARE NURSING DIVISIONS

International

International Labour Office
  Geneva 22, Switzerland
International Red Cross
  7 Avenue de la Paix
  1211 Geneva, Switzerland
World Health Organization
  Avenue Appia
  Geneva, Switzerland

National (United States)

American Cancer Society
  777 Third Avenue
  New York, N.Y. 10017
American Health Care Association
  1200 15th Street, N.W.
  Washington, D.C.
American Heart Association
  7320 Greenville Avenue
  Dallas, Tex. 75231
American Hospital Association
  840 North Lake Shore Drive
  Chicago, Ill. 60611
American National Red Cross
  17th & D Streets
  Washington, D.C. 20006
American Public Health Association
  1015 18th Street, N.W.
  Washington, D.C. 20006
American Society of Childbirth Educators
  10948 North 56 Street
  Tampa, Fla. 33617

American Urological Association Allied
  111 East 210 Street
  Bronx, N.Y. 10467
Association for the Care of Children in Hospitals
  P.O. Box H
  Union, W. Va. 24983
Association for Practitioners in Infection Control
  Box 4342
  Euclid, Ohio 44132
Catholic Hospital Association
  1438 South Grand Boulevard
  St. Louis, Mo. 63104
National Education Association, Department of School Nurses
  1201 Sixteenth Street, N.W.
  Washington, D.C.
National Joint Practice Commission
  875 North Michigan Avenue
  Chicago, Ill. 60611
Society for Total Emergency Programs (STEP)
  693 Portland Avenue
  Rochester, N.Y. 14621

Regional (United States)

New England Board of Higher Education
  40 Grove Street
  Wellesley, Mass. 02181
Southern Regional Education Board
  130 6th Street, N.W.
  Atlanta, Ga. 30313
Western Interstate Commission for Higher Education
  Drawer P
  Boulder, Colo. 80302

Index

Page numbers in **boldface** indicate illustrations; *n.* indicates footnote; *t.* indicates table

Proper names are not included in this Index except when they relate to a program or system, a process, a test, or a product, as for example the Kaiser-Permanente program, the Heimlich maneuver, Benedict's test on urine, or Harris flush tube.

DATE DUE
